CLINICAL PATHOLOGY PANELS (Continued)

Newborn Screening (NY State)

Phenylalanine (phenylketonuria)
Leucine (branched-chain ketonuria)
Galactose-1-phosphate uridyl transferase (galactosemia)
Methionine (homocystinuria)
Thyroxine, TSH (hypothyroidism)
Hemoglobin electrophoresis (sickle cell)
Biotinidase (biotinidase deficiency)

Pancreatic

Amylase	Lipase
Calcium (total and ionized)	Glucose
Triglycerides	

Parathyroid

Albumin	Protein, total
Alkaline phosphatase	Calcium (total and ionized)
Magnesium	Phosphorus
Creatinine	Urinary calcium

PTH (whole molecule, amino terminal)

Prenatal Screening

CBC	Glucose
BUN	Creatinine
Uric acid	Free T_4
ABO and Rh typing	Antibody screen
Urinalysis	Urine culture
Toxoplasmosis Ab	Rubella titer
CMV Ab	VDRL
Hepatitis B surface Ag	Herpes simplex I & II Ab

Cervical Pap smear
Cervical cultures for GC, *Chlamydia*, group B streptococci

Renal

Chem. Path. 7	Calcium (total and ionized)
Magnesium	Phosphorus
Albumin	Protein, total
24-hr urine protein	24-hr urine creatinine
Creatinine clearance	CBC

Thyroid Screening

Thyroxine (free T_4)	TSH (third or fourth generation)

Toxicology Screening (urine)

Amphetamines	Barbiturates
Benzodiazepines	Cocaine metabolites
Marijuana metabolites	Methadone
Methaqualone	Opiate metabolites
Phencyclidine	Propoxyphene

Transplant

HIV Ab	HTLV-1 Ab
CMV Ab	VDRL
HSV I and II Ab	EBV capsid Ag and IgG Ab
ABO and Rh typing	Antibody screen
Hepatitis B surface Ag	Hepatitis C Ab

Rubella immune status
Hepatitis A Ab total and IgM
HLA typing: A, B, DR, and crossmatch
Lymphocytotoxic antibody screen

Final selection for ambulatory and inpatient use of the most cost-effective, sensitive, and specific measurements for each panel should be based on available laboratory technology and appropriate medical staff consultation with the Director of Laboratories in the context of relevant Practice Parameters* and Practice Guidelines. Use for hospitalized patients may be incorporated into "critical pathways" that are evolving.

References

*Department of Practice Parameters: Principles of Practice Parameters. Chicago, American Medical Association, 1995, pp 1–18.
Glenn GC: Practice Parameter on Laboratory Panel Testing for Screening and Case Finding in Asymptomatic Adults (in press).
Henry JB: Focused profiling: Selection of laboratory measurements and examinations. Videotape or 35-mm slides. Wilmington, E.I. du Pont DeNemours & Co., 1982.
Henry JB, Arras MJ: Organ panels: An innovation in health care delivery. Med Times 1970; 98:106.
Henry JB, Howantiz PJ: Organ panels and the relationship of the laboratory to the physician. *In* Young DS, Uddin D, Nipper H, et al (eds), King JS (exec ed): Clinician and Chemist: Proceedings of the First Arnold O. Beckman Conference in Clinical Chemistry. Washington, DC, American Association for Clinical Chemistry, 1979.
Henry JB, Howanitz PJ: Organ panels and the relationship of the laboratory to the physician. *In* AMA Council on Scientific Affairs: Laboratory Tests in Medical Practice. Chicago, 1980.

*Order number OP271693
American Medical Association
P.O. Box 7046
Dover, DE 19903

Clinical Diagnosis *and* Management *by* Laboratory Methods

NINETEENTH EDITION

• Associate Editors •

Frederick R. Davey, M.D.
Professor and Chair, Department of Pathology
Vice Dean for Clinical Affairs
SUNY Health Science Center at Syracuse
Syracuse, NY

Robert M. Nakamura, M.D.
Chair Emeritus
Department of Pathology
Scripps Clinic and Research Foundation
La Jolla, CA

Matthew R. Pincus, M.D., Ph.D.
Professor of Pathology
SUNY Health Science Center
Chair, Department of Pathology and Laboratory Medicine
Veterans Affairs Medical Center
Brooklyn, NY

Gail L. Woods, M.D.
Professor of Pathology
Director, Division of Microbiology
University of Texas Medical Branch
Galveston, TX

• Assistant Editors •

David J. Bylund, M.D.
Adjunct Assistant Member
Department of Molecular and Experimental Medicine
The Scripps Research Institute
Laboratory Director
Scripps Reference Laboratory
La Jolla, CA

Howard S. Fox, M.D., Ph.D.
Assistant Member
Department of Neuropharmacology
The Scripps Research Institute
Consulting Pathologist
Scripps Clinic and Research Foundation
La Jolla, CA

Sanford A. Stass, M.D.
Professor of Pathology and Medicine
Director, Laboratories of Pathology
University of Maryland School of Medicine
and University of Maryland Medical System
Baltimore, MD

Clinical Diagnosis *and* Management *by* Laboratory Methods

NINETEENTH EDITION

[edited by]

JOHN BERNARD HENRY, M.D.

Professor of Pathology
Director, Pathology 200 and 5214
Deputy Director, Blood Bank and Transfusion Medicine
Department of Pathology
State University of New York Health Science Center at Syracuse
Syracuse, New York

W.B. SAUNDERS COMPANY
A Division of Harcourt Brace & Company
Philadelphia London Toronto Montreal Sydney Tokyo

W.B. SAUNDERS COMPANY
A Division of Harcourt Brace & Company

The Curtis Center
Independence Square West
Philadelphia, Pennsylvania 19106

Library of Congress Cataloging-in-Publication Data

Clinical diagnosis and management by laboratory methods. — 19th ed./
[edited by] John Bernard Henry.

p. cm.

Includes bibliographical references and index.

ISBN 0–7216–6030–4

1. Diagnosis, Laboratory. I. Henry, John Bernard
[DNLM: 1. Diagnosis, Laboratory. QY 4 C6405 1996]
RB37.C54 1996 616.07′56—dc20

DNLM/DLC 95-33534

Clinical Diagnosis and Management by Laboratory Methods ISBN 0–7216–6030–4

Printed in the United States

Last digit is the print number: 9 8 7 6 5 4 3 2

To

Georgette,

my best friend and wife of 43
years and mother of our six children,
Maureen Henry Mayer, Julie Patricia Henry, M.D.,
Capt. William Bernard Henry, U.S.M.C., Paul Bernard Henry,
John Bernard Henry, Jr., and Thomas David Henry;
our sons-in-law Thom A. Mayer, M.D. and Peter J. Paganussi, M.D.;

and our grandchildren,

Gregory, Joshua and Kevin Mayer
and Caroline, Claire and Matthew Paganussi
all of whom accepted patiently the inconvenience
and separation associated with my preoccupation
with this work, which, without their sustained
support and understanding,
could not have been completed.

TODD-SANFORD-DAVIDSOHN:

A Tribute

Todd and Sanford is a legend among medical textbooks. It has spanned 87 years and has served as a resource for thousands of physicians, scientists, students, and medical technologists. This textbook has its roots in the first edition, published in 1908 as **A Manual of Clinical Diagnosis** by James C. Todd, M.D. Dr. Todd was the author of the first six editions, though he was in ill health in his final years; he died in 1928 at the age of 54.

The sixth edition was edited by Dr. Todd and Arthur H. Sanford, M.D. Dr. Sanford continued with four more editions on his own. He had the assistance of George G. Stilwell, M.D., as a collaborator on the eleventh edition, and Benjamin B. Wells, M.D., as coeditor on the twelfth edition. Dr. Sanford died in 1959 at age 77.

The thirteenth edition, **Clinical Diagnosis by Laboratory Methods,** was edited by Israel Davidsohn, M.D., and Dr. Wells. I joined Dr. Davidsohn with the fourteenth edition, published in 1969. We shared the fifteenth edition, published in 1974. Israel Davidsohn, M.D., died in 1979, at the age of 84. I have continued as editor for the subsequent editions. The title of the sixteenth edition, **Clinical Diagnosis and Management by Laboratory Methods,** was augmented to reflect major current use of laboratory measurements and examinations in patient care management as well as diagnostic applications. The nineteenth edition represents my sixth edition.

Although the names of Todd, Sanford, and Davidsohn are no longer visible on the cover, their presence will always be with this textbook. We stand on the shoulders of giants and can account for whatever contributions we have made as individuals because of the tremendous effort and commitment of those who have preceded us.

It is with deep humility and respect that I pause to reflect and point out to the reader the history of this remarkable text. After more than 87 years, it can take its place among the most significant textbook contributions in modern medicine as attested by the durability of its readership for these many years.

Personally, I have greatly missed working with Dr. Davidsohn over the past four editions, and can only encourage the reader who has an interest in history to read "The History of a Book and of a Medical Specialty, Todd and Sanford (1908–1969)," written by Israel Davidsohn, M.D., in the fourteenth edition of **Clinical Diagnosis by Laboratory Methods,** edited by Davidsohn and Henry, published in 1969.

The memory and contributions of Todd, Sanford, and Davidsohn should never be forgotten. I am and always will be indebted to each of them. May you share my feelings of respect and gratitude for these leaders in medicine and pathology.

JOHN BERNARD HENRY, M.D.

Contributors

Naif Z. Abraham, Jr., M.D., Ph.D.
Attending Pathologist,
Baton Rouge General Medical Center,
Baton Rouge, Louisiana
Toxicology and Therapeutic Drug Monitoring

Lynne V. Abruzzo, M.D., Ph.D.
Assistant Professor, Department of Pathology,
University of Maryland School of Medicine,
Baltimore, Maryland
Molecular Genetics of Hematopoietic Neoplasms

Daniel R. Alexander, M.D.
Assistant, Department of Pathology, State University of New York, Health Science Center, Syracuse, New York
Evaluation of Endocrine Function; Laboratory Diagnosis of Gastrointestinal Tract and Exocrine Pancreatic Disorders

Raymond D. Aller, M.D.
Professor of Pathology and of Medical Informatics,
Director, Hospital Clinical Laboratories,
University of Utah Health Sciences Center,
Department of Pathology and Associated Regional and University Pathologists, Inc., Salt Lake City, Utah
Informatics, Imaging, and the Pathologist's Workstation

Chester A. Alper, M.D.
Professor of Pediatrics, Harvard Medical School;
Vice President, The Center for Blood Research,
Boston, Massachusetts
The Major Histocompatibility Complex and Disease

Leona W. Ayers, M.D.
Director, Division of Clinical Microbiology and Department of Hospital Epidemiology; Hospital Epidemiologist; Associate Professor of Pathology and Allied Health Sciences, Ohio State University, Columbus, Ohio
Medical Bacteriology

Paul S. Bachorik, Ph.D.
Professor of Pediatrics and Associate Professor of Pathology, The Johns Hopkins University School of Medicine, Baltimore, Maryland
Lipids and Dyslipoproteinemia

Ulysses J. Balis, M.D.
Medical Director, Image Processing and Analysis Laboratory, University of Utah, Department of Pathology and Associated Regional and University Pathologists, Inc., Salt Lake City, Utah
Informatics, Imaging, and the Pathologist's Workstation

Nimrat Bawa, M.D.
Assistant, Department of Pathology and Laboratory Medicine, University of Wisconsin Hospital/Clinics, Madison, Wisconsin
Laboratory Evaluation of Immunoglobulin Function and Humoral Immunity

Wendy V. Beadling, M.S., MT(ASCP)SBB
Assistant Professor, College of Health-Related Professions, SUNY Health Science Center at Syracuse; Blood Bank Teaching Supervisor, University Hospital, SUNY Health Science Center at Syracuse, Syracuse, New York
Immunohematology

Leonard I. Boral, M.D., M.B.A.
Associate Professor of Clinical Laboratory Medicine and Pathology, University of Medicine and Dentistry of New Jersey; Director of Laboratories, Newark Beth Israel Medical Center, Newark, New Jersey
Transfusion Medicine

Paul W. Brandt-Rauf, M.D., Sc.D., Dr.P.H.
Professor and Director of Occupational and Environmental Medicine, Columbia University School of Public Health, New York, New York
Cell Biology and Early Tumor Detection

David J. Bylund, M.D.
Adjunct Assistant Member, Department of Molecular and Experimental Medicine; Laboratory Director, Scripps Reference Laboratory, The Scripps Research Institute, La Jolla, California
Vasculitis; Organ-Directed Autoimmune Diseases

Martin G. Cormican, M.D.
Fellow, Department of Pathology, University of Iowa Hospitals and Clinics, Iowa City, Iowa
Molecular Pathology of Infectious Diseases

Deyanira Corzo, M.D.
Resident in Pediatrics, Maimonides Medical Center, Brooklyn, New York; Former Postdoctoral Research Fellow in Pathology, Division of Immunogenetics, Dana-Farber Cancer Institute Department of Pathology, Harvard Medical School
The Major Histocompatibility Complex and Disease

Michael Costello, Ph.D.
Associate Director—Microbiology, Lutheran General Hospital, Park Ridge, Illinois
Viral Infections

Susanna Cunningham-Rundles, Ph.D.
Associate Professor of Immunology, Cornell University Medical College; Director, The Immunology Research Laboratory, Department of Pediatrics, The New York Hospital–Cornell Medical Center, New York, New York
Laboratory Evaluation of the Cellular Immune System

Frederick R. Davey, M.D.
Professor and Chair, Department of Pathology, College of Medicine, SUNY Health Science Center; Vice Dean, Clinical Affairs, SUNY Health Science Center, Syracuse, New York
Basic Examination of Blood; Hematopoiesis; Erythrocytic Disorders; Leukocytic Disorders

M. Tarek Elghetany, M.D.
Assistant Professor of Pathology and Associate Director of Hematopathology, University of Texas Medical Branch, Galveston, Texas
Erythrocytic Disorders

Clifford D. Eng, M.D.
Clinical Assistant Professor of Pathology, Uniformed Services University of the Health Sciences; Medical Director and Head of Clinical Chemistry, National Naval Medical Center, Bethesda, Maryland
Evaluation of Endocrine Function

Andrea Ferreira-Gonzalez, M.S., Ph.D.
Assistant Professor, Pathology Department; Molecular Diagnostics Specialist, Division of Molecular Diagnostics, Medical College of Virginia, Virginia Commonwealth University, Richmond, Virginia
Establishing a Molecular Diagnostics Laboratory

Stuart D. Flynn, M.D.
Associate Professor; Director, Flow Cytometry and Molecular Pathology, Department of Pathology, Yale University School of Medicine, New Haven, Connecticut
Clinical Application of Human Chorionic Gonadotropin

Howard S. Fox, M.D., Ph.D.
Assistant Member, Department of Neuropharmacology, The Scripps Research Institute; Consulting Pathologist, Scripps Clinic and Research Foundation, La Jolla, California
Overview of the Immune System; Cytokines and Cell Adhesion Molecules

Michael M. Frank, M.D.
Professor of Pediatrics, Immunology, and Medicine, Chairman of Pediatrics, Duke University Medical Center, Durham, North Carolina
Complement and Kinins: Mediators of Inflammation

Thomas R. Fritsche, M.D., Ph.D.
Associate Professor of Laboratory Medicine and Microbiology, University of Washington School of Medicine; Director, Clinical Microbiology, University of Washington Medical Center, Seattle, Washington
Medical Parasitology

Carleton T. Garrett, M.D., Ph.D.
Professor of Pathology and Chairman, Division of Molecular Diagnostics, Department of Pathology, Medical College of Virginia, Virginia Commonwealth University, Richmond, Virginia
Establishing a Molecular Diagnostics Laboratory

Wayne W. Grody, M.D., Ph.D.
Associate Professor, Divisions of Molecular Pathology and Medical Genetics, Departments of Pathology & Laboratory Medicine and Pediatrics, UCLA School of Medicine; Director, Diagnostic Molecular Pathology Laboratory, UCLA Medical Center, Los Angeles, California
Molecular Diagnosis of Genetic Diseases

Robert J. Hartzman, CAPT, MC, USN, M.D.
Director, C. W. Bill Young Marrow Donor Recruitment and Research Program, Naval Medical Research Institute, Bethesda, Maryland
Human Leukocyte Antigen (HLA): The Major Histocompatibility Complex of Humans and Transplantation Immunology

John Bernard Henry, M.D.
Professor of Pathology, College of Medicine; Attending Pathologist and Deputy Director, Blood Bank and Transfusion Medicine, University Hospital, State University of New York, Health Science Center at Syracuse, New York
The Clinical Laboratory: Organization, Purposes, and Practice; Principles of Instrumentation; Quality Management; Evaluation of Renal Function, Water, Electrolytes, Acid-Base Balance, and Blood Gases; Metabolic Intermediates and Inorganic Ions; Carbohydrates; Clinical Enzymology; Evaluation of Endocrine Function; Basic Examination of Urine; Andrology Laboratory and Fertility Assessment; Immunohematology; Transfusion Medicine; Appendices 1 to 4

Erik K. Hofmeister, D.V.M., Ph.D.
Department of Laboratory Medicine and Pathology, Mayo Clinic and Foundation, Rochester, Minnesota
Spirochete Infections

Henry A. Homburger, M.D.
Professor of Laboratory Medicine, Mayo Medical School, Mayo Foundation; Consultant, Mayo Clinic, Rochester, Minnesota
Allergic Diseases

Richard Hong, M.D.
Professor of Pediatrics, University of Vermont Medical School; Attending Physician, Fletcher Allen Health Care Medical Center Hospital of Vermont Campus, Burlington, Vermont
Immunodeficiency Disorders

Carolyn Katovich Hurley, Ph.D.
Professor, Department of Microbiology, Georgetown University Medical Center, Washington, D.C.
Human Leukocyte Antigen (HLA): The Major Histocompatibility Complex of Humans and Transplantation Immunology

Robert E. Hutchison, M.D.
Associate Professor, Department of Pathology; Director of Hematology, Division of Clinical Pathology, State University of New York Health Science Center, Syracuse, New York
Hematopoiesis; Leukocytic Disorders

Armead H. Johnson, Ph.D.
Professor, Departments of Pediatrics and Pathology, Georgetown University Medical School; Director—Clinical HLA Laboratory, Georgetown University Hospital, Washington, D.C.
Human Leukocyte Antigen (HLA): The Major Histocompatibility Complex of Humans and Transplantation Immunology

Yuan S. Kao, M.D., FCAP
Professor of Pathology, Louisiana State University Medical Center; Visiting Pathologist, Medical Center of Louisiana, Consultant, Children's Hospital, New Orleans, Louisiana
Laboratory Diagnosis of Gastrointestinal Tract and Exocrine Pancreatic Disorders

Yasushi Kasahara, Ph.D., D.M.Sc.
Managing Director, Diagnostics Research & Development, Fujirebio, Inc., Tokyo, Japan
Immunoassays and Immunochemistry

Wasiuddin Ahmed Khan, Ph.D.
Research Associate, Department of Pediatrics, Duke University Medical Center, Durham, North Carolina
Complement and Kinins: Mediators of Inflammation

Carl R. Kjeldsberg, M.D.
Professor of Pathology and Medicine, University of Utah School of Medicine; Chairman, Department of Pathology, University of Utah Health Sciences Center, Salt Lake City, Utah
Cerebrospinal, Synovial, and Serous Body Fluids

Bruce E. Kloster, M.D.
Assistant Professor, Department of Pathology; Director, Blood Bank and Transfusion Medicine, SUNY Health Science Center, Syracuse, New York
Transfusion Medicine

Anthony S. Kurec, M.S., H(ASCP)DLM
Clinical Associate Professor, Department of Medical Technology, College of Health-Related Professions, State University of New York; Assistant Department Manager of Anatomic Pathology, Department of Pathology, University Hospital, State University of New York, Health Science Center, Syracuse, New York
The Clinical Laboratory: Organization, Purposes, and Practice

Peter O. Kwiterovich, Jr, M.D.
Professor of Pediatrics and Medicine, The Johns Hopkins University School of Medicine; Pediatrician, Johns Hopkins Hospital, Baltimore, Maryland
Lipids and Dyslipoproteinemia

Reginaldo B. Lauzon, M.S., MT(ASCP)
Assistant Professor, Education Coordinator, Graduate Program; Assistant Chair, Undergraduate Program, Department of Medical Technology, College of Health-Related Professions, SUNY Health Science Center, Syracuse, New York
Basic Examination of Urine

H. Peter Lehmann, Ph.D.
Professor, Department of Pathology, Professor of Medical Technology, Department of Medical Technology, Louisiana State University Medical Center, New Orleans, Louisiana
Appendix 4

Frank Ju-Feng Liu, M.D., FCAP
Associate Professor of Laboratory Medicine; Associate Pathologist, Division of Laboratory Medicine, The University of Texas M.D. Anderson Cancer Center, Houston, Texas
Laboratory Diagnosis of Gastrointestinal Tract and Exocrine Pancreatic Disorders

Linda M. Mann, Ph.D.
Assistant Professor, Departments of Pathology and Pediatrics; Associate Director, Clinical Microbiology Laboratory, University of Texas Medical Branch at Galveston, Galveston, Texas
Spirochete Infections

Rex M. McCallum, M.D.
Associate Professor of Medicine, Division of Rheumatology, Allergy, and Clinical Immunology, Duke University Medical School; Vice Chair for Clinical Services, Department of Medicine, Duke University Arthritis Center, Duke University Medical Center, Durham, North Carolina
Vasculitis

Richard A. McPherson, M.D.
Professor of Pathology and Chairman, Division of Clinical Pathology; Director of Laboratories, Medical College of Virginia Hospitals, Virginia Commonwealth University, Richmond, Virginia
Specific Proteins

Jonathan L. Miller, M.D., Ph.D.
Professor of Pathology, College of Medicine; Director of Clinical Pathology, SUNY Health Science Center at Syracuse, Syracuse, New York
Blood Platelets; Blood Coagulation and Fibrinolysis

Michael W. Morris, M.S., DLM(ASCP)SH
Professor of Medical Technology, College of Health-Related Professions; Manager, Department of Pathology, University Hospital, SUNY Health Science Center at Syracuse, Syracuse, New York
Basic Examination of Blood

Robert M. Nakamura, M.D.
Chairman Emeritus, Department of Pathology, Scripps Clinic and Research Foundation, La Jolla, California
Immunoassays and Immunochemistry; Clinical and Laboratory Evaluation of Systemic Rheumatic Diseases; Organ-Related Autoimmune Diseases; Molecular Pathology: An Introduction

Andy N. D. Nguyen, MSME M.D.
Assistant Professor of Pathology, University of Texas Medical School at Houston; Director of Clinical Chemistry, Lyndon B. Johnson General Hospital, Houston, Texas
Principles of Instrumentation

Walter W. Noll, M.D.
Professor of Pathology, Dartmouth Medical School, Hanover, New Hampshire; Director, Clinical Chemistry and Molecular Genetics Diagnostic Laboratories, Dartmouth-Hitchcock Medical Center, Lebanon, New Hampshire
Molecular Diagnosis of Genetic Diseases

David Nostro, M.S., MT(ASCP)
Director of Quality Assurance, Department of Pathology and Laboratory Medicine, Department of Veterans Affairs Medical Center, Brooklyn, New York
Cell Biology and Early Tumor Detection

Maurice R. G. O'Gorman, M.Sc., Ph.D., D(ABMLI)
Assistant Professor—Pediatrics, Northwestern University Medical School; Director, Diagnostic Immunology and Flow Cytometry Laboratories, The Children's Memorial Hospital, Chicago, Illinois
Laboratory Evaluation of the Cellular Immune System

Helene Paxton, M.S., MT(ASCP)
President, Research Director, Integrated Diagnostics, Inc, Baltimore, Maryland
Laboratory Evaluation of the Cellular Immune System

David H. Persing, M.D., Ph.D.
Associate Professor of Laboratory Medicine; Director, Molecular Microbiology Laboratory, Mayo Clinic, Mayo Foundation for Medical Education and Research, Rochester, Minnesota
Spirochete Infections

Michael A. Pfaller, M.D.
Professor, Department of Pathology, University of Iowa College of Medicine; Co-Director, Clinical Microbiology and Molecular Pathology Laboratories, University of Iowa Hospitals and Clinics, Iowa City, Iowa
Molecular Pathology of Infectious Diseases

Matthew R. Pincus, M.D., Ph.D.
Professor of Pathology, SUNY Health Science Center; Chairman, Department of Pathology and Laboratory Medicine, Veterans Affairs Medical Center, Brooklyn, New York
Interpreting Laboratory Results: Reference Values and Decision Making; Evaluation of Renal Function, Water, Electrolytes, Acid-Base Balance, and Blood Gases; Assessment of Liver Function; Clinical Enzymology; Cell Biology and Early Tumor Detection; Toxicology and Therapeutic Drug Monitoring

Margaret A. Piper, Ph.D.
Adjunct Professor, Department of Pathology and Laboratory Medicine, Emory University, Atlanta, Georgia
Molecular Diagnostics: Basic Principles and Techniques

Herbert F. Polesky, M.D.
Director, Memorial Blood Centers of Minnesota; Professor Department of Laboratory Medicine and Pathology, University of Minnesota School of Medicine, Minneapolis, Minnesota
Blood Groups, Human Leukocyte Antigens and DNA Polymorphism, and Parentage Testing

Harry G. Preuss, M.D.
Professor of Medicine and Pathology, Georgetown University Medical Center, Washington, D.C.
Evaluation of Renal Function, Water, Electrolytes, Acid-Base Balance, and Blood Gases

Basil M. Rifkind, M.D., FRCP
Senior Scientific Advisor, National Institutes of Health, National Heart, Lung, and Blood Institute, Division of Heart and Vascular Disease, Vascular Research Program, Bethesda, Maryland
Lipids and Dyslipoproteinemia

Zeev Ronai, Ph.D.
Associate Professor, Department of Microbiology and Immunology and Department of Pathology, New York Medical College; Head, Molecular Carcinogenesis, American Health Foundation, Valhalla, New York
Polymerase Chain Reaction in Early Detection and Monitoring of Cancer

Jerald M. Rosenbaum, M.D.
Associate Clinical Professor of Pathology, Tufts University School of Medicine, Boston, Massachusetts; Chief, Clinical Pathology, Baystate Medical Center, Springfield, Massachusetts
Examination of Amniotic Fluid

Siddhartha Sarkar, Ph.D.
Clinical Associate Professor of Pathology, College of Medicine; Director of Andrology, University Hospital, SUNY Health Science Center, Syracuse, New York
Andrology Laboratory and Fertility Assessment

John A. Schaffner, M.D.
Associate Professor of Medicine, Rush Medical College; Director, Clinical Gastroenterology, Rush–Presbyterian–St. Luke Medical Center, Chicago, Illinois
Assessment of Liver Function

G. Berry Schumann, M.D.
Adjunct Associate Professor, University of Connecticut, School of Allied Health Professions, Storrs, Connecticut; Director, Cytopathology and Cytotechnology, Dianon Systems, Inc., Stratford, Connecticut
Basic Examination of Urine

David B. Seifer, M.D.
Associate Professor, Division Director of Reproductive Endocrinology and Infertility, The Ohio State University Medical Center, Columbus, Ohio
Clinical Application of Human Chorionic Gonadotropin

Gregory P. Smith, M.D.
Assistant Professor of Pathology, University of Utah School of Medicine; Staff Pathologist, St. Mark's Hospital, Salt Lake City, Utah
Cerebrospinal, Synovial, and Serous Body Fluids

James W. Smith, M.D.
Professor and Chair, Department of Pathology and Laboratory Medicine, Indiana University School of Medicine, Indianapolis, Indiana
Medical Parasitology

Sanford A. Stass, M.D.
Professor of Pathology and Medicine, Director, Laboratories of Pathology, University of Maryland School of Medicine and University of Maryland Medical System, Department of Pathology, Baltimore, Maryland
Molecular Pathology: An Introduction; Molecular Genetics of Hematopoietic Neoplasms

Mark H. Stoler, M.D.
Associate Professor of Pathology, University of Virginia Health Sciences Center, Charlottesville, Virginia
Tissue In Situ *Hybridization*

Robert L. Sunheimer, M.S., MT(ASCP)SC
Associate Professor, Department of Medical Technology, College of Health Related Professions, SUNY Health Science Center at Syracuse, Syracuse, New York
Principles of Instrumentation

Susan L. Swarner, M.P.H. (Forensic Science)
Supervisory DNA Analyst, Armed Forces DNA Identification Laboratory, DoD DNA Registry, Office of the Armed Forces Medical Examiner, Armed Forces Institute of Pathology, Washington, D.C.
Forensic Identity Testing by DNA Analysis

Gregory A. Threatte, M.D.
Associate Professor, Department of Pathology; Director, Clinical Chemistry, Division of Clinical Pathology, University Hospital, SUNY Health Science Center, Syracuse, New York
Physician Office Laboratories; Carbohydrates

Christopher P. Tirabassi, M.B.A., MT(ASCP)DLM
Clinical Associate Professor, Department of Medical Technology, College of Health-Related Professions, State University of New York, Health Science Center at Syracuse; Administrator, Internist Associates of Central New York, PC, Syracuse, New York
Physician Office Laboratories

Russell H. Tomar, M.D.
Professor, Pathology and Laboratory Medicine, University of Wisconsin—Madison; Director, Immunopathology Laboratory, University of Wisconsin Hospital and Clinics, Madison, Wisconsin
Laboratory Evaluation of Immunoglobulin Function and Humoral Immunity

Elizabeth R. Unger, Ph.D., M.D.
Associate Professor, Department of Pathology and Laboratory Medicine, Emory University School of Medicine, Atlanta, Georgia
Molecular Diagnostics: Basic Principles and Techniques

David H. Walker, M.D.
Professor and Chairman, Department of Pathology, University of Texas—Medical Branch, Galveston, Texas
Chlamydial, Rickettsial, and Mycoplasmal Infections

John A. Washington, M.D.
Professor, Department of Pathology, The Cleveland Clinic Foundation Health Sciences Center of The Ohio State University, Ohio State University, Columbus, Ohio; Vice Chairman, Division of Pathology and Laboratory Medicine, Chairman, Department of Clinical Pathology, Head, Section of Microbiology, The Cleveland Clinic Foundation, Cleveland, Ohio
Medical Bacteriology; In Vitro *Testing of Antimicrobial Agents*

Victor Walter Weedn, Lieutenant Colonel, U.S. Army, M.D., J.D.
Chief Deputy Medical Examiner for DoD DNA Registry, Armed Forces DNA Identification Laboratory, Rockville, Maryland
Forensic Identity Testing by DNA Analysis

Robert E. Wenk, M.D., M.S.
Clinical Professor of Pathology, Milton S. Hershey Medical Center, Pennsylvania State University, Hershey, Pennsylvania; Clinical Associate Professor of Human Genetics, University of Maryland; Assistant Professor of Pathology, The Johns Hopkins University; Director, Clinical Laboratories and Blood Bank, Sinai Hospital; Director, Baltimore Rh Typing Laboratory, Baltimore, Maryland
Examination of Amniotic Fluid

Fred W. Westenfeld, MT(ASCP)SM
Clinical Instructor, Department of Biomedical Technologies, University of Vermont; Special Microbiology Team Leader, Fletcher Allen Health Care Center, Burlington, Vermont
Mycotic Diseases

Delbert R. Wigfall, M.D.
Assistant Professor of Pediatrics, Duke University Medical Center, Durham, North Carolina
Complement and Kinins: Mediators of Inflammation

Washington C. Winn, Jr., M.D., M.B.A.
Professor, Department of Pathology, University of Vermont Medical School; Director, Clinical Microbiology Laboratory, Fletcher Allen Health Care, Medical Center Hospital of Vermont Campus, Burlington, Vermont
Mycotic Diseases

Jannie Woo, Ph.D.
Professor of Pathology, SUNY Health Science Center, Syracuse, New York
Quality Management; Metabolic Intermediates and Inorganic Ions

Gail L. Woods, M.D.
Professor of Pathology; Director, Division of Microbiology, University of Texas, Medical Branch, Galveston, Texas
Chlamydial, Rickettsial, and Mycoplasmal Infections; Medical Bacteriology; In Vitro *Testing of Antimicrobial Agents; Spirochete Infections; Mycobacteria; Specimen Collection and Handling for Diagnosis of Infectious Diseases*

James T. Wu, Ph.D.
Professor of Pathology, University of Utah Medical Center; Medical Director of Special Chemistry Laboratory, Associated Regional and University Pathologists, Inc. (ARUP), Salt Lake City, Utah
Diagnosis and Management of Cancer Using Serologic Tumor Markers

Margaret Yungbluth, M.D.
Assistant Professor of Pathology, Northwestern University Medical School, Department of Pathology; Staff Pathologist, St. Joseph Hospital, Chicago, Illinois
Viral Infections

Edmond J. Yunis, M.D.
Professor of Pathology, Harvard Medical School; Chief, Division of Immunogenetics, Medical Director, HLA Laboratory, Dana-Farber Cancer Institute, Boston, Massachusetts
The Major Histocompatibility Complex and Disease

Hyman J. Zimmerman, M.D., MACP
Professor of Medicine Emeritus, George Washington University Medical Center and Distinguished Scientist Emeritus, Armed Forces Institute of Pathology, Washington, D.C.
Clinical Enzymology

Preface

Clinical pathology and laboratory medicine contribute more hard scientific objective data and information to a patient's medical care and medical record and database than any other single source. The most use of clinical laboratory measurements and examinations today (approximately two thirds) is in clinical and therapeutic management and monitoring, with the remainder used mostly for confirming or ruling out a diagnosis, followed by case finding or screening to detect disease or risk factors to promote health; last, such determinations are used for assessment of prognosis or magnitude or extent of existing disease. Over the past decade, an explosion in biomedical information and technology, and the new biology of medicine (cell and molecular biology, genetics, immunology, and reproductive biology) have been translated into patient care primarily through the clinical laboratory. These trends will continue to transform the practice of medicine and the clinical laboratory and clinical pathology itself into the next century. The 19th edition of this book, which has become synonymous with clinical pathology and laboratory medicine for over 85 years, will sustain and assist physicians and others in this new era of medicine that has been undergoing change as a result of the biomedical information explosion and health care reform in a competitive, regulated, and resource-limited environment.

The objective of the 19th edition is to provide a scientific information resource in virtually all aspects of clinical pathology and laboratory medicine relevant to patient care, health promotion, and disease prevention to promote understanding and facilitate learning with critical analysis. It also includes:

1. Identification of appropriate measurements and examinations for diagnosis, for confirmation of a clinical impression, for guiding therapy or patient management, for prognosis, and for case finding or screening to identify risk factors in health promotion and disease prevention.
2. Delineation of the order, sequence, or grouping of determinations, when appropriate, and circumstances in which such measurements and examinations should be requested.
3. Interpretation and translation or explanation of laboratory measurements and examinations in light of a patient's particular medical problem and progress.
4. Promotion of the understanding and clarification of pathophysiology or natural history of disease as reflected by clinical pathology information/data.
5. Recognition of pitfalls, problems, and limitations of laboratory data, including quality control (sensitivity, precision, accuracy, specificity), drug interaction, and predictive values, as well as relative merits of an assay in terms of methodology, turnabout time, patient preparation, communication, and cost effectiveness.
6. Appreciation and understanding of the importance of laboratory quality management for efficient and cost-effective medical and health care delivery.

However, the thrust of this 19th edition remains the same as in earlier editions but also encompasses the new biology of medicine manifest primarily in molecular pathology (Part 7); immunopathology (Part 5); clinical chemistry (Part 2); hematology, coagulation, and transfusion medicine (Part 4); medical microbiology (Part 6); and urine and other body fluids (Part 3). The andrology laboratory and fertility assessment (Chap. 22) are presented for the first time, along with other chapters on clinical applications of human chorionic gonadotropin measurement (Chap. 20), examination of amniotic fluid (Chap. 21), and evaluation of endocrine function (Chap. 16) in order to bring reproductive biology to the forefront.

This edition begins in Part 1 with an examination of the clinical laboratory, including its organization, purposes, and practice, that is, operations management so crucial to laboratory service. The structure of the central laboratory in a hospital also serving outpatients persists amidst the pull and push of near patient care/alternative site testing (AST); physician office laboratories, or POLs (Chap. 2); and regional laboratories. All of these sites are experiencing the impact of new and renewed technology (Chap. 3), not only in terms of productivity (increased volume and variety of complex measurements/examinations) but also in selecting the most expeditious laboratory service responsive to providers' and patients' needs in terms of access, cost, and quality. This is a challenge to pathologists and all laboratorians to thrive in managed care with capitation and discounted service contracts. Quality management (Chap. 6) and informatics, imaging and pathologist's work stations (Chap. 5), including telemedicine and telepathology, are key to quality in laboratory medicine in all 63 current, updated and augmented, strengthened chapters that embrace each topic in a compelling manner from patient specimen collection and processing to results reporting. A new chapter (Chap. 4) describes the selection and interpretation of laboratory information and data results to achieve the most cost-effective, efficient medical problem-solving with clinical laboratory testing.

For the first time, molecular pathology and molecular diagnostics are presented in depth (Chaps. 55 to 63). These sections embrace basic principles and techniques, establishing a molecular diagnostics laboratory, molecular diagnosis and pathology of infectious and genetic diseases and hematopoietic neoplasms, tissue *in situ* hybridization, and forensic identity, as well as comprehensive paternity testing through DNA fingerprinting.

Similarly, oncology with cell biology and early tumor detection have been expanded for better understanding and application of serologic tumor markers (Chap. 45), polymerase chain reaction (PCR) for oncogenes (Chap. 14), and oncoproteins in body fluids and tissues (Chap. 15) plus genetics (Chaps. 58 and 59) in the diagnosis, management, early detection, and monitoring of cancer.

Immunology and immunopathology is renewed and enhanced through updating and expansion to include cytokines and adhesion molecules (Chap. 37), major histocompatibility complex (MHC), transplantation and specific disease associations (Chap. 38 and 39), vascular inflammatory disease (Chap. 42), organ-directed autoimmune diseases (Chap. 43), rheumatic diseases (Chap. 41), allergic diseases (Chap. 44), and serologic tumor markers (Chap. 45) relevant to cancer monitoring.

The section on transfusion medicine (Chaps. 30 and 31) addresses pretransfusion testing and problem-solving of untoward/unexpected reactions, as well as therapy with blood products (components and derivatives) and therapeutic applications of apheresis including collection, processing, and dispensing stem cells from bone marrow, peripheral, and cord blood.

Part 6, entitled Medical Microbiology, begins with a chapter on viral infections (Chap. 46) and other vectors of infection (Chlamydial, Rickettsial and Mycoplasmal [Chap. 47]) before continuing with classic medical bacteriology (Chap. 48) plus a chapter on mycobacteria (Chap. 51), underscoring tuberculosis with emerging drug resistance and widespread infection among immunosuppressed patients. Spirochete infections (Chap. 50) and mycology (Chap. 52) with medical parasitology (Chap. 53) and antimicrobial in vitro testing (Chap. 49) also are covered in a comprehensive, succinct manner. Because of its special importance in achieving maximum patient and physician benefit from the laboratory, the chapter on specimen collection and handling for diagnosis of infectious diseases (Chap. 54) concludes this part.

The advent of managed care and a greater emphasis on primary care, with awareness of the emergence of practice parameters and practice guidelines through text, tables, and images, continue to require increased consolidation and focus on essential information that is relevant to early diagnosis and more cost-effective and efficient clinical management through laboratory methods. Clinical pathology organ panels with diagnostic and management applications have been expanded and updated, along with the guidelines for ordering blood for elective surgery within the inside covers of the book.

This approach in seven parts and 63 chapters should assist not only virtually all clinicians, especially primary care physicians and pathologists, but also undergraduate medical students, medical technology students, and graduate medical education trainees and residents in pathology and related disciplines to attain information in the knowledge management and learning process for specific resource reference and continuous reading to promote continuing medical education and life long learning.

Although individual authors deserve full credit for their contributions, I accept full responsibility for any errors of omission or commission and enthusiastically welcome any comments, reactions, or suggestions regarding this book to make the next edition even better.

It is a privilege and honor to serve as editor of this 19th edition.

JOHN BERNARD HENRY, M.D.

Acknowledgments

It is with sincere gratitude and pleasure that I acknowledge the collaboration of my esteemed colleagues as new associate editors: Frederick R. Davey, M.D., Robert M. Nakamura, M.D., Mathew R. Pincus, M.D., Ph.D., and Gail L. Woods, M.D., and assistant editors David J. Bylund, M.D., Howard S. Fox, M.D., Ph.D., and Sanford A. Stass, M.D. Each has been most gracious, diligent, and resourceful in their efforts to accomplish our task of renewal and enhancement for the revision of this book. A work of multiple authors requires a willingness of the contributors to accept the guidance of the editor. Our contributors have been responsible and responsive in this regard and also have my respect and thanks for a job well done.

Special thanks are due to Vincent P. Perna, M.D., Dan R. Alexander, M.D., and Lesley A. Winters, M.D. for their assistance in reviewing and critiquing chapter manuscripts and follow through. In addition, I am grateful to Sharad Mathur, M.D., John Ninos, M.D., Michael Nolan, M.D., and Felicitas Lacbawan, M.D. for their much-needed assistance in proofreading chapters. Constance K. Stein, Ph.D., Antony Shrimpton, Ph.D., and Celeste M. Lamberson, M.S., MT(ASCP) gave me special assistance and guidance in the field of molecular pathology and genetics.

Paul Bachner, M.D.'s critical review and contribution to Chapter 2, Physician Office Laboratories, and Richard McPherson, M.D.'s critical review and comments overall and in targeted areas were especially valuable and most appreciated. Peter J. Howanitz, M.D., and Joan H. Howanitz, M.D., authors of "Evaluation of Endocrine Function," took this chapter over from me after the 14th and 15th editions for the 16th, 17th, and 18th editions, and they laid the foundation for our efforts in this edition. Hence, they have my gratitude for a solid foundation and review of Chapter 16.

In addition, I wish to acknowledge and express my eternal gratitude to my former associate editors, Douglas A. Nelson, M.D., Russell H. Tomar, M.D., and John A. Washington, M.D., who worked with me on the 16th, 17th, and 18th editions, as well as to Gregory A. Threatte, M.D., who served as assistant editor on the 18th edition. Although their presence and association were missed in this edition, the impact of their efforts was sustained.

I also acknowledge with gratitude the stimulus of all the medical technology, medical students, residents, and colleagues who have helped in so many ways over the years to improve this text. Likewise, I am most grateful to all the physicians but especially all my colleagues in pathology who have written or commented to me on how to make the book better. I ask the forgiveness of each for not identifying them individually here, lest I expand the text inordinately and possibly omit someone. However, each can take pride in their contributions, and that is most important.

For her sustained loyalty and extra effort, I express my deepest gratitude and sincere appreciation to my associate, Ms. Joan A. Hough, who has been most supportive with meticulous attention to detail and with a creative commitment and dedication in helping me move this edition forward in a timely manner. Our association for nearly a decade at the SUNY Health Science Center at Syracuse has made it possible for me to undertake this project as well as participate in so many other related activities that have enhanced this effort.

To our entire SUNY Health Science Center Library staff, under the direction of Ms. Suzanne Murray, and especially Mr. Peter Uva, I am most appreciative and grateful for all their assistance in validating references and conducting literature searches. Having access to and support from a superb Biomedical Information Resource Center/Medical Library and staff, especially Rosemary Bundy and Diane Hawkins, is an essential prerequisite to writing. I would also like to give recognition and thanks to our talented and professional staff in the Educational Communications Department, directed by Mr. Joseph Smith and, in particular, Winthrop H. Rice, III, Ph.D., who have helped me prepare teaching materials and have taught me to appreciate and apply the desktop computer as a tool for learning.

Special thanks and gratitude are due to the associate editors' spouses: Doris Davey, Raymond P. Latimer, husband of Gail L. Woods, M.D, Jane Nakamura, and Naomi Pincus. I would also like to thank the assistant editors' spouses: Audrey Bylund, Nora Sarvetnick, wife of Howard S. Fox, M.D., Ph.D., and Ann Stass. Without their understanding and faithful support, the contributions of my associate and assistant editors would not have been possible. I am also grateful to the families of the author contributors, who made it possible for our authors to fulfill their assignments in a timely manner.

To my deceased colleagues and friends, Israel Davidsohn, M.D., and James Patterson, M.D., I am and always will be grateful for their encouragement, guidance, and collaboration. Without them and their confidence in me, I would not have been able to celebrate this, my sixth edition of this text.

In addition, there are associates, colleagues, friends, and others who have taught me much over the years and from whom I continue to learn. I acknowledge their sustained support, and will always be grateful to them. There are many others who, in various ways, have contributed to and assisted in this work. I express my sincere thanks to them, although they are not identified.

I sincerely appreciate the cooperation and guidance of Lisette Bralow, Medical Book Editor-in-Chief, Lesley Day, Editor, Janice Gaillard, Developmental Editor, Ms. Sandra Won, Assistant Developmental Editor, and Mr. Michael Carcel, Production Manager, as well as the entire staff of W.B. Saunders Company who shared and supported this endeavor.

Writing and editing a book is truly a labor of love that makes one feel humble and grateful to countless individuals who have made it possible. Hence, I am forever grateful to those I have identified and others not recognized here.

JOHN BERNARD HENRY, M.D.

Contents

Color plates are found after pages 456, 472, 584, 616, 648, 680, 1160, 1208, 1224, and 1256.

Part 1

THE CLINICAL LABORATORY

Edited by
John Bernard Henry, M.D.

Chapter 1

The Clinical Laboratory: Organization, Purposes, and Practice

John Bernard Henry, M.D.
Anthony S. Kurec, M.S., H(ASCP)DLM

The purpose and function of laboratorians through clinical pathology and laboratory medicine are to assist clinicians in (1) confirming or rejecting a diagnosis, (2) providing guidelines in patient management, (3) establishing a prognosis, (4) detecting disease through case finding or screening, and (5) monitoring follow-up therapy. Satisfaction in laboratory performance is attained through quality assurance, which mandates maximal contributions to benefit patients and to assist health care providers in an effective, efficient, and economic manner. Although accuracy and precision have always been prerequisites to good laboratory service, promptness of a lucid result report is equally critical to overall excellence in patient care. The generation of quality laboratory values must be inherent by explicit adherence to basic laboratory principles through proper collection, handling, and processing of *each* patient specimen. This is best accomplished by implementing appropriate quality assurance programs that identify optimal utilization of space, equipment, reagents, and personnel with outcome measurements. Other aspects to consider include hiring and training qualified staff, employing sound management practices, and providing a safe and healthy environment. These systems must be adhered to by thoroughly understanding and responding to laboratory measurements and examinations by all participants in the management process of patient care.

This chapter reviews fundamental knowledge important in the preparation, acquisition, and analysis of patient material submitted for laboratory measurement and examination, keeping in mind why specimens are submitted and how activities within a laboratory accomplish this service (Table 1–1). We also provide an overview of clinical pathology and laboratory medicine at a time when transformation is occurring with the introduction of health care reform and managed care concepts.

ORGANIZATION AND OPERATION OF THE LABORATORY

Operational Standards and Organization

The operation of a clinical laboratory and effective delivery of service to clinicians, patients, and public requires a complex interdigitation of (1) expertise in medical, scientific, and technical areas; (2) resources in the form of personnel, laboratory and data processing equipment, supplies, and facilities; and (3) skills in organization, management, and communication. All laboratory personnel, especially those in leadership and management, must be aware of current accreditation and governmental regulations and evolving practice guidelines and parameters that relate to laboratory services. The increasing costs of medical care mandate that the responsibility of laboratory utilization falls on the laboratory and clinical colleagues while providing the best services for patients. Misuse of laboratory determinations and diagnostic procedures has been reviewed (Adams, 1992; Axt-Adam, 1993) and means to improve the efficiency in laboratory utilization and performance have been proposed (Watts, 1988). Selectively reducing overutilization of laboratory services may have a negative impact on quality care, and administrative intervention often improves test ordering beyond that achieved through education alone. Panels of selected measurements and examinations that reflect an organ or specific disease are especially beneficial to medical problem solving; they can also provide the most cost-effective and current utilization management in conjunction with practice guidelines. Other studies have shown that initiating a feedback system to the individual physician may be an effective self-monitoring mechanism (Hasman, 1993). This requires good management and communication skills at all levels in the laboratory.

In Figure 1–1, laboratory medicine can be viewed as a

Table 1–1. SCHEMATIC OUTLINE OF ACTIVITIES IN PATHOLOGY AND LABORATORY MEDICINE

	Leadership and Management Administration	
	Patient Care Services	
Indications and selection	Technology and generation	Interpretation and translation
	TEACHING	
	RESEARCH	

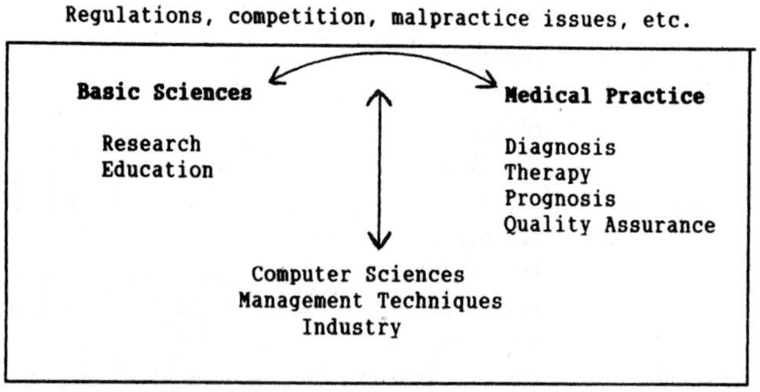

Figure 1–1. A concept of the practice of pathology and laboratory medicine.

bridging endeavor linking basic biological and physical sciences with medical principles. This bridging is not complete without the appropriate support mechanisms of modern equipment; good reagents, interfaced through computer technology and informatics; and greater understanding of the laboratory by industry and vendors. Regulatory and financial controls have significantly altered the way laboratories operate and have changed them from revenue generators to cost centers. In response, there is a shift from hospital to free-standing and ambulatory sites to maximize revenue and reduce costs.

Integrated into the fabric of laboratory medicine is the need for education and research. It is imperative for laboratories to assume a significant level of responsibility in educating all health care providers so that utilization and test ordering patterns are implemented in the best interest of the patient and clinician decision making at an appropriate cost. The team approach to patient management that includes the laboratory professional staff enhances the level of care provided and economically utilizes available resources. Clinicians, patients, students, industry partners, and others associated with health care are now viewed as customers (Montebello, 1994). Furthermore, continuing education for laboratory personnel is essential to promoting a quality service and good employee morale. The laboratory and entire organization reap the benefits as each member of the team enhances his or her knowledge base. Congruent to education is the need for a well-developed research program. Through sustained efforts in research management, new technologies and procedures are developed and implemented to provide the highest level in patient diagnosis and clinical management.

The future of pathology and laboratory medicine through clinical laboratory services is evident in four directions: (1) molecular pathology diagnostics (polymerase chain reaction [PCR], DNA probes, restriction fragment length polymorphism [RFLP], genetics) (Inhorn, 1994); (2) point-of-care (POC)/alternate-site testing (Friedman, 1994); (3) automation through enhanced informatics and robotics (O'Bryan, 1994); and (4) telemedicine. The use of telecommunication in Pathology (Telepathology) as part of Telemedicine ranges from the use of simple ISDN (International Standardized Digital Network; Kayser, 1993) image transfer to technology that incorporates image processing through the use of parallel computers, clusters of high-performance work stations, high-resolution video equipment, and multigigabit-per-second telecommunications. Digitization and high-speed transmission of images, three-dimensional reconstruction of cell and tissue morphology, and the use of intelligence/neural networks are in development at different sites across the country (Corona, 1994). These systems are part of a telemedicine project that will link hospitals, clinics, extended care facilities, and other health care provider offices. Communication links will provide real-time, robotic microscopy for consultations, preventive evaluations; aid in forensic activities; enhance educational endeavors; promote videoconferencing; and assist in the development of regional health care facilities. Development of these regional systems will increase access to health care services, improve medical education, and provide continuity in individual health care maintenance. Table 1–2 identifies the new biology of medicine that promotes and permeates patient care through a transformation in clinical laboratory service and that will continue to have a favorable impact on patient care.

Leadership and Management

Whereas leadership provides the direction of where one (or an organization) is going, management provides the steps of how to get there. If you do not know where you are going, any road will get you there. Hence, goals for direction and objectives for steps are crucial to an organization (Table 1–3). Likewise, effective management uses good communication skills to work with and through people to get things done. It requires an optimal mix of people-oriented and task-oriented leaders who make good decisions, are skilled communicators and negotiators, are sensitive to the needs of others, and care about the outcome. Continuing education through the College of American Pathologists (CAP), American Society of Clinical Pathologists (ASCP), American College of Physician Executives (ACPE), and Clinical Laboratory Management Association (CLMA) provides ample opportunities to acquire, reaffirm and improve, and maintain current knowledge and skills in leadership and management.

The efficient operation and effective delivery of laboratory services are dependent on modern equipment, well-trained staff, adequate and well-designed physical environment, and a good management team. Implementation of total quality management (TQM) and continuous quality improvement (CQI) techniques have been recognized as useful tools in establishing quality leadership (Juran, 1988; Deming, 1986). One particular instrument used in establishing quality management is the FOCUS-PDCA process (Baralden, 1989), as shown in Table 1–4. This process has been successfully used to solve problems within the laboratory environment (Denington, 1993). It may also be used in response to many of the responsibilities facing laboratory managers (Table 1–5). Although these issues and others are beyond the scope of this book, an excellent source is *Administration and Supervision in Laboratory Medicine* by John Snyder and David Wilkinson (1995).

Table 1–2. NEW BIOLOGY OF MEDICINE

Cell biology
Molecular biology
Neurobiology
Reproductive biology
Immunology

Table 1–3. LEADERSHIP VERSUS MANAGEMENT: GOALS INDICATE DIRECTION AND OBJECTIVES

Leadership
Goals: Where
Management
Objectives: How Steps 1. Organize 2. Plan 3. Direct 4. Control 5. Staff

Facilities and Design

A cost-effective and successful laboratory service is one that comes from planning and design to meet current and foreseeable needs for personnel, equipment, and space. Organization of the clinical laboratory includes both structure and process, where structure refers to framework and process to interactive relationships and systems. Three key elements to organization within the laboratory are the workplace, staff, and tasks to be performed. These existing or anticipated elements provide the foundation for the most effective use of space, personnel, and finances. Five main steps (Table 1–6) to complete this process include preparation, developing and understanding the function, schematic design, design development, and construction process (Koenig, 1989).

The process of designing a new or refurbishing an existing laboratory involves many decisions and requires a number of professionals to assist in the development and implementation of such projects. Laboratorians must provide constant feedback to the designers to ensure optimal placement of utilities and that integrity of space functionality is maintained. Some considerations (Painter, 1993) in the

Table 1–4. QUALITY MANAGEMENT PROCESS OF TOTAL QUALITY MANAGEMENT (TQM)

Find a problem or process to improve
Organize a team
Clarify what is known about the process
Understand causes of the problem/variation
Select the way the process is to be improved
Plan implementation of improvements to be made
Do what is appropriate to implement
Check data collected from monitoring—customer outcome
Act to maintain and continue the process

Modified with permission from Columbia/HCA Hospital Corporation, Nashville, TN 37202.

Table 1–5. BASIC MANAGERIAL RESPONSIBILITIES

Quality leadership
Personnel management
Policy and procedure manuals
Criteria-based job descriptions
Recruitment and staffing
Orientation
In-service and continuing education
Staff meetings
Personnel records
Performance evaluation/appraisals
Discipline and dismissal
Legislative/regulatory issues
Medical-legal concerns
Financial management
Marketing
Benchmarking
Productivity assessment

Table 1–6. FACILITY DESIGN PROCESS

Phase	Concerns
Preparation	Needs assessment
	Staffing needs/requirements
	Technologic changes, current and anticipated
	Identify team players (architect, laboratory staff, medical staff, interior designer)
Function	Activities to be performed
	Flow of people and materials
	Storage
	Equipment used
	Utilities
	Specific laboratory sectional needs
Schematic design	Structural design
	Identify construction materials
	Architectural design
	Cost
	System options (plumbing, electricity, heating/ventilation/air conditioning)
Design development	Interior design
	Colors, fabric, texture, finish, etc.
Construction	Bidding/negotiating contracts
	Legal documentation
	Actual construction
	Completion and occupancy

planning process are listed in Table 1–7. Current and future laboratory needs must be determined for the next three to five years to fully capitalize on resources. A well-planned laboratory is essential to efficient use of staff and equipment in a cost-effective manner. Achieving flexibility in the design process, including plumbing, electrical lines, and ventilation, and anticipating future changes in equipment design and development of new technologies, are key to meeting these needs.

Technologic advances have overlapped traditional functions and responsibilities among different laboratory sections; thus the *open laboratory concept* is frequently implemented. This provides the opportunity to share equipment, use staff more effectively, and reduce redundant purchases of equipment and supplies. Such consolidation measures affect overall operational costs. Functional characteristics of each laboratory section must be considered and planned for appropriately, in addition to recognizing the trend for consolidation to a centralized laboratory, while experiencing forces of decentralization with point-of-care (POC) testing. Phlebotomy areas and patient examination rooms (if appropriate) should be *customer friendly* and accessible. Specimen processing, patient registration, and laboratory information system (LIS) should be close to each other. Spatial requirements in relationship to other hospital services must be considered: proximity to emergency department, intensive care units, and operating rooms. Regulatory and safety mandates must be carefully reviewed and implemented appropriately. Robotics, pneumatic tubes, computers, and facsimile machines are the new tools used in modern laboratories and must be accounted for in the design plans. Adequate electri-

Table 1–7. CONSIDERATIONS IN LABORATORY DESIGN

1. In developing a needs assessment, identify space for offices, personal facilities, storage, conference/library area, and students.
2. Routinely review all floor plans and elevations for appropriate usage and ensure space and function are related. Handicap accessibility may be required.
3. Develop and use a *project schedule*.
4. Fumehoods and biological safety cabinets must be located away from high traffic areas and doorways.
5. Modular furniture is generally more expensive than conventional but allows for flexibility in moving or reconfiguration of the laboratory according to current and anticipated needs.
6. Conventional laboratory fixtures may be considered in building depreciation, whereas modular furniture is not.
7. Base cabinets (under lab counters) provide 20% to 30% more storage space than suspended cabinets.
8. Noise control in open labs may be obtained by installing a drop ceiling. Installation of utilities above a drop ceiling adds to flexibility in their placement.
9. In general, space requirements are 150 to 200 net square feet (excludes hallways, walls, custodial closets, etc.) per FTE, or 27 to 40 net square feet per hospital bed.
10. Suggested standard dimensions in planning and designing a laboratory:
    - lab counter width: 2′6″
    - lab counter to wall clearance: 4′
    - lab counter to counter clearance: 7′
    - desk height: 30″
    - keyboard drawer height: 25–27″
    - human body standing: 4 square feet
    - human body sitting: 6 square feet
    - desk space: 3 square feet

Modified with permission from Painter P: Laboratory Design Workshop, Clinical Laboratory Management Association Annual Meeting, 1993; San Antonio, TX.

cal power (including emergency power), temperature control, and ventilation must be in place.

POINT-OF-CARE TESTING (NEAR-PATIENT TESTING, ALTERNATE-SITE TESTING)

Role of Laboratory

Point-of-care (POC) testing (also known as near-patient testing, alternate-site testing (AST), patient-focused testing) is used in a variety of settings such as the emergency department, operating suites, clinics, health maintenance organizations (HMOs), physician offices, and nursing homes (Kurec, 1993). POC brings laboratory testing to the site of the patient rather than obtaining a specimen and sending it to the laboratory. Real-time measurements of a patient's status may be obtained in a short period of time allowing the health care provider to address acute patient needs (Zaloga, 1991; Woo, 1993). The so-called biological half-life of laboratory data for chronically ill patients generally shows minimal changes, whereas the clinical conditions of acutely ill patients are more variable (Geyer, 1992). A POC program must involve the laboratory in the development, maintenance, and decision-making process. POC is recognized by the Joint Commission on Accreditation of Healthcare Organizations (JCAHO; PA 6.4), College of American Pathologists (CAP; Ancillary Testing; section 30.0), and Clinical Laboratory Improvement Act of 1988 (CLIA'88; Federal Register 55CFR, 1990; 57CFR, 1992). Selection of test methodology and instrumentation should be determined by laboratory staff in conjunction with hospital staff. Reasonably reliable instrumentation for POC is available, with improved options and increased test menus to come. Table 1–8 outlines actions to be taken in the development of a POC program. Handorf (1994) and colleagues provide a comprehensive review of POC/alternate-site testing.

Table 1–8. POINT-OF-CARE TESTING CHECKLIST

Action	Date
Needs assessment	
Select method or instrument	
Gain commitment from laboratory, nursing, and medical staff, and any other departments, including top administration (total quality management [TQM] process)	
Identify patient type to be tested	
Identify instrument users (lab staff, nursing staff, operating room staff)	
Research and develop test procedure (accuracy and precision studies)	
Establish quality control/assurance procedures	
Develop guidelines for staff training (qualification, skills checklist, accountability)	
Develop risk management protocols	
Monitor and get feedback	
Make changes and improvements	

Technology Evolution

POC is driven by technology. Microcomputer chips and sensors are incorporated into instrumentation, making it portable and readily accessible. Instrumentation includes portable chemistry analyzers, glucose meters, blood gas analyzers, hemoglobin meters, and coagulation testing. Criteria to follow in selecting appropriate instrumentation are cost, accuracy, ease of maintenance, ability to self-calibrate, quality control functions, reporting capabilities, and safety. Instrumentation should be durable, simple to use, cost-effective, and capable of rapid throughput (turn-around time, TAT).

Team Building

To successfully implement POC testing, a collaborative team effort is required. Often nonlaboratory personnel from nursing, surgery technicians, respiratory therapists, and others may be responsible for actual patient testing. Appropriate training in instrument performance, maintenance, and quality control procedures are essential for quality patient care. Cooperation and acceptance from top administrators to the medical staff and to all others involved are necessary to provide a quality service in a cost-effective manner. It is critical that the laboratory take a leading role in developing and maintaining POC practices (Kurec, 1993).

A POC service is clearly a major evolution in the delivery of health care; the extent and magnitude of application may well challenge conventional laboratory operations. As technology expands and improves, site delivery of laboratory services will be rendered by those responsible for POC. The favorable impact by decreasing TAT of laboratory procedures and prompt medical attention and decision in expediting patient care has yet to be fully appreciated, although our experience with I-Stat (I-Stat Corp., Kanata, Canada) in the Emergency Department has been most positive (Woo, 1993).

Future Direction

Moving laboratory measurements and evaluations closer to the patient's bedside is, and will continue to become, an important part of providing quality patient care. Use of biosensors and noninvasive techniques, such as transcutaneous monitoring, could clearly enhance the caregiver's ability to provide real-time care in a prompt and cost-effective manner (Woo, 1994). As POC technology develops further, its use in patient-focused hospitals and arenas will have a significant impact on personnel and how that care is provided (Cousar, 1994). Nonlaboratorians cross-trained to perform POC testing (and other multidisciplinary functions) and the need for appropriate training and monitoring by laboratory personnel are critical in maintaining a high level of efficiency and quality (Allred, 1994).

PREANALYTICAL TESTING

Measurement/Examination (Test) Requisition

The clinician initiates the request for a laboratory measurement and examination by completing a written order for desired laboratory measurements or examinations in the patient's medical record or chart. This information is conveyed through written or computer order entry. Physician direct order entry and result acquisition through user-friendly computers that are interfaced and networked are realistic approaches to provide prompt and accurate patient care (see Chap. 5). Patient demographics include the patient's name, sex, age, date of birth (DOB), date of admission, date measurement and examination ordered, hospital number, room number, physician, and physician's pharmacy code number. Computer-generated blood collection lists and specimen labels with appropriate patient information (accession number, draw time, tube type, and test name) assist the phlebotomist in the timely and accurate procurement of specimens (Slockbower, 1982; Finn, 1988). Hand-held phlebotomy workstation terminals (Intellihand, Sunquest, Tuscon, AZ) are computer devices that allow uploading and downloading of collection list data. This type of system provides the phlebotomist with a real-time entry of time, technician identification, patient verification, and specimen-type collection. Information can be collected using a bar code reader or an alphanumeric key pad. These data may be uploaded to the LIS to complete collection verification. Monitoring accurate and expedient delivery of measurement and examination requisitions to the laboratory should be an indispensable component of the quality assurance program if the laboratory is to provide prompt delivery of services.

Preparation of the Patient

In preparing a patient for phlebotomy, care should be taken to minimize factors related to activities that might influence laboratory determinations. These factors include diurnal variation, exercise, fasting, diet, ethanol consumption, tobacco smoking, drug ingestion, and posture. Diurnal variation may be encountered when testing for cortisol, serum iron, or neutrophil counts. Physical activity has transient and long-term effects on laboratory determinations. Transient changes may include an initial decrease followed by an increase in free fatty acids—as much as 180% increase in alanine and 300% increase in lactate. Exercise may elevate creatine phosphokinase (CPK), aspartate aminotransferase (AST), and lactate dehydrogenase (LD), and may activate coagulation, fibrinolysis, and platelets (Garza, 1989). These changes are related to increased metabolic activities for energy purposes and usually return to pre-exercise levels soon after exercise cessation (Statland, 1973a). Long-term effects of exercise may increase creatine kinase (CK), aldolase, AST, and LD values. Sex hormones, including plasma testosterone, androstenedione, and luteinizing hormone levels, have been shown to be increased with long-term physical training (Remes, 1979).

After 48 hours of fasting, serum bilirubin concentrations may increase. Fasting 72 hours decreased plasma glucose levels in healthy women to 45 mg/dL (2.5 mmol/L), while a study in men showed an increase in plasma triglycerides, glycerol, and free fatty acids, with no significant change in plasma cholesterol (Statland, 1977). When determining blood constituents such as glucose, triglycerides, cholesterol, and electrolytes, collection should be in the basal state (Garza, 1989). Eating a meal, depending on fat content, may elevate plasma potassium, triglycerides, and alkaline phosphatase. Blood type O or B positive, Lewis-positive secretors may yield especially high levels of the latter (Statland, 1973b). In addition, physiologic changes may include hyperchylomicronemia, thus increasing turbidity of the serum and plasma and potentially interfering with instrument readings. Certain foods or diet regimens may affect serum or urine constituents. A high meat or other protein-rich diet may increase serum urea, ammonia, and urate levels. Food with high unsaturated to saturated fatty acid ratio may show decreased serum cholesterol, whereas a diet rich in purines may show an increased urate value. Foods such as bananas, pineapples, tomatoes, and avocados are rich in serotonin. When ingested, elevated urine excretion of 5-hydroxyindoleacetic acid may be observed. Beverages rich in caffeine elevate plasma free fatty acids and cause release of catecholamines from the adrenal medulla and from brain tissue. Ingestion of ethanol will increase plasma lactate, urate, and triglyceride concentrations. Elevated high-density lipoprotein (HDL) cholesterol, gamma-glutamyl transferase (GGT), urate, and mean corpuscular volume (MCV) have been associated with chronic alcohol abuse. Tobacco smokers have high blood carboxyhemoglobin levels, plasma catecholamines, and serum cortisol. Changes in these hormones often result in decreased numbers of eosinophils, whereas neutrophils, monocytes, and plasma fatty free acids increase. Chronic effects of smoking lead to increased hemoglobin concentration, erythrocyte count (RBC), MCV, and increased leukocyte count (WBC).

Drug interferences are of two types: (1) physiologic *in vivo* effects of the drug and its metabolites on the quantity to be measured, and (2) *in vitro* effects that result from some physical or chemical property that interferes with the assay. A comprehensive list of drug-assay interactions may be found in Young (1975). Table 1–9 lists some drugs associated with hepatic changes, ultimately affecting liver function assays. Table 1–10 is an abridged compilation of the drugs affecting clinical chemistry tests. Some physical attributes to consider when obtaining blood specimens include posture and incorrect tourniquet application. As a patient moves from supine to a standing position, there is a hydrostatic efflux of water and filterable substances from the intravascular space to the dependent interstitial fluid of the extracellular space. Nonfilterable substances, such as proteins, cellular elements, and compounds associated with either, will increase in concentration in the intravascular space. Albumin and calcium levels may become elevated as one changes position from supine to upright. Elements that are effected by postural changes are albumin, total protein, enzymes, calcium, bilirubin, cholesterol, triglycerides, and drugs bound to proteins. Hematocrit, hemoglobin, and leukocyte levels may also rise. Incorrect application of the tourniquet and fist exercise can result in erroneous test results. Using a tourniquet to collect blood to determine lactate concentration may increase the lactate to falsely high levels. Prolonged tourniquet application may also increase serum enzymes, proteins, and protein-bound substances, including cholesterol, calcium, and triglycerides. Stress, anxiety, and hyperventilation may affect

Table 1–9. SELECTED MEASUREMENTS OF HEPATIC FUNCTION AND A LIST OF DRUGS IMPLICATED IN PHARMACOLOGIC INTERFERENCE

Effects on Liver Function Tests	
Urine:	Bilirubin: increased
Serum:	Alkaline phosphatase: increased
	Bilirubin: increased
	Bromsulphalein (BSP): increased
	Glucose: decreased
	Alanine aminotransferase (ALT) and aspartate aminotransferase (AST): increased

Drugs That May Affect Liver Function Tests	
Acetohexamide	Methylthiouracil
Allopurinol	Nicotinic acid
Aminosalicylic acid	Nitrofurantoin
Amodiaquine	Novobiocin
Amphotericin B	Oleandomycin
Anabolic agents	Oxazepam
Androgens	Oxyphenbutazone
Chlorpropamide	Paraldehyde
Cyclophosphamide	Paramethadione
Desipramine	Phenacemide
Erythromycin	Phenacetin
Glycopyrrolate	Phenothiazines
Haloperidol	Phenylbutazone
Halothane	Progestins
Hydrazine	Progestins-estrogens (oral contraceptives)
Imipramine	Propylthiouracil
Indomethacin	Quinacrine (mepacrine)
Isoniazid	Sulfonamides
Lincomycin	Tetracyclines
MAO inhibitors	Thiosemicarbazones
Mercaptopurine	Thiothixene
Metaxalone	Tolazamide
Methoxsalen	Tolbutamide
Methoxyflurane	Trimethadione
Methyldopa	Uracil mustard

Modified from Martin TJ: The Pharmacologic Interactions with Laboratory Test Values, 1970: 596 Burnhamthorpe, Etobiocoke, Ontario, Canada.

hormone secretions and acid-base balance, and may elevate leukocyte counts, serum lactate, or free fatty acids. In general, patients scheduled for phlebotomy should refrain from strenuous physical activity, alcohol, drugs, or changes in diet for 24 hours prior to procedure. The patient should go to bed at the usual time and rise no later than one hour before anticipated specimen collection (Alström, 1993).

Before Specimen Collection

Venipuncture is accomplished using a needle attached to an evacuated glass test tube with a rubber stopper. Rubber stoppers are color-coded to distinguish whether the tube contains a specific anticoagulant, is a plain tube, or a special tube made chemically clean (e.g., for lead or iron determinations). Listed in Table 1–11 are the most frequently used anticoagulants based on color-coded tube stoppers. The system makes direct sampling from a vein economical and efficient. Tubes come in various sizes (2, 5, 7, and 10 mL) with disposable needles. The use of anticoagulants allows for analysis of whole-blood specimens or plasma constituents obtained by centrifugation and separation of the plasma. Plasma contains fibrinogens, which is missing from serum. Tubes also come sterile or nonsterile, and silicone coated or nonsilicone coated. Nonglycerin coated tops are available for lipid analysis. Heparin in the form of a lithium salt is an effective anticoagulant in small quantities without significant effect on many determinations and is the ideal universal anticoagulant for blood (Table 1–12). Availability of plastic collection tubes with piercing sampler (Venoject II, Terumo Medical Corp, Somerset, NJ) permits the blood smear to be prepared without removing the stopper. In addition, it diminishes the potential for splattering, is shatterproof, is lighter in weight (thus reduces waste removal costs compared with heavier glass tubes), and incinerates with no poisonous residues.

For glucose measurements, fluoride may be added to heparin. Fluoride inhibits glycolysis of the blood cells, which may otherwise destroy glucose at the rate of about 5%/hour. In the presence of bacterial contamination of blood specimens, fluoride inhibition of glycolysis is neither adequate nor effective in preserving glucose concentration. Furthermore, prompt separation of plasma or serum from cells is important to yield a proper specimen for most chemical determinations and precludes movement of intracellular constituents (Ca^{+2}, K^{+2}, and certain enzymes). Physiologic pumps within viable red blood cells maintain a higher concentration of intracellular potassium and extracellular sodium.

Integrated serum separator tubes are available for isolating serum from whole blood. During centrifugation, blood is forced into a silicone gel material located at the base of the tube, causing a temporary change in viscosity. The specific gravity of the gel is intermediate to that of the red cells and serum, so that the gel rises and lodges between the packed cells and the top serum layer (Chan, 1988). The gel hardens and forms an inert barrier. Pediatric-sized tubes are also available with the same concept. Advantages of serum separator tubes are (1) ease of use, (2) shorter processing time through clot activation, (3) higher serum yield, (4) minimal liberation of potentially hazardous aerosols, (5) only one centrifugation step, (6) use of the same tube as that into which the patient specimen was drawn, and (7) use of a single label. A unique advantage is that centrifuged specimens can be transported without disturbing the separation. Angle-head centrifuges do not produce a horizontal barrier and may allow red blood cells to escape back into the serum in a relatively short time. Some silica gel serum separation tubes give rise to minute particles that cause flow problems in continuous flow analyzers. Filtering the serum solves the problem.

The use of anticoagulants may cause variable dilution owing to water transport or osmotic pressure change from cells of the blood to the plasma and should be considered a source of bias. Anticoagulants that act as calcium chelators will inhibit various plasma enzyme activities if calcium is not added later. Amylase activity may be inhibited by oxalate or citrate, while lactate dehydrogenase and acid phosphatase are inhibited by oxalate. The sodium or potassium salt of fluoride, heparin, or ethylenediaminetetraacetate (EDTA) will interfere with the accurate determination of the

Table 1–10. SOME DRUGS WITH PHYSIOLOGIC EFFECTS ON AND/OR CHEMICAL INTERFERENCE WITH COMMONLY ORDERED CONSTITUENTS IN BLOOD AND URINE

Constituent in Blood	Drugs Causing Physiologic Effect	Type of Effect*	Drugs with Chemical Interference	Type of Effect*
Acid phosphatase (ACP)	Androgens (in women)	I	Fluorides	D
			Oxalates	D
Alkaline phosphatase (ALP)	(Refer to Table 1–9)	I	Albumin from placental sources	I
	Phenytoin		Fluorides	D
			Oxalates	D
			Theophylline	D
Ammonia			Isoniazid	I
Amylase (AMS)	Cholinergics	I	Citrate	D
	Ethanol	I	Oxalate	D
	Narcotics	I	Fluorides	D
Bilirubin	(Refer to Table 1–9)		Dextran	I
	Chlordiazepoxide	I	Novobiocin	I
	Gallbladder dyes	I	Ascorbic acid	D
	Phenobarbital	D	Caffeine	D
			Theophylline	D
Bromsulphalein (BSP)	(Refer to Table 1–9)		Heparin	I
	Barbiturate	I	Phenazopyridine	I
	Clofibrate	I	Phenolphthalein	I
	Narcotics (opiates–meperidine and methadone)	I	Phenolsulfonphthalein	I
	Phenytoin	I		
	Probenecid	I		
Calcium	Androgens	I	Citrate salts	D
	Calciferol-activated calcium salts	I	EDTA (interferes with dye-binding methods)	D
	Dihydrotachysterol	I		
	Progestins-estrogens	I		
	Thiazide diuretics	I		
	Acetazolamide	D		
	Corticosteroids	D		
	Mithramycin	D		
Chloride	Acetazolamides	I	Bromide	I
	Chlorides	I		
	Oxyphenbutazone	I		
	Phenylbutazone	I		
	ACTH, corticosteroids	D		
	Ethacrynic acid	D		
	Furosemide	D		
	Mercurial diuretics	D		
	Triamterene	D		
Cholesterol	ACTH	I	Bromide	I
	Bile salts	I		
	Chlorpromazine	I		
	Heparin	D		
	Thyroxine	D		
Cortisol			Chlordiazepoxide	I
			Dexamethasone	I
			Digoxin	I
			Methenamine	I
			Thorazine	I
Creatine kinase (CK)	Carbenoxolone	I		
	Clofibrate	I		
	Codeine	I		
	Dexamethasone	I		
	Digoxin	I		
	Ethanol	I		
	Furosemide	I		
	Glutethimide	I		
	Halothane anesthesia	I		
	Heroin	I		
	Imipramine	I		
	Lithium carbonate	I		
	Meperidine hydrochloride	I		
	Morphine sulfate	I		
	Phenobarbital	I		
	Suxamethonium	I		

Table 1–10. SOME DRUGS WITH PHYSIOLOGIC EFFECTS ON AND/OR CHEMICAL INTERFERENCE WITH COMMONLY ORDERED CONSTITUENTS IN BLOOD AND URINE *Continued*

Constituent in Blood	Drugs Causing Physiologic Effect	Type of Effect*	Drugs with Chemical Interference	Type of Effect*
Creatinine	Amphotericin B	I	Ascorbic acid	I
	Kanamycin	I	Barbiturates	I
			Cephalosporins	I
			Glucose	I
			Levodopa	I
			Methyldopa	I
			BSP and phenolsulfonphthalein	I
Glucose	ACTH, corticosteroids	I	Acetaminophen	I
	Epinephrine	I	Aminosalicylic acid (para-aminosalicylic acid)	I
	Ethacrynic acid	I	Ascorbic acid	I
	Furosemide	I	Dextran	I or D
	Thiazides	I	Hydralazine	I
	Phenytoin	I	Isoproterenol	I
	Propranolol	D	Levodopa	I
			Mercaptopurine	I
			Methimazole	I
			Methyldopa	I
			Nalidixic acid	I
			Oxazepam	I
			Propylthiouracil	I
Lactate dehydrogenase	Clofibrate	D	Oxalate	D
			Theophylline	D
Lipase	Cholinergics	I	Bilirubin	I
	Ethanol	I		
	Narcotics	I		
Phosphate	Calciferol-activated methicillin	I		
	Tetracyclines	I		
	Aluminum hydroxide	D		
	Glucose infusion	D		
	Insulin	D		
	Mithramycin	D		
Potassium	Heparin	I	Calcium	I
	Potassium	I	Penicillin G	I
	Spironolactone	I		
	ACTH, corticosteroids	D		
	Amphotericin	D		
	Glucose infusion	D		
	Insulin	D		
	Oral diuretics	D		
	Salicylates	D		
	Tetracycline	D		
Total protein	ACTH, corticosteroids	I	BSP dye	I
	Anabolic/androgenic steroids	I	Bilirubin	I
			Dextran	I
			Phenazopyridine	I
			Acetylsalicylic acid	D
Transferases	(Refer to Table 1–9)		*For spectrophotometric assay of AST:*	
AST (GOT) and ALT (GPT)	Ampicillin	I	Ascorbic acid	I
	Cephalothin	I	Erythromycin	I
	Clofibrate	I	Isoniazid	I
	Colchicine	I	Levodopa	I
	Gentamicin	I	Para-aminosalicylic acid	I
	Methyltestosterone	I		
	Nafcillin	I		
	Opiates	I		
	Oxacillin	I		
Sodium	Androgens	I		
	Rauwolfia alkaloids	I		
	Corticosteroids	I		
	Mannitol	I		
	Methyldopa	I		
	Oxyphenbutazone	I		
	Phenylbutazone	I		
	Ammonium chloride	D		

Table continued on following page

Table 1–10. SOME DRUGS WITH PHYSIOLOGIC EFFECTS ON AND/OR CHEMICAL INTERFERENCE WITH COMMONLY ORDERED CONSTITUENTS IN BLOOD AND URINE *Continued*

Constituent in Blood	Drugs Causing Physiologic Effect	Type of Effect*	Drugs with Chemical Interference	Type of Effect*
	Heparin	D		
	Oral diuretics	D		
	Mercurial diuretics	D		
	Spironolactone	D		
Urea	Alkaline antacids	I	Chloral hydrate	I
	Antimony salts	I	Chlorobutanol	I
	Arsenicals	I	Guanethidine	I
	Cephaloridine	I		
	Furosemide	I		
	Gentamicin	I		
	Kanamycin	I		
	Methyldopa	I		
	Neomycin	I		
Urate	Adrenocortical steroids	I	Ascorbic acid	I
	Busulfan	I	Glucose	I
	Ethacrynic acid	I	Methyldopa	I
	Nitrogen mustard	I	Theophylline	I
	Purine analogue antimetabolites	I		
	Pyrazinamide	I		
	Quinethazone	I		
	Thiazides	I		
	Vincristine sulfate	I		
	Acetylsalicylic acid	D		
	Allopurinol	D		
	Chlorpromazine	D		
	Chlorprothixene	D		
	Oxyphenbutazone	D		
	Phenylbutazone	D		
	Probenecid	D		

Constituent in Urine	Drugs Causing Physiologic Effect	Type of Effect*	Drugs with Chemical Interference	Type of Effect*
Catecholamines	Nitroglycerin	I	B-vitamin (high dose)	I
	Phenothiazines	I	Erythromycin	I
	MAO inhibitors	D	Hydralazine	I
			Levodopa	I
			Methenamine hippurate	I
			Methenamine mandelate	I
			Methyldopa	I
			Nicotinic acid	I
			Quinine-quinidine	I
			Salicylate	I
			Tetracyclines	I
Chloride			Bromide	I
Creatinine			Ascorbic acid	I
			Levodopa	I
			Methyldopa	I
			Nitrofuran derivatives	I
Glucose				
1. Enzymatic method (Clinistix, Tes Tape)			Ascorbic acid	D
			Levodopa	D
2. Benedict's solution of Clinitest			Ascorbic acid	I
			Cephalosporins	I
			Chloral hydrate	I
			Nitrofuran derivatives	I
Porphyrins	Progestins-estrogens	I	Acriflavine	I
			Ethoxazene	I
			Phenazopyridine	I
			Procaine	I
			Sulfonamides	I
Hydroxyindoleacetic acid (5-HIAA)	Reserpine	I	Mephenesin	I
			Methocarbamol	I
			Phenothiazines	D
17-Hydroxycorticosteroids = (17-OH)				
17-Ketogenic steroids = (17-KGS)				
17-Ketosteroids = (17-KS)				

Table 1–10. SOME DRUGS WITH PHYSIOLOGIC EFFECTS ON AND/OR CHEMICAL INTERFERENCE WITH COMMONLY ORDERED CONSTITUENTS IN BLOOD AND URINE *Continued*

Constituent in Urine	Drugs Causing Physiologic Effect	Type of Effect*	Drugs with Chemical Interference	Type of Effect*
(17-KS)	Anabolic steroids	I		
(17-KS, 17-OH)	Phenytoin	D		
(17-KS, 17-OH)	Estrogens	D		
(17-KS)	Ethacrynic acid	D		
(17-KS, 17-KGS)	Penicillin	D		
(17-KS)	Probenecid	D		
(17-OH)	Thiazide diuretics	D		
(17-OH, 17-KS, 17-KGS)	Meprobamate	I		
(17-OH, 17-KS, 17-KGS)	Phenothiazines	I		
(17-OH, 17-KS, 17-KGS)	Spironolactone	I		
(17-OH, 17-KS, 17-KGS)	Penicillin G	I		
(17-OH)	Ascorbic acid	I		
(17-OH)	Chloral hydrate	I		
(17-OH)	Chlordiazepoxide	I		
(17-OH)	Hydroxyzine	I		
(17-OH)	Inorganic iodides	I		
(17-OH)	Methenamine	I		
(17-KS)			Phenothiazines	I
(17-OH)			Quinidine, quinine	I
(17-OH)			Reserpine	I
(17-KS)			Ethinamate	D
(17-OH, 17-KS, 17-KGS)			Nalidixic acid	D
Pregnanediol			Mandelamine	I
Phenolsulfonphthalein	Penicillin	D		
	Probenecid	D		
	Salicylates	D		
	Sulfonamides	D		
	Thiazide diuretics	D		
Vanillylmandelic acid	Epinephrine	I	Anileridine	I
	Lithium carbonate	I	Caffeine	I
	Nitroglycerin	I	Mandelamine	I
	Chlorpromazine	D	Methocarbamol	I
	Guanethidine	D	Salicylates	I
	MAO inhibitors	D		
	Reserpine	D		

*I indicates an increase and D a decrease.

Modified from Martin TJ: The Pharmacologic Interactions with Laboratory Test Values. Washington DC, Bureau of Standards, Circular 547, US Department of Commerce, 1954; and Young DS, Pestaner LC, Gibberman V: Effects of drugs on clinical laboratory tests. Clin Chem 1975; 21:1D.

electrolyte involved. Fluoride is used as an anticoagulant for glucose determinations, but it inhibits glucose oxidase activity in enzymatic glucose reaction measurements, diminishes acid phosphatase activity, and increases amylase activity. Table 1–12 serves as a guide to appropriate blood specimen collection.

Blood may also be collected in a syringe and transferred to an appropriate specimen container (evacuated tube system). Use of a syringe may be particularly useful when procuring a specimen from the hand, ankle, or a small child. In addition, patients with small or poor veins may experience collapse of veins with use of an evacuated tube system. However, the latter system is recommended to limit the phebotomist's exposure to accidental needle sticks. Use of tube closures consisting of a rubber stopper and a plastic shield with the evacuated tube have been designed to protect laboratory personnel from noncontained blood (on outside of tube) and aerosol. Problems associated with blood collection

Table 1–11. COLOR-CODED TUBE SELECTION OF ANTICOAGULANTS COMMONLY USED

Stopper Color	Additive	Notes
Red	No additive	Collection of serum
Lavender	EDTA (Versene)	Collection of whole blood; binds calcium
Green	Heparin	Inhibits thrombin activation
Blue	Buffered citrate	Coagulation studies; binds calcium
Black	Buffered sodium citrate	Westergren ESR
Gray	Contains glycolytic inhibitor for glucose	Glucose determinations
Yellow	Citrate dextrose (ACD)	Preserves red cells

Table 1–12. GUIDE TO SUGGESTED SPECIMEN COLLECTION*

Blood Bank

- 7-mL plain tube (red top)
  - Antibody detection/identification (2 tubes)
  - Antiglobulin (direct and indirect)
  - Erythrocyte typing (ABO, Rh, extended)
  - Open-heart work-up (2 tubes)
  - Prenatal work-up (2 tubes)
- 7-mL Na Heparin (green top)
  - HLA typing
  - Mixed lymphocyte cultures (MLC)

Chemistry

- 7-mL plain tube (red top)
  - Acetaminophen (μg/mL)
  - Acetone
  - Albumin (g/dL)
  - Alanine aminotransferase (ALT; U/L)
  - Alkaline phosphatase (U/L @ 37°C)
  - Amylase (U/L)
  - Aspartate aminotransferase (AST; U/L)
  - Barbiturate screen
  - Bilirubin (mg/gL)
  - Blood urea nitrogen (BUN; mg/dL)
  - Calcium (mEq/L)
  - Calcium, ionized (mmol/L)
  - Carbamazepine (μg/mL)
  - CEA (ng/mL)
  - Chloride, sweat (mmol/L)
  - Cholesterol (mg/dL)
  - Cortisol (μg/dL)
  - Creatine kinase (CK; U/L)
  - CKMB (ng/mL)
  - Creatinine (mg/dL)
  - Cyclosporine (ng/mL)
  - Digoxin (ng/mL)
  - Electrolytes (mmol/L)
    - Chloride
    - CO_2
    - Potassium
    - Sodium
  - Ethosuximide (Zarontin; μg/mL)
  - Ethanol (do not use alcohol swabs)
  - Ferritin (ng/mL)
  - Follicle-stimulating hormone (mIU/mL)
  - Folic acid (ng/mL)
  - Free thyroxine (free T_4)
  - Gentamicin (μg/mL)
  - Glucose (mg/dL)
  - Growth hormone (ng/mL)
  - hCG (mIU/L)
  - Hemoglobin A_{1c} (%)
  - Iron (μg/dL)
  - Lactic acid (mmol/L)
  - Lactate dehydrogenase (LD; U/L)
  - Luteinizing hormone (LH; mU/mL)
  - Lithium (mmol/L)
  - Lipase (U/L)
  - Magnesium (mEq/L)
  - Osmolality, serum (mOsm/kg)
  - Phenobarbital (μg/mL)
  - Phenytoin (Dilantin; μg/mL)
  - Phosphorus (mg/dL)
  - Primidone (μg/mL)
  - Procainamide (μg/mL)
  - Prolactin (ng/dL)
  - Prostate-specific antigen (ng/mL)
  - Protein (g/dL)
  - Salicylate (mg/dL)
  - Theophylline (μg/mL)
  - Thiocyanate (mg/dL)
  - Tobramycin (μg/mL)
  - Thyroid-stimulating hormone (μU/mL)
  - Triglyceride (mg/dL)
  - Triiodothyronine (T_3; ng/dL)
  - Thyroxine (T_4; μg/mL)
  - Uric acid (mg/dL)
  - Valproic acid (μg/mL)
  - Vancomycin (mg/dL)
  - Vitamin B_{12} (pg/mL)
  - Zinc (μg/mL)
- Heparin (5-mL green top tube)
  - Ammonia (on ice; μmol/L)
  - Carboxyhemoglobin/O_2 saturation
  - Methemoglobin
  - Hemoglobin, plasma (mg/dL)
- NaF Oxalate (5-mL gray top tube)
  - Glucose
  - Glucose tolerance
  - Lactate (on ice)
  - Lactose tolerance
- EDTA (Versene; 7-mL lavender top tube)
  - Carcinoembryonic antigen (CEA; ng/mL)
  - Lead (μg/dL)

Hematology

- EDTA (Versene; 7-mL lavender top tube)
  - Complete blood count (CBC)
  - WBC differential
  - Erythrocyte sedimentation rate (mm/h)
  - G-6-PD (IU/g)
  - Hgb electrophoresis
  - Reticulocyte count
  - Platelet count
  - Sickle cell preparation
- Na Citrate (4.5-mL blue top tube)
  - Factor assays
  - Fibrinogen
  - Prothrombin time (PT)
  - Partial thromboplastin time (PTT)
  - Thrombin time
- Plain tube (7-mL red top tube)
  - Haptoglobin
  - LE preparation
  - Serum viscosity (3 tubes)

Immunology

- Plain tube (7-mL red top tube)
  - All antibody tests
- EDTA (Versene; 7-mL lavender top tube)
  - Lymphocyte subsets
- Heparin (7-mL green top tube)
  - Lymphocyte subsets
  - Lymphoma/leukemia panel
  - Nitroblue tetrazolium (NBT)
  - Phagocytosis (2 tubes)

*Two to three tests can be done per tube, unless otherwise specified.

CEA = Carcinoembryonic antigen; CKMB = creatine kinase muscle band; hCG = human chorionic gonadotropin.

are short draws (excessive EDTA may affect red blood cell [RBC] morphology; excessive anticoagulant prolongs coagulation times), hemolysis (traumatized specimen, excessive heat during transport), and clotted specimens (incomplete mixing with anticoagulant).

Anticoagulants

Anticoagulants may also be a source of error. Potassium oxalate may cause variable dilution of plasma due to water transport from cells to the plasma. Calcium chelator anticoagulants may inhibit different enzyme activities if calcium is not added as part of the respective analyses. Oxalate and citrate may inhibit amylase, LD, and acid phosphatase activities. Oxalate, citrate, and EDTA cause decreased calcium levels when evaluated by spectrophotometry but not by atomic absorption. Sodium or potassium salts, when incorporated into an anticoagulant, affect the respective assay.

Icteric or lactescent serum provide additional challenges in laboratory evaluations. When serum bilirubin approaches 430 μmoles/L (25 mg/L), interference may be observed in assays for albumin (HABA [4-hydroxyazobenzene-2-carboxylic acid] procedure), cholesterol (using ferric chloride reagents), glucose (*o*-toluidine method), and total protein (biuret procedure). Artefactually induced values in some laboratory determinations result when triglyceride levels are elevated (turbidity) based on absorbance of light of various lipid particles. Lactescence occurs when serum triglyceride levels exceed 4.6 mmol/L (400 mg/dL). Inhibition of amylase, urate, urea, CK, bilirubin, and total protein may be observed. To correct for artefactual absorbance readings, so-called blanking procedures (the blank contains serum, but lacks a crucial element to complete the assay) or dual wavelength methods may be used. A blanking process may not be effective in some cases of turbidity, thus ultracentrifugation may be necessary.

Specimen Receptacles for Arterial Blood Gases

Many types of blood specimen collection receptacles have been evaluated and recommended for blood gas determinations. One of the first and still preferred is the glass syringe, which is particularly better in preserving blood samples with high Po_2 (Pretto, 1994). Regular and specialized plastic syringes, vacuum tubes, and capillary tubes should be compared with glass syringes. The glass syringe and plunger should be matched for best fit. Approximately 1 mL of heparin (1000 or 5000 U/mL, depending on syringe volume) is drawn into the syringe and the barrel lubricated. The plunger is tested to ensure easy mobility, and the heparin should be expelled, leaving the dead space filled with residual heparin. Advantages of the glass syringe include the most accurate results attainable, a glass plunger that moves upward because of arterial pressure (if 23-gauge or larger needle is used), and reusability. Disadvantages of the glass syringe include relatively high initial cost, need for proper sterilization for reuse between patients, concerns of blood-borne disease transmission, and easy breakage. Plastic syringes eliminate the need for resterilization and are low in cost, readily available in any hospital setting, and relatively unbreakable. Unfortunately, standard plastic syringes have their own disadvantages. A valid question concerns accuracy because of gas leakage through the plastic. A major technical disadvantage is that the plunger often does not move from arterial pressure, and a minor problem is that air bubbles are harder to remove.

Leakage of gases through plastic can pose problems depending on the type of plastic and the oxygen and carbon dioxide tensions of the blood specimen collected. The greater the difference between the partial pressures of oxygen and carbon dioxide in the blood and the partial pressures in room air, the larger the leakage. Use of plastic syringes may alter Po_2 levels and, if used, should be analyzed within 15 minutes (Muller-Plathe, 1992). Polypropylene plastic syringes are superior to polystyrene plastic syringes. Plastic syringes featuring a plunger that rises due to arterial pressure have replaced the standard glass or plastic syringes in many institutions. Numerous brands are available. The use of these newer syringes has alleviated the major disadvantage of the plastic syringe (the plunger not rising due to arterial pressure) and the major disadvantages of the glass syringe (the easy breakage and need of sterilization).

Another type of blood gas syringe is a preheparinized needle-syringe assembly with a vented plunger. An example is OMNISTIK (Marquest Medical Products, Englewood, CO). Petty (1981) has reported that OMNISTIK showed no significant analytical errors introduced by gas exchange at the advancing blood-air interface. Small-volume specimens may be collected in syringes containing crystalline heparin because Pco_2 dilution artifact is eliminated. Fleisher (1971) reported the successful use of a special Vacutainer tube (Becton-Dickinson and Company, Rutherford, NJ) filled with nitrogen gas at a pressure of 152 mm Hg and containing 143 units of sodium heparin. A special adapter was used to collect specimens for arterial blood gases. Although these specialized vacuum tubes were shown to produce accurate results, the large air space at the top of standard heparin vacuum tubes can produce erroneous measurements by equilibrating with the blood.

The last type of acceptable container for blood collection and transport (skin puncture blood) is special capillary tubes (Caraway, 1972). However, their accuracy and deficiencies cannot easily be separated from the arterialized capillary blood that they contain. Use of a butterfly infusion set may cause falsely elevated Po_2 (Garza, 1989).

Specimen Collection and Processing

Blood

Blood is the most frequent body fluid used for analytical purposes. Three general procedures for obtaining blood are (1) venipuncture, (2) arterial puncture, and (3) skin puncture. The technique used to obtain the blood specimen is critical in order to maintain its integrity. Even so, arterial and venous blood differ in important respects. Blood oxygenated by the lungs is pumped from the heart to all organs and tissues to meet metabolic needs. Arterial blood is essentially uniform in composition throughout the body. The composition of venous blood varies and is dependent on metabolic activity of the perfused organ or tissue. Site of collection can affect the venous composition (Pryce, 1980). Venous blood is oxygen deficient relative to arterial blood, but also differs in pH, carbon dioxide concentration, and packed cell volume. Glucose, lactic acid, chloride, and ammonia concentrations also may vary. Blood obtained by skin puncture (sometimes incorrectly called capillary blood) is an admixture of blood from arterioles, venules, and capillaries. Increased pressure in the arterioles yields a specimen enriched in arterial blood. Skin puncture blood also contains interstitial and intracellular fluids.

Venous Puncture

The relative ease of obtaining venous blood makes this a primary source of specimen for clinical laboratory analyses.

TECHNIQUE FOR VENOUS PUNCTURE (NCCLS Pub. H3-A3, 1991)

1. Verify that computer-printed labels match requisitions.
2. Check patient identification band against labels and requisition forms. Ask the patient for his or her full name or verify identity from another reliable source as established by protocol. If the patient's identity is unknown or questionable, give the patient a temporary identification. *Do not draw any specimen without properly identifying the patient.*
3. If a fasting specimen is required, confirm that the fasting order has been followed.
4. Address the patient, and inform the patient what is to be done. Reassure the patient to avoid as much tension as possible. Identification of phlebotomist should be evident to the patient (i.e., ID card should be visible).
5. Position the patient properly, depending on whether the patient is sitting or prone, for easy, comfortable access to the antecubital fossa.
6. Assemble equipment and supplies, including collection tubes, tourniquet, preparations for cleansing the area, syringes if necessary, sterile blood collection needle, and holder used to secure the needle (for evacuated collection tube system). Gloves and laboratory coat must be worn according to established policy (see section on safety).
7. Ask the patient to make a fist so veins are more palpable.
8. Select a suitable vein for puncture. Veins of the antecubital fossa, in particular, the median cubital and cephalic veins, are preferred. Wrist, ankle, and hand veins may also be used. If one arm has an intravenous line, use the other arm to draw a blood specimen.
9. Cleanse the venipuncture site with 70% isopropanol alcohol solution or 1% iodine-saturated swabstick. Begin at the puncture site, and cleanse outward in a circular motion. Allow the area to dry. Do not touch the swabbed area with any unsterile object.
10. Apply a tourniquet several inches above the puncture site. Never leave the tourniquet in place longer than one minute.
11. Anchor the vein firmly, both above and below the puncture site. Use either the thumb and middle finger or thumb and index finger.
12. Perform the venipuncture. (a) Enter the skin with the needle at approximately a 15-degree angle to the arm, with the bevel of the needle up. Follow the geography of the vein with the needle. (b) Insert the needle smoothly and fairly rapidly to minimize patient discomfort. Do not bury the needle. (c) If using a syringe, pull back on the barrel with a slow, even tension as blood flows into the syringe. Do not pull back too quickly to avoid hemolysis or collapsing the vein. (d) If using an evacuated system, as soon as the needle is in the vein, ease the tube forward in the holder as far as it will go, firmly securing the needle holder in place. When the tube has filled, remove it by grasping the end of the tube and pull gently to withdraw.
13. Release the tourniquet when blood begins to flow. Never withdraw the needle without removing the tourniquet.
14. After all blood has been drawn, have the patient relax his or her fist. Do not allow the patient to pump the hand.
15. Place a clean sterile cotton ball or gauze lightly over the site. Withdraw the needle, then apply pressure to the site.
16. Apply an adhesive bandage strip over the cotton ball or gauze to adequately stop bleeding and avoid a hematoma.
17. Mix and invert tubes with anticoagulant; do **not** shake the tube. For syringe-drawn specimens, transfer blood to appropriate tubes, taking caution not to hemolyze the specimen(s) and observing needle safety. Follow any special handling procedures, e.g., chilling certain specimens.
18. Check condition of the patient, e.g., whether patient is faint and that bleeding is under control. Always anticipate that a syncope episode may occur.
19. Dispose of contaminated material such as needles, syringes, and cotton, in designated hard-cased containers (sharps container). Do not recap or remove the needle by hand but use appropriate device designed for this function (i.e., needle resheather; Datar, Inc., Long Lake, MN).
20. Initial the labels and record the time specimens were drawn. Deliver tubes of blood for testing to appropriate laboratory section or central receiving and processing area.

COMPLICATIONS

The prolonged application of a tourniquet produces a measurable increase in blood cell concentration (hemoconcentration). Failure to obtain blood includes (1) a missed vein, which may result in a hematoma; (2) excessive pull on syringe plunger may collapse a small vein; (3) patient syncope; (4) excessive bleeding; (5) thrombosis of the vein, and (6) infection of the site where blood was drawn. Failure to obtain blood after two attempts is an indication that another phlebotomist should make an attempt. To avoid unwanted clotted specimens, ensure adequate and prompt tube inversion with mixing of blood and additive. When multiple tubes of blood are to be obtained, follow the recommended order of draw to avoid possible contamination. Draw specimens into nonadditive tubes before tubes with additives. Fill additive-containing tubes in the following order: (1) blood culture tubes, (2) red stopper tubes, (3) blue stopper tubes, (4) green stopper tubes, (5) lavender stopper tubes, and (6) gray stopper tubes (McCall, 1993; see Table 1–11).

Arterial Puncture (NCCLS Publication H11-A2, 1992)

Arterial blood is used to measure oxygen and carbon dioxide tension, as well as pH (arterial blood gases [ABGs]). These blood gas measurements are critical in the assessment of oxygenation problems encountered in patients with pneumonia, pneumonitis, and pulmonary embolism. Patients on prolonged oxygen therapy or mechanical ventilation are monitored to avoid extremes in oxygenation that produce either anoxia with respiratory acidosis or oxygen toxicity. Critically ill cardiovascular patients and patients undergoing major surgery, especially cardiac or pulmonary surgery, are closely monitored for hypoxemia.

Arterial punctures are technically more difficult to perform than venous punctures. Increased pressure in the arteries makes it more difficult to stop bleeding with the undesired development of a hematoma. Arterial selection includes radial, brachial, and femoral arteries in order of choice. Sites not to be selected are irritated, edematous, near a wound, or in an area of an arteriovenous (AV) shunt or fistula (McCall, 1993). Arterial spasm is a reflex constriction that restricts blood flow with possible severe consequences on circulation and tissue perfusion. Patients may complain of considerable discomfort associated with radial artery puncture. Symptoms of temporary discomfort may be expressed as aching, throbbing, tenderness, sharp sensation, and cramping. At times, it is either impractical or impossible to obtain arterial blood from a patient for blood gas analysis. Under these circumstances, another source of blood can be obtained, recognizing that arterial blood provides a more accurate result. Although venous blood is more readily obtained, it usually reflects the acid-base status of an extremity, not the body as a whole. Venous blood properly collected yields adequate pH values, but venous blood yields incorrect values for arterial oxygen saturation and alveolar P_{CO_2} (Gambino, 1961).

COLLECTION TECHNIQUE AND PATIENT PREPARATION FOR ARTERIAL BLOOD (NCCLS Pub. H11-A2, 1992)

1. The radial and brachial arteries are the preferred vessels for arterial puncture. The femoral artery is relatively large and easy to puncture, but care must be taken in older individuals, in whom the femoral artery tends to bleed more than the radial or brachial. Because the bleeding site is hidden by bed covers, it may not be noticed until bleeding is massive. The radial artery is more difficult to puncture but exhibits a lower incidence of complications.
2. When using the radial artery, it is essential to assess the collateral circulation (blood supplied from more than one artery, i.e., radial and ulnar arteries) of the hand using the Allen test. The Allen test consists of elevating and occluding both the radial and ulnar arteries simultaneously to empty them of blood, making the hand appear blanched. Lowering the hand and releasing pressure on the ulnar artery allows return of blood flow through the ulnar artery. This test ensures collateral circulation should the radial artery become occluded as a consequence of manipulation or puncture. If the Allen test is negative (the hand does not flush pink with presumption of collateral circulation insufficiency), another site should be used. The major complications of arterial puncture include thrombosis, hemorrhage, and possible infection. Petty (1966) reported no complications except for minimal hematomas with 475 arterial punctures, whereas Sackner (1971) found no morbidity in 1541 radial artery punctures.
3. The artery to be punctured is identified by its pulsations and cleansed with 70% aqueous isopropanol solution followed by iodine.
4. Although a local anesthetic wheal may be made, it is not usually required. An unanesthetized arterial puncture provides an accurate measurement of resting pH and P_{CO_2} in spite of the theoretical error possible from patient hyperventilation caused by the pain of the arterial puncture. The use of butterfly infusion sets is not recommended. Using 19-gauge versus 25-gauge needles does not vary the P_{CO_2} or P_{O_2} more than 1 mm Hg.
5. Prepare the ABG syringe as directed earlier. The needle (18- to 20-gauge for brachial artery) should pierce the skin at an angle of approximately 45 to 60 degrees (90 degrees for femoral artery) in a slow and deliberate manner. Some degree of dorsiflexion of the wrist is necessary with the radial artery, for which a 23- to 25-gauge needle is used.
6. The pulsations of blood into the syringe confirm that it will fill by arterial pressure alone. If the plunger is pulled back and air is aspirated, immediately withdraw the syringe.
7. After the blood specimen is collected, the needle is removed using a needle resheather and an airtight cap (Luer tip cap) placed over the tip of the syringe. Gently rotate syringe, mixing blood and heparin. Place in ice water (or other coolant that will maintain a temperature of 1°C to 5°C) to minimize leukocyte consumption of oxygen. Historically, it has been common practice to force the point of the needle into a cork or rubber stopper. However, this should be avoided to prevent accidental needle puncture while handling the specimen.
8. After the arterial puncture, compression with a sterile gauze pad on the puncture site should be applied for a minimum of two minutes and preferably for five minutes (timed).

The recommended volume of arterial blood obtained varies, but certainly the greater the specimen volume, the less dilution effect from the heparin. With a 10-mL syringe, the dead space is 1.2% to 2.4% of the maximal volume. The heparin dilution primarily affects the P_{CO_2}. Dilution errors up to a 28% fall in P_{CO_2} may occur. Use of preheparinized syringes for blood gas analysis presents a more convenient and rapid method of blood collection. Excess heparin solution must be expelled prior to collection and the prescribed volume of blood (3 mL) must be obtained to minimize dilutional error. Use of syringes containing lyophilized (freeze-dried) heparin does not introduce dilutional errors if syringe is underfilled.

Blood gases obtained by skin puncture may be collected from the finger as a suitable substitute for arterial blood for pH and Pco_2 but may not be acceptable for Po_2. In order for it to be a satisfactory substitute for arterial blood, some estimation of the Po_2 must be available. The recommended site for obtaining arterialized capillary blood is the earlobe (Pitkin, 1994) because of its vascularity, its low metabolic requirements, and the ease with which it can be arterialized.

Skin Puncture

Skin puncture is the method of choice in pediatric patients, especially infants. The large amount of blood required from repeated venipunctures may cause anemia (iatrogenic), especially in premature infants. Venipuncture of deep veins in pediatric patients may also rarely cause (1) cardiac arrest, (2) hemorrhage, (3) thrombosis, (4) venous constriction followed by gangrene of an extremity, (5) damage to organs or tissues accidentally punctured, and (6) infection. However, accessible veins in sick infants must be reserved exclusively for parenteral therapy. Skin puncture is useful in adults with (1) extreme obesity, (2) severe burns, and (3) thrombotic tendencies. Skin puncture is often preferred in geriatric patients because of thinness of skin and the loss of elasticity.

The earlobe can be arterialized (Phelan, 1993) by heat (paper towel saturated with warm water, 39 to 42°C), by flicking with the index finger until definite flushing is observed, or by chemical means with Trafuril paste (Ciba A-G, Basel, Switzerland). The earlobe is cleansed with 70% aqueous isopropanol solution and punctured. The puncture area should be adequate to obtain a free flow of blood and the lobe wiped dry. Two heparinized capillary tubes (100 μL) are placed in the center of the drop and filled to capacity without air bubbles, which may alter oxygen partial pressure (Po_2). Both ends are sealed in clay after the insertion of a rust-proof metal stirrer (flea type). Blood in the tubes is stirred by the use of a magnet, thus mixing the specimen with heparin. Whenever cardiac output is severely restricted, systolic pressure is less than 95 mm Hg, or vasoconstriction is present, skin puncture blood may yield unreliable data.

The greatest value of skin puncture blood is in the pediatric age group. In the older pediatric population, earlobe blood is available, but in neonates and infants, in whom it is impractical to sample the earlobe, the heel is often used. A deep heel prick is made at the distal edge of the calcaneal protuberance following a five- to ten-minute exposure period of prewarmed water. The specimen is then handled as described for the earlobe specimen. Skin puncture blood obtained in this manner is unacceptable for Pco_2 and Po_2 determination in the first day of life, probably owing to vasoconstriction and poor perfusion of the extremities. In infants with respiratory distress syndrome, heel blood deviates significantly from arterial blood in all parameters except base excess and standard bicarbonate (Bigen, 1975). The best method for blood gas collection in the newborn still remains the indwelling umbilical artery catheter.

TECHNIQUE FOR SKIN PUNCTURE
(NCCLS Pub. H4-A3, 1991)

1. Select an appropriate puncture site. For infants, this is most usually the lateral or medial plantar heel surface. In older infants, the palmar surface of the last digit of the second, third, or fourth fingers may be used. Other sites for skin puncture are the plantar surface of the big toe, the lateral side of a finger adjacent to the nail, and the earlobe. The site of puncture must not be edematous or a previous puncture site.
2. Warm the puncture site with a warm, moist towel no hotter than 42°C; this increases the blood flow through arterioles and capillaries and results in arterial-enriched blood.
3. Cleanse the puncture site with 70% aqueous isopropanol solution. Allow the area to dry. Do not touch the swabbed area with any unsterile object.
4. Make the puncture with a sterile lancet, using a single deliberate motion nearly perpendicular to the skin surface. For a heel puncture, hold the heel with forefinger at the arch and thumb proximal to the puncture site at the ankle. Use a lancet with blade no longer than 2.4 mm to avoid injury to the calcaneus (heel bone). Meites (1988) evaluated the use of a lancet with a puncturing tip length of 1.8 mm for newborns and found no apparent diminution of blood volume obtained. Alternatively, devices are available (Tenderfoot, ITC Commercial Group, Edison, NJ) containing a spring-loaded surgical blade that allows for a clean incision with minimal skin trauma (incision ranges available from 0.85 to 2.0 mm deep and 1.75 to 3.0 mm in length).
5. Discard the first drop of blood by wiping it away with a sterile pad. Regulate further blood flow by gentle thumb pressure. Do not milk the site, because this may hemolyze the specimen and introduce excess tissue fluid.
6. Collect the specimen in a suitable container (NCCLS Pub. H14-A2, 1990) by capillary action. Closed systems are available for collection of non-anticoagulated blood and with additives for whole analysis (Unopette, Becton-Dickinson, Rutherford, NJ; Capijet, Terumo Corp., Elkton, MD). Open-ended, narrow-bore disposable glass micropipettes are most often used up to volumes of 200 μL. The bore may be uniform or tapered at one end (Caraway and Natelson pipettes). Both heparinized and nonheparinized micropipettes are available. Oral aspiration of blood is discouraged for obvious safety and health risk reasons; manual aspirators are recommended. Plastic and clay compounds are available to seal the pipettes. Test tubes are available up to 1000 μL capacity, without anticoagulant. Serum separator tubes with an inert polyester barrier material are also available in various tube sizes.
7. Seal the specimen container, e.g., insert clay into each end of the micropipettes.
8. Label the specimen container with date, time of collection, and patient demographics.
9. Indicate in the report that test results are from skin

puncture blood, bearing in mind that differences may exist in concentrations of glucose, potassium, total protein, and calcium between skin puncture and venous serum specimens (Meites, 1988).

Transcutaneous Monitoring

Transcutaneous monitoring allows for continuous measurement of blood gases in a simple and effective way (Rooke, 1992). The skin is arterialized by using electric heat, causing dilatation of the microvasculature, thus increasing capillary flow, which is similar in nature to arterial blood. Oxygen and carbon dioxide diffuse through the skin, providing a noninvasive medium for the measurement of arterial blood gases. Transcutaneous monitoring has become common in newborn infants; by the fetal scalp (with Europe); and in adult intensive care patients. Transmucous membrane oxygen monitoring has been advocated intraoperatively (Czech, 1979). Poor correlation is seen in adult patients undergoing surgery when transcutaneous monitoring is used owing to many factors, which may include thickness of skin, oxygenation, local perfusion, state of vasodilatation, and skin metabolism. The use of transcutaneous oxygen measurement has been the standard accepted practice using a Clark electrode and an electric heater. Transcutaneous carbon dioxide measurement usually involves the use of a modified Severinghaus electrode with a heater. The usefulness of transcutaneous monitoring in obstetric care has been demonstrated by Huch (1979 a and b).

A study by Cabal (1981) concluded that patients with intact hemodynamic function have close agreement between $P_{TC}O_2$ and arterial blood tensions. Unheated $P_{TC}CO_2$ sensors measure tissue carbon dioxide. When a high $P_{TC}O_2$ was observed without a clinically apparent cause, the patients later developed manifestations of inadequate tissue perfusion. In patients with hemodynamic compromise, a $P_{TC}O_2$ rise was often the only indication of altered tissue perfusion. In abnormal tissue, circulation persists and the $P_{TC}O_2$ further increases, ultimately compromising oxygen delivery, resulting in a lower $P_{TC}O_2$ than arterial oxygen. Therefore, in cardiovascular compromise, the $P_{TC}CO_2$ reflected tissue perfusion and the $P_{TC}O_2$ monitored oxygen delivery to the tissues. In patients with ventilatory problems without cardiovascular alterations, $P_{TC}O_2$ and $P_{TC}co_2$ reliably reflect arterial values. Conditions such as severe hypovolemia (blood volume <58 mL/kg), arterial hypotension (systolic blood pressure 10 to 33 mm Hg), anemic hypoxemia (hematocrit 5% to 23%), or acidemia (pH 6.72 or less) were associated with poor $P_{TC}O_2$ and arterial oxygen correlation (Versmold, 1979). A minor complication that may be associated with transcutaneous monitoring of blood gases is a mild, localized erythema at the site of the heated electrode, which usually disappears within a few hours of sensor removal. This can be minimized by limiting temperature to $<44°C$ and changing the site every four hours (Shapiro, 1989).

The management of neonatal bilirubin can be accomplished using a transcutaneous approach and filter paper. This technique is simple, noninvasive, and reliable; however, reference ranges must be adjusted to accommodate skin pigment, gestational age, and use of phototherapy (Kumar, 1992). Correlations between serum bilirubin (BI) results and transcutaneous results (BI_{TC}) have been shown to be acceptable until critical serum levels are reached.

Indwelling Lines and Catheter Access

Indwelling catheters (such as central venous lines) provide ready access to the patient's circulation, eliminating multiple phlebotomies, and are especially useful in critical care and surgical situations. Arterial catheters most often are placed in the radial artery. Indwelling catheters are surgically inserted in the cephalic vein (or internal jugular, subclavian, or femoral veins) and positioned. They are especially useful in selected patients for drawing venous blood, administering drugs or blood products, and providing total parenteral nutrition. Continuous, real-time intra-arterial monitoring of blood gases and acid-base status using fiberoptic channels containing fluorescent and absorbent chemical analytes has been used successfully (Smith, 1992).

Placement of indwelling catheters, although not a routine laboratory function, is of primary concern to the laboratorian; blood specimens drawn from catheters may be contaminated with whatever was administered or infused via the catheter. The solution (usually heparin) used to maintain patency of the vein must also be cleared. Sufficient blood (minimum of 2 to 3 mL) must be withdrawn to clear the line so laboratory data are reliable. To obtain a blood specimen from the indwelling catheter, first draw 6 mL of intravenous fluid from the line and discard. In a separate syringe, withdraw the amount of blood required for requested laboratory procedures. Follow strict aseptic technique to avoid site or catheter contamination or both. Coagulation measurements (prothrombin time, activated partial thromboplastin time, and thrombin time) are extremely sensitive to heparin interference, so that even larger volumes of presample blood must be withdrawn before the laboratory results are acceptable. The appropriate volume to be discarded should be established by each laboratory. When performing prothrombin times (PT) and activated partial thromboplastin times (APTT), a minimum of 5.3 mL discard volume should be used (Konopad, 1992). The laboratory is sometimes asked to perform blood culture studies on blood drawn from indwelling catheters. This procedure is not recommended because organisms that grow on the walls of the catheter can contaminate the blood specimen.

SPECIMEN INTERFERENCES

The collection of specimens depends on proper identification of the patient, the appropriate collecting method to procure the specimen, and the correct collection tubes. Timed collections must be verified to ensure accuracy in generating laboratory data that will be used in the diagnosis or management of a patient. The site of collection is generally not critical except for glucose tolerance test, in which it has been reported that capillary glucose is 10% to 30% higher than venous blood glucose (Larsson-Cohn, 1976). Additionally, blood specimens collected from an extremity with any type of catheter delivering parenteral solutions can generate artefactual results. If this type of collection cannot be avoided, the venipuncture must be performed distal to the intravenous needle site, with the tourniquet between the two. Blood-drawing equipment must be void of any residual detergents, plasticizers, or other material that may interfere with laboratory determinations. Examples include specimens for lead analysis, which must be collected in acid-washed, lead-free containers, and contamination from tissue thromboplastin that may interfere with specific coagulation assays if a double-syringe technique (first 5 mL of blood is discarded) is not used.

Lysis of red blood cells during the collection process or after phlebotomy, before analysis is performed, can contaminate the serum (or plasma) and alter results (in vitro hemolysis). Overzealous mixing of blood in collection tubes, residual alcohol left when cleansing skin, prolonged exposure of tubes to heat or extreme cold (freezing), and inadequate removal of red cells during centrifugation may cause hemolysis. Even small amounts of lysed erythrocytes may have a significant impact on blood plasma and serum analyte concentrations (Table 1–13; Caraway, 1972). *In vitro* hemolysis results may show increased levels of serum acid phosphatase, zinc, magnesium, albumin, potassium, bilirubin (spectrophotometrically determined), and CK. Thrombolysis can result in elevated serum potassium, magnesium, acid phosphatase, and aldolase. Granulocytosis releases muramidase (lysozyme), phosphohexose isomerase, arginase, glucose-6-phosphatase (G6PD), and glutamate dehydrogenase (Swartz, 1973). Hemolysis may alter spectrophotometric readings, such as those used in coagulation studies or hemoglobin evaluations.

Urine Specimen Collection

Collection and preservation of urine for analytical testing must follow a carefully prescribed procedure to ensure valid results (NCCLS Pub. GP16-T, 1992). Laboratory testing of urine generally falls under three categories, i.e., chemical, bacteriologic, and microscopic examination. There are also three kinds of collection for urine specimens: (1) random, (2) timed, and (3) 24-hour total volume. Random specimens may be collected any time, but a first morning voided aliquot is optimal for constituent concentration. Laboratory results from a random urine collection are expressed per unit volume if the result is a quantitative analysis. Result reporting of a random collection is expressed as positive or negative, indicating the presence or absence of a particular constituent, such as glucose. Random urine specimens should be collected in a chemically clean receptacle, either glass or plastic. A clean-catch midstream specimen is most desirable for bacteriologic examinations. The vessel is tightly sealed, labeled with the patient's name and date of collection, and submitted for analysis. A first morning urine specimen is generally the most concentrated and considered a better specimen for evaluation. Timed specimens are obtained at designated intervals, starting from time zero, and are noted on each subsequent container time of collection. Urine specimens for a 24-hour total volume collection are most difficult to obtain and require cooperation from the patient. Incomplete collection is the major problem. In some instances, overcollection occurs. Because in-hospital collection is usually under the supervision of the nursing staff, it is more reliable than outpatient collections. Collection of urine specimens from pediatric patients requires special attention to avoid contamination from the stool. One can avoid problems by giving patients complete written and verbal instructions with a warning that the test can be invalidated by incorrect collection technique. If specimen is to be collected on an outpatient basis, exercise care and instruct patient's parents to keep the specimen out of the reach of children, especially if concentrated acid is used as a preservative. An unbreakable, 4 L (approximately) plastic, chemically clean container with the correct preservative already added is preferred. One should remind the patient to *discard* the first morning specimen, record the time, and collect every subsequent voiding for the next 24 hours, with the last to be 24 hours after timing commenced. Overcollection occurs if the first morning specimen is included in this routine. Measure the total volume collected, record the information on the request form, thoroughly mix the entire 24-hour collection, and submit for analysis. A 40-mL aliquot is adequate for this purpose. Completeness of collection is difficult to determine. If results appear clinically invalid, this is cause for suspicion. Because creatinine excretion is based on muscle mass, and because a patient's muscle mass is relatively constant, creatinine excretion is also reasonably constant. Therefore, one should measure creatinine on several 24-hour collections and keep this as part of the patient's record. Another approach is to express results relative to the concentration of creatinine when collecting a specimen other than a 24-hour one. One-

Table 1–13. CHANGES IN THE SERUM CONCENTRATION (OR ACTIVITIES) OF SELECTED CONSTITUENTS DUE TO LYSIS OF ERYTHROCYTES (RBC)

Constituent	Ratio of Concentration (or Activity) in RBC to Concentration (or Activity) in Serum	Change of Concentration (or Activity) in Serum After Lysis of 1% RBC, Assuming a Hematocrit of 0.50 (%)
Lactate dehydrogenase	160:1	+272.0
Aspartate aminotransferase (AST or GOT)	40:1	+220.0
Potassium	23:1	+24.4
Alanine aminotransferase (ALT or GPT)	6.7:1	+55.0
Glucose	0.82:1	−5.0
Inorganic phosphate	0.78:1	÷9.1
Sodium	0.11:1	−1.0
Calcium	0.10:1	÷2.9

Modified from Caraway, 1972; and Laessig, 1976a.

and two-hour timed collection specimens may suffice in some instances.

SPECIAL URINE COLLECTION TECHNIQUES

Catheterization of the bladder may cause infection but is necessary in some patients. Catheterization also is used for urine collection when patients are unable to void or control micturition. *Suprapubic aspiration* is performed with a syringe and needle above the symphysis pubis, through the abdominal wall, into a full bladder. This method is used to obtain otherwise problematic anaerobic cultures. Ureteral catheters are inserted via a cystoscope into the ureter. Bladder urine is collected first, followed by a bladder washing. Ureteral urine specimens are useful in differentiating bladder from kidney infection or for differential ureteral analysis, and may be obtained separately from each kidney pelvis (labeled left and right). First morning urine samples for cytologic examination are optimal.

Other Body Fluids

CEREBROSPINAL FLUID

Lumbar punctures (LPs) are performed to collect cerebrospinal fluid (CSF) that may be evaluated in the laboratory to establish a diagnosis of infection (bacterial, fungal, mycobacterial, or amebic meningitis), malignancy, subarachnoid hemorrhage, multiple sclerosis, or demyelinating disorders. A serious complication of an LP is cerebellar tonsillar herniation in patients with elevated intracranial pressure and should be avoided unless CSF findings are expected to improve treatment or outcome. Patients with spinal cord tumors with paresis may progress to paralysis following LP. To avoid introduction of infection, patients with sepsis in the lumbar region (skin infection, cellulitis, or epidural abscess) should not have an LP performed to avoid introduction of infection. Other complications of lumbar puncture include asphyxiation in infants due to hyperextending the head forward, thus occluding the trachea; paresthesia; headache; and rarely, hematomas.

Before collection of CSF begins, the pressure, measured by allowing fluid to rise in a sterile, graduated manometer, should be between 90 and 180 mm Hg. Breath holding, abdominal compression, congestive heart failure, inflammation of the meninges, obstruction of intracranial venous sinuses, mass lesions, and cerebral edema may cause the pressure to be elevated (above 180 mm Hg). Initially, only 1 to 2 mL of CSF should be removed. A marked decrease in pressure following this procedure suggests cerebellar herniation or spinal cord compression, thus no additional CSF should be collected. Patients with partial or complete spinal block may have low pressure (<80 mm Hg), falling to zero after removal of only 1 mL. Again, no additional fluid should be removed. If pressure is normal and does not fall after several milliliters are removed, additional fluid may be taken. Three aliquots are generally collected in separate, sterile tubes labeled appropriately with name, date, and sequential tube collection number and distributed for chemical and immunologic studies (#1), microbiologic studies (#2), and cell count and differential (#3). Closing pressure of 40 to 90 mm Hg is common after 10 to 20 mL of CSF has been removed.

SYNOVIAL FLUID

Synovial fluid is produced by dialysis of plasma across the synovial membrane and secretion of a hyaluronate-protein complex. This fluid is collected using careful, aseptic technique, avoiding aspiration from patients with bacteremia or extra-articular soft tissue infection. Collection of synovial fluid (arthrocentesis) should be performed after six hours of fasting into a syringe containing about 25 units of heparin per milliliter of synovial fluid collected. Generally, less than 2.0 mL of fluid is collected unless an effusion is present and therapeutic collection is continued. Using additional syringes, larger amounts may be collected when appropriate for microbiologic and other studies.

PLEURAL FLUID, PERICARDIAL FLUID, AND PERITONEAL FLUID

The lubricating fluids found between potential spaces of pleura, from the pericardial sac, or from the peritoneum, may accumulate excessively. Thoracentesis is a surgical procedure that is performed to drain accumulated fluids (effusions) from the thoracic cavity and is helpful in the diagnosis of inflammation or neoplastic diseases in the lung or pleura. Likewise, pericardiocentesis and peritoneocentesis refer to the collection of fluid from the pericardium and the peritoneal cavities, respectively.

The patient, sitting in an upright position, with arms and head extended on an overbed table, is prepared with a local anesthetic after appropriate cleansing of the site. A 50-mL syringe is fitted with a stopcock and rubber tubing to assist in the aseptic collection process. Specimens are obtained for chemical, microbiological, and cytologic examination and measurements and are transferred to collecting tubes with appropriate additive(s). For most chemical evaluations, no additive is used and specimen is allowed to clot. Bacteriologic and cytologic specimens may be collected in EDTA or sterile sodium heparin (without preservatives). Special studies for *Mycobacterium*, anaerobic bacteria, or viruses may require special handling procedures, which are planned and reviewed prior to collection.

Specimen Transport

Transport of blood, urine, and other body fluids and tissue specimens from collection site to the laboratory is an important component of processing. For blood samples, it comprises approximately one third of the total TAT (Howanitz, 1992). Specimens should be received by the laboratory staff within 45 minutes of collection to allow timely completion of specimen processing (Rosen, 1989). Avoid agitation of blood specimens to minimize hemolysis. Specimens should be protected from direct exposure to light, which causes breakdown of certain analytes, e.g., bilirubin. For analysis of unstable constituents, such as ammonia, plasma renin activity, and acid phosphatase, specimens must be kept at 4°C immediately after collection and they should be transported on ice. Blood gas specimens should be handled as described earlier.

Routine urine samples are collected in sterile, disposable, 200-mL plastic containers. Pediatric urine collectors are flexible, polyethylene bags, which may be sealed for transportation. All laboratory specimens must be transported in a safe and convenient manner to prevent biohazard exposure or contamination of the specimen. Broken or leaking specimens are a biohazard to those who may come in contact with them, and the problem requires recollection of a new specimen; this procedure can delay treatment of the patient and add to the cost. The stability for the constituents must be determined prior to transporting specimens. Such information is usually provided by the laboratory, along with instructions for specimen preparation and shipping. Polystyrene or other high-impact plastic-type containers are commonly used. Specimens requiring refrigeration must be maintained between 2° and 10°C and can be appropriately carried in an insulated container. Large-volume urine specimens should be collected in a leak-proof, 3-L container. Stool specimens are transported in a cardboard container and placed in a polyethylene bag. To mail a specimen in the frozen state, solid carbon dioxide (dry ice) may be packed in a styrofoam container with the specimen, which can be kept frozen at temperatures as low as −70°C (Kalish, 1983). Some reference laboratories offer contractual agreements that include courier services for specimen transport.

For local, on-site transport, pneumatic tube systems provide a rapid, efficient, and cost-effective way of transporting laboratory specimens to a specific location. A pneumatic tube consists of a vertically and horizontally branched tube system that is available in 4- or 6-inch diameter, or 4- × 7-inch oblong size capable of transporting blood specimens, requisitions, pharmaceutical orders and drugs, medical reports, and limited medical supplies, using a microcomputer system to direct and secure transported material (Jones, 1983). For laboratory use, blood specimens are placed in a carrier with liners to prevent leakage and padding, to ensure that specimen containers remain intact. Using positive and negative air pressure, the carriers travel through the tube at a rate of about 25 feet/sec, thus requiring a soft, cushioned landing. The advantages of a pneumatic tube system are improved TAT, reliability, and minimal training to use, with low maintenance, availability 24 h/day, 7 days/week, and improved staff utilization. Average time in payback in labor cost savings has been estimated to be 2.6 years (Baer, 1993). Computerized pneumatic tube systems (TransLogic, Denver, CO 80239) provide a bidirectional transport of specimens in a safe and economical fashion. System improvements now minimize hemolysis, along with subsequent biochemical and hematologic changes. Studies have shown that most routine chemical and hematologic evaluations are not substantially affected by rapid transport, including blood gases, red cell packs, and LH values (Hardin, 1990; Keshgegian, 1992). TAT for some determinations may be improved by 25% with the use of a pneumatic tube system (Keshgegian, 1992).

BLOOD SPECIMEN PRESERVATION

During storage, the concentration of a blood constituent in the specimen may change as a result of various processes, including adsorption on glass or plastic tube, protein denaturation, evaporation of volatile compounds, and continuing metabolic activities of leukocytes and erythrocytes. Frozen specimens may also undergo changes for certain metabolites or cellular constituents. Enzymatic reactions may be particularly sensitive to storage conditions. Folic acid, for example, is unstable at −20°C. Control specimens stored at −20°C can degrade, causing changes in concentration with long-term storage and can be observed as gradually decreasing values on control charts. The effect of freeze-thaw cycles on constituent stability is an important consideration. In plasma or serum specimens, the ice crystals formed cause shear effects that are disruptive to molecular structure(s), particularly to large protein molecules. Slow freezing allows larger crystals to form, causing more serious degradable effects. Thus, quick freezing is recommended for optimal stability.

PRESERVATION OF URINE SPECIMENS

Preservation of a urine specimen is essential in order to maintain its integrity. Unpreserved urine specimens are subject both to microbiologic decomposition and to inherent chemical changes. Table 1–14 lists common changes seen in urine as it decomposes. To prevent growth of microbes, the specimen should be refrigerated promptly after collection and, when necessary, contain the indicated chemical preservative. For some determinations, the addition of a chemical preservative could affect assay outcome, thus refrigeration may be more appropriate. The preservative is added to the empty bottle, and a warning label is placed on the bottle as well. Warnings are necessary, e.g., acid burns to patient's genitals are not an unknown occurrence with the use of concentrated acids as preservatives. Light-sensitive compounds are protected in either amber glass bottles or plastic bottles wrapped in aluminum foil. Precipitation of calcium and phosphorus occurs unless the urine is acidified adequately before analysis.

It is particularly important to use *freshly* voided and concentrated urine to identify casts, RBCs, and WBCs, because these elements undergo decomposition on storage at room temperature or decreased concentration and osmolality (<1.015 specific gravity). They disappear rapidly in hypotonic and alkaline urine samples. Bilirubin and urobilinogen decrease, especially after exposure to light. Glucose and ketones may be used, whereas bacterial contamination and loss

Table 1–14. CHANGES THAT OCCUR IN URINE AS IT DECOMPOSES

Result	Reason
Changes in color	Breakdown or alteration of chromogen or other urine constituent (e.g., hemoglobin or homogentisic acid)
Changes in odor	Bacterial growth, decomposition
Increased turbidity	Increased bacteriuria, crystal formation, precipitation of amorphous material
Falsely low pH	Glucose converted to acids and alcohols by bacteria and yeast
Falsely elevated pH	Breakdown of urea by bacteria, producing ammonia
	CO_2 lost
False-negative glucose	Utilization by bacteria (glycolysis)
False-negative ketone	Volatilization of acetone
	Breakdown of acetoacetate by bacteria
False-negative bilirubin	Destroyed by light
	Oxidized to biliverdin
False-negative urobilinogen	Destroyed by light
False-positive nitrite	Nitrite produced by bacteria after specimen is voided
False-negative nitrite	Nitrite converted to nitrogen, which evaporates
Increased bacteriuria	Bacteria multiply in specimen
Disintegration of cells/casts	Unstable environment, especially when urine is alkaline, hypotonic, or both

of CO_2 increases the pH. Turbidity, precipitates, and color changes occur. One should deliver specimens for these measurements to the laboratory within one hour of collection. A useful guide for the collection and preservation of urine specimens according to the chemical analyte measured is presented in Table 1–15.

Urine may be frozen in aliquots to be assayed at a later date. When repeat testing is expected, store the specimen in multiple aliquots to circumvent specimen degradation as a result of repeated freeze-thawing of a single specimen. Preservatives may also be added, depending on the substance to be tested. Sodium fluoride added to 24-hour urines for glucose determinations inhibits bacterial growth and cell glycolysis, but not yeast. About 0.5 g of sodium fluoride is added to a 3- to 4-L container. Use of a reagent (enzyme embedded) strip test for glucose may be inhibited by sodium fluoride but not the copper reduction test. Tablets containing formaldehyde, mercury, and benzoate (95-mg tablet/20-mL urine) have also

Table 1–15. URINE DETERMINATION WITH RECOMMENDED COLLECTION AND PRESERVATION

Determination	Collection*	No Preservative	Boric Acid (10–15 g)	Glacial Acetic Acid (15 mL)	Hydrochloric Acid (15 mL)	Refrigeration—No Preservative
Albumin	24		X			
Aldosterone	24			X		
α-amino nitrogen	24		X			
Amino acids	24		X			
Amylase	2					X
Arsenic	24	X				
Barbiturates	R					X
Bence Jones protein	24		X			X
Calcium	24				X	
Catecholamines	24			X		
Chloride	24		X			
Chorionic gonadotropin	24					X
Copper	24	X				
Coproporphyrin (see under porphyrins)						
Cortisol	24		X			
Creatine	24		X			
Creatinine	24		X			
δ-Aminolevulinic acid (ALA)	24				X	
Drug abuse screen	R					X
Electrolytes (Cl, K, Na)	24					X
Estriol, pregnancy	24	X	X(Kober)			
Estrogens, total	24		X			
Follicle-stimulating hormone	24					X
Glucose	24		X			
Heavy metals	24	X				
17-Hydroxycorticosteroids (17-OH)	24			X		
5-Hydroxyindoleacetic acid (5-HIAA)	24		X			
Hydroxyproline	24		X			
17-Ketogenic steroids (17-KGS)	24			X		
17-Ketosteroids (17-KS)	24			X		
Lead	24	X				
Lithium	24			X		
Mercury	24	X				
Metanephrines	24			X		
Osmolality	24					X
Phosphorus	24				X	
Porphobilinogen (see under porphyrins)						
Porphyrins, Total	24					
Coproporphyrin	24	5 g Na_2CO_3				
Porphobilinogen	24	(protect from light)				
Protoporphyrin	24					
Uroporphyrin	24					
Potassium	24					X
Pregnanediol	24			X		
Pregnanetriol	24			X		
Protein	24		X			X
Protoporphyrin (see under porphyrins)						
Sodium	24					X
Tetrahydro compound "S" (THS)	24			X		
Uric acid	24		X			
Uroporphyrin (see under porphyrins)						
Vanillylmandelic acid (VMA)	24			X		

*Time of collection: 24 = 24 hour; 2 = 2 hour; R = random.

been used; however, specific gravity may be elevated (0.002/one tablet/20 mL). Boric acid in a concentration of 1 g/dL preserves urine elements such as estriol and estrogen for up to seven days. Glyceroboric acid (0.5 mL) with sodium formate buffer minimizes bacterial growth for 24 hours without refrigeration. A pH of 1 to 2 (add 30 mL of 6N HCl to a 3- to 4-L container) is appropriate for catecholamines, vanillylmandelic acid (VMA), or 5-hydroxyindoleacetic acid (5-HIAA) urine collection. For amino acid evaluation, a pH of 3 is required using HCl. Twenty-four–hour urine specimens collected for porphyrins, porphobilinogen, and δ-aminolevulinic acid determinations must be maintained at a pH of 6 to 7 using acetic acid or sodium bicarbonate. Such specimens are collected in dark containers and refrigerated. Urine is collected for cytologic identification of tumor cells into equal volume of 50% alcohol. Alternatively, urine may be collected into Saccomanno's fixative (490 mL of 50% ethanol + 10 mL carbowax [polyethylene glycol 1500]).

Specimen Processing

Processing of specimens includes three distinct phases: precentrifugation, centrifugation, and postcentrifugation (NCCLS pub. H18-A, 1990). Continuing appraisal of all specimen handling activities is an important preanalytical component to total quality control. Appropriate guidelines must be established and adhered to by laboratory personnel in each phase of specimen handling to ensure the generation of reliable and medically meaningful measurement and examination results. Assessing specimen pathways improves workflow and quality in the specimen processing (Kaufman, 1992).

PRECENTRIFUGATION PHASE

SPECIMEN TYPE. Ideally, all measurements should be performed within one hour after collection. Whenever this is not practical, the specimen should be processed to a point at which it can be properly stored in order to preclude alterations of constituents to be measured. With the exception of blood gases and ammonia determinations, plasma or serum is preferred for most determinations because many constituents are distributed differently in erythrocytes compared with serum or plasma. In clinical chemistry, serum and plasma are interchangeable except for a few measurements, such as ACTH and resin assays. Serum is required for protein electrophoresis and immunofixation assays, just as plasma is necessary for fibrinogen and other coagulation measurements. Serum is the specimen of choice, owing to its simplicity in collection and handling. Additionally, interference from anticoagulants is obviated. Plasma, if collected appropriately, may be used in medical emergencies when expedited analysis is indicated, because plasma preparation does not require completion of coagulation prior to centrifugation. Usually, a greater volume of plasma than serum is obtained from a given volume of whole blood due to the clot formation process. Urine and other body fluids may be centrifuged to concentrate particulate matter in order to minimize interference, while the sediment may be submitted to microscopic examination.

A blood specimen should ideally be centrifuged as soon as clot formation is complete (about 20 minutes at room temperature). In practice, a time interval of two hours between blood collection and serum separation is acceptable (Burtis, 1994). Prolonged contact of serum with cell clot beyond two hours can cause significant changes in certain constituents, such as glucose, potassium, phosphorus, creatinine, AST, and alanine aminotransferase (ALT) (Rehak, 1988).

Blood should be kept in the original stoppered container until it is ready for separation. For plasma preparation, centrifuge blood within one hour after collection, for 10 minutes at a relative centrifugal force (RCF) of 850 to 1000 × gravity (× g), keeping the container stoppered to prevent evaporation of plasma or serum water. Allow adequate time for clotting to prevent latent fibrin formation, which may cause undesirable clogging of automated chemistry analyzers. This problem may be resolved with the use of plasma after the addition of lithium heparin to the specimen. Loosening the clot by trimming or ringing the tube may cause some hemolysis and should be done only when necessary. When glass tubes are used, they should be centrifuged in an aerosol-contained vessel. Centrifuge blood for 10 minutes at an RCF of 850 to 1000 × g in stoppered container. If analysis is to be delayed for more than four hours, store serum or plasma at 4° to 6°C until analysis. Retention of such specimens for seven days permits additional measurements or confirmations to be performed at a later date.

CENTRIFUGATION PHASE

A centrifuge uses centrifugal force to separate phases of suspensions by different densities. It is most frequently used in processing blood to derive plasma or serum fractions. Conditions for centrifugation should specify both the time and the centrifugal force. In selecting a centrifuge, one should look for the highest possible centrifugal force and not the rotational speed. Measuring the radius (r) of the centrifuge head, the calculation of the relative centrifugal force (g) may be made from a nomogram (Fig. 1–2) or by the use of the following formula:

$$RCF = 1.118 \times 10^{-5} \times r \times (rpm)^2 \qquad (1\text{-}1)$$

in which *RCF* is the relative centrifugal force in units of g, i.e., multiples of the gravitational force; 1.118×10^{-5} is a constant; *r* is the radius, expressed in centimeters, between the axis of rotation and the center of the centrifuge tube; and *rpm* is the speed in revolutions per minute. Several principles must be observed to avoid damage to the centrifuge or the specimen and danger to personnel. Tubes, carriers, or shields of equal weight, shape, and size should be placed in opposing positions in the centrifuge head to achieve appropriate balance. Specimens must be placed with regard for a geometrically symmetric arrangement, using water-filled tubes to attain balance.

EQUIPMENT

A wide variety of centrifuges and accessories are available to meet specific needs in the clinical laboratory. These include tabletop, general laboratory centrifuges; fixed-angle, high-speed centrifuges; portable floor models; undercounter models; microcentrifuges; refrigerated and unrefrigerated types; and ultracentrifuge models. Capacities vary with model type and centrifuge head. Specimen volume (per tube), number of tubes to be centrifuged, speed required for adequate separation, and durability of equipment should be considered.

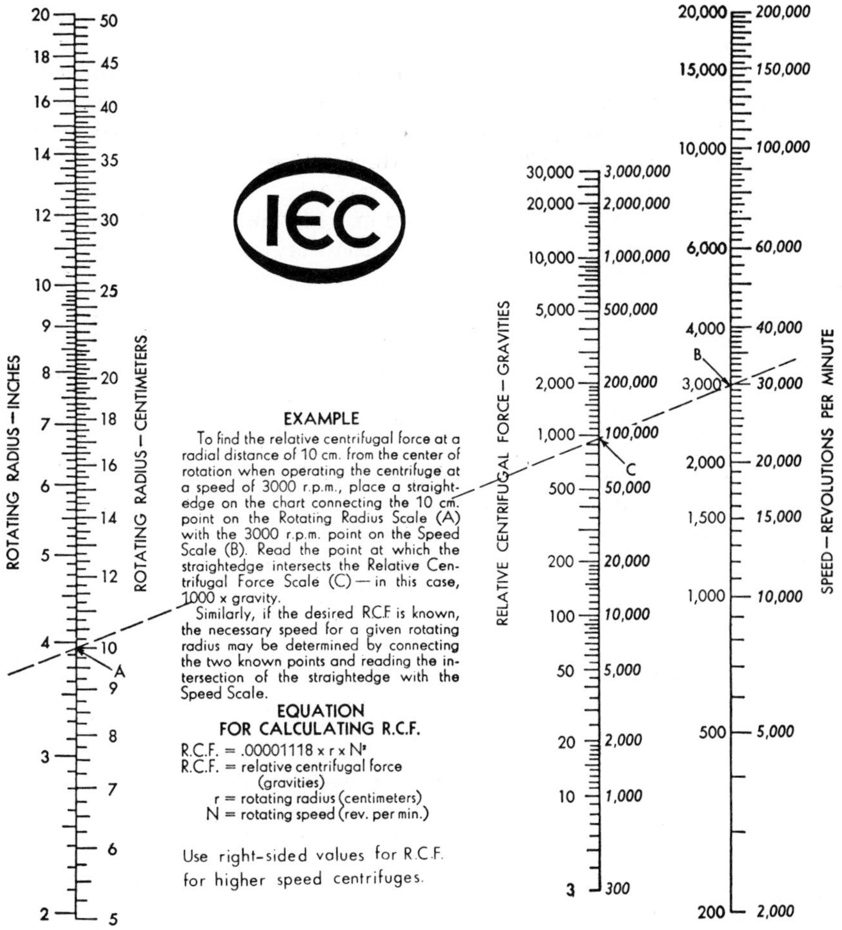
ROTATING RADIUS—INCHES
ROTATING RADIUS—CENTIMETERS
IEC
EXAMPLE
To find the relative centrifugal force at a radial distance of 10 cm. from the center of rotation when operating the centrifuge at a speed of 3000 r.p.m., place a straightedge on the chart connecting the 10 cm. point on the Rotating Radius Scale (A) with the 3000 r.p.m. point on the Speed Scale (B). Read the point at which the straightedge intersects the Relative Centrifugal Force Scale (C)—in this case, 1000 x gravity.
Similarly, if the desired R.C.F. is known, the necessary speed for a given rotating radius may be determined by connecting the two known points and reading the intersection of the straightedge with the Speed Scale.
EQUATION
FOR CALCULATING R.C.F.
R.C.F. = .00001118 x r x N²
R.C.F. = relative centrifugal force (gravities)
r = rotating radius (centimeters)
N = rotating speed (rev. per min.)
Use right-sided values for R.C.F. for higher speed centrifuges.
RELATIVE CENTRIFUGAL FORCE—GRAVITIES
SPEED—REVOLUTIONS PER MINUTE
A
B
C

Figure 1–2. Nomogram for calculation of relative centrifugal force (RCF) in g.

CALIBRATION OF CENTRIFUGE. For every laboratory procedure requiring centrifuge operation, a written specification identifying centrifuge type, what temperature, the g forces required, and the length of centrifugation time is to be noted in the procedure manual. Calibration of the centrifuge must be part of the quality assurance process. Koenig (1982) provides an excellent review of function, verification, and adjustment for a centrifuge. In general, speed and timer must be tested under similar conditions (same number of tubes with same volume) for each time tested to ensure consistency. Any significant changes indicate deterioration effects, such as wearing of brushes, bearing problems, or a defective timer.

ROBOTICS

Advances in technology have led to the development of mechanically driven laboratory instruments interfaced with supporting computer hardware and software (Felder, 1990). Use of robotics may increase productivity, decrease biohazard exposure, decrease labor costs, enhance TAT, and offer a level of procedural consistency. As much as 50% to 70% of laboratory time consumed in the analysis of a specimen is expended on specimen sample preparation (Schoeny, 1991). Modern laboratory equipment now includes automated sampling and aliquoting devices, scanning devices, pipetting stations, or specimen and aliquot transfer. Motorized microscope stages and mechanical arms are integrated with laboratory equipment to make the process more efficient and improve workflow. Robots have been described as cartesian (three degrees of freedom of the X, Y, and Z axes), cylindrical (four degrees of freedom that includes rotation), and articulated (5 or 6 degrees of freedom that include bending or gripper movements) and driven by a programmable controller (Markin, 1992 and 1993). Automated guided vehicles and conveyor systems have been used to transport specimens to work stations.

BAR CODING

Bar code reading capabilities are widely used in modern clinical laboratory instruments found in chemistry, hematology, immunology, microbiology, and blood banks (Kasten, 1992). Bar code readers have become an integral part of many instruments and LIS. Bar coding has been useful in identifying patients and patient demographics, types of specimens to be collected, and tests to be performed (Neeley, 1990). Bar coding consists of pairs of lines (a character) and spaces of varying widths. Each character represents a number, letter, or some other graphic symbol. A laser light source in the form of a light pen, wand, hand-held scanner or fixed scanner, reads the black lines (absorbs light) and spaces (reflects light), transforms the analog patterns into electrical pulses, and translates them into binary computer code.

Integration of bar coding into the laboratory and other departments of the hospital clearly identifies patients when laboratory work is to be completed, when blood-drawing lists are to be created, and during transfer of patient data to the LIS or internal instrument computer systems. Bar coding eliminates secondary labeling of tubes (decanting, aliquoting, or storage of tubes), decreases labeling errors, and enhances turn-around time (Kasten, 1993). By improving accuracy, productivity, and workflow, patient care and cost savings may be significantly enhanced. Advantages of bar coding data entry over handwritten data entry are "keyless data entry, automatic time-stamping, standardization of documentation, legibility of medical record, and point-of-care data capture" (Chua, 1993).

ANALYTICAL STAGE

The validity of clinical laboratory data is dependent not only on proper manipulation of equipment but also on use of specific reagents, quality of materials, and environmental control. An understanding of these fundamental issues embracing materials and essential measurements is a prelude to an appreciation of analytical procedures.

Reagents

GRADES. Chemicals exist in varying degrees of purity. Meticulous attention to the label on a bottle as well as to the supplier's catalogue frequently reveal the maximum limits of impurities in chemicals. The content actual analysis is often provided on the label so one may identify the type and amount of an impurity present. The use of reagent-grade chemicals, although more expensive than less pure grades of chemicals, is essential for accuracy. Chemicals identified as spectrograde, hanograde, HPLC grade, or ACS, have met the established standards of highest purity by the American Chemical Society (ACS) and are readily identified on a label or in a catalogue. Less pure grades are referred to as purified and technical. Chemicals labeled as USP and NF grade represent a level of purity as stipulated in the United States Pharmacopeia or the National Formulary. Although adequate for human consumption, they may not be pure enough for specific chemical applications.

The National Bureau of Standards (NBS), through the Office of Standard Reference Materials (Alvarez, 1982), the College of American Pathologists (CAP), and the National Committee for Clinical Laboratory Standards (NCCLS), also identifies clinical laboratory standards for chemicals. These standards, in addition to the listing provided by suppliers (Medical Safety Data Sheets [MDS]), are preferred sources for information and use in medical chemistry.

Proprietary reagents of undisclosed composition should be carefully evaluated. With abnormal specimens or under abnormal conditions, confusing results as well as invalid data may be produced if purity or constituents of certain reagents are not provided. It is important to know what compounds are being used in a specific determination to understand what reaction is taking place and to identify as well as anticipate and evaluate abnormal reactions or interferences.

TECHNIQUES OF USE AND STORAGE. Once a container is opened, steps must be taken to ensure that the chemical or reagent is handled under optimal conditions. It is extremely important to read the label for proper storage. Although most chemical compounds are stable at room temperature without desiccation, some must be refrigerated, frozen, or even stored at −70°C. Light-sensitive chemicals and reagents must be stored in brown bottles. Advances in materials technologies have made possible prepackaged reagents as packets, thin films, or tablets. They can be loaded directly into automated analyzers for use without an operator's intervention. Use of these reagents eliminates labor-intensive reagent reconstitution and minimizes reagent waste.

Commercially available kits used in immunoassays, both isotopic and nonisotopic (enzyme, fluorescence, chemiluminescence, or electrochemical tags are used in place of radioisotope as the labeled moleculed), include all essential reagents, standards, diluents, radiolabeled antigens, antibodies, plus any other ancillary reagents. When compared with radioimmunoassays, nonisotopic kits are more stable, provide equivalent assay sensitivity, and pose less safety hazards. The reliability of such kits are dependent on the supplier to produce and maintain appropriate quality control. It is essential that each laboratory first evaluate a kit according to an established protocol (NCCLS EP7-P, 1986; EP9-T, 1993; EP10-T2, 1993). Many of the analytes measured by immunochemical methods, such as hormones, are available as reference preparations from the World Health Organization (WHO) or the National Institutes of Health (NIH).

Water

Purification

The two methods in general use for preparation of laboratory reagent grade water are distillation and deionization. Reagent water is obtained by purifying distilled water by deionization. Deionizers work on the principle of ion exchange. Insoluble resin polymers are prepared with acid or amine functional groups on the molecule. A cation exchange resin, for example, a phenolformaldehyde polymer with ;bsSO_3H_3, ;bsCH_2COOH, ;bsCOOH, or ;bsOH radicals, reacts in the following manner, with R;bs representing the insoluble backbone of the polymer, and Na^+ as an example:

$$(1)\ R\ O\ S\ O\ OH + Na^+ \rightleftarrows R\ O\ S\ O\ O\ Na + H^+ \qquad (1\text{-}2)$$

In this reaction, sodium ions are removed from solution and hydrogen ions are ejected into solution, thus initiating hydrogen for sodium ions. In a similar manner, an anion exchange resin such as that formed by the condensation of formaldehyde with various amines, for example, *m*-phenylenediamine and urea, exchanges hydroxyl ions for negatively charged ions in solution. One such reaction is:

$$(2)\ R_4NOH + Cl^- \rightleftarrows R_4NCl + OH^- \qquad (1\text{-}3)$$

Commercially installed systems use a cationic exchange resin, followed by an anionic exchange resin, a charcoal filter to remove organic compounds, and a final filter to remove particulate matter. This type can be monitored at 1 megohm per cm specific resistance with a light to indicate that the system is producing water at least equal to the indicated quality. At peak operation, this system generates water at 10 megohms per cm specific resistance or better.

Specifications set by the CAP (Hamlin, 1978) define three

Table 1–16. RESISTANCE SPECIFICATIONS OF REAGENT WATER

Specification	Type I	Type II	Type III
Specific resistance* megohms @ 25°C, minimum	In-line 10	Effluent 2.0	(As used) 0.1

*Specific resistance is the resistance in ohms of a column of solution 1 cm long and 1 cm² in cross-sectional area.

grades of water: Types I, II, and III, with resistance specifications shown in Table 1–16. Each test established in the laboratory must be judged for the type of water necessary to avoid interference with specificity, accuracy, and precision. For example, metal contaminants can have profound effects on enzyme values.

TYPE I REAGENT WATER. For procedures that require maximum water purity: (1) Preparation of standard solutions, (2) ultramicrochemical analyses, (3) measurements at nanogram or subnanogram concentrations, and (4) tissue or cell culture methods, or both.

TYPE II REAGENT WATER. For most laboratory determinations in chemistry, hematology, microbiology, immunology, and other clinical laboratory areas.

TYPE III REAGENT WATER. For most qualitative measurements/examinations; most procedures in urinalysis, parasitology, and histology; washing glassware; in general, any laboratory procedures not requiring Type I or II reagent water. Carbon dioxide (CO_2)–free water (reagent water, free of CO_2) is used when such gases as CO_2, ammonia, and oxygen may affect analysis. Boiled Type II water is adequate for such use.

Measurement of Mass

Measurement of mass is a fundamental process in the preparation of standards, reagents, gravimetric analysis, or calibration of volumetric equipment, requiring use of analytical balances. The basic principle in the measurement of mass is to balance an unknown mass with a known mass. Analytical balances, though extremely sophisticated, use the basic concept of a simple lever that pivots on a knife-edge fulcrum placed at the lever's center of gravity. From this concept, balances are designed in a variety of ways. *Two pans* of equal mass may be suspended from the ends of the lever, or beam. *Calibrated* weights are placed on one pan to counterbalance an object of unknown mass on the other. A rider or a chain weight device, or both, is generally used to avoid fractional weights. Motion of the beam is indicated by a pointer traversing a scale much like a ruler. Macrobalances of this sort generally have a capacity of 200 g and a sensitivity of 0.1 mg.

Single-pan balances offer the speed and accuracy necessary in the clinical laboratory. These balances encompass a range from 1 μg to 1000 g in both analytical and top-loading balances. Although single-pan balances work on the principle of weighing by substitution, they still use the basic concept of a lever and fulcrum. The balance is first set at the zero point. The sample is placed on the pan, and the selector knobs are adjusted by removing weights until the zero point is again reached. These weights are nonmagnetic chrome-nickel steel rings or cylinders standardized against prototype weights at the NBS. Therefore, the mass of the sample is exactly substituted for an equivalent mass of weights originally on the sample side of the beam.

The sequence in weighing a sample using a single-pan balance is as follows:

1. The balance is leveled by checking the level indicator and adjusting the feet.
2. Observe that the balance is not in direct sunlight and is in a draft-free location.
3. Set the balance to its zero point. If taring (compensating for the weight of the weighing vehicle, i.e., weighing paper, weighing boat) is used, set the read-out at zero. For the analytical balance, this setting is made with the sliding windows closed and the beam resting on the knife edge.
4. Lock the beam of the analytical balance. Open the window of the balance case and place the object to be weighed on the pan. Close the window.
5. Set the beam arrest knob in the intermediate position.
6. Make gross weight changes until the weight of the object is in the range of the optical scale.
7. Fully release the beam and allow the pan to come to its final point of rest.
8. Record the mass of the object.
9. Fully arrest the beam and remove the object from the pan.

Analytical balances are delicate instruments that require care and proper maintenance. Damage to the knife-edged fulcrum can occur by lowering the beam too hard, overloading, or applying excessive vibration. Make gross weight changes with the balance in the beam arrest position and release gently. Clean chemical spills immediately, and never weigh a sample directly on the pan. Materials difficult to weigh, such as hygroscopic and volatile materials, can be weighed in bottles with ground-glass stoppers.

Calibration

The weights in a typical single-pan analytical balance meet individual and group tolerances for Class S weights established by the NBS (Washington, DC; NBS Circular 547, Lasof, 1954). Class S calibration tolerances are available in a variety of fractional weights (1 mg to 500 mg). These weights must be handled with forceps supplied with the set to avoid oils from the skin or powder from gloves. A balance out of calibration usually requires a specialist for adjustment and realignment.

Top-Loading Balances

Single-pan top-loading balances operate on the same principle as single-pan analytical balances, i.e., weighing by substitution. Damping is magnetic rather than air-release. These balances are especially suitable for rapidly weighing larger masses (up to 10,000 g) that do not require as much analytical precision, such as large volume reagent preparation.

Electronic Balances

Modern electronic balances couple the advantage of ease of use with very high resolution. Resolution is an expression of sensitivity in relation to the total dynamic range, defined in points. A scale with 130-kg capacity that reads accurately to 0.5 kg has a resolution of 260 points. An electronic semimicro balance has a resolution of 3 million points (30 g accurate to 0.01 mg). An electronic balance operates on the principle of electromagnetic force compensation. A coil, placed between the poles of a cylindrical electromagnet, is mechanically connected to a weighing pan. Mass placed on the pan produces a force that displaces the coil within the magnetic field. A regulator generates a compensation current just sufficient to return the coil to its original position. The more mass placed on the pan, the larger the deflecting force and the stronger the current required to correct the deflection of the coil. The measuring principle is based on a strict linear relationship between compensation current and force produced by the load placed on the pan.

Measurement of Volume

Types of Glassware

The most common type of glassware encountered in volume measurements is borosilicate glass. This glass is characterized by a high degree of thermal resistance, has a low alkali content, and is free from the magnesia-lime-zinc group of elements, heavy metals, arsenic, and antimony. Commercial brands are known as Pyrex (Corning, Corning, NY) and Kimax (Kimble, Vineland, NJ). The caustic conditions in storing concentrated alkaline solutions in borosilicate glass will etch or dissolve the glass and destroy the calibration. Frozen glass stoppers are difficult to remove without breaking the neck of the flask. Borosilicate glassware with heavy walls, such as bottles, jars, and even larger beakers, should not be heated with a direct flame or hot plate. Glass should not be heated above its strain point (Pyrex is 515°C) because rapid cooling strains and cracks glass easily when heated again. In the case of volumetric glassware, heating can destroy the calibration.

Corex (Corning, Corning, NY) brand glassware is a special alumina-silicate glass strengthened chemically rather than thermally. Corex is six times stronger than borosilicate glass (e.g., Corex pipettes have a typical strength of 30,000 psi, compared with 2000 to 5000 psi for borosilicate pipettes) and will outlast conventional glassware by 10 times. Corex also resists clouding and scratching better. Alkali-resistant glassware should be used to handle strongly alkaline solutions. However, it has only about half the thermal shock resistance of Pyrex glassware and, therefore, must be heated and cooled more carefully. Low actinic glassware is a glass of high thermal resistance with a red color added as an integral part of the glass. The density of the red color is adjusted to permit adequate visibility of the contents yet give maximum protection to light-sensitive materials, such as bilirubin standards.

SPECIFICATIONS

Volumetric glassware is classed as A, B, and student grade. The tolerances for accuracy of Class A glassware meet or exceed the strict requirements specified by the NBS in Circular C-602. Only Class A volumetric glassware is acceptable by the CAP for use in an approved clinical laboratory.

PIPETTES

There are many kinds of pipettes available for use in a clinical laboratory, each intended to serve a specific function. In general, pipettes fall into two classes: volumetric or transfer pipettes and graduated or measuring pipettes. The volumetric pipette is calibrated for one specified volume measurement, either "to deliver" (T.D.) or "to contain" (T.C.). For Class A pipettes, this distinction is clearly indicated on the pipette. A "to deliver" pipette calibrated for blowout has an opaque ring near the top. In this case, the small amount of liquid remaining in the tip after free delivery has ceased is blown out and added to the initial volume. "To deliver" pipettes are calibrated for the volume delivered, with no attempt to wash out the film that adheres to the inside glass surface. "To contain" pipettes are calibrated for the total volume of liquid held in the pipette and must be washed out completely for delivery of the correct volume. Most micropipettes, in the range up to 0.5 mL, are calibrated "to contain." Graduated pipettes are long, cylindrical tubes drawn out to a tip and are calibrated in uniform fractional volume measurements. The Mohr type is calibrated between two marks on the stem, whereas the serologic type is calibrated to the tip. All serologic pipettes therefore are calibrated for blowout, and accordingly have an opaque ring at the top for identification. Ensure pipettes are the correct size, clean, and free of chips before using. Without careful inspection, a broken tip may go unnoticed. To avoid ingestion of body fluids, caustic chemicals, or other infectious agents, mouth pipetting is not permitted under any circumstances. Use of a rubber-bulb or Pipet-Aid (Drummond Scientific, Broomall, PA) for all pipetting is recommended.

The steps in good pipetting procedure include the following:

1. Place safety pipette filler on the stem of the pipette.
2. Lower the pipette into the solution. Allow sufficient depth to fill the pipette above the calibration mark.
3. Apply suction using pipette bulb and load the pipette to a point above the calibration mark. In cases of a critically low volume of solution, fill the pipette slowly and watch carefully to avoid aspiration of air.
4. Remove the pipette from the solution. Wipe the tip with a tissue or gauze.
5. Hold the pipette in a vertical position. Empty the pipette slowly until the lower meniscus just touches the calibration mark. Pay attention to parallax errors.
6. Touch the tip to a clean, dry receptacle to remove any pendant drop.
7. Drain the pipette freely in a vertical position. The pipette has been calibrated to deliver its specified volume in a vertical position with a constant rate of delivery. Changing the angle of the pipette changes the rate of delivery and hence the volume of liquid left behind in the pipette. For the same reason, do not attempt to force the liquid from the pipette at a faster rate than free drainage permits.
8. When the liquid enters the stem just below the bulb, touch the tip to the side of the receiving vessel, but not into the liquid. Allow several seconds for the pipette to drain. For blowout pipettes, manipulate the small bulb of the safety pipette filler to force a gentle blast of air

through the pipette. This removes the last bit of liquid from the tip.

SEMIAUTOMATIC AND AUTOMATIC PIPETTES

Automatic pipetting devices (Oxford Pipetters, Sherwood Medical Co., St. Louis, MO) permit rapid, repetitive measurement and delivery of equal volumes. Commercial automatic pipettes are either of the sampling type, usually manually operated, or of the sampling-diluting type, usually electrically operated. Manually operated automatic pipettes are generally of the air-displacement variety, with a range in volume capacity from 1 to 6000 μL. Tip-ejector models, variable-setting digital pipettes, and repetitive-dispensing pipettes are available for added convenience. Because proper care and calibration are essential to precise, accurate sampling, it is important to read and follow the manufacturer's instructions. Two common errors include allowing a sample to aspirate into the barrel of the pipette and ignoring lubrication of the piston. The sampling-dispensing automatic pipettes fall into two general classes: (1) the peristaltic type and (2) the piston type. Automatic sampler-diluters are available with sampling volume ranges from 0.1 to 5000 μL and diluting volumes from 0.2 to 25 mL. For maximum accuracy and precision, diluent volumes up to 5000 μL are best.

Automatic pipettes remove much of the tedium associated with repetitive sampling and dilution. Even for a limited number of samples, the speed of an automatic pipette is an advantage. Because operator fatigue is minimized, precision of multiple sampling and dilution is often improved with the automatic pipette. The microautomatic pipettes, which can sample as little as 2 to 5 μL, offer a unique advantage, especially for radioimmunoassay.

Manufacturers generally claim a pipetting and dilution accuracy in the range of 0.0% to 1.0%. However, it is essential that automatic pipettes be calibrated when new and at regular intervals thereafter. Never assume that factory calibrations are accurate! The random analytical variation of an automatic manual pipette can be established by repetitive pipetting of a radioactive solution and counting the activity of each sample. Calculations are made to determine the mean and standard deviation of the counts. The total variance includes both the variance of the counter and the variance of the pipette. The variances are additive. Therefore, the variance of pipetting is calculated as:

$$\sigma^2 \text{ Total} = \sigma^2 \text{ Counter} + \sigma^2 \text{ Pipetting} \qquad (1\text{-}4)$$

A second method involves the gravimetric evaluation of an aliquot of deionized, distilled water. The volume of water can be calculated using the weight of water at a known temperature. The process is as follows:

1. Set pipettor to the desired dispensing volume.
2. Weigh an empty beaker that will accommodate 10 dispensed sample volumes. Do not touch the beaker once it has been weighed.
3. Dispense set volume 10 times into beaker, noting weight after *each* addition.
4. Record temperature of the water and note water density as listed in Figure 1–3.

Temperature (°C)	Density (g/mL)
17	0.99880
18	0.99862
19	0.99843
20	0.99823
21	0.99802
22	0.99780
23	0.99756
24	0.99732
25	0.99707

Figure 1–3. Relative density of water at various room temperatures.

5. Calculate the weight of each aliquot. Record all data.
   a. $\dfrac{\text{Mean weight of aliquot (g)}}{\text{Density of } H_2O \text{ @ temperature recorded (g/mL)}} = \text{Mean volume (mL)}$
   b. Mean volume − expected volume (as set on pipettor) = Volume error (mL)
   c. $\dfrac{\text{Volume error (mL)}}{\text{Expected volume (mL)}} \times 100 = \text{Volume error in \%}$
   d. Acceptable volume error = $<3\%$

In using an automatic pipette, the tip-wiping technique is important in obtaining reproducibility. Aspirate the sample into the tip, and wipe with absorbent cloth or tissue with two downward strokes at 90 degrees with respect to one another. Each stroke should start above the level that the tip was immersed into the fluid sample and proceed downward past the tip. Do not actually touch the fluid in the tip, because this will draw the fluid out of the tip.

When a sample from an automatic pipet is introduced into the tip, diffusion of sample occurs leading to possible carryover. The washout by diluent may be insufficient to remove all the sample, and this becomes mixed with the succeeding sample. The result is that any analyses performed on the first sample dilution are too low, and those done on the second are too high. In general, the ratio of diluent to sample must be at least 5:1 for quantitative washout. This must be increased if the sample is viscous or oily and the diluent is of an aqueous base. Also, certain components are adsorbed by the tip construction, and the washout must be increased. In general, a Teflon tip absorbs less than a glass tip. Some hormones and drugs, for example, have a high affinity for glass.

VOLUMETRIC FLASKS

Inspect the flask to be sure that it is clean, dry, and not cracked. For glass-stoppered flasks, be sure the stopper fits properly so it does not leak.

The steps in using a volumetric flask are as follows:

1. Add to the flask the solution to be diluted or the solid to be dissolved and diluted to volume. A solid is best added to the flask by having first weighed the material in a beaker. Then add enough solvent/diluent to the beaker to dissolve the solid. Hold a glass rod across the beaker with one end over the lip. Tip the beaker and allow the solution to pour down the glass rod into the opening of the flask. Keep adding small volumes of

solvent to wash the beaker. This procedure will result in a quantitative transfer to the flask.

2. Bring nearly to volume with solvent or diluent.
3. Use a Pasteur pipette to wet the neck of the flask. Add solvent drop by drop to bring the meniscus to the final calibration mark.
4. Stopper the flask and mix thoroughly. For adequate mixing, turn the flask upside down and shake. Then turn the flask upright. Repeat this four more times. In the case of solutions that foam, mixing must be done more slowly with many more revolutions of the flask. In extreme cases of foaming, the flask can only be rotated, not tipped upside down. Magnetic stir bars and plates may be used.

CALIBRATION

According to the strictest of standards, every piece of volumetric glassware in the clinical laboratory should be coded and a record kept of its calibration. Any piece of glassware that does not meet Class A tolerance should be rejected. To prepare a piece of glassware for calibration, rinse with tap water, followed by a thorough rinsing with reagent grade water.

CLEANING OF GLASSWARE

Glassware used in the general laboratory should be rinsed and immediately placed into a weak detergent solution. Corrosive chemicals should never be kept in glassware that may be spilled by unsuspecting personnel. Glassware must be rinsed, prewashed, washed, rinsed, and finally rinsed with reagent grade water before use. The surface of a thoroughly clean glass apparatus becomes uniformly wet, with no adhering water droplets. Special treatment is required in cases of stubborn grease and other organic residues. Let the glassware stand overnight in a sulfuric acid–dichromate mixture, prepared by pouring 1000 mL of concentrated sulfuric acid into 35 mL of saturated sodium dichromate. Avoid contact with the skin or clothing. Rinse the glassware *thoroughly* after removal from the mixture.

Bacteriologic glassware should be soaked in 2% to 4% cresol solution, followed by autoclaving and a thorough washing procedure. Glassware used for iron determinations must be soaked in hydrochloric acid solution (concentrated HCl diluted 1:2) or nitric acid solution (concentrated HNO_3 diluted 1:3) and then rinsed with reagent grade water.

Control of Temperature

Precise temperature control and recording is essential for all sections of the laboratory. The dependence of enzyme activity on temperature and the requirement for precise temperature control is a classic example.

Constant Temperature Baths

For general clinical laboratory use, constant temperature water baths must offer variable temperature control from +5°C above ambient temperature to 100°C, with accurate control to ±0.2°C. No refrigeration capabilities are required in this type of unit. For precise temperature control at room temperatures or below, refrigeration is necessary. Baths are available with a temperature range from −30°C to 100°C, accurate to ±0.02°C. A compressor and heater work in tandem to offer temperature control over this range. An important consideration in the selection of a constant temperature bath is that the model be large enough to accommodate the desired working volume. Models that have independent controlled agitation to maintain a uniform bath temperature are desirable. Heating blocks are more useful for high temperature use.

Maintenance

Maintenance of a constant temperature water bath is improved by filling it with distilled or deionized water. This prevents the accumulation of mineral deposits from regular tap water, which can affect the temperature sensing elements and generally lead to poor heat transfer. However, if an accumulation of these minerals does occur, a weak hydrochloric acid solution dissolves the deposits. Frequent cleaning and use of fresh water prevent overgrowth of bacteria and algae. Overheating and subsequent damage can occur if the bath goes dry. At higher temperatures, the bath should be covered, both to maintain proper temperature control and to prevent rapid evaporation to dryness.

Quality Control

Accurately calibrated thermometers are issued by the NBS. These thermometers have an auxiliary ice-point scale from −0.20°C to +0.20°C to check the calibration. A thermometer calibrated against another certified by the NBS must be a component of any constant temperature bath. The temperature should be noted and recorded for each assay. This function by the operator ensures that indeed the temperature of the bath is the same as the reading of the thermometer.

Evaporation and Specimen Concentration

Evaporation as a batch or unit process is an essential step in many analytical procedures. Solvent extraction is almost always followed by evaporation of solvent to recover the extracted material for further processing. CSF, urine, and serum specimens may need to be concentrated to bring certain constituents within the range of analytical sensitivity.

Large-volume solvent evaporation is best accomplished with a thin-film rotary vacuum evaporator. Evaporation of test-tube quantities of solvent, in the range of 10 to 15 mL or less, is handled conveniently in an evaporator that concentrates by blowing a stream of an inert gas, usually nitrogen, across the surface of the solvent. Freeze-drying (lyophilization), a process best used for preservation of unstable reagents, is used especially in clinical chemistry for the preparation of control materials.

Polymer films, or membranes, constructed with an effective pore size to retain solutes above a selected molecular weight, can be used to concentrate proteins, including enzymes, isoenzymes, and hormones. Typical molecular weight cut-off (MWCO) values for these ultrafiltration membranes are 15,000, 25,000, 75,000, and 125,000. Amicon Corporation (Lexington, MA) uses these films in the construction of clinical specimen concentrators. Ultrafiltration membranes constructed in a tube and placed in a centrifuge, drive liquid and solute past the membrane, below a critical molecular weight cut-off value. Protein-free filtrates can be prepared with this technique. Therefore, it becomes possible to determine the free, or nonprotein bound, fraction of blood components.

Filtration

Filtration may be used in place of centrifugation to separate solids from liquids. This is performed with filter paper circle, folded in half and then folded again, and a funnel. A funnel containing glass wool may be substituted for paper when acids or bases too strong for filter paper require filtering. Many types of filter paper (Whatman, Clifton, NJ 07014) with different degrees of porosity are available for selection according to requirements of separation by filtration.

Dialysis

Dialysis is a technique for the separation of substances in molecular or ionic solution from colloidally dispersed molecules. A dialyzing membrane is a porous diaphragm that acts like a sieve. When an aqueous system to be dialyzed is placed on one side of the membrane and pure water is placed on the other side, the substances in molecular or ionic solution diffuse through the pores of the membrane. Colloidally dispersed molecules are too large to pass through the pores and, therefore, are held back. Diffusion of the smaller molecules or ions continues until at equilibrium with respective concentrations on either side. The material that passes through the membrane during the process of dialysis is referred to as diffusate, or dialysate. The term *retentate* applies to the substance that does not pass through the membrane. Membranes used in dialysis are most commonly made of regenerated cellulose, using cotton linters for the source of cellulose. The membrane may be constructed as a tube or sheet (Spectr/Por, Spectrum Medical Industries, Los Angeles, CA). Cellulose membranes are available with a molecular weight specification ranging from 1000 to 50,000 MWCO. The 12,000 MWCO film has an average pore diameter of 4.8 nanometers. The 12,000- to 14,000-MWCO membrane has a dialysis rate about three times that of the 6000- to 8000-MWCO membrane. After processing, cellulose membranes have glycerol added as a humectant to keep the film supple. Small amounts (0.1%) of polysulfides are also generally present as a contaminant. Both the glycerol and polysulfide may be removed by proper washing.

Extraction

Theory

Extraction is a separation technique in which a solute is transferred from one solvent to a second immiscible solvent by allowing the solute to form an equilibrium distribution between the two solvent phases. For increased separation efficiency, the solute is transferred in fractions by a series of single extractions. The distribution of solute between the two immiscible solvents is quantitatively expressed by the distribution, or partition, coefficient, K, according to equation (5):

$$K = \text{concentration of A in solvent 1}/\text{concentration of A in solvent 2} \quad (1\text{-}5)$$

Consider X_0 g of compound A is being extracted from V mL of solution by repeated extraction with v mL of an immiscible solvent. The number of grams, X_n, of compound A remaining in solution after n extractions can be shown to be

$$X_n = X_0\,(KV/[KV + v])^n \quad (1\text{-}6)$$

where K is the partition coefficient. This illustrates that extraction with several smaller volumes of an extracting solvent is more efficient than using the same total volume of solvent in one extraction.

Technique

A separatory funnel is commonly used in the laboratory for extraction, especially for larger volumes. Screw-capped or glass-stoppered centrifuge tubes are convenient for extraction involving large numbers of samples. An entire rack of tubes can be placed in a shaker to rapidly equilibrate the solute being extracted. A problem in using screw-capped or glass-stoppered centrifuge tubes for extraction is leakage during the shaking operation. Caps of screw-capped tubes must be lined with Teflon and the rim of the glass tube must not be chipped. Caps of screw-capped tubes must be lined with Teflon. The glass tube must be inspected for defects, and the rim must not be chipped. Glass-fitted stoppers must fit properly and must be held firmly in place during shaking. If both layers must be saved, use a glass transfer pipette to draw off the top layer; otherwise, aspirate.

Column extraction technique is widely used in the clinical laboratory especially in toxicology. Various types of column materials are (1) diatomaceous earth, (2) silica gel, (3) C-18 bonded silica gel, and (4) ion-exchange resins. Drugs in solution are adsorbed on the surface of the column packing in an extremely thin film of liquid, approaching a monolayer. An extremely large surface area is exposed to the eluting solvent, with single-pass extraction efficiencies from 75% to 95%. High-performance liquid chromatography (HPLC) offers advantages of high resolution with fast, accurate quantitation for polar, nonpolar, and heat-labile compounds and is further discussed in Chapter 3.

Mixing

Mixing is an operation intended to form a homogeneous mass or create a uniform heterogeneous system. Mixing is used to bring solids into solution; to bring phases into intimate contact, for instance, in extraction procedures; to wash suspended solids; to homogenize liquid phases; and to perform many other operations. Mixing and centrifuging accomplish opposite objectives. A serious consequence of inadequate mixing can be failure to completely resuspend protein that settles out under long-term frozen storage of serum controls, resulting in invalid data. In some instances, excessive mixing may cause denaturation of protein or hemolysis. A phase separation occurs when serum (or plasma) specimens stand for a period of time and must be thoroughly mixed before analysis. The concentration of even small molecules in such a system will be heterogeneous as proteins settle and become more concentrated, thus effective water concentration decreases in this layer. This produces a water concentration gradient throughout the system and, consequently, a concentration gradient of all components.

Single-Tube Mixers

A vortex mixer is capable of a variable speed oscillation that results in a swirling motion to liquid contents of a test tube or other container. The angle of contact and degree of pressure can be regulated for optimal mixing action. A very effective mixing action is created by a multiple touch sequence, i.e., touching and withdrawing the tube from the neoprene oscillating cup of the mixer. The operator must be careful not to fill the container too full or to mix the liquid contents too fast, because spillage can occur.

Multiple-Tube Mixers

Various mixers are available that handle a number of tubes, tube sizes, and with different types of mixing motions. A Thermolyne Maxi-Mix (Sybron Corporation, Dubuque, IA) can conveniently be used for vortex, mixing one tube or several tubes at one time. Mixing action is varied by changing the pressure of the container against the replaceable foam rubber top. Circular motion on a tilted disc provides continuous inversion of contents in tubes, which are clipmounted at the circumference of the rotating disc. Rotational speed can be varied to provide gentle or more vigorous mixing. Control sera are conveniently reconstituted in this type of mixer. Tube shakers that tilt back and forth at variable speeds provide thorough mixing of whole blood samples.

Detection of Analytical Response

For every analytical procedure, there is a concentration-response curve, also referred to as a dose-response curve. The response per unit of concentration is the analytical sensitivity. Every measurement system requires a mechanism to detect a response. To achieve maximum sensitivity with accuracy and precision requires optimal response of the detection system. For example, lamps, mirrors, and slits on a spectrophotometer must be properly aligned and cleaned at regular intervals. The pulse height analyzer of a scintillation counter must be adjusted to the correct "window" settings. Much of what is gained by meticulous detail to all other steps of the analytical process may be lost by improper calibration and maintenance of the detection system.

Calculation of Results

Errors in patient or specimen identification as well as transcription errors may well constitute major problems, but errors in arithmetic warrant equal attention. A brief review of the mathematics most frequently used by laboratory personnel should clarify and identify principles so essential for accurate work (Campbell, 1984).

Significant Figures

In addition, subtraction, multiplication, and division, calculations of data should retain as many significant figures as are contained in the quantity having the least number of significant figures.

Example: Sum of

65.12
2.115
1.2222
68.4572

Answer: 68.46

Exponents

The use of exponential forms permits simple calculation involving large or small numbers.

$5^2 = 5 \times 5 = 25$ $\quad$ $5^{-2} = 5 \times 10^{-2} = 0.05$

$5^0 = 1$ $\quad$ $5^2 \times 5^3 = 5^5$

$5^{1/2} = 1\sqrt{5^1} = \sqrt{5} = 2.23$ $\quad$ $5^{2/3} = \sqrt[3]{5^2} = \sqrt[3]{25} = 2.92$

Logarithms

The common logarithm of a number is the exponent that must be applied to base 10 in order to produce the number.

Example: $10^3 = 1000$. The exponent 3 is the common logarithm of 1000, since 3 applied as an exponent to 10 = 1000.

In logs, this is written as follows: $\log_{10} 1000 = 3$ (logarithm of 1000 to the base 10 equals 3)

Exponents and Logarithms

$\log_{10} 1 = 0$	or	$1 = 10^0$
$\log_{10} 10 = 1$	or	$10 = 10^1$
$\log_{10} 100 = 2$	or	$100 = 10^2$
$\log_{10} 1000 = 3$	or	$1000 = 10^3$
$\log_{10} 0.1 = -1$	or	$0.1 = 10^{-1}$
$\log_{10} 0.01 = -2$	or	$0.01 = 10^{-2}$

A logarithm is composed of two parts: mantissa (found in logarithm tables), which is placed to the right of the decimal point, and the characteristic, which is placed to the left of the decimal point. The mantissa gives the antilogarithm, or the number of which it is the logarithm. The characteristic identifies the decimal point in the antilogarithm. Logs simplify arithmetic calculations.

To find the log of 768:

Characteristic (digits to the left of decimal point minus one): 768

Characteristic is: 2

Mantissa (from log table) = 0.8854

The log of 768 = 2.8854

For example:

1. To multiply two or more numbers, add their logs, then look up the antilog (antilog is the number that corresponds to a log).
2. To divide, subtract logs, then look up the antilog.
3. For roots and fractional exponents, multiply the log by the fractional exponent, then look up the antilog (many scientific calculators perform this function).

Examples:

$\log(5.5 \times 73) = \log 5.5 + \log 73 = 0.7404 + 1.8633 = 2.6037$
antilog 2.6037 = 401.5

$\log 47/2 = \log 47 - \log 2 = 1.6721 - 0.3010 = 1.3711$
antilog 1.3711 = 23.5

$\log 76^{3/8} = 3/8 \log 76 = 3/8\ (1.8808) = 1.4178$
antilog 1.4178 = 26.2

Aqueous Solution

The concentration of a solution may be expressed as molarity (M), normality (N), and weight/volume (w/v). These are concentrations based on volume. Solutions based on weight and expressed as molality and weight/weight (w/w) are used less frequently in the laboratory (Burtis, 1994).

Molarity (M) is equal to the number of moles of solute per liter of solution (solvent). One gram molecular weight of a substance (GMW) is also called 1 mole of the substance. One mole (1 M) of water (H_2O) = 18.015 g of H_2O. Mole = g/GMW

A 1-molar (M) solution contains 1 mole of solute per liter of finished/final solution.

$$\text{Molarity} = \text{moles/liter} = \text{grams/liter/GMW}$$

A millimole (mmole) is 1/1000 of a mole.

$$\text{Millimoles per liter} = \text{milligrams/liter/GMW}$$

$$\begin{aligned}\text{Avogadro's number} &= \text{number of molecules per g-mole}\\ &= \text{number of atoms per g-atom}\\ &= \text{number of ions per g-ion}\\ &= 6.023 \times 10^{23}\end{aligned}$$

In practice, one Avogadro's number of particles (e.g., 1 g-mole, 1 g-atom, or 1 g-ion) is called a mole regardless of whether the substance is ionic, monoatomic, or molecular in nature. Thus, 39.0 g of K^+ ion may be called a mole, instead of a gram-ion. To make 1 L of a 1 M NaCl solution (mol. wt. = 58.5), 58.5 g of NaCl is dissolved in a quantity sufficient (qs) of water to make 1 L.

When small concentrations are used, they are frequently expressed in millimoles/liter (1000 millimoles = 1 mole). For example, to prepare 10 mL of a 10 mM (0.01 M) NaOH solution, 4 mg NaOH are diluted to 10 mL.

Normality (N) is equal to the number of gram equivalents of solute per liter of solution and is dependent on type of reaction involved (acid-base, oxidation). One gram equivalent weight of an element or compound equals the gram molecular weight divided by valence.

$$\text{Gram equivalents} = \text{GMW/valence}$$
$$1\text{ N} = \text{Number of gram equivalents of solute/Liter of solution}$$

Examples:

$Ca(OH)_2$ (GMW = 74)
Equivalent wt. = 74/2 = 37
1 mole = 2 equivalents

H_2SO_4 (GMW = 98)
Equivalent wt. = 98/2 = 49
1 mole = 2 equivalents

Therefore, one equivalent (i.e., the equivalent weight) of an acid or base is the weight that contains 1 g-atom (1 mole) of replaceable hydrogen, or 1 g-ion (1 mole) of replaceable hydroxyl. To prepare 1 L of 1 N H_2SO_4 from pure (96.2%) concentrated sulfuric acid having a specific gravity of 1.84, dilute 27.7 mL H_2SO_4 to 1 L (specific gravity = weight in g/volume in mL). Appendix 1 contains useful information about various acids and bases commonly used in the laboratory.

Weight/volume per cent (% w/v) is equal to the number of grams of a solid dissolved in enough solvent to bring the final volume to 100 mL. A 10% NaOH solution is prepared by dissolving 10 g NaOH in enough water to make a *final* volume of 100 mL.

A molal solution contains 1 mole of solute in 1 kg of solvent. A molal solution is used in certain physical chemical calculations, e.g., calculations of boiling-point elevation and freezing-point depression.

Weight/weight per cent (% w/w) is equal to the weight in g of a solute per 100 g of solution. The concentrations of many commercial acids are given in terms of % w/w.

When solutions are diluted, volume increases and concentrations decrease.

$$\text{Concentration A} \times \text{Volume A} = \text{Concentration B} \times \text{Volume B}$$

5M NaCl × 10 mL = 2M NaCl × Volume B;
Answer: Volume B = 25 mL

To get 2M NaCl from 5M NaCl, add 15 mL of diluent to get a total volume of 25 mL

Acids, Alkalis, and pH

An acid molecule yields hydrogen ions (protons) in aqueous solutions; an alkali accepts these. At room temperature in pure water:

$$[H^+] = [OH^-] = 1 \times 10^{-7}\text{ molar}$$

In all aqueous solutions, both acid and alkaline:

$$K_w = [H^+] \times [OH^-] = 10^{-14}$$

In an acid solution, $[H^+]$ is greater than 10^{-7} M. In an alkaline solution, $[H^+]$ is less than 10^{-7} M. pH is the exponent that must be applied to 10 in order to give the value of $1/H^+$. That is,

$$pH = \log_{10} 1/H^+$$

When pH is 1; H^+ is 10^{+1} and OH^- is 10^{-13}
2; 10^{-2} 10^{-12}
4; 10^{-4} 10^{-10}
6; 10^{-6} 10^{-8}
10; 10^{-10} 10^{-4}
13; 10^{-13} 10^{-1}

A change of one pH unit indicates a tenfold change in H^+ concentration.

Buffer Solutions

The theory of buffers and their preparation can be found in Appendix 1. A more extensive description of various buffer solutions is reviewed by Gomori (1955).

POSTANALYTICAL STAGE

Reporting/Laboratory Information System (LIS)

Clinically useful data generated by the laboratory must be reported promptly and accurately to optimize patient management. Delay in reporting can make data useless, as, for example, reporting out an acetaminophen concentration in serum 24 hours after the test was requested. The ability to provide accessibility to laboratory data and its timely reporting is heavily dependent on the LIS (see Chap. 3).

Quality Assurance/Quality Control

Retention of Reports/Slides

Record-keeping (Baer, 1993) is part of laboratory management and is mandated by the Joint Commission on Accreditation of Healthcare Organizations, the CAP, and the Health Care Financing Administration (HCFA) through the Clinical Laboratory Improvement Act (CLIA '88). Local governing agencies may supersede other agencies' mandates and must be consulted to ensure appropriate compliance. Table 1–17 offers guidelines regarding report and specimen disposal based primarily on CAP and CLIA '88 regulations. In general, most records are required to be kept only two years, except for blood bank records, which are kept for five years. Records documenting instrument or equipment maintenance must be retained for the life of the instrument. General laboratory reports may be disposed of after two years. Procedures and former procedures must be kept on file. Retired procedures should be kept an additional two years before disposal. Documentation of test requests and results should be kept for two years; however, a patient's medical record also contains this information. Those reports that provide actual diagnosis are retained for at least 20 years. It is suggested that cytogenetic reports be kept for 25 years (in response to number of child-bearing years frequently observed). Personnel records, including training, health records, personal exposure testing, and any other related issue, may be required to be retained for 30 years, especially those related to chemical or biohazard exposures (mandated by the Occupational Safety and Health Administration; Federal Register 56, 29CFR, 1990; 55, 29CFR, 1992; OSHA). Specimen retention varies as to the nature of the specimen and its diagnostic value after an extended period of time. The CAP recommends that blood smears be retained for only seven days, yet it is the practice of some laboratories to retain all blood smears for one year. Bone marrow, abnormal cytology slides, and other pathology slides must be retained for 20 years. Paraffin tissue blocks are to be kept for at least five years; however 20-year retention will keep laboratories on the safe side in medical-legal cases.

Electronic record keeping on computer disks, magnetic tapes, microfilm, microfiche, or optical disks are acceptable. They require considerably less physical space and provide rapid retrieval of information. Optical disk technology is a particularly attractive mechanism for long-term data storage. One 5.25-inch, double-sided optical disk can hold 500,000 document pages. Document-based management retrieval systems appear to be more efficient and less costly to operate: they eliminate the need to upgrade computer hard disc memory, avoid microfilm and microfiche processing, decrease paper usage, and obviate the need for extensive document storage (Brzezicki, 1994).

Table 1–17. SUGGESTED GUIDELINES FOR RECORD AND SPECIMEN RETENTION*

	Record Type	Retention
Records	Test Records	2 years
	Requisition	2 years
	Quality Control	2 years
	Procedures/Manuals	2 years
	Proficiency Testing	2 years
	Remedial Actions	2 years
	Instrument Maintenance	2 years
	Personnel Records	30 years
	Blood Bank Donor/recipient Records	Indefinitely
	Blood Bank Employee Signatures/ Initial	Indefinitely
	Blood Bank Quality Control Records	5 years
	Plasmaphoresis Records	5 years
	Permanently Deferred Donors	Indefinitely
Reports	Lab Reports	2 years
	Autopsy	10 years
	Pathology	10 years
	Bone Marrow	10 years
	Cytopathology	10 years
	Cytogenetic	25 years
Specimens	Serum/other Body Fluids	24 hours
	Blood smears–routine	7 days
	Blood smears–non-routine	(1 year)
	Bone Marrow slides	10 years
	Microbiology smears	7 days
	Cytology negative slides	5 years
	Cytology positive slides	5 years
	FNA Slides	10 years
	Wet Tissue–Surgical	2 weeks after report
	Wet Tissue–Autopsy	3 months after final report
	Paraffin Blocks	5 years
	Pathology Slides	10 years
	Blood Bank Donor/recipient Specimens	7 days post Transfusion
	Cytogenetic Slides	6 years
	Cytogenetic Photographs	25 years

*College of American Pathologists (CAP), 1995, Northfield, IL and/or CLIA '88 guidelines (Federal Register 55, 1990; 57, 1992) with additional suggestions; check with regional or other regulatory agencies for local codes.

LABORATORY SAFETY

The Psychology of Safety

Laboratory safety is a concern for all personnel. Injuries affect the morale and threaten the emotional and physical health of the individual involved and his or her coworkers. Injuries are expensive in terms of lost work days and wages, damaged equipment, and medical treatment. An injured person may be absent for an indefinite period of time and often cannot work at peak efficiency on return. Preventive measures as practiced in the laboratory are essential to the well-being of employees. Such measures include annual safety reviews, disaster drills, and general consciousness raising by employees of maintaining a safe work environment. Although inexperience may cause some accidents, others may be a result of ignoring known risks, haste, carelessness, fatigue, or mental preoccupation (failure to focus attention or concentrate on what is at hand). Appropriate orientation to safety rules, frequent review of these rules, and management's insistence in providing clear guidelines and a safe work environment will diminish unnecessary exposures to health and safety risks. Each laboratory must assume responsibility to develop biological exposure and chemical exposure plans (response action procedures) for the protection of employees (Gile, 1990, 1992).

Biohazards/Universal Precautions

The spread of hepatitis B virus (HBV) and human immunodeficiency virus (HIV) has focused the responsibility on the health care organization to protect its employees from infection. Concern about HIV has prompted the Centers for Disease Control (CDC) in 1987 to update its 1983 *Guidelines for Isolation Precautions in Hospitals* (Garner, 1983) with the release of its Universal Precautions, which recommends that blood and body fluid precautions be consistently used for all patients regardless of their blood-borne infection status (CDC Recommendations and Reports, 1989). Such guidelines are meant to minimize employees' occupational exposures. OSHA defines occupational exposures as "reasonably anticipated skin, eye, mucous membrane, or parenteral contact with blood or other potentially infectious materials that may result from the performance of an employee's duties" (Federal Register, 29CFR, 1910.1030; 1992). Blood and most other body fluids including semen, vaginal secretions, pericardial fluid, peritoneal fluid, synovial fluid, pleural fluid, amniotic fluid, saliva, tears, cerebrospinal fluid, urine, and breast milk of all patients may be considered potentially infectious for HIV, HBV, and other blood-borne pathogens (NCCLS Pub. M29-T2, 1991). In addition, any unfixed tissues, organs, or blood slides may also be considered potentially infectious.

Precautions include appropriate barriers, such as gloves, gowns, or laboratory coats, masks, and eyewear that must be worn to prevent skin and mucous membrane exposure when contact with blood or other body fluids of any patient is anticipated. Every laboratory must have appropriate biohazard policies and procedures and develop plans for use in their laboratories (Gile, 1992). Appropriate engineering controls (devices or equipment that minimize or remove hazards) must also be supplied and include shields, sharps containers, biohazard hoods, centrifuge bucket containers, mechanical pipetting devices, and air respirators, when appropriate.

Although many laboratories require gloves to be worn when an employee performs phlebotomies, OSHA recommendations state that gloves are needed when the health care worker has cuts or other open wounds on his or her skin; when the worker anticipates hand contamination; when performing skin punctures; or during phlebotomy training (OSHA Correspondence, 1991). All other phlebotomy access procedures may require use of gloves as determined by local policy. Employees must wash their hands after removal of gloves, after any contact with blood or body fluids, and between patients. The practice of washing and reusing gloves between patients is discouraged because microorganisms that adhere to the gloves are difficult to remove (Doebbeling, 1988). All protective equipment that has potential of coming in contact with infectious material, including laboratory coats, must be removed before leaving the laboratory area and never taken home or outside the laboratory (such as at lunch or on personnel breaks). Many laboratories require a second laboratory coat be used when the employees perform phlebotomies outside the laboratory. Cleaning of laboratory coats must be done on site or handled professionally. Eating, drinking, smoking, applying cosmetics, or touching contact lenses is prohibited in working laboratory areas. It is helpful for all employees to know what areas are designated as laboratory work areas and those that are not (offices, conference rooms, and lounges).

Infective agents may be inactivated by conventional sterilization techniques such as heat sterilization (250°C for 15 min), ethylene oxide (450 to 500 mg/L at 55 to 60°C), 2% glutaraldehyde, 10% hydrogen peroxide, 10% formaldehyde, and 5.25% hypochlorite (bleach). A 10% solution (v/v with tap water, made daily) of common household bleach makes a very effective and economical disinfectant, inactivating HBV in 10 minutes and HIV in 2 minutes (NCCLS Pub. M29-T2, 1991). Prewashing removes concentrated amounts of proteins, which is required before effective decontamination is achieved. Furthermore, all laboratory surfaces must be made of nonporous material that allows for easy cleaning and decontamination.

Vaccination against HBV is another safety precaution recommended by the CDC's advisory committee on immunization practices, specifically for medical technologists, phlebotomists, and pathologists (NCCLS Pub. M29-T2, 1991). OSHA mandates that an employer make this available to those employees with occupational exposure (Federal Register 55, 29CFR, 1990). Efforts are also made by reagent and instrument manufacturers in offering products designed to reduce exposure of laboratory personnel to blood and blood products that would cause HIV, HBV, or other infections.

Safety Against Exposure to Toxic Chemicals

To minimize the incidence of chemically related occupational illnesses and injuries in workplaces, OSHA published its Hazard Communication Standard in 1983 (Federal Register, 29CFR 1910.1200, 1983), requiring the manufacturers of chemicals to evaluate the hazards of the chemicals they produce and to develop hazard communication programs for employees exposed to the hazardous chemicals. This standard was designed to reduce the hazards faced by manufacturing workers handling chemicals without adequate knowledge or understanding about the physical and health hazards of the chemicals, safe handling precautions, and emergency and first aid procedures. OSHA (Federal Register 56, 1992) requires clinical laboratories to develop and institute a chemical hygiene plan (Gile, 1990). Many states have also developed individual guidelines and regulations mandating the employers to develop and implement safety and toxic chemical information programs for their workers, e.g., the Right-to-Know Law in New York State (Chap. 551, Art. 48, 12 NYCRR Part 820).

Under OSHA regulations and often state law, hospitals and laboratories are obligated to maintain an inventory of all hazardous substances used in the workplace. The hazardous nature of a chemical may be determined on the basis of evaluations made by manufacturers, which are summarized in the Material Safety Data Sheets (MSDS). To be in compliance, the employer must maintain and update its inventory of toxic chemicals periodically and to communicate the hazards to employees. Communication may be achieved by (1) labeling the containers and posting warnings, (2) informing employees of employer's responsibilities and training employees regarding the nature and the safe handling of hazardous chemicals, and (3) developing and implementing a written program of hazard communication (i.e., making MSDS available to employees upon request). The program must specify (1) how the employer has fulfilled its responsibilities and (2) employees' rights to request and receive all information concerning hazards of toxic substances in the workplace and to be free from retaliation for exercising this right. The employee may refuse to work with, handle, or remain in risk of exposure to a toxic substance that the employee has requested information on but not received a written reply (within 72 hours of its receipt by the employer).

Americans with Disabilities Act

The Americans with Disabilities Act (ADA) of 1990 (42 USC§12101; 12111; 1990; 1992; Bureau of National Affairs, Washington, DC) was signed into law January 26, 1992. This law prohibits employment discrimination against qualified individuals with disabilities in the public and private sectors. Individuals seeking specific employment must possess the appropriate skills, experience, education, and any other job-related requirements, and cannot be discriminated based on potential inability to do the job. This law protects individuals with physical or mental impairments that significantly limit one or more life's major activities (walking, breathing, speaking, hearing, seeing, learning, and performing manual tasks).

Disabilities may include recovery from drug addict, HIV-positive individual (or living with an HIV-positive person), disfiguring scar, deafness, blindness, alcoholism, epilepsy, diabetes mellitus, dyslexia, mental illness, stress or depression, overeating, obesity, and infertility. Under the ADA, an employer may not ask about the existence, severity, or nature of a disability, and may not ask for a medical examination until after a job offer has been made. During the preoffer stage, an employer may ask if an applicant can perform certain job-related functions. If an applicant voluntarily discloses a disability and requests reasonable accommodations to perform the job, further inquiry at the preoffer stage regarding the type of accommodation needed is discouraged. After a conditional offer is made, an employer may require a medical examination and make disability-related inquiries if it is done for all new employees within that job category. Supervisors, managers, and employers may be held accountable for any inappropriate questions or actions.

Job descriptions must be specific and contain only the *minimum* requirements acceptable in fulfilling the duties and functions considered essential to performing the job with or without reasonable accommodations. *Essential functions* are those that change the job category if they are removed from the job description. Job requirements may have to be reviewed and restructured to accommodate an otherwise qualified applicant. In addition, one may have to identify those parts of the job that could be performed by other employees. However, those changes that create undue hardship for the employer related to costs, extensive modifications, or disruption to business, may be eligible for exemption. It is essential that clear documentation of accurate job descriptions identifying essential functions and performance standards are in place prior to any job offerings and that the job description is shared with the incumbent. Consistency in the hiring process using established standards and questions when interviewing will protect employers and employees.

Cumulative Trauma Disorders

Ergonomic hazards in the workplace have been addressed by OSHA (Federal Register 54 (29), 1989; OSHA #3123, 1991), who has presented guidelines to assist in preventing work-related problems. Cumulative trauma disorders are a collective group of injuries involving the musculoskeletal or nervous systems, or both, in response to long-term, repetitive twisting, bending, lifting, or assuming static postures (Riggle, 1991). These injuries may evolve from environmental factors such as constant or excessive repetitive actions, mechanical pressure, vibrations, or compressive forces on the arms, hands, neck, or back. Human error may also be a causative factor when individuals push themselves beyond their limits or when productivity limits are set too high.

Some common cumulative trauma disorders are listed in Table 1–18 (Gile, 1994). Prevention is the key to managing these disorders. Use of engineering controls such as ergonomically correct seating, table heights, padded edges (wrist pads and elbow pads), or mechanical-assisted lifting devices should be promoted. In addition, job rotation, job-site modifications, proper orientation and training, and continuing education of all employees are essential to promoting a safe work environment.

Table 1–18. CUMULATIVE TRAUMA DISORDERS AMONG LABORATORY PERSONNEL

Disorder	Symptom	Affects or Caused By
Carpal tunnel syndrome	Compression and entrapment of nerve from wrist to hand	Repetitive pipetting, keyboard use, transcription
De Quervain's disease	Inflammation between two thumb tendons	Twisting or forceful gripping—seen in morgue assistants
Joint and disk degeneration	Microscopic stretching, tearing, or raveling	Cumulative microdamage from repetitive bending, lifting, or any other normal activity
Raynaud's syndrome	Damaged blood vessels in hand	Extended exposure to vibration, intensified when exposed to cold
Tendinitis	Inflammation of tendon	Repetitive pipetting, keyboard use, transcription
Tenosynovitis	Inflammation or injury to synovial sheath	Repetitive pipetting
Trigger finger	Creation of groove in flexing tendon of finger	Causing snapping/jerking movements; associated with sharp-edged tools like autopsy scissors

Modified with permission from Gile T: Clin Lab Manage Rev 1994; 8:5–18.

Table 1–19. CHAIN OF CUSTODY FORM

Hospital Name
Street
City
Director of Laboratories

Patient Name: ______________________ Date: __________
ID Number: ______________________ Location: __________
Ordering Physician: ______________________

Specimen Type				
Amount Collected				
Color				
Collection Site				
	Print Name	**Signature**	**Date**	**Time**
Collected by				
Witnessed by				
Received by				
Received by				
Received by				
Tests Performed by				
Disposition of Specimen				

Laboratory Director or Designee ______________________ **Date:**

MEDICAL-LEGAL CONCERNS

Consent

A major liability risk for laboratories is that of procuring informed consent from the patient. Informed consent refers to the patient agreeing to and understanding the nature of the measurement and examination to be performed, what will be done with the results, and what will be done with the specimen. Generally, the consent for a simple venipuncture is implied when the patient enters the hospital or seeks care from a health care provider when routine procedures are performed. For more complex procedures, such as apheresis techniques, bone marrow aspiration, lumbar puncture, and fine-needle aspiration, a signed informed consent authorization by the patient or guardian should be obtained.

Confidentiality

Patients are entitled to strict confidentiality concerning their health care including types of laboratory measurements and examinations and results. Release of any patient information must be authorized by the patient, especially to non–health care entities (insurance companies, lawyers, and friends of the patient). Discussions and written documents regarding any one patient's laboratory results must be limited to authorized parties involved in the caregiving to the patient. Breech of this confidentiality, even accidently, can result in litigation against institutions or individuals. More recently, the issues of confidentiality in regard to patients with AIDS or HIV-positive blood examinations have caused specific legislation to be passed in many states to ensure the protection of these patients and their families.

Chain of Custody

Chain of custody involves any procedure or specimen that requires detailed tracking of its integrity and handling, from the moment of specimen collection to the time it is analyzed and reported (Chamberlain, 1989). Laboratory evaluations, including alcohol levels, various drug levels, other toxicologic assays, specimens collected from rape victims, paternity evaluations, or tissues submitted from medical examiner cases, are examples that most often require this level of documentation. The National Institute on Drug Abuse has developed mandatory guidelines for the Federal Workplace Testing Programs. Table 1–19 outlines some of these application guidelines.

Adams JG Jr, Weigelt JA, Poulos E: Usefulness of preoperative laboratory assessment of patients undergoing elective herniorrhaphy. Arch Surg 1992; 127:801–804.

Allred TJ, Steiner L: Alternate-site testing. Consider the analyst. Clin Lab Med 1994; 14:569–604.

Alström T, Gräsbeck R, Lindbald B, et al: Establishing reference values from adults: Recommendation on procedures for the preparation of individuals, collection of blood, and handling of storage specimens. Scand J Clin Lab Invest 1993; 53:649–652.

Alvarez R, Rasberry SD, Uriano GA: N.B.S. Standard Reference Materials: Update 1982. Anal Chem 1982; 54:1226A.

Axt-Adam P, van der Wouden JC, van der Does E: Influencing behavior of physicians ordering laboratory tests: A literature study. Med Care 1993; 31:784–794.

Baer DM: Patient records: What to save, how to save, how long to save it. Med Lab Observ 1993; 25:22–27.

Baralden PB: HCA Q100 training manual. Knoxville, TN, Hospital Corporation of America, 1989.
Bigen R, Racine T, Roy JC: Value of capillary blood gas analysis in the management of acute respiratory distress. Am Rev Respir Dis 1975; 112:879.
Brzezicki LA: Move over microfiche, optical disk is here to stay. Adv Adminis Lab 1994; 3:49–51.
Bureau of National Affairs, 42 USC §12101, Americans with Disabilities Act, 1990.
Bureau of National Affairs, 42 USC §12111, Americans with Disabilities Act, 1992.
Burtis CA, Ashwood ER, eds: Tietz's Textbook of Clinical Chemistry, 2nd ed. Philadelphia, WB Saunders Company, 1994.
Cabal L, Hodgman J, Siassi B, Plajstek C: Factors affecting heated transcutaneous PO_2 and unheated transcutaneous PO_2 in preterm infants. Crit Care Med 1981; 9:298.
Campbell JM, Campbell JB: Laboratory Mathematics. Medical and Biological Applications. 3rd ed. St. Louis, C.V. Mosby, 1984.
Caraway WT, Kammeyer CW: Chemical interference by drugs and other substances with clinical laboratory test procedures. Clin Chem Acta 1972; 41:395.
Centers for Disease Control: Recommendations and reports: Guidelines for prevention of transmission of human immunodeficiency virus and hepatitis B virus to health care and public-safety workers. MMWR 1989; 38, No. S-6.
Chamberlain RT: Chain of custody: Its importance and requirements for clinical laboratory specimens. Lab Med 1989; 20:477–480.
Chan KM, Daft M, Koenig JW, et al: Plasma separation tube of Becton Dickinson evaluated. Clin Chem 1988; 34:2158.
Chua RV, Cordell WH, Ernsting KL, et al: Accuracy of bar codes versus handwriting for recording trauma resuscitation events. Ann Emerg Med 1993; 22:1545–1550.
College of American Pathologists; Northfield, IL 60093-2750: CAP Inspection Checklist, Ancillary Testing, 1994.
Corona R: Telepathology, SUNY Health Science Center Telemedicine Consortium, Syracuse, NY, personal communication, 1994.
Cousar JB, Peters TH Jr.: Laboratories in patient-centered units. Clin Lab Med 1994; 14:525–538.
Czech K, Lackner F, Porges P: Intraoperative transmucous PO_2 monitoring ($tmPO_2$). Birth Defects 1979; 15:551.
Deming WE: Out of Crisis. Cambridge, MA: MIT, Center for Advanced Engineering Study, 1986.
Dennington SR, Wilkinson DS: CQI in action in the Central Lab Laboratory. Clin Lab Manage Rev 1993; 7:516–519.
Doebbeling BN, Pfaller MA, Houston AK, Wenzel RP: Removal of nosocomial pathogens from the contaminated glove. Ann Intern Med 1988; 109:394.
Federal Register, 54, 29CFR 1910; Ergonomic Safety and Health Program Management Guidelines, 1989.
Federal Register, 55, 42CFR 493; Clinical Laboratory Improvement Act, 1990.
Federal Register, 55, 29CFR 1910; Occupational Exposure to Hazardous Chemicals in Laboratories, 1990.
Federal Register, 56, CFR 1910.1030; Occupational Exposure to Blood Borne Pathogens, 1992.
Federal Register, 57, 42CFR 493; Clinical Laboratory Improvement Act, 1992.
Felder RA, Boyd JC, Margrey K, et al: Robotics in the medical laboratory. Clin Chem 1990; 36:1534–1543.
Finn AF, Valenstein PN, Burke D: Alteration of physicians' orders by nonphysicians. JAMA 1988; 259:2549.
Fleisher M, Schwartz MK: Use of evacuated collection tubes for routine determination of arterial blood gases and pH. Clin Chem 1971; 17:610.
Friedman BA: The laboratory information float, time-based competition, and point-of-care testing. Clin Lab Manage Rev 1994; 8:509–514.
Gambino SR: Collection of capillary blood for simultaneous determinations of arterial pH, CO_2 content, PCO_2 and oxygen saturation. Am J Clin Path 1961; 35:175.
Garner JS, Simmons BP: Guidelines for isolation precautions in hospitals. Infect Control 1983; 4:245.
Garza D, Beacon-McBride K: Phlebotomy Handbook, 2nd ed. Norwalk, Conn., Appleton & Lange, 1989, pp 79–82.
Geyer SJ: Joining the technological evolution of healthcare. Med Lab Observ 1992; 24(9S):2–7.
Gile TJ: A Model Exposure Control Plan for Laboratories. Malvern, PA, Clinical Laboratory Management Association, 1992.
Gile TJ: A Model Chemical Hygiene Plan for Laboratories. Malvern, PA, Clinical Laboratory Management Association, 1990.
Gile TJ: Ergonomics for the laboratory. Clin Lab Manage Rev 1994; 8:5–18.
Gomori G: Preparation of buffers for use in enzyme studies. Methol Enzymol 1955; 1:138.
Hamlin WB: Reagent Water Specifications. Commission on Laboratory Inspection and Accreditation. Skokie, IL, College of American Pathologists, 1978.
Handorf CR: Quality control and quality management of alternate site testing. Clin Lab Med 1994; 14: 539–557.
Hardin G, Quick G, Ladd DJ: Emergency transport of AS-1 cell units by pneumatic tube system. J Trauma 1990; 30:346–348.
Hasman A, Pop P, Winkens RAG, Blom JL: To test or not to test, that is the question. Clin Chim Acta 1993; 222:49–56.
Howanitz PJ, Steindel SJ, Cembrowski GS, et al: Emergency department stat turn-around times. A College of American Pathologists' Q-Probes study for potassium and hemoglobin. Arch Pathol Lab Med 1992; 116:122–128.
Huch A, Huch R, Schneidor H: Fetal transcutaneous PO_2—current knowledge. Birth Defects 1979a; 15:185.
Huch R, Fallenstein F, Seiler D, Lubbers D, Hutch A: $tcPCO_2$—state of development. Birth Defects 1979b; 15:413.
Inhorn SL: Molecular genetic testing. Clin Lab Manage Rev 1994; 8:492–498.
Joint Commission on the Accreditation for Healthcare Organizations (JCAHO): Accreditation Manual for Pathology and Laboratory Services. 1993; PA 6.4.
Jones JD: Transport of blood specimens by pneumatic tube. *In* Slockbower J, Blumenfeld TA: Collection and Handling of Laboratory Specimens: A Practical Guide. Philadelphia: J.B. Lippincott, 1983, pp 151–171.
Juran J: Juran on Planning for Quality. New York, The Free Press, 1988.
Kalish RI, Cheskin HS, Blumenfeld TA: *In* Stockbower J, Blumenfeld TA: Collection and Handling of Laboratory Specimens: A Practical Guide. Philadelphia: J.B. Lippincott, 1983, pp 114–125.
Kasten BL, Schrand P, Disney M: Joining the bar code revolution. Med Lab Observ 1992; 24:22–27.
Kasten BL: Bar coding: the ideal system. Med Lab Observ 1993; 25:40–43.
Kaufman HW: Specimen pathway analysis aids quality and efficiency. Med Lab Observ 1992; 24:33–39.
Kayser K: Progress in telepathology. In Vivo 1993; 7:331–333.
Keshgegian AA, Bull GE: Evaluation of a soft-handling computerized pneumatic tube specimen delivery system. Am J Clin Pathol 1992; 97:535–540.
Koenig AS, Day JC, Sodeman TM, Alpert NL: Laboratory Instrument Verification and Maintenance Manual. Skokie, IL, College of American Pathologists, 1982.
Koenig AS: Medical Laboratory Planning and Design. Northfield, IL, College of American Pathologists, 1989, pp 1–186.
Konopad E, Grace M, Johnston R, et al: Comparison of PT and aPTT values drawn by venipuncture and arterial line using discard volumes. Am J Crit Care 1992; 1:94–101.
Kumar A: Micro-invasive management of neonatal bilirubinemia. Indian Pediatr 1992; 29:1101–1106.
Kurec AS: Implementing point-of-care. Clin Lab Sci 1993; 6:225–227.
Laessig RH, Hassemer DJ, Paskay TA, et al: The effects of 0.1 and 1.0 percent erythrocytes and hemolysis on serum chemistry values. Am J Clin Pathol 1976; 66:639–644.
Larsson-Cohn U: Differences between capillary and venous blood glucose during oral glucose tolerance tests. Scand J Clin Lab Invest 1976; 36:805.
Lasof TW, Macurdy LB: Precision Laboratory Standards of Mass and Laboratory Weights. Washington DC, National Bureau of Standards US Dept Commerce, Circular 547, 1954.
Markin RS: Clinical laboratory automation: A paradigm shift. Clin Lab Manage Rev 1993; 7:243–251.
Markin RS: A laboratory automation platform: The next robotic step. Med Lab Observ 1992; 24:24–28.
Martin TJ: The Pharmacologic Interactions with Laboratory Test Values, August 1970. 596 Burnhamthorpe Etobiocoke, Ontario, Canada.
McCall RE, Tankersley CM: Phlebotomy Essentials. Philadelphia, J.B. Lippincott, 1993, pp 202–206.
Meites, S.: Skin-puncture and blood-collecting technique for infants: Update and problems. Clin Chem 1988; 34:1890.
Montebello AR: Teamwork in health care: Opportunities for gains in quality, productivity, and competitive advantage. Clin Lab Manage Rev 1994; 8:91–110.
Mullerr-Plathe O, Hayduck S: Stability of blood gases, electrolytes and haemoglobin in heparinized whole blood samples: Influence of the type of syringe. Eur J Clin Chem Clin Biochem 1992; 30:349–355.
National Committee for Clinical Laboratory Standards Publication EP7-P: Interference testing in clinical chemistry. Villanova, PA, NCCLS, 1986.
National Committee for Clinical Laboratory Standards Publication EP9-T: Method comparison and bias estimation using patient samples. Villanova, PA, NCCLS, 1993.
National Committee for Clinical Laboratory Standards Publication EP10-T2: Preliminary evaluation of quantitative clinical laboratory methods. Villanova, PA, NCCLS, 1993.
National Committee for Clinical Laboratory Standards Publication GP-16T: Collection and preservation of timed urine specimens. Villanova, PA, NCCLS, 1992.
National Committee for Clinical Laboratory Standards Publication H4-A3:

Procedures for the collection of diagnostic blood specimen by skin puncture, 3rd ed. Villanova, PA, NCCLS, 1991.

National Committee for Clinical Laboratory Standards Publication H11-A2: Percutaneous collection of arterial blood for laboratory analysis, 2nd ed. Villanova, PA, NCCLS, 1992.

National Committee for Clinical Laboratory Standards Publication H14-A2: Use of devices for collection of skin puncture blood specimens, 2nd ed. Villanova, PA, NCCLS, 1990.

National Committee for Clinical Laboratory Standards Publication H18-A: Procedures for the handling and processing of blood specimens. Villanova, PA, NCCLS, 1990.

National Committee for Clinical Laboratory Standards Publication H3-A3: Procedures for collection of diagnostic blood specimens by venipuncture, 3rd ed. Villanova, PA, NCCLS, 1991.

National Committee for Clinical Laboratory Standards Publication M29-T2: Protection of Laboratory workers from infectious disease transmitted by blood, body fluids, and tissue, 2nd ed. Villanova, PA, NCCLS, 1991.

Neeley W: Heighten efficiency with an integrated bar code system. Med Lab Observ 1990; 22:22–27.

New York State Public Health Law, Chapter 551, Article 48 of the Article 28 of the New York State Labor Laws, Part 820 Title 12 of the New York Codes, Rules and Regulations, Right-to-Know Law, 1987.

O'Bryan D: Robotics: A way to link the "islands of automation." Clin Manage Rev 1994; 8:446–460.

Occupational Safety and Health Administration Regulations 29CFR1910.1200, Hazard Communications Standard; 1983.

Occupational Safety and Health Administration Regulations CPL 2.244B, Glove Wearing: 1991.

Painter P: Laboratory Design Workshop. Clinical Laboratory Management Association Annual Meeting, 1993, San Antonio, TX.

Petty TL, Bailey D: A new, versatile blood gas syringe. Heart Lung 1981; 10:672.

Petty TL, Bigelow DB, Levine BE: The simplicity and safety of arterial puncture. JAMA 1966; 195:181.

Phelan S: Phlebotomy Techniques: A Laboratory Workbook. Chicago: Chicago, IL, ASCP Press, 1993, pp 224–230.

Pitkin AD, Roberts CM, Wedzicha JA: Arterialised earlobe blood gas analysis: An underused technique. Thorax 1994; 49:364–366.

Pretto JJ, Rockford PD: Effects of sample storage time, temperature and syringe type on blood gas tensions with high oxygen partial pressures. Thorax 1994; 49:610–612.

Rehak NN, Chiang BT: Storage of whole blood: Effect of temperature on the measured concentration of analytes in serum. Clin Chem 1988; 34:2111.

Remes K, Kuoppasalmi K, Aldercreutz H: Effects of long term physical training on plasma testosterone, androstenedione, luteinizing hormone and sex-hormone–binding globulin capacity. Scand J Clin Lab Invest 1994; 39:743.

Riggle M: Cumulative trauma in the workplace. Physical Therapy Forum 1991; April, 11–12.

Rooke TW: The use of transcutaneous oximetry in the non-invasive vascular laboratory. Int Angiol 1992; 11:36–40.

Rosen P, Hedges J: Emergency department stat laboratory: A solution or a problem? Emerg Med 1989; 7:401–402.

Sackner MA, Avery WG, Sokolowski J: Arterial punctures by nurses. Chest 1971; 59:97.

Schoeny DE, Rollheiser JJ: The automated analytical laboratory: introduction of a new approach to laboratory robotics. Am Lab 1991; September, 42–47.

Shapiro BA, Cane RD: Blood gas monitoring: Yesterday, today, and tomorrow. Crit Care Med 1989; 17:573.

Slockbower JM: Blood collection problems: Factors in specimen collection that contribute to laboratory error. Am Assoc Clin Chem, 1982; October: 1–26.

Smith BE, King PH, Schlain L: Clinical evaluation—continuous real-time intra-arterial blood gas monitoring during anesthesia and surgery by fiber-optic sensor. J Clin Monit Comput 1992; 9:45–52.

Snyder JR, Wilkinson D: Administration and Supervision in Laboratory Medicine, 3rd ed. Philadelphia, J.B. Lippincott, 1995.

Statland BE, Winkel P, Bokelund H: Factors contributing to intra-individual variation of serum constituents: 2. Effects of exercise and diet on variation of serum constituents in healthy subjects. Clin Chem 1973a; 19:1380.

Statland BE, Winkel P, Bokelund H: Serum alkaline phosphatase after fatty meals: The effect of substrate on the assay procedure. Clin Chim Acta 1973b; 49:299.

Statland BE, Winkel P, Bokelund H: Factors contributing to intra-individual variation of serum constituents: 4. Effects of posture and tourniquet application on variation of serum constituents in healthy subjects. Clin Chem 1974; 20:1513.

Swartz MK: Interferences in diagnostic biochemical procedures. Adv Clin Chem 1973; 16:1.

Versmold HT, Linderkamp O, Holzmann M, et al: Transcutaneous monitoring of PO_2 in newborn infants: Where are the limits? Influence of blood pressure, blood volume, blood flow, viscosity and acid base state. Birth Defects 1979; 15:285.

Watts NB: Medical relevance of laboratory tests. A clinical perspective. Arch Pathol Lab Med 1988; 112:379.

Woo J, Henry JB: The advance of technology as a prelude to the laboratory of the twenty-first century. Clin Lab Med 1994; 459–471.

Woo J, McCabe JB, Chauncey D, et al: The evaluation of a portable clinical analyzer in the emergency department. Am J Clin Pathol 1993; 100: 599–605.

Young DS, Pestaner LC, Gibberman V: Effects of drugs on clinical laboratory tests. Clin Chem 1975; 21:1D.

Zaloga GP: Monitoring versus testing technologies: present and future. Med Lab Observ 1991; 23(9S):20–31.

Chapter 2

Physician Office Laboratories

Gregory A. Threatte, M.D.
Christopher P. Tirabassi, M.B.A., MT(ASCP)DLM

Advances in medical technology, such as prepackaged reagent systems, microprocessor-controlled reactions and calibrations, and miniaturization of components, have led to a modern generation of laboratory instrumentation that requires less technical skill on the part of the operator. Increased competitiveness among primary care physicians has led to greater concern about patient convenience. Many physicians have chosen to reduce the difficulties associated with issues such as parking near the laboratories of major medical centers, turn-around time, and the need for second office visits when laboratory measurements are referred. The estimated revenue from laboratory measurements and examinations (Fig. 2–1) and the imbalance in reimbursement between intellectual evaluation and management patient interactions and procedural encounters such as laboratory determinations (Hsiao, 1988) have also been incentives for office laboratory measurements and examinations in many situations. There may be compelling medical value in physicians' having laboratory results in the shortest time interval possible. This improved efficiency and patient convenience must be balanced against cost-effectiveness and the exposure of the physician office to a set of problems that the physician and staff may not be adequately trained to handle efficiently and effectively. For these reasons, as well as others, pathologists and other laboratory professionals will increasingly be called on as consultants and supervisors in the creation, design, and management of physician office laboratories (POLs).

Several chapters in Part I, especially Chapters 1, 3, and 6, complement and supplement information in this chapter. Most of the regulatory information in this chapter was taken directly from the Survey Procedures and Interpretive Guidelines for Laboratory Services published by the National Technical Information Service.*

*Contact the National Technical Information Service, US Department of Commerce, Springfield, VA 22161, (703) 487-4650.

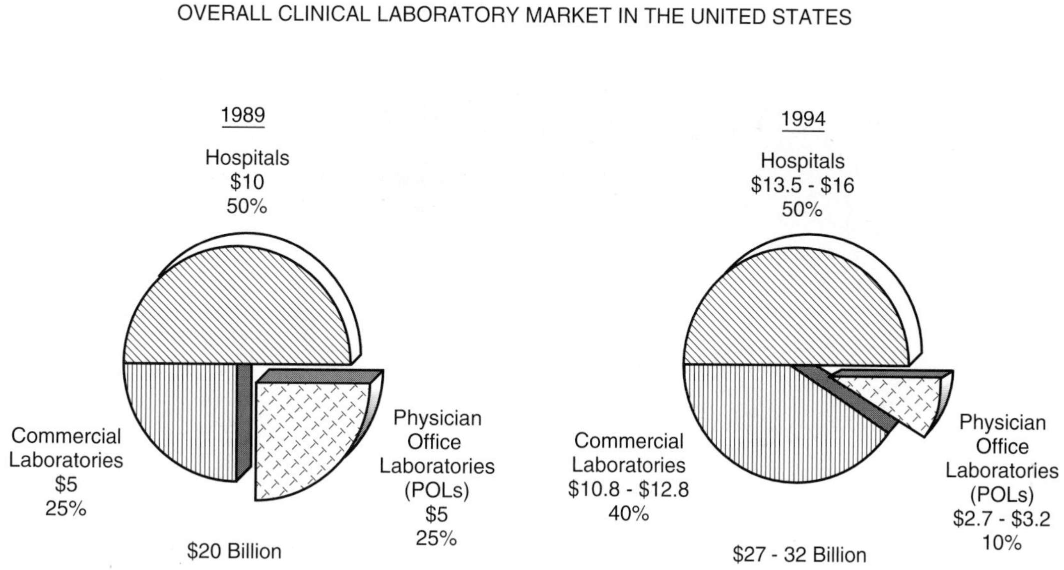

Figure 2–1. Estimated revenue from laboratory measurements and examinations in 1989 and 1994. Commercial laboratories' share of market has grown, and physician office laboratories' (POLs) share of market has decreased, with approximately 110,000 POLs in 1989 and 70,000 in 1994. (Courtesy of V. P. Perna, M.D., SmithKline Beecham Clinical Laboratories.)

CHANGED LABORATORY REGULATION

The definition of a POL varies, but in general, this category refers to those laboratories whose laboratory services are limited to a physician or physician group's own patients or consultations. Under the Clinical Laboratories Improvement Act of 1967 (CLIA-67) and in most states, POLs remained unregulated until recently. Under CLIA-67 and Medicare—Conditions for Coverage, POLs were excluded from federal regulation and licensure requirements if (1) these laboratory services were not advertised in telephone listings or listed on letterhead or office signs, or (2) fewer than 100 patient specimens in one of six categories were accepted on referral from other physicians. To be considered part of a physician's practice, laboratory testing had to be done in conjunction with a history and physical examination of the patient.

The total number of previously unregulated POLs is not clear, but in a Maryland survey, POLs accounted for more than a quarter of all laboratory measurements and examinations (DeBoy, 1988). The growth rate of these determinations was estimated to be at 15% per year. In this survey, it was also found that 88 different laboratory measurements and examinations were performed, yet more than 70% of POLs possessed medical laboratory instruments that were operated by people with no formal education, training, or experience in laboratory science. Studies of proficiency surveys in Idaho and Illinois found persistent differences in accuracy and variability between small office laboratories and large commercial or hospital laboratories (Crawley, 1986; Lunz, 1987). In a Pennsylvania study, 17 out of 67 office laboratories demonstrated error rates of greater than 20% in a state-mandated proficiency program (Bloch, 1988). Presumably because of both the magnitude of this unregulated industry and concerns about its quality and unknown costs, Congress enacted the Clinical Laboratories Improvement Act of 1988 (CLIA-88) extending laboratory regulation to POLs.

CLIA registrations as of April, 1995 are indicated in Figure 2–2; POLs constituted approximately 60% of all 151,888 laboratories that had registered with the Health Care Financing Administration (HCFA) as a result of CLIA-88 process. Figure 2–3 shows that of these 83,328 POLs, more than half are performing only waived tests or tests in the Physician (Provider) Performed Microscopy Procedures category. Approximately 30% opted for certificate status via inspection by a state agency acting on behalf of HCFA, and the remaining 10% have sought private accreditation predominantly from the Commission for Office Laboratory Accreditation (COLA) (Bachner, 1995).

Figure 2–4 shows the frequency of performance of the most commonly performed tests in POLs. It is of interest to note that seven of the 12 tests may now be performed as waived tests (Bachner, 1995).

Clinical Laboratories Improvement Act of 1988

CLIA-88, first published May 20, 1990, prohibits any laboratory from soliciting or accepting human specimens for analysis unless it holds a certificate issued by the Secretary of the Department of Health and Human Services (HHS) for each category of testing that is to be performed. This certification must be in compliance with the performance standards derived from the new law or by proof of accreditation by a private accrediting agency, or deemed authority, approved by HHS. By definition, a laboratory is "A facility for the . . . examination of materials derived from the human body for the purpose of providing information for the diagnosis, prevention, or treatment of any disease or impairment of, or the assessment of the health of, human beings." Effective September 1, 1992, all

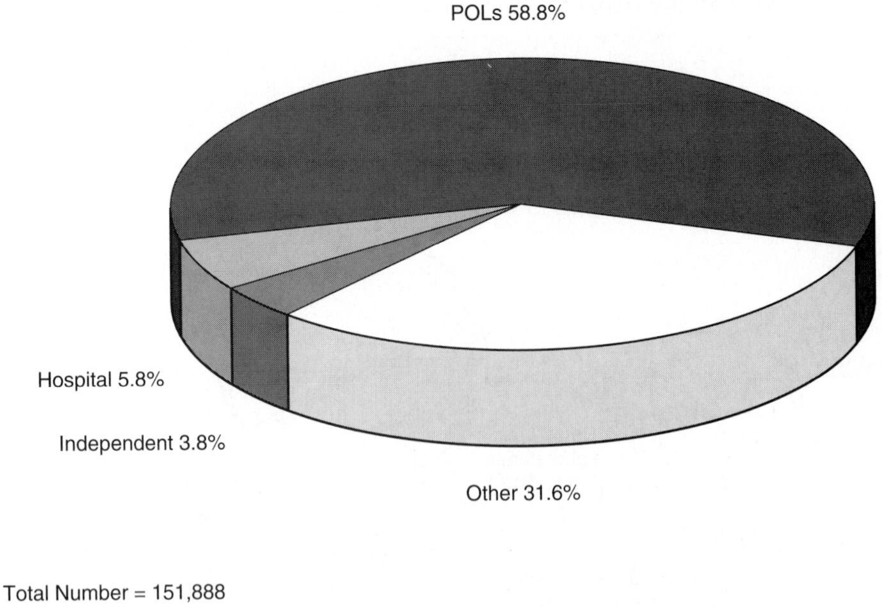

Figure 2–2. CLIA laboratories by type. (Courtesy of Ms. Judy Yost, Director, Division of Laboratory Standards and Performance Health Standards & Quality Bureau, Health Care Financing Administration.)

laboratories were required to be registered with the federal government and have a valid CLIA identification number before performing any laboratory analysis used in patient care. For office laboratories, CLIA-88 mandates a new era of accreditation and registration fees; documentation of procedures; quality control and assurance monitoring; proficiency testing; unannounced, or usually, announced inspections; and potential fines for those found in violation of the law.

Certification and Licensing Requirements

For all laboratories, CLIA-88 relies heavily on outcome measures such as satisfactory performance in proficiency testing. Personnel standards vary according to the complexity of the measurements performed. Simple tests that HHS has determined to have low patient risk, even if they are performed incorrectly, are categorized as waived and exempt from most regulations. These types of procedures include those that have been approved by the Food and Drug Administration (FDA) for home use or are so simple and accurate as to render the likelihood of erroneous results negligible. All laboratories must be certified or receive a certificate of waiver based on the complexity of the tests performed.

A three-tiered approach was initially implemented, classifying all laboratory tests based on the complexity of testing. The three categories are certificate of waiver, or waived tests; moderate complexity tests; and high complexity testing. Laboratories performing only waived tests would be exempt from personnel, proficiency testing, and quality assurance requirements. HHS retains the right to conduct spot checks to

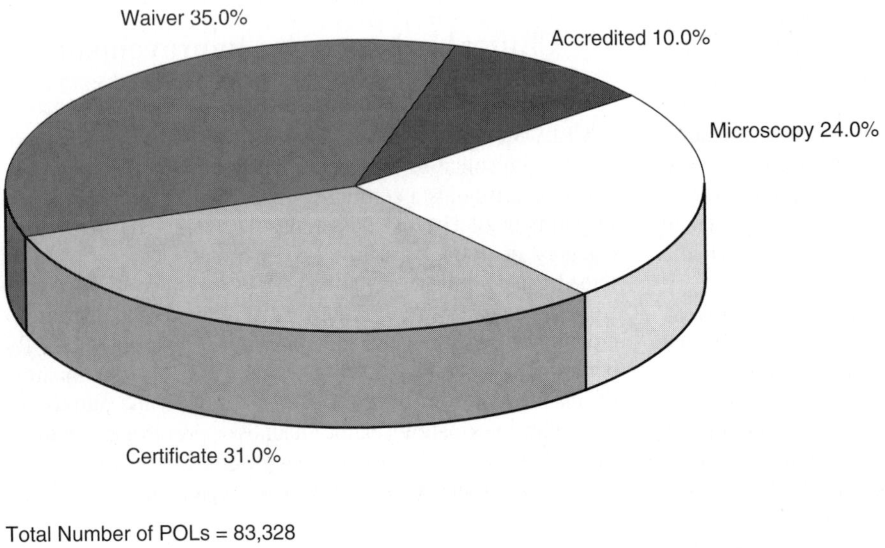

Figure 2–3. Distribution of POLs by type. (Courtesy of Ms. Judy Yost, Director, Division of Laboratory Standards and Performance Health Standards & Quality Bureau, Health Care Financing Administration.)

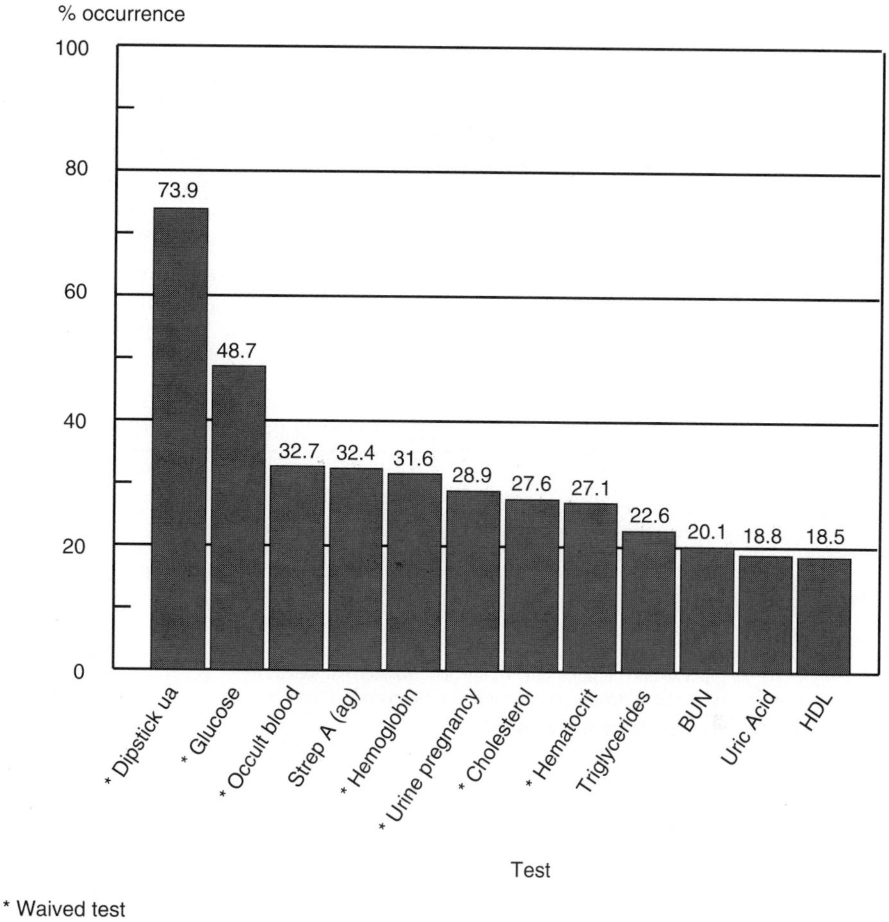

Figure 2–4. Most common tests performed in POLs. (Courtesy of Ms. Judy Yost, Director, Division of Laboratory Standards and Performance Health Standards & Quality Bureau, Health Care Financing Administration.)

make sure that these laboratories are performing only waived tests. At this time, the exempt tests include urinalysis dipstick or tablet reagent analysis of pH, specific gravity, glucose, protein, bilirubin, hemoglobin, ketone, leukocytes, nitrite, and urobilinogen (see Chap. 18). Also exempt are whole blood glucose (see Chap. 9) using devices approved by the FDA specifically for home use, spun microhematocrits (see Chap. 24), hemoglobin by copper sulfate method or by self-contained single-analyte instruments with direct measurement and readout (e.g., HemoCue), fecal occult blood (see Chap. 23), urine pregnancy tests by visual color comparison (see Chaps. 20 and 22), visual color ovulation tests for human luteinizing hormone, and the erythrocyte sedimentation rate (see Chap. 24). In April 1995, a single-analyte (glucose) instrument with direct measurement and readout (HemoCue) and a similar device for measuring total cholesterol (AccuMeter, ChemTrak) were added to the waived list of tests. Laboratories performing only waived tests must register and pay a biennial fee.

A fourth category, physician-performed microscopy (PPM), was created and published in the *Federal Register* on January 19, 1993. This category includes six procedures—wet mounts, including preparations of vaginal, cervical, or skin specimens; potassium hydroxide preparations; pinworm examinations (see Chap. 53); fern tests; postcoital direct, qualitative examinations of vaginal and cervical mucus; and urine sediment examinations (see Chap. 18). Initially, only physicians were permitted to perform the procedures under this category, which was exempt from on-site inspections. However, moderate complexity testing standards would need to be adhered to for proficiency testing, quality control, and quality assurance as described later in this chapter. In the *Federal Register* as of April 24, 1995, this category has been removed and provider-performed microscopy procedures (PPM), including work done by midlevel practitioners (nurse practitioners, nurse-midwives, and physician assistants) as well as dentists, were added. In addition, examination for nasal granulocytes, fecal leukocytes, and qualitative semen analysis (presence or absence of sperm and detection of motility) are now included in PPM.

A fifth category called accurate and precise testing (APT) has been proposed by the Centers for Disease Control (CDC). This category will be a hybrid of waived and moderately complex testing that would permit reduced regulation of testing based on operational characteristics of the method and field-validated performance criteria including instrumentation (ASCP, 1993). Manufacturers would be permitted to submit specific tests with supporting data for inclusion into this category. The CDC would determine whether a test or method qualified based on strict criteria. Quality assurance, proficiency testing, and quality control would be required; however, personnel standards would be established that would permit manufacturer's representatives to serve as technical consultants. Unless a complaint or failed proficiency testing occurred, inspections would be done on a random basis only. APT (originally called robust testing) was not endorsed by CLIA because the category was opposed by professional laboratory groups as an additional dilution of the concepts of site-neutrality (the level playing field) and not supported by industry or physician groups who expected much greater regulatory relief from the 103rd Congress as part of the failed Clinton health care reform process (Bachner, 1995). The CDC remains in favor of creation of the APT category, and it may yet be a part of so-called final, final rulemaking (Bachner, 1995).

A laboratory is classified as moderately complex if it performs only waived tests and one or more tests designated as moderately complex by the FDA. This category is the primary focus of this chapter and includes most of the laboratory measurements and examinations actually performed in a POL. To determine whether a particular measurement has been categorized, refer to the Specific List for Categorization of Laboratory Test Systems, Assays, and Examinations by Complexity; Notice as published in the *Federal Register*, May 15, 1995. Manufacturers of moderately complex tests must submit their testing system to the FDA for classification. Therefore, this list will be continuously updated and at the time of this publication includes methodologies summarized in Table 2–1.

HHS requires that moderate complexity laboratories be di-

Table 2–1. ABBREVIATED LIST OF METHODS BY COMPLEXITY

Certificate of Waiver

1. Dipstick or tablet reagent analysis of pH, specific gravity, glucose, protein, bilirubin, hemoglobin, ketone, leukocytes, nitrite, and urobilinogen
2. Whole-blood glucose using devices approved by the FDA specifically for home use
3. Spun microhematocrits, hemoglobin by copper sulfate method
4. Fecal occult blood
5. Urine pregnancy tests by visual color comparison
6. Visual color ovulation tests for human luteinizing hormone
7. Erythrocyte sedimentation rate
8. Single analyte glucose and hemoglobin (HemoCue, Mission Viejo, CA)
9. Single analyte cholesterol (ChemTrak AccuMeter, Sunnyvale, CA)

Physician (Provider)–Performed Microscopy

1. Wet mounts, including preparations of prostate, vaginal, cervical, or skin specimens
2. Potassium hydroxide preparations
3. Pinworm examinations
4. Postcoital direct, qualitative examinations of vaginal and cervical mucus
5. Fern tests
6. Urine sediment examinations
7. Nasal granulocytes
8. Fecal leukocytes
9. Qualitative semen analysis

Hematology Methodology*

Moderate Complexity

1. Automated hematology analyzer profiles, with and without platelet count and differential, that have direct readout results and require no operator interpretation
2. Automated and/or direct readout prothrombin time, partial thromboplastin time, thrombin time, and activated clotting time methods
3. Rapid solubility tests for hemoglobin S
4. Manual differentials that exclude the interpretation of atypical cells (e.g., blasts, red cell morphology)
5. Duke bleeding time

High Complexity

1. Manual methods for cell counts and coagulation
2. Platelet aggregometry
3. Differentials that include interpretation of atypical cells

Microbiology Methodology*

Primary culture inoculations can be performed if the culture is then referred to a certified laboratory for identification

Moderate complexity

1. Tests for the presence or absence of bacteria, dermatophytes, *Trichomonas vaginalis, Neisseria gonorrhoeae*, and other organisms if performed directly on selective media and/or identified by color or turbidity change
2. Direct acid-fast smears that do not involve concentration of specimen
3. Gram's stains from urethral sources and endocervical smears
4. Darkfield examination for *Treponema pallidum*

High Complexity

1. All procedures requiring identification or susceptibility determination of organisms after transfer from primary culture medium
2. Gram's stains from sources other than urethral or endocervical origin

Chemistry, Drug Monitoring, Immunology, and Endocrinology*

1. Automated methods of moderate complexity are available in nearly all routine areas
2. Maternal α-fetoprotein and electrophoresis methods that require interpretation by the operator are high complexity

Blood Bank Methodology*

1. Direct antiglobulin (Coombs' test), ABO group, and ABO group confirmation are moderate complexity
2. Most nonautomated methods requiring end-point interpretation are high complexity

*All moderately complex methods must be reviewed and designated as such by the FDA. The performance of one or more high complexity methods requires certification as a high complexity laboratory.

Table 2–2. QUALIFICATION REQUIREMENTS FOR LABORATORY DIRECTOR OR TECHNICAL CONSULTANT

1. The laboratory director must have a current license as a laboratory director issued by the state in which the laboratory is located.
2. If the laboratory director is a licensed doctor of medicine or osteopathy, he or she must
   a. Have at least 20 credit hours of continuing medical education in laboratory practice commensurate with the director's responsibilities, or
   b. Have at least one year of experience directing, supervising, or performing nonwaived testing on human samples, or
   c. Have laboratory training in a board approved residency that includes directing or supervising laboratory personnel, or performing diagnostic tests on patient specimens, or
   d. Be board eligible or certified in anatomic and clinical pathology.
3. If the laboratory director holds an earned doctorate in a chemical, physical, biological, or clinical laboratory science from an accredited institution, he or she must
   a. Be certified by either the American Board of Medical Microbiology, American Association of Clinical Chemistry, American Board of Bioanalysts, or the American Board of Medical Laboratory Immunology, or
   b. Have at least one year of experience directing, supervising, or performing nonwaived testing on human samples.
4. If the laboratory director holds an earned master's degree in a chemical, physical, biological, or clinical laboratory science from an accredited institution, he or she must
   a. Have at least one year of laboratory training or experience, and
   b. In addition, have at least one year of laboratory supervisory experience.
5. If the laboratory director holds an earned bachelor's degree in a chemical, physical, biological, or clinical laboratory science from an accredited institution, he or she must
   a. Have at least two years of laboratory training or experience, and
   b. In addition, have at least two years of laboratory supervisory experience.

rected by a laboratory director or a laboratory consultant, or both, with at least the credentials listed in Table 2–2. This director is to be responsible for determining the qualifications of individuals performing and reporting test results, as well as ensuring compliance with all applicable regulations. The director is also responsible for the analytical performance of all assays. (This is of importance because characteristics not directly related to the difficulty of performing the test, such as inherent inaccuracy and imprecision, are not included in the explicit criteria used by the FDA for grading tests by complexity.) If more than one individual in the practice qualifies as a laboratory director, the laboratory is required to designate one as being responsible. It must be demonstrated that the laboratory director is providing effective direction over the operation of the laboratory, and if he or she does not provide on-site direction, he or she must provide consultation by phone or delegate to qualified personnel specific responsibility as required by regulation. Technical consultants must be used on a full-time or part-time basis if the laboratory director does not have experience or training in any specialty or subspecialty area.

In a high complexity laboratory, one or more tests not specifically listed or included in the waived or moderately complex categories are performed. In addition to meeting all standards for moderately complex laboratories, high complexity laboratories must comply with personnel and quality assurance standards similar to those of current Medicare certified hospital or commercial laboratories. These standards include more stringent requirements for procedure manuals and guidelines for the implementation of new tests as well as more rigorous requirements for adequate space and ventilation, water quality, temperature, and humidity.

Laboratories must submit an application to HHS or its designee on a form prescribed by HHS detailing the number, type, and methodologies employed for each measurement or examination, as well as the qualifications of the persons directing, supervising, and performing these procedures. Each laboratory location must complete a separate application except for mobile sites, not-for-profit and governmental agencies, and multiple laboratories that share the same street address under common direction. Certificates may be valid for up to two years, and any changes in the information required in the application must be submitted to HHS or its designee within 30 days of any change in ownership, name, location, or director. Changes in methodology require notification within six months of the change. This application may be through an approved accrediting body or state agency if the accrediting standards of the agency have been deemed by HHS to be equal to or more stringent than those of HHS and if the agency is authorized to inspect the laboratory as frequently as required and submit to HHS required records and information. The regulations implementing CLIA are complex and detailed. Subsequent to the publication of the final rule in February 1992, technical corrections have been published and additional changes are anticipated. The interested reader is referred to additional publications (Bachner, 1993a; CAP, 1994).

Cytology Services

The negative publicity about cytology services was one of the primary forces driving passage of CLIA-88; cytology services became subject to increased regulation that is beyond the scope of this chapter but described in greater detail elsewhere (Bachner, 1993a). The most important of these were limits on the number of slides that may be screened on a daily basis by a cytotechnologist. In addition, these regulations include mandatory record keeping on the number of slides screened per laboratory individual, proficiency testing and grading of each individual, procedural rescreening criteria, and on-site screening and slide retention requirements.

SELECTION OF MEASUREMENTS

Volume

The first and most important consideration in method selection is the volume of patient samples that will be measured. Infrequently performed assays are difficult to control for quality and can lead to outdating of expensive reagents. Some estimate of which measurements are most frequently ordered by the physician clientele is absolutely necessary. Ongoing monitoring of usage statistics in an established laboratory is also necessary. Even university hospitals, which generally attempt to provide full service, require special circumstances before providing an assay that is ordered less than 10 times per week. Low-volume assays can easily degrade to a situation in which controls, standards, and calibrators and repeats outnumber actual specimens at a ratio of greater than 2:1.

A useful tool for estimating volume has been developed by James and Barrett (1987) and modified as shown in Table 2–3. When this tool is implemented with the aid of a computer spreadsheet, labor requirements and reagent consumption can be estimated if proper factors are included for controls and calibrators per billable measurement. Data should be monitored over several months to reduce seasonal variations.

Reference Laboratory Selection

Care must be taken in selecting a reference laboratory for measurements not performed in the POL. A transport and reporting mechanism should be maintained, because turnaround time will be largely a function of this mechanism for most specimens. A lost patient specimen and problem specimen log should be maintained, because when specimen problems become excessive, it is time to consider shifting to a new referral laboratory after appropriate inquiries and checks. A correlation on split-specimen aliquots comparing results of analytes measured in the POL with those of the reference laboratory should be conducted so that back-up is available when illness, staff leave, or instrument malfunction disables the POL service. This back-up is especially useful when troubleshooting suspicious results and troublesome lots of reagents. Confirmation by the reference laboratory gives more confidence in what the expected result should be. Good communication between the POL staff and the laboratory professionals of the re-

Table 2–3. ASSESSING LABORATORY TESTING NEEDS

Category	Specific Procedure	Number Ordered per Month	Controls and Calibrations (from Vendor)	Labor Units (a)	Cost per Measurement (from Vendor)	Total (b) Labor (min)	Reagent Cost per Result (c)
Specimen collection	Phlebotomy (venipuncture)			4.0			
	Urine (clean catch)			5.0			
Urinalysis	Biochemical			4.0			
	Full urinalysis			6.0			
	Pregnancy testing			5.0			
Hematology	Sedimentation rate			4.0			
	Hemoglobin and hematocrit			8.0			
	WBC(d) and differential			11.0			
	Platelet count			9.0			
	Prothrombin time and/or PTT(e)			8 (ea.)			
Chemistry	Glucose			8.0			
	Potassium/electrolytes			12 (ea.)			
	BUN(f)/creatinine			7 (ea.)			
	Bilirubin, liver enzymes			15 (ea.)			
	Amylase			10.0			
	Cholesterol, triglycerides			10 (ea.)			
	Therapeutic drug monitoring			2.2			
Microbiology	Urine screening culture			7.7			
	Strep screening			11.4			
	Wound culture			26.8			
	STD(g) cultures			16.4			
Immunohematology	Type Rh, antibody screen			7.0			
	Antenatal Rh immune globulin			17.0			
Miscellaneous	Occult blood			4.0			
	Mononucleosis			5.0			
	Rheumatoid factor			5.0			
	RPR(h)			3.0			
	Rubella immunity			7.0			
General screening	CBC(i)/Platelets			3.0			
	Chemistry profile			3.0			
	TSH(j), T_4, T_3U			4 (ea.)			

(a) Labor units = minutes of time needed to perform task.
(b) Total labor = labor units × (# ordered + controls and calib.)
(c) Reagent cost per result = cost per measurement × (# ordered + controls and calib.)
(d) WBC = white blood cell count
(e) PTT = partial thromboplastin time
(f) BUN = blood urea nitrogen
(g) STD = sexually transmitted diseases
(h) RPR = rapid plasma reagin screening for syphilis
(i) CBC = complete blood count
(j) TSH = thyroid-stimulating hormone; T_3U = T_3 uptake
Modified from James K, Barrett DA II: Establishing a physician's office laboratory. Med Clin North Am 1987; 71:691.

ferral laboratory about troubleshooting issues, in-service training, and other support should be negotiated as part of the referral package contract. It is important for the POL to avoid accepting any equipment or supplies from the reference laboratory beyond those needed for normal operation or in the normal course of business. In addition, the reference laboratory must not provide any instrument or provide any service or personnel to referring clients for which it does not receive reasonable reimbursement. The Medicare and Medicaid fraud and abuse, or anti-kickback, statutes provide for criminal penalties for those providing or receiving direct or indirect remuneration for inducing business reimbursed under these two programs. Cook (1994) has suggested eight criteria for evaluating and selecting a reference laboratory; these include quality, scope of testing, ease of requisitioning, turn-around time, cost, result reporting, marketing support, and specimen transport.

SELECTION OF OFFICE INSTRUMENTATION

Once an estimate has been made of the expected number of patient specimens and the corresponding volume of measurements and examinations, acquisition costs, operating costs, and technical expertise required become the most important factors in the selection of instrumentation and methodologies for the POL. These three factors must be considered, with priority given to the most frequently performed measurements. It is unwise to acquire an instrument with an expensive and cumbersome glucose methodology merely because it has a method for measuring human chorionic gonadotropin, which might be ordered only once per week. Once appropriate instrumentation is selected for high-volume assays, if that instrumentation also performs additional low-volume measurements, these may be added to the POL menu with minimal incremental cost.

It is also necessary to consider whether the revenue generated from POL testing will be sufficient to pay for office instrumentation throughout its useful lifespan. Reimbursement rates for laboratory tests continue to be an HCFA target, and rate controls are used in an attempt to contain overall health care costs. When profiles or panels are performed on automated instruments, many Medicare carriers will require that some or all tests in a panel have clinical relevance to the specific patient for whom they are ordered. Furthermore, a laboratory must not bill for individual measurements if they are part of a panel or profile performed on a single instrument. If the laboratory is found guilty of such a practice, a heavy fine may be levied. As a result, financial calculations that may demonstrate generated revenue for the office based on outdated reimbursement schedules and not including the costs of laboratory registration and regulation may turn a long-term instrument commitment into a financial burden.

Hematology Methodology

Hematology office analyzers tend to be similar in basic operation, using electrical impedance to size and count blood cells, producing two to eight parameters. Alternative capillary tube density gradient methods exist that measure red blood cells, white blood cells, and platelets in a manner similar to the centrifuged microhematocrit. The best decision is based on whether the instrument has sufficient capacity for the projected volume, is easy to operate, and is sufficiently reproducible (see Chap. 24).

The prothrombin time becomes a consideration only if a sufficient number of patients on warfarin therapy are being followed (see Chap. 29). Mennemeyer and Winkleman (1993) have shown by a review of Medicare records that in POLs that performed fewer than 40 tests of prothrombin time a month, the rate of stroke, myocardial infarction, or death within six days of measurement increased nearly two-fold when compared with that in patients whose testing was performed in hospital or commercial laboratories. This increased morbidity and mortality rate is presumed to be due to incorrect results obtained by inexperienced operators of equipment.

The white blood cell differential is classified as a high complexity test if not performed as a direct readout from an automated instrument or if atypical cells are identified. By including the white blood cell differential in the test menu, the POL incurs an increased level of necessary staff training, quality control, proficiency surveys, and continuing education. This examination appears to be overutilized in clinical practice, because it has been shown that the differential does not change significantly unless the white cell count either halves or doubles (Brecher, 1980). An efficient small office strategy would be to refer blood specimens when the white blood cell count is abnormal initially or significantly changed. Turn-around time is generally tolerable, and unwarranted differentials usually are avoided.

Chemistry Methodology

Selection of chemistry instrumentation requires knowledge of available methodology and equipment. Expert, impartial advice from a clinical pathologist who keeps abreast of the latest technologic advances is strongly recommended concerning the choice and evaluation of chemistry laboratory equipment. Modern instrumentation should have multiple applications. It should be compact, with minimal reagent preparation and adequate capacity to handle the projected specimen volume. It must be understood that sensitivity, specificity, accuracy, and precision are not part of the explicit criteria used by the FDA or CDC for grading tests by complexity and therefore must be independently verified. By reviewing the performance of individual analyzers in external proficiency surveys, the expert consultant should have some idea of the instrument's reproducibility when different operators are employed. Even when all resources are employed and best judgment is exercised, today's top-performing analyzer may be outdated or become technologically surpassed by a hand-held biosensor in the subsequent six months or year. The current movement to alternate-site testing or near patient care clinical laboratory services is substantial. Hence, a number of new instruments and technologies are rapidly evolving to meet this perceived need (Woo, 1993).

Urinalysis

Urinalysis is presented in Chapter 18. POLs should ensure that each person involved in the reading of macroscopic reagent strips has been examined for color blindness. Documentation of this examination should be placed in their personnel files. In addition, procedures for confirming positive reagent strip results should be established and implemented. The protein reagent strip is based on the principle of the protein error of pH indicators and can be falsely activated by a high or alkaline pH, such as quaternary ammonium cleaning compounds and fabric softeners. Using Triton X-100, a quaternary ammonium salt, added to a pooled negative urine in a proficiency survey, Bloch and colleagues (1988) have demonstrated that 95% of POLs omitted positive urine confirmations that were mandated by state regulation.

Therapeutic Drug Monitoring

The volume of drug assays performed in the office laboratory rarely justifies the acquisition of an analyzer solely for therapeutic drug monitoring (see Chap. 17). When drug assays are included as an additional feature of a routine chemistry analyzer, care must be taken before the assay is set up. When reagent kits come in 100-test packages, the reagent will frequently become contaminated or outdated before the kit is used completely, wasting hundreds of dollars in supplies. Individually packaged reagents allowing single measurements reduce wastage but are usually obtained at higher costs. Calibrations and control costs can become prohibitive with low-volume single measurements and should be avoided unless indicated by both the clinical need and the ease of obtaining an accurate and reproducible result.

Microbiology Methodology

Primary culture inoculations in the POL are not considered a complete test and are permitted in the POL if the culture is referred to a certified laboratory for identification of colonies. If the culture is kept in the office and read as no growth, classification as a moderate complexity laboratory is required. No growth means that there are no bacterial colonies on the media after incubation. The identification of normal flora, contaminants, or any pathogenic or nonpathogenic organism requires high complexity certification. Gram's stains of urethral sources and endocervical smears are moderately complex, whereas all other Gram's stains are high complexity. Direct acid-fast smears that do not involve concentration of the specimen are moderately complex. Selective media systems and antigen detection systems that, when used for identification, in most cases will identify an organism without further biochemical or physiologic testing may also qualify as moderately complex testing. Additional office methods are dependent on complexity classification, but methods that require identification or susceptibility determinations, or both, on organisms after transfer from primary culture medium likely fall into the category of highly complex.

Rapid Streptococcal Antigen

Although faster than traditional cultures, rapid streptococcal antigen (RSA) methods are by no means cheaper and not necessarily easier to perform and maintain than routine cultures (see Chaps. 48 and 54). If the assay is not of sufficient sensitivity, an appropriate strategy would be to screen all cases of pharyngitis with the RSA. When the RSA is positive, treatment is indicated; when negative, a routine throat culture is performed. The latter component of this strategy not only identifies false-negative results but also allows correct diagnosis of pneumococcal, staphylococcal, meningococcal, and *Haemophilus influenzae* colonization and pharyngitis.

Urinary Tract Infections and Sexually Transmitted Diseases

Methods exist for the rapid detection of urinary tract infections and sexually transmitted diseases. Leukocyte esterase and nitrite-detecting reagent strips, urine filtration systems, and bioluminescence detection of ATP have all been used in the diagnosis of urinary tract infections and found to have low sensitivity or both low specificity and predictive value (Stribling, 1988). In contrast to streptococcal throat infections, in which a single pathogen with known antibiotic sensitivity accounts for a significant proportion of disease, routine urine cultures for identification and sensitivities are virtually always necessary for proper management. With specific sexually transmitted pathogens such as *Neisseria gonorrhoeae*, *Chlamydia trachomatis*, and herpes simplex virus, antigenic or nucleic acid detection is possible. However, the social consequences and implied liability of both false-positive and false-negative results make the selection of an appropriate assay more difficult for a POL.

COST ACCOUNTING

Cost accounting is essential in the decision as to whether an assay is to be performed in the office or referred to an outside laboratory. In the POL, expenses associated with instrumentation, space, interest, depreciation, specimen collection and processing, instrument maintenance, quality control, and proficiency testing, as well as analytical and clerical supplies, should be appropriately proportioned over each measurement performed. The cost of compliance with regulatory mandates such as CLIA, Americans with Disabilities Act, and the Occupational Safety and Health Administration Standards also must be captured and allocated to the laboratory service (Tirabassi, 1994).

Labor in the office laboratory can be a special case because office staff frequently perform other functions. Office staff time could possibly be divided into three categories—analysis time, nonlaboratory time, and coverage. Analysis time would include time spent in instrument setup, maintenance, measurement, quality control, reporting, and record keeping. Nonlaboratory time is time spent on other physician office functions or roles. Coverage is the idle time that a person hired primarily to perform laboratory functions spends waiting for specimens to arrive. Personnel who are functionally on call to perform *ad libitum* laboratory measurements will spend more time in coverage than if assays are performed in scheduled batches. Analysis and coverage time should be apportioned in the cost per test, and nonlaboratory time should be excluded. Coverage is a good parameter to estimate and monitor. When it is excessive, new assays should be considered. When coverage time approaches nil, capacity and the ability to respond to volume peaks or unusual circumstances are limited.

Spreadsheet-based cost accounting programs are probably the most effective in the POL setting. Spreadsheet models can be more easily adapted to the individual setting. Small office laboratories can be extremely sensitive to changes in volume and reassignment of office staff function. The ability to project changes in reimbursement, supply expenses, volume, and staffing may prevent costly decisions. Although cost-accounting studies are important and should be performed, the final decision to implement, continue, expand, or halt testing may be heavily influenced by physician and patient preference and consideration of practice competitiveness.

PERSONNEL AND TRAINING REQUIREMENTS

CLIA-88 requires that laboratories employ personnel who meet established qualifications in training, experience, job performance, and competency (Halper, 1989). In the assignment of methods to complexity levels, HHS considers the methodologies, difficulty in calibration and operation, degree of calculations, and analyst training, knowledge, experience, and independent judgment involved, as well as quality control of the instruments employed. These methodology and analyst-based requirements cannot be exclusively based on an obtained academic degree. For example, it is estimated that Maryland alone has more than 1861 small office laboratories (DeBoy, 1988). To require that each be staffed by a medical technologist or medical laboratory technician would increase the severity of the current shortage of laboratory technical staff. Instead, the focus probably will be on strict documentation of the formal and informal training and experience of persons employed.

With waived tests, there are no personnel requirements. With moderately complex tests, the minimum requirement is a high school diploma or equivalent, as long as there is documented training appropriate for the testing performed. This training must be sufficient to ensure that the individual has the skills necessary for specimen collecting, identifying, processing, and performing each measurement. Manufacturers of moderately complex methods may provide instrument calibration, preventive maintenance, and assay methodology, as well as quality control training. But the laboratory director must ensure that employees have training in preanalytic processing and reporting methods. The Occupational Safety and Health Administration requires training in chemical hazards as well as in the handling of infectious material, which is reviewed in Chapter 1. In-service training acquired at local hospitals or provided by local laboratory professionals is acceptable, if it has been documented.

Personnel Records

Employee records should detail education, training, and level of competency and certification of each person who performs laboratory measurements. Copies of degrees and the length and evidence of accreditation of any nondegree training, in-service, or continuing education program should be maintained, and registration numbers of any certifications should be kept on file. Vaccination records, including declinations, for hepatitis B, rubella, and tetanus should be maintained. In addition, letters from former employers may be needed to document that a particular experience requirement has been met.

In-Service Education

A regular program of in-service education should be in place. Incentives such as paid time while in attendance and support to attend meetings or conferences can supplement such continuing education. Small office laboratories should make arrangements with larger laboratories so that staff can take part in the latter's in-service activities. Workshops and user groups sponsored by manufacturers of office equipment may also be used. All in-service activities have to be documented to be considered valid, and each staff person's attendance should be included in the individual's personnel file to supplement documentation. Continuing education positively affects both performance and morale, and is well worth the added expense.

LABORATORY PROCEDURE MANUALS

Procedure manuals document most important laboratory functions. These manuals should be simple, easy to follow, and functional rather than a collection of articles, package inserts, and instrument protocols that are too disorganized for the inexperienced operator to follow. The procedure manual should include specimen requirements, procedures for specimen collection, identification and processing, assay methodology, reference intervals, quality control, and reporting methods. A written standard operating procedure (SOP) must be available for every test performed in the laboratory, regardless of who performs it. Such written procedures are available commercially through professional consultants or the National Committee for Clinical Laboratory Standards (NCCLS).*

Specimen Collection and Identification

A system of written policies and procedures for positive patient-specimen aliquot identification and specimen and reagent handling must be established. Included in this system should be proper procedures for the collection, transportation, and storage of specimens. If the specimens are not analyzed within two hours, particular attention must be paid to the preservation of the specimen. In the development of these procedures, concern should be taken where indicated concerning various preanalytic errors, which are discussed in Chapters 1 and 6. A procedure that sets criteria for acceptable specimens and provides proper notification on receipt when a

*Located at 771 E. Lancaster Avenue, Villanova, PA 19085; (215) 525-2435.

specimen is not properly labeled or has insufficient quantity is required. The laboratory must perform testing only at the written or electronic request of an authorized person, and the test requisition or medical chart containing the requisition must be retained for two years.

Methodologies

CLIA requires a specific premarket approval process for all moderate complexity testing, and the laboratory must follow the manufacturer's instructions for the instruments and test systems used. A copy of the procedure should be made available at each workbench as a resource for the less experienced operator. A common cause of imprecision is when different operators use a slightly different technique because of excessive concern for speed or lack of understanding about proper technique. As part of the procedure, reagents must be dated and initialed when received, opened, and prepared and routinely checked for outdating. Calibration procedures, linearity protocols, and preventive maintenance procedures are usually specified by the manufacturer but, unless spelled out in the procedure, frequently are forgotten or lost. Because procedures can have manufacturer-initiated analytical changes as well as changes that naturally evolve in office practice, each method should be reviewed and compared with recent package inserts on an annual basis.

Reference Ranges

The sensitivity, specificity, and reference ranges provided by the instrument manufacturer may be derived from statistical measures of an inadequate or nonrepresentative spectrum of patients. A systematic analysis of data collected from the practitioner's patient population is possible and indicated for refinement of reference ranges after implementation (see Chap. 6). For analytes such as cholesterol, for which a national standard reference range is operative, a comparison with the consensus in an external proficiency survey may be appropriate in validating the reference range (see Chap. 10).

Quality Control

Each laboratory must establish and maintain a quality control and quality assurance program that is "adequate and appropriate for the validity and reliability" of the procedures performed (Halper, 1989). CLIA inspections specifically focus on these issues. Evidence exists that office-based laboratories have a greater problem with poor quality control than hospital and independent commercial laboratories (Lunz, 1987). Although less sophisticated instrumentation and operators with less training contribute to this problem, a clearly defined protocol for quality control derived from principles reviewed elsewhere in Part I can greatly enhance performance (see Chaps. 1 and 6).

A good source of procedure and required frequency of control measurements is the manufacturer of the reagents for the method being used. All manufacturers were required to revise product information to meet CLIA standards by 1994, and compliance with the manufacturer's procedure reduces problems. All calibrations must be performed at the manufacturer's recommendation and must be documented. However, the laboratory is responsible for the interpretation of quality control data.

When a problem occurs, it should be investigated and corrected. If possible, steps should be taken to prevent its recurrence. If problems recur, replacement of the methodology or instrumentation should be considered. Problematic methodologies can be a cause of low staff morale and high staff turnover. Frequent staff turnover and the associated training costs can be one of the office laboratory's largest expenses.

Controls are used to document reproducibility, and at least two levels, normal and abnormal, must be performed in each run. A run is defined by HHS as an interval within which the accuracy and precision of a testing system is expected to be stable but cannot be greater than 24 hours. Target values for controls are determined by repetitive testing and the use of statistical methods described in Chapter 6. A minimum of 20 replicate tests is needed to establish statistical limits. If control results detect drift or error, remedial action must be performed and documented. All patient test results obtained in the unacceptable test run and since the last acceptable run must be evaluated to determine whether patient test results have been adversely affected, and corrected results must be issued promptly if such are identified.

Much confusion exists about the use of unassayed versus the more expensive assayed controls. A year or more's supply of unassayed control can quantitatively document precision using standard statistical quality control techniques (see Chap. 6). If a quarterly external proficiency program is used to validate accuracy during this interval, then both accuracy and precision can be documented without the use of expensive assayed controls. Each physician in the group should be made aware of the coefficient of variation (CV) of in-office laboratory measurements to ensure that they are adequate for clinically useful decision making. For instance, at 95% confidence limits, if potassium has a CV of 7%, a 4.8 mEq/L level could range from 4.1 to 5.5 and be analytically "correct" but clinically misleading.

Quality control results should be charted or analyzed by computer such that each result is compared with expected and previous results. Each result should be analyzed, not just the best results of the day. Analysis of trends can be conducted visually because results are plotted on standard Levi-Jennings type plots. Deviations and adverse trends indicate that something is changing in the analytical system. If a computerized system is used, it must be capable of detecting deviations and trends, or it gives only a false sense of security. Action must be taken as deviations and trends appear. Merely to collect data that are not actively monitored as they are derived is a waste of time and reagent. Records of quality control activities must be retained for a minimum of two years.

Preventive Maintenance

In addition to preventive maintenance required by the manufacturer to maintain the moderately complex status of its method, a temperature log for each temperature-dependent piece of equipment must be maintained. Refrigerator, incubator, and freezer temperatures must be recorded daily or continuously monitored if this equipment is used for reagent storage or if any part of an assay depends on it. Instrument and water bath temperatures should be recorded each day of use. Each instrument should have its own equipment maintenance, linearity, and troubleshooting log. The instrument log should include the manufacturer's name, address, phone number, model and serial numbers, and date of purchase. Instrument logs should be maintained for the life of the instrument and readily available for an inspector's review. Centrifuges should be maintained by a professional qualified service agent so that operating speeds are checked and brushes are changed periodically.

Quality Assurance

An ongoing quality assurance process is necessary for moderate and high complexity laboratories to assess various facets of their technical and nontechnical performance. This involves setting a quality target, measuring whether the target has been reached, and instituting corrective action if it has not. Potential areas for quality assurance monitoring include assessment of specimen quality, identification and handling, timeliness and accuracy of reporting systems, as well as timeliness of personnel evaluations.

ACCREDITATION

Accreditation and certification must be obtained from HHS or an organization deemed by HHS. Table 2–4 lists currently deemed organizations, as well as those whose applications for deemed status are pending at the time of this publication. One of the most active is COLA. COLA is a not-for-profit voluntary education and accreditation program for POLs. Jointly sponsored by the American Academy of Family Physicians, American Society of Internal Medicine, College of American Pathologists, and the American Medical Association, it provides a system of standards, checklists, inspections, and accreditation for the POL. COLA accredits over 6800 office laboratories.* With the exception of validation inspections performed on 5% of COLA-inspected laboratories, all federal inspection requirements are met. Standards include requirements for sufficient space, personnel training and continuing education, appropriateness of methodologies, records, preventive maintenance, and quality control, as well as enrollment in a proficiency testing program. The College of American Pathologists, American Society of Internal Medicine, American Association of Bioanalysts, and other organizations provide approved proficiency testing programs designed to be useful for the POL. It is expected that these programs will remain current with federal standards as additional CLIA-88 regulations are implemented or changed.

Table 2–4. ALTERNATIVE CLIA ACCREDITATION

Organizations and Agencies with Deemed Status
State of Washington
Commission for Office Laboratory Accreditation (COLA)
College of American Pathologists
American Society of Histocompatibility & Immunogenetics
Joint Commission on Accreditation of Healthcare Organizations
New York State Health Department
American Association of Blood Banks
American Osteopathic Association
Organizations with Pending Applications for Deemed Status
Puerto Rico

*COLA offers a toll-free number (1-800-298-8044) to assist existing and prospective clients.

PROFICIENCY TESTING REQUIREMENTS

All laboratories performing moderate or highly complex testing must participate in an accredited proficiency program and be tested in every analyte for which the laboratory is certified except for nonregulated analytes. Laboratories that were not regulated prior to CLIA-88 were required to participate in an HHS-approved proficiency testing program prior to January 1, 1994, with successful performance by 1995. A score of greater than 80% is needed for a single testing event for most analytes. "Unsatisfactory participation" is defined as failure to pass two out of three consecutive testing events for any analyte or specialty.

Proficiency samples must be treated in the same way that specimens are treated in the ordinary course of testing. If a laboratory is identified that refers its proficiency samples to another laboratory for analysis, it may have its certificate revoked for one year and it will be subject to fines and other penalties.

INSPECTION REQUIREMENTS

Inspections of certified laboratories shall be conducted on a biannual basis or more frequently if HHS determines a need to ensure compliance with requirements and standards. Inspections may be announced or unannounced, and full access to all facilities and relevant information is required.

RECORD KEEPING

Daily Log

A worksheet or daily log that documents each batch of specimens analyzed and quality control results associated with the batch, along with time of day and identification of the person who performed the measurements, should be maintained in a systematic manner.

Sendout Log

A log of reference laboratory sendout specimens should be maintained that indicates specimen number, patient name, collection date and time, date sent, and date result received, as well as measurements requested. This log facilitates tracking of sendout specimens, saving valuable time otherwise spent on the phone. It also serves as a quality control check of the reference laboratory because inordinate delays in the "date result received" column will be noticed each time the log book is used.

Master Log

An efficient and error-free procedure for the reporting of test results is necessary. A master test log in which all requests and all results are recorded is frequently required of licensed laboratories and should be maintained on site for three months. Some legally reproduced record of each test result must be kept for at least two years.

American Society of Clinical Pathology: Washington Report, December 22, 1993, 11:23.

Bachner P: Personal communication. May 12, 1995.

Bachner P, Hamlin W: Federal regulation of clinical laboratories and the clinical laboratory improvement amendments of 1988—Part II. Clin Lab Med 1993a; 13:987.

Bachner P, Hamlin W: Federal regulation of clinical laboratories and the clinical laboratory improvement amendments of 1988—Part I. Clin Lab Med 1993b; 13:739.

Bloch MJ, Cembrowski GS, Lembesis GJ: Longitudinal study of error prevalence in Pennsylvania physicians' office laboratories. JAMA 1988; 260:230.

Brecher G, Anderson RE, McMullen PD: When to do diffs: How often should differential counts be repeated. Blood Cells 1980; 6:431.

College of American Pathologists: Comparison Chart of the CLIA February 28, 1994, Final Rules, Major Regulatory Revisions/Clarifications Following Publication of the Final Rules and CLIAC Recommendations (available from CAP, Div. of Government and Professional Affairs, Washington, DC 20005; 202-371-6617).

Cook J: Choosing a reference lab. Advance for Administrators of the Laboratory 1994; 3:8.

Crawley R, Belsey R, Brock D, Baer D: Regulation of physicians-office laboratories: The Idaho experience. JAMA 1986; 255:374.

DeBoy JM, Wajda MJ, Shanoltz EC: Unregulated physician office laboratories in Maryland. Report on a study conducted for the Maryland General Assembly, 1988.

Halper HR, Foster HS: Aspen Systems Laboratory Regulation Manual. Rockville, MD, Aspen Publishers, Inc, 1989.

Hsiao WC, Braun P, Dunn D, Becker ER, DeNicola M, Ketcham TR: Results and policy implications of the resource-based relative-value study. N Engl J Med 1988; 319:881.

James K, Barrett DA II: Establishing a physician's office laboratory. Med Clin North Am 1987; 71:691.

Lunz ME, Castleberry BM, James K, Stahl J: The impact of the quality of laboratory staff on the accuracy of laboratory results. JAMA 1987, 258:361.

Mennemeyer ST, Winkelman JW: Searching for inaccuracy in clinical laboratory testing using Medicare data. JAMA 1993; 269:1030.

Stribling MD, Cohen MS: The urologic office laboratory. Urol Clin North Am 1988; 15:635.

Tirabassi CP: Cost accounting in the POL. POL Adviser 1994; 2:1.

US Department of Health and Human Services, Health Care Financing Administration: Specific List for Categorization of Laboratory Test Systems, Assays, and Examinations by Complexity; Notice. Federal Register 1995; 60:25943.

Woo J, McCabe JB, Chauncey D, Schug T, Henry JB: The evaluation of a portable clinical analyzer in the emergency department. Am J Clin Pathol 1993; 100:599.

Principles of Instrumentation

Andy N.D. Nguyen, MSME, M.D.
John Bernard Henry, M.D.
Robert L. Sunheimer, M.S., MT(ASCP)SC

INTRODUCTION TO CLINICAL INSTRUMENTATION

The initial growth phase of clinical laboratory instrumentation started in the early 1950s. This period emphasized the classic techniques of quantitative analytical chemistry and manual cell counting. Training focused on the manual skills of pipetting and rigid conformance to protocols. Simple photometers and pH meters often represented the only instruments in the clinical laboratory. Because many laboratories still made their own reagents, pH meters were essential. The analysis of sodium and potassium using flame photometers was just beginning in this decade. Much more common in the clinical laboratory was protein fractionation by electrophoresis. Developments were started on liquid chromatography for amino acids, gas chromatography for volatile substances, and low-pressure column chromatography for many substances using ion exchange and gel permeation. All the described instruments required manual pipetting of specimens and samples and were labor intensive.

The commercial development of the Technicon* AutoAnalyzer system in 1957 established the continuous flow technique as a viable technology for routine clinical analysis. Coulter† Company developed particle counters that enabled routine cell counting in the standard complete blood count (CBC). The Coulter design incorporated size discrimination capability using an impedance method. This approach has served the clinical hematology laboratory for over 40 years.

In the early 1960s, the single-channel analyzers expanded into multichannel analyzers that adapted to a variety of laboratory settings. A successful application of multichannel analysis was the Technicon SMA 12/60 system. Since then, chemistry profiles have become an integral part of routine testing for inpatient admissions and outpatient visits. The DuPont* aca I was first introduced in 1968. This discrete analyzer incorporated the reagents into compartments with temporary seals. One or two reagent packs were used depending on the analyte being measured.

In the 1970s, microprocessors started to be integrated into many analytical analyzers. Onboard microprocessors captured changes in absorbance and converted them to concentrations. By the end of that decade, most manufacturers incorporated communication ports (RS 232) into their instruments to interact with a variety of available laboratory information systems. Another development that came to the forefront early in that decade was the successful application of ion-selective electrodes for routine analysis of sodium and potassium. Progress was also made in automated white blood cell

*Miles, Inc., Tarrytown, NY.
†Coulter Company, Hialeah, FL.

*DuPont Medical Products, Wilmington, DE.

differential counting. The inclusion of a laser (light amplification by stimulated emission of radiation) into cell counters and flow cytometers greatly helped cell differential measurements. The continuous-flow Hemalog-D system from Technicon used cytochemical stains to differentiate the cell populations with light scattering technique. Instead of the usual manual count of 100 leukocytes on a slide, the instrument could examine 30,000 cells per specimen aliquot. The laser was also used as the light source for turbidimetric and nephelometric measurements, using specific antibodies to improve accuracy of specific protein quantitation.

A new type of automated system, the random-access analyzer, made its appearance in the 1980s. They generally had on-board storage for up to 30 different assays, and the operator could select any combination of determinations on a given specimen aliquot depending on reagent availability. Developers of these systems took advantage of a variety of technologies to offer random-access capability to the analyzers. One interesting approach was developed for the Kodak Ektachem* system that used multilayer film slide technology for a variety of assays. Reaction of reagent and specimen in this system was accomplished by the diffusion of specimen aliquots through a series of film layers, and the concentration was measured by reflectance photometry. Extra-high-voltage capillary electrophoresis (CE) instruments were also developed in this decade. Specimen aliquots of only a few picoliters in volume could be measured with capillary electrophoresis. This technique has been applied to measuring nucleic acids and peptides. The late 1980s was characterized by the rapid development of compact instruments that decentralized laboratory measurements. Many laboratory measurements were performed in the doctor's office, at the patient's bedside, or intensive care units with the introduction of these testing modalities.

The goal of this chapter is to provide the reader with a brief and broad description of the essential principles of analytical instruments in the clinical laboratory. For a more comprehensive review of this topic, the reader is referred to references on clinical instrumentation at the end of this chapter.

PRINCIPLES OF INSTRUMENTATION

Spectrophotometry

Many determinations made in the clinical laboratory are based on the measurements of radiant energy absorbed or transmitted under controlled conditions. The device used to measure the absorbed or transmitted light energy is the spectrophotometer. Electromagnetic radiation (EMR) is the flow of energy through space at the universal speed of light as electric and magnetic fields that make up an electromagnetic wave. EMR exists as Maxwell's waves and as streams of particles called photons. These photons or packets of energy ($h\nu$) have unique frequencies. The spectrum of frequencies of EMR extends from very low values over the range of radio waves to visible light and beyond to the higher values of ultraviolet (UV) light, x-rays, and gamma rays. Photons of radiant energy are exchanged whenever electrically charged subatomic particles interact. When these electrons move from one orbit to another, some energy is either absorbed or released. In the visible spectrum near the yellow region, the energy of a photon is about 2.2 eV (electron volt). Compare this with the photon energy of x-rays, which is 200–100,000 eV. Clearly, large differences may exist in the energies of photons within the electromagnetic spectrum. The wavelength of light is the distance between successive peaks. Frequency is the number of waves that pass an observation point in one unit of time. The wavelength is inversely related to frequency and energy, that is, the shorter the wavelength, the higher the frequency and energy and vice versa. The relationship between the energy of the photons and their frequency is given by the following equation:

$$E = h\nu \quad (3\text{-}1)$$

where E refers to the energy (in ergs), h is Planck's constant (6.62×10^{-27} erg·second), and ν is the frequency (Hertz). The frequency of light is related to the wavelength by:

$$\nu = c/\lambda \quad (3\text{-}2)$$

where c is the speed of light in a vacuum (3×10^{10} cm/sec) and λ is the wavelength (cm). If one substitutes the expression of ν from this equation into the previous one, the following is obtained:

$$E = hc/\lambda \quad (3\text{-}3)$$

This equation shows that the energy is inversely proportional to the wavelength. Table 3–1 shows the relationship between the types of electromagnetic radiation, wavelength, and source of radiation. In the clinical laboratory, the wavelengths of primary interest in spectrophotometric measurement fall between 150 nm and 2500 nm. This corresponds to the UV, the visible, and the near infrared (IR) regions. The visible region is further subdivided into various color regions (Table 3–2).

The term photometer is often used in its generic sense as any instrument that measures light intensity. Photometric instruments measure light in a variety of ways. Besides molecular absorption spectrophotometers, there are flame photometers (atomic emission spectrophotometer), atomic absorption photometers, and fluorometers (molecular emission spectrophotometer). Specifically, a spectrophotometer measures the absorption of monochromatic light produced by a grating monochromator. A flame photometer measures the light emitted by single atoms burned in a flame. An atomic absorption photometer measures the light absorbed by atoms dissociated by heat. A fluorometer measures the light of a specific wavelength emitted by a molecule after it has been ex-

Table 3–1. ELECTROMAGNETIC RADIATION SPECTRUM

Radiant Energy	Wavelength (nm)*
Gamma rays	0.1
X-rays	1
Ultraviolet (UV)	180
Visible light	390
Infrared (IR)	780
Microwave	400,000

*The wavelength where the lowest type of respective radiant energy occurs.
From Kaplan LA, Pesce AJ: Clinical Chemistry: Theory, Analysis and Correlation. St. Louis, Mosby–Year Book, 1989.

*Eastman Kodak Co., Rochester, NY.

Table 3–2. COLORS AND COMPLEMENTARY COLORS OF THE VISIBLE SPECTRUM*

Wavelength (nm)	Color Absorbed	Complementary Color
350–430	Violet	Yellow-blue
430–475	Blue	Yellow
475–495	Green-blue	Orange
495–505	Blue-green	Red
505–555	Green	Purple
555–575	Yellow-green	Violet
575–600	Yellow	Blue
600–650	Orange	Green-blue
650–700	Red	Blue-green

*If a solution absorbs light of a certain color (second column), the observed color of the solution is the complementary color (third column).

From Kaplan LA, Pesce AJ: Clinical Chemistry: Theory, Analysis and Correlation. St. Louis, Mosby–Year Book, 1989.

cited by electromagnetic radiation of a given energy. Energy released as the electrons return to lower vibrational level is lower than their original energy level. Spectroscopy can be classified into four main categories: absorption or emission by molecules, and absorption or emission by atoms.

The **Beer-Lambert law** states that the concentration of a substance is directly proportional to the amount of light absorbed or inversely proportional to the logarithm of transmitted light. This law can be expressed by the following equation:

$$A = abc = \log(100/\%T) \quad (3\text{-}4)$$

where

A = absorbance
a = absorptivity of the compound under standard conditions
b = light path of the solution
c = concentration of the compound
%T = per cent transmittance

This law is an idea mathematical relationship that has some limitations in practice. Essentially, this law will be followed only if the incident radiation is monochromatic, the solvent absorption is insignificant compared with the solute absorbance, the solute concentration is within linearity limits, and a chemical reaction does not occur between the molecules of interest and other solute or solvent molecules.

Components of a Spectrophotometer

Basic components of a spectrophotometer consist of the exciter lamp, the entrance slit, the monochromator, the analytical cell or cuvette, and the photodetector (Fig. 3–1). An exciter lamp provides electromagnetic radiation as visible, infrared, or UV light that will pass through the monochromator to be separated into discrete wavelengths. Light of a selected wavelength will be incident on the cuvette containing the solution of which the absorption is to be measured. For spectrophotometric work in the visible and near-infrared ranges, tungsten and halogen quartz lamps are good sources of radiant energy. Several types of vapor lamps are available for ultraviolet range. The hydrogen lamp is widely used. A mercury lamp is less desirable owing to its uneven emission spectrum. A xenon lamp gives a brilliant light that is ideal for applications requiring a narrow slit, but it is not suited for routine application owing to problems with stray light. For infrared spectrophotometry, a silicone carbide rod heated to 1200°C works well. Collimating lenses are often inserted between the exciter lamp and the entrance slit to focus the light into a beam of parallel light rays.

The function of the entrance slit is to reduce stray light and prevent scattered light from entering the monochromator. If stray light were allowed to pass through the analytical cell, this would cause a deviation from the Beer-Lambert law. The result would cause a significant error in the measurement.

A monochromator is a device that produces light of specific wavelengths from a light source. Types of monochromators include prism, diffraction grating, and interference filter. Prisms are wedge-shaped pieces of glass, quartz, or sodium chloride. When white light strikes a prism, it is dispersed to form a spectrum due to different angles of refraction by different wavelength at the air-prism interface.

Diffraction gratings are made by cutting tiny grooves or slits into an aluminized surface of a flat piece of crown glass. These grooves are cut at a precise angle and at an equal distance from each other. There are usually 1000 to 50,000 grooves to the inch. Each of these grooves acts both as a prism to refract white light and as a slit to diffract it into several spectra. Each spectrum is at a different angle from the grating. The brightest of these is called the first-order spectrum that is to be used for measurement. Usually, gratings are capable of better resolution than prisms. Gratings also have the additional advantage of covering all essential wavelengths, in contrast to the glass or quartz prisms, which cannot be used in the ultraviolet region. Because high-quality gratings can now be produced economically, most spectrophotometers incorporate diffraction gratings.

Interference filters are made by placing semitransparent silver films on both sides of a dielectric such as magnesium fluoride (Fig. 3–2). When light perpendicular to the silvered surface enters the filter, it passes through the dielectric and is

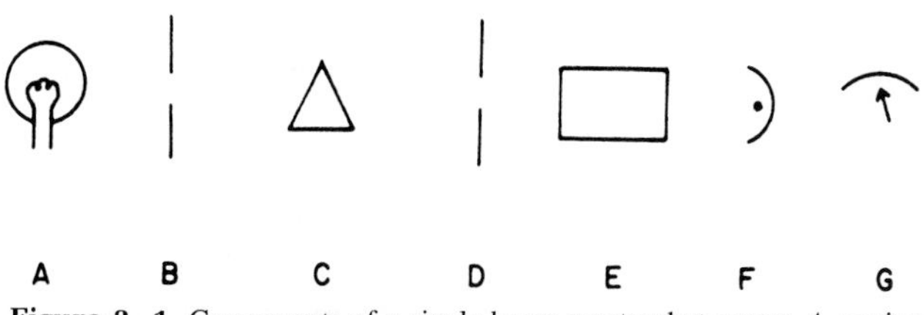

Figure 3–1. Components of a single-beam spectrophotometer. *A*, exciter lamp; *B*, entrance slit; *C*, monochromator; *D*, exit slit; *E*, cuvette; *F*, photodetector; *G*, meter.

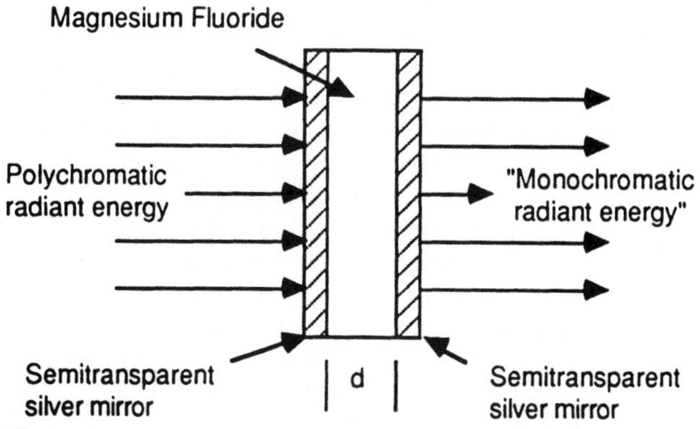

Figure 3–2. An interference filter. (Reproduced with permission from Bender GT: Principles of Chemical Instrumentation. Philadelphia, W. B. Saunders Company, 1987.)

reflected from the second silvered surface back to the first surface. This process repeats itself until the light is finally transmitted through the filter and into the analytical cell. Constructive and destructive interferences occur as the light is reflected between the silver films. Interference filters allow transmission of 40% to 60% of the incident light, with a bandwidth between 10 nm and 20 nm. By definition, a bandpass is the range of wavelengths between the points at which transmittance is one half peak transmittance. The dielectric thickness may be varied to produce filters of different bandpasses.

The cuvette or analytical cell holds the solution of which the absorption is to be measured. Cuvettes are made of soft glass, borosilicate glass, quartz, or plastic. Soft glass cuvettes are preferable for acidic solutions that do not etch glass. Strong alkaline solutions should be measured in borosilicate cuvettes because of their high resistance to alkali. Only quartz or plastics that do not absorb ultraviolet radiation may be appropriate for wavelengths below 320 nm. A rectangular cuvette, which presents a flat surface to the incident light, has less radiant energy loss from reflection than does a round cuvette. For routine work, this loss is usually not significant, accounting for about 4% of the incident energy for most round cuvettes. Room light entering the cuvette may cause measurement errors. A light shield should be placed over the cuvette well when a spectrophotometric reading is being made.

Types of photodetectors include barrier-layer cell, phototube, photomultiplier tube (PMT), and a variety of semiconductor photodetectors. All of these devices use photosensitive materials in their cathodes that release electrons when they are exposed to light energy. The anodes attract or collect electrons emitted from the cathode. If a closed electrical circuit is provided, the free electrons produce a current.

Barrier layer cells generate their own electrical output directly from light energy and do not need an external power source. Selenium coated with silver serves as the negative electrode while the iron base serves as the positive electrode. The spectral response of a barrier layer cell is in the range of 380 to 700 nm. These cells are found in older model colorimeters and spectrophotometers.

The widely used phototube has a curved sheet of photosensitive material that serves as the cathode and a positively charged thin tube that serves as the anode. A limitation of the phototube is the small amount of photocurrent generated.

PMTs consist of a photoemissive cathode, an anode, and an internal electron-multiplying series of dynodes. Many photomultiplier tubes have 9 to 16 photosensitive dynodes (Fig. 3–3). All of these components are encased in a glass evacuated tube. When radiant energy strikes the cathode, the emitted electrons are attracted to the first adjacent dynode. On striking the dynode, each electron causes the emission of several other electrons. The electrons emitted from the first dynode are subsequently attracted to the second dynode, where the same emission cycle is repeated. This process continues through the entire series of dynodes, resulting in a multiplication of the number of electrons, until the anode is reached. The amplification factor achieved by a photomultiplier tube may be as high as 10^6. Because of their excellent sensitivity and rapid response, all stray light and room light must be carefully shielded from the photomultiplier tube to prevent burn out.

Semiconductor detectors including photoresistor, photodiode, and phototransistor have virtually replaced conven-

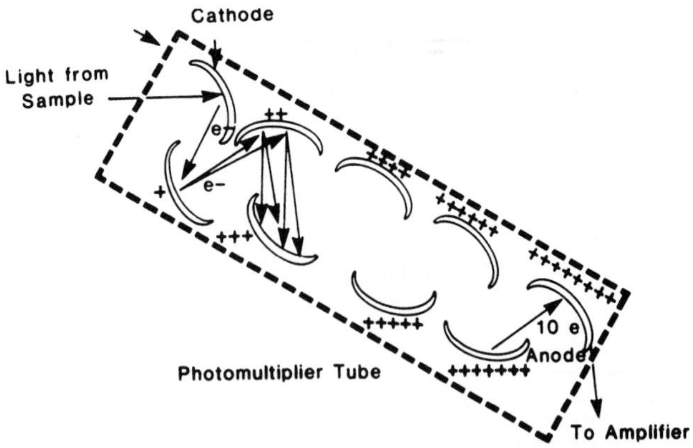

Figure 3–3. Schematic of a photomultiplier tube. (Reprinted from Simonson MG: *In* Kaplan LA, Pesce AJ [eds]: Nonisotopic alternatives to radioimmunoassay. New York, Dekker, 1981.)

tional phototubes in modern laboratory instruments. A semiconductor is used in an electrical circuit to regulate the current by changing its internal resistance. This is accomplished by changing the potential bias across its semiconductor junction. Unlike conventional semiconductors that respond to changes in voltage, semiconductor photodetectors respond to bias changes resulting from absorption of radiant energy.

DOUBLE-BEAM SPECTROPHOTOMETER. In a double-beam system monochromatic light from either a single or two identical monochromators pass through both a reference and sample compartment. The intensity of these two light beams is then measured by one or two photodetectors. The sample beam intensity is compared with the reference one as a ratio. Double-beam designs include double beam in space and double beam in time.

In a double beam in space spectrophotometer (Fig. 3–4), the light is split with a half-silvered mirror, called a dichroic mirror. The dichroic mirror splits the beam so half the light passes through the specimen aliquot and the other half to the reference cell. Both beams pass simultaneously through different components separated in space. This arrangement compensates for changes in intensity of the light source. However, photodetectors may age differently, resulting in different responses. This design also does not compensate for fluctuation in the photodetector output.

In a double beam in time spectrophotometer (Fig. 3–5), the light beam is split with a rotating chopper that alternately

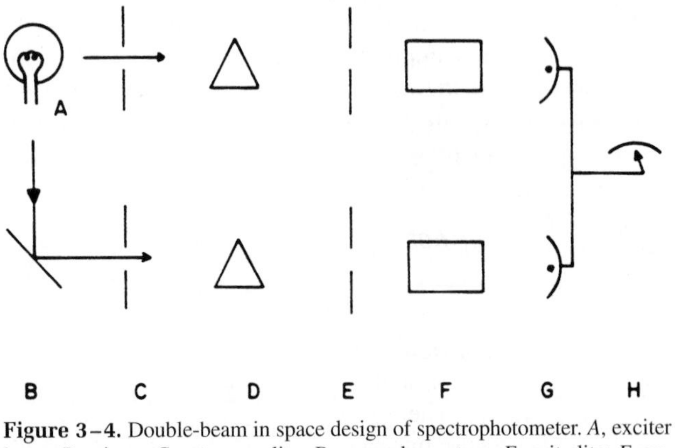

Figure 3–4. Double-beam in space design of spectrophotometer. *A*, exciter lamp; *B*, mirror, *C*, entrance slits; *D*, monochromators; *E*, exit slits; *F*, cuvettes; *G*, photodetectors; *H*, meter.

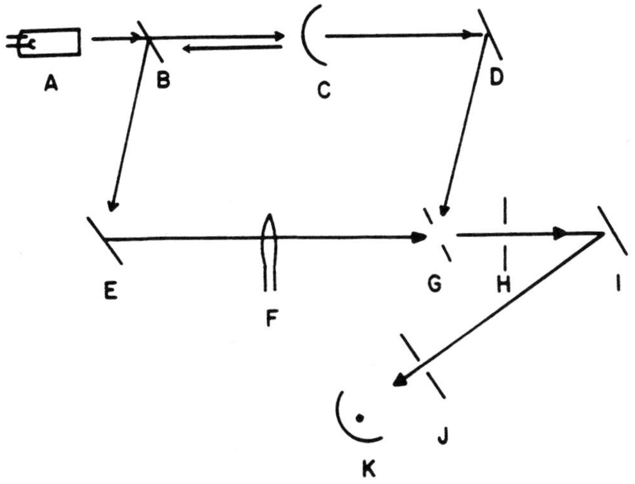

Figure 3–5. Double-beam in time design of an atomic absorption spectrophotometer. *A*, Hollow cathode lamp; *B*, half-silvered mirror; *C*, chopper; *D* and *E*, mirrors; *F*, flame; *G*, half-silvered mirror; *H*, slit; *I*, grating; *J*, slit; *K*, photodetector.

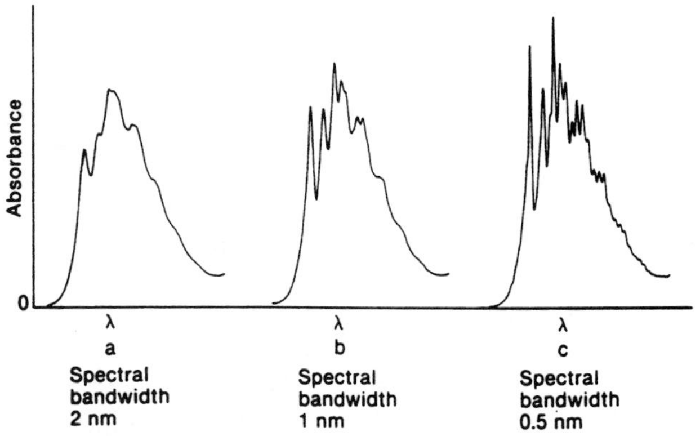

Figure 3–6. Absorption spectra of toluene at three different bandwidths. (Reproduced with permission from Bender GT: Principles of Chemical Instrumentation. Philadelphia, W. B. Saunders Company, 1987.)

presents a mirror and an opening. One beam passes through the sample and the other through a reference solution or blank. The open part of the chopper passes the beam directly to one path, while the mirrored part reflects the beam to the second path. Each beam, consisting of a pulse of electromagnetic radiation separated in time by a dark interval, is directed onto a photodetector. The output of the detector is an alternating current that has an amplitude proportional to the difference in intensity of the two beams.

To produce a spectral absorbance curve, a drive motor is geared to the diffraction grating. It is turned slowly in the light path so that light of various wavelengths pass through the exit slit of the monochromator. The light is passed through the cuvette compartment in succession. Spectral scans require adequate resolution for interpretation. To resolve absorbance peaks, the bandpass must be short (Fig. 3–6). Often, a very sharp, narrow peak may be characteristic of a compound. This peak may be completely missed if a wide bandpass were selected. It is possible to use, as a calibrating standard, almost any substance that has a spectral absorbance curve.

It is sound practice to calibrate at more than one wavelength on any spectrophotometers. Didymium is a commercially available calibration material. Its principal absorption peak is around 500 nm, and there are four wavelength maxima that may be chosen as calibration points. Another widely used wavelength calibration material is holmium oxide glass. It has about 10 sharp major absorption peaks. Two frequently used wavelengths are 360 and 536 nm. Therefore, an advantage of using this filter is that your spectrophotometer can be calibrated near the UV region.

Common Spectrophotometers in Use

With the introduction of integrated circuits and microprocessors, it has become commonplace to design spectrophotometers that do a variety of calculations, cycle through programmed sequences, and even automatically monitor their own performance. There is also a trend back to single-beam instruments because microprocessors can store reference data and continually compensate for variations. These new instruments are faster, more accurate, and more compact. A few typical spectrophotometers are listed here for reference (Schoeff, 1993).

Coleman* Model 35 Digital Spectrophotometer has a wavelength range of 335 to 825 nm, a bandpass of 8 nm, a quartz halogen lamp, and stray light that accounts for less than 0.1% T at 340 nm.

Gilford† Micro-Sample Spectrophotometer is an early version of an instrument designed primarily for microsamples. Sample volumes of 500 μL will create a 1 cm light path. The spectral range is 340 to 700 nm, with a bandpass of 8 nm.

Beckman‡ DU-70 Scanning Spectrophotometer is a highly sophisticated, computer-driven spectrophotometer. This single-beam spectrophotometer has automatic zeroing, blank subtraction, wavelength range selection from UV to visible light, and a wavelength bandpass of 2 nm. The computer module includes a high-resolution video graphic display for presentation of spectral data.

Atomic Emission Spectrophotometry (Emission Flame Photometry)

When a metallic salt is burned in a flame, the heat energy that the atom absorbs drives one or more of the electrons out of their usual orbits. As the excited electrons return to a lower or ground electronic state, they emit electromagnetic radiation. The heat energy absorbed and the light emitted are characteristic of the atom under consideration. Each metal has its own emission spectrum showing emission at characteristic wavelengths.

Components of an Atomic Emission Spectrophotometer

The atomizer-burner breaks up the specimen aliquot into fine droplets so that the atoms will absorb heat energy from the flame (Fig. 3–7*A*). In a total consumption burner, a fuel gas (propane) with an oxidizing agent (compressed air) is

*Perkin-Elmer Corp., Norwalk, CT.
†Ciba Corning Diagnostics Corporation, Medfield, MA.
‡Beckman Instruments, Brea, CA.

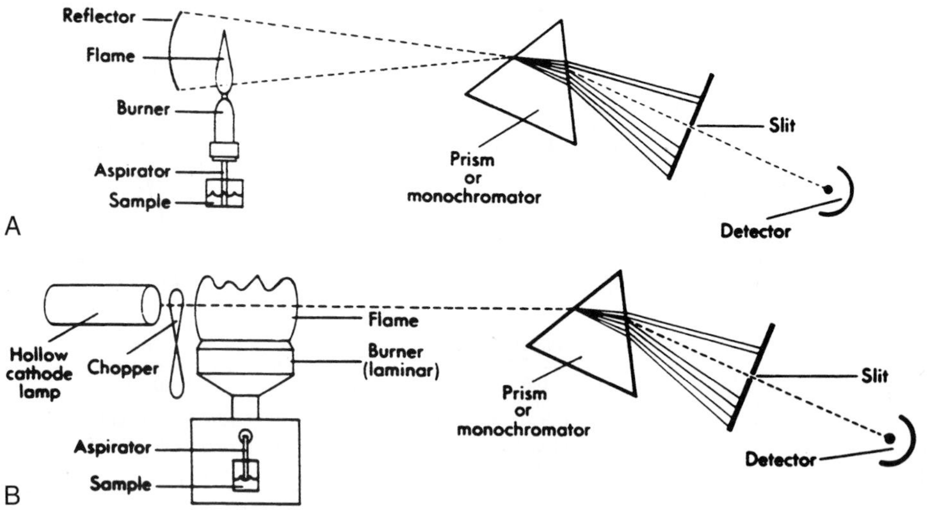

Figure 3–7. Atomic spectrophotometer. *A*, Atomic emission spectrophotometer. *B*, Atomic absorption spectrophotometer. (Reproduced with permission from Schoeff LE, Williams RH: Principles of Laboratory Instruments. St. Louis, Mosby, 1993.)

burned to produce the flame. A diluted specimen is drawn into the flame as compressed air passes over the end of a capillary tube or sample probe. This is known as Venturi action. In total consumption burners, gases are rushing past the tip of the capillary, nebulizing the specimen aliquot and spraying it in a fine mist within a closed chamber located beneath the flame. The larger droplets fall to the floor of the chamber, and only the very fine droplets are carried upward by the gas flow into the flame. In the base of the flame, the element absorbs heat energy. As the element rises within the flame, it moves into the cooler part of the flame and releases its energy as light. Less than 5% of the ions passing through the flame are energized in flame photometers. The fuel content, and the pressure and moisture content of the gas mixture are critical in maintaining a constant flame temperature. Otherwise, the accuracy of measurement can be seriously impaired. The instrument must be designed to detect a very small light signal because the light intensity of the flame is much less than that of an exciter lamp. Variations in sample aspiration rate, atomization rate, and solution viscosity are compensated for by use of an internal standard. An internal standard, usually a salt of lithium, is mixed with each sample. Internal standards contain known concentration of an element whose emission peak differs from that of the element to be measured such that the two can be readily differentiated. The internal standard and the specimen solution are affected similarly in emission flame photometry. Later models of flame photometers use cesium as an internal standard. Cesium has an absorption peak at 852 nm and allows the operator to measure sodium, potassium, and lithium directly.

Common Atomic Emission Spectrophotometers in Use

Although the ion-selective electrodes (ISEs) have virtually replaced atomic emission photometers in routine measurements of sodium, potassium, and lithium, clinical laboratories still use atomic emission spectrophotometers for a few specific applications. They offer more reliable sodium and potassium levels in urine, especially at low concentrations, because these instruments are not affected by interferences such as urine constituents, as seen with ion selective electrodes. Instrumentation Laboratory is the only major manufacturer of atomic emission photometers. The IL 943* is the only model that this company markets. It is an upgraded instrument that replaced the previous IL 643 model. Improved electronics and software have resulted in less maintenance and greater measurement accuracy.

Atomic Absorption Spectrophotometry

In atomic absorption spectrophotometry, the analytical reaction is essentially the reverse of that in atomic emission spectrophotometry. The atom under consideration is dissociated from its chemical bonds, then it absorbs light of a specific wavelength in its ground state. Initially, the best way found to dissociate the atoms from their chemical bonds was to heat it in a flame to convert the ions into an atomic vapor. However, the flame can be replaced by other atomization processes that result in even greater sensitivity of measurement. One process applicable to mercury analysis uses a chemical reaction to convert mercury to an atomic vapor. The most advanced technique for atomic absorption is the graphite furnace. In this technique, a small volume of sample solution is placed in a graphite tube, where the sample vaporizes in an inert atmosphere when electric current passes through the tube.

Components of an Atomic Absorption Spectrophotometer

Because a dissociative atom absorbs the same amount of energy that an excited atom of the same element emits, it is logical to produce the required energy by heating this element using a hollow cathode lamp. The hollow cathode lamp is neon or argon with a cathode made of the metal under consideration. This lamp emits only the electromagnetic radiation

*Instrumentation Laboratory, Lexington, MA.

spectrum of the heated metal plus that of the contained gas. More than one element may be present in a cathode such that one lamp can be used to measure two or more elements. The emitted light is directed to the flame containing the metal. Atoms of the metal absorb this light energy. In its simplest form, the atomic absorption spectrophotometer consists of a hollow cathode lamp, a chopper, an atomizer-burner, a monochromator, and a photodetector (Fig. 3–7*B*). The most critical components in the instrument are the flame and its associated nebulizer. A steady flame is essential, and tight control of gas flows is required for both oxidant and fuel. As the flame burns the sample, approximately 1% to 2% of all the atoms are excited and emit light of the same wavelength as that from the hollow cathode lamp. To eliminate this source of error, the beam from the lamp is modulated either mechanically, using choppers, or electronically to differentiate it from the flame emission. Only the modulated light from the lamp is measured. The monochromator must be of high quality because the emission bands to be measured are very narrow.

Common Atomic Absorption Spectrophotometers in Use

More Perkin-Elmer atomic absorption spectrophotometers are found today in clinical laboratories than any other type. Their products range from the basic Model 3100 to the more advanced Model 5100 PC. Both models have double-beam optics and adapt to all the common sampling techniques including flame, mercury/hydride, and graphite furnace. Varian Techtron* is another major manufacturer of atomic absorption spectrophotometers. This company offers the single-beam SpectrAA-10 and the double-beam SpectrAA-20 with varying degrees of automation for flame, furnace, and hydride analysis. Varian now markets their most advanced instrument, the SpectrAA-400. This model features multiple element analysis. An automated run sequence of up to 12 elements can be selected for specimens.

Fluorometry (Molecular Emission Spectrophotometry)

Fluorometry is based on an energy exchange process that occurs when certain compounds absorb electromagnetic radiation, become excited, and return to an energy level higher than or equal to their original level. Because some energy is lost before emission from the excited state by collision with the solvent or other molecules, the wavelength of the emitted light is longer than that of the exciting light. Most uncharged molecules contain even numbers of electrons in the ground state. The electrons fill molecular orbits in pairs with their spins in opposite directions. No electron energies can be detected by application of a magnetic field to such spin patterns, and this electronic state is called the singlet state. Similarly, if an electron becomes excited by electromagnetic radiation and its spin remains paired with the ground state, it creates a singlet excited stated. The lifetime of the excited state is the average length of time the molecule remains excited before emission of light. For a singlet excited state, the lifetime of the excited state is on the order of 10^{-9} to 10^{-6} seconds. The light emission from a singlet excited state is called *fluorescence*. When the spins of the electrons in the excited state are unpaired, the electron energy levels will be split if a magnetic field is applied, and this electronic state is called a triplet state. Triplet state lifetimes range from 10^{-4} to 10 second (Willard, 1988). Light emission from an excited triplet state is called *phosphorescence*. The remainder of this review will focus on fluorescence, the more common of the two processes in clinical laboratory application.

Components of a Fluorometer

Instruments designed for fluorescence measurement have the following basic components: a light source, an excitation (primary) monochromator, cuvette, an emission (secondary) monochromator, and a photodetector (Fig. 3–8). The exciter lamp is a high-intensity light source such as a mercury vapor lamp or a xenon arc lamp. Simple instruments use mercury vapor lamps that do not require any special power supply. Mercury vapor lamps produce discrete and intense resonance lines that are not ideal for compounds with absorption bands at wavelengths not coinciding with these emission bands. For such compounds, xenon arc lamps producing a continuous spectrum between 250 nm and 600 nm are appropriate. A disadvantage of xenon arc lamps is their requirement of a special power supply to produce a stable output. In fluorescence measurements, the emitted light is detected at a right angle to the incident light to eliminate potential interference by the excitation signal. Phototubes or photomultiplier tubes are required for fluoresence measurements because signals are generally of low intensity.

An advantage of fluorescence is its extremely high sensitivity, which is approximately 100 to 1000 times that of absorption measurements. For applications requiring high sensitivity and for which the spectral properties of the fluorophore are known, a simple fluorometer may be the optimal approach. Fluorescence measurements are affected by operating variables including light scattering, self-quenching,

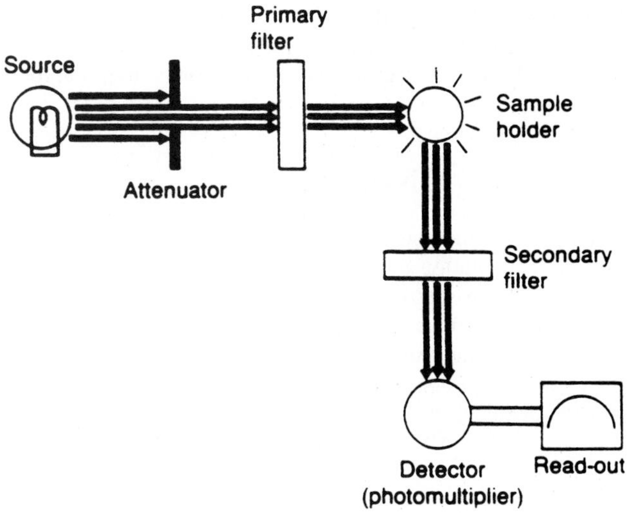

Figure 3–8. Components of a fluorometer. (Reproduced with permission from Bishop ML, Duben-Engelkirk JL, Fody EP: Clinical Chemistry: Principles, Procedures, Correlations. Philadelphia, J. B. Lippincott, 1992.)

*Varian Techtron, Melbourne, Australia.

self-absorption, and changes in temperature and pH. Scattering of the excitation light into the photodetector can occur even with the detector positioned at a right angle to the incident light. As the absorbance in a sample with a high fluorophore concentration increases, more of the excitation light is absorbed before it reaches the molecules near the center of the cuvette. This process is called self-quenching and results in less fluorescence from the center of the cuvette. Similarly, if the fluorophore concentration is high, light emission from the center of the cuvette may be absorbed before it exits the sample. This type of quenching is called self-absorption. Finally, at high concentrations, some fluorophores can form complexes with themselves or with other molecules. In both instances, these complexes lead to a decrease in fluorescence intensity.

Common Fluorometers in Use

A common fluorometer used in clinical laboratories is the TURNER* Model 111. Their Model 112 is an upgrade with solid-state electronics and digital readout display but with the same basic design (Schoeff, 1993). Both excitation and emission lights are modulated, resulting in an alternating current as the photomultiplier tube output. The difference in intensity between the two light signals is directly related to the fluorescence of the sample. This dual-path design eliminates variations in line voltage, lamp intensity, and photomultiplier tube sensitivity. Although the general, multipurpose fluorometers continue to be widely used, many applications of fluorescence have used instruments modified to meet the demands of the application. An example is the Abbott TD_X† based on *fluorescence polarization.* In this method, a polarizing filter produces vertically polarized light, which is used to excite the sample. The emitted light is partially depolarized depending on the amount of rotation occurring in the molecules of the sample. Emitted light passes through another polarizing filter, which polarizes the light in a vertical plane. Polarized light from the first filter is then rotated 90°, and measurements are taken to find out the extent of depolarization. A phototube detects the vertical polarized light. Fluorescence polarization methods measure the rate of rotation of fluorophores in the excited state as a function of light depolarization. Rapidly rotating molecules emit more depolarized light. Large fluorophores or fluorophores attached to macromolecules would be expected to rotate more slowly and therefore be less depolarized.

Nephelometry

Two useful methods available for measuring the concentration of a solution that contains particles too large for absorption spectroscopy are nephelometry and turbidimetry. These nonabsorptive methods may be suitable for quantitative assays using antigen-antibody complexes or measuring the amount of proteins in fluids.

To understand the principles of nephelometry and turbidimetry, the idea of radiation scattering by particles in solution must first be reviewed. When a collimated light beam strikes a particle in suspension, portions of the light are absorbed, reflected, scattered, and transmitted. Nephelometry is the measurement of the light scattered by a particulate solution. Three types of light scatters occur based on the relative size of the light wavelength (Gauldie, 1981). If the wavelength (λ) of light is much larger than the diameter (d) of the particle, where $d < 0.1\ \lambda$, the light scatter is symmetric around the particle. Minimum light scatter occurs at 90° to the incident beam and was described by Rayleigh (Rayleigh, 1885). If the light wavelength is much smaller than the particle diameter, where $d > 10\ \lambda$, the light scatters forward owing to the destructive out-of-phase back-scatter, as described by the Mie theory. If the wavelength of light is approximately the same amount as the particle size, more light scatters in the forward direction than in other directions, as defined by the Rayleigh-Debye theory. A common application of nephelometry is the measurement of antigen-antibody reactions. Because most antigen-antibody complexes have a diameter of 250 to 1500 nm and the wavelengths used are 320 to 650 nm, the light scatter is essentially of the Rayleigh-Debye type.

Components of a Nephelometer

A typical nephelometer consists of a light source, a collimator, a monochromator, a sample cuvette, stray light trap, and a photodetector. Light scattered by particles is measured at an angle, typically 15–90° to the beam incident on the cuvette. Figure 3–9 shows two possible optical arrangements for a nephelometer. Light scattering depends on the light wavelength and the particle size. For macromolecules with size close to or larger than the light wavelength, measurement of the forward light scatter increases the sensitivity of nephelometry. Light sources include a mercury-arc lamp, a tungsten-filament lamp, a light-emitting diode, and a laser.

Lasers produce stable, nearly ideal monochromatic light of narrow linewidth. It emits radiant energy that is coherent, parallel, and polarized. A laser beam can be maintained as a very slim cylinder only a few micrometers in cross section (Willard, 1988). A typical helium-neon laser lamp consists of a helium-pumping electrode (cathode) and a hollow glass laser core surrounded by a laser plasma tube (anode). Both the plasma tube and the core are filled with free helium and neon gases. The electrical discharge between the cathode and the anode is confined to the hollow glass core to keep it concentrated for maximum energy transfer. Two mirrors are positioned at the ends of the laser tube. One of them is fully reflective and the other partially transparent. When the electrode is charged, the helium atoms are excited to a higher energy state and then transfer this energy to the neon atoms by collision. In turn, the excited neon atoms emit photons. Photons bounce back and forth between the two end mirrors, stimulating other atoms to emit further photons, resulting in an amplification process. The amplified light eventually emerges as a laser beam through the partially transparent mirror. With the high intensity monochromatic beam, a substantial increase in sensitivity has been seen with lasers over conventional instruments. Disadvantages of laser sources include cost, safety problems, limited availability of wavelengths, and substantial cooling requirements for all but the smallest lasers.

*TURNER, Santa Clara, CA.

†Abbott Laboratories, Abbott Park, IL.

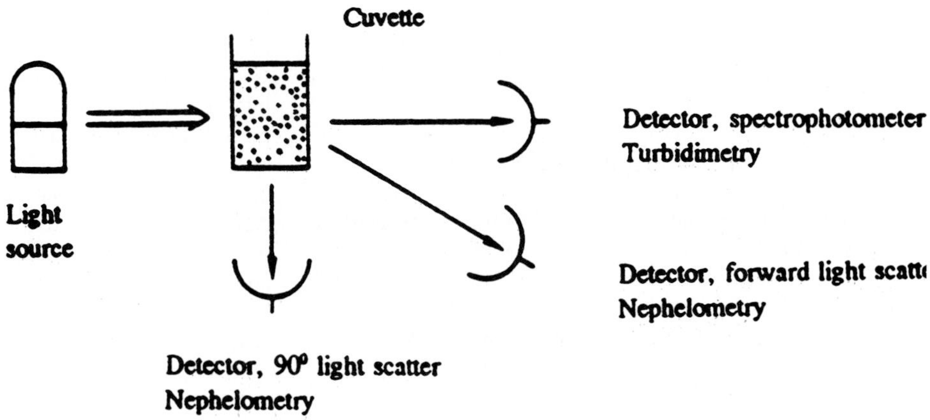

Figure 3–9. Optical arrangements of nephelometry and turbidimetry. (Reproduced with permission from Bishop ML, Duben-Engelkirk JL, Fody EP: Clinical Chemistry: Principles, Procedures, Correlations. Philadelphia, J. B. Lippincott, 1992.)

Common Nephelometers in Use

At present, the single most common uses of nephelometry is the measurement of antigen-antibody complexes formed in enzyme immunoassays. A typical nephelometer in this category is the Beckman Array 360 Protein/Drug System. This instrument measures the formation rate of insoluble immunoprecipitation products resulting from a specific antigen combining with a specific antibody. The Array model allows random access, fully automated testing of many proteins, such as apolipoproteins, immunoglobulins, prealbumin, and therapeutic drugs such as theophylline.

Turbidimetry

Turbidimetry is the measurement of the reduction in light transmission caused by particle formation. Light transmitted in the forward direction is detected. The amount of light absorbed by a suspension of particles depends on the specimen concentration and on the particle size. Solutions requiring quantitation by turbidimetry are measured using visible photometers or visible spectrophotometers (see Fig. 3–9). High sensitivity has been achieved through photodetectors that can quantify small changes in signals. Sensitivity comparable to nephelometry can be attained using low wavelengths and high-quality spectrophotometers. Many clinical applications exist for turbidimetry. Various microbiology analyzers measure turbidity of samples to detect bacterial growth in broth cultures. Turbidimetry is routinely used to measure the antibiotic sensitivity from such cultures. In coagulation analyzers, turbidimetric measurements detect clot formation in the sample cuvettes. Turbidimetric assays have long been available in clinical chemistry to quantitate protein concentration in biological fluids, such as urine and cerebrospinal fluid.

Refractometry

Refractometry is based on light refraction. When light passes from one medium into another, the light beam changes its direction at the boundary surface if its speed in the second medium is different from that in the first. The ability of a substance to bend light is called refractivity. The refractivity of a liquid depends on the wavelength of the incident light, the temperature, the nature of the liquid medium, and the concentration of the solute dissolved in the medium. If the first three factors are held constant, the refractivity of a solution is an indirect measurement of the solute concentration. Refractometry has been applied to various measurements, for example, total serum protein concentration, specific gravity of urine (Chap. 18), and column effluent of high-performance liquid chromatography analysis.

Osmometry

Osmometry is the measurement of the osmolality of an aqueous solution such as serum, plasma, or urine. As osmotically active particles are added to a solution causing its osmolality to increase, four other properties of the solution are also affected. These properties are osmotic pressure, boiling point, freezing point, and vapor pressure. They are called colligative properties of the solution because they can be related to each other and to the osmolality. As the osmolality of a solution increases, (1) the osmotic pressure increases, (2) the boiling point is elevated, (3) the freezing point is depressed, and (4) the vapor pressure is depressed. Osmometry is based on measuring changes in the colligative properties of solutions that occur owing to variations in particle concentration. Freezing-point depression osmometry is the most commonly used method for measuring the changes in colligative properties of a solution. Therefore, only components of a freezing-point osmometer are described in detail. A freezing-point osmometer consists of a sample chamber containing a stirrer and a thermistor (temperature-sensing device) connected to a readout device. The sample is rapidly supercooled to several degrees below its freezing point in a refrigeration chamber containing antifreeze. The sample is then agitated with the stirrer to initiate freezing. As the ice crystals form, heat of fusion is released from the solution. The rate of heat of fusion released from the ice being formed rapidly reaches equilibrium with the rate of heat removed by the colder temperature of the sample chamber. This equilibrium temperature, known as the freezing point of the solution, stays constant for several minutes once it is reached. This freezing point is detected by the thermistor, and the osmolality of the sample is displayed in units of milliosmoles per kilogram of water.

Freezing-point osmometers in common use include the Micro Osmette* and Osmette II models. The Micro Osmette

*Precision Systems Inc., Natick, MA.

model measures samples of 50 μL in volume, and the Osmette II measures samples of 200 μL in volume. Both models have a measurement time of 180 seconds.

Flow Cytometry

Flow cytometry measures the properties of cells suspended in a moving fluid medium. All cells pass single file through a sensing point, where they are intercepted typically by either water or air cooled argon laser beam. The transmitted light consists of both scattered light (forward and 90°) and fluorescent light. The light is directed by lenses and focused onto appropriate PMT. An analogue signal from the PMT is converted to a digital signal that the computer can use for quantitation.

Components of a Flow Cytometer

A typical laser-based flow cytometer includes a cell transportation system, a laser light source, a flow chamber, monochromatic filters, lenses, dichroic mirrors, photomultiplier tubes, and a computer for data analysis (Fig. 3–10). Samples to be analyzed are prepared depending on the source, and they are suspended in a medium. The cell suspension aliquots are introduced into the flow chamber using air pressure. As the cells pass through the flow chamber, they are surrounded by a low-pressure sheath fluid. This outer fluid stream creates a laminar flow forcing the specimen to the center, and results in a single-file alignment of the individual cells. This process is known as hydrodynamic focusing. Each cell sample is then intersected by a laser beam. The forward light scatter is proportional to the cell size, and the 90° or right angle scatter is related to the cell granularity and density. If the cells are labeled with appropriate fluorochromes, fluorescent signals can be measured. Commercial fluorochromes are available over the entire ultraviolet and the visible spectra. Excitation and emission spectra of each fluorochrome, and the wavelength of the exciting light, need to be carefully evaluated to ensure differentiation between the excitation and emission wavelengths in measurements.

Forward light scatter is directed to the forward scatter photodetector. At right angle to the laser beam are mirrors that divide the right-angle light scatter among the remaining photomultiplier tubes (right-angle scatter detector and fluorescence detectors). Simultaneous analysis of forward and right-angle light scatter allows for separation of granulocytes, monocytes, and lymphocytes based on their size and granularity. Electronic gating may also help delineate the desired cell population for further study.

Flow cytometers may be designed as cell sorters to physically sort the cells from the liquid suspension. In cell sorters (see Fig. 3–10), the cells of interest are identified with electronic gating and are given an electrical charge. The droplets containing the desired cells are electrically charged with a

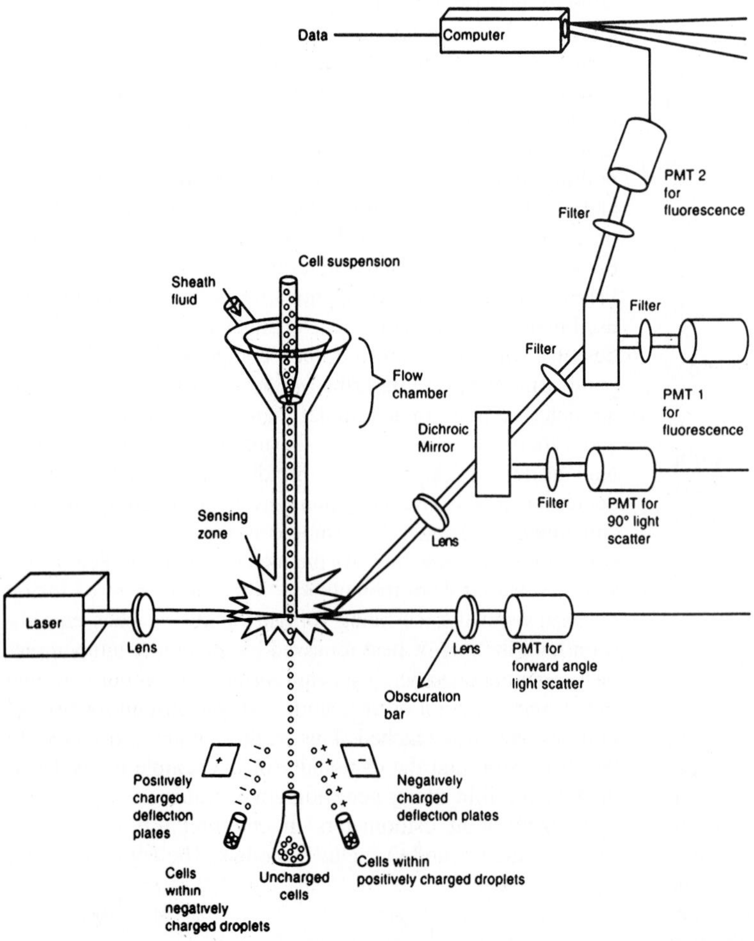

Figure 3–10. Components of a flow cytometer and a cell sorter. (Reproduced with permission from Ward KM, Lehmann CA, Leiken AM: Clinical Laboratory Instrumentation and Automation; Principles, Applications, and Selection. Philadelphia, W. B. Saunders Company, 1994.)

voltage pulse and enter an electrical field and are deflected into suitable collection containers for further analysis. The unwanted cells are not charged and pass through the field undeflected.

Common Flow Cytometers in Use

Application of flow cytometry in clinical and research laboratories has been extensive. Modern high-speed flow cytometers can handle up to 70,000 events per second. Multiparameter analyses include the number of cells, cell size, and presence of surface and cytoplasmic markers. Fluorochromes with a diversity of excitation and emission wavelengths and their conjugation to monoclonal antibodies have contributed to the widespread application of flow cytometry to immunophenotyping in leukemia, lymphoma, and monitoring of immune status. Flow cytometry can also be used in cell cycle analysis by staining the cells with a fluorescent dye such as propidium iodide that binds DNA and by quantifying the number of cells in components of the cycle (Coons, 1991). A common clinical laboratory flow cytometer is the FACScan* that has a 15-mW laser. This model combines the high performance of larger instruments with a compact design and relative ease of operation, making it suitable for clinical use. Other manufacturers including Coulter and Ortho make similar instruments. A modified model of the FACScan is also available that will sort cells using a mechanical sorting arm FACSort. Flow cytometry has also been successfully applied to hematology analyzers. Technicon H-1 is currently a widely used model using flow cytometric technique and can perform complete blood counts for red blood cells, white blood cells, and platelets, along with five-part differential for leukocytes.

Electrical Impedance

Electrical impedance measurement is based on the change in electrical resistance across an aperture when a particle in conductive liquid passes through this aperture. Electrical impedance is used primarily in the hematology laboratory to enumerate leukocytes, erythrocytes, and platelets (see Chap. 24). In a typical electrical impedance instrument by Coulter, aspirated blood is divided into two separate volumes for measurements. One volume is mixed with diluent and delivered to the cell bath, where erythrocyte and platelet counts are performed. As the blood passes through the aperture, the electric current between the electrodes changes each time a cell passes through. This produces a voltage pulse, the size of which is proportional to the cell size. The number of pulses is directly related to the cell count. Particles measuring between 2 and 20 fL are counted as platelets, whereas those measuring greater than 36 fL are counted as erythrocytes. The other blood volume is mixed with diluent and a cytochemical-lytic reagent. A leukocyte count is performed as cells pass through an aperture. Particles greater than 35 fL are recorded as leukocytes. Among the manufacturers of hematology analyzers, Coulter has long been a leader. Electrical impedance remains the basis for its current hematology instruments. The popular Coulter STKS model was first introduced in 1987. This model features three simultaneous measurements: volumetric impedance for cell size, high-frequency electromagnetic energy for nuclear constituents, and laser scattering for cell shape and granularity (see Chap. 24).

*Becton Dickinson, Mountain View, CA.

Electrochemistry

Electrochemistry involves the measurement of the current or voltage generated by the activity of specific ion species. Analytical electrochemistry for the clinical laboratory includes potentiometry, coulometry, and amperometry.

POTENTIOMETRY. The measurement of potential (voltage) between two electrodes in a solution forms the basis for a variety of procedures for measuring analyte concentration. Electrical potentials are produced at the interface between a metal and ions of that metal in a solution. Such potentials also exist when different concentrations of an ion are separated by a membrane semipermeable to that ion. To measure the electrode potential, a constant-voltage source is needed as the reference potential. The electrode with a constant voltage is called the reference electrode, whereas the measuring electrode is termed the indicator electrode. Concentration of ions in a solution can be calculated from the measured potential difference between the two electrodes.

The measured cell potential is related to the molar concentration by the Nernst equation:

$$E = E^\circ - (0.059/z) \log (C_{red}/C_{ox}) \qquad (3\text{-}5)$$

where

E = the cell potential measured at 25°C
E° = the standard reduction potential
z = the number of electrons involved in the reaction
C_{ox} = the molar concentration of the oxidized form
C_{red} = the molar concentration of the reduced form

If either of the concentrations (oxidized or reduced form) is known, the unknown concentration can be calculated from the above-mentioned equation.

Reference Electrodes. Different types of reference electrodes are available. These electrodes include standard hydrogen electrode, saturated calomel electrode, and silver–silver chloride electrode. The standard hydrogen electrode is the international standard but is seldom used for routine work as other more convenient types with reliable calibration buffers are available. Saturated calomel electrodes are widely used as reference electrodes. However, it becomes unstable at high temperatures (above 80°C) in which case the silver–silver chloride electrode should be used.

pH Electrode. Glass electrodes were the first and are still the most common electrode for measuring hydrogen ion activity (pH or negative log of the hydrogen ion concentration). A pH electrode consists of a small bulb made of layers of hydrated and nonhydrated glass, which contains a chloride ion buffer solution. The buffer has a known hydrogen ion concentration. An internal electrode, usually silver–silver chloride, serves as a reference electrode. One theory suggests that the sodium ions in the hydrated glass layer drift out. Sodium ions have a large ionic radius. Specimens containing hydrogen ions, which have a smaller ionic radius, replace the sodium ions. The result is a net increase in the external membrane potential. This potential propagates through the thin, dry membrane to the inner hydrated surface of the glass. Chloride ions in the inner buffer solution respond by migrating to the internal glass layer. Potentials generated at the pH electrode are referenced to the external reference electrode (saturated calomel), and the difference or change is displayed as pH units.

pCO_2 Electrode. The pCO_2 electrode is a pH electrode contained within plastic jacket. This plastic jacket is filled with a sodium bicarbonate buffer and has a gas permeable membrane (Teflon or silicone) across its opening. When whole blood containing dissolved CO_2 contacts the Teflon membrane, CO_2 from the blood passes through and mixes with the buffer. A chemical reaction, shown here, occurs that results in a decrease in pH. The hydrogen ion activity is measured by a potentiometric pH indicator system.

$$CO_2 + H_2O \rightarrow HCO_3^- + H^+ \qquad (3\text{-}6)$$

Ion-selective Electrode. An ISE is an electrochemical transducer capable of responding to one given ion. ISEs are very sensitive and selective for the ion it measures. An ISE consists of a membrane separating a reference solution and a reference electrode from the solution to be analyzed. The complexity of ion selective electrode design depends on the membrane composition that determines its ionic selectivity. Many types of ion selective electrodes are available including glass electrode, liquid membrane electrode, precipitate-impregnated membrane electrode, solid-state electrode, gas electrode, and enzyme electrode.

COULOMETRY AND AMPEROMETRY. Coulometry is an electrochemical titration in which the titrant is electrochemically generated and the endpoint is detected by amperometry. Coulometry is based on Faraday's law, which relates electrical charge (Q), current (I), and time (t), according to the following equation:

$$Q = It \qquad (3\text{-}7)$$

Amperometry is the measurement of the electrical current at a single applied potential. These two electrochemical principles are combined in the coulometric titrator used for measuring chloride ion concentration in biological fluids. Many laboratories are using the coulometric titrator (chloridometer) to assay sweat samples, urine, and cerebrospinal fluid (CSF). In measuring chloride using coulometry, a constant current is applied across the two silver electrodes, which liberate silver ions into the specimen at a constant rate. Chloride ions in the sample will combine with the released silver ions to produce insoluble silver chloride. A pair of indicator and reference electrodes senses the excess silver ions and stops the titration. The number of silver ions released by ionization, which is exactly equal to that of chloride ions in the sample, can be calculated from Faraday's law:

$$Q = It = znF \qquad (3\text{-}8)$$

where

z = the number of electrons involved in the reaction
n = the number of moles of analyte in the sample
F = Faraday's constant (96,487 coulombs/mole of electrons)

pO_2 Gas-Sensing Electrode. The most widely used oxygen sensing electrodes use an amperometric or current-sensing electrolytic cell as the indicator system. The pO_2 electrode uses a gas-permeable membrane, usually polypropylene, which allows dissolved oxygen to pass through. This membrane also prevents other blood constituents from passing through, which may interfere with the electrode. The dissolved oxygen diffuses through the oxygen permeable membrane. It mixes in a phosphate buffer solution and reacts with the polarized platinum cathode, resulting in the following reaction:

$$O_2 + 2H_2O + 4e^- \longrightarrow 4OH^- \qquad (3\text{-}9)$$

Electrons produced change the current through the cell, and the change is directly proportional to the partial pressure of oxygen present in the specimen. The silver anode provides the oxidizing electrode to complete the circuit.

Common Electrochemical Analyzers in Use

Electrochemistry has been applied to measurements of pH and a variety of electrolytes and gases. Electrochemical analysis has made it possible to use microliter sample volumes and measure analytes with concentrations between 10^{-8} and 10^{-3} moles/L. These techniques exhibit a high degree of precision, ease of operation, and a remarkably short analysis time. ISEs have been successfully developed for physiologically important alkali and alkaline earth cations (e.g., K^+, Na^+, Ca^{+2}, Li^+, and H^+). Many electrochemical analyzers are multichannel systems used for measuring electrolytes and blood gases. Some analyzers may be configured to include the measurement of additional chemistry analytes. A typical system is the NOVA 11* Electrolyte Analyzer. This desktop system is fully automatic with three channels to measure sodium, potassium, and lithium. The electrodes used for these analytes are glass electrode, valinomycin liquid membrane, and neutral carrier liquid-membrane, respectively. It is direct-reading with digital readout. Throughput ranges from about 45 samples per hour in single measurement mode to around 60 samples per hour using an automatic sampler upgrade. Sample types include whole blood, plasma, serum, and urine.

The Corning Model 925 Chloride Analyzer† is widely used for the measurement of chloride in body fluids, such as urine and CSF. It can also be used to measure chloride concentration in sweat to aid in the diagnosis of cystic fibrosis. Specimen volumes are 20 or 100 μL and titration time is around 20 seconds. It has a direct readout with digital display. The partial pressure of oxygen measured by the Radiometer‡ ABL-3 uses a pO_2 gas-sensing electrode. Specimen volumes are less than 200 μL. Time of analysis for one specimen is less than three minutes.

---

*NOVA Biomedical, Waltham, MA.
†Corning Medical and Scientific, Medfield, MA.
‡Radiometer America Inc., Westlake, OH.

Electrophoresis

Electrophoresis is the separation of charged compounds based on their electrical charge. When a voltage is applied to a salt solution (usually sodium chloride), an electrical current is produced by the flow of ions: cations toward the cathode, and anions toward the anode. Conductivity of a solution increases with its total ionic concentration. The greater the net charges of a compound, the faster it moves through the solution toward the oppositely charged electrode. The net charge of a compound, in turn, depends on the solution pH. Electrophoresis separations often require high voltages (50–200V DC); therefore, the power supply should supply a constant DC voltage at these levels. The buffer solution must have a carefully controlled ionic strength. A dilute buffer causes heat to be generated in the cell while a high ionic strength does not allow good separation of the fractions. Common support media for electrophoresis in clinical work include cellulose acetate, agarose, and polyacrylamide gels. Total volume of specimen applied depends on the sensitivity of the detection method. For clinical work, 1 μL of serum may be applied. Once the electrophoresis is completed, the support medium is treated with a dye to identify the separated fractions. The most common dyes used for the visualization step include Amido Black, Ponceau S, Fat Red 7B, and Sudan Black B. To obtain a quantitative profile of the separated fractions, densitometry is performed on the stained support medium.

The most common applications of electrophoresis include serum proteins (see Chap. 11), hemoglobins (see Chap. 26), and isoenzymes (see Chap. 13). The isoenzymes include creatine kinase (CK), lactate dehydrogenase (LD), and alkaline phosphatase (AP). Manufacturers of the electrophoresis instruments and consumable supplies include Beckman Instruments and Helena Laboratories.*

Isoelectric Focusing

Proteins are polymers of amino acids that can be anions or cations depending on the pH environment. At a specific pH, a protein will have a net charge of zero when the positive charge and the negative charge of its amino acids cancel each other out. At this pH value, known as the protein's isoelectric point (pI), the protein is isoelectric. Isoelectric focusing (IEF) technique is performed similarly as other electrophoretic methods except that the separating molecules migrate through a pH gradient. This pH gradient is created by adding acid to the anodic area of the electrolyte cell and adding base to the cathode area (Fig. 3–11). A solution of ampholytes (mixtures of small amphoteric ions with different pIs) is placed between the two electrodes. These ampholytes have high buffering capacity at their respective isoelectric points. The ampholytes close to the anode carry a net positive charge, and those close to the cathode carry a net negative charge. When an electrical voltage is applied, each ampholyte will rapidly migrate to the area where the pH is equal to its isoelectric point. With their high buffering capacity, the ampholytes create stable pH zones for the more slowly migrating

*Helena Laboratories, Beaumont, TX.

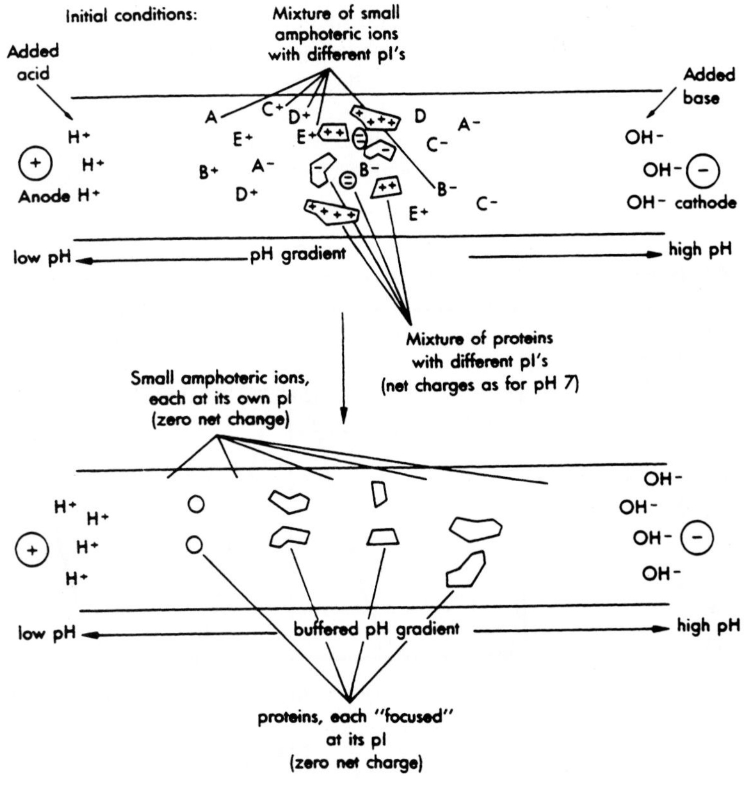

Figure 3–11. Isoelectric focusing (see text). (Reproduced with permission from Schoeff LE, Williams RH: Principles of Laboratory Instruments. St. Louis, Mosby, 1993.)

proteins. The advantage of isoelectric focusing techniques lies in its ability to resolve mixtures of proteins. Using narrow-range ampholytes, macromolecules differing in isoelectric point by only 0.02 pH units can be identified. Isoelectric focusing has been useful in measuring serum acid phosphatase isoenzymes. Its application has also been extended to detect oligoclonal immunoglobulin bands in cerebrospinal fluid and isoenzymes of creatine kinase and alkaline phosphatase in serum.

Densitometry

Densitometry is basically an absorbance measurement. A densitometer measures the absorbance of the stain on a support medium. The basic components of a densitometer include a light source, a monochromator, a movable carriage to scan the medium over the entire area, an optical system, and a photodetector. Signals detected by the photodetector are related to the absorbance of the sample stain on the support, which is proportional to the specimen concentration. The support medium is moved through the light beam at a fixed rate so that a graph may be constructed that represents multiple density readings taken at different points.

Most modern densitometers have a built-in integrator to find the area under the curve so that all sample fractions can be quantified. The Beckman Appraise is an example of a densitometer widely used in the clinical laboratory. This model has an elaborate database management system for reporting and interpreting patient results.

Chromatography

Chromatography is a separation method based on the different interactions of the specimen compounds with the mobile phase and with the stationary phase, as the compounds travel through a support medium. The compounds interacting more strongly with the stationary phase are retained longer in the medium than those that favor the mobile phase. Chromatographic techniques may be classified according to their mobile phase: gas chromatography, and liquid chromatography. Figure 3–12 shows a typical chromatogram representing the concentration of each detectable compound eluting from the column as a function of time. Retention time (t_R) is the time it takes a compound to elute. This value is characteristic of a compound and is related to the strength of its interaction with the stationary phase and the mobile phase. The retention time therefore can be used to determine a compound's identity. In this example, two compounds are separated and their retention times are represented by (t_{R1}) and (t_{R2}). These are uncorrected retention times and are measured from the injection time, $t = 0$. A column's ability to separate two compounds depends on two factors: (1) the difference in retention of the compounds or capacity factor, k', and (2) the width of their peaks, W_b. The value of k' can be calculated by the following equation:

$$k' = (t_{R1} - t_m)/t_m \text{ or } t_{R1}'/t_m \quad (3\text{-}10)$$

where

t_m is the retention time of a nonretained compound
t_{R1}' is the corrected retention time

Another measurement derived from the calculated capacity factor is the selectivity factor (α) or relative retention of two solutes. A ratio of both capacity factors is used to calculate the selectivity factor. To measure the width of each peak, draw tangents along the sides of the peak to the baseline. The distance between the two intersected lines is represented by W_b. To calculate the number of theoretical plates (N), use the following equation:

$$N = 16\,(t_R/W_b)^2 \quad (3\text{-}11)$$

A plate number has no units and the larger the value of (N) for a column, the greater its separation efficiency. The combined effects of solvent efficiency and column efficiency are expressed in the resolution (R_s) of the column:

$$R_s = 2\,(t_{R2} - t_{R1})/(W_{b1} + W_{b2}) \quad (3\text{-}12)$$

The concentration of unknown compound is found out from

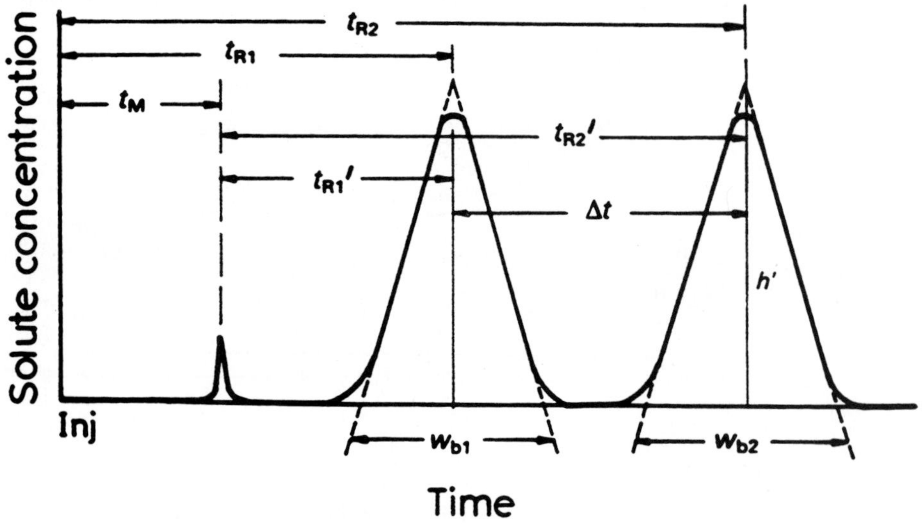

Figure 3–12. Chromatogram for the separation of two compounds (see text for explanation of terms). (Reproduced with permission from Ravindranath B: Principles and Practice of Chromatography. United Kingdom, Ellis Horwood Ltd., 1989.)

the peak height (h′) and may be calculated using an integrator or the method of internal standardization.

Gas Chromatography

Gas chromatography (GC) is useful for compounds that are naturally volatile or can be easily converted into a volatile form. GC has been a widely used method for decades owing to its high resolution, low detection limits, accuracy, and short analytical time. Applications include various organic molecules including many drugs (see Chap. 17). Retention of a compound in GC is determined by its vapor pressure and volatility, which, in turn, depend on its interaction with the stationary phase. Two types of stationary phases commonly used in GC are solid absorbent (gas-solid chromatography [GSC]) and liquids coated on solid supports (gas-liquid chromatograph [GLC]). In GSC, the same material (usually alumina, silica, or activated carbon) acts as both the stationary phase and the support phase. Although this was the first type of stationary phase developed, it is not as widely used as other types primarily because of the strong retention of polar and low volatile solutes by the column (Ravindranath, 1989). GLC uses liquid phases such as polymers, hydrocarbons, fluorocarbons, liquid crystals and molten organic salts to coat the solid support material. Calcine diatomaceous earth graded into appropriate size ranges is often used as a stationary phase because it is a stable inorganic substance. The use of fused silica capillary columns in which the stationary phase is chemically bonded on to the inner surface of the column has become very popular with chromatographers. The advantage of this type of column is that the stationary phase does not leave the solid support and bleed into the detector, and a uniform monomolecular layer of the stationary phase is obtained through the bonding procedure.

Components of a typical GC system are illustrated in Figure 3–13. Its basic design consists of five components: a gas cylinder as a mobile phase source, a sample injector, a column, a detector, and a computer for data acquisition. These systems may be automated to provide the user with a more precise and efficient separation. The mobile phase (carrier gas) used in gas chromatography is usually an inert gas such as nitrogen, helium, hydrogen, or argon. Other substances used as mobile phases include steam and supercritical fluids. Examples of these are carbon dioxide, nitrous oxide, and ammonia. The carrier gas should be of high purity, and the flow must be tightly controlled to ensure optimum column efficiency and reproducibility of test results. Samples are introduced into the GC using a hypodermic syringe or an automated sampler. A needle pierces an elastic septum contained within the injector port. Each injection port is heated to very high temperatures. Samples are vaporized and swept onto the column. If the molecule of interest is not volatile enough for direct injection, it is necessary to derivatize it into a more volatile form. Most derivatization reactions belong to one of three groups: silylation, alkylation, and acylation. Silylation is the most common technique that replaces active hydrogens on the compounds with alkylsilyl groups. This substitution results in a more volatile form that is also less polar and more thermally stable. Examples of other sampling techniques are headspace sampling and pyrolysis.

Retention of compounds in a GC column can also be adjusted by changing the column temperature. The column temperature affects the volatility of the compounds and thus the degree of their interaction with the stationary phase. By proper selection of the starting temperature and temperature gradient during the procedure, good resolution of both weakly and strongly retained compounds may be achieved. The GC column, enclosed in a temperature-controlled oven, can be a packed column or capillary column. Packed columns are usually 1 to 5 m long and 2 to 4 mm in diameter, and are filled with a stationary phase. Capillary columns range from 5 to 100 m in length, 0.1 to 0.8 mm in diameter, and have a stationary phase located on their interior surface (Bartle, 1993). Capillary columns generally have higher efficiency and better detection limits. However, packed columns have a larger specimen or sample capacity, making them more useful in purification work. Examples of detectors used in GC include a flame ionization detector, a thermal conductivity detector, a nitrogen-phosphorous detector, an electron capture detector, a flame photometric detector, and a mass spectrometric detector. *Flame ionization detectors* (FID) are widely used and are capable of detecting almost all organic compounds and many inorganic compounds. This type of detector measures the ions produced by the compounds when burned in a hydrogen-air flame. The ions are collected by an electrode producing an electric current. Generating results from the analogue signal

Figure 3–13. Components of a gas chromatographic system. G = Gas cylinder; PR1 and PR2 = regulators; PG = pressure gauge; NV = valve for adjusting the gas flow rate. (Reproduced with permission from Ravindranath B: Principles and Practice of Chromatography. United Kingdom, Ellis Horwood Ltd., 1989.)

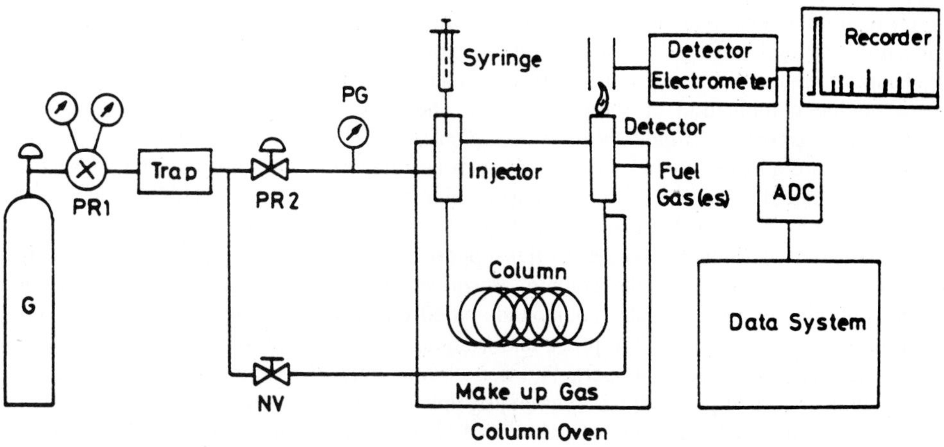

produced by the detector can be accomplished in two ways (Tipler, 1993):

1. The recorder output can be connected to a strip chart recorder, and a chromatogram is traced on the chart paper. Manual methods may be employed to quantitate the amount of analyte in the sample. These methods include figuring out peak areas, cutting out each peak and weighing it, measuring the peak width and height, and calculating half their product or using a planimeter.
2. More superior means to manipulate the data is to use microprocessor-based systems. They may be personal integrators, work stations, or laboratory automation systems.

Liquid Chromatography

GC as a separation technique has some restrictions that make liquid chromatography a suitable alternative. Many organic compounds are too unstable or are insufficiently volatile to be assayed by GC without prior chemical derivitization. Liquid chromatography techniques use lower temperatures for separation, thereby achieving better separation of thermolabile compounds. These two factors allow liquid chromatography to separate compounds that cannot be separated by GC. Finally, it is easier to recover a sample in liquid chromatography than in gas chromatography. The mobile phase can be removed, and the sample can be processed further or reanalyzed under different conditions.

There are many forms of liquid chromatography available, and the selection of an appropriate form depends upon a variety of factors. These factors include analysis time, type of compound, and detection limits. Paper, thin-layer, ion exchange, and exclusion liquid chromatography often result in poor column efficiency and a very long analysis time owing to low mobile phase flow rates. High-performance liquid chromatography (HPLC) emerged in the late 1960s as a viable form of liquid chromatography that provided advantages over other forms of liquid chromatography and gas chromatography. HPLC uses small, rigid supports and special mechanical pumps producing high pressure to pass the mobile phase through the column. HPLC columns can be used many times without regeneration. The resolution achieved with HPLC columns is superior to that of other forms of liquid chromatography, analysis times are usually much shorter, and reproducibility is greatly improved. All of these attributes of HPLC render it a better method of separation over other forms of liquid chromatography.

There are five commonly used separation techniques in liquid chromatography. They include adsorption, partition, ion exchange, affinity, and size exclusion. Each is characterized by a unique combination of stationary phase and mobile phase. In *adsorption (liquid-solid) chromatography*, the compounds are adsorbed to a solid support such as silica or alumina. Although this was the first type of column liquid chromatography developed, it is not widely used owing to the strong retention of many compounds by the supports, making them difficult to elute from the column. *Partition (liquid-liquid) chromatography* separates compounds based on their partition between a liquid mobile phase and a liquid stationary phase coated on a solid support. Partition chromatography includes normal-phase liquid chromatography, which uses a polar liquid stationary phase, and reverse-phase liquid chromatography, which uses a nonpolar stationary phase. *Ion-exchange chromatography* uses column packings that have charge-bearing functional groups attached to a polymer matrix. The mechanism in this type of chromatography is the exchange of sample ions and mobile-phase ions with the charged group of the stationary phase. *Affinity chromatography* uses immobilized biochemical ligands as the stationary phase to separate a few solutes from other unretained solutes. This type of separation uses the so-called lock and key binding that is widely present in biological systems. *Size exclusion chromatography* separates molecules according to the difference in their size. The support material has a certain range of pore sizes. As solutes travel through, the small molecules can enter the pores, whereas the larger ones cannot and will elute first from the column.

Liquid chromatography is similar in many aspects to GC, and therefore, the instrumentation is similar. A typical liquid chromatography system consists of a liquid mobile phase, a sample injector (manual or automatic), a mechanical pump, a column, a detector, and a data recorder. The liquid mobile phase is pumped from a solvent reservoir through the column. A mechanical pump must provide precise and accurate flow, often working at high pressures (typically up to 6000 psi). The pump also must have low internal volume and be constructed of material that does not react with the solvent. Sample injection is achieved using a syringe and depositing the sample into a loop. The injection may be performed manually or automatically using a microprocessor control autosampler. Most analytical separations are performed using packed column. There are many types of packing material available. Selection of the appropriate packing material is largely dependent on the type of compound(s) to be separated. In liquid chromatography, the physical properties of the sample and mobile phase are often very similar. Two basic types of detectors have been developed. One is based on the differential measurement of a physical property common to both the sample and mobile phase; examples include refractive index, conductivity and electrochemical detectors. The other is based on the measurement of a physical property that is specific to the sample, either with or without the mobile phase; examples include absorbance and fluorescent detectors.

Mass Spectrometry

Mass spectrometry (MS) is based on fragmentation and ionization of molecules using a suitable source of energy. The resulting fragment masses and their relative abundances yield the characteristic mass spectrum of the parent molecule. Before a compound can be detected and quantitated by mass spectrometry it must be isolated by another method, usually GC. Great specificity and sensitivity are achieved by this GC/MS combination. A typical mass spectrometry system is composed of an inlet unit, an ion source unit, a mass analyzer, an ion detector, and a data unit. The inlet unit admits samples to the mass spectrometer. When the instrument is part of a GC/MS arrangement, the inlet unit must be heated to maintain the volatile compounds in the vapor state on coming into the ion source unit. It must also strip away most of the carrier gas to adapt to the high vacuum condition required for mass spectrometry operation.

The ion source unit is maintained at high temperature and vacuum to provide adequate conditions for ionizing the vaporized sample molecules. Several types of energy sources are available to ionize the sample molecules in mass spectrometry. One commonly used source is a beam of electrons produced by a heated filament. The process of bombarding the sample with electrons is called *electron-impact ionization*. Other processes of ionization include (1) *chemical ionization*, in which the sample molecules are ionized by a reagent gas that has been ionized by an electron beam, and (2) *fast atom bombardment* in which a solid sample is ionized by a beam of atoms such as argon. A mass spectrometer sorts the parent molecular ions and their fragment ions according to their mass-to-change ratio. Mass spectrometers are of three different types: magnetic sector, quadrupole, and ion trap. In the magnetic sector mass spectrometer, a very high voltage accelerates the ions out of the ion source unit onto a magnetic field. The exiting path curvature of an ion depends on its mass-to-charge ratio, the magnetic field strength, and the applied voltage. The magnetic field or the voltage can be varied to allow selective ions to exit the magnetic field. In the *quadrupole mass spectrometer* (Fig. 3–14*A*), direct electrical current and radiofrequency voltages of selected magnitudes are applied to two pairs of metallic rods. Only ions of specific mass-to-charge ratio can pass undeflected to the end of the rods, where they are detected. All other ions have unstable trajectories along the path and are deflected toward the rods, never reaching the detector. A more modern form of mass analyzer now in widespread use is the *ion-trap mass spectrometer* (Fig. 3–14*B*). It functions as a mass analyzer and an ion source unit. Three electrodes, in a ring shape and two end caps, produce ions in the cavity until selectively ejected to the ion detector as the scanning radiofrequency voltage on the ring electrode varies. A major advantage of the ion-trap analyzer is its ability to get full mass spectra at very low sample concentrations (Karasek, 1988). The ion detector in mass spectrometry is usually an electron multiplier or an ion-photon conversion detector. In an *electron multiplier*, the ions strike the detector's first dynode, which triggers the release of secondary electrons. A cascade of electrons occurs similarly to that in a PMT, resulting in an amplification of about a millionfold. In an *ion-photon conversion detector*, the ions strike a phosphor that emits a photon for each corresponding ion. A conventional PMT then amplifies the signal in the usual fashion. The computerized data unit is an indispensable part of any modern mass spectrometer. It controls the multiple operating parameters of the instrument components, and stores and analyzes a vast amount of acquired data. The built-in libraries of reference mass spectra for known compounds can be searched by computer and compared with the sample spectrum for identification. In recent years, several bench-top mass spectrometers have been introduced for routine clinical and toxicology measurements. A typical instrument of the quadrupole type is the Hewlett Packard* model 5971 MSD. Typical instruments of the ion-trap type include Finnigan† MAT, and the Varian Instruments‡ Saturn 3 GC/MS.

*Hewlett Packard Co., Wilmington, DE.
†Finnigan MAT, San Jose, CA.
‡Varian Instruments, Walnut Creek, CA.

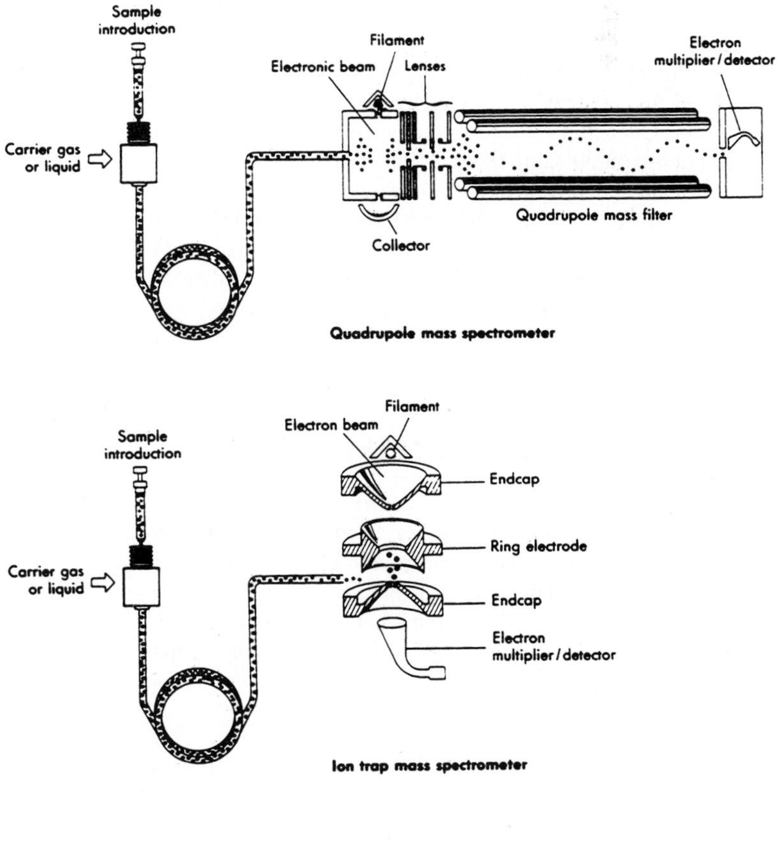

Figure 3–14. Mass spectrometer. *A*, Quadrupole type. *B*, Ion-trap type. (Courtesy of Finnegan MAT in Schoeff LE, Williams RH: Principles of Laboratory Instruments. St. Louis, Mosby, 1993.)

Scintillation Counter

Scintillations are flashes of light that occur when gamma rays or charged particles interact with matter. Chemicals used to convert their energy into light energy are called scintillators. If gamma rays or ionizing particles are absorbed in a scintillator, some energy absorbed by the scintillator is emitted as a pulse of visible light or near-UV radiation. Light is detected by a PMT, either directly or through an internally reflecting optic fiber. A scintillation counter is an instrument that detects scintillations using a PMT tube and counts the electrical impulses produced by the scintillations. An important application of scintillation counting is radioimmunoassay (RIA) for hormones. Two types of scintillation methods exist: crystal scintillation and liquid scintillation.

CRYSTAL SCINTILLATION. Crystal scintillation generally is used to detect gamma radiation. When a gamma ray penetrates the sodium iodide (NaI) crystal, which contains 1% thallium, it excites the electrons of iodine atoms and raises them to higher energy states. When the electrons return to ground state, energy is emitted as UV radiation. The UV radiation is promptly absorbed by the thallium atoms and emitted as photons in the visible or near-UV range. The photons pass through the crystal and are detected by a PMT. A pulse-height analyzer sorts out the pulse signals from the PMT according to their pulse height and allows only those within a restricted range to reach the rate meter for counting.

LIQUID SCINTILLATION. Liquid scintillation counters are primarily used to count radionuclides that emit beta particles. A sample is suspended in a solution or "cocktail" consisting of a solvent such as toluene, a primary scintillator such as 2,5-diphenyloxazole (PPO), and a secondary scintillator such as 2,2′-*p*-phenylenebis(5-phenyloxazole), or POPOP. Beta particles from the radioactive sample ionize the primary scintillator of the solvent. A secondary scintillator absorbs the photons emitted by the primary scintillator and re-emits them at a longer wavelength. The secondary scintillator facilitates more effective energy transmission from the beta particles, especially when a large amount of quenching is present. Quenching is a process that results in a reduction of the photon output from the sample. This phenomenon may be due to chemical quenching, in which impurities in the sample compete with the scintillators for energy transfer, or color quenching, in which colored substances such as hemoglobin absorbs the light photons produced by scintillation. The light photons produced in the sample are detected and amplified by the photomultiplier tubes in the same manner as for the crystal scintillation counter.

AUTOMATED ANALYZERS

Automated analyzers allow laboratories to process a large volume or number of tests quickly. This is accomplished owing to the increased speed of analysis. Hundreds or even thousands of tests can be done in an hour by these automated analyzers. This increase in test throughput has been made possible by automating many manual steps. Some manual steps automated include

1. Identifying the sample and patient
2. Measuring and adding reagents
3. Mixing the sample and reagents
4. Incubating the sample mixture
5. Calibrating the assay
6. Measuring and reading the sample reaction
7. Recording, analyzing, and storing sample data

Automation has allowed the laboratory to improve the precision of the assays. Automated instruments are designed to perform repetitive functions without deviation if they are properly maintained.

There are a variety of classification schemes in the literature to describe automated analyzers, especially, chemistry analyzers. Most automated analyzers are either continuous flow or discrete. In continuous flow the samples flow through a common reaction vessel or pathway. Samples in discrete analyzers travel through the instrument in its own reaction vessel. The design of the analyzer pathway that the samples travel may be sequential, parallel, batch, or random access (Karselis, 1994):

Sequential testing: multiple tests analyzed one after another on a given specimen.
Batch testing: all samples are loaded at the same time, and a single test is conducted on each sample.
Parallel testing: more than one test is analyzed concurrently on a given clinical specimen.
Random access testing: any test that can be performed on any sample in any sequence.

In 1957, Dr. Leonard Skeggs, in cooperation with Technicon, released the first automated chemistry analyze, the AutoAnalyzer. This system was a continuous flow chemistry analyzer capable of analyzing one analyte at a time. As the volume of testing increased, Technicon began to develop sequential multichannel analyzers (SMAs) using continuous flow analysis. This system performed all tests on all samples, even if they were not requested. This method of analysis was inefficient because the analyzer conducted tests that were not requested and the reagent volumes were large. These problems led to the development of analyzers that could only perform tests requested by the operator. Most of these automated analyzers were discrete systems.

Major Components of Automated Analyzers

PATIENT IDENTIFICATION. Before the use of laboratory computers, patient identification was accomplished by transcribing patient information onto sample cups and printouts of test results. With the arrival of computers, the operator could input patient information into the analyzer's computer and then upload the information to the laboratory computer. In the past few years, instrument manufacturers have designed bar code labeling systems for use on many of their analyzers. The bar code was read and would match patient data with test results. The use of bar code labels has served to reduce errors in matching test results with the proper patient.

SAMPLING. Sampling of biological fluids in automated systems is usually accomplished by syringe pipette or aspirating probe. The specimens are transferred to a sample cup, and the sample pickup device aspirates the specimen. In continuous flow analyzers, the aspirating probe is dipped into the sample cup and the specimen is drawn up using a peristaltic pump. The reagents are also transferred from their containers into the sample stream by this pump. Discrete analyzers employ a variety of syringe pipettes to aspirate and dispense sample and reagents. An important consideration for any sampling device is specimen carry-over and therefore it should be designed to reduce this problem.

SAMPLE AND SPECIMEN TRANSPORT. In continuous flow analyzers, specimen transport is accomplished using the peristaltic pump. Air bubbles separate aliquots of the same sample and isolate one specimen from another. Sample transport in discrete analyzers is accomplished in many ways. In the DuPont aca, the sample reagent pack is transported throughout the analyzer with a chain-driven pulley system. Some analyzers use a motorized carousel, for example, the Olympus Demand,* to move the reaction vessel in a circular path within the instrument. The Kodak Ektachem† analyzers meters the sample aliquot, by use of a disposable sample tip secured by an apparatus called a proboscis, onto a slide for transport to incubation chambers and detectors.

DILUTION. Sample and reagent dilutions are usually accomplished with the syringe pipettes and pumps. These pumps may be peristaltic or pneumatic in design. The pumps must be designed to aspirate and deliver precise volumes of fluid. The dilution volumes may be adjusted by use of a cam (Technicon Autoanalyzers) or programmed via a microprocessor as seen in many discrete analyzers.

MIXING. In an automated system such as continuous flow analyzer mixing of a sample and reagents is accomplished using a glass coil inserted into the flow path. As the sample mixture passes through the coil, it is inverted and mixed via gravity. Mixing in discrete analyzers is done in a variety of ways. In the Beckman ASTRA systems, a magnetically driven Teflon stirring bar located in the bottom of the reaction chamber is used. The DuPont aca employs a breaker mixer that mechanically vibrates and shakes the pack. Many centrifugal analyzers use acceleration and deceleration of the rotor to transfer the reagents and sample from one chamber to another, mixing them in the process.

INCUBATION. Reaction mixtures that require incubation must be conducted at constant temperatures without significant fluctuations. A variety of methods are available to maintain proper temperatures. These methods include heating the air around the cuvet, heating metal blocks, and using water baths. Sophisticated electronic circuits are required to monitor and maintain the temperatures of these devices within a narrow tolerance range.

REACTION VESSELS. The types of reaction vessels vary widely in automated analyzers. In continuous flow systems the tubing serves as the reaction vessel. The DuPont aca uses a sealed plastic bag that also serves as the cuvette. The Teflon or plastic rotors in centrifugal analyzers serve as reaction vessels. Many analyzers such as the Hitachi‡ series and Baxter§ Paramax 720 ZX use plastic cuvettes. Eastman Kodak Ektachem uses a multilayer thin film slide. Each slide is impregnated with reagents. Samples are transferred from a sample cup via a disposable pipette tip onto the slide that also serves as the cuvette for the reflectance or electrochemical measurement.

ANALYSIS OF MEASUREMENT. Most automated chemistry analyzers use photometric methods of analysis such as spectrophotometry, fluorometry, nephelometry, and reflectometry. Some analytes, for example sodium and potassium, require the use of electrochemistry for analysis. Instrument manufacturers have designed electrochemical devices based on coulometry, amperometry, and potentiometry to measure these and other analytes. Automated systems based on colorimetry use narrow-band interference filters for the isolation of specific wavelengths. The filters are contained in a circular disk, called a filter wheel, that rotates into the light path. A computer controls the rotation of the filter wheel and multiple wavelengths can be used to analyze a specimen.

DATA ANALYSIS. Light-emitting diodes offer direct readout of absorbance or concentration and replace the earlier recorders that used an ink pen to trace the response of the phototube on paper. The emergence of computers in laboratory instrumentation allowed users to display results in a variety of formats and printers allowed users to provide a hard copy of patient's results. Calculations, calibration curves, and quality control are performed by the computers, thus reducing errors and providing more accurate results than a noncomputerized instrument.

THE EMERGING TECHNOLOGIES

Capillary Electrophoresis

CE represents a new breakthrough in separation techniques. A typical capillary electrophoresis system, as shown in Figure 3–15, consists of a fused silica capillary, two electrolyte buffer reservoirs, a high-voltage power supply, and a detector linked to a data acquisition unit. The sample is introduced into the capillary inlet. When a high voltage is applied across the capillary ends, the sample molecules are separated by electroosmotic flow, a bulk flow resulting from excess positive ions at the inner capillary surface moving toward the cathode. The positive ions in the specimen emerge early at the capillary outlet because the electroosmotic flow and the ion movement are in the same direction. Negative ions in the specimen also move toward the capillary outlet but at a slower rate. As the sample ions migrate toward the capillary outlet, they may be detected by different types of detectors, including optical, conductivity, electrochemical, mass spectroscopy, or radioactivity detectors. Advantages of CE over conventional electrophoresis and HPLC are its short analytical time, resolving power, and micro sample volumes (Love, 1994). Using nanoliter quantities of specimen, complex mixtures of molecules can be separated with a theoretical plate number approaching one million. Separations may be completed in less than 10 minutes with very high applied voltage. The application of high voltage is made possible by the capillary's high surface-to-volume ratio that allows for efficient heat transfer through the capillary wall. Potential applications of capillary electrophoresis in the future include separation of serum proteins and hemoglobin variants.

*Olympus Corp., Lake Success, NY.
†Eastman Kodak, Rochester, NY.
‡Boehringer Mannheim Diagnostics, Indianapolis, IN.
§Baxter Diagnostics, Irvine, CA.

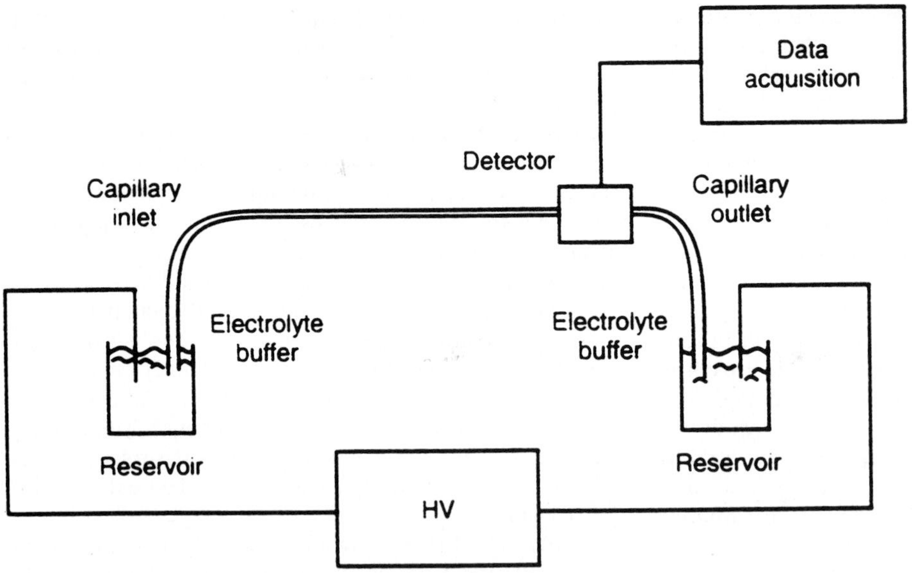

Figure 3–15. Capillary electrophoresis system. HV = High-voltage source. (Reproduced with permission from Ward KM, Lehmann CA, Leiken AM: Clinical Laboratory Instrumentation and Automation: Principles, Applications, and Selection. Philadelphia, W. B. Saunders Company, 1994.)

Point-of-Care Analyzers

After the introduction of bench-top analyzers in the early 1980s, a new generation of more compact instruments has emerged that are more automated and user-friendly. There are now many compact analyzers available for bedside testing, screening projects, wellness centers, emergency rooms, operating rooms, and physician office laboratories. These point-of-care (POC) analyzers have extensive test menus and provide rapid laboratory test results to expedite a patient's diagnosis and treatment. The fast growth of POC chemistry analyzers has been made possible by advances in microprocessors, stable reagents, ion-specific electrodes, and other advanced medical technologies. Depending on specific models, POC chemistry analyzers may be manual, semiautomated, or fully automated and may use serum, plasma, or preferably whole blood for analysis. Most POC chemistry analyzers use samples of less than 50 μL in volume, with turnaround time of less than 10 minutes. Many of these instruments have ready-to-use reagents, controls, and calibrators with a shelf life of 12 months or more. Common POC chemistry analyzers that use dry reagents include Seralyzer III Blood Chemistry Analyzer,* Eastman Kodak DT System, Boehringer Mannheim Reflotron System, and Du Pont Analyst. A common POC chemistry analyzer that uses wet reagents is Abbott Vision System. Hand-held chemistry analyzers are also available for whole blood glucose. Typical instruments include Lifescan One Touch II† and Boehringer Mannheim Accu-Chek II. Hematology analyzers for POC testing may be semiautomated or fully automated and usually need less than 50 μL of blood to measure erythrocyte count, platelet count, hemoglobin, and hematocrit. The more sophisticated analyzers can also measure platelet count and erythrocyte indices. Common hematology analyzers for POC testing include Boehringer Mannheim Hemo-W, and Coulter CBC-5. The current state-of-the-art technology in POC testing is shown in the i-STAT* Portable Clinical Analyzer (Woo, 1993). This hand-held, microprocessor-controlled instrument has a liquid crystal display, and a disposable multianalyte sensor array packaged into a single-use cartridge. Its test menu currently includes sodium, potassium, chloride, glucose, urea, nitrogen, hematocrit, and calculated hemoglobin. This analyzer is self-calibrated and requires only 65 μL of whole blood, which is added to a capillary port in the cartridge (Maclin, 1994).

*Miles Inc., Tarrytown, NY.
†Lifescan Inc., Milpitas, CA.

Sample Processing Automation

Most clinical laboratories use a manual system for specimen processing. This type of system requires many steps and is very labor intensive, contributing to long turnaround time and potential human errors. Specimens must be sorted, centrifuged, transferred to aliquot containers, and placed in the analyzers. A few large reference laboratories are currently developing automated specimen processing systems. Conveyer belts, bar codes, and robotics (for sorters, centrifuges, aliquotters) are the essential features of such systems. The aliquotter reads the bar code from the original sample tube, generates labels, puts these labels on the aliquot tubes, and pipettes from the original tube into the aliquot tubes. This process can reduce errors by maintaining a complete chain of custody from the original specimen to the aliquots. An ideal automated system should integrate several different technologies including serial centrifugation, automated specimen storage, and a conveyance mechanism routing individual specimens in random access to different testing stations. At present, there are only a few systems available for clinical laboratories. The Coulter Laboratory Automation System† facilitates concurrent testing in chemistry, hematology, coagulation, urinalysis, and immunochemistry. It is designed as

*i-STAT Corp., Princeton, NJ.
†IDS, Kumamoto, Japan.

modular components that can be assembled in different configurations. This system can adapt to various testing and space requirements, and can be modified for future expansion. Other automated specimen processing systems include AutoMed* ASHS, Boehringer Mannheim BM/D Hitachi Clinical Laboratory Integration System, OASYS,† and Automated Aliquot System.‡

SUMMARY

The applications of laboratory instrumentation broaden as the rate of technology development accelerates. Clinical instruments range from the hand-held analyzers at patients' bedside to the extremely sophisticated ones in large centralized laboratories. No field in medicine has expanded more rapidly with technology than laboratory medicine, especially in the area of instrument automation. With tremendous advances in technology it is difficult for this chapter to be comprehensive and current on all laboratory instrumentation. What may be state-of-the-art technology today, seen only as ideas on drawing boards or prototypes in research laboratories, can become reality in clinical laboratories in a matter of months. Clinical laboratories are expected to be affected in the current health care reform system being subjected to the cost review process. At this time, it is still not possible to forecast the impact of new technologies on lowering the operating costs while still providing timely laboratory data to clinicians in this era of cost containment. Federal regulations on clinical laboratories (Clinical Laboratory Improvement Act, 1988) impose quality control for all clinical laboratory procedures. This has created a great impact on POC testing, in which fewer accurate instruments, inadequate use of quality control, and insufficient laboratory expertise has been a potential problem. POC analyzers are expected to evolve into even smaller, easier to operate, and more accurate to conform to the new laboratory regulations. One cannot predict the future, but the brief review of instrumentation conveys a theme of constant change in the development and use of instrumentation in the clinical laboratory. This will inevitably support and promote both decentralization and centralization in laboratory medicine (Woo, 1994).

*Arden Hills, MN.
†Olympus America Inc., Lake Success, NY.
‡Biomedical Devices Co., Pontiac, MI.

Bartle KD: Introduction to the theory of chromatographic separations with reference to gas chromatography. *In* Baugh PJ (ed): Gas Chromatography; A Practical Approach, 1st ed. New York, Oxford University Press, 1993, pp 9–10.

Coons JS, Weinstein RS: Diagnostic Flow Cytometry. Baltimore, Williams & Wilkins, 1991.

Gauldie J: Principles and Clinical Applications of Nephelometry. *In* Kaplan LA, Pesce AJ (ed): Nonisotopic Alternatives to Radioimmunoassay. New York, Marcel Dekker, Inc., 1981, pp 289–291.

Karasek FW, Clement RE: Basic Gas Chromatography–Mass Spectrometry; Principles and Techniques. Amsterdam, Elsevier, 1988.

Karselis TC: The Pocket Guide to Clinical Laboratory Instrumentation. Philadelphia, FA Davis, 1994.

Love JE, Ward KM: Electrophoretic instrumentation systems. *In* Ward KM, Lehmann CA, Leiken AM (eds): Clinical Laboratory Instrumentation and Automation; Principles, Applications, and Selection. Philadelphia, W.B. Saunders, 1994, pp 173–174.

Maclin E, Young DS: Automation in the Clinical Laboratory. *In* Burtis CA, Ashwood ER (eds): Tietz Textbook of Clinical Chemistry, 2nd ed. Philadelphia, W.B. Saunders, 1994, pp 321–324.

Ravindranath B: Principles and Practice of Chromatography. Chichester, England, Ellis Horwood, 1989, pp 89–127.

Rayleigh, Lord B: On waves propagated along the plane surface of an elastic solid. Proc London Math Soc xviv:4–11, 1885.

Schoeff LE, Williams RH: Principles of Laboratory Instruments. St. Louis, Mosby, 1993.

Tipler A: Gas chromatography instrumentation, operation, and experimental considerations. *In* Baugh PJ (ed): Gas Chromatography; A Practical Approach, 1st ed. New York, Oxford Univ Press, 1993, pp 63–67.

Willard HH, Merritt LL, Dean JA, et al: Instrumental Methods of Analysis. Belmont, CA, Wadsworth, Inc., 1988.

Woo J, Henry JB: The advances of technology as a prelude to the laboratory of the twenty-first century. Clin Lab Med, 1994; 14:3; 459–471.

Woo J, McCabe JB, Chauncey D, et al: The evaluation of a portable clinical analyzer in an emergency department. Am J Clin Pathol, 1993; 100:599–605.

Chapter 4

Interpreting Laboratory Results: Reference Values and Decision Making

Matthew R. Pincus, M.D., Ph.D.

The major purpose of performing analyte determinations in the clinical laboratory is to aid in the diagnosis and management of patients with disease and individuals in health assessment. It is therefore important to understand how reference values are arrived at for each analyte whose level is being determined. Once values of the levels of specific analytes have been determined to be abnormal, it is then important to be aware of how reliable these abnormal values are in the diagnosis of specific disease states. For example, if a patient is found to have elevated levels of serum amylase, with what degree of confidence can we make the diagnosis of pancreatitis? Finally, if laboratory values are found to be abnormal, what possible clinical diagnoses are likely, based on these findings? In this chapter, each of these topics is discussed in turn.

TEST VALUES, VALUE RANGES, AND RELIABILITY OF TEST VALUES

Reference Values and Reference Intervals

Interpretation of laboratory measurements depends on a knowledge of the normal, expected ranges for these values. For example, serum sodium in most laboratories ranges between 137 and 144 mEq/L, with the mean reference value at or close to 140 mEq/L. It is important to understand how these ranges and means are ascertained.

To determine the reference interval for a given analyte, it is the general practice to perform a specific measurement on a large number of individuals, often grouped by age and sex, who are normal—that is, who are not known to have any disease (Winkel, 1972). Important factors should be standardized. In particular, most values should be determined under fasting conditions; the phlebotomy technique (discussed in Chapter 1) should be the same for all of the normal volunteers, and of course, the actual method of determination in the laboratory should be the same.

Among normal individuals, one might expect the values for the levels of a given analyte, in their sera or other body fluid, to exhibit some variation that reflects random fluctuations from person to person. If these fluctuations are truly random, then the values will follow what is referred to as the normal or gaussian distribution. The gaussian distribution for a specific value is given by the following formula:

$$P(x) = \left[1/\left(\sigma\sqrt{2\pi}\right)\right]e^{-[(x-\mu)^2/2\sigma^2]} \qquad (4\text{-}1)$$

where P(x) is the probability that the value x will be observed, e is the base of the natural logarithm system (= 2.71828), π is 3.14159, σ is a constant called the standard deviation, and μ is the mean or average value. To compute the probability that

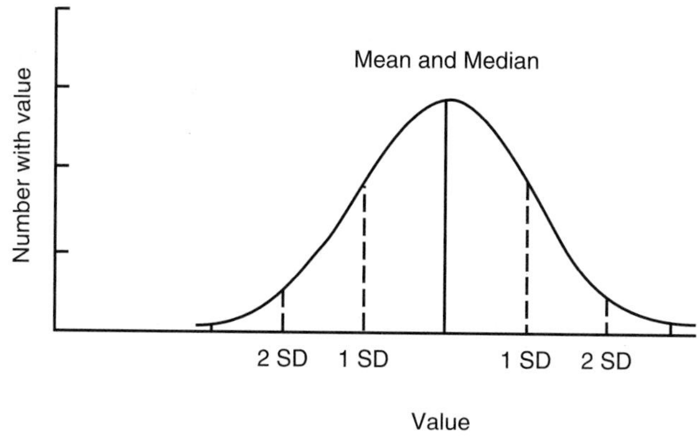

Figure 4–1. Gaussian distribution showing typical bell-shaped curve. The most probable value is the center solid line, which coincides with the mean or average value and the median value. The dashed vertical lines show one and two standard deviations from the mean as indicated on the abscissa.

a value will be less than or equal to some value, x in equation 4-1 is integrated as

$$\int_{-\infty}^{x} P(x)dx$$

Figure 4–1 is a plot of this equation and shows the typical bell-shaped curve. Shown in this plot is the mean or average value that coincides with the most probable value and with the median value, or that value at which the values for half the population are greater than the median and half are less than the median.

The width of the curve at half the maximum value gives a value range that represents one standard deviation, or σ, from the mean, as shown in Figure 4–1. Two standard deviations from the mean, or 2σ, encompass a wider area under the gaussian curve (see Fig. 4–1). If the values obtained using a particular method follow a gaussian distribution, then values will fall within ± two standard deviations from the mean 95% of the time. Most laboratories use two standard deviations as the limits of the acceptable range for a given value of an analyte (Harris, 1981).

If one actually determines analyte levels in serum for a large number of normal individuals in a given group, one finds that the values often do not conform to a true gaussian distribution because of such factors as differences in specimen collection and processing and preparation of the patient (Statland, 1977). Thus, the concept of the standard deviation becomes nonapplicable. In these instances, we use so-called nonparametric statistics, a multisyllabic way of saying that we take arbitrary cuts to define the reference interval. Thus, we may simply take the entire range found for the normal group as the reference interval. Often, the values that lie between the third and 97th percentiles are chosen to be the ones that define the reference interval.

PRECISION AND ACCURACY IN VALUE DETERMINATION

There are numerous methods for quantitating the levels of a particular analyte in body fluids. It is important to see how these values compare with one another with respect both to the reliability of the values and to their reproducibility.

Accuracy

Accuracy refers to the reliability of the method in determining the real or true value of the level of the analyte. Generally, there is a particular method that serves as the gold standard for determination of this real value. The results of other methods are then compared with those obtained with the gold standard method to determine their reliability. The tolerable limits of difference between methods is somewhat arbitrary and depends on the analyte whose levels are being determined. For example, a systematic difference between serum sodium levels of greater than 3 mEq/L would be deemed unacceptable. On the other hand, major differences between levels of some hormones determined by immunoassay by different antibodies are tolerated because the use of different antibody preparations produce different matrix effects. In these instances, different reference intervals are established for different assays for the same hormone.

Comparison of a new method with the reference method is best expressed as a correlation plot where each method is used to determine the value for the analyte for each aliquot of specimen or reference control sample. These values are then plotted against one another. The least squares best fit line, described in Chapter 6, is then determined for this plot. The slope and intercept of this line are computed. Most importantly, the correlation coefficient for the plot is determined. This number gives an overall measure as to how closely the least square best fit line fits all of the data points. Correlation coefficients of over 0.9 are usually deemed acceptable and indicate that the new method agrees satisfactorily with the reference method.

Precision

Precision refers to the reproducibility of the method. This reproducibility is measured in several ways. The first is to measure the value of a particular analyte on the *same* sample or specimen several times on the same day in the same batch load of samples. Then, the values are measured on the same sample on successive days. The variation of the values so measured will generally follow a gaussian distribution, provided the method of measurement is stable.

For each type of determination, the average value (x_{av}) for the measurements is determined, and the difference of each measured value (x_i) from this average is determined and squared. The standard deviation σ is then the square root of the sum of these squares divided by the number of points N minus one, as given in equation 2:

$$\sigma = [\Sigma(x_i - x_{av})^2/(N-1)]^{1/2} \quad (4\text{-}2)$$

The standard deviation divided by the average is referred as the coefficient of variation, or CV—that is, a measure of the variation of values from the average value of the repetitive measurement of the same specimen or sample solution.

Awareness of the CV allows one to determine what represents a change in the individual versus expected fluctuations in laboratory determinations. For example, daily hemoglobin and hematocrit values may be determined to ascertain blood loss (progressive anemia) and blood product transfusion needs.

Precision or reproducibility is therefore measured for the determinations on the same day and the same batch run, the so-called within-run CV. The day-to-day variation is measured by the between-run CV. Generally, these CVs should not exceed 5%, although on some types of measurements, especially some enzyme levels in serum and for some immunoassays, 10% is acceptable.

A good analogy for the difference between precision and accuracy is shooting at a target. The shooter may hit a site repeatedly and consistently, but this site may be far removed from the bull's-eye. Thus, the shots are precise but not accurate. A shooter who repeatedly hits the bull's-eye or sites near it exhibits both precision *and* accuracy.

Random and Systematic Error

When the values for a particular analyte are determined over the time periods described in the preceding section, and these values are plotted as a function of time, then values may distribute themselves randomly about the mean or they may fall away from the mean, exhibiting a systematic pattern. Random deviations are thus called random error, whereas deviations that show a pattern are called systematic errors. The latter may indicate an underlying correctable fault in the methodology, such as a leaky ion selective electrode or diminishing lamp power in spectrophotometric assays.

Method Sensitivity

Method sensitivity refers simply to the lowest level of an analyte that can be detected by a given method with low CVs. This sensitivity of detection must be distinguished from the sensitivity of the method used in detecting disease states, a topic to which we now turn.

SENSITIVITY, SPECIFICITY, AND PREDICTIVE VALUE

Many of the measurements performed in the clinical laboratory are used as diagnostic markers (Galen, 1975). For example, elevations in the enzyme alanine aminotransferase (ALT) are used as markers for liver disease; elevations in the MB fraction of the enzyme creatinine phosphokinase (CK) are used to diagnose myocardial infarction. Many of these marker tests are discussed subsequently. The question always arises as to how reliable a specific result of a measurement is. When elevated, how often does it accurately predict disease? When depressed, how often will individuals *not* have the disease?

Sensitivity

Sensitivity measures how many individuals who *are known to have a disease* will be picked up by a given method as having that disease. If the number of individuals with a particular disease is NP and we apply our test to this group, the test results will be either truly positive (TP) or falsely negative (FN). The total number of individuals in the study will be TP + FN. Then the sensitivity of the test is defined as the total number of individuals with the disease *who are found to be positive (TP) by the test* divided by the total number of individuals with the disease (TP + FN), some of whom may be found to be falsely negative. The sensitivity of the test is, therefore,

$$\text{Sensitivity} = \text{TP}/(\text{TP} + \text{FN}) \qquad (4\text{-}3)$$

Specificity

Specificity measures how specific a test is for a certain disease. Suppose we have a test that is always positive. Then it will be 100% sensitive, but it will also falsely identify many normal persons as having the disease. Thus, the specificity of a test measures how many truly negative (TN) individuals there are in a population *without* the disease. The total number of individuals in this population will be the number found to be truly negative and those found to be falsely positive (FP). Thus, the specificity is defined as

$$\text{Specificity} = \text{TN}/(\text{TN} + \text{FP}) \qquad (4\text{-}4)$$

Predictive Value

Now suppose the test is applied to a random population, in which the disease exists but not all of the individuals have the disease. How good is the test in predicting which individuals have the disease? One way to measure this quantitatively is to determine the number of individuals who are truly positive divided by the total number of individuals who are found to be positive, some of whom may be falsely positive. Thus, the *positive predictive value,* or PPV, is defined as

$$\text{PPV} = \text{TP}/(\text{TP} + \text{FP}) \qquad (4\text{-}5)$$

Now this population contains the number of individuals, NP, who have the disease and the number of individuals, NN, who do not have the disease. The total number of individuals in the population, N, is NP+NN.

Of the NP individuals, the number of true positives will be NP times the sensitivity (sens). Of the NN individuals who do not have the disease, the number of these individuals who will be found by the test to be truly negative will be NN times the specificity (spec). Of these NN individuals, $\text{NN} - \text{spec} \times \text{NN}$ or $\text{NN}(1 - \text{spec})$ will therefore be found to be *falsely positive.* NN is the number of negative individuals or N minus the number of "positives," NP. Then the number of false positives is $(\text{N} - \text{NP})(1 - \text{spec})$. In equation 4-5, we can substitute for TP and FP to obtain

$$\text{PPV} = \text{sens} \times \text{NP}/[\text{sens} \times \text{NP} + (\text{N} - \text{NP})(1 - \text{spec})] \qquad (4\text{-}6)$$

If the numerator and denominator of this equation are now divided by the total number of individuals, N, in the population being screened, we obtain

$$\text{PPV} = \text{sens} \times \text{NP/N}/[\text{sens} \times (\text{NP/N}) + (1 - (\text{NP/N}))(1 - \text{spec})] \qquad (4\text{-}7)$$

Note that NP/N is the *prevalence* (prev) of the disease—that is, the fraction of the total number of individuals who have the disease. Thus, equation 4-7 can be rewritten as

$$PPV = sens \times prev/[(sens \times prev) + (1 - prev)(1 - spec)] \quad (4\text{-}8)$$

It is of vital importance to note that the positive predictive value heavily depends on the *prevalence of the disease* in the population being screened. Even a superb test with a high sensitivity and a high specificity will have a low predictive value if the prevalence of the disease being screened for is low. In equation 4-8, this conclusion may easily be demonstrated by setting the prevalence to 0. The PPV then also goes to 0!

Thus, in using a test for screening purposes, always select a population at risk, that is, one in which the prevalence will be high. For example, if we wish to screen for individuals with myocardial infarctions using elevated levels of CK-MB as the indicator, we would choose an older population in which many of the individuals would have anginal episodes rather than a population of young athletes, for example.

With regard to such screening, it is now generally recognized that case finding (e.g., referrals to physicians for evaluation of clinical conditions) is more cost-effective than screening diverse populations without complaints or illness for the presence of disease. Case referrals are preselected populations who are more likely to have a particular disease. One poignant example of this is screening individuals for prostate carcinoma using prostatic-specific antigen (PSA—see Chapters 13 and 45). This test is better performed on individuals who present to a physician with a history of urinary obstruction and an enlarged prostate than used as a general screening tool for all individuals in a given community.

It is of great interest that, overall, two thirds of all clinical laboratory testing is employed to follow the course of disease in individuals with established diagnoses, whereas one third is employed to establish new diagnoses.

INTERPRETING AND CORRELATING ABNORMAL LABORATORY VALUES

General Considerations

One of the most important functions of the clinical pathologist is to interpret abnormal laboratory values. Often, clinicians who order a battery of laboratory tests on their patients are confronted with vast, almost bewildering sets of numbers that can be difficult to evaluate. Frequently, therefore, consultation with clinical pathologists or other experts in the field of laboratory medicine are sought. Besides advising in interpretation of the values, clinical pathologists also can recommend the most appropriate selection of laboratory measurements and examinations that should be ordered in the diagnostic workup of a patient for a particular medical problem (Martin, 1982; Pauker, 1987; Statland, 1988).

In addition to answering questions about specific laboratory values from clinicians, the clinical pathologist must also be aware of unusual test results on patients in the hospital and must evaluate these even without requests for consultation. Frequently, conditions in patients that might cause such abnormal results may be overlooked. Confirming a result by repeating measurement(s) on the same (original) specimen and on a new specimen within 24 hours of original collection should clarify the values that are not consistent with the patient's physician's interpretation or the clinical pathologist's assessment. The clinical pathologist may have to order further tests to pin down the diagnosis for a given patient. Thus, it is important for clinical pathologists to check results on patients that are unusual or sets of results that do not seem to correlate with one another.

In this respect, the laboratory computer is an invaluable aid. On the Sunquest Health Information Computer System, for example, daily checks for patient values that lie significantly outside of their established reference intervals or that have undergone large changes over a 24-hour period are reported as failed delta checks. Thus, patients with significantly abnormal laboratory findings can be identified. In addition, programs are now available that can evaluate clinical and laboratory findings to generate differential diagnoses (Myers, 1986).

An approach to interpretation of laboratory values is presented here that enables laboratorians to help establish clinical diagnoses and assist in clinical management. This discussion is by no means comprehensive and cannot possibly cover every conceivable illness afflicting patients. Rather, this presentation is concerned with general approaches to interpreting abnormal values and discussion of the most common causes of such findings.

In contrast with earlier editions of this book (Winkel, 1991), in which this chapter was concerned with general approaches to problem-based decision-making processes, we now present specific approaches to diagnosing the more common disease states. The reader may prefer to complete the Clinical Chemistry (Part II) and Hematology (Part IV) sections of this book before reading this section, which gives an overview of both of these vital diagnostic areas. Alternatively, the reader may decide to read this chapter to obtain the overview before reading the several chapters in chemistry and hematology (Parts II and IV, respectively).

Fundamental Principles in Interpretation of Values

Before embarking on a discussion of specific conditions giving rise to abnormal values, certain precepts should always be followed, encapsulated as follows:

1. Never rely on a single value to make a diagnosis. It is vital to establish a *trend* in values. A single sodium value of, for example, 130 mEq/L does not necessarily indicate hyponatremia. This single abnormal value may be spurious and may reflect such factors as improper phlebotomy technique or laboratory variability. Rather, a series of low sodium values in successive serum samples from a given patient do indicate hyponatremia. Thus, it is vital to follow trends in particular values. Much as in navigation, in which several (at least three) points must be obtained for triangulation to establish location, more than one laboratory value should be obtained to firmly establish a diagnosis.
2. *Osler's rule.* If the patient is under the age of 60 years, try to attribute all abnormal laboratory findings to a single cause. Only if there is no possible way to correlate all possible abnormal findings should the possibility of multiple diagnoses be entertained.
3. Abnormal laboratory values should be repeated so that the abnormal result is confirmed. It is also important to

determine if there is a consistent trend in the results of the particular laboratory tests, as in number 1 above. It may also be desirable to check the quality control for the particular analyte, as discussed in Chapter 6.

Interpretation of Laboratory Results

The first section of a laboratory report often contains the hematology profile, including the complete blood count (CBC). Comprehensive discussions of clinical hematopathology are given in Part IV. Here, we discuss very basic patterns of abnormalities to provide an overall reference frame for interpreting values and for the ordering of further examinations. Although this part of the book is concerned with clinical chemistry or chemical pathology, we discuss some aspects of hematology because the interpretation of hemato-pathologic results often depends on the results of quantitative determinations performed in clinical chemistry.

Hematology

Red Blood Cell Mass

This value is the key to determining whether a patient has anemia. If, in the absence of evidence of hemodilution, the value lies below approximately 4×10^6 red cells per liter, the patient, by definition, has anemia. Backing up this diagnosis, the hematocrit and hemoglobin should also both be low. Normal hematocrits are generally around 40% to 45%, whereas normal hemoglobin levels range around 12 to 15 g/dL. Remember that, in numeric value, the hematocrit is always about three times the hemoglobin concentration. Thus, if one of these quantities is known, the other may be accurately estimated.

If anemia has been diagnosed, it is then mandatory to determine the cause of the anemia. To accomplish this task, a particularly useful approach is to use the so-called red cell indices (i.e., the red cell size) called the mean corpuscular volume (MCV) and the mean hemoglobin concentration per cell or the mean corpuscular hemoglobin concentration (MCHC). It is the intracellular hemoglobin concentration that determines the observed color of erythrocytes. Thus, for example, cells with low hemoglobin concentration will appear hypochromic (i.e., their color will be lessened).

Overall, therefore, the MCV and the MCHC reflect the cell size and chromicity—that is, whether the red cells are macrocytic, normocytic, or microcytic and whether they are hyperchromic, normochromic, or hypochromic, as would be observed from direct microscopic viewing. Given the three characteristics of erythrocytes with respect to cell size and color, one might expect nine possible combinations of these characteristics (e.g., hyperchromic macrocytic, hyperchromic normocytic, and so on). As it turns out, only three of these nine combinations occur commonly in anemia, as indicated in Table 4–1: hypochromic, microcytic; normochromic, normocytic; and macrocytic anemias. If an anemia is macrocytic, the chromicity usually is unimportant.

Hypochromic, Microcytic Anemia

There are two basic causes of these conditions: iron deficiency anemia (IDA), the most common cause of which is blood loss, and the anemia of chronic disease (ACD). The defective production of the $\alpha\beta$-chains of hemoglobin, as occurs in thalassemia minor, gives rise to a hypochromic, microcytic state, but the red cell mass is usually increased, and the hemoglobin and hematocrit are often within the reference interval. Thus, thalassemia minor can be readily diagnosed.

Table 4–1. THREE COMMON TYPES OF ANEMIAS AND THEIR DIAGNOSTIC WORKUPS*

Anemia	Cause	Analyte Abnormality
1. Hypochromic, microcytic	Iron deficiency	Low ferritin Increased IBC Reduced Fe/TIBC ratio Increased RDW
2. Hypochromic, microcytic	Anemia of chronic disease	Normal or high ferritin Normal IBC Normal Fe/TIBC ratio Generally normal RDW
3. Normochromic, normocytic	Consumption hemolytic anemia	Schistocytosis, Burr cells Low haptoglobin Elevated CO Elevated indirect bilirubin
4. Normochromic, normocytic	Bone marrow hemolytic anemia	Schistocytosis, Burr cells Low haptoglobin Elevated CO Elevated indirect bilirubin Leukoerythroblastic picture
5. Normochromic, normocytic	Renal failure	Elevated BUN and creatinine Low erythropoietin
6. Macrocytic, megaloblastic	B_{12} and folate deficiency; hypothyroidism	Low B_{12} and folate; hyperlobulated neutrophils (hypersegmentation) Low T_4 and free T_4 Release of erythrocyte precursors

*In this table, low is equivalent to depressed, and high is equivalent to elevated. Ferritin, haptoglobin, bilirubin, BUN, creatinine, erythropoietin, T_3, and T_4 are all expressed as concentrations. CO is measured as a concentration of carboxyhemoglobin. All of these analytes are measured in serum.
BUN, blood urea nitrogen; CO, carbon monoxide; Fe, iron; IBC, iron-binding capacity; RDW, red cell distribution width; TIBC, total IBC.

To distinguish between IDA and ACD, a number of different laboratory measurements are very useful. Because IDA is always accompanied by loss of iron that is stored bound to the protein ferritin in macrophages in bone marrow, the diagnosis can always in principle be made with a bone marrow biopsy with an iron stain that shows absence of iron in marrow. This procedure is, of course, invasive and should only be performed as a last resort.

Ferritin Levels

There is an equilibrium, however, between intracellular and extracellular ferritin. The lower the stored iron becomes, the lower is the intracellular ferritin and, consequently, the lower the extracellular ferritin becomes. The level of extracellular ferritin can be directly measured by determining the serum ferritin level, which is readily and accurately performed on serum aliquots, now using nonradioactive enzyme-linked immunosorbent assay (ELISA) techniques such as on the Abbott (North Chicago, IL) ImX analyzers. Overall, therefore, serum ferritin levels give an excellent measure of available iron stores, noninvasively. Because, in ACD, iron stores are usually normal, serum ferritin levels are also normal. Thus, an excellent way of distinguishing iron deficiency from ACD is serum ferritin level determination.

One caveat in using serum ferritin values to make this distinction is the fact that ferritin also happens to be an acute phase reactant. Acute phase reactants are proteins (discussed in Chapter 11) that rise in response to an acute process, usually an acute inflammatory condition. So, if a patient has an acute infection and, at the same time, suffers acute blood loss, the ferritin levels may fall because of the loss of stored iron but may rise because of the acute inflammatory process. The net effect may be a ferritin in the reference interval. Usually, in these instances, this level is in the *low* reference range.

Use of Serum Iron and Iron-Binding Capacity

In addition to ferritin levels, serum iron and serum iron-binding capacity (IBC) can be measured. On average, serum iron is, of course, reduced in iron deficiency anemia and is normal or sometimes low in ACD. The IBC is a direct measure of the protein transferrin, which transports iron as Fe^{+2} from the gut to iron storage sites in bone marrow. In IDA, the serum iron is reduced, and the IBC increases. However, both serum iron and transferrin are subject to wide fluctuations because of such factors as diet and do not always reliably reflect iron stores. Also, transferrin is a β-protein—that is, it migrates in the β-region in serum protein electrophoresis and is a negative acute phase reactant. Thus, it may also rise in inflammatory conditions. There is considerable overlap between serum levels of iron and IBC in IDA and ACD. A somewhat more reliable discriminating measure of IDA is the *ratio* of serum iron to the total IBC (TIBC). This ratio is around 1:3 for normal individuals; in IDA, it is significantly reduced to values of around 1:5 or lower. Again, there is considerable overlap even in this ratio for patients with IDA and ACD, so the values should always be interpreted with care.

Use of Red Blood Cell Distribution Width

Finally, use of automated procedures for determination of cell counts and indices have enabled us to obtain average erythrocyte sizes and size distributions. In IDA, there is a marked dispersion in cell volumes (sizes) so that the *red blood cell distribution width (RDW)* increases, whereas it generally remains within normal limits in ACD. Normal RDWs are 11.5% to 14.5%. Unfortunately, the standard deviations for normals and for patients with IDA or ACD overlap greatly, tending to limit the validity of using the RDW for distinguishing between these conditions. For example, in a study of several hundred patients with differing types of anemias conducted from 1986 to 1987 at Bellevue Hospital in New York City, no significant differences could be found for the RDWs among these groups (Thompson, 1986).

Note that most of the major tests used to distinguish IDA from ACD are performed in the clinical chemistry laboratory. This emphasizes the strong interdependence of both of these services in obtaining definitive diagnoses through laboratory measurements.

Normochromic, Normocytic Anemias

There are many causes of this condition, as discussed in Chapter 26. One important cause of *persistent* normochromic, normocytic anemia is hemolytic anemia. Occasionally, renal failure can cause this condition because of diminished production of erythropoietin. Here, we emphasize the term persistent because hypochromic, microcytic anemias often begin as normochromic, normocytic anemias and then progress to the hypochromic, microcytic state. Thus, as was noted earlier, it is crucial to follow *trends* in the cell indices in patients with anemia. (This emphasizes rule 1, given earlier, of not relying on a single value to make a diagnosis.)

In this chapter, for the purpose of simplification, a functional distinction is made between two types of hemolytic anemias: *consumption* and *bone marrow (hypoplasia/aplasia)* hemolytic anemias. The first type is due to intravascular or extravascular hemolysis secondary to such causes as antibodies to red cell antigens (e.g., as in hemolytic transfusion reactions, fixation of immune complexes on red cell membranes with complement, hereditary conditions such as glucose-6-phosphate dehydrogenase deficiency, sickle cell anemia, hereditary spherocytosis, paroxysmal nocturnal hemoglobinuria). The second type is caused by lesions in the microvasculature of bone marrow causing suppression of the production of erythrocytes and red cell deformities. In both types of anemias, abnormal erythrocytes undergo membrane lysis either intravascularly or in the spleen (extravascularly). These cells appear as markedly abnormal fragmented or crenated forms, or they appear as schistocytes, teardrop cells, burr cells, echinocytes (shaped like starfish), and acanthocytes. There is also a noticeable difference in the sizes (anisocytosis) and shapes (poikilocytosis) of cells due to the presence of damaged erythrocytes. The extent of these patterns depends on splenic function. In individuals with normal or especially in those with enlarged spleens, this pattern may not be pronounced. In asplenic or hyposplenic patients, however, many abnormal red cell forms can be seen on the peripheral smear. Because of the often-marked anisocytosis, the RDW is markedly elevated.

Because there is increased destruction of red blood cells peripherally, the bone marrow responds by increasing red blood cell production and releases erythrocyte precursor forms, mainly reticulocytes and occasionally nucleated red blood cells.

Thus, consumptive hemolytic anemia is accompanied by reticulocytosis.

Specific laboratory measurements that readily confirm the diagnosis of consumptive hemolytic anemia are based on the natural events that occur subsequent to hemolysis. After erythrocyte membrane breakdown, hemoglobin is extruded. This hemoglobin becomes bound to the α_2-fraction protein, haptoglobin. The hemoglobin-haptoglobin complex becomes catabolized by macrophages that engulf these complexes by receptor-mediated endocytosis. Thus, an excellent laboratory test for hemolytic anemia is a *low* haptoglobin value. Extremely sensitive and rapid ELISAs for haptoglobin are available for this purpose.

When hemoglobin is extruded, large amounts of it become oxidized to methemoglobin. The heme portion dissociates and then becomes oxidized ultimately to bilirubin. The first step in this process is the oxidative opening of the porphyrin ring of heme with the attendant liberation of carbon monoxide (CO). CO may be measured easily by gas chromatographic techniques or even more conveniently by co-oximetry, based on spectrophotometry (see Chap. 3), as carboxyhemoglobin. Elevated CO levels in normochromic, normocytic anemias are an excellent indicator of hemolytic anemia.

Because there is an increased production of bilirubin, which is unconjugated (see Chap. 12), serum indirect bilirubin will be at least transiently elevated. This elevation, in the presence of normal liver function, will be modest, usually in the range of about 2 to 2.5 mg/dL. (The upper limit of normal is around 1.2 mg/dL.)

Thus, the serum levels of at least three different analytes—haptoglobin, CO, and bilirubin—often performed in the clinical chemistry laboratory can be conveniently used to confirm the diagnosis of hemolytic anemia in addition to the hematologic findings, such as schistocytosis, reticulocytosis, anisocytosis, and poikilocytosis.

Bone Marrow (Hypoplasia/Aplasia) Hemolytic Anemias

Schistocytosis with burr cells and echinocytes can also result from problems of *production* of red cells in the microvasculature of bone marrow. The cause of red cell damage is either microvascular disease or space-occupying lesions that compress and/or destroy the small vessels of bone marrow where erythrocytes, myeloid line cells such as neutrophils and lymphocytes, are produced. Both of these causes result not only in damaged erythrocytes but—peculiar to this condition—in the release of many precursor red *and* white cell forms such as nucleated red blood cells, myelocytes, metamyelocytes, and band forms. This pattern is referred to as the leukoerythroblastic pattern. If the laboratory report shows a consistent normochromic, normocytic anemia that, together with the results of the measurements considered earlier, suggests hemolytic anemia *and* the report shows the presence of a leukoerythroblastic picture, then a bone marrow (hypoplasia/aplasia) hemolytic anemia can be diagnosed. This type of hemolytic anemia, because it results from a disease condition in the *microvasculature* of the bone marrow, is called microangiopathic hemolytic anemia.

The most common causes of microangiopathic hemolytic anemias are immune-mediated small vessel endothelial cell disease; disseminated intravascular coagulopathy (DIC), discussed subsequently; fibrosis of bone marrow (myelofibrosis with extramedullary hematopoiesis, discussed in Part IV); chronic myelogenous leukemia and any other conditions involving a neoplastic proliferation of cells in marrow, such as metastatic carcinoma, lymphoma, and plasmacytoma; and infectious causes, such as gram-negative sepsis, tuberculosis, and viral infiltration.

With regard to small vessel disease, two conditions give rise to the microangiopathic hemolytic anemic, leukoerythroblastic pattern: thrombotic, thrombocytopenic purpura (TTP) and the hemolytic uremic syndrome (HUS). In both of these conditions, because the small vessel disease is not confined to marrow and because it affects such extramedullary tissue as kidney, there will be evidence of renal failure with a rise of blood urea nitrogen (BUN) and creatinine, as discussed subsequently. Note that in TTP, there is also a marked decrease in platelet count, and the small vessel disease is more widespread, often affecting the central nervous system with attendant changes in mentation, paresthesias, movement disorders, and behavioral abnormalities. Thrombocytopenia is less frequently observed in HUS.

Macrocytic Anemias

By far the most common cause of macrocytosis in erythrocytes is nutritional deficiency, specifically in vitamin B_{12} or folate, or both. Because of the large erythroblastic forms seen on bone marrow aspirates and biopsies, this condition is also referred to as megaloblastic anemia. Accompanying the macrocytosis is the presence of hyperlobated neutrophils (five-lobed nuclei in more than 5% of the neutrophils or any neutrophil with six or more nuclear lobes). As soon as the laboratory confirms an anemia with a pattern of higher-than-normal MCV, B_{12} and folate levels should immediately be ordered. If these return as normal, tests for thyroid function should be performed because hypothyroidism can also be a cause of macrocytosis.

In this era of automated CBCs, it is possible also that red cell precursor forms, such as reticulocytes and nucleated red blood cells, may be counted as mature erythrocytes. Therefore, in a patient with a so-called macrocytic anemia with normal B_{12}, folate, and thyroid hormone levels, it is important to check the reticulocyte and nucleated red blood cell count to determine if these are significantly elevated. If so, the possibility of a hemolytic anemia should be considered. Thus, the diagnostic workup for hemolytic anemia described in the preceding section should be instituted. Note again that the definitive tests for confirming the diagnosis of macrocytic anemia are often performed in the clinical chemistry section.

Table 4–1 summarizes each of these three types of anemias and the specific determinations used to distinguish the types (such as IDA from ACD) and to confirm the diagnosis. Note that this table is a guide as to what specific tests should be ordered and, by implication, what need not be ordered. For example, a hypochromic, microcytic anemia should be worked up with orders for ferritin levels, TIBC, and Fe/TIBC ratios, but there is no need to order measurements of B_{12} and folate levels. Conversely, there is no need to order such tests as ferritin levels and TIBC for macrocytic anemia, for which measurement of B_{12} and folate levels should be ordered.

Coagulation Disorders

This vast and complex topic is discussed in Part IV. For our review, we focus on three hematologic parameters that may be important in correlation with test results in chemistry determinations: the platelet count, the activated partial thromboplastin time (aPTT), reflecting the function of the intrinsic coagulation system, and the prothrombin time (PT), reflecting the function of the extrinsic coagulation system. Diminished values of the platelet count or abnormalities in platelet aggregation, or both, can lead to abnormal bleeding times. Elevated PTs and aPTTs are not generally associated with abnormal bleeding times except in Factor VIII deficiency with concomitant deficiency of von Willebrand factor. This latter factor is needed for platelet aggregation.

Remember that the anticoagulant heparin, which accelerates the inactivation of thrombin and other coagulation factors (XIIa, XIa, Xa, IXa) by antithrombin III, preferentially blocks the intrinsic system, leading to prolonged aPTTs but not significant elevations in PTs. On the other hand, the vitamin K antagonist, warfarin (Coumadin), preferentially blocks Factor VII in the extrinsic system, leading to prolonged PTs but not aPTTs.

If the PT or the aPTT becomes elevated, but the platelet count is normal, it is important to perform mixing studies of the patient's plasma with normal plasma to determine if the coagulation time normalizes (i.e., whether there is a factor deficiency). A not-infrequent cause of factor deficiency is liver failure, discussed subsequently and in Chapter 12. Thus, liver function measurements should also be checked in these instances. If mixing studies do not completely correct the prolonged coagulation times, the presence of coagulation inhibitors, such as circulating lupus-anticoagulant or antifactor antibodies, should be suspected.

If the platelet count diminishes and the aPTT and PT rise, the diagnosis of DIC should be entertained. This diagnosis is confirmed by the finding of elevated fibrin split products (FSPs) due to the fibrinolytic action of plasmin on the fibrin clot that forms. DIC is an extremely dangerous condition and must be diagnosed rapidly. In this condition, there is an abnormal activation of *both* coagulation cascades and a consumption of platelets. This activation, which may be secondary to gram-negative sepsis (activation of the cascades may be from bacterial endotoxins), cancer, or chronic inflammatory states such as collagen vascular diseases, causes the formation of microemboli that can result in widespread tissue infarction or ischemia with attendant abnormal chemical values (e.g., elevated liver function enzymes, elevated BUN and creatinine suggestive of renal failure, even elevation of cardiac enzymes such as creatine phosphokinase and its cardiac-specific MB fraction, indicative of myocardial damage). Thus, low platelet counts and elevated aPTT and PT, together with chemical abnormalities suggestive of multisystem dysfunction, strongly suggest DIC. Anticoagulant therapy must be instituted rapidly to block further embolization and tissue destruction.

White Blood Cell Abnormalities

Again, this prodigious topic is discussed at length in Part IV. Here, we note several simple patterns that correlate with abnormal chemical findings. The white blood cell count consists of two types of cells: myeloid (mostly neutrophils) and lymphoid (mainly lymphocytes). Some eosinophils, monocytes, and occasional basophils may be observed.

HIGH WHITE BLOOD CELL COUNTS

Elevated white blood cell counts over about 10,000/μL up to about 20,000/μL point to an infectious process. In bacterial infections, the preponderance of white cells are neutrophils, whereas in viral infections, they are lymphocytes and monocytes. Exceptions to the neutrophilia seen in bacterial infections are tuberculosis, brucellosis, pertussis (wherein the predominant cells are lymphocytes), and infections, mainly in newborns, with *Listeria monocytogenes* (for which a monocytic response is predominant). In acute bacterial diseases in which neutrophilia is present, there is often an increase in band forms of neutrophils, giving rise to the so-called shift-to-the-left pattern and toxic granulation of neutrophils.

If the white blood cell count *exceeds 20,000/μL* and is uniformly lymphocytic, the possibility of *chronic lymphocytic leukemia* must be considered. Generally, but not always, this condition is accompanied by *lymphadenopathy and hepatosplenomegaly,* which, in turn, can cause *anemia and thrombocytopenia.* In patients with *high white blood cell counts* and with a *leukoerythroblastic picture* but in whom, in addition to myelocytes and metamyelocytes, there are *myeloblasts and promyelocytes and an abnormally elevated basophil count, chronic myelogenous leukemia* is likely. Cytogenetic studies are indicated in which a search is made for the Philadelphia chromosome. Often, in this condition, basophilia is also present.

LOW WHITE BLOOD CELL COUNTS

Low white blood cell counts, if accompanied by anemia and thrombocytopenia, may be part of *generalized pancytopenia secondary to marrow failure.* This condition may be secondary to drug therapy (e.g., chemotherapy or other marrow-suppressive drugs). *Isolated, consistently low white blood cell counts* are most commonly seen in *gram-negative sepsis.* Interestingly, gram-negative sepsis with low white blood cell counts is often accompanied by a cholestatic pattern in liver (i.e., a *mild rise in bilirubin and alkaline phosphatase*).

Abnormalities in Clinical Chemistry: Chemical Pathology

Electrolyte Abnormalities

Figure 4–2 summarizes the basic mechanisms by which the kidneys control electrolyte and water balance. Keep in mind that, functionally, *the purpose of the kidneys is to conserve fluids or, tantamount to this, to concentrate the urine.* The mechanism by which this conservation of fluids is effected is by the building up of high sodium chloride gradients in the interstitial space between the descending and ascending limbs of the loop of Henle using the counter-current exchange mechanism. In this mechanism, chloride ion is extruded into the interstitial space such that NaCl concentrations become greater toward the tip of the loop of Henle. The ascending limb of the loop of Henle is impermeable to water, as is the distal convoluted tubule. However, under the effect

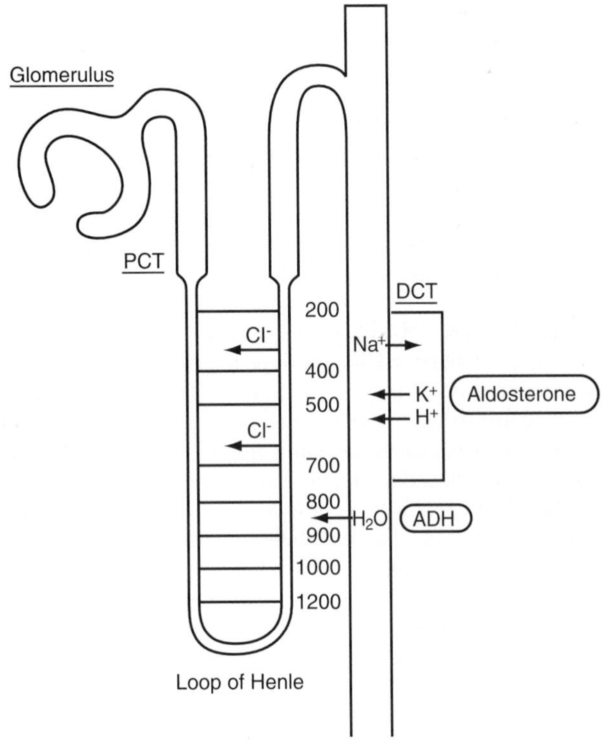

Figure 4–2. A schematic representation of a nephron showing the fundamental mechanism of water and salt conservation by the kidneys. Filtration occurs at the glomerulus (*upper left*), and the filtrate passes through the proximal convoluted tubule (PCT), where about 70% of the total filtered sodium is reabsorbed. In the loop of Henle, the countercurrent multiplier mechanism is operative. Chloride ion is extruded from the ascending limb into the interstitial space (shown in the upper middle part of the figure). Sodium ion passively follows. The cells of the ascending loop of Henle are impermeable to water, and the cells of the descending limb of the loop of Henle are impermeable to chloride ions. The result of this system is that high concentrations of NaCl are built-up at the tip of the loop of Henle. The numbers along the loop of Henle are osmolalities at different levels along the loop. The hypertonic interstitium allows water to diffuse in from the distal convoluted tubule (DCT) provided that antidiuretic hormone (ADH in the figure) is secreted. More sodium ion can be conserved in the DCT provided aldosterone is secreted resulting in the one-to-one exchange of Na^+ for K^+ and H^+.

of antidiuretic hormone (ADH), discussed in Chapters 7, 8, and 16, the distal convoluted tubule is made permeable to water, allowing it to flow into the interstitial space and to penetrate the vasa recta. The entire driving force for this process is the high concentrations of NaCl in the interstitium. Any interference with the counter-current multiplier will prevent water from being reabsorbed because the ion gradients are eliminated.

As also shown in Figure 4–2, sodium ion, 70% of which is reabsorbed in the proximal convoluted tubule, can be further reabsorbed in the distal convoluted tubule under the effect of aldosterone from the zona glomerulosa of the adrenal cortex. This hormone promotes the 1:1 exchange of sodium for potassium or hydrogen ion. Sodium levels in serum depend almost completely on the interplay between aldosterone and ADH. With these simple considerations in mind, the most common causes of hyponatremia and hypernatremia are now summarized with an explanation of how to identify them. Normal renal function is assumed.

HYPONATREMIA

The four *most common causes* of hyponatremia are given in Table 4–2, together with a fifth, rare cause, Bartter's syndrome. In all forms of hyponatremia, the chloride ion concentration also should be low, because chloride is the chief counter-ion for sodium. If chloride ion is not decreased, either a specimen or, less likely, a laboratory error should be suspected, or another source of chloride ion must be present (such as ammonium chloride).

BASIC PRINCIPLE. All confirmed serum sodium abnormalities must be followed up with urinalysis on the patient, who should be under fluid restriction. This urinalysis should include the urine sodium and urine osmolality. For all of these conditions, except for Bartter's syndrome, the serum sodium tends to correct over a 24-hour period when the patient is under fluid restriction.

OVERHYDRATION. In this condition, the most common cause of which is the consumption of large amounts of water or hypotonic fluids because of such conditions as psychogenic polydipsia, serum sodium is reduced below 135 mEq/L. Because the consumed water is excreted by the kidneys, the urine is also dilute in this ion. In fact, *the osmolality of urine will be low (i.e., <300 mOsm).* Often accompanying hyponatremia in overhydration are *low values of the hematocrit and low values of BUN,* discussed subsequently. This triad of findings strongly suggests overhydration as the cause. Urinalysis in the fluid-restricted patient reveals urinary sodiums of less than 25 mEq/L and low osmolalities. The potassium may also be low, although it often remains within the reference range. Because mainly water is excreted in urine in this condition, the total 24-hour sodium excretion will be low (cause no. 1 in Table 4–2).

USE AND ABUSE OF DIURETICS. Loop diuretics block the chloride pump in the loop of Henle, thereby blocking the formation of the ion gradients via the counter-current multiplier, necessary for water conservation. Thus, water is lost. Also, because sodium is no longer retained because it follows

Table 4–2. COMMON CAUSES OF HYPONATREMIA AND ELECTROLYTE PATTERNS IN SERUM AND URINE WITH NORMAL RENAL FUNCTION*

Cause	Serum Na	Urine Na	Urine Osm	Serum K	24-Hour UNa
1. Overhydration	Low	Low	Low	Normal or low	Low
2. Diuretics	Low	Low	Low	Low	High
3. SIADH	Low	High	High	Normal or low	High
4. Adrenal failure	Low	Mildly elevated	Normal	High	High
5. Bartter's syndrome	Low	Low	Low	Low	High

*All Na and K values are concentrations except for 24-hour UNa, which is the total number of milliequivalents of Na excreted in 24 hours in the urine.
SIADH, secretion of inappropriate levels of antidiuretic hormone.

chloride in the loop, it also is depleted from serum. The 24-hour sodium excretion is high, unlike in overhydration (cause no. 2 in Table 4–2). The pattern resembles overhydration (dilute serum and urine) except that loop diuretics cause severe potassium depletion unless the diuretic is combined with a potassium-sparing diuretic such as triamterene. Combined hyponatremia and hypokalemia with a high urinary sodium and potassium 24-hour excretion point to diuretic use. Of course, a history generally also reveals use of diuretics.

SYNDROME OF INAPPROPRIATE ADH (SIADH) SECRETION. In this condition, secondary to head trauma, seizures, other central nervous system diseases, and neoplastic conditions, especially lung, breast, and ovarian cancers, that secrete ADH-like hormones, the serum sodium is depressed because of the excess retention of water in the distal convoluted tubule. This results in depletion of water in the renal tubules, thereby concentrating the urine. Therefore, although the serum is dilute in sodium (hypotonic), the urine is concentrated to levels exceeding 40 mEq/L, and the urine osmolality exceeds 300 mOsm while the serum osmolality remains below 280 mOsm. This pattern clearly is diagnostic of SIADH.

ALDOSTERONE DEFICIT. This condition is secondary to Addison's disease and AIDS-related hypoadrenalism. Without aldosterone, the Na-K and Na-H^+ exchange in the distal convoluted tubule does not occur. Therefore, serum sodium concentration is reduced while serum potassium concentration increases, and there is a mild metabolic acidosis. Urinary sodium increases but not to the high levels seen in SIADH, and the osmolality of urine is also not as elevated as it is in SIADH.

BARTTER'S SYNDROME. This condition resembles diuretic use except that the hyponatremia is not corrected with fluid restriction. The cause of this rare condition is unknown. It is suspected that there is a deficit in reabsorption of potassium in the proximal convoluted tubule. This results in retention of chloride ion that is not available for the countercurrent mechanism. Thus, the ion gradients that normally form in the Loop of Henle cannot exist. In this condition, there is a persistent hyponatremia, hypokalemia, and a high 24-hour sodium and potassium excretion.

HYPERNATREMIA

Table 4–3 summarizes the three basic causes of hypernatremia. Note that each cause is the counterpart of a cause for hyponatremia. These causes are summarized in the following section.

DEHYDRATION. This can be caused by excess renal loss with high positive free water clearance (i.e., loss of water in excess of NaCl), excessive sweating, and low water intake. The serum sodium is elevated, as is the hematocrit (possibly masking a true anemia), *and* the urine sodium is high because of increased renal excretion of NaCl.

DIABETES INSIPIDUS. Functionally, this condition is the reverse of SIADH (i.e., water retention in the tubules is not adequate). Although this condition is not completely understood, it may result from inadequate levels of ADH from the pituitary or from receptor defects in the renal tubules (a form of nephrogenic diabetes insipidus) (DeVita, 1993). The pattern is characterized by elevated serum sodium but dilute urinary sodium due to the functionally inadequate levels of ADH.

HYPERALDOSTERONISM. This condition may result from adrenal hyperplasia, Cushing's syndrome, and Cushing's disease. The levels of circulating aldosterone are inappropriately high, causing excessive reabsorption of Na and excretion of K^+ and H^+ ions. The patient is hypernatremic and hypokalemic and exhibits mild metabolic alkalosis.

Renal Disease

There are four analytes that aid in the diagnosis of this condition: BUN, creatinine, calcium, and phosphate. It is amazing that neither BUN nor creatinine has any inherent relationship to kidney function, but both fortuitously are superb indicators of renal condition.

BUN

BUN is blood urea nitrogen. The formula for urea is H_2N-CO-NH_2. There are two moles of nitrogen per mole of urea. This is the end product of NH_3 metabolism in the liver, as discussed in Chapter 8. Urea is secreted by the renal tubules at a rate that is proportional to the glomerular filtration rate (GFR). Note, therefore, that the *retained* urea (i.e., plasma or serum urea or BUN) is *inversely* proportional to the GFR—that is,

$$\text{BUN} \propto 1/\text{GFR} \qquad (4\text{-}9)$$

CREATININE

Creatinine is secreted but is also reabsorbed to an equal extent so that the *net* effect is that the amount filtered is the amount excreted. The total amount of creatinine filtered, then, is its urinary concentration, $U_{cr} \times$ the volume of urine, V, over a given time. The total plasma volume that delivered this quantity of creatinine to the glomerulus is the total amount of creatinine filtered divided by the plasma concentration, P_{cr}. This quantity is also the creatinine clearance, C_{cr}. So the GFR is

$$\text{GFR} = C_{cr} = U_{cr} \times V/P_{cr} \qquad (4\text{-}10)$$

Suppose the BUN is abnormally high (reference range = 10 to 20 mg/mL). There are two possible reasons for this. The first is *prerenal,* wherein renal plasma flow is reduced from such lesions as renal artery stenosis and renal vein thrombo-

Table 4–3. COMMON CAUSES OF HYPERNATREMIA AND ELECTROLYTE PATTERNS IN SERUM AND URINE WITH NORMAL RENAL FUNCTION*

Cause	Serum Na	Urine Na	Urine Osm	Serum K	24-Hour UNa
1. Dehydration	High	High	High	Normal	Low
2. Diabetes insipidus	High	Low	Low	Normal	Low
3. Cushing's disease or syndrome	High	Low	Normal	Low	Low

*In this table, low is equivalent to depressed, and high is equivalent to elevated. All Na and K values are concentrations except for 24-hour UNa, which is the total number of milliequivalents of Na excreted in 24 hours in the urine.

sis. This causes a reduction in the GFR. From equation 4-9, the BUN then rises. However, the serum creatinine levels (P_{cr} in equation 4-10), for which the reference range is 0.5 to 1.0 mg/dL, generally remains within normal limits or may be mildly elevated because, from equation 4-10, low GFR results in lower urine flow (V in equation 4-10). P_{cr} and U_{cr} remain generally within normal limits. Thus, BUN rises disproportionately over creatinine. The normal BUN/creatinine ratio is 10:1 to 20:1; in prerenal disease, it rises to well above 20:1.

The second cause of elevated BUN is true *renal* disease. Here again there is a rise in BUN owing to low GFRs. Now, however, creatinine filtration is compromised so that its serum level rises correspondingly. Thus, in true renal disease, *both* BUN and creatinine rise together, maintaining the BUN:creatinine ratio at 10:1 to 20:1.

PINPOINTING THE LESION. Suppose a patient is found to have a BUN of, say, 60 mg/dL and a creatinine of 3.5 mg/dL. True renal failure therefore can be diagnosed. Now consider the kidney to be two compartments, one a filtration compartment (glomerulus) and the other a concentration compartment (renal tubules). If renal failure is present, where is the lesion—in the filtration or in the concentration compartment?

As discussed previously, the function of the kidneys is to *conserve* fluids or to concentrate the urine. Therefore, if a patient is on a fluid-restricted diet, the osmolality of urine (Uosm) should be significantly higher than the osmolality of plasma (Posm). In fact, Uosm/Posm is greater than 1.2 for normal individuals. If a 24-hour urine specimen collection from the above-mentioned patient on a fluid-restricted diet is measured for Uosm, we can determine where the lesion has occurred. If Uosm/Posm is less than 1.2, then the urine is not being concentrated so that there *must* be a tubular lesion. On the other hand, if there is a normal ratio, then, by exclusion, the lesion must be glomerular. Causes of glomerular lesions are many: glomerulonephritis, pyelonephritis, diabetes, and infarction number among these; tubular lesions also have many causes, including pyelonephritis, diabetes, papillary necrosis, acute tubular necrosis (ATN), infarction, shock, and ischemia. It is remarkable that from a blood specimen of only 100 μl and several urine aliquots, not only can we determine the presence of renal failure, but we can localize the lesion, and all of this can be done virtually noninvasively.

CALCIUM AND PHOSPHATE

The kidneys are important to the regulation of calcium levels. In renal failure, calcium levels tend to fall while phosphate levels correspondingly tend to rise. The topic of calcium and phosphorous metabolism is discussed in detail in the endocrine section, Chapter 16. Here, we discuss these two analytes for diagnostic purposes.

Remember that calcium is the most abundant cation in the body, most of it stored in bone as a calcium hydroxyphosphate in hydroxyapatite. Calcium complexes with phosphate in several different forms, depending on the ionization state of phosphate—that is,

$$H_3PO_4 \leftrightarrows Ca(H_2PO_4)_2 + H^+ \leftrightarrows Ca(HPO_4) + H^+ \leftrightarrows Ca_3(PO_4)_2 + H^+ \quad (4\text{-}11)$$

The most insoluble calcium phosphate forms are those toward the right of this equation. Thus, alkaline conditions promote calcium deposition in bone, whereas acidic conditions promote leaching of calcium from bone. Thus, alkalosis promotes hypocalcemia, whereas acidosis promotes hypercalcemia.

Note also that there is an equilibrium between soluble calcium phosphate and insoluble calcium phosphate in bone. We represent this equilibrium as

$$Ca + P \leftrightarrows (CaP)\text{ insoluble} \quad (4\text{-}12)$$

where the left side is all soluble calcium phosphate salts and the right side is the insoluble salt forms. The equilibrium constant, Ksp, for this equilibrium is

$$Ksp = (Ca) \times (P)/(CaP)\text{insoluble} \quad (4\text{-}13)$$

Because (CaP)insoluble is constant in concentration, the soluble Ca $\times$ P is a constant (called the solubility constant, Ksp). Thus, there is an *inverse* relationship between Ca and P. Hypocalcemic states are almost always accompanied by hyperphosphatemic states and *vice versa*.

Of the soluble calcium, in the numerator of equation 4-13, there are two forms, calcium bound to albumin and globulin in chelate form and so-called ionized or nonchelated calcium. Biologically active calcium is in the ionized form. Therefore, serum levels of ionized calcium are considered to be the best measure of hypocalcemia, normocalcemia, and hypercalcemia.

The kidneys are vital in calcium metabolism and regulate calcium levels in two ways: parathyroid hormone stimulates the renal tubules to *excrete phosphate*. According to equation 4-13, the serum calcium level must then rise. Also, the kidneys are vital to the formation of active vitamin D in the synthesis of 1,25-dihydroxycholecalciferol, which is necessary for the absorption of calcium in the gut.

In renal disease, tubular failure causes phosphate excretion to be inhibited because of the nonresponsiveness of the tubules to parathyroid hormone. Therefore, phosphate levels rise while calcium levels fall. In addition, active vitamin D production is reduced, lowering absorbed calcium. *Hypocalcemia and hyperphosphatemia,* in the face of elevated BUN and creatinine, indicative of renal disease, strongly suggest *tubular failure.*

OTHER CAUSES OF HYPOCALCEMIA. Besides alkalosis and renal failure, hypocalcemia may be caused by hypoparathyroidism, also leading to hyperphosphatemia. Rarely, such as in medullary thyroid carcinomas and other amine precursor uptake and decarboxylase activity (APUD) cell tumors, the elaboration of calcitonin, a well-known calcium lowering hormone, may lead to decreased serum calcium levels.

CAUSES OF HYPERCALCEMIA. Besides acidosis, the possible causes of this condition may be summarized by Bakerman's CHIMPS mnemonic (Bakerman, 1994), or *C*ancer, *H*yperthyroidism, *I*atrogenic causes, *M*ultiple myeloma, *P*arathyroidism, and *S*arcoidosis.

Blood Gas Abnormalities

We have discussed the effects of acidosis and alkalosis on serum calcium levels. The actual diagnosis of acidosis or alkalosis, however, depends on measurement of the pH of arterial blood. The topic of arterial blood gases and their methods of measurement are discussed in Chapters 3 and 7. Here we focus on how to interpret abnormal results and to correlate them with other laboratory findings.

Blood gas determinations refer to the quantitative measurement of the pH of arterial blood, the P_{CO_2}, the bicarbonate, the P_{O_2}, oxygen saturation, and base excess. Three of these quantities are interdependent (i.e., the P_{CO_2}, the bicarbonate, and the pH) by the Henderson-Hasselbalch equation:

$$pH = 6.1 + \log[(HCO_3^-)/(H_2CO_3)] \quad (4\text{-}14)$$

Because the H_2CO_3 concentration in blood is directly proportional to the P_{CO_2} (i.e., at room temperature, $H_2CO_3 = 0.03 \times P_{CO_2}$) (equation 4-15), equation 4-14 can be written as

$$pH = 6.1 + \log[(HCO_3^-)/(0.03 \times P_{CO_2})] \quad (4\text{-}15)$$

Note that if bicarbonate, in the numerator of equation 4-15, becomes consumed as in metabolic acidosis, by increasing the respiratory rate, thereby decreasing the P_{CO_2}, the denominator of this equation falls to compensate. If the P_{CO_2} increases as in respiratory acidosis, the kidneys retain bicarbonate so that *both* numerator and denominator increase so as to maintain the ratio relatively constant (i.e., buffering capacity).

In interpreting blood gas results, the first number to note is the pH. Regardless of the values of the bicarbonate and P_{CO_2}, if the pH is less than 7.4, the patient is acidotic; if it is greater than 7.4, the patient is alkalotic; if it is equal to 7.4, the patient is neither. Once acidosis or alkalosis is diagnosed, then the bicarbonate or the P_{CO_2} can be used to decide whether the condition is of metabolic or respiratory origin.

Table 4–4 summarizes the four basic abnormal states: metabolic and respiratory acidosis and metabolic and respiratory alkalosis. In metabolic acidosis, the primary problem is production of acid as in diabetic ketoacidosis, lactic acidosis (e.g., from gram-negative sepsis), and renal failure. This acid is buffered by bicarbonate, which is therefore consumed. To compensate for the bicarbonate loss, the breathing rate increases to lower the P_{CO_2}. Thus, a low pH combined with a low bicarbonate and a low P_{CO_2} point to metabolic acidosis as shown in condition 1 of this table. As shown in condition 2 of Table 4–4, the opposite condition, metabolic alkalosis, results in reversal of the levels shown in condition 1. The most common cause of metabolic alkalosis is vomiting with a loss of HCl from the stomach and an attendant rise in bicarbonate.

When CO_2 is abnormally retained by the lungs as in chronic obstructive pulmonic disease (COPD), the denominator of equation 4-15 increases, causing the pH of blood to fall. To compensate, the kidneys retain bicarbonate to increase the numerator of this equation. If the blood pH is below 7.4 and the CO_2 and bicarbonate are both *increased* (condition 3 in Table 4–4), the acidosis is of respiratory origin. Note the mirror-image condition (opposite levels) for respiratory alkalosis in condition 4 of this table. Besides COPD, the major causes of respiratory acidosis include diseases such as myasthenia gravis in which there is partial paralysis of the accessory muscles of breathing, pneumonia, and central nervous system diseases affecting the brainstem in areas involved in respiratory control. Respiratory alkalosis is mainly due to hyperventilation, often of psychogenic origin. Here, the P_{CO_2} is reduced because of the rapidity of breathing.

The pH of blood can affect the levels of electrolytes in serum. In acidosis, besides bicarbonate buffering, red cells also buffer the excess H^+ ions by exchanging these for intracellular K^+ ions, the net effect being mild hyperkalemia. An attendant hypokalemia occurs in alkalosis. Remember also that acidosis can cause mild hypercalcemia; alkalosis can cause mild hypocalcemia and especially affect the ionized calcium moiety concentration.

ANION GAP

All sodium ions must be neutralized by counter-ions, most of which are constituted by chloride and bicarbonate ions, and to a lesser degree, by phosphate, sulfate, and protein carboxylate groups. Normal serum sodium is about 140 mEq/L, chloride is usually around 100 mEq/L, and bicarbonate is around 24 mEq/L. The anion gap is then defined as $Na^+ - (Cl^- + HCO_3^-)$, which, for normal individuals, is around 16. This 16 mEq/L is really composed of the other counter-ions that neutralize sodium but are not measured in serum.

If an individual has metabolic acidosis, in which HCl is retained, then the bicarbonate value decreases but there is a 1 : 1 increase in chloride ion, so that the anion gap does not change. If the metabolic acidosis is due to the presence of an acid whose counter-ion is not Cl^-, such as acetoacetic acid (in diabetic acidosis) or lactic acid as in sepsis or hypoperfusion, then bicarbonate is reduced, but there is no corresponding increase in Cl^-. Therefore, there is an increase in the anion gap, which can reach values of 25 to 30 mEq/L. The presence of a widened anion gap signifies the presence of metabolic acidosis due to a non–chloride-containing acid.

LOW ANION GAPS. *Consistently* low anion gaps, typically in the range of 1 to 3 mEq/L, signify the presence of high levels of basic protein, often a myeloma protein. Basic protein contains ammonium ions, the counter-ions for which are chloride. Now the invisible ion is ammonium, whereas there is a measurable increase in chloride ion. This tends to decrease the anion gap. Persistently low anion gaps are a serious sign of possible malignancy (i.e., myeloma).

OXYGENATION

Blood gases also give an excellent measurement of tissue perfusion through measurement of the P_{O_2} and the oxygen saturation of hemoglobin. Normal P_{O_2} values should be 90 to 100 mm Hg, whereas O_2 saturation should be 100%. Low

Table 4–4. PATTERNS OF pH, P_{CO_2}, AND BICARBONATE IN DIFFERENT CONDITIONS

Condition	pH	Bicarbonate	P_{CO_2}	Typical Causes
1. Metabolic acidosis	<7.40	Low	Low	Diabetic ketoacidosis; lactic acidosis
2. Metabolic alkalosis	>7.40	High	High	Vomiting
3. Respiratory acidosis	<7.40	High	High	COPD; paralysis of respiratory muscles
4. Respiratory alkalosis	>7.40	Low	Low	Anxiety; acute pain

COPD, chronic obstructive pulmonary disease.

values of either or both of these numbers indicate an underlying pathology. The major causes of low values for these measurements are myocardial infarction, pulmonary embolus, and tissue anoxic states secondary to hypoperfusion, as in septicemia and severe congestive heart failure. In pulmonary embolus, there is blockage of the pulmonary circulation by the embolus despite adequate ventilation, giving rise to ventilation/perfusion inequalities.

ARTERIAL BLOOD GAS PATTERNS IN PATIENTS WITH MYOCARDIAL INFARCTION AND PULMONARY EMBOLISM

The chief findings are a drop in the Po_2 and a metabolic acidosis. The drop in Po_2 in myocardial infarction (MI) is caused by diminished circulation times—that is, the *rate* of oxygenation of venous blood is *reduced*. In pulmonary embolism (PE), the low Po_2 is caused by direct blockage of blood flow into the pulmonary circuit. The acidosis in MI is caused by low tissue perfusion of oxygenated blood due to compromised cardiac output. In PE, the acidosis is caused by low oxygen saturation in the lungs with consequent diminished oxygen delivery to tissues. Both conditions result in tissue hypoxia.

HYPERCAPNIA AS A CAUSE OF HYPOXIA

Another major cause of hypoxic states in arterial blood is CO_2-retentive states, such as severe COPD. This occurs because, as CO_2 builds up in alveoli, it reduces the volume of O_2 in the air space. At Pco_2 values of over 50 mm Hg, the effect on alveolar Po_2, represented as P_ACO_2, becomes important, as illustrated in Figure 4–3. Oxygen, unlike CO_2, is not soluble in water or membranes, so that there is a difference of about 10 to 15 mm Hg pressure between alveolar and arterial O_2 (represented as P_aCO_2), called the A-a gradient. It is important to remember that the total oxygen breathed in, called the $P{\rm IO}_2$, is *partitioned*, therefore, between the alveolar sac and the arterial blood. This relationship may be written as

$$P{\rm IO}_2 = P_AO_2 + P_aO_2 \qquad (4\text{-}16)$$

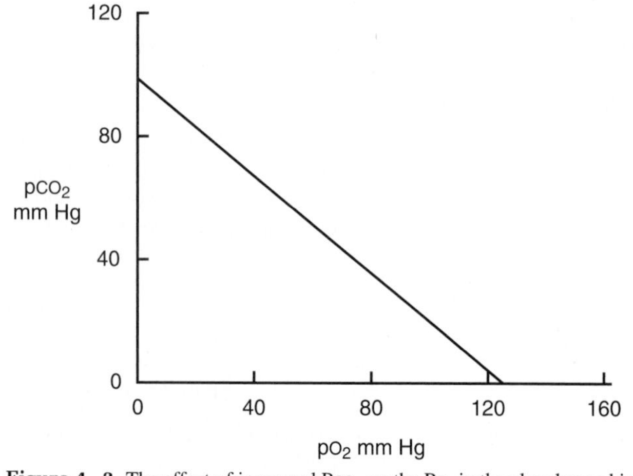

Figure 4–3. The effect of increased Pco_2 on the Po_2 in the alveolus and in arterial blood. This figure demonstrates that as the Pco_2 increases, there is a greater than a one-to-one decrease of Po_2.

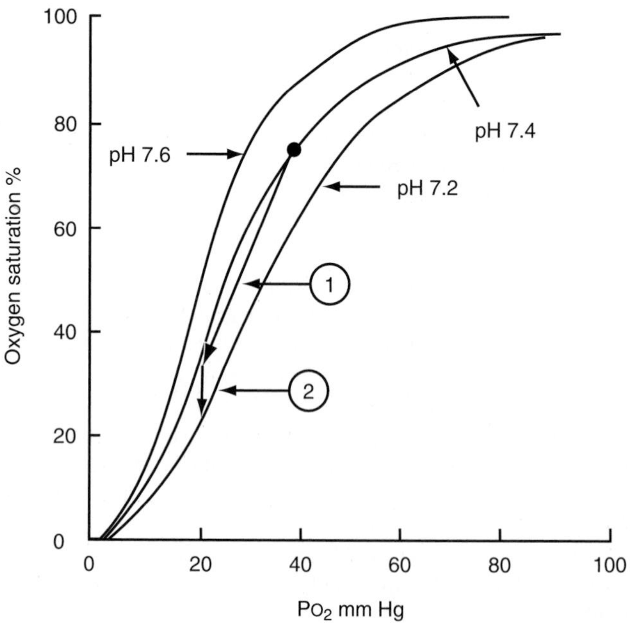

Figure 4–4. The effects of decreasing Po_2 in the allosteric zone of the oxygen-hemoglobin dissociation curve. On the pH 7.4 curve, if the Po_2 drops from 80 to 60, there is little effect on the oxygen saturation. However, a drop from 40 to 20 mm Hg results in a large drop in oxygen saturation from about 80 to 30% (arrow 1 in the figure). With this low oxygen saturation, there is a marked tissue lactic acidosis from anaerobic metabolism. The increased acidosis results in a drop in blood pH to 7.2, shifting the oxygen-hemoglobin dissociation to the right (pH 7.2 curve). Now, for a Po_2 of 30, the oxygen saturation drops even further (arrow 2 in the figure) to about 20%, setting a vicious cycle in motion.

For each mole of O_2 consumed, approximately 0.8 mole of CO_2 is produced. The ratio of CO_2 produced to O_2 consumed is called the respiratory quotient, or the RQ. The P_aO_2 may be written as P_aCO_2/RQ. Overall, equation 4-16 can be rewritten as

$$P_AO_2 = P{\rm IO}_2 - P_aCO_2/RQ \qquad (4\text{-}17)$$

This equation states that *for each increment in the P_aCO_2, there will be a more than one-to-one decrease in the P_AO_2.* This will result in severe oxygen deficits.

Figure 4–4 is the oxygen-hemoglobin dissociation curve. Note that the curve is sigmoidal because of the allosteric nature of the binding of oxygen to hemoglobin. For Po_2 values between 70 and 100 mm Hg, the saturation of hemoglobin is close to 100%. But at Po_2 values below 70 mm Hg, there is a *steep* drop in the saturation fraction so that small drops in Po_2 lead to large decreases in the percentage of saturation. Compounding this effect is the disproportionate decrease in Po_2 whenever Pco_2 increases as described previously.

While these detrimental events transpire, tissue perfusion severely diminishes because of the diminished oxygen saturation of arterial blood. The result is tissue acidosis (mainly from lactic acid as a result of anaerobic metabolism). Acidosis shifts the oxygen-hemoglobin dissociation to the right as in Figure 4–4, causing even lower saturation for a given Po_2, causing further diminished tissue perfusion and more tissue acidosis. This vicious circle can be corrected by placing the patient on a respirator to cause increased expiration of CO_2.

The pattern of arterial blood gas determinations for this

type of patient are low arterial blood pH, low Po_2, low oxygen saturation, high Pco_2, and low bicarbonate. This pattern is not typical of the four basic patterns given in Table 4–4 because, on top of a fundamental respiratory acidosis (high Pco_2), there is a superimposed tissue metabolic lactic acidosis, causing low bicarbonate. These findings, together with the low Po_2, indicate the immediate need for ventilation of the patient on a respirator.

Unlike myocardial infarction and pulmonary embolus, described earlier, the acute hypercapnic state is *not* treated with oxygen administration *unless* the patient is being adequately ventilated. Hypercapnia induces a CO_2-induced inhibition of the respiratory centers in the pons and the medulla oblongata in the brainstem. In fact, the only impetus to breathe is the hypercapnia-induced hypoxia, causing chemoreceptors in the aortic arch to send signals to the respiratory center in the brain to continue breathing. *Administration of oxygen to patients with this condition without ventilation can cause cessation of respiration and the acute demise of the patient.*

Glucose Abnormalities

The normal reference interval for fasting serum glucose is generally between 70 and 110 mg/dL. As described in Chapter 9, the two basic abnormalities that occur with serum glucose levels are hyperglycemia, almost always associated with diabetes mellitus, and hypoglycemia due to iatrogenic (overdose with insulin in the diabetic patient) or to other underlying causes (e.g., reactive hypoglycemia due to hypersensitivity to insulin or insulinoma). To establish hyperglycemia, it is vital to determine whether the patient has *serum glucose levels that are greater than 140 mg/dL on a series of random fasting serum samples.* If this is found to be the case, diabetes mellitus can be diagnosed provisionally.

Another manner of establishing the diagnosis of diabetes mellitus is the use of the glucose tolerance test, also described in Chapter 9. In this process, after giving a well-defined amount of glucose orally to the patient, who has not eaten for 12 hours overnight, the blood and urine glucose levels are followed. Normally, serum glucose levels rise and then fall within about a two-hour period. If the glucose levels remain elevated, however, diabetes mellitus may again be diagnosed. Also, detection of glucose in the urine at any point is evidence for this condition, although absence of urinary glucose does not rule out diabetes mellitus in any way.

High levels of serum glucose also result in the glycosylation of hemoglobin. Glycated hemoglobin levels tend to increase over time. A number of elegant methods have been devised to measure glycated hemoglobin levels in whole blood rapidly, including the Abbott Laboratories new ion capture method. Of all of the methods for diagnosing diabetes mellitus and for following the efficacy of therapy, measurement of glycated hemoglobin levels is perhaps the most accurate and should be performed in conjunction with blood glucose determinations.

OTHER ABNORMAL LABORATORY FINDINGS IN DIABETES MELLITUS

Under the influence of insulin, whenever glucose is transported into the cell, it is accompanied by potassium. In diabetes, in the absence of insulin, blood glucose is elevated, as is potassium. Because of increased metabolism of fats, there is a build up of acetoacetic acid, leading to a metabolic acidosis. In diabetes, wherein the blood glucose becomes exceptionally elevated (i.e., >300 mg/dL) the serum osmolality becomes dangerously high and can cause nonketotic, hyperosmolar coma. In this condition, red (and white) blood cell water flows from the cells into the vascular volume, tending to dilute analytes such as sodium. Thus, the patient with nonketotic, hyperosmolar coma may have a hyperosmolar serum, hyperglycemia, hyperkalemia, and hyponatremia. In ketotic states, the patient also has metabolic acidosis and a large anion gap.

In hypoglycemia, serum glucose levels of less than 60 mg/dL on a series of random fasting serum specimens strongly indicate this condition. Glucose tolerance tests show that after an initial sharp rise of serum glucose levels, there is an abnormally rapid drop to levels substantially below 60 mg/dL. If hypoglycemia is suspected, it is advisable to give the patient a five-hour glucose tolerance test, because the so-called hypoglycemic dip often is not seen until after three hours. Glucose tolerance tests on patients with suspected hypoglycemia should be performed with great caution because the procedure can induce severe reactive hypoglycemia, causing loss of consciousness and even shock.

Liver Function Tests

The immense topic of liver function tests is discussed in depth in Chapter 12, which gives a detailed breakdown of different patterns in abnormal liver function tests. The reader will find it virtually impossible to memorize these patterns without a basic understanding of the underlying principles. We can reduce the most common liver test abnormalities to a set of six conditions summarized in Table 4–5. The principles for these patterns are explained as follows.

Table 4–5. SIX FUNDAMENTAL PATTERNS OF LIVER FUNCTION TESTS

Condition	AST	ALT	LD	ALP	TP	Alb	Bilirubin	Ammonia
1. Hepatitis	H	H	H	H	N	N	H	N
2. Cirrhosis	N	N	N	N-sl H	L	L	H	H
3. Biliary obstruction	N	N	N	H	N	N	H	N
4. Space-occupying lesion	N or H	N or H	H	H	N	N	N-H	N
5. Passive congestion	sl H	sl H	sl H	N-sl H	N	N	N-sl H	N
6. Fulminant failure	very H	H	H	H	L	L	H	H

H, N, L, high, normal, low; AST, aspartate aminotransferase; ALT, alanine aminotransferase; LD, lactate dehydrogenase; ALP, alkaline phosphatase; TP, total protein; Alb, albumin; sl, slightly.

1. All acute injuries and/or necrotic lesions in the liver *primarily cause a marked rise in the levels of the aminotransferases, aspartate aminotransferase (AST) and alanine aminotransferase (ALT).* Cell injury and necrosis also cause the rise of other enzymes such as lactate dehydrogenase (LD). These include hepatitis (both infectious and chemically induced), infarction, and trauma. The biliary tract is always affected so that direct bilirubin rises from interference with bile flow. Because of biliary tract injury, the enzyme alkaline phosphatase rises along with gamma-glutamyl transferase (GGT) and 5′-nucleotidase (5′-N). Hepatocyte injury causes loss of conjugation of transported bilirubin, so that indirect (unconjugated) bilirubin also rises.

   Because, generally, in hepatitis, much less than 80% of the liver is destroyed, total regeneration occurs and enough tissue is present to enable adequate levels of protein synthesis and ammonia fixation as urea. Therefore, the total protein and albumin and ammonia levels remain normal. These typical results are summarized in condition 1 of Table 4–5.
2. Cirrhosis of the liver is characterized by two cardinal features: fibrosis, preventing regeneration of liver tissue wherever this has occurred, and nodules of regenerating liver tissue, which are the only source of any kind of hepatocytic function. Thus, in cirrhosis, almost the *reverse* pattern occurs from the one seen in Table 4–5 for hepatitis. Because, in panhepatic cirrhosis, there is destruction of more than 80% of liver tissue, with no regeneration of all damaged liver tissue, the AST/ALT aminotransferases and LD levels (all from the regenerating nodules) tend to be normal or low or occasionally mildly elevated. However, the total protein and albumin both are abnormally low. The ammonia levels are elevated. Because there is insufficient viable liver tissue remaining, and because fibrosis destroys the cholangioles, both indirect and direct bilirubin tend to be elevated. These findings are summarized in condition 2 of Table 4–5.
3. Biliary obstruction caused by stones in the biliary tree or by neoplasms that block bile excretion cause elevations in direct bilirubin and biliary tract alkaline phosphatase, along with the enzymes, GGT, and 5′-N (see no. 1). All other liver function test results are normal. For simple biliary obstruction, therefore, the pattern is as shown in condition 3 of Table 4–5.
4. Space-occupying lesions of the liver are characterized, for reasons that are not well understood, by isolated elevations of the enzymes, alkaline phosphatase, and LD. This pattern is shown in condition 4 of Table 4–5. The most common cause of this condition is metastatic carcinoma to the liver.
5. Passive congestion of the liver is characterized by a mild elevation of aminotransferases (AST/ALT) and LD and, in more severe cases, elevations of total bilirubin and alkaline phosphatase. This pattern is also seen in infectious mononucleosis, wherein the rise in bilirubin may be marked. The general passive congestion pattern is shown in condition 5 of Table 4–5.
6. Acute fulminant hepatic failure from a variety of causes, which include Reye's syndrome, is discussed in Chapter 12. This condition is *total liver failure.* The overall pattern, which has been described (Sunheimer, 1994) and is shown in condition 6 of Table 4–5, appears as a *combination* of hepatitis and cirrhosis. Here, AST and ALT reach exceptionally high values, often in excess of 10,000 IU/L. At the same time, total protein and albumin are markedly reduced, and the ammonia levels are abnormally elevated, causing hepatic encephalopathy. LD, alkaline phosphatase, and bilirubin are also elevated. Besides the marked rise in AST and ALT, combined with hyperammonemia, there is a characteristic disproportional rise of AST over ALT, further confirming the diagnosis. It is vital to recognize this pattern because the underlying condition is a medical emergency that must be treated promptly.

CORRELATIONS OF LIVER FUNCTION TEST RESULTS WITH OTHER LABORATORY FINDINGS

In severe liver failure, secondary to cirrhosis or to fulminant hepatic failure, it is not uncommon to find electrolyte abnormalities and abnormalities in renal function tests and in the coagulation profile. Patients with either condition 2 or 6 in Table 4–5 often have ascites, with marked third-space fluid loss. This results in increased levels of both ADH and aldosterone to retain intravascular water. Depending on which levels "win out," the patient may become hyponatremic or hypernatremic.

Severe liver failure can also cause the hepatorenal syndrome—that is, renal dysfunction secondary to hepatic failure. This disease is characterized by the typical patterns shown in conditions 2 and 6 in Table 4–5. Renal failure results in elevations in BUN and creatinine with a 10:1 to 20:1 ratio, indicative of renal failure. The Uosm/Posm is less than 1.2:1, indicating tubular dysfunction.

Severe coagulopathies with elevated aPTTs and PTs may be seen because of the absence of production of coagulation factors. Not infrequently, DIC accompanies the liver failure. This condition must be distinguished from low coagulation factor production combined with hepatosplenomegaly due to portal hypertension, as in cirrhosis. The splenomegaly may result in sequestration of platelets, so that the overall pattern may resemble DIC but not be true DIC. To clinch the diagnosis of DIC, the FSP level should be elevated. Also, in severe liver failure, abnormal red cell forms, called target cells, may be seen in the peripheral blood smear.

Patients with cirrhosis and acute fulminant hepatic failure tend to be immunocompromised. Many of these patients have defective T-cell function but produce an excess of (ineffective) immunoglobulin. Thus, these patients tend to have low serum albumin levels from diminished albumin synthesis but elevated serum immunoglobulins.

Cardiac Function Tests—Diagnosis of Myocardial Infarction

Cardiac function tests are discussed at length in Chapter 13. The salient features of the laboratory findings that characterize this disease are summarized here. There are three enzymes that have characteristic time courses of elevations followed by decreases in MI: creatine phosphokinase (CK), AST, and LD. In MI, CK rises within 12 hours, peaks within 24 hours, and then falls to normal. AST elevations are rarely used as a means to diagnose MI, although if CK, AST, and LD levels are all elevated simultaneously, MI should be considered in the differential diagnosis. AST levels characteristically rise to a maximum in 24 hours in MI and then decline to normal levels in about 48 hours. LD values peak around 48 hours and then decline to normal within several days.

CK has three isoforms composed of two chains (called the M and B chains), which are MM, MB, and BB. The MB fraction is predominantly found in cardiac muscle. To diagnose MI from CK-MB serum levels, it is important to show both a rise in the *concentration* of CK-MB and a rise in the *ratio of CK-MB to total CK* (Thompson, 1988). Furthermore, it is important to obtain serial values of CK-MB and total CK from a patient with suspected MI to demonstrate a consistent rise or fall in these values. Typically, CK-MB begins to rise in two to six hours after the initial event and peaks within 12 hours, and it can be used to establish the *diagnosis* of MI.

Like CK, LD contains two chains, H and M, that comprise tetramers. Cardiac muscle contains predominantly the H_4 and H_3M forms, called LD_1 and LD_2, respectively. Normally, LD_2 is greater than LD_1, but this ratio reverses in MI about 24 to 36 hours after the initial insult. The finding of a so-called flipped LD_1/LD_2 ratio *confirms* the diagnosis of MI but is not used to diagnose this condition because of the long postacute MI time periods over which this ratio reverses.

Pancreatic Function Tests

Elevations in serum pancreatic amylase and lipase are definitive markers for pancreatic disease. The most common cause for such increases in the serum levels of these enzymes is pancreatitis. In acute pancreatitis, both enzymes are elevated. Because amylase can also be produced by the salivary glands, amylase is slightly less specific as a marker for pancreatitis than lipase is. Elevations in the lipase are definitive for pancreatic disease.

Markers for Inflammatory Conditions

As discussed previously under Hematology, increases in the white blood cell count, especially with a predominance of neutrophils, indicate acute infection. In most acute inflammatory conditions, acute phase reactant proteins are also increased. These proteins occur in the α and β fractions, identified in the serum protein electrophoretogram, as discussed in Chapter 11 on serum protein electrophoresis. Fibrinogen, also an acute phase reactant, may also increase. Often, the platelet count tends to rise, and platelets themselves have been considered acute phase reactants.

In addition, in both acute and chronic inflammatory conditions, erythrocytes exhibit increased mobilities. Thus, there is an increase in the erythrocyte sedimentation rate. This is described in Chapter 24.

Finally, one common cause of acute inflammation is gout (i.e., hyperuricemia, or elevations of uric acid in serum). Uric acid crystals cause a severe, acute arthritic condition (gout). Serum levels of uric acid above 7.5 mg/dL are indicative of this condition. Less constant findings are the presence of uric acid crystals in the urinary sediment (see Chap. 18) or in joint fluid (see Chap. 19).

EXAMPLES OF CLINICAL CASES WITH CLINICOPATHOLOGIC CORRELATIONS

Having provided an overview of many salient features of the causes of the more common abnormal laboratory findings, the laboratory results from three patients illustrate how analyte levels change in different disease states.

EXAMPLE A. A 64-year-old white man was found unconscious in his home after suffering a cerebrovascular accident (CVA) and brought to the Emergency Medicine Department. His hematocrit was 44%, but his red blood cell count was 4.3 million/L (lower limit of normal, 4.6 million/μL) with an MCV of 104 fL; a series of serum sodium values ranged from 164 to 175 mEq/μL; admission BUN was 33 mg/dL; and creatinine was 1.5 mg/dL. The total serum osmolality was 357 mOsm (upper limit of normal, 295), whereas the urine osmolality was 1008 mOsm (upper limit of normal, 1000 mOsm) and the random urine sodium was 228 mEq/L.

A liver panel showed a marginally elevated AST at 41 IU/L (upper limit of normal, 39 IU/L), elevated but continually decreasing LD (admission value of 426 IU/L, upper limit of normal, 200 IU/L), GGT of 72 IU/L (upper limit of normal, 43 IU/L), total protein of 7.8 g/dL (normal) but a low albumin of 2.8 g/dL (normal 3.5 to 5.0 g/dL). Lipase was mildly elevated at 127 IU/L (upper limit of normal, 60 IU/L). Occult blood was found in his stool, which was found positive for *Clostridium difficile*. Urine was nitrite positive (indicative of bacteriuria) and was markedly positive for hemoglobin, red blood cells, and white blood cells.

After infusion of half-normal saline, the hematocrit was reduced to 34% but then rose to 38% with a persistently elevated MCV. The sodium and the BUN were reduced to within the reference range.

Evaluation. This patient was dehydrated as shown by the markedly elevated serum sodium (average value of 169 mEq/L), high normal hematocrit, and elevated BUN. Note that the diagnosis of dehydration was confirmed by the finding of a high serum (228 mEq/L) sodium and a high urinary osmolality of 1008 mOsm (see Table 4–3).

The red blood cell count was low, which seems to contradict the high-normal hematocrit. This apparent discrepancy may be explained by the macrocytosis, causing each erythrocyte to occupy a greater than normal volume. Yet the total number of cells was reduced. The low red blood cell count indicates true anemia. The macrocytosis was caused by a nutritional (vitamin B_{12}) deficiency. All of these findings may be attributed to malnutrition and insufficient fluid consumption, a not-uncommon finding in the elderly, especially in this stroke victim.

Note that the BUN and creatinine were mildly elevated in a pattern with a ratio exceeding 20:1, suggesting a prerenal (low perfusion) etiology. The renal tubules were evidently functioning well, as evidenced by the high urine-to-serum osmolality ratio (1008/357 = 2.8, which is greater than 1.2:1). Hypoperfusion may have also caused the mild abnormalities found in some of the liver function tests and the elevated pancreatic lipase.

Note also that the total protein was normal even though the

albumin, the most abundant serum protein, was low. Because of possibly two infectious diseases identified in urine and stool examinations, the patient may have had elevated levels of immunoglobulins.

Accompanying the CVA was a peptic ulcer, so-called Cushing's ulcer, known to be associated with this condition; hence, the occult blood in this patient's stool. *C. difficile* is known to infect patients with chronic debilitating disease. The urinary tract infection was responsible for the high red blood cell count and hemoglobin in this patient's urine.

EXAMPLE B. A 31-year-old white man with known juvenile-onset diabetes mellitus, end-stage renal disease secondary to diabetic nephropathy, and a history of alcoholism was admitted with acute abdominal pain in the mid-epigastrium, with a serum glucose of 736 mg/dL, which rose as high as 933 mg/dL; serum sodium of 134 mEq/L, which decreased to as low as 124 mEq/L; potassium of 7.1 mEq/L; BUN of 64 mg/dL; and a creatinine of 18 mg/dL. These values were confirmed and found to follow a consistent trend. Serum osmolality was 316 mOsm. Blood gas values on admission were pH of 7.58, Po_2 of 121 mm Hg, O_2 saturation of 99%, Pco_2 of 20 mm Hg, and bicarbonate of 20 mEq/L. The anion gap rose in one day from 13 (high end of normal) to 20. Serum lipase was elevated at 469 IU/L (upper limit of normal is 60 IU/L). There was no urine output, and the patient was subjected to peritoneal dialysis.

Evaluation. This diabetic patient was evidently in a hyperosmolar state due to abnormally elevated glucose levels. The low serum sodium and high serum potassium levels might appear to be due to low circulating aldosterone or renal tubular failure. However, there was no urine output, so no filtration could occur. The end-stage renal disease is reflected in the BUN and especially in the creatinine value (18 mg/dL). The BUN/creatinine ratio of about 4 confirms the diagnosis of true renal failure.

As noted in the discussion on glucose, in diabetes mellitus with high serum glucose levels, there is an efflux of cell water that causes dilution of serum analytes such as sodium. Whenever glucose is transported into cells under the influence of insulin, it is accompanied by potassium. Low insulin levels can therefore result in hyperkalemia. This mechanism was operative in this patient. Although the anion gap increased after admission, it was normal on admission. Thus, this patient was in a nonketotic, hyperosmolar state but subsequently became ketotic.

The admission blood gas picture suggests respiratory alkalosis because the Pco_2 was low at 20 mm Hg and the bicarbonate was low at 20 mEq/L (condition 4 in Table 4–4). This is an unusual finding in a patient with diabetes mellitus, in whom a finding of metabolic acidosis is more common.

An explanation for this finding may be found in the serum lipase, which was markedly elevated, denoting pancreatitis, a common finding in patients with a history of alcoholism. The sharp epigastric pain caused increased respiration (respiratory rate on admission was 25/min), precipitating a *lowering* of the Pco_2, which was partially compensated for by a lowering of the bicarbonate.

Treatment of this patient with dialysis, hydration, and insulin corrected the abnormal laboratory findings, and the patient was discharged on chronic dialysis.

EXAMPLE C. A 38-year-old white woman, with a past medical history of multiple abdominal surgical procedures over a seven-year period, sporadic alcohol abuse, pancreatitis, and a 30 pack-year history of smoking, was brought to the emergency department in shock and acute abdominal distress. Significant laboratory values included a white blood cell count of $12.1 \times 10^3/\mu L$, a red blood cell count of $3.07 \times 10^6/\mu L$, hematocrit of 34.6%, and red blood cell indices that showed macrocytosis and hypochromia. Vitamin B_{12} and folate levels were normal. The peripheral blood smear showed a leukoerythroblastic pattern. Serum glucose was low at 38 mg/dL; total protein was 4.3 g/dL; and albumin was 1.5 g/dL. Lactate levels were elevated. The alkaline phosphatase level was elevated at 241 IU/L (upper limit of normal, 129 IU/L), and the bilirubin level was mildly elevated at 1.6 mg/dL (upper limit of normal, 1.2 mg/dL). Serum ammonia level was found to be elevated at 146 μM (upper limit of normal, 30 μM). Screens for hepatitis A, B, and C were all negative. Multiple blood, urine, and throat cultures were negative. Exploratory laparotomy revealed abdominal adhesions and cholestasis. Postoperatively, the patient became encephalopathic; her liver function deteriorated, as evidenced by dramatic elevations of AST and ALT from normal levels to 1660 and 545 IU/L, respectively; of LD to 2190 IU/L; of bilirubin to 14.5 mg/dL; and of ammonia to 177 μM. A liver-spleen scan performed on the fifth hospital day showed no dye uptake in the liver, which is consistent with functional liver failure. The serum sodium, which was normal on admission, increased within five days to 166 mEq/L, together with chloride levels that rose to 123 mEq/L, a pattern that persisted throughout the patient's hospital course despite aggressive intravenous infusion of half-normal saline. Serum potassium was consistently less than 3.5 mEq/L. The BUN and creatinine both rose to abnormally high levels with a ratio of less than 20:1, suggesting renal failure. Plasma aldosterone was elevated at 13.2 ng/dL (upper limit of normal, 8.5 ng/dL). The platelet count dropped rapidly, whereas the aPTT and PT rose to values at least twice those of the corresponding normal controls while her level of FSPs became abnormally elevated. Her condition worsened, and the patient expired on the eighth hospital day.

Evaluation. Although a complex patient presentation, the fundamental problem with this patient lay in the dramatically abnormal liver function test profile. Note how there was an acute elevation in the aminotransferases (transaminases) with the AST/ALT ratios significantly greater than 1. There were concurrent rapid elevations in the bilirubin and the LD. At the same time, the total protein and albumin were abnormally low. The ammonia levels rose rapidly (despite high doses of lactulose). The pattern is that of fulminant hepatic failure, as shown in condition 6 in Table 4–5. This condition is a medical emergency and is associated with fatal encephalopathy and severe DIC, as evidenced by the low platelet counts and elevated PT and aPTT and FSP levels. This condition can cause multiple system infarcts, resulting in multiple organ failure.

The patient's peripheral blood picture showed macrocytosis but, concurrently, a leukoerythroblastic picture. This pattern suggests that the macrocytosis was caused by an increased number of erythrocyte precursor forms. It is not completely clear as to the cause of this condition, but, with the persistently elevated white cell count and the elevated lactate levels, gram-negative sepsis affecting bone marrow must be considered a prime cause of this pattern. Although cultures were consistently negative, the patient was being treated with broad-spectrum antibiotics, the effects of which may have blocked growth of the organism(s) in culture. As noted previously, patients with liver failure from either cirrhosis or acute fulminant hepatic failure are generally immunocompromised.

In both panhepatic cirrhosis and fulminant hepatic failure, severe third-space fluid loss associated with ascites invariably develops. We noted previously that, to retain vascular volume, both aldosterone and ADH rise. It appears that aldosterone became elevated to markedly high values, causing abnormal sodium retention and potassium loss in this patient.

Almost always accompanying both cirrhosis and acute fulminant hepatic failure is renal failure, generally manifested by the hepatorenal syndrome. In fulminant hepatic failure, an additional possible cause is acute tubular necrosis.

Bakerman S, Strausbauch P: ABC's of Interpretive Laboratory Data. 2nd ed. Myrtle Beach, SC, Interpretive Laboratory Data, 1994.

DeVita MV, Michelis MF: Perturbations in sodium balance. Clin Lab Med 1993; 13:135–148.

Galen RS, Gambino SR: Beyond Normality: The Predictive Value and Efficiency of Medical Diagnosis. New York, John Wiley & Sons, 1975.

Harris EK: Statistical aspects of reference values in clinical pathology. *In* Stefani M, Benson ES (eds): Progress in Clinical Pathology. Vol. 8. New York, Grune & Stratton, 1981, p 45.

Martin AR: Common and correctable errors in diagnostic testing ordering. West J Med 1982; 136:456.

Martin HF, Gudzinowicz BJ, Fanger H: Normal Values in Clinical Chemistry: A Guide to Statistical Analysis of Laboratory Data. New York, Marcel Dekker, 1975.

Myers JD: The computer as a diagnostic consultant, with emphasis on use of laboratory data. Clin Chem 1986; 32:1714.

Pauker SG, Kassier JP: Medical progress: Decision analysis. N Engl J Med 1987; 316:250–258.

Statland BE: Clinical Decision Levels for Lab Tests. Oradell, NJ, Medical Economics, 1988.

Statland BE, Winkel P: Effects of non-analytical factors on the intra-individual variation of analytes in the blood of healthy subjects: Consideration of preparation of the subject and time of venipuncture. CRC Crit Rev Clin Lab Sci 1977; 8:105.

Sunheimer R, Capaldo G, Kashanian F, et al: Serum analyte pattern characteristic of fulminant hepatic failure. Ann Clin Lab Sci 1994; 24: 101–109.

Thompson WG, Mahr RG, Yohannan W, Pincus MR: Use of creatine kinase MB isoenzyme for diagnosing myocardial infarction when total creatine kinase activity is high. Clin Chem 1988; 34:2208–2210.

Winkel P, Lyngebye J, Jorgensen K: The normal region: A multivariate problem. Scand J Clin Lab Invest 1972; 30:339.

Winkel P, Statland B: Interpreting labarataory results: Reference values and decision making. *In* Henry JB (ed): Clinical Diagnosis and Management by Laboratory Methods. 18th ed. Philadelphia, W. B. Saunders, 1991.

Chapter 5

Informatics, Imaging, and the Pathologist's Workstation

Raymond D. Aller, M.D.
Ulysses J. Balis, M.D.

FUNDAMENTAL CONCEPTS OF INFORMATION MANAGEMENT IN LABORATORY MEDICINE

A Key Tool and Standard of Practice

Information is the primary, and in most cases sole, product of the work of the medical laboratory. Medicine as a whole is an information-centered activity; indeed, Friedman (1988) has suggested that pathologists are best described as information brokers. Although physicians have been managing information for more than a century, new tools have emerged in the past few decades to improve the accuracy and speed of this information management. These tools have enabled us to address issues that have been present since the beginning but that were unapproachable until the advent of automated information systems.

The most important benefit of computerized information processing is improvement in accuracy. When only humans were relied on, the 3% error rate inherent in human information processing was acceptable. Now that automated systems can eliminate transcription, calculation, and other such errors, this error rate is no longer acceptable. One would not patronize a bank in which one's account balance was calculated incorrectly 3% of the time. Why do physicians and the public continue to tolerate manual information processing in hospitals, where one can get the wrong medication, or the wrong dose, or the wrong time, 3% of the time?

With the low cost of powerful computer hardware and the ready availability of a wide range of commercially supported software packages to automate the processing of clinical laboratory data, every clinical laboratory in this country, whether it processes 10 samples or 1000 samples a day, should be using a computerized laboratory information system (LIS). That is to say, the use of a computerized LIS is now the *standard of practice* for clinical laboratories in the United States.

Focus on Information Management

This chapter focuses on information processing in medicine, with particular attention to laboratory medicine. It is crucial to recognize that information management is different from computer technology. It happens that computers are a useful tool to automate information handling. However, many of the important issues in informatics have little or nothing to do with computers and existed long before computers were available. Therefore, this chapter discusses computers only to the extent that they provide a useful tool in information management, rather than devoting attention to computer-specific issues and technology. Most of the principles discussed in this chapter would apply equally well if one were attempting to operate a laboratory without a computer; however, as emphasized previously, it is rarely appropriate (given today's tools) to process laboratory data manually.

Vocabulary

Modern informatics relies on many technologic tools, which are far too complex and detailed to be covered here. Just as in any other specialty of medicine, there is a large, complex vocabulary; in addition, rapid technologic advancement causes relatively rapid evolution of this vocabulary. With one exception (image management), this chapter does not attempt to teach the vocabulary of informatics. It does rely on the reader's familiarity with this vocabulary. The reader should pursue the following to become familiar with the definition and significance of the terms listed in Table 5–1:

1. Symposia, books, periodicals (Aller, 1983 and 1991; CAP TODAY; Elevitch, 1989; Friedman, 1992)
2. Purchase and use a personal computer (IBM-compatible, Macintosh, or possibly another variety)
3. Take introductory computer courses as offered at such places as your local library, adult education centers, high school
4. Read popular-level computer magazines (e.g., *PC Computing, MacUser, MacWorld, PC World, PC Magazine*)

Table 5–1. INFORMATICS: A NEW VOCABULARY/LANGUAGE

Hardware Terms

Data quantity/storage: bit, byte, kilobyte (KB), megabyte (MB), ASCII, RAM, ROM
CPU: Intel series (8086, 80286, 386, 486, Pentium), Motorola series (68000, 68030, 68040), RISC chips (e.g., PowerPC, DEC Alpha)
Speed: megahertz, MIPS, Specmarcs
Communications: modem, baud, RS232, parallel, LAN, Ethernet, TCP/IP, ATM
User interfaces: keyboard, monitor, terminal, CRT, VDU, workstation touch screen, mouse, digitizer pad, lightpen, voice I/O
Disk: magnetic (floppy, hard), optical (analog video disc, digital CD; read-only vs. writable, rewritable)
Magnetic tape: 9-track, cartridge, digital, DAT
Printers: dot matrix, inkjet, laser; fonts; TrueType, HP PCL, PostScript
Barcode: symbologies (Codabar, Code39, Code128, 16K, PDF), scanners (wand, CCD, laser), printers (e.g., thermal, thermal transfer)

Software Terms

Programming languages: FORTRAN, COBOL, MUMPS (M), C, C++, 4th generation (4GLs)
Operating systems: MS/DOS, OS/2, Finder, UNIX, VMS, VM, Windows NT, NextStep, others
Application programs, utilities, drivers
Databases: hierarchic, relational (SQL; Oracle, Sybase, MS Sequel Server), object-oriented
Database flags, dictionaries/tables
User interface design: bookmarking, graphic user interfaces (GUIs)
Security: Passwords, dialback modems, encryption, viruses, worms
Safety/hazard analysis, software testing, validation
Rapid prototyping, change control
Bugs, undocumented features, documented unfeatures, bit bucket
Software licensing, public domain, shareware
Fritterware (software that takes more time to learn than it would have taken to do the whole job by hand)
Download, upload
Clinical information processing scenarios (nonstandard but frequent)

Key Concepts for the Practicing Pathologist

Define and Solve the Problem

One should never computerize for its own sake. The problem must be precisely stated and the requirements clearly defined so that the solution to one problem does not disrupt other aspects of the manual and automated information processing systems.

Focus on the Information Needed

Clinicians are today deluged with words and numbers but often at a loss for information (data in context). Practitioners of laboratory medicine must ensure that the clinician has the information (without extraneous data) needed to care for the patient, when and where it is most helpful. The data available as a byproduct of the LIS should be used to continually improve the quality of laboratory performance. The laboratory database must be under the control of the laboratory director, and detailed data on test orders and results must remain available for years, for both patient care and laboratory management.

You Are the Expert

It is much easier to teach laboratorians what they need to know about computer technology than it is to teach a computer expert about the relevant aspects of laboratory practice (Elevitch, 1989). Although one must master a new and unfamiliar vocabulary, there is far more inherent complexity in the departmental operations of a laboratory than there is in the basic capabilities and characteristics of computer technology. Just as the laboratorian need not know how to design and construct a chemistry analyzer but only how to use and troubleshoot it, the pathologist does not have to have a degree in computer science to effectively use a commercially supported LIS.

Reliability Is a Two-Edged Sword

Computer programs perform much more reliably than human beings do. However, they are extremely literal and require detailed instructions. Because of their complexity, all medical computer programs contain so-called bugs, which cannot be eliminated by even exhaustive testing; therefore, laboratorians must learn to live with software problems and defects (Beizer, 1986). Although LIS managers may call these bugs mysterious evil forces, vendors have been known to refer to them (not entirely tongue in cheek) as undocumented features. It is essential that humans retain a healthy skepticism and not place undue reliance on the apparent judgment of the computer. Likewise, computer hardware is now extremely reliable but still fails at the most inconvenient time. Optimally, systems central to patient care functions should be fully redundant—at least two of every component, of which one will continue running if the other fails. Daily back-up copies of patient and operational data are essential and must be periodically rotated to another building (to enable recovery from a physical disaster in the computer room). Copies of all transactions must be journalized to enable complete recreation of the database without ever requiring manual re-entry.

Productivity and quality improvements are maximized if data is recorded once, directly into the computer. However, such a strategy is difficult to implement unless the physician, nurse, and other health care professionals can be assured that manual re-entry will never be required.

Personal versus Laboratory Computers

Personal computers fulfill an important role in the practice of laboratory medicine (see the subsequent discussion of the pathologist's workstation), both as single-user systems with advanced user interfaces and as tools for running standardized applications, such as word processing and spreadsheet what-if scenarios. Although important, an individual application may be optional or can be readily shifted to another computer if the primary personal computer is unavailable.

LISs, and beyond them clinical and community health information networks, emphasize multiple concurrent use of a shared database; disk contention, record locking, and network speed become critical issues. Applications are complex, interwoven, and custom tailored to an individual institution's patient mix and style of practice. Because the development and testing cycle is so prolonged, most useful systems today rely on primitive user interfaces (character-based terminals); efforts to migrate these systems to fully graphic user interfaces (like those of typical PC software) will take years. The LIS is a mission-critical tool—unlike the personal computer, the laboratory simply cannot run for more than a few hours without the LIS. We are relying more and more on these systems as time goes on. As bedside-based clinical information systems become more prevalent, even a few hours of downtime severely impairs the delivery of patient care; a new generation of systems is being designed that will involve no scheduled downtime.

Despite the apparent clarity of the distinction between personal computer applications and the laboratory-wide information system, many institutions are still afflicted by individuals suffering from "micromania and the instant expert syndrome" (McAlister, 1981), who believe that knowledge of a personal computer automatically conveys detailed understanding of the complexities of a full-fledged LIS.

Evolution and Revolution

To use the tool of information technology, one must both follow the rapid evolution of existing technologies and take notice of the introduction of revolutionary new technologies. The evolutionary increase in central processing unit (CPU) power and speed, in memory capacity, and in magnetic disk capacity have enabled software developers to continually increase the capability of software packages. Revolutions are occurring with more effective tools to craft software (client-server computing), low-cost publishing media such as CD-ROM, hardware and software adapted to image management, and new data acquisition technologies such as voice recognition.

Scope of Medical Informatics

Medical informatics is a diverse discipline that incorporates many aspects of the application of automated information technology to the advancement of medical science and practice (Shortliffe, 1990; Springer-Verlag series). The remainder of this chapter focuses on two of these aspects: clinical informatics and image processing. However, it is important to recognize the critical contributions of medical informatics to many other areas, such as physiologic modeling and the creation of medical instrumentation (Clark, 1992), medical education and training (Henry, 1990), and the fascinating detective story of the human genome project and the genetic epidemiology of disease (Skolnick, 1990).

CLINICAL INFORMATICS

American Board of Pathology Definition

The American Board of Pathology has defined clinical laboratory informatics as "that aspect of the practice of pathology which focuses on the management (generation, collection, organization, validation, processing, storage, integration, interpretation, communication, and presentation) of information and systems in support of patient care decision-making, education, and research" (Balis, 1993, page 545). This is in every respect as complex and demanding a scope of study as transfusion medicine or medical microbiology but without the benefit of 50 years of intellectual development. Nevertheless, it will constitute an ever-expanding portion of the practice of clinical pathology in the coming decades.

Generation

Data come to us from many different sources—from the primary patient encounter as the history and physical examination, from physician and nursing observations, from outcome measurements such as patient satisfaction questionnaires, from human-interpreted morphologic studies, from laboratory instruments, and from automated analyses of waveforms and images. Part of the role of the clinical pathologist is to help the clinician determine which of these data sources (e.g., diagnostic tests) will be most effective in the diagnosis and management of his or her patient.

Collection

Effective use of automated information processing tools requires that the data needed for clinical decision-making be converted into electronic form—if possible, *directly from the primary source*. Physicians (Bria, 1992), nurses, patients, and others making observations must interact directly with the computer in a structured fashion. Direct order entry by physicians reduces cost of care (Tierney, 1993) and malpractice claims. Input modalities are now widely diverse; they include keyboard, barcode, touch screen, mouse, optical character recognition (OCR), handwriting recognition, and voice input. Each of these could in itself be a useful chapter in a textbook on efficient and accurate medical care. Barcode technology has proved to be a particularly high-yield, low-cost application in the laboratory (Aller, 1994a; Dito, 1992), and the ASTM E1466–92 standard for its use has been published (ASTM, 1995).

Often, the information needed can be acquired from another computer (e.g., hospital admitting system) or electronic device (e.g., laboratory instrument). Many components of the electronic medical record (Institute of Medicine, 1991) can be assembled today by simply gathering together data that are already in electronic form somewhere in the institution. In striving to continually lower the error rates in health care, a good case can be made for interfacing *every* instrument in the laboratory that can send results to the LIS.

Organization

As noted earlier, information must be organized and structured for it to be used by computer programs. The basic element of organization in a patient-centered clinical information system is a unique identification of the patient. Amazingly, such a basic item as a permanent, nationwide patient identification number seems to remain a holy grail; it has been estimated that it would cost several billion dollars to issue a new national health identification number. Therefore, despite its shortcomings, the social security number will probably have to serve this purpose for several years. Any procedure or observation on a patient must be unequivocally linked to the correct patient's record. At present, the most practical technology to accomplish this in the inpatient setting seems to be a wristband containing a barcoded patient number, together with barcode-reading personal work systems carried (and *used*) by everyone who provides care to that patient. In the outpatient setting, requesting a picture ID when drawing blood may be appropriate; in the longer term, new biometric devices such as electronic thumbprint or iris scanners may become feasible.

A second fundamental of information organization is the structuring of diagnostic and procedural coding. The systems commonly required for governmental reporting and billing (ICD-9-CM and CPT) were originally designed for classifying causes of death and for requesting payment for medical procedures; these systems are far too aggregated to be used for electronic medical records. The Systematized Nomenclature of Medicine (SNOMED International) (Cote, 1993) is the most promising tool for detailed recording of findings, diagnoses, and procedures.

Validation

Validation presents a dual challenge: to ensure that the patient-related information flowing into laboratory and clinical information systems is valid, and to ensure that the systems themselves have been thoroughly tested. Quality control and assurance are reviewed in Chapter 6, and the reader is referred to the extensive published literature on regulation and validation of medical information systems (Aller, 1992; Brannigan, 1992; Steane, 1989–1994).

Processing

Computers are very useful and effective for some applications (information retrieval, calculations, data transmission), whereas humans are far more effective for others (judgment, reasoning from incomplete data). Systems should be predicated on this, rather than devoting undue emphasis to artificial intelligence. Structured, rule-based decision support systems will be very helpful in improving the quality of care; on the other hand, systems should continue to support human judgment. Ongoing challenges in health care information processing include keeping multiple diverse computer databases synchronized and conveying knowledge of critical logic paths from a domain expert to a computer programmer (knowledge engineering). Some areas, such as the conversion of textual information to structured knowledge, remain the domain of basic research in computer science and informatics.

Important architectural issues include the concept of open systems as well as client-server computing; object-oriented analysis, design, and programming; and networking and communications technology (Tapscott, 1993).

Storage

Long-term storage of patient data is no longer an issue of the physical capacity of storage devices but rather of the ability to retrieve these data in a complete yet focused and structured manner. The overnight conversion of all medical records to electronic form by scanning-in images of all the paper documents would be a disaster for American health care. For care of an individual patient, the system must be able to rapidly retrieve a few key facts pertinent to a particular problem out of several million characters of data that could accumulate in even a short, acute-care hospitalization. The medical record also serves an important medical-legal and regulatory role, and the electronic implementations must satisfy authentication and retention requirements.

Eventually, these patient-specific databases will evolve into the electronic medical record (Ball, 1992; Institute of Medicine, 1991). Already, some physicians' offices have reduced physical retrievals of the paper chart by 75%, and others have completely eliminated the paper medical record.

The pathologist and other clinicians must also be conversant with local and national databases containing information on groups of patients, on the opinions of experts (American Medical Association, 1995), and on the medical literature (MEDLINE). Database design and structure (relational, hierarchic, object-oriented) must become familiar concepts, as must the tools to access them (particularly the System/Structured Query Language, or SQL).

Integration

As an informaticist, the clinical pathologist must move beyond the boundaries of the laboratory and become conversant with the distinct information processing requirements of many other areas in the hospital: radiology/imaging, respiratory therapy, nutrition and dietary, operating room, anesthesia, pharmacy, medical transcription and records, quality improvement, delivery room, emergency department, and dozens of others. The pathologist must move even further, beyond the doors of the hospital, and recognize the seemingly unique needs of group practices, physician's offices, managed care organizations, and home health.

But why? To a very real degree, the pathologist's practice will be guided by the needs of the health care–wide information network. In its responsibility to the clinician to provide relevant information for patient care, the laboratory must collate laboratory data with those produced in many other disciplines. Not only must the clinician have an integrated, longitudinal view of all data on a patient (to avoid "hunting and gathering" of data), the clinical pathologist must provide automated guidance on diagnostic and therapeutic choices and must automate correlation of key results with clinical follow-up. The pathologist must ensure that the loop has been closed—it is no longer acceptable to send out a thyroid stimulating hormone result which is pathognomonic of hypothyroidism and merely assume that the clinician will see and act on this information. Such laboratory results can be electronically correlated with discharge diagnoses, ambulatory problem lists, and pharmaceutical orders to ensure that results have been appropriately recognized and acted on.

Interpretation

Interpretation of laboratory findings has long been recognized as a key professional role of the pathologist. Information tools now automate some of this process, and they make meaningful and useful interpretive information much more widely available. Practice parameters, flow charts, algorithms, panels, and even administrative procedures are more uniformly implemented with computer-based reminders. Knowledge-based systems have made great strides, and their dissemination will be facilitated by the standardized ASTM E1460–92 (Arden) syntax for sharing of medical knowledge rules (ASTM, 1995). More sophisticated techniques, including neural networks, decision analysis, Bayesian analysis, and fuzzy logic, are being implemented in specific domains. Statistical tools, receiver-operating-characteristic curves, and other techniques are achieving wider acceptance.

As noted earlier, the pathologist not only must interpret laboratory findings but he or she must ensure that appropriate action ensues. Informatics provides a wide selection of new effector mechanisms:

- Reflexive testing, in which the results of one or more analyses trigger the performance of a confirmatory or supplementary test, may even be built into the analytical instrument
- Reminders can be provided as part of the routine laboratory report
- Clinical alerts can be communicated more rapidly to the clinician, as discussed subsequently

Communications and Standards

No one seems to notice the road, except when it is full of potholes. By the same token, the communications infrastructure of medicine must be transparent to the user. To enable this, a wide variety of physical and logical communication protocols have been established (e.g., Ethernet, TCP/IP, Token Ring). Standards for packaging of information have been developed, such as the Standard Generalized Markup Language (SGML), which many feel will be the core of future electronic medical records systems. The need for record format and content standards has become glaringly apparent as medical informaticists have attempted to connect diverse medical systems. In a pessimistic view, the wonderful thing about standards is that there are so many to choose from. In reality, health care has come to remarkable agreement on a number of communications standards, as listed in Table 5–2.

Advances in communications technology have provided many innovative methods for communicating laboratory results to the clinician in addition to the traditional printed reports: inquiry/display terminals, voice output, beeper activation, fax, office and home computers, and wireless links to hand-held workstations.

Electronic mail is a key management tool within the laboratory (to enable reliable communication with all staff members, on three shifts, seven days a week). It will be even more critical to the practice of laboratory medicine, because access from one's desktop to the Internet will make a worldwide network of consultants immediately available to even the most geographically isolated solo practitioner of clinical pathology.

Presentation

The formatting of printed reports and screen displays (Connelly, 1995) is an entire science in itself (Tufte, 1990), and deserves far more attention by the pathologist and other laboratorians than it has traditionally received. The clinician must be able to quickly look at a report and gather the most significant information from it without being distracted or confused by reference ranges, units, or extraneous data. Reports should be organized in a pathophysiologic fashion—thus, ferritin should be listed with complete blood count

Table 5–2. EXAMPLES OF STANDARDS FOR HEALTH CARE INFORMATION SYSTEMS

HL7—admission/discharge/transfer, orders, others
ASTM E1238-94—clinical observations
ACR/NEMA DICOM 3.0—images
ANSI X12—billing
HIBCC (Health Industries Business Communication Council)—barcode
EUCLIDES, LOINC—naming of clinical laboratory tests

All of these standards are coordinated through the Healthcare Information Standards Planning Panel, American National Standards Institute, New York, NY.

(CBC), mean corpuscular volume (MCV), iron, and vitamin B_{12}, rather than with immunoassays. The chart output from the SMA-12 instrument, popular in the 1970s, allowed the clinician to understand the results of a chemistry profile far more rapidly than currently available tabular listings of numeric values; the use of graphic and semigraphic displays in future versions of LISs will increase.

High-quality, low-cost hardcopy output devices are now readily available—laser and other technologies allow resolution of 300 dots per inch (DPI) or higher for well under $500; for selected types of graphic data presentation, color printers enable us to convey information more effectively. To achieve the best results, the information system should make full use of a downloaded printer programming language, such as PostScript. The high quality thus achievable can now be electronically mapped onto a fax transmission. Despite the battle cry to do away with the paper chart, laboratories will have to produce paper reports of their results for many years to come.

Screen displays offer many advantages, including the ability to customize the format and content to the needs of the individual user. However, one must be careful to not go overboard and use 20 different colors or thousands of different, obscure icons. Likewise, the maintenance overhead to support customized views for hundreds of different physicians may be excessive. As physicians' workstations become more common, the art of screen design will increase in importance.

Safeguarding of Patient Data

Security and access control (Donaldson, 1994) are crucial components of clinical informatics. Patients expect health care professionals to treat their information confidentially; this requires the use of tools that do not compromise this confidentiality. At the same time, the informaticist must ensure the integrity and safety of the data; clinicians will use a system for their primary medical records only if they can be assured that no data will be lost. Safeguarding incorporates system integrity and reliability (discussed previously), access control (password protection and limited access to modification of the database, security against phone line or network access by hackers), and patient confidentiality (e.g., limiting access to only those with a need to know and logging all who have inquired on each patient's data). Again, this domain is not limited to computer use but includes the use of paper shredders to destroy handwritten records before they are sent to the paper recycler.

Systems Selection, Implementation, and Management

The first step in acquisition of an automated information system, as noted earlier, is to define the objectives of that system. Next, one must analyze the economic and quality aspects to justify the cost. Selection of a vendor, contracting, implementation, and ongoing management of the system complete the process.

Definition of Objectives; Systems Analysis

Before embarking on selection and implementation of an LIS, the laboratory staff must clearly define what is to be accomplished by the project. What problems are being addressed, and what are the objectives? This can only be accomplished by a careful analysis of the present (manual or computerized) laboratory system—what are its shortcomings, and what are its benefits? If the present manual system has been operating without problems or significant limitations, computerization is likely to worsen the situation. However, manual systems invariably *do* have important limitations—not the least of which is inability to detect most errors of omission. Laboratories of *any* size can now benefit from computerized LISs. Table 5–3 lists some possible benefits of installing a computerized LIS. However, one cannot assume that implementation of a computer system will automatically solve a laboratory's organizational problems. Introduction of a computer system into a poorly organized environment may even worsen operations. On the other hand, it also forces one to confront and deal with problems that may have been ignored previously.

Selection and implementation of the LIS should involve as many of the laboratory staff members as possible. In addition, other members of the hospital staff, including the medical, nursing, medical records, and information systems staffs, should participate in and support the project. A key decision is to select the most capable member of your technical staff, a person who is thoroughly familiar with the operation of the laboratory, to be system manager and project leader.

Cost Justification

Having compiled an analysis of the specific benefits a computer system will provide to the laboratory, one must then show how these benefits will justify purchase and ongoing maintenance of such a system.

Typically, information systems increase the productivity of laboratory personnel. In some settings, it is possible to decrease personnel levels enough to pay for the system (Hendricks, 1985); in others, staffing levels are dictated by shift and departmental coverage requirements, and it is therefore difficult to reduce the staff. In either case, the laboratory will be able to increase its capacity as repetitive clerical tasks are streamlined and attention can be devoted to tasks requiring human interpretation.

Table 5–3. BENEFITS OF INSTALLING A COMPUTERIZED LABORATORY INFORMATION SYSTEM

Reduced errors
Mischarted reports
Specimen mix-ups
Calculation errors
Transcription errors
Errors of omission
Reduction in lost charges (improved revenue)
Improved staff productivity
More rapid availability of results for phone inquiries
Transmission of laboratory results to remote locations
Improved turnaround time
Improved patient reports
Legibility
Multiple copies
Cumulative
Interpretive
Graphic
Improved information for management
Better data for quality assurance

An important caveat must be observed: not all commercially available LISs improve productivity. Indeed, some require considerably *more* staff time (e.g., clerical entry area) than the manual system they replace. For example, the number of keystrokes (and amount of staff time) required to enter the order for a 7 A.M. hemoglobin varies fourfold or more between different vendors' systems. Therefore, efficiency should be an important selection criterion in the evaluation of vendors.

Another major justification deserves more attention than it traditionally receives. An important characteristic of computerized information systems is their ability to reduce errors. As attention is devoted to deriving the maximum benefit from every health care dollar spent, error prevention may become the primary justification for many systems.

Finally, computerized information systems provide us with some abilities not otherwise feasible—particularly in the areas of result reporting and management analysis. Appropriate interpretive comments can be automatically attached to reports, reflex tests can be automatically performed, and results can be transmitted to printers hundreds of miles away. Ongoing monitoring of laboratory performance, such as turnaround times, no longer requires a prohibitive investment of time and clerical effort. Capture of data for laboratory management may be the most clearly definable benefit. Systems also provide the detailed record-keeping and audit trails required by regulatory agencies.

Make or Buy?

Some laboratorians, enchanted by the power of the newest PC database tools, will conclude that they should proceed to design and implement a comprehensive LIS themselves. In other settings, the hospital data processing department will insist that the laboratory can be implemented on the reserve capacity of the hospital financial computer. Neither course of action is advisable in the present environment. Instead, choose a vendor-developed and vendor-supported system designed to optimize laboratory function, for a variety of reasons:

Clinical laboratories, and the information systems designed to serve them, are tremendously complex operations. For example, one popular LIS contains more than 7000 distinct modules. Another contains more than 10 million lines of COBOL code.

Successful development of a fully functional system is unlikely; there is an extremely high risk of failure, and an unpredictably high cost.

The *de novo* creator of an LIS is committed to ongoing maintenance and upgrades of that system as the laboratory's requirements evolve. Experience has shown that this maintenance and evolutionary process is often more complex and costly than the design and implementation of the first version of the system.

Design input from a broad base of users (from many different institutions) results in systems with far broader and deeper capabilities than a system designed from the point of view of only one institution.

A laboratory with a so-called home grown system must bear the costs of any necessary program updates and new instrument interfaces by itself instead of being able to split these costs among several users.

A responsible vendor, serving dozens of laboratories, will continue updating its system to keep up with changing requirements and will be able to maintain a much larger staff than would be financially feasible for any individual laboratory.

The laboratory with a home grown system becomes dependent on maintaining an in-house programming staff and may be crippled if a key staff member moves on to another job.

Vendors now serve a wide variety of laboratory types and needs, and most laboratories should be able to find a vendor that fits well with their strategic plan and environmental constraints. The old adage "there is nothing new under the sun" is operative, and a previously installed software module comes with significant debugging already performed. However, an agreement should be worked out with the vendor to allow you to do some program development without interfering with the evolution of the rest of the system. Indeed, larger and more complex laboratories may well seek a cooperative, alpha- or beta-site relationship with their chosen software vendor in which laboratory staff members can enhance the software and the vendor can incorporate these enhancements into its standard software package.

Vendor Selection

In choosing an LIS vendor, one is entering into a long-term partnership, with great impact on the future ability of the laboratory to grow, to provide top quality services to the patient, and to compete in the laboratory marketplace. Therefore, it is crucial that one choose a partner who will be well equipped to support the laboratory's needs and goals in the long term. Since the 1980s, there has been an overemphasis on selecting systems with a given checklist of characteristics (e.g., a detailed scoring system, which emphasizes that vendor A has subfeature 1.653, whereas vendor B lacks this) and often too little consideration for the vendor's corporate philosophy, attitude toward its users, and the like.

To begin gathering information, first consult published lists of vendors. *CAP TODAY* (College of American Pathologists, 325 Waukegan Road, Northfield, IL 60093-2750) publishes five surveys per year, each focusing on a different type of laboratory or clinical information system. Most vendors exhibit at the American Society of Clinical Pathologists/College of American Pathologists fall national meetings and other meetings (Table 5–4). Visit other laboratories to gain some general ideas of how they are supported by their vendors.

The next step is to prepare a brief summary of your laboratory and its requirements, and send this summary to 10 or 15 of the more promising vendors, as a request for information, or a request for quotation—this request should ask for a *complete* list of user sites. The vendors' responses to this request, plus telephone reference checks with a number of sites, should allow you to further narrow the field to four to six semi-finalists, all of whom appear to have the ability and experience to support your laboratory.

Table 5–4. WHERE TO FIND INFORMATION

National meetings: ASCP/CAP, other laboratory meetings (AABB, CLMA, AACC), American Medical Informatics Association (AMIA), Healthcare Information and Management Systems Society (HIMSS)
Journals: *CAP TODAY*, other standard lab journals, plus the journals of the AMIA and the HIMSS, and newsletters: *Inside Healthcare Computing, National Report on Computers and Health.*
National informatics courses: University of Michigan, Harvard, Stanford, Utah
User group meetings (annual and regional)
Colleagues (local, at national meetings, via E-mail)
The Internet and other online services:
CompuServe MedSig
PathInfo (contact: Spackman@ohsu.edu)
User-group-specific list servers (e.g., CernerUG@lists.utah.edu)
Technical magazines:
PC, PC World, InfoWorld
MacUser, MacWorld, MacWeek
Vendor training
Site visits
CAP and AABB inspections (inspector or inspectee)
Residency training
Preceptorships, fellowships

Site visits are the most valuable tool in the selection of the finalists. Ideally, the visiting team should include bench-level technologists and clerks as well as supervisors, managers, and pathologists; it is also desirable to include representatives of the hospital information systems department and the hospital vice president or administrator responsible for the laboratory. A group of four to eight is an appropriate size.

The prospective customer should be permitted to visit any site on the user list—if the vendor objects, is this because the site is unhappy with the vendor and its service? In selecting sites to visit, choose those of approximately the same size as your own laboratory. Some systems that function well in the smaller laboratory suffer unacceptable performance degradation when transaction volume exceeds a certain critical figure; for example, the system may pass all transactions through a single process, which becomes a bottleneck at a certain transaction rate. Likewise, some systems appropriate for large laboratories turn out to have large amounts of personnel overhead (e.g., required database maintenance) that is unacceptable to the smaller laboratory. Some of these larger systems have so many interacting options and control tables that full-time system manager attention is required to keep the system operational.

A productive technique is to arrange to have dinner with the director the preceding evening and ask permission to visit the evening shift; evening shift members are more often independent and are generally willing to tell an attentive listener about shortcomings as well as advantages. When one is equipped with this insight, the official site visit beginning the next morning can be much more informative. Free exchange of opinions and observations can be inhibited by the presence of a vendor representative. Likewise, after the initial introductions, the visiting chiefs (director, laboratory manager) should sit down with the site's chiefs (who chose this system and may be unwilling to admit that they bought a lemon), while the other staff on the site visit team disperse into the laboratory to talk to the bench technologists and find out how well the system *really* works.

A single site visit is *not* sufficient to evaluate fully a vendor or its system; even a disastrous visit could have been to an outlier laboratory that is not making proper use of the software. Likewise, a very positive site visit to a site carefully selected by the vendor may represent close personal (or even financial) links between vendor and site.

Pay particular attention to how well the system adapts to each laboratory that you visit. If each laboratory seems to function in exactly the same manner, this may reflect rigidity of the software—the laboratory had to change its operation to fit the computer.

You should also determine if the systems of particular interest have an active users' group; talk to the officers of that users' group. Such groups can be useful in guiding ongoing development of a vendor's product.

Having narrowed your field to two or three finalists, you may wish to send out a formal request for proposal (RFP). In the past, this was standard practice; unfortunately, laboratories began sending 250-page wish lists to 15 vendors. Many vendors could not afford to reply to these massive (and often ambiguous) questionnaires. Laboratories often eliminated some vendors on a few key points and did not even read the reams of paper a vendor had spent thousands of dollars to compile. Therefore, if you do choose to send an RFP, it should be only at the final stage of vendor evaluation (the vendors should be informed that they are one of three, not one of 15), and it should be *brief.* The RFP is, in essence, your business plan for this large new investment—so even if you choose not to send it out, you should probably write one. Lincoln (1991) has provided a sample outline for an RFP, but do not feel obligated to write a page, or even a paragraph, on each topic. Emphasize key and unique features about the laboratory and its needs; do not rehash capabilities that you already know are standard in all three vendors' products. If the RFP document is longer than 30 or 40 pages, you should condense it. Again, the RFP responses will provide valuable supplemental information, but the primary data source for the final vendor decision should be the site visits.

You should consider the stability and long-term viability of both the hardware and the software vendors. One is generally best advised to choose a system running on a standard, widely installed hardware line (e.g., Hewlett Packard, SUN, DEC, IBM, Apple Macintosh, IBM-compatible PCs ["Industry Standard Architecture"]). On the other hand, the history of laboratory *software* support by large hardware vendors has been dismal: IBM, DEC, Honeywell, and Control Data have all at one time marketed a laboratory software product, then dropped or sold that division.

A final consideration is the federal government requirements for registration of certain LIS software as a medical device. This is particularly a concern for software to be used in a blood bank or transfusion service. This area is in a state of great flux; you should verify that your vendor of choice has registered and tested its software to the extent required by current (and potential) regulations and guidelines (Table 5–5). When the Food and Drug Administration (FDA) first began regulating blood bank software, they approached the field with the expectation that software suppliers had built their systems, five or ten years previously, with formal specification, validation, and change control procedures typical of those used in the pharmaceutical industry. The FDA has since expressed an interest in regulating other areas of medical soft-

Table 5-5. AGENCIES, ORGANIZATIONS, AND REGULATIONS THAT AFFECT CLINICAL INFORMATION SYSTEMS

College of American Pathologists Laboratory Accreditation Program, section I
American Association of Blood Banks
Food and Drug Administration
Joint Commission on Accreditation of Healthcare Organizations (information management section)
Clinical Laboratory Improvement Act (CLIA-88), especially the cytology section

ware. It would therefore seem prudent to apply the blood bank standards of software validation (Steane, 1989–1994) to general LISs.

Contracting

Having decided on the vendor of choice, one must negotiate a contract with that vendor. The vendor will no doubt have a draft ready to present to you. You should seek the advice of legal counsel, preferably someone familiar with computer law, and negotiate toward a balanced contract that does not unduly favor either the vendor or the client. Please consult Lincoln (1991) and Elevitch (1992) for detailed coverage, but important points and common clauses include the following:

1. Ground rules for acceptance and for payment for hardware, software, training, and implementation: The system should be accepted, and paid for, in at least three parts:

- Hardware, systems software, and general utilities
- Applications software, utilities, and training (the laboratory system)
- Live operation of the system in *your* laboratory, including both proper function and adequate performance (e.g., response time of less than 2 seconds 95% of the time during peak load conditions and with a fully loaded database [several months of "live" data])

As implementation progresses, each of these components is accepted and paid for. The final 25% of payment should be withheld until all contractual obligations have been satisfied and the system has been operating satisfactorily in a so-called live mode for at least 60 days. All vendors have a responsibility to test proper operation of software; although federal regulations in some areas (e.g., blood banking) are beginning to assure an acceptable level of reliability, most laboratory software users are still well advised to use the principle of *caveat emptor*—let the buyer beware! It remains the user's responsibility to fully validate proper operation of the system.

2. Hardware and software warrantee: For at least 90 days after live date, preferably for one year, any errors identified in that time will be fixed free of extra charge.

3. Guarantee of maintenance availability: The vendor guarantees that hardware and software will be maintained for at least five years after live date, and vendor staff will be available for emergency problems 24 hours a day, 7 days a week, 365 days per year. The details of software maintenance, including cost, are covered in a separate maintenance agreement, commonly included as an appendix or attachment to the contract. Another common provision is that the cost of software maintenance will increase by no more than $x\%$ per year—x is usually tied to the Consumer Price Index to correct for inflation. Interestingly, some vendors, recognizing that the laboratory is actually contracting for an ongoing service (software function) rather than purchasing a static set of software, no longer charge an initial software license fee. These vendors now rely entirely on a monthly software use and maintenance fee, equivalent to a rental. However, they may also charge a hefty installation and training fee.

4. Source code availability: If the vendor becomes unable or unwilling to maintain the system, how will the laboratory obtain maintenance? In the absence of source code (the original computer programs used to create the operational computer system), this can be exceedingly difficult. The best solution is for the laboratory to be given a set of the source code, maintained on-site; typically, the contract includes a nondisclosure clause, preventing the laboratory from distributing this source code to others. However, given the complexity of design, implementation, and maintenance of a modern LIS, the source code would be of rather little use to a competitor. A much less desirable alternative is for the source code to be held in an escrow account, by an independent third party (such as an attorney); the contract then provides that the source code be given to the laboratory if the vendor is unable to provide maintenance services for a set time period (e.g., 72 hours of unresponsiveness). In either case, it is essential that the copy of the source code held by the laboratory, or by the third party, be continually updated.

5. Required modifications and enhancements in the system: Frequently, in evaluating a vendor's system, the laboratory finds that there are a few slight modifications that would enhance function. If the vendor and user agree on these, and they can be integrated into the standard system (e.g., controlled by database flags, so they only appear if the flags are set), then they should be listed in an attachment to the contract. However, the number of these modifications should be minimized—the history of LISs is replete with laboratories paying tens of thousands of dollars for modifications, then installing the system and finding that the standard system renders the special capabilities unnecessary.

6. Standard system: The standard system clause states that the software being installed, including modifications just noted, will be the vendor's standard system. The vendor will endeavor to install this same software in all its sites. Any future enhancements or releases of the software made by the vendor will be on this platform, so that it will be easy for the laboratory to install future releases.

7. Performance guarantee: This specifies that the system will provide certain maximum response times, print times, and other performance benchmarks over some projected time period (e.g., three years) that is based on assumptions about volume growth and system use. This avoids the scenario of the vendor who has quoted an intentionally too-small computer configuration to make their system price more competitive. Even with appropriate initial sizing, system performance has been a problematic area. New releases of software are often far less efficient than the preceding release, and it may be necessary for the client site to budget for hardware upgrades every two years simply to accommodate the decreasing efficiency of vendor software.

8. RFP response is a part of this contract: The vendor was selected, in part, on the basis of responses made to an RFP. This clause gives the vendor's guarantee that all statements made in the response are accurate. For example, if the response states that the vendor's system can produce a report doing A, B, and C, and the user installs the vendor's system, only to discover that the report fails to do C, the vendor is then obligated without additional charge to modify the program so that it has the claimed capability.

9. Software efficacy as demonstrated in site visits: One of the best and abbreviated ways to ensure efficacy in a system is to require that functions demonstrated during a site visit (or set of visits) will be included in the system installed in the user site.

10. Ongoing upgrades and enhancements: As a vendor continues to develop its system and install it in new sites, the software will continue to evolve. All sites running the software should periodically (usually yearly) be brought up to date to the current version. This update should be done as a part of the regular software maintenance agreement, without an extra charge, and should include all enhancements made for the modules the laboratory is running. (Although such enhancements may be expected to affect system performance to some degree, the vendor has a duty to avoid major degradation of system performance when introducing new features.) If the vendor introduces a brand new module (e.g., blood bank, radiology), this would reasonably require an additional license fee.

11. The vendor guarantees to keep its system in compliance with current and future state and federal requirements and with requirements of accrediting agencies (such as the CAP and AABB); all sites paying regular maintenance fees will receive such updates without additional charge.

If the proper vendor has been selected and the laboratory is reasonable and fair in its approach to the vendor, you should be able to sign the contract, put it on the shelf, and never have to look at it again. The basis of a good user-vendor relationship is communication and mutual trust and respect. If you cannot trust the vendor, the most finely honed contract in the world will not rescue the situation. However, a properly worded contract can avoid future misunderstandings between the parties.

Implementation, Maintenance, and Evaluation

Now that the system is justified, the vendor is selected, and the contract is signed, the most important part has just begun! Perhaps this is a bit overstated, but it points out that implementation is the key to the success of your system. As observed earlier, your most capable staff member should be appointed system manager—computer knowledge is not important; knowledge of the laboratory practices, policies, and procedures is.

System configuration decisions must be made; this may be a good time to make one or two additional site visits to see how successful users of the system have set up their dictionaries and operation. The final location of workstations and printers must be decided.

The vendor will train the laboratory staff on construction of the dictionaries that describe the laboratory and its operation. After this training, the entire laboratory must be encoded into this unfamiliar format, then entered into a computer; often, the vendor will provide a small "loaner" system at this time to enable keying of the dictionaries before the main laboratory computer has been installed.

Site preparation means making the laboratory environment ready for computer installation. In the past, this was an extremely costly prospect, entailing locked, air-conditioned rooms with raised flooring, special power supplies, and cabling. Environmental requirements for modern hardware are becoming less stringent, but clean, consistent power is still a necessity, and investing in an uninterruptable power supply is usually worthwhile. Physically, the computer can be placed within the main laboratory room but avoid areas where reagents or water may be splashed into it! If the computer is in a separate room, a fire suppression system is an appropriate investment. LIS data storage is more secure than manual data, because an additional (back-up) copy of the data may be kept at a remote site, immune from even a devastating fire.

As with any other laboratory instrument, the operation and maintenance of the LIS are best placed under the control of the laboratory. Because it is a computer and may have special environmental requirements, the hardware is often placed in a central hospital computer room. However, if computer operations are managed outside the laboratory, the challenge of maintaining communication and ensuring that the system is optimally supporting the function of the laboratory is greater. In general, the greater the degree to which the laboratory feels a sense of ownership of the system, the more satisfactorily the system will function.

Requisitions and report forms must be designed, and these and other supplies needed for computer operations must be ordered.

When the hardware is installed, the vendor will verify that it is functioning properly and correct any problems. The vendor-specific laboratory software is then loaded, and the training of the laboratory staff can begin. In some cases, a few key laboratory staff members are trained at the vendor's headquarters; in other cases, this is done at the user's site. In either instance, it is expected that the key laboratory staff members will, in turn, train all other laboratory staff members; it is best to have at least one, and preferably two, key individuals on each shift and in each major department. The work schedule must allow for adequate time for training and practice.

As a part of the implementation procedure, laboratory staff members must verify and validate proper operation of the major vendor software modules. This should follow a formal protocol, including normal, abnormal, *and* invalid data for all fields, and the validation should be carefully documented (to be available for future laboratory inspections). The parallel test is *not* sufficient for this purpose but may still be advisable. However, the length of time for parallel operation should be minimized, because the system will not be fully utilized until there is no alternative.

A detailed account of the many activities necessary to ensure continued operation of the laboratory computer is beyond the scope of this chapter. However, these activities should include the following:

1. New procedures must be established to ensure proper operation of the new laboratory instrument—the computer. In most cases, rather than simply reproducing the

vendor's materials, it is appropriate to prepare laboratory-specific user manuals. For sections that already have established procedure manuals (e.g., hematology), these materials can consist of additional notes attached to each procedure, describing, for example, how worklists for that procedure are printed, how results are entered, and the handling of critical values. Brand new procedure manuals must be prepared for computer operations, such as making back-up copies of the database (typically done daily) and printing patient reports.
2. A plan must be developed and periodically practiced to ensure continuing laboratory operations and provision of laboratory service even when the computer is temporarily out of operation.
3. Security policies must be defined and implemented to protect laboratory data against both unauthorized modification and inappropriate access and breach of patient confidentiality.

Excellent reference sources that list the standard operating procedures needed for the computer include the CAP Laboratory Accreditation Program (College of American Pathologists, 1995), and section 14 of the AABB Accreditation Requirements Manual (Sazama, 1995).

Workers outside the laboratory must be trained on the new system as well—even if nurses will not be entering laboratory orders into the hospital computer, they must be trained to use the new test request forms that usually accompany a new system. Medical staff members must be educated about the new laboratory reports; even so, after six months of speaking at medical staff meetings, papering the hospital with notices and examples of the new reports, and an all-staff mailing two weeks before implementation, do not be surprised if a few physicians walk into your office the day after you go live, demanding to know "What's this?"

The first few days, or sometimes weeks, after implementation of a new LIS are often traumatic. Errors in the dictionary descriptions of laboratory activities are discovered and must be rapidly corrected. If the vendor has made additions to its software as part of the laboratory's contract, these new features will often prove problematic at first. Nursing and medical staff members will have questions about test ordering and report interpretation. Laboratory workers will still be relatively unfamiliar with the new computer functions and so will work more slowly. However, within a few weeks after implementation, a well-engineered system will typically smooth out, and the laboratory staff will soon begin asking themselves how they ever got along without it.

After implementation, the system must be maintained—not only must printers be periodically vacuumed to remove paper dust and ribbons changed so reports remain readable, but the dictionary files must be continuously updated to reflect the current operation of the laboratory. Whenever a new test is established, all the required elements must be defined in the dictionary; as reference ranges or test methods change, these must be updated. Periodically, prices are updated, and the laboratory files must keep pace. Dictionary updates are particularly challenging and critical when two systems (e.g., hospital information system and LIS) must be kept in synchronization. In a large laboratory, the job of system manager can easily occupy a technologist's full time. Even in the smaller laboratory, it is important to allocate some time specifically to these activities, or the laboratory will begin to suffer as the system tables no longer match laboratory practice.

Having expended dollars and time to select, purchase, and install an LIS, one should evaluate the final product (Anderson, 1994). Six to nine months after implementation, determine if the objectives that had been defined at the beginning have been met. Have errors been reduced? Is productivity improving? Are reports easier to read, and are result inquiries handled more promptly? Has turnaround time improved?

From the time of implementation, there is a need for almost continuous software upgrade and expansion of system capacity (e.g., additional workstations, printers, software modules). Fortunately, such upgrades are often possible within the capacity of the original central hardware configuration; this is a potent argument against beginning operation of an LIS on a fully utilized machine with no spare capacity. Part of the ongoing evaluation of the LIS should be assessment of its present capacity and prediction of when major additions to capacity will be needed. Within two to three years of implementation, if the original computer was appropriately sized, the laboratory should begin planning for a major hardware upgrade. Hardware cost is now decreasing so rapidly that it is unwise to buy too much excess capacity initially. Also, the annual maintenance costs on older hardware can quickly exceed the entire purchase price of a newer, higher-capacity set of hardware. Even if testing volume does not increase, the laboratory will gradually make more complete use of computer functions as all staff members become more familiar with them. As the database grows, more computer resources will be required. Functionality, as well as its evolution, should also be evaluated. If the computer system is becoming an impediment to laboratory operation because of faulty software design or poor vendor support, the search for another software vendor should begin. With the prolonged capital equipment cycles found in many hospitals (up to two years is typical), hardware or software replacement budgeting should begin when the first hint of a problem appears, not when the laboratory's function is being severely impaired.

Regulatory and Accreditation Issues

In recent years, the attention of regulatory agencies and accrediting organizations (see Table 5–5) to medical information systems has increased greatly. Obtain and read a copy of the standards and requirements from each of these agencies and organizations. Even when the focus appears to be different, most aspects of the computer requirements are useful (e.g., the AABB requirements are helpful in evaluating management of the microbiology computer system).

Clinical Informatics in the Practice of Medicine

The tools and techniques discussed in this chapter are becoming central to the practice of medicine (Aller, 1994a; Lincoln, 1980). Clinical informaticists are responsible for designing, selecting, and implementing systems to support and enhance patient care. Physician informaticists must build on the tools provided by standard systems to further benefit patients. Information processing lies at the very core of medicine; in order to have control over medical decision-making, the physician must retain control over automated information systems (Friedman, 1990). The clinical informaticist not only selects systems but in his or her daily practice of medicine pioneers innovative uses of these systems for individual patient care decisions. Just as the general internist has worked with the radiologist to learn the art of reading a chest radiograph, the clinical informaticist must teach his or her clinical colleagues the use of informatics tools in patient care decision-making. In their role as laboratory directors, clinical pathologists use systems to formulate policy decisions that will affect many patients. To close the loop, the informaticist can apply the practical lessons learned in using these systems for patient care and health care management to improve the capability and scope of the next generation of systems.

Clinical Informatics as a Medical Specialty

Although it will be many years before an official board certification in informatics is available through the American Board of Medical Specialties (ABMS), clinical informatics is rapidly being recognized as a specific area of expertise within many specialties. There is a distinct body of knowledge, which is briefly summarized in this chapter (see Table 5–4 for additional sources of self-education), together with a unique vocabulary. Practitioners come from many medical specialties, such as internal medicine, anesthesiology, and cardiac surgery, although a greater percentage of pathologists practice informatics than do most other specialists. Several national organizations focus on informatics, the most prominent being the American Medical Informatics Association. A number of medical schools and many hospitals have separate departments of medical informatics. Most pathology residency programs (Balis, 1993) and many other specialty residencies include informatics in their curriculum. Opportunities for advanced training (e.g., fellowship programs, graduate degrees) are available. Informatics has become a part of the board examinations in pathology, with the appointment of a Test Committee on Informatics. Just as pathology groups have traditionally acknowledged and sought new associates with expertise in cytology, hematopathology, or transfusion medicine, increasing numbers of groups are explicitly recruiting (or designating) associates to be the experts in informatics. The informaticist not only improves the efficiency of his or her colleagues in pathology but also provides tools to assist the clinician in diagnosis and treatment, is a pivotal player in quality improvement, and generates new knowledge about cost-effective medical practice.

Board certification in clinical informatics will most likely first occur as a special competence under an existing Board of the ABMS; under this provision, a physician already certified in any ABMS-recognized primary specialty could take an additional examination in clinical informatics (e.g., an internist could take the examination administered by the American Board of Pathology). However, ABMS approval of this new certification is unlikely to occur before the year 2000.

Career Opportunities in Clinical Informatics

Most practitioners of informatics will pursue this as a part-time vocation in conjunction with or in addition to other activities (e.g., surgical pathology, clinical pathology, transfusion medicine). Indeed, experience has shown that better quality and relevance of contribution results when the designer has to use the fruits of his or her design efforts in clinical practice. Less than 5% of practitioners will pursue informatics as a full-time occupation in a hospital, HMO, or other provider setting; in a medical school; as an employee/director of an information systems vendor; as a consultant; or in government service.

The practitioner of informatics faces some formidable challenges: One must maintain expertise in at least two extremely volatile fields—that is, information technology and pathology—both of which are moving at accelerating rates. Unfortunately, many colleagues still view the field as playing with computers or as engineering, not medicine. Ignorance may translate into resentment or fear. There may be a lack of respect and support, even though the very survival of the laboratory and pathology practice depends on the information systems. Therefore, in discussing informatics with colleagues in pathology, it is important to avoid jargon, use analogies from other basic sciences, and educate incessantly.

LABORATORY INFORMATION PROCESSING

The Laboratory as an Information Engine

The laboratory (with the exception of issuing blood components) exists for the sole purpose of providing diagnostic and management information for the physician to aid in the care of the patient. Although this chapter focuses on automated information handling, the laboratory director must never forget that the human resource is the laboratory's most valuable asset. Oral communication and sensitive personnel management must not be neglected in the pursuit of high technology.

From the point of view of those outside the laboratory, the laboratory is a so-called black box into which the physician or nurse puts test requests, specimens, or both and from which emerges reports of test results. Clinicians, nurses, and administrators have no concept of the complexity of processing that occurs within that black box—indeed, it is the laboratory's responsibility to provide information in such a way that outside users do not have to concern themselves with learning about that complexity. The laboratory director is responsible for the entire path from input (test order conceived by clinician) to output (test result understood by physician)—whether or not he or she actually has control over the intermediate steps. It is clearly to our benefit to control as many steps in this pathway as possible to ensure a flawless and rapid process. In a large institution, literally dozens of people may be involved in this loop (Krieg, 1978). With each additional step, an opportunity is introduced for delay and error; additional feedback loops must be added to improve the accuracy of operations. Large medical institutions resemble multicellular organisms in that they must devote an increasing proportion of their resources to the internal task of circulation and information transfer. Fortunately, automated information technology provides tools to eliminate some of these steps and to ensure loop closure where multiple steps must remain.

While ensuring the reliable, immediate flow of individual patient information to the clinician, the pathologist must remain aware of the importance of integrating laboratory information with other patient data (e.g., pharmacy profiles, problem lists, vital signs), to better place the laboratory findings into clinical context, to improve laboratory utilization, and to support patient outcome studies.

Tools for Communication

Within the Laboratory

Within the laboratory, the staff must be aware of policies, standard operating procedures, and updates to those practices. Procedure manuals are moving from paper to electronic form but remain critically important. Electronic broadcast to all workstations permits immediate notification (e.g., of arrival of the FDA inspector!), whereas electronic mail helps ensure that every employee is made aware of changes, even if he or she has been on vacation for two weeks. Computer tools can also enforce policies, such as documentation of who was called with a critical value. Regular staff meetings (section, shift, or entire laboratory) remain important, even in the electronic age. When devoted to the rapid communication of items relevant and important to all those in attendance or to an opportunity for staff feedback on items of concern, this time is well spent—but meetings held for their own sake destroy productivity. More valuable is the pathologist, as laboratory director, making a daily practice of walking around in the laboratory to remain aware of its activities and the staff's concerns.

Communications with Our Clients

Communication with our clients is critical to ensuring that the laboratory is providing the services needed. Communicate with them through the laboratory report (which can contain notices on such matters as test changes in addition to the results themselves), the laboratory handbook or user's manual (which has traditionally been paper and immediately out of date, but which is rapidly evolving to an online electronic document residing on the hospital clinical information network), and laboratory newsletters (which are also evolving from paper to an electronic message given when clinicians sign on, or when they order a particular test that has been updated).

Opportunities for Interaction

More crucial than one-way communications are opportunities for interaction with the medical staff (during division meetings, in hallway "curbside consults," and in the physician's dining room at lunch), as well as other laboratory users (especially during nursing unit rounds). Always ask "are you getting all the help you need from the laboratory?" Be receptive to any and all comments, and avoid defensive attitudes and immediate excuses. The most valuable laboratory quality assurance tools are comments from vocal clinicians, whom some laboratory staff members may consider troublesome or picky. In fact, these vocal individuals are your best friends in that they identify problems requiring attention. Often, these are the clinicians who pay the most careful attention to the quality, consistency, and timeliness of laboratory findings. The individuals most essential to successful laboratory function are often those with the least amount of training and lowest status in the organization: the nursing unit clerk, the laboratory clerk, and the phlebotomist. The best analytical instruments and staff in the world are useless unless these people understand and carefully execute their tasks.

Point-of-Use Communication

Point-of-use communication has traditionally occurred when an unusual or unclear order is received by the laboratory; the pathologist calls the clinician, providing education and consultation pertinent to the particular patient being cared for. Computerized order entry systems now provide help with common problems (e.g., a carcino-embryonic antigen (CEA) was ordered on this patient yesterday—do you really want another one? Do you want to transfuse platelets?—the patient's platelet count is 150,000). The principal limitation today is sociologic, not technologic—persuading clinicians of the benefits of direct computerized order entry (Bria, 1992). In the long term, direct entry of orders by the physician has great potential for providing information at the point of decision and thereby improving utilization of laboratory tests.

Information Flow in a Typical Laboratory

Patient Identification

When a patient is first registered, the identifying information must be entered into the laboratory computer database. A unique patient identification number, permanently assigned to that patient, should be used as a primary identifier; this medical record number is the standard of practice in hospitals. In outpatient and independent laboratories, such identifiers may be unavailable—this is of little concern for most chemistry, hematology, and microbiology procedures, in which appropriate values can usually be reported without knowing the patient's history. However, record linkage is of critical importance in a blood bank (searching for previous atypical antibodies, the computerized crossmatch), surgical pathology, hematopathology, and cytology. In these settings, it is particularly important to gather date of birth and sex (and, wherever possible, social security number) in addition to patient name, because accurate linkage is often impossible on patient name alone (in cytology databases, the maiden name of the patient's mother is a better tool than the patient's last name). Additional data typically gathered at this time include billing information, patient location (room number), physician (attending, admitting), and diagnosis. If contact with the laboratory will extend beyond the immediate time of patient registration (e.g., inpatient settings, outpatient transfusions), a wrist band with patient identification number must be applied. This wrist band should be machine-readable (e.g., HIBCC/Code39 barcode) (HIBCC, 1992), and should be used by *all* hospital departments for patient identification.

In terms of patient identification and in many other ways, the challenges faced by the outpatient and independent laboratories, and in ambulatory care information systems in general, are distinct from those encountered within hospitals (Matson, 1990).

Test Requests and Specimen Collection

After patient identification, test requests are entered, indicating when the specimen was (or will be) collected, who collected it, the time of collection, what tests are to be performed, and who ordered the tests. Test requests may be entered as short alphabetic mnemonics (e.g., CBC, CEA, Na) or by numeric codes; although faster to key, numeric codes require more training.

In many hospitals, laboratory tests are requested on paper requisitions, which are physically sent to the laboratory for entry. Typically, these are full-page sheets, having replaced the partial-page multipart forms used for ordering, reporting, and billing in the previous manual system (however, the multipart forms may be retained as a manual back-up reporting system).

Other hospitals now enter test requests on the nursing units into the hospital information system (HIS); the training requirements for such an approach are greater than when laboratory orders are entered by a small fraction of the laboratory staff. These requests are then transferred across an "order entry interface" into the LIS. If the HIS lacks the cross-checking and order validation routines found in a comprehensive LIS, this validation must be done at the level of the interface; in such instances, the interface may require extremely complex programming. Even after the bugs have been worked out, such interfaces require a great deal of monitoring by the laboratory staff. In addition, the tables or dictionaries of orderable tests on the HIS must be periodically checked against those on the laboratory computer.

Whether orders are sent on paper requisitions or on a computerized interface, major advantages accrue if the *physician* actually completes the order form or screen. This greatly facilitates the introduction of more appropriate diagnostic profiles and the removal of obsolete tests, because the physician is presented a choice of currently orderable options. Otherwise, physician orders must be translated by nonphysicians to fit available testing packages. Indeed, important cost and quality benefits have been shown to accrue when physician order entry becomes the standard (Sittig, 1994).

When test requests are entered into or received by the laboratory computer system, they are typically assigned an accession number, which serves to identify the specimen. A single accession number may be used for several tubes, some of which will be processed in chemistry, others in hematology. In other laboratories, separate accession number series are used for separate departments; in the latter case, order labels must be carefully coordinated so the patient is not stuck with a needle (phlebotomized) several times in a few hours.

Test requests typically fall into two categories: (1) requests with accompanying specimen, which can be logged in directly (as discussed later), and (2) requests for the laboratory to obtain the specimen, which introduce complexity. In the hospital setting, test requests received in advance are entered into the LIS and can then be grouped into routine phlebotomy batches. Shortly before the scheduled time of collection, labels are printed, listing all the patients from whom blood is to be drawn, and preprinted labels are provided for the blood tubes needed. These labels include all the information that will be needed to collect and process the specimen properly, such as required specimen/aliquot volumes and special handling instructions. Blood tube labels should be barcoded to allow bedside verification (with a hand-held phlebotomist workstation) of proper patient identification (scanning first the wrist band, then blood tubes) and accurate time-clocking of the time collection. Comments on such matters as patient availability and uncollected portions of a specimen can be keyed into such readers. Collection labels are printed in the order in which the phlebotomist should draw the specimens — urgent specimens first, then others in geographic sequence. Alternatively, the entire phlebotomist work queue can be stored in the workstation, and labels can be generated at the bedside as tubes are being drawn.

Whenever a specimen is collected, the phlebotomist, nurse, physician, or other person responsible for specimen collection *must* ensure proper patient identification by checking the patient's wrist band (a band on the foot of the bed is *not* an acceptable alternative) and must ensure that the specimen is fully labeled with patient name, hospital number, date and time, and the phlebotomist's initials before leaving the patient's bedside (see Chap. 1).

When the specimens are returned to the laboratory, the actual collection of the ordered specimens must be confirmed. The most efficient process is to plug the portable barcode scanners directly into the laboratory computer. Short of this, the best approach is batch entry ("I collected all of batch 516, except the PT on Mr. Smith").

For orders received with a specimen, the computer-printed label is applied to the specimen shortly after the order has been entered into the laboratory computer; this carries a risk that the wrong computer label will be applied to a patient tube. Unless the original tube label contains a patient number barcode that can be directly read, mislabeling can be prevented only by careful human attention to detail.

Specimen Processing

After confirmation of specimen receipt, some specimens (e.g., EDTA tubes for CBC) can be sent directly to that workstation (see Chap. 1). Clotted blood must be centrifuged, and the serum must be separated and aliquotted. This remains a labor-intensive step in most laboratories, although automated equipment to perform some of these functions is now available. Again, each aliquotting step has the potential of specimen mix-up; labels for the aliquot tubes should be computer-printed. With barcode labeling of all tubes and scanning at the time of aliquotting (or total avoidance of aliquotting with instruments using primary tube sampling), the number of errors will be reduced.

When specimens arrive at the various laboratory workstations, there must be a mechanism for organizing the work to be performed at that workstation. For some workstations at which single specimens are being run as they arrive (e.g., CBCs on a cell counter, chemistry panels), the specimen itself can serve this purpose. As specimens are received in the laboratory, the computer automatically downloads the orders to the instrument. Alternatively, using the host query mode, the instrument reads the sample's barcoded accession number and inquires of the laboratory computer what tests are to be performed on the specimen. Periodically, a "pending test list" can be checked on the workstation screen to verify that no specimens have been overlooked. Newer "random access" instruments in hematology, chemistry, and immunoassay now permit most workstations to function this way.

When the design of the instrument or the organization of workflow requires batch processing, it may be necessary to print a worklist, including not only the specimens to be run but also a list of controls and standards required for the run. Printed worklists avoid transcription errors resulting from manually copying load lists from a display-only terminal. Content of these worklists (e.g., what tests, controls, and standards are included) should be under laboratory control. In some cases, a test should be routed to one workstation at some times of the day or on some days of the week and to others at different times. Stat and routine tests are typically routed differently. For tests performed manually or on noninterfaced instruments, the worklist should have a space for writing the test results; the technologist then keys these results into the laboratory computer. Although it is unlikely that worklists will soon be extinct, their use will rapidly diminish as random-access instruments that can sample barcoded primary tubes replace the older, obsolete instruments still in use in many laboratories.

Result Entry and Automated Instruments

For manual workstations performing relatively standardized assays, a particularly effective mode of entry is to assign phrases and concepts to single keys on the workstation keyboard. This has proved to be effective in microbiology, blood bank, hematology (differential counts and morphology), microscopy, and cytology. Other approaches, which do not require adaptation of the LIS software, include loading of key sequences into shifted function keys on the terminal, barcoded phrases read by a wand (Aller, 1994b), and macro key definitions when a PC is used as a workstation or terminal emulator.

When specimens are to be sent to an outside laboratory for processing, the laboratory computer should transfer specimen identification and orders directly to the computer serving the reference laboratory; likewise, results can be electronically sent from the outside laboratory back to the laboratory computer (McDonald, 1994). Reference laboratories without direct electronic linkages typically place a modem and printer in the client laboratory to which the reference laboratories transmit results for printing.

Automated instruments with a random-access test menu (e.g., run sodium on one specimen, bilirubin and alkaline phosphatase on the next) and the ability to read barcoded primary specimen tubes should be bidirectionally interfaced with the LIS, so that the LIS can transfer test orders for each specimen directly into the instrument.

Generally, it is effective to interface an automated instrument to the laboratory computer whenever specimen identification can be directly collated with results at the instrument. Ideally, this is done by the instrument itself via a barcoded identification label on the original specimen tube. A second choice is keying in the accession number as the specimen is presented to or loaded onto the instrument (e.g., specimen no. 1234 is in cup 1, no. 2247 in cup 2). The results, collated with specimen identification, are automatically transferred to the LIS. After a technologist verifies the quality controls and outlier results, the results can be released for reporting.

Even when an instrument processes a relatively low volume of assays, it should be interfaced with the LIS. The medical consequences of a transcription error are so severe that the 1% error rate of manual transcription processes is not acceptable.

In the future, LIS vendors will empower the customer laboratory to interface new instruments by setting flags and variables in a standard dictionary; in addition, ASTM Standards E1381-91 and E1394-91 (ASTM, 1995) for instrument interface have been defined and implemented in newer instruments. Until these tools become widespread realities, interface processors will be very helpful to convert diverse instrument outputs into a standardized data stream (Aller, 1995).

Bedside-based analysis systems with integrated barcode readers are becoming available. After scanning the patient wristband, collecting a patient specimen, and analyzing it immediately, these systems transmit collated patient identification and results to the central LIS via a wireless (radio frequency or infrared) link.

As results are entered into the laboratory computer, either via keyboard or via instrument, the computer performs a wide variety of validity checks. Results that should be numeric are checked; required numbers of decimal places are verified. Reference ranges, specific for the patient's age and sex (and, where available, other factors, including medication and diagnoses), are compared with the result. For laboratories performing veterinary work, species-specific reference ranges are required. Results are compared with previous results on the patient to see if the amount of change is reasonable (so-called delta check). Coded comments are checked to be sure the code is listed in the proper dictionary. Critical (panic) values are flagged, and the technologist is required to enter a comment indicating to whom the results were called. Some results are processed through laboratory-defined calculation routines or algorithms to generate interpretive comments (Pribor, 1992). Certain results may cause a test to be ordered as a matter of course (e.g., a low MCV generates a ferritin order) to expedite diagnostic workups, improve patient care, and reduce unnecessary testing (e.g., having the computer order direct bilirubin only if the total bilirubin is elevated).

Quality control values are checked against defined limits for that particular test method, lot number, and level of control, and complex multirule algorithms can readily be applied.

As noted earlier, one of the most important advantages of an LIS is that it closes the loop between the test order and the result entry: an order without corresponding result should appear on the incomplete test list, compelling the technologist to seek out and resolve the discrepancy.

Result Reporting

Results are reported to the ordering physician in a wide variety of ways, and there are many important considerations in the formatting of such reports. Manual reports, color-coded by laboratory department and shingled onto carrier sheets, have been replaced by computer-printed reports; unfortunately, certain advantages and features can be lost in this transition if the new reports are not designed properly. Printed reports may contain only the most recent results, the results for a single specimen, or cumulative results, including all the specimens since the patient was admitted to the hospital. Readability of these reports has been improved dramatically by the introduction of laser printers, which allow rapid printing of a variety of high-quality fonts. The report should include the name, telephone number, and electronic mail address of the laboratory director to facilitate consultation between the clinician and the pathologist and to help improve laboratory service.

An important issue in modern laboratory medicine is information overload, such that clinicians may fail to recognize or properly interpret laboratory findings of critical significance to a patient's well-being. Altshuler (1983) found that the diagnosis of hypothyroidism was missed in one third of patients with laboratory findings pathognomonic of that condition; few data suggest that the situation has improved since then. Therefore, interpretive reports to ensure that the clinician recognizes such findings are an essential component of laboratory practice. In this capacity, the computer may be used as a clerical tool for transmission of pathologist-generated comments; as an "algorithm interpreter," applying simple flow charts; or as a complex expert system, suggesting interpretive comments to the pathologist. Full potential of these systems in medical quality assurance will be realized only when the full cycle, including clinician action taken, is recorded in a structured fashion on information systems, allowing the computer to verify that a pathognomonic laboratory result actually resulted in appropriate therapeutic intervention.

Traditionally, reports were printed in the laboratory and carried by hand, pneumatic tube, or courier to the nursing unit or physician's office. Communications technology now allows transmission of results via telephone modem or wire to a printer in the patient care area. Even laboratories without flexible computer systems can take advantage of fax transmission, because an image of a piece of paper can appear across town (or across the nation) in a matter of seconds.

Frequently, the physician or nurse calls the laboratory to obtain test results—for tests with a longer turnaround time, when the patient is critically ill, or (in some cases) when the report has been lost between the laboratory and the physician's office chart. In most laboratories, staff members key the patient identifier into a workstation, repeat the patient name, then read the results to the inquiring clinician—or inform him or her of specimen status, if results are not yet available. Efficiency and accuracy are gained if the physician or nurse can look up this information directly on his or her own workstation—on the nursing unit, in the physician's dining room, or even via dial-up modem access from the physician's home computer. In one institution, even though the laboratory lacked the staff to deliver or chart laboratory results, patient care continued unabated with interns using laboratory result inquiry workstations located on each nursing unit.

In critical care areas such as operating rooms, display units similar to those in airports can be used to show results; the most recent report to that location appears at the bottom of the screen, pushing previous reports up and off the top of the screen; this may be a general display, or it may be patient specific at each bedside. More complex displays may show a variety of relevant determinations (Connelly, 1995).

Physician's office computers connect directly (or via telephone modem) to the laboratory computer or hospital network to inquire about results. For physicians without a display unit, telephoning a voice response system allows the laboratory computer to read the results to them over the telephone, after the physician has entered his or her password and the patient's identification number on his touch-tone telephone. Storing laboratory results and information in computer memory is futile if physician and hospital staff access to this information is time consuming and cumbersome. Good public relations for both the computer and the laboratory are enhanced when access is efficient. Imaginative solutions to information access and communications are a major remaining challenge in laboratory computing.

Laboratory Management and Quality Assurance

As already emphasized, the operation of a laboratory is complex. To keep a laboratory operating at peak efficiency and effectiveness, the pathologist or his or her designee must have reliable and up-to-date information on exactly what is going on. Drawing from its database and time-stamped audit trails of what has happened to every specimen at each step of processing, the laboratory computer can produce extremely detailed and accurate accounts of laboratory activities, including the following:

- Turnaround time, by test, shift, technologist, ordering locations
- Laboratory workload distribution, by time of day and day of week
- Hour-to-hour and day-to-day variations in inquiry activity

In addition, a variety of department-specific result review and outlier reports should be produced—these must be so-called reports by exception, highlighting significant or atypical findings in one to three pages, rather than dumping three inches of computer printout on the pathologist's or supervisor's desk each morning.

Particularly valuable management byproducts of LISs are workload recording, productivity assessment, and management index reports (e.g., the Laboratory Management Index Program, College of American Pathologists, Northfield, IL). These reports can be used for tracking internal, longitudinal trends and for comparing laboratory fiscal performance with that of comparable laboratories.

A critically important function of the LIS in most institutions is its production of billing transactions for every test performed. These may be issued at the time of test order, specimen collection or receipt, or report completion. In practice environments in which billings have some correlation with income (e.g., non-HMO outpatient services), improvement in billing accuracy and completeness can be a realistic and appropriate justification for LIS purchase. Billing transactions can be sent, via magnetic tape or electronic communication, to a separate computer for printing of the patient or client bill and accounts-receivable management. Such electronic billing can expedite and enhance cash flow. As a byproduct, this billing information should also be used in management reports and analyses.

In addition to the reports preprogrammed by the LIS vendor, the laboratory staff will need to pull up *ad hoc* reports—for example, "Give me all the patients with sodium of greater than 150, between the ages of 62 and 75, who were on the oncology ward." This *ad hoc* query capacity should be able to address all fields in any of the files in the database—both dictionary and operational—and should be able to format its output for downloading into a personal computer. Although programs on the main laboratory computer are needed to extract the data, single-user workstations are better suited for detailed statistical analysis, graphics, and spreadsheets.

As discussed previously, the LIS's security functions also constitute an important laboratory management tool, ensuring that each staff member has access to only those functions appropriate for his or her job duties, training, and level of licensure and providing an extensive audit trail, including each individual involved with specimen log-in, processing, resulting, reporting, inquiry, and client service.

The laboratory computer database and other clinically oriented computers throughout the hospital are powerful tools for medical quality assurance. Without detailed information on patient condition (severity) and outcome, it is impossible to assess the appropriateness of laboratory use or the true cost-effectiveness of laboratory testing. Quality assurance software packages (e.g., Medical Information Data Analysis System, MIDS Inc., Tucson, AZ) that combine outcome, severity, and complication data from computer-stored medical records with other components of electronic information, such as the laboratory computer database, are now making it feasible for us to address these issues.

Requirements of Individual Laboratory Sections

Each laboratory section has unique data management requirements; a few such specialized needs are summarized here very briefly. Each area could easily be the subject of an entire chapter. With some of these sections, particularly the blood bank, surgical pathology, and cytology, one must consider the relative merits of integrating all functions into one LIS or purchasing specialized software modules to address the needs of the particular section, as well as interfacing these modules into the software package that serves the remainder of the clinical laboratory (Skinner, 1994).

Chemistry, hematology, and immunology require many instrument interfaces. Indeed, similarities in function are causing these three sections to become one in many laboratories. Sophisticated numeric quality-control techniques, patient-mean-value controls, blind duplicate delta checks, and the like are necessary. Instruments that do not provide a final, patient-reportable result are rapidly disappearing from clinical laboratories; where they remain, data reduction is typically performed on a PC, not on the main laboratory computer. Specialized keyboard programming for WBC differentials, smear morphology, and urinalysis have already been mentioned.

Microbiology must have an efficient method of entering organism names and antimicrobial sensitivities (including instrument interfaces). Paperless microbiology systems, in which all observations (e.g., colonial morphology, biochemical results) are entered, must be very carefully designed—if not, they can result in an excessive number of keystrokes and decreased productivity (rather than increasing productivity, as one would hope with paper elimination). The microbiology database is structured and must be analyzed differently from that used in chemistry/hematology; a single specimen can result in multiple organism isolates, each of which can have one or more sets of biochemical characterizations (for internal use) and susceptibility results (for external reporting). Susceptibility reporting is often formatted to influence clinical practice; for example, expensive and toxic antimicrobials may be omitted from the report if the organism is susceptible to inexpensive and safe agents. Epidemiology reports, antimicrobial susceptibility patterns, and other specialized summaries are needed.

The blood bank must track not just patient specimens but also blood components and the matching of these two. Blood component and derivative unit inventories, with careful attention to expiration dates and special characteristics of each unit (e.g., special antigen typing), must be maintained. Special units for special patients (autologous and directed units) have imposed complex new record-keeping and cross-checking requirements. The possible status of a unit in inventory may vary widely (e.g., just received from regional supplier, ABO retested and available, allocated to a patient [or, in blood shortages, crossmatched with multiple different patients at once], issued to a patient, quarantined for a variety of reasons). Before blood can be issued, a unit tag must be attached to the unit, confirming the identity of the patient for whom this blood is intended. On issue, records must be kept of reinspection of unit appearance, who picked up the unit, and so on. Patient histories must be maintained for prolonged periods, particularly on problem patients, to avoid infusing incompatible blood into a patient who has temporarily lost his or her atypical blood group antibodies. A whole additional set of requirements apply for the donor center, including maintenance of a donor database and permanent deferral lists, processing and testing of donor units, more extensive inventory functions, and many other requirements. As noted earlier, particular attention must be devoted to the software, dictionary, and system validation, as well as to other FDA regulatory requirements (see Table 5–5), for any activity that involves the blood bank—including interfaces with chemistry instruments that process donor screening tests (hepatitis, HIV, and other assays for infectious disease).

Surgical pathology must provide for word processing and text reporting, both for long-term history-keeping and structured diagnosis retrieval. One of the most difficult aspects is linkage of all data on a single patient, particularly when the department's historical files have not been linked by a permanent patient medical record number. Outpatient, outside, and consultation specimens typically lack a medical record number identifier. Diagnoses must be retrievable not only for an individual patient but for all patients with a given diagnosis. The most generally applicable tool for diagnosis retrieval is SNOMED International (Cote, 1993). Several LIS vendors now provide for automatic encoding of English-language diagnoses.

Cytology information systems require specially designed quality assessment, patient follow-up, and cytology/histology correlation functions. Specialized software packages are also available to serve the information processing needs of autopsy pathology and for management of forensic pathology practices and coroners' offices.

Flow cytometry is an important new tool in immunology, surgical pathology, and cytopathology. Cell cycle analysis and interpretation of the data from such studies require sophisticated numeric models, usually processed on PC workstations.

Other specialized laboratory sections, including histocompatibility (human leukocyte antigen, or HLA), stem cell, apheresis, cytogenetics, molecular diagnostics, and paternity testing, have unique requirements as well.

IMAGE TECHNOLOGY

Although pathology is a medical specialty that makes significant use of images, *standardized* application of digital imaging technology has been minimal in this field. This contrasts sharply with specialties such as radiology, cardiology, and nuclear medicine, which have actively incorporated digital imaging into the setting of routine daily activities. This disparity can be explained, at least in part, by the need for *color*. Until the innovations of the mid-1990s, the implementation of color digital imaging systems was technically challenging and extremely expensive, even with relatively poor image quality. Conversely, the black-and-white digital imaging systems prevalent in other medical specialties had been in place for over a decade and represented a relatively mature segment of the imaging technologies.

Table 5–6. ESSENTIAL TERMINOLOGY IN IMAGE TECHNOLOGY

Pixel: Short for picture element, each pixel represents one unit point on a digital image. The greater the density of pixels per arc-field-of-view, the greater the resolution.

Voxel: A volumetric pixel encountered in three-dimensional image data sets, such as those seen in sequential-plane confocal microscopy.

Resolution: A generally misleading term; true digital system resolution is a function of total vertical and horizontal pixels, the physical size of the rendered image, and the distance from which the image is viewed. Thus, without proper categorization, the term resolution is essentially meaningless. Buyers should be warned when encountering systems claiming high-resolution or ultra-high-resolution capability without accompanying specifications.

Digitizer: An electronic device capable of converting the analog values of pixels obtained from a camera to a numeric format that a computer can use. An image represented by numbers is what is meant by a digital image. Typically, imaging systems use 8-, 10-, or 12-bit digitizers. The greater the number of bits, the greater the dynamic range (from dark to bright) the system possesses. An 8-bit system has 2^8 (256) brightness levels, whereas a 12-bit system has 2^{12} (4096) levels. An increase in bit number increases both system performance and overall system expense.

Frame buffer: An electronics device capable of rendering a digital image to a computer monitor. For color systems, these devices are three separate systems, each for a separate color channel. Color digital systems use the additive color scheme with red, green, and blue as the three primary colors. This system is the same as that used in human vision. Typically, each channel has its own 8 bits. Thus, the typical color system is a 24-bit system.

General Technologic Overview

With the advent of extremely inexpensive and high-capacity memory chips, it has become possible to fabricate inexpensive graphic display systems that offer outstanding performance. Also, the maturation of the charge-coupled device (CCD) camera has turned reliable and consistent digital imaging from a mystical to a relatively hands-off process. As manufacturers continue to exploit improvements in available graphics system component technology, the pathologist can expect to see regular and significant improvements in imaging systems designed for gross and microscopic imaging. Image management and display will become as important a component of the practice of pathology as they have become in many other fields (Aston, 1994).

Overview of the "Prototypic" Imaging System

The typical imaging system (Table 5–6 presents the terminology) incorporates some type of camera, digitizer, and frame buffer. A computer is used to link the functions of these devices and provide enhanced functionality. Typically, the software on a given system determines the overall system capabilities. The most crucial component of any imaging system is the camera. Without sufficient image quality, the capabilities of all subsequent devices are compromised. Correspondingly, the camera has been and continues to be the single most expensive component of any imaging system. The overall system may be attached to either a color or a black-and-white photorealistic printer.

Cameras

The CCD camera (Table 5–7) has vastly changed the world of computer imaging. The CCD (Figs. 5–1, 5–2) is actually an integrated circuit (a large silicon wafer in a package with a clear window) with special light-sensitive properties. Instead of scanning an antimony-trisulfide or silicon surface with an electron beam, as in the case of a conventional video tube, the CCD generates its image by using a charge-coupled area (usually square) for every image position (pixel). This area produces a voltage increase proportional to the quantity of photons striking it per unit of time. An analog-to-digital converter, ideally placed adjacent to the CCD, converts these accumulated voltages to digital values. Each of these pixel-values are recognized as *unique* locations by the computer (or digitizer) that scans the CCD. As a result, pixel jitter, a severe artifact inherent to analog conventional video in which one pixel may be interpreted as having come from any of several scan lines, does not occur with CCDs that are digitally scanned. One should be aware, however, that many CCD cameras convert their digital output to conventional analog

Table 5–7. ATTRIBUTES OF THE IDEAL CHARGE–COUPLED DEVICE (CCD) CAMERA

Full-frame transfer high-resolution CCD (at least 1K × 1K)
Thermoelectric cooling
Integrated analog-to-digital converter
All-digital interface
Computer-controlled shutter time

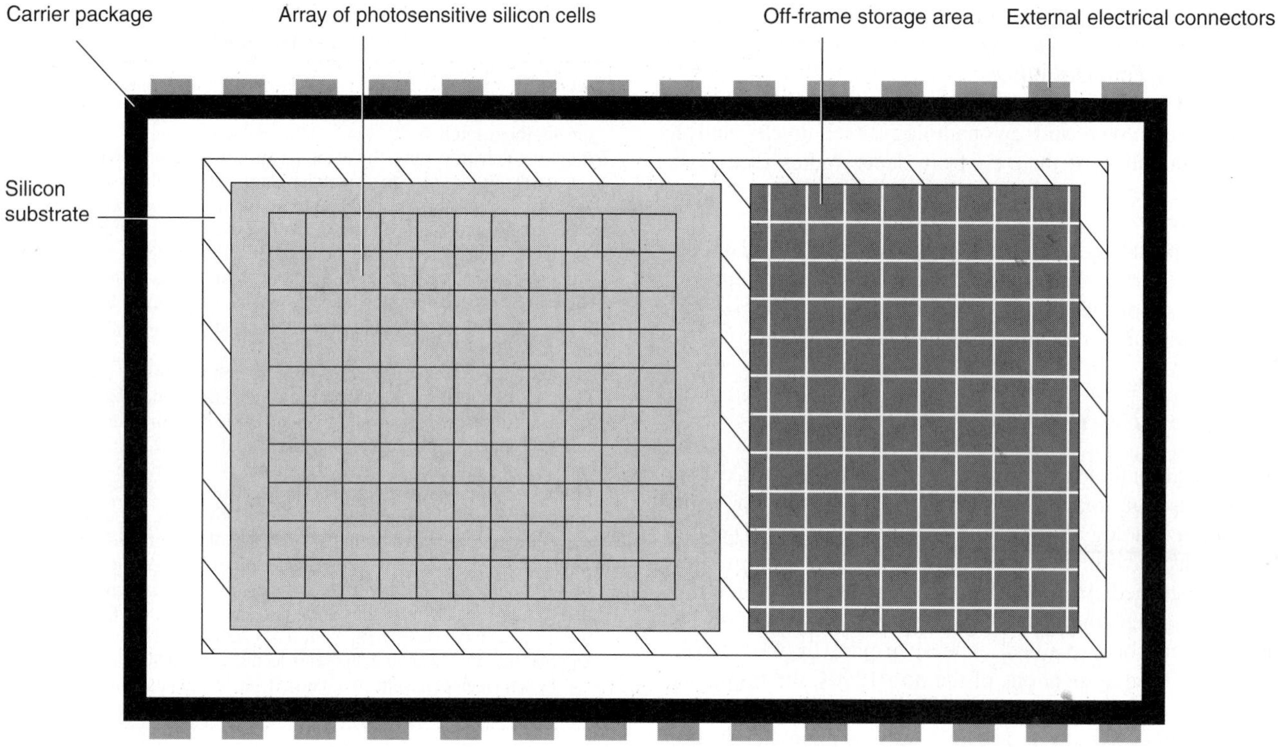

Figure 5-1. Frame-transfer design CCD.

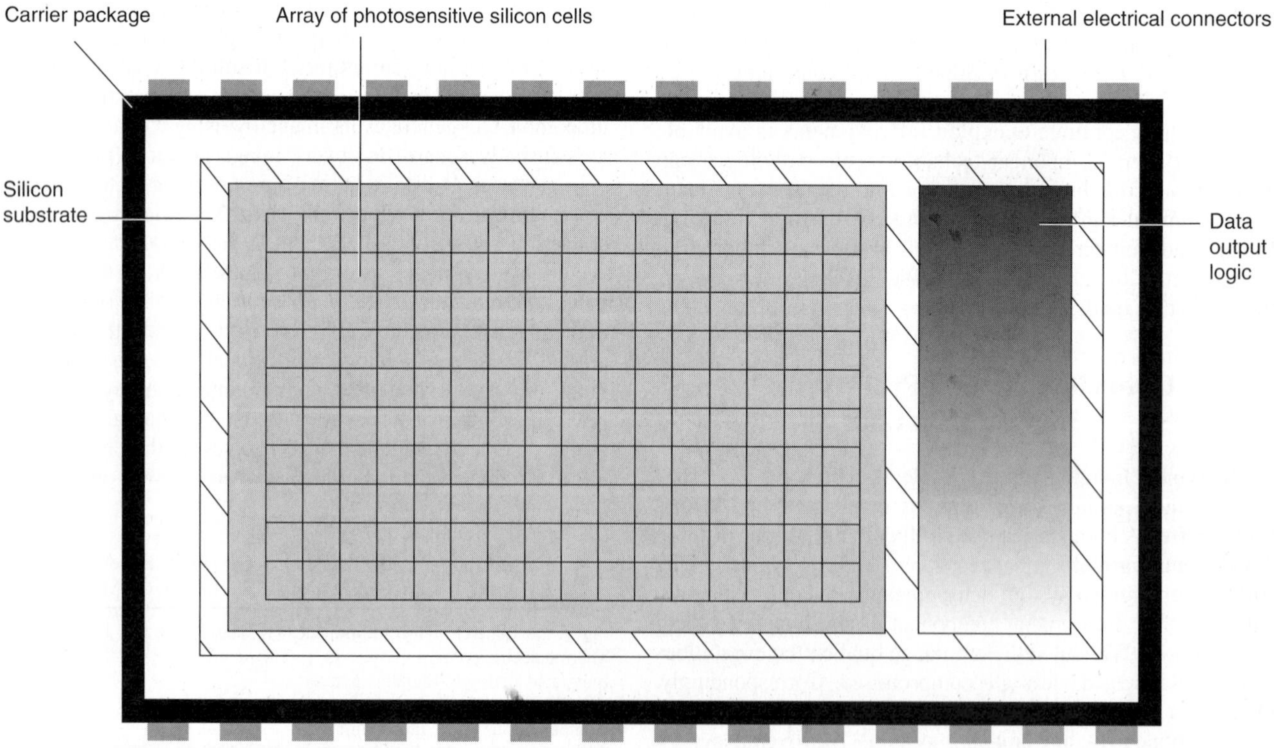

Figure 5-2. Full-frame design CCD.

National Television Systems Committee (NTSC—a U.S. standard for video) format for compatibility with existing video monitors and digitizers. This conversion effectively loses most benefits of the native digital nature of the CCD. It is unfortunate that manufacturers choose to label NTSC-format cameras as digital devices when in actuality they are not.

CCDs come in many formats. Aside from the obvious variation of resolution, light sensitivity, linearity, noise floor, and homogeneity are additional factors. From a design viewpoint, CCDs are either full-frame or interline. Full-frame CCDs use 100% of their surface area for light gathering. Thus, the pixels touch each other on all four sides. This is the best possible geometry for quality imaging, but it is also a more expensive technology, because the wires used to get the information to the outside of the chip must be fabricated *underneath* the imaging cells. In contrast, an interline CCD has its imaging cells spaced vertically and horizontally by some finite distance; the cells *do not* touch each other. In this interpixel space are placed the wires connecting the cells to the outside world. Thus, light-sensitive surface area is traded for a flat, inexpensive fabrication topology. Interline CCDs are typically one third to one fifth the cost of full-frame CCDs.

Another design issue of CCDs is the method in which the image information will be stored until the digitizer is ready to acquire. The two basic methods are frame-transfer CCDs and nontransfer CCDs. Frame-transfer CCDs are the more sophisticated of the two implementations. In this system, after some finite exposure period, the acquired image is rapidly transferred to another memory storage location on the CCD chip itself. This secondary storage location is light-insensitive. As such, subsequent changes in lighting following the specified exposure period will have no effect on the captured image. By altering the time period of exposure, followed by the rapid transfer phase, camera designers have been able to incorporate electronic shutters into their designs, all without mechanical assistance. An added feature of the frame-transfer CCD is the removal of a problem known as pixel blur. To understand pixel blur, one should understand the nontransfer CCD. Being a simpler device, the nontransfer CCD has only one storage area; it is one and the same with the image-sensitive area of the chip. As such, the device is sensitive to light at all times other than the erase cycle. Without proper design, this simplicity may lead to several artifacts. Information is read from a CCD serially—that is, one pixel at a time (some newer devices may actually have *four or more* serial channels) and via a method known as shifting. In this system, the entire row of analog voltage values is shifted one location, with the value on the end being read in the process. As this shifting takes some finite time, the intrinsic voltages of any *a priori* pixel address are subjected to the light-intensity features present at each pixel address on their journey out of the CCD. Thus, if light continues to reach the CCD once the shift stage of the CCD has commenced, each voltage value will be tainted with additional voltages of every pixel situated between the pixel in question and the output of the device. This contamination of the original pixel voltage is known as pixel blur. The obvious solution is to equip the camera with a mechanical shutter that physically prevents light from reaching the camera during the shift phase. As the frame-transfer CCD rapidly moves this data to a light-insensitive area *en bloc,* the issue of pixel blur is moot, as is the need for a mechanical shutter. Frame-transfer CCDs do have disadvantages. The act of moving image data, while still in analog format, from one location to another imposes a small but quantifiable noise artifact on the actual voltage level. When extremely accurate light intensity measurements are necessary, this may be unacceptable. Additionally, the need for additional off-frame storage circuitry can double the cost of the device.

The way in which color images are captured is equally variable. For real-time color, the best and most expensive approach is the three-CCD camera. In this format, focused light reaches a three-way splitting prism with special color filters (interference filters) laminated to its three outputs, so that each of the output facets pass relatively pure red, green, and blue light. Adjacent to each facet is a monochromatic CCD, positioned correctly for shift and rotation relative to the other two CCDs, to provide correct color and spatial registration. This three-CCD module (Fig. 5–3) tends to be expensive to manufacture and calibrate and usually is found on high-end cameras. The most common alternative approach to attain real-time color images makes use of the inline color CCD. In this scheme, a conventional monochromatic CCD is bonded with a plastic filter of alternating red, green, and blue vertical stripes (Fig. 5–4) such that each stripe is correlated with a column of pixels. Thus, as the CCD is read from left to right, alternating red, green, and blue pixels are obtained. This creates color data from a *single CCD* at the expense of decreasing horizontal resolution by two thirds. Some specialized inline color CCDs decrease this shortcoming by vastly increasing the number of horizontal pixels. Other vendors bypass this shortcoming by using tiny piezoelectric transducers to physically shift the entire imaging surface, thus registering the three colors with three passes. A final approach to color imaging involves the use of a single CCD with a bank of computer-selectable interference filters. In this scheme, a single monochromatic image is taken when each filter is mechanically positioned in the light path. This system excels in both potential clarity and resolution, because only *a single* high-resolution CCD is needed to obtain color images. An obvious drawback with this final system is the inability to generate real-time color images, because it takes some finite length of time to switch filters.

The topic of camera interfaces is also paramount to effective digital imaging. Although the specifics are beyond the scope of this chapter, it is sufficient to say that an all-digital interface is preferable to an analog interface. Thus, better cameras will contain the analog-to-digital converter within the camera head itself, minimizing noise and signal loss that can be encountered along even a short length of analog signal path. It has also been shown that thermoelectric cooling can significantly reduce the noise (known as dark current) inherent in the charge-coupled cell's behavior. High-performance CCD sensors are less imperative when image archival of bright images, and not analysis or low-light imaging, is the task at hand. In such cases, resolution, cooling, and full-frame transfer may not be as important.

Image Archival

Image archival may be the most immediately realizable benefit of digital imaging. Current methods rely heavily on film-based recording technologies for long-term archival.

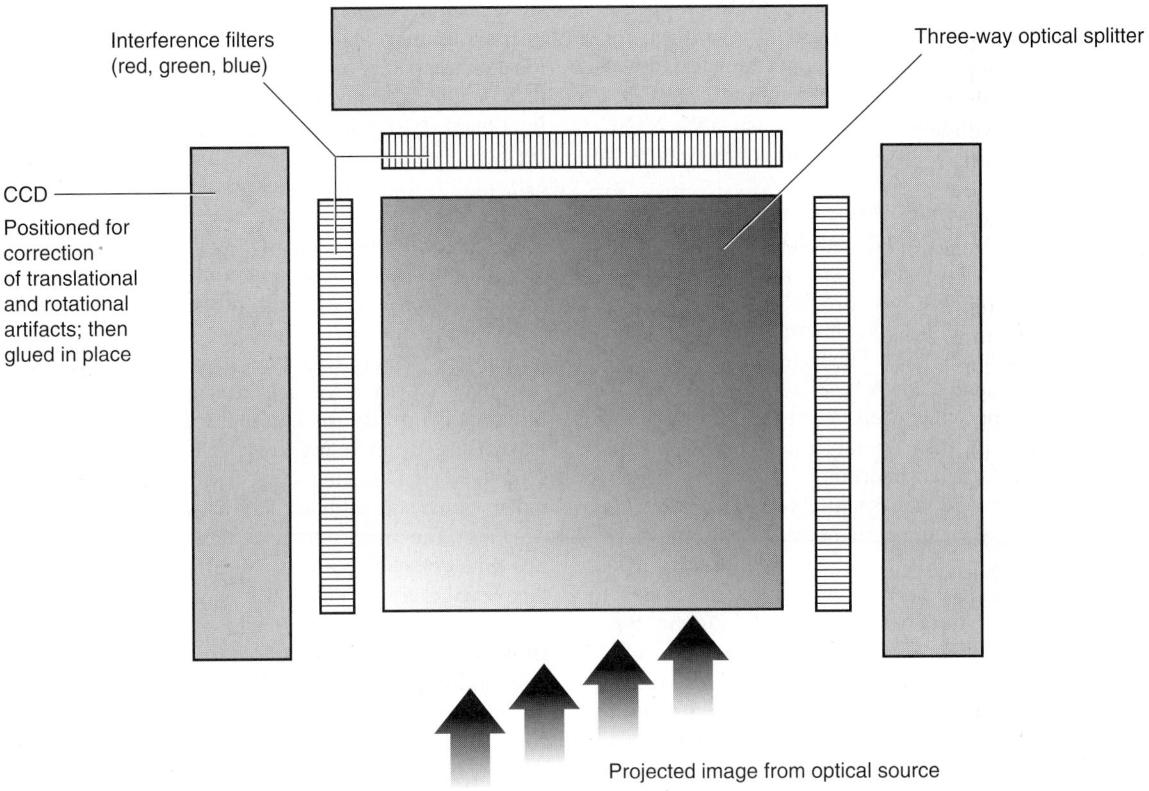

Figure 5–3. 3-CCD color image sensor.

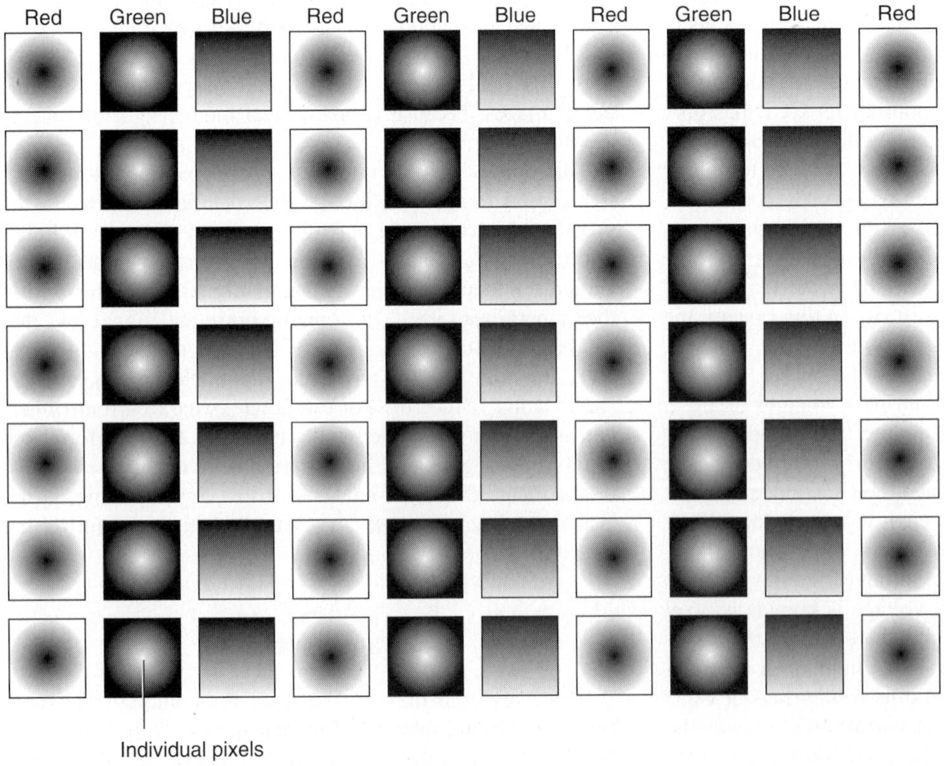

Figure 5–4. Single inline color CCD sensor layout.

Film has the benefit of relatively high image resolution and an established cadre of support services such as local graphic arts houses. Its pitfalls include but are not limited to expense associated with materials, expense of development and duplication, unavoidable aging and deterioration of media, inflexibility with respect to modification and overlaying, inflexibility in combining of text and graphics for publication proofs, space needed for storage, lack of immediacy of acquired image adequacy evaluation, and difficulty of incorporation into a computerized database for immediate and simplified image retrieval. Digital image archival counters these limitations in that it offers unlimited storage life without *any* deterioration, indelibility of storage (if a write-once optical drive is used, pertinent to medical-legal aspects of pathology), flexibility with respect to modification and overlays, simplicity with text/image integration for publication documents, and ease of in-house production without expensive services or consultants. Digital archival has the disadvantages of an expensive initial set-up cost as compared with film-based technology and its increased technical demands compared with film for those unfamiliar with digital methodologies.

Image Databases

As already mentioned, digital image archival facilitates the implementation of efficient and functional databases for immediate recall of one or numerous images from a file of thousands (e.g., Fetch, Aldus, Seattle, WA). The advantages of computerized databases over conventional filing techniques include the ability to conduct searches by more than one variable (such as accession number) and the ability to generate topic-specific reports in minimal time. This could be an invaluable feature to individuals conducting clinical research or desiring to retrieve a number of similar cases for patient care conferences such as a weekly tumor board.

Video Disc

Although this chapter emphasizes the use and advantages of digital image capture and storage, at least one analog storage format continues to be useful in medical practice and teaching. Video disc inscribes an analog representation of a video signal on a single spiral track on an optical disk. It is possible to represent more than 54,000 high-quality color video images on a single 12-inch disk, a much higher density than is possible with CD-ROM. Video disc has been widely used for publication of image libraries for various specialties in medicine.

THE INTERNET

Originally started as a joint project between the National Science Foundation and the Department of Defense as a method of exchanging defense project information, the Internet has grown to a level of sophistication that makes it the most complex and widespread network in the world (Gilster, 1994; Hahn, 1994), with perhaps the single exception of the worldwide telephone network. In many ways, this distinction is becoming obscured, because many Internet connections and links are accomplished via the telephone system itself.

In its simplest definition, the Internet is an interconnected collection of addresses, all with the capability of reaching any other address on the network. What makes the Internet a special network is its absolute and total incorporation into many aspects of academic, corporate, governmental, and organizational intercommunication and intracommunication. To this effect, it provides a unique window to the outside world. The visible horizon is already enormous, and estimates in early 1995 indicate that the Internet is growing at a rate exceeding 10% per month.

Tools available on the Internet include a wide array of protocols to allow for simple and rapid exchange of information between specific points. Because the network operates in real time, it is possible for two remotely located computer systems to interact without a perceivable delay. The major tools in use to accomplish this feat are known as Telnet and file transfer protocol (FTP).

Telnet

As the name implies, Telnet allows a computer user on the Internet to telephone across the net in order to establish an interactive text-based log on session with some remote host computer site. Being a real-time protocol, Telnet allows any computer user to interactively use any other computer in the entire world, provided that both are on the Internet. The implications of this to telemedicine are clear. The computer-stored patient record (CPR) (Institute of Medicine, 1991), an emerging digital standard, can be stored entirely in electronic format. With widespread implementation of the CPR by the turn of the century, it will become possible to rapidly transfer comprehensive patient records anywhere in the world. This is attractive as compared with current methods, which often involve use of fax and mail. The Internet transmission rate is significantly higher than that of a conventional facsimile message, and significant flexibility is gained by the receiving site obtaining the record in electronic format as opposed to printed format. Searches for a particular diagnosis or finding are relatively straightforward for an electronic text document, but they are virtually impossible if the document has been transmitted and stored as a fax image. For this paradigm to reach its highest level of functionality, the current concept of the medical record will need to be modified. Handwritten entries such as progress notes and orders will need to be transcribed into electronic format; handwriting recognition software such as that available on Apple's *Newton* and other personal digital assistants (PDAs) may eventually fulfill this need.

Anonymous FTP

File transfer protocol, or FTP as it is commonly called, is a powerful and effective tool to accomplish real-time format-independent information transfer across the Internet. For example, a user of FTP in North America could easily access digitized gel electrophoretic images from Europe, with the total time for file transfer being less than a minute. Conventional FTP, however, requires that the remote user have both a user ID and a password for the site being accessed. Early on, architects of the Internet realized that some type of *public access* provisions had to be established for data intended for global on-demand distribution. The answer to this need was the creation of *anonymous FTP.* When using anonymous FTP, the remote user uses the log-in ID of "anonymous" and then his or her actual Internet ID as a password. This paradigm serves two functions. First, a remote user may access data on a computer system without having a specific ID for that system. Second, the FTP server receives general information concerning destination of database information. Such information may be useful in further refining the demographic targeting of the database or identifying areas of users on the Internet who have a similar interest in the content of the database. The overall notion of anonymous FTP is the provision for worldwide *sharing* of data.

A local system administrator may base a decision to allow or disallow anonymous FTP service from a particular machine on the type and content of its data. Without this service, FTP may still reside, but it will require specific user names and passwords for data access. The limiting or disallowing of specific services is known as a firewall. At present, most academic centers, including the health sciences, offer at least one anonymous FTP server within their respective institutions. Such FTP addresses may be found in various documents including the Internet Phone Book. These addresses also may be found by use of Gopher, Veronica, WAIS, or Archie, all tools available on the Internet.

As the Internet's total information throughput increases, and as software and hardware technology mature to a point allowing effective and reliable telepathology applications, the issue of standards will become paramount (Mattheus, 1992 and 1993). The medical specialty of radiology realized a similar technologic crisis in the early 1980s, as many vendors started providing radiologic imaging equipment with *vendor-specific* image exchange capability. Coordinated and sweeping measures executed by the American College of Radiology in concert with the National Electrical Manufacturer's Association and the American National Standards Institute halted the continued development of multiple, noninteroperable protocols. Rather, the Digital Image Communications in Medicine (DICOM) standard was established to allow for a common interface protocol between all vendors. This standard has been recently opened to all medical specialties, and imaging modalities such as angiographic cine and endoscopy have been added to the DICOM repertoire. One of us (Balis) chairs the Image Exchange Committee of the College of American Pathologists; we anticipate that a standard for both telepathology and digital encoding of glass slides will be established by mid-1996. This standard also addresses issues intrinsic to the practice of clinical pathology and the clinical laboratory. Items that may need to be included within the CPR are images of electrophoretic and chromatographic gels, bacterial and fungal culture plates, cytogenetics, and immunofluorescent microscopy. Formulated as an extension to the existing DICOM 3.0 standard, this all-encompassing standard, Pathology and Laboratory Extensions to DICOM (PLEXCOM), is being positioned to become the framework on which future modalities and formats of pathology imaging are added as they appear.

The Internet as an Information Source

Besides its obvious use as a fast telecommunications medium, the Internet is also a vast compendium of information sources. As a resource, the topics span the gamut of humanity itself, with significant representation in the sciences. To this effect, many Internet locations, including academic, commercial, and governmental sites, have placed on-line databases on the Internet for public access. As the Internet has grown in complexity since the 1980s, so has the multitude of methods available for the access and interchange of these data.

E-Mail

As perhaps the most fundamentally useful aspect of the Internet, electronic mail (E-mail) allows Internet users to send messages to one or many members of the Internet throughout the world. As the Simple Mail Transfer Protocol (SMTP) is now largely real-time, most E-mail reaches its target address in minutes if not seconds. Because E-mail is a text-transfer protocol, various extensions have been developed for sending images and programs via E-mail. Common examples are MIME and UUencode. With MIME, the source file is encoded into a series of fixed-length text lines and then subsequently sent as a standard text E-mail message. On the receiving end, this text file is decoded by a similar MIME-aware program to derive the original file. More sophisticated protocols, such as FTP and KERMIT, can accomplish file transfer without the encoding-decoding steps, because they are intended for use with all types of file formats. The attractiveness of E-mail file exchange lies in that many Internet users have only access to E-mail and not the other, more advanced file-exchange applications.

UseNet

Foremost in value within the Internet is an entity known as UseNet. This is a news service. Unlike conventional news services, in which a central organization or entity decides on the content of the news, UseNet is a news service entirely supplied by Internet users. As such, *any* Internet subscriber can both read and post messages to UseNet. To prevent complete pandemonium, UseNet has been divided by topics into segments known as Newsgroups. In this manner, messages may be posted to readerships with a shared interest. Internet users may roam UseNet either by alphabetical listing or by topic search. The Newsgroups present on UseNet at any given moment reflect the interests of the current worldwide Internet usership. Because the Internet is expanding at a rate of greater than 10% per month, a similar but less rapid expansion is also being experienced in the quantity of messages and the number of Newsgroups. From a medical perspective, UseNet is a wonderful opportunity for pathologists to share information with the general medical and pathology communities and to target difficult inquiries at a specific audience, thus increasing the chance of effective information sharing. As a greater fraction of the global pathology community joins the Internet, the enormous power of this tool will be realized. Even now, the sum total of health care professionals on the Internet represents an invaluable resource.

Gopher

Developed at the University of Minnesota, Gopher represents the logical evolution in tools that simplify navigation throughout the Internet. With Gopher, the user may search for other systems and Gopher servers in the Internet, both geographically on a worldwide basis and by topic. As a primary function, Gopher will identify all available machines in Internet space and translate necessary protocols so that the user may interact with any machine by a standard command interface. Gopher will identify a number of categories of Internet entities. These include institutional phone books, computers available for log-on by Telnet, addresses available for anonymous or conventional FTP, and other Gopher servers. A Gopher server is merely the Gopher server application running on a remote computer that is attached to the Internet. This remote Gopher may present its menus in a manner more suited to the users of that remote system. Once a system is selected, Gopher will assist with initiating and executing file transfer, obtaining text or other information such as phone book entries, or initiating a Telnet log-on session.

Veronica

Veronica is a tool commonly executed from within Gopher, or Gopherspace, as it is also commonly referred to. Veronica allows the user to search all of Gopherspace, and indeed the Internet, for a particular keyword or set of search parameters within Gopher menus. One possible search might include the keywords *blood bank* and *utilization.* Within seconds to minutes of initiating such a search, Veronica will return all the worldwide Gopher entries that match this search. If a very large number of entries are encountered, Veronica will usually truncate to the first 50 or so unless otherwise directed. This tool is a very real source of immediate and specialized information for those interested in clinical pathology and informatics, because many specialists have already entered the Internet with Gopher servers.

World Wide Web (WWW)

With the creation of Internet browse and search tools such as Gopher, it became obvious to many that the full impact of telecommunications could be realized if hypertext was available on a worldwide basis in real time. In its simplest definition, hypertext is the implementation of text, images, sound, video, and interactive linking of information. The migration of hypertext to the Internet resulted largely from the efforts of CERN, the European Laboratory for Particle Physics. Their product, HyperText Markup Language (HTML), allowed for the creation of documents with hypertext attributes and links with other hypertext documents. Collectively, the presence of hypertext servers on the Internet is known as the World Wide Web, or WWW for short. As the name implies, the WWW is a diffuse conglomeration of HTML servers throughout the world, linked by references within any *a priori* HTML document, thus creating one uninterrupted web. The overall web has no particular focal point or central command center; it is entirely distributed. To allow one to view HTML documents and to traverse the links that they contain, a family of programs has developed, known as WWW browsers, which offer unprecedented ease and access to data anywhere in the world. A key aspect of these browsing tools is their interactive nature; they operate in real time in a client-server paradigm. One popular browsing tool is the program MOSAIC, which is produced by the National Center for Supercomputing Applications, a center of the University of Illinois at Urbana-Champaign. This browsing tool has been ported to many computer platforms and is constantly being updated. Another popular browsing tool is a program called NetScape. Produced by Netscape Communications, it offers a simplified user interface and has many enhancements that allow it to operate more efficiently over slower telephone links to the Internet, such as serial line Internet protocol (SLIP) and point-to-point protocol (PPP). It is anticipated that telemedicine and telepathology will be based on this type of interface.

Other Information Providers

Although the Internet remains a large, if not the largest portion of the noncommercial worldwide telecommunications network, a number of additional commercial services that also provide valuable information access are of immediate importance to the specialty of pathology. These networks include, but are not limited to, CompuServe (compuserve.com), America OnLine (aol.com), Prodigy (prodigy.com), Genie (genie.geis.com), and Bixnet (bix.com). Large information providers such as CompuServe make available to their users a multitude of other databases and networks, including Paperchase, the Internet E-mail system, UseNet, and FTP.

THE PATHOLOGIST'S WORKSTATION: A DIGITAL DESKTOP

The Pathologist's Microscope for the 21st Century: An Assembly of Tools

As the pathologist is called on to assume an ever-expanding role in information management, he or she needs a set of tools to facilitate this. These tools are assembled—either by an individual or by a commercial supplier—in the form of a workstation.

The pathologist's workstation is a combination of hardware, software, databases, and interfaces, providing at least certain minimal capabilities, designed to facilitate the pathologist's time and expertise in providing appropriate patient care. Its primary goal is to facilitate the work of a general pathologist (or subspecialist) to do the following:

1. Increase the quality of patient work
2. Increase service to clinicians
3. Improve effectiveness of the lab and the larger organization
4. Increase personal efficiency and effectiveness

Clearly, a desktop computer simply connected to a microscope, video camera, and a bit of image annotation software does not constitute a pathologist's workstation. On the other hand, a workstation incorporating *all* the capabilities listed in Table 5–8 may be a Holy Grail rather than an achievable, practical reality. As much as possible, the workstation should be constructed using commercially available, general-purpose software tools.

Capabilities

Table 5–8 lists desirable capabilities of a pathologist's workstation. To define a minimal set of capabilities worthy of the name pathologist's workstation is not feasible at present. Each pathologist may need a different combination of these capabilities or prefer to use different tools to achieve them. Thus, the workstation suppliers need to provide considerable flexibility to the end-user.

The workstation should provide transparent, unified, easy-to-use, simultaneous, seamless access to, integration of, and presentation of multiple data sources, with the ability to show multiple text and image windows on the screen. One must be able to immediately switch tasks, then rapidly return to one's previous activity. Automatic communication and acquisition and downloading of data from a wide variety of information sources are required. A particularly helpful feature is the ability to automatically pull up data on the same patient from different systems. However, the inconsistent command structures of different systems should be concealed behind a standard, intuitive command set. The learning curve must be minimized, so that the time and effort involved in accessing the various functions and databases cease to be any impediment to their use. Likewise, very rapid interaction, with subsecond response time for commonly used functions, will encourage use. One useful technique is for the workstation to anticipate the pathologist's next request with advance fetching of data.

For anatomic pathology, the workstation should facilitate generation of accurate and timely reports more conveniently and rapidly than the system it replaces. These capabilities sometimes require replacement of an existing surgical pathology information system. In others, the existing system may provide sufficiently robust hooks and speed to interact with an intelligent pathologist's workstation. Although a complete description of functions for anatomic pathology is beyond the scope of this discussion, a few features to consider include the following: barcodes to pull up each case, voice recognition and transcription, the ability to capture the image currently under the microscope to file with the case, the ability to show laboratory data and radiology images *pertinent* to this particular specimen (keyed off specimen source), verification/electronic signature at the workstation while showing the complete report on-screen, and the ability to shadow the information on a case displayed on a secretary's terminal onto the pathologist's terminal (i.e., the secretary has received a call inquiring about a report and transfers the call in to the pathologist for further discussion).

The workstation can also facilitate the practice of clinical pathology in laboratory leadership and consultation. This requires ready access to data in LIS, HIS, and regional medical information systems. Management reports should be produced automatically or on demand. The system must collate data on an individual patient quickly and in the most useful form, including patient demographics, history, physical examination, therapy, previous diagnoses, problem list, an image of the laboratory requisition slip, the test orders as entered in the laboratory computer, ordering physician (with telephone number), collection information, results (numeric, text, images such as cytogenetics, and patterns such as electrophoretograms), and laboratory notes. Also useful are timing and chronology of the specimen (collection, receipt, processing, when reports were produced) and previous results on the patient. The ability to define rule-based decision logic into the workstation will aid consultative practice and will drive alarm and alert functions for circumstances worthy of the pathologist's attention.

Context-specific help information should provide views into one's own in-house laboratory manual and procedures (test selection, interpretation, patient and specimen preparation, testing schedules, test charges, costs), as well as into manuals from reference laboratories, published textbooks, practice parameters, guidelines, and diagnostic and monitoring algorithms.

Flexibility is a key characteristic, enabling easy and extensive customization so that each pathologist can tailor the workstation to his or her particular work patterns and readjust personal features at will. This includes the ability to build and maintain personal databases and to integrate commercial databases; create an index of articles, images, and so on by one's own keywords; and include random notes, diagnostic lists, and outlined information. The functionality of the workstation should be expandable so that modules or features peculiar to each practice can be added and newly developed tools can be easily and inexpensively integrated into the system.

Personal information management functions include a tickler (e.g., *remind* me to check on this case tomorrow morning), calendar and alarm, meeting scheduling (coordination among several pathologists), shared meeting agendas, and diagnosis-driven and results-driven scheduling systems. Telephone handling is a particularly useful function. At a basic level, the system can maintain telephone number lists and autodial the number when desired. At a more advanced level, when one receives a phone call, the system would automatically call up on the screen the characteristics of the per-

Table 5–8. DESIRABLE CAPABILITIES OF A PATHOLOGIST'S WORKSTATION

1. Transparent integration of multiple data sources (see Table 5–9)
2. A unified multiwindow graphic user interface
3. Anatomic pathology report production and inquiry on data relevant to case
4. Facilitates the practice of clinical pathology (lab leadership and consultation)
5. Rule-based systems
6. Context-specific help
7. Flexibility and expandability
8. Personal information management
9. Portability of workstation functions to the bedside and conference room
10. Image management
11. Electronic mail
12. Automatic collation and organization of data from multiple sources
13. Standard/commercial tabletop computing productivity tools

son calling (e.g., medical specialty, list of current inpatients, recent problems and follow-ups)—either by the pathologist's entry of a name or by the caller ID function on the telephone. Finally, the workstation could maintain a private, professional, automatic log of pathologist consultative activities (e.g., phone inquiries from clinicians, substrate for billing, private notebook for future reference). However, one must avoid overdocumenting—such a log must be marked "not [an official?] part of the medical record." This log could be automatically produced as a byproduct (e.g., when the phone rings, enter the name of the clinician, and the workstation keeps track of all patients and items you have looked at).

A workstation is most helpful when it is always available. Therefore, the pathologist must have access to at least a subset of workstation functions at all times, even when up on the nursing unit on hospital rounds. Most of the database could be contained within a laptop computer carried by the pathologist at all times or accessed via wireless modem access from other locations. Some are attempting to incorporate workstation functions into even smaller PDAs. The challenges of a separate laptop or PDA database include keeping the database synchronized with the main workstation, software compatibility, and building the necessary communications infrastructure (such as wireless modems).

Image capabilities of the workstation include the capture of high-resolution color images from macroscopic sources (such as the surgical pathology gross bench and electrophoretic plates), from the microscope, from other patient image sources (such as radiology and endoscopy), and from both analog (video disc) and digital (CD-ROM) image databases. The pathologist must be able to annotate these images with text, freehand drawing, and voice, then store them in a long-term, well-indexed database (Foley, 1982). Images can be integrated with printed reports, used to create 35-mm Kodachrome slides or PhotoCDs for offsite presentations, or images can be transmitted electronically to the conference room. More sophisticated capabilities, including image processing and analysis, are discussed subsequently; some workstations will be able to drive an automated microscope.

Electronic mail must be automatically retrieved from LISs, HISs, the Internet, and other incompatible systems by the workstation, and the user must be alerted as it arrives. In some cases (e.g., the pathologist is out of the office for a few days), it may be desirable to reroute the messages to other modalities (fax, beeper, voice synthesis, voicemail).

A key feature of the workstation is its ability to seek and gather data from multiple data sources automatically (e.g., three times daily) and assemble this gathering into usable information. This may be in predefined ways, programmed by the workstation vendors, or in programmable fashion, as defined by the user.

Finally, the system should incorporate standard, commercially available tabletop computing productivity tools rather than reinvent the wheel. Even in the mid-1980s, the capabilities of these tools in meeting clinical laboratory needs was widely recognized; McNeeley (1987) has articulated these applications well.

Recent innovation in computer and telecommunications technology has made the paperless office feasible. Aside from the fact that it conserves trees, implementation of an all-electronic office is attractive in that it provides a work environment in which all information items may be tracked by a computer and an associated database. In such a setting, the likelihood of data loss or failure of adequate case follow-up is significantly reduced. For purposes of total quality management, comprehensive computer tracking is ideal, because specialized queries can be fabricated with little effort. Storing such data in a comprehensive database management system (DBMS) enables retrieval by multiple keys in addition to simple storage of data. Resulting database reports will be more complete and reflective of the actual state of data-flow within the laboratory. Documentation of quality control may also be more readily accessed for state and federal certifications, as needed.

Resources Available

A wide variety of knowledge resources are readily available to the pathologist; in addition to hundreds of sources on the Internet, some of the more important and commonly used are listed in Table 5–9. This list is for illustration only and is not complete; for one thing, the resources available will expand markedly over the next several years.

Table 5–9. RESOURCES FOR THE PATHOLOGIST'S WORKSTATION

1. Local computer systems
   a. LIS—lab data
   b. HIS—demographics, orders, financial, medical staff directory, etc.
   c. Radiology—reports
   d. Radiology picture archiving and communications systems (PACS)
   e. Pharmacy—medication profiles, drug interaction, etc.
   f. Transcription system—history and physicals, discharge summary
   g. Departmental local area networks (LANs)
   h. Databases derived from personal and hospital experience—surgical path, autopsy data, hospital-wide, test costing data
   i. Any database capable of accepting SQL queries
2. CD-ROMs
   a. MEDLINE—15–20 vendors (Aires, CD Plus, SilverPlatter, etc.)
   b. Other indexes (National Library of Medicine [NLM]—HLTH, non-NLM)
   c. Full-text journals
   d. Electronic textbooks—*SciAm Medicine, MAXX*, etc.
   e. Practice parameters
   f. Other resources—government regulations, lists, etc.
3. Video disc atlases
   a. ASCP, Image PSL, Slice of Life, University of Washington, etc.
   b. Use with screen grabber/digitizer
4. Electronic publishing
   a. Keyboard Publishing, Inc. full-text and hypercard stacks
   b. Government regulations
   c. Pathologist-oriented expert systems
      i. Commercially available—e.g., Nathwani's IntelliPath
      ii. Personal, group, institutional
5. Electronic bulletin boards—e.g., AACC
6. Online services—CompuServe, Prodigy, America Online, etc.
7. Online database vendors
   a. NLM—Grateful Med, PDQ, others
   b. Commercial—Paperchase, HealthCare Information Services, Dialog, etc.
8. Internet resources
   a. FTP sites
   b. Gopher
   c. WWW/Mosaic/NetScape servers
9. Images captured by video cameras, scanners, and so on
10. Entered by keyboard or optical character recognition from printed materials (e.g., self-assessment, recertification tests)

(Table continued on following page)

Table 5–9. RESOURCES FOR THE PATHOLOGIST'S WORKSTATION *(Continued)*

Company Addresses:

Aires Systems Corporation
200 Sutton Street
North Andover, MA 01845
(508) 975-7570

CD Plus
333 Seventh Avenue, 4th Floor
New York, NY 10001
(800) 950-2035

SilverPlatter Information, Inc.
100 River Ridge Drive
Norwood, MA 02062-5043
(800) 343-0064

Scientific American Medicine
415 Madison Ave
New York, NY 10017
(800) 545-0554

MAXX
c/o Little, Brown and Company
34 Beacon Street
Boston, MA 02108
(617) 859-0629

ASCP
2100 W. Harrison
Chicago, IL 60612
(800) 621-4142

Image Premastering Services, Ltd.
724 North 1st Street, Lower Level
Minneapolis, MN 55401
(800) 966-2932

Slice of Life
Eccles Health Sciences Library
University of Utah, Bldg #589
Salt Lake City, UT 84112-1185
(801) 581-8694

University of Washington
Health Sciences Center for Educational Resources
Health Sciences Bldg. T252, Mail Stop SB56
Seattle, WA 98195
(206) 685-1186

Keyboard Publishing, Inc.
482 Norristown Road, Suite 111
Blue Bell, PA 19422
(610) 832-0945

Intellipath
2828 East Foothill Blvd., Suite 204
Pasadena, CA 91107
(818) 585-9825

CompuServe
5000 Arlington Centre Blvd.
P.O. Box 20212
Columbus, OH 43220
(800) 848-8990

Prodigy
Corporate Headquarters
445 Hamilton Ave
White Plains, NY 10601
(800) 776-0845

America Online
8619 Westwood Center Drive
Vienna, Virginia 22181
(800) 827-6364

National Library of Medicine
8600 Rockville Pike
Bethesda, MD 20894
(301) 496-4671

Paperchase
350 Longwood Avenue
Boston, MA 02115
(800) 722-2075

HealthCare Information Services, Inc.
2335 American River Dr., #307
Sacramento, CA 95825
(800) 468-1128

Dialog Data Star
now: **Knight-Ridder Information, Inc.**
3460 Hillview Ave
Palo Alto, CA 94304
(800) 334-2564

An Example of Hardware Configuration

Table 5–10 lists, and Fig. 5–5 depicts, some hardware components that might form part of a pathologist's workstation. Again, evolving technology and locally available expertise are likely to make large changes in these components.

A digital desktop is made possible by several key elements. These usually include a personal computer, a high-speed fax modem, a flatbed page scanner, a direct digital camera, OCR software, a dedicated phone line, a link to the LIS, off-line back-up storage, a CD-ROM, and, optionally, a printer. With the juxtaposition of these components, it becomes possible to enter and generate documents without generating paper. This paperless office, as it is called, is attractive because the computer replaces conventional filing storage strategies. As already mentioned, with all files in digital format, not only can specialized searches be constructed, they can be performed in a fraction of the time that would be required to review a large file room.

As programs, operating systems, and data recording responsibilities become more complex, it becomes advantageous to use a machine with significant memory and hard disk space. An appropriate implementation (see Table 5–10) might include at least 32 megabytes of RAM and 1 gigabyte of hard disk space. With the doubling time of computer capability being approximately 18 months, it is reasonable to assume that a 64-megabyte memory/4-gigabyte hard disk desktop computer system will soon be commonplace.

For sites without direct access to the Internet by high-speed fiberoptic or coaxial cable, a high-speed modem is essential. Additionally, a modem may provide access to a number of commercial data service providers. Recent telecommunication standards provide for fast data rates (28.8 KBaud) via protocols such as V.Fast and V.34. The transmission rate of text files can be up to four times faster, owing to integral compression/decompression within the hardware of the modem. Many modems now incorporate fax capability and allow any computer to send or receive fax files without requiring or generating paper. This technology further speeds the advent of the paperless office.

Flatbed page scanners provide a quick and convenient method of entering images or printed matter into digital for-

Table 5–10. HARDWARE/SOFTWARE/SUPPORT OF THE PATHOLOGIST'S WORKSTATION

1. **Operating systems:** Mac, DOS, Windows, OS/2, UNIX, NextStep, Windows NT, Novell, etc.
2. **Hardware platform:** PC (486 or Pentium), Mac (PowerPC), UNIX (RISC chips), etc.
3. **Large-screen, high-resolution color monitor**
4. **Pointing devices:** mouse, light pen, touch screen, touch pad, etc.
   a. Future: Data glove (virtual reality), eyeball motion tracking
5. **Input devices**
   a. Keyboard
   b. Handwriting recognition/input
   c. Microphone for voice input
   d. Flatbed scanner
   e. Direct digital camera (microscope and copystand)
6. **Connections to LIS, HIS, Internet**
7. **Modem:** 14.4 KBaud or faster
8. **CD-ROM**
9. **1000+ MB magnetic disk**
10. **The following are often shared resources:**
    a. Backup device: tape, network
    b. Other image capture devices (e.g., slide scanners)
    c. Image output: slidemaker, overhead or projector
11. **Standard and specialized software**
    a. Word processor
    b. Spreadsheet
    c. Presentation graphics
    d. Statistical tools
    e. Communications programs
    f. Parser tools (e.g., Monarch)
    g. Outline processors (e.g., Maxthink)
    h. Database manager, indexing tools
    i. Programming tools (e.g., Visual Basic)
    j. Virus protection, locking software
12. **Staff to provide support!**—critical, often overlooked

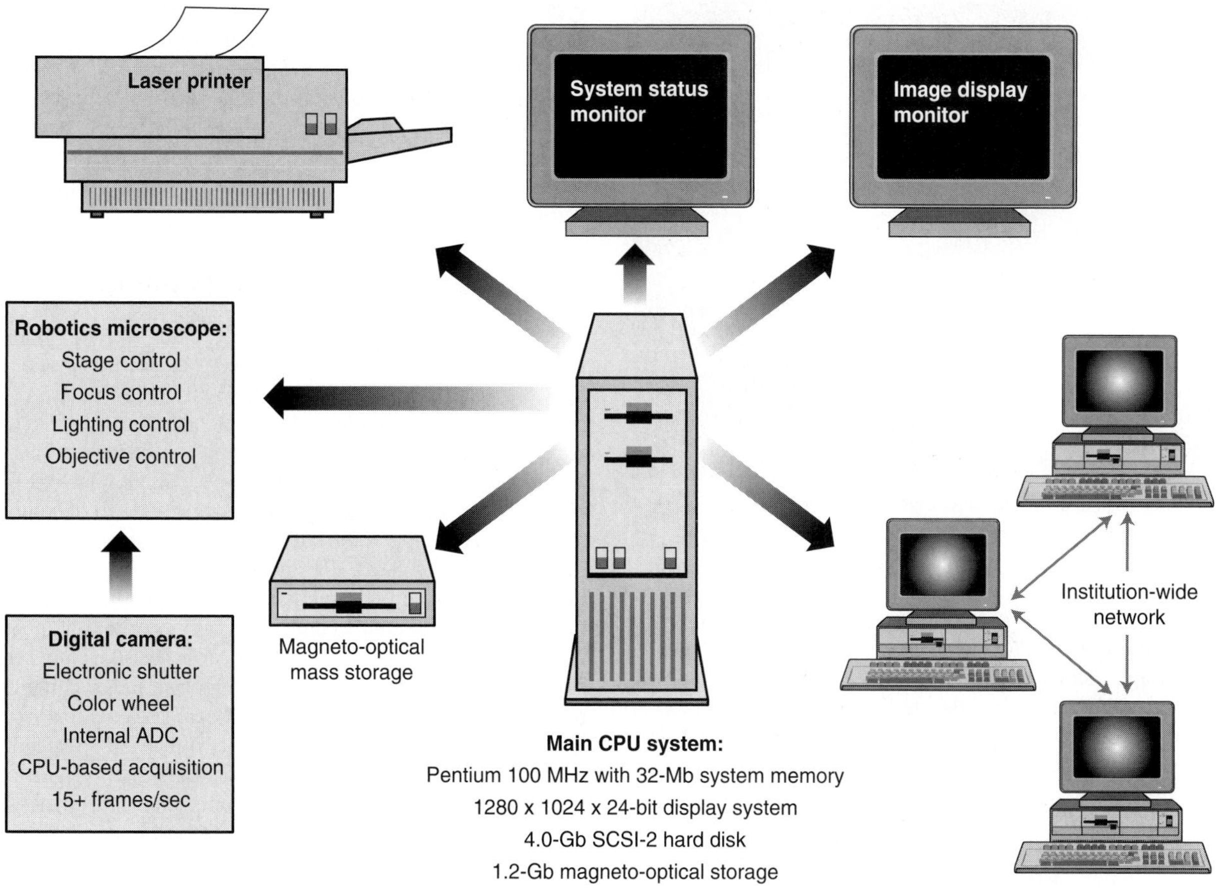

Figure 5–5. Typical pathologist workstation components.

mat for subsequent incorporation into documents and reports. With the addition of a transilluminator, it is also possible to scan slides, negatives, and even gels into digital format. A variation on this device, the slide scanner, is specifically designed to digitize 35-mm slides and negatives. Although somewhat more constrained in input versatility, it often provides for higher resolution and may be a useful tool in those applications requiring frequent and rapid digitization of large slide collections in which image fidelity is of utmost concern. Because this technology has matured in recent years, it is now possible to obtain a color scanner with 2700 DPI resolution for less than $2000.

The addition of a direct digital camera may be seen as a logical extension to the use of a flatbed page scanner. With a camera, it becomes possible to capture images from all types of settings, including microscopy, forensic documentation, and laboratory result documentation. Direct digital CCD cameras are preferable to the older analog counterparts in that they provide outstanding image fidelity and complete computer control of color balance, exposure, and linearity. The number of types of these devices is rapidly increasing alongside a concomitant precipitous decline in their overall expense.

Because some images may involve text, the use of a flatbed page scanner in conjunction with OCR software provides a powerful tool for entering printed matter into computer-readable text format. Some current packages recognize the text *and* layout information, such as columns, underlining, and italics. With this tool, the need for retyping documents from preprinted matter may be significantly reduced if not completely eliminated.

Hardcopy generation may be a necessary component of the workstation, depending on surrounding network topology. Current laser-electrostatic printers offer resolution between 600 and 2400 DPI with a vast array of features. Of note are the class of laser printers that incorporate the Postscript (Adobe) language. These printers offer maximal flexibility and printing capability with wide acceptance within the industry. Printer control language (PCL)–based printers, such as those manufactured by Hewlett Packard, are also widely supported by software. As a printer's DPI rating increases, so does its ability to render black-and-white and grayscale images. Grayscales are rendered on black-and-white output devices by a process known as halftoning. Grids of dots are assigned to each pixel on the source image. Light areas leave most of the dots white, whereas darker areas fill in with black increasing areas of the individual grid elements. When viewed at arm's length, the poor acuity of the human visual system blends these collections of dots together to form shades of gray. Color hardcopy generation has been available for some time in the form of inkjet printers. Although adequate for color graphic generation, they are less than ideal for generating true-color images. A recent entry to the true-color

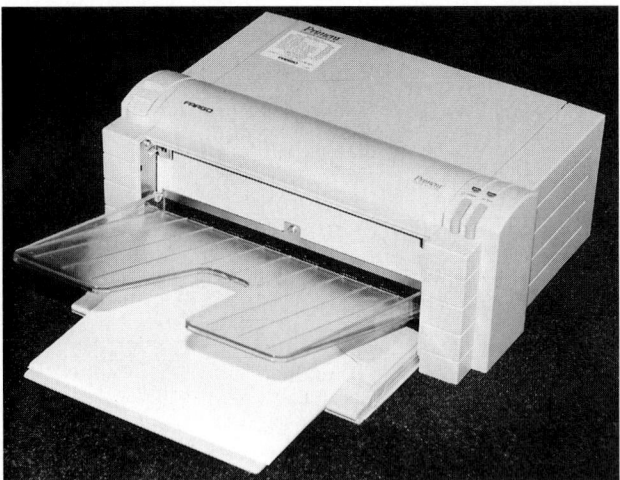

Figure 5–6. Dye sublimation true-color printer.

arena has been the dye sublimation printer. These devices (Fig. 5–6) can generate 24-bit, true-color printed images by using a three-color ribbon that deposits dye proportionally to the quantity of heat applied during the print process. The cost of these printers has fallen below $1000, making them accessible for most clinical laboratories.

Incorporation of Images into the Pathology Report

Applying the system just discussed to pathology creates an environment in which a pathologist could look up a case within seconds and have the computer display the archetypal images that were stored when the case was originally signed out. Numerous facts could be incorporated into the database, along with the pertinent gross and microscopic images. These could include patient name and demographics, medical record number, date, accession number, grossing physician/technologist, signing pathologist, gross and microscopic descriptions, diagnosis, SNOMED codes, CPT codes, hospital codes, and any additional comments that the pathologist believed it necessary to include. A number of LIS companies have started to offer these features as value-added features of their LIS. As technology improves and becomes less expensive, the digital image archival feature will become a standard and essential component of all pathology LIS packages.

Digital Imaging as a Cost-Effective Replacement for Film-Based Documentation

The standard method for image archival within the realm of pathology has been and continues to be the glass slide itself and the 35-mm slide. Of these two formats, the 35-mm slide is essentially the mainstay for compilation of teaching and lecture sets. Depending on the volume of photographs taken, it may be cost-effective to switch from film-based documentation to digital documentation and storage (Aubry, 1988; Lemke, 1993). Certainly, the initial cost of a digital imaging system is higher than a typical microscope camera. However, as the number of images acquired with the system increases, one will ultimately reach a break-even point at which the costs of the film has equaled the cost of the imaging system. The cost of any digital image is essentially nil; long-term storage on floppy disks would cost about 2.5 cents per image. This is considerably less than the cost of current film and development charges.

Digital Image Presentations

As already mentioned, a significant advantage of imaging in the digital domain is the *plasticity* that is gained in terms of image composition and manipulation. With digital images, it becomes possible to compile a slide presentation without slides in which the pathologist is free to overlay text, juxtapose images, and reorder images, all without having a single piece of film. Numerous commercial programs are available to accomplish this with ease (e.g., *Photoshop,* Adobe, Mountain View, CA; *Powerpoint,* Microsoft, Redmond, WA; *Persuasion,* Aldus, Seattle, WA). When the final slide presentation is compiled, it then may be presented to audiences by use of any number of high-resolution video projectors that can render the output from computers. These are becoming common in larger conference rooms and auditoriums. For a tumor board presentation, for example, the pathologist would arrive with a laptop computer containing the preselected and preordered digital images, connect it to the video projector or liquid-crystal display panel on a high-power overhead projector, and proceed. In this setting, the need for film would be completely eliminated.

Telepathology

An interesting development made possible by digital imaging is telepathology. Initially, these systems were analog video and poor in image quality. As digital systems have come into being, it has become possible to rapidly send a high-quality, color image over the phone line or other communications link. Telepathology implementations are beginning to appear within the domain of the Internet. The standard Internet information packet transfer protocol, TCP/IP, can be used as a wrapper for both real-time and still-frame image information. Both paradigms have successfully used TCP/IP to exchange histopathologic images for diagnostic and educational applications. Standardized Internet applications for image exchange are starting to appear, such as "C U, See Me," a protocol designed primarily for video teleconferencing over the network.

It remains to be seen whether telepathology applications will rely mainly on point-to-point connection (via high speed lines or the telephone network) or on a shared network such as the Internet. In either case, this field of pathology will mature rapidly in the next decade, a change facilitated by improving technology and driven by the needs of the solo or geographically isolated pathologist.

IMAGE PROCESSING

As the name implies, image processing reflects an operation in which a source image is to be acted on (processed), producing an *output image*. This is not that same as image analysis, in which a source image is mathematically examined to produce (nonimage) data. A technology inspired by satellite and reconnaissance photography, image processing is most often concerned with the removal of a known (or unknown) artifact or the rendering of the image to a *more useful state* by some set of functions (Gonzalez, 1992; Russ, 1992; Watkins, 1993).

Photographic Issues

Photomicrography can be a challenging task. Inherent problems include focus, color temperature, exposure, contrast, depth of field, color inaccuracy due to film variation, color bleeding (chromatic aberration) due to poor optics, vignetting (spherical aberration) due to nonplanar optics, nonuniform lighting, and dust. The reversal of these and other artifacts is a task well-suited for image processing.

Exposure and Contrast

In performing photomicrography, one is acutely aware of ensuring correct exposure. The use of color film compounds this need, because it possesses significantly less dynamic range than black-and-white film does. Typically, an overexposed or underexposed photograph will need to be retaken. When working with images in the digital domain, there is no added expense for taking additional photographs. Thus, if one is obtaining images directly from a digital camera, the electronic shutter time can be adjusted until the exposure is perfect. In the setting of an improperly exposed print or negative, image processing can offer its greatest impact. High-resolution flatbed color scanners have become affordable (e.g., those made by Hewlett Packard, Palo Alto, CA; Epson, Torrance, CA; and Apple, Cupertino, CA). With them, it is possible to take any print, negative, or slide and convert it to the digital domain. Once in the digital format, an image may be easily manipulated to compensate for overexposure or underexposure. This typically involves multiplying each color component (red, green, blue) of a pixel by some constant. This constant is chosen such that it expands or compresses the dynamic range of the image to appropriate contrast levels. This is followed by an addition or subtraction step, which places the image in the correct brightness range. In many ways, this is like the brightness and contrast controls of any television. The only real difference is that the operations are done in a digital domain and are thus much more immune to cumulative system noise. The final result is a better image. Also, because of the real-time nature of image processing, the final image is immediately available for critique. If it is not satisfactory, the processing parameters may be modified until an acceptable image is obtained.

Color Systems

Although humans perceive color to be a continuum from the deep red to the violet, the reality is that our perception is based on the combination of photoreceptors sensitive to three specific wavelength bandpasses: Red, green, and blue. These three colors, known as *the primary colors,* form the basis of our perception of color. The primary color system is based on the premise of an emissive light source—that is, situations in which light is being produced as opposed to being absorbed. Conversely, the secondary color system applies to situations in which an absorptive color source is in place, such as printed color images. The three secondary colors are cyan, magenta, and yellow, or CMY (for four-process printing, black may be included—CMYK). Deposition of these colors on paper or film in varying ratios will produce any color of the spectrum. Distinction of color system is essential for both image processing and analysis. Most, if not all, digital color cameras generate a color image by obtaining a monochromatic image in the red, green, and blue bands. Conversely, most color hardcopy generation systems employ CMY generation. As such, the imaging system must be able to perform the appropriate matrix transformation to convert between these color systems. Neither the RGB nor the CMY system is always the optimal color image representation for either image processing or analysis. Because actual perceived color is a function of *the ratio* of the three primary colors, changing the brightness or saturation of a color within the RGB system, without changing the hue, can become complex. To alleviate this difficulty, the hue-saturation-intensity (HSI) system was developed. With this representation, it becomes possible to change any one of the aforementioned color properties without affecting the other two. From a computational perspective, this is ideal, because the image may be edited in more naturally such that hue is the color itself, saturation is the color's deviation from gray, and intensity is the color's brightness, ranging from black to white. Selection of an imaging system with RGB, HSI, and CMY color schemes is desirable. Most desktop color production systems now offer these color representations; some offer even additional ones (e.g., HSY and Y/C).

Color Temperature

The use of a tungsten filament for a light source is problematic. As voltage is increased to the filament, the light intensity increases. Unfortunately, this increase is not uniform across the visible spectrum. The notion of *color temperature* has been developed to deal with this fact. Hotter filaments have a higher color temperature, whereas cooler filaments have a lower color temperature. Higher color temperatures have a greater predominance of blue, whereas lower color temperatures have a higher predominance of red. Thus, the color response of color film, which also has red and blue layers, will depend on filament temperature. It is not uncommon to take many photomicrographs only to later discover that they are all too red or too blue. This situation usually results in rephotographing the slides with the filament intensity appropriately modified (or so one hopes). With a digital camera, this problem is minimized, because color temperature can be corrected in real time, as one observes the digital image. Again, as in the example given earlier, if the image is already a print or slide, a flatbed scanner can be used to enter the digital domain. The digital correction of color temperature is a close relative of the contrast and brightness functions. Specific operators are applied individually to the red, green, and blue channels to obtain the correct tint. Thus, if an image were too blue, the blue components of each pixel would be divided by some value, the green would be left unchanged, and the red components would be multiplied by some value. Again, the analogy of the television holds true, with this processing operation being similar to *tint*.

Film Variation

Not all films are created equal. Not all films respond to light in the same manner. With current multilayer film technology, there appears to be significant variation in spectral response, depending on film brand and speed. This results in subtle color variations between film types that extends beyond simple color temperature variations. By going to the digital domain and individually modifying the separate red, green, and blue multipliers and divisors, it is possible to compensate for just about any type of color film artifact. In the case of direct digital imaging, this is not an issue, because most cameras provide individual color channel gain control.

Poor Optics

Microscope image aberrations caused by low-grade or improperly coupled optics include both spatial and chromatic aberrations. In an attempt to compensate for these refractive errors, manufacturers have developed plan (two-color correcting) and plan-apo (three-color correcting) objectives. This has resulted in superior image quality as seen at the binocular eyepiece. Unfortunately, this is not always the case at the film or CCD image plane. Often, camera coupling systems make use of the secondary image plane as opposed to the primary image plane. This may introduce unnecessary optics. The lenses in these adapters may or may not have three-color correction, as with the primary objective. If they do not, both chromatic and spherical aberrations *will* occur. If the image recording device is film-based, these artifacts are essentially irreversible. If the imaging device is a digital CCD, essentially every artifact can be numerically reversed. Polynomial warping, a technique developed to patch together satellite photographs, is a technique of transforming images with a known spherical aberration (i.e., the moon is round) to a hypothetic flat domain. In this setting, all images are normalized to a "flat" world in which no stretch or compression occurs.

Polynomial warping can just as easily be applied to a spherically defective microscopic image with remarkable success. Correcting chromatic aberration is almost as simple. The red-blue color-fringing of chromatic aberration is due to different degrees of spherical aberration (i.e., refraction) at different wavelengths. Thus, if each channel of a color CCD were to be warped separately, with appropriate transformations for each color, *both spherical and chromatic* defects would be removed. Finally, problems of unflat focus field may be corrected by applying a specialized *finite response filter* to reverse the lens defect. This is the same technique as used to initially correct the Hubble telescope's defective mirror artifact before corrective optics could be inserted. Without going into further detail, suffice it to say that a number of commercial image archival and analysis packages offer automated correction of all the artifacts discussed.

Nonuniform Light

Even a correctly aligned microscope substage condenser and light assembly produces nonuniform lighting. This is sometimes a problem with low-magnification micrography. A digital CCD can be used to completely avoid this problem. If the background variation is known for every point in the image, a compensatory function can be applied to an image projected via this nonuniform light source. This leads to the notion of a subtraction, or background, image. An initial so-called white background image is taken. The variation in pixels is noted and stored. When a test image is later taken, each pixel in this test image is normalized by the local domain differences in the background image. The final image exhibits uniform background intensity characteristics.

IMAGE ANALYSIS

As already mentioned, image analysis is that field concerned with extracting some type of useful data from an image. Often, this is as simple as a single numeric value. In biology, image analysis is primarily concerned with identifying cells and then determining what qualitative and quantitative features are present in these cells.

Basic Tools and Applications of Image Analysis

Thresholding

This technique converts a color image into a two-tone black-and-white image (Fig. 5–7). Thresholding is important in that it provides a platform for subsequent image analysis operations. The advantage of a thresholded image is that it is binary; colors are either black (0) or white (1). In such a situation, the operators of Boolean algebra can be directly applied to the image. Thresholding is an important first step for operators involved with counting items, such as cell counting. This makes sense, because cells are often darker than their surrounding area (e.g., a cervical cytology smear).

Erosions/Dilations (Opening Function)

Once an image is thresholded, this process may be used to separate cells that are touching. Thus, the computer can identify each cell as a separate, *individually quantifiable* entity. This is important when it is desirable to attain accurate counts of cells with a unique feature, such as immunoperoxidase positivity.

Color Space Evaluation

In the preceding example, cell identification was not the only function employed. With the use of immunoperoxidase, it is clear that the computer will need to identify a specific color—in this case, brown. As it turns out, evaluating and identifying color in red-green-blue space is cumbersome and slow. Modeled after the additive color system, a three-dimensional colorspace has been developed that separates hue, saturation, and intensity. This is known as the HSI system. In this colorspace, it is possible to specify a color with a single value: hue. The saturation is a parameter indicating the deviation from neutral gray, and the intensity is the lightness value of the color between black and white. To search for the brown of an immunohistochemical stain, a hue (color) and an intensity must be selected. This is followed by the selection of a saturation range (a range of browns that could be very washed-out to very rich); this sets the guidelines for what types of browns will be considered immunohistochemically positive. This method is simpler for a computer than attempting to analyze varying ratios of red, green, and blue as the intensity changes. Image analysis systems that cannot perform HSI calculations offer greatly decreased flexibility and effectiveness.

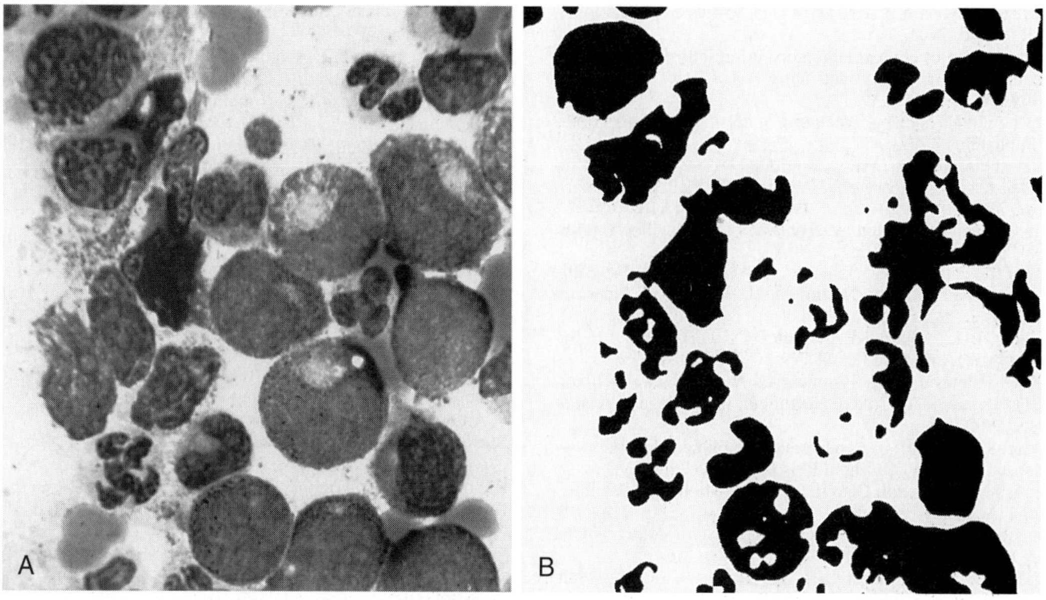

Figure 5–7. Basic illustration of thresholding: Original gray-scale digital image (*A*) is compared on a pixel by pixel basis with any arbitrary threshold value. Those pixels brighter than this value are assigned white; all other pixels are assigned a color of black. The resulting image (*B*) is a thresholded image, being suitable for many image analysis and processing operations not easily performed on original images.

Optical Density Integration

The Feulgen stain, discovered in Germany in the 1920s, is valuable in that it binds with DNA stoichiometrically (at least theoretically). An interesting consequence of this property is that optical density (absorbance) for any given point in the cross-sectional image of a Feulgen-stained cell is proportional to total DNA content for that area. Thus, if optical densities are taken for all points within the cross-sectional area of the cell, an integrated DNA content will be obtained. This is the basis of most, if not all, image-based DNA cytometers. Typically, this is a monochromatic measurement and often requires greater than the usual 8 bits of dynamic range (generally, at least 12-bit CCDs are needed to cover the dynamic range [four absorbance units] of typical Feulgen staining). Often, DNA analysis by image is helpful when material is insufficient for flow-cytometric analysis.

Cellularity Determination in Bone Marrow Biopsies

Taking a ratio of cellular to acellular areas seen on a bone marrow biopsy has proven helpful in generating quantitative cellularity values. This is of particular value in patients who have undergone bone marrow transplantation, in whom a precise cellularity determination is helpful in assessing engraftment course. Variation in human performance can be essentially removed.

The Virtual Reality Slide

With the large storage capabilities offered by the CD-ROM, it has become possible to encode the entire three-dimensional information of a glass slide and compress it to fit within the space of a CD-ROM (about 600 megabytes). Thus, a pathologist could wander around a slide, focus up and down, and change magnifications, all without ever having the glass itself. Proficiency testing for cytopathology is a prime candidate for this technology; CD-ROMs could be sent to proficiency participants in lieu of slides. The advantages of such a system include unlimited same slide, no attrition or loss of slides, it is inexpensive to write CD-ROMs ($2.00 apiece), and CD-ROMs are easily extended to thousands of new proficiency sites as CLIA '88 guidelines for cytology proficiency testing begin to be enforced. The use of this technology for cytology proficiency testing is being considered because CLIA '88 recommendations make it impractical to continue with a slide-based national testing program serving an increasing number of participants.

Aller RD: Clinical informatics as a medical subspecialty. Health Care Information Management 1994a; 7(4):11.

Aller RD: The laboratory information system as a medical device: inspection and accreditation issues. Clinical Laboratory Management Review 1992 (Jan/Feb); 6(1):58.

Aller RD, deWitt C: Cytology result entry without using the keyboard. Acta Cytol 1994b; 38:739.

Aller RD, Elevitch ER (eds): Symposium on computers in the clinical laboratory. Clin Lab Med 1983; 3(1): entire issue.

Aller RD, Elevitch FR (eds): Symposium on laboratory and hospital information systems. Clin Lab Med 1991; 11(1): entire issue.

Aller RD, Weilert M: Instrument interface subsystems. CAP TODAY 1995 (June); 9(6):636.

Altshuler CH: Building a database for monitoring and facilitating health care. Clin Lab Med 1983; 3(1):179.

American Medical Association: Practice Guidelines on CD-ROM. Chicago, AMA, 1995.

Anderson JG, Aydin CE, Jay SJ: Evaluating Health Care Information Systems, Methods and Applications. Thousand Oaks, CA, Sage Publications, 1994.

ASTM Standards, Volume 14.01, Philadelphia, American Society for Testing and Materials, 1995.

Aston R, Schwarz J: Multimedia—Gateway to the Next Millenium. Boston, Academic Press, 1994.

Aubry F, Badaoui S, Kaplan H, et al: Design and implementation of a biomedical image database (BDIM). Med Inf (Lond) 1988; 13(4):241.

Balis UJ, Aller RD, Ashwood ER: Informatics training in U.S. pathology residency programs. Results of a survey. Am J Clin Pathol 1993; 100(4 Suppl 1):S44–7.

Ball MJ, Collen MF: Computers in Health Care, Aspects of the Computer-based Patient Record. New York, Springer-Verlag, 1992.

Beizer B: The Frozen Keyboard, Living with Bad Software. Philadelphia, Van Nostrand Reinhold, 1986.

Brannigan VM: Regulation of clinical laboratory information systems after the 1990 amendments to the Food and Drug Act. Clinical Laboratory Management Review 1992; 6(1):49.

Bria WF, Rydell RL: The Physician-Computer Connection. Chicago, American Hospital Publishing, 1992.

CAP TODAY: Newsbytes column, every issue. Articles and surveys on informatics in at least six issues per year, Northfield, IL, College of American Pathologists, 1987–ongoing.

Clark JS, Voterri B, Ariagno R: Noninvasive assessment of blood gases. Am Rev Respir Dis 1992; 145:220.

College of American Pathologists: Laboratory Accreditation Program. Checklist for General Laboratory. Northfield, IL, College of American Pathologists, 1995.

Connelly DP, Sielaff BH, Willard KE: A clinician's workstation for improving laboratory use. Am J Clin Pathol 1995; 104:243.

Cote R, Rothwell D, Palotay J, et al: Systematized Nomenclature of Medicine (SNOMED International), 3rd ed. Northfield, IL, College of American Pathologists, 1993.

Dito WR, McIntire S, Leano J: Bar codes and the clinical laboratory—adaptation perspectives. Clin Lab Mgmt Rev 1992; 6(1):72.

Donaldson M, Lohr K (eds): Health Data in the Information Age. Washington, DC, National Academy Press, 1994.

Elevitch FR: Negotiating a laboratory information system contract. Clin Lab Mgmt Rev 1992; 6(1):30.

Elevitch FR, Aller RD: The ABCs of LIS, Revised ed. Chicago, ASCP Press, 1989.

Foley JD, VanDam A: Fundamentals of Interactive Computer Graphics. Reading, MA, Addison-Wesley, 1982.

Friedman BA: The impact of new features of laboratory information systems on quality assurance in anatomic pathology. Arch Pathol Lab Med 1988; 112:1189.

Friedman BA: The potential role of the physician in the management of hospital information systems. Clin Lab Med 1990: 10(1):239.

Friedman BA, Dito WR (eds): Laboratory Information Systems—A Focus Issue. Clin Lab Mgmt Rev 1992: 6(1):entire issue.

Gilster P: The Internet Navigator. New York, John Wiley and Sons, 1994.

Gonzalez RC, Woods RE: Digital Image Processing. Reading, MA, Addison-Wesley, 1992.

Hahn H, Stout RO: The Internet Yellow Pages. Berkeley, McGraw-Hill, 1994.

Hendricks EJ: Laboratory computers: Tools for increased productivity. Clin Lab Med 1985: 5(4):709.

Henry JB: Computers in medical education. Hum Pathol 1990; 21:998.

HIBCC: Provider Applications Standard. Phoenix, AZ, Health Industries Business Communications Council, 1992.

Institute of Medicine: The Computer-Based Patient Record. Washington, DC, National Academy Press, 1991.

Krieg AF: Laboratory Communication: Getting Your Message Through. Oradell, NJ, Medical Economics Press, 1978.

Lemke HU: Future directions in electronic image handling. Invest Radiol 1993; 28(Suppl 3):S79.

Lincoln TL, Aller RD: Acquiring a laboratory computer system—vendor selection and contracting. Clin Lab Med 1991; 11(1):21.

Lincoln TL, Korpman RA: Computers, health care, and medical information science. Science 1980; 210(4467):257.

Matson TA, McDougall MD: Information Systems for Ambulatory Care. Chicago, American Hospital Publishing, 1990.

Mattheus R: European standardization efforts: An important framework for medical imaging. Eur J Radiol 1993; 17(1):28.

Mattheus R, Noothoven van Goor JM: The European Community: Standardization in medical informatics and imaging. Comput Methods Programs Biomed 1992; 37(4):333.

McAlister NH, Covvey HD: Micromania and the instant expert syndrome. Computers in Hospitals, 1981 (Nov/Dec); 2(6):36.

McDonald C (Chairman): ASTM Committee on Interlaboratory Data Exchange: Specification for Transferring Clinical Observations Messages Between Independent Computer Systems, E1238-94. Philadelphia, American Society for Testing and Materials, 1994.

McNeeley MD: Microcomputer Applications in the Clinical Laboratory. Chicago, ASCP Press, 1987.

Pribor HC: The Laboratory Consultant. Philadelphia, Lea & Febiger, 1992.

Russ JC: The Image Processing Handbook. Boca Raton, FL, CRC Press, 1992.

Sazama K: Accreditation Requirements Manual, 6th ed. Bethesda, MD, American Association of Blood Banks, 1995.

Shortliffe EH, Perreault LE, Wiederhold G, Fagan LM: Medical Informatics: Computer Applications in Health Care. Reading, MA, Addison-Wesley, 1990.

Sittig DF, Stead WW: Computer-based physician order entry: The state of the art. J Am Med Informatics Assoc 1994; 1(2):108.

Skinner M, Aller RD, Weilert M: Anatomic pathology computer systems survey: To integrate or stand alone. CAP Today 1994; 8(2):227.

Skolnick MH, Cannon-Albright LA, Ward JH, et al: Inheritance of proliferative breast disease in breast cancer kindreds. Science 1990; 250:1715.

Springer-Verlag Series on Computers in Medicine (Orthner H, series editor) and on Computers in Health Care (Hannah K, Ball M, series editors). New York, Springer-Verlag, 1986–ongoing.

Steane S (Chairman): American Association of Blood Banks Information Systems Committee, Guidelines for Implementation and Validation of Blood Bank Computer Systems. Arlington, VA, AABB, several sections published 1989–1994.

Tapscott D, Caston A: Paradigm Shift, The New Promise of Information Technology. New York, McGraw-Hill, 1993.

Tierney WM, Miller ME, Overhage JM, McDonald CJ: Physician inpatient order writing on microcomputer workstations: Effects on resource utilization. JAMA 1993; 269:379.

Tufte ER: Envisioning Information. Cheshire, CT, Graphics Press, 1990.

Watkins C: Modern Image Processing: Warping, Morphing, and Classical Techniques. Cambridge, MA, Academic Press, 1993.

Quality Management

Jannie Woo, Ph.D.
John Bernard Henry, M.D.

Clinicians depend on clinical laboratory data to assist them with

1. Screening for disease or case finding
2. Diagnosis of disease
3. Therapeutic monitoring

The analytical requirements of a laboratory result differ for each category of use. Analytical precision influences the usefulness of a test result in recognizing day-to-day changes in a patient versus a change in the laboratory result (i.e., therapeutic monitoring). Both analytical precision and accuracy to achieve clinical utility are required in the diagnosis of disease. For screening or case-finding purposes, clinical sensitivity and specificity are critical factors. Case finding applies to disease or risk factor identification among patients who have had the benefit of prior physician or other health professional assessment with measurement selection and a need for special determinations thus identified. Although screening because of population selected and disease prevalence may offer less benefit in terms of cost, case finding is more cost-effective. Hence, screening for disease has diminished compared with case finding.

QUALITY ASSURANCE AND QUALITY CONTROL

Quality assurance (QA) is defined by the National Committee for Clinical Laboratory Standards (NCCLS)* as "the practice which encompasses all endeavors, procedures, formats, and activities directed towards ensuring that a specified quality or product is achieved and maintained." When applied to the clinical laboratory, QA includes maneuvers encountered in the preanalytic, analytic, and postanalytic phases of laboratory testing. More specifically, QA monitors quality performance starting from the ordering of a laboratory determination to its reporting, the interpretation of results, and their application in patient care. QA may be modeled after Deming's (1986) concept of total quality control, which requires constant attention of all involved with the process or system. This is discussed further in Chapter 1.

Statistical quality control (QC) is concerned with the analytical phase of QA. It monitors the overall reliability of labo-

*NCCLS, 771 E. Lancaster Avenue, Villanova, PA 19085.

ratory results in terms of accuracy and precision according to the criteria specified for each measurement/examination. Its success relies on the diligent and persistent execution of the following QC-associated activities, all of which are part and parcel of quality management and QA:

1. Assay of control samples
2. Instrument maintenance
3. Statistical data analysis
4. Proficiency testing survey

Analytical Bias

A basic premise of QC is that reported laboratory values should correspond to the correct or expected values—that is, the reported values should fall along a line of slope 1.00 when graphed as shown in Figure 6–1*A*. However, all procedures are subject to a variety of analytical variations and inaccuracies, or biases. Figure 6–1*B* illustrates the effects of a proportional bias in which the reported values are higher than the expected values. Figure 6–1*C* illustrates the effect of a constant bias, wherein the reported values are higher than the expected values by a constant amount at all concentrations of analyte.

Many analytical procedures are subject to either constant or proportional bias, or to both. Figure 6–1*D* illustrates how combined constant and proportional biases may affect the correlation of reported and expected values.

Charts such as those shown in Figure 6–1 have been called operational charts, and the lines on which the reported values fall have been called operational lines, because every laboratory produces results that tend to fall along some line when graphed as shown in Figure 6–1 (Grannis, 1972). That is, each laboratory for each analytical procedure customarily operates with a certain degree of bias that causes its results to be distributed along some operational line, as shown in Figure 6–1. Ideally, all laboratories would have an operational line of slope 1.00 (see Fig. 6–1*A*) so that their reported values would be unbiased and correspond exactly to the known values. But if this ideal cannot be attained, then the laboratory's customary operational line should at least be maintained in a reproducible manner.

Random Analytical Variability

In addition to analytical biases, laboratory analyses are also subject to imprecision, or random variability. The effects of random variation on analyses are illustrated in Figure 6–2,

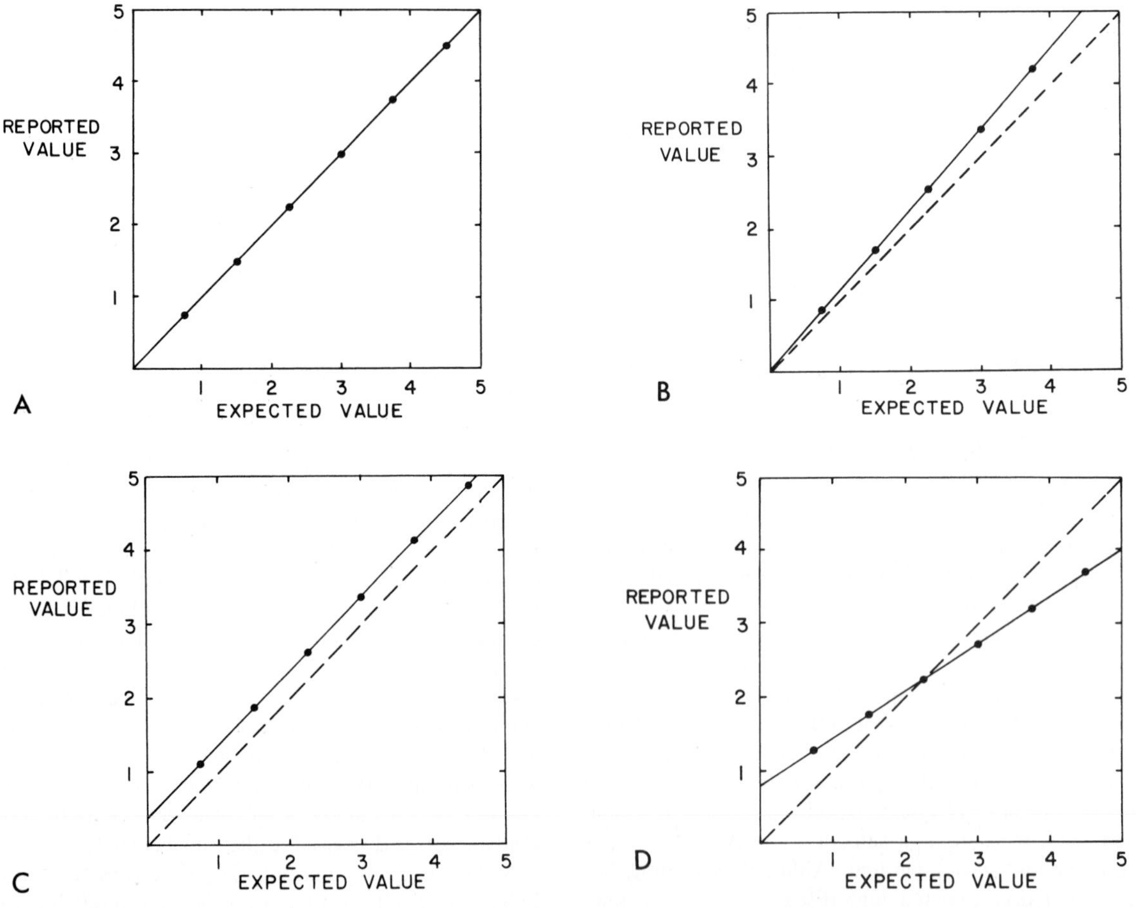

Figure 6–1. Illustration of the concept of the "operational line" when the laboratory's reported values for a series of specimens are plotted against the expected values. *A* shows an ideal situation, in which the reported values fall along the straight line of slope 1.0. However, variations from the ideal condition occur with all laboratory procedures. *B* illustrates the occurrence of proportional bials. *C* illustrates constant bias. *D* shows the occurrence of both proportional and constant biases.

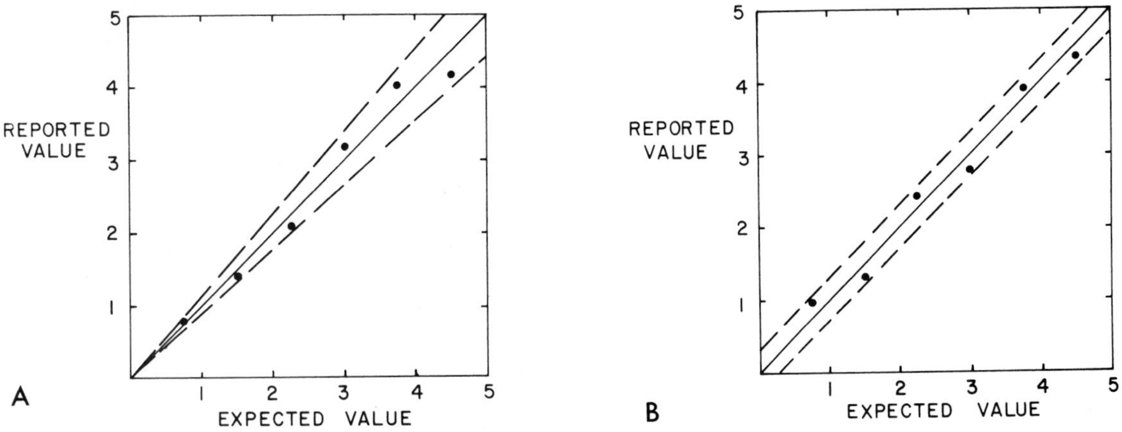

Figure 6–2. Illustration of the effect of random variations on laboratory results. *A* shows random variation that increases in proportion to the mean analyte concentration, whereas *B* shows random variation that may be constant at all analyte concentrations.

which shows how a laboratory's results may, on the average, fall along some operational line even though the individual results are distributed about the line within certain limits of variability. Figure 6–2*A* illustrates limits of variability that increase in proportion to the mean analyte concentration, whereas Figure 6–2*B* illustrates limits of variability that are constant at all concentrations of analyte.

Knowledge of the kinds of bias and random variability that affect an analytical system is helpful in identifying their causes. For example, proportional limits of variability are commonly caused by a bias in volumetric dispensing of the specimen aliquot. An automatic pipettor is a mechanical device, and as such there may be a certain amount of variation in the operation of its parts, which may increase as the parts become worn. Variation in the amount of specimen measured by such a pipettor introduces variation in the analytical results that is proportional to the analyte concentration of the specimen, and causes proportional variability as shown in Figure 6–2*A*. Similarly, constant limits of variability are commonly observed in analytical procedures that are influenced by the turbidity of the specimen. Specimen turbidity is usually independent of analyte concentration but may vary from specimen to specimen, thus causing results to be distributed between constant limits, as shown in Figure 6–2*B*. Thus, knowledge of how various sources of analytical bias and variability affect the accuracy and precision of the operational line can be most helpful in identifying and in correcting analytical problems as they arise.

Errors

In addition to analytical factors that introduce bias and random variability into the analytical procedure, laboratory analyses are also subject to errors. It is sometimes difficult to determine whether an erroneous result was due to an analytical factor or to an error, but the differentiation is important if the cause of a problem is to be identified and corrected. Analytical errors are usually systematic. That is, they are caused by some factor in the analytical system that can affect a series of analyses. For example, an erroneously calibrated pipettor might cause a systematic proportional bias, whereas a pipettor that operates imprecisely causes random variability of analyses. Such personnel or operator errors occur rather seldomly, however, and usually affect only a few analyses. A specimen might be mislabeled, the analytical result might be assigned to the wrong specimen, or the numbers in the analytical value might be transposed. These incidents are due to human carelessness rather than to deficiencies in the analytical system.

One important aspect of QC is to identify those steps in the analytical process in which the likelihood of error is high and to consider ways to minimize that likelihood.

Accuracy

Accuracy is defined as the extent to which the mean measurement is close to the true value. The accuracy of a method is generally reflected by its ability to reproduce the values of reference samples of known concentrations. Sometimes, the accuracy of a determination for an analyte is impossible to achieve or can be acquired only at the expense of lengthy turn-around time. Examples are the determination of blood glucose prior to the era of specific enzymatic glucose assays, the determination of creatinine before the advent of initial rate reaction, or the measurement of suppressed thyroid-stimulating hormone (TSH) levels of hyperthyroid patients using a first-generation TSH assay. It is critical that the user or clinician be made aware of the analytical performance of each assay so that due allowance may be made in the clinical interpretation of the results. Accuracy sufficient for clinical use, as well as for analytical accuracy, should be recognized.

Precision

The distribution of results of a given assay in the laboratory, when performed multiple times, may be graphically depicted by a frequency curve. Most statistical techniques are based on the assumption that such distributions are usually symmetric and bell-shaped, the so-called normal or gaussian curve. As shown in Figure 6–3, if the total area under the

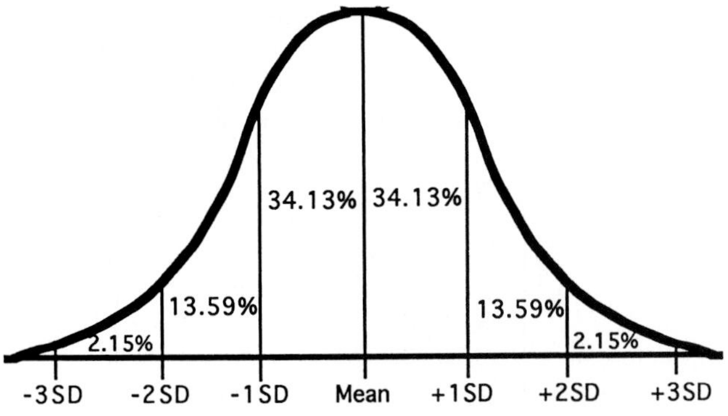

Figure 6–3. Normal frequency or gaussian curve.

curve is equal to all the results plotted, then 68% of the values fall within one standard deviation (SD) around the mean, 95.5% of the values fall within 2 SDs around the mean, and 99.7% of the values fall within three SDs around the mean. SD is a measure of dispersion of the values and may be calculated as follows:

$$SD = (\Sigma(\overline{X} - X)^2/(n-1))^{1/2} \qquad (6\text{-}1)$$

Where $\overline{X}$ = mean of all observed values
= $\Sigma X/n$
X = observed values
n = number of observations

Precision is a measure of random variability. It is defined as the reproducibility of a laboratory determination when it is run repeatedly under identical conditions. Precision is independent of accuracy; an inaccurate result can be extremely precise. Precision is commonly expressed in terms of SD, which can be determined using the formula described previously. For practical convenience, SD is converted to the coefficient of variation (CV), which is calculated as follows:

$$CV = (SD/X) \times 100 \qquad (6\text{-}2)$$

where X = the concentration of the analyte in question.

Use of CV to express precision is adequate for most routine clinical laboratory determinations when SD is proportional to the concentration range of interest.

Most laboratories choose the 95% confidence limit in expressing precision (i.e., mean ± 2 SD), taking 95% of the area under the gaussian curve to be the limit of precision or expected variation.

INTRODUCTION TO QUALITY CONTROL TECHNIQUES

QC can be divided into two major types: internal QC (intralaboratory QC), which primarily monitors the day-to-day performance of laboratory tests, namely *precision*, and external QC (interlaboratory QC), which monitors primarily the *accuracy* of laboratory tests. Intralaboratory QC can be based either on the results of control specimens or on the results of patient specimens.

INTRALABORATORY PRECISION MONITORING BASED ON CONTROL SPECIMENS

A variety of statistical control techniques use control charts to display the control observation (or a calculated statistic) as a function of time (date, run number). The Levey-Jennings chart (Barger, 1992) provided an early description of the use of statistical QC for improvement of laboratory performance. A so-called multi-rule technique developed by Westgard (1981) is now widely used both manually and implemented in automatic chemistry analyzers. A cumulative sum technique developed by Woodard (1964) has shown good sensitivity in detecting bias but has not been widely applied in clinical laboratories. Other QC formats in use include the mean and range techniques, the trend analysis techniques, and the analysis of variance technique.

Quality Control Materials

The use of samples obtained from the same pool for the comparison of laboratory analyses was the first method introduced and is still the most direct and widely applied QA technique (Henry, 1952). When samples (assumed to be identical) of aqueous solutions of analytes, or of liquid serum or urine, were distributed to several laboratories for analysis, the results revealed clear evidence of substantial systematic differences among the laboratories (Belk, 1947). This established the important principle that a laboratory's analyses could be compared with those of other laboratories, or with its own prior analyses, simply by periodically analyzing samples that had been reserved from a large serum pool. The studies of Belk and Sunderman (1947) led directly to the establishment of interlaboratory comparison programs, and the studies of Levey led to the establishment of intralaboratory QC programs.

However, the development of these programs was not without difficulty. In order to be effective, the samples had to be essentially equivalent to one another, the analytes in the sample had to be stable in storage over a substantial period of time, and enough of the material had to be available to be used by many laboratories or by a single laboratory for a long period of time. Most QC materials used today are lyophilized products prepared from large pools of serum.

To enhance clinical usefulness, commercial suppliers of control sera are advised to target the values of analytes at or near the clinical decision levels (Statland, 1983). Moreover, the clinician should be informed as to the analytical performance at or near those values at which clinical decisions will be made.

Levey-Jennings Control Chart

The control results are plotted on the ordinate (y-axis) versus time on the abscissa (x-axis), as illustrated in Figure 6–4. This chart shows the expected mean value by the solid line in the center and indicates the control limits or range of

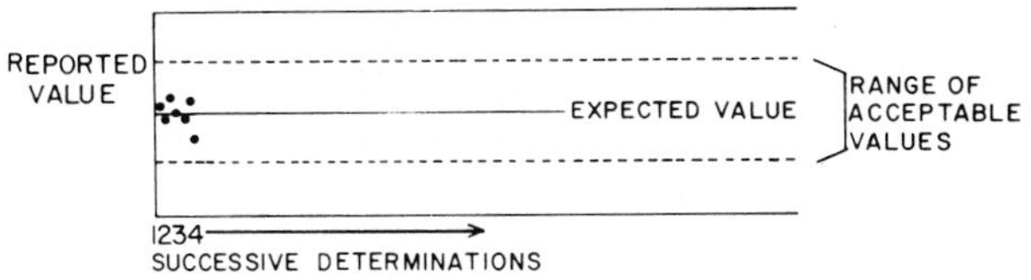

Figure 6–4. Illustration of a Levey-Jennings control chart. The control results are plotted on the ordinate (Y axis) against time on the abscissa (X axis).

acceptable values by the interrupted or dashed lines. The usual way of interpreting this control chart is to consider the run to be in control when the control values fall within the control limits and to be out of control when a result exceeds the control limits. Control limits are commonly set either at ± 2 SD or ± 3 SD around the mean.

When changes in control data indicate that the performance of an analytical method has deteriorated, the analyst must determine the cause of the problem. It is generally useful first to try to classify the error as random or systematic, because the different kinds of errors suggest different sources. As seen in Figure 6–5, random error shows a wider range of scatter of the points on the control chart. Systematic error can be seen when the points drift or shift to one side of the central solid line. Further information on the nature of the systematic error can be obtained by remembering the concept of the operational line. Each control material provides one point along the operational line. When data from two or more materials are available, they may be assessed to determine if the error is constant, proportional, or mixed.

Westgard's Multi-Rule Technique

Analysts who do not have years of experience interpreting control charts may find it difficult to interpret the more subtle changes occurring in control data. To help uncover these problems, a series of control rules can be applied, some which are sensitive to random error and some which are sensitive to systematic error. The control data are plotted in the same manner as for a Levey-Jennings chart; however, the control chart has several limit lines (drawn at the mean ± 1 SD, 2 SD, and 3 SD) to permit application of additional control rules.

For manual implementation, the 1:2s rule (occurrence of control values outside ± 2 SD) is recommended as a warning to trigger inspection of the control data, using other rules as rejection criteria. The other rules can be selected to have a very low probability for false rejection; thus, the overall false rejection level can be suitably low. The rules can also be chosen for their sensitivity in detecting either random or systematic errors and can therefore provide improved error detection.

The set of rules recommended by Westgard (1981) includes the following:

1:3s—reject when one observation exceeds the mean ± 3 SD limit

2:2s—reject when two consecutive observations exceed the same mean + 2 SD limit or the same mean − 2 SD limit

R:4s—reject when one control observation in the run exceeds its mean + 2 SD limit, and another exceeds its mean − 2 SD limit

4:1s—reject when four consecutive control observations exceed the same mean + 1 SD limit or the same mean − 1 SD limit

10:mean—reject when 10 consecutive control observations fall on one side of the mean

The procedure for employing the multi-rule analysis is outlined by the logic diagram shown in Figure 6–6. When there are no control observations in a run that exceeds a 2s limit, the run can be accepted without further inspection. It is theoretically possible that a 4:1s or 10:mean rule could still be violated, but it is pragmatic with manual implementation to accept the run without further inspection. (With computer-

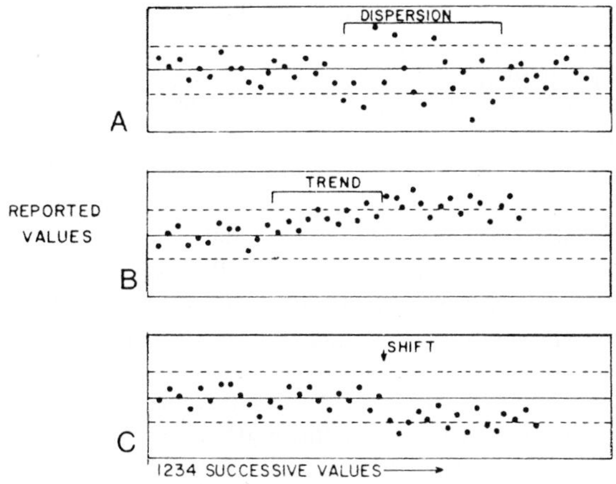

Figure 6–5. Illustration of three common patterns of control data resulting from random and/or systematic errors. Random error usually causes *dispersion*, whereas systematic error may produce a *trend* (a progressive drift of values) or a *shift* (an abrupt change from the established mean value).

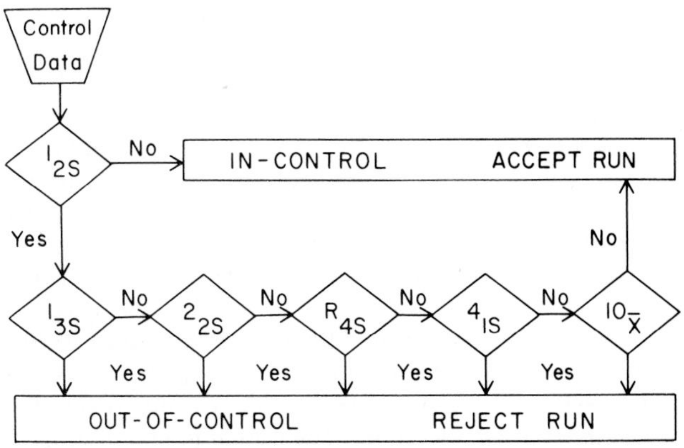

Figure 6–6. Logic diagram for applying the multi-rule control technique. (Adapted from Westgard JO, Barry PL, Hunt M, Groth T: Clin Chem, 27:493, 1981.)

ized implementation, the 1:2s warning rule can be omitted and all the rules applied automatically.) When any one of the control observations exceeds a 2s limit, it is interpreted as a warning of possible problems. The control data are inspected by applying each of the rules in sequence. If any one rule indicates a rejection, the run should be rejected. If none of the rules indicates a rejection, the run should be accepted.

The multi-rule technique can be applied to QC materials both within a run and across runs. For example, when collecting two control observations per run, one each on normal and on elevated materials, the 2:2s rule can be used to test the two observations obtained within the run (within-run and across QC materials), or it can be used to test each of the last two observations on each material by looking back to a previous run (within QC material and across runs). This can improve error detection by increasing the number of control observations available for inspection, and it makes possible the differentiation of systematic errors, such as a systematic shift occurring throughout the analytical range from a shift occurring in one part of the analytical range. A baseline shift may be detected by observing that the two observations within the run both exceed the same 2s limit (2:2s across QC materials, within-run). A loss of linearity at the high end of the analytical range may be detected by observing that the current observation is low by more than 2s and that the observation from the previous run was also low by more than 2s (2:2s within QC material, across runs).

The multi-rule technique has been recommended for number of observations from 2 to 4, with 5 being the maximum number of observations to be used. For these N's, the probability for false rejection is much lower than observed for the 1:2s rule alone. When the multi-rule technique is compared with the 1:3s rule, error detection is improved because of the effects of the R:4s, 4:1s, and 10:mean rules.

In addition to the improved performance characteristics, multi-rule analysis can provide some indication of the type of error occurring. The 1:3s and R:4s rules generally suggest random error, whereas the 2:2s, 4:1s, and 10:mean rules generally suggest systematic error. With large systematic errors, the 1:3s rule may also be violated, and with very large random errors, all rules have shown an increased probability for rejection.

Cumulative Sum Technique (CUSUM)

Systematic errors can be observed qualitatively by noticing whether the control points scatter randomly about the expected mean. Counting the number of consecutive observations falling on one side of the mean (or one side of some other limit) is another way of assessing systematic errors. A more exact and quantitative way is to calculate the actual differences between the individual values and the expected mean value, then sum those differences to determine the cumulative effect for all control observations collected. Woodard (1964) introduced techniques for accomplishing this, which have found widespread application in industrial laboratories.

The calculation of CUSUM for a set of control data is illustrated in Table 6–1. CUSUM values can be plotted versus time, as is done with other control charts. However, there is a major difference in the CUSUM control chart in that control status is generally based on the angle or slope of the CUSUM line. When control data are randomly scattered about their expected mean value, the CUSUM value wanders above and below zero, yielding a horizontal line on the CUSUM chart. When a systematic error is present, the CUSUM values steadily increase. The slope of the line will be related to the size of the systematic error that is occurring—the larger the error, the steeper the angle of the CUSUM line. At a certain size, the error will be too large to be acceptable and the method will be considered out of control. The slope, therefore, becomes the criterion by which control status is determined.

Table 6–1. CALCULATION OF CUMULATIVE SUMS FOR DAILY OBSERVED VALUES IN CONTROL SPECIMENS OF SERUM CHLORIDE

Day No.	Serum Chloride (mmol/Liter)	Assigned Value	Daily Difference	CUSUM*
1	100	100	0	0
2	98	100	−2	−2
3	102	100	+2	0
4	99	100	−1	−1
5	101	100	+1	0
6	100	100	0	0
7	98	100	−2	−2
8	101	100	+1	−1
9	97	100	−3	−4
10	99	100	−1	−5
11	98	100	−2	−7
12	101	100	+1	−6
13	100	100	0	−6
14	99	100	−1	−7
15	99	100	−1	−8
16	101	100	+1	−7
17	97	100	−3	−10
18	100	100	0	−10
19	101	100	+1	−9
20	99	100	−1	−10

*CUSUM on day n = daily difference + CUSUM on day (n − 1).

In the use of CUSUM techniques in clinical laboratories, the slope of the line has generally been assessed visually. The criterion, therefore, has been qualitative and difficult to employ on a uniform basis when many analysts are involved in assessing control status. This difficulty limited the application of CUSUM control charts in clinical laboratories.

Even when CUSUM charts are employed, it is recommended that a Levey-Jennings chart still be used. CUSUM responds primarily to systematic errors. Random errors must be monitored by some other technique, such as a Levey-Jennings chart with a 1:3s rule.

CUSUM techniques generally provide better detection of systematic errors than can be obtained from a Levey-Jennings chart. The multi-rule technique provides nearly as good detection of systematic errors, which should not be too surprising in view of how the 2:2s, 4:1s, and 10:mean rules accumulate differences. (In addition, the multi-rule technique has criteria for monitoring random error.) False rejections can be minimized by proper choice of conditions; thus, good performance can be expected from CUSUM techniques. In spite of these capabilities, the CUSUM technique has not been widely used. This is perhaps due to the difficulty of establishing the technique when used manually in busy service laboratories. With the advent of computerization, however, such limitations are less prohibitive. Furthermore, the CUSUM scheme has been found to be a near-optimal QC tool for all types of error detection (Bishop, 1993).

Other techniques have also been used for precision monitoring, but none appears to be superior to those described.

INTRALABORATORY PRECISION MONITORING BASED ON PATIENT SPECIMENS

The reference specimen approach to QC (i.e., the use of identical specimen aliquots over a long period of time) is widely used because it provides the laboratory with a rather constant frame of reference for the evaluation of its performance. However, commercial control specimens do not exactly simulate genuine clinical specimens, and occasionally changes in the control specimen (e.g., a loss of glucose) may incorrectly lead the laboratory personnel to believe that their analytical method is out of control. In addition, the analytical biases observed with clinical specimens may not be identical to those observed with control specimens.

In the case of patient specimens, one must take into account the preinstrumental sources of variation, including specimen collection, specimen transport, and specimen preparation. These same sources of variation are not present in the case of control material. For these reasons, a number of approaches of QC assessment using the results observed on patient specimens have been proposed. They include determining the daily mean of certain patient results, using one or more arithmetic checks on multiple results obtained on the same specimen, comparing the present result with any previous results from the same patient, noting apparently absurd results and so-called alert values, evaluating the combination of multiple results for unusual patterns, and assaying randomized duplicate patient specimens. Each of these approaches is reviewed subsequently.

Average of Normals

The average of normals method for QC was first advocated by Hoffmann and Waid (1965). The basic assumptions are that (1) the overall distribution of patient results displays a marked stability under stable laboratory conditions, and (2) most specimens analyzed in the clinical laboratory are normal with respect to many tests, particularly the electrolytes. They proposed several techniques for detecting changes in the frequency distribution of the clinical assay values. Although these procedures are basically attractive because they deal with clinical specimens, they have not been widely adopted. Several studies have shown the methods to be relatively insensitive to changes in analytical bias (Frankel, 1967; Kilgariff, 1968). The reason these methods are insensitive may be understood by considering that for many analytes, the clinical assays include values both above and below the reference interval. When either constant or proportional biases are introduced, some clinical assays will move into the reference interval whereas others will move out, and the number of values within the central portion of the distribution curve will tend to remain constant (Kilgariff, 1968). In addition, many analytical systems employ the technique known as single-point calibration. This technique is subject to combined constant and proportional systematic biases, and the operational line may pivot about the calibration value (see Fig. 6–1*D*). Because the calibration point is often near the mean value of the clinical specimens, most clinical assays are relatively unchanged, even when the method is clearly biased at other concentrations. It is possible that in the routine operation of the clinical laboratory, a subtle combination of compensatory biases affects the clinical assays, making the detection of the biases from examination of the clinical data difficult. Nevertheless, a number of authors have reported successful application of the techniques, particularly when large biases were present (Begtrup, 1971; Cembrowski, 1984; Dixon, 1970). Woo and colleagues (1988) reported the successful use of a version of average of normals to resolve assay discrepancies with CO_2 determination that the traditional QC program appeared incapable of detecting. They found the mean of patients within the reference range to be a sensitive indicator of systematic bias and the percentage of patients within the reference interval to be a good indicator of random imprecision.

Delta Check

Delta check (Ladenson, 1975) compares the result obtained for one specimen with the previous result(s) obtained for the same patient. Limits for the usual differences between specimens are entered into the computer program, and specimens having differences greater than these limits are listed for review by laboratory personnel. Knowledge of the magnitude of the total (physiologic and analytical) intraindividual variation under various conditions is critical. The limits can be based solely on a statistical model, and the width of the interval depends on the probability value that one is using to decide if a measurement is outside the limits. Of course, finding such a result does not necessarily indicate an analytical error. In fact, such a finding usually is associated with a change in the patient's disease course or a change in therapy.

Pattern Recognition

Lindberg (1965) has described the use of pattern recognition techniques to detect unlikely combinations of values. As examples, (1) urea, creatinine, and uric acid values or (2) sodium, potassium, chloride, and bicarbonate values are found to occur in clinical specimens in distinctive combinations, and the frequency of these various combinations can be calculated. The laboratory director should be aware of unusual combinations, such as grossly elevated serum alanine aminotransferase (ALT) in association with a normal serum aspartate aminotransferase (AST) level. An additional example is when the results of the visual inspection of erythrocytes in a blood smear do not correspond to the values of red blood cell indices (see Chap. 24). When such unusual combinations occur, the possibility of laboratory error should be considered.

In all the cases presented, the laboratory-based computer may be programmed to detect unusual combinations of laboratory values. These various data analysis procedures are basically systems for checking and cross-checking the clinical determinations for known internal consistencies and for identifying unusual values.

Randomized Duplicate Specimens

An additional technique, which is useful for *occasional* checks of the reproducibility of a laboratory's analyses, is the use of randomized duplicate specimens (Bokelund, 1974). This technique is applied to serum analytes as follows: (1) Two blood specimens are obtained per venipuncture. (2) Each specimen is uniquely labeled and uniquely processed. (3) All specimens in a batch are placed in randomized order. (4) The technologist is not informed as to which two samples are members of a duplicate pair. (5) The specimens are assayed for the analyte(s) of interest, and the results are recorded. (6) The within-batch random analytical variation is computed on the basis of the difference of duplicates approach. (7) Whenever the absolute difference in duplicate values for any particular pair of results is greater than a predefined limit, both specimens are reassayed. The limit is based on the calculated SD. (8) If the difference of the reassayed duplicates is still greater than the limit, the cause for the apparent discrepancy is sought. (9) If the difference is within the limit, the average of two replicates is computed and the resultant mean value is reported to the requesting physician.

The use of randomized duplicates for monitoring within-batch QA has certain advantages. Randomization of the specimens within a batch (as compared with the case wherein one replicate specimen follows the other) should overcome any possible correlation between time of assay and the order of the specimen—that is, any general analytic drift occurring during the assaying of the batch of specimens will be included. In addition, the use of duplicates obtained at venipuncture allows estimation of the *total* (preinstrumental and instrumental) within-batch analytical variation. Thus, this approach realistically assesses total variability in the entire analytical process and should give a greater degree of confidence in the quality of each particular measurement reported from the laboratory. Of course, the cost-benefit of this approach may be questioned; however, the availability of laboratory-based computers and analyzers with very high throughputs should make this method cost-effective, especially for intermittent application.

EXTRALABORATORY ACCURACY MONITORING

At present, there are two principal types of programs in which laboratories may compare their analytical results. There are proficiency testing (PT) survey programs, in which large numbers of laboratories analyze the same specimens several times each year, and there are regional QC programs, in which a group of laboratories in a geographic region use the same lots of QC specimens each day for their internal QC programs. The first of the survey programs was initiated in the late 1940s by Sunderman, and the most successful of these, The College of American Pathologists (CAP) Survey Program, has grown to include more than 25,000 clinical laboratories with more than 140,000 individual Survey subscriptions (CAP, 1994).* The first regional QC program was started by Preston in 1967 (Lawson, 1976). Many such regional programs are now used by laboratories in the United States.

Regional Quality Control Programs

These programs are available from the major manufacturers of QC specimens, as well as from various professional societies. In a typical program, each participant receives a stock of QC serum that is to be analyzed daily over a period of about one year. The analytical results are sent weekly or monthly to the supplier of the program for entry into a computer, and the participant receives a monthly report that compares the mean value and SD of his or her analyses with those of peer laboratories—that is, laboratories that use a comparable analytical method. Most of these programs also supply computer-generated Levey-Jennings graphs of the data with ample room for the laboratory personnel to manually plot current results. This type of program is very useful to smaller laboratories that lack the personnel or computer facilities to perform the statistical calculations or to prepare the graphs that are necessary to maintain their internal QC program.

Regional QC programs are necessarily limited in size because of limitations in the volume of serum that can be processed to prepare such QC specimens. However, some of these regional QC programs have been integrated through the CAP Computer Center. That is, the data from various regional programs are processed by the CAP Computer Center. In this way, the data from the various programs, even though based on the use of several different serum pools, may be combined for detailed statistical analyses. These data may be used by the individual laboratories in evaluating their acceptable limits for QC specimens in their internal control program as well as being an indicator of the current level of performance of laboratories using their own comparisons with others throughout the country.

Proficiency Testing Survey

Although many clinical chemistry survey programs are available to laboratories through governmental, private, and professional agencies, the program developed by the CAP is the largest in scope and the most comprehensive. The CAP first began its interlaboratory comparison survey following a model set forth by Belk and Sunderman (1947). It was initially perceived as a tool to enable participating laboratories to obtain an unbiased and critical assessment of its proficiency in relation to peer laboratories throughout the United States and abroad, and its basic purpose was laboratory improvement. In an effort to optimize evaluation criteria, various schemes of assigning the true values to survey specimens have been experimented with and evolved by CAP throughout the years. Initially, a single referee system was

*CAP (College of American Pathologists), 325 Waukegan Road, Northfield, IL 60093-2750

used to produce target values for survey samples. It was soon realized that with the large volume of participants using this program, their results could serve as reference values for PT survey samples. This marked the introduction of the so-called all participants, all methods system, which was used until it became apparent that certain instrument or method systems would produce results that might be at variance with the all participants, all methods mean and could still generate medically useful, accurate patient results. This discrepancy has now been attributed to "matrix effects" exhibited by PT survey materials on certain analytical systems (Eckfeldt 1993; Rej, 1994). To circumvent this problem, selected peer groups now assign appropriate survey specimens values for specific instruments.

Participants in the program receive survey specimens several times each year for analysis and return their results to the CAP Computer Center. Shortly thereafter, each participant receives a report that compares this reported value with the mean and SD obtained by peer laboratories, the number of peer laboratories, and the standard deviation interval (SDI) of the reported value. (The SDI is the difference between the reported value and mean value, divided by the SD. For example, an SDI of −0.4 means that the reported value is 0.4 SD units below the group mean value).

In compliance with the CLIA '67 regulations, participants are graded as acceptable (within ± 2 SD), needs improvement (between ± 2 and 3 SD), or unacceptable (exceeding ± 3 SD). It was sometimes found that when a laboratory failed to be within ± 3 SD on some analytes whose designated ranges of ± 3 SD were hard to attain, it would be graded unacceptable but would still be within medically useful limits. To resolve this, a fixed-limits criteria system was introduced. Although somewhat empirical, this system is an attempt to combine medical decision making and instrument capabilities as components in assessing performance of the survey sample. The difficulty with incorporating medical decision in interlaboratory comparison as elaborated earlier by Batsakis (1982) is still acutely present today.

In addition, each participant receives a concise summary of the performance of all methods for each analyte covered in the survey. The summary lists results according to all method and instrument combinations that were used by 20 or more laboratories. The complete participant report includes data for each of more than 20 analytes. This kind of report provides an overview of the field at the time of each survey and is valuable to participants because it indicates the popularity of various methods and the relative bias and variability of the various methods as they are actually used in the field. Because such summaries are provided with each survey, the popularity and performance characteristics of each method over a period of time are continuously documented. An additional bonus from the CAP survey program is the availability of survey specimens that are manufactured in excess of survey needs. After each survey is completed, the excess serum is made available as a survey-validated reference material (SVRM). This reference serum, with consensus mean values assigned for more than 20 analytes and for all methods used by 20 or more laboratories, has many practical uses for troubleshooting analytical problems, comparing methods, or checking analytic values assigned to other reference, calibration, or QC products.

The advent of CLIA '88 is placing greater emphasis on the performance of PT. The Health Care Financing Administration (HCFA), the regulatory agency responsible for CLIA implementation, has specified that satisfactory PT is a condition for laboratory accreditation. Criteria for acceptable PT performance have been defined in terms of total error, which encompasses both random error (imprecision) and systematic error (inaccuracy). These criteria are used in setting PT limits that laboratories must achieve a pass rate of 80% for successful performance. The number of annual PT events is reduced from four to three, but each event would continue to contain five challenges. The HCFA-specified minimum performance limits have also been changed somewhat (e.g., most of the 3 SD limits in routine chemistry have been changed to fixed limits). To assist laboratories to optimally meet accreditation requirements, Westgard has developed operational process specification charts (Westgard, 1992) that enable laboratories to design QC programs that would monitor laboratory performance to be within the allowable inaccuracy and imprecision to satisfy PT criteria. Ehrmeyer and Laessig (1990) demonstrated that the probability of passing PT is directly correlated with the imprecision and inaccuracy (bias) achievable within a laboratory. They recommend that to pass the 80% PT rule, laboratories should aim at reducing bias to a minimum with careful instrument calibration and decrease imprecision of each analyte to one third of the federally mandated performance limit. There is also concern that the HCFA's use of the broader and more lenient fixed PT limits in lieu of the earlier SDI criteria for many analytes may reduce the incentive of laboratories to identify significant out-liers to improve analytical process (Cembrowski, 1993).

ANALYTICAL GOAL SETTING IN CLINICAL ASSAYS

Precision and Accuracy Goals

Ideally, quantitative clinical laboratory measurements should be highly accurate and precise to meet the need of different medical situations. Since the 1960s, different approaches have been taken in defining analytical goals toward optimizing patient care. Tonks (1963) proposed that allowable imprecision should not exceed one fourth of the reference interval or mean of reference interval. Barnett (1968) introduced the medically useful criteria judged by clinicians as desirable standards. Another group proposed that analytical goals be set according to state-of-the-art instrument capability. Cotlove (1970) proposed that the tolerable analytical variability be less than one half of the intrinsic biological variation. The first official attempt at setting analytical goals in the clinical laboratory was made in 1976 by the CAP, which recommended that analytical goals be defined in terms of the needs of patient care (Elevitch, 1976). The recommended standard for group screening is that the CV should be equal to or less than half of the within-subject plus between-subject variations, whereas for individual testing the CV should be equal to or less than half the within-subject variation. Experts thus appeared to reach a consensus in favor of setting tolerable imprecision on the basis of biological variation, although it was also recognized that analytical performance could affect clinical decision making.

Although substantial data are available on biological variation (Fraser, 1989, 1992; Ross, 1982), laboratories have been slow to adhere to the CAP recommendation, and Tonks' rule and Barnett's approach are still very much in use. The heterogeneity found in within-patient biological variation and its variability relative to within-subject variation in healthy individuals, the unusually stringent biological variation of some analytes (e.g., Na and Ca), the effect of preanalytical errors (e.g., triglycerides), the module's insensitivity to bias, and excessive distractive debates over the setting of performance standards are cited as reasons for the less than universal application of standards based on biological variation (Fraser, 1993). This, and the fact that adherence to setting standards by biological variation would result in an increase of test result variation by 11.8%, has prompted a move toward setting standards based on assessment of medical needs—that is, adopting the magnitude of changes in test results to which clinicians will react (Lott, 1991; Skendzel, 1985). Nonetheless, this approach has problems as well. A major difficulty is that laboratory tests are used in many different clinical situations such as in screening and case finding, diagnostic, or therapeutic monitoring; each has different requirements of precision and accuracy. Moreover, changes due to analytical imprecision and bias, as well as within-patient biological and preanalytical variation, are not accounted for. Finally, because the median of responses is used, not all clinical situations can be satisfied (Hyltoft Petersen, 1994).

Analytical goal setting is further complicated by the advent of CLIA '88, which emphasizes PT as a criterion for accreditation. The HCFA rules (Federal Register, 1992) have specified acceptable performance standards for over 80 tests that are based directly on state-of-the-art technology without consideration of biological variation or clinical significance.

Laboratory professionals must now cope with more than one set of desirable performance standards formulated on different concepts. The CLIA-specified standards reflect the state-of-the-art technology needed to achieve laboratory certification and to maintain accreditation. On the other hand, desirable performance goals that encompass medical usefulness and biological variation are prerequisites to everyday patient care endeavors. With the use of operating specification charts (Westgard, 1992), Westgard and associates (1994) have developed a means of comparing the desirable performance goals based on biological variation and medical usefulness with goals set by CLIA. These authors found the CLIA outcome criteria to be more demanding than the clinical outcome criteria for many common clinical chemistry tests. Westgard's study also suggests that medically relevant criteria for PT can be established.

It is believed that the process of theoretical goal setting based on clinical or biological variation, or both, has failed to consider the state-of-the-art technology that reflects current analytical standards. Thus, the theoretically derived standards are not always attainable with existing techniques and equipment. This inconsistency may explain why these goal-setting approaches have not been wholeheartedly endorsed by the PT agencies. The establishment of increased awareness of clinicians on laboratory aspects and better knowledge of laboratory staff on how medical decisions are made are considered essential before clinical opinions can be adequately translated into desirable performance standards for laboratory testing (Fraser, 1993). A call for the integration and harmonization of quality standards for both PT and clinical needs to effect a unified set of outcome criteria is urged (Hyltoft Petersen, 1994).

Impact of CLIA '88 Implementation

CLIA '88 was created as a result of media attention to allegations of inaccurate "Pap" or cervical cytology examinations. The intent of CLIA '88 was to bring all clinical laboratory measurements/examinations under federal regulation irrespective of site, scope, volume, or frequency in an effort to provide laboratory tests of predictably high quality to all individuals in this country. This amendment was enacted into law in October 1988 (CLIA, 1988).

The status of CLIA '88 applies to all clinical laboratories that perform patient care activities, inclusive of research laboratories and physicians' office laboratories (POLs) (see Chap. 2). Furthermore, CLIA '88 contains very specific regulatory requirements on QC and PT that had previously been left to regulatory agencies. The first proposed regulations on CLIA '88 were published on May 2, 1990 (Federal Register, 1990). This was followed by several other proposed regulations dealing with fees, sanctions and enforcement procedures, categories of tests classified by complexity, and the granting and withdrawal of deeming authority. These regulations essentially combined the Medicare, Medicaid, and interstate rules into one body of regulation. The complexity and the controversial nature of the proposed regulations generated unprecedented public response and raised practical concern over access to testing, introduction and use of new technologies, personnel standards, cost, and PT and QC requirements. Over 60,000 mostly negative comments were received and reviewed by the HCFA prior to the publication of the final version on February 28, 1992 (Federal Register, 1992). The final rule extends federal regulation from 12,000 hospital and independent laboratories to 140,000 facilities, most of which have not been previously subject to any regulation.

The major framework of CLIA '88 consists of a complexity model that categorizes all testing procedures into three groups: (1) the waived tests, (2) moderate-complexity tests, and (3) high-complexity tests. Waived tests, which account for less than 1% of tests performed, require no specified PT, QC, or personnel standards. Tests of both moderate complexity (about 75% of tests performed) and high complexity (about 25% of tests performed) are subject to similar PT, QC, and personnel regulations specified by the HCFA.

The CLIA '88 regulations on QC, PT, and personnel standards acutely affect management of the laboratory. (The effect of personnel regulations is discussed in Chapters 1 and 2.) The QC requirements have also been modified. The HCFA has more stringent requirements now on validation of methods; instrument calibration and calibration checks; performance characteristics in terms of precision, accuracy, specificity, and sensitivity; and reference intervals. Linearity is not required, and emphasis is now on accuracy throughout the reported range of each analyte. Under CLIA '88, each lab-

Table 6–2. HCFA–APPROVED PROFICIENCY TESTING (PT) PROVIDERS FOR 1995*

Accutest
American Academy of Family Physicians
American Academy of Pediatrics
American Association for Bioanalysts
American Osteopathic Association
American Proficiency Institute
American Society of Internal Medicine
American Thoracic Society
California Thoracic Society
College of American Pathologists/Excel
College of American Pathologists/Surveys
Commonwealth of Pennsylvania
Commonwealth of Puerto Rico
Pacific Biometrics Research Foundation
Solomon Park Research Institute
State of Idaho
State of New Jersey
State of New York
State of Ohio
Wisconsin State Laboratory of Hygiene

*Not all programs offer PT for all analytes.

oratory must enroll in a PT program, approved by the Department of Health and Human Services (HHS), for each of the specialties and subspecialties for which it performs testing. To date, the HCFA has approved 19 PT providers for 1995 (see Tables 2–4 and 6–2). (The regulatory aspect of PT requirements were discussed in the previous section, Proficiency Testing Survey.) Some state governments and accrediting bodies have initiated legislative and regulatory efforts to increase their oversight of clinical laboratory testing. Some of them are also revising their rules in terms of the HCFA's requirements in an effort to obtain deemed status or equivalency with the CLIA '88 standards from the HCFA. Laboratories accredited by such an approved organization will be considered in compliance with CLIA '88. The state of Washington was the first to receive such status in October 1993. The HCFA has since granted deemed status to the CAP, the Commission of Office Laboratory Accreditation (COLA), the Joint Commission on Accreditation of Health Care Organization (JCAHO), and the American Society of Histocompatibility and Immunogenetics (ASHI).

Impact of CLIA '88 on the Physician Office Laboratory

(see Chap. 2)

Because CLIA '88 regulations apply to all sites performing patient care activities, POLs, which had been spared from either state or federal regulations in the past, must now prepare themselves to meet HCFA-mandated requirements for certification and accreditation. The exponential increase in popularity of POLs has been a combination of economic impact of fixed reimbursement by diagnosis-related groups (DRGs) that shifted laboratory tests to doctor's offices and the availability of sophisticated instrumentation that could generate rapid and accurate tests (Handorf, 1994). The personnel requirement was minimal because instruments were user-friendly, self-contained, and designed for office use and did not require formally trained technologists.

Most POLs perform tests of moderate complexity: 59% perform microbiology, 78% perform chemistry, 90% perform hematology, and 95% perform immunology (Kroger, 1994). Several surveys (Loschen, 1992) have shown that about one third of POLs had participated voluntarily in some forms of PT, and over 50% employed nonlaboratory trained personnel. Despite initial frustration and confusion caused by the impending CLIA regulation, physicians are establishing CLIA-compliant QA programs in their POLs. QA programs generally include policies and procedures for QC, equipment maintenance and record-keeping, and participation in a PT program. Over 80,000 POLs have now received registration (certification of accreditation) from the HCFA, and most POLs are awaiting their first official inspection. COLA, a nonprofit peer-review accrediting program for the POL, has modified its program to meet CLIA requirements and has been granted "deemed status" by the HCFA (see Chap. 2). COLA has provided valuable guidance to POLs in their undertaking to become CLIA-certified laboratories.

CONCLUSIONS

QA, emphasizing a system approach to individual actions and activities that make up a laboratory determination, provides powerful quality management when coupled with a variety of QC techniques. When this is incorporated into total quality management (TQM) that extends from patient and health care provider to clinical laboratory professionals and back to patient and physician, the public, patients, and professionals all benefit. This is especially true now in an era of health care reform that is focused on cost, access, and quality of medical and health care. However, "re-engineering" appears to be a new thrust to "right size" or down-size an organization. It may replace or strengthen further TQM. With re-engineering, there is an analysis and reassessment of all systems and operations within an organization or service to achieve minimal cost and be most cost-effective and competitive in a managed care environment with new and different forms of reimbursement, such as capitation per patient/individual and bundling of all related services within a single procedure or DRG. Just as new technology is integrating the analyses of specimens (part of patient) and dissolving the functional barriers or walls that separate the clinical laboratory sections of pathology and laboratory medicine (e.g., anatomic pathology and clinical pathology, chemistry, immunology, molecular pathology, hematology), so too must various clinical services—the primary care, medical, and surgical disciplines, along with the supporting services of anesthesiology, emergency medicine, pathology, radiology, and others (clinic, office, or hospital)—integrate for a new cost-effective continuity of care and accessibility coupled with health/wellness promotion and preventive medicine.

Barger JD: Levey and Jennings revisited. Arch Path Lab Med 1992; 116:799–803.

Barnett RN: Medical significance of laboratory results. Am J Clin Pathol 1968; 50:671–676.

Batsakis JG: Analytical goals and the College of American Pathologists. Am J Clin Pathol 1982; 78(Suppl):678–680.

Begtrup H, Leroy S, Thyregod P, Wallow-Hansen P: Average of normals used as control of accuracy, and a comparison with other controls. Scand J Clin Lab Invest 1971; 27:247.

Belk WP, Sunderman FW: A survey on the accuracy of chemical analysis in clinical laboratories. Am J Clin Pathol 1947; 17:854.

Bishop J, Nix ABJ: Comparison of quality-control rules used in clinical chemistry laboratories. Clin Chem 1993; 39:1638–1649.

Bokelund H, Winkel P, Statland BE: Factors contributing to intraindividual variation of serum constituents: 3. Use of randomized duplicates to evaluate sources of analytic error. Clin Chem 1974; 20:1507.

CAP Survey Manual (1994), College of American Pathologists, 325 Waukegan Road, Northfield, IL 60093-2750.

Cembrowski GS, Chandler EP, Westgard JO: Assessment of "average of normals" quality control procedures and guidelines for implementation Am J Clin Pathol 1984; 81:492–499.

Cembrowski GS, Hackney JR, Carey N: The detection of problem analytes in a single proficiency test challenge in the absence of the Health Care Financing Administration Rule Violation. Arch Pathol Lab Med 1993; 117:437–443.

Cembrowski GS, Westgard JO, Eggert AA, Toren EC Jr: Trend detection in control data: Optimization and interpretation of Trigg's technique for trend analysis. Clin Chem 1975; 21:1396.

Clinical Laboratory Improvement Amendments of 1988. Pub No. 100-578. Washington, DC, US Government Printing Office.

Cotlove E, Harris EK, Williams GZ: Biological and analytic components of variation in long-term studies of serum constituents in normal subjects: III. Physiological and medical implications. Clin Chem 1970; 16:1028–1032.

Deming WE: Out of the Crisis. Cambridge, MA, MIT Press, 1986.

Dixon K, Northam BE: Quality control using the daily mean. Clin Chim Acta 1970; 30:453.

Eckfeldt JH, Copeland KR: Accuracy verification and identification of matrix effects. The College of American Pathologists' protocol. Arch Pathol Lab Med 1993; 117:381–386.

Ehrmeyer SS, Laessig RH, Leinweber JE, Oryall JJ: Medicare/CLIA final rules for proficiency testing: Minimum intralaboratory performance characteristics (CV and bias) needed to pass. Clin Chem 1990; 36:1736–1740.

Elevitch F: Proceedings of the 1976 Aspen Conference on Analytical Goals in Clinical Chemistry. Skokie, IL, College of American Pathologists, 1977.

Frankel S, Ahrlen RC: An evaluation of the number plus method of quality control. Am J Clin Pathol 1967; 37:248.

Fraser CG: Biological variation in clinical chemistry. An update: Collated data (1988–1991). Arch Pathol Lab Med 1992; 116:916–923.

Fraser CG, Harris EK: Generation and application of data on biological variation in clinical chemistry. Crit Rev Clin Lab Sc 1989; 27:409–437.

Fraser CG, Hyltoft Petersen P: Desirable standards for laboratory tests if they are to fulfill medical needs. Clin Chem 1993; 39:1447–1455.

Grannis GF, Gruemer HD, Lott JA, et al: Proficiency evaluation of clinical chemistry laboratories. Clin Chem 1972; 18:222.

Handorf CR: Background-setting the stage for alternate-site laboratory testing. Clin Lab Med 1994; 14:451–458.

Henry RJ, Segalove M: The running of standards in clinical chemistry and the use of the control chart. J Clin Pathol 1952; 5:305.

Hoffmann RG, Waid ME: The "average of normals" method of quality control. Am J Clin Pathol 1965; 43:134.

Hyltoft Petersen P, Fraser GC: Setting quality standards in clinical chemistry: Can competing models based on analytical, biological, and clinical outcomes be harmonized? [editorial]. Clin Chem 1994; 40:1865–1868.

Kilgariff M, Owen JA: An assessment of the "average of normals" quality control method. Clin Chim Acta 1968; 19:175.

Kroger JS: Coping with CLIA [editorial]. JAMA 1994; 271:1621–1622.

Ladenson JH: Patients as their own controls: Use of the computer to identify "laboratory error." Clin Chem 1975; 21:1648.

Lawson NS, Haven GT: The role of regional quality control programs in the practice of laboratory medicine in the United States. Am J Clin Pathol 1976; 66:286.

Lindberg DA, Van Peenen HJ, Couch R: Patterns in clinical chemistry. Am J Clin Pathol 1965; 44:315.

Loschen DJ: The impact of new regulations on laboratory testing in physicians' offices. Clin Chem 1992; 38:1273–1279.

Lott JA, Surufka N, Massion GC: Proficiency testing of serum enzymes based on medical-needs criteria. Arch Pathol Lab Med 1991; 115:11–14.

Rej R: Proficiency testing, matrix effects, and method evaluation [editorial]. Clin Chem 1994; 40:345–346.

Ross JW: Evaluation of precision. *In* Werner M (ed): Handbook of Clinical Chemistry. Vol. 1. Boca Raton, FL, CRC Press, 1982, pp 391–422.

Skendzel LP, Barnett RN, Platt R: Medically useful criteria for analytic performance of laboratory tests. Am J Clin Pathol 1985; 83:200–205.

Statland BE: Decision Levels for Laboratory Testing. Oradell, NJ, Medical Economics Company, 1983.

Tonks DB: A study of the accuracy and precision of clinical chemistry determinations in 170 Canadian laboratories. Clin Chem 1963; 9:217–233.

US Dept of Health and Human Services, Health Care Financing Administration, Laboratory requirements: Final rule and regulations. Federal Register 1992; 57:7002–7288, 33992–34021.

US Dept of Health and Human Services, Health Care Financing Administration, Regulations implementing the Clinical Laboratory Improvement Amendments of 1988: Proposed rule. Federal Register 1990; 55:20896–20959.

Westgard JO, Barry PL, Hunt M, Groth T: A multi-rule Shewhart chart for quality control in clinical chemistry. Clin Chem, 1981; 27:493.

Westgard JO: Charts of operational process specifications ("OPSpecs Charts") for assessing the precision, accuracy, and quality control needed to satisfy proficiency testing performance criteria. Clin Chem 1992; 38:1226–1233.

Westgard JO, Seehafer JJ, Barry PL: Allowable imprecision for laboratory tests based on clinical and analytical test outcome criteria. Clin Chem 1994; 40:1909–1914.

Woo J, LeFever D, Winkelman JW: Use of "average of normals" quality control procedure in the detection and resolution of assay discrepancies. Am J Clin Pathol 1988; 89:125–129.

Woodard RH, Goldsmith PL: Cumulative Sum Techniques. ICI Monograph No. 3. Edinburgh, Oliver and Boyd, 1964.

Part 2

CLINICAL CHEMISTRY

Edited by
Matthew R. Pincus, M.D., Ph.D.,
John Bernard Henry, M.D.

2

Chapter 7

Evaluation of Renal Function, Water, Electrolytes, Acid-Base Balance, and Blood Gases

Matthew R. Pincus, M.D., Ph.D.
Harry G. Preuss, M.D.
John Bernard Henry, M.D.

2

As discussed in Chapter 4, the fundamental purpose of the kidneys is to conserve fluids by concentrating the urine. In addition to this basic function, the kidney has three additional major functions: (1) elimination of toxic substances produced during metabolism or ingested directly, (2) regulation of the internal fluid environment, and (3) production of hormones (Preuss, 1993a). Any of these functions may be used to assess the renal status. As kidneys fail, either acutely or chronically, end products of nitrogen metabolism accumulate, increasing levels of nonprotein nitrogen (NPN), reflected in a rise of blood urea nitrogen (BUN) and creatinine. Buildup of the nitrogenous products leads to azotemia. Symptoms associated with azotemia result in a state called uremia, in which the kidneys fail to eliminate waste products of metabolism. The kidneys regulate tonicity, volume, acid-base balance, and chemical composition of body fluid. In order that intracellular metabolic processes occur at maximal efficiency, the internal cellular composition has to be controlled within narrow limits. Intracellular fluid is influenced greatly by the composition of surrounding extracellular fluid (ECF), which is precisely regulated by the respiratory and renal systems via exchange with the intravascular fluid compartment. The lungs establish partial pressures and concentrations of the blood gases, the respiratory component of the acid-base system. The kidneys regulate concentrations of nonvolatile substances. It follows that abnormalities of water balance, electrolyte concentrations, and acid-base status may reflect disturbances in renal function. Finally, kidneys also participate in endocrine functions such as the formation of $1,25-(OH)_2$ vitamin D_3 and the synthesis of erythropoietin. They also play a vital role in the renin-angiotensin system. Perturbations in calcium and phosphorus concentrations or red blood cell mass suggest renal inadequacies. Accordingly, assessment of many different functions often contributes to a better understanding of a renal disorder and its ultimate prognosis.

RENAL FUNCTION

The initial and most cost-effective screening evaluation of renal function is the measurement of BUN and creatinine in serum. As noted in Chapter 4 and discussed subsequently, elevated BUN and creatinine with a ratio of BUN to creatinine of 20 or less, indicate renal failure. Renal failure can be further investigated with urinalysis (see Chap. 18) (Geyer, 1993). The urinary supernatant can be used for measuring urinary osmolality, sodium, potassium, chloride, calcium, protein, albumin, glucose, creatinine, bilirubin, and hemoglobin. Timed urine specimens with simultaneously collected blood specimens can be used for measurement of clearance with other analytes in serum and urine to detect subtle abnormalities and estimate the magnitude or resolution of renal disease. The urinary sediment can be evaluated for cells, crystals, and casts. Serum and urine protein electrophoresis with quantitative immunoglobulins (Chap. 11) and blood lipid analyses (Chap. 10) may also yield crucial clinical diagnostic and prognostic information.

Provocative testing and concentration-dilution studies can also be performed on timed urine collections. If there is a significant reduction in the glomerular filtration rate (azotemia with or without uremia), measurements of electrolytic and acid-base status are in order. Serum potassium is critically important to evaluate because of the significant adverse consequences of hyperkalemia and hypokalemia. Further documentation of renal failure and its causes can be obtained from excretory urographic and retrograde pyelographic contrast, ultrasound and angiographic studies, radionuclide scans, and renal biopsies.

Evaluation and management of patients with chronic disorders of renal function are achieved by periodic measurements of urinary volume; urinalysis, with special attention to protein excretion (Moore, 1993); creatinine; electrolyte determinations; and clearance studies (Duarte, 1993). These parameters, used alone or combined, aid in the determination of appropriate fluid and electrolyte replacement as well as deciding the frequency of dialysis and the constitution of dialysate.

Renal Clearance Studies

Normal kidney function depends on four aspects of renal physiology:

1. The renal blood flow must be appropriate.
2. Glomerular filtration should be adequate.
3. Renal tubular function should be normal.
4. There must be no significant obstruction to urine outflow.

Overall renal function and some aspects of its physiology can be assessed by determination of renal clearance. By measuring substances such as creatinine in the urine (U) and the volume of urine formed during a timed collection (V), as well as the concentration of the substance in serum (S) or plasma (P) from a midperiod blood collection, the volume of serum (plasma) that contained the measured substance excreted into the urine per unit of time (usually one minute) can be calculated. This volume, expressed in milliliters per minute, is defined as renal clearance. The formula for calculating renal clearance is

$$\text{Clearance (mL/min)} = \text{U(mg/dL)} \times \frac{\text{V(mL/min)}}{\text{S(mg/dL)}} \qquad (7\text{-}1)$$

It is necessary that the concentration units for U and S be identical for calculation. Milligrams per deciliter are used above, because this is the commonly reported value for creatinine. Serum clearance is proportional to the total number and size of glomeruli, which are proportional to renal parenchymal mass. It is customary to standardize the absolute clearance by a factor, 1.73/A, which represents the external surface area (m^2) of the average-size person (standard surface area) divided by the body surface area of the subject (determined from nomograms (see Appendix 2) or from formulas that relate weight and height to surface area), that is,

$$\text{Clearance (mL/min/std. surface area)} = \frac{\text{U} \times \text{V}}{\text{S}} \times \frac{1.73}{\text{A}} \qquad (7\text{-}2)$$

The clearance of small molecules that are not bound to protein and, therefore, are freely filtered by glomeruli and neither reabsorbed nor secreted by the tubules is a measure of the glomerular filtration rate (GFR), that is, the amount of ultrafiltrate passing from the blood into the renal tubular lumen over a given period of time.

Inulin, a polysaccharide with a molecular weight of 5100 daltons, is an ideal substance to measure GFR, but it is not routinely employed in a clinical setting because of the necessity for continuous intravenous infusion and the need for manual measurement. The latter disadvantage can be compensated for by use of [^{14}C] inulin or other equally inert radiolabeled substances such as [^{51}Cr] ethylenediaminetetraacetic acid (EDTA) (Favre, 1968; Granerus, 1981), [^{169}Yb] diethylenetriaminepentaacetic acid (DPTA), [^{125}I] diatri-zoate (Farmer, 1967), [^{125}I] iothalamate (Elwood, 1967; Sigman, 1965), and radioactive B_{12} (Breckenridge, 1965; Farmer, 1967; Nelp, 1964).

Generally, however, measurement of inulin clearance is the reference method in comparing other assessments of GFR. Inulin is measured spectrophotometrically. The average inulin clearance is 125 mL/min/1.73 m^2 for men and 110 mL/min/1.73 m^2 for women. The difference between the sexes is due to the larger renal mass in men. GFRs are lower in neonates (even when corrected for surface area) until the age of three to five months (West, 1948) because of the physiologic and anatomic immaturity of glomeruli as they develop from germinal epithelium of the visceral surface. The GFRs usually decrease steadily as individuals pass middle age (Wesson, 1969). For the most part, this is due to a progressive decrease in the number of glomeruli due to arteriolonephrosclerosis.

During pregnancy, the GFR increases approximately 50% and returns to normal after delivery (Semple, 1974). This results from increased blood volume and renal plasma flow. In addition, a direct hormonal (placental) influence on the kidneys is possible (Matthews, 1960). Increased GFRs and overall renal mass have been demonstrated in early juvenile diabetics (Morgensen, 1973). The approximately 25% augmentation results from increased glomerular size. Enhanced renal growth in patients with diabetes mellitus has been attributed, at least in part, to high circulating glucose concentrations. Adequate control with insulin results in the return of GFR and renal mass back toward baseline values (Seyer-Hansen, 1976). GFRs are increased in patients with major burns, perhaps owing to both hypoproteinemia and increased renal blood flow secondary to extensive volume replacement (Loirat, 1978).

Because of the necessity of intravenous infusion of inulin and the necessity for measuring its concentration manually, it is preferred to substitute an easily measured substance that is endogenous to the body to approximate GFR. The endogenous substance used most commonly in the clinical assessment of GFR is creatinine (Tobias, 1962).

CLEARANCE MEASURED WITH CREATININE. Creatinine, the cyclized form of creatine, is formed at a relatively constant rate by muscle, the major storage site of creatine phosphate. Thus, creatinine production and excretion relate directly to muscle mass. Accordingly, males and muscular athletes produce greater amounts of creatinine than do unconditioned women, children, and elderly individuals (Jackson, 1966). Creatinine assays (over 110 million assays per year performed in hospital laboratories) are among the most frequently performed clinical assays, ranking behind only glucose, $[K^+]$, and BUN.

Creatinine excretion is not routinely affected by diet. However, large quantities of creatinine are present in sterilized canned meats (Jackson, 1966) and cooked meats (Camara, 1951). If excessive quantities (i.e., >75 g) of these meat sources of exogenous creatinine are consumed, both serum and clearance values of creatinine will be increased for 48 hours (Camara, 1951).

Besides free glomerular filtration, there is also active tubular secretion of creatinine in humans that may result in an overestimation of the actual GFR when compared with inulin clearance. However, this secretion is counterbalanced by reabsorption of creatinine in the renal tubules. If the GFR is within the normal range, the creatinine clearance estimated by true creatinine (*vide infra*) exceeds the inulin clearance by 5 to 10% (Renkin, 1974). As the GFR decreases in renal disease, tubular secretion relative to glomerular load becomes a larger proportion of the clearance, making the estimate of GFR by creatinine clearance more uncertain. It has also been shown that glomerular filtration of creatinine is increased in patients with nephrotic syndrome (Carrie, 1980). As a result, the "true" creatinine clearance may at times exceed the actual GFR by 50% or more (Renkin, 1974). Another variable to be considered in evaluation of creatinine clearance is drug interference. Salicylates (Burry, 1976), cimetidine (Tagamet) (Larrson, 1980), trimethoprim (Lee, 1981), triamterene (Kampmann, 1981), spironolactone (Kampmann, 1981), and amiloride (Kampmann, 1981) interfere with tubular secretion of creatinine. Thus, although GFR may not change, the creatinine clearance is lowered and may confuse the interpretation of GFR. In spite of the many variables that influence creatinine clearance, this estimate of GFR has good clinical utility, especially because reliable creatinine methods are available in the clinical laboratory.

METHODS OF MEASUREMENT. These methods are based on the Jaffe reaction, which is the colorimetric determination of a complex of creatinine with picric acid. This measurement can be performed either as an end-point method or a kinetic assay. Most automated chemistry instruments use the kinetic Jaffe assay because of its low cost, speed, and simplicity. These determinations are linear to 20 mg/dL. Considering that the usual upper limit of normal for serum creatinine is on the order of 1 mg/dL, this linearity range is sufficient. Specificity is obtained by measuring the product in a narrow time window between production of early and late interferents. Acid blanking and bichromatic measurement have also been used to improve the assay specificity. Bilirubin is a signifi-cant negative interferent. Further, chromagens present in plasma, unless specifically removed, may give a falsely high reading of serum creatinine, that is, lower calculated clearance of creatinine.

Another method, available on the Ektachem chemistry analyzer (Eastman Kodak, Rochester, NY), which avoids some of these problems, uses enzymatic degradation of creatinine with creatinase. Ammonium ion generated in this reaction interacts with bromphenol blue, and the reaction is monitored by reflectance spectrophotometry. Interference from bilirubin in this method is negligible.

For all methods, falsely low values are obtained if the collected urine is not refrigerated or a bacterial inhibitor (e.g., thymol) is not added to the collection container. Changes in the acidity or alkalinity of the urine (a result of bacterial metabolism) may promote the conversion of creatinine to creatine. Bacteria may also produce creatinases, which degrade creatinine.

CLINICAL DETERMINATION OF CREATININE CLEARANCE. Serial measurements for creatinine clearance can demonstrate progression of renal disease or response to therapy. However, precisely timed and complete urine collections are required. The usual urine collection is over 24 hours, with blood being drawn for convenience at the beginning or end of the collection. Many now prefer a hydrated clearance over two hours (three periods of 40 minutes), with blood drawn at the midpoint of the second urine collection. Hydration is accomplished by giving the patient 20 mL H_2O/kg body weight at the initiation of the test and replacing urine volume throughout. Routinely, the assessment should be performed within a given time of the day for comparative purposes because of the well-known diurnal variation in GFR. Reference values for GFR based on creatinine clearance are 85 to 125 mL/min/1.73 m^2 for males and 75 to 115 mL/min/1.73 m^2 for females. Ideally, the urine creatinine concentration should be determined immediately but no later than 24 hours after collection.

If a specific method that removes chromagens, which may absorb at the same wavelength as the creatinine-picrate complex, is used to measure true creatinine concentrations, these ranges become 97 to 137 mL/min/1.73 m^2 for males and 88 to 128 mL/min/1.73 m^2 for females.

To obviate the well-known difficulties in obtaining a complete urine collection, nomograms have been developed to estimate glomerular filtration rate using creatinine clearance (C_{Cr}) by considering the serum value of creatinine (S_{Cr}), body weight, age, and gender. A popular formulation was devised by Cockcroft and Gault (Cockcroft, 1976).

$$C_{Cr} = \frac{(140 - \text{age}) \times \text{weight in kg}}{72\ S_{Cr}} \qquad (7\text{-}2A)$$

For females, $C_{Cr} = 0.85 \times C_{Cr}$ obtained in the equations given earlier for males.

Using this equation does not resolve the uncertainties related to creatinine metabolism (Levey, 1991), and studies have demonstrated that prediction of GFR by this method has a greater range of error than the Standard C_{Cr} (Lerner, 1985).

Because the reciprocal of S_{Cr} ($1/S_{Cr}$) declines in a linear fashion with progressive renal failure, the resulting slope has been used to determine and predict the rate of progressive renal failure (Mitch, 1976). Unfortunately, studies comparing this method with simultaneous measurements of GFR demonstrate that $1/S_{Cr}$ frequently is a misleading predictor of the progression of renal failure (Walser, 1989).

UREA AS AN INDICATOR OF RENAL DISEASE. As discussed in Chapter 8, renal function can also be assessed by determining serum concentrations of urea as blood urea nitrogen (BUN). Urea is the major end product of protein and nucleic acid metabolism and constitutes approximately 80% of the nitrogen excreted. Urea is predominantly handled by the kidneys via reabsorption as well as filtration, the latter being influenced by urinary flow. Therefore, BUN clearance does not give reliable estimates of the GFR. In addition, urea production is strongly affected by ingestion, catabolism, and loss of proteins into the gastrointestinal tract.

A rise in BUN in serum can result from prerenal causes (excess urea production, diminished renal blood flow, or both), from postrenal causes (obstruction along the genitourinary tract), or from true renal causes (e.g., parenchymal kidney damage). If excessive production is the only factor elevating urea, the BUN rarely exceeds 40 mg/dL. Values above this level usually indicate renal damage, urinary tract obstruction, or diminished renal blood flow.

The urea clearance test is an infrequently used and often difficult-to-interpret measurement of total renal function (i.e., glomerular and tubular function). Urea, having a very small molecular weight of 60 daltons, is freely filtered by the glomerulus but variably reabsorbed by the tubules. Reabsorption depends on the transit time of filtrate in the tubules. Accordingly, interpretation of urea clearance is evaluated keeping the urine flow rate in mind. If the flow rate is 2 mL/min or greater, the normal urea clearance is 65 to 100 mL/min. This is referred to as the maximal clearance (C_m). If the flow rate is less than 2 mL/min, the normal urea clearance is 40 to 70 mL/min. This is referred to as the standard clearance (C_s). The standard clearance is calculated by substituting the square root of V for V in the formula for clearance. Mathematically, these two clearance values can be compared by dividing each by the average value for each respective clearance (i.e., mean $C_m = 75$ mL/min; mean $C_s = 54$ mL/min) and converting to percent by multiplying by 100. The reference intervals for both clearances expressed as percent of normal are 75% to 125%. As the number of functioning nephrons decreases in chronic renal disease, less urea is reabsorbed and the urea clearance approaches the inulin clearance. Because of the many factors influencing urea clearance (see Chap. 8), this test has been replaced by the creatinine clearance. The urea clearance, however, may have some value when interpreted with the creatinine clearance in severe renal failure (i.e., GFR less than 20 mL/min). The difference between the urea and inulin clearances is approximately the same as the difference between the creatinine and inulin clearances (Lubowitz, 1967). Therefore, an average of urea and creatinine clearances may be a better approximation of the actual GFR in advanced renal disease.

METHODS OF MEASUREMENTS. BUN is usually measured by an indirect method, which generates NH_4^+ from urea through the use of the bacterial enzyme urease. Ammonium ion produced can be detected in a coupled reaction in which glutamate dehydrogenase converts α-ketoglutarate to glutamate with simultaneous oxidation of NADH to NAD. The reaction is quantitated by measuring decreased absorption at a wavelength of 340 nm. This method is usually linear to greater than 100 mg/dL concentration. Citrate or fluoride can inhibit urease, resulting in negative interference. Endogenous ammonia can give falsely elevated results. Another commonly used laboratory method for measuring urea concentration in serum is the condensation of urea with a diacetyl group to form a chromagen whose concentration can be measured spectrophotometrically.

Characteristically, especially for the urease reaction, the concentration is expressed as urea nitrogen (BUN-blood, PUN-plasma, or SUN-sera). Nitrogen comprises 47% of the molecular weight of urea; therefore, urea concentrations can be approximated by doubling the values found for urea nitrogen.

BUN AS AN INDICATOR OF RENAL FAILURE. Serum creatinine concentrations are considered to be better indicators of glomerular function than urea. Compared with urea, creatinine concentrations are less influenced by diet and prerenal and postrenal factors, which alter renal tubular handling, as mentioned earlier. However, there are other considerations when using serum creatinine concentrations to estimate renal function. With aging, there is a decrease in the GFR, but there is also a loss of muscle mass. The net result of these divergent factors may result in a serum creatinine that is elevated only minimally or not at all, even though the creatinine clearance may fall substantially in patients from 50 to 80 years of age (Lindeman, 1986).

The relationship between the clearances of urea and creatinine at a constant production rate describes a rectangular hyperbola (Fig. 7–1). This means that the circulating concentrations of urea and creatinine show little relative change until a great deal of renal mass has been lost (>50%). In contrast, a small loss of filtration when the GFR is already low causes a marked rise in the concentration. Although most clinicians favor serum creatinine over BUN as a single test to assess renal functioning, there are cogent arguments for measuring both. First, one assay may confirm the implications of the other, and second, the ratio derived from both measurements (BUN/creatinine) may suggest an etiology for a perturbation (Dossetor, 1966).

The ratio of BUN to serum creatinine is generally between 10 : 1 and 20 : 1. When renal parenchymal damage occurs, BUN and serum creatinine characteristically rise in concert and maintain a similar ratio. An altered ratio suggests other abnormalities. The most important cause of an increased BUN to serum creatinine ratio is compromised blood flow resulting in low urine flow rates that enhance urea reabsorption without decreasing creatinine secretion proportionately. A low urine flow may result from dehydration, congestive heart failure, hepatorenal syndrome, or obstruction of the urinary tract. Other possible causes include excess urea production from gastrointestinal bleeding, fever, or catabolic drugs (Preuss, 1988b).

Low ratios are commonly seen in patients consuming low-protein diets. They may also be observed in patients undergoing chronic hemodialysis, because urea is more efficiently dialyzed than creatinine. During pregnancy, the ratio tends to decrease because of increased GFR, which has a greater effect on urea excretion relative to creatinine excretion. A final reason for measuring both urea and creatinine is that urea

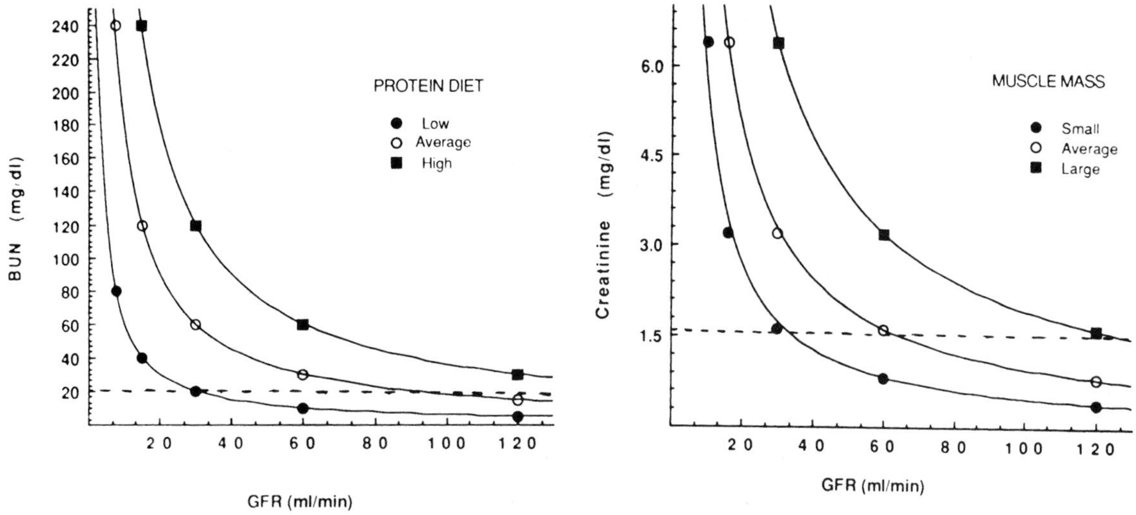

Figure 7–1. Use of blood urea nitrogen (BUN) and serum creatinine measurements as an estimate of glomerular filtration rate (GFR). In the first depiction, BUN is compared with GFR in patients ingesting three different levels of dietary protein. The interrupted line represents the upper limit of normality for BUN used by most clinical laboratories. It can be seen that the subject consuming a high-protein diet exceeds the upper limit of normality at a GFR of 120 mL /min, whereas that individual on a low-protein diet does not exceed this upper limit until his or her GFR decreases below 30 mL /min. In the second depiction, serum creatinine is compared with GFR in three individuals of different sizes. The upper limit of normal for this measurement, as arbitrarily judged by the clinical laboratory, is depicted by the interrupted line. The subject with the large muscle mass hovers around the upper limit of normal even though the GFR is 120 mL /min, whereas the small person will only exceed the upper limit when his or her GFR decreases below 30 mL /min.

concentrations may correlate better with uremic symptoms than creatinine concentrations.

A better understanding of a patient's prognosis can be gained from serial determinations of BUN and serum creatinine. A consistent increase of either that is not explicable by other causes suggests deteriorating renal function. Rapid changes suggest an acute illness or exacerbation of a chronic disorder. In contrast, a reduction in the BUN or creatinine concentration may indicate improvement.

Although clearance studies are technically demanding, requiring accurately timed and complete urine collections, they are very sensitive indices of kidney function. Measurements of plasma metabolic waste substances alone may be insufficient. A steep hyperbolic relationship between clearance values and plasma concentrations exists. In many instances, 65% to 75% of renal function must be lost before the various nonprotein nitrogenous substances exceed the reference intervals. BUN/creatinine serum ratios, however, can be very useful guidelines in differentiating the various etiologies of azotemia (see Chap. 8).

In summary, accurately timed and complete urine collections can provide sensitive indices of renal function even though clearance studies are technically demanding. Measurements of plasma metabolic waste substances alone may be insufficient. Elevations of either urea or creatinine may signal renal failure; however, in normal individuals, approximately 50% of renal function may be lost before the tests exceed the upper limits of normal (see Fig. 7–1). In addition, wide variations in production and renal handling may exist among individuals. As an example, a normal person on a low-protein diet has a baseline BUN of 8 mg/dL (see Fig. 7–1). If the production rate is unchanged, destruction of one half of the kidney mass would raise the BUN to 16 mg/dL, a value considered within the reference interval. Although the relationships between serum creatinine and GFR are influenced less by differences in production, people with a small muscle mass have a lower baseline serum creatinine at normal GFR. A serum creatinine of 1.2 mg/dL, which would be considered within a normal range in standard tables, represents a loss of two thirds of kidney function in a very slight person who normally has a baseline serum creatinine of 0.4 mg/dL (see Fig. 7–1). Thus, if any doubt exists about renal function, even though serum concentrations of urea or creatinine are within the reference interval, a creatinine clearance (or other index of GFR) should be measured. The BUN and serum creatinine are less useful to assess subtle changes in renal function than is the creatinine clearance. On the other hand, if the BUN and serum creatinine both markedly exceed the upper limits of their reference intervals, there is usually little reason to obtain a confirming clearance study.

Measurements of Urinary Solute Concentration

The ability of kidneys to maintain both the tonicity and water balance of the ECF requires that the tubules be functional and responsive to antidiuretic hormone (ADH) or vasopressin. These specific functions can be evaluated by measuring the solute concentrations of the urine either randomly or under well-controlled conditions (i.e., concentration and dilution tests). Additional important information concerning renal function, pathology, and the cause of hydration and electrolyte perturbations can be obtained when urinary and serum measurements are compared. Solute concentrations of fluid are most conveniently and economically quantitated in the clinical laboratory by measuring either specific gravity, refractive index, or osmolality (Davis, 1993).

SPECIFIC GRAVITY. Specific gravity is the ratio of the

mass of a solution compared with the mass of an equal volume of water. Because this is actually a comparison of weights, it does not measure the exact number of solute particles. However, there is a good correlation between specific gravity and osmolality under most circumstances. The specific gravity of plasma is fairly constant and ranges from 1.010 to 1.012. Urine specific gravity varies from 1.003 to 1.035, reflecting either dilution or concentration of the glomerular ultrafiltrate. Urine specific gravity is measured with a calibrated hydrometer, called a urinometer, or more commonly, a temperature-compensated refractometer calibrated in specific gravity units. Both of these techniques are discussed in detail in Chapter 18.

OSMOLALITY. Osmolality is a measure of the number of dissolved particles in solution (Chap. 3). Unlike specific gravity, which depends on both the nature and number of particles, osmolality depends only on the number of particles. Dissolved solutes change four physical properties of solutions. These colligative properties are osmotic pressure, vapor pressure, boiling point, and freezing point. It is worth repeating that the extent of these changes at a constant temperature is determined only by the number and *not* by the nature or mass of the particles in solution. One gram molecular weight (mole) of a nonelectrolyte (e.g., glucose) which contains 6.023×10^{23} particles (Avogadro's number), if dissolved in 1 kg of water, will increase the boiling point of water 0.52°C and the osmotic pressure 17,000 mm Hg, and lower the vapor pressure 0.3 mm Hg and the freezing point 1.858°C. This solution is defined as having an osmolality of 1 (or 1 osmol/kg H_2O). A related expression is osmolarity, defined as 1 osmol of a nonelectrolyte dissolved in 1 L of distilled water. Osmolality is the preferred unit of measurement because it is a constant weight/weight relationship. In contrast, osmolarity varies because of the volume-expanding effect of dissolved solute and the direct proportional effect of temperature on fluid volume.

The osmolality of a one-molal solution of an electrolyte (e.g., NaCl) is greater than 1 owing to the dissociation of electrolyte into component atoms when in solution. The osmolality of an electrolyte solution is determined by the following formula:

$$\text{Osmolality} = \phi n C \qquad (7\text{-}3),$$

where n is the number of atoms that dissociate in solution, C is the concentration of the electrolyte in moles/kg H_2O, and ϕ is the osmotic coefficient.

Differing coefficients for each electrolyte arise because the dissociation of an electrolyte into individual atoms is not complete and the individual particles may form secondary chemical bonds with solvent molecules. The osmotic coefficient ϕ is derived from dividing the measured osmolality by the theoretical osmolality of the electrolyte solution. ϕ for NaCl is 0.93.

The electrolytes Na^+, Cl^-, and HCO_3^-, because they are present in high concentrations in the ECF, contribute to over 92% of the serum osmolality. The other ECF electrolytes, serum proteins, glucose, and urea are responsible for the remaining 8%. The normal osmolality of the serum is between 285 and 319 mOsm/kg H_2O. Many simple formulas have been devised to convert serum solute concentration to osmolality (Weisberg, 1975). The formula with good clinical utility and most easily remembered is

$$\text{Osmolality (mOsm/kg } H_2O) = 2\,(Na^+) + \frac{(\text{Glucose})}{20} + \frac{(\text{BUN})}{3} \qquad (7\text{-}4),$$

which is a simplification of the formula

$$\text{Osmolality (mOsm/kg } H_2O) = 1.86\,(Na^+) + \frac{(\text{Glucose})}{18} + \frac{(\text{BUN})}{2.8} \qquad (7\text{-}4A).$$

The number 1.86 is derived from 0.93×2 (ϕn), because each Na^+ in solution is balanced by a corresponding anion (CL^- or HCO_3^-). The number 18 is used because the molecular mass of glucose is 180 daltons and the expression $\frac{(\text{Glucose})}{18}$ converts the units from mg/dL to mmol/L. Similarly, 2.8 is used because the molecular mass of the two nitrogen atoms in urea is 28 daltons and the expression $\frac{(\text{BUN})}{2.8}$ converts the units from mg/dL to mmol/L.

Urine osmolality varies, of course, depending on the state of hydration. Maximally diluted and concentrated urine shows osmolalities between 50 and 1400 mOsm/kg H_2O. Urine osmolality corresponds well with urinary specific gravity in nondisease states. However, the correlation is less reliable in renal disease states owing to the greater contribution of high-molecular-weight substances such as glucose and protein to specific gravity than to osmolality (Holmes, 1962). One may be perplexed by the high urine specific gravity found after intravenous pyelogram (IVP) studies; this is due to the dye in the urine.

OSMOMETRY. Osmolality can be estimated by measuring the freezing point depression of a solution using an osmometer or cryoscope (Chaps. 3 and 18). Serum or heparinized plasma may be used, but plasma anticoagulated with chelating or precipitating agents is unsuitable. Urine is centrifuged to remove all large particulate matter. The solution is supercooled (i.e., cooled below its freezing point) in an insulated freezing bath and then crystallized, using a vibrator that agitates the solution. As crystallization occurs, heat of fusion is produced and the temperature is compared with plateau temperatures obtained with known standards; therefore, no correction factor is necessary. The temperature changes are measured by a thermistor and converted to mOsm/kg H_2O.

An alternative method for measuring osmolality is to use a vapor-pressure or dew-point osmometer. The sample to be tested is absorbed into a small disk of filter paper, which is inserted into a sample holder and then sealed in an enclosed chamber. A temperature-sensitive thermocouple is incorporated into the chamber. Initially, the thermocouple is cooled electrically below the dew point. Water in the chamber air condenses and forms a thin film on the surface of the thermocouple. The dew point is the temperature of the atmosphere at which water begins to condense. As water condenses on the junction, heat of condensation is given off, the thermocouple temperature is increased to the dew-point temperature, and water ceases to condense.

When this temperature is stabilized, it is compared with the initial chamber temperature. This measured temperature change is proportional to the vapor pressure of the evaporating fluid in the filter disk and is calibrated in mOsm/kg H_2O by use of known standards.

Vapor-pressure osmometers are simpler in design than the freezing-point instruments and use smaller sample volumes. Although both instruments give identical results with clear serum and urine, there is a positive bias with the dew-point instruments if the serum is lipemic (Mercier, 1978). The reason for this difference is not well understood but may be either kinetic or thermodynamic in origin. Comparison studies have indicated that dew-point instruments are less precise than the freezing-point instruments (Juel, 1977). Another major difference between the two instrument types is that dew-point instruments cannot detect the presence of volatile agents (e.g., alcohols) in solution, whereas freezing-point instruments can (Rocco, 1976; Weisberg, 1975). This occurs because *volatile* solute increases the total vapor pressure of solutions, eliminating the direct solute depression of vapor pressure (Barlow, 1976). If significantly different values are obtained by the two methods, the presence of a volatile substance should be suspected.

Clinical Utility of Osmolality Studies

Hyperosmolality of the serum (or plasma) is commonly associated with excessive water loss when water replacement is inadequate. Accordingly, it is commonly seen in infants and the elderly. Increased solute intake is less likely to be a cause. In contrast, hyposmolality of serum is due to increased water intake with or without an increased solute load. This is associated with conditions referred to as primary polydipsia, psychogenic water drinking, psychotic water drinking, and drug-induced polydipsia (Davis, 1988), as well as excessive intravenous fluid hydration in hospitalized patients.

Comparison of measured and calculated serum osmolality has clinical significance. Calculated osmolalities of serum (and plasma) are usually a little lower than measured osmolalities (Weisberg, 1975). This is referred to as the delta-osmolality. If this calculation is more than 40 mOsm/kg H_2O in critically ill patients, there is a poor prognosis (Weisberg, 1975); the difference arises from the accumulation of osmotically active metabolites, including lactic and keto acids. The delta-osmolality also may be helpful in evaluating acutely ill or comatose patients. An increased gap between the measured (freezing-point instrument) and calculated osmolality may indicate the presence of an ingested volatile substance or poison. Common causes of increased gap are ethanol overdose and azotemia (Loeb, 1974). Other important considerations, if ethanol and azotemia can be ruled out, are methanol, isopropanol, and ethylene glycol poisoning.

In the evaluation of renal function, the ratio of urine to serum (plasma) osmolality (U/S or U/P osmol ratio) together with urinary electrolyte studies can be especially useful (Levinsky, 1976). Under usual circumstances, the ratio of urine osmolality to serum (plasma) osmolality is between 1 and 3. In acute tubular dysfunction (including necrosis) and in chronic renal insufficiency, the U/S or U/P osmol ratio is equal to or less than 1.2 and the urinary Na^+ is greater than 20 mEq/L (mmol/L). In diseases in which the GFR is primarily impaired (e.g., congestive heart failure, acute glomerulonephritis, acute obstructive uropathy), the U/S (or U/P) ratio is greater than 1.2 and the urinary Na^+ is less than 20 mEq/L (mmol/L).

More recently, physicians confronted with the differentiation of prerenal and parenchymal acute renal failure have turned to the renal failure index (RFI) or the fractional sodium excretion (FeNa) for more complete differentiation. The RFI is defined as

$$\text{RFI} = \text{Urine Na} \div \text{Urine Cr/Plasma Cr} \qquad (7\text{-}5).$$

FeNa is defined as

$$\text{FeNa} = \frac{\text{Na clearance}}{\text{Creatinine clearance}} \times 100 = \frac{\text{Urine Na} \times \text{Plasma Cr}}{\text{Urine Cr} \times \text{Plasma Na}} \times 100 \qquad (7\text{-}6).$$

An RFI or FeNa below 1.0 indicates prerenal failure, and a level above 2.0 suggests acute tubular necrosis. These simple tests more clearly differentiate the type of renal failure better than osmolality or sodium excretion alone (Espinel, 1976).

The U/S osmol ratio can differentiate among etiologies of polyuria. The U/S osmol ratio is greater than 1 in osmotic diuresis and less than 1 in water diuresis. In complete central or nephrogenic diabetes insipidus, the ratio is less than 1 and remains unchanged with water deprivation. In patients with incomplete or partial (i.e., decreased release of ADH) central diabetes insipidus and in psychogenic diabetes insipidus, the ratio will increase and be greater than 1 with fluid restriction (Ruddy, 1981). After ADH or vasopressin (Pitressin) administration, the ratio increases significantly in patients with severe central diabetes insipidus. In addition, the urine osmolality increases at least 50% above that obtained by fluid restriction alone (Ruddy, 1981). Patients with partial defects of ADH release show a smaller increment, between 10% and 50%. In patients with nephrogenic diabetes insipidus, an important cause of which is the absence of ADH receptors or the presence of defective receptors in the distal convoluted tubule, there is no increase in either the U/S osmol ratio or urine osmolality after ADH administration due to the lack of receptor binding. If hypertonic saline is administered to patients with psychogenic diabetes insipidus, there is a sharp decline in free water clearance (*vide infra*) when the serum osmolality is less than 290 mOsm/kg H_2O (Ruddy, 1981). In patients with partial diabetes insipidus, there is a similar response but only when the serum osmolality is greater than 290 mOsm/kg H_2O. No change, however, is noted in those individuals with complete central or nephrogenic diabetes insipidus. Partial central diabetes insipidus may respond to chlorpropamide, which stimulates ADH release and augments the renal tubular response to ADH.

Urine osmolality studies are the best method to determine maximal concentration and dilution of urine. The simplest test to evaluate concentrating ability is to withhold fluids overnight. In normal subjects, the specific gravity should exceed 1.025 after 16 hours of fluid deprivation. Urine osmolality must exceed 800 mOsm/kg water or the ratio of urine to serum osmolality (U/S) must exceed 3.0 to be considered

Table 7–1. A METHOD TO EVALUATE CONCENTRATING ABILITY

1. Patient consumes evening meal.
2. After 6:00 P.M., patient is deprived of all fluid intake but is allowed to consume solid food. The patient voids at 8:00 A.M. next day.
3. At 10:00 A.M., serum (S) osmolality and urine (U) osmolality are determined. If U/S is greater than 3.0 (or urine osmolality exceeds 850 mOsm), the test response is considered normal and no vasopressin (Pitressin) is needed. Test is terminated.
4. If U/S is less than 3.0 (or urine osmolality is below 850 mOsm), 5 units of Pitressin tannate in oil are given subcutaneously.
5. Urine and serum osmolality are then determined at 2:00 P.M. (20 hours) and, if necessary, at 6:00 P.M. (24 hours).
6. If U/S osmolality ratio reaches or exceeds 3.0 (or urine osmolality exceeds 850 mOsm) at any time, test is immediately terminated and patient is allowed fluids.
7. If patient does not attain an osmolality of 850 mOsm/kg or a U/S of 3.0 by 6:00 P.M., test is terminated regardless.
8. Urine osmolality is determined on A.M. specimen the next day.

normal (Isaacson, 1960). A specific gravity of 1.020 approximates 700 mOsm/kg. One common method used to assess concentrating ability is described in Table 7–1.

Nephrogenic diabetes insipidus is present when the renal tubular concentrating mechanism does not respond adequately to ADH. Nephrogenic diabetes insipidus may be produced by drugs such as lithium or demeclocycline. Hypokalemia and hypercalcemia are often associated with similar problems. Other causes for nephrogenic diabetes are interstitial nephritis, arterionephrosclerosis, and chronic renal disease. Concentrating ability is one of the first functions to be impaired as a result of renal tubular damage.

Maximal urinary dilution can be evaluated by observing the change in urine osmolality after water loading. The accepted response in already normally hydrated subjects after drinking 500 mL of water is a reduction in the urine osmolality to 40 to 80 mOsm/kg H_2O (Schreiner, 1971). This test is not considered a useful procedure to elucidate the etiology of hyponatremia (van Ypersele, 1979).

To challenge the diluting mechanism in a more precise manner, the following procedure is used. An oral water load of 20 mL/kg body weight is given, and the subsequent urine volume is replaced with an equal amount of water. With maximal water diuresis, urine osmolality decreases to 50 to 100 mOsm/kg. The normal kidney response is to excrete water in excess of salt and other osmotically active substances such that the serum osmolality is returned toward normal.

A slightly different approach to evaluate concentration and diluting capacities of the kidneys is to calculate osmolar and free water clearances. The U/S (or U/P) osmol ratio can be converted to a clearance value when it is multiplied by the urinary volume (V).

$$C_{osmol} = \frac{U_{osmol} \times V}{S_{osmol}} \quad (7\text{-}7).$$

The osmol clearance is a measure of the amount of water that is cleared from the plasma resulting in urine that has the same osmolality as plasma. The difference between the total urine volume and osmol clearance is called the free water clearance (C_{H_2O}).

$$C_{H_2O} = V - C_{osmol} \quad (7\text{-}8).$$

If the value is positive, this indicates that the urine is dilute compared with serum; conversely, if the value is negative, it indicates that the urine is more concentrated than serum.

The highest free water clearance is 10–15 mL/min. To maximally dilute urine, the ascending limb of Henle's loop must function properly and ADH release must be inhibited. A decrease in NaCl delivery to the distal diluting site can be caused by diminished GFR (myxedema) and excessive proximal tubular sodium reabsorption (congestive heart failure or liver disease) and may decrease C_{H_2O}. Generally, diuretics such as furosemide and ethacrynic acid, which block the chloride pump in the ascending limb of the loop of Henle, inhibit the ability of the nephron to concentrate the urine. Use of diuretics generally gives rise to a positive free water clearance.

WATER BALANCE

Serum and urinary osmolality studies are also valuable in evaluating the course(s) of both hypernatremia and hyponatremia (sodium, *vide infra*). Water balance is controlled by mechanisms responsive to the tonicity and volume of the ECF. They are (1) the effect of ADH on the collecting tubules, (2) the renin-angiotensin-aldosterone system, and (3) the thirst center. Disorders of these mechanisms and, hence, water balance are seen frequently in clinical medicine.

If water losses exceed replacement, dehydration with hypovolemia develops. Sodium (Na^+) is usually lost with water, but the relative concentration of Na^+ varies depending on the type of fluid lost. The more common causes of volume depletion are vomiting, diarrhea, surgical drainage, internal pooling (third spacing) of the fluids (e.g., peritonitis, ileus), renal disease, diuretic administration, fever, excessive sweating, and hypoadrenocorticism (i.e., Addison's disease).

There are no laboratory measurements that can quantitate the amount of fluid loss. Laboratory evaluations (concentration measurements) are relative (i.e., comparison of amounts of substances in specific volumes of fluid). The hematocrit and serum protein concentrations can fluctuate. Nevertheless, these changes may be helpful in estimating the status of plasma volume. The BUN is usually increased to a greater extent than serum creatinine during a dehydrated state (prerenal failure). The U/S osmol ratio is greater than 1, and the urine Na^+ concentrations are less than 20 mEq/L (mmol/L), except in Addison's disease and renal diseases, in which there is Na^+ loss. The diagnosis of dehydration and hypovolemia is made clinically (tissue turgor, cardiac and renal dynamics), and treatment consists of administering appropriate fluids to correct both fluid and electrolyte losses.

The opposite situation, an increase in total body H_2O or volume overload is usually associated with an increase in total body Na^+. This occurs frequently in cardiac failure and in conditions associated with hypoalbuminemia such as cirrhosis or the nephrotic syndrome. The common denominator in the latter conditions is so-called forward failure, that is, a decrease in renal blood flow. In turn, this causes increased aldosterone and ADH production with Na^+ and H_2O retention. More H_2O than Na^+ is retained. As a result of the impaired hemodynamics, fluid may accumulate in the interstitial spaces, resulting in edema, ascites, and pleural effusions.

For the reason discussed earlier, there is no practical laboratory measurement to quantitate the amount of overhydration. Assessment is made clinically, and treatment is directed toward correcting the underlying pathology and, in some cases, includes the use of diuretics.

ELECTROLYTES AND ELECTROLYTIC BALANCE

Electrolytes are ions that exist in body fluids. In the ECF, the major cation is Na^+ and the major anions are Cl^- and HCO_3^- (DeVita, 1993). Metabolic events are affected, to some degree, by the relative and absolute concentrations of these electrolytes, which are important determinants of osmolality, state of hydration, and pH of both the intracellular fluid (ICF) and the ECF. In addition, membrane potentials and normal functioning of nervous tissue and muscle (including cardiac muscle) are regulated by the concentration differences between ICF and ECF electrolytes. Electrolyte concentrations are expressed either as milliequivalents per liter (mEq/L) or in Standard International (SI) units, that is, millimoles per liter or mmol/L (Lehmann, 1976). Because 1 mEq is equal to 1 mmol for monovalent ions, the numerical values for the four major electrolytes are the same using either system of units.

Sodium

Na^+ is the major cation in the ECF and the principal osmotic particle outside the cell. Active cation transport systems at the cellular membrane maintain high Na^+ levels in the extracellular space, whereas K^+ is concentrated within cells. The Na^+ is freely filtered at the glomerulus, and roughly 70% of the amount filtered is reabsorbed isotonically in the proximal tubule. Both Na^+ and Cl^- are reabsorbed in the loop of Henle. Na^+ reabsorption also occurs throughout the remaining segments of the distal nephron, in part, secondary to an aldosterone effect. Changes in extracellular Na^+ concentration result in increases or decreases in the osmolality of the extracellular fluid, which, in turn, influence the distribution of body water.

Serum Na^+ concentration varies between 136 and 145 mmol/L in healthy individuals. The normal daily intake of Na^+ is 100 to 250 mmol. Ordinarily, the amount of Na^+ loss is balanced by the daily intake. The usual Na^+ excretion level in urine varies from 30 to 280 mmol/day. Hyponatremia, or decreased serum Na^+, is one of the most common electrolyte disorders encountered in clinical medicine. The symptoms of hyponatremia can vary from very subtle changes in mentation or level of energy to profound neurologic abnormalities including generalized convulsions. The rate of decrease of serum Na^+ is directly proportional to the severity of symptoms noted. Those patients whose serum Na^+ falls slowly, over days or weeks, may exhibit lassitude, slow mental or physical responses, nausea, muscle cramps, and nonspecific complaints of not feeling well. When serum Na^+ falls quickly, over hours, or one or two days, the abnormalities can include marked disorientation, confusion, coma, and convulsions.

Hyponatremia may occur in a variety of conditions. It can occur with Na^+ (solute) loss or H_2O (solvent) excess. In these situations, the serum osmolality is decreased. Excess Na^+ loss relative to water loss can occur via renal or extrarenal routes. Renal etiologies behind hyponatremia include (1) overhydration, such as in psychogenic polydipsia; (2) diuretic therapy; (3) salt-wasting nephropathies; (4) adrenal insufficiency; (5) bicarbonaturia; and (6) ketonuria. The urinary Na^+ concentration is usually greater than 20 mmol/L despite the presence of hyponatremia. Extrarenal etiologies include (1) overhydration, (2) vomiting, (3) diarrhea, (4) "third-space" losses, and (5) burns. The urinary Na^+ concentration is less than 10 mmol/L. Therapy to correct this electrolyte imbalance includes Na^+ and fluid replacement.

Excess total body water (edema) is present in (1) the nephrotic syndrome, (2) cirrhosis, (3) cardiac failure, and (4) acute and chronic renal failure. Total body Na^+ is also increased, but the excess of retained water is greater. The urinary Na^+ concentration is less than 10 mmol/L except in renal failure, in which the value may exceed 20 mmol/L. Hyponatremia *without* a visible increase in ECF volume (euvolemia) can be seen in (1) hypothyroidism, (2) glucocorticoid deficiency, (3) chronic disease, and (4) persistent or inappropriate secretion of ADH (SIADH). Patients with hypothyroidism are not able to dilute their urine maximally (Derubertis, 1971). They may also secrete increased levels of ADH (Skowsky, 1978). Free water excretion is inhibited in patients with glucocorticoid deficiency (i.e., Addison's disease). The explanation for this inhibition is not understood. Hyponatremia is common in patients with chronic diseases and is believed to be a result of the secretion of ADH, which is stimulated despite lower-than-normal plasma osmolalities. SIADH has been demonstrated in patients under severe emotional or physical stress or who are in pain, and in some receiving various medications, such as central nervous system–acting agents, antineoplastic drugs, and diuretics (Ruddy, 1981).

SIADH refers to the continued secretion of ADH even though the plasma osmolality is subnormal and the plasma volume is normal or increased (Cooke, 1979). This syndrome is associated with a wide variety of neoplasms, inflammatory pulmonary disorders, and inflammatory, traumatic, and metabolic central nervous system disorders, including head trauma and seizures. Therapy for situations in which hyponatremia with excess total body water or euvolemia exists includes water restriction. In situations in which acute water intoxication is a possibility, administration of loop diuretics with sodium replacement may be necessary. Lithium and demeclocycline base also have been used by some physicians.

Artifactual hyponatremia is encountered in the laboratory in two situations. Hyperglycemia increases serum osmolality, with a subsequent shift of ICF to the ECF, decreasing ECF electrolyte concentration. Roughly, for each 100 mg/dL increase in blood glucose, there is a 1.6 mmol/L decrease in the serum Na^+ concentration (Schrier, 1981). Hyponatremia (pseudohyponatremia) may also be present if the serum specimens are lipemic or contain abnormally large amounts of protein (e.g., Waldenström's macroglobulinemia). Na^+ concentrations are restricted to the water space, which is proportionately decreased by the lipid or protein volume. Na^+ concentration in the serum and plasma volume is correspondingly less.

Most often, pseudohyponatremia occurs when sodium concentration is measured by methods like flame photometry that measure the number of moles of Na^+ in the sample and then divide by the *total* volume of sample, which includes the nonsodium (lipid) volume. Pseudohyponatremia is less likely to be encountered by methods based on ion-selective electrodes.

Importantly, when pseudohyponatremia does occur, the serum osmolality is normal. Actual or true Na^+ values can be found by redrawing the serum after fasting or by using ultracentrifuge (165,000 g for 10 minutes) to separate the aqueous from the lipid or protein phases (Steffes, 1976).

Hypernatremia, or increased serum Na^+, is seen when there is an excessive loss of H_2O, relative to Na^+, from the body and when the total amount of Na^+ in the body is increased. Hypotonic fluid loss may occur via renal or extrarenal routes. Renal losses occur because of osmotic diuresis, in which case the urine osmolality is low or normal and its Na^+ concentration is greater than 20 mmol/L. Extrarenal etiologies are (1) profuse sweating and (2) diarrhea in children without adequate fluid replacement. In these situations, the urine has an increased osmolality and an Na^+ concentration less than 10 mmol/L.

Hypernatremia can also result from loss of H_2O alone. Renal losses occur because of (1) central diabetes insipidus or (2) nephrogenic diabetes insipidus. In the latter condition, the kidneys are not able to respond to circulating ADH. Etiologies are diverse and include parenchymal diseases affecting the renal medulla, electrolyte disturbances such as hypercalcemia and hypokalemia, and drug therapy such as lithium (Ruddy, 1981). Hereditary nephrogenic diabetes insipidus, a sex-linked disease with variable penetrance, is much rarer (Ruddy, 1981). The osmolality of the urine is either normal or decreased (see the section entitled Osmolality).

Purely extrarenal water losses are primarily insensible losses from the lungs and skin (e.g., fever). The osmolality of the urine in these conditions is increased.

Significant hypernatremia may also be observed in Cushing's syndrome, which involves hyperaldosteronism, leading to increased renal Na^+ reabsorption and renal secretion of hydrogen and potassium ions in the distal convoluted tubule, leading to mild hypokalemic metabolic alkalosis.

Excessive Na^+ intake may also result in hypernatremia. This is occasionally encountered in clinical medicine (e.g., $NaHCO_3$ administration during a cardiac arrest). The urine osmolality in these situations is normal or increased.

Therapy for hypernatremia consists of appropriate fluid replacement combined with the use of diuretics to rid the body of excess Na^+. Knowledge concerning the renal handling of Na^+ can be helpful in assessment. The renal tubules reabsorb roughly 99% of the filtered Na^+. In edematous states, such as congestive heart failure, cirrhosis, and nephrotic syndrome, relatively more Na^+ is reabsorbed. In some disease states, such as polycystic kidneys, medullary cystic disease, tubulointerstitial diseases, and chronic renal failure, urinary Na^+ wasting may become a severe complication.

Deficiency in the ability of tubules to regulate Na^+ excretion can be tested either by increasing or decreasing the intake of Na^+ and relating it to urinary excretion. The patient initially receives a normal diet containing a known quantity of Na^+, e.g., 100 mmol/day, and the daily urinary excretion is measured. Na^+ excretion should approximate 15 mmol/day less than the intake, which allows for loss of Na^+ in sweat and feces. After three days, the dietary intake of Na^+ is reduced to 10 mmol/day, which is the usual content of a hospital salt-free diet. Within 7 to 10 days, urinary Na^+ excretion should be less than 10 mmol/day. Another measure of tubular ability to control Na^+ excretion is obtained by allowing the patient to have a normal diet and giving a mineralocorticoid twice a day for two or three days. The urinary excretion of Na^+ should fall below 10 mmol/day. Daily decreases in body weight despite an adequate caloric intake suggest loss of Na^+ and water. Postural hypotension, signs of dehydration, or edema are indications to halt these tests.

Frequently, consultations are requested to determine the cause of a rising concentration of nitrogenous products in the circulation or oliguria. We have alluded to the individual use of various laboratory tests for diagnostic purposes earlier in the chapter. However, combining all these measurements can provide a more comprehensive and definitive means to differentiate prerenal, renal, and postrenal etiologies (Table 7–2).

Potassium

Potassium (K^+) is the major intracellular cation; only 2% of the total body K^+ is extracellular (Perez, 1988). The expected range of serum [K^+] is 3.8 to 5.5 mmol/L. An average diet contains 50 to 150 mmol K^+/day, whereon the kidneys usually excrete 80% to 90% of the ingested K^+. In normal subjects, this amounts to a daily urinary excretion of 25 to 125 mmol. Unlike Na^+, however, there is no renal threshold for K^+, and some K^+ continues to be excreted into the urine even in K^+-depleted states (10 to 20 mmol/day).

Hypokalemia, or decreased serum K^+, can occur even when the total amount of K^+ in the body is normal (Latta, 1993). Intracellular movement from the ECF into the ICF occurs during alkalemia, insulin therapy, and periodic paralysis. The latter condition can also occur associated with hyperkalemia. Hypokalemic, or hyperkalemic, periodic paralysis is a familial disease with autosomal dominant inheritance characterized by intermittent attacks of weakness or paralysis of limb and trunk muscles when the serum K^+ is markedly decreased or increased by the potassium ion intracellular shift.

Depletion of total body K^+ stores and hypokalemia occur as a result of (1) gastrointestinal fluid losses due to vomiting or diarrhea or (2) renal losses. Diuretics are the most important cause of renal losses. Other important renal etiologies are losses secondary to metabolic alkalosis, renal tubular acidosis (RTA) (*vide infra*), and mineralocorticoid excess.

As mentioned earlier, even with low plasma [K^+], the kidneys cannot completely conserve K^+, and urinary [K^+] rarely drops below 5 to 10 mmol/L. In the hypokalemic patient, a spot urinary [K^+] greater than 20 mmol/L suggests that the kidney may be the source of K^+ loss or that the hypokalemia

Table 7–2. HELPFUL LABORATORY EVALUATIONS TO ASSESS OLIGURIA

Diagnostic Test	Prerenal	Renal	Postrenal
Urine volume	<500 mL/day	<500 mL/day	Variable
BUN/creatinine ratio in serum	>20:1	10:1	Variable
Urine/plasma urea concentration	>10:1	<10:1	About 15:1
Urine/plasma creatinine concentration	>20:1	<20:1	<20:1
Urine specific gravity	>1.020	About 1.010	About 1.010
Urine osmolality	>600 mOsm/kg	About 300 mOsm/kg	About 300 mOsm/kg
Urine/plasma osmolality	>2:1	<1.2:1	Variable
Urine sodium concentration	<20 mEq/L	>30 mEq/L	>30 mEq/L
Fractional excretion Na	>1.0	>1.0	>1.0
Renal failure index	<1.0	>1.0	>1.0

$$\text{Fractional Excretion Na} = \frac{[\text{urine Na}] \times [\text{plasma creatinine}]}{[\text{plasma Na}] \times [\text{urine creatinine}]} \times 100$$

$$\text{Renal Failure Index} = \frac{[\text{urine Na}] \times [\text{plasma creatinine}]}{[\text{urine creatinine}]} \times 100$$

is acute, because the kidney takes one to three weeks to effectively conserve K^+. If, under the same circumstances, the $[K^+]$ is less than 20 mEq/L, then the kidney is probably not the major source of K^+ loss and the hypokalemia is of several weeks' duration.

Hyperkalemia, or increased serum $[K^+]$, can result from transfer of K^+ from the ICF to the ECF and from an actual increase in total body K^+. Cellular efflux occurs in acidemia and from cellular damage (e.g., fever, hemolysis, rhabdomyolysis). Increased total body potassium and hyperkalemia occur typically in acute and chronic renal failure and in mineralocorticoid deficiency (e.g., Addison's disease).

Artifactual hyperkalemia may be encountered when the platelet count is elevated (Weismann, 1974). As clotting occurs in the test tube, intraplatelet K^+ is released and measured in the serum. To overcome this problem, heparinized plasma can be used for $[K^+]$ determination. False high $[K^+]$ values are also seen if a prolonged tourniquet application causes juxtavenular cellular injury producing leakage of K^+ into the plasma. An increase in muscular activity, such as if the fist is repeatedly clenched prior to and during drawing, may cause an elevated $[K^+]$ value. A hemolyzed specimen yields an elevated $[K^+]$ value owing to the high concentration of K^+ within erythrocytes (105 mmol/L). Special care should be taken to avoid contamination of samples with K^+ EDTA. This may be accomplished by collecting samples for $[K^+]$ prior to that for the complete blood count (CBC).

Elevated and depressed serum $[K^+]$ may have profound adverse effects on the neuromuscular system, including apathy, weakness, and paralysis. Effects on the myocardium include serious arrhythmias, which may cause death. This makes $[K^+]$ one of the most important clinical analytes. Hypokalemia is treated by parenteral or nonparenteral administration of K^+. The symptoms and signs of acute hyperkalemia are treated by Ca^{+2} infusion, which antagonizes the effect of K^+ on cardiac tissue; by $NaHCO_3$ infusion, which causes the movement of K^+ into cells; by glucose infusion, which stimulates insulin production with resultant intracellular sequestration of glucose and K^+; by oral or rectal administration of the cation exchange resin Kayexalate, which binds K^+ (removing it from the ECF); and by dialysis. Chronic hyperkalemia is treated by use of oral sodium polystyrene sulfonate (Kayexalate), diuretics, and reduction of dietary K^+.

Measurement of Na^+ and K^+

The most frequent means for measuring Na^+ and K^+ in the clinical laboratory are emission photometry and ion-selective electrodes (Chap. 3). The alkali metals lithium and cesium are used as internal standards in flame photometry. Cesium is used in instruments that quantitate lithium.

Ion-selective electrodes have been incorporated into many automated systems. The most practical Na^+ electrode is made of specialized glass, selective for Na^+. A liquid ion-exchange membrane electrode, incorporating the antibiotic valinomycin as the K^+ binder, is the most selective for K^+.

It has been demonstrated in intralaboratory (Ladenson, 1979) and interlaboratory surveys (MacDonald, 1981) that the potentiometric instruments give values approximately 1% to 3% higher than those from flame-emission instruments. This difference is not great enough to interfere with clinical correlations. The difference may result from the physiochemical properties of the two analytical techniques because ion-selective electrodes are not affected, to the same extent, by variations in plasma water from increased protein or lipid content (Ladenson, 1979).

Chloride

Chloride (Cl^-) is the major extracellular anion. Most ingested Cl^- is absorbed, and the excess is excreted in the urine. The normal serum concentration is 98 to 106 mmol/L. Slightly lower values are observed in postprandial serum specimens. This occurs from increased synthesis of hydrochloric acid (HCl) by the parietal cells of the stomach. The usual daily urinary output of Cl^- is 110 to 250 mmol/L.

Hypochloridemia, or low serum Cl^-, is seen when there is excessive loss of Cl^- from the body, such as that occurring with (1) gastrointestinal (HCl) losses, (2) diabetic ketoacidosis, (3) mineralocorticoid excess, and (4) salt-losing renal diseases. Low serum values may also be encountered in diseases in which there is a high serum $[HCO_3^-]$ concentration (e.g., compensated respiratory acidosis, metabolic alkalosis). This is a result of the intracellular shift and increased renal excretion of Cl^- in these conditions. Finally, hypochloridemia is seen with low serum $[Na^+]$ in chronic diseases.

Hyperchloridemia may occur during metabolic acidosis resulting from excess loss of HCO_3 due to (1) losses from the lower gastrointestinal tract in diarrhea, (2) renal tubular acidosis (*vide infra*), and (3) mineralocorticoid deficiency. Infrequently, excess administration of NH_4Cl or acidic salts of amino acids (during hyperalimentation) can cause hyperchloridemia. Elevated serum Cl^- values have been reported in some cases of hyperparathyroidism (Wells, 1971). This may be a result of parathyroid hormones (PTHs) decreasing proximal renal tubular reabsorption of HCO_3^- and augmenting chloride reabsorption (Karlinsky, 1974).

Measurement of $[Cl^-]$ in sweat is useful in diagnosing the exocrine glandular disorder cystic fibrosis (Littlewood, 1980). The secretion of sweat Cl^- is increased above the reference range, which is approximately 5 to 45 mmol/L in children (Shwachman, 1981) and slightly higher in adults. Affected infants characteristically have concentrations greater than 60 mmol/L, and affected adults have levels in excess of 70 mmol/L. When the disease is mild, it may not be diagnosed until adult life (Boye, 1980). The patient is induced to sweat by iontophoresis or the introduction of pilocarpine into the skin (method of Gibson and Cooke). Sweat Cl^- activity is measured directly using ion-selective electrodes, or the $[Cl^-]$ is measured after the sweat is weighed. It is recommended that the sweat $[Na^+]$ also be quantitated. This serves as an internal quality control check because the $[Na^+]$ and $[Cl^-]$ should be within 10 mmol/L of each other. Repeat studies with clinical and cytogenetic correlations are recommended to rule out false-positive results.

Measurement of Cl^-

Cl^- is measured in the laboratory by mercurimetric titration, by coulometric titration, by colorimetry using $Hg(SCN)_2$, and by the use of ion-selective electrodes.

In the mercurimetric method, Cl^- combines with added Hg^{+2} to form the soluble complex $HgCl_2$. Excess added Hg^{+2} combines with the indicator diphenylcarbazone to form a blue color, the endpoint of the titration.

Coulometric titration is described in Chapter 3. This is very accurate; small volumes are required; and it is suitable for pediatric work, including sweat Cl^- determination.

In the automated thiocyanate method, $Hg(SCN)_2$ is added to the sample and dissociates owing to the complexing of Hg^{+2} with Cl^-. The free thiocyanate ion (SCN^-) reacts with added Fe^{+3} to form the colored complex $Fe(SCN)_3$, which is measured photometrically. Cl^- electrodes are solid-state electrodes using membranes composed of AgCl.

All chloride methods measure bromide to some extent (Driscoll, 1966; Elin, 1981). The electrode methods are influenced to the greatest extent; and the mercurimetric and coulometric methods the least. Patients with bromide toxicity will likely have increased chloride levels as determined by colorimetric and ion-selective electrode methods. The levels will be less elevated if they are determined by mercurimetric and coulometric methods.

Surveys have demonstrated that all methods provide comparable clinical data (Geisinger, 1980). However, ion-selective electrodes are the most precise and the manual mercurimetric methods are the least precise.

Total CO_2

HCO_3^- is quantitatively the second most important anionic fraction in serum. Its production in the body results from the dissociation of H_2CO_3 produced from the formation of CO_2 during metabolism (Table 7–3). HCO_3^- is reconverted to H_2CO_3 and, hence, to H_2O and CO_2 as the blood perfuses the lungs. HCO_3^- is filtered freely by the kidneys, but little or no HCO_3^- is present in the urine ($pH < 6.1$) when the diet is acidic. Most HCO_3^- is reabsorbed by the proximal tubules (about 85%), and a small amount (about 15%) is reabsorbed by the distal tubules. HCO_3^- in serum or plasma can be measured directly by titration with acid or indirectly by using the measured P_{CO_2} and $[H^+]$ in an equation (see Table 7–3) or a nomogram. However, HCO_3^- is most commonly measured with other combined forms of CO_2 (CO_2, H_2CO_3, carbamino groups) as total CO_2. This value approximates the HCO_3^- very closely, because 89% to 90% of all the CO_2 that can be liberated from serum is in the form of HCO_3^-. The reference intervals for total CO_2 are 19 to 25 mmol/L for arterial blood and 23 to 30 mmol/L for venous blood.

Total CO_2 determinations are useful, along with pH and P_{CO_2} measurements, in evaluating acid-base disorders. Discussion of high and low values and their etiologies are included in this chapter in the section entitled Acid-Base Balance.

Measurement of Total CO_2

Total CO_2 measurements are performed in the clinical laboratory volumetrically, manometrically, or colorimetrically, or by using a P_{CO_2} electrode to measure the rate of formation of released CO_2.

A syringe containing a reaction chamber in which serum and acid are mixed and a calibrated barrel has been found to be convenient and also to have suitable clinical accuracy and precision (Lam, 1978). The heights to which the acid-liberated CO_2 pushes the barrel are compared between specimen and standard, and the ratio is converted to mmol/L.

Automated methods have been developed that measure pressure (by means of a pressure-transducer) of the acid-released CO_2, which is vacuum-extracted into an enclosed space. Another automated method (Technicon; Miles, Tarrytown, N.Y.) measures the liberated CO_2 after it permeates a

Table 7–3. THE BICARBONATE BUFFER SYSTEM

$$H^+ + HCO_3^- = H_2CO_3 = CO_2 + H_2O$$

Why is normal $[H^+]$ 40 nmol/L?

Normal Acid-Base Values

Blood Pa_{CO_2} = 38–42 mm Hg

Plasma HCO_3^- = 24–28 mmol/L

Henderson Equation

$$[H^+]\ (\text{nmol/L}) = \frac{24\ P_{CO_2}\ (\text{mm Hg})}{HCO_3^-\ (\text{mmol/L})}$$

$$[H^+] = \frac{24 \times 40}{24} = 40\ \text{nmol/L}$$

silicon rubber membrane into a recipient stream containing the pH indicator phenolphthalein and TRIS buffer. The intensity of the color produced from acidification of the buffer is proportional to the total amount of CO_2 present. A third automated method (Beckman Instruments, Fullerton, CA) uses two Pco_2 electrodes to monitor the rate of formation of acid-released CO_2 gas. One electrode is the reference electrode. The resulting voltage change is converted to a digital readout in millimoles per liter. The principle of the CO_2 electrode is discussed in Chapter 3.

The specimen to be analyzed must be handled anaerobically to minimize atmosphere losses of CO_2 and HCO_3^- (converted to CO_2), which would cause a falsely low total CO_2 value. In the laboratory, this can be accomplished by covering the specimen container with plastic or Parafilm M (American National Can, Greenwich, CT). Another method to prevent loss of CO_2 is to add one drop of 1 N (NH_4OH) to both standards and samples, decreasing the Pco_2 in the sample to that of the atmosphere, thereby preventing loss of CO_2 and a reduction of HCO_3^- (Gambino, 1966).

Anion Gap

The anion gap (AG) is a mathematical approximation of the difference between the anions and cations routinely measured in serum (Fig. 7–2). Routine electrolyte measurements include Na^+, K^+, Cl^-, and HCO_3^- (as total CO_2). The unmeasured cations (i.e., Ca^{+2}, Mg^{+2}) average 7 mmol/L, and

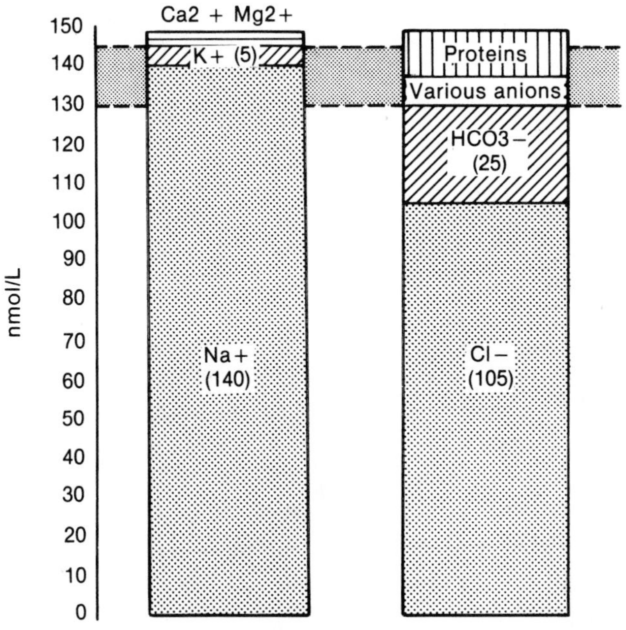

Figure 7–2. Anion gap. Depiction of the quantities of anions and cations in the circulating blood. The positive charges equal the negative charges to maintain electrical neutrality. However, only Na^+, K^+, Cl^-, and HCO_3^- are routinely measured. The sum of the measured positive charges (Na^+, K^+) (top interrupted line) normally exceeds the sum of the measured negative charges ($Cl^- + HCO_3^-$) (bottom interrupted line). This difference, which is known as the anion gap, is depicted by shading outside the histogram.

the unmeasured anions (i.e., PO_4^{-3}, SO_4^{-2}, protein$^-$, and the anions of organic acids) average 24 mmol/L. If the Cl^- and the total CO_2 concentrations are summed and subtracted from the Na^+ concentration (and, in some laboratories, the $Na^+ + K^+$ concentrations), the difference should be less than 17 mmol/L. If the anion gap exceeds 17 mmol/L, this usually indicates significantly increased concentrations of unmeasured anions. Causes for this condition are (1) uremia with retention of fixed acid anions such as PO_4^{-3} and SO_4^{-2}; (2) ketotic states, as in diabetes, alcoholism, or starvation; (3) lactic acidosis, as in shock; (4) ingestion of toxins, such as methanol, salicylate, ethylene glycol, and paraldehyde; and (5) increased plasma proteins as occurs in dehydration. An increased anion gap occurs occasionally in metabolic alkalosis (Madias, 1979). This is believed to be due to the titration of plasma proteins resulting in loss of H^+ and the consequent increase in the net negatively charged proteins.

Decreased anion gaps (<10 mmol/L) can result from either an increase in unmeasured cations or a decrease in unmeasured anions. An increase in unmeasured cations can be seen in (1) Li^+ intoxication, (2) hypermagnesemia, (3) multiple myeloma, (4) polyclonal gammopathy, and (5) polymyxin B therapy, because this drug is polycationic (O'Connor, 1978). Gamma globulins have a net positive charge at physiologic pH (Keshgegian, 1978; Murray, 1975). Decreased unmeasured anions occur in (1) hypoalbuminemia and (2) hyponatremia with normal or increased ECF (e.g., SIADH) (Oh, 1978). This is postulated to result from the selective renal excretion of unmeasured anions in this condition. Finally, interference in measured Cl^- caused by bromide intoxication can cause a spurious decrease in the calculated gap (see the section entitled Chloride).

In some forms of acidosis, the fall in HCO_3^- is balanced by an elevation in Cl^- owing to a loss of HCO_3^--rich, Cl^--poor fluids and retention of dietary Cl^-. The anion gap remains within normal limits. These so-called hyperchloridemic acidoses are associated with loss of HCO_3^- through the gastrointestinal tract or kidneys. An increased anion gap (AG) develops in lactic, diabetic, or uremic acidosis or secondary to ingestion of foreign acids. In these conditions, there is minimal rise or even a slight depression in Cl^- and the difference between Na^+ and ($Cl^- + HCO_3^-$) exceeds 17 mmol/L. The increased anion gap seen during chronic renal failure rarely exceeds 20 to 25 mmol/L. Retention of phosphates, sulfates, and organic anions constitutes the unmeasured anions causing the excessive gap in renal failure. The presence or absence of an increased AG is characteristic of certain disorders. Therefore, it is helpful in diagnosing the underlying etiology of metabolic acidosis. The increased AG in metabolic alkalosis may be moderately increased owing to hemoconcentration, increased blood lactate (from lactate infusion), or increased negative charges on circulating proteins, as discussed earlier. Serum Cl^- is usually decreased. Thus, modest increases of the AG are not diagnostic. Nevertheless, when the AG exceeds 30 mmol/L, the presence of an organic acidosis is highly likely.

In organic acidoses, the increase in the blood acid anion concentration parallels the increase in the AG, and both values closely approximate the decrement in plasma HCO_3^-. An AG/HCO_3^- ratio considerably greater than 1.0 suggests a su-

2

perimposed metabolic alkalosis, and a ratio less than 0.8 is consistent with a hyperchloridemic component of the acidosis (Perez, 1986).

The AG is useful also for quality control of laboratory results for Na^+, K^+, Cl^-, and total CO_2. If an increased or decreased AG is calculated for a set of electrolytes from a healthy individual, this would indicate that one or more of the laboratory results are erroneous. Another possible explanation is that a mixed acid-base disturbance is present.

ACID-BASE BALANCE

A large quantity of acid is ingested daily in the normal diet and produced endogenously as a result of metabolism. Thirteen thousand to 20,000 mmol of CO_2 largely converted to carbonic acid (H_2CO_3) is formed resulting from oxidation of carbohydrates, proteins, and fats (Valtin, 1973). Ketoacids from incomplete oxidation of lipids, and sulfuric and phosphoric acid from oxidation of sulfur-containing amino acids and phosphorus-containing compounds account for an additional 40 to 60 mmol of acid (Valtin, 1973).

H_2CO_3 is called a volatile acid because it can be converted to CO_2, which can be excreted by the lungs. However, the other acids produced by the body cannot be converted to a gaseous state and are called nonvolatile or fixed acids. The latter must be excreted in the urine.

Many metabolic reactions are catalyzed by enzymes, which function at optimal pH. Accordingly, it is necessary that the body possess efficient mechanisms to maintain the pH of both the ECF and ICF within narrow limits, usually 7.35 to 7.45. These mechanisms include buffering the blood, respiration (*vide infra*), and renal mechanisms.

A buffer is a weak acid in solution with its conjugate base, which is in the form of a salt. When acid is added to a solution, it combines with the conjugate base to form a weaker acid. The result is a smaller decrease in pH. The ECF buffers, which account for a little less than half of the systemic buffering capacity, are, in descending order of buffering capacity, (1) bicarbonate/carbonic acid, (2) hemoglobin, (3) plasma proteins, (4) erythrocytes, and (5) plasma phosphates. The bicarbonate/carbonic acid equilibrium ($H_2O + CO_2 \rightleftarrows H_2CO_3 \rightleftarrows H^+ + HCO_3^-$) can be conveniently expressed using the Henderson-Hasselbalch equation:

$$pH = pK_a + \log \frac{[HCO_3^-]}{H_2CO_3} \qquad (7\text{-}9),$$

where pK_a is the negative logarithm of the dissociation constant K'_a of H_2CO_3. The pK' of normal plasma at 37°C is 6.1. The pK' varies inversely with both pH and ionic strength and directly with temperature. This equation can also be expressed as

$$pH = pK'_a + \log \frac{(\text{total } CO_2) - 0.03\ Pco_2}{0.03\ Pco_2} \qquad (7\text{-}10).$$

In normal plasma, 0.03 is the solubility coefficient of CO_2 gas at 37°C. This value (0.03) times the Pco_2 is equivalent to the small amount of H_2CO_3 found dissolved in plasma. The solubility coefficient varies inversely with temperature or concentration, or both, of salt or protein and varies directly with lipid concentration. The product, $0.03 \times Pco_2$, subtracted from the total CO_2 values, is a close approximation of the HCO_3^-. Although the pK'_a of this buffer system is low (6.1) compared with the pH of plasma (7.4), it is an extremely effective buffer because the ratio of base to acid is finely regulated by respiration.

It is easier to think of acid-base balances in terms of $[H^+]$ (normally 40 nmol/L) (Preuss, 1993b). Because a pH is actually measured in and reported from the laboratory, a conversion from pH to $[H^+]$ is made. There exists a close inverse relationship of pH to $[H^+]$ between pH 7.25 and 7.50 (Fig. 7–3). An increase of 0.01 pH unit represents a decrease in $[H^+]$ of approximately 1 nmol/L, and a decrease of 0.01 pH unit represents an increase in $[H^+]$ of 1 nmol/L. For example, at pH 7.30, $[H^+] = 50$ nmol/L, and at pH 7.50, $[H^+] = 30$ nmol/L. After conversion, the Henderson equation is used to evaluate acid-base perturbations (see Table 7–3):

$$[H^+]\ \text{nmol/L} = \frac{24\ Pco_2\ (\text{mm Hg})}{[HCO_3^-]\ \text{mmol/L}} \qquad (7\text{-}11).$$

Hemoglobin is the second most important blood buffer, owing to the fact that each hemoglobin molecule contains 38 histidine residues that are able to bind with H^+ and owing to its relatively high concentration (15 g/dL) in whole blood. Plasma proteins act as buffers because both their free carboxyl and amino groups are able to bind H^+.

Least important is the buffering capacity of the inorganic and organic phosphates present in blood. At a pH of 7.4, the $(HPO_4)^{-2}/(H_2PO_4)^{-1}$ ratio is 4:1.

The sum of all blood buffers is called the buffer base. The reference values are between 46 and 52 mmol/L, with an average value of 49 mmol/L. If this average value is subtracted from the actual buffer base, base excess is derived. The reference interval for base excess is ±3.0 mmol/L. A

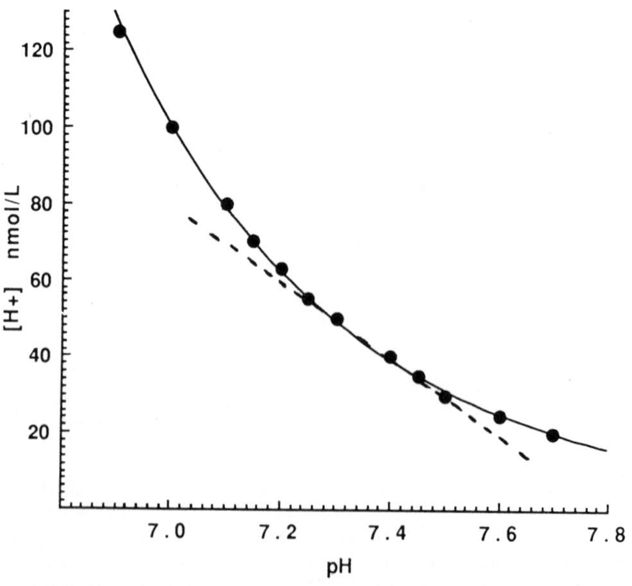

Figure 7–3. Correlation between pH and $[H^+]$. Between pH 7.25 and pH 7.50, the line of correlation (represented by an interrupted line) is relatively straight. Within this range, pH can be easily converted into $[H^+]$ by the formula described in the text.

negative base excess, or decrease in blood buffering capacity, is sometimes referred to as base deficit.

OTHER WAYS OF COMPUTING THE BASE EXCESS. The basic purpose of computing base excess is to estimate how much base (usually in the form of bicarbonate) must be given to an acidotic patient to cause the pH of the patient's blood to return to 7.4. Much less commonly, it gives an estimate of how much acid to administer to an alkalotic patient to change the blood pH to 7.4. Rather than using the estimation presented earlier, a more accurate method for performing this computation is to compute the amount of bicarbonate that must increase in the numerator of equation 7-9, that is

$$7.4 = 6.1 + \log \frac{[(HCO_3^- + X)]}{0.03 \times Pco_2} \qquad (7\text{-}12).$$

In equation 7-12, the bicarbonate HCO_3^- is the current value *prior to* addition of base. X is the concentration of bicarbonate that must be added to restore the pH to 7.4, as on the left side of the equation. This equation is based on the assumption that pulmonary function remains constant at the level prior to treatment and that the Pco_2 is directly measured. This equation can be solved for X, that is,

$$X = 0.6 \times Pco_2 - HCO_3^- \qquad (7\text{-}13).$$

If only the pH and the total CO_2 are known, the base excess must be computed from the following considerations. The pH of the arterial blood *prior to* correction, pHo, is

$$pHo = 6.1 + \log \frac{(HCO_3^-)}{0.03 \times Pco_2} \qquad (7\text{-}13A).$$

The total CO_2 is given by the expression

$$\text{total } CO_2 = TC = HCO_3^- + 0.03 \times Pco_2 \qquad (7\text{-}13B).$$

The amount of HCO_3^- that must be added to change the blood pH to 7.4 is given by equation 7-12. The three equations 7-12, 7-13A, and 7-13B contain three unknowns, Pco_2, HCO_3^-, and X. Solving these equations for X in terms of TC and pHo,

$$X = \frac{TC(20 - 10^{(pHo\text{-}6.1)})}{(1 + 10^{(pHo\text{-}6.1)})} \qquad (7\text{-}13C).$$

Equations 7-13 and 7-13C are used to compute the amount of bicarbonate that must be administered to an acidotic patient to return the blood pH to 7.4. Most blood gas analyzers are equipped with computer processors that perform these computations and give the base excess as a calculated value.

COMPENSATION FOR ACIDOSIS AND ALKALOSIS. Although the blood buffers act instantaneously to minimize the change in pH, their capacity to do so is limited. Respiratory compensation is prompt, but ultimate regulation of acid-base balance, with regeneration of free buffers, is a function of the renal tubular cells. Renal compensation is gradual and occurs over a three- to four-day period after the acid-base imbalance occurs. HCO_3^- is freely filtered by the glomeruli and, at normal plasma levels, is completely reabsorbed by the renal tubules with approximately 85% being absorbed by the proximal tubules. There is a renal threshold for HCO_3^-, and this electrolyte will normally be present in the urine when the total plasma CO_2 (HCO_3^-) is greater than 30 mmol/L (Stenzel, 1981). The respiratory compensation in simple metabolic disturbances and the renal HCO_3^- compensation in simple respiratory disturbances can be estimated (Table 7–4). Deviations from this formula suggest the presence of coexisting acid-base perturbations. The compensatory mechanisms are also summarized in Chapter 4.

Table 7–4. EQUATIONS USED TO PREDICT COMPENSATORY RESPONSES

Metabolic acidosis	
	$\Delta Pco_2 = 1.2\ \Delta HCO_3^-$
Metabolic alkalosis	
	$\Delta Pco_2 = 0.5\ \Delta HCO_3^-$
Respiratory acidosis	
Acute	$\Delta HCO_3^- = 0.10\ \Delta Pco_2$
Chronic	$\Delta HCO_3^- = 0.35\ \Delta Pco_2$
Respiratory alkalosis	
Acute	$\Delta HCO_3^- = 0.20\ \Delta Pco_2$
Chronic	$\Delta HCO_3^- = 0.50\ \Delta Pco_2$

During the process of HCO_3^- reabsorption, H^+ is excreted by the proximal tubules into the urine. H^+ is also excreted by the distal tubules. Filtered dibasic phosphate (HPO_4^-) combines with H^+ to form monobasic phosphate. This is referred to as titratable acidity. H^+ also combines with NH_3 to form NH_4^+. NH_3 is produced in the proximal tubular cells from the deamination of glutamine and other amino acids by glutaminase, glutamate dehydrogenase, or both (Preuss, 1980). The total amount of H^+ excreted by these mechanisms is 1 to 2 mmol/kg body weight (Stenzel, 1981). The mechanisms of respiration that control the Pco_2 (and therefore, the H_2CO_3 concentration) are discussed subsequently.

Laboratory Measurement of Acid-Base Parameters

In order to evaluate the acid-base status of the patient and to identify causes (i.e., metabolic, respiratory, or both) responsible for imbalances, it is necessary to determine, besides pH [H^+], one or both of the following parameters: (1) total CO_2 (really, the bicarbonate) and (2) Pco_2. In addition, the AG determination can be useful if metabolic acidosis is present (see the section entitled Anion Gap). Finally, renal function studies that measure the ability of the kidneys either to excrete an acid load or to reabsorb an alkali load are useful for confirming renal tubular diseases resulting in hyperchloridemic acidosis. These diseases are discussed in the section entitled Renal Tubular Acidosis.

Acid-Base Imbalances

ACIDEMIA. Acidemia is defined as a blood pH of less than 7.35, $[H^+] > 45$ nmol/L. It can result from the accumulation of CO_2 in the body. This is called respiratory acidosis because it is a result of hypoventilation or ventilation/perfusion inequalities (*vide infra*). By reabsorbing HCO_3^-, the kidneys are able to compensate somewhat, the degree of compensation depending on the chronicity of the ventilatory insufficiency and the functional capacity of the renal tubules. This is reflected by an increase in total CO_2 and in HCO_3^-.

Acidemia can also occur from an accumulation of fixed acids or a loss in HCO_3^-. This results in a primary decrease in

2

total CO_2 and is referred to as metabolic acidosis. Clinically, metabolic acidosis can be divided into two types: acidemia with an increased AG (>17 mmol/L) and acidemia with a normal AG (<17 mmol/L). The latter is often referred to as hyperchloridemic metabolic acidosis. Causes of metabolic acidosis with an increased AG have been listed previously (Preuss, 1988a). Likewise, etiologies resulting in hyperchloridemic acidosis also have been reviewed previously. Renal tubular acidosis is discussed in greater detail later in the section entitled Renal Tubular Acidosis. As a result of metabolic acidosis, the rate and depth of respiration compensate by increasing, with the degree of compensation dependent on the adequacy of respiratory function. Treatment of acidemia is directed at correction of the underlying disease process(es), with the administration of HCO_3^- to acutely ill and symptomatic patients, and simultaneous correction of existing electrolyte and fluid imbalances.

ALKALEMIA. Alkalemia is defined as a blood pH greater than 7.45, $[H^+]$ less than 35 nmol/L. Alkalemia can occur from decreased P_{CO_2} concentrations in the blood. This is called respiratory alkalosis because it is secondary to hyperventilation. Etiologies are discussed in Chapter 4 and subsequently. As a result of respiratory alkalosis, the kidneys compensate to varying degrees, depending on the chronicity of the alkalemia, by decreasing the reabsorption of HCO_3^-. Correspondingly, the total circulating HCO_3^- is decreased from baseline by this renal compensatory response.

Alkalemia also occurs when there is loss of fixed acids or an increase in blood alkali such as HCO_3^-. The primary increase in HCO_3^- is referred to as metabolic alkalosis. Loss of fixed acids is most often due to prolonged vomiting or to nasogastric suctioning. Alkali excess can occur in excessive ingestion of basic substances, such as antacids. Metabolic alkalosis can also occur in disease states in which there is excessive intracellular movement of H^+ from the extracellular space (often induced by hypokalemia) or excess excretion of H^+ into the urine, or both. The latter occurs with mineralocorticoid excess syndromes such as hyperaldosteronism, Cushing's syndrome, or prolonged administration of corticosteroids. Respiratory rate decreases in metabolic alkalosis, with a compensatory increase of P_{CO_2}. As in all acid-base imbalances, treatment is directed toward the correction of the underlying disease process(es) with the replacement of K^+ defects with KCl and the correction of fluid imbalances.

Mixed Acid-Base Disturbances

Because respiratory disturbances are frequently associated with simultaneous metabolic perturbations, mixed acid-base disturbances are commonly encountered. These can be detected if the compensatory response falls short or exceeds that expected or if the AG or the ratio change in anion gap to that of HCO_3^- (AG/HCO_3^-) is abnormal. The mixed disturbance can lessen the $[H^+]$ disturbance or worsen it.

Common Combinations Making H^+ Perturbation Worse

RESPIRATORY ACIDOSIS AND METABOLIC ACIDOSIS. *Example:* Acute pulmonary edema and cardiorespiratory arrest causing both poor tissue perfusion (lactic acidosis) and pulmonary edema (poor alveolar ventilation).

RESPIRATORY ALKALOSIS AND METABOLIC ALKALOSIS. *Example:* Patients who are vomiting and hyperventilating secondary to such disturbances as pain or psychogenic stress.

Common Combinations Lessening H^+ Perturbations

RESPIRATORY ACIDOSIS AND METABOLIC ALKALOSIS. *Example:* Patients with chronic obstructive pulmonary disease receiving diuretics.

METABOLIC ACIDOSIS AND RESPIRATORY ALKALOSIS. *Example:* Patients with chronic renal failure and hyperventilation.

METABOLIC ACIDOSIS AND METABOLIC ALKALOSIS. *Example:* Patients with chronic renal failure complicated by severe vomiting or nasogastric suction.

In the two examples making H^+ perturbations worse, perturbations in P_{CO_2} and HCO_3^- are exaggerated and, in the three examples lessening H^+ perturbations, would be decreased. In fact, pH, P_{CO_2} and $[HCO_3^-]$ may be normal and the only clue to an acid-base disturbance would be an increased AG. The medical history of the patient as well as the clinical setting are often clues to the possibility of a mixed acid-base disturbance, as suggested previously. Laboratory data may also provide a clue. The existence of a large AG indicates the presence of an organic acidosis even if acidemia is not present. Organic acidoses are associated with a ratio AG/HCO_3^- of one.

Hypokalemia and hypochloridemia are common findings in metabolic alkalosis. Hyperkalemia or hyperchloridemia, or both, occur in some but not all forms of metabolic acidosis. In acute respiratory acidosis and alkalosis, the $[HCO_3^-]$ rarely deviates more than 4 mmol/L from baseline, that is, lower than 20 mmol/L or higher than 30 mmol/L. In acid-base disturbances, the adequacy of the compensatory response can be assessed by simple equations (see Table 7–4) or an acid-base map.

Renal Tubular Acidosis

Renal tubular acidosis (RTA) is defined as defective secretion of H^+ by the renal tubules in the presence of a normal or near-normal GFR (Lash, 1993; Quintanilla, 1980). Either the distal elements such as the collecting ducts or the proximal tubules can be responsible. If the collecting ducts are to blame, this is referred to as distal or type 1 RTA. Proximal defects (pRTA) are type 2 RTA. Both types of tubular defects can result from primary (both sporadic and familial) tubular defects or secondary defects, which result from a variety of unrelated diseases.

In the complete form of type 1 RTA, there is impaired excretion of H^+, resulting in a urinary pH that is inappropriately high (>pH 5.3) even though acidemia is present. The distal tubular defect may result from a gradient or secretory defect (Arruda, 1977). The acidemia that develops in this condition results in extensive buffering by $CaCO_3$ in bone with resultant osteomalacia, hypercalcemia, and nephrocalcinosis. Hypokalemia also develops owing to increased renal excretion of K^+ enhanced by increased aldosterone secretion resulting from decreased ECF. An incomplete form of type 1 RTA has been identified; patients have osteomalacia, hypercalciuria, and renal stones, but acidemia is not present. Acidemia, however, develops when these individuals are challenged with an acid load. Apparently, the tubular defect is mild, and the retained H^+ is completely buffered. Secondary causes of type 1 RTA are many and include (1) cirrhosis, (2) renal diseases resulting from nephrocalcinosis and nephrotoxic drugs (e.g., amphotericin B, Li^+), (3) kidney transplant rejection, and (4) diseases characterized by hypergammaglobulinemia (Quintanilla, 1980). In cirrhosis, there is decreased urinary filtration of Na^+ which results in reduced H^+ secretion.

In type 2 RTA, there is reduced proximal reabsorption of HCO_3^- resulting in a significant bicarbonaturia. However, the tubules are able to reabsorb all of the filtered HCO_3^- if the plasma HCO_3^- falls below 14 mmol/L. In other words, a lesser HCO_3^- challenge can be handled competently by some kidneys. Type 2 RTA may be associated with a more generalized dysfunction of the proximal tubules called Fanconi's syndrome. Therefore, glycosuria, phosphaturia, aminoaciduria, and uricosuria may be associated with loss of HCO_3^-. Mild hypokalemia is not frequently seen in type 2 RTA. When mild hypokalemia occurs, it results from increased exchange of K^+ for the increased Na^+ delivered with the nonabsorbed HCO_3^- to the distal tubules and collecting ducts. In contrast to type 1 RTA, nephrocalcinosis is rare, probably due to hypercitruria, which binds Ca^{+2}. The hypercitruria occurs secondary to poor proximal reabsorption of citrate. Secondary causes of type 2 RTA include (1) multiple myeloma, (2) renal diseases (e.g., medullary cystic disease, transplant rejection), (3) proximal tubular defects associated with diseases of inborn errors of metabolism (e.g., cystinosis, Wilson's disease), and (4) drugs and toxins (e.g., outdated tetracycline, heavy metal intoxication) (Quintanilla, 1980).

Combined type 1 and type 2 defects are referred to as type 3 RTA. Another category of RTA is referred to as type 4 RTA (Sebastian, 1977). This condition is characterized by mild to moderate renal insufficiency, hyperchloridemic acidosis, and hyperkalemia. Many of these patients have reduced mineralocorticoid secretion or decreased renal tubular responsiveness to mineralocorticoids. This condition is probably due, at least in part, to the decreased renal ammoniagenesis resulting from hyperkalemia (Sleeper, 1982; Szylman, 1976) and the diminished mineralocorticoid secretion or diminished responsiveness to circulating mineralocorticoids.

Treatment of RTA is individualized and involves administration of alkalinizing salts and K^+ (for types 1 and 2 RTA). If possible, secondary causes should be identified and treated.

Laboratory Diagnosis of Renal Tubular Acidosis

The initial laboratory evaluation in diagnosing RTA includes simultaneous measurement of the serum HCO_3^-, P_{CO_2}, and $[H^+]$ and urinary pH (Lash, 1993).

Four tests described subsequently, that is, acid challenge, bicarbonate titration, $(U\text{-}A)P_{CO_2}$, and sulfate or phosphate infusions, are frequently used in various combinations for the complete workup of RTA—distal, proximal, or type 4.

For an acute acid challenge, NH_4Cl is administered orally (0.1 g/kg) in a gelatin capsule. It is important that NH_4Cl be given in a form that is readily absorbed from the gastrointestinal tract. If NH_4Cl is contraindicated by liver disease, $CaCl_2$ (0.1 g/kg) can be substituted. NH_4Cl results in increased $[H^+]$ through hepatic metabolism, and the $CaCl_2$ binds HCO_3^- in the gastrointestinal tract. Between four and eight hours after acute acid challenge, urine pH should normally decrease to 5.3 or lower (a detailed test is described in Table 7–5).

To challenge acid excretion maximally, NH_4Cl (0.1 g/kg) can be given for four to five consecutive days in divided doses. On the fifth day, the urinary pH should be 5.0 or lower and the total acid excretion should exceed 120 mEq/day. The total acid excreted is the sum of excreted NH_4^+ plus titratable acid minus bicarbonate. The titratable acid is equal to the quantity of alkali in millimoles required to titrate the urine to pH 7.4.

A urine pH greater than 5.3 following acute acid challenge when the blood pH is low and the serum $[HCO_3^-]$ is less than 22 mmol/L establishes the diagnosis of distal RTA. Heavy urinary HCO_3^- loss associated with hyperchloridemic acidosis suggests proximal RTA. It is important to make sure that urea-splitting organisms like *Proteus* are not responsible for the alkaline pH (normal pH should not exceed 7.8). A urinary tract infection must be treated before an accurate assessment of urinary pH can be made.

A more specific test of renal HCO_3^- handling can be performed by infusing 7.5% $NaHCO_3$ (0.9 M) at the rate of 2 mL/min for two to three hours and producing a stepwise increment of serum HCO_3^-. The serum $[HCO_3^-]$ at which HCO_3^- first appears in the urine is noted. Care must be taken to prevent an increase of serum HCO_3^- of more than 2 mmol/L in each 15-minute period. In normal individuals, urinary $[HCO_3^-]$ does not appear until a serum concentration of 24 to 26 mmol/L is reached. Accordingly, the appearance of HCO_3^- excretion at a low serum $[HCO_3^-]$ suggests type 2 RTA.

Table 7–5. TEST TO EVALUATE ABILITY OF KIDNEYS TO HANDLE ACUTE ACID CHALLENGE

1. Be sure that patient is well hydrated after breakfast. Draw blood for initial set of electrolytes.
2. From 8:00 to 10:00 A.M., collect baseline urine for pH, NH_4^+, titratable acidity (TA) (rate and amount for NH_4^+ and TA).
3. At 10:00 A.M., patient receives 100 mg/kg NH_4Cl orally over ½ hour (should be taken on a relatively full stomach). Volume is recorded for each specimen.
4. Urine is then collected approximately every two hours for pH, TA, and NH_4^+ as in step 2.
5. At 2:00 P.M., draw blood for electrolytes (Na^+, K^+, Cl^-, HCO_3^-).
6. During the entire procedure, the patient should be encouraged to drink fluids.
7. Test terminates six hours after NH_4Cl at 4:00 P.M.
8. For results to be normal, urine pH should be 5.3 or below, NH_4^+ excretion should exceed 35 mEq/min, and TA should exceed 25 mEq/min.

In practicality, urine HCO_3^- does not necessarily have to be measured. It can be assumed that if urine pH rises to 6.1 or above, HCO_3^- is being excreted. An approximation of the tubular HCO_3^- reabsorption threshold can be accomplished by giving increasing doses of oral HCO_3^- and measuring the urinary pH at regular intervals (Greenhill, 1976). When the urine pH is found to be 6.1 or greater, a sample of blood plasma is drawn and its [HCO_3^-] is measured. This value approximates the HCO_3^- excretion threshold, which normally is 25 to 28 mmol/L and is decreased in type 2 RTA.

An additional confirmatory test for the presence of type 1 RTA is the measurement of the difference between urinary and blood P_{CO_2} (Halperin, 1974). The test is performed by giving orally 0.5 to 2.0 mmol $NaHCO_3$/kg and measuring P_{CO_2} in blood and urine samples collected one hour later.

CO_2 is normally present in alkaline urine, because carbonic anhydrase is lacking in the luminal borders of the distal tubular cells. Approximately 15% of filtered HCO_3^- reaches the distal segment of nephrons. Hydrogen ion reacts with HCO_3^- to form H_2CO_3, but CO_2 formation is delayed for lack of enzyme (see Table 7–3). To test CO_2 excretion, $NaHCO_3$ is administered to raise the urinary pH above 7.4 (see method of giving bicarbonate under HCO_3^- titration). Alkaline urine normally contains some CO_2 because of this delay in conversion. HCO_3^- is eventually formed in areas of the genitourinary tract where back diffusion into the circulatory system essentially does not occur. In control subjects, the usual range of (urinary-arterial), that is (U-A)P_{CO_2}, is 40 to 70 mm Hg.

For valid measurements of urinary P_{CO_2} or HCO_3^-, urine must be collected anaerobically to prevent loss of CO_2 to the ambient air. This usually can be done by syringe aspiration directly from a catheter or immediately drawing the urine collected under oil into an air-free syringe. The inability to excrete sufficient P_{CO_2} in a maximally alkalotic urine (pH 7.4 to 7.8) suggests a distal tubular defect in hydrogen elimination. Factors known to influence the (U-A)P_{CO_2} are arterial P_{CO_2}, serum K^+, and urine P and HCO_3^- concentrations. A low (U-A)P_{CO_2}, however, does not distinguish a secretory (production defect) from a gradient (backleakage defect) cause. To determine whether low (U-A)P_{CO_2} concentrations are due to abnormalities in distal hydrogen production or backleakage, a sodium sulfate or sodium phosphate infusion is performed.

Infusion of sulfate or phosphate increases distal Na^+ delivery, allowing for greater exchange with hydrogen. Because doubly charged anions are not readily absorbed, they capture hydrogen and prevent the backleakage into blood seen with gradient defects. Prior to a sulfate infusion, 1 mg of fludrocortisone can be given orally on the night preceding the test to enhance Na^+ avidity. After a baseline collection, 500 mL of 4% sodium sulfate is infused over one hour. Collections of blood and urine are made over the next four hours. With sulfate infusion, titratable acidity will increase, and urine pH should decrease below 5.5 to be considered normal. In the case of neutral phosphate infusion, a solution of 0.2 M neutral phosphate (pH 7.4) is infused at a rate of 1 to 1.5 mL/min for two to three hours. The bound urinary hydrogen is eventually released to react with HCO_3^- and increase the P_{CO_2}. P_{CO_2} measurements are made at two, three, and four hours after initiation of infusion. If the urine pH is close to 6.8, the (U-A)P_{CO_2} in normal subjects increases from 5 to 30 mm Hg. With a secretory defect, no significant increase in titratable acidity or P_{CO_2} will be noted after either sulfate or phosphate infusion, a distinguishing feature from normal individuals and those with gradient defects.

Any pathologic process that alters tubular function may limit the ability of the kidneys to excrete a maximal acid load. This is a frequent finding in chronic renal disease and in causes of chronic interstitial nephritis such as pyelonephritis.

ARTERIAL BLOOD GASES, PULMONARY FUNCTION, AND ACID-BASE BALANCE

Regulation of acid-base balance in the body is accomplished by cooperative interactions between the kidneys and the lungs. The pulmonary-renal axis serves to maintain normal blood pH at 7.40 by controlling the concentration of arterial CO_2 (lung) and the bicarbonate ion concentration (kidney) such as to maintain blood pH at a value of 7.40. The role of the kidney has been discussed in this process; the role of the lungs is now discussed.

To understand pulmonary function in the regulation of acid-base balance, it is necessary to review the role of the lungs in gas exchange. In the alveolar sac, inspired oxygen diffuses into the pulmonary capillary while carbon dioxide diffuses out of the capillary into the sac, where it is expired into the atmosphere. There is an intricate relationship between oxygen diffusion into and carbon dioxide diffusion out from the pulmonary capillary circuit that ultimately determines the concentrations of these gases in blood and the acid-base status of the individual. Blood gas measurements comprise pH, P_{O_2}, P_{CO_2}, bicarbonate (by calculation from the Henderson-Hasselbalch equation), and O_2 saturation. The base excess is also computed as discussed previously.

These quantities are measured in arterial blood because these measurements best reflect the state of gas exchange and the overall metabolic status of an individual. The amount of each gas that is exchanged in the lungs depends on its partial pressure.

HENRY'S LAW. The partial pressure of a gas is the pressure exerted by a particular gas in a mixture and, using O_2 as an example, is represented as

$$P_{O_2} = P_T \times F_{O_2} \quad (7\text{-}14),$$

where the P_{O_2} = partial pressure of O_2, P_T = the total pressure of the gas mixture, and F_{O_2} represents the mole fraction of O_2 in the gas mixture.

The concentration of a gas dissolved in a liquid in equilibrium with the gas is proportional to the partial pressure of the gas in the gas phase above the liquid (Henry's Law). The partial pressure of a gas in the liquid phase is equal to the partial pressure of the gas in the gas phase.

OXYGEN EXCHANGE. For oxygen, which is only sparingly soluble in water (and therefore in serum), Henry's Law is

$$C_{O_2} = 0.003 \times P_{O_2} \quad (7\text{-}15),$$

where C_{O_2} is the concentration of O_2 dissolved in aqueous solution.

To be transported to the erythrocyte, oxygen must diffuse across the alveolar basement membrane, across the capillary endothelium, into serum, across the erythrocyte membrane, and finally bind to hemoglobin. Over 99% of the total oxygen in blood is bound to hemoglobin.

The actual amount of oxygen bound to hemoglobin depends on the oxygen-hemoglobin dissociation curve, shown in Figure 4–4 of Chapter 4. In this figure, the curve at pH 7.40 is sigmoidal, reflecting the allosteric nature of the binding, as discussed in Chapter 4. At low values for Po_2, there is a low oxygen saturation of hemoglobin. At Po_2s between 20 and 40 mm Hg, there is a steep increase in oxygen saturation. Conversely, as the partial pressure of oxygen decreases below 50 mm Hg, there is a dramatic decrease in oxygen saturation for small decreases in Po_2. This has major physiologic implications, as discussed in Chapter 4 and discussed further subsequently. For normal subjects, the lower limit of Po_2 giving 100% saturation is about 80 mm Hg.

It should be noted that it is not necessary to measure the O_2 saturation, or O_2 sat, from the oxygen-hemoglobin dissociation curve. O_2 sat can be directly measured noninvasively by the technique of pulse oximetry, in which the absorbance of light at 660 nm (oxyhemoglobin) and 940 nm (reduced hemoglobin) is measured simultaneously in the capillaries of the finger or the ear. Corrections are made for background tissue absorbance by measuring kinetically the pulsatile (arterial) component of the absorbance at both wavelengths. The ratio of oxyhemoglobin to total hemoglobin is the direct measure of the saturation fraction. High levels of carboxyhemoglobin or methemoglobin, or both, can lead to errors using this technique.

Because of the insolubility of oxygen in serum and its prolonged diffusion path between the alveolar membrane and the erythrocyte, there is normally a gradient in Po_2 between the alveolus (A) and arterial blood (a), referred to as the A-a gradient, which is normally around 10 mm Hg, that is,

$$P_AO_2 - P_aO_2 = 10 \text{ mm Hg} \quad (7\text{-}16).$$

Increased A-a gradients often signify a defect in oxygen diffusion or other important underlying pathologic conditions. These conditions include pulmonary fibrosis; alveolar capillary block syndrome; any thickening of the interstitium, as in acute respiratory distress syndrome and in interstitial pneumonitis; loss of diffusive surface area, as in chronic obstructive pulmonary disease; and, ironically, high cardiac output states (as in exercise), in which the time for exchange of gases in the alveoli is reduced, resulting in decreased oxygenation. Most commonly, in addition to physical blockade of gas exchange, there are two other major causes of increased A-a gradients: ventilation-perfusion inequalities and right-to-left shunting.

VENTILATION-PERFUSION INEQUALITIES. The perfusion of alveoli is unequal throughout the lung, being greatest at the base, due to gravity, and least at the apices. Thus, the ventilation (V) to perfusion (Q) ratio is greatest at the apices and least at the bases. The V/Q ratios for the apices, mid-portions, and bases of the lungs are 3.3, 0.9, and 0.6, respectively. As it happens, the bases of the lungs, which are the most perfused and the most underventilated, contribute the most mass to the lungs. Thus, oxygenation of blood is lower than would be expected from uniform gas exchange. Regional V/Q inequalities thus contribute to the A-a gradient. In chronic obstructive pulmonary disease, especially in the so-called blue-bloater form of emphysema, large regions of the lungs are perfused but do not exchange gas, giving rise to large increases in the A-a gradient.

RIGHT-TO-LEFT SHUNTING. Normally, 3% to 5% of cardiac output is returned to the left heart (via, for example, the thebesian veins) without gas exchange. In shock, pulmonary edema, atelectasis, and sometimes pneumonia, not only are regions of the lungs perfused but not ventilated but arteriovenous anastomoses are formed, resulting in the mixing of large volumes of unoxygenated blood with oxygenated blood and greatly lowering the pO_2 of arterial blood. This lowering results from the oxygen-hemoglobin dissociation curve. To illustrate how this occurs, suppose equal volumes of blood are mixed, one with a pO_2 of 120 mm Hg and the other with a pO_2 of 40 mm Hg at pH 7.40. From the middle curve in Figure 4–4, oxygen saturation at a pO_2 of 120 mm Hg is about 100%, while at a pO_2 of 40 mm Hg, it is about 76%. The average O_2 saturation is therefore (100 + 76)/2 or 88%. From the same curve, an O_2 saturation of 88% corresponds to a pO_2 of 61 mm Hg. Note that if the two solutions were mixed without oxygen's having to bind to hemoglobin, the pO_2 of the combined solutions would be simply (120 + 40)/2 = 80 mm Hg, which is substantially higher than 61 mm Hg.

EFFECT OF CARDIAC OUTPUT ON SHUNTING. The Fick equation states that oxygen consumption per unit of time ($\dot{V}o_2$) by the tissues is measured by the difference between the O_2 content of arterial blood (C_ao_2) minus that of venous blood (C_vo_2) per unit of time. Stated formally,

$$\dot{V}o_2 = (C_ao_2 - C_vo_2) \times Q \quad (7\text{-}17),$$

where Q is the cardiac output and measures blood flow. If cardiac output decreases while O_2 consumption remains the same, the ($C_ao_2 - C_vo_2$) difference must become greater, owing to increased tissue oxygen extraction. This results in lower oxygenation of venous blood. Right-to-left shunting of this blood results then in a *further* lowering of the pO_2 of the mixed arterial blood and an increase in the A-a gradient.

MEASURING THE A-a GRADIENT. To measure the A-a gradient, the PAo_2 and Pao_2 must be measured. Pao_2 is measured by the oxygen electrode, as described in Chapter 3. PAo_2 must be calculated from the simplified alveolar air equation, described in Chapter 4, equations 4-17 and 4-18. For a given Po_2 of inspired air,

$$P_Io_2 = PAo_2 + \frac{pACo_2}{R} \quad (7\text{-}18),$$

where PAo_2 is the partial pressure of oxygen in the alveolus, $pACo_2$ is the partial pressure of CO_2 in the alveolus, and R is the respiratory quotient (ratio of CO_2 produced to O_2 consumed), which is usually around 0.8. Because both P_Io_2 and $pACo_2$ are known, the PAo_2 can be computed from equation 7-18.

Once the A-a gradient is known, there are three approaches to evaluating its significance. These are measurement of the $PAo_2 - Pao_2$ difference, the Pao_2/PAo_2 ratio, and the so-called venous admixture ratio. The A-a difference varies widely depending on the P_Io_2. On room air, the reference range is 5 to 20 mm Hg. On 100% O_2, the value rises to about 50 mm Hg, although higher values in normal individuals have been reported.

The most commonly used measurement for the A-a gra-

2

dient is the ratio, which for most normal individuals lies in the range of 0.75. This value remains approximately constant for wide ranges of inspired fractions of O_2 ranging between 20% and 100%.

VENOUS ADMIXTURE RATIO (VAD). This ratio, which is often used in intensive care units, is defined as

$$VAD = \frac{(Cco_2 - Cao_2)}{(Cco_2 - Cvo_2)} \quad (7\text{-}19),$$

where Cco_2 is the concentration of O_2 in the pulmonary capillaries (assumed to be the same as PAo_2), Cao_2 is the arterial oxygen concentration, and Cvo_2 is the concentration of oxygen in mixed venous blood. To compute the O_2 concentration in arterial and venous blood, the hemoglobin concentration is multiplied by the O_2 sat times a factor 1.39 that gives the molar concentration and accounts for the fact that there are four oxygen-combining sites per hemoglobin molecule. To this is added the term $0.003 \times Po_2$ for the small amount of oxygen dissolved in plasma. For the capillary oxygen concentration, for patients who are receiving high amounts of oxygen, it is assumed that the capillary oxygen has saturated the hemoglobin. The capillary oxygen concentration is then computed as 1.39 × hemoglobin concentration + 0.003 × PAo_2, obtained from the alveolar air equation (7-18).

Because the ratio depends on the capillary minus the venous difference in oxygen concentration, it depends on cardiac output, from the Fick equation (7-17). Especially in cases in which right-to-left shunting occurs, the difference in oxygen concentration between saturated capillary blood and arterial blood (numerator of equation 7-19) is large while, because of the mixing of arterial and venous blood, the difference in oxygen concentration between arterial and venous blood (denominator in equation 7-19) becomes smaller, causing the VAD to increase. However, the VAD depends on the P_Io_2 and reaches a minimum at a P_Io_2 of around 0.4. The denominator of equation 7-19 may also be expressed as $(Cco_2 - Cao_2 + AV)$, where AV is the arteriovenous difference in oxygen concentration between arterial and venous blood, which is usually around the value of 3.5 volumes % (Cain, 1988).

THE SIGNIFICANCE OF HYPOXEMIA. The most important cause of hypoxemia is hypoventilation. Reduced gas exchange in the alveoli is much more likely to reduce Po_2 than to raise Pco_2 significantly because of the relatively low diffusion of O_2 and the necessity for O_2 to bind to hemoglobin. At Po_2 values of <50 mm Hg, small decreases in this value lead to large decreases in O_2 sat. The same does not hold for CO_2, which is freely diffusible and does not require a saturation mechanism for transport.

Hypoventilation may result from mechanical problems such as alveolar block secondary to interstitial processes (e.g., pneumonia) and decreased V/Q ratios. Hypoxemia may also result from low or excessively high cardiac output and right-to-left shunting, as in COPD and shock, especially when the Po_2 is reduced to 50 mm Hg or below. With the consequent major decrease in the O_2 sat, tissue perfusion diminishes, leading to anaerobic metabolism and metabolic lactic acidosis. The acidosis causes a shift to the right of the oxygen-hemoglobin dissociation, leading to a further drop in the O_2 sat, setting in motion a vicious cycle, as discussed in Chapter 4 and shown in Figure 4–4.

It is vital to recognize that hypoxemia is a life-threatening condition and should be corrected on an emergent basis. For all conditions other than hypercapnia, which occurs most frequently in chronic obstructive pulmonary disease, administration of oxygen-enriched inspired gases is the requisite treatment. In the event of hypoxemia secondary to hypercapnia, as discussed in Chapter 4, it is vital to reduce the Pco_2. Oxygen administration in this condition is *contraindicated.*

Effects of Carbon Dioxide on Acid-Base Balance and Gas Exchange

The effects of CO_2 on acid-base balance have been discussed previously in this chapter and in Chapter 4. The effect of elevated Pco_2 is to increase the denominator of the Henderson-Hasselbalch equation, causing a respiratory acidosis, whereas the reverse is true for low values of the Pco_2. The lungs can compensate for metabolic acidosis by increasing exhalation of increased amounts of CO_2 and, for metabolic alkalosis, by decreasing CO_2 excretion.

CO_2 AND ALVEOLAR VENTILATION. CO_2 exhalation can be increased merely by increasing the breathing rate. This is due to the fact that the volume of CO_2 expired per unit of time, $\dot{V}co_2$, is directly proportional to the alveolar ventilation rate, $\dot{V}A$, i.e.,

$$\dot{V}co_2 = \frac{1}{0.863} \times \dot{V}_A \times PAco_2 \quad (7\text{-}20),$$

where $PAco_2$ is the partial pressure in the alveolus. Because there is no diffusion barrier for CO_2, the alveolar CO_2 ($PAco_2$) is the same as the arterial CO_2 ($Paco_2$).

In diseases in which ventilation-perfusion inequalities exist, increasing the ventilation of functional alveoli directly increases CO_2 expiration. This mechanism does *not* occur to the same extent with oxygen because, by increasing P_Io_2, blood perfusing ventilated alveoli will eventually become saturated with oxygen (100% saturation of hemoglobin). Further increasing the ventilation of these units will then not result in major increases in Po_2 except for the small amount of O_2 directly dissolved in plasma. Thus, one of the first signs of hypoventilation is hypoxemia. More severe hypoventilation must occur in order for hypercapnic states to result.

The effect of ventilation on CO_2 expiration is shown in Figure 7–4. The hyperbolic curve is steep on the left where ventilation is low. For a given $\dot{V}co_2$, generally around 200 mL/min, small increases in ventilation cause large decreases in $PAco_2$, up to $PAco_2$ values of 40 mm Hg. The curve then flattens out so that further increases in ventilation result in only small changes in $PAco_2$.

The causes of hypercapnia are chronic obstructive pulmonary disease, especially centrilobular emphysema (so-called blue-bloater syndrome); partial or complete paralysis of the accessory muscles of breathing, most commonly occurring in myasthenia gravis and in some demyelinating diseases; depression of the brainstem neural centers of breathing in the medulla and pons secondary to head injury and stroke; occasionally pneumonia; and severe kyphoscoliosis. Virtually all hypercapnic states are accompanied by hypoxemia because of the increased sensitivity of Po_2 to hypoventilation and because, as CO_2 builds up in alveoli, O_2 diffusion into

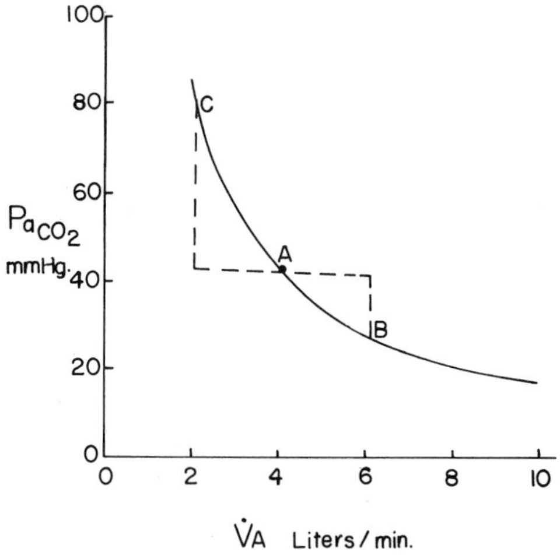

Figure 7–4. Effect of ventilation ($\dot{V}$A) on $Paco_2$. $Paco_2$ is plotted on the ordinate while alveolar ventilation is plotted on the abscissa. From point C to point A, at high Pco_2 values, small increases in alveolar ventilation cause large drops in Pco_2. From point A to point B, at high ventilation rates, $Paco_2$ is relatively insensitive to the alveolar ventilation.

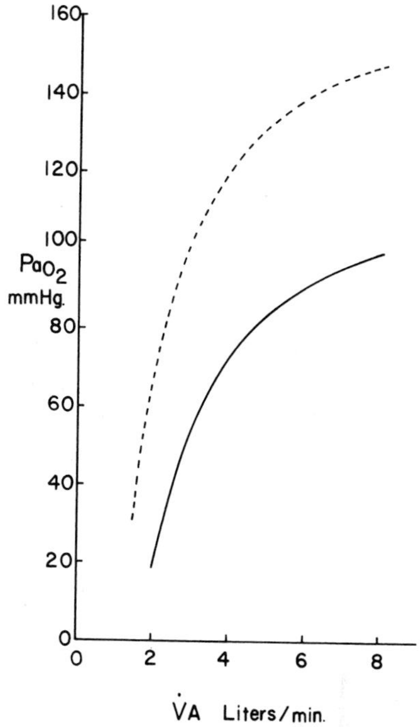

Figure 7–5. Plot of equation 7-21, the combined alveolar air equation (equation 7-18), and the Pco_2–alveolar ventilation equation (equation 7-20). Pao_2 is plotted on the ordinate, and alveolar ventilation is plotted on the abscissa. The solid curve is for F_Io_2 of 21% (room air) and an A-a gradient of 20 mm Hg, whereas the dotted curve is for F_Io_2 of 30% and an A-a gradient of 35 mm Hg.

the alveolar sac is impaired. As discussed in Chapter 4, hypercapnia with a Pco_2 of greater than 50 mm Hg can cause depression of the respiratory centers of the central nervous system. The main stimulus to breathing is hypoxia. Thus, oxygen administration will remove this stimulus to breathing. The appropriate therapy is assisted increased ventilation to reduce the Pco_2.

RELATIONSHIP BETWEEN O_2 AND CO_2. Solving equation 7-20 for $PAco_2$ and substituting it into the alveolar air equation, 7-18,

$$PAo_2 = P_Io_2 - \frac{0.863 \times \dot{V}co_2}{R \times \dot{V}_A} \quad (7\text{-}21).$$

This equation states that, for a given $\dot{V}co_2$, increasing ventilation increases PAo_2. This relationship is plotted in Figure 7–5 for two situations. The first (solid curve) is for a mole fraction of O_2, of F_Io_2, in room air of 21% and an A-a gradient of 20 mm Hg, while the second (dotted) curve is for F_Io_2 of 30% and an A-a gradient of 35 mm Hg. Note that for small decreases in $\dot{V}_a$ below 4 L/min, there are large decreases in Pao_2. Further, comparing Figures 7–4 and 7–5, it can be seen that ventilation rates of over 4 L/min are necessary in breathing room air to reach a saturating Pao_2 of 80 mm Hg, whereas at 4 L/min, a normal PCO_2 is reached. Increasing the F_Io_2 significantly helps in reaching saturating levels of O_2 at lower $\dot{V}_A$ values.

From the alveolar air equation as plotted in Figure 4–3 in Chapter 4, there is a negative linear relationship between Pao_2 and $PAco_2$. The slope of this line is 1/R, R being the respiratory quotient, usually 0.8. Thus, each unit increase in pco_2 is accompanied by a corresponding 1.25 (1/0.8) unit decrease in Po_2. At alveolar ventilation rates of under 4 L/min, there is a sharp increase in $Paco_2$ but an even sharper decrease in Pao_2. Thus, the result of the hypercapnia is severe hypoxemia. The hypoxemia then leads to tissue acidosis and a shift in the hemoglobin-oxygen dissociation curve to the right, resulting in lower O_2 saturation and more tissue acidosis. This is the vicious cycle referred to previously.

Arterial Blood Gases in Disease States

There are a number of conditions in which arterial blood gases must be measured in order to evaluate the overall metabolic status of an individual and to measure the efficacy of therapeutic modalities. Blood gas patterns do not necessarily reflect specific disease entities. There is considerable overlap between the arterial blood gas patterns found among different disease states. However, there are certain stereotypic blood gas patterns that are often observed in particular diseases. Several of these patterns are summarized here.

MYOCARDIAL INFARCTION. Typically, because of the diminished cardiac output and the low tissue perfusion, the Po_2 is significantly reduced (hypoxemia), and a metabolic acidosis ensues. The pco_2 is usually normal or low to compensate for the metabolic acidosis.

PULMONARY EMBOLUS. The major finding is low Po_2 (hypoxemia), and because of the effort to compensate by increased breathing, a respiratory alkalosis often results. The Pco_2 is usually normal.

SEPTIC SHOCK. Septic shock is due mainly to the splanchnic pooling of blood and the formation of arteriovenous anastomoses. The result is often increased venous return to the heart and high-output failure. Because tissue perfusion is low, metabolic acidosis results and is a cardinal feature of this condition. Because pulmonary transit times are reduced, hypoxemia may result. In the absence of respiratory failure, the Pco_2 is low to compensate for the metabolic acidosis.

CHRONIC OBSTRUCTIVE PULMONARY DISEASE. This refers to a group of conditions such as severe bronchitis, asthma, and emphysema. All share an inability to expire CO_2 because of low elasticity in the alveolar wall or because of spasmodic contractions in the smooth muscle of the respiratory bronchioles. These conditions lead to accumulation of CO_2 in the alveoli and a consequent increase in Pco_2. In panacinar emphysema, the so-called pink-puffer syndrome, there is destruction of both alveolar capillary walls *and* the elastic tissue of alveoli (often due to deficiency of α_1-antitrypsin). Thus, both ventilation and perfusion decrease together such that the V/Q ratio remains relatively normal. However, gas exchange is impaired so that hypoxemia develops. Often, the increased demand for oxygen leads to an increased respiratory rate and a resulting respiratory alkalosis. Eventually, CO_2 accumulates in compromised alveoli that may still be perfused, and a respiratory acidosis may ensue.

In centriacinar emphysema, or the so-called blue-bloater syndrome, secondary to such causes as smoking, only the alveolar wall is compromised, but perfusion of the alveoli still occurs, leading to large V/Q abnormalities, that is, V/Q decreases. CO_2 is retained, often causing severe hypercapnia and respiratory acidosis. Because of the inability of the affected alveoli to exchange gases, the patient becomes hypoxemic. The accessory muscles of respiration become hypertrophic to help expel CO_2 and to increase lung capacity. The patient consequently becomes barrel-chested. The patient is cyanotic (blue) because of the continuing hypoxemia. Thus, the cardinal features of centriacinar emphysema are hypercapnia, respiratory acidosis, and hypoxemia. Ultimately, metabolic (tissue) acidosis ensues, as described previously.

In asthma and bronchitis, depending on the severity of the disease, the patient in an acute attack may become acutely hypoxemic due to decreased functional lung volume. The acute need for oxygen can lead to an increased respiratory rate and respiratory alkalosis. In severe cases, CO_2 accumulates, resulting in respiratory acidosis and hypoxemia.

PNEUMONIA. Generally, bronchial or lobar pneumonias do not result in blood gas disorders. In severe pneumonias, hypoxemia may result with some CO_2 retention, leading to respiratory acidosis. In interstitial pneumonia and other conditions resulting in thickening of the interstitial space, hypoxemia can develop. In pulmonary edema, the hypoxemia can be severe enough to induce metabolic acidosis. Retention of CO_2 (hypercapnia) results in a superimposed respiratory acidosis. Generally, in these situations, the bicarbonate is lower than normal.

ASPIRIN INTOXICATION. Overdose of aspirin or acetylsalicylate occurs most often in children. If the acid form of this drug is ingested, metabolic acidosis results. To compensate, the Pco_2 is reduced. However, the salicylate anion stimulates central nervous system respiratory centers to increase breathing, leading ultimately to a superimposed respiratory alkalosis. The salicylate anion is also a metabolic inhibitor. As a result, metabolic acidosis ensues.

If the salicylate anion is ingested, respiratory alkalosis occurs first, followed by mild metabolic acidosis. Overall, there may be a reduced or normal pH. Children with normal blood pH and low values for Pco_2 should be suspected of having salicylate poisoning.

ADULT RESPIRATORY SYNDROME. This condition resembles interstitial disease resulting in hypoxemia and respiratory alkalosis. Late in the disease, the hypoxemia leads to metabolic acidosis, and respiratory acidosis develops owing to hypercapnia.

Arruda JAL, Kurtzman NA: Metabolic acidosis and alkalosis. Clin Nephrol 1977; 7:201.

Barlow, WK: Volatiles and osmometry (continued). Clin Chem 1976; 22:1230.

Boye NP, Skarpass IJ, Fausa O: Cystic fibrosis in adult patients. Eur J Respir Dis 1980; 6:227.

Breckenridge A, Metcalfe-Gibson A: Methods of measuring glomerular filtration rate. A comparison of inulin, vitamin B_{12} and creatinine clearances. Lancet 1965; 2:265.

Burry HC, Dieppe PA: Apparent reduction of endogenous creatinine clearance by salicylate treatment. BMJ 1976; 12:16.

Cain RD, Shapiro BA, Templin R, Walther K: Unreliability of oxygen-tension–based indices in reflecting intrapulmonary shunting in critically ill patients. Crit Care Med 1988; 16:1243.

Camara AA, Arn KD, Reimer A, Newburgh LH: The twenty-four hourly endogenous creatinine clearance as a clinical measure of the functional state of the kidneys. J Lab Clin Med 1951; 37:743.

Carrie BJ, Golbetz HV, Michaels AS, Myers BD: Creatinine: An inadequate filtration marker in glomerular diseases. Am J Med 1980; 69:177.

Cockcroft DW, Gault MH: Prediction of creatine clearance from serum creatinine. Nephron 1976; 16:31.

Cooke CR, Turim MD, Walker WG: The syndrome of inappropriate antidiuretic hormone secretion (SIADH): Pathophysiologic mechanisms in solute and volume regulation. Medicine 1979; 58:240.

Davis BB, Michelis MF: Polyuria and nocturia. *In* Preuss HG (ed): Management of Common Problems in Renal Disease. New York, Macmillan Publishing Company, 1988, p 102.

Davis BB, Zenser TV: Evaluation of renal concentrating and diluting ability. *In* Preuss HG (ed): Clinics in Laboratory Medicine: Renal Function. Philadelphia, W.B. Saunders Company, 1993, p 131.

DeVita MV, Michelis MF: Perturbations in sodium balance: Hyponatremia and hypernatremia. *In* Preuss HG (ed): Clinics in Laboratory Medicine: Renal Function. Philadelphia, W.B. Saunders Company, 1993, p 134.

Derubertis FR, Michelis MF, Bloom ME, et al: Impaired water excretion in myxedema. Am J Med 1971; 51:41.

Dossetor JB: Creatininemia versus uremia. Ann Intern Med 1966; 65:1287.

Driscoll JL, Martin HF: Detection of bromism by an automated chloride method. Clin Chem 1966; 12:314.

Duarte CG: Assessment of renal function—glomerular and tubular. *In* Preuss HG (ed): Clinics in Laboratory Medicine: Renal Function. Philadelphia, W.B. Saunders Company, 1993, p 330.

Elin RJ, Robertson EA, Johnson E: Bromide interferes with determination of chloride by each of four methods. Clin Chem 1981; 27:778.

Elwood CM, Sigman EM: The measurement of glomerular filtration rate and effective renal plasma flow in man by iothalamate ^{125}I and iodopyracet ^{131}I. Circulation 1967; 36:441.

Espinel CH: The FeNa test. JAMA 1976; 236:579.

Farmer CD, Tauxe WN, Hunt JC: Measurement of renal function with radioiodinated diatrizoate and o-iodohippurate. Am J Clin Path 1967; 47:9.

Favre HR, Wing AJ: Simultaneous ^{51}Cr edetic acid, inulin, and endogenous creatinine clearance in 20 patients with renal diseases. Br Med J 1968; 1:84.

Gambino SR, Schreiber H: The measurement of CO_2 content with the AutoAnalyzer. Am J Clin Pathol 1966; 45:406.

Geisinger KF, Wakely PE Jr, Batsakis JG: Serum chloride: A CAP survey. Am J Clin Pathol (Suppl) 1980; 74:546.

Geyer SJ: Urinalysis and urinary sediment in patients with renal disease. *In* Preuss HG (ed): Clinics in Laboratory Medicine: Renal Function. Philadelphia, W.B. Saunders Company, 1993, p 130.

Gill JR Jr, Bartter FC: Evidence for a prostaglandin-independent defect in chloride reabsorption in the loop of Henle as a proximal cause of Bartter's syndrome. Am J Med 1978; 65:766.

Granerus G, Aurell M: Reference values for ^{51}Cr-EDTA clearance as a measure of glomerular filtration rate. Scand J Clin Lab Invest 1981; 41:611.

Greenhill A, Grusk AB: Laboratory evaluation of renal function. Pediatr Clin North Am 1976; 23:661.

Groth T, Tengstrom B: A simple method for the estimation of glomerular filtration rate. Scand J Clin Lab Invest 1977; 37:39.

Halperin ML, Goldstein MB, Haig A, et al: Studies on the pathogenesis of type 1 (distal) renal tubular acidosis as revealed by the urinary PCO_2 tensions. J Clin Invest 1974; 53:669.

Holmes JH: Measurement of osmolality in serum, urine, and other biological fluids by the freezing point determination. *In* Workshop Manual on Urinalysis and Renal Function Studies, ASCP—Commission on Continuing Education, 1962.

Isaacson LC: Urinary osmolality in thirsting normal subjects. Lancet 1960; 1:467.

Jackson S: Creatinine in urine as an index of urinary excretion rate. Health Phys 1966; 12:843.
Juel R: Serum osmolality: A CAP survey analysis. Am J Clin Pathol 1977; 68:165.
Kamel SK, Ethier JH, Richardson RMA, et al: Urine electrolytes and osmolality: When and how to use them. Am J Nephrol 1990; 10:89.
Kampmann JP, Hanson JM: Glomerular filtration rate and creatinine clearance. Br J Clin Pharmacol 1981; 12:7.
Karlinsky ML, Sager DS, Pillay VK: Effect of parathyroid hormone and cyclic adenosine monophosphate on renal bicarbonate reabsorption. Am J Physiol 1974; 227:1226.
Keshgegian AA: Decreased anion gap in diffuse polyclonal hypergammaglobulinemia. N Engl J Med 1978; 299:99.
Ladenson JH: Evaluation of an instrument (Nova-1) for direct potentiometric analysis of sodium and potassium in blood and their indirect potentiometric determination in urine. Clin Chem 1979; 25:757.
Lam CWK, Tau IK: Evaluation of the Harleco micro CO_2 system for measurement of total CO_2 in serum or plasma. Clin Chem 1978; 34:143.
Larrson R, Bodemar G, Kagedal B, Walon A: The effects of cimetidine (Tagamet) on renal function in patients with renal failure. Acta Med Scand 1980; 208:27.
Lash JP, Arruda JAL: Laboratory Evaluation of Renal Tubular Acidosis. *In* Preuss HG (ed): Clinics in Laboratory Medicine: Renal Function. Philadelphia, W.B. Saunders Company, 1993, p 117.
Latta K, Hisano S, Chan JCM: Perturbations in potassium balance. *In* Preuss HG (ed): Clinics in Laboratory Medicine: Renal Function. Philadelphia, W.B. Saunders Company, 1993, p 149.
Lee J, Hollyer R, Rodelas R, Preuss HG: Influence of trimethoprim, sulfamethoxazole, and creatinine on renal organic anion and cation transport in rat kidney tissue. Toxicol Appl Pharmacol 1981; 58:184.
Lehmann HP: Metrication of clinical laboratory data in SI units. Am J Clin Pathol 1976; 65:2.
Lerner A, DeLosAngeles A, Goldstein S, et al: Correlation of predicted glomerular filtration rate (PGFR) with measured creatinine and insulin clearance (abstract). Kidney Int 1985; 27:145.
Levey AS, Madaio MP, Perrone RD: Laboratory assessment of renal diseases: Clearance, urinalysis, and renal biopsy. *In* Brenner BM, Rector FC Jr (eds): The Kidney, 4th ed. Philadelphia, W.B. Saunders Company, 1991, p 919.
Levinsky NG, Alexander EA: Acute renal failure. *In* Brenner BM, Rector FC (eds): The Kidney. Philadelphia, W.B. Saunders Company, 1976, p 806.
Lindeman RD, Preuss HG: Renal physiology and pathophysiology of aging. *In* Preuss HG (ed): Geriatric Nephrology. New York, Field and Rich, 1986, p 5.
Littlewood JM: The diagnosis of cystic fibrosis. Practitioner 1980; 224:305.
Loeb JN: The hyperosmolar state. N Engl J Med 1974; 290:1184.
Loirat P, et al: Increased glomerular filtration rate in patients with major burns and its effect on the pharmacokinetics of tobramycin. N Engl J Med 1978; 299:915.
Lubowitz H, Slatopolsky E, Shankel S, et al: Glomerular filtration rate determination in patients with chronic renal disease. JAMA 1967; 199: 252.
MacDonald NF: Sodium and potassium measurements: Direct potentiometry and flame photometry. Am J Clin Pathol 1981; 76(CAP Suppl):575.
Madias NE, et al: Increased anion gap in metabolic alkalosis: The role of plasma-protein equivalency. N Engl J Med 1979; 300:1421.
Matthews BF: Effects of pregnancy on inulin and para-aminohippurate clearances in the anesthetized rat. J Physiol 1960; 151:385.
Mercier DC, Feld RD, Witte DC: Comparison of dewpoint and freezing point osmometry. Am J Med Technol 1978; 44:1066.
Mitch WE, Buffington J, Lemann J, et al: A simple method of estimating progression of chronic renal failure. Lancet 1976; 2:326.
Moore J Jr, Carome MA: Proteinuria. Clin Lab Med 1993; p 21 .
Morgensen CE: Elevated glomerular filtration rate in insulin-treated short-term diabetes: Nondependence on blood sugar value. Acta Med Scand 1973; 194:559.
Murray T, Long W, Narins RG: Multiple myeloma and the anion gap. N Engl J Med 1975; 292:574.
Narins RG (ed): Maxwell and Kleeman's Clinical Disorders of Fluid and Electrolyte Metabolism, 5th ed. McGraw-Hill, New York, 1994, pp 886–887.
Nelp WB: Renal excretion of vitamin B_{12} and its use in measurement of glomerular filtration rate in man. J Lab Clin Med 1964; 63:480.
O'Connor DT, Stone RA: Hyperchloremia and negative anion gap associated with polymyxin B administration. Arch Intern Med 1978; 138: 478.
Oh MS, Carroll HJ: Decreased anion gap and hyponatremia. N Engl J Med 1978; 298:111.
Perez GO, Oster JR: Use of AG/HCO_3^- in the evaluation of acid-base disorders: A patient management problem. South Med J 1986; 79:882.
Perez G, Delaney V, Bourke E (eds): Hypo and hyperkalemia. *In* Preuss HG (ed): Management of Common Problems in Renal Disease. New York, Macmillan Publishing Company, 1988, p 128.
Preuss HG: Regulation of renal ammoniagenesis during acidosis: The pyridine nucleotide hypothesis revisited. Life Sci 1980; 27:2293.
Preuss HG, Perez G: Systemic acidosis and alkalosis. *In* Preuss HG (ed): Management of Common Problems in Renal Disease. New York, Macmillan Publishing Company, 1988a, p 70.
Preuss HG, Rodelas R, Terlinsky A, Gelfond M: Effects of glipizide on water and electrolyte handling in water-loaded humans. Renal Physiol 1981; 4:173.
Preuss HG, Zelman SJ: Azotemia and uremia. *In* Preuss HG (ed): Management of Common Problems in Renal Disease. New York, Macmillan Publishing Company, 1988b, p 1.
Preuss HG: Basics of renal anatomy and physiology. *In* Preuss HG (ed): Clinics in Laboratory Medicine: Renal Function. Philadelphia, W.B. Saunders, 1993a, p 1.
Preuss HG: Fundamentals of clinical acid-base evaluation. *In* Preuss HG (ed): Clinics in Laboratory Medicine: Renal Function. Philadelphia, W.B. Saunders Company, 1993b, p 103.
Quintanilla AP: Renal tubular acidosis: Mechanisms and management. Postgrad Med 1980; 67(4):60.
Renkin EM, Robinson RR: Glomerular filtration. N Engl J Med 1974; 290:785.
Rocco WV: Volatiles and osmometry. Clin Chem 1976; 22:399.
Ruddy MC, Stenzel KH: Disorders of water, sodium and potassium metabolism. *In* Cheigh JS, Stenzel KH, Rubin AL (eds): Manual of Clinical Nephrology. Martinus Nijhoff, 1981, pp 30–67.
Schreiner G: Renal biopsy. *In* Strauss MB, Welt LG (eds): Diseases of the Kidney. Boston, Little, Brown and Co., 1971, pp 197–210.
Schrier RW: The patient with hyponatremia or hypernatremia. *In* Schrier RW (ed): Manual of Nephrology. Boston, Little, Brown and Co., 1981, pp 15–30.
Sebastian A, Morris RC Jr: Renal tubular acidosis. Clin Nephrol 1977; 7:216.
Semple PF, Carswell PF, Carswell W, Boyle JA: Serial studies of the renal clearance of urate and insulin during pregnancy and after the puerperium in normal women. Clin Sci Mol Med 1974; 47:559.
Seyer-Hansen K: Renal hypertrophy in streptozotocin diabetic rats. Clin Sci Mol Med 1976; 51:551.
Shwachman H, Mahmoodian A, Neff RK: The sweat test: Sodium and chloride values. J Pediatr 1981; 98:576.
Sigman EM, Elwood CM, Knox F: The measurement of glomerular filtration rate in man with sodium iothalamate ^{131}I (Conray). J Nucl Med 1966; 7:60.
Skowsky RW, Kikuchi TA: The role of vasopressin in the impaired water excretion of myxedema. Am J Med 1978; 64:613.
Sleeper RS, Belanger P, Lemieux G, Preuss HG: Effects of in vitro potassium on ammoniagenesis in rat and canine kidney tissue. Kidney Int 1982; 21:345.
Steffes MW, Frier EF: A simple and precise method of determining true sodium, potassium and chloride concentrations in hyperlipemia. J Lab Clin Med 1976; 88:683.
Stenzel KH: Acid-base disturbances. *In* Cheigh JS, Stenzel KH, Rubin AL (eds): Manual of Clinical Nephrology. Martinus Nijhoff, 1981.
Szylman P, Better OS, Chaimowitz C, Rosler A: Role of hyperkalemia in the metabolic acidosis of isolated hypoaldosteronism. N Engl J Med 1976; 294:361.
Tobias GJ, McLaughlin RF Jr, Hopper J Jr: Endogenous creatinine clearance. N Engl J Med 1962; 266:317.
Valtin H: Renal Function: Mechanisms Preserving Fluid and Solute Balance in Health. Boston, Little, Brown and Co., 1973.
van Ypersele C, Bodart P, Dardenne A: General techniques in clinical nephrology. *In* Hamburger J (ed): Nephrology. New York, Wiley-Flammarion, 1979, pp 103–156.
Walser M, Drew HH, LaFrance MD: Reciprocal creatinine slopes often give erroneous estimates of progression of chronic renal failure. Kidney Int 1989; 36(Suppl 27):S81.
Ward PC: Renal dysfunction 1: Urea and creatinine. Postgrad Med 1981; 69(5):93.
Weisberg HF: Osmolality-calculated, "delta," and more formulas. Clin Chem 1975; 21:1182.
Weissman N, Pileggi VJ: Inorganic ions. *In* Henry RJ (ed): Clinical Chemistry, Principles and Technics, 2nd ed. Hagerstown, MD, Harper and Row Publishers, Inc., 1974, p 645.
Wells MR: Value of plasma chloride concentration and acid-base status in the differential diagnosis of hyperparathyroidism from other causes of hypercalcemia. J Clin Pathol 1971; 24:219.
Wesson LG: Renal hemodynamics in physiological states. *In* Wesson LG (ed): Physiology of the Human Kidney. New York, Grune and Stratton, 1969, p 109.
West JR, Smith HW, Chasis H: Glomerular filtration rate, effective renal blood flow, and maximal tubular excretory capacity in infancy. J Pediatr 1948; 32:10.

Chapter 8

Metabolic Intermediates and Inorganic Ions

Jannie Woo, Ph.D.
John Bernard Henry, M.D.

NONPROTEIN NITROGENOUS COMPOUNDS

There are more than 15 different nonprotein nitrogenous (NPN) compounds in plasma with a total nitrogen concentration of 250 to 400 mg/L. The NPN of whole blood is approximately 75% greater than that of plasma, largely because of the high glutathione content of erythrocytes. Urea is the major NPN constituent in plasma and constitutes about 45% of the total. Other major constituents in decreasing order of nitrogen contribution are amino acids, uric acid, creatinine, creatine, and ammonia. The NPN determination was previously used as an index of renal function. Increased concentrations of several of the major components—that is, urea, uric acid, and creatinine—do occur as a consequence of diminished renal function. The NPN, however, is a relatively nonspecific index of renal disease because other diseases can cause significant alterations in the plasma concentrations of the various constituents. For example, gout or excessive catabolism of purines increases the uric acid concentration in plasma. Liver disease can cause diminished amino acid metabolism and a corresponding rise in plasma amino acid nitrogen. In contrast, urea synthesis is diminished in severe liver disease. Consequently, NPN determinations are no longer performed in the laboratory. Instead, serum concentrations of the following constituents that are of clinical importance are offered: urea nitrogen and creatinine, uric acid, creatine, ammonia, and α-amino acid nitrogen.

Urea

Physiologic Chemistry

Urea is the major end product of protein and amino acid catabolism and is generated in the liver through the urea cycle. From the liver, urea enters the blood to be distributed to all intracellular and extracellular fluids, because urea is freely diffusible across most cell membranes. Most of the urea is ultimately excreted by the kidneys, but minimal amounts are also excreted in sweat and degraded by bacteria in the intestines.

Urea is freely filtered by the glomeruli. Depending on the state of hydration and therefore the rate of urine flow, 40% to 80% of the filtered urea is passively reabsorbed with water, mostly in the proximal tubules. There does not appear to be active tubular reabsorption or secretion of urea by mammalian kidneys. Urea ordinarily constitutes about half (25 g) of the total urinary solids and 80% to 90% of the total urinary nitrogen. Although most cell membranes and capillary walls in the body are freely permeable to urea, the renal nephrons can concentrate urea with a gradient of up to 50-fold greater than plasma.

The analytical measurement of urea is still termed by convention as blood urea nitrogen (BUN), although urea determination is actually performed on serum or plasma. The SI system recommends that results be expressed as units of urea itself in millimoles per liter. Nevertheless, urea concentration is often expressed as units of urea nitrogen in blood, in milligrams per deciliter. The molecular weight of urea is 60, including two nitrogen atoms with a weight of 28. Consequently, BUN can be converted to urea by multiplying by 60/28, or 2.14. Conversely, the factor 28/60, or 0.467, converts urea to BUN. The reference range for BUN is about 6 to 20 mg/dL (2.1 to 7.1 mmol/L).

Clinicopathologic Correlations

The serum concentration of urea varies rather widely in health and is influenced by such diverse factors as dietary intake of protein and the state of hydration. Glucocorticoids have an antianabolic effect, and thyroid hormones have a catabolic effect on protein and thus tend to raise the BUN. Androgens and growth hormone have an anabolic effect and thus decrease the formation of urea.

Azotemia is a biochemical designation referring to any significant increase in the plasma concentration of NPN compounds, principally urea and creatinine. Azotemia is frequently categorized as prerenal, renal, and postrenal. *Prerenal azotemia* is the result of inadequate perfusion of the kidneys and, therefore, diminished glomerular filtration in the presence of otherwise normal renal function. Important etiologies include dehydration, shock, diminished blood volume, and congestive heart failure. Although the increased serum urea or BUN accompanying many cases of massive gastrointestinal hemorrhage is sometimes explained on the basis of greatly increased absorption of amino acids following the digestion of blood proteins, it is probable that hypovolemia resulting from the hemorrhage is the single most important factor. An additional cause of increased serum urea (BUN) is increased protein catabolism, for example, with fever, stress, and burns.

The pathogenesis of *renal azotemia* is primarily diminished glomerular filtration and, therefore, urea retention as a consequence of acute or chronic renal disease. Other complicating factors frequently present are dehydration or edema, which causes diminished renal perfusion, increased catabolism of proteins, and the general antianabolic effect of glucocorticoids. *Uremia* is a clinical syndrome that can occur with protracted severe azotemia and includes acidosis, water and electrolyte imbalance, nausea, vomiting, anemia, neuropsychiatric changes, and a variety of other clinical manifestations, including coma. The elevated BUN varies in magnitude but usually is in excess of 100 mg/dL, or approaching 200 mg/dL with deep coma or stupor. The progressively rising but at times fluctuating BUN is in contrast to the more slowly rising creatinine value, which rarely exceeds 20 mg/dL, and to uric acid, which in the absence of gout does not usually rise above 12 mg/dL in chronic renal failure. *Postrenal azotemia* is usually the result of urinary tract obstruction, so that urea is reabsorbed into the circulation. An uncommon cause is perforation of the lower urinary tract with extravasation of urine into soft tissues.

From the foregoing discussion, it is evident that the BUN can at best be a rough guide to renal function. Even in the presence of normal dietary intake, hydration, renal perfusion, and integrity of the lower urinary tract, BUN will ordinarily not be significantly increased until the glomerular filtration is decreased by at least 50%. This is a reflection of the fact that the glomerular filtration rate is related to the BUN in a hyperbolic instead of a linear fashion (see Fig. 7–1).

A significantly decreased BUN or serum urea occurs in only a few conditions. Poor nutrition, high fluid intake, or excessive administration of intravenous fluids (overhydration) in the presence of normal renal function will result in a decreased BUN level because relatively little urea will be reabsorbed by the renal tubules. A tendency to a decreased BUN level in pregnancy is probably the result of an augmented glomerular filtration rate. Severe liver disease can cause a decrease in urea synthesis because of diminished activity of the urea cycle.

There is some advantage in terms of clinical interpretation to determine both the serum urea and the creatinine concentration and to calculate the BUN/creatinine (B/C) ratio. Creatinine is affected very little by diet and minimally if at all by the state of hydration. Ordinarily the B/C ratio is about 10 to 20. A high B/C ratio is typically associated with prerenal azotemia because of augmented tubular reabsorption of urea in the presence of diminished glomerular filtration. Postrenal azotemia also results in a high B/C ratio because urea is reabsorbed to a much greater extent than creatinine, whether from the urinary tract in the case of acute obstructive uropathy or from the tissues in the case of extravasation of urine. The ratio may be affected by the degree of specificity of the methods used for BUN and creatinine determination. In patients with reduced muscle mass, creatinine production is subnormal and the B/C ratio will be high. A high ratio can also occur in patients with compromised renal function who have a high protein diet, tissue destruction, thyrotoxicosis, or Cushing's syndrome.

A decreased B/C ratio can occur in any of the previously mentioned conditions in which urea production is decreased. Because of their greater creatinine formation, muscular individuals who develop renal failure can also have a low ratio. Renal dialysis causes a decreased ratio because urea is more readily dialyzed than creatinine.

Analytical Techniques

There are two general procedures used to determine urea nitrogen in biologic fluids. A direct method involves the formation of diacetyl from diacetyl monoxime and the subsequent condensation of diacetyl with urea to form a colored chromogen diazine, which can be quantitated by photometry. The liberated hydroxylamine accompanying diacetyl formation interferes with quantitation and is usually eliminated with appropriate oxidizing agents such as ferric ammonium sulfate, potassium persulfate, or arsenic acid. The diacetyl reaction, although simple to perform, lacks specificity. Other limitations include instability of the reaction color; deviation from Beer's law; and the irritating odor of the reagents, which can necessitate working in a fume hood. The alternative, indirect procedure uses the action of enzyme urease on urea to produce ultimately ammonia and carbonic acid.

Various methodologies have been developed for the measurement of the liberated ammonia, including acidimetric titration, colometric titration with hypobromite nesslerization, and the indophenol reaction of Berthelot. In the Berthelot procedure, catalysts such as nitroprusside are added to facilitate the conversion of ammonia to indophenol.

For ease of adaptation to automation, the ammonia released from the urease reaction is reacted with α-ketoglutaric acid in the presence of glutamic dehydrogenase. The decrease

2

of absorbance at 340 nm, corresponding to the oxidation of nicotinamide adenine dinucleotide (NADH) reduced to nicotinamide adenine dinucleotide (NAD), is proportional to the ammonium concentration. This procedure is currently used on most automated analyzers.

Semiautomated procedures for the determination of urea nitrogen include (1) the conductivity rate measurement of NH_4^+ and HCO_3^- generated from the action of urease on urea, and (2) the measurement of ammonia eluted from immobilized urease with use of an ammonia-sensing electrode. Because ammonia may be present in the urine, care must be taken to ensure removal of preformed ammonia prior to assay.

Because hemoglobin causes colorimetric interference, measurement of urea nitrogen using serum or plasma is preferred over measurement using whole blood. The urease reaction has also been shown to be inhibited by a high concentration of sodium fluoride. Although urea is stable in plasma, serum, or urine for several days under refrigeration, samples, especially urine, should be assayed within a few hours to avoid bacterial contamination, which can result in rapid loss of urea.

Creatine and Creatinine

Physiologic Chemistry

Creatine is important in muscle metabolism in that it provides storage of high-energy phosphate through synthesis of phosphocreatine. Creatine is synthesized in a two-step process involving the initial synthesis of guanidoacetate (glycocyamine), which takes place in the kidneys, small intestinal mucosa, pancreas, and probably the liver. This reaction between glycine and arginine is catalyzed by a transaminidase, which is subject to feedback inhibition by increased creatine. Guanidoacetate is transported to the liver, where it is methylated to creatine. Creatine then enters the blood to be widely distributed, chiefly to muscle cells, which contain about 98% of the total body creatine pool. The body content of creatine is proportional to the muscle mass.

Creatinine is formed as a result of nonenzymatic dehydration of muscle creatine. Free creatinine is not reused in the body's metabolism and thus functions solely as a waste product of creatine. Creatinine turnover rates in normal men are reasonably constant, and 1.6% to 1.7% of the creatine is so transformed every 24 hours. Consequently, creatinine formation also has a direct relationship to muscle mass.

Creatine is filtered by the glomeruli but is largely or completely reabsorbed by the proximal tubules. Consequently, there is only a very small net excretion, that is, from 0 to 40 mg/24 h (0 to 0.35 mmol/24 h) for adult males and 0 to 100 mg/24 h (0 to 0.88 mmol/24 h) for adult females. Creatinine is also freely filtered by the glomeruli but is not reabsorbed to any appreciable extent under normal circumstances. However, tubular reabsorption of creatinine has been observed under certain clinical conditions, including severe congestive heart failure and uncontrolled diabetes mellitus. A substantial fraction of creatinine excretion by the kidney is the result of proximal tubular secretion. Thus, in normal individuals, creatinine clearance may regularly exceed inulin clearance by 10% to 40%. In patients with severe renal insufficiency, as much as 60% of urinary creatinine may be derived from tubular secretion (Perrone, 1992). Tubular creatinine secretion may be inhibited by drugs, such as cimetidine, probenecid, and trimethroprim. Although ranges are frequently quoted for total creatinine excretion—for example, 1.0 to 2.0 g/24 h (8.8 to 17.6 mmol/24 h) for adult males and 0.6 to 1.5 g/24 h (5.3 to 13.2 mmol/24 h) for adult females—a better index would relate creatinine excretion to muscle mass or lean body weight. A reasonable compromise is to relate creatinine excretion to total body weight—that is, 21 to 26 mg/kg body weight/24 h (0.18 to 0.23 mmol/kg/24 h) for adult males and 16 to 22 mg/kg body weight/24 h (0.14 to 0.19 mmol/kg/24 h) for adult females. Severe exercise and a high-meat diet causes significantly increased creatinine excretion. Total creatinine measurement is commonly used as an index of the completeness of 24-hour urine collections.

The serum concentration of creatinine is relatively constant and somewhat greater in males than in females—that is, 0.6 to 1.2 mg/dL (53 to 106 μmol/L) for males and 0.5 to 1.0 mg/dL (44 to 88 μmol/L) for females. Serum creatinine concentration is often interpreted as a measure of glomerular filtration rate and is used as an index of renal function in clinical practice. It should be remembered that a variety of other factors also influence serum creatinine concentration; they include the renal handling and metabolism of creatinine, and methods of measurement. Furthermore, the effects of aging, pregnancy, diabetes mellitus, drug administration, and acute and chronic renal failure must be correctly interpreted when using serum creatinine as an index of renal function (Levey, 1988; Perrone, 1992).

The serum creatine concentration is more variable than creatinine and is higher in females than in males—that is, 0.2 to 0.6 mg/dL (15 to 45 μmol/L) for males and 0.6 to 1.0 mg/dL (45 to 76 μmol/L) for females.

Clinicopathologic Correlations

Serum or plasma creatine concentration and urinary creatine excretion are increased significantly by skeletal muscle necrosis or atrophy (Pennington, 1971), such as trauma, the rapidly progressing muscular dystrophies, poliomyelitis, amyotrophic lateral sclerosis, amyotonia congenita, dermatomyositis, myasthenia gravis, and starvation. Methyltestosterone stimulates increased creatine synthesis by the liver. Increased creatine is also associated with hyperthyroidism, diabetic acidosis, and the puerperium.

Both serum creatinine and urine creatinine have been used as indices of renal function because of the constancy of creatinine formation. However, because of the interfering chromogens in plasma, most methods used in the clinical laboratories overestimate the serum creatinine (Scre) and underestimate the clearance of creatinine (Ccre). Under normal conditions, this is balanced by the opposite effect of tubular creatinine secretion, resulting in a Ccre closely approximating the clearance of inulin. However, these two effects are completely unrelated and they are influenced independently by numerous variables, including renal function and drugs. As GFR decreases, contribution of creatinine secretion to Ccre increases. Thus, change in Ccre may not adequately reflect a change in glomerular filtration rate (GFR). The use of Scre as a renal function index is also subject to difficulties on the basis that increased tubular creatinine secretion during reduced GFR has resulted in a much smaller increase in Scre; thus the sensitivity of Scre as a marker may be compromised (Perrone, 1992). Nevertheless, the finding of decreased Ccre and increased Scre is certainly indicative of decreased renal function.

By virtue of its relative independence from such factors as diet (protein intake), degree of hydration, and protein metabolism, the plasma creatinine is a significantly more reliable screening test or index of renal function than is the BUN. The plasma creatinine tends to increase somewhat more slowly than the BUN in renal disease but also decreases more slowly with hemodialysis. The usefulness of plasma creatinine and the creatinine clearance test are discussed in detail in Chapter 7.

Analytical Techniques

Creatinine may be measured in serum, plasma, or urine. There is no systematic differences between serum and plasma creatinine. Most of the commonly used methods for the determination of creatinine and creatine are based on the Jaffe reaction, in which creatinine is treated with an alkaline picrate solution to yield a bright orange-red complex. Unfortunately, this simple procedure is subject to interferences from a variety of substances—e.g., glucose, proteins, acetoacetate, pyruvate, uric acid, fructose, and ascorbic acid. The reaction is also sensitive to temperature and pH changes. The presence of these noncreatinine chromogens causes an increase of up to 20% over the true creatinine value. In addition, bilirubin and other compounds in the serum of jaundiced patients exhibit a negative interference in the Jaffe reaction.

More specific methods based on principles other than the Jaffe reaction have been developed. Lloyd's reagent, an aluminum silicate, has been used to separate creatinine from other chromogens prior to the Jaffe reaction. Colorimetric determination of complexes formed with 3,5-dinitrobenzoic acid and with *o*-nitrobenzaldehyde has also been used. Creatinine determinations based on enzyme reactions and on kinetic rate reactions have found universal applications in clinical practice. The procedure used on the Ektachem analyzer (Kodak, Rochester, NY) is based on the enzymatic reaction of creatinine with creatinine imidohydrolase to form *N*-methylhydantoin and ammonium ion; the latter is measured by reflectance spectrophotometry. Interfering substances for this reaction include glucose, 5-flucytosine, and environmental ammonia. Kinetic assays are modifications of the Jaffe reaction, and they are adaptable to automated chemistry analyzers. These assays make use of the differential rate of color development of noncreatinine chromogens compared with creatinine, thus allowing a rate-dependent separation of creatinine from interfering substances. However, some of these methods are still subject to interferences by α-keto compounds, bilirubin, and its metabolites. A new methodology using blank correction has eliminated the bilirubin interference (Boot, 1994).

Creatine is usually measured by the difference in creatinine before and after conversion of creatine to creatinine, generally by heat.

Because considerable amounts of noncreatinine chromogens are present in the erythrocytes, plasma and serum are preferred over whole blood for measuring creatinine. Although hemolysis does not affect the determination of creatinine, it increases the creatine value by 100% to 200%. Because of the lability of creatine and creatinine, fresh specimens are recommended. Also, specimens should be maintained at pH 7 during storage to minimize interconversion. Substances that can interfere with creatinine determination by Jaffe's reaction include acetoacetate, acetone, barbiturates, phenolsulfonphthalein, sulfobromophthalein, and protein.

2

Uric Acid

Physiologic Chemistry

Uric acid is the major product of purine catabolism in humans and the anthropoid apes, and is formed from xanthine by the action of xanthine oxidase. In lower mammals, uric acid is further oxidized by the action of uricase to allantoin, which is their main excretory product of purine catabolism. Interestingly, birds and reptiles synthesize uric acid as an end product of both purine and protein catabolism, with the distinct advantage that these animals can excrete the sparingly soluble uric acid as crystals and thereby conserve water. The metabolism of uric acid has been reviewed by Conger (1990).

The average adult has a total body content of about 1.2 g of uric acid, which may be considered to be a miscible pool with high turnover. Uric acid in this pool is derived from three sources: (1) catabolism of ingested nucleoproteins, (2) catabolism of endogenous nucleoproteins, and (3) direct transformation of endogenous purine nucleotides (Ryckewaert, 1974). Approximately 60% of this pool is replaced daily by concomitant formation and excretion. Most uric acid formation occurs in the liver, which has a high activity of xanthine oxidase, as does the intestinal mucosa. Only traces of xanthine oxidase are present in other tissues. On a low-purine diet, about 275 to 600 mg of uric acid is excreted by the average adult in a 24-hour period. This is somewhat less than the amount formed by endogenous metabolism. It is probable that most, if not all, of the remaining uric acid excretion occurs through biliary, pancreatic, and gastrointestinal secretions, followed by degradation by the intestinal flora. Human tissues have very limited uricolytic capability.

Uric acid is a weak acid with a pKa_1 of 5.75 and a pKa_2 of 10.3. Consequently, at the pH of body fluids, uric acid exists almost entirely as the urate anion. Although there is some difference of opinion, it appears that urate binding to plasma proteins is minimal. The stated reference interval for serum or plasma urate varies considerably as a consequence of differences in analytical methods and in age, sex, racial, social, and geographic factors. One study of 1419 clinically healthy Americans revealed a 95% nonparametric normal range of 4.0 to 8.5 mg/dL (0.24 to 0.51 mmol/L) for males and 2.7 to 7.3 mg/dL (0.16 to 0.43 mmol/L) for females when uric acid was analyzed by a phosphotungstate method. This study included adult subjects from age 20 to old age, but there was no statistically significant effect of age except for an increased upper limit of normal of about 0.5 mg/dL for females at the time of menopause. Urate concentration in male children is approximately 1 mg/dL less than that in adult males, but this difference disappears between ages 15 and 20 (Ryckewaert, 1974).

The average adult excretes approximately 0.4 to 0.8 g of uric acid in the urine every 24 hours. On a low-purine diet, about 275 to 600 mg of uric acid will still be excreted as a result of catabolism of endogenous purines (Ryckewaert, 1974). Uric acid excretion can exceed 1.0 g/24 h as a consequence of a high-purine diet or any of the various causes for increased synthesis or catabolism of endogenous purines. The renal handling of urate is complex and may best be described by a four-component model that includes glomerular filtration, proximal tubular reabsorption, tubular secretion, and postsecretory reabsorption. Urate is freely filtered by the glomerulus. Tubular reabsorption is an active transport process by which greater than 90% of filtered uric acid, as well as the subsequently secreted uric acid, is reabsorbed (Becker, 1988). The physiologic role of uric acid as an antioxidant has recently been advocated.

Clinicopathologic Correlations

Numerous diseases, physiologic conditions, biochemical changes, and even social and behavioral factors are associated with alterations in the urate concentration of plasma. Increased serum urate concentration is much more frequent and clinically more significant than decreased concentration. Among the most common etiologies of hyperuricemia are renal failure, ketoacidosis, lactate excess, toxemia of pregnancy with increased lactic acid, and the use of diuretics. Hyperuricemia also has a positive relationship to hyperlipidemia, obesity, atherosclerosis, diabetes mellitus, hypertension, social class, exercise, and achievement-oriented behavior. In hypertensive patients, the reduced renal blood flow and increased vascular resistance may be responsible for the decreased filtration fraction for urate. Dietary intake of purine-rich foods, such as meat, viscera, leguminous vegetables, and yeast, causes mild hyperuricemia as well as significantly increased urinary excretion of urate.

Gout is a disorder of purine metabolism or renal excretion of uric acid characterized by (1) hyperuricemia; (2) precipitation of monosodium urate as deposits (tophi) throughout the body except for the central nervous system but with a special predilection for joints and the periarticular cartilage, bone, bursae, and subcutaneous tissue; (3) recurrent clinical attacks of arthritis, which typically respond to colchicine or nonsteroidal anti-inflammatory agents; and (4) nephropathy and frequently nephrolithiasis. Although genetic in origin, fewer than one third of all patients have a family history of clinical gout. Hyperuricemia is frequently found in asymptomatic close relatives. Although some investigators have considered gout to be an autosomal dominant trait with incomplete penetrance, the mode of inheritance is not known with certainty. Gout may well be of polygenic origin. Males constitute more than 90% of all cases. Gout is uncommon in females prior to menopause. The peak age of onset is in the fifth decade, and the disease is very rare prior to age 20.

Gout is frequently categorized as primary or secondary on the basis of whether the disease is presumed to be an inborn error of metabolism directly involving uric acid synthesis or excretion or whether it is associated with hyperuricemia from any of numerous other etiologies. The miscible pool of uric acid is greatly increased in gout and can exceed 30 g. The concentration of urate in plasma is roughly correlated with clinical severity, but it is not known why one individual will have clinical gout while another in the same kinship with an equally elevated concentration of urate in the plasma can be asymptomatic. The increased body burden of uric acid is a result of increased *de novo* purine synthesis, increased purine nucleotide degradation, diminished renal excretion of urate, or a combination of these defects (Garcia, 1994). In the past, most investigators have emphasized the importance of overproduction of uric acid in the pathogenesis of gout. In fact, the great majority of patients with gout suffer from both overproduction and underexcretion of urate. The pathogenesis of the acute inflammation accompanying uric acid deposits in gout is unclear. It is possible that the monosodium urate crystals enhance bradykinin synthesis through activation of the Hageman factor.

Two sex chromosome–linked enzyme defects have been identified as etiologies for primary gout: hypoxanthine-guanine phosphoribosyl-transferase (HGPRT) deficiency and phosphoribosyl pyrophosphate (PRPP) synthetase overactivity (Becker, 1988). HGPRT normally is present in all tissues. It converts hypoxanthine and guanine to their respective nucleotides—isosinic acid and guanylic acid. A deficiency in HGPRT is frequently associated with gross endogenous overproduction of purine and marked accumulation of uric acid. PRPP synthetase catalyzes the production of PRPP, which is an important regulator in the rate of *de novo* purine synthesis. Increased synthesis of PRPP that is due to a mutation of its synthetase is also associated with overproduction of urate. Individuals with severely aberrant enzymes may present with sensorineural deafness and neurodevelopmental impairment in PRPP synthetase overactivity, and with the Lesch-Nyhan syndrome in HGPRT deficiency. This syndrome is characterized by mental retardation, choreoathetosis, spastic cerebral palsy, aggressive behavior, and compulsive self-mutilation, in addition to the pathologic manifestation of hyperuricemia, gouty arthritis, tophi, nephrolithiasis, and nephropathy (Nyhan, 1974).

Urate retention and hyperuricemia are early consequences of azotemic renal disease. Although previously considered to be a reflection of decreased glomerular filtration, the urate retention is more likely the result of decreased tubular secretion of urate or altered postsecretory reabsorption of both factors. The plasma urate concentration seldom increases much above 10 mg/dL in renal failure, probably because of increased gastrointestinal secretion and uricolysis. Clinical gout is an uncommon complication of the hyperuricemia of renal disease and occurs in fewer than 5% of all cases. There are two interesting exceptions, however. Chronic lead nephropathy is associated with gout (saturnine gout) in about half of all cases. Polycystic kidney disease predisposes an individual to both hyperuricemia and secondary gout even before renal function deteriorates enough to cause azotemia.

Various drugs and chemical substances interfere with renal excretion of urate. Ethacrynic acid, furosemide, and the benzothiadiazide diuretics have a definite antiuricosuric effect. *p*-Aminohippurate, lactate, acetoacetate, and β-hydroxybutyrate competitively inhibit tubular secretion of urate. Some drugs such as salicylate, probenecid, sulfinpyrazone, and phenylbutazone are of particular interest in that they inhibit uric acid excretion in low doses but have a marked uricosuric effect in high doses. This is explained by the fact that these drugs inhibit tubular secretion of urate in low doses but are able to inhibit tubular reabsorption only at significantly higher levels.

Increased nucleoprotein production and catabolism are important in the hyperuricemia that occurs with leukemia, lymphoma, macroglobulinemia, polycythemia, multiple myeloma, neuroblastoma, and various other widely disseminated neoplasms. Chemotherapeutic agents and ionizing radiation therapy of malignant neoplasms can greatly increase the formation of uric acid. Psoriasis is also associated with hyperuricemia, which is the result of increased proliferation of epidermal cells. Hyperuricemia occurs frequently in sickle cell anemia.

Ethanol ingestion frequently increases the plasma concentration of urate and can cause attacks of gout in susceptible patients. Ethanol alters uric acid metabolism both by increasing urate production through an acetate-mediated adenine nucleotide catabolism and by suppression of renal uric acid excretion. The latter is a result of lactate excess, produced by the oxidation of ethanol to acetaldehyde, which competitively inhibits renal tubular urate secretion. Lactate excess is also associated with hyperuricemia in severe exercise, toxemia of pregnancy, and ethylene glycol intoxication. Increased acetoacetate and β-hydroxybutyrate similarly contribute to hyperuricemia in diabetic ketoacidosis and starvation. Glycogen storage disease type 1 is regularly accompanied by hyperuricemia as a consequence of both lacticacidemia and increased formation of purines.

Hyperuricemia occurs in many other conditions in which the pathogenetic relationship is less well defined. Included are Down syndrome, barbiturate overdose, chloroform, carbon monoxide, ammonia and beryllium poisoning, hypoparathyroidism, acromegaly, nephrogenic diabetes insipidus, sarcoidosis, and liver disease.

Causes of hypouricemia are relatively few. Renal tubular reabsorption defects, either congenital, as in the Fanconi's syndrome and Wilson's disease, or acquired, particularly through toxic damage, can cause increased urinary loss of urate and low plasma levels. Hypouricemia has also been described in association with malignant disorders, such as Hodgkin's disease, multiple myeloma, and bronchogenic carcinoma. Xanthinuria, a rare condition, is caused by a congenital deficiency of xanthine oxidase so that xanthine and hypoxanthine are excreted instead of uric acid. Vigorous treatment of gout with the xanthine oxidase inhibitor allopurinol can have a similar effect. Another rare congenital condition, phosphoribosyl-pyrophosphatase deficiency, also causes extremely low plasma urate concentrations. Severe liver disease can seriously impair the conversion of xanthine to uric acid. An alkaline urine solubilizes uric acid, thus calculi do not evolve or form in the urinary tract.

Uric acid is an important constituent of renal calculi, but only a small minority of patients with either primary or secondary gout form renal calculi. The risk in primary gout is estimated to be 10% to 30%. Hyperuricosuria, from dietary purine excess or from endogenous overproduction, and low urine pH can promote the formation of stones that are pure uric acid or mixed calcium oxalate and uric acid.

Analytical Techniques

Most methods are based on the oxidation of uric acid to allantoin by either chemical or enzymatic means. The older methods are mainly photometric procedures involving the reduction of tungstate to a blue complex. The most commonly used oxidizing agent is alkaline phosphotungstate, the reduction product of which, tungsten blue, can be measured photometrically at 70 nm. However, there are several inherent difficulties with this method, including the coprecipitation of uric acid with plasma proteins, the formation of turbidity during color development, and the presence of endogenous, potentially interfering substances such as ascorbic acid, free thiols, methylated purines, homogentisic acid, and glucose in very high concentrations. The use of a protein-free filtrate for color formation has eliminated most of the interferences. The sodium carbonate reagent initially used to provide the alkaline medium has been replaced by sodium cyanide in order to increase assay sensitivity. Furthermore, the inclusion of urea has been shown to reduce turbidity in the final color solution.

In spite of numerous modifications of the basic colorimetric method aimed at improving specificity, the oxidation of uric acid to allantoin using the enzyme uricase remains the most specific method available. Because uric acid, but not allantoin, absorbs at 293 nm, the difference in absorbance before and after treatment of the sample with uricase is proportional to the uric acid concentration. The advantages of this method are that it avoids protein precipitation and has superior sensitivity and specificity. It is adapted for use on most automated analyzers.

Several modifications making use of the H_2O_2 formed during the enzymatic reaction include the formation of chromogen via coupling with the enzyme catalase and the formation of fluorescent compounds either by self-coupling of *p*-hydroxyphenylacetic acid or by the oxidation of homovanillic acid. Other methods of quantitation include the measurement of oxygen uptake during the formation of H_2O_2, colometric titration, and chromatographic determinations.

Uric acid is stable in both serum and urine for about three days at room temperature. Stability can be increased with the addition of fluoride or thymol. All anticoagulants can be used except potassium oxalate, which forms insoluble potassium phosphotungstate, resulting in turbidity.

Ammonia

Physiologic Chemistry

Ammonia is a product of amino acid metabolism and therefore of protein catabolism. Considerable ammonia is also absorbed from the intestinal tract, where it is formed by bacterial degradation of dietary proteins and the urea present in gastrointestinal secretions. Ammonia is formed principally in the liver by the oxidative deamination of amino acids, chiefly by the glutamic dehydrogenase–catalyzed deamination of L-glutamate to form α-ketoglutarate. Net synthesis of L-glutamate occurs as a result of transamination involving other amino acids, which are transformed in the reaction to their corresponding α-keto acids. Smaller amounts of ammonia are formed by nonoxidative deamination of amino acids and aerobic oxidation of various physiologic amines, such as epinephrine and dopamine.

Most ammonia is ultimately disposed of as urea, which is formed in the urea cycle subsequent to the synthesis of carbamyl phosphate. Glutamine is the principal source of renal ammoniagenesis. It is formed from glutamic acid principally

2

in the liver but also to some extent in the brain and in skeletal muscle. The kidneys take up glutamine from plasma and form ammonium ions by the action of glutaminase. The classic view is that glutamine breakdown results in generation of ammonia that diffuses into the tubular lumen and is excreted in the urine as one of the two most important urine buffers of hydrogen ions. This traditional view has been questioned, because at physiologic pH, hydrolysis of glutamine yields NH_4^+ instead of NH_3; the former can no longer act as a proton acceptor. Evidence appears to favor direct NH_4^+ transport in the kidney as a major pathway in the renal regulation of ammonia (Knepper, 1991). Available studies suggest that NH_4^+ accumulates in the renal medullary interstitium as a result of active NH_4^+ absorption in the thick ascending limb of Henle's loop prior to excretion in the urine. The human kidneys excrete about 30 to 50 mmol of ammonia each day, accounting for about 5% to 10% of all nitrogen excreted and buffering most of the 40 to 80 mmol of metabolic acid produced and excreted by the body (Goldstein, 1976).

Ammonia concentration in plasma is ordinarily less than 120 μg/dL (67 μmol/L).

Clinicopathologic Correlations

The most frequent etiology of altered ammonia metabolism is severe liver disease. It is also elevated in Reye's syndrome. When liver function is no longer adequate to metabolize ammonia, the plasma concentration increases, with various toxic manifestations, particularly in the brain. This is discussed in more detail in Chapter 12.

Inborn errors of the urea cycle are more common than is generally recognized. They are known to occur at each step in the urea cycle—that is, carbamyl phosphate synthetase, ornithine transcarbamylase, argininosuccinic acid synthetase, argininosuccinase, and arginase—and can cause increased plasma ammonia (Walter, 1987).

In metabolic acidosis, the renal excretion of ammonia rises precipitously, provided that normal renal function is maintained. In chronic renal disease, the ability of the kidneys to excrete ammonia and, therefore, to excrete metabolic acid is compromised. This problem is discussed further in Chapter 7.

Analytical Techniques

The measurement of ammonia in blood involves the conversion of NH_4^+ to gaseous NH_3. This initial reaction can be conducted directly in blood or in a protein-free filtrate. The liberated NH_3 can be separated from the plasma or serum by reabsorption on a cation exchange resin followed by quantitation either with Nessler's reagent or by the indophenol reaction, in which NH_4^+ reacts with sodium phenoxide in the presence of hypochlorite and nitroprusside to yield a stable blue color. An alternative and more widely used procedure in separating ammonia from blood or plasma is isothermal diffusion. The isolated NH_3 can be measured by acidimetric titration, nesslerization, photometric determination of the color produced with ninhydrin or with the indophenol reaction, colometric titration with electrolytically produced hydrobromite, or a variety of other means. Another approach for determining blood ammonia is the enzymatic reaction of ammonia with α-ketoglutaric acid in the presence of glutamic dehydrogenase. The decrease of absorbance at 340 nm from the corresponding conversion of NADH to NAD is proportional to the ammonia concentration.

The *in vitro* formation of ammonia in blood, which results from enzymatic action on labile amides such as glutamine, poses a problem in ammonia determinations. The ammonia content in freshly drawn blood increases at the rate of 0.003 μg/mL blood/min at room temperature. The ammonia concentration will remain constant for at least 24 hours if the sample is frozen at −20°C. If analysis is delayed for more than a few minutes, quick freezing of arterial rather than venous plasma samples in dry ice and acetone is recommended.

Amino Acids

Physiologic Chemistry

An examination of Figure 8–1 reveals that the α-amino acid molecule contains an amino group ($-NH_2$); a carboxyl group ($-COOH$); and an R group or side chain, which is responsible for specific characteristics of the particular amino acid. Although more than 150 different amino acids are known biologically, only 21 are present in the body as significant constituents of proteins. Some of these amino acids must be supplied by dietary intake, whereas others can be synthesized by various metabolic pathways. Those amino acids that have to be supplied by dietary intake because endogenous synthesis is inadequate to meet normal requirements are termed essential amino acids. This distinction implies only a necessity for supply from an external source and does not imply that these amino acids are more important for metabolism and growth than the remaining nonessential amino acids. The essential and nonessential amino acids are shown in Table 8–1.

Amino acids that possess an asymmetric carbon atom, that is, those with four different substituent groups, have dextrorotatory (D) and levorotatory (L) optical specificity. All amino acids in human proteins are of the L configuration, which is diagrammatically shown in Figure 8–1.

Amino acids in their crystalline state have melting points above 190°C and are more soluble in water than in other less polar solvents. At a pH that is specific for each amino acid, the molecule is doubly charged, that is, the carboxyl group is negatively charged and the amino group is positively charged, thus resulting in a net charge of zero. Dipolar ions of this type are referred to as zwitterions (Fig. 8–1). Amino

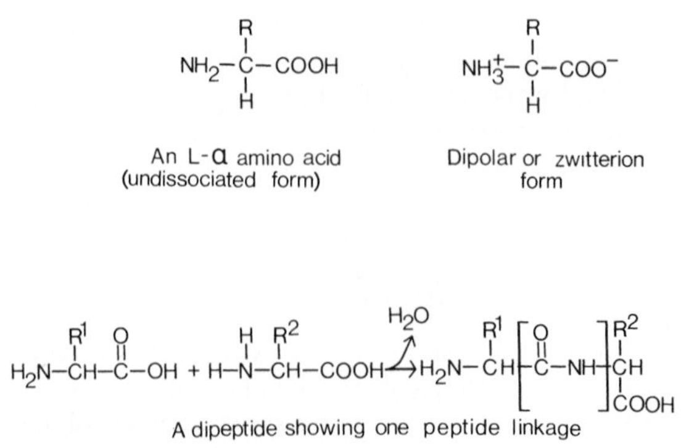

Figure 8–1. Chemical characteristics of amino acids.

Table 8–1. AMINO ACIDS AS SIGNIFICANT CONSTITUENTS OF BODY PROTEINS

Essential	Nonessential
Valine	Glycine
Leucine	Alanine
Isoleucine	Serine
Methionine	Cysteine
Threonine	Cystine
Arginine	Aspartic acid
Lysine	Glutamic acid
Phenylalanine	Hydroxylysine
Histidine	Tyrosine
Tryptophan	Proline
	Hydroxyproline

acids thus behave as both weak acids and weak bases—that is, they are amphoteric.

Proteins are composed of long chains of amino acids joined by peptide linkage (see Chap. 11). The peptide or amide linkage is formed by the condensation of the α-amino group of one amino acid with the carboxyl group of another. A molecule of water is removed in the formation of the amide bond (see Fig. 8–1). After the peptide linkage has been formed, a carboxyl group of one amino acid and the amino group of the other are still available to form additional peptide linkages.

Proteins in ingested foods are not absorbed intact to any significant degree. In the process of digestion, enzymatic cleavage of peptide linkages occurs. In the stomach and proximal small intestine, endopeptidases hydrolyze the inner portions of the polypeptide chains, while exopeptidases attack the terminal linkages.

The action of the endopeptidases, pepsin, trypsin, chymotrypsin, and elastase, and the exopeptidases, carboxypeptidases A and B, results in a mixture of amino acids and small peptides, which can be absorbed by the intestine. After absorption into the microvilli, further enzymatic hydrolysis converts oligopeptides into the constituent amino acids. The molecules of essentially all the amino acids are much too large to diffuse passively through the membrane pores of the intestinal mucosal cells. The amino acids are absorbed by at least three stereospecific active transport systems: (1) neutral amino acids are absorbed competitively by a single transport system; (2) basic amino acids are absorbed, but at a slower rate, by a second active transport system; and (3) proline and hydroxyproline are absorbed by a third transport system. After absorption, amino acids enter the portal venous blood to be transported to the liver, where some are used for protein synthesis, while others enter the systemic amino acid pool. Protein synthesis throughout the body uses amino acids from the systemic pool, while protein catabolism contributes additional amino acids. The usual process of catabolism involves initial removal of the amino group. The resultant keto acids enter the Krebs aerobic cycle to be oxidized to CO_2 and water with the production of energy, which can be stored as adenosine triphosphate (ATP). Amino acids exist in the systemic circulatory pool but cannot be stored as such. The adult normal range of plasma amino acids varies according to the method of analysis. Reference concentrations of individual amino acids in healthy subjects by high-pressure liquid chromatography (HPLC) technique have been reported by Teerlink (1994).

Amino acids are filtered by renal glomeruli and are very efficiently reabsorbed by active transport processes in the proximal tubules. Ordinarily less than 5% of the filtered amino acids are not reabsorbed and are thus excreted in the urine. In the normal adult, urinary excretion of amino acids is fairly constant and averages 200 mg of α-amino nitrogen per 24 hours.

Clinicopathologic Correlations

Amino acids are the second largest constituent of the plasma nonprotein nitrogen. Significant decreases in either the plasma concentration of amino acids or the urinary excretion rate are rare. Even in severe cachexia, the plasma amino acid pool is relatively well maintained as a consequence of the catabolism of intrinsic body proteins.

Increased concentrations of plasma amino acids and especially their urinary excretion rates are of considerable medical importance, particularly in newborns and children. More than 50 hereditary diseases of amino acid metabolism have now been described, most of which have an autosomal recessive mode of inheritance. All of these diseases are uncommon to extremely rare, which is fortunate in view of the fact that many of the diseases are associated with mental retardation, severe metabolic derangements, and failure to thrive. Typically, a hereditary amino acid disorder is directly related to the absence of an enzyme involved in the metabolism of one or more amino acids, so that these amino acids increase greatly in both plasma concentrations and urinary excretion rates. Phenylketonuria, for example, is the result of an inherited deficiency or absence of phenylalanine hydroxylase, which is necessary for the metabolic conversion of phenylalanine to tyrosine, with a resulting increase in both phenylalanine and its deaminated metabolite, phenylpyruvic acid, in plasma and urine. Phenylketonuria is one of the most common hereditary amino acid disorders and affects about one in 10,000 newborns. Early diagnosis is essential so that diets lacking in phenylalanine can be instituted and thereby decrease or avoid the cerebral damage that otherwise invariably occurs.

Increased concentrations of amino acids in plasma can be categorized as primary (hereditary) metabolic defects and secondary metabolic responses. Secondary responses involve virtually all amino acids. Significant increases are usually a consequence of severe liver disease that inhibits the oxidative deamination of amino acids. Small increases in the plasma concentration of many amino acids occur after ingestion of a protein-rich meal.

In general, measurement of urinary concentration of amino acids is of a more clinical value than plasma concentrations. Increased urinary excretion of amino acids is of two major types—overflow and renal. Overflow aminoacidurias are those that accompany increased plasma concentrations of amino acids when normally functioning kidney tubules are unable to reabsorb the increased concentrations of amino acids in the glomerular filtrate, that is, the renal tubular maximum reabsorption capacity is exceeded. Specific aminoacidurias are discussed in Chapter 18.

Renal aminoacidurias are those conditions associated with increased urinary excretion of one or more amino acids while plasma amino acid concentrations are normal. These various conditions have in common a defect in the renal tubular transport mechanism that causes decreased reabsorption of amino acids from the glomerular filtrate. Primary or hereditary renal aminoacidurias are those involving a hereditary defect in renal tubular transport of one or several amino acids. For example, cystinuria results in an inability of the renal tubules to reabsorb not only cysteine but also lysine, arginine, ornithine, and occasionally other amino acids as well. Secondary renal aminoacidurias are those resulting from acquired renal tubular disease, often of a toxic etiology, such as heavy metal poisoning. Other etiologies include acute renal tubular necrosis, severe malnutrition, and various metabolic diseases otherwise unrelated to amino acid metabolism, such as galactosemia, hereditary fructose intolerance, and Wilson's disease. The renal threshold for amino acid excretion is lowered in pregnancy and in newborns.

Other than in plasma and urine, amino acid analysis is of no significant clinical importance except for the quantitation of glutamine in cerebrospinal fluid. Glutamine, the most abundant amino acid in plasma, is of major importance as a source of ammonia in the renal tubules for buffering hydrogen ion in urine.

Analytical Techniques

Analytical techniques are of two basic types in terms of the information generated—(1) those that quantitate total amino acids and (2) those that separate and quantitate individual amino acids or groups of amino acids. Analytical methods for total amino acids rely on the unique reactivity of the amino group attached to the alpha carbon of the basic amino acid structure. The classic reference method for the measurement of α-amino nitrogen is the gasometric Ninhydrin procedure of Van Slyke, but this method is technically demanding and seldom used in spite of its exquisite reliability. Other reliable methods have since been developed. These procedures generally are applicable to both serum and urine.

In many metabolic disturbances, the knowledge of altered concentration of one amino acid or a group of related amino acids is essential in correct diagnosis. In many such instances, a urinary screen for amino acids may be performed with use of chromatographic techniques, particularly by HPLC. The amino acids in serum or urine can be separated on an automated HPLC system (amino acid analyzer) using an ion-exchange resin followed by gradient elution. In the original amino acid analyzer, quantitation was achieved by spectrophotometric analysis following Ninhydrin derivatization. Refinements in the original procedure, particularly improved column technology such as precolumn derivatization and the development of new fluorescent detection systems (fluorescamine and phthaldealdehyde) on HPLC, have resulted in increased sensitivity and reduced analysis time (Teerlink, 1994).

Reasonably specific methods that avoid the high cost of column chromatography have been developed for some amino acids, including thyroxine, triiodothyronine, hydroxyproline, glutamine, phenylalanine, and tyrosine. Thyroxine and triiodothyronine, although structurally amino acids, are important as thyroid hormones and not as protein constituents. They are discussed in Chapter 16. Hydroxyproline excretion in urine is an important index of collagen catabolism and is discussed later in this chapter. Cerebrospinal fluid glutamine is discussed in Chapter 19.

By virtue of its application to biochemical screening of the newborn, phenylalanine is frequently determined in plasma during the first few days after birth. The Guthrie screening test is a microbiologic assay that measures the ability of phenylalanine in the test sample to overcome the metabolic inhibition of β-2-thienylalanine on a strain of *Bacillus subtilis*. A more commonly performed assay today involves a fluorometric reaction between phenylalanine, copper, and Ninhydrin with enhancement by any of several dipeptides. Other chemical methods include gas-liquid chromatography and ultraviolet spectrophotometry. Phenylalanine and phenylketonuria are discussed further in Chapter 18.

Tyrosine can be quantitated fluorometrically following its reaction with 1-nitroso-2 naphthol. The procedure is adaptable to automated continuous flow analysis.

PORPHYRINS

Physiologic Chemistry

The porphyrins are metabolic intermediates in the biosynthetic pathway that has heme as its principal product. The basic structure common to all porphyrins is the porphin nucleus, which consists of one pyrrolenine, one maleimide, and two pyrrole-type rings. These rings are joined together by four methene bridges, as shown in Figure 8–2. The porphyrins are differentiated by the substituents found in the eight peripheral positions. There are many kinds of porphyrins known, but very few are found in nature and only three are of clinical significance: uroporphyrins, coproporphyrins, and protoporphyrins. Four isomeric forms can exist for each porphyrin. All naturally occurring porphyrins are of either the I or III isomer type. Only the type III isomers have been shown to play a functional role in the biosynthesis of heme.

A brief sequence of the heme biosynthetic pathway is shown in Figure 8–3. The initial rate-limiting step in hepatic porphyrin synthesis is the formation of δ-aminolevulinic acid (ALA), which requires the presence of pyridoxal phosphate and involves the enzyme ALA synthetase. The condensation of ALA to porphobilinogen (PBG) involves ALA dehydratase, which is present in relatively high levels in both hepatic and bone marrow cells. The formation of uroporphyrinogens I and III from PBG occurs under the influence of enzymes uroporphyrinogen I synthetase and uroporphyrinogen III co-

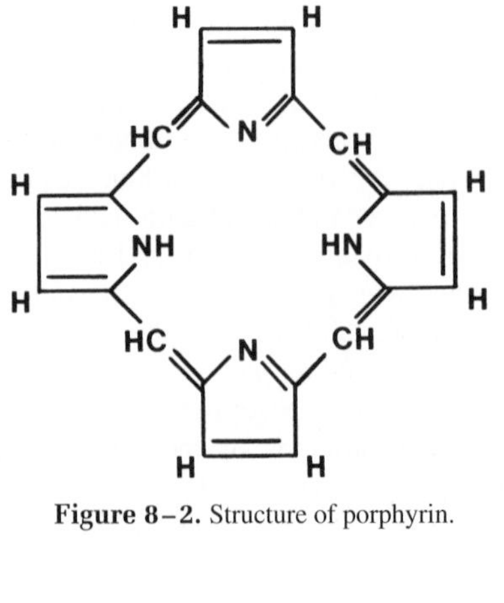

Figure 8–2. Structure of porphyrin.

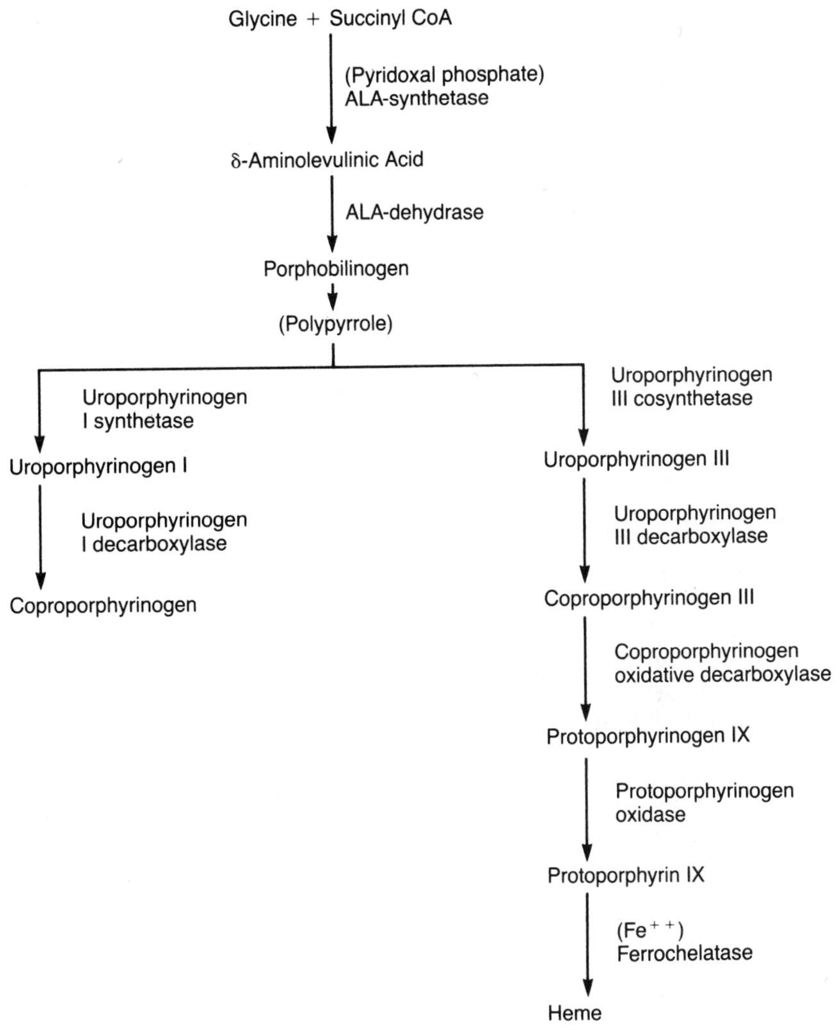

Figure 8–3. Biosynthetic pathway of heme.

synthetase. Both isomers undergo decarboxylation to yield the respective coproporphyrinogens. The type III isomer undergoes oxidative decarboxylation to form protoporphyrin, which reacts with ferrous ion to produce heme.

It is worth noting that the biosynthetic intermediates between PBG and protoporphyrin are not porphyrins but rather their reduced forms, the porphyrinogens. They are colorless nonfluorescent compounds readily converted to porphyrins by weak oxidizing agents, such as air in the presence of light. Thus uroporphyrin and coproporphyrin are merely the oxidation of their respective porphyrinogens, which are the true substrates in the biosynthetic pathway.

Clinicopathologic Correlations

The porphyrias comprise a group of inherited and acquired disorders characterized by aberrations in the activities of specific enzymes of the heme biosynthetic pathway, culminating in the excess secretion of porphyrins or porphyrin precursors. Advances in the understanding of the porphyrias have led to the conclusion that the principal control of the heme biosynthetic pathway lies at the level of ALA synthetase, the activity of which is normally low, but is readily inducible by drugs and steroids and is susceptible to negative feedback by heme. It is further recognized that a secondary control point resides with the activity of uroporphyrinogen I synthetase. Disease manifestations appear to depend on the type of porphyrin oversecretion. Afflicted individuals with an accumulation of ALA and PBG usually exhibit neuropsychiatric presentations, while excess secretion of the porphyrin intermediates is associated with cutaneous manifestations. In patients with oversecretion of both porphyrin intermediates and their precursors, the manifestations are both neuropsychiatric and cutaneous (Tefferi, 1994). Accordingly porphyrias are differentiated into acute porphyrias and nonacute porphyrias on the basis of their clinical manifestation as well as the pattern of production and excretion of porphyrins and their precursors. Acute intermittent porphyria (AIP), hereditary coproporphyria (HCP), and variegate porphyria (VP) are grouped as acute porphyrias because they display similar abdominal, autonomic, and neuropsychiatric features; whereas porphyria cutanea tarda (PCT), erythropoietic protoporphyria (EPP), and congenital erythropoietic porphyria (CEP), typically associated with solar photosensitivity of the skin, are classified as nonacute porphyrias.

Acute Intermittent Porphyria

AIP is the most common of the inherited porphyrias. It is transmitted as an autosomal dominant trait but affects three females to every two males. Numerous drugs can precipitate attacks, including barbiturates, diazepam, chlordiazepoxide, methyldopa, and oral contraceptives. This disease typically presents with colicky abdominal pain often associated with vomiting, constipation, fever, and leukocytosis, leading all too frequently to exploratory laparotomy. Hypertension, peripheral neuritis, behavioral changes, and frank psychosis can occur. Enzyme defects have been shown to include decreased levels of PBG deaminase and ALA dehydratase. Laboratory findings include elevated urinary ALA and PBG; inappropriate secretion of antidiuretic hormone; and overt liver function abnormalities, such as transient elevation of bilirubin and alkaline phosphatase.

Hereditary Coproporphyria

This hepatic porphyria is transmitted as an autosomal dominant trait. Affected patients either are asymptomatic or present with mild neurologic, abdominal, or psychiatric symptoms. Acute attacks have also been reported. Coproporphyrin III is excreted virtually constantly in the feces, whereas coproporphyrin, ALA, and PBG appear intermittently in the urine. Deficient coproporphyrinogen oxidase has been implicated in the mechanism of this condition. The substrate accumulation may serve to allosterically inhibit PBG deaminase activity, resulting in ALA and PBG elevations.

Variegate Porphyria

This autosomal dominant porphyria affects females and males equally and is particularly prevalent in the white population of South Africa. The disease onset is usually in the third or fourth decade of life and is somewhat variable in its clinical manifestations. In addition to the symptoms and signs of acute attacks that are similar to those of acute intermittent porphyria, afflicted patients commonly also present with cutaneous lesions. Elevated urinary ALA, PBG, porphyrins and highly elevated fecal porphyrins can be found during acute attacks. Decreased protoporphyrinogen oxidase and subsequent protoporphyrinogen inhibition of PBG deaminase activity have been implicated in this disorder.

Congenital Erythropoietic Porphyria

This extremely rare autosomal recessive disorder develops shortly after birth. It is associated with red-pigmented urine, erythrodontia, hemolytic anemia, and severe cutaneous photosensitivity. Splenomegaly and hemolytic anemia typically develop, and early death usually occurs. The red urine is the result of excessive excretion of coproporphyrin and uroporphyrin, mainly of type I. The responsible enzyme defects have been attributed to increased activity of ALA synthetase and decreased activity of uroporphyrinogen III cosynthetase.

Erythrohepatic Protoporphyria

Thus far, EPP appears to be the only known inherited disorder in which the biochemical lesions are localized in both hepatic and erythropoietic cells. Transmitted as an autosomal dominant trait, it is associated with mild skin photosensitivity. The onset of disease occurs during the first few years of life or adulthood. Laboratory findings are those of abnormally high protoporphyrin in circulating erythrocytes and elevated fecal coproporphyrin and protoporphyrin, which cause the feces to be fluorescent. Overactivity of ALA synthetase appears to be important in the pathogenesis of this disease. It has been proposed that deficient synthesis of heme from protoporphyrin results in deficient production of a specific heme protein that is important in a feedback suppression of ALA synthetase.

Porphyria Cutanea Tarda

Except for rare familial cases, this group of porphyrias is acquired. Skin lesions are the most obvious clinical feature. The condition has been reported in association with liver disease, particularly with alcohol as the inciting agent; with estrogen therapy; and with ingestion of hexachlorobenzene. A characteristic biochemical finding is elevated urinary uroporphyrin, which is attributed to decreased erythrocyte uroporphyrinogen decarboxylase; excretion of PBG and ALA is usually normal.

Lead Intoxication

Many of the clinical features of lead poisoning, such as abdominal pain, constipation, and other manifestations of neuropathy, are similar to those of the acute porphyrias, such as erythropoietic protoporphyria. Lead has an inhibitory effect on ferrochelatase activity in the final phase of heme synthesis, resulting in marked elevation of erythrocyte Zn protoporphyrin (ZPP). Unlike the metal-free protoporphyrin present in erythropoietic protoporphyria, this compound does not lead to photosensitivity. Thus, measurement of ZPP provides a means of differentiating acute porphyria from lead intoxication. Other characteristic laboratory findings include elevated urinary ALA and coproporphyrin. The clinical manifestations and laboratory tests of lead intoxication are further discussed in Chapter 17.

Analytical Techniques

A complete laboratory investigation of any disorder of porphyrin generally begins with screening tests for porphyrins or their precursors, ALA and PBG, in urine, feces, and blood. This is usually followed by the appropriate quantitative determinations should the preliminary investigation suggest further study. The typical biochemical findings associated with disorders of porphyrin metabolism are shown in Table 8–2.

All porphyrins have in common a characteristic type of absorption spectrum in the near-ultraviolet and visible region, resulting primarily from the conjugated bond system of the tetrapyrrole ring. Hence, all porphyrins have an intense absorption band near 400 nm, known as the Soret band. When irradiated with light of this wavelength, all free porphyrins exhibit an intense red fluorescence. This property enables porphyrins to be detected and quantitated in the laboratory at concentrations of 2×10^{-4} μmol/L. Reference values for porphyrins and their precursors are listed in Table 8–3. A study using fluorescence emission maximum in saline-diluted plasma at 626 nm has been found to be more effective in detecting latent VP (sensitivity of 86%) than the tradi-

Table 8–2. TYPICAL BIOCHEMICAL FINDINGS ASSOCIATED WITH DISORDERS OF PORPHYRIN METABOLISM

	Erythrocyte			Urine				Feces		
Disorders	***UP***	***CP***	***PP***	***ALA***	***PBG***	***UP***	***CP***	***UP***	***CP***	***PP***
Acute intermittent porphyria (AIP)	N	N	N	↑↑	↑↑	↑	↑ or N	N	N	N
Hereditary coproporphyria	N	N	N	↑	↑	N	↑	N	↑	N
Variegate porphyria (acute attacks)	N	N	N	↑	↑	↑ or N	↑ or N	N	↑	↑↑
Congenital erythropoietic porphyria	↑↑	↑↑	↑	N	N	↑↑	↑	N	↑	N
Erythropoietic protoporphyria	N	N	↑↑	N	N	N	N	N	↑	↑
Symptomatic porphyria	N	N	N	N	N	↑↑	↑	N	↑ or N	↑ or N
Lead poisoning	N	↑ or N	↑	↑	↑ or N	N	↑	N	N	N

ALA = δ-aminolevulinic acid; UP = uroporphyrin; CP = coproporphyrin; PP = protoporphyrin; PBG = porphobilinogen; ↑ = increased; ↑↑ = large increase; N = normal.

tional fecal porphyrin measurement (sensitivity = 36%) (Long, 1993).

With the advent of HPLC, screening by this technique has enabled rapid fractionation of porphyrins in a variety of biological fluids for the detection of elevated components. Because the solubility of both the porphyrins and their precursors decreases with decreasing number of hydroxyl and carboxylic groups, PBG and uroporphyrin are excreted mainly in the urine, whereas protoporphyrin is excreted exclusively in the bile and thus appears in the feces. Coproporphyrin is excreted mainly in the bile but also in urine as coproporphyrinogen. Thus, the solubility difference plays an important role in the choice of specimen to be analyzed and in the method of measurement. Although urine and blood screening is the routine procedure, bile porphyrin analysis has been shown to be more effective than fecal determination in the detection of VP (Logan, 1991). A recent study also suggested that bile porphyrin analysis can facilitate the diagnosis of EPP, especially in orthotopic liver transplants, because of its extremely high protoporphyrin concentration (Beukeveld, 1994).

ALA and PBG

The most widely used screening procedure for excess ALA and PBG was first introduced by Watson (1941). PBG condenses with *p*-dimethylaminobenzaldehyde in hydrochloric acid (Ehrlich's reagent) to form a magenta-colored complex (Chapter 18).

Table 8–3. REFERENCE VALUES OF PORPHYRINS AND THEIR PRECURSORS

Analyte	**Reference Interval**
Erythrocyte	
Coproporphyrin	0.5–2.0 μg/dL (0.75–3.00 nmol/L)
Protoporphyrin	4–52 μg/dL (7.2–93.6 nmol/L)
Urine	
ALA	1.5–7.5 mL/24 h (11.2–57.2 μmol/24 h)
PBG	<1.0 mg/24 h (<4.4 μmol/24 h)
Coproporphyrin	50–160 μg/24 h (0.075–0.24 μmol/24 h)
Uroporphyrin	10–30 μg/24 h (0.012–0.037 μmol/24 h)
Feces	
Coproporphyrin	0–500 μg/24 h (0–0.75 μmol/24 h)
Protoporphyrin	0–600 μg/24 h (0–1.08 μmol/24 h)

ALA = δ-aminolevulinic acid; PBG = porphobilinogen.

Porphyrins

The characteristic red fluorescence exhibited by all porphyrins serves as the basis for the screening tests of porphyrins in urine, feces, and blood. The traditional screening procedure involves the extraction of porphyrins into an organic solvent system, such as acetic acid–ethyl acetate, followed by re-extraction into HCl. The fluorescence is read with an ultraviolet light source. Most quantitative measurements of porphyrins are based on preliminary extraction and differentiation by solvent partition followed by spectrophotometric or fluorometric measurement. Although improved resolution of porphyrin fractionation has been achieved in recent years by electrophoresis and by thin-layer chromatography after extraction and esterification, these methods are nevertheless technically demanding and time consuming. The advent of HPLC has made rapid identification and quantification of porphyrins possible in urine, blood, and feces (Beukeveld, 1987).

Although the determination of ALA dehydratase has been emphasized as a diagnostic test for lead intoxication, it has met with limited acceptance. Zn protoporphyrin determination in circulating erythrocyte is now the recommended primary screening test for lead poisoning (Piomelli, 1987). The protoporphyrin is extracted in acetone followed by quantitation with a hematofluorometer. With this method, the Zn remains attached to the porphyrin, thus allowing differentiation of erythropoietic protoporphyria from lead poisoning. When the test is positive—that is, greater than 35 μg/dL—confirmation by blood lead determination is recommended. Zn protoporphyrin results are best expressed in μg/dL of packed red cells or in μg/g of hemoglobin. If results are expressed in terms of concentration in whole blood, elevation of protoporphyrin can be missed if there is an associated anemia.

ALA Dehydratase

Clinical tests that have been used for the diagnosis of lead intoxication include blood lead, coproporphyrin, and ALA. Greater specificity is achieved by the determination of ALA dehydratase, because the inhibitory action by lead on this enzyme occurs long before other biological effects are measurable. The procedure of choice for measurement of ALA dehydratase appears to be that of Bonsignore or its modifications. This method measures the amount of PBG formed in the crude enzyme assay. However, partial conversion of PBG to porphyrin during the crude enzyme assay has been shown to result in underestimation of its activity and an alternate procedure of measuring the ALA consumed has been proposed (Tomokuni, 1974).

CALCIUM AND PHOSPHORUS

Physiologic Chemistry

Calcium Homeostasis

Calcium is the fifth most abundant mineral element in the human body. Approximately 98% of the 1000 to 1200 g of calcium in the adult is present in the skeleton, primarily as hydroxyapatite, which is a crystal lattice composed of calcium, phosphorus, and hydroxide. Of the remaining calcium, about half is present in extracellular fluid and the remainder is present in a variety of tissues, particularly skeletal muscle. Of critical importance to calcium homeostasis is the fact that only about 1% of the total skeletal reservoir of calcium is readily exchangeable with extracellular fluid. In addition to its obvious importance in skeletal mineralization, calcium plays a vital role in such basic physiologic processes as blood coagulation, neural transmission, enzyme activity, maintenance of normal tone, and excitability of skeletal and cardiac muscle. Calcium is also involved in the glandular synthesis and regulation of exocrine and endocrine glands, as well as preservation of cell membrane integrity and permeability, particularly in terms of sodium and potassium exchange.

Calcium in the blood is present almost exclusively in the plasma, the extracellular to intracellular calcium gradient being on the order of 10^4:1. The low intracellular concentration is maintained by an ion pump and exchange mechanism. Calmodulin, an intracellular calcium receptor, appears to play a key role in the process. Extracellularly, calcium in serum is maintained within a narrow range of about 9.0 to 10.0 mg/dL (4.5 to 5.0 mEq/L or 2.25 to 2.5 mmol/L) in healthy individuals. Quoted reference intervals vary among laboratories, partly as a result of different analytical methods. Each laboratory should establish a reference interval for its own population and methodology used. Calcium exists in serum (or plasma) in three distinct forms: (1) free or ionized calcium, which is the physiologically active form, accounts for about 50% of total calcium; (2) about 5% of total calcium is complexed with a variety of anions, particularly phosphate and citrate; (3) the remaining 45% of calcium is bound to plasma proteins, especially to albumin but also to globulin to a limited extent. Both ionized calcium and the calcium complexes are freely dialyzable. The relative distributions of the three forms are altered as a result of change either in pH of the extracellular fluids or in the protein concentration. Acidosis promotes an increase in ionized calcium, whereas alkalosis causes a corresponding decrease. If ionized calcium is to remain within its normal physiologic range, an increased concentration of plasma proteins will result in a corresponding increase in total calcium, which reflects an increase in bound calcium. Similarly, decreased plasma protein concentration will ordinarily result in decreased total calcium.

The binding of calcium to plasma proteins is a freely reversible process, which is governed by a dissociation constant. Thus, the process is analogous to the dissociation of a weak acid or base. This was long ago recognized by McLean and Hastings (1935), who represented the relationship as follows:

$$\frac{[Ca^{2+}][Pr^{=}]}{[CaPr]} = K \qquad (8\text{-}1)$$

where $[Ca^{2+}]$ is the concentration of ionized calcium; [CaPr] is the concentration of protein-bound calcium; $[Pr^{=}]$ is the concentration of free protein capable of binding calcium; and K is a constant, which is specific for each protein species and varies with pH and temperature. Simple transposition of this equation serves to emphasize that the concentration of ionized calcium will remain constant and is thus independent of the absolute value of bound calcium as long as the ratio of the concentrations of protein-bound calcium to free protein remains constant:

$$[Ca^{2+}] = \frac{K\,[CaPr]}{[Pr^{=}]} \qquad (8\text{-}2)$$

Use has been made of this relationship to construct various equations and nomograms for estimating ionized calcium from measurements of total calcium and protein concentrations. Although this approach has worked reasonably well with some patients, nomogram-predicted calcium and ionized calcium correlation has been less than satisfactory in the newborns, older children, and adolescents, and the direct measurement of ionized calcium is preferred. Ionized calcium is also more useful in certain clinical conditions. They include disorders of acid-base balance, in which ionized calcium is altered without affecting total calcium concentration; hemodialysis, in which change in protein concentration may affect total calcium but not ionized calcium; myeloma; renal failure; cirrhosis; treatment with thiazide diuretics; patients with sepsis or other cardiovascular instabilities; patients who have received massive transfusions and citrated blood product transfusions; patients having a citrate infusion with plasma exchange (plasmapheresis); and patients undergoing cardiopulmonary bypass or liver transplantation. Ionized calcium is also superior in the diagnosis of hyperparathyroidism, because calcium elevation in some patients is subtle and the mild acidosis in primary hyperparathyroidism shifts the equilibrium toward increased ionization (Forman, 1991).

Maintenance of calcium homeostasis involves the participation of three major organs—the small intestine, the kidneys, and the skeleton. The mammary gland is also important during lactation, as are the placenta and fetus during gestation. Although the sweat glands are usually ignored in balance studies, they are responsible for a small but significant excretion of calcium. In the adult, there is no persistent net gain or loss of calcium in health. During growth and pregnancy, a positive calcium balance must be maintained. Calcium homeostasis is regulated by various hormones that act principally on the major organs involved in calcium metabolism. The most important hormones are parathyroid hormone and the 1,25-dihydroxycholecalciferol hormones derived from renal metabolism of vitamin D_3, notably. Calcitonin possibly plays a role in the regulating process, although its significance in humans is controversial. Other hormones that affect calcium metabolism but whose secretions are not primarily affected by changes in plasma calcium and phosphate include thyroid hormones, growth hormone, adrenal gluco-

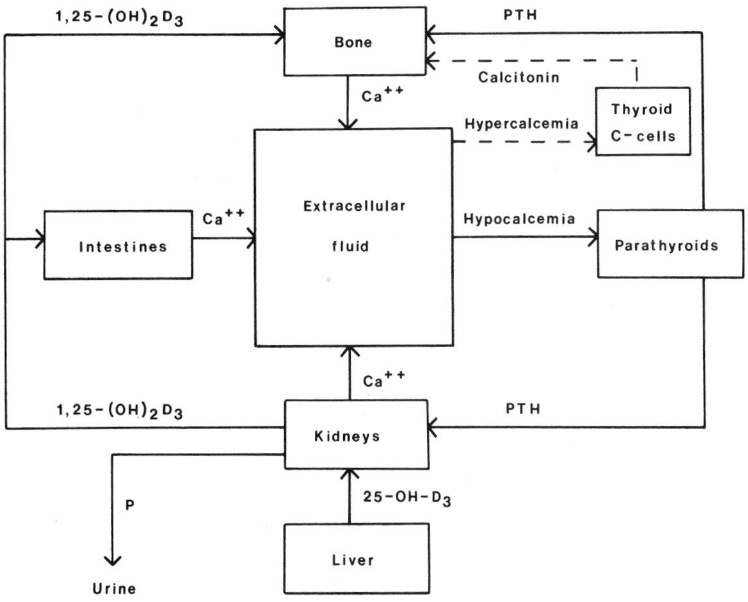

Figure 8–4. Major hormonal regulators of calcium metabolism.

corticoids, and gonadal steroids. Present concepts of the major hormonal regulations of calcium metabolism are summarized in Figure 8–4.

Intake of dietary calcium varies widely for adults from about 200 to 1500 mg/day, most of which in the American diet is derived from milk or other dairy products. The minimum daily dietary requirement for calcium is commonly stated to be 800 mg, but it has been sufficiently demonstrated that calcium balance can be maintained in adults who ingest as little as 200 to 400 mg of calcium daily. It is commonly recommended that the daily dietary intake of calcium should be about 1200 mg during pregnancy and lactation and 800 to 1200 mg during childhood. Considerable emphasis is now placed on calcium supplementation for older persons, particularly postmenopausal females, in order to prevent or at least delay the manifestations of osteoporosis. Many physicians recommend at least 1000 mg of calcium supplement daily.

Calcium is absorbed by an active transport process that occurs mostly in the duodenum and upper jejunum. The major stimulus of calcium absorption is vitamin D. Absorption is also enhanced by growth hormone, an acid medium in the intestines, and increased dietary protein. The ratio of calcium to phosphorus in the intestinal contents is also important in that a ratio greater than two tends to inhibit calcium absorption because of the formation of insoluble calcium phosphates. Phytic acid derived from various cereal grains can also form insoluble calcium compounds, as can dietary oxalate and fatty acids. Cortisol and excessive alkalinity of the intestinal contents are both inhibitory to calcium absorption. The net absorption of calcium from the intestinal tract is only about 10–20% of dietary intake. However, this approximation is grossly misleading because considerable calcium is actively secreted into the intestines.

Estimates of the daily calcium excretion in sweat vary widely—from 15 mg to more than 100 mg. The loss can greatly exceed this range during extreme environmental conditions. The major net loss of calcium is urinary excretion, which accounts for 50 to 200 mg or more each day, depending on dietary intake. Urinary calcium excretion is enhanced by hypercalcemia, phosphate deprivation, acidosis, and glucocorticoids. Urinary calcium excretion is diminished by parathyroid hormone, certain diuretics, and probably vitamin D. The physiology of calcium, its regulating hormones, and the alteration of calcium homeostasis in disease have been extensively reviewed (Boden, 1990).

Phosphorus Homeostasis

Phosphorus is also an abundant element in the body and is omnipresent in its distribution. About 85% of the 500 to 600 g of phosphorus (measured as inorganic phosphorus) in the adult is present in bone as hydroxyapatite crystals. The remaining phosphorus is mostly combined with lipids, proteins, carbohydrates, and other organic substances to fill vital roles as phospholipids, nucleic acids, nucleotides, constituents of cell membranes and cell cytoplasm, and compounds that are important in biochemical energy storage and exchange.

Most of the phosphorus in extracellular fluid is inorganic, predominantly as two species: HPO_4^{2-} and $H_2PO_4^-$. Negligible amounts of PO_4^{3-} exist in the physiologic pH range. The relative amounts of the two phosphate ions are obviously pH dependent (Table 8–4). At pH 7.4, the ratio of HPO_4^{2-} to $H_2PO_4^-$ is about 4:1. Because of the effect of pH on the relative concentrations of the two phosphate species, serum phosphorus should be expressed as milligrams per deciliter. In health, serum phosphorus varies over a rather wide range of 2.5 to 4.8 mg/dL (0.80 to 1.54 mmol/L). Higher phosphorus levels occur in growing children (4 to 7 mg/dL or 1.30 to 2.25 mmol/L). Ingestion of food can significantly alter serum phosphorus concentration. Ingestion of phosphate-rich food can increase serum phosphorus concentration, whereas a high-carbohydrate meal can cause a significant decrease. Adult values are lower than normal during menstruation.

Three major organs are involved in phosphorus homeostasis: the small intestine; the kidneys; and the skeleton, which functions as a storage reservoir. Phosphorus is present in virtually all foods. Consequently, dietary deficiencies do not occur. The average dietary intake for adults is about 800 to

Table 8–4. pH CONVERSION FACTORS FOR INORGANIC PHOSPHORUS*

pH	Factor
7.10	0.537
7.15	0.546
7.20	0.555
7.25	0.563
7.30	0.570
7.35	0.577
7.40	0.583
7.45	0.589
7.50	0.594
7.55	0.599
7.60	0.603
7.70	0.611

*Milligrams per deciliter × factor = mEq per liter.
From Sunderman FW Sr: Inorganic Phosphorus. Proficiency Test Service. Institute for Clinical Science, Inc., Philadelphia, April 1973, p. 3.

1000 mg, most of which is derived from milk and dairy products. About two thirds of ingested phosphate is absorbed, mostly in the jejunum. The remaining dietary phosphate is excreted in the feces, mostly as insoluble calcium compounds. Intestinal absorption of phosphate is an active, energy-dependent process. Absorption is increased in association with decreased dietary calcium and increased acidity of the intestinal contents. Absorption is also augmented by the action of vitamin D and growth hormone. The action of parathyroid hormone on the intestinal absorption of phosphate is probably purely indirect through its effect on the metabolism of vitamin D.

Most of the phosphorus absorbed from the intestines of adults who are in phosphorus balance is excreted in the urine. This is equivalent to about 0.35 to 1.0 g of inorganic phosphorus daily. About 90% of plasma phosphorus is filterable by the glomeruli. Ordinarily about 85% to 95% of the filtered phosphate is reabsorbed. Parathyroid hormone inhibits renal tubular reabsorption of phosphate.

Parathyroid Hormone

Parathyroid hormone (PTH) is secreted primarily as a single-chain polypeptide consisting of 84 amino acids with a molecular mass of 9500 daltons. It is derived from a larger precursor, Pre-ProPTH, of 115 amino acids, which undergoes two successive cleavages both at the amino-terminal sequences to yield, first, an intermediate precursor, ProPTH, and then the hormone itself.

Circulating PTH exists as a mixture of heterogeneous forms, principally as the middle and carboxyl terminal fragments. Biologically active intact PTH has a short half-life of minutes and is present in very low concentration in the circulation. In contrast, the biologically inactive middle and carboxyl terminal fragments, which are cleared by the kidneys, have half-lives of hours and even days, especially during renal insufficiency.

The primary physiologic function of PTH is to regulate the concentration of ionized calcium in extracellular fluids. PTH secretion ordinarily causes a rise in serum ionized calcium concentration and a fall in phosphorus concentration. By way of an effective negative feedback mechanism, hypercalcemia leads to PTH suppression. PTH secretion may also be mediated by the magnesium concentration. In severe hypomagnesemia, for example, PTH secretion is impaired. Patients with low serum magnesium concentration often require magnesium to increase the serum PTH levels before the serum calcium concentration can be restored to the desired interval.

The best-known effect of PTH is bone resorption to restore extracellular fluid calcium concentration. The site of action of PTH on bone appears to be directed primarily to the stable or established component of bone rather than to the labile component. Bone resorption induced by PTH is mediated by increased activity of osteoclasts. Increased conversion of osteoprogenitor cells to osteoclasts occurs as a consequence of more prolonged PTH stimulation. Additional effects of PTH on bone are increased formation of collagenase, which degrades the matrix of bone, and increased breakdown of the ground substance of bone. The end result of PTH action on bone is thus true bone resorption and not simply demineralization.

The major actions of PTH on the kidneys are the simultaneous reduced reabsorption of sodium, phosphorus, calcium, and bicarbonate ions in the proximal tubule and the enhanced reabsorption of calcium at the distal tubule. The net effect is a rise in serum calcium concentration, phosphaturia, and mild metabolic acidosis. The action of PTH in kidney and bone is mediated through the stimulation of adenyl cyclase activity, which ultimately leads to enhanced cyclic AMP production. These effects precede and presumably mediate changes in phosphorus and calcium transport in kidney and in bone.

The effect of PTH on intestinal absorption of dietary calcium is indirect. PTH stimulates the renal synthesis of the active vitamin D metabolite, 1,25-$(OH)_2D_3$, which, in turn, acts as a regulator of intestinal calcium absorption.

Vitamin D Compounds

Vitamin D is a generic designation for a group of fat-soluble, structurally similar sterols, several of which are vitally important in calcium and phosphorus metabolism. Some of these sterols appropriately are termed provitamins because they can be transformed into physiologically active compounds by irradiation with ultraviolet light. The two most important vitamins are vitamin D_2, or ergosterol, and vitamin D_3, or cholecalciferol. Ergocalciferol is present in yeast and a variety of plant substances and can be transformed into the antirachitic ergocalciferol by irradiation. Ergocalciferol is the active vitamin D in various commercial vitamin preparations and in irradiated bread. Cholecalciferol, in contrast, is found in certain animal tissues and products, particularly fish livers, the livers of fish-eating mammals, and irradiated milk. Approximately 94% of the vitamins D_2 and D_3 in plasma are bound to serum alpha globulin, which has a molecular mass of 60,000 daltons. Excess vitamin D can be stored in tissues, metabolized to inactive products, or excreted in the bile. One reduction product, dihydrotachysterol, is formed from either ergocalciferol or cholecalciferol and has therapeutic uses.

In addition to dietary sources, cholecalciferol is synthesized in the skin by ultraviolet irradiation of 7-dehydrocholesterol. Cholecalciferol is transported to the liver, where it undergoes hydroxylation to produce 25-hydroxycholecalciferol (25-$[OH]D_3$). Although 25-$(OH)D_3$ has limited biological activity, it is the major circulating metabolite of vitamin D_3. In the kidney, 25-$(OH)D_3$ undergoes further hydroxylation to form dihydroxy metabolites 1,25-$(OH)_2D_3$, 23,25-$(OH)_2D_3$, and 24,25-$(OH)_2D_3$. The 23-metabolite is biologically inert, and its function is still unknown. It undergoes further oxidation to form 26-lactone. The 24-hydroxylation is induced under circumstances when 1-hydroxylation is suppressed. It is believed that the formation of the 24-metabolite is the initial event in the inactivation of vitamin D (DeLuca, 1988).

The production of 1,25-$(OH)_2D_3$ is regulated by a negative feedback mechanism depending on the need for calcium and phosphorus in the circulation. Decreased blood calcium stimulates the parathyroid glands to secrete PTH, which, in turn, increases production of 1,25-$(OH)_2D_3$ in the renal proximal tubules. Conversely, a rise in blood calcium suppresses PTH secretion, which lowers the production of 1,25-$(OH)_2D_3$. Although PTH is required for the mobilization of calcium from bone and for the renal conservation of calcium, stimulation of intestinal reabsorption of calcium is achieved by 1,25-$(OH)_2D_3$ independently of PTH. The ability of the vitamin D hormone to facilitate calcium transport across the intestinal membrane provides a successful means of administering exogenous vitamin D hormone and adequate dietary calcium to patients with hyperparathyroidism and pseudohypoparathyroidism. Administration of the vitamin D hormone has also been shown to be effective in the therapeutic management and prevention of postmenopausal and age-related osteoporosis. Production of 1,25-$(OH)_2D_3$ is also stimulated by hypophosphatemia.

The demonstration that the locations of 1,25-$(OH)_2D_3$ are not limited to its target tissues, namely the intestine, bone, and kidney, has expanded the therapeutic function of vitamin D. There is evidence that besides its calciotropic properties, vitamin D may also be a developmental hormone with differentiative activity. The therapeutic usefulness of 1,25-$(OH)_2D_3$ in treating psoriasis, female reproduction, and certain malignant diseases is entirely possible if the hypercalcemic activity can be suppressed. The development of analogues of vitamin D compounds to achieve such properties has been reported (DeLuca, 1992).

Calcitonin

Calcitonin (CT) is a peptide hormone produced and secreted by specialized C cells (parafollicular cells) in the lateral lobes of the thyroid gland. Circulating immunoreactive CT is derived from a larger precursor and the monomeric form is the only biologically active entity. CT monomer is a 32 amino acid peptide with a molecular mass of 3500 daltons. Structural differences in the hormone among humans, rats, cows, pigs, and salmon are reflected in differences in their relative potency. Response of CT to calcium infusion, which is a measure of the secretory capacity, does not appear to change with age. Postmenopausal osteoporosis is not associated with CT deficiency. C cell response to a hypercalcemic stimulus to elicit basal or stimulated CT secretion is poor in primary hyperparathyroidism but is significant in tumor-induced hypercalcemia (Body, 1993).

Although CT was viewed as a major calcium-regulating factor because of its calcium-lowering and phosphorus-lowering properties, its precise physiologic role is unknown. In humans, it plays a minor role in calcium homeostasis. Serum calcium does not appear to be affected by either total thyroidectomy or inappropriately high levels of CT as in medullary thyroid carcinoma. Secretion of CT is stimulated by an increase in ionic calcium concentration.

The pharmacologic action of CT is more definitive. By inhibiting osteoclastic bone resorption, CT causes a decrease in urinary excretion of hydroxyproline. The administration of CT decreases renal tubular resorption of calcium and phosphorus, as well as sodium, potassium, and magnesium. CT decreases gastrin and gastric acid secretion and increases small bowel secretion of sodium, potassium, chloride, and water. CT administered nasally may have value both in the long-term treatment of Paget's disease and osteoporosis and in the short-term treatment of hypercalcemia of malignancy.

Biochemical Markers of Bone Turnover

Although bone metabolic homeostasis is regulated by hormones and other mediators, they do not reflect the metabolic changes in diseased bone tissues. Three major diagnostic procedures are available for the evaluation of metabolic bone diseases: bone density, bone biopsy, and the biochemical markers of bone turnover. Bone density does not provide information on the dynamics of bone formation and bone resorption. Although bone biopsy allows such assessment, it is an invasive procedure and is not amenable to routine patient management of osteoporosis. Because of its noninvasive nature, the laboratory assessment of biochemical markers to investigate bone diseases, particularly osteoporosis, has been the focus of much attention in recent years. Because the abnormality of bone formation and bone resorption leading to bone loss in osteoporosis is subtle, the conventional markers, such as calcium and PTH, are usually normal.

Bone metabolism is characterized by two opposing activities, the formation of new bone by osteoblasts and the resorption of old bone by osteoclasts (Manolagas, 1995). Bone formation may be assessed with the measurement of serum bone-specific alkaline phosphatase, osteocalcin, and type I collagen extension peptides, whereas bone resorption may be recognized with the determination of urinary hydroxyproline, urinary pyridinium cross-links, pyridinoline (Pyr) and deoxypyridinoline (D-pyr), and serum tartrate–resistant acid phosphatase activity. These markers have unequal sensitivity and specificity toward different bone disease states, and some have not been fully investigated and characterized in terms of their metabolic clearance and their technique of measurement. Thus, their clinical significance in the diagnosis and monitoring of therapy of bone diseases is not fully established.

OSTEOCALCIN. Osteocalcin (OC) is a noncollagenous vitamin K–dependent 49 amino acid protein. It is synthesized by osteoblasts and incorporated into the bone matrix, but a fragment of the newly synthesized molecule is released into the circulation, where it can be measured by immunoassay. It is measured in serum as an indicator of osteoblastic activity and metabolic turnover in bone. Assays for OC are available using radiolabeled, enzyme-labeled, or chemiluminescent-labeled immunoassays with monoclonal or polyclonal antibodies, and are used widely in many clinical settings. Increased OC is associated with primary hyperparathyroidism (PHPT), Paget's disease, chronic renal failure, and some cases of osteoporosis, whereas decreased OC is found in pregnancy and in glucocorticoid treatment. Nonetheless, major discrepancies have been reported in OC results between laboratories and between kits that failed to be resolved even with use of common reference materials. Immunoheterogeneity of the OC molecule and strong dependence of the assays on calcium concentration have been suggested as possible causes (Masters, 1994). Degradation of OC with storage during preanalytical sample handling was also cited as a possible source of variation. In most cases, however, serum OC appears to be a valid marker of bone turnover when resorption and formation are coupled and a specific marker of bone formation whenever formation and resorption are uncoupled (Delmas, 1993).

ALKALINE PHOSPHATASE. Because of the hepatic isoenzyme, measurement of total alkaline phosphatase ALP lacks sensitivity and specificity for the investigation of osteoporosis. The bone-specific fraction of ALP (B-ALP) can be separated and determined with use of heat, activators, inhibitors, and electrophoresis, but most procedures are tedious and nonspecific. An immunoradiometric monoclonal assay that is specific for B-ALP has been developed (Garnero, 1993). This assay has a low cross-reactivity with liver isoenzyme, giving specific and direct measurement of B-ALP.

B-ALP increases with age, demonstrating an age-related increase of bone turnover. B-ALP is also increased in Paget's disease, PHPT and chronic renal failure. Decreased B-ALP is associated with treatment of bisphosphonate pamidronate reflecting decreased bone remodeling, suggesting that B-ALP may be a sensitive marker of bone formation for the investigation of osteoporosis.

PROCOLLAGEN I EXTENSION PEPTIDES. Type I collagen is a major component of bone accounting for $>90\%$ of bone matrix protein content. During extracellular processing, some peptide fragments of type I collagen are cleaved in the circulation; its serum concentration may thus correlate with the rate of bone formation. Radioimmunoassays for procollagen I extension peptides (PCIEP) are now available. However, one study reported poor correlation of PCIEP with serum OC and B-ALP in several metabolic bone diseases. This may be due to nonspecificity arising from variable uptake by the liver. Lack of specificity may be another limitation because PCIEP represents all procollagen peptides released from other sites in addition to bone (Linkhart, 1993).

URINARY HYDROXYPROLINE. Found mainly in collagen, urinary hydroxyproline (HP) represents about 13% of the amino acid content. It is considered to be a marker for bone resorption because 50% of human collagen resides in bone. However, about 90% of HP released during collagen breakdown is metabolized in the liver. Thus, urinary HP represents only 10% of total collagen catabolism. Not surprisingly, it correlates poorly with bone resorption, as determined by bone histomorphometry and by calcium kinetics (Delmas, 1993).

URINARY HYDROXYLYSINE GLYCOSIDES. Derived mostly from type I collagen of bone, urinary hydroxylysine glycosides (HYLG) is present in part as galactosylhydroxylysine and in part as glucosylgalactosyl hydroxylysine. The relative ratio of HYLGs released differs in bone and soft tissue. They are more specific than hydroxyproline and thus may be a potential marker for osteoporosis. It is presently limited by its HPLC assay technology, which is not amenable to rapid and batch analysis.

URINARY PYRIDINIUM CROSS-LINKS. Urinary pyridinoline (Pyr) and deoxypyridinoline (D-Pyr) are nonreducible cross-links that stabilize the collagen chain within the extracellular matrix. They may be the most sensitive and specific new markers of bone resorption. The relative ratio of Pyr and D-Pyr in human bone is 2:3. Available data suggest that they are excreted in urine in free form (40%) and in peptide-bound form (60%). D-Pyr is reported to be strongly correlated with bone turnover when compared with calcium kinetics and with bone histomorphometry. Both urinary Pyr and D-Pyr appear to be more sensitive than hydroxyproline in the assessment of the extent of bone involvement in Paget's disease of bone, in PHPT, and in humoral hypercalcemia of malignancy, with decreased values in response to treatment. Urinary Pyr and D-Pyr are also elevated in osteomalacia and in hyperthyroidism (Delmas, 1993).

Presently, HPLC assay is the method in use, but more convenient immunoassays with specific antibodies are emerging.

Clinicopathologic Correlations

In the last two decades, the detection of hypercalcemia has been greatly facilitated by the inclusion of a calcium determination in most automated multichannel chemistry screen and panel testing. Although the differential diagnosis of hypercalcemia has now expanded to over 25 disease states (Lafferty, 1991), PHPT and malignancy account for 80–90% of the hypercalcemic patients. Malignancy is the most frequent cause of hypercalcemia in the hospital inpatient population, and PHPT is the major cause of calcium elevation in ambulatory patients. Some of the more frequently occurring diseases affecting calcium and phosphorus metabolism are shown in Table 8–5.

It is noteworthy that dietary inadequacies of calcium and phosphorus are seldom the cause of significant metabolic derangements. The high phosphate content of cow's milk can result in deficient calcium absorption and tetany in the newborn. Other factors incriminated in neonatal hypocalcemia include prematurity, vitamin D deficiency, transient physiologic hypoparathyroidism, and decreased ability of the kidneys to excrete inorganic phosphate. A rare dietary problem affecting calcium and phosphorus metabolism is vitamin D intoxication, which is usually the result of excessive intake of vitamin supplements over a prolonged period of time. Large amounts of vitamin D can be stored in the body, because it is fat soluble. Clinically, vitamin D intoxication is manifested by weakness, irritability, nausea, vomiting, and diarrhea. Plasma calcium concentration is typically elevated, whereas the level of inorganic phosphorus is variable. The hypercalcemia is the result of both increased intestinal absorption of calcium and increased mobilization from bone. Metastatic calcification of soft tissues and viscera, compromised renal function with frank azotemia, and osteoporosis can occur.

Useful laboratory measurements have expanded to encompass not only serum total calcium, ionized calcium, phosphorus, alkaline phosphatase, urinary calcium, and phosphorus but also intact serum PTH, 25-$(OH)D_3$, 1,25-$(OH)_2D_3$, chloride, and cyclic AMP. Ionized calcium determinations are increasingly available now. Determination of various

Table 8–5. TYPICAL CHEMICAL PATHOLOGIC FINDINGS IN METABOLIC BONE DISEASES

	Serum				Urine	
Disease	Ca^{2+}	HPO_4^-	*PTH*	*Alkaline Phosphatase*	Ca^{++}	$H_2PO_4^-$
Primary hyperparathyroidism	↑	↓	↑	N, ↑	↑	↑
Renal osteodystrophy	↓, N	↑	↑	↑	↓	↓
Vitamin D deficiency (rickets or osteomalacia)	N, ↓	↓	↑	↑	↓	↑
Hypoparathyroidism	↓	↑	↓	N	↓	↓
Pseudohypoparathyroidism	↓	↑	↑	N	↓	↓
Vitamin D–resistant rickets	N, ↓	↓	N, ↑	↑	↓	↑
Renal tubular acidosis	N, ↓	↓	N, ↑	↑	↑	↑
Fanconi's syndrome	N, ↓	↓	N, ↑	↑	↑	↑
Idiopathic osteoporosis	N	N	N, ↑	N	N, ↑	N
Paget's disease	N, ↑	N	N	↑	N, ↑	N
Hypophosphatasia	N, ↑	N	—	↓↓	N	N
Vitamin D intoxication	↑	N, ↕	↓	N	↑	↑
Fibrous dysplasia	N	N	N	↑	N	N
Osteogenesis imperfecta	N	N	—	N	N	N
Osteopetrosis	N	N	—	N	↓	N

↑ = increase; N = normal; ↕ = increase or decrease; ↓ = decrease; ↓↓ = great decrease.

2

other analytes can provide valuable information in selected cases—e.g., growth hormone, cortisol, vitamin D metabolites, and urinary hydroxyproline. Meaningful interpretation of the relevant laboratory data often requires various special studies in addition to a complete history and physical examination. Abstinence from thiazides, large doses of vitamin A, vitamin D, lithium, or theophylline must be observed before undertaking specialized testing. Patient immobilization should be noted. A history of tuberculosis or fungal infection should also be identified. Familial hypocalciuria hypercalcemia or multiple endocrine neoplasms should be ruled out. Roentgenographic examinations can also provide valuable information regarding both the etiology and extent of disease. Renal function tests and studies of acid-base balance may be indicated. Histopathologic examination of bone biopsy specimens from appropriate sites such as the iliac crest in generalized bone disease or directly from localized lesions can be of unique value in selected cases.

Parathyroid Diseases

PHPT is characterized by excessive secretion of PTH in the absence of an appropriate physiologic stimulus. The availability of automated chemical screening testing that includes calcium determination has helped in establishing PHPT as a relatively common often asymptomatic disease of persistent hypersecretion of PTH coexisting with chronic hypercalcemia. Current perspective has replaced the pre-1960s concept of characterizing PHPT based on kidney stones, bone loss, bone fracture, and ectopic calcification. Approximately 100,000 cases of PHPT occur each year in the United States, and the incidence increases with age. The disease affects women twice as frequently as it affects men. Single parathyroid adenomas account for the majority of cases of PHPT. Other causes include multiple adenomas, hyperplasia, and rarely carcinoma. Hypercalcemia in PHPT is characteristically associated with decreased serum phosphorus due to PTH-induced phosphate diuresis and is frequently accompanied by mild acidosis from decreased renal reabsorption of bicarbonate. The hypercalcemia is attributed to (1) the direct action of PTH on bone to cause increased resorption, (2) PTH-activated renal tubular reabsorption, and (3) PTH-stimulated increased renal biosynthesis of 1,25-$(OH)_2D_3$, which increases intestinal absorption of calcium (Boden, 1990). Clues leading to the diagnosis of PHPT include kidney stones, chronic constipation, mental depression, neuromuscular dysfunction, recurrent pancreatitis, peptic ulcer, and unexplained or premature osteopenia (Deftos, 1993).

A test in which the total calcium level exceeds the upper reference limit should always be repeated. Ionized calcium is preferred especially in patients with abnormal concentrations of total serum proteins or albumin. Confirmatory tests to follow should include fasting serum phosphorus and PTH determination. Serum phosphorus is not a reliable marker in the diagnosis of PHPT because its concentration is diet dependent. Studies have also shown that fewer than 50% of PHPT patients had serum phosphorus below the reference interval (Kao, 1992). Detection of excessive phosphate diuresis is sometimes helpful in distinguishing PHPT from other etiologies of hypercalcemia. This can be achieved by determining the tubular reabsorption of phosphate (TRP) or the renal phosphate clearance (C_p). The TRP is normally 80% to 90%, whereas the C_p is normally 5 to 15 mL/min. In hyperparathyroidism, the TRP is usually less than 78%, whereas the C_p is greater than 18 mL/min. The TRP is not applicable even in mild azotemia. Reliable PTH assays now include measurements for the carboxy-terminal fragments, midregion molecule, and intact PTH. Although all these assays are useful for diagnosing hyperparathyroidism, the use of intact PTH assay is preferred in patients with renal disease, because carboxy-terminal fragments accumulate with decreased renal function. Because of overlap in PTH values between patients with hyperparathyroidism and healthy individuals particularly in carboxy-terminal assays, serum PTH values obtained may not differentiate between the two groups. This discrepancy is resolved in most cases, however, when serum PTH values are compared with plasma ionized calcium concentrations. The discrimination is made on the basis that, in a healthy individual, serum calcium concentration bears an inverse relationship to the PTH concentration. Thus, although the serum PTH values may be within the reference range for patients with PHPT, this level is inappropriately high when it is coexistent with hypercalcemia. Hence, the demonstration of detectable amounts of circulating PTH in the presence of elevated calcium is strongly indicative of PHPT.

The definitive treatment of patients with signs and symptoms of PHPT is always surgery. Although preoperative localization of the abnormal gland is superior, the use of preoperative imaging technique on computer-enhanced densitometry for evaluating skeletal status is emerging and spreading as the accuracy continues to improve. Conversely, management for patients with asymptomatic PHPT is far from unanimous, and medical nonsurgical surveillance is considered justified for asymptomatic patients with mild hypercalcemia and with normal renal and bone status. A unified protocol in the diagnosis and management of asymptomatic PHPT is being formulated (Deftos, 1993).

PTH elevation in hyperparathyroidism may result in dramatically increased bone resorption leading to osteitis fibrosa cystica. These extensive fibroblastic proliferations occur in the marrow spaces and can cause cystic lesions. Bone pain, skeletal deformities, and fractures can result.

Secondary hyperparathyroidism is characterized by an appropriately excessive secretion of PTH in response to chronic hypocalcemia. In the United States and Europe, most cases of chronic hypocalcemia are the result of either vitamin D deficiency or renal disease; hypocalcemia is rarely caused by an inadequate dietary intake of calcium. Vitamin D deficiency leads to decreased absorption of both calcium and phosphate, so that both the serum calcium and inorganic phosphorus are low. Increased PTH secretion tends to increase calcium concentration toward normal but suppress inorganic phosphorus even further because of the increased renal loss of phosphate under the influence of PTH (see Table 8–5).

Chronic renal failure can result in compensatory hyperparathyroidism, which, in turn, causes diffuse bone disease, including osteoporosis, osteomalacia, osteosclerosis (areas of increased bone density), osteitis fibrosa cystica, and metastatic calcification. The disease complex is sometimes termed renal osteodystrophy or, when it occurs in children, renal rickets. The bone manifestations of chronic renal disease are seen more often now that life is prolonged with maintenance hemodialysis. The interrelationships in hyperparathyroidism secondary to chronic renal disease are very complex, as shown in Figure 8–5. The pathogenesis varies somewhat, depending on the nature and severity of the renal disease. Decreased renal excretion of phosphate as a consequence of impaired glomerular filtration is paramount. Diminished responsiveness to vitamin D and probably decreased renal biosynthesis of 1,25-$(OH)_2D_3$ are also important. The effectiveness of PTH is compromised by the functional deficiency of vitamin D and the inability of the renal tubules to respond with a phosphate diuresis. Increased fecal loss of calcium also occurs. There is evidence that normal calcification is impeded by circulating inhibitors.

Hypoparathyroidism is usually the result of parathyroidectomy, frequently as an unintentional consequence of thyroidectomy. Uncommonly it can result from an idiopathic lack of parathyroid function. Lack of parathyroid hormone from whatever cause leads to a fall in plasma calcium and a corresponding rise in plasma inorganic phosphorus concentration. The biosynthesis of 1,25-$(OH)_2D_3$ can be impaired as a result of PTH deficiency and perhaps also hyperphosphatemia. The most important clinical manifestations are directly attributable to decreased ionized calcium concentrations, which can cause increased neuromuscular excitability and tetany.

Pseudohypoparathyroidism (PHP) is a rare genetic disorder characterized by signs and symptoms of hypoparathyroidism. It is, however, distinguishable from true hypoparathyroidism in that serum calcium concentration is low despite an increased concentration of serum PTH. Moreover, whereas infusion of PTH into patients with hypoparathyroidism generally results in a marked increase in both urinary cyclic AMP and phosphaturia, patients with PHP usually respond with subnormal urinary phosphate excretion and cyclic

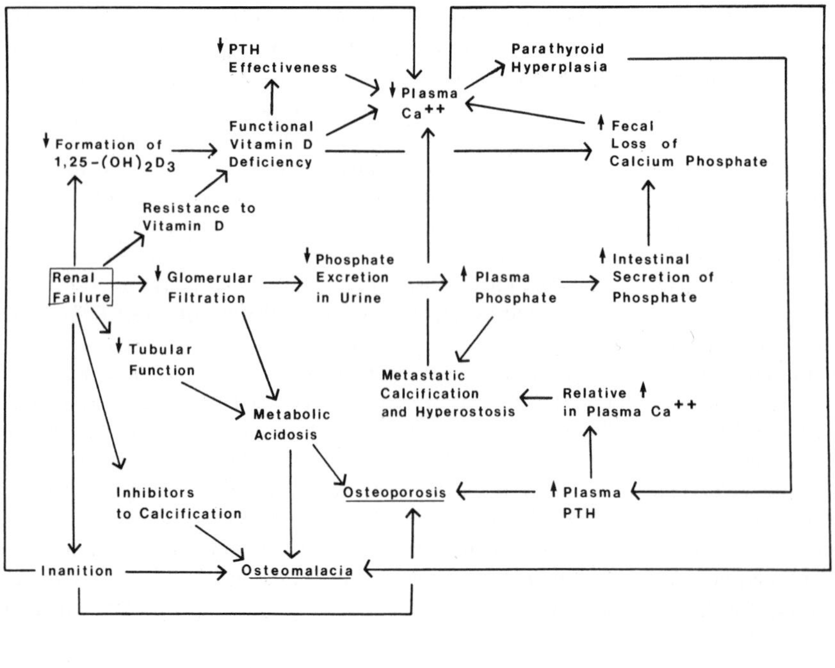

Figure 8–5. Pathophysiologic interrelationships in hyperparathyroidism associated with chronic renal disease.

AMP production. This is due to a defect in the stimulatory G protein of adenylate cyclase that is necessary for the action of PTH. Pseudo-pseudohypoparathyroidism (PPHP) is a related genetic variant, which differs from PHP in its lack of PTH resistance; thus patients with PPHP are normocalcemic. Both PHP and PPHP patients exhibit characteristic phenotypic abnormalities, which include round face, short stature, and possibly mental retardation (Trueb, 1993).

Malignancy-Associated Hypercalcemia

First described in 1921, malignancy-associated hypercalcemia MAHC can be divided into two main subtypes. The first category of calcium elevation, known as local osteolytic hypercalcemia, occurs in the presence of bone metastases or a primary hematologic malignancy that is caused by local paracrine factors mediating accelerated bone resorption. The tumors involved are typically multiple myeloma, breast carcinoma, or lymphoma. The second subtype of hypercalcemia, known as humoral hypercalcemia of malignancy (HHM), occurs in patients without bony metastases, in whom the tumor produces a humoral factor that acts on the skeleton to promote bone resorption and on the kidney to inhibit calcium excretion. HHM associated also with pain and pathologic fractures is frequently found in patients with squamous cell carcinoma of the lung and other epithelial cancers, including prostate, breast and renal cortical carcinoma; other sources of bone metastases include pancreas, gastrointestinal, genitourinary, liver, thyroid, and melanoma. The prevalence of HHM in malignancy is up to 80%.

The humoral factor that causes the distal calcium-mobilizing effect in HHM was first thought to be PTH itself or a PTH-related humoral agent, and the term pseudohyperparathyroidism was formerly used to describe patients with HHM. It is now recognized that PTH-related protein (PTHrP), secreted mainly from solid tumors, is responsible for the hypercalcemia mediated primarily via an increased renal reabsorption of calcium and secondarily by bone resorption. This protein has since been isolated, structurally sequenced, and cloned (Burtis, 1992). Biochemically, HHM is characterized by hypercalcemia, hypophosphatemia, increased nephrogenous cAMP excretion, and suppressed intact PTH and 1,25-$(OH)_2D_3$ levels. The partial resemblance of the HHM profile to PHPT, that is, hypercalcemia, hypophosphatemia and elevated nephrogenous cAMP excretion, may be explained by the N-terminal sequence homology of PTHrP to PTH. However, bone histomorphometry studies in HHM patients show markedly increased osteoclastic bone resorption with suppressed osteoblastic bone formation, which stands in vivid contrast to the coupled resorption and formation observed in PHPT. The suppressed intact PTH and 1,25-$(OH)_2D_3$ in HHM are consistent with decreased reabsorption of calcium and increased calcium excretion. The suppressed bone formation explains the typically severe hypercalcemia found in patients with HHM (Wysolmerski, 1994). Reports of chronic myeloid leukemia complicated by hypercalcemia have also been attributed to the presence of PTHrP (Seymour, 1993). Furthermore, PTHrP has been detected immunohistochemically in normal adult and fetal tissues and organs, including the keratinocytes, placenta, and fetal parathyroid gland. The recently improved immunoassay technology may solidify the role of PTHrP in the differential diagnosis and therapy of hypercalcemia, as well as defining its possible physiologic and endocrine function in the fetus (Birkeland, 1992).

The discriminatory immunoassays now available for intact PTH, which is low or low normal in HHM but high or high normal in PHPT, are useful tools for the differential diagnosis of PHP and HHM. Nevertheless, it may still be equivocal at times because intact PTH may not be elevated in all patients with PHPT, thus the lack of intact PTH elevation may not always rule out PHPT. Although not definitive, the presence of elevated chloride and 1,25-$(OH)_2D_3$ also favors PHPT over HHM. The most specific confirmatory test is the determination PTHrP, which allows the differentiation of not only HHM from PHP but also other hypercalcemic states in which serum PTH is suppressed. Several PTHrP assays of good specificity are now available commercially.

2

Bone Disease

Most of the body content of calcium and phosphorus is present in bone as a highly structured crystal lattice similar to hydroxyapatite, the general formula of which is $Ca_{10}(PO_4)_6(OH)_2$. Bone minerals also include 70% of the body content of magnesium; 30% of the sodium; and smaller amounts of potassium, carbonate, citrate, and fluoride. The dry weight of compact bone consists of approximately 75% inorganic mineral salts and 25% organic matrix, as shown in Table 8–6. Mineralization of bone matrix is not a simple precipitation of salts but rather is a complex, incompletely understood physicochemical process (Parfitt, 1976). In previous times, the importance to bone mineralization of the solubility product of calcium phosphate, $Ca^{2+} \times HPO_4^{2-}$, was emphasized. Although the initial salt that is formed may well be $CaHPO_4$, the solubility product explanation is overly simplistic, particularly because extracellular fluid is supersaturated with these ions.

Even in adult life, bone is in a dynamic state, as evidenced by the fact that perhaps 3% to 5% of the bone mass is undergoing active remodeling at any one time. The processes of bone formation and resorption with remodeling continuously during adulthood are controlled by various hormonal and metabolic influences (Deftos, 1975) and local factors (Manolagas, 1995). Bone is formed by the action of osteoblasts, the activity of which is reflected in the alkaline phosphatase level in serum. Bone resorption occurs predominantly as a result of

Table 8–6. COMPOSITION OF BONE

Mineral inorganic crystalline salts (75% of dry weight)	Phosphate and carbonate salts of calcium (compressional strength) Small amounts of magnesium, sodium, potassium, hydroxide, fluoride, and sulfate
Organic matrix (25% of dry weight)	94% collagen fibers (tensile strength) (hydroxyproline and proline constitute a third of total amino acid composition of collagen fibrils) 5% ground substance: Extracellular fluid Mucoprotein Chondroitin sulfate Hyaluronic acid 1% citrate

Table 8–7. ELEVATION OF URINARY HYDROXYPROLINE IN DISEASE

Marked
Paget's disease
Fibrous dysplasia
Osteomalacia
Neoplastic bone disease
Rickets
Hyperthyroidism
Hyperparathyroidism (primary and secondary)
Severe burns
Acute osteomyelitis
Congenital hypophosphatasia
Moderate
Acromegaly
Marfan's syndrome
Active rheumatoid arthritis
Active scleroderma
Normal to slight
Inflammatory skin diseases
Osteoporosis
Pregnancy
Aseptic bone necrosis
Diabetes mellitus
Renal disease

From Niejadlik DC: Postgrad. med., *51*(no. 5):214, 1972.

Table 8–8. ETIOLOGIC CLASSIFICATION OF OSTEOPOROSIS

Primary (idiopathic, postmenopausal, and senile)
Secondary
Hyperparathyroidism
Cushing's syndrome
Hyperthyroidism
Acromegaly
Heparin therapy (prolonged high dosage)
Vitamin D excess
Immobilization
Pregnancy (rare cause)
Miscellaneous (diabetes, liver disease, sickle cell anemia, various lipid or carbohydrate storage diseases)

the action of osteoclasts and ordinarily involves dissolution of both minerals and organic matrix. The urinary excretion of hydroxyproline is elevated in association with increased bone resorption, as it is in other etiologies of increased collagen turnover (Table 8–7). This is a result of the fact that collagen is the only mammalian protein that contains significant amounts of hydroxyproline.

Osteoporosis is the most common metabolic disease of bone. It is not a single etiologic entity but rather is associated with a variety of epidemiologic, clinical, and biochemical factors that result in decreased bone mass. The term bone atrophy is sometimes applied to this pathologic process, but this term is imprecise because osteoporosis can occur as a consequence of increased bone resorption, decreased bone formation, or a combination of both factors. Normal mineralization of existing osteoid is a critical feature that distinguishes osteoporosis from osteomalacia. The roentgenographic appearance of diffusely diminished bone density is reflected in the histopathologic appearance of thinned bone cortices and delicate trabeculae. Skeletal deformities; fractures, especially compression fractures of the vertebral bodies; and bone pain are common sequelae.

The various etiologies of osteoporosis are shown in Table 8–8. The most common types by far include postmenopausal and senile osteoporosis. Manolagas (1995) has emphasized that osteoporosis is a reduction in skeletal mass caused by an imbalance between bone resorption (osteoclasts) and bone formation (osteoblasts) related to bone marrow. Postmenopausal bone loss appears to be associated with excessive osteoclastic activity while bone loss that accompanies aging appears to be associated with a progressive decline in the supply or number of osteoblasts in proportion to demand for them. Furthermore, postmenopausal bone loss occurs primarily in trabecular bone, whereas the aging-associated bone loss primarily affects cortical bone (Manolagas, 1995). There are various theories as to other etiologic or contributory factors in senile osteoporosis, including diminished physical activity, deficiency of gonadal hormones, and dietary inadequacies. Urinary calcium and hydroxyproline excretions are frequently increased. Other parameters of calcium and phosphorus metabolism are usually normal. In contrast, both calcium and inorganic phosphate in plasma can be elevated in rapidly developing osteoporosis of disuse, such as occurs following immobilization or paralysis in a previously active individual.

Osteomalacia refers to deficient mineralization of bone resulting from various disturbances in calcium and phosphorus metabolism. Osteoid formation continues, but the bones become softened. Weakness, skeletal pain and deformities, and fractures can occur as the disease progresses. Roentgenographic examination reveals generalized rarefaction of the skeleton with an accentuated trabecular pattern. Rickets is the designation for osteomalacia that occurs prior to cessation of growth, that is, closure of the epiphyses of bones. The skeletal deformities in rickets are accentuated as a consequence of compensatory overgrowth of epiphyseal cartilage, wide bands of which remain unmineralized and unresorbed. In severe cases of rickets, decreased growth can be associated with such evident deformities as swellings of the costochondral junctions of the ribs (rachitic rosary), a protuberant sternum, frontal bossing, and delayed closure of the anterior fontanelle.

There are various etiologies of osteomalacia. Vitamin D deficiency is particularly important in childhood and can be caused by inadequate dietary intake, intestinal malabsorption, or diminished synthesis of active metabolites as a consequence of inadequate exposure to sunlight. Dietary deficiency is very uncommon in the United States because of the widespread use of fortified milk and bread and vitamin supplements. When vitamin D deficiency occurs in adults, it is usually a consequence of malabsorption. Because vitamin D is a fat-soluble vitamin, its absorption is impaired in sprue, biliary or pancreatic disease, or steatorrhea from other causes. A systemic resistance to vitamin D can be of major importance in the osteomalacia that accompanies chronic renal disease. Dietary inadequacy of calcium is a rare cause of osteomalacia, whereas dietary deficiencies of phosphorus do not occur. Increased loss of inorganic phosphorus in the urine occurs in various renal tubular disorders and can result in osteomalacia. These diseases include vitamin D–resistant rickets (phosphate diabetes), renal tubular acidosis, and Fanconi's syndrome.

A rare cause of osteomalacia is hypophosphatasia, an inherited autosomal recessive disease characterized by a significant depression of alkaline phosphatase in both plasma and tissues. Concentrations of calcium and phosphorus in plasma are normal or increased. Urinary excretion of hydroxyproline is decreased. A curious finding is the presence of significant amounts of phosphoethanolamine in urine.

It is not currently possible to designate a common denominator in the pathogenesis of osteomalacia. Formerly, the criticality of the solubility product of calcium phosphate, $Ca^{2+} \times HPO_4^{2-}$, was emphasized. In chronic renal disease, however, osteomalacia can progress in the presence of a normal or even elevated solubility product. Other etiologies, including vitamin D deficiency, can cause severe osteomalacia in the presence of normal or only slightly decreased serum calcium concentration. Phosphate depletion is probably of greater importance than decreased calcium.

Osteitis deformans, or Paget's disease of bone, is a disorder of varying severity, which can involve only one bone or be more or less generalized. Osteoclastic resorption of bone; extensive production of abnormal, poorly mineralized osteoid; and fibrous tissue proliferation result in bone that is structurally weak and prone to deformities and fractures. Osteogenic sarcoma is a late complication in a small percentage of cases. Serum calcium and inorganic phosphorus concentrations are usually normal but occasionally are elevated. Of particular significance is the greatly elevated alkaline phosphatase activity in plasma, which reflects the active but pathologic osteoblastic proliferation. Urinary excretion of calcium and phosphorus is normal or increased, whereas excretion of hydroxyproline is usually significantly increased. Osteitis deformans frequently responds both clinically and pathologically to therapeutic administration of CT (calcitonin).

Renal Diseases

Chronic renal failure, discussed previously as an important etiology of secondary hyperparathyroidism, is by far the most important renal disease affecting calcium and phosphorus metabolism. In addition, however, several uncommon or rare renal tubular defects can significantly affect calcium and phosphorus metabolism.

Vitamin D–resistant rickets, also termed familial hypophosphatemia and phosphate diabetes, is inherited, usually as a sex-linked dominant character. The exact pathogenesis of the disease is not known with certainty but is believed to be a primary defect in the ability of the renal tubules to reabsorb inorganic phosphorus. Renal phosphate clearance is definitely increased and accounts for the associated hypophosphatemia. Plasma calcium concentration is usually normal, whereas alkaline phosphatase is moderately elevated. The disease can be asymptomatic or manifested by severe osteomalacia or rickets and growth retardation. The disease can be treated with some success using dietary phosphorus supplementation and high doses of vitamin D.

Renal tubular acidosis consists of both inherited and acquired conditions having in common a metabolic acidosis resulting from decreased ability of the renal tubules to secrete hydrogen ions. The defect can involve primarily either the proximal or distal tubules. The disease inherited as an autosomal dominant trait and involving the distal tubules is of particular importance to calcium and phosphorus metabolism. Increased calcium excretion occurs, but plasma calcium concentration is usually normal, probably as a consequence of compensatory stimulation of the parathyroids to secrete PTH. Increased phosphate excretion typically leads to low plasma inorganic phosphorus. These factors lead to osteomalacia, which is aggravated by the systemic acidosis. Renal calculi are common sequelae.

The Fanconi syndrome consists of inherited renal diseases characterized by increased urinary excretion of phosphate, glucose, and amino acids; low plasma inorganic phosphorus; and systemic acidosis. Acquired diseases can have identical manifestations. The pathogenesis of the osteomalacia that develops is not well understood.

2

Calcitonin and Other Hormones

No essential physiologic role has yet been established for CT. The only known cause for excessive secretion of CT is medullary carcinoma of the thyroid, which originates from the parafollicular C cells. This neoplasm is frequently familial, and kindred of affected patients frequently have elevated levels of CT in their plasma (Dunn, 1993). The elevated levels of CT are associated with decreased skeletal remodeling, but there is no appreciable effect on plasma calcium and phosphorus. Other disease states associated with increased concentration of CT include the Zollinger-Ellison syndrome, pyknodysostosis, chronic hypocalcemia, carcinoid neoplasms, and nonthyroidal neoplasms such as breast cancer and oat cell and squamous cell carcinomas of the lung.

Hyperthyroidism is associated with hypercalciuria, hyperphosphatemia, elevated alkaline phosphatase activity, and occasionally hypercalcemia. There is marked increase in bone turnover and in skeletal remodeling. It is believed that thyroxine acts directly on bone to cause greater bone resorption than formation. This results in decreased PTH secretion, which accounts for the diminished activity of PTH and vitamin D.

The effect of growth hormone on skeletal growth has been revealed to be mediated indirectly via somatomedin. In adults, growth hormone is not necessary for the maintenance of mineral homeostasis. Growth hormone induces an increase in both intestinal absorption and renal reabsorption of calcium and phosphorus. Because of this positive balance with regard to skeletal mass, growth hormone has been proposed as a therapeutic agent for the treatment of osteoporosis.

Administration of glucocorticoids results in a decrease in both intestinal absorption and renal tubular reabsorption of calcium. Consequently, PTH secretion is stimulated and increased bone resorption occurs. Osteoporosis is indeed a prominent sign of Cushing's disease. However, the mode of action of cortisol, either in bone or in the intestine, is still unclear.

For postmenopausal women, estrogen is still the best therapy in the prevention of bone loss as well as in decreasing the incidence of vertebral and femoral fractures. Although estrogen is most frequently used alone or supplemented with calcium, progesterone is an additive to provide a more nearly physiologic milieu. Nonetheless such a combination may counteract the benefit of estrogen, such as the risk of cardiovascular diseases. The indication for estrogen treatment and its optimal time course still depend on individual factors such as age, medical history, cost, and potential side effects (Belchetz, 1994).

Analytical Techniques

Total Calcium

The oldest procedure for the determination of total serum calcium concentration is that of Clark and Collip. Calcium in serum is precipitated as calcium oxalate, which is subsequently redissolved with acidification. The resulting oxalic acid is titrated against potassium permanganate in a redox reaction, in which the purple $Mn_2O_7^{=}$ is reduced to the colorless Mn^{2+}. This method, although highly reliable and regarded for many years as the reference procedure, requires meticulous attention in order to achieve good accuracy and is time consuming. The Clark-Collip procedure has been replaced by the more convenient and accurate methods involving photometry, fluorometry, and atomic absorption spectrophotometry.

The first direct determination of serum calcium involved titration with the calcium-chelating agent ethylenediamine-tetra-acetic acid (EDTA), using a fluorescent indicator, calcein, to which calcium is complexed. Alternatively, the fluorometric determination of calcium-calcein complex provided a sensitive method for calcium determination that is suitable for pediatric specimens. However, this method is susceptible to interferences by copper, iron, zinc, and certain drugs such as sulfadiazine, heparin, and acetylsalicylic acid.

Attempts at determining serum calcium concentration by flame photometry have not met with much success because of positive interference by sodium and potassium, inhibitory interference by phosphates and sulfates, and the fact that excitation of the calcium atom itself is difficult. Isolation of calcium as the oxalate to eliminate interfering substances has not been successful because oxalate itself lowers the emission, probably as a result of the introduction of degradation products with low excitation potential.

With the advent of the automated analyzers, simple chemical methods for the determination of calcium based on color complex formation have found wide application. For example, color complex formation between calcium and *o*-cresolphthalein complex and its subsequent spectrophotometric quantitation is now the most popular automated method. In this procedure, 8-hydroxyquinoline is added to bind magnesium, which otherwise would cause interference. Other automated methods include color complex formation of calcium with alizarin, subsequent quantitation by spectrophotometry, and complex formation of calcium with Arsenazo III dye at pH 5.5. Under this condition, magnesium does not interfere with the reaction. The precision obtained with automated instruments is on the magnitude of $\pm 3-5\%$.

In terms of accuracy, precision, and speed, the determination of serum calcium concentration by atomic absorption spectrophotometry is undoubtedly the method of choice both for routine analysis and as a reference procedure. Calcium in serum and urine is diluted sufficiently with lanthanum chloride solution, which binds interfering substances such as protein and phosphates. When introduced into a flame, the dissociated free calcium atom absorbs light from the characteristic wavelengths (e.g., 422.7 nm) produced by a hollow cathode lamp with a calcium filament. A small fraction of calcium atoms (about 1/1000) is raised to a high energy level and, on returning to the ground state, emits radiation, the intensity of which is proportional to the calcium concentration in the sample. Precision achievable on standard instruments is about $\pm 3.5\%$. Serum calcium determination has been extensively reviewed by Robertson (1979).

In general, specimens for total calcium determination should be serum or heparinized plasma collected in the fasting state. Oxalate and EDTA interfere with most determinations, because the former causes precipitation and the latter results in chelation of calcium, thus rendering it unavailable for analysis. Total calcium concentrations are known to be affected also by prolonged venous occlusion and by posture. The former leads to hemoconcentration, thereby causing an increase in the calcium values; whereas patients in a recumbent posture have lower calcium concentrations. Both factors, however, appear to affect mainly the protein-bound fraction of the calcium concentration.

Ionized Calcium

A prerequisite for the determination of ionized calcium is that the equilibrium between ionized and protein-bound calcium in serum not be affected at all stages of the procedure. The development of a calcium ion selective electrode for the measurement of ionized calcium has largely replaced the earlier colorimetric methods that used the calcium-sensitive dyes murexide and tetramethyl murexide, because the ion-selective electrode technique offers speed, simplicity, and improved assay precision. Commercially available ionized calcium analyzers include: Orion (Cambridge, MA), Applied Medical Technology (Menlo Park, CA), Nova Biomedical (Newton, MA), and Radiometer (Copenhagen, Denmark). Although each differs in its ion selectivity characteristics, all appear to operate satisfactorily in serum and, in some cases, in blood and give moderately fast and fairly accurate ionized calcium results. Automated systems, consisting of a flow-through electrode with a liquid ion-exchange–impregnated membrane, permit simple and rapid determinations on relatively small sample volumes (0.15 to 0.5 mL) and are amenable to emergency response and performance. Assay time per sample ranged from 1.3 to 6 minutes. The between-run precision is generally within the range of 2% CV. The reference interval is about 1.0 to 1.2 mmol/L. It varies with different systems, with variations attributed to the selectivities of electrode and to sample preparation.

Because the ionized calcium fraction is pH dependent, the most important condition throughout the analysis is the maintenance of a constant pH. Unless the specimen aliquot is analyzed promptly on an instrument that permits re-equilibration of pH, blood collection and specimen handling procedures should be conducted anaerobically, and the red cells separated as soon as clotting is complete to obviate pH changes. Variations in serum ionized calcium concentration due to the effect of pH changes can be corrected for, provided that the values both at the time of collection of the blood sample and at the time of analysis are known. However, such a situation should be avoided because ionized calcium obtained in this manner may not reflect its *in vivo* condition. Hyperventilation sufficient to cause an increase of 0.1 to 0.2 pH unit of blood pH is known to produce up to a 10% reduction in ionized calcium concentration. It is therefore imperative that the state of ventilation be normal during sampling. Prolonged venous occlusion will influence the total serum calcium concentration if pH changes occur as a result.

Ionized calcium in serum is also temperature dependent, and measurement at 37°C is recommended. Although serum, plasma, and blood are all purported to be acceptable specimens for ionized calcium determination, common anticoagulants, e.g., heparin, EDTA, oxalate and citrate, have been shown to decrease ionized calcium concentration. However, the effect is insignificant if heparin of up to 15 IU/mL of blood is used in the specimen collection procedure (Forman, 1991). Because the ion-selective electrode responds to the presence of other ions in the sample, a serum or aqueous standard should contain ionic compositions of sodium and magnesium similar to those in the serum of healthy individuals.

Phosphorus

Most methods for phosphorus determination are based on the principle that under suitable conditions, molybdates react with phosphate to form various heteropoly compounds, such as ammonium phosphomolybdate, which is believed to have the formula $(NH_4)_3[PO_4(MoO_3)_{12}]$. Different techniques have been employed in the quantitation of this complex. An ultramicromethod has been described in which the phosphomolybdate is determined by acidimetric titration. Direct measurement of this complex at 340 nm is now adapted for use as an automated procedure. To improve assay sensitivity, the phosphomolybdate has also been extracted into xylene-isobutanol prior to spectrophotometric determination at 310 nm. However, most of the techniques for the determination of phosphorus involve photometric measurement of the molybdenum blue formed by reduction of phosphomolybdate under conditions that do not reduce the excess molybdate present. Various reducing agents have been introduced, including stannous chloride, *p*-aminonaphtholsulfonic acid, ascorbic acid, *p*-methylaminophenolsulfate (Elon), *N*-phenyl-*p*-phenylenediamine, and ferrous sulfate. Most procedures involve proteinization with trichloroacetic acid. The protein-free filtrate is mixed with molybdic acid to form phosphomolybdate, which is reduced with the appropriate reducing agent to produce molybdenum blue. Quantitation is usually carried out at 660 nm. A modification using iron (Fe^{2+}) and thiourea is the method of choice because of its color stability, improved sensitivity, and conformity to Beer's law over a wide range of concentrations. The precision of this method is reported to be in the range of $\pm 5\%$.

Complex formation between phosphomolybdate and the triphenylmethane dye malachite green appears to be the most sensitive procedure known for phosphorus determination. Unfortunately, the high acidity at which the complex is formed also causes hydrolysis of organic phosphates. An enzymatic method for phosphorus determination is also described whereby phosphorus undergoes successive enzymatic reactions catalyzed by glycogen phosphorylase, phosphoglucomutase, and glucose-6-phosphate dehydrogenase. The NADPH produced can be quantitated fluorometrically or spectrophotometrically. The reaction takes place at neutral pH, thus permitting the measurement of inorganic phosphorus in the presence of unstable organic phosphates. Because organic phosphates exist principally in the erythrocytes, it is important to separate serum from the red cells as soon as clotting is complete.

Hydroxyproline

Because more than 90% of the hydroxyproline in urine is present as a component of oligopeptides, almost all laboratory procedures begin with acid hydrolysis of the sample. The liberated hydroxyproline is then oxidized by chloramine T to pyrrole, which reacts with Ehrlich's reagent to form a red chromogen that is determined colorimetrically. However, most hydrolysates of urine also contain ammonium chloride, glucose, and mannitol, which interfere with color formation. Various modifications to this procedure have been developed in an effort to improve assay specificity. For example, the use of a cation-exchange resin is recommended for the separation of hydroxyproline from interfering contaminants prior to hydrolysis, oxidation, and color development. Alternately, the isolation of the oxidized product by distillation or extraction with toluene has successfully eliminated interferences caused by nonvolatile color compounds produced by tyrosine and tryptophan. This procedure is found to yield accurate results, provided that care is taken to avoid loss of the volatile oxidation products.

HPLC methods involving precolumn derivatization have been developed (Reed, 1991). Results obtained with HPLC procedures are more specific, cover a wider assay range, and compare well with the colorimetric method.

Parathyroid Hormone

Although the measurement of PTH by radioimmunoassay (RIA) was first described in 1963, this assay has now found widespread clinical application. The theoretical and technical problems contributing to this delay are many. The most important complication has been the heterogeneous nature of the hormone in circulation as a result of PTH metabolism peripherally or within the parathyroid glands. The biologically active intact hormone represents only a small portion of the total PTH immunoreactivity and is present in very low concentration. In contrast, the biologically inactive C-terminal and midregion fragments are cleared less rapidly from the circulation and are present in higher concentrations. Since the late 1970s, greater understanding of PTH physiology and improved technology have helped in the production of antisera of desired regional specificity, enabling the detection and measurement of different species of circulating immunoreactive PTH fragments.

The most widely used assays are those directed against the midregion and the C-terminal part of the hormone. These assays are very useful in differentiating patients with primary hyperparathyroidism from healthy subjects. However, in patients with renal dysfunction, elevated results from these assays are difficult to interpret because these fragments are cleared from the circulation by glomerular filtration. Assays for biologically active N-terminal or intact PTH are less dependent on renal function. However, overlap between these two groups can be appreciable, and detection of primary hyperparathyroidism using N-terminal/intact PTH assay relies on the use of simultaneous determination of calcium and the formal discriminate analysis of calcium versus PTH. Furthermore, most RIAs, including the midregion and C-terminal assays, are not sufficiently sensitive to distinguish subnormal from normal levels, nor can they reliably differentiate HHM from PHPT.

Intact PTH assays of improved sensitivity and specificity have been developed using a two-site immunoradiometric assay (IRMA) technique, which involves use of two groups of affinity-purified antibodies (Blind, 1988). The N-terminal (1 to 34)–directed antibodies, or so-called signal antibodies, are labeled with ^{125}I, while the C-terminal (39 to 84)–directed antibodies are immunoabsorbed to a solid support. Although both intact PTH and midregion or C-terminal fragments are bound to the antisera on the solid support, the intact hormone alone has binding affinity for the ^{125}I-labeled N-terminal antisera. Similarly, immunochemiluminometric assays for intact PTH, using the IRMA technique, but labeling the signal antibodies with a chemiluminescent compound, have also been developed (Kao, 1992). The IRMA technique has several advantages over the conventional RIA: increased sensitivity and specificity, extended assay concentration range, and decreased incubation time. Using these assays, detection of hypoparathyroidism and separation of hyperparathyroidism from hypercalcemia of malignancy are achievable. The intact hormone assay is also useful in assessing glandular secretion as well as in the venous catheterization procedure for the preoperative localization of parathyroid adenomas. Unlike RIAs, these IRMA assays can suppress PTH levels in sera of patients with HHM, allowing a more definitive diagnosis of hypercalcemia of malignancy.

Vitamin D Compounds

The laborious classic bioassay of vitamin D, the rat-line test, which measures the concentrations of all vitamin D precursors and metabolites, has been replaced by specific assays for the individual metabolites.

Because 25-(OH)D_3 is the most abundant metabolite in the circulation, several competitive protein-binding methods using high-affinity binding protein to this metabolite have been developed. These techniques provide exquisite sensitivity, require small sample volume, and are amenable to assaying a large number of samples simultaneously. Unfortunately, interference from other metabolites that compete with the binding protein compromises method precision; therefore, partial chromatographic separation prior to assay is necessary. HPLC is rapidly becoming the technique of choice for measuring 25-(OH)D_3 levels in biological fluids because this method offers sensitivity, precision, and specificity without being technically cumbersome. As the major circulating metabolite, 25-(OH)D_3 provides an index of vitamin D status. The reference intervals, however, are subject to seasonal variations because concentrations of 25-(OH)D_3 are affected by solar exposure. Circulating 25-(OH)D_3 levels are also affected by prior administration of vitamin D. Although both reduced 25-(OH)D_3 and osteomalacia are encountered in anticonvulsant therapy, lowered 25-(OH)D_3 level itself does not appear to cause osteomalacia because these drugs directly inhibit calcium transport in bone and intestine. Measurement of 25-(OH)D_3 is of limited use in patients with renal disorders because of interference in the conversion to 1,25-$(OH)_2D_3$ in the kidney. Although increased levels of 25-(OH)D_3 are associated with vitamin D intoxication, a precise level at which intoxication occurs has not been established.

Much attention has been focused on the determination of 1,25-$(OH)_2D_3$ because of its physiologic importance as well as its clinical uses. Patients with disturbed calcium metabolism tend to show significantly different mean values compared with those of healthy individuals. Lowered 1,25-$(OH)_2D_3$ concentrations are associated with renal osteodystrophy, vitamin D–resistant rickets, hypoparathyroidism, rickets, and pseudohypoparathyroidism. Elevated levels of 1,25-$(OH)_2D_3$ are found in hyperparathyroidism and in acromegaly. The low circulating level of this metabolite necessitates extensive purification prior to its measurement. RIA has been attempted, but the lack of antibody specificity precludes its use in distinguishing 1,25-$(OH)_2D_3$ from other metabolites. Quantitative separation of 25-(OH)D_3, 24,25-$(OH)_2D_3$, and 1,25-$(OH)_2D_3$ from the same sample by HPLC followed by individual measurement of these metabolites using appropriate competitive protein-binding assays has been reported. One source of specific cytosolic receptor for assaying 1,25-$(OH)_2D_3$ is from the intestinal mucosa of a rachitic chick; the preparation of the receptor protein requires three distinct chromatographic steps. This assay is available in several specialized reference laboratories and medical centers. The reference values are in the range of 30 pg/mL. The clinical implications of measurements of circulating vitamin D metabolites have been reviewed by Igbal (1994).

Calcitonin

CT was previously measured by a bioassay based on the ability of CT to lower serum calcium concentration in rats. This method was subsequently replaced by the more sensitive RIAs, which use antisera prepared against CT from extracts of medullary thyroid carcinoma. Earlier RIAs, however, still failed to detect CT in most healthy individuals. The availability of synthetic human CT in recent years has increased assay sensitivity to enable definitive measurement of CT levels in healthy individuals (reference interval < 100 pg/mL). Nevertheless, extremely variable reference intervals of up to 600 pg/mL have also been reported. The issue is further complicated by the finding that heterogeneity of immunoreactive CT occurs in patients with medullary carcinoma, which adds uncertainty to the interpretation of assay results. Other techniques for measuring CT have also been reported. They include a specific receptor assay that uses cell membrane preparation from renal tissue, and a CT receptor assay linked to an adenylate cyclase system. However, sensitivity by either assay does not appear adequate for routine use. An extraction procedure has recently been incorporated to a monoclonal antibody assay that measures the monomeric form with a sensitivity of 1 pg/mL. CT in women measured with this assay appears to be 4–5 fold lower than in men (Body, 1993).

The most valuable aspect of the CT assay is in the diagnosis and management of medullary carcinoma of the thyroid. This neoplasm is CT producing and is familial. In a significant number of patients affected with the disease, the baseline levels of CT are normal. However, stimulation with an appropriate secretagogue, such as calcium infusion or pentagastrin injection, or both, usually results in an abnormally large increase in serum CT levels. These provocative tests have proved useful in the diagnosis of medullary thyroid carcinoma, even in the premalignant and hyperplastic phase of the disease, and facilitate identification of individuals with abnormal C-cell mass at a sufficiently early stage (Dunn, 1993). It is recommended that the stimulation test be conducted on kindreds of affected patients. In case of a normal response, the procedure should be repeated periodically.

Cyclic AMP

Sensitive assays are available for the determination of urinary cyclic AMP. A competitive protein-binding procedure uses a binding protein from either the muscle or the adrenal cortex, which is presumably cyclic AMP–activated protein kinase. The assay is based on the competition between cyclic AMP and the radioiodinated nucleotide for binding sites on the binder. Assay sensitivity is 0.05 to 0.1 pmole. The binder, however, cross-reacts with cyclic GMP, which can be removed by separation on a Dowex 1 ion-exchange column. The chromatographic separation step can be eliminated if the measurement is performed using RIA because antisera prepared for this purpose have shown adequate specificity for cyclic AMP (Steiner, 1969). Assay sensitivity has been reported to be 0.01 pmole. Both assays are now available commercially in kit packages. However, cyclic AMP measurements have not proved to be as useful as anticipated for hyperparathyroidism.

OTHER INORGANIC IONS

Magnesium

Physiologic Chemistry

Magnesium is the fourth most abundant cation in the body and is essential to many physicochemical processes. As an intracellular cation, magnesium is second in abundance only to potassium, and its concentration in intracellular fluid is about 10 times that in the extracellular fluid. Magnesium is an activator of various enzymes, including phosphatases, transphosphorylases, pyrophosphatases, carboxylases, and hexokinase. Magnesium is also essential for the preservation of the macromolecular structure of DNA, RNA, and ribosomes.

The body of an adult contains about 1 mole of magnesium (24 g), 50% of which is present in bone and the other 50% in soft tissue. Less than 1% of total magnesium is present in the blood. One third of serum magnesium is bound to protein, mostly albumin. The other two thirds is ultrafiltratable, existing predominantly as the free ion with a small percentage as a complex of anions. About 40% of the average adult daily dietary intake (300 mg) is absorbed in the small intestine and excreted in the urine. The absorption process appears to be poorly controlled, and homeostasis is maintained largely by renal excretion, which is regulated by tubular reabsorption.

The dynamics of magnesium exchange and homeostasis are not as well understood as for other common elements in the body. This is mainly attributable to the fact that most investigative work on magnesium has been directed to extracellular aspects, whereas the physiologic role of magnesium is primarily intracellular. Assessment of magnesium status cannot be made with a routine clinical laboratory assay of total serum magnesium because it has little correlation with intracellular magnesium, and information on free magnesium is presently insufficient. Nonetheless, assays for ionized magnesium in serum and whole blood (Altura, 1992; van Ingen, 1994) and intracellular magnesium (Murphy, 1993) are emerging. The availability of such assays should facilitate the diagnosis of magnesium deficiency, which at present relies on a careful history and physical examination, assisted by the EKG and laboratory tests, such as serum magnesium, 24-hour urine excretion, and retention of magnesium following parenteral administration. The metabolism of magnesium is extensively reviewed by Elin (1988).

Reference serum levels vary somewhat depending on the analytical method employed. Using atomic absorption spectrometry, the reference range is 1.3 to 2.1 mEq/L (0.7 to 1.1 mmol/L). There appears to be no sex difference, and the concentration in newborns is essentially the same as in adults; both serum and red cell magnesium do not vary significantly between the ages of 11–75 years. Erythrocyte magnesium is about three times that of serum. The magnesium concentration in cerebrospinal fluid is 2.0 to 2.7 mEq/L (1.0 to 1.4 mmol/L).

2

Clinicopathologic Correlations

Magnesium depletion is clinically more significant and frequent than an excess, with a prevalence of 11% in hospitalized patients. Signs and symptoms of magnesium depletion do not usually appear until extracellular levels have fallen to 1 mEq/L (0.5 mmol/L) or less. Manifestations of significant magnesium depletion include weakness, muscle fasciculations, depression, agitation, seizures, hypocalcemia, hypokalemia, and cardiac arrhythmias. Causes for symptomatic hypomagnesemia include malabsorption, severe diarrhea, nasogastric suction with administration of magnesium-free parenteral fluids, alcoholism, acute pancreatitis, early chronic renal disease, dietary malnutrition, excessive lactation, chronic dialysis, digitalis intoxication, hyper- and hypoparathyroidism, hyperaldosteronism, diabetes mellitus, pregnancy at term (toxemia/eclampsia), Paget's disease, diuretic therapy (mercurial diuretics, thiazides, and ammonium chloride), and porphyria with inappropriate secretion of antidiuretic hormone.

The prevalence of hypermagnesemia in hospitalized patients is about 9.3%. Signs of magnesium toxicity include anesthesia, flaccidity, paralysis of voluntary muscles, and hypotension. Symptomatic hypermagnesemia can be caused by advanced renal failure, acute diabetic acidosis, Addison's disease, severe dehydration, overly aggressive administration of magnesium sulfate enemas, or ingestion of excessive amounts of magnesium-containing antacids.

The role of magnesium as a mediator of PTH secretion has long been recognized. Endogenous PTH affects both the ionized and the intracellular magnesium concentration, but it has no significant influence on plasma magnesium (Elin, 1990).

Analytical Techniques

TOTAL SERUM MAGNESIUM. Serum is preferred over plasma for magnesium determination because anticoagulant interferes with most procedures. The oldest method for the determination of magnesium in biological fluids, but one that is occasionally still used, involves precipitation of magnesium as the ammonium phosphate salt after removal of calcium as calcium oxalate. Phosphorus in the precipitate is then quantitated by any of several methods, usually photometry as molybdenum blue or as the molybdivanadate complex. Precipitation of magnesium with 8-hydroxyquinoline is the basis for many procedures. The precipitate is quantitated by titrimetry, colorimetry, flame photometry, or fluorometry. Calcium, which will interfere, is eliminated by complexing with ethylene bis(oxyethylenenitrilo) tetra-acetic acid (EGTA).

In terms of accuracy, the determination of magnesium by atomic absorption spectrophotometry is the method of choice. After deproteinization and removal of phosphate ions with a lanthanum salt, the diluted filtrate is analyzed using the 285.2 nm line of a magnesium hollow cathode lamp.

Most clinical laboratories now routinely use colorimetric methods for magnesium determination on automated analyzers using chromophores such as calmagite, methylthymol blue, formazan dye, and magon. Methodologies for serum magnesium determination in the clinical laboratory have been reviewed by Elin (1992).

IONIZED MAGNESIUM. Ion-selective electrode technology is used exclusively in the determination of ionized magnesium in serum and in whole blood. One recently evaluated assay for ionized magnesium using a neutral carrier, liquid-membrane–based ion-selective electrode (van Ingen, 1994) was reported to be rapid and precise with precision of 2% to 4%. This assay is not influenced by calcium and can measure ionized magnesium to 0.3 mmol/L. The reference interval is 0.56 ± 0.5 mmol/L. However, the nonlinearity at the low range of concentration limits its use in assessing magnesium status in patients with severe hypomagnesemia.

INTRACELLULAR MAGNESIUM. Significant methodologic advances in intracellular magnesium (iMg) measurement have allowed greater understanding of magnesium homeostasis. iMg can now be assayed by fluorescence measurement using furaptra, which is a magnesium binder; by nuclear magnetic resonance spectroscopy; by ion-selective microelectrode; and by electroprobe microanalysis (Murphy, 1993).

Iron

Physiologic Chemistry

Iron is essential to most living organisms and participates in a variety of vital processes varying from cellular oxidative mechanisms to the transport of oxygen to the tissues. It is a constituent of the oxygen-carrying chromoproteins, hemoglobin and myoglobin, as well as various enzymes, such as cytochrome oxidase, xanthine oxidase, peroxidase, and catalase. The remaining body iron is present in the flavoproteins (NADH dehydrogenase and succinic dehydrogenase), the iron-sulfur proteins, as well as the storage (ferritin) and transport (transferrin) forms of iron. The approximate distribution of iron in the normal adult male is presented in Table 8–9.

Unlike that of other trace elements, iron homeostasis is unique in that it is regulated primarily by absorption and not by excretion. Because the capacity of the body to excrete iron is very limited, its absorption from the intestine must be controlled so that tissue accumulations do not reach toxic levels. Iron metabolism in hematologic disorders is also reviewed in Chapter 26. Salient features of iron homeostasis are presented in Figure 8–6.

In adult males, iron is lost by way of the gastrointestinal tract (0.6 mg), sweat and exfoliation of squamous cells (0.2 mg), and the urinary tract (0.1 mg), for a total of 0.9 mg daily. In the female, losses through normal menstruation add an additional average daily increment of 0.4 mg, giving a total daily loss of 1.3 mg. During pregnancy and lactation, additional demands of up to 4 mg/day are placed on maternal iron stores.

Table 8–9. APPROXIMATE DISTRIBUTION OF IRON IN THE NORMAL ADULT MALE

Compound	Iron Content (mg)	Percent
Hemoglobin	2800	68.3
Myoglobin	135	3.30
Ferritin	520	12.7
Hemosiderin	480	11.7
Transferrin	7	0.17
Enzyme iron	8	0.19
Remaining organic iron (by difference)	150	3.65
Total	4100	100

The recommended allowance of 10 mg/day for adult males is readily obtainable from a well-balanced diet. It is difficult for women to obtain the recommended allowances (18 mg/day) from dietary sources unless fortified foods or supplements are included. The richest dietary source of iron is animal viscera, e.g., liver, kidney, heart, and spleen. Other good sources include egg yolks, fish, oysters, clams, and dried legumes.

Because the body conserves iron extremely well, only 6% to 12% of dietary intake needs to be absorbed in order to maintain iron equilibrium. However, in iron deficiency states and during growth and pregnancy, the normal gastrointestinal absorption will be increased from 1.3 mg daily to perhaps 4 mg/day (Jacobs, 1977).

Aside from a small amount of iron that is absorbed from the stomach, most iron absorption takes place in the duodenum and jejunum. In order to be absorbed, iron must be in its reduced or ferrous form. The acid pH of the stomach, along with reducing substances and ascorbic acid, enhances iron absorption by maintaining iron in a reduced, more soluble form and by forming a chelate with ferric iron, which remains soluble as the pH rises in the small intestine. The regulation of iron absorption is largely carried out by the intestinal epithelial cells, and a mucosal control mechanism has been proposed in which solubilized ionic iron in the intestinal lumen adsorbs to specific receptors in the brush border of the mucosal cells. The iron then passes from these receptors into the cytosol of the mucosal cell by an energy-dependent process. Controversy still exists concerning the mechanism of transport across the mucosal cell to the serosal surface. Several possible explanations of the process have been proposed. In addition to the classic apoferritin theory, it has been suggested that iron is solubilized by chelation to low-molecular-weight endogenous substances, and that transport of iron across the cell is effected by chelation to amino acids. Most absorbed iron becomes attached to the plasma protein, transferrin, for transport in the plasma. Any remaining iron is retained within the cell, where it combines with the protein apoferritin (molecular weight, 460,000) to form ferritin. Ferritin also occurs in hepatic parenchymal cells and reticuloendothelial cells of the bone marrow, liver, and spleen. If the

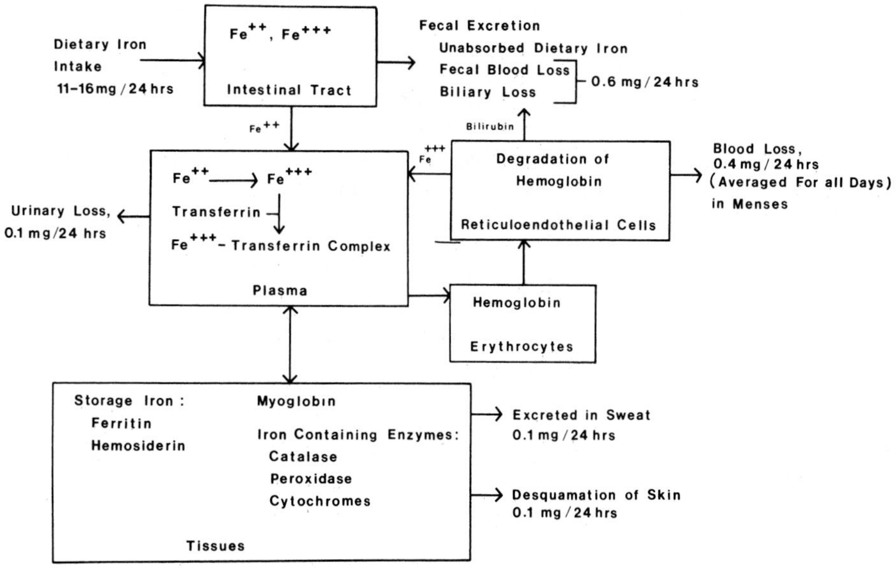

Figure 8-6. Interrelationships in iron homeostasis.

2

amount of apoferritin is insufficient to bind the remaining iron, it is deposited in tissues as small iron oxide granules known as hemosiderin. Approximately 25% of the iron in the body is in the storage forms of ferritin and hemosiderin. These storage forms represent a ready reserve of iron that can be mobilized to meet homeostatic needs.

The plasma iron transport protein, transferrin (formerly known as siderophilin), has the electrophoretic mobility of a β_1-globulin and is formed in the liver. It has a molecular weight of approximately 90,000. Each molecule is able to bind two atoms of ferric iron. The half-life of this protein is about 10 days. By contrast, the iron in the plasma pool has a half-life of 60 to 120 minutes.

Iron is carried to storage sites and to the bone marrow. Transferrin is not itself assimilated by the target tissues. Indeed, transferrin may bind briefly to normoblast membranes, where the iron is passed directly into the developing erythrocyte for incorporation into heme. Subsequently, transferrin returns to plasma to take up unbound iron. From effete erythrocytes, iron is split from hemoglobin by reticuloendothelial system cells and returns to plasma, where it is again bound to transferrin. A small portion of the emergent iron may enter the plasma in the form of ferritin. Free iron is extremely toxic, and little, if any, is present in the body.

Clinicopathologic Correlations

Serum iron reflects principally the amount of iron bound to transferrin. Serum transferrin represents the maximal amount of iron that can be bound, which is referred to as total iron-binding capacity (TIBC). Normally, only one third of the binding sites of transferrin are occupied. The unsaturated iron-binding capacity (UIBC), obtained by subtracting serum iron from TIBC, is a measure of reserve iron-binding capacity of transferrin. Measurement of serum iron alone is of limited value, because decreased levels of serum iron are usually associated with both iron deficiency anemia and the anemia of chronic disease. Concomitant determination of serum iron and transferrin allows the computation of transferrin saturation, which is expressed as (serum iron/TIBC) $\times$ 100. This ratio is a better index of iron storage than serum iron alone, and it is useful in the differentiation of the common causes of anemia, because TIBC normally increases in response to decreased serum iron in iron deficiency, whereas it is usually normal in chronic inflammatory disorders. The relationship among serum iron, transferrin (TIBC), and transferrin saturation as it occurs in various conditions and diseases is presented in Table 8-10. Additional clinicopathologic correlations are reviewed in Chapter 26.

Normal values for the TIBC in healthy adults average between 300 and 360 μg/dL (54 to 64 μmol/L). There is no diurnal variation in the level of the TIBC as there is for serum iron. TIBC values tend to decrease with age (250 μg/dL or 48 μmol/L in individuals above 70 years of age). At birth, the average newborn levels are about 275 μg/dL or 49 μmol/L and reach a peak by the eighth month.

Table 8-10. SERUM IRON, TIBC,* AND PERCENT SATURATION IN VARIOUS CONDITIONS

	Serum Fe (μg/dL)	TIBC (μg/dL)	Saturation (Percent)
Normal	*60-150*	*300-360*	*20-50*
Iron deficiency	↓	↑	↓
Chronic infections	↓	↓	↓
Malignancy	↓	↓	↓
Menstruation	↓	N	↓
Iron poisoning	↑	↓	↑
Hemolytic anemia	Var	Var	Var
Hemochromatosis	↑	N, ↓	↑
Myocardial infarction	↓	N	↓
Late pregnancy	↓	↑	↓
Oral contraceptives	N, ↑	↑	N
Viral hepatitis	↑	↑	N, ↑
Nephrosis	↓	↓	↑
Kwashiorkor	↓	↓	Var
Thalassemia	↑	↓	↑

↓ = decrease; ↑ = increase; N = normal; Var = variable.
*TIBC = total iron-binding capacity.

Despite methodologic sophistication, positive demonstration of iron deficiency from human behavioral alterations has yet to be realized. At present, no single laboratory test can adequately characterize the iron status of an individual, and multiple testing using a battery of specific iron-related determinations is commonly employed in iron storage assessment. Acceptable tests include hematocrit, hemoglobin, transferrin saturation, erythrocyte protoporphyrin (EP), and serum ferritin. Based on current understanding of iron metabolism, the progressive severity of iron reduction has been grouped into three stages (Lozoff, 1988). Iron depletion has been associated with a decrease in ferritin levels without concomitant abnormalities in other tests used for iron status assessment. The term iron deficiency without anemia has been used to denote additional decrease in iron storage that may limit heme production. Abnormal laboratory results include decreased levels of both ferritin and transferrin saturation and elevated EP. Iron deficiency anemia has been used to designate a further diminution of total body iron. This condition is usually associated with decreased hemoglobin levels accompanied by increased EP, and decreased levels of both ferritin and transferrin saturation.

Common causes for an increase in TIBC include iron deficiency anemia, infancy, ingestion of oral contraceptives, and possibly hepatitis (see Table 8–10). Decreased transferrin and, therefore, TIBC can be found in association with a generalized decrease in plasma proteins from various causes, e.g., reduced protein synthesis, nephrosis or other direct loss, and increased catabolism (malignancy or starvation). In common with albumin, but unlike many of the glycoproteins of plasma, transferrin tends to be decreased by inflammatory conditions. Patients with iron overload from repeated blood transfusions also have a depression of transferrin. The average serum iron level is about 125 μg/dL in adult males and 100 μg/dL in adult females. The range varies between 60 and 150 μg/dL (11 to 27 μmol/L). There is no seasonal variation in iron levels, although a diurnal variation has been observed. Serum iron levels can be one third higher in the morning than at night. The average plasma and serum iron levels at birth approach 200 μg/dL. There is a drop to about 45 μg/dL during the first few hours of life and then an increase to 125 μg/dL after the first three weeks of life. In the elderly, the serum iron level decreases to 40 to 80 μg/dL (7 to 14 μmol/L). In pathologic states, elevations of serum iron can be seen in (1) conditions of increased erythrocyte destruction (hemolytic anemia), (2) decreased blood formation (lead poisoning or pyridoxine deficiency), (3) increased release of iron from the body stores (release of ferritin in acute hepatic cell necrosis), (4) defective iron storage (pernicious anemia), and (5) increased rate of absorption (hemochromatosis and transfusion siderosis).

Decreased serum iron occurs in association with (1) generalized iron deficiency (lack of sufficient dietary iron), inadequate absorption, or chronic loss as a result of bleeding or nephrosis; and (2) impaired release of iron from the reticuloendothelial system (infection). Moderate depression of serum iron can occur in association with conditions such as malignancies and rheumatoid arthritis.

The ratio of serum iron level to plasma transferrin level (percentage saturation) is altered in various diseases (see Table 8–10). An increase in the saturation can occur in conditions of decreased circulating protein (chronic liver disease, nephrosis, kwashiorkor), in conditions associated with ineffective erythropoiesis or blocks in hemoglobin synthesis (thalassemia, lead poisoning, pyridoxine deficiency anemia), in disease associated with iron overload (idiopathic hemochromatosis and hemosiderosis), and in acute blood loss. A decrease in the percentage of saturation (less than 15%) is present in iron deficiency anemia and in late pregnancy. In conditions such as infection and malignancies, both serum iron and TIBC are decreased, but the serum iron depression is proportionately greater, so that the percentage of saturation is lower.

In evaluating patients for iron deficiency or iron overload, the workup should include a complete hematologic profile, including an examination of peripheral blood smear, as well as measurements of serum ferritin, serum iron, and TIBC, with calculation of percentage saturation. A single measurement of serum iron, except in iron poisoning, is inadequate for confirmation of iron overload or iron deficiency.

Analytical Techniques

SERUM IRON. The assessment of iron stores has traditionally been dependent on the colorimetric determination of serum iron. The first step in any analytic procedure for iron is the dissociation of iron from its binding proteins by exposure to strong acids. In manual methods, this is accomplished either by removal of proteins by precipitation with hot trichloroacetic acid or by providing conditions that allow the protein to remain in solution without interfering with subsequent analytical manipulations. In automated methods, iron is dialyzed from the transferrin. The next step in most procedures is the reaction of the reduced iron with a chromogen to produce an iron-chromogen complex. Reagents with superior sensitivity for complexation with iron include sulfonated bathophenanthroline 2,4,6-tripyridyl-S-triazine (TPTZ), ferrozine, and terosite. Addition of the color reagent results in the formation of a deeply colored Fe-chromogen complex with an absorbance maximum in the visible region. A recent study (Tietz, 1994) comparing five commercially available automated methods against the 1990 ICSH Reference Method reported a negative intercept of between 15 and 217 mg/L. In light of the significant result variations observed, the authors posted concern on the reliability of routine iron methods for confirmation of iron deficiency.

The determination of serum iron by atomic absorption spectrophotometry has had only limited success, primarily because of the relatively low sensitivity and the interference from other iron-containing compounds such as hemoglobin-Fe and dextran-Fe. Thus all samples must first be deproteinized prior to measurement. Other attempts at serum iron determination include emission spectrography, flameless atomic absorption spectrophotometry, and x-ray fluorescence spectrometry (Zak, 1980).

TOTAL IRON-BINDING CAPACITY (TIBC). TIBC is routinely determined by saturating the transferrin with iron, removing the excess unbound iron with an iron absorbent, and measuring the iron in the filtrate. Absorbents serve to remove any unbound iron excess and ideally should not remove iron that has become bound to the transferrin molecule.

Effective absorbents include activated charcoal, magnesium carbonate, and Amberlite resin. UIBC may be obtained by subtracting serum iron from TIBC. Serum transferrin can now be determined directly by a two-site enzyme immunoassay with use of monoclonal antibodies. Good correlation between serum transferrin and TIBC determined by the conventional method has been reported (Guindi, 1988). Other advantages of using this assay include small sample requirement (20 μL) and nonsusceptibility to iron contamination.

SERUM FERRITIN. Because the concentration of circulating ferritin in healthy individuals is proportional to the size of iron stores, serum ferritin is a sensitive indicator of iron deficiency. However, increased serum ferritin levels are found in a large number of chronic disorders, including inflammation, infection, viral hepatitis, and malignancy. Thus, in patients with iron deficiency in conjunction with any of these disorders, serum ferritin levels may be misleadingly normal. Iron overload, such as that found in idiopathic hemochromatosis or thalassemia major, is associated with increased serum ferritin concentration. Serum ferritin can be reliably determined by RIA, enzyme immunoassay, immunoradiometric assay, or chemiluminescence immunoassay. Very small sample volume is required (20 to 100 μL).

Copper

Physiologic Chemistry

Copper is an essential trace element that is a constituent of certain metalloenzymes and proteins. It is required for hemoglobin synthesis and is a constituent of cytochrome oxidase, tyrosinase, monoamine oxidase, ascorbic acid oxidase, uricase, galactose oxidase, and amino-levulinate dehydratase.

The major portion of copper in the erythrocyte (at least 80%) occurs as a constituent of the enzyme superoxide dismutase (erythrocuprein). This enzyme, also found in liver (hepatocuprein) and brain (cerebrocuprein), has the unique role of protecting cells by catalytically scavenging the toxic-free radical superoxide ion (O_2^-) generated during aerobic metabolism. The remainder of erythrocyte copper is dialyzable and is believed to consist of complexes with amino acids, which function to maintain dismutase activity. The total copper content of erythrocytes tends to remain constant, on the average 98 μg/dL (15 μmol/L), despite deficiencies of dietary copper or increases in plasma or hepatic copper (Burch, 1975).

The concentration of copper in the plasma is somewhat higher than in the erythrocyte. The normal range for serum copper in adults is 70 to 140 μg/dL (11 to 22 μmol/L) for males and 80 to 155 μg/dL (13 to 24 μmol/L) for females. Copper in plasma occurs in two main forms—one loosely bound and the other firmly bound to plasma proteins. Only trace amounts of copper remain free or dialyzable in plasma. Loosely bound copper is a minor fraction and includes copper bound predominantly to serum albumin.

The albumin-bound copper probably represents copper in transit and increases promptly after copper is ingested, then falls exponentially as a result of hepatic uptake. Firmly bound copper, composing 80% to 95% of the total plasma copper, is incorporated into an α_2-globulin, which is called ceruloplasmin because of its blue color. Serum ceruloplasmin concentration increases as albumin-bound copper decreases. Ceruloplasmin, a multifunctional enzyme, aids in the mobilization of iron from storage sites and functions as a ferroxidase enzyme during the ferrous-ferric conversion of iron. Reference values for ceruloplasmin range from 25 to 43 mg/dL (250 to 430 mg/L).

Clinicopathologic Correlations

The most important abnormality in copper metabolism is Wilson's disease, or hepatolenticular degeneration. This disease is of autosomal recessive inheritance with onset usually in the second or third decade but occasionally as early as four or five years of age. The disease is characterized by degenerative changes, particularly in the liver and the basal ganglia of the brain, as a result of excessive deposition of copper. The most common presenting signs and symptoms are those of central nervous involvement—rigidity, dysarthria, dysphagia, tremor, incoordination, choreoathetotic movements, and ataxia. Some patients, especially those in the younger age ranges, may present with liver insufficiency ranging from weakness and anorexia to jaundice and progressing to ascites and other features of portal hypertension as a consequence of cirrhosis. Other patients present with a combination of central nervous system and hepatic disease. A pathognomonic finding is a brown ring near the limbus of the cornea, termed the Kayser-Fleischer ring, which results from deposition of copper in Descemet's membrane (Clayton, 1980).

Plasma ceruloplasmin in Wilson's disease is ordinarily greatly decreased, usually to less than 20 mg/dL. It is unlikely, however, that the depression of ceruloplasmin is a causative factor in the disease because a few patients with Wilson's disease have normal levels of ceruloplasmin. Furthermore, 10% to 20% of heterozygote carriers and other patients with the nephrotic syndrome or sprue have significantly decreased ceruloplasmin but are free of the manifestations of Wilson's disease. Plasma copper is correspondingly decreased. Patients with Wilson's disease have a persistently positive copper balance in spite of increased renal excretion. The fact that biliary and, therefore, fecal excretion of copper is abnormally low may be of pathogenetic importance. Copper is also increased in the cerebrospinal fluid.

Prompt diagnosis of Wilson's disease is important so that therapy can be instituted. Progression of the disease can be abated and manifestations at least partially reversed by a diet low in copper and therapy with D-penicillamine, which promotes copper excretion (Evans, 1981).

Hypercupremia is usually observed during pregnancy, with ceruloplasmin concentrations in serum reaching values at parturition that are twice those found in nonpregnant women. Extremely high concentrations of ceruloplasmin, and therefore of copper, have been found in various lymphomas, particularly Hodgkin's disease. Increased ceruloplasmin also occurs in acute and chronic infections, rheumatoid arthritis, biliary cirrhosis, and thyrotoxicosis.

There are several other conditions in which subnormal concentrations of copper are found in the serum. Hypocupremia has been observed in conditions associated with hypoproteinemia, such as protein malnutrition (kwashiorkor), protein malabsorption syndrome (sprue), and nephrosis.

Hypocupremia is also a characteristic feature of Menkes' kinky hair syndrome, or trichopoliodystrophy, a sex-linked recessive disorder characterized by progressive mental deterioration, retardation of growth, defective keratinization and pigmentation of hair (kinky hair, or pili torti), hypothermia, degenerative changes in aortic elastic, scorbutic bone changes, and cerebral gliosis with cystic degeneration. In addition to hypocupremia, this syndrome is associated with profound hypoceruloplasminemia and diminished concentrations of copper in the hair. The copper deficiency may be responsible for the alterations in the elastic fibers of arterial walls and the scorbutic bone deformities, as well as the changes in hair. Although orally administered copper has been ineffective in treating this syndrome, parenteral administration of copper was therapeutically beneficial as a result of stimulation of ceruloplasmin formation.

Analytical Techniques

Colorimetric methods for measuring copper are prone to interference. These methods also lack sensitivity and specificity. Atomic absorption spectrometry remains the method of choice for the determination of copper in serum, plasma, or urine. Atomic absorption spectrometry provides speed and ease of analysis required for routine clinical use. Methods of sample preparation for measurements of copper in serum, plasma, and whole blood by flame atomic absorption include (1) simple dilution and aspiration in the flame, (2) dissociation of copper from the proteins (albumin and ceruloplasmin) by treatment with acid followed by protein precipitation and aspiration of the supernatant, and (3) liberation of plasma and erythrocyte copper by acid digestion followed by chelation and extraction into an organic solvent for flame atomic absorption measurement. Copper determination may also be performed by graphite furnace atomic absorption spectroscopy (AAS), which offers greater sensitivity and requires smaller sample volume.

It should be noted that copper nutrition status may not be adequately assessed with the use of serum copper or ceruloplasmin concentration alone. Copper-containing enzymes such as erythrocyte superoxide dismutase and platelet or leukocyte cytochrome c oxidase may be better indicators of metabolically active copper storage (Milne, 1994).

Zinc

Zinc is a nutrient. It is an essential component of many important enzymes, including alcohol dehydrogenase, carbonic anhydrase, alkaline phosphatase, procarboxypeptides, and superoxide dismutase. It is also important as an antioxidant or free radical scavenger. The importance of zinc in several diseases has now been clearly established.

Low plasma levels of zinc occur as a nonspecific finding in association with a variety of diseases, including alcoholic cirrhosis, sickle-cell anemia, carcinoma of the lung, acute myocardial infarction, chronic renal failure, cutaneous burns, corticosteroid therapy, and oral contraceptive therapy (Prasad, 1981). Improvement in healing of extensive burns or wounds has been observed following administration of zinc sulfate to patients with zinc depletion or dietary inadequacy. Zinc deficiency in children is associated with anorexia, impaired taste perception, pica, lethargy, failure to thrive as infants, growth retardation of older children, and delayed sexual maturation.

Acrodermatitis enteropathica is a disease with onset in early childhood characterized by various gastrointestinal and cutaneous manifestations including alopecia, diarrhea, and vesiculopustulous dermatitis, particularly of the extremities and around mucous membranes. This disease, inherited as an autosomal recessive trait, has been attributed to a defect related to zinc metabolism (Clayton, 1980).

Although deficiencies of zinc have received greater attention than overdoses, acute zinc intoxications from industrial exposure, consumption of acidic foods or beverages from galvanized containers, illicit spirits, and children's toys have been reported. Symptoms from accidental ingestion include gastrointestinal irritation with fever, nausea, vomiting, diarrhea, abdominal pain, and a metallic taste. With industrial exposure via inhalation, metal fume fever is the predominant symptom. Other toxic effects include dry throat, cough and chest discomfort, tachycardia, hypertension, and pulmonary edema. Considerable discrepancies exist in the literature concerning normal zinc levels. Improper specimen collection and/or nonspecific colorimetric methods explain part of the disparity. The normal plasma concentration of zinc by atomic absorption is approximately 100 μg/dL, with a range of 55 to 150 μg/dL (8.42 to 22.95 μmol/L). Platelet disintegration is thought to account for the higher level in serum. Plasma levels of zinc can be affected by its binding affinity to albumin, exogenous steroid administration, and hemolysis (Solomons, 1979).

Although plasma zinc concentration is used as an indicator of zinc deficiency, it is not reliable for assessment of zinc status, because it does not appear sensitive to changes in dietary zinc. The latter has been shown to correlate well with plasma metallothionine concentration. Measurement of both plasma zinc and plasma metallothionine may differentiate dietary zinc deficiency from other causes such as stress, infection, or other metabolic conditions (King, 1990).

Chromium

Although chromium as a component of several enzyme systems may be important in nucleic acid metabolism, its physiologic role in humans remains unclear. Chromium appears to potentiate the action of insulin, and a trivalent chromium nicotinic acid complex has been referred to as "glucose tolerance factor." Improved insulin efficiency appeared to be associated with an optimal amount of chromium (Mertz, 1993). Available data suggest that improved chromium nutrition leads to improved glucose metabolism in hypoglycemics, hyperglycemics, and diabetics.

Chromium toxicity is seen primarily in occupational exposure to chromium compounds. Toxic exposure to the skin results in dermatitis and persistent ulceration. Accidental ingestion has resulted in vertigo, abdominal pain, vomiting, anuria, convulsions, shock, and coma. Chromium levels in blood are extremely low. A serum level of 1.58 ± 0.08 μg/L in a group of 15 healthy adults was reported. Levels of chromium in hair are substantially higher than in serum and may be used as an index of chromium nutrition.

Altura BT, Altura BM: Measurement of ionized magnesium in whole blood, plasma and serum with a new ion-selective electrode in healthy and diseased human subjects. Magnes Trace Elem 1992; 10:90.

Becker MA: Clinical aspects of monosodium urate monohydrate crystal deposition disease (gout). Rheum Dis Clin North Am 1988; 14:377.

Belchetz PE: Hormonal treatment of postmenopausal women. New Engl J Med 1994; 330:1062.

Beukeveld GJJ, Meerman L, Huizenga JR, et al: Determination of porphyrins in bile using high performance liquid chromatography and some clinical applications. Eur J Clin Chem Clin Biochem 1994; 32:153.

Birkeland KI, Gallefoss F, Olsson S, et al: Primary hyperparathyroidism or hypercalcaemia of malignancy? Scand J Clin Lab Invest 1992; 52:347.

Blind E, Schmidt-Gayk H, Scharla S, et al: Two-site assay of intact parathyroid hormone in the investigation of primary hyperparathyroidism and other disorders of calcium metabolism compared with a midregion assay. J Clin Endocrinol Metab 1988; 67:353.

Boden SD, Kaplan FS: Calcium homeostasis. Orthop Clin North Am 1990; 21:31.

Body JJ: Calcitonin: From the determination of circulating levels in various physiological and pathological conditions to the demonstration of lymphocyte receptors. Horm Res 1993; 39:166.

Boot S, LaRoch N, Legg EF: Elimination of bilirubin interference in creatinine assays by routine techniques: Comparison with a HPLC method. Ann Clin Biochem 1994; 31:262.

Burch RE, Hahn HKJ, Sullivan JF: Newer aspects of the roles of zinc, manganese, and copper in human nutrition. Clin Chem 1975; 21:501.

Burtis WJ: Parathyroid hormone–related protein: Structure, function, and measurement. Clin Chem 1992; 38:2171.

Clayton BE: Clinical chemistry of trace elements. Adv Clin Chem 1980; 21:147.

Conger JD: Acute uric acid nephropathy. Med Clin North Am 1990; 74:859.

Deftos LJ, Roos BA, Parthemore JG: Calcium and skeletal metabolism. West J Med 1975; 123:447.

Deftos LJ, Parethemore JG, Stabile BE: Management of primary hyperparathyroidism. Annu Rev Med 1993; 44:19.

Delmas PD: Biochemical markers of bone turnover. J Bone Miner Res 1993; 8(Suppl 2):S549.

DeLuca HF: The vitamin D story: A collaborative effort of basic science and clinical medicine. FASEB J 1988; 2:22.

DeLuca HF: New concepts of vitamin D functions. Ann N Y Acad Sci 1992; 669:59.

Dunn JM, Farndon JR: Medullary thyroid carcinoma. Br J Surg 1993; 80:6.

Elin RJ: Magnesium metabolism in health and disease. Dis Mon 1988; 34:161.

Elin RJ: Determination of serum magnesium concentration by clinical laboratories. Magnes Trace Elem 1992; 10:60.

Elin RJ, Hosseini JM, Fitzpatrick L, et al: Blood magnesium status of patients with parathyroid disease. Magnes Trace Elem 1990; 9:119.

Evans GW: The role of copper in metabolic disorders. Adv Exp Med Biol 1981; 135:121.

Forman DT, Lorenzo L: Ionized calcium: Its significance and clinical usefulness. Ann Clin Lab Sci 1991; 21:297.

Garcia PJ, Mateos FA: Clinical and biochemical aspects of uric acid overproduction. Pharm World Science 1994; 16:40.

Garnero P, Delmas PD: Assessment of the serum levels of bone alkaline phosphatase with a new immunoradiometric assay in patients with metabolic bone disease. J Clin Endocrinol Metab 1993; 77:1046.

Goldstein L: Ammonia production and excretion in the mammalian kidney. *In* Thurau K (ed): Kidney and Urinary Tract Physiology II. Baltimore, University Park Press, 1976.

Guindi ME, Skikne BS, Covell AM, et al: An immunoassay for human transferrin. Am J Clin Nutr 1988; 47:37.

Igbal SJ: Vitamin D metabolism and the clinical aspects of measuring metabolites. Ann Clin Biochem 1994; 31:109.

Jacobs A: Serum ferritin and iron stores. Fed Proc 1977; 36:2024.

Kao CP, Grnat CS, Klee GG, et al: Clinical performance of parathyroid hormone immunometric assays. Mayo Clin Proc 1992; 67:637.

King JC: Assessment of zinc status. J Nutrition 1990; 120(Suppl 11):1474.

Knepper KA: NH_4^+ transport in the kidney. Kidney Int 1991; 40(Suppl 33):S95.

Lafferty FW: Differential diagnosis of hypercalcemia. J Bone Miner Res 1991; 6:S51.

Levey AS, Perrone RD, Madias NE: Serum creatinine and renal function. Annu Rev Med 1988; 39:465.

Linkhart SG, Linkhart TA, Taylor AK, et al: Synthetic peptide–based immunoassay for amino-terminal propeptide of type 1 procollagen: Application for evaluation of bone formation. Clin Chem 1993; 39:2254.

Logan GM, Weimer MK, Ellefson M, et al: Bile porphyrin analysis in the evaluation of variegate porphyria. N Eng J Med 1991; 324:1408.

Long C, Smyth SJ, Woolf J, et al: Detection of latent variegate porphyria by fluorescence emission spectroscopy of plasma. Br J Dermatol 1993; 129:9.

Lozoff B: Behavioral alterations in iron deficiency. Adv Pediatr 1988; 35:331.

Manolagas SC, Jilka RL: Mechanisms of disease: Bone marrow, cytokines, and bone remodeling—emerging insights into the pathophysiology of osteoporosis. New Engl J Med 1995; 332:305.

Masters PW, Jones RG, Purves DA, et al: Commercial assays for serum osteocalcin give clinically discordant results. Clin Chem 1994; 40:358.

McLean FC, Hastings AB: The state of calcium in the fluids of the body. 1. The conditions affecting the ionization of calcium. J Biol Chem 1935; 108:285.

Mertz W: Chromium in human nutrition: A review. J Nutr 1993; 123:626.

Milne DB: Assessment of copper nutritional status. Clin Chem 1994; 40:1479.

Murphy E: Measurement of intracellular ionized magnesium. Miner Electrolyte Metab 1993; 19(4-5):250.

Nyhan WL: The Lesch-Nyhan syndrome. Adv Nephrol 1974; 3:59.

Parfitt AM: The actions of parathyroid hormone on bone: Relation to bone remodeling and turnover, calcium homeostasis, and metabolic bone disease. Part III. PTH and osteoblasts: The relationship between bone turnover and bone loss, and the state of the bones in primary hyperparathyroidism. Metabolism 1976; 25:1033.

Pennington RJ: Biochemical aspects of muscle disease. Adv Clin Chem 1971; 14:409.

Perrone RD, Madias NE, Levey AS: Serum creatinine as an index of renal function: New insights into old concepts. Clin Chem 1992; 38:1933.

Piomelli S: The diagnostic utility of measurements of erythrocyte porphyrins. Pediatr Hemat 1987; 1:419.

Prasad AS: Zinc deficiency in human subjects. Prog Clin Biol Res 1981; 77:165.

Reed P, Holbrook IB, Gardner MLG, et al: Simple, optimized liquid-chromatographic method for measuring total hydroxyproline in urine evaluated. Clin Chem 1991; 37:285–290.

Robertson WG, Marshall RW: Calcium measurements in serum and plasma—total and ionized. CRC Crit Rev Clin Lab Sci 1979; 11:271.

Ryckewaert A, Kuntz D: Etiologic varieties of hyperuricemia and gout. Adv Nephrol 1974; 3:29.

Seymour JF, Grill V, Martin TJ, et al: Hypercalcemia in the blastic phase of chronic myeloid leukemia associated with elevated parathyroid hormone–related protein. Leukemia 1993; 7:162.

Solomons NW: On the assessment of zinc and copper nutriture in man. Am J Clin Nutr 1979; 32:856.

Steiner AL, Kipnis DM, Utiger R, et al: Radioimmunoassay for the measurement of adenosine 3′,5′-cyclic phosphate. Proc Natl Acad Sci U S A 1969; 64:367.

Teerlink T, van Leeuwen PAM, Houdijk A: Plasma amino acids determined by liquid chromatography within 17 minutes. Clin Chem 1994; 40:245.

Tefferi A, Solberg Jr, LA, Ellefson RD: Porphyrias: Clinical evaluation and interpretation of laboratory tests. Mayo Clin Proc 1994; 69:289–290.

Tietz NW, Rinker AD, Morrison SR: When is a serum iron really a serum iron? The status of serum iron measurements. Clin Chem 1994; 40:546.

Tomokuni K: New method for determination of aminolaevulinate dehydratase activity of human erythrocytes as an index of lead exposure. Clin Chem 1974; 20:1287.

Trueb RM, Panizzon RG, Burg G: Cutaneous ossification in Albright's hereditary osteodystrophy. Dermatology 1993; 186:205.

van Ingen HE, Huijgen HJ, Kok WT, et al: Analytical evaluation of Kone Microlyte determination of ionized magnesium. Clin Chem 1994; 40:52.

Walter JH, Leonard JV: Inborn errors of urea cycle. Br J Hosp Med 1987; 176.

Watson CJ, Schwartz S: A simple test for urinary porphobilinogen. Proc Soc Exp Biol Med 1941; 47:393.

Wysolmerski JJ, Broadus AE: Hypercalcemia of malignancy: The central role of parathyroid hormone–related protein. Annu Rev Med 1994; 45:189.

Zak B, Baginski ES, Emanuel E: Modern iron ligands useful for the measurement of serum iron. Ann Clin Lab Sci 1980; 10:276.

2

Chapter 9

Carbohydrates

Gregory A. Threatte, M.D.
John Bernard Henry, M.D.

Carbohydrates are compounds of carbon, hydrogen, and oxygen, usually with hydrogen and oxygen in a proportion of two hydrogen atoms to one oxygen atom, as in water. These "carbohydrates" (carbon hydrates) have the general formula $C_n(H_2O)_n$. The medically important carbohydrates that contain six carbons (hexoses) are glucose, fructose, and galactose. Lactose (glucose and galactose) and sucrose (glucose and fructose) are important disaccharides.

Abnormalities in the quantity or structure of enzymes involved in carbohydrate metabolism are numerous; the most important are discussed under disorders of fructose, galactose, and glycogen metabolism.

Carbohydrates are measured using whole blood, serum, or plasma. In addition, measurements of glucose in urine, cerebrospinal fluid, and other body fluids are important clinically; these are discussed in Chapters 18 and 19. The concentration of carbohydrates in blood is controlled within narrow limits by many hormones, the most important of which are produced by the endocrine pancreas.

PANCREATIC HORMONES

The cells of the endocrine pancreas secrete three major hormones that are involved in glucose homeostasis: insulin, glucagon, and somatostatin. Each hormone is made by an individual cell type physically contiguous with the other types of hormone-producing cells. The primary function of pancreatic somatostatin likely is regulation of glucagon while insulin and glucagon regulate metabolism by stimulating the anabolism or catabolism of carbohydrates. It is thought that secretion of a hormone by one cell type can influence secretion of the other cells.

Under physiologic circumstances, the intermittent availability of food and energy sources necessitates release of insulin or glucagon, which have a reciprocal relationship. Insulin acts to store carbohydrates as energy and inhibit mobilization of energy stores from endogenous sources, such as liver, fat, and muscle. In contrast, during fasting periods, glucagon enhances catabolic functions such as hepatic glycogenolysis, and, in conjunction with other catabolic hormones, stimulates the formation of glucose. This bihormonal control of glucose regulation requires appropriate secretion of varying amounts of these two hormones, which act on adipose tissue, liver, and muscle to maintain a relatively steady concentration of plasma glucose. Somatostatin acts locally to regulate the release of insulin and glucagon from the pancreas. Additionally, maintenance of plasma glucose concentrations is affected by adrenergic, cholinergic, and possibly peptidergic mechanisms.

Insulin

Insulin is a small peptide with a mass of about 6000 daltons consisting of an A-chain of 21 amino acids and a B-chain of 30 amino acids connected by two disulfide bonds. A polypeptide precursor of insulin, called proinsulin, is synthesized in the microsomal fraction of the pancreatic β cell as a long single chain with a mass of 9000 daltons. During the storage of proinsulin in the cell, two disulfide bonds are formed within the chain. It is converted to a double-chain molecule by a proteolytic process that removes the 31-amino-acid C-pep-

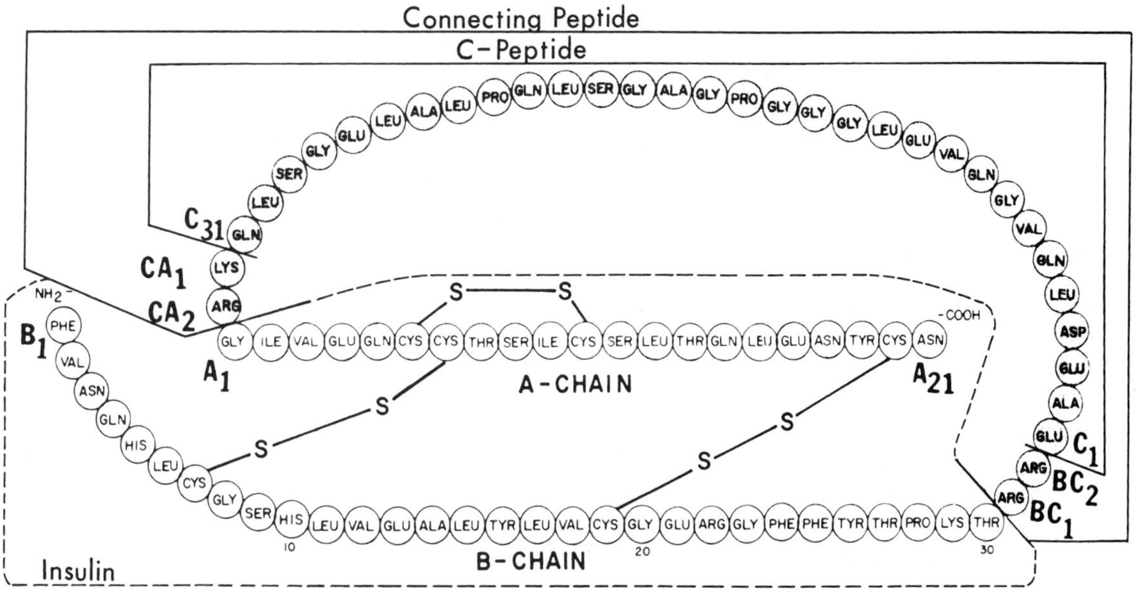

Figure 9–1. Proposed amino acid sequence of human proinsulin. Connecting peptide is the amino acid residue connecting the carboxy end of the B chain to the amino end of the A chain of insulin. "C" peptide is formed when two basic residues BC_1–BC_2 and CA_1–CA_2 have been removed from connecting peptide. Insulin (*broken line*) consists of the A and B chains. (Modified from Kitabchi, AE: Proinsulin and C-peptide: A review. Metabolism 1977; 26:547.)

tide, thus forming insulin (Fig. 9–1). A molecule even larger than proinsulin with 24 additional amino acids has been identified and called pre-proinsulin: this is most likely a precursor of proinsulin. With stimulation, equimolar amounts of C-peptide and native insulin are secreted into the blood. In the fasting state, insulin secretion is minimal, and proinsulin secretion is only about 15% that of insulin. This ratio stays about the same when there is an acute stimulus to insulin secretion. However, the percentage of circulating proinsulin is increased in older patients, pregnant diabetics, obese diabetics, patients with insulinomas, some patients with functional hypoglycemia, and those with a rare syndrome called hyperproinsulinemia. *In vivo* studies of proinsulin have shown that it has less than 10% of the biological activity of insulin; however, it has a half-life three times as long.

The reference interval for fasting serum insulin by radioimmunoassay usually ranges from 2 to 25 μU/mL, but this depends on the antibody used in the assay. Antibodies used in the radioimmunoassay of insulin cross-react with proinsulin. The extent of cross-reactivity depends on the individual antibody but usually is in the range of 30%. Measurement of insulin appears to have little clinical value except in diagnosis of spontaneous hypoglycemia (Marks, 1976). The utility of the assay is discussed later. In general, the sensitivity of the insulin radioimmunoassay is such that it is impossible to differentiate low insulin levels from those within the reference interval. Assays for proinsulin are not readily available.

Although the secretory ratio of C-peptide to insulin is 1:1, the ratio in serum is about 5:1 to 15:1. This occurs because 50% of insulin is rapidly removed by its initial passage through the liver, but hepatic extraction of C-peptide is negligible. Circulating C-peptide does not appear to have any significant biological activity (Wojcikowski, 1990).

C-peptide is measured in a few clinical settings (Table 9–1). In certain hypoglycemic states due to increased β-cell activity, such as insulinoma, C-peptide is elevated. A diagnostic test for insulinoma involves injection of insulin and quantitation of C-peptide (discussed in the section on insulinoma). In addition, because insulin measurements in diabetics can be confounded by anti-insulin antibodies developed as a result of therapy, C-peptide measurements may be the best indicator of residual islet cell function. The most important use of C-peptide measurements is in the diagnosis of surreptitious injection of insulin resulting in "factitious" hypoglycemia. Because C-peptide is removed during purification of commercial insulin preparations, patients who have injected insulin will have demonstrable insulin by radioimmunoassay but no C-peptide. The absence of C-peptide, high serum insulin, and hypoglycemia point to injection of exogenous insulin. Other uses of C-peptide assays include follow-up evaluation of total pancreatectomy for carcinoma and demonstration of the remission phase of "recovery" from diabetes. Patients with complete loss of β-cell capacity have no C-peptide and are frequently "brittle" diabetics, whereas diabetics with residual β-cell function, and thus C-peptide, tend to have more stable diabetes mellitus.

Fasting serum C-peptide concentrations in healthy subjects

Table 9–1. CLINICAL INDICATIONS FOR C-PEPTIDE MEASUREMENT

Hypoglycemic states
Diagnosis of insulinoma
Diagnosis of surreptitious injection of insulin
Euglycemic states
Demonstration of remission phase or "recovery" from diabetes
Hyperglycemic states
Follow-up evaluation after pancreatectomy
Evaluation of the "brittle" diabetic patient

range from 1.0 to 2.0 ng/mL. After administration of a glucose load, levels rise fivefold to sixfold. In insulin-dependent diabetics, C-peptide may be decreased or undetectable; in diabetic ketoacidosis, C-peptide is not measurable. In the usual C-peptide assays, cross-reactivity with proinsulin may be as high as 20%. However, because the serum concentration of proinsulin in a reference population is about 10% that of C-peptide, cross-reactivity of proinsulin in C-peptide assays usually is negligible. In insulin-requiring diabetics, endogenous insulin antibodies are produced that bind proinsulin. In the presence of these antibodies, residual β-cell function results in accumulation of proinsulin in the circulation. In some diabetics, up to 80% of measured C-peptide is due to proinsulin cross-reactivity. Thus, the presence of C-peptide indicates only that β-cell secretion is taking place, and values that are obtained cannot be compared with those in a reference population to quantitate insulin secretion (Horwitz, 1976).

Glucagon

Glucagon is formed by the α_2 (or A cells) that make up about 25% of the islet cells of the pancreas. Glucagon-like polypeptides of varying molecular weights also are formed by the gastrointestinal tract. The naming of these polypeptides is based on reactivity with glucagon antibodies: Polypeptides that react with both C- and N-terminal antibodies are called immunoreactive glucagon (IRG), whereas polypeptides that react only with N-terminal specific antibodies are said to have glucagon-like immunoreactivity (GLI) (Conlon, 1980). According to this classification, IRG is associated with the pancreas and GLI with the gut. Thus, measurements of pancreatic glucagon in serum require antibody that is specific for the C-terminal region of glucagon.

The circulating plasma pancreatic glucagons apparently are heterogeneous. The four fractions that are found include a component with a mass of 160,000 daltons ("big plasma glucagon"), others with masses of 9000 and 3500 daltons, and one component with a mass less than 2000 daltons. The last of these is thought to be a degradation product of glucagon. The largest molecule is probably an original precursor that contains glucagon as one of its fragments as well as a family of related proteins. Glicentin is a fragment that is released by the small bowel during the absorption of glucose. There is both sequence homology and immunologic cross-reactivity between fragments.

In healthy individuals, fasting plasma pancreatic glucagon concentrations are about 50 to 150 pg/mL, with the 160,000-dalton component accounting for 54% and the 3500-dalton fraction accounting for the remainder. The various components show marked differences in response to agents that are known to stimulate or suppress plasma pancreatic glucagon secretion. Hypoglycemia results in a twofold to threefold increase, whereas hyperglycemia results in a decrease in plasma glucagon levels by one half. In patients with renal failure, glucagon levels are increased by up to five times, with the 9000-dalton component predominating because the kidneys are responsible for removal of this fraction. Although not characterized chemically, the 3500-dalton glucagon is thought to be the physiologically important fraction; the functions of the remaining fragments may be diverse.

Glucagon concentrations are important in the diagnosis of A-cell tumors of the pancreas (glucagonomas). This tumor is associated with mild diabetes mellitus and plasma glucagon concentrations ranging from 900 to 7800 pg/mL. A very high glucagon level in a diabetic suggests this diagnosis. Clinically, these patients present with a characteristic necrotizing migratory rash, weight loss, anemia, stomatitis, and glossitis, and about two thirds of patients have metastases at presentation. In familial hyperglucagonemia, an autosomal dominant disorder, glucagon is elevated mainly because of the increase of the 9000-dalton component.

In insulin-dependent diabetics, IRG levels are within the reference interval but inappropriate for plasma glucose concentrations and show an exaggerated response to such stimuli as protein loading. Because evidence has indicated that glucagon is stable, precautions such as collection in cold tubes containing a protease inhibitor such as aprotinin (Trasylol) and immediate centrifugation at 4°C may be superfluous (Hendriks, 1981).

Somatostatin

Somatostatin, a tetradecapeptide with a disulfide bond, first was isolated from the hypothalamus. Somatostatin was originally considered a strictly hypothalamic hormone that inhibited growth hormone secretion, but the discovery of somatostatin in the islets of Langerhans prompted further investigation of its function in the endocrine pancreas. Subsequently, somatostatin was also found in gastric mucosa and intestine. It inhibits pituitary, gastrointestinal, and pancreatic hormones as well as possessing nonendocrinologic functions (Table 9–2).

The D cells of the pancreas, which make up 10% of the total islet mass, are thought to be the site of somatostatin synthesis. The D cells are distributed asymmetrically such that they are close to glucagon-producing or A cells and thus can affect glucagon by diminishing its release. Somatostatin's short half-life of one minute, its diverse actions, and the failure to detect it in peripheral circulation argue against its function as a circulating hormone and point to its action as a local modulator. Somatostatin is measured by radioimmunoassay, but the assay is not widely available.

A few tumors of somatostatin-producing D cells of the pancreas have been described; in these cases, patients present with hyperglycemia, hypoglucagonemia, malabsorption, and achlorhydria.

Table 9–2. FUNCTIONS OF SOMATOSTATIN

Endocrine	Nonendocrine
Inhibition of secretion or diminution of:	
Growth hormone	Gastric acid secretion
Thyrotropin	Gastric emptying time
Gastrin	Gallbladder contraction
Secretin	Pancreatic bicarbonate release
Vasointestinal peptide	Pancreatic enzyme release
Glucagon	Acetylcholine release from peripheral nerve endings
Insulin	

GLUCOSE MEASUREMENTS

Specimen Considerations

Diagnosis of disorders of carbohydrate metabolism rests in part on the measurement of plasma glucose, either in the fasting state or following stimulation or suppression tests. Venous blood is the specimen of choice for glucose analysis, but capillary blood can be used in infants and others in whom venipuncture is difficult. After an overnight fast, capillary blood glucose values are only 2 to 3 mg/dL (0.1 to 0.2 mmol/L) higher than venous concentrations, but after carbohydrate loading, capillary values may be 20 to 30 mg/dL (1.1 to 1.7 mmol/L) higher. Glucose concentrations in arterial and capillary blood are similar.

Although early manual laboratory determinations of glucose were performed using whole blood, these measurements are no longer used. However, because some criteria for the laboratory diagnosis of diabetes mellitus were developed using whole blood glucose values, it is important to have at least some knowledge of these determinations. In addition, whole blood measurements have new importance because bedside glucose monitors and home glucose monitoring devices use whole blood specimens.

Another problem with whole blood glucose levels is that they vary with the hematocrit. Furthermore, there is no readily automated method. Saccharides, substances from erythrocytes that do not reduce glucose, interfere with measurement; also, an inhibitor of glycolysis must be included in the specimen to prevent erythrocytes and leukocytes from metabolizing glucose.

At room temperature, glucose in whole blood specimens without added inhibitors of glycolysis is metabolized at approximately 7 mg/dL/h (0.4 mmol/L/h); at 4°C, the loss is approximately 2 mg/dL/h (0.1 mmol/L/h) (Weissman, 1958). Although erythrocytes and platelets use glucose, leukocytes and bacterial contamination are the usual agents of glycolysis. A serum specimen is appropriate for glucose analysis if serum is separated from the cells within 30 minutes, but if serum is in contact with cells for longer than 30 minutes, a preservative such as fluoride that inhibits glycolysis should be added. However, in serum specimens without bacterial contamination or leukocytosis, results remain clinically acceptable even after a delay of up to 90 minutes before separation of serum and cells. If whole blood is refrigerated, 2 mg of sodium fluoride per milliliter of whole blood prevents glycolysis for up to 48 hours (Chan, 1989). When refrigerated, glucose is stable in serum or plasma for 48 hours. With long-term specimen storage, even at −20°C, glucose values decrease significantly and progressively.

Glucose Methods

Glucose methods can be divided into two groups—chemical and enzymatic. Most chemical measurements of glucose depend on its reducing properties; most are no longer used because of lack of specificity. Ortho-toluidine is the only chemical method still used widely and is based on the condensation of aldosaccharides, such as glucose, with an aromatic amine and glacial acetic acid. The stable green color that develops then is measured spectrophotometrically. This method can be used for plasma, urine, or cerebrospinal fluid without protein precipitation. Galactose and mannose react as well as glucose; lactose, maltose, sucrose, and fructose also react, but to a much lesser extent. Hence, values for this method are slightly higher than for more specific enzymatic methods; in patients with uremia, this difference is even more marked. A major disadvantage of ortho-toluidine is the corrosiveness of the reagent to laboratory equipment as well as its toxicity. Other infrequently used chemical methods are reviewed in Chapter 7 of the 16th edition of this book.

2

Enzymatic methods yield maximum specificity for glucose measurements. Glucose can be measured by its reaction with glucose oxidase, in which gluconic acid and hydrogen peroxide (H_2O_2) are generated. Hydrogen peroxide then reacts with an oxygen acceptor, such as ortho-dianisidine, phenylamine-phenazone (Trinder's reagent), or other chromogenic oxygen acceptors, in a reaction catalyzed by peroxidase to form a color:

$$\beta\text{-D-Glucose} + O_2 \xrightarrow[\text{oxidase}]{\text{glucose}} \text{gluconolactone} \xrightarrow[O_2]{H_2O} \text{gluconic acid} + H_2O_2 \quad (9\text{-}1)$$

$$H_2O_2 + \begin{matrix}\text{Ortho-dianisidine } (or) \\ \text{phenylamine-phenazone} \\ (\text{chromogenic } O_2 \text{ acceptor})\end{matrix} \xrightarrow{\text{peroxidase}} \text{color (chromogen)} + H_2O \quad (9\text{-}2)$$

Glucose oxidase is highly specific for β-D-glucose, and any glucose present in the α form must be converted to the β form before reacting. Some preparations of glucose oxidase contain the enzyme mutarotase, which accelerates this process. The second step involving peroxidase is less specific than the first, and numerous reducing substances inhibit oxidation of the chromogens used in the peroxidase reaction. Although uric acid and creatinine cause little interference in most of these methods, ascorbic acid can lead to spuriously decreased values. One of the chief advantages of a glucose oxidase method is its low cost.

Another useful approach to glucose methodology has been the glucose oxidase-oxygen electrode method. In this method, an oxygen-sensing electrode monitors reaction of glucose with oxygen while generated H_2O_2 is removed by reaction with ethanol and iodide. By determining the rate of oxygen consumption, one can accurately estimate glucose. This method is precise, linear, and free from important interferences. Results approximate those of the hexokinase glucose method.

A hexokinase method that provides a high degree of specificity for estimating glucose is the generally accepted reference method for glucose. In this method, glucose is measured by quantitating reduced nicotinamide adenine dinucleotide phosphate (NADPH) formation from the following reactions:

$$\text{Glucose} + \text{ATP} \xrightarrow[Mg^{+2}]{\text{hexokinase}} \text{glucose 6-phosphate} + \text{ADP} \quad (9\text{-}3)$$

$$\text{Glucose 6-phosphate} + \text{NADP} \xrightarrow{\text{G6PD}} \text{6-phosphogluconolactone} + \text{NADPH} + H^+ \quad (9\text{-}4)$$

The main disadvantage of hexokinase is its cost; however, in an extended comparison, it produced the best between-run and within-run precision. No major interferences have been demonstrated with a large number of substances that are known to interfere with other methods.

Fasting Plasma Glucose

Plasma specimens collected after a 12- to 14-hour fast vary less among individuals than do specimens collected at other times. Plasma glucose results can be classified as either hyperglycemic or hypoglycemic, but both of these definitions are rather arbitrary, with no clear-cut distinction between what is normal and abnormal. An overnight fasting glucose concentration between 50 and 110 mg/dL (2.8 to 6.2 mmol/L) is accepted by most workers as within the reference interval. Many syndromes and diseases are associated with inappropriately high fasting plasma glucose levels. Some of them are listed in Table 9–3, wherein they are separated into primary (diabetes mellitus) and secondary causes. Hyperglycemia may result from a total absence of insulin secretion, such as after surgical pancreatectomy; it may occur from infiltration of the pancreas, as in hemochromatosis; or it may occur intermittently during periods of stress, such as with severe infection, dehydration, or pregnancy. Hyperglycemia may be secondary to other endocrine diseases or even due to an antibody to the insulin receptor. Some drugs, such as propranolol, thiazide diuretics, and phenytoin, can block insulin release and cause hyperglycemia.

Table 9–3. CLASSIFICATION OF HYPERGLYCEMIA

Primary
Insulin-dependent diabetes mellitus
Non–insulin-dependent diabetes mellitus
Secondary
Hyperglycemia resulting from disease of the pancreas
Inflammation
Acute pancreatitis (rare)
Chronic pancreatitis
Pancreatitis due to mumps
? Cell damage due to coxsackievirus B_4 infection
? Autoimmune disease
Pancreatectomy
Pancreatic infiltration
Hemochromatosis
Tumors
Trauma to pancreas (rare)
Hyperglycemia related to other major endocrine diseases
Acromegaly
Cushing's syndrome
Thyrotoxicosis
Pheochromocytoma
Hyperaldosteronism
Glucagonoma
Somatostatinoma
Hyperglycemia caused by drugs
Steroids
Thiazide diuretics, propranolol, phenytoin, and diazoxide
Oral contraceptives
Alloxan and streptozotocin
Hyperglycemia related to other major disease states
Chronic renal failure
Chronic liver disease
Infection
Miscellaneous hyperglycemia
Pregnancy
Related to insulin receptor antibodies (acanthosis nigricans)
Abnormal insulin

Diabetes mellitus can be diagnosed by measurement of plasma glucose when the patient is fasting. A fasting plasma glucose level greater than 140 mg/dL (7.8 mmol/L) is considered abnormal. If the plasma glucose is above this level on two or more occasions, diabetes mellitus can be diagnosed in accordance with criteria of the National Diabetes Data Group (NDDG).

Diabetes mellitus is a chronic disease characterized by abnormally high concentrations of plasma glucose and glucosuria and disordered carbohydrate, protein, and fat metabolism associated with impaired insulin secretion or insulin resistance. Diabetes mellitus affects about 10 million Americans (5% of the population) and is the third leading cause of death in the United States. Individuals with diabetes have an increased risk of blindness, kidney disease, peripheral vascular disease, and heart disease.

Clinically, diabetes mellitus is a heterogeneous disorder, especially when gestational diabetes and patients with impaired glucose tolerance are also considered. Patients with impaired glucose tolerance have fasting glucose or glucose tolerance test (GTT) levels that lie between normal and NDDG criteria and may represent an early stage in the natural history of diabetes. Patients who meet NDDG criteria are generally divided into two groups: non–insulin-dependent diabetes mellitus (NIDDM) and insulin-dependent diabetes mellitus (IDDM). Patients with IDDM classically present at an early age (usually before 30) and have a rapid onset of the disorder, occasional remissions, and episodes of ketosis. In contrast, patients with NIDDM are commonly obese and present at an older age; the onset is insidious, and ketosis is rare. In insulin-dependent diabetics, there is an increased incidence of histocompatibility antigens (see Chap. 39) HLA-DR3, DR4, and DQ, whereas DR2 and B7 seem to resist affliction with IDDM. There is also evidence that individuals who inherit both DR3 and DR4 genes are at greater risk than those with two copies of DR3 or DR4 (Svejgaard, 1980). Having two or more first-degree relatives with either IDDM or NIDDM strongly increases the risk of developing diabetes mellitus; however, NIDDM and HLA have not been linked except in specific population groups with a high incidence of NIDDM in children and adolescents.

Hypoglycemia is defined as a syndrome characterized by low plasma glucose and an associated group of symptoms that are relieved by ingestion of food or carbohydrate. Overnight fasting plasma glucose levels below 45 mg/dL (2.5 mmol/L) are clearly abnormal, whereas those above 55 mg/dL (3.1 mmol/L) usually are accepted as normal. During the first week of life, hypoglycemia is defined as plasma glucose concentrations of less than 25 mg/dL (1.4 mmol/L) in the preterm or low birth weight infant. In the full term infant, plasma glucose values of less than 35 mg/dL (1.9 mmol/L) from birth to 72 hours of age and of less than 45 mg/dL (2.5 mmol/L) thereafter are considered to represent hypoglycemia. Not all pediatricians agree with these statistical definitions and thus vigorously treat patients when plasma glucose is less than 40 mg/dL (2.2 mmol/L) (Aynsley-Green, 1982).

In adults, two different groups of symptoms occur, depending on whether the hypoglycemia is acute or chronic. If plasma glucose becomes low rapidly, homeostatic mechanisms release epinephrine and produce symptoms of sweating, shakiness, trembling, weakness, and anxiety. If plasma glucose is reduced slowly, headache, irritability, lethargy, and other central nervous system symptoms predominate. If the hypoglycemia can be documented, its cause must be investigated fully.

Fasting values also need to be interpreted in relationship to the preparation of the patient. For instance, Felig (1982) has shown that when fasting healthy individuals are exercised to exhaustion, their plasma glucose values commonly are considered hypoglycemic; some were lower than 35 mg/dL (1.9 mmol/L). Merimee (1974) has attempted to define the criteria for laboratory diagnosis of hypoglycemia during extended fasting. In a group of healthy subjects who had fasted for 24 hours, lower reference limits of plasma glucose were found to be 55 mg/dL (3.1 mmol/L) in men and 35 mg/dL (1.9 mmol/L) in young women. Men who fasted for 72 hours had plasma glucose values as low as 50 mg/dL (2.8 mmol/L). It became virtually impossible to define a reference plasma glucose value that was meaningful for discrimination of hypoglycemia in premenopausal women who had fasted more than 36 hours. In these studies, after a 72-hour fast, plasma glucose in this reference population was found to be as low as 15 mg/dL (0.8 mmol/L). These and other studies have raised a question of the definition of hypoglycemia. Merimee (1977) concluded that what has been called "functional" hypoglycemia (a variety of hypoglycemia provoked by modest withholding of food) is in fact normal, and in this instance false standards may have created a false disease.

The causes of syndromes presenting with hypoglycemia are classified in Table 9–4. In the first group, there is no anatomic lesion; hypoglycemia usually occurs in relationship to a meal, and fasting plasma glucose is within the reference interval. The causes of reactive hypoglycemia fall into this category and may be evaluated by five-hour glucose tolerance testing (see later).

Ethanol and other drugs can cause fasting hypoglycemia.

Table 9–4. CLASSIFICATION OF SOME OF THE MORE COMMON CAUSES OF HYPOGLYCEMIA

No anatomic lesion present
Fasting plasma glucose normal
Reactive hypoglycemia
Functional hypoglycemia
Alimentary hypoglycemia
Diabetic and impaired glucose tolerance
Fasting plasma glucose low
Ethanol-induced hypoglycemia
Drug-induced hypoglycemia
Sulfonylurea
Phenformin*
Insulin
Ethanol
Salicylates
Combinations of the above
Factitious—fasting glucose normal or low
Anatomic lesion present
Insulinoma
Extrapancreatic neoplasms
Adrenocortical insufficiency
Hypopituitarism
Massive liver disease

*No longer available in the United States.

Ethanol-induced hypoglycemia occurs only after prolonged ingestion of alcohol and when the liver supply of glycogen is depleted concurrently. The most common causes of drug-induced hypoglycemia are hypoglycemic agents (e.g., sulfonylureas, insulin), which account for more than half of the drug-induced causes; others are salicylates, sulfonamides, propranolol, or a combination of these. Factitious hypoglycemia is another phenomenon that can be unrelated to meals.

Insulinomas or other tumors such as mesotheliomas, hepatic carcinomas, adrenocortical tumors, and gastrointestinal carcinomas may cause hypoglycemia. The hypoglycemia caused by lesions such as tumors generally is profound and unremitting. About 30% to 50% of tumors, such as large mesenchymal tumors, hepatomas, and adrenocortical carcinomas, produce insulin-like substances that cause hypoglycemia. The activity of these substances is not suppressed by insulin antibodies *in vitro;* therefore, this material has been called nonsuppressible insulin-like activity. Other diseases that commonly present with hypoglycemia include adrenocortical insufficiency, hypopituitarism, and diffuse liver disease.

2

Random Plasma Glucose

In healthy individuals, plasma glucose concentrations vary only slightly throughout the day and generally are in the range of 45 to 130 mg/dL (2.5 to 7.2 mmol/L). The only rise is found following a meal, but even then it rarely exceeds 10 to 15 mg/dL (0.6 to 0.8 mmol/L). This degree of elevation is different from that obtained during a GTT. When healthy middle-aged and older subjects are given a glucose load, plasma glucose concentrations may range from 20 to 50 mg/dL (1.1 to 2.8 mmol/L) higher than when the same subjects are given a breakfast with 75 g of carbohydrate.

In IDDM diabetics, plasma glucose concentrations may be grossly abnormal during the day, with fluctuations in plasma glucose as great as 150 mg/dL (8.3 mmol/L). Although 130 mg/dL (7.2 mmol/L) is considered the upper limit of normal for a random plasma glucose concentration, values for healthy individuals who are over 65 years old can range up to 180 mg/dL (10.0 mmol/L).

Random plasma glucose levels below 45 mg/dL (2.5 mmol/L) are unusual and warrant further investigation, especially if the individual is symptomatic. Low values may reflect normal physiologic response in plasma glucose concentrations such as occur following a meal, or they could be the first and only clue to a disorder in glucose homeostasis. It is unlikely that symptoms attributable to hypoglycemia occur when plasma glucose concentrations are greater than 45 mg/dL (2.5 mmol/L).

INSULINOMA

The most important cause of hypoglycemia is excessive and inappropriate secretion of insulin by pancreatic β-cell tumors. These tumors, called insulinomas, have been reported to occur in every age group, but they are most common in the fourth to sixth decades of life. The many clinical features associated with these tumors are caused by the hypoglycemia that they induce. The diagnosis of hypoglycemia should be made using the criteria known as Whipple's triad: (1) hypoglycemic attacks precipitated by fasting, (2) plasma glucose below 45 mg/dL (2.5 mmol/L) during the attack, and (3) symptoms relieved promptly by the administration of glucose. Approximately 80% of insulinomas are benign, 10% are multiple, and another 10% are malignant. Malignant insulinomas also have been reported to produce other hormones, including ACTH, glucagon, and gastrin.

Because hypoglycemia is caused by excessive and inappropriate production of insulin, the insulin radioimmunoassay is essential in confirming this diagnosis. Normally, fasting is associated with a progressive fall in serum insulin concentrations; however, patients with insulinomas usually do not have a diminished level of insulin even with hypoglycemia. Although the absolute insulin concentration in a patient with an insulinoma may actually be within the reference interval, the value is inappropriately high for the degree of hypoglycemia. An overnight fast may not be sufficient to demonstrate inappropriate insulin secretion in patients with tumors; however, three consecutive overnight fasts, or a fast for up to 72 hours, identifies almost all insulinoma patients. Apart from factitious hypoglycemia, the only other disorder in which inappropriate insulin secretion has been documented during fasting is idiopathic hypoglycemia of childhood.

As the glucose concentration falls during a fast, serum insulin values decline steadily to reach low levels. The ratio of immunoreactive insulin (μU/mL) to glucose (mg/dL) after an overnight fast, or during a 72-hour fast, usually is less than 0.30 μU/ml–mg/dL (Fajans, 1976). Insulin-to-glucose ratios have become important in the definition of inappropriate insulin secretion and the definition of hypoglycemia.

A ratio of insulin to glucose has been developed that corrects for technical problems involved in the insulin assay and has led to an "amended" insulin-to-glucose ratio. Because insulin secretion from the healthy β cell is reduced to basal levels with hypoglycemia, insulin will be undetectable by radioimmunoassay at glucose concentrations of about 30 mg/dL (1.7 mmol/L). Therefore, a value of 30 mg/dL is subtracted from the glucose value. This amended ratio is seen as follows (in μU/mg):

$$\frac{\text{Insulin } (\mu\text{U/mL})}{\text{glucose (mg/dL} - 30 \text{ (mg/dL)}} \times 100 \qquad (9\text{-}5)$$

In a reference population, the amended ratio extends up to 100 μU/mg; in insulinoma patients, the mean ratio was 180 μU/mg (Frerichs, 1976). A similar study by Fajans (1976) suggested that an amended ratio up to 50 μU/mg is normal. In both studies, a few patients with insulinomas were found to have normal amended ratios. Some workers have not found these formulas clinically useful and simply use a serum insulin level of greater than 10 μU/mL in the presence of fasting hypoglycemia as diagnostic of an insulinoma.

For patients in whom the diagnosis cannot be confirmed during a 72-hour fast, stimulatory procedures can be used. Manifestations of inappropriate insulin release are exaggerated by responses to insulin secretagogues such as tolbutamide, an oral hypoglycemic agent. When given as a rapid intravenous infusion, tolbutamide causes an immediate release of insulin, resulting in hypoglycemia. The depth and length of hypoglycemia have been used to indicate the presence of an insulinoma. The criteria used are as follows: (1) a decrease in plasma glucose of more than 65% or to levels below 30 mg/dL (1.7 mmol/L), (2) plasma glucose of less than 40 mg/dL (2.2 mmol/L) persisting for at least 180 minutes, and (3) significant increase of serum insulin concentrations above the reference interval (Frerichs, 1976). Tolbutamide test results sometimes are falsely positive in obese subjects and patients with nesidioblastosis, whereas results are falsely negative in up to 50% of patients with insulinomas. A stimulatory test using the amino acid leucine causes insulin release in about 50% of insulinoma patients. Although other secretagogues such as glucagon and calcium infusions have been used, experience with them is limited, and results are inconsistent. False-positive results for leucine and glucagon procedures may approach 40%. The GTT is of little use in diagnosis of an insulinoma, because no diagnostic pattern is found.

Use of the C-peptide assay also has been helpful in the diagnosis of insulinomas; the suppressibility of β-cell secretion with insulin-induced hypoglycemia maintained for one hour is monitored by C-peptide measurements. Because C-peptide is removed during purification of commercial insulin preparations, presence of C-peptide levels in the circulation is good evidence of autonomous insulin secretion. C-peptide secretion is suppressed to less than 1.2 ng/mL in healthy persons, whereas patients with insulinomas have C-peptide concentrations of greater than 1.9 ng/mL (Service, 1977). C-peptide secretion is decreased or absent in some patients with insulinomas, however.

GLUCOSE TOLERANCE TESTING

When fasting plasma glucose levels are less than 140 mg/dL (7.8 mmol/L) in patients with suspected glucose intolerance, an oral GTT may be indicated. Furthermore, because diabetes mellitus during pregnancy may be associated with increased morbidity and mortality, the increased sensitivity of a GTT may be needed. In this test, the response of a patient to a glucose load or challenge is measured by assaying glucose at postchallenge intervals. This challenge has been standardized: after either an oral or an intravenous load of glucose, plasma glucose values are determined. Although the GTT is sensitive, it suffers from lack of specificity. It is abnormal in a wide variety of diseases and is influenced by diet as well as other variables.

Preparatory Phase

If test data are to be meaningful, test conditions must be controlled rigidly. For three days prior to the GTT, the patient's diet must contain at least 150 g of carbohydrate per day. Two additional days of this diet are essential if the patient has not been on a diet with sufficient carbohydrates previously. Anorexia or any other condition precluding adequate food intake automatically invalidates the test. Inactivity, such as bed rest, has been reported to impair glucose tolerance; thus, a GTT should not be performed in nonambulatory patients. During the 12 hours prior to a test, the patient must fast and avoid even black coffee. In addition, smoking and even mild exercise are not permitted. The test should not be performed in patients who have been ill during the prior two weeks. Endocrine disorders such as acromegaly, hyperthyroidism, or Cushing's syndrome frequently are associated with abnormal glucose tolerance. Thus, dysfunction of the endocrine system should be evaluated and corrected before a GTT is performed. Many drugs such as salicylates, diuretics, and anticonvulsants decrease insulin secretion; they should be avoided for at least three days prior to the performance of the test, as should all nonessential medications. Oral contraceptives will both cause insulin resistance and alter the half-life of insulin (Godsland, 1992).

Procedures

The size of the glucose load employed varies; a 50-g, 75-g, or 100-g load currently is used. A 75-g load for nonpregnant adults and a pediatric glucose load of 1.75 g/kg body weight (up to 75 g) is recommended. In gestational diabetes, a 100-mg dose is used for patients who have an elevated glucose level in a specimen drawn one hour following a 50-g screening dose (Narayanan, 1991). Higher doses are more sensitive and reproducible but lead to more nausea and vomiting, which may invalidate the results. An alternative to glucose monomers used in the challenge is to use a glucose polymer (Polycose, Ross Laboratories, Columbus OH). Several studies have compared glucose polymer with glucose monomer and found equivalent glucose kinetics (Murphy, 1994; Philipson, 1992; Reece, 1989). However, because the osmotic load of the polymer is only a fifth of that found with the monomer, adverse symptoms related to the ingestion of glucose were halved (Bergus, 1992).

Between 7 and 9 A.M. and after 30 minutes of rest, a blood sample for baseline glucose is obtained, and the patient ingests the glucose load within 5 minutes of the fasting sample. The glucose is ingested over 5 minutes, and the first blood specimen is drawn at a specified time after baseline, depending on the criteria used for interpretation (Table 9–5). If nausea, fainting, sweating, or other autonomic nervous system overactivity occurs, a specimen for glucose should be drawn immediately and the procedure discontinued and repeated at a later date if indicated. Because of the diurnal variation in glucose tolerance, if a GTT is performed in the morning and repeated 12 hours later, some patients who are judged normal in the morning would be classified as diabetic with the evening test. Other patients tested on different days may be found to have a GTT consistent with diabetes on one day but not on the second day.

Evaluation of Results

Most of the data used to establish criteria for glucose tolerance testing are based on measurements of whole blood glucose. However, diagnostic glucose currently is determined only on serum or plasma specimens. Many different glucose methods have been used in determining reference intervals for the GTT; these different methods result in dissimilar glucose values and add further confusion to the interpretation of results. The most widely used criteria are those of the Wilkerson point system, those of Fajans-Conn, those of Siperstein, and those proposed by the NDDG. Many other criteria have been proposed, but for the sake of brevity they have been omitted. The Fajans-Conn criteria were developed using whole blood as the specimen source but have been modified so that plasma values exceeding 185 mg/dL (10.3 mmol/L) at one hour, exceeding 160 mg/dL (8.9 mmol/L) at one and a half hours, and exceeding 140 mg/dL (7.8 mmol/L) at two hours are used as the criteria to diagnose diabetes. Diagnostic interpretation can depend on the criteria used.

Siperstein criticized the GTT in 1975. He points out that the reference population used for the Fajans-Conn criteria were young subjects; that glucose intolerance increases with age; and that if these criteria are accepted, 35% to 60% of the general population over age 40 would be labeled diabetic. Siperstein recommends that a glucose concentration of greater than 260 mg/dL (14.4 mmol/L) at one hour and 220 mg/dL (12.2 mmol/L) at two hours be the criteria used for the diagnosis of diabetes mellitus. He recommends that a fasting plasma glucose level of 140 mg/dL (7.8 mmol/L) or greater on two and preferably three separate occasions also can be used to establish the diagnosis of diabetes mellitus. Some workers even recommend that the GTT be abandoned, and the trend has been away from criteria established by Fajans and Conn toward more liberal criteria. The criteria proposed by the NDDG (1979) reflect this trend and have been endorsed by the American Diabetes Association as well as the World Health Organization (WHO). They recommend that diabetes mellitus be diagnosed only when (1) fasting plasma glucose exceeds 140 mg/dL (7.8 mmol/L), (2) the two-hour value is equal to or more than 200 mg/dL (11.1 mmol/L), and (3) a level between 0 and two hours exceeds 200 mg/dL (11.1 mmol/L). The WHO criteria do not require the latter abnormal level between 0 and two hours. The glucose levels of the reference population of nonpregnant adults during fasting, at

Table 9–5. ORAL GTT DIAGNOSTIC CRITERIA FOR DIABETES MELLITUS

	Criteria Based on Plasma Glucose mg/dL (mmol/L)
National Diabetes Data Group: 75 g to all nonpregnant subjects	Diabetes = fasting ≥140 (7.8) 2 h and ½, 1, or 1½ hr > 200 (11.1)
Fajans and Conn	1 h—>185 (10.3) 1½ h—>160 (8.9) 2 h—>140 (7.8) All three values together abnormal for diagnosis
Wilkerson point system	Fasting—>125 (6.9) = 1 point 1 h—>195 (10.8) = ½ point 2 h—>145 (8.0) = ½ point 3 h—>125 (6.9) = 1 point 3 h—>125 (6.9) = 1 point Points for abnormal values: 2 points for diagnosis
Siperstein	Fasting—>140 (7.8) 1 h—>260 (14.4) 2 h—>220 (12.2) Elevated fasting levels on two occasions or abnormal 1- and 2-h values
Pregnancy: O'Sullivan: 100 g to all subjects National Diabetes Data Group: 75 g carbohydrate load	Fasting—>105 (5.8) 1 h—>190 (10.6) 2 h—>165 (9.2) 3 h—>145 (8.0) Two or more values abnormal for diagnosis of gestational diabetes

2

two hours, and at intermediate times are greater than 115, 140, and 200 mg/dL (6.4, 7.8, and 11.1 mmol/L), respectively. Patients whose glucose values are between those of the reference and diabetic groups are placed in a category called "impaired glucose tolerance."

In many laboratories, urine is collected frequently during the GTT for measurement of glucose. Although this practice may be of some value in detection of renal glycosuria, it is of no value in the diagnosis of diabetes mellitus and may actually be an additional stress on the patient, thereby adversely affecting the test. For these reasons, such practice is not recommended.

It is important to identify mild gestational diabetic women, because perinatal mortality in infants of these patients exceeds that observed in infants of nondiabetics, and treatment significantly decreases this loss. In pregnancy, diabetic patients are identified by the presence of an abnormal glucose tolerance using a 100-g glucose load. Throughout pregnancy, the fasting glucose concentration normally is lower, but glucose intolerance increases during the second and third trimesters. O'Sullivan (1964) established reference values during pregnancy as a fasting plasma glucose level of up to 105 mg/dL (5.8 mmol/L) and one-, two-, and three-hour levels of up to 190, 165, and 145 mg/dL (10.6, 9.2, and 8.0 mmol/L), respectively. If two of these values are exceeded, gestational diabetes is diagnosed (see Table 9–5). A one-hour plasma glucose value exceeding 155 mg/dL (8.6 mmol/L) following a 50-g oral glucose load has generally been used as the screening criterion for performing the GTT in pregnant women, but studies have used a level as low as 130 mg/dL as the cut-off for using the three-hour GTT (Super, 1991).

Additional Diagnostic Procedures

Although a three-hour GTT has been used for the diagnosis of hyperglycemia, a five-hour GTT traditionally has been used for the diagnosis of reactive hypoglycemia. Because symptoms of hypoglycemia are so transient, specimens are obtained every 30 minutes along with a specimen drawn when the patient becomes symptomatic. During a five-hour GTT, 2.5% of asymptomatic patients have glucose concentrations of less than 40 mg/dL (2.2 mmol/L); therefore, chemical hypoglycemia may be considered to occur when the plasma glucose falls below this level. During the five-hour GTT, about one fourth of healthy individuals have plasma glucose values of less than 60 mg/dL (3.3 mmol/L), and diabetics have about the same incidence. These groups occasionally include patients with plasma values of less than 40 mg/dL (2.2 mmol/L).

Hypoglycemia that occurs following a meal is classified as "reactive" hypoglycemia and has been divided traditionally into (1) alimentary, (2) functional, and (3) that in diabetics and in those with impaired glucose tolerance. Alimentary hypoglycemia usually occurs in patients who have undergone gastrointestinal surgery. Accelerated absorption of a glucose load leads to marked postprandial hyperglycemia with a corresponding exaggerated insulin release; the ensuing hypoglycemia typically occurs from one and one half to three hours after eating. This pattern of glucose intolerance and a history of gastrointestinal surgery suggest the diagnosis. Diabetics or patients with impaired glucose tolerance may also experience reactive hypoglycemia. In these patients, hypoglycemia occurs later than in the group with an alimentary disorder, and insulin response is delayed and exaggerated.

Functional hypoglycemia is perceived to be common in adults; it may be characterized by abnormally low plasma glucose and symptoms of lightheadedness, shakiness, diaphoresis, weakness, and fatigue occurring with the modest withholding of food. Complaints suggestive of this syndrome are common in persons with emotional problems. However, when the five-hour GTT is used to diagnose this disorder, the latter patients are indistinguishable from healthy individuals. Because these patients have unremarkable plasma glucose values during the occurrence of symptoms, the five-hour GTT seems unreliable for the diagnosis of functional hypoglycemia (Johnson, 1980). Patients with functional hypoglycemia do not develop diabetes mellitus more often than does the general population.

It is exceedingly important to obtain plasma for a glucose determination if and when symptoms occur. During the GTT, a significant number of patients will experience the symptoms that resulted in their referral, but these symptoms may not be related to low plasma glucose values. These patients should be evaluated for anxiety states and should receive supportive therapy with deemphasis of hypoglycemia. These patients often improve when their food intake is divided so that they eat many small meals rather than several large ones.

Insulin determinations have been suggested in conjunction with glucose measurements in order to improve the diagnostic accuracy of the GTT. They have not been widely used, however. The expense of performing multiple insulin measurements and difficulties in data interpretation probably have been responsible for the lack of widespread use. The extreme variability of the insulin response to identical glucose loads also has cast doubt on the appropriateness of insulin measurements during a GTT.

The intravenous GTT has been used to diagnose diabetes mellitus in patients with gastrointestinal disorders. In this test, 0.5 g of glucose per kilogram of body weight is given as a rapid intravenous infusion within 3 minutes. Blood is drawn for glucose before infusion and at 1, 3, 5, 10, 20, 30, 40, 60, and 120 minutes following the end of the infusion. Glucose disappearance constants (k values) are calculated from a plot of the log of the glucose concentration in relationship to time. A k value of less than 1.2 is considered to be diagnostic of diabetes mellitus. In a comparison of the oral GTT and the intravenous test, Olefsky (1973) found that these two tests gave different diagnostic information 40% of the time, and it was concluded that the intravenous GTT is a poor method for estimating glucose disposal. However, Martin (1992) and Lillioja (1993) have used variations of the intravenous GTT, including computer modeling of results, and have found it to be predictive of a subsequent onset of NIDDM in high-risk populations.

Another test of glucose tolerance involves the use of cortisone and glucose (cortisone GTT). Because cortisone promotes gluconeogenesis, it may accentuate carbohydrate intolerance in latent or mild diabetics. After two doses of cortisone, an oral GTT is performed. A two-hour specimen yielding a plasma glucose value exceeding 165 mg/dL (9.2 mmol/L) is used to discriminate between diabetics and nondiabetics. This single two-hour value has been an unreliable upper reference limit, because it results in a diagnosis of diabetes mellitus in a large number of people. The prognostic implication of this test is uncertain, not only in the elderly but also in other age groups.

Two-Hour Postprandial Plasma Glucose

Two-hour postprandial plasma glucose levels have been used to case find or screen for diabetes mellitus, to diagnose diabetes mellitus, and to monitor glucose control. The maximum increase in plasma glucose following a meal usually occurs at about 60 to 90 minutes, and by two hours the levels are similar to the fasting values. In older persons, however, the two-hour level may be slightly higher than the fasting glucose level. Many studies have shown that the two-hour postprandial plasma glucose is the most sensitive of the values of the GTT in establishing a diagnosis of diabetes.

The significance of the two-hour postprandial value is limited by the lack of rigidly controlled conditions such as the amount of carbohydrate, the age of the patient, and intercurrent infection. These factors are responsible for the differences in the interpretation of the results. As with the GTT, the diagnostic value of the two-hour postprandial glucose is debatable. However, if it is to be used, some workers suggest that a formal GTT be performed when a two-hour postprandial plasma glucose level is greater than 140 mg/dL (7.8 mmol/L). Good control of diabetes has been defined as a two-hour plasma glucose value of less than 130 mg/dL (7.2 mmol/L).

HEMOGLOBIN A_{1c}

Current methods of assessing control in patients with diabetes mellitus include measurement of blood and plasma glucose. Urine glucose measurements are no longer recommended. These glucose measurements reflect acute changes and not the long-term aspects of diabetic control. A more useful technique for assessing the control of diabetes is using the measurement of glycosylated hemoglobins—that is, hemoglobins with glucose or glucose phosphate moieties bound to the amino terminal valine of one or both β chains. Although many other proteins such as albumin are glycosylated, glycosylated hemoglobins are numerous enough and have a long enough half-life to be used routinely to monitor patients for long-term glucose control.

When hemolysates of human red cells are chromatographed using cation-exchange resins, three or more small peaks named hemoglobin A_{1a}, A_{1b}, and A_{1c} elute before the main hemoglobin A peak. These hemoglobins are made by postsynthetic modification of hemoglobin A at a slow rate directly dependent on the glucose concentration during the 120-day life span of the red cell. Hemoglobin A_{1c}, which composes 3% to 6% of the total hemoglobin in healthy individuals, may double or even triple in diabetics, depending on the level of hyperglycemia. Other hemoglobin variants, Hb A_{1a} and Hb A_{1b}, usually account for about 1.6% and 0.8% of the total hemoglobin, respectively; these hemoglobins also are increased in diabetics. When the total fraction of Hb_{1a}, Hb_{1b}, and Hb_{1c} is measured as a group (fast hemoglobins), the total fraction is referred to as hemoglobin A_1 or A_{1ac}.

Increased synthesis of hemoglobin A_{1c} correlates with lack of glucose control; in diabetics with good glucose control, the amount of hemoglobin A_{1c} returns to the reference interval. Hemoglobin A_{1c} is proportional to the time-average concentration of glucose; thus, A_{1c} assays are a useful means of evaluating the success of long-term diabetic control.

The validity of hemoglobin A_{1c} measurements depends in part on the method used. Methods of measurement include electrophoresis, isoelectric focusing, radioimmunoassay, chromatography, and colorimetry, with the latter two being the most common. A new method, ion capture, by Abbott Laboratories (North Chicago, IL), has proved to be an excellent and rapid method for determining glycosylated hemoglobin. With most column chromatography methods, methemoglobin, hemoglobin F, and hemoglobin Wayne co-elute with the glycohemoglobins, whereas hemoglobin S or methemoglobin can obscure or falsely elevate electrophoretic measurements. Isoelectric focusing methods avoid interference from abnormal hemoglobins but are tedious to perform. Column methods that measure "fast hemoglobins" also measure pre-A_{1c}, a labile intermediate in the synthesis of hemoglobin A_{1c}. This component may constitute up to 25% of the fast hemoglobins and can change significantly within 12 to 48 hours following alterations in plasma glucose concentrations. These rapid changes may reduce the degree of correlation between glycosylated hemoglobins and diabetic control. At present, none of the methods available for quantitating glycosylated hemoglobins is ideal, nor is there consensus on either a reference method or a glycosylated hemoglobin standard (Bruns, 1992). Currently, the trend is toward automated glycated hemoglobin methods that are calibrated to report a hemoglobin A_{1c} that is referent to ion exchange HPLC methods (Tiran, 1994). One of these is the ion capture method in which borate derivatives of the carbohydrates attached to hemoglobin are trapped on a cationic resin. The amount of hemoglobin trapped is then estimated by its ability to quench the fluorescence of umbellyferate esters.

HOME GLUCOSE MONITORING

Control of diabetes mellitus in patients is based on the triad of diet, exercise, and appropriate medication. Diabetic control has been improved substantially with the self-monitoring of blood glucose by patients at home. Self-monitoring has allowed many patients to maintain a lower mean glucose level with a corresponding expectation that reduced renal, retinal, and neuropathic complications should result. Further benefits include the ability to evaluate hypoglycemic reactions immediately, alert patients to impending preacidosis or acidosis, and adjust insulin doses and prescribe multiple insulin doses for the patient in whom glucose control is more difficult.

There are many commercial manufacturers of these instruments, which can be hand held, operator friendly, and reasonably priced. They usually require a drop of whole blood obtained by fingerstick to be applied to a reagent test strip. After appropriate incubation for color development, the test strip is read by a reflectance photometer contained within the hand-held unit. The strips usually use a glucose oxidase enzymatic method embedded in the test strip.

Methodologic variability is inherent with the test strip. With high hematocrits, as plasma is absorbed from the drop of whole blood, cells, protein, and other less permeable constituents undergo hemoconcentration at the test strip surface, blocking further diffusion. Conversely, when hematocrit or protein is low, relatively more glucose diffuses into and reacts with the strip. The reagent strip thus tends to measure the glucose content of the absorbed fluid rather than the glucose concentration of the aliquot of blood. With otherwise healthy ambulatory patients, the hematocrit, lipid, and protein concentrations are relatively uniform, and these instruments can be calibrated to provide reliable glucose measurements. Because these blood constituents vary much more widely in hospitalized patients, variability and error have increased when these same instruments have been used as bedside glucose monitors. Extensive training and quality control programs have been proposed and implemented in an attempt to control the incidence of inconsistent results.

DISORDERS OF FRUCTOSE METABOLISM

Fructose is a ketohexose as opposed to glucose, which is an aldohexose. Disorders of fructose metabolism are divided into three groups: essential fructosuria, hereditary fructose intolerance, and fructose-1,6-diphosphatase deficiency. All are transmitted as autosomal recessive traits. Only in essential fructosuria are there no outward signs or symptoms, and the patient leads an essentially normal life.

Normally, fructose is found in small quantities in serum, usually in the range of 1 to 6 mg/dL (55 to 333 μmol/L). A major source of fructose is the disaccharide sucrose, which contains one molecule of glucose and one molecule of fructose and is present in table sugar, fruits, and vegetables. The relationship of the enzymes involved in fructose metabolism is shown in Figure 9–2. After fructose loading, values as high as 100 mg/dL (5550 μmol/L) are seen in patients with disorders of fructose metabolism.

Essential fructosuria is a benign condition resulting from a relative lack of hepatic fructokinase. This deficiency results in high serum fructose levels after meals containing either sucrose or fructose. The reducing sugar fructose can be detected in urine by nonspecific glucose methods. Neither serum glucose nor serum phosphorus falls in these patients following a fructose load.

Hereditary fructose intolerance is characterized by the development of nausea, abdominal pain, hypoglycemia, aminoaciduria, hyperuricemia, uricosuria, and fructosuria following ingestion of fructose, sucrose (glucose and fructose), or sorbitol (an alcohol that is converted to sucrose). Infants with hereditary fructose intolerance develop normally as long as they are fed only human or cow's milk; however, they may become acutely ill, exhibiting vomiting and hypoglycemia, when fed formulas high in fructose or fruit juices. Hereditary fructose intolerance is diagnosed by the intravenous fructose tolerance test. After the intravenous infusion of 0.25 g/kg body weight of fructose, blood is obtained at frequent intervals, such as 0, 10, 20, 30, 45, 60, 75, and 90 minutes, and glucose as well as phosphorus is measured. Healthy individuals respond with only a small, short-lived fall in phosphorus concentrations. Patients with hereditary fructose intolerance show a persistent decrease in the plasma concentrations of glucose and phosphorus and usually become hypoglycemic. A definitive diagnosis can be made by liver biopsy and the measurement of fructose-1-phosphate aldolase, the enzyme that is markedly decreased in this disease. In newborns, the fructose tolerance test may not be as helpful as in adults. Biopsies may not be necessary if there is a clear response to a fructose-free diet following an abnormal intravenous fructose tolerance test result.

Other enzymatic defects have been associated with hereditary fructose intolerance and account for hypoglycemia (see Fig. 9–2). Renal tubular acidosis (Type I, or the distal type) has been described in some patients, whereas in others a proximal defect (Type II) occurs during periods of hyperfructosemia as a result of fructose-1-phosphate accumulation in renal tubular cells (see Chap. 7).

The symptoms of patients presenting with fructose-1,6-diphosphatase deficiency tend to be indistinguishable from those of type I glycogen storage disease. Lactic acidosis, ketoacidosis, hyperlipidemia, hyperuricemia, and hepatomegaly occur, but skeletal and mental growth are normal. This disease results from a total lack of functioning fructose-1,6-diphosphatase. Because fructose-1,6-diphosphatase is absent, fructose-6-phosphate cannot be formed, and glyconeogenesis

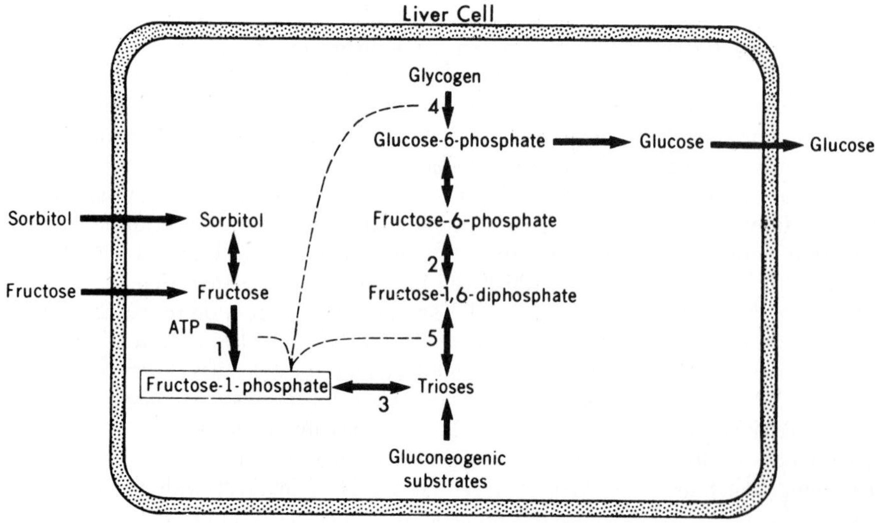

Figure 9–2. Hereditary defects in fructose metabolism:
1-Primary defect in fructosuria (fructokinase).
2-Primary defect in fructose-1, 6-diphosphatase.
3-Primary defect in hereditary fructose intolerance (fructose diphosphate aldolase).
Defects secondary to accumulation of fructose-1-phosphate:
1-Fructokinase.
4-Phosphorylase and phosphoglucomutase.
5-Fructose diphosphate aldolase.
(Modified from Steiner, G, Wilson, D, and Vranic, M: Studies of glucose turnover and renal function in an unusual case of hereditary fructose intolerance. Am J Med 1977; 62:150.)

cannot occur. The liver can produce glucose as long as glycogen is present, but once glycogen is depleted, the child becomes hypoglycemic. Symptoms usually occur in response to an infection or a prolonged fast. Fructosuria and hypoglycemia without vomiting may occur in response to a large fructose load. Lactic acidosis is found, because fructose enters the glycolytic scheme below the enzyme deficiency. Once the disease is recognized, the patient is treated with frequent meals.

GALACTOSEMIA

Galactosemia is a rare genetic disorder transmitted as an autosomal recessive trait. It is characterized by low plasma glucose and inability to metabolize galactose, a monosaccharide that is contained in milk as a constituent of the disaccharide lactose. The classic syndrome develops in infants who appear normal at birth but, after ingestion of milk, develop vomiting, diarrhea, jaundice, failure to thrive, cirrhosis, cataracts, and mental retardation. Many states now require galactosemia screening for newborns; the New York State experience has been described (Kelly, 1980). The metabolism of galactose involves the following three enzymatic steps:

1. $\text{Galactose} + \text{ATP} \xrightarrow{\text{I}} \text{galactose 1-PO}_4 + \text{ADP}$ (9-6)

2. $\text{Galactose 1-PO}_4 + \text{UDP glucose} \xrightarrow{\text{II}} \text{UDP galactose} + \text{glucose 1-PO}_4$ (9-7)

3. $\text{UDP galactose} \xrightarrow{\text{III}} \text{UDP glucose}$ (9-8)

The three enzymes involved in the metabolism of galactose are galactokinase (I), P-gal uridyl transferase (II), and UDP-Gal-4-epimerase (III), with almost all defects involving the transferase. Symptoms of classic transferase (II) deficiency include mental retardation, failure to thrive, jaundice, and juvenile cataracts, whereas with galactokinase (I) deficiency, juvenile cataracts are the only manifestation. Epimerase (III) deficiency is rare and relatively asymptomatic. There is some evidence that the liver and lens changes that occur in the transferase deficiency are reversible, but that mental retardation resulting from low glucose is not. It is imperative that the diagnosis be documented early in the course of the disease, because dietary restriction of galactose intake is an effective treatment if started before irreversible damage has occurred. The laboratory diagnosis of the homozygotic state is suggested by the presence of a reducing sugar that is not glucose as detected by specific enzymatic glucose methods in plasma and urine.

Widespread screening programs for galactosemia are based on measuring transferase (II) activity in red blood cells using the method of Beutler (1966). The enzyme is monitored by the generation of fluorescent NADPH with a coupled enzymatic reaction. Glucose-1-phosphate formed by the transferase is converted to glucose-6-phosphate and then to 6-phosphogluconate with formation of NADPH. Absence of transferase results in failure to produce glucose-1-phosphate and subsequently fluorescent NADPH. With this method, false-positive results (absence of fluorescent NADPH) occur with a frequency of 1 in 100 to 1 in 5000. Some of these false-positive results are due to the presence of other enzyme deficiencies, such as glucose-6-phosphate dehydrogenase or phosphoglucomutase, two enzymes that are required in the coupled enzymatic assay for NADPH formation. False-positive results may be caused by heat inactivation of the transferase during shipping of the specimen to a central laboratory. Specimens from asymptomatic individuals who have enzymatic variants give abnormally low assay results. For confirmation of the diagnosis, a positive result by this method requires quantitative measurement of galactose or galactose-1-phosphate.

If a patient has clinical findings compatible with galactosemia and transferase activity is present, an elevated serum galactose concentration can be used to diagnose galactokinase deficiency. The Guthrie or the Paigen test, each of which monitors growth of *Escherichia coli* in the presence of elevated galactose concentrations, is used. Measurement of the enzyme galactokinase is a more specific technique for making this diagnosis. Management of transferase deficiency involves monitoring the level of erythrocyte galactose-1-phosphate: levels exceeding 110 μg/g of hemoglobin indicate dietary noncompliance (reference interval >40 μg/g hemoglobin) (Pesce, 1982). Galactosemia can be diagnosed prenatally by measuring transferase activity in cultured amniotic cells (Shin, 1983) or by measuring galactitol in amniotic fluid (Jakobs, 1984).

2

GLYCOGEN STORAGE DISEASES

Glycogen storage diseases result from specific deficiencies of enzymes involved in metabolism of glycogen. As a consequence of these deficiencies, glycogen accumulates in the liver, but with some defects this deposition is generalized. The incidence of all forms of glycogen storage diseases combined is about 1 in 40,000. There are many types of glycogen storage disease; however, several are extremely rare. Most are inherited as autosomal recessive traits, with only a few also exhibiting other forms of inheritance. The classification presented in Table 9–6 employs Roman numerals for the most common types. In many descriptions of these diseases, eponyms are used; they also are listed.

Those diseases that can be detected by the intramuscular injection of 100 μg/kg of glucagon (1 mg maximum) include Type I (von Gierke), Type III (Cori-Forbes), and Type VI (Hers). Serial blood specimens are collected for two hours at 15-minute intervals. Normal response is a glucose rise of 60 to 80 mg/dL (3.3 to 4.4 mmol/L) in 15 to 30 minutes with no change in lactate. In Type I, fasting patients show no increase in glucose during this procedure, and lactate levels rise sharply within 30 to 60 minutes. In Type II or III, glucose response fails and lactate response is normal. With refeeding and retesting two hours later, the responses of patients with Type III are similar to those of the reference population. During the glucagon test, plasma lactate increases to more than 27 mg/dL ($>$ 3 mmol/L) in patients with Type I (von Gierke) disease. Laboratory diagnosis of McArdle disease is made by applying a blood pressure cuff on an exercising forearm and sampling blood lactate one minute after the exercise has begun. In this disease, blood lactate does not rise. In all glycogen storage diseases, the definitive diagnosis can be made by assay of the enzyme from the appropriate tissue and by the

Table 9–6. GLYCOGEN STORAGE DISEASES

Type	Major Clinical Features	Enzyme Deficiency (Tissue Affected)	Plasma Glucose Response to IM Glucagon (0.5 mg)
I Von Gierke	Hepatomegaly, lactic acidosis, hyperlipidemia, severe fasting hypoglycemia	Glucose-6-phosphatase (Liver, kidney)	No response
II Pompe	a. Cardiomegaly, muscle weakness, death in infancy b. Adult	α-1,4-Glucosidase (All tissues) (Muscle)	Normal Normal
III Cori-Forbes	Variable degrees of hepatomegaly, muscle weakness, fasting hypoglycemia	Debrancher (All tissues)	Normal after food; poor after fasting
IV Andersen	Portal cirrhosis; usually death in infancy	Brancher (All tissues)	Normal
V McArdle	Pain and stiffness after exertion; myoglobinuria in 50% of cases	Phosphorylase (Muscle)	Normal
VI Hers	Hepatomegaly, mild fasting hypoglycemia	Phosphorylase (Liver)	No response fasting or after food
VII Tarui	Pain and stiffness on exertion	Phosphofructokinase (Muscle, ? liver)	Normal
VIII	Spasticity, decerebration, high urinary catecholamines, death in infancy	Adenyl kinase (Liver, brain)	Normal
IX	Hepatomegaly, occasional fasting hypoglycemia	Phosphorylase kinase (Liver)	Normal, poor
X	Hepatomegaly only	Cyclic AMP–dependent kinase (Liver, muscle)	Normal

characteristic microscopic appearance of the affected tissues. A prenatal diagnosis can be made in those disorders in which the defect is present in all tissues. Generally, in those cases in which the defect is present in only one or two tissues, a prenatal diagnosis is not possible. Glycogen storage diseases have been reviewed extensively; for further details, see Hers (1989).

L-LACTATE

Lactic acid, which is a strong acid with a pK of 3.9, is dissociated at physiologic pH. Therefore, practically all of plasma L-lactic acid is in the form of L-lactate and hydrogen ion. Lactate is the end product of anaerobic metabolism, and its level is related to oxygen availability. When the supply of oxygen is limited, the cytochrome system is unable to function as an intermediate in transfer of hydrogen to molecular oxygen. In this situation, reduced nicotinamide adenine dinucleotide (NADH) accumulates and is oxidized by lactate dehydrogenase with production of lactate by the following reaction:

$$\text{Pyruvate} + \text{NADH} + H^+ \leftrightarrow \text{L-lactate} + \text{NAD} \qquad (9\text{-}9)$$

Lactate is a dead-end branch of the energy metabolism chain and, following its accumulation, is metabolized back to pyruvate when oxygen again becomes abundant. As lactate increases in tissues (skeletal muscle, liver, and erythrocytes), it begins to diffuse out of these tissues, and blood lactate begins to rise. In nonexercising humans, liver and to a certain extent kidneys are the chief organs responsible for lactate metabolism to glucose or oxidation to CO_2 and H_2O. When concentrations are elevated, cardiac and skeletal muscle also may oxidize lactate.

Shock is perhaps the most widely recognized cause of lactic acidosis; however, excess lactate production sometimes precedes shock. Such conditions as myocardial infarction, severe congestive heart failure, pulmonary edema, and blood loss are common causes of shock associated with lactic acidosis. The oral hypoglycemic drug phenformin is no longer available in the United States because of frequent reports of its inducing lactic acidosis. Other causes of lactic acidosis include intravenous infusion of substances such as fructose, sorbitol, or epinephrine and large doses of drugs such as ethanol or acetaminophen (Table 9–7). Hepatic necrosis, neoplasms, lymphomas, and various forms of leukemia have been reported to cause lactic acidosis. In diabetic coma, lactic acidosis is common. In some of these cases, lactic acidosis is secondary to causes such as shock, phenformin ingestion, or epinephrine release, but in other instances it has been reported secondary to ketoacidosis. A few cases with D-lactic acidosis due to abnormal gut flora have been described (Stolberg, 1982).

An elevated anion gap in a patient with metabolic acidosis suggests the diagnosis of lactic acidosis. It can be suspected when the sum of anions minus the sum of cations $[(Na^+ + K^+) - (Cl^- + HCO_3)]$ exceeds 18 mEq/L (18 mmol/L) in the absence of other causes of an increased anion gap, such as renal failure, salicylate ingestion, methanol poisoning, or significant ketonemia.

Lactate values are determined by enzymatic methods employing lactate dehydrogenase; however, several precautions are necessary in collection of a satisfactory specimen for lactate analysis. Although a venous blood specimen may yield higher results than an arterial specimen, venous specimens often are used for convenience. If the patient remains at complete rest prior to specimen withdrawal, venous and arterial levels are the same. Venostasis formed by applying a tourni-

Table 9–7. COMMON CAUSES OF L-LACTIC ACIDOSIS

Shock
Exercise
Drugs
Phenformin*
Sorbitol
Fructose
Ethanol
Epinephrine
Acetaminophen
Seizures
Hepatic disease
Neoplasms
Diabetic ketoacidosis
Idiopathic
Congenital
Glucose-6-phosphatase deficiency (Type I glycogen storage disease)
Fructose-1,6-diphosphatase deficiency

*No longer available in the United States.

quet has little effect, but such minor movements as hand clenching can raise blood lactate levels significantly. Blood may be collected in a syringe and deproteinized immediately by adding the blood to a tube containing perchloric acid. Plasma kept at 25°C is also a satisfactory specimen if tubes containing sodium fluoride and potassium oxalate are used for the blood collection and the plasma is separated completely within 15 minutes, or when specimens are collected and stored in 0.5 g/L of iodoacetate for up to two hours. If blood is not collected by these or comparable methods, lactate will increase rapidly from glycolysis by red cell enzymes. When the specimen is not collected in the correct tube, lactate increases may be as great as 20% in 3 minutes or 70% within 30 minutes at 25°C.

Plasma lactate concentration has a reference interval of 8.1 to 15.3 mg/dL (0.9 to 1.7 mmol/L) for venous blood, but even mild exercise will increase lactate levels substantially. In lactic acidosis, values exceeding 63 to 72 mEq/L (7 to 8 mmol/L) are usually associated with fatal outcome. The absence of a rise in lactate levels after mild exercise is an important criterion in the diagnosis of patients with McArdle disease (Type V glycogen storage disease), as discussed earlier. The finding of elevated lactate in cerebrospinal fluid can discriminate between meningitis of bacterial and of viral etiology. Its measurement can also aid in differentiating septic from other forms of monarticular arthritis. For further information, see Chapter 19.

Aynsley-Green A: Hypoglycaemia in infants and children. Clin Endocrinol Metab 1982; 11:159.

Bergus GR, Murphy NJ: Screening for gestational diabetes mellitus: Comparison of a glucose polymer and a glucose monomer test beverage. J Am Board Fam Pract 1992; 5:241.

Beutler E, Baluda MC: A simple spot screening test for galactosemia. J Lab Clin Med 1966; 68:137.

Bruns DE: Standardization, calibration, and care of diabetic patients. Clin Chem 1992; 38:2363.

Chan AYW, Swaminathan R, Cockram CS: Effectiveness of sodium flouride as a preservative of glucose in blood. Clin Chem 1989; 35:315.

Conlon JM: The glucagon-like polypeptides—order out of chaos? Diabetologia 1980; 18:85.

Fajans SS, Floyd JC: Fasting hypoglycemia in adults. N Engl J Med 1976; 294:766.

Felig P, Cherif A, Minagawa A, et al: Hypoglycemia during prolonged exercise in normal men. N Engl J Med 1982; 306:895.

Frerichs H, Creutzfeldt W: Hypoglycaemia: 1. Insulin secreting tumours. Clin Endocrinol Metab 1976; 5:747.

Godsland IF, Walton C, Felton C, et al: Insulin resistance, secretion, and metabolism in users of oral contraceptives. J Clin Endocrinol Metab 1992; 74:64.

Hendriks T, Benraad TJ: On the stability of immunoreactive glucagon in plasma samples. Diabetologia 1981; 20:553.

Hers HG, Van Hoof F, de Barsy T: Glycogen storage diseases. *In* Scriver CR, Beaudet AL, Sly WS, Valle D (eds): The Metabolic Basis of Inherited Disease. New York, McGraw-Hill, 1989, p 425.

Horwitz DL, Kuzuya H, Rubenstein AH: Circulating serum C-peptide: A brief review of diagnostic implications. N Engl J Med 1976; 295:207.

Jakobs C, Warner TG, Sweetman L, et al: Stable isotope dilution analysis of galactitol in amniotic fluid: An accurate approach to the prenatal diagnosis of galactosemia. Pediatr Res 1984; 18:714.

Johnson DD, Dorr KE, Swenson WM, et al: Reactive hypoglycemia. JAMA 1980; 243:1151.

Kelly S: Galactosemia identified in newborn screening program: Clinical and biochemical characteristics. NY State J Med 1980; 80:1836.

Kitabchi AE: Proinsulin and C-peptide: A review. Metabolism 1977; 26:547.

Lev-Ran A, Anderson RW: The diagnosis of postprandial hypoglycemia. Diabetes 1981; 30:996.

Lillioja S, Mott DM, Spraul, M, et al: Insulin resistance and insulin secretory dysfunction as precursors of non-insulin-dependent diabetes mellitus: Prospective studies of Pima Indians. N Engl J Med 1993; 329:1988.

Marks V, Alberti, KGMM: Selected tests of carbohydrate metabolism. Clin Endocrinol Metab 1976; 5:805.

Martin BC, Warram JH, Krolewski AS, et al: Role of glucose and insulin resistance in development of type 2 diabetes mellitus: Results of a 25-year follow-up study. Lancet 1992; 340:925.

Merimee TJ: Spontaneous hypoglycemia in man. Adv Intern Med 1977; 22:301.

Merimee TJ, Tyson JE: Stabilization of plasma glucose during fasting: Normal variations in two separate studies. N Engl J Med 1974; 291:1275.

Murphy NJ, Meyer BA, O'Kell RT, et al: Carbohydrate sourced for gestational diabetes mellitus screening. A comparison. J Reprod Med 1994; 39:977.

Narayanan S: Laboratory monitoring of gestational diabetes. Ann Clin Lab Sci 1991; 21:392.

National Diabetes Data Group: Classification and diagnosis of diabetes mellitus and other categories of glucose intolerance. Diabetes 1979; 28:1039.

Olefsky JM, Farquhar JW, Reaven GM: Do the oral and intravenous glucose tolerance tests provide similar diagnostic information in patients with chemical diabetes mellitus? Diabetes 1973; 22:202.

O'Sullivan JB, Mahan CM: Criteria for the oral glucose tolerance test in pregnancy. Diabetes 1964; 13:278.

Pesce MA, Bodourian SH: Clinical significance of plasma galactose and erythrocyte galactose-1-phosphate measurements in transferase-deficient galactosemia and in individuals with below-normal transferase activity. Clin Chem 1982; 28:301.

Philipson EH, Rossi KQ, Isaac RM, et al: Glucose, insulin, gastric inhibitory polypeptide, and pancreatic polypeptide responses to polycose during pregnancy. Obstet Gynecol 1992; 79:592.

Reece EA, Gabrielli S, Abdalla M, et al: Diagnosis of gestational diabetes by use of a glucose polymer. Am J Obstet Gynecol 1989; 160:383.

Service FJ, Horwitz DL, Rubenstein AH, et al: C-peptide suppression test for insulinoma. J Lab Clin Med 1977; 90:180.

Shin YS, Endres W, Rieth M, et al: Prenatal diagnosis of galactosemia and properties of galactose-1-phosphate uridyltransferase in erythrocytes of galactosemic variants as well as in human fetal and adult organs. Clin Chim Acta 1983; 128:271.

Siperstein MD: The glucose tolerance test: A pitfall in the diagnosis of diabetes mellitus. Adv Intern Med 1975; 20:297.

Steiner G, Wilson D, Vranic M: Studies of glucose turnover and renal function in an unusual case of hereditary fructose intolerance. Am J Med 1977; 62:150.

Stolberg L, Rolfe R, Gitlin N, et al: D-Lactic acidosis due to abnormal gut flora. N Engl J Med 1982; 306:1344.

Super DM, Edelberg SC, Philipson EH, et al: Diagnosis of gestational diabetes in early pregnancy. Diabetes Care 1991; 14:288.

Svejgaard A, Platz P, Ryder LP: Insulin dependent diabetes mellitus, joint results of the 8th workshop study. *In* Terasaki PI (ed): Histocompatibility Testing. Los Angeles, UCLA, 1980, p 947.

Tiran A, Pieber T, Tiran B, et al: Automated determination of glycated hemoglobin: Comparative evaluation of five assay systems. J Clin Lab Analysis 1994; 8:128.

Weissman M, Klein B: Evaluation of glucose determinations in untreated serum samples. Clin Chem 1958; 4:420.

Wojcikowski C, Blackman J, Ostrega D, et al: Lack of effect of high dose biosynthetic human C-peptide on pancreatic hormone release in normal subjects. Metabolism 1990; 39:827.

Chapter 10

Lipids and Dyslipoproteinemia

Paul S. Bachorik, Ph.D.
Basil M. Rifkind, M.D., FRCP
Peter O. Kwiterovich, Jr., M.D.

PLASMA LIPOPROTEINS, APOLIPOPROTEINS, AND ENZYMES OF LIPOPROTEIN METABOLISM

Plasma Lipoproteins

Plasma lipoproteins transport essentially all of the cholesterol and esterified lipids in the blood. Four major lipoprotein classes (chylomicrons, very low density lipoproteins [VLDL], low density lipoproteins [LDL], and high density lipoproteins [HDL]) and two quantitatively minor lipoproteins (intermediate density lipoproteins [IDL], lipoprotein [a] [Lp(a)]) can be identified based on particle size, chemical composition, physicochemical and flotation characteristics, and electrophoretic mobility (Tables 10–1 to 10–3).

The protein moiety of the lipoproteins is composed of several specific proteins called apolipoproteins. Each lipoprotein fraction has a particular and more or less constant apolipoprotein composition. The apolipoproteins play important roles in lipid transport by activating or inhibiting enzymes involved in lipid metabolism, binding lipoproteins to cell surface lipoprotein receptors, or both. The apolipoprotein composition of the various lipoprotein fractions is summarized in Table 10–3. A useful alphabetical classification was introduced by Alaupovic (1971) and is now the most commonly used nomenclature for apolipoproteins (discussed later).

Chylomicrons

Chylomicrons are large particles produced by the intestine that are very rich (85% to 95%) in triglycerides of exogenous (dietary) origin and relatively poor in free cholesterol and phospholipids; chylomicrons contain about 1% to 2% protein (by weight). Because of the very high lipid/protein ratio, the chylomicron is considerably less dense than water and floats even without centrifugation. High chylomicron content results in a "milky" plasma in which the chylomicrons accumulate as a floating creamy layer when left undisturbed for several hours. The apolipoproteins in chylomicrons include

This chapter was written by Dr. Basil M. Rifkind in his private capacity. No official support or endorsement by the NIH is intended and none should be inferred.

Table 10–1. MAJOR CLASSES OF HUMAN PLASMA LIPOPROTEINS: PHYSICOCHEMICAL CHARACTERISTICS

	Diameter (Å)	Density (kg/L)	Sf	Electrophoretic Mobility*
Chylomicrons	750–12,000	<0.95	>400	Origin
VLDL	300–700	0.95–1.006	20–400	Pre-β
IDL		1.006–1.019	12–20	β or pre-β
LDL	180–300	1.019–1.063	0–12	β
HDL_2		1.063–1.125		
	50–120			α_1
HDL_3		1.125–1.210		
Lp(a)		1.045–1.080		Pre-β

*Agarose-gel electrophoresis.

apoB-48, apoA-I, and apoA-IV, which are present in newly secreted particles, and apoC-I, apoC-II, apoC-III, and apoE, which are acquired from other lipoproteins in the circulation. Interaction of chylomicrons and lipoprotein lipase results in a smaller particle, depleted in triglycerides and some surface elements, which is referred to as the chylomicron remnant.

Very Low Density Lipoproteins

VLDL particles are smaller than chylomicrons and also are rich in triglycerides, though to a lesser extent. They have a lower lipid/protein ratio and thus "float" at a somewhat higher density. Like chylomicrons, the particles are large enough to scatter light, and when excessive amounts of VLDL are present, the plasma is turbid. VLDL triglycerides are of endogenous, mainly hepatic origin and constitute about half the particle mass. Cholesterol and phospholipids make up about 40% of the particle, and about 10% of the mass is protein, mostly apoB-100 and apoC but also some apoE (see Tables 10–2 and 10–3). VLDL particle sizes vary widely, with a concomitant variation of the chemical composition; the larger particles are richer in triglycerides and in apoC, and the smaller particles are poorer in these two components. Smaller particles depleted of triglyceride and surface material result from the hydrolysis of VLDL by lipoprotein lipase. These particles are often referred to as VLDL remnants and intermediate density lipoproteins (IDL) (see Table 10–1).

Low Density Lipoproteins

LDL constitute about 50% of the total lipoprotein mass in human plasma. LDL particles are much smaller than the triglyceride-rich lipoproteins; even greatly increased concentrations of LDL do not scatter light or alter the clarity of plasma. Cholesterol, most of which is esterified, accounts for about half of LDL mass. About 25% of LDL mass is protein, mostly apoB-100 with traces of apoC. (For details, see Tables 10–1 to 10–3.)

Discrete subfractions of LDL have been identified that differ somewhat in their size and chemical composition. The smaller species of LDL contain lower amounts of cholesterol ester, resulting in a lower ratio of cholesterol to apoB in these particles than in larger species of LDL. Increased amounts of the smaller particles have been found in patients with several common forms of dyslipoproteinemia that are associated with coronary artery disease (discussed later).

High Density Lipoproteins

HDL are small particles consisting of 50% protein (mostly apoA-I and apoA-II, but also some apoC and apoE), 20% cholesterol (mostly esterified), 30% phospholipids, and only traces of triglycerides. HDL can be separated into two major subclasses, HDL_2 and HDL_3, which differ in their density, particle size, and composition (see Table 10–1). As with LDL, a number of discrete subpopulations of HDL have been separated based on their size or charge differences (Blanché, 1981; MacKenzie, 1973; Sundarum, 1974). In addition, immunochemical separation techniques have been used to subfractionate HDL into particles that contain apoA-I but not apoA-II and those that contain both apoA-I and apoA-II (Fruchart, 1992; von Eckardstein, 1994). The physiologic function of these particles and the relation of low levels of apoA-I–only particles to cardiovascular disease are of current interest; the laboratory measurements of such particles may eventually prove to be clinically useful.

Lp(a) Lipoprotein

This lipoprotein is found primarily in the density range 1.055 to 1.085 kg/L. It is composed of 27% protein, 65% lipid, and 8% carbohydrate and thus has a composition similar to that of LDL but is generally present in much lower concentrations. The apolipoprotein components of Lp(a) are apoB and apo(a), which are bound to each other through disulfide bonds (Fless, 1984, 1985; Gaubatz, 1983). The elec-

Table 10–2. MAJOR CLASSES OF HUMAN PLASMA LIPOPROTEINS: CHEMICAL COMPOSITION

	Protein (%)*	Cholesterol (%)	Cholesteryl Esters (%)	Triglyceride (%)	Phospholipid (%)
Chylomicrons	1–2	1–3	2–4	80–95	3–6
VLDL	6–10	4–8	16–22	45–65	15–20
IDL			*intermediate between VLDL and LDL*		
LDL	18–22	6–8	45–50	4–8	18–24
HDL	45–55	3–5	15–20	2–7	26–32

*Percentage of dry weight.
Data from Albers (1974); Fless (1986); Gaubatz (1983); Gotto (1986); Gries (1988).

Table 10–3. MAJOR CLASSES OF HUMAN PLASMA LIPOPROTEINS: APOLIPOPROTEIN COMPOSITION

			Plasma Concentration		% Distribution† Among:			
	Mr* (kD)	Located on Chromosome	*(umol/L)*	*(mg/dL)*	*Chylomicrons*	*VLDL*	*LDL*	*HDL*
A-I	29	11	32–46	90–130	1	—	—	90‡
A-II	17.4	1	18–29	30–50	—	—	—	95
A-IV	44.5	11			+	—	—	+
B-100	512.7	2	1.5–1.8	80–100	—	<10	90	—
B-48	240.8	2	<0.2	<5	100	—	—	—
C-I	6.6	19	6.1–10.8	4–7	Major	Major	Minor	Minor
C-II	8.9	19	3.4–9.1	3–8	Major	Major	Minor	Minor
C-III	8.8	11	9.1–17.1	8–15	Minor	25	Minor	60
D	19	3			—	—	—	+
E	34.1	19	0.8–1.6	3–6	Minor	Major	Minor	Minor

*Mr, relative molecular mass.
†Percentage of total plasma apolipoprotein.
‡Up to 10% of apoA-I is found complexed with phospholipid in the density range 1.21–1.25 kg/L and has been called very high density lipoprotein (VHDL).

trophoretic mobility of Lp(a) is usually pre-β but can vary between that of LDL and that of albumin. Apo(a) is a polymorphic protein in which the molecular weights of the various polyforms vary from about 350 kD to 700 kD. Apo(a) has a high degree of homology with plasminogen due to a variable number of repeating amino acid sequences homologous to the kringle 4 region of plasminogen (McLean, 1987; Scanu, 1988). The number of kringle 4–like repeat sequences in Lp(a) in any given individual is genetically determined (Gaw, 1994) and ranges from 12 to 51 repeats. The Kringle 4 region of plasminogen contains the protease domain and is activated by tissue plasminogen activator or urokinase, but apo(a) has a serine for arginine substitution at the point at which plasminogen is activated, and itself does not acquire plasmin-like activity on treatment with plasminogen activators (McLean, 1987).

Lp(a) concentrations in normal subjects may vary from less than 0.05 to 1.90 mmol/L (<20 to 1500 mg/L) or more, and increased levels are familial with autosomal dominant inheritance. When concentrations in the plasma are increased above 200 to 300 mg/L, Lp(a) appears electrophoretically as a lipid-staining pre-β band in the plasma fraction containing lipoproteins of density greater than 1.006 g/mL.

LpX Lipoprotein

LpX is an abnormal lipoprotein found in patients with obstructive biliary disease. Lipids account for more than 90% of its weight (mostly phospholipids, unesterified cholesterol, and very little esterified cholesterol). Proteins, primarily apoC and some albumin, constitute less than 10% of LpX by weight.

β-VLDL ("floating β" lipoprotein) is an abnormal lipoprotein that accumulates in Type III hyperlipoproteinemia. It is richer in cholesterol than typical VLDL and apparently results from the defective catabolism of VLDL. The particle is found in the VLDL density range but migrates electrophoretically with or near LDL. Typically, however, in Type III hyperlipoproteinemia, there is a broad band that spans both the VLDL and LDL bands and is diagnostic of this condition when accompanied by a VLDL-cholesterol : triglyceride ratio exceeding 0.3, and characteristic physical findings (*vide infra*).

Apolipoproteins

As mentioned earlier, the apolipoproteins are most commonly referred to using the nomenclature introduced by Alaupovic (1971).

Apolipoproteins A (ApoA). The A apolipoproteins are the major protein components of HDL. The two major components of apoA are apoA-I and apoA-II.

ApoA-I. ApoA-I constitutes about 75% of apoA in HDL. It consists of 243 to 245 amino acids with a molecular weight of 29,000. ApoA-I is synthesized in the liver and intestine and is an activator of the enzyme lecithin:cholesterol acyltransferase (LCAT—see later discussion), which esterifies cholesterol in plasma.

ApoA-II. ApoA-II constitutes about 20% of apoA in HDL. It consists of 154 amino acids and has a molecular weight of 17,400. In the human, each apoA-II molecule consists of two identical peptides linked by a single disulfide bond. The physiologic role of apoA-II is not known.

Apolipoprotein B (ApoB). ApoB is the major protein constituent (95%) of LDL and also constitutes about 40% of the protein moiety of VLDL and chylomicrons. It has been very difficult to study the physical and chemical characteristics of apoB because it is insoluble in water. Several forms of apoB occur (Kane, 1980). The major component is apoB-100. It is synthesized by the liver and found in lipoproteins of endogenous origin (VLDL and LDL). The complete amino acid sequence of apoB was deduced from molecular biologic studies of the apoB gene (Cladaras, 1986; Hospattankar, 1986; Knott, 1986; Law, 1986; Yang, 1986; Young, 1986a). It is one of the longest proteins known, consisting of a single chain of 4536 amino acids, and it has a molecular weight of about 513,000 (see Table 10–3). ApoB-100 is secreted in VLDL and is the recognition signal that targets LDL to the LDL (apoB,E) receptor through a receptor recognition domain in the carboxyl terminal portion of the molecule. ApoB-48, with a molecular weight of approximately 241,000 (see Table 10–3), is of intestinal origin and is found in chylomicrons. The synthesis of both apoB-48 and apoB-100 is directed by the same gene (Hospattankar, 1986; Young, 1986a), and various studies revealed that apoB-48 is the same as the amino terminal half of apoB-100 (Hardman, 1986;

Marcel, 1987). Because the apoB,E receptor–binding region of apoB-100 is in the carboxyl terminal third of the protein (Knott, 1986; Marcel, 1987), apoB-48 does not bind to the LDL receptors (Hui, 1984; Mahley, 1983, 1984). The two forms of apoB result from the presence of two species of mRNA, one of which codes for apoB-100 and the other of which contains a premature stop codon and codes for apoB-48 (Higuchi, 1988; Powell, 1987). The conversion of apoB-100 mRNA to apoB-48 mRNA is catalyzed by an apoB-mRNA editing protein (REPR). Cells that do not express the *REPR* gene do not make apoB-48 but can be induced to do so when the *REPR* gene is transfected into them (Giannoni, 1994; Yao, 1994).

Apolipoprotein C (ApoC). ApoC is a major protein component of VLDL and is a minor constituent of HDL and LDL. Three different groups of C apolipoproteins occur:

ApoC-I. ApoC-I consists of 57 amino acid residues and has a molecular weight of 6500. It is a minor constituent of chylomicrons and VLDL and HDL proteins. Its function is not entirely clear, but it may activate LCAT, which catalyzes the esterification of cholesterol in the circulation (discussed later).

ApoC-II. ApoC-II has a molecular weight of 8900 and consists of 78 or 79 amino acid residues. It constitutes 5% to 10% of VLDL protein and less than 2% of HDL protein. ApoC-II is a potent activator of the enzyme lipoprotein lipase (LPL) (LaRosa, 1970) and, when deficient, results in the reduced clearance of triglyceride-rich lipoproteins from the plasma (Brechenridge, 1978; Gotto, 1986).

ApoC-III. Several forms of apoC-III exist, differing in the molar content of sialic acid residues. ApoC-III is a major component of VLDL protein (25% to 30%). It is also the main form of apoC in HDL, constituting about 2% of its protein moiety. Its molecular weight is 8800, and it consists of 79 amino acid residues. The physiologic role of apoC-III is not completely clear, but it appears to inhibit the lipolysis of triglyceride-rich lipoproteins and seems to be involved in regulating the rate of clearance of triglyceride-rich lipoprotein remnant particles.

Minor Apolipoproteins. ApoD is a minor constituent of HDL protein (5% or less). It is also present in very small amounts in other lipoproteins. The molecular weight of apoD is about 32,000. ApoD was shown to activate the LCAT reaction, possibly by serving as a specific lysolecithin carrier. ApoA-IV has a molecular weight of about 44,500 (see Table 10–3) and is found in the $d > 1.21$ fraction of plasma, in HDL, and in very small amounts as a constituent of chylomicrons. Its function is unknown, but it may be a cofactor for LCAT.

Apolipoprotein E (ApoE). This arginine-rich apolipoprotein is found in VLDL, IDL, remnant lipoproteins, chylomicrons, and HDL. ApoE exists in several forms that can be separated by isoelectric focusing and that are designated as E-2, E-3, and E-4 isoforms (Pagnan, 1977; Utermann, 1975). ApoE-3 is the most common isoform and contains a cysteine residue at position 112 and an arginine at position 158. In apoE-2, position 158 is substituted with a cysteine residue, which reduces its ability to bind to the B-E receptor. ApoE-4, on the other hand, contains an arginine for cysteine substitution at position 112, which has the opposite effect; this isoform binds to the B-E receptor with a higher affinity than apoE-3 does, leading to increased uptake of cholesterol by the cell, down-regulation of the apoB,E receptor (discussed later), and higher plasma levels of LDL. Several post-translational modifications of the major E isoproteins, which differ in the number of sialic acid residues in the carbohydrate side chains of the polypeptides, can also be identified using two-dimensional isoelectric focusing (Zannis, 1980, 1981). The molecular weight of apoE is 34,000 (see Table 10–3), and it consists of 299 amino acid residues. The synthesis of the various apoE isoforms is under genetic control (see discussion under dysbetalipoproteinemia), and apoE is believed to be the recognition factor that targets chylomicron and VLDL remnants to the hepatic receptor. It also binds to cell surface LDL receptors (Green, 1981; Sherrill, 1980). Of vital importance, apoE protein has been found to have a crucial role in the pathogenesis of Alzheimer's disease and may be involved in the formation of neural plaques in the central nervous system (Corder, 1993; Poirier, 1993; Saunders, 1993; Scott, 1993).

2

Enzymes Participating in Lipoprotein Metabolism

The major enzymatic systems that are known to participate in plasma lipoprotein metabolism are the lipolytic enzymes and LCAT.

Lipolytic Enzymes. In fasting human plasma, lipolytic activity is barely detectable. A few minutes following the intravenous injection of heparin, several lipolytic activities are discerned. At least two triglyceride hydrolases, lipoprotein lipase and hepatic triglyceride lipase, are detected in post-heparin plasma. They differ in their pH optima, inhibition by protamine or concentrated salt solution, activation by specific apolipoprotein cofactors, and substrate specificity.

Lipoprotein Lipase (LPL). This enzyme, derived mainly from adipose tissue, hydrolyzes triglycerides in chylomicrons and VLDL. LPL is normally located on the surface of capillary endothelial cells of adipose tissue and of skeletal and heart muscles. Chylomicron triglyceride is hydrolyzed following the attachment of these particles to the capillary endothelial cells. Phospholipids and apoC-II are essential cofactors for triglyceride hydrolysis by LPL.

Hepatic Triglyceride Lipase. Hepatic triglyceride lipase (HTGL) is secreted by hepatocytes and associates with the surface membrane of nonparenchymal liver cells. The function of the enzyme is not entirely clear. It has only a limited capacity to hydrolyze triglycerides in intact chylomicrons and VLDL, and it does not require apoC-II as a cofactor. HTGL may participate in the conversion of VLDL remnants and IDL to LDL (Clay, 1989; Eisenberg, 1976; Havel, 1984). The enzyme seems to be most active in hydrolysis of phospholipids and triglycerides of HDL_2 and may play a role in HDL metabolism (Tikkanen, 1981).

Lecithin:Cholesterol Acyltransferase (LCAT). Normally present in human plasma, this enzyme system catalyzes the esterification of cholesterol by promoting transfer of fatty acids from lecithin to cholesterol, which results in the formation of lysolecithin and cholesterol ester. The enzyme is synthesized in the liver and circulates in plasma associated with HDL, which seems to be its preferred substrate. It has been suggested that this enzyme system also plays a role in removing surface material of chylomicrons and VLDL. LCAT may also be involved in removal of excess free cholesterol and lecithin from the circulation (discussed later).

ApoA-I is an activator of LCAT, but enzyme activity can be detected even in the absence of apoA-I. LCAT in plasma can be measured either in terms of its enzymatic activity or in terms of its mass, using specific antibodies to the enzyme (Albers, 1981).

LIPOPROTEIN METABOLISM

Lipid Transport in Lipoproteins

The major function of the plasma lipoproteins appears to be the transport of triglycerides and cholesterol from sites of origin in the intestine (exogenous origin: 0.079 to 0.113 mol [70 to 100 g] triglycerides per day, and 0.779 to 2.597 mmol [300 to up to 1000 mg] cholesterol per day) and the liver (endogenous origin: 0.028 to 0.056 mol [25 to 50 g] triglycerides per day) to sites of energy storage and utilization.

Triglycerides and cholesterol enter the plasma in the form of triglyceride-rich lipoprotein particles (chylomicrons and VLDL) that supply the tissues with fatty acids for energy requirements and storage. Exogenous dietary fat is transported from its intestinal absorption site in chylomicrons. Endogenously synthesized triglyceride is transported from the liver in VLDL. The general structures of the two triglyceride-rich particles are similar, but they differ in size, triglyceride content, and apolipoprotein content (see previous discussion). ApoB is the major protein component in both, but, as mentioned previously, apoB-48 is present in chylomicrons, whereas apoB-100 is present in lipoproteins of hepatic origin. Both particles contain the E apolipoproteins and acquire the C apolipoproteins in the plasma, but only chylomicrons include the A apolipoproteins as major surface protein components. Chylomicrons and VLDL undergo intravascular change almost immediately after their entry into the circulation through the action of lipoprotein lipase, which hydrolyzes triglycerides and diglycerides. This hydrolysis is stimulated by apoC-II, which is present in the triglyceride-rich particles. During this process, the chylomicron loses over 95% of its mass, primarily as triglyceride, as well as the A and C apolipoproteins. Both surface lipid and apolipoproteins are transferred to HDL. The depleted chylomicron particle, or remnant as it is called, contains apoB and apoE as the major apolipoproteins. It subsequently binds to the surface of hepatocytes and is then internalized by means of a highly rapid and specific receptor-mediated endocytotic process, and then it is degraded. ApoE apparently targets the chylomicron remnant to its receptor. The other C apolipoproteins seem to inhibit the uptake of chylomicrons themselves, allowing them to remain in the circulation long enough to complete the hydrolysis of triglycerides. In the fasting state, the intestine continues to make apoB and secretes "intestinal VLDL" (small chylomicrons). These particles may constitute up to 10% or 20% of the circulating VLDL (Byers, 1960; Ceredella, 1974; Risser, 1978); they are probably metabolized as chylomicrons (Green, 1981).

VLDL is synthesized in the liver. It is catabolized in part by lipoprotein lipase and converted to cholesterol-enriched VLDL remnants, some of which are removed by the liver remnant receptor, and some of which are further catabolized to IDL (Bachorik, 1988). Surface materials, including free cholesterol, phospholipids, and apolipoproteins, are transferred from VLDL to HDL, which then interact with LCAT to form cholesterol esters and lysolecithin. The cholesterol esters are subsequently transferred from HDL to IDL, a process catalyzed by a specific plasma protein, cholesterol ester transfer protein (CETP). IDL is then converted to LDL. LDL is thus an end product of intravascular VLDL metabolism. LDL carries most of the circulating cholesterol in humans and transports cholesterol into tissues via LDL receptor–mediated endocytosis, which takes place in hepatic as well as extrahepatic tissues (Brown, 1981). LDL binds to the LDL-receptor (i.e., apoB) and is subsequently internalized and directed to the lysosome, where apoB-100 is degraded and cholesterol ester and other lipids are hydrolyzed. The LDL receptor itself moves back to the cell membrane and is reused to transport more LDL. The unesterified cholesterol produced becomes available for membrane synthesis, and excess cholesterol is re-esterified by the microsomal enzyme acyl:cholesterol acyl transferase (ACAT) and is stored until it is needed; it is then hydrolyzed by a neutral cholesteryl ester hydrolase (CEH). Cellular cholesterol, when present in sufficient quantity, down-regulates the LDL-receptor, reducing the number of cell membrane receptors and consequently the uptake of LDL. Under conditions of cholesterol excess, the rate-limiting enzyme of cholesterol biosynthesis, hydroxymethylglutaryl CoA (HmG CoA) reductase is also down-regulated, slowing cellular cholesterol biosynthesis.

About two thirds of the plasma LDL is removed via hepatic LDL-receptors. Unlike most other tissues, which can only use cholesterol for membrane synthesis or store it as cholesterol ester, the liver can also dispose of cholesterol in several ways. Part of the sterol is excreted into the bile both as unesterified cholesterol and after conversion to bile acids. Cholesterol is also reused for lipoprotein synthesis and is secreted to the circulation as in VLDL. Steroid-secreting tissues use cholesterol as a precursor of the steroid hormones.

HDL is secreted from both the liver and the intestine as nascent, disk-shaped particles that contain cholesterol and phospholipid (Havel, 1980; Oppenheimer, 1987; Oram, 1986; Scanu, 1982). HDL is thought to be the vehicle for reverse cholesterol transport, the process by which excess cholesterol is removed from tissues peripheral to the liver and transported back to the liver for reuse or disposal in the bile. HDL accumulates cholesterol from cell membranes and other lipoproteins and is converted to a spherical particle in the circulation through the action of LCAT and the movement of the cholesterol esters formed into the core of the HDL particle. In humans, HDL-cholesteryl esters are then transferred to VLDL and IDL and are removed with these lipoproteins. This transfer is catalyzed by CETP, which is found in plasma and catalyzes the exchange of cholesterol esters for triglyceride (Tall, 1990). As a consequence, HDL become somewhat enriched in triglycerides and their size increases. This process appears to operate in the conversion of HDL_3 to HDL_2. Cholesteryl esters may also be delivered directly to the liver from HDL (Bachorik, 1987; Glass, 1983; Stein, 1984). In addition, a portion of HDL appears to arise *de novo* in the circulation from the excess surface material (e.g., free cholesterol, apolipoproteins A-I, A-II, C-I, C-II, C-III, phospholipid) removed from the triglyceride-rich lipoproteins as they are catabolized.

Lp(a) is synthesized in the liver, but the details of its metabolism are poorly understood. Lp(a) binds to the LDL receptor by virtue of its apoB component, albeit with lower affinity than LDL (Armstrong, 1985; Floren, 1981). The removal of apo(a) from Lp(a) increases the affinity of the residual apoB-containing particle for the LDL receptor (Armstrong, 1985), and it has been suggested that apo(a) may interfere with the uptake of apoB-100 particles (Scanu, 1988). By virtue of its similarity to plasminogen, Lp(a) or apo(a) might interfere with normal thrombolysis, which may account for the association between elevated Lp(a) levels and cardiovascular disease. This has indeed been demonstrated *in vitro*, but there appears to be no relation between plasma Lp(a) levels and various indicators of thrombolysis *in vivo*, and the *in vitro* and *in vivo* observations remain to be reconciled (Bachorik, 1993). Plasminogen binds to endothelial cells and, to a lesser extent, fibroblasts (Hajjar, 1986), apparently through regions of the molecule with which Lp(a) shares homology. It has been suggested that if Lp(a) binds similarly, it might afford a pathway by which cholesterol-rich particles might enter the arterial wall (Scanu, 1988). At present, neither the function of Lp(a) nor its coronary atherogenic properties and association with cerebrovascular disease and stroke are understood.

LIPID AND LIPOPROTEIN MEASUREMENT

Lipoprotein concentrations have been expressed in several ways. When expressed in terms of particle mass, the values account for the contributions of both the protein and the lipid components of the particles. Mass concentrations are generally determined with the analytical ultracentrifuge or from chemical measurements of the protein and each of the major classes of lipids. Neither of these technically demanding approaches is easily applied for screening or routine clinical purposes.

Because the cholesterol composition of each lipoprotein class is generally similar from individual to individual, lipoprotein cholesterol is most commonly determined as a measure of lipoprotein concentration. Lipoprotein-cholesterol concentrations correlate fairly well with analytical ultracentrifuge values; in most population studies, these values were determined when relating lipoprotein concentration to cardiovascular risk. More recently, the growing interest in measuring the apolipoproteins acknowledges their role in lipoprotein metabolism and the link between apolipoprotein abnormalities and clinically identifiable problems. Furthermore, measurements of apolipoproteins, particularly apoA-I and apoB, can supplement the measurement of other lipoprotein components and increase their ability to identify individuals who are at increased risk for coronary heart disease and perhaps other kinds of arteriosclerosis (Albers, 1989a; Bachorik, 1988).

The analysis of plasma lipoproteins usually requires, first, the separation of the lipoprotein classes, and second, measurement of the lipoprotein or lipoprotein component of interest. Both steps contribute to the error in the measurements; as a rule, the more complicated the analytical procedures, the greater the variability of the analyses. Lipoprotein measurements must therefore be monitored using some formal system of quality control, and it is useful for individuals who must interpret lipid and lipoprotein data to have some idea of the uncertainty of the measurements. Consider the example of how laboratory variability affects the results reported for a plasma sample with a known cholesterol concentration of 6.494 mmol/L (250 mg/dL). If a laboratory operating with a coefficient of variation (CV) of 3% were to analyze the sample once, in 95% of the cases that laboratory would report a value ranging between 6.104 and 6.883 mmol/L (235 and 265 mg/dL). Using modern computer-controlled automatic analyzers, most laboratories can analyze cholesterol with a CV of 2% or less, and the variation in reported values attributable to analytical error is actually somewhat smaller. Three points should be made. First, as mentioned previously, lipoprotein-cholesterol analyses will generally be more variable than total cholesterol analyses because of the additional manipulations required to prepare the lipoprotein-containing fractions. Second, as to be discussed in detail, a number of factors other than analytical error contribute to the measured lipid and lipoprotein levels. Some of these factors operate before the sample reaches the laboratory. In the broadest sense, "quality control" begins outside the laboratory and runs as a common theme through all phases of lipoprotein analysis regardless of the method used or components measured. Finally, plasma lipoprotein concentrations can change as a result of normal physiologic variation. The physiologic variations of cholesterol, triglyceride, and lipoproteins have been examined in a number of studies (Bookstein, 1990; Brown, 1990; Demacker, 1982; Kafonek, 1992; Warnick, 1975). For cholesterol, the coefficient of physiologic variation (CV_p) within an individual averages about 6.5% but can be higher in certain individuals. Thus, when measured in serial samples from the same person, the cholesterol levels in 95% of the samples will vary by about 13% above or below that person's mean level. Physiologic variation is therefore several times greater than analytical error, and measurements must be made in several blood samples taken at least a week apart in order to establish the individual's usual lipoprotein concentration.

Table 10–4 shows the CV_p for several lipids, lipoproteins, and apolipoproteins as estimated in a study on patients in a lipid clinic (Kafonek, 1992). Estimates of physiologic variation have varied somewhat in different studies, and Table 10–4 also shows the estimates used by the National Choles-

2

Table 10–4. PHYSIOLOGIC VARIATION OF PLASMA LIPIDS, LIPOPROTEINS, AND APOLIPOPROTEINS

Component	CV_p (%)*	CV_p (%)†
Total cholesterol	5.0	6.4
Triglycerides	17.8	23.7
LDL-cholesterol	7.8	8.2
HDL-cholesterol	7.1	7.5
ApoA-I	7.1	—
ApoB	6.4	—

CV_p = coefficient of physiologic variation.
*Data from patients of a lipid clinic (Kafonek, 1992).
†Data from the National Cholesterol Education Program (NCEP) 1995 Working Group on Lipoprotein Measurement.

terol Education Program (NCEP) Working Group on Lipoprotein Measurement on developing guidelines for reliable LDL, HDL, and triglyceride measurements (NCEP Working Group on Lipoprotein Measurement Recommendations, 1995).

Blood Sampling and Storage

Certain kinds of physiologic variations and errors can be introduced before or during venipuncture, or when the specimens are handled and stored before analysis (Bachorik, 1982), and it is important to standardize as much as possible the conditions under which blood specimens are drawn and prepared for analysis.

Ideally, the patient is requested to fast for 12 hours before venipuncture. Chylomicrons are usually present in postprandial plasma and, depending on the type and amount of food ingested, can markedly increase the plasma triglyceride concentration. The concentrations of LDL- and HDL-cholesterol also decline transiently, in part as a consequence of CETP-mediated compositional changes that occur during the catabolism of chylomicrons (Cohn, 1988). Chylomicrons are almost completely cleared within 6 to 9 hours, and their presence after a 12-hour fast is considered abnormal. Fasting has little effect on plasma total cholesterol levels. The NCEP Adult Treatment Panel II (1993) has recommended that patients be requested to fast for at least 9 hours before blood specimens are taken for lipid and lipoprotein analysis. This recommendation accommodates patients who may be unable or unwilling to fast for 12 hours. The shorter fasting period would be expected to produce only minor and for the most part clinically insignificant errors in the estimation of the patient's usual triglyceride, LDL-cholesterol, and HDL-cholesterol levels, but a 12-hour fasting period is appropriate when making lipoprotein measurements in clinical and epidemiologic studies.

When a standing patient reclines, extravascular water transfers to the vascular system and dilutes nondiffusible plasma constituents. Decreases of as much as 10% in the concentrations of total cholesterol, LDL-cholesterol, HDL-cholesterol, and apolipoproteins A-I and B (Miller, 1992) have been observed after a 20-minute period of recumbence. The decrease in triglycerides is about 50% greater, suggesting that factors other than simple hemodilution may be involved. These effects are about half as great in a standing subject who sits (Miller, 1992). Postural changes are reversible when the patient resumes the standing position. The position of the patient should therefore be standardized for venipuncture, preferably to the sitting position, which is most commonly used. If it is necessary to use the recumbent position, this position should be used each time the patient is sampled to minimize postural change. Prolonged application of a tourniquet during venipuncture can increase apparent lipid concentrations, and the tourniquet should be released within a minute or two, if possible.

Either plasma or serum can be used when only cholesterol, triglyceride, and HDL-cholesterol are to be measured and LDL-cholesterol is calculated from the three measurements (discussed later). Plasma is preferred when the lipoproteins will be measured by ultracentrifugal or electrophoretic methods, because the samples can be cooled to 4°C immediately to retard changes that can occur in the lipoproteins at room temperature. The choice of anticoagulant is important, however. Some anticoagulants such as citrate exert rather large osmotic effects that result in artifactually low plasma lipid and lipoprotein concentrations. Heparin, because of its relatively large molecular weight, has little effect on plasma volume, but it can alter the electrophoretic mobilities of the lipoproteins. EDTA is the preferred anticoagulant, even though cholesterol and triglyceride concentrations in EDTA plasma are about 3% lower than in serum (Laboratory Methods Committee, 1977). This anticoagulant retards certain kinds of oxidative and enzymatic alterations that can occur in the lipoproteins during storage. When plasma is to be used, blood is cooled in an ice bath as soon as it is drawn, and the cells are removed as soon as possible, generally within three hours. Plasma should not remain in contact with the cells overnight. The plasma is then stored at 4°C until it is analyzed. Despite the presence of the anticoagulant, however, protein can aggregate in plasma that is stored in the refrigerator for a few days or frozen for longer periods. This can make it difficult to obtain a homogeneous aliquot for analysis and, furthermore, can interfere with the flow of sample in automatic analyzers, resulting in inaccurate or variable results. Protein aggregates less frequently in serum, and serum has been used under certain circumstances, such as when it is necessary to store samples for weeks or months before analysis. Cholesterol, triglycerides, and HDL can be satisfactorily analyzed in frozen samples, and LDL concentrations can be estimated with the Friedewald equation (Friedewald, 1972). Apolipoproteins can also be measured in frozen samples (discussed later). Frozen samples are not appropriate for ultracentrifugal analysis, however, because the triglyceride-rich lipoproteins do not withstand freezing.

Storage. When serum or plasma is to be stored for long periods, it should be maintained at temperatures of −70°C or lower. For short-term storage (up to a month or two), the samples can be kept at −20°C, but they should not be stored in a self-defrosting freezer. The temperature in a self-defrosting freezer actually cycles between about −20°C and −2°C during the defrost cycle and effectively subjects the samples to daily freeze-thaw cycles, which can hasten their deterioration and cause the lipid and lipoprotein measurements to become variable (i.e., less reproducible).

Estimation of Plasma Lipids

Cholesterol and triglycerides are the plasma lipids of most interest in the diagnosis and management of lipoprotein disorders. Phospholipid analyses are seldom required because they generally provide little additional information, but they may be requested occasionally in cases of obstructive liver disease or disorders associated with abnormally low lipoprotein levels.

Cholesterol. Cholesterol accounts for almost all of the sterol in plasma. It exists as a mixture of unesterified (30% to 40%) and esterified (60% to 70%) forms, and the proportion of the two forms is fairly constant within and between normal individuals. Total cholesterol and lipoprotein-cholesterol concentrations are usually expressed in terms of the sterol nucleus without distinguishing the esterified and unesterified fractions. In general, it is not necessary to distinguish the two forms except when the contribution of the fatty acid moiety to cholesteryl ester mass must be accounted for, or when the cholesterol/cholesteryl ester mass ratio is of interest.

The present discussion considers primarily the enzymatic methods, which have virtually replaced the chemical methods that were used for most clinical and research purposes (Bachorik, 1979; Lipid Research Clinics Program, 1982; Wood, 1980). However, one of the chemical methods, a modification of the Abell-Kendall method (Abell, 1952) continues as the basis for the Centers for Disease Control and Prevention (CDC) reference method for cholesterol (Myers, 1989). In the Abell-Kendall method, cholesteryl esters are hydrolyzed with alcoholic KOH, and unesterified cholesterol is extracted with petroleum ether and measured with the Liebermann-Burchard reagent using purified cholesterol standards. This method can be accurate to within about 0.5% of true value and has been transferred to the National Reference Method Laboratory Network, which was established in 1989 as a means for laboratories and manufacturers of cholesterol reagents and calibration materials to maintain traceability to the CDC reference method for measuring cholesterol.

Enzymatic Methods. Enzymatic methods for cholesterol analysis were developed in the 1970s and have since replaced the chemical methods almost entirely. In these methods (Allain, 1974), total cholesterol is determined directly in plasma or serum in a series of reactions in which cholesteryl esters are hydrolyzed; the 3-OH group of cholesterol is oxidized; and hydrogen peroxide, which is one of the reaction products, is determined enzymatically:

$$\text{Cholesteryl ester} + H_2O \xrightarrow[\text{hydrolase}]{\text{cholesteryl ester}} \text{cholesterol} + \text{fatty acid} \quad (10\text{-}1)$$

$$\text{Cholesterol} + O_2 \xrightarrow[\text{oxidase}]{\text{cholesterol}} \text{cholest-4-en-3-one} + H_2O_2 \quad (10\text{-}2)$$

$$H_2O_2 + \text{phenol} + \text{4-aminoantipyrine} \xrightarrow{\text{peroxidase}} \text{quinoneimine dye} + 2H_2O \quad (10\text{-}3)$$

The absorbance of the dye is measured at 500 nm.

The enzymatic methods are less subject to interference by nonsterol substances that react in the chemical methods. However, they are not absolutely specific for cholesterol, because cholesterol oxidase can react with other sterols that have been reported as being present in plasma and with plant sterols present in appreciable concentrations in the circulation of patients with β-sitosterolemia. However, these sterols also contributed to the measured values with most chemical methods for estimating cholesterol. Reducing substances such as ascorbic acid and bilirubin can interfere with the measurements by consuming H_2O_2 (Naito, 1984; Witte, 1978). Interference by bilirubin is complex and, depending on the reagent concentrations, can produce artifactually high or low cholesterol values. Bilirubin itself absorbs light at 500 nm, which would tend to increase the assayed cholesterol values. It is, however, oxidized by H_2O_2. Furthermore, when oxidized, bilirubin loses its absorbance at 500 nm. This complicates the application of a serum blank to correct for bilirubin absorbance. Bilirubin may also interfere directly by reacting with an intermediate in the peroxidase reaction. Interference by bilirubin seems to be significant only at concentrations exceeding 5 mg/dL, at which level it has been reported to decrease apparent cholesterol values by 5% to 15% (Deacon, 1979; Naito, 1984; Pesce, 1977). Sample turbidity as a result of elevated triglyceride concentrations can also interfere with the enzymatic methods (Pesce, 1977). Uric acid, hemoglobin, and many other substances in abnormally high concentrations apparently do not affect the cholesterol measurements (Deacon, 1979; Naito, 1984).

The enzymatic methods consume only microliter quantities of sample and do not require a preliminary extraction step. They are rapid and, if cholesteryl ester hydrolase is omitted, also provide a measurement of unesterified cholesterol. Finally, the enzymatic methods appear to be precise, with CVs generally in the range of 1% to 2%. For the most part, these methods employ stabilized pure cholesterol standards or serum calibration standards, for which the stated values are traceable to the CDC reference method for cholesterol (Cooper, 1982). Enzymatic values generally agree with reference values to within 1% or 2% when measured in a laboratory setting with modern equipment.

Triglycerides. A wide variety of methods have been used to measure plasma triglycerides (Bachorik, 1977), but the methods most commonly used for clinical or epidemiologic purposes are based on the hydrolysis of triglycerides and the measurement of glycerol that is released in the reaction:

$$\text{Triglyceride} + 3H_2O \xrightarrow{\text{lipase}} \underset{\text{Glycerol}}{\begin{array}{c} H_2COH \\ | \\ HCOH \\ | \\ H_2COH \end{array}} + \underset{\text{Fatty acid}}{3RC\begin{array}{l} {/\!\!/}O \\ \backslash OH \end{array}} \quad (10\text{-}4)$$

The reactions are almost universally performed enzymatically; as with cholesterol, the enzymatic methods have replaced the earlier chemical methods (Kessler, 1966; Lipid Research Clinics Program, 1982). One chemical method is still used as the CDC reference method for triglycerides (Myers, 1989). The CDC reference method uses a chloroform extraction procedure followed by silicic acid chromatography to isolate the triglycerides (Myers, 1989). Glycerol is released by saponification and oxidized with sodium periodate:

$$\text{Glycerol} + NaIO_4 \longrightarrow \underset{\text{Formaldehyde}}{2HC\begin{array}{l} {/\!\!/}O \\ \backslash H \end{array}} + \underset{\text{Formic acid}}{HC\begin{array}{l} {/\!\!/}O \\ \backslash OH \end{array}} \quad (10\text{-}5)$$

The formaldehyde produced is measured by reaction with a sulfuric acid solution of chromotropic acid to produce a pink chromophore.

Periodate oxidation is not specific for glycerol. Formaldehyde is also formed from substances such as glucose, which have vicinal hydroxyl groups, or from substances with hydroxyl and amino groups on adjacent carbon atoms. Formaldehyde is also produced from glycerol-containing phospholipids such as phosphatidylcholine, which upon alkaline hydrolysis produces α-glycerophosphate. α-Glycerophosphate is also oxidized by periodate to form formaldehyde.

These kinds of substances are removed during the extraction and adsorption steps and do not interfere with triglyceride measurements made with the CDC reference method.

Enzymatic Methods. Enzymatic methods (Bucolo, 1973) are now universally used for triglyceride analysis. They are relatively specific, rapid, and easy to use. The analyses are performed directly in plasma or serum and are not subject to interference by phospholipids or glucose. In one series of reactions, triglycerides are hydrolyzed, and the glycerol formed is converted to glycerophosphate and measured as follows:

$$\text{Triglycerides} \xrightarrow{\text{lipase}} \text{glycerol} + \text{fatty acids} \quad (10\text{-}6)$$

$$\text{Glycerol} + \text{ATP} \xrightarrow{\text{glycerokinase}} \text{glycerophosphate} + \text{ADP} \quad (10\text{-}7)$$

$$\text{Glycerophosphate} + \text{NAD} + \xrightarrow[\text{dehydrogenase}]{\text{glycerophosphate}} \text{dihydroxyacetone phosphate} + \text{NADH} + \text{H}^+ \quad (10\text{-}8)$$

$$\text{NADH} + \text{tetrazolium dye} \xrightarrow{\text{diaphorase}} \text{formazan} + \text{NAD}^+ \quad (10\text{-}9)$$

The NADH formed in reaction 10-8 can be measured spectrophotometrically. In other methods, reaction 10-9 has been added so that the absorbance readings can be made in the spectral region of 500 to 600 nm using instruments that are commonly available in the clinical laboratory. In a more common variation, the glycerophosphate formed in reaction 10-7 is oxidized by the action of glycerophosphate oxidase:

$$\text{Glycerophosphate} + O_2 \xrightarrow[\text{oxidase}]{\text{glycerophosphate}} \text{dihydroxyacetone} + H_2O_2 \quad (10\text{-}10)$$

The H_2O_2 produced is measured as described previously for cholesterol methods.

In a third approach, ADP, rather than glycerophosphate as formed in reaction 10-7, is quantitated:

$$\text{ADP} + \text{phosphoenol pyruvate} \xrightarrow[\text{kinase}]{\text{pyruvate}} \text{ATP} + \text{pyruvate} \quad (10\text{-}11)$$

$$\text{Pyruvate} + \text{NADH} + \text{H}^+ \xrightarrow[\text{dehydrogenase}]{\text{lactate}} \text{lactate} + \text{NAD}^+ \quad (10\text{-}12)$$

In this case, the disappearance of NADH is measured at 340 nm.

Enzymatic triglyceride methods generally perform well. The reagents are available commercially as lyophilized preparations that need only be reconstituted before use. Judged from recent College of American Pathologists (CAP) surveys (1993 CAP Surveys, 1993), enzymatic triglyceride methods give values that, on average, agree with CDC reference values within a few milligrams per deciliter; the interlaboratory CVs for triglyceride measurement in about 5500 participating laboratories, using a variety of enzymatic methods, was on the order of 5% to 6%. Nonetheless, before selecting an enzymatic method, it is prudent to evaluate its accuracy and precision over the range of triglyceride concentrations likely to be encountered most frequently (1.299 to 12.987 mmol/L; 50 to 500 mg/dL).

Triglyceride Blanks. The estimation of triglyceride blanks continues to be an area of uncertainty in triglyceride measurements. Increased blank readings can arise from a number of sources, depending on the samples, the methods used, or the physiologic state of the patient. Calculations should account for the nonglyceride substances that would add to the triglyceride measurements. As mentioned earlier, phospholipids and glucose do not interfere with enzymatic methods. Free glycerol, on the other hand, does. Glycerol is normally present in plasma in concentrations below 0.163 mmol/L (1.5 mg/dL), equivalent to a triglyceride concentration of about 14 mg/dL, but it can be present in higher concentrations after extremely vigorous exercise, in some patients with uncontrolled diabetes, by chance contamination with the glycerol lubricant used on the stoppers of some blood collection tubes, after recent ingestion of glycerol-containing medications, or in a relatively rare disorder, hyperglycerolemia.

It is common practice to determine triglyceride blanks by omitting the hydrolysis step. In an alternative procedure, free glycerol is consumed in a preliminary reaction before initiating triglyceride hydrolysis. In this case, the equivalent of a blanked triglyceride is measured directly. These procedures are satisfactory for correcting blanks that arise from many nonglyceride sources. Partial glycerides are generally present in very low concentrations in fresh plasma or serum, but they can form from the slow hydrolysis of triglycerides when samples are stored. It is not clear whether partial glycerides present in fresh plasma should be subtracted, but those that may form during storage should not be subtracted because they arise from triglycerides that were originally present in the sample.

Fortunately, as complex as the blanking problem is, it is usually of little practical importance, and blanks are not determined routinely in many laboratories. The magnitude of the blanks encountered in most fresh samples is on the order of about 0.056 to 0.112 mmol/L (5 to 10 mg/dL), expressed as triglyceride, although it can be higher (e.g., 0.224 mmol/L [20 mg/dL]) in samples with high triglyceride concentrations. However, blanks can assume importance in the standardization and quality control of triglyceride measurements, because they can be on the order of 0.226 to 0.339 mmol/L (20 to 30 mg/dL) or more in serum pools used for these purposes, probably owing in part to the partial hydrolysis of triglycerides during the preparation of the pools. In the reference methods, triglycerides are isolated before analysis; the reference values reflect the actual concentrations of triglycerides at the time of analysis and do not include the partial glycerides or glycerol that may have been produced during the preparation of the pools. Methods in which free glycerol is measured along with triglycerides would therefore give higher results if blanks are not analyzed.

Phospholipids. Phosphatidyl choline and sphingomyelin constitute over 90% of the phospholipids in human plasma, and of this, about 80% is phosphatidyl choline. The remaining phospholipids include phosphatidyl serine and phosphatidyl ethanolamine (3% to 6%) and lysophosphatidyl choline (4% to 9%). Although phospholipid analyses usually provide little additional information with respect to dyslipoproteinemia, it may be desirable on occasion to determine total phospholipids or individual phospholipid classes in patients with certain kinds of disorders such as obstructive jaundice, abetalipoproteinemia or hypobetalipoproteinemia, Tangier disease, or LCAT deficiency, in which the concentration, composition, or lipoprotein distribution of the phospholipids, or some combination of these, is altered.

Total phospholipids can be most conveniently determined by measuring phospholipid phosphorus. Lipids are extracted from the sample and oxidized completely to convert phospholipid phosphorus to inorganic phosphate, which is then determined colorimetrically. Various extraction media have proved to be satisfactory, such as ethanol-diethylether (Ellefson, 1976) or chloroform-methanol used as described by Folch (1957). Oxidation is generally performed with concentrated H_2SO_4 used in conjunction with H_2O_2 or perchloric acid at temperatures of 150°C to 250°C (Bartlett, 1959; Ellefson, 1976). The released phosphate is converted to phosphomolybdate by reaction with ammonium molybdate, and the mixture is treated with a mild reducing agent (aminonaphthalsulfonic acid, p-methylaminophenol, stannous chloride, or one of several others) to form heteropolymolybdenum blue, which has an intense blue color. The procedures are reproducible and sensitive and can be adapted to measure total phospholipid phosphorus in 100 μL or less of plasma or serum. Each mole of phosphorus contributes about 4% to the total phospholipid mass and, if expressed in milligrams per deciliter, can be converted to total phospholipid mass by multiplying the phosphorus concentration by 25.

Serum or plasma phospholipids can also be measured enzymatically using commercially available methods. In the method available from WAKO Pure Chemical Industries, Ltd. (Osaka, Japan), lecithin, sphingomyelin, and lysolecithin are hydrolyzed using phospholipase D, and the choline liberated is oxidized.

$$\text{phospholipid} \xrightarrow{\text{phospholipase D}} \text{choline} \qquad (10\text{-}13)$$

$$\text{choline} \xrightarrow[\text{oxidase}]{\text{choline}} H_2O_2 + \text{betaine} \qquad (10\text{-}14)$$

The H_2O_2 produced is measured in a manner similar to that shown in reaction 10-3.

Analysis of individual phospholipid classes is seldom required for the evaluation of the dyslipoproteinemias and is not discussed in this chapter.

Desk-Top Analyzers

Since the mid-1980s, small, portable, and relatively inexpensive desk-top instruments have been introduced with which a number of blood analytes can be measured, including cholesterol, triglycerides, and HDL-cholesterol (Bachorik, 1994a). These analyzers use enzymatic methods similar to those described previously for measuring cholesterol and triglycerides and were originally designed for use in nonlaboratory environments such as the physician's office. They have also been used extensively in cholesterol-screening programs conducted at field sites such as shopping malls and other nontraditional locations, although such use has apparently declined in recent years as more people have become aware of their cholesterol levels and have sought appropriate treatment. Some of these instruments are "dry-chemistry" analyzers. They use reagent-impregnated test strips or slides to which 10 to 30 μL of sample are applied. The sample diffuses to the reagent-impregnated zone, where it dissolves the reagents and allows the enzymatic reactions to proceed. The reaction conditions are controlled by the analyzer. At the end of the incubation period, a light source illuminates the strip, and the reflectance of the reaction mixture is measured. The readings are converted to concentration units and are displayed on a digital readout or paper tape.

Many of the desk-top methods require separate blood samples for cholesterol, triglycerides, and HDL-cholesterol, but at least one analyzer (the one available from Cholestech, Inc., Hayward, CA) can measure all three analytes in a single sample. This is accomplished by diverting portions of the sample to three different reagent regions, one for cholesterol, one for triglycerides, and one for HDL. The path to the HDL region contains a precipitant to remove apoB-containing lipoproteins so that HDL-cholesterol can be measured without having to remove the apoB-containing lipoproteins manually.

2

Other instruments use solutions of reagents rather than impregnated test strips, and the absorbance of the sample is measured. Several of these analyzers can measure plasma lipids in whole blood, as well as in serum or plasma, but most require the preliminary removal of cells.

All of the instruments use microliter quantities of sample obtained either by venipuncture or by fingerstick and provide results within about three to eight minutes. In addition, many of them require only periodic calibration (e.g., once every two to three months) rather than each time the instrument is used. Generally, they can be used by operators without formal laboratory training, although this is not recommended, because the accuracy and precision of the analyses are related to the training and experience of the operators (Belsey, 1987a, 1987b; Lunz, 1987). When these instruments are properly calibrated and operated, the analyses can be reasonably accurate and precise (Bachorik, 1989, 1994; Belsey, 1987a, 1987b; Boerma, 1988; El-Dering, 1986; Koch, 1987; Schultz, 1985; Sedor, 1988; Stavljenic, 1987). Notwithstanding their simplicity and ease of operation, however, the procedures involve steps in which errors can occur and that trained technologists are more likely to detect.

There have been efforts to develop cholesterol screening tests that do not require the use of an analyzer. The first such test became available to the general public for home use in 1994 (Acumeter Cholesterol Test, marketed by Johnson and Johnson). This is a dry chemistry enzymatic test that relies on chemistry similar to that shown in equations 10-1 to 10-3. The H_2O_2 produced in reaction 10-3, however, moves into a linear color development zone, producing a colored bar the length of which depends on the amount of H_2O_2 produced and thus on the cholesterol concentration of the sample. The length of the colored bar is measured visually against a scale of arbitrary units that can be converted to milligrams per deciliter using a conversion table supplied with the test and calibrated to the nearest 5 mg/dL. The test is supplied as a single-use cassette, can be used with whole blood, plasma, or serum, and includes instructions that can be understood by the layperson. It is intended for screening use only, but it has the potential to be used as an adherence aid for the patient undergoing treatment for hypercholesterolemia. The test could be misused by the layman who fails to follow up a higher reading by seeking appropriate medical care, who attempts a program of self-treatment without adequate medical evaluation, or who substitutes this screening tool for more reliable laboratory measurements.

Finally, the question arises as to whether fingerstick samples should be used with these analyzers. Although it is generally assumed that venous and capillary samples are equivalent, the available information at present is limited and somewhat contradictory. Some investigators have found that cholesterol measurements in the two kinds of samples agree within about 4% (Koch, 1987) or less (Bachorik, 1989; Boerma, 1988), but others have reported differences of 8% to 12% (El-Dering, 1986; Katan, 1988; Kupke, 1979). In general, however, the measurements in capillary blood samples seem to be a little lower than in venous samples. In addition, measurements in fingerstick samples tend to be more variable than measurements in venous samples obtained at the same time (Bachorik, 1990). The reasons for capillary-venous sample differences are not clear. There is no reason to suspect that the physical-chemical properties of fingerstick or venous samples might differ so as to affect their diffusion or other characteristics that might affect any of the desk-top or noninstrumental systems. It is more likely that such differences, particularly the greater variability of the measurements in fingerstick samples, actually arises from preanalytical factors, such as the techniques used to collect the sample, application of sufficient volume of sample to the test strip, biologic variations in lipoprotein concentrations in fingerstick samples arising from such factors as the temperature of the patient's finger, and differences in postural effects on venous and fingerstick samples. The biologic component of intersubject variations has been estimated for lipid, lipoprotein, and apolipoprotein concentrations in venous samples, but apparently no such data are currently available for fingerstick samples. Although the use of capillary samples may be unavoidable under some conditions, it is well to keep in mind first, that the epidemiologic data on which risk levels for lipids and lipoproteins are based on measurements in venous samples, and second, that for various physiologic and methodologic reasons, the measurements in the two kinds of samples may differ.

Estimation of Lipoproteins

Because the lipoproteins share common lipid and apolipoprotein components, one problem in lipoprotein analysis is the separation of the lipoprotein classes from each other. The methods that have been applied to lipoprotein separation include ultracentrifugation, adsorption, gel filtration, affinity chromatography, electrophoresis in various media, polyanion and alcohol precipitation, immunochemical procedures, and various combinations of methods. Some of these methods require special skills and equipment and are not easily adapted for clinical or epidemiologic purposes. This discussion is limited to several procedures that have been used by the routine or special clinical laboratory that assists with the diagnosis and management of disorders of lipoprotein metabolism.

Ultracentrifugal Methods. Ultracentrifugal methods take advantage of two properties of the lipoproteins. First, by virtue of their lipid content, they have lower densities than the other plasma macromolecules. Second, each class of lipoproteins has a different density. Thus, chylomicrons and VLDL float at d 1.006 kg/L, the density of plasma; LDL and HDL are sedimented at this density. LDL and VLDL both float at d 1.063 kg/L, and these lipoproteins, as well as HDL, float at d 1.21 kg/L. In contrast, other plasma proteins have densities above 1.3 kg/L. The lipoproteins can thus be separated from the other plasma proteins, and from each other, by ultracentrifugation at the appropriate density or densities.

Analytical Ultracentrifugation: The "Reference Method." The lipoproteins have classically been defined in terms of their rates of flotation under specified conditions in the analytical ultracentrifuge (Lindgren, 1972). Although this method is not used in most clinical laboratories or in very many research laboratories, analytical ultracentrifugation has been considered the reference method with which other methods are compared (discussed later). It can break down the lipoprotein spectrum (especially VLDL, LDL, and HDL) into several different subclasses that can be accurately quantified.

The lipoproteins are first isolated from plasma by preparative ultracentrifugation and then centrifuged in the analytical ultracentrifuge—VLDL and LDL at d 1.063 kg/L and HDL at d 1.21 kg/L. The lipoprotein classes and subclasses migrate at different rates depending on their densities, and their movement and concentrations can be measured using Schlieren optics, which detect the concentration-dependent changes in refractive index as the particles migrate in the centrifugal field. Lipoprotein concentrations are expressed in terms of total lipoprotein mass using calculations that account for the empirically determined relationships between refractive index and dry weight for each of the major lipoprotein classes. Conditions of sample preparation, temperature, density adjustments, and other factors must be controlled rigorously, and the measurements must be corrected for various effects, such as variations in flotation rate with concentration, Ogston-Johnson effects, the redistribution of salts that changes the background density during ultracentrifugation, and correction of the measurements to standard conditions of temperature and density. The calculations are complex and generally performed by computer.

Preparative Ultracentrifugation. Individual classes of lipoproteins can be quantitatively separated by ultracentrifugation at different densities (Havel, 1955). The separated lipoproteins are then measured in various ways, commonly in terms of their cholesterol content. In one approach, plasma is centrifuged sequentially at d 1.006 kg/L and d 1.063 kg/L. The cholesterol concentrations of the respective floating VLDL and LDL fractions are measured as an index of the concentrations of these lipoproteins. Cholesterol in the d 1.063 kg/L infranatant is associated almost entirely with HDL, and the cholesterol concentration of this fraction can be measured without separating HDL from the other plasma proteins. If it is desirable to isolate HDL, the d 1.063 kg/L infranatant is adjusted to d 1.21 kg/L, and HDL is removed in the same way. With appropriate density adjustment, similar procedures can be used to determine subclasses of lipoproteins—for example, IDL (d 1.006 to d 1.019 kg/L), HDL_2 (d 1.063 to 1.12 kg/L), and HDL_3 (d 1.12 to 1.21 kg/L).

Another approach is to centrifuge aliquots of the plasma simultaneously at d 1.006 kg/L, d 1.063 kg/L, and d 1.21 kg/L. The cholesterol contents of the floating layers are determined, and the individual lipoprotein concentrations are calculated by difference.

Preparative ultracentrifugation can provide reasonably accurate estimates of the concentrations of VLDL, LDL, and HDL in samples that do not contain appreciable concentrations of IDL, Lp(a), or other unusual lipoproteins, or in which the densities of the major lipoproteins are not altered. Lp(a) overlaps the LDL and HDL density ranges and would contribute to cholesterol in both fractions. Similarly, IDL can overlap the VLDL-LDL density range. β-VLDL, or so-called floating beta lipoprotein, manifested in Type III hyperlipoproteinemia, is rich in cholesterol, floats at d 1.006 kg/L, and, when present, greatly increases the cholesterol concentration of the VLDL fraction.

Electrophoretic Methods. Electrophoresis had been widely used in the routine clinical laboratory to separate and measure lipoproteins, but the limitations of this method (which will be discussed subsequently) and the realization that it is not really needed for diagnosis of most dyslipoproteinemias have considerably limited the use of lipoprotein electrophoresis for routine clinical practice. The most commonly used support medium is agarose gel because of its speed, sensitivity, and resolution of the lipoprotein classes. Chylomicrons, if present, remain at the origin, and the other major lipoproteins migrate at rates that increase in the order of HDL > VLDL > LDL. The electrophoretically separated lipoproteins have been named according to their mobilities: HDL (α-lipoprotein) moves with the α_1-globulins, LDL (β-lipoprotein) migrates with the β-globulins, and VLDL (pre-β lipoprotein) migrates with the α_2-globulins. Different properties of the lipoproteins form the basis for electrophoretic and ultracentrifugal separation, and analogous fractions separated by the two techniques may not be identical. For example, β-VLDL is isolated with VLDL by ultracentrifugation but moves electrophoretically with LDL. In the absence of additional information, a sample containing β-VLDL would appear to have an elevated VLDL-cholesterol concentration by ultracentrifugation and an increased LDL concentration by electrophoresis. Another example is Lp(a); ultracentrifugally, it is isolated in the LDL-HDL density range, but it has an electrophoretic mobility similar to that of VLDL. This dichotomy is why Lp(a) is called sinking pre-β lipoprotein.

Lipoprotein electrophoretograms are usually visualized with a lipid-staining dye such as Oil Red O, Fat Red 7B, or Sudan Black B, and electrophoresis can be performed in unfractionated plasma or in plasma fractions that contain other serum proteins. These lipid stains react primarily with the ester bonds in triglycerides and cholesteryl esters. Lipoproteins rich in free cholesterol and phospholipids (such as LpX) stain very poorly and thus are grossly underestimated by electrophoretic techniques.

Attempts have been made to quantitate the lipoproteins by densitometry. Lipoprotein levels have been expressed in terms of the percentage of distribution of lipid-staining material in β-lipoproteins, pre-β lipoproteins, and α-lipoproteins, or these levels have been converted to lipoprotein-cholesterol concentrations according to calculations that incorporate assumptions about cholesterol content and dye uptake of the lipoproteins. In general, these approaches have not been successful for reasons that include incomplete resolution of β-lipoproteins and pre-β lipoproteins, the presence of minor or unusual lipoproteins, and differences in the intensity of staining. Electrophoresis has been most successfully used in conjunction with other methods.

Polyanion Precipitation Methods. Lipoproteins are precipitated with polyanions, such as heparin sulfate, dextran sulfate, phosphotungstate, and others, in the presence of divalent cations, such as Ca^{2+}, Mg^{2+}, and Mn^{2+}. Precipitation is influenced by factors such as reagent concentration, pH, ionic strength, the presence of other serum proteins and anticoagulants, the relative amounts of lipid and protein in the lipoprotein particles, and the duration and conditions of sample storage. Conditions have been established in which the major classes of lipoproteins can be precipitated in stepwise fashion beginning with the lower-density, lipid-rich lipoproteins (Burstein, 1982). The more dissimilar the lipoproteins, the more satisfactorily they can be separated from each other. Thus, although apoB-containing lipoproteins can be precipitated from most samples under conditions in which virtually all the HDL remains soluble, it is more difficult to separate VLDL from LDL. Similarly, HDL can be isolated from the lower density lipoproteins much more satisfactorily than HDL_2 can be separated from HDL_3. In part, the more similar in composition the lipoprotein classes or subclasses to be separated are, the more critically the conditions of precipitation must be controlled to separate them. Therefore, the likelihood increases that a reagent concentration suitable for some samples may not be suitable for others, and the frequency of inadequate separations becomes unacceptably high. Although theoretically attractive, lipoprotein quantitation schemes based entirely on precipitation methods have not gained wide acceptance, and polyanion precipitation is most commonly used to remove apoB-containing lipoproteins prior to the analysis of HDL-cholesterol.

Methods for Determining HDL-Cholesterol Values. In the methods most commonly used, apoB-containing lipoproteins (chylomicrons, VLDL, IDL, LDL, Lp[a]) are removed by polyanion-divalent cation precipitation, and HDL-cholesterol is analyzed directly in the supernatant. Several combinations of polyanion-divalent cations have been used, and not all of them give precisely the same results. HDL-cholesterol values determined with heparan sulfate–Mn^{2+} procedures agree closely with those obtained with the analytical or preparative ultracentrifuge (Bachorik, 1976; Warnick, 1979). Dextran sulfate (Mr-50,000)–Mg^{2+} and sodium phosphotungstate–Mg^{2+} apparently give results about 5% lower than those obtained with ultracentrifugation, and heparin-Ca^{2+} appears to give results that are about 10% higher. The differences arise, in part, from the extent to which apoB-containing lipoproteins remain unprecipitated and can lead to a gross overestimation of HDL-cholesterol. In other cases, some HDL may be precipitated and cause an underestimation of HDL-cholesterol. In addition, the adequacy of separation may also be influenced by factors such as the concentration of apoB-containing lipoproteins in the sample and the age of the sample. It should be mentioned that the heparan sulfate–Mn^{2+} method was widely used in major population surveys and epidemiologic studies in which the relationship between plasma HDL-cholesterol concentration and cardiovascular risk was established. However, Mn^{2+} has been reported to interfere with some enzymatic cholesterol methods, and modifications, such as removal of excess Mn^{2+} by precipitation with $NaHCO_3$ or addition of EDTA to the enzymatic cholesterol reagent to complex excess

Mn^{2+} remaining in the HDL-containing supernatant, have been introduced to obviate this problem. Heparin–$MnCl_2$ is not routinely used any more in the clinical laboratory. Other precipitants, particularly dextran sulfate–Mg^{2+} or phosphotungstate–Mg^{2+}, are now most commonly used because they do not interfere with enzymatic cholesterol methods. In addition, agreement of those methods with the heparin-Mn^{2+} method has improved, partly because of refinement of the methods themselves and the materials used to calibrate HDL procedures. The heparin-Mn^{2+} method, however, remains as the standard by which other methods are assessed.

Combined Methods. Evaluation of the hyperlipidemic patient can include measurements of plasma cholesterol, VLDL, LDL, HDL, and triglyceride levels; an assessment of whether the patient has chylomicrons in the fasting state; and an assessment of the presence or absence of β-VLDL (floating beta lipoproteins, characteristic of overt Type III hyperlipoproteinemia). In addition, Lp(a) has become more widely appreciated as an independent risk factor for coronary disease (Berg, 1979; Dahlen, 1983; Kostner, 1981; Murai, 1986), at least in certain kinds of patients (discussed in Bachorik, 1992, 1993). It may also be necessary on occasion to assess the activity of lipoprotein lipase or the presence and nature of one or more of the apoproteins. Two approaches to lipoprotein measurement are in common use. The more extensive of the two employs a combination of preparative ultracentrifugation, polyanion precipitation, and electrophoresis (Fredrickson, 1968; Lipid Research Clinics Laboratory Manual, 1982).

Plasma total cholesterol, HDL-cholesterol, and triglyceride (TG) concentrations are determined as described previously. A separate aliquot of plasma is ultracentrifuged without density adjustment. The floating layer containing VLDL (Fig. 10–1*A*) (and, if present, chylomicrons and β-VLDL [Fig. 10–1*B*]) and the infranatant fraction, which contains LDL, Lp(a), and HDL (see Fig. 10–1*A*), are quantitatively recovered. The cholesterol content of the infranatant fraction is determined. The lipoprotein cholesterol concentrations are calculated as follows:

1. HDL-cholesterol, measured directly
2. LDL-cholesterol = [infranatant cholesterol] – [HDL-cholesterol]
3. VLDL-cholesterol = [total cholesterol] – [infranatant cholesterol]

As discussed earlier, Lp(a) is found in the LDL-HDL density range. However, it is precipitated with the apoB-containing lipoproteins, and the LDL-cholesterol measurement includes the contribution of Lp(a)-cholesterol, which in most people is on the order of 2 to 4 mg/dL.

A simplified procedure that does not require the ultracentrifuge was described by Friedewald (1972):

4. $[\text{LDL-cholesterol}] = [\text{total cholesterol}] - [\text{HDL-cholesterol}] - \dfrac{[\text{PlasmaTG}]}{2.175}$

where the concentrations are expressed in millimoles per liter. The factor $\dfrac{\text{plasma TG}}{5}$ is used when concentrations are expressed in milligrams per deciliter.

In this method, the plasma total cholesterol, triglyceride, and HDL-cholesterol concentrations are determined as described. Because most of the plasma triglycerides are carried in VLDL, VLDL-cholesterol concentration is estimated from the ratio of triglyceride to cholesterol in VLDL:

$$\text{VLDL-cholesterol} = \frac{\text{plasma TG}}{2.175} \qquad (10\text{-}15)$$

It has been reported that the factor [plasma TG]/2.825 gives a more nearly accurate estimate of VLDL-cholesterol (DeLong, 1986). This is equivalent to:

$$\frac{\text{plasma TG}}{6.5} \qquad (10\text{-}16)$$

when concentrations are expressed in mg/dL.

It has been found, however, that the factor that gives the best estimate of VLDL-cholesterol, and therefore the best estimate of LDL-cholesterol, can vary with the population studied and with the triglyceride methods used; on balance, the NCEP Working Group on Lipoprotein Measurement felt it best to use the unmodified Friedewald equation.

This assay should be performed on a fasting sample. The method assumes that essentially all the plasma triglycerides are carried in VLDL and that the TG/cholesterol ratio of VLDL is invariant. Neither assumption is entirely true, and both can lead to fairly large percentage errors in estimates of VLDL-cholesterol. However, this does not normally produce errors of more than 0.130 to 0.260 mmol/L (5 to 10 mg/dL) in LDL-cholesterol measurements because VLDL generally carries only about 25% of the plasma total cholesterol. There are some limitations on the kinds of samples to which the equation can be applied. It is not suitable for use with samples in which triglyceride concentrations exceed 10.390 mmol/L (400 mg/dL). The error in LDL-cholesterol actually becomes noticeable at triglyceride levels above 5.195 mmol/L (200 mg/dL) but is thought to become unacceptably large at triglyceride levels above 10.390 mmol/L (400 mg/dL). The method is similarly unsuitable for samples that have chylomicrons or β-VLDL. Compared with VLDL, the ratio of triglycerides to cholesterol in chylomicrons is much higher, and the use of the factor $\dfrac{\text{TG}}{2.175}$ can overestimate the amount of cholesterol in VLDL, leading to an underestimate of LDL-cholesterol. Similarly, the ratio of triglyceride to cholesterol in β-VLDL is much lower than in VLDL, and the use of the factor $\dfrac{\text{TG}}{2.175}$ can underestimate VLDL-cholesterol and thus overestimate LDL-cholesterol. Thus, a patient with Type III hypolipoproteinemia can be misclassified as having elevated LDL-cholesterol. It is important to distinguish the two conditions, because their treatments differ. Provided that its limitations are appreciated, the Friedewald equation has broad usefulness, both as a screening tool and for following patients whose lipoprotein patterns are known from more extensive analyses.

VLDL-cholesterol can be measured directly in the $d < 1.006$ g/mL fraction, but the result tends to be inaccurate because of the difficulty in recovering VLDL quantitatively.

Standing Plasma Test. Chylomicrons, if present in appreciable quantities, are detected using the "standing plasma" test. An aliquot of plasma (2 mL) is placed into a 10×75 mm test tube and allowed to stand in the refrigerator at 4°C undisturbed overnight. Chylomicrons accumulate as a floating "cream" layer and can be detected visually. The

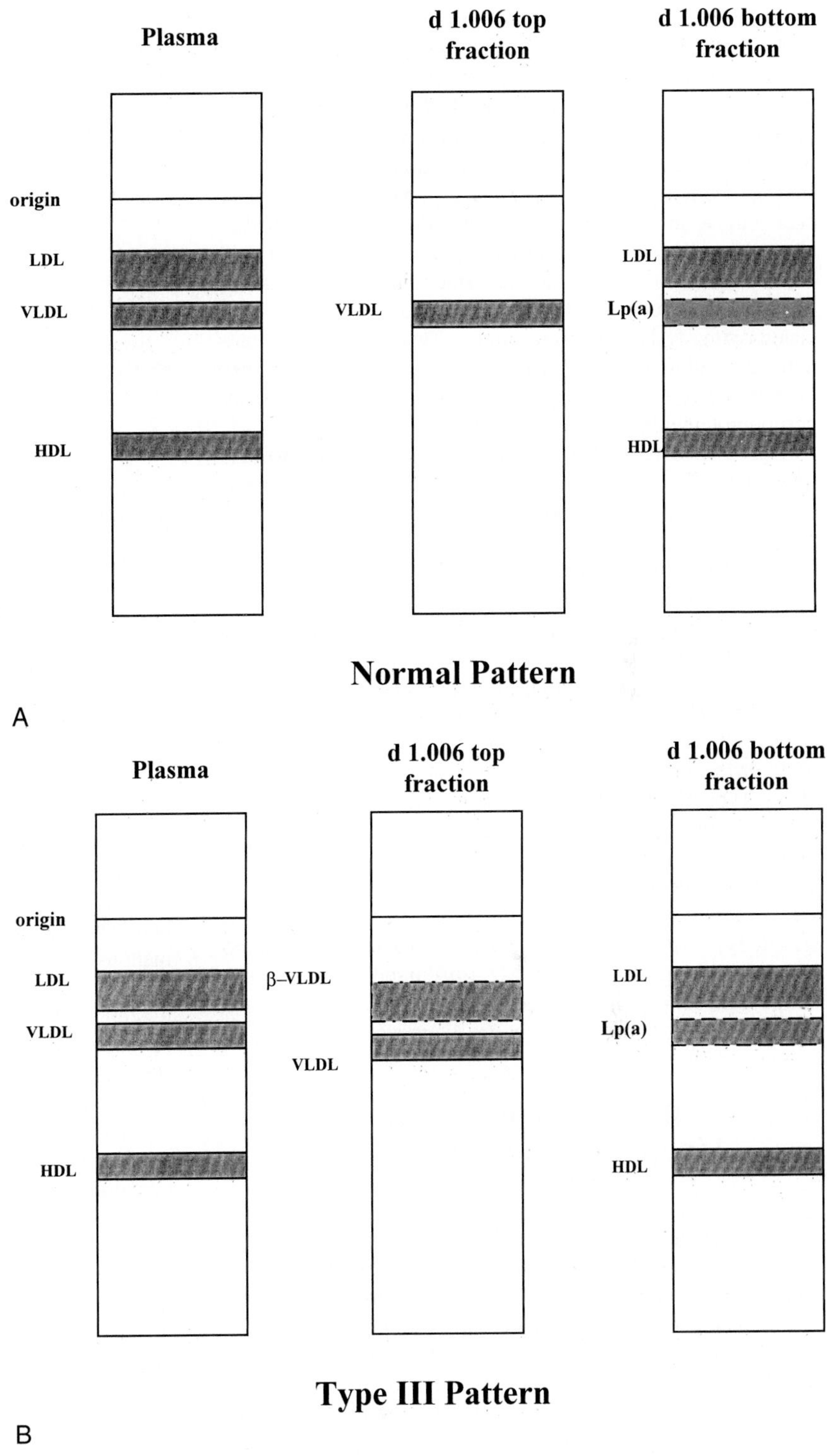

Figure 10–1. Representation of lipoprotein electrophoretic patterns in unfractionated plasma and in ultracentrifugal fractions. *A*, Normal lipoprotein pattern. *B*, Pattern seen in Type III hyperlipoproteinemia.

presence of chylomicrons in fasting plasma is considered abnormal. A plasma sample that remains turbid after standing overnight contains excessive amounts of VLDL, and if a floating cream layer is detected, chylomicrons are present also.

Detection of β-VLDL and Lp(a). The ultracentrifugal fraction of d $<$ 1.006 kg/L is examined electrophoretically for the presence of β-VLDL (floating beta lipoproteins), and the d $>$ 1.006 g/mL protein can be examined similarly for the presence of Lp(a) (Bachorik, 1980). In practice, unfractionated plasma and both ultracentrifugal fractions are examined at the same time; each sample thus serves as its own control to establish the relative migration of the lipoprotein bands. In normal plasma, the β-lipoprotein, pre-β lipoprotein, and α-lipoprotein bands are visible in unfractionated plasma. Only the pre-β band is present in the d $<$ 1.006 kg/L fraction, and the β-lipoprotein and α-lipoprotein bands are seen only in the d > 1.006 kg/L fraction. In addition, when Lp(a) is present in concentrations exceeding 20 to 30 mg/dL (i.e., when they contribute more than about 10 mg/dL to the LDL-cholesterol measurement), an additional band with pre-β mobility is also observed in the d > 1.006 kg/L fraction (hence the name sinking pre-β lipoprotein. Under such conditions, the physician may wish to request a quantitative Lp(a) measurement also. When present, β-VLDL is observed as a band with β-mobility in the d < 1.006 kg/L fraction (see Fig. 10–1*B*). Its presence is considered abnormal, and it is usually associated with dysbetalipoproteinemia (Type III hyperlipoproteinemia), although it is occasionally seen in other disorders as well. Chylomicrons, which are often seen in Type III hyperlipoproteinemia, remain at the origin on agarose gel.

VLDL-Cholesterol/Plasma Triglyceride Ratio. The ratio of VLDL-cholesterol to plasma triglycerides is also calculated. This ratio (mol/mol [mass/mass]) is generally in the range of 0.230 to 0.575 (0.1 to 0.25) in samples without β-VLDL, depending on the relative amounts of VLDL, LDL, and HDL present and on the errors inherent in the VLDL-cholesterol and plasma triglyceride measurements. Type III hyperlipoproteinemia subjects manifest ratios greater than 0.689 (0.3), usually in the range of 0.689 to 0.919 (0.3 to 0.4), although higher ratios can be observed. Again, because of the error in the measurements, the observation of a ratio of 0.689 (0.3) on a single occasion may or may not be significant. Overt Type III hyperlipoproteinemia patients manifest both β-VLDL and a VLDL-cholesterol/plasma triglyceride ratio of 0.689 (0.3) or greater.

Occasionally, a lipid disorder treatment clinic may request the assessment of apoE phenotype to supplement the diagnosis of Type III hyperlipoproteinemia (discussed later), because homozygosity for apoE-2 (discussed later) is associated with this disorder. This is not a routine chemical test, however, and is not required for the diagnosis.

Reliability of Lipid and Lipoprotein Measurements—NCEP Guidelines

Blood cholesterol concentrations were originally interpreted in terms of normal ranges defined from measured cholesterol levels in normal populations. It has long been appreciated that cardiovascular risk is a continuous function of cholesterol concentration, and that individuals in the upper normal range are at greater risk than those in the lower normal range. In 1988, the Adult Treatment Panel of the NCEP published guidelines for recognizing and treating hypercholesterolemia in adults; these guidelines were updated in 1993 (Expert Panel, 1988, 1993). They included a redefinition of cholesterol, LDL-cholesterol, and HDL-cholesterol levels in terms of cardiovascular risk (discussed later). Risk-based cut-off points for cholesterol, triglycerides, HDL-cholesterol, and LDL-cholesterol were established (Expert Panel, 1993) from studies in which the accuracy of the measurements approximates those made with reference methods. The Adult Treatment Panel recommendations thus require the adoption of a single set of cut-off points regardless of which laboratory or other facility makes the measurements.

Table 10–5. NCEP GUIDELINES FOR LIPID AND LIPOPROTEIN MEASUREMENT

Analyte	Total Error	Consistent with: *Bias*	*CV**
Cholesterol	≤ 9%	≤ 3%	≤ 3%
Triglyceride	≤ 15%	≤ 5%	≤ 5%
HDL-cholesterol	≤ 22%†	≤ 10%	≤ 6%‡
LDL-cholesterol	≤ 12%	≤ 4%	≤ 4%

*Coefficient of variation defined as standard deviation/mean × 100.

†To be reduced to ≤ 13% by 1998, providing analytical methods to achieve this are then available.

‡Precision criteria applied to HDL-cholesterol levels of 42 mg/dL (1.09 mmol/L) and higher. At lower levels, CV is not used; rather, standard deviation should not exceed 2.5 mg/dL (0.065 mmol/L).

The value of interpreting cholesterol levels in terms of risk rather than arbitrarily defined normal ranges is obvious, but the adoption of a single set of cut-off points by the entire medical community imposes on the laboratories the mandate to measure lipids and lipoproteins accurately. The Laboratory Standardization Panel of the NCEP released its recommendations for cholesterol measurement in the United States in 1990 (Laboratory Standardization Panel, 1990). Its report recommends that current cholesterol measurements be accurate to within 3% and that the reproducibility of the measurements, as measured by the CV, not exceed 3% (Table 10–5). The basis for accuracy is the CDC reference method for cholesterol, which has been validated with a definitive method that employs mass spectrometry. At present, most laboratories meet these criteria. Furthermore, the Panel made *no distinction* in the criteria to be applied to laboratory-based and non-laboratory-based measurements or to the kinds of equipment used to make the measurements. The combined cooperation of the laboratories, various government agencies, professional clinical chemistry organizations, and manufacturers of reagents, calibration and quality control materials, and instrumentation were required to attain these goals. There have been major efforts to standardize lipid and lipoprotein measurements and to define cardiovascular risk–based lipid and lipoprotein cut-off points that do not depend on local laboratory definitions of normal ranges. The usefulness of a single set of risk-based cut-off points for lipids and lipoproteins presupposes the ability to make the measurements accurately regardless of where or how they are made. This section summarizes current recommendations for reliability in lipid and lipoprotein measurements. These recommendations were developed by the NCEP Laboratory Standardization Panel (Cholesterol) and the NCEP Working Group on Lipoprotein Measurement (Triglycerides, HDL-cholesterol, LDL-cholesterol) after considering the medical requirements of accuracy and precision; the technology available for the measurements; various biologic, preanalytical, and analytical factors that can affect the measured values; and the resources available to improve the reliability of the measurements in the United States.

Triglycerides, HDL-Cholesterol, and LDL-Cholesterol

Recommendations for the measurement of triglycerides, HDL-cholesterol, and LDL-cholesterol were completed by the NCEP Working Group on Lipoprotein Measurement

(1995). The development of these recommendations was complicated by a number of considerations.

First, unlike cholesterol, none of these analytes has a unique chemical structure. The two classes of lipoproteins each consists of a population of similar molecules, the individual members of which differ somewhat in their size and composition, and the fatty acyl residues of triglyceride can vary somewhat according to diet and other factors. By virtue of these characteristics, there are no true reference methods for any of these components, and each must be defined functionally in terms of the methods used to analyze it.

Second, in the case of LDL, the clinical and epidemiologic database in which estimates of coronary risk are based was primarily established using either the combined ultracentrifugation-polyanion precipitation or the Friedewald methods described earlier. Furthermore, the HDL method used for this purpose was primarily the heparin-Mn^{2+} procedure.

Third, with either the combination method or the Friedewald equation, some non-LDL lipoproteins, primarily IDL and Lp(a), which are also atherogenic, are included in the measurement. Thus, the relationship between "LDL-cholesterol" and cardiovascular risk includes the contribution of these lipoproteins, and LDL-cholesterol measured with these methods actually represents the concentration of potentially atherogenic apoB-containing lipoproteins. Of course, LDL contributes most of the cholesterol to the measurement; in the general population, IDL and Lp(a) contribute only a few milligrams per deciliter each. It is well to keep in mind, however, that these lipoproteins can contribute considerably more cholesterol to the measurement when the measurements are made in some hyperlipidemic patients or in those with coronary artery disease. For example, an adult patient whose sample was analyzed in one of our laboratories (PSB) had an LDL-cholesterol level of about 160 mg/dL, which is in the high-risk range. This patient was found to have an Lp(a) concentration of 150 mg/dL, which would contribute about 45 mg/dL to the LDL-cholesterol measurement. When corrected for this contribution, the LDL-cholesterol value was actually in the desirable concentration range, and the apparently elevated LDL concentration was due to a high Lp(a) level.

It has been suggested that in order to estimate LDL-cholesterol more accurately, it is necessary to correct the value for the contribution of Lp(a) cholesterol (Kostner, 1981). As mentioned earlier, however, doing so could produce a less sensitive indicator of risk because the value would not include the contribution of one of the atherogenic particles. Nonetheless, as was just illustrated, Lp(a) measurements are helpful because they can clarify a potentially important contribution to the measured "LDL-cholesterol" value. In addition, because Lp(a) levels are not lowered by a number of treatments that effectively lower LDL levels, Lp(a) measurements can sometimes reveal why a particular patient may be less responsive to LDL-lowering therapy. The following relationship has been used to estimate the contribution of Lp(a) cholesterol to the measured LDL-cholesterol value (Kostner, 1981):

$$\text{Lp(a)-cholesterol} = 0.3 \times [\text{Lp(a) mass}] \qquad (10\text{-}17)$$

$$\text{LDL-cholesterol} = \text{total cholesterol} - [\text{HDL-cholesterol}] - \frac{\text{ETG3}}{5} - (0.3[\text{Lp(a) mass}])$$

where the values are given in milligrams per deciliter.

After considering these and a number of other factors, the NCEP Lipoprotein Measurement Working Group made the following recommendations. The measured values should be linked to the epidemiologic and clinical databases on which the association between lipoprotein level and cardiovascular risk were established. To achieve this, the measurements should be traceable to CDC reference methods (Myers, 1989), and in the absence of any true reference method for triglycerides or HDL-cholesterol, the basis for accuracy should be as defined by those methods. The working group also recommended the development of a standardization program for LDL-cholesterol based on the existing programs for total cholesterol, triglycerides, and HDL-cholesterol.

The specifications for reliable measurements were established after considering the current CDC lipid and lipoprotein standardization criteria, levels of performance that could reasonably be expected in competent laboratories using modern equipment, generally accepted criteria for the maximum contribution of analytical error to a useful medical test, and the current state of the art in lipoprotein measurement. These guidelines reaffirm the decision of the NCEP Laboratory Standardization Panel to recommend a single set of performance guidelines that does not distinguish laboratory-based from non–laboratory-based measurements.

NCEP guidelines for reliable lipid and lipoprotein measurement are shown in Table 10–5. This table requires some comment.

First, the NCEP Laboratory Standardization Panel recommendations for cholesterol used separate specifications for bias and precision (expressed in terms of CV) and noted that they were consistent with a total error of 8.9% or less (or approximately 9%). The NCEP Working Group on Lipoprotein Measurement recommendations are set in terms of a single value, total error, which considers both bias and imprecision at the same time. Total error can be calculated as follows:

$$\%\ \text{total error} = \%\ \text{bias} + 1.96\ (\%\text{CV}) \qquad (10\text{-}18)$$

The biases and CVs shown are considered examples of conditions that would satisfy the total error criteria and were included because laboratory performance has been traditionally expressed in this way and the terms are more familiar. The advantage of using a total error criterion, however, is more easily understood using an example that compares the two methods. Consider total cholesterol. For a laboratory to satisfy NCEP criteria for reliable cholesterol measurement, it would have to maintain a bias of 3% or less and a CV of 3% or less; both criteria would have to be met. A laboratory operating at these limits would have a total error of 8.9%. Another laboratory that had a bias of 3.5% and a CV of 2% would not meet NCEP criteria because the bias limit was exceeded. The total error in this case, however, would be only 7.5% (i.e., 3.5% + 1.96 × 2%). Using a total error criterion, both laboratories would satisfy the recommendations, and either bias or imprecision could exceed the specifications slightly, providing that the other was sufficiently small to maintain the total error within the guideline.

Second, the recommendations shown in Table 10–5 for HDL-cholesterol apply to levels of 42 mg/dL (1.09 mmol/L) and higher. Below this level, the absolute reproducibility of the cholesterol measurements themselves becomes limiting, and the recommendations call for the stan-

2

dard deviation of the measurements not to exceed 2.5 mg/dL (0.065 mmol/L).

Third, more rigorous guidelines for HDL-cholesterol measurement were suggested for adoption by 1998 *provided* that an HDL-cholesterol measurement method is then available to accomplish this. Those suggestions are for a total error not exceeding 13% at levels of 42 mg/dL (1.09 mmol/L) and higher, and standard deviation of 1.5 mg/dL or less (0.039 mmol/L). This level of performance was thought to be beyond the capability of currently used methods.

Apolipoprotein Analysis

Quantitation of apolipoproteins is now performed as a somewhat routine clinical procedure. A number of studies have indicated that apolipoproteins A-I and B are better discriminators of atherosclerotic disease than lipid or lipoprotein determinations (Albers, 1989a; Bachorik, 1988). In general, the evidence for this has been more consistent for apoB than for apoA-I, but the reason for this is not clear. Most of the quantitation methods are based on immunologic identification of the apolipoproteins. Immunoreactivity must then be related to mass, determined by other means. Simple chemical determination of total protein in a particular lipoprotein fraction is not very useful, because even carefully separated lipoprotein fractions contain more than one apolipoprotein, and the chemical determination will not discriminate between the various determinants. ApoB can be determined chemically in a "narrow" cut of LDL (d 1.030 to 1.050 kg/L) because LDL does not contain significant amounts of other apolipoproteins in this density range. ApoA-I measurements are ultimately based on standards of purified apoA-I. These procedures were used to develop the currently available World Health Organization/International Federation for Clinical Chemistry (WHO-IFCC) First International Reference Materials for Apolipoproteins A-I and B.

Apolipoprotein Immunoassays. These determinations are based on recognition of the apolipoprotein antigen by an antibody or a group of antibodies against one or more of the antigenic sites on the molecule. Automation of immunoassays generally uses nonisotopic labels (e.g., enzyme, fluorescence, and chemiluminescence). A number of different kinds of immunoassays have been used, and the advantages and disadvantages of each have been discussed by Stein (1994).

Radioimmunoassay (RIA). Sensitive RIAs have been described for measurement of apoA-I (Schonfeld, 1974), apoA-II (Schonfeld, 1977), apoB (Albers, 1975), apoC-II and apoC-III (Schonfeld, 1979), apoE (Falko, 1980), and Lp(a) (Albers, 1977). RIA is a competition assay. In this procedure, conditions are first selected in which the radioiodinated antigen is approximately 50% precipitated by the specific antibody. These conditions are arbitrarily assigned a value of "100% precipitation" when unlabeled antigen (in standards or samples) is not present. When added, the unlabeled antigen competes with the radiolabeled apolipoprotein for the antibody, and the degree of competition is a measure of the concentration of the unlabeled antigen. Standard curves that use varying amounts of unlabeled antigen are then used to calculate the concentration of apolipoprotein in the samples being measured. The advantages of this technique are its sensitivity and its need for only small amounts of antibody. Furthermore, the method can be automated. However, RIAs require special and expensive equipment and create radioactive waste. Radiolabeling may also damage the antigen, shorten its shelf-life, and cause the labeled standard to react differently from the apolipoprotein in the unlabeled standard or the clinical specimen.

Radial Immunodiffusion (RID). This is a relatively simple method in which an antigen is allowed to diffuse from a well into the surrounding gel (usually agarose), which contains an antibody to it, and thus forms a disk of precipitation. The area of the disk is proportional to the amount of antigen in the sample. RID does not require complicated and expensive equipment; however, it is not amenable to automation and thus cannot be performed on a very large scale. Because the procedure is manual, it can be less precise than automated assays. It also requires one to three days to reach completion and uses large amounts of antibody. Another problem that limits the usefulness of this method is the size-related diffusion differences between the various particles containing the antigen. RID for apoB, for instance, may be accurate for measurement of LDL apoB, but it may underestimate VLDL apoB and thus be inaccurate for lipemic samples as a result of slow and incomplete diffusion of the large VLDL particles by the time the readings are made. Although this characteristic of RID can produce a systematic underestimate of apoB when the aim is to measure the total concentration of this apolipoprotein in serum or plasma, it can be useful in principle when the aim is to estimate apoB concentrations in LDL, because the method has a degree of selectivity for smaller apoB-containing particles (Sniderman, 1980).

Electroimmunoassay. This is a rather simple and relatively accurate method based on principles similar to those for the RID, except that the samples are subject to electrophoresis and the areas of precipitation are in the form of "rockets" rather than disks. Most of the advantages and disadvantages of RID also apply to this method. Electrophoresis improves the movement of large particles into the gel, but it also has its own inherent problems. Electroimmunoassays have been described for most of the A (Curry, 1976a), B (Curry, 1978), C (Curry, 1980, 1981), D (Curry, 1977), and E (Curry, 1976b) apolipoproteins.

Immunonephelometry. This method is based on measurement of the turbidity caused by the apolipoprotein-antibody complex (Lopes-Virella, 1980). Either the final amount of turbidity that forms after the antigen-antibody reaction reaches completion (end-point assay) or the rate of antigen-antibody complex formation (rate assay) can be measured. A major advantage of these methods is that they are readily automated and can provide results within a few minutes compared with hours or days with other methods. Nephelometry can be subdivided into immunoturbidmetric methods (ITA) and immunonephelometric methods (INA). In both, a small aliquot (i.e., 20 μL) of sample is appropriately diluted, mixed with antibody to the apolipoprotein of interest, and incubated for an appropriate period. The primary distinction between ITA and INA is in the instrumentation used to measure sample turbidity. In ITA, a beam of light (840 nm) impinges on the reaction mixture, and the reduction in transmitted light is measured and converted to units of concentration using standards of known concentration. ITA methods can be performed using a spectrophotometer or an automated clinical chemistry analyzer used for spectrophotometric assays. In INA methods, light that has been scattered by the antigen-antibody complex is detected and converted to units of concentration, again through the use of standards of known concentrations. INA methods require the use of a nephelometer; automated INA methods for apoA-I and apoB are now available from several manufacturers, such as Beckmann Instruments (Palo Alto, CA) and Behring Diagnostics (Somerville, NJ). One potential limitation of the ITA and INA methods stems from the inherent turbidity of lipemic samples or even nonlipemic samples subjected to repeated freezing and thawing. The automated systems described can, within useful limits, correct for such sample-caused or lipoprotein-caused turbidity. Bachorik (1994b) has described the use of rate INA for measuring apoA-I and apoB distributions in a large sample of the noninstitutionalized U.S. population. The measurements were made in the Third National Health and Nutrition Examination Survey (NHANES III) and are traceable to the WHO-IFCC international reference materials for apoA-I and apoB.

Enzyme-Linked and Fluorescence Immunoassays. Enzyme-linked immunosorbent assays (ELISA) and fluorescence immunoassays have been developed for apolipoprotein analysis (Fruchart, 1978) and are useful for clinical application. They, like RIA, are competitive binding assays but they do not require radiolabeled reagents. The assay is commonly performed by first coating a series of reaction tubes or titer plates with monospecific or monoclonal antibodies to the apolipoprotein of interest. The standards or samples are then added and incubated for some period, during which the "capture antibody" binds the antigen. The amount of antigen bound is a function of the antigen concentration. The reaction mixture is then removed, the plate is washed extensively to remove unbound antigen, and a second, "detection antibody" is added. The detection antibody, which is also specific for the bound apolipoprotein, is first conjugated with an enzyme such as peroxidase or alkaline phosphatase or with a fluorescent label. The amount of bound detection antibody depends on the amount of bound antigen. After the second incubation, the excess detection antibody is removed, the plate is washed extensively, and the amount of bound detection antibody is quantitated by measuring the activity of the conjugated enzyme or the fluorescence of the conjugated label. Again, the standard curves are constructed using solutions containing known concentrations of the antigen. In another variation, the sample or standard solution is incubated with antibody in a tube that has been precoated with the antigen. The amount of antibody in the solution available for binding to the precoated-tube antigen depends on the sample antigen concentration. The higher the sample antigen concentration, the more antibody is bound, and the less of it is left to react with the precoated antigen on the tube. The tube-bound antibody is then reacted with a second antibody that reacts with the first antibody. The second antibody, which has been previously labeled, is measured by quantitating the label as described earlier. The assays are as sensitive as RIA; are amenable to automation, usually using well-characterized antibodies; and lack some of the problems inherent in the use of radiolabeled reagents. Several investigators have developed ELISA methods for apoB that use monoclonal capture antibodies to apoB (Albers, 1989b; Young, 1986b). Such methods distinguish between apoB-48 and apoB-100 through the use of at least two antibodies, one that detects only apoB-100 and one that detects both apoB-48 and apoB-100. ELISA has also been widely used to measure Lp(a) using monoclonal capture antibodies that recognize the multiple polyforms of apo(a) and polyclonal detection antibodies.

Problems with Apolipoprotein Immunoassays. At present, there is no standard reference method for apolipoprotein analysis. One problem, particularly for apolipoproteins such as apoB that are present in more than one lipoprotein fraction, is that their immunoreactivity can differ in different lipoprotein fractions. Thus, purified LDL, which is currently used as the basis for assigning values to standards and quality control pools, is most satisfactorily applied to measuring apoB concentrations in similarly isolated LDL preparations but may not be the appropriate standard for VLDL-apoB measurement. This can affect the measurement of the total plasma apolipoprotein concentrations. Various approaches have been used to circumvent this problem, such as pretreating samples with lipase or detergents in an effort to render all apoB-containing particles equally immunoreactive. A more recent approach has been to develop mixtures of monoclonal antibodies that are specific for apolipoprotein epitopes that are expressed in all lipoprotein classes. Such a method has been suggested as a candidate reference method for apoB (Albers, 1989b) and appears to detect apoB equally well in the various lipoprotein classes.

Apolipoprotein Standardization

Some of the issues that complicate the development of guidelines for reliable lipoprotein measurement also apply to apolipoproteins. The location of apoA-I and apoB in several lipoprotein subfractions, differential abilities to detect the apolipoproteins in different fractions, the lack of true reference methods for either apolipoprotein, uncertainties related to the assignment of values to calibration materials, and other factors have made it difficult to measure the two apolipoproteins reliably or to compare results obtained in different studies using different or, for that matter, even similar methods. These problems led to a cooperative effort by a number of groups, including the CDC, WHO, IFCC, manufacturers of instrumentation and diagnostic materials, academic investigators, and others, to understand and define the nature of the problem and to develop materials and procedures that will lead to standardized apolipoprotein measurement methods. Such efforts have been discussed (Bachorik, 1994; Marcovina, 1990, 1991; Stein, 1994). Although not all these problems have been resolved, the development of the WHO-IFCC First International Reference Materials for Apolipoproteins A-I and B represents an important advance. These materials are intended for use as calibrators to allow manufacturers a common basis for assigning values to calibration and quality control materials supplied for use with different methods. The values assigned to the WHO-IFCC reference materials are based on the use of highly purified preparations of apoA-I and narrow-cut LDL used as primary standards. Values were assigned to these "primary standards" using a well-defined version (Henderson, 1990) of the chemical method of Lowry (1952).

Work continues to develop reference methods and a standardization program for apoA-I and apoB comparable with the CDC standardization programs for cholesterol, triglycerides, and HDL-cholesterol. Nonetheless, the availability of internationally agreed-on reference materials for the two apolipoproteins will increase the reliability of the measurements with different methods and the comparability of values determined in different laboratories.

Qualitative Apolipoprotein Analysis. Several qualitative analyses of apolipoproteins may supply important information to the researcher or the clinician. A simple immunodiffusion technique can determine the presence or absence of a given apolipoprotein. This can be useful in evaluating certain lipoprotein disorders in which a particular apolipoprotein may not be present in the circulation (e.g., Tangier disease, abetalipoproteinemia, apoC-II deficiency). Gel electrophoresis techniques (in polyacrylamide, agarose, or other media), which separate apolipoproteins by molecular weight; isoelectric focusing, which separates them by charge; and especially the combination of the two in a bidimensional system have considerably improved our understanding of dysbetalipoproteinemia and some of the lipoprotein-deficiency states (Utermann, 1975; Zannis, 1980, 1981). (For detailed description, see the later section on dysbetalipoproteinemia [Type III hyperlipoproteinemia].) Application of these techniques is sometimes clinically important.

FACTORS AFFECTING VARIATION OF PLASMA LIPID AND LIPOPROTEIN CONCENTRATIONS IN INDIVIDUALS AND IN POPULATIONS

Plasma lipid and lipoprotein concentrations vary within and among populations and under different conditions within a given individual. Technical factors may also account for variation in values obtained in measurement. Such variability poses problems for the selection of cut-off points for the diagnosis and treatment of hyperlipidemia. Thus, the selection of a cholesterol level of 6.234 mmol/L (240 mg/dL) to identify high blood cholesterol by the Expert Panel on Detection, Evaluation, and Treatment of High Blood Cholesterol in Adults (1988) was partly based on its defining the upper quartile of the U.S. adult cholesterol distribution. Use of this cut-off point in other populations in which cholesterol distributions differ would lead to a greater or lesser proportion of individuals being so defined.

In considering various influences on an individual's cholesterol level, the NCEP Laboratory Standardization Panel (1990) and the Working Group on Lipoprotein Measurement (1995) described *factors that contribute to the patient's usual lipid and lipoprotein levels.* These factors include age, sex, and body weight; behavioral factors such as diet, alcohol use, and exercise; genetic factors such as primary dyslipoproteinemia; and chronic disorders such as hypothyroidism, obstructive liver disease, or kidney disease.

Cholesterol concentrations rise with age from early adulthood in both sexes. Females have lower levels than males except in childhood and after the early fifties. The variation with age is why the NCEP recommended that cholesterol screening be repeated every five years. Cholesterol varies slightly with the season in that cholesterol levels are higher in the winter (Gordon, 1987).

The dietary intake of saturated fat and cholesterol are important influences on plasma cholesterol levels, the effects taking one to two weeks to become apparent. To ascertain a person's usual cholesterol level, it is important that he or she be on his or her usual diet for two weeks or so before the measurement and is neither gaining nor losing weight.

Several medications can alter lipid levels. Some of these are used by a high proportion of the population, including oral contraceptives, postmenopausal estrogens, and various antihypertensive drugs. The main disorders that can lead to secondary dyslipoproteinemia, such as thyroid, hepatic, and kidney disease, are usually readily detectable. Subsequent management of the hyperlipidemia is predominantly a function of treatment of the underlying disorder.

The NCEP Laboratory Standardization Panel (1990) and the Working Group on Lipoprotein Measurement (1995) also identified *factors that alter the patient's usual cholesterol level.* These include fasting, posture, venous occlusion, anticoagulants, recent myocardial infarction, stroke, cardiac catheterization, trauma, acute infection, and pregnancy. Total cholesterol and HDL-cholesterol levels can be measured in nonfasting individuals, greatly facilitating screening and monitoring, although nonfasting HDL-cholesterol levels can be a few milligrams per deciliter lower than fasting levels. This would not lead to misclassification of patients with low HDL levels, however. It is only when triglycerides and LDL-cholesterol are also being measured that fasting becomes a requirement, because a recent fatty meal results in the appearance of triglyceride-rich chylomicrons in the plasma and in compositional changes in LDL. Both factors lead to the underestimation of LDL-cholesterol and can result in the misclassification of truly affected patients.

As discussed earlier, posture significantly influences the plasma lipid and lipoprotein level. Blood should be drawn only after the patient has been sitting quietly for about five minutes. It is important to avoid prolonged venous occlusion before venipuncture, because it can lead to hemoconcentration and cholesterol increases of 10% to 15%. The effects of various anticoagulants have already been discussed.

The association of hospitalization for recent myocardial infarction, stroke, and cardiac catheterization with falls in cholesterol and LDL-cholesterol levels has been well documented. Increased VLDL levels have also been observed after a myocardial infarction. Depressions in cholesterol levels have also been observed after trauma, and acute bacterial and viral infection leads to transiently altered cholesterol and HDL-cholesterol levels. Lipoprotein measurements should be made no sooner than eight weeks after any form of trauma or acute bacterial or viral infection. Pregnancy consistently raises cholesterol levels, and measurements should be deferred until three to four months after delivery.

NCEP Guidelines

Adults

Guidelines for the Detection, Evaluation and Treatment of High Blood Cholesterol in Adults have been developed by an

Table 10–6. INITIAL CLASSIFICATION OF ADULTS BASED ON TOTAL CHOLESTEROL AND HDL-CHOLESTEROL

Total Cholesterol	
Desirable blood cholesterol	<200 mg/dL
Borderline-high blood cholesterol	200–239 mg/dL
High blood cholesterol	≥240 mg/dL
HDL-Cholesterol	
Low HDL-cholesterol	<35 mg/dL

Expert Panel of the National Cholesterol Education Program and have been widely promulgated (NCEP Summary, 1993). They identify LDL-cholesterol as the primary target of cholesterol-lowering therapy. To this end, serum cholesterol levels should be measured in all adults 20 years of age and older at least once every five years; HDL-cholesterol should be measured at the same time if accurate results are available. As mentioned earlier, these measurements may be made in the nonfasting state. Although screening programs specifically intended to invite the public to receive the tests can be used, the preferred approach is case-finding by using the opportunity to perform a total cholesterol (and HDL-cholesterol [HDL-C]) test in the setting of a medical examination that also assesses other coronary heart disease (CHD) risk factors. In individuals free of CHD, total cholesterol levels below 200 mg/dL are classified as desirable blood cholesterol, those of 200 to 239 mg/dL as borderline-high blood cholesterol, and those of 240 mg/dL and above as high blood cholesterol (Table 10–6).

In individuals with desirable cholesterol levels, the HDL-cholesterol level determines the appropriate follow-up; those with an HDL-cholesterol level of less than 35 mg/dL should proceed to lipoprotein analyses. Patients with borderline levels should also proceed to lipoprotein analyses if they have an HDL-cholesterol level below 35 mg/dL or at least two other risk factors for CHD. Lipoprotein analyses are also required for those with high cholesterol levels. It includes measurement of fasting levels of total cholesterol, total triglyceride, and HDL-cholesterol. LDL-cholesterol is then calculated

$$\text{LDL-cholesterol} = \text{total cholesterol} - \text{HDL-cholesterol} - \frac{\text{triglyceride}}{5} \quad (10\text{-}19)$$

where the concentrations are expressed in milligrams per deciliter. The limitations of using this equation have been discussed.

Levels of LDL-cholesterol are classified as "high risk" when above 160 mg/dL, as "borderline" when in the range of 130 to 159 mg/dL, and as "desirable" when below 100 mg/dL (Table 10–7).

The approach to patients with a history of CHD is based on different criteria because, at a given level of cholesterol, their risk of a new event is much greater than for those without such a history. For these patients, a lipoprotein analysis should be done at the onset of their evaluation. The "optimal" level of LDL-cholesterol is below 100 mg/dL in this important group; a level above this is considered "suboptimal." Although the LDL-cholesterol level is important in assessing patients with or without CHD, the decision of whether and how to treat also is based on whether there is prior CHD, whether other risk factors are present (Table 10–8), and general clinical assessment.

Hypertriglyceridemia. The NIH Consensus Conference on Hypertriglyceridemia (1984) recommended that triglyceride values about 5.650 mmol/L (500 mg/dL) be considered abnormally high and that values below 2.825 mmol/L (250 mg/dL) be regarded as generally normal. The Consensus Conference suggested that persons with fasting plasma triglyceride levels between 2.825 and 5.650 mmol/L (250 and 500 mg/dL) presented a different problem because, in the aggregate, such levels are associated with an approximate twofold excess of cardiovascular disease. These are the cases with higher cholesterol (e.g., Type IIB—conditions associated with the presence or elevated levels of remnants and IDL). In an individual patient, these triglyceride levels may be normal or a marker for increased risk. If confirmed by repeated measurement, they warrant further investigation in the patient who has a family history of premature cardiovascular disease or other heart disease risk factors such as high cholesterol levels, hypertension, cigarette smoking, obesity, or a secondary cause for elevated triglycerides. Some of these persons will be found to have dyslipoproteinemia; others will ultimately be considered normal.

Although there are many links between high triglyceride levels and CHD, our understanding of the risk relationships is poor, so that reducing triglyceride levels to prevent CHD has not been generally advocated and is much less important than reducing LDL-cholesterol levels. The NCEP Adult Treatment Panel II report (NCEP Summary, 1993) classified triglyceride levels below 200 mg/dL as normal, levels of

Table 10–7. TREATMENT DECISIONS BASED ON LDL-CHOLESTEROL

Diet Therapy		
	Initiation Level	***LDL Goal***
Without CHD and with fewer than two risk factors	≥ 160 mg/dL	< 160 mg/dL
Without CHD and with two or more risk factors	≥130 mg/dL	< 130 mg/dL
With CHD	> 100 mg/dL	≤ 100 mg/dL
Drug Treatment		
	Consideration Level	***LDL Goal***
Without CHD and with fewer than two risk factors	≥ 190 mg/dL	< 160 mg/dL
Without CHD and with two or more risk factors	≥ 160 mg/dL	< 130 mg/dL
With CHD	≥ 130 mg/dL	≤ 100 mg/dL

CHD, coronary heart disease.

Table 10–8. RISK STATUS BASED ON PRESENCE OF CHD RISK FACTORS OTHER THAN LDL-CHOLESTEROL

Positive Risk Factors

- Age:
  - Male: ≥ 45 years
  - Female: ≥ 55 years or premature menopause without estrogen replacement therapy
- Family history of premature CHD (definite myocardial infarction or sudden death before 55 years of age in father or other male first-degree relative or before 65 years of age in mother or other female first-degree relative)
- Current cigarette smoking
- Hypertension (≥ 140/90 mmHg or on antihypertensive medication)
- Low HDL-cholesterol (> 35 mg/dL)
- Diabetes mellitus

Negative Risk Factor

- High HDL-cholesterol (≥ 60 mg/dL)

200 to 400 mg/dL as borderline high, levels of 400 to 1000 mg/dL as high, and levels above 1000 mg/dL as very high.

Children

Guidelines for approaching children and adolescents have also been developed by the NCEP (NCEP Expert Panel on Children and Adolescents, 1993). They recommend selective screening, in the context of health care, of children and adolescents who have a family history of premature cardiovascular disease or at least one parent with high blood cholesterol. The classification of these children by their total and LDL-cholesterol levels is given in Table 10–9. For young people being tested because they have at least one parent with high blood cholesterol, the initial measurement should be of total cholesterol. A level above 200 mg/dL is "high" and should lead to a lipoprotein analysis. A total cholesterol level of 170 to 199 mg/dL is "borderline" and should lead to a repeat measurement. If the average is borderline or high, a lipoprotein analysis is warranted. For young people being tested because of a history of premature cardiovascular disease in a parent or a grandparent, the initial test should be a lipoprotein analysis, because a high proportion of these children have some lipoprotein abnormality.

In both cases, once a lipoprotein analysis has been obtained, it should be repeated to determine the average LDL-cholesterol level, which will determine the recommended steps for risk assessment and treatment. The LDL-cholesterol level is acceptable if it is under 110 mg/dL, borderline if it is 110 to 129 mg/dL, and high if it is 130 mg/dL or above.

Table 10–9. CLASSIFICATION OF TOTAL AND LDL-CHOLESTEROL LEVELS IN CHILDREN AND ADOLESCENTS FROM FAMILIES WITH HYPERCHOLESTEROLEMIA OR PREMATURE CARDIOVASCULAR DISEASE

Category	Total Cholesterol (mg/dL)	LDL-Cholesterol (mg/dL)
Acceptable	< 170	< 110
Borderline	170–199	110–129
High	≥ 200	≥ 130

LIPIDS, LIPOPROTEINS, AND DISEASE

Lipoproteins and their lipids, especially cholesterol, are measured primarily because of their association with atherosclerotic cardiovascular disease. Furthermore, altering lipid and lipoprotein levels by dietary and drug intervention can dramatically alter cardiovascular disease.

Today, the question is when and what to measure and how to treat the hyperlipidemic patient. This has led to the publication of guidelines on the diagnosis and treatment of blood cholesterol disorders (NCEP Summary, 1993), as well as specific recommendations for improved laboratory lipid and lipoprotein measurements as discussed.

The plasma levels of lipids, apolipoproteins, and lipoproteins vary considerably and reflect the expression of exogenous (diet, medication, and hormones) and endogenous (genetic and metabolic) factors. Lipoprotein disorders were for a number of years classified into the six major types as suggested by Fredrickson (1967). As our understanding of the biochemical and genetic bases of the various lipoprotein disorders has increased, the focus has changed to consideration of the underlying biochemical lesions responsible for these disorders, and the Fredrickson classification system is less widely used. The six lipoprotein phenotypes are still useful, however, as a convenient way of referring to the patterns of lipoprotein elevations seen in patients with hyperlipoproteinemia. These patterns are summarized in Table 10–10.

Although the biochemical and genetic bases for the inherited disorders of lipid and lipoprotein metabolism differ considerably (Breslow, 1989), one can gain significant insight into the basis for their dietary and drug treatment by understanding the pathophysiology of these genetic defects. Their clinical complications generally include premature atherosclerosis and deposition of lipid in various tissues (Table 10–11). In patients with marked hypertriglyceridemia, pancreatitis can be a problem (see Table 10–11).

The inherited disorders of lipid and lipoprotein metabolism may be classified into four major categories: (1) those in the exogenous lipoprotein pathway, (2) those in the endogenous lipoprotein pathway, (3) those in both of these pathways, and (4) those in the reverse cholesterol transport pathway (see Table 10–11).

Table 10–10. BLOOD LIPOPROTEIN PATTERNS IN PATIENTS WITH HYPERLIPOPROTEINEMIA

Type	Lipoprotein Pattern*
I	Extremely elevated TG due to presence of chylomicrons
IIa	Elevated LDL
IIb	Elevated LDL and VLDL
III	Elevated cholesterol, TG; presence of β-VLDL; VLDL-cholesterol/plasma TG ratio > 0.3
IV	Elevated VLDL
V	Elevated VLDL and presence of chylomicrons

*Patterns observed in plasma obtained after a 12-hour fasting period.

Table 10–11. DISORDERS OF LIPID AND LIPOPROTEIN METABOLISM

	Lipoprotein Phenotype	Premature CAD	Xanthomas	Pancreatitis
I. Disorders in exogenous lipoprotein pathway				
A. Defective or absent lipoprotein lipase	I	No	Eruptive	Yes
B. Deficiency of apolipoprotein C-II	I or V	No	Eruptive	Yes
II. Disorders of endogenous lipoprotein pathway				
A. Familial combined hyperlipidemia	IIa, IIIB, IV (rarely V)	Yes	Isolated xanthelasma	Rarely
1. Hyperapobetalipoproteinemia	N, IV	Yes	Isolated xanthelasma	No
B. Familial hypertriglyceridemia	IV (occasionally V)	Can occur	No (occasionally eruptive)	Occasionally
C. Familial hypercholesterolemia	IIa (occasionally IIb)	Yes	Tendon, tuberous	No
D. Familial defective, apoB-100	N, IIa	Yes	Occasionally tendon	No
III. Disorders of both exogenous and endogenous lipoprotein pathway				
A. Type V hyperlipoproteinemia	V	Can occur	Eruptive	Yes
B. Dysbetalipoproteinemia (Type III hyperlipoproteinemia)	III	Yes	Yes	No
C. Deficiencies of apoB-containing lipoproteins				
1. Abetalipoproteinemia	Hypobeta or abeta	No	No	No
2. Hypobetalipoproteinemia	Hypobeta	Decreased	No	No
IV. Disorders of reverse cholesterol transport pathway				
A. Decreased synthesis of HDL (apolipoprotein A-I)	Hypo α	Yes	Planar	No
B. Increased catabolism of HDL				
1. Apolipoprotein A-I variants	Hypo α	No	No	No
2. Tangier disease	Hypo α	Can occur	No	No
C. Lecithin cholesterol acyltransferase (LCAT) deficiency	Hypo α	Can occur	No	No
D. Cholesterol ester transferase protein (CETP) deficiency	Hyper	Decreased	No	No

N = Normal.

2

Disorders of the Exogenous Lipoprotein Pathway

The term exogenous lipoprotein pathway refers to the metabolism of intestinal lipoproteins, primarily those formed in response to dietary fat (i.e., chylomicrons).

Genetic defects in either lipoprotein lipase (LPL) or apoC-II can lead to significant hyperchylomicronemia and hypertriglyceridemia (Brunzell, 1989).

Defective or Missing LPL. This genetic condition is ordinarily accompanied by massive increases in chylomicrons with marked hypertriglyceridemia (as high as 10,000 mg/dL). The marked chylomicronemia, indicative of an inability to clear dietary fat, is manifested by a thick creamy layer over a clear infranate in a tube of plasma left to stand overnight at 4°C (Type I pattern). Hypercholesterolemia is normally present, but the ratio of triglyceride to cholesterol is usually 10 or higher. VLDL-cholesterol is normal, but HDL-cholesterol and LDL-cholesterol levels are low. In individuals with functional LPL, the intravenous injection of heparin releases membrane-bound LPL into the bloodstream (this is called the post-heparin lipolytic activity test, or PHLA test). PHLA is absent from the plasma of affected patients (and also from adipose tissue when tested). The cofactor for LPL, apoC-II, is present in normal concentrations, however.

This pediatric disorder ordinarily presents before the age of 10 years. Abdominal pain is usually the initial symptom, presenting as colic in the first year of life or as an acute abdominal condition later in childhood. Other clinical features may include eruptive xanthomas, hepatosplenomegaly, and lipemia retinalis. The absence of atherosclerosis in LPL deficiencies suggests that chylomicrons, unlike chylomicron remnants, are not atherogenic.

This disorder is rare and is due to the homozygous state for a mutant allele. The human *LPL* gene is approximately 30 kb in length and consists of 10 exons interrupted by nine introns. Missense mutations typically predominate in the *LPL* gene, with a preferential location in exons 3, 4, and 5; mutations have been described in the catalytic triad, Asp_{158}, His_{241}, and Ser_{132} (Brunzell, 1989). Once the mutation has been elucidated in the affected proband, the DNA from the members of these rare families can be screened for a similar mutation. Parents or siblings who are obligate heterozygous carriers for the defect in the *LPL* gene can have mild dyslipidemia, which can present as hypercholesterolemia alone, hypertriglyceridemia alone, or both lipids elevated; an isolated low HDL-cholesterol level has also been described. The pleiotropic presentation in obligate heterozygous carriers for LPL deficiency led to the hypothesis that such patients may reflect a subset of familial combined hyperlipidemia (FCHL) (Kwiterovich, 1993a).

Deficiency of ApoC-II. When apoC-II (the cofactor for LPL) is deficient, hypertriglyceridemia can vary from 800 to almost 10,000 mg/dL. A massive increase of chylomicrons alone may occur or can also be accompanied by an increase in VLDL (see later). Cholesterol levels range from approximately 150 to 1000 mg/dL. LDL-cholesterol and HDL-cholesterol levels are below the fifth percentile for normal individuals. PHLA activity is absent or very low. However, addition of apoC-II to plasma of these patients *in vitro* or by blood or plasma transfusion *in vivo* allows normal PHLA activity. ApoC-II levels, when measured immunochemically, are present in only trace amounts. The problem usually presents in adulthood with pancreatitis, although one patient developed pancreatitis as early as age six.

The disorder is rare and inherited as an autosomal recessive trait. A number of abnormalities in APOC-II have been described. They are usually caused by either small deletions or a splice site mutation (Breslow, 1989; Brunzell, 1989).

Disorders of the Endogenous Lipoprotein Pathway

The endogenous lipoprotein pathway refers to lipoproteins and apolipoproteins that are synthesized in tissues other than the intestine, predominantly in the liver.

Genetic defects have been described at various points along the VLDL-endogenous lipoprotein pathway, IDL-endogenous lipoprotein pathway, and LDL-endogenous lipoprotein pathway. Such defects are primarily related to (1) increased hepatic production of apoB-100, leading to a group of closely related syndromes of VLDL apoB overproduction, (2) increased synthesis of VLDL triglyceride without a concomitant increase in apoB production, leading to the secretion of a triglyceride-enriched VLDL, or (3) catabolic defects in the removal of LDL, either through the defect in the LDL receptor itself or a defect in the ligand for the LDL receptor, namely, apoB-100.

Familial Combined Hyperlipidemia (FCHL). One of the first disorders of VLDL apoB overproduction was described in families of survivors of premature myocardial infarction (Kwiterovich, 1993a). Overproduction of apolipoprotein B and VLDL lead to the overproduction of VLDL remnants, IDL and LDL (Kane and Havel, 1989). Depending on the activity of LPL, the patient may present with an elevated level of VLDL alone (Type IV lipoprotein phenotype), an elevated level of LDL alone (Type IIa lipoprotein phenotype), or an elevated level of both VLDL and LDL (Type IIb lipoprotein phenotype). Tendon and tuberous xanthomas are *not* part of the clinical presentation of FCHL, although corneal arcus, vertical ear creases, and isolated xanthelasma can be. This disorder is probably inherited as an autosomal dominant trait, and ordinarily the diagnosis is made by finding at least one first-degree relative who has a lipoprotein phenotype distinctly different from the proband. Expression of the disorder is delayed, but it is not unusual to see FCHL, or one of its metabolic variants, presenting in children and adolescents from families with premature CHD (Cortner, 1990).

Other variants of FCHL, which are also characterized by the presence of small, dense LDL particles, include hyperapobetalipoproteinemia (hyperapoB), LDL subclass pattern B, familial dyslipidemic hypertension, and syndrome X (Kwiterovich, 1993a). In addition to small, dense LDL particles, these syndromes tend to share other characteristics, such as hyperinsulinism, glucose intolerance (and adult-onset diabetes mellitus), hypertension, and low levels of HDL, particularly when hypertriglyceridemia is part of the phenotype.

The genetic defects underlying FCHL are not known, but FCHL is undoubtedly genetically heterogeneous. A number of candidate genes for FCHL and its related syndromes have been proposed. These include defects in the regulatory or structural portion of the *APOB* gene (although evidence from three laboratories indicates that a defect in this gene is highly unlikely as a common etiology of FCHL); the *trans* DNA-binding protein for *APOB*; heterozygous carriers for a defect in the *LPL* gene (although recent data indicate that this is unlikely to be a common cause of FCHL); the *APOA*-I/C-III/A-IV gene complex (e.g., increased levels of apoC-III may inhibit lipolysis, or a defect in apoA-IV may interfere with its proposed role in facilitating the transfer of apoC-II to chylomicrons); the *ATHS* gene on chromosome 19; the insulin receptor gene; the gene for the putative basic protein receptor; and mutations in the genes for several basic serum proteins that play a role in cellular lipid acylation (Kwiterovich, 1993a).

Several laboratories have shown evidence that there is a cellular defect in cultured fibroblasts from patients with hyperapo-B to the normal response to serum basic proteins I and II on the production of cellular triglyceride and cholesteryl esters, respectively (Kwiterovich, 1993a).

Overproduction of Triglyceride-Enriched VLDL. In some patients with endogenous hypertriglyceridemia, hepatic triglycerides are oversynthesized, but apoB is not, leading to the secretion of triglyceride-enriched VLDL (Kane, 1989). Such patients usually present with hypertriglyceridemia and low levels of LDL-cholesterol and HDL-cholesterol. The disorder is believed to be due to the inability of LPL to hydrolyze normally such large, triglyceride-enriched VLDL. In contrast with FCHL, such patients and their affected family relatives do not have elevations in LDL, and treatment of such familial hypertriglyceridemic patients (FHTs) with diet, weight loss, and medication will *not* produce a "flip-flop pattern" with a conversion from a Type IV to a Type IIa or Type IIb pattern (see Table 10–11), as can occur in FCHL. CAD appears less prevalent in such patients, compared with patients with Type IV lipoprotein patterns from FCHL families in whom the Type IV pattern is often accompanied by above-average levels of LDL-cholesterol and significant elevations in LDL apoB. In families in whom FHT breeds true, the adults often have glucose intolerance, obesity, hyperuricemia, and peripheral vascular disease. This disorder is probably inherited as an autosomal dominant trait with reduced penetrance in that the phenotype is expressed in only one of five children under the age of 20 years born to an affected parent.

Familial Hypercholesterolemia. Familial hypercholesterolemia (FH) is an autosomal dominantly inherited condition that has a gene-dosage effect (Hobbs, 1992). FH heterozygotes have plasma concentrations of total and LDL-cholesterol that are elevated two to three times above normal; FH homozygotes have levels that are elevated by five to six times. FH is completely expressed at birth and early in childhood, and the frequency of FH heterozygotes is about 1 in 500 (Kwiterovich, 1993b). The triglyceride and HDL-cholesterol levels are often normal in FH heterozygotes, but persons with FH can have modest hypertriglyceridemia and a lower HDL-cholesterol level.

The heterozygous FH child is clinically asymptomatic in the first decade of life; 10% to 15% of these children develop tendon xanthomas during the second decade of life, most commonly in the Achilles tendon and extensor tendons of the hands (Kwiterovich, 1993b). However, children with heterozygous FH manifest endothelial cell dysfunction in the first decade of life (Celemajer, 1992). CAD is present in about 20% of males by age 40 and in 50% by age 50; such early CAD is delayed 10 years in females with heterozygous FH. Homozygous FH children have cholesterol levels that range from 600 to 1000 mg/dL. Planar xanthomas—flat, orange-colored skin lesions—may be present at birth and usually occur by five years of age. Planar xanthomas can be found on the buttocks, between the webbings of the fingers, and in the popliteal fossa. Tendon and tuberous xanthomas often develop between the ages of 5 and 15 years. Angina pectoris and myocardial infarction are common in the second decade of life and have occurred as early as six years of age. Generalized atherosclerosis affects the aortic valve and the aorta, leading to aortic stenosis that is often life threatening.

The fundamental defect in FH has been elegantly elaborated by Goldstein, Brown, and coworkers (Hobbs, 1992). Over 150 genetic mutations have been described in the locus that specifies the LDL receptor protein. The LDL receptor gene has been mapped to chromosome 19. The defects in the LDL receptor gene include insertions, deletions, missense, and nonsense mutations. The synthesis, intracellular transport, clustering in coated pits on the cell surface, ability to bind and internalize LDL, and recycling of the LDL receptor can each be affected by a mutation in the LDL receptor gene. A number of patients with the clinical phenotype of homozygous FH are true genetic compounds—that is, they have two different mutant alleles at the LDL receptor locus that results in nonfunctional or markedly defective LDL receptors.

Familial Defective ApoB-100. In 1 of about 20 families, the presence of high LDL-cholesterol levels and xanthomas is not due to FH; LDL receptor activity is normal, but a defect in the ligand apoB is present, in which glutamine is substituted for arginine at residue 3500 (Myant, 1991). The mutant apoB in this disorder, familial defective apoB-100, is not bound normally by the LDL receptor, often leading to elevated LDL-cholesterol levels. However, most patients with familial defective apoB-100 do not have tendon xanthomas, and the LDL-cholesterol levels in children or adults with this disorder can be normal or moderately elevated (Myant, 1991). The defect appears to account for only a small proportion (perhaps 1% to 2%) of premature CAD. For the purpose of treatment, it does not appear necessary to distinguish FH from familial defective apoB-100.

Disorders of Both the Endogenous and the Exogenous Lipoprotein Pathways

Type V Hyperlipoproteinemia. Patients with a Type V lipoprotein phenotype have marked hypertriglyceridemia secondary to increased levels of both VLDL and chylomicrons. Such patients may reflect the extreme expression of either FCHL or, more commonly, FHT (see earlier). Those with a deficiency of apoC-II may also present with a Type V lipoprotein pattern. Despite the genetic heterogeneity, patients with the Type V lipoprotein phenotype share certain common clinical findings, namely, pancreatitis, eruptive xanthomas, lipemia retinalis, abnormal glucose tolerance, and hyperinsulinism (Brunzell, 1989). The atherosclerosis associated with some of the other disorders of the endogenous lipoprotein pathway is not as prevalent in those with Type V, although some of these patients may have premature peripheral vascular or coronary artery disease.

The increased VLDL in Type V may be due to increased synthesis, decreased clearance of VLDL, or a combination of both, leading to a more extreme elevation of VLDL, which may then impinge on the normal clearance of chylomicrons by saturating the LPL pathway. There is a delayed expression of Type V phenotype, and only a few preadolescent children have been described with this condition. The genetic defects are not known, but a pattern of autosomal dominant inheritance has been found in some families, with variable presentation as Type IV and Type V phenotypes.

Dysbetalipoproteinemia (Type III Hyperlipoproteinemia). Another disorder that involves both endogenous and exogenous pathways of lipoprotein metabolism is dysbetalipoproteinemia (or Type III hyperlipoproteinemia) (Mahley, 1989). This dyslipoproteinemia is usually defined by plasma VLDL that are enriched in cholesterol, and the ratio of VLDL-cholesterol to total triglyceride is usually greater than 0.3 (see Table 10–10). The VLDL in Type III hyperlipoproteinemia usually has β rather than pre-β electrophoretic mobility (see earlier); β-VLDL reflects the increased quantities of remnant lipoproteins that have accumulated as a result of delayed clearance. Dysbetalipoproteinemia is usually accompanied by both hypercholesterolemia and hypertriglyceridemia, sometimes in approximately equal amounts (i.e., plasma cholesterol and triglyceride levels can be about the same when the two lipid concentrations are expressed in milligrams per deciliter; the levels of LDL and HDL are usually low or average). The marked hyperlipidemia and clinical features of Type III are usually delayed until adulthood, when affected patients often develop xanthomas, particularly yellowish deposits in the creases of the palms, as well as tuberous and tuberoeruptive xanthomas over the elbows, knees, and buttocks. Tendon xanthomas are less frequent. Premature atherosclerosis of the coronary, aortic, abdominal, and femoral arteries is very prevalent. Hyperuricemia and glucose intolerance occur in up to half of patients with this syndrome.

Normally, the apoE on chylomicron remnants binds to the putative chylomicron remnant receptor, and the apoE on VLDL remnants binds to the LDL (B,E) receptor, leading to the hepatic uptake of these remnant triglyceride-rich lipoproteins. The VLDL and chylomicron remnants accumulate, a process resulting from defects involving a polymorphic genetic locus that specifies the structure of apoE. Human apoE exists as three major isoforms (E-2, E-3, and E-4), each of which is specified by an independent allele within the locus of the *APOE* gene. The most common allele is APOE3 and the rarest APOE2. As discussed, an apoE-3 isoform has an arginine at residue 158 and a cysteine at residue 112. An apoE-2 isoform has a cysteine at both residues 158 and 112, whereas the apoE-4 isoform has an arginine at both residues (Mahley, 1989). One in 100 persons is homozygous for the apoE-2 allele. Most patients with dysbetalipoproteinemia are apoE-2 homozygotes. However, the prevalence of Type III hyperlipoproteinemia is only 1 in 2000, and another modifying factor, perhaps a so-called hyperlipidemia gene, seems to be necessary for expression of the complete clinical syndrome. ApoE-2 may also be genotypically heterogeneous, and a number of other isoforms have been described, all involving a substitution of a neutral amino acid for either lysine or arginine. An apparent absence of apoE has also been reported.

Deficiencies in ApoB-Containing Lipoproteins. In

addition to hyperlipidemia, which can result from abnormalities involving both the exogenous and the endogenous pathways, there are several other unusual genetic defects involving both these pathways which, in contrast, cause *hypo*lipidemia.

Abetalipoproteinemia (Bassen-Kornzweig Syndrome). Abetalipoproteinemia is a rare autosomal recessive disorder; its clinical expression in childhood includes fat malabsorption, severe hypolipidemia, retinitis pigmentosa, cerebellar ataxia, and acanthocytosis (Kane, 1989). As well, there are large intracellular fat particles in biopsy specimens of the jejunum and a failure to form chylomicrons following a meal. Three of the four major lipoprotein classes (i.e., the apoB-containing lipoproteins, chylomicrons, VLDL, and LDL) are absent from plasma. Concentrations of both cholesterol and triglyceride are low, and both apoB-48 and apoB-100 are absent from plasma.

The pathophysiology of abetalipoproteinemia is important because the clinical findings result from defects in absorption and transport of lipids, especially the fat-soluble vitamins A, D, E, and K (Rader, 1993). Digestion of dietary triglyceride and uptake of free fatty acids (FFA) and monoglyceride proceed normally, but the cells fail to make chylomicrons, presumably because apoB-48 is not available. Jejunal cells become fat laden, and most of the dietary fat is excreted in the stool. Most patients with abetalipoproteinemia do not have a clinical deficiency in vitamin D, because vitamin D does not depend on lipoproteins for absorption or transport. Deficits in vitamins A and K do occur because these vitamins are absorbed from the intestine and transported to the liver via the chylomicron pathway. However, once they have reached the liver, vitamins A and K are not secreted on VLDL, and they have their own independent transport systems. In contrast, vitamin E requires chylomicrons to reach the liver and then is secreted on VLDL and subsequently ends up in LDL. Significant impairment of delivery of vitamin E to peripheral tissues appears to be the most clinically important vitamin deficiency in patients with abetalipoproteinemia (Rader, 1993). Most of the major symptoms in this disorder, particularly in the retina and nervous system, appear to be due to vitamin E deficiency.

Abetalipoproteinemia is not due to a defect in the *APOB* gene. A microsomal triglyceride transfer protein from liver and intestine has been found that mediates the intracellular transport of membrane-associated lipids. Microsomal triglyceride transfer protein and activity were absent in the intestines of patients with abetalipoproteinemia (Rader, 1993). These observations indicate that the molecular defect, in at least some patients with abetalipoproteinemia, may reside in the gene for microsomal transfer protein, leading to the inability to secrete either apoB 48 or apoB 100.

Hypobetalipoproteinemia. Hypobetalipoproteinemia is characterized by very low levels of LDL-cholesterol, usually less than the fifth percentile of the normal distribution. The total cholesterol level is low, and the VLDL-cholesterol and total triglyceride levels are low or normal. Familial hypobetalipoproteinemia may confirm a decreased risk for CAD. This disorder is inherited as an autosomal dominant trait. At least 25 mutations in the *APOB* gene causing hypobetalipoproteinemia have been described (Linton, 1993). Almost all of the mutations are either nonsense mutations or frame-shift mutations, resulting from the deletion of one to five base pairs, creating a premature stop codon. Truncated forms of apoB are usually found in the plasma.

Homozygous Hypobetalipoproteinemia. The clinical presentation of children with this disorder depends on whether they are homozygous for null alleles in the *APOB* gene (i.e., they make no detectable apoB) or compound heterozygous for other alleles leading to the production of lipoproteins that contain small amounts of apoB or truncated apoB. Null-allele homozygotes are similar phenotypically to persons with abetalipoproteinemia (see earlier) and may, on clinical presentation, prominently show fat malabsorption, neurologic disease, and hematologic abnormalities (Kane, 1989). However, the parents of these children are heterozygotes for hypobetalipoproteinemia. Patients with homozygous hypobetalipoproteinemia may develop less marked ocular and neuromuscular manifestations and do so at a later age than do those with abetalipoproteinemia. Concentrations of fat-soluble vitamins are low. In homozygotes whose plasma contains small amounts of apoB, the total and LDL-cholesterol values are as low as they are in persons with the null alleles, but the triglyceride levels, in contrast, are normal.

Chylomicron Retention Disease. A syndrome known as chylomicron retention disease, or Andersen disease, is characterized by a selective inability to secrete apoB from the intestinal cells, leading to fat malabsorption and neurologic disease (Pessah, 1991). The basic defect is not known, but appears distinct from that of abetalipoproteinemia and hypobetalipoproteinemia.

Disorders of the Reverse Cholesterol Transport Pathway

A number of defects can occur in the reverse cholesterol transport pathway (Breslow, 1989). These may involve (1) decreased synthesis of HDL, involving mutations in the *APOA*-I/C-III/A-IV gene complex, (2) accelerated removal of HDL, (3) defects in the *LCAT* gene, and (4) defects in the cholesteryl ester transfer protein (*CETP*) gene. The first three classes of defects lead to low HDL levels, whereas the fourth defect causes high HDL levels.

Phenotype of Hypoalphalipoproteinemia

Many relatives from families with premature CAD will have a low HDL-cholesterol level; however, this will not be the primary abnormality but will accompany the pleiotropic presentation of one of the disorders of the endogenous pathway of the lipoprotein metabolism (see earlier). Some patients with hypoalphalipoproteinemia, particularly if the HDL-cholesterol and apoA-I levels are severely depressed, may have a defect in the reverse cholesterol transport pathway.

Decreased Synthesis of HDL—Defects in the *APOA-I/C-III/A-IV* Gene Complex. Examples of two such defects are distinguished by clinical and laboratory findings. In patients with apoA-I and apoC-III deficiency, very low HDL levels are accompanied by corneal clouding and premature CAD; HDL production is defective, because these homozygotes are unable to synthesize apoA-I. Examples of such mutations include a rearrangement of the apolipoprotein gene locus that inactivates both apoA-I and apoC-III; deletion of the entire locus, producing deficiency in apoA-I/C-III/A-IV; and a small insertion of the *APOA*-I gene (Breslow, 1989). Heterozygotes with one mutant allele have HDL levels that are above 50% normal. The variation of such defects involves patients with HDL deficiency with planar xanthomas, the clinical findings of whom are similar to those of apoA-I and apoC-III deficiency, but this syndrome is distinguished by an elevated (not deficient) level of apoC-III.

Increased Catabolism of HDL–apoA-I Variants. A number of distinct apoA-I variants, such as apoA-I Milano, have been described (Breslow, 1989). These apoA-I variants were detected by isoelectric focusing of apoA-I and each have a specific amino acid substitution. For example, apoA-I Milano results from a mutation in the *APOA*-I gene in codon 173, changing arginine to cysteine. Heterozygous carriers for such a codominant trait often have low levels of HDL-cholesterol but are usually asymptomatic in regard to premature CAD. A mutant apoA-I variant can be catabolized more rapidly in plasma than the normal apoA-I can.

Tangier Disease. Tangier disease is a rare metabolic disorder in which the plasma HDL is both abnormal and present in severely reduced concentration. The compositions and amounts of the other lipoproteins are also abnormal (Breslow, 1989). The total cholesterol is decreased with normal or elevated total triglyceride levels. These lipoprotein abnormalities are accompanied by striking deposition of cholesteryl esters in different tissues. Major clinical manifestations reflect the lipid storage, and include enlarged orange tonsils, splenomegaly, and a relapsing peripheral neuropathy. Mild hepatomegaly, lymphadenopathy, and corneal clouding (in adulthood) may also occur. Foam cells can be demonstrated by biopsy of the skin, bone marrow, peripheral nerves, or rectum. The disorder can be detected in children, but the age range for detection is 3 to 40 years. Tangier homozygotes have apoA-I levels that are less than 3% of normal, but immunochemically detectable apoA-I is synthesized by intestinal cells and rapidly catabolized in plasma. The *APOA*-I gene is normal in Tangier disease, and the fundamental defect is not well understood.

Lecithin:Cholesterol Acyltransferase Deficiency. In blood, LCAT esterifies cholesterol through association with HDL (α-LCAT) or, to a lesser extent, with VLDL/LDL (β-LCAT). In classic LCAT deficiency, both α-LCAT and β-LCAT activities are virtually absent, resulting in a markedly reduced plasma cholesterol esterification rate, a low plasma cholesterol ester content, and an abnormal lipoprotein profile with very low HDL. Clinical findings include glomerulosclerosis, normochromic anemia, corneal opacities (it can be detected in childhood), and premature peripheral atherosclerosis. Specific defects in the LCAT gene, including stop codons and amino acid substitutions, have been elucidated in several kindreds with LCAT deficiency (Klein, 1993a). Fish eye disease is a phenotypically distinct syndrome of LCAT deficiency, in which most, but not all, patients appear to have a selective defect in β-LCAT activity that is accompanied similarly by dense corneal opacities; HDL-cholesterol is low, but premature atherosclerosis is not present (Klein, 1993b). Similar molecular defects have been described in the *LCAT* gene of patients with fish eye disease, but an interesting mutation ($LCAT^{300del}$) has led to the postulate that the heterogeneity in the phenotypic syndromes of LCAT deficiency may be related to the residual amounts of total plasma LCAT activity (Klein, 1993b).

Phenotype of Hyperalphalipoproteinemia

In contrast with hypoalphalipoproteinemia, some individuals have very high HDL-cholesterol levels (greater than the 95th percentile), a condition called hyperalphalipoproteinemia. The total cholesterol is elevated as a result of the high HDL-cholesterol level, the LDL-cholesterol level is usually normal, and the triglyceride level is normal or low. Hyperalphalipoproteinemia is associated with longevity and decreased risk of CAD.

2

***CETP* Gene Defects.** Several mutations have been described in the *CETP* gene, which is particularly prevalent in the Japanese population, leading to hyperalphalipoproteinemia and longevity (Breslow, 1989). Genetic defects in other individuals with high HDL-cholesterol levels have not yet been elucidated.

Abell LL, Levy BB, Brodie BB, et al: A simplified method for the estimation of total cholesterol in serum and demonstration of its specificity. J Biol Chem 1992; 195:357.

Alaupovic P: Apolipoproteins and lipoproteins. Atheroscler 1971; 13:141.

Albers JJ, Adolphson JL, Chen CH: Radioimmunoassay of human plasma lecithin:cholesterol acyltransferase. J Clin Invest 1981; 67:141.

Albers JJ, Adolphson JL, Hazzard WR: Radioimmunoassay of human plasma Lp(a) lipoprotein. J Lipid Res 1977; 189:331.

Albers JJ, Brunzell JD, Knopp RH: Apoprotein measurement and their clinical application. Clin Lab Med 1989a; 9:137.

Albers JJ, Cabana VG, Hazzard WR: Immunoassay of human plasma apolipoprotein B. Metabolism 1975; 24:1339.

Albers JJ, Hazzard WR: Immunochemical quantification of human plasma Lp(a) lipoprotein. Lipids 1974; 9:15.

Albers JJ, Lodge MS, Curtiss LK: Evaluation of a monoclonal antibody based enzyme-linked immunosorbant assay as a candidate reference method for the measurement of apoprotein B-100. J Lipid Res 1989b; 30:1445.

Allain CC, Poon LS, Chan CSG, et al: Enzymatic determination of total serum cholesterol. Clin Chem 1974; 20:470.

Armstrong VW, Walli AK, Seidel D: Isolation, characterization, and uptake in human fibroblasts of an apo(a)-free lipoprotein obtained on reduction of lipoprotein (a)1. J Lipid Res 1985; 26:1314.

Bachorik PS: Electrophoresis in the determination of plasma lipoprotein patterns. *In* Lewis LA, Opplt JA (eds): CRC Handbook of Electrophoresis, Vol. 2. Boca Raton, Florida, CRC Press, 1980.

Bachorik PS: Collection of blood samples for lipoprotein analysis. Clin Chem 1982; 28:1375.

Bachorik PS: The elusive connection between lipoprotein (a) and thrombosis *in vivo*. Curr Opin Lipidol 1993; 4:19.

Bachorik PS: Lipid and lipoprotein analysis with desk-top analyzers. *In* Rifai N, Warnick GR (eds): Laboratory Measurement of Lipids, Lipoproteins and Apolipoproteins. Washington, DC, AACC Press, 1994a.

Bachorik PS: Cardiovascular disease and hyperlipidaemia. Curr Opin Lipidol 1994b; 5:U150.

Bachorik PS, Kwiterovich PO Jr: Apolipoprotein measurements in clinical biochemistry and their utility vis-a-vis conventional assays. Clin Chim Acta 1988; 178:1.

Bachorik PS, Wood PDS: Laboratory considerations in the diagnosis and management of hyperlipoproteinemia. *In* Rifkind BM, Levy RI (eds): Hyperlipidemia: Diagnosis and Therapy. New York, Grune & Stratton, 1977.

Bachorik PS, Bradford RH, Cole T, et al: Accuracy and precision of analyses for total cholesterol performed with the Reflotron cholesterol method. Clin Chem 1989; 35:1734.

Bachorik PS, Rock R, Cloey T, et al: Cholesterol screening: Comparative evaluation of on-site and laboratory-based measurements. Clin Chem 1990; 36:255.

Bachorik PS, Virgil DG, Kwiterovich PO: Effect of apolipoprotein E-free high density lipoproteins on cholesterol metabolism in cultured pig hepatocytes. J Biol Chem 1987; 262:13636.

Bachorik PS, Wood PDS, Albers JJ, et al: Plasma high-density lipoprotein cholesterol concentrations determined after removal of other lipoproteins by heparin/manganese precipitation or by ultracentrifugation. Clin Chem 1976; 22:1828.

Bachorik PS, Wood PDS, Williams J, et al: Automated determination of to-

tal plasma cholesterol: A serum calibration technique. Clin Chim Acta 1979; 96:145.
Bartlett GR: Phosphorus assay in column chromatography. J Biol Chem 1959; 234:466.
Belsey R, Goitien RK, Baer DM: Evaluation of a laboratory system intended for use in physicians' offices. I. Reliability of results produced by trained laboratory technologists. JAMA 1987a; 258:353.
Belsey R, Vandernbark M, Goitien RK, Baer DM: Evaluation of a laboratory system intended for use in physicians' offices. II. Reliability of results produced by health care workers without formal or professional laboratory training. JAMA 1987b; 258:357.
Berg K, Dahlen G, Borresen AL: Lp(a) phenotypes, other lipoprotein parameters and family history of heart disease in middle aged males. Clin Genet 1979; 16:347.
Blanche PJ, Gong EL, Forte TM, et al: Characterization of human high density lipoproteins by gradient gel electrophoresis. Biochim Biophys Acta 1981; 665:408.
Boerma GJM, van Gorp I, Liem TL, et al: Revised calibration of the Reflotron cholesterol assay evaluated. Clin Chem 1988; 34:1124.
Bookstein L, Gidding SS, Donovan M, Smith FA: Day-to-day variability of serum cholesterol, triglyceride and high density lipoprotein cholesterol levels. Arch Intern Med 1990; 150:1653.
Breckenridge WC, Little LA, Steiner G, et al: Hypertriglyceridemia associated with deficiency of apolipoprotein CII. N Engl J Med 1978; 298:1265.
Breslow JL: Genetic basis of lipoprotein disorders. J Clin Invest 1989; 84:373.
Brown MS, Kovanen PT, Goldstein JL: Regulation of plasma cholesterol by lipoprotein receptors. Science 1981; 212:628.
Brown SA, Boerwinkle E, Kashanian FK, et al: Variation in concentrations of lipids, lipoprotein lipids, and apolipoproteins A-I and B in plasma from healthy women. Clin Chem 1990; 36:207.
Brunzell JD: Familial lipoprotein lipase deficiency and other causes of the chylomicronemia syndrome. *In* Scriver CR, Beaudet AL, Sly WS, Valle D (eds): The Metabolic Basis of Inherited Disease, 6th ed. New York, McGraw-Hill, 1989.
Bucolo G, David H: Quantitative determination of serum triglycerides by the use of enzymes. Clin Chem 1973; 19:476.
Burstein M, Legmann P: Lipoprotein precipitation. *In* Clarkson TB, Kritchevsky D, Pollak OJ (eds): Monographs on Atherosclerosis, Vol. II. Basel, S Karger AG, 1982.
Byers SO, Friedman M: Site of origin of plasma triglyceride. Am J Physiol 1960; 198:629.
Celemajer DS, Sorensen KE, Gooch VM, et al: Noninvasive detection of endothelial dysfunction in children and adults at risk of atherosclerosis. Lancet 1992; 340:1111.
Ceredella RJ, Crouthamel WG, Mengoll MF: Intestinal versus hepatic contribution to circulating triglyceride levels. Lipids 1974; 9:35.
Cladaras C, Hadzopoulou-Cladaras M, Nolte RT, et al: The complete sequence and structural analysis of human apolipoprotein B-100: Relationship between apoB-100 and apoB-48 forms. EMBO J 1986; 5:3495.
Clay HA, Hopkins GJ, Enholm C, et al: The rabbit as an animal model of hepatic lipase deficiency. Biochim Biophys Acta 1989; 1002:173.
Cohn JS, McNamara JR, Schaefer EJ: Lipoprotein cholesterol concentrations in plasma of human subjects as measured in the fed and fasted states. Clin Chem 1988; 34:2456.
Cooper GR, Duncan PH, Hazlehurset JS, et al: Cholesterol, enzymic method. *In* Faulkner WR, Meites S (eds): Selected Methods of Clinical Chemistry, Vol. 9. Washington, DC, American Association for Clinical Chemistry, 1982.
Corder EH, Saunders AM, Strittmatter WJ, et al: Gene dose of apolipoprotein E type 4 allele and the risk of Alzheimer's disease in late onset families. Science 1993; 216:921–923.
Cortner JA, Coates PM, Gallagher PR: Prevalence and expression of familial combined hyperlipidemia in childhood. J Pediatr 1990; 116:514.
Curry MD, Alaupovic P, Suenram CA: Determination of apolipoprotein A and its constitutive A-I and A-II polypeptides by separate electroimmunoassays. Clin Chem 1976a; 22:315.
Curry MD, Gustafson A, Alaupovic P, et al: Electroimmunoassay, radioimmunoassay, and radial immunodiffusion assay evaluated for quantification of human apolipoprotein B. Clin Chem 1978; 24:280.
Curry MD, McConathy WJ, Alaupovic P, et al: Determination of human apolipoprotein E by electroimmunoassay. Biochim Biophys Acta 1976b; 439:413.
Curry MD, McConathy WJ, Alaupovic P: Quantitative determination of human apolipoprotein D by electroimmunoassay and radial immunodiffusion. Biochim Biophys Acta 1977; 491:232.
Curry MD, McConathy WJ, Fesmire JD, et al: Quantitative determination of human apolipoprotein C-III by electroimmunoassay. Biochim Biophys Acta 1980; 617:503.
Curry MD, McConathy WJ, Fesmire JD, Alaupovic P: Quantitative determination of apolipoproteins C-I and C-II in human plasma by separate electroimmunoassays. Clin Chem 1981; 27:543.
Dahlen GH, Atar M, Guyton IR, et al: Lipoprotein(a) and coronary artery disease. Arterioscler 1983; 3:478a.
Deacon AC, Dawson PJG: Enzymic assay of total cholesterol involving chemical or enzymic hydrolysis—a comparison of methods. Clin Chem 1979; 25:976.
DeLong DM, DeLong ER, Wood PD, et al: A comparison of methods for the estimation of plasma low-and very low-density lipoprotein cholesterol. The Lipid Research Clinics Prevalence Study. JAMA 1986; 256:2372.
Demacker PNM, Schade RWB, Jansen RTP, et al: Intra-individual variation of serum cholesterol, triglycerides, and high density lipoprotein cholesterol in normal humans. Atherosclerosis 1982; 45:259.
Eisenberg S, Levy RI: Lipoprotein metabolism. Adv Lipid Res 1976; 13:1.
El-Dering S, Ng RH, Staatland BE: Evaluation of the Kodak Ektachem DT60 Analzyer. Clin Chem 1986; 32:1415.
Ellefson RD, Caraway WT: Lipids and lipoproteins. *In* Tietz NW (ed): Fundamentals of Clinical Chemistry. Philadelphia, W. B. Saunders, 1976.
Expert Panel on Detection, Evaluation, and Treatment of High Blood Cholesterol in Adults: Report of the National Cholesterol Education Program Expert Panel on detection, evaluation, and treatment of high blood cholesterol in adults. Arch Intern Med 1988; 148:36.
Falko JM, Schonfeld G, Witztum JL, et al: Effects of diet on apoprotein E levels and on the apoprotein E subspecies in human plasma lipoproteins. J Clin Endocrinol Metab 1980; 50:521.
Fless GM, Rolih CQ, Scanu AM: Heterogeneity of human plasma lipoprotein(a). Isolation and characterization of the lipoprotein subspecies and their apoproteins. J Biol Chem 1984; 259:11470.
Fless GM, ZumMallen ME, Scanu AM: Isolation of apolipoprotein(a) from lipoprotein(a). J Lipid Res 1985; 26:1224.
Floren C-H, Albers JJ, Bierman EL: Uptake of Lp(a) lipoprotein by cultured fibroblasts. Biochem Biophys Res Commun 1981; 102:636.
Folch J, Lees M, Sloan-Stanley GH: A simple method for the isolation and purification of total lipids from animal tissues. J Biol Chem 1957; 226:497.
Fredrickson DS, Levy RI, Lees RS: Fat transportation in lipoproteins—an integrated approach to mechanisms and disorders. N Engl J Med 1967; 276:32,94,148,215,273.
Fredrickson DS, Levy RI, Lindgren FT: A comparison of heritable abnormal lipoprotein in patterns as defined by two different techniques. J Clin Invest 1968; 47:2446.
Friedewald WT, Levy RI, Fredrickson DS: Estimation of the concentration of low density lipoprotein cholesterol in plasma without use of the preparative ultracentrifuge. Clin Chem 1972; 18:499.
Fruchart JC, Ailhaud G: Apolipoprotein A-containing particles: Physiologic role, quantification and clinical significance. Clin Chem 1992; 38:793.
Fruchart JC, Desreumaux C, Dewailly P, et al: Enzyme immunoassay of human apolipoprotein B, the major protein moiety of low-density and very-low-density lipoproteins. Clin Chem 1978; 24:455.
Gaubatz JW, Heideman C, Gotto AM Jr, et al: Human plasma lipoprotein(a). Structural properties. J Biol Chem 1983; 258:4582.
Gaw A, Hobbs HH: Molecular genetics of lipoprotein (a): New pieces to the puzzle. Curr Opin Lipidol 1994; 5:149.
Giannoni F, Bonen DK, Funahashi T, et al: Complementation of Apolipoprotein B mRNA editing by human liver accompanied by secretion of Apolipoprotein B48. J Biol Chem 1994; 269:5932.
Glass C, Pittman RC, Weinstein DB, et al: Dissociation of tissue uptake of cholesterol ester from that of apoprotein A-I of rat plasma high density lipoprotein: Selective delivery of cholesterol ester to liver, adrenal and gonad. Proc Natl Acad Sci U S A 1983; 80:5435.
Gordon DJ, Trost DC, Hyde J, et al: Seasonal cholesterol cycles: The Lipid Research Clinics Coronary Primary Prevention Trial placebo group. Circulation 1987; 76:1224.
Gotto AM Jr, Pownall HJ, Havel RJ: Introduction to the plasma lipoproteins. Meth Enzymol 1986; 128:3.
Green PHR, Glickman RM: Intestinal lipoprotein metabolism. J Lipid Res 1981; 22:1153.
Gries A, Fievet C, Marcovina S, et al: Interaction of LDL, Lp(a), and reduced Lp(a) with monoclonal antibodies against apoB. J Lipid Res 1988; 29:1.
Hajjar KA, Harpel PC, Jaffe EA, et al: Binding of plasminogen to cultured human endothelial cells. J Biol Chem 1986; 261:11656.
Hardman DA, Kane JP: Isolation and characterization of apolipoprotein B-48. Meth Enzymol 1986; 128:262.
Havel RJ: Lipoprotein biosynthesis and metabolism. Ann N Y Acad Sci 1980; 348:16.
Havel RJ: The formation of LDL: Mechanisms and regulation. J Lipid Res 1984; 25:1570.
Havel RJ, Eder HA, Bragdon JH: The distribution and chemical composition of ultracentrifugally separated lipoproteins in human serum. J Clin Invest 1955; 34:1345.
Henderson LO, Powell MK, Smith SJ, et al: Impact of protein measurements on standardization of assays of apolipoproteins AI and B. Clin Chem 1990; 36:1911.
Higuchi K, Hospattankar AV, Law SW, et al: Human apolipoprotein B

(apoB): Identification of two distinct apoB mRNAs, an mRNA with the apoB-100 sequence and an apoB mRNA containing a premature in-frame translational stop codon, in both liver and intestine. Proc Natl Acad Sci U S A 1988; 85:1772.

Hobbs HH, Brown MS, Goldstein JL: Molecular genetics of the LDL receptor gene in familial hypercholesterolemia. Hum Mutation 1992; 1:445.

Hospattankar AV, Fairwell T, Meng M, et al: Identification of sequence homology between human plasma apolipoprotein B-100 and apolipoprotein B-48. J Biol Chem 1986; 261:9102.

Hui DY, Innerarity TL, Milne RW, et al: Binding of chylomicron remnants and β-VLDL to hepatic and extra-hepatic lipoprotein receptors: A process independent of apolipoprotein B-48. J Biol Chem 1984; 259:15060.

Kafonek SD, Derby CA, Bachorik PS: Biological variability of lipoproteins and apolipoproteins in patients referred to a Lipid Clinic. Clin Chem 1992; 38:864.

Kane JP, Hardman DA, Paulus HE: Heterogeneity of apolipoprotein B: Isolation of a new species from human chylomicrons. Proc Natl Acad Sci U S A 1980; 77:2465.

Kane JP, Havel RF. Disorders of the biogenesis and secretion of lipoproteins containing the B apolipoproteins. *In* Scriver CR, Beaudet AL, Sly WS, Valle D (eds): The Metabolic Basis of Inherited Disease, 6th ed. New York, McGraw-Hill, 1989.

Kessler G, Lederer H: Fluorometric measurement of triglycerides. *In* Skeggs LT (ed): Automation in Clinical Chemistry, Technicon Symposia. New York, Mediad, 1966.

Klein HG, Lohse P, Duverger N, et al: Two different allelic mutations in the lecithin:cholesterol acyltransferase (LCAT) gene resulting in classic LCAT deficiency: LCAT (try^{83} → stop) and LCAT (try^{156} → asn). J Lipid Res 1993a; 34:49.

Klein HG, Santamarina-Fojo S, Duverger N, et al: Fish Eye Syndrome: A molecular defect in the lecithin-cholesterol acyltransferase (LCAT) gene associated with normal α-LCAT-specific-activity. J Clin Invest 1993b; 92:479.

Knott TJ, Pease RJ, Powell LM, et al: Complete protein sequence and identification of structural domains of human apolipoprotein B. Nature 1986; 323:734.

Koch TR, Mehta V, Lee H, et al: Bias and precision of cholesterol analysis of physician's office analyzers. Clin Chem 1987; 33:2262.

Kwiterovich PO Jr: Genetics and molecular biology of familial combined hyperlipidemia. Curr Opin Lipidol 1993a; 4:133.

Kwiterovich PO Jr: Identification and treatment of heterozygous familial hypercholesterolemia in children and adolescents. Am J Card (Suppl) 1993b; 72:D30.

Laboratory Methods Committee of the Lipid Research Clinics Program: Cholesterol and triglyceride concentrations in serum/plasma pairs. Clin Chem 1977; 23:60.

Laboratory Standardization Panel, National Cholesterol Education Program, National Heart, Lung, and Blood Institute: A report on current status of blood cholesterol measurement in clinical laboratories in the United States. Clin Chem 1988; 34:193.

LaRosa JC, Levy RI, Herbert P, et al: A specific apoprotein activator for lipoprotein lipase. Biochem Biophys Res Commun 1970; 41:57.

Law SW, Grant SM, Higuchi K, et al: Human liver apolipoprotein B-100 cDNA: Complete nucleic acid and derived amino acid sequence. Proc Natl Acad Sci U S A 1986; 83:8142.

Li Z, McNamara JR, Ordovas JM, et al: Analysis of high density lipoproteins by a modified gradient gel electrophoresis method. FASEB J 1993; 7:A730.

Lindgren FT, Jensen LC, Hatch FT: The isolation and quantitative analysis of serum lipoproteins. *In* Nelson GJ (ed): Blood Lipids and Lipoproteins—Quantitation, Composition and Metabolism. New York, Wiley-Interscience, 1972.

Linton MF, Farese RV, Young SG: Familial hypobetalipoproteinemia. J Lipid Res 1993; 34:521.

Lipid Research Clinics Program: Manual of laboratory operations. Lipid and lipoprotein analysis. U.S. Department of Health and Human Services, Publication No. (NIH) 75. Revised September, 1982.

Lopes-Virella MFL, Virella G, Evangs G, Malenkos SB, et al: Immunonephelometric assay of human apolipoprotein A-I. Clin Chem 1980; 26:1205.

Lowry OH, Rosebrough NJ, Farr AL, et al: Protein measurement with the Folin phenol reagent. J Biol Chem 1951; 193:265.

Lunz ME, Castleberry BM, James K, et al: The impact of the quality of laboratory staff on the accuracy of laboratory results. JAMA 1987; 258:361.

MacKenzie SL, Sundarum GS, Sodhi HS: Heterogeneity of human high density lipoprotein (HDL2). Clin Chim Acta 1973; 43:223.

Mahley RW, Innerarity TL: Lipoprotein receptors and cholesterol homeostasis. Biochim Biophys Acta 1983; 737:197.

Mahley RW, Innerarity TL, Rall SC Jr, et al: Plasma lipoproteins: Apolipoprotein structure and function. J Lipid Res 1984; 25:1277.

Mahley RW, Rall SC Jr: Type III hyperlipoproteinemia (dysbetalipoproteinemia): The role of apolipoprotein E in normal and abnormal metabolism. *In* Scriver CR, Beaudet AL, Sly WS, Valle D (eds): The Metabolic Basis of Inherited Disease, 6th ed. New York, McGraw-Hill, 1989.

Marcel YL, Innerarity TL, Spilman C, et al: Mapping of human apolipoprotein B antigenic determinants. Arteriosclerosis 1987; 7:166.

Marcovina S, Albers JJ: Apolipoprotein assays: Standardization and quality control. Scand J Clin Lab Invest 1990; 50:58.

Marcovina SM, Albers JJ: International Federation of Clinical Chemistry Study on the Standardization of apolipoproteins AI and B. Curr Opin Lipidol 1991; 2:355.

McLean JW, Tomlinson JE, Kuang, W-J, et al: cDNA sequence of human apolipoprotein(a) is homologous to plasminogen. Nature 1987; 330:132.

Miller M, Bachorik PS, Cloey TA: Normal variation of plasma lipoproteins: Postural effects on plasma concentrations of lipids, lipoproteins and apolipoproteins. Clin Chem 1992; 38:569.

Murai A, Miyahara T, Fujimoto N, et al: Lp(a) lipoprotein as a risk factor for coronary heart disease and cerebral infarction. Atherosclerosis 1986; 59:199.

Myant NB, Gallagher JJ, Knight BL, et al: Clinical signs of familial hypercholesterolemia in patients with familial defective apolipoprotein B-100 and normal low density lipoprotein receptor function. Arterioscler Thromb 1991; 11:691.

Myers GL, Cooper GR, Winn CL, et al: The Centers for Disease Control—National Heart, Lung and Blood Institute Lipid Standardization Program. An approach to accurate and precise lipid measurements. Clin Lab Med 1989; 9:105.

Naito HK, David JA: Laboratory considerations: Determination of cholesterol, triglyceride, phospholipid, and other lipids in blood and tissues. *In* Lipid Research Methodology. New York, Alan R. Liss, 1984.

National Cholesterol Education Program: Recommendations for improving cholesterol measurement. A report from the Laboratory Standardization Panel of the National Cholesterol Education Program. NIH Publication No. 90-2964, Bethesda, Maryland, February, 1990.

National Cholesterol Education Program: Summary of the Second Report of the National Cholesterol Education Program (NCEP) Expert Panel on Detection, Evaluation, and Treatment of High Blood Cholesterol in Adults (Adult Treatment Panel II): JAMA 1993; 269:3015.

National Cholesterol Education Program: Expert Panel on Blood Cholesterol Levels in Children and Adolescents. National Cholesterol Education Program (NCEP): Highlights of the Report of the Expert Panel on Blood Cholesterol Levels in Children and Adolescents. Pediatrics 1992; 89:494.

National Cholesterol Education Program Working Group on Lipoprotein Measurement: Recommendations for Measurement of LDL-Cholesterol, HDL-Cholesterol and Triglycerides. NIH publication (in press, 1995).

National Institutes of Health (NIH) Consensus Conference: Treatment of hypertriglyceridemia. JAMA 1984; 251:1196.

Oppenheimer MJ, Oram JF, Bierman EL: Down regulation of high density lipoprotein receptor activity of cultured fibroblasts by platelet-derived growth factor. Arteriosclerosis 1987; 7:325.

Oram JF: Receptor-mediated transport of cholesterol between cultured cells and high-density lipoproteins. Meth Enzymol 1986; 129:645.

Pagnan A, Havel RJ, Kane JP, et al: Characterization of human very low density lipoproteins containing two electrophoretic populations: Double pre-beta lipoproteinemia and primary dysbetalipoproteinemia. J Lipid Res 1977; 18:613.

Pesce MA, Bodourian SH: Interference with the enzymatic measurement of cholesterol in serum by use of five reagent kits. Clin Chem 1977; 23:757.

Pessah M, Benlian P, Beucler I, et al: Andersen's disease: Genetic exclusion of the apolipoprotein-B gene in two families. J Clin Invest 1991; 87:367.

Poirier J, Davignon J, Bouthiller D, et al: Apolipoprotein E polymorphism and Alzheimer's disease. Lancet 1993; 342:697–699.

Powell LM, Wallis SC, Pease RJ, et al: A novel form of tissue-specific RNA processing produces apolipoprotein B-48 in intestine. Cell 1987; 50:831.

Rader DJ, Brewer HB: Abetalipoproteinemia. New insights into lipoprotein assembly and Vitamin E metabolism from a rare genetic disease. JAMA 1993; 270:865.

Risser TR, Reaven GM, Reaven EP: Intestinal contribution to secretion of very low density lipoproteins into plasma. Am J Physiol 1978; 234:E277.

Saunders AM, Schmader K, Brietner JCS, et al: Apolipoprotein E ϵ4 allele distributions in late-onset Alzheimer's disease and in other amyloid-forming diseases. Lancet 1993; 342:710–711.

Scanu AM: Lipoprotein(a). A potential bridge between the fields of atherosclerosis and thrombosis. Arch Pathol Lab Med 1988; 112:1045.

Scanu AM, Byrne RE, Mihovilovic M: Functional roles of plasma high density lipoproteins. CRC Crit Rev Biochem 1982; 13:109.

Schonfeld G, Pfleger B: The structure of human high density lipoprotein and the levels of apolipoprotein A-I in plasma as determined by radioimmunoassay. J Clin Invest 1974; 54:236.

Schonfeld G, George PK, Miller J, et al: Apolipoprotein C-II and C-III levels in hyperlipoproteinemia. Metabolism 1979; 28:1001.

Schultz SG, Holen JT, Donohue TP, et al: Two dimensional centrifugation for desk top clinical chemistry. Clin Chem 1985; 31:1457.

Scott J: Apolipoprotein E and Alzheimer's disease. Lancet 1993; 342:696.
Sedor FA, Holleman CM, Heyden S, et al: Reflotron cholesterol measurement evaluated as a screening technique. Clin Chem 1988; 34:2542.
Sherrill BC, Innerarity TL, Mahley RW: Rapid hepatic clearance of the canine lipoproteins containing only the E apoprotein by a high affinity receptor. J Biol Chem 1980; 255:1804.
Sniderman AD, Shapiro S, Marpole D, et al: Association of coronary atherosclerosis with hyperapobetalipoproteinemia (increased protein but normal cholesterol levels in human plasma low density lipoproteins). Proc Natl Acad Sci U S A 1980; 77:604.
Stavljenic A, Vrkic N, Herak C, et al: Analytical performance of the Vision system evaluation. Clin Chem 1987; 33:1672.
Stein EA: Clinical Significance and Measurement of Apolipoproteins AI and B. *In* Rifai N, Warnick GR (eds): Laboratory Measurement of Lipids, Lipoproteins and Apolipoproteins. Washington, DC, AACC Press, 1994.
Stein O, Stein Y, Coetzee GA, Van der Westhuyzen DR: Metabolic fate of low density lipoprotein and high density lipoprotein labeled with an ether analogue of cholesteryl ester. Klin Wochenschr 1984; 62:1151.
Sundarum GS, MacKenzie SL, Sodhie HS: Preparative iso-electric focusing of human serum high density lipoprotein (HPL3). Biochem Biophys Acta 1974; 337:196.
Tall AR: Plasma high density lipoproteins: Metabolism and relationship to atherogenesis. J Clin Invest 1990; 86:379.
Tikkanen M, Nikkila EA, Sipinen S: Reduction of plasma high-density lipoprotein-2 (HDL2) and increase in postheparin plasma hepatic lipase activity during progestin treatment. Clin Chim Acta 1981; 115:63.
Utermann G, Jaeschke M, Menzel J: Familial hyperlipoproteinemia Type III —deficiency of a specific apolipoprotein (apoE-III) in the very low density lipoproteins. FEBS Lett 1975; 56:352.
von Eckardstein A, Huang Y, Assmann G: Physiologic role and clinical relevance of high density lipoprotein subclasses. Curr Opin Lipidol 1994; 5:404.
Warnick GR, Albers JJ: Physiologic and analytical variation in cholesterol and triglycerides. Lipids 1975; 11:203.
Warnick GR, Cheung MC, Albers JJ: Comparison of current methods for high-density lipoprotein cholesterol quantitation. Clin Chem 1979; 25:596.
Witte DL, Brown LF, Feld RD: Effects of bilirubin on the detection of hydrogen peroxide by use of peroxidase. Clin Chem 1978; 24:1778.
Wood PD, Bachorik PS, Albers JJ, et al: An investigation of the effects of sample aging on total cholesterol values determined by the automated ferric choloride–sulfuric acid and Liebermann-Burchard procedures. Clin Chem 1980; 26:592.
Yang, C-Y, Chen, S-H, Gianturco S, et al: Sequence, structure, receptor-binding domains and internal repeats of human apolipoprotein B-100. Nature 1986; 323:738.
Yao Z, McLeod RS: Synthesis and secretion of hepatic apolipoprotein B-containing lipoproteins. Biochim Biophys Acta 1994; 1212:152.
Young SG, Berties SJ, Scott TM, et al: Parallel expression of the MB19 genetic polymorphism apoprotein B-100 and apoprotein B-48. Evidence that both apoproteins are products of the same gene. J Biol Chem 1986a; 261:2995.
Young SG, Smith RS, Hogle DM, et al: Two new monoclonal antibody-based enzyme-linked assays for apolipoprotein B. Clin Chem 1986b; 32:1484.
Zannis VI, Breslow JL: Human very low density lipoprotein apolipoprotein E variant associated with Type III hyperlipoproteinemia. J Biol Chem 1980; 255:1759.
Zannis VI, Breslow JL: Human very low density lipoprotein apolipoprotein E isoprotein polymorphism is explained by genetic variation and post-translational modification. Biochem 1981; 20:1033.
1993 CAP Surveys, Chemistry Series 1, Series 2. The College of American Pathologists. Northfield, Illinois, 1993.

Chapter 11

Specific Proteins

Richard A. McPherson, M.D.

2

Examination of the proteins in plasma can provide information reflecting disease states in many organ systems. The most frequently performed measurement, that for total protein, is usually performed on serum, which has no fibrinogen and no anticoagulant that may slightly dilute proteins in plasma. Although total protein determination gives the physician some information as to a patient's general status regarding nutrition or severe organ disease (as in protein-losing states), further fractionations yield far more clinically useful information.

Additional quantitation of albumin, for example, is more informative regarding nutritional status, liver synthetic capacity, or protein-losing nephropathy. It also allows the clinician to interpret high or low calcium and magnesium levels, because albumin binds about one half of each of those ions on a molar basis. Calculations of the difference between total protein and albumin yield the value of all globulins, a mixture of the other fractions that individually can rise severalfold in severe disorders.

Protein electrophoresis separates the globulins from albumin and resolves the major proteins of serum into patterns that may be highly specific for some diseases. High-resolution techniques can provide a display of all the components in concentrations down to about 1 g/L (0.1 g/dL in traditional units); however, at that level, quantitation by scanning of stained proteins is not highly reliable and alternative methods should be employed. Such techniques, involving immunologic detection of individual proteins, have the dual advantages of specificity and sensitivity over electrophoresis.

Yet there is much to be appreciated from visual inspection of an electrophoretogram of proteins, because the human eye is still the best scanning device for detecting subtle variations in patterns. Identification of these patterns is a useful screening method to be followed by more specific confirmatory procedures. Protein electrophoresis also can be a useful tool for monitoring patients over long periods of time when there are marked alterations in levels of particular proteins such as in myeloma, nephrotic syndrome, cirrhosis, or extensive body burn.

This chapter reviews protein structure, methodologies of measurement and separation, the major plasma proteins (except for coagulation factors, immunoglobulins, and the complement system, which are covered elsewhere), and some of the patterns encountered in particular disease states.

PROTEIN STRUCTURE

The backbone of all protein molecules is a continuous chain of carbon and nitrogen atoms joined together through *peptide bonds* between adjacent *amino acids.* At one end (the amino terminus), there is a free amino group, and at the other end (the carboxy terminus), there is a free carboxyl group. Whereas the peptide backbone is qualitatively invariant between different proteins (its total length is equivalent to the total number of amino acids in a particular protein), proteins have structural identity by virtue of the side groups of residues of the constituent amino acids. The average molecular weight of an amino acid is 120 daltons. Serum proteins range in size from roughly 66 kilodaltons (kDa) to over 700 kDa. These amino acid side chains are conventionally grouped according to chemical nature (*hydrogen:* glycine; *aliphatic*: alanine, valine, leucine, and isoleucine; *hydroxyamino*: serine and threonine; *aromatic*: tyrosine, phenylalanine, and tryptophan; *imino*: proline and hydroxyproline; *acidic*: aspartate and glutamate; *basic*: arginine, histidine, and lysine; *amides*: asparagine and glutamine; *sulfur-containing*: cysteine and methionine).

The linear sequence of the amino acids in a protein is called its *primary structure*. This primary sequence of amino acids is what determines the identity of a protein, what its molecular structure is, what functions it can perform, how it can bind to other molecules, and how it can participate in processes of recognition between molecules and cells. These biological interactions are guided by reactivities between charged groups on one molecule and those on another and similarly by hydrophobic interactions between molecules. Analytic processes such as chromatography, electrophoresis, dye binding, light absorbance, and others also depend on the primary amino acid sequence.

The *secondary*, or regular, *structure* refers to specific three-dimensional structures into which portions of the polypeptide chain fold. There are three such structures. First is the α-helix, in which the chain forms a regular helix such that the backbone C=O of the ith peptide group hydrogen bonds to the N-H of the $(i + 4)$th peptide unit. The second is β-pleated sheets in fully extended structures, in which the chain forms a flat structure such that the side chains of adjacent amino acids point in opposite directions; in this configuration, two or more extended chains can associate so that the maximum number of C=O · · · HN bonds form between them. Finally, a third grouping of regular structures is the bend conformation, in which the direction of the polypeptide chain reverses itself.

Plasma proteins typically contain both α and β portions that give rise to additional unique qualities that influence intermolecular actions. On degradation of some proteins (e.g., serum amyloid–associated protein, immunoglobulin light chains, prealbumin), there is release of fragments rich in beta regions. These fragments are capable of coming together *in vivo* to form deposits of beta forms in fibrils that constitute amyloid. Recent work has shown an association between the genotype of apoliprotein E (especially the allele ApoE4) and the progression of late-onset Alzheimer's disease, in which cerebral plaques of amyloid form within the brain. These genetic findings suggest that Alzheimer's disease may be understood and treated as a disease that has a biochemical basis in β-pleated sheet generation (Roses, 1994).

Molecular regions with clusters of hydrophobic side groups tend to remain inside a protein that is soluble in water, whereas those regions with clusters of charges or other hydrophilic moieties tend to appear on the protein's surface. Conversely, proteins that are membrane bound usually have a distinct hydrophobic segment sticking out to anchor the protein molecule in the lipid phase of the membrane. The actual three-dimensional structure or folding pattern of the protein, uniquely determined by its amino acid sequence, is termed its *tertiary structure.* Individual proteins or monomeric subunits may form more stable complexes, such as dimers, trimers, tetramers, which is termed *quaternary structure*.

The sulfhydryl group on a cysteine residue can form a *disulfide* (covalent) bond with another cysteine within the same protein to hold different segments tightly together. This action helps stabilize the whole structure from disruption by mechanical, thermal, or other forces. These intramolecular disulfide bonds most likely form after spontaneous protein folding along the linear amino acid sequence into thermodynamically most stable conformations.

The acidic and basic amino acids determine the net charge on a protein and hence its electrophoretic mobility. The charge on carboxyl and amino groups is a function of pH (i.e., whether a hydrogen ion is attached or dissociated from the group). Combining all the different side groups and their different degrees of dissociation, the pH at which a particular protein has net charge equal to zero is called its *isoelectric point (pI)*. Proteins with pI less than 7 are acidic and tend to have carboxyl side groups exposed; whereas those with pI greater than 7 are basic (e.g., histones that, in turn, bind to the external helical structure of DNA that is negatively charged with phosphate groups).

Proteins are synthesized from the amino end to the carboxyl end by ribosomes translating from the information encoded in messenger RNA. The initial translation product of some proteins is acted on before secretion by proteolytic enzymes that convert a preform to the mature protein by removal of a signal peptide (generally hydrophobic) that otherwise holds the new protein molecule to the endoplasmic reticulum. Additional modifications to protein structures occur post-translationally (i.e., after joining of the amino acids is complete) (Harding, 1985). *Phosphorylation* consists of the enzymatically regulated attachment of phosphate groups to serine or threonine groups in the peptide backbone, thereby forming phosphoproteins with a more negative charge. *Glycosylation* can occur either spontaneously, in the presence of sugar molecules, or in a directed manner under enzymatic control in which oligosaccharides, frequently terminating with sialic acid (which carries a negative charge), are attached to the protein. These species of molecules are termed glycoproteins. Linkages are generally to asparagine residues through *N*-acetylglucosamine or to serine and threonine residues through *N*-acetylgalactosamine. *Proteolysis* results in the cleavage or removal of short segments of the peptide backbone that can open up catalytic sites of a zymogen (e.g., plasminogen to plasmin) or facilitate recognition by a receptor molecule (e.g., proinsulin to insulin). These molecular changes in the structure of proteins determine their antigenicity, specific chemical or catalytic activities, abilities to bind to receptors, and electrophoretic mobility.

TECHNIQUES OF PROTEIN SEPARATION

Electrophoresis

Modern understanding of the protein composition of serum and plasma derives from the electrophoretic techniques introduced by Tiselius. He separated proteins dissolved in an electrolyte solution by application of an electric current through a U-shaped quartz tube that held the protein solution. At pH 7.6, four serum protein fractions designated albumin, α, β, and γ were identified and quantified optically by change in refractive index at the boundaries among these bands. Because separation was achieved in a homogeneous solution without solid support medium, convective forces prevented resolution into distinct zones. Hence, this technique has been termed *moving boundary* or *frontal electrophoresis*. Introduction of filter paper as an anticonvection support medium permitted separation of the protein fractions into discrete bands or zones in a process termed *zonal electrophoresis*. On solid support medium and at pH 8.6, the α fraction further splits into two groups of proteins, α_1 and α_2.

Other support media have been used, such as cellulose acetate membrane, agarose gel, starch gel, and polyacrylamide gel. Cellulose acetate and agarose have predominated in the clinical laboratory because of ease of use, low cost, and commercial availability (Jeppsson, 1979).

Application of samples can be done in wells that are cut into the gel, but this process typically leaves an artifact that can interfere with the scan. A method to get around this problem involves soaking the sample into the gel by means of an overlying template. Each end of the gel is then immersed into separate buffer chambers in which electrodes are mounted. A voltage is applied between the electrodes generating a current that passes through the gel, usually for a period of about 30 minutes, to achieve desired resolution. The ionic strength of the buffer determines the amount of current and the movement of the proteins for a fixed voltage. If ionic strength is low, relatively more current is carried by the charged proteins. If the ionic strength is high, less current is carried by the proteins, which move a shorter distance. If the electrodes are not properly aligned, the current may be denser on one side of the gel than on the other; proteins will migrate further on the side with more current. If the electrophoresis proceeds too long, the proteins may migrate off the gel into the buffer. If there is a break in the electrical circuit and no current passes, the proteins will not move from the point of application.

Following electrophoresis, the gel is treated with a mild fixative, such as acetic acid, that precipitates the proteins at the positions to which they have migrated. They are then stained, and the gel is dried and cleared. Protein patterns can be inspected visually for qualitative identification of abnormal proteins. Densitometric scanners are used to generate tracings and quantitate the relative percentages of protein in each fraction. Those percentages are then multiplied by the total protein (separately measured) in the sample to yield the concentration of protein in each fraction.

When an electrophoretic support medium has a negative charge, the electromotive force to which it is subjected tends to move it toward the anode (positive pole). However, the solid support medium is fixed and so it cannot move. The complementary positively charged ions in the surrounding buffer are free to move under the electromotive force, and they carry with them molecules of the solvent water, which are clustered around their charges. The net result is flow of buffer toward the cathode. This buffer flow is termed *electro-osmosis* or *endosmosis*, which also carries the proteins with it to some extent by mechanical flow, not by charge. The actual distance traveled by a particular protein migrating in an electrical field is determined by the combined magnitudes of the electromotive force (a feature of the protein itself and the pH) and the electro-osmotic force (a function primarily of the support medium). When the electro-osmotic force is greater than the electrophoretic force acting on weakly anionic proteins (e.g., γ-globulins), those proteins move from the application point toward the cathode, even though their charge is slightly negative.

Through critical manipulations of buffer salt composition, endosmotic properties of the medium, and means of sample application, commercially available electrophoretic agarose plates now achieve consistently high-resolution qualities that allow routine separation of all the major serum protein species (Fig. 11–1). Because of variability in chemical formulations of gels, it should not necessarily be expected that each manufacturer's electrophoretic system will yield identical protein separation patterns. Furthermore, optimal separation of isoenzymes generally requires different buffer and gel composition compared with the conditions for best resolution of serum proteins versus lipoproteins versus hemoglobins. A significant variation in conditions for protein electrophoresis is that for optimizing the separation of the gamma region to resolve and detect oligoclonal bands of immunoglobulin in cerebrospinal fluid. In this case, the endosmosis is set high to maximize the cathodal movement of immunoglobulins from the point of application over a span of the gel that is convenient for visual inspection.

Polyacrylamide is an inert support whose porosity is easily adjusted by changing the composition of acrylamide prior to polymerization. Although *polyacrylamide gel electrophoresis* (PAGE) is applicable to standard separation of native proteins, it can also be used for separating proteins according to molecular weight when they are denatured in the presence of sodium dodecyl sulfate (SDS). SDS-PAGE is at present the most widely used protein electrophoretic technique for research in molecular biology. However, its very power for resolving proteins and separating them into multitudinous subunits has virtually excluded it from routine use in the clinical laboratory. Nevertheless, there is promise for clinical application of *two-dimensional electrophoresis* (2-DE), which uses standard separation in one direction followed by SDS-PAGE in the perpendicular direction. 2-DE results in perhaps hundreds of identifiable protein peaks from which it may be possible to obtain important diagnostic information by sophisticated pattern analysis.

Isoelectric focusing affords superior resolution of closely migrating proteins or various forms of a single protein that differ in charge owing to minor modifications (e.g., post-translational). By this technique, proteins migrate through a gel containing a gradient of pH established with a mixture of ampholytes. As each protein reaches the gel location where the pH is equal to its pI, the net charge on it becomes zero. It no longer has electromotive force acting on it, and it comes to rest. Thus the final pattern is strictly according to pI.

Precipitation

Chemical precipitations of serum proteins have been devised to resolve albumin and the globulins into two or more fractions that can then be measured for protein content. With the addition of sodium sulfate, sodium sulfite, ammonium sulfate, or methanol, the globulins tend to precipitate, leaving albumin in solution. By measuring total protein in the original serum and protein in either the precipitate or the supernatant, values for albumin and globulin can be derived. The ratio of these values (A/G ratio) has been used extensively because it accentuates abnormalities in serum protein composition, which in disease generally involve depression of albumin and elevation of one or more globulin fractions. Albumin may be depressed owing to either decreased synthesis (malnutrition, malabsorption, liver failure, diversion to synthesis of other proteins) or increased loss (proteinuria, accumulation of ascites fluid, enteropathy). Globulins may be elevated owing to increased synthesis of many different proteins as

2

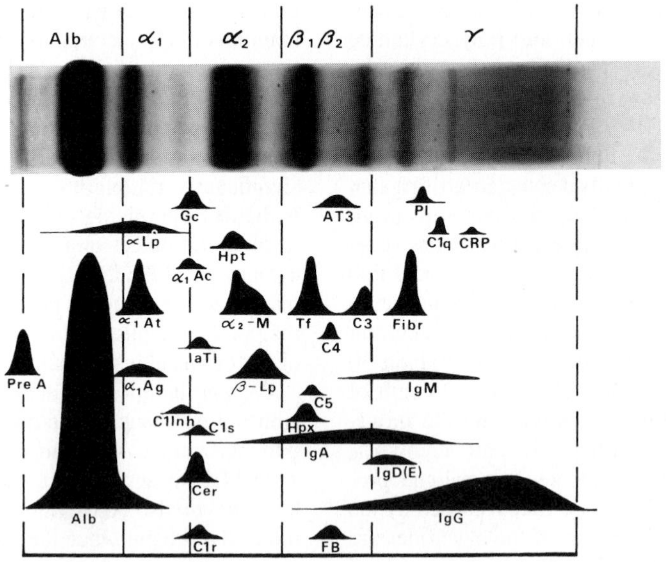

Figure 11–1. Plasma protein electrophoresis pattern in agarose gel is composed of five fractions, each composed of many individual species (see Fig. 11–2). Some of the major proteins are shown here in an artist's rendition for clarity. (Adapted from Laurell C B: Electrophoresis, specific protein assays, or both in measurement of plasma proteins? Clin Chem 1973; 19:99.)

α_1Ac = Alpha-1-antichymotrypsin
α_1Ag = Alpha-1-acid glycoprotein
α_1At = Alpha-1-antitrypsin
α_2-M = Alpha-2-macroglobulin
α-LP = Alpha lipoprotein
Alb = Albumin
AT3 = Antithrombin III
β-Lp = Beta lipoprotein
Complement components:
Clq, Clr, Cls, C3, C4, C5 = As designated
ClInh = Cl esterase inhibitor
Cer = Ceruloplasmin
CRP = C-reactive protein
Gc = Gc-globulin (vitamin D-binding protein)
FB = Factor B
Fibr = Fibrinogen
Hpt = Haptoglobin
Hpx = Hemopexin
Immunoglobulins:
IgA, IgD, IgE, IgG, IgM 6 = As designated
Pl = Plasminogen
Pre A = Prealbumin
Tf = Transferrin

part of acute or chronic reactions to disease. The lowering of albumin and elevation of globulins tend to occur simultaneously in disease, thus leading to exaggerated changes in the A/G ratio as the numerator and denominator move in opposite directions. Precipitation methods are not as accurate as zonal electrophoresis, because some alpha globulins may fail to precipitate and thus lead to an overestimate of the albumin fraction.

Preparative procedures for the isolation of a single minor protein constituent usually begin with a precipitation step to remove the bulk of other undesired serum proteins. The next step in protein isolation is typically a column that separates on the basis of molecular size (gel filtration) or charge (ion exchange).

Column Separations

Gel filtration media such as Sephadex or agarose beads are rated according to pore sizes, which, in turn, determine what size molecules can pass through the interior of each bead or particle of the column. After application of a sample composed of various sized proteins in aqueous solvent containing buffer and salt, more of the buffer is applied to drive the sample through the column. Very large molecules tend to flow through interstices of the column without entering the beads and emerge first from the bottom of the column in the void volume. Slightly smaller molecules enter the largest pores before being washed through and so are slightly retarded in passing through the column. Small protein molecules pass into still smaller pores and are retained still longer. Finally, particles the size of dissolved salt penetrate farthest into the interior of gel filtration beads and come out after all the proteins have emerged in an amount of applied buffer called the salt volume. Thus, in gel filtration, the order of protein elution is by molecular weight or size from largest first to smallest last. Because all protein species continuously move through a gel filtration column all at the same time but with different rates, it is necessary to apply the sample in a small and uniform volume in order to optimize separation between peaks. Gel filtration requires that the medium be inert and not interact chemically or by charge with the proteins. It is not a method to be employed for high-resolution separation.

Ion exchange chromatography, on the other hand, takes advantage of the charge on proteins to bind them to beads of a charged support medium such as DEAE or QAE. In *anion exchange chromatography,* proteins are usually applied at a basic pH such as 8.6, at which they are either negatively charged (albumin and α_1-, α_2-, and β-globulins are anions) or have no net charge (γ-globulins). The neutral proteins pass immediately through an anion exchange column, whereas the anionic ones stick to the positively charged column matrix. If a buffer with a higher salt concentration is washed through, anions of the salt displace the anionic proteins and exchange for them by binding to the support medium. The proteins then elute from the column. By using a steadily increasing gradient of salt concentration in the eluting buffer, the proteins can be resolved according to charge. The ones with a small amount of charge will elute first, whereas those with the greatest charge (e.g., albumin) elute only when displaced by higher salt levels.

Alternatively, if pH is lowered while salt concentration is held low, anionic proteins acquire a net neutral or slightly positive charge and pass through the column. A gradient of falling pH can be used to resolve anionic proteins, with the order of elution being roughly β-, α_2-, and α_1-globulins, and albumin. Note that this order of elution is the reverse order of electrophoretic migration at pH 8.6, because in anion exchange chromatography, mobility is retarded according to net negative charge, whereas in electrophoresis the mobility is enhanced by that charge.

Cation exchange chromatography begins at an acid pH with the proteins having positive charge (cations) and adhering to a negatively charged column matrix such as carboxymethylcellulose. They can be displaced by the cations of high salt in an eluting buffer or by increasing the pH, which will reverse the charge on the proteins to negative. By cation exchange, albumin should elute first, followed by α_1-, α_2-, β-, and γ-globulins.

Another separation modality by column is *hydrophobic chromatography*, in which samples are applied at high salt and eluted with low salt. The support medium interacts with proteins according to hydrophobic nature and is a good complementary technique to follow ion exchange chromatography, in which the sample was eluted with high salt.

Affinity chromatography is based on specific binding between a protein of interest and another protein that has been covalently linked to the solid support medium of a column. For example, coagulation Factor VIII complexed with von Willebrand factor (vWF) can be selectively removed from the other plasma proteins by passing plasma through a column that contains monoclonal anti-vWF antibody linked to the solid phase matrix. The Factor VIII–vWF complex selectively binds to the column as other plasma proteins wash through. The Factor VIII is then dissociated from the vWF thereby allowing it to elute in a purified fraction suitable for transfusion therapy. Such antigen-antibody interactions may be disrupted by high salt concentration, change in pH, or a chemical denaturant, such as urea, in different applications. Other affinity chromatography gels use a binding phenomenon that mimics naturally occurring molecular interactions. Thus, some dyes coupled to agarose are able to bind albumin thereby removing it selectively from serum. Immunoglobulins can also be absorbed from a sample by staphylococcal protein A coupled to the gel matrix. Many other separation schemes exist that effect a high degree of purification in a single step with affinity chromatography medium coupled to dyes, drugs, nucleotide cofactors, and sugars. The most widespread clinical testing using affinity chromatography is quantitation of glycosylated hemoglobin using a dihydroxyboronate affinity matrix that selectively binds molecular species of hemoglobin to which glucose has been covalently attached, while allowing the nonglycosylated forms to pass through the column. The glycosylated hemoglobin is then separately eluted and quantitated.

PROTEIN DETECTION AND QUANTITATION

The ultimate reference method for determining concentration of protein is the analysis for *nitrogen content*. Nitrogen is present uniformly along the peptide bonds throughout the length of a protein and more irregularly in the side groups wherever tryptophan, arginine, lysine, histidine, asparagine, or glutamine is present. The Kjeldahl technique consists of an acid digestion to release ammonium ions from nitrogen-containing compounds. The ammonium can then be quantitated by conversion to ammonia gas and titration as a base or by nesslerization, in which double iodides (potassium and mercuric) form a colored complex with ammonia in alkali. Although determination of nitrogen content can be extremely precise, its use for calculation of protein concentration depends on the exact protein composition of a sample, since each protein has a somewhat different nitrogen content according to amino acid composition. However, for a sample of a purified protein, nitrogen content is highly accurate for estimating protein concentration when the nitrogen content on a molar basis is already known for that purified protein. Knowledge of a protein's exact amino acid sequence allows an accurate calculation of what the nitrogen content should be. Because clinical samples consist of unpredictable mixtures of different proteins and measurement of nitrogen content is not a simple procedure, it is not commonly used in clinical laboratories.

Refractive index can be accurate for measuring serum protein concentration as dissolved solute for levels above 2.5 g/dL. Hemolysis, lipemia, icterus, and azotemia produce erroneously high results. Refractive index cannot be used for urine protein measurements because of excess amounts of solutes in relation to the protein.

Specific gravity (and thus, by inference, protein content) can be estimated by pipetting drops of serum or blood into a graded series of copper sulfate solutions. A protein-copper shell forms about the drop to prevent dissolution for a short interval, during which the drop falls to the bottom, remains stationary, or rises to the top. The protein concentration of a sample is estimated from the specific gravity of the copper sulfate solution in which the drop remains stationary. This technique is simple and has been used widely as a screening test for hemoglobin concentration in whole blood.

Proteins in solution *absorb ultraviolet light* at 280 nm (A280), owing mostly to tryptophan but also owing to tyrosine and phenylalanine (Layne, 1957). For accurate conversion of A280 readings to protein concentration, the molar absorptivity must be used, because each protein contains a different amount of these three amino acids. However, the A280 of a mixture of proteins is not an accurate measure of protein content, because molar absorptivities vary greatly between different proteins. Because nucleic acids (which absorb strongly at 260 nm and also somewhat at 280 nm) may be present in protein preparations, a better estimate of protein concentration in the presence of nucleic acids is given by the formula:

$$\text{Protein concentration (mg/mL)} = 1.55 \times A_{280} - 0.76 \times A_{260}$$

Direct measurements of absorbance can be used for quantitating proteins in the range of 0.05 to 1.5 mg/mL.

Turbidimetric methods are often used for a similar concentration range in cerebrospinal fluid (CSF) or urine. Protein forms precipitate on the addition of trichloroacetic acid, sulfosalicylic acid, or other acid reagent. The resulting turbidity can be used for protein quantitation by increment in optical density in comparison with similarly treated standards. However, these techniques are not specific to proteins, because other acid-insoluble substances such as nucleic acids can also precipitate.

A *colorimetric* technique highly specific for proteins and peptides is the *biuret* method by which copper salts in alkaline solution form a purple complex with substances containing two or more peptide bonds. Interferences are minimal, although ammonium ion may acidify the reaction, while hemoglobin and bilirubin absorb in the same region as the biuret complex (540 to 560 nm). The biuret method is extensively used in clinical laboratories, particularly in automated analyzers in which protein concentration can be measured down to 10 or 15 mg/dL.

Greater sensitivity can be obtained using the *Folin-Ciocalteu reagent* (or phenol reagent, phosphotungstomolybdic acid), which oxidizes phenolic compounds such as tyrosine and, in addition, tryptophan and histidine to give a deep blue color.

Lowry (1951) used the biuret method followed by the phenol reagent, which greatly enhanced color formation, because the phenol reagent can react with biuret complexes involving all the peptide bonds. The *Lowry assay* has been extensively used for consistently accurate determinations of protein concentration.

Further sensitivity for detection of down to 1 μg of protein can be obtained using *Coomassie brilliant blue dye*, which is free of interferences from a very wide range of substances.

Comparable sensitivity is also obtained with *ninhydrin*, which develops a violet color by reacting with primary amines. This reagent is widely used for detection of peptides and amino acids after paper chromatography and amino acid analyses from ion exchange columns.

Quantitation of albumin in the presence of other proteins is possible by virtue of the specific binding of albumin to certain dyes such as bromphenol blue, methyl orange, HABA, bromcresol purple, and bromcresol green (BCG). BCG is extensively used in automatic analyzers for determining serum albumin in parallel with biuret reagent for total protein. Dyes bound to albumin absorb maximally at slightly different wavelengths, thus allowing direct spectrophotometric quantitation of the albumin.

The standard dyes used for staining in electrophoresis are Coomassie brilliant blue, ponceau S, and amido black. For detection of minor components in high-resolution gels, silver staining is very sensitive down to nanogram quantities (Merril, 1981).

In addition, special dyes, such as Oil Red O and Sudan black, stain lipoproteins and periodic acid–Schiff stains glycoproteins separated in special electrophoretic applications.

Because electrophoresis followed by staining does not afford explicit identification of serum proteins, immunologic measurements have been instituted for quantitation of individual proteins (Laurell, 1966; Fig. 11–2). Nephelometry detects the turbidity produced usually within minutes or less by

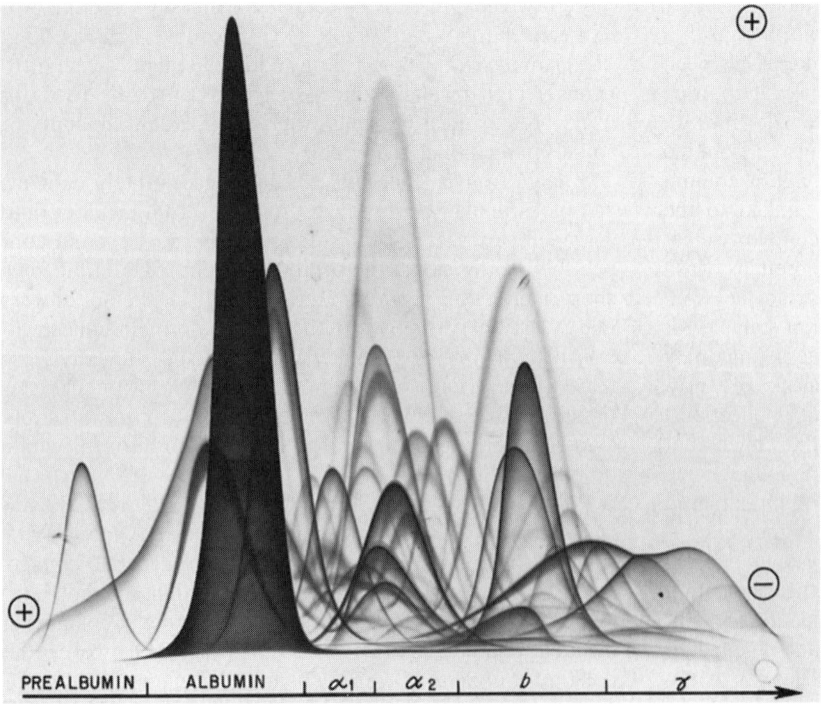

Figure 11–2. Two-dimensional crossed immunoelectrophoresis in a gel containing high-quality anti–whole serum shows a complex population of proteins spread from prealbumin to gamma globulin. Each electrophoretic fraction can be seen to contain all or part of many individual species each identified as a separate "rocket." The dense peak at left is albumin, and the broadest peak at the right is IgG. Without specific studies, it is impossible to unequivocally identify any of the others. (Plate courtesy of DAKOPATTES, A-F, DK-2000, Copenhagen, Denmark.)

the precipitation of a reagent antibody with its target protein in a serum sample. The major serum proteins are now widely measured by this method on automated immunochemistry analyzers that have supplanted former measurements by radial immunodiffusion. Owing to the specificity of the antibody reagent, nephelometry has great specificity for quantitating individual proteins even in the presence of others. Proteins present in lower concentrations may also be quantitated by immunologic methods, such as radioimmunoassay or enzyme-linked immunosorbent assay (ELISA).

SPECIFIC PLASMA PROTEINS

Major Components

The major serum proteins are those components that are readily resolved and detected on electrophoretic gels stained by conventional clinical laboratory techniques (Table 11–1).

PREALBUMIN. Prealbumin is defined electrophoretically as the fraction that migrates in a position faster than albumin toward the anode. Prealbumin has a tetrameric structure with total molecular weight of 62,000 daltons, making it one of the smaller serum proteins. Each monomer can bind a molecule of thyroxine. As such, it is also called thyroxine-binding prealbumin (TBPA) or transthyretin (TTR), although only a small fraction of thyroxine is actually bound to TBPA in normal individuals, because thyroxine-binding globulin has a 100-fold greater affinity for thyroxine (Oppenheimer, 1968). However, there is at least one molecular variant of prealbumin, inherited in a familial pattern, that has a greatly increased affinity for thyroxine resulting in elevated serum thyroxine content, although those individuals have normal free thyroxine concentrations and so are euthyroid (Moses, 1982).

Prealbumin plays a significant role in the metabolism of vitamin A by complexing with the retinol-binding protein (RBP), which, in turn, complexes with vitamin A to transport it through the body (Peterson, 1971). RBP is a small protein of only 182 amino acids, and so it would be rapidly removed from the circulation by filtration through the kidney if it were not held in the plasma by the larger protein prealbumin, which is not cleared into the glomerular filtrate.

Prealbumin is rich in tryptophan (sometimes called tryptophan-rich prealbumin) and also has considerable β-pleated sheet conformation. A portion of prealbumin is the source of the beta-fibrillar amyloid component in type I familial amyloidotic polyneuropathy (Glenner, 1980). This hereditary amyloidosis derives from a mutation in the prealbumin gene that results in a protein (e.g., TTR met 30 variant) susceptible to proteolytic cleavage creating the beta structured fragments that are the building blocks of amyloid in nerve fibers (Li, 1991; Saraiva, 1989). This pathogenetic variant of prealbumin cannot be distinguished from normal by standard protein electrophoresis. Current diganosis is based on analysis at the DNA level.

Prealbumin has a relatively short half-life in the circulation (roughly two days) compared with other major serum proteins. Its synthetic rate is also exquisitely sensitive to intake of adequate nutrition and to alterations in hepatic function where it is produced. Therefore, prealbumin concentrations in serum fluctuate more rapidly in response to alterations in synthetic rate than do those of other proteins such as albumin. For that reason, quantitation of serum prealbumin has major clinical utility as a marker for nutritional status (Gofferje, 1978). Because of the rapid dynamics of its synthesis and clearance, prealbumin is considered to be a better early indicator of change in nutritional status than other commonly used markers, such as albumin and transferrin, which are more abundant but whose levels respond to other factors as well and at slower time scales.

Because of its compactness, prealbumin crosses more easily into the CSF than do the other serum proteins. Therefore, concentrating CSF prior to electrophoresis allows visualization of a distinct prealbumin band in CSF. CSF normally contains a major peak of albumin plus prealbu-min and a small amount of transferrin. Electrophoresis of CSF is usually requested for detection of oligoclonal bands of immunoglobulin, and the presence of a distinct band of prealbumin is used only as a landmark to confirm that the specimen was likely CSF. True prealbumin is generally below the level of detection by serum electrophoresis; instead it is best quantified by immunologic measurements such as nephelometry. A protein band frequently appears in the prealbumin position of patients who have had heparin therapy. In the circulation,

2

Table 11–1. CHARACTERISTICS OF MAJOR PLASMA PROTEINS

Protein	Concentration Range (g/L)	Molecular Weight	Actions
Prealbumin	0.15–0.36	62,000	Binds thyroxine: transports vitamin A
Albumin	39–51	66,000	Oncotic pressure: amino acid reservoir: carries small molecules
α_1-Antitrypsin	2.0–4.0	54,000	Protease inhibitor
α_2-Macroglobulin	1.5–3.5	725,000	Protease inhibitor
Haptoglobulin	0.4–2.9	1,000,000 (Type 1–1)	Binds hemoglobin
β-Lipoprotein	2.7–7.4	380,000	Lipid transport
Transferrin	2.0–4.0	80,000	Transports iron
C3	0.6–1.4	185,000	Component of complement system
Fibrinogen	1.0–4.0	340,000	Clot formation
Immunoglobulin A	0.4–3.5	160,000	Surface immunity
Immunoglobulin D	0.1–0.4	180,000	
Immunoglobulin E	50–600 (μg/L)	180,000	Binds to mast cells: hypersensitivity reactions
Immunoglobulin G	7–15	150,000	Humoral immunity
Immunoglobulin M	0.25–2.0	850,000	Humoral immunity primary response

heparin activates and releases lipoprotein lipase activity, which attacks triglycerides in lipoprotein fractions, thereby greatly enhancing their electrophoretic migration anodally. Protein stain reveals the apolipoproteins in the prealbumin position but no beta lipoprotein fraction. This is an *in vivo* effect that does not occur if heparin is added to samples already collected.

ALBUMIN. The single most abundant protein in normal plasma is albumin, usually constituting up to two thirds of total plasma protein (Peters, 1975). For that reason, depressions in albumin level due to impaired synthesis (e.g., malnutrition, malabsorption, hepatic dysfunction) (Rothschild, 1972) or to losses (e.g., ascites or protein-losing nephropathy or enteropathy) result in serious imbalance of intravascular oncotic pressure. This loss is manifested clinically by the development of peripheral edema (Slater, 1975). However, the congenital absence of albumin (analbuminemia) generally does not lead to such problems, presumably because of lifelong compensatory mechanisms that control hydrostatic pressures (Waldmann, 1964). Albumin also serves as a mobile repository of amino acids from the liver, where it is synthesized, to other tissues, where it is broken down intracellularly into free amino acids for incorporation into other proteins. A third function ascribed to albumin is that of a general transport or carrier protein. Many organic and inorganic ligands (e.g., thyroxine, bilirubin, penicillin, cortisol, estrogen, free fatty acids, warfarin [Coumadin], calcium, magnesium, and heme) complex with different regions of the albumin molecule in either covalent (e.g., delta bilirubin) (Lauff, 1982) or dissociable binding (Koch-Weser, 1976). These binding in-teractions with very different ligands are possible because of a wide variety of binding sites on the albumin molecule, which consists of 585 amino acids arranged in nine loops held together by the disulfide bonds between cysteine residues (Meloun, 1975). The primary sequence of albumin contains three major regions with three peptide loops each, suggesting that it arose from gene duplication of some ancestral gene in a tandem rearrangement process (Peters, 1977; Sevall, 1986). It is also interesting to note that α-fetoprotein has regions of homology with serum albumin, which may indicate a common ancestral gene origin for these two proteins.

In addition to the genetic abnormality of analbuminemia, there are many hereditary variants of albumin that differ from the most common allotype, albumin A, by single amino acid substitutions. These variants can be either rapid or slow migrating compared with albumin A, leading to two distinct albumin peaks (bisalbuminemia) in the heterozygous state. None of the variant albumins appear to affect health, but a recently described variant does have greatly enhanced affinity for thyroxine, which leads to elevated thyroxine content in the serum of such persons, who nevertheless remain euthyroid (Ruiz, 1982). Up to 8% of albumin circulating in normal persons becomes glucosylated nonenzymatically, whereas up to 25% becomes glucosylated during hyperglycemia in analogy with glucosylated hemoglobin (Guthrow, 1979). The half-life of circulating albumin is about 17 days, so that measurements of the glucosylated form may be useful in monitoring diabetic control during a short interval.

Analysis of newly synthesized albumin from intracellular sites has revealed the existence of a precursor proalbumin, which has an additional hexapeptide at its amino terminal end. The primary structure of albumin has 35 cysteine residues, of which 34 form intramolecular disulfide bonds and one remains free. On storage for many days, albumin forms covalently linked dimers through the free cysteines, resulting occasionally in an extra band of albumin on electrophoresis.

Clinical measurements of albumin are very frequent, with determinations of total protein and albumin often included in chemistry panel profiles. Elevations of serum albumin concentration are infrequent, although they do occur in dehydration as the plasma water phase shrinks. Following rehydration, the albumin level should fall to within the normal reference range. Elevation of serum albumin may also occur artifactually as the result of prolonged application of a tourniquet for venipuncture. In that instance, the increased hydrodynamic pressure from venous backup forces water and small solutes out of the intravascular space, thereby concentrating cellular elements, micellar forms of lipoproteins, and proteins such as albumin.

Depression of albumin concentrations are frequent in sick individuals, and a review of hospitalized patients reveals a substantial proportion of albumin measurements that are below healthy reference ranges. Although some of these decreases are likely dilutional owing to the administration of intravenous fluids, others are caused by loss of albumin into urine, ascites fluid, or the gastrointestinal tract in enteropathies or by decreased synthesis in the liver due to either hepatic disease such as cirrhosis or to the secondary effect on synthesis from compromised nutrition or diversion of synthetic capacity to other proteins. Measurements of albumin concentrations are vital to the understanding and interpretation of calcium and magnesium levels because these ions are bound to albumin, and so decreases of albumin are directly responsible for depression of their concentrations, too. In some disease states, decreases in albumin are at least partially compensated for by increases in other serum proteins, thereby stabilizing oncotic pressures intravascularly. In particular, cirrhosis shows a major polyclonal increase of immunoglobulins in the gamma fraction and nephrotic syndrome shows high levels of α_2-macroglobulin (AMG).

Body fluids that form normally, such as CSF, or pathologically, such as filtrates of plasma (e.g., ascites), contain albumin as the major component with very little contribution from other plasma proteins. The presence of albumin in the urine is generally considered abnormal even in trace amounts, although some healthy individuals exhibit albuminuria following intense exercise. Progression of diabetic nephropathy can be assessed by the quantitative measurement of albuminuria, as it tends to appear ahead of the other serum proteins in urine during the course of renal glomerular damage. The immunologic measurement of microalbumin in urine is now considered a standard of care for management of diabetes mellitus and the early detection of diabetic complications.

α_1-ANTITRYPSIN. The major component of the α_1-globulins is the protease inhibitor α_1-antitrypsin (AAT), which has the capacity to combine with and inactivate trypsin (Eriksson, 1965; Berninger, 1985). The first clue to this function came with the discovery that the serum of some young adults with pulmonary emphysema was deficient in α_1-globulin. Further investigations revealed a similar deficiency of AAT in children with cirrhosis (Sveger, 1976). Usually, there are no appreciable circulating levels of trypsin in blood, but other related proteases, such as elastase, are released from leukocytes responding to irritants or inflammation. AAT is able to neutralize the activity of these proteases, too, and hence is an intrinsic factor in the homeostatic mechanism modulating endogenous proteolysis within the body and preventing inappropriately severe biochemical response to inflammation (Cow, 1986).

The majority of people are homozygous for the normal fully active M allele of AAT, or phenotype MM (Lieberman, 1972). About 10% of whites (and fewer of other races) are heterozygous for M and some other allele of the protease inhibitor or Pi system. More than 2% carry the PiZ allele and exhibit the phenotype MZ. Although these individuals have somewhat reduced levels of trypsin inhibitory capacity in serum, they are asymptomatic; however, their homozygous ZZ offspring are susceptible to pulmonary or hepatic disease. The ZZ phenotype occurs in about 1 in 4000 individuals. Serum protein electrophoresis may be used to screen for AAT deficiency, but confirmation must be made with ancillary tests such as trypsin inhibitory capacity (TIC) and phenotyping by cross-electrophoresis or isoelectric focusing (Jeppsson, 1982) in order to rule out the presence of some other alleles, such as PiS or PiF, which migrate differently. These alleles result in a lower TIC but probably are sufficient to prevent the abnormalities seen with the ZZ phenotype, which has a very low TIC corresponding to low concentration of antigenic AAT. Screening can also be conducted in suspected cases by nephelometry to quantitate serum levels of AAT. Only the ZZ phenotype yields markedly low levels of AAT. Definitive typing may require analysis of the DNA sequence for the *AAT* gene. At least 75 different alleles exist for AAT. About 17 alleles have sufficiently low protein production to lead to pulmonary disease, and only a few are responsible for liver disease (Cow, 1986).

Therapy for pulmonary emphysema secondary to AAT deficiency has been greatly advanced with intravenous replacement of AAT, using concentrates or recombinant protein, to bring circulating levels into ranges sufficient for anti-elastase protection to the lungs (Snider, 1989). Further replacement has also been successful with AAT inhalation for patients in whom pulmonary disease has not yet become extensive (Hubbard, 1989). Avoidance of cigarette smoking by homozygous individuals is essential, because cigarette smoke is a major source of irritants that trigger leukocytes in the lung to release proteases (Gelb, 1976). The cirrhosis in young children is treated by hepatic transplant, because the liver is the site of AAT synthesis. An interesting aspect of cirrhosis and the ZZ phenotype is the presence of unsialylated mutant type AAT granules in the hepatocytes, implying a defect of secretion in those alleles. Cirrhosis secondary to AAT abnormality has not been improved by replacement therapy. Children with this disorder can develop progressive, severe cholestasis prompting liver transplantation. Following transplant, the recipient takes on the AAT phenotype of the donor.

AAT is one of the serum glycoproteins that rise in response to acute inflammation, but such elevations lack clinical specificity. The α_1-fraction never appears completely empty in AAT deficiency, because other proteins (e.g., α-lipoprotein, α_1-acid glycoprotein) migrate there but do not resolve into distinct bands.

α_2-MACROGLOBULIN. AMG is one of the largest, non-immunoglobulin proteins in plasma, with a molecular weight of 725,000 daltons (Roberts, 1985). The serum concentration in normal individuals is comparable to the other major protease inhibitor AAT, although women have higher levels than men in response to estrogen (Horne, 1970). The concentration of AMG rises tenfold or more in the nephrotic syndrome when other lower molecular weight proteins are lost (Beetham, 1993). The loss of AMG into urine is prevented by its large size. The net result is that AMG reaches serum levels equal to or greater than albumin (about 2 to 3 g/dL) in the nephrotic syndrome, which has the effect of maintaining oncotic pressure. There may also be enhanced synthesis of AMG in nephrotic syndrome, which accounts for its absolute increase in concentration. AMG inactivates proteases by complexing with them and forming covalent bonds to them. Its own conformation is thereby altered, which enhances clearance by the reticuloendothelial system. There are at least four molecular forms of AMG that differ in sialic acid, mannose, and galactose content and that can be separated by isoelectric focusing. Other molecular variations probably are the result of proteases linked to AMG prior to removal from the circulation. The spectrum of inhibition by AMG is very wide, including virtually all types of serine, carboxyl, thiol, and metal proteases. Although AMG function is certainly important for maintaining balance in the ebb and flow of proteolysis, no specific deficiency state with associated disease has been recognized, and there is no disease state generally attributed to low concentrations of AMG. Mild but distinct elevations of AMG can be observed on serum protein electrophoresis early in the course of diabetic nephropathy.

HAPTOGLOBIN. The other major protein migrating in the α_2-region is haptoglobin, which has the function of combining with hemoglobin released by lysis of red cells in order to preserve body iron and protein stores. The circulating half-life of haptoglobin, free of hemoglobin, is roughly four days. Hemoglobin-haptoglobin complexes are removed from the circulation within minutes by the reticuloendothelial system, where the hemoglobin is broken down into globin and heme, which further degrades to iron and bilirubin. When the hemoglobin-binding capacity of haptoglobin is exceeded, the free hemoglobin enters the glomerular filtrate as alpha chain–beta chain dimers that are subsequently reabsorbed in the proximal renal tubules and converted to hemosiderin.

Haptoglobin has two heavy chains and two light chains linked by disulfide bonds in analogy to the basic structure of immunoglobins. Some persons have a light chain gene that is duplicated in a head-to-tail arrangement (Type 2). Normal haptoglobin (Type 1–1) gives rise to a single molecular species of molecular weight 100,000. Heterozygous individuals (1–2) have, in addition to Type 1–1 haptoglobin, a series of multimers (e.g., dimers, trimers) by virtue of intermolecular disulfide linkages through the duplicated light chain. Type 2–2 haptoglobin consists of a different series of multimers, because Type 2 light chain has a different molecular weight from the Type 1 light chain (Konigsberg, 1974).

Haptoglobin can be quantitated in terms of its hemoglobin-binding capacity or by immunologic means, especially nephelometry. Owing to steric hindrance between molecular sites on the multimers, the different phenotypes of haptoglobin yield measurements of antigen- or hemoglobin-binding capacity that may be discrepant with the absolute amount of haptoglobin protein present in a sample. Accordingly, the reference range for haptoglobin is broader for an entire population of different phenotypes than within individual phenotypes. For that reason, interpretation of haptoglobin concentrations is soundest for serial measurements in the same individual. However, very high levels can readily be distinguished from very low ones, which can be important in the first-time evaluation of a patient for hemolysis.

Serum haptoglobin rises in response to stress, infection, acute inflammation, or tissue necrosis, probably by stimulation of synthesis (see the section entitled Acute Phase Reactants, later). After a hemolytic episode, haptoglobin concentrations fall as the complexes with hemoglobin are cleared from the circulation. This effect is dramatic following massive hemolysis in situations of hemolytic transfusion reaction, thermal burns, or autoimmune hemolytic anemia. It is also a useful measurement for serially monitoring patients who have a slow but steady rate of red cell breakdown such as by mechanical heart valves, hemoglobinopathies, or exercise-associated trauma. Low haptoglobin concentrations may accompany liver disease when hepatic synthetic capacity is impaired. There are also individuals with congenital deficiency of haptoglobin who apparently use other mechanisms to conserve body iron stores. Serum samples from blood hemolyzed *in vitro* during phlebotomy or processing show a displaced band of haptoglobin-hemoglobin complex on protein electrophoresis.

It should be noted that myoglobin does not bind to haptoglobin, and therefore, release of large amounts of myoglobin by rhabdomyolysis does not diminish haptoglobin levels in serum. This difference can be useful in the workup of a positive dipstick test for blood (actually a test for pseudo-peroxidase activity of heme in hemoglobin or myoglobin) in urine with no coexisting red cells. In that case, low serum haptoglobin suggests hemoglobinuria (hemolysis), and high serum haptoglobin suggests myoglobinuria. Lactate dehydrogenase (LD) isoenzyme 1 in serum is also associated with hemolysis, whereas LD5 is released in rhabdomyolysis.

β-LIPOPROTEIN. β-Lipoprotein (low-density lipoprotein, LDL) migrates with a characteristic sharp leading cathodal edge and feathery trailing region more anodally. Although it is better quantitated by stains for lipid, there is sufficient apoprotein content to be a distinct band on staining for protein. The exact position of the β-lipoprotein band is sensitive to recent ingestion of fatty foods, and so, samples from fasting versus postprandial collections will show the β-lipoprotein in slightly different positions. The other lipoproteins (VLDL, HDL, and chylomicrons) are relatively small in intensity, and they occur in overlapping electrophoretic positions with other serum proteins so that these fractions are generally not appreciated on protein stain. Administration of heparin activates post-heparin lipoprotein lipase, which degrades triglycerides in the circulating lipoprotein fractions. Consequently, heparinized patients frequently demonstrate a transiently anomalous band of β-lipoprotein that can migrate very rapidly and also unevenly across the electrophoretic path, even into the prealbumin region. Elevations of LDL, with greater staining intensity to the β-lipoprotein band, occur in hypercholesterolemia. Lipoproteins are discussed more thoroughly in Chapter 10.

TRANSFERRIN. The major β-globulin is transferrin (siderophilin), which transports ferric ions from the iron stores of intracellular or mucosal ferritin to bone marrow, where erythrocyte precursors and lymphocytes have transferrin receptors on their surfaces (Irie, 1987).

Transferrin consists of 687 amino acids with a calculated molecular weight of 79,550 daltons (MacGillivray, 1982). Analysis of the amino acid sequence shows that transferrin has two homologous domains that may have arisen by contiguous duplication of an ancestral transferrin gene. Each domain has a binding site with very high affinity for iron. Transcription of mRNA for transferrin synthesis in the liver is regulated by the concentration of iron in the circulation and surrounding the hepatocytes.

In normal serum, transferrin ranges in concentration from 200 to 400 mg/dL, which is conveniently measured as iron-binding capacity (IBC) (Tsung, 1975). In response to short-term iron deficiency, transferrin levels rise markedly to twice normal levels or higher. Because transferrin is a single molecular species with a tight electrophoretic mobility, an elevated level can have the appearance of a paraprotein (pseudoparaproteinemia) in cases of severe iron deficiency (Zawadzki, 1970). At least some iron deficiency and elevation of transferrin should be expected with pregnancy (Mendenhall, 1970). Administration of iron to deficient patients increases the saturation followed by return of transferrin to normal.

Chronic saturation of transferrin occurs in idiopathic hemochromatosis and transfusional hemosiderosis. Because there is almost no unsaturated IBC in those syndromes, iron cannot be mobilized normally for excretion, resulting in the disorders of deposition that also occur in congenital deficiency of transferrin. Current strategies to screen for hemochromatosis include measurement of serum iron and serum transferrin (usually by nephelometric immunoassay), with the calculation of percent saturation as the best index for identifying previously unrecognized cases. Hemochromatosis is a hereditary disorder that results in cirrhosis, diabetes, cardiomyopathy, arthritis, and other endocrine disorders owing to the toxic effects of excess free iron. Screening for hemochromatosis is desirable because the disease progression can be halted by lowering the body burden of iron by such means as phlebotomy or chelation therapy.

Transferrin may also demonstrate an antibacterial effect by complexing iron and removing it from bacteria that require iron for growth (McFarlane, 1970; Weinberg, 1978).

In protein-losing nephropathy of sufficient severity, transferrin is lost from the circulation into the urine, carrying iron with it. This loss may contribute to the development of hypochromic anemia.

In addition to prealbumin and albumin, CSF contains a small peak of normal transferrin plus an altered transferrin with a more cathodal electrophoretic mobility due to a difference in carbohydrate content (sialic acid). This altered transferrin may be useful as a confirmatory marker for identifying CSF (e.g., in cases of rhinorrhea).

Electrophoretic variants of transferrin occur occasionally in serum owing to allotypic variation in the amino acid sequence and hence have a different charge on the molecule. In that case, the heterozygous state shows a doublet in place of a single electrophoretic band for transferrin.

COMPLEMENT. A separate fraction of β-globulin consists of the C3 component of complement. Although this protein can be resolved easily with a fresh serum sample, in stored specimens and commercial control serum that has been lyophilized, C3 is cleaved to form C3c, which migrates anodally to native C3 as a band nondistinct from other beta globulins. Depression of C3 occurs in autoimmune disorders when the complement system is activated and C3 becomes bound to immune complexes deposited in tissues, thereby removing them from plasma. Thus, C3 (and also C4) concentration is a convenient marker for assessing disease activity in the rheumatic disorders such as lupus erythematosus and rheumatoid arthritis. C4 is not appreciated on serum protein electrophoresis because its concentration is normally only about one fifth that of C3. Both C3 and C4 are now easily quantitated by nephelometry for monitoring rheumatic disease activity. No particular diagnostic significance is ascribed to higher than normal levels of C3 or C4 except as mild indicators of an acute phase response. The complement system and its inhibitors are discussed further in Chapter 36.

FIBRINOGEN. Plasma contains 100 to 400 mg/dL of fibrinogen, which is the most abundant of the coagulation factors and which forms the fibrin clot. With an overall molecular weight of 340,000 daltons, fibrinogen is a dimer consisting of three pairs of peptide chains (A-α, B-β, and γ) linked with multiple disulfide bonds near their amino terminal ends (Doolittle, 1975). This region of the molecule is termed the E domain or disulfide knot (DSK). The chains extend outward into two other identical domains (D) at their carboxyl ends, where all three chains are intertwined. Thrombin cleaves fibrinopeptides A and B from the amino ends of the A-α and B-β chains, thereby resulting in a fibrin monomer that polymerizes into fibrils that macroscopically form a fibrin clot. Factor XIII then produces covalent bonds between lysine and glutamine residues on adjacent gamma chains of different fibrin molecules, making the fibrin clot essentially a single molecule. A cross-linked clot is refractory to dissolution by chemical denaturants and is mechanically very stable.

Numerous hereditary variants of fibrinogen (dysfibrinogenemias) have been identified, in which a functionally abnormal fibrinogen molecule is synthesized with altered amino acid sequence owing to genetic mutation. Some dysfibrinogenemias exhibit impairment of clotting and a hemorrhagic diathesis, whereas others show increased tendency to thrombosis (Menache, 1973). Congenital afibrinogenemia, in which essentially no fibrinogen is synthesized, results in a hemorrhagic disorder, which paradoxically is not as severe as the hemophilias in terms of joint abnormalities secondary to hemorrhage (hemarthroses).

Fibrinogen levels become elevated with the other acute phase reactants, occasionally to over 1.0 g/L. In such instances, the erythrocyte sedimentation is also markedly elevated owing to fibrinogen content directly. Fibrinogen levels also rise with pregnancy and use of contraceptive medications. Low levels generally indicate extensive activation of coagulation with consumption of fibrinogen. During this process, plasminogen is also activated into plasmin, which degrades fibrin and fibrinogen into split products that are measured for the assessment of intravascular coagulation. Normally, clots that form are removed by action of plasmin, which, in turn, is inactivated by antiplasmin and the other protease inhibitors.

Fibrinogen is absent from normal serum but should appear in plasma electrophoresis as a distinct band between the beta and gamma globulins. Not infrequently, blood drawn from heparinized patients does not fully clot, so that a fibrinogen band is present on electrophoresis. It can be distinguished by examining the specimen for a fine clot and by repeat electrophoresis of a thoroughly clotted sample. This maneuver is important to distinguish a residual fibrinogen band from a monoclonal spike of immunoglobulin that can migrate in the same electrophoretic position.

Minor Components

The next group of individual proteins are those not usually detected by standard protein electrophoresis owing to low levels in serum. Their quantitation is typically performed by immunologic methods.

CERULOPLASMIN. Migrating with the α_2-globulins is a copper-binding protein, ceruloplasmin, whose precise physiologic function is unknown, although it does exhibit oxidase activity in the laboratory. Synthesized in the liver, it has a molecular weight of 132,000 daltons and consists of a single polypeptide chain. Although lower at birth (Al-Rashid, 1971), serum levels are 20 to 40 mg/dL in normal adults, with twofold elevations found in oral contraceptive therapy and pregnancy (Burrows, 1971), or as an acute phase reactant. Each molecule of ceruloplasmin can bind six atoms of copper, which imparts a blue color to the protein. The combination of this blue with the yellow from other chromogens of plasma imparts a greenish color to plasma with elevated ceruloplasmin concentrations (Schenker, 1971). Iron is oxidized from ferrous to ferric ions by ceruloplasmin, which may be a means of releasing iron from ferritin for binding to transferrin (Roeser, 1970).

Wilson's disease (hepatolenticular degeneration) results from disordered copper metabolism, in which hepatic excretion of copper into the bile is impaired leading to toxic deposition of copper in tissues. The primary biochemical defect responsible for Wilson's disease is not known, although the gene for the disease has been mapped to chromosome 13. Ceruloplasmin levels are reduced in Wilson's disease, most likely secondary to decreased rate of transcription from the ceruloplasmin gene. Diagnosis of Wilson's disease is based on physical findings (liver disease, neurologic signs, Kayser-Fleischer ring in the cornea), measurement of low serum ceruloplasmin level, and increased copper concentrations in urine and on liver biopsy. The oxidase activity of ceruloplasmin can be used in a colorimetric assay, with *p*-phenylenediamine as substrate, for quantitation. Additionally, immunochemical methods are used, because the band is too faint to be used reliably on protein electrophoresis.

Gc-GLOBULIN. Vitamin D binds to the group-specific component (Gc) globulin (vitamin D–binding protein, DBP) (Daiger, 1975; Bikle, 1986), which migrates as an α_1-globulin and has a molecular weight of about 51,000 daltons. Normal serum concentration is 20 to 55 mg/dL. It may be decreased in severe liver disease. Gc-globulin has two autosomal codominant alleles expressed as three phenotypes: 1–1, 2–2, and 1–2 (Giblett, 1969). Congenital absence of this protein may be a lethal mutation, owing to impairment of vitamin D transport, because vitamin D has low solubility in aqueous medium. Gc-globulin binds vitamin D and its metabolites on a mole-per-mole basis, but in plasma, it probably is not fully saturated. Nephrotic syndrome results in urinary loss of DBP, some of which is complexed with vitamin D. This loss of vitamin D may contribute to subsequent problems of calcium metabolism encountered in nephrotic syndrome (Goldstein, 1981). As a minor component of plasma proteins, Gc-globulin must be quantitated by radioimmunoassay, radioimmunodiffusion, or rocket immunoelectrophoresis (Walsh, 1982; Westwood, 1986).

HEMOPEXIN. The β-migrating globulin hemopexin binds heme released by degradation of hemoglobin (Muller-Eberhard, 1970). By this means, this small porphyrin molecule with its iron atom is protected from excretion, thereby contributing to the preservation of body iron stores. Normal serum concentration is 50 to 120 mg/dL so that it must be quantitated by immunologic means. It has a molecular weight of 70,000 daltons, of which 20% is carbohydrate and consists of a single polypeptide chain. Although low levels of hemopexin can occur with nonspecific urinary loss or due to decreased synthesis in liver failure, the most profound decreases occur following intravascular hemolysis when the amount of free hemoglobin exceeds the binding capacity of haptoglobin. The circulating plasma hemoglobin can then degrade to release heme, which is bound molecule per molecule by hemopexin. Heme-hemopexin complexes are cleared from the circulation by hepatocytes, which markedly lowers hemopexin concentration in serum. Excess heme then binds to albumin as methemalbumin. As more hemopexin is made available by new synthesis, heme passes from methemalbumin to hemopexin, which continues to depress the hemopexin level. As such, it can be an additional aid for diagnosing hemolysis at an earlier time, after haptoglobin levels have returned to normal but before full clearance of the heme (Wochner, 1974).

α_1-ACID GLYCOPROTEIN. This protein, also known as orosomucoid, has a very high carbohydrate content, which minimizes its visualization by standard protein stains (Alvan, 1986). With a molecular weight of roughly 44,000 daltons, it passes into the glomerular filtrate to a large extent, resulting in a half-life of only about five days in the circulation. Serum levels are normally 40 to 105 mg/dL with elevations during pregnancy (Schmid, 1975). It is an acute phase reactant, but its biological function is not known. As a binder of progesterone, it may be important in the transport or metabolism of that steroid hormone. It also binds some drugs (e.g., lidocaine) and keeps them in an inactive circulating pool. Measurements of this protein have clinical utility in interpreting levels of drugs, such as lidocaine, that may achieve high serum concentrations without expected therapeutic effect owing to being complexed in inactive form to higher than normal amounts of α_1-acid glycoprotein. There are also some genetic polymorphisms of this protein that may be additionally complicated by isomorphic forms from specific tissue sources, although the primary site of its synthesis appears to be the liver.

C-REACTIVE PROTEIN. This serum constituent was discovered by interacting the serum of patients, who had recovered from pneumococcal infections, with C-polysaccharide of that bacterium. Visible flocculates formed, which allowed extensive study and purification of this C-reactive protein (CRP) from serum in the 1940s. It was found that CRP is present in the serum of patients with disorders other than pneumococcal infections, but that it rises strikingly whenever there is tissue necrosis. Many other substances react with CRP, such as DNA, nucleotides, various lipids, and other polysaccharides (Hokama, 1982). Thus, it appears to serve as a general scavenger molecule. Its molecular weight is between 118,000 and 144,000 daltons with substantial carbohydrate content. The normal serum concentrations are about 100 ng/mL at birth, 170 ng/mL in children, and 470 to 1340 ng/mL in adults. Despite these low concentrations, CRP has major significance as a highly sensitive acute phase reactant (Deodhar, 1989). It is generally measured by its capacity to precipitate C-substance or by immunologic methods, including nephelometry, precipitations, RIA, and enzyme immunoassay (Saxstad, 1970; Claus, 1976). By electrophoresis, CRP is a gamma-migrating protein that may form a distinct monoclonal-appearing band in patients having a severe inflammatory response. CRP levels are sometimes used as a rapid test for presumptive diagnosis of bacterial infection (high CRP) versus viral infection (low CRP). CRP is often used by rheumatologists to monitor the progression or remission of autoimmune disease. The gene for CRP has been localized to human chromosome 1 (Whitehead, 1983).

Protease Inhibitors

In addition to α_1-antitrypsin and α_2-macroglobulin, which have already been considered, other distinct inhibitors of different proteases are present in plasma. They include α_1-antichymotrypsin (AAC) (Berninger, 1985), inter-α-trypsin inhibitor (IATI) (Daniels, 1975), anti-thrombin III (AT3), antiplasmin, CI esterase inhibitor (Prograis, 1985), protein C (Stenflo, 1984), and plasminogen activator inhibitor-1 (Nilsson, 1984). None of these five proteins attains plasma concentrations appreciable on stained protein electrophoresis. Whereas the other inhibitors show inhibition over a rather wide range of proteases, AAC is highly specific for neutralizing chymotrypsin, which cleaves peptide bonds at the carboxyl side of tyrosine and phenylalanine residues. AAC has a molecular weight of 68,000 daltons with about 25% carbohydrate content. Normal serum concentration is 40 to 60 mg/dL, but AAC can rise rapidly to five times normal as an acute phase reactant that remains elevated throughout a period of inflammation (Kosaka, 1976). It can be lost along with other low-molecular-weight serum proteins in the proteinuria of nephrotic syndrome.

IATI is a glycoprotein of molecular weight 160,000 daltons. Its concentration normally is about 50 mg/dL. IATI does not rise appreciably as an acute phase reactant. Its role in disease states is probably similar to that of the major protease inhibitors in preventing autodigestion of tissues by endogenous cellular enzymes (Daniels, 1975).

AT3 is of special clinical interest because of the role it plays in neutralizing thrombin, which normally becomes activated intravascularly from prothrombin during clot formation. This 62,000-dalton protein forms a covalently bonded complex with thrombin over a period of several minutes when mixed in solution. On addition of heparin, the complex formation occurs almost instantaneously (Rosenberg, 1975,

1985, 1987). Although AT3 is probably essential for successful therapeutic administration of heparin, only those rare individuals with marked deficiencies seem to have thrombotic disorders (Carvalho, 1976). The action of AT3 extends to other coagulation factors (IX, X, XI, XII, and kallikrein). Serum levels of AT3 may be depressed in severe liver disease or in protein-losing disorders when the similar-sized molecule albumin is lost, and also in disseminated intravascular coagulopathy (DIC). A new experimental protocol for treating DIC involves replacing AT3, by infusion of concentrates, when the patient's AT3 level falls to very low concentrations as part of the consumptive coagulopathy. Presumably, return to normal levels of AT3 has the effect of blocking further thrombosis systemically. AT3 levels are lower in heparin therapy and slightly elevated in oral anticoagulant therapy owing to reduced turnover.

Although AAT, AMG, and AT3 provide the bulk of plasmin-neutralizing activity in serum (Harpel, 1976), there is a distinct antiplasmin that migrates as an α_2-globulin (Lijnen 1985). This cross-reactivity of serum protease inhibitors for plasmin illustrates the difficulty in sorting out the precise physiologic function of each molecular species, because each one appears capable of substituting for another in different instances. However, antiplasmin binds quantitatively to the majority of plasmin that is generated from plasminogen in human plasma that undergoes clotting. Antiplasmin thus serves as one of the critical checks within the joint coagulation-fibrinolytic system, which maintains hemostasis by balancing clot formation against dissolution. By this mechanism, clot formation and breakdown are generally contained within local regions of the vasculature without extending to the entire circulation. Hereditary deficiency of antiplasmin results in a bleeding disorder owing to relatively unlimited fibrinolysis.

Plasminogen activator inhibitor-1 (PAI-1) acts to prevent activation of plasminogen, thereby blocking fibrinolysis at an early step. Deficiency of PAI-1 results in less inhibition leading to greater fibrinolysis and potentially a bleeding disorder. Elevated levels of PAI-1 prevent fibrinolysis, leading to thrombotic disorders and interestingly also to the progression of atherosclerosis. Protein C (with its cofactor protein S) inactivates activated coagulation factors V and VIII. Deficiency of protein C or S (Griffin, 1987) allows prolonged activity *in vivo* of procoagulant factors leading to thrombotic disorders.

The C1 esterase inhibitor is capable of inhibiting activated complement components C1r and C1s plus some other coagulation and fibrinolytic factors. It rises as an acute phase reactant. Hereditary deficiency of C1 esterase inhibitor allows activation of complement to proceed relatively unabated, a disorder termed hereditary angioedema. The complement system and its inhibitors are described in depth in a subsequent chapter.

Acute Phase Reactants

The acute phase reactant proteins share the property of showing elevations in concentrations in response to stressful or inflammatory states that occur with infection, injury, surgery, trauma, or other tissue necrosis (Daniels, 1974; Laurell, 1975; Downton, 1988). They include AAT, α_1-acid glycoprotein, haptoglobin, ceruloplasmin, fibrinogen, serum amyloid A protein, and CRP. Others are Factor VIII, ferritin, lipoproteins, complement proteins, and immunoglobulins. It is easy to see how such a response of the plasma proteins would be advantageous to the body: inflammation causes release from leukocytes of proteolytic enzymes in tissue that must be neutralized by enzyme inhibitors to limit their extent of destruction; scavenger proteins (haptoglobin, CRP) help collect and transport cellular debris and breakdown products to phagocytic cells (reticuloendothelial system) to process them and conserve vital substances (e.g., iron); healing of wounds requires a large amount of fibrin, which arrives via the circulation as fibrinogen. Thus, the humoral response of the acute phase reactants can be viewed as a phenomenon that is geared to handle extensive insult each time it is triggered even though not all components will be needed on every occasion. The elevation of acute phase reactants is likely a response to the cytokines including interleukin-1, tumor necrosis factor, interferon-γ, and interleukin-6. The total physiologic response includes induction of fever, recruitment of leukocytes, catabolism of muscle, and a shift in protein synthesis patterns with reduction in albumin production.

For clinical use in diagnosis, other parameters may in fact be as sensitive as these and far easier to measure (e.g., fever, leukocytosis, or erythrocyte sedimentation rate). However, these proteins provide another dimension of quantitation that can be useful for monitoring the course of a patient by serial determinations (van Oss, 1975). Of course, those patients with congenital deficiencies (Gitlin, 1975), those with other impairment of synthesis due to drugs or organ disease, or newborns who normally have lower levels of many constituents (Gitlin, 1969) may not show the dramatic increases expected. However, a generally useful acute phase reactant for monitoring response is CRP, which is the fastest rising acute phase reactant and one that returns to normal quickly following successful therapies (Fisher, 1976). CRP is frequently applied to the detection and preliminary classification of occult infection, because bacterial infections can stimulate much higher levels of CRP than viral ones. It is also widely used for assessing disease activity in autoimmune disorders, because it is rarely elevated persistently without continued inflammatory response. Elevations of CRP can be up to 1000 times normal levels, which greatly assists in detecting abnormal states compared with the other acute phase reactants that may rise at most only severalfold in such responses, although ferritin levels may occasionally rise to values of over 20,000 ng/mL.

PATTERNS OF PROTEIN ABNORMALITIES

Some of the most frequently encountered patterns of protein abnormalities in electrophoresis are shown by actual stained gel appearance in Figure 11–3 and as densitometric scans in Figure 11–4. Scanning allows quantitation of each fraction, but visual inspection of the electrophoretic strip provides more detailed information abut individual proteins separated in high-resolution systems (Ritzmann, 1975). Interpretation of electrophoretic results depends on visual inspection to identify abnormal patterns or aberrant bands and on

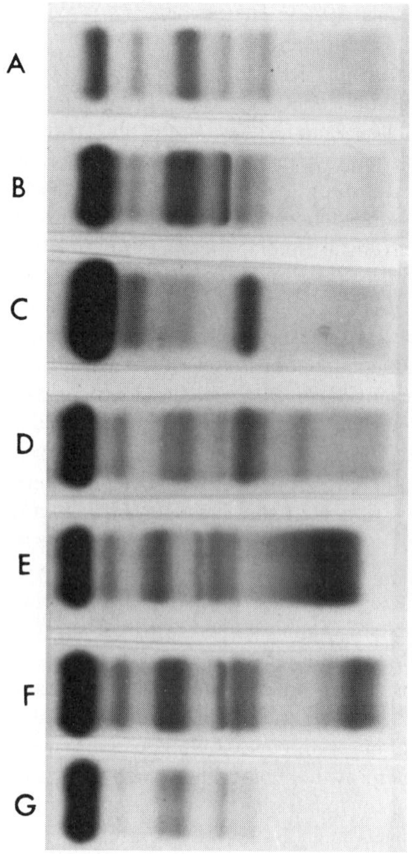

Figure 11–3. Abnormal protein patterns by agarose gel electrophoresis. Anode is to the left; fractions are as labeled in Figure 11–1; all samples are serum except for C. *A*, Inanition in an elderly patient with low total protein and markedly depressed albumin. *B*, Nephrotic syndrome with elevated α_2-macroglobulin and beta lipoprotein. *C*, Urine from protein-losing nephropathy. *D*, Iron deficiency with elevated transferrin. *E*, Broadly elevated gamma and low albumin due to liver disease. *F*, Oligoclonal gamma fraction in patient with renal disease. *G*, Hypogammaglobulinemia.

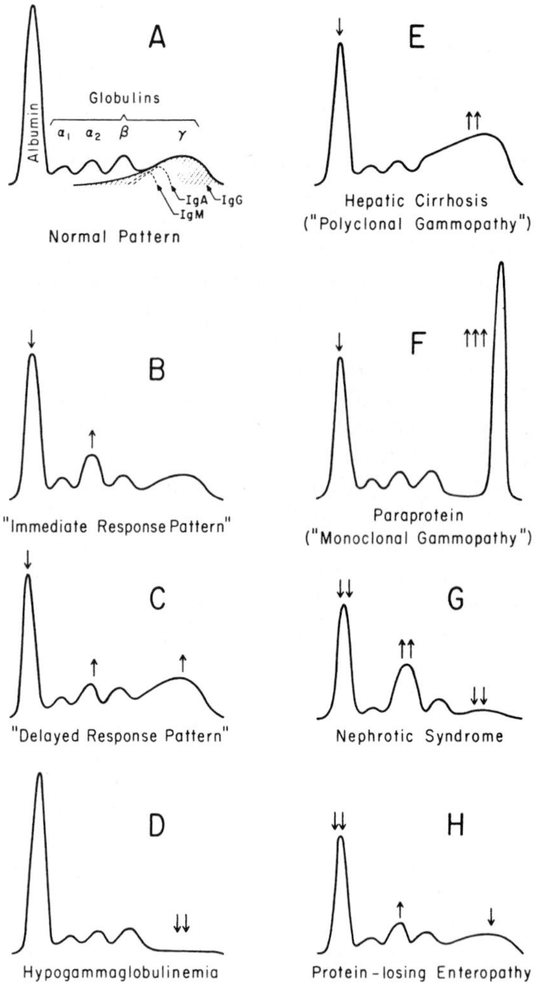

Figure 11–4. Serum protein electrophoresis: clinicopathologic correlations. (Courtesy of Dr. A. F. Krieg.)

quantitation by scan to gauge the relative quantities of individual fractions.

Patterns of *hypoproteinemia* due to malnutrition or gross loss of protein show decreases in all fractions, but the most dramatic reduction is often seen in albumin compared with its normally high value as the most abundant serum protein (see Fig. 11–3*A*, inanition in an elderly patient). Severe starvation, malabsorption, or the inanition associated with severe chronic disease will show marked reduction in albumin to levels below 20 g/L. The other serum proteins appear even fainter on electrophoresis including AAT, AMG, haptoglobin, transferrin, and C3. Reduction of staining intensity for the β-lipoprotein parallels a marked decrease in serum cholesterol concentration. The immune system is strongly affected by severe starvation with decreased synthesis of immunoglobulins resulting in hypogammaglobulinemia and impaired resistance to bacterial and other infections. Protein-losing enteropathy (see Fig. 11–4*H*) shows a variation on the hypoproteinemia pattern in which most fractions are diminished owing to the combination of decreased synthesis and increased loss, although α_2 may be relatively higher owing to a coexisting acute phase response (haptoglobin) or to preferential retention of larger molecules (α_2-macroglobulin).

Specific loss of proteins into the urine such as in *nephrotic syndrome* occurs on a molecular weight basis, with smaller proteins being lost more rapidly than larger ones. Accordingly albumin appears early in the course of protein-losing nephropathies followed by smaller amounts of AAT, transferrin, and ultimately, immunoglobulins. The very large molecule AMG is retained, as are the large micelles of β-lipoprotein. The result is complementary patterns of proteins in the serum (see Figs. 11–3*B* and 11–4*G*, decreases in albumin and alpha-1, beta, and gamma globulins; increased α_2-macroglobulin and elevated beta lipoprotein) versus those in urine (see Fig. 11–3*C*, glomerular proteinuria with albumin, α-1, β, and γ fractions present but without α_2-macroglobulin in the urine sample). Tubular proteinuria that is due to impaired renal tubular reabsorption of small proteins shows a pattern of α, β, and γ in the urine with only minimal albumin loss into the urine (Killingsworth, 1982).

Acute phase or *immediate response* patterns have greatest effect on serum protein electrophoresis by increasing the amount of haptoglobin while slightly decreasing the concentration of albumin. Increases in haptoglobin usually indicate some form of response, whether acute or chronic, to stressful stimuli (see Fig. 11–4*B* and *C*). Other proteins such as AAT can contribute in this response; the minor components such as CRP do not contribute significantly to this protein stain pattern, although immunologic measurement of CRP may show up to 1000-fold elevations. If the haptoglobin has been depleted in a patient as a result of active hemolysis, there can be an independent band of hemoglobin migrating in the β- or α_2-region. Hemolysis of a sample *in vitro* may show a red-colored band of the haptoglobin-hemoglobin complex that migrates differently from hemoglobin alone. The pattern of delayed response or chronic pattern is an extension of the acute phase response (high haptoglobin, slight reduction in albumin) with greater decrease of albumin and polyclonal increase of immunoglobulins broadening the gamma region.

A striking elevation of transferrin in the beta region sometimes occurs in patients suffering from *iron deficiency anemia* (see Fig. 11–3*D*). The increase of transferrin corresponds to increased IBC, and the percent saturation is low (Koerper, 1977). This variation may be confused with a myeloma protein because the transferrin band forms a narrow, clonal-appearing band.

Cirrhosis of the liver creates a protein pattern that is recognizable (see Figs. 11–3*E* and 11–4*E*). Hepatocellular damage from cirrhosis results in diminished capacity to synthesize albumin. Furthermore, the imbalance of hemodynamic pressures in portal hypertension secondary to cirrhosis leads to the formation of ascites fluid, which contains almost exclusively albumin. Thus decreased synthesis, coupled with increased loss, greatly reduces serum albumin concentrations. The loss of albumin is balanced to some extent by marked polyclonal increase in immunoglobulins with a gamma fraction that may contribute significantly to oncotic pressures. The increase in gamma globulin involves all immunoglobulins; the increase of IgA in the slow β-region shows a continuum with the γ (also termed β-γ bridging).

In contrast to polyclonal increases, *oligoclonal bands* consist of only a few clones of distinct immunoglobulins that migrate in defined positions (see Fig. 11–3*F*). This pattern is seen in serum in cases in which immunologic disorder is present or in some patients treated with chronic immunosuppression for organ transplantation (Myara, 1991). Oligoclonal bands in the CSF are used to indicate immunologic activity in the central nervous system and occur in infectious diseases or autoimmune or demyelinating disorders.

Hypogammaglobulinemia is manifested as a nearly to completely absent gamma fraction (see Figs. 11–3*G*, and 11–4*D*). It occurs normally in neonates prior to maturation of the immune system. It also occurs in some congenital immunodeficiency states such as Bruton's agammaglobulinemia and other states involving B-cell function. Perhaps more commonly, this pattern is seen in adults with lymphoreticular disorders in whom normal plasma cells have been displaced by lymphocytic proliferations and also to some extent after chemotherapy for eradication of malignancies.

The single most important and widespread clinical application of serum protein electrophoresis is for the detection of *monoclonal gammopathies*. This very explicit pattern comes from a paraprotein (immunoglobulin) secreted by a monoclonal proliferation of plasma cells and is generally found without normal amounts of polyclonal gamma as normal plasma cells are replaced by the malignant clone (see Fig. 11–4*F*). Presence of a paraprotein with normal polyclonal gamma suggests a possible plasmacytoma that has not yet spread throughout the bone marrow. The laboratory evaluation of myeloma should include serum and urine protein electrophoreses to detect aberrant clonal bands, immunoelectrophoresis or immunofixation to type the heavy and light chains of the paraprotein, and quantitation of immunoglobulins to provide a baseline for monitoring the patient's response to therapy or disease progression. Other proteins that may sometimes be mistaken for monoclonal bands of immunoglobulin on serum protein electrophoresis include haptoglobin-hemoglobin complexes, C3 and its variants, β-lipoprotein, transferrin, fibrinogen, immune complexes, CRP, and occasionally, α_2-macroglobulin.

Immunoglobulins, disorders of the immune system, and abnormalities of complement are discussed further in Chapters 32, 33, and 36 in Part V.

2

Al-Rashid RA, Spangler J: Neonatal copper deficiency. N Engl J Med 1971; 285:841.

Alvan G: Other protein variants with pharmacogenetic consequences: Albumin and orosomucoid. Prog Clin Biol Res 1986; 214:345.

Beetham R, Cattell WR: Proteinuria: pathophysiology, significance and recommendations for measurement in clinical practice. Ann Clin Biochem 1993; 30:425.

Berninger RW: Protease inhibitors of human plasma. Alpha 1-antitrypsin. J Med 1985; 16:23.

Berninger RW: Protease inhibitors of human plasma. Alpha 1-antichymotrypsin. J Med 1985; 16:101.

Bikle DD, Halloran BP, Gee E, et al: Free 25-hydroxyvitamin D levels are normal in subjects with liver disease and reduced total 25-hydroxyvitamin D levels. J Clin Invest 1986; 78:748.

Burrows S, Pekala B: Serum copper and ceruloplasmin in pregnancy. Am J Obstet Gynecol 1971; 109:907.

Carvalho A, Ellman L: Hereditary antithrombin III deficiency. Effect of antithrombin on platelet function. Am J Med 1976; 61:179.

Claus DR, Osmand AP, Gewurz H: Radioimmunoassay of human C-reactive protein and levels in normal sera. J Lab Clin Med 1976; 87:120.

Cow DW: Clinical and molecular studies of alpha 1-antitrypsin deficiency. Prog Clin Biol Res 1986; 214:373.

Daiger SP, Schanfield MS, Cavalli-Sforza LL: Group-specific component (Gc) proteins bind vitamin D and 25-hydroxy-vitamin D. Proc Natl Acad Sci U S A. 1975; 72:2076.

Daniels JC: Abnormalities of protease inhibitors. *In* Ritzmann SE, Daniels JC (eds): Serum Protein Abnormalities, Diagnostic and Clinical Aspects. Boston, Little, Brown and Company, 1975.

Daniels JC, Larson DL, Abston S, Ritzmann SE: Serum protein profiles in thermal burns. II. Protease inhibitors, complement factors and C-reactive proteins. J Trauma 1974; 14:153.

Deodhar SD: C-reactive protein: The best laboratory indicator available for monitoring disease activity. Cleveland Clin J Med 1989; 56:126.

Doolittle RF: Fibrinogen and fibrin. *In* Putnam FW (ed): The Plasma Proteins, Vol. II, 2nd ed. New York, Academic Press, 1975, p 110.

Downton SR, Colten HR: Acute phase reactants in inflammation and infection. Semin Hematol 1988; 25:84.

Eriksson S: Studies in alpha 1-antitrypsin deficiency. Acta Med Scand 1965; 177(Suppl):432.

Fisher CL, Gill C, Forrester MG, Nakamura R: Quantitation of "acute phase proteins" postoperatively. Value in detection and monitoring of complications. Am J Clin Pathol 1976; 66:840.

Gelb AF, Klein E, Lieberman F: Pulmonary function in nonsmoking subjects with alpha-1-antitrypsin deficiency (MZ phenotype). Am J Med 1976; 62:93.

Giblett ER (ed): Genetic Markers in Human Blood. Oxford, Blackwell Scientific, 1969.

Gitlin D, Biasucci A: Development of gamma G, gamma A, gamma M, C'1 esterase inhibitor, ceruloplasmin, transferrin, hemopexin, haptoglobin, fibrinogen, plasminogen, alpha 1-antitrypsin, orosomucoid, beta-lipoprotein, alpha 2-macroglobulin, and prealbumin in the human conceptus. J Clin Invest 1969; 48:1433.

Gitlin D, Gitlin JD: Genetic alterations in the plasma proteins of man. *In* Putnam FW (ed): The Plasma Proteins, Vol. II, 2nd ed. New York, Academic Press, 1975, p 321.

Glenner GG: Amyloid deposits and amyloidosis. The beta-fibrilloses. N Engl J Med 1980; 302:1283.

Gofferje H: Prealbumin and retinol binding protein, highly sensitive parameters for the nutritional state in respect to protein. Med Lab 1978; 5:38.

Goldstein DA, Haldimann B, Sherman D, et al: Vitamin D metabolites and calcium metabolism in patients with nephrotic syndrome and normal renal function. J Clin Endocrinol Metab 1981; 52:116.

Griffin JH, Heeb MJ, Schwarz HP: Plasma protein S deficiency and thromboembolic disease. Prog Hematol 1987; 15:39.

Guthrow CE, Morris MA, Day JF, et al: Enhanced nonenzymatic glucosylation of human serum albumin in diabetes mellitus. Proc Natl Acad Sci U S A 1979; 76:4258.

Harding JJ: Nonenzymatic covalent posttranslational modification of proteins in vivo. Adv Protein Chem 1985; 37:247.

Harpel PC, Rosenberg RD: Alpha-2-macroglobulin and antithrombin-heparin cofactor: Modulators of hemostatic and inflammatory reactions. *In* Spaet TH (ed): Progress in Hemostasis and Thrombosis, Vol. 3. New York, Grune & Stratton, 1976, p 145.

Hokama Y: Methods of assay and role of acute phase C-reactive protein in human diseases. *In* Nakamura RM, Dito WR, Tucker ES (eds): Immunologic Analysis. Recent Progress in Diagnostic Laboratory Immunology. New York, Masson Publishing U.S.A., Inc., 1982, p 239.

Horne CHW, Weir RJ, Howie PW, Goudie RB: Effect of combined oestrogen-progesterone oral contraceptives on serum levels of alpha-2-macroglobulin, transferrin, albumin and IgG. Lancet 1970; 1:49.

Hubbard RC, Brantly ML, Sellers S, et al: Anti-neutrophil-elastase defenses of the lower respiratory tract in alpha 1-antitrypsin deficiency directly augmented with an aerosol of alpha 1-antitrypsin. Ann Intern Med, 1989: 111:206.

Irie S, Tavassoli M: Transferrin-mediated cellular iron uptake. J Med Sci 1987; 293:103.

Jeppsson J-O, Laurell CB, Franzen B: Agarose gel electrophoresis. Clin Chem 1979; 25:629.

Jeppsson J-O, Franzen B: Typing of genetic variants of alpha-1-antitrypsin by electrofocusing. Clin Chem 1982; 28:219.

Killingsworth LM: Clinical applications of protein determinations in biological fluids other than blood. Clin Chem 1982; 28:1093.

Koch-Weser J, Sellers EM: Drug therapy. Binding of drugs to serum albumin. N Engl J Med 1976; 294:311.

Koerper MA, Dallman PR: Serum iron concentration and transferrin saturation in the diagnosis of iron deficiency in children: Normal developmental changes. J Pediatr 1977; 91:870.

Konigsberg W: Molecular diseases. *In* Bondy PK, Roenberg LE (eds): Duncan's Diseases of Metabolism, 7th ed. Philadelphia, W.B. Saunders Company, 1974, p 86.

Kosaka S, Tazawa M: Alpha-1-antichymotrypsin in rheumatoid arthritis. Tohoku J. Exp Med 1976; 119:369.

Lauff JJ, Kasper ME, Wu TW, Ambrose RT: Isolation and preliminary characterization of a fraction of bilirubin in serum that is firmly bound to protein. Clin Chem 1982; 28:629.

Laurell CB: Quantitative estimation of proteins by electrophoresis in agarose gel containing antibodies. Anal Biochem 1966; 15:45.

Laurell CB: Electrophoresis, specific protein assays, or both in measurement of plasma proteins? Clin Chem 1973; 19:99.

Laurell CB, Jeppsson J-O: Protease inhibitors in plasma. *In* Putnam FW (ed): The Plasma Proteins, Vol. I, 2nd ed. New York, Academic Press, 1975, p 299.

Layne E: Spectrophotometric and turbidimetric methods for measuring proteins. *In* Colowick SP, Kaplan NO (eds): Methods in Enzymology, Vol. III. New York, Academic Press, 1957, p 447.

Li S, Minnerath S, Li K, et al: Two-tiered DNA-based diagnosis of transthyretin amyloidosis reveals two novel point mutations. Neurology 1991; 41:893.

Lieberman J, Gaidulis L, Garoutte B, Mittman C: Identification and characteristics of the common alpha-1-antitrypsin phenotypes. Chest 1972; 62:557.

Lijnen HR, Collen D: Protease inhibitors of human plasma. Alpha 2-antiplasmin. J Med 1985; 16:225.

Lowry OH, Rosebrough NJ, Farr L, Randall RJ: Protein measurement with Folin phenol reagent. J Biol Chem 1951; 193:265.

MacGillivray RTA, Mendez E, Sinha S, et al: The complete amino acid sequence of human serum transferrin. Proc Natl Acad Sci U S A 1982; 79:2504.

McFarlane H, Reddy S, Adcock KJ, et al: Immunity, transferrin, and survival in kwashiorkor. BMJ 1970; 4:268.

Meloun B, Moravek L, Kostka V: Complete amino acid sequence of human serum albumin. FEBS Letters 1975; 58:134.

Menache D: Abnormal fibrinogens: A review. Thromb Diath Haemorrh 1973; 29:525.

Mendenhall HW: Serum protein concentrations in pregnancy. I. Concentrations in maternal serum. Am J Obstet Gynecol 1970; 106:388.

Merril CR, Goldman D, Sedman SA, Ebert MH: Ultrasensitive stain for proteins in polyacrylamide gels shows regional variation in cerebrospinal fluid proteins. Science 1981; 211:1437.

Moses AC, Lawlor J, Hallow J, Jackson IMD: Familial euthyroid hyperthyroxinemia resulting from increased thyroxine binding to thyroxine-binding prealbumin. N Engl J Med 1982; 306:966.

Muller-Eberhard U: Hemopexin. N Engl J Med 1970; 283:1090.

Myara I, Quenum G, Storogenko M, et al: Monoclonal and oligoclonal gammopathies in hearttransplant recipients. Clin Chem 1991; 37:1334.

Nilsson IM, Tengborn LA: A family with thrombosis associated with high level of tissue plasminogen activator inhibitor. Haemostasis 1984; 14:24.

Oppenheimer JH: Role of plasma proteins in the binding, distribution and metabolism of the thyroid hormones. N Engl J Med 1968; 278:1153.

Peters T, Jr: Serum albumin. *In* Putnam FW (ed): The Plasma Proteins, Vol. I, 2nd ed. New York, Academic Press, 1975, p 133.

Peters T: Serum albumin: Recent progress in the understanding of its structure and biosynthesis. Clin Chem 1977; 23:5.

Peterson PA: Studies on interaction between pre-albumin, retinolbinding protein and vitamin A. J Biol Chem 1971; 246:44.

Prograis LJ, Brickman CM, Frank MM: Protease inhibitors of human plasma. Cl-inhibitor (Cl-Inh). J Med 1985; 16:303.

Ritzmann SE, Daniels JC (eds): Serum Protein Abnormalities. Diagnostic and Clinical Aspects. Boston, Little, Brown and Company, 1975.

Roberts RC: Protease inhibitors of human plasma. Alpha 2-macroglobulin. J Med 1985; 16:129.

Roeser HP, Lee GR, Nacht S, Cartwright GE: The role of ceruloplasmin in iron metabolism. J Clin Invest 1970; 49:2408.

Rosenberg RD: Actions and interactions of antithrombin and heparin. N Engl J Med 1975; 292:146.

Rosenberg RD, Bauer KA: Thrombosis in inherited deficiencies of antithrombin, protein C, and protein S. Hum Pathol 1987; 18:253.

Rosenberg RD, Bauer KA, Marcum JA: Protease inhibitors of human plasma. Antithrombin-III: The heparin-antithrombin system. J Med 1985; 16:351.

Roses AD: Apoliprotein E is a genetic locus that affects the rate of Alzheimer disease expression. Neuropsychopharmacology 1994; 10:55.

Rothschild MA, Oratz M, Schreiber SS: Albumin synthesis. N Engl J Med 1972; 286:748, 816.

Ruiz M, Rajatanavin R, Yound RA, et al: Familial dysalbuminemic hyperthyroxinemia. A syndrome that can be confused with thyrotoxicosis. N Engl J Med 1982; 306:635.

Saraiva M, Alves IL, Costa PP: Simplified method for screening populations at risk for transthyretin met 30 associated familial amyloidotic polyneuropathy. Clin Chem 1989; 35:1.

Saxstad J, Nilsson L-A, Hanson LA: C-reactive protein in serum from infants as determined with immunodiffusion techniques. Acta Paediatr Scand 1970; 59:676.

Schenker JG, Jungreis E, Polishuk WZ: Oral contraceptives and serum copper concentration. Obstet Gynecol 1971; 37:233.

Schmid K: Alpha-1-acid glycoprotein. *In* Putnam FW (ed): The Plasma Proteins, Vol. I, 2nd ed. New York, Academic Press, 1975.

Sevall JS: The albumin gene: DNA-protein interaction. Fed Proc 1986; 45:2412.

Slater L, Carter PM, Hobbs JR: Measurement of albumin in the sera of patients. Ann Clin Biochem 1975; 12:33.

Snider GL: Pulmonary disease in alpha$_1$-antitrypsin deficiency. Ann Intern Med 1989; 111:957.

Stenflo J: Structure and function of protein C. Semin Thromb Hemost 1984; 10:109.

Sveger T: Liver disease in alpha 1-antitrypsin deficiency detected by screening of 200,000 infants. N Engl J Med 1976; 294:1316.

Tsung SH, Rosenthal WA, Milewski KA: Immunological measurement of transferrin compared with chemical measurement of total iron-binding capacity. Clin Chem 1975; 21:1063.

van Oss CJ, Bronson PM, Border JR: Changes in the serum alpha glycoprotein distribution in trauma patients. J Trauma 1975; 15:451.

Waldmann TA, Gordon RS, Rosse W: Studies on the metabolism of the serum proteins and lipids in patients with analbuminemia. Am J Med 1964; 37:960.

Walsh PG, Haddad JG: "Rocket" immunoelectrophoresis assay of vitamin D-binding protein (Gc globulin) in human serum. Clin Chem 1982; 28:1781.

Weinberg ED: Iron and infection. Microbiol Rev 1978; 42:45.

Westwood SA, Werrett DJ: Group-specific component: A review of the isoelectric focusing methods and auxillary methods available for the separation of its phenotypes. Forensic Sci Int 1986; 32:135.

Whitehead AS, Bruns GAP, Markham AF, et al: Isolation of human C-reactive protein complementary DNA and localization of the gene to chromosome 1. Science 1983; 221:69.

Wochner RD, Spilberg I, Atsushi I, et al: Hemopexin metabolism in sickle cell disease, porphyrias and control subjects: Effect of heme injection. N Engl J Med 1974; 290:822.

Zawadzki Z, Edwards G: Pseudoparaproteinemia due to hypertransferrinemia. Am J Clin Pathol 1970; 54:802.

Chapter 12

Assessment of Liver Function

Matthew R. Pincus, M.D., Ph.D.
John A. Schaffner, M.D.

2

OVERVIEW OF LABORATORY TESTING FOR HEPATOBILIARY FUNCTION

One of the areas in which laboratory medicine has made fundamentally important contributions to our ability to diagnose pathologic conditions noninvasively is in the evaluation of liver function. Chapter 4 presents an overview of liver function testing. Liver function tests become easier to interpret when one understands that the liver really encompasses three systems: the hepatocyte, involved in fundamental biochemical processes; the biliary tract, concerned with excretion of bilirubin; and the reticuloendothelial system, involving hemoglobin and bilirubin metabolism. The serum levels of specific analytes reflect disorders in one or more of these three systems.

With regard to hepatocyte function, it is important to remember that, in the body, over 90% of all proteins and 100% of specific proteins, such as albumin and many of the coagulation factors, are synthesized in the liver. Thus, serum levels of total protein and albumin become important gauges of liver function. Also, all of the known metabolic pathways occur in the hepatocyte, including the citric acid (Krebs) cycle, glycolysis, gluconeogenesis, the hexose-monophosphate shunt, fatty acid synthesis and breakdown, lipoprotein metabolism, and amino acid and nucleic acid metabolism. Especially important in these biochemical processes are two general metabolic pathways. First, there are the amino acid–carbohydrate interconversion pathways involving the aminotransferases, alanine amino transferase (ALT) and aspartate amino transferase (AST). The reactions catalyzed by these enzymes are shown in equation 13-7 in Chapter 13. Of these two enzymes, ALT occurs predominantly in the liver and is an excellent marker for liver injury or necrosis. Second, there is the urea cycle (Krebs-Henseleit cycle) in which ammonia, a byproduct of amino acid and nucleic acid metabolism, is detoxified by being converted into urea, which is excreted via the kidneys. Most of the enzymes involved in the urea cycle are unique to the liver, especially the enzyme involved in the rate-limiting step in this cycle, ornithine carbamoyl transferase (OCT). Elevations of serum ammonia point to severe liver disease. Elevations in OCT often reflect acute liver dysfunction.

A unique feature of liver tissue is its ability to regenerate. To abolish liver tissue function, over 80% of the liver must first be destroyed. In acute conditions of the liver, such as hepatitis or trauma, most of the liver is generally unaffected, so that normal liver function is easily regenerated. During the acute process, however, enough hepatocytes undergo injury or necrosis that their intracellular contents, such as the enzymes AST, ALT, and OCT, become extruded into the local circulation. The serum levels of these enzymes then become abnormally elevated.

On the other hand, if most of the liver is destroyed as a result of such conditions as cirrhosis, the serum levels of these enzymes are generally either normal or low because little liver tissue remains. Because the liver has ceased to function, the urea cycle enzymes are no longer present, resulting in the toxic buildup of ammonia. Protein synthesis, especially of albumin, also is diminished significantly, resulting in hypoproteinemia and hypoalbuminemia.

Bilirubin metabolism depends on its rate of synthesis from the breakdown of hemoglobin (reticuloendothelial system) and its rate of excretion via the bile canaliculi and bile ducts (biliary system) in the liver. Before it can be excreted, bilirubin becomes conjugated to glucuronic acid, mostly as the diglucuronide, in the smooth endoplasmic reticulum of the hepatocyte. Overly rapid production of bilirubin, as in hemolytic anemia, will result in an increase in unconjugated bilirubin in serum, whereas blocks in bilirubin excretion will result in abnormally elevated levels of conjugated bilirubin in serum.

In this chapter, we discuss how abnormal functioning in any or all three systems in the liver can be rapidly and specifically diagnosed using serum levels of analytes such as the aminotransferases, total protein and albumin, ammonia, bilirubin, and other analytes.

HEPATOCYTE FUNCTION

Enzymes

Aminotransferases (Transaminases)

There are two vitally important enzymes in this category: AST, also known as serum glutamate oxaloacetate transaminase (SGOT) and ALT, formerly called serum glutamate pyruvate transaminase (SGPT). The prototypical reactions catalyzed by these enzymes are shown in equation 13-7 in Chapter 13. These enzymes catalyze reversibly the reductive transfer of an amino group of either aspartate or alanine to α-ketoglutarate to yield glutamate plus the corresponding keto acid of the starting amino acid (i.e., oxaloacetate or pyruvate). Both enzymes require pyridoxal phosphate (vitamin B_6) as a cofactor. AST and ALT have blood half-lives of 17 and 47 hours, respectively. AST is ubiquitously distributed in the body tissues, including the heart and muscle, whereas ALT is found primarily in the liver, although significant amounts are also present in kidney. Approximately 80% of AST in hepatocytes appears to be located in mitochondria, whereas ALT is thought to be predominantly nonmitochondrial. It has been postulated that, in mild hepatocellular injury, when the hepatocyte plasma but not the mitochondrial membrane is damaged, cytoplasmic AST and ALT are released into serum. With more severe hepatocellular injury, mitochondrial membrane damage may result in the release of mitochondrial AST, elevating the AST/ALT ratio. Serum mitochondrial AST has been measured in cirrhotic and noncirrhotic patients who abuse alcohol (Nalpas, 1986). Patients who chronically abused alcohol, regardless of the extent of their underlying liver disease, had more consistent mitochondrial AST elevations than other patients; values dropped more than 50% with abstinence for more than one week. The ratio of mitochondrial AST to total AST does appear to discriminate alcoholic hepatitis from other liver diseases (Panteghini, 1983). The ratio of AST to ALT, or DeRitis quotient, which normally is 1 or slightly more, has been used diagnostically in alcoholic liver disease, with which a value of 3 : 1 to 4 : 1 can be found when the ALT is near normal. The exact reason for this is unknown, but two possible explanations are (1) that alcohol is a mitochondrial toxin and (2) that pyridoxine is deficient in alcoholics. Pyridoxal 5′-phosphate deficiency is rate limiting in the assay for ALT (Vanderlinde, 1986); treatment of either the patient or the assay *in vitro* with pyridoxal 5′-phosphate tends to normalize the ratio.

ALT is usually increased more than AST in patients with acute or chronic viral hepatitis. The AST/ALT ratio is generally 1 or less in patients with acute hepatocellular injury. ALT activity is more specific for detecting liver disease in nonalcoholic, asymptomatic patients. For example, donor blood is routinely screened for elevation of ALT prior to transfusion in an attempt to exclude patients with viral hepatitis. Values above 55 IU (see Chap. 13 for definition of enzyme units) in a standardized test with an upper limit of normal of 50 IU lead to exclusion of that unit of blood. AST is used for monitoring therapy with potentially hepatotoxic drugs; a result more than three times the upper border of normal should signal that therapy has been stopped. Chronic elevation of aminotransferase activities in asymptomatic patients may have several causes, including alcohol or medication use, chronic viral hepatitis, or nonalcoholic fatty liver disease. Weight reduction may lower ALT in overweight patients whose ALT is elevated (Palmer, 1989). Ursodeoxycholic acid lowers ALT as well as γ-glutamyl transferase (discussed later; see also Chap. 13) when these aminotransferases are elevated in blood donors (Bellentani, 1989).

Lactate Dehydrogenase

As shown in Chapter 13, lactate dehydrogenase (LD), a vital cytosolic glycolytic enzyme, catalyzes the reversible oxidation of lactate to pyruvate. As summarized in Tables 13–8 and 13–9 in Chapter 13, five LD isoenzymes have been isolated. LD_1 and LD_2 predominate in cardiac muscle, kidney, and erythrocytes. LD_4 and LD_5 are the major isoenzymes in liver and skeletal muscle. Total LD activity is significantly elevated in hepatitis.

Of great importance is the large increase of total LD to levels of 500 IU/L or more combined with a significant increase in alkaline phosphatase (ALP), discussed subsequently and in Chapter 13, to levels above 250 IU/L in the *absence* of other dramatic abnormalities in liver function enzyme levels, especially the transaminases. These selective increases almost always accompany space-occupying lesions of the liver, most often metastatic carcinoma. Other space-occupying lesions include primary hepatocellular carcinoma (HCC), or, rarely, benign lesions such as hemangiomata. The source of the LD, most often the LD_5 isozyme, is not clear because LD can originate from hepatocytes, from the tumor, or from both. The rise in ALP is due to blockage of local canaliculi and ductules by the masses in the liver as discussed subsequently and in Chapter 13.

Alkaline Phosphatase (ALP)

ALP is present in several tissues, including liver, bone, kidney, intestine, and placenta. ALP in the liver exists predominantly in the biliary tract and is therefore a marker for biliary dysfunction. Total ALP in serum is mainly present in the unbound form and, to a lesser extent, complexed with lipoproteins or rarely with immunoglobulins.

As explained in Chapter 13, bone, biliary tract, intestinal

and placental forms are distinct isozymes that can be separated from one another by electrophoresis. The bone isozyme is particularly heat-labile, allowing it to be distinguished from the other three major forms. In addition, small intestinal and placental ALP are antigenically distinct from liver, bone, and kidney ALP. The bulk of ALP in the serum of normal patients is made up of liver and bone ALP. Determining activities of the different isoenzymes is most valuable when liver and bone diseases coexist (Moss, 1987). The reason for the high levels of ALP in the biliary tract is not clear.

In obstruction of the biliary tract from stones in the ducts or ductules, infectious processes resulting in ascending cholangitis, or space-occupying lesions, biliary tract ALP rises rapidly to values sometimes in excess of 10 times the upper limit of normal. The reasons for this increase are probably a combination of increased synthesis and decreased excretion of ALP. In obstructive cholestasis, ALP most commonly rises to twice the upper limit of normal or greater, roughly paralleling the rate of rise in serum bilirubin. If obstruction is partial, ALP usually increases as much as with complete obstruction, often out of proportion to the increase in conjugated bilirubin (dissociated jaundice). Passive congestion of the liver can also result in moderate ALP elevations, more so than abnormal bilirubin levels. ALP is also moderately elevated in most instances of jaundice resulting from hepatic injury. When the resulting cholestasis is relieved, serum ALP levels fall to normal more slowly than bilirubin does.

A high-molecular-weight ALP appears in serum in cholestasis. This ALP is different from the isoenzymes originating from the liver plasma membrane (DeBroe, 1985). The exact mechanism for its release is unclear. The most accepted explanation is that cholestasis induces membrane-bound enzyme activity. Bile salts solubilize the enzymes from the sinusoidal and canalicular membranes. In serum, the membrane-bound enzymes aggregate with lipids and lipoproteins. This may explain the relationship that has been observed, for instance, with lipoprotein-X (see Chap. 10). Another form of high-molecular-weight ALP, which migrates differently on electrophoresis from the isozyme just described, has been found in malignant disease involving the liver (Viot, 1983).

Intestinal ALP is increased in a variety of disorders of the intestinal tract and in cirrhosis. Serum intestinal ALP is detected in over 80% of cirrhotic patients as compared with 10% of normal controls. The measurement of this enzyme activity was suggested as one method of discriminating intrahepatic from extrahepatic jaundice, because intestinal ALP may be absent in extrahepatic obstruction, but it lacks adequate sensitivity and specificity (Collin, 1987).

γ-Glutamyl Transferase

γ-Glutamyl transferase (GGT) regulates the transport of amino acids across cell membranes by catalyzing the transfer of a glutamyl group from glutathione to a free amino acid. Its major use is to discriminate the source of elevated ALP (i.e., if ALP is elevated and GGT is correspondingly elevated, the source of the elevated ALP must be biliary tract). The highest values, often greater than 10 times the upper limit of normal, may be found in chronic cholestasis due to primary biliary cirrhosis or sclerosing cholangitis. The serum assay for this enzyme is discussed in Chapter 13.

The gene for human GGT has been cloned and the nucleotide sequence identified (Rajpert-DeMeyts, 1988). GGT can be detected in three major forms in serum (Wenham, 1985), but such determinations are not readily available. A high-molecular-weight form is present in normal serum as well as in biliary obstruction and more frequently in malignant infiltration of the liver. An intermediate-molecular-weight form consists of two fractions, the major one detected in liver diseases and the other one found in biliary obstruction. Determination of these fractions lacks both sufficient sensitivity and sufficient specificity to be worthwhile (Collin, 1987). The third form is a low-molecular-weight compound of uncertain importance.

2

Serum levels of GGT differ from those of ALP during pregnancy, in which GGT remains normal even during cholestasis in pregnancy. GGT is often increased in alcoholics even without liver disease, in some obese people, in the presence of high concentrations of therapeutic drugs such as acetaminophen, and even in the absence of any apparent liver injury. Possibly, GGT increases to restore glutathione used in the metabolism of these drugs, which may account for the elevated GGT. Glutathione is conjugated to these drugs via the glutathione S-transferase system, and the complex is then excreted.

Other Enzymes

5′-Nucleotidase activity (see Chap. 13) is increased in cholestatic disorders with virtually no increase in activity in patients with bone disease. Measurement of 5′-nucleotidase can corroborate the elevation of ALP from a hepatic source. Other enzymes, such as leucine aminopeptidase (LAP), can also be used for the same purpose but rarely are. Isocitrate dehydrogenase and OCT activities are elevated in hepatocellular injury and parallel ALT and AST activities, but they are not specific for liver. Again, like LAP, they are rarely used in routine laboratory assays.

Proteins Related to Liver Function

Two vital measurements of liver function are total protein and albumin levels in serum. The liver is the site of more than 90% of all protein and 100% of albumin synthesis. Thus, extensive destruction of liver tissue will result in low serum levels of these two analytes. It should be noted that other major causes of low serum total protein and albumin are renal disease, malnutrition, protein-losing enteropathies, and, less commonly, chronic inflammatory diseases. These alternative causes must always be considered when evaluating liver function status.

Determination of serum protein levels is based usually on the biuret method. This method reflects the ability of the peptide backbone C=O groups of proteins to form color complexes with copper that absorb strongly at 540 nm. Some methods utilize a dye-binding method in which the proteins form a complex with the dye Coomassie blue. Albumin forms a unique color complex with the dye bromcresol green, the absorption of which can be determined at 630 nm.

Total serum protein consists of albumin and globulins. As discussed in Chapter 11 on electrophoresis of serum proteins, the globulins consist grossly of α_1, α_2, and β proteins and the γ-immune globulins. Normal total serum protein levels are generally in the range of 6 to 7.8 g/dL. At least 60% of this protein should be albumin, the normal range for which is about 3.2 to 4.5 g/dL. Serum proteins that are important in evaluating liver function will now be discussed.

Albumin

This protein is the major osmotically active component of the vascular system. It is also a transport protein for many endogenous (e.g., bilirubin and thyroid hormone) and exogenous (e.g., drugs) substances. The liver can synthesize approximately 120 mg/kg of albumin daily. This rate can approximately be doubled if serum albumin falls, because of either loss (e.g., from the kidneys) or serodilution.

Low serum albumin levels due to liver disease are almost always caused by massive destruction of liver tissue and are seen primarily in cirrhosis, most often secondary to alcoholism. The diminution in albumin is paralleled by a fall in total serum protein. Because albumin is the osmotically active intravascular colloid, hypoalbuminemia often results in edema. In cirrhosis, wherein destruction of sinusoids causes portal hypertension, the combined effect of elevated hydrostatic pressure in the portal system and the low colloid osmotic pressure results in ascites.

It is interesting that, in cirrhosis, while the serum albumin falls, the serum immunoglobulin levels increase, reversing the albumin/globulin ratio. Patients with this condition, however, are generally in an immunosuppressed state. This pattern is typical of cirrhosis (especially alcoholic cirrhosis), acquired immunodeficiency syndrome (AIDS), and sometimes diabetes. A common finding in each of these conditions is diminished CD4-positive T-cell function. Characteristically, in cirrhosis, serum protein electrophoresis reveals that the albumin is low, the γ-globulin is high, and there is the typical β-γ bridging pattern as described in Chapter 11.

γ-Globulins

Polyclonal elevations of these immune globulins are never specific for liver disease. When hypergammaglobulinemia does occur in patients with liver disease, it usually reflects the severity of the disease, although this correlation does not always hold. In autoimmune chronic hepatitis, markedly elevated values range from around 2.5 g/dL to over 6 g/dL. At the higher levels, hyperviscosity of blood may occur. Chronic active hepatitis B is often accompanied by mild elevations in γ-globulin, mainly IgG. Chronic alcoholic liver disease may result in similar elevations due to *both* IgA and IgG. IgA is also elevated in biliary obstruction. On the other hand, primary biliary cirrhosis is associated with marked elevations in IgM.

Special Serum Proteins

α_1-Antitrypsin

α_1-Antitrypsin (AAT), which constitutes about 90% of the α_1 band on serum protein electrophoresis (see Chap. 11), is a circulating serine protease inhibitor that blocks the degradative action of trypsin on tissue proteins. It is also an acute phase reactant. Deficiency of AAT is associated with lung and liver disease. In the former, it is associated with centrilobular emphysema, which becomes progressively worse with time. Patients with AAT deficiency are also predisposed to cholestasis in childhood and to cirrhosis, usually in adolescence or adult life.

There are three known AAT proteins, called M, S, and Z. All are encoded on allelic genes. In the United States, the overwhelming genotype is Pi^{MM}, where Pi is protease inhibitor. The other genotypes, Pi^{ZZ}, Pi^{SS}, Pi^{SZ}, Pi^{MZ}, and Pi^{MS}, all contain measurable activity of antiprotease except a rare null genotype Pi^{-}. If the antiprotease activity of the MM phenotype is used as the reference, the activity in phenotype ZZ is 15%, SS is 60%, MZ is 57.5%, and MS 80%. Adults with Pi^{ZZ} are the most prone to develop emphysema relatively early in life as a result of uninhibited trypsin activity on alveolar wall elastin. Patients with Z protein tend to accumulate the Z protein in periportal hepatocytes, where it forms discrete cytoplasmic bodies.

Ceruloplasmin

Ceruloplasmin is a copper-containing oxidase that is a glycoprotein synthesized in the liver. In Wilson's (hepatolenticular) disease, ceruloplasmin is low, most likely secondary to a defect in hepatic synthesis. Thus, patients with Wilson's disease accumulate copper, which becomes elevated both in serum and in urine. Detection in urine is usually the method of choice for screening patients with this disease. The excess copper becomes deposited in lysosomes in hepatocytes, leading ultimately to cell necrosis and cirrhosis or, rarely, fulminant hepatic failure. It also becomes deposited in the cornea (Kayser-Fleischer ring) and the lenticular nucleus of the basal ganglia in the central nervous system. Serum ceruloplasmin can also be low in severe hepatocellular disease and may be elevated in chronic cholestasis.

α-Fetoprotein

α-Fetoprotein (AFP) is synthesized by embryonic hepatocytes and fetal yolk sac cells and peaks in the second trimester of pregnancy, eventually constituting up to one third of fetal serum protein. The function of AFP is not known. It may be immunosuppressive, preventing fetal destruction by circulating maternal antibodies.

As noted in Chapter 21, AFP becomes abnormally elevated in fetal neural tube defects. The reasons for this correlation are unclear. It is important to note that normal AFP levels vary considerably with gestational age. Therefore, the decision that the serum level of this protein is abnormally high will depend on the reference interval for the gestational age of the patient.

Shortly after birth, AFP levels fall, reaching the adult normal range at around one year of age. After acute hepatic injury, AFP from regenerating hepatocytes usually rises (typically 100 to 200 ng/dL). Often, however, these typical elevations after acute hepatic insults do not occur after surgical resection of the liver. Regeneration is therefore not enough to cause elevated AFP levels.

AFP is an important marker for hepatocellular carcinoma (HCC). Elevated levels occur in over 90% of patients with this disease. As noted earlier, levels can become elevated after acute liver disease, making this marker somewhat nonspecific. However, at levels exceeding 400 ng/dL, there is a high probability of HCC, but at these levels of AFP, the tumor is widespread so that its use as an early detector of HCC is limited. Serum levels of AFP in HCC also depend on the extent and degree of differentiation of the tumor and the age of the patient.

Fibronectin

Plasma fibronectin is a glycoprotein synthesized in the liver and is important in the removal of particulate debris, such as membranes, from the circulation (Mosher, 1986). Plasma fibronectin is decreased in hepatocellular disease, such as cirrhosis and fulminant hepatic failure (discussed later; see also Chap. 4). Marked decreases in fibronectin suggest a poor prognosis in alcoholic cirrhosis (Naveau, 1985). Determination of fibronectin levels may become important in assessing the status of the liver, especially in shock when it is being considered as a donor organ for transplantation.

Type III Collagen

Connective tissue biosynthesis greatly increases in hepatocellular disease such as chronic hepatitis and cirrhosis. A major component of connective tissue is collagen. Type III collagen is first synthesized in a procollagen form that is then split by a peptidase into Type III collagen and an amino terminal procollagen Type III peptide, called PIIIP, some of which is extruded into serum, where it may be detected by immunoassay (Hahn, 1984; Teare, 1993). Serum levels of PIIIP are elevated in alcoholic hepatitis and active cirrhosis (Teare, 1993; Weigand, 1984), although the correlation between the PIIIP level and the degree of fibrosis is reportedly poor in patients with inactive cirrhosis (Heredia, 1985). High levels of PIIIP also have been found in chronic forms of hepatitis B and in biliary cirrhosis (Teare, 1993). In alcoholic hepatitis, the increased levels of PIIIP appear to correlate with the activity of vitamin C–dependent hepatic prolylhydroxylase, the enzyme responsible for the formation of hydroxyproline necessary for synthesis of collagen (Torres-Salinas, 1986).

PIIIP may be useful for monitoring the effects of drugs such as methotrexate (Risteli, 1988) and as a prognostic factor. PIIIP levels have been reported not to correlate with the degree of hepatic fibrosis in patients with idiopathic hemochromatosis (Roberts, 1986). Serum levels of PIIIP may be elevated in patients with viral hepatitis but normalize as the infection subsides. Continued elevated levels of PIIIP after a viral infection may indicate chronic hepatitis. It was once thought that PIIIP levels could distinguish between chronic active hepatitis and chronic persistent hepatitis (Annoni, 1986). However, it has been found that PIIIP cannot distinguish between chronic viral hepatitis subgroups (Teare, 1993).

Clotting Factors

(see also Chaps. 4 and 29)

Except for Factor VIII, including the von Willebrand factor, which is made by endothelial cells (including those in the liver [Wion, 1985]), coagulation proteins are synthesized in the liver. Also, inhibitors of coagulation, such as antithrombin III, α_2-macroglobulin, α_1-antitrypsin, C1 esterase inhibitor, and protein C, are synthesized in the liver. Low levels of antithrombin III in patients with cirrhosis and hepatitis may be caused by decreased synthesis, increased consumption, or an alteration in the transcapillary flux ratio (Kelly, 1987).

Patients with liver disease may also manifest platelet deficiency or dysfunction. Thrombocytopenia may result from splenic sequestration in patients with hepatosplenomegaly. Occasionally, it results from the presence of platelet antibodies. Alcoholism and (rarely) acute viral hepatitis can cause thrombocytopenia. Alcohol is known to suppress the marrow, leading to this condition.

Disseminated intravascular coagulation (DIC), characterized by an increased consumption of clotting factors and platelets, may accompany cirrhosis and acute fulminant hepatic failure. The mechanism has been postulated to be decreased synthesis of clotting inhibitory factors, decreased clearance of activated clotting factors, or release of tissue thromboplastin from hepatocytes (Kelly, 1986). Fibrin split products, detected in DIC, have been found in up to 80% of patients with liver disease without evidence of fibrinolysis (Van de Water, 1986).

In patients with cholestasis, absorption of the fat-soluble vitamin K from the gut may be impaired because of low levels of bile salts that allow membrane transport of this vitamin. Because Factors II, VII, IX, and X depend on this vitamin for activation via carboxylation, coagulation abnormalities often result. Thus, in patients with cholestasis but not cirrhosis or fulminant hepatic failure, serum levels of inactive precursor forms of these four coagulation factors are normal. Prothrombin time usually can be corrected by the administration of vitamin K when Factor V is normal in patients with cholestatic liver disease.

Coagulation abnormalities in patients with liver disease are often an important cause of bleeding. In cirrhosis, another important cause of bleeding is portal hypertension, which results in varices throughout the entire gastrointestinal tract and abdomen. The most frequent sites of variceal bleeding in these patients are the esophagus and the stomach. Patients with liver disease also have increased incidence of gastritis and peptic ulcer disease as well as portal hypertensive gastropathy, which may appear as a "watermelon" stomach.

Ammonia and Amino Acids

Ammonia is produced endogenously in the body as the end product of amino acid and nucleic acid metabolism. Some ammonia is also liberated from metabolic reactions such as the action of the enzyme glutaminase on glutamine, resulting in the production of glutamic acid and ammonia. Ammonia is highly toxic to the central nervous system for a variety of reasons. For example, one major effect of ammonia is to cause the conversion of glutamic acid to glutamine via reversal of the glutaminase-catalyzed reaction referred to earlier. Normally, decarboxylation of glutamic acid yields γ-aminobutyric acid (GABA), an extremely important neurotransmitter. Because ammonia decreases the concentration of glutamic acid by reacting with it to form glutamine, the concentration of GABA is lowered in the central nervous system.

Liver is the only tissue that can detoxify ammonia by converting it to urea in the urea cycle. In this cycle, ammonia is condensed with CO_2 and ATP to form carbamoyl phosphate in the presence of the widely distributed enzyme, carbamoyl phosphate synthetase. In the next, rate-limiting, step, which is unique to the liver, carbamoyl phosphate is condensed with the amino acid ornithine to form citrulline in the presence of the enzyme ornithine carbamoyl transferase (OCT). Citrulline is then itself condensed with aspartate to yield argininosuccinic acid that is cleaved to yield arginine and fumarate. The latter is metabolized in the Krebs cycle, while the former is then degraded by the enzyme arginase to form urea and ornithine that is then recycled in the urea cycle.

If more than 80% of liver tissue is destroyed, as in cirrhosis or fulminant hepatic failure, ammonia cannot be detoxified. Also, in the process of hepatic necrosis, some of the amino acid intermediates in the urea cycle that have known neurotoxic effects, such as arginine, may accumulate. The result is the buildup of ammonia and these amino acid intermediates in the circulation and in the central nervous system, giving rise to hepatic encephalopathy. In addition, in most cirrhotics, intrahepatic portal-systemic shunting occurs, thereby causing ammonia to bypass the liver and resulting in elevated serum ammonia concentrations.

In patients with cirrhosis or fulminant hepatic failure, there is some dispute as to whether ammonia itself is the cause of the observed metabolic encephalopathy; other toxins that accumulate as a result of absent hepatic detoxification are a possible cause. One of the arguments often used is that the severity of the encephalopathy does not correlate clearly with the serum ammonia concentrations. Countering this argument is the finding that in patients with cirrhosis or fulminant hepatic failure, lowering the serum ammonia invariably diminishes the severity of the encephalopathy. This finding, combined with the known ammonia-induced inhibition of neurotransmitter synthesis in the central system, suggests that ammonia is critical as a cause of encephalopathy (Pincus, 1991). Because ammonia causes the accumulation of glutamine in the central nervous system, serum or cerebrospinal fluid levels of glutamine are sometimes used in the diagnosis and management of hepatic encephalopathy.

Elevated serum ammonia concentrations in hepatic encephalopathy usually are reduced with the agent lactulose, which is metabolized by specific gut bacteria to lactic acid. The acid so produced in the intestinal lumen traps ammonia as ammonium ion, which can no longer diffuse across the intestinal membrane and is thus excreted. Ammonia-producing bacteria in the intestine are removed by treatment with antibiotics such as neomycin.

Measurement of Ammonia Concentrations in Serum and Other Body Fluids

A number of methods have been devised for measuring ammonia concentrations in serum and other body fluids. All require prompt analysis of a chilled, fresh specimen. One of these is enzymatic, in which ammonia is used in the reductive amination of a keto acid to form the amino acid. In this reaction, NADH is converted to NAD. The most widely used method involves the reaction of α-ketoglutarate with ammonia and NADH to form glutamate and NAD in the presence of the enzyme glutamate dehydrogenase. The decrease in absorbance at 340 nm, from the conversion of NADH to NAD, is measured to quantitate the ammonia present.

Amino Acidopathies in Liver Disease

Patients with hepatic encephalopathy sometimes have increased concentrations of methionine and the aromatic amino acids tyrosine, tryptophan, and phenylalanine and decreased concentrations of branched-chain amino acids such as valine and isoleucine. Excess aromatic amino acids in the central nervous system may be converted to neurotransmitters, neurotransmitter inhibitors, or both that may help to cause and exacerbate the hepatic encephalopathy. The ratio of branched-chain amino acids to aromatic amino acids is decreased in chronic liver disease such as cirrhosis. If the ratio falls below 1 in fulminant hepatic failure, it is considered a poor prognostic sign (Steigman, 1984). Amino acid concentrations in serum are rarely used in evaluation of hepatic disease states.

HEPATOBILIARY SYSTEM

Bilirubin and Other Pigments

Bilirubin is the major metabolic product of heme from hemoglobin, about 70% of which is derived from senescent red cells (Crawford, 1988). About 15% derives from hepatic sources, and a minor amount derives from kidney and bone marrow. Bilirubin production in healthy adults averages 250 to 350 mg per day (Muraca, 1988). Various amounts of serum bilirubin circulates in plasma bound to albumin, so-called δ-bilirubin (Lauff, 1982), which becomes elevated particularly in patients with cholestatic jaundice (Van Hootegem, 1985). With recovery, δ-bilirubin takes longer to clear than other bilirubin fractions not bound to albumin.

In the spleen and in the reticuloendothelial system, methemoglobin is metabolized to give free globin chains and heme. The heme porphyrin ring (Fig. 12–1) is then oxidized to the open chain form, called biliverdin, resulting in the release of iron in the Fe^{+3} state. This reaction is catalyzed by a microsomal heme oxygenase system. In the ring opening reaction, one mole of carbon monoxide (CO) is released, which is transported ultimately as carboxyhemoglobin. Biliverdin is then reduced to bilirubin (see Fig. 12–1) by the NADPH-dependent enzyme, biliverdin reductase. Bilirubin is then transported mainly in the portal system to the liver, where it enters the hepatocyte on its membrane surface in contact with the sinusoids, as shown in Figure 12–2.

Bilirubin enters hepatocytes by two mechanisms: one is by passive diffusion and the other is by receptor-mediated endocytosis. As summarized in Figure 12–2, once in the hepatocyte, bilirubin is "handed-off" from one protein complex to another in a chain. First, it complexes with the so-called Y and Z proteins and then binds sequentially to a protein complex called ligandin. From this complex, it is transported to the smooth endoplasmic reticulum (SER). In the SER, bilirubin becomes the substrate of the enzyme, glucuronyl transferase, which catalyzes the esterification of the propionic acid side chains of bilirubin with glucuronic acid (present as uridine diphosphate glucuronic acid) to form mainly the diglucuronide conjugate, shown in Figure 12–1 (Chowdhury, 1988). Some monoglucuronide and a small amount of triglucuronide also form. The ratio of monoconjugated to diconjugated pigment in bile is 1:4, whereas the ratio is nearly 1:1 in plasma, suggesting that monoconjugates reflux into plasma more readily.

As schematized in Figure 12–2, the conjugated bilirubin is then transported to the membrane surface opposite the sinusoidal face, which is in contact with bile canaliculi. Conjugated bilirubin can be directly excreted into the canaliculi, whereas unconjugated bilirubin cannot traverse this membrane. Once bilirubin is excreted into the canaliculi and ultimately into the

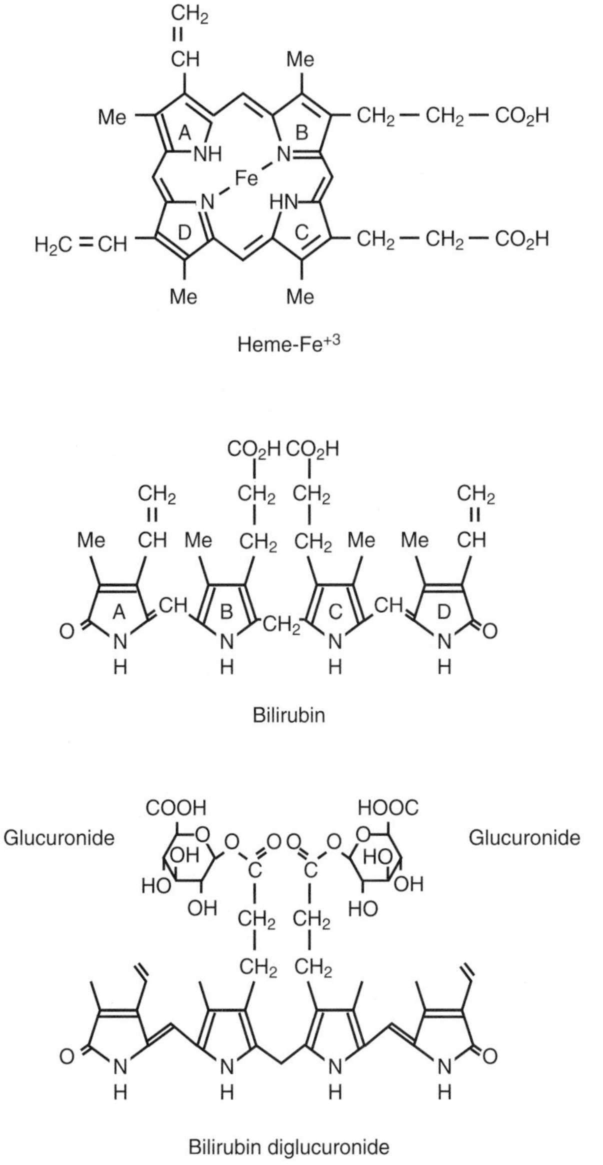

Figure 12–1. Structures of critical molecules in the conversion of heme bound to ferric ion (Heme-Fe^{+3}) to bilirubin and the metabolism of bilirubin to its diglucuronide. Bilirubin is transported into the hepatocyte, where it is converted into the diglucuronide form and secreted into canaliculi. (Adapted from Crawford JM, Hauser SC, Gollan JL: Formation, hepatic metabolism, and transport of bile pigments: A status report. Semin Liver Dis 1988; 8:105.)

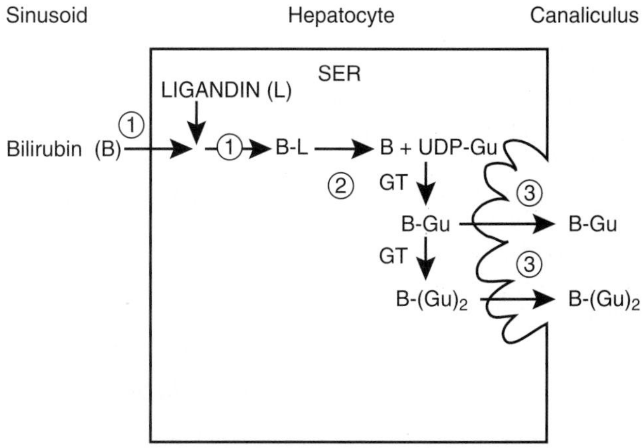

Figure 12–2. Schematic summary of the pathway of bilirubin (B) transport and metabolism. After hemoglobin (Fe^{+2}) is split into heme-Fe^{+3} and globin, the ferric ion is removed from the heme protoporphyrin ring. This ring is oxidized to biliverdin and thence to bilirubin in the reticuloendothelial system. The bilirubin is transported to the hepatocyte, where it can diffuse and be transported into this cell. In the cytosol, it complexes with ligandin (L) and is further transported to the smooth endoplasmic reticulum (SER), where it dissociates from ligandin and reacts with uridine diphosphoglucuronic acid (UDP-Gu) to form the monoglucuronide (B-Gu) and the diglucuronide (B-Gu_2) in the presence of the enzyme glucuronyl transferase (GT). The latter two compounds are then secreted into the canaliculus as conjugated bilirubin. There are several steps at which the process of transport and secretion can be blocked in inborn errors of metabolism. At step 1, transport of bilirubin into the hepatocyte and/or its complexing with ligandin may be deficient. This condition results in increased concentrations of unconjugated bilirubin in serum, such as Gilbert's disease. At step 2, glucuronyl transferase may be deficient, leading to a severe unconjugated hyperbilirubinemia, the Crigler-Najjar syndrome. At step 3, blockage of the secretion of conjugated bilirubin leads to a conjugated hyperbilirubinemia, in the Dubin-Johnson or the Rotor syndrome.

intestinal tract, it is further metabolized by intestinal bacteria, which effect its deconjugation and oxidation or reduction with the formation of compounds collectively called urobilinogen and urobilin, which can then be reabsorbed from the gut. Most absorbed urobilinogen is re-excreted by the liver. A minor fraction may be excreted in the urine. Larger quantities are found in the urine in conditions leading to hyperbilirubinemia or in conditions in which the liver cannot readily secrete urobilinogen absorbed from the gut.

Methods of Measurement

From the earlier discussion, it is clear that there are two forms of bilirubin that can exist in serum: conjugated, the major component of so-called *direct* bilirubin, and unconjugated, the major component of so-called *indirect* bilirubin (Muraco, 1988). Bilirubin is measured by conjugating it to an appropriate diazonium salt, most often diazotized sulfanilic acid. The resulting azo dye absorbs strongly at 540 nm. This is known as the van den Bergh method.

Historically, it was noted that the reaction of azo dye with bilirubin was biphasic (i.e., a fast phase followed by a more prolonged phase). Investigation of this reaction revealed that the fast reaction component was due mainly to the soluble conjugated bilirubin, whereas the slow component was due predominantly to the less soluble, unconjugated bilirubin. Most current methods, such as the most commonly used Jendrassik-Grof method, use solubilizing agents such as theophylline and methanol to ensure that both conjugated and unconjugated bilirubin are fully solubilized and react rapidly with the diazonium salt. This reaction then gives the total bilirubin. If the solubilizing agents are omitted from the reaction, the rapid color change that is observed measures the immediately reacting, direct, bilirubin. The total bilirubin minus the direct bilirubin gives the indirect or unconjugated bilirubin. Using this method, total bilirubin levels in normal individuals should not exceed about 1.2 to 1.5 mg/dL, over 70% of which is indirect (unconjugated) bilirubin (Sieg, 1986). It should be realized that normal bilirubin ranges depend on age and sex. In a study at Columbia Presbyterian Medical Center of a large patient population with normal serum bilirubin levels, the overall mean for males was found to be 0.5 mg/dL, whereas for females it was 0.3 mg/dL (Rosenthal, 1983). The lower levels in females may be the result of more efficient conjugation of bilirubin (Fevery, 1986).

Most interference with the accurate determination of serum levels of bilirubin measured by the method just described is due to hemoglobin. At hemoglobin levels between 1 and 5 g/dL, the method overestimates bilirubin levels, whereas at higher levels of hemoglobin, the method underestimates bilirubin levels. Thus, in hemolyzed blood specimens, either from *in vivo* or *in vitro* hemolysis, accurate determinations of bilirubin may be compromised.

Derangements of Bilirubin Metabolism

As shown in Figure 12–2, in each step in the excretion of bilirubin, there is a possible lesion leading to elevated serum levels of bilirubin. Each of these is discussed in turn.

HEMOLYSIS

In hemolytic anemias, unconjugated bilirubin rises because of abnormally high levels of hemoglobin released from erythrocytes. If the rate of bilirubin formation exceeds the rate of the liver to conjugate it, the bilirubin level in serum will rise. Virtually all of this bilirubin will be *indirect* bilirubin. Thus, one manner of confirming a diagnosis of hemolytic anemia in adults is the finding of elevated indirect bilirubin levels in serum. Usually, these levels are not dramatically elevated and are generally in the range of 1.5 to 3.0 mg/dL.

GILBERT'S SYNDROME—BILIRUBIN TRANSPORT DEFICIT

A significant number of persons have a transport deficit in the sinusoidal membrane of the hepatocyte. Transport of bilirubin into hepatocytes is thus compromised, resulting in an elevation in *indirect* bilirubin. This hereditary condition is called Gilbert's syndrome. Because bilirubin passively diffuses into hepatocytes, this condition is rarely serious and may result in mild elevations of bilirubin such as those seen in hemolytic anemia as described earlier.

Gilbert's syndrome has perhaps been overdiagnosed. This condition is most frequently diagnosed in young adults ranging in age from 20 to 30 years. However, we have found (Rosenthal, 1983) that normal bilirubin ranges are age-dependent and actually reach their highest levels in this age group (for males, > 0.6 mg/mL).

CONJUGATION DEFICIT—CRIGLER-NAJJAR SYNDROME

Much more serious is an inborn error of metabolism, called the Crigler-Najjar syndrome, in which the enzyme glucuronyl transferase is absent or defective. This condition results in low or no conjugation of bilirubin to glucuronic acid so that bilirubin cannot be excreted into the canaliculi. Indirect bilirubin builds up within hepatocytes and then back-diffuses into the sinusoids and thence into the circulation, where it is detected in serum.

Newborns with this disease become jaundiced (bilirubin levels > 5 mg/dL). Of great danger in this condition is the condition of kernicterus, wherein unconjugated bilirubin becomes deposited in the lenticular nucleus of the basal ganglia of the central nervous system, causing severe motor dysfunction and retardation (see Chaps. 21, 26, and 30). This condition, if not corrected immediately, is uniformly fatal. Kernicterus becomes a danger when indirect bilirubin levels exceed 15 mg/dL; kernicterus is a certainty at levels exceeding 20 mg/dL. It is vital to treat these infants with phototherapy to cause excretion of the unconjugated bilirubin. Phototherapy causes a change in the conformation of the bilirubin molecule, making it more compact and soluble.

EXCRETION DEFICITS: DUBIN-JOHNSON SYNDROME

In another inborn error of metabolism, called the Dubin-Johnson syndrome, there is a blockade of the excretion of bilirubin into the canaliculi, possibly caused by defects in the hepatocyte membrane. Thus, *conjugated* bilirubin accumulates within the hepatocyte and eventually back-diffuses into the circulation, where it is detected in serum. This inborn error can sometimes be confused with the Rotor syndrome, of viral origin, where there is also a block in the excretion of conjugated bilirubin. In these cases, liver biopsy often will reveal cytosolic inclusion bodies within hepatocytes.

BILIARY OBSTRUCTION

In adults, cholelithiasis is the most common cause of hyperbilirubinemia. This condition results from the presence of bile stones (that are composed of either bilirubin or cholesterol) anywhere in the biliary tree (i.e., the gall bladder and the cystic duct, the common bile duct, and the right, left, and common hepatic ducts). Most frequently, patients presenting with this condition are parous white females in early middle age (giving rise to the semi-mnemonic, "fair, fecund, fortyish female"). Biliary obstruction due to cholelithiasis always results in the elevation of total bilirubin, more than 90% of which is direct bilirubin. In over 90% of such patients, there is a concomitant rise in ALP. The levels of this enzyme are variable but are frequently above 300 IU/L.

Inflammatory conditions of the biliary tract also give rise to elevated serum levels of direct bilirubin and ALP. In hepatitis, in which there is toxic destruction of hepatocytes due to viral, chemical, or traumatic causes, focal necrosis, cellular injury, or both cause blocking of conjugation of bilirubin and excretion of conjugated bilirubin. Thus, *both* direct and indirect bilirubin are elevated. Serum levels of bilirubin vary with the severity of infection and the extent of disease. In viral hepatitis, such as hepatitis B, as discussed subsequently, serum bilirubin levels may reach levels of 5 to 10 mg/dL.

In contrast, inflammation of the biliary tract itself, mainly in the condition of ascending cholangitis, results in the elevation predominantly of direct bilirubin and ALP. The rise in direct bilirubin often exceeds 5 mg/dL. In gram-negative sepsis, what appears to be a mild inflammation of the biliary tract can result in mild elevations of direct bilirubin to levels of 2 to 3 mg/dL. There is a concomitant elevation of ALP to levels of 200 to 300 IU/L.

Cholesterol and Other Lipids

(see Chap. 10)

Because the liver is vital in lipoprotein metabolism, hepatic disorders cause derangements in lipoprotein metabolism. These include altered lipoprotein distributions, deficiency of lecithin-cholesterol acyltransferase (LCAT—the enzyme that esterifies cholesterol), lipolytic defects that result in hypertriglyceridemia (triglyceride levels ranging from 250 to 500 mg/dL) due to low levels of lipoprotein lipase, and elevations of biliary lipids into plasma (Seidel, 1987).

The elevated triglycerides in patients with hepatocellular injury are usually found in an abnormal low-density lipoprotein (LDL) fraction, the so-called abnormally migrating β lipoprotein, typical of Type III hyperlipoproteinemia. Fatty liver with obesity or diabetes mellitus is also associated with hypertriglyceridemia. The hypertriglyceridemia in these individuals is mainly carbohydrate-induced, whereas in the alcoholic it results mainly from decreased lipoprotein lipase activity. Injection of a test dose of heparin enhances lipoprotein lipase activity but not in acute alcoholic hepatitis.

Another major abnormality in patients with hepatocellular injury is a decrease in the percentage of cholesteryl esters, a result of LCAT deficiency. These patients also have an increase in lecithin, a decrease in lysolecithin, and marked elevations in unesterified cholesterol. Conversely, in cirrhotics, poorly nourished patients may have low levels of cholesterol (<100 mg/dL).

Furthermore, in patients with hepatocellular injury, there is often an increase in phospholipids in very-low-density lipoproteins (VLDL) and a decrease in the cholesteryl esters of high-density lipoproteins (HDL). HDL subpopulations are variably reduced in chronic liver disease. HDL_3 is reduced, whereas HDL_2 may be unaffected. HDL_3 concentration may be elevated in alcoholic patients if alcohol ingestion continues (Chang, 1986).

Many patients with cholestatic liver disease show the same patterns as do patients with hepatocellular injury. In addition, other lipoproteins, notably lipoprotein-X, appear. One possible explanation for the origin of lipoprotein-X is regurgitation of biliary lipids. Another is the accumulation of substrates because of the LCAT deficiency, although LCAT deficiency is more variable in cholestatic disease than in hepatocellular injury. Patients with primary biliary cirrhosis have very high levels of HDL, presumably as a result of some lipoprotein-X being included in this fraction (Siede, 1983).

The apo A1 protein in the HDL fraction is significantly decreased in chronic diseases of the liver, especially in cirrhosis (Teare, 1993). As discussed subsequently, if apo A1 levels are combined with γ-glutamyl transferase activity and the prothrombin time (the so-called PGA index), alcoholic hepatitis and cirrhosis can be diagnosed without the necessity of liver biopsy.

Bile Acids and Salts

Bile salts are products of cholesterol metabolism. They are not usually used in the diagnosis of abnormal liver function but are important in that they account for a substantial amount of bile in bilirubin excretion and can therefore be of use in diagnosing cholestasis. Also, in severe biliary obstruction, the buildup of bile salts in serum causes symptomatic illness in the form of intractable itching. The primary bile acids, cholic and chenodeoxycholic, are produced in the liver. These bile acids are further metabolized to deoxycholate and lithocholate, respectively, when they are excreted into the intestine via the enterohepatic system (Carey, 1988) by bacterial 7-α-dehydroxylation in the intestinal lumen. Ursodeoxycholic acid, an end product of bile salt metabolism in humans, is produced by isomerization of secondary bile acids. These bile salts are conjugated to glycine and taurine and are also sulfated and glucuronidated. Conjugation of bile salts to taurine and as sulfates increases with the severity of cholestasis in conditions causing obstruction to bile outflow. Recirculation of bile salts to the liver occurs by reabsorption from the terminal ileum where deoxycholate is almost completely reabsorbed, and chenodeoxycholate is about 75% reabsorbed.

2

Renal clearance of bile acids is negligible in normal patients, but in cholestasis, renal excretion of bile salts, mainly in the form of sulfates and glucuronides, is enhanced. Fasting bile acids, when normal, can exclude the presence of parenchymal liver disease in patients with Gilbert's syndrome (Vierling, 1982), as discussed earlier. It should also be recognized that defective production of bile salts, which help solubilize the contents of bile, in the liver may predispose to the formation of bilirubinate or cholesterol stones and posthepatic biliary obstruction.

SPECIAL MARKERS IN HEPATIC AND HEPATOBILIARY DISEASE

(see Chaps. 41 and 43)

The liver is often involved in systemic diseases, especially in the autoimmune diseases such as systemic lupus erythematosus (SLE). Thus, elevated serum concentrations of the transaminases and LD with a significantly elevated titer of antinuclear double-stranded DNA antibody (ANA) suggest SLE as the cause of the abnormal liver function. In fact, one important cause of chronic active hepatitis is SLE. It should also be noted that primary liver disease can also cause systemic disease, such as the hepatorenal syndrome (see Chap. 4). Chronic active hepatitis with persistent circulating hepatitis B surface antigen, discussed subsequently, may also cause renal failure. The specific serologic markers for liver disease will now be discussed.

Antimitochondrial Antibodies (Primary Biliary Cirrhosis)

Biliary cirrhosis has two forms, primary and secondary. In the former, the bile canaliculi and ductules undergo fibrosis in the portal triads. Bile eventually seeps into hepatocytes, causing necrosis. Granulation tissue replaces hepatocytes so that the fibrosis eventually spreads into the liver parenchyma, giving rise to the pattern of fibrosis and regenerating nodules. Secondary biliary cirrhosis involves a similar course as a result of other underlying conditions such as choledocholithiasis, carcinoma of the head of the pancreas, and occasionally hepatitis and sepsis.

A vital difference between primary and secondary biliary cirrhosis is that the former uniquely appears to be part of a generalized autoimmune condition. Serum antibodies react with liver, kidney, stomach, and thyroid tissue in over 90% of patients with primary biliary cirrhosis. These circulating antibodies are directed against mitochondrial antigens from the inner mitochondrial membrane, called M2, which has been found to be dihydrolipoamide acetyltransferase, a component of the pyruvate dehydrogenase multienzyme complex (Coppel, 1988; Kaplan, 1984; Krams, 1989).

Antimitochondrial antibodies (AMAs) have been found in a variety of disease states, but there are two anti-M2 antibodies in primary biliary cirrhosis that uniquely react with either a protein of molecular mass 48 kilodaltons or a protein of molecular mass 62 kilodaltons (Fussey, 1988; Manns, 1987). In other disorders, anti-M1 has been found in syphilis, anti-M5 in collagen vascular diseases, anti-M6 in iproniazid-induced hepatitis, and anti-M7 in cardiomyopathies (Berg, 1986). AMAs with anti-M2 specificity are 100% specific for primary biliary cirrhosis.

Serologic Markers for Infectious Hepatitis

Many infectious agents can cause hepatitis. The three most important are hepatitis A, B, and C, caused by distinct viruses, which are discussed subsequently. Other causes that will be mentioned are the herpesviruses (i.e., cytomegalovirus and the Epstein-Barr virus as in infectious mononucleosis). Common to all acute virally induced hepatitis is a rapid rise in aminotransferase activity. Both ALT and AST rise to values often into the range of 300 to 500 IU/L and maintain a ratio of 1 or a ratio that slightly favors ALT.

It should be noted that the presence of hepatitis A, B, and C is detected serologically (i.e., viral antigens or antibodies to the virus-specific antigens are detected in the serum of the patient). In the assays for circulating viral antigens, a "capture" antibody is usually bound to a solid support. The patient's serum is then added to this system, and the captured antigen from the patient's serum is then identified by a second labeled antiantigen antibody in a "sandwich" technique in the ELISA assay as described in Chapter 33. To detect antibody to viral antigen in serum, the viral antigen is generally bound to a solid support and incubated with the patient's serum, and the antibody is detected again using the ELISA assay. Acute infection is detected by the presence of viral particles or by the presence of elevated antivirus IgM. Chronic infection or exposure to the virus is detected by elevated antiviral IgG.

Hepatitis A is caused by enterovirus 72 in the family of the RNA Picornaviridae. The virus is referred to as the hepatitis A virus (HAV). There are approximately 150,000 new cases of this disease per year in the United States. The most common mode of transmission of this virus is the fecal-oral route. The incubation time is 15 to 50 days (mean 28 days). The excretion of HAV precedes the onset of symptoms and rise in aminotransferase activity. In the early acute phase, which lasts for about two weeks and in which the patient becomes symptomatic and the aminotransferases are elevated, anti-HAV IgM is elevated and is an excellent marker for the disease. It remains detectable in serum for about three to six months. By the end of the early acute phase, the patient is no longer considered to be infectious even though the aminotransferases and bilirubin may continue to be elevated. Anti-HAV IgG rises within the first two weeks of the early acute phase and remains elevated for the remainder of the patient's life. The surface hepatitis A viral antigen can be detected both in the incubation period and in the early acute phase in the patient's serum and stool wherein whole viral particles may also

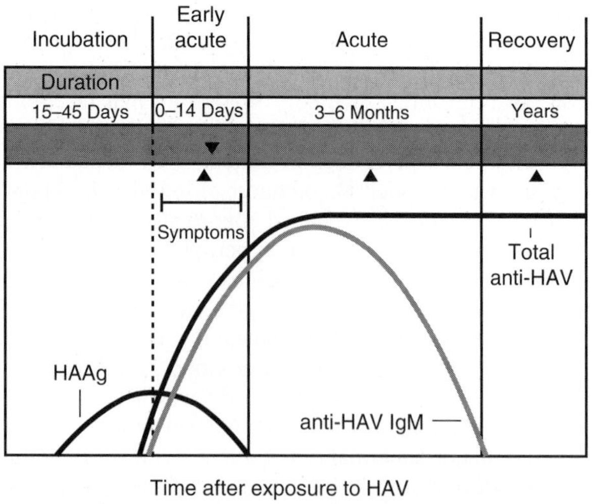

Figure 12–3. Typical time course for appearance of viral antigens and antiviral antibodies in hepatitis A viral (HAV) infection. The appearance of the hepatitis A antigen, HAAg, occurs early and is no longer present during the acute phase. The most effective diagnostic determination of acute hepatitis A infection is the detection of anti-HAV IgM. Not shown in this figure is the rise of the aminotransferases, AST and ALT, which occurs at the beginning of the early acute phase and lasts for several weeks to a month. The patient ceases to be infectious after anti-HAV IgM falls to undetectable levels in 3–6 months post–early phase. Permanent anti-HAV IgG rises over several months and lasts for many years, conferring immunity on the exposed or infected individual. (Reproduction of figure from "Hepatitis A Diagnostic Profile" has been granted with approval of Abbott Laboratories; all rights reserved by Abbott Laboratories.)

be detected. Procedures for detecting these particles are rarely performed given the ease of detecting anti-HAV IgM and IgG. Figure 12–3 summarizes the course of HAV infections in humans.

Hepatitis B is caused by a member of the Hepadnaviridae family, which are DNA viruses. The hepatitis B virus (HBV) is the 42-nm Dane particle that contains three viral protein antigens that are detected serologically: the hepatitis B surface antigen (HBsAg), the inner hepatitis B core antigen (HBcAg), and the e antigen (HBeAg), which may be a breakdown product of HBcAg and whose presence denotes infectivity. It is also possible to detect the Dane particle in acutely infected patients and to detect HBV DNA and its DNA polymerase. HBV DNA can be detected by hybridization or the polymerase chain reaction. Sometimes associated with HBV is an RNA virus called the hepatitis D virus, a 35-nm to 37-nm virus that contains the HBsAg and a core D antigen, called HDAg. This virus cannot replicate without the presence of the HBsAg of HBV. Together with HBV, the D-particle or δ-particle is a highly infectious agent and causes severe hepatitis.

HBV infection is transmitted mainly via blood contamination through open wounds. It is also transmitted by intravenous drug abuse (use of dirty, contaminated needles) and can be transmitted sexually. The virus can cross the placenta and causes neonatal hepatitis, often leading to chronic active hepatitis. There are approximately 750,000 to 1 million cases of hepatitis B in the United States. The fatality rate from HBV is 1.4%.

Figure 12–4 summarizes the course of HBV infections. The incubation period is 4 to 15 weeks. HBsAg rises at the

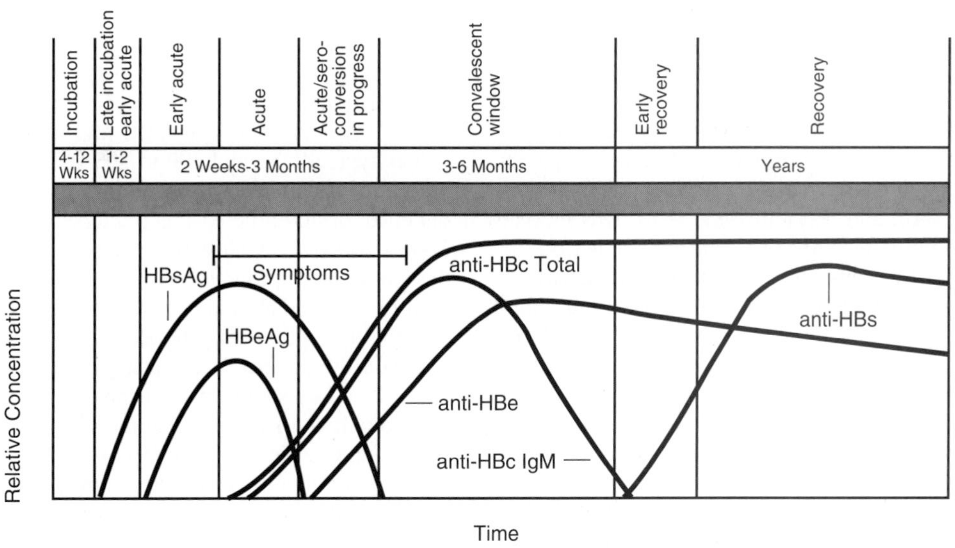

Figure 12–4. Typical time course for appearance of viral antigens and anti-viral antibodies in hepatitis B viral (HBV) infection. In the early acute phase, the HBV surface antigen (HBsAg) appears and lasts for several months. Detection of this antigen signifies acute HBV infection. Between the time the titer of HBsAg falls and the titer of anti-HBV IgG, which confers immunity, rises, there is a gap of about six months. In this time period, the titers of anti-HBV core antigen (anti-HBc) IgM and IgG rise, indicating acute HBV infection. This is the so-called core window. IgG anti-HBV e antigen (anti-HBe) also rises during this core window period. Permanent immunity is conferred by anti-HBsAg IgG (anti-HBs in the figure). It is difficult to determine the time at which the patient is no longer infectious. Generally, an individual is considered noninfectious when no HBsAg, HBeAg, and anti-HBcAg IgM can be detected, and the anti-HBsAg IgG has plateaued. Not shown in this figure is the pattern of AST and ALT elevations. These elevations occur in the early acute phase, slightly after HBsAg rises. AST and ALT levels may remain elevated for several weeks to several months, after which time they decline. In chronic HBV active hepatitis, HBsAg is present continuously. AST and ALT generally remain elevated although they can oscillate throughout the course of the disease. (Reproduction of figure from "Hepatitis B Diagnostic Profile" has been granted with approval of Abbott Laboratories; all rights reserved by Abbott Laboratories.)

end of the incubation period and at the beginning of the early acute phase. Not shown in this figure is the elevation of aminotransferases, which occurs in the early acute phase, about six weeks after infection, after HBsAg begins to rise. In the average patient with HBV, HBsAg persists for about three months after the incubation period. HBeAg persists throughout the early acute phase for about three months after the incubation period. After about three months, HBsAg disappears, but the patient is still in the infectious phase of the disease. During the acute phase of the disease, anti-HBcAg IgM rises and persists for about six months. Concurrently, anti-HBcAg IgG rises in the acute phase and persists for years after infection. Detection of anti-HBcAg IgM or total antibody (IgM + IgG) even in the absence of HBsAg indicates acute infection and infectivity of the patient. Within six months after infection, anti-HBsAG IgG rises and persists for many years. The rise of the latter antibody indicates recent infection or recent exposure. The period of time after which HBsAg disappears and anti-HBsAg IgG rises is referred as the "core window" during which the HBV infection can be diagnosed by detecting antibody to the core antigen, HBcAg.

It is important to note that, until well after anti-HBsAg IgG rises into the early recovery phase, the patient is considered potentially infectious. A chronic carrier state develops in 6% to 10% of adults, 25% to 50% of children, and 70% to 90% of infants with HBV infection. These individuals are found to have HBsAg for a prolonged period of time. If symptoms of hepatitis persist, these patients are said to have chronic active hepatitis. In asymptomatic patients with persistent HBsAg, the condition is referred to as chronic persistent hepatitis. In either condition, eventual liver damage occurs in a high percentage of these patients, and they are at risk for developing cirrhosis or HCC.

In **hepatitis B-δ**, with the hepatitis D viral co-infection, there is a major risk of severe hepatitis that may progress to fulminant hepatic failure (Sunheimer, 1994). The mortality rate for combined hepatitis B and D is 30%. Hepatitis D is diagnosed by detection of the D-antigen (HDAg) or the IgM or IgG antibody against it.

Hepatitis C is most commonly acquired from blood transfusions. It is also transmitted by intravenous drug abuse. Many cases of hepatitis C are cryptogenic, with no predisposing causes. Hepatitis C virus, or HCV, belongs to the Flavivirus family and contains a single strand of RNA with about 10,000 nucleotides covered by viral proteins. The entire genome of this virus has been cloned, and the antigens, called c-100-3, HC-31, and HC-34, have been overexpressed in *Escherichia coli*. Antibodies to these antigens can be detected in patients' sera, which develop within the incubation time of 2 to 26 weeks, using the Abbott Corporation (North Chicago, IL) EIA 2.0 ELISA method. Over 75% of infected individuals become chronically infected with the virus. The fatality rate is 1% to 2%. Often, in the carrier state, the serum ALT activity remains elevated for prolonged periods of time. Screening for hepatitis C carriers for blood transfusions by measuring ALT activity and anti-HCV antibodies in donor blood has reduced the risk of transmission of HCV from 21% to less than 1%.

Hepatitis E is a small RNA enterovirus that may belong to the Picornaviridae or Caliciviridae family and causes hepatitis mainly in Africa, Asia, Mexico, and increasingly in the

United States. Clinical manifestations are similar to those caused by HAV. Infection is acquired through the fecal-oral route, and the incubation period is about three to six weeks. Onset of symptoms is abrupt. The fatality rate is 1% to 2% except in pregnant women, for whom mortality reaches 20%.

Other Hepatitides. Other viral infectious agents, especially those among the herpesvirus family, in particular cytomegalovirus (CMV) and Epstein-Barr virus (EBV), can cause generally mild hepatitis. The incubation period for these viruses prior to symptoms varies from several days to several months. Symptoms generally are abrupt and short-lived and cause a mild elevation of the aminotransferases and hyperbilirubinemia, often manifested as frank jaundice (total bilirubin is greater than 2 mg/dL). CMV infection most often occurs in pregnant women and in patients on immunosuppressive therapy, especially for transplants. EBV infection occurs in the postpubescent college-age population and causes mononucleosis, a component of which may be mild hepatitis. Acute CMV infection is detected either by assays for anti-CMV IgM or a fourfold rise in the titer of anti-CMV IgG over a six-week period. Acute EBV infection is detected by a variety of techniques, including anti-EBV serum antibodies and specific anti-EBV IgM in the heterophile agglutination assay described in Chapter 27.

DIAGNOSIS OF LIVER DISEASES

Chapter 4 summarizes the fundamental patterns of laboratory findings in liver function abnormalities, which are encapsulated in Table 4–5. In this section, the major hepatic disorders are discussed with emphasis on laboratory evaluations that enable diagnosis, often without the need to perform invasive procedures such as liver biopsies.

It is important to remember that in acute hepatitis, the principal changes are significant elevations of aminotransferases; in cirrhosis, these tend to remain normal or become slightly elevated while the total protein and albumin are depressed, and ammonia concentrations in serum are elevated. In post-hepatic biliary obstruction, bilirubin and ALP become elevated; and in space-occupying diseases of the liver, ALP and LD are elevated. In fulminant hepatic failure, the aminotransferases and ammonia are elevated while total protein and albumin are depressed.

Hepatitis

Hepatitis usually first manifests itself clinically with the symptoms of fatigue and anorexia. Jaundice may be present. Generally, jaundice is first seen as scleral icterus when the patient has total serum bilirubin concentrations above 2 mg/dL. The cause of acute hepatitis is almost always viral, although chemical exposure such as to carbon tetrachloride or chloroform or to drugs such as acetaminophen, especially in children, should be considered. A special category of toxin-induced hepatitis is that induced by alcohol, discussed subsequently.

The cardinal finding in hepatitis is a rise in the aminotransferases to values of more than 200 IU/L and often to 500 or even 1000 IU/L. The AST/ALT ratio is close to 1 or may slightly favor ALT. The bilirubin is invariably elevated and is composed of both direct and indirect types. Elevations of indirect bilirubin are due to the inability of injured hepatocytes to conjugate bilirubin, whereas the rise of direct bilirubin is due to the blockage of compromised canaliculi secondary to the inflammatory process that occurs in the acute phase. Because of hepatocyte damage, LD levels are mildly elevated to values typically around 300 to 500 IU/L. Because of inflammation of canaliculi and ductules, necrosis of canaliculi and ductules, or both, the ALP is often also elevated to values of 200 to 500 IU/L. Unless the hepatitis is severe and involves the whole liver, progressing to fulminant hepatic failure, the total protein and albumin are within their normal ranges. The γ-globulin fractions may be elevated as a result of infection.

Given the pattern of the analytes suggestive of hepatitis, specific causes should be screened for (i.e., a determination of serologic markers for hepatitis A, B, and C). Screening for anti-hepatitis A IgM and for HBsAg can be performed within one day. If either of these tests is positive, the diagnosis is established. If they are negative, further screening for hepatitis B should be undertaken (i.e., determination of serum titers of anti-HBcAg IgM and IgG [core window] and anti-HBsAg IgG). If only the latter screen is positive, it may be difficult to establish whether hepatitis B is the cause of the infection or whether the patient has been exposed to the virus in the past. Unless the patient has chronic active or persistent hepatitis, in which case HBsAg is continuously present, titers of anti-HBsAg IgG are elevated long after the aminotransferases return to normal levels. If hepatitis B can be ruled out, screening for antibodies to hepatitis C should be performed. If this screen is negative, other viral causes should be sought (e.g., CMV and EBV). Other causes, such as chemical toxins, should also be considered, especially when a viral hepatitis screen is negative.

In **alcoholic hepatitis**, the described pattern of abnormal analyte concentrations holds except that AST often becomes disproportionately elevated over ALT. In addition, there are marked elevations of the enzyme GGT, often out of proportion to elevations in ALP. It has been postulated that alcohol causes damage to mitochondria in hepatocytes, resulting in the release of AST, a mitochondrial enzyme (ALT is non-mitochondrial), resulting in the higher serum levels of AST. Unless the alcoholic patient is malnourished, the total protein and albumin will be within their reference ranges.

Chronic Passive Congestion

In chronic passive congestion of the liver, most often secondary to congestive heart failure, back pressure from the right side of the heart is transmitted to the hepatic sinusoids from the inferior vena cava and hepatic veins. Increased pressure causes sinusoidal dilatation, which may cause some physical damage to hepatocytes. The result is a mild increase in the amino transferases and occasionally a mild hyperbilirubinemia. Other analytes that measure liver function are within their reference ranges.

Cirrhosis

Cirrhosis of the liver results in parenchymal fibrosis and hepatocytic nodular regeneration and can be caused by alcoholism (micronodular or Laennec's cirrhosis), panhepatic hepatitis, chronic active hepatitis, toxins and drugs, and diseases of the biliary tract as in primary and secondary biliary cirrhosis. Furthermore, systemic diseases can predispose to cirrhosis. In hemochromatosis, for example, excess iron becomes deposited in a variety of tissues including liver and becomes toxic to hepatocytes, causing cirrhosis. In Wilson's disease, in which the copper-binding oxidase, ceruloplasmin, is deficient, copper deposits in liver are also toxic and can also lead to a form of chronic active hepatitis and cirrhosis. This condition can be diagnosed from detecting low serum levels of ceruloplasmin and elevated urine levels of copper. In α_1-antitrypsin deficiency, patients have a significantly increased propensity to develop cirrhosis. In general, irrespective of the cause, cirrhosis is a chronic but gradually worsening condition. At its inception, it is often focal and may not be evident clinically.

A study of cirrhotic patients at different levels of progression of the disease (Teare, 1993) suggests that this condition can be diagnosed early using what is called the PGA index. This index (Poynard, 1991) is computed from the prothrombin time (PT) and from serum levels of γ-glutamyl transferase and apolipoprotein A1. Ranges of values for each of these analytes are divided into categories, numbered 0 to 4, in increasing order of severity. For example, GGT values between 20 and 49 are scored as 1, values between 50 and 99 are scored as 2, etc. For apo A1, increasing severity of disease correlates with *decreasing* concentration of this protein in serum. The prothrombin time increases with severity of disease because the liver is responsible for synthesis of coagulation factors. Details of this method are described by Poynard (1991). The scores for each of the three analytes are then summed to give a total PGA score or index. This index correlates well with the level of procollagen Type III propeptide (PIIIP) in serum, also used to follow active cirrhosis. Higher PGA scores correlate closely with the degree of hepatic fibrosis and with the severity of cirrhosis as judged both by clinical (Child's) grading and from liver biopsies. Thus, the PGA score and the PIIIP level aid diagnosis of cirrhosis and following the course of this disease. This simple index significantly reduces the need for liver biopsy (Teare, 1993).

As cirrhosis progresses to involve most of the liver parenchyma (>80%), liver function becomes compromised. Total protein synthesis drops to low levels, as does synthesis of albumin. Sclerosis of sinusoids in the liver causing portal hypertension, together with the drop in colloid osmotic pressure, results in ascites and even anasarca. Fibrosis of the intrahepatic bile ductules and cholangioles results in diminished excretion of bilirubin and bile salts, causing hyperbilirubinemia and a rise in ALP, GGT, and 5′-nucleotidase. If nodular regeneration is minimal, the serum concentrations of hepatocytic enzymes, such as AST, ALT, and LD, are either normal or diminished. If regeneration is more widespread, the levels of these enzymes in serum may become mildly elevated.

In all forms of cirrhosis, serum ammonia levels become significantly elevated and correlate roughly with the degree of encephalopathy. There are four clinically graded levels of hepatic encephalopathy: motor tremors detected as asterixis, in which the hands of the patient when pressed back and then released move back and forth in a flapping motion; a lethargic, stuporous state; severe obtundation; and frank coma. Lowering ammonia levels reduces the degree of encephalopathy.

Because the liver is the site of synthesis of all of the coagulation factors except Factor VIII, and because synthesis of these factors diminishes significantly in cirrhosis, coagulation disorders result. Accelerated partial thromboplastin and prothrombin times become prolonged, often accompanied by diminished platelet counts. The latter may be caused by splenic sequestration due to splenomegaly caused by portal hypertension. However, disseminated intravascular coagulopathy may occur in cirrhosis as evidenced by high levels of fibrin split products in serum and may be the cause of the diminished platelet count. Because of derangements in lipid metabolism in the liver, fats enter the circulation and become deposited in erythrocyte membranes, causing these cells to appear as target cells.

Loss of vascular volume from ascites and anasarca can cause low tissue perfusion and lactic acidosis. Volume receptors, sensitive to volume loss, stimulate the secretion of antidiuretic hormone (ADH). The retained water causes serodilution, leading to hyponatremia. However, the urine becomes concentrated, leading to the diagnosis of secretion of inappropriate amounts of ADH (SIADH), which, however, are really appropriate in the face of volume depletion.

Cirrhosis of the liver is often associated with renal failure as a result of the hepatorenal syndrome. In this condition, which is not well understood, renal tubular function is compromised. Serum BUN and creatinine rise to markedly elevated levels, indicating renal failure. Low tissue perfusion may also cause acute tubular necrosis. In hepatorenal syndrome, restoration of liver function will reverse renal failure.

Primary and secondary biliary cirrhosis are discussed earlier in this chapter. These conditions are difficult to diagnose because of the changing pattern of serum analyte concentrations used to evaluate liver status. Usually beginning as a posthepatic obstructive pattern, in which bilirubin and ALP are elevated (or, sometimes an isolated elevation of ALP is observed), the pattern progresses to one that resembles hepatitis due to the toxic effects of bile salts on hepatocytic function. With time, this pattern gives way to a cirrhotic pattern in which the aminotransferases decrease, total protein and albumin decrease, and ammonia rises. In patients with a persistent obstructive pattern indicated by laboratory results with no evidence of mass lesions or stones causing blockage of bile flow, the presence of anti-M2 AMA should be tested for. Increased titers of this antibody are virtually 100% diagnostic of biliary cirrhosis.

Survival for patients with primary biliary cirrhosis may be computed using an empirical formula that utilizes the age of the patient, the serum albumin and bilirubin, the prothrombin time, and the extent of edema (Dickson, 1989). This formula estimates the time limit within which the patient may undergo liver transplantation.

Biliary Tract Obstruction

Posthepatic biliary obstruction refers to blockage of the intrahepatic, extrahepatic, or cystic ducts and/or to blockage of bilirubin excretion from the hepatocyte into the canaliculi. All of these conditions lead to back-flow of bile into the hepatocyte and ultimately into the circulation; or to both. The most common cause of this condition is cholelithiasis. Other causes include inflammation of the biliary tract, as occurs in ascending cholangitis and in gram-negative sepsis. Drugs, such as the neuroleptics (e.g., chlorpromazine), can cause cholestatic jaundice. Mass lesions such as carcinoma of the head of the pancreas or lymphoma can also cause posthepatic biliary obstruction by blocking the common bile duct at the porta hepatis. Often, especially in inflammatory conditions in the biliary tract, bile flow is obstructed incompletely, permitting partial flow of bile. Under these conditions, bilirubin remains normal or is only mildly increased. Because of the inflammation, however, ALP becomes markedly elevated.

Occasionally, hyperbilirubinemia is observed in patients who are otherwise normal. The bilirubin is of the indirect type and most often results from hemolysis, most often in hemolytic anemia. Hemolytic anemias may be triggered by hepatic disease. For example, viral hepatitis may precipitate hemolysis in patients with glucose-6-phosphate dehydrogenase deficiency. In Zieve's syndrome, hemolysis occurs in conjunction with alcoholic hepatitis and hyperlipidemia. Wilson's disease is sometimes associated with acute hemolysis. Patients with chronic hepatitis secondary to autoimmune disease may develop severe hemolytic disease, sometimes requiring splenectomy.

Space-Occupying Lesions

In space-occupying lesions of the liver—a high percentage of which are due to metastatic cancer, a smaller percentage of which are due to lymphoma, primary HCC, angiosarcoma, and benign hemangiomas—the cardinal finding is isolated increases in the two enzymes, LD and ALP. Increases in ALP are caused by encroachments of the masses on canaliculi and cholangioles and even on the main bile ducts. The reasons for increases in LD are not clear. Most commonly, the LD_5 fraction is responsible for the increase. This fraction may be produced by the liver but also may be produced by the tumor. Typically, the values are 500 to 1000 IU/L or more for LD and above 500 IU/L for ALP. If a malignant tumor spreads widely through the liver, the aminotransferases may be elevated mildly, along with hyperbilirubinemia due to bile duct obstruction, and low protein and albumin. The latter findings may not be caused as much by liver dysfunction as by generalized cachexia associated with tumor spread.

Fulminant Hepatic Failure

In fulminant hepatic failure, an uncommon but highly fatal condition, massive necrosis of the liver results in complete liver failure. Depending on the nature and extent of the necrosis, ultimate liver regeneration frequently does not occur, although if the necrosis is limited and if hepatocytes can recover from the acute injury, normal liver function may return. The causes of this condition are largely unknown. Reye's syndrome is an example of this condition in which a child has an acute viral infection with fever and is treated with aspirin. Within one to two weeks after the infection and fever have dissipated, the child suddenly becomes encephalopathic secondary to acute hepatic failure. An adult form of Reye's syndrome has also been described. Other possible causes of fulminant hepatic failure include acute hepatitis B with hepatitis D superinfection, Budd-Chiari syndrome and other hepatic vein thrombotic conditions, vascular hypoperfusion of the liver, ileojejunal bypass for obesity, Tylenol intoxication, alcoholism, and cirrhosis. Another significant predisposing condition is the fatty liver of pregnancy.

There are two histopathologic forms of fulminant hepatic failure: panhepatic necrosis, in which all hepatocytes have become necrotic, and microvesicular steatosis, in which there is sinusoidal enlargement and cholestasis. The latter is most common in Reye's syndrome and the fatty liver of pregnancy. It is important to note that because the microvesicular steatosis pattern often shows only minimal changes histologically, liver biopsy is unrevealing. It is necessary to rely on laboratory analysis of liver function for a definitive diagnosis, as described subsequently.

Many of the pathophysiologic sequelae of cirrhosis also occur in fulminant hepatic failure. Patients develop ascites and become encephalopathic because of hyperammonemia. Total serum protein and serum albumin are depressed. Virtually all of the patients with fulminant hepatic failure exhibit severe coagulopathies, particularly disseminated intravascular coagulopathy, and virtually all are anemic. All develop renal failure because of the hepatorenal syndrome and acute tubular necrosis.

Furthermore, many of these patients become hypoglycemic, possibly because of the inability of the liver to break down glycogen. Lactic acidosis also develops because of poor tissue perfusion. Interestingly, unlike cirrhosis, in which the patients become hyponatremic, fulminant hepatic failure always leads to *hyper*natremia and hypokalemia. This observation may be explained by the finding that circulating levels of aldosterone in the serum of some of these patients are high. Perhaps the failure of the liver to clear aldosterone from the circulation results in the observed high levels of this hormone.

Diagnostic laboratory findings for fulminant hepatic failure (Sunheimer, 1994) are rapid increases in serum levels of the aminotransferases to levels often greater than 1000 IU/L such that AST is at least 1.5 times greater in value than ALT. While these enzymes rise, the total protein and albumin become markedly depressed. Overall, this pattern resembles hepatitis and cirrhosis combined except that in all forms of acute hepatitis, save alcoholic hepatitis, AST and ALT rise in a ratio of about 1:1 or in a ratio that favors ALT. Shortly after these patterns occur, serum ammonia increases rapidly, leading to encephalopathy. LD, ALP, and bilirubin all increase markedly. All of the changes described previously occur over a period of about one week. After another week, the serum AST and ALT return to low, sometimes undetectable levels. This finding signifies complete destruction of all viable liver tissue.

Patients whose AST and ALT values undergo the stereotypic changes described should be observed closely for fulminant hepatic failure, especially if there is any indication of encephalopathy. Though supportive therapy can sometimes restore normal liver function, for most patients in fulminant hepatic failure, the only ultimate cure is liver transplantation.

Annoni G, Cargnel A, Colombo M, Hahn EG: Persistent elevation of the aminoterminal peptide of procollagen type III in serum of patients with acute viral hepatitis distinguishes chronic active hepatitis from resolving chronic persistent hepatitis. J Hepatol 1986; 2:379.

Bellentani S, Tabarroni G, Barchi T, et al: Effect of ursodeoxycholic acid treatment on alanine aminotransferase and γ-glutamyltranspeptidase serum levels in patients with hypertransaminasemia. J Hepatol 1989; 8:7.
Berg PA, Klein R, Fotinos JL: Antimitochondrial antibodies in primary biliary cirrhosis. J Hepatol 1986; 2:123.
Carey MC, Cahalane MJ: Enterohepatic circulation. *In* Arias IM, Jakoby WB, Popper H, Schachter D, Shafritz, DA (eds): The Liver: Biology and Pathobiology, 2nd ed. New York, Raven Press, 1988.
Chang L, Clifton P, Barter P, Mackinnon M: High density lipoprotein subpopulations in chronic liver disease. Hepatology 1986; 6:46.
Chowdhury JR, Wolkoff AW, Arias IM: Heme and bile pigment metabolism. *In* Arias IM, Jakoby WB, Popper H, et al (eds): The Liver: Biology and Pathobiology, 2nd ed. New York, Raven Press, 1988.
Collin D, Goold MF, Rosalki SB, et al: Plasma intestinal alkaline phosphatase and intermediate molecular mass gamma glutamyltransferase activities in the differential diagnosis of jaundice. J Clin Pathol 1987; 40:1252.
Coppel RL, McNeilage LJ, Surh CD, et al: Primary structure of the human M2 mitochondrial autoantigen of primary biliary cirrhosis: Dihydrolipoamide acetyl transferase. Proc Natl Acad Sci U S A 1988; 85:7317.
Crawford JM, Hauser SC, Gollan JL: Formation, hepatic metabolism, and transport of bile pigments: A status report. Semin Liver Dis 1988; 8:105.
DeBroe ME, Roels F, Nouwen EJ, et al: Liver plasma membrane: The source of high molecular weight alkaline phosphatase in human serum. Hepatology 1985; 5:118.
Dickson ER, Grambsch PM, Fleming TH, et al: Prognosis in primary biliary cirrhosis: Model for decision making. Hepatology 1989; 10:1.
Fevery J, Blanckaert N: What can we learn from analysis of serum bilirubin? J Hepatol 1986; 2:113.
Fussey SPM, Guest JR, James OFW, et al: Identification and analysis of the major M2 autoantigens in primary biliary cirrhosis. Proc Natl Acad Sci U S A 1988; 85:8654.
Hahn EG: Blood analysis for liver fibrosis. J Hepatol 1984; 1:67.
Heredia D, Caballeria J, Pares A, et al: Serum procollagen type III peptide does not reflect hepatic collagen content in alcoholics with inactive cirrhosis. J Hepatol Suppl 1985; 2:S252.
Kaplan MM, Gandolfo JV, Quaroni EG: An enzyme-linked immunosorbent assay (ELISA) for detecting antimitochondrial antibody. Hepatology 1984; 4:727.
Kelly DA, Summerfield JA: Hemostasis in liver disease. Semin Liver Dis 1987; 7:182.
Kelly DA, Tuddenham EGD: Haemostatic problems in liver disease. Gut 1986; 27:339.
Krams SM, Surh CD, Coppel RL, et al: Immunization of experimental animals with dihydrolipoamide acetyltransferase, as a purified recombinant polypeptide, generates mitochondrial antibodies but not primary biliary cirrhosis. Hepatology 1989; 9:411.
Lauff JJ, Kasper ME, Wu TW, Ambrose RT: Isolation and preliminary characterization of a fraction of bilirubin that is firmly bound to protein. Clin Chem 1982; 28:629.
Manns M, Gerken G, Kyriatsoulis A, et al: Two different subtypes of antimitochondrial antibodies are associated with primary biliary cirrhosis: Identification and characterization by radioimmunoassay and immunoblotting. Hepatology 1987; 7:893.
Mosher DF: Fibronectin and liver disease. Hepatology 1986; 6:1419.
Moss DW: Diagnostic aspects of alkaline phosphatase and its isoenzymes. Clin Biochem 1987; 20:225.
Muraca M, Fevery J, Blanckaert N: Analytic aspects and clinical interpretation of serum bilirubins. Semin Liver Dis 1988; 8:137.
Nalpas B, Vassault A, Charpin S, et al: Serum mitochondrial aspartate aminotransferase as a marker of chronic alcoholism: Diagnostic value and interpretation in a liver unit. Hepatology 1986; 6:608.
Naveau S, Poynard T, Abella A, et al: Prognostic value of serum fibronectin concentration in alcoholic cirrhotic patients. Hepatology 1985; 5:819.
Palmer M, Schaffner F: Effect of weight reduction on hepatic abnormalities in overweight patients [abstract]. Gastroenterology 1990; 99:1408–1413.
Panteghini M, Falsetti F, Chiari E, Malchiodi A: Determination of aspartate aminotransferase isoenzymes in hepatic diseases: Preliminary findings. Clin Chim Acta 1983; 128:133.
Pincus JH, Cohan JL, Glaser GH: Neurologic Complications of Internal Disease. *In* Baker AB, Baker LH (eds): Clinical Neurology. New York, Harper & Row, 1991, pp 10–13.
Poynard T, Aubert A, Bedossa P, et al: A simple biological index for detection of alcoholic liver disease in drinkers. Gastroenterology 1991; 100:1397–1402.
Rajpert-DeMeyts E, Heisterkamp N, Groffen J: Cloning and nucleotide sequence of γ-glutamyl transpeptidase. Proc Natl Acad Sci U S A 1988; 85:8840.
Risteli J, Søgaard H, Oikarinen A, et al: Aminoterminal propeptide of type III procollagen in methotrexate-induced liver fibrosis and cirrhosis. Br J Dermatol 1988; 119:321.
Roberts FD, Sandford NL, Bradbear RA, et al: Serum procollagen-III-peptide: Failure to reflect the extent of hepatic fibrosis. Journal of Gastroenterology and Hepatology 1986; 1:27.
Rosenthal P, Pincus MR, Fink D: Serum bilirubin is strongly influenced by age and sex in humans. Hepatology 1983; 3:799.
Seidel D: Lipoproteins in liver disease. J Clin Chem Clin Biochem 1987; 25:541.
Siede WH, Seiffert UB: Relative merits of the biliary alkaline phosphatase isoenzyme and lipoprotein-X in diagnosis of cholestasis. Clin Chem 1983; 29:698.
Sieg A, Stiehl A, Raedsch R, et al: Gilbert's syndrome: Diagnosis by typical serum bilirubin pattern. Clin Chim Acta 1986; 154:41.
Steigman F, Szanto PB, Poulos A, et al: Significance of serum aminograms in diagnosis and prognosis of liver diseases. J Clin Gastroenterol 1984; 6:453.
Sunheimer R, Capaldo G, Kashanian F, et al: Serum analyte pattern characteristic of fulminant hepatic failure. Ann Clin Lab Sci 1994; 24:101–109.
Teare JP, Sherman D, Greenfield SM, et al: Comparison of serum procollagen III peptide concentrations and PGA index for assessment of hepatic fibrosis. Lancet 1993; 342:895–898.
Torres-Salinas M, Pares A, Caballeria J, et al: Serum procollagen type III peptide as a marker of hepatic fibrogenesis in alcoholic hepatitis. Gastroenterology 1986; 90:1241.
Vanderlinde RE: Review of pyridoxal phosphate and the transaminases in liver disease. Ann Clin Lab Sci 1986; 16:79.
Van de Water L, Carr JM, Aronson D, McDonagh J: Analysis of elevated fibrinogen degradation product levels in patients with liver disease. Blood 1986; 67:1468.
Van Hootegem P, Fevery J, Blanckaert N: Serum bilirubins in hepatobiliary disease: Comparison with other liver function tests and changes in the post obstructive period. Hepatology 1985; 5:112.
Vierling JM, Berk PD, Hoffman AF, et al: Normal fasting-state levels of serum cholyl-conjugated bile acids in Gilbert's syndrome: An aid to the diagnosis. Hepatology 1982; 2:340.
Viot M, Thyss A, Schneider M, et al: Isoenzyme of alkaline phosphatases. Clinical importance and value for the detection of liver metastases. Cancer 1983; 52:140.
Weigand K, Zaugg PY, Frei A, Zimmerman A: Long-term follow-up of serum N-terminal propeptide of collagen Type III levels in patients with chronic liver disease. Hepatology 1984; 4:835.
Wenham PR, Horn DB, Smith AF: Multiple forms of γ-glutamyl-transferase: A clinical study. Clin Chem 1985; 31:569.
Wion K, Kelly DA, Summerfield JAS, et al: Distribution of Factor VIII MRNA and antigen in human liver and other tissues. Nature 1985; 317:726.

Chapter 13

Clinical Enzymology

Matthew R. Pincus, M.D., Ph.D.
Hyman J. Zimmerman, M.D.
John Bernard Henry, M.D.

Enzymes, protein catalysts that are responsible for most of the chemical reactions of the body, are found in all tissues. Some have been identified in the plasma (or serum), to which they gain access from injured cells or even perhaps from intact cells that have been subjected to stress. Some are released from blocks in their metabolism or excretion. Clinicians became interested in serum enzymes more than a half century ago with the demonstration of the usefulness of alkaline phosphatase levels in the diagnosis of osseous and hepatobiliary disease, of acid phosphatase levels in the diagnosis of carcinoma of the prostate, and of amylase and lipase levels for the diagnosis of pancreatic disease. Despite the clinical usefulness of these parameters of disease and the demonstration, during the next 25 years, of a number of other enzymes in the serum, clinical interest in serum enzymology remained relatively dormant until 1953. The demonstration in that year of serum glutamate oxaloacetate transaminase (SGOT; now called aspartate aminotransferase [AST]) in the serum of normals and the subsequent observations that increased levels of this enzyme helped to diagnose cardiac and hepatic disease led to an intensification of interest in serum enzymology.

By now, many enzymes have been identified in the serum. The levels of many of these enzymes have been studied extensively in a variety of conditions. Table 13–1 lists the main conditions in which abnormal values of the enzymes listed are found.

Enzyme activities or concentrations in serum can become elevated by a number of factors. In most disease states in which enzyme elevations occur, the cause is increased membrane permeability, usually secondary to cell injury or necrosis. These intracellular enzymes diffuse into capillaries and thence into the general circulation. Occasionally, increased enzyme levels in serum are caused by increased rates of intracellular synthesis and the subsequent diffusion of these secreted enzymes into the circulation.

The degree of damage to cells leads to the elevation of different enzymes in serum. For example, damage to hepatocytes but not to their mitochondria will result in the preferential elevation of the enzyme alanine aminotransferase (ALT)

Table 13–1. CLASSIFICATION OF ENZYMES DEMONSTRATED IN SERUM WITH TYPE AND DEGREE* OF ABNORMALITY IN DISEASE

Type of Enzyme	Condition†								Comments or Other Abnormalities
	Hepatitis	*Inf. Mono.*	*Cirrhosis*	*Met. Ca.*	*Obst. Jaundice*	*Heart Failure*	*Myocard. Infarct.*	*Prog. Musc. Dyst.*	
I. Carbohydrate metabolism									
A. Glycolytic									
1. Phosphoglucomutase	uuu		N	u	u				
2. Phosphohexoisomerase (PHI)	uuu	uu	u	u	u	u	uu	u	
3. Fructose 1,6-diphosphate aldolase (ALS)	uuu	u	u	u	N or u	u	uu	uuu	
4. Fructose-P-aldolase	uuu		N	N		N	N	N	
5. Lactate dehydrogenase (LD)	u	uu	u	uu	N or u	u	uu	uu	
6. Pyruvate kinase (PK)	uu			uu					
7. Enolase	u						u		
8. Triose-P-isomerase				u					
9. Glyceraldehyde 3-P-dehydrogenase	u	u							
B. Hexose monophosphate shunt (pentose phosphate pathway)									
1. Glucose-6-phosphate dehydrogenase (GPD)	N		N		N		uu		Fig. 13–10
2. 6-P-Gluconate dehydrogenase (6-P-GD)	u	u							
3. 5-Phosphoriboisomerase	N		uu	uu	u				
4. Transketolase	u								
C. Citric acid cycle									
1. Malate dehydrogenase (MD)	uuu	u	u	u	u	u	uu		
2. Isocitrate dehydrogenase (ICD)	uuu	u	N or u	uu	N or u	u	N	N	
3. Fumarase	u		u						
D. Other									
1. Amylase (AMS)	N	N	N or d	N	N	N	N	N	Chapter 23
2. β-Glucuronidase	uu						N or u		Cancer, pregnancy
3. Iditol dehydrogenase (ID)	uuu	u	u	N or u	N or u		N	N	
II. Esterases									
A. Lipid									
1. Lipase (LPS)	N	N	N	N	N	N	N	N	Chapter 23
2. Aliesterase	N	N	N	N	N	N	N	N	Acute pancreatitis
3. Cholesterol esterase	d		d	N or d	N				
4. Lipoprotein lipase (LPL)	uu		uu						
5. Lecithinase	N		N	N	N				Acute pancreatitis
6. Lecithin-cholesterol acyl transferase									

Table continued on following page

Table 13–1. CLASSIFICATION OF ENZYMES DEMONSTRATED IN SERUM WITH TYPE AND DEGREE* OF ABNORMALITY IN DISEASE (*Continued*)

	Condition†								
Type of Enzyme	*Hepatitis*	*Inf. Mono.*	*Cirrhosis*	*Met. Ca.*	*Obst. Jaundice*	*Heart Failure*	*Myocard. Infarct.*	*Prog. Musc. Dyst.*	**Comments or Other Abnormalities**
II. Esterases (*continued*)									
B. Nonlipid									
1. Cholinesterase (pseudo)	d	d	d		N or u	N or u		N	Fig. 13–9
2. Phosphates									Increase in bone disease, Table 13–3
a. Alkaline phosphatase (ALP)	u	u	u	uu	uuu	u	N	N	
b. Acid phosphatase (ACP)	N	N	N	N	N	N	N	N	Cancer of prostate
c. Nucleotidase (5′-N)	u		u	uu	uuu				Normal in bone disease
d. Adenosine triphosphatase (ATPase)	u		u	u	uu				Elevated in bone disease
3. Deoxyribonuclease I (DNase)	u	±			N			N	Acute hemorrhagic pancreatitis
4. Ribonuclease (RNase)	N		N	N	N	u	u		Uremia, myeloma, pancreatitis, pancreatic cancer
5. Adenosine deaminase‡	uu	uuu	uu	uuu		uu	N		Leukemia
III. Protein and amino acid enzymes									
A. Proteolytic enzymes (trypsin)									Acute pancreatitis
B. Peptidases									
1. Leucine aminopeptide (LAP)	u	uuu	u	uu	uuu	uu	N	N	Pregnancy, cancer of pancreas, pancreatitis
2. Aminotripeptidase	uu	uu	u	uu	uu				
3. γ-Glutamyl transpeptidase (GGTP) (γ-Glutamyl transferase [GGT])	u		u	uuu	uu	u	uu		
C. Pepsinogen									Duodenal ulcer
D. Amino acid substrate									
1. Aminotransferase (transaminase)									
a. Aspartate aminotransferase (AST) (glutamate oxaloacetate transminase [GOT])	uuu	uu	u	u	u	u	uu	uu	Chapter 12, Fig. 13–6
b. Alanine aminotransferase (ALT) (glutamate pyruvate transaminase [GPT])	uuu	uu	u	u	u	u	N or u	uu	Chapter 12
c. Glutamate dehydrogenase (GD)	uu	N	N or u	N	N	N	N	N	

2. Urea cycle									
a. Ornithine carbamoyl transferase (OCT)	uuu		u	uu					Acute cholecystitis
b. Arginase	uu		u						
IV. Other enzymes									
A. Glutathione reductase (GR)	uu		u	uu			u		
B. Ceruloplasmin	uu		u	uu	uu				Wilson's disease
C. Creatine kinase (CK) (creatine phosphokinase [CPK])	N		N	N	N	N	uuu	uuu	Dermatomyositis
D. Benzidine oxidase	u		u	uuu	uu	u	uuu		
E. Hydroxybutyrate dehydrogenase (HBD)	u	u	±	u	±	u	uuu	±	Isoenzyme of LD
F. Guanase	uuu	u	u	u	u				
G. Alcohol dehydrogenase									
H. Acylase	uu		N	N	N	N	N	N	
I. Angiontensin-converting enzyme (ACE)									Elevated in sarcoidosis
J. Catalase									
K. Amine oxidase									
L. Prolyl hydroxylase									
M. Lysozyme (muramidase)									Elevated in monocytic leukemias

*u Slight increase
uu Moderate increase
uuu Marked increase
d Slight decrease
N No change
± Variable
† Inf. Mono.—Infectious mononucleosis
Met. Ca.—metastatic carcinoma
Obst. Jaundice—obstructive jaundice
Myocard. Infarct.—myocardial infarction
Prog. Musc. Dyst.—progressive muscular dystrophy
‡ Not an esterase. This is properly a deaminase.

while, with mitochondrial damage, AST tends to become elevated more in serum. When subjected to stress, injury or necrosis, certain tissues release into serum specific enzymes or specific isozymes of these enzymes that reflect the tissue in which a disease process is taking place.

The usefulness of several serum enzymes—alkaline phosphatase, SGOT (now called AST), and serum glutamate pyruvate transaminase (SGPT), now called ALT—in the diagnosis of hepatic disease and of several other enzymes (amylase, lipase) in the diagnosis of pancreatic disease is considered in the chapters devoted to the liver (Chap. 12) and pancreas (Chap. 23). This chapter considers the more general aspects of serum enzymology. The principles of the methods for measuring enzyme activity are discussed, the possible factors responsible for abnormal values are analyzed, and special attention is devoted to a few of the enzymes found in the serum. Brief reference is made to enzymes of other body fluids and to the clinical significance of enzymes in the formed elements of the blood.

Nomenclature

The numerical designation for each enzyme consists of four numbers separated by periods (e.g., EC 1.1.1.27 for lactate dehydrogenase). EC stands for "Enzyme Commission"; the first number defines the class (one of six reactions) to which the enzyme belongs, whereas the next two numbers indicate the subclass and sub-subclass to which the enzyme is assigned. A specific serial number is the last number given each enzyme in its sub-subclass.

Properties of Enzymes

All enzymes are proteins—that is, polypeptide chains with specific amino sequences that determine their ultimate three-dimensional structure. This structure then determines the specificity of the enzyme for its substrate. Often, enzymes, like many other proteins, have a number of different forms that differ in a few amino acids. These different forms are referred to as isozymes. As discussed later, a number of enzymes contain two or more polypeptide chains in a multimeric complex. Each multimeric complex contains the same number of chains, but the chain composition can differ. These different forms of the multimeric enzyme are also referred to as isozymes. Often, injured tissue will release enzymes that are specific for that tissue, such as ALT, which is specific for liver, so that detection of elevated levels of the enzyme will enable rapid diagnosis. Even for enzymes that are not tissue specific, their isozymes often are tissue specific, so that determination of elevated levels of these particular isozymes in body fluids again allows rapid diagnosis. An example is the MB hybrid dimer isozyme of creatine phosphokinase (CK), which is an excellent marker for myocardial infarction.

Most enzymes catalyze specific reactions with reactive groups at their active sites but often also contain nonprotein cofactors such as nicotinamide adenine dinucleotide (NAD), as occurs with the enzyme lactate dehydrogenase (LD). The protein portion of the enzyme-cofactor complex is called the apoenzyme, whereas the entire complex is called the holoenzyme.

Enzymes, like all proteins, are susceptible to denaturation due to physical and chemical agents and may thus lose their activities. They may also bind to molecules other than the substrate that may reduce or enhance their activities. These molecules are referred as inhibitors and activators, respectively.

Enzymes display specificity with regard to substrate (substance that is acted on) and effect (chemical action). For example, LD catalyzes the reversible reaction,

$$\text{Lactate} + \text{NAD}^+ \rightleftharpoons \text{pyruvate} + \text{NADH} + \text{H}^+ \quad (13\text{-}1)$$

This enzyme acts virtually only on L-lactic acid and pyruvic acid as substrates and catalyzes the reversible transfer of hydrogen between lactate and NAD. Other enzymes are required for the decarboxylation or amination of pyruvic acid.

Many chemical and physical agents influence enzymes significantly. Temperature and hydrogen ion concentration are probably the two best-studied agents. Most enzymes are inactivated in the neighborhood of 65°C. Low temperature or freezing, however, does not usually destroy enzymes. Two exceptions to this rule are CK and LD. Freezing the former enzyme at −20° destroys its activity, whereas freezing at −70°C does not. On the other hand, LD cannot be stored at 4°C without its losing its activity.

For each 10°C rise in temperature (Q_{10}), some enzymes will demonstrate a twofold increase in activity, but the increase in denaturation may be even greater. Hence, the temperature activity curve for an enzyme will show a maximum, depending on the opposed activating and denaturing effects of rising temperature. Although there is not complete agreement, 37°C appears to be the best single choice of reaction temperature, followed by 30°C for most clinical serum enzyme assays. Statland (1977) has reviewed the arguments regarding one temperature versus another. These fall into chemical, technical, and economic categories.

A bell-shaped curve will also often describe the optimal pH for an enzyme (Fig. 13–1). This phenomenon occurs usually because two catalytic groups are involved, one in the basic form and the other in the acid form. At low pH, the basic catalytic group is protonated, so that catalytic efficiency decreases; at high pH, the acid group dissociates a proton, decreasing its efficiency in acid catalysis.

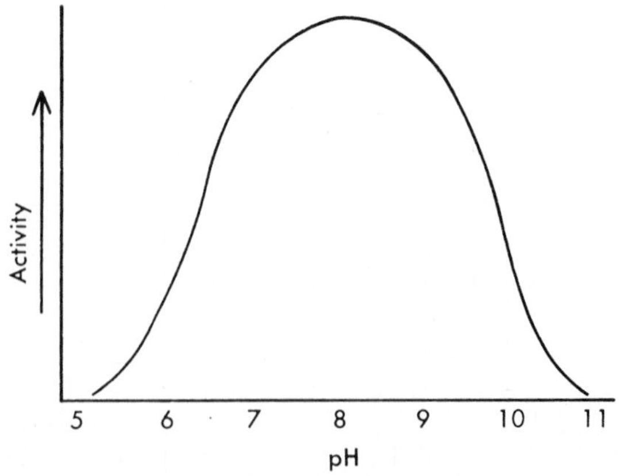

Figure 13–1. Typical curve of activity versus pH for an enzymatic reaction. (From Henry JB: Fundamentals of clinical enzyme determinations. Postgrad Med 1963; 33:A–66, Thieme Medical Publishers, Inc.)

PRINCIPLES OF ENZYME ACTIVITY DETERMINATIONS

Enzymes are unique in that their presence in serum can be detected quantitatively simply by adding specific substrates, almost always small molecules, to the serum and detecting their rates of conversion to product. Often, enzyme concentrations are expressed in units of their activities rather than their concentrations. Enzyme activity is expressed in units that usually represent one of the following: (1) increase in concentration of one of the products, (2) decrease in concentration of substrate, or (3) change in concentration of coenzyme. The rate of change of any of these is a measure of the rate of reaction. The level of enzymes in serum can be determined in terms of their catalytic rates, which, under the right conditions, are directly proportional to their concentrations. Absolute enzyme concentrations can be measured using immunochemical methods. For example, immunoassays for serum levels of isoenzymes of LD and CK using immunochemical procedures are now well established.

Although an enzyme reaction represents complex mechanisms that are not fully understood, it can be stated that an enzyme (E) reversibly forms at least one noncovalent complex with its substrate (S). Functional groups of coenzymes or prosthetic groups or both may play a role in the formation of this enzyme-substrate (ES) complex. The ES complex decomposes to enzyme and product (P). The enzyme is not altered in the overall reaction. The Michaelis-Menten hypothesis describes this sequence of events, as follows:

$$E + S \underset{k_2}{\overset{k_1}{\rightleftarrows}} (ES) \xrightarrow{k_3} E + P \qquad (13\text{-}2)$$

where k_1 = forward rate constant, k_2 = reverse rate constant, and k_3 = covalent catalytic constant.

ENZYME ASSAYS ARE BASED ON MICHAELIS-MENTEN KINETICS

Enzyme-catalyzed reactions are unique in that they exhibit large rate enhancements over the uncatalyzed reactions and show saturation kinetics—that is, the rate of the reaction reaches a maximal value at a particular concentration of substrate, and higher concentrations of substrate do not result in increased rates of reaction. To explain this phenomenon, the scheme shown in equation 13–2 was proposed by Michaelis and Menten. The essential feature of this scheme is the formation of an enzyme-substrate complex in which the substrate binds to the enzyme and is stabilized by noncovalent, nonbonded interactions between enzyme and substrate (Pincus, 1981). This enzyme-substrate complex can either dissociate or break down to product and free enzyme (provided that the product has a low affinity for the enzyme). Saturation is achieved when the substrate concentration exceeds the value of the Michaelis constant, K_m. The Michaelis-Menten scheme is described by a fundamental kinetic equation (to be discussed) on which enzyme assays are based.

It should be noted that enzymes do not change the equilibrium constant for the equilibrium between substrate and products but affect only the rate of the interconversion. The rate enhancement is due to the lowering of the energy of activation of the reaction by the enzyme. This lowering of the energy of activation is achieved by critical positioning of catalytic groups at the active site of the enzyme. These catalytic groups are usually involved in general acid-base catalysis. For a number of enzymes, a transient covalent complex is formed between the enzyme and the substrate as, for example, is found for the serine proteases (e.g., trypsin, chymotrypsin, elastase), in which an acyl-enzyme complex can be isolated.

It is almost always assumed that the noncovalent ES complex exists in a steady state—that is, the rate of its formation in the k_1 rate step in equation 13–2 equals the rate of its breakdown to E + S (eq. 13–2) and to P. Thus, the rate of change of ES with time, or d(ES)/dt, is 0. Given this assumption, it is possible to derive the following law governing the rate of formation of product, P:

$$v = \text{rate} = dP/dt = \frac{k_3 \times E_0 \times S}{K_m + S} \qquad (13\text{-}3)$$

where dP/dt is the rate of formation of product with time; k_3 is as defined in equation 13–2; E_0 is the total concentration of enzyme present in a given reaction mixture; S is the free substrate concentration (unbound to enzyme); and K_m, called the Michaelis constant, is defined as

$$K_m = \frac{k_2 + k_3}{k_1} \qquad (13\text{-}4)$$

where k_1, k_2, and k_3 are as defined in equation 13–2. It is almost always true, that $k_2 >> k_3$, $K_m = k_2/k_1$—that is, it is the equilibrium constant for dissociation of the ES complex. The term k_3E_0 is called V_{max}, as discussed subsequently.

If the rate is plotted against substrate concentration, a curve such as that shown on Figure 13–2 is obtained. The plateau segment occurs where the enzyme is saturated with substrate, as will be discussed. It is important to note that the rate plotted is always taken as the *initial* rate of the reaction for a given initial substrate concentration. If the initial rate is not plotted, the kinetics of the reaction may become complex from such effects as end-product inhibition of the reaction, so that accurate determination of the substrate concentration may no longer be possible.

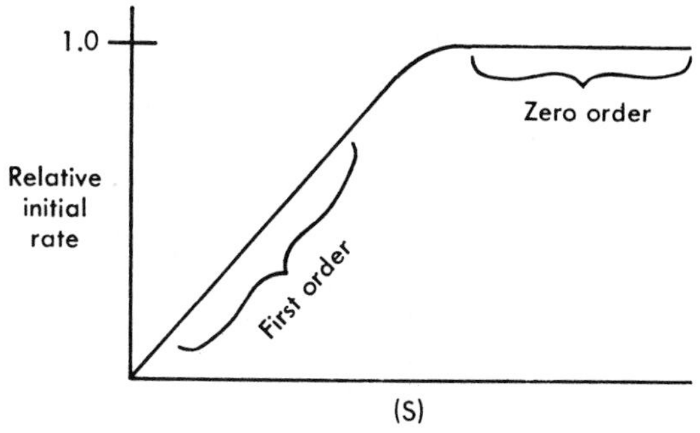

Figure 13–2. Relative rate of reaction expressed as function of substrate concentration (*S*). (From Henry JB: Fundamentals of clinical enzyme determinations. Postgrad Med 1963; 33:A–66.)

The Michaelis-Menten equation can be linearized by taking the reciprocals of both sides of equation 13–3 to give

$$\frac{1}{V} = \frac{K_m}{V_{max}} \times \frac{1}{S} + \frac{1}{V_{max}} \qquad (13\text{-}5)$$

Plots of 1/v versus 1/S, called Lineweaver-Burk plots, should yield straight lines, the intercepts being equal to $1/V_{max}$ and the slopes being equal to K_m/V_{max}.

Equation 13–3 has fundamental consequences for enzyme-catalyzed reactions. Most important is the fact that if $S >> K_m$—that is, the free substrate concentration is much greater than the numerical value of K_m, the Michaelis constant—the rate of the enzyme-catalyzed reaction is constant because it becomes equal to k_3E_0. This term is often called V_{max}, the maximal rate of the reaction that is directly proportional to the total enzyme concentration. This is the rate observed when all enzyme molecules in solution become saturated with substrate. This rate occurs where the curve of rate (or V) versus S in Figure 13–2 becomes flat, the plateau or "zero order" part of the curve. Because the rate of product formation at saturation is constant and the concentration of product formed is directly proportional to the time, as shown in Figure 13–3, this plateau region of the curve is called zero order (rate independent of concentration of reactants). In the event that $S << K_m$, then from equation 13–3,

$$\frac{dP}{dt} = \frac{k_3 \times E_0 \times S}{K_m} \qquad (13\text{-}6)$$

Because k_3, E_0, and K_m are constants, the rate of the reaction is proportional to the substrate concentration and is thus said to be "first order" in substrate. If a reaction is first order in substrate, the time taken for half of the substrate to be converted to products is independent of the initial concentration of substrate—that is, the $t_{1/2}$, or half-time, is constant. The constancy of the half-time is an intrinsic feature of all first order reactions.

Equation 13–2 clearly shows that if one wishes to determine the concentration of an enzyme in serum, this concentration is best measured at saturating concentrations of specific substrate. In this event, the rate of the reaction is directly proportional to the total enzyme concentration. If the value of k_3 is known and the rate at saturation is known, the enzyme concentration can be determined directly. However, because usually more than one isozyme of the enzyme being assayed is present, each with a different value for k_3, it is not practical to determine total enzyme concentration in this manner. Rather, the total enzymatic activity, V_{max}, is determined and is given in terms of international units, IU. An IU is defined as one micromole of substrate converted per minute. Of profound importance in this definition of enzyme activity is the fact that it is substrate dependent. Two assays using two different substrates for a given enzyme will in general yield different results in IU. Thus, the method (substrate) used in an enzyme assay must be specified. Note also that the *volume* of the reaction must also be specified. Generally, if the activity of an enzyme is expressed in IU, the volume will be 1 L, so that the activity of the enzyme will be expressed in IU/L. If the activity is in mIU, the activity is expressed in mIU/mL.

In an enzyme assay, one may measure activity as increase in product (ΔP in Fig. 13–3) or decrease in substrate (ΔS in Fig. 13–3), depending on which is more convenient analytically (see Fig. 13–3). Many enzymes bind to cofactors, such as NAD, which undergo spectrophotometric changes as a result of the reaction catalyzed by the enzyme. For example, LD catalyzes the reduction of pyruvate to lactate, a reaction in which NADH is oxidized to NAD. NADH absorbs strongly at 340 mm, whereas NAD does not absorb at this wavelength. Thus, this absorbance change (decrease at 340 mm) is a direct measure of ΔS (see Fig. 13–3).

Coupled Reactions

Often, the detection of enzyme activity can be measured by using the product of the enzyme-catalyzed reaction as the substrate for a second, "marker" enzyme–catalyzed reaction. For example, to measure the activity of the aminotransferase, aspartate aminotransferase (AST or SGOT), the product of the reaction is glutamate and oxaloacetate. Either may be measured by coupling to an appropriate enzyme. For example, oxaloacetate is reduced to malate by the enzyme ma-

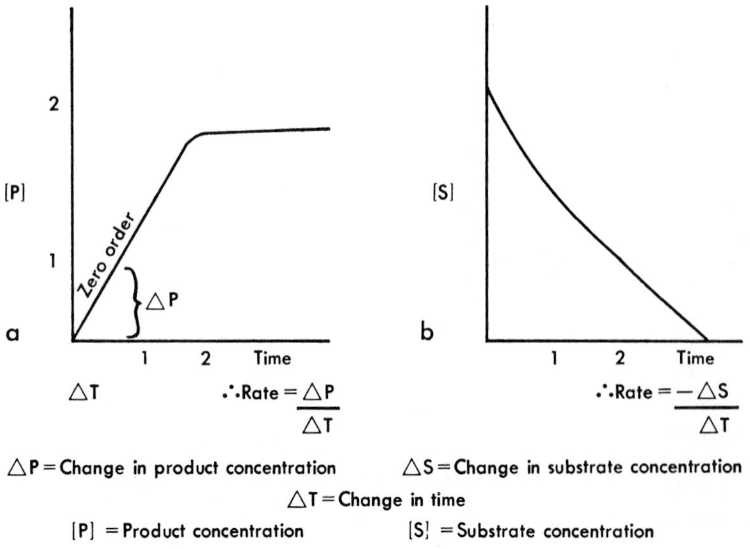

Figure 13–3. Rate of product formation (*a*) and substrate disappearance (*b*). (From Henry JB: Fundamentals of clinical enzyme determinations. Postgrad Med 1963; 33:A–68.)

late dehydrogenase wherein NADH is oxidized to NAD. Thus, by adding malate dehydrogenase to the reaction mixture, one can measure the decrease in absorbance at 340 mm. Because the amount of product formed is not in the saturating region for the second marker enzyme, high concentrations of the latter are used to ensure that any product formed will be immediately converted to the next product in the chain (i.e., conditions are such that the first step is rate-limiting and the second step is virtually instantaneous).

Enzyme Inhibition

Enzymes can be inhibited (or activated) in a number of different ways, each of which affects the kinetics of the reaction. For example, if an assay for LD is being performed in which pyruvate is converted to lactate on serum from a patient with lactic acidosis, the endogenous lactate in the serum can competitively inhibit the enzyme, giving falsely low values. There are three forms of enzyme inhibition for simple Michaelis-Menten kinetics (eq. 13–2): competitive, noncompetitive, and uncompetitive. In competitive inhibition, the substrate and inhibitor compete for the same active site of the enzyme, and the inhibition can be overcome by high concentrations of substrate. The parameter V_{max} is therefore unaffected, whereas the apparent K_m is raised as a result of competitive binding. Examples of this phenomenon abound. α-Ketoglutarate at high levels can compete with L-aspartate at the active site of AST. Sulfonamides compete with *p*-aminobenzoic acid for folate synthetase in bacteria, which are then unable to synthesize folic acid. In noncompetitive inhibition, binding of the inhibitor to the enzyme lowers the affinity of the enzyme for the substrate and V_{max}. The inhibition of enolase by fluoride is an example of this type of inhibition. In uncompetitive inhibition, the affinity of the enzyme for the substrate is unchanged, but V_{max} is lowered. An example is the inhibition of placental and intestinal alkaline phosphatase by L-phenylalanine. In the latter two types of inhibition, the inhibitor occupies a site on the enzyme that may be different from the active site of substrate binding.

Table 13–2. THREE TYPES OF ENZYME INHIBITION AND THEIR EFFECTS ON THE DOUBLE RECIPROCAL EQUATION*

Inhibition Type	Double Reciprocal Equation
1. None	$\frac{1}{v} = \frac{K_m}{V_{max}} \times \frac{1}{S} + \frac{1}{V_{max}}$
2. Competitive	$\frac{1}{v} = \frac{K_m}{V_{max}} \times \left(1 + \frac{I}{K_I}\right) \times \frac{1}{S} + \frac{1}{V_{max}}$
3. Noncompetitive	$\frac{1}{v} = \frac{K_m}{V_{max}} \times \left(1 + \frac{I}{K_I}\right) \times \frac{1}{S} + \frac{1}{V_{max}} \times \left(1 + \frac{I}{K_I}\right)$
4. Uncompetitive	$\frac{1}{v} = \frac{K_m}{V_{max}} \times \frac{1}{S} + \frac{1}{V_{max}} \times \left(1 + \frac{I}{K_I}\right)$

*All symbols are defined as in the text. "I" is the concentration of inhibitor (assumed to be constant), and K_I is the equilibrium constant for the reaction $E + I \rightleftarrows EI$, where EI is the noncovalent enzyme-inhibitor complex.

Table 13–2 lists the effects of three different types of inhibition on the form of the double reciprocal expression, equation 13–5, and the effects of these types of inhibition on the Lineweaver-Burk plots are shown in Figure 13–4. It is to be emphasized that in each expression, the concentration of inhibitor is assumed to be constant in the course of an experiment.

2

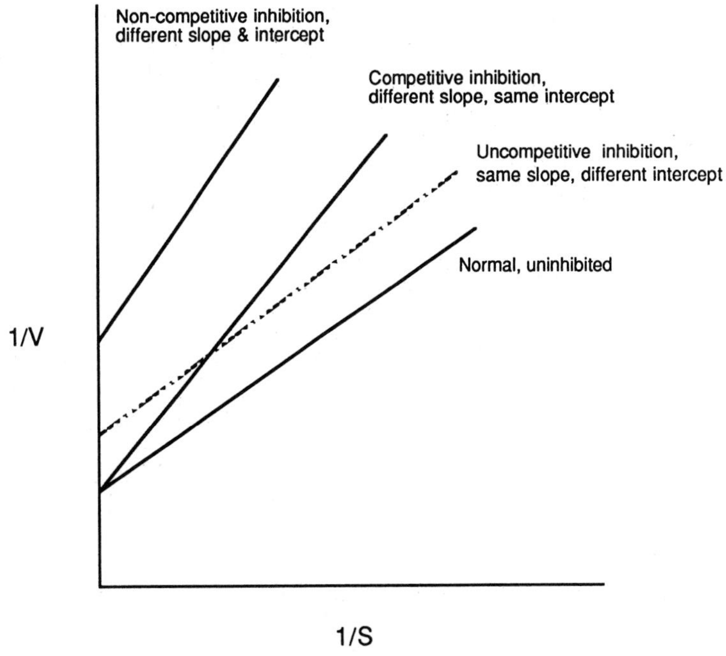

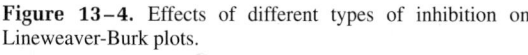

Figure 13–4. Effects of different types of inhibition on Lineweaver-Burk plots.

Performance of Enzyme Assays

To determine the level of an enzyme present in serum, in most commercial systems, a substrate specific for the enzyme is added so that its concentration is saturating ($S >> K_m$). The initial rate is then determined. For example, to assay for total LD activity, pyruvate is added at saturating concentration, and the decrease in absorbance at 340 mm is measured over a time course. The decrease in absorbance is measured at several time points in this interval to ensure that the change is linear—that is, it obeys zero-order kinetics. If only one time point is used to measure enzyme activity, there is no assurance that ΔP (see Fig. 13–3*A*) is linear in time. Possible pitfalls that can occur using a single time point are summarized in Figure 13–5.

Immunochemical Assays

A number of immunoassays are available for the determination of enzyme activity. These assays are used primarily to determine the level of a specific isozyme of the enzyme (e.g., the MB fraction of CK or the LD_1 isozyme of LD). These methods depend on the fact that the isozymes of an enzyme have local differences in amino acid sequences. For CK-MB and LD_1, these methods also depend on antibodies that recognize unique interfaces between subunits (e.g., between the M and B subunits of CK-MB). These sequences can be recognized by different antibodies that can therefore be used to quantitate the level of specific isozyme. Currently, immunoassays for CK-MB, such as on the Abbott (North Chicago, IL) IMX or the Baxter (Miami, FL) Stratus analyzer, can be performed on a stat basis, requiring 8 to 20 minutes per assay.

An example of an immunoassay combined with activity measurement for quantitating CK-MB isozymes is a Roche (Nutley, NJ) two-step assay in which two antibodies are used. The first is an anti-M antibody that precipitates all isozymes of CK in serum containing the M subunit—that is, MM and MB. The immunoprecipitate is then redissolved in buffer, and a second anti-M monoclonal antibody is added to the solution of MM and MB isozymes. This antibody completely blocks the activity of the M subunit, so that all CK activity in the buffer is due to the B fraction of the MB isozyme. The total MB activity is then twice the activity of the measured B activity.

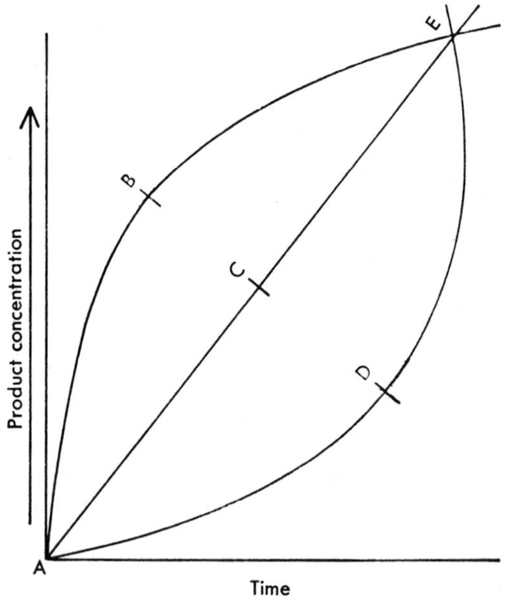

Figure 13–5. Illustration of potential hazards of using a single determination in enzyme assays. Line *ACE* is a zero-order reaction that permits accurate determination of enzyme activity for the entire reaction time. Curve *ABE* shows initial zero-order reaction of high rate followed by falling off of rate of reaction. This is possibly due to exhaustion of substrate prior to termination of assay at point *E*. Curve *ADE* reveals an initial lag phase that masks true activity. (From Henry JB: Fundamentals of clinical enzyme determinations. Postgrad Med 1963; 33:A–72.)

Pitfalls in Conventional Enzyme Assays

Numerous pitfalls are encountered in enzyme assays in the clinical laboratory. Hemolysis may be associated with the release of enzymes from red blood cells into the serum, causing falsely high serum values. Because of the adverse effects on enzyme activity of various anticoagulants, serum rather than plasma is the preferred specimen for clinical enzyme assays. Lactescence, or milky serum, may result in variable absorbance readings in spectrophotometric assays. Most enzymes in biological fluids are stable at 6°C (with the exception of LD, as noted earlier) for at least 24 hours and at room temperature for lesser periods. For prolonged storage, temperatures must be at −20°C or lower to ensure preservation of enzyme activity. Heat lability must be considered with respect to each enzyme to be assayed as well as to other components in the entire enzyme system, especially coenzymes and substrates. Accuracy in timing each assay and use of meticulously clean glassware are essential. In addition, it is vital that the pH of the reaction be maintained constant. For example, in assaying for LD, using pyruvate or lactate as substrate, the equilibrium favors reduction of pyruvate to lactate at a pH of 7 to 8, whereas at pH 9 to 10, the reverse is true. Thus, control of pH is essential in performing enzyme assays.

To ensure accuracy and precision in clinical enzyme determinations, one must be aware of the pitfalls and informed regarding the principles of enzyme assays. A quality control program for clinical enzyme assays should include the following: (1) adherence to zero-order kinetics, (2) proportionality studies with increments of sample, (3) use of pooled frozen serum or stable reference materials (lyophilized) as control solutions, and (4) replicate measurements to evaluate precision of assay.

The serum enzymes discussed in detail in this chapter have been of the greatest clinical usefulness or interest in the past or hold the most promise. Particular attention is given to the phosphatases, aminotransferases, LD and its isoenzymes, and cholinesterase. Many of the other serum enzymes are described, and their clinical relevance is discussed.

SPECIFIC ENZYMES

Phosphatases

The phosphatases of the blood, more properly called phosphomonoesterases or orthophosphoric ester monohydrolases, include two main types. The "alkaline phosphatase" has a pH optimum of approximately 9, whereas the "acid phosphatase" has its optimal activity at a pH of approximately 5. Although there is evidence that alkaline and acid phosphatases each include several different enzymes (isoenzymes), it has been convenient for clinical purposes to consider each as a single enzyme.

Alkaline Phosphatase (ALP) (EC 3.1.3.1)

The application of ALP determination to the study of hepatic disease is discussed in Chapter 12. The demonstration that bone is rich in alkaline phosphatase and that normal plasma (or serum) contains the same or a similar enzyme led to the study of serum ALP levels in patients with diseases of bone. ALP levels are elevated in patients with bone diseases characterized by increased osteoblastic activity (Table 13–3). These include osteitis deformans, rickets, osteomalacia, hyperparathyroidism, healing fractures, and osteoblastic bone tumors, both primary and secondary. Growing children and pregnant women in the third trimester have "physiologically" elevated serum ALP levels. Lower than normal levels are observed in patients with hypophosphatasia (an inborn error of metabolism) and in malnourished patients.

ISOENZYMES OF ALKALINE PHOSPHATASE

Studies of the properties of ALP isolated from various tissues (liver, bone, spleen, kidney, intestine) indicate that each differs from the others. Total serum ALP in normals consists of isoenzymes contributed by liver, bone, placenta, and intestine (especially in individuals with blood group types B and O who are secretors). Placental ALP characteristically rises during the first and second trimester of pregnancy and reaches a peak in the third trimester, so that it constitutes 40% to 65% of the total ALP, returning to normal in about one month post partum. One outstanding characteristic of the placental isoenzyme is its stability to heat. Heating this isozyme to 65°C for 30 minutes causes only minimal denaturation. Isoenzymes from these four sources have thus been distinguished from each other by electrophoretic analysis, differential inhibition by chemicals and heat, and immunochemically, although there are also differences in substrate dependence and reaction kinetics.

The degrees of inhibition of isoenzymes of hepatic, osseous, intestinal, and placental origin produced by heating to 56°C for 15 minutes, exposure to 3 M urea for 18 minutes, and incubation with 5×10^{-3} M L-phenylalanine, as well as the relative electrophoretic migration of these isoenzymes, are shown in Table 13–4. It is interesting that the Regan isoenzyme of alkaline phosphatase, observed in about 5% of persons with carcinomas, is strikingly similar to the placental form and is now thought to be due to derepression of the gene coding for this protein in these malignancies. The placental isozyme (called PLAP) is also markedly elevated in germ cell tumors, especially testicular carcinoma and primary germ cell tumors of the brain. The methods outlined in Table 13–4 help to identify placental and intestinal ALP (both phenylalanine inhibited) and in distinguishing them from hepatic and bone isoenzymes. Distinction of hepatic from osseous ALP is aided by heat or urea inhibition, but the overlapping effects lead to imprecision. Nevertheless, the susceptibility of the osseous isoenzyme to heat inactivation has been applied widely to distinguish it from the hepatic isoenzyme. Electrophoretic analysis of ALP isoenzymes employing acrylamide gel usually will also permit identification of the main isoenzyme contributing to an elevated level. Quantitation of the fractions, however, is prevented by the lack of distinct separation of the two rapidly moving isoenzymes (hepatic and osseous). A modification of cellulose acetate or polyacrylamide gel electrophoresis has been successful in separating these isoenzymes. In this modification, treatment of the ALP isoenzymes with neuraminidase from *Vibrio cholerae* for short times allows better separation of bone from liver ALP (Moss and Edwards, 1984). A limit digest of the ALP isoenzymes with neuraminidase is useful in

Table 13–4. CHARACTERISTICS OF ISOENZYMES OF ALKALINE PHOSPHATASE

	Inhibition* by		
Source of Enzyme	***L-Phenylalanine†*** **(%)**	***Heat‡ or Ureas§*** **(%)**	**Order Anodal Migration**
Liver	10	60	1
Bone	10	90	2
Intestine	75	60	4
Placenta	80	0	3
Regan (carcinoma)	80	0	3

*Approximate figures.
†L-Phenylalanine (5×10^{-3} M).
‡56°C for 15 minutes.
§3M concentration.

2

Table 13–3. CONDITIONS IN WHICH THE SERUM ALKALINE PHOSPHATASE LEVEL IS INCREASED*

Hepatobiliary Disease		**Bone Disease**		**Other Conditions**	
Obstructive jaundice	↑↑↑	Osteitis deformans	↑↑↑	Healing fractures	↑
Biliary cirrhosis	↑↑↑	Rickets	↑↑	Normal growth	↑
Intrahepatic cholestasis	↑↑↑	Osteomalacia	↑↑	Pregnancy (last trimester)	↑
Space-occupying lesions (granuloma, abscess, metastatic carcinoma)	↑↑	Hyperparathyroidism	↑↑		
		Metastatic bone disease	↑↑		
		Osteogenic sarcoma	↑↑↑		
Viral hepatitis	↑				
Infectious mononucleosis	↑↑				
Cirrhosis (alcoholic)	↑				

*Degree of increase indicated by number of arrows. Depressed values: hypophosphatasia, malnutrition.

Table 13–5. RELATIVE VALUES* FOR ALKALINE PHOSPHATASE AND ENZYMES THAT REFLECT ITS HEPATIC ISOENZYMES IN SEVERAL CLINICAL SETTINGS

	Hepatobiliary Disease				
	Hepatocellular	*Cholestatic or Posthepatic*	*Infiltrative*	*Osseous Disease*	**Alcoholism or Inducing Drugs**
Alkaline phosphatase	1+	3+	3+	1–3+	±
5′-Nucleotidase	1+	3+	3+	—	—
Leucine aminopeptidase	1+	3+	3+	—	—
γ-Glutamyl transferase	1+	3+	3+	—	1–3+

*Number of +'s indicates relative degree of elevation.

identifying the placental form because it contains no sialic acid residues and is not cleaved by neuraminidase, and therefore its mobility on electrophoresis is unaffected (Moss and Edwards, 1984).

As discussed in Chapter 12, the probable hepatic origin of an elevated serum ALP level can be recognized by assay of leucine amino peptidase (LAP), 5′-N, or γ-glutamyl transferase activity. Values for these enzymes are high in patients whose hepatobiliary disease leads to high ALP levels but not in those with osseous disease responsible for this increased phosphatase value (Table 13–5).

METHODS FOR ASSAYING ALKALINE PHOSPHATASE

Originally, total serum ALP was assayed using the Kay and Bodansky method, in which β-glycerophosphate was used as the substrate and the inorganic phosphate liberated was measured as a function of time. This method was superseded by the King-Armstrong method, in which phenylphosphate was converted by the enzyme to phenol + phosphate. The phenol liberated can be measured spectrophotometrically. This method has now been largely replaced with one using the substrate *p*-nitrophenyl phosphate, which is colorless and is cleaved by ALP to the strongly chromogenic *p*-nitrophenoxide anion, at alkaline pH, and P_i. The former reaction product can be measured conveniently at 405 nm.

Acid Phosphatase (ACP) (EC 3.1.3.2)

This enzyme, first demonstrated in the urine in 1925, was found to be much more prevalent in male than in female urine. It was soon shown that prostatic tissue contains this enzyme in high concentration. Another ACP, which differs from that found in the prostate (Table 13–6), is present in erythrocytes and platelets.

Patients with prostatic carcinoma that has metastasized have elevated serum levels of ACP. One half to three fourths of patients with carcinoma of the prostate that has extended beyond the capsule have elevated ACP levels. Patients with prostatic carcinoma still confined within the capsule usually have normal serum levels of this enzyme. However, patients with benign prostatic hypertrophy may have slight elevations of the serum ACP level after vigorous prostatic "massage." Thus, ACP determination is useful in diagnosing metastatic carcinoma of the prostate but is of little value in diagnosing resectable prostatic carcinoma. Because other tissues, such as erythrocytes, may also release ACP into the serum, minor elevations of enzyme levels may reflect such an origin rather than the prostate. Accordingly, efforts have been made to distinguish "prostatic" ACP from the isoenzymes that are of erythrocyte and other origin. The efforts to distinguish prostatic ACP from erythrocyte ACP have been based on the differential effect of various substrates and various inhibitors on enzymes from these two sources (see Table 13–6). The inhibition of prostatic ACP by tartrate and the lack of inhibition by cupric ion, compared with the lack of inhibition of erythrocyte ACP by tartrate and the inhibition by cupric ion, are the properties most commonly utilized (see Table 13–6). ACP released from platelets, however, resembles the prostatic enzyme in its response to inhibitors (Wilkinson, 1976).

ACP may also be elevated in diseases of bone such as Paget's disease and in cancers, such as breast, lung, thyroid, and prostate cancers, that metastasize to bone. These conditions result in abnormal deposition of bone, causing osteoblastic lesions. The ACP in these conditions is usually, but not always, tartrate resistant and is thought to originate from osteoclasts.

Elevated levels of this enzyme are also frequently seen in metabolic disorders such as Gaucher's disease and Niemann-Pick disease. Elevated levels of tartrate-resistant ACP are found in hairy cell leukemia, an important diagnostic aid for this condition. ACP is present in significant amounts in seminal fluid and has been found useful forensically in the diagnosis of rape because vaginal ACP activity is low (< 10 IU/L), whereas postcoitally it reaches values exceeding 50 IU/L (Schumann, 1976).

METHODS FOR MEASURING ACID PHOSPHATASE

Acid phosphatase can be measured in several ways. The substrate thymolphthalein monophosphate appears to be selective for ACP and is hydrolyzed by the enzyme to yield thymol, whose concentration is determined spectrophotomet-

Table 13–6. EFFECT OF INHIBITORS ON ACID PHOSPHATASE OF PROSTATE AND OTHER TISSUES*

Inhibitor	Inhibition of Prostatic Phosphatase	Inhibition of Erythrocyte Phosphatase
L(+)–Tartaric acid 0.02 M	+	–
Formaldehyde 2%	–	+
Cupric sulfate 0.001 M	–	+

*+ represents marked inhibition.
– represents minimal inhibition.

rically at 595 nm. Nitrophenyl phosphate substrate, discussed later, can also be used. In this case, the total ACP and the tartrate-inhibitable phosphatase activity are measured, usually at pH 5.4. Also available are immunochemical methods that are specific for prostatic ACP.

5′-Nucleotidase (5′-N) (EC 3.1.3.5)

Significantly elevated levels of this enzyme occur specifically in hepatobiliary disease. The highest values are observed in patients with posthepatic jaundice, intrahepatic cholestasis, and infiltrative lesions of the liver. Mildly elevated levels are observed in patients with hepatocellular disease. Measurement of 5′-N also has been proposed as a diagnostic aid, more specific than ALP, in patients with hepatobiliary disease (see Table 13–5). Measurement of this enzyme utilizes the specific substrate adenosine 5′-monophosphate (5′-AMP), which is converted to adenosine and P_i. Either the P_i produced can be measured using the phosphomolybdate color reaction, or the adenosine liberated can be measured using coupled reactions. In the iatter case, the adenosine is deaminated by adenosine deaminase. The ammonia liberated can be measured either titrimetrically or in a further coupled reaction in which α-ketoglutarate is converted reductively to glutamate, a reaction in which NADH is converted to NAD. The decrease in absorbance at 340 nm can be directly monitored. It is important to note that measurement of the activity of 5′-nucleotidase is complicated by phosphatases that also catalyze the preceding reaction, 5′-AMP → adenosine + P_i. Because 5′-N can be selectively inhibited by Ni^{+} ions or by concanavalin A, the rates of reaction with and without inhibitors can be measured, and the difference in rates is that due to 5′-N activity.

γ-Glutamyl Transferase (γ–Glutamyl Transpeptidase, GGT) (EC 2.3.2.1)

This enzyme catalyzes the transfer of a γ-glutamyl group from a γ-glutamyl peptide to another peptide or an amino acid. It is present in the cell membrane and microsomal fractions and may be involved in amino acid transport across cell membranes and in glutathione metabolism. Kidney and, to a lesser extent, liver and pancreas are rich in GGT. A number of other tissues contain small amounts. Different forms of this enzyme appear to result from post-translational modification and are probably not true isoenzymes.

The chief clinical value of measuring GGT is in the study of hepatobiliary disease. Values parallel those of ALP, LAP, and 5′-N in obstructive (posthepatic) jaundice and infiltrative disease of the liver. Accordingly, assay of GGT, like that of 5′-N and LAP, estimates the level of the hepatic isoenzyme of ALP. Because GGT is a microsomal enzyme, its tissue levels increase in response to microsomal enzyme induction. This phenomenon may explain the elevated serum levels in chronic alcoholics and in patients taking drugs (e.g., phenytoin) known to induce the microsomal enzyme system (Rosalki, 1975). Serum GGT has thus been advocated in the evaluation of patients with alcoholism. Specifically, the alcoholic who has become abstinent should show a reduction of previously elevated GGT levels. The activity of this enzyme is measured in the reaction of γ-glutamyl-*p*-nitroanilide + glycylglycine, yielding γ-glutamyl-glycyl-glycine + *p*-nitroaniline. The concentration of *p*-nitroaniline liberated is readily measured at 405 nm.

Aminotransferases (Transaminases)

These critical enzymes are involved in the interconversion of metabolites of carbohydrate and protein catabolic pathways. The two major aminotransferases are aspartate amino transferase (AST, formerly called SGOT) and alanine amino transferase (ALT, formerly called SGPT). The reaction catalyzed by ALT is:

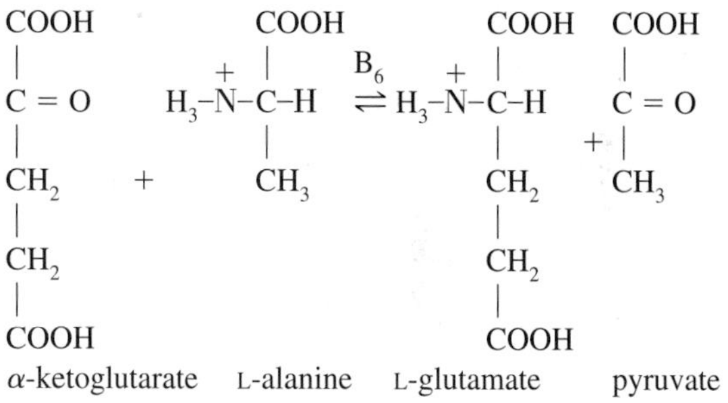

(13-7)

For AST, the L-alanine is replaced with aspartate and the pyruvate with oxaloacetate.

Aspartate Aminotransferase (AST) (Glutamate Oxaloacetate Transaminase) (EC 2.6.1.1)

This enzyme is elevated in diseases involving the tissues that are rich in it. Table 13–7 lists the tissues with the highest AST concentrations, the categories of disease that may show abnormal levels, and the range of values seen in many of these conditions. The AST levels in patients with liver disease are discussed in Chapter 12.

Extensive studies have shown that patients with acute myocardial infarction have elevated serum AST levels, if measured at the proper interval after infarction (West, 1966). The values are usually 4 to 10 times the upper limit of normal. These elevations usually develop within 12 hours of the time of infarction and reach the peak by the second day; the levels usually return to normal by the fifth day after infarction (Fig. 13–6). Secondary rises may reflect extension or recurrence of myocardial infarction. Experimental work with animals suggests that the degree of rise of serum AST is related to the extent of myocardial necrosis.

There is a stereotypical elevation of three enzymes in myocardial infarction that follows a specific time course (see Fig. 13–6). Note that CK, a muscle-specific enzyme, rises to a peak within 24 hours after infarction; AST then follows, rising to a peak within 48 hours; the enzyme LD is the last to rise, peaking within 72 hours. Although this pattern is almost pathognomonic for myocardial infarction, it cannot be used diagnostically because of the prolonged times for enzyme elevations. CK and LD isozymes are used for the diagnosis and confirmation of myocardial infarction, respectively (Galen, 1975a, 1975b). This is discussed later in more detail.

Table 13–7. TISSUES RICH IN AST AND CONDITIONS IN WHICH THE SERUM ENZYME IS ABNORMAL*

A. Tissue content of AST (descending order of concentration)	
1. Heart	
2. Liver	
3. Skeletal muscle	
4. Kidney	
5. Brain	
6. Pancreas	
7. Spleen	
8. Lung	
9. Serum	
B. Conditions in which serum AST is elevated	**Usual Values (U/L)**
1. *Cardiac disease*	
Myocardial infarction	20–200
Pericarditis	<100
Cardiac arrhythmias	<200
Acute rheumatic fever (?)	<100
Postcardiac surgery and catheterization	<100
Heart failure	<100
2. *Hepatic disease*	
Acute hepatitis (viral, toxic)	500–4000
Infectious mononucleosis	50–800
Cirrhosis	<100
Hepatic congestion	<100
Space-occupying lesions (granuloma, metastatic carcinoma)	<200
Obstructive jaundice	<200
3. *Other diseases*	
Shock	20–1000
Pulmonary infarction	<50
Acute pancreatitis	20–1000
Renal infarction (experimental animals)	<200
Cerebral necrosis	<50
Dermatomyositis	<200
Progressive muscular dystrophy	<200
Delirium tremens	<100
Hemolysis (slight)	<50
Gangrene (slight)	<50
C. Conditions in which serum AST is depressed	
1. Pregnancy	0–6

*In acute hepatitis, values above 300 U/L are usual and above 500 U/L are frequent. In all the other conditions shown, the levels are usually below this value, although higher values are occasionally observed in infectious mononucleosis, myocardial infarction, pancreatitis, and shock. Almost all patients with acute myocardial infarction have elevated values during the first few days. In the other cardiac diseases listed, elevations are less frequent and usually are slight.

Because of its ubiquitous distribution and the lack of a myocardial-specific isozyme, AST is not routinely used for the diagnosis of myocardial infarction. Laboratory diagnosis of myocardial infarction is more specifically made by following the serum levels of CK, CK isoenzymes, LD, and LD isoenzymes.

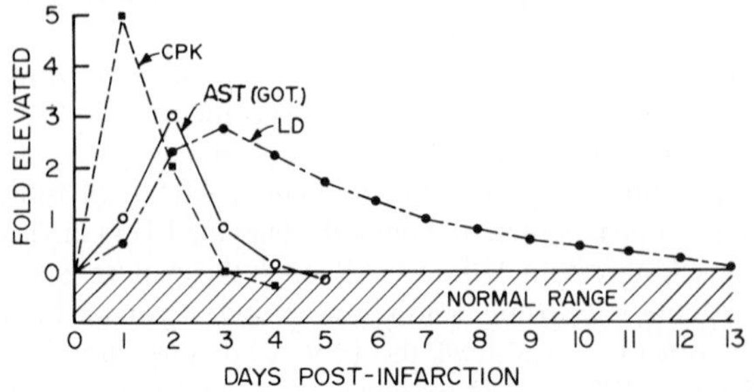

Figure 13–6. CK, AST (GOT), and LD levels after myocardial infarction (means of values for 200 patients). Note that the CK rise is earliest, the LD rise is latest, and the LD elevations are present longer than those of CK and AST (GOT).

In patients with electrocardiographic and clinical criteria of "coronary insufficiency" rather than myocardial infarction, serum AST levels may become elevated. It is not clear whether this phenomenon represents myocardial necrosis that has not been recognized by other means or "leakage" of the enzyme into the serum even without frank myocardial necrosis.

Mild elevations of the serum AST levels have been reported in some patients with pulmonary infarction. The incidence has varied from 0% to 30%, and the elevations are slight to moderate. Animal studies have also yielded inconclusive results on the occurrence of elevated serum AST levels in experimental pulmonary infarction. The incidence of increased values in humans is low, the degree of abnormality slight, and the rise delayed for three to five days after the onset of pain.

In patients with congestive heart failure or marked tachycardia, AST levels may become mildly to moderately elevated. This has been attributed to the hepatic necrosis secondary to hepatic congestion. A 50% incidence of slightly elevated AST levels also has been reported for patients with pericarditis. The incidence and mechanism of occurrence of elevated enzyme levels in patients with rheumatic fever are not clear. Slight serum AST elevations have been reported after cardiac catheterization and mitral commissurotomy (Galen, 1975a).

Determination of AST or other enzyme levels is not necessary for the diagnosis of myocardial infarction in most patients with classic clinical and electrocardiographic evidence of this condition. Enzyme determinations are of value in patients whose electrocardiographic changes are insufficiently helpful (e.g., those with left bundle branch block or Wolff-Parkinson-White syndrome or in those with electrocardiographic abnormalities remaining from previous infarction, which may obscure acute changes). Measurement of serum enzymes is also of value in recognizing the recurrence or extension of an infarction during convalescence. Normal values obtained on three successive serum specimens collected at intervals four hours apart are of value in excluding a diagnosis of myocardial infarction.

Patients with disease or injury producing inflammation or destruction of skeletal muscle may also have elevated serum AST levels. Patients with progressive muscular dystrophy, dermatomyositis, and trichinosis may have elevated levels, whereas those with amyotrophic lateral sclerosis, myasthenia gravis, and nerve section do not. Gangrene of the extremities and surgical or other trauma may produce slight AST elevations. Serum AST is elevated in less than 50% of patients with cerebrovascular accidents.

Levels may be elevated in acute pancreatitis. It has been suggested that obstruction of the biliary tree by the edematous pancreas and the presence of associated hepatic disease or of delirium tremens may contribute to the elevated AST levels in these patients.

Alanine Aminotransferase (ALT) (Serum Glutamate Pyruvate Transaminase) (EC 2.6.1.2)

This enzyme is discussed in detail in Chapter 12. In patients with myocardial infarction, elevations of the serum levels of ALT are slight or absent. The chief application of determination of this serum enzyme is in the diagnosis of hepatocellular disease.

In hepatocellular disease, both AST and ALT are markedly

elevated, often reaching 20 to 50, and sometimes 100, times the upper limit of normal. In viral hepatitis, peak values of AST and ALT occur about one to two weeks after the onset of infection and then decrease in the third to the fifth week. In hepatocellular disease other than viral hepatitis, amino transferase elevation is such that the ratio of ALT to AST is less than 1. This ratio, called the DeRitis ratio (DeRitis, 1956), is often reversed in viral hepatitis, facilitating the diagnosis. Values for these enzymes may be somewhat elevated in cirrhosis, depending on the degree of ongoing necrosis. In terminal cirrhosis, the values are often normal or low. In biliary disease, both intrahepatic and extrahepatic, the amino transferase levels are usually normal but sometimes are mildly elevated. In metastatic carcinoma to liver, the pattern may be similar to that in biliary disease, depending on the extent of parenchymal involvement (the greater involvement leading generally to greater elevations, at least initially). Persistently elevated ALT has proved to be useful in diagnosing the presence of hepatitis C.

Enzyme Assays

Several coupled enzymatic assays can be employed. One is to add saturating concentrations of specific substrate such as alanine to drive the reaction in equation 13–7 to the right. L-Glutamate formed can be directly measured using glutamate dehydrogenase, a reaction in which NADH is converted to NAD so that decrease in absorbance at 340 nm can be measured. In the case of AST, addition of saturating concentrations of aspartate will yield glutamate that is measured in the same way. Alternatively, in the case of ALT, the oxaloacetate (OAA) produced can be measured using malate dehydrogenase in which OAA is reduced to malate and, again, NADH is converted to NAD. It should be noted that both amino transferases absolutely require pyridoxal phosphate, vitamin B_6, the cofactor that undergoes sequential reactions with each substrate and is converted to pyridoxine as an intermediate. Thus, vitamin B_6 should always be in the reaction mixture.

Lactate Dehydrogenase (LD) (EC 1.1.1.27)

LD, which catalyzes the reversible oxidation of lactate to pyruvate with the oxidation of NADH to NAD, is widely distributed in mammalian tissues, being rich in myocardium, kidney, liver, and muscle. Serum levels of LD are elevated in a variety of conditions (Fig. 13–7). Fundamentally, elevated serum levels of LD are used to diagnose myocardial infarc-

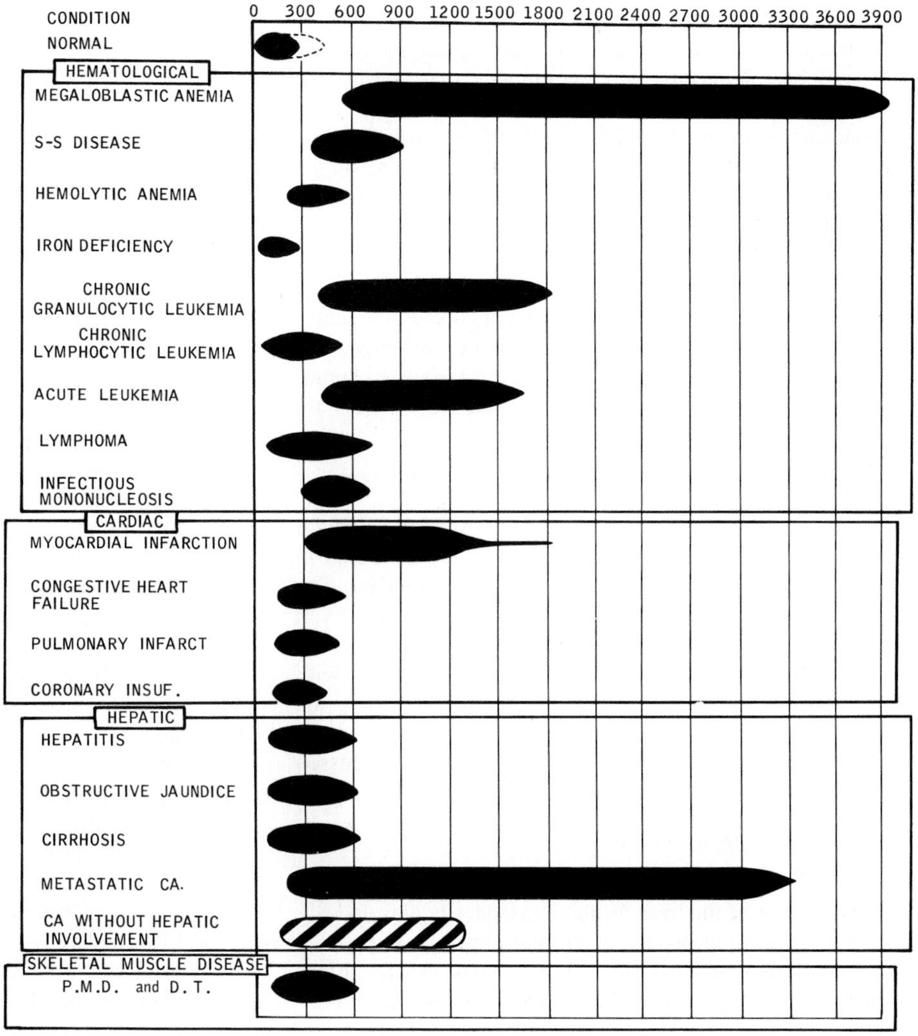

Figure 13–7. Lactate dehydrogenase values (U/L or Units/liter) in normals (dotted line represents higher values in children) and in patients with various diseases. Equivalent degrees of elevation of ALS and PHI occur in all these conditions with the exceptions of megaloblastic anemia, in which levels of LD are relatively higher, and acute hepatitis, in which levels of LD are relatively lower than those of PHI and ALS. Values for ALS are higher than those of PHI and LD in muscle disease.

tion and liver dysfunction. The former condition will be discussed later under the topic of isozymes of LD, whereas the latter is discussed in Chapters 4 and 12.

In general, the highest values (twofold to 40-fold elevations) are seen in patients with megaloblastic anemia, in those with extensive carcinomatosis, and in those with severe shock and hypoxia. Moderate (twofold to fourfold) elevations occur in patients with myocardial infarction, pulmonary infarction, granulocytic or acute leukemia, Hodgkin's disease, hemolytic anemia, infectious mononucleosis, and progressive muscular dystrophy. Relatively slight elevations occur in patients with hepatitis, obstructive jaundice, or cirrhosis, but values are higher in those with delirium tremens. Values also are increased in patients with chronic renal disease, especially those with nephrotic syndrome or hemolytic anemia. In patients with myxedema, the LD values are also elevated, presumably because of muscle abnormality.

Pulmonary Infarction

Most patients with pulmonary infarction have elevated levels of LD, usually within 24 hours of the onset of pain. The pattern of normal AST and elevated LD levels within one or two days after an episode of chest pain is suggestive evidence of pulmonary infarction.

Megaloblastic Anemia

LD levels are elevated in almost all patients with megaloblastic anemia. Often the values are strikingly increased. Possible factors in the production of the high values include the large number of megaloblasts, presumably rich in LD, and the intramedullary destruction of these cells. As the anemia responds to treatment, the LD levels return to normal. Hemolytic anemias yield variably elevated levels, depending on the extent of hemolysis. Values usually are normal in patients with aplastic and iron deficiency anemias.

White Cell Disorders

LD levels are moderately elevated in patients with granulocytic and acute leukemia. In lymphocytic leukemia, the values are usually normal, unless there is an associated hemolytic state. In patients with Hodgkin's disease, LD levels are often strikingly elevated.

Neoplastic Conditions

LD levels usually are normal in patients and animals with small, localized carcinomas, whereas levels are increased in those with distant metastases or even local extension. The highest values occur in patients with metastases to the liver, although increased levels are also found in some patients with only extrahepatic metastases or extension. In patients with Hodgkin's disease, abdominal tumors, and lung tumors, the LD levels are elevated, and the LD_5 isoenzyme is the predominantly elevated one. The isoenzymes of LD are discussed later. In germ cell tumors, LD_1 is markedly elevated.

Hepatic Dysfunction

Elevations of total LD are large in patients with space-occupying lesions of the liver. Values are modestly elevated (by one or two times) in patients with viral hepatitis. In patients with infectious mononucleosis, LD levels are usually somewhat higher, perhaps released from the aggregates of immature mononuclear cells throughout the body. Values are only slightly increased in patients with obstructive jaundice and sometimes in those with cirrhosis.

Muscle Disorders

Interestingly, LD values are increased in almost all patients with delirium tremens; perhaps the skeletal muscle is the origin of this increase because, as with the elevated LD levels of progressive muscular dystrophy, these elevations are accompanied by increased serum levels of creatine kinase.

Myocardial Disease

The pattern of elevated serum LD levels in patients with myocardial infarction is characteristic. High levels are observed in almost all patients within 24 hours of the apparent onset of infarction. Levels peak generally at 72 hours after the onset of infarction (see Fig. 13–6). Although the degree of elevation is not so striking as that of AST, the elevated levels persist longer (10 to 14 days). The characteristically prolonged period of elevated LD values with an increase of LD isoenzymes—that is, LD_1 higher than LD_2 ("flipped" LD), as described subsequently—yields a pattern that is useful in the laboratory diagnosis of myocardial infarction (Galen, 1975a). The flipped LD pattern usually appears within 12 to 24 hours and is present within 48 hours in the sera of 80% of patients with a myocardial infarction (Galen, 1975a).

Assay Methods

Spectrophotometric, fluorometric, and colorimetric methods have been applied to the assay of LD. The spectrophotometric method determines the rate of change in concentration of NADH. The reaction may be measured by following the disappearance of NADH at 340 nm (pyruvate + NADH→ lactate + NAD) at a pH of 7.4 or by following the appearance of NADH in the reverse reaction (lactate + NAD→pyruvate + NADH) at 340 nm at a pH of 8.8 or higher. The results should be expressed as the disappearance or the appearance of NADH at 340 nm in U/L (i.e., mmol/min of NADH consumed or formed per liter of specimen assayed).

Isoenzymes of Lactate Dehydrogenase

The LD of normal human serum can be separated into five different components by appropriate electrophoretic techniques. Each of these isoenzymes is distinguishable from the others by serologic, electrophoretic, and various other chemical procedures (Table 13–8). Indeed, the great current interest in isoenzymology derives from the observations on the multiple molecular forms of LD. The isoenzymes of LD are designated according to their electrophoretic mobility. The fraction with the greatest mobility (anodic) is called LD_1, the one with least anodic mobility is called LD_5, and the other three are designated accordingly as LD_2, LD_3, and LD_4, respectively.

The five LD isoenzymes have the same molecular weight (135,000) but differ in the charge that they carry. Each isoenzyme is a tetramer made up of four subunits, each of 34,000 daltons. There are two types of these subunits, designated H and M, for heart polypeptide chain (H) and skeletal muscle chain (M). The five isoenzymes of LD consist of the five possible combinations of monomers H and M (see Table 13–8). Hence, there are two homotetramers (LD_1 and LD_5) and three

Table 13–8. NOMENCLATURE, COMPOSITION, ISOENZYMES, AND TISSUE SOURCE OF LACTATE DEHYDROGENASE FOUND IN HUMAN SERUM BY ELECTROPHORETIC TECHNIQUES

Nomenclature of Isoenzyme Starting with Most Anodic	Composition Proportion of Monomers* in Each Isoenzyme	Relative Content† of Isoenzyme					
		Myocardium	*Liver*	*Skeletal Muscle*	*Brain*	*Kidney*	*RBC*
1	HHHH	++++	±	±	++	+	+++
2	HHHM	++++	±	±	++	+	+++
3	HHMM	+	+	+	++	++	+
4	HMMM	±	++	++	++	++	±
5	MMMM	±	++++	++++	±	++	±

*Monomer H (myocardial); monomer M (skeletal muscle).
†Content grades from ±, which represents almost no activity, to ++++, which represents high activity.

hybrids. The H and M chains differ significantly in their amino acid composition and thus in their structural and kinetic properties; they are probably controlled by two distinct genes.

Tissue LD consists of the five isoenzymes in varying proportions, and the LD activity of each tissue has a characteristic isoenzyme composition (see Table 13–8). The LD of myocardium and erythrocytes consists largely of the fastest moving isoenzymes (LD_1 and LD_2).

In liver and skeletal muscle, the principal isoenzymes are LD_4 and LD_5. In general, tissues exhibiting aerobic metabolism demonstrate predominantly faster-moving isoenzymes (LD_1) with more H subunits, whereas tissues exhibiting anaerobic metabolism demonstrate predominantly slower-moving isoenzymes (LD_5) with more M units. The H subunit exhibits a much higher affinity for lactate than pyruvate, whereas the reverse is true for the M subunit. Isozymes with predominantly H subunits tend to cause buildup of pyruvate that can be converted to acetyl-CoA (via the pyruvate decarboxylase complex), which is then used in the Krebs cycle (aerobic metabolism) to generate high levels of ATP. Thus, cardiac tissue, whose need for energy is constant, contains almost exclusively LD_1 and LD_2 (i.e., a vast preponderance of H chains). A number of tissues (lung, spleen, pancreas, thyroid, adrenals, and lymph nodes) consist mainly of LD_3. The relative concentration of the several isoenzymes in normal serum is LD_2, LD_1, LD_3, LD_4, and LD_5, in descending order. Normal serum LD has been presumed to derive mainly from erythrocytes, with LD_2 higher than LD_1.

Studies of the isoenzyme composition of the elevated serum LD levels of various diseases have revealed abnormal patterns that reflect the tissues involved (Table 13–9). In cardiac muscle, the LD_1/LD_2 ratio is less than 1 and is generally around 0.5 to 0.75. In acute myocardial infarction, the elevated serum LD levels consist largely of LD_1 and LD_2, and this ratio often reverses or becomes close to 1. When the LD_1/LD_2 ratio is greater than 1, the so-called flipped pattern, the most likely diagnosis is myocardial infarction. Two other diagnostic possibilities are acute renal infarction and acute hemolysis as in hemolytic anemia. LD_1 is the chief erythrocytic LD isozyme. Following acute myocardial infarction, the LD isoenzymes assume the flipped profile within 12 to 24 hours, with LD_1 greater than LD_2 in over 50% of cases. "Flipped LD" is present in 80% of patients with myocardial infarction within 48 hours after the acute episode. It is not necessarily maintained, because it is present in less than half of such patients (who earlier had a flipped LD) at the end of a week, even though the serum LD is elevated (Galen, 1975a). Likewise, increased LD_5 indicates either hepatic or skeletal muscle injury. LD patterns with intermediate hybrid fractions

Table 13–9. RELATIVE DEGREE OF INCREASE OF LACTATE DEHYDROGENASE AND PATTERN OF ABNORMALITY OF ISOENZYME IN VARIOUS DISEASES

Disease	Relative Degree of Increased Total LD Activity	Isoenzyme Fraction Most Abnormal				
		Most Anodic (+)				(−)
		LD_1	LD_2	LD_3	LD_4	LD_5
Myocardial infarction	↑↑	X	X			
Pulmonary infarction*	↑				X	X
Congestive heart failure	↑				X	X
Viral hepatitis	↑				X	X
Toxic hepatitis	↑				X	X
Cirrhosis	↑				X	X
Leukemia, granulocytic	↑↑		X	X		
Pancreatitis	↑		X	X		
Carcinomatosis (extensive)	↑↑↑		X	X		
Megaloblastic anemia	↑↑↑↑	X	X			
Hemolytic anemia	↑	X	X			
Muscular dystrophy†	↑	X	X			

*In pulmonary infarction, LD_3 may be elevated.
†In muscular dystrophy, LD_1 and LD_2 are elevated only in a relative sense, because LD_4 and LD_5 are depressed.

are found in several pathologic conditions but are less specific than the homotetramer elevations and, thus, are less diagnostic. Such patterns are seen in pulmonary embolism as well as in disease states in which levels of all five isoenzymes are increased, but their relationship to one another is virtually unchanged (isomorphic elevation). In acute viral hepatitis, the serum LD shows a higher proportion of LD_4 and LD_5 than normal. Some of the isoenzyme patterns observed in other diseases are indicated in Table 13–9.

Methods

Electrophoresis employing cellulose acetate or agarose is the best way to determine LD isoenzymes. The isozyme levels may then be quantitated by incubating the electrophoretic gels with substrate (e.g., pyruvate and NAD). In the presence of the enzyme catalase, tetrazolium dye reduction, by generated NADH, permits visual display and measurement of LD isoenzymes by scanning.

LD_1 levels may be determined directly in serum using immunochemical techniques based on antibodies specific for LD_1. Levels above a given cut-off value suggest myocardial disease. This method does not offer the advantage of measuring the ratio of LD_1 to LD_2 and may therefore not be as sensitive as the electrophoretic method.

LD_1, the myocardial isoenzyme, also may be approximated by techniques that are as simple as the measurement of total LD activity. Isoenzyme LD_1 resists denaturation at 65°C for 30 minutes, whereas the activity of the other four isoenzymes is destroyed under these conditions. Accordingly, the relative amounts of LD_1 can be estimated by comparing the heat-stable LD with the total LD activity. The serum level of LD_1 can also be estimated by measuring the level of α-hydroxybutyrate dehydrogenase (HBD). At one time considered to be the activity of a separate enzyme, HBD activity is now recognized to represent that of isoenzymes of LD—largely LD_1, with smaller amounts of other isoenzymes. HBD activity is measured by a technique similar to that just described for measuring LD. Normally, the LD/HBD ratio varies between 1.2 and 1.6. In myocardial infarction, this ratio decreases to 0.8 to 1.2. These latter two methods have given ground to the electrophoretic and immunochemical approaches.

LD Isozymes in Cerebrospinal Fluid

In cerebrospinal fluid, the distribution of isoenzymes is $LD_1 > LD_2 > LD_3 > LD_4 > LD_5$, whereas in some neurologic disorders, such as hydrocephalus and seizure disorders, $LD_2 > LD_1$ and the remainder of the pattern remains the same (Kjeldsberg, 1993). In bacterial meningitis, the order exactly reverses—that is, $LD_5 > LD_4 > LD_3 > LD_2 > LD_1$, making this technique, although seldom employed, excellent for confirmation.

Creatine Kinase (CK) (Creatine Phosphokinase [CPK]) (EC 2.7.3.2)

CK, also referred to as ATP-creatine-N-phosphotransferase, catalyzes the reversible reaction shown in Figure 13–8. Its concentration in skeletal muscle and myocardium is very high. Appreciable amounts are found in the brain. It is also found in intestine and lung. None is found in the liver. Many studies have shown that CK values are high in patients with myocardial infarction, progressive muscular dystrophy, alcoholic myopathy, rhabdomyolysis (Beressi, 1994) and delirium tremens, but normal in patients with hepatitis and other forms of liver disease. The high values in patients with hypothyroidism reflect the muscle changes in this condition. CK is found in skeletal muscle and myocardium. Other causes of CK elevation include exercise, intramuscular injections, and acute psychotic reactions. Coxsackie B4 viral infection associated with the acquired immunodeficiency syndrome (AIDS) has been found to cause dramatic elevations of CK (Beressi, 1994). In myocardial infarction, CK rises to high levels within 24 hours after infarct as noted previously and as shown in Figure 13–6. Most useful in the acute diagnosis of myocardial infarction is the isozyme distribution as discussed subsequently.

Methods of Measurement

From the reversible reaction catalyzed by CK shown in Figure 13–8, if ADP and creatine phosphate are added in saturating concentrations, ATP will be formed. This ATP is then incubated with glucose, hexokinase, glucose-6-phosphate dehydrogenase, and NADP to form glucose-6-phosphate and then gluconic acid-6-phosphate plus NADPH. The latter compound absorbs at 340 nm, allowing detection of product of the CK reaction. This is an example of the use of coupled reactions to determine enzyme activity levels as discussed earlier.

Isoenzymes of CK

CK exists as a dimer—that is, CK is, in turn, composed of three combinations of two chains, called M (originally for muscle) and B (originally for brain), as follows: MM, MB, and BB (Roberts, 1979). These three forms can be separated by electrophoresis. The BB form, also called CK_1, migrates the most anodally; the MM form, also called CK_3, migrates the most cathodally; and the MB form, also called CK_2, migrates in between. About 99% of total CK in skeletal muscle is the MM dimer, whereas in brain a high percentage (about 90%) of the CK is the BB dimer. In cardiac muscle, about 80% of the total CK is in the MM form, whereas about 20% is in the MB heterodimeric form. A small percentage of the CK of skeletal muscle is in the MB form, which can become important with major skeletal muscle conditions.

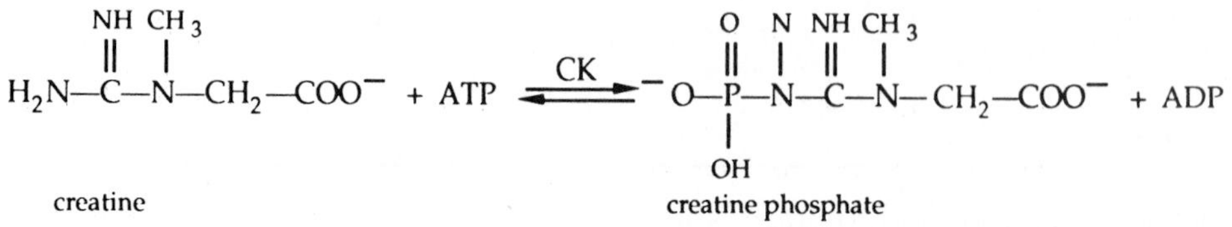

Figure 13–8. Reaction catalyzed by creatine phosphokinase (CK).

Both M and B isoenzymes can complex with immunoglobulins to form "macro-CK," which migrates between CK_1 and CK_2. Other forms are sometimes observed that are oligomeric forms of the mitochondrial form of CK, called CK-Mt. The MM (CK_3) isoenzyme undergoes post-translational modification in serum to a small extent and can appear between MB and BB fractions.

The isozymes of CK can also be determined immunochemically as discussed previously. Monoclonal antibodies that recognize the MB interface can be used to determine the concentration of CK-MB directly and form the basis for rapid immunoassays for CK-MB such as on the Abbott (North Chicago, IL) IMX and the Baxter (Miami, FL) Stratus analyzers.

Elevated levels of CK_2 (MB) in sera indicate damage to the myocardium; such elevations occur during the 48 hours following acute myocardial infarction in all patients (Galen, 1975a). In fact, after acute myocardial infarction, CK_2 (MB) appears within approximately 4 to 8 hours and peaks at 12 to 24 hours; it may persist throughout the initial 72-hour period. CK_2 (MB) activity never exceeds 40% of the total CK serum activity, with the remainder being CK_3 (MM) (Galen, 1975a). However, the CK_3 (MM) level of serum remains elevated for four to five days following the onset of chest pain (Galen, 1975a). CK isoenzyme determinations performed after day four, even with an elevated total CK level, will reveal only CK_3 (MM) activity, and the origin of CK_3 (MM) in heart or muscle cannot be established.

High levels of CK-MB are found less commonly in patients with severe angina and coronary insufficiency without evidence of infarction. CK_3 (MM) is found in the sera of patients with muscle trauma, including intramuscular injections, shock, and postoperatively following major surgical procedures.

Caveats in Interpretation of Elevated CK-MB Levels

Because there is a small amount of CK-MB in skeletal muscle, diseases of skeletal muscle that cause the level of CK-MM to rise to high values will also cause the levels of CK-MB to rise to high *absolute* concentrations in serum. For example, if CK-MB accounts for about 1% of the total CK in skeletal muscle, and the total CK rises to 100,000 IU/L because of, say, rhabdomyolysis, the CK-MB value will be 1000 IU/L, which is markedly elevated yet not diagnostic of myocardial infarction. Thus, a measurement showing that the CK-MB level is high in serum does not necessarily signify myocardial damage. It is also necessary to establish that the relative concentration of CK-MB in serum (ratio of CK-MB to total CK) is high.

This conclusion is especially true of the immunochemical determination of absolute concentrations of CK-MB, for which the manufacturer has determined that the values for CK-MB over a certain cut-off value are diagnostic of myocardial infarction. For example, the Roche (Nutley, NJ) combined immunoassay-activity assay recommends 10 IU/L as the cut-off for CK-MB. The Baxter-Stratus (Miami, FL) cut-off is around 4 ng/mL.

To determine the critical ratio of CK-MB to total CK that is diagnostic of myocardial infarction, given that the absolute concentration of CK-MB is over the cut-off, it is necessary to determine the CK-MB/total CK ratios for a group of patients who carry the diagnosis of myocardial infarction and whose sera have CK-MB concentrations above the cut-off. The maximal value for the ratio is selected such that no patient with myocardial infarction would be misdiagnosed as not having this condition. This method ensures that the sensitivity of the CK-MB assay is 100% (no false-negative results) and that the specificity of the method remains as high as possible, minimizing the number of false-positive results. (It is better to overdiagnose than to underdiagnose myocardial infarction.) Thus, to diagnose myocardial infarction, it is necessary to find CK-MB levels that are higher than a given cut-off value *and* to find that the ratio of CK-MB to total CK is greater than or equal to the experimentally determined cut-off ratio, often referred to as the cardiac index (Woo, 1992).

False-positive results for myocardial infarction with elevated CK-MB are found in any condition in which rhabdomyolysis is significant (Thompson, 1988) and have been found in hypothermia and hyperthermia, uremia, diabetic ketoacidosis, and septic shock. If the total CK is greater than 1000 IU/L, the cardiac index at which myocardial infarction could be diagnosed is 2% (Thompson, 1988) using the Roche (Nutley, NJ) diagnostic assay. In other studies (Woo, 1992), using the Stratus CK-MB immunoassay, a cut-off of CK-MB concentration of 3.5 ng/mL and a cardiac index of 0.37 were found to allow diagnosis of myocardial infarction with 100% sensitivity and the maximal corresponding specificity. The latter index differs from the former in that it involves a ratio of the absolute concentration of CK-MB to the total activity of CK, whereas the former involves the ratio of CK-MB activity to total CK activity.

Regardless of the method used and the levels found with a single specimen, *serial* determinations of MB fraction that show a progressive rise that reaches a peak, followed by a fall to low levels, are virtually 100% diagnostic of myocardial infarction (Lott, 1984). Blood specimens collected at intervals of 3 to 4 hours over a period of 12 to 16 hours may be required to confirm early diagnosis of myocardial infarction.

Elevations of the BB Isozyme

Significant serum levels of BB (CK_1) can be detected following head injury and crush injury of the anterior chest wall. These elevations result from cerebral BB and possibly lung BB fractions, respectively. Interestingly, in subarachnoid hemorrhage, wherein one expects the CK-BB fraction to be elevated, the MB (CK_2) fraction frequently is elevated, suggesting possible myocardial damage. CK (BB) has also been noted in the sera of patients with carcinoma of prostate, colon, lung, and esophagus.

Cholinesterase (CHS) (EC 3.1.1.8)

The cholinesterase of the serum has been referred to as pseudocholinesterase to distinguish it from the true cholinesterase (AcCHS) (EC 3.1.1.7) of erythrocytes and nerve tissue. The tissue enzyme acts optimally on acetylcholine and on acetyl-β-methylcholine but not on benzoylcholine, whereas the serum enzyme hydrolyzes acetylcholine and other choline esters even more rapidly (Fig. 13–9; Table 13–10) but not acetyl-β-methylcholine. Alkylphosphates are potent in-

2

$$RCOOCH_2CH_2N^+(CH_3)_3Cl^- + H_2O \xrightarrow{CHS} RCOOH + HOCH_2CH_2N^+(CH_3)_3Cl^-$$

R = CH_3 optimally for acetylcholinesterase.
R = CH_3 and many other alkyl or aryl groups for cholinesterase.
Method of assay is based on pH change (electrometric titration) that results from acid liberated.
Tissue content: acetylcholinesterase, RBC, nerve cells, synapses, and motor end plates. *Cholinesterase (pseudo):* serum or plasma, pancreas, and liver.
Conditions characterized by abnormal levels:

Depressed		*Elevated*	
Insecticide poisoning	↓	Nephrotic syndrome	↑
Hepatitis	↓		
Cirrhosis	↓		
Abscess	↓		
Metastatic carcinoma	↓ or N		
Obstructive jaundice	↓ or N		
Malnutrition	↓		
Anemias	↓		
Acute infections	↓		
Myocardial infarction	↓		
Dermatomyositis	↓		
Genetic acholinesterasemia	↓		

Figure 13–9. Reaction catalyzed by cholinesterases (CHS), principle of assay, and list of conditions that cause decreased (down arrow) or increased (up arrow) serum levels.

hibitors of both serum and tissue cholinesterase. Both enzymes react covalently with di-isopropylfluorophosphate (DIFP) and are inactivated by it.

Serum CHS values are characteristically depressed in patients with parenchymatous liver disease, including viral hepatitis, cirrhosis, metastatic carcinoma, the hepatic congestion of heart failure, and amebic hepatitis and abscess. In acute hepatitis, levels of the enzyme are lowest at the peak of the disease. Because, with recovery, the CHS level returns to normal, it has been suggested that the enzyme level may serve as an index of recovery and prognosis. In cirrhosis with jaundice, ascites, or other evidence of parenchymal insufficiency, CHS levels are usually depressed. In cirrhotics without these manifestations, the enzyme levels may be normal. Persistent depression of the CHS level in cirrhotics has been considered a poor prognostic sign.

In patients with obstructive jaundice, serum cholinesterase (CHS) levels are often normal. After prolonged obstruction, or when there is cholangitis, the level of CHS may be low.

Low values are also observed in patients with malnutrition, acute infections, anemias, myocardial infarction, and dermatomyositis (see Fig. 13–9). In these nonhepatic diseases and in hepatic disease, the CHS level is depressed in patients who also have a low serum level of albumin. Accordingly, it has been suggested that the low CHS level reflects impaired hepatic protein synthesis. Some support for this concept is derived from the observation that patients with the nephrotic syndrome, in whom the rate of albumin synthesis is increased, may have increased CHS levels, even though serum albumin levels are low.

As a measure of hepatic function and status, the determination of CHS is hardly used today. It is not sufficiently consistent to be useful in the differential diagnosis of jaundice. As an index of parenchymal function during the course of hepatic disease, it appears to add little to more commonly used laboratory measurements.

Assay of serum CHS has found several applications other than in the diagnosis of hepatic disease. The organophosphorous insecticides are potent inhibitors of the cholinesterases. Depression of the acetylcholinesterase of the tissue (reflected in levels of erythrocyte AcCHS) and of the pseudocholinesterase of the serum CHS occurs. Serum CHS, which is depressed before erythrocyte AcCHS, is a sensitive measure of overexposure to these agents. Severe exposure is usually reflected in depression of both erythrocyte AcCHS and serum CHS. Serum levels appear to return to normal earlier than do the erythrocyte values.

The genetic control of serum CHS activity has been of great theoretical interest and is of some practical importance. At least two forms of serum CHS have been recognized. One has been called "normal" and the other "atypical." The genes controlling their synthesis are allelic to each other. Persons homozygous for the atypical gene can be distinguished readily from the homozygous normal. The homozygous abnormal patient has very low CHS levels, and the abnormal CHS is not inhibited by dibucaine. The ho-

Table 13–10. SUBSTRATE RELATIONSHIP OF BLOOD CHOLINESTERASES

Enzyme	Source in Blood	Substrates Hydrolyzed: *Acetylcholine*	*Acetyl-β-Methylcholine*	*Butyrylcholine*	*Benzoylcholine*	Kinetics with Acetylcholine: *Optimal Concentration*	*Inhibition by Excess*
Acetylcholinesterase (true cholinesterase)	RBC	+	+	–	–	3×10^{-3}	+
Cholinesterase (pseudocholinesterase)	Plasma or serum	+	–	+	+	2×10^{-2}	–

mozygous normal has much higher levels of CHS activity, inhibitable by dibucaine, whereas the heterozygote has intermediate levels and an intermediate response to the inhibitors. Fluoride shows the same inhibition pattern. Typical dibucaine numbers for normals, heterozygotes, and homozygotes are 78%, 60%, and 16%, respectively, using benzoylcholine as the substrate (Tietz, 1993). Not only is hereditary hypocholinesterasemia an interesting genetic state to study but it is also of clinical importance in regard to the administration of muscle relaxants (succinylcholine). Homozygous abnormals may develop prolonged apnea after they receive succinylcholine. Accordingly, patients who become apneic under these circumstances should undergo CHS studies. Indeed, it has been proposed that one of the simple screening methods for CHS be performed prior to administration of an acetylcholine antagonist in order to exclude subjects who should not receive the agent.

AcCHS levels are now most commonly measured using a convenient colorimetric method in which propionyl thiocholine is hydrolyzed by the enzyme to form thiocholine and acetate. The thiocholine reacts with the Ellman reagent (5,5′-dithiobis-(2-nitrobenzoic acid)) to form a colored disulfide product monitored at 410 nm.

Angiotensin-Converting Enzyme (ACE) (EC 3.4.15.1)

ACE, also called peptidyldipeptide hydrolase, converts angiotensin 1 to angiotensin 2 by splitting off the carboxyl terminal dipeptide of the dodecapeptide, angiotensin 1. ACE usually is assayed by employing a synthetic substrate, benzoyl-glycyl-histidyl-leucine, and measuring spectrophotometrically the rate of release of benzoylglycine (hippuric acid). This method is a manual one. A radioassay is also available. An automated procedure using the substrate furoylacroyl-Phe-Gly-Gly has been developed (Beneteau, 1986). This peptide is also a substrate for chymotrypsin. An automated spectrophotometric method for assay of ACE, based on coupled enzyme reactions, has also been developed (Haskins, 1991) in which the specific ACE substrate, hippuryl-His-Leu, is hydrolyzed to hippuric acid and His-Leu. The His-Leu is then cleaved by leucine amino peptidase to yield free His, which is then cleaved by histidase to yield ammonia and urocanic acid. The ammonia generated is then reacted with α-ketoglutarate to yield glutamate in the presence of glutamate dehydrogenase, a reaction in which NADH is converted to NAD. The decrease in absorbance at 340 nm is then directly measured.

The main source of ACE is lung, particularly the endothelial cells of the pulmonary artery (Velletri, 1985). The testes are also a major source of this enzyme (Velletri, 1985). A brain isozyme of ACE has been discovered (Strittmatter, 1985) and has been found to be a possible indicator of neuronal dysfunction in such conditions as Alzheimer's disease when measured in CSF (Zubenko, 1985). ACE levels are elevated in primary liver disease (Johnson, 1987). In an age in which hypertensive patients are being treated with ACE inhibitors, artificially low values of this enzyme can be traced to the presence of these inhibitors.

Serum levels are elevated in patients with active sarcoidosis and leprosy. Values are particularly high in patients with active pulmonary sarcoidosis and usually are normal in inactive disease, as well as in other granulomatous disease of the lung, including tuberculosis, mycotic infections, and berylliosis (Rohrbach, 1982).

ACE values also are high in patients with Gaucher's disease, a phenomenon attributed to increased synthesis in Gaucher's or other macrophage-derived cells in this disease (Silverstein, 1978). Other conditions with increased levels of ACE are primary biliary cirrhosis and amyloidosis (Rohrbach, 1982).

2

Pancreatic Enzymes

(see also Chap. 23)

Amylase (EC 3.2.1.1)

Amylase, predominantly of pancreatic (P-form) and salivary gland (S-form) origin, hydrolyzes the α-1,4-linked glucose units in glycogen and amylopectin. It does not split the α-1,6-glucosyl bonds of these molecules. It can hydrolyze poly-α-1,4-glucose to maltose (i.e., the disaccharide). Levels are elevated in pancreatitis, salivary gland lesions (such as mumps), perforated peptic ulcers, appendicitis, ruptured ectopic pregnancy, dissecting aortic aneurysm, and biliary tract disease. In acute pancreatitis, the level of amylase can reach four to six times the upper reference limit of normal and returns to normal within three to four days. With the formation of pancreatic pseudocyst, the levels frequently remain elevated. Amylase is the only protein that can be cleared by the kidneys. In pancreatitis, the clearance of amylase is increased. The ratio of amylase clearance to creatinine clearance (which is constant in individuals with normal renal function) is usually elevated in acute pancreatitis. Although reference ranges for this ratio vary for normals, the usual value is 2% to 5%; values over 8% are common in acute pancreatitis. However, values are similarly elevated in burns, renal insufficiency, myeloma, march hemoglobinuria, and other conditions. In renal failure, serum levels of amylase are elevated as a result of decreased renal clearance. In macroamylasemia, amylase is bound to immunoglobulin, and the complex is too large to be filtered by the glomeruli. Thus, this condition gives rise to apparent hyperamylasemia (called macroamylasemia), which does not indicate disease. In pancreatic carcinoma, the levels are elevated if the tumor causes obstruction of the main pancreatic duct. Otherwise, the levels are normal and can even be low (Tietz, 1993). Amylase may be elevated in neoplastic disease. Tumors of the lung and ovaries can cause elevation of amylase, which appears to be of the S-type.

MEASUREMENT OF AMYLASE

A number of methods are available for measuring amylase activity and are divided into starch substrate–based methods and defined-substrate methods. In the former, using starch, a heterogeneous polymer, decreases in turbidity as a function of time can be measured nephelometrically. In addition, because starch forms a blue-colored complex with iodine, the disappearance of this color as a function of time can be measured. It has been reported that an unknown substance in serum can interfere with the starch-iodine complex formation, a finding that detracts from the validity of the method. In another method, triazine dyes are linked covalently to amylopectin or starch to form an insoluble chromophobic suspension. Hydrolysis of the polymers into soluble oligomers results in soluble dye in solution. After centrifugation, this soluble dye can be measured spectrophotometrically.

A number of specific-substrate methods, which are preferable to the starch-based methods because they contain well defined substrates rather than heterogeneous polymers, are available. In the Beckman (Fullerton, CA) assay, maltotetrose is hydrolyzed to two maltose units. This reaction is coupled to maltose phosphorylase, which converts maltose to glucose-1-phosphate and glucose. This reaction is, in turn, coupled to phosphohexoisomerase, which converts glucose-1-phosphate to glucose-6-phosphate. In the last step, glucose-6-phosphate is oxidized by glucose-6-phosphate dehydrogenase to gluconolactone-6-phosphate wherein NADP is converted to NADPH, the indicator reaction monitored at 340 nm. Other methods, using nitrophenyl saccharide substrates, are also available.

ISOENZYMES OF AMYLASE

Isoenzymes of amylase are broadly separated into P (pancreatic) and S (salivary gland) isoenzymes. However, at least six isoenzymes appear to exist on cellulose acetate (40°C, discontinuous buffer system) (Legaz, 1976). Three fast-moving (toward the cathode) isoenzymes were identified as being of salivary origin (labeled S1, S2, and S3), whereas three slower-moving ones were identified as of pancreatic origin (labeled P1, P2, and P3). Interestingly, P3 was present only in the serum of patients with acute or chronic pancreatitis and in those with renal insufficiency. S-type amylase activity is strongly inhibited by a protein isolated from wheat (Huang, 1982; O'Donnell, 1977), which has been used to differentiate amylase activities on automated analyzers.

Lipase

This enzyme, produced predominantly in the pancreas, hydrolyzes triglycerides to monoglycerides that contain the acyl-link at the 2-position of the glycerol moiety. Lipase hydrolyzes triglycerides that are present in micelles, often with cholic and deoxycholic acid. The enzyme does not directly attach itself to these micelles but interacts with them through co-lipase, a smaller protein that binds to the micelles and with high affinity to lipase. Co-lipase, being a small protein, is cleared by the kidneys. Lipase is elevated in pancreatic disorders, especially in acute and often in chronic pancreatitis. Because co-lipase is filtered by the kidney at a rate proportional to its concentration, levels of co-lipase do not rise concomitantly with lipase in pancreatitis. Lipase is essentially a specific marker for pancreatic disease and becomes elevated within the first 12 hours of the onset of pancreatitis. The rise of serum levels of this enzyme does not always coincide with the rise of pancreatic amylase in pancreatic disease. Therefore, it is recommended that serum levels of both lipase and amylase be measured in diagnosing disorders of the pancreas.

There are two general methods for measuring lipase: titrimetric and turbidimetric. In both, a triglyceride, such as triolein, or a mixture of triglycerides such as occurs in olive oil, is hydrolyzed to monoglycerides and diglycerides and free fatty acids. The free fatty acids dissociate hydrogen ions, which can be directly measured titrimetrically. In addition, because triglycerides form emulsions that scatter light, hydrolysis of these triglycerides to soluble monoesters and glycerol results in a decrease in light scattering, which is easily monitored spectrophotometrically.

There are a number of lipases, other than pancreatic lipase, whose activities may also be monitored using the preceding assay systems, in particular, serum lipoprotein lipase, which hydrolyzes triglycerides in chylomicrons and in the β-lipoprotein fractions and which is activated by heparin; aliesterases, which hydrolyze short chain triglycerides and fatty acid esters; and aryl-esterase, which hydrolyzes arylesters of short chain acids. However, these latter enzymes have low hydrolytic activities when the substrates are present in micelles such as with cholate and other bile acids. Pancreatic lipase, however, is highly active against the micelle-bound substrates, provided that co-lipase is present. More recently developed assays incorporate the addition of bile acids and co-lipase that effectively eliminates the activity of the other esterases (Tietz, 1993). These modified methods also appear to eliminate measurement of postheparin lipoprotein lipase activity.

Other Serum Enzymes

Many other enzymes have been demonstrated in the serum (see Table 13–1). These are too numerous for individual description in this discussion, but a few warrant special mention. These include guanase, an enzyme that has been reported to reflect, sensitively and specifically, hepatic disease; β-glucuronidase, considered a biochemical clue to neoplastic, hepatic, and other disease; alcohol dehydrogenase, proposed as a measure of hepatic disease; plasma pepsinogen, an enzyme precursor that reflects function and disease of the stomach (high levels in patients with peptic ulcer, low levels in patients with pernicious anemia); and ceruloplasmin, a copper-carrying protein that is also an enzyme, the serum levels of which are depressed in patients with hepatolenticular degeneration (Wilson's disease). Ceruloplasmin measurement is useful in the diagnosis of Wilson's disease. The practical role of the other enzymes cited and of those listed in Table 13–1 in clinical medicine remains to be demonstrated.

CLINICAL APPLICATION OF SERUM ENZYME ASSAYS

Serum enzymology provides aids in making the diagnosis, monitoring the course, and demonstrating subclinical evidence of disease. Diseases that are characterized by distinctly abnormal values of one or more enzymes (see Table 13–1) can be readily distinguished from clinically similar states in which values for the respective enzymes remain normal. The diagnostic circumstances that are most clearly aided by serum enzymology are the distinction of myocardial infarction from other causes of chest pain, the differential diagnosis of hepatobiliary and muscle disease, the diagnosis of pancreatitis, and the recognition of metastases of neoplastic disease to bone or liver.

Thus, osteoblastic lesions lead to elevations of ALP values that range from slight to marked. Obstruction of the biliary tree (or intrahepatic cholestasis) leads to markedly elevated values of ALP, LAP, nucleotidase (5′-N), and GGT; relatively slightly elevated values of the aminotransferases, ALT and AST, and other liver-specific enzymes such as ornithine carbamoyl transferase (OCT); and normal values for CK. Hepatic necrosis leads to lesser values of ALP, LAP, 5′-N, and GGT, but very high values of AST, ALT, and OCT, and normal values for CK. Myocardial necrosis leads to moderately elevated levels of AST, LD, and CK. Skeletal muscle disease of the progressively degenerative or inflammatory type (progressive muscular dystrophy, dermatomyositis, trichinosis) leads to striking elevations of CK and LD levels and moderate elevations of fructose 1,6-diphosphate aldolase (ALS), phosphohexo isomerase (PHI), and malate dehydrogenase (MD), with more modest increase in the AST level and even lesser values of ALT and normal levels of the other enzymes listed in Table 13–1. Neoplastic disease is characterized by increased values of LD, ALS, PHI, and MD, with the increase seemingly dependent on the tumor having reached sufficient total mass. Reports of GGT suggest that this enzyme is also increased in the serum of patients with carcinomatosis. Metastatic carcinoma of the liver leads to moderate or marked elevations of LD and of ALP, LAP, 5′-N, and GGT and to slightly or moderately elevated values of AST and ALT. These abnormalities are also seen with other space-occupying lesions of the liver (granuloma, abscess, amyloidosis, and hemangioma). The pattern of serum enzyme abnormality of hepatic metastases also includes increased values of enzymes that reflect neoplastic growth. Metastases to various sites from prostatic carcinoma lead to high ACP levels. Metastases of carcinoma to the bone, if osteoblastic, lead to high ALP levels but to normal values of AST and ALT.

Monitoring the course of disease by serial determinations of serum enzyme levels is useful in the management of hepatitis, in the chemotherapy of neoplastic disease, in the treatment of dermatomyositis, and in the recognition of recurrent infarction or other complications during convalescence from acute myocardial infarction. Detection of subclinical disease by serum enzyme assay is exemplified by the use of serum aldolase or CK levels to recognize persons destined to develop progressive muscular dystrophy and by the employment of AST, ALT, or ALP to monitor patients exposed to known or potentially hepatotoxic agents and ALT to monitor hepatitis.

Serum Enzymes in Myocardial Infarction

The typical time courses for the rise of the three cardiac enzyme markers—CK, AST, and LD—are shown in Figure 13–6. Myocardial infarction is thus usually distinguishable from pulmonary infarction, which is characterized by elevated LD levels and usually by normal AST and CK values. In a small proportion of patients with pulmonary embolism, values for AST are elevated for three or four days after the bout of chest pain. The complication of myocardial infarction by shock leads to higher values of AST and LD and to abnormal levels of enzymes that reflect hepatic injury such as ALT.

Within the first 48 hours after an acute myocardial infarction, CK-MB, also called CK_2, is significantly elevated with respect to both its concentration or activity and its cardiac index, defined earlier, in virtually all patients with myocardial infarction, as well as in some cases of severe coronary insufficiency (Galen, 1975a). *Importantly, CK-MB often rises within the first 4 to 6 hours after the onset of myocardial infarction, so the diagnosis can be made in this time period and thrombolytic therapy can be instituted.* A newer, more sensitive method for diagnosis of acute myocardial infarction is discussed later.

Additionally, the measurement of LD isoenzymes further refines laboratory assessment of patients with myocardial infarction. However, the flipped LD ($LD_1 > LD_2$) is a more variable phenomenon, which may become evident at 12 hours (at the earliest) and be present in approximately 80% of patients with myocardial infarction within the first 48 hours (Galen, 1975a).

2

Combined Criteria Isoenzyme Analysis

Overall, CK levels and significant levels of CK_2 (MB) appear to be the most sensitive and specific tests for the diagnosis of acute myocardial infarction (Fisher, 1983). The simultaneous use of CK and LD isoenzyme determinations combines the high degree of sensitivity offered by CK with the high degree of specificity offered by LD (Galen, 1975a) (Table 13–11). Combined criteria are met when there is a flipped LD pattern ($LD_1 > LD_2$) in a patient exhibiting CK_2 (MB) in specimens drawn during the first 48 hours following an acute episode of suspected myocardial infarction (Galen, 1975a). Ideally, three separate specimens are collected—the first on admission, the second at 24 hours, and the third at 48 hours. Both CK and LD serum assays are measured. If total enzyme activity is elevated, isoenzymes are analyzed. The flipped LD comes after the appearance of CK_2 (MB). It should also be noted that the criteria do not have to be demonstrated in a single specimen. Indeed, they are frequently met by examining serum patterns in 24-hour and 48-hour specimens together. Table 13–11 describes how to interpret combined isoenzyme data during the initial 48-hour period (Galen, 1975a).

To be used most efficiently, the combined criteria must be evaluated during the initial 48 hours of suspected onset of ischemic heart disease. Once diagnostic criteria are met, further determinations are not needed to document the diagnosis. Indeed, if at 24 hours both criteria are met, the diagnosis is affirmed (Galen, 1975a). A CK_2 (MB) determination may then be done to estimate the infarct size or detect extension or reinfarction (Roberts, 1979). If combined criteria are not met by 48 hours, the diagnosis is then presumptively not myocardial infarction (see Table 13–11). It should be emphasized, however, that the combined criteria after a 48-hour interval do not rule out myocardial infarction with the same high de-

Table 13–11. COMBINED ISOENZYME ANALYSIS: RULE OUT MYOCARDIAL INFARCTION (MI)*

CK-MB Absent	CK-MB Present Usual LD	CK-MB Present Flipped-LD
100% predictive value that there is no MI	Both MI and non-MI cases†	100% predictive value that there is MI

*During acute 48-hour period following episode.
†Non-MI cases reflect clinical and electrocardiographic evidence of ischemia.
From Galen RS: The enzyme diagnosis of myocardial infarction. Hum Pathol 1975; 6:141–155. With permission of R.S. Galen, M.D.

gree of certainty present during the acute phase (initial 48-hour period) of potential ischemic injury. Indeed, a myocardial infarction could cause significant levels of CK_2 (MB) and the usual LD profile on day four.

Galen has also emphasized the application of combined isoenzyme analysis to special conditions in which confirmation of acute myocardial infarction is hampered by nonspecific enzyme elevation. In electroshock cardioversion, there is no CK_2 (MB). Major operative procedures usually lead to no elevation of CK_2 (MB) but only to that of the MM. However, as noted earlier, a variety of conditions, including rhabdomyolysis, Duchenne's muscular dystrophy, intravenous drug abuse, septic shock, and even some cases of AIDS, result in elevated CK_2 (MB) levels, having no apparent relationship to myocardial damage (Lott, 1984; Thompson, 1988). In addition, patients undergoing cardiopulmonary bypass procedures in open heart surgery for valve replacements or bypass grafts have elevated MB fractions that reflect the procedure rather than inherent myocardial damage (Galen, 1975a; Lott, 1984; Thompson, 1988). It should further be noted that LD patterns are flipped in 25% of patients without myocardial infarction secondary to hemolysis from extracorporeal circulation (Galen, 1975a).

CK-MB Subforms

The only isozyme of CK-MB in cardiac muscle is the CK-MB_2 form. However, in serum, this enzyme is cleaved by lysine carboxypeptidase to yield a des-lysyl CK-MB molecule that is now more negatively charged, called CK-MB_1. Because of this unique difference in charges between the two proteins, they can be separated from one another, and each form quantitated, using high-voltage electrophoresis. In normal persons, the total concentration of both forms is on the order of 0.5 to 1.0 U/L. It has been shown that in acute myocardial infarction, within six hours after the onset of symptoms, CK-MB_2 increases to values greater than 1 IU/L, with a ratio of CK-MB_2 to CK-MB_1 greater than 1.5 (Puleo, 1994). The sensitivity of the method was 97%, and the specificity was 94%. These results may be compared with those for use of total CK-MB to diagnose myocardial infarction within the same time period (i.e., sensitivity of 48% and specificity of 94%). It thus appears that the newer approach significantly improves the early diagnosis of myocardial infarction and dramatically reduces the number of false-negative results in the first six hours after onset of symptoms.

Other Analytes Diagnostic of Myocardial Infarction

Two other analytes, myoglobin and troponin, have been found to be useful in the diagnosis of acute myocardial infarction. Myoglobin is present in cardiac, skeletal, and smooth muscle. In myolytic diseases, the serum concentrations of this protein are therefore increased. Often, in rhabdomyolysis, myoglobinuria is observed (Beressi, 1994). Elevated myoglobin levels in serum, determined using the ELISA assay, have been used to screen patients for myocardial infarction, because myoglobin is released from damaged cardiac muscle within two hours after the onset of symptoms. The specificity of the method is limited because myoglobin can be elevated in serum from non–cardiac-related conditions. However, serum myoglobin determination holds promise in early screening for myocardial infarction in symptomatic patients.

Troponin is a complex of three proteins that regulate the interaction of myosin with actin in the contractile process: troponin T, which binds the complex to tropomyosin; troponin C, which binds calcium in the initiation of contraction; and troponin I, an inhibitor that blocks contraction in the absence of calcium. The amino acid sequences of these proteins in cardiac muscle differ locally from the corresponding sequences for the homologous proteins in skeletal muscle. Therefore, it has been possible to differentiate between troponins of cardiac and skeletal muscle immunochemically. An ELISA assay for cardiac troponin T is available for this purpose (Wu, 1994).

In myocardial infarction, the rise of cardiac troponin T parallels that of CK-MB, but the rise of troponin T is much greater (up to 80 times the upper limit of normal) than that of CK-MB. The reference range is 0 to 0.1 ng/mL. This rise is prolonged, allowing detection of myocardial infarction even 10 days after the onset of symptoms. After the onset of symptoms, within the first four hours, the levels of troponin T rise sharply, followed by a decline, corresponding to reperfusion, and then rise again about four days later, corresponding to release of bound troponin in necrotic myocytes. Thus, troponin is useful in the early diagnosis of myocardial infarction, allowing the early institution of thrombolytic therapy.

The sensitivity of cardiac troponin T (single determination) is approximately the same as that for CK-MB (multiple determinations) in the first four days after onset of symptoms: 82% in the first 11 hours, and about 99% from 12 to 95 hours after the onset of symptoms. After 96 hours, sensitivity remains at about 93%, whereas the sensitivity of CK-MB declines to about 10%. The specificity of the troponin T assay approaches 100%. Cardiac troponin is also useful in predicting the outcome of patients with unstable angina, for whom the serum levels of CK-MB may be too low to be of use. High levels of cardiac troponin T correlate with worsening prognosis.

Serum Enzymes in Liver Disease

The enzymologic approach to liver disease is discussed in Chapters 4 and 12. The four most commonly used enzymes in evaluating liver function are AST, ALT, ALP, and LD. Marked elevations in the two amino transferases, AST and ALT, to values over 500 IU/L suggest an acute hepatitic process. In this condition, the other two enzymes are also generally elevated to moderate levels, although with a panhepatitic process, these enzymes may be markedly elevated. Isolated elevations of ALP suggest biliary disease. The biliary tract source of this enzyme can be confirmed by elevated bilirubin levels and elevations in the two enzymes, GGT and 5′N. Isolated elevations of ALP and LD to values greater than 500 IU/L suggest the presence of space-occupying lesions in the liver. Among the four enzymes listed, ALT is the most specific for the presence of liver disease. The liver is the only tissue that can detoxify ammonia as urea via the urea cycle. The rate-determining step in this process is the one involving the enzyme OCT, which is unique to liver. Elevations of this enzyme signal liver dysfunction. However, it is far more convenient to assay ALT.

Serum Enzymes in Muscle Disease

Measurement of serum enzyme levels has become a major component of the diagnostic approach to muscle disease. The enzymes that have been studied most extensively are CK, aldolase (ALS), AST, and LD. CK, composed almost entirely of the MM fraction, is the most reliable measure of skeletal muscle disease. Aldolase levels are as sensitive to disease of muscle, although somewhat less specific.

In the progressive muscular dystrophies, especially the Duchenne type, the values are particularly high. Values are moderately or markedly elevated in dermatomyositis, in polymyositis, in scleroderma with an associated myositis, and in trichinosis. These enzymes also are slightly or moderately increased in myotonic dystrophy, in myotonia congenita, in the crush syndrome, and in McArdle disease. Values of these and other enzymes are high in patients with delirium tremens, irrespective of associated hepatic disease, and presumably arise in muscle (LD_5 and CK_3). The muscle involvement of myxedema appears to be responsible for the elevated serum enzyme levels in this condition. Strenuous muscle activity in untrained persons also leads to increased levels of these enzymes. Serum enzyme levels are normal in patients with neurogenic muscle disease. High levels of CK are also seen in McLeod's syndrome, a rare condition characterized by absence of the Kell red cell antigen, leukocyte bactericidal deficiencies, and neurologic deficits.

Prostatic Specific Antigen, a Protease Specific for Prostate Disease

A unique protease, prostate-specific antigen (PSA), a 34-kd glycoprotein, is located in the acinar and ductal cells of the prostate and in seminal fluid but has not been located in any other tissue. In diseases of the prostate, including benign prostatic hypertrophy and prostatic carcinoma, serum levels of this protein become elevated. Most PSA that circulates in serum is protein-bound, mainly to α_1 antichymotrypsin and to α_2 macroglobulin.

Both polyclonal and monoclonal antibodies against PSA have been produced, allowing for quantitative detection of this protease in serum using ELISA technology. The reference range for this protein in serum among normals is generally accepted as 0 to 4 ng/mL. It is important to note that values of PSA that barely exceed 4 ng/mL are not diagnostic of pathologic conditions, and the assay should be repeated on new serum specimens from the patient prior to further investigation. One of the major uses of PSA is in the early detection of prostatic carcinoma. This disease is the most common visceral cancer in American men and the second most common cause of cancer-related deaths in the United States. Thus, PSA has been the subject of intense study for use in the early detection of this disease.

PSA values in the range of 4 to 25 ng/mL have been found to indicate some form of prostate disease but are not definitive for the diagnosis of prostate cancer and may be caused by benign prostatic hypertrophy. The probability of carcinoma of the prostate for PSA values in this range is about 20% to 50%. Nonetheless, PSA values of at least 4 ng/mL warrant further investigation for possible prostatic malignancy.

In patients with biopsy-proven prostate cancer, the serum levels of PSA do not correlate with the stage or size of the tumor or the extent of the disease unless the tumor has broken through the prostatic capsule, has become metastatic, or both. Furthermore, undifferentiated tumors do not always elaborate PSA and can give rise to false-negative results. Thus, low serum values of PSA do not rule out prostatic carcinoma definitively.

However, elevated PSA levels in serum are proving to be the most reliable indicator of patients who have this disease. For example, in a study of over 6000 male volunteers 50 years of age or older, serum values of PSA greater than 4 ng/mL were considered to indicate possible prostatic carcinoma (Catalona, 1994). It was found that the positive predictive value (see Chap. 4) using this criterion was 32%. Using digital rectal examination to detect this disease, the positive predictive value was significantly lower at 21%. Of biopsy-proved carcinomas in this study, 82% were detected using PSA and the 4 ng/mL cut-off alone. Importantly, PSA levels were positive in 75% of patients with proved *organ-confined* cancers. The diagnostic yield could be further improved if the PSA results were combined with results from digital rectal examination. Of great interest was the finding that using PSA alone or with digital rectal examination dramatically increased the tumor detection rate over that obtained from transrectal ultrasonography. It therefore appears that combining serum levels of PSA with the digital rectal examination is the most effective means of identifying the existence of prostatic carcinoma in patients.

ENZYMES OF THE FORMED ELEMENTS OF THE BLOOD

Assays for red and white cell enzymes have proved useful in the diagnosis of a variety of disorders in these cells, most of them being genetic in origin. The major conditions are summarized here.

Hemolytic Anemia Associated with Deficiency of Erythrocyte Enzymes

Genetic defects in erythrocyte metabolism have been found or suspected to be responsible for well over a dozen forms of hemolytic anemia (Table 13–12). Some of the demonstrated or assumed enzymatic defects relate to the hexose monophosphate shunt (G-6-PD, 6-PGD, glutathione reductase [GR], glutathione [GSH]-synthetase, GSH-peroxidase), and some of the enzymatic defects relate to the anaerobic glycolytic pathway (HK, PHI, PFK, ALS, TPI, 2,3-DPGM, PGK, PK) and ATPase. The hemolytic syndromes associated with enzymatic defects are listed in Table 13–12 and are discussed further in Chapter 26.

Table 13–12. TYPES OF HEREDITARY NONSPHEROCYTIC HEMOLYTIC ANEMIA (HNHA) THAT ARE KNOWN OR SUSPECTED TO BE DUE TO ENZYMATIC DEFECTS OF ERYTHROCYTES*

Most important and frequent conditions
1. Glucose-6-phosphate dehydrogenase (G-6-PD) deficiency
2. Pyruvate kinase (PK) deficiency
3. Phosphohexoisomerase (PHI) (glucose phosphate isomerase) deficiency
Rare conditions
4. Hexokinase (HK) deficiency
5. Phosphofructokinase (PFK) deficiency
6. Triosephosphate isomerase (TPI) deficiency
7. Phosphoglycerate kinase (PGK) deficiency
Very rare conditions
8. Pyrimidine-5′-P-nucleotidase (5-5′-PN) deficiency
9. Aldolase deficiency†
10. GSH synthetase deficiency
11. GSH peroxidase deficiency
Very rare or equivocal conditions
12. Glutathione reductase (GR) deficiency
13. Glyceraldehyde phosphate dehydrogenase deficiency
14. 6-Phosphoglycerate dehydrogenase (6-PGD) deficiency
15. 2,3-Diphosphoglycerate mutase (2,3-DPGM) deficiency
16. ATPase deficiency
17. Adenylate kinase (AK) deficiency
18. Diphosphoglycerate phosphatase (DPGP) deficiency
19. Enolase deficiency

*See Beutler, 1976.

†At one time aldolase deficiency was considered to be responsible for familial spherocytic anemia, now known not to be true.

Hemolytic Anemia Secondary to Glucose-6-Phosphate Dehydrogenase (G-6-PD) Deficiency

Deficiency of erythrocyte G-6-PD activity has been estimated to involve 2% to 3% of the world population and to be responsible for almost one third of the cases of chronic or recurrent nonspherocytic hemolytic anemia. The defect is sex-linked and appears in a number of genetic variants. The first to be recognized is the relatively mild condition observed almost exclusively in blacks and characterized by deficient concentration in leukocytes and platelets. These persons develop hemolysis on exposure to a number of drugs, including primaquine, sulfonamides, and other agents, and to other stresses, including various infections. Common to all of these agents is oxidative stress on the red cell (i.e., drugs and infectious agents induce oxidation of red cell membrane lipids), causing hemolysis. Normally, the effects of these agents are countered by glutathione, which itself becomes oxidized, thereby preventing oxidation of the membrane lipids. Oxidized glutathione is then reduced by NADPH, which is generated by the oxidation of glucose-6-phosphate by G-6-PD in the hexose monophosphate shunt in the presence of the enzyme glutathione reductase (GR). Thus, a deficiency of either of these enzymes, G-6-PD and GR, will result in the lack of reduced glutathione, allowing for oxidation of membrane lipids. The basic pathways involved in these reductive processes are summarized in Figure 13–10.

A more severe form of G-6-PD deficiency, characterized by deficiency of the enzyme in leukocytes and erythrocytes, by more severe anemia, and by sensitivity to fava beans and to various drugs, is seen in whites, particularly Sephardic Jews; other ethnic groups of the Mediterranean littoral; American Indians; and Asians. Studies of the various forms of G-6-PD deficiency have shown not only differences in the severity of the clinical illness and the degree of depression of enzyme levels of erythrocytes and leukocytes but also that there are different molecular variants (isoenzymes) of G-6-PD.

Assay of G-6-PD activity has become a routine procedure in patients with hemolytic anemia, especially if it occurs after administration of a drug or during an acute illness. A precise assay of G-6-PD activity of hemolysate involves measuring the rate at which NADP is reduced in the presence of glu-

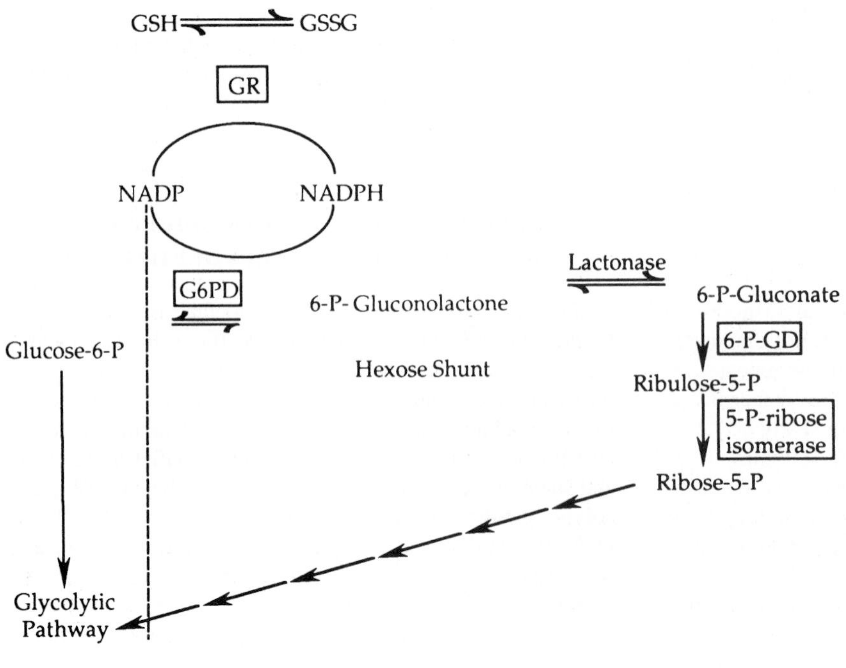

Figure 13–10. Initial reactions of hexose monophosphate shunt showing the role of generation of NADPH in maintaining reduced glutathione. Enzymes in boxes (GR, G-6-PD, 6-P-GD, 5-P-ribose isomerase) may be found in serum. Transketolase (not shown) also was reported in serum. (Carson PE, Frischer H: Glucose-6-phosphate dehydrogenase deficiency and related disorders of the pentose phosphate pathway. Am J Med 1966;41:744.)

cose-6-phosphate. Simplified assays suitable for screening large populations are available.

Hemolytic Anemia Secondary to Deficiency of Glutathione Reductase (GR), Glutathione Peroxidase (GSH-Px), or Glutathione Synthetase

A few instances of mild hemolytic anemia have been reported in patients with genetic deficiency in erythrocyte levels of GR. Some have been instances of chronic hemolysis and others of hemolytic anemia after exposure to drugs such as primaquine. Thus far, the condition appears to be rare and primarily of genetic interest. In several genera, glutathione has been almost completely absent from erythrocytes as a genetic abnormality. The deficiency of glutathione in these persons appears to be transmitted as an autosomal recessive trait and presumably results from subnormal glutathione synthetase activity. The erythrocytes of patients with GSH deficiency, like those of patients with G-6-PD and GR deficiency, are susceptible to drug-induced hemolysis. A similar syndrome has been attributed to deficiency of glutathione-peroxidase (GSH-Px), the enzyme presumed to be mainly responsible for destroying H_2O_2 in human erythrocytes.

Hemolytic Anemias Secondary to Deficiency in Glycolytic Enzymes

Pyruvate kinase (PK) deficiency is the most frequent and important form of hemolytic anemia that is due to deficiency of glycolytic enzymes in the erythrocyte. It is transmitted as an autosomal recessive trait and is characterized by a nonspherocytic, chronic hemolytic anemia. The hemolysis is attributable to the inability of the PK-deficient erythrocyte to maintain normal ATP levels and the resulting membrane defect. Enzyme activity of the erythrocyte can be assayed by measuring the ability of hemolysate to form pyruvate from ADP and phosphoenol pyruvate. The pyruvate formed can then be coupled to the LD reaction in which NADH is oxidized to NAD, and the pyruvate can be followed by the rate of decrease in absorbance at 340 nm.

Similar syndromes appear to result from deficient erythrocyte content of other glycolytic enzymes such as hexokinase, phosphohexoisomerase, phosphofructokinase, triose phosphate isomerase, 2,3-diphosphoglycerate mutase, phosphoglycerate kinase, and ATPase and other enzymes. These are rare syndromes and are, at present, of little clinical importance.

Systemic Diseases Reflected in Abnormal Erythrocyte and Leukocyte Enzymes

Several genetic diseases are reflected by abnormal levels of enzymes in the erythrocytes (Table 13–13). Acatalasia, also called Takahara disease or oral gangrene, is a condition characterized by marked deficiency in the concentration of catalase in the tissues and in the erythrocytes. Deficiency of catalase, an enzyme that destroys hydrogen peroxide in the reaction, $2H_2O_2 \rightarrow 2H_2O + O_2$, leads to the accumulation of hydrogen peroxide. This condition is mostly asymptomatic and becomes of clinical importance only in some patients with oral sepsis, in whose oral cavities peroxide formed by bacteria can accumulate and lead to gangrene. It is a self-limiting state that disappears after the teeth are lost. Transmitted as an autosomal recessive trait, the condition is of greater genetic interest than clinical importance. Homozygous abnormals who have almost no catalase in the erythrocytes can be distinguished from the heterozygotes whose values are midway between the homozygote abnormal and normal values.

Hereditary methemoglobinemia secondary to deficiency of erythrocyte NADH-methemoglobin reductase (diaphorase) is a rare oligosymptomatic condition that is transmitted as an autosomal recessive trait. The methemoglobinemia leads to cyanosis.

Glycogenosis of Types III, IV, and VII and hypophosphatasia can be identified by measuring the leukocyte content of the relevant enzyme. Confirmation of the diagnosis of Type IV glycogenosis, which is due to *hepatophosphorylase* deficiency, can be obtained by measuring the phosphorylase activity of leukocytes. Type III glycogenosis, which is a manifestation of deficiency of the glycogen *debrancher* enzyme (amylo-1-6-glucosidase), can also be diagnosed by measuring the leukocyte content of that enzyme. Type VII glycogenosis, which is associated with a hemolytic anemia, can be identified by demonstrating deficient phosphofructokinase

Table 13–13. SYSTEMIC DISEASES IN WHICH DIAGNOSIS CAN BE ESTABLISHED BY ANALYSIS OF ENZYME ACTIVITY OF FORMED ELEMENT OF BLOOD

Condition	Formed Element	Enzyme Assay
Genetic		
Methemoglobinemia	RBC	NADH-methemoglobin reductase
Acatalasemia	RBC	Catalase
Galactosemia	RBC	Gal-1-P-uridyl transferase
Glycogenosis (Type III)	WBC	Amylo-1,6-glucosidase
(Type IV)	WBC	Phosphorylase
(Type VII)	RBC	Phosphofructokinase
Hypophosphatasia	WBC	Alkaline phosphatase
Lipid storage diseases		
Gaucher's	WBC	β-Glucosidase
Niemann-Pick	WBC	Sphingomyelinase
Krabbe's leukodystrophy (globoid)	WBC	β-Galactosidase
Metachromatic leukodystrophy	WBC	Sulfatidase
Fabry's disease	WBC	α-Galactosidase
Tay-Sachs disease	WBC	Hexosaminidase
Acquired		
Thiamine deficiency	RBC	Transketolase
Pyridoxine deficiency	RBC	Alanine aminotransferase
Hyperthyroidism	RBC	Carbonic anhydrase
Leukemia, granulocytic	WBC	Alkaline phosphatase
Lead poisoning	RBC	δ-Aminolevulinic acid dehydrase

activity in the erythrocytes. *Hypophosphatasia* is characterized by a genetic deficiency of ALP content of tissues and blood. ALP levels of the leukocytes can be measured in the proper clinical setting to help establish the diagnosis.

Galactosemia is an inborn error of metabolism characterized by a specific defect in the utilization of galactose that results in widespread tissue damage. The defect has been found to be deficiency of the enzyme phosphogalactose-uridyltransferase. The resulting accumulation of galactose-1-phosphate is considered responsible for the development of cataracts, liver disease, renal disease, and other abnormalities. The hereditary enzyme deficiency can be demonstrated by studying the erythrocyte. The ability of hemolysate to catalyze the conversion of galactose-1-phosphate to UDP-galactose in the presence of UDP-glucose is measured by following the disappearance of UDP-glucose. The assay, which can be readily performed, yields very low values in patients with galactosemia, who are homozygous for the abnormal gene. Heterozygote carriers can usually be identified by this assay, which yields values intermediate between the normal and the homozygous abnormal values.

A number of lipid storage diseases can be identified by demonstrating deficient activity of the related enzyme in circulating leukocytes (see Table 13–13). Several acquired diseases can also be identified by studying enzyme activity of the formed elements. Thiamine deficiency can be confirmed by demonstrating depressed transketolase activity of hemolysate. Pyridoxine deficiency can be demonstrated by measuring the ALT activity of erythrocytes before and after incubation with pyridoxal-5-phosphate. Abnormal levels of cholinesterase, carbonic anhydrase, and several other enzymes have been demonstrated in the erythrocytes of patients with a variety of acquired systemic diseases, but these are of pathophysiologic rather than diagnostic importance. The description of depressed erythrocyte levels of δ-aminolevulinic acid dehydrase as a measure of blood levels of lead suggests that measurement of this enzyme may be useful in the diagnosis of lead poisoning. Measurement of leukocyte ALP helps in distinguishing granulocytic leukemia from leukemoid states. ALP levels are very low in the leukocytes of granulocytic leukemia, but they are normal or elevated in patients with nonleukemic leukocytosis.

ENZYME CONCENTRATIONS IN OTHER BODY FLUIDS

Measurement of enzyme activity in serous effusions, gastrointestinal juices, cerebrospinal fluid, and urine has been applied to the diagnosis of various diseases. Localized release of enzyme from neoplastic cells has been considered responsible for the high levels of LD (and other glycolytic enzymes) in malignant pleural and peritoneal effusions, in the gastric juice of patients with carcinoma of the stomach, and in the urine of patients with renal carcinoma. The glucuronidase in the urine of patients with carcinoma of the bladder and in the vaginal fluid of patients with carcinoma of the cervix may also be considered to be enzyme shed by neoplastic cells.

Determination of levels of LD in serous cavity effusions has been proposed as a method of demonstrating neoplastic involvement of serosal surfaces. In such circumstances, the serous fluid usually shows higher levels of LD than does the serum. However, LD levels are also higher in patients with inflammatory and hemorrhagic effusions. Levels of LD in ascitic fluid that are greater than 500 sigma units indicate possible malignant effusion. If the ratio of the LD level in the fluid to that in serum is greater than 0.6, there is high probability (about 80%) that the effusion is malignant (Kjeldsberg, 1993).

The demonstration of a high amylase value in pleural or ascitic fluid is useful in diagnosing pancreatitis. The demonstration of increased levels of amylase in the urine is also a useful supplement to the measurement of serum levels of the enzyme in the diagnosis of pancreatitis, as discussed previously.

The CK_1 (BB) fraction of CK has been found in significant concentration in the serum and pleural fluid of patients with carcinoma of the lung and prostate. If the ratio of CK_1 (BB isozyme) in pleural effusion fluid to that in serum is greater than 3.7, the probability is high that a malignant tumor is the cause. The ratio of patients with a benign course of pleural effusions was less than 1.6 (Petterson, 1981).

Cerebrospinal fluid enzyme levels are relatively independent of the serum levels. Spinal fluid levels of aspartate amino transferase, LD, ribonuclease, and glutathione reductase have been increased in patients with various diseases of the central nervous system. The levels of one or more of these enzymes are increased in patients with cerebrovascular hemorrhage, thrombosis or embolism, meningitis, and neoplasms of the central nervous system. The pattern of LD isozymes in some of these conditions was discussed earlier. The clinical application and value of spinal fluid enzyme determinations remain to be established (see Chap. 19).

General References

Kjeldsberg CR, Knight JA: Body fluids, 2nd ed. Chicago, American Society of Clinical Pathology, 1993.

Pincus MR, Scheraga HA: Theoretical calculations on enzyme-substrate complexes: The basis of molecular recognition and catalysis. Accnt Chem Res 1981; 20:3960.

Statland BE: The case for standardizing enzyme assays. Lab Mngmt 1977; 15:46.

Tietz NW: Textbook of Clinical Chemistry. Philadelphia, WB Saunders, 1993.

Wilkinson JH: The Principles and Practice of Diagnostic Enzymology. London, Edward Arnold, 1976.

Serum Enzyme Levels in Liver Disease

Moss DW, Edwards RK: Improved electrophoretic resolution of bone and liver alkaline phosphatases resulting from partial digestion with neuraminidase. Clin Chem Acta 1984; 143:177.

Creatine Kinase and Other Enzymes in Myocardial Infarction and Muscle Disease

Beressi A, Sunheimer RL, Huish S, et al: Acute severe rhabdomyolysis in an human immunodeficiency virus-seropositive patient associated with rising anti-coxsackie B viral titers. Ann Clin Lab Sci 1994; 24:278–281.

Fisher MD, Carliner NH, Becker LC, et al: Serum creatine kinase in the diagnosis of acute myocardial infarction. Optimal sampling frequency. JAMA 1983; 249:393.

Galen RS: The enzyme diagnosis of myocardial infarction. Hum Pathol 1975a; 6:141.

Galen RS, Reiffel JA, Gambino SR: Diagnosis of acute myocardial infarction: Relative efficiency of serum enzyme and isoenzyme measurement. JAMA 1975b; 232:145.

Lott JA: Serum enzyme determinations in the diagnosis of acute myocardial infarction: An update. Hum Pathol 1984; 15:706.

Puleo PR, Meyer D, Wathen C, et al: Use of a rapid assay of subforms of creatine kinase MB to diagnose or rule out acute myocardial infarction. N Engl J Med 1994; 331:561–566.
Roberts R: Creatine kinase isozymes as diagnostic and prognostic indices of myocardial infarction. *In* Rattazzi M, Scandallos JG, Whitt GS (eds): Isozymes: Current Topics in Biological and Medicine Research, Vol 3. New York, Alan R. Liss, 1979, pp 115–154.
Thompson WG, Mahr RG, Yohannan W, Pincus MR: Use of creatine kinase MB isozyme for diagnosing myocardial infarction when total creatine kinase activity is high. J Clin Chem 1988; 34:2208.
West M, Eshchar J, Zimmerman HJ: Serum enzymology in the diagnosis of myocardial infarction and related cardiovascular conditions. Med Clin North Am 1966; 50:171.
Woo J, Zaman S, Patel L: The diagnostic value of specific CK-MB assay in acute myocardial infarction. *In* Miyai K, Kanino T, Ishikawa E (eds): Progress in Clinical Biochemistry. New York, Elsevier Science Publishers, 1992, pp 243–246.
Wu AHB, Valdes R, Apple FS, et al: Cardiac troponin T immunoassay for diagnosis of acute myocardial infarction. Clin Chem 1994; 40:900–907.

Phosphatases

Schumann GB, Badawy S, Peglow A, Henry JB: Prostatic acid phosphatase. Current assessment in vaginal fluid of alleged rape victims. Am J Clin Pathol 1976; 66:6.

γ-Glutamyltransferase

Rosalki SB: Enzyme tests in diseases of the liver and hepatobiliary tract. *In* Wilkinson JH (ed): The Principles and Practice of Diagnostic Enzymology. London, Edward Arnold, 1975, p 303.

Aminotransferases (Transaminases)

DeRitis F, Coltori M, Giusti C: Diagnostic value and pathogenic significance of transaminase activity changes in viral hepatitis. Minerva Med 1956; 47:101.

Angiotensin-Converting Enzyme

Beneteau B, Baudin B, Morgant G, et al: Automated kinetic assay of angiotensin-converting enzyme in serum. Clin Chem 1986; 32:884.
Haskins C, Mukerjee H, Pincus MR: An automated assay for angiotensin converting enzyme. American Association of Clinical Chemistry, 43rd National Meeting, Washington, DC, 1991, p 663.
Johnson DA, Diehl AM, Sjogren MH, et al: Serum angiotensin converting activity in evaluation of patients with liver disease. Am J Med 1987; 83:256.
Rohrbach MS, DeRemee RA: Pulmonary sarcoidosis and angiotensin converting enzyme. Mayo Clin Proc 1982; 57:64.
Silverstein E, Friedland J, Vuletin JC: Marked elevation of serum angiotensin-converting enzyme and hepatic fibrosis containing long-spacing collagen fibrils in Type 2 acute neuronopathic Gaucher's disease. Am J Clin Pathol 1978; 69:457.
Strittmatter SM, Thiele EA, Kapiloff MS, Snyder SH: A rat brain isozyme of angiotensin converting enzyme. Unique specificity for amidated peptide substrates. J Biol Chem 1985; 260:9825.
Velletri P: Testicular angiotensin I—converting enzyme. Life Sci 1985; 36:1597.
Zubenko GS, Volicer L, Direnfeld LK, et al: Cerebrospinal fluid levels of angiotensin converting enzyme in Alzheimer's disease, Parkinson's disease and progressive supranuclear palsy. Brain Res 1985; 238:215.

2

Pancreatic Enzymes

Huang WY, Tietz NW: Determination of amylase isoenzymes in serum by use of a selective inhibitor. Clin Chem 1982; 28:1525.
Legaz ME, Kenney MA: Electrophoretic amylase fractionation as an aid in diagnosis of pancreatic disease. Clin Chem 1976; 22:57.
O'Donnell MD, Fitzgerald O, McGreeney KF: Amylase determination by use of an inhibitor and design of a routine procedure. Clin Chem 1977; 23:560.

Tumor Markers

Catalona WJ, Richie JP, Ahmann FR, et al: Comparison of digital rectal examination and serum prostate specific antigen in the early detection of prostate cancer: Results of a multicenter clinical trial of 6630 men. J Urology 1994; 151, 1283–1290.
Petterson T, Weber TH, Ojala K: Creatine kinase isozyme BB as a tumor marker in pleural effusions. Clin Chem 1981; 27:1147.

Enzymes of the Formed Elements of the Blood

Beutler E: Enzyme tests in hematological diseases. *In* Wilkinson IH (ed): The Principles and Practice of Diagnostic Enzymology. Chicago, Year Book Medical Publishers, 1976, pp 423–454.
Carson PE, Frischer H: Glucose-6-phosphate dehydrogenase deficiency and related disorders of the pentose phosphate pathway. Am J Med 1966; 41:744–761.

Chapter 14

Polymerase Chain Reaction in Early Detection and Monitoring of Cancer

Zeev Ronai, Ph.D.

The principles of and methodologies for the polymerase chain reaction (PCR) have been extensively reviewed (Arnheim, 1992; Grompe 1993; Mullis, 1990). The purpose of this chapter is to provide an up-to-date summary of the use of PCR-based methodologies with various technical modifications for early detection and monitoring of cancer. Being a multistep process, cancer development involves multiple genetic lesions that change both genotype and phenotype. These genetic changes include mutations, activating dominant cellular proto-oncogenes, as well as those inactivating recessive tumor suppressor genes, that play a key role in the control of cell growth and in cell differentiation. Among these genes are protein kinases, key modulators of signal transduction pathways, proteins involved in cell cycle control as well as in transcription factors. The subsets of genomic alterations required for transformation have been well documented in the case of lung and colon cancer. Although in both cases multiple genomic changes are required, their chronologic order is not always defined, as illustrated in Figure 14–1. The presence of genomic alterations at very early stages of the multistage carcinogenesis process could serve as a good indicator for previous exposure or, alternatively, for an improper cellular repair of DNA damage. Accordingly, detection of such genomic alterations at early stages when there is no histopathologic evidence for dysplasia or hyperplasia requires highly sensitive techniques that are based on PCR methods. The major principles and precautions to be considered in selecting PCR reactions for these purposes are also briefly outlined. It is anticipated that PCR-based techniques will become routine diagnostic procedures in both screening for cancer predisposition and monitoring cancer patients for planning treatment and medical management.

POLYMERASE CHAIN REACTION—GENERAL OVERVIEW

Principle

The PCR is an *in vitro* method for amplifying selected nucleic acid sequences. It consists of repetitive cycles of DNA denaturation, primer annealing, and extension by DNA polymerase (Fig. 14–2). To target the amplification to a specific DNA segment, two primers, bearing the complementary sequence of the target gene, are used. These two primers hybridize to opposite strands of the target DNA and are in opposite orientation thus enabling DNA polymerase to extend the sequences between them. Each cycle produces complemen-

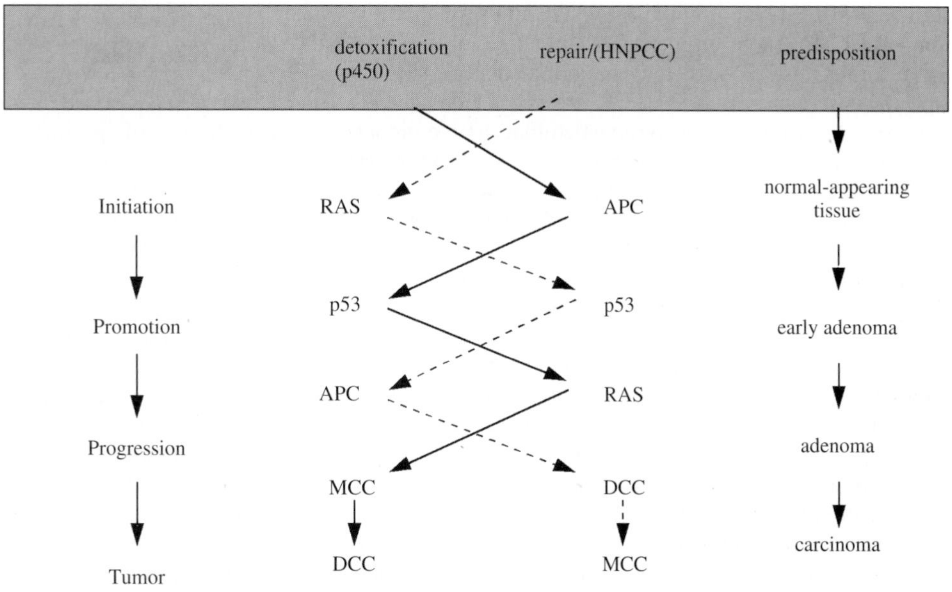

Figure 14–1. Outline of the amplification process accomplished *via* the polymerase chain reaction (PCR). Template DNA is incubated with primers that anneal to a specific DNA sequence, determining the boundaries of the amplification. Each primer promotes synthesis of the complementary strand, generating two copies from each molecule of template DNA in a given cycle. The exponential increase in the number of copies enables generation of 10^6 copies within 20 cycles (which may take 3 to 180 minutes, depending on the type of equipment used for these repetitive amplification cycles).

tary DNA strands to which the primers bind before the polymerase affects another extension in the next cycle of amplification. As such, the products of each cycle are doubled, generating an exponential increase in the overall number of copies synthesized. This results in a highly sensitive method that allows multiple reactions from a very small number of initial DNA sequences.

One of the critical components of the PCR reaction mixture is the polymerase. To date, several thermostable DNA polymerases have been identified and are available for use in these reactions. However, they vary in their fidelity, efficiency, and proofreading ability (Gelfand, 1990). Most important is their fidelity—the rate of misincorporating a base pair during the polymerase action. The presently available polymerases have an error rate of 1/10,000 to 1/100,000, pending the enzyme to be used (Krawczak, 1989). Exclusion of errors is critically important when an assay is aimed at identifying a single point mutation, so start with plenty of target/template DNA or duplicate analysis.

Primer selection is highly dependent on the application and the PCR methodology, as is discussed below. Usually, a 20-bp primer (a single-stranded DNA complementary to the 5′ end of a single copy sequence within the target DNA), which confers specific homology to the target DNA, is adequate to achieve specific annealing and, thus, amplification. In recent years, several computer programs have become available for the design of the optimal primer (Nash, 1993). These programs analyze the most important parameters to be considered, including (1) the secondary structure of the primer itself, (2) GC content should be as close as possible to AT content (3) primer-dimer formation (undesirable annealing of the two primers to themselves at a higher affinity than that of the primer to the template DNA), (4) matched Tm (to ensure that the optimal annealing temperature is similar for both primers), and (5) specificity (that the selected primers will amplify only the desired target gene). The sequence of these primers is aligned with those stored in the computerized databases to allow identification of the matched sequences and determine the degree of their homology. One of the most important criteria in designing primers is the need to ensure complete homology at their 3′ ends from which synthesis must proceed.

A serious problem in PCR amplification is contamination

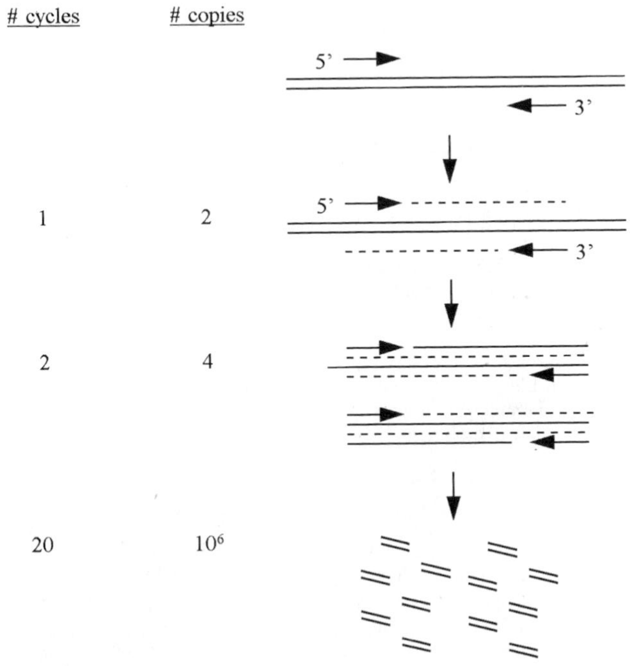

Figure 14–2. Multiple genomic alterations in the course of colon cancer development. Although the occurrence of multiple genomic alterations during the multistage carcinogenesis process is well documented, the order in which alterations appear varies. Two examples of possible sequences of mutant accumulation are shown, both of which originate from an existing predisposition, yet they lead to a different subset of mutations in normal-appearing tissues. In all, the accumulation of mutant tumor suppressor genes and oncogenes promote the development of subsequent steps, that is, early adenoma progression to adenoma as part of the promotion stage of cancer development. The respective stage is outlined on the left; the right side shows the respective morphologic and clinical staging.

(Prince, 1992). Owing to the high sensitivity of this reaction, either exogenous or previously amplified DNA can easily generate false signals. It is important that all solutions and all plasticware used for PCR are strictly dedicated to this reaction. It is highly recommended that sample preparation take place in a laboratory that is separate from the one used for the setup of the PCR reaction to avoid cross contamination. The latter is critical when the reaction is for diagnostic purposes.

The limitations of PCR technologies are at three levels: (1) Components used in the reaction such as thermostable polymerases have their characteristic rate of misincorporation (fidelity), which requires limiting the total number of cycles to a minimum, especially when analysis of a point mutation is performed. (2) Reaction primers with high sensitivity for binding to target sequences may also bind nonspecifically to other genomic DNA sequences, giving rise to several undesired coamplification products. (3) The overall yield of amplified material is limited to a few micrograms, which necessitates the use of additional related technologies to enable proper analysis.

POLYMERASE CHAIN REACTION METHODOLOGIES

Several PCR-based methodologies are available to amplify aliquots of specimen for possible diagnostic and monitoring purposes. Each of the PCR-based techniques offers certain advantages (Table 14–1). The methodologies differ in (1) the principal method of selection and (2) detection; they can be divided into two major categories—those that provide very high sensitivity and those that do not. Some clinical applications of PCR require high sensitivity, which is of major importance for diagnosis. For example, some of the desirable applications include early detection of point mutations in oncogenes or in tumor suppressor genes in specimens that are of normal appearance according to histopathologic analysis. The frequency of mutations in normal tissues is expected to be very low, because they are present only in a very small fraction of the overall cell population analyzed (Kumar, 1990), unlike in tumor tissues where mutant alleles are expected to appear at very high frequency. Thus, in performing PCR on normal tissues, the amplified material is expected to

Table 14–1. PCR METHODS FOR DIAGNOSTIC PURPOSES

Method	Advantages	Disadvantages	Primary Use	Reference(s)
Direct PCR	Easy, quick, good for identifying presence of given DNA in test sample	May encounter false-positive results	Identifying presence of a specific DNA fragment (i.e., virus; bacteria)	Grompe, 1993; Bej, 1991
RFLP	Relatively quick, adds assurance of the specificity of amplification	Relies on enzyme efficiencies	Achieves greater sensitivity (i.e., identify specific strain)	Felley-Bosco, 1991; Jiang, 1989
MAMA	Highly sensitive, quick, and relatively easy ($1/10^{-5}$)	Requires special setup for each mutation, may give false-positive results owing to run-through of polymerase; must be carefully controlled	Enables identification of specific point mutations present at very low frequencies without preselection	Cha, 1992
RFLP-PCR	Highly sensitive quantitative assay	Relies on enzyme efficiencies; requires cloning into phage and depends on hybridization efficiency	Quantification of mutant alleles present at low frequencies	Pourzand, 1993
Enriched PCR	Sensitive two-stage assay to identify specific point mutations ($1/10^{-4}$)	Relies on enzyme efficiencies; two-step reaction which requires careful setup and analysis	Identification of specific point mutations present at low frequencies	Kahn, 1991
SSC	Enables detection of mutation at unknown site	Requires confirmation under different conditions and preferably through sequencing	Identification of mutant at unknown site within a defined segment	Orita, 1989
PCR-based dot blot hybridization	A sensitive and specific assay for single base pair substitution (1/250–1/500)	Two-step procedure that requires careful monitoring of amplification yield and hybridization signal. Caution should be used *via* appropriate set of negative controls to rule out false-positive results	Identify single point mutations or general conformation for amplified sequences	Dolnick, 1992
DGGE	High sensitivity to identify mutations at unknown sites	Complicated, needs careful setup and monitoring	Identification of point mutation at unknown sites over a relatively large DNA fragment (2Kb)	Smith-Sorensen, 1993

DGGE = Denaturated gradient gel electrophoresis; MAMA = mismatch amplification mutation assay; PCR = polymerase chain reaction; RFLP = restriction fragment length polymorphism; SSC = single strand confirmation.

represent the most predominant sequences, which, in this case, will be normal rather than mutant. This explains the need for sensitive methods that offer selection of the mutant alleles over the normal ones. Several approaches have been developed and successfully used for analysis of mutant alleles that are present at low frequencies. These approaches include the following:

MISMATCHED AMPLIFICATION MUTATION ASSAY. Mismatched amplification mutation assay (MAMA) (Cha, 1992), also known as amplification refractory mutation analysis (ARMS), is based on the concept that a mismatch at the 3′ end of the primer does not allow proper amplification (Fig. 14–3). However, the efficiency of the amplification varies when different base pairs are used for these mismatches. As such, using selective primers that provide a greater mismatch at the 3′ end (two base pairs rather than one) improves the ability to amplify preferentially mutant rather than (at substantially lower efficiency) normal sequences. The MAMA was shown to exhibit a sensitivity of 1/100,000, which was successfully used to reveal the presence of background *RAS* mutation in normal tissues of rats (Cha, 1994). Interestingly, the frequency of background mutation identified in the MAMA reaction resembles the spontaneous mutation frequency identified in the lac I operon in transgenic animals (Sullivan, 1993).

ENRICHED POLYMERASE CHAIN REACTION. Enriched PCR is a different concept for providing selective amplification of the mutant allele; it relies on the effective elimination of most of the normal alleles of a given gene before amplification, thus enriching the fraction of mutant gene that is available for the amplification (Kahn, 1991). This is accomplished by using restriction endonucleases, which specifically cleave the normal but not the mutant allele (Fig. 14–4). The enzyme site therefore is restricted to the point of mutation, which distinguishes the normal from the mutant allele. Yet, few sites harbor a naturally occurring restriction enzyme that enables such reaction. Therefore, a two-stage procedure has been devised to adopt the methodology to any possible mutation. The first stage uses primers that were designed to create a restriction site within the normal but not the mutant allele. Accordingly, following 10 to 20 rounds of amplification, an aliquot of the amplified material is taken for restriction enzyme digestion, which cleaves only normal alleles. An aliquot of the cleaved material is then used as a template for second-stage amplification, which is subsequently analyzed via restriction fragment length polymorphism (RFLP). Although most of the amplified material is enriched for the mutant form, a small amount of normal allele could also reamplify (due to noncomplete digestion, single-strand DNA, or original genomic DNA, which could also serve as a template in the second round of amplification). This approach allows the identification of 1/1000–1/10,000 mutant alleles (Kahn, 1991). This method was used successfully to detect mutant *RAS* alleles in NMU-treated rats three weeks after carcinogen administration (Ronai, 1991), and in normal-appearing colonic mucosa of human patients with colorectal cancer (Minamoto, 1994; Ronai, 1994). The enriched PCR was also useful in enabling detection of mutant ras in colonic washings obtained from patients without colon cancer, yet who were at risk for developing it (Tobi, 1994).

LIGASE CHAIN REACTION–POLYMERASE CHAIN REACTION. The combination of ligase chain reaction with PCR has been shown to yield the highest sensitivity (up to $1/10^8$) (Wiedmann, 1994). It is based on the concept that specific primers are designed to overlap only mutant alleles but not normal alleles; thus, ligation occurs only at the mutant sites. Subsequent PCR allows selective amplification of the mutant alleles that were ligated in the first step.

Other PCR methodologies are designed to identify mutations at unknown sites, which is a characteristic of mutation in tumor suppressor genes. Although these methodologies lack, at this point, the sensitivity of the procedures mentioned previously, they are not restricted to a specific site. Among the mutation screening methods are the following.

SINGLE-STRAND CONFIRMATION POLYMORPHISM. Single-strand confirmation polymorphism (SSC) is based on the concept that a mutant allele migrates as single-stranded DNA to a different extent than its normal counterpart (Fig. 14–5), owing to a different conformation (Orita, 1989). This method has been successfully applied in the search for mutations in PCR products of less than 400 bp, and is expected to enable identification of over 80% of mutations (Grompe, 1993). It is most efficient in analyzing PCR products if they are less than 200 bp.

CHEMICAL MISMATCH. Chemical mismatch is based on the concept that single-stranded DNA that harbors a mutation can form a heteroduplex with the normal allele (Fig. 14–6). In subsequent steps, the chemistry used for the

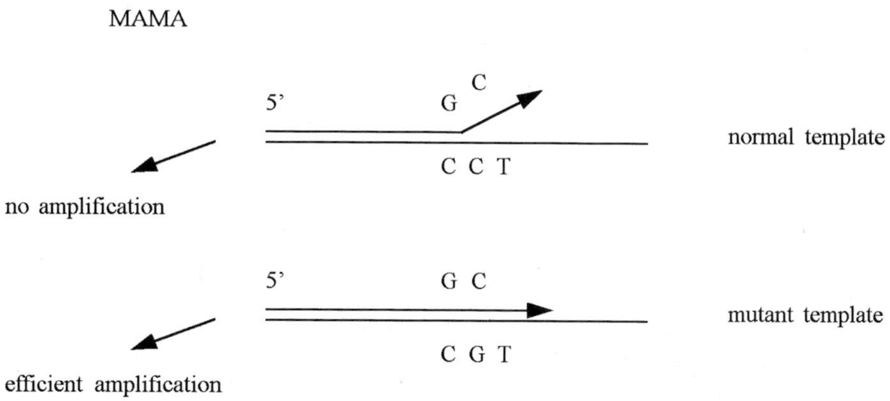

Figure 14–3. Mismatch amplification mutation assay (MAMA). One of the crucial requirements for the efficient PCR amplification is the complete match between the 3′ end of the primer and its template DNA sequence. This is the concept underlying the MAMA reaction, which uses primers that were modified on their 3′ end to match or mismatch mutant and normal template sequences. As shown, a primer that contains the sequence of a mutant form on its 3′ end does not permit efficient amplification from normal templates, but allows efficient amplification from mutant sequences, enabling selective amplification of the desired mutant alleles.

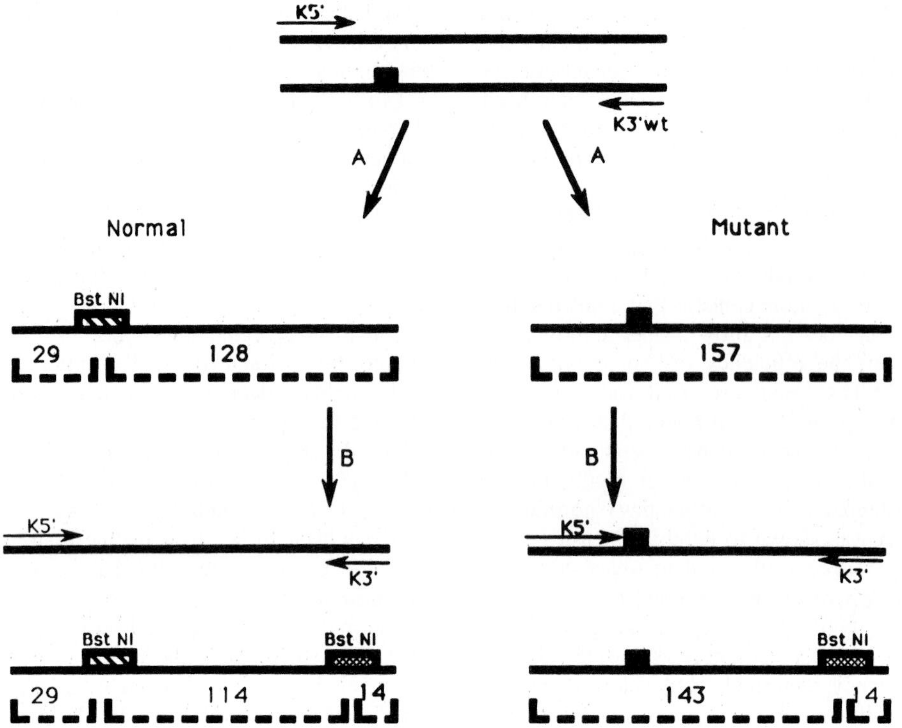

Figure 14–4. RFLP and enriched PCR. The use of specific restriction enzymes during or after PCR reactions enables verification of the nature of the amplified product as well as distinction of variants of the amplification (as per subsequences or mutations within the amplified region). On the basis of this concept, simple amplification (A) of template DNA, followed by restriction enzyme cleavage, allows us to determine the existence of mutation as shown here for the *KRAS* codon 12 mutation when the BstNI enzyme is used. Shown is a schematic diagram of the two-stage procedure for the "enriched" amplification of mutant human K-ras codon 12 sequences. In the first round of amplification (A), primers K5′ and K3′wt are used for the synthesis of a 157 nt fragment including codon 12 sequences. K5′ contains a nucleotide substitution at the first positive of codon 11, creating a BstNI restriction site (*C*CTGG) overlapping the first two nucleotides of wild-type codon 12 (hatched box). Digestion of PCR-amplified sequences from the first round with BstNI leaves uncleaved products enriched in mutant codon 12 sequences (black box). These uncleaved products are subject to a second round of amplification (B) using primers K5′ and K3′ (containing a control BstNI site; cross-hatched box). On RFLP analysis with BstNI, sequences derived from a mutant codon 12 allele show bands of 143 and 14nt, whereas amplified wild type allele remnants are cleaved to generate fragments of 114, 29, and 14nt. Because mostly mutant DNA retains its complete size, the second amplification enriches the population of mutant alleles, enabling detection of mutant alleles that were present in 1/10,000 cells of the original test material. Analysis is then performed through ethidium bromide–stained gels.

Maxam and Gilbert (1977) reaction has been applied, in part, to allow the cleavage of a mismatched site (Forrest, 1991).

DENATURING GRADIENT GEL ELECTROPHORESIS. Denaturing gradient gel electrophoresis (DGGE) separates DNA molecules that differ by a single base change and identifies whether there is a mutation, and if so, where it is localized (Fig. 14–7). To achieve this sensitivity, the method requires GC-rich clamps (40 bp) coupled to the ends of the primers used in these reactions (Saleeba, 1992). One reaction can screen up to 2000 bp, which encompass more than the complete cDNA of p53 and a significant portion of other tumor suppressor genes (Saleeba, 1992).

RESTRICTION FRAGMENT LENGTH POLYMORPHISM–POLYMERASE CHAIN REACTION. A variation of RFLP-PCR has been developed to enable genotype mutation analysis. In this method, a wild-type DNA is restricted selectively (thus not affecting the mutant sequence) before PCR amplification is performed (Felley-Bosco, 1991). Following amplification, the fragment is cloned into the phage gt 10. (Plaques containing DNA wt and mutant alleles are quantitated by hybridization with specific oligonucleotide probes.) This approach identifies one mutant allele in the presence of 10^7 to 10^8 wild-type sequences (Pourzand, 1993). Although highly sensitive, this approach requires the presence of naturally occurring restriction enzyme sites (Aguilar, 1993).

BIOMARKERS FOR EARLY DETECTION AND MONITORING OF CANCER

The detection of cancer-related genes has been a major focus of PCR applications. To date, several dozen genes that were shown to undergo genomic changes have been identified and specific PCR reactions have been designed to enable their detection. A partial list of neoplastic diseases that can be detected or monitored via PCR-based methodologies is present in Table 14–2. Generally, cancer-related genes can be divided into those that feature gross genomic alterations (deletions; rearrangements; translocations) and those with lesser changes such as small deletions, or point mutations. Biomarkers that can assist in early detection and monitoring of cancer should (1) be prevalent (i.e., present in a significant percentage of the diseased population and (2) be present at early stages of the multistage carcinogenesis process.

Two types of biomarkers could be envisioned. The first consists of genes that are modulated during our lifetime (i.e.,

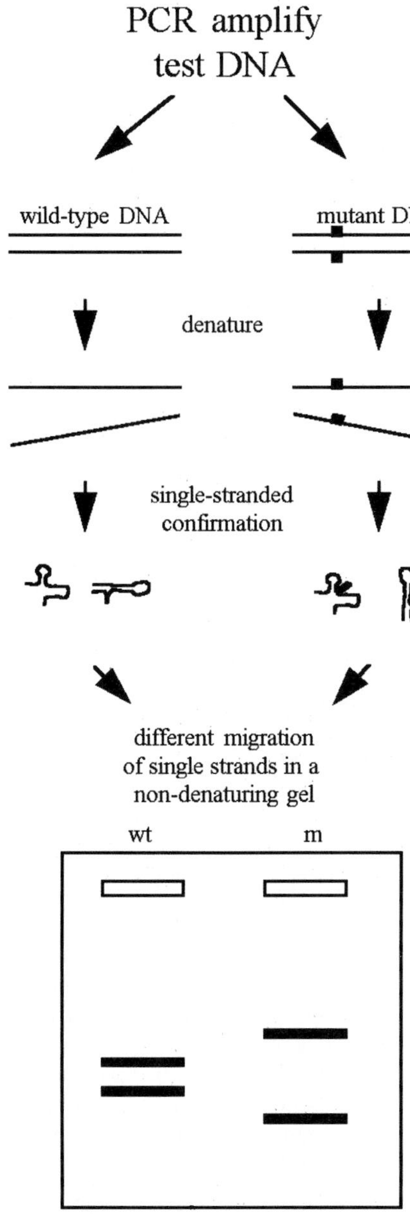

Figure 14–5. Single strand confirmation (SSC) methodology relies on the differences toward confirmation that are generated by normal DNA or mutant DNA (when present) on separation on a nondenaturing gel when it occurs as single-strand DNA. In this procedure, amplified DNA is denatured *in vitro* and separated on nondenaturing polyacrylamide gel electrophoresis. The pattern of migration generated by mutant versus normal alleles allows the identification of sequences that harbor single base pair substitutions.

somatic mutations). Within this category are genes that play an important role in the regulation of normal growth and differentiation, as well as in the response to stress and DNA damage. Alteration of these genes results in deregulated cell cycle control and increased growth rate, and in many cases, involves activation of oncogenes and inactivation of tumor suppressor genes. These changes often result in the accumulation of minor and gross genomic abnormalities, including chromosomal translocation and various types of mutations as time progresses.

An example of a genomic alteration that serves as a good biomarker are translocations that are characteristic of B-cell and T-cell neoplasia; these can be detected at high sensitivity via the use of primers that match different chromosomes within areas that correspond to the breakpoint regions; thus, there would be no amplification where there is no translocation. Such primers are, therefore, highly specific and can be used in routine diagnosis of various lymphatic neoplasia (see Table 14–2) (Allieri, 1992; Jacobson, 1994; Liang 1993; Ono, 1993; Zaccaria, 1991).

A different genomic alteration that has been associated

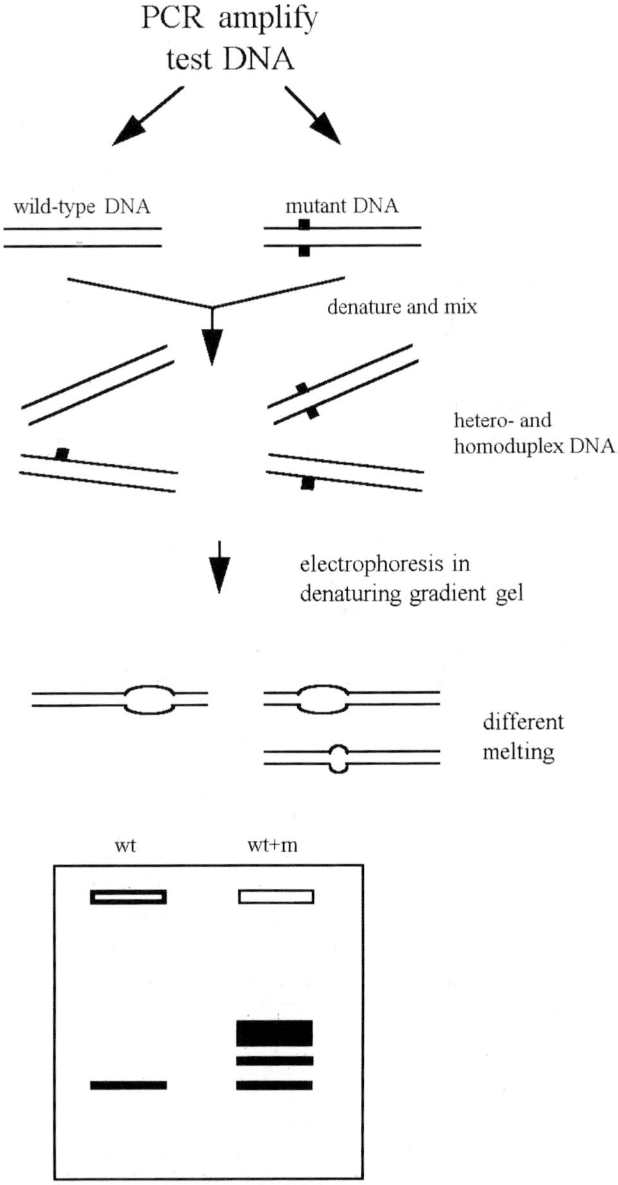

Figure 14–6. Denaturing gradient gel electrophoresis (DGGE). The principle of the SSC is further developed to enable detection of point mutations within large DNA fragments. Amplified DNA is mixed with nonmutated templates, generating homoduplexes and heteroduplexes, which are then separated on gels that vary in composition from denaturing to nondenaturing conditions. To enable correct identification of small changes within large sequences, a GC clamp (e.g., primer sequences used for the amplification contain 40 GC repeats) is added to the primers so that the reaction products will join more strongly at their ends. (Adapted from Grompe M: Rapid detection of unknown mutations in nucleic acids. Nature Genet 1993; 5:111–117.)

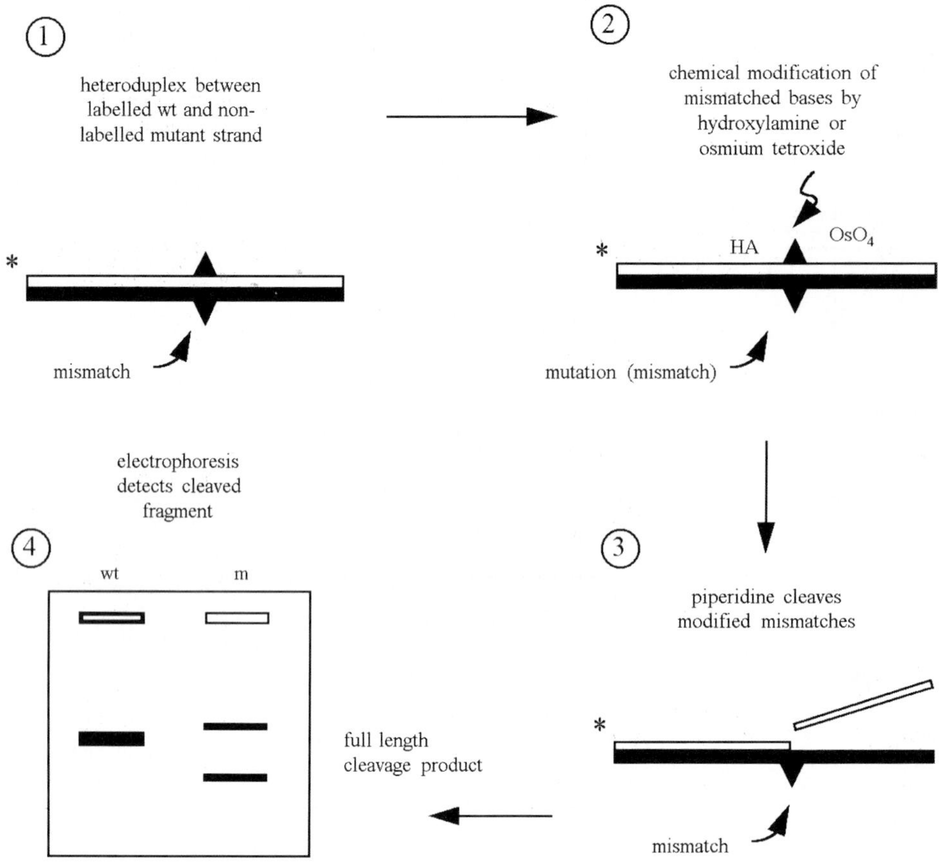

Figure 14–7. Chemical mismatch cleavage (CME). Homoduplex and Heteroduplex DNA generated in the PCR reactions, as outlined for DGGE, are subjected to generation of nicks at the mismatched sites using hydroxylamine or osmium tetroxide. The nicked DNA is cleaved with the aid of piperidine, thus generating fragments of different length when normal-normal and normal-mutant duplexes are compared. Analysis of cleaved products on nondenaturing gel allows us to identify such differences. (Adapted from Grompe M: Rapid detection of unknown mutations in nucleic acids. Nature Genet 1993; 5:111–117.)

with tumor suppressor genes in certain types of cancer is that of deletions (i.e., deleted in colon cancer [DCC]). These are detected through the analysis of the amplified fragment on gels, leading to the identification of a smaller fragment than anticipated (Cho, 1994; Simon, 1994). The second genomic alteration is that of genes that are inherited (i.e., germline mutations), thus leading to a potential predisposition. In recent years, several examples of such genes were reported. They include mismatch repair genes, whose mutation is expected to incur a higher frequency of errors than would accumulate during the lifetime, as well as impaired genomic integrity (Ionov, 1993; Leach, 1993a; Stand, 1993). One of the indications for a mutation in a mismatched repair gene is the change in the length of dinucleotide or trinucleotide repeats (van Leeuwen, 1991; Wada, 1994). As such, the length of these repeats may enhance the mutation's utility as a biomarker for predisposition toward genomic instability.

Among the minor alterations, point mutations in oncogenes and tumor suppressor genes are the most thoroughly studied events. Point mutations can be detected by a variety of PCR methods (see Table 14–1). These mutations can be categorized as those that occur at known sites, that is, *RAS* oncogenes, which harbor mutations in codon 12, 13, or 61 (Fearon, 1993; Ronai, 1992), and those that appear at unknown sites; the latter is characteristic of tumor suppressor genes, as shown for p53 (Hollstein, 1991), *APC* (Nakamura, 1991, 1992; Varesco, 1993), *DCC* (Cho, 1994), *MCC* (van Leeuwen, 1991). Although earlier methodologies enabled the identification of such genomic alterations within tumors without high sensitivity, recently developed PCR-based methods have greatly increased this sensitivity (see Table 14–1), so that some mutations can now be detected, even when present at very low frequencies. Because some of these mutations have the potential to serve as biomarkers of exposure, their early detection is of diagnostic and possibly also preventive value. A summary of markers used for cancer diagnosis *via* PCR based methodologies is shown in Table 14–2.

RAS Oncogene as a Potential Biomarker in Colon, Pancreas, and Lung Tumors

RAS is a family of genes that share many similarities and accumulate mutations at specific sites during the early stages of the transformation. These mutations are confined, in most cases, to codons 12, 13, or 61. *RAS* mutation has been shown to serve as a good pathogenic and potential diagnostic marker in human colorectal cancer. The prevalence of mutations in aberrant crypt foci and in normal-appearing tissues of high-risk patients provide strong support for such diagnostic potential in cancers of the gastrointestinal tract (Pretlow, 1993; Ronai, 1994a; Tobi, 1994; Urban, 1993). Mutated *RAS* has been extensively studied in both animal models and human cancer. Although it is mutated in 15% of all human tumors, its incidence is substantially higher in certain types of human tumors, including neoplasms of the pancreas (>90%) (Urban, 1993), colon (50%) (Pretlow, 1993), and lung

Table 14–2. PCR IN DIAGNOSIS OF CANCER

Disease	Marker	Reference(s)
Non-Hodgkin's lymphomas and leukemias	Ig rearrangement	Inghirami, 1993
Chronic lymphocytic leukemia	Ig rearrangement trisomy 12	Liang, 1993
Acute lymphoblastic leukemia	*RAS* mutation, *BCR-ABL* translocation	Jacobson, 1994; Allieri, 1992
Acute myeloid leukemia	*NRAS*	Lubbert, 1990
Adult T-cell lymphoma	HTLV sequences	Zucker-Franklin, 1994
B cell lymphoma	JH rearrangement	Liang, 1992
Chronic myeloid leukemia	Philadelphia chromosome, Ig rearrangement PCR of breakpoint region	Zaccaria, 1991; Wada, 1994
Bladder carcinoma	*HRAS* mutations, p53	Saito, 1992; Fujimoto, 1992
Breast cancer	p53 mutations, Her-2/neu amplification	Li, 1994a; Runnebaum, 1991; Tsuda, 1994
Lung cancer	p53 and ras mutations, HPV infection, RFLP chromosome 3. Microsatellite repeats	Husgafvel-Pursiainen, 1993; Shamanin, 1994; Ganly, 1992; Taylor, 1994; Mao, 1994; Merlo, 1994
Gastric malignant lymphoma	Ig heavy chain rearrangements	Ono, 1993
Colorectal cancer	*KRAS* mutation, *DCC* and *APC* deletion and p53 mutation, mutS mutation and changes in microsatellite repeats	Tobi, 1994; Ronai, 1994a; Leach, 1993a; Fearon, 1993; Nakamura, 1992; Parsons, 1993; Varesco, 1993
Pancreatic cancer	CEA detection, *RAS* p53 and *DCC* mutations	Gerhard, 1994; Shen, 1991; Simon, 1994; Urban, 1993; Tada, 1993
Hepatocellular carcinoma	HBV, p53	Hsu, 1991; 1993; Oda, 1992
Esophageal cancer	p53, *DCC* mutations	Hollstein, 1990; Miyake, 1993
Ovarian cancer	p53 mutation	Kupryjanczyk, 1993
Skin cancer	p53, *RAS* and *DCC* mutations, HPV sequence	Pirceall, 1993; Nakazawa, 1994
Cervical cancer	HPV sequences	Zhang, 1991; Nawa, 1993
Prostate cancer	DNA polymerase B, p53 mutation	Dobashi, 1994; Mocoska, 1993; Tornaletti, 1994
Peripheral primitive neuroectodermal tumors	fEWS/FL-I fusion transcripts	Sorensen, 1993

CEA = carcinoembryonic antigen; HPV = human papillomavirus; HTLV = human T-cell lymphotrophic virus; PCR = polymerase chain reaction; RFLP = restriction fragment length polymorphism.

($>60\%$) (Husgafvel-Pursiainen, 1993). Mutant alleles of *RAS* oncogenes have been identified not only at the tumor site but also in pancreatic juice and in serum of patients with pancreatic tumors (Taka, 1993) as well as in the stool of patients with colorectal cancer (Sidransky, 1992). *RAS* mutations were even identified in the sputum of patients with lung cancer (Mao, 1994; Takeda, 1993). It should, therefore, also be possible to detect *RAS* mutation in a small fraction of cells that are shed into other body fluids.

One of the critical requirements for a biomarker as a diagnostic tool, as outlined previously, is the ability to detect it before a tumor appears. To achieve this goal, one needs to overcome the technical obstacle of the low frequency of mutations expected at such early stages of the multistep carcinogenetic process. The concept we have used to enable sensitive detection of *RAS* mutation was to eliminate all normal alleles before amplification toward the final analysis is carried out.

This was achieved with the aid of the enriched PCR, which enabled us to detect codon 12 K-ras mutations in normal-appearing mucosa of patients who have colorectal cancer (Minamoto, 1994; Ronai, 1994). In two independent studies normal-appearing mucosa was obtained from over 90 patients with colorectal cancer. In all cases, both the normal and the tumor tissues were obtained (the normal tissue specimens were taken more than 10 cm away from the tumor site). The analysis of mutant *RAS* revealed that 30 to 50% of the patients harbored mutated *KRAS* codon 12 alleles at their tumor site, whereas only 5% to 18% were found to have this mutation in their normal-appearing mucosa (Ronai, 1994a; Minamoto, 1994). The variation in the frequency of mutant *RAS* alleles found in the two studies was attributed to sampling error. Indeed, when multiple samples of normal-appearing tissue were collected from different parts of the colon, only a few were found to harbor this mutation (usually 1/4 to 1/6) (Minamoto, 1994). This indicates that the mutant alleles may be localized in certain regions within the colon. As such, it was of major importance to test multiple samples from different parts of the colon. As one practical option, we have considered using cells that were shed from different parts of the colon as a representative sample for a more accurate analysis. This was tested by analyzing colonic effluent samples from patients who are free of colorectal cancer. These effluents were obtained as the last enema, prior to colonoscopy. Analysis of 39 cases revealed that 40% of patients who were at high risk for colon cancer (because they have a first-degree relative with a history of colon cancer or had themselves had previous resection of colorectal neoplasms) harbor this mutation (Tobi, 1994). None of the patients who were diagnosed with inflammatory bowel disorders were found to be positive for this mutation. Interestingly, follow-up of those found to harbor the *RAS* mutation revealed that one patient developed colorectal cancer four years after the identification of the mutant allele in his effluent sample. These results indicate that the *RAS* mutation potentially could be used as a biomarker to identify patients who are at a higher risk for developing colorectal cancer. That this mutation can be detected with a noninvasive procedure further supports its diagnostic potential. The presence of mutant alleles in shed cells suggests that it should be possible to use body fluids for analysis at early stages when histopathologic evidence for abnormal tissue development does not yet exist. The frequency of mutant *RAS* alleles found in various tumors and related specimens is shown in Table 14–3.

Tumor Suppressor Genes as Markers for Early Detection of Cancer

The growing list of tumor suppressor genes that play an important role in tumor development led to extensive examination of the potential use of each of them for diagnostic purposes. A characteristic of tumor suppressor genes is the wide distribution of mutation, almost throughout the overall coding region. The latter makes it substantially more difficult to develop highly sensitive and selective methods to detect such mutations at early stages. This obstacle has not yet been overcome. Of the numerous tumor suppressor genes identified so far, including p53, *APC, DCC, BRCA1,* and *BRCA2,* the one that has been most extensively studied is p53.

The tumor suppressor gene p53 is found to be mutated in about half of all human cancers (Dobashi, 1994; Fujimoto, 1992; Hollstein, 1990, 1991; Mitsudomi, 1993; Nakazawa, 1994; Oda, 1992; Tsuda, 1994). It is also of interest that even

Table 14–3. BIOMARKERS FOR EARLY DETECTION OF CANCER IN TUMORS AND RELATED SPECIMENS VIA PCR

Tissue	Specimen	Gene	Percent Positive	Reference
Colon	Tumor	*RAS*	50	Forrester, 1987; Vogelstein, 1988
	Normal mucosa		5–18	Minamoto, 1994
	Stool		40	Sidransky, 1992a and b
	Washing	p53	40*	Tobi, 1994
	Tumor		14	Han, 1991
Lung	Tumor	*RAS*	25–60	Reichel, 1994; Casson, 1994; Husgafvel-Pursiainen, 1993; Li, 1994b
	Bronchial biopsy		1/5	Mitsudomi, 1993
	Sputum		20	Takeda, 1993; Mao, 1994
	Tumor/sputum	p53	46	Kishimoto, 1992
	Tumor	microsatellite instability	45	Merlo, 1994
Pancreas	Tumor	*RAS*	90	Trumper, 1994
	Pancreatic juice		35	Tada, 1993
	Serum			Trumper, 1994
	Tumor	p53	80	Berrozpe, 1994
	Precancerous lesions			Shiao, 1994
Breast	Tumor		36	Runnebaum, 1991
	Normal tissue		51	Sidransky, 1992
Oral	Tumor		63	Sakai, 1992
	Cheek	p53	1/1	Koch, 1994
Soft tissue	Sarcoma	p53	30	Leach, 1993b
Bladder	Tumor	p53	61	Sidransky, 1991
	Urine		3/3	Sidransky, 1991
Blood	Lymphocytes	*IG* rearrangement		
	Follicular lymphoma	t(14:18)	57	Corbally, 1992
	Diffuse lymphoma		21	Segal, 1994
	Leukemia	*AMLI-ETO* t(8:21)	90	Zhang, 1994
	Acute promyelocytic leukemia	t(15:17)	<90	Lo Coco, 1994
	Chronic myeloid leukemia	*BCR-ABL*	20	Qian, 1993
	Acute myelogenous leukemia	*RAS*	20	Neubauer, 1994

*Of patients at risk. PCR = Polymerase chain reactions.

though the mutations in this and in other tumor suppressor genes are spread throughout the coding region (Hollstein, 1991), several hot spots with higher accumulations of these mutations were identified. Such hot spots are the preferred candidates to serve as useful biomarkers. For example, 31% of 52 large cell and squamous cell cancers from uranium miners with high radon exposure were found to contain AGG to ATG transversion at codon 249. This so-called radon-associated p53 hot spot was reported in only 1 of 241 published p53 mutations from lung cancers (Taylor, 1994). Similarly, specific hot spots in the p53 gene were reported in skin tumors. CC to TT mutations were detected in 74% of these tumors and were found to localize at codons 245,247/248 of the p53 gene; only 1/20 samples from non–sun-exposed sites contained such a mutation (Nakazawa, 1994). A high frequency of p53 mutations was also found in liver tumors induced by aflatoxin; in these cases, most mutations were localized at codon 248 (Hsu, 1991). In addition to their use as diagnostic biomarkers, these mutations also indicate the potential of creating personal fingerprints as exposure profiles, thus providing a highly valuable tool for modern molecular epidemiology. The mutation pattern of the p53 gene proved to be useful as a diagnostic marker for multiple hepatocellular carcinomas, because it enables identification of the origin of multiple tumors when multiple nodules are compared (Oda, 1992). Although these hot spots may satisfy the need for a high-frequency mutation, the overall occurrence of p53 mutation during the multistage carcinogenesis process has not been well established, mainly due to technical obstacles.

In studying the timing of p53 alterations in gastric tumorigenesis, including precancerous (chronic atrophic gastritis, intestinal metaplasia and dysplasia) and cancerous lesions, mutations in p53 were detected in 37.5% of the metaplasia cases, in 58.3% of the dysplasia cases, as well as in 66% of cases with carcinomas (Shiao, 1994). This study suggests that the p53 mutation is an early event in stomach tumorigenesis. Additional support for the presence of p53 mutation at early stages of tumor formation comes from the ability to detect p53 mutations in normal-appearing liver tissues of aflatoxin B1 exposed people (Aguilar, 1994).

Mutations in tumor suppressor genes have also been implicated as potential prognostic markers. Frequent p53 mutation was associated with invasive bladder cancer (Fujimoto, 1992). Similarly, aggressive phenotypes in breast cancer were associated with p53 mutation (Tsuda, 1994). Mutations of the p53 gene were also predictive of poor prognosis in patients with non-small-cell lung cancer (Mitsudomi, 1993). Li-Fraumeni syndrome families have an inherited p53 germline mutation.

Among the tumor suppressor genes associated with colorectal cancer development are *DCC* and *APC*. Both point mutations and deletions were reported in these two tumor suppressor genes; they can be detected *via* PCR of the 29 exons present in the *DCC* gene (Cho, 1994). Frequent alterations of the *DCC* gene were also reported in 7 of 12 pancreatic carcinoma cell lines that were analyzed. It is of interest to note that the latter were also associated with changes in p53 and *KRAS* oncogene (Simon, 1994). *DCC* mutation and allelic detection were also reported in esophageal carcinoma; the latter were related to the degree of lymph node metastasis and the degree of differentiation (Miyake, 1994). *DCC* alterations were also reported in 50% of endometrial carcinomas, as part of the loss of chromosome 18 q (Gima, 1994). This information suggests that the development of adequate methods to screen large gene segments such as *DCC* will make them useful biomarkers.

APC is the putative tumor suppressor gene responsible for adenomatous polyposis coli, an inherited autosomal dominant predisposition to colon cancer, which is also implicated in the development of sporadic colorectal tumors. Interestingly, 10 of 12 patients with adenomatous polyposis that were found to harbor *APC* alteration have been found to have a 5 bp deletion at one of two defined positions (93183-3187 and 3926-3930), indicating the mutational hot spots at these two sites (Varesco, 1993). Frequency of p53 mutation in tumors and related specimens is outlined in Table 14–3.

2

Early Detection of Cancer-Related Viral Infection

Numerous DNA and RNA viruses including retroviruses are implicated in the etiology of malignancies such as lymphomas, leukemias, sarcomas and carcinomas. Such viruses have also been associated with autoimmune diseases, such as rheumatoid arthritis and lupus erythematosus, and with cytopathic diseases that lead to anemia and immunodeficiency states. Common to retroviral infection is its relatively long latent period. Symptoms usually occur many years after infection.

PCR has provided support to the molecular epidemiology of these diseases because it can assist in identifying the different viruses in general populations. This has been the case with HTLV-I and HTLV-II and, more recently, with HIV, HPV, and HBV (Golpalkrishna, 1992; Kaneko, 1990; Kaye, 1991; Tuke, 1992). Now a focus on viruses that contribute to tumor formation is presented.

HEPATITIS B VIRUS. Identification of hepatitis B virus (HBV) infection has relied on the presence of specific viral antigens or antibodies and immunoassays such as radioimmunoassay (RIA) or enzyme-linked immunosorbent assay (ELISA). Yet, in some cases HBV-DNA cannot be detected in serum because of the low levels of the virus (Kaneko, 1990). PCR-based methodology using HBV-related sequences allows selective amplification of the viral genes at a sensitivity that is at least 10 times greater. Association between HBV infection and the susceptibility to develop hepatomas has been well established.

The detection of other strains of hepatitis such as Hepatitis C Virus (HCV) and Hepatitis D Virus (HDV) was also made possible through the use of specific PCR-related primers (Cristiano, 1992; Lecot, 1993).

HUMAN PAPILLOMAVIRUS. Over 20 types of human papillomavirus (HPV) are associated with certain neoplasms, such as cervical and oral cancers. Selective primers allow amplification and analysis for the distinction between most of these HPV strains (Gopalkrishna, 1992; Kinoshita, 1993; McNicol, 1992; Vandenvelde, 1990). Analyses of 140 cases of cervical cancer *in situ*, including severe dysplasia, invasive cervical carcinoma, mild cervical dysplasia, and moderate cervical dysplasia, revealed that 25% to 70% were found to harbor the HPV sequences, indicating close association between cervical cancer and HPV 16 infection (Zhang, 1991). In a separate study, HPV 16 was detected in 47% and HPV 18 in 20% of cervical cancer patients. Fifty percent were also found to harbor the HPV sequences in their lymph nodes (Nawa, 1993). HPV 16 was reported in nonmelanoma skin cancer, in 19% of squamous cell carcinomas, and in 19% of basal cell carcinomas (Pirceall, 1993).

EPSTEIN-BARR VIRUS. Epstein-Barr virus (EBV) has been associated with Burkitt's lymphoma, as well as several other types of lymphomas (Saito, 1989). Using a small aliquot of lymphocytes, EBV can be easily detected in biopsies of patients with Sjögren's syndrome and Hodgkin's lymphoma, as well as in immunocompromised patients (Bignon, 1990; Knecht, 1990; Saito, 1989). The titer and presence of EBV can be associated with some lymphoproliferative disorders occurring during immunosuppression. Recent reports have indicated that EBV was also identified in the nucleus of gastric cancer cells (Leoncini, 1993).

Overall screening for viral sequences is easier than for a single point mutation. Another important advantage in the analysis of viral DNA is that viral sequences are not part of the human genome; therefore, their identification serves as a clear indication of infection. However, similar to the detection of mutation in oncogenes or tumor suppressor genes, detection of viral sequences does not necessarily imply that the patient will suffer from the viral disease. In many cases, close follow-up with multiple analyses to determine viral titer (i.e., quantitative PCR) is required. Overall, identification of viral sequences serves as a good indicator for the presence of an etiologic agent associated with specific types of cancer.

EARLY DIAGNOSIS OF HEREDITARY DISORDERS

The potential presence of a hereditary disorder can be identified with significantly enhanced sensitivity using PCR-based approaches. In most cases, early diagnosis can be achieved through a simple blood specimen analysis. For example, genomic rearrangements can be readily identified using site-specific primers that would amplify only rearranged regions. This enables identification of translocations that are characteristic of lymphomas and leukemias. In this category, recent findings identified several repair genes that appear to contain genomic alterations in the form of mutations or deletions. The best characterized so far is the MSH2 homologue, which causes the condition known as hereditary nonpolyposis colorectal cancer (HNPCC) (Leach, 1993). As a mutated mismatch repair gene, it is thought to produce destabilization of tracts of simple repetitive DNA in yeast (Stand, 1993) and in humans (Wada, 1994). Associated with the mutation in mutS homologue genes is the replication errors (RER) phenotype, which results in genomic instability of microsatellite repeats (Goldberg, 1993; Leach, 1993; van Leeuwen, 1991; Warner, 1993). About 12% of colorectal carcinomas carry somatic deletions in poly (dA/dT) sequences and other simple repeats. Such mutations can also be identified in all neoplastic regions of multiple tumors, including adenomas, from the same patient (Ionov, 1993). DNA from an affected member of a New Zealand HNPCC family was shown to contain one hMSH2 allele with a C to T transition within a highly conserved region. Although 11 additional affected members of this same kindred had the same germline mutation, 10 unaffected family members had two normal alleles, thus showing perfect segregation from the disease (Jass, 1994). Genomic instability of microsatellite repeats was also demonstrated for other types of cancer including chronic myelogenous leukemia (Wada, 1994), and small cell lung cancer (Merlo, 1994). It appears that mutations in repair genes could confer a certain predisposition toward cancer development.

The ongoing human genome project identifies numerous genes that are associated with hereditary disorders. To this fast-growing list one can add the recently identified *BRCA1* and *BRCA2* genes (Futreal, 1994), which are targets for extensive examination for clinical diagnostic purposes among patients at risk for breast cancer. Indications for the possible p53 germline mutations were also seen in children and adults with second malignant neoplasms (Malkin, 1992). Among other hereditary components that could contribute toward a potential predisposition are genes that actively participate in metabolism or detoxification of carcinogens. This has been shown for p450 *CYP2E1*, which generates a unique pattern of RFLP in lung cancer patients (Hirvonen, 1993), and which can be identified *via* RFLP-based PCR analysis using the respective flanking regions.

DETECTING ENVIRONMENTAL EXPOSURE

Dosimetry of mutations in oncogenes and tumor suppressor genes has been suggested as one possible tool toward the identification of the type of carcinogenic agent that has caused these changes. A good example comes from the type and position of mutations identified within the p53 tumor suppressor gene. Having mutations throughout the coding region, it appears that some are localized in hot spots and may correlate with the type of exposure. This was demonstrated for p53 mutation in skin cancer related to ultraviolet light (Nakazawa, 1994) and aflatoxin-related p53 mutation in liver cancer (Aguilar, 1994) Other examples relate to lung carcinogens present in cigarette smoke. In most cases, these carcinogens yield the same type of base pair substitutions in both the p53 gene and in codon 12 of the *KRAS* oncogene (D'Amico, 1992; Husgafvel-Pursiainen, 1993), which is associated with the type of exposure (i.e., as smoking and occupational exposure to asbestos) (Husgafvel-Pursiainen, 1993). Nevertheless, the nature of the mutation cannot always reveal the etiologic exposure. For example, mutations found in human colon cancer lack association with any known (or hypothesized) colon carcinogens (Ronai, 1994b). This finding supports the hypothesis that other factors such as endogenous carcinogens in combination with certain predispositions may provide the critical factors in the etiology of cancer.

SUMMARY

The current status of early detection is our ability to identify patients at risk of developing specific types of tumors based on predisposition and accumulation of mutations in key regulatory genes. The battery of assays will certainly grow in coming years, and so will the interpretable information. The next critically needed step is to identify preventive measures that can be prescribed for the high-risk population. Legal and ethical problems that may arise from the use of the new powerful diagnostic tools have to be addressed as well.

Aguilar F, Harris CC, Sun T, et al: Geographic variation of p53 mutational profile in nonmalignant human liver. Science 1994; 264:1317–1319.

Aguilar F, Hussain SP, Cerutti P: Aflatoxin B1 induces the transversion of G-->T in codon 249 of the p53 tumor suppressor gene in human hepatocytes. Proc Natl Acad Sci USA 1993; 90:8586–8590.

Allieri MA, Fabrega S, Ozsahin H, et al: Detection of BCR/ABL translocation by polymerase chain reaction in leukemic progenitor cell (ALL-CFU) from patients with acute lymphoblastic leukemia (ALL). Exp Hematol 1992; 20:312–314.

Arnheim N, Erlich H: Polymerase chain reaction strategy. Annu Rev Biochem 1992; 61:131–156.

Bej AK, Mahbubani MH, Atlas RM: Amplification of nucleic acids by polymerase chain reaction and other methods and their application. Crit Rev Biochem Mol Biol 1991; 26:301–334.

Berrozpe G, Schaeffer J, Peinado MA, et al: Comparative analysis of mutations in the p53 and K-ras genes in pancreatic cancer. Int J Cancer 1994; 58:185–191.

Bignon Y, Bernard D, Cure H, et al: Detection of Epstein-Barr viral genomes in lymph nodes of Hodgkin's disease patients. Mol Carcinog 1990; 3:9.

Casson AG, McCuaig S, Graig I, et al: Prognostic value and clinicopathologic correlation of p53 gene mutations and nuclear DNA content in human lung cancer: a prospective study. J Surg Oncol 1994; 56:13–20.

Cha RS, Thilly WG, Zarbl H, et al: *N*-Nitroso-*N*-methylurea-induced rat mammary tumors arise from cells with preexisting oncogenic Hras1 gene mutations. Proc Natl Acad Sci USA 1994; 91:3749–3753.

Cha RS, Zarbl H, Keohavong P, et al: Mismatch amplification mutation assay (MAMA): application to the c-H-*ras* gene. PCR Methods Appl 1992; 2:14–20.

Cho KR, Oliner JD, Simons JW, et al: The DCC gene: structural analysis and mutations in colorectal carcinomas. Genomics 1994; 19:525–531.

Corbally N, Grogan L, Dervan PA, Carnery DN: The detection of specific gene rearrangements in non-Hodgkin's lymphoma using the polymerase chain reaction. Br J Cancer 1992; 66:805–808.

Cristiano K, Di Bisceglie AM, Hoofnagle JH, et al: Hepatitis C viral RNA in serum of patients with chronic non-A, non-B hepatitis: detection by the polymerase chain reaction using multiple primer sets. Arch Virol Suppl 1992; 4:172–178.

D'Amico D, Carbone D, Mitsudomi T, et al: High frequency of somatically acquired p53 mutations in small-cell lung cancer cell lines and tumors. Oncogene 1992; 7:339–346.

Dobashi Y, Shuin T, Tsuruga H, et al: DNA polymerase beta gene mutation in human prostate cancer. Cancer Res 1994; 54:2827–2829.

Dolnick BJ, Zhang ZG, Hines JD, et al: Quantitation of dihydrofolate reductase and thymidylate synthase mRNAs in vivo and in vitro by polymerase chain reaction. Oncol Res 1992; 4:65–72.

Fearon ER: K-ras gene mutation as a pathogenetic and diagnostic marker in human cancer. J Natl Cancer Inst 1993; 85:1978–1980.

Felley-Bosco E, Pourzand C, Zijlstra J, et al: A genotypic mutation system measuring mutations in restriction recognition sequences. Nucleic Acids Res 1991; 19:2913–2919.

Forrest SM, Dahl HH, Howells DW, et al: Mutation detection in phenylketonuria by using chemical cleavage of mismatch: Importance of using probes from both normal and patient samples. Am J Hum Genet 1991; 49:175–183.

Forrester K, Almoguera C, Han K, et al: Detection of high incidence of K-ras oncogenes during human colon tumorigenesis. Nature 1987; 327: 298–303.

Fujimoto K, Yamada Y, Okajima E, et al: Frequent association of p53 gene mutation in invasive bladder cancer. Cancer Res 1992; 52:1393–1398.

Futreal PA, Liu Q, Shattuck-Eidens D, Cochran C, Frye C, et al: BRCA1 mutations in primary breast and ovarian carcinomas. Science 1994; 266:120–122.

Ganly PS, Jarad N, Rudd RM, et al: PCR-based RFLP analysis allows genotyping of the short arm of chromosome 3 in small biopsies from patients with lung cancer. Genomics 1992; 12:221–228.

Gelfand DH, While TJ: Thermostable DNA Polymerases. *In* Innis M, (ed): PCR Protocols: A Guide to Methods and Applications. New York, Academic Press, 1990, p 129.

Gerhard M, Juhl H, Kalthoff HW, et al: Specific detection of carcinoembryonic antigen-expressing tumor cells in bone marrow aspirates by polymerase chain reaction. J Clin Oncol 1994; 12:725–729.

Gima T, Kato H, Honda T, et al: DCC gene alteration in human endometrial carcinomas. Int J Cancer 1994; 57:480–485.

Goldberg YP, Andrew SE, Clarke LA, et al: A PCR method for accurate assessment of trinucleotide repeat expansion in Huntington disease. Hum Mol Genet 1993; 2:635–636.

Gopalkrishna V, Francis A, Sharma JK, et al: A simple and rapid method of high quantity DNA isolation from cervical scrapes for detection of human papillomavirus infecton. J Virol Methods 1992; 36:63–72.

Grompe M: Rapid detection of unknown mutations in nucleic acids. Nature Genet 1993; 5:111–117.

Han ES, Moyer MP, Sakaguchi AY: Mutation in the TP53 gene in colorectal carcinoma detected by polymerase chain reaction. Genes Chrom Cancer 1991; 3:313–317.

Hirvonen A, Husgafvel-Pursiainen K, Anttila S, et al: The human CYP2E1 gene and lung cancer: DraI and RsaI restriction fragment length polymorphisms in a Finnish study population. Carcinogenesis 1993; 14:85–88.

Hollstein MC, Metcalf RA, Welsh JA, et al: Frequent mutation of the p53 gene in human esophageal cancer. Proc Natl Acad Sci USA 1990; 87:9958–9961.

Hollstein M, Sidransky D, Vogelstein B, Harris CC: p53 mutations in human cancer. Science 1991; 253: 49–53.

Hsu IC, Metcalf RA, Sun T, et al: Mutational hotspot in the p53 gene in human hepatocellular carcinomas. Nature 1991; 350: 427–428.

Hsu IC, Tokiwa T, Bennett W, et al: p53 gene mutation and integrated hepatitis B viral DNA sequences in human liver cancer cell lines. Carcinogenesis 1993; 14:987–992.

Husgafvel-Pursiainen K, Hackman P, Ridanpaa M, et al: K-ras mutations in human adenocarcinoma of the lung: Association with smoking and occupational exposure to asbestos. Int J Cancer 1993; 53:250–256.

Inghirami G, Szabolcs MJ, Yee HT, et al: Detecton of immunoglobulin gene rearrangement of B cell non-Hodgkin's lymphomas and leukemias in fresh, unfixed and formalin-fixed, paraffin-embedded tissue by polymerase chain reaction. Lab Invest 1993; 68:746–757.

Ionov Y, Peinado MA, Malkhosyan S, et al: Ubiquitous somatic mutations in simple repeated sequences reveal a new mechanism for colonic carcinogenesis. Nature 1993; 363:558–561.

Jacobson DR, Mills NE: A highly sensitive assay for mutant *ras* genes and its application to the study of presentation and relapse genotypes in acute leukemia. Oncogene 1994; 9:553–563.

Jass JR, Stewart SM, Stewart J, et al: Hereditary nonpolyposis colorectal cancer—morphologies, genes and mutations. Mutat Res 1994; 310:125–133.

Jiang W, Kahn S, Guillem J, et al: Rapid detection of ras oncogenes in human tumors: Applications to colon, esophageal, and gastric cancer. Oncogene 1989; 4:923–928.

Kahn SM, Jiang W, Culbertson TA, et al: Rapid and sensitive nonradioactive detection of mutant K-*ras* genes via 'enriched' PCR amplification. Oncogene 1991; 6:1079–1083.

Kaneko S, Miller RH, Di Bisceglie AM, et al: Detection of hepatitis B virus DNA in serum by polymerase chain reaction. Application for clinical diagnosis. Gastroenterology 1990; 99:799–804.

Kaye S, Loveday C. Tedder RS: Storage and preservation of whole blood samples for use in detection of human immunodeficiency virus type-1 by the polymerase chain reaction. J Virol Methods 1991; 35:217–226.

Kinoshita M, Shin S, Aono T: A sensitive and quantitative method for the determination of number of HPV 16 DNA copies by using the competitive polymerase chain reaction. Genet Anal Tech Appl 1993; 10:116–121.

Kishimoto Y, Murakami Y, Shiraishi M, et al: Aberrations of the p53 tumor supressor gene in human non-small cell carcinomas of the lung. Cancer Res 1992; 52:4799–4804.

Knecht H, Sahli R, Shaw P, et al: Detection of Epstein-Barr virus DNA by polymerase chain reaction in lymph node biopsies from patients with angioimmunoblastic lymphadenopathy. Br J Haematol 1990; 75:610–614.

Koch WM, Boyle JO, Mao L, et al: p53 gene mutations as markers of tumor spread in synchronous oral cancers. Arch Otolaryngol 1994; 120: 943–947.

Krawczak M, Reiss J, Schmidtke J, et al: Polymerase chain reaction: replication errors and reliability of gene diagnosis. Nucleic Acids Res 1989; 17:6.

Kumar R, Medina D, Sukumar S: Activation of H-ras oncogenes in preneoplastic mouse mammary tissues. Oncogene 1990: 5:1271–1277.

Kupryjanczyk J, Thor AD, Beauchamp R, et al: p53 gene mutations and protein accumulaton in human ovarian cancer. Proc Natl Acad Sci USA 1993; 90:4961–4965.

Leach FS, Nicolaides NC, Papadopoulos N, et al: Mutations of a mutS homology in hereditary nonpolyposis colorectal cancer. Cell 1993a; 75:1215–1225.

Leach FS, Tokino T, Meltzer P, et al: p53 mutation and MDM2 amplification in human soft tissue sarcomas. Cancer Res 1993b; 53:2213–2234.

Lecot C, Jeantils V, Ovaguimian L, et al: Polymerase chain reaction-based detection of hepatitis D virus RNA in patients infected with human immunodeficiency virus. Prog Clin Biol Res 1993; 382:329–335.

Leoncini L, Vindigni C, Megha T, et al: Epstein-Barr virus and gastric cancer: data and unanswered questions. Int J Cancer 1993; 53:898–901.

Li BD, Harlow SP, Budnick RM, et al: Detection of HER-2/neu oncogene amplification in flow cytometry-sorted breast ductal cells by competitive polymerase chain reaction. Cancer 1994a; 73:2771–2778.

Li S, Rosell R, Urban A, et al: K-*ras* gene point mutation: a stable tumor marker in non-small cell lung carcinoma. Lung Cancer 1994b; 11:19–27.

Liang R, Chan V, Chan TK, et al: Detection of immunoglobulin gene rearrangement in lymphoid malignancies of B-cell lineage by seminested polymerase chain reaction gene amplification. Am J Hematol 1993; 43:24–28.

Lo Coco F, Pelicci PG, Biondi A: Clinical relevance of the PML/RAR-a gene rearrangement in acute promyelocytic leukaemia. Leuk Lymphoma 1994; 12:327–332.

Malkin D, Jolly KW, Barbier N, et al: Germline mutations of the p53 tumor-suppressor gene in children and young adults with second malignant neoplasms. N Engl J Med 1992; 326;1309–1315.

Mao L, Hruban RH, Boyle JO, et al: Detection of oncogene mutations in sputum precedes diagnosis of lung cancer. Cancer Res 1994; 54: 1634–1637.

Maxam AM, Gilbert W: A new method for sequencing DNA. Proc Natl Acad Sci USA 1977; 74:560.

McNicol P, Guijon F, Brunham R, et al: Laboratory diagnosis of latent human papillomavirus infection. Diagn Microbiol Infect Dis 1992; 15:679–683.

Merlo A, Mary M, Gabrielson E, et al: Frequent microsatellite instability in primary small cell lung cancer. Cancer Res 1994; 54:2098–2101.

Minamoto T, Ronai Z, Yamashita N, et al: Detection of Ki-ras mutation in non-neoplastic mucosa of Japanese patients with colorectal cancers. Int J Oncol 1994; 4:397–401.

Mitsudomi T, Lam S, Shirakusa T, Gazdar AF: Detection and sequencing of p53 gene mutations in bronchial biopsy samples in patients with lung cancer. Chest 1993; 104:362–365.

Mitsudomi T, Oyama T, Kusano T, et al: Mutations of the p53 gene as a predictor of poor prognosis in patients with non-small-cell lung cancer. J Natl Cancer Inst 1993; 85:2018–2023.

Miyake S, Nagai K, Yoshino K, et al: Point mutations and allelic deletion of tumor suppressor gene DCC in human esophageal squamous cell carcinomas and their relation to metastasis. Cancer Res 1994; 54: 3007–3010.

Mullis, KB: The unusual origin of the polymerase chain reaction. Scientific American April, 1990, pp 56–65.

Nakamura Y, Nishisho I, Kinzler KW, et al: Mutations of the adenomatous polyposis coli gene in familial polyposis coli patients and sporadic colorectal tumors. Princess Takematsu Symp 1991; 22:285–292.

Nakamura Y, Nishisho I, Kinzler KW, et al: Mutations of the APC (adenomatous polyposis coli) gene in FAP (familial polyposis coli) patients and in sporadic colorectal tumors. Tohoku J Exp Med 1992; 168:141–147.

Nakazawa H, English D, Randell PL, et al: UV and skin cancer: specific p53 gene mutation in normal skin as a biologically relevant exposure measurement. Proc Natl Acad Sci USA 1994; 91:360–364.

Nash JH: A computer program to calculate and design oligonucleotide primers from amino acid sequences. Comput Appl Biosci 1993; 9: 469–471.

Nawa A, Nishiyama Y, Kikkawa F, et al: Detection of human papillomaviruses from histologically normal lymph nodes of Japanese cervical cancer patients by nested polymerase chain-reaction assay. Int J Cancer 1993; 53:932–937.

Neubauer A, Dodge RK, George SL, et al: Prognostic importance of mutations in the ras proto-oncogenes in de novo acute myeloid leukemia. Blood 1994; 83:1603–1611.

Oda T, Tsuda H, Scarpa A, et al: Mutation pattern of the p53 gene as a diagnostic marker for multiple hepatocellular carcinoma. Cancer Res 1992; 52:3674–3678.

Ono H, Kondo H, Saito D, et al: Rapid diagnosis of gastric malignant lymphoma from biopsy specimens: detection of immunoglobulin heavy chain rearrangement by polymerase chain reaction. Jpn J Cancer Res 1993; 84:813–817.

Orita M, Suzuki Y, Sekiya T, et al: Rapid and sensitive detection point mutations and DNA polymorphisms using the polymerase chain reaction. Genomics 1989; 5:874–879.

Parsons R, Li GM, Longley MJ, et al: Hypermutability and mismatch repair deficiency in RER^+ tumor cells. Cell 1993; 75:1227–1236.

Pirceall WE, Goldberg LH, Ananthaswamy HN: Presence of human papilloma virus type 16 DNA sequences in human nonmelanoma skin cancers. J Invest Dermatol 1993; 97:880–884.

Pourzand C, Cerutti P: Genotypic mutation analysis by RFLP/PCR. Mutat Res 1993; 288:113–121.

Pretlow TP, Brasitus TA, Fulton NC, et al: K-ras mutations in putative preneoplastic lesions in human colon. J Nat Cancer Inst 1993; 85:2004–2007.

Prince AM, Andrus L: PCR: How to kill unwanted DNA. Biotechniques 1992; 12:258–260.

Qian XH, Yang AD, Fei HB, Wang CC: Detection of the BCR/ABL fusion gene in chronic myeloid leukemia by RNA polymerase chain reaction. J Tongji Med Univ 1993; 13:129–133.

Reichel MB, Ohgaki H, Petersen I, Kleihues P: p53 mutations in primary human lung tumors and their metastases. Mol Carcinog 1994; 9:105–109.

Ronai Z, Lau Y, Cohen LA: Dietary N-3 fatty acids do not affect induction of Ha-ras mutations in mammary glands of NMU-treated rats. Mol Carcinog 1991; 4:120.

Ronai Z, Luo F-C, Gradia S, et al: Detection of K-ras mutation in normal and malignant colonic tissues by an enriched PCR method. Int J Oncol 1994a; 4:391–396.

Ronai Z: Ras oncogene detection in pre-neoplastic lesions: possible applications for diagnosis and prevention. Oncology Res 1992; 4:45–48.

Ronai Z: Heterocyclic amines and colon carcinogenicity. Jpn J Cancer Res 1994b; 85:1312–1313.

Runnebaum IB, Nagarajan M, Bowman M, et al: Mutations in p53 as potential molecular markers for human breast cancer. Proc Natl Acad Sci USA 1991; 88:10657–10661.

Saito I, Servenius B, Compton T, et al: Detection of Epstein-Barr virus DNA by polymerase chain reaction in blood and tissue biopsies from patients with Sjögren's syndrome. J Exp Med 1989; 169:2191–2198.

Saito S: Detection of H-ras gene point mutations in transitional cell carcinoma of human urinary bladder using polymerase chain reaction. Keio J Med 1992; 41:80–86.

Sakai E, Rikimaru M, Ueda M, et al: The p53 tumor-suppressor gene and ras oncogene mutations in oral squamous-cell carcinoma. Int J Cancer 1992; 52:867–872.

Saleeba JA, Ramua SJ, Cotton RGHI: Complete mutation detection using unlabeled chemical cleavage. Hum Mut 1992; 1:63–69.

Segal GH, Scott M, Jorgensen T, Braylan RC: Standard polymerase chain reaction analysis does not detect t(14;18) in reactive lymphoid hyperplasia. Arch Pathol Lab Med 1994; 118:791–794.

Shamanin V, Delius H, de Villiers EM: Development of a broad spectrum PCR assay for papillomaviruses and its application in screening lung cancer biopsies. J Gen Virol 1994; 75:1149–1156.

Shen C, Chang JG, Lee LS, et al: Analysis of ras gene mutations in gastrointestinal cancers. J Formos Med Assoc 1991; 90:1149–1154.

Shiao YH, Rugge M, Correa P, et al: p53 alteration in gastric precancerous lesions. Am J Pathol 1994; 144:511–517.

Sidransky D, Tokino T, Hamilton SR, et al: Identification of ras oncogene mutation in the stool of patients with curable colorectal tumors. Science 1992a; 256:102–105.

Sidransky D, Tokino T, Helzlsouer K, et al: Inherited p53 gene mutations in breast cancer. Cancer Res 1992b; 52:2984–2986.

Sidransky D, Von Eschenbach A, Tsai YC, et al: Identification of p53 gene mutations in bladder cancers and urine samples. Science 1991; 252:706–709.

Simon B, Weinel R, Hohne M, et al: Frequent alterations of the tumor suppressor genes p53 and DCC in human pancreatic carcinoma. Gastroenterology 1994; 106:1645–1651.

Smith-Sorensen B, Gebhardt MC, Kloen P, et al: Screening for TP53 mutations in osteosarcomas using constant denaturant gel electrophoresis (CDGE). Hum Mutat 1993; 2:274–285.

Sorensen PH, Liu XF, Delattre O, et al: Reverse transcriptase PCR amplification of EWS/FLI-1 fusion transcripts as a diagnostic test for peripheral primitive euroectodermal tumors of childhood. Diagn Mol Pathol 1993; 2:147–157.

Stand M, Prolla TA, Liskay RM, et al: Destabilisation of tracts of simple repetitive DNA in yeast by mutation affecting DNA mismatch repair. Nature 1993; 365:274–276.

Sullivan N, Gatehouse D, Tweats D: Mutation, cancer and transgenic models: Relevance to the toxicology industry. Mutagenesis 1993; 8:167–174.

Taka M, Omata M, Kawai S, et al: Detection of ras gene mutations in pancreatic juice and peripheral blood of patients with pancreatic adenocarcinoma. Cancer Res 1993; 53:2472–2474.

Takeda S, Ichii S, Nakamura Y: Detection of K-ras mutation in sputum by mutant-allele-specific amplification (MASA). Hum Mutat 1993; 2: 112–117.

Taylor JA, Watson MA, Devereux TR, et al: p53 mutation hotspot in radon-associated lung cancer. Lancet 1994; 343:86–87.

Tobi M, Luo FC, Ronai Z: Detection of K-ras mutation in colonic effluent samples from patients without evidence of colorectal carcinoma. J Natl Cancer Inst 1994; 86:1007–1010.

Trumper LH, Burger B, von Bonin F, et al: Diagnosis of pancreatic adenocarcinoma by polymerase chain reaction from pancreatic secretions. Br J Cancer 1994; 70:278–284.

Tsuda H, Hirohashi S: Association among p53 gene mutation, nuclear accumulation of the p53 protein and aggressive phenotypes in breast cancer. Int J Cancer 1994; 57:498–503.

Tuke PW, Luton P, Garson JA, et al: Differential diagnosis of HTLV-I and HTLV-II infections by restriction enzyme analysis of 'nested' PCR products. J Virol Methods 1992; 40:163–173.

Urban T, Ricci S, Grange JD, et al: Detection of c-Ki-ras mutation by PCR/RFLP analysis and diagnosis of pancreatic adenocarcinomas. J Nat Cancer Inst 1993; 85:2008–2012.
van Leeuwen C, Tops C, Breukel H, et al: CA repeat polymorphism within the MCC (mutated in colorectal cancer) gene. Nucleic Acids Res 1991; 19:5805.
Vandenvelde C, Verstraete M, Van Beers D: Fast multiplex polymerase chain reaction on boiled clinical samples for rapid viral diagnosis. J Virol Methods 1990; 30:214–227.
Varesco L, Gismondi V, James R, et al: Identification of APC gene mutations in Italian adenomatous polyposis coli patients by PCR-SSCP analysis. Am J Hum Genet 1993; 52:280–285.
Vogelstein B, Fearon ER, Hamilton SR, et al: Genetic alterations during colorectal-tumor development. N Engl J Med 1988; 319: 525–532.
Wada C, Shinoya S, Fujino Y, et al: Genomic instability of microsatellite repeats and its association with the evolution of chronic myelogenous leukemia. Blood 1994; 83:3449–3456.
Warner JP, Barron LH, Brock DJ: A new polymerase chain reaction (PCR) assay for the trinucleotide repeat that is unstable and expanded on Huntington's disease chromosomes. Mol Cell Probes 1993; 7:235–239.
Wiedmann M, Wilson WJ, Czajka J, et al: Ligase chain reaction (LCR)—overview and applications. PCR Methods Appl 1994; 3:S51–S64.
Zaccaria A, Tassinari A, Guerrasio A, et al: Molecular diagnosis of Philadelphia chromosome-positive chronic myeloid leukemia. Haematologica 1991; 76:183–187.
Zhang T, Hillion J, Tong JH, et al: AML-1 gene rearrangement and AML-1-ETO gene expression as molecular markers of acute myeloblastic leukemia with t(8;21). Leukemia 1994; 8:729–734.
Zhang W, Sun Y, Jin S, et al: The association between cervical carcinoma and human papilloma virus (HPV) in Xiangyuan country. Chin Med Sci J 1991; 6:74–77.
Zucker-Franklin D, Pancake BA: The role of human T-cell lymphotropic viruses (HTLV-I and II) in cutaneous T-cell lymphomas. Semin Dermatol 1994; 13:160–165.

Chapter 15

Cell Biology and Early Tumor Detection

Matthew R. Pincus, M.D., Ph.D.
Paul W. Brandt-Rauf, M.D., Sc.D., Dr.P.H.
David Nostro, M.S., MT(ASCP)

CELL BIOLOGY AND MITOGENESIS—TUMOR MARKERS

The preceding chapter presented methods for detecting oncogenes in body fluids and tissues. All of these genes act by encoding proteins that are critical in regulating the cell cycle. Malfunctioning of any of these proteins results ultimately in the loss of control over the process of mitosis, which then occurs continually, giving rise to malignant tumor cells. In this chapter, we discuss how detection of these oncogenic *proteins*, or oncoproteins, that occur in the serum of patients with malignant tumors enables us to diagnose malignancy, often at an early stage of tumor development. Because elevated levels of any of these oncoproteins or mutated forms of these proteins in human serum indicate the presence of a malignant tumor, these proteins are also referred to in this chapter as tumor markers.

The preceding chapter noted that oncogenesis, the process by which normal cells become malignant, involves multiple steps. As noted in Chapter 17, these steps can be broadly classified into tumor initiation and tumor promotion. As discussed in this chapter, mitogenesis is a multistep process that commences at the cell membrane as a result of the activation of a growth factor receptor, which then activates other membrane and cytosolic proteins and second messenger molecules that transduce the mitogenic "signal" to the nucleus. Lesions in more than one of these intracellular components may be sufficient to remove cellular controls on the mitogenic pathways. The more of these lesions that occur, the more likely it is that the cell will become malignant. Thus, progressive lesions in the mitogenic pathways may correspond to the multiple steps in carcinogenesis.

Signal Transduction Pathways

Growth Factors and Growth Factor Receptors

Mitogenesis is often initiated at the cell membrane when a growth factor, such as epidermal growth factor (EGF), fibroblast growth factor (FGF), transforming growth factors α and β, platelet-derived growth factor (PDGF), or insulin, binds to its receptor. The receptor itself consists of three domains: The extracellular binding domain, a transmembrane domain, and an intracytoplasmic domain. Binding of the growth factor to the receptor causes the latter to become activated. Activation of the receptor results in the triggering of the sequential activation of membrane and cytosolic proteins in cascades that ultimately cause stimulation of mitosis. The cascades that begin at the cell membrane and terminate in nuclear mitogenic signals are referred to as signal transduction pathways.

Prominent among the growth factor receptors are the members of the oncogene-encoded ERBB family (cellular homologues of one of the viral oncogenes responsible for cellular transformation in the avian erythroblastosis model, hence the name), including the ERBB oncogene-encoded EGF receptor, a protein of molecular mass 170 kd, the p170 protein, and the ERBB2 oncogene-encoded growth factor receptor protein of molecular mass 185 kd, or the p185 protein. The latter was originally cloned from a neuroblastoma, hence the designation NEU. In humans, this oncogene is referred to as *HER2* and is strongly associated with breast cancer (Slamon, 1989).

G Proteins

Figure 15–1 emphasizes that many growth factor receptors rely on activation of G proteins. One vital G protein that is of great importance in mitogenic signaling is the *RAS* oncogene–encoded p21 protein. The p21 protein, like all G

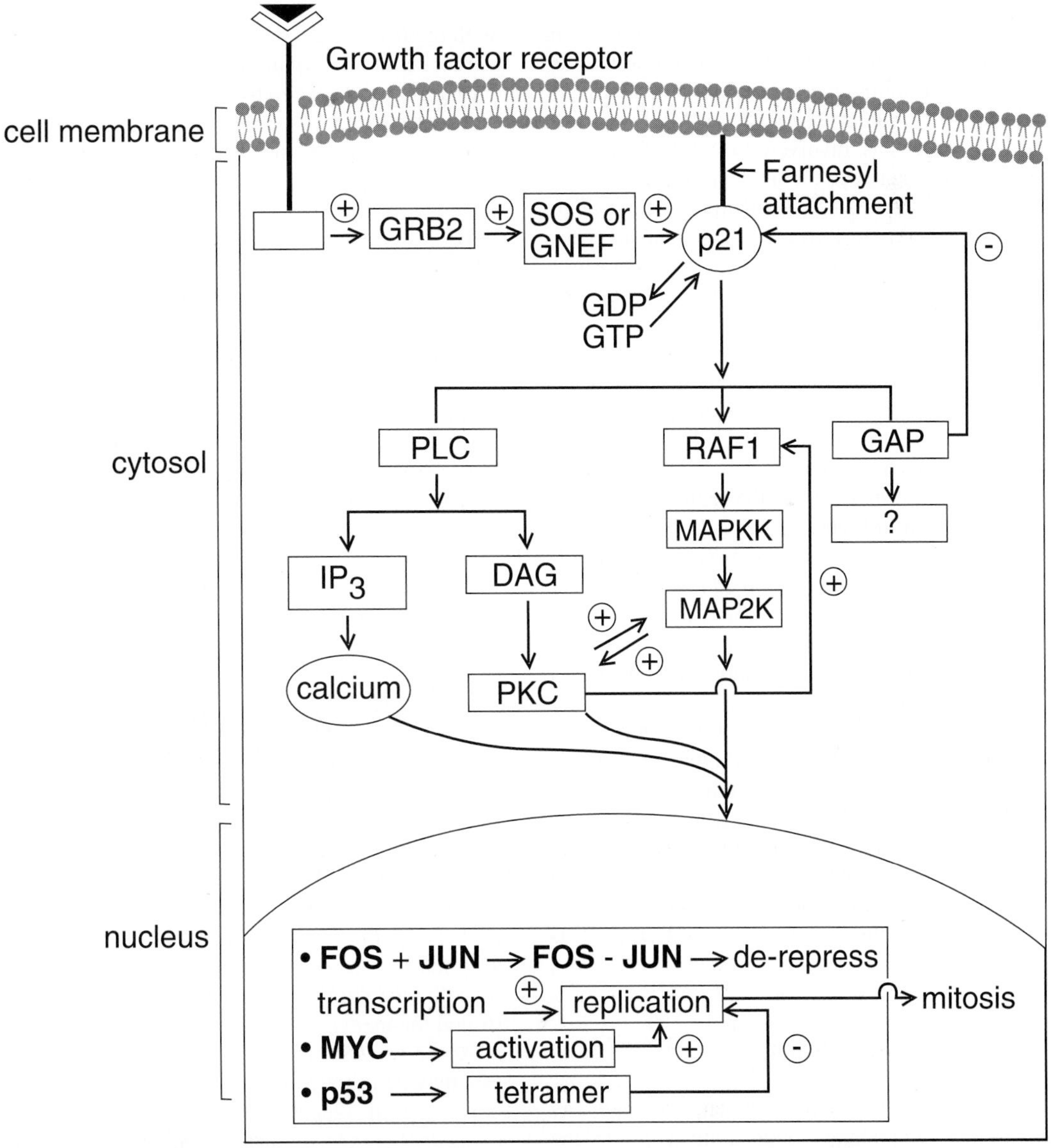

Figure 15–1. Scheme of some of the known components of the *ras* signal transduction pathway beginning (*top, left*) when a growth factor binds to its cell receptor. The remainder of events is explained in the text. The following abbreviations are used: *GRB*-2 is the adaptor protein that concurrently binds growth factor receptor and the guanine nucleotide exchange protein or factor (GNEF), or SOS; *RAS*-p21 protein is defined in the text; PLC is phospholipase C; DAG is diacylglycerol; PKC is protein kinase C; IP3 is inositol triphosphate; *RAF*-1 is the oncogene-encoded p74 protein, which functions as a kinase that phosphorylates another kinase of molecular mass 43 kd, called MAP2 kinase kinase (MAPKK in the figure). MAP2 kinase is mitogen-activated protein kinase or microtubule-associated protein kinase-2 (MAP2K in the figure). GAP is GTPase-activating protein (GAP), which promotes hydrolysis of GTP to GDP bound to p21. *MYC, FOS*, and *JUN* are all nuclear oncogenes that code for nuclear proteins that are transcription factors.

proteins, is bound to guanosine diphosphate (GDP) in an inactive state and is activated by exchanging GDP for guanosine tri-phosphate (GTP). In its activated state, it sets in motion a cascade of activation processes that ultimately trigger cell division.

As shown in Figure 15–1, for mitogenic pathways involving the RAS-p21 protein, activation of a cellular receptor causes the binding of the intracytoplasmic domain of the receptor to the protein GRB2; this protein, in turn, binds to a guanine nucleotide exchange factor, called SOS, which, in turn, activates the *RAS* oncogene–encoded p21 protein, a G protein, causing it to exchange GTP for GDP. When activated, p21 binds, in the membrane, to the amino terminus of another oncogene-encoded protein, the RAF1 p74 protein, which is a kinase that phosphorylates another kinase of molecular mass 43 kd, called MAP2 kinase kinase (MAPKK in Fig. 15–1) (Moodie, 1993; Stokoe, 1994). This protein, in turn, serves as a kinase for the centrally important protein kinase, MAP2 kinase or mitogen-activated protein kinase or microtubule-associated protein kinase-2 (MAP2K in Fig. 15–1). The latter protein is involved in cytoskeletal rearrangements and shuttles between the nucleus and the cytosol. In addition, other proteins become sequentially activated by the p21 protein: Phospholipase C becomes activated and catalyzes the synthesis of diacylglycerol (DAG), which, in turn, activates protein kinase C (PKC), a critical protein on the signal transduction pathway (Pincus, 1992).

As shown in Figure 15–1, it is vital that the p21 protein be bound to the cell membrane in order to function. This binding is caused by the farnesylation of (addition of farnesyl pyrophosphate onto) the critical cysteine 186 residue in the presence of the enzyme farnesyl transferase.

Another critical protein involved in the regulation of activated p21 protein, shown in Figure 15–1, is GTPase activating protein (GAP), which binds to p21 in its GTP-bound state and promotes GTP hydrolysis to GDP. In addition to being a regulatory protein, this protein may serve as another target of activated p21. In neurofibromatosis, overexpression of a form of the *GAP* gene is known to occur and is responsible for the pathogenesis of this condition.

Many growth factors and growth factor receptors, once activated, transduce their mitogenic signals to the RAS-p21 protein. These include insulin, transforming growth factors α and β, EGF, and PDGF. In addition, the *SRC* oncogene–encoded tyrosine kinase protein exerts its mitogenic effects via RAS. As noted previously, RAS-p21 itself activates RAF-p74. Thus, many oncogene-encoded proteins are closely interrelated on the mitogenic signal transduction pathway.

Nuclear Events

As shown in Figure 15–1, the signal transduction pathway ultimately leads, by incompletely understood steps, to the nucleus, where specific oncogene-encoded nuclear proteins become activated. These include FOS, JUN, and MYC proteins. The FOS and JUN proteins form complexes with one another in the α-helical regions of each, which associate to form dimers (i.e., the FOS-JUN complex). The helical regions of each protein that associate contain "leucine zipper" consensus sequences, wherein every seventh amino acid residue in the sequence is leucine. In the dimeric complex, FOS-JUN intercalates with DNA to allow expression (derepression) of genes that encode other proteins involved with cell replication. Mutations in the leucine zipper region of the JUN protein results in its inactivation.

The *MYC* gene codes for a protein of molecular mass 64 kd whose function is largely unknown. There is strong evidence that it is a transcription factor that, when activated, derepresses expression of other genes that encode proteins involved in replication. This oncogene is overexpressed in a number of tumors, including Burkitt's lymphoma, wherein the *MYC* gene on chromosome 8 is translocated to a long-terminal repeat-like region of an immunoglobulin-coding region of chromosome 14. Long-terminal repeat regions allow constitutive expression of genes that are adjacent to them. Interestingly, there are cell lines that, when transfected either with the *RAS* oncogene or with the *MYC* oncogene, do not undergo cell transformation, but, when transfected with *both* oncogenes simultaneously, do undergo cell transformation. These results indicate that the cellular effects of *RAS* and *MYC* may be interdependent. Also, this type of experiment is an excellent prototypical example of the multistage nature of oncogenesis.

Besides oncogene-encoded proteins, antioncogenic regulatory proteins are also present in the nucleus, the best-studied of which is the p53 protein. The p53 protein is known to function as a homotetramer and, in this form, binds to specific sequences of DNA. The effect is to repress the mitotic process. Thus, p53 is an antioncogene protein. As noted in Chapter 14, mutations can occur in p53 that inactivate it. This inactivation can itself be oncogenic because the vital control that this protein exerts over mitogenesis is removed. Among the inactivating mutations are deletions of the whole gene, as occurs in a number of colon cancers. Mutations in the p53 gene can cause amino acid substitutions in the protein that, as in the p21 protein, cause conformational changes in the protein that result in its inability to perform its antioncogenic function in the cell.

MECHANISMS FOR ONCOPROTEIN-INDUCED CARCINOGENESIS

As summarized in Table 15–1, proteins involved with regulation of the cell cycle become oncogenic by a number of mechanisms. At the growth factor level, the cell may constitutively synthesize autocrine growth factors, which are then secreted into its surroundings. The growth factor then binds to cell receptors and stimulates mitogenesis in an uncontrolled manner.

At the growth factor receptor level, uncontrolled mitogenesis may be initiated by several mechanisms (Fig. 15–2). For both the EGF receptor and the *NEU (HER2)* oncogene–encoded p185 growth factor receptor protein, strongly associated with breast cancer (Slamon, 1989), the receptor dimerizes and activates tyrosine kinases that are involved in the phosphorylation of proteins that transduce the mitogenic signal to the nucleus. Three known pathologic mechanisms can result in abnormally prolonged receptor dimerization that in turn results in continuous mitogenic signaling. These are loss of the extracellular binding domain, mutations in the trans-

Table 15–1. MECHANISMS FOR INDUCTION OF CARCINOGENESIS BY MITOGENIC PATHWAY ELEMENTS

Pathway Element	Mechanism of Action
1. Growth factors	a. Overproduction by cell into surroundings
	b. Interaction of growth factors with high-affinity receptors
2. Growth factor receptors	a. Overexpression leading to high concentration of dimers
	b. Loss of extracellular domain resulting in permanent dimerization of growth factor receptor and continuous signaling
	c. Amino acid substitutions in transmembrane domain leading to permanent dimerization
3. Cytosolic proteins: G proteins and kinases	a. Overexpression of normal protein
	b. Amino acid substitutions that permanently change conformation to activated form
	c. Mutations that remove regulatory domains of kinases
4. Nuclear oncoproteins	a. Overexpression of transcription and replication proteins
	b. Mutations in antioncogene proteins that inactivate them

membrane domain that promote dimerization (Brandt-Rauf, 1990), and overexpression of the receptor.

At the level of signaling proteins and their downstream target proteins, overexpression of the proteins (i.e., elevation of their intracellular concentrations) can become sufficient to stimulate cell division continuously. Of fundamental importance in oncogenesis, the protein can become mutated such that the protein contains amino acid substitutions at critical positions in the polypeptide chain. These amino acid substitutions cause the protein to undergo conformational changes that result in its becoming permanently activated to stimulate cell division (Pincus, 1983, 1992).

This mechanism has been well documented for the *RAS* oncogene–encoded p21 protein, for which substitutions of most amino acids for glycine 12 or glutamine 61 result in an oncogenic protein. Many p21 proteins with such substitutions have been cloned and directly microinjected into normal cells in culture, such as NIH 3T3 cells (Barbacid, 1987). The cells undergo malignant transformation that lasts until the added mutant protein is metabolized and cleared from the cells.

Mutations can also occur in negatively regulating proteins, encoded by *anti*oncogenes such as the p53 protein, resulting in their inactivation. Without inhibition of stimulation of cell division, mitogenesis occurs continuously, resulting in malignancy.

Oncoproteins in Tumor Detection

These general mechanisms are summarized because each mechanism gives rise to abnormal proteins whose presence or whose abnormal concentration in body fluids, mostly in serum, can be detected. Positive results suggest the presence of a malignant tumor. Many assays for different oncoproteins are now available in kit form, including enzyme-linked immunosorbent assay (ELISA) assays for the growth factors TGF-α and FGF, the growth factor receptor proteins EGFR and NEU/HER2, and the nuclear protein p53 from such companies as Oncogene Science (Uniondale, NY) and Triton Bioscience (Houston, TX).

Figure 15–3 presents an overview of the results of serum assays for growth factors and proteins on mitogenic signal transduction pathways in patients who have been diagnosed with different types of cancer or in patients who first have been found to have elevated serum levels or mutant forms of one of these proteins and who then have developed cancer. In this three-dimensional figure, the tumor type is plotted on one axis, the serum marker is plotted on a second axis, and the frequency of occurrence of each marker in each tumor type is plotted as a histogram on the third axis.

Numerous studies have documented alterations in oncogenes, or oncoprotein or growth factor expression in terms of mRNA or protein, in tumor tissue compared with normal tissue (Pimentel, 1989). Several studies have examined oncoprotein or growth factor expression in biological fluids such as urine or effusions (Niman, 1985; Yeh, 1989). The results of these studies are highly promising but will not be considered further here. Rather, this chapter will focus on the identification of differences in oncoproteins and growth factors in *serum* or *plasma* in patients with cancer or who are at risk for cancer. As indicated in Figure 15–3, this approach is proving to be highly effective for early tumor detection.

The results of assays for different oncoproteins in human serum are presented in the order of the sequence of events listed in Table 15–1 (i.e., beginning with growth factors, progressing to growth factor receptors, then to G proteins and other signal transduction elements, and finally to nuclear proteins). A summary of some of the many (over 50) known oncogenes and their functions in the cell is given in Table 15–2. The oncogenes in Table 15–2 for which assays are available are labeled with an asterisk.

GROWTH FACTORS

Because various growth factors are believed to play a role in influencing cellular proliferation during tumorigenesis and because growth factors are actively secreted into the extracellular environment, they are potentially attractive targets for detection in blood during cancer development. Several studies to date have demonstrated differences in blood levels of growth factors in cancer patients and controls without cancer.

Transforming Growth Factors α and β

Transforming growth factor α is a polypeptide with 50 amino acids that binds to the EGF receptor, which dimerizes upon binding to EGF. TGF-β is a family of proteins labeled β_1 through β_5. TGF-β_1 is a homodimer of two 12-kd subunits linked together by disulfide bonds. Although TGF-β has been found to be elaborated by many different types of human malignant tumors, serum levels of this growth factor usually are elevated in cancers of the liver and bladder. Interestingly, TGF-β *inhibits* mitosis in specific cell lines in culture, such as mink bronchial epithelial cells. Thus, the serum of patients who have tumors elaborating this growth factor can be as-

2

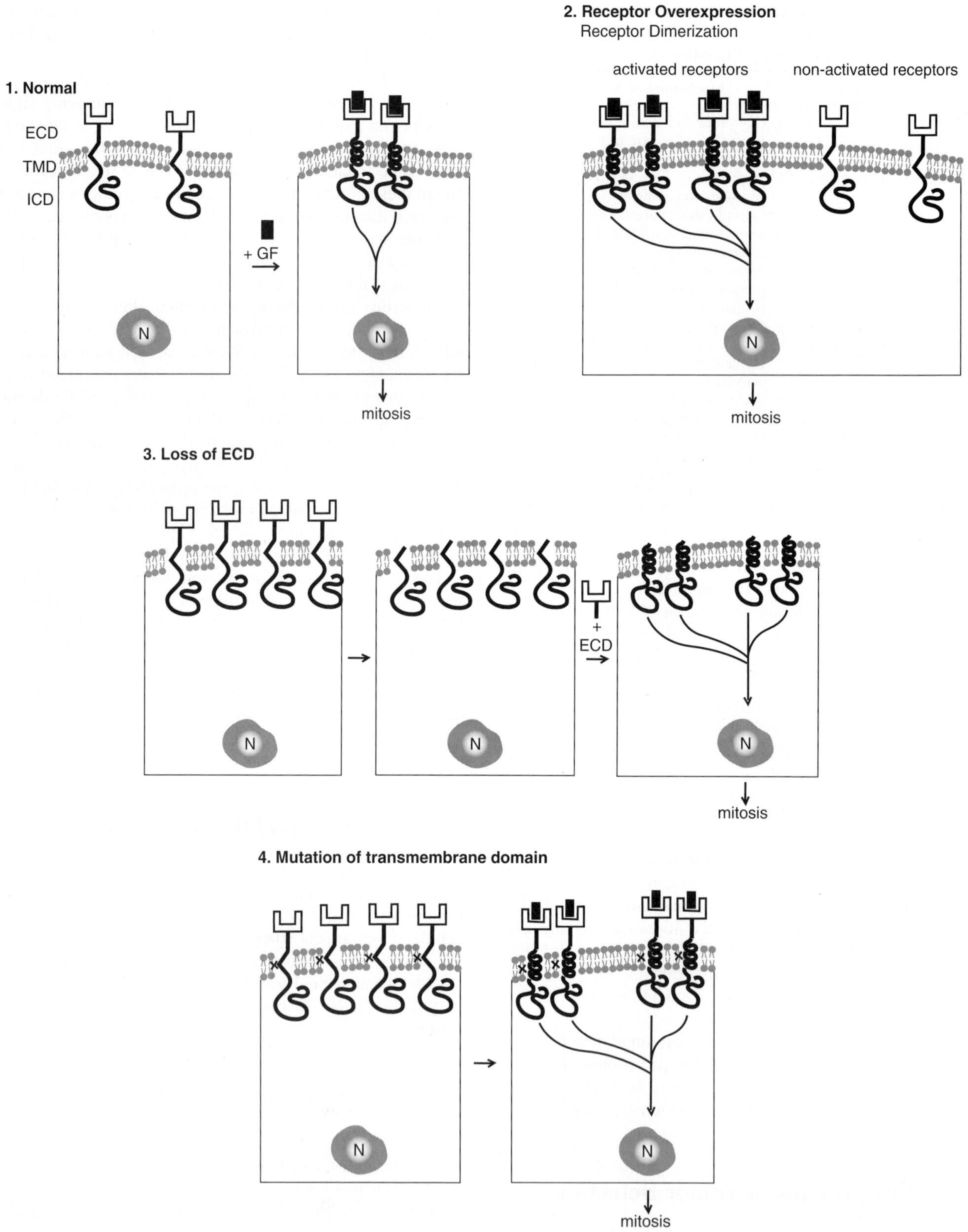

Figure 15–2. Mechanisms for continuous mitogenic signaling by growth factors receptors.

Scheme 1 shows that these receptors have three domains: an extracellular, growth factor–binding domain (ECD); a transmembrane domain (TMD) and an intracytoplasmic domain (ICD). A growth factor (GF) binds to the receptor, causing it to dimerize and setting in motion a cascade of intracellular events that are transduced to the nucleus (N) described in Figure 15–1. There are three known ways in which continuous cell signaling by the growth factor receptor can occur, resulting in malignant transformation of cells.

Scheme 2 depicts the first of these: overexpression of the receptor that results in many activation processes and continuous signaling to the nucleus.

Scheme 3 shows the second mechanism wherein the ECD is either absent or cleaved off by intracellular proteases leading to spontaneous dimerization.

Scheme 4 shows the third mechanism in which a mutation in the growth factor receptor gene results in an amino acid substitution (X in the figure) in the transmembrane domain leading to formation of α-helices that associate (Brandt-Rauf, 1990) resulting in spontaneous dimerization.

sayed for it by measuring the extent of inhibition of cell growth.

TGF-β activity, determined using this technique, has been found to be markedly elevated in patients with hepatocellular carcinoma but not in age-matched controls (Shirai, 1992). In the sera of patients who have undergone surgical resection of these tumors, the activity of TGF-β is barely detectable, suggesting that the tumor was the source of the elevated levels of growth factor in serum. Additionally, use of an ELISA assay with a monoclonal antibody directed against TGF-β_2 has revealed that TGF-β_2 is elevated in a high proportion of patients with invasive bladder cancer but not in patients with noninvasive bladder cancers or in cancer-free patients (Klocker, 1994).

Thus, serum assays for TGF-β are highly useful in diagnosing and following hepatocellular carcinoma. They are less useful in the diagnosis of carcinoma of the bladder, although this growth factor is highly sensitive and specific for invasive bladder cancer.

TGF-α has been found to be elevated in a large number of patients with epithelial cell tumors (Chakrabarty, 1994; Katoh, 1990), predominantly breast (almost 100%), stomach, colon, and liver. In contrast, normal individuals have very low serum levels. TGF-α thus appears to be an excellent marker for the presence of malignancy. Unlike the case with TGF-β, these elevations are not tumor-specific. Nonetheless, it is clear that TGF-α is extremely useful in screening patients for the presence of malignant tumors.

Platelet-Derived Growth Factor

Platelet-derived growth factor (PDGF), a protein of molecular mass 28 kd, exists as a dimer of A and B chains as the A–A, A–B, or B–B dimer forms. Either chain can be glycosylated, increasing the molecular mass to 30 kd. This growth factor, originally isolated from platelets, binds to a transmembrane growth factor receptor. The B chain is encoded by the *SIS* oncogene. It has been found to be a potent mitogen in lymphoid, myeloid, and fibroblastic cell lines. It has also been examined in the blood of cancer patients. Overall, this growth factor has been found to be significantly elevated in over 15% of patients with carcinomas, sarcomas, and lymphomas but not at all in normal individuals. In patients with breast cancer, the stage of the cancer correlates well with the serum level of the growth factor (Ariad, 1991). Higher levels predict shorter survivals.

Basic Fibroblast Growth Factor

Basic fibroblast growth factor (bFGF) is a protein containing 155 amino acids. It is a growth factor for mesenchymal cells but has also been found in relatively high concentrations in the central nervous system. Interestingly, bFGF has been found to be high concentrated in the sera of patients with epithelial cell tumors. Prominent among these tumors is renal cell carcinoma. Over 50% of patients with this disease have markedly elevated serum levels of bFGF (Fujimoto, 1991; Ii, 1993) as determined either by ELISA or by enhanced chemiluminescent assays. This growth factor is also elevated in the sera of over 50% of patients with central nervous system tumors, 90% of patients with lung cancers (Ii, 1993), and over 60% of patients with lymphomas (Kurobe, 1993). It is not elevated, however, in the sera of large populations of normal (control) individuals (see Fig. 15–3*A*).

Thus, TGF-α and TGF-β, PDGF, and bFGF all appear to be elevated in the sera of a significant number of patients with epithelial cell tumors but are not completely tumor-specific. TGF-α has some specificity for breast cancer and TGF-β for hepatocellular carcinoma. bFGF is elevated in a variety of malignancies, including nonepithelial cell tumors, such as CNS tumors and lymphomas. PDGF shows little specificity for tumor type, but high levels in serum indicate the presence of malignancy.

2

Other Growth Factors

Epidermal growth factor has been found to be elevated in the serum of some patients with stomach cancer (Pawlikowski, 1989) and cancer of the tongue (Bhatavdekar, 1993) but has been found to be unchanged or decreased in other cancers (Nedvidkova, 1992). Elevated serum levels of hepatocyte growth factor have been reported in hepatocellular carcinoma. However, this growth factor appears to be unique in that levels also are elevated in nonmalignant liver diseases (Hioki, 1993), which diminishes its utility as a tumor marker.

GROWTH FACTOR RECEPTORS

Transmembrane growth factor receptors encoded by the *ERBB* family of oncogenes (i.e., *ERBB,* which encodes the EGF receptor, also called EGFR, and NEU/HER2 [ERBB2]) are particularly attractive targets for detection in blood during cancer development because, in human cancers induced by these receptors, the mechanism appears to be proteolysis of the extracellular receptor-binding domain (see Fig. 15–2, third illustration). The liberated extracellular domains, called ECD, then enter the circulation and can be readily detected in serum using conventional immunoassay techniques (Brandt-Rauf, 1994a, 1994b).

EGF-Receptor (EGFR)

Elevations of circulating levels of the ECD of EGFR have been studied in patients with asbestosis (Brandt-Rauf, 1992), which is known to predispose to malignancies. Such patients with ECD serum levels of 636 fmol/mL or higher either have an asbestos-associated malignancy (carcinoma of the lung or mesothelioma) or *subsequently* develop such a malignancy. Many normal individuals have been found to have much lower serum ECD levels. Thus, EGFR appears to be an excellent marker for asbestos-induced tumors. These results are also of interest because they suggest that the primary effect of asbestos as a carcinogen is to cause mutations in the *EGFR* gene.

NEU/HER2 Receptor

Because of the documented strong association between breast cancer and mutations in the *NEU/HER2* gene, many studies have examined the p185 ERBB2 ECD in the blood of cancer patients, particularly breast cancer. Prior studies on *NEU*-oncogene–induced overexpression of the p185 protein

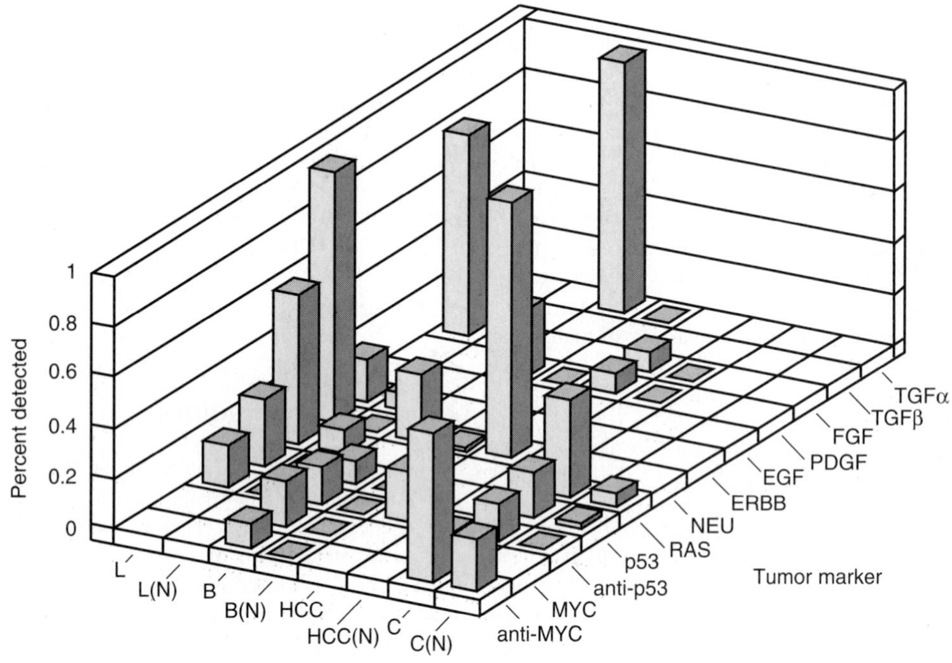

A

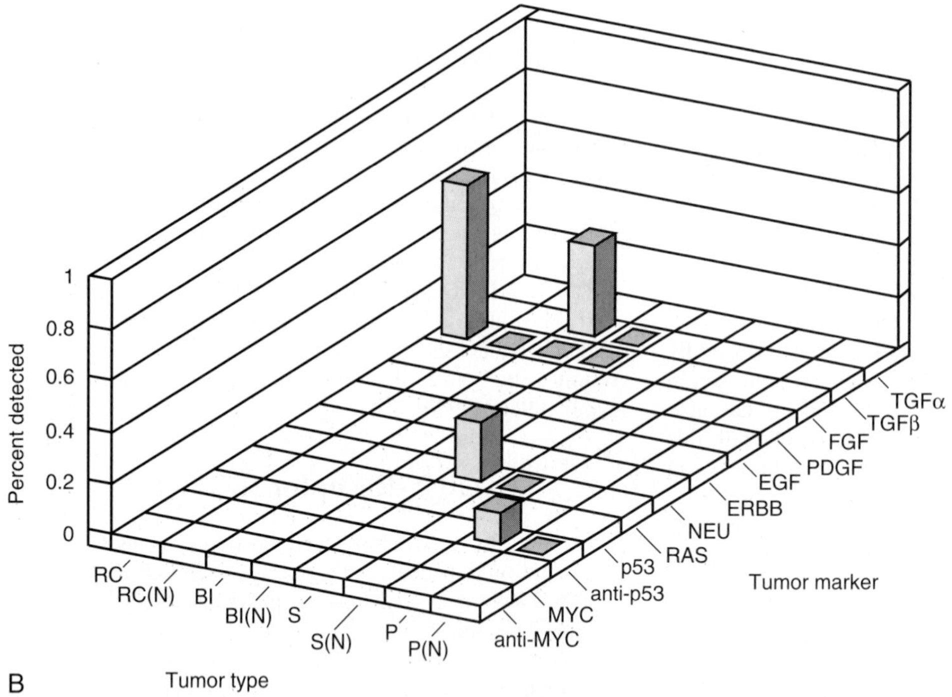

B

Figure 15–3 *A* to *B*. Summary of results of serum assays for different components of mitogenic signaling pathways. These are three-dimensional plots of tumor type on one axis, pathway component (tumor marker) on another axis and the percent detected or the frequency of finding each of the pathway components elevated in the serum of patients with each tumor type on the perpendicular vertical axis. Next to the results for each tumor type, the results for control groups are given. These controls are always represented as the abbreviated tumor type with an added (N) to indicate normal, that is, individuals who were tumor free. The abbreviation label for each pathway component corresponds to the box beginning at the lower left and proceeding to the upper right along the tumor marker axis.

In *A* to *C*, the oncoproteins assayed for are abbreviated as follows: TGF_{α}, TFG_{β}, FGF, PDGF, and EGF represent transforming growth factor α, transforming growth factor β, fibroblast growth factor, platelet-derived growth factor, and epidermal growth factor, respectively; ERBB is the epidermal growth factor (EGF) receptor; NEU is the p185 protein, which is similar to the ERBB protein and is also called ERBB2 and HER-2; RAS is the p21 protein; p53 is an antioncogene protein; anti-p53 is anti-p53 antibody; *MYC* is a nuclear oncogene that encodes the MYC protein; and anti-MYC is antibody to the MYC protein.

In *A*, the tumor types are abbreviated as follows: L = lung; B = breast; HCC = hepatocellular carcinoma; C = colon. The various assayed components of mitogenic signal transduction pathways are plotted on the tumor marker axis.

In *B*, the following abbreviations are used for the different tumor types; RC = renal cell carcinoma; Bl = bladder; S = stomach; and P = pancreas. The tumor marker axis contains the assayed pathway components.

(Slamon, 1989) found that the level of expression of the *NEU* oncogene in breast cancer biopsy tissue correlated with the extent of the tumor and was the best prognostic indicator of survival rates, exceeding extent of lymph node involvement as a prognostic indicator.

Results on quantitation of p185 ECD in the serum of patients with breast cancer parallel those of the prior genetic results. Serum levels of p185 ECD have been markedly elevated in 25% to 50% of patients with Stage 3 or 4 breast cancer (40 to 190 times higher than in the sera of normal control individuals) (Carney, 1991; Kath, 1993; Mori, 1990). When tumor biopsy material is available, serum ECD levels correlate well with tissue level of expression (Breuer 1993, 1994). Levels of serum ECD also correlate well with recurrent disease.

Because serum levels of p185 ECD correlate with tumor load and stage, detection of incipient breast cancer by observing elevated serum levels of p185 ECD is less effective for these patients. Overall, the rate of detection of Stages 1 and 2 breast cancers using serum levels of ECD, based on conventional ELISA assay techniques, ranges from 10% to 15%. However, use of a sensitive ELISA for p185 ECD in

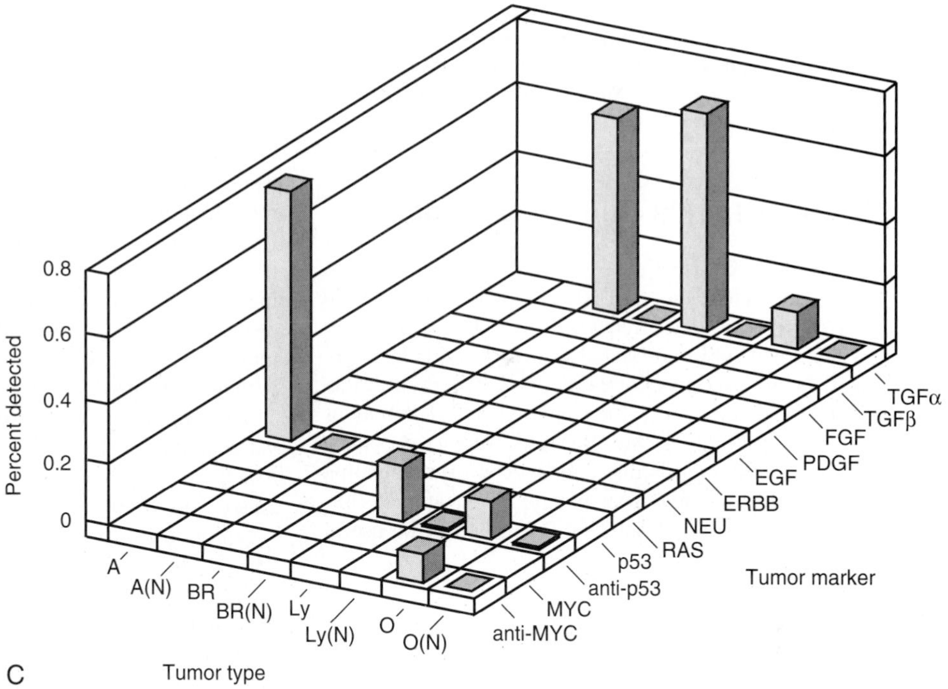

Figure 15–3 *C*. In *C*, the following abbreviations are used for the different tumor types: A = angiosarcoma of the liver; BR = brain and central nervous system; Ly = lymphoma; and O = ovarian cancer. The tumor marker axis contains the assayed pathway components.

breast cancer patients resulted in discovery of carcinoma in situ in 43% of patients with this disease (Breuer, 1993). This latter result indicates that more sensitive assays for p185 ECD identify a significant increase in the number of patients with carcinoma in situ.

Pulmonary Neoplasms

p185 ECD is also elevated in a high percentage of patients with pulmonary cancer. Serum levels of p185 ECD have been used to screen patients with known predisposition, such as pneumoconioses, for developing these cancers. In 45% of patients with pneumoconioses, elevated serum p185 ECD levels have been found *prior to* the onset of frank malignancy. In over 70% of patients with this predisposing factor who have cancer of the lung, serum p185 ECD is markedly elevated (Brandt-Rauf, 1994). Clearly, this protein is an excellent marker for pulmonary cancers. No elevations of p185 ECD have been found in the sera of large numbers of normal individuals (see Fig. 15–3*A*).

Hepatocellular Carcinomas

It was noted previously that the growth factor TGF-β may be a good marker for hepatocellular carcinoma. There are now strong indications that p185 ECD is also an excellent marker for this disease. Serum p185 ECD has been found to be elevated in over 33% of Orientals who have known risk

Table 15–2. SUMMARY OF SOME IMPORTANT ONCOGENES AND THEIR PROTEIN PRODUCTS*

Oncogene	Protein Product	Function
1. *ERBB*†	EGF receptor	Binds to EGF; dimerizes; activates tyrosine kinases in signal transduction; may work through *RAS*
2. *ERBB2*†	GF receptor	Very similar to EGF receptor but uses different GF; may work through *RAS*
3. *SIS*†	β-chain of PDGF	Growth factor receptor; may work through *RAS*
4. *SRC*†	Tyrosine kinase	Transduces signal through *RAS*
5. *RAS*†	p21 proteins: H-, K-, and N- forms	G proteins; bind to cell membrane and transduce signals through second messengers and *RAF*, PKC, PLC, and GAP proteins
6. *RAP*1A	Anti-*RAS* oncogene; in *RAS* family	Blocks *RAS* action in cells
7. *RAF*	74 kd protein	Phosphorylates MAP kinase kinase that then phosphorylates MAP kinase
8. *ERK*1 and *ERK*2	MAP kinase family	43-kd proteins involved in cytoskeletal rearrangements and nuclear signaling
9. *MYC*†	62/64 kd nuclear	Turns on transcription factors involved in replication
10. *JUN*	Nuclear protein	Forms complex with *FOS*
11. *FOS*	Nuclear protein	Forms complex with *JUN*; *FOS-JUN* complex activates transcription factors
12. p53† antioncogene	53-kd nuclear protein	Forms tetramers, then binds DNA segments to block transcription and replication

*Only a few of the many (more than 50) oncogenes are listed in this table. The ones that are listed here encode proteins for which assays have been developed or are closely related to these proteins. No growth factors except PDGF are included in this table. The following abbreviations are used: GF, growth factor; EGF, epidermal growth factor; PKC, protein kinase C; PLC, phospholipase C; GAP, GTPase activating protein; MAP kinase, mitogen-activated protein kinase. The names of the oncogenes are commonly used and relate to the sources from which they were originally discovered. For example, *RAS* is an abbreviation for rat sarcoma viral oncogene.

†Oncogene-encoded proteins are ones for which assays have been performed on human serum.

factors for developing this disease (Luo, 1993; Yu, 1994). However, no such elevations have been observed in normal individuals of similar age and race or in those with exposure to risk factors for this disease but who did not subsequently develop cancer.

ERBB2 (p185) ECD in Other Tumors

Serum ERBB2 ECD levels have been elevated in patients with colorectal, pancreatic, prostatic, hepatic, and ovarian cancers (Wu, 1993) at lower frequencies of detection (15% to 20%). Serum levels have correlated well with tissue levels in these cases. There is a direct correlation between serum levels of p185 ECD and tumor size for premalignant adenomas of the colon (Brandt-Rauf, 1994). Because colonic neoplasia usually progresses through well defined steps from adenoma to carcinoma with the malignant potential of adenomas increasing with size, serum ERBB2 ECD levels may be useful in monitoring this progression.

G PROTEINS

As noted previously, the *RAS* oncogene–encoded p21 proteins are 21-kd, membrane-associated G proteins with GTPase activity that have been implicated in the growth signal transduction process from the cell membrane to cytoplasmic kinases. Qualitative changes (i.e., point mutations) and quantitative changes (i.e., overexpression) in p21 have been identified as contributing to human carcinogenesis (Barbacid, 1987). By as-yet undefined mechanisms, p21 proteins gain access to the extracellular environment. Thus, increased amounts of p21 or point-mutated forms of p21 can be detected by immunoblotting with monoclonal antibodies in the supernatant of cells in culture known to overexpress p21 or to express mutant p21, respectively (Brandt-Rauf, 1991). Some aspects of these studies are outlined in Chapter 17.

Similarly, mice bearing tumors that overexpress p21 or express mutant p21 are found by immunoblotting to have increased amounts of p21 or mutant forms of p21 in their serum, respectively (Hamer, 1991). These results suggest that the detection of increased p21 or mutant p21 in blood is possible in humans.

Because of its central role in mitogenic signal transduction, overexpressed p21 protein, mutated p21 protein, or both might be expected in a wide variety of human tumors. Indeed, elevated serum p21 has been identified in the serum of up to 68% of patients with many different cancers, including breast, prostate, colon, lung, and liver cancer. On the other hand, serum levels are detectable in only a small percentage of normal individuals (Weissfeld, 1994).

As noted in Chapter 14, the incidence of the oncogenic form of the *KRAS* gene in human pancreatic and colonic cancers is very high. New assays based on the polymerase chain reaction (PCR) have detected the *RAS* oncogene in the stool of a high percentage of patients with colonic cancer. Further similarly encouraging results have been obtained using the sputum of patients with lung cancer. The ELISA for the p21 protein using the serum of patients with lung and colonic carcinoma also has yielded similar results. Elevated levels (fivefold over controls) of serum p21 have been found in up to 83% of lung cancer patients, whereas only low levels were found in the sera of normal individuals (Brandt-Rauf, 1991).

In the earlier discussion of the NEU oncogene-encoded p185 protein, it was noted that serum levels of this protein were elevated in patients with pneumoconioses who then progressed to develop frank malignancies. Serum p21 levels has been similarly studied in patients with pneumoconioses. Immunoblotting (Western blotting) detected elevated serum levels of the p21 protein in 39% of patients with this predisposing condition. Almost all of these patients developed a malignant lung tumor *subsequent to* the observed elevations of the p21 protein. Thus, like p185 ECD, elevated serum p21 may be a biomarker of early malignant disease in patients with a known predisposition.

The preceding studies are concerned with detecting elevated serum levels of p21 in serum as an indicator of malignancy. As noted previously, a major mechanism for oncogenesis induced by the RAS-p21 protein is amino acid substitutions in its sequence that result in its permanent activation. Mutant *RAS* genes have been identified by PCR and direct sequencing of DNA isolated from the serum or plasma of three patients with pancreatic cancer (Sorenson, 1994), but the direct detection of mutant p21 protein has only recently been reported in human blood. Now, however, oncogenic amino acid substitutions in the p21 protein can be identified through the use of monoclonal antibodies that recognize specific oncogenic substitutions.

Mutated p21 has been found in the serum of patients with a known history of exposure to the carcinogen vinyl chloride. This chemical has been shown to predispose individuals to angiosarcomas. Tissue studies of these angiosarcomas reveal a mutant *RAS* gene in the tumor cells that codes for aspartic acid in place of the normally occurring glycine at position 13 in the polypeptide chain. A specific monoclonal antibody that recognizes the ASP13 form of the p21 protein has been obtained. This mutant p21 protein has been identified in the sera of 80% of patients with vinyl chloride–induced angiosarcoma of the liver but not in normal individuals (DeVivo, 1994). Moreover, the degree of exposure of patients to vinyl chloride correlates directly with the probability of discovering the oncogenic form of the protein in their serum.

A number of other highly specific antimutant p21 monoclonal antibodies recognize specific amino acid substitutions at positions 12, 13, 59, and 61. Use of these antibodies on the sera of patients with known risk factors for cancer appears to offer much promise for early tumor detection in the future.

NUCLEAR ONCOPROTEINS

As noted previously, two important nuclear proteins appear to be critical to the regulation of cell growth and division: The tumor suppressor gene protein p53 and the p62/64 protein of the *CMYC* oncogene, for which serum assays have been developed. Many different point mutations in p53 have been identified in human tumors (Soussi, 1994). The effect of these mutations is to cause a loss of the normal growth inhibitory function of p53; at the same time, some of these mutations result in p53 proteins with considerably increased half-lives so that the mutant proteins accumulate in the transformed cells (Soussi, 1994). The CMYC oncoprotein is activated to cause cell transformation by overexpression, so it too accumulates in transformed cells (Field, 1990). Thus, for both p53 and p62/64 *MYC*, levels of the proteins are increased in transformed cells and human tumors (Field, 1990; Soussi, 1994). It is unknown how these nuclear proteins gain access to the extracellular environment, but they apparently do in some cases, because some cancer patients develop antibodies to p53 or p62/64 *MYC*. Therefore, increased amounts of p53 or p62/64 (or antibodies to these proteins) in blood also are potential markers for the study of human carcinogenesis.

Detection of Malignancies by Assaying for p53 Protein

Hepatocellular Carcinoma

Increased levels of mutant p53 in serum by ELISA (>0.3 ng/mL, the upper limit of 100 normals) have been found in 20% of patients with hepatocellular carcinoma and 30% of patients with cirrhosis, a group known to be at increased risk for hepatocellular carcinoma (Virji, 1992). Because patients with cirrhosis have high levels of p53 in their sera and a known risk factor for developing hepatocellular carcinoma, the elevated p53 levels may be an early indicator of tumorigenesis.

Breast and Lung Cancers

There have been few studies on p53 as a tumor marker in the sera of patients with breast and lung cancers. Elevated serum mutant p53 levels determined by ELISA have been reported in 8% of breast cancer patients, with levels decreasing following surgical resection of the tumors (Rosanelli, 1993), indicating that the tumors were the source of the elevated p53. Elevations of p53 protein have not been observed in the sera of any normal individuals.

For lung cancer, serum mutant p53 levels as determined by ELISA and immunoblotting have been elevated in up to 34% of lung cancer patients but not in normal individuals (Fontanini, 1994). For the cancer patients, immunohistochemical staining of subsequently obtained biopsy tissue showed elevated p53 levels, correlating with the serum findings.

Colon Cancer

As noted in Chapter 14, an important mechanism believed to be operative in the development of colonic carcinoma is the deletion of the normal p53 gene or mutation of the gene, leading to a nonfunctional antioncogenic protein. Elevated serum mutant p53 levels have been determined by ELISA in about one in five patients with colon carcinoma and in approximately 1 in 10 patients with colon adenoma. Serum p53 protein was not found in normal persons. These results show relatively low sensitivity of this marker for colon cancer, possibly because the p53 gene was deleted in a high percentage of the tumors studied.

Circulating Anti-p53 Antibodies in Tumor Detection

A unique aspect of nuclear proteins is that, because they are normally sequestered in the nucleus, if they are released into the circulation, they are often detected by the immune system as foreign. Serum antibodies against p53, in fact, have been reported frequently in patients with several types of cancer. In several major studies (including a large study of 1392 cancer patients), serum levels of anti-p53 antibodies were elevated in patients with ovarian and colon cancers (15%), lung cancers, including small cell tumors (up to 25%), and breast cancers, including intraductal carcinoma (up to 15%). Serum levels of these antibodies were not elevated in normal persons (Angelopolou, 1994). In a significant number of patients who have been followed for the presence of anti-p53 antibodies in their sera, these antibodies have been found prior to the occurrence of malignant tumors.

Anti-p53 antibodies are also found in over 20% of patients with bladder cancer, in a high proportion of patients with pancreatic and hepatocellular carcinomas, and in childhood lymphomas.

2

MYC-Oncogene–Encoded Protein in Tumor Detection

CMYC-related proteins and antibodies to the CMYC protein have likewise been identified in the serum of cancer patients. Detection of this 62-kd to 64-kd protein is hampered by its short half-life in serum. However, immunoblotting can be used to detect a specific CMYC-related p40 protein in the serum of these patients. The highest frequencies of occurrence of MYC protein in human serum have been found in breast cancer (about 20%) and in colon cancer. Treatment of both types of cancer results in marked diminution in the serum levels of this protein. Recurrences result in elevated levels. CMYC protein is therefore potentially useful in following the course of malignant tumors. It has not been detected in the sera of normal individuals.

Serum Anti-MYC Protein Antibodies in Tumor Detection

Serum levels of anti-CMYC antibodies have been elevated in patients with colorectal cancer (55% to 65%) and in patients with both myeloid leukemias and Burkitt's lymphoma. Lower occurrences of elevated antibodies have been reported in patients with breast cancer (around 10%) and ovarian cancer (10%). Anti-CMYC antibodies have not been found in the sera of normal individuals.

EVALUATION AND CONCLUSIONS

The pathways for mitogenic signal transduction between the membrane and the nucleus of cells are well defined. These pathways consist mainly of proteins, mutations in which or overexpression of which can give rise to uncontrolled mitogenic signaling and cancer.

Diagnostic Efficacy of Serum Oncoproteins

From Figure 15–3, it is clear that, with the proteins studied thus far, positivity rates are high in certain cancers, whereas these rates are low in control groups. For example, the growth factor TGF-α is elevated in many breast cancers; FGF is elevated in a high proportion of lung cancers; the p185 ECD (NEU) protein is elevated in the sera of many patients with lung and hepatocellular carcinomas; p21 protein is elevated in hepatocellular carcinomas, angiosarcomas of the liver, and lung cancers; p53 is elevated in lung cancers; and anti-MYC protein is elevated in colon cancers. For these proteins, the sensitivity for disease detection is high. Also, these growth factors or oncoproteins have been rare in the sera of individuals who do not have cancer in every study performed to date on several thousand patients. Therefore, the specificity of using growth factors and oncoproteins as tumor markers is also high. This conclusion does not imply that absence of a given oncoprotein in the serum of a patient implies absence of a malignancy. Because of the multistep nature of carcinogenesis, many potential oncoproteins may become abnormal. Any one or group of *other* oncoproteins may therefore be present in the patient's serum.

Indeed, Figure 15–3 also indicates that the frequency of detection of certain oncoproteins in the sera of patients who have a given type of tumor can be relatively low. For example, from Figure 15–3*A*, CMYC has been found to be elevated in the sera of about 8% of patients with breast cancer; p185 ECD (NEU) protein has been found in up to 25% of patients with breast cancer. The low rates of detection of these oncoproteins in these tumor types result from the large number of possible steps on the pathway in which aberrant proteins or growth factors can be produced. Thus, the tumors that occur in a given tissue may have a multiplicity of different causes leading to the production of different aberrant proteins in the chain. The next step, therefore, in using these oncoprotein markers in the early diagnosis of cancer is to assay for multiple markers on a given patient's serum. Discovery of at least one aberrant component of the signal transduction pathway thus becomes far more likely.

Origins of Malignancies

Figure 15–3 also indicates that discovery of elevated levels of an oncoprotein in the serum of a patient does not give information as to the source of the malignancy. For example, from Figure 15–3*A*, p21 has been found to be elevated in colon, lung, and angiosarcomas of the liver; NEU/HER2 (CERBB2) p185 ECD has been found to be elevated in colon, lung, and breast cancers. Because the signal transduction pathways in most cells are remarkably similar, a rise in any oncoprotein can signify malignancy in a number of different cell types.

Additionally, many studies on the correlations between the presence of tumors and serum levels of oncoproteins remain to be performed. For example, there are no published data on detectable forms of mutant p21 protein in the serum of patients with pancreatic carcinoma with control groups consisting of age-matched and sex-matched controls and with groups containing patients with pancreatitis but no tumors.

One way of using serum oncoproteins to detect specific tumors at an early stage in tumor progression is on populations known to be at risk for specific cancers from a history of exposure to carcinogens or mutagens, as in occupational exposure or from preexisting medical conditions, as seen from the examples of vinyl chloride exposure associated with angiosarcoma of the liver, pneumoconioses associated with lung cancer, and both conditions associated with elevated serum levels of RAS-p21 protein.

Another way of using serum oncoproteins to detect early cancers is to test for the expression of a wide variety of oncoproteins in patients' sera. If at least one positive result is found, the patient can be followed for signs of a tumor.

Tumor Size and Oncoprotein Levels

Currently, there is little information on the minimal size of a tumor that gives rise to serum elevations of oncoproteins. However, there are indications that small lesions may give rise to significant levels of certain oncoproteins.

First, in a significant number of patients with known cancer risks, oncoproteins were discovered in their sera *prior to* the development of detectable cancer. Thus, in patients with asbestosis, the ECD of the p185 ERBB protein became elevated before lung tumors were diagnosed. The p185 ECD was overexpressed in a number of patients prior to the diagnosis of breast cancer. Oriental patients who had high serum levels of p185 ECD went on to develop hepatocellular carcinoma. Patients with pneumoconioses and elevated levels of p185 ECD and/or p21 protein subsequently developed lung carcinomas. Mutant (ASP13-)p21 protein was discovered in the sera of a high percentage of patients exposed to vinyl chloride who subsequently developed angiosarcoma. Anti-p53 antibodies were found in the sera of persons who subsequently developed angiosarcomas or lung cancers. All of these studies suggest that malignant lesions that are undetectable by conventional techniques may be detected by measuring the serum levels of oncoproteins, especially in patients with known exposures or risk factors for cancer.

Second, in some patients, serum levels of marker oncoproteins correlate well with tumor size, level of expression of the marker in the tumor tissue itself, or both. In this regard, some small adenomas ($<$ 1 cm) have given rise to elevated levels of p185 ECD or RAS-p21 in these patients' sera. Larger adenomas and carcinomas may give rise to even higher levels of these proteins. For both RAS-p21 protein and ERBB2-p185 ECD, the serum level of these markers correlates well with the pretreatment and post-treatment clinical status of the patient. Nonetheless, substantially more studies of the correlation between tumor size and serum level of oncoproteins are needed. One confounding factor may be that a small tumor may produce large amounts of the marker, whereas larger tumors may produce smaller amounts.

Despite the foregoing caveats in interpretations of elevations of serum levels of oncoproteins or the detection of abnormal forms of these proteins in serum and the need for further correlation studies, assays for the presence of oncoproteins in serum show exceptional promise for detection of malignant tumors at an early stage and for monitoring their progression, response to therapy, remission, and recurrence.

Angelopolou K, Diamandis EP, Sutherland DJA, et al: Prevalence of serum antibodies against the p53 tumor suppressor gene protein in various cancers. Int J Cancer 1994; 58:480–487.
Ariad S, Seymour L, Bezwoda WR: Platelet-derived growth factor (PDGF) in plasma of breast cancer patients: Correlation with stage and rate of progression. Breast Cancer Res Treat 1991; 20:11–17.
Barbacid M: Ras genes. Annu Rev Biochem 1987; 56:779–827.

Bhatavdekar JM, Patel DD, Vora HH, et al: Circulating markers and growth factors as prognosticators in men with advanced tongue cancer. Tumour Biol 1993; 14:55–58.

Brandt-Rauf PW: Oncogene proteins as biomarkers in the molecular epidemiology of occupational carcinogenesis: The example of the ras oncogene encoded p21 protein. Int Arch Occup Environ Health 1991; 63:1–8.

Brandt-Rauf PW, Pincus MR, Carney WP: The c-erbB-2 protein in oncogenesis: Molecular structure to molecular epidemiology. Crit Rev Oncog 1994a; 5:313–329.

Brandt-Rauf PW, Rackovsky S, Pincus MR: Correlation of the Transmembrane Domain of the *Neu*-Oncogene-Encoded p185 Protein with its Function. Proc Natl Acad Sci U S A 1990; 87:8660–8664.

Brandt-Rauf PW, Luo JC, Carney WP, et al: The detection of increased amounts of the extracellular domain of the c-erbB-2 oncoprotein in serum during pulmonary carcinogenesis in humans. Int J Cancer 1994b; 56:383–386.

Brandt-Rauf PW, Smith S, Hemminki K, et al: Serum oncoproteins and growth factors in asbestosis and silicosis patients. Int J Cancer 1992; 50:881–885.

Breuer B, DeVivo I, Luo JC, et al: ErbB-2 and myc oncoproteins in sera and tumors of breast cancer patients. Cancer Epidemiol Biomarkers Prev 1994; 3:63–66.

Breuer B, Luo JC, DeVivo I, et al: Detection of elevated c-erbB-2 oncoprotein in the serum and tissue in breast cancer. Med Sci Res 1993; 21:383–384.

Carney WP, Hamer PJ, Petit D, et al: Detection and quantitation of the human neu oncoprotein. Tumor Marker Oncol 1991; 6:53–72.

Chakrabarty S, Huang S, Moskal TL, et al: Elevated serum levels of transforming growth factor-α in breast cancer patients. Cancer Lett 1994; 79:157–160.

DeVivo I, Marion MJ, Smith SJ, et al: Mutant c-Ki-ras p21 protein in chemical carcinogenesis in humans exposed to vinyl chloride. Cancer Causes Control 1994; 5:273–278.

Field JK, Spandidos DA: The role of ras and myc oncogenes in human solid tumours and their relevance in diagnosis. Anticancer Res 1990; 10:1–22.

Fontanini G, Fiore L, Bigini D, et al: Levels of p53 antigen in serum of non-small lung cancer patients correlate with positive p53 immunohistochemistry on tumor sections, tumor necrosis and nodal involvement. Int J Oncol 1994; 5:553–558.

Fujimoto K, Ichimori Y, Kakizoe T, et al: Increased serum levels of basic fibroblast growth factor in patients with renal cell carcinoma. Biochem Biophys Res Commun 1991; 180:386–392.

Hamer PJ, LaVecchio J, Ng S, et al: Activated Val-12 ras p21 in cell culture fluids and mouse plasma. Oncogene 1991; 6:1609–1615.

Hioki O, Watanabe A, Minemura M, et al: Clinical significance of serum hepatocyte growth factor levels in liver diseases. J Med 1993; 24:35–46.

Ii M, Yoshida H, Aramaki Y, et al: Improved enzyme immunoassay for human basic fibroblast growth factor using a new enhanced chemiluminescence system. Biochem Biophys Res Commun 1993; 193:540–545.

Kath R, Hoffken K, Otte C, et al: The neu-oncogene product in serum and tissue of patients with breast carcinoma. Ann Oncol 1993; 4:585–590.

Katoh M, Inagaki H, Kurosawa-Ohsawa K, et al: Detection of transforming growth factor alpha in human urine and plasma. Biochem Biophys Res Commun 1990; 167:1065–1072.

Klocker EI, Stenzl A, Cronauer MV, et al: Quantitative determination of transforming growth factor-β in serum and urine in patients with bladder cancer and its expression in malignant and non-malignant primary epithelial cells. Proc Am Assoc Cancer Res 1994; 35:A261.

Kurobe M, Takei Y, Ezawa H, et al: Increased level of basic fibroblast growth factor (bFGF) in sera of patients with malignant tumors. Horm Metab Res 1993; 25:395–396.

Luo JC, Yu MW, Chen CJ, et al: Serum c-erbB-2 oncopeptide in hepatocellular carcinogenesis. Med Sci Res 1993; 21:305–307.

Moodie SA, Willumsen BM, Weber MJ, Wolfman A: Complexes of Ras·GTP with Raf-1 and mitogen-activated protein kinase kinase. Science 1993; 260:1588.

Mori S, Mori Y, Mukaiyama T, et al: In vitro and in vivo release of soluble erbB-2 protein from human carcinoma cells. Jpn J Cancer Res 1990; 81:489–494.

Nedvidkova J, Nemec J, Stolba P, et al: Epidermal growth factor (EGF) in serum of patients with differentiated carcinoma of thyroid. Neoplasma 1992; 39:11–14.

Niman HL, Thompson AMH, Yu A, et al: Anti-peptide antibodies detect oncogene-related proteins in urine. Proc Natl Acad Sci U S A 1985; 82:7924–7928.

Pawlikowski M, Cicslak D, Stepien H, et al: Elevated blood serum levels of epidermal growth factor in some patients with gastric cancer. Endokrynol Pol 1989; 40:149–153.

Pimentel E: Oncogenes, 2nd ed. Boca Raton, Florida, CRC Press, 1989.

Pincus MR, Chung DL, Dykes DC, et al: Pathways for activation of the *ras*-oncogene-encoded p21 protein. Ann Clin Lab Sci 1992; 22: 323–342.

Pincus MR, van Renswoude J, Harford JB, et al: Prediction of the three-dimensional structure of the transforming region of the EJ/T24 human bladder oncogene product and its normal cellular homologue. Proc Natl Acad Sci U S A 1983; 80:5253.

Rosanelli GP, Wirnsberger GH, Purstner P, et al: DNA flow cytometry and immunohistochemical demonstration of mutant p53 protein versus TPS and mutant p53 protein serum levels in human breast cancer. Proc Am Assoc Cancer Res 1993; 34:A1353.

Shirai Y, Kawata S, Ito N, et al: Elevated levels of plasma transforming growth factor-β in patients with hepatocellular carcinoma. Jpn J Cancer Res 1992; 83:676–679.

Slamon DJ, Godolphin W, Jones LA, et al: Studies on the HER-2/*neu* proto-oncogene in human breast and ovarian cancer. Science 1989; 224:707–712.

Sorenson GD, Pribish DM, Valone FH, et al: Soluble normal and mutated DNA sequences from single-copy genes in human blood. Cancer Epidemiol Biomarkers Prev 1994; 3:67–71.

Soussi T, Legros Y, Lubin R, et al: Multifactorial analysis of p53 alteration in human cancer: A review. Int J Cancer 1994; 57:1–9.

Stokoe D, MacDonald SG, Cadwallader K, et al: Activation of Raf as a result of recruitment to the plasma membrane. Science 1994; 264:1463.

Virji MA, Rosendale B, Piper M, et al: Circulating levels of a mutant p53 protein in patients with hepatocellular carcinoma. Proc Am Assoc Cancer Res 1992; 33:A1508.

Weissfeld JL, Larsen RD, Niman HL, et al: Evaluation of oncogene-related proteins in serum. Cancer Epidemiol Biomarkers Prev 1994; 3:57–62.

Wu JT, Astill ME, Zhang P: Detection of the extracellular domain of c-erbB-2 oncoprotein in sera from patients with various carcinomas: Correlation with tumor markers. J Clin Lab Anal 1993; 7:31–40.

Yeh J, Yeh JC: Transforming growth factor α and human cancer. Biomed Pharmacother 1989; 43:651–660.

Yu MW, Luo JC, Brandt-Rauf PW, et al: Correlations of chronic hepatitis B virus infection and cigarette smoking with elevated expression of the neu oncoprotein in the development of hepatocellular carcinoma. Proc Am Assoc Cancer Res 1994; 35:A1754.

Chapter 16

Evaluation of Endocrine Function

John Bernard Henry, M.D.
Daniel R. Alexander, M.D.
Clifford D. Eng, M.D.

Most of the hormones of the endocrine system are discussed in this chapter, although the following hormones are described elsewhere: the hormones of calcium metabolism; parathyroid hormone and calcitonin (see Chap. 8), the hormones of glucose metabolism produced by pancreatic islet cells; insulin, glucagon, and somatostatin (see Chap. 9), hormones produced by neoplastic cells (see Chap. 45), human chorionic gonadotropin (Chap. 20), and hormones of the gastrointestinal tract (see Chap. 23). Cytokines (see Chaps. 36 and 37) are becoming increasingly recognized both as regulators and mediators of endocrine secretion as well as humoral factors themselves.

PITUITARY GLAND

The pituitary is a small gland that extends below the hypothalamus of the brain and lies within the sella turcica bones at the base of the skull. It is formed by fusion of two embryologically distinct tissues (Fig. 16–1). Neural tissue from the hypothalamus forms the infundibular stalk and the posterior pituitary (neurohypophysis). Glandular tissue from the anterior wall of Rathke's pouch forms the anterior pituitary (adenohypophysis). A rudimentary intermediate lobe derived from the posterior wall of Rathke's pouch is a vestigial gland with little known function. Because of their separate embryologic origins, the anterior and posterior lobes have different physiology in health and are each subject to unique pathologic processes.

The hypothalamus controls the secretion of hormones from the posterior and anterior lobes of the pituitary by different mechanisms (Pelletier, 1991). The secretion of posterior pituitary hormones into the blood is stimulated directly by nerve action potentials transmitted from neuron cell bodies within the hypothalamus along axons that extend down through the infundibular stalk and form nerve terminals. Oxytocin or antidiuretic hormone (vasopressin) are then stored and released from the posterior pituitary. The anterior pituitary, on the other hand, is not directly innervated by the hypothalamus. Instead, it is controlled by hypophyseotropic hormones from the hypothalamus that are delivered by the hypothalamic-hypophyseal microvascular portal plexus. The secretion of anterior and posterior pituitary hormones is regulated both by the hypothalamus and by humoral and physiologic feedback from the target organ. Thus, pituitary endocrinopathies may either be classified as primary to the pituitary gland itself or secondary to the hypothalamus or end-organ feedback mechanisms.

Anterior Pituitary Hormones

The hormones of the anterior pituitary gland are listed in Table 16–1. In addition to these six major hormones, the anterior pituitary, along with the rudimentary intermediate lobe, also produces small amounts of other neuroendocrine factors whose functions are not completely understood (Houben,

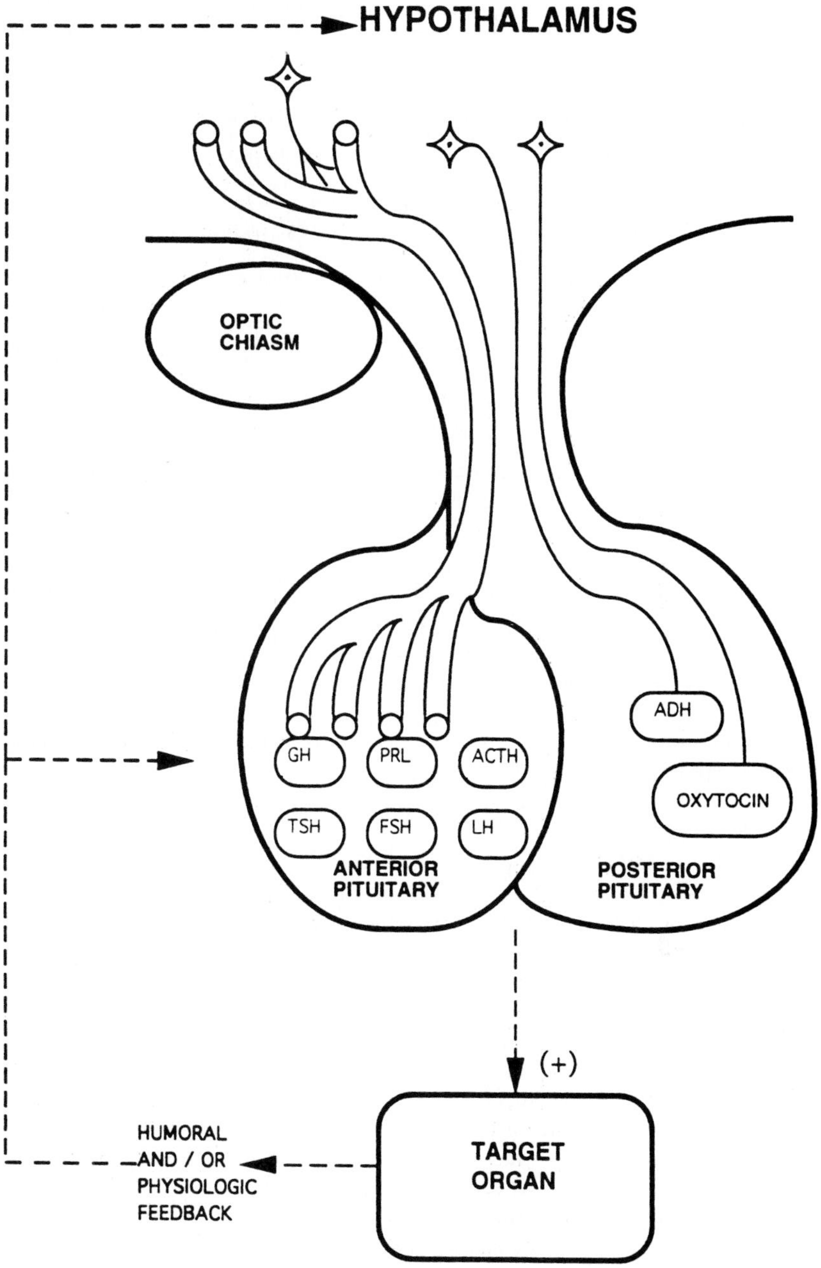

Figure 16–1. Hypothalamic neurons regulating the secretion of 1. anterior pituitary hormones by hypothalamic hormones delivered through the hypothalamic-hypophyseal portal venous plexus. 2. Posterior pituitary hormones released by neural action potentials carried along axons ending in nerve terminals in the posterior pituitary.

1994). These include β-lipotropin, β-melanocyte-stimulating hormone, endorphins, and enkephalins. These peptides are formed along with adrenocorticotropic hormone (ACTH) from the common precursor polypeptide proopiomelanocortin (POMC), as illustrated in Figure 16–2. Because of their uncertain clinical significance, these minor neuroendocrine peptides are not routinely assayed in the clinical laboratory. Growth hormone and prolactin are described here; the remaining anterior pituitary hormones are included in the discussions of their respective target organs.

Growth Hormone

Growth hormone (GH), also known as somatotropin for its growth-promoting effects on the body, is the most abundant hormone of the anterior pituitary. The major physiologic effects of GH are anabolic, promoting protein synthesis; lipolytic, stimulating fat breakdown; lactogenic; and diabetogenic by increasing resistance to insulin. Paradoxically, it also has intrinsic insulin-like hypoglycemic activity. In addition, GH stimulates the secretion of somatomedins by the liver, which along with GH itself and thyroid hormone are chondrogenic in children, stimulating linear skeletal growth. Because of its effects on linear bone growth along the epiphyseal plate, the clinical manifestations of GH secretory disorders in children may be profound. Complete absence of GH slows the rate of growth to only one third to one half of normal. Abnormally elevated levels lead to gigantism. In the adult patient with GH excess, no effects are seen in the long bones after the epiphyseal growth plates have fused. Instead, GH excess gradually produces acromegaly, a coarse thicken-

Table 16–1. HORMONES OF THE ANTERIOR PITUITARY GLAND

Hypothalamic Hormone	Pituitary Hormone	Biochemistry	Target Organ	Physiologic Effects	Feedback Hormone
GHRH (+) SS (−)	GH	polypeptide: 191a.a. 22 kDa M.W., & other molecular forms	Whole body	(+) Bone growth, (+) Protein synthesis, lipolytic, lactogenic.	IGF I (−)
Dopamine (−)	PRL	polypeptide: 199a.a. 23 kDa M.W.	Mammary gland	(+) Proliferate glandular epithelium, initiation of milk secretion.	Neural suckling reflex (+)
CRH (+) ADH (−)	ACTH	polypeptide: 39a.a. 4.5 kDa M.W.	Adrenal cortex	(+) Adrenal corticoid formation & secretion.	Cortisol (−)
TRH (+)	TSH	Glycoprotein dimer*: (α) subunit 89a.a. (β) subunit 112a.a. 28 kDa M.W.	Thyroid gland	(+) Thyroid hormone formation & secretion.	Thyroid hormones (−)
LHRH (+)	FSH	Glycoprotein dimer*: (α) subunit 89a.a. (β) subunit 115a.a. 29 kDa M.W.	Ovary Testes	(+) Growth of follicles, ovulation, secretion of estrogens. (+) Development of seminiferous tubules, spermatogenesis.	Inhibin, estradiol (−) Testosterone (−)
LHRH (+)	LH	Glycoprotein dimer*: (α) subunit 89a.a. (β) subunit 115a.a. 29 kDa M.W.	Ovary Testes	(+) Ovulation, formation of corpora leutea, secretion of progesterone. (+) Secretion of androgens.	Estradiol (−) Testosterone (−)

*Glycoprotein hormone α subunits are identical; differences in β subunits confer hormone specificity.
(+) = stimulatory; (−) = inhibitory.
GH = growth hormone; PRL = prolactin; ACTH = adrenocorticotrophic hormone; TSH = thryoid stimulating hormone; FSH = follicle stimulating hormone; LH = luteinizing hormone; GHRH = GH-releasing hormone; SS = somatostatin; CRH = corticotropin-releasing hormone; ADH = antidiuretic hormone; TRH = thyrotropin-releasing hormone; LHRH = LH-releasing hormone; IGF I = insulin-like growth factor I.

ing of the bones of the skull, hands, and feet over the course of years to decades. GH excess in adults also may be detected in the workup for diabetes mellitus. GH deficiency in adults tends to produce vague symptoms that often go unrecognized; however, when correctly diagnosed, these patients may benefit from replacement therapy (De Boer, 1995). GH hyposecretory and hypersecretory disorders are most often detected in the evaluation of lesions affecting the optic chiasm or other pituitary disorders.

The first tests developed for measuring serum GH levels were by bioassay. The most widely used bioassay still in existence employs cultures of GH-sensitive rat lymphoma cells (Nb2 cells) (Tanaka, 1980). Since this bioassay system was first described, it has been modified to improve both its specificity and sensitivity (Dattani, 1993, 1994). The bioassay remains clinically useful in determining the functional activity of variant forms of GH, including recombinant human GH. In most clinical laboratories today, the standard method for measuring serum GH levels is by radioimmunoassay (RIA) or immunoradiometric assay (IRMA). More recently, nonradioisotopic immunoassays also have been developed. Immunoassays measure the number of immunoreactive GH molecules per unit volume rather than biologic activity. Wide variations in measured GH levels have been found not only between different test methodologies, but also among different commercial kits employing similar methodology that use antibodies of differing specificities. The reason for this appears to be that different tests measure different aspects of GH biochemistry or physiology. Thus, the correct interpretation of measurements of GH either by bioassay or immunoassay requires consideration of a number of variable factors:

1. The specimen: Serum samples collected from the same patient at different times over the course of a day may show GH levels varying from undetectable to dramatically high owing to the pulsatile nature of GH secretion, its short half-life (<30 min), and the effects of physiologic factors such as sleeping, eating, and exercise.
2. The bioassay or immunoassay system: Variability in serum levels of different biochemical forms of GH, formation of GH oligomers, and the presence of cross-reacting GH variant molecules all may have different effects on test results.
3. GH-binding proteins (GHBPs): Affect not only circulating GH levels, but may also affect assay results, and in some circumstances, abnormalities of GHBPs themselves are of diagnostic importance in GH-resistant conditions.

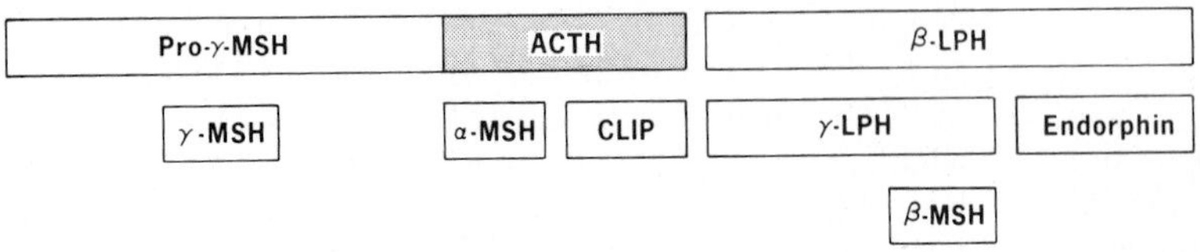

Figure 16–2. Structure of pro-opiocortin and peptides derived from it. MSH indicates melanocyte-stimulating hormone; β-LPH, lipotropin: CLIP, corticotropin-like intermediate lobe peptide.

4. Somatomedin levels: These cytokines, also known as insulin-like growth factors (IGFs) are principally affected by GH, insulin, and IGF-binding proteins; their levels, at least in part, reflect target organ responses to GH.

Thus, correct interpretation of GH levels by any of the various test methodologies currently available requires a basic knowledge of GH biochemistry and physiology.

THE SPECIMEN FOR GH LEVELS

The secretion of GH from the anterior pituitary is regulated by the hypothalamus from above, as well as by humoral and physiologic feedback from target organs below. Hypothalamic neurons secrete both GH-releasing hormone (GHRH), which stimulates the synthesis and secretion of GH and somatostatin, which inhibits GH release. These two hypothalamic hormones travel to the anterior pituitary through hypothalamic-hypophyseal portal venous plexus. GH released from the anterior pituitary also circulates back through the portal plexus to the hypothalamus, where it may reciprocally exert negative feedback inhibition. Once secreted, GH exerts its effects both directly on target organs such as bone and muscle, as well as indirectly, through the somatomedins, a family of insulin-like growth factor (IGF) hormones produced mainly by the liver. In particular, somatomedin C (IGF-I) is essential for bone growth during childhood. The importance of IGF in promoting skeletal growth is demonstrated by a subclass of dwarfs first described by Laron (1966) who were found to have elevated GH but markedly decreased IGF levels. IGFs also circulate back to the pituitary and hypothalamus, where they exert negative-feedback inhibition on GH release (Trainer, 1994). Clinically, IGF levels are commonly measured along with GH, not only to exclude Laron dwarfism but also because they act as an in vivo bioassay reflecting target organ response to GH.

In addition to the humoral feedback pathways that regulate GH secretion, a number of physiologic mechanisms also affect the release of GH from the anterior pituitary (Hartman, 1993). GH secretion follows a circadian rhythm characterized by discontinuous, pulsatile secretory bursts with intervening periods during the day when GH levels are undetectable. Sleep may be the strongest physiologic stimulus for GH secretion. At night, there are typically one or two major bursts of GH secretion that begin one to two hours after the onset of sleep. Other physiologic stimuli or GH secretion include physical and emotional stress, exercise, surgery, high-protein meals, and hypoglycemia. Hyperglycemia inhibits GH secretion. In children affected by emotional deprivation, GH secretion is inhibited, resulting in growth retardation. Age is another important factor; GH secretion is high at birth and generally declines with age, with the exception of a second increase in secretion during the growth spurt of early adolescence. Gender is also important; young women typically have serum GH levels that are 50% higher than that of age-matched males. Moreover, GH levels in women tend to be much higher during the late follicular phase of the menstrual cycle than at other times of the month.

Because of the pulsatile and sporadic nature of GH secretion during the course of a day and its short half-life, single random serum levels for GH generally do not yield clinically useful information. To overcome this problem, GH can be measured in terms of total micrograms secreted/24 hours. To do this, blood must be collected every 20 to 30 mins, the serum immediately separated and frozen until the time of assay. By this rather cumbersome technique, detailed information about not only the total 24-hour secretion but also the diurnal pattern of secretion can be obtained. However, in the low-normal range, considerable overlap in total 24-hour serum GH levels may occur between normal and hypopituitary patients (Reutens, 1995).

In order to avoid this time-consuming and labor-intensive specimen collection process, strategies have been developed to obtain meaningful information about GH levels from a more limited number of collected blood specimens. One way of doing this is by using urine as a reflection of the serum levels over the previous several hours (Aman, 1994; Main, 1994). There have been concerns about applying RIA and IRMA test kits intended for use on serum samples for GH determinations in urine, in part because urinary GH levels are only a small fraction of those in serum and also because GH is not only excreted but also metabolized by the kidney. However, using an IRMA test kit specific for the 22-kDa form of GH, the GH detected in urine was found to have the same elution pattern as the GH control standards (Mauri, 1993). In that study, urinary GH levels predictably correlated with serum levels in both normal and acromegalic patients, suggesting that urinary GH levels may be useful clinically as a simple screening tests for acromegaly. Similarly, a nonradioisotopic assay of urinary GH levels showed good correlation with serum levels and also demonstrated reliable clinical utility in distinguishing normal from acromegalic patients (Turner, 1993). When using a single urine sample to identify GH deficiency in children, a diagnostic sensitivity of 70% and specificity of 96% has been reported (Skinner, 1993); a major source of variation in measured urinary GH levels was found to be related to physiologic variations in total renal protein excretion. Both the sensitivity and specificity of the assay could be improved by making determinations on multiple urine specimens.

Another alternative to collecting multiple serum specimens for GH levels is the use of various provocative tests that employ physiologic or pharmacologic stimuli to induce GH secretion. Insulin-induced hypoglycemia is a strong stimulus for GH secretion that is used in clinical testing. After determining baseline levels of glucose and GH, intravenous insulin is administered to an endpoint of serum glucose of less than 40 mg/dL or symptomatic hypoglycemia. Fifty-percent dextrose solutions should be readily available to reverse severe hypoglycemic symptoms. Three consecutive blood samples are then collected at 30-minute intervals for GH and glucose determinations. An inadequate rise in GH levels suggests GH insufficiency but does not distinguish between hypothalamic and pituitary lesions. The sensitivity and specificity of this test has been reported to be 64% and 70%, respectively (Dattani, 1992). To distinguish between hypothalamic and pituitary etiologies of GH deficiency, L-dopa, which stimulates release of GHRH from the hypothalamus, and GHRH, a potent direct-acting GH secretagogue can also be used as differential stimuli in provocative GH testing (Chevenne, 1993). Other tests employ exercise or intravenous arginine infusion as secretory stimuli to compare post-stimulation GH levels to baseline.

Alternatively, the physiologic suppressive effect of hyperglycemia may be used to confirm GH hypersecretion. After drawing fasting baseline GH and glucose levels, a 100-gram dose of glucose is administered orally, followed by subsequent blood levels drawn one and two hours later. Failure of GH levels to drop is consistent with autonomous hypersecretion. The cutoff levels for both provocative and suppressive tests of GH secretion used to distinguish normal from abnormal results need to be established separately for each laboratory depending on the GH assay method used. The reason for this procedure is that the different antibodies used in immunoassays have varying specificities for the different heterogeneous forms of GH (Banfi, 1991), as described subsequently.

ASSAY TECHNIQUES FOR GH

Biochemically, several forms of GH are known to occur in humans. GH variants may differ in molecular weight and the number of amino acid residues. They may differ by amino acid side chain glycosylation, acylation, or desamidation. In addition, GH molecules may occur as monomeric peptides or form dimers, trimers, or larger oligomers. They may circulate free in the serum, or bound to a number of different GH-binding proteins. Additional GH variants produced by the placenta share amino acid homology with the major form of GH produced by the pituitary; they have similar affinity for GH-binding proteins (Evain-Brion, 1994), and similar somatotropic biological activities (MacLeod, 1991). Placental GH variants can be distinguished from pituitary GH by immunoassays using specific monoclonal antibodies. However, they may compete with pituitary GH for binding to the polyclonal antibodies used in some RIA kits. Low levels of placental GH in pregnancy correlate with intrauterine growth retardation.

At least five different forms of GH that vary in molecular weight and number of amino acid residues have been identified (Lewis, 1994). The major form of GH produced by the pituitary is 191 amino acid residues in length, with a molecular weight of 22 kDa. This form, which possesses all of the known biological activities of GH, is often but not always the predominant form found in serum. A 20-kDa form, produced by alternative splicing of precursor mRNA, has nearly the same direct acting growth-promoting and lactogenic biological activity. It is almost as active as the 22-kDa form in its ability to increase serum IGF-1 levels in hypophysectomized rats (Kostyo, 1987). However, it binds to GH receptors on human liver only very weakly (McCarter, 1990), and has only a fraction of the insulin-like activity of the 22-kDa form (Smal, 1986). Moreover, the 20-kDa variant may be carried in the circulation on a different binding protein than the one that carries the 22-kDa form (Baumann, 1990). In acromegaly and other conditions in which GH secretion is increased, it appears that the 22-kDa and 20-kD forms are secreted in a relatively constant proportion of approximately 5:1 (Baumann, 1986b). A comparison of two immunoenzymometric assays using either monoclonal antibodies specific for 22-kDa GH only or for both the 22-kDa and 20-kDa forms demonstrated a correlation coefficient of 0.99 between the two tests, with no diagnostic discrepancies in distinguishing patients with growth retardation or acromegaly from normal individuals (Vieira, 1992).

Under unstimulated, basal conditions between secretory bursts of GH from the pituitary, other GH variants may predominate in the circulation (Baumann, 1985). In particular, about 85% of GH molecules measured in serum specimens drawn during the day are 17-kDa fragments (Warner, 1993). Because the 17-kDa form accounts for less than 1% of the GH in the pituitary, it has been hypothesized that it may be formed by proteolytic cleavage of the 22-kDa form after it has been secreted (Sinha, 1994). The 17-kDa form exhibits much stronger activity in blocking the effects of insulin as compared with the 22-kDa form, while completely lacking its growth-promoting and insulin-like effects. Physiologically, it may act to help maintain blood glucose levels in the fasting state. In excess, it may contribute to the pathogenesis of insulin-resistant forms of diabetes. An immunoassay using antibodies specific for 17-kDa GH but not other GH forms has been developed (Sinha, 1994). However, its use in clinical diagnosis awaits further advances in our understanding of the role of 17-kDa GH in health and disease. Depending on the nature of the antibodies used in the various commercially available immunoassay kits, 17-kDa GH may or may not be detected along with the somatotropically active forms of GH. Other minor forms of GH in the serum include a glycosylated 27-kDa form and a 5-kDa fragment. Deamidated and acylated acidic variants of the 22-kDa GH molecule account for about 8% of serum GH.

GH molecules may circulate either as monomeric peptides or as dimers, trimers, or larger high molecular weight oligomers. Oligomeric peptides of GH generally form by noncovalent binding after being released from the pituitary, although some may occur as covalently bound dimers formed within the pituitary. Homodimers (20 to 20 kDa, 22 to 22 kDa) as well as heterodimers (20 to 22 kDa) may form (Brostedt, 1989). Most GH molecules circulate as monomers; about 45% occur as dimers or larger oligomers. The biological significance of the oligomeric forms of GH is uncertain; they may have increased circulating half-lives owing to delayed metabolic clearance. Synthetic GH dimers appear to have significantly less biological activity than monomeric forms (Becker, 1987). Of diagnostic significance, measured concentrations of native and recombinant GH samples containing mixtures of monomeric and dimeric GH forms using different commercially available RIA and IRMA kits gave results that varied with the cross-reactivity of dimeric form (Bowsher, 1990). The polyclonal RIA kits tested in that study gave higher results than the monoclonal IRMA kit (Hybritech, San Diego, CA), which showed higher specificity for the more biologically active monomeric form. However, the Hybritech kit, in contrast to other IRMAs, does not detect the 20-kDa GH variant (Celniker, 1989).

THE ROLE OF GH-BINDING PROTEINS

Other higher-molecular weight forms of circulating GH occur by complexing with GH-binding proteins (GHBP). GHBPs share amino acid homology with cellular GH receptors and have slightly lower GH-binding affinity. Laron dwarfs have decreased levels of both cellular GH receptors and circulating GHBPs, suggesting that they are both encoded by a common gene (Carlsson, 1994b; Rosenfeld, 1994). Different mutations producing subtypes of Laron dwarfism characterized by either quantitatively decreased or qualitatively abnormal GH receptors and GHBPs have been described (Francke, 1993), and tests for detecting heterozygous carriers by restriction fragment length polymorphism analysis have been developed (Berg, 1994). The receptor-like GHBP, as well as GH receptors on the liver, which both have a high affinity for 22-kDa GH, only very weakly bind to the 20-kDa form. Instead, about 25% of the 20-kDa form circulates bound to a different protein that does not have affinity for 22-kDa GH (Baumann, 1990). This 20-kDa GHBP is present in normal levels in Laron dwarfs. The GH receptor–like GHBP is a 61-kDa glycoprotein; when complexed with GH, its apparent mass increases to 80 to 85 kDa (Baumann, 1986a). About 45% of serum 22-kDa GH is bound to GHBPs; the rest circulate as free monomers, dimers, or other oligomers. The placental GH variant also binds to GHBP with an affinity similar to that of the 22-kDa pituitary GH (Baumann, 1991). The serum levels of total GHBP are stable over the course of a day; however, the relative proportion that forms GH-GHBP complexes varies with secretory bursts of GH (Carlsson, 1993). In patients with acromegaly, GHBP levels may be normal (Baumann, 1993) or decreased (Amit, 1992; Mercado, 1993). The biological significance of these GHBPs is unclear. The major effect may be to increase GH bioactivity by prolonging its half life; it has been estimated that the circulating half-life of free GH is about 7 minutes, whereas the half-life of GHBP-bound GH is about 29 minutes, with a combined half-life of mixed bound and free GH *in vivo* of about 18 minutes (Veldhuis, 1993). GHBPs may act by retaining GH in the serum, preventing its metabolism and clearance and keeping it from extravasating into the interstitial space (Herington, 1991). A secondary minor effect of circulating GHBPs is that they compete with cellular GH receptors for GH; thus, only unbound GH is biologically active (Mannor, 1991). The levels of GH-binding protein have been found to vary considerably between individuals. Neither RIA nor IRMA immunoassays are significantly affected by the presence of GHBPs because the antibodies used in these assays generally have a much higher affinity for GH than do GHBPs, and so they tend to measure the total amount of GH present in the sample (Jan, 1991). However, another study did report interference from GHBPs when GH immunoassays were performed (Chapman, 1994). GHBPs are known to cause decreases in GH levels determined by radioreceptor assays, which have a similar binding affinity for GH as the GHBPs.

GHBPs may be assayed in the evaluation of Laron dwarfism and other GH-resistant conditions. Moreover, studies of serum GHBP may be used as an indirect reflection of cellular GH receptor abnormalities or deficiencies without obtaining a liver biopsy. GHBP may be assayed by incubating serum with radiolabeled GH and then separating the bound and unbound GH; GHBP concentration and binding affinity can then be determined by Scatchard analysis (Baumann, 1994). Ligand-mediated immunofunctional assay (Carlsson, 1991) and RIA (Carmignac, 1992) studies of GHBPs have also been developed. The normal range of serum GHBPs varies widely among normal adults and depends on test methodology (Mercado, 1993). A comparative analysis of these different GHBP assay systems is described in a review by Carlsson (1994a).

In summary, laboratory methods of assaying serum GH levels include bioassay, radioreceptor assay, radioimmunoassay, immunometric radioassay, and sandwich enzyme-linked immunosorbent assay (ELISA). Bioassays, alluded to previously, remain in use as a research tool but generally are not available through clinical reference laboratories. Instead, commercial laboratories now use a variety of immunoassays. Competitive radioimmunoassay kits employ a known quantity of radiolabeled GH that competes with an unknown quantity of GH in the serum sample for limited number of binding sites on either polyclonal or monoclonal antibodies. RIA kits using antibodies specific for different GH epitopes may yield varying results on the same specimen partly because epitopes may be concealed by the formation of GH dimers or GH-GHBP complexes (Chatelain, 1990).

2

GH molecules have a number of different antigenic epitopes, some of which are associated with its biological activity (Strasburger, 1994). The biologically active epitopes can be detected by radioreceptor assays (RRA), which are a sort of hybrid between the biological assay and RIA, in which biologically active epitopes on a known quantity of radiolabeled GH compete with an unknown quantity of GH of unknown antigenic structure in the serum sample for binding to cellular GH receptors *in situ* (Friesen, 1990). Case reports of abnormal GH forms in pituitary dwarfs that do not bind to cellular receptors (low levels by RRA) but retain immunoreactive epitopes detectable as normal levels by RIA have been described (Valenta, 1985). However, these cases of discrepancies between RRA and RIA measurements are decidedly rare (Ilondo, 1991).

The sensitivity and specificity of immunoassays can be increased by using a sandwich with one antibody bound to a solid substrate to capture the hormone and a second labeled soluble antibody to detect it. The soluble antibody may be labeled with a radioisotope (IRMA), an enzyme (ELISA), or a chemiluminescent marker. A comparison of some commercial kits using these different techniques is shown in Table 16–2. The most recently developed GH immunoassays give a one- to two-log improvement in the lower limits of sensitivity, down to as low as 1 to 2 ng/L. These high-sensitivity tests include a sandwich ELISA specific for the 22-kDa form of GH (Yuki, 1994) and a modified version of the commercially available Nichols Luma Tag GH chemiluminescence immunometric assay (Chapman, 1994). However, given the amount of overlap that occurs in the 100- to 300-ng/L range between some normal and hypopituitary patient populations (Reutens, 1995), the added diagnostic value of these high-sensitivity tests remains uncertain.

Differences in GH immunoassay results due to serum or buffer matrix effects and to different calibration standards have also been reported (Celnicker, 1989). Pituitary-derived reference standards are composed of a mixture of GH forms, whereas recombinant GH consists only of purified monomeric 22-kDa GH. To control for these differences, purified 22-kDa GH monomer has been recommended as a reference standard for calibrating different assay systems regardless of whether or not they are specific for the 22-kDa form only (Banfi, 1992). As with most other tests, individual laboratories must establish their own reference intervals for the particular GH assay used and how it is performed.

Finally, one must be aware of the potential for endogenously occurring antibodies in a patient's specimen that may cross-react in immunoassays, yielding anomalous results. In some circumstances, these autoantibodies may have impor-

Table 16–2. COMPARISON OF COMMERCIAL GH IMMUNOASSAY KITS

Assay Kit	Antibody	Measures Free 22-kDa Monomers?	Measures 20 kDa GH?	Measures GH Bound To GHBP?	Measures GH Dimers and Other Oligomers?
Cambridge RIA, Billerica, MA	Polyclonal	Yes	Yes[1]	Yes[2]	Yes[4]
Kallestad RIA, Austin, TX	Polyclonal	Yes	Yes[1]	?	Partly[4]
Hybritech, IRMA, San Diego, CA	Monoclonal	Yes	No[1]	Yes[2]	No[4]
Nichols IRMA, San Juan Capistrano, CA	Monoclonal	Yes	Partly[1]	Yes[2]/No[3]	?

Data compiled from 1. Celnicker, 1989; 2. Jan, 1991; 3. Chapman, 1994; and 4. Bowsher, 1990.

tant pathologic significance; their presence may be demonstrated by displacement radiobinding assay or ELISA. Autoantibodies may cause GH-deficiency if they are directed against the GH molecule (Llera, 1993), or they may produce the clinical manifestations of GH excess by acting as a GH agonist if they have specificity for GH receptors (Campino, 1992). With the advent of recombinant (r) GH for therapeutic use, antibodies directed against methionyl-rGH may form (Massa, 1993), whereas the nonmethionylated authentic rGH has much lower immunogenicity (Lundin, 1991).

THE SOMATOMEDINS

The somatomedins, or IGFs, are a family of cytokines induced by GH that mediate the chondrogenic effects of GH in promoting long bone growth and also feed back to the hypothalamic-pituitary axis, where they inhibit GH secretion. Thus, normal levels of IGF suggest normal GH levels. High IGF levels reflect increased GH secretion occurring independently of regulatory controls. Low IGF levels may reflect either low GH levels, biologically inactive GH forms, or unresponsiveness of the target cells to normal GH, usually due to a GH receptor defect as in Laron dwarfism. Because of this physiologic link between GH and IGF, they may be assayed together in the evaluation of suspected GH secretory disorders. As the name implies, IGFs have partial amino acid homology with the proinsulin peptide and also have insulin-like bioactivity, which may become important in the treatment of insulin-resistant diabetics, as well as in the treatment of GH-resistant conditions.

The biochemistry and physiology of IGFs is at least as complex as that of GH; there are two major forms, IGF I and IGF II that interact with a family of six different binding proteins, IGFBP-1 through IGFBP-6 (Jones, 1995). IGFs are produced by the liver and many other cells, including osteoblasts. Physiologic stimuli and hormones other than GH also affect serum IGF I levels. Because IGF I levels are not exclusively regulated by GH, the ability of IGF-I to distinguish between GH deficient and normal patients may have diagnostic limitations (Reutens, 1995). Serum levels of IGF I are probably of greatest diagnostic value in identifying GH-resistant conditions and in predicting and monitoring a patient's response to GH replacement therapy (Blum, 1994).

GH stimulates the release of IGF I, the more somatotropically active somatomedin, predominantly from the liver. In the blood, IGF I circulates mainly bound to IGFBP-3, which prolongs its half-life and influences its biological activity. Assays for both IGF I and IGF II, as well as for the IGFBPs, are commercially available for use in clinical diagnosis. Because IGFs and IGFBPs bind to each other, they mutually occupy biologically important antigenic epitopes and interfere with most immunoassays. Therefore, various separation techniques have been developed for isolating IGFs from IGFBPs in the serum specimen (Holly, 1994). IGF levels can then be determined using RIA, IRMA, or ELISA techniques that have specificity for IGF I or IGF II. Similar techniques may be applied to determining IGFBP levels. However, IGFs may reciprocally interfere with the IGFBP assay. Because IGFs and IGFBPs interfere with each others' measurement, the accuracy of immunoassays must be validated by demonstrating parallelism of serial dilutions with a standard reference curve or by other confirmatory tests (Bang, 1995).

Prolactin

Prolactin occurs as a number of heterogeneic biochemical forms that share partial amino acid homology with growth hormone and the placental GH variant (placental lactogen). Accordingly, it also shares many of the physiologic properties of these previously described hormones. In nonpregnant women, both prolactin and GH contribute to the total serum lactogenic activity as determined by bioassay. In pregnant women, placental lactogen is the main source of total serum lactogenic bioactivity (Maddox, 1991).

Prolactin's main target organ is the adult female mammary gland. During pregnancy, it helps promote glandular enlargement; after delivery, it initiates and maintains lactation. Increased prolactin bioactivity stimulated by breast feeding acts to suppress ovulation. In males, prolactin may play a role in the growth and development of the prostate (Costello, 1994). Prolactin may also have a physiologic role in immunoregulation (Lindstedt, 1994); practical applications for this aspect of prolactin's biological activity have already been put to use in the Nb2 rat lymphoma cell bioassay (Tanaka, 1980).

Pathologic hypersecretion of prolactin is associated with hypogonadism in both sexes. In women, ovulation may be suppressed with resultant oligomenorrhea or amenorrhea and infertility. Galactorrhea is also common. In men, inhibition of testosterone synthesis by hyperprolactinemia may lead to decreased spermatogenesis and infertility. Galactorrhea may also occasionally occur in affected males. Other metabolic manifestations of hyperprolactinemia include decreased bone density, hyperinsulinemia, glucose intolerance, and psychiatric disturbances, including anxiety disorders and depression. Prolactin deficiency may be associated with impaired lactation following childbirth (Falk, 1992). Otherwise, there are no distinctive clinical syndromes associated with hypoprolactinemia, a condition that is most often recognized in the evaluation of other hypopituitary conditions.

Prolactin secretion is inhibited by dopamine released from hypothalamic neurons and is induced by afferent neurons traveling up ascending tracts of the spinal cord that are stimulated by breast feeding. Ultimately, these afferent stimuli activate serotonergic pathways within the hypothalamus that produce prolactin-releasing factors, including vasoactive intestinal peptide (VIP), thyrotropin-releasing hormone (TRH), and other neuroendocrine factors that are carried by portal vessels to the anterior pituitary (Moltich, 1992). Accordingly, medications such as dopamine blockers and serotonin reuptake inhibitors increase prolactin levels, whereas the dopamine agonist bromocriptine is used to decrease prolactin sercretion. Lesions affecting the hypothalamus or infundibular stalk lead to disinhibition of prolactin secretion that is normally suppressed by dopamine, resulting in hyperprolactinemia associated with deficiencies of other anterior pituitary hormones. Thus, in hyperprolactinemia associated with the radiologic finding of a lesion involving the pituitary, one may not be able to distinguish between the differential diagnosis of a true prolactinoma and disinhibition of the hypothalamic-pituitary axis (Smith, 1994).

Measurement of serum prolactin levels have been used in testing for a recent unwitnessed generalized seizure or in distinguishing seizures from pseudoseizures. Essentially all generalized tonic-clonic seizures, most complex partial seizures, and some simple partial seizures cause a rise in serum prolactin levels above the upper limit of normal (Pritchard, 1991). On the other hand, absence seizures, myoclonic seizures, and pseudoseizures do not cause a significant rise in prolactin levels. A study of epileptic children demonstrated postseizure prolactin levels of 28.6 ± 2.3 ng/mL as compared with 9.8 ± 2.6 ng/mL in controls and 10.4 ± 3.8 ng/mL after a pseudoseizure (Singh, 1994).

Hyperprolactinemia may also occur in conditions in which TRH secretion is increased, as in primary hypothyroidism. The stimulatory effect of intravenous TRH has been used clinically as a provocative test of prolactin secretion. The causes of elevated serum prolactin levels are summarized in Table 16–3.

Table 16–3. CAUSES OF ELEVATED SERUM PROLACTIN LEVELS

Physiologic	Pathologic	Iatrogenic (Medications)
Exercise	Acromegaly	Metoclopramide
Neonate	Cirrhosis (alcoholic)	Methyldopa
Nursing	Empty sella syndrome	Reserpine
Pregnancy	Hypothalamic lesions	Verapamil
Sleep	1° Hypothyroidism	TRH
Stress	Nelson's syndrome	Cimetidine (intravenous)
Dietary protein	Neurogenic	Estrogens
Hypoglycemia	Pituitary prolactinomas	Opioid narcotics
	Pituitary stalk lesions	Chlorpromazine
	Renal failure	Haloperidol
	VIPoma	Serotonin-reuptake inhibitors
	Generalized seizures	

TRH = Thyrotropin-releasing hormone.

THE SPECIMEN FOR PROLACTIN LEVELS

Prolactin levels within a given individual typically fluctuate over the course of a day. Physiologic stimuli that are known to increase prolactin secretion include pregnancy (mediated by estrogen), breast feeding, sleep, dietary protein ingestion, hypoglycemia, exercise, and stress. The minor stress of venipuncture is not sufficient to alter serum levels of prolactin (Maddox, 1992a). Under basal conditions, bursts of prolactin secretion occur approximately every 95 minutes during the day, with larger bursts released shortly after the onset of sleep. Because prolactin secretory bursts occur at regular intervals and the half-life is sufficiently long (~50 minutes), a single fasting morning blood specimen may be adequate diagnostic material in evaluating hyperprolactinemia. However, single determinations of moderately increased or moderately decreased levels cannot be distinguished from normal fluctuations. These fluctuations have been found to be more widely variant in women of reproductive age than in postmenopausal women (Koenig, 1993). In these cases, a limited number of additional blood specimens drawn at different times of the day may be necessary.

Determinations of prolactin levels in urine and amniotic fluid have also been studied. The concentration of prolactin in urine is about 3 to 4 orders of magnitude lower than that of serum. However, by using concentrated urine specimens and a high sensitivity immunoassay, accurate determinations of the biologically active form of prolactin can be made (Keely, 1994). Using this technique, patients with hyperprolactinemia can be reliably distinguished from normals. In amniotic fluid, the variant forms of prolactin have been characterized (Fukuoka, 1991) and a range of reference values has been determined (Demir, 1992). However, clinical guidelines for the use of amniotic fluid prolactin measurements in diagnostic testing have not been established.

ASSAY TECHNIQUES FOR PROLACTIN

Prolactin, initially characterized as a single peptide hormone, is now being recognized as a large family of hormones of remarkable biochemical and physiologic heterogeneity. It therefore comes as no surprise that no single assay technique can always accurately reflect prolactin levels in all patients. This fact is illustrated by a study that compared measurements of serum samples for luteinizing hormone (LH), follicle-stimulating hormone (FSH), estradiol, progesterone, and prolactin made by RIA and chemiluminescence immunoassay. The correlation coefficient (r) between results of the two assays for prolactin was only 0.81, whereas for all the other hormones tested it was between 0.92 and 0.98 (Rojanasakul, 1994). Thus, a biochemical property unique to prolactin must be responsible for the unusually high disparity in results between immunoassay methods. This interassay variability can be almost completely eliminated by using monoclonal sandwich immunoassays that are calibrated against the same reference standard (Bodner, 1991; Navarro

Moreno, 1991). Thus, it is relatively easy to standardize different assays to measure the same biochemical property of the different forms of prolactin in a sample. In that case, the question must be asked, what if any additional prolactin forms in the sample are both assay systems missing?

The interpretation of immunoassays for prolactin, which measure hormone amount, is based on the assumption that the measurements closely reflect the hormone's biological activity *in vivo*. In healthy men and women who are not pregnant or lactating, prolactin measured by bioassay has been found to be consistently about 1.5 times higher than its immunoreactivity measured by IRMA, thus validating the correlation between the two tests (Maddox, 1991). However, this is not always the case. A subset of lactating women in whom postpartum ovulation was not suppressed by elevated immunoreactive prolactin levels has been identified (Campino, 1994). In these patients, prolactin measured by bioassay was significantly lower than in other lactating women whose ovulation was suppressed by similar immunoreactive prolactin levels. This suggests that either different bioactive forms of prolactin with similar immunoreactivity are present or that a second substance is enhancing the bioactivity of prolactin in one group or inhibiting it in the other. This finding may also have important clinical implications in patients breast cancer. Although prolactin levels determined by IRMA were similar between postmenopausal breast cancer patients and healthy controls, they were significantly higher by bioassay in the breast cancer group (Maddox, 1992b). In the patients with breast cancer, prolactin levels measured by bioassay were ~2.9 times higher than by IRMA, whereas the ratio of bioassay : IRMA results was ~1.3 in the healthy control group. Similarly, discrepant results in prolactin levels found to be higher by bioassay than by RIA have been reported in patients with prolactinomas (Peabody, 1992). Again, it is not known whether these discrepant results are due to prolactin variants with different bioactivities or biomodulating factors distinct from prolactin. These findings do, however, identify subsets of patients in whom immunoassay for prolactin may be considered to be unreliable and a bioassay preferable.

Prolactin hormones are known to occur as a number of different sized variants, the predominant form being 199 amino acid residues in length with a molecular weight of 23 kDa, which possesses full prolactin bioactivity. Other size variants with differing biological activities, including 16-kDa and 26-kDa (Fonseca, 1991), 27-kDa to 125-kDa (Lohrke, 1993), 150-kDa to 170-kDa (Bjoro, 1993), and 291-kD and 669-kD forms (Carlson, 1992), have also been described. The 16-kDa fragment may uniquely possess antiangiogenic bioactivity (Clapp, 1993). At least some of the higher molecular weight forms, which are detectible by RIA, have no activity measurable by the Nb2 lymphoma cells bioassay as compared with the 23-kDa form of prolactin, which is both immunoreactive and bioactive (Subramanian, 1991).

Prolactin may circulate as a monomeric peptide or may form dimers (M.W. ~50 kDa) or larger oligomers (M.W. >100 kDa). Some of the larger forms may be bound to circulating immunoglobulins (Hattori, 1992; Leite, 1992). These different forms are likely to possess different biological activities and may be produced in differing amounts in various physiologic and pathologic conditions. Larger prolactin forms are more likely to be retained intravascularly and to have delayed metabolic clearance (Carlson, 1992). These two physiologic features attributable to larger size may have opposing effects on prolactin bioactivity *in vivo* that may not be appreciable by *in vitro* bioassays. The relative amounts of the different-sized forms present may vary following pharmacologic stimulation of prolactin secretion (Bjoro, 1993) or with physiologic influences associated with advancing gestation (Fonseca, 1991) and lactation in the postpartum period (Kamel, 1993). Moreover, the predominant form of prolactin secreted in pathologic conditions of hyperprolactinemia may change following treatment (Moran, 1994). Thus, depending on the ability of a given assay to detect these different sized prolactin forms, comparisons of prolactin measurements made at different times on the same patient may or may not be reliable.

Amino acid side chains of prolactin molecules may undergo phosphorylation, sulfation, deamidation, or glycosylation. The glycosylated forms of prolactin are about 50% less bioactive and 68% less immunoreactive than nonglycosylated forms (Hoffmann, 1992). Most prolactin *in vivo* in both healthy people and in those with prolactinomas is in the nonglycosylated form. Using an immunoassay with monoclonal antibodies specific for glycosylated epitopes on the prolactin molecule, the relative amount of nonglycosylated prolactin has been found to increase slightly as pregnancy advances, from ~76% in non-pregnant and first trimester patients up to ~85% in the last trimester of pregnancy (Brue, 1992). Similarly, when prolactin is secreted in other stimulatory conditions, either during spontaneous or pharmacologically induced secretory bursts, the proportion of non-glycosylated prolactin is slightly higher (~81 to 88%) than during unstimulated periods (~71%).

Pituitary prolactin forms also share biochemical and physiologic similarities to placental lactogen. Although it is not generally a problem in immunoassays, cross-reactivity with placental lactogen in bioassays for prolactin may produce spurious results. Prolactin is also produced by cells of the decidual endometrium, which is stimulated by increased progesterone secretion during days 22 to 28 of the menstrual cycle (Handwerger, 1991). This extrapituitary source of prolactin may contribute to the finding that women in their reproductive years generally have higher prolactin levels than postmenopausal women. Accordingly, diagnostic testing must take into account a number of variables in order to arrive at a clinically useful interpretation of serum prolactin levels.

Other factors that are also known to result in anomalous or aberrant immunoassay measurements of prolactin levels should be considered. These include the possible presence of antiprolactin autoantibodies in the serum sample, and the prozone effect. The prozone or so-called "hook" effect may occur, whereby very high prolactin levels appear low or undetectable until the serum is diluted. This phenomenon has been reported to occur in immunoassays using two antibodies in a sandwich technique (Comtois, 1993; Haller, 1992). Finally, antiprolactin autoantibodies have been detected in some patients as a cause of biochemical hyperprolactinemia, which may or may not be associated with clinical signs of excess prolactin bioactivity. The biological roles of antiprolactin antibodies that have been speculated on but not proven include a low affinity intravascular prolactin storage reservoir, a regulator of prolactin's immunomodulatory function, or a manifestation of a pathologic autoimmune process. In some cases, it may be a functionally benign phenomenon similar to macroamylasemia. In any case, there is little doubt that to varying degrees, these autoantibodies compete with the antibodies used in some immunoassay systems to yield falsely low prolactin levels (Hattori, 1994). Antiprolactin autoantibodies are detectible in serum either by immunosorbent radioassay or the polyethylene-glycol precipitation assay, in which the autoantibody is first dissociated from any endogenous prolactin that may be bound to it and then assayed for by adding exogenous radiolabeled prolactin. It has been suggested that an assay for antiprolactin autoantibodies be performed on every specimen yielding elevated prolactin levels (Lindstedt, 1994). Continued improvements in clinical laboratory studies of prolactin await further advances in our understanding of its complex and diverse biochemistry and physiology.

Posterior Pituitary Hormones

Oxytocin and vasopressin are the two major hormones of the posterior pituitary. They each have distinct physiologic roles, with partly overlapping effects in stimulating smooth muscle contraction and in maintaining water homeostasis. They are both small oligopeptides, each composed of nine amino acid residues, with a total mass of about 1 kDa. They are synthesized in nerve cell bodies within the hypothalamus and are transported along axons to nerve terminals within the posterior pituitary, where they are stored in secretory granules. Neural action potentials conducted along these nerve tracts from the hypothalamus cause the storage vesicles within the nerve terminals of the posterior pituitary to degranulate and release oxytocin and vasopressin into the circulation. It must be kept in mind that unlike the anterior pituitary, the posterior pituitary is little more than a storage site where hormones are held until they are secreted. Accordingly, traumatic disruption of the infundibular stalk or destruction or removal of the posterior pituitary does not necessarily result in complete loss of these hormones, which are produced in the hypothalamus.

Oxytocin

Oxytocin secretion is stimulated by stretching of the uterus during labor and delivery and by breast feeding. In addition, some of the stimuli known to cause vasopressin release may also cause secretion of oxytocin. Oxytocin's main effect is to stimulate smooth muscle contraction. In women of reproductive age, its effects are directed toward the uterus during labor and delivery, and toward the myoepithelial cells of mammary gland ducts to cause milk ejection. Extrapituitary synthesis of oxytocin by the amnion, chorion, and decidua may also play a role in the normal physiology of parturition (Chibbar, 1993). In males, oxytocin appears to have a role in gonadal and sexual functions (Argiolas, 1993; Nicholson, 1993).

Pathologic conditions associated with oxytocin excess or deficiency necessitating its measurement in the laboratory are rare. It may be a useful test in some pregnant patients for predicting premature onset of labor (Behrens, 1991). Oxytocin levels have also been found to increase following a seizure (Meierkord, 1994); this may be useful, along with other pituitary hormones, as a marker for an unwitnessed seizure. Finally, tumors that produce ectopic oxytocin have been identified, including oat cell carcinoma of the lung and adenocarcinoma of the pancreas (North, 1993).

Oxytocin is secreted in pulsatile bursts during delivery and lactation. Under basal conditions however, pulsatile secretion does not occur (Challinor, 1994), making single random blood samples adequate specimens for oxytocin levels. In women of reproductive age, plasma oxytocin levels do not vary significantly with the menstrual cycle but are likely to be higher and more variable during pregnancy (Stock, 1991). Given its limited role, oxytocin deficiency is probably not recognized as a clinical syndrome; however, its secretion can be stimulated by using insulin-induced hypoglycemia as a provocative test (Chiodera, 1992).

2

Oxytocin has a half-life of only 3 to 5 minutes in plasma and is subject to rapid degradation by oxytocinase. Therefore, once collected, blood samples for oxytocin levels should be transported to the laboratory on ice, and the serum separated and frozen until the assay is performed. Because the normal serum level of oxytocin may be as low as 1 ng/L, it is often undetectable without a preceding extraction procedure such as by affinity chromatography (Torok, 1994). Oxytocin in serum can be quantified by bioassay or RIA.

Vasopressin

Vasopressin is also known as antidiuretic hormone (ADH), and in accordance with these two names, it has two important physiologic functions. It has vasopressor effects mediated by contraction of arterial smooth muscle, and it also has antidiuretic effects mediated by promoting renal water reabsorbtion from the cortical collecting ducts. In addition, it also promotes reabsorbtion of sodium and chloride in the thick ascending limb of the loop of Henle. The regulation of ADH secretion is controlled by osmoreceptors within the central nervous system (CNS) and low- and high-pressure baroreceptors located in the right atrium and carotid sinuses, respectively. In concert with atrial natriuretic factor and the renin-angiotensin-aldosterone axis, these hormones all work together to maintain blood pressure, volume, and tonicity. Accordingly, when evaluating a patient for a disorder of water homeostasis, these multiple interactive factors need to be taken into consideration (see Chaps. 4 and 7).

Biochemically, ADH is very similar to oxytocin, differing by only two amino acid substitutions. One of these is in position 8, where ADH has an L-arginine residue, hence the name arginine vasopressin (AVP). This feature distinguishes human ADH from the porcine ADH, which has a lysine residue at that position, and also from the synthetic form, which has a D-arginine substitution at that position, giving it decreased vasopressor effects. Deamination makes D-AVP more resistant to metabolic degradation. This synthetic form of ADH, known as dD-AVP, which has greater antidiuretic activity and less vasopressor activity than native human ADH, is clinically useful as a long-acting therapeutic agent.

Disturbances in water metabolism due to disorders of ADH excess or deficiency are classically manifested as the syndrome of inappropriate ADH secretion (SIADH) and diabetes insipidus, respectively. The differential diagnosis of these two conditions by laboratory testing is summarized in Table 16–4.

Table 16–4. TESTS IN THE DIFFERENTIAL DIAGNOSIS OF DISORDERS OF WATER HOMEOSTASIS

	Baseline			After 12 Hour Fluid Restriction			
Disorder	*Serum Na^+ and Osm*	*Urine Na^+ and Osm*	*Serum ADH*	*Serum Na^+ and Osm*	*Urine Na^+ and Osm*	*Serum ADH*	*Urine Osm Post AVP Challenge*
Normal Control	N	N	N	N	High	High	Same
SIADH	Low	N–High	High	Low–N	High	High	Same
Neurogenic DI	N–High	Low	Low	High	Low–N	Low	Increased
Nephrogenic DI	N–High	Low	N–High	High	Low–N	High	Same
Psychogenic Polydipsia	Low–N	Low	Low	N	N–High	N–High	Same

SIADH = Syndrome of inappropriate antidiuretic hormone secretion; DI = diabetes insipidus; Osm = osmolality; ADH = antidiuretic hormone; AVP = arginine vasopressin; N = normal.

The patient with SIADH presents with severe hyponatremia associated with inappropriately high urine osmolality. This most often occurs as a paraneoplastic syndrome associated with a number of different malignancies, especially lung cancer, but may also occur with other lung diseases, CNS trauma or infection, or secondary to other endocrine disorders (North, 1993). Medications including vinca alkaloids, cyclophosphamide, carbamazepine, clofibrate, tricyclic antidepressants, and MAO inhibitors may also cause excess ADH secretion. Physiologic stimuli known to increase ADH secretion include nausea, pregnancy, hypoglycemia, intracranial hypertension, mechanical ventilation, and hypoxia. In SIADH, the serum levels of ADH may be variably increased, usually out of proportion to serum osmolality. In the right clinical setting, the diagnosis of SIADH can often be confidently made based on serum and urine electrolytes determinations alone.

Diabetes insipidus (DI) is the inverse situation, in which decreased ADH leads to excessive water loss from the kidney, resulting in hypertonic plasma associated with dilute urine. DI may be neurogenic, due to impaired secretion of ADH from the neurohypophysis, or nephrogenic, due to renal insensitivity to its presence. In both circumstances, the serum osmolality is increased, with inappropriately low urine osmolality. The two can be distinguished, however, by the response to either endogenous or exogenous vasopressin. In neurogenic DI, ADH levels are low, and the kidney rapidly acts to conserve water once exogenous ADH is administered. In contrast, nephrogenic DI is associated with normal or increased ADH levels, and administration of additional ADH has no significant effect on renal water reabsorbtion.

Nephrogenic DI may either be congenital, due most often to an X-linked receptor defect, or acquired, most commonly secondary to medications (Holtzman, 1994). Drugs known to be associated with acquired nephrogenic DI include lithium, demeclocyline, and methoxyflurane anesthetics. Other causes of acquired nephrogenic DI include hypercalcemia, hypokalemia, and amyloidosis.

Neurogenic DI may result from any number of lesions affecting the hypothalamus, including primary and metastatic tumors, trauma, stroke, or sarcoidosis. Medications that may cause neurogenic DI by suppressing ADH release from the pituitary include phenytoin, chlorpromazine, atrial natriuretic factor, alcohol, and α-adrenergic agonists. It has been speculated that autoantibodies directed against the ADH-producing cells of the hypothalamus may be responsible for some cases of idiopathic neurogenic DI (De Bellis, 1994). These antibodies are detectable by indirect immunofluorescence assay.

Another common condition in which decreased ADH levels have been found is primary nocturnal enuresis in children. Although these patients have ADH levels only slightly lower than controls (2.9 ng/L versus 3.6 ng/L), the clinical symptoms are reliably ameliorated by vasopressin supplementation therapy (Wille, 1994). Determinations of ADH levels in diagnosing this condition are not always helpful because of moderate overlap in borderline levels between enuretic and normal children. Instead, determination of first morning urine specific gravity is a more reliable test for identifying children who may benefit from ADH supplementation in the treatment of nocturnal eneuresis. Eneuretic children consistently have a urine specific gravity below 1.015, whereas nonbedwetters are able to concentrate their morning urine to a specific gravity above 1.015 (Mevorach, 1995).

ADH levels usually do not need to be measured directly because the patient's own body can be used as an *in vivo* bioassay system to test the biological response to exogenous ADH and osmotic challenges. These *in vivo* tests first require that other potentially confounding factors be excluded, so that ideally, only one factor affecting water homeostasis is being tested. Some of the confounding factors that are known to hamper the interpretation of these tests include concurrent kidney or urinary disorders, adrenal insufficiency, diabetes mellitus, thyroid disorders, and diuretics or other medications known to affect ADH secretion or function. Because these tests have the potential to exacerbate the condition being tested for, close monitoring of the patient during and shortly after testing is essential.

In SIADH, the patient's ability to suppress ADH secretion is tested by challenging with a water load to induce a hypotonic state. This test must be conducted cautiously in a controlled environment; if a moderately hyponatremic patient is challenged with a large water load, severe hyponatremia may occur. The water load test for SIADH is described subsequently. Conversely, the patient suspected of having DI is challenged by restricting water intake to test the ability to concentrate the urine by secreting and responding to ADH. Similarly, cautious monitoring is essential to avoid severe dehydration in the DI patient with persistent uncontrolled diuresis who is denied access to water. The dehydration test for DI is also described subsequently. Finally, in differentiating between neurogenic and nephrogenic DI, the ability of the kidney to respond to ADH can be tested by administering exogenous ADH and measuring the change in urine osmolality.

*Water load test for SIADH**

1. Baseline serum Na^+ must be 125 to 150 mmol/L.
2. The patient is given 20 mL of water per kilogram of body weight (max. = 1500 mL) to drink in less than 30 minutes.
3. With the patient maintained in a recumbent position, urine output is collected every hour for the next 5 hours.
4. The volume and osmolality is measured on each sample separately.
5. Interpretation:
   Normal: Greater than 65% of water load excreted after 4 hours, or greater than 80% excreted after 5 hours, with the lowest urine osmolality less than 100 mOsm/kg. Failure to meet these criteria in the absence of medications or other conditions that may impair diuresis is consistent with SIADH by exclusion.

Dehydration test for DI

1. Immediately before beginning the test, collect baseline urine and blood for osmolality measurements.
2. Withhold fluids beginning at time zero.
3. Collect urine samples for volume and osmolality measurements every hour for 6 to 12 hours or until the osmolality is stable for three consecutive hours.
4. Draw blood to confirm that serum osmolality is greater than 288 mmol/kg before proceeding to the next step.
5. Administer 5 units aqueous AVP subcutaneously.
6. One hour after AVP challenge, collect a urine sample for osmolality.
7. Interpretation:
   Normal: Final urine osmolality before AVP challenge is higher than serum, and after AVP challenge, it is less than 10% higher than the maximal urinary osmolality achieved by water restriction alone.
   Neurogenic DI: Urine remains dilute even with dehydration, and becomes concentrated by more than a 10% increase in osmolality following exogenous AVP.
   Nephrogenic DI: Urine remains dilute even with dehydration and does not become more concentrated following exogenous AVP.
   Psychogenic polydipsia: Urine gradually becomes more and more concentrated during 12 hours of water restriction, and urine osmolality rises by less than 10% after exogenous AVP.

Direct measurement of ADH in serum or urine by immunoassay may be helpful to confirm the diagnosis of pathologic ADH excess or deficiency in the presence of a second known or suspected disorder of renal function or fluid and electrolyte homeostasis, or when a patient is unable to tolerate a physiologic stress test. It may also be helpful in cases of partial ADH deficiency or partial renal insensitivity to ADH. Direct measurement of ADH levels may be used to demonstrate disorders of osmoreceptor regulation of ADH secretion. In cases of congenital DI, family members who are heterozygous carriers of ADH gene mutations may be identified by demonstrating decreased ADH levels, which may be the only subclinical manifestation of ADH deficiency (Robertson, 1994).

Because ADH secretion varies with osmotic, volume, and blood pressure changes, these variables must be simultaneously determined at the time blood is drawn for ADH levels. When attempting to rule out SIADH, the patient should not be hypovolemic or hypernatremic, because these are both strong physiologic stimuli for ADH secretion. Conversely, when attempting to rule out DI, it is best to restrict fluids for several hours before the blood sample is drawn, so as not to suppress endogenous ADH secretion. It is also important to determine if any medications the patient may be taking have known effects on ADH secretion. Simultaneous serum and urine samples for osmolality must be submitted, along with the sample for ADH levels.

ADH levels are measured in the clinical laboratory by RIA. However, the RIA results for ADH determinations have not been as reliable as for other hormones because of the presence of interfering substances in the plasma obscuring the very low concentrations of ADH that are normally present. An extraction procedure to concentrate the serum and remove interfering substances has been developed to increase the sensitivity of the RIA for detecting ADH (Penny, 1992). The use of an extraction procedure performed before RIA measurement can give a lower limit of test sensitivity as low as 0.3 ng/L. This allows one to distinguish normal levels (~1.9 to 2.5 ng/L) from physiologic ADH suppression by water loading (~1.4 to 1.8 ng/L) (Gerbes, 1992). More important, a distinction can be made between suppressed ADH levels and true pathologic absence of ADH.

Finally, it must be re-emphasized that under no circumstances can any assay for ADH be interpreted without simultaneous knowledge of the patient's serum osmolality, urine osmolality, intravascular volume status, and blood pressure. The importance of correlating these physiologic variables with ADH immunoassay results is illustrated by a case of markedly elevated ADH levels in a patient with only mild hyponatremia. Evaluation of these discrepant findings demonstrated that a malignant tumor secreted large amounts of an abnormal form of ADH with low biological activity, along with lesser amounts of authentic ADH (Mizobuchi, 1994). In addition, the possibility exists, at least with urine specimens, that ADH immunoassays may also measure biologically inactive ADH metabolites, giving falsely high results (Claybaugh, 1993).

THE THYROID GLAND

Physiology

The follicles of the thyroid gland contain colloid, the main constituent of which is thyroglobulin. Thyroglobulin is the storage site of the thyroid hormones. Iodide is actively taken up by thyroid cells; iodination of tyrosine residues in thyroglobulin results in formation of monoiodotyrosine (MIT) and diiodotyrosine (DIT). When two DIT residues couple, thyroxine (T_4) is formed. When one DIT residue couples with one MIT residue, triiodothyronine (T_3) is formed. Thyroxine and

*Patients with renal insufficiency or adrenal insufficiency are excluded.

2

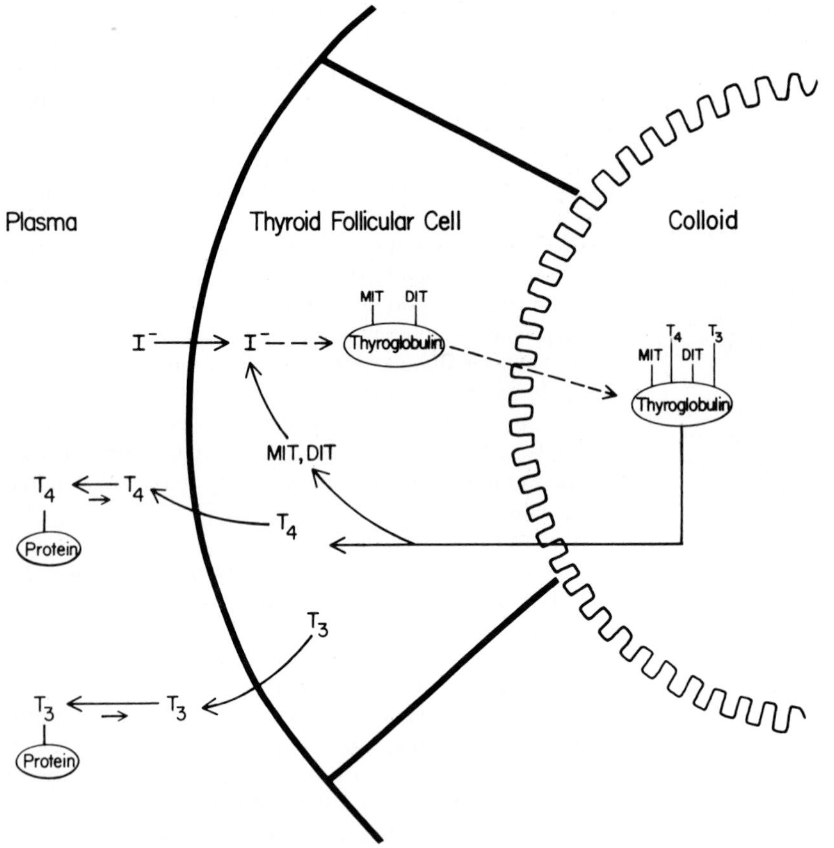

Figure 16–3. Schematic diagram of a thyroid cell outlining formation and release of T_4 and T_3.

triiodothyronine are cleaved from thyroglobulin before secretion from the thyroid gland (Fig. 16–3). Under usual circumstances, T_4 secretion predominates and some thyroglobulin may leak into the circulation.

Most thyroid hormones circulate attached to plasma proteins: about 70% of T_4 noncovalently binds to thyroxine-binding globulin (TBG), 20% to transthyretin (also known as thyroxine-binding prealbumin), and 10% to albumin, whereas most T_3 is bound to TBG. Up to 5% of T_4 may be associated with lipoproteins, IgM, and IgG (i.e., anti-T_4 in autoimmune diseases) (Bartalena, 1990a). A small percentage of the total thyroid hormones circulate in the free form—about 0.03% of T_4 and approximately 0.3% of T_3. The free fraction presumably is the active hormonal form. The majority of T_3 arises by peripheral deiodination, with the liver and the kidney having an important role in this transformation. About 35% of T_4 is monodeiodinated to T_3; 15% to 20% is changed to tetraiodothyroacetic acid (Tetrac) or is conjugated and excreted in urine or bile. The remainder of T_4 is deiodinated to 3,3′,5′-triiodothyronine (reverse T_3, or rT_3) (Fig. 16–4). Further deiodination then occurs: 3,3′-diiodothyronine (T_2) is formed from both T_3 and rT_3.

Biosynthesis and release of thyroid hormones from thyroglobulin are controlled by thyrotropin (thyroid-stimulating

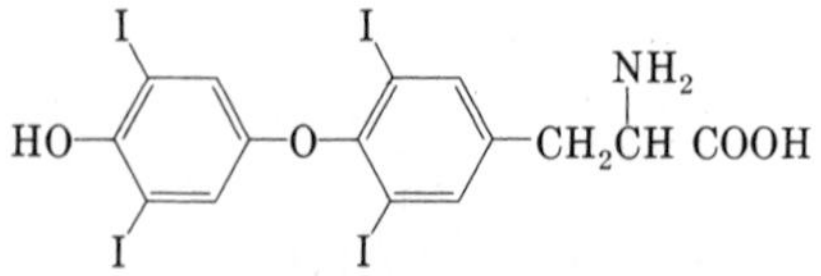

3,5,3′,5′-Tetraiodothyronine (T_4 or Thyroxine)

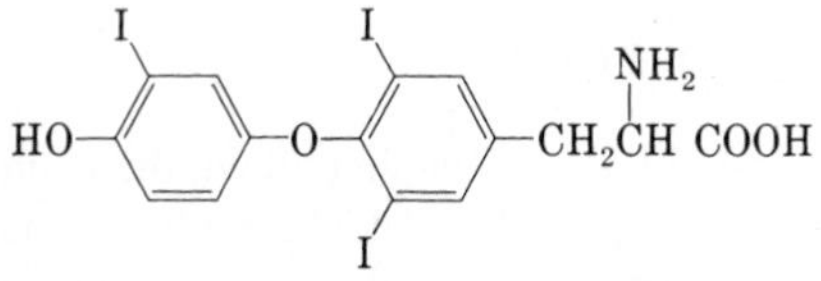

3,5,3′-Triiodothyronine (T_3)

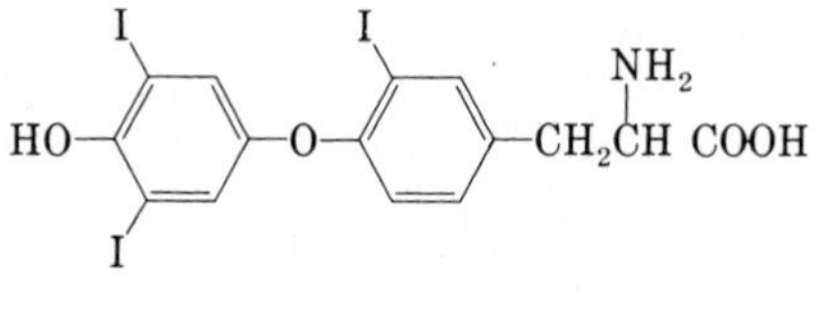

3,3′,5′-Triiodothyronine (Reverse T_3)

Figure 16–4. Structure of T_4, T_3, and reverse T_3 (rT_3).

hormone [TSH]), a glycoprotein hormone synthesized and secreted from the anterior pituitary gland. TSH secretion, in turn, is regulated by the hypothalamus through the thyrotropin-releasing hormone (TRH) and possibly somatostatin, as well as negative feedback from the thyroid hormones. An in-depth review on thyroid physiology and diseases from the clinical pathology viewpoint is available for further reading (Klee, 1993).

Thyroid Disease

Thyroid disease may be classified on a functional basis into hyperthyroidism, hypothyroidism, and euthyroidism. Hyperthyroidism usually results when tissues are exposed to excessive quantities of thyroid hormones. Classic signs and symptoms include heat intolerance, tachycardia, weight loss, weakness, emotional lability, and tremor. The most common causes of hyperthyroidism are autoimmune disorders such as Graves' disease, which is due to circulating antibodies to the TSH receptor (see the section on thyroid autoimmune antibodies). Typically, there is a diffuse goiter that hypersecretes T_3 and T_4. The underlying defect appears to be a defect in suppressor T lymphocytes that allows production of an antibody to this receptor (Strakosch, 1982). Other disorders that lead to hyperthyroidism include toxic multinodular goiter, toxic adenoma, and rarely, TSH-secreting pituitary adenoma (2° hyperthyroidism) and thyroid carcinoma. Moreover, the long term lithium treatment for manic depression, which more commonly is associated with hypothyroidism can also lead to hyperthyroidism (Barclay, 1994). Pituitary adenomas secreting excess TSH can have normal levels of TSH but have excess α-subunits (Gesundheit, 1989). However, there has been a reported case in which the α-subunits remain within reference range, but the TSH increases (Korn, 1994).

Hypothyroidism results from a lack of thyroid hormone action on tissues. Signs and symptoms include bradycardia, hoarseness, cold sensitivity, dry skin, and muscle weakness. Myxedema coma is an advanced stage of thyroid hormone deficiency characterized by progressive stupor, hypothermia, and hypoventilation. Cretinism is the term employed for functional failure of the thyroid in the newborn period. Failure of the thyroid itself to secrete an adequate amount of thyroid hormone is called primary hypothyroidism and most commonly is due to destruction or ablation of the gland. Secondary hypothyroidism results when TSH secretion is decreased as a result of pituitary gland or hypothalamic disorders. A rare cause of hypothyroidism is selective familial TSH deficiency (α and β chains fail to join because of an abnormal TSH β gene).

A variety of diseases of the thyroid usually are characterized by euthyroidism. These include goiter, benign tumors such as follicular adenomas, and malignant tumors. Thyroid function tests are normal in these conditions.

In conjunction with the clinical evaluation of the patient, laboratory determinations are valuable in diagnosing and following the course of a patient with hyperthyroidism or hypothyroidism. The patient's serum thyroid hormone-binding capacity, age, drug therapy, and intercurrent illness can all influence results of various laboratory determinations of thyroid function (*vide infra*). In addition to diagnostic testing, thyroid function measurements are a part of case finding or screening panels, especially at academic centers in the United States. In contrast, the Canadian Task Force (1990) recommended screening tests only for congenital hypothyroidism. Small (1990) concluded that nondiscriminant thyroid screening for acute medical admissions is unwarranted because of the low detection of new clinically inapparent thyroid disease. Thyroid function determinations are, however, appropriate in the elderly population, in which clinical symptoms may be masked or less apparent because of the presence of other illnesses and use of medications.

Laboratory Measurements

Thyroxine

Estimation of circulation levels of thyroid hormones became possible when, in the 1940s, the protein-bound iodine (PBI) method was developed. Small amounts of nonhormonal iodine are present in the serum of healthy subjects; under most clinical circumstances, 80% to 90% of the PBI is derived from thyroxine. The PBI is largely a reflection of the serum T_4 concentration. The major problem with the PBI determination is a spurious elevation due to inorganic or organic iodine contamination that invalidates the estimate of circulating thyroxine.

Serum T_4 by competitive protein binding (CPB) or displacement analysis, which was developed in the 1960s, is based on specific binding properties of TBG, thus allowing determination of T_4 independent of its iodine content. CPB is subject to a number of limitations. These include variability in the extraction step used to eliminate interference by endogenous thyroxine-binding proteins. The PBI and CPB have been supplanted by better methods.

Modern serum T_4 methods begin with radioimmunoassays (T_4 RIA), that employs a radioactive-labeled thyroxine that competes with the patient's T_4. Antisera to T_4 can be produced readily and have satisfactory specificity for T_4 but commonly cross-react with D-thyroxine. To quantitate total levels, T_4 must be released from its endogenous binding proteins. This may be accomplished by use of blocking agents, such as 8-anilino-1-naphthalene sulfonic acid (ANS) or heat denaturation. Advantages of serum T_4 RIA include its sensitivity and elimination of the extraction step. The reference interval for serum T_4 RIA in adults is approximately 5.5 to 12.5 μg/dL (72 to 163 nmol/L) expressed as thyroxine.

Serum T_4 measurements, once the primary means of biochemically diagnosing patients suspected of having hyperthyroidism or hypothyroidism, have been displaced in importance by third-generation TSH assays at many institutions. Serum T_4 remains an inexpensive test, but TSH has become more specific and sensitive as the assay improved (de los Santos, 1989). Compared with TSH, total T_4 (TT_4) has a sensitivity of 93% but a specificity of only 68%, using a cutoff of 7 μg/dL. The receiver operator curve indicates moderate diagnostic accuracy (Schectman, 1990). In fact, altered protein-binding characteristics account for more cases of out-of-reference T_4 levels than thyroid dysgenesis (Hay, 1991). Table 16–5 shows the test characteristics with various disease states. Although these are the common responses, not all patients can be easily characterized. Most patients with hyperthyroidism have elevated serum T_4 and T_3 values. Hyperthy-

Table 16–5. CHANGES IN THYROID FUNCTION TESTS WITH VARIOUS DISEASE STATES

	TSH	T_4	FT_4	T_3
Hyperthyroidism	↓	↑	↑	↑
T_3 toxicosis	nl/↑			↑
Factitious (T_3)	↓	↓	↓	↑
Factitious (T_4)	↓	↑	↑	↑
Hypothyroidism first degree	↑	↓	↓	nl/↓
Second-degree pituitary/hypothalamic	↑	↓	↓	↓
Second-degree selective deficiency	nl	↓	↓	↓
Nonthyroidal illness	↓/nl	↓/nl/↑	nl	↓
Psychiatric NTI		↑	↑	↑
Peripheral hormone resistance	nl	↑	↑	↑
Familial dysalbuminemic hyperthyroxinemia (FDH)	nl	↑	nl	nl
TBG deficiency	nl	↓	nl	↓
FDH + TBG deficiency	nl	nl	nl	↓
HIV+	nl	nl	nl	nl
AIDS with secondary infection	nl	nl	nl	↓

nl = Normal.

Table 16–7. SOME CAUSES OF ABNORMALITIES IN PROTEIN-BINDING CAPACITY

	Increased Binding Capacity	Decreased Binding Capacity
Thyroxine-binding globulin (TBG)	Acute intermittent porphyria	Active acromegaly
	Estrogens	Androgens
	Genetic	Genetic
	Hepatic disease	Hepatic disease
	Hypothyroidism	Nephrotic syndrome
	Newborn infants	Phenytoin
	Oral contraceptives	Prednisone
	Perphenazine	Severe illness or surgical stress
	Pregnancy	Thyrotoxicosis
Thyroxine-binding prealbumin (TBPA)	Active acromegaly	Nephrotic syndrome
	Androgens	Salicylates
	Prednisone	Severe illness or surgical stress
		Thyrotoxicosis

roidism has been reported in patients with serum T_4 values within the reference interval and elevated serum T_3, so-called T_3 thyrotoxicosis. Some patients with hyperthyroidism may have an elevated serum T_4 but have serum T_3 levels that are within the reference interval or low. This so-called T_4 thyrotoxicosis can occur in patients with iodine-induced thyrotoxicosis and in patients with nonthyroidal illness. Other patients with nonthyroidal illness have these findings for thyroid function tests but are clinically euthyroid (*vide infra*). Increased serum T_4 levels can occur as a result of a variety of other causes (Table 16–6). In these clinical situations, the patients generally are euthyroid but further laboratory determinations are necessary to confirm these patients' metabolic status.

Table 16–6. SOME CAUSES OF INCREASED SERUM T_4

Cause	Comment
Increased serum-binding proteins	See Table 16–7
Isolated hyperthyroxinemia	Some patients with non-thyroidal illness (↑ T_4 but T_3 not increased)
Familial dysalbuminemic hyperthyroxinemia	Increased affinity of albumin for T_4
Familial euthyroid thyroxine excess	Increased affinity of thyroxine-binding prealbumin (TBPA) for T_4
Psychiatric disease	? Mechanism
Target organ resistance (a) familial (Refetoff), (b) acquired	Intracellular resistance to thyroid hormone
Other syndromes: (for example, decreased peripheral T_3 production)	(Miscellaneous: ? inhibition of T_4 transport into tissues or reduced T_4 to T_3 conversion)
Spurious	Circulating antibody to T_4
Drugs (excluding those that ↑ thyroxine-binding globulin [TBG]); amiodarone,* amphetamine, heparin, heroin, iodine-containing radiocontrast media,* propranolol*	

*Indicates those drugs that block T_4 to T_3 conversion. For further information, see Wenzel (1981) and Cavalieri (1981).

Serum T_4 levels are affected by changes in serum T_4-binding proteins. In situations in which drugs or other factors cause increased protein binding, there is an increased serum T_4 level; when decreased binding capacity occurs, there is a decreased serum T_4 (Table 16–7). These effects, however, are not reflected at the physiologic level, and in these situations, the free or unbound concentration of T_4 correlates better with thyroid functional status than total levels of serum T_4. It is presumably the free fraction that is the active form of T_4 and the moiety that is homeostatically controlled.

In addition to patients with increased TBG, several types of familial euthyroid hyperthyroxinemia have been described, including peripheral resistance to thyroid hormone (Refetoff, 1993), albumin with increased affinity for T_4 (familial dysalbuminemic hyperthyroxinemia), and TBPA with increased affinity for T_4. It is interesting that the lack of albumin or a variant called bisalbumin have no effect on T_4. Although serum T_4 is usually within the reference interval in patients with nonthyroidal illness, many patients have a decreased serum T_4 level, and less commonly, serum T_4 may be increased. In hospitalized patients, isolated hyperthyroxinemia in euthyroid patients is about as common as true hyperthyroidism. Patients with acute hepatitis may have increased serum T_4 levels secondary to increases in TBG (Gardner, 1982).

Evaluation of serum T_4 values in infants is complicated by TBG elevations in the neonatal period and a TSH surge occurring at the time of birth, both of which lead to increased levels that may remain elevated for a number of weeks (Larsen, 1975). At birth, healthy infants have been reported to have serum T_4 concentrations in the range of 7.8 to 16 μg/dL (101 to 208 nmol/L) (Burman, 1976). Serum T_4 concentrations are remarkably constant throughout the day in hypothyroid patients chronically treated with T_4 (Saberi, 1974). Patients treated with T_3 preparations have very low or undetectable serum T_4 levels.

Triiodothyronine

Serum T_3 levels usually are measured by immunoassay using highly specific T_3 antisera with little T_4 cross-reactivity and a blocking agent, such as sodium salicylate, to eliminate endogenous T_3 protein binding. The reference interval for serum T_3 varies widely among laboratories but is typically in the range of 60 to 160 ng/dL (0.92 to 2.46 nmol/L). T_3 is much less tightly bound to serum proteins than T_4; a relatively greater proportion of T_3 than T_4 exists in the free, diffusible state. It is estimated that approximately 0.3% of T_3 is free (nonprotein bound). Serum free T_3 has been measured by methods analogous to those used for serum free T_4 (FT_4).

In over 90% of patients with hyperthyroidism, both serum T_3 and T_4 values are increased, with the increase in serum T_3 usually greater than the increase in serum T_4. Serum T_3 levels, however, may be within the reference interval or low in patients with hyperthyroidism and coexistent nonthyroidal illness. For example, as HIV infection proceeds to AIDS and then to AIDS with secondary infections, the T_3 and FT_3 index fall to abnormal values but the rT_3, TSH, and FT_4 all remain within reference range (Grunfeld, 1993). As with TT_4, the newer assays for TSH and FT_4 have supplanted T_3 in most cases.

The principle application of T_3 is in diagnosing T_3 thyrotoxicosis, which accounts for about 5% of hyperthyroidism cases. It is more common in regions of iodine deficiency. The patient may appear hyperthyroid with a suppressed TSH but the T_4 and free T_4 values are within their respective reference intervals. The serum T_3 level, however, is elevated. Thyrotropin may not always be suppressed because the feedback mechanisms are based on T_4 levels. Although most of the patients with T_3 thyrotoxicosis have Graves' disease, other causes of thyrotoxicosis are toxic nodular goiter or toxic adenoma. Elevated serum T_3 and T_4 levels within the usual reference interval also may occur in patients with hyperthyroidism early in the course of treatment with antithyroid drugs or during relapse after treatment. In clinically euthyroid patients, there are a number of situations in which serum T_3 concentrations are elevated in the presence of increased TSH levels; for example, this is seen in some patients with endemic iodine deficiency in the presence of low serum T_4 concentrations. Elevated T_3 levels occur in patients with elevated TBG levels.

Qualitatively, T_3 can provide the clinician a sense of the severity and recovery from hyperthyroidism. Although TSH makes the diagnosis for most cases, T_3 tends to increase more than T_4, going up to several hundred nanograms per deciliter (ng/dL) while the T_4 attains levels only in the high teens (μg/dL). During treatment, the T_3 decreases faster than the other parameters.

Generally, serum T_3 levels are not useful in diagnosing patients suspected of having hypothyroidism, because serum T_3 levels are within the reference interval in 20% to 30% of hypothyroid patients. Serum T_3 levels are depressed only in patients who are severely hypothyroid—that is, those with serum T_4 levels less than about 2 μg/dL (26 nmol/L) (Bigos, 1978). In addition, low values for serum T_3 along with other changes in thyroid function tests may occur in patients with a wide variety of severe nonthyroidal illnesses (Table 16–8). In patients with acute illness such as myocardial infarction, the decrease in serum T_3 occurs rapidly, declining to about 50% of the reference value within three or four days (Utiger, 1980). Serum T_3 concentrations also are low in cord blood but increase rapidly during the first few hours of life, attaining values higher than those in healthy adults (Abuid, 1974). There appears to be a progressive decrease in T_3 concentrations with advancing age.

Table 16–8. NONTHYROIDAL ILLNESS: TYPICAL FINDINGS FOR THYROID FUNCTION TESTS

Determination	Findings
T_4	Within reference interval or, if severe, low
Free thyroxine index (FTI), or free T_4	Method dependent
T_3	Decreased
Reverse T_3 (rT_3)	Increased
Thyroid-stimulating hormone (TSH)	Variable, depending on stage of illness

2

Patients receiving thyroid preparations containing T_3, such as desiccated thyroid and synthetic T_3 and T_4 combinations, or those patients treated with T_3 alone will have uninterpretable serum T_3 results unless the time of the hormone administration is known. Administration of T_3 results in a rise in T_3 concentrations, with peak serum values occurring between two and four hours. In patients treated with daily doses of T_4 alone, serum T_3 levels do not show a peak after ingestion of the medication. Stable levels of serum T_3 from the peripheral conversion of the T_4 are reached only after weeks of treatment.

Reverse T_3

rT_3 is a major metabolite of thyroxine produced by 5-deiodination of T_4. Although it is thought to have little or no metabolic activity, rT_3 is a measure of tissue utilization of T_4. The reference interval for serum rT_3, which is measured by radioimmunoassay, is in the range of about 10 to 50 ng/dL (0.15 to 0.77 nmol/L). In general, the specificity of the radioimmunoassay for rT_3 is such that cross-reactivity with T_3 assays is not significant.

In many clinical situations, serum T_3 and serum rT_3 have been found to vary reciprocally. Serum rT_3 often is elevated in patients with nonthyroidal illness in whom serum T_3 concentrations are decreased; this mainly is due to decreased rT_3 degradation to 3,3′-diiodothyronine. Serum rT_3 is increased in healthy newborns and in patients with hyperthyroidism. Drugs, including amiodarone and propranolol, cause increases in serum rT_3 levels (Cavalieri, 1981).

Serum rT_3 is infrequently used to assess thyroid function. It has usefulness in assessing peripheral resistance because it is not increased despite elevated T_4 levels and a normal TSH level. Also in determining whether the patient has a nonthyroidal illness or hypothyroidism, serum rT_3 is decreased in the hyperthyroidism (Chopra, 1979) but normal or increased in nonthyroidal illness (Utiger, 1980).

Free Thyroxine

T_4 lacks specificity when there are changes in thyroxine-binding proteins or their binding characteristics (see Table 16–7). High or low levels of serum thyroxine that occur incorrectly reflect the clinical state. In these situations, free thyroxine (FT_4) is more closely correlated with the patient's clinical status.

There are three methods of assessing FT_4. The most often used at least cost is the free thyroxine index (FTI or T7). The FTI is a calculated estimate of FT_4 ($T_4 \times TU$ or T_3U), where FT_4 is free thyroxine, T_4 is thyroxine, and TU is thyroxine uptake. Thyroxine uptake may use T_3 or T_4 as a signal. The T_3 or T_4 uptake provides information about free binding sites on TBG; the T_3 or T_4 refers to the signal label used in the determination and not to the measurement of serum T_3 or T_4 levels. Although this method is generally successful, shortcomings are apparent in cases in which other proteins or immunoglobulins compete with TBG for the tracer, that is, familial dysalbuminemic hyperthyroxinemia affects T_4U but *not* T_3U. In efforts to reduce the confusion surrounding the interpretation of TU and to standardize measurements among methods and institutions, the American Thyroid Association now calls TU the thyroid hormone–binding ratio (THBR). Patient results are normalized to a control pool used by the testing laboratory (THBR = TU [patient]/TU [pool]) (Larsen, 1987), and the THBR reference range is 0.85 to 1.15. The T_4 to TBG ratio (T_4/TBG) also has been employed to correct for changes in binding proteins (Attwood, 1978; Faix, 1995).

FT_4 quantitated using equilibrium dialysis is the gold standard but is considered too time consuming and technically demanding for routine clinical use. Variability can be substantial with these assays. The temperature at which the assay is conducted can considerably alter the FT_4 measurement (van der Sluijs Veer, 1992) and fatty acids can cause a positive interference (Liewendahl, 1992; Lim, 1991).

The third category of FT_4 assays are direct immunoassays for FT_4. These include the one step labeled T_4 antibody, the two step immunoextraction and the one step labeled T_4 analog. The theoretical foundations are discussed in great detail by Ekins (1993). Figure 16–5 highlights the concepts of the two-step immunoextraction and the one-step analogue methods. These assays tend to underestimate the direct equilibrium dialysis values and have a protein bound dependence. The T_4 analogues are usually the most affected and the two-step immunoextractions are much less so but still significant (Beckett, 1990; Nelson, 1994); more recently, Christofides (1995a, 1995b) demonstrated great improvements in one T_4 analogue kit. Most analogue methods greatly overestimate the FT_4 in familial dysalbuminemic hyperthyroxinemia. However, for most clinical situations, these assays are useful and offer improvement over the FTI in cases of nonthyroidal illness (NTI).

Increases or decreases in serum T_4 without concomitant changes in the metabolic state result from alterations in protein binding by certain drugs or from what is commonly known as euthyroid or nonthyroidal illness. Prolonged administration of phenytoin results in a 15% to 30% decrease in both serum T_4 and FT_4. Carbamazepine has been reported to have similar effects (Cavalieri, 1981). Within a half hour, drugs like heparin and salicylate cause an increase in FT_4 by displacing T_4 from its protein-binding sites and are accompanied by a decrease in TSH (Faber, 1993).

In certain clinical circumstances, FT_4 results will differ, depending on the method employed. The FTI may be low in patients with NTI, whereas FT_4 values as determined by equilibrium dialysis are either within the reference interval or higher (Chopra, 1979). It was hypothesized that an inhibitor in the serum of some critically ill individuals altered protein binding, ultimately leading to a low FTI. Mendel (1991) could not find evidence for such an inhibitor but showed that when TBG is desialylated, a marked decrease in avidity for T_4 occurred with no change in T_3 avidity. This would explain the poor performance of T_3U assays in NTI, hence the low FTI. Values for FT_4 are mostly within the reference interval. However even with the gold standard (FT_4 equilibrium dialysis),

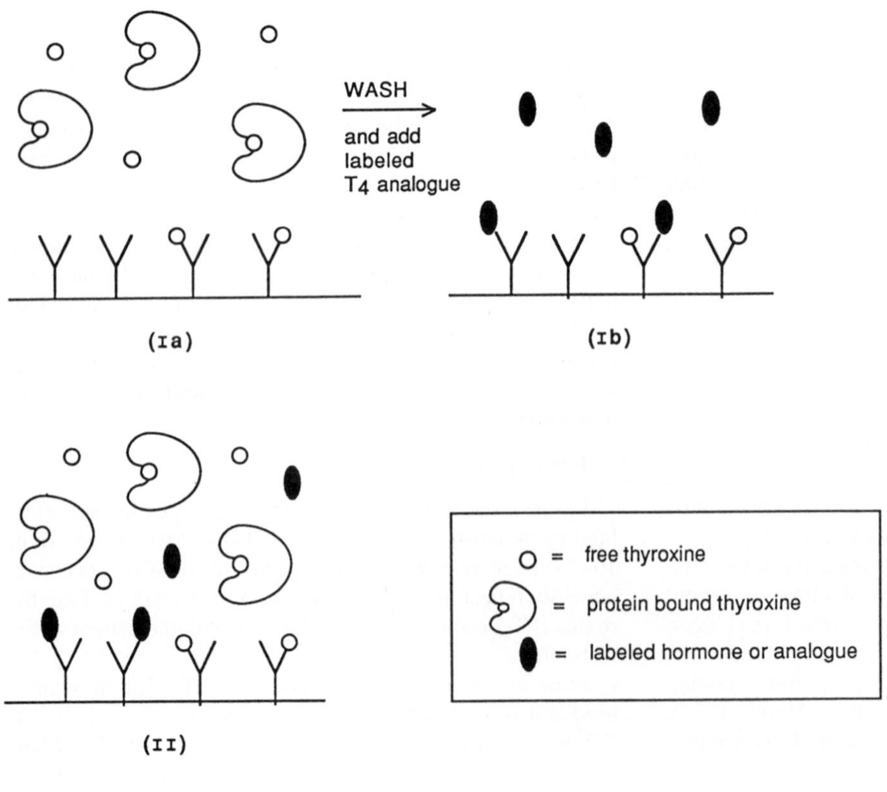

Figure 16–5. Principles of two free thyroxine assays. *Ia*, Serum in contact with capture antibody, 1% to 5% of free T_4 is bound to Ab. *Ib*, In the second step, the sample is washed and labeled T_4 analogue or antiidiotypic Ab is added, which adsorbs to the free binding sites. The remaining tracer is washed, and the bound tracer is measured by any number of techniques such as radioactivity, enzyme conversion of dye, or chemiluminescence. *II*, In the one-step analogue method, the tracer analogue is added with the sample. After incubation, the excess is washed and the captured analogue is measured.

substantial numbers of NTI patients can have high or low FT_4 (Faber, 1993). Hence, third- and fourth-generation TSH assays have been advocated as the single best test for use on patients without neuropsychiatric or pituitary disease (Klee, 1993). Although a variety of changes in thyroid function tests occur in patients with nonthyroidal illness (see Table 16–8), most clinicians agree that the majority of these patients are euthyroid. When the results are out of line with the clinical picture, the presence of a laboratory artifact must be considered such as antithyroid hormone antibodies (John, 1990; Kabadi, 1994; Ritter, 1993; Sapin, 1995; Zweig, 1987, 1991).

FT_4 measured by equilibrium dialysis and FTI do not yield comparable results in patients with familial dysalbuminemic hyperthyroxinemia. Patients with this disorder are clinically euthyroid, but they have a high serum T_4 level as a result of increased binding of thyroxine by a protein that migrates similarly to albumin on electrophoresis. These patients have FT_4 levels within the reference interval as measured by equilibrium dialysis, but they have elevated values for FTI (Ruiz, 1982).

FT_4 clinically has some limitations in that some patients with suppressed TSH exhibit FT_4 levels within the reference range and yet have hyperthyroid symptoms. These patients are believed to have a lower setpoint. No test is perfect because the distribution between the nondiseased population and the population of disease overlaps (see Chap. 6).

Thyrotropin (Thyroid-Stimulating Hormone)

TSH is measured by immunoassay, with first-generation TSH assays having a reference interval of less than about 5 to 7 μU/mL (5 to 7 mU/L). Conventional first-generation TSH assays are useful in detecting primary hypothyroidism, but they are not useful in detecting hyperthyroidism. With first generation TSH assays, undetectable results occur not only with hyperthyroidism but also in 20% or more of euthyroid individuals. Second-generation immunoassays for TSH were introduced in the mid 1980s and have a slightly lower reference interval than older assays; they could detect 0.1 to 0.2 μU/L. There is also considerable variation in the lower detection limit of second generation TSH assays. Hence, venders report their lowest sensitivity as what is distinguishable from the zero calibrator. In practice, the functional sensitivity is much higher. The mean TSH in hyperthyroid individuals is in the range of 0.05 to 0.11 μU/mL (0.05 to 0.11 mU/L) (Hershman, 1988). With the third- and fourth-generation assays now available, TSH can be detected below this range (functional sensitivities—0.01 to 0.02 and 0.001 to 0.002 respectively) (Spencer, 1993).

Generally, results from sensitive TSH assays that are within the reference interval exclude thyroid dysfunction, but results outside these limits do not always indicate thyroid disease. For example, clinically euthyroid persons over 60 years old with normal T_4 or FTI can have TSH levels less than 0.1 mU/L, which is usually considered suppressed (Sawin, 1991). A low TSH alone in this population had a predictive value of only 12% while adding T_4 or FTI raised the predictive value five fold. At least in older people, this is counter to the theory that a suppressed TSH with a normal FTI is indicative of a subclinical hyperthyroid state. Hyperthyroid patients have suppressed TSH values, with the exception of those rare individuals who have hyperthyroidism caused by a TSH-producing pituitary tumor. In addition, TSH is suppressed in individuals treated with exogenous thyroid hormone, and this may eventually prove useful in the assessment of long-term suppressive hormone therapy (Bartalena, 1987).

In most patients with primary hypothyroidism, serum TSH results are markedly elevated, but results are low in individuals with hypothyroidism caused by pituitary disorders. In individuals with hypothyroidism secondary to hypothalamic lesions, TSH results may be within the reference range or elevated, with the elevated values thought to be caused by immunoactive but bioinactive hormone. TSH levels also are increased in patients with compensated hypothyroidism as well as in the newborn.

2

An elevated TSH without clinical correlation should lead one to suspect assay artifact. Some patients develop antibodies to the animal from which the antibodies for the immunoassay were raised (Iitaka, 1992; Zweig, 1987, 1991). The prevalence of this phenomenon is roughly 5% to 8% and is the same in both healthy subjects and in patients with autoimmune thyroid disease. Analyzing the specimen with different animal antibodies or the addition of animal antibody (i.e., mouse) to the kit usually exposes this type of interference.

An important cause of both increased and decreased TSH results is nonthyroidal illness. Patients with nonthyroidal illness tend to have low TSH results during their acute illness, then TSH rises to within or above the reference range, with resolution of the underlying illness (Brent, 1986). The situation is complicated because drugs, including glucocorticoids and dopamine, also suppress TSH.

The new third- and fourth-generation TSH assays have simplified the biochemical diagnosis for confirmation of hyperthyroidism. Together with its previous role in confirming hypothyroidism, TSH may be the *single* best measurement for screening patients suspected of having either hypothyroidism or hyperthyroidism. However, other determinations (e.g., FT_4, T_4) are useful adjuncts in special situations such as pituitary or hypothalamic etiologies of thyroid dysfunction, psychogenic NTI, and in the elderly. One should keep in mind that clinical evaluation alone detects most cases of thyroid dysfunction in the outpatient setting.

TRH Tests

Prior to the development of TSH assays that could measure suppressed levels, the TRH stimulation test was the primary determination to confirm hyperthyroidism. Now the TRH test is reserved for investigating central hypothyroidism and resolving unclear thyroid function tests. The third- and fourth-generation TSH assays quantitate suppressed TSH levels and correlate with the TRH stimulation test when the hypothalamic-pituitary axis is intact (Spencer, 1993).

A TRH test may be performed in a number of ways. Usually a single bolus of TRH (200 to 500 μg) is administered intravenously after blood has been drawn for a baseline TSH. Additional specimens for TSH are obtained at 20, 30, or 60 minutes after TRH administration. Within about 5 minutes of intravenous administration, TRH causes a rise in serum TSH that reaches a peak in 20 to 30 minutes and returns to baseline in two to four hours (Fig. 16–6). A typical response to intravenous injection of 500 μg of TRH (maximal stimulation) is a rise in serum TSH to a concentration of about 16 to 26 μU/L in women (slightly lower in men) from a mean value of about

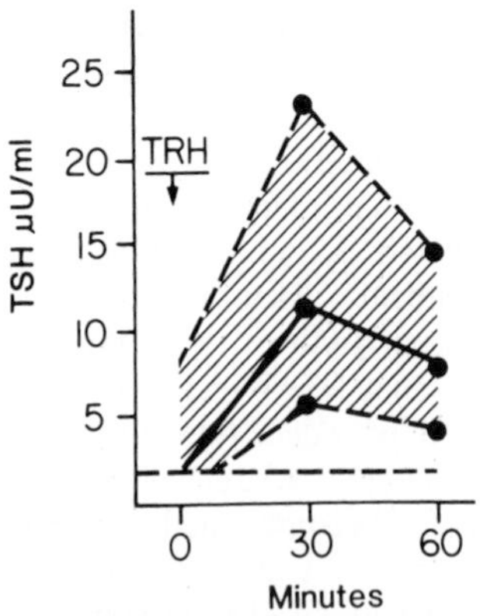

Figure 16–6. The TSH response to 500 μg of intravenous TRH in healthy subjects. (Modified from Jackson IMD: Reprinted by permission of the New England Journal of Medicine 1982; 306:145.)

6 μU/L (Sterling, 1977). The rise in TSH is proportional to the basal TSH. Alternatively, the so-called fold increase over the basal TSH is a better measure of response than the absolute increase. The fold increase to TRH in euthyroid patients is 8.5 ± 0.2, absent in hyperthyroidism, and attenuated in hypothyroidism (2.5 ± 0.4) (Spencer, 1993). Moreover, the fold increase is independent of age, sex, and nonthyroidal illness.

In euthyroid subjects, serum T_3 increases to about 70% above baseline levels one to four hours after administration of TRH, and serum T_4 also increases but to a lesser extent. TRH usually stimulates prolactin secretion and causes GH release in patients with a variety of conditions, including acromegaly. Serum T_3, T_4, prolactin, and GH usually are not measured during a TRH test.

The response of TSH to TRH usually is suppressed in hyperthyroid patients. Although the presence of an impaired response to TRH commonly is due to hyperthyroidism, it may occur in a number of conditions, including patients with multinodular goiter or patients with Graves' disease who are euthyroid after therapy. A number of other disorders may give rise to a suppressed or blunted TSH response, including renal failure, Cushing's syndrome, and depression. Chronic renal failure may have an element of central hypothyroidism because there is also a failure to produce a nocturnal surge in TSH that seems necessary to maintain homeostasis (Bartalena, 1990b). The TSH response to TRH also is blunted by a number of drugs, including corticosteroids, L-dopa, and large doses of salicylate (Lamberg, 1978). There is a significant time interval following withdrawal of long-term thyroid hormone therapy before the normal response to TRH is restored (Burger, 1977).

Patients with primary hypothyroidism have a high basal serum TSH level and an exaggerated serum TSH response to TRH. In patients with hypothyroidism secondary to pituitary or hypothalamic disease, basal serum TSH levels usually are within the reference interval; however, some patients with hypothalamic hypothyroidism may have slightly elevated basal serum TSH values. Absent TSH response to TRH in a patient who does not have hyperthyroidism suggests a pituitary rather than hypothalamic lesion, but an intact response of TSH to TRH may be seen in patients with pituitary disease (Burger, 1977). The response to TRH in patients with hypothalamic disease is usually within normal limits or exaggerated, and it may be prolonged (Lamberg, 1978). The frequency with which aberrant responses to TRH occur reduces its usefulness in distinguishing between hypothalamic and pituitary disorders (Jackson, 1982).

Thyroxine-Binding Globulin (TBG)

Thyroxine-binding globulin (TBG) is the principal serum carrier protein for T_4 and T_3; levels in healthy individuals are in the range of 12 to 30 μg/mL. The thyroxine-binding capacity of TBG can be determined using immunoassays, electrophoresis, or an ion-exchange resin method. Table 16–7 summarizes some of the causes of binding capacity changes in TBG. Estrogen influences the level of binding proteins, whereas some drugs compete with T_4 for binding sites, decreasing bound T_4. Two inherited defects of transport proteins can confuse the interpretation of thyroid function tests (TFTs) (Langsteger, 1994).

Measurement of TBG is rarely indicated. It may be helpful in patients who have serum T_3 and T_4 levels that do not agree with other laboratory parameters of thyroid function, or that are not compatible with clinical findings. TBG:T_4 ratios have been used for diagnosis of hyperthyroidism and hypothyroidism in patients with binding protein abnormalities prior to the new TSH assays.

Thyroglobulin

Thyroglobulin, which usually is measured by immunoassay, is present in serum of most healthy individuals, with levels ranging up to about 30 to 40 ng/mL.

Although thyroglobulin can be elevated with adenomas, goiters, thyroiditis, and even nonthyroid malignancies, its primary medical use is in following patients with papillary and follicular carcinoma after total thyroidectomy. Typically, after total thyroidectomy and ^{131}I treatment, thyroglobulin should be less than 10 ng/mL. However, lung or bone metastases can result in values in the thousands (Pacini, 1980). Because thyroglobulin is dependent on TSH, thyroglobulin increases when thyroxine is withdrawn to prepare for a body scan. During treatment with exogenous thyroid hormone, Ashcraft (1981) found that no metastases occurred in thyroidectomized patients with undetectable thyroglobulin levels (<1 ng/mL), whereas detectable thyroglobulin levels (even as low as 4.2 ng/mL) occasionally were associated with metastases. In an 18-year study, Ozata (1994) found that 95% of the time, a thyroglobulin less than 5 ng/mL during suppressive therapy meant there was no residual tumor. Moreover, patients do not need to become hypothyroid (TSH stimulation to maximize thyroglobulin production) in order for them to be adequately monitored for recurrence or metastasis. After withdrawal of T_4 treatment in these patients, thyroglobulin levels less than 10 ng/mL were found to be indicative of successful therapy for thyroid carcinoma, whereas levels greater than 10 ng/mL suggested the presence of metastases in three quarters of patients, even in individuals with negative ^{131}I total body scans. In one study, serum thyroglobulin showed a sensitivity of 88%, a specificity of 99%, and an accuracy of 96.5% (Lubin, 1994). The body scan in the same study only found 55% of the metastatic cases. A tumor that has a low thyroglobulin level with a negative body scan suggests dedifferentiation and hence a poorer prognosis.

Thyroglobulin levels also have been used to identify individuals with factitious thyrotoxicosis. These patients have undetectable thyroglobulin levels, in contrast to elevated levels found in patients with hyperthyroidism due to a wide variety of other causes (Mariotti, 1982).

Thyroid Autoimmune Antibodies

There are several types of antibodies of clinical significance. TSH receptor antibodies is the preferred term for autoantibodies to the TSH receptor. Previously, these antibodies were known by such terms as thyroid-stimulating immunoglobulins or long-acting thyroid stimulator (LATS) (Larsen, 1987). The antibodies fall into two general categories—stimulatory and blocking. In patients with Graves' disease, TSH receptor antibodies usually act as agonists, activating cyclic AMP and causing hyperthyroidism. Patients with Graves' disease also may have blocking antibodies called thyrotropin-binding inhibitor immunoglobulin (TBII) that usually cause no symptoms but, in a few cases, may lead to hypothyroidism. Measurements of TSH receptor antibodies have been used to predict the outcome of patients with Graves' disease treated with drug therapy; detectable TSH receptor antibodies following drug treatment therapy predict relapse of thyrotoxicosis (Smith, 1988). Monitoring TBII and TSH during antithyroid drug treatments can prevent overtreatment (Cho, 1992). The length of treatment can be arbitrary. Cho and colleagues found that when TBII was normalized, they could safely reduce their standard two-year treatment regimen by as much as over a year. In addition, measurement of TSH receptor antibodies have been used to predict the risk of thyroid dysfunction in newborns of mothers with Graves' disease and as a diagnostic tool in difficult cases in which Graves' disease is a consideration.

Antibodies to thyroid peroxidase (TPO), known previously as thyroid microsomal antigen, is one of the main laboratory markers of Hashimoto's (goiterous lymphocytic) thyroiditis and is also prevalent among patients with Graves' disease. Anti-TPO antibodies are associated with destruction of the thyroid in Hashimoto's disease. The level of antithyroid antibodies against TPO and TSH receptors may be a function of thyroid status (Rieu, 1994). Thyroxine replacement decreased the circulating antibodies. A cutoff of 100 IU/mL in a system with recombinant TPO had a sensitivity of 90.5% and a specificity of 95% for autoimmune disease (Haubruck, 1993). The ELISA based on TPO appear to fair better than the hemagglutination method for microsomal antigens (Laurberg, 1992) but did not seem to be as specific as the Haubruck assay.

Thyroglobulin antibodies can be found in patients with differentiated thyroid carcinoma. These antibodies can interfere with thyroglobulin assays used to survey these patients, thus nullifying the clinical usefulness. In patients with TgAb, Rubello (1992) found that disappearance of TgAb after treatment signified a favorable outcome. The continued presence of TgAb offered no additional prognostication. Both anti-TPO and TgAbs can be associated with hypothyroidism in patients with endogenous depression (Custro, 1994). These patients have subclinical hypothyroidism from autoimmune thyroiditis.

Screening Programs for Detection of Neonatal Hypothyroidism

Neonatal hypothyroidism is estimated to occur in about one of 3500 to 4000 live births. Treatment of hypothyroidism within one month of birth eliminates the development of severe mental retardation. Various approaches to screening have been employed, including T_4 and TSH measurements using dry blood spots or cord serum. Screening has been performed using T_4 alone, TSH alone, and various combinations of T_4 and TSH, that is, T_4 with testing of TSH on those specimens with the lowest T_4 levels and visa versa.

Originally, screening programs relied on estimation of T_4 using either cord blood or dried blood spots collected for phenylketonuria tests. Measurement of only T_4 can lead to a high false-positive rate with too conservative a cutoff, necessitating recall of a large number of infants for retesting. Causes of false-positive results include low T_4 levels, which occur in both premature infants and those with congenital deficiency of TBG. Screening with only T_4 may miss infants with compensated or partial thyroid insufficiency. About 15% of infants with primary thyroid disorders have compensated hypothyroidism—that is, they have the serum T_4 within the reference interval and an elevated TSH. A marked increase in T_4 occurs during the first 24 hours of life as a result of TSH surge at delivery, but in hypothyroid infants, T_4 levels do not increase during this period.

The strategy favored in Canada and the United States is to use T_4 initially, followed by TSH if the measured T_4 is below an assigned cutoff, such as 10% of the lowest T_4 (AAP section, 1993). Verkerk (1993) confirmed a 10% cutoff as cost effective. Using a cutoff of 2.1 standard deviation (SD) below the geometric mean of the run, only one case in 93,000 newborns was missed (Dussault, 1993). The second strategy that is used in Europe and Japan is TSH first followed by T_4 if the TSH is elevated (Grüters, 1994). Elevated TSH is theoretically the most sensitive test for the diagnosis of congenital hypothyroidism; however, false-positive results are occasionally seen—for example, in premature or severely stressed infants. Screening with TSH alone can also miss cases of hypothalamic-pituitary hypothyroidism, hypothyroxinemia with delayed TSH elevation, and TBG deficiency. Moreover, with hospital stays shortened to 24 to 48 hours, there will be a high recall rate because of normally higher TSH levels during this time. Age-adjusted cutoffs may minimize the effect. Because some infants will still be missed by these algorithms, another approach used by some state agencies requires a second blood specimen between two to six weeks postpartum. In this manner, an additional 10% of hypothyroid cases have been picked up (AAP section, 1993).

Eighty-nine percent of congenital hypothyroid patients are permanent forms, that is, hypoplasia and agenesis of thyroid gland (Dussault, 1993). Eleven percent are transient, with unknown etiology being the largest category. However, a small portion of this group is caused by transplacental passage of antibodies such as TBII and TGBI (Dussault, 1993). In fact, a low T_4 with normal TSH may indicate maternal Graves' disease (Slyper, 1993). Despite a normal screen, if the infant fails to thrive, transient hypothalamic hypothyroidism (Jain, 1994) and hypopituitary etiologies need to be considered, in which case a TRH stimulation test is appropriate. Although

TRH stimulation has been advocated by Rapaport (1993) in the case of mildly abnormal thyroid function tests, the meaning of a hyperresponsive TSH (>35 mU/L) is not known.

Recently, the concern for loss of potential due to severe hypothyroidism at birth (Tillotson, 1994) has led to treatments of the fetus *in utero* (Davidson, 1991; Perelman, 1990; Van Wassernaer, 1993). Suspected cases are derived from ultrasound study showing goiters and maternal history of Graves' Disease.

ADRENAL GLAND

Hormones of the Adrenal Medulla

The adrenal medulla is embryologically derived from the neuroectoderm and functions as a neuroendocrine organ. It is under direct sympathetic control from the CNS. The main function of the adrenal medulla is to secrete the catecholamines dopamine, norepinephrine, and epinephrine in response to acutely stressful fight or flight situations. The catecholamines are synthesized in chromaffin cells (pheochromocytes), named for the unique brown color produced as the catecholamines become oxidized by staining with chromic acid. In the pheochromocytes, catecholamines are stored along with ATP, calcium and magnesium ions, chromogranin A, and other proteins within electron-dense chromaffin granules. Release of these products from the chromaffin granules in pheochromocytes is controlled by preganglionic as well as postganglionic innervation.

Catecholamine Pharmacology and Biochemistry

Pharmacologically, catecholamines possess potent α- and β-adrenergic effects, which produce vasopressor effects on peripheral arterioles, and positive inotropic and chronotropic effects on the heart, respectively. The net result of both these actions is to acutely increase blood pressure. Other effects include dilation of pupils, lipolysis, and hyperglycemia by increasing gluconeogenesis in the liver and by inhibiting insulin release from the pancreas.

Biochemically, the catecholamines are small endocrine compounds, derived from the amino acid tyrosine. The biochemical pathways by which catecholamines are synthesized and metabolized are shown in Figure 16–7. Two enzymes are important for catecholamine metabolism: monoamine oxidase (MAO), which catalyzes oxidative deamination, and catechol-*O*-methyltransferase (COMT), which catalyzes *O*-methylation. The major metabolites of epinephrine and norepinephrine are metanephrine and normetanephrine, respectively. The final metabolic end product of both epinephrine and norepinephrine is vanillylmandelic acid (VMA). The metabolite 3-methoxy-4-hydroxyphenylethylene glycol (MHPG), which appears in the urine as well, may be preferentially derived from brain norepinephrine. In addition, small amounts of epinephrine and norepinephrine are excreted in the urine both in the free form and as inactive conjugates of sulfates or glucuronides. Similarly, metanephrine and normetanephrine may also be excreted either free or conjugated. Dopamine is metabolized to 3,4-dihydroxyphenylacetic acid (DOPAc) or 3-methoxydopamine, and then to homovanillic acid (HVA). A small amount of intact dopamine is also present in urine. Less than 5% of all plasma catecholamines are excreted directly into the urine without undergoing metabolic degradation or conjugation.

When catecholamines are released from neural tissues other than the adrenal medulla, the primary means of inactivation is by reuptake into presynaptic nerve endings by active transport mechanisms and metabolic degradation by MAO. Circulating catecholamines, on the other hand, are metabolized by COMT and conjugating enzymes present in the liver, kidney, and other organs. In the laboratory diagnosis of disorders of catecholamine excess, measurement of the more stable catecholamine metabolites metanephrine, normetanephrine, and HVA is used as a reflection of the overall secretion of the short-lived parent compounds epinephrine, norepinephrine, and dopamine, respectively.

Disorders of Catecholamine Deficiency and Excess

Adrenal medullary insufficiency may be secondary to surgery, bilateral adrenal lesions, sympathectomy, or neuropathies. The manifestations are usually clinically silent, but hypoglycemia may result if adrenal medullary insufficiency coexists with glucagon deficiency, as in type I diabetes. A subset of patients with severe orthostatic hypotension due to the absence of vascular sympathetic tone have been found to be deficient in dopamine β-hydroxylase, the enzyme that converts dopamine to norepinephrine (Gentric, 1993). Even though dopamine β-hydroxylase deficiency also results in adrenal medullary insufficiency, which may lead to hypoglycemia, the symptoms of severe orthostatic hypotension are attributable nearly exclusively to extramedullary autonomic insufficiency. This condition is suggested by the finding of decreased or absent plasma norepinephrine levels that fail to increase when the patient changes position from recumbency to the upright position. Dopamine levels are relatively increased in these patients because they accumulate as a precursor just before the block in the biosynthetic pathway (Robertson, 1991).

The predominant disorder associated with catecholamine excess is pheochromocytoma, a neoplasm of the adrenal medullary chromaffin cells. These rare tumors are diagnosed most often in people aged 30 to 60. A minority of pheochromocytomas arise from extra-adrenal rests of chromaffin cells in paraspinal sympathetic ganglia. Most of the extra-adrenal pheochromocytomas (paragangliomas) occur below the diaphragm, with a common site being the organ of Zuckerkandl, a sympathetic neural ganglion located anterior to the abdominal aorta which is prominent only in infancy.

Epinephrine is the predominant catecholamine of the adrenal medulla, in contrast to the brain, where norepinephrine and dopamine are the major catecholamine neurotransmitters. However, in pheochromocytomas of the adrenal medulla, norepinephrine is usually the predominant catecholamine secreted. A minority of pheochromocytomas produce epinephrine as the predominant catecholamine, in which case diastolic hypertension may not be seen due to epinephrine's preferential β-adrenergic vasodilatory effects on peripheral vascular beds. In addition, pheochromocytomas may also produce a number of other hormones including calcitonin, GHRH, VIP, and ACTH.

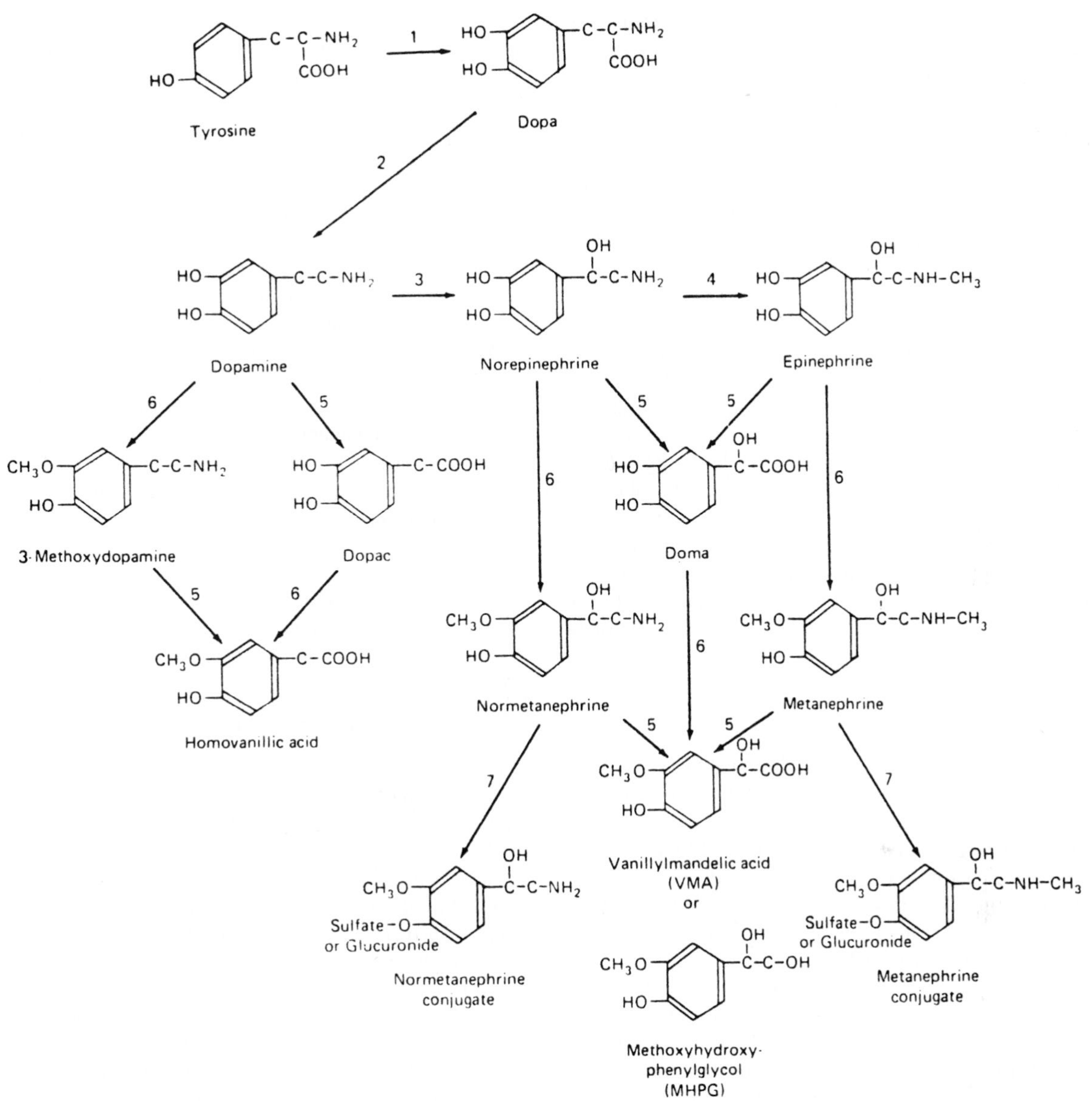

Figure 16–7. Metabolic pathways of catecholamine synthesis and degradation. Enzymes: 1. tyrosine hydroxylase, 2. decarboxylase, 3. dopamine β-hydroxylase, 4. phenylethanolamine N-methyltransferase (PNMT), 5. monoamine oxidase (MAO) & aldehyde dehydrogenase, 6. catechol-O-methyltransferase (COMT), 7. conjugating enzymes. (Modified from Manger WM, Gifford RW: Catecholamine metabolism: Biosynthesis, storage, release, and inactivation. *In* Manger WM, Gifford RW (eds): Pheochromocytoma, New York, Springer-Verlag, 1977, p 10.)

Clinically, patients with a pheochromocytoma display paroxysmal attacks of headache, diaphoresis, tachycardia, nervousness, and tremors. These attacks may occur as variably as once in several weeks to several times per day, or may be persistent. Other signs of pheochromocytoma include hyperglycemia, hyperthermia, weight loss, hypertension, and orthostatic hypotension. If undiagnosed, patients may eventually present with the catastrophic consequences of malignant hypertension, including aortic dissection, stroke, renal failure, or myocardial infarction.

Pheochromocytomas occur at a prevalence rate of approximately 0.1% in hypertensive patients, with an annual incidence rate of about 2 cases per 1,000,000 people per year for the general population (Fernandez-Calvet, 1994; Stenstrom, 1986). Because of the very low prevalence of this tumor, routine screening of all newly diagnosed hypertensive patients has a low positive predictive value. Instead, patients should be selected for testing based on an increased index of suspicion aroused by a history of familial endocrine tumors or the clinical presentation.

Pheochromocytomas are usually benign and most often occur unilaterally. Although most are sporadic, the finding of juvenile, familial, or bilateral pheochromocytomas should prompt a workup for von Recklinghausen neurofibromatosis, von Hipple–Lindau disease, tuberous sclerosis, and multiple endocrine neoplasia (MEN) types 2A and 2B. Once a proband case of pheochromocytoma associated with a familial syndrome is identified, genetic testing for oncogene mutations can be performed to identify other family members who may share an identical mutation (Raue, 1994). This allows other high-risk individuals to be identified and closely monitored for tumor formation. Patients who undergo surgical resection of benign pheochromocytomas are cured in more than 90% of cases.

About 10% of pheochromocytomas are malignant, as demonstrated by metastatic tumor spread or extensive local invasion. Histologic examination alone is not reliable in distinguishing benign pheochromocytomas from those that are malignant (Ram, 1995). DNA flow cytometry studies on these tumors demonstrate that tetraploidy or aneuploidy are commonly found in malignant pheochromocytomas, whereas the benign forms are most often diploid but may also be tetraploid or aneuploid (Lai, 1994; Nativ, 1992). A rare case of a malignant pheochromocytoma having diploid DNA content has also been reported (Jung, 1992). The distinction between benign and malignant pheochromocytomas has been blurred by the finding of both local and distant tumor recurrence several years after resection of solitary localized pheochromocytomas presumed to be benign at the time of diagnosis (Van Heerden, 1990). Given the often indistinguishable histologic features and DNA ploidy contents common to both benign and malignant pheochromocytomas, it is likely that some of the tumors thought to be benign at the time of diagnosis may actually have a low malignant potential. Thus, the DNA ploidy may be a useful indicator of the tumor's long-term behavior, with the finding of nondiploid DNA content in pheochromocytoma being an unfavorable prognostic sign, warranting close follow-up (Pang, 1993).

Other neuroendocrine tumors that may secrete excess catecholamines include neuroblastomas and ganglioneuromas. Neuroblastoma is a common malignancy of infancy that arises from neural crest cells in the adrenal medulla or along the sympathetic chain in the retroperitoneum and posterior mediastinum. It usually presents as a mass lesion that causes symptoms of compression or obstruction either at the primary site or at metastatic foci such as liver and bone marrow. Symptoms suggestive of catecholamine excess such as hypertension are often mild or absent. These tumors produce norepinephrine, or more characteristically, dopamine; but not epinephrine. However, the catecholamines are usually degraded before they are secreted, thus they are best diagnosed by measuring urinary normetanephrines, HVA, and VMA (Candito, 1992). If the metabolites are elevated at the time of diagnosis, they may be used as a tumor marker to follow response to treatment or to diagnose a relapse. Ganglioneuromas are well-differentiated, benign neural tumors that arise from sympathetic ganglia in older children and young adults. These tumors almost exclusively secrete norepinephrine and are amenable to surgical resection.

Functional hypersecretion of catecholamines may be related to the pathophysiology of essential hypertension and has been found to occur in so-called white coat hypertension, a psychogenic reaction which occurs in some physicians' offices or clinics. In particular, plasma norepinephrine levels have been found to be elevated in white coat hypertensives (Weber, 1994), which may overlap with the upper limits of normal and also with the lower range seen in some patients with pheochromocytoma.

The selection of laboratory measurements used in the diagnosis of pheochromocytoma should be guided by the clinical presentation of the individual patient. If the patient presents with sustained hypertension and other persistent features, plasma epinephrine and norepinephrine are the determinations of choice. However, given the very short plasma half-life of the catecholamines (about two minutes), detection of elevated plasma epinephrine and norepinephrine levels could easily miss a secretory burst. More often, paroxysmal attacks occur intermittently, or the patient may be asymptomatic (adrenal incidentaloma). Then, the assay of choice is a 24-hour urine collection for metanephrines and normetanephrines (Gerlo, 1994). If the paroxysmal secretory bursts are very infrequent, the catecholamine metabolites may be diluted out or missed entirely in a 24-hour urine collection aliquot. In such a case, the patient may be given a urine container to keep on hand in the outpatient setting. Following a rare paroxysmal attack, the first urine specimen passed is collected, immediately refrigerated, and sent to the laboratory as the diagnostic material for metanephrine analysis. If an extramedullary tumor is suspected of producing dopamine, urine should be assayed for HVA. Urine assays for HVA and VMA are best suited for testing for neuroblastoma. However, when testing for pheochromocytoma, urinary HVA, VMA, and free catecholamines are less sensitive as diagnostic tests and are generally not recommended for initial screening. Dietary restriction prior to specimen collection for VMA warrants attention to the elimination of bananas, chocolate, coffee, tea and vanilla (Young, 1993).

Diagnosis of Catecholamine Excess

STUDIES ON URINE

The diagnosis of pheochromocytoma or neuroblastoma can be made by demonstrating increases in catecholamine metabolites from an aliquot of a patient's 24-hour urine specimen. When testing for neuroblastoma, the analytes of choice are dopamine, HVA, normetanephrine, and VMA. Measurement of urinary VMA, the final common metabolite of both epinephrine and norepinephrine may be used as a measure of total urinary catecholamines; however, it does not distinguish between excess epinephrine and norepinephrine. Instead, urinary metanephrine and normetanephrine levels are cited as the single most useful clinical laboratory determination for diagnosing or excluding pheochromocytoma (Peplinski, 1994). The sensitivity and specificity of testing for the urinary metanephrines in this setting are greater than 99% and 95%, respectively.

Urine specimens for catecholamine analysis may be collected over 24 hours, overnight, or by random sampling. Random urine specimens may miss sporadic secretory bursts and, therefore, may not be an accurate representation of total catecholamine secretion over the course of a day. On the other hand, a urine sample collected shortly after a clinically evident secretory burst of catecholamines may be sufficient diagnostic material. The urine collection container should be opaque to light, contain acid (10 mL of 6N HCl) to prevent degradation of the catecholamine metabolites, and refrigerated until the collection is complete and the assay can be performed (see Chap. 1). The total 24-hour urine volume is then measured, and an aliquot is either assayed immediately or frozen until testing can be performed.

Dopamine is the major intact catecholamine present in the urine; its quantification is most useful in diagnosing neuroblastoma, but it may also be elevated in pheochromocytoma. Epinephrine and norepinephrine can also be quantified in the urine and used in the diagnosis of pheochromocytoma. They are excreted into the urine either in the unconjugated (free) form or conjugated with glucuronide or sulfate. More than half of the catecholamines in the urine are in the conjugated form. Total catecholamines, both conjugated and unconjugated, can be measured by removing glucuronide or sulfate groups from the conjugated catecholamines by a hydrolysis step prior to assay. However, there are several disadvantages to measuring total urinary catecholamines; for example, the wide reference interval may obscure the diagnosis of a minimally secreting tumor. In addition, dietary catecholamines, which occur in the conjugated form, may bias the total catecholamine measurements. For these reasons, urinary free epinephrine and norepinephrine measurements are preferred, and may be more specific particularly when interference from dietary catechols is a concern.

Laboratory methods for measuring catecholamines and their metabolites include fluorometry, spectrophotometry, gas chromatography, liquid chromatography, radioenzymatic assay, immunoassay, and HPLC with electrochemical detection, the latter being the standard methodology in most reference laboratories.

Urinary free catecholamines may be assayed by a modification of the trihydroxyindole fluorometric technique or by HPLC. The fluorometric assay is performed by oxidizing catecholamines to trihydroxyindole compounds, which fluoresce in proportion to the initial catecholamine concentrations in the urine. This method may also be used to assay epinephrine and norepinephrine separately by the different fluorescent wavelengths they produce. HPLC detection of free catecholamines in urine involves ion-exchange or reversed-phase chromatography to separate dopamine, norepinephrine, and epinephrine in the specimen, followed by electrochemical or fluorescent detection. The usual reference interval for urinary free catecholamines is up to about 100 μg/24 h; the reference intervals for epinephrine and intervals for epinephrine and norepinephrine separately is less than 20 μg/24 h and less than 80 μg/24 h, respectively. However, urinary free catecholamine levels are much more variable in the pediatric age group, and the reference interval should be adjusted accordingly (Nunez, 1994).

Urinary metanephrines and normetanephrines may be assayed by either spectrophotometry, fluorometry, gas chromatography, immunoassay, radioenzymatic methods, or HPLC. In contrast to conjugated forms of epinephrine and norepinephrine, conjugated forms of the metanephrine metabolites are derived only from endogenous catecholamine production, and not dietary sources. Therefore, it is desirable to measure the total amount of both the conjugated and unconjugated metanephrines and normetanephrines in the urine. This is accomplished by an acid hydrolysis step, which removes the glucuronide or sulfate conjugate groups, thus transforming all the metanephrines present into the unconjugated form before the assay is performed. The spectrophotometric assay for the metanephrines is performed by extraction and then subsequent oxidation of the compounds to form vanillin which can then be measured by ultraviolet spectrophotometry (Pisano method) or by coupling it to indole to form a colored product. Spectrophotometry along with most of the other chemical techniques have given way to HPLC, which is the method of choice in most laboratories because of its technical simplicity and reliability. The measured urine metanephrines may be expressed as a total amount per 24-hour excretion, as a concentration if it is from a single urine specimen, or as a ratio of metanephrine : creatinine excretion.

Measurement of VMA and HVA in the urine is generally reserved for patients suspected of having neuroblastoma. The Pisano spectrophotometric method has been used in the detection of VMA. However, HPLC is now the preferred assay method for both of these compounds. The adult reference interval for VMA is less than 8 mg/24 h. In patients with renal insufficiency, or those not in normal fluid balance, urinary VMA measurements need to be correlated with creatinine excretion.

STUDIES ON PLASMA

Determination of plasma catecholamines in the diagnosis of pheochromocytoma have several advantages over some of the other tests commonly employed. If the tumor persistently secretes excess catecholamines, it is the most direct test for establishing a diagnosis. Diagnostic blood specimens can also be obtained immediately following a symptomatic attack. Furthermore, even if the diagnosis of pheochromocytoma has already been made by elevated urinary catecholamine metabolites, follow-up measurement of serum catecholamines may be helpful in localizing the tumor because pathologically elevated plasma epinephrine levels occur nearly exclusively in pheochromocytomas originating within the adrenal medulla (Karet, 1994). The disadvantages of plasma catecholamine determinations include performing the assay on specimens collected when catecholamine secretion is low or on blood specimens drawn from a patient during an acutely stressful event, because there may be considerable overlap in values between physiologic and pathologic secretion of catecholamines.

Because catecholamine levels in plasma are dependent on the sampling technique, certain precautions must be taken to obtain reliable, interpretable results. When testing for plasma catecholamines, secretory stimulants including exercise, smoking, standing upright, and volume depletion should be avoided. The venipuncture procedure alone often causes sufficient emotional anxiety to elevate catecholamine secretion significantly above baseline, and it should be performed at least half an hour before the specimen is collected. During the time between venipuncture and specimen collection, the patient should remain calm and quiet in a recumbent position. The specimen should be collected in a tube containing heparin and transported to the laboratory on ice to prevent degradation. Erythrocytes contain COMT, which at room temperature, will metabolize catecholamines present in the blood. If a long delay in analysis is anticipated, the plasma should be separated and frozen.

Circulating catecholamines are rapidly taken up by most of the tissues they perfuse. Therefore, the concentration of epinephrine in the venous circulation is about half that in the arterial circulation. For norepinephrine, the situation is more complex because peripheral sympathetic neurons release about as much norepinephrine back into the blood as is taken up by the tissues. Accordingly, under baseline conditions, about half of the norepinephrine present in venous blood is from extra-adrenal sympathetic neurons (Cryer, 1992). When interpreting norepinephrine levels in blood, the component derived from peripheral autonomic neural activity is indistinguishable from that secreted from the adrenal medulla except by selective venous sampling.

Normally, 60% to 80% of epinephrine and norepinephrine in the blood are conjugated. Some of the circulating conjugated catecholamines may be dietary in origin. In renal failure, excretion of conjugated metabolites may be impaired, leading to persistently elevated plasma levels, which may be a source of false-positive catecholamine elevations. Moreover, only the free catecholamines are biologically active, therefore no special efforts are made to include the conjugated forms in measurements of plasma catecholamines.

Epinephrine and norepinephrine in plasma can be measured using fluorometry, radioenzymatic assay, or HPLC. All of these methods usually require an extraction and concentration procedure on the plasma before the assay is performed. About 50% to 60% of circulating catecholamines are loosely bound to albumin, globulins, and other serum proteins. However, this generally has no bearing on radioenzymatic and HPLC assays that measure both bound and unbound catecholamines.

The fluorometric techniques involve either chemical oxidation of the catecholamines to fluorescent trihydroxyindole compounds or a condensation reaction with ethylenediamine. The measured fluorescence produced by either of these reactions is directly proportional to the amount of epinephrine and norepinephrine in the sample. This technique is no longer in common use because the sensitivity and specificity of fluorometry is less than that of radioenzymatic and HPLC assays.

Radioenzymatic isotope derivative assays use partially purified COMT enzyme preparations to transfer a tritium-labeled methyl group to the catecholamine molecule. COMT catalyzes the transfer of a labeled methyl group from ^{3}H-S-adenosylmethionine (SAM) to dopamine, norepinephrine, and epinephrine present in the specimen, with the subsequent formation of tritiated 3-methoxytyramine, normetanephrine, and metanephrine, respectively. The labeled products are then extracted and separated chromatographically. Measurement of the radioactivity of the 3-methoxytyramine fraction gives a direct estimate of the dopamine content of the specimen. The labeled metanephrine and normetanephrine that remain are then oxidized to form tritiated vanillin, which is then counted, and the norepinephrine and epinephrine catecholamine concentrations in the plasma are determined from a standard curve. Another radioenzymatic assay specific for norepinephrine only uses phenylethanolamine-N-methyltransferase (PNMT) to catalyze the transfer of a tritium-labeled methyl group from SAM to the amino group of norepinephrine. The labeled product is isolated chromatographically, eluted, and counted. Shortcomings of the radioenzymatic assay include the time-consuming and labor-intensive nature of the method and problems with precision in test results both within and between laboratories. Because of these problems, this method is being replaced in many laboratories by HPLC techniques.

The HPLC techniques involve an initial alumina extraction and concentration step, often with an ion exchange procedure followed by reverse-phase or ion-exchange HPLC separation of dopamine, norepinephrine, and epinephrine. As each catecholamine fraction elutes off the column, it is oxidized and an electric current is generated that is detected by amperometric or coulometric measurement. Fluorogenic and chemiluminescent detection methods for use in catecholamine determinations by HPLC have also been described that may have improved sensitivity and specificity (Alberts, 1992; Prados, 1994).

For healthy subjects, plasma norepinephrine values range up to about 500 ng/L, and plasma epinephrine levels range up to about 100 ng/L. These reference values are used by most clinical laboratories. The major source of variability in plasma catecholamine test results is related to true fluctuations in circulating levels, not to test methodology (Rosano, 1991). In young children, plasma catecholamine levels are generally higher and more widely variable, which may obscure the diagnostic distinction between normal and pathologic catecholamine secretion (Candito, 1993). In general, total plasma catecholamine results greater than 2000 ng/L are seen almost exclusively in pheochromocytoma; levels below 1000 ng/L generally exclude the diagnosis.

In borderline cases, administration of 0.3 mg of the α-adrenergic agonist clonidine suppresses catecholamine release in normal patients but not in those with autonomously secreting pheochromocytomas. The clonidine suppression test compares plasma epinephine levels before to three hours after administration of clonidine under stable conditions, which should produce at least a 50% decrease. However, either false-positive or false-negative results may occur if catecholamine secretion is erratic or the patient is taking other medications that have an effect on the cardiovascular system (Sjoberg, 1992). Pentolinium has been substituted for clonidine because of its more potent sympatholytic effects and shorter half-life. Provocative tests for pheochromocytomas, however, have been largely abandoned owing to the risks associated with inducing an acute hypertensive crisis.

Another confirmatory test in diagnosing pheochromocytoma in patients with borderline catecholamine levels is by assaying plasma for chromogranin A, a soluble protein secreted along with the catecholamines from chromaffin granules. Chromogranin A levels in plasma have been reported to have a diagnostic sensitivity and specificity for pheochromocytoma of 83% and 96%, respectively (Hsiao, 1991). High chromogranin A levels may occur in patients with renal insufficiency, which accounts for a major source of false positive results (Canale, 1994). Chromogranin levels reliably decline following surgical resection of pheochromocytomas, which may then be used as a marker to follow response to treatment (Grondal, 1991).

Additional Follow-Up Testing

Once diagnosed by biochemical studies, pheochromocytomas need to be localized by CT scan or T_2-weighted MRI in anticipation of surgical resection. If the tumor cannot be found, or if metastatic deposits are suspected, scintillation scanning can be performed using ^{131}I-labeled meta-iodobenzylguanidine (MIBG), a catecholamine analogue that is sequestered in sympathetic tissue by active reuptake mechanisms. Individual adrenal gland tumors suspicious for pheochromocytoma and extramedullary pheochromocytomas may also be diagnosed *in vivo* by fluoroscopically guided selective venous blood sampling for epinephrine and norepinephrine secretion. Although the invasive nature of this test speaks against it, this test has been found to be more sensitive and more specific than both radiologic and nuclear medicine studies in successfully locating catecholamine-secreting pheochromocytomas and paragangliomas (Chew, 1994). Selective venous sampling is usually reserved for patients suspected of having multiple tumor foci. Following successful tumor resection, the prognosis is usually excellent. Urinary metanephrines should be retested several weeks after surgery to ensure completeness of resection and also periodically thereafter as an early marker of recurrence (Werbel, 1995).

Hormones of the Adrenal Cortex

The adrenal cortex is composed of three distinct zones. The most superficial is the zona glomerulosa, the primary source of the mineralocorticoid aldosterone, which promotes reabsorption of salt and water by the kidney to help maintain blood pressure and tonicity. In addition, the precursor molecules 11-deoxycorticosterone (DOC) and 11-deoxycortisol also have mineralocorticoid activity, which in excess, are responsible for hypertension seen in some of the congenital adrenal hyperplasia syndromes. Next is the zona fasciculata, where the glucocorticoid cortisol is produced. The glucocorticoids are 21 carbon steroid compounds with a hydroxyl group on carbon 17, hence the synonym 17-hydroxycorticosteroids. These hormones are needed in times of stress to maintain blood glucose levels and prevent shock. Cortisol regulates its own secretion by a negative feedback effect on the hypothalamic-pituitary axis, inhibiting release of ACTH from the pituitary gland. Although cortisol is the most important glucocorticoid, corticosterone, which is a hormone of the mineralocorticoid pathway, also has glucocorticoid activity. Closest to the medulla is the zona reticularis, where the sex hormones testosterone and estradiol are synthesized. The androgens are 18-carbon steroids with saturated A rings, in contrast to the estrogens, which are 17-carbon steroids with unsaturated A rings. The functions of these hormones are summarized in Table 16–9.

Congenital Disorders of Adrenal Cortical Enzyme Deficiencies

2

The different hormones of the adrenal cortex are all steroid derivatives synthesized from cholesterol, as illustrated in Figure 16–8. The enzymes that catalyze the synthetic reactions in these pathways are of four general types: hydroxylases, dehydrogenases, desmolases, and isomerases. Because most of the inborn errors of metabolism affecting steroid hormone synthesis in the adrenal cortex involve deficiencies of the hydrolases, they constitute the most clinically important group of enzymes.

At least eight different metabolic defects in the synthesis of cortisol and aldosterone have been described, each characterized by a deficiency of a specific adrenal enzyme. Most of these enzymatic deficiencies are inherited as autosomal recessive traits with variable degrees of penetrance. Depending on the severity and location of the enzymatic defect in the metabolic pathway, deficiencies of glucocorticoids, mineralocorticoids, or sex hormones occur, with clinical manifestations of shock, salt wasting, or anomalous sexual development, respectively. Other findings may occur as a result of hormone excess caused by mass action shunting of steroid hormone synthesis down one pathway when another is blocked by an enzyme deficiency. Thus, hypertension may result from excess accumulation of mineralocorticoids, or virilization is seen if the pathway is shunted toward testosterone

Table 16–9. EFFECTS OF ADRENOCORTICAL HORMONES

Representative Hormone	Biological Effects
Cortisol (as a representative glucocorticoid)	Protein nitrogen catabolism increased
	Gluconeogenesis
	Increased blood glucose concentration
	Decreased glucose tolerance
	Increased liver glycogen
	Increased liver glycogenolysis
	Decreased peripheral uptake and utilization of glucose
	Decreased synthesis of acid-sulfated mucopolysaccharides
	Fat synthesis and redistribution
	Cellular or tissue effects
	Anti-inflammatory (retardation of inflammatory reactions)
	Dissolution of lymphoid tissue
	Lymphopenia
	Eosinopenia
	Increased erythropoiesis
	Alteration of cellular permeability, especially decreased membrane permeability to water
	Increased gastritis (HCl and pepsin) secretion
Aldosterone (as a representative mineralocorticoid)	Electrolyte regulation
	Sodium (Na^+) retention
	Potassium (K^+) excretion
	Retension of water and expansion of extracellular fluid volume
	Increases in blood pressure
Androgens (as representative sex hormones)	Protein nitrogen anabolism
	Growth and maturation—osseous and muscular
	Body hair (pubic and axillary)
	Seborrhea

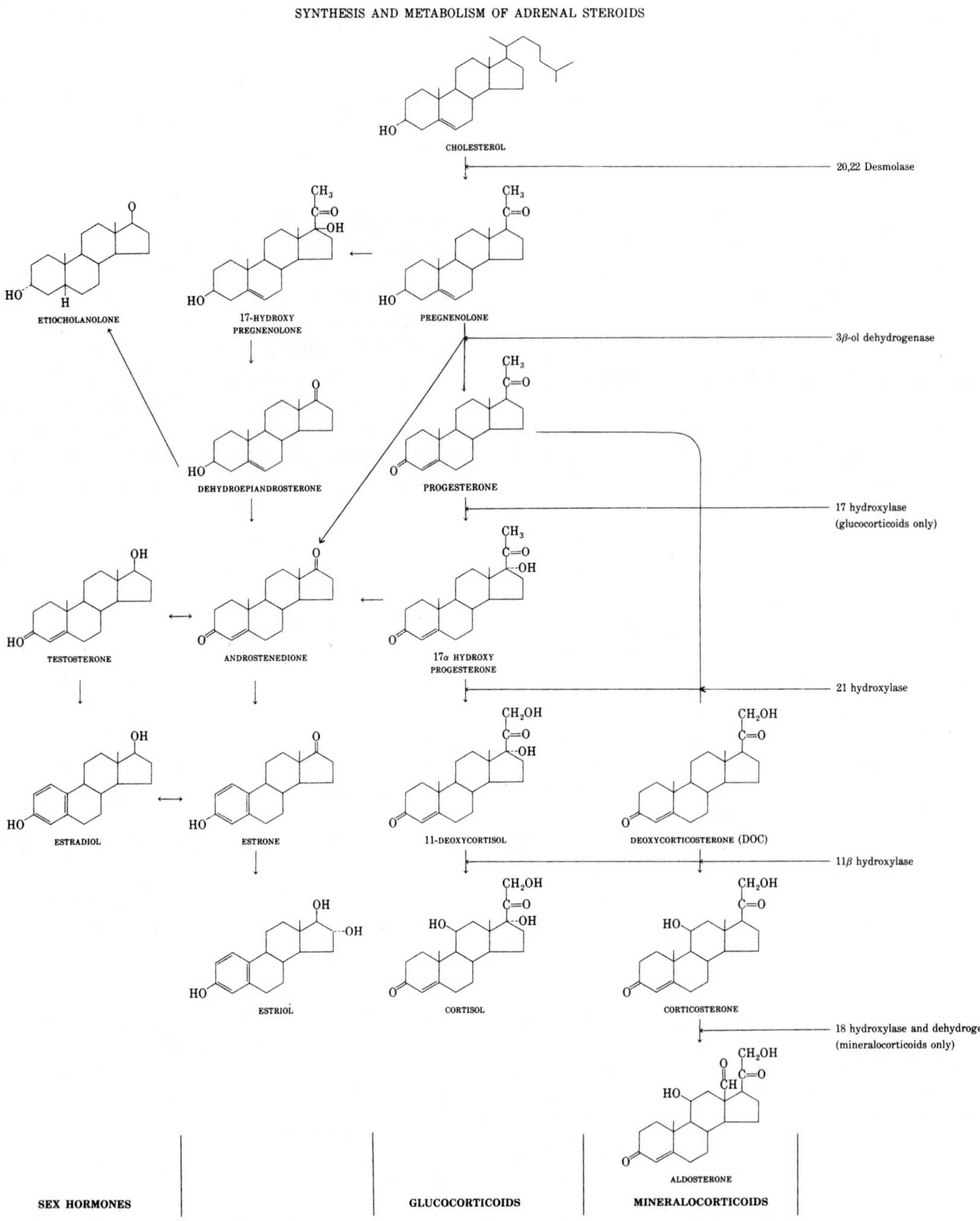

Figure 16–8. Simplified pathways of adrenocortical hormone synthesis and metabolism.

synthesis. Sometimes, as in partial enzyme deficiencies of cortisol synthesis, near-adequate hormone synthesis may be possible if hypersecretion of ACTH from the pituitary is able to stimulate adrenal hyperplasia to compensate for the deficiency. The clinical manifestations of various adrenal cortical enzyme deficiencies and their associated laboratory findings are summarized in Table 16–10.

About 95% of all cases of congenital enzyme deficiencies of the adrenal cortex are due to a single enzyme defect: 21-hydroxylase (21-OH) deficiency. Screening of newborns using capillary heel blood on paper filter disks has identified this disorder in ~1 in 10,000 persons in North America and Europe, and as high as 1 in 300 in Yupik Eskimos of Alaska. 21-OH is involved in the pathway that converts 17-α-hydroxyprogesterone (17-OHP) to 11-deoxycortisol, and progesterone to 11-deoxycorticosterone. This defect results in the shunting away from cortisol and aldosterone synthesis toward testosterone. Depending on the degree of 21-OH deficiency, the patient may be asymptomatic except in times of stress or may present in infancy with severe salt wasting, hypoglycemia, and in females, virilization. The deficiency of aldosterone and cortisol is associated with excess levels of the precursors 17-hydroxyprogesterone (17-OHP) and pregnanitriol in the urine and also elevated 17-OHP in the serum. Partial 21-OH deficiency, as may occur in heterozygotes, can be confirmed by comparing serum 17-OHP levels before and 60

Table 16–10. CONGENITAL ENZYME DISORDERS OF THE ADRENAL: CLINICAL AND BIOCHEMICAL FEATURES

Enzyme Deficiency	Virilization	Adrenocortical Insufficiency (Salt Losing)	Hypertension	Anomalous Sexual Development	Laboratory Findings
21-Hydroxylase	Present	Present in <1/3	Absent	Female virilized	Greatly increased urinary pregnanetriol and 17-KS; increased plasma 17-OHP
11-Hydroxylase	Present	Absent	Present in majority	Female virilized	Increased serum 11-deoxycortisol and urinary 17-OHCS and 17-KS
3-β-hydroxysteroid dehydrogenase	Slight (in female)	Present	Absent	Female normal or slight virilization	Increased dehydroepiandrosterone; increased 17-KS
17-Hydroxylase	Absent	Absent	Present	Absent secondary sex characteristics	Metabolites of corticosterone and DOC increased; urinary 17-OHCS, 17-KS decreased
20,22-Desmolase	Absent	Present	Absent	Lack of masculinization	All urine and plasma adrenal steroids decreased
18-Hydroxylase and 18-hydroxysteroid dehydrogenase	Absent	Present	Absent	Normal	Metabolites of corticosterone and 11-deoxycorticosterone increased; 17-OCHS increased in 18-dehydrogenase defect

17-KS = 17-ketosteroids; 17-OHP = 17-α-hydroxyprogesterone; 17-OHCS = 17-hydroxycorticosteroids; DOC = 11-deoxycorticosterone.

minutes after administering 0.25 mg ACTH to stimulate hormone synthesis. If a partial deficiency exists, 17-OHP levels should increase. However, if a proband is available, genetic testing is superior to these older biochemical tests in identifying heterozygotes (Honour, 1993). The goal of glucocorticoid and mineralocorticoid replacement therapy in patients with 21-OH deficiency is to keep 17-OHP levels below 2.0 μg/L and ACTH levels under 100 ng/L, and to prevent shunting toward testosterone synthesis, as demonstrated by normal levels of β-4-androstenendione. The gene responsible for 21-OH deficiency, CYP21, has been identified and used in prenatal diagnostic testing by PCR and Southern blotting on chorionic villous samples (New, 1994; White, 1994a).

The second most common enzyme deficiency of the adrenal cortex is 11-β-hydroxylase (11-OH) deficiency. This defect blocks the final conversion of 11-deoxycortisol to cortisol and deoxycorticosterone (DOC) to corticosterone. As with 21-OH deficiency, there is again mass action shunting of precursor steroids toward testosterone synthesis, with resulting virilization. However, DOC has mineralocorticoid activity, so that its accumulation results in hypertension by a similar mechanism as in hyperaldosteronism. In some circumstances, 11-OH deficiency may only affect the synthesis of cortisol. Prenatal diagnosis is made by measuring levels of 11-deoxycortisol in maternal urine or amniotic fluid. DOC levels are also elevated in these patients. Mutations in the genes CYP11B 1 and 2 have been identified in patients with 11-OH deficiency (White, 1994b).

Deficiency of 20,22 desmolase results in severe clinical manifestations involving all three groups of adrenal cortical hormones because the steroid synthetic pathway is blocked at the earliest step in the conversion of cholesterol to pregnenolone. Pathologically, the adrenal cortex shows marked accumulation of cholesterol and other lipids, which is the primary distinguishing feature from congenital adrenal hypoplasia. This condition may be diagnosed by the absence of testosterone, cortisol, and aldosterone, as well as the clinical manifestations thereof.

Deficiency of 3-β-hydroxysteroid dehydrogenase, the second enzymatic step in the pathway, blocks the synthesis of cortisol, aldosterone, and androgens. The gene that codes for this enzyme has been identified, and a point mutation associated with deficiency in its activity has been described (Rheaume, 1994; Simard, 1993). Excess pregnenolone, 17-OH-pregnenolone, and dehydroepiandrosterone accumulate and are detectable in the urine. Affected males have incomplete masculinization and females have clitoromegaly, along with the other manifestations of adrenal insufficiency.

17-Hydroxylase deficiency blocks the conversion of progesterone to 17-hydroxy derivatives, causing shunting from testosterone and cortisol synthesis to aldosterone. Accordingly, these patients develop hypertension and hypokalemic alkalosis in association with incomplete masculinization and decreased testosterone and cortisol levels. 17-OH deficiency is diagnosed by demonstrating high DOC levels, along with decreased urinary 17-ketosteroids and 17-hydroxycorticosteroids in these patients. The gene associated with this condition, CYP17, has been located on chromosome 10 (Kater, 1994).

Isolated enzyme deficiency of the final step of the synthetic pathway catalyzed by 18-hydroxysteroid dehydrogenase and hydroxylase to produce aldosterone leads to salt wasting. This condition may be diagnosed by demonstrating the presence of metabolites of corticosterone and 11-deoxycorticosterone in the urine.

Cortisol and the Glucocorticoids

Secretion of cortisol by the adrenal cortex occurs in response to three identifiable influences: ACTH, a diurnal rhythm, and stress. ACTH and other corticotropin-related peptides compose a family of simple peptides that are synthesized in a single chain as part of a large prohormone with a mass of about 31,000 daltons (see Fig. 16–2). This prohormone has been referred to by a variety of names, including POMC, ACTH-endorphin precursor, and ACTH/β-LPH precursor. In the anterior pituitary gland, POMC is processed predominantly to ACTH and β-lipotropin (β-LPH); β-LPH is subject to proteolytic cleavage to yield γ-LPH and β-endorphin. Within the ACTH sequence are α-MSH and the corticotropin-like intermediate lobe peptide (CLIP). The endorphin peptide appears to act on neurons in the brain and comprises a distinct peptidergic system related to pain perception. Although β-endorphin is secreted in parallel with ACTH, the significance of this is unknown.

ACTH consists of 39 amino acid residues, with the amino terminal end of amino acid residues 1 to 24 possessing full steroidogenic activity. Occasionally, processing of POMC is incomplete; other forms of ACTH thus occur, which usually have little biological activity. These forms may predominate in malignant conditions such as ectopic production by primary or metastatic lung carcinoma, and in some patients with Nelson's syndrome, a disorder characterized by the occurrence of a pituitary tumor and skin pigmentation following bilateral adrenalectomy for adrenal hyperplasia. POMC cleavage enzyme defects may also be responsible for rare forms of isolated ACTH deficiency (Nussey, 1993).

Secretion of ACTH from the pituitary is stimulated by corticotropin-releasing hormone (CRH) produced by the hypothalamus. CRH is released in a circadian pattern and in response to physiologic stimuli such as stress and hypoglycemia. Synthetic forms of CRH are used in testing anterior pituitary reserves of ACTH by comparing plasma ACTH or cortisol before and one hour after CRH stimulation (Grodum, 1993). This test is useful in distinguishing between lesions affecting the hypothalamus, pituitary, and adrenal gland (Fukata, 1993). If the lesion is in the hypothalamus, ACTH levels rise after a time delay following CRH administration. If it is in the pituitary, there is no significant ACTH response. If there is primary adrenal insufficiency, administration of CRH causes a further rise in already elevated ACTH levels.

By direct action on the pituitary, cortisol inhibits ACTH directly and probably inhibits the release of CRH as well. When plasma cortisol becomes elevated, it suppresses release of ACTH (and probably CRH), thereby ultimately lowering cortisol. Conversely, when serum cortisol reaches a nadir, the pituitary responds by increasing ACTH production, resulting in stimulation of cortisol formation. By this mechanism, ACTH and cortisol control the concentration of each other within a very narrow range, and a small change in one results in a concomitant change in the other. When the adrenal is unable to respond to ACTH because of damage or disease, cortisol levels are low and ACTH levels are high. In those conditions in which the pituitary is destroyed, ACTH is not formed and cortisol levels are consequently low. If the pituitary-adrenal axis is interrupted by the administration of large amounts of exogenous glucocorticoids, they will have an inhibitory effect on the hypothalamus and pituitary, suppressing ACTH secretion. If this suppression continues over a period of weeks, the pituitary may become persistently suppressed, and the adrenals may become atrophied in the absence of ACTH. The pituitary-adrenal axis is then unable to secrete cortisol, even when stressed.

The second influence on plasma cortisol levels is the diurnal pattern, which, in turn, is due to a circadian pattern of ACTH release. There is a major increase in secretion between 4:00 A.M. and 8:00 A.M., followed by a decrease in ACTH during the rest of the day. In subjects with a normal sleep-wake schedule, the lowest ACTH concentrations are found shortly after midnight (Fig. 16–9). Sudden changes in sleep-wake patterns have little effect on the diurnal pattern, but permanent changes in daily sleeping habits result in a gradual change in diurnal secretory patterns. Superimposed on the circadian periodicity is an ultradian rhythm of 5 to 10 secretory bursts. Although cortisol generally follows ACTH, it cannot be assumed that serum cortisol concentration is always a direct reflection of ACTH levels. An occasional ACTH surge may not result in a rise of cortisol because of the episodic secretion of ACTH and the lag of cortisol secretion, and also because of differences in half-lives (the half-life of ACTH is ~5 minutes, and it is ~65 minutes for cortisol).

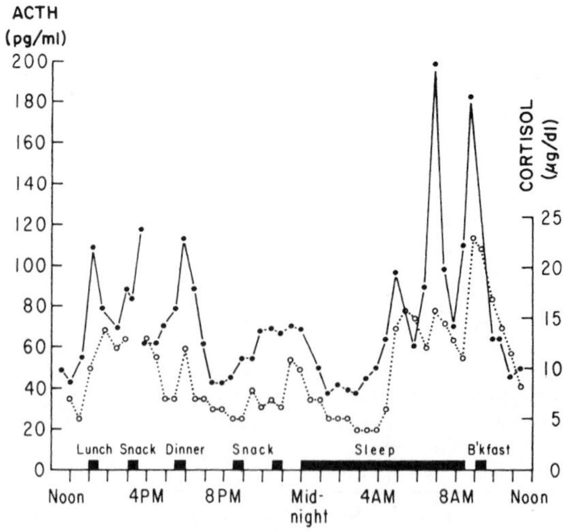

Figure 16–9. Circadian periodicity of plasma cortisol and plasma ACTH levels over a 24-hour period as determined by half-hourly sampling. ACTH and cortisol are lowest at about 4 A.M. and rise to highest level when awakening. Solid line indicates ACTH; dotted line indicates cortisol. (Modified from Krieger DT, et al: J Clin Endocrinol Metabol 1971; 32:266. © by the Endocrine Soc.)

The third important influence on cortisol secretion is stress. Stimuli such as surgical trauma, pyrogens, hypoglycemia, and hemorrhage are capable of bringing about an acute increase in ACTH and cortisol secretion. Response to stress may be absent or decreased in magnitude in patients in whom large doses of steroids have been administered for some time. The initiation of any stressful response also is dependent on an intact nervous system. For example, trauma results in the acute release of ACTH and cortisol; however, in patients with spinal cord transections, the same trauma applied to an extremity will not elicit any ACTH or cortisol response. There is evidence that the stress response of cortisol is mediated through excitatory and inhibitory inputs that become integrated at the level of the hypothalamus and modulate CRH secretion.

Most disorders of cortisol secretion can be classified by the patterns of three test results: ACTH, plasma cortisol, and urinary free cortisol (Snow, 1992).

LABORATORY MEASUREMENTS OF ACTH

The first peptide hormone measured by RIA was ACTH; however, widespread popularity and utility of ACTH measurements in clinical medicine have not occurred. Although ACTH by RIA has diagnostic usefulness, technical and practical limitations, as well as cost, have limited its use. Of these, instability of ACTH in plasma probably has been the greatest limitation of its use. ACTH appears to be rapidly deactivated by proteolytic enzymes in plasma, and even addition of the proteolytic inhibitor aprotinin (Trasylol) has little effect on its preservation. *N*-ethylmaleimide (NEM), an inhibitor of

SH-peptidases, has been used in Great Britain; it has been reported to inhibit degradation of plasma ACTH for up to 72 hours. Although no current method completely arrests the destruction of ACTH, storing specimens at 4°C greatly reduces enzymatic degradation of ACTH. Specimens should not be allowed to have contact with glass during collection, storage, and assay because ACTH becomes adsorbed to glass (Reinazartz, 1993).

Timing of specimen collection is important because of the circadian variation in ACTH. If plasma cannot be analyzed immediately, it should be stored below −20°C. Other problems associated with the measurement of ACTH are incubation damage during assay, poor sensitivity, and poor precision of the assay at low concentrations. Plasma ACTH concentrations in healthy subjects are usually less than 50 ng/L, whereas stressed individuals may have values up to about 500 ng/L.

ACTH levels are useful in differentiating primary from secondary adrenal insufficiency. In primary adrenal insufficiency, low cortisol concentrations are found, along with increased ACTH levels. In adrenal insufficiency secondary to decreased ACTH production from the pituitary, both ACTH and cortisol are expected to be low. Although in the past, stimulatory tests such as cosyntropin and ACTH infusions have been used, a single ACTH level will distinguish between primary and secondary adrenal insufficiency. In the primary disorder, ACTH levels are usually greater than 200 ng/L, whereas in pituitary insufficiency, ACTH concentrations are usually less than 50 ng/L. ACTH levels best discriminate between healthy individuals and those with adrenal insufficiency when specimens for ACTH are collected between 8:00 A.M. and 10:00 A.M.

ACTH measurements may be of great value in establishing the differential diagnosis of patients with Cushing's syndrome. Those patients with ectopic ACTH-secreting tumors characteristically have elevated plasma ACTH (usually >200 ng/L) and an elevated serum cortisol. Occasionally, neoplasms may be occult, and because of diagnostic difficulties, ACTH measurements using blood specimens obtained by selective venous sampling may be useful in localization of the lesion.

In patients with increased levels of circulating glucocorticoids due to adrenal adenomas or carcinomas, ACTH secretion is inhibited; hence, circulating ACTH levels are low or undetectable. In patients with pituitary-induced adrenal hyperplasia, plasma ACTH may be at or above the upper reference interval at 9:00 A.M., but fail to show the expected fall after midnight. It should be emphasized that ACTH best discriminates between patients with suspected Cushing's syndrome and healthy individuals when the blood specimens are obtained between 9:00 P.M. and midnight. Another use of ACTH assays is in the determination of adequacy of cortisol replacement in congenital adrenal hyperplasia syndromes. When replacement therapy is optimal, ACTH values are similar to those seen in a reference population.

ACTH levels can be measured by RIA or IRMA (Tabarin, 1992). Nonisotopic methods such as chemiluminescent immunoassays have been developed (Raff, 1994). These immunoassays all have specificity for epitopes on the biologically active amino-terminal end of the ACTH polypeptide.

SERUM CORTISOL MEASUREMENTS

About 90% of circulating cortisol is bound to serum protein, whereas the remainder is free. It is estimated that 10% to 20% is loosely bound to albumin, and the remainder is bound to the glycoprotein transcortin (cortisol-binding globulin), an α_1-globulin. It is believed that only free cortisol is active, and that the protein-bound fraction is metabolically inert, probably serving as a reservoir of free cortisol. Protein binding also may protect cortisol from deactivation by the liver or filtration by the kidney.

2

One of the earliest and simplest methods used to determine serum cortisol was a fluorometric assay. By this method, cortisol was extracted from serum with dichloromethane, acidified in an acid-alcohol mixture, and the fluorescence was measured. Corticosterone is the most important interfering substance in this assay, contributing about 40 μg/L, with other adrenal steroids such as dihydroepiandrosterone, testosterone, and 11-desoxycortisol, contributing about 20 μg/L. Spironolactone, tetracycline, and birth control pills containing estrogen also lead to spuriously high cortisol levels when measured by the fluorometric assay technique.

Cortisol can also be determined by competitive protein binding (CPB), but this technique lacks specificity. CPB assays make use of the naturally occurring cortisol-binding protein transcortin from various species. The specificity of the method depends on the binding characteristics of transcortin. Cortisone and 11-deoxycortisol compete equally well with some of the binding proteins. Progesterone, which is present in increased amounts in pregnancy, also competes with cortisol for transcortin. The CPB method has a major advantage in that 11-deoxycortisol can be extracted with carbon tetrachloride and subsequently measured in the assay. The CPB technique gives results that are about 25% lower than those measured in the Porter-Silber reaction and 25% to 50% lower than those obtained by the fluorometric procedure.

A more specific method for cortisol estimation is immunoassay. Advantages of immunoassay include small specimen volume and rapid turn-around time. When radioimmunoassay is used, cortisol must first be released from its endogenous binding proteins by blocking agents such as 8-anilino-1-naphthalene sulfonic acid (ANS). Some of the antibodies that are used show a large degree of cross-reactivity with other steroids such as 11-deoxycortisol, desoxycorticosterone, and synthetic steroids such as dexamethasone. Although cross-reactivity does not pose a problem with baseline testing, in stimulatory and suppressive maneuvers such as metyrapone or dexamethasone suppression, this can lead to spuriously high measurements. With deterioration of renal function, various steroids and their glucuronides accumulate in the blood. Because of their structure, conjugates may cross-react with some cortisol antibodies, producing an interference that can be of the same magnitude as the actual cortisol concentration. In congenital adrenal hyperplasia, high concentrations of cortisol precursors occur in the serum because of an enzyme defect. Because these precursors cross-react with assay antibodies, spurious elevations of cortisol concentrations are found; the degree of interference varies with the assay used and cannot be predicted easily. Nonisotopic immunoassay methods using organometallic tracers, fluorescence polarization, and enzyme immunoassay techniques have also been developed for cortisol determinations (Bacarese-Hamilton, 1992; Lentjes, 1993; Philomin, 1994). The major disadvantage of cortisol assays continues to be lack of specificity; however, the specificity of the immunoassay is better than that of either fluorometric or the CPB method.

HPLC assays appear to offer the ultimate in specificity. Most HPLC systems for cortisol measurements use reverse-phase liquid chromatography with ultraviolet detection (Volin, 1992). This method is both sensitive and free from many of the sources of interference encountered in immunoassays (Samaan, 1993). Other advantages of this technique include its amenability to automation and the ability to perform simultaneous determinations of other steroids, such as occur in congenital adrenal hyperplasia or following metyrapone testing.

Reference values for serum cortisol are in the range of 50 to 250 μg/L at 0800 to 1000 hours, which drop to about 20 to 120 μg/L by 2000 hours. There also is less clinical reliance on absolute cortisol values than on most other laboratory determinations because the diurnal and circadian variation is large. Serum cortisol assays are most useful in evaluating responses to adrenal stimulation or suppression tests.

DETERMINATION OF GLUCOCORTICOIDS IN URINE

One of the first procedures for estimation of glucocorticoids in urine was the method described by Porter (1950). When phenylhydrazine and sulfuric acid are added to urine, those steroids that contain 21 carbons and have a characteristic dihydroxyacetone side chain produce a color with a peak absorption at 410 nm (Porter-Silber chromogens). Methodologic improvements, such as extractions with various organic solvents, purification of urine extracts by chromatography, and the correction for a high blank (Allen corrections), have all increased the accuracy of this measurement. Because most glucocorticoids are excreted in urine as conjugates, hydrolysis with a glucuronidase is performed prior to measurement. The glucocorticoids that are measured include 11-deoxycortisol, cortisol, and cortisone (a metabolite of cortisol). Other metabolites of cortisol and cortisone, in which the A ring of the steroid is saturated (tetrahydro derivatives), also are included in this measurement. Although this method has been used to estimate 17-hydroxycorticosteroids (17-OHCS) in urine, in certain pathologic states it does not measure all of the 17-OHCS that are excreted. For example, compounds such as pregnanetriol (a metabolite of 17-OH progesterone) and certain 20-OH compounds may be extremely elevated but are not measured by this technique. Many drugs, including reserpine, chlorpromazine, meprobamate, and spironolactone, interfere with the measurement Porter-Silber chromagens. Elevated 17-OHCS being replaced by urinary free cortisol (*vide infra*) have been reported in patients treated with carbamazepine; this occurs because of formation of a metabolite that reacts with assay reagents. In newborns or neonates with congenital adrenal hyperplasia, this measurement is relatively unreliable; this is due to interference by steroids and their metabolites that usually are not present in the urine but that are excreted in large amounts in these patients.

Reference intervals for urine 17-OHCS measurements are 5 to 15 mg per 24 hours for adult males, and 5 to 13 mg/24 h for adult females. Values for 17-OHCS may be low or within the reference interval in pituitary insufficiency and adrenal insufficiency, whereas in adrenocortical hyperfunction, they may be increased. More definitive diagnostic information is obtained by using these determinations in conjunction with dexamethasone suppression. The Porter-Silber method usually is not used for glucocorticoid estimations in serum because of its lack of specificity, requirements for large serum volumes, and the need for a prior extraction step. The diagnostic accuracy of urinary 17-hydroxycorticosteroid determinations in distinguishing patients with Cushing's syndrome from normal individuals shows a sensitivity and specificity of 73% and 94%, respectively (Mengden, 1992). This is in contrast to urinary free cortisol determinations, which have a diagnostic sensitivity of 100% and specificity of 98% for the same groups of patients (Rudd 1985).

URINARY FREE CORTISOL MEASUREMENTS

Only 1% of the total adrenal secretion appears in the urine as cortisol, but it is this fraction that provides a valuable aid in diagnosis of adrenal disease. In the kidney, glomerular filtration of free cortisol is followed by passive tubular reabsorption without a demonstrable reabsorption maximum. Urine collected over 24 hours is the best specimen to submit because it provides an integrated profile of total cortisol secretion. The reliability of the test may be further improved by submitting urine collected over 2 or 3 days because day-to-day fluctuations in cortisol excretion are known to occur.

At serum cortisol levels of about 200 to 250 μg/L (the upper 0800-hour reference value), the binding capacity of transcortin is exceeded; this leads to a very rapid and disproportionate increase in the unbound fraction compared with the total serum cortisol. For example, a doubling of the cortisol from 200 to 400 μg/L results in at least a fivefold increase in the unbound cortisol in serum. At these levels, free cortisol clearance by the kidneys is directly proportional to the unbound serum cortisol concentration and leads to a steep rise in cortisol clearance. Thus, when urinary free cortisol excretion rather than serum cortisol is used, it is easier to discriminate patients with adrenal hyperfunction from a reference population.

Urinary free cortisol levels are unaffected by alterations of hepatic metabolism of cortisol. Although total cortisol production and urinary 17-OHCS may be increased, the serum cortisol and urinary free cortisol remain within the reference interval. As a result of the increased serum concentration of transcortin in pregnancy and estrogen therapy, serum cortisol is increased. This increase is not reflected by an elevation of cortisol metabolites in urine, but urinary free cortisol may be increased. Because the renal clearance of cortisol is dependent on normal kidney function, it is not surprising that patients with renal disease may have low urinary values. Conditions in which spuriously elevated values occur include starvation, application of topical steroids, and perhaps hydration in the form of water loading.

The techniques used for urinary free cortisol measurements include CPB, RIA, and HPLC, which is considered the reference method by many. The specificity of the CPB technique is limited by the specificity of the transcortin used as the binding protein. Similarly, the measurement of urinary free cortisol using RIA is dependent on the antibody used. Reference intervals for urinary free cortisol by RIA or CPB are 20 to 90 μg/24 hours. When measuring free cortisol in urine by RIA, reference intervals have been found to vary with patient gender (men had higher reference intervals than women), the use of an extraction procedure, and the RIA test kit used (Lamb, 1994). For increased specificity, RIA is performed following chromatography or extraction of urine specimens. Without chromatography to purify the urinary steroids, CPB and RIA methods overestimate the amount of cortisol present. For example, when antigenically interfering compounds are removed by HPLC, followed by RIA quantification, a reference interval of 10 to 42 mg/24 h is obtained. Measurement of urinary free cortisol by CPB or RIA methods can yield an accurate reflection of adrenocortical function provided that there are no gross metabolic abnormalities present and that the reference interval is established carefully for each method used. The most specific assay method for determination of urinary free cortisol is by HPLC, which has a lower reference interval than RIA measurements.

A low urinary free cortisol value is suggestive of adrenal hypofunction, such as occurs in Addison's disease, but overlap of values with the reference interval is large. The greatest use of urinary free cortisol determinations is for states of adrenal hyperfunction, such as Cushing's syndrome, in which patients have urinary free cortisol values greater than the reference interval.

HYPERCORTISOLISM: CUSHING'S SYNDROME

Cushing's syndrome is a group of clinical and metabolic disorders characterized by adrenocortical hyperfunction; it is associated with excess production of glucocorticoids, or glucocorticoids and androgens. Patients with severe forms of the syndrome are easily recognizable when the disorder is florid. In less severely afflicted individuals, the vague signs and symptoms that occur may not be easily recognized as caused by hypercortisolism. Although many patients with ectopic ACTH-producing tumors have elevated ACTH and glucocorticoids, the patient's demise may occur before clinical signs of the syndrome appear because of the rapid growth of these tumors.

Laboratory findings in Cushing's syndrome are (1) excessive and persistent production of cortisol measured as elevated serum cortisol, urinary free cortisol, or 17-OHCS; (2) loss of usual circadian rhythm of ACTH and cortisol; (3) loss of suppression of cortisol production by administration of the synthetic glucocorticoid dexamethasone; and (4) hyperglycemia. Of the clinical findings that suggest Cushing's syndrome, the most common are obesity, hypertension, and hirsutism.

Cushing's disease or pituitary Cushing's syndrome, the most common disorder of glucocorticoid excess, occurs as a result of an ACTH-secreting tumor of the pituitary. If the pituitary is the source of excess ACTH secretion, this can be demonstrated directly by selective sampling of the inferior petrosal sinus blood, an invasive procedure that has a relatively high cost and complication rate. The ACTH concentration in the petrosal sinus blood should exceed twice that of peripheral venous blood to ensure a diagnostic sensitivity and specificity of 100% (Orth, 1995).

Cushing's disease is to be distinguished from Cushing's syndrome due to an ectopic tumor producing corticotropin-releasing hormone (CRH), indirectly leading to pituitary ACTH hypersecretion, and also from an ectopic tumor releasing excess ACTH. In patients with either pituitary or ectopic ACTH-secreting tumors, CRH levels by immunoassay are suppressed; whereas in ectopic CRH syndrome, they are elevated. Administration of exogenous CRH to patients with an ACTH-producing pituitary adenoma will produce a rise in ACTH that is not completely suppressible by high dose dexamethasone. However, in pure ectopic CRH syndrome, the exogenous CRH-induced rise in ACTH can be suppressed by high-dose dexamethasone.

2

Adrenal Cushing's syndrome is a primary disorder of excess autonomous cortisol production, with the hypothalamic-pituitary axis being suppressed. Adrenal Cushing's (adenoma or carcinoma) accounts for less than 20% of the cases, whereas pituitary Cushing's accounts for about 68%, and ectopic production of ACTH outside the pituitary-adrenal axis is the cause of about 12% of cases (Orth, 1995). Because the therapeutic modality and prognosis differ depending on location of the cause, it is important that a specific diagnosis be reached.

Serum cortisol concentrations greater than 300 μg/L at 0800 hours and greater than 150 μg/L at 1600 hours provide useful guidelines for selecting patients for further diagnostic evaluation. Cushing's syndrome may then be confirmed by suppressive or provocative testing. Suppressive testing usually involves oral administration of dexamethasone, a steroid that has at least 25 times more glucocorticoid potency than cortisol. It is administered in small quantities to suppress ACTH but provokes little interference with glucocorticoid measurements by any of the commonly used methods. Suppressive testing procedures are divided into two groups: (1) those in which only a serum cortisol value is obtained and (2) those in which a 24-hour urine collection prior to and following doses of dexamethasone is obtained. Because of difficulty in collection of a complete 24-hour urine sample and in administration of dexamethasone on a regularly scheduled basis, those tests that involve urine collection are usually reserved for hospitalized patients. The response of serum and urine determination to dexamethasone suppression is shown in Tables 16–11 and 16–12.

A simple screening test is the overnight dexamethasone suppression test. One milligram of dexamethasone is ingested by the patient at 2300 hours, and the following morning at 0800 hours, a serum cortisol level is obtained. In healthy individuals a serum cortisol level of less than 50 μg/L is observed, but in patients with Cushing's syndrome, there is rarely suppression to less than 100 μg/L. Other causes of nonsuppressed cortisol levels include psychiatric disease, alcoholism, and stress. Because phenytoin causes increased metabolism of dexamethasone, cortisol may not become fully suppressed, causing false-positive dexamethasone suppression test results. Drugs such as estrogen, which increase serum transcortin, the cortisol-binding protein, may also result in elevated cortisol levels. Because of these and possibly other factors, about 1% of healthy individuals, 13% of obese patients, and 25% of hospitalized and chronically ill patients show false positive overnight dexamethasone suppression tests. False-negative results, on the other hand, occur in less than 2% of patients.

Table 16–11. SERUM CORTICOSTEROID RESPONSES TO DIAGNOSTIC MANEUVERS DESIGNED TO DEMONSTRATE NONAUTONOMY OR AUTONOMY OF ADRENAL FUNCTION

	Serum Cortisol Concentrations					
Condition	*Basal (0800-Hour)*	*Circadian Variation*	*0800-Hour Response to Dexamethasone (1 mg at 2300 hours)*	*Response to Aqueous Pitressin (10 Units IM)*	*Response to Cosyntropin*	**0800-Hour Plasma ACTH**
Normal	10–25 μg/dL (276–690 nmol/L)	A.M. greater than P.M.	<6 μg/dL (166 nmol/L	≥15 μg/dL (414 nmol/L) increase above baseline	Doubling of baseline value	20–100 pg/mL (4.4–22 pmol/L)
Adrenal hyperplasia	Normal or increased	Absent	>6 μg/dL (166 nmol/L)	Increased	Increased	Normal or increased
Adrenal adenoma	Normal or increased	Absent	>6 μg/dL (166 nmol/L)	Absent	None or normal	Decreased
Adrenal carcinoma	Increased	Absent	>6 μg/dL (166 nmol/L)	Absent	None	Decreased
Pituitary tumor	Increased	Absent	>6 μg/dL (166 nmol/L)	Absent	None to slight	Markedly increased
Ectopic ACTH syndrome	Increased	Absent	>6 μg/dL (166 nmol/L)	Absent	Usually none	Markedly increased

Modified from Krieger, 1976.

Low-dose dexamethasone is used to differentiate healthy individuals from those with Cushing's syndrome. At least two baseline 24-hour urine collections are obtained for 17-OHCS (reference interval: 3 to 11 mg/24 h). For two days, 0.5 mg of dexamethasone is given orally every 6 hours and the response of urinary 17-OHCS or urinary free cortisol is measured. On the second day of dexamethasone, a reference group population suppresses urinary 17-OHCS to less than 3 mg/24 h and urinary free cortisol to less than 20 μg/24 h, whereas patients with Cushing's syndrome fail to suppress to this level. However, a number of patients with Cushing's syndrome have been described whose response is within the reference interval.

The high-dose dexamethasone suppression test (2 mg given orally every 6 hours for two days) is used to differentiate patients with adrenal hyperplasia from others with hypercortisolism. A reference population and those with adrenal hyperplasia show urinary 17-OHCS levels that are less than 50% of the initial value and urinary free cortisol less than 20% of baseline. However, occasionally a paradoxical response of nonsuppression occurs in patients with adrenal hyperplasia. Most patients with adrenal adenomas, carcinomas, or ectopic ACTH syndromes do not show suppression. Patients with adrenal carcinoma usually have 17-keto-steroids above 20 mg/24 hr and signs of virilization in contrast with those patients with adrenal adenomas. Pituitary and ectopic tumors can then be localized by radiographic procedures. Although urinary 17-OHCS may be elevated in obesity, urinary free cortisol and serum cortisol are within the reference interval and suppress in response to overnight dexa-

Table 16–12. URINARY CORTICOSTEROID RESPONSES TO DIAGNOSTIC MANEUVERS DESIGNED TO DEMONSTRATE NONAUTONOMY OR AUTONOMY OF ADRENAL FUNCTION

	Urinary 17-Hydroxycorticosteroids				Urinary 17-Ketosteroids
		Suppression with Dexamethasone			
Condition	*Basal*	*2 mg*	*8 mg*	*ACTH Stimulation*	*Basal*
Normal	3–10 mg/24 h (8.3–27.6 μmol/day)	<3 mg/24 h (8.3 μmol/day)	<50% initial value	Two- to threefold baseline increase	Female: 5–15 mg/24 h (13.8–41.4 μmol/day) Male: 8–20 mg/24 h (22.1–55.2 μmol/day)
Adrenal hyperplasia	Increased	Not suppressed	<50% initial value, occasional "paradoxical" response	Hyperresponsive	Normal or increased
Adrenal adenoma	Increased	Not suppressed	Not suppressed	None or normal response	Decreased or normal
Adrenal carcinoma	Markedly increased	Not suppressed	Not suppressed (rare exceptions)	No response (rare exceptions)	Markedly increased
Pituitary tumor	Markedly increased	Not suppressed	Not suppressed	No to slight response	Increased
Ectopic ACTH syndrome	Markedly increased	Not suppressed	Usually not suppressed	Usually no response	Increased

Modified from Krieger, 1976.

methasone. This response and the usual circadian variation of plasma cortisol make it possible to differentiate obese individuals from patients with Cushing's syndrome.

The diagnosis of Cushing's syndrome can be made following dexamethasone suppression tests by measuring either serum or urine cortisol. During the second day of the suppression test, nonsuppressed cortisol levels at 1600 hours are those greater than 50 μg/L with low-dose dexamethasone and greater than 100 μg/L with high-dose dexamethasone. In those patients whose serum cortisol values were nonsuppressible, a baseline dehydroepiandrosterone value at 0800 hours below 0.4 mg/L is suggestive of an adrenal adenoma. The laboratory findings in patients with hypercortisolism are summarized in Tables 16–11 and 16–12.

Vasopressin, which releases ACTH probably because its structure is similar to that of CRH, has been of value in the diagnosis of adrenal and pituitary disease. A normal response following administration of 10 units of vasopressin intramuscularly is a doubling of ACTH levels and an increase in serum cortisol of 150 μg/L over baseline values. In patients with adrenal carcinoma, adenoma, or pituitary tumor, high circulating levels of cortisol from the autonomously secreting lesion suppress the intact hypothalamic-pituitary axis; therefore a response to vasopressin does not occur. Another aid to localization of the lesion responsible for Cushing's syndrome is the cortisol response to stimulatory testing. Those patients whose Cushing's syndrome is due to adrenal hyperplasia have an increased response of serum cortisol to vasopressin and cosyntropin, a synthetic ACTH analogue. Patients with other forms of the syndrome have little or no response to these stimuli.

Two modifications of the dexamethasone suppression test result in improved accuracy in the diagnosis of Cushing's syndrome. When the dose of dexamethasone is administered in terms of body weight (i.e., 5 μg/kg/6 h for the low dose) and urinary excretion of 17-OHCS is expressed in milligrams or grams creatinine, better discrimination between Cushing's syndrome and a reference population can be made.

Plasma ACTH levels are suppressed in patients with adrenal tumors, and are elevated to over 200 ng/L in most patients with ectopic ACTH production. In about half the patients with pituitary Cushing's syndrome, ACTH levels may be within the reference interval despite the presence of hypercortisolism.

HYPERCORTISOLISM AND THE DEXAMETHASONE SUPPRESSION TEST IN DEPRESSION

Excess activity of the hypothalamic-pituitary axis similar to that seen in pituitary Cushing's syndrome has been demonstrated in some patients with primary affective disorders. This phenomenon is sometimes referred to as pseudo-Cushing's syndrome because of the similar findings of elevated cortisol levels which do not follow a diurnal rhythm (Murphy, 1991). The suppression of this axis by dexamethasone has been used as a biochemical indicator of endogenous depression.

A common protocol for the dexamethasone suppression test in the diagnosis of depression is as follows: The patient ingests 1 mg of dexamethasone at 2300 hours, and serum cortisol measurements are obtained at 1600 and 2300 hours the following day. Approximately 50% of depressed patients demonstrate abnormal early escape from suppression (i.e., serum cortisol levels > 50 μg/L by CPB at 1600 or 2300 hours). If, for practical reasons, sampling is limited to only the 1600-hour specimen, there is about a 20% loss in procedure sensitivity. Depressed patients who fail to suppress cortisol secretion in response to dexamethasone also show an impaired ACTH response to exogenous CRH (Thalen, 1993).

Many drugs interfere with interpretation of this test, including methyldopa, meprobamate, spironolactone, reserpine, and cyproheptadine. Other drugs such as phenobarbital and phenytoin interfere by accelerating the metabolism of dexamethasone. Illnesses such as cardiac failure, uncontrolled diabetes mellitus, pulmonary disease, fever, and anorexia also interfere with test results. A few patients with psychiatric disease such as dementia, schizophrenia, character disorders, and bipolar disorders may also show nonsuppression.

HYPOCORTISOLISM: ADDISON'S DISEASE AND PITUITARY INSUFFICIENCY

Primary adrenocortical insufficiency (Addison's disease) occurs most commonly from an autoimmune process and less often from tuberculosis and iatrogenic causes (Davenport, 1991). When hypocortisolism results from a pituitary lesion, it is termed secondary adrenal insufficiency. Patients with primary adrenal insufficiency have deficiencies of both glucocorticoids and mineralocorticoids in contrast to individuals with secondary adrenal insufficiency who have only a glucocorticoid deficiency. Because mineralocorticoid-deficient patients have a higher plasma renin activity than those with only a glucocorticoid deficiency, renin measurements may be of some value in diagnosis. Although most patients with hypocortisolism have low serum cortisol levels, a value within the reference interval obtained from a specimen drawn during a time of stress does not exclude the diagnosis. Rather, it may support this diagnosis because a suboptimal cortisol level may have risen into the reference interval in response to a very high ACTH level induced by stress.

Both primary and secondary adrenal insufficiency can be demonstrated by failure of the adrenal to respond to various stimulatory procedures. The most convenient procedure for studying patients suspected of having hypocortisolism is the injection of a commercially available ACTH analogue, cosyntropin. This peptide is the biologically active amino-terminal end of the ACTH molecule and contains amino acids 1 to 24. Serum specimens for cortisol determinations are drawn as a baseline as well as 30 and 60 minutes following cosyntropin injection. A normal response is a doubling of serum cortisol, but more stringent criteria such as a baseline of 50 μg/L, with an increase of at least 70 μg/L at 30 minutes and 110 μg/L at 60 minutes, or the 30-minute level exceeding 180 μg/L have been applied. Evidence indicates that the cosyntropin test accurately reflects integrated hypothalamic, pituitary, and adrenal function. The diagnosis of pituitary or adrenal insufficiency, or both, made by the insulin tolerance test (ITT). When compared with the cosyntropin procedure, the ITT is equally accurate for the diagnosis of hypocortisolism.

Other stimulatory testing involves infusion of ACTH or its analogues for two to five days, with the response of 17-hydroxysteroids or urinary free cortisol measured. Patients with either primary or secondary adrenal insufficiency may present with low serum cortisol and may not respond to cosyntropin. To substantiate the diagnosis of primary or secondary adrenal insufficiency indisputably, prolonged exposure of the adrenal to ACTH is essential. An intravenous infusion of ACTH or its analogues for two days appears to be the most advantageous in this regard. With this procedure, a normal response is an elevation of urinary 17-hydroxycorticoids three to five times higher than baseline, whereas patients with primary adrenal insufficiency have extremely low baseline values that fail to exhibit this degree of stimulation. Patients with secondary adrenocortical insufficiency (hypopituitarism) or patients receiving suppressive doses of steroids for a prolonged period of time usually have an inadequate or absent response in urinary 17-hydroxycorticosteroids on the first day of testing and a slight rise on the second day to about 10 mg/24 h. It should be noted that the ACTH infusion test can be performed on patients presenting with signs of acute adrenal insufficiency, a medical emergency. If this diagnosis is suspected, a baseline cortisol and ACTH should be obtained and a stimulation test performed over two days, with dexamethasone used to provide the patient with an immediate source of glucocorticoids.

Metyrapone has been used to assess pituitary ACTH reserve. For the performance of this test, metyrapone is ingested in divided doses over two days and urinary excretion of glucocorticoids is measured. Because metyrapone is an inhibitor of the 11-hydroxylase enzyme, it blocks the formation of cortisol from 11-deoxycortisol, causing cortisol levels to fall and ACTH levels to rise. If metyrapone is continued for a period of time, the blockade is overcome and glucocorticoids rise. Patients with reduced pituitary reserves such as those with pituitary tumors are unable to increase ACTH secretion to maintain cortisol levels. These patients may suffer from acute adrenal insufficiency during testing if exogenous glucocorticoids are not provided. In contrast to the rapid evaluation of pituitary reserve provided by insulin tolerance or cosyntropin testing, this provocative test requires three days to perform. Because of this and the severe side effects that may occur, the metyrapone test has fallen into disfavor. However, metyrapone remains in use as an overnight procedure performed by administering a single dose of 30 mg/kg body weight given at bedtime. The following morning, plasma 11-deoxycortisol and ACTH are measured. In a reference population, 11-deoxycortisol increases to above 70 μg/L and ACTH to over 100 ng/L, whereas in those patients with secondary adrenal insufficiency, the response is much lower. The overnight metyrapone test may be superior to the high-dose dexamethasone suppression test in the differential diagnosis of Cushing's syndrome. When testing the pituitary's ability to secrete ACTH, the overnight metyrapone test is comparable to the CRH stimulation test (Riddick, 1994).

The majority of severely ill patients in intensive care units have elevated serum cortisol levels. Similar to Cushing's syndrome patients, hypercortisolism in patients in septic shock is not suppressible by dexamethasone (Perrot, 1993). Critically ill patients whose cortisol levels are below 130 μg/L have a particularly poor prognosis.

The use of steroids for the treatment of many malignant and immunologic disorders is a common iatrogenic cause of adrenal insufficiency. The degree of adrenal suppression is dependent on the specific glucocorticoid dose, duration, frequency, and route of administration. To assess adrenal function in a patient being tapered off exogenous steroids, the morning glucocorticoid dose is omitted and the 0800-hour cortisol level is measured. If it is above 100 μg/L, routine supplementation of steroids can be ended. Because the adrenal cortex lags behind the pituitary in recovery from steroid suppression, complete adrenal recovery can also be demonstrated by an appropriate rise in serum cortisol following an 0800-hour cosyntropin infusion.

RENIN-ALDOSTERONE AXIS

Hypertension is a major affliction of modern society, striking at least 10% to 15% of adults in industrialized nations. At least 20 million people in the United States have hypertension, with 90% to 98% of the cases classified as essential hypertension. The mortality and morbidity from associated myocardial, cerebrovascular, and renal complications necessitate treating this disorder. Investigation of the etiology of hypertension revealed the importance of the renin-angiotensin-aldosterone system, not only in the origin and persistence of hypertension but also as a guide to its treatment. The role of the renin-aldosterone axis is to maintain blood pressure within normal limits by sensing the plasma volume and then adjusting it.

Renin is a proteolytic enzyme formed and stored by juxtaglomerular cells of the kidney and released into the lymph and the renal venous blood. There are several isoenzymes of renin. Their release is regulated by cAMP. Prorenin, the precursor of renin, enters the circulation unregulated but may regulate vascular tone locally. Renin acts on renin substrate or angiotensinogen, an α_2-globulin made by the liver, to split off the decapeptide, angiotensin I. Angiotensin I is converted within the circulation into an octapeptide, angiotensin II, by a converting enzyme system found mainly in the lung. It is believed that angiotensin II is the peptide responsible for the physiologic effects on target tissues. Evidence indicates that the octapeptide angiotensin II is further split to a heptapeptide, angiotensin III, or that angiotensin I may be changed directly to angiotensin III without being converted to angiotensin II. Although there is still speculation about the functions of angiotensin III, it appears to modulate aldosterone secretion. The active angiotensins are rapidly cleared by various aminopeptidases (angiotensinases) within the circulation and during transit through tissues. These relationships are shown in Fig. 16–10. Renin is synthesized in a larger form (prorenin or big renin) and converted to its active form within the juxtaglomerular cell. Circulating prorenin has been associated with some renal tumors, and has been found to increase in parallel with renin in patients undergoing various diagnostic and therapeutic maneuvers. Baxter (1995) provides a more complete description of renin physiology and synthesis.

Renin, through its product, angiotensin II, directly stimulates the synthesis and secretion of aldosterone by the adrenal zona glomerulosa. Renin release is dependent on changes in effective plasma volume, which, in turn, is dependent on tubular reabsorption of serum sodium by the kidney. Low plasma volume and low serum sodium stimulate the secretion of renin, resulting in aldosterone release, which causes sodium retention with an increase in plasma volume, and elevated blood pressure and potassium loss. Conversely, in-

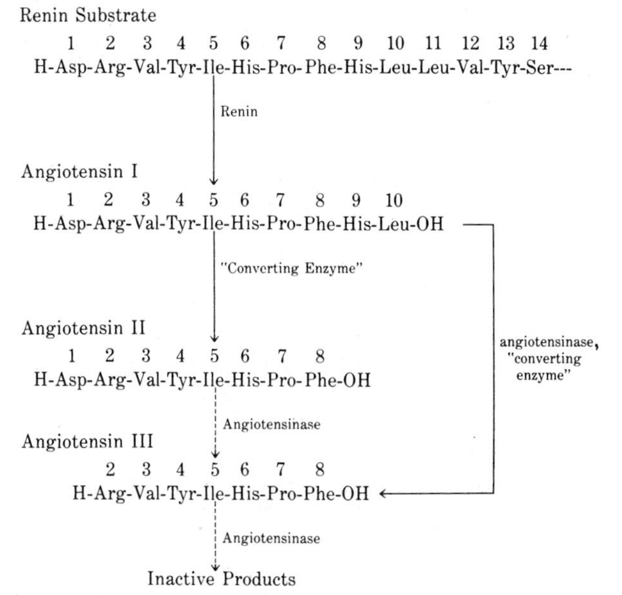

Figure 16–10. The renin-angiotensin system. Angiotensin II is thought to modulate vasoconstriction and is formed from angiotensin I by "converting enzyme." Angiotensin III is formed from angiotensin II; however, it can also be formed from the action of an angiotensinase and converting enzyme without being converted to angiotensin II. (Modified with permission from Oparil, S.: Clinical Chemistry, Volume 22 [1976], page 583.)

creased effective blood volume or acute elevation in blood pressure results in low renin, low angiotensin II, low aldosterone, and subsequent sodium loss. Potassium loss stimulates aldosterone secretion and suppresses renin release, whereas elevated potassium has the opposite effect. A number of studies have demonstrated that ACTH stimulates aldosterone secretion. Subsequently, it has been found that potassium and the renin-angiotensin system in the control of aldosterone production are more important. The exception is the rare abnormality of glucocorticoid-remediable aldosteronism (Dluhy, 1994).

Renin and Hypertension

The work of Laragh (1972, 1993) has indicated that essential hypertension can be classified on the basis of renin measurements as high, low, or normal renin and that drug selection can be based on this classification. About 15% of patients with essential hypertension have high-renin hypertension. Excessive renin, which can be secondary to kidney pathology or its vascular supply, ultimately leads to increased aldosterone production and subsequent retention of sodium and enhanced potassium excretion. Patients with this condition are hypovolemic, intensely vasoconstrictive, and are more prone to ischemic injury. Renin profiling has shown renin to be an independent risk factor for myocardial infarction. Even if the pressures are controlled by antihypertensives, if they do not address plasma renin activity, such patients fare worse than people with lower renin levels (Alderman, 1991). The increased aldosterone (secondary aldosteronism) may contribute significantly to the symptoms and course of high-renin hypertension. Some of the causes of high-renin hypertension are listed in Table 16–13.

Table 16–13. SOME CAUSES OF HYPERTENSION ASSOCIATED WITH HIGH LEVELS OF PLASMA RENIN

Renin-secreting tumor
Malignant accelerated hypertension
Renovascular hypertension
Major arterial lesions
Segmental lesions
Chronic renal failure
End stage
Transplant rejection
Cushing's syndrome
Iatrogenic
Volume-depleting agents
Vasodilating agents
Glucocorticoids
Estrogens

Renin-secreting tumors are an extremely rare finding and are not easy to diagnose. They can be benign or malignant. They can also be renal or extrarenal. The most common location is the juxtaglomerular apparatus. A young patient with markedly elevated plasma renin, hyperaldosteronism and hypokalemia in the absence of a renovascular lesion typifies the classic clinical case (Corvol, 1994). Malignant hypertension is associated with high plasma renin activity and aldosterone. When such patients are given angiotensin-converting enzyme inhibitors such as captopril, the renin activity usually can be reduced to the reference interval. This is called the captopril test. A positive test leads to renal vein angiograms and catheterization for selective blood sampling. In unilateral renal disease, both plasma renin and aldosterone are elevated. The most firmly established clinical application of the renin assay occurs in these patients. Asymmetry in the renin levels obtained during renal vein catheterization offers one of the best measurements to judge the likelihood of blood pressure response to corrective surgery. It has been established that when the ratio of plasma renin in the renal vein of the affected to nonaffected side is at least 1.5 to 1, surgery may lead to improvement. With suppression of renin release from the nonaffected side, renal vein renin levels approximating those found in blood specimens obtained from the inferior vena cava also indicate probable success of curative surgery. However, almost 40% of these patients have peripheral blood plasma renin activity that is within the reference interval (Streeten, 1979). Consequently, peripheral plasma renin is a poor predictor of response to surgery. Renin secretion can be found in lung cancers, hepatic hamartoma, and other unusual conditions (Anderson, 1989).

When there is an acceleration of hypertension, renin is usually markedly increased; however, with chronic renal failure, almost any renin level can be expected. A small number of hypertensive patients on dialysis have intractable, accelerated hypertension. In those patients in whom dialysis cannot control the hypertension, markedly elevated plasma renin levels can be lowered by nephrectomy. In those renal transplant patients with rejection, elevated plasma renin may be indicative of renal ischemia. Systemic hypertension has been found to be present in patients with Cushing's syndrome. In some of these patients, plasma renin and renin substrate are increased

(Krakoff, 1975). In other patients with Cushing's syndrome and hypokalemia, it has been found that the secretion of a minor mineralocorticoid such as DOC or corticosterone is responsible for the hypertension. A suppressed plasma renin in a patient with Cushing's syndrome is presumptive evidence that a mineralocorticoid is present in excess. Other causes of high-renin hypertension include treatment with medications such as diuretics, vasodilators, or antihypertensives. Hormonal agents such as glucocorticoids as well as some estrogen-containing oral contraceptives have been found to increase renin substrate activity.

Although plasma renin, aldosterone, and urinary sodium excretion may be normal in 60% of hypertensive patients, evidence has accumulated that indicates that renin-angiotensin plays a significant part in normal-renin hypertension. The response of many hypertensive patients with normal renin to converting enzyme inhibitors or angiotensin II antagonists (saralasin) has implicated renin and angiotensin II in sustaining hypertension in these patients. Moreover, Ames (1965) showed that once the blood pressure was increased by angiotensin infusion, it could be maintained with only one fifth of the original dose.

It was found that low-renin essential hypertension, which involves chronic expansion of plasma and extracellular fluid volume, is characterized by aldosterone oversecretion and responds to diuretic therapy. At least 25% of patients with essential hypertension are found to have low-renin hypertension. Most investigators have characterized this state as hyporesponsive, meaning that low-renin–hypertensive patients fail to respond as well as healthy subjects do with upright posture, sodium restriction, diuretics, vasodilators, or a combination of these. Atrial natriuretic peptide may be elevated in these patients, along with an exaggerated response of aldosterone to renin (Sergev, 1990). It has been found that renin suppression increases with age, appears to be more common in women, and is more frequently found in older black individuals.

Listed in Table 16–14 are a group of syndromes associated with low levels of plasma renin. These have been divided into a subgroup that is of adrenal origin (primary) and a subgroup that is nonadrenal or secondary in origin. Primary aldosteronism is uncommon compared with renin hypertension. It is characterized by (1) systolic and diastolic hypertension caused by oversecretion of aldosterone by an adrenal adenoma or hyperplasia, (2) low renin or a high aldosterone to renin ratio (>50), (3) potassium wastage, and (4) sodium retention. Forty percent of patients have proteinuria. Several potential screening tests to detect primary aldosteronism and to separate unilateral aldosterone-producing adenomas from other causes of primary aldosteronism have been used. Low-salt diet (<2 g/day), stress, upright posture, and diuretics all increase plasma aldosterone, whereas a high-salt diet and lying in a supine position suppress aldosterone secretion in healthy subjects. Combinations of these maneuvers are used in diagnosis of excessive aldosterone secretion. When healthy subjects are placed on a high-salt diet and lie in the supine position, they suppress their plasma aldosterone levels to less than 10 ng/dL (278 pmol/L).

Table 16–14. SOME CAUSES OF HYPERTENSION ASSOCIATED WITH LOW LEVELS OF PLASMA RENIN

"Primary" excess of mineralocorticoids
Primary aldosteronism
Pseudoprimary (idiopathic) aldosteronism
Glucocorticoid-suppressible aldosteronism
11-Deoxycorticosterone excess
18-Hydroxy-11-deoxycorticosterone excess
Adrenal carcinoma (mineralocorticoid excess)
"Secondary" excess of mineralocorticoids
Licorice ingestion
Excess unsupervised sodium intake
Low renin, low aldosterone syndrome
1. Longstanding essential hypertension
2. Diabetes mellitus

The algorithm proposed by Blumenfeld (1994) for evaluating hypertensive patients suspected of having primary hyperaldosteronism is to measure the serum potassium initially. If it is less than 3.6 mmol/L, then plasma renin activity is measured. A plasma renin activity of 1.0 ng/mL/h or less leads to a 24-hour urine collection for aldosterone and potassium excretion. Findings of potassium excretion greater than 40 mmol/24 h and aldosterone greater than 15 μg/24 h lead to localization of adrenal pathology. Equivocal cases also should have a postural stimulation test, as well as 18-oxocortisol and 18-hydroxycortisol determinations. In Blumenfeld's sample of 15 patients with adrenal adenomas, 13 had 18-oxocortisol greater than 15 μg/dL and 15 had 18-hydroxycortisol greater than 60 μg/dL. One out of nine hyperplasia patients also had similar values. Measuring urinary aldosterone during salt loading has been advocated in evaluating equivocal cases (Bravo, 1994). The more common adenoma differs from hyperplasia by more extreme blood pressures, greater potassium wasting, higher atrial natriuretic peptide levels, and higher urinary 18-oxocortisol and 18-hydroxycortisol excretion. Also, a positive postural stimulation test (plasma aldosterone: ambulating < 130% of supine) has a moderate sensitivity and specificity for adenoma but not for hyperplasia. CT scan or adrenal vein sampling, or both, for aldosterone can reveal disease confined to one adrenal gland. Removal of the adenoma is curative in 35% of cases and leads to improvement in another 55% (Blumenfeld, 1994). Hyperplasia is not always bilateral. Surgery can cure or improve the hypertension in patients with unilateral disease. For those in whom the disease is bilateral, medical treatment with drugs such as spironolactone leads to improvement in 76% of cases. In addition, renin may be suppressed by ingestion of licorice which has a high content of glycyrrhizic acid, chewing tobacco, carbenoxolone, excessive sodium intake, and the syndrome of low renin and low aldosterone, which is most commonly seen in patients with diabetes mellitus and renal disease.

Secondary aldosteronism results from nonadrenal disease, in which both adrenal glands are stimulated. Typically, these patients are not hypertensive. Such conditions as nephrosis, cirrhosis, and heart failure are usual causes. In all of these conditions, both renin and aldosterone are increased. The response of the renin-aldosterone system in pregnancy is especially complex; there appears to be increased renin, renin substrate, angiotensin II, and aldosterone.

The gene responsible for renin is on chromosome 1. Efforts to relate hypertension to this gene are in its infancy in research and have yet to prove fruitful (Lezin, 1993). Angiotensinogen gene variants may be related to hypertension in some patients (Jeunemaitre, 1992). However, there is evidence to suggest that hypertension is not dependent on a known variant and may be in a region of the chromosome near the angiotensinogen gene (Caulfield, 1994). Families with glucocorticoid remediable aldosteronism have well-documented mendelian inheritance (Kurtz, 1993; Lifton, 1992).

Aldosterone Measurements

Because the concentration of aldosterone in plasma is low (1000-fold lower than cortisol), it has been difficult to measure. Developments have made it possible to measure aldosterone directly from plasma after treatment to remove aldosterone from plasma proteins but cross-reactivity may make traditional purification techniques necessary. An isolated aldosterone measurement with no attention to patient preparation, however, is of little clinical value. Even when time of sampling, posture, and dietary sodium and potassium are controlled, it is difficult to discriminate with certainty between primary aldosteronism and other forms of hypertension by using plasma aldosterone measurements. Direct aldosterone assays without chromatography are available in kits using ^{125}I. In a reference population, plasma aldosterone concentrations are of the order of 10 ng/dL (278 pmol/L) and urinary aldosterone concentrations usually are 6 to 25 μg/24 h (16.6 to 69.4 nmol/24 h).

Renin Measurements

There are important technical differences in the determination of renin using current methodology. Renin measurements are of two types: plasma renin activity and plasma renin concentration. In the past, bioassays of the precursor activity of angiotensin were used, but now radioimmunoassay of generated angiotensin I is commonly employed. A plasma specimen containing renin is allowed to react with its substrate; then, after a specified period of time, the reaction is terminated and measurement of generated angiotensin I (or II) made. Given the lability of angiotensin, the blood is drawn into an EDTA tube which inactivates enzyme activity (e.g. angiotensenases); the plasma should be separated promptly from the cells and frozen until analysis. Acid and specific enzyme inhibitors have also been used in addition to chelators (e.g., EDTA).

For the estimation of what has become known as plasma renin activity (PRA), the endogenous substrate is not eliminated. Therefore, the rate of generation of angiotensin I is influenced by both the concentration of endogenous renin and its substrate. This type of assay is the most widely used method for the determination of renin. Comparison of results among laboratories is an impossibility because of procedural differences such as variations of pH, ionic strength, the length of the assay, the angiotensinase inhibitor, lack of a specific reference preparation, and the conditions under which the specimen was obtained. In addition, literature on renin assays reveals confusion regarding units of measurements employed, and even when an attempt is made to express the many arbitrary units in the same terms (nanograms of angiotensin liberated per milliliter per hour), there are wide ranges reported for human plasma renin activity in reference populations.

When measuring renin concentration rather than PRA, the effect of substrate is eliminated. To accomplish this, the specimen may be treated in a number of ways; for example, the plasma may be incubated at a low pH, denaturing the substrate. Then highly active bovine substrate is added, and because substrate is in excess, angiotensin I generation occurs linearly with increasing renin concentrations. Under these conditions, angiotensin generation is independent of substrate concentration and proportional to renin concentration (zero-order kinetics). An international reference standard has been developed for this method, and PRA, which is expressed in Goldblat units/dL (GU/dL), can be compared among different laboratories.

Assays of PRA and plasma renin concentration provide similar information except in a few clinical situations. With oral contraceptive administration, plasma renin concentration remains within the reference interval, whereas PRA increases owing to the increase in substrate. Other procedures such as freezing, thawing, and acidification have been found to convert prorenin to renin and thereby increase values in plasma renin concentration assays.

The direct measurement of renin substrate, angiotensin I, or angiotensin II is not used widely in clinical practice because of tedious extraction or concentration steps as well as difficulty in eliminating formation or degradation of these compounds by proteases and other enzymes involved in the renin system.

Because renin release is controlled by many physiologic and pharmacologic variables, it is extremely important to know the conditions under which the blood specimen was obtained. Such conditions as upright posture, the administration of diuretics, or low sodium diets are potent stimuli of renin release and should be adequately controlled prior to the measurement of plasma renin. Renin also appears to be extremely labile, so that the variables involved in specimen processing should be vigorously controlled. Blood should be drawn into iced tubes containing chelating agents for inactivation of enzymes (angiotensinases) and centrifuged in the cold, and the plasma frozen to avoid substantial losses from angiotensinase activity; with this technique, the specimen is stable for several months at −20°C.

Plasma renin has been interpreted in individuals relative to a simultaneous 24-hour urine sodium excretion after several days on a stable sodium intake and off diuretics. With normal kidney function, urinary sodium excretion is related to the extracellular or fluid volume and inversely related to the plasma concentration of renin (Fig. 16–11). From this nomogram, it should be possible to distinguish low, normal, and high plasma renin groups.

Because the 24-hour renin-sodium profile is cumbersome, various stimuli for renin release have been used. One of the simplest is the procedure described by Kaplan (1976); PRA is determined in fasting subjects after 30 minutes in an upright position following 40 mg of furosemide (Lasix) given intravenously. This test does not require hospitalization, a special diet, or prolonged standing. In this study, a reference

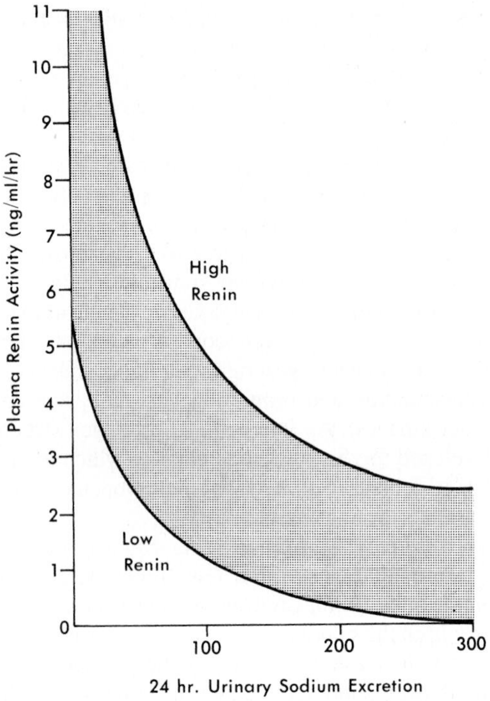

Figure 16–11. Plasma renin activity as a function of the 24-hour urinary sodium excretion. Normal renin hypertension is represented by shaded area. (Modified from Brunner, H.R., et al.: Reprinted by permission of the New England Journal of Medicine 1972; 286:441.)

population of whites and blacks had PRAs greater than 1.0 and 0.5 ng/mL/h, respectively, whereas low-renin hypertensive patients were unable to respond as well. Although different methods of renin categorization do not always similarly classify the same patients, this test correlates well with other procedures being used to identify low-renin hypertensives.

Angiotensin-Converting Enzyme Activity

The measurement of angiotensin-converting enzyme activity, although of limited usefulness in diagnosis and treatment of hypertension, has been found to be helpful in other circumstances. Increased enzyme activity values have been found in patients with active sarcoid. However, patients with other granulomatous diseases and in those whose sarcoid is dormant, the enzyme activity is within the reference interval. Diagnostic usefulness of this determination, however, has been decreased by the finding of elevated serum activity in a number of other disorders. For example, serum angiotensin-converting activity has been shown to be increased in many liver diseases, including chronic persistent hepatitis, chronic active hepatitis, fatty liver, and obstructive jaundice. Other diseases such as neonatal respiratory distress, silicosis, asbestosis, hyperthyroidism, diabetic retinopathy, Gaucher's disease, and leprosy also may give rise to elevated serum enzyme activity. For further information on methods of measurement, see Rohrbach (1982).

GONADOTROPINS AND SEX HORMONES

Luteinizing Hormone and Follicle-Stimulating Hormone

The hypothalamus secretes the gonadotropin-releasing hormone (GnRH), a single peptide releasing hormone that controls secretion of the gonadotropins, luteinizing hormone (LH), and follicle-stimulating hormone (FSH) from the anterior pituitary. GnRH, a decapeptide, releases both LH and FSH from the same population of pituitary cells. An earlier or older name for GnRH is luteinizing-releasing hormone (LRH).

Both LH and FSH consist of a glycopeptide framework to which carbohydrate side chains are attached. Structurally, LH and FSH are related to the other glycoprotein hormones, thyrotropin (TSH) and human chorionic gonadotropin (hCG). These hormones are made from two different noncovalently bound, biologically inactive subunits designated α and β. It has been found that α- and β-subunits can be separated and then recombined to give an active hormone. The α-subunit is nearly identical for all glycoprotein hormones, but the β-unit differs for each, that is, this subunit confers hormone specificity. Stimulation with GnRH causes release of free α-subunits, LH, FSH, and TSH (Samuels, 1990). LH and FSH are secreted from the pituitary and are carried in the blood to their sites of action, the testes or ovary.

During infancy, serum levels of both gonadotropins are low and relatively constant. In children of both sexes, serum FSH levels are higher than LH, and the FSH response to GnRH is greater than LH. During puberty, both gonadotropins increase, with FSH reaching a plateau during midpuberty and LH reaching a maximum at the end of puberty. In pubertal children, a major increment in serum LH concentrations first occurs in an episodic pattern during sleep. In general, these episodes closely follow onset of non-REM (rapid eye movement) sleep and terminate in relation to REM sleep. As puberty proceeds, daytime secretory episodes also begin, and by completion of puberty, sleep and wake patterns are equivalent.

In men, secretion of LH and to a lesser degree FSH is episodic, with 9 to 14 such secretory surges of LH per 24 hours corresponding to a 200% to 300% increase over the mean value. FSH also is secreted in a pulsatile manner, but the oscillations are of low magnitude, representing only 25% of the mean. The principle reason for the differences in amplitude is the half-life of FSH is several fold longer than LH (Catt, 1991).

In women, all ovulatory menstrual cycles have a pattern of LH and FSH similar to that seen in Figure 16–12. The female menstrual cycle is divided into a follicular phase and a luteal phase by the midcycle surge of the pituitary gonadotropins. There is a single major sharp peak in LH concentration at about midcycle near the time of ovulation. The peak in FSH concentration occurs coincident with the peak of LH, but is of lesser magnitude and briefer duration. Both gonadotropin levels are generally higher during the preovulatory period than during the luteal phase; however, as the follicular phase progresses, FSH concentration falls. FSH levels generally are

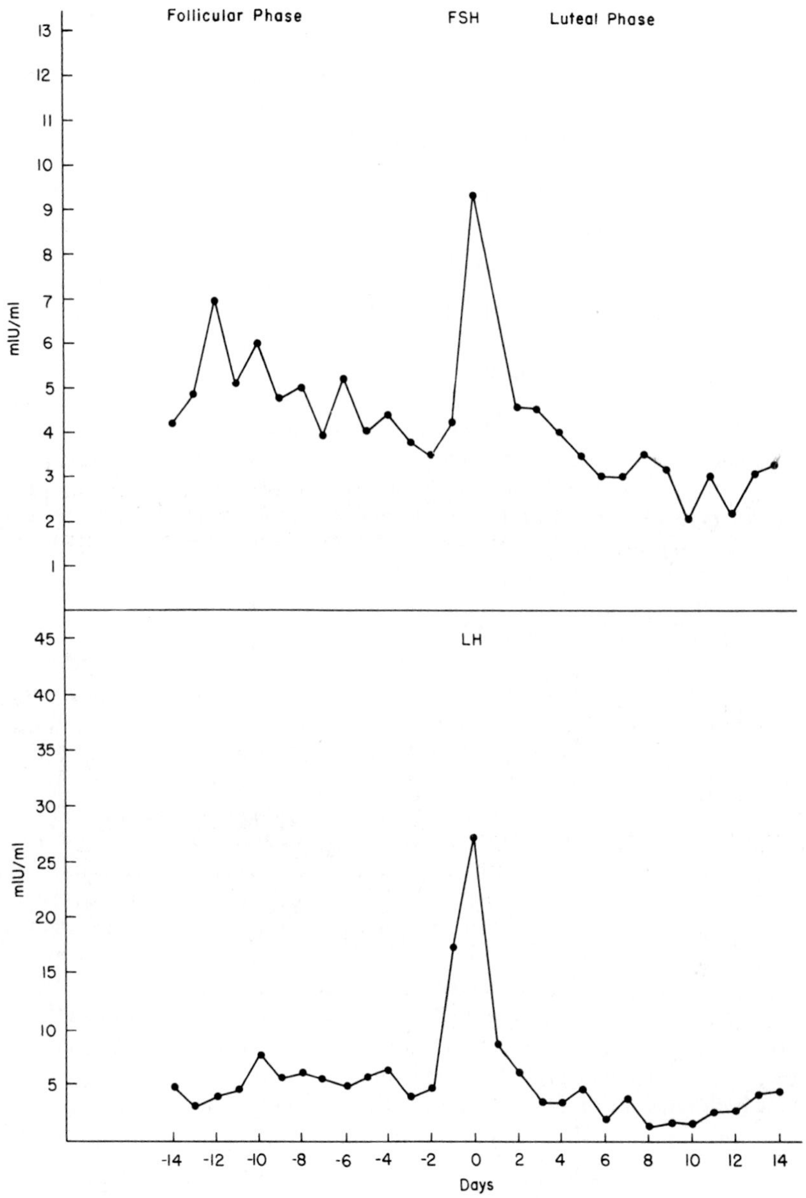

Figure 16–12. Dynamics of serum FSH and LH levels during the course of the menstrual cycle.

higher during the follicular phase than during the luteal phase. Following the midcycle surge of LH and FSH, there is a drop in the concentration of both hormones to lower, more irregular levels with occasional spikes of LH unaccompanied by spikes of FSH. The sleep-associated pulsatile nature of LH and hence GnRH seems to be required for normal cycling. The lack or alteration of this may contribute to the loss of menses among some women athletes (Loucks, 1989). At and after menopause, the gonadotropins continue to be secreted in episodic fashion. FSH levels, however, are higher than those seen during the course of the menstrual cycle; this probably is due to lack of granulosa cell production of inhibin, which is responsible for the feedback suppression of FSH (Buckler, 1991). Furthermore, administration of estrogens to such women do not affect FSH because of the loss of inhibin production. Serum LH levels after menopause may be similar to or slightly higher than those during the menstrual cycle; this may be a reflection of the persistence of the episodic pattern of LH release as well as a suppressive effect of estradiol, which is secreted from the adrenal.

In men, at about the sixth decade, there is a gradual increase in LH and FSH; however, there are large individual variations. Testosterone exerts negative feedback effects on the gonadotropins at the hypothalamic and pituitary levels. In addition, testosterone is aromatized into estradiol, which also inhibits secretion at the same sites.

FSH and LH can be measured by bioassay or immunoassay. Because of the many different glycated isoforms of these hormones, bioassays were preferable to the immunologically recognized hormone. Depending on the time in the menstrual cycle, different amounts of carbohydrate became part of the hormone and each isoform had a different half-life. Furthermore, the glycoprotein hormones are structurally similar and antibody cross-reactivity may be a problem. As a result, a ratio of biological to immunologic measurements were used. However, this is no longer an issue because the newer sandwich assays correlate well with the bioassays (Santen 1995). The pulsatile pattern of gonadotropin release results in the uncertainty that an isolated sample can represent either the peak or nadir of secretion. The LH can vary 60% from the daily mean in the course of a day, whereas FSH can vary 20%. For these reasons, some clinicians have advocated obtaining at least six serum specimens for LH over a six-hour period. The specimens may be assayed individually or pooled. However, in those patients in whom gonadotropins are high, such as those with anorchism or testicular failure or those who are postmenopausal, only one specimen may be necessary. Measurement of the gonadotropins in timed urine specimens has been advocated by some clinicians as an alternative to pooling serum specimens and when there are borderline results.

Reference values for serum LH are up to 12 mIU/mL (12 IU/L) for children, up to 15 mIU/mL (15 IU/L) for men, and between 30 and 200 mIU/mL (30 to 200 IU/L) in postmenopausal women. In menstruating women, LH values of up to 10 mIU/mL (10 IU/L) occur, except during the midcycle peak, when they may reach 80 mIU/mL (80 IU/L). Reference values for FSH are up to 12 mIU/mL (12 IU/L) for children, up to 15 mIU/mL (15 IU/L) for men, and up to 200 mIU/mL (200 IU/L) for postmenopausal women. Menstruating women have FSH values up to 10 mIU/mL (10 IU/L) except during the midcycle peak, when FSH values as high as 20 mIU/mL (20 IU/L) may occur. In patients with ovarian failure, such as occurs with menopause, high levels of FSH (>40 mIU/mL [40 IU/L]) and LH occur, with FSH almost always exceeding LH. Absolute levels of LH and FSH can be used to aid in the diagnosis of polycystic ovary syndrome, in which elevated levels of LH (>35 mIU/mL [35 IU/L]) and normal or depressed (<15 mIU/mL [15 IU/L]) levels of FSH are found. Patients with hypogonadotropin-hypoestrogenic states, such as psychogenic amenorrhea or anorexia nervosa, have gonadotropin levels that are depressed, with FSH being slightly higher than LH. In a series of patients with pituitary tumors, about 20% were found to have high levels of FSH, although serum LH levels were either within or below the reference interval (Snyder, 1979). LH and FSH measurements also have been used for the diagnosis of ectopic tumor production.

Patients with abnormalities in gonadotropin concentrations are classified as having hypergonadotropinism or hypogonadotropinism. Hypogonadotropinism (low GnRH, or decreased or no pulse frequency) is a very common cause of secondary amenorrhea as well as delayed menarche. Hypergonadotropinism can result in precocious puberty. The findings in some disorders in males of the hypothalamic-pituitary-gonadal axis are summarized in Table 16–15. Like other endocrine systems, acute illness affects this axis. Luteinizing hormone, FSH, and testosterone decrease in proportion to the severity of the disease in men and postmenopausal women with either rebound or gradual return to preillness levels at the end of the disease. Spratt (1993) attributes this to suppression centrally and at the target organ.

Dynamic Testing

There are three tests that can be used to evaluate the hypothalamic/pituitary portion of the axis. One of the most commonly used is clomiphene testing. Clomiphene, an antiestrogen, has uses as a diagnostic and a therapeutic agent. It blocks the uptake of estrogens by the hypothalamus, thus nullifying the normal feedback on the hypothalamic-pituitary system. In women, this results in secretion of larger amounts of LH, FSH, and up-regulation of FSH and LH receptors. The increase in FSH, in turn, induces follicular growth and initiates an ovulatory cycle.

Table 16–15. BASAL HORMONE LEVELS IN DISORDERS OF THE HYPOTHALAMIC-PITUITARY-GONADAL AXIS IN MEN

Diagnosis	LH	FSH	Testosterone	Estradiol
Hypothalamus and pituitary (hypogonadotropic syndromes)				
Hypopituitarism	↓ or N*	↓ or N	↓ or N	↓ or N
Kallmann syndrome	↓ or N	↓ or N	↓ or N	↓ or N
Isolated gonadotropin deficiency	↓ or N	↓ or N	↓ or N	↓ or N
Simple delayed puberty	↓ or N	↓ or N	↓	↓
Gonad (hypergonadotropic syndromes)				
Primary testicular failure	↑	↑	↓	↓ or N
Anorchism	↑	↑	↓	↓ or N
Cryptorchidism	N	N or ↑	N	N
Azoospermia and oligospermia	N or ↑	N or ↑	N	N
Variocele	N	N	N	N
Klinefelter's syndrome	↑ or N	↑	↓ or N	N or ↑
Complete testicular feminization syndrome	↑	↑ or N	N or ↑	↑
Precocious puberty				
Idiopathic or central nervous system lesion	↑	↑	↑	↑
Adrenal tumors or congenital adrenal hyperplasia	↓	↓	↑	↑ or N

*Normal represented by N, increases and decreases by arrows.

Modified from Marshall JC: Clin Endocrinol Metab, 1975; 4:545. © by The Endocrine Soc.

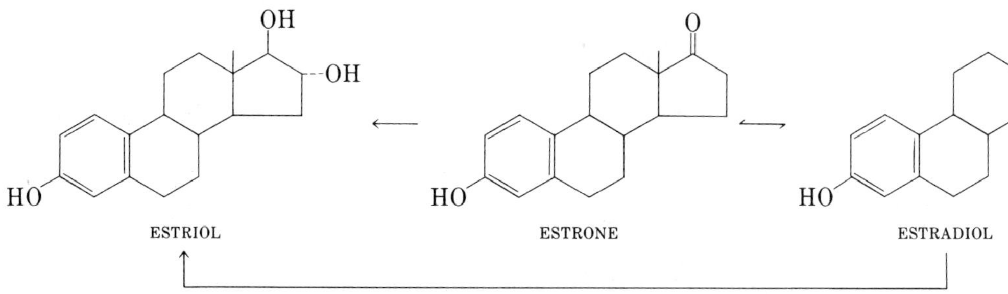

A functioning hypothalamic-pituitary-ovarian axis is essential for successful therapy with clomiphene. Therefore clomiphene is indicated in anovulatory women in whom there is evidence of follicular function and adequate estrogen production (in that they menstruate after administration of progesterone). Patients suspected of having polycystic ovaries may need progesterone along with clomiphene to create the proper milieu.

Clomiphene citrate usually is given in a dosage of 50 to 100 mg daily for five to 10 days. Therapy is usually begun at the lower dose and duration, and if the patient fails to ovulate after two or three cycles, the dose or the length of therapy is increased. A convenient starting point is the fifth day of menstrual bleeding induced by progesterone administration.

A reference population (those with adequate pituitary gonadotropin reserve) shows a 100% increase of LH over baseline and a 50% increase of FSH over baseline on the last day of a seven-day clomiphene test (Santen, 1995). Clomiphene stimulates production of estrogen by the ovaries, which, in turn, negatively feeds back to the pituitary. An abnormal test is one in which there is insufficient estrogen produced, which, in turn, fails to suppress the normal rise in FSH. FSH is measured on day 3 and day 10 after the drug is given (Scott, 1995).

GnRH can be used to test the capacity of gonadotrophs to release LH and FSH. It provides greater stimulation of the pituitary than clomiphene. The intravenous administration of GnRH in healthy individuals results in prompt increases in serum LH, with maximal levels occurring in about 30 minutes. Serum LH then declines gradually over the next few hours. A similar response of FSH also occurs, but it is not as marked and is more variable between individuals. However, if the gonadotrophs have not been maintained by endogenous GnRH, the response will be limited.

The third test available is constant stimulation by hCG for five days. At the end of the test, testosterone levels should rise to twice that of the baseline (Wang, 1992).

Estrogens

The estrogens are responsible for female secondary characteristics. They are steroids that have an A ring containing three unsaturated double bonds. Although over 30 estrogens have been identified, measurements of only three estrogens—estradiol (E_2), estrone (E_1), and estriol (E_3)—are used in clinical practice. Estriol is the metabolite of estradiol. Its measurement has been used to assess the fetoplacental unit and is discussed in Chapter 20. The structure of the three common estrogens and their interrelationships are shown above. A detailed account of these hormones can be found in Carr (1992).

The ovaries, the testes, and the adrenal glands have the capacity to synthesize estrogens from the androgens androstenedione and testosterone. During the follicular phase of the menstrual cycle, ovarian secretion represents only one third of total estrogen production. The ovary secretes almost all the estradiol, while most of the estrone forms from the peripheral conversion of androstenedione and from estradiol metabolism. In healthy postmenopausal women, the ovaries atrophy, leaving virtually all estrogen production from the peripheral conversion of androstenedione made by the adrenal gland. Although estradiol is the most abundant estrogen in premenopausal women, estrone is the estrogen in highest concentration in postmenopausal women.

In men, about one third of all estradiol is produced by the testes which also produces small amounts of estrone. The remainder arises from extraglandular conversion of testosterone and estrone. Thus, the testes are indirectly responsible for most of the estrogen production.

A wide range of organs in the body, including skin, fat, red blood cells, uterus, and liver, have enzymes that metabolize estrogens, but the liver plays the most important role. Estradiol and estrone are conjugated in the liver and excreted as sulfates and glucuronates. Estrone sulfate and other estrogen conjugates are excreted in the bile and then hydrolyzed in the gut and reabsorbed into the peripheral circulation. The metabolic pattern or rate of estrogen metabolism apparently does not change during various disease states.

Estradiol, estriol, and estrone are bound to sex hormone–binding globulin (SHBG), the same carrier protein that binds testosterone. In serum, estradiol is largely in the conjugated form and 60% is found bound to albumin, 38% to SHBG and 3% is free (Rosner, 1991). In contrast, most serum estrone is present as estrone sulfate.

Measurements of serum and urinary estrogen concentrations are far less useful than LH and FSH in assessing disorders of the menstrual cycle or fertility. This is because the effect of estrogen on secondary female characteristics, the cervical mucosa (Pap smear), and on the use of progestin withdrawal to assess actual uterine bleeding produce clearer indications. Some clinicians use estrogen levels to confirm menopause; others find clinical assessment adequate and possibly high levels of FSH and LH. FSH has also been found to be a better predictor of ovarian reserve than estrogen (Scott, 1995).

Progesterone is more useful in assessing ovulation than estrogen. The measurements of estrogen remain useful in diagnosing hyperestrogen states.

As an historical note, urinary estrogens were measured when immunoassays lacked sensitivity and specificity. Estrogens occur in urine as water-soluble conjugates of glucuronate or sulfate; these groups must be hydrolyzed before the estrogens are extracted with organic solvents. Following extraction, the method of Brown (1968) usually is used to estimate total estrogens in urine. The end-point reaction depends on the ability of the phenolic group of estrogens to react with Kober reagent (a mixture of phenol and sulfuric acid) to produce a pink color.

For estimation of total estrogens in serum, the method of Brown usually is too insensitive for most purposes and often an immunoassay of estradiol is used. Like other steroid hormones measured by radioimmunoassay, estradiol usually is quantitated after extraction and chromatographic purification. Nonisotopic assays have been developed that do not require the extraction step. Antibody prepared with estradiol-conjugated protein at the C-3 or 17 position may show up to 30% to 50% cross-reactivity with other estrogens, whereas antibody produced using conjugation at the C-6 position is more specific.

When measurement of serum estradiol was compared with total estrogens in urine, serum estradiol determinations were found to be a more accurate reflection of ovarian function than urinary excretion of total estrogens. When ovarian secretion of estradiol is high, correlation between serum and urinary levels is good, but if the ovarian secretion is low, correlation is poor. When urinary estrogen measurements are compared with serum estradiol to monitor ovulation, the peaks and nadirs of the urinary measurements are delayed one to two days with respect to the corresponding serum profiles (Roger, 1980).

Estradiol is the most potent of the estrogens and is present in concentrations less than 50 pg/mL (18.4 pmol/L) in the preovulatory period. Concentrations rise during the second half of the follicular phase and reach a peak of 150 to 500 pg/mL (550 to 1836 pmol/L) on the day prior to or the day of the LH surge. The midcycle surge of LH may be related to these rising estrogen levels if they are present for the appropriate amount of time. Following the LH surge, serum estradiol drops precipitously, almost to preovulatory levels, but then rises slightly to 100 to 200 pg/mL (367 to 734 pmol/L) during the luteal phase (Fig. 16–13). During menopause, estradiol concentrations steadily decrease to approximately 15% of premenopausal levels, and estrone, primarily produced by peripheral aromatization of adrenal androsterone, becomes the predominant estrogen. Estrone concentration in the late follicular phase is in the range of 150 to 200 pg/mL (550 to 730 pmol/L), whereas levels in postmenopausal women are approximately 35 pg/ml (130 pmol/L).

In prepubertal children, reference values for estradiol by RIA are up to 20 pg/mL (73.4 pmol/L); in men, they are usually 10 to 80 pg/mL (36.7 to 293.7 pmol/L). A few patients with Leydig cell tumors of the testes present with secondary female characteristics; these patients have elevated serum estrogen levels. For further information on the elevated estrogen levels produced by these tumors, see Perez (1980). The most common tumors producing signs of estrogen excess in women are the granulosa-thecal cell tumors. In order to determine whether hypogonadism is present, estrogen determinations usually are interpreted with gonadotropin measurements (see the section entitled Luteinizing Hormone and Follicle-Stimulating Hormone).

Progesterone

In menstruating women, progesterone is secreted mainly by the corpus luteum of the ovary; it is partially responsible for cyclic changes in the endometrium that are necessary for attachment and growth of an embryo. Progesterone levels are low prior to the midcycle gonadotropin surge. Shortly after the gonadotropin surge, they begin to rise rapidly, reaching peak levels during the middle of the luteal phase. Therefore, a progressive fall occurs with barely detectable progesterone levels reached prior to menses (see Fig. 16–13). Although progesterone in large amounts produces a negative feedback on gonadotropin secretion, it is not the major component in the negative feedback system for ovarian steroids.

The small amounts of progesterone in men and nonmenstruating women are derived mainly from extraglandular conversion of adrenal pregnenolone and pregnenolone sulfate to progesterone, and by secretion of progesterone by the adrenals. In serum, about 18% of progesterone is bound to cortisol-binding globulin and 79% to albumin, whereas the remainder is free (unbound).

Progesterone production by the corpus luteum can be indirectly assessed by measurement of the basal body temperature. During the luteal phase, there is about a 0.5°C rise in body temperature, which lasts about 10 to 12 days (hyperthermic portion of the luteal phase) and parallels the increase in progesterone concentration. For information on progesterone measurements during pregnancy, see Chapter 20.

Function of the corpus luteum can be assessed by measuring serum progesterone concentration. On days 21 to 22 of the menstrual cycle, an elevated progesterone is indicative of ovulation. Although conventional radioimmunoassays involving extraction of progesterone with organic solvents have been used, more recent approaches that employ nonisotopic immunoassays include displacement of progesterone from binding sites with danazol or ANS, freeing progesterone for assay without extraction. With radioimmunoassay methods, serum progesterone concentrations of less than 1 ng/mL (3.2 nmol/L) are found during the preovulatory phase. At the time of the LH surge, serum progesterone levels begin to rise and about four to six days later reach a peak of about 10 to 20 ng/mL (31.8 to 63.6 nmol/L). After remaining more or less stable for about one week, progesterone concentrations drop rapidly to about 1 ng/mL (3.2 nmol/L) a short time before the onset of menstruation. A midluteal phase serum progesterone concentration of 5 ng/mL (15.9 nmol/L) or more is a satisfactory index of ovulation. In men, progesterone levels are usually less than 1 ng/mL (3.2 nmol/L); levels are fairly constant and slightly lower than those in women during the follicular phase of the menstrual cycle. In children, progesterone concentrations are about 0.3 to 0.4 ng/mL (10.5 to 12.8 nmol/L) until the second half of puberty, at which time they rise by about 50%.

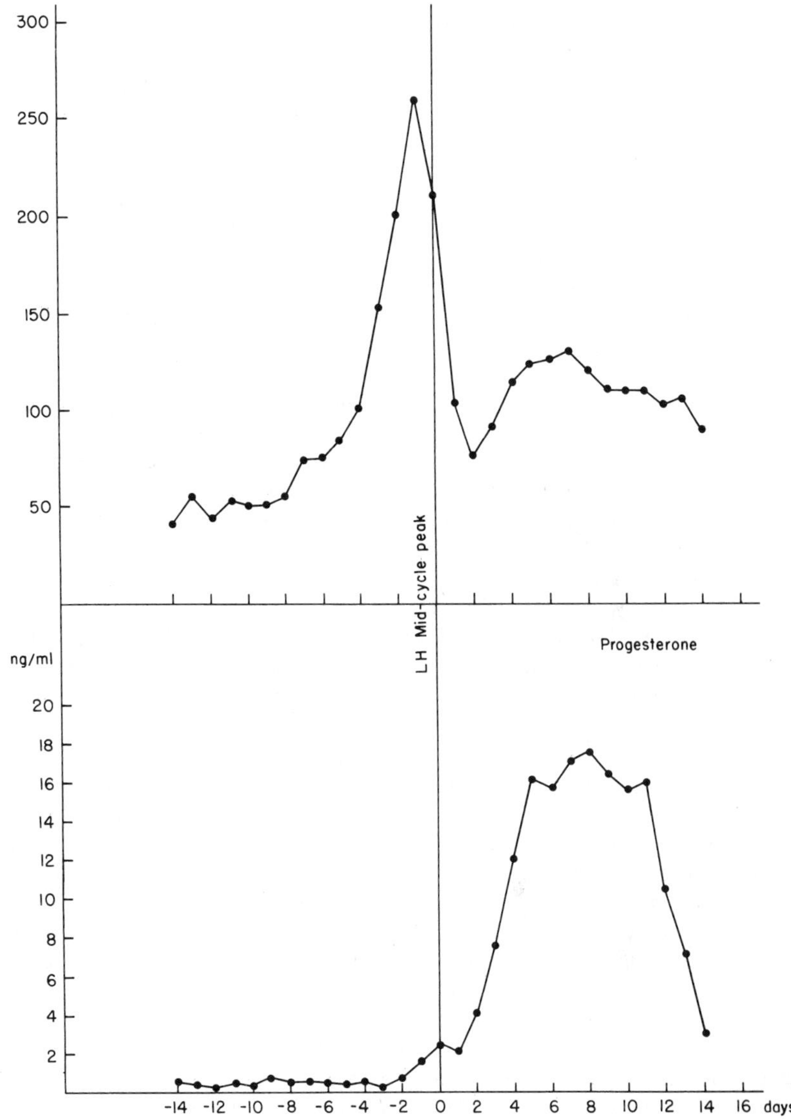

Figure 16–13. Evolution of progesterone and 17-β estradiol during the course of the menstrual cycle.

Luteal function has been assessed by measuring progesterone in a serum specimen drawn during the midluteal phase; a value of 10 ng/mL (31.8 nmol/L) delineated adequate from inadequate luteal function (Jordan, 1994). However, because of a large overlap of progesterone levels in individuals with normal and abnormal luteal function, this demarcation has been questioned and endometrial biopsies are still required in half the cases (Kusuhara, 1992). Kusuhara also recommended that serum specimens be obtained during the early, mid-, and late luteal phase to increase the detection of luteal phase defects. In a large study of 753 infertile women, by using stimulation tests, Aisaka (1992) found that the principle underlying cause of low progesterone was hyperprolactinemia, followed by the hyper-LH syndrome, in which the LH to FSH ratio is greater than one. Luteal phase defects may be demonstrated in a wide variety of patients, including those who present with habitual miscarriages, infertile women (March, 1995), and those receiving clomiphene.

The ability of the corpus luteum to secrete steroids can be assessed by the administration of hCG. Starting on the third day of the hyperthermic portion of the luteal phase, a dose of 3 mg of dexamethasone is given daily for six consecutive days. On the first, third, and fifth days, 5000 units of hCG is injected intramuscularly. Baseline and post-hCG urinary or serum steroids are measured; serum estradiol or progesterone, urinary estrogens, or urinary pregnanediol may be used. The normal response is a doubling of the baseline value on the last (sixth) day of dexamethasone administration (Franchimont, 1974).

Progesterone can be monitored indirectly by measuring its metabolite pregnanediol in urine. Because progesterone can now be directly measured, this assay is of historical note. Urinary pregnanediol, which is essentially all conjugated to glucuronide, is hydrolyzed and measured by colorimetry or gas chromatography, or measured directly by radioimmunoassay using an antibody highly specific for the conjugate. Serum progesterone or urinary pregnanediol has been found to be elevated in those rare patients with feminizing interstitial (Leydig) cell tumor of the testes (see the section entitled Estrogens).

Androgens

Testosterone

The testes have two main functions: (1) spermatogenesis, the production of germ cells; and (2) steroidogenesis, the synthesis and subsequent secretion of the androgenic hormones. In men, LH binds to testicular Leydig cell receptors, enhancing conversion of cholesterol to testosterone (see Fig. 16–8). Once testosterone is formed in the Leydig cell, capillaries and veins carry it to the periphery, or it traverses testicular myoid cells and enters the seminiferous tubules, where it is involved in spermatogenesis. FSH is responsible for activation of the seminiferous tubules, resulting in production of sperm (see Chap. 22) as well as the conversion of testosterone to estradiol. The testosterone that diffuses from the Leydig cell into the seminiferous tubules is bound to a binding protein and occurs in concentrations 20 times that of the peripheral circulation. In the seminiferous tubules, testosterone stimulates primary spermatocytes to form secondary spermatocytes and finally young spermatocytes. Testicular secretion accounts for 95% of the circulating testosterone present in men. In addition to testosterone, the testes also secrete dihydrotestosterone, progesterone; 17-hydroxyprogesterone, and androstenedione.

In women, the majority of testosterone in the blood derives from the metabolism of androstenedione. Small amounts of testosterone are secreted directly by the ovary and adrenal glands.

About 60% of circulating testosterone binds strongly to SHBG, a β-globulin synthesized in the liver, which also binds but with less affinity, estradiol, and other steroids containing a 17-β hydroxy substitution. It has been postulated that free testosterone feeds back on LH at the level of the pituitary and hypothalamus, and that testosterone metabolites may have similar feedback effects. Almost 40% of testosterone is bound loosely to albumin, and about 2% is free (unbound). One study has indicated that not only free testosterone but also the albumin-bound fraction is able to traverse the blood-brain barrier.

Hormones and drugs that affect testosterone binding are important because they may lead to changes in free testosterone. (When there is a decrease in SHBG, an increased concentration of free hormone occurs, and an increase in the binding protein leads to a decrease in free hormone concentration.) Excess thyroid hormones and growth hormone decrease the concentration of SHBG and concentration of androgens, whereas estrogens and hypothyroidism increase SHBG. Anticonvulsants increase SHBG and decrease free testosterone levels (Dana-Haeri, 1982).

Testosterone is metabolized by the enzyme 5α-reductase to another biologically active androgen, dihydrotestosterone. Other testosterone metabolites include androsterone, etiocholanolone, and their sulfates and glucuronides as well as estradiol. In men, 70% of serum dihydrotestosterone is derived from testosterone, but in women, most of the dihydrotestosterone comes from androstenedione.

The androgens have widespread effects on sexual and nonsexual tissue. Testosterone is the dominant androgen in brain, pituitary, kidney, and testes, whereas dihydrotestosterone is the major androgen in skin, prostate, seminal vesicles, and epididymis. Androgens cause an increase in total body mass, with such tissues as muscle, bones, kidney, and larynx relatively sensitive to their effects. The androgens also have specific effects on hair growth. Under the influence of the androgens, hair at specific sites become replaced with longer, coarser, and darker terminal hair. The amount of androgen necessary for the change depends on the race, sex, and age of the individual, as well as the site of the hair follicle.

There is a circadian pattern of testosterone secretion, with highest levels occurring at about the time of awakening, but this pattern disappears with advancing age. During periods of stress such as illness, serum testosterone values decrease, but the mechanism for this decrease is not known. Although studies have demonstrated an age-related decrease in serum testosterone in men, healthy individuals probably show no significant age-related decrease.

Excessive growth of body hair is called hirsutism, which is a visible biological indicator of inordinate testosterone secretion or its precursor androstenedione. Etiologically, the two categories of hirsutism—androgen-dependent and androgen-independent hirsutism—can be separated by hair distribution over the body. Androgen-dependent hirsutism is restricted to the chin, upper lip, chest, and other androgen-sensitive areas; whereas these areas as well as the forehead, abdomen, arms, and legs are involved in androgen-independent hirsutism. Causes of androgen-independent hirsutism include acromegaly, chronic skin irritation, and anabolic drugs.

Listed in Table 16–16 are most causes of androgen-dependent hirsutism. Polycystic ovary disease is the most common etiology. In these patients free testosterone is usually elevated; other measurements of lesser reliability are serum testosterone and dihydrotestosterone, serum androstenedione, dehydroepiandrosterone sulfate (DHEAS),

Table 16–16. CAUSES OF ANDROGEN-DEPENDENT HIRSUTISM

Ovarian causes
Neoplastic
Sertoli-Leydig cell tumors (arrhenoblastoma)
Granulosa-stromal cell tumors
Gonadoblastoma
Lipoid cell tumor
Non-neoplastic
Polycystic ovarian disease
Hyperthecosis
Idiopathic hirsutism
Adrenal abnormalities
Neoplastic
Adrenocortical carcinoma
Virilizing adrenal adenoma
Non-neoplastic
Congenital adrenal hyperplasia
21-Hydroxylase deficiency
11-Hydroxylase deficiency
Cushing's disease
Medications
Androgens (danazol, fluoxymesterone [Halotestin])
19-Nortestosterone derivatives

and urinary 17-ketosteroids. However, by definition, the patient with hirsutism is presenting with a symptom of hyperandrogenism. Also, patients can have normal serum testosterone levels but increased androgen effect at the hair follicle due to excessive 5-α-reductase activity such as in idiopathic hirsutism.

Measurement of serum total testosterone levels is the first step in testing because it can exclude adrenal carcinoma in these patients. Typically, this rare etiology of hirsutism is characterized by high basal testosterone ($>$200 ng/dL) and DHEAS ($>$700 μg/dL) levels. Most of the time, dexamethasone suppression fails to normalize DHEAS or urinary 17-ketosteroids in carcinoma (Derksen, 1994). Dynamic testing involving dexamethasone suppression has been used in diagnosis and treatment, but results have been conflicting. A series has been reported by Abraham (1981). Likewise the same can be said about ACTH stimulation with the exception of detecting 21-hydroxylase deficiency. However, in a small series, Siegel (1990) found that ACTH stimulation was more useful than basal levels of hormones in determining the etiology of the hirsutism, such as late-onset congenital adrenal hyperplasia. They suggested that it leads to superior detection of subtle defects in steroidogenesis. Among the majority of our endocrinologists, the mainstay of treatment appears to include antiandrogens regardless of benign etiologies. Hence, the main objective is to rule out tumor and then treat with antiandrogens. Measurement of serum total testosterone and DHEAS levels will rule out tumor. Measurement of prolactin levels will help rule out a pituitary adenoma, if the patient has menstrual dysfunction.

Total testosterone can be measured directly by RIA by using agents to displace the bound hormone from proteins, which is similar in principle to the assay for progesterone. Alternatively, an extraction step to purify the specimen prior to measurement can be used. Although this procedure is more time consuming, it also is far less susceptible to SHBG and other interferences. Reagent antibodies used for measurements of testosterone are subject to major cross-reactivity by dihydrotestosterone. This does not represent a problem if the androgen assessment is desired. Moreover, testosterone exists in much higher quantities than testosterone metabolites. Danazol, a synthetic androgen used for treatment of endometriosis, also has been reported to cross-react with some antibodies used for testosterone estimation, thereby elevating values (Sharp, 1981). In assays in which this cross-reactivity does not occur, low values have been reported because danazol displaces testosterone from SHBG. Other synthetic steroids that displace testosterone from SHBG are methyltestosterone, fluoxymesterone, and norgestrel. Reference intervals for prepubertal children are less than 1.0 ng/mL (3.5 nmol/L) for men and less than 0.4 ng/mL (1.4 nmol/L) for women. In adults, reference values are less than 3.0 ng/mL, (10.4 nmol/L) for men and $<$0.8 ng/mL (2.8 nmol/L) for women.

Low values in a male are suggestive of hypogonadism such as occurs with Klinefelter's syndrome; they warrant further evaluation with gonadotropin measurements to localize the cause of hypogonadism. In women, testosterone values above 1.6 ng/mL (5.5 nmol/L) usually are reflected by virilization. Although virilized women with androgen-producing adrenal and ovarian tumors generally have serum testosterone levels higher than 2.5 ng/mL (8.7 nmol/L), some patients have been reported who have serum concentrations less than this value (Muechler, 1978). In the differential of high results, interference with the assay has to be considered (Young, 1990). The direct assay can be checked against a method that employs an extraction step such as another immunoassay, HPLC, or GC-MS.

Free serum testosterone measurements are favored by some people because they correlate better with biological activity than does total testosterone. However, as stated before, clinical assessment shows hyperandrogenism. Salivary testosterone was proposed as alternative sample (Osredkar, 1989), because of the ease of collection and it theoretically would be a physiologic protein-free testosterone measurement. Problems such as the salivary testosterone exceeding the serum free testosterone have not inspired much use of this method (Ruutiainen, 1987). Many indirect methods have been used whereby free testosterone is estimated as the product of total serum concentration and the fraction of testosterone free in serum, but most of these methods have one or more shortcomings. The most commonly reported methods involve equilibrium dialysis or ultrafiltration. A typical range of free testosterone concentrations in healthy individuals as found by Moll (1981) are 1.5 to 11.4 pg/mL (5.2 to 39.5 pmol/L) for menstruating women and 56 to 240 pg/mL (204 to 832 pmol/L) for men. Bioavailable testosterone measurement has supplanted free and total testosterone assays at some institutions (Howanitz, 1995).

17-Ketosteroids

The 17-ketosteroids (17-KS) are a group of steroid compounds that have a ketone at position C-17 of the steroid nucleus. This class is considered essentially the same as the 17-hydroxycorticosteroids, with the exception of a small fraction of C21-methyl and C20-keto compounds measured by the Porter-Silber reaction. Historically, they marked great time savings over bioassays for adrenal corticoids. However, along with 17-hydroxycorticoids, they should be retired. The development of specific immunoassays for cortisol, testosterone, dehydroepiandrosterone, and others are more specific and sensitive markers (Rudd, 1985). In women, the adrenal glands secrete almost all of these compounds, whereas in men, the adrenal glands are responsible for two thirds and the testes the remainder. Measurement of 17-KS was important because of their androgenic properties. The principal contribution to 17-KS is from dehydroepiandrosterone sulfate (DHEA-sulfate), which can be directly measured by immunoassays. Hence, DHEA-sulfate is now used as a replacement for 17-KS determinations (Howanitz, 1995). The 17-KS are not specific for androgens, let alone the most important androgens. For example, the androgens androsterone and dehydroepiandrosterone are measured as 17-KS, whereas etiocholanolone, although measured, lacks androgenic properties. The structures of these compounds are shown on page 368. The most potent androgens testosterone and dihydrotestosterone fail to be measured as 17-ketosteroids. Although compounds such as the estrogens are theoretically measurable, they are not in practice because they are removed during the extraction procedure.

2

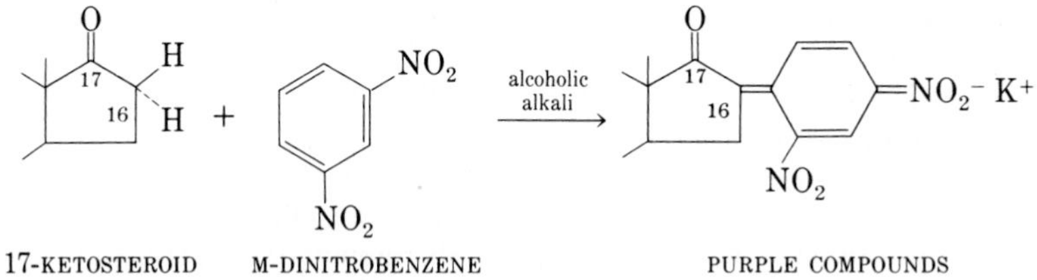

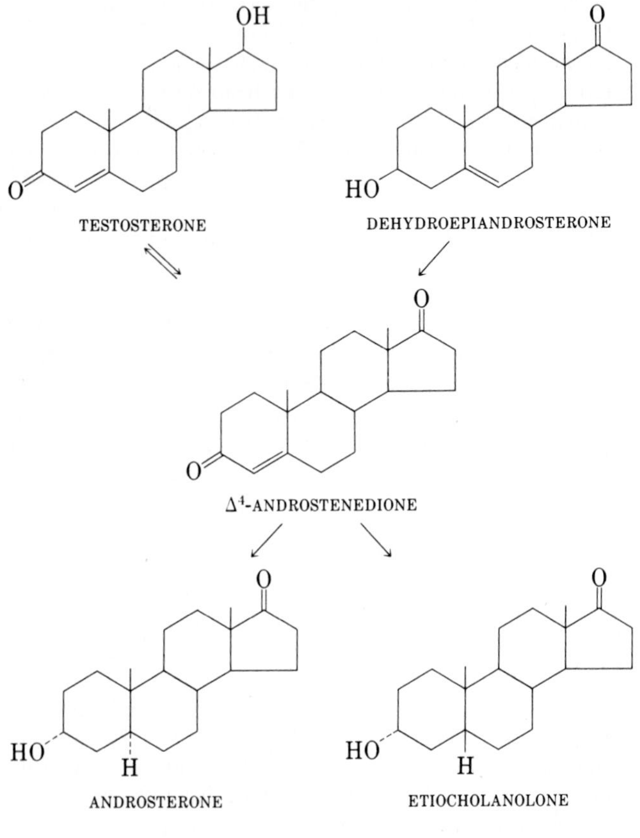

Measurement of the 17-KS involves selective oxidation and reduction of steroids. Most 17-KS are excreted as sulfate or glucuronide conjugates. Prior to extraction, the conjugates are cleaved by acid and reacted with m-dinitrobenzene and alcoholic alkali to produce a red-purple color that absorbs light maximally at 520 nm (Zimmermann reaction). When a keto group occurs on another carbon, such as the 3-keto group in progesterone, a less intense color with a different absorption maximum occurs with the Zimmermann reaction.

The interference by other chromogens led to methods to improve the specificity. Extractions that remove interfering chromogens have been used, and the use of a mathematical formula relating to the different wavelengths near the absorption peak (Allen correction) minimizes this problem. Still, a variety of drugs spuriously increase or decrease 17-KS values, including carbamazepine, cephalothin, and tiaprofenic acid (Nahoul, 1979).

Elevated urine 17-KS are associated with some adrenal, testicular, and ovarian tumors; Cushing's syndrome; some congenital adrenal hyperplasia syndromes (see the section entitled Congenital Enzyme Disorders of the Adrenal); and pregnancy. However, detecting sexual precocity due to Leydig cell tumors and congenital adrenal hyperplasia is poor. Decreased urinary 17-KS occur with adrenalectomy, castration, Addison's disease, nephrotic syndrome, and hypothyroidism.

AAP Section on Endocrinology and Committee on Genetics and American Thyroid Association Committee on Public Health: Newborn screening for congenital hypothyroidism: Recommended guidelines. Pediatrics 1993; 91:1203.

Abraham GE, Maroulis GB, Boyers SP et al: Dexamethasone suppression test in the management of hyperandrogenized patients. Obstet Gynecol 1981; 57:158.

Abuid J, Klein AH, Foley TP, Larson PR: Total and free triiodothyronine and thyroxine in early infancy. J Clin Endocrinol Metab 1974; 39:2630.

Aisaka K, Yoshida K, Mori H: Analysis of clinical backgrounds and pathogenesis of luteal-phase defect. Horm Res 1992; 37(Suppl 1):41.

Alberts G, Boomsma R, Veld AJ, et al: Simultaneous determination of catecholamines and dobutamine in human plasma and urine by high-performance liquid chromatography with fluorimetric detection. J Chromatog 1992; 583:236.

Alderman MH, Hadhavan S, Oor WL, et al: Association of the renin-sodium profile with the risk of myocardial infarction in patients with hypertension. N Engl J Med 1991; 324:1098.

Aman J, Jones I: Urinary growth hormone determination in prepubertal children using a modification of a commercial kit designed for determination of growth hormone in serum. Scand J Clin Lab Invest 1994; 54:227.

Ames RP, Borkowski AJ, Sicinski AM, et al: Prolonged infusions of angiotensin II and norepinephrine and blood pressure, electrolyte balance, aldosterone and cortisol secretion in normal man and in cirrhosis with ascites. J Clin Invest 1965, 44:1171.

Amit T, Ish-Shalom S, Glaser B, et al: Growth-hormone binding protein in patients with acromegaly. Horm Res 1992; 37:205.

Anderson PW, Macaulay L, Do YS, et al: Extrarenal renin-secreting tumors: Insights into hypertension and ovarian renin production. Medicine 1989; 68:257.

Argiolas A, Melis MR, Stancampiano R: Role of central oxytocinergic pathways in the expression of penile erection. Regul Peptides 1993; 45:139.

Ashcraft MW, Van Herle AJ: The comparative value of serum thyroglobulin measurements in iodine 131 total body scans in the follow-up study of patients with treated differentiated thyroid cancer. Am J Med 1981; 71:806.

Attwood EC, Seddon RM, Probert DE: The T_4/TBG ratio and the investigation of thyroid function. Clin Biochem 1978; 11:218.

Bacarese-Hamilton T, Cattini R, Shandley C, et al: A fully automated enzyme immunoassay for the measurement of cortisol in biological fluids. Eur J Clin Chem Clin Biochem 1992; 30:531.

Banfi G, Marinelli M, Casari E, et al: Isotopic and nonisotopic assays for measuring somatotropin compared: Re-evaluation of cutoff value in provocative tests. Clin Chem 1991; 37:273.

Banfi G, Marinelli M, Pontillo M, et al: Standardization with synthetic 22-kDa monomer human growth hormone reduces discrepancies between two monoclonal immunoradiometric assay kits. Clin Chem 1992; 38:2107.

Bang P, Baxter RC, Blum WF: Valid measurements of total IGF concentrations in biological fluids. Recommendations from the 3rd international symposium on insulin-like growth factors. Endocrinology 1995; 136:816.

Barclay ML, Brownlie BEW, Turnover JG, et al: Lithium associated thyro-

toxicosis: A report of 14 cases, with statistical analysis of incidence. Clin Endocrinol 1994; 40:759.
Bartalena L, Martino E, Falcone M, et al: Evaluation of the nocturnal serum thyrotropin (TSH) surge, as assessed by TSH ultrasensitive assay in patients receiving long term L-thyroxine suppression therapy and in patients with various thyroid disorders. J Clin Endocrinol Metab 1987, 65:1265.
Bartalena L: Recent achievements in studies on thyroid hormone–binding proteins. Endocr Rev 1990a; 11:47.
Bartalena L, Pacchiarotti A, Palla R, et al: Lack of nocturnal serum thyrotrophin (TSH) surge in patients with chronic renal failure undergoing regular maintenance hemofiltration: A case of central hypothyroidism. Clin Nephrol 1990b; 34:30.
Baumann G: Growth hormone–binding proteins. Proc Soc Exp Biol Med 1993; 202:392.
Baumann G: Growth hormone binding proteins: State of the art. J Endocrinol 1994; 141:1.
Baumann G, Davila N, Shaw MA, et al: Binding of human growth hormone (GH)–variant (placental GH) to GH-binding proteins in human plasma. J Clin Endocrinol Metab 1991; 73:1175.
Baumann G, Shaw MA: Plasma transport of the 20,000-dalton variant of human growth hormone (20K): Evidence for a 20 K–specific binding site. J Clin Endocrinol Metab 1990; 71:1339.
Baumann G, Stolar MW, Amburn K, et al: A specific growth hormone–binding protein in human plasma: Initial characterization. J Clin Endocrinol Metab 1986a; 62:134.
Baumann G, Stolar, MW: Molecular forms of human growth hormone secreted in vivo: Nonspecificity of secretory stimuli. J Clin Endocrinol Metab 1986b; 62:789.
Baumann G, Stolar MW, Amburn K: Molecular forms of circulating growth hormone during spontaneous secretory episodes and in the basal state. J Clin Endocrinol Metab 1985; 60:1216.
Baxter JD, Perloff D, Hsueh W, et al: The endocrinology of hypertension. *In* Felig P, Baxter JD, Frohman LA (eds): Endocrinology and Metabolism, 3rd ed. New York, McGraw-Hill, 1995.
Becker GW, Bowsher RR, Mackellar WC, et al: Chemical, physical, and biological characterization of a dimeric form of biosynthetic human growth hormone. Biotechnol Appl Biochem 1987; 9:478.
Beckett GJ, Ratcliffe WA, Chapman B, et al: Non-isotopic, two-step free thyroxine immunoassay: A better measure of free thyroxine than analogue radioimmunoassay. Ann Clin Biochem 1990; 27:581.
Behrens O, Bohmer S, Goeschen K, et al: Plasma oxytocin but not prostaglandin F2 alpha metabolite levels at cerclage may predict preterm delivery. Obstet Gynecol 1991; 77:879.
Berg MA, Peoples R, Perez-Jurado L, et al: Receptor mutations and haplotypes in growth hormone receptor deficiency: A global survey and identification of the Ecuadorean E180 splice mutation in an oriental Jewish patient. Acta Paediatr 1994; 399(Suppl):112.
Bigos ST, Ridgway EC, Kourides IA, Maloof F: Spectrum of pituitary alterations with mild and severe thyroid impairment. J Clin Endocrinol Metab 1978; 46:317.
Bjoro T, Johansen E, Frey HH, et al: Different responses in little and bigbig prolactin to metoclopramide in subjects with hyperprolactinemia due to 150-170kD (bigbig) prolactin. Acta Endocrinol 1993; 128:308.
Blum WF, Cotterill AM, Postel-Vinay MC: Improvement of diagnostic criteria in growth hormone insensitivity syndrome: Solutions and pitfalls. Acta Paediatr 1994; 399(Suppl):117.
Blumenfeld JD, Sealey JE, Schlussel Y, et al: Diagnosis and treatment of primary hyperaldosteronism. Ann Intern Med 1994; 121:877.
Bodner JB, Klein L, Baar JG, et al: Automated immunoassay for prolactin with the Abbott IMx analyzer. Clin Chem 1991; 37:291.
Bowsher R, Apathy J, Ferguson A, et al: Cross-reactivity of monomeric and dimeric biosynthetic human growth hormone in commercial immunoassays. Clin Chem, 1990; 36:362.
Bravo EL: Primary aldosteronism. Endocrinol Metab Clin North Am 1994; 23:271.
Brent GH, Hershman JM, Braustein GD: Patients with severe nonthyroidal illness and serum thyrotropin concentrations in the hypothyroid range. Am J Med 1986; 81:463.
Brostedt P, Roos P: Isolation of dimeric forms of human pituitary growth hormone. Prep Biochem 1989; 19:217.
Brown JB, MacLeod SC, MacNaughtan C, et al: A rapid method for estimating oestrogens in urine using semi-automatic extractor. J Endocrinol 1968; 42:5.
Brue T, Caruso E, Morange I, et al: Immunoradiometric analysis of circulating human glycosylated and nonglycosylated prolactin forms: Spontaneous and stimulated secretions. J Clin Endocrinol Metab 1992; 75:1338.
Buckler HM, Evans C, Mamtora H, et al: Gonadotropin, steroid, and inhibin levels in women with incipient ovarian failure during anovulatory and ovulatory rebound cycles. J Clin Endo Metab 1992; 72:116–124.
Burger HG, Patel YC: Thyrotrophin-releasing hormone—TSH. Clin Endocrinol Metab 1977; 6:83.
Burman KD, Read J, Dimond RC, et al: Measurement of 3,3′,5′-triiodothyronine (reverse T3), 3,3′-1-diiodothyronine, T_3, and T_4 in human amniotic fluid and in cord and maternal serum. J Clin Endocrinol Metab 1976; 43:1351.
Campino C, Ampuero S, Diaz S, et al: Prolactin bioactivity and the duration of lactational amenorrhea. J Clin Endocrinol Metab 1994; 79:970.
Campino C, Szecowka J, Lopez JM, et al: Growth hormone (GH) receptor antibodies with GH-like activity occur spontaneously in acromegaly. J Clin Endocrinol Metab 1992; 74:751.
Canadian Task Force on the Periodic Health Examination: Periodic health examination, 1990 update: 1. Early detection of hyperthyroidism and hypothroidism in adults and screening of newborns for congenital hypothyroidism. Can Med Assoc J 1990; 142:955.
Canale MP, Bravo EL: Diagnostic specificity of serum chromogranin-A for pheochromocytoma in patients with renal dysfunction. J Clin Endocrinol Metab 1994; 78:1139.
Candito M, Albertini M, Politano S, et al: Plasma catecholamine levels in children. J Chromatogr, 1993; 617:304.
Candito M, Thyss A, Albertini M, et al: Methylated catecholamine metabolites for the diagnosis of neuroblastoma. Med Pediatr Oncol 1992; 20:215.
Carlson HE, Markoff E, Lee DW: On the nature of serum prolactin in two patients with macroprolactinemia. Fertil Steril 1992; 58:78.
Carlsson L, Mercado M, Baumann G, et al: Assay systems for the growth hormone–binding protein. Proc Soc Exp Biol Med 1994a; 206:312.
Carlsson LM, Attie KM, Compton PG, et al: Reduced concentration of serum growth hormone–binding protein in children with idiopathic short stature. National Cooperative Growth Study. J Clin Endocrinol Metab 1994b; 78:1325.
Carlsson LM, Rosberg S, Vitangcol RV, et al: Analysis of 24-hour plasma profiles of growth hormone (GH)–binding protein GH/GH-binding protein complex, and GH in healthy children. J Clin Endocrinol Metab 1993; 77:356.
Carlsson LM, Rowland AM, Clark RG, et al: Ligand-mediated immunofunctional assay for quantitation of growth hormone–binding protein in human blood. J Clin Endocrinol Metab 1991; 73:1216.
Carmignac DF, Wells T, Carlsson LM, et al: Growth hormone (GH)–binding protein in normal and GH-deficient dwarf rats. J Endocrinol 1992; 135:447.
Catt KJ, Dufau ML: Gonadotropic hormone biosynthesis, secretion, receptors and actions. *In* Yen SSC, Jaffe RB (eds): Reproductive Endocrinology, Physiology, Pathophysiology and Clinical Management. (pp 105–155). Philadelphia, W.B. Saunders Company, 1991, pp 105–155.
Caulfield M, Lavender P, Farrall M, et al: Linkage of the angiotensinogen gene to essential hypertension. N Engl J Med 1994; 330:1629.
Cavalieri RR, Pitt-Rivers R: The effects of drugs on the distribution and metabolism of thyroid hormones. Pharmacol Rev 1981; 33:55.
Celniker DC, Chen AB, Wert RM, et al: Variability in quantitation of circulating growth hormone using commercial immunoassays. J Clin Endocrinol Metab 1989, 68:469.
Challinor SM, Winters SJ, Amico JA: Patterns of oxytocin concentrations in the peripheral blood of healthy women and men: Effect of the menstrual cycle and short-term fasting. Endocrinol Res 1994; 20:117.
Chapman IM, Hartman ML, Straume M, et al: Enhanced sensitivity growth hormone (GH) chemiluminescence assay reveals lower postglucose nadir GH concentrations in men than women. J Clin Endocrinol Metab 1994; 78:1312.
Chatelain P, Bouillat B, Cohen R, et al: Assay of growth hormone levels in human plasma using commercial kits: Analysis of some factors influencing the results. Acta Pediatr Scand 1990; 370(Suppl):56.
Chevenne D, Beau N, Leger J, et al: Variability of serum human growth hormone levels in different commercial assays: Specificity of growth hormone–releasing hormone stimulation. Horm Res 1993; 40:168.
Chew SL, Dacie JE, Reznek RH, et al: Bilateral phaeochromocytomas in von Hippel–Lindau disease: Diagnosis of adrenal vein sampling and catecholamine assay. Q J Med 1994; 87:49.
Chibbar R, Miller, FD, Mitchell BF: Synthesis of oxytocin in amnion, chorion, and decidua may influence the timing of human parturition. J Clin Invest 1993; 91:185.
Chiodera P, Volpi R, Capretti L, et al: Hypoglycemia-induced arginine vasopressin and oxytocin release is mediated by glucoreceptors located within the blood-brain barrier. Neuroendocrinology 1992; 55:655.
Cho BY, Shong MH, Yi KH, et al: Evaluation of serum basal thyrotrophin levels and thyrotrophin receptor antibody activities as prognostic markers for discontinuation of antithyroid drug treatment in patients with Graves' disease. Clin Endocrinol 1992; 36:585.
Chopra IJ, Solomon DH, Hepner GW, Morgenstein AA: Misleadingly low free thyroxine index and usefulness of reverse triiodothyronine measurement in nonthyroidal illness. Ann Intern Med 1979; 90:905.
Christofides ND, Sheehan CP: Enhanced chemiluminescence-labeled–antibody immunoassay (Amerlite-MAB) for free thyroxine: Design, development, and technical validation. Clin Chem 1995a; 41:17.
Christofides ND, Sheehan CP: Multicenter evaluation of enhanced chemiluminescence labeled-antibody immunoassay (Amerlite-MAB) for free thyroxine. Clin Chem 1995b; 41:24.
Clapp C, Martial JA, Guzman RC, et al: The 16-kilodalton N-terminal frag-

ment of human prolactin is a potent inhibitor of angiogenesis. Endocrinology 1993; 133:1292.
Claybaugh JR, Uyehara CFT: Metabolism of neurohypophysial hormones. Ann NY Acad Sci 1993; 689:250.
Comtois R, Robert F, Hardy J: Immunoradiometric assays may miss high prolactin levels. Ann Intern Med 1993; 119:173.
Corvol P, Pinet F, Plouin PF, et al: Renin-secreting tumors. Endocrinol Metab Clin North Am 1994; 23:255.
Costello LC, Franklin RB: Effect of prolactin on the prostate. Prostate 1994; 24:162.
Cryer PE: Pheochromocytoma. West J Med 1992; 156:399.
Custro N, Scafidi V, LoBaido R, et al: Subclinical hypothyroidism resulting from autoimmune thyroiditis in female patients with endogenous depression. J Endocrinol Invest 1994; 17:641.
Dana-Haeri J, Oxley J, Richens A: Reduction of free testosterone by antiepileptic drugs. Br Med J 1982; 1:85.
Dattani MT, Hindmarsh PC, Brook CG, et al: Enhancement of growth hormone bioactivity by zinc in the eluted stain assay system. Endocrinology, 1993; 133:2803.
Dattani MT, Hindmarsh PC, Brook CG, et al: Inhibition of growth hormone bioactivity by recombinant human growth hormone–binding protein in the eluted stain assay system. J Endocrinol 1994; 140:445.
Dattani MT, Pringle PJ, Hindmarsh PC, et al: What is a normal stimulated growth hormone concentration? J Endocrinol 1992; 133:447.
Davenport J, Kellerman C, Reiss D, et al: Addison's disease. Am Fam Physician 1991; 43:1338.
Davidson KM, Richards DS, Schatz DS, et al: Successful in utero treatment of fetal goiter and hypothyroidism. N Engl J Med 1991; 324:543.
De Bellis A, Bizzarro A, Amoresano Paglionico V, et al: Detection of vasopressin cell antibodies in some patients with autoimmune endocrine diseases without overt diabetes insipidus. Clin Endocrinol 1994; 40:173.
De Boer H, Blok G, Van Der Veen E: Clinical aspects of growth hormone deficiency in adults. Endocr Rev 1995; 16:63.
de los Santos ET, Tarich GH, Mazzaferri EL: Sensitivity, specificity, and cost-effectiveness of the sensitive thyrotropin assay in the diagnosis of thyroid disease in ambulatory patients. Arch Intern Med 1989; 149:526.
Demir N, Celiloglu M, Thomassen PA, et al: Prolactin and amniotic fluid electrolytes. Acta Obstet Gynecol Scand 1992; 71:197.
Derksen J, Nagesser SK, Meinders AE, et al: Identification of virilizing adrenal tumors in hirsute women. N Engl J Med 1994; 331:968.
Dluhy RG, Lifton RP: Glucocorticoid-remediable aldosteronism. Endocrinol Metab Clin North Am 1994; 23:285.
Dussault JH: Neonatal screening for congenital hypothyroidism. Clin Lab Med 1993; 13:645.
Ekins R: Analytic measurements of free thyroxine. Clin Lab Med 1993; 13:599.
Evain-Brion D, Alsat E, Igout A, et al: Placental growth hormone variant: Assay and clinical aspects. Acta Paediatr 1994; 399(Suppl):49.
Faber J, Waetjen I, Siersbaek-Nielsen K: Free thyroxine measured in undiluted serum by dialysis and ultrafiltration effects of non-thyroidal illness, and an acute load of salicylate or heparin. Clin Chim Acta 1993; 223:159.
Faix JD, Rosen HN, Velazquez FR: Indirect estimates of thyroid hormone–binding proteins to calculate free thyroxine index: Comparison of nonisotopic methods that use labeled thyroxine ("t-uptake"). Clin Chem 1995; 41:41.
Falk RJ: Isolated prolactin deficiency: A case report. Fertil Steril 1992; 58:1060.
Felig P, Baxter JD, Frohman LA: Endocrinology and Metabolism, 3rd ed. New York, McGraw-Hill, 1995.
Fernandez-Calvert L, Garcia-Mayor RV: Incidence of pheochromocytoma in South Galicia, Spain. J Intern Med 1994; 236:675.
Fonseca ME, Ochoa R, Moran C, et al: Variations in molecular forms of prolactin during the menstrual cycle, pregnancy, and lactation. J Endocrinol Invest 1991; 14:907.
Franchimont P, Valcke JC, Lambotte R: Female gonadal dysfunction. Clin Endocrinol Metab 1974; 3:533.
Francke U, Berg MA: Genetic heterogeneity in Laron syndrome. Acta Paediatr 1993; 391(Suppl):3.
Friesen HG: Receptor assays for growth hormone. Acta Paediatr Scand 1990; 370(Suppl):87.
Fukata J, Shimizu N, Imura H, et al: Human corticotropin-releasing hormone test in patients with hypothalamo-pituitary-adrenocortical disorders. Endocr J 1993; 40:597.
Fukuoka H, Hamamoto R, Higurashi M: Heterogeneity of serum and amniotic fluid prolactin in humans. Horm Res 1991; 35(Suppl 1):58.
Gardner DF, Carithers RL, Utiger RD: Thyroid function tests in patients with acute and resolved hepatitis B virus infection. Ann Intern Med 1982; 96:450.
Gentric A, Fouilhoux A, Caroff M, et al: Dopamine β hydroxylase deficiency responsible for severe dysautonomic orthostatic hypotension in an elderly patient. J Am Geriatr Soc 1993; 41:550.
Gerbes AL, Witthaut R, Samson WK, et al: A highly sensitive and rapid radioimmunoassay for the determination of argenine 8-vasopressin. Eur J Clin Chem Clin Biochem 1992; 30:229.
Gerlo EA, Sevens C: Urinary and plasma catecholamines and urinary catecholamine metabolites in pheochromocytoma: Diagnostic value in 19 cases. Clin Chem 1994; 40:250.
Gesundheit N, Petrick PA, Nissim M, et al: Thyrotropin-secreting pituitary adenomas: Clinical and biochemical heterogeneity. Ann Intern Med 1989; 111:827.
Grodum E, Petersen PH, Hangaard J, et al: Biological description of the cortisol responses to corticotropin-releasing hormone (CRH) stimulation. An optimization and simplification of the test. Ups J Med Sci 1993; 98:311.
Grondal S, Eriksson B, Hamberger B, et al: Plasma chromogranin A + B, neuropeptide Y and catecholamines in pheochromocytoma patients. J Intern Med 1991; 229:453.
Grunfeld C, Pang M, Doerrler W, et al: Indices of thyroid function and weight loss in human immunodeficiency virus infection and the acquired immunodeficiency syndrome. Metabolism 1993; 42:1270.
Grüters A, Delange F, Givannelli G, et al: Guidelines for neonatal screening programs for congenital hypothyroidism. Horm Res 1994; 41:1.
Haller BL, Fuller KA, Brown WS, et al: Two automated prolactin immunoassays evaluated with demonstration of a high dose "hook effect" in one. Clin Chem 1992; 38:437.
Handwerger S, Markoff E, Richards R: Regulation of the synthesis and release of decidual prolactin by placental and autocrine/paracrine factors. Placenta 1991; 12:121.
Hartman ML, Veldhuis JD, Thorner MO: Normal control of growth hormone secretion. Horm Res 1993; 40:37.
Hattori N, Ikekubo K, Ishihara T, et al: Effects of antiprolactin autoantibodies on serum prolactin measurements. Eur J Endocrinol 1994; 130:437.
Hattori N, Ishihara T, Ikekubo K, et al: Autoantibody to human prolactin in patients with idiopathic hyperprolactinemia. J Clin Endocrinol Metab 1992; 75:1226.
Haubruck H, Mauch L, Cook NJ, et al: Expression of recombinant human thyroid peroxidase by the baculovirus system and its use in ELISA screening for diagnosis of autoimmune thyroid disease. Autoimmunity 1993; 15:275.
Hay ID, Bayer MF, Kaplan MM, et al: American Thyroid Association assessment of current free thyroid hormone and thyrotropin measurements and guideline for future clinical assays. Clin Chem 1991; 37:2002.
Herington AC, Ymer SI, Tiong TS: Does the serum binding protein for growth hormone have a functional role? Acta Endocrinol 1991; 124S:14.
Hershman JM, Pekary AE, Smith V, et al: Evaluation of five high-sensitivity American thyrotropin assays. Mayo Clin Proc 1988; 63:1133.
Hoffmann T, Gunz G, Brue T, et al: Prolactin isoforms secreted by human prolactinomas. Horm Res 1992; 38:164.
Holly JMP, Hughes SC: Measuring insulin-like growth factors: Why, where, and how? J Endocrinol 1994; 140:165.
Holtzman EJ, Ausiello DA: Nephrogenic diabetes insipidus: Causes revealed. Hosp Pract 1994; 29:89.
Honour JW, Rumsby G; Problems in diagnosis and management of congenital adrenal hyperplasia due to 21-hydroxylase deficiency. J Steroid Biochem Mol Biol 1993; 45:69.
Houben H, Denef C: Bioactive peptides in anterior pituitary cells. Peptides 1994; 15:547.
Howanitz PJ: Personal communication. August 2, 1995.
Hsiao RJ, Parmer RJ, Takiyyuddin MA, et al: Chromogranin A storage and secretion: Sensitivity and specificity for the diagnosis of pheochromocytoma. Medicine 1991; 70:33.
Iitaka M, Kitahama S, Fukasawa N, et al: Incidence of anti-mouse IgG in normal subjects and patients with autoimmune thyroid disease. Intern Med 1992; 31:984.
Ilondo MM, Vanderschueren-Lodeweyckx M, De Meyts P: Measuring growth hormone activity through receptor and binding protein assays. Horm Res 1991; 36(Suppl 1):21.
Jackson IMD: Thyrotropin-releasing hormone. N Engl J Med 1982; 306:145.
Jain R, Isaac RM, Gottschalk ME, et al: Transient central hypothyroidism as a cause of failure to thrive in newborns and infants. J Endocrinol Invest 1994; 17:631.
Jan T, Shaw MA, Baumann G: Effects of growth hormone–binding proteins on serum growth hormone measurements. J Clin Endocrinol Metab 1991; 72:387.
Jeunemaitre X, Soubrier F, Kotelevtsev VY, et al: Molecular basis of human hypertension: Role of angiotensinogen. Cell 1992; 71:169.
John R, Henley R, Shankland D: Concentration of free thyroxin and free triiodothyronine in serum of patients with thyroxin- and triiodothyronine-binding antibodies. Clin Chem 1990; 36:470.
Jones J, Clemmons DR: Insulin-like growth factors and their binding proteins: Biological actions. Endocrin Rev 1995; 16:3.
Jordan J, Craig K, Clifton DK, Soules MR. Luteal phase defect: The sensi-

tivity and specificity of diagnostic methods in common clinical use. Fertil Steril 1994; 62:54–62.
Jung WH, Yang WI, Park C, et al: DNA flow cytometry in pheochromocytoma and paraganglioma. Yonsei Med J 1992; 33:249.
Kabadi UM, Fox IS, Cook P: Falsely low serum thyroxine concentration measured with the Abbott Tdx. (Letter.) Clin Chem 1994; 40:337.
Kamel, MA, Neulen J, Sayed GH, et al: Heterogeneity of human prolactin levels in serum during the early postpartum period. Gynecol Endocrin, 1993; 7:173.
Kaplan NM, Kem DC, Holand OB, et al: The intravenous furosemide test: A simple way to evaluate renin responsiveness. Ann Intern Med 1976; 84:639.
Karet FE, Brown MJ: Phaeochromocytoma: Diagnosis and management. Postgrad Med J 1994; 70:326.
Kater CE, Biglieri EG: Disorders of steroid 17 alpha-hydroxylase deficiency. Endocrinol Metab Clin North Am 1994; 23:341.
Keely EJ, Faiman C: Measurement of human urinary prolactin as a noninvasive study tool. Clin Chem 1994; 40:2017.
Klee GG (ed): Pathophysiology of thyroid disease. Clin Lab Med 1993a; 13:531.
Klee GG, Hay ID: Role of thyrotropin measurements in the diagnosis and management of thyroid disease. Clin in Lab Med 1993b; 13:673–682.
Koenig KL, Tonilo P, Bruning PF: Reliability of serum prolactin measurements in women. Cancer Epidemiol Biomarkers Prev 1993; 2:411.
Korn EA, Gaich G, Brines M, et al: Thyrotropin-secreting adenoma in an adolescent girl without increased serum thyrotropin-alpha. Horm Res 1994; 42:120.
Kostyo JL, Skottner A, Brostedt et al: Biological characterization of purified native 20-kDa human growth hormone. Biochim Biophys Acta 1987; 925:314.
Krakoff L, Nicolis G, Amsel B: Pathogenesis of hypertension in Cushing's syndrome. Am J Med 1975; 58:216.
Kurtz TW, Spence MA: Genetics of essential hypertension. Am J Med 1993; 94:77.
Kusuhara K: Clinical importance of endometrial histology and progesterone level assessment in luteal-phase defect. Horm Res 1992; 37(Suppl 1):53.
Lai MK, Sun CF, Chen CS, et al: Deoxyribonucleic acid flow cytometry study in pheochromocytomas and its correlation with clinical parameters. Urology 1994; 44:185.
Lamb EJ, Noonan KA, Burrin JM: Urine-free cortisol excretion: Evidence of sex-dependence. Ann Clin Biochem 1994; 31:455.
Lamberg BA, Gordin A: Abnormalities of thyrotropin secretion and clinical implications of the thyrotropin-releasing hormone stimulation test. Ann Clin Res 1978; 10:171.
Langsteger W, Stockigt JR, Docter R, et al: Familial dysalbuminaemic hyperthyroxinaemia and inherited partial TBG deficiency: First report. Clin Endocrinol 1994; 40:751.
Laragh JH, Baer L, Brunner HR, et al: Renin, angiotensin and aldosterone system in pathogenesis and management of hypertensive vascular disease. Am J Med 1972; 52:633.
Laragh JH: Renin profiling for diagnosis, risk assessment, and the treatment of hypertension. Kidney Int 1993; 44:1163.
Laron Z, Pertzelan A, Mannheimer S: Genetic pituitary dwarfism with high serum concentration of growth hormone—a new inborn error of metabolism? Isr J Med Sci 1966; 2:152.
Larsen PR: Tests of thyroid function. Med Clin North Am 1975; 59:1063.
Larsen PR, Alexander NM, Chopra IJ: Revised nomenclature for thyroid hormones and thyroid-related proteins in serum. J Clin Encodrinol Metab 1987; 64:1089.
Laurberg P, Pedersen KM, Vittinghus E, et al: Sensitive enzyme-linked immunosorbent assay for measurement of autoantibodies to human thyroid peroxidase. Scand J Clin Lab Invest 1992; 52:663.
Leite V, Cosby H, Sobrinho LG, et al: Characterization of big, big prolactin in patients with hyperprolactinemia. Clin Endocrinol 1992; 37:365.
Lentjes EG, Romijn F, Massen RJ, et al: Free cortisol in serum assayed by temperature-controlled ultrafiltration before fluorescence polarization immunoassay. Clin Chem, 1993; 39:2518.
Lewis UJ, Sinha YN, Haro LS: Variant forms and fragments of human growth hormone in serum. Acta Paediatr 1994; 399(Suppl):29.
Lezin EMS, Kurtz TW: The renin gene and hypertension. Semin Nephrol 1993; 13:581.
Liewendahl K, Helenius T, Näveri H, et al: Fatty acid–induced increase in serum dialyzable free thyroxine after physical exercise: Implication for nonthyroidal illness. J Clin Endocrinol Metab 1992; 74:1361.
Lifton RP, Dluhy RG, Powers M: A chimeric 11 β hydroxylase/aldosterone synthase gene causes glucocorticoid remediable aldosteronism and human hypertension. Nature, 1992; 355:264.
Lim CF, Curtis AJ, Barlow JW, et al: Interactions between oleic acid and drug competitors influence specific binding of thyroxine in serum. J Clin Endocrinol Metab 1991; 73:1106.
Lindstedt G: Endogenous antibodies against prolactin—a new cause of hyperprolactinemia. Eur J Endocrinol 1994; 130:429.
Llera AS, Cardoso AI, Stumpo RDR, et al: Detection of autoantibodies against hGH in sera of idiopathic hypopituitary children. Clin Immunol Immunopathol 1993; 66:114.
Lohrke B, Kunkel S, Kowitz J, et al: Prolactin heterogeneity: A limitation on the evaluation of results from prolactin assays due to differences in immunoassays and the different bioactivities of prolactin forms. Eur J Clin Chem Clin Biochem 1993; 31:815.
Loucks AB, Mortola JF, Girton L, et al: Alterations in the hypothalamic-pituitary-ovarian and the hypothalamic-pituitary-adrenal axes in athletic women. J Clin Endocrinol Metab 1989; 68:402.
Lubin E, Mechlis-Frish S, Zatz S, et al: Serum thyroglobulin and iodine-131 whole-body scan in the diagnosis and assessment of treatment for metastatic differentiated thyroid carcinoma. J Nucl Med 1994; 35:257.
Lundin K, Berger L, Blomberg F: Development of anti-hGH antibodies during therapy with authentic human growth hormone. Acta Paediatr Scand 1991; 372(Suppl):167.
MacLeod JN, Worsley I, Ray J, et al: Human growth hormone variant is a biologically active somatogen and lactogen. Endocrinology 1991; 128:1298.
Maddox PR, Jones DL, Mansel RE: Bioactive and immunoactive prolactin levels after TRH-stimulation in the sera of normal women. Horm Metab Res 1992a; 24:181.
Maddox PR, Jones DL, Mansel RE: Prolactin and total lactogenic hormone measured by microbioassay and immunoassay in breast cancer. Br J Cancer 1992b; 65:456.
Maddox PR, Jones DL, Mansel RE: Basal prolactin and total lactogenic hormone levels by microbioassay and immunoassay in normal human serum. Acta Endocrinol 1991; 125:621.
Main KM, Jarden M, Angelo L, et al: The impact of gender and puberty on reference values for urinary growth hormone excretion: a study of 3 morning urine samples in 517 healthy children and adults. J Clin Endocrinol Metab 1994; 79:865.
Mannor DA, Winer LM, Shaw MA, et al: Plasma growth hormone (GH)–binding proteins: Effect on GH binding to receptors and GH action. J Clin Endocrinol Metab 1991; 73:30.
March CM, Shoupe D: Luteal phase defects. *In* Mishell DR, Davajan V, Lobo RA (eds): Infertility, Contraception, and Reproductive Endocrinology. Boston, Blackwell Scientific Publications, 1995, pp 793–806.
Mariotti S, Martino E, Cupini C, et al: Low serum thyroglobulin as a clue to the diagnosis of thyrotoxicosis factitia. N Engl J Med 1982; 307:410.
Massa G, Vanderschueren-Lodeweyckx M, Bouillon R: Five year follow-up of growth hormone antibodies in growth hormone deficient children treated with recombinant human growth hormone. Clin Endocrinol 1993; 38:137.
Mauri M, Pico AM, Alfayate R, et al: Usefulness of urinary growth hormone (GH) measurement for evaluating endogenous GH secretion in acromegaly. Horm Res 1993; 39:13.
McCarter J, Shaw MA, Winer LA, et al: The 20,000 Da variant of human growth hormone does not bind to growth hormone receptors in the liver. Mol Cell Endocrinol 1990; 73:11.
Meierkord H, Shorvon S, Lightman SL: Plasma concentrations of prolactin, noradrenalin, vasopressin and oxytocin during and after a prolonged epileptic seizure. Acta Neurol Scand 1994; 90:73.
Mendel CM, Laughton CW, McMahon FA, Cavalieri RR: Inability to detect an inhibitor of thyroxine-serum protein binding in sera from patients with nonthyroid illness. Metabolism 1991; 40:491–502.
Mengden T, Hubmann P, Muller J, et al: Urinary free cortisol versus 17-hydroxycorticosteroids: A comparative study of their diagnostic value in Cushing's syndrome. Clin Investig 1992; 70:545.
Mercado M, Carlsson L, Vitangcol R, et al: Growth hormone–binding protein in plasma: A comparison of immunofunctional and growth hormone-binding assays. J Clin Endocrinol Metab 1993; 76:1291.
Mevorach RA, Bogaert GA, Kogan BA: Urine concentration and enuresis in health preschool children. Arch Pediatr Adolesc Med 1995; 149:259.
Mizobuchi M, Kunishige M, Kubo K, et al: Syndrome of inappropriate secretion of ADH (SIADH) due to small cell lung cancer with extremely high plasma vasopressin level. Intern Med, 1994; 33:501.
Moll GW, Rosenfield RL, Helke JH: Estradiol-testosterone binding interactions and free plasma estradiol under physiological conditions. J Clin Endocrinol Metab 1981; 52:868.
Moltich ME: Pathologic hyperprolactinemia. Endocrinol Metab Clin North Am 1992; 21:877.
Moran C, Tena G, Fonseca ME, et al: Changes in the prolactin serum isoforms secreted by a pituitary adenoma associated with therapy. Arch Med Res 1994; 25:1.
Muechler EK, Grove S, Kohler D: Steroid hormones in ovarian vein and cyst fluid of a virilizing stromal tumor. Obstet Gynecol 1978; 52:609.
Murphy BE: Steroids and depression. J Steroid Biochem Mol Biol 1991; 38:537.
Nahoul K, Dehennin L, Scholler R: Interference of tiaprofenic acid in Zimmermann reaction. J Steroid Biochem 1979; 10:471.
Nativ O, Grant CS, Sheps SG, et al: The clinical significance of nuclear DNA ploidy pattern in 184 patients with pheochromocytoma. Cancer, 1992, 69:2683.
Navarro Moreno MA, Rivera-Coll A, Huguet Ballester J, et al: Evaluation

of the measurement of prolactin in serum with Enzymun-Test System ES-600. Eur J Clin Chem Clin Biochem 1991; 29:569.

Nelson JC, Weiss RM, Wilcox RB: Underestimates of serum-free thyroxine (T_4) concentrations by free T_4 immunoassays. J Clin Endocrinol Metab 1994; 79:76.

New MI: 21-hydroxylase deficiency congenital adrenal hyperplasia. J Steroid Biochem Mol Biol 1994; 48:15.

Nicholson HD, Pickering BT: Oxytocin, a male intragonadal hormone. Regul Pept 1993; 45:253.

North WG, Friedmann AS, Yu X: Tumor biosynthesis of vasopressin and oxytocin. Ann N Y Acad Sci 1993; 689:107.

Nunez C, Ortiz-Apodaca MA: Excretion of free catecholamines by children. Eur J Clin Chem Clin Biochem 1994; 32:461.

Nussey SS, Soo SC, Gibson S, et al: Isolated congenital ACTH deficiency: A cleavage enzyme defect? Clin Endocrinol 1993; 39:381.

Orth DN: Cushing's syndrome. N Engl J Med 1995; 332:791.

Osredkar J, Vrhovec I, Jesenovec N, et al: Salivary-free testosterone in hirsutism. Ann Clin Biochem 1989; 26:522.

Ozata M, Suzuki S, Miyamoto T, et al: Serum thyroglobulin in the follow-up of patients with treated differentiated thyroid cancer. J Clin Endocrinol Metab 1994; 79:98.

Pacini F, Pinchera A, Giani C, et al: Serum thyroglobulin in thyroid carcinoma and other thyroid disorders. J Endocrinol Invest 1980; 3:283.

Pang LC, Tsao KC: Flow cytometric DNA analysis for the determination of malignant potential in adrenal and extra-adrenal pheochromocytomas or paragangliomas. Arch Pathol Lab Med 1993; 117:1142.

Peabody CA, Schultz PN, Warner MD, et al: Prolactin bioassay and hyperprolactinemia. J Endocrinol Invest 1992; 15:497.

Pelletier G: Anatomy of the hypothalamic-pituitary axis. Methods Achieve Exp Pathol 1991; 14:1.

Penny MD, Hampton D, Oleesky DA, et al: Radioimmunoassays of arginine vasopressin and atrial natriuretic peptide: Application of a common protocol for plasma extraction using Sep-Pak C18 cartridges. Ann Clin Biochem 1992; 29:652.

Peplinski GR, Norton JA: The predictive value of diagnostic tests for pheochromocytoma. Surgery 1994; 116:1101.

Perelman AH, Johnson RL, Clemons RD, et al: Intrauterine diagnosis and treatment of fetal goitrous hypothyroidism. J Clin Endocrinol Metab 1990; 71:618.

Perez C, Novoa J, Alcañiz J, et al: Leydig cell tumour of the testis with gynaecomastia and elevated oestrogen, progesterone and prolactin levels. Case report. Clin Endocrinol 1980; 13:409.

Perrot D, Bonneton A, Dechaud H, et al: Hypercortisolism in septic shock is not suppressible by dexamethasone infusion. Crit Care Med 1993, 21:396.

Philomin V, Vessieres A, Jaouen G: New applications of carbonylmetalloimmunoassay (CMIA): A non-radioisotopic approach to cortisol assay. J Immunol Methods 1994; 171:201.

Porter CC, Silber RH: A quantitative color reaction for cortisone and related 17,21-dihydroxy-20-ketosteroids. J Biol Chem 1950; 185:201.

Prados P, Higashidate S, Imai K: A fully automated HPLC method for the determination of catecholamines in biological samples utilizing ethylenediamine condensation and peroxyoxalate chemiluminescence detection. Biomed Chromatogr 1994; 8:1.

Pritchard PB: The effect of seizures on hormones. Epilepsia 1991; 32:546.

Raff H, Shaker JL, Nelson DK, et al: Rapid measurement of corticotropin (ACTH) with a modified immunochemiluminescent assay. Clin Chem 1994; 40:1344.

Ram CVS, Fierro-Carrion GA: Pheochromocytoma. Semin Nephrol 1995, 15:126.

Rapaport R, Sills I, Patel U, et al: Thyrotropin-releasing hormone stimulation tests in infants. J Clin Endocrinol Metab 1993; 77:889.

Raue F, Frank-Raue K, Grauer A: Multiple endocrine neoplasia type 2. Clinical features and screening. Endocrinol Metab Clin N Am 1994; 23:137.

Refetoff S: Resistance to thyroid hormone. Clin Lab Med 1993; 13:563.

Reinazartz JJ, Ramey ML, Fowler MC, et al: Plastic vs glass SST evacuated serum-separator blood-drawing tubes for endocrinologic analytes. (Letter.) Clin Chem 1993; 39:2535.

Reutens AT, Hoffman DM, Kin-Chuen L, et al: Evaluation and application of a highly sensitive assay for serum growth hormone (GH) in the study of adult GH deficiency. J Clin Endocrinol Metab 1995; 80:480.

Rheaume E, Sanchez R, Simard J, et al: Molecular basis of congenital adrenal hyperplasia in two siblings with classical nonsalt-losing 3 beta-hydroxysteroid dehydrogenase deficiency. J Clin Endocrinol Metab 1994; 79:1012.

Riddick L, Chrousos GP, Jeffries S, et al: Comparison of adrenocorticotropin and adrenal steroid responses to corticotropin-releasing hormone versus metyrapone testing in patients with hypopituitarism. Pediatr Res 1994; 36:215.

Rieu M, Richard A, Rosilio M, et al: Effects of thyroid status on thyroid autoimmunity expression in euthyroid and hypothyroid patients with Hashimoto's thyroiditis. Clin Endocrinol 1994; 40:529.

Ritter D, Stott R, Grant N, et al: Endogenous antibodies that interfere with thyroxine fluoresce polarization assay but not with radioimmunoassay or EMIT. Clin Chem 1993; 39:508.

Robertson D, Haile V, Perry SE, et al: Dopamine beta-hydroxylase deficiency. A genetic disorder of cardiovascular regulation. Hypertension 1991; 18:1.

Robertson GL: The use of vasopressin assays in physiology and pathophysiology. Semin Nephrol 1994; 14:368.

Roger M, Grenier J, Houlbert C, et al: Rapid radioimmunoassays of plasma LH and estradiol-17β for the prediction of ovulation. J Steroid Biochem 1980; 12:403.

Rohrbach MS, DeRemee RA: Measurement of angiotensin converting enzyme activity in serum in the diagnosis and management of sarcoidosis. Clin Lab Annu 1982; 1:435.

Rojanasakul A, Udomsubpayakul U, Chinsomboon S: Chemiluminescence immunoassay versus radioimmunoassay for the measurement of reproductive hormones. Int J Gynecol Obstet 1994; 45:141.

Rosano TG, Swift TA, Hayes LW: Advances in catecholamine and metabolite measurements for diagnosis of pheochromocytoma. Clin Chem 1991; 37:1854.

Rosenfeld RG, Rosenbloom AL, Guevara-Aguirre J: Growth hormone (GH) insensitivity due to GH receptor deficiency. Endocrinol Rev 1994; 15:369.

Rosner W: Plasma steroid-bind proteins. Endocrinol Metab Clin North Am 1991; 20:697.

Rubello D, Casara D, Girelli ME, et al: Clinical meaning of circulating anti-thyroglobulin antibodies in differentiated thyroid cancer: A prospective study. J Nucl Med 1992; 33:1478.

Rudd BT: Measurement of urine 17-oxogenic steroids, 17-hydroxycorticosteroids, and 17-oxosteroids has been superseded by better tests. BMJ, 1985; 291:805.

Ruiz M, Rajatanavin R, Young RA, et al: Familial dyalbuminemic hyperthyroxinemia. A syndrome that can be confused with thyrotoxicosis. N Engl J Med 1982; 306:635.

Ruutiainen K, Sannikka E, Santti R, et al: Salivary testosterone in hirsutism: Correlations with serum testosterone and the degree of hair growth. J Clin Endocrinol Metab 1987; 64:1015.

Saberi M, Utiger RD: Serum thyroid hormone and thyrotropin concentrations during thyroxine and triiodothyronine therapy. J Clin Endocrinol Metab 1974; 39:923.

Samaan GJ, Porquet D, Demelier JF, et al: Determination of cortisol and associated glucocorticoids in serum and urine by an automated lipid chromatographic assay. Clin Biochem 1993; 26:153.

Samuels MH, Veldhuis JD, Henry P, et al: Pathophysiology of pulsatile and copulsatile release of thyroid-stimulating hormone, luteinizing hormone, follicle-stimulating hormone, and alpha subunit. J Clin Endocrinol Metab 1990; 71:425.

Santen RJ: The testis. *In* Felig P, Baxter JD, Frohman LA: Endocrinology and Metabolism, 3rd ed. New York, McGraw Hill, 1995, pp 855–972.

Sapin R, Gasser F, Boehn A, et al: Spuriously high concentration of serum-free thyroxine due to anti-triiodothyronine antibodies. Clin Chem 1995; 41:117.

Sawin CT, Geller A, Kaplan MM, et al: Low serum thyrotropin (thyroid-stimulating hormone) in older persons without hyperthyroidism. Arch Intern Med 1991; 151:165.

Schectman JM, Pawlson G: The cost-effectiveness of three thyroid function testing strategies for suspicion of hypothyroidism in a primary care setting. J Gen Intern Med 1990; 5:9.

Scott RT, Hofmann GE: Prognostic assessment of ovarian reserve. Fertil Steril 1995; 63:1.

Sergev O, Racz K, Varga I, et al: Atrial natriuretic peptide in normal and low renin essential hypertension. Kidney Int 1990; 38:S.

Sharp AM, Fraser IS, Robertson S, Turtle JR: Positive interference by danazol in a testosterone radioimmunoassay kit procedure. Clin Chem 1981; 27:603.

Siegel SF, Finegold DN, Lanes R, et al: ACTH stimulation tests and plasma dehydroepiandrosterone sulfate levels in women with hirsutism. N Engl J Med 1990; 323:849.

Simard J, Rheaume E, Sanchez R, et al: Molecular basis of congenital adrenal hyperplasia due to 3 beta hydroxysteroid dehydrogenase deficiency. Mol Endocrinol 1993; 7:716.

Singh UK, Jana UK: Plasma prolactin in epilepsy and pseudoseizures. Ind Pediatr 1994; 31:667.

Sinha YN, Jacobsen BP: Human growth hormone (hGH), a reportedly diabetogenic fragment of hGH, circulates in human blood: Measurement by radioimmunoassay. J Clin Endocrinol Metab 1994; 78:1411.

Sjoberg RJ, Simcic KJ, Kidd GS: The clonidine suppression test for pheochromocytoma. A review of its utility and pitfalls. Arch Intern Med 1992; 152:1193.

Skinner AM, Clayton PE, Price DA, et al: Variability in the urinary excretion of growth hormone in children: A comparison with other urinary proteins. J Endocrinol 1993; 138:337.

Slyper AH, Shaker JL: Neonatal hypothyroxinemia with normal thyrotropin. Clin Pediatr 1993; 32:121.

Smal J, Closset J, Hennen G, et al: The receptor binding properties of the 20K variant of human growth hormone explain its discrepant insulin-like and growth promoting activities. Biochem Biophys Res Commun 1986; 134:159.

Small M, Buchanan L, Evans R: Value of screening thyroid function in acute medical admissions to hospital. Clin Endocrinol 1990; 32:185.

Smith BR, McLachlan SM, Furmaniak J: Autoantibodies to the thyrotropin receptor. Endocr Rev 1988; 9:106.

Smith MV, Laws ER: Magnetic resonance imaging measurements of pituitary stalk compression and deviation in patients with nonprolactin-secreting intrasellar and parasellar tumors: Lack of correlation with serum prolactin levels. Neurosurgury 1994; 34:834.

Snow K, Jiang N, Kao PC, et al: Biochemical evolution of adrenal dysfunction: The laboratory perspective. Mayo Clin Proc 1992; 67:1055.

Snyder PJ, Bigdeli H, Gardner DF: Gonadal function in fifty men with untreated pituitary adenomas. J Clin Endocrinol Metab 1979; 48:309.

Spencer CA, Schwarzbein D, Guttler RB, et al: Thyrotropin (TSH)–releasing hormone stimulation test responses employing third and fourth generation TSH assays. J Clin Endocrinol Metab 1993; 76:494.

Spratt DI, Cox P, Orav J, et al: Reproductive axis suppression in acute illness is related to disease severity. J Clin Endocrinol Metab 1993; 76:1548.

Stenstrom G, Svardsudd K: Pheochromocytoma in Sweden 1958–1981. An analysis of the National Cancer Registry Data. Acta Med Scand 1986; 220:225.

Sterling K, Lazarus JH: The thyroid and its control. Ann Rev Physiol 1977; 39:349.

Stock S, Bremme K, Uvnas-Moberg K: Plasma levels of oxytocin during the menstrual cycle, pregnancy and following treatment with HMG. Hum Reprod 1991; 6:1056.

Strakosch CR, Wenzel BE, Row VV, Volpe R: Immunology of autoimmune thyroid diseases. N Engl J Med 1982; 307:1499.

Strasburger CJ: Implications of investigating the structure-function relationship of human growth hormone in clinical diagnosis and therapy. Horm Res 1994; 41(Suppl): 113.

Streeten DHP, Tomycz N, Anderson GH: Reliability of screening methods for the diagnosis of primary aldosteronism. Am J Med 1979; 67:403.

Subramanian MG, Sacco AG, Moghissi KS, et al: Prolactin size heterogeneity in human follicular fluid: A preliminary study. Int J Fertil 1991; 36:367.

Tabarin A, Corcuff JB, Rashedi M, et al: Comparative value of plasma ACTH and beta-endorphin measurement with three different commercial kits for the etiological diagnosis of ACTH-dependent Cushing's syndrome. Acta Endocrinol 1992; 126:308.

Tanaka T, Shiu R, Gout P, et al: A new sensitive and specific assay for lactogenic hormones: Measurement of prolactin and growth hormone in human serum. J Clin Endocrinol Metab 1980; 51:1058.

Thalen BE, Kjellman BF, Ljunggren JG, et al: Release of corticotropin after administration of corticotropin-releasing hormone in depressed patients in relation to the dexamethasone suppression test. Acta Psychiatr Scand 1993; 87:133.

Tillotson SL, Fuggle PW, Smith I, et al: Relation between biochemical severity and intelligence in early treated congenital hypothyroidism: A threshold effect. BMJ 1994; 309:440.

Torok A, Vecsernyes M, Penke B: Affinity chromatographic method for the extraction of ocytocin from human and rat plasma. Eur J Clin Chem Clin Biochem 1994; 32:595.

Trainer PJ: Effect of insulin-like growth factor I on anterior pituitary function. Acta Paediatr 1994; 399(Suppl):173.

Turner G, Brown RC, Weeks I, et al: Urinary growth hormone excretion as measured by a sensitive immunochemiluminometric assay. Ann Clin Biochem 1993; 30:180.

Utiger RD: Increased extrathyroidal triiodothyronine production in nonthyroidal illness: Benefit or harm? Am J Med 1980; 69:807.

Valenta LJ, Sigel MB, Lesniak MA, et al: Pituitary dwarfism in a patient with circulating abnormal growth hormone polymers. N Engl J Med 1985; 312:214.

Van Heerden JA, Roland CF, Carney JA, et al: Long-term evaluation following resection of apparently benign pheochromocytoma(s)/paraganglioma(s). World J Surg 1990; 14:325.

van der Sluijs Veer G, Vermes I, Bonte HA, et al: Temperature effects on free-thyroxine measurements: Analytical and clinical consequences. Clin Chem 1992; 38:1327.

Van Wassemaer AG, Kok JH, Endert E, et al: Thyroxine administration to infants of less than 30 weeks' gestational age does not increase plasma triiodothyronine concentration. Acta Endocrinol 1993; 129:139.

Veldhuis JD, Johnson ML, Faunt LM, et al: Influence of the high-affinity growth hormone (GH)–binding protein on plasma profiles of free and bound GH and on the apparent half-life of GH. Modeling analysis and clinical applications. J Clin Invest 1993; 91:629.

Verkerk PH, Buitendijk SE, Verloove-Vanhorick SP: Congenital hypothyroidism screening and the cutoff for thyrotropin measurement: Recommendations from the Netherlands. Am J Public Health 1993; 83:868.

Vieira JG, Ando MH, Nishida SK, et al: Clinical utility of a 22-kDa growth hormone–specific assay. Brazil J Med Biol Res 1992; 25:243.

Volin P: Simultaneous determination of serum cortisol and cortisone by reversed-phase liquid chromatography with ultraviolet detection. J Chromatogr 1992; 584:147.

Warner MD, Sinha YN, Peabody CA: Growth hormone and prolactin variants in normal subjects. Relative proportions in morning and afternoon samples. Horm Metab Res 1993; 25:425.

Weber MA, Neutel JM, Smith DH, et al: Diagnosis of mild hypertension by ambulatory blood pressure monitoring. Circulation 1994; 90:2291.

Wenzel KW: Pharmacological interference with in vitro tests of thyroid function. Metabolism 1981; 30:717.

Werbel SS, Ober KP: Pheochromocytoma. Update on diagnosis, localization, and management. Med Clin North Am 1995; 79:131.

White PC, Curnow KM, Pascoe L: Disorders of steroid 11 beta-hydroxylase isoenzymes. Endocr Rev 1994b; 15:421.

White PC, Tusie-Luna MT, New MI, et al: Mutations in steroid 21-hydroxylase (CYP21). Hum Mutat 1994a; 3:373.

Wille S, Aili M, Harris A, et al: Plasma and urinary levels of vasopressin in enuretic and non-enuretic children. Scand J Urol Nephrol 1994; 28:119.

Young DS: Effects of Drugs on Clinical Laboratory Tests, 3rd ed. Washington, DC, AACC Press, 1990, pp 218–219.

Young DS: Effects of Preanalytical Variables on Clinical Laboratory Tests. Washington, DC, AACC Press, (1993); 3:312.

Yuki Y, Kato K: A 22-kDa human growth hormone–specific enzyme-linked immunosorbent assay. Biol Pharm Bull 1994; 17:977.

Zweig MH, Csako G, Benson CC, et al: Interference by anti-immunoglobulin G antibodies in immunoradiometric assays of thyrotropin involving mouse monoclonal antibodies. Clin Chem 1987; 33:840.

Zweig MH, Csako G, Reynolds JC, et al: Interference by iatrogenically induced anti-mouse IgG antibodies in a two-site immunometric assay for thyrotropin. Arch Pathol Lab Med 1991; 115:164.

Chapter 17

Toxicology and Therapeutic Drug Monitoring

Matthew R. Pincus, M.D., Ph.D.
Naif Z. Abraham, Jr., M.D., Ph.D.

Toxicology is the study of substances introduced exogenously into the body. Elsewhere in this textbook, all of the analytical methods discussed are concerned with determining the presence and levels of natural substances involved in normal body function. In this chapter, we discuss the biological effects and methods for detection of exogenous chemical compounds that profoundly influence bodily functions, often in a deleterious way but also for therapeutic benefit.

Vast changes have occurred in this field in view of the revolution that has taken place in such widely disparate areas as chemotherapy and new antibiotic therapy, both of which demand the frequent, accurate determination of the levels of drugs in patients treated for neoplasia or infectious diseases. Unfortunately, major changes have occurred in the area of drug abuse, especially in the development of new and potent forms of mood-lifting drugs such as "crack," the free-base form of cocaine, leading to the demise of large segments of the population.

As it has evolved over the past several years, toxicology has been divided into four areas. The first two areas are the detection of drugs of abuse and the determination of the levels of therapeutic drugs being administered to patients. Also, it has been recognized that certain environmental compounds that are mutagens and carcinogens such as benzpyrene and acetylaminofluorene cause mutations in critical sequences of human DNA, leading to the frank development of cancer. A whole methodology has therefore been devised to detect carcinogen levels in individuals who are suspected of having been exposed to them. In the ongoing revolution in molecular biology, this field has now expanded into the detection of certain markers such as abnormal DNA sequences or abnormal protein sequences whose presence in individuals indicates early-on the development of neoplasia.

Finally, there are a variety of toxins to which individuals become exposed such as carbon monoxide, cyanide, metals, and so forth, and for which detection is vital in order for physicians to be able to reverse the adverse acute physiologic effects. In this chapter, we discuss each of these divisions of toxicology with special reference to new developments in techniques for detecting drugs in body fluids and with respect to the rapidly developing field of early tumor detection (Henderson, 1989).

BASIC TECHNIQUES FOR DETECTING DRUGS IN SERUM AND URINE

The techniques involved in detecting the presence and the level of particular drugs, whether they are drugs of abuse or therapeutic drugs, are of two basic types: immunochemical and chromatographic. Although both of these techniques are explained elsewhere in this volume (see Chaps. 3 and 33), there are special adaptations of these methods that warrant discussion in this chapter.

Immunochemical Methods

Much drug testing today is performed using the so-called homogeneous immunoassay. The term homogeneous refers to the fact that these assays are all performed in a single step—that is, only one antibody is used in the procedure. This technology has revolutionized toxicology because it allows performance of rapid, stat analyses of blood and urine constituents. The technique is shown schematically in Figure 17–1*A*. Notice that there are two types of assays. In the first, the enzyme-mediated (or multiplied) immunologic technique (EMIT), the drug itself is covalently attached to an enzyme such as alkaline phosphatase. When the drug-enzyme complex is incubated with an antibody (usually monoclonal) to the drug, the enzyme activity is markedly decreased as a result of the blocking of the active site of the enzyme by the antibody. When, as in Figure 17–1*A*, exogenous drug (such as in serum) is added to the immune complex, this exogenous drug competes with the drug-enzyme for the antibody. Liberated drug-enzyme results in increased enzymatic activity. Increasing concentrations of drug in serum result in increased observed enzymatic activity. This ingenious and sensitive method has been pioneered largely by the Syva Corporation (Palo Alto, CA) and has been applied both to therapeutic drug monitoring and to the detection of drugs of abuse.

Fluorescence polarization immunoassay (FPIA) is the second type of homogeneous drug assay, as shown in Figure 17–1*B*. This method is particularly sensitive and elegant. Rather than being linked to an enzyme, as in Figure 17–1*A*, the drug is covalently attached to a fluorescent probe molecule. If a fluorescent molecule is excited with polarized light, if the molecule is stationary—that is, it does not "tumble" in solution—it will emit polarized light as a fluorophore. If a fluorophore tumbles freely in solution, however, the polarization is lost. However, if the fluorophore is bound to a macromolecule, like an antibody, the polarization is strong because, being attached to the nontumbling antibody, it remains relatively stationary. In these assays, the probe-labeled drug is incubated with the antibody. The fluorescence polarization of the probe-labeled drug is, of course, high because the fluorescent probe is relatively immobilized, bound to the antibody directed against it. Addition of exogenous drug, as in serum, to the incubated mixture results in displacement of some of the fluorescent probe–labeled drug molecules, as shown in Figure 17–1*B*. These displaced molecules can now tumble freely in solution. The result is a *decrease* in fluorescence polarization. This decrease is directly related to the concentration of drug in serum.

This assay can detect drug levels in the nanomolar range and is both highly sensitive and specific. Both Abbott Laboratories (Chicago, IL), with the TDX analyzers, and Roche Diagnostic Laboratories (Nutley, NJ), with the COBAS analyzer, have pioneered this most effective technique in monitoring a wide variety of therapeutic drugs and also drugs of abuse.

2

Drug Binding to Antibodies

In both of the homogeneous methods discussed previously, there is a nonlinear relationship between the concentration of drug in serum and the response of the system—that is, the color that results from the enzymatic reaction (see Fig. 17–1*A*) or the decrease in fluorescence polarization (see Fig. 17–1*B*). This nonlinearity in response is due to the phenomenon of binding—that is, the drug must bind to antibody before it is detected. This phenomenon may be expressed by the following equilibrium:

$$D + D^* - Ab \rightleftarrows D - Ab + D^* \qquad (17\text{-}1),$$

where D is the drug concentration in serum, D* is the so-called marker drug (i.e., a drug labeled with an enzyme or a fluorescent probe), and Ab is the antibody. The concentration of free D* is a measure of D − Ab, because both are equimolar. The concentration of D − Ab is, in turn, related to D—the more D present, the more D − Ab formed. However, because the concentration of Ab is fixed in a given experiment, at sufficiently high concentrations of D, all of the Ab is saturated, so that at higher concentrations of D, no further D − Ab can form. The relationship between D and D − Ab is given by the Langmuir expression:

$$r = (D - Ab)/(Ab_o) = nkD/(kD + 1) \qquad (17\text{-}2),$$

where (Ab_o) is the total concentration of antibody, k is the equilibrium constant for formation of the D − Ab complex, n is the number of antibody-binding sites per molecule of antibody, and D is defined earlier. Equation 17-2 is very similar to the Michaelis-Menten equation discussed in Chapter 13, except that there is no catalytic step here. This equation shows that the concentration of D − Ab is nonlinear in D except where $kD << 1$. Where $kD >> 1$, saturation is achieved. This equation can be linearized in the form used for a Scatchard plot—that is,

$$r/D = nk - kr \qquad (17\text{-}3),$$

where r/D is plotted versus r. Given the results for a set of experiments, a least-squares–best-fit line is drawn through the points, and the values of n and k are determined. Once values

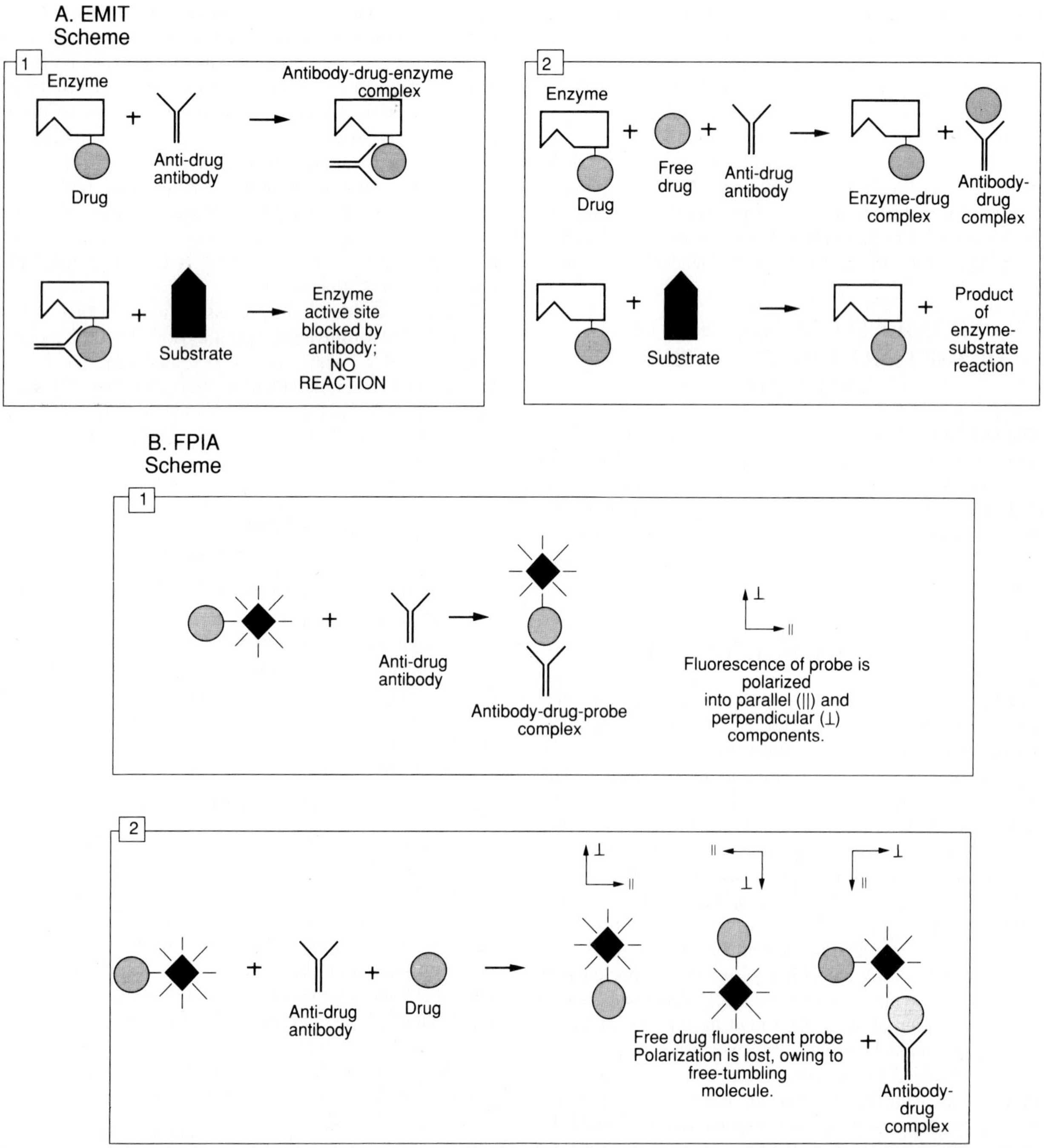

Figure 17–1. Homogeneous methods for detecting qualitatively or quantitatively the levels of drugs in body fluids. *A,* In the EMIT method, a drug-enzyme complex is used as the marker. When bound to the anti-drug antibody, the active site of the enzyme (linked to the drug) is blocked. Therefore, when substrate is added, no reaction will occur, as shown in Part 1. However, if free drug (as in serum) is present, some or most of the enzyme-drug complex is displaced from the anti-drug antibody. Now the active sites of the liberated enzyme-drug complexes are free, and the substrate undergoes reactions as indicated in Part 2. *B,* In the fluorescence polarization method (FPIA), the same general approach is used as in *A* except that in this method the drug is attached to a fluorescent label. When the drug-label complex is bound to the anti-drug antibody, its fluorescence is polarized into parallel and perpendicular components. When displaced by free drug, as in serum or urine, the drug-probe complex is displaced from the anti-drug antibody, resulting in diminished fluorescence polarization.

for n and k are known, the value of D for any measured value of r can be *directly computed* from Equation 17-3. The purpose of the calibration procedures on various analyzers is to determine n and k so that the drug concentration in serum can be computed for a given value of r.

Two problems that arise in using Equation 17-3 are that often the antibodies are nonhomogeneous, so that the Scatchard plot is nonlinear, and possible blockage of free antibody sites may occur because of drug molecules in solid-phase immunoassays. The first problem has been solved by Rodbard (1971), wherein the analysis mentioned previously has been applied to multiple-binding equilibria. This analysis is used commonly in microprocessors that analyze the calibration curves in immunoassays. The second problem has been analyzed using a different theoretical approach (Pincus, 1981). Equation 17-3 illustrates the basic principle of how the results of the drug immunoassay on serum are converted into drug concentrations in serum.

Chromatographic Techniques

Chromatographic procedures have been applied mainly to the qualitative detection of drugs of abuse and toxins and less to the determination of the levels of therapeutic drugs. The three major methods are thin-layer chromatography (TLC), high-performance liquid chromatography (HPLC), and gas chromatography–mass spectroscopy (GC-MS).

THIN-LAYER CHROMATOGRAPHY. This technique is described in Chapter 3. Briefly, compounds are separated from one another in this method, based on their relative affinities for a polar solid stationary phase (usually a hydrated silicate) and a mobile liquid phase that is nonpolar (such as 10% methanol in chloroform). Depending on these affinities, different compounds adsorb to the hydrated silicate at different positions as the nonpolar solvent migrates up the stationary hydrated silicate. The principle is illustrated in Figure 17–2. For a given solvent system, the ratio of the distance traversed by the compound to the distance traversed by the solvent front is a constant for the compound and can be used to identify the compound in a mixture. This ratio is called the r_f. This technique is central to identifying different drugs of abuse, all of which can be separated from one another using TLC. The method has now been packaged in the form of Toxi-lab (Irvine, CA) kits, in which the user is supplied with discrete strips of silicate, extraction solvents, and color-developing solutions.

TOXI-LAB PROCEDURES. The procedures of processing specimens using this technique summarize the essential features of drug identification. First, the best specimen for drug detection is urine because large quantities of this body fluid can be collected noninvasively. Once a urine specimen is collected, it is subjected to extraction procedures. In these procedures, acidic drugs are separated from basic ones. Almost all drugs of abuse are basic drugs, all of which are amine derivatives. The important so-called acid drugs comprise the barbiturates almost exclusively. In aqueous solution, the basic drugs are charged because of the equilibrium, as shown in Equation 17-4a:

$$R - NH_2 + H^+ \rightleftarrows R - NH^{3+} \qquad (17\text{-}4a)$$

$$RNH^{3+} + OH^- \rightleftarrows RNH_2 + H_2O \qquad (17\text{-}4b),$$

in which a primary amine (secondary and tertiary amines exhibit the same equilibrium) is represented by RNH_2. The ammonium ion form (right side of Equation 17-4a) is soluble in water but not in nonpolar organic solvents. However, the amine-free base (left side of Equation 17-4a) is soluble in nonpolar organic solvents. Extraction procedures to isolate the basic drugs are aimed at treating the urine with base so that significant amounts of the basic drugs will be uncharged as the amine-free base (Equation 17-4b). This form can then be extracted into a nonpolar organic phase and then applied to the silicate strip. The reverse process is carried out for acidic drugs—that is, these are treated with acid and extracted into nonpolar solvents. In practice, a small paper disk is added to the organic extraction mixture, and the solvent is then evaporated so that all basic drugs adsorb onto the paper disk. This disk is then applied to one end of the silicate strip, and the strip is placed in the migrating nonpolar solvent. A separate strip is used for each extraction, the A strip being used for basic drugs and the B strip for acidic drugs. The chief utility of the B strip is in identifying the barbiturates, as discussed subsequently.

IDENTIFICATION OF SPECIFIC DRUGS. After the drugs are separated on the plate, it is necessary to identify them. This objective is achieved by subjecting the drugs to color reactions for each separate compound. Toxi-lab has the added feature of subjecting the separated compounds to a series of color reactions that further assist in identification of drugs. In

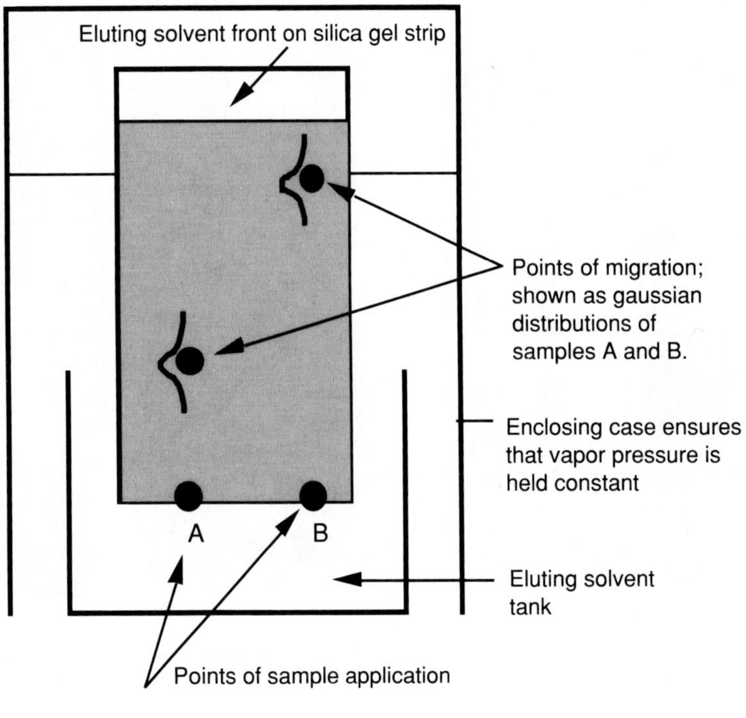

Figure 17–2. Illustration of the principle of thin-layer chromatography (TLC). Two solutes, A and B, are applied to the polar silicate strip. A is more polar than B and has a higher affinity, therefore, for the polar stationary phase than for the non-polar mobile phase (usually methanol in chloroform). This relative affinity of A is, moreover, higher than the affinity of B for the polar phase. Therefore, A separates out first on the strip and B migrates further on the strip. Notice that for both solutes the band of separation is really bell shaped (gaussian distribution for each compound), as it would be in column chromatography.

this procedure for basic drugs, the strip is simply dipped successively in three different solvents, which result in characteristic color patterns for each drug. The strip is also subjected to ultraviolet light, which excites fluorescence in selected compounds. Similar procedures are used for the acidic drugs extracted onto the B strip. As shown in Figure 17–3*A*, which is from the Toxi-lab reference pattern book, each drug can be identified not only by its r_f but also by its color and characteristic color change in different reagents. These patterns are reinforced by the fluorescence characteristics. As an example, notice in Figure 17–3*A* that heroin has a characteristic r_f of 0.14 and, not shown, a characteristic dark red color in the first solvent that disappears in the second solvent, water. It is nonfluorescent. If one or more of these characteristics differ from this pattern, strong doubt about identification of the spot as heroin would exist. If all criteria are met, the sensitivity and specificity of the method are increased.

RELIABILITY OF THE METHOD. Because the identification of each drug depends on use of qualitative color changes or the presence of fluorescence, or both, the sensitivity of the method is limited by the ability of the naked eye to detect these changes. Practically, the level of detection is on the order of 1 μg/mL of compound present on the strip. The chief value of the chromatographic method is confirmatory—that is, confirmation of a positive immunoassay test result. The two methods are often performed together on a single specimen.

The major problems that occur with this method are that extraction procedures are occasionally inefficient, so that insufficient amounts of drug are adsorbed onto the disk. Also, the extraction and evaporation procedures are somewhat time consuming, requiring approximately half an hour for full processing. Furthermore, cocaine has a number of metabolites that are polar (e.g., ecgonine) and that barely migrate from the origin, so that it is sometimes difficult to detect the presence of this drug of abuse because it has been converted completely to the polar metabolites prior to excretion. Some difficulty may also be encountered in distinguishing among various opiates, such as between morphine and other opiates because the r_f values of these drugs can be close to one another (see Fig. 17–3*A*). However, experienced personnel can make this distinction in most cases. Also, some nontoxic drugs may give characteristic color changes and r_f values that are similar to those for the drug of abuse. For example, certain antihistamines that appear on the A strip are very similar to amphetamines.

HIGH-PERFORMANCE LIQUID CHROMATOGRAPHY. Thin-layer chromatography allows direct qualitative detection of drugs in a panoramic way, but HPLC allows quantitative detection of drugs and allows sharper separation of

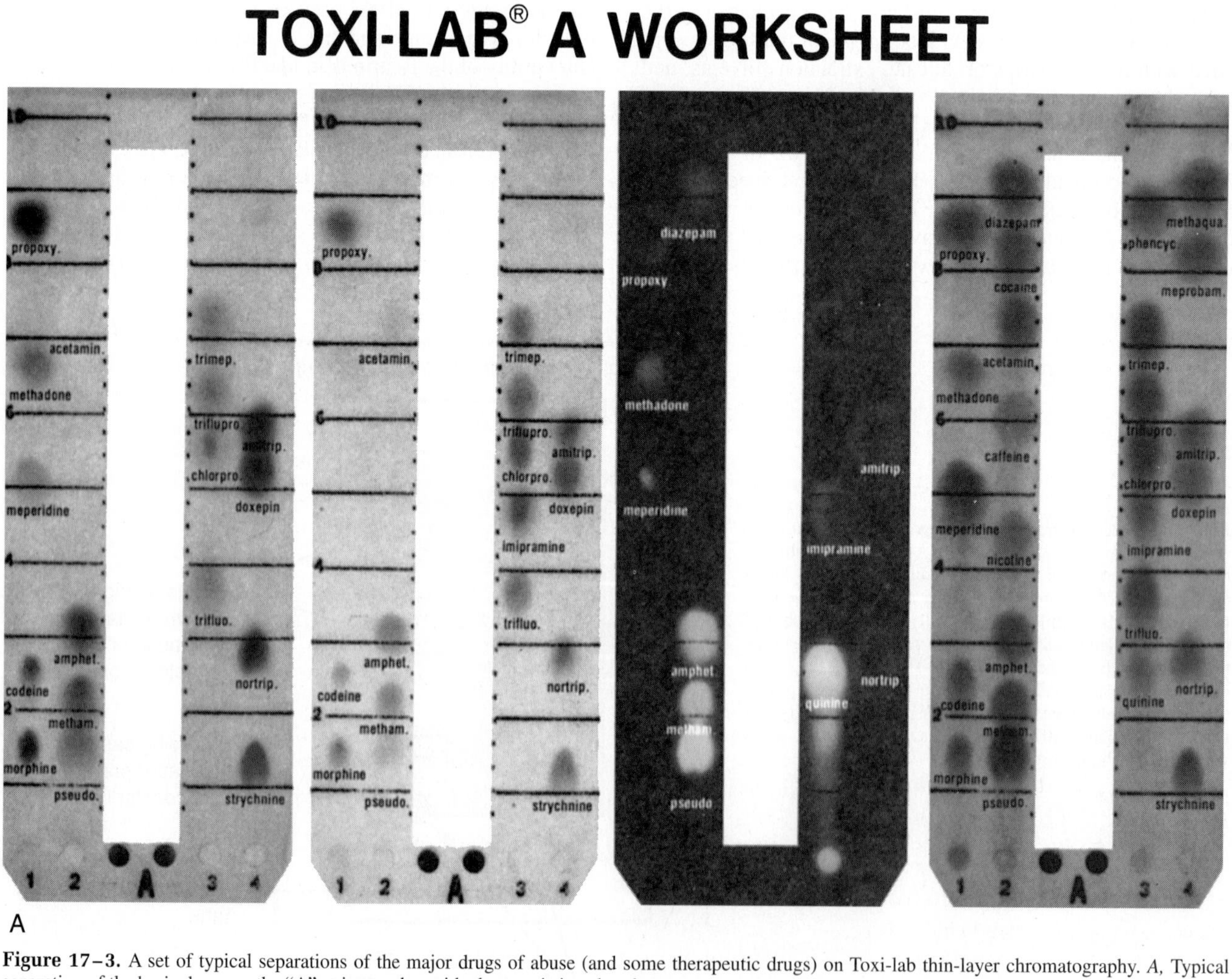

A

Figure 17–3. A set of typical separations of the major drugs of abuse (and some therapeutic drugs) on Toxi-lab thin-layer chromatography. *A*, Typical separation of the basic drugs on the "A" strip together with characteristic color changes.

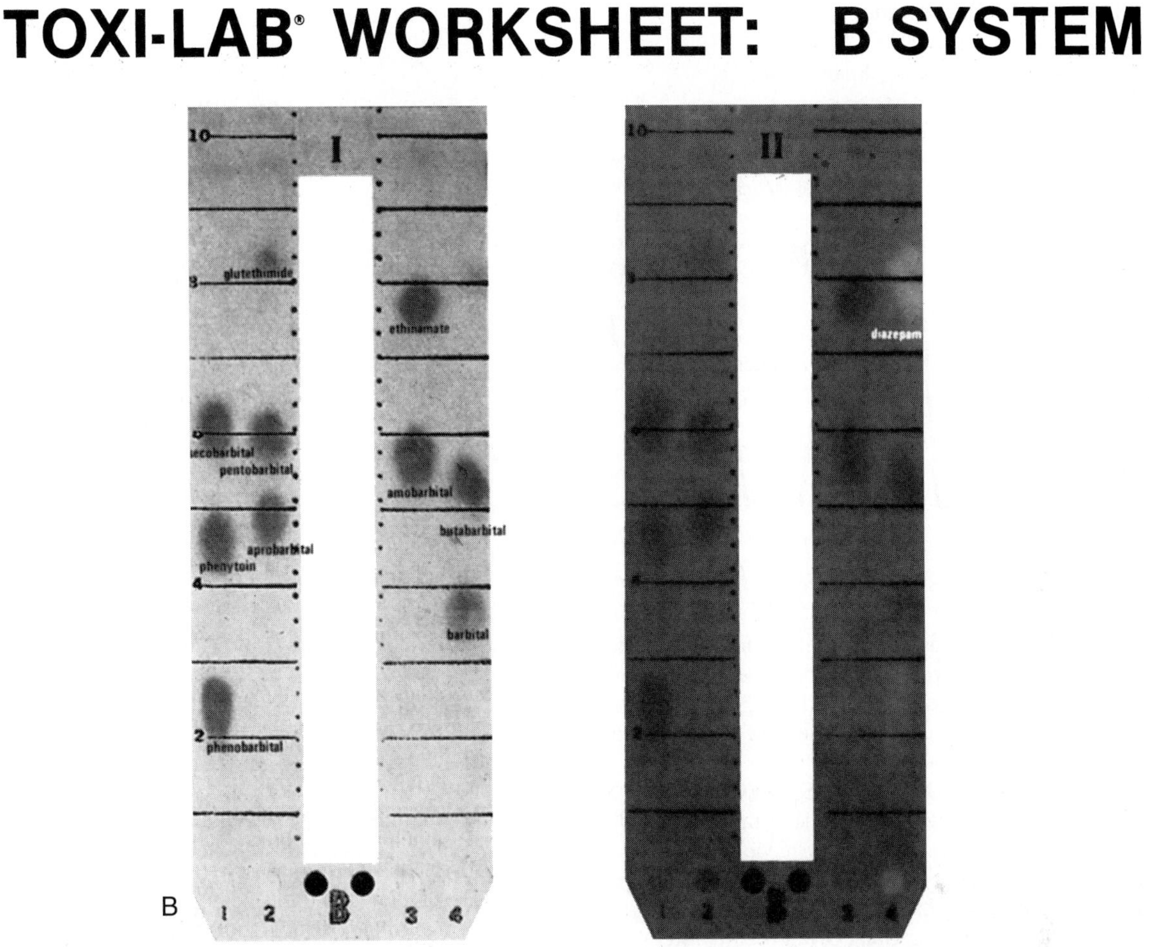

Figure 17–3 *Continued B,* Typical separation of the more acidic drugs on the "B" strip with characteristic color changes. The major use of the "B" strip is to identify the presence of barbiturates.

these same drugs. In HPLC (as discussed in Chap. 3), the stationary phase, which can be *either* polar (silicic acid) or nonpolar (such as the C-18 columns), in reverse-phase chromatography is composed of uniform, ultrafine particles that vastly increase its adsorptive surface area. This stationary phase is packed into a column. The resistance to flow in this column is high, so that large pressures are required to deliver constant reasonable flow rates. In the Waters HPLC instrument (Millipore Corporation, Medford, MA), a constant pressure head is delivered to the column by the use of two pumps that operate so that as one withdraws, the other pushes forward (i.e., the two operate 180 degrees out of phase). The eluate from the column is monitored by a variety of detectors ranging from ultraviolet multiwavelength detectors to redox potential electrode detectors. It is the usual practice in performance of quantitative HPLC to use an internal standard—that is, a compound similar in structure to the drug(s) of interest, which is added to the specimen to be analyzed in a known concentration. By knowing how much of this marker compound or internal standard is placed on the column and how much is recovered from the column in the eluate, the percentage recovery from the column can be calculated for this compound and, by extrapolation, for all of the drugs of interest for which concentrations are being quantitated. Thus, losses owing to the column (in addition to losses in extraction procedures) can be corrected for using this technique. Generally, HPLC has been used for the quantitation of specific therapeutic drugs but has found use in detection of cocaine and heroin in urine. The sensitivity of the method is in the nanomolar to micromolar range.

One of the most frequent uses of HPLC is in the separation and quantitation of the tricyclic antidepressants and their metabolites. These are among the most commonly prescribed drugs and are also used in excess as drugs of abuse in suicide attempts. It is often necessary to determine the levels not only of the parent tricyclic antidepressant but also of its active and inactive metabolites reviewed subsequently. Figure 17–4 shows a typical separation on a silicate column. Protriptyline, an inactive tricyclic compound, is the internal standard. It is clear that the separation among the metabolites and parent compounds is sharp. This separation is completely reproducible.

A recent variant of TLC that includes the advantages of HPLC is capillary electrophoresis (Shihabi, 1993). In this method, a capillary tube, lined with silicate, 10 to 100 μm in diameter and 100 to 1000 mm in length is used as the solid support in an electrophoresis apparatus. Here, the driving force for separation is the voltage (on the order of 25 kV) rather than pressure, as in HPLC. Because of the vast surface area, separations are sharp. The system is highly versatile and can be used to separate serum proteins and small molecules. This method has been applied successfully to quantitative de-

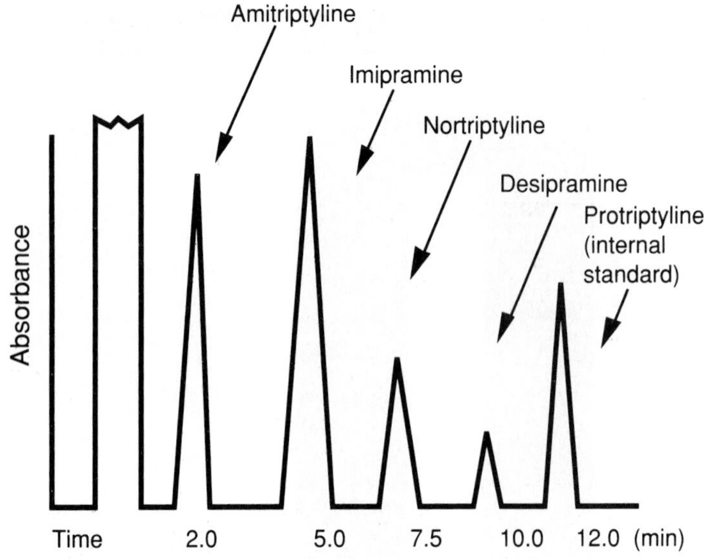

Figure 17–4. Sketch of a typical separation of the major tricyclic antidepressants on high-performance liquid chromatography (HPLC). A complete separation can be effected in 12 minutes. The concentration of each drug is on the order of 100 μg/mL.

termination of drugs such as pentobarbital (an intermediate-acting barbiturate). However, chiefly because of laborious necessary deproteinization of samples, the technique has not enjoyed widespread use as compared with the immunoassay techniques discussed previously.

GAS CHROMATOGRAPHY–MASS SPECTROSCOPY. Testing for drugs of abuse has become one of the most rapidly developing areas in the clinical laboratory in view of the widespread and ever-expanding use of these drugs among large segments of the working population. In view of the increasing requirements for routine drug screening, it has become necessary to have a gold standard for techniques to confirm the results obtained using screening methods such as EMIT and TLC.

GC-MS has proved to be such a gold standard because of its great sensitivity and its reliability. This methodology, as its name implies, involves two techniques: gas-liquid chromatography and mass spectroscopy. In gas-liquid chromatography, compounds are directly heated into the gas phase or are derivatized to make them labile to facilitate heating them into the gas phase. They are then passed over a column containing the stationary phase, which often consists of a liquid, usually a hydrocarbon or silicone oil, that coats a solid support in the column and offers a large surface area for absorption. Separation is based, much as in TLC, on the ability of each compound to adsorb to the stationary phase, which partially depends on the relative solubilities of the compound in the gas versus the liquid phase. Normally, the compounds eluting from the column could be detected by conventional techniques, as discussed previously, except that once the compounds are in the gas phase, in which they are heated, advantage can be taken of another feature of the system—the ability of compounds that are heated to high temperatures to lose or gain electrons.

At high temperatures, the highest energy electrons of a compound—that is, the ones of lowest ionization potential—can be excited such that the molecule can lose or gain electrons and become charged. This process may be aided by such techniques as electron bombardment in a specially designed chamber that directly creates molecule-ions. Most of these resulting molecule-ions are single cations. Different molecule-ions in general have different sizes and different molecular weights. These molecule-ions decompose into characteristic fragments whose ratios with respect to one another and whose positions of migration relative to one another are also constant. The molecule-ions are then passed through an electrical field generated by four rods that are subjected to rapidly alternating currents, the so-called quadrupole detector. Depending on how the field is tuned, certain molecule-ions with specific mass-to-charge ratios can pass through the field to a detector. Thus, the molecule-ions can be separated on the basis of molecular weight or, more exactly, on their mass-to-charge ratios. The overall design of GC-MS is shown in Figure 17–5.

The presence of the molecule-ion on the plate is detected by a charge multiplier detector system very similar to the ones in optical systems discussed in Chapter 3. The technique of GC-MS has become highly refined. Each molecule-ion created in the gas phase can undergo further changes, such as elimination reactions and rearrangements and further degradation to small fragments that, in turn, ionize and give characteristic decomposition patterns. The patterns of thousands of compounds have now been determined. The position of the parent molecule-ion of the compound and the decomposition fragments give rise to a fingerprint-like pattern unique to the compound. These patterns are stored in a computer so that when a pattern for an unknown compound or group of compounds is obtained, the pattern is compared with the stored patterns to identify the compounds of interest. The entire methodology has been highly successful in detecting even low levels of cocaine or its metabolites, or both, in body fluids. A typical cocaine pattern is shown in Figure 17–6. Because single ion-molecule species give rise to significant currents in the detector, it is possible to detect very low levels of drugs, making this technique the ultimate reference method and the best confirmatory testing procedure available at present.

Screening for Drugs of Abuse

In most states of the United States, two levels of testing for drugs of abuse have become recognized: emergency room testing and forensic testing. The former involves rapid, stat

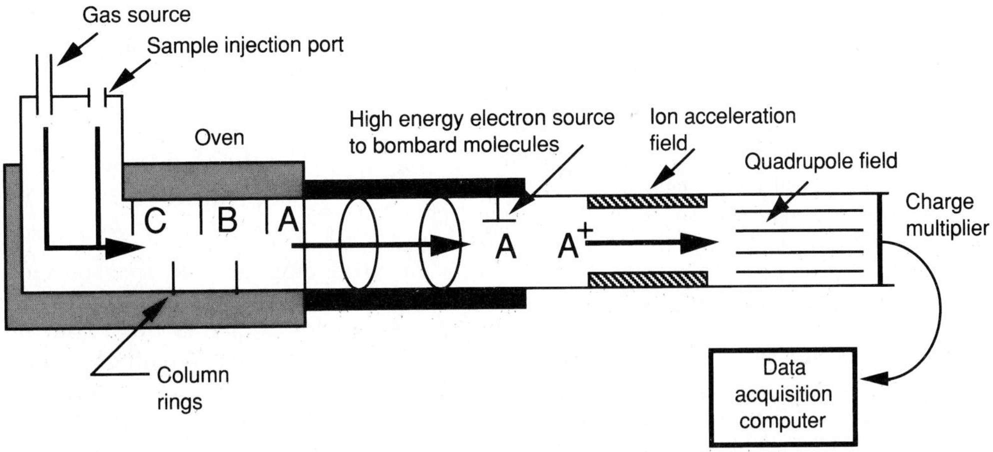

Figure 17–5. A schematic view of the components of gas chromatography–mass spectroscopy (GC-MS) instrumentation. On the left of the figure is the gas chromatographic system, where a volatilized compound is moved over a column consisting of rings coated with a liquid by an inert gas. Compounds C, B, and A separate on this column and are maintained in the gas phase by the oven that surrounds the column. The separated compounds then enter the mass spectrometer on the right side of the figure, where they are subjected to bombardment by electrons, resulting in molecule ion species. These ionic species then are accelerated in a field and then passed through an electrical quadrupole field. Only those ions with a narrow range of mass-to-charge ratio (m/e ratios) will pass through the tuned field so that they strike the detector. The electrical currents that result are digitalized and stored in a computer that analyzes the data. (See Davis, 1989.)

screening methods, in particular EMIT (or FPIA) and TLC. The purpose of this type of screening test is to detect the presence of a drug or several drugs of abuse in the patient's urine. Rarely are the more sophisticated chromatographic procedures like HPLC and GC-MS used for this purpose. Forensic testing, on the other hand, requires not only a screen but also an independent confirmatory method, which is almost always GC-MS or, less commonly, HPLC. It should be noted that, strictly by law, any confirmatory method is valid provided it is a completely different method from the primary one. Thus, TLC can confirm EMIT, whereas FPIA cannot confirm it because both EMIT and FPIA are immunochemical methods.

Another important legalistic development that has occurred in forensic testing is the so-called chain-of-custody. This process is used in the collection of urine from the individual from whom the specimen is taken. It may begin by observation of specimen collection by one person. Then, that person or another specifically designated individual, usually a police officer (in the case of prisoners or suspects) or some other designated official, accompanies the messenger who brings the specimen from the individual to the laboratory. This individual is a witness to the testing (and must sign a legal docu-

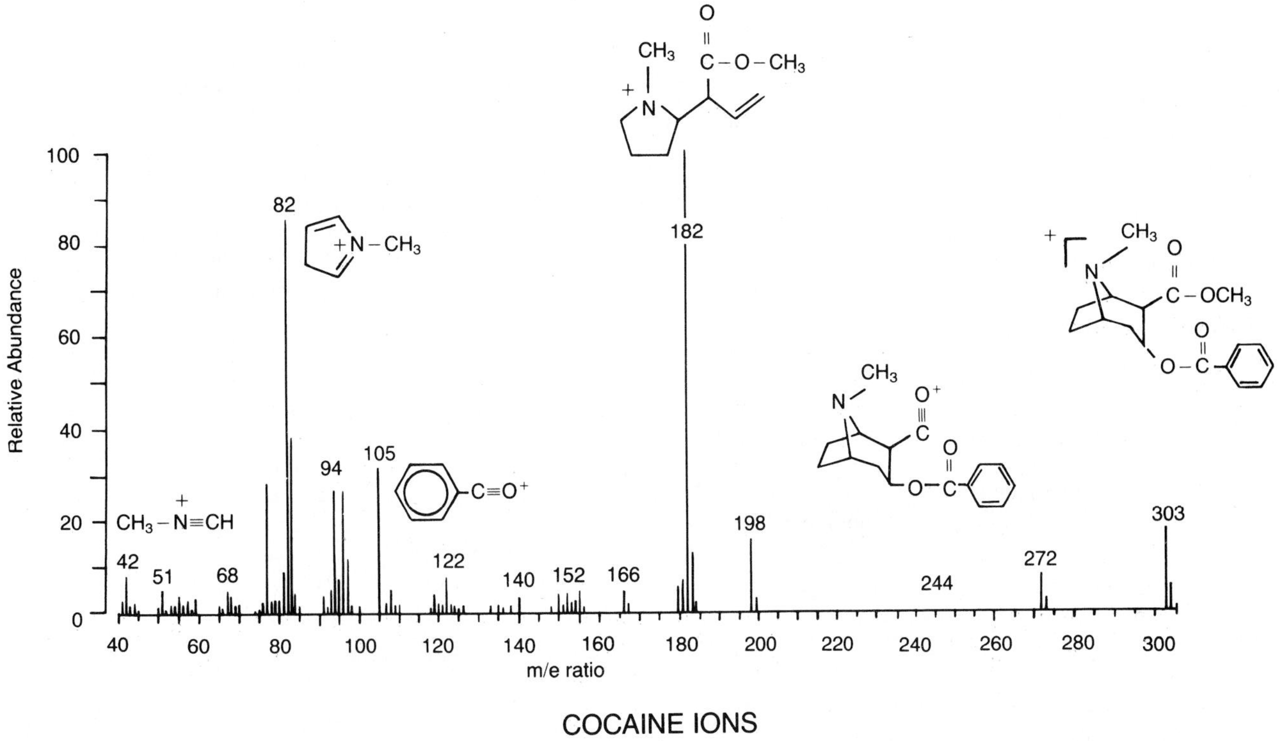

Figure 17–6. Fragmentogram for cocaine using gas chromatography–mass spectroscopy (GC-MS). The specimen is urine. This figure shows the characteristic peaks for cocaine metabolites. (Courtesy of Dr. Chip Walls, Onondaga County, NY, Medical Examiner's Office.)

ment to this effect) of the specific urine sample collected. More than one designated individual may be involved as the witness in this chain. The proliferation of rules and regulations regarding the detection of drugs of abuse has substantially complicated testing in this area, and a concise discussion is provided by DeCresce (1989). Far more important than these rules are the biological and clinical effects of the major drugs of abuse, which we now discuss.

THE DRUGS OF ABUSE

Although it is true that, as the adage goes, too much of anything is bad for the health, the consumption of even small amounts of any of a number of biogenic compounds causes enormously deleterious effects on human function. Hence, it is important to consider a number of different drugs of abuse, the results of which are commonly seen in emergency rooms, especially of large city hospitals.

General Aspects of the Mechanisms of Action

The major drugs of abuse are shown in Figure 17–7. As may be seen in this figure, these drugs, with the exception of the barbiturates, are all from basic amino group–containing compounds that also all contain benzene rings. The steric relationship of the amino group with respect to the aromatic benzene rings is rather similar, especially in cocaine, the opiates, and methadone. As might be expected,

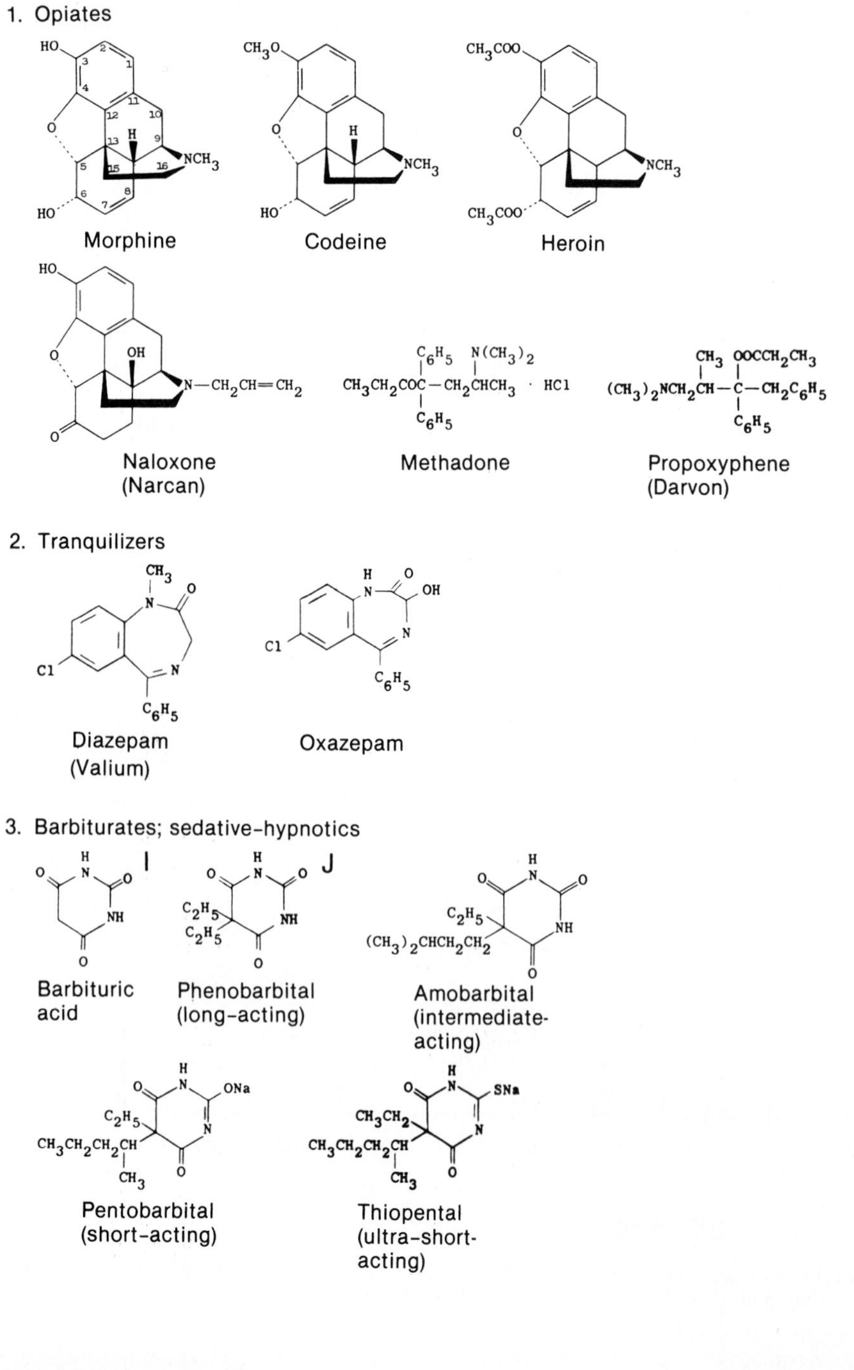

Figure 17–7. Chemical structures for the major drugs of abuse. All of the opiates are seen to be basic compounds that are tertiary amines and that contain benzene rings. Notice that, in the barbiturate series, barbituric acid may be considered as a condensation product of urea and malonic acid. (Structures reproduced from *The Merck Index*, Eleventh Edition, [1989], S. Budavari, M. J. O'Neil, A. Smith, P. E. Heckelman, Eds., by permission of copyright owner, Merck & Co., Inc., Rahway, NJ, U.S.A. © Merck & Co., Inc., 1989.)

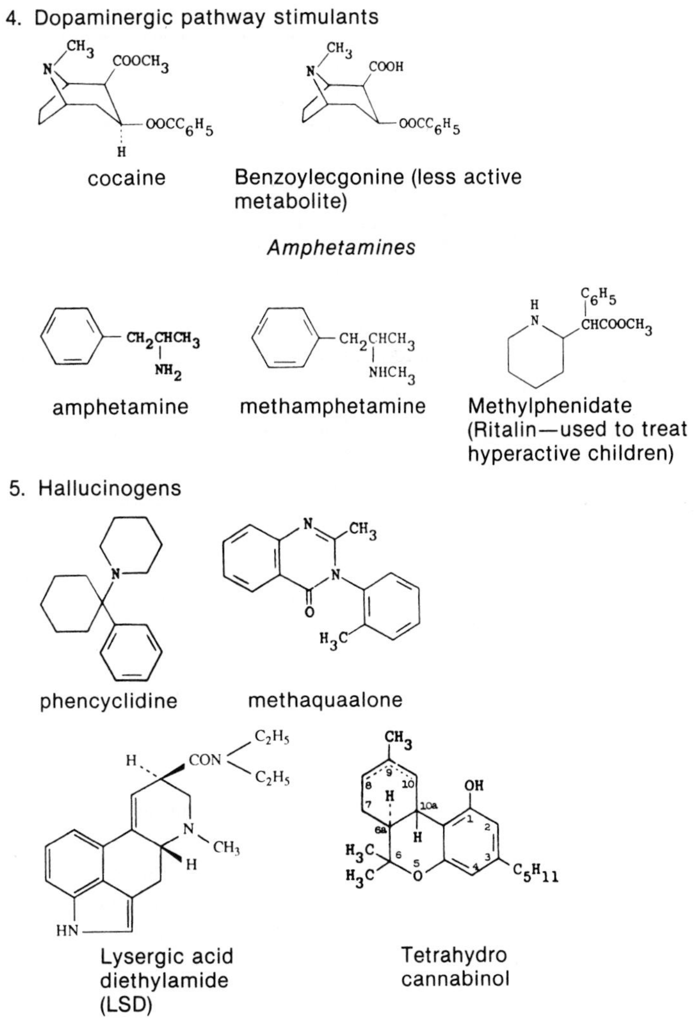

Figure 17–7 *Continued*

these compounds can cross-react with each other's target receptors.

The primary physiologic mechanisms of action of these drugs are not known, but some rudimentary knowledge has been gained over the past several years as to some of the main targets of these drugs. Many of these drugs act directly on dopaminergic neurotransmitter systems, especially the limbic system (sometimes referred to as the smell brain). This system is a more primitive one associated with pleasure seeking. In Figure 17–8, we show possible effects of several of the most important drugs on this system. It appears that the amphetamines, which are closely related structurally to dopamine and the catecholamines, can both directly act as neurotransmitters at critical synapses in dopaminergic pathways *and* can cause release of dopamine from the vesicles at the axonal side of the synapse. Cocaine further appears to stimulate release of dopamine in this system, which may partially be responsible for its producing a pleasant sensation (so-called high) in many individuals (Hurd, 1988). The tricyclic antidepressants also stimulate the dopaminergic pathways except that rather than promoting release of the neurotransmitters, they block reuptake of dopamine into the vesicles on the axonal side of the synapse. It is of great interest that paradoxically the tricyclic antidepressants such as imipramine (Tofranil) have been used successfully to treat the effects of cocaine. The major tranquilizers such as haloperidol (Haldol) and chlorpromazine appear to block attachment of dopamine to the dendritic receptors in the synapse, thereby blocking the stimulatory effects of dopamine. Associated with many dopaminergic neurons are inhibitory neurons that use γ-aminobutyric acid (GABA) as their neurotransmitters. It appears that many benzodiazepine receptors exist on these neurons, causing the release of GABA at the synapses in this system, reducing the dopaminergic effects of the stimulatory pathways on the limbic system. Thus, some of the tranquilizing effects of diazepam (Valium) and other benzodiazepines can be explained.

Widely distributed throughout the brain are a variety of opiate receptors classified mainly as μ-, γ-, and ϵ-receptors. The μ-receptors appear to be highly specific for morphine and heroin, both of which produce a general analgesic state. At the moment, there appears to be no direct relationship between these receptors and the dopaminergic pathways. Interestingly, the naturally produced opiate peptide met-enkephalin, whose amino acid sequence is Tyr-Gly-Gly-Phe-Met, cross-reacts significantly with μ-receptors, although its primary "target" is ϵ-receptors. It has been shown that Valium may be structurally related to enkephalin, which in turn

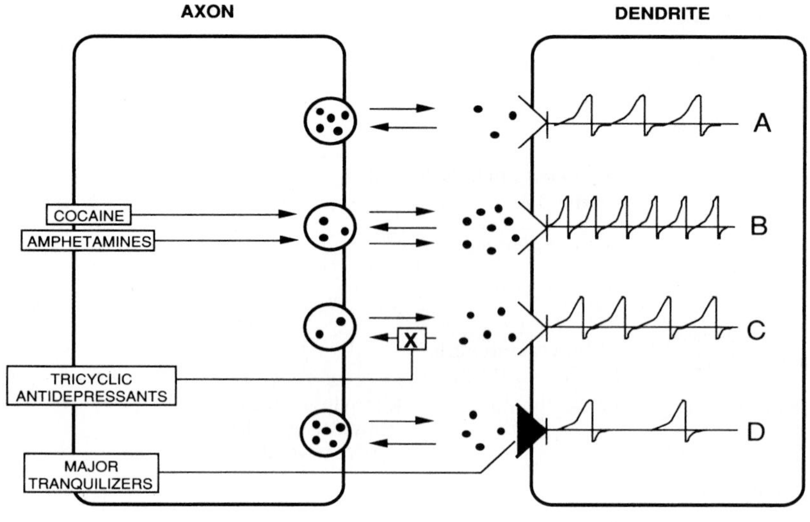

Figure 17–8. Illustration of the possible mechanisms of action of drugs of abuse and some therapeutic drugs on dopaminergic pathways. *A,* Normal neural transmission. A nerve impulse is conducted down the axon to the terminal boutons at the nerve ending. Vesicles, represented by large circles, release their contents of neurotransmitter, here dopamine, represented by small black circles. Dopamine molecules traverse the synaptic cleft and bind to dendritic receptors, initiating action potentials in the dendrites. Notice the arrows showing that dopamine is both released and taken up by the vesicles. *B,* In the presence of cocaine and amphetamines, enhanced release of neurotransmitter from vesicles occurs, increasing the rate of firing in the dendrites. Amphetamines can also directly act as neurotransmitters. *C,* Tricyclic antidepressants block the reuptake of the neurotransmitter (arrow with x), causing more dopamine to "recycle" to the dendritic receptors, causing increased firing. *D,* Some of the neuroleptics act by blocking postsynaptic dendritic receptors for dopamine, causing decreased firing.

may be structurally related to morphine (Pincus, 1987; Murphy, 1992). It is therefore possible that these compounds have the same effect, at least indirectly, on the dopaminergic pathways. The described possible general interrelationships of some of the major drugs of abuse permit consideration of these drugs specifically.

Cocaine

Cocaine is derived from the coca plant and has enjoyed much popularity as an additive to certain foods. At the beginning of the twentieth century, it was used in Coca-Cola, but owing to its addictive effects, this practice was discontinued. Cocaine is a derivative of the alkaloid ecgonine—that is, the methyl ester of benzoylecgonine, as shown in Figure 17–7. Unfortunately, use of cocaine has now been rediscovered in a particularly perverse way in modern times. There has been a virtual epidemic of cocaine abuse and addiction in the United States. It is estimated that there are at least 5 million known addicts in the United States and a reported 30 million overall users of this drug (DeCresce, 1989). Fatalities from cocaine abuse are now a major cause of death in the United States. These fatalities result from two factors: direct toxicity of the drug (Johanson, 1989) and crime related to the illicit acquisition of the drug. The normal route of administration of cocaine is nasal—that is, inhalation, so-called snorting, such that the drug passes through the nasal membranes. The prevalent form of cocaine currently used, called crack, is the free-base form that passes rapidly across the nasal membranes and is highly potent for that reason—that is, for a given dose, most or all of it enters the bloodstream rapidly. Its half-life is 1 to 2 hours, and the parent compound and its metabolites are usually cleared from the body within two days.

Cocaine is used medically to induce local anesthesia during nasopharyngeal surgery. However, in large doses, it induces a euphoric state (the so-called high experienced by the user) and may also induce hallucinatory states. It can also promote violent behavior. Many of these results can be explained by cocaine's dopaminergic effects. One study (Azmitia, 1990) suggests that cocaine induces increased calcium ion influxes in dopaminergic neurons. The increased intracellular calcium activates phospholipases that possibly act as second messengers in causing ultimate release of dopamine in synapses. Prolonged action of phospholipases, however, ultimately causes cell death. In the previously mentioned study, in fact, cocaine was found to be neurotoxic. It also has a general cytotoxic effect from formation of an *N*-oxide free radical produced in the metabolism of this compound in the liver. It appears then that, over time, cocaine induces neuronal loss.

Studies (Lange, 1989) further indicate that prolonged use of cocaine results in cardiotoxicity—that is, cocaine causes constriction of the coronary arteries that can, in turn, induce myocardial ischemia and sometimes frank infarction. The pathogenesis of cocaine-induced coronary artery disease is not known. At Bellevue Hospital in New York City, high proportions of cocaine-positive patients seen in the emergency room have significant rises in the MB fraction of creatine phosphokinase (CK; see Chap. 13), possibly indicating myocardial damage. This finding, however, must be tempered by the fact that the total CK was also high, indicating severe noncardiac rhabdomyolysis (Thompson, 1988). One highly disturbing aspect of cocaine abuse is the fact that it passes readily across the placenta and also into the lactating mammary gland, and is readily passed from mothers to nursing infants. Often in the hospital setting, mothers receive the drug from dealers and breast feed their newborn babies, who are therefore maintained on this drug. Cocaine causes mental retardation, delayed development, and strong drug dependence in newborns. It can also produce malformations *in utero.*

Cocaine classically has not been considered to be an addictive drug, because it does not cause the true physical dependence typical of abusers of barbiturates and opiates. However, the high produced by the drug is extraordinarily reinforcing, so that the drug-seeking behavior of the cocaine abuser and the opiate abuser is similar. Clinically, patients who are overdosed with cocaine may become violent and irrational, requiring sedation. Interestingly, many new users of this drug find themselves in a hyperexcitable state with palpitations and use large quantities of Valium to calm themselves. Thus, it is not uncommon to find cocaine and Valium in the urine of cocaine addicts. Occasionally, overdosed patients become obtunded or comatose. The treatment for these patients is usually supportive. It has been found, as noted in the previous section, that antidepressants, including the tricyclics and fluoxetine (Prozac), have been found to inhibit the actions of cocaine. Thus, treatment with these drugs is often instituted.

METABOLISM. The half-life of cocaine, as stated previously, is approximately 1 to 2 hours. It is metabolized to more polar compounds that have significantly less potency than the parent compound. These metabolites have longer half-lives and, with techniques such as GC-MS, can be detected up to 48 hours after administration of the drug. The immunoassay methods can detect the drug for about 24 to 36 hours after administration. With the crack epidemic, it is possible to detect the parent compound, cocaine, by TLC up to several hours after administration, owing to the high doses of drug present.

The Opiates (Morphine, Codeine, Heroin)

The structures for these drugs are shown in Figure 17–7 and are similar to one another. Morphine is used as a powerful analgesic and acts by binding to μ-receptors in the central nervous system (CNS) and has become important in treating acute congestive heart failure by lowering venous return to the heart—that is, it is a powerful preload reducer by causing increased splanchnic pooling of blood. Codeine is used as a mild analgesic and as an antitussive. Heroin induces a pleasant, euphoric state and is highly addictive both physically and psychologically. Withdrawal from this drug is exceedingly difficult, with a myriad of symptoms such as hypothermia, palpitations, cold sweats, and nightmares. This class of compounds exhibits certain important paradoxical effects on the parasympathetic nervous system. These drugs exert a procholinergic effect on the eyes and blood vessels in the periphery—that is, they cause constriction of pupils and peripheral vasodilation. In contrast, in the gut they lower gastrointestinal (GI) motility—that is, they exhibit anticholinergic effects in the GI tract. This fact enables rapid diagnosis of heroin or, in general, opiate abuse in a patient brought to the emergency room in an obtunded or a comatose state. These patients typically have severe miosis (pupilloconstriction). Although the sign is not useful in acute diagnosis, constipation commonly occurs in these patients.

Administration of heroin occurs via the intravenous route. Addicts are readily recognized by the presence of needle tracks on their arms and hands and by extensive thrombosis of their peripheral veins. The half-life of heroin via the intravenous route is about three minutes, and the effects of the drug last approximately three hours. The major metabolites are *N*-acetylmorphine and morphine. The half-life of morphine is about three hours.

Overdoses of heroin are extremely dangerous and can cause severe obtundation, coma, respiratory arrest, and cardiac arrhythmias. One of the most common therapeutic modalities for heroin overdose is treatment intravenously with naloxone (Narcan), a strong competitive antagonist to the action of heroin. The structure of naloxone is shown in Figure 17–7. Heroin addiction, as a chronic problem, is treated pharmacologically with a partial agonist of heroin, methadone.

Methadone

This interesting compound, whose structure is shown in Figure 17–7, is a nonbicyclic drug that binds competitively with morphine to μ-receptors in the brain. However, although it can become addictive, the addictive effects are less than those of equivalent concentrations of heroin. Thus, administration of methadone to heroin addicts allows them to experience the effects of heroin but in a modulated manner. By gradually lowering the methadone dose, physical dependence becomes reduced and it appears that a trough serum methadone level greater than 100 ng/mL is adequate for effective methadone maintenance (Bell, 1988). However, it should be noted that addiction to methadone can also occur. In toxicology laboratories, the most common request received for methadone screens comes from methadone clinics to test whether a patient is administering methadone or has relapsed into taking heroin. As can be seen in Figure 17–3, it is a simple matter to distinguish methadone from the opiates. Similarly, EMIT or FPIA detects each drug with high specificity.

2

Amphetamines

These compounds, as can be seen in Figure 17–7, bear an uncanny resemblance to the adrenergic amines such as epinephrine and norepinephrine and may be expected to exert sympathomimetic effects. They also resemble dopamine and may also be expected to have effects on dopaminergic pathways. The predominant effects of the amphetamines on these latter pathways have been considered. Indeed, the amphetamines cause euphoria and increased mental alertness that may be attributed to their effects on these pathways. This group of drugs, however, also exerts pronounced stimulatory effects on α- and β-receptors in the cardiovascular system and in the kidneys to cause pronounced adrenergic effects such as increased heart rate, increased blood pressure, palpitations, bronchodilation, anxiety, pallor, and tremulousness. Studies indicate that amphetamines are also competitive inhibitors of the enzyme monoamine oxidase, which inactivates adrenergic neurotransmitters by oxidatively removing their amino groups. Blockage of this enzyme prolongs the effect of epinephrine and norepinephrine, with the attendant neurologic and cardiovascular sequelae.

CLINICAL SYMPTOMS. The pharmacologic action of amphetamines includes CNS and respiratory stimulation and sympathomimetic activity (e.g., bronchodilation, pressor response, and mydriasis). Loss of weight may also occur as a result of an anorectic effect. Psychic stimulation and excitability, leading to a temporary increase in mental and physical activity, can occur, and nervousness can also be produced.

ACUTE TOXICITY. Initial manifestations of an overdose may be cardiovascular in nature; symptoms may include flushing or pallor, tachypnea, palpitation, tremor, labile pulse rate and blood pressure (hypertension and hypotension), cardiac arrhythmias, heart block, circulatory collapse, and angina. Mental disturbances such as delirium, confusion, delusions, disorientation, and hallucinations may occur. Acute psychotic syndromes may occur characterized by vivid auditory and visual hallucinations, restlessness, homicidal or suicidal tendencies, panic state, paranoid ideation, loosening of associations, combativeness, and changes in affect. A frequent and potential sign of acute intoxication is hyperpyrexia; rhabdomyolysis has also been associated with acute amphetamine overdose. Cardiovascular collapse is the usual cause of death.

CHRONIC USAGE. Tolerance may be produced within a few weeks, and possibly physical or psychic dependence may occur with prolonged usage. Symptoms of chronic abuse include emotional lability, somnolence, loss of appetite, occupational deterioration, mental impairment, and social withdrawal. Trauma and ulcer of the tongue and lip may occur as a result of continuing chewing or teeth-grinding movements. A syndrome with the characteristics of paranoid schizophrenia can occur with prolonged high-dosage usage. Aplastic anemia and fatal pancytopenia are rare complications.

TREATMENT. No specific antidote for amphetamine overdosage exists, and treatment of overdosage is symptomatic with general physiologic supportive measures immediately implemented. For cardiovascular symptoms, administration of propranolol (Inderal), discussed subsequently under therapeutic drugs, can be used as an antidote.

DETECTION. Both Toxi-lab (Irvine, CA) and EMIT-FPIA (Palo Alto, CA) procedures are effective in detecting these drugs of abuse. Occasionally, on the Toxi-lab A strip, amphetamines may be confused with antihistamines like diphenhydramine.

Benzodiazepines

Among this group of drugs, shown in Figure 17–7, the most prominent is Valium; they are used therapeutically, as so-called minor tranquilizers. Their mechanisms of action appear to be induction of the secretion of GABA, a neurotransmitter that inhibits conduction in dopaminergic neurons. Usually used as a therapeutic drug to produce calming effects at doses between 2.5 and 10 mg and to produce muscle-relaxing effects at higher doses, Valium has been used by drug addicts in high dosage to counter the excitatory effects of other drugs of abuse or as a means of inducing tranquil states. A number of drug abusers have become addicted to Valium when using high doses several times each day. Acutely, benzodiazepine overdose may produce somnolence, confusion, seizures, and coma. Rarely, hypotension, respiratory depression, and cardiac arrest may occur. Chronically, physical and psychological dependence occur. Sudden discontinuance of the drug may lead to anxiety, sweating, irritability, hallucinations, diarrhea, and seizures. Treatment is supportive. Gradual diminution of the benzodiazepine removes physical dependence. The half-life of Valium is 20 to 70 hours, but the half-life of one of its active metabolites is 50 to 100 hours.

Phencyclidine

Phencyclidine (PCP), shown in Figure 17–7, has numerous effects on a variety of different neural pathways. Used almost exclusively as a drug of abuse, this drug is traded on the streets under the name of angel dust or angel hair. It is peculiar that the use of this drug appears to be periodic. At Bellevue Hospital in New York City, where over 50 drug screens per day are performed, mainly on patients in the emergency room, the appearance of this drug in the urine of these patients is seasonal, occurring mostly in the early spring, before and after which time little or no drug has been detected in urine screens.

The physiologic effects of PCP appear to be analgesic and anesthetic and, paradoxically, stimulatory. This drug has been found to interact with cholinergic, adrenergic, GABA-secreting, serotoninergic, and opiate neuronal receptors. Thus, a wide variety of bizarre and apparently paradoxical symptoms can be seen in the same patient. This drug has been shown to bind to specific regions of the inner chloride channels of neurons, apparently profoundly affecting chloride transport. It has also been found to bind strongly to a newly discovered class of neural receptors, the σ-receptor, which has now been isolated (Schuster, 1994). This receptor also binds strongly to the neuroleptic, antipsychotic drug haloperidol (Haldol), a finding that may implicate the σ-receptor in some of the clinical findings of severe psychosis in patients suffering from overdose with PCP.

Because of its varied actions, clinically acute manifestations vary from depression to euphoria and can involve catatonia, violence, rage, and auditory and visual hallucinations. Vomiting, hyperventilation, tachycardia, shivering, seizures, coma, and death are also among the common occurrences that result from abuse of this drug. Most fatalities occur from the hypertensive effects of the drug, especially on the large cerebral arteries (Bayorh, 1984). As can be inferred from this spectrum of possible symptoms, diagnosis based on clinical findings is impossible. Only the results of a drug screen can be diagnostic. Treatment of drug abuse with PCP is supportive, with the patient kept in isolation in a darkened, quiet room. Acidification of the urine increases the rate of PCP excretion. As might be expected from the findings regarding the σ-receptor, treatment with Haldol results in sedation of the violent, hallucinating patient.

Barbiturates: Sedative-Hypnotics

There is an almost bewildering variety of these major sedative drugs. However, all are derivatives of barbituric acid, which may be regarded as the condensation product of urea and malonic acid, as indicated in Figure 17–7. Depending on the substituents on the $—CH_2$ group of the malonic acid portion, the particular drug may be long acting, as is phenobarbital, with a benzene ring and ethyl group substituents on this carbon; short acting, as is pentobarbital, with neopentyl and ethyl groups at this position; or ultra short acting, as is the case with thiopental. The long-acting barbiturate phenobarbital is a therapeutic drug used as an anticonvulsant, unlike the short-acting and ultra-short-acting drugs, and is discussed subsequently under therapeutic drugs.

All of the barbiturates are fat soluble and therefore pass easily across the blood-brain barrier. All of them seem to stabilize membranes such that depolarization of the membranes becomes more difficult. For unknown reasons, the short-acting and ultra-short-acting barbiturates seem to inhibit selectively the reticular-activating system, which is involved with arousal; hence, their sedative and hypnotic effects. The ultra-short-acting barbiturates rapidly diffuse out of the CNS, accounting for their rapid action. Phenobarbital, however, selectively reduces the excitability of rapidly firing neurons and is therefore a highly effective antiseizure drug. It may be more than coincidental that phenobarbital and the equally effective anticonvulsant phenytoin (Dilantin) bear structural resemblance to one another and may exert similar effects on rapidly firing neurons. The mechanism of action of Dilantin is discussed subsequently.

Clinically, at low doses, the short-acting and ultra-short-acting barbiturates produce sedation, drowsiness, and sleep. They also impair judgment. At higher doses, anesthesia is produced. At very high dose, these drugs can cause stupor, coma, and death. The toxic manifestations of these drugs are depression, Cheyne-Stokes respiration, cyanosis, hypothermia, hypotension, tachycardia, areflexia, and pupilloconstriction.

The treatment of drug overdose is supportive and includes the standard treatment for shock. When administered within 30 minutes of drug ingestion, activated charcoal is an effective barbiturate chemoadsorbent.

Diagnosis of drug abuse with short-acting and ultra-short-acting barbiturates is by immunoassay and TLC screening procedures. HPLC has found some use in this regard but is not a standard method. The barbiturates are weak acids, the N—H protons being somewhat acidic, so that they are acid extracted and placed on the B strip in Toxi-lab (Irvine, CA) procedures. Their presence is easily detected by Toxi-lab TLC, as shown in Figure 17–3*B*. Immunoassays for those drugs are also excellent, the one caveat being that high levels of phenobarbital in urine cross-react with the antibodies against the short-acting barbiturates. Thus, it is important that TLC confirm a positive immunoassay result for sedative-hypnotic barbiturates.

Propoxyphene (Darvon)

This analgesic drug has very similar pharmacologic properties to those of the opiates like morphine. This drug can be taken orally so that the sedated, good feelings induced by opiates can be induced without having to have recourse to the intravenous apparatus needed for infusion of heroin. A major cause of drug-related deaths is propoxyphene overdose, either alone or in combination with CNS depressants like barbiturates and alcohol. Toxic symptoms are similar to those seen with overdoses of opiates—viz., respiratory depression, cardiac arrhythmias, seizures, pulmonary edema, and coma. Nephrogenic diabetes insipidus may also occur. The treatment for propoxyphene overdose is mainly supportive. Administration of Narcan reverses the toxic effect of the drug.

Methaqualone (Quaalude)

Methaqualone is a 2,3-disubstituted quinazoline that has sedative-hypnotic properties. This compound also possesses anticonvulsant, antispasmodic, local anesthetic, antitussive, and weak antihistamine actions. Oral administration leads to rapid and complete absorption of the drug, with approximately 80% bound to plasma protein. Peak plasma concentrations are reached in approximately 2 to 3 hours, and almost all of the drug appears to be metabolized by the hepatic cytochrome P-450 microsomal enzyme system, with only a small percentage (<5%) excreted unchanged in the urine. The serum half-life ranges from 20 to 60 hours.

The dosages that are used for its hypnotic-sedative actions are 150 to 300 mg daily. Toxic serum concentrations are generally reached at 10 μg/mL. Tolerance to some of its actions, as well as dependence, occurs, such that abusive dosages can be up to six to seven times greater than those employed therapeutically.

Symptoms of overdosage can be similar to barbiturate toxicity and produce CNS depression with lethargy, respiratory depression, coma, and death. However, unlike barbiturate overdosage, muscle spasms, convulsions, and pyramidal signs (hypertonicity, hyperreflexia, and myoclonus) can result from severe methaqualone intoxication. Treatment for overdose includes supportive therapy as well as delaying absorption of remaining drug with activated charcoal and drug removal by gastric lavage.

Marijuana (Cannabis)

This is one of the oldest and most widely used of the mind-altering drugs. Marijuana is a mixture of cut, dried, and ground portions of the hemp plant *Cannabis sativa.* Hashish refers to a more potent product produced by extraction of the resin from the plant. The principal psychoactive agent in marijuana is considered to be δ-9-tetrahydrocannabinol (THC), a lipid-soluble compound that readily enters the brain and may act by producing cell membrane changes. Marijuana may be introduced either through the lungs by smoking or through the GI tract by oral ingestion in food. Once THC enters the body, it is readily stored in body fat and has a half-life of approximately one week. Biotransformation is complex and extensive, and less than 1% of a dose is excreted unchanged. About one third is excreted in the urine as, primarily, δ-9-carboxy-THC and 11-hydroxy-δ-9-THC. These metabolites may be detected in the urine from one to four weeks after the last ingestion, depending on both dosage and frequency of ingestion.

Marijuana does not appear to cause physiologic dependence, but tolerance and psychological dependence do seem to occur (Reynolds, 1989). Two major physiologic effects of marijuana are reddening of the conjunctivae and an increased pulse rate. Muscle weakness and deterioration in motor coordination can also occur. The preponderant changes seen with cannabis intoxication are perceptual and psychic changes. These range from euphoria, relaxation, passiveness, and altered time perception, which is seen at low doses, to adverse reactions such as paranoia, delusions, and disorientation, which can be seen at high doses in psychologically susceptible individuals. The dosage, the route of administration, the individual's psychological make-up, and the setting are important determinants in each individual's reaction to cannabis intoxication. Thus, high doses in an individual unprepared or unaware of drug consumption may produce a disturbing experience. More commonly, experienced users report mild euphoria, enhancement or alteration of the physical senses, introspection with altered emphasis or importance of ideas, and heightening of subjective experiences. Heavy chronic use may produce bronchopulmonary disorders, and although the relative safety of chronic use is controversial, acute panic reactions, delirium, and psychoses occur rarely (Bryson, 1989; Reynolds, 1989). Few users seek treatment, and when this

2

occurs in a distressed patient, medical intervention generally is conservative. However, following an acute episode, psychological evaluation may be necessary in an individual with an underlying psychiatric disturbance.

Rarely, marijuana may be ingested by intravenous infusion of a boiled concentrate. Severe multisystem toxicity may be produced by this route of administration. Symptoms may include acute renal failure, gastroenteritis, hepatitis, anemia, and thrombocytopenia.

Lysergic Acid Diethylamide

Lysergic acid diethylamide (LSD, lysergide) is a semisynthetic indolalkylamine and a hallucinogen. It is one of the most potent pharmacologic materials known, producing effects at doses as low as 20 μg, and is equally effective by injection or oral administration. LSD is believed to affect multiple sites in the CNS and may act on a presynaptic serotonin receptor, decreasing the activity of serotonin by inhibiting its release. This process, in turn, may produce a state of CNS hyperarousal. Both the sympathetic and parasympathetic nervous systems are affected. However, the sympathetic effect appears to be greater and initial symptoms include hypertension, tachycardia, mydriasis, and piloerection.

The usual dosage of LSD is 1 to 2 μg/kg; LSD produces an experience that begins within an hour of ingestion, usually peaks at two to three hours, and generally lasts eight to 12 hours after ingestion. Metabolism occurs in the liver, whereas excretion occurs mainly in the bile.

LSD is the most commonly abused drug in its class and is believed by its users to provide insights and new ways of solving problems. The psychic effects are usually intense, and vary, depending upon the user's personality, expectations, and circumstances. LSD acts upon all the body senses, but visual effects are most intense. Common perceptual abnormalities include changes in the sense of time, organized visual illusions or hallucinations, blurred or "undulating" vision, and synesthesias. Mood may become very labile, and dissolution and detachment of ego may occur. LSD toxicity levels are low, and deaths are generally due to trauma secondary to errors in the user's judgment. Panic reactions—a "bad trip"—are the most common adverse reactions. These may occur in any user and cannot be reliably predicted or prevented. Borderline psychotic and depressed individuals are at risk for the precipitation of suicide or a prolonged psychotic episode by the usage of LSD. Flashbacks, which are poorly understood, also occur days to months after ingestion. This occurs when the user experiences recurrences of a previous hallucinogenic experience in the absence of drug ingestion.

Acute panic reactions may be treated by frequent reassurance and a quiet and calm environment; diazepam may also be effective. However, except for treating specific complications, LSD abuse has no systematic program of treatment.

THERAPEUTIC DRUG MONITORING

It has become recognized that it is critical that the serum levels of many of the therapeutic drugs administered to patients be frequently determined, both because of the possible toxic side effects of many of these medications and because, often, lack of patient compliance results in subtherapeutic levels of the drug. Furthermore, it is important for the physician, when initiating drug therapy, to ascertain when the serum levels of the drug have achieved a stable therapeutic level. It becomes important, therefore, to understand the principles on which drug therapy is based—that is, pharmacokinetics. Some of the basic principles of pharmacokinetics and then the physiologic effects of specific classes of therapeutic drugs are presented in this section. The ones discussed are those whose specific levels are most commonly followed by clinicians and are most commonly assayed in clinical laboratories. It should be noted that virtually all therapeutic drugs are assayed from specimens of serum, not urine, most commonly using immunoassay techniques such as FPIA.

Pharmacokinetics

Figure 17–9 summarizes the two ways in which a therapeutic drug is administered to a patient: discontinuously or continuously. The former method is the most common one. Most patients are treated with medications taken orally at fixed periods. For example, to achieve anti-inflammatory effects, two aspirin tablets of 350 mg each are taken every four to six hours. In this case, the aspirin is taken at discrete times between which a certain amount is excreted before the next dose is given. Sometimes, a patient is infused with a drug intravenously, such as with lidocaine (Xylocaine) in the intensive care unit (ICU) for a cardiac arrhythmia or with heparin to prevent thromboembolic events. In this case, while the drug is metabolized, a constant amount of the drug is being infused.

For both discontinuous and continuous infusions, the ultimate drug level is determined by a battle between the amount

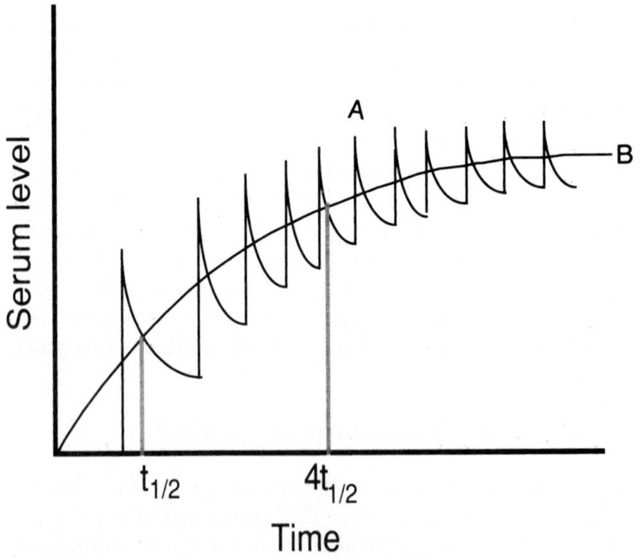

Figure 17–9. Illustration of the time course of drug levels as a function of method of administration. *A,* Discontinuous method. A constant dose is administered at each half-life for the drug. After four half-lives, close approach to the steady-state level is reached. *B,* Continuous method (IV infusion). Convergence to the steady-state limit achieved in *A.*

infused and the amount excreted. All drugs are eventually excreted. They can be excreted unchanged in urine, or excreted in urine as metabolites of the parent drug. These metabolic conversions occur in the liver. Occasionally, some drugs enter the enterohepatic circulation and are excreted in stool. Regardless of their mode of excretion, many drugs have a half-life that is more or less independent of their concentrations. The half-life of a drug is the time taken for half the drug that was initially present in serum to be excreted. The reason that the half-life of a drug is independent of its concentration is that many drugs are excreted according to so-called first-order kinetics. This process may be summarized as follows:

$$D \xrightarrow{k} E \quad (17\text{-}5),$$

where D is the drug concentration and E is the excreted form of the drug. The constant, k, is the rate constant for the disappearance of D. The half-life, called $t_{1/2}$, is related to the rate constant, k, by the following relationship:

$$t_{1/2} = 0.693/k \quad (17\text{-}6).$$

As can be seen from this equation, $t_{1/2}$ is a constant and does not depend on drug concentration.

The object of all drug therapy is to achieve a constant serum level of the drug that will be therapeutic. If the half-life for a drug is known, it is possible to compute the divided dose of the drug that should be given and the time interval between doses so that this level is achieved. As can be seen in Figure 17–9, at the beginning of drug administration, there are wide fluctuations of the drug level until, after a given period, the fluctuations converge to a constant level. In general, for discontinuous doses, the drug level can be expressed as the sum of a geometric series:

$$D = (D_o/r \times r^n - D_o/r)/(r - 1) \quad (17\text{-}7),$$

where D_o is the desired steady-state level of the drug; r is the fraction of drug remaining after the constant time interval between doses; and n is the number of the dose—that is, the second dose, third dose, and so on. If the time interval between doses is chosen as the $t_{1/2}$, r = 1/2. If the time interval is chosen to be that for 3/4 of the drug to remain, r = 3/4. (This time can be calculated directly from the $t_{1/2}$ as 1/2 $t_{1/2}$.) After four timed doses, if, for example, r = 1/2, the first term in the numerator of Equation 17-7 is small and, in effect,

$$D = (D_o/1/2)/(1/2) = D_o \quad (17\text{-}8),$$

that is, after four half-lives, the steady-state level is reached.

For continuous infusions, for the simplest case in which drug distribution is instantaneous, it can be shown that the drug level at any time is given by the following:

$$D = k_1(1 - e^{-k_2 t}) \quad (17\text{-}9),$$

where D is the drug concentration, k_1 is the constant infusion rate, k_2 is the rate constant for excretion of the drug, and t is the time. Because, as shown previously in Equation 17-6, $k_2 = 0.693/t_{1/2}$, after four half-lives when $t = 4t_{1/2}$,

$$D = k_1(1 - e^{-2.772}) \quad (17\text{-}10),$$

where, in effect, D is close to k_1. Thus, for continuous infusions, assuming no loading dose is given, the amount of drug infused per unit of time is the desired steady-state level.

There are two major points from this presentation. First, it is a good rule of thumb to wait for four half-lives to achieve the steady-state level of a drug. Second, results of an assay for a drug level in the time period during which this steady state is being achieved should be interpreted with extreme caution, a rule often forgotten in clinical practice. Notice from Figure 17–9 that if assays are performed in the pre–steady-state period, highly erratic results are obtained owing to the fluctuations in drug concentrations for the discontinuous case, and rising but persistently low values for the continuous case.

VOLUME OF DISTRIBUTION. When one is administering drugs, it is of vital importance to know whether the drug is stored in fat or other tissue or whether it is all present in serum. Because a given dose of a drug is known and the concentration of the drug in serum can be determined, one can measure the total volume of body fluid in which the drug is dissolved by the following relation:

$$D = D_o/V_d, \text{ or } V_d = D_o/D \quad (17\text{-}11),$$

where D is the concentration of drug in serum, D_o is the amount of drug administered, and V_d is the volume in which D_o must be dissolved to give the concentration D. This volume V_d is referred to as the volume of distribution. If all of the drug is present in serum, V_d is the blood volume that can be determined from conversion tables relating body weight to blood volume. If, however, some of the drug is stored in body tissue, a smaller amount is present in serum, so that the denominator in equation 17-11 ($V_d = D_o/D$) is reduced and V_d will be larger than the expected blood volume, indicating that some drug is being stored in tissue. If this result occurs, it means that the drug is being released continuously from storage depots (i.e., tissues), which can raise anomalously the level of drug in serum, potentially to toxic levels. Thus, before any drug is administered, the volume of distribution should be known.

METABOLISM IN THE LIVER. Many drugs are converted to metabolites, some of which are pharmacologically active and some inactive. Much of this conversion occurs in the extramitochondrial, microsomal system present in hepatocytes. This metabolic system is mainly an oxidative one that uses a series of oxidative enzymes that, in turn, use a special cytochrome system: cytochrome P-450 (Gilman, 1985). This extremely critical cytochrome system has now been strongly implicated as predisposing certain individuals to developing cancer by metabolizing certain environmental compounds such as benzpyrene into frank carcinogens (*vide infra*). The excretion of many drugs depends on the integrity of the liver and the cytochrome P-450 system. In patients with liver failure due to passive congestion, hepatitis, and cirrhosis, the effective half-life of the drug is increased, making it necessary to *lower* the divided dose of the drug. Conversely, some drugs induce the intracellular synthesis of the microsomal enzymes, leading to *diminished* half-life values, so that it may be necessary to *raise* the divided dose.

One example of drug induction of microsomal enzymes is phenobarbital. This drug induces its own metabolism (so that its concentration levels do not obey first-order kinetics). In instances in which the levels of a drug metabolized in the liver are higher than the highest therapeutic value, reductions in the levels may be induced by administering low levels of phenobarbital to induce the microsomal system.

Table 17–1. DIGOXIN

Purpose:	Treatment of congestive heart failure and atrial fibrillation-flutter
General adult dose:	Oral: 0.75–1.5 mg for digitalization, 0.125–0.5 mg/day for maintenance
Usual bioavailability:	~60%–85% for tablet or elixir; 90%–100% for liquid-filled capsules
Half-life:	~35–40 hours; however, prolonged in patients with decreased renal function
General therapeutic range:	0.5–2 ng/mL
General toxic level:	>2 ng/mL, but somewhat variable
Transport:	~20%–25% plasma protein bound
Metabolism:	Generally, only small amounts are metabolized (liver, lumen of large intestine)
Elimination:	~50%–75% unchanged in urine
Steady state:	~7 days in undigitalized patients with normal renal function
Mechanism of action:	Causes release of Ca^{2+} ions in T-system of myocardium
Toxic effects:	Gastric disturbances, nausea, vomiting, atrial and ventricular arrhythmias (irregular pulse)

Table 17–3. PHENOBARBITAL

Purpose:	Treatment of generalized tonic-clonic seizures, simple partial seizures, anxiety, insomnia
General adult dose:	Oral: 100–200 mg/day for seizure control; 30–120 mg/day for anxiety; 100–320 mg for sleep induction
Usual bioavailability:	~90%–100%
Half-life:	~5–6 days in adults; ~3–4 days in children
General therapeutic range:	15–30 μg/mL for epilepsy control
General toxic level:	>40 μg/mL, although tolerance may develop
Transport:	~40%–60% plasma protein bound
Metabolism:	~75% hepatic: p-hydroxyphenobarbital, inactive
Elimination:	~25% unchanged in urine
Steady state:	~14–21 days
Mechanism of action:	Stabilizes damaged membranes and raises threshold for neuronal membrane depolarization
Toxic effects:	Drowsiness, depression, respiratory depression, coma, sedation, hypotension. Respiratory depression may be caused by rapid intravenous administration

This summary of some of the general principles of drug administration should be helpful in the interpretation of values clinically and permit a better understanding of the subsequent discussion of specific therapeutic drugs, most commonly measured or determined in the laboratory. Tables 17–1 to 17–7 summarize the critical pharmacologic data for the most commonly assayed drugs.

Cardiotropics

These drugs are the ones most commonly used to treat congestive heart failure and cardiac arrhythmias.

The *digitalis glycosides* have complex cardiovascular actions and are used in the treatment of congestive heart failure and atrial fibrillation and flutter (to slow ventricular response). Their direct positive inotropic effect may increase cardiac output in cardiac failure, whereas prolongation of the atrioventricular (AV) nodal conduction time and functional refractory period is important in antiarrhythmia therapy.

The mechanism of action of the digitalis glycosides is via inhibition of sodium-potassium-ATPase and inactivation of the myocardial membrane sodium pump. These effects, in turn, decrease intracellular potassium concentration and increase intracellular sodium concentration, and are also accompanied by increased cellular influx of calcium ion and its increased release into the T system of the myocardium. These changes in ionic concentration are believed to be responsible for the positive inotropic effect and the direct electrophysiologic, as well as toxic, effects seen with these drugs.

Digoxin (see Table 17–1) has a rapid onset of action (within one to two hours when given orally) and a relatively short half-life (35 to 40 hours). Most patients excrete approximately 50% to 75% of a dose unchanged in the urine.

Table 17–2. PROCAINAMIDE

Purpose:	Treatment of supraventricular or ventricular arrhythmias
General adult dose:	Oral: 4 g/day, in divided doses, for maintenance therapy
Usual bioavailability:	75%–95%
Half-life:	~3.5 hours in patients with normal renal function
General therapeutic range:	4–10 μg/mL
General toxic level:	>12 μg/mL
Transport:	~15% plasma protein bound
Metabolism:	Hepatic: *N*-acetylprocainamide (active), with $t_{1/2}$ ~7 hours in patients with normal renal function
Elimination:	~50%–60% unchanged in urine
Steady state:	Minimum of 12 hours
Mechanism of action:	Prolongation of atrial refractory period and decreased myocardial excitability
Toxic effects:	Reversible lupus erythematosus–like syndrome, irregular pulse, hypotension, rash, agranulocytosis

Table 17–4. PHENYTOIN (DILANTIN)

Purpose:	Treatment of generalized tonic-clonic seizures, simple partial seizures, complex partial seizures
General adult dose:	Oral: 300–400 mg/day maintenance dose
Usual bioavailability:	Variable: 30%–95%
Half-life:	24 ± 12 hours, and dose-dependent
General therapeutic range:	10–20 μg/mL
General toxic level:	>20 μg/mL
Transport:	~90%–95% plasma protein bound
Metabolism:	Hepatic: 5-(p-hydroxyphenyl)5-phenylhydantoin, inactive
Elimination:	~5% unchanged in urine
Steady state:	~7–8 days
Mechanism of action:	Appears to block sodium and calcium ion influxes into repeatedly depolarizing CNS neurons
Toxic effects:	Nystagmus, ataxia, diplopia, drowsiness, coma; rapid intravenous administration may produce cardiovascular collapse and/or CNS depression

Table 17–5. CARBAMAZEPINE (TEGRETOL)

Purpose:	Treatment of generalized tonic-clonic seizures, simple partial seizures, complex partial seizures; trigeminal neuralgia and glossopharyngeal neuralgia
General adult dose:	Oral: 800 mg–1.2 g/day maintenance for seizure control; 200 mg–1.2 g/day for neuralgia
Usual bioavailability:	~70%
Half-life:	Initially ~35 hours; ~8–20 hours after 3–4 weeks of administration
General therapeutic range:	4–12 μg/mL
General toxic level:	>12 μg/mL
Transport:	~60%–70% plasma protein bound
Metabolism:	Hepatic: carbamazepine-10,11-epoxide, active; carbamazepine-10,11-transdihydrodiol (inactive)
Elimination:	~1%–2% unchanged in urine
Steady state:	~3–7 days
Mechanism of action:	Decreases sodium and calcium ion influx into repeatedly depolarizing CNS neurons; reduces excitatory synaptic transmission in the spinal trigeminal nucleus
Toxic effects:	Drowsiness, ataxia, dizziness, nausea, vomiting, involuntary movements, abnormal reflexes, irregular pulse

Table 17–6. THEOPHYLLINE

Purpose:	Treatment and prevention of moderate to severe asthma
General adult dose:	Depends on body weight, route of administration, and age and condition of patient
Usual bioavailability:	Varies according to form, with ~100% for oral liquids and uncoated tablets
Half-life:	Varies: ~8–9 hours in non-smoking adults, 5–6 hours in adults who smoke, and 3–4 hours in children, but may vary widely
General therapeutic range:	10–20 μg/mL
General toxic level:	>20 μg/mL
Transport:	~60% plasma protein bound
Metabolism:	Hepatic: caffeine; 1,3-dimethyluric acid; 1-methyluric acid; 3-methylxanthine
Elimination:	~10% unchanged in urine
Steady state:	~5 half-lives; ~90% of steady state reached in three half-lives
Mechanism of action:	Increases intracellular cAMP by inhibiting phosphodiesterase; this causes the smooth muscle of the bronchial airways and pulmonary blood vessels to relax
Toxic effects:	Hypotension, syncope, tachycardia, arrhythmias, seizures, gastrointestinal bleeding

The general range of therapeutic serum levels is from 0.5 to 2 ng/mL. High concentrations of the drug are found in skeletal and cardiac muscle as well as in liver, brain, and kidneys.

In contrast, *digitoxin* has a longer half-life (four to six days) with a relatively slower onset of action (within one to four hours when given orally, with maximal effect in eight hours). Ninety to one hundred percent of a dose is absorbed, with approximately 95% bound to plasma protein. The general range of therapeutic serum levels is from 9 to 25 ng/mL. The drug is extensively metabolized in the liver (90%), with digoxin being the active metabolite.

Toxic side effects of the digitalis glycosides include gastric disturbances, nausea, vomiting, and atrial and ventricular arrhythmias. It is crucial that levels of digoxin (or digitoxin) be monitored closely and accurately while the patient is initially being given this drug. As we mentioned earlier, the therapeutic range for digoxin is from 0.5 to 2 ng/mL—that is, the range is narrow. Toxic levels exceed 3 ng/mL, so the difference between therapeutic and toxic doses is small. This difference necessitates careful digoxin assay.

Procainamide (Pronestyl) (see Table 17–2) is an antiarrhythmic drug that is useful in treating supraventricular or ventricular arrhythmias. Its actions are based on increased refractoriness of the atrium and decreased myocardial excitability. The bioavailability of procainamide is 75% to 95%. Approximately 15% is bound to plasma protein and approximately 50% is excreted by the kidneys. The half-life is approximately 3.5 hours, with a general range of therapeutic serum level of 4 to 8 ng/mL. *N*-acetylation to the major active metabolite *N*-acetylprocainamide (NAPA) is the major metabolic pathway of biotransformation. Toxic side effects include a reversible lupus-like syndrome with elevated antinuclear antibody (ANA) titers, urticaria, rash, agranulocytosis, and nephrotic syndrome.

The lupus-like syndrome may be initiated by leukocyte metabolism of procainamide to a chemically reactive metabolite that could then covalently bind to monocyte and macrophage membrane proteins to stimulate production of autoantibodies. In addition, the tertiary-amino moiety of the covalently bound procainamide metabolite might mimic a portion of histone protein and result in the production of antihistone antinuclear antibody (Uetrecht, 1988).

Table 17–7. METHOTREXATE

Condition	Usual Dose	Serum Level
Psoriasis	IM or IV: 7.5–50 mg/week Oral: 7.5–30 mg/week	$<1 \times 10^{-8}$ M (see Roenigk, 1988)
Refractory rheumatoid arthritis	IM: 5–25 mg/week Oral: 7.5–15 mg/week	*(see Tugwell, 1987a and b)
Malignant neoplastic diseases†	IM or IV: 25 mg/M^2, 1–2 ×/week Oral: 2.5–5 mg/day	
	High-dose IV: 1.5 g/M^2 with rescue every 3 weeks (different regimens are available)	Approximately 5×10^{-8} M

*Baseline monitoring of patient parameters (hemoglobin; white blood cell count; mean corpuscular volume; platelet count; urinalysis; blood urea nitrogen; and serum creatinine, transaminase, and alkaline phosphatase levels) is advocated.

†With high-dose therapy, methotrexate levels are followed and leucovorin doses are adjusted until serum methotrexate levels are less than 5×10^{-8} M (see Wittes, 1989).

Quinidine is used to treat supraventricular and ventricular arrhythmias and tachyarrhythmias. The prevention of ventricular tachycardia or frequent premature ventricular contractions and the maintenance of sinus rhythm after the conversion of atrial flutter or atrial fibrillation are its two major uses. Its mechanism of action is through decreased myocardial contractility.

The bioavailability of quinidine is 90% to 100%, with approximately 85% of the drug bound to plasma protein. Quinidine is 60% to 85% metabolized in the liver via hydroxylation reactions, with some metabolites being active. Urinary excretion is approximately 20%. The half-life of quinidine is 5 to 12 hours, and the general therapeutic range is 2.3 to 5 ng/mL. Maximal serum levels are reached in one to three hours. Toxic side effects of quinidine include cinchonism (vertigo, tinnitus, headache, visual disturbances, and disorientation), fever, hepatitis, and blood dyscrasia. Ventricular arrhythmias, AV block, and ventricular fibrillation lead to syncope, and sudden death can occur.

Lidocaine (Xylocaine) can be used as an antiarrhythmic and as a local anesthetic. Its major use as an antiarrhythmic is in the acute control and prevention of ventricular arrhythmias after acute myocardial infarction. Its mechanism of action is through a decreased rate of ventricular diastolic depolarization.

A loading intravenous dose of 50 to 100 mg is given over two to three minutes to treat ventricular arrhythmias in adults. These dosages may be repeated in 5- to 10-minute intervals of 25 to 50 mg, up to a maximum of 300 mg in a one-hour period. Following loading, infusion is then continued at a rate of 1.4 to 3.5 mg/min for a 70-kg man. In children, 0.5 to 1 mg/kg can be given every five minutes for a maximum of three doses.

Lidocaine is neither highly protein bound nor appreciably stored in body tissues; it has a half-life of approximately two hours and a therapeutic serum range of 1.2 to 5.5 μg/mL. It generally takes five to eight hours for the drug to reach its maximal serum level. Ninety percent of a dose of lidocaine is metabolized in the liver via *N*-dealkylation. Urinary excretion is 10%. Toxic side effects include convulsions, coma, and respiratory depression (CNS effects), as well as bradycardia and hypotension.

Propranolol is used in the treatment of angina pectoris; hypertension; symptomatic coronary artery disease, particularly after an acute myocardial infarction; and arrhythmias. Oral dosages vary from 40 mg to 320 mg daily in adults for antiarrhythmic activity to as high as 480 mg daily in the control of hypertension. Propranolol acts as a nonselective β-adrenergic blocker, antagonizing the effects of epinephrine on the heart, on the arteries and arterioles of skeletal muscles, and on the bronchi. Blockade of cardiac (β_1) receptors reduces heart rate, myocardial contractility and output, AV conduction time, and cardiac automaticity. Both supine and standing blood pressure are also reduced.

Bioavailability of propranolol is approximately 30%. The half-life of propranolol is three hours, with a therapeutic serum range of 50 to 100 ng/mL and with maximal serum levels reached in approximately six hours. Approximately 93% is protein bound. Propranolol is metabolized in the liver, with 0.5% excreted in the urine unchanged. Toxic effects include bradycardia, arterial insufficiency (Raynaud's type), hypotension, AV block, nausea, vomiting, pharyngitis, bronchospasm, and thrombotic thrombocytopenic purpura. Marrow suppression occurs rarely.

Anticonvulsants

Anticonvulsants are used in the treatment of seizure disorders, in particular grand mal, petit mal, and psychomotor seizures and other specialized seizure disorders such as tic douloureux (trigeminal neuralgia).

Phenobarbital (see Table 17–3), a long-acting barbiturate, is used in the treatment of generalized tonic-clonic seizures and simple partial seizures with motor or somatosensory symptoms, as well as for anxiety and insomnia. It is not used in the treatment of absence seizure—that is, petit mal, which may be exacerbated with phenobarbital; nor for complex partial seizures, which do not respond well. Phenobarbital is also given for withdrawal symptoms in infants born to opiate-addicted or barbiturate-addicted mothers. Because phenobarbital enhances the metabolism of bilirubin by enzyme induction, it has been used to treat cases of congenital hyperbilirubinemia (familial nonhemolytic, nonobstructive jaundice). In addition to induction of hepatic microsomal enzymes, barbiturates are believed to stabilize damaged membranes as well as to raise the threshold for neuronal membrane depolarization.

The oral dose of phenobarbital for anxiety in adults is 30 to 120 mg daily in divided doses; for sleep induction in adults, 100 to 320 mg daily generally is used. For seizure control, divided doses of 100 to 200 mg per day in adults or 30 to 100 mg per day in children generally are used.

Phenobarbital has a long half-life of four to six days. Oral doses are almost completely absorbed (90% to 100% bioavailability), and the optimal serum concentration for seizure control is generally 15 to 30 μg/mL. Forty to sixty percent is metabolized in the liver, whereas 10% to 40% may be eliminated unchanged in the urine. Approximately 40% to 60% is plasma protein bound, and the main site of storage is the brain. A steady state is reached in 14 to 21 days. Toxic side effects include nystagmus, ataxia, stupor, respiratory depression, coma, and hypotension. Barbiturates are contraindicated in patients with acute intermittent porphyria, partial porphobilinogen deaminase deficiency, because barbiturates enhance the synthesis of δ-aminolevulinic acid synthetase and thus the synthesis of heme pathway intermediates in the liver.

Phenytoin (Dilantin) is used to treat generalized tonic-clonic, simple partial, and complex partial seizures (see Table 17–4). It is ineffective in treating myoclonic, absence (petit mal), and atonic seizures. It is usually given intravenously in addition to intravenous diazepam to terminate status epilepticus. Data on the mechanism of action of this drug strongly suggest that Dilantin blocks sodium and calcium influxes into repeatedly depolarizing neurons in the CNS and also into neurons that are partially depolarized. By reducing sodium and calcium influx into these cells, it reduces their excitability and prolongs their refractory period (Yaari, 1986). Remarkably, Dilantin has no apparent effects on resting neurons or on normally firing neurons. It is thus specific for epileptogenic foci in the CNS (Yaari, 1986). Interestingly, carbamazepine (Tegretol) exerts similar effects, as discussed later.

Although the average daily maintenance dose in adults is 300 to 400 mg, dosage must be tailored to the patient's response and serum drug concentrations. The usual therapeutic serum concentration is 10 to 20 μg/mL, with a steady state reached in 5 to 10 days (for plateau, see Fig. 17–9). The serum half-life is generally 24 hours, but it is dose dependent. Thus, its excretion is not a first-order process. Phenytoin is stored in the brain, metabolized in the liver (95%), and is approximately 90% to 95% bound to plasma protein. Both aspirin and phenylbutazone can displace phenytoin from serum albumin and can significantly increase the serum concentration of phenytoin. Because phenytoin, like phenobarbital, is a relatively potent enzyme inducer, certain antibiotics, oral anticoagulants, quinidine, and oral contraceptives may be more rapidly metabolized, thus decreasing their effectiveness.

Because the relationship between serum concentrations and daily dosage is not linear, small increases in dosage can greatly increase therapeutic serum concentrations. Symptoms of toxicity generally occur at serum concentrations greater than 20 μg/mL. Toxic side effects include nystagmus, ataxia, stupor, and coma. Arrhythmias can be produced by rapid intravenous administration.

Primidone (Mysoline) is used to treat generalized tonic-clonic, simple partial, and complex partial seizures. Its chemical structure is closely related to the barbiturates, and it is metabolized in the liver into two active metabolites: phenobarbital and phenylethylmalonamide (PEMA). The mechanism of action of this drug is not definitely known, but it may increase the threshold of membrane depolarization within the CNS.

Oral doses range from 250 mg daily to 2 g/day in divided doses. Absorption is rapid and complete (100%), with the usual therapeutic serum concentration being 5 to 21 μg/mL. A steady state is reached in four to seven days, and the half-life is approximately 12 hours. Plasma protein binding is relatively low (20%), with most of the drug remaining free in the serum and with little drug being stored in body tissues.

Sedation is a common toxic side effect. Dizziness, ataxia, and skin rashes have also been observed. Primidone, like phenobarbital, is contraindicated in patients with acute intermittent porphyria.

Ethosuximide (Zarontin) is the drug of choice for absence (petit mal) seizures unaccompanied by other types of seizures. It is preferred over valproic acid (*vide infra*), at least initially, because hepatotoxicity is a rare but serious side effect of valproic acid. Ethosuximide may depress the motor cortex and may reduce the frequency of neuronal firing, but its molecular site of action is poorly understood.

The oral dosage in adults is generally 500 to 1000 mg daily. Absorption is fairly rapid and complete (100%), with peak serum concentrations occurring in one to four hours. A steady state is reached in 8 to 10 days. The usual therapeutic serum concentration is 40 to 100 μg/mL, but can be as high as 170 to 190 μg/mL in children. The serum half-life is generally 60 hours in adults and 30 hours in children. Ethosuximide is essentially free in serum and not protein bound. It is mainly metabolized in the liver (60% to 90%) to desmethylmethsuximide. GI disturbances are among the most common toxic effects and include nausea, vomiting, and gastric distress. Other effects include drowsiness and ataxia. Rare serious side effects, such as systemic lupus erythematosus (SLE), aplastic anemia, and pancytopenia have been reported.

Carbamazepine (Tegretol) (see Table 17–5) is a primary antiepileptic drug and is used in the treatment of generalized tonic-clonic seizures and simple partial and complex partial seizures, as well as in combinations of these seizure types. Absence (petit mal), myoclonic, and atonic seizures may be exacerbated by this drug. This drug is also used to treat tic douloureux (trigeminal neuralgia) and glossopharyngeal neuralgia, and is, in fact, the drug of choice in the treatment of these neuralgias.

Carbamazepine is a tricyclic compound (i.e., iminostilbene) and is chemically related to imipramine, a tricyclic antidepressant. It is believed that a reduction of excitatory synaptic transmission in the spinal trigeminal nucleus is the basis for this drug's antineuralgic action. Its antiepileptic action is similar to that of Dilantin—that is, it decreases sodium and calcium influx into hyperexcitable neurons (Yaari, 1986).

Oral doses of carbamazepine are completely absorbed, and the usual adult maintenance dose is 800 mg to 1.2 g per day. Ninety-eight percent is biotransformed in the liver into two metabolites: a 10,11-epoxide form and a 10,11-dihydroxy form of carbamazepine. The usual therapeutic serum concentration is 4 to 12 μg/mL with a steady state reached in three to four days. The serum half-life of Tegretol is 8 to 20 hours, and 60% to 70% is plasma protein bound. The more common toxic reactions seen with this drug include drowsiness, ataxia, dizziness, nausea and vomiting, and lightheadedness. Rare hematologic reactions may occur and can be very serious; they include aplastic anemia, thrombocytopenia, and agranulocytosis.

Valproic acid (Depakene) is commonly used in the treatment of generalized tonic-clonic, absence, myoclonic, and atonic seizures. It is not effective for the treatment of infantile spasms. Although the mechanism of action is not definitely known, valproic acid is thought to enhance the activity of the GABA-mediated inhibitory system.

Absorption of valproic acid is rapid and complete. The average daily maintenance dose of valproic acid in adults is 15 to 30 mg/kg, when used alone, and 30 to 45 mg/kg in combination with other antiepileptic drugs. The usual therapeutic serum concentration is 50 to 100 μg/mL, and a steady state is reached in one to four days. Most (90% to 100%) of the drug is metabolized in the liver, whereas a high percentage (90%) of the drug is plasma protein bound. The serum half-life is 8 to 15 hours. Valproic acid has been shown to produce teratogenic effects in experimental animals; these included developmental abnormalities and skeletal defects. Thus, valproic acid should be used with caution in pregnant women. Toxic side effects include sedation, gastric disturbances, hematologic reactions, ataxia, somnolence, and coma. Rare fatal hepatotoxicity has occurred, and severe or fatal pancreatitis has been reported.

Antiasthmatics

Asthma is a form of chronic obstructive pulmonary disease that has a variety of causes, some of them allergic in nature. Many different therapeutic modalities are now available for treating this condition, ranging from antihistamines to phosphodiesterase inhibitors like theophylline (allowing high levels of cyclic adenosine monophosphate [3′, 5′-cAMP] to build up, promoting bronchodilation) and more recent bronchodilators such as albuterol (Ventolin). Steroids such as prednisone have been found to be highly effective against asthma. By far, however, the most commonly prescribed antiasthmatic drug is theophylline, and this is the drug whose levels are the most commonly monitored.

Theophylline (see Table 17–6) is used as a bronchodilator for the treatment of moderate or severe asthma, both for the prevention of attacks and for the treatment of symptomatic exacerbations. Theophylline also exerts additional actions, including vasodilation, diuresis, positive cardiac inotropic effects, and the stimulation of diaphragmatic contraction. Owing to the stimulating effect on the diaphragm, theophylline may be of some benefit to some patients with emphysema. Theophylline has also been effective in the treatment of primary apnea of prematurity, in which the absence of respiratory effort lasts more than 20 seconds in newborn infants. The mechanism of action of primary apnea is thought to be due to medullary stimulation by the drug. Its bronchodilator effect comes about from an increase in intracellular cAMP as a result of the inhibition, by theophylline, of the enzyme phosphodiesterase. This increase, in turn, causes relaxation of the smooth muscle of the bronchial airways and pulmonary blood vessels.

In the treatment of asthma, dosage is calculated on the basis of body weight and depends on the route of administration and the age of the patient. Because the therapeutic index (i.e., the closeness of toxic levels to the therapeutic levels) of theophylline is low, cautious dosage determination is essential. Careful monitoring of patient response and serum theophylline levels is required because theophylline is metabolized at different rates for each patient. For example, for intravenous (IV) treatment of acute bronchospasm in healthy adults, an initial loading dose of 4.7 mg/kg (anhydrous theophylline equivalents) may be given, followed by a maintenance dosage of approximately 0.5 mg/kg per hour for the next 12 hours, which is then changed to approximately 0.4 mg/kg per hour maintenance dosage. If, during chronic therapy (i.e., after three days), the recommended maximal dosage is exceeded, peak serum theophylline levels should be measured to adjust dosage. These levels can be estimated at one hour after IV administration, one to two hours after oral administration, or generally three to eight hours after extended-release administration from appropriately drawn blood samples.

The therapeutic serum level is 10 to 20 μg/mL, and the mean half-life is approximately 8.7 hours in nonsmoking adults (5.5 hours in smoking adults). However, the half-life may vary widely among individuals, again indicating the need for close supervision of the patient and appropriate monitoring of serum concentrations in each patient. Approximately 60% of the drug is protein bound, and about 90% is metabolized in the liver, with caffeine being one of the inactive metabolites produced.

Theophylline crosses the placenta, and may be teratogenic in pregnant females. Other common side effects include tachycardia, arrhythmias, seizures, and GI bleeding.

Anti-inflammatory Drugs

The drugs discussed in this section are some of the nonsteroidal anti-inflammatory drugs. Although many drugs in this category, such as naproxen (Naprosyn) and ibuprofen (Motrin) have become available, and these drugs are widely prescribed, only two drugs—Tylenol and aspirin—are monitored extensively in serum. We thus discuss these two drugs here.

Acetaminophen (Tylenol) is used as an analgesic and antipyretic to treat fever, headache, and mild-to-moderate myalgia and arthralgia. However, acetaminophen does not possess potent anti-inflammatory activity and is unsatisfactory for such conditions (e.g., rheumatic disease). Although acetaminophen is as effective as aspirin in its analgesic and antipyretic actions, it is preferred over aspirin in patients with a bleeding or coagulation disorder or in children requiring only antipyretics or analgesics because no association between acetaminophen and the incidence of Reye's syndrome in children has been demonstrated. Furthermore, an accidental overdose in children may be less toxic than with aspirin, because hepatotoxicity is rarely associated with acetaminophen overdosage in children under the age of six years.

Oral doses of acetaminophen are rapidly and essentially completely absorbed from the GI tract. Generally, 325 to 650 mg at four-hour intervals is prescribed for adults and children over 12 years of age, with a maximum of 4 g daily. The plasma half-life is approximately two hours, with peak plasma levels of 5 to 20 mg/mL occurring in 30 to 60 minutes. The percentage of plasma protein binding is not significant (approximately 20%) with therapeutic doses. The major metabolites of acetaminophen produced by the liver are glucuronide and sulfate conjugates, with minor metabolites being deacetylated and hydroxylated derivatives. The latter metabolite is thought to produce hepatotoxicity with overdosage.

The mechanism of action of acetaminophen appears to be related to the central inhibition of prostaglandin cyclo-oxygenase. Its effect on peripheral prostaglandin synthetase appears to be less, and its peripheral action appears to be mainly related to the blockage of pain impulse generation. Inhibition of prostaglandin synthetase within the hypothalamus probably accounts for its antipyretic action.

Acute manifestations of toxic doses generally occur within two to three hours after ingestion and include nausea, vomiting, and abdominal pain. A characteristic sign of toxicity is cyanosis of the skin, mucosa, and fingernails due to the production of methemoglobinemia. However, this is seen more frequently with phenacetin poisoning. CNS stimulation followed by CNS depression may occur in severe poisoning with vascular collapse, shock, and total seizures occurring. Coma usually precedes death. Hepatic necrosis may also occur, with maximal liver damage not becoming apparent until two to four days after drug ingestion.

Chronic acetaminophen abuse may produce chronic toxicity and death. Anemia, renal damage, and GI disturbances are usually associated with chronic toxicity.

Acetylsalicylic acid (aspirin) is a nonsteroidal anti-inflammatory compound and is used as an analgesic, an antipyretic and, in larger doses, an anti-inflammatory agent. In lower doses, it exhibits its anticoagulant activity. It can be effective in the treatment of fever, neuralgia, headache, myalgia, and arthralgia, and in the management of some rheumatic diseases.

The mechanism of action of aspirin is similar to that of acetaminophen, in that aspirin inhibits the enzyme prostaglandin synthetase. Unlike acetaminophen, however, it inhibits prostaglandin synthetase both centrally and peripherally, and it is this latter action that appears to produce its anti-inflammatory effect.

Oral dosages of aspirin that are generally used for analgesia and antipyresis in adults range from 500 mg as necessary, to a maximum of 4 g daily. Increased dosages (3.5 to 5.5 g daily) are used for rheumatoid arthritis and osteoarthritis in adults and for juvenile arthritis (up to 3.5 g daily) in children.

The small intestine is the primary site of aspirin absorption, and absorption usually occurs rapidly following oral administration, with peak plasma levels established within one to two hours. Before entering the system's circulation, aspirin is rapidly hydrolyzed to acetic acid and salicylic acid. Hydrolysis occurs partly by plasma esterase and partly by the liver. Both aspirin and salicylic acid enter the CNS.

Approximately 70% to 90% of salicylic acid is plasma protein bound. The serum half-life is dose dependent and increases with the dose: from approximately three hours with 500 mg to approximately 15 hours with 4 g. Salicylic acid is cleared not only by metabolism but also by urinary excretion, and as the half-life increases, the rate of urinary excretion decreases. This can produce toxic effects if the dosage interval is not increased appropriately (Fig. 17–10). However, the rate of elimination can vary widely with the patient, necessitating individualization of dosage for large amounts of drug. Tinnitus, muffled hearing, and a sensation of fullness in the ears are the most common signs of chronic aspirin toxicity. In infants, young children, and patients with pre-existing hearing loss, otic symptoms do not occur, and hyperventilation is the most common sign of overdosage. It is important to note that overdoses of aspirin can cause metabolic acidosis. However, salicylate itself stimulates central respiratory centers to cause an increased breathing rate, leading to a respiratory alkalosis.

Acute aspirin intoxication is a common cause of fatal drug poisoning in children. Toxic doses produce acid-base disturbances, direct CNS stimulation of respiration, hyperpyrexia

2

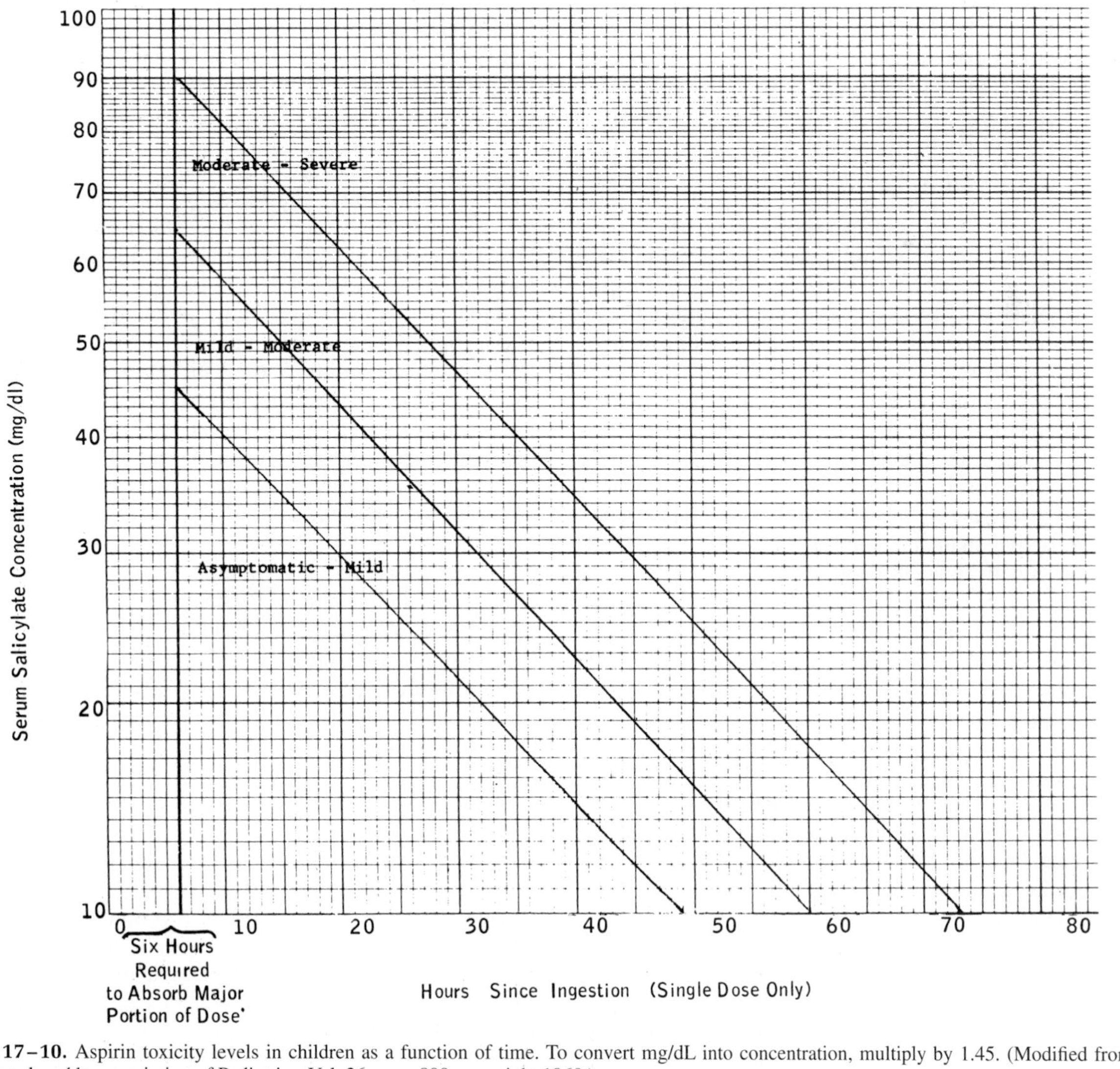

Figure 17–10. Aspirin toxicity levels in children as a function of time. To convert mg/dL into concentration, multiply by 1.45. (Modified from Done, AK: Reproduced by permission of Pediatrics, Vol. 26, page 800, copyright 1960.)

and hypoglycemia, GI bleeding, and nausea and vomiting. Acute renal failure, CNS dysfunction with stupor and coma, and pulmonary edema may develop. Figure 17–10 summarizes the toxic levels of aspirin in children as a function of time after the toxic dose was taken.

Immunosuppressives

Drugs in this class are used in the treatment of autoimmune diseases to reduce inflammation and include prednisone, a steroid, and cyclophosphamide (Cytoxan), a cytotoxic drug. One immunosuppressive drug for which there is now a great demand in terms of drug monitoring is cyclosporine, which is used for patients undergoing transplants.

Cyclosporine is a cyclic polypeptide containing 11 amino acids that is believed to inhibit selectively T-helper cell function with sparing and augmentation of T-suppressor cell populations (see Chap. 38). The augmentation of T-suppressor cell populations appears to be important in maintaining an unresponsive state to allografts, because these cells appear to play a role in down-regulating T-helper cell activation. The inhibition of T-helper cell production of interleukin-2 (IL-2) appears to be a critical immunosuppressive effect of cyclosporine (Kahan, 1989; Hess, 1988). Maximal suppression with cyclosporine occurs during the first 24 hours of antigen stimulation by the allograft. Thus, cyclosporine must be administered in the early phase of the immune response for optimal suppression of T-cell function and increased success of transplantation. Cyclosporine is indicated to prevent organ rejection in kidney, heart, and liver allogeneic transplants and is the drug of choice for maintenance of kidney, liver, heart, and heart-lung allografts. Cyclosporine is being investigated for treatment of established graft-versus-host disease (GVHD) in bone marrow transplant patients, to prevent bone marrow transplant rejection, and in the treatment of a number of autoimmune diseases.

Because cyclosporine is variably absorbed from the GI tract, the optimal dose must be carefully determined for each patient individually, and blood levels should be monitored frequently. It has been occasionally found that, although serum levels of the parent drug are low, the metabolites, some of which are active, maintain a therapeutic drug level. Therefore, in patients with apparently low levels of the parent drug, it is necessary to determine the levels of metabolites. Peak blood concentrations occur at approximately 3.5 hours after administration. About 20% to 40% of a given dose of cyclosporine is absorbed, and it is metabolized on the first pass through the liver. Human cytochrome P-450 III A3 of the P-450 III gene family appears to be the primary enzyme responsible for cyclosporine metabolism. Because a number of drugs either may induce or may be metabolized by this cytochrome P-450 isoenzyme, coadministration of these drugs may be responsible for alterations in cyclosporine levels that can complicate cyclosporine therapy (Kronbach, 1988). Trough whole blood or plasma concentrations, at 24 hours, of 250 to 800 ng/mL or 50 to 300 ng/mL, respectively (as determined by radioimmunoassay [RIA]), are believed to minimize graft rejection and toxic effects.

Trough serum levels (determined by RIA) greater than 500 ng/mL are associated with cyclosporine-induced nephrotoxicity, which is the most frequent toxic reaction seen with cyclosporine. Other toxic effects include hypertension, tremor, hirsutism, gingival hyperplasia, diarrhea, nausea and vomiting, anorexia, and infectious complications. An increased risk of lymphoma and CNS lymphoma may also be associated with immunosuppression with cyclosporine. Intravenous cyclosporine is reserved for patients unable to tolerate oral administration because of a small (0.1%) but definite risk of anaphylaxis. This has not been reported following administration of cyclosporine oral solution.

It should be noted that until recently, the levels of cyclosporine were monitored by RIA methods or by HPLC. Both methods yield levels of parent compound and metabolites. At present, however, rapid and accurate FPIA methods exist, such as with the Abbott IMX analyzer, that are capable of determining the total level of cyclosporine and all of its metabolites.

Drugs Used in the Treatment of Manic-Depression: Lithium and the Tricyclic Antidepressants

Both lithium and the tricyclic antidepressants are used in the treatment of psychiatric affective disorders.

LITHIUM. Lithium is a monovalent cation, a member of the group of alkali metals, and is available commercially as the citrate and carbonate salts. Lithium salts are considered to be anti-manic agents and are used for the prophylaxis and treatment of bipolar disorder (manic-depressive psychosis). In addition, lithium is considered by some investigators to be the drug of choice for the prevention of chronic cluster headache, and it may also be effective in episodic or periodic forms of cluster headache.

Initial oral dosages of lithium for acute mania range from 600 mg to 1.8 g daily (maximum of 2.4 g) to produce a therapeutic serum level of 0.75 to 1.5 mEq/L. Once the attack subsides, the dose is reduced rapidly to produce a serum concentration of 0.4 to 1.0 mEq/L. Oral adult dosages for cluster headaches generally range from 600 mg to 1200 mg daily in divided doses. In general, serum levels and patient response are used to individualize dosage and must be monitored carefully.

Complete absorption of lithium occurs six to eight hours after oral administration. Plasma half-life varies from 17 to 36 hours, and the onset of action is slow (5 to 10 days). Elimination occurs almost entirely by the kidneys, and about 80% of filtered lithium is reabsorbed. Lithium is not protein bound and is distributed in total body water, but shows delayed and varied tissue distribution. Thus, symptoms of acute intoxication may not correlate well with serum levels, because the distribution of the drug into different organs may be slow or varied.

The exact mechanism of action of lithium is unknown, but lithium, as a monovalent cation, competes with other monovalent and divalent cations (such as sodium, potassium, calcium, and magnesium) at ion channels in cell membranes; competes at intracellular and extracellular protein-binding sites, including, possibly, membrane receptors; and competes for binding to protein and peptide transport molecules and enzymes. Many of these molecular processes are critical to the synthesis, storage, release, and uptake of central neurotransmitters, and lithium may exert its effect through any of these processes within the CNS.

Toxicity may occur acutely, as the result of a single toxic dose, or chronically, from high or prolonged dosages or changes in lithium pharmacokinetics. Water loss (resulting from fever, decreased intake, abnormal GI conditions such as diarrhea, vomiting, diuresis, or pyelonephritis) is the main contributing factor underlying chronic intoxication.

The severity of intoxication is not clearly related to serum lithium levels. However, an imprecise prediction of severity of intoxication may be attempted from serum lithium levels obtained 12 hours after the last dose: slight to moderate intoxication with 1.5 to 2.5 mEq/L, severe intoxication with 2.5 to 3.5 mEq/L, and potentially lethal intoxication if greater than 3.5 mEq/L. The severity of lithium intoxication also depends on the length of time that the serum concentration remains at toxic levels.

The most common symptoms of mild to moderate intoxication include nausea, malaise, diarrhea, and fine hand tremor. In addition, thirst, polydipsia, and polyuria, as well as drowsiness, muscle weakness, ataxia, and slurred speech may occur. Symptoms of moderate to severe toxicity include hyperactive deep tendon reflexes, choreoathetoid movements, persistent nausea and vomiting, fasciculations, generalized seizures, and clonic movements of whole limbs. These may progress rapidly to generalized seizures, oliguria, circulatory failure, and death with serum levels greater than 3.5 mEq/L.

TRICYCLIC ANTIDEPRESSANTS. The structures of these compounds are shown in Figure 17–11. The mechanism of action—blockage of the reuptake of adrenergic and dopaminergic neurotransmitters—is discussed under drugs of abuse. The action of these excitatory neurotransmitters is thereby prolonged by allowing them to remain at their receptor sites. Besides stimulating dopaminergic pathways, the tricyclics, especially amitriptyline, have anticholinergic effects.

The pharmacologic side effects of the tricyclic antidepressants in fact reflect their anticholinergic activities. These include dry mouth, constipation, blurred vision, hyperthermia, adynamic ileus, urinary retention, and delayed micturition. Other CNS effects include drowsiness, weakness, fatigue, and lethargy, which are most common, as well as agitation, restlessness, insomnia, and confusion. Seizures and coma can also occur. Extrapyramidal symptoms may also occur and include a persistent fine tremor, rigidity, dystonia, and opisthotonos.

It is important to realize that the tricyclic antidepressants are frequently used in suicide attempts by depressed individuals who are being treated for depression with these drugs. The cardinal signs of tricyclic antidepressant overdose are anticholinergic symptoms: dilated pupils and dry skin. Pupil dilation is an extremely important clue of tricyclic overdose in the obtunded or comatose patient.

TOXICITY. Overdose produces symptoms that are primarily extensions of common adverse reactions with excess CNS stimulation and anticholinergic activity. These include seizures, coma, hypotension, respiratory depression, areflexia, shock, and cardiorespiratory arrest. Agitation, confusion, hypertension, and the parkinsonian syndrome may also occur, as well as hallucinations and delirium. Occasional manifestations include ataxia, renal failure, dysarthria, and vomiting.

TREATMENT. Symptomatic and supportive care are general modes of treatment. Gastric lavage, accompanied by instillation of activated charcoal, is usually recommended for removal of the tricyclic from the GI tract. Seizures are generally treated with intravenous diazepam. Cardiac arrhythmias, conductive disturbance, and hypotension may respond to phenytoin, lidocaine (Xylocaine), or propranolol. For overdoses with amitriptyline (see Fig. 17–11), use of cholinesterase inhibitors such as neostigmine has proved to be effective in reversing the anticholinergic symptoms.

The Neuroleptics, Antipsychotic Major Tranquilizers

These drugs are used mainly in the treatment of acute schizophrenia and result in suppression of the agitated state. There are two general classes of these drugs: the phenothiazines, typified by chlorpromazine; and the butyrophenones, typified by haloperidol (Haldol). Both of these drugs appear to block the postsynaptic (dendritic) receptors of dopamine and serotonin in the excitatory pathways using these neurotransmitters (see Fig. 17–8). Haldol is known also to bind with high affinity to σ-receptors in the CNS, and this action may stimulate inhibitory pathways that modulate the activity of the dopaminergic pathways.

It has been difficult to monitor the levels of either drug in serum because of the large number of metabolites for each drug, which results from extensive metabolism in the liver. Chlorpromazine, for example, has approximately 150 metabolites. The therapeutic efficacy of most of these metabolites is unknown. It is, therefore, difficult to establish ranges for nor-

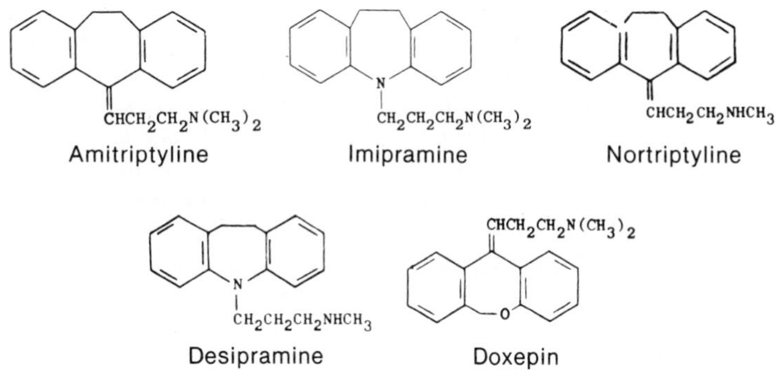

Figure 17–11. Structures of the most commonly used tricyclic antidepressants.

mal serum levels of these drugs. Methods for assay include FPIA and HPLC. It is not clear in FPIA which, if any, metabolites cross-react with the antibody. For chlorpromazine, the estimated therapeutic range is wide, between 50 and 300 ng/mL. The half-life of the drug is 16 to 30 hours, and its bioavailability is 25% to 35%. Normal doses for chlorpromazine are 200 to 600 mg daily in divided doses. Other drugs in the phenothiazine series include thioridazine and fluphenazine (Prolixin).

The chief toxic side effects of the preceding neuroleptic drugs are tardive dyskinesia and parkinsonian effects—that is, antiextrapyramidal systemic effects in the CNS. Also, orthostatic hypotension, cholestasis, and rarely, aplastic anemia have been known to occur as toxic side effects. Occasionally, contact dermatitis has been reported to occur with phenothiazines. Of great importance is the subset of patients who have been chronically treated with these drugs and develop tardive dyskinesia. In most of these patients, these motor disturbances are irreversible.

Chemotherapeutic Agents: Methotrexate

Many drugs have been developed that are aimed at specific targets in the cell to block the cell from dividing (see Table 17–7). These drugs are used as antineoplastic agents. Some of these agents are aimed at blocking replication of DNA, and others are designed as antimetabolites and are aimed at blocking specific steps in metabolism that ultimately block DNA synthesis and cell division. Often, these agents are used in combination in treating specific neoplasms. Serum levels of these drugs generally are not followed routinely except when clinical indications suggest drug toxicity. However, it is important to monitor the level of some of these drugs to determine whether they are present in lethal concentrations. One of the most commonly used antineoplastic drugs for which this consideration applies is methotrexate, a mixture containing no less than 85% 4-amino-10-methylfolic acid and related compounds. This drug, a folic acid antagonist, inhibits the enzyme dihydrofolate reductase. Inhibition of this enzyme blocks formation of tetrahydrofolic acid, which is needed for the formation of N-5,10-tetrahydrofolate, an intermediate in the transfer of a methyl group to deoxyuridylate to form thymidylate, which is needed in DNA synthesis. It has also been suggested that methotrexate also may cause a rise in the intracellular levels of adenosine triphosphatase (ATP), which blocks ribonucleotide reduction, also resulting in the blocking of DNA synthesis. Methotrexate also appears to inhibit polynucleotide ligase involved in DNA synthesis and repair.

Methotrexate as an important immunosuppressive agent is used in the treatment of psoriasis, rheumatoid arthritis, and some of the collagen vascular diseases. Depending on the specific disease entity being treated, dosages given will vary, as will the therapeutic level of the drug. In Table 17–7, the doses and therapeutic drug levels for several different conditions are noted. The serum levels were determined by FPIA.

The kinetics of steady-state levels of this drug are biphasic: a rapid phase with $t_{1/2}$ = two to three hours and a slow phase with $t_{1/2} = 8$ to 10 hours. Excretion of the drug is also biphasic: 92% is excreted within 24 hours, and the remainder over a period of days. Approximately 50% of the drug in blood is bound to serum proteins.

The toxic effects of methotrexate include hematologic effects, such as leukopenia and thrombocytopenia; GI effects, such as ulceration, glossitis, stomatitis, nausea, vomiting; hepatic lesions, such as cirrhosis; pulmonary lesions, such as pulmonary fibrosis; dermatologic effects, such as urticaria and vasculitis; and CNS effects from intrathecal methotrexate, including arachnoiditis, leukoencephalopathy, and increased cerebrospinal fluid pressure.

It is occasionally necessary to administer high doses of methotrexate to individuals with tumors that do not respond to normal doses of this drug. In these cases, the drug leucovorin (citrovorum factor) is given 18 to 36 hours after the initial methotrexate dose. Leucovorin is N5-formyltetrahydrofolate, which is the product of dihydrofolate reductase. Thus, this compound overcomes the blockage caused by methotrexate. The rationale for this regimen is that the rapidly proliferating tumor cells will be killed by the high dose of methotrexate, while many normal cells that are not dividing often can be rescued by leucovorin. Especially in this type of drug regimen, it is essential to monitor the serum levels of methotrexate carefully. In addition, leucovorin should be immediately administered to a patient receiving low-dose methotrexate when methotrexate overdose is suspected (Roenigk, 1988).

The drugs discussed previously are the ones most commonly monitored. Overdosages of any of these drugs cause symptoms that must be diagnosed so that blood levels of the overdosed therapeutic drug can be determined.

Exposure to high levels of other agents that may cause no acute symptoms but have lethal effects on the body warrant further discussion. These are the toxins, which are divided into the environmental carcinogens and chemical toxins.

ENVIRONMENTAL CARCINOGENESIS

General Considerations

Over the past decade or so, great attention has been focused on the effects of chemical and physical agents in the atmosphere that predispose individuals exposed to them to develop tumors in various tissues where these agents accumulate. The chemical agents are referred to as carcinogens. Many of the individuals who are exposed to these agents work in industries where these agents are produced. Benzpyrene, an aromatic compound produced in cigarettes and also produced in the exhaust of engines, is a known potent carcinogen and has been implicated in lung cancer. Nitrites, used as preservatives in red meats, have been associated with colon cancer. Aflatoxin, produced by the fungus *Aspergillus,* has been implicated in causing hepatocellular carcinoma. Aromatic hydrocarbons such as benzene and ionizing radiation have been implicated in causing acute leukemias. Vinyl chloride and the formerly used dye Thorotrast have been linked to angiosarcoma. Benzidine dyes, β-naphthylamine, dimethylbenzanthracene, and other aromatic compounds have been linked to multiple malignancies occurring in humans. Exposure to asbestos has been strongly implicated as a carcinogen in lung cancer. In animal studies, polychlorinated biphenyls

(PCBs), produced in fires, and dioxin have been strongly implicated as causing a variety of cancers.

Hence, much interest has now been focused on workers in occupations in which carcinogens are present in significant amounts. Steel foundries, shipbuilding and rubber plants, and other industrial plants may produce such carcinogens in significant amounts. In some of these industries, certain cancers occur at rates higher than in the general population (Brandt-Rauf, 1982). Thus, in these exposed populations, it has become desirable to determine the levels of exposure to certain known carcinogens.

Methods for Detecting Environmental Carcinogens

Because of the vast range of potential carcinogens and the relatively small numbers of individuals whose body fluids have thus far been tested for them, few standard assays exist for these carcinogens. The method of choice is GC-MS. For certain carcinogenic compounds like PCBs, the method of electron capture is used. Halogenated compounds like PCBs are separated on a GC column using an ionized gas as the carrier. Halogenated compounds capture electrons conducted through the carrier gas and are thus detected by the reduced currents.

WESTERN (IMMUNO) BLOTTING. Often, the presence of carcinogens in blood or urine is hard to detect directly. The carcinogens, however, may be bound to proteins or to DNA intracellularly. As discussed subsequently, in cohorts known to be exposed to carcinogens, there is evidence that strongly suggests that certain oncogene-encoded proteins increase in the serum and urine of these individuals. Thus, it is desirable to test for their presence.

At present, the most sensitive methods are adaptations of the enzyme-linked immunosorbent assay (ELISA) technology that are referred to as Western blotting. In these assays, easily obtainable cells like peripheral lymphocytes are harvested from an individual and lysed. The protein or nucleic acid fractions are isolated by standard techniques and then mixed with the denaturing agent, sodium dodecyl sulfate (SDS). The mixture is then placed on a polyacrylamide gel and subjected to electrophoresis (SDS-PAGE). DNA or protein molecules separate on the gel according to molecular weight under these conditions. For oncogene-encoded proteins, body fluids can be used directly; cells are not necessary.

As discussed subsequently, monoclonal antibodies to carcinogen adducts to DNA and protein have been prepared. Also, numerous monoclonal antibodies have been prepared against oncogene-encoded proteins. To identify a carcinogen adduct or an oncogene-encoded protein, the specific antibody is incubated with the separated DNA or protein bands to determine which, if any, of the bands contains the sought-after molecules. Because it is technically difficult to incubate the gel with the antibody, the bands on the gel are blotted onto nitrocellulose strips, much as they are in Northern and Southern blots. The nitrocellulose blot is then incubated with antibody. The antibody-treated blot is then washed and incubated with a second anti-IgG antibody coupled to an enzyme such as horseradish peroxidase. The blot is washed again, and substrate is added. The visible appearance of colored product at specific bands indicates the presence of the carcinogen or oncoprotein. This technique is sensitive to nanogram quantities of the protein or nucleic acid.

Carcinogenesis and Mutagenesis

It happens that carcinogens often cause mutagenesis by binding to DNA, causing errors in replication and transcription of m-RNA. The resulting mistranscribed RNA codes for proteins that are mutated, resulting in their causing measurable altered cell function. This phenomenon has been quantitated in the Ames assay (Ames, 1973, 1975). In this assay, *Salmonella* bacteria, which are histidine dependent and which have permeable cell walls and defective DNA repair enzymes, are exposed to a potential mutagen or suspected carcinogen. Mutagenesis results in colonies that no longer have the cell permeability deficits. By measuring the number of back-mutated colonies after a specific period of time, a measure of the efficiency of the mutagen can be obtained. The mutagen is also tested for its ability to produce tumors in animals.

The mutagenicity is then plotted against the carcinogenicity of the compound. For a related series of mutagens, a straight line is obtained, indicating a good correlation between the two indices. Overall, of 73 known carcinogens and noncarcinogenic compounds, 45% of the known carcinogens were found to be mutagens, whereas 86% of noncarcinogens were nonmutagenic (Santella, 1987). The low overall correlation between carcinogens and mutagens across-the-board is caused by three different phenomena. First, many so-called carcinogens are themselves not true carcinogens but become carcinogenic only after they are metabolized. This metabolism occurs in the cytochrome P-450–dependent oxidases in the microsomal fraction in the liver. Many different isoenzymes of cytochrome P-450 have been isolated and sequenced. Some of these isoenzymes are highly active in the oxidation reactions that convert compounds into carcinogens, whereas others are much less active (Cheng, 1986). Thus, certain parent compounds are noncarcinogens and do not mutagenize bacteria and have different effects in different individuals, depending on the nature of liver metabolism.

One excellent example of this phenomenon is benzpyrene, a heterocyclic aromatic compound found in cigarette smoke and in the exhaust from engines. This compound is successively converted in the liver to an epoxide and then into benzpyrene diol epoxide, which then reacts with DNA. It is the latter diol epoxide compound that is the carcinogen. The parent compound benzpyrene is itself noncarcinogenic.

A second reason for the lack of overall correlation between mutagenicity and carcinogenicity relates to specific observable changes in *Salmonella*. Not all mutagens may produce an effect on these bacteria.

A third reason for the lack of correlation may relate to the phenomenon of tumor initiators versus tumor promoters. It is now thought that normal cells transform into malignant ones via a series of steps, not in a single step. These steps are divided into tumor initiation—that is, the production of a premalignant lesion; and tumor promotion—that is, the enhancement of the initial lesion to cause ultimate unregulated cell division. Many mutagens are tumor initiators but are not promoters, whereas some carcinogens are known to be tumor promoters and are not mutagens.

One use of the Ames assay is to screen body fluids like urine in individuals who have some history of exposure to carcinogens. The assay itself is now automated. In urine screens, the problem of absence of metabolites that are carcinogenic is removed because most of the metabolites of carcinogen parent compounds are entirely excreted in the urine. This consideration increases the sensitivity of the method.

Detection of the Presence of Carcinogens and Oncogenic Proteins in Body Fluids and Cells

It has been found that exposure of animals to specific carcinogens results in activation of proto-oncogenes in cells. Proto-oncogenes code for proteins that are involved in control of the cell cycle. If mutations occur in these genes or in their controller regions, mutated or overexpressed proteins result that continuously signal the cell to divide. One excellent example of oncogene-induced cell transformation is the *RAS* oncogene that codes for the p21 protein (protein of molecular weight 21 kDa). A single base change in the twelfth coding triplet, for example, from GGC to GTC, in the *RAS* proto-oncogene, results in a protein that contains a valine in place of the glycine that occurs in the normal protein (Barbacid, 1987). This protein is oncogenic (Stacey, 1984), and in fact, p21 proteins with any amino acid except proline at position 12 cause malignant transformation of cells.

The normal p21 protein is activated by binding GTP—that is, it is a G protein. Hydrolysis of the GTP to GDP and Pi inactivates the protein. Oncogenic p21 proteins appear to be permanently activated. This activation is caused by a change in the three-dimensional structure of the protein that allows it to interact with target proteins intracellularly (Chen, 1989; Pincus, 1983, 1985). Although the mechanism for the stimulation of cell division by the p21 protein is not completely understood (see Chaps. 14 and 15), it is known that the p21 protein is a signal-transducing protein that activates second messenger molecules like diacylglycerol and phosphatidylinositol. An important target of the action of p21 appears to be activation of both protein kinase C (Chung, 1992; Pincus, 1992) and phospholipase c (Smith, 1990). It should be noted that high levels of expression of the normal p21 protein also result in cell transformation.

Thus, it is desirable, in screening specific populations exposed to carcinogens, as discussed previously, to detect proteins, like the p21 protein, encoded by oncogenes. If there are oncoproteins discovered in cells or in body fluids like urine, in a particular individual, such an individual is at high risk for developing or has already developed cancer. The patients must therefore be examined carefully for the presence of a malignancy.

Studies involving Western blots of serum and urine for oncogenes in a large population have revealed the presence of cancer (Niman, 1985). Here, results in screening cells and body fluids both for oncogenes and oncoproteins and for carcinogens that are implicated in activating these genes and proteins are discussed.

CELL STUDIES. One of the most convenient assay systems for oncogenes is the NIH 3T3 cell culture system. These cells are mouse fibroblasts into which oncogenes can be transfected or into which oncogenic proteins can be microinjected (Barbacid, 1987). For example, when the *RAS* oncogene is treated with calcium phosphate and incubated with these cells in monolayer culture, the DNA becomes transfected into the cells and ultimately becomes incorporated into the host cells' genome. The cells then transform into malignant cells and heap up on top of one another—that is, lose contact inhibition. The result is plaques or foci of malignant cells in the culture dish.

This system has been used to study the effects of mutagens on NIH 3T3 cells. Incubation of the cells with nitrous acid resulted in cell transformation. Several oncogenes were isolated, all from the *RAS* family, each coding for proteins with single substitutions at specific portions—that is, Gly 13, Gln 61, and Glu 63 (Fasano, 1984). This pioneering study indicates the potential utility of NIH 3T3 cells to assay for the effects of putative carcinogens.

ANIMAL STUDIES. Exposure of mice to the carcinogen nitrosourea over a relatively short time resulted in mammary tumors. Screens for activated oncogenes revealed the presence of both oncogenic p21 protein and elevated expression of the *NEU* oncogene (Barbacid, 1987). Exposure of the skin of mice to the carcinogen dimethylbenzanthracene resulted in skin tumors after a short period of exposure. Restriction fragment length polymorphism (RFLP) analysis of the DNA taken from these tumors revealed the presence of the *HRAS* oncogene with substitutions at position 12 (Balmain, 1983). Exposure of mice to plutonium and its daughters (lower atomic mass radioactive fragments) resulted in lung carcinomas for which the *KRAS* oncogene was found (Frazier, 1986).

On the other hand, exposure of the skin of mice to certain known tumor promoters like phorbol esters did not result in tumor formation. Only if the animals were first exposed to such initiating events as ultraviolet light and then exposed to phorbol esters did tumors develop in the skin of these animals. This latter finding illustrates that a carcinogen may not by itself induce a tumor without other accompanying cellular changes. It is of interest that phorbol esters act as second messengers and activate protein kinase c, actions also thought to be promoted by the p21 protein.

HUMAN STUDIES. It is important to diagnose carcinogen-induced cancer early in individuals who may be at risk for developing these cancers. Several studies have indicated that such screening is now possible. Brandt-Rauf (1990) performed a study of 18 workers who had been exposed to benzpyrene in varying doses. These workers were divided into groups based on their levels of exposure: high, medium, and low. Nonexposed controls constituted a fourth group. The presence of benzpyrene adducts to DNA can be conveniently detected in peripheral blood lymphocytes using a monoclonal antibody to benzpyrene-DNA adducts (Perera, 1988). At the same time, the presence of oncogenes in the serum of these patients can be monitored by Western blotting as described previously in this chapter and in Chapter 15 (Niman, 1985).

Of great interest was the finding that the workers in the high-exposure group were found to have high levels of benzpyrene-DNA adducts in their peripheral blood lymphocytes. Much lower levels were found in the members of the other groups. All of the high-exposure group patients were found to have elevated levels of two oncoproteins in their sera: *RAS*-p21 protein and *FES* protein. No oncoproteins were found, however, in the lower exposure groups. Similar results were found in a cohort of workers with known diagnoses of silicosis and asbestosis (Brandt-Rauf, 1992). A group of individuals, all of whom had known exposures to the agent vinyl chloride, were followed for the presence of a mutated p21 protein in their sera (De Vivo, 1995). Vinyl chloride predisposes to the development of angiosarcoma of the liver and is known to induce base changes in codon 13 of the *RAS* gene (reviewed in De Vivo, 1995), resulting in the oncogenic substitution of an Asp for the naturally occurring Gly at this position in the amino acid sequence. The Asp 13-p21 protein can be detected by a monoclonal antibody that specifically recognizes this amino acid at position 13 (De Vivo, 1995). All but one of the patients in this study expressed this protein at high levels in their sera and were found *subsequently* to develop angiosarcomas.

These studies illustrate the new developments in testing for exposure to carcinogens and the effects of these carcinogens in terms of oncogene and oncoprotein production. Increasingly, toxicology laboratories are being called on to assay for these products and to become involved in the early detection of cancer. The newer techniques outlined in this discussion may be expected to become important features of clinical laboratories in the near future.

TOXINS AND ACUTE POISONING

Having reviewed toxins that cause cancer after chronic exposure, it is important to consider toxins that are acute or chronic metabolic poisons. It is imperative to understand the signs and symptoms caused by specific toxins to enable rapid diagnoses to be made and to institute immediate effective therapy.

Cyanide

The cyanide anion binds avidly to iron in the ferric or trivalent state. Because cyanide forms a relatively stable cyanoferric complex, it is able to inactivate iron-containing enzymes that cycle between the ferrous and ferric states in oxidation-reduction reactions.

Cyanide produces tissue and cellular hypoxia primarily by reversibly binding to cytochrome A_3 and by inhibiting its reoxidation. This inhibits the electron transport system and prevents cellular respiration and ATP (high-energy phosphate) formation. This blockade prevents the utilization of oxygen and aerobic metabolism, producing severe metabolic (lactic) acidosis.

Although cyanide binds preferentially to the ferric form of iron, it can also bind to the ferrous iron of hemoglobin, producing cyanohemoglobin, which cannot transport oxygen. Cyanide also forms complexes with other iron-containing enzymes, but its acute poisonous effect is attributable to the inhibition of electron transport and cell death, predominantly in the CNS.

The principal symptoms of cyanide overdose are tachypnea (initially) followed by respiratory depression and cyanosis, hypotension, convulsions, and coma. Death may occur in a matter of minutes because cyanide is a fast-acting toxin. Diagnosis may be difficult, and a high index of suspicion is needed to make the correct diagnosis. Clues include the odor of bitter almonds, the occurrence of an altered mental status and tachypnea in the absence of cyanosis, and an unexplained metabolic acidosis (with an increased anion gap).

Antidotal therapy is based on a two-step strategy. First, to pull the CN^- ions away from cytochrome A_3, hemoglobin is converted to methemoglobin (Fe^3 state) by using specific oxidants—that is, amyl nitrite and sodium nitrite. Amyl nitrite is given first because it can be inhaled. Methemoglobin directly competes with ferricytochrome A_3 to form a methemoglobin-CN^- complex. This cyanomethemoglobin complex is relatively nontoxic. In a second step, sodium thiosulfate is given intravenously. This reagent reacts with cyanomethemoglobin to form thiocyanate, which is harmless and is excreted in urine. The first step is necessary simply to remove CN^- from the respiratory chain. Approximately 25% to 40% of the patient's total hemoglobin is converted to methemoglobin in this step; this methemoglobin is rapidly reconverted to oxyhemoglobin by red cell enzymes. The antidotes that are involved in each step are now sold commercially as a cyanide antidote package by Eli Lilly and Company (Indianapolis, IN).

Carbon Monoxide

Carbon monoxide (CO) intoxication produces tissue hypoxia as a result of decreased oxygen transport. Carbon monoxide disrupts oxygen transport by binding to hemoglobin to form a reversible complex, carboxyhemoglobin. It also produces toxicity by decreasing or inhibiting oxyhemoglobin saturation by shifting the oxyhemoglobin dissociation curve to the right and by binding to other heme-containing proteins such as myoglobin and cytochrome A_3. Binding to cytochrome A_3 inhibits cellular respiration and electron transport, whereas binding to hemoglobin decreases the oxygen reserve available to cardiac and skeletal muscle, with cardiac muscle being more severely affected.

Because the brain and heart are most susceptible to carbon monoxide poisoning, carbon monoxide intoxication is commonly manifested through respiratory, neurologic, and cardiac symptoms, with dyspnea being a principal symptom. Others include headache, visual disturbances, tachycardia, syncope, tachypnea, coma, convulsions, and death. Symptoms correlate somewhat with blood carboxyhemoglobin concentrations. However, diagnosis is difficult, because no pathognomonic symptoms occur except for a cherry red color of the face that is a strong clue to acute CO poisoning. CO poisoning should enter into the differential diagnosis of an acute encephalopathic state in the appropriate circumstances or setting.

A co-oximeter is used to make the definitive diagnosis by measuring the concentration of blood carboxyhemoglobin. This instrument is a dedicated spectrophotometer that measures total hemoglobin and the percentage of carboxyhemoglobin, oxyhemoglobin, and methemoglobin by screening at four different wavelengths simultaneously. This accurate and rapid analysis is mandatory to establish the diagnosis and should be performed with minimal delay after CO exposure.

Treatment is mainly with 100% oxygen, with additional supportive treatment given as necessary.

Alcohols and Glycols

Methanol (wood alcohol) poisoning occurs in patients who ingest methylated spirits or methanol-containing antifreeze. It is rapidly absorbed from the GI tract and is metabolized and excreted at approximately 20% of the rate of ethanol. The toxic range is thought to be 60 to 250 mL, although as little as 15 mL has caused death. Alcohol dehydrogenase metabolizes methanol to formaldehyde and formic acid, which is responsible for ocular toxicity (diminished light sensation or frank blindness), and anion gap metabolic acidosis, which are the principal symptoms of intoxication. Other symptoms include nausea, vomiting, headache, seizures, and coma. GC-MS is used to measure blood methanol levels, with a peak level greater than 50 mg/dL considered to be toxic. In addition, serum osmolality levels are increased to levels greater than 300 mOsm. Methanol (or ethylene glycol) poisoning should be considered in acutely ill patients with hyperosmolarity, metabolic acidosis, and increased anion gap.

Ethylene glycol (1, 2-ethanediol) is used in car radiator antifreeze. It has a half-life of approximately three hours and is metabolized to three major toxic compounds: glycolaldehyde, glycolic acid, and glyoxylic acid. The oxidation of ethylene glycol to glycolaldehyde is catalyzed by liver alcohol dehydrogenase. Both oxalic acid and formic acid are formed in smaller amounts. Oxalic acid itself is a highly toxic compound, which can rapidly precipitate as calcium oxalate in various tissues as well as in urine. The formation of these crystals in urine, although not a constant finding, is an important diagnostic clue to ethylene glycol poisoning. The metabolite that accumulates in the highest concentrations in the blood is glycolic acid, and its concentration in blood and urine appears to correlate directly with symptoms and mortality. It is the major contributor to the high anion gap seen in metabolic acidosis. The fatal dose of ethylene glycol is approximately 100 g, and anuria and necrosis are the principal symptoms of acute poisoning. Other symptoms include nausea and vomiting, myoclonus, seizures, convulsions, depressed reflexes, and coma. Definitive diagnosis of ethylene glycol intoxication can be made by measuring serum ethylene glycol and glycolic acid by HPLC.

Treatment of both ethylene glycol and methanol toxicity is similar and is based on the patient's symptoms and serum level. The mainstay of treatment is ethanol therapy, because ethanol competes with both methanol and ethylene glycol in metabolism by alcohol dehydrogenase. If this enzyme is saturated by ethanol, methanol and ethylene glycol metabolism is decreased, their toxic products do not build up in the tissues, and the parent compounds may be excreted unchanged in the urine. In addition to ethanol, intravenous alkali (bicarbonate) therapy is generally begun in the acidotic patient, to correct the metabolic acidosis. Dialysis, either hemodialysis or peritoneal dialysis, is also used to remove either parent compound and its corresponding toxic metabolic products.

Ethanol (Table 17–8) is probably the most common drug of abuse and is frequently responsible for the presentation of patients with altered mental status to hospitals and emergency rooms. Ethanol is rapidly absorbed from the GI tract, has a volume of distribution approximately equal to that of total body water, and diffuses freely in body tissues. It is predominantly metabolized by hepatic alcohol dehydrogenase to acetaldehyde and acetic acid and then, by way of the Krebs cycle, to carbon dioxide and water. The fatal dose is generally 300 to 400 mL of pure ethanol (600 to 800 mL of 100 proof whiskey) consumed in less than one hour. Peak plasma concentrations usually are reached within one hour after ingestion. Table 17–8 summarizes the effects of different levels of ethanol in serum on human function.

Ethanol acts as a sedative-hypnotic and depresses the CNS irregularly in descending order from cortex to medulla. Acute intoxication may be manifested by decreased inhibitions, incoordination, blurred vision, slurred speech, stupor, coma, seizures, and death. Most fatal intoxications occur at blood concentrations greater than 400 mg/dL. Capillary and arterial blood samples most accurately reflect brain ethanol concentrations. Serum ethanol concentrations are usually determined by enzymatic, gas chromatographic, or electrochemical oxidation techniques. In the most accurate assays for ethanol, serum is incubated with alcohol dehydrogenase, which oxidizes ethanol to acetaldehyde, and NAD is converted to NADH. Thus, simple monitoring of the absorbance of the incubated serum at 340 nm gives a direct determination of alcohol present. Acute poisoning is generally treated by supportive therapy, gastric lavage with tap water, or hemodialysis, if indicated (>500 mg/dL). Symptoms of chronic intoxication, such as acute alcoholic mania, may be treated with diazepam. Phenytoin may be used in patients with a history of seizures.

Isopropyl alcohol has a half-life of approximately three hours and a volume of distribution similar to that of ethanol. It

Table 17–8. INFLUENCE OF ACUTE ETHANOL INGESTION ON ETHANOL LEVELS AND BEHAVIOR

Whiskey (Ounces)	Blood Concentration	Influence
1–2	10–50 mg/dL (2.2–10.9 mmol/L)	None to mild euphoria
3–4	50–100 mg/dL (10.9–21.7 mmol/L) or greater	Mild influence on stereoscopic vision and dark adaptation
	100 mg/dL (21.7 mmol/L)	Legally intoxicated
4–6	100–150 mg/dL (21.7–32.6 mmol/L)	Euphoria; disappearance of inhibition; prolonged reaction time
6–7	150–200 mg/dL (32.6–43.4 mmol/L)	Moderately severe poisoning; reaction time greatly prolonged; loss of inhibition and slight disturbances in equilibrium and coordination
8–9	200–250 mg/dL (43.4–54.3 mmol/L)	Severe degree of poisoning; disturbances of equilibrium and coordination; retardation of the thought processes and clouding of consciousness
10–15	250–400 mg/dL (54.3–86.8 mmol/L)	Deep, possibly fatal coma

is readily absorbed through the GI tract and is metabolized at approximately 50% of the rate of ethanol. The metabolism of isopropanol occurs mainly by alcohol dehydrogenase to produce acetone, carbon dioxide, and water. The fatal dose of ingestion is 250 mL. Both isopropyl alcohol and its major metabolite, acetone, are CNS depressants.

CNS depression is the principal symptom of acute isopropanol intoxication. In addition, it produces significant GI irritation, which may be manifested by nausea and vomiting, including hematemesis, abdominal pain, and gastritis, as well as melena. Other symptoms include confusion, coma, hypertension, respiratory failure, and death.

The diagnosis of isopropanol intoxication is difficult to make. Clues to the diagnosis include acetonuria, acetonemia and hyperosmolarity without glycosuria, hyperglycemia, or acidosis. Gas chromatography is generally considered to be the best technique to determine isopropanol blood concentrations. Treatment includes supportive care, activated charcoal with gastric lavage, and hemodialysis in severe poisoning.

Arsenic

Arsenic is used in ant poisons, rodenticides, herbicides and weed killers, insecticides, paints, wood preservatives, ceramics, in the production of various metal alloys, in livestock feed, as a tanning agent, and in medicines. Inorganic arsenicals, including sodium arsenate and lead or copper arsenite; organic arsenicals, such as carbarsone and tryparsamide; and arsine gas are the major toxicologic forms of arsenic. Arsine gas poisoning generally occurs in the industrial setting, where its production arises from the action of acid or water on arsenic-bearing metals.

Arsenic is readily absorbed through the GI tract and lungs, whereas absorption through the skin occurs more slowly. Twenty-four hours after ingestion, arsenic is distributed to all body tissues. The major route of excretion is through the kidneys. Arsenic can cross the placenta.

The major concern with arsenic ingestion is systemic poisoning, presumably through its reversible interaction with multiple enzyme sulfhydryl groups. This, in turn, leads to the disruption of multiple metabolic systems.

Arsine gas, the most dangerous form of arsenic, may irreversibly attach to sulfhydryl groups of hemoglobin, causing intravascular hemolysis, hemoglobinemia, and consequent acute renal failure, as well as direct nephrotoxicity.

The acute fatal dosage of arsenic trioxide is approximately 120 mg, whereas less than 30 parts per million (ppm) of arsenic gas can produce poisoning. Organic arsenicals release arsenic slowly and have a fatal dose of approximately 0.1 to 0.5 g/kg.

Acute toxicity is usually manifested within the first hour of ingestion, and generally reflects multiorgan involvement. GI symptoms are the most common presentation, with burning and dryness of the mouth and throat, difficulty in swallowing, vomiting, and watery or bloody diarrhea containing shreds of intestinal lining or mucus. There may be the odor of garlic on the breath, and a metallic taste in the patient's mouth. Cyanosis, hypotension, tachycardia, and ventricular arrhythmias may develop. Neuropathy usually occurs late (approximately one to two weeks) after ingestion, or it may become most intense during this time period. Severe volume depletion and acute renal tubular necrosis may occur, with death resulting from circulatory failure. Symptoms of poisoning with arsine gas usually manifest approximately 2 to 24 hours after exposure and may initially include nausea and vomiting, headache, anorexia, and paresthesias. Hematemesis and abdominal pain are also common, and acute renal failure, cardiac damage, anemia and hemolysis, or pulmonary edema may also occur. The diagnosis of chronic intoxication is usually difficult and should be considered in patients with a combination of GI symptoms; neuropathy; and cutaneous, cardiovascular, and renal disturbances.

2

Analysis of urine, hair, and nails, using ion emission spectroscopy, is important for the diagnosis of chronic arsenic poisoning. Treatment of acute poisoning includes removal of residual arsenic by gastric lavage or emesis, and treatment with dimercaprol, or British antilewisite (BAL), which combines with arsenic through its sulfhydryl groups to produce cyclic water-soluble complexes. However, the inherent toxicity of this compound limits its therapeutic usefulness. Less toxic derivatives of BAL have recently been synthesized, and one compound, 2, 3-dithioerythritol, appears to be less toxic in cell culture while showing greater efficacy than BAL at rescuing arsenical poisoned cells in culture (Boyd, 1989). In severe poisoning, hemodialysis can be used to remove the arsenic-dimercaprol complexes.

Mercury

Mercury compounds exist in four different forms with different toxicologic potential: elemental or metallic (Hg°); mercurous (Hg^{+}); mercuric (Hg^{2+}); and alkyl mercury—that is, organomercurials.

Elemental mercury is poorly absorbed from the GI tract if mucosal integrity is preserved, and it shows no toxic effect unless it is converted to the divalent form. This may occur slowly by oxidation-reduction with water and chloride ion if a GI site for mercury stasis exists, but this scenario is uncommon. Significant poisoning occurs with elemental mercury when it is inhaled or absorbed through the skin. It can pass through the blood-brain barrier and can accumulate in the CNS, where oxidation produces mercuric ion; thus, primarily pulmonary and CNS toxicities are produced.

Of the two inorganic salts of mercury, mercurous (Hg^{+}) salts are poorly soluble and thus poorly absorbed. However, the mercuric (Hg^{2+}) salt is readily soluble and is readily absorbed after oral ingestion or inhalation. Severe inflammation of the mouth as well as other GI symptoms can result. The kidney is also a preferred site of accumulation of inorganic mercuric compounds, where acute renal tubular and glomerular damage can ensue. Both elemental mercury and the inorganic mercury compounds are excreted mainly in urine.

In contrast to elemental and inorganic mercury, organic mercury compounds, containing alkyl, aryl, and alkoxyalkyl moieties, are environmental pollutants. These compounds contain at least one covalent mercury-carbon bond. Both the alkoxyalkyl and aryl mercurial compounds undergo metabolic breakdown and biotransformation to produce inorganic mercury, which toxicologically acts and manifests intoxication as would the above-mentioned inorganic mercury compounds. In contrast, the mercury-carbon bonds that occur within the methyl-forms and ethyl-forms are extremely stable and produce greater toxicity than the aryl and the alkoxyalkyl forms. The alkyl forms are more lipid soluble, pass readily through biological membranes and, on ingestion, show generally greater absorption into the body. Their major chemical effect is on the CNS, and they show a biological half-life of 70 to 90 days. Because bile is the major route of excretion, methyl-mercury can be reabsorbed into the blood, accounting, in part, for its extended half-life.

The major mechanism of action of mercury poisoning is through covalent bonding with protein sulfhydryl groups, producing widespread and nonspecific enzyme dysfunction, inactivation, and denaturation.

Mercury, depending on its form, may cause systemic toxicity or local skin and mucous membrane lesions. Both organic and elemental mercury can cause CNS effects, whereas GI symptoms primarily occur with inorganic salts. Elemental mercury may also produce severe pulmonary reactions.

In general, acute toxicity, with elemental, inorganic, or most organic forms, can be diagnosed from 24-hour urine levels. Blood levels may rise rapidly after acute exposure but fall rapidly and may not reflect total body burden. In contrast, because the short chain alkyl organic mercuric compounds are mainly excreted in the bile, blood levels are better indicators of tissue levels and significant acute exposure. Hair analysis for mercury may help identify chronic mercury exposure.

Treatment includes gastric lavage or emesis to remove the ingested poison, as well as the use of dimercaprol and penicillamine. However, in methyl-mercury and alkyl-mercury poisoning, dimercaprol is contraindicated because it has been found to increase the concentration of these compounds in the brain (Bryson, 1989). In these cases, treatment is symptomatic, although new agents are being evaluated clinically.

Iron

Acute iron poisoning is common in young children and is usually the result of ingestion of iron-containing products. Although ferric ions from food are usually reduced to ferrous ions and absorbed in the stomach, the large and small bowel can rapidly absorb toxic amounts (>30 mg/kg) of elemental iron. Once absorbed into the body, iron removal is difficult. Large doses of iron are thought to cause acute mucosal cell damage, and significant absorption of iron occurs once the binding capacity of transferrin is exceeded. Unbound iron in the serum causes toxicity by hepatic cell damage, shock, and production of lactic acidosis.

Vomiting appears to be an early manifestation of iron intoxication, along with severe gastroenteritis, melena, abdominal pain, and hematemesis. This occurs up to six hours after ingestion. For up to the next 10 hours, the patient may appear to improve. This is deceptive because manifestations of systemic toxicity (cyanosis, convulsions, shock, coagulopathy, renal and hepatic failure) may occur, producing death. Both patients who develop severe systemic symptoms and those who do not may develop late complications, including GI obstructions or strictures.

Definitive diagnosis is made with measurements of serum iron concentration and the total iron-binding capacity (TIBC) of transferrin. In addition to supportive treatment, emesis or gastric lavage with sodium bicarbonate is used to prevent iron absorption. Chelation therapy with deferoxamine is also used if the acute intoxication is severe.

Lead

Both organic and inorganic compounds of lead may be highly toxic, with their most serious effects occurring in the central and peripheral nervous system. Absorption may occur by either inhalation or ingestion. If greater than 0.5 mg of lead is absorbed per day, lead accumulation and toxicity are believed to occur, whereas 0.5 g of absorbed lead is considered a fatal dose. However, acute toxicity is uncommon and is generally observed in patients who have been exposed to high concentrations of lead dusts. Lead poisoning is seen in children in large cities who consume lead in the form of paint (pica). Acute manifestations are primarily CNS symptoms (encephalopathy, convulsions, stupor), and GI symptoms such as colic. Chronic toxicity with lead accumulating in blood, soft tissues, and bone is more common. The largest body compartment of lead is bone, which contains approximately 96% of the total body burden. The half-life of lead in bone is 32 years, and bone may act as a reservoir for endogenous intoxication. Chronic toxicity may be manifested by a wide range of systemic effects, including general malaise, weight loss, anorexia, constipation; lead encephalopathy exhibited by malaise with apathy, drowsiness, stupor, and seizures; peripheral neuropathy with wrist drop or foot drop; and lead nephrosis with albuminuria, hematuria, and pyuria and anemia (hypochromic, normocytic) with basophilic stippling, the latter finding often a strong clue.

In addition, recent reports suggest that lead-induced pathologic changes may occur at even low levels of lead exposure. Needleman and Gatsonis (1990) reviewed 24 recent studies of childhood lead exposure to provide statistical evidence that low doses of lead may produce an intellectual deficit in children. Schwartz and colleagues (1990) examined lead-induced anemia in children one to five years of age, using a cross-sectional epidemiologic study. They found a relationship between age, blood lead level, and hematocrit such that younger children had an increased risk of anemia at lower blood levels than children only a few years older. It thus appears that lead may produce deleterious effects, especially in children, at low levels of exposure. Generally, serum lead levels greater than 25 μg/mL are considered to be toxic if present chronically in children.

Organolead compounds, such as tetraethyl and tetramethyl lead, are lipid soluble and, like the organomercurials discussed previously, produce their major toxic effects on the CNS. Lead encephalopathy may occur early in the onset of intoxication, and does not correlate well with blood lead concentrations. Hyperactive deep tendon reflexes, intention tremor, abnormal jaw jerk, and abnormalities of stance and gait are the most consistently observed neurologic manifestations of organolead toxicity.

Lead appears to interact with thiol, carboxylic, and phosphate groups to form stable complexes with enzymes and proteins (Bryson, 1989). This is particularly well known for heme synthesis, in which lead blocks the action of δ-aminolevulinic acid (ALA) synthetase, δ-ALA dehydratase (ALAD), coproporphyrinogen decarboxylase, and ferrochelatase, producing anemia. These disruptions in heme synthesis allow for objective testing for inorganic lead exposure. Increased amounts of ALA in urine, decreased ALAD activity in red blood cells, increased amounts of free erythrocyte protoporphyrin, and elevated amounts of zinc protoporphyrin are found with inorganic lead poisoning. The assay for zinc protoporphyrin is a particularly simple fluorimetric one that is widely used and is an excellent screening test. The most sensitive screening test for organolead poisoning is decreased ALAD activity in urine because changes in the other enzymes and products of heme synthesis are not consistent. Although whole blood lead concentrations are a reliable indicator of recent lead exposure, the short half-life of circulating lead in blood makes estimates of total body burden unreliable.

Treatment of poisoning includes supportive therapy, as well as removal of soluble lead compounds by gastric lavage. Dilute magnesium sulfate or sodium sulfate solutions are commonly used. In addition, chelating agents such as dimercaprol, calcium disodium edetate, and penicillamine may be used, if necessary.

QUANTITATION OF LEAD IN SERUM. Lead levels in serum may be determined directly using either atomic absorption spectroscopy or a newer, more readily accessible method called anode stripping. In the first method, the sample is heated to temperatures wherein the outer shell electrons of lead atoms absorb ultraviolet light. The absorption of light is proportional to the concentration of lead in the sample.

In the second method, a voltaic cell is set up such that the anode consists of a mercury-coated graphite rod. When a negative potential is applied to this anode, cationic metals, such as lead, become deposited in their metallic forms on the anode. The applied voltage is then stopped. Because there is an excess of electrons on the anode, current flows to the cathode. Each of the metals deposited on the anode will therefore become oxidized back to its respective ionic form, that is, be stripped from the anode. The metals with lowest oxidation potentials strip first. Each metal strips from the anode in the order of oxidation potential, recorded as the half-wave potential (as described in Chap. 3), which is a constant for a given metal. The total current associated with the stripping of each metal is proportional to the concentration of that metal.

Organophosphates and Carbamates

The organophosphates are esters of phosphoric acid or thiophosphoric acid, whereas the carbamates are synthetic derivatives of carbamic acid. Although these are two distinctly different types of compounds, they both interfere with neurotransmission and are widely used as pesticides in agriculture. Both compounds inhibit the enzyme acetylcholinesterase (AchE), which normally hydrolyzes the neurotransmitter acetylcholine (Ach) after Ach has effected an action potential and has been released from its receptor site. Both compounds produce inhibition by reacting with the active site of AchE. This occurs by phosphorylation with the organophosphates to produce a relatively stable phosphate ester bond; and by carbamoylation with the carbamates to form a more labile, and hence more easily reversible, carbamate ester bond. Both compounds thus cause accumulation of Ach at neuronal synapses and myoneural junctions to produce toxicity.

Ach is an important neurotransmitter in both the peripheral and central nervous systems. It is located at a number of different synapses in the CNS, at the ganglionic synapses between the sympathetic and parasympathetic preganglionic and postganglionic fibers, at the junctions between parasympathetic postganglionic fibers and effector organs, and at the junctions between somatic motor neurons and skeletal muscle cells. Thus, signs and symptoms of organophosphate poisoning include parasympathetic manifestations such as salivation, lacrimation, urination, and defecation (SLUD); pupillary constriction; bradycardia; and bronchoconstriction, which may predominate at low-dose poisoning. Autonomic ganglionic and somatic motor manifestations (such as muscular weakness, twitching, areflexia, tachycardia, and hypertension) and CNS manifestations (such as confusion, slurred speech, ataxia, convulsions, and respiratory and cardiovascular center depression) may predominate in severe intoxication. Death usually results from respiratory failure as a result of a combination of central depression, bronchospasm, excessive bronchial secretions, and respiratory muscle paralysis.

It should be noted that rates of morbidity and mortality due to carbamate poisoning are lower, because carbamates do not penetrate the CNS as effectively as organophosphates and central cholinergic effects are thus minimal. In addition, the much greater lability of the carbamate ester bond allows for spontaneous reactivation of AchE. This, in turn, decreases the slope of the toxicity dose-response curve, as compared with the curve for organophosphates, such that small increments in carbamate dose are less likely to produce severe increases in toxicity.

In addition to acute poisoning, organophosphates may produce a so-called intermediate syndrome occurring one to four days after poisoning, as well as delayed neurotoxicity usually occurring two to five weeks after acute exposure. The intermediate syndrome develops after acute cholinergic crisis and appears to involve cranial nerve palsies, proximal limb weakness, and respiratory paralysis, with the patient requiring ventilatory support (Senanayake, 1987). In contrast, delayed neurotoxicity, which is not seen with all organophosphate compounds, appears to be due to neurotoxic esterase inhibition and usually produces a distal and symmetric sensorimotor polyneuropathy of the extremities (Davies, 1987; Tafuri, 1987).

Diagnosis of organophosphate poisoning depends on a history of exposure shortly before the onset of illness, signs and symptoms of diffuse parasympathetic stimulation, and laboratory confirmation of exposure by measurement of erythrocyte acetylcholinesterase and plasma pseudocholinesterase activities. Whereas AchE is found primarily in nervous tissue and erythrocytes, pseudocholinesterase is found in plasma. The latter enzyme is much more nonspecific in its action than AchE, in that in addition to hydrolysis of Ach, pseudocholinesterase can hydrolyze many other natural and synthetic esters. Both activities may be decreased, and both activities can be measured in the laboratory. However, only inhibition of AchE is considered specific for organophosphate poisoning because a number of conditions may produce a low plasma pseudocholinesterase level (Tafuri, 1987). Thus, the latter measurement is more sensitive but less specific than the red blood cell cholinesterase level for organophosphate poisoning. Generally, levels 30% to 50% of normal indicate exposure, and toxic manifestations occur with greater than 50% inhibition; however, symptoms may not appear until levels are 20% or less of normal. In actuality, confirmation of poisoning, rather than diagnosis, occurs by laboratory determinations. Because baseline values of cholinesterase levels prior to exposure are unlikely to be available, sequential postexposure cholinesterase determinations appear to be the best way to confirm organophosphate poisoning (Coye, 1987).

Treatment of acute poisoning includes respiratory support, if necessary, decontamination of the patient, and gastric lavage or emesis. In the presence of symptoms, atropine is given to ameliorate excessive parasympathetic stimulation by competitively blocking the action of Ach at muscarinic receptors. Pralidoxime also may be given as a specific antidote for organophosphate poisoning. If pralidoxime is given within 24 to 36 hours of exposure, it may reactivate phosphorylated cholinesterase by removal of the covalently bound phosphate group from the enzyme's active site. Chronic poisoning is usually treated by avoidance of further exposure until cholinesterase levels become normal.

General References

Bryson PD: Comprehensive Review in Toxicology. Rockville, MD, Aspen Publishers, 1989.

Budavari S, O'Neil MJ, Smith A, Heckelman PE: The Merck Index: An Encyclopedia of Chemicals, Drugs and Biologicals, 11th ed. Rahway, Merck and Co, 1989.

Reynolds JEF: Martindale, the Extra Pharmacopoeia, 29th ed. London, The Pharmaceutical Press, 1989.

Drugs of Abuse: Drug Assay Methods

Azmitia EC, Murphy RB, Whitaker-Azmitia PM: MDMA (ecstasy) effects on cultured serotonergic neurons: Evidence for Ca^{2+}-dependent toxicity linked to release. Brain Res 1990; 510:97–103.

Bayorh MA, Zokowska-Grojec Z, Palkovits M, Kopin IJ: Effect of phencyclidine (PCP) on blood pressure and catecholamine levels in discrete brain nuclei. Brain Res 1984; 321:315.

Bell J, Seres V, Bowron P, et al: The use of serum methadone levels in patients receiving methadone maintenance. Clin Pharmacol Ther 1988; 43:623.

Davis IM, Bousquet RW, Childs PS: Gas chromatography/mass spectroscopy in clinical and forensic toxicology. Service Training and Continuing Education 1989; 10(12):7–21.

DeCresce RP, Mazura AC, Lifshitz MS, Tilson JE: Drug Testing in the Workplace. Chicago, American Society of Clinical Pathology Press, 1989.

Hurd YL, Kehr J, Ungerstedt U: In vivo microdialysis as a technique to monitor drug transport: Correlation of extracellular cocaine levels and dopamine outflow in the rat brain. J Neurochem 1988; 51:1314.

Johanson C-E, Fischman MW: The pharmacology of cocaine related to its abuse. Pharmac Rev 1989; 41:3.

Lange RA, Cigarroc RO, Yancy CW Jr, et al: Cocaine-induced coronary artery vasoconstriction. N Engl J Med 1989; 321:1557.

Murphy RB, Pincus MR, Beinfeld MC, et al: Enkephalin is a competitive antagonist of cholecystokinin in the gastrointestinal tract, as predicted from prior conformational analysis. J Protein Chem 1992; 11:731–737.

Pincus MR, Carty RP, Chen JM, et al: On the biologically active structures of cholecystokinin, little gastrin and enkephalin in the gastrointestinal system and in brain. Proc Natl Acad Sci USA 1987; 84:4821.

Pincus MR, Rendell M: General quantitative treatment for the binding of divalent antibodies to antigens immobilized on a solid phase. Proc Natl Acad Sci USA 1981; 78:5924.

Rodbard D, Ruder HJ, Vaitukaitis J, Jacobs HS: Mathematical analysis of kinetics of radioligand assays: Improved sensitivity obtained by delayed addition of labeled ligand. J Clin Endocrinol Metab 1971; 33:343.

Schuster DI, Ehrlich GK, Murphy RB: Purification and partial amino acid sequence of 28 kda cyclophilin-like component of the rat liver sigma receptor. Life Sci 1994; 55:1–6.

Thompson WG, Mahr RG, Yohannan W, Pincus MR: Use of creatine kinase MB isozyme for diagnosing myocardial infarction when total creatine kinase activity is high. J Clin Chem 1988; 34:2208.

Therapeutic Drugs

Gilman AG, Goodman LS, Rall TW, Murad F: The Pharmacological Basis of Therapeutics. New York, Macmillan Publishing Co, 1985.

Hess AD, Esa AH, Colombani PM: Mechanisms of action of cyclosporine: Effect on cells of the immune system and on subcellular events in T cell activation. Transplant Proc 1988; 22(Suppl. 2):29.

Kahan BD: Pharmacokinetics and pharmacodynamics of cyclosporine. Transplant Proc 1989; 21(Suppl 1):9.

Kronbach T, Fischer V, Meyer VA: Cyclosporine metabolism in human liver: Identification of a cytochrome P-450 III gene family as the major cyclosporine-metabolizing enzyme explains interactions of cyclosporine with other drugs. Clin Pharmacol Ther 1988; 43:630.

Roenigk HH, Auerbach R, Maibach HI, Weinstein GD: Methotrexate in psoriasis: Revised guidelines. J Am Acad Dermatol 1988; 19:145.

Tugwell P, Bennett K, Gent M: Methotrexate in rheumatoid arthritis: Indications, contraindications, efficacy, and safety. Ann Intern Med 1987a; 107:358.

Tugwell P, Bennett K, Gent M: Position paper: Methotrexate in rheumatoid arthritis. Ann Intern Med 1987b; 107:418.

Uetrecht JP: Mechanism of drug-induced lupus. Chem Res Toxicol 1988; 1:133.

Wittes RE, Leyland-Jones B, Fortner C, Hubbard SM: Chemotherapy: The properties and uses of single agents: Methotrexate. *In* Wittes RE (ed): Manual of Oncologic Therapeutics 1989/1990. Philadelphia, JB Lippincott, 1989, pp 134–138.

Yaari Y, Selzer ME, Pincus JH: Phenytoin: Mechanism of its anticonvulsant action. Ann Neurol 1986; 20:171.

Environmental Carcinogenesis

Ames BN, Durston WE, Yamasaki E, Lee FD: Carcinogens are mutagens: A simple test system combining liver homogenates for activation and bacteria for detection. Proc Natl Acad Sci USA 1973; 70:2281.

Ames BN, McCann J, Yamasaki E: Methods for detecting carcinogens and mutagens with *Salmonella*/mammalian microsome mutagenicity test. Mutation Res 1975; 31:447.

Balmain A, Pragnell IB: Mouse skin carcinomas induced *in vitro* by chemical carcinogens have a transforming Harvey *ras*-oncogene. Nature (London) 1983; 303:72.

Barbacid M: *ras*-Genes. Annu Rev Biochem 1987; 56:779.

Brandt-Rauf PW, Pincus MR, Adelson SP: Carcinoma of the gall bladder. A study of 42 cases. Hum Pathol 1982; 13:48.

Brandt-Rauf PW, Smith S, Niman H, et al: Serum oncogene proteins in foundry workers. J Soc Occup Med 1990; 40:11–14.

Brandt-Rauf PW, Smith S, Hemminki K, et al: Serum oncoproteins and growth factors in asbestosis and silicosis patients. Int J Cancer 1992; 50:881–885.

Chen JM, Lee G, Murphy RB, et al: Comparison of the computed structures for the phosphate-binding loop of the p21 protein containing oncogenic site Gly 12 with the x-ray crystallographic structures for this region in the p21 protein with EFtu. A model for the structure of the p21 protein in its oncogenic form. J Biomol Structure Dynamics 1989; 6:859.

Cheng KC, Krutsch HC, Park SS, et al: Amino-terminal sequence and structure of monoclonal antibody–immunopurified cytochrome P-450. Biochemistry 1986; 25:2397.

Chung DL, Brandt-Rauf PW, Weinstein IB, et al: Evidence that the *ras*-oncogene-encoded p21 protein induces oocyte maturation *via* activation of protein kinase c. Proc Natl Acad Sci USA 1993–1996; 1992.

De Vivo M, Marion MJ, Smith SJ, et al: Mutant c-K-*ras*-p21 in chemical carcinogenesis in humans exposed to vinyl chloride. Cancer Causes and Control 1995; 5:273–278.

Fasano O, Aldrich T, Tamanoi F, et al: Analysis of the transforming potential of the human H-*ras* gene by random mutagenesis. Proc Natl Acad Sci USA 1984; 81:4008.

Frazier ME, Lyndberg RA, Mueller DM: Oncogene involvement in plutonium-induced carcinogenesis. Int J Rad Biol 1986; 49:542.

Henderson RF, Bechtold WE, Bond JA, Sun JD: The use of biological markers in toxicology. Crit Rev Toxicol 1989; 20:65.

Niman HL, Thompson AMH, Yu A, et al: Anti-peptide antibodies detect oncogene-related proteins in urine. Proc Natl Acad Sci USA 1985; 82:7924.

Perera F, Hemminki K, Young T, et al: Detection of polycyclic aromatic hydrocarbon-DNA adducts in white blood cells. Cancer Res 1988; 48:2888.

Pincus MR, Brandt-Rauf PW: Protein structure and cancer. Cancer Invest 1985; 4:185.

Pincus MR, van Renswoude J, Harford JB, et al: Prediction of the three-dimensional structure of the transforming region of the EJ/T24 human bladder oncogene product and its normal cellular homologue. Proc Natl Acad Sci USA 1983; 80:5253.

Pincus MR, Chung DL, Dykes DC, et al: Pathways for activation of the *ras*-oncogene-encoded p21 protein. Ann Clin Lab Sci 1992; 22:323–342.

Santella R, Hatch M, Pirastu R, Brandt-Rauf PW: Carcinogen evaluation: In vitro testing, in vivo testing, and epidemiology. Semin Occupational Med 1987; 2:245.

Smith MR, Liu Y-L, Kim H, et al: Inhibition of serum- and *ras*-stimulated

DNA synthesis by antibodies to phospholipase C. Science 1990; 247: 1074–1077.
Stacey DW, Kung H-F: Transformation of NIH 3T3 cells by microinjection of Ha-*ras*-p21 protein. Nature (London) 1984; 310:508–511.

Toxins and Acute Poisoning

Boyd VL, Harbell JW, O'Connor RJ, McGown EL: 2,3-Dithioerythritol, a possible new arsenic antidote. Chem Res Toxicol 1989; 2:301.
Coye MJ, Barnett PG, Midtling JE, et al: Clinical confirmation of organophosphate poisoning by serial cholinesterase analyses. Arch Intern Med 1987; 147:438.
Davies JE: Changing profile of pesticide poisoning. N Engl J Med 1987; 316:807.
Dreisbach RH, Robertson WO: Handbook of Poisoning. Norwalk, CT, Appleton and Lange, 1987.
Klaasen CD, Amdur MO, Doull J: Casarett and Doull's Toxicology: The Basic Science of Poisons, 3rd ed. New York, Macmillan Publishing Co, 1986.
Needleman MD, Gatsonis CA: Low-level lead exposure and the IQ of children: A meta-analysis of modern studies. JAMA 1990; 263:673.
Schwartz J, Landrigan PJ, Baker EL Jr, et al: Lead-induced anemia: Dose-response relationships and evidence for a threshold. Am J Public Health 1990; 80:165.
Senanayake N, Karalliedde L: Neurotoxic effects of organophosphorus insecticides: An intermediate syndrome. N Engl J Med 1987; 316:761.
Shihabi ZK: Applications of Capillary Electrophoresis in the Clinical Laboratory. Check Sample, Vol. 33. Clinical Chemistry No. CC 94–4 (CC-242). Chicago, American Society of Clinical Pathologists, 1993.
Tafuri J, Roberts J: Organophosphate poisoning. Ann Emerg Med 1987; 16:193.
Zwiener RJ, Ginsburg CM: Organophosphate and carbamate poisoning in infants and children. Pediatrics 1988; 81:121.

2

Part 3

URINE AND OTHER BODY FLUIDS

Edited by
John Bernard Henry, M.D.

Chapter 18

Basic Examination of Urine

John Bernard Henry, M.D.
Reginaldo B. Lauzon, M.S., MT(ASCP)
G. Berry Schumann, M.D.

The examination of urine provides a wide variety of useful medical information regarding the diseases involving the kidney and lower urinary tract. Both functional (physiologic) and structural (anatomic) disorders of the kidney and lower urinary tract may be elucidated, and diagnostic, monitoring, and prognostic information may be gathered as well. When properly performed, urine testing provides data and interpretations obtained without pain, danger, and with only minimal distress to the patient. We believe laboratory urine tests will remain an essential part of clinical medicine.

Many clinical laboratory disciplines are involved in the evaluation of urine. These include chemistry, microbiology, routine wet urinalysis, cytology, and other specialty sections. New technologies, including immunocytochemistry, molecular and genetic biology, DNA ploidy, and cell cycle analysis, will continue to expand potential diagnostic and prognostic information. It is important that users of urine laboratory tests distinguish the clinical utility of individual tests. Table 18–1 lists the benefits (i.e., for screening, diagnosis, monitoring, or prognosis) of common urine laboratory tests.

The purpose of this chapter is to discuss information produced from urinalysis. At present, three types of urinalysis are performed and they include (1) a reagent strip (dipstick) urinalysis for screening laboratories, physician offices, and patient home testing; (2) a screening wet urinalysis commonly referred to as a routine or basic urinalysis; and (3) a urinalysis that is a specialized, cytologic approach to the urine sediment. The dipstick urinalysis remains a valuable front-line test for the early detection and monitoring of patients for chemical abnormalities and is a part of every urine assessment.

Reagent strip urinalysis encompasses the physiochemical analysis of urine. It requires less sophisticated training of personnel, is easily performed in multiple settings, and provides accurate information in several clinical situations. Wet routine urinalysis provides a reliable, cost-effective screening test for urinary system disorders. Wet urinalysis procedures consist of two major components: (1) macroscopic urinalysis, or physicochemical determinations (appearance, specific gravity, and multiparameter reagent strip measurements of several chemical constituents), and (2) a brightfield or phase contrast microscopic examination of urine sediment for evidence of hematuria, pyuria, cylindruria (casts), and crystalluria. Cytodiagnostic urinalysis has gained medical acceptance as a more sensitive pathologic test for evaluating urine sediment in several renal and lower urinary tract disorders. This specialized urine cytology test has replaced the quantitative Addis count method and provides sequential information regarding the progression or regression of many urinary system conditions.

We believe that this spectrum of urinalysis meets the needs of our multidimensional health care system. Each laboratory is encouraged to identify their own unique requirements based on the patient population served and to then select the most cost-effective use of urine tests.

Table 18–1. BENEFITS OF COMMON URINE LABORATORY TESTS

		Clinical Utility			
Type of Test	**Aims**	***Screen***	***Diagnosis***	***Monitor***	***Prognosis***
Urine chemistry (Reagent strip)	Glucosuria Proteinuria Hematuria Leukocyturia Infection	+++	+/−	+	+
Wet urinalysis (routine)	Diabetes Proteinuria Hematuria Leukocyturia Infections Cylindruria Crystalluria	++++	++	++	+
Urine microbiology	Infections	++	++++	++	+
Urine cytology (conventional)	Cancer Inflammation Viral infections	+	++	+	−
Cytodiagnostic urinalysis	Glomerular and renal tubular disorders LUT disorders Nonbacterial Infections Lithiasis	+	++++	+++	++
Image cytometry and DNA analysis	Urothelial cancer	−	++	+++	+++
Flow cytometry	Urothelial cancer	−	+	+++	++

LUT = Lower urinary tract.

Courtesy of G. Berry Schumann, MD, Janet L. Schumann, CT(ASCP), and Niels Marcussen, MD, from the book *Cytodiagnostic Urinalysis of Renal and Lower Urinary Tract Disorders,* Igaku-Shoin Medical Publishers, New York, NY, 1995.

URINE FORMATION

The kidneys have the remarkable ability to select and retain essential substances while excreting end products of metabolism and excess substances from the diet. They maintain water and electrolyte balance and substantially contribute to acid-base homeostasis. To accomplish this balance, the composition of urine is varied with water and salt intake, protein intake, and metabolic status. This variability creates a practical problem in the timing of collection of urine specimens and in the use of random specimens as representative samples of urinary output. Timed (2-, 12-, 24-hour) urinary collections are therefore preferred to random specimens for quantitative tests.

In a normal adult, 25% of the cardiac output, or more than a liter of blood, perfuses the two kidneys each minute, and an ultrafiltrate of the plasma passes through each glomerular capillary tuft into Bowman's capsule. The filtrate has a pH of 7.4 and an osmolality similar to that of plasma (about 285 mOsm/kg water). The specific gravity is about 1.010. Modification of this filtrate to produce excreted urine occurs in the tubules and collecting duct of each nephron. Final concentrations depend on the state of hydration. Entering the collecting ducts, the pH is usually about 6 with a typical Western diet, and the osmolality may be increased to 800 to 1200 mOsm/kg water. In a very well-hydrated person, the osmolality is much lower because the kidneys excrete a dilute urine. The glomerular filtrate volume of about 180 L in 24 hours (for an 80-kg man) has been reduced to about 1 or 2 L, and water and sodium have been conserved. This is now urine. It passes from the collecting ducts into the kidney pelvis, ureters, bladder, and urethra to be voided. In disease states, this fluid is altered chemically and cytologically.

COMPONENTS OF BASIC (ROUTINE) URINALYSIS

A basic (routine) urinalysis is composed of four parts: specimen evaluation, gross/physical examination, chemical screening, and sediment examination.

Specimen Evaluation

Before one proceeds with any testing, the urine specimen must be evaluated in terms of its acceptability. Considerations include proper labeling, proper specimen for requested test, proper receptacle, storage conditions (time, temperature) and preservative, visible signs of contamination, and any transportation delays in moving the specimen to the laboratory. Each laboratory should have written and enforced guidelines for the acceptance or rejection of specimens. A properly labeled specimen must have the patient's full name and the date and time of collection. Additional information may be required, but these three essentials constitute minimum labeling requirements.

If only one specimen is submitted for multiple testing, bacteriologic examination should be performed first, provided that the urine has been properly collected. With pediatric patients and persons in acute renal failure, it may be necessary to process a volume of urine less than the standardized volume. In such cases, a notation should be made and tests most pertinent to the diagnosis should be performed first.

Gross/Physical Examination

Appearance

COLOR

The yellow color of urine is due largely to the pigment urochrome and to small amounts of urobilins and uroerythrin. Urochrome excretion is thought to be proportional to the metabolic rate and is increased during fever, thyrotoxicosis, and starvation. The pink pigment (uroerythrin) may be deposited in uric acid or urate crystals (brick dust deposit), and these should not be confused with blood. Pale or colorless urine in a normal person follows high fluid intake. Darker urine may be seen when fluids are withheld. Thus, the color roughly indicates the degree of hydration and urine concentration, which should correlate with urine specific gravity. Note that pale urine of high specific gravity may be found in diabetes mellitus and after the use of radiographic media.

Normal concentrated urine may show a sedimentary deposit if allowed to stand after cooling from body temperature. Precipitation due to phosphates or urates may then occur. Mucus from the urinary and genital tracts is seen as small cloudy patches (nubeculae) in normal urine.

Certain food and candy dyes color the urine (Levin, 1965), as do drugs used for investigation and therapy. An innocuous red urine associated with ingestion of beets is seen in genetically susceptible persons.

Some of the more important changes in the gross appearance of urine are described in this section. For color changes in urine in pediatric patients, see Cone (1968). A comprehensive list is provided in Table 18–2.

RED URINE. The most common abnormal color is red or red-brown. When it is seen in females, contamination with menstrual flow should be considered. The urine in hematuria

3

Table 18–2. APPEARANCE AND COLOR OF URINE

Appearance	Cause	Remarks
Colorless	Very dilute urine	Polyuria, diabetes insipidus
Cloudy	Phosphates, carbonates	Soluble in dilute acetic acid
	Urates, uric acid	Dissolve at 60°C and in alkali
	Leukocytes	Insoluble in dilute acetic acid
	Red cells ("smoky")	Lyse in dilute acetic acid
	Bacteria, yeasts	Insoluble in dilute acetic acid
	Spermatozoa	Insoluble in dilute acetic acid
	Prostatic fluid	
	Mucin, mucous threads	May be flocculent
	Calculi, "gravel"	Phosphates, oxalates
	Clumps, pus, tissue	
	Fecal contamination	Rectovesical fistula
	Radiographic dye	In acid urine
Milky	Many neutrophils (pyuria)	Insoluble in dilute acetic acid
	Fat	
	Lipiduria, opalescent	Nephrosis, crush injury—soluble in ether
	Chyluria, milky	Lymphatic obstruction—soluble in ether
	Emulsified paraffin	Vaginal creams
Yellow	Acriflavine	Green fluorescence
Yellow-orange	Concentrated urine	Dehydration, fever
	Urobilin in excess	No yellow foam
	Bilirubin	Yellow foam if sufficient bilirubin
Yellow-green	Bilirubin-biliverdin	Yellow foam
Yellow-brown	Bilirubin-biliverdin	"Beer" brown, yellow foam
Red	Hemoglobin	Positive } reagent strip for blood
	Erythrocytes	Positive } reagent strip for blood
	Myoglobin	Positive } reagent strip for blood
	Porphyrin	May be colorless
	Fuscin, aniline dye	Foods, candy
	Beets	Yellow alkaline, genetic
	Menstrual contamination	Clots, mucus
Red-purple	Porphyrins	May be colorless
Red-brown	Erythrocytes	
	Hemoglobin on standing	
	Methemoglobin	Acid pH
	Myoglobin	Muscle injury
	Bilifuscin (dipyrrole)	Result of unstable hemoglobin
Brown-black	Methemoglobin	Blood, acid pH
	Homogentisic acid	On standing, alkaline; alkaptonuria
	Melanin	On standing, rare
Blue-green	Indicans	Small intestine infections
	Pseudomonas infections	
	Chlorophyll	Mouth deodorants

(presence of red blood cells) may appear cloudy, smoky, pink, red, or brown. The urine in hemoglobinuria may be clear red, clear red-brown, or dark brown. Methemoglobin is dark brown and develops in bladder urine of acid pH or in acid urine on standing. Blood and blood pigments are easily detected by means of a reagent strip. A positive test result indicates the presence of hemoglobin or myoglobin (see Blood, Hemoglobin, and Myoglobin in Urine).

In the porphyrias, the urine may be normal, red, or purple. It is usually red in congenital erythropoietic porphyria and the cutanea tarda form of porphyria. In acute intermittent hepatic porphyria, it is normal but darkens on standing. In lead porphyrinuria, the urine color is normal. Red urine also may be associated with the use of drugs and dyes in diagnostic tests—for example, phenolsulfonphthalein (PSP), which is sometimes used in testing renal function, causes a red color in alkaline urine. In the presence of unstable hemoglobin, such as hemoglobin Köln, the urine is red-brown and does not give a positive test result for hemoglobin or for bilirubin. The pigment is probably a dipyrrole or bilifuscin.

YELLOW-BROWN OR GREEN-BROWN URINE. Yellow-brown or green-brown urine is most often associated with bile pigments, chiefly bilirubin. On shaking the urine specimen, a yellow foam may be seen, which distinguishes bilirubin from a normal, dark, concentrated urine, which has white foam. In severe obstructive jaundice, the urine may be dark green.

ORANGE-RED OR ORANGE-BROWN URINE. Urine containing large amounts of urobilin may resemble a dark, concentrated normal urine. Excreted urobilinogen is colorless but is converted in the presence of light and acid pH to urobilin, which is dark yellow or orange. Urobilin does not color the foam on shaking a urine sample. Urinary analgesics (phenazopyridines) cause an orange color and color any foam present.

DARK BROWN OR BLACK URINE. Acid urine containing hemoglobin darkens on standing because of the formation of methemoglobin. Other, rarer causes of dark brown urine are homogentisic acid (alkaptonuria) and melanin. Colorless melanogens are converted in acid urine to melanin. Urine containing homogentisic acid darkens more rapidly when alkaline. Dark brown or cola-colored urine is seen in some patients taking levodopa. See Table 18–1 for causes of colored urines and Table 18–3 for a list of common drugs causing colored urine.

Table 18–3. URINE COLOR CHANGES WITH COMMONLY USED DRUGS*

Drug	Color
Alcohol, ethyl	Pale, diuresis
Anthraquinone laxatives (senna, cascara)	Reddish, alkaline; yellow-brown, acid
Chlorzoxazone (Paraflex) (muscle relaxant)	Red
Deferoxamine mesylate (Desferal) (chelates iron)	Red
Ethoxazene (Serenium) (urinary analgesic)	Orange, red
Fluorescein sodium (given IV)	Yellow
Furazolidone (Furoxone) (Tricofuron) (an antibacterial, antiprotozoal nitrofuran)	Brown
Indigo carmine dye (renal function, cytoscopy)	Blue
Iron sorbitol (Jectofer) (possibly other iron compounds forming iron sulfide in urine)	Brown on standing
Levodopa (L-dopa) (for parkinsonism)	Red then brown, alkaline
Mepacrine (Atabrine) (antimalarial) (intestinal worms, *Giardia*)	Yellow
Methocarbamol (Robaxin) (muscle relaxant)	Green-brown
Methyldopa (Aldomet) (antihypertensive)	Darken; if oxidizing agents present, red to brown
Methylene blue (used to delineate fistulas)	Blue, blue-green
Metronidazole (Flagyl) (for *Trichomonas* infection, amebiasis, *Giardia*)	Darkening, reddish brown
Nitrofurantoin (Furadantin) (antibacterial)	Brown-yellow
Phenazopyridine (Pyridium) (urinary analgesic), also compounded with sulfonamides (Azo Gantrisin, etc.)	Orange-red, acid pH
Phenindione (Hedulin) (anticoagulant) (important to distinguish from hematuria)	Orange, alkaline; color disappears on acidifying
Phenol poisoning	Brown; oxidized to quinones (green)
Phenolphthalein (purgative)	Red-purple, alkaline pH
Phenolsulfonphthalein (also sulfobromophthalein)	Pink-red, alkaline pH
Rifampin (Rifadin, Rimactane) (tuberculosis therapy)	Bright orange-red
Riboflavin (multivitamins)	Bright yellow
Sulfasalazine (Azulfidine) for ulcerative colitis)	Orange-yellow, alkaline pH

*Other commonly used drugs have been noted to produce color change once or occasionally: amitriptyline (Elavil)—blue-green; phenothiazines—red; triamterene (Dyrenium)—pale blue (blue fluorescence in acid urine). An extensive list may be found in Young et al: Clin Chem 1975; 21:379.

Character (Clarity)

Normal urine is essentially clear, and the presence of particulate matter in unspun urine needs to be explained microscopically. Cloudy urine is not necessarily pathologic. The turbidity may be due to the precipitation of crystals or nonpathologic salts referred to as amorphous. Phosphate (and occasionally carbonate) precipitates in alkaline urine; the phosphates and carbonates redissolve when acetic acid is added. Uric acid and urates cause a white, pink, or orange cloud in acid urine and redissolve on warming to 60°C. Ammonium urates occur in neutral and alkaline urine and dissolve in acetic acid. Leukocytes may form a white cloud similar to that caused by phosphates, but in this case the cloud remains after the addition of dilute acetic acid; the presence of leukocytes is confirmed by microscopic examination of the sediment. Bacterial growth causes a uniform opalescence that is not removed by acidification or by filtering through paper.

Turbidity or smokiness may be due to red blood cells as seen in gross hematuria. This turbidity does not clear on warming, and the presence of erythrocytes may be confirmed microscopically. The presence of increased numbers of epithelial cells may also account for turbidity. Spermatozoa and prostatic fluid may cause turbidity not cleared by acidification or heating. Prostatic fluid normally contains a few leukocytes and other formed elements. Mucus from the urinary passages may cause a fluffy, bulky deposit; this is increased in inflammatory states of the lower urinary tract or genital tract. Turbidity due to blood clots, menstrual discharge, and other particular material such as pieces of tissue, small calculi, clumps of pus, and fecal material is sometimes seen. Fecal material in urine may result from a fistula between the colon or rectum and bladder. Contamination with powders or with antiseptics that become opaque with water (phenols) also causes turbid urine.

CHYLURIA. This is rare. The urine contains lymph. It is associated with obstruction to lymph flow and rupture of lymphatic vessels into the renal pelvis, ureters, bladder, or urethra. Filariasis (late in the disease), abdominal lymph node enlargement, and tumors have been associated with chyluria. Even with filariasis, this is a rare event.

The appearance of the urine varies with the amount of lymph present. It may appear normal, opalescent, or milky. Clots may form. If sufficient lymph is present after a meal, the urine may layer, showing the chylomicrons on top and fibrin and cells beneath. Large numbers of red blood cells may cause a pink discoloration. Chylomicrons may not be apparent microscopically unless they have coalesced as microglobules. This fat can be extracted from urine using an equal volume of ether or chloroform. If urine is turbid as a result of phosphates, it does not clear. The protein test result is positive; leukocytes and red blood cells are present (Sanjurjo, 1970). Pseudochyluria occurs with the use of paraffin-based vaginal creams for the treatment of *Candida* infections (Blank, 1982).

LIPIDURIA. Oily contaminants such as paraffin float on the urine surface as well as endogenous lipids. Fat globules appear in the urine most often with the nephrotic syndrome; these are neutral fats (triglycerides) and cholesterol. Cholesterol esters polarize.

Lipiduria is also present in a significant number of patients who have sustained major skeletal trauma with one or more fractures to major long bones or the pelvis. The source of lipid presumably is exposed fatty marrow. Microscopic examination of the urine may be required to screen for these fatty materials as Oil Red O–positive fat droplets.

Odor

Normal urine has a faint, aromatic odor of undetermined source. Odor is chiefly important in the recognition of specimens that, owing to bacterial contamination on standing, are ammoniacal, fetid, and unsuitable for laboratory examination. Lack of odor in urine from patients with acute renal failure coincides with acute tubular necrosis rather than prerenal failure (Najarian, 1980).

Characteristic urine odors are produced after ingestion of asparagus or thymol. Urine odors associated with amino acid disorders include the following:

Isovaleric acidemia and glutaric acidemia	Sweaty feet
Maple syrup urine disease (MSUD)	Maple syrup
Methionine malabsorption	Cabbage, hops
Phenylketonuria	Mousy
Trimethylaminuria	Rotting fish
Tyrosinemia	Rancid

Urine Volume

Under ordinary physiologic conditions, the chief determinant of urine volume is the intake of water. The average daily urine volume in a normal adult ranges from about 600 to 2000 mL. The night urine is generally not in excess of 400 mL. In normal pregnancy, the usual diurnal variation is reversed, causing nocturia and the excretion of dilute urine. Young children, unlike adults, excrete about three to four times as much urine per kilogram of body weight. Measurement of the urine volume during timed intervals may be a valuable aid in clinical diagnosis.

INCREASES IN URINE VOLUME

A volume of more than 2000 mL in 24 hours is termed polyuria. Any increase in urine volume, even though transitory, is called diuresis.

Excessive intake of water (polydipsia) results in polyuria that may be confused with diabetes insipidus. Certain drugs exert a diuretic effect. Among these are caffeine, alcohol, thiazides, and other diuretics. Intravenous saline or glucose solutions may increase the urine output. Increased salt intake and high-protein diets also require more water for excretion.

Classic pathologic states characterized by continuous polyuria are diabetes insipidus and diabetes mellitus. They result in excessive thirst and in excessive water intake. Patients with pituitary diabetes insipidus have a deficiency of antidiuretic hormone, and polyuria with nocturia is marked, up to 15 L/day. An excessive amount of glucose is excreted in diabetes mellitus, causing a solute diuresis. Compulsive water drinkers have variable polyuria.

In chronic progressive renal failure, functioning renal tissue is lost and the kidneys gradually lose their ability to concentrate urine. In order to excrete the daily renal load, an increase in urine volume is inevitable. The urine eventually becomes iso-osmotic with the plasma ultrafiltrate; the normal day and night volume ratio (2:1) of urine is lost. Nocturia is arbitrarily defined as the excretion by an adult of more than 500 mL of urine with a specific gravity of less than 1.018 at night. Polyuria may also result when tubular damage causes sodium wasting or with impairment of the countercurrent mechanism. High volumes of urine result in a low specific gravity.

DECREASES IN URINE VOLUME

Oliguria is the excretion of less than 500 mL of urine daily, and anuria is virtually complete suppression of urine formation. Water deprivation causes a decrease in urine volume even before signs of dehydration appear.

Decreases in urine volume to oliguric levels occur under pathologic circumstances such as the following:

DEHYDRATION. In prolonged vomiting, diarrhea, or excessive sweating, such as may occur in febrile states, loss of body water without adequate replacement results in dehydration and hemoconcentration. Oliguria ensues, and retention of nitrogenous waste products (azotemia) may even occur as a result of a decrease in the glomerular filtration rate (see Chap. 8). Urinary specific gravity is elevated to about 1.030. Oliguria also occurs when water is shifted from intravascular to extravascular compartments with edema.

RENAL ISCHEMIA. With a poor blood supply to the kidneys due to heart failure or hypotension, oliguria and then anuria occur. This represents a common cause of acute tubular necrosis and acute renal failure. These prerenal causes are associated with low sodium excretion and urine of high specific gravity. Similar findings are observed with decreased filtration in acute glomerulonephritis. Anuria (or oliguria) also follows major hemolytic transfusion reactions and accompanies the crush syndrome. Anuria in these conditions is thought to be related to loss of functioning renal mass.

RENAL DISEASE. When oliguria with uremia (azotemia plus acidemia and electrolyte imbalance) results from progressive renal disease, urinary specific gravity is low; sodium concentration is elevated; and proteinuria, casts, and renal cells may be evident. Pyelonephritis or interstitial nephritis causes predominantly tubular dysfunction with polyuria early in the disease, but oliguria of chronic renal failure occurs later. Toxic agents, such as mercury bichloride, carbon tetrachloride, and diethylene glycol, may result in anuria secondary to acute tubular necrosis.

OBSTRUCTION. Bilateral hydronephrosis, resulting from high-grade or longstanding obstruction of the urinary tract, may be associated with a marked decrease in urine flow and even anuria. This occurs with prostatic hyperplasia and carcinoma. Bilateral ureteral obstruction due to stones, clots, and sloughed tissue and urethral obstruction due to stricture or valves are other forms of obstruction. The anuria associated with sulfonamide therapy and dehydration is due to obstruction caused by the precipitation of crystals in the renal tubules when the urinary pH is acidic.

Specific Gravity and Osmolality

The volume of excreted urine and its concentration of solute are varied by the kidneys to maintain homeostasis of body fluid and electrolytes. In order to achieve this, the kidneys produce urine with specific gravity that ranges from 1.005 to 1.035. Inability to concentrate or dilute urine is an indication of renal disease or hormonal deficiency (antidiuretic hormone). See Chapter 7 for a discussion of the concentrating ability of the kidneys.

Urine of low specific gravity is called hyposthenuric, the specific gravity being less than 1.007. Urine of fixed specific gravity of about 1.010 is known as isosthenuric. The specific gravity of the protein-free glomerular filtrate is about 1.010. Its osmolal concentration is about 285 mOsm, or the osmolality of protein-free plasma (the plasma protein makes little contribution to the total osmolality of the plasma, only about 2 mOsm).

The measurement of specific gravity or osmolality should give an indication of the urinary total solute concentration. In critical circumstances, the measurement of osmolality of urine and plasma is preferred to the measurement of specific gravity. Readers should refer to Chapter 7 for a discussion of osmolality versus specific gravity of urine.

SPECIFIC GRAVITY

Useful clinical information can be obtained from the measurement of maximal specific gravity. Urea (20%), sodium chloride (25%), sulfate, and phosphate contribute most to the specific gravity of normal urine. Normal adults with normal diets and normal fluid intake produce urine of specific gravity 1.016 to 1.022 during a 24-hour period. If a random specimen of urine has a specific gravity of 1.023 or more, concentrating ability can be considered normal.

Urinary specific gravity after taking no fluids for 12 hours overnight should be about 1.022, and after 24 hours without fluid, 1.026 or higher.

Minimum specific gravity after a standard water load should be less than 1.003. For details of concentration and dilution tests, see Chapter 7.

METHODS. Several methods are available to measure specific gravity—refractometer, reagent strip, and urinometer (hydrometer).

Salt solutions have much lower readings on the urine specific gravity scale of the refractometer when compared with the urinometer readings. The refractometer specific gravity scale is valid only for urine and cannot be used to indicate the specific gravity of salt or sugar solutions. This should be borne in mind if salt solutions are to be used for calibration. A 5% NaCl solution has a calculated specific gravity of 1.035, but a 7.5% NaCl solution w/v is required to give a reading of 1.035 on the refractometer scale. Special graphs or tables are required to convert refractive index scale numbers to solute concentration in aqueous solutions if this should be required (American Optical Catalog number 10403).

Refractometer. The refractive index of a solution is related to the content of dissolved solids present. It is the ratio of the velocity of light in air to the velocity of light in a solution. This ratio varies directly with the number of dissolved particles in solution. Measurement of refractive index of urine became feasible and convenient with the development of a clinical refractometer. This device requires only a few drops of urine (unlike the minimum 15 mL of urine necessary with the urinometer). Although the refractometer measures refractive index of a solution, scale readings of the instrument have been calibrated in terms of specific gravity for human urine total solids and for serum protein levels. The specific gravity reading on the refractometer is generally slightly lower than a urinometer reading on the same urine specimen by about 0.002.

Procedure. A temperature-compensated hand model is available. The instrument is temperature compensated between 16° to 38°C. It is damaged by heat above 66°C and by immersion of the eyepiece and focusing ring in water. It should read zero with distilled water; the zero reading can be reset if necessary by breaking the seal over the setscrew, turning it with a small screwdriver, and resealing. To prevent dropping and lens damage, a stand is recommended to support the refractometer. Always check calibration daily.

To make a specific gravity determination of urine, first clean the surfaces of the cover and prism with a drop of distilled water and a damp cloth and then dry. Close the cover. Hold horizontally and apply a drop of urine at the notched bottom of the cover so that it flows over the prism surface by capillary action.

Point the instrument toward a light source at an angle that gives optimal contrast. Rotate the eyepiece until the scale is in focus. Read directly on the specific gravity scale the sharp dividing line between light and dark contrast.

The entire procedure should be repeated with a second drop of urine from the same specimen of urine.

Urinometer. This is a hydrometer adapted to measure the specific gravity of urine at room temperature. It should be checked each day by measuring the specific gravity of distilled water; it should approximate a specific gravity of 1.000. If the urinometer does not give a reading of 1.000, an appropriate correction must be applied to all readings taken with that urinometer. The accuracy of a urinometer may be further checked in solutions of known specific gravity—for example, a solution of potassium sulfate with a specific gravity of 1.015 may be prepared by diluting 20.29 g potassium sulfate to 1 L with distilled water.

Procedure. The urinometer vessel is filled three fourths full with urine (minimum volume of urine required is about 15 mL). The urinometer is inserted with a spinning motion to make sure that it is floating freely. (When reading the urinometer, be sure that it is not touching the sides or the bottom of the cylinder. Avoid surface bubbles, which obscure the meniscus.) Read the bottom of the meniscus.

Because temperature influences the specific gravity, urine samples should be allowed to come to room temperature before a reading is made, or a correction of 0.001 should be made for each 3°C above or below the calibration temperature indicated on the urinometer, usually 20°C.

For accurate determinations of specific gravity in concentration-dilution tests, corrections are made for protein or glucose present. Subtract 0.003 for every 1 g/100 mL of protein and 0.004 for every 1 g/100 mL of glucose.

COLORIMETRIC METHOD. Specific gravity can be estimated chemically by reagent strip methods. The principle of the specific gravity area is based on a pKa change of certain pretreated polyelectrolytes in relation to ionic concentration. The reagent is sensitive to the number of ions in the urine specimen. An indicator changes color in relation to ionic concentration and is translated to specific gravity values.

In addition, specific gravity can be determined by sound wave frequency or by the falling drop method in some automated instruments.

OSMOLALITY

A normal adult on a normal diet with a normal fluid intake produces urine of about 500 to 850 mOsm/kg water. A normal kidney is able to produce urine of osmolality in the range of 800 to 1400 mOsm/kg water in dehydration and a minimal osmolality of 40 to 80 mOsm/kg water during water diuresis. After a period of dehydration, the osmolality of the urine should be three to four times that of the plasma (e.g., with a normal plasma osmolality of 285 mOsm/kg water, the urine osmolality should be at least 855 mOsm/kg water).

METHODS. The freezing point depression method is commonly used. A solution containing 1 osmol or 1000 mOsm/kg water depresses the freezing point 1.86°C below the freezing point of water (for method, see Chaps. 3 and 7).

Chemical Screening

Reagent Strip Method

The reagent strip method represents the main focus of the chemical examination of urine. Confirmatory tests and other methods may be required for certain patient populations or under special circumstances. The chemical tests most commonly found on multiple reagent strips are discussed first, with less commonly tested chemical parameters following. The clinical application of each analyte is discussed before reagent strips and other methods. Confirmatory tests are included when available and necessary.

REAGENT STRIP PRECAUTIONS

The complexity of reagent strip testing must not be overlooked. Although they are easily used, reagent strips represent complex, multiple, state-of-the-art chemical reactions. Table 18–4 lists recommendations for both the storage and the use of reagent strips.

It should be noted that reagent strip methods are changed periodically, sensitivities and color reactions altered, and new tests added. Manufacturers supply tables of common interfering substances, and these should be consulted. Problems with ascorbic acid and drugs producing colored urine such as phenazopyridine (Pyridium) and other azo compounds and methylene blue are most frequently encountered. As much as 3 g/day of ascorbic acid may be administered in parenteral vitamin preparations with maintenance fluid therapy in an adult. More detailed information on drug interference is listed in Hansen (1979) and Young (1975). For a listing of urine constituents detected by some available reagent strips and tablet tests, see Table 18–5.

pH of Urine

The pH of urine is a reflection of the ability of the kidneys to maintain normal hydrogen ion concentration in plasma and extracellular fluid. The metabolic activity of the body produces nonvolatile acids that cannot be extracted by the lungs—principally sulfuric, phosphoric, and hydrochloric acids but also small amounts of pyruvic, lactic, and citric acids and some ketone bodies. These acids are excreted by the glomeruli with cations, chiefly sodium. Bicarbonate is re-

Table 18–4. RECOMMENDATIONS FOR REAGENT STRIPS

Storage
Protect from moisture and excessive heat.
Store in cool, dry area but not in a refrigerator.
Check for discoloration with each use; discoloration may indicate loss of reactivity. Do not use discolored strips or tablets.
Keep container tightly stoppered.
Check manufacturer's directions with each new lot number for changes in procedure.
Testing
Test urine as soon as possible after receipt.
Remove only enough strips for immediate use; recap tightly.
Test a well-mixed, unspun urine sample.
Urine samples must be at room temperature before testing.
Do not touch the test area with fingers.
Do not use reagent strips in the presence of volatile acids or alkaline fumes.
Dip reagent strip into urine briefly—no longer than one second.
Drain excess urine off—run edge of strip along rim of tube or blot edge on absorbent paper.
Do not allow reagents to run together.
Do not lay reagent strip directly on workbench surface.
Follow exact timing recommendations for each chemical test.
Hold reagent strip close to the color chart and read under good lighting.
Know sources of error, sensitivity, and specificity of each test on the reagent strip.
Think! Make correlations between patient history and individual test, then follow through.

Table 18–5. COMMERCIAL PRODUCTS FOR DETECTION OF URINE CONSTITUENTS

Product	pH	Glucose	Protein	Blood	Ketone	Bilirubin	Urobilinogen	Nitrite	Leukocyte Esterase	Specific Gravity	Reducing Substances	Ascorbic Acid
Multistix 10 SG*	X	X	X	X	X	X	X	X	X	X		
Rapignost Total Screen L†	X	X	X	X	X	X	X	X	X			X
Chemstrip 10 S-UA‡	X	X	X	X	X	X	X	X	X	X		

Other reagent strips or tablets are available to detect one or a combination of analytes (e.g., Chemstrip G‡/Diastix*—detects only glucose, Uristix*/Chemstrip GP‡—detects protein and glucose only).

*Trademark of Ames Division, Miles Laboratories, Elkhart, IN.
†Trademark of Behring Diagnostics, Inc., Somerville, NJ.
‡Trademark of Boehringer Mannheim Corporation, Indianapolis, IN.

absorbed. The tubular cells exchange hydrogen ions for sodium of the glomerular filtrate, and the urine becomes acid in reaction. Hydrogen ions are also excreted as ammonium ions (NH_4). For a discussion of this exchange process, see Chapter 7.

NORMAL pH. An average adult on a normal diet excretes about 50 to 100 mEq of hydrogen ions in 24 hours to produce urine of about pH 6. In health, urine pH may vary from 4.6 to 8. When protein intake is high, more phosphates and sulfates are produced, resulting in more acid urine. On a predominantly vegetable diet, as in many non-Western countries, the urine may have a pH higher than 6. The urine becomes less acid after a meal as a result of secretion of acid into the stomach (the so-called alkaline tide). At night, during the mild respiratory acidosis of sleep, a more acid urine may be formed.

ACID URINE. Acid urine may be produced by a diet high in meat protein and in some fruits such as cranberries. Ammonium chloride, methionine, methenamine mandelate, or acid phosphate is used to produce acid urine in treatment of some calculi. Acid phosphates with or without antibacterials help keep calcium in solution. Acidifiers are useful for ammonium magnesium stone prevention, because these stones form in alkaline urine.

ALKALINE URINE. Alkaline urine may be induced by use of a diet high in certain fruits and vegetables, especially citrus fruits. Sodium bicarbonate, potassium citrate, and acetazolamide may be used to alkalize urine in the treatment of some calculi. They may also be used in some urinary tract infections (the antibiotics neomycin, kanamycin, and streptomycin are more active in alkaline urine), in sulfonamide therapy, and in the treatment of salicylate poisoning.

INTERPRETATION OF URINE pH IN PATHOLOGIC STATES. The capacity to exchange hydrogen ion for cation and the formation of ammonia is decreased when tubular function is impaired. In classic renal tubular acidosis, glomerular filtration is normal but distal tubular ability to form ammonia and exchange hydrogen ions for cations is defective. Systemic acidosis results. The urine is relatively alkaline, and the pH cannot be lowered below pH of 6 to 6.5, even with the administration of an acid-loading substance. Titratable acidity and the concentration of ammonium are decreased. In proximal renal tubular acidosis, bicarbonate wasting occurs, as in proximal tubular diseases such as Fanconi's syndrome.

In metabolic acid-base disturbances, the pH of the urine may reflect attempts at compensation by the kidneys. In metabolic acidosis, acid urine is produced and titratable acidity and ammonium ion concentrations are increased. In chronic acidosis, as in diabetic ketoacidosis, very large amounts of hydrogen ions are excreted, much of it as ammonium ion. In metabolic alkalosis, alkaline urine with higher levels of bicarbonate is produced and ammonia production is decreased. The kidneys may produce urine with a pH as high as 7.8. In respiratory acidosis, acid urine is formed and the amount of ammonium excreted is increased; in respiratory alkalosis, alkaline urine is produced and is associated with increased excretion of bicarbonate. In potassium depletion such as in hypokalemic alkalosis of prolonged vomiting or in hypercorticism or with prolonged use of diuretics, paradoxical aciduria may occur with slightly acid urine in the presence of a metabolic alkalosis.

METHODS

REAGENT STRIP. Indicators methyl red and bromthymol blue give a range of orange, green, and blue as the pH rises. The test permits differentiation of pH values to half a unit within the range of 5 to 9. It should be read immediately, but time is not critical.

pH is not affected by the urinary buffer concentration. Bacterial growth in a specimen may cause a marked alkaline shift (pH $>$ 8.0) and render it unsuitable for testing, usually because of urea conversion to ammonia. Care should be taken not to have excessively wet strips where acid buffer from the protein patch runs into the pH patch, causing it to become orange.

Precautions. Measurement of urine pH and acidity must always be made on freshly voided specimens. If precise measurements are required, the container should be filled and the urine covered tightly to minimize the amount of dead space. The container should be kept cold, preferably on ice, but not frozen. On standing, the pH tends to rise because of loss of carbon dioxide (the Pco_2 of freshly voided urine is approximately 40 mm Hg, that of normal plasma) and because bacterial growth produces ammonia from urea.

pH ELECTRODE. A rough estimate of the pH is usually sufficient and may be made with indicator paper. In patients with disturbances of acid-base balance, urinary pH may be accurately measured with a pH meter with a glass electrode (see Chap. 3).

Procedure. Urinary pH may be measured by means of a closed glass electrode and read directly from the scale of a pH meter. Because the pH meter may tend to drift, it must be standardized with three buffers of known pH immediately before use. After standardization, spray the electrodes with distilled water, clean, and dry with tissue. Immerse the electrodes in the urine sample. Report the pH of urine at the temperature of measurement.

TITRATABLE ACIDITY OF URINE. The pH of the urine is largely dependent on the amount of mono- and dibasic phosphate present. Titratable acidity is measured by titrating an aliquot of 24-hour urine (collected on ice) with 0.1 N NaOH with pH 7.4 as an end point. The test may be used together with urinary ammonia determination in patients with chronic acidosis of obscure origin.

Procedure. To 25 mL of urine in a flask, add 10 g of powdered potassium oxalate (to precipitate calcium). Mix well. Titrate to pH 7.4 using 0.1 N NaOH with a pH meter and glass electrode. Three reference buffers are used to standardize the pH meter.

Titratable acidity is usually reported as number of milliliters of 0.1 N NaOH required to neutralize a 24-hour specimen:

$$= \frac{\text{mL NaOH} \times \text{24-hour volume in mL}}{\text{25 mL}}$$

For milliequivalents per 24 hours, multiply by the normality of NaOH (0.1). Normal titratable acidity is in the range of 200 to 500 mL 0.1 N NaOH (or 6 mL 0.1 N NaOH per kilogram of body weight), or 20 to 40 mEq/24 hours.

3

Protein in Urine

Normally there is a scant amount of protein in urine, up to about 150 mg/24 hour or 10 mg/dL, depending on urine volume (Kim, 1988; Ward, 1989). The proteins are derived from plasma and the urinary tract. About one third is albumin, and the remaining plasma proteins include many small globulins. Plasma proteins with molecular weight less than 50,000 to 60,000 pass through the glomerular membrane and are normally reabsorbed by proximal tubular cells. Albumin, molecular weight 69,000, is apparently filtered but only in very small amounts. Retinol binding, β_2-microglobulin, immunoglobulin light chains, and lysozyme are excreted in small amounts. Tamm-Horsfall glycoprotein (uromucoid), secreted by distal tubular cells and cells of the ascending loop of Henle, constitutes about one third or more of the total normal protein loss. Immunoglobulin A in secretions of the urinary tract, enzymes and proteins from tubular epithelial cells, and other desquamated cells and leukocytes are other proteins found in very small amounts in normal urine. Anderson (1979) has demonstrated more than 200 urinary proteins.

Healthy persons may exceed normal levels during exercise or with dehydration. Proteinuria is a consistent finding after strenuous exercise. Proteinuria can occur in the absence of urinary tract disease in patients with hemorrhage or salt depletion and in febrile illnesses. These may cause dehydration and relative renal ischemia.

Screening tests are required to differentiate normal protein excretion from abnormal and therefore should not detect less than about 8 to 10 mg/dL in a normal adult with a normal rate of urine flow. It should be noted that a very dilute random specimen of urine may have a falsely low protein value. Because a positive result for protein is significant, it should be confirmed by a second, different method and on repeated specimens. The reagent strip method is sensitive to albumin; the acid precipitation tests detect all proteins and therefore indicate the presence of globulins, as well as albumin.

Detection of an abnormal amount of protein in urine is a reliable indicator of renal disease because protein has a very low maximal tubular rate (Tm) of reabsorption; thus, increased filtration or production quickly saturates the reabsorptive mechanism. When proteinuria is confirmed, a 24-hour collection to measure protein excretion is made. This indicates the degree of proteinuria. Repeated measurements may be needed to decide whether the proteinuria is intermittent or persistent. Depending on the history and examination, confirmatory tests for protein are usually accompanied by tests of renal function, examination of the urine sediment, and urine culture. Errors in quantitative protein determinations result from poor collections of 24-hour specimens and variable methods (see Chap. 1—Urine Specimen Collection). To detect the kinds of protein present in urine requires electrophoretic separation of serum and urine proteins. Based on these and on clinical findings, proteinuria may be separated into a glomerular pattern and tubular pattern, indicating which part of the nephron is primarily involved. However, these anatomic entities tend to merge as disease progresses. A third type has been designated overflow proteinuria because the protein material initially results from disease elsewhere—for example, hemoglobin, after intravascular hemolysis.

GLOMERULAR PATTERN

By definition, glomerular disease causes proteinuria. A loss or reduction of the fixed negative charge on the glomerular capillary wall allows albumin to permeate into Bowman's space in large quantities, more than can be reabsorbed by the proximal tubular cells (Brenner, 1978). Glomerular disease often causes heavy proteinuria, greater than 3 to 4 g/day. Small amounts of albumin found in urine of insulin-dependent diabetic patients correlate with very early diabetic nephropathy.

When serum albumin is lost in urine, other proteins of similar size or charge are also lost—for example, antithrombin, transferrin, prealbumin, α_1-acid glycoprotein, and α_1-antitrypsin—that is, proteins that are usually retained in the plasma. Large proteins are not found in urine while the glomerulus is still selective—for example, α_2-macroglobulin and β-lipoprotein. Because tubular function may still be normal, very small plasma proteins are largely reabsorbed. When only albumin or smaller proteins are found, the pattern indicates minimal change disease and generally augurs a more favorable prognosis. As larger proteins appear, the proteinuria is less selective, indicating greater morphologic changes—for example, with membranous nephropathy and proliferative glomerulonephritis.

Nephrotic syndrome is principally associated with glomerular diseases and is diagnosed when the protein excretion is greater than 3.0 to 3.5 g/day or 2 g/m^2/24 hours. Losses of 10 to 20 g/day are found. In addition to heavy proteinuria, the classic syndrome is characterized by low serum albumin level, generalized edema, and increased serum lipids (cholesterol, triglycerides, and phosphatides). Lipoproteins, low density and very low density, are increased in serum, whereas high-density lipoprotein, a smaller molecule, has been demonstrated in urine (de Mendoza, 1976). It has been suggested that loss of lipoprotein lipase in urine contributes to the rise of serum lipid levels. Gamma globulin is lost in urine. This contributes to susceptibility to bacterial infections commonly found in the nephrotic syndrome. When lipid is lost in urine, many granular casts, fatty casts, and fat-filled renal tubular epithelial cells (oval fat bodies) are found in the sediment. Cholesterol ester droplets may be demonstrable by polarization. Common causes of the nephrotic syndrome are mentioned later under Heavy Proteinuria.

TUBULAR PATTERN

A tubular pattern is associated with loss of urinary protein that would otherwise be largely reabsorbed. These proteins are usually of low molecular weight—for example, α_1-microglobulin, β-globulin such as β_2-microglobulin, light-chain immunoglobulins, and lysozyme. By radioimmunoassay, β_2-microglobulin excretion has been measured in microgram amounts in urine as an indication of tubular damage; its normal excretion is about 100 μg/day. A tubular pattern proteinuria occurs with renal tubular disease such as Fanconi's syndrome, cystinosis, Wilson's disease, and pyelonephritis and with renal transplantation rejection. The amount of proteinuria is lower than with glomerular diseases and is about 1 to 2 g/day.

Tubular proteinuria may be missed by the reagent strip test because of absent or very low amounts of albumin but may be detected by acid precipitation or by a relevant and more sensitive assay.

OVERFLOW PROTEINURIA

Excessive production or overflow proteinuria is due to hemoglobin, myoglobin, or immunoglobulin loss into the urine. These proteins are not initially associated with glomerular or tubular disease but may cause renal disease. Myoglobin causes acute tubular necrosis (see Myoglobinuria). Hemoglobin is not thought to be toxic unless a patient is dehydrated.

BENCE JONES PROTEINURIA

Bence Jones proteinuria is associated with multiple myeloma, macroglobulinemia, and malignant lymphomas. The incidence of Bence Jones proteinuria in multiple myeloma has been estimated to be 50% to 80%; however, its demonstration depends greatly on the technique used. Electrophoresis and immunofixation electrophoresis (IFE) methods are best. Bence Jones protein may be missed altogether if only a reagent strip test for protein is used (see Measurement of Proteinuria).

Excretion of Bence Jones protein in large amounts, sometimes several grams per 24 hours, causes the tubular cells to become degenerated because of the high levels of protein reabsorbed. Inclusions may form in the cells. Desquamated cells form casts in the tubular lumen. Casts also form from immunoglobulin and Tamm-Horsfall protein mixtures. With renal failure, less protein is reabsorbed and more Bence Jones protein and other proteins appear in the urine. The damaged kidney is sometimes called a myeloma kidney, and the nephrotic syndrome may follow.

More useful information for diagnosis of kidney disease and for monitoring response to treatment is obtained by quantitatively analyzing the amount of protein excreted during a 24-hour period. It should be noted that the accuracy of test results of any quantitative urine determination depends on the adequacy and completeness of the urine collection. Errors in the results are often related to collection problems.

HEAVY PROTEINURIA (>3 TO 4 G/DAY)

Heavy protein loss is characteristic of the nephrotic syndrome. The syndrome is associated with (1) primary renal diseases, including idiopathic disease, and (2) systemic diseases causing renal involvement. Transient or mechanical causes are severe congestive heart failure, constrictive pericarditis, and renal vein thrombosis. The last is also a consequence of the nephrotic syndrome because of losses of anticlotting factors in urine and elevation of serum fibrinogen. A common cause of heavy proteinuria is minimal change (also known as nil lesion, idiopathic) nephrotic syndrome. This is a steroid-responsive disease usually encountered in young children. In adults, diabetes mellitus and lupus erythematosus are frequent causes of heavy proteinuria. In Africa, malaria is a frequent cause of childhood nephrotic syndrome. Acute, rapidly progressive, and chronic glomerulonephritis are causes of heavy proteinuria. Protein and lipids may then be accompanied by erythrocytes in the urine. Erythrocyte casts are sometimes seen. The sediment may be telescoped—that is, display all kinds of cells and casts in lupus nephritis or with a hypersensitivity reaction. Malignant hypertension, toxemia of pregnancy, heavy metals (gold, mercury), drugs (penicillamine), neoplasia in general, amyloidosis (primary, secondary, and with multiple myeloma), sickle-cell disease, and renal transplant rejection all are causes of heavy proteinuria.

MODERATE PROTEINURIA (1.0 TO 3 OR 4 G/DAY)

Moderate proteinuria may be found in a large number of renal diseases, primarily glomerular, including those mentioned previously, and nephrosclerosis, multiple myeloma, and various toxic nephropathies, including radiation nephritis.

MINIMAL PROTEINURIA (<1.0 G/DAY)

Minimal proteinuria may be noted in chronic pyelonephritis, in which case it may be intermittent, and in relatively inactive phases of glomerular diseases. It is also noted with nephrosclerosis, chronic interstitial nephritis, congenital diseases such as polycystic disease and medullary cystic disease, and renal tubular diseases. The urinary sediment is usually not abnormal, but erythrocytes, leukocytes, and tubular cells may be seen with interstitial nephritis. However, as to be mentioned, significant sediment findings may sometimes accompany trace protein results. Minimal proteinuria is present in benign postural proteinurias and transient proteinuria.

Proteinuria may be absent in phases of acute pyelonephritis, in chronic pyelonephritis, and in the presence of obstructive nephropathy, kidney stones, kidney tumors, and congenital malformations. Cells and casts can be found in the urine in significant numbers when the protein reagent strip screening test has negative results.

POSTURAL PROTEINURIA

Postural proteinuria (orthostatic) occurs in 3% to 5% of apparently healthy young adults. In these persons, proteinuria is found during the day but not at night, when a recumbent position is assumed. Persistent proteinuria may develop in some of these healthy subjects at a later date, and renal biopsy specimens have shown abnormalities of the glomerulus in a few cases (Robinson, 1961). Proteinuria is apparently related to an exaggerated lordotic position and may result from renal congestion or ischemia. The total daily excretion of protein rarely exceeds 1 g. In most instances, no other evidence of renal disease develops.

To evaluate the possibility of postural proteinuria, the patient is instructed to empty his or her bladder on going to bed in the evening and to discard the specimen. Immediately on rising in the morning, the patient voids and saves this specimen. After two hours of standing and walking about, the patient voids again and saves the specimen. The two urine specimens are tested for protein. If the first is negative and the second positive, the patient may have postural proteinuria. Frequent examination of the patient should be made to re-evaluate this condition.

INTERMITTENT, TRANSIENT PROTEINURIA

The history, physical examination findings, and renal function test results are normal. Except for occasional proteinuria, results of routine urinalysis are normal. These patients are monitored every six months to check for hypertension or other abnormalities. The prognosis is favorable. Transient proteinuria may occur in normal pregnancy, but any proteinuria in pregnancy is an important finding and requires investigation.

PERSISTENT PROTEINURIA
(1 TO 2 G/DAY)

Persistent proteinuria in an asymptomatic person or when accompanied by hematuria has a poorer prognosis than intermittent (transient) or postural proteinuria (Thompson, 1970; Rytand, 1981).

FUNCTIONAL PROTEINURIA

Functional proteinuria is usually less than 0.5 g/day. It is encountered with heavy exercise (e.g., long-distance running, hockey, racquetball) and accompanies congestive heart failure, cold exposure, and fever. Dehydration contributes to the level of protein measured in urine. With strenuous exercise, a mixture of high- and low-molecular-weight proteins appears, and many casts, both hyaline and granular, are seen (Bailey, 1976). Functional proteinuria resolves with appropriate treatment or rest within two to three days.

METHODS

REAGENT STRIP. Tests are based on the principle of protein error of pH indicators. Because proteins carry a charge at physiologic pH, their presence elicits a pH change. The test area is buffered to a constant low pH, and thus color changes reflect only the presence and concentration of proteins.

Results may be read in a plus system with any plus value indicating significant proteinuria. In concentrated specimens from healthy persons, a trace result may occur with physiologic normal excretion of protein.

The reagent strip is impregnated with tetrabromphenol blue buffered to an acid pH of 3, or tetrachlorophenol-tetrabromosulfophthalein. This area is yellow in the absence of protein but changes to a shade of green, depending on the type and concentration of protein present, in 30 to 60 seconds. It is important to match the colors closely with the reacted strip.

Five to 20 mg of albumin per deciliter of urine may be detected. The test area is more sensitive to albumin than to globulin, Bence Jones protein, or mucoprotein. For an evaluation, see James (1978a; see also Hindmarsh, 1988; McKenna, 1987).

High salt levels lower results (Gyure, 1977). Exceptionally alkaline or highly buffered urine samples may give positive results in the absence of significant proteinuria, such as with a patient on alkaline medication or with bacterial contamination. Leaching of the acid buffer by excessive wetting causes false-positive results. False-positive results also occur with quaternary ammonium compounds used for cleaning containers and skin (Zephiran) and with amidoamines in fabric softeners and chlorhexidine. The test results are unaffected by urine turbidity, radiographic media, and most drugs or their metabolites (Table 18–6).

MEASUREMENT OF PROTEINURIA. Qualitative, semiquantitative, and quantitative methods are available for analysis of protein in urine. Because the positive result of a screening test may have grave significance, it is important to be able to confirm it by a second, different method.

A comparison of reagent strips and the sulfosalicylic acid method shows that with reagent strips, accurate results are obtained only when albumin is measured. Changes in urinary solute concentration affect the reagent strip results but not the sulfosalicylic acid method. High salt levels lower the reagent strip result (Gyure, 1977).

Table 18–6. SCREENING TEST FOR DETECTION OF PROTEINURIA

Urine Constituents or Condition	Reagent Strip	Acid Precipitation
Highly buffered alkaline urine	May cause FP	May cause FN
Drug metabolites	No effect	May cause FP
Radiocontrast media	No effect	May cause FP
Turbidity	No effect	May cause FP
Quarternary ammonium groups or chlorohexidine	May cause FP	No effect

FP = false positive; FN = false negative.

Although not as sensitive as precipitation tests, the reagent strip has the advantage of avoiding false-positive reactions with organic iodides, such as those used for x-ray contrast and tolbutamides or other drugs (see Table 18–5). Reagent strip results should not be used to predict the absence or degree of proteinuria.

Most other qualitative screening tests rely on protein precipitation—for example, with heat and acetic acid, with nitric acid, and with sulfosalicylic acid (SSA) and trichloroacetic acids (TCA). These methods also precipitate globulins as well as albumin. In practice, negative reagent strips with positive SSA test results in urine specimens are attributable to x-ray dye, to penicillins, and rarely to globulins. SSA and TCA are used to precipitate protein in the cold and are used as convenient screening tests. The sensitivity may be as low as 0.25 mg/dL, depending on the techniques used.

Because of a lack of sensitivity of the reagent strip to globulins, it may be necessary to use an acid precipitation test for screening purposes. This depends on the patient population and the diseases under investigation.

OTHER QUALITATIVE OR
SEMI-QUANTITATIVE METHODS

SULFOSALICYLIC ACID METHOD—QUALITATIVE. Different concentrations and proportions of SSA have been used in the qualitative test and provide different ranges of results.

Specimens should be centrifuged, and a clear supernatant used.

Procedure. To approximately 3 mL of supernatant urine aliquot (about 1 inch) in a 16 × 125 mm test tube, add an equal amount of 3% SSA. Invert to mix. Let stand exactly 10 minutes. Invert again twice. Using ordinary room light (not a lamp), observe the degree of precipitation, and grade the results according to the following descriptions:

Negative—no turbidity or no increase in turbidity (approximately 0.005 g/dL or less)
Trace—perceptible turbidity (approximately 0.020 g/dL)
1+—Distinct turbidity but no discrete granulation (approximately 0.050 g/dL)
2+—Turbidity with granulation but no flocculation (approximately 0.20 g/dL)
3+—Turbidity with granulation and flocculation (approximately 0.5 g/dL)
4+—Clumps of precipitated protein or solid precipitate (approximately 1.0 g/dL or more)

The method detects about 5 to 10 mg/dL. Albumin, globulins, glycoproteins, and Bence Jones proteins are detected. High levels of detergents may decrease the result.

When radiographic dye is present, the specific gravity of the urine is usually greater than 1.035 and the SSA precipitate increases on standing. Typical crystals are seen on the microscopic examination of the precipitate; a protein precipitate is amorphous. Another urine specimen from the patient should be tested. However, the effects of the radiographic media may persist as long as three days. A reagent strip test may be substituted, or the heat and acetic acid test used. In the acetic acid test, radiographic contrast media clear with heat, whereas protein increases.

SEMI-QUANTITATIVE METHODS. Commercial standards are available to increase the sensitivity of standard SSA procedures. A set of gelled standards that correspond to 10, 20, 30, 40, 50, 75, and 100 mg/dL are provided. Urine is mixed with SSA, allowed to sit, then compared visually with the standards. Results are reported in mg/dL versus 1+, 2+, and so on.

CONFIRMATORY TESTS. SSA and TCA are commonly used as precipitants; the resultant turbidity is measured by a photometer or nephelometer or by eye and compared with known standards. With SSA, the turbidity produced with albumin is 2.4 times that produced with globulin (Henry, 1956). Polypeptides, glycoproteins, and Bence Jones proteins are also precipitated. Exton's reagent (1925) contains SSA, sodium sulfate, and an indicator—bromphenol blue. TCA is a protein precipitant that causes gamma globulin to be precipitated with greater turbidity than albumin. However, the difference is not marked (Henry, 1956). More precise measurements especially suitable for smaller amounts of protein are available. In these tests, a TCA precipitate is dissolved in sodium hydroxide and measured by use of the biuret reaction (Kibrick, 1958). For a comparison of biuret methods with the SSA turbidity test, see Lizana (1977). For comparisons with the dye-binding methods, Coomassie blue, Ponceau S, and benzethonium turbidity, see McElderry (1982).

Very small amounts of proteins, such as albumin and β_2-microglobulin, are measured by immunologic means using antibodies to the proteins and nephelometric methods or by radioimmunoassay (Brodows, 1986; Lee, 1989; Hindmarsh, 1988). Microalbuminuria has been suggested as a predictor of clinical nephropathy in insulin-dependent diabetes mellitus (Mogensen, 1984a, 1984b; Viberti, 1982).

Automated methods for total urine protein include automation of biuret techniques. An automated turbidimetric method using benzethonium chloride in an alkaline medium is available (Dupont-ACA).

Methods used to quantitate urinary protein have not been satisfactory. Participants in the College of American Pathologists proficiency testing surveys are aware that these test results show that the mean values reported vary twofold between methods, with the SSA method producing high values. Precision is poor, and the SSA turbidimetric method shows the poorest coefficient of variation. The TCA-biuret, Coomassie blue, and TCA turbidity tests show closer agreement and about half the coefficient of variation of the SSA method. Problems arise from nonstandardized methods. With turbidity tests, these include different acid concentrations and timing, as well as variation in the protein standard. Variability also occurs in the proteins excreted, and a primary standard representing this variable mixture of proteins is not possible.

The quantitative TCA-biuret method (Henry, 1984) is tedious but gives good precision. A color correction blank is used. Bovine albumin assayed by the Kjeldahl's technique is used as the protein standard.

SULFOSALICYLIC ACID TURBIDITY METHOD—SEMI-QUANTITATIVE

Principle. SSA precipitates protein in urine with a turbidity that is approximately proportional to the concentration of protein in a solution. The turbidity may be measured with a photometer (see Henry, 1979).

Bence Jones Proteinuria. The best method for detection of Bence Jones protein in urine is protein electrophoresis. The presence of Bence Jones globulin or clonal production of immunoglobulin is indicated by a single sharp peak in the globulin region on protein electrophoresis. Bence Jones globulin represents either the kappa or lambda immunoglobulin light chain identified with IFE.

Measurement of Bence Jones Protein. Globulins are not sensitive to the reagent strip test for protein, which screens predominantly for albumin (Bowie, 1977). Many techniques have been proposed, most of them based on the unusual heat solubility properties of Bence Jones protein. This protein precipitates at temperatures between 40° and 60°C and redissolves near 100°C (Henry, 1984). Other tests depend on precipitation in the cold with salts, ammonium sulfate, and acids.

In the presence of marked Bence Jones proteinuria, most tests yield positive results. When only a small amount of Bence Jones protein is present or when other globulins are present, results may be doubtful. False-positive reactions are seen when other globulins are precipitated by acetic acid in the heat precipitation method. A false-negative reaction may occur if the Bence Jones protein is too concentrated and the precipitate does not redissolve on boiling.

Glucose in Urine

Glucose may appear in the urine at different blood glucose levels, varying in individuals. The blood level, glomerular blood flow, tubular reabsorption rate, and urine flow influence its appearance. Glucosuria usually occurs when the blood level is more than 180 to 200 mg/dL.

DIABETES MELLITUS

The level and duration of hyperglycemia required to make a diagnosis of diabetes mellitus are variously interpreted by groups in different parts of the world. Although hyperglycemia alone is not necessarily indicative of diabetes mellitus, the appearance of glucose in the urine is regarded as a hallmark of the disease and requires that a patient receive a workup for diabetes mellitus.

A patient diagnosed as having diabetes mellitus has hyperglycemia that results in glucosuria when the renal threshold for glucose is exceeded. Glucosuria is attended by polyuria and an increase in thirst. With the need to metabolize protein and then fats, ketone levels rise in the blood and urine, and with the excretion of ketones and the accompanying base, metabolic acidosis ensues.

For diabetic patients, the advantage of a urine test over a

blood test for glucose is that it is painless and inexpensive. However, reagent strips are difficult to interpret at the 1 g/dL (1%) and 2 g/dL (2%) glucose levels, and the Clinitest method is preferred by many to try to offset this problem. Newer reagent strips that discriminate between high urinary glucose levels to 5 g/dL may help. With the Clinitest method, diabetic patients are able to estimate reducing substance levels in urine to about 10 g/dL, using one drop of specimen rather than two or five drops.

Urine glucose tests are generally useful for patients who do not have to make frequent insulin dose adjustments. In insulin-dependent diabetes, a negative urine test result could correspond to a wide range of blood glucose levels (Malone, 1976); this is attributed to a great variation in renal threshold for glucose in diabetic patients. In unstable diabetic patients, therefore, urine test results may be misleading and home blood glucose monitoring is advocated.

In some clinics, the 24-hour urine glucose measurement is found to be useful for monitoring patients. It represents a defined longer time period, and with blood levels of glycosylated hemoglobin, it contributes to the regular overall long-term management of the disease.

Glucosuria with hyperglycemia is also encountered in endocrine disorders other than diabetes mellitus—for example, in pituitary and adrenal disorders such as acromegaly and in Cushing's syndrome or hyperadrenocorticism, and with functioning α- or β-cell pancreatic tumors, hyperthyroidism, and pheochromocytoma. Pancreatic disease with loss of functioning islets is also associated with glucosuria—for example, hemochromatosis, carcinoma, pancreatitis, and cystic fibrosis.

Glucosuria and hyperglycemia may accompany central nervous system disorders, brain tumor or hemorrhage, hypothalamic disease, asphyxia, and disturbances of metabolism associated with burns, infection, fractures, myocardial infarction, and uremia. Liver disease, glycogen storage diseases, obesity, and feeding after starvation are also associated with glucosuria, as are certain drugs (e.g., thiazides, corticosteroids and adrenocorticotropic hormone, and birth control pills).

Pregnant women have an increase in glomerular filtration rate, and all of the filtered glucose may not be reabsorbed; thus, glucosuria may appear at relatively low blood glucose levels. Persistent or greater than trace amounts of glucosuria should be investigated. In some patients, diabetes occurs only during pregnancy. A decrease in glucose tolerance occurs in the aged, especially when the patients have a poor intake of carbohydrate, but this is not necessarily accompanied by glucosuria.

Glucosuria without hyperglycemia is usually associated with renal tubular dysfunction. True inherited renal glucosuria is uncommon; it is associated with reduced glucose reabsorption. In renal tubular transport diseases, glucosuria is not a major finding but one of many. Water, amino acid, bicarbonate, phosphate, and sodium reabsorption is impaired, a pattern seen in Fanconi's syndrome. Galactosemia, cystinosis, lead poisoning, and myeloma are examples of conditions associated with renal tubular dysfunction and possible glucosuria.

METHODS

Reagent Strip. Tests are based on a specific glucose oxidase and peroxidase method, a double sequential enzyme reaction. Reagent strips differ in the chromogen used. The reagent strips may be used for semi-quantitative results. Results should be reported as approximate grams per deciliter (g/dL) to avoid confusion about the relative amounts of glucose represented by the plus systems used in the many glucose and sugar tests available. Diabetic patients commonly use a combination glucose and ketone reagent strip. This not only detects ketonuria but also helps detect the suppression of glucose reaction by ketones occurring with some reagent strips.

CHEMISTRY

$$\text{Glucose} + O_2 \xrightarrow{\text{glucose oxidase}} \text{gluconic acid} + H_2O_2$$

$$H_2O_2 + \text{chromogen} \xrightarrow{\text{peroxidase}} \underset{\text{(color change)}}{\text{oxidized chromogen}} + H_2O$$

The glucose oxidase test is specific for glucose; it does not react with lactose, galactose, fructose, or reducing metabolites of drugs. False-positive readings may be produced by strongly oxidizing cleaning agents in the urine container. Use of sodium fluoride as a preservative causes false-negative readings (Table 18–7). High specific gravity decreases color development. All strips should be carefully protected against humidity, which reduces reactivity. It is important to have the urine at room temperature for these enzyme reactions.

Clinistix—*o*-Toluidine Chromogen. Color changes from pink to purple. This formulation detects 100 mg/dL of glucose and is more sensitive to interfering substances such as ascorbic acid than are the tests listed next.

Multistix—Potassium Iodide Chromogen. Color changes from blue to brown at 30 seconds. Brown shades are difficult to distinguish.

Chemstrip—An Aminopropyl-Carbazol Chromogen. Color changes from yellow to orange-brown at 60 seconds.

Chemstrip uGc. Reagent pads have different sensitivities to urine glucose, ranging from 60 mg/dL to 5 g/dL. The chromogen is tetramethylbenzidine. Strips are read at two to three minutes and produce results close to a quantitative hexokinase method (Bandi, 1982).

Other Sugar Tests. Glucose and other reducing substances in urine are detected by a copper reduction test. Comments on other sugars follow. The glucose oxidase reagent strip test was described earlier.

Copper Reduction Tests. As a screening test, the glucose oxidase test does not detect increased levels of galactose or other sugars in urine. It is therefore important that a copper reduction test be used especially for young pediatric patients.

Of the copper reduction tests (Clinitest) used for screening purposes, the qualitative Benedict test (1909) is more sensitive to reducing substances in urine than the single-tablet copper reduction test (Cook, 1953). Urine samples containing nonglucose reducing substances may give positive results in healthy persons. Many substances in urine, metabolites, or drug-related metabolites influence urinary sugar test results (see Table 18–6). Strong reducing substances such as ascorbic acid, gentisic acid, or homogentisic acid may inhibit the enzyme test results while contributing to positive results of the copper reduction test. The tablet test is not affected as much as the Benedict's test. According to Smith (1977b),

Table 18–7. REACTIONS OF SUBSTANCES TO TEST FOR GLUCOSURIA

Constituent	Glucose Oxidase Reagent Strip	Copper Reduction Tablet Test
Glucose	Positive	Positive
Sugars other than glucose		
Fructose, Galactose, Lactose, Maltose, Pentose	No effect	Positive
Sucrose	No effect	No effect
Ketones (large amounts)	May depress color	No effect
Creatine, Uric acid	No effect	May cause false positive
Homogentisic acid (alkaptonuria)	No effect	Positive
Drugs*		
Ascorbic acid (large amounts)	May delay color	Trace positive
Cephalosporins (Keflin), etc.	No effect	Positive, brown color
L-Dopa (large)	False negative	No effect
Nalidixic acid glucuronide	No effect	Positive
Probenecid	No effect	Positive
Pyridium	Orange color may affect result	
Salicylate (large)	May lower reading	No effect
X-ray dye (diatrizoates)	No effect	Black color
Contaminants		
Hydrogen peroxide	False positive	May inhibit positive test
Hypochlorite (bleach)	False positive	
Sodium fluoride	False negative	No effect

*Other drugs implicated in copper reduction are amino acids, caronamide, chloral, chloroform, chloramphenicol, formaldehyde, hippuric acid, isoniazid, thiazides, oxytetracycline, *p*-aminosalicylic acid, penicillin, phenols, streptomycin, phenothiazine, and sulfonamides.

Data from Caraway (1962); Wirth (1965); Young (1975).

very large doses of ascorbic acid do not affect results of the two-drop copper reduction test. In those instances when the copper test result is positive and the glucose oxidase test is negative, glucosuria is ruled out; however, before investigating for other sugars, the clinical findings and drug history should be evaluated. Although the Clinitest detects nonglucose reducing sugars, the yield for these sugars is extremely low. Drugs give false-positive results or unusual colors with Clinitest, especially the cephalosporins such as cephalexin (Keflex) and radiographic media. Although large doses of ascorbic acid do not affect the two-drop Clinitest results for sugars (i.e., do not cause false-positive results) (Smith, 1977b), delay may occur in color development with the glucose oxidase test. Note that glycolytic enzymes from cells and bacteria reduce glucose levels in urine; prompt refrigeration or testing is essential.

Reference Values. Using these tests, the urine of normal children and adults is negative for glucose. Normal neonates during the first 10 to 14 days of life may excrete urine giving a positive reaction owing to glucose, galactose, fructose, and lactose (Bickel, 1961). Normal pregnant and postpartum women may give positive reactions because of the presence of lactose.

Copper Reduction Tablet Test. Clinitest tablets react with sufficient quantities of any reducing substances in the urine, including reducing sugars such as lactose, fructose, galactose, maltose, and the pentoses.

Both a five-drop and a two-drop Clinitest method have been described (Belmonte, 1967), and corresponding color charts are available for both. The two-drop method was developed in response to a so-called pass-through phenomenon, which may occur if more than 2 g/dL of sugar is present in the urine. In the pass-through phenomenon, the solution that results after addition of the Clinitest tablet goes through the entire range of colors and back to a dark greenish brown. This final color does not compare with any section of the color chart; however, it corresponds most closely to a significantly lower result. It is important to observe the entire reaction and for 15 seconds after boiling inside the tube has stopped so that the reversion to a different color is not missed and a falsely low result reported.

Chemistry. Copper sulfate, sodium hydroxide, sodium carbonate, and citric acid are incorporated into a tablet. Copper sulfate reacts with reducing substances in the urine, converting cupric sulfate to cuprous oxide. Based on Benedict's copper reduction reaction,

$$Cu^{++} \xrightarrow{\text{hot alkaline solution}} Cu^{+}$$
$$Cu^{+} + OH^{-} \rightarrow CuOH\ (\text{yellow})$$
$$2CuOH \xrightarrow{\text{heat}} Cu_2O\ (\text{red}) + H_2O$$

Heat is caused by the reaction of sodium hydroxide with water and citric acid.

Procedure

FIVE-DROP METHOD. Place 5 drops of urine in a dry test tube and add 10 drops of water. Add one Clinitest tablet by easing it into the tube without touching it—it contains strong alkali. Watch while boiling takes place but do not shake or touch the bottom of the tube—it is hot. Wait for 15 seconds after boiling stops, then shake the tube gently, and immediately compare the color of the solution with the color scale. Results correspond to the following approximate concentrations: negative; 0.25 g/dL; 0.5 g/dL; 0.75 g/dL; 1.0 g/dL; 2.0 g/dL; pass through. It is important to watch the solution carefully while it is boiling. If at this time the solution passes through orange to a dark shade of greenish brown, it indicates that more than 2 g/dL sugar is present, and this should be recorded as greater than 2 g/dL without reference to the color scale. Urine samples showing this pass-through phenomenon should be retested with the two-drop method.

TWO-DROP METHOD. Place 2 drops of urine in a test tube and add 10 drops of water. Add one Clinitest tablet. Watch while boiling takes place but do not shake. Wait 15 seconds after the boiling stops, then shake the tube gently, and compare the color of the solution with the color scale supplied for the two-drop method. The pass-through phenomenon may also occur with the two-drop test with large concentrations of sugar, more than 5 g/dL. Therefore, it is important to watch the test throughout the entire reaction and waiting period. Report results as 1 g/dL, 2 g/dL, 3 g/dL, 5 g/dL, and more than 5 g/dL if a pass-through reaction occurs. Negative or low-level results should have the five-drop method performed.

Clinitest reagent tablets detect 150 to 250 mg glucose per deciliter of urine. See Table 18–6 for reactions of sugars and drugs to glucose oxidase and copper reduction.

PRECAUTIONS. Observe the precautions in the literature supplied with the Clinitest tablets. The bottle must be kept tightly closed at all times to prevent absorption of moisture and kept away from direct heat and sunlight in a cool, dry place. The tablets normally have a spotted bluish white color. If not stored properly, they absorb moisture or deteriorate from heat, turning dark blue or brown. In this condition, they do not give reliable results. They are also available individually packaged in aluminum foil to help prevent this absorption of moisture. Although more expensive, such packaging is useful when a limited number of tests are performed.

Other Sugars in Urine

Some hexoses and pentoses cause positive copper reduction test results in urine when the glucose oxidase test is negative. In some rare cases, it is important to identify the sugars in patients with persistent mellituria by copper reduction. Fructose, galactose, lactose, maltose, and L-xylulose are found in urine in patients with inherited metabolic disorders (Scriver, 1989). It should be noted that many drug metabolites (e.g., in the form of glucuronides) also give positive copper reduction test results. If an inherited disorder is suspected, the sugar may be identified by thin-layer chromatography (Young, 1970). Qualitative confirmatory tests are generally not satisfactory for sugars.

Small amounts of disaccharides are normally excreted in the urine, about 50 mg in 24 hours. With intestinal diseases such as severe sprue or acute enteritis, the level may rise to 250 mg or more. With high levels of sugars in the gut as in lactose intolerance, lactose is absorbed and excreted unchanged in the urine.

GALACTOSE

Galactose is found in the urine in genetic disorders of galactose metabolism associated with a deficiency of galactose-1-phosphate uridyl transferase or galactokinase. In these diseases, galactose derived from dietary lactose is not converted to glucose. Early detection followed by dietary restriction may control the disease and avoid untoward sequelae (see Chap. 9).

SCREENING FOR GALACTOSE. Urine is tested with the glucose oxidase reagent strip and a copper reduction test. The presence of a reducing substance without glucose in the urine of newborns may suggest galactosemia. Thin-layer chromatography is used to identify galactose in urine. However, the disease is usually identified by erythrocyte enzyme assay when suspected (see Chap. 9).

LACTOSE

Lactose may appear in the urine late in normal pregnancy or during lactation.

SCREENING FOR LACTOSE. A positive result with the copper reduction test coupled with a negative glucose test result may be due to lactose or other reducing sugars. A qualitative lactose test may also be used. Lactose is identified using thin-layer chromatography.

LACTOSE TEST (Rubner, 1884). To 15 mL of urine in a test tube, add 3 g lead acetate. Shake and filter. Boil filtrate, add 2 mL of concentrated NH_4OH, and boil. Lactose causes the formation of a brick-red solution and then a red precipitate with clear supernatant. Glucose causes a yellow solution and yellow precipitate.

FRUCTOSE

Fructose appears in urine during parenteral feedings with fructose and in association with inherited enzyme deficiencies that cause benign essential fructosuria and serious fructose intolerance associated with severe vomiting and liver and kidney disease. Fructose is identified by thin-layer chromatography. A qualitative test, a resorcinol test, is found to be useful by some investigators (see Henry, 1984).

PENTOSE

Pentosuria may follow the ingestion of large amounts of fruits, causing the excretion of L-xylose and L-arabinose in amounts up to 0.1 g/day. L-Xylulose is excreted in benign essential pentosuria in amounts of 1 to 4 g/day. At concentrations of 250 to 300 mg/dL, L-xylulose reduces Benedict's qualitative reagent at 50°C (water bath) within 10 minutes or at room temperature in several hours. Fructose also reduces Benedict's reagent at low temperatures (see Henry, 1979). The pentoses are identified by thin-layer chromatography.

SUCROSE

Sucrose may appear in the urine after ingestion of very large amounts of sucrose. Sucrase deficiency is associated with intestinal diseases such as sprue in the same manner as lactase deficiency. Sucrose intolerance is an inherited disorder associated with sucrase and α-dextrinase (isomaltase) deficiencies. Symptoms are similar to those of lactase deficiency and occur in the first few weeks of life when sweetened food is ingested. Tolerance may develop, but sucrose may have to be avoided permanently.

Factitious sucrosuria may create high-specific-gravity urine with negative results of glucose oxidase and negative copper reduction tests. (Sucrose is not a reducing sugar.) Sucrose ferments yeast and can be separated by chromatography but needs to be stained with a substance not dependent on reducing properties.

Ketones in Urine

Ketone bodies are the products of incomplete fat metabolism, and their presence may be indicative of acidosis.

In ketonuria, the three ketone bodies present in the urine are acetoacetic (diacetic) acid (20%), acetone (2%), and 3-hydroxybutyrate (about 78%) (Henry, 1974). Acetone is formed nonreversibly from acetoacetic acid. β-Hydroxybutyric acid (3-hydroxybutyrate) forms reversibly from acetoacetic acid.

$$\text{Acetoacetic acid} \xrightarrow{-CO_2} \text{acetone}$$

$$\text{Acetoacetic acid} \underset{-2H}{\overset{+2H}{\rightleftharpoons}} \text{3-hydroxybutyrate}$$

Ketonemia and ketonuria are commonly encountered in uncontrolled diabetes mellitus. In urine, reagent strips and tablets react to 10 mg of acetoacetic acid per deciliter and are less sensitive to acetone. In plasma, about the same amounts of ketone bodies are detectable. When a patient is being monitored with repeated determinations of acetone and acetoacetic acid, the concentrations of these compounds may start at a high level and fall but still give elevated results. Therefore, repeated reports of elevations would not reflect the change taking place. In such an instance, semi-quantitative results can be obtained with either the reagent strip or Rothera's tablet test by testing several different dilutions of each specimen. Reagent strips correlate only moderately well with quantitative acetoacetate in plasma and poorly with total blood ketones (Alberti, 1972).

NONDIABETIC KETONURIA

In infants and children, ketonuria commonly occurs in various conditions, such as acute febrile diseases and toxic states accompanied by vomiting or diarrhea (Riekers, 1958). Ketonuria is also present in vomiting of pregnancy, in cachexia, and after anesthesia. In these cases, it is related most probably to increased tissue (especially fat) catabolism in the presence of limited food intake. In pregnancy, a normal patient may have a low fasting blood glucose level and mild ketonuria. The use of a low-carbohydrate diet for weight reduction produces ketonuria. Ketonuria is occasionally noted after exposure to cold or severe exercise.

Inherited metabolic disease should be suspected in neonates with severe ketoacidosis.

DIABETIC KETONURIA

The presence of ketonuria indicates the presence of ketoacidosis (ketosis) and may provide a warning of impending coma. Up to 50 mg of acetoacetic acid per deciliter may be present without clinical evidence of ketosis (Killander, 1962). Diabetic children and young adults are prone to episodes of ketosis, often associated with infection as well as with other problems in management. It is the usual practice in the management of diabetes to test for ketonuria when the urine, on qualitative examination, displays more than 1 to 2 g/dL of glucose. Combination glucose and ketone reagent strips are useful for patients. Large amounts of ketones depress the glucose oxidase test results and give falsely low results for glucose on some glucose oxidase strips. The urine of diabetic patients controlled with oral hypoglycemic agents should be tested regularly for ketone bodies as well as for glucose, especially in the presence of infection, because insulin may then be required for control. Ketonuria should also be watched for when changes in diabetic therapy are prescribed.

Whereas large amounts of ketones and glucose are noted in the urine of patients with diabetic ketoacidosis, ketonuria is not found with the hyperosmolar hyperglycemic coma sometimes occurring in older diabetic patients.

LACTIC ACIDOSIS

Lactic acidosis occurs with shock and with diabetes mellitus, renal failure, liver disease, and infections and in response to certain drugs, especially phenformin and salicylate poisoning. Levels of both acetoacetate and 3-hydroxybutyrate may be highly elevated in lactic acidosis. Usually the butyrate is high and acetoacetate is low, and it may not be detected by the nitroprusside test (Cohen, 1976; Hansen, 1978).

METHODS FOR DETECTION

REAGENT STRIP. The test is based on a nitroprusside (sodium nitroferricyanide) reaction for ketones. The reagent is very sensitive to moisture and quickly becomes nonreactive. With elevated (3+) results, urine may be diluted and retested, reporting a moderate result and the dilution factor.

Chemstrip contains sodium nitroferricyanide and glycine, which react with acetoacetic acid and acetone in an alkaline medium to form a violet dye. A positive result is indicated by a color change from beige to violet, which is read at 60 seconds. The test detects about 10 mg/dL of acetoacetic acid and 70 mg/dL of acetone. The sensitivity and reaction of the reagent strip are similar to those of the tablet (Acetest), described later.

Multistix contains buffers and sodium nitroferricyanide, which react with acetoacetic acid, producing a pink-maroon color in 15 seconds. The reagent area detects 5 to 10 mg acetoacetic acid per deciliter of urine. It does not react with acetone.

Color reactions (false positives) occur after the use of phthaleins (sulfobromophthalein [BSP] or PSP dyes), in the presence of extremely large amounts of phenylketones, and with the preservative 8-hydroxyquinoline, or L-dopa metabolites. Acetylcysteine (aerosol) produces a strong red color. The antihypertensive drugs methyldopa and captopril give positive results. False-negative results occur because of loss of reagent reactivity. These tests do not measure the predominant ketone body, 3-hydroxybutyrate.

OTHER TESTS FOR KETONES. Different tests measure acetoacetic acid or both acetone and acetoacetic acid. Commonly used nitroprusside strip and tablet tests based on the Rothera's method detect acetoacetic acid and acetone but not 3-hydroxybutyrate. Ferric chloride (Gerhardt's test) is a wet test that detects acetoacetic acid, and one nitroprusside strip test (Ames') detects only acetoacetic acid and does not detect acetone. These reagents are markedly subject to deterioration with humidity and become nonreactive.

Problems occur with false-negative results because of unstable reagents and labile ketones. Specimens need to be refrigerated if not tested immediately but should be brought to room temperature for testing. Preservatives do not prevent decay of ketones. If results are unexpected, fresh reagents, checked against known positive and negative controls, should be used.

Gerhardt's ferric chloride test has been used for many years as a test for acetoacetic acid. Ferric chloride tests are not very specific, however, and the sensitivity is low, about 25 to 50 mg/dL. The ferric chloride test gives positive results with salicylate and L-dopa.

Acetone and acetoacetic acid react with sodium nitroprusside (nitroferricyanide) in the presence of alkali to produce a purple complex. This reaction was described by Legal (1883) in diabetic urine specimens. In the simplest form of the nitroprusside test, reagent strips impregnated with sodium nitroprusside and alkali are used (discussed earlier). A tablet form of the test with similar sensitivity is available. A reagent strip without alkali reacts to acetoacetic acid and not to acetone. The blood level of ketone bodies may be estimated by the nitroprusside test at the bedside. This is especially helpful in determining the severity of ketosis in the treatment of diabetic acidosis, provided that the reagents are fresh.

Stability of Ketones. In urine, bacterial action causes loss of acetoacetic acid. This may happen *in vivo* as well as *in vitro*. Acetone is lost at room temperature but not if kept in a closed container in a refrigerator. If a sample cannot be tested immediately, it should be refrigerated.

Reference Values. Depending on the methods used, total ketone bodies (as acetone) range from 17 to 42 mg/dL (Henry, 1964). According to Killander (1962), up to 2 mg acetoacetic acid per deciliter is normal.

Nitroprusside Tablet Test. A tablet test method may be useful if the urine has an interfering color. The tablets are very sensitive to humidity and deteriorate if not stored properly. The Acetest tablet contains sodium nitroprusside, glycine, and a strongly alkaline buffer. It can be used to test whole blood, plasma, serum or urine.

Procedure. Place the tablet on a clean surface, preferably a piece of white paper. Place 1 drop of urine, serum, plasma, or whole blood on the tablet. For urine testing, compare the color of the tablet with a color chart 30 seconds after application of the specimen. For serum or plasma testing, compare the color of the tablet with the color chart two minutes after application of specimen. For whole blood testing, 10 minutes after application of the specimen, remove clotted blood from the tablet and compare the color of the tablet with the color chart.

If acetone and acetoacetic acid are present, the tablet shows a color varying from lavender to deep purple. Report the results as negative, small, moderate, or large. If large, a dilution may be made. Report these analyses in a form such as this: undiluted "large," 1:2 dilution "large," 1:4 dilution "moderate," and so on.

Acetest detects 5 to 10 mg of acetoacetic acid per deciliter of urine and 20 to 25 mg acetone per deciliter of urine. Like the reagent strips, it does not react with 3-hydroxybutyrate. It gives positive results with L-dopa and large amounts of phenylketones and with BSP and PSP dyes, which react with the alkali in the tablets.

Rothera's Test—Urine (see Henry, 1979). The test tube nitroprusside test of Rothera (1908) is sensitive to acetoacetic acid, about 1 to 5 mg/dL, and to acetone with a sensitivity of 10 to 25 mg/dL.

Blood, Hemoglobin, and Myoglobin in Urine

HEMATURIA

The presence of an abnormal number of blood cells in urine is known as hematuria, whereas the term hemoglobinuria indicates the presence of hemoglobin in solution in urine (Corwin, 1988). Hematuria is relatively common, hemoglobinuria uncommon, and myoglobinuria rare.

Because of the diagnostic importance of small amounts of hematuria and because of the tendency of erythrocytes to undergo lysis in urine, a screening test for heme is a useful adjunct to the microscopic examination of the sediment (Shenoy, 1986). However, a common problem with the test is inhibition of the heme reagent strip test, often owing to ascorbic acid, when erythrocytes are present. This problem emphasizes the need for routine microscopic tests in order to make a diagnosis of hematuria.

Because true hemoglobinuria is uncommon, a positive test result for hemoglobin with a normal urinary sediment suggests that a fresh urine sample should be examined for erythrocytes. Urine specific gravity of 1.010 or less may cause lysis of erythrocytes, as does alkaline pH.

Hematuria occurs with disease or trauma anywhere in the kidneys or urinary tract, with bleeding diseases and anticoagulants, and with the use of drugs such as cyclophosphamide. Hematuria is also noted in health persons undertaking excessive exercise (marathon runners), in whom bleeding emanates from the bladder mucosa.

HEMOGLOBINURIA

Any cause of hemolysis has the potential for causing hemoglobinuria, but the presence of hemoglobinuria indicates significant intravascular hemolysis as opposed to extravascular hemolysis. Free hemoglobin binds to plasma haptoglobin, and once this binding capacity is saturated, dissociated hemoglobin passes through the glomerulus as $\alpha\beta$ dimers with a molecular weight of 32,000. Some hemoglobin is reabsorbed by proximal tubular cells, and the remaining hemoglobin is excreted.

Hemoglobinuria may follow activities in which the small blood vessels suffer direct trauma as in marching, jogging, karate, or bongo drum playing. Many other causes of acute erythrocyte lysis are summarized in the next section. A comparison of expected urine and plasma findings with moderate and marked hemolysis is shown in Table 18–8. Plasma appears pink at levels of about 50 mg/dL of hemoglobin. With

Table 18–8. URINE AND PLASMA FINDINGS WITH INTRAVASCULAR HEMOLYSIS

Test	Moderate Hemolysis	Marked Hemolysis
Urine		
Bilirubin (conjugated)	Absent	Absent
Urobilinogen	Normal or elevated	Elevated
Hemoglobin	Absent	Present
Hemosiderin	Absent	Present (late)
Plasma		
Bilirubin (conjugated)	Elevated	Elevated
Haptoglobin	Decreased	Absent
Hemoglobin	Elevated	Elevated (marked)

marked hemolysis, plasma levels reach 1 g/dL. The plasma hemoglobin level is more often increased in severe acquired hemolytic anemias than in hereditary hemolytic anemias. However, moderately elevated levels occur with sickle-cell disease and homozygous thalassemias. Note that unstable hemoglobins (e.g., hemoglobin Köln) cause a brown-pigmented urine, but this is not due to hemoglobin. It is thought to be a dipyrrole or bilifuscin and does not react with the reagent strip test for heme.

SOME CAUSES OF HEMOLYSIS AND HEMOGLOBINURIA

Trauma to erythrocytes. Prosthetic cardiac valves (especially aortic), ostium primum repair with patch causing turbulence, extensive burns, strenuous exercise, marching, severe trauma to muscle and other vascular tissues (Daum, 1988).

Organisms. Malaria, *Bartonella*, *Clostridium welchii* toxin, brown recluse spider bite.

Erythrocyte enzyme-deficient (glucose-6-phosphate dehydrogenase [G6PD]) individuals. With oxidant drugs: acetanilid, sulfamethoxazole, nitrofurantoin, antimalarials (primaquine, and others); with fava beans (*Vicia fava*) in susceptible groups; with diabetic acidosis; with infections.

Unstable hemoglobin diseases and oxidant drugs.

Normal individuals, oxidative hemolysis due to drugs. Large doses or exposure to naphthalene (mothballs), some sulfonamides, sulfones, nitrofurantoin.

Immune mediated (see Chaps. 26 and 31). Severe hemolytic-uremic syndrome in children, thrombotic thrombocytopenic purpura. Incompatible blood transfusions. Warm antibodies: autoimmune—transient after infection, drug-induced. Cold antibodies: IgM—viral anti-i, mycoplasma anti-I; IgG—paroxysmal, Donath-Landsteiner anti-P; may be associated with congenital and acquired syphilis. Membrane sensitivity, complement mediated: paroxysmal nocturnal hemoglobinuria. Drugs: as haptens (penicillins), immune complex (quinidine, phenacetin), α-methyldopa.

MYOGLOBINURIA

With acute destruction of muscle fibers (rhabdomyolysis), myoglobin is released, rapidly cleared from blood, and excreted in the urine as a red-brown pigment. If large amounts of myoglobin are presented to the kidneys, anuria may result from renal damage.

Free myoglobin, a monomer with molecular weight of 17,000, is excreted quickly, whereas the hemoglobin-haptoglobin complex is slowly removed and hemoglobin is excreted mostly as dimers of 38,000 molecular weight. Urinary acid pH affects the stability of myoglobin. The specimen should be neutralized and refrigerated as soon as possible.

The distinction between hemoglobinuria and myoglobinuria is difficult to make on examination of the urine. Immunochemical tests may prove to be more useful than qualitative tests.

The diagnosis of rhabdomyolysis and myoglobinuria is usually made from the history and other laboratory findings as follows. Myoglobinuria has been noted after a number of strenuous exercises, in the military, and with marathon running and karate. Patients typically have muscle tenderness or cramps and void red-brown urine within a day or two after exertion. The reagent strip urine test for heme is markedly positive, and protein and a few red blood cells are present. Serum is clear and has markedly elevated creatine kinase (CK > 100,000 IU/L is typical) and elevated serum aldolase levels but normal haptoglobin level. Serum creatinine may be slightly increased. The urine usually clears in two to three days, and the serum CK level slowly declines. The serum measurements and history help distinguish myoglobinuria from hemoglobinuria. Proteinuria; hematuria; myoglobinuria; and hyaline, granular, and pigmented casts all are seen after severe exercise, especially in untrained persons (Bailey, 1976). Myoglobin appears to be more toxic to the kidneys than hemoglobin.

REAGENT STRIP FOR HEME COMPOUNDS (HEMOGLOBIN, MYOGLOBIN)

The test is based on the liberation of oxygen from peroxide in the reagent strip by the peroxidase-like activity of heme from free hemoglobin, lysed erythrocytes, or myoglobin. Intact erythrocytes are lysed on the strip, causing the hemoglobin to react. Therefore, well-mixed urine must be tested, because intact erythrocytes are missed if only supernatant urine is used. Because of its reducing properties, ascorbic acid interference is a problem with certain reagent strips. Hematuria may be missed if only the reagent strip test is used and a microscopic examination is omitted.

The reagent area is impregnated with a buffered mixture of an organic peroxide and the chromogen tetramethylbenzidine.

$$H_2O_2 + \text{chromogen} \xrightarrow[\text{Peroxidase activity}]{\text{Heme}} \underset{\text{(color change)}}{\text{oxidized chromogen}} + H_2O$$

Heme catalyzes the oxidation of tetramethylbenzidine to produce a green color. The test zone is yellow in the absence of blood and green to blue-green in the presence of blood. Timing is important.

Multistix and Chemstrip detect 0.015 to 0.062 mg hemoglobin per deciliter of urine. This hemoglobin concentration is equivalent to approximately 5 to 20 intact red blood cells per microliter of urine. It is assumed that these are normal erythrocytes containing approximately 30 picograms of hemoglobin per cell. Excretion of less than 5 RBCs per microliter may be not be detected. Read at 60 seconds.

Sensitivity is reduced in urine specimens with high specific gravity, in which erythrocyte lysis may not occur, and when protein levels are high. Ascorbic acid in larger concentrations may depress results by approximately one color block. The presence of nitrite in large amounts delays the test reaction, and formalin used as a urine preservative may cause falsely low or negative reactions. Oxidizing contaminants such as hypochlorites (bleach) may produce false-positive results. Microbial peroxidase, associated with urinary tract infection, potentially causes a false-positive reading.

OTHER TESTS FOR HEMOGLOBIN AND MYOGLOBIN

HEMOGLOBIN AND MYOGLOBIN. The distinction between hemoglobinuria and myoglobinuria is difficult to make on examination of the urine. In both cases, the urine is dark red or brown and some erythrocytes are seen in the sediment.

3

Table 18–9. DIFFERENTIATION OF HEMATURIA, HEMOGLOBINURIA, AND MYOGLOBINURIA

Condition	Plasma Findings	Urine Findings
Hematuria	Color—normal	Color—normal, smoky, pink, red, brown Erythrocytes—many Renal—red blood cell casts Protein—marked increase Lower urinary tract—no casts Protein—present or absent
Hemoglobinuria	Color—pink (early) Haptoglobin—low	Color—pink, red, brown Erythrocytes—occasional Pigment casts—occasional Protein—present or absent Hemosiderin—late
Myoglobinuria	Color—normal Haptoglobin—normal Creatine kinase—marked increase Aldolase—increased	Color—red, brown Erythrocytes—occasional Dense brown casts—occasional Protein—present or absent

Pigment casts may be found; these may be dark brown with myoglobin. Table 18–9 compares the findings of hemoglobinuria, myoglobinuria, and hematuria.

The reagent strip test for blood is positive with hemoglobin and myoglobin. If serum can be examined, it is often pink with hemoglobinemia but a normal color with myoglobinemia because this pigment is cleared so rapidly. None of the qualitative tests have been satisfactory in separating myoglobin and hemoglobin, both of which may be present after crush injuries. The salt precipitation method of Blondheim (1958) has been used, as have spectroscopic methods. According to Boesken (1979), hemoglobin and some myoglobin are bound to proteins in urine, and this contributes to the difficulty of separating them by salt precipitation or acetate electrophoresis.

Immunochemical tests with antisera to human myoglobin require a human myoglobin standard from muscle or from urine containing myoglobin and an antiserum that does not cross-react with hemoglobin (Kagen, 1967; Markowitz, 1977). The myoglobin antigen is not very stable (Boesken, 1979), but these tests are specific and are preferred. End-point and rate nephelometric methods are available.

QUALITATIVE TEST FOR MYOGLOBIN. (Blondheim, 1958)

1. Use a fresh urine specimen. Observe the color of the urine. Urine with myoglobinuria is characteristically red when fresh and turns brown on standing, but some myoglobin may be present without color change. Myoglobin is less stable at an acid pH. Neutralize and refrigerate the specimen pending testing.
2. Mix 1 mL of urine and 3 mL of 3% sulfosalicylic acid to test for protein. If the pigment is precipitated, it is a protein. Filter. If the filtrate is a normal color, no abnormal nonprotein pigment is present. (Note: The heat and acetic acid test does not precipitate myoglobin or hemoglobin.)
3. To 5 mL of urine in a test tube, add 2.8 g of ammonium sulfate. Dissolve by mixing. The urine is now 80% saturated with ammonium sulfate. This is optimal for precipitation of hemoglobin. Filter or centrifuge. If the supernatant shows a normal color, the precipitated pigment is hemoglobin. If the supernatant fluid is colored, this is presumptive evidence of myoglobin.

Note that with muscle injury, both pigments may be present.

HEMOSIDERIN

Free hemoglobin is readily filtered out by the glomeruli (Fig. 18–1). Filtered hemoglobin is reabsorbed by proximal tubular cells and catabolized into ferritin and hemosiderin, which can later be detected in the urinary sediment with Prussian blue stain in desquamated cells and in casts (see Table 18–7).

Thus, the presence of hemosiderin in urine, usually two to three days after the acute hemolytic episode, is an indication of significant intravascular hemolysis. Note that hemosiderinuria is also found with diseases causing siderosis of the kidneys—namely, hemochromatosis.

Because of the intermittent presence of hemosiderinuria, urinary iron levels may be quantitated to establish the presence of chronic intravascular hemolysis. Normal urinary iron excretion is about 0.1 mg/day. It is increased with hemochromatosis and in association with erythrocytes traumatized by prosthetic heart valves. Urinary iron levels are normal with pernicious anemia and in hereditary spherocytosis.

Hemosiderin appears in the urine sediment in diseases involving a true siderosis of the kidney parenchyma (hemochromatosis). It is also present two to three days after an acute hemolytic episode that caused hemoglobinuria. At this time, the reagent strip test result for hemoglobin is often negative. Hemosiderin is found as yellow-brown granules that are free or in epithelial cells and occasionally in casts (Plate 18–1). The Prussian blue reaction is used to demonstrated iron in hemosiderin (Plate 18–2). A wet preparation (Rous) and a dry smear (Cartwright) are alternative methods.

WET PROCEDURE (Rous, 1918)

1. Centrifuge a complete morning specimen or random urine samples at 450 g for 5 minutes and pool the sediment. Examine several drops of sediment microscopically, searching for coarse yellow-brown granules, especially within renal tubular epithelial cells or casts.

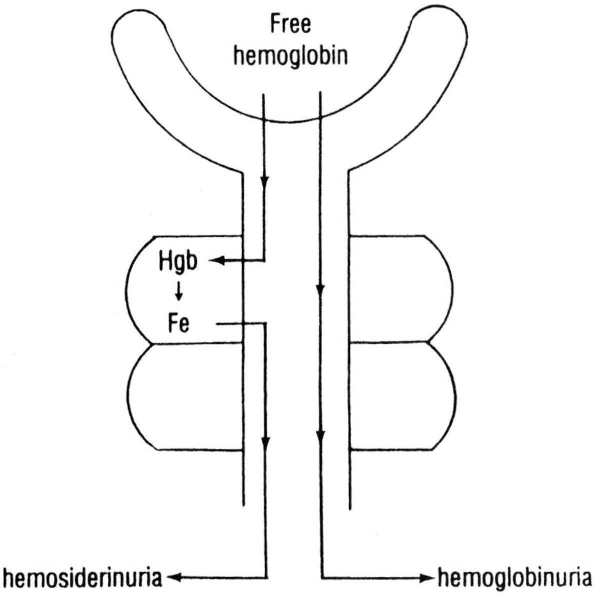

Figure 18–1. Renal processing of filtered hemoglobin.

2. If such granules are seen, suspend the rest of the sediment in a fresh mixture of 5 mL of 2% potassium ferrocyanide solution and 5 mL of 1% HCl and allow to stand for 10 minutes.
3. Centrifuge the specimen and discard the supernatant. Examine the sediment microscopically. Coarse granules of hemosiderin appear blue in this preparation (Plate 18–1) in cells, casts, and amorphous material. If granules do not stain, re-examine after 30 minutes (occasionally the reaction is delayed).

DRY PROCEDURE (Cartwright, 1968). When stained, hemosiderin appears as blue granules, 1 to 3 μm, singly or in groups, in renal tubular epithelial cells, as amorphous sediment, or as blue granules in casts. An iron stain used for siderocytes in blood or bone marrow is also suitable. Urine is collected overnight in an iron-free glass container. Let stand for two hours. Decant three fourths of it. Centrifuge the remainder. Make a smear(s) of the sediment. Air-dry.

Reagents. The Prussian blue reagent is made fresh.

1. Potassium ferrocyanide, 20% in demineralized water. Store in a dark bottle (iron free) at room temperature. Stable for three weeks.
2. Concentrated HCl.
3. Prussian blue stain: Add concentrated HCl to an aliquot of the potassium ferrocyanide solution until a white precipitate forms that remains stable on shaking. Filter through Whatman's number 5 filter paper.
4. Safranin O, 0.5 g in 100 mL distilled water. Stable stock solution.
5. Phosphate buffer pH 6.4 to 6.7 for counterstain.
6. Working counterstain. Dilute 1 mL safranin O stain to 50 mL with phosphate buffer.

Procedure

1. Fix the smear in methyl alcohol for 10 minutes.
2. Rinse with iron-free water (demineralized) and air-dry.
3. Stain with Prussian blue reagent for 30 minutes.
4. Wash gently for at least four minutes with iron-free water and air-dry.
5. Counterstain with safranin O for one to five minutes.
6. Rinse with iron-free water. Air-dry.
7. Mount a coverslip using a drop of immersion oil.
   Note: All glassware, slides, coverslips, and so on should be iron free. Water should be demineralized.

Bilirubin in Urine

Bilirubin is a breakdown product of hemoglobin formed in the reticuloendothelial cells of the spleen, liver, and bone marrow and carried in the blood by protein. Unconjugated bilirubin in the blood is not able to pass through the glomerular barrier of the kidneys. When bilirubin is conjugated in the liver with glucuronic acid to bilirubin glucuronide, it becomes water soluble and is able to pass through the glomeruli of the kidneys into the urine. Normal adult urine contains about 0.02 mg of bilirubin per deciliter (With, 1954), and this is not detected by the usual tests. For a review of bilirubin metabolism, see Chapter 12.

3

Conjugated bilirubin is normally excreted in the bile into the duodenum. Conjugated bilirubin appearing in urine suggests obstruction to bile outflow from the liver—for example, gallstones in the common bile duct or carcinoma of the head of the pancreas. The urine is dark and may have a yellow foam. Bilirubinuria is associated with elevated serum bilirubin (conjugated), jaundice, and pale-colored feces. These acholic stools are so called because of the absence of bilirubin-derived pigment. Bilirubin is also found in the urine when intracanalicular pressure rises because of periportal inflammation or fibrosis and from swelling of liver cells. Bilirubin may, for example, appear in the urine in acute viral hepatitis or drug-induced cholestasis before the appearance of jaundice. The test is helpful in diagnosis and in monitoring the course of infectious hepatitis. A positive test result for urinary bilirubin with a negative test result for urobilinogen in urine is indicative of intrahepatic or extrahepatic biliary obstruction. The test is, therefore, of value in the differential diagnosis of jaundice, because bilirubinuria is not found with hemolytic jaundice (Table 18–10).

In congenital hyperbilirubinemias, bilirubin appears in the urine in the Dubin-Johnson type and the Rotor type. It does not appear with Gilbert's disease or Crigler-Najjar disease. In persons exposed to toxins and ingesting certain drugs, a positive test result for bilirubinuria may be an early indication of cholestasis or liver damage. Bilirubinuria is found with jaundice of acute alcoholic hepatitis.

Excretion of bilirubin is enhanced by alkalosis.

A test for bilirubin in urine should be performed when the dark color of the urine or the presence of yellow foam indicates its possibility.

METHODS FOR DETECTION

REAGENT STRIP. The test for bilirubin is based on a diazo reaction, and tests differ in the diazonium salt used. Urine must be fresh because bilirubin glucuronide in urine quickly hydrolyzes to less-reactive bilirubin. Then, oxidation of bilirubin in specimens that have stood too long, especially when exposed to light, results in false-negative findings. With use of this method, normal urine contains no detectable bilirubin (see the section entitled Diazo Tablet Method).

Table 18–10. URINE AND FECAL FINDINGS IN JAUNDICE

Finding	Normal	Obstruction to Bile Flow	Hemolysis, Hemolytic Anemia	Liver Damage, Hepatitis, Cholestasis
Urinary bilirubin	Absent	Increased, dark urine	Absent	Increased early
Urinary urobilinogen	Present	Neoplasm—low or absent; gallstones—variable	Increased	Decreased early; increased late
Fecal color	Dark	Pale; intermittent with gallstones in common bile duct; persistent with neoplasm in duct or pancreas	Dark	Pale early and dark late in hepatitis; pale with cholestasis

The reaction is based on the coupling reaction of bilirubin with a diazonium salt in acid medium.

Multistix—Diazotized 2,4-Dichloroaniline. Color changes from cream-buff to tan at 20 seconds and detects 0.8 mg/dL urine. Colors are hard to read.

Chemstrip — 2,6-Dichlorobenzene-Diazonium Tetrafluoroborate. Color changes from pink to violet at 30 to 60 seconds and detects 0.5 mg/dL urine.

Large amounts of ascorbic acid and nitrite lower bilirubin results. Metabolites of drugs such as phenazopyridine give a reddish color at the low pH of the strip and mask the result. Rifampin and large amounts of chlorpromazine metabolites may give positive results. Salicylates do not interfere. Urobilinogen does not affect the result.

Confirmatory Bilirubin Tests. The diazo test method, in which bilirubin is coupled to *p*-nitrobenzene diazonium *p*-toluene sulfonate to form a blue or purple color (in the form of a tablet or reagent strip), is commonly used. Another test uses a ferric chloride reagent to oxidize bilirubin to a green biliverdin (Watson, 1946; see Henry, 1979).

The reagent strip test is much less reactive to the free bilirubin than the tablet test; thus, a difference in results becomes more apparent as the urine ages. See the section that follows for the interpretation of the bilirubin and urobilinogen tests. The reagent strip method was described earlier.

Diazo Tablet Method (Free, 1953)

REAGENTS. Tablets containing *p*-nitrobenzene diazonium *p*-toluene are used. The tablets also contain sulfosalicylic acid and sodium bicarbonate to provide an acid medium for the reaction and an effervescent mixture that ensures the solution of a portion of the tablet when water is added. (Ictotest kit, including asbestos-cellulose mats and reagent tablets, is available through Ames Company, Elkhart, IN.)

PROCEDURE

1. Place 10 drops of specimen on an asbestos-cellulose mat provided with the kit. Bilirubin, if present, is adsorbed onto the mat surface.
2. Place a reagent tablet on the moistened area of the mat.
3. Allow two drops of water to flow over the tablet onto the mat. If bilirubin is present, bilirubin couples with *p*-nitrobenzene diazonium *p*-toluene sulfonate from the tablet, as shown by the formation of a blue to purple color within 30 seconds. Pink or red represents a negative result. The tablet should be moved to reveal the purple reaction.

The diazo test reacts positively to bilirubin in amounts of 0.05 to 0.1 mg/dL. No purple reaction occurs with urobilin or other pigments or with any other known constituent of normal urine. High levels of urobilin or indican give a red color. Azo compounds cause an atypical color (e.g., phenazopyridine). Rifampin may interfere. Chlorpromazine metabolites in large amounts produce a purple color. Metabolites of the anti-inflammatory drugs mefenamic and flufenamic acid cause false-positive results.

WASH-THROUGH TABLET METHOD (Free, 1978). When false-positive reactions are suspected (e.g., with chlorpromazine), the contaminant is diluted out with water in the mat. Prepare duplicate mats with 10 drops of urine on each. Add 10 drops of water to one mat. Place a reagent tablet on each mat and then 2 drops of water onto each tablet. Bilirubin, if present, is adsorbed into the mat fibers and appears the same on each mat; an interfering substance produces a light color or no color on the mat with the extra water.

STABILITY OF REAGENT. Ictotest reagent tablets are effervescent and somewhat hygroscopic, and accordingly, they should be protected from moisture or high humidity. The tablets are packed in a brown bottle, because prolonged direct exposure to strong light results in decomposition of the stabilized diazonium compound. Prolonged exposure of several weeks to temperatures of 38°C or more may also result in deterioration of the tablets. A brown discoloration indicates deterioration, and brown tablets should not be used. When each new bottle is opened, tablets should be checked for positive and negative reactions.

Urobilinogen in Urine

After conjugation in the liver cells, bilirubin diglucuronide reaches the duodenum complexed with cholesterol, bile salts, and phospholipids. The conjugated bilirubin is not absorbed from the small intestine. In the colon, glucuronidases from bacteria hydrolyze the conjugate. The free bilirubin is reduced to urobilinogen, mesobilirubinogen, and stercobilinogen. Most of the pigment is excreted in feces as colored urobilins or stercobilin formed after further removal of hydrogen. A small amount of urobilinogen is absorbed into the portal circulation from the colon and travels to the liver, where it is re-excreted, unconjugated, in the bile. A small amount normally reaches the kidneys.

Urobilinogen in urine represents more than one closely related tetrapyrrole derived from bilirubin. They are normally present, are colorless and labile, and react to form red-purple compounds with Ehrlich's aldehyde reagent. Urobilins are orange oxidation products of urobilinogen that do not react with Ehrlich's reagent but react with Schlesinger's zinc reagent. Urobilins impart color to normal urine.

Normal output of urobilinogen is 0.5 to 2.5 mg or units/24 hours. Tubular reabsorption is decreased and output is increased in alkaline urine, such as with the alkaline tide after meals. The level is decreased in acid urine. Because a mixture of substances is measured, the term units is frequently used instead of milligram terminology. They are roughly equivalent. For quantitative comparative purposes in the same patient, a two-hour test is used. Urine is collected from 2 to 4 P.M. after lunch, making sure that the patient is well hydrated. The period after the meal coincides with more excretion of urobilinogen when the pH of the urine is more nearly neutral. Other two-hour periods may be selected, provided that they are the same for each patient, for purposes of comparison.

In patients with liver damage or dysfunction, more urobilinogen than normal is excreted through the kidneys. With liver cell damage due to viral hepatitis, with drugs or toxic substances, or in some cases of portal cirrhosis, recirculated urobilinogen is not re-excreted in the bile and appears in urine. With congestive cardiac failure and liver congestion, urobilinogen handling and re-excretion in bile are impaired. With an infection, such as cholangitis associated with obstruction, large amounts of urobilinogen are excreted in urine together with bilirubin. Urobilinogen is also increased in urine of patients with fever; some of this increase is associated with dehydration and concentrated urine.

Persistent excess urobilinogen in urine with negative bilirubin is seen with jaundice due to hemolytic anemias. These jaundiced patients have dark-colored stools. For a comparison of urinary and fecal findings in jaundice, see Table 18–10. Urobilinogen is increased after acute lysis of erythrocytes and with the destruction of erythrocyte precursors in the bone marrow with megaloblastic anemias. Increased urobilinogen also accompanies bleeding into tissues and the subsequent formation of excess bilirubin. Persistent absence of urinary urobilinogen occurs with complete obstruction of the common bile duct and is associated with pale stools. It should be noted that an absence of urobilinogen cannot be detected by reagent strips. When also accompanied by blood in feces, carcinoma of the pancreas or the ampulla of Vater is likely. Broad-spectrum antibiotics cause reduction of urobilinogen formation in the colon and therefore reduce its excretion in feces and urine.

Mesobilifuscin is a dipyrrole that normally contributes to fecal and urine color. It is not derived from bilirubin, like urobilinogen, but is probably a byproduct of heme synthesis. It causes dark brown urine whenever Heinz bodies form in erythrocytes (e.g., with the unstable hemoglobins). This brown pigment in urine also occurs in cases of homozygous β-thalassemia. It does not react to tests for blood or bilirubin.

METHODS FOR DETECTION

REAGENT STRIP. Urobilinogen is normally present in urine. The test is based on Ehrlich's aldehyde reaction or the formation of a red azo dye from a diazonium compound. Urine must be fresh and at room temperature. Urobilinogen is very labile in acid urine and, with light, forms nonreactive urobilin; a negative result is not significant. Normally, 1 Ehrlich unit/dL or 1 mg/dL may be present. Urobilinogen is often designated in units because it represents a mixture of more than one substance (see Tables 18–8 and 18–10 for urobilinogenuria).

Multistix impregnated with *p*-dimethyl-amino-benzaldehyde produces a reddish brown color with urobilinogen. The test is read in Ehrlich units per deciliter. Color blocks representing 0.2 to 12 Ehrlich units per deciliter are provided. Color varies from light yellow to shades of brown.

The Multistix reagent strip is not specific for urobilinogen and reacts with substances known to react with the Ehrlich's reagent. These include porphobilinogen, *p*-aminosalicylic acid metabolites, sulfonamides, procaine, 5-hydroxyindoleacetic acid, indole, and methyldopa (Aldomet). The test is not a reliable method for the detection of porphobilinogen. Porphobilinogen and intermediate Ehrlich-reacting substances can be detected by using the Watson-Schwartz test (described later).

Chemstrip impregnated with 4-methoxybenzene-diazonium-tetrafluoroborate couples with urobilinogen in an acid medium to form a red azo dye. Values are read at 10 to 30 seconds. The test detects approximately 0.4 mg/dL. Values up to 1 mg/dL are considered normal. Nitrite or formalin may reduce the color reaction. This test is specific for urobilinogen.

Both reagent strips are affected by the metabolites of drugs such as phenazopyridine, which colors the urine orange red in an acid medium, and other compounds such as Azo Gantrisin. These may mask the reaction with urobilinogen or give a false-positive result. Interfering substances often react faster than urobilinogen.

Bilirubin and blood do not usually affect the results, but bilirubin may occasionally cause a green color.

OTHER UROBILINOGEN AND PORPHOBILINOGEN TESTS

Urobilinogen. The qualitative test for urobilinogen and porphobilinogen may be performed as a confirmatory test when more than 1 Ehrlich unit is shown on the reagent strip test. The Watson-Schwartz test is used to separate causes of a positive Ehrlich-reacting strip test and to give an indication of large amounts of urobilinogen or the presence of porphobilinogen. Quantitative tests for urobilinogen in urine are seldom performed. Consult Henry (1979) for two-hour quantitative urobilinogen method and Davidsohn (1974) or Schwartz (1944) for 24-hour quantitation.

Normal adult urine contains from about .05 to 2.5 mg of urobilinogen in a 24-hour collection; less than 1 Ehrlich unit in two hours is excreted as measured by a semi-quantitative method (Balikov, 1957).

The strip test for urinary urobilinogen that uses the Ehrlich's aldehyde should not be used to screen for the presence of urinary porphobilinogen. The reagent strip is not a reliable method for detecting porphobilinogen in urine. A positive result for porphobilinogen in the Watson-Schwartz test is confirmed by Hoesch's test, because the Watson-Schwartz test may show false-positive results for porphobilinogen as a result of drugs such as methyldopa. Very large amounts are needed to cause false-positive results in the Hoesch test. When a qualitative porphobilinogen test is requested or a known porphyric patient is being monitored, the simpler Hoesch's test is used instead of the Watson-Schwartz test.

The urine specimen for urobilinogen or porphobilinogen must be fresh. If the test cannot be performed at once, the pH should be adjusted to near neutral (pH 7) and the specimen stored in a refrigerator, where it is stable for about one week (With, 1980). Urine may darken if the patient has porphyria, especially if left at room temperature.

The Ehrlich's aldehyde reaction and Watson-Schwartz tests are based on solubility differences between urobilinogen and porphobilinogen. Urobilinogen can be extracted by chloroform or butanol, whereas porphobilinogen remains in an aqueous phase (Henry, 1984; Watson, 1941).

Procedure: Watson-Schwartz Test

1. To 2.5 mL fresh urine, add 2.5 mL Ehrlich's reagent and mix.
2. Add 5 mL saturated sodium acetate and mix. Check with pH paper to confirm that the solution is in the pH range of 4 to 5. Adjust pH if necessary.
3. Add 5 mL of chloroform; invert and shake vigorously for one minute. Permit the phases to separate.
4. Examine the upper (aqueous) phase. If the color is absent, consider the result of the screening test to be negative and stop.
5. If color is present, separate the upper (aqueous) phase and add 5 mL of butanol. Insert the stopper and shake vigorously for one minute. Allow phases to separate.
6. A pink to rose-red color in the lower aqueous layer indicates a positive result and suggests a concentration of porphobilinogen that is several times normal. A color in the upper butanol layer indicates an increase in urobilinogen concentration (Fig. 18–2).

Hoesch's Test. Hoesch's test is based on the inverse Ehrlich's reaction (i.e., of maintaining an acid solution by adding a small urine volume to a relatively large reagent volume), eliminating the problem of urobilinogen reaction. The urine specimen must be fresh or stored at neutral pH in a refrigerator. The urine specimen from a patient having an acute porphyric attack may become dark red; dilute 1:10 with water and test (Henry, 1984; Hoesch, 1947).

The sensitivity is similar to that of the Watson-Schwartz test, but the reaction is for porphobilinogen (see Hoesch, 1947). The test detects about 20 to 100 mg/L of porphobilinogen. A yellow color is caused by urea. Urobilinogen in amounts up to 200 mg/L does not cause a red color.

According to Pierach (1977), the Watson-Schwartz test is more sensitive than Hoesch's test for porphobilinogen, and therefore it may yield a positive result between attacks of acute intermittent porphyria. The Watson-Schwartz test detects greater than 6 mg/L and Hoesch's test greater than 11 mg/L of porphobilinogen. Large doses of methyldopa (Aldomet) gave positive results, as did indoles in some patients with intestinal ileus, and the drug phenazopyridine, which becomes orange with hydrochloric acid. Very large amounts of urobilinogen are needed to give a positive Hoesch's test result, and this is not a practical problem.

A quantitative porphobilinogen test is necessary if either the Watson-Schwartz test or the Hoesch's test result is questionable; this situation may arise because of the instability of porphobilinogen.

The urorosein urinary pigment related to indoleacetic acid produces a positive Hoesch's test result (in response to strong HCl), and the rose color may be confused with a positive porphobilinogen result. Some of the false-positive problems may be excluded by testing the specimen with concentrated HCl (12 mol/L) separately in conjunction with Hoesch's test.

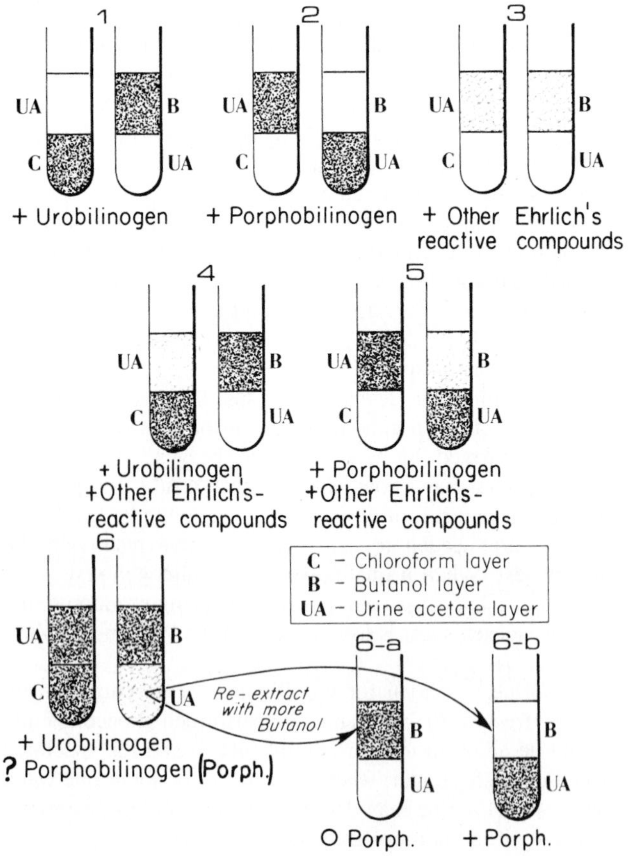

Figure 18–2. Watson-Schwartz test. Interpretation of screening method for urine urobilinogen and porphobilinogen.

Nitrite in Urine

A positive nitrite test result indicates that bacteria that reduce urinary nitrate to nitrite are present in significant numbers. Many enteric gram-negative organisms give positive results when their number is greater than 10^6/mL of bladder urine. If the test result is positive, a culture should be considered, provided that the specimen was properly collected and stored before testing. A first morning, clean, midstream specimen is best. False-positive results occur with poorly collected and stored specimens because of contaminants and bacterial proliferation.

According to Kunin (1975), self-administered repeated nitrite tests (three tests) in a small group of patients revealed about 70% overall positive results when compared with cultures. When only *Escherichia coli* was present, bacteriuria detected by a positive nitrite test result in any of the three first morning specimens showed 93% agreement with culture results. There were no significant false-positive nitrite results in his large test group.

METHODS FOR DETECTION

REAGENT STRIP. The test depends on the conversion of nitrate to nitrite by certain bacterial action in the urine. Because the test requires an overnight (minimum of four hours) bladder bacterial population to convert urinary nitrate to nitrite, a first morning specimen is best. Most Enterobacteriaceae bacteria are able to form nitrite from nitrate, but not all bacteria in bladder urine convert nitrate to nitrite (e.g., *Enterococcus*). Known nitrate-reducing organisms at significant levels may produce negative results. These organisms reduce nitrate to ammonia, nitric and nitrous oxide, hydroxylamine, and nitrogen and therefore give a negative nitrite test result. A positive result is a possible indication for culture, unless the specimen has been improperly stored after collection, allowing bacterial growth. A fresh specimen is essential.

MULTISTIX. At an acid pH, nitrite, if present, reacts with *p*-arsanilic acid to give a diazonium salt, which by coupling with benzoquinoline forms a pink azo dye. It detects 0.075 mg of nitrite per deciliter in solution. Read at 40 seconds.

Chemstrip contains a benzoquinoline and sulfanilamide, which produce a pink azo dye with nitrite at 30 seconds. It detects 0.05 mg of nitrite per deciliter.

False-positive readings may be produced by medication that colors the urine red or turns red in an acid medium (e.g., phenazopyridine). Pink spots or edges are interpreted as negative. False-negative results occur with nitrite tests as a result of ascorbic acid, urobilinogen, or low pH (<6) (James, 1978b).

False-negative results occur because some nitrate-reducing organisms form compounds other than nitrite and are not detected. Random specimens collected during the day and urine from patients with draining catheters do not show good correlation between the nitrite test and significant bacteriuria, presumably because of the time required for the chemical reduction to nitrite in the bladder urine.

Leukocyte Esterase in Urine

Esterase activity has been demonstrated in the azurophilic or primary granules of the neutrophil series of leukocytes and is used as a marker for these cells by means of the chloroacetate stain. Extracts of human azurophil neutrophil granules contained up to 10 proteins showing esterolytic activity (Dewald, 1975). Because neutrophils and other cells are labile in urine (Triger, 1966), this test is thought to be useful in detecting the enzyme remnants of cells that are not visible microscopically. It is also assumed that granulocytes are the only source of these esterases in urine.

Healthy persons excrete blood cells in urine. A difficulty has arisen in determining suitable cut-off points for normal and abnormal numbers of these cells. Because quantitative counts are so low when compared with those of blood, precision is poor (see Quantitative Counts and Differential Counts). Attempts to correlate low urinary chamber cell counts with estimates on sediments and with esterase tests are fraught with difficulties. Values of $10/\mu L$ to $30/\mu L$ of leukocytes have been used as cut-off points using clinical correlates, usually infection (Stansfeld, 1953; Houston, 1963). Using fresh clean-catch or catheter specimens, Kusumi (1981) found that the esterase test gives a reasonably good indication of the presence of neutrophil esterases when about 10 or more cells per microliter is used as an indication of pyuria. Using a concentrated (10:1) urine sediment and a cytocentrifuged stained preparation, Avent (1983) showed that a negative reagent strip test result is associated with fewer than 100 neutrophils in 10 high-power fields (hpf) ($\times 450$).

The esterase test is a useful adjunct to the microscopic examination of the urine sediment. Test results are probably more reliable when clean-catch midstream specimens are collected. Contamination with vaginal fluid may result in positive results. The presence of large numbers of squamous epithelial cells and bacteria, indicating vaginal contamination, is easily detected microscopically.

It should be noted that the common finding of leukocytes in urine is not as reliable an indication of urinary tract infection as the detection of bacteriuria by Gram's stain or culture of a fresh midstream specimen. In a series of 32,000 tests, Washington (1981) found 94% sensitivity and 90% specificity for the microscopic examination of the Gram's stain when compared with significant culture results. A positive microscopic test result is defined as even distribution of at least two organisms per oil immersion field throughout at least 20 oil immersion fields. The microscopic examination was accomplished quickly but required a carefully collected clean-catch midstream specimen with experienced personnel assisting the patient. The negative predictive value of this test was 99%, and the positive predictive value was 90%.

METHODS FOR DETECTION

3

REAGENT STRIP. Neutrophil granulocytes contain many esterases, which catalyze the hydrolysis of an ester to produce its alcohol and acid. The test is similar in principle to the naphthol chloroacetate test used for granulocyte esterases in hematology. The esterase level in urine correlates with the number of neutrophils present. Cells from the urinary tract and erythrocytes do not contribute to this esterase level. The test should be used in conjunction with the microscopic appraisal for leukocytes.

A substrate, indoxyl carbonic acid ester, is catalyzed to indoxyl and by oxidation from atmospheric oxygen forms indigo, a blue color. Reaction time for this formulation is 15 minutes. The reagent has been modified with the addition of a diazonium salt to produce a faster reaction, with the indoxyl reacting with diazonium to form a purple reaction in 1 to 2 minutes.

Positive results correlate with significant numbers of neutrophils either intact or lysed. With the use of a chamber count of about 10 neutrophils per microliter of fresh urine as a cut-off point, the number of false-negative and false-positive results was low (Gillenwater, 1981).

Interference. Hematuria and bacteriuria affect the reaction. Protein inhibits the test. Oxidizing agents give false-positive colors. Very large amounts of ascorbic acid may inhibit the reaction. Formalin inhibits the reaction. Nitrofurantoin and other strong colors affect color interpretation. *Trichomonas* and eosinophils may represent sources of esterases causing a false-positive result.

CONFIRMATORY TESTS FOR LEUKOCYTE ESTERASE AND BACTERIURIA. Microscopic urinalysis serves as a rapid confirmatory test for the presence of leukocytes and bacteria. Bacteriologic culture is the definitive test for bacteriuria.

Miscellaneous Chemical Screening Tests

ASCORBIC ACID

Because of its reducing properties, a large urinary concentration of ascorbic acid from therapeutic doses of vitamin C or preparations containing ascorbic acid may inhibit several reagent strip reactions (i.e., glucose, blood, bilirubin, nitrite, and leukocyte esterase). Manufacturers differ in their reagent strip susceptibility to ascorbic acid. It is useful to check for the presence of ascorbic acid when the microscopic examination of a urine sediment shows more than two erythrocytes per high-power field and the screening test result for blood on the uncentrifuged urine specimen is negative.

Urine tests for ascorbic acid have been used as an indication of adequate ascorbic acid therapy. With an adequate diet, 2 to 10 mg/dL is excreted daily. After ingestion of large amounts of ascorbic acid, levels in urine are about 200 mg/dL. Metabolites of ascorbic acid are sulfate and oxalate. With a large intake, 1 g or more per day, oxalate stones may form in susceptible persons.

C-Stix reagent strips have a reagent-impregnated area consisting of phosphomolybdates buffered in an acid medium. Phosphomolybdates are reduced by ascorbic acid to molybdenum blue. This test detects 5 mg/dL of ascorbic acid in urine after 10 seconds. Gentisic acid and L-dopa may cause false-positive results.

Stix reagent strips are not as sensitive as C-Stix. They detect about 25 mg/dL of ascorbic acid at 60 seconds. The reagent is methylene green, which is reduced to its colorless form with ascorbic acid. Neutral red provides a background color, and the overall color changes from blue to purple at levels of 150 mg/dL. This test is also part of the Multistix multiple reagent strips. Large amounts of bilirubin and pH greater than 7.5 interfere with the color. False-positive results are not seen with urates, salicylates, gentisic acid, or creatinine.

PROCEDURE. Dip the test end of the strip into the specimen. Compare the color of the reagent area of the strip with the color chart supplied by the manufacturer and report as indicated on the chart.

5-HYDROXYINDOLEACETIC ACID

Serotonin (5-hydroxytryptamine) is produced by the argentaffin cells of the intestines from tryptophan and is carried in the blood by platelets.

Carcinoid tumors (argentaffinoma) arising from the argentaffin cells produce excessive amounts of serotonin, especially when metastatic. Serotonin causes intestinal disturbances, vasomotor disturbances, and bronchoconstriction. Edema, right-side valvular heart disease, and neurologic symptoms are seen. The screening test (Sjoerdsma, 1955) is useful for the detection of the serotonin metabolite 5-hydroxyindoleacetic acid in the urine if it appears in fairly large amounts. The quantitative method is more sensitive, because it eliminates the interfering ketoacids and indoleacetic acid (Udenfriend, 1955).

Normal excretion of 5-hydroxyindoleacetic acid in 24 hours is 1 to 5 mg. A random specimen of urine is usually sufficient for screening purposes; if a 24-hour collection is made, it should be acidified with HCl (see Collection of Urine). Boric acid may also be used as a preservative. Patients should not take any drugs for 72 hours before the test; phenothiazines, acetanilid drugs, and mephenesin, a muscle relaxant, interfere with this test.

The principle of the test is based on the development of a purple color specific for 5-hydroxyindoles with nitrous acid and 1-nitroso-2-naphthol. Ethylene dichloride is used to remove interfering chromogens (for procedure, see Henry, 1984).

MELANIN

Melanin is a pigment derived from tyrosine, which is normally present in hair and skin and in the eyes. Two metabolic pathways for the conversion of tyrosine to melanin are recognized: the eumelanin (brown or black) and the pheomelanin (yellow-red) pathways. Normal melanocytes in skin convert tyrosine to dihydroxyphenylalanine (DOPA) and then to dopaquinone and by oxidative steps to eumelanin. The enzyme tyrosinase is required for the first step and is found in the specific organelles of melanocytes called melanosomes. Its formation is stimulated by melanin-stimulating hormone. The number of granules present is related to the amount of pigmentation seen. Melanosomes with pigment are normally transferred from melanocytes to skin and mucous membrane cells. Large melanosomes are found in tumor cells (e.g., nevus, melanoma).

Urinary excretion of melanin metabolites increases as malignant melanoma metastasizes. These are called urinary melanogens and include indoles, catechols, and catecholamines. DOPA does not appear in large amounts in urine from melanotic patients, and it is unusual to find a dark color even after standing at room temperature for 24 hours.

Rarely, cells containing melanin pigment are seen in urine sediment when melanuria follows pigment uptake by renal tubular cells and when melanoma is metastatic to the bladder (Piva, 1964). A ferrous ion uptake stain can be used to color the melanin in cells dark blue.

Screening tests for melanin should be made on fresh specimens of urine. Ferric chloride, Ehrlich's aldehyde reagent, and nitroferricyanide give nonspecific color reactions with melanin. There is no simple specific test for melanuria. Procedures for the ferric chloride and nitroferricyanide tests for melanin can be found in Henry (1984).

A column cation-exchange chromatographic method that has been described allows detection of abnormal metabolites in urine and the early detection of liver metastases (Banda, 1977). Another approach is to measure DOPA-oxidase levels in urine. The enzyme is increased in the urine of patients with melanoma and is markedly increased with liver metastases (Roguljic, 1975).

PORPHYRINS

The porphyrias are a group of diseases resulting from defects in the synthesis of heme. These are inherited enzyme deficiencies in which the enzyme substrate is usually excreted in excess in urine or feces.

A description of the chemistry and synthesis of porphyrins with clinical pathologic correlation and analytical techniques is given in Chapter 8.

The patterns of excretion of the various porphyrins vary with the different diseases. These and the clinical findings help establish the diagnosis. Skin photosensitivity and skin lesions frequently accompany high levels of porphyrins. The one entity without skin lesions is acute intermittent porphyria. Patients presenting with neurologic disease and acute abdominal pain—the hepatic group—have increased production and excretion of δ-aminolevulinic acid (ALA) and porphobilinogen during the acute porphyric attack. There is probably increased activity of ALA synthase and subsequent increased production of the precursors. Exacerbations of the hepatic diseases are precipitated by drugs known to induce liver enzyme activity (e.g., barbiturates and certain steroids).

SCREENING TESTS. In patients suspected of having an acute porphyric attack, porphobilinogen is sought in a urine specimen using the Watson-Schwartz test. Porphobilinogen is insoluble in chloroform or butanol and remains in the aqueous phase of the separation. Hoesch's test is used as a second confirmatory test. During the acute attack, high levels of porphobilinogen are excreted, but the urine is not always colored because about 500 μg/L of porphyrins can be present without causing a red-purple color (Henry, 1974). Between attacks, levels of porphobilinogen may be increased but may also be normal.

Uroporphyrin and coproporphyrin are detected by fluorescence. An orange-red fluorescence is seen if the specimen is placed near an ultraviolet light source. The porphyrins are excreted in most of the porphyrias and in lead poisoning. Coproporphyrin and uroporphyrin can also be separated by thin-layer chromatography or by extraction and fluorometry and quantitated using ion-exchange columns.

Screening tests together with the clinical findings indicate whether quantitative tests should be carried out. These are usually performed by reference or research laboratories.

The urine specimen for quantitative porphobilinogen should be kept at near neutral pH (between 6 and 7) and protected from light (Bossenmaier, 1968). Frozen specimens are fairly stable. ALA is more stable if the urine is acidic. However, if both substances are to be tested, the near neutral pH is preferred and the urine aliquot is frozen. These substances are quantitated by eluting from different columns and reacting with Ehrlich's reagent.

A urine specimen for quantitative porphyrins is collected in a dark container containing 5 g sodium carbonate for a 24-hour specimen to give a concentration of 0.1% sodium carbonate or to produce urine of neutral pH. Urine buffered at pH 7 is preferred to prevent formation of porphyrin from porphobilinogen (Fogstrup, 1979).

Fecal porphyrins can be qualitatively estimated using extraction and ultraviolet (UV) light, or quantitated. In protoporphyria, the fecal specimen may fluoresce, owing to high protoporphyrin levels. In some porphyrias, erythrocytes may show fluorescence when an unstained blood smear is examined microscopically. The nucleated bone marrow erythrocytes give greater fluorescence.

In lead poisoning, blood and urinary lead levels, ALA levels in serum and urine, and coproporphyrin levels in urine all are used to help make a diagnosis.

Screening Procedure for Porphyrin. The urine is acidified, and the extracted porphyrin exposed to UV light.

1. Place 5 mL urine in a stoppered glass centrifuge tube. Add 3 mL of a mixture of one part glacial acetic acid with four parts of ethyl acetate.
2. Shake and allow to separate. Centrifuging accelerates the separation.
3. Using a Wood's lamp, observe the upper layer for fluorescence. Inspect the tube in a dark room with UV reflected light. A lavender to violet color indicates the presence of porphyrins; pink to red fluorescence indicates higher levels of porphyrin. Pale blue with no pink tinge is a negative result. Normal urine may fluoresce blue.

To increase the sensitivity of the test and remove interfering drug metabolites, transfer the upper layer to a glass tube and acidify with 0.5 mL of 3 M HCl (25 mL concentrated HCl diluted to 100 mL with water). Shake. Porphyrins are extracted into the lower aqueous layer and give a red-orange fluorescence (Haining, 1969).

An alternative screening method uses an anion-exchange resin column. Porphyrins are adsorbed, eluted, and exposed to fluorescent light. This method removes interfering substances and is similar in principle to the quantitative method for total porphyrins (Fogstrup, 1979) and for coproporphyrin and uroporphyrin (Leahy, 1982). Urinary porphyrin profiles demonstrating more metabolites are detected by high-performance liquid chromatography.

EXAMINATION OF URINE SEDIMENT

Microscopic examination of urine is the most common laboratory procedure used for the detection of renal or urinary tract disease. Interpretation of urine sediment requires time, skill, training, and experience acquired through constant use of various microscopic methods and continuous pathophysiologic correlation of the sediment findings with the macroscopic results and clinical status of the patient. In order to practice with competence, one must be knowledgeable about numerous morphologic entities (e.g., organisms, hematopoietic and epithelial cells, casts). Also, microscopists must be alert about the clinical relevance of urine findings as well as the common chemical abnormalities associated with microscopic interpretations. For a more detailed discussion of urinary findings in urinary system diseases, readers are referred to Haber (1981), Schumann (1980, 1981b), Ross (1983), Mandal (1988), and relevant textbooks.

Formed Elements of Urine

Centrifuged urine sediment contains all the insoluble materials (commonly referred to as formed elements) that have accumulated in the urine in the process of glomerular filtration and during passage of fluid through the tubules of the kidneys and lower urinary tract. Cells found in urine come from two sources: (1) desquamation or spontaneous exfoliation of epithelial cells lining the upper (kidney) and lower urinary tract and adjacent structures and (2) cells from the circulating blood (leukocytes and erythrocytes). Casts formed in the renal tubules and collecting ducts are the other formed elements frequently seen.

Organisms (bacteria, fungi, viral inclusion cells, parasites) and neoplastic cells represent elements foreign to the urinary system, and proper identification of these elements may provide important diagnostic clues to the cause of certain urinary system disorders.

Normal or reference values for formed elements vary from one laboratory to another because of (1) the variation in concentration of random urine specimens as voided and (2) the different methods used to concentrate the sediment by centrifugation. Individual laboratories have established their own reference values, often in conjunction with nephrologists and nephropathologists.

Microscopic Components in Urine Sediment

Cells

ERYTHROCYTES

Under high power, unstained erythrocytes or red blood cells appear as pale disks. They vary somewhat in size but are usually about 7 μm in diameter. If the specimen is not fresh when it is examined, the cells appear as faint, colorless circles or shadow cells, because the hemoglobin may dissolve out. These membranes are more obvious with phase-contrast microscopy. They may become crenated in hypertonic urine and appear as small, rough cells with crinkly edges. Smooth, folded, and crenated cells may be seen in the same specimen. On occasion, erythrocytes may be confused with oil droplets or yeast cells. Oil droplets, however, exhibit a great variation in size and are highly refractile. Yeast cells usually show budding and do not stain. If there is doubt about identification, two preparations may be made and a few drops of acetic acid added to one. Erythrocytes are lysed in the acidified preparation.

Erythrocytes are found in small numbers in normal urine. How these cells enter the urine is not known.

In normal individuals, occasional red blood cells (0 to 2/hpf or 3 to 12/μL) may be seen on microscopic examination of the sediment.

DYSMORPHIC ERYTHROCYTES. When increased numbers of erythrocytes are found in the urine in conjunction with erythrocyte casts, bleeding may be assumed to be renal in origin. In the absence of casts or proteinuria, increased erythrocytes suggest a bleeding site distal to the kidney. Fairley (1982) has observed that aberrant or dysmorphic erythrocyte morphology is specific in detecting glomerular bleeding (Plate 18–3). These distorted cells are also more readily observed using phase-contrast microscopy. When 80% or more of red blood cells are undistorted and uniform, these are regarded as nonglomerular (i.e., from a tubular source or associated with calculi or lower urinary tract disease). Normal persons also have a mixture of distorted and undistorted erythrocytes in urine (Fassett, 1982).

Increased numbers of erythrocytes in the urine may be present in (1) renal disease, including glomerulonephritis, lupus nephritis, interstitial nephritis associated with drug reactions, calculus, tumor, acute infection, tuberculosis, infarction, renal vein thrombosis, trauma (including renal biopsy), hydronephrosis, polycystic kidney, and occasionally acute tubular necrosis and malignant nephrosclerosis; (2) lower urinary tract disease, including acute and chronic infection, calculus, tumor, stricture, and hemorrhagic cystitis following cyclophosphamide therapy; (3) extrarenal disease, including acute appendicitis, salpingitis, diverticulitis, and tumors of the colon, rectum, and pelvis (Table 18–11); acute febrile episodes, malaria, subacute bacterial endocarditis, polyarteritis nodosa, malignant hypertension, blood dyscrasias, and scurvy; (4) toxic reactions due to drugs such as sulfonamides, salicylates, methenamine, and anticoagulant therapy; and (5) physiologic causes, including exercise.

LEUKOCYTES

NEUTROPHILIC LEUKOCYTES. Under high power, neutrophilic leukocytes appear as granular spheres about 12 μm in diameter. In freshly voided urine, nuclear detail is not well defined. Nuclear segments may appear as small round discrete nuclei. When cellular degeneration has begun, nuclear detail may be lost. Neutrophils may then become difficult to distinguish from renal tubular epithelial cells. By allowing a small drop of dilute acetic acid to run under the coverslip, one may enhance nuclear detail so that definition may still be possible (Plate 18–4). Ultimately, however, with continued degeneration, neutrophilic nuclear segments fuse, making distinction from mononuclear cells difficult or impossible.

Supravital staining may also be helpful in emphasizing nuclear detail. With crystal-violet safranin, neutrophilic nuclei appear reddish purple and cytoplasmic granules violet. Cytochemical definition of neutrophils using the peroxidase reaction has been found to be especially useful in distinguishing neutrophils from tubular cells (Bradley, 1968). The stain is described later.

In dilute or hypotonic urine, neutrophils swell and cytoplasmic granules exhibit brownian movement. Because of the refractility of the moving granules, neutrophils in this setting are known as glitter cells. These cells take supravital stains poorly, if at all. Papanicolaou's stain also reflects the swelling of neutrophils in hypotonic urine. In addition, the neutrophils show loss of nuclear segmentation (Palmieri, 1977). Clinical studies have shown that leukocyte esterase reagent strips with a sensitivity of 81% to 94% and a specificity of 69% to 83% are valuable in the confirmation of pyuria in hypotonic urine specimens (Avent, 1983).

PYURIA. Increased numbers of leukocytes in the urine, principally neutrophils, are found in almost all renal diseases and diseases of the urinary tract. They may also be transiently increased during fevers and after strenuous exercise. When accompanied by leukocyte casts or mixed leukocyte-epithelial cell casts, increased urinary leukocytes are considered to be renal in origin.

The presence of many leukocytes (>20/hpf using a standardized slide) or clumps of leukocytes in the sediment is considered abnormal. Counts greater than 30/hpf suggest an acute infection. Repeated sterile cultures in this setting may indicate tuberculosis or a nephritis. Gross pyuria may reflect rupture of a renal or urinary tract abscess.

Moderate numbers of leukocytes in conjunction with leukocyte casts may reflect either bacterial (acute and chronic pyelonephritis) or nonbacterial (acute glomerulonephritis, nephritis) renal disease. Calculous disease at any level may give rise to increased numbers of urinary leukocytes because of either stasis-induced ascending infection or localized mucosal inflammatory response. Bladder tumors, as well as various acute or chronic localized inflammatory processes, may also cause leukocytes to be increased in the urine. The latter disorders include cystitis, prostatitis, urethritis, and balanitis. In women, the acute urethral syndrome or dysuria-pyuria syndrome is regularly associated with neutrophils in excess of 8/μL in clean-catch urine specimens; however, bacterial colony counts are lower than expected. *Chlamydia trachomatis* as well as staphylococci and coliforms was the causative agent (Stamm, 1981). It should be recognized that even in normal circumstances, some leukocytes are found in the secretions of the male and female genital tracts and appear in urine.

Finally, leukocytes are rapidly lysed in hypotonic or alka-

Table 18–11. VARIOUS URINARY SYSTEM DISEASES AND CORRESPONDING URINALYSIS ABNORMALITIES

Diseases	Macroscopic Urinalysis	Microscopic Urinalysis
Acute glomerulonephritis	Gross hematuria "Smoky" turbidity Proteinuria	Erythrocyte and blood casts Epithelial casts Hyaline and granular casts Waxy casts Neutrophils Erythrocytes
Chronic glomerulonephritis	Hematuria Proteinuria	Granular and waxy casts Occasional blood casts Erythrocytes Leukocytes Epithelial casts Lipid droplets
Acute pyelonephritis	Turbid Occasional odor Occasional proteinuria	Numerous neutrophils (many in clumps) Few lymphocytes and histiocytes Leukocyte casts Epithelial casts Renal epithelial cells Erythrocytes Granular and waxy casts Bacteria
Chronic pyelonephritis	Occasional proteinuria	Leukocytes Broad waxy casts Granular and epithelial casts Occasional leukocyte cast Bacteria Erythrocytes
Nephrotic syndrome	Proteinuria Fat droplets	Fatty and waxy casts Cellular and granular casts Oval fat bodies and/or vacuolated renal epithelial cells occurring singly or as cellular clusters
Acute tubular necrosis	Hematuria Occasional proteinuria	Necrotic or degenerated renal epithelial cells Neutrophils and erythrocytes Granular and epithelial casts Waxy casts Broad casts Epithelial tissue fragments
Cystitis	Hematuria	Numerous leukocytes Erythrocytes Transitional epithelial cells occurring singly or as fragments Histiocytes and giant cells Bacteria Absence of casts
Dysuria-pyuria syndrome	Slightly turbid	Numerous leukocytes, bacteria Erythrocytes No casts
Acute renal allograft rejection (lower nephrosis)	Hematuria Occasional proteinuria	Renal epithelial cells Lymphocytes and plasma cells Neutrophils Renal epithelial casts Renal epithelial fragments Granular, bloody, and waxy casts
Urinary tract neoplasia	Hematuria	Atypical mononuclear cells with enlarged, irregular hyperchromatic nuclei and sometimes containing prominent nucleoli that occur singly or as tissue fragments Neutrophils Erythrocytes Transitional epithelial cells
Viral infection	Hematuria Occasional proteinuria	Enlarged mononuclear cells and/or multinucleated cells with prominent intranuclear and/or cytoplasmic inclusions Neutrophils Lymphocytes and plasma cells Erythrocytes

line urine. Approximately 50% are lost after two to three hours of standing at room temperature (Triger, 1966). The need for prompt examination of the urinary sediment after collection is thus dramatized.

EOSINOPHILS (Plate 18–5). If clinically indicated, leukocyturia should be further analyzed for the presence of eosinophils (Schumann, 1980). A cytocentrifuge preparation with Wright's, Diff-Quik, or Papanicolaou's stain may be used to demonstrate eosinophils in urine. Hansel's secretion stain (methylene blue and eosin-Y in methanol, Libe Labs,

Florissant, MO) has been shown to be an excellent stain for recognition of eosinophiluria (Nolan, 1988). Appropriately stained, bilobed eosinophils may be noted in patients with tubulointerstitial disease associated with hypersensitivity to drugs such as penicillin and its analogues (Lombardo, 1980). Eosinophiluria is also seen in other acute disorders of the genitourinary tract (Nolan, 1988). Eosinophils are difficult to find in the cell sediment if the total number of leukocytes is low. Helgason (1972) collected specimens by suprapubic aspiration and prepared cytocentrifuged smears. A total leukocyte count of 10 or more cells per microliter gave satisfactory smear results. The cell pattern in allergic interstitial nephritis usually includes many erythrocytes and some renal tubular epithelial cells.

LYMPHOCYTES AND MONONUCLEAR LEUKOCYTES. Small lymphocytes are normally present in urine, although they are not routinely recognized. These cells and histiocytes are more easily differentiated in stained smears. When mononuclear cells (histiocytes, lymphocytes, or plasma cells) constitute 30% or more of a differential count, chronic inflammation is suggested (Lindqvist, 1975). Many small lymphocytes may be found in urine during renal transplant rejection. Plasma cells and atypical lymphocytes should be noted when present, and further investigation is essential.

RENAL EPITHELIAL CELLS

RENAL TUBULAR EPITHELIAL CELLS (Plates 18–6 and 18–7). Small numbers of tubular cells may be seen in normal urine, reflecting the normal sloughing of aging cells. They are present in somewhat larger numbers in the urine of normal newborns (Cruikshank, 1967).

Papanicolaou's stain has been shown to be especially useful in distinguishing renal tubular cells from other mononuclear cells in urine. Using this method, renal tubular cells from the proximal and distal convoluted tubules have been identified and may be semi-quantitated. Renal epithelial cells from the proximal and distal convoluted tubules occur singly and are large (14 to 60 μm), oblong or egg-shaped cells with characteristic coarsely granular eosinophilic cytoplasm. Nuclei may be multiple but are small, with dense chromatin and rare nucleoli. Increased numbers of proximal and distal convoluted renal epithelial cells are seen in cases of acute tubular necrosis and certain drug or heavy metal toxicity (Schumann, 1981b).

Epithelial cells from the small and large collecting duct measure 12 to 20 μm and are identified by their characteristic cuboidal or polygonal shape and large, usually slightly eccentric nucleus. Cytoplasmic properties include a basophilic endo-ecto plasmic rim commonly found in transitional epithelial cells. Increased numbers of collecting duct epithelial cells are found in renal transplant rejection, acute tubular necrosis (diuretic phase), and other ischemic injuries of the kidneys. They may also be found in increased numbers in malignant nephrosclerosis as well as in cases of acute glomerulonephritis accompanied by tubular damage. Ingestion of various drugs and chemicals may cause significant tubular desquamation. Collecting duct tubular cells are easily found in the urine after salicylate intoxication.

Renal epithelial fragments of collecting duct origin have been described. Proximal and distal convoluted tubular cells are not found in fragment form. Three or more renal cells of collecting duct origin constitute a renal epithelial fragment and indicate a more severe form of renal tubular injury with basement membrane disruption. Renal epithelial fragments are indicative of ischemic necrosis and are usually found accompanying varying degrees of renal tubular injury and pathologic casts. Five common configurations of renal epithelial fragments have been described (Schumann, 1981a). Proper identification of renal epithelial fragments is essential not only in the diagnosis of a more severe form of renal tubular injury but also in avoiding a false-positive diagnosis of low-grade transitional cell carcinoma.

Lipids in Renal Tubular Epithelial Cells. Oval fat bodies are tubular cells that have absorbed lipoproteins with cholesterol and triglycerides leaked from nephrotic glomeruli (Plate 18–8). Oval fat bodies therefore constitute one form of lipiduria. Lipids may also appear in the urine as free fatty droplets. Histiocytes may also ingest lipids and become impossible to distinguish from oval fat bodies. Their clinical significance, however, is similar. The presence of any or all of these lipid forms accompanied by marked proteinuria is characteristic of the nephrotic syndrome.

Positive identification of lipid is required before reporting lipiduria. When free or incorporated droplets contain large amounts of cholesterol, they exhibit Maltese cross formation under polarized light (Plate 18–9*A* and *B*). When they contain large amounts of triglycerides, fat stains (Oil Red O or Sudan III) are required for positive lipid identification.

Pigment in Renal Tubular Epithelial Cells. With hemoglobinuria or myoglobinuria, heme pigment is absorbed into the cells and converted to hemosiderin. The iron-laden cells are desquamated and found in the urine sediment. Granules appear yellow brown and stain for iron with Prussian blue. These cells are also incorporated into casts (Plates 18–1 and 18–2).

Melanin granules are absorbed into the tubular cells in rare cases of melanuria. The desquamated pigmented cells may be demonstrated in the sediment. Pigmented tumor cells are also found in patients with melanoma metastases to the bladder (Piva, 1964).

Bilirubin pigment colors all of the elements of the sediment, including renal tubular epithelial cells and casts. Note that urobilin does not color cells and casts.

LOWER URINARY TRACT EPITHELIAL CELLS

TRANSITIONAL (UROTHELIAL) EPITHELIAL CELLS. These cells line the urinary tract from the renal pelvis to the proximal two thirds of the urethra. In the urine, their size ranges from 40 to 200 μm, and they are round or pear shaped. The nuclei are round and central. These cells may occasionally be binucleate. A few are present in normal urine, reflecting normal desquamation. The presence of large clumps or sheets of these cells in the absence of instrumentation (i.e., catheterization) suggests the need for cytologic examination with Papanicolaou's stain because of possible transitional cell carcinoma anywhere from the renal pelvis to the bladder.

When stained, transitional cells have dark blue nuclei with variable amounts of pale blue cytoplasm (Plate 18–10). Another helpful clue to the proper identification of transitional cells is a characteristic "endo-ecto cytoplasmic" rim.

SQUAMOUS EPITHELIAL CELLS. The distal one third of the urethra is lined by squamous epithelial cells. In the urine, these cells are large and flat, with abundant cytoplasm and small round central nuclei (Plate 18–11). Their margins are often folded. The cells are occasionally rolled into cylinders. Many of the squamous cells present in female urine may derive from the vagina or vulva. When stained with crystal-violet safranin, nuclei are purple and cytoplasm pink to violet. By and large, squamous cells in female urine have little diagnostic significance. Large numbers in women and uncircumcised men may be a source of contamination.

Casts

Casts are formed as translucent, colorless gels from protein in the tubules of nephrons. In a normal person, very few are seen in the urinary sediment. In kidney diseases, they may appear in large numbers and in many forms (Table 18–12). Increased numbers of casts usually indicate that kidney disease is widespread and that many nephrons are involved. With chronic renal diseases, some casts become denser in appearance and are known as waxy. Large numbers of casts may also be seen in healthy persons after strenuous exercise, accompanying the proteinuria of exercise.

Normal urine has a very small amount of protein—about 150 mg/24 hours. Albumin and small molecular plasma globulins constitute about two thirds of the protein, and about one third is the glycoprotein secreted by the thick part of the ascending loop of Henle and possibly the distal tubule. This is known as Tamm-Horsfall protein. It is generally held that Tamm-Horsfall protein forms the matrix of all casts. The protein forms a meshwork of fibrils that may trap cells, cell fragments, or granular material. Cast formation increases with lower pH and increased ionic concentration and with stasis or obstruction of the nephron by cells or cell debris. Casts begin to disintegrate in dilute and alkaline urine or in the presence of bacteria that probably contribute to the alkalinity.

Cast formation is increased when larger than normal amounts of plasma proteins enter the tubules. The protein in excess usually is albumin, but globulins such as the Bence Jones immunoglobulin cause cast formation, as do hemoglobin and myoglobin. The plasma proteins possibly react or combine with Tamm-Horsfall protein to form less translucent casts and granular casts.

Table 18–12. CLASSIFICATION OF CASTS

Matrix
Hyaline—variable size
Waxy—often broad in use
Inclusions
Granules—proteins, cell debris
Fat globules—triglycerides, cholesterol esters
Hemosiderin granules
Crystals—uncommon
Melanin granules—rare
Pigments
Hemoglobin, myoglobin, bilirubin, drugs
Cells
Erythrocytes and red blood cell remnants
Leukocytes—neutrophils, lymphocytes, monocytes, and histiocytes
Renal tubular epithelial cells
Mixed cells—erythrocytes, neutrophils, and renal tubular cells
Bacteria

The size and shape of casts depend on the site of formation. Large casts are seen in dilated tubules or with stasis in collecting ducts. Thin casts occur in tubules compressed by swollen interstitial tissue or because of disintegration. Casts are sometimes convoluted and occasionally show a branch. They may be short and stubby or long. Long, convoluted casts appear when diuresis occurs after urinary stasis. Casts have parallel sides and usually have blunt ends. With age they may begin to disintegrate and show thinning and irregularities. Fibrils separate, causing a frayed appearance. Tails and tapering ends are seen, and these disintegrating forms have been referred to as cylindroids (see Wenk, 1981; Haber, 1975; and Mandal, 1988).

Casts may be classified according to their matrix, inclusions, pigments, and cells (see Table 18–11). A detailed discussion, including clinical significance, follows.

3

CAST MATRIX

HYALINE CASTS. Hyaline casts are translucent with brightfield microscopy but are easily seen with phase-contrast microscopy (Plate 18–12*A* and *B*). With phase contrast, the typical hyaline cast is seen to contain some fine granules. However, these casts are currently reported as hyaline rather than granular. Increased numbers are found with renal diseases and transiently with exercise, fever, congestive heart failure, and diuretic therapy (Imhof, 1972).

WAXY CASTS. These differ from hyaline casts in that they are easily visualized because of their high refractive index. Early waxy casts are believed by some investigators to reflect the final phase of dissolution of the fine granules of granular casts (Plate 18–13). Because time is required for granules to undergo lysis, waxy casts imply localized nephron obstruction and oliguria.

With brightfield microscopy, waxy casts are homogeneously smooth in appearance (Plate 18–14). Their margins are sharp even in subdued light. Their ends are blunt, and cracks or convolutions are frequently seen along the lateral margins, indicating a measure of brittleness. Waxy casts are commonly associated with tubular inflammation and degeneration. They are observed most frequently in patients with chronic renal failure. They are also found during acute and chronic renal allograft rejection. When waxy casts are unusually broad, they are known as renal failure casts. These casts carry the implication of advanced tubular atrophy or dilation, in turn reflecting end-stage renal disease.

INCLUSION CASTS

Granules, small (fine) and large (coarse), represent plasma protein aggregates that pass into the tubules from damaged glomeruli and cellular remnants from leukocytes, erythrocyte remnants, or damaged renal tubular cells and possibly fine salt precipitates. Protein aggregates include fibrinogen, immune complexes, and globulins. Lipid droplets are sometimes mistaken for large granules. With prolonged stasis, large granules in casts may become smaller.

GRANULAR CASTS (Plate 18–15). These are common. There appears to be no advantage to separating kinds of granular casts. Granular casts appear with glomerular and tubular diseases but are also a feature of tubulointerstitial disease and renal allograft rejection. Granular casts accompany pyelonephritis, viral infections, and chronic lead poisoning. Coarsely granular casts occur, with hematuria, in cases of renal papillary necrosis. It is possible that some fine granules represent calcium phosphate precipitants in hyperparathyroidism. These fine granules disappear from the hyaline matrix as a patient's urine is acidified by giving ammonium chloride and return when the urine is allowed to become more alkaline (Albright, 1935).

FATTY CASTS (Plates 18–16 and 18–17). Fatty material is incorporated into the cast matrix from lipid-laden renal tubular cells. Visible fat droplets are triglycerides or cholesterol esters. These are common in the presence of heavy proteinuria and are a feature of the nephrotic syndrome (see Renal Tubular Epithelial Cell Casts).

HEMOSIDERIN CASTS. Hemosiderin granules in casts derive from pigment-laden renal tubular cells.

CRYSTAL CASTS. Casts containing urates, calcium oxalate, and sulfonamides (sulfamethoxazole) are occasionally seen. A matrix is visible in a true crystal cast. The crystals may polarize and are readily identifiable in and around the cast. Crystal casts should be carefully distinguished from clumps of crystals forming at room or refrigerator temperatures. These casts indicate deposition of crystals in the tubule or collecting duct. Obstruction occurs, and hematuria, possibly related to tubular damage, is regularly seen with crystal casts. Hyaline casts incorporating calcium deposits have been reported in hyperparathyroidism.

PIGMENTED CASTS

HEMOGLOBIN (BLOOD) CASTS (Plate 18–18). Hemoglobin casts appear yellow to red; the color is sometimes very pale and difficult to interpret. Hemoglobin casts, also known as blood casts, most often accompany erythrocyte casts and glomerular disease. Less commonly, they are seen with tubular bleeding and rarely with hemoglobinuria (see under Hemosiderin).

MYOGLOBIN CASTS. These casts are red brown and occur with myoglobinuria following acute muscle damage. These may be associated with acute renal failure.

BILIRUBIN AND OTHER DRUG CASTS. Bilirubin, seen in urine of patients with obstructive jaundice, colors casts a deep yellow brown. Drugs such as phenazopyridine cause a bright yellow to orange color in acid urine and color casts and cells.

CELLULAR CASTS

ERYTHROCYTE (RED BLOOD CELL) CASTS. Finding these casts in the urine is of singular importance. By and large they are diagnostic of glomerular disease or renal parenchymal bleeding. Glomerular damage (most frequently due to immune injury) allows erythrocytes to escape into the tubule. With concomitant proteinuria and if conditions are optimal for cast formation, red blood cell casts form in the distal nephron. In urine, these casts appear yellow under the low-power objectives. A prerequisite for the identification of an erythrocyte cast is that red blood cell outlines be sharply defined in at least part of the cast (Plate 18–19). If many red blood cells are present, the matrix may not be visible. However, there may also be delicate hyaline casts with one or two red blood cells visible in the matrix. These are best seen with phase-contrast microscopy. With supravital staining, the erythrocytes are colorless or lavender in a pink matrix. When stasis has occurred in the nephron, a red blood cell cast may degenerate and appear in the urine as a reddish brown, coarsely granular cast. Such a cast is known as a blood (see Plate 18–18) or hemoglobin cast. In the absence of concomitant bilirubinuria or phenazopyridine therapy (both of which spontaneously color formed elements in the urine), a pigmented, coarsely granular cast should raise the suspicion of a blood cast. Rarely seen are myoglobin casts with red-brown pigment resembling blood casts. These occur with rhabdomyolysis.

Disorders reflected in the presence of erythrocyte casts in the sediment include many acute glomerulonephritides, IgA nephropathy, lupus nephritis, subacute bacterial endocarditis, and renal infarction. Rarely, tubulointerstitial disease may allow transtubular entry of erythrocytes with subsequent incorporation into a cast. This may occur in severe pyelonephritis (Haber, 1975).

LEUKOCYTE (WHITE BLOOD CELL) CASTS. Leukocytes usually enter tubular lumina from the interstitium. They enter through and between tubular epithelial cells (Haber, 1975). Hence, diseases that might be expected to be associated with leukocyte cell casts (Plate 18–20) in the urine are those in which neutrophilic exudates and interstitial inflammation are present in the kidney. The most common disease satisfying these criteria is pyelonephritis. It is also true that leukocyte casts may be present in glomerular disease owing to the chemotactic effect of complement, interstitial nephritis, and lupus nephritis and even in the nephrotic syndrome (Schreiner, 1957). By and large, leukocyte casts reflect tubulointerstitial disease.

With brightfield microscopy, leukocyte casts (Plate 18–21) may be difficult to identify as such, particularly if stasis and nuclear fragmentation or fusion have occurred. Phase-contrast microscopy may be helpful in delineating nuclear segments.

RENAL TUBULAR EPITHELIAL CELL CASTS. The difficulties encountered in distinguishing leukocytes from tubular cells are amplified when one is trying to identify casts in which either or both of these cell types occur. Supravital staining, phase-contrast microscopy, and Papanicolaou's stain (Plate 18–22) are helpful in separating tubular epithelial casts from leukocyte casts.

Renal tubular epithelial cell casts are seen in urine with acute tubular necrosis, viral disease (e.g., cytomegalovirus disease), or exposure to various drugs. Heavy metal poisoning and ethylene glycol and salicylate intoxication may cause tubular cells and casts to appear in the urine. In transplant units, these cells and casts constitute one of the more reliable criteria for detecting acute allograft rejection after the third postoperative day (Schumann, 1980, 1986).

MIXED CELLULAR CASTS. When two distinct cell types are present within a cast, the resulting hybrid is called a mixed cast (Mandal, 1988). Examples are leukocyte/renal, erythrocyte/leukocyte, eosinophil/renal, and so on (Plate 18–23). When the cell type cannot be established with certainty, the resulting cast is known as a cellular cast (Plate 18–24). Some inferences about cell type may be drawn from the dominant population of free cells in the surrounding sediment. If not, the differential diagnosis is additive (e.g., that of leukocyte casts and tubular epithelial cell casts).

BROAD CASTS. Broad casts are defined as those with a

diameter two to six times that of normal casts. They indicate tubular dilatation or stasis in the distal collecting duct. They are typically seen in individuals with chronic renal failure and represent a poor prognosis. Any type of cast may be broad.

OTHER MISCELLANEOUS CASTS OR CASTLIKE STRUCTURES. Bacteria on occasion may be embedded in cast matrices. On supravital staining, they appear dark purple in a pale pink matrix. Mucous threads are commonly confused with casts. However, they are larger, long, and ribbonlike, with poorly defined edges and pointed or split ends. They are readily apparent in the background of the sediment when phase-contrast microscopy is used.

New types of casts are being identified using Papanicolaou-stained preparations. Cytodiagnostic urinalysis allows for greater accuracy in identifying and quantitating types of casts and any inclusions present (Eggensperger, 1988; Schumann, 1986). Immunocytologic methods are being developed to analyze urine sediments using monoclonal antibodies (Segasothy, 1988).

TELESCOPED SEDIMENT. This term is used to describe the simultaneous occurrence of elements of acute and chronic glomerulonephritis as well as those of the nephrotic syndrome in the same urine specimen. A telescoped sediment might therefore include red blood cells, red blood cell casts, cellular casts, broad waxy casts, lipid droplets, oval fat bodies, and fatty casts. Such sediment may be found in collagen vascular disease (notably lupus nephritis) and subacute bacterial endocarditis.

Abnormal Cells and Other Formed Elements

TUMOR CELLS. Malignant tumor cells exfoliated from the renal pelvis, ureter, bladder wall, and urethra are best identified using cytologic techniques. When present, kidney and metastatic tumor cells may be diagnosed with this method. Myeloma cells have been described with and without apparent renal involvement (Riggs, 1975). For a comprehensive discussion of collection methods, cellular features, and types of disease, one should review a standard urinary cytology textbook (Tweeddale, 1977; Schumann, 1981b).

VIRAL INCLUSION CELLS. Epithelial cells with inclusion bodies may be found in the urine sediment in certain viral diseases (Dewall, 1966). Syncytial giant cells containing eosinophilic, intranuclear inclusion are seen in patients during herpetic infections. In children or immunosuppressed patients with cytomegalic inclusion disease, epithelioid cells with basophilic intranuclear inclusion or cytoplasmic bodies may be found in the urine sediment. Cytologic techniques are more sensitive than conventional urine microscopy in detecting virally infected cells (Schumann, 1980).

PLATELETS. These have been demonstrated in urine. Up to 30,000/μL were found in urine of patients with hemolytic-uremic syndrome before and after therapy. These were found by phase-contrast microscopy and confirmed by electron microscopy (Sutor, 1976).

BACTERIA. Bacteria may or may not be significant, depending on the method of urine collection and how soon after collection of the specimen the examination takes place (Fang, 1988). Well-mixed uncentrifuged urine may be examined with Gram's stain. If bacteria are identified in the uncentrifuged specimen under an oil-immersion lens, more than 100,000 organisms per milliliter are probably present (i.e., significant bacteriuria). Rod-shaped bacteria are most commonly seen, because the enteric organisms are most often found in urinary tract infection. If urinary tract infection is present, many leukocytes are usually seen in the sediment.

Using direct immunofluorescence as a means of visualizing antibody complexed with the bacteria in the urine, Thomas (1974) found a significant correlation between the presence or absence of antibody-coated bacteria and the localization of the infection in the kidneys or the bladder, respectively.

Acid-fast staining of the urine sediment may reveal tubercle bacilli, but because the urethra may contain nonpathogenic acid-fast organisms, the presence of tubercle bacilli in urine must be substantiated by culture.

FUNGI. Yeast cells (*Candida*) are found in urinary tract infection (e.g., in diabetes mellitus), but yeasts are also common contaminants from skin and air. They may be confused with erythrocytes; budding is usually seen and helps to identify them as yeast cells (Plate 18–25). Pseudomycelial forms of *Candida* are occasionally found (Plate 18–26).

PARASITES. Parasites and parasitic ova may be seen in urine sediments as a result of fecal or vaginal contamination. When these are noted, the examination should be repeated on a fresh, clean-voided urine specimen. In patients with schistosomiasis due to *Schistosoma haematobium*, typical ova are shed directly into the urine accompanied by erythrocytes from the urinary bladder. Trichomonads may be present in urine as a result of vaginal contamination. When urethral or bladder infection is suspected, the protozoa should be searched for immediately in a wet preparation of the sediment; the motility of the organism is helpful in making the appropriate identification. Amebas are rarely seen in the urine; these may reach the bladder from lymphatics or more likely from fecal contamination of the urethra. The pathogenic *Entamoeba histolytica* is usually accompanied by erythrocytes and leukocytes.

Contaminants and Artifacts

Partly digested muscle fibers or vegetable cells may be found when there is fecal contamination (Plate 18–27). Spermatozoa are occasionally present in the urine of men and are occasionally seen in the urine of women. They are easily recognized. Pollen grains contaminate specimens seasonally.

Cotton, hair, and other fibers may be seen and are easily identified. Wood fibers from applicator sticks may be found if sticks are used to mix the sediment. Short fibers from disposable diapers are easily confused with casts. Unlike casts, these fibers polarize brightly.

Granules of starch appear bright and faintly striated and should not be confused with cells. They have an irregular outline and a central depression. With crossed polarizing filters, starch granules exhibit a typical Maltese cross pattern. However, because they are large, several times larger than an erythrocyte, they are not likely to be confused with cholesterol droplets. Starch from surgical gloves is the most common contaminant of urine and other body fluids.

Oil droplets from catheter lubricants may be confused with cells, especially red blood cells, but are structureless. Lipid material from vaginal creams also forms droplets in urine and may aggregate into large amorphous shapes.

Crystals

By and large, crystals in the urine are of limited clinical significance. Phosphates, urates, and oxalates are especially common and occur in normal urine sediment. Their presence often deflects attention from more important formed elements. A few crystals, however, are important. For the purposes of separating these from more commonly occurring nuisance crystals, a summary of crystal morphology is presented (Table 18–13).

A prerequisite for the positive identification of crystals is a knowledge of the urinary pH. This helps with the preliminary separation.

CRYSTALS FOUND IN NORMAL ACID URINE

AMORPHOUS URATES (CALCIUM, MAGNESIUM, SODIUM, AND POTASSIUM URATES). The amorphous material precipitates often on sanding in concentrated urine of a slightly acid pH as yellow-brown small granules. The gross urine specimen precipitate may appear pink orange to reddish brown and is sometimes called brick dust. Granules form clumps and adhere to fibers and mucous threads. They convert to uric acid crystals with acidification with acetic acid and dissolve with warmth (60°C) and with dilute alkali.

CRYSTALLINE URATES (SODIUM, POTASSIUM, AND AMMONIUM). These biurates and acid urates form small brown spheres (Plate 18–28) or colorless needles in slightly acid urine. Spheres cluster in pairs and triplets. They slowly revert to uric acid plates on acidification with acetic acid on the microscope slide.

CRYSTALLINE URIC ACID. Uric acid crystals occur at low pH, 5 to 5.5. Various shapes are seen, and the crystals are usually colored. They typically are four-sided, flat, yellow or reddish brown. Other shapes are rhombic plates or prisms, oval forms with pointed ends (lemon shaped), wedges, rosettes, and irregular plates (Plate 18–29 and 18–30). Rarely they are colorless and hexagonal like cystine (Plate 18–31*A*). Uric acid crystals polarize and show interference colors (Plate 18–31*B*).

CALCIUM OXALATES. Dihydrates appear at pH 6 or in neutral urine. They typically are small, colorless octahedrons that resemble envelopes (Plate 18–32). Also seen are large crystals, sometimes in clusters. They are insoluble in acetic acid. Rarely dumbbell, ovoid forms (Plate 18–33), or longer forms of calcium oxalate monohydrate are seen.

CRYSTALS FOUND IN NORMAL ALKALINE URINE

Phosphates form soluble sodium and potassium salts and less soluble calcium and magnesium salts. Calcium and magnesium phosphate are the least soluble in alkaline urine; calcium and magnesium monohydrogen phosphate are not very soluble, but the dihydrogen phosphates are soluble at alkaline pH. Phosphates, in general, dissolve in acids such as dilute hydrochloric and nitric acids and vary in solubility in acetic acid. They do not dissolve in dilute sodium hydroxide solutions or alcohol.

AMORPHOUS PHOSPHATES (CALCIUM AND MAGNESIUM). These colorless amorphous granules are found in urine of an alkaline or slightly acidic pH. Clumps or masses are seen (Plate 18–34). They typically form a fine or lacy precipitate macroscopically.

CRYSTALLINE PHOSPHATES. Triple phosphate (ammonium magnesium phosphate) crystals form at alkaline pH, often with infection present. They commonly show a variation in size. Colorless, three- to six-sided prisms with oblique ends are referred to as coffin lids, less often flat fern forms (Plate 18–35). They may form colorless sheets or flakes. Dicalcium hydrogen phosphate crystals are long, three-sided prisms with pointed ends. They are seen in neutral or slightly acidic urine. They form clusters or rosettes. Magnesium phosphate forms colorless rhomboids, some with notched ends or corners. They are seldom recognized.

CALCIUM CARBONATE. These uncommon crystals are small granules or colorless spheres. They form pairs or fours in alkaline urine. Calcium carbonate produces carbon dioxide with acids.

AMMONIUM BIURATE. Crystalline urate forms in alkaline urine. These are also seen in neutral and occasionally in slightly acid urine. They usually are seen with phosphate crystals and amorphous phosphates. Yellow-brown spheres are referred to as thorn apples, showing radial or concentric striations and irregular projections or thorns or horns (Plate 18–36). They dissolve with heat at 60°C and with acetic acid, reappearing as typical uric acid crystals after about 20 minutes.

CRYSTALS FOUND IN ABNORMAL URINE

Always check a patient's drug therapy when unusual crystals are found.

CYSTINE. Cystine crystals are found at acid pH. They are colorless, refractile, hexagonal plates (Plate 18–37), sometimes twinned. They are soluble in water at pH less than 2 or greater than 8. They may be confused with hexagonal forms of uric acid (Plate 18–31*A*). Whereas uric acid crystals polarize (Plate 18–30*B*), thin cystine crystals do not, although thick laminated forms do polarize. The diagnosis can be confirmed with the cyanide-nitroprusside reaction (see Cystinuria). Both cystine and uric acid are soluble in ammonia water, but cystine also dissolves in dilute hydrochloric acid and uric acid does not.

TYROSINE. Tyrosine crystals are uncommon fine, silky needles that may be arranged in sheaves or clumps, especially after refrigeration. They are colorless or yellow, appearing black as the microscope is focused (Plate 18–38). They are soluble in alkali (ammonia and potassium hydroxide) and in dilute hydrochloric acid. They are not soluble in alcohol or ether. They are less soluble than leucine and therefore are more often precipitated in urine (see Nitrosonaphthol Test for Tyrosine).

LEUCINE. These rare, yellow, oily-appearing spheres have radial and concentric striations. Leucine and tyrosine crystals may occur together. Leucine may be precipitated with tyrosine crystals if alcohol is added to the urine. They are soluble in acids and alkalis. Unlike fat globules, leucine is not soluble in ether and may be differentiated from fat.

SULFONAMIDE (SULFADIAZINE) CRYSTALS. These are seen in urine of acid pH, usually less than 6. Various forms are seen, depending on the form of drug involved. They occasionally are colorless but usually are yellow-brown. They resemble sheaves of wheat with central bindings, striated sheaves with eccentric bindings (Plate 18–39), rosettes, arrowheads, petals, needles, and round forms with

3

Table 18–13. CHARACTERISTICS OF AMORPHOUS AND CRYSTALLINE URINARY SEDIMENTS

Substance	Description	Urine pH Where Found			Solubility Characteristics and Comments
		Acid	*Neutral*	*Alkaline*	
Ampicillin	Uncommon—from high dose; colorless; long prisms that form clusters, sheaves	+	–	–	
Bilirubin	Reddish brown; amorphous needles, rhombic plates, or cubes; may color uric acid crystals	+	–	–	Soluble in alkali, acid, acetone, and chloroform
Cholesterol	Rare; colorless; flat plate with corner notch; accompanies fatty casts and oval fat bodies	+	+	–	Very soluble in chloroform, ether, and hot alcohol
Calcium carbonate	Colorless; small granules in pairs, fours; spheres; rarely needles	–	+	+	Soluble in acetic acid with effervescence
Calcium oxalate	Dihydrate—common; colorless; small refractile octahedron Monohydrate—uncommon; dumbbell and ovoid rectangle	+	+	–	Soluble in dilute HCl
Cystine	Colorless; hexagonal plates, often laminated; rapidly destroyed by bacteria; may be confused with uric acid, but cystine is soluble in dilute hydrochloric acid	+	–	–	Soluble in alkali (especially ammonia) and dilute HCl; insoluble in boiling water, acetic acid, alcohol, ether; apply cyanide-nitroprusside reaction
Hematin	Small, biconvex "whetstone" seen with hemoglobinuria	+	–	–	
Hemosiderin	Golden brown; granules in clumps, in cells, casts	+	+	–	Blue with Prussian blue
Hippuric acid	Rare; colorless; needles, rhombic plates and four-sided prisms; distinguish from phosphates	+	+	+	Soluble with hot water and alkali; insoluble in acetic acid
Indigotin	Rare; blue; amorphous or small crystals; colors other crystals	+	+	+	Very soluble in chloroform; soluble in ether; insoluble in acetone
Phosphates					
Amorphous phosphate (magnesium, calcium)	Colorless; fine, granular precipitate	–	+	+	Insoluble with heat; soluble with acetic acid, dilute HCl
Calcium hydrogen phosphate	Less common; colorless, star-shaped or long, thin prisms or needles; form rosettes	sl	+	sl	Slightly soluble in dilute acetic acid, soluble in dilute HCl
Triple phosphate (ammonium, magnesium)	Common form: colorless; three- to six-sided prisms, "coffin lids" Less often: flat, fern leaf form, sheets, flakes	–	+	+	Soluble in dilute acetic acid
Radiographic media (meglumine diatrizoate)	Intravenous: colorless; thin, rhombic plates, some with notch, resemble cholesterol plates; elongated crystals Retrograde: colorless; long, pointed crystals	+	–	–	Soluble in 10% NaOH: insoluble in ether and chloroform; high specific gravity in urine; polarizes with interference colors
Sulfonamides					
Acetylsulfadiazine	Wheat sheaves with eccentric binding	+	–	–	
Acetylsulfamethoxazole	Brown; dense spheres or irregular divided spheres	+	–	–	
Sulfadiazine	Brown; dense globules	+	–	–	Soluble in acetone
Tyrosine	Rare; colorless or yellow, appears black with focusing; fine silky needles in sheaves or rosettes	+	–	–	Soluble in alkali, dilute mineral acid, relatively heat soluble; insoluble in alcohol, ether
Urates					
Amorphous (calcium, magnesium, sodium, potassium)	Common; colorless to yellow-brown; amorphous, granular precipitate	+	+	–	Soluble in dilute alkali; soluble at 60°C or lower; change to uric acid crystal with concentrated HCl or acetic acid
Monosodium urate	Colorless; needles or amorphous precipitate	+	–	–	
Urates (sodium, potassium, ammonium)	Brown; small, spherical; clusters resemble biurates	sl	+	–	Soluble at 60°C; change to uric acid with glacial acetic acid
Ammonium biurate	Common in "old" urine; dark yellow or brown; spheres or "thorn apples" (spheres with horns)	–	+	+	Soluble at 60°C with acetic acid; soluble strong alkali; change to uric acid with concentrated hydrochloric or acetic acid
Uric acid	Common; yellow, red-brown, brown; large variety of shapes—rhombic, four-sided plates, rosettes, "whetstones" lemon shapes; rarely, colorless hexagonals	+	–	–	Soluble in alkali; insoluble in alcohol and acids; polarizes with interference colors
Xanthine	Rare; colorless; small, rhombic plates	+	+	–	Soluble in alkali, soluble with heat; insoluble in acetic acid

sl = Slight.

radial striations. Apply the diazo reaction to confirm the type. The lignin test is not reliable.

AMPICILLIN (HIGH DOSE). These crystals occur at acid pH. Long, fine, colorless crystals (Plate 18–40) form coarse sheaves after refrigeration.

RADIOGRAPHIC MEDIA (MEGLUMINE DIATRIZOATE). These crystals are found at acid pH briefly after intravenous radiographic studies. Flat, clear, colorless notched rhombic plates or longer, slender rectangles are seen. They are easily polarized, showing interference colors (Plate 18–41*A* and 18–41*B*). They are also seen after retrograde cystograms as long, colorless needles, forming clusters after refrigeration. The presence of radiographic crystals should correlate with a high specific gravity (> 1.040).

CLINICAL SIGNIFICANCE

Little significance can be attached to crystals detected in urine standing at room temperature. When urine is heated to 37°C, most crystals disappear. Those still present at 37°C might have some significance when correlated with clinical symptoms.

Phosphate crystals have little if any clinical significance. They are often seen in infected urine of alkaline pH. Large numbers of uric acid crystals and urates may reflect increased nucleoprotein turnover, especially during chemotherapy of leukemias or lymphoma. They may provide circumstantial evidence for the nature of small stones lodged in the ureters, especially when radiolucent and found in conjunction with raised serum uric acid levels. They may also herald the urate nephropathy of gout. Oxalate crystals in large numbers may reflect severe chronic renal disease or ethylene glycol or methoxyflurane toxicity. Oxaluria has come into prominence as a reflection of the increased absorption of oxalates from food after small bowel diseases and resection, notably for Crohn's disease (Dobbins, 1977). However, oxalates may be confused with hexagonal forms of uric acid (Plate 18–31*A*). Cystine crystals are among the most important found in the urine. Whereas uric acid crystals polarize (Plate 18–31*B*), thin cystine crystals do not, although thick or laminated forms do polarize. They occur in patients with cystinuria and may be associated with cystine calculi. Tyrosine and leucine crystals are occasionally seen in the urine of patients with severe liver disease (see Urinary Screening for Inherited Metabolic Diseases). With the advent of soluble sulfonamides, sulfa crystals (Plate 18–39) are not as frequently found in urine, especially when the urine is examined at 37°C (Alfthan, 1972). However, sulfamethoxazole (Bactrim, Septra) is seen with some regularity. Urinary crystals follow radiographic examinations with diatrizoate dyes (Plate 18–41*A* and 18–41*B*). Ampicillin may crystallize in the urine under conditions of high doses (Plate 18–40). Other drugs are occasionally reported to cause crystalluria when administered in high-dose schedules or after overdose. Examples include high-dose 6-mercaptopurine therapy (Duttera, 1972), primidone overdosage (Bailey, 1972), and dihydroxyadenine from massive blood transfusion (Falk, 1972) (see Urinary Calculi).

Methods for Examining Urine Sediment

SPECIMEN

For screening purposes, a randomly collected specimen of urine is usually satisfactory. For evaluation of renal disease, a first morning urine sample is recommended. Contamination with vaginal elements is less likely to occur in women if the urine is collected as a midstream specimen.

The urine specimen must be examined while fresh, because cells and casts begin to lyse within two hours. Refrigeration (2° to 8°C) helps prevent the lysis of pathologic entities. If the urine cannot be examined within two hours of voiding, it should be refrigerated before and after transportation or preserved with a suitable sediment preservative.

BRIGHTFIELD MICROSCOPY OF UNSTAINED URINE

Subdued light is needed to delineate the more translucent formed elements of the urine such as hyaline casts, crystals, and mucous threads. Identification of leukocytes (neutrophils, eosinophils, lymphocytes), histiocytes, renal epithelial cells, viral inclusion cells, neoplastic cells, and cellular casts may be very difficult in unstained preparations. Phase-contrast microscopy is strongly recommended for the detection of casts.

BRIGHTFIELD MICROSCOPY WITH SUPRAVITAL STAINING

Cellular detail is best seen with stained sediments. A crystal-violet safranin stain (Sternheimer, 1951) may be used to aid in the identification of cellular elements.

REAGENTS

Solution I:	Crystal violet	3.0 g
	Ethyl alcohol (95%)	20.0 mL
	Ammonium oxalate	0.8 g
Solution II:	Safranin O	1.0 g
	Ethyl alcohol (95%)	40.0 mL
	Distilled water	400.0 mL

Three parts of solution I and 97 parts of solution II are mixed and filtered. The mixture should be clarified by filtering every two weeks. Discard after three months. Separately, solutions I and II keep indefinitely at room temperature. In highly alkaline urine specimens, the stain precipitates. A similar stain is also available commercially as Sedi-Stain (Clay-Adams), Kova-Stain (ICL Scientific), and others.

PROCEDURE. Add one or two drops of crystal-violet safranin stain to approximately 1 mL of concentrated urine sediment. Mix with a pipette and place a drop of this suspension on a slide and coverslip.

A 2% solution of methylene blue and toluidine blue (Holmquist, 1980) may also be used as a simple, quick supravital stain. An improved supravital stain that facilitates identification of cells, casts, and their inclusions is also recommended (Sternheimer, 1975).

PHASE-CONTRAST AND INTERFERENCE MICROSCOPY

Many laboratory personnel prefer to use phase-contrast microscopy for the detection of more translucent formed elements of the urinary sediment. Such elements, notably casts (but also mucous threads and bacilli), may escape detection using ordinary brightfield microscopy. Phase-contrast microscopy has the advantage of hardening the outlines of even the most ephemeral formed elements, making detection simple (Plate 18–12*A* and 18–12*B*) (Brody, 1968). A microscope equipped with 10× and 40× phase objectives plus a 40× brightfield objective and the appropriate rotating phase/brightfield condenser is most useful. Scanning time is decreased and the yield is increased. Even greater morphologic detail of formed elements (notably casts and cells) is afforded by interference-contrast microscopy (Haber, 1972). This technique, however, is time consuming and not in common use.

POLARIZED MICROSCOPY

Polarized microscopy is used to distinguish crystals and fibers from cellular or protein cast material. Sterols, such as cholesterol droplets, form Maltese crosses with crossed polars. With the addition of a retardation plate, crystals may be further identified as positively or negatively birefringent (see the section entitled Synovial Fluid, Microscopic Examination).

CYTODIAGNOSTIC URINALYSIS

Cytodiagnostic urinalysis is a combined cytocentrifugation (Cytospin, Shandon Southern Instruments, Sewickley, PA) and Papanicolaou's staining method used to identify and quantitate changes in the urine sediment in renal parenchymal diseases (Schumann, 1981b). Use of cytocentrifugation permits a simple, rapid, reproducible, and semi-quantitative method for concentrating urine sediments. Cellular casts, mononuclear cells (plasma cells, lymphocytes, histiocytes, and so on), tissue fragments, and neoplastic cells may be clearly demonstrated with this method.

QUANTITATIVE COUNTS AND DIFFERENTIAL COUNTS

In some laboratories, a hemotocytometer is used for quantifying urine sediment findings from random and timed urine specimens. For example, cells and casts from undiluted well-mixed urine are counted in a hemotocytometer and reported as the number of cells per microliter. Gadeholt (1964) describes and reviews factors affecting the quantitative cell count. For example, very low specific gravity (<1.012) causes a marked reduction in erythrocytes, as does alkaline pH. Recovery of cells may differ slightly with different centrifuge speeds.

Normal values for neutrophils vary from 5 to 30/μL, according to different workers; upper limits for erythrocytes vary from 3 to 20/μL (Fassett, 1982) and casts as few as 1 to 2/mL (Wenk, 1981). Freni (1977) used centrifugal force of 1230 g for nine minutes and evaluated stained smears of the sediment in a consistent fashion to determine an upper limit for erythrocytes of 20,000/mL in men age 50 to 65 years. Kesson (1978) provided evidence that chamber counts on centrifuged urine sediments are more reliable in predicting renal functional abnormalities than is a conventional method using cells per high-power field. He used white blood cell values of 2000/mL, red blood cells of 500/mL, and casts of 15/mL as upper limits of normal on clean-catch midstream urine specimens. These correspond to daily urine volumes of 1250 mL and a calculated leukocyte excretion rate of 100,000/24 hours.

Whereas quantitated cell counts differentiate between healthy persons and those with disease, differential counts using phase-contrast microscopy or stained cytocentrifuged sediments help discriminate among diseases (Wahlin, 1977).

Methods for Microscopic Urinalysis

Basic (Routine)

1. Pour 10, 12, or 15 mL of a well-mixed urine specimen (casts tend to settle) into a graduated disposable centrifuge tube. Perform physical/chemical evaluations. Centrifuge at 450 g for five minutes.
2. Carefully remove and save the supernatant. The final volume used to resuspend the sediment may vary with the standardized system used but should remain a constant within any given laboratory. Use a disposable pipette, specialized tube, or pipette system to concentrate the sediment.
3. Gently resuspend the sediment in the remaining supernatant, and add one half to one drop of stain if desired. Using an appropriate pipette, load/charge the examination chamber of a standardized slide. Allow the urine to settle for 30 to 60 seconds.
4. Examine with low- and high-power objectives. Subdued light or phase-contrast illumination is required to detect sediment entities with a low refractive index. The fine focus should be varied continuously while scanning. Systematically progress around the entire examination chamber, being careful to examine along the edges for casts.
5. Count the number of casts in at least 10 low-power fields, average, and report the number of casts per low-power field. A reasonable range may be used in reporting (i.e., 0 to 2, 2 to 5, 5 to 10, and so on). Use high power to identify casts by type. Casts will not be missed if phase-contrast microscopy is used (Plates 18–12*A* and 18–12*B*).
6. Identify and count erythrocytes, leukocytes, and renal epithelial cells using the high-power objective. Count at least 10 hpf, average, and report as cells/hpf. A reasonable range may be used for reporting.
7. Comment on:
   a. Squamous and transitional cells if present in large numbers or as fragments (transitional cells).
   b. Bacteria, yeast, microorganisms. Bacteriuria detectable on low power should be reported as at least 2+.
   c. Crystals are quantitated under low power. The presence of abnormal crystals should be confirmed chemically and correlated with the patient's history.
   d. Large amounts of mucus.
8. The authors recommend confirming the following results with cytodiagnostic urinalysis or specific chemical tests (crystals):
   a. More than two renal epithelial cells per high-power field.
   b. Pathologic casts.
   c. Atypical mononuclear cells.
   d. Tissue fragments.
   e. Pathologic crystals.
9. Review the entire report, including physical, chemical, and microscopic data, and correlate with available clinical information. Discrepancies should be resolved before releasing the report. Normal values for the procedure are red blood cells, 0 to 10/hpf; white blood cells, 0 to 10/hpf;

hyaline casts, 0 to 2/hpf. Values vary, depending on the standardized system used.

Cytodiagnostic Urinalysis (Eggensperger, 1988; Schumann, 1986)

When possible, first morning urine specimens are collected (volumes ranging from 10 to 30 mL). The container is immediately delivered to the laboratory or refrigerated. An accompanying requisition form noting pertinent patient history is required.

PROCEDURE

1. Pour 10 mL of urine into an optically clear centrifuge tube. Perform a physical and chemical examination of the urine (see Gross/Physical Examination and Chemical Screening).
2. Centrifuge capped tubes at 1500 rpm ($490 \times g$) for 10 minutes.
3. Remove the supernatant and concentrate the sediment to exactly 1 mL.
4. Using a cytocentrifuge, prepare four slides using 250 μL of resuspended sediment per chamber. Cytocentrifuge at 750 rpm ($65 \times g$) for 6 minutes. If the sediment is hypercellular, use a smaller amount of sediment and decrease centrifugation time.
5. After cytocentrifuging, discard the filter card and immediately add one to two drops of Parlodion to the cell button.
6. Fix slides for 15 minutes in Saccomanno's fixative, in 95% ethyl alcohol or ethanol, or in acetic acid-alcohol.
7. Stain slides using modified Papanicolaou's technique.
8. Screen all four slides completely, noting background pattern, cellularity, viral inclusions, tissue fragments, and abnormal cells.
9. Count erythrocytes, leukocytes, lymphocytes, casts, and renal tubular epithelial cells in 10 hpf. Casts and renal epithelial cells are differentiated by type.
10. If more than two eosinophils per high-power field are seen, count 200 granulocytes and report eosinophils as a percentage of neutrophils.
11. Review the report, including physical, chemical, and microscopic data, and correlate with the clinical history. Discrepancies must be resolved before reporting.
12. Sign out the report with pathologist/physician specialist.

Lipiduria

METHOD FOR EXAMINING REFRACTILE BODIES IN URINE

Lipid droplets or spherocrystals containing cholesterol esters are anisotropic in polarized light, show up brightly against a dark field, and appear to be divided into four quadrants. This appearance resembles a Maltese cross. Visible evidence of anisotropy depends on the orientation of the crystal in the field; not all will be seen. Crystals, hair, and clothing fibers also show up brightly but do not exhibit Maltese cross forms. Fatty acids and triglyceride do not form liquid spherocrystals and do not show anisotropy, but glycosphingolipids in Fabry's disease are birefringent and may be seen in urinary sediments.

A polarizing microscope with a rotating stage may be used in this examination. If one is not available, an ordinary light microscope can be easily made usable by adding suitable filters. Polaroid filters, consisting of an analyzer circle and a polarizer circle, are used. Install the analyzer disk in the ocular lens of a microscope by unscrewing the eye lens assembly. Insert the polarizer disk in the slotted opening under the substage condenser. Components are available for the binocular microscopes in common use (e.g., American Optical). A turret can be inserted in the microscope below the binocular head; it carries a polarizing filter (analyzer) and can be rotated in or out. A second detachable polarizing filter with an attached retardation plate is centered over the field lamp below the condenser. The set of filters is useful for identifying of synovial fluid crystals but can also be used for crystals and lipids in urine.

Sediment from a fresh urine sample is examined. Using high-power magnification and brightfield illumination, turn one polarizing filter until a maximum darkening of the field is produced. Birefringent crystals and fibers are seen white against a black background. If cholesterol is present, small refractile bodies will have the typical Maltese cross form in cells, casts, or free. If a red retardation plate is inserted, the cholesterol droplet shows typical blue and yellow quadrants against a red background. Starch granules have a similar appearance when polarized but are much larger.

Automated Urinalysis

Instrumentation is now available to automate routine urinalysis partially or completely. In addition to enhancing production, automation can also standardize some aspects of manual urinalysis. Most of these instruments can be interfaced with laboratory information systems, facilitating reporting and prior result retrieval.

The Yellow IRIS Urinalysis work station combines several automated subsystems to perform a complete urinalysis (Carlson, 1988; Roe, 1986). Specific gravity is measured by a mass gravity meter, urine chemistries are measured by a standard reflectance spectrophotometer, and microscopic analysis is facilitated with an automated intelligent microscopy system. No centrifugation is involved, and the handling of the specimen is minimal. A touch-sensitive video screen eliminates keyboard entry. In the analysis, the urine specimen is poured into the instrument's entry port over a urine chemistry reagent strip. This reagent strip is then placed in the reflectance photometer reader platform. The urine chemistry values are automatically timed, read, and collated by the internal computer. A portion of the specimen is diverted to the harmonic oscillator mass gravity meter for specific gravity determination, and the rest of the specimen is then stained and passed into a laminar flow chamber, where the formed elements are detected and imaged by a video camera mounted to a microscope and a stroboscopic lamp that allows stop-motion images. Electronic centrifugation takes place as the computer recognizes and discards empty images. Images that contain the cells, casts, crystals, yeast, and bacteria that are usually found in the sediment are then sorted by size and presented to the operator on the touch-sensitive screen for identification. Because the volume of the laminar flow chamber is known, the images can be counted and related to a volume of urine with a precision that exceeds that which can be obtained with a centrifuged specimen, glass slide, and coverslip. The computer then consolidates the report for printing or transmission to the laboratory information system.

If urine microscopic examination is to be performed the traditional way, the use of automatic urine chemistry strip readers can standardize strip interpretation. These are available from several manufacturers and are generally reflectance spectrophotometers that analyze the color and intensity of the light reflected from the reagent area.

URINARY CALCULI

Kidney stones are common, with about 5 in 1000 persons affected; in the United States, the average age of onset of common calcium stones is in the thirties (Coe, 1981). Males are more often affected with calcium stones than females. Children are not often affected with calcium stones. Subsequent recurrences are frequent, but with appropriate identification of the stones and the risk factors associated with them, stone formation may be greatly reduced. Upper (renal) stones are common in Western industrialized countries, whereas bladder stones are uncommon. Most of the stones received for analysis are very small calcium oxalate stones; the larger phosphate stones, cystine stones, and uric acid stones are occasionally submitted.

The passage of stones down the ureter produces renal colic, which is characterized by severe pain in the back radiating to the groin. Stones may also be passed through the urethra with great pain. Hematuria is a common urinary finding when symptoms of stones are present. If stones obstruct the pelvis of the kidney or ureter, hydronephrosis results. Infection is a common consequence.

Calcium oxalate is the most commonly found constituent of urinary calculi. It precipitates at acid or neutral pH. Calcium phosphate (hydroxyapatite $Ca_{10}(PO_4)_6(OH)_2$ forms calculi at the normal urinary pH of 6.0 to 6.5. Less commonly, uric acid, which is not very soluble, crystallizes at a low pH (5.3) and forms stones. Magnesium ammonium phosphate (struvite) forms stones at alkaline pH, when the ammonium level is high. They form in the pelvis of the kidney but apparently are not attached to papillae, as are the calcium stones. They may, however, develop on pre-existing nuclei when infection from organisms such as *Proteus* causes alkalization of the urine. These stones become large, forming casts of the kidney pelvis and showing staghorns. Mixed stones occur because calcium or uric acid crystals or stones may cause obstruction followed by infection and the subsequent deposition of ammonium salts. With the inherited renal tubular transport disease cystinuria, cystine stones form. Patients with renal tubular acidosis may form calcium phosphate stones; conversely, patients with renal nephrocalcinosis and stones may have subsequent renal tubular damage resulting in renal tubular acidosis.

In Prien's series (1963), calcium oxalate or a mixture of oxalate and calcium phosphate was most often found in stones (80% to 84%). Mixed calcium phosphate, magnesium ammonium phosphate, and uric acid were the next most common constituents (3% to 10% each), and these were followed by cystine (1% to 2%). Carbonate, which is frequently detected in chemical analysis, probably results from adsorption of carbon dioxide to the calcium phosphate crystal. Rarely, calculi containing sulfonamides are found, and silica calculi have been reported in patients ingesting silica gel over a long period (Levison, 1982). Triamterene (Dyazide, Dyrenium), a relatively insoluble diuretic, contributes to stone formation. It forms 1- to 2-mm mustard-colored stones, giving a bright blue fluorescence when dissolved in butanol and with exposure to UV light (Ettinger, 1979). Although it was anticipated that adenine stones would be found after multiple blood transfusions using an acid-citrate-dextrose-adenine blood preservative, this has not yet been the case. Crystals were found only after enormous amounts of blood were given—118 units (Falk, 1972). Rare adenine stones have been described in children with an inherited enzyme deficiency disorder and hyperuricemia (Simmonds, 1979). Xanthine stones are uncommon and may be associated with a genetic disorder with an absence of liver xanthine oxidase (Scriver, 1989).

3

Monitoring Patients

For the common calcium stones, large amounts of fluids and thiazide diuretics are used for treatment. Thiazides plus allopurinol are used for patients who have calcium stones and increased levels of calcium and uric acid in urine. Urine calcium levels are monitored and reduced to less than 4 mg/kg/24 hours and urate excretion to less than 700 mg/24 hours (male) and 650 mg/24 hours (female) (Coe, 1981). There is some disagreement about the need for drug therapy in all of these patients. When applicable for uric acid stones, urinary pH is raised with bicarbonate to 6 to 6.5, or diuretics and allopurinol may be used to reduce hyperuricemia and hyperuricosuria. Alkalizing urine sufficiently for cystine stone formers is difficult, and large fluid intake is used for treatment. Stones resulting from infection contain bacteria and are removed surgically and the appropriate fluids and antibiotic therapy instituted.

Laboratory Tests Used to Investigate Stone Formers

1. Urine examinations. (a) Routine urinalysis, qualitative test for cystine, and urine culture. (b) Twenty-four-hour urine specimen: sodium, calcium, phosphorus, uric acid, oxalate, and creatinine clearance. Quantitative urine studies may have to be repeated. (c) Urine pH determination on a fresh specimen is important in determining the kinds of crystals likely to be precipitated—for example, uric acid with low pH (5 to 5.5) and triple phosphate with alkaline urine.
2. Serum chemistry. Calcium, phosphorus, uric acid, and electrolytes.
3. Stone analysis.
4. Radiologic examination. Asymptomatic stones are sometimes found. All stones are radiopaque except pure uric acid and the rare xanthine; cystine stones are opaque because of their sulfur content.

Urinalysis Reveals Hematuria

Hematuria is a constant finding when stones are present, even when they are asymptomatic. Erythrocyte casts are not found; other casts are unusual. Leukocytes are increased when infection is present. Multiple clusters of nonmalignant transitional cells may be found in the urine of patients with calculous disease and may be helpful in the diagnosis of unsuspected calculi (Highman, 1982).

Proteinuria is usually not a feature of calculous disease, but with renal tubular damage there may be increased excretion of low-molecular-weight plasma proteins such as β_2-microglobulin, as well as some albumin.

Crystals may or may not be found when stones are present. Large calcium oxalate crystals in clusters are said to be associated with stone formation. Both the dihydrate and the monohydrate forms are found. Calcium phosphate (apatite) appears as fine granules, whereas calcium hydrogen phosphate (brushite) is seen as colorless, long, thin flat crystals, and triple phosphate in alkaline urine as colorless coffin lids. Uric acid forms fine granules and various crystal shapes, usually yellow to brown. Cystine classically presents as hexagonal, colorless flat crystals at an acid pH.

Calcium Stones

Calcium oxalate stones are the most common. Calcium stones form with excess oxalate and uric acid in urine. The uric acid crystals may provide a nidus for stone formation.

Newly formed calcium oxalate aggregates are about 20 to 25 μm in diameter, much smaller than the outlet of the collecting ducts. Adherence to the surface apparently allows them to grow rather than be excreted. Calcium salts as opposed to uric acid, cystine, and triple phosphate tend to plug the nephrons. Calcium hydrogen phosphate (as brushite) crystallizes more readily in stone formers and may form a nucleus for calcium oxalate stones and for calcium phosphate stones largely composed of the hydroxyapatite form of calcium phosphate. Calcium phosphate stone formation rather than oxalate is favored by a less acid urine, as in renal tubular acidosis, with infection, and in persons consuming large amounts of alkali. Calcium phosphate stones are also found in primary hyperparathyroidism, although the urine is in the normal pH range. In a patient exposed to heat and dehydration, these may contribute to a rise in urinary solute levels, followed by crystallization and stone formation.

Causes of Hypercalciuria

Calcium homeostasis is maintained by parathyroid hormone (PTH) and 1,25-dihydroxycholecalciferol [1,25-(OH) 2D]. Low serum ionized calcium levels cause increased PTH secretion, and low serum phosphorus levels stimulate 1,25-(OH)2D synthesis. Both affect bone resorption by osteoclasts. PTH causes a diminution of phosphorus reabsorption and an increase in calcium reabsorption by renal tubular cells. PTH also causes increased synthesis of 1,25-(OH)2D, which acts on the small intestinal mucosa, causing increased absorption of calcium and phosphorus (see Chap. 8).

Increased calcium in urine results from an increase in intestinal calcium absorption, a lack of appropriate renal tubular reabsorption of calcium, resorption or loss of calcium from bone, or a combination of these. About 10 g of calcium is filtered by the kidneys each day, and all but a small fraction is normally reabsorbed by renal tubular cells.

About 40% of patients with calcium stones have hypercalciuria. Urine calcium levels of more than 300 mg/day in men or 250 mg/day in women are regarded as excessive when the patients are receiving a test diet containing 1 g of calcium per day.

Dietary hypercalciuria is not a common cause of calcium stones; it is associated with large calcium intake, on the order of 3 to 4 g/day, and with high protein intake. About 800 mg/day is a normal recommended adult intake.

Increased absorption of calcium from the gut and hypercalciuria occur when there is excessive loss of phosphorus from the kidneys and low serum phosphorus levels, when there is increased serum 1,25-(OH)2D with normal serum phosphorus levels, and in a group of individuals with normal serum factors, when the cause is unknown.

Patients with renal loss of calcium as a result of a defect in renal tubular calcium resorption have increased calcium resorption from the gut. Furosemide, a diuretic, also causes renal hypercalciuria.

Increased resorption of bone causes hypercalciuria. This occurs with immobilization of the skeleton, rapidly progressive bone disease, thyrotoxicosis, and Cushing's disease. Calcium is lost from bone as a result of osteolytic tumors and in the presence of renal disease such as distal renal tubular acidosis and medullary sponge kidney.

Therefore, excessive loss of calcium in urine and the possibility of stone formation are secondary to a number of diseases, including sarcoidosis and vitamin D excess, but also to unknown causes.

Primary hyperparathyroidism causing increased mineral turnover in bone and hypercalcemia is an important cause of hypercalciuria. It often presents with stone symptoms, and calcium phosphate deposits may be found in the renal tissue, cornea, and other organs. About 5% to 10% of calcium stones are associated with primary hyperparathyroidism. Patients with intermittent hypercalcemia may also have persistent hypercalciuria and stones (Stewart, 1981).

Causes of Hyperoxaluria

The majority of calcium stones (70% to 80%) contain oxalate. Some of the oxalate in urine is dietary in origin from beverages (tea, cocoa, coffee, cola), vegetables (beans, rhubarb, spinach), nuts, berries, and citrus fruits. Oxalate is also derived from ascorbic acid. Diseases of the small bowel such as Crohn's disease, ileal resection, and intestinal bypass surgery result in excessive oxalate absorption, probably in the colon, and excretion in the urine. Oxalate absorption increases when calcium and magnesium intakes are decreased. Malabsorption with steatorrhea causes loss of calcium as soaps, and malabsorption with increased bile salts remaining in the gut is thought to promote oxalate absorption in the colon. Pyridoxine deficiency is associated with oxalate stones. Primary hyperoxaluria is a rare inherited autosomal recessive disease with oxoglutarate carboligase deficiency. Systemic oxalosis and renal failure occur in young adulthood. Renal transplantation and large doses of pyridoxine or nicotinamide have been tried for the treatment of these patients (Coe, 1978; Brown, 1982).

Causes of Hyperuricuria

Uric acid is a weak acid and at pH 5.5 forms free, insoluble, undissociated uric acid and a urate that is more soluble with some sodium and potassium present. The amount of free uric acid present in urine decreases as the pH rises. At pH 7, uric acid is more soluble as urate, but with high salt concentrations the urate becomes less soluble. Solute concentration as well as pH appears to be important in the solubility of uric acid and urate. Whereas large quantities of uric acid crystals are regularly found in urinary sediment, uric acid stone formation is not common. Uric acid crystals form a sludge that may obstruct the nephron without forming a stone. On the other hand, uric acid and sodium acid urate crystals are found as nuclei for calcium stones. Average uric acid excretion by adults is 500 to 600 mg/24 hours. If the urine volume is low, solubility of uric acid at acid pH is exceeded. Most normal persons with a pH of 6 have urine saturated with uric acid but do not form stones. Further acidity or dehydration is apparently required to engender stone formation.

Excessive excretion of uric acid relates to excessive dietary intake of purines (liver, dried beans, some fish, meat). Endogenous uric acid production is increased in gout, glycogen storage diseases, Lesch-Nyhan syndrome, myelogenous leukemia, acute leukemia in childhood, and treated tumors with associated cell necrosis. Chemotherapy and irradiation cause cell necrosis. Increased breakdown of tumor cells (nucleotide/purine forms uric acid) has caused acute renal failure because of tubular and ureter obstruction by masses of uric acid crystals. In gout, about 20% of patients form stones, most of which are pure uric acid and others uric acid and calcium. Heat and dehydration and unusually acid urine contribute to stone formation. Gouty nephropathy occurs with sodium urate deposits in the medulla even when stones are not present, and masses of crystals may cause obstruction of terminal collecting ducts in the kidneys (Cameron, 1979).

Normally, about one third of the uric acid formed is degraded by bacteria in the colon. Absence of bacteria or intestinal diversions cause increased absorption of uric acid from the gut. Because patients having undergone ileostomy lose large amounts of alkaline fluid from the intestine, they excrete concentrated acidic urine and are likely to produce uric acid stones. Uricosuric drugs cause potential problems with massive uric acid output in the first three to four days of treatment.

Cystinuria

Cystine stones form in patients with an inherited amino acid transport disorder for cystine, ornithine, lysine, and arginine and subsequent excretion of large amounts of these amino acids in the urine. Only cystine forms crystals and stones. Cystine does not become soluble until the urine pH is 7.4, and stones form over a range of normal urinary pH. Heterozygous carriers for the disease have increased amounts of cystine in urine but do not form stones. Homozygotes are stone formers. A 24-hour quantitative urine cystine measurement is needed to detect the potential stone formers and should always be performed when crystals are found in random specimens.

Analysis of Calculi

Gross Appearance

Calculi may be of various sizes, commonly described as sand, gravel, or stone. Large round stones are characteristic of those found in the bladder; however, large rounded and staghorn shapes derive from the kidney pelvis. The physical characteristics of the various calculi rarely suffice for their identification, but a few points are worth noting. Uric acid and urate stones are always yellow to brownish red and are moderately hard. Phosphate stones are usually pale and friable. Calcium oxalate stones are very hard, are often a dark color, and typically have a rough surface. Cystine stones are the color of old yellow-brown soap and feel somewhat greasy.

Several methods are available for the analysis of calculi, such as optical crystallography, x-ray diffraction, and infrared spectroscopy. Electron beam analysis and mass spectroscopy are also used. A simplified method for analysis of renal calculi is presented by Farrington (1980). Most laboratories refer specimens for calculi analysis to more specialized laboratories.

A quantitative method for five of eight frequently measured substances has been described using available clinical chemistry methods: calcium, phosphorus, magnesium, ammonium, and uric acid. Cystine, oxalate, and carbonate are detected by qualitative means and interpreted with the quantitative results to characterize the stones (Westbury, 1970).

3

Qualitative Analysis of Urinary Calculi

(adapted from Winer 1943, 1959)

GROSS EXAMINATION OF CALCULI

1. If not done previously, wash the stone(s) free from blood, mucus, preservation solution, and so on. Stones submitted after sonic disintegration have adherent blood and tissue and are difficult to clean. Place the stones in a beaker, cover the beaker with several thicknesses of gauze held firmly in place with rubber bands, and wash under cold running water. Drain, remove the gauze carefully, and dry the beaker and stones in an oven. Rinse tiny stones with water from a squeeze bottle (not running water).
2. Record the dimension of the stone.
3. Describe briefly the color and texture of the stone's exterior surface. The stone may be photographed for record purposes.
4. Cut, saw, or break the stone to examine the interior. Note whether there is a foreign body that may have acted as a nucleus for its formation. Describe the color and texture of the interior and layers, if present.
5. Reduce small stones to a fine powder by pulverizing with a mortar and pestle.
6. If possible, if the stone is very large, it may be advisable to make separate analyses of layers that appear to have different constituents.

FOR RARE STONES

1. 0.1% sodium nitrite ($NaNO_2$)—prepared fresh on alternate days for sulfonamide test.
2. 0.5% ammonium sulfamate for sulfonamide test.
3. Sulfa dye reagent: 0.1% (w/v) *N*-(1-naphthyl) ethylenediamine dihydrochloride. The dye is more soluble in warm water. Store this solution in a dark bottle. Refrigerate.
4. Concentrated nitric acid—xanthine test.

5. Concentrated sulfuric acid—cholesterol test.
6. Acetic anhydride—cholesterol test.
7. Chloroform—cholesterol test.

CONTROLS

Use known stones. It is important to have known positive material to test the reagents.

SEQUENCE OF CHEMICAL DETERMINATIONS IN URINARY CALCULI

Because most small calculi consist of calcium oxalate, the best way to analyze them is to put all available powder in one test tube. (If the stone is very tiny, it may be placed directly in the test tube and crushed with a spatula.) Add HCl, pour off the supernatant for the calcium, and add manganese oxide to the residue for the oxalate. If the stone is a little larger, some of the powder could be used to test for phosphates.

URINARY SCREENING FOR INHERITED METABOLIC DISEASES

Urine has been used for many years to screen for metabolic diseases, including those determined by genetic inheritance. In these diseases, an abnormal metabolite or a larger than normal amount of a normal metabolite is often excreted in the urine, although the kidneys themselves are not always involved. Many of these diseases are associated with mental retardation, degeneration of the nervous system, and failure to thrive.

Although a number of inborn errors of metabolism have been identified, this section describes only some of the more common diseases encountered in the urinalysis section of the laboratory. These conditions are uncommon and often have nonspecific symptoms, but some may be treatable if early diagnosis is confirmed; therefore, blood and urine should be analyzed using techniques that are highly selective and sensitive.

See Burtis (1996) for analytical techniques and Scriver (1989) for details of individual diseases.

Aminoacidurias

The excretion of one or more amino acids in the urine may be an expression of a block in a major metabolic pathway (overflow type) or a deficiency in renal tubular function (renal type).

With an enzyme deficiency affecting amino acid metabolism, the substrate and other metabolites in the pathway accumulate, causing increased body fluid levels and increased substrate excretion in urine. Phenylketonuria is an example of this type of overflow aminoaciduria.

The renal type of aminoacidurias is not characterized by high levels of the amino acids in the blood because the primary defect is in the renal tubular reabsorption mechanism. An example of renal transport aminoaciduria is cystinuria.

Phenylketonuria

Phenylketonuria is an autosomal recessive inherited disease associated with an absence of active liver enzyme phenylalanine hydroxylase. Because dietary L-phenylalanine is not converted to tyrosine, phenylalanine and other metabolites accumulate. Both sexes are affected equally, with an incidence of about 1 in 11,000, with most cases occurring in individuals of northern European ancestry. Several types of disease occur, varying in severity. Mental retardation is the major clinical finding. Dietary restriction of phenylalanine has shown good results.

This disease is marked by an accumulation of normal metabolites in abnormal amounts. Plasma phenylalanine and phenylpyruvic acid levels are elevated; urinary phenylpyruvic acid (highest), phenylacetic acid, and phenylalanine are increased. Urinary indoleacetic acid and other indoles arising from altered tryptophan metabolism and indican (an indole) are also increased. The excretion of 5-hydroxyindoleacetic acid is diminished, paralleling the low level of serum 5-hydroxytryptamine.

A characteristic odor is due to phenylacetic acid in urine and sweat and is described as mousy or musty.

REAGENT STRIP TEST. Phenistix reagent strips contain ferric ammonium sulfate, magnesium sulfate, and cyclohexylsulfamic acid. The cyclohexylsulfamic acid provides optimal acidity for the reaction.

Procedure. Dip the reagent-impregnated portion of the strip into the urine and remove it immediately or press it against a wet diaper. At 30 seconds, compare the color of the dipped end of the strip with the color chart provided. A positive test result is a gray to gray-green reaction. Report as positive or negative. The test detects 5 to 10 mg/100 mL. (See Kelly, 1977, for a comparison of ferric chloride results and reagent strip results with numerous metabolites.) Salicylates and metabolites of phenothiazine derivatives may cause a pink to purple reaction.

Alkaptonuria

Homogentisic acid (dihydroxyphenylacetic acid) is excreted in the urine in large quantities in a rare hereditary disease, alkaptonuria. Phenylalanine and tyrosine are normally metabolized to homogentisic acid, which is then oxidized to maleylacetoacetic acid. With a deficiency of the liver enzyme homogentisic acid oxidase, homogentisic acid accumulates.

Patients with alkaptonuria develop dark blue to black pigmentation in cartilage and connective tissue. The disease may not be diagnosed until arthritis develops. A dark color on diapers has been noted in infants (Vaughan, 1979).

SCREENING. Screening test procedures may be found in Henry (1984).

FERRIC CHLORIDE TEST. A transient, very dark blue color is seen as 2 drops of 10% ferric chloride solution are added to about 2 mL of urine.

SILVER NITRATE TEST. Add 4 mL of 3% silver nitrate to 0.5 mL urine. Mix, then add several drops of 10% NH_4OH. Homogentisic acid causes the development of a black color.

Identification of homogentisic acid is made by using paper or thin-layer chromatography. It should be distinguished from gentisic acid, an aspirin metabolite. Normally, no homogentisic acid is present in urine.

Tyrosinuria

Tyrosinemia with tyrosinuria occurs as a result of abnormal metabolism of tyrosine derived from the diet or from phenylalanine. This may be part of a generalized amino acid disorder associated with liver disease or may be a transitory tyrosinemia in premature or low-weight infants or, rarely, in the syndrome of hereditary tyrosinemia. The genetic disease tyrosinosis is extremely rare.

Transitory hypertyrosinemia occurs in infants of low birth weight and is found in asymptomatic infants tested in screening programs. No liver or renal disease is present, and the entity is benign. The elevated tyrosine levels may on occasion be accompanied by transiently elevated phenylalanine levels. Tyrosine and the phenolic acids *p*-hydroxyphenyllactic and *p*-hydroxyphenylpyruvic acids are excreted in larger than normal amounts in the urine.

Hereditary tyrosinemia Type I or tyrosinosis is accompanied by a generalized aminoacidemia with a marked loss of *p*-hydroxyphenyllactic acid, glucosuria, ketonuria, proteinuria, and loss of phosphate. Tyrosine level is elevated in blood and urine. Cirrhosis of the liver, renal dysfunction, and rickets are the principal findings. Hepatoma occurs in childhood. The clinical entity in some respects resembles that of hereditary fructosemia and galactosemia, characterized by liver and kidney involvement and a generalized aminoaciduria because of renal tubular damage. Children do not survive the first decade of life.

TYROSINE CRYSTALS. Very fine, silky crystals are seen in the urinary sediment in severe liver disease. They are scattered in the field or aggregated to form sheaves. The crystals appear brown to black while focusing. Leucine crystals may accompany the tyrosine. The crystals precipitate at acid pH and are soluble in alkali.

NITROSONAPHTHOL TEST FOR TYROSINE. This is a nonspecific screening test and should be confirmed by chromatography or quantitative serum assay of tyrosine. Tyrosine and tyramine form soluble red complexes with nitrosonaphthol. Normal urine contains tyrosine. In tyrosinosis, levels are about 100 times normal.

Maple Syrup Urine Disease

MSUD is one of a group of diseases associated with abnormal branched-chain amino acid metabolism. These include hypervalinemia, isovaleric acidemia causing sweaty feet odor, and other rare diseases. In some of these diseases such as MSUD, the amino acids accumulate and are measured in serum and urine; in others, accumulated organic acids are measured by gas chromatography alone or coupled with mass spectrometry.

There are several forms of MSUD. The severe form is marked by severe neonatal vomiting, seizures and stupor, and often episodes of hypoglycemia. Leucine, isoleucine, valine, and their corresponding keto acids are elevated in the plasma and are excreted in the urine because deficient decarboxylases and other enzymes prevent the conversion of the keto amino acids to fatty acids. The urine has an odor resembling maple syrup, caramelized sugar, or curry, the source of which is not certain. The urinary keto acids are demonstrable by the first week of life. A screening test with dinitrophenylhydrazine demonstrates keto acids and their transformation into keto acid phenylhydrazones. A microbiologic blood screening test for the elevated leucine is used for mass screening.

DINITROPHENYLHYDRAZINE TEST. This test detects α-keto amino acids in the urine. Insoluble hydrazones form from the reaction of carbonyl groups with dinitrophenylhydrazine. A positive result is seen with MSUD and possibly in phenylketonuria (phenylpyruvic acid), histidinemia (imidazole pyruvic acid), and methionine malabsorption (oasthouse syndrome). The test result is positive with ketonuria due to other inherited diseases and other causes. A preliminary screening test for ketones should be performed.

Reagent. Use 100 mg of 2,4-dinitrophenylhydrazine in 100 mL of 2 N HCl. The reagent should be stored in a brown bottle in the refrigerator.

Procedure

1. Reagent and control should be at room temperature.
2. Add 10 drops of reagent to 1 mL of clear urine.
3. After or within 10 minutes, a yellow or chalky white precipitate indicates a positive reaction. It should be the same as or greater than the control precipitate.

Control. Use ketoglutaric acid, 25 mg in 100 mL of normal urine. Freeze in small aliquots.

3

Cystinuria

The defective transport of cystine by the epithelial cells of the renal tubules and gut is transmitted as an autosomal recessive trait. The basic defect is not known. Although large amounts of the dibasic acids, ornithine, lysine, and arginine, are also excreted in this disease, cystine is the only one that crystallizes out. Stone formation is a clinical manifestation.

Cystinuria is a common amino acid disorder. It occurs equally in both sexes, with an incidence estimated at about 1 per 10,000 (homozygous) and in larger numbers for heterozygotes. In mass screening programs for infants, the homozygous form is detected at about the same rate as phenylketonuria. Cystinuria is sometimes detected in patients with renal tubular disease. It is excreted with other amino acids in Wilson's disease, in Lowe's disease, and with the aminoaciduria of Hartnup's disease. The cyanide nitroprusside test, to be described, has a positive result in cystinuria.

The classic form of homocystinuria is due to deficiency of the liver enzyme cystathionine β-synthase, which catalyzes the formation of cystathionine from homocystine and serine in the methionine pathway. Homocysteine is rapidly oxidized to homocystine, which accumulates along with methionine and is excreted in the urine. Children with this disease may have seizures and thromboses and become mentally retarded. Urine for testing must be fresh because homocystine is labile. Quantitative urinalysis reveals high levels of homocystine, methionine, and cysteine-homocysteine disulfide. Results of the cyanide nitroprusside test are positive. Urine levels are checked to monitor the effects of the methionine-restricted diet used to treat the disease.

Cystinosis, a recessively inherited disorder of unknown cause, is characterized by cystine crystal deposition in lysosomes in cells. Crystals accumulate in the kidneys, eyes, bone marrow, and spleen. The severe form is marked by photophobia, renal failure, rickets, and growth failure. With renal tubular involvement, Fanconi's syndrome develops and patients have generalized aminoaciduria and glucosuria. Unlike cystinuria, the cystine loss in cystinosis parallels the loss of other amino acids in the urine.

CYSTINE CRYSTALS. Examine a first morning urine specimen for colorless, hexagonal crystals of cystine. Urine is of acid pH. Note that the solubility of cystine is less in water than in urine, and cystine may not always crystallize in a concentrated urine although present in large amounts (Ettinger, 1971).

CYANIDE-NITROPRUSSIDE TEST. This test is Brand's modification of Legal's nitroprusside reaction (Brand, 1930; Legal, 1883). Cystine is reduced to cysteine by sodium cyanide, and the free sulfhydryl groups then react with nitroprusside to produce a red-purple reaction. Freeing of sulfhydryl groups takes time. Cysteine, cystine, homocystine, and ketones (dark red) give positive reactions. Smith (1977a) evaluated the qualitative test for cystinuria and found that it separated normal, heterozygote, and homozygote ranges of excretion. The lower limit of the test was 35 to 60 μmol of cystine per mole of creatinine, and this corresponded to the heterozygote range. Homozygous stone formers usually excrete more than 300 mg/g of creatinine and are detected by this test.

Specimen. A concentrated early morning specimen gives best results. Dilute specimens may be falsely negative. Refrigerate until tested.

Procedure. Place 3 to 5 mL of urine in a test tube, add 2.0 mL of sodium cyanide solution (5 g/dL water), and allow to stand for 10 minutes. Timing is important. Treat a control solution in the same way. Sodium cyanide solution is stable for three months when stored in a refrigerator.

Add fresh aqueous sodium nitroprusside solution (5 g/dL) by drops (about 5 drops), and mix. (In some laboratories, the nitroprusside solution is made weekly and refrigerated.) A stable red-purple color develops with cystine.

Read immediately as positive or negative. Trace results may also be reported. A concentrated normal specimen could give a weakly positive trace result.

Further identification of cystine is made by chromatography and quantitative amino acid analysis.

Positive Control. Use 5 mg of cystine dissolved in 10 mL 0.1 N HCl, diluted to 100 mL with normal urine. Freeze aliquots. To save positive urine specimens, acidify with 0.1 N HCl to pH 1 or 2 and freeze.

Alberti KGMM, Hockaday TDR: Rapid blood ketone body estimation in the diagnosis of diabetic ketoacidosis. Br Med J 1972; 2:565.

Albright F, Bloomberg E: Hyperparathyroidism and renal disease with a note as to the formation of calcium casts in this disease. J Urol 1935; 34:1.

Alfthan OS, Liewendahl K: Investigation of sulfonamide crystalluria in man. Scand J Urol Nephrol 1972; 6:44.

Anderson NG, Anderson NL, Tollaksen SL: Proteins of human urine. I. Concentration and analysis by two-dimensional electrophoresis. Clin Chem 1979; 25:119.

Avent J, Schumann GB, Vars L: Comparison of the Chemstrip[c] leukocyte test with a standardized Papanicolaou-stained urine sediment evaluation. Lab Med 1983; 14:163.

Bailey DN, Jatlow PI: Chemical analysis of massive crystalluria following primidone overdose. Am J Clin Pathol 1972; 58:583.

Bailey RR, Dann E, Gillies AHB, et al: What the urine contains following athletic competition. N Z Med J 1976; 83:309.

Balikov B: Urobilinogen excretion in normal adults; results of assays with notes on methodology. Clin Chem 1957; 3:145.

Banda PW, Sherry AE, Blois MS: Column cation-exchange separation of melanin-related metabolites in urine from cases of melanoma. Clin Chem 1977; 23:1397.

Bandi ZL, Meyers JL, Bee DE, James GP: Evaluation of determination of glucose in urine with some commercially available dipsticks and tablets. Clin Chem 1982; 28:2110.

Belmonte MM, Sarkozy E, Harpur E: Urine sugar determination by the two drop Clinitest[a] method. Diabetes 1967; 16:557.

Benedict SR: A reagent for the detection of reducing sugars. J Biol Chem 1909; 5:485.

Benham L, O'Kell RT: Urinalysis: Minimizing microscopy. Clin Chem 1982; 28:1722.

Bickel H: Mellituria, a paper chromatographic study. J Pediatr 1961; 59:641.

Blank DW, Frohlich J: Pseudochyluria caused by vaginal cream. Clin Chem 1982; 28:2181.

Blondheim SH, Margoliash E, Shafur E: A simple test for myohemoglobinuria (myoglobinuria). JAMA 1958; 167:453.

Boesken WH, Boesken S, Marmier A: Myoglobinuria. Immunochemical quantitation and electrophoretic separation of free and protein-bound myoglobin (Mb). *In* Dubach VC, Schmidt V (eds): Diagnostic Significance of Enzymes and Proteins in Urine. Current Problems in Clinical Biochemistry, 9. Bern, Huber, 1979.

Bossenmaier I, Cardinal R: Stability of {delta}-aminolevulinic acid and porphobilinogen in urine under varying conditions. Clin Chem 1968; 14:610.

Bowie L, Smith S, Gochman N: Characteristics of binding between reagent-strip indicators and urinary proteins. Clin Chem 1977; 23:128.

Bradley GM: Differentiating epithelial cells from leukocytes in urine. Postgrad Med 1968; 43:245.

Brand E, Harris MM, Biloon S: Cystinuria: The excretion of cystine complex which decomposes in the urine with the liberation of free cystine. J Biol Chem 1930; 86:315.

Brenner BM, Hostetter TH, Humes HD: Molecular basis of proteinuria of glomerular origin. N Engl J Med 1978; 298:826.

Brodows RG, Nichols D, Shaker G, et al: Evaluation of a new radioimmunoassay for urinary albumin. Diabetes Care 1986; 9:189.

Brody LH, Webster MC, Kark RM: Identification of elements of urinary sediment with phase-contrast microscopy. JAMA 1968; 206:1977.

Brown DC: Kidney stones. Current issues in diagnosis and therapy. Postgrad Med 1982; 72:124.

Burtis CA, Ashwood ER: Fundamentals of Clinical Chemistry, 4th ed. Philadelphia, W.B. Saunders Company, 1996.

Cameron JS, Simmonds HA: Gout and crystal related nephropathy. Contrib Nephrol 1979; 16:147.

Caraway WT: Chemical and diagnostic specificity of laboratory tests. Am J Clin Path 37:445, 1962.

Carlson DA, Statland BE: Automated urinalysis. Clin Lab Med 1988; 8:449.

Cartwright GE: Diagnostic Laboratory Hematology. New York, Grune & Stratton, 1968.

Coe FL: Nephrolithiasis. Pathogenesis and Treatment. Chicago, Year Book Medical Publishers, 1978.

Coe FL: The patient with renal stones. *In* Schrier RW (ed): Manual of Nephrology. Boston, Little, Brown and Co., 1981.

Cohen RD, Woods HF: Clinical and Biochemical Aspects of Lactic Acidosis. London, Blackwell Scientific Publishers, 1976.

Cone TE Jr: Diagnosis and treatment: Some syndromes, diseases and conditions associated with abnormal coloration of the urine or diaper. Pediatrics 1968; 41:654.

Cook MH, Free AH, Giordano AS: The accuracy of urine sugar tests. Am J Med Technol 1953; 19:283.

Corwin HL, Silverstein MD: Microscopic hematuria. Clin Lab Med 1988; 8:601.

Cruikshank G, Edmond E: "Clean catch" urine in the newborn—bacteriology and cell excretion patterns in the first week of life. Br Med J 1967; 4:704.

Daum GS, Krolikowski FJ, Reuter KL, et al: Dipstick evaluation of hematuria in abdominal trauma. Am J Clin Pathol 1988; 89:538.

Davidsohn I, Henry JB (eds): Todd-Sanford Clinical Diagnosis by Laboratory Methods, 15th ed. Philadelphia, W.B. Saunders Co., 1974.

de Mendoza SG, Kashyap ML, Chen CY, Lutmer RF: High density lipoproteinuria in nephrotic syndrome. Metabolism 1976; 25:1143.

Dewald B, Rindler-Ludwig R, Bretz V, Baggiolini M: Subcellular localization and heterogeneity of neutral proteases in neutrophilic polymorphonuclear leukocytes. J Exp Med 1975; 141:709.

Dewall CP, Casazza AR, Grimley PM, et al: Recovery of cytomegalovirus from adults with neoplastic disease. Ann Intern Med 1966; 64:531.

Dobbins JW, Binder HJ: Importance of the colon in enteric hyperoxaluria. N Engl J Med 1977; 296:298.

Duttera MJ, Carolla RL, Galleli JF, et al: Hematuria and crystalluria after high-dose 6-mercaptopurine administration. N Engl J Med 1972; 287:292.

Eggensperger D, Schweitzer S, Ferriol E, et al: The utility of cytodiagnostic urinalysis for monitoring renal allograft injury. Am J Nephrol 1988; 8:27.

Ettinger B, Kolb FO: Factors involved in crystal formation in cystinuria; in vivo and in vitro crystallization dynamics and a simple, quantitative colorimetric assay for cystine. J Urol 1971; 106:106.

Ettinger B, Weil E, Mandel NS, Darling S: Triamterene-induced nephrolithiasis. Ann Intern Med 1979; 91:745.

Exton WG: A simple and rapid quantitative test for albumin in urine. J Lab Clin Med 1925; 10:722.

Fairley KF, Birch DF: Hematuria: A simple method for identifying glomerular bleeding. Kidney Int 1982; 21:105.

Falk JS, Lindblad GTO, Westman JM: Histopathologic studies on kidneys from patients treated with large amounts of blood preserved with ACD-adenine. Transfusion 1972; 12:376.

Fang LST: Urinalysis in the diagnosis of urinary tract infections. Clin Lab Med 1988; 8:567.

Farrington CJ, Liddy ML, Chalmers AH: A simplified sensitive method for analysis of renal calculi. Am J Clin Pathol 1980; 73:96.

Fassett RG, Horgan BA, Mathew TH: Detection of glomerular bleeding by phase-contrast microscopy. Lancet 1982; 1:1432.

Fogstrup J, With TK: Urinary total porphyrins by ion exchange analysis: Reference values for the normal range and remarks on preformed porphyrins in acute porphyria tarda. J Clin Pathol 1979; 32:109.

Fraser CG, Smith BC, Peake MJ: Effectiveness of an outpatient urine screening program. Clin Chem 1977; 23:2216.

Free AH, Free HM: A simple test for urine bilirubin. Gastroenterology 1953; 24:414.

Free AH, Free HM: Urinalysis in Clinical Laboratory Practice. Cleveland, CRC Press, 1975.

Free AH, Free HM: Rapid convenience urine tests: Their use and misuse. Lab Med 1978; 9:9.

Freni SC, Dalderup LM, Oudegeest JJ, Wensveen N: Erythrocyturia, smoking and occupation. J Clin Pathol 1977; 30:341.

Gadeholt H: Quantitative estimation of urinary sediment with special regard to sources of error. Br Med J 1964; 1:1547.

Gillenwater JY: Detection of urinary leukocytes by Chemstrip[c]-I. J Urol 1981; 125:383.

Gyure WL: Comparison of several methods for semiquantitative determination of urinary protein. Clin Chem 1977; 23:876.

Haber MH: Interference contrast microscopy for identification of urinary sediments. Am J Clin Pathol 1972; 57:316.

Haber MH: Urine Casts, Their Microscopy and Clinical Significance. Chicago, American Society of Clinical Pathologists, 1975.

Haber MH: Urinary Sediment: A Textbook Atlas. Chicago, American Society of Clinical Pathologists, 1981.

Haber MH: Pisse prophecy: A brief history of urinalysis. Clin Lab Med 1988a; 8:415.

Haber MH: Quality assurance in urinalysis. Clin Lab Med 1988b; 8:431.

Haining R, Hulse T, Labbe R: Rapid porphyrin screening of urine, stool and blood. Clin Chem 1969; 15:400.

Hansen JL, Freier EF: Direct assays of lactate, pyruvate, {beta}-hydroxybutyrate and acetoacetate with a centrifugal analyzer. Clin Chem 1978; 24:475.

Hansen OH, Hansen A, Vibild O, et al: The relationship of lipuria to the fat embolism syndrome. Acta Chir Scand 1973; 139:421.

Hansen PD: Drug Interactions, 4th ed. Philadelphia, Lea and Febiger, 1979.

Helgason S, Lindquist B: Eosinophiluria. Scand J Urol Nephrol 1972; 6:257.

Henry JB (ed): Clinical Diagnosis and Management by Laboratory Methods, 16th ed. Philadelphia, W.B. Saunders Co., 1979.

Henry JB (ed): Clinical Diagnosis and Management by Laboratory Methods, 17th ed. Philadelphia, W.B. Saunders Co., 1984.

Henry RJ: Clinical Chemistry: Principles and Techniques. New York, Harper & Row, 1964.

Henry RJ, et al: Clinical Chemistry: Principles and Techniques, 2nd ed. New York, Harper & Row, 1974.

Henry RJ, Sobel C, Segalove M: Turbidometric determination of proteins with sulfosalicylic and trichloroacetic acids. Proc Soc Exp Biol Med 1956; 92:748.

Highman W, Wilson E: Urine cytology in patients with calculi. J Clin Pathol 1982; 35:350.

Hindmarsh JT: Microalbuminuria. Clin Lab Med 1988; 8:611.

Hoesch K: Über die Auswertung der Urobilinogenurie und die umgekehrte Urobilinogenreaktion. Dtsch Med Wochenschr 1947; 72:704.

Holmquist N: Detection of cancer with urinary sediment. J Urol 1980; 123:188.

Houston IB: Pus cell and bacterial counts in diagnosis of urinary tract infections in childhood. Arch Dis Child 1963; 38:600.

Imhof PR, Hushak S, Schumann G: Excretion of urinary casts after the administration of diuretics. Br Med J 1972; 2:199.

James GP, Bee DE, Fuller JB: Proteinuria: Accuracy and precision of laboratory diagnosis by dip-stick analysis. Clin Chem 1978a; 24:1934.

James GP, Paul KL, Fuller JB: Urinary nitrite and urinary-tract infection. Am J Clin Pathol 1978b; 70:671.

Kagen LJ: Immunologic detection of myoglobinuria after cardiac surgery. Ann Intern Med 1967; 67:1183.

Kelly S: Biochemical Methods in Medical Genetics. Springfield, IL, Charles C Thomas, 1977.

Kesson AM, Talbolt JM, Gyory AZ: Microscopic examination of urine. Lancet 1978; 2:809.

Kibrick AC: Extended use of the Kingsley biuret reagent. Clin Chem 1958; 4:232.

Killander J, Sjolin S, Zaar B: Rapid tests for ketonuria. Scand J Clin Lab Invest 1962; 14:311.

Kim MS: Proteinuria. Clin Lab Med 1988; 8:527.

Kunin CM, Degroot JE: Self-screening for significant bacteriuria. JAMA 1975; 231:1349.

Kusumi RK, Grover PJ, Kunin CM: Rapid detection of pyuria by leukocyte esterase activity. JAMA 1981; 245:1653.

Leahy DT, Brien TG: A simple method for the separation and quantification of urinary porphyrins. J Clin Pathol 1982; 35:1232.

Lee C: An enzyme immunoassay for urinary albumin at low concentrations. Lab Med 1989; 20:564–566.

Legal E: Regarding a new acetone reaction and its use in urinalysis. Chemisch Zentralbl 1883; 13:652.

Levin S: Red urine: The Monday morning disorder of children. Pediatrics 1965; 36:134.

Levison DA, Crocker PR, Banim S, Wallace DMA: Silica stones in the urinary bladder. Lancet 1982; 1:704.

Lindqvist B, Wahlin A: Differential count of urinary leukocytes and renal epithelial cells by phase contrast microscopy. Acta Med Scand 1975; 198:505.

Lizana J, Brito M, Davis MR: Assessment of five quantitative methods for determination of total proteins in urine. Clin Biochem 1977; 10:89.

Lombardo JV, Terlinsky A, Chester AC, Preuss HG: Tubulointerstitial diseases. Am Fam Physician 1980; 21:128.

Malone JI, Rosenbloom AL, Grgic A, Weber FT: The role of urine sugar in diabetic management. Am J Dis Child 1976; 130:1324.

Mandal AK: Analysis of urinary sediment by transmission electron microscopy. An innovative approach to diagnosis and prognosis in renal disease. Clin Lab Med 1988; 8:463–481.

Markowitz H, Wobig G: Quantitative method for estimating myoglobin in urine. Clin Chem 1977; 9:1689.

McElderry LA, Tarbit IF, Cassells-Smith AJ: Six methods for urinary protein compared. Clin Chem 1982; 28:356.

McKenna M, Amin V, Feldkamp C, et al: Albumin excretion rate is the preferred way to report microalbuminuria—a study in normal people. J Clin Immunoassay 1987; 10:151.

Mogensen CE: Microalbuminuria predicts clinical proteinuria and early mortality in maturity-onset diabetes. N Engl J Med 1984a; 310:356.

Mogensen CE, Christensen CK: Predicting diabetic nephropathy in insulin-dependent patients. N Engl J Med 1984b; 311:89.

Najarian JS: The diagnostic importance of the odor of urine. N Engl J Med 1980; 303:1128.

Nolan CR, Kelleher SP: Eosinophiluria. Clin Lab Med 1988; 8:555–565.

Palmieri LJ, Schumann GB: Osmotic effects on neutrophil segmentation. An *in vitro* phenomenon. Acta Cytol 1977; 21:2.

Pierach CA, Cardinal R, Bossenmaier I, Watson CJ: Comparison of the Hoesch and Watson-Schwartz tests for urinary porphobilinogen. Clin Chem 1977; 23:1666.

Piva AE, Koss LG: Cytologic diagnosis of metastatic malignant melanoma in urinary sediment. Acta Cytol 1964; 8:398.

Prien EL: Crystallographic analysis of urinary calculi: A 23 year survey study. J Urol 1963; 89:917.

Riekers H, Miale JB: Ketonuria. An evaluation of tests and some clinical implications. Am J Clin Pathol 1958; 30:530.

Riggs SA, Minuth AN, Nottebohm GA, et al: Plasma cells in urine. Occurrence in multiple myeloma. Arch Intern Med 1975; 135:1245.

Robinson RR, Glover SN, Phillippi PJ, et al: Fixed and reproducible orthostatic proteinuria. Am J Pathol 1961; 39:291.

Roe CE, Carlson DA, Daigneault RW, Statland BE: Evaluation of the Yellow IRIS. An automated method for urinalysis. Am J Clin Pathol 1986; 86:661.

Roguljic A, Ruzdic I: The DOPA-oxidase activity in urine and its diagnostic importance for malignant melanoma. Clin Chem 1975; 21:1025.

Ross DL, Neely AE: Textbook of Urinalysis and Body Fluids. Norwalk, CT, Appleton-Century-Crofts, 1983.

Rothera ACH: Note on the sodium nitroprusside reaction for acetone. J Physiol 1908; 37:491.

Rous P: Urinary siderosis. J Exp Med 1918; 28:645.

Rubner M: Über die Einwirkung von Bleiacetat auf Trauben- und Milchzucker. Z Biol 1884; 20:397.

Rytand DA: Prognosis in postural (orthostatic) proteinuria. N Engl J Med 1981; 305:618.

Sanjurjo LA: Parasitic diseases of the genitourinary system. *In* Campbell MF, Harrison JH (eds): Urology, 3rd ed. Philadelphia, W.B. Saunders Co., 1970.

Schreiner GE: Identification and significance of casts. Arch Intern Med 1957; 99:956.

Schumann GB: Urine Sediment Examination. Baltimore, Williams and Wilkins, 1980.

Schumann GB: Cytodiagnostic urinalysis for the nephrology practice. Semin Nephrol 1986; 6:308.

Schumann GB, Greenberg NF: Usefulness of macroscopic urinalysis as a screening procedure. A preliminary report. Am J Clin Pathol 1979; 71:452.

Schumann GB, Johnston JL, Weiss MA: Renal epithelial fragments in urine sediment. Acta Cytol 1981a; 25:147.

Schumann GB, Schumann JL, Marcussen N. Cytodiagnostic urinalysis of renal and lower urinary tract disorders. New York, Igaku-Shoin, 1995, pp 3–4.

Schumann GB, Schumann JL, Schweitzer S: The urine sediment examination. A coordinated approach. Lab Management 1983; 21:45.
Schumann GB, Weiss MA: Atlas of Renal and Urinary Tract Cytology and Its Histopathologic Bases. Philadelphia, J.B. Lippincott, 1981b.
Schwartz S, Shorov V, Watson CJ: Studies of urobilinogen. IV. Quantitative determination of urobilinogen by means of Evelyn photoelectric colorimeter. Am J Clin Pathol 1944; 14:598.
Scriver CR, Beaudet AL, Sly WS, Valle D: Metabolic Basis of Inherited Diseases, 6th ed. New York, McGraw-Hill, 1989.
Segasothy M, Lau TM, Birch DF, et al: Immunocytologic dissection of the urine sediment using monoclonal antibodies. Am J Clin Pathol 1988; 90:691.
Shenoy UA, Schumann GB, DeBellis CC: Prevalence of hematuria in urothelial neoplasia. Am J Clin Pathol 1986; 85:80.
Simmonds HA: 2,8-Dihydroxyadeninuria—or when is a uric acid stone not a uric acid stone? Clin Nephrol 1979; 12:196.
Sjoerdsma A, Weissbach H, Udenfriend S: Simple tests for diagnosis of metastatic carcinoid. JAMA 1955; 159:397.
Smith A: Evaluation of the nitroprusside test for the diagnosis of cystinuria. Med J Aust 1977a; 2:153.
Smith D, Young WW: Effect of large dose ascorbic acid on the two-drop Clinitest[a] determination. Am J Hosp Pharm 1977b; 34:1347.
Stamm WE, Running K, McKeirtt M, et al: Treatment of the acute urethral syndrome. N Engl J Med 1981; 304:956.
Stansfeld JM, Webb JKG: Observations on pyuria in children. Arch Dis Child 1953; 28:386.
Sternheimer R: A supravital cytodiagnostic stain for urinary sediments. JAMA 1975; 231:8.
Sternheimer R, Malbin B: Clinical recognition of pyelonephritis with a new stain for urinary sediments. Am J Med 1951; 11:312.
Stewart AF, Broadus AE: The regulation of renal calcium excretion. An approach to hypercalciuria. Annu Rev Med 1981; 32:457.
Sutor AH, Ketelson VP, Schindera F: Platelets in the urine: Further evidence. Thromb Haemost 1976; 36:647.
Thomas V, Shelokov A, Forland M: Antibody-coated bacteria in the urine and the site of urinary-tract infection. N Engl J Med 1974; 290:11.
Thompson AL, Durrett RR, Robinson RR: Fixed and reproducible orthostatic proteinuria. Ann Intern Med 1970; 73:235.
Triger DR, Smith JWC: Survival of urinary leucocytes. J Clin Pathol 1966; 19:443.
Tweeddale DN: Urinary Cytology. Boston, Little, Brown and Co., 1977.
Udenfriend S, Titus E, Weissbach H: The identification of 5-hydroxy-3-indoleacetic acid in normal urine and a method for its assay. J Biol Chem 1955; 216:299.
Vaughan VC III, McKay RJ, Behrman RE (eds): Nelson Textbook of Pediatrics, 11th ed. Philadelphia, W.B. Saunders Co., 1979.
Viberti GC, Jarrett RJ, Mahmud U, et al: Microalbuminuria as a predictor of clinical nephropathy in insulin-dependent diabetes mellitus. Lancet 1982; 1:1430.
Wahlin A: Differential count of urinary leukocytes and renal epithelial cells. Upsala J Med Sci 1977; 82:43.
Ward KM: Microalbuminuria: Clinical laboratory aspects. Clin Lab Sci 1989; 2:212.
Washington JA, White CM, Laganiere M, Smith LH: Detection of significant bacteriuria by microscopic examination of the urine. Lab Med 1981; 12:294.
Watson CJ, Hawkinson V: Semiquantitative estimation of bilirubin in the urine by means of barium strip modification of Harrison's test. J Lab Clin Med 1946; 31:914.
Watson CJ, Schwartz S: A simple test for urinary porphobilinogen. Proc Soc Exp Biol Med 1941; 47:393.
Wenk RE, Bhagavan BS, Rudert J: Tamm-Horsfall uromucoprotein and the pathogenesis of casts, reflux nephropathy and nephritides. Pathol Annu 1981; 11:229–257.
Westbury EJ, Omenogor P: A quantitative approach to the analysis of renal calculi. J Med Lab Technol 1970; 27:462.
Winer J: Practical value of analysis of urinary calculi. JAMA 1959; 169:1715.
Winer J, Mattic MR: Routine analysis of urinary calculi: Rapid, simple method using spot tests. J Lab Clin Med 1943; 28:989.
Wirth WA, Thompson RL: The effect of various conditions and substances on the results of laboratory procedures. Am J Clin Pathol 1965; 43:579.
With TK: Biology of Bile Pigments, Including a Review of Their Chemistry and a Discussion of Analytical Methods. Copenhagen, Arne Frost-Hansen, 1954.
With TK: Diagnostic tests for porphyria. Lab Med 1980; 11:446.
Young D, Jackson A: Thin layer chromatography of urinary carbohydrates: A comparative evaluation of procedures. Clin Chem 1970; 16:954.
Young DS, Pestaner LC, Gibberman V: Effects of drugs on clinical laboratory tests. Clin Chem 1975; 21:386D.

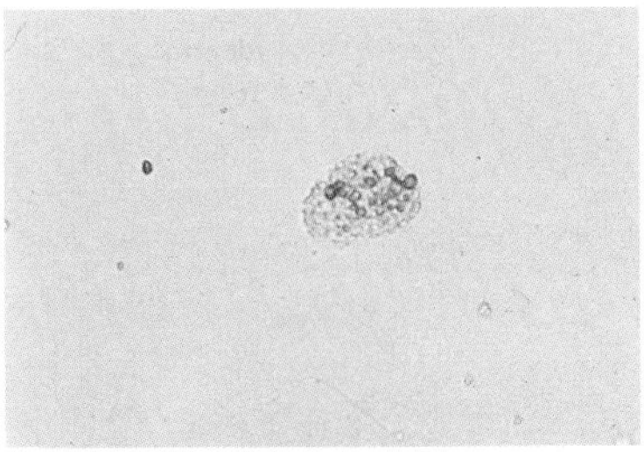

Plate 18–1

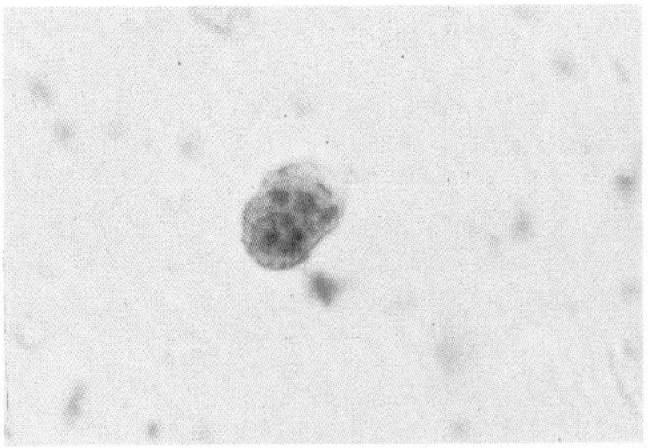

Plate 18–2

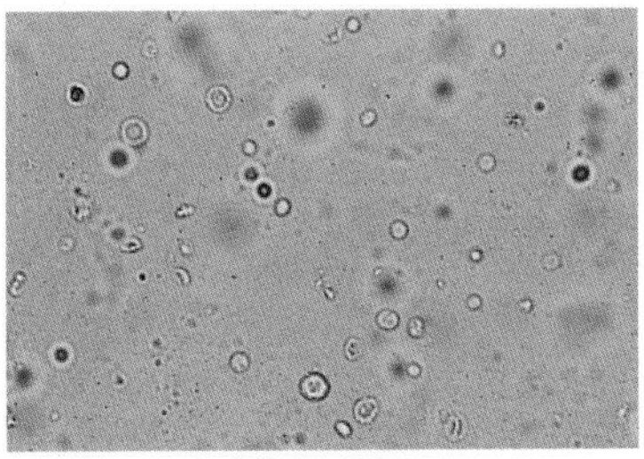

Plate 18–3

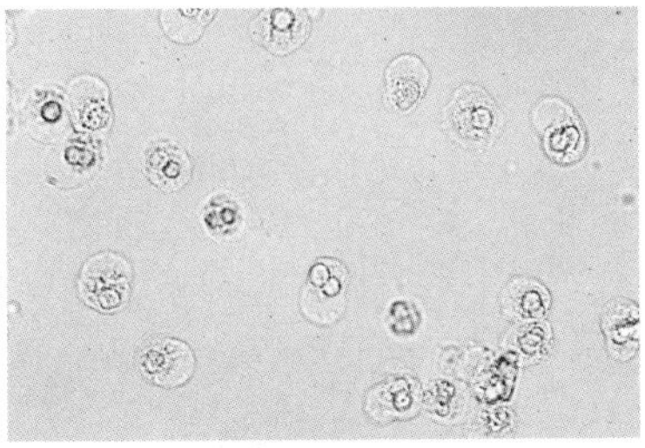

Plate 18–4

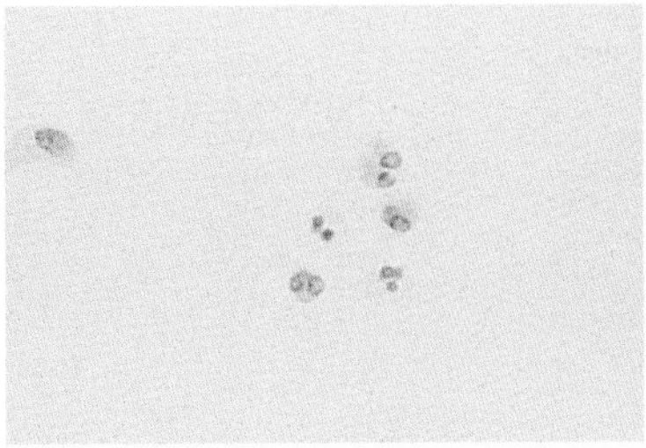

Plate 18–5

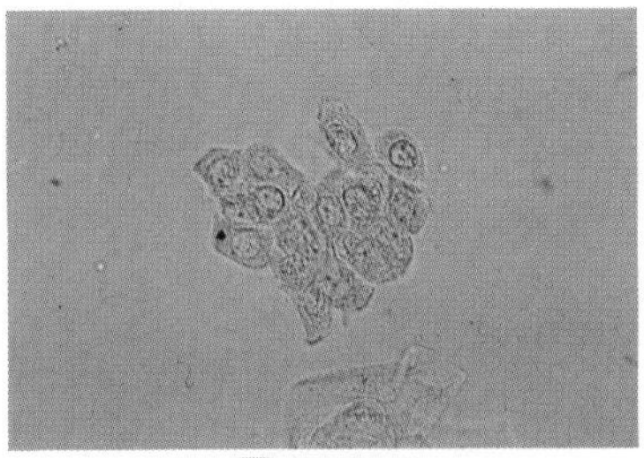

Plate 18–6

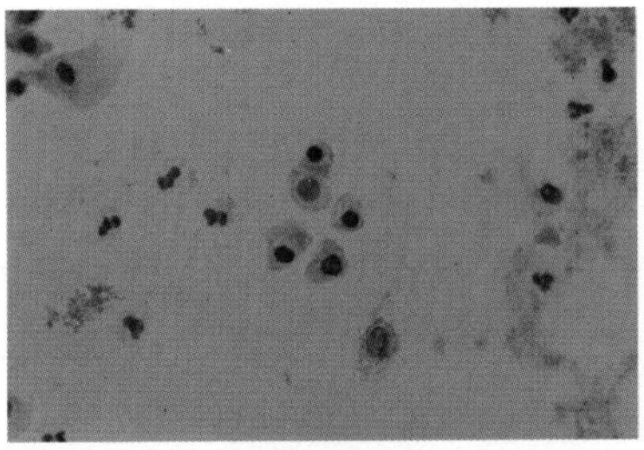

Plate 18–7

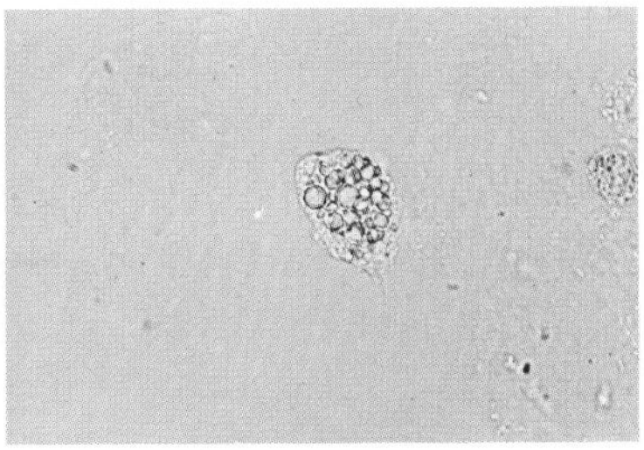

Plate 18–8

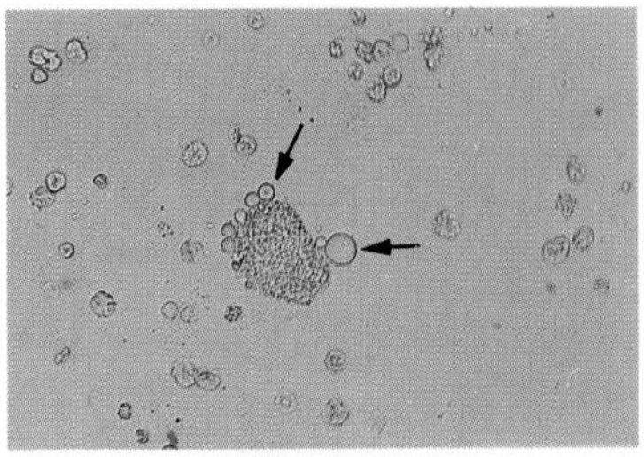

Plate 18–9A

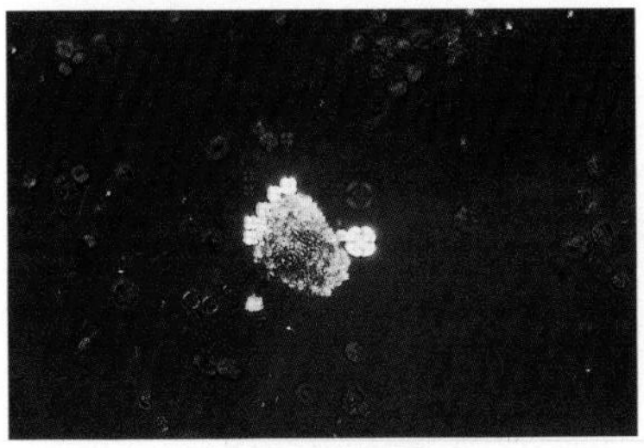

Plate 18–9B

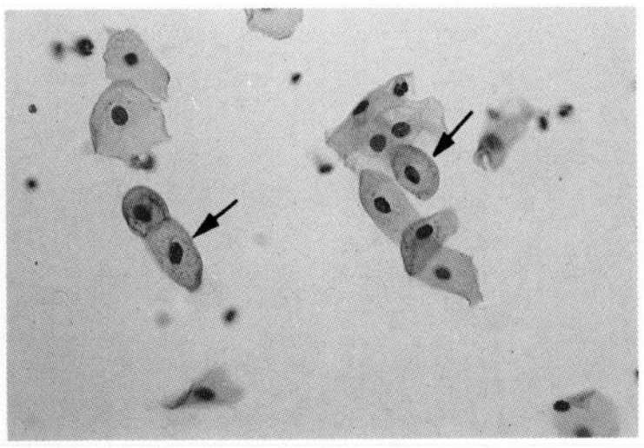

Plate 18–10

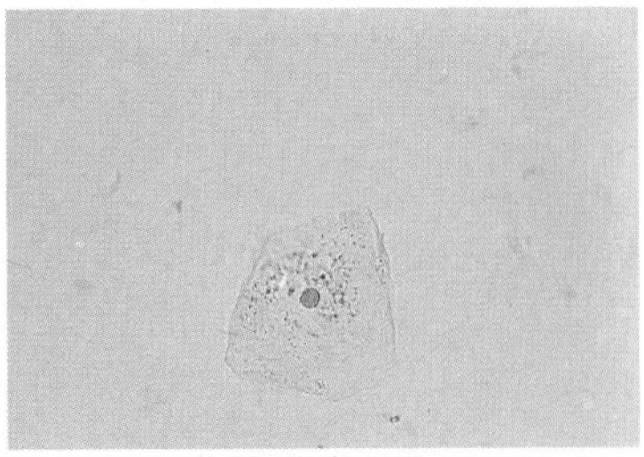

Plate 18–11

Plate 18–1. Renal tubular epithelial cell (unstained) containing brown pigment, iron (× 260). **Plate 18–2.** Renal tubular epithelial cell positive with Prussian blue stain, hemosiderin (× 260). **Plate 18–3.** Dysmorphic erythrocytes (× 160). **Plate 18–4.** Neutrophils with dilute acetic acid (× 200). **Plate 18–5.** Eosinophils (× 500). **Plate 18–6.** Renal tubular epithelial cells (× 200). **Plate 18–7.** Renal tubular epithelial cells and neutrophils. Papanicolaou stain (× 430). **Plate 18–8.** Oval fat body (× 160). **Plate 18–9.** *A*, Oval fat body with attached fat droplets. Brightfield (× 160). *B*, Oval fat body with attached fat droplets—polarized (× 160). **Plate 18–10.** Transitional epithelial cells. Papanicolaou stain (× 430). **Plate 18–11.** Squamous epithelial cell. Pyridium stained (× 200).

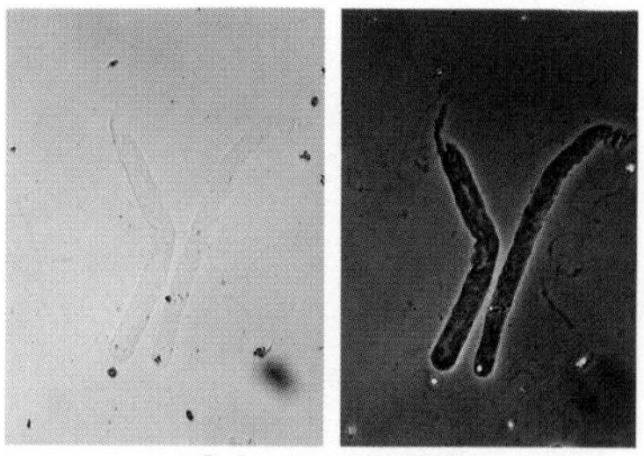

Plate 18–12 A&B

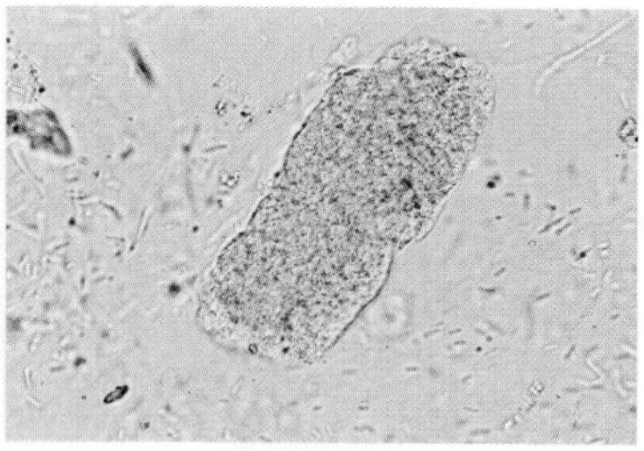

Plate 18–13

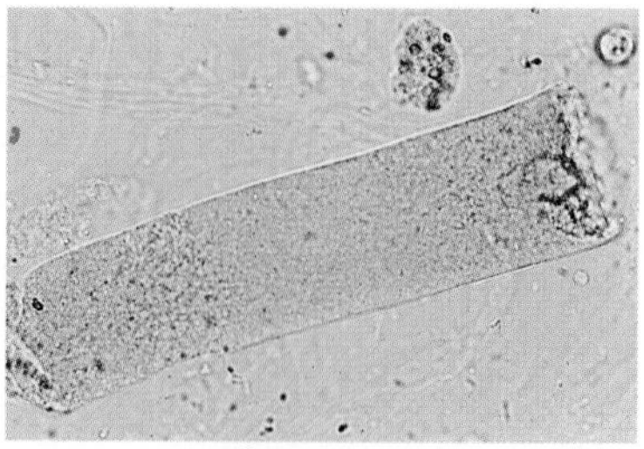

Plate 18–14

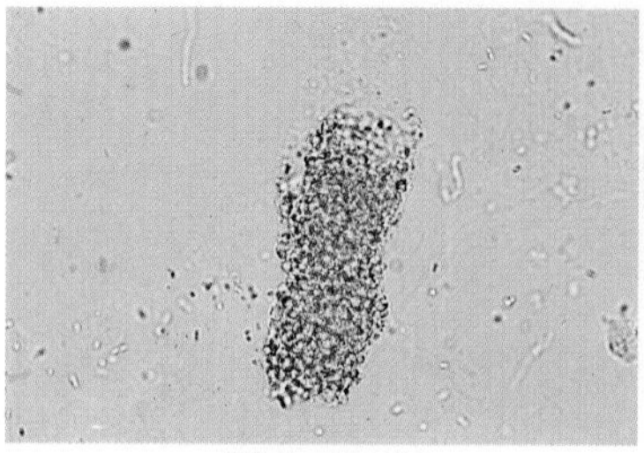

Plate 18–15

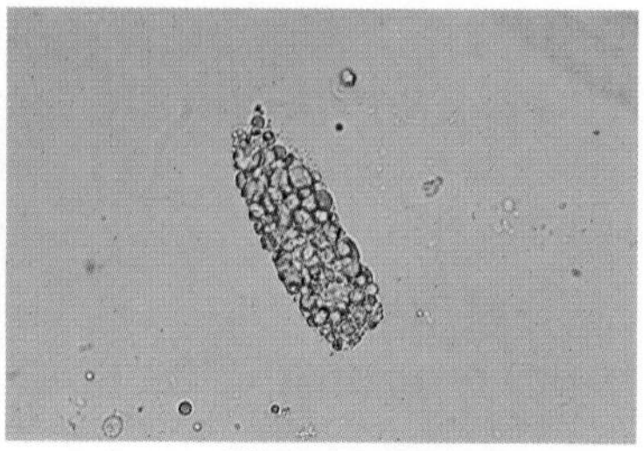

Plate 18–16

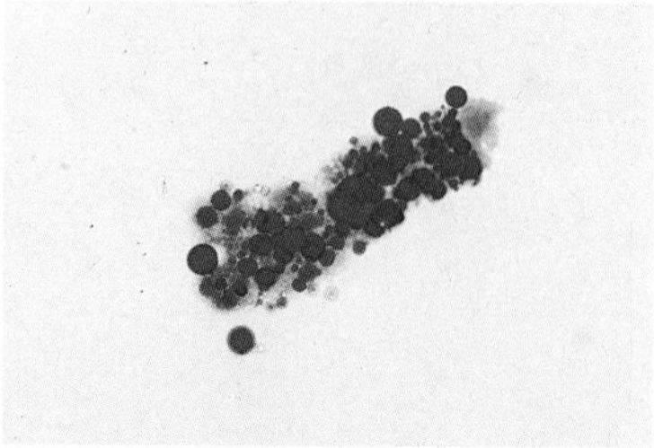

Plate 18–17

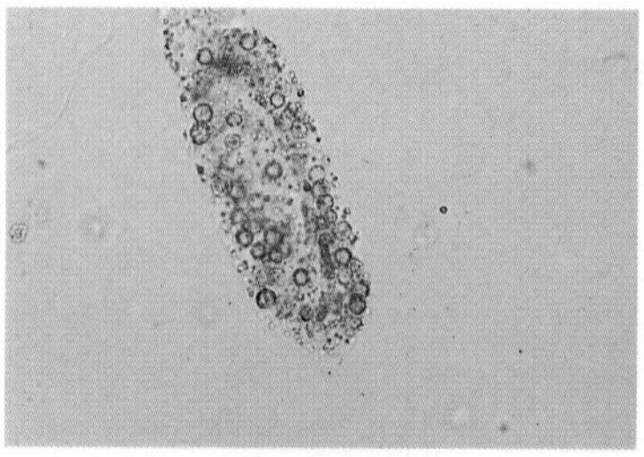

Plate 18–18

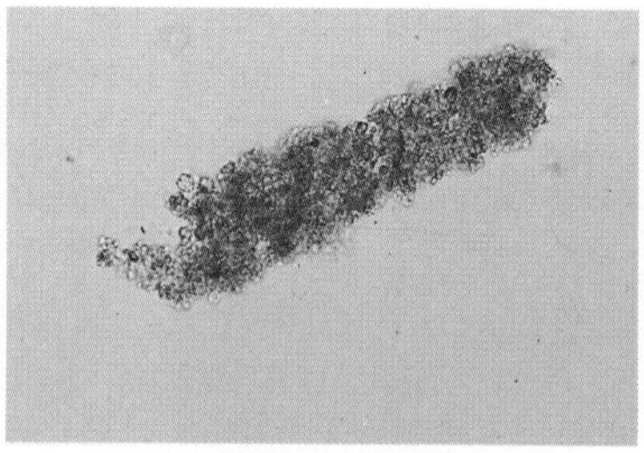

Plate 18–19

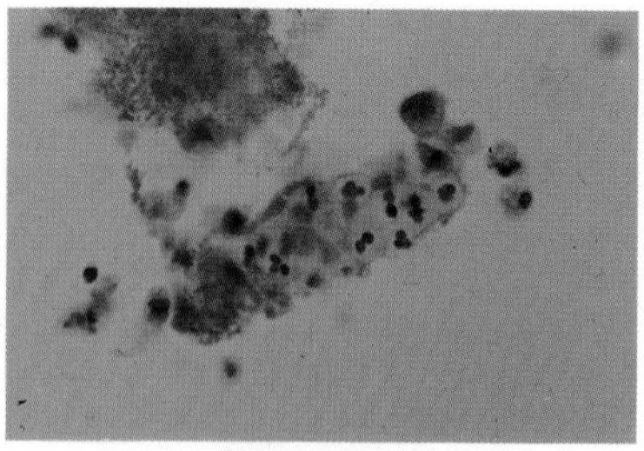

Plate 18–20

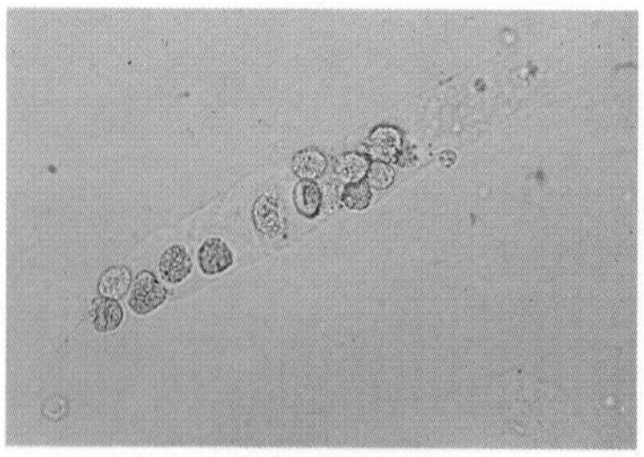

Plate 18–21

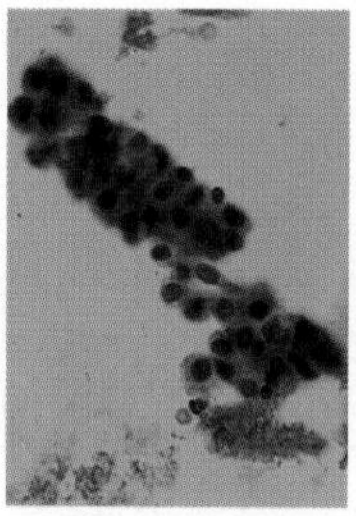

Plate 18–22

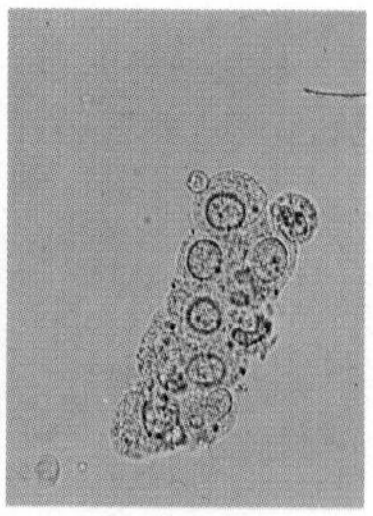

Plate 18–23

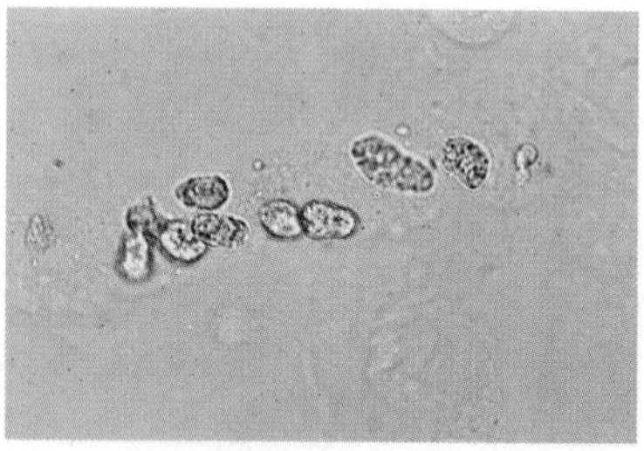

Plate 18–24

Plate 18–12. *A*, Hyaline casts. Brightfield (× 100). *B*, Hyaline casts. Phase contrast microscopy (× 100). **Plate 18–13.** Fine granular cast becoming waxy (× 200). **Plate 18–14.** Waxy cast (× 200). **Plate 18–15.** Granular cast (× 200). **Plate 18–16.** Fatty cast. Brightfield, nonpolarized (× 160). **Plate 18–17.** Fatty cast—positive Oil red O (× 200). **Plate 18–18.** Erythrocyte cast (× 200). **Plate 18–19.** Hemoglobin cast (× 200). **Plate 18–20.** Leukocyte cast. Papanicolaou stained (× 200). **Plate 18–21.** Cellular cast (× 200). **Plate 18–22.** Renal tubular epithelial cell cast. Papanicolaou stained (× 430). **Plate 18–23.** Mixed (leukocyte and renal tubular epithelial cell) cast (× 200). **Plate 18–24.** Cellular cast (× 200).

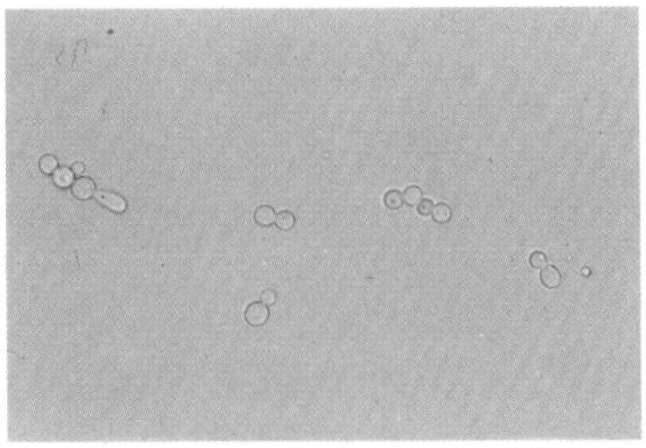

Plate 18–25

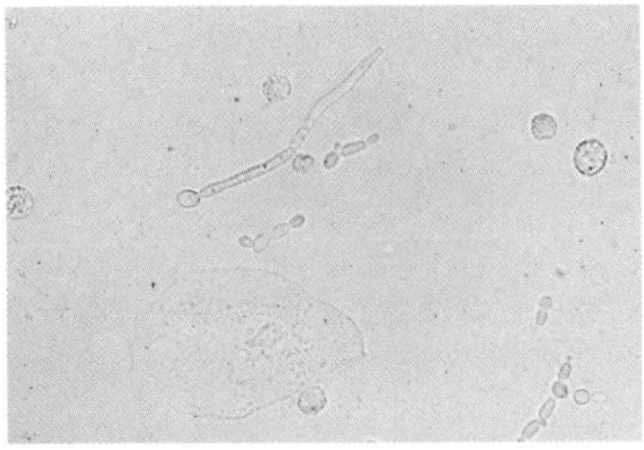

Plate 18–26

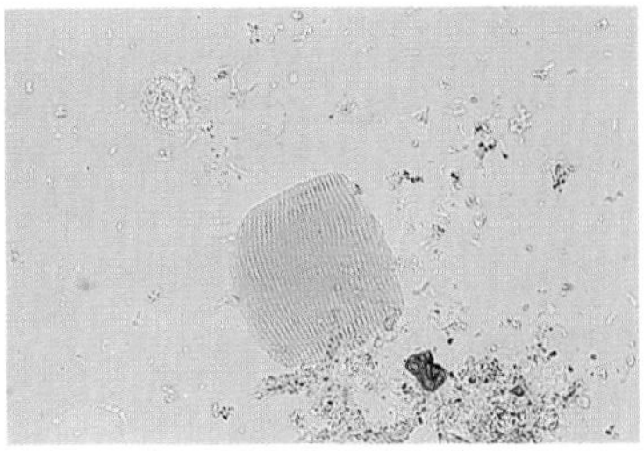

Plate 18–27

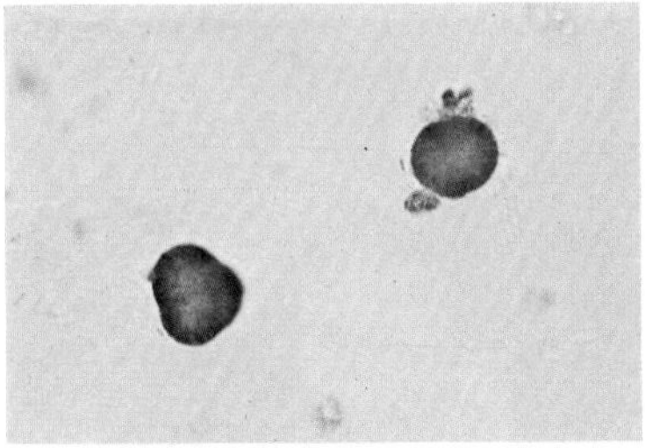

Plate 18–28

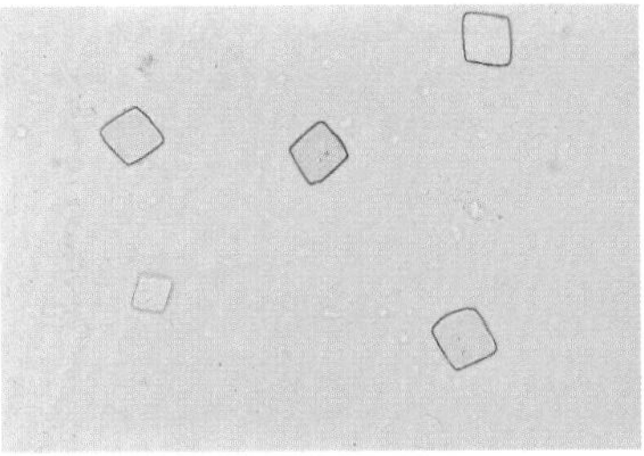

Plate 18–29

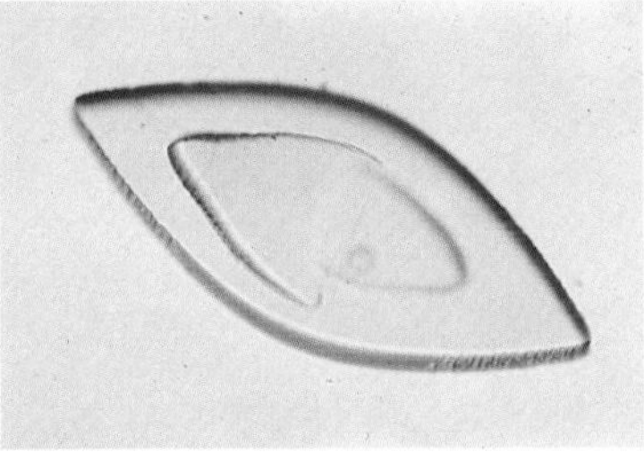

Plate 18–30

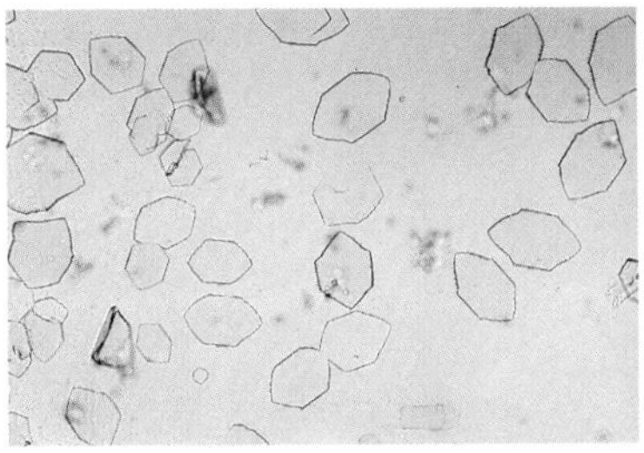

Plate 18–31A

Plate 18–31B

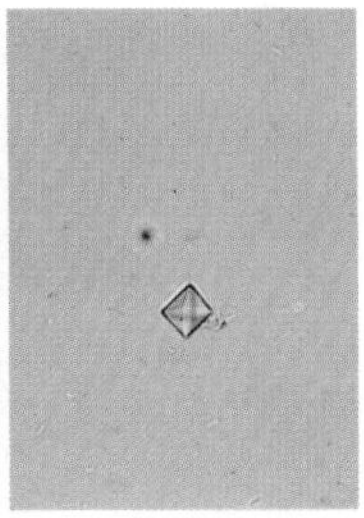

Plate 18–32

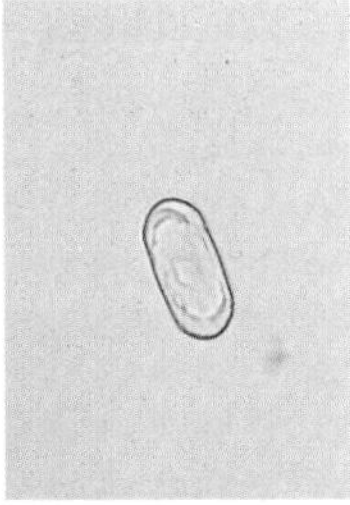

Plate 18–33

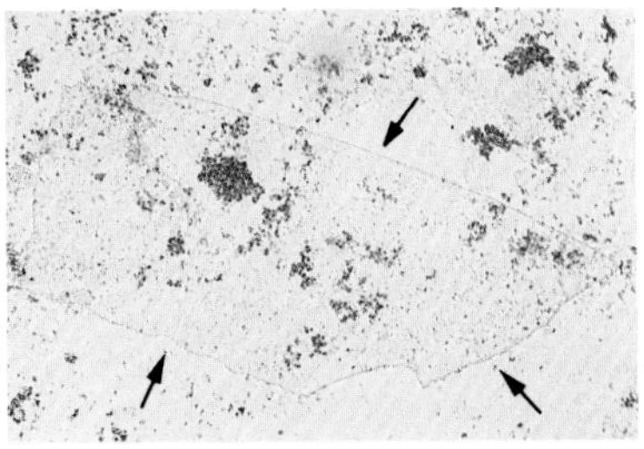

Plate 18–34

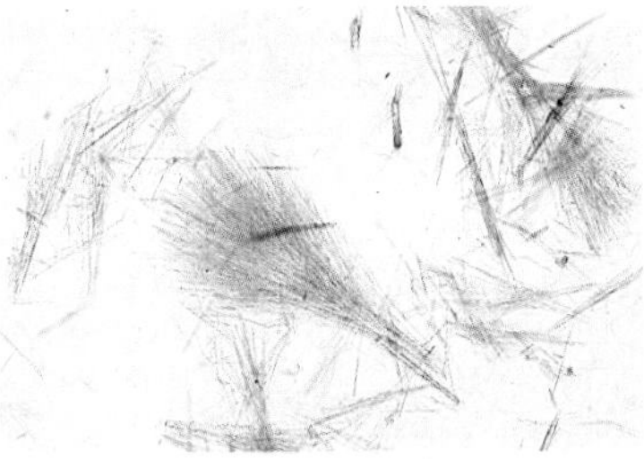

Plate 18–35

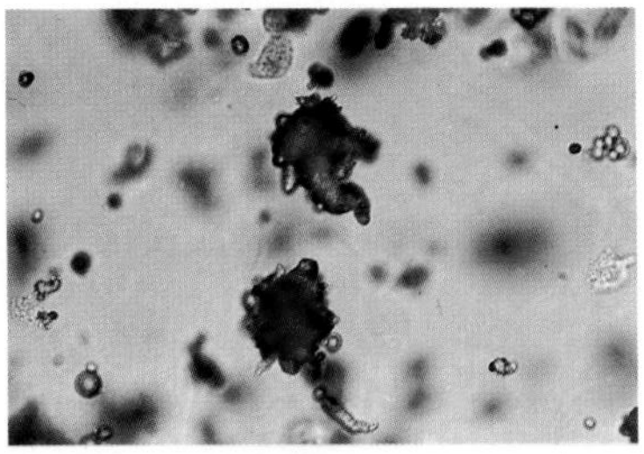

Plate 18–36

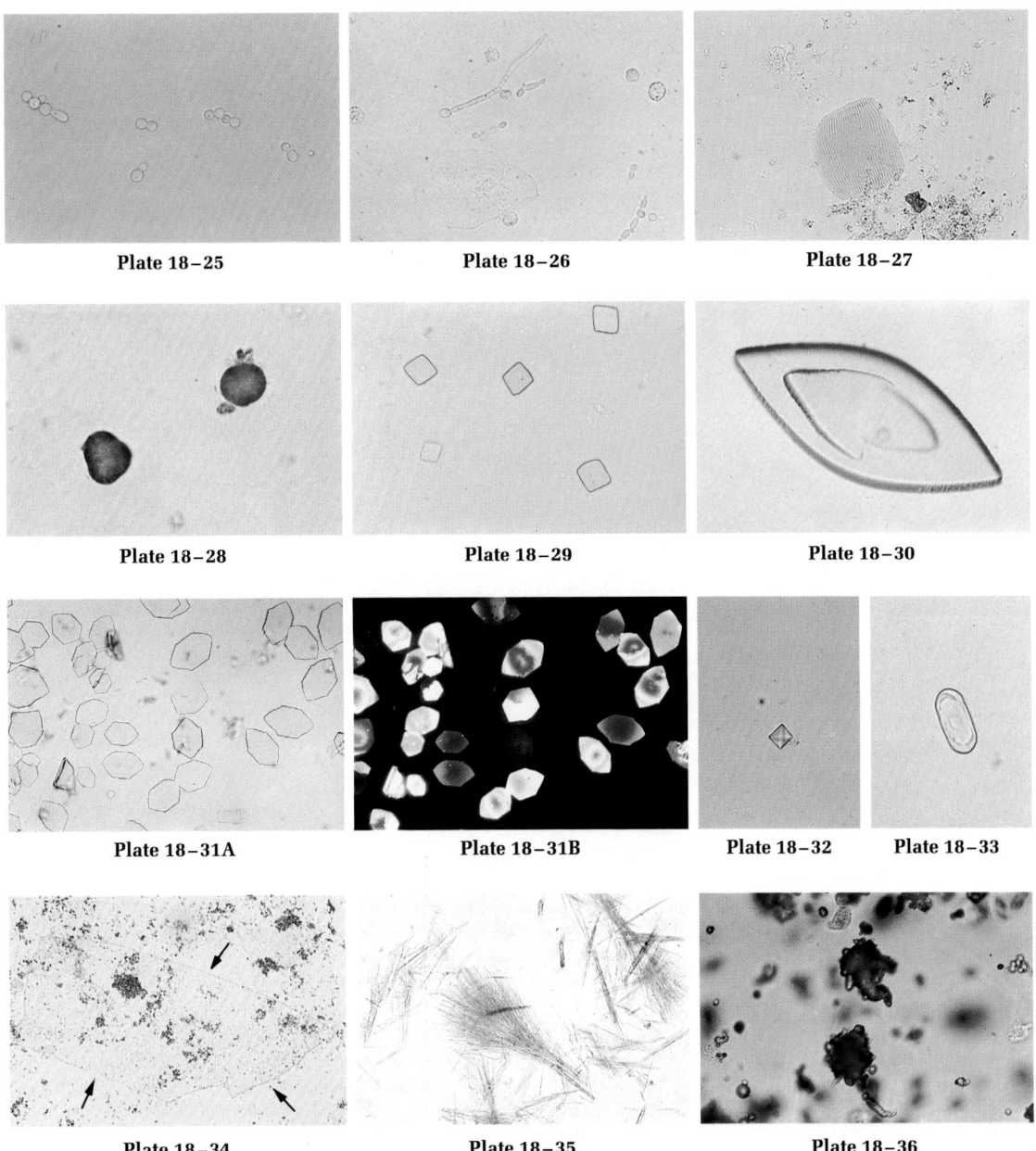

Plate 18–25. Candida. Budding yeasts (× 200). **Plate 18–26.** Candida. Pseudohyphae (× 160). **Plate 18–27.** Muscle fiber (× 200). **Plate 18–28.** Acid urates (× 160). **Plate 18–29.** Uric acid crystals (× 160). **Plate 18–30.** Large uric acid plate. Laminated (× 160). **Plate 18–31.** *A*, Hexagonal uric acid crystals. Brightfield (× 50). *B*, Hexagonal uric acid crystals. Polarized (× 50). **Plate 18–32.** Calcium oxalate crystal (× 200). **Plate 18–33.** Calcium oxalate. Unusual oval form (× 200). **Plate 18–34.** Calcium phosphate (large clear plate). Also amorphous phosphates (× 64). **Plate 18–35.** Calcium phosphate (fine sheaves) (× 160). **Plate 18–36.** Ammonium biurate (× 160).

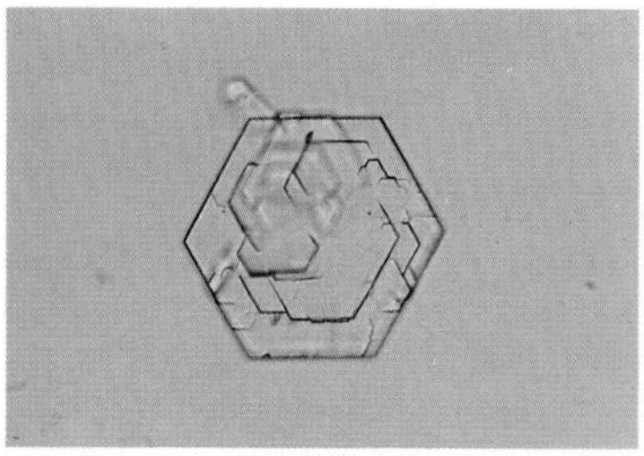

Plate 18–37

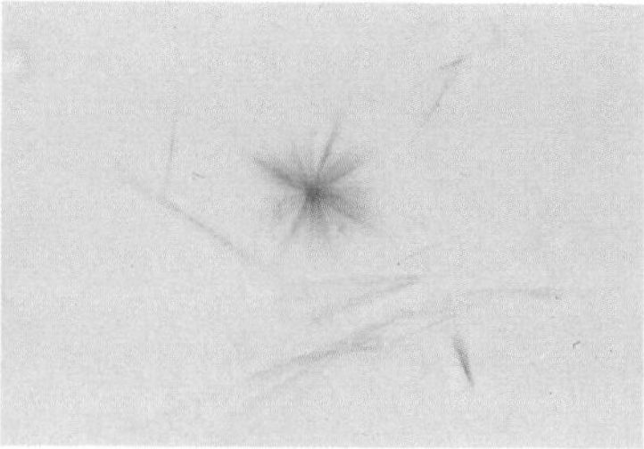

Plate 18–38

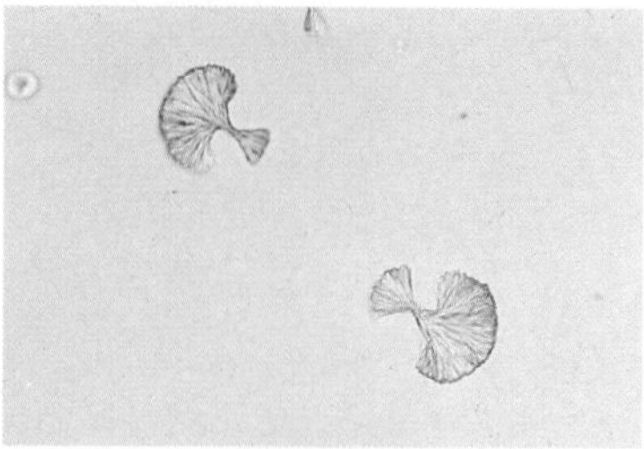

Plate 18–39

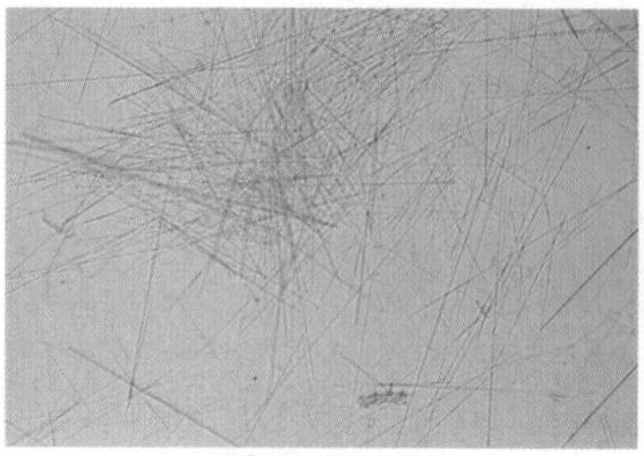

Plate 18–40

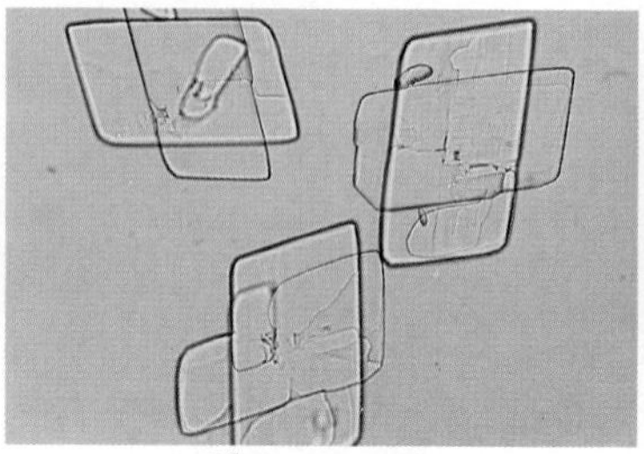

Plate 18–41A

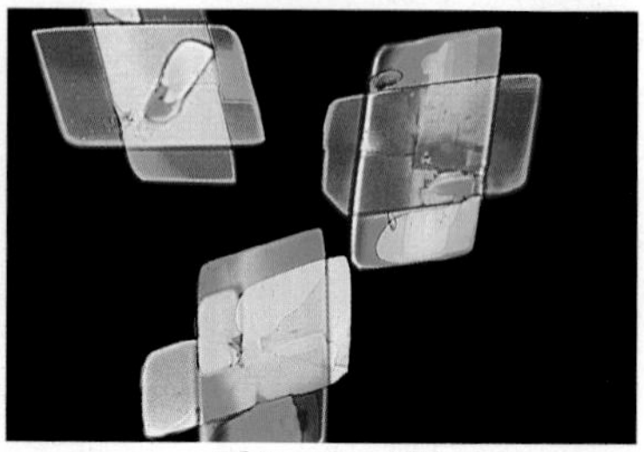

Plate 18–41B

Plate 18–37. Cystine (hexagonal, laminated) (× 200). **Plate 18–38.** Tyrosine crystals (× 160). **Plate 18–39.** Sulfadiazine (× 160). **Plate 18–40.** Ampicillin (× 160). **Plate 18–41.** *A,* Renografin (meglumine diatrizoate). Brightfield (× 160). *B,* Renografin (meglumine diatrizoate). Polarized (× 160).

Chapter 19

Cerebrospinal, Synovial, and Serous Body Fluids

Gregory P. Smith, M.D.
Carl R. Kjeldsberg, M.D.

3

CEREBROSPINAL FLUID

Cerebrospinal fluid (CSF) is produced at a rate of approximately 500 mL/day, about 70% of which is derived by ultrafiltration and secretion through the choroid plexuses. The ependymal lining of the ventricles and cerebral subarachnoid space account for the remainder. It leaves the ventricular system through the medial and lateral foramina, flowing over the brain and spinal cord surfaces within the subarachnoid space (Fig. 19–1). It acts to collect wastes, circulate nutrients, and cushion and lubricate the central nervous system. Resorption of CSF occurs at the arachnoid villi (Fishman, 1992). Total CSF volumes are 90 to 150 mL in adults and 10 to 60 mL in neonates.

The blood-brain barrier is a *concept* derived from dye-exclusion studies. It consists of two morphologically distinct components: a unique capillary endothelium held together by intercellular tight junctions, and the choroid plexus, where a single layer of specialized choroidal ependyma cells connected by tight junctions overlie fenestrated capillaries. Certain substances in the CSF are tightly regulated by specific transport systems (e.g., H^+, K^+, Ca^{2+}, Mg^{2+}, bicarbonate), whereas others like glucose, urea, and creatinine diffuse freely but take several hours to equilibrate. Proteins cross by passive diffusion at a rate dependent on the plasma-to-CSF concentration gradient and inversely proportional to the molecular weight and hydrodynamic volume (Fishman, 1992). Thus, the blood-brain barrier maintains the relative homeostasis of the CNS environment during acute perturbations of plasma components.

Specimen Collection and Opening Pressure

Cerebrospinal fluid may be obtained by lumbar puncture, cisternal puncture, lateral cervical puncture, or through ventricular cannulas or shunts. Details of the performance of lumbar puncture are described elsewhere (Herndon, 1989; Ward, 1992). Respiratory compromise may occur in young infants if the head is flexed (Ward, 1992). A manometer should be attached before any fluid is removed to record the opening pressure.

The normal opening pressure in adults is 90 to 180 mm of water in the lateral position, slightly higher if the patient is sitting up or is markedly obese, and varies up to 10 mm with

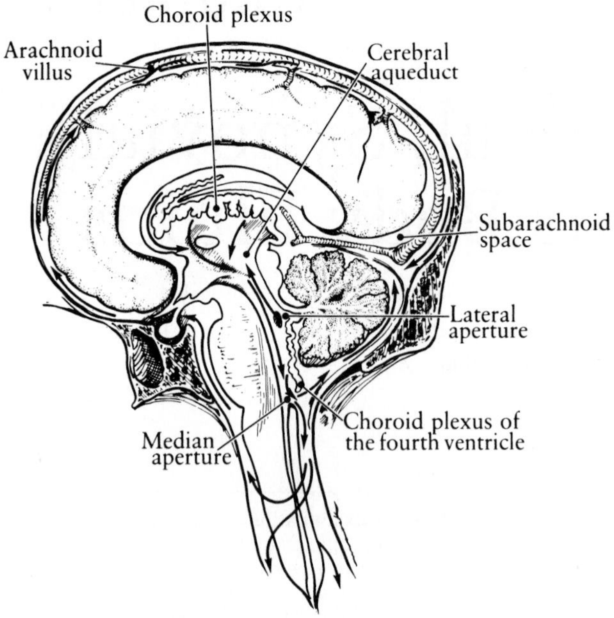

Figure 19–1. Cerebrospinal fluid (CSF) flow. (Reproduced with permission from Kjeldsberg CR, Knight JA: Body Fluids: Laboratory Examination of Amniotic, Cerebrospinal, Seminal, Serous and Synovial Fluids, 3rd ed. © 1993 by the American Society of Clinical Pathologists, Chicago.)

respiration. In infants and young children the normal range is 10 to 100 mm H_2O, attaining the adult range by the age of six to eight years (Fishman, 1992). If the opening pressure is greater than 200 mm in a relaxed patient, no more than 2 mL of fluid should be withdrawn.

Elevated pressures may be seen in patients who are tense or straining and in those with congestive heart failure, meningitis, superior vena cava syndrome, thrombosis of the venous sinuses, cerebral edema, mass lesions, hypo-osmolality, or conditions inhibiting CSF absorption. Elevation of the opening CSF pressure may be the only abnormality found in patients with cryptococcal meningitis and pseudotumor cerebri (Hayward, 1987).

Decreased CSF pressure may be seen in spinal-subarachnoid block, dehydration, circulatory collapse, and CSF leakage (Kjeldsberg, 1993). A dramatic pressure drop after removal of 1 to 2 mL suggests herniation or spinal block above the puncture site; no further fluid should be withdrawn in such cases.

Up to 20 mL of spinal fluid may normally be removed. The clinician should be aware of the quantity of CSF required for the ordered tests to ensure that a sufficient sample is obtained and should provide an appropriate clinical history to the laboratory. The sample site (lumbar, cisternal, etc.) should be noted because cytologic and chemical parameters vary at different sites.

Ordinarily, the specimen is divided into three sterile tubes: tube 1 for chemistry and immunology studies, tube 2 for microbiologic examination, and tube 3 for cell count and differential. An additional tube may be inserted in the No. 3 position for cytology if malignancy is suspected. Avoid glass tubes because cell adhesion to the glass affects the cell count and differential. Specimens need to be received in the laboratory and processed *quickly* to minimize cellular degradation, which begins as soon as one hour after collection. Refrigeration is contraindicated for culture specimens because fastidious organisms like *Haemophilus influenzae* and *Neisseria meningitidis* will not survive.

Indications and Recommended Tests

Indications for lumbar puncture can be divided into four major disease categories: meningeal infection, subarachnoid hemorrhage, CNS malignancy, and demyelinating diseases (American College of Physicians, 1986) (Table 19–1). Identification of infectious meningitis, particularly bacterial, is the most important indication for CSF examination. Recommended laboratory tests are directed toward identification of these disorders (Table 19–2). In other disorders examination of the CSF is less helpful and provides only supportive evidence of a clinical diagnosis or helps to rule out other diseases. Limited routine studies followed by retrospective ordering of the more focused tests (as needed) on the stored specimen has been advocated as a way of improving test efficiency (Albright, 1988).

Gross Examination

Normal CSF is clear and colorless and has a viscosity similar to water. Turbidity or cloudiness begins to appear with leukocyte counts of over 200 cells/μL or red cell (RBC) counts of 400 cells/μL. Microorganisms (bacteria, fungi, amebas), radiographic contrast material, aspirated epidural fat, and elevated protein level may also cause cloudiness. Experienced observers may be able to detect cell counts of less than 50 cells/μL with the unaided eye by observing for Tyndall's effect (Simon, 1978). *Direct sunlight* directed on the tube at a 90-degree angle from the observer will impart a "sparkling" or "snowy" appearance as suspended particles scatter the light.

Clot formation may be seen in patients with traumatic taps, complete spinal block (Froin's syndrome), or suppurative or tuberculous meningitis. It is not seen in patients with subarachnoid hemorrhage. Fine surface pellicles may be observed after refrigeration for 12 to 24 hours. Clots may interfere with cell count accuracy by entrapping inflammatory cells.

Table 19–1. DISEASE DETECTED BY LABORATORY EXAMINATION OF CSF

High sensitivity, high specificity
Bacterial, tuberculous and fungal meningitis
High sensitivity, moderate specificity
Viral meningitis
Subarachnoid hemorrhage
Multiple sclerosis
Central nervous system syphilis
Infectious polyneuritis
Paraspinal abscess
Moderate sensitivity, high specificity
Meningeal malignancy
Moderate sensitivity, moderate specificity
Intracranial hemorrhage
Viral encephalitis
Subdural hematoma

Sensitivity = the ability of a test to detect disease when it is present; specificity = the ability of a test to exclude disease when it is not present.

From American College of Physicians, Health and Public Policy Committee: The diagnostic spinal tap. Ann Intern Med 1986; 104:880–885.

Table 19–2. RECOMMENDED LABORATORY TESTS ON CSF

Routine
Opening CSF pressure
Total cell count
Differential cell count (stained smear)
Glucose (CSF/plasma ratio)
Protein
Useful in certain circumstances
Cultures (bacteria, fungi, viruses, *Mycobacterium tuberculosis*)
Gram's stain, acid-fast stains
Fungal and bacterial antigens
Cytology
Protein electrophoresis
VDRL test for syphilis
Fibrin-derivitive D-dimer

Modified from Kjeldsberg CR, Knight JA: Body Fluids: Laboratory Examination of Amniotic, Cerebrospinal, Seminal, Serous and Synovial Fluids, 3rd ed. © American Society of Clinical Pathologists, Chicago, 1993.

Viscous CSF may be encountered in patients with metastatic mucin-producing adenocarcinomas, cryptococcal meningitis due to capsular polysaccharide, or liquid nucleus pulposus resulting from needle injury to the annulus fibrosus.

Pink-red CSF usually indicates the presence of blood. The CSF becomes grossly bloody when the red cell count exceeds 6000/μL; blood may originate from subarachnoid hemorrhage, intracerebral hemorrhage, infarct, or traumatic tap.

XANTHOCHROMIA. The CSF is centrifuged, and the supernatant fluid is compared with a tube of distilled water. Xanthochromic CSF is pink, orange, or yellow owing to RBC lysis and hemoglobin breakdown. Pale pink to orange xanthochromia from released oxyhemoglobin is usually detected by lumbar puncture performed 2 to 4 hours after the onset of subarachnoid hemorrhage, but it may take as long as 12 hours. Peak intensity occurs at about 24 to 36 hours, gradually disappearing in about four to eight days. Yellow xanthochromia is derived from bilirubin. It develops 12 hours after a subarachnoid bleed, peaks at two to four days, and may persist for two to four weeks.

Visible CSF xanthochromia may also be due to: (1) oxyhemoglobin resulting from artifactual red cell lysis caused by detergent contamination of the needle or tube or a delay of more than one hour without refrigeration before examination; (2) bilirubin (bilirhachia) in jaundiced patients; (3) CSF protein levels of over 150 mg/dL, which are seen in very bloody traumatic taps (over 100,000 RBCs/μL) or in pathologic states such as complete spinal block, polyneuritis, and meningitis; (4) Merthiolate disinfectant contamination; (5) carotinoids (orange), found in people with dietary hypercarotenemia; (6) melanin (brownish), from meningeal metastatic melanoma; and (7) rifampin therapy (red-orange).

Spectral absorbance scans provide an objective record of xanthochromia, but careful gross inspection of the CSF has comparable sensitivity (Britton, 1983). Spectrophotometry can help to differentiate hemoglobin-derived pigments from other xanthochromic pigments with different maximal absorption peaks.

DIFFERENTIAL OF BLOODY CSF. Distinction of a traumatic tap from pathologic hemorrhage is of vital importance. Although the presence of crenated RBCs is not useful, certain observations help to distinguish the two forms of bleeding.

1. When bloody fluid is obtained it usually clears between the first and third tubes collected in a traumatic tap but remains relatively uniform in subarachnoid hemorrhage.
2. Xanthochromia, microscopic evidence of erythrophagocytosis, or hemosiderin-laden macrophages indicate a subarachnoid bleed in the absence of a prior traumatic tap. RBC lysis begins as early as one to two hours after a traumatic tap, however, so rapid evaluation is necessary to avoid false-positive results.
3. A commercially available latex agglutination immunoassay for cross-linked fibrin derivative D-dimer is specific for fibrin degradation and is negative in traumatic taps (Lang, 1990). False-positive results might be expected in conditions such as disseminated intravascular coagulation, fibrinolysis, and trauma from repeated lumbar punctures.

Microscopic Examination

TOTAL CELL COUNT. Cell counts are performed on undiluted CSF in a manual counting chamber. Automated counting of leukocytes and erythrocytes has been described (Talstad, 1984), but precision is poor in the low counts normally encountered in the CSF. The inherent precision of manual counts is also limited. For example, using 18 large squares (1 mm^2 each) in a Fuchs-Rosenthal type chamber with a depth of 0.2 mm, a total volume of 3.6 μL (18 × 0.2 μL per square) is examined. With 5 cells/μL a total of 18 cells is counted. The coefficient of variation (CV), defined as 100 divided by the square root of the number of cells counted, is $100/\sqrt{18}$, or 24%. Therefore, ±2 CV is about ±48%. A Neubauer hemacytometer with nine 1 mm^2 squares with a depth of 0.1 mm has a CV of 45% (±90% for 2 CV) with the same cell concentration.

The normal leukocyte cell count in adults is 0 to 5 cells/μL. It is higher in neonates, ranging from 0 to 30 cells/μL, with the upper limit of normal decreasing to adult values by adolescence.

Red cell counts of CSF have limited diagnostic value but may allow a useful *approximation* of the true CSF leukocyte (WBC) count or total protein in the presence of traumatic puncture by correcting for leukocytes or protein introduced by the bleed. To be valid, all measurements (RBC, WBC, protein) must be performed on the same tube. This procedure also assumes that the blood is derived *exclusively* from the traumatic tap. The corrected WBC count is:

$$WBC_{corr} = WBC_{obs} - WBC_{added}$$

where:

$$WBC_{added} = \frac{WBC_{BLD} \times RBC_{CSF}}{RBC_{BLD}}$$

and

WBC_{obs} = leukocyte count in CSF
WBC_{added} = leukocytes added to CSF by traumatic tap
WBC_{BLD} = leukocyte count in peripheral blood
RBC_{CSF} = erythrocyte count in CSF
RBC_{BLD} = erythrocyte count in peripheral blood.

An analogous formula may be used to correct for "added protein":

$$TP_{added} = [TP_{serum} \times (1 - HCT)] \times RBC_{CSF}/RBC_{BLD}$$

In the presence of a normal peripheral blood RBC count and serum protein, these corrections amount to 1 WBC added for every 700 RBCs, and about 8 mg/dL protein for every 10,000 RBC/μL. The accuracy of these corrections is limited by the precision of the CSF RBC count, which can significantly limit its value (Novak, 1984; Mayefsky, 1987).

An observed-to-expected (added) WBC count ratio greater than 10 has a sensitivity of 88% and a specificity of 90% for bacterial meningitis (Mayefsky, 1987). When the predicted WBC is below the observed count the probability of bacterial meningitis appears to be low (Mayefsky, 1987; Bonadio, 1990).

DIFFERENTIAL COUNT. Suggested reference ranges are given in Table 19–3. A differential performed in a counting chamber is unsatisfactory because the low cell numbers have poor precision, and identifying the cell type beyond granulocytes and "mononuclears" is difficult in a wet preparation. Direct smears of the centrifuged CSF sediment are subject to much error from cellular distortion and fragmentation. Different methods have been developed to improve precision and accuracy. Variable cell loss precludes their use for cell counts, however.

The *cytocentrifuge* is rapid, requires minimal training, and allows Wright's staining of air-dried cytospins. It is the recommended method for all body fluids (Rabinovitch, 1994). Cell yield and preservation are better than with simple centrifugation. From 30 to 50 cells can be concentrated from 0.5 mL of "normal" CSF. Variable artifactual distortion may be seen, but this is minimized when the specimen is fresh, albumin is added to the specimen (2 drops of 22% bovine serum albumin), and the cell concentration is adjusted to about 300 WBC/L prior to centrifugation (Kjeldsberg, 1993).

Filtration methods provide excellent cell recovery and slightly better preservation than the cytocentrifuge but are more costly and time-consuming and require considerably more skill to prepare a satisfactory specimen. Romanowsky's stains cannot be used with this method. Advantages are the ability to concentrate large volumes of CSF for cytologic examination or culture while retaining the fluid filtrate for additional studies.

Sedimentation methods provide high-quality smears, but the yield is not as high as filtration methods, and these methods are more cumbersome than cytocentrifugation.

The CSF normally contains a small number of lymphocytes and monocytes in a ratio of approximately 70:30 in adults. A higher proportion of monocytes is present in young children, in whom up to 80% may be normal (Pappu, 1982). Erythrocytes due to minor traumatic bleeding are commonly seen, especially in infants. Small numbers of neutrophils (PMNs) may be seen in "normal" CSF specimens, most likely as a result of minor hemorrhage (Hayward, 1988) and improved cell concentration methods. No general consensus regarding an upper limit of normal for PMNs has been established. We accept up to 7% neutrophils with a normal WBC count. Sixty percent neutrophils has been reported in high-risk neonates without meningitis (Sarff, 1976). The number of PMNs may be decreased by as much as 68% within the first two hours after lumbar puncture owing to cell lysis (Steele, 1986).

Ependymal cells and choroid plexus cells may be seen rarely (Plate 19–1). Traumatic puncture may result in bone marrow cells, cartilage cells, squamous cells, ganglion cells, and soft tissue elements in the CSF. Blastlike primitive cell clusters, most likely of germinal matrix origin, are sometimes found in premature infants with intraventricular hemorrhage (Plate 19–2).

Increased *neutrophils* may occur in conditions summarized in Table 19–4. In early bacterial meningitis the proportion of PMNs usually exceeds 60%, but in about one-quarter of cases of early viral meningitis the proportion of PMNs also exceeds 60%. Viral-induced neutrophilia usually changes to a lymphocytic pleocytosis within two to three days. A total PMN count of over 1180 cells/μL (or more than 2000 WBC/μL) has a 99% predictive value for bacterial meningitis (Spanos, 1989). Persistent neutrophilic meningitis (over one week) may be noninfectious or may be due to less common pathogens like *Nocardia*, *Actinomyces*, *Aspergillus*, and the zygomycetes (Peacock, 1984).

Increased *lymphocytes* have been reported in conditions summarized in Table 19–5. Lymphocytosis (>50%) is not uncommon in acute bacterial meningitis when the CSF WBC count is under 1000/μL (Powers, 1985). Atypical, reactive, lymphoplasmacytoid and immunoblastic variants may be present (Plate 19–3). Blastlike lymphocytes may be seen admixed with small and large lymphocytes in the CSF of neonates.

Plasma cells are not normally present in the CSF but appear in a variety of inflammatory conditions (Table 19–6) along with large and small lymphocytes and in association with malignant brain tumors (Fishman, 1992). Multiple myeloma may rarely involve the meninges (Oda, 1991).

Table 19–3. REFERENCE INTERVALS FOR CSF DIFFERENTIAL COUNTS BY CYTOCENTRIFUGE

Cell Type	Adults (%)	Neonates (%)
Lymphocytes	62 ± 34	20 ± 18
Monocytes	36 ± 20	72 ± 22
Neutrophils	2 ± 5	3 ± 5
Histocytes	Rare	5 ± 4
Ependymal cells	Rare	Rare
Eosinophils	Rare	Rare

Table 19–4. CAUSES FOR INCREASED NEUTROPHILS IN CSF

- Meningitis
  - Bacterial meningitis
  - Early viral meningoencephalitis
  - Early tuberculous meningitis
  - Early mycotic meningitis
  - Amebic encephalomyelitis
- Other infections
  - Cerebral abscess
  - Subdural empyema
- Following seizures
- Following CNS hemorrhage
  - Subarachnoid hemorrhage
  - Intracerebral hemorrhage
- Following CNS infarct
- Reaction to repeated lumbar puncture
- Injection of foreign materials into subarachnoid space (e.g., methotrexate, contrast media)
- Metastatic tumor in contact with CSF

Table 19–5. CAUSES FOR INCREASED LYMPHOCYTES IN CSF

Meningitis
Viral meningitis
Tuberculous meningitis
Fungal meningitis
Syphilitic meningoencephalitis
Leptospiral meningitis
Bacterial meningitis due to unusual organisms—e.g., *Listeria monocytogenes*
Parasitic infestations of the CNS—e.g., cysticercosis, trichinosis, toxoplasmosis
Aseptic meningitis due to septic focus adjacent to meninges
Degenerative disorders
Subacute sclerosing panencephalitis
Multiple sclerosis
Encephalopathy due to drug abuse
Guillain-Barré syndrome
Acute disseminated encephalomyelitis
Other inflammatory conditions
Sarcoidosis of meninges
Polyneuritis
Periarteritis involving the CNS

Table 19–7. CAUSES OF CSF EOSINOPHILIC PLEOCYTOSIS

Commonly associated with
Parasitic infections
Fungal infections
Reaction to foreign material in CNS (drugs, shunts)
Acute polyneuritis
Idiopathic hypereosinophilic syndrome
Idiopathic eosinophilic meningitis
Infrequently associated with
Bacterial meningitis
Tuberculous meningoencephalitis
Viral meningitis
Rickettsial infection (Rocky Mountain spotted fever)
Leukemia, lymphoma
Myeloproliferative disorders
Primary brain tumors
Neurosarcoidosis

Modified with permission from Kjeldsberg CR, Knight JA: Body Fluids: Laboratory Examination of Amniotic, Cerebrospinal, Seminal, Serous and Synovial Fluids, 3rd ed. © American Society of Clinical Pathologists, Chicago, 1993.

3

Eosinophils may rarely be seen in normal CSF; increased eosinophil counts are associated with a variety of infectious and noninfectious conditions (Table 19–7). The eosinophilia is frequently mild (1% to 4%) and is part of a general inflammatory response. A suggested criterion for eosinophilic meningitis is 10% eosinophils (Kuberski, 1981). Parasitic invasion of the CNS is the most common cause worldwide. *Coccidioides immitis* fungal infections are a significant cause of CSF eosinophilia in endemic regions of the United States (Ragland, 1993).

Increased *monocytes* lack diagnostic specificity and are usually part of a "mixed cell reaction" that includes neutrophils, lymphocytes, and plasma cells. Tuberculous and fungal meningitis, chronic bacterial meningitis, leptospiral meningitis, ruptured brain abscess, *Toxoplasma* meningitis, and amebic encephalomeningitis show this pattern. A mixed cell pattern without neutrophils is characteristic of viral and syphilitic meningoencephalitis.

Macrophages with phagocytosed erythrocytes *(erythrophages)* appear from 12 to 48 hours following subarachnoid hemorrhage or traumatic tap. Hemosiderin-laden macrophages *(siderophages)* begin to appear after 48 hours and may persist for weeks (Plate 19–4). Brownish yellow or red hematoidin crystals may form after a few days.

Cerebrospinal fluid examination for tumor cells has moderate sensitivity and high specificity (97% to 98%) (Marton and Gean, 1986). Sensitivity depends on the type of tumor; CSF examination of leukemic patients has the highest sensitivity (about 70%), followed by examination of patients with metastatic carcinoma (20% to 60%) and primary CNS malignancies (30%). Sensitivity may be optimized by using filtration methods with larger fluid volumes or by performing serial punctures in patients in whom tumor is strongly suspected.

Table 19–6. CAUSES FOR PLASMACYTOSIS IN CSF

Tuberculous meningitis
Syphilitic meningoencephalitis
Multiple sclerosis
Parasitic infestations of CNS
Subacute sclerosing panencephalitis
Guillain-Barré syndrome
Sarcoidosis
Acute viral infections

Leukemic involvement of the meninges is more frequent in patients with acute lymphoblastic leukemia (ALL) than in those with acute myeloblastic leukemia (AML), both of which are far more common than CNS involvement in the chronic leukemias. A WBC count of over 5 cells/μL with unequivocal lymphoblasts on cytocentrifuged preparations is commonly accepted as evidence of CSF involvement. The incidence of CNS relapse in children with lymphoblasts but cell counts of less than 6 cells/μL appears to be low and is not significantly different from cases in which no blasts are identified (Odom, 1990; Tubergen, 1994).

Non-Hodgkin's lymphomas involving the leptomeninges are usually high-grade tumors (lymphoblastic, large cell immunoblastic, small noncleaved); low-grade lymphomas and Hodgkin's disease are far less common (Bigner, 1992; Walts, 1992). T lymphocytes predominate in normal and inflammatory conditions, whereas most lymphomas, especially those occurring in immunocompromised hosts, are of B-lymphocyte lineage. The most common T-lymphocytic lymphoma is lymphoblastic lymphoma, which can be detected by terminal deoxynucleotidyl transferase (TdT) stain.

The polymerase chain reaction (PCR) is a promising technique ideally suited for low cell samples like CSF because of its ability to amplify very small quantities of specific DNA. It may be useful in detecting monoclonal gene rearrangements or in identifying tumor-specific chromosome translocations (Shibata, 1990), but the utility of this highly sensitive test for predicting clinical CNS involvement needs further evaluation.

Amebas, fungi (especially *Cryptococcus neoformans*), and *Toxoplasma gondii* organisms may be present on cytocentrifuge specimens but can be difficult to recognize without confirmatory stains.

Chemical Analysis

Reference values for lumbar cerebrospinal fluid in adults are listed in Table 19–8.

TOTAL PROTEIN. Over 80 of CSF protein content is derived from the plasma, in concentrations of less than 1% of the blood level (Table 19–9). Although some authors have argued against routine measurement of total protein (American College of Physicians, 1986), an increase in protein serves as a useful but nonspecific indicator of disease.

Turbidimetric methods, commonly based on trichloroacetic acid (TCA) or sulfosalicylic acid (SSA) and sodium sulfate for protein precipitation, are popular because they are simple, rapid, and require no special instrumentation. They are, however, temperature sensitive and require much larger specimen volumes (about 0.5 mL), and some methods are prone to significant variation from changes in the albumin/globulin ratio (Schriever, 1965). A false elevation of protein may be observed using TCA methods in the presence of methotrexate (Kasper, 1988). Benzethonium chloride or benzalkonium chloride have been used as precipitating agents in automated or micromethods (Luxton, 1989; Shephard, 1992).

Colorimetric methods include the Lowry method, dye-binding methods using Coomassie brilliant blue (CBB) or Ponceau S, and the modified biuret method. The CBB method is moderately popular because it is rapid and highly sensitive and can be used with small sample sizes. Immunologic methods measure specific proteins, require only 25 to 50 μL of CSF, and are relatively simple to perform once conditions and reagents have been standardized. Automated methods are increasing in use and often show good correlation with standard methods (Lott, 1989).

Reference ranges for CSF total protein vary considerably between laboratories owing to differences of methodology, instrumentation, and type of reference standard used (College of American Pathologists CSF chemistry survey, Set M-B, 1991; Gerbaut, 1986). Protein concentration normally increases caudally from the ventricles (15 mg/dL) to the cisterns (25 mg/dL) and the lumbar sac. Mean lumbar values in adults range from 23 to 38 mg/dL with a generally accepted range of 15 to 45 mg/dL (Silverman, 1994). Each laboratory must establish its own reference intervals. The upper limit of normal for neonates is 150 mg/dL (1.5 g/L) and may be as high as 500 mg/dL (4.0 g/L) in premature infants.

Elevated CSF protein levels may be caused by increased permeability of the blood-brain barrier, decreased resorption at the arachnoid villi, mechanical obstruction of CSF flow due to spinal block above the site of puncture, or an increase in intrathecal immunoglobulin synthesis. Common conditions associated with elevated lumbar CSF protein values (over 65 mg/dL) are summarized in Table 19–10.

Low lumbar CSF total protein levels (<20 mg/dL) occur normally in some young children between six months and two years of age and in patients with conditions associated with increased CSF turnover. These include (1) removal of large volumes of CSF; (2) CSF leaks induced by trauma or lumbar puncture; (3) increased intracranial pressure, probably due to an increased rate of protein resorption by the arachnoid villi; and (4) hyperthyroidism, for unknown reasons (Fishman, 1992).

Protein electrophoresis of concentrated normal CSF reveals two distinct differences from serum: a prominent transthyretin band, and two transferrin bands. Transthyretin is relatively high because of its dual synthesis by the liver and choroid plexus. The second transferrin band, referred to as β_2-transferrin or tau-protein, migrates more slowly than its serum equivalent owing to cerebral neuraminidase digestion of sialic acid residues.

DIAGNOSIS OF CSF LEAKAGE. Cerebrospinal fluid leakage usually presents as otorrhea or rhinorrhea following trauma, in some cases beginning months to years after the in-

Table 19–8. REFERENCE VALUES FOR LUMBAR CEREBROSPINAL FLUID IN ADULTS

	Conventional Units	SI Units
Protein	15–45 mg/dL	0.15–0.45 g/L
Prealbumin	2–7%	
Albumin	56–76%	
α_1-Globulin	2–7%	
α_2-Globulin	4–12%	
β-Globulin	8–18%	
γ-Globulin	3–12%	
Electrolytes		
Osmolality	280–300 mOsm/L	280–300 mmol/L
Sodium	135–150 mEq/L	135–150 mmol/L
Potassium	2.6–3.0 mEq/L	2.6–3.0 mmol/L
Chloride	115–130 mEq/L	115–130 mmol/L
Carbon dioxide content	20–25 mEq/L	20–25 mmol/L
Calcium	2.0–2.8 mEq/L	1.00–1.40 mmol/L
Magnesium	2.4–3.0 mEq/L	1.2–1.5 mmol/L
Lactate	10–22 mg/dL	1.1–2.4 mmol/L
pH		
Lumbar fluid	7.28–7.32	
Cisternal fluid	7.32–7.34	
P_{CO_2}		
Lumbar fluid	44–50 mm Hg	
Cisternal fluid	40–46 mm Hg	
P_{O_2}	40–44 mm Hg	
Other constituents		
Ammonia	10–35 μg/dL	6–20 μmol/L
Glutamine	5–20 mg/dL	0.3–1.4 mmol/L
Creatinine	0.6–1.2 mg/dL	45–92 μmol/L
Glucose	50–80 mg/dL	2.8–4.4 mmol/L
Iron	1–2 μg/dL	0.2–0.4 μmol/L
Phosphorus	1.2–2.0 mg/dL	0.4–0.7 mmol/L
Total lipid	1–2 mg/dL	0.01–0.02 g/L
Urea	6–16 mg/dL	2.0–5.7 mmol/L
Urate	0.5–3.0 mg/dL	30–180 μmol/L
Zinc	2–6 μg/dL	0.3–0.9 μmol/L

Table 19–9. CONCENTRATIONS OF PROTEINS IN PLASMA AND CEREBROSPINAL FLUID

Protein	CSF Concentration (mg/L)	Plasma/CSF Ratio
Prealbumin	17.3	14
Albumin	155.0	236
Transferrin	14.4	142
Ceruloplasmin	1.0	366
IgG	12.3	802
IgA	1.3	1346
α_2-Macroglobulin	2.0	1111
Fibrinogen	0.6	4940
IgM	0.6	1167
β-Lipoprotein	0.6	6213

Adapted from Felgenhauer K: Klin Wochenschr 1974; 52:1158.

Table 19–10. CONDITIONS ASSOCIATED WITH INCREASED CSF TOTAL PROTEIN

- Traumatic spinal tap
- *Increased blood-CSF permeability*
  - Arachnoiditis (e.g., following methotrexate therapy)
  - Meningitis (bacterial, fungal, viral, tuberculous, etc.)
  - Hemorrhage (subarachnoid, intracerebral)
  - Endocrine/metabolic disorders
    - Milk alkali syndrome with hypercalcemia
    - Diabetic neuropathy
    - Hereditary neuropathies and myelopathies
    - Decreased endocrine function (thyroid, parathyroid)
    - Other disorders (uremia, dehydration)
  - Drug toxicity
    - Ethanol, phenothiazines, phenytoin
- *CSF circulation defects*
  - Mechanical obstruction (tumor, abscess, herniated disk)
  - Loculated CSF effusion
- *Increased IgG synthesis*
  - Neurosyphilis, multiple sclerosis
  - Subacute sclerosing panencephalitis (SSPE)
- *Increased IgG synthesis and blood-CSF permeability*
  - Guillain-Barré syndrome
  - Collagen vascular diseases (e.g., lupus, periarteritis)
  - Chronic inflammatory demyelinating polyradiculopathy

jury. Recurrent meningitis is a serious complication making accurate identification of the leaking fluid important. In this regard glucose measurements are too nonspecific to be of value. Protein electrophoresis with immunofixation for transferrin is recommended. It is a noninvasive, rapid, and inexpensive test of high sensitivity and specificity that requires as little as 0.1 mL of fluid (Ryall, 1992). Cerebrospinal fluid shows two isoform bands, whereas other body fluids and secretions lack the second isoform. A polypeptide allelic variant of transferrin that migrates like β_2-transferrin may produce false-positive results (Sloman, 1993).

MEASUREMENT OF ALBUMIN AND IgG. The permeability of the blood-brain barrier may be assessed by accurate immunochemical quantification of the CSF albumin-to-serum albumin ratio in grams per deciliter (g/dL). The normal ratio of 1:230 (Tourtellotte, 1985) yields an unwieldy decimal of 0.004, which has prompted use of a CSF/serum *albumin index*, which uses CSF albumin values in milligrams per deciliter:

$$\text{CSF/serum albumin index} = \frac{\text{albumin}_{\text{CSF}}\ \text{mg/dL}}{\text{albumin}_{\text{serum}}\ \text{g/dL}}$$

An index of less than 9 (or a ratio of under 0.009) is consistent with an intact barrier. Slight impairment is considered with index values of 9 to 14, moderate impairment with values of 14 to 30, and severe impairment at values of 30 to 100 (Silverman, 1994). The index is slightly elevated in infants up to 6 months of age, reflecting the immaturity of the blood-brain barrier, and increases gradually after the age of 40. A traumatic tap invalidates calculation of the index.

Increased intrathecal IgG synthesis is reflected by an increase in the CSF/serum IgG ratio:

$$\text{CSF/serum IgG ratio} = \frac{\text{IgG}_{\text{CSF}}\ \text{g/dL}}{\text{IgG}_{\text{serum}}\ \text{g/dL}}$$

The normal ratio is 1:390, or 0.003 (Tourtellotte, 1985). Like the albumin index, a CSF/serum IgG *index* may be obtained by using milligrams per deciliter for the value for IgG_{CSF}. The normal range of the CSF/serum IgG index is 3 to 8.

The CSF/serum IgG index can be elevated by intrathecal IgG synthesis or increased plasma IgG cross-over from breakdown of the blood-brain barrier. Immunoglobulin derived from plasma cross-over may be corrected by dividing the CSF/serum IgG index by the CSF/albumin index to yield the CSF *IgG index*:

$$\text{IgG index} = \frac{\text{IgG}_{\text{CSF}}\ \text{mg/dL}}{\text{IgG}_{\text{serum}}\ \text{g/dL}} \bigg/ \frac{\text{albumin}_{\text{CSF}}\ \text{mg/dL}}{\text{albumin}_{\text{serum}}\ \text{g/dL}} \quad \text{or}$$

$$\text{IgG index} = \frac{\text{IgG}_{\text{CSF}}\ \text{mg/dL} \times \text{albumin}_{\text{serum}}\ \text{g/dL}}{\text{IgG}_{\text{serum}}\ \text{g/dL} \times \text{albumin}_{\text{CSF}}\ \text{mg/dL}}$$

The normal reference range for the IgG index varies, reflecting variations in determination of the four index components. A reasonable upper limit of normal is 0.8 (Souverijn, 1989). Each laboratory should determine its own critical ratio.

The *IgG synthesis rate* is calculated by an empirical formula (Tourtellotte, 1985):

IgG synthesis (mg/day) =

$$\left[\left(\text{IgG}_{\text{CSF}} - \frac{\text{IgG}_{\text{serum}}}{369}\right) - \left(\text{alb}_{\text{CSF}} - \frac{\text{alb}_{\text{serum}}}{230}\right) \times \left(\frac{\text{IgG}_{\text{serum}}}{\text{alb}_{\text{serum}}}\right) \times 0.43\right] \times 5\ \text{dL/day}$$

All protein concentrations are expressed in milligrams per deciliter. The first bracketed term represents the difference between the measured CSF IgG and the IgG *expected* from diffusion across a normal blood-brain barrier, and 369 is the normal serum/CSF ratio. The second bracketed term represents the difference between measured CSF albumin and expected albumin if the blood-brain barrier is intact and 230 is the normal serum/CSF albumin ratio. This CSF albumin excess is multiplied by the IgG/albumin ratio and the molecular weight ratio of IgG to albumin (0.43) to correct for changes in CSF IgG due to increased barrier permeability. The number 5 converts the result from a concentration to a daily amount, assuming an average daily CSF production of 500 mL (5 dL). The formula does not consider variations in CSF production or immunoglobulin consumption. It assumes that the IgG/albumin ratio remains constant over various degrees of blood-brain barrier impairment, a concept that may lead to variable error (Lefvert and Link, 1985). The normal reference interval for the synthesis rate is − 9.9 to + 3.3 mg/day (Silverman, 1994).

The CSF IgG index and IgG synthesis rate have a sensitivity of 90% in patients with definite multiple sclerosis (MS), but sensitivity is lower in patients with possible MS in whom test accuracy is most needed (Marton, 1986). Specificity for MS is only moderate because increased intrathecal IgG synthesis occurs in many other inflammatory neurologic diseases.

The immunoglobulin index and synthesis rate calculations may be applied to IgM, IgA, immunoglobulin light chains, and specific antibodies to infectious microorganisms. For example, increased synthesis of IgM and free kappa light chains have been suggested as markers for MS (Rudick, 1989; Lolli, 1991).

ELECTROPHORESIS. Agarose gel electrophoresis of concentrated CSF is widely used in laboratories to look for *oligoclonal bands*, defined as two or more discrete bands in the gamma region that are absent or of lesser intensity in the concurrently run patient's serum. CBB or paragon violet stains can resolve oligoclonal bands in only 5μg of IgG (Silverman, 1994). *Silver staining* is 20 to 50 times more sensitive than CBB and can be used on unconcentrated CSF but is a more complex procedure. *Immunofixation electrophoresis* (IFE) is popular because of its better resolution and ability to identify specific immunoglobulin bands.

CSF oligoclonal bands have been identified in 83% to 94% of patients with definite MS, 40% to 60% of those with probable disease, and 20% to 30% of possible MS cases. They are also seen in nearly all patients with subacute sclerosing panencephalitis and in 25% to 50% of patients with various viral CNS infections, neurosyphilis, neuroborreliosis, cryptococcal meningitis, Guillain-Barré syndrome, transverse myelitis, meningeal carcinomatosis, gliobastoma multiforme, Burkitt's lymphoma, chronic relapsing polyneuropathy, Behçet's disease, cysticercosis, and trypanosomiasis, among others (Trotter, 1989; Chalmers, 1990; Fishman, 1992; Hall, 1992). *In summary, elevated IgG indices and the presence of oligoclonal bands are complementary findings useful in the diagnosis of multiple sclerosis, but the positive predictive value of these tests is largely dependent on the degree of clinical suspicion (prevalence).*

OTHER CSF PROTEINS. Approximately 300 different proteins have been identified in CSF using two-dimensional electrophoresis and silver staining.

***β_2-Microglobulin* (B_2M).** This protein is part of the HLA-Class I molecule on the surface of all nucleated cells. CSF levels above 1.8 mg/L are associated with leptomeningeal leukemia and lymphoma but are not highly specific (Weller, 1992) in that they have a maximal predictive value positive of 78% in cases with a positive cytology (Jeffrey, 1990). Viral infections (including HIV-1), various inflammatory conditions, and other malignancies also produce elevated levels. Measurement of B_2M remains primarily investigational.

C-Reactive Protein (CRP). Increased levels of this acute-phase reactant have been advocated as a way of differentiating bacterial from viral meningitis (Abramson, 1985) but other studies have failed to show good sensitivity (Benjamin, 1984). CSF measurements are seldom used for clinical diagnosis.

Fibronectin. High CSF levels of this large glycoprotein involved in cellular adhesion have been observed in patients with lymphoblastic leukemia, Burkitt's lymphoma (Rajantie, 1989), some metastatic solid tumors, astrocytomas, and bacterial meningitis (Weller, 1990; Torre, 1991). Relatively low levels have been observed in viral meningitis (Torre, 1991). The value of fibronectin measurement in diagnosis requires further investigation.

GLUCOSE. Derived from blood glucose, fasting CSF glucose levels are normally 50 to 80 mg/dL (2.8 to 4.4 mmol/L), 60% of plasma values. Results should be compared with plasma levels, ideally following a 4-hour fast, for adequate clinical interpretation. The normal CSF/plasma glucose ratio may vary from 0.3 to 0.9 with fluctuations of blood levels because of the lag in CSF glucose equilibration time.

CSF values below 40 mg/dL (2.2 mmol/L) or ratios below 0.3 are considered abnormal. Hypoglycorrhachia is a characteristic finding of bacterial, tuberculous, and fungal meningitis. However, sensitivity can be as low as 55% for bacterial meningitis (Hayward, 1987), so a normal level does not exclude these conditions. Some cases of viral meningoencephalitis also have low glucose levels but generally not to the degree seen in bacterial meningitis. Meningeal involvement by malignant tumor, sarcoidosis, cysticercosis, trichinosis, and ameba (*Naegleria*), acute syphilitic meningitis, intrathecal administration of radioiodinated serum albumin, subarachnoid hemorrhage, symptomatic hypoglycemia, and rheumatoid meningitis may also produce low CSF glucose levels (Fishman, 1992).

Decreased CSF glucose results from increased use via anaerobic glycolysis by brain tissue and leukocytes and impaired transport into the CSF. Bacteria are usually present in insufficient concentrations to be a major contributor.

Increased CSF glucose is of no clinical significance, reflecting increased blood glucose levels within 2 hours of lumbar puncture. Traumatic tap may also cause a spurious increase.

LACTATE. CSF and blood lactate levels are largely independent of each other. Reference intervals for older children and adults are 9.0 to 26.0 mg/dL (1.0 to 2.9 mmol/L) (Knight, 1981). Newborns have higher levels, ranging from about 10 to 60 mg/dL (1.1 to 6.7 mmol/L) for the first 2 days to 10 to 40 mg/dL (1.1 to 4.4 mmol/L) for days 3 to 10 (McGuinness, 1983). Elevated CSF lactate levels reflect anaerobic metabolism within the CNS due to tissue hypoxia.

Lactate measurement is used as an adjunctive test in differentiating viral meningitis from bacterial, mycoplasma, fungal, and tuberculous meningitis in cases in which routine parameters yield equivocal results. In patients with viral meningitis lactate levels are usually below 25 mg/dL (2.8 mmol/L) and nearly always under 35 mg/dL (3.9 mmol/L), whereas bacterial meningitis typically has levels above 35 mg/dL (Bailey, 1990; Cameron, 1993). Sensitivity and specificity are about 80% to 90% in infectious meningitis cases using 30 to 36 mg/dL as a cut-off. Viral meningitis, partially treated bacterial meningitis, and tuberculous meningitis often have intermediate lactate levels that overlap each other, limiting the use of lactate measurements in this differential.

Persistently elevated ventricular CSF lactate levels are associated with a poor prognosis in patients with severe head injury (DeSalles, 1986).

ENZYMES. A wide variety of enzymes have been described in the CSF, derived from brain tissue, blood, or cellular elements within the CSF. Generally speaking, CSF enzyme assays have not proved to be of practical use in clinical laboratory diagnosis.

Lactate dehydrogenase (LD) is normally present in CSF, with 40 U/L a reasonable upper limit of normal for adults and 70 U/L for neonates (Donald, 1986; Engelke, 1986). LD values may help in differentiating traumatic tap from intracranial hemorrhage because fresh traumatic taps with intact RBCs do not significantly elevate the LD level (Engelke, 1986). Sensitivity and specificity are about 70% to 85% depending on the cut-off value used.

As with lactate, LD activity is significantly higher in bacterial meningitis than in aseptic meningitis (Donald, 1986; Engelke, 1986), with a sensitivity of about 86% and a specificity of 93% using a cut-off value of 40 U/L.

Elevated LD levels 76 hours following resuscitation predict a poor outcome in patients with hypoxic brain injury (Kärkelä, 1992).

Creatine kinase (CK) is normally present in the CSF at a concentration less than 5 U/L, predominantly in the CK-BB (brain) isoform with small contributions by CK-MB and CK-MM. The latter two substances are most likely secondary to blood contamination. Elevations of CK-BB are seen in patients with demyelinating diseases, seizures, stroke, malignant tumors, meningitis, and head injury. Brain injury also releases *mitochondrial CK* (CK-mt) into CSF.

CK-BB measurements may provide prognostic information in patients with global brain injury from ischemia or anoxia (Kärkelä, 1992). CSF CK-BB levels must not be obtained for at least 24 hours following cardiac or pulmonary arrest.

AMMONIA AND AMINES. Ammonia levels in the CSF are between one-third and one-half the values in blood. Elevated values are generally proportional to the degree of existing hepatic encephalopathy but are difficult to quantitate. α-Ketoglutarate combines with ammonia in brain tissue to form *glutamine*, which protects the CNS from ammonia toxicity. Glutamine levels therefore reflect brain ammonia. Reference intervals are method dependent, with an upper limit of normal or about 20 mg/dL. Glutamine values of over 35 mg/dL are almost invariably associated with hepatic encephalopathy (Fishman, 1992). Elevated CSF glutamine levels may also be seen in patients with encephalopathy secondary to hypercapnia or sepsis (Mizock, 1989).

ELECTROLYTES AND ACID-BASE BALANCE. There are no clinically useful indications for the measurement of *sodium*, *potassium*, *chloride*, *calcium*, or *magnesium* in cerebrospinal fluid. Measurements of CSF *pH*, Pco_2, and *bicarbonate* are not practical for patient care (Fishman, 1992).

TUMOR MARKERS. The value of most of these tests in routine clinical practice has not been established. *Carcinoembryonic protein* (CEA) is an oncofetal protein produced by a variety of carcinomas. Elevated CSF levels of CEA have a sensitivity of only 31% and a specificity of 90% for detecting metastatic carcinoma of the leptomeninges (Klee, 1986; Twijnstra, 1986).

Other oncofetal proteins include *human chorionic gonadotropin*, produced by choriocarcinoma and malignant germ cell tumors with a trophoblastic component, and α-*fetoprotein*, a glycoprotein produced by yolk sac elements of germ cell tumors.

Elevation of CSF *ferritin* is a sensitive indicator of CNS malignancy but has low specificity because it is also increased in patients with inflammatory neurologic diseases (Zandman-Goddard, 1986).

Microbiologic Examination

Diagnosis of CNS infection is the most compelling reason for examining the CSF because delay may result in significant mortality or morbidity. Changes in opening pressure, cell count, differential, protein, and glucose allow a tentative diagnosis in most cases (Table 19–11), but specific etiologic diagnosis requires more directed tests.

BACTERIAL MENINGITIS. The most common agents of bacterial meningitis are group B streptococcus and gram-negative rods (most prevalent in neonates from birth to one month old); *Haemophilus influenzae* (1 month to 5 years); *Neisseria meningitidis* (5 to 29 years old); *Streptococcus pneumoniae* (29 years and older); and *Listeria monocytogenes* (newborns, elderly, and immunosuppressed patients) (Graves, 1989; Wenger, 1990). Other streptococci, staphylococci, and anaerobes are rare causes of bacterial meningitis.

Gram's stain has a sensitivity of 60% to 90% in experienced hands, depending on the number and type of organisms present. Its sensitivity for *Listeria*, gram-negative organisms, and anaerobes is 50% or less (Greenlee, 1990). Detection limit is about 10^5 colony-forming units (CFU)/mL. Sensitivity may be improved by sedimenting the specimen at 1500 g for 15 minutes, using a cytospin concentration and acridine orange fluorochrome staining for screening.

Cultures have a sensitivity of 80% to 90% but drop 30% in partially treated cases (Greenlee, 1990).

Rapid bacterial antigen tests using *latex agglutination* (LA) are popular because of their great sensitivity, ease of use, and commercial availability. Sensitivity for *H. influenzae* is about 90%, for *S. pneumoniae* about 60%, for *N. meningitidis* about 50%, and for group B streptococcus about 90%. False-positive results due to rheumatoid factor may be eliminated by treating the specimen with a sulfhydryl reagent and by heating it prior to the test (Graves, 1989). Latex agglutination antigen tests are best applied in cases of partially treated meningitis in which Gram's stain has been negative. *Enzyme-linked immunosorbent assays* (ELISA), which have a 100-fold greater sensitivity than LA methods, are highly promising but are not widely used in clinical laboratories for common bacteria (Edberg, 1986).

The *Limulus lysate assay* identifies essentially all cases of gram-negative bacterial meningitis and has been particularly useful as a rapid test in the newborn (Dyson, 1976).

NEUROSYPHILIS. *Darkfield microscopy* has long been used to identify spirochetes in the CSF but is largely unavailable because of the rarity of neurosyphilis and the high technical expertise and experience required for accurate diagnosis.

CSF *fluorescent treponemal antibody with absorption* (CSF FTA-ABS) is essentially 100% sensitive for neurosyphilis but may be *too* sensitive for such a critical diagnosis because specificity is about 96% to 97%. Increased blood-brain barrier permeability resulting from inflammation, or as little as 0.8 μL of blood per milliliter of CSF (4000 CSF RBCs/μL) produces false-positive results (Davis, 1989). A nonreactive *serum* FTA-ABS test rules out neurosyphilis. Negative CSF FTA-ABS and positive serum FTA-ABS tests in a patient with neurologic signs make acute neurosyphilis highly unlikely.

The CSF *Venereal Disease Research Laboratory test* (CSF VDRL) has a sensitivity of only 50% to 60% but is highly specific: a positive test rules in neurosyphilis (Davis, 1989; Albright, 1991). CSF VDRL is inappropriate as a screening test for neurosyphilis; it should be performed only if serum FTA-ABS tests are positive (Davis, 1989; Albright, 1991).

The *rapid plasma reagin* (RPR) test is unsuitable for CSF

Table 19–11. CEREBROSPINAL FLUID FINDINGS IN MENINGITIS

Meningitis	Opening Pressure	Leukocytes/μL	Protein (mg/dL)	Glucose (mg/dL)*	Comments
Acute bacterial	Usually increased	1000–10,000 or more; occasionally <100 PMNs	Most 100–500	Usually <40	Partially treated cases may convert to lymphocytosis; most retain the other abnormalities
Viral	Normal to moderate increase	5–300; some >1000; lymphocytes and PMNs may predominate in first 24–36 hr	Normal to mildly increased (most <100)	Normal	Reduced glucose seen in 25% of cases of mumps, some HSV
Fungal	Increased	40–400; lymphocytes and/or PMNs predominate; eosinophilia may be found in *Coccidioides*	50–300; average about 100	Decreased	Neutrophilic pleocytosis most common with mycelial fungal forms
Tuberculous	Increased; decreased with spinal block	100–600 up to 1200. Mixed or lymphocytic; PMNs often predominate early	50–300 marked increase with spinal block	Decreased; <45 in many cases	Findings vary depending on clinical stage
Acute syphilitic	Increased	Average 500; lymphocytic, rarely neutrophilic	Increased, usually no more than 100	Normal	Up to 15% have normal CSF parameters
Amebic (*Naegleria*)	Increased	Mildly increased to grossly purulent (>20,000); PMNs	Increased, may reach 1000	Normal to decreased	RBCs suggest hemorrhagic brain necrosis
Lyme disease (Stage II findings)	Increased	5–400; lymphocytes predominate	Normal to increased, most <300	Normal to decreased	CSF normal in early infection (Stage I)
Carcinomatous	Normal to increased	0 to hundreds; lymphocytes predominate; variable number of tumor cells may be seen	Usually increased; most <500	Decreased in most cases	Marked neutrophilic pleocytosis may be seen in large necrotic tumors

*In presence of normal serum levels

Adapted from Fishman RA: Cerebrospinal Fluid in Diseases of the Nervous System, 2nd ed. Philadelphia, W. B. Saunders, 1992.

because it has a higher false-positive than the VDRL (Fishman, 1992).

Assessment of intrathecal immunoglobulin synthesis through calculation of the IgG index, IgM index, or *Treponema pallidum* specific IgG index using quantitative FTA-ABS titers may help rule out disease in equivocal cases (Muller, 1983; Hische, 1988). Oligoclonal bands do not correlate with disease activity and may persist after successful therapy. Their use in diagnosis has not been proven (Jones, 1990).

VIRAL MENINGITIS. Enteroviruses (echoviruses, coxsackie viruses, polio viruses) are responsible for up to 80% of cases of viral meningitis, which has a seasonal peak in late summer. Diagnosis of viral meningitis is mostly a matter of exclusion; specific etiologic diagnosis by viral culture or immunologic methods is rarely necessary in uncomplicated cases. Sensitivity of CSF viral cultures varies from a high of 72% for enterovirus to a low of 5% for herpes simplex virus (HSV) (Marton, 1986). Retrospective epidemiologic studies are made by serologic methods.

Viral inclusions (cytomegalovirus, HSV) may rarely be seen in the CSF and may be demonstrated by immunostains. Diagnosis of herpes simplex encephalitis generally requires brain biopsy. PCR amplification of HSV DNA in CSF has shown excellent promise as a rapid diagnostic test in several preliminary studies.

HUMAN IMMUNODEFICIENCY VIRUS (HIV). A wide variety of CSF abnormalities may be found in HIV-positive patients with or without neurologic disease (Chalmers, 1990; Hall, 1992), including lymphocytic pleocytosis, elevated IgG indexes, and oligoclonal bands. Identification of opportunistic infections is the most important reason for examining the CSF. Serious fungal infections may exist in the presence of little or no CSF abnormalities.

FUNGAL MENINGITIS. India ink or nigrosin stains for cryptococcal capsular halos have a sensitivity of about 25%, increasing to up to 53% with multiple lumbar punctures (Marton, 1986). False-positive results may be minimized by identifying narrow-based budding and a refractile cell wall. Culture sensitivity is about 60% with a single attempt. Cultures require large volumes of CSF (40 to 50 mL) for best results and may take weeks to grow.

Cryptococcal antigen tests using latex agglutination are rapid and have established diagnostic use (Kaufman, 1976). Sensitivity varies from 60% to 95%; higher values are seen with repeated punctures and in AIDS patients (Kaufman, 1976; Marton, 1986). False-negative results due to a prozone effect may occur, requiring a 1:10 dilution for confirmation. Early disease, intraparenchymal infection, infection with nonencapsulated *Cryptococcus neoformans* variants, and immune complexes (corrected with pronase treatment) also produce false-negative results. Rheumatoid factor and *Klebsiella* infections may produce false-positive results (Graves, 1989).

Complement-fixing antibodies are found in the CSF of up to 95% of patients with coccidioidal meningitis (Bouza, 1981).

TUBERCULOUS MENINGITIS. Early diagnosis of this disease is extremely difficult. A reasonable sensitivity of acid-fast stains in hospital laboratories is only 10% to 12% (Greenlee, 1990). Fluorescent auramine-rhodamine stains are recommended for higher sensitivity (Woods, 1994). Positive fluorescent stains should be confirmed with an acid-fast stain, which can be performed on the same slide.

Large volumes of CSF are recommended to ensure maximal culture sensitivity, which is 75% to 90% (Marton, 1986).

Adenosine deaminase levels are significantly higher in tuberculous meningitis than in other types of meningitis and CNS disorders and have a sensitivity of 87% and a specificity of 84% (Blake, 1982). This test is not widely available for clinical use, however.

ELISA techniques for *Mycobacterium tuberculosis* antigens or antibodies have been reported to have a sensitivity of about 50% to 82% and a specificity of 90% to 100% but are not standardized or widely available (Greenlee, 1990; Radhakrishnan, 1990). Molecular amplification techniques are becoming commercially available but at present are not recommended for use in diagnosis (CDC, 1993).

PRIMARY AMEBIC MENINGOENCEPHALITIS (PAM). This rare disease is caused by the free-living ameba *Naegleria fowleri* or *Acanthamoeba* species. *Naegleria* is more likely to cause an acute inflammatory response, whereas *Acanthamoeba* more often produces a granulomatous meningitis. Motile *Naegleria* trophozoites may be visualized by light or phase-contrast microscopy in direct wet mounts, allowing rapid diagnosis. Intact and degenerating organisms may be identified on Wright's or Geimsa-stained cytospin slides but must be distinguished from macrophages (dos Santos, 1970; Benson, 1985). Acridine orange stain will help to differentiate ameba (brick red) from leukocytes (bright green) (Medley, 1980).

SYNOVIAL FLUID

Synovium refers to the tissue lining synovial tendon sheaths, bursae, and diarthrodial joints except for the articular surface. It is composed of one to three cell layers that form a discontinuous surface overlying fatty, fibrous, or periosteal joint tissue.

Synovial fluid (synovia, SF) is an imperfect ultrafiltrate of plasma combined with hyaluronic acid produced by the synovial cells (Sledge, 1989). Small ions and molecules like glucose and urea cross easily into the joint space and are therefore similar in concentration to plasma, but large molecules are absent or are present in only trace amounts (Weinberger, 1989). Resorption is accomplished by the lymphatics and is not size dependent. Synovial fluid acts as a lubricant and adhesive and provides nutrients for the avascular articular cartilage.

Specimen Collection

Joint fluid aspiration (arthrocentesis) is indicated in a patient with an undiagnosed effusion or a clinical change related to a known effusion. It should be performed by an experienced operator using good sterile technique. Caution is necessary to avoid aspirating a sterile joint in someone with bacteremia or aspirating through a cutaneous or periarticular soft tissue infection into a sterile joint. The procedure used for various joints has been described elsewhere (Gatter, 1991). Even large joints like the knee normally contain no more than 4 mL of synovia, so a small sample size is common unless an effusion is present.

Synovial fluid is collected with sterile, disposable needles and plastic syringes to avoid contamination by birefringent particulates. The syringe may be heparinized with 25 units of *sodium* heparin per milliliter of SF in routine arthrocentesis. Oxalate, powdered ethylenediaminetetra-acetic acid (EDTA), and lithium heparin anticoagulants should be avoided because they form crystal artifacts that may be misleading during examination. The joint should be turned or manipulated prior to aspiration to ensure mixing of its contents.

Ideally the specimen should be separated into three parts: 5 to 10 mL is placed in a sterile heparinized tube or syringe for microbiologic studies; 2 to 5 mL is placed in an anticoagulant tube (sodium heparin or liquid EDTA) for microscopic examination; and about 5 mL is put into a plain (no anticoagulant) "red top" tube and allowed to clot (normal SF does not clot). Concentrations of heparin greater than 125 U/mL have an inhibitory effect on some pathogenic bacteria (Rosett, 1980). Specimens for culture should therefore be at least 1 to 2 mL in volume if they are submitted in "green top" heparin tubes (Becton Dickinson, Rutherford, NJ) containing 143 U/tube of heparin, or they can be submitted in recapped syringes after the needle and excess air have been removed.

"Dry taps" may still have fluid within the needle, which may be sufficient for the most critical tests. Such specimens should be submitted with the needle still on the syringe, its tip stuck into a sterile cork.

Recommended Tests

Diagnosis of infectious arthritis and synovial fluid crystals is the most compelling reason for SF analysis. Routine tests, therefore, are directed toward the diagnosis of these disorders (Table 19–12). *It is vital that they be performed well* because they can provide highly specific diagnostic information. High-quality performance is, unfortunately, inconstant (Hasselbacher, 1987; Rabinovitch, 1994). Other tests are not of practical value for routine use but may provide diagnostic information under certain circumstances.

Gross Examination

Total volume should be recorded at the bedside, especially if the sample is to be divided for submission to different laboratory sections.

Table 19–12. RECOMMENDED TESTS FOR SYNOVIAL FLUID

Routine
Gross examination (color and clarity)
Total leukocyte count and differential
Gram's stain and bacterial culture (aerobic and anaerobic)
Crystal examination with polarizing microscope and compensator
Useful in certain circumstances
Fungal and acid-fast stains and cultures
Countercurrent immunoelectrophoresis for bacterial antigens
Serum-synovial fluid glucose differential
Lactate
Complement
Enzymes

Adapted from Kjeldsberg CR, Knight JA: Body Fluids: Laboratory Examination of Amniotic, Cerebrospinal, Seminal, Serous and Synovial Fluids, 3rd ed. © American Society of Clinical Pathologists, Chicago, 1993.

Color is evaluated in a clear glass tube against a white background. Normal SF is colorless to pale yellow owing to diapedesis of a few RBCs associated with even mild trauma. Noninflammatory and inflammatory disorders are usually straw to yellow in color (xanthochromia). Septic fluid may be yellow, brown, or green, depending on the chromogens produced by the offending organism and the host response, including WBCs and RBCs.

Traumatic tap produces an uneven distribution of blood during arthrocentesis or streaking in the syringe. Although pale yellow xanthochromia is difficult to distinguish from normal, a red-brown color following centrifugation is good evidence of pathologic hemarthrosis.

Clarity relates to the number and type of particles within the synovia. Normal SF is transparent; newsprint is easily read through the tube. Translucent fluid obscures details, but black and white areas can be distinguished, whereas opaque fluid completely obscures the background.

Leukocytes are most commonly responsible for changes in clarity, but massive numbers of crystals may produce an opaque, milky opalescent fluid without white cells. A shimmering, oily-appearing specimen suggests an abundance of cholesterol crystals, which may look like pus.

Increased turbidity is less often due to concentrations of fibrin, free-floating "rice bodies" (fragments of degenerating proliferative synovial cells or microinfarcted synovium), metal and plastic particles from patients with joint prostheses, or cartilage fragments in patients with osteoarthritis. A "ground pepper" appearance resulting from pigmented cartilage fragments is a sign of ochronosis.

Microscopic Examination

TOTAL CELL COUNT. Total leukocyte counts should be performed promptly to avoid degenerative cell loss, which begins as soon as one hour following arthrocentesis. Tubes must be inverted before sampling to ensure uniform mixing. Counts are usually performed in a standard hemocytometer. Automated cell counters may be used, but these risk clogging the machine aperture or obtaining spuriously high cell counts from non-WBC particles (crystals and fat globules), especially in multichannel machines. A wet-prep slide count of 0 to 2 leukocytes per high-power field (hpf) (averaged over 10 fields) predicts less than 1300 WBCs by cell count (Clayburne, 1992). Leukocyte counts of over 50,000/μL require dilution, which should be done with saline, *not* acetic acid, to avoid mucin clot formation and cell clumping.

Highly viscous SF should be incubated with hyaluronidase before it is counted, specially if automated cell counters are used.

Red cells should be counted unless it is an obvious traumatic tap. If a large number of red cells interferes with the WBC count, they may be lysed by dilution with 0.3 N saline, 0.1 N HCl, or 1% saponin in saline.

The upper limit of normal for SF leukocytes in clinical specimens is 150 to 200/μL (Kjeldsberg, 1993). Elevated cell counts are used to help divide the findings into different disease categories (see later under Clinical Correlations) but are nonspecific for any particular disease because of extensive overlap.

DIFFERENTIAL COUNT. Cytospin preparations are preferred over smears of centrifuged SF because they have better cell morphology (Rabinovitch, 1994). Treatment with hyaluronidase may be necessary to produce thin smears in viscous specimens.

Neutrophils normally account for about 20% of SF leukocytes. Using 75% as a cut-off point, the sensitivity for an inflammatory process is 75% and the specificity is 92% (Shmerling, 1990). SF from patients with urate gout or rheumatoid arthritis (RA) may also have high percentages. Neutrophils frequently exhibit pyknosis and karyorrhexis and may contain bacteria, crystals, lipid droplets, vacuoles, or dark blue inclusions (ragocytes, RA cells).

Lymphocytes, normally comprising about 15% of the differential, are prominent in early RA, chronic infections, and collagen disorders (Amor, 1984). Reactive forms, including immunoblasts, may be seen.

Monocytes and *macrophages* account for approximately 65% of the normal cell count. Monocytosis may be self-limited in patients with viral arthritis or serum sickness or more chronic in those with lupus erythematosus.

Eosinophilia, defined as over 2% of the leukocyte count, has been reported in rheumatoid arthritis, rheumatic fever, metastatic carcinoma, Lyme disease, parasitic infections, chronic urticaria, angioedema, and following arthrography and irradiation (Podell, 1980; Kay, 1988).

Synovial cells have no pathologic significance. They look like mesothelial cells and may be difficult to differentiate from monocytes.

Lipid bodies are associated with trauma, aseptic necrosis, and RA. These droplets often form Maltese crosses under polarized light, can be associated with a leukocytic response, and may cause spurious elevations of the automated WBC count (Wise, 1987).

CRYSTAL EXAMINATION. *Gout* refers to the process of crystal deposition in articular tissue. An inflammatory response to crystal deposition is referred to as gouty arthritis. The most common types of endogenous crystals responsible for gouty arthritis are monosodium urate monohydrate (urate gout); calcium pyrophosphate dihydrate (pyrophosphate gout, chondrocalcinosis, or "pseudogout"); apatite and other basic calcium phosphates (BCP; apatite gout); calcium oxalate (oxalate gout); and lipids (lipid gout).

Except for BCP, all of these crystals can be detected by polarized light microscopy. A high-quality polarizing microscope with a first-order red plate compensator should be used. The polarizer filter is placed directly above the light source. The analyzer (another polarizing filter) is placed between the specimen slide and microscope oculars and is oriented 90 degrees from the polarizer to produce a dark background. The compensator is placed between the polarizer and the analyzer, usually oriented 45 degrees (half way) between the planes of the two polarizing filters.

Initial examination should be performed on a wet preparation using polarized light. Phase contrast microscopy enhances crystal detection. The slide and coverslip need to be cleaned and carefully dried immediately before use to avoid birefringent dust particulate artifacts. The edges of the coverslip are sealed with nail polish, which retards but does not prevent evaporation. The edge of the coverslip is used to find the proper plane of focus, but crystals in this location are ignored because they are most likely artifacts. Most crystals are scanned with a 10× objective and evaluated at 40×, concentrating especially on cellular areas. Complete examination requires 100× oil immersion, however, because apparently negative fluids on scanning may contain a large population of small crystals (Gatter, 1991). Aligning the crystal's orientation to the compensator by rotating the microscope stage or the compensator facilitates recognition and identification. Crystal morphology, the strength and sign of any birefringence, and the extinction angle are noted.

Monosodium urate crystals (MSU) appear as needle-shaped rods 5 to 20 μm long but may be only 1 to 2 μm in length (Plate 19–5). They are strongly birefringent: yellow when oriented parallel to the compensator, blue with perpendicular orientation (negative birefringence or elongation). *Extinction*, the point at which the crystal loses birefringence and becomes rose-colored like the background, is rapid and complete at the same angle as the polarizer and analyzer (axial or parallel extinction) (Fig. 19–2*A*). A control slide of MSU crystals should always be used for comparison.

3

MSU crystals are found in 90% of cases of acute urate gout and in about 75% of patients between attacks (Kjeldsberg, 1993). Intracellular MSU crystals are characteristic of acute urate gout. They are occasionally observed as a result of inflammation in septic arthritis (McCarty, 1988).

Calcium pyrophosphate dihydrate crystals (CPPD) are found in a group of conditions collectively known as CPPD crystal deposition disease. These crystals appear as rhomboids, rods, or rectangles 1 to 20 μm in length (Plate 19–6). CPPD crystals are no more than weakly birefringent with positive elongation (blue when aligned with compensator axis). Many are too small to polarize the light, so they may be hard to detect without the added help of phase-contrast microscopy. Extinction is incomplete and occurs at 20 to 30 degrees from the angle of the polarizer and analyzer (oblique or inclined extinction) (Fig. 19–2*B*).

CPPD crystals are associated with degenerative arthritis and arthritides associated with hypomagnesemia, hemochromatosis, hyperparathyroidism, and hypothyroidism (Jones, 1992).

Hydroxyapatite and the other BCP crystals are typically too small and nonbirefringent to be seen with light microscopy unless they are clumped into 1- to 50-μm spherical microaggregates. *Alizarin red S* dye may be used to stain these and other calcium-containing crystals (Lazcano, 1993). At present, identification of BCP crystals is not important for diagnosis, prognosis, or guidance in treatment.

Calcium oxalate dihydrate crystals are 5 to 30 μm in diameter and are bipyramidal "envelopes" with variable birefringence and positive elongation. They are seen in arthropathy associated with chronic renal dialysis and primary oxalosis, a rare inborn error of metabolism (Rosenthal, 1988; Gatter, 1991). The monohydrate form is birefringent but nondescript in shape.

Lipid crystals are spheres 1 to 20 μm in diameter with a Maltese cross appearance and positive birefringence under compensated polarized light. They have been implicated as a cause of acute arthritis (McCarty, 1988).

Crystalline corticosteroids for intra-articular injection may appear similar to MSU or CPPD crystals. Most often they have blunt, jagged edges with no clear crystal structure be-

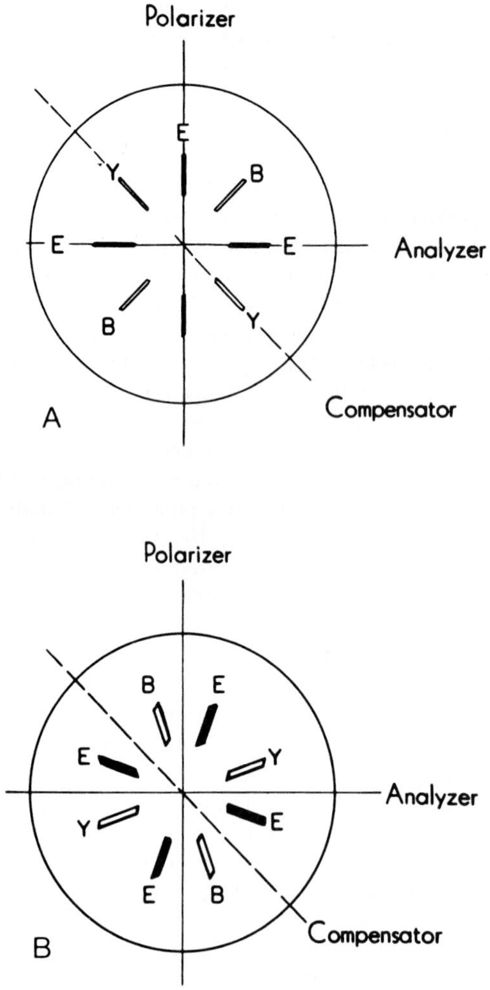

Figure 19–2. *A*, Monosodium urate (MSU) crystals by compensated polarized light. Maximal brightness occurs when the long axis of the MSU crystal is oriented 45 degrees off the axis of either the polarizer or analyzer. Birefringence is lost (extinction, *E*) when the crystal is oriented parallel to the axis of the polarizer or analyzer. MSU crystals appear yellow *(Y)* when oriented parallel to the compensator, and they are blue *(B)* when aligned perpendicular to the compensator (negative birefringence). *B*, Calcium pyrophosphate dihydrate (CPPD) by compensated polarized light. The larger crystals have weak, positive birefringence (blue when oriented parallel to the compensator) and show inclined extinction, off the axis of the polarizer and analyzer. (Reproduced with permission from McCarty DJ: Crystal identification in human synovial fluids. Rheum Dis Clin North Am 1988; 14:253.)

cause they are prepared by grinding up larger crystalline forms (Plate 19–7). Triamcinolone hexacetonide is negatively birefringent, but most others show positive birefringence.

Cholesterol crystals typically appear as irregular birefringent plates with notched margins (Plate 19–8). In chronic effusions like tuberculous arthritis or RA, needle- or rhomboid-shaped crystals similar to MSU or CPPD may be present (Ettlinger, 1979). Cholesterol crystals are, however, ethanol or ether soluble and are not phagocytosed by leukocytes.

Glove powder introduced during joint surgery appears as round, strongly birefringent particles 5 to 30 μm in diameter with a Maltese cross appearance when polarized.

A variety of other crystals or particulates may be seen in SF. These include monoclonal immunoglobulin crystals or cryoglobulins, Charcot-Leyden crystals, amyloid fragments, cartilage fragments, collagen fibrils and fibrin strands, hematoidin crystals from prior hemorrhage, crystals from certain anticoagulants, nail polish, prosthetic fragments, and dust particles (Gatter, 1991).

Chemical Analysis

Chemical analyses of SF tend to offer only information that supports the routine tests (Shmerling, 1990). High viscosity may be remedied by dilution with normal saline, sonication, or hyaluronidase treatment (Baker, 1991). Reference intervals are shown in Table 19–13.

MUCIN CLOT TEST. Addition of acetic acid to SF precipitates hyaluronate into a mucin clot, which may be graded as good, fair, or poor. A fair to poor mucin clot reflects dilution and depolymerization of hyaluronic acid, a nonspecific finding characteristic of several inflammatory arthritides. Although of historical significance, the mucin clot test has little clinical use (Baker, 1991).

GLUCOSE. Proper interpretation of SF glucose values requires comparison with serum levels, ideally preceded by a fast of 8 hours to allow glucose to equilibrate across the synovial membrane (Gatter, 1991). The serum-synovia differential is less than 10 mg/dL in normal and many noninflammatory conditions. In septic arthritis this difference ranges from 20 to 60 mg/dL but overlaps significantly with other inflammatory conditions, limiting its clinical usefulness (Baker, 1991). The sensitivity of low glucose values for detecting inflammatory joint disease is only 20% and the specificity is 84%, using a cut-off value of 75 mg/dL (Shmerling, 1990).

Glycolysis by large numbers of leukocytes *in vitro* may falsely reduce SF glucose values unless testing is performed within one hour of collection or tubes containing sodium fluoride inhibitor are used.

PROTEIN. The mean normal protein concentration is 1.38 g/dL in living volunteers (Weinberger, 1989). With increasing inflammation, larger proteins like fibrinogen enter the synovia. Spontaneous clot formation may be detected in nonanticoagulated specimen tubes (fibrin clot test). Measurement of SF protein has a sensitivity of 52% and a specificity of 56% for inflammatory disorders and seldom affects diagnosis, treatment, or outcome (Shmerling, 1990).

Table 19–13. REFERENCE INTERVALS FOR CONSTITUENTS OF SYNOVIAL FLUID

	Synovial Fluid	Plasma
Protein	1–3 g/dL	6–8 g/dL
Albumin	55–70%	50–65%
α_1-Globulin	6–8%	3–5%
α_2-Globulin	5–7%	7–13%
β-Globulin	8–10%	8–14%
γ-Globulin	10–14%	12–22%
Hyaluronate	0.3–0.4 g/dL	
Glucose	70–110 mg/dL	70–110 mg/dL
Uric acid	2–8 mg/dL	2–8 mg/dL

ENZYMES. Enzyme activities are generally of little clinical value in the evaluation of joint effusions. *Lactate dehydrogenase* is elevated in RA, gout, and infectious arthritis but most likely reflects the leukocyte infiltrate (Kjeldsberg, 1993). Elevated *acid phosphatase* may have negative prognostic value in RA but is not specific (Luukkainen, 1989).

LACTATE. Levels exceeding 250 mg/dL (27.8 mmol/L, about 10 times normal) are typically associated with septic arthritis (Borenstein, 1982). Intermediate levels neither rule in nor rule out infection, however, and gonococcal arthritis is notorious for not elevating SF lactate (Curtis, 1983). RA is also associated with increased levels (Curtis, 1983). An elevated lactate level may provide rapid provisional evidence of infection in specimens with negative Gram's stain.

URIC ACID. SF levels of uric acid generally parallel serum levels and have no clinical value in the diagnosis of urate gout (Baker, 1991).

LIPIDS. SF lipid abnormalities include (1) rare cholesterol-rich pseudochylous effusions typically associated with chronic RA; (2) lipid droplets, usually the result of trauma; and (3) extremely rare chylous effusions seen in association with RA, systemic lupus erythematosus, filariasis, pancreatitis, and trauma (Wise, 1987). These can usually be differentiated clinically and by gross and microscopic examination; quantification of lipids currently has no clinical value in joint fluid analysis.

Immunologic Studies

Rheumatoid factor (RF) is found in synovia of about 60% of RA patients, usually at a titer equal to or slightly lower than that of serum. Its presence, however, is nonspecific, and measurements are generally not helpful for diagnosis or prognosis.

Antinuclear antibodies (ANA), found in the SF of about 70% of patients with systemic lupus erythematosus and 20% of patients with RA, have little disease specificity (Cohen, 1985).

Complement levels in SF are normally about 10% of serum levels because of size exclusion. With inflammation this increases to 40% to 70% of serum activity, proportional to the increase in protein exudation. Exceptions are systemic lupus erythematosus and RA, in which complement consumption leads to levels of less than 30% of serum complement. This is most consistently associated with RF-positive RA (Wolf, 1978). Complement is also decreased in some cases of bacterial or crystal-induced arthritis, so measurement is impractical for routine diagnosis.

Microbiologic Examination

Rapid transportation of joint fluid and good communication of clinical suspicions to the laboratory maximize the chances of identifying an infectious agent.

Gram's stain should always be performed as part of the routine evaluation of SF. Sensitivity varies from 75% for staphylococcal infections to 50% for most gram-negative infections to under 25% for gonococcal infections (Goldenberg, 1985). Specificity is very high in experienced hands.

Ziehl-Neelsen or *Kinyoun* stains for acid-fast bacteria have a sensitivity of about 20%. Synovial biopsy is recommended for suspected tuberculous arthritis to provide rapid diagnosis. PCR kits for detection of tuberculous infection are becoming commercially available, but at present are not recommended for routine diagnostic use (CDC, 1993).

Arthritis develops in approximately 60% of patients with Lyme disease. The PCR test for *Borrelia burgdorferi* DNA in SF is positive in 96% of untreated cases (Nocton, 1994) but is not yet available for routine laboratory use. ELISA blood serology appears to be the test of choice because it has an optimal sensitivity of 94% and a specificity of 97% (Golightly, 1993). The predictive value of a positive result is only 6.1% when the test is used as a screening test, however, because of the low prevalence of Lyme disease (Golightly, 1993). To be practical, laboratory testing must be confined to patients with a strong clinical suspicion of Lyme disease.

Synovial fluid culture has a sensitivity of 75% to 95% for nongonococcal joint infections in patients who have not received antibiotics; for patients with gonococcal infections the sensitivity is only around 10% to 50% (Shmerling, 1994). Aerobic and anaerobic bacterial cultures should be routine; fungal and mycobacterial cultures should be performed only in clinically suspicious cases. Cultures for *M. tuberculosis* are positive in about 80% of proven cases but require 4 to 6 weeks for completion (Kjeldsberg, 1993).

Detection of microbial metabolites by *gas-liquid chromatography* may be useful in identifying partially treated cases in which Gram's stain and cultures are negative (Borenstein, 1982).

Identification of microbial antigens or nucleic acids by counter immunoelectrophoresis (CIE), latex agglutination, or molecular studies (nucleic acid probes and PCR) are limited in the evaluation of synovial fluids (Borenstein, 1991).

Clinical Correlation

Gross and microscopic findings of SF examination have traditionally been divided into "reaction types," as depicted in Table 19–14.

Noninflammatory effusions (Group I) typically have leukocyte counts of less than 3000 cells/μL, with a minority of neutrophils. Osteoarthritis, traumatic arthritis, neuropathic osteoarthropathy, pigmented villonodular synovitis, and early rheumatic fever, among others, appear in this way, but early RA or early bacterial infections may occasionally appear as noninflammatory effusions.

Inflammatory effusions (Group II) have leukocyte counts of between 3000 and 75,000, with neutrophils accounting for over half the cell population. RA, lupus erythematosus, Reiter's syndrome, rheumatic fever, acute crystal-induced arthritis, arthritis associated with inflammatory bowel disease, psoriatic arthritis, and fat droplet synovitis are examples of this reaction group.

Purulent (infectious) effusions (Group III) have leukocyte counts of more than 50,000, of which over 90% are neutrophils. Bacterial, fungal, and tuberculous joint infections appear this way.

Hemorrhagic effusions (Group IV) may be seen in association with traumatic arthritis, pigmented villonodular synovitis, synovial hemangioma, neuropathic osteoarthropathy,

Table 19–14. SYNOVIAL FLUID FINDINGS BY DISEASE CATEGORY

	Category				
Finding	*Normal*	*Group I (Noninflammatory)*	*Group II (Inflammatory)*	*Group III (Infectious)*	*Group IV (Hemorrhagic)*
Appearance	Clear to straw colored	Yellow, transparent	Yellow, cloudy, turbid, or bloody	Yellow, purulent	Red-brown or xanthochromic
WBCs/mL	0–150 (0–0.15 $\times 10^9$/L)	<3000 (0–3 $\times 10^9$/L)	3000–75,000 (3–75 $\times 10^9$/L)	50,000–200,000 (50–200 $\times 10^9$/L)	50–10,000 (0.05–10 $\times 10^9$/L)
Neutrophils (%)	<25	<30	>50	>90	<50
RBCs present	No	No	No	Yes	Yes
Glucose (blood-SF difference in mg/dL)	0–10 (0–0.56 mmol/L)	0–10 (0–0.56 mmol/L)	0–40 (0–2.22 mmol/L)	20–100 (1.11–5.55 mmol/L)	0–20 (0–1.11 mmol/L)

Note: Values in parentheses are SI units.

Adapted from Kjeldsberg CR, Knight JA: Body Fluids: Laboratory Examination of Amniotic, Cerebrospinal, Seminal, Serous and Synovial Fluids, 3rd ed. © American Society of Clinical Pathologists, Chicago, 1993.

joint prostheses, and hematologic disorders (hemophilia, thrombocytopenia, anticoagulant therapy, sickle cell disease or trait, myeloproliferative syndrome).

These groups are largely descriptive, and there is much overlap between groups. *Except for Gram's stain, culture, and crystal examination, most findings of SF examination are nonspecific and need to be integrated into the clinical context.*

PLEURAL FLUID

The pleural cavity is a potential space lined by mesothelium of the visceral and parietal pleura. The pleural cavity normally contains a small amount of fluid that facilitates movement of the two membranes against each other. This fluid is a plasma filtrate derived from capillaries of the parietal (outer) pleura. It is produced continuously at a rate that depends on capillary hydrostatic pressure, plasma oncotic pressure, and capillary permeability. Pleural fluid is reabsorbed through the lymphatics and venules of the visceral pleura.

An accumulation of fluid is called an *effusion*, which results from an imbalance of fluid production and reabsorption. In the pleural, pericardial, and peritoneal cavities this accumulation is known as a *serous effusion*.

Specimen Collection

Thoracentesis is indicated for any undiagnosed pleural effusion or for therapeutic purposes in patients with massive symptomatic effusions (American College of Physicians, 1985; American Thoracic Society, 1989). Except for an EDTA tube for cell counts and differential, the specimen should be collected in heparinized tubes to avoid clotting. If malignancy, fungal infection, or mycobacterial infection is suspected, all remaining fluid (100 mL or more) should be submitted to the laboratory in heparinized containers to maximize the yield of stains and culture. Serous effusions are more forgiving than CSF in maintaining cellular integrity; if necessary, fresh specimens for cytology may be stored up to 48 hours in the refrigerator with satisfactory results. For pH measurements the fluid should be collected anaerobically in a heparinized syringe and submitted to the laboratory on ice. Grossly purulent specimens may clog the analyzer, however.

Transudates and Exudates

Normal pleural fluid is a transudate. Transudative effusions are usually bilateral owing to systemic conditions leading to increased capillary hydrostatic pressure or decreased plasma oncotic pressure (Table 19–15).

Exudates are more often unilateral and are associated with localized disorders that increase vascular permeability or interfere with lymphatic resorption (see Table 19–15).

The criteria of Light and colleagues (Light, 1972) suggest that an exudate should meet one or more of the following criteria: (1) pleural fluid/serum protein ratio greater than 0.5; (2) pleural fluid/serum LD ratio greater than 0.6; and (3) pleural fluid LD greater than two-thirds of the serum upper

Table 19–15. CLASSIFICATION OF PLEURAL EFFUSIONS

Transudates: increased hydrostatic pressure or decreased plasma oncotic pressure
- Congestive heart failure
- Hepatic cirrhosis
- Hypoproteinemia (e.g., nephrotic syndrome)

Exudates: increased capillary permeability or decreased lymphatic resorption
- Infections
  - Tuberculosis
  - Bacterial pneumonia
  - Viral or mycoplasma pneumonia
- Neoplasms
  - Bronchogenic carcinoma
  - Metastatic carcinoma
  - Lymphoma
  - Mesothelioma (increased hyaluronate content of effusion fluid)
- Pulmonary infarct (may be associated with hemorrhagic effusion)
- Noninfectious inflammatory disease involving pleura
  - Rheumatoid disease (low pleural fluid glucose in most cases)
  - Systemic lupus erythematosus (LE cells occasionally present)

Fluid from extrapleural sources
- Pancreatitis (elevated amylase activity in effusion fluid)
- Ruptured esophagus (elevated amylase activity and low pH)
- Urinothorax (elevated creatinine and low pH)

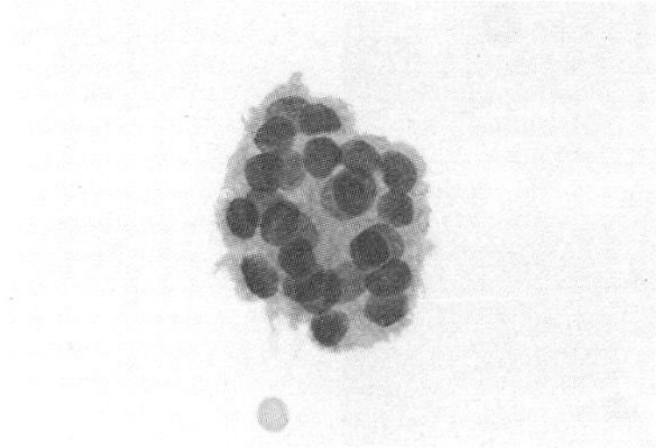

Plate 19–1

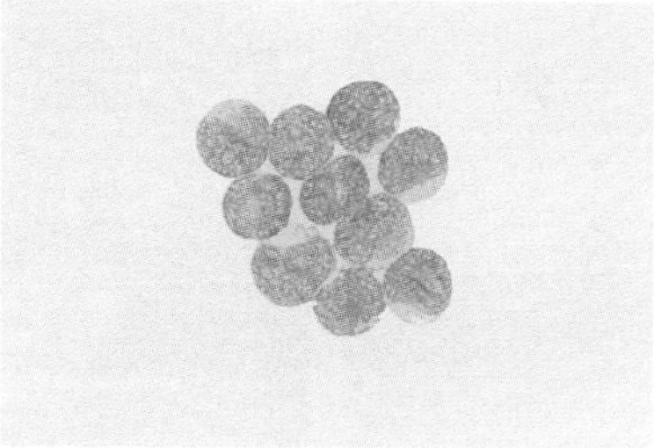

Plate 19–2

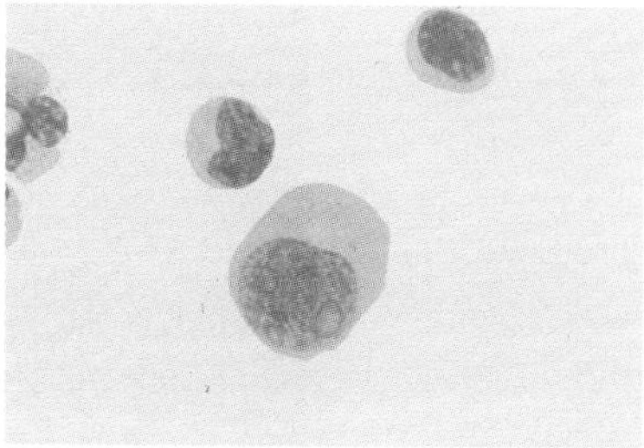

Plate 19–3

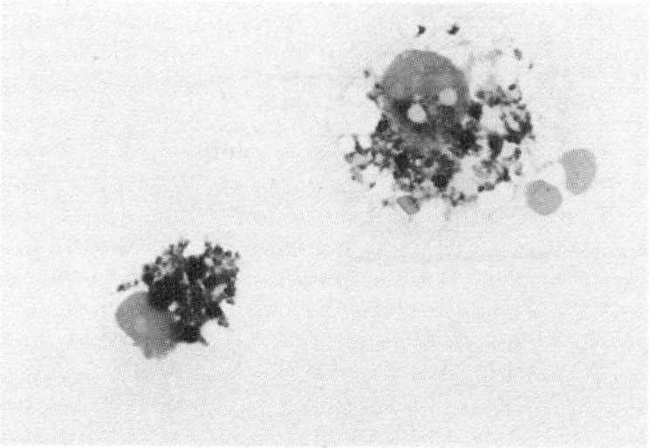

Plate 19–4

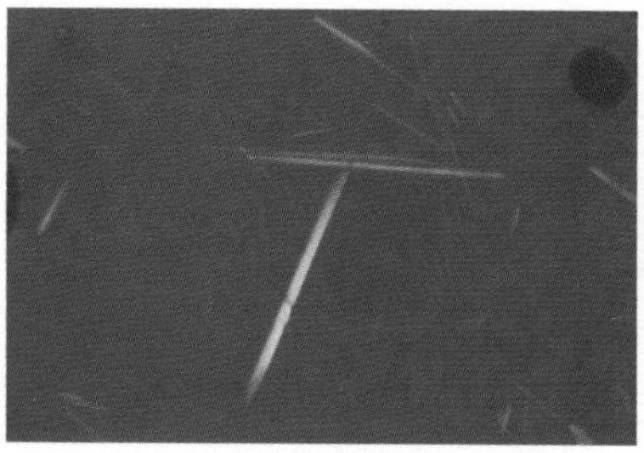

Plate 19–5

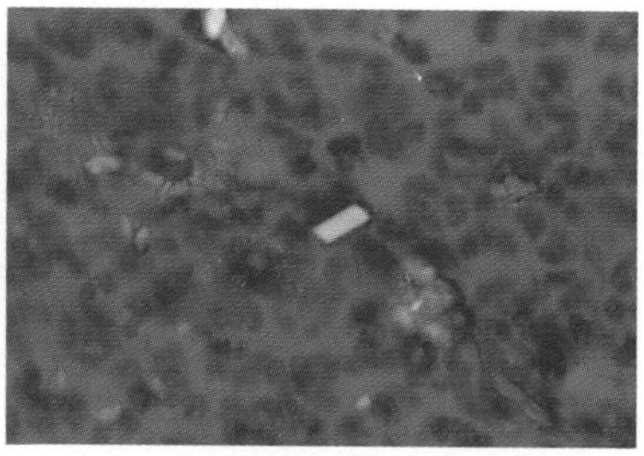

Plate 19–6

Plate 19–1. Choroid plexus cells in CSF. (Reproduced with permission from Kjeldsberg CR, Knight JA: Body Fluids: Laboratory Examination of Amniotic, Cerebrospinal, Seminal, Serous and Synovial Fluids, 3rd ed. © 1993 by the American Society of Clinical Pathologists, Chicago.) **Plate 19–2.** Blastlike cell cluster of probable germinal matrix origin from the CSF of neonate. **Plate 19–3.** Atypical lymphocyte (immunoblast) in CSF. **Plate 19–4.** Hemosiderin-laden macrophages (siderophages) from the CSF of a patient with subarachnoid hemorrhage. Hematoidin crystals (golden yellow) are also present. **Plate 19–5.** Monosodium urate (MSU) crystals in synovial fluid from a patient with urate gout. Compensated polarized light. (Reproduced with permission from Kjeldsberg CR, Knight JA: Body Fluids: Laboratory Examination of Amniotic, Cerebrospinal, Seminal, Serous and Synovial Fluids, 3rd ed. © 1993 by the American Society of Clinical Pathologists, Chicago.) **Plate 19–6.** Calcium pyrophosphate dihydrate (CPPD) crystals in synovial fluid. Compensated polarized light.

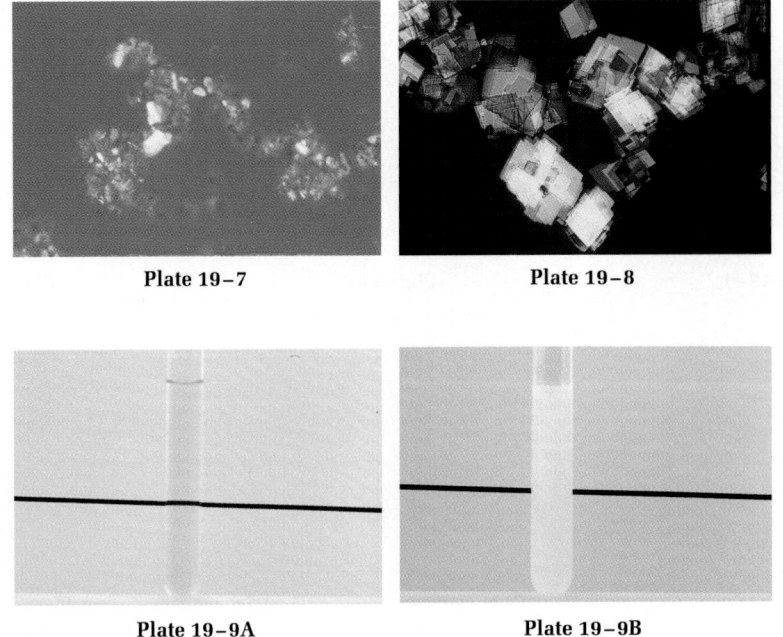

Plate 19–7

Plate 19–8

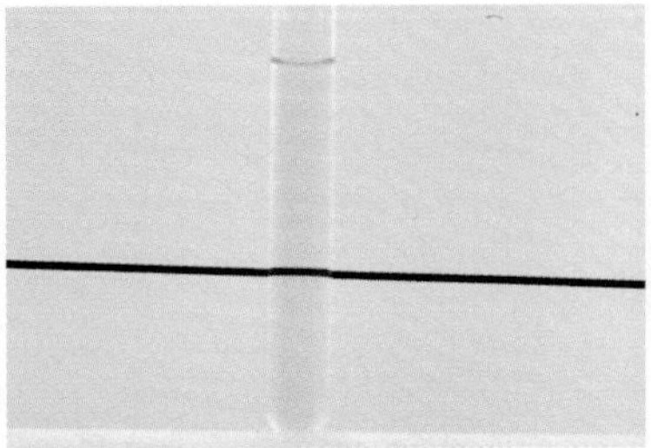

Plate 19–9A

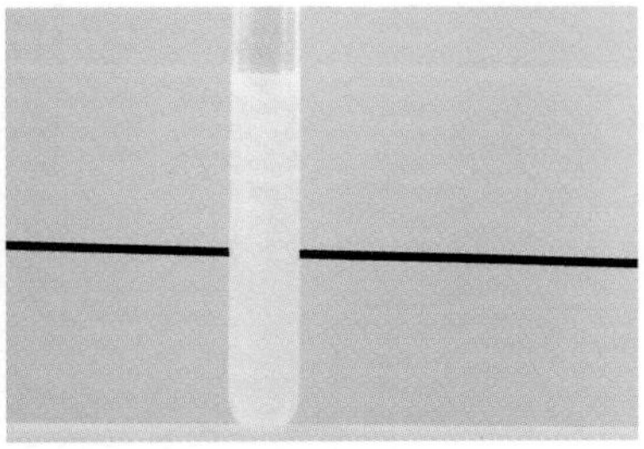

Plate 19–9B

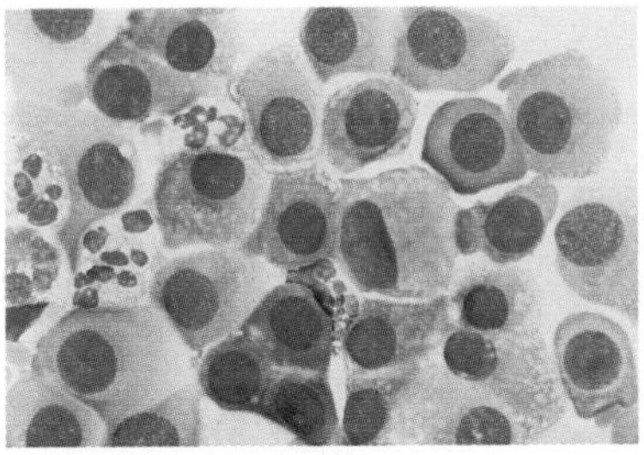

Plate 19–10

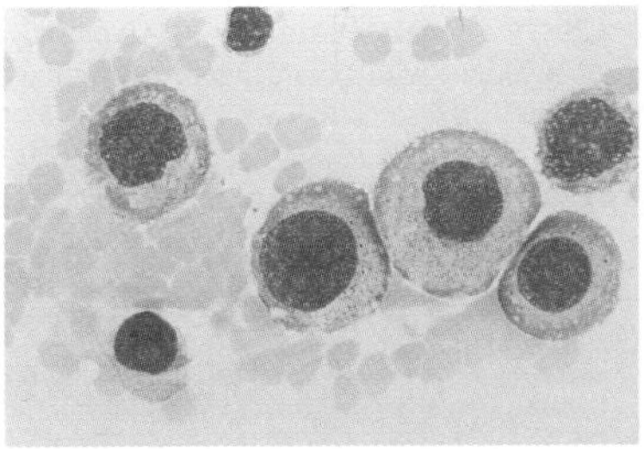

Plate 19–11

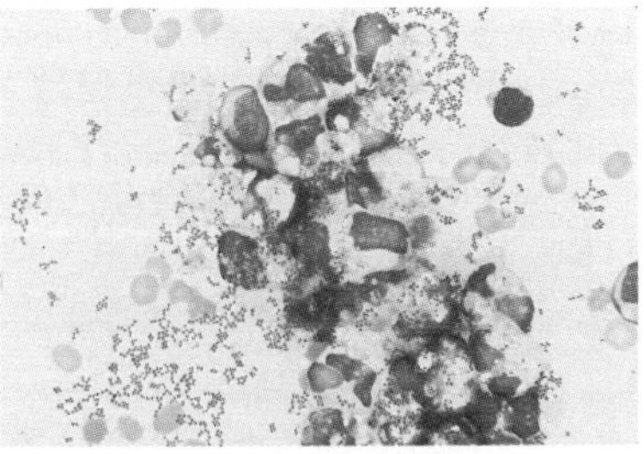

Plate 19–12

Plate 19–7. Corticosteroid crystals in synovial fluid. Compensated polarized light. **Plate 19–8.** Cholesterol crystals in synovial fluid. Polarized light. (Reproduced with permission from Kjeldsberg CR, Knight JA: Body Fluids: Laboratory Examination of Amniotic, Cerebrospinal, Seminal, Serous and Synovial Fluids, 3rd ed. © 1993 by the American Society of Clinical Pathologists, Chicago.) **Plate 19–9.** *A*, clear, pale yellow transudative pleural fluid; *B*, milky, opaque chylous pleural fluid. **Plate 19–10.** Mesothelial cells, pleural fluid. (Reproduced with permission from Kjeldsberg CR, Knight JA: Body Fluids: Laboratory Examination of Amniotic, Cerebrospinal, Seminal, Serous and Synovial Fluids, 3rd ed. © 1993 by the American Society of Clinical Pathologists, Chicago.) **Plate 19–11.** Adenocarcinoma cells in the pleural fluid of a patient with metastatic breast cancer. **Plate 19–12.** Bacterial peritonitis. Neutrophils often show degenerative changes.

Table 19–16. PLEURAL FLUID LABORATORY DIFFERENTIATION OF TRANSUDATES AND EXUDATES

	Transudate	Exudate
Appearance	Clear, pale yellow	Cloudy, turbid, purulent or bloody
Pleural fluid/serum protein ratio	<0.5	>0.5
Pleural fluid/serum LD ratio	<0.6	>0.6
Pleural fluid cholesterol	<60 mg/dL (<1.55 mmol/L)	>60 mg/dL (>1.55 mmol/L)
Pleural fluid/serum cholesterol ratio	<0.3	>0.3
Pleural fluid/serum bilirubin ratio	<0.6	>0.6

Values in parentheses are SI units.

Adapted from Kjeldsberg CR, Knight JA: Body Fluids: Laboratory Examination of Amniotic, Cerebrospinal, Seminal, Serous and Synovial Fluids, 3rd ed. © American Society of Clinical Pathologists, Chicago, 1993.

limit of normal (usually > 200 U/mL). Sensitivity is 98% and specificity is 77% for exudates (Romero, 1993).

Specificity may be improved by measuring pleural fluid cholesterol or bilirubin. A pleural fluid *cholesterol* level of more than 60 mg/dL, a *pleural fluid/serum cholesterol ratio* of more than 0.3, or a *pleural fluid/serum total bilirubin ratio* of 0.6 or more is associated with exudates (Hamm, 1987; Meisel, 1990; Valdés, 1991). Cholesterol concentrations with or without bilirubin measurements are recommended when protein and LD results are equivocal. These criteria are summarized in Table 19–16. None are 100% accurate in separating transudates from exudates.

Recommended Tests

The evaluation of serous body fluids (pleural, pericardial, peritoneal) is directed toward (1) differentiating transudative from exudative effusions; (2) identifying malignancy or infection in exudative effusions; and (3) establishing a specific diagnosis. Routine tests screen the effusion for an exudative process, an important characterization in pleural fluid because transudates generally do not require further evaluation. Further analysis of exudates is directed toward ruling out malignancy and infection. Cytology and appropriate cultures are the most useful tests in this regard. Recommended tests for the evaluation of pleural effusions are summarized in Table 19–17. The type of tests ordered and the interpretation of test results should always be correlated with the clinical findings and differential diagnosis. Total leukocyte counts and red cell counts are of limited use in the evaluation of serous effusions (Light, 1973b; Dines, 1975; Cheson, 1985).

Gross Examination

Transudates are typically clear, pale yellow to straw colored, odorless, and do not clot (Plate 19–9*A*). Approximately 15% of transudates may be blood-tinged (Light, 1990).

A bloody pleural effusion (hematocrit over 1%) suggests trauma, malignancy, or pulmonary infarction (Jay, 1986). A traumatic tap is suggested by uneven blood distribution,

Table 19–17. RECOMMENDED TESTS IN PLEURAL EFFUSION

Routine
- Gross examination
- Pleural fluid/serum protein ratio
- Pleural fluid/serum LD ratio
- Examination of stained smear

Useful in most patients
- Stains and cultures for microorganisms
- Cytology
- Pleural fluid cholesterol
- Pleural fluid/serum cholesterol ratio

Useful in certain circumstances
- pH
- Lactate
- Amylase
- Pleural biopsy
- Lipid analysis
- Immunologic studies
- Tumor markers
- Pleural fluid/serum bilirubin ratio

Adapted from Kjeldsberg CR, Knight JA: Body Fluids: Laboratory Examination of Amniotic, Cerebrospinal, Seminal, Serous and Synovial Fluids, 3rd ed. © American Society of Clinical Pathologists, Chicago, 1993.

3

clearing of the fluid with continued aspiration, or formation of small blood clots. A pleural fluid hematocrit of more than 50% of the blood hematocrit is good evidence of a hemothorax (Light, 1990).

Exudative processes may look like transudates, but most show variable degrees of cloudiness or turbidity and often clot if not heparinized. A feculent odor may be detected in patients with anaerobic infections. Turbid, milky, or bloody specimens should be centrifuged and the supernatant examined. If the supernatant is clear, the turbidity is mostly likely due to cellular elements or debris. If turbidity persists after centrifugation, a *chylous* or *pseudochylous* effusion is likely.

True chylous effusions are produced by leakage from the thoracic duct by lymphatic obstruction due to lymphoma or carcinoma, or by traumatic disruption (Plate 19–9*B*). A creamy top layer of chylomicrons may form if the specimen is allowed to stand. Idiopathic congenital chylothorax is the most common form of pleural effusion in the newborn.

Pseudochylous or chyliform effusions may have a milky, greenish, or "gold paint" appearance. They accumulate gradually through the breakdown of cellular lipids in long-standing effusions such as rheumatoid pleuritis, tuberculosis, or myxedema (Light, 1990). Features that distinguish true chylous from pseudochylous effusions are summarized in Table 19–18.

Microscopic Examination

CELL COUNTS. A leukocyte count of 1000 cells/μL has been used as a cut-off point between transudates (less than 1000 cells/μL) and exudates (over 1000 cells/μL), but considerable overlap makes this criterion unreliable: Red cell counts of more than 100,000 cells/μL are highly suggestive of malignancy, trauma, or pulmonary infarction. Formal cell counts have little practical value.

DIFFERENTIAL COUNT AND CYTOLOGY. Examination should be performed on a stained smear, preferably pre-

Table 19–18. DISTINGUISHING FEATURES IN CHYLOUS AND PSEUDOCHYLOUS EFFUSIONS

	Chylous	Pseudochylous
Onset	Sudden	Gradual
Appearance	Milky-white, or yellow-bloody	Milky or greenish, metallic sheen
Microscopic examination	Lymphocytosis	Mixed cellular reaction, cholesterol crystals
Triglycerides	>110 mg/dL (>1.24 mmol/L)	<50 mg/dL (<0.56 mmol/L)*
Lipoprotein electrophoresis	Chylomicrons present	Chylomicrons absent

*Some pseudochylous effusions have triglyceride levels higher than 110 mg/dL. Values in parentheses are SI units.

Modified from Kjeldsberg CR, Knight JA: Body Fluids: Laboratory Examination of Amniotic, Cerebrospinal, Seminal, Serous and Synovial Fluids, 3rd ed. © American Society of Clinical Pathologists, Chicago, 1993.

pared by cytocentrifugation and an air-dried Romanowsky's stain (Venrick, 1993). Filtration methods with Papanicolaou's stain may also be used, especially if there is concern about cell loss. Preparation of cell blocks is unnecessary except for effusions in which malignancy is a consideration (Jonasson, 1990).

Mesothelial cells are common in pleural fluids from inflammatory processes (Plate 19–10). They are however conspicuously scarce in patients with tuberculous pleurisy, empyema, or rheumatoid pleuritis and those who have had pleurodesis because fibrin deposition and fibrosis prevent exfoliation of the mesothelial cells (Kjeldsberg, 1993). Carcinoma cells may closely mimic mesothelial cells (Plate 19–11) and may require a panel of immunocytochemical stains for confirmation (Kjeldsberg, 1993).

Neutrophils predominate in pleural fluid from patients with inflammation of the pleura (Table 19–19). Over 10% of transudates also show a predominance of neutrophils, but this has no clinical significance.

Lymphocytes predominate in the disorders summarized in Table 19–19. Most are small, but medium, large, and reactive (transformed) variants may be seen. Nucleoli and nuclear cleaving are more prominent in effusions than in the peripheral blood. *Plasma cells* may also be observed. Lymphocytosis associated with transudates is of no clinical significance.

Low-grade non-Hodgkin's lymphomas or CLL may be difficult to distinguish from benign lymphocyte-rich effusions. Immunophenotyping by flow cytometry or immunocytochemistry, used in conjunction with cellular morphology, is usually helpful for making a correct diagnosis (Katz, 1987). However, the relative proportions of T cells, B cells, and light chains are by themselves not definitive for separating benign from malignant exudates (Ibrahim, 1989).

An eosinophilic effusion is defined as an effusion that has more than 10% eosinophils. The most common causes are related to the presence of air or blood in the pleural cavity (see Table 19–19). In about 35% of patients the cause is unknown (Adelman, 1984). A small number of *mast cells* or *basophils* often accompany the eosinophils. Eosinophil-derived *Charcot-Leyden* crystals may be seen.

Lupus erythematosus (LE) cells and related Tart cells may be found in a minority of effusions from patients with systemic lupus erythematosus (Naylor, 1992).

Table 19–19. CELLULAR DIFFERENTIAL OF PLEURAL EFFUSIONS

Neutrophilia (>50%)
Bacterial pneumonia (parapneumonic effusion)
Pulmonary infarction
Pancreatitis
Subphrenic abscess
Early tuberculosis
Transudates (over 10%)
Lymphocytosis (>50%)
Tuberculosis (mesothelial cells rare)
Viral infection
Malignancy
True chylothorax
Rheumatoid pleuritis
Systemic lupus erythematosus
Uremic effusions
Transudates (approximately 30%)
Eosinophilia (>10%)
Air in pleural space
Trauma
Pulmonary infarction
Congestive heart failure
Infection (especially parasitic, fungal)
Hypersensitivity syndromes
Drug reaction
Rheumatologic diseases
Hodgkin's disease
Idiopathic

Chemical Analysis

PROTEIN. Measurement of pleural fluid total protein has little clinical usefulness except when it is combined with other parameters to differentiate exudates from transudates. Protein electrophoresis shows a pattern similar to that of serum protein except for a higher proportion of albumin and has little value for differential diagnosis (Light, 1990).

GLUCOSE. The glucose level of normal pleural fluid, transudates, and most exudates is similar to serum glucose levels. Decreased pleural fluid glucose, accepted as a level below 60 mg/dL (3.33 mmol/L) or a pleural fluid/serum glucose ratio of less than 0.5 (Sahn, 1982), is most consistent and dramatic in rheumatoid pleuritis and grossly purulent parapneumonic exudates. Effusions due to malignancy, tuberculosis, nonpurulent bacterial infections, lupus pleuritis, and esophageal rupture have low glucose levels in a minority of cases (sensitivity 15% to 25%) (Light, 1973a; Sahn, 1980).

LACTATE. Pleural fluid levels of lactate can be a useful adjunct in the rapid diagnosis of infectious pleuritis. Levels are significantly higher in patients with bacterial and tuberculous pleural infections than in those with other pleural effusions; moderate elevations are observed in malignant effusions (Brook, 1980). Values greater than 90 mg/dL (10 mmol/L) have a positive predictive value for infectious pleuritis of 94% and a negative predictive value of 100% (Gästrin, 1988).

ENZYMES. Elevations of *amylase* activity above the

serum level (usually 1.5 to 2.0 times greater or more) indicate the presence of pancreatitis, esophageal rupture, or malignant effusion (Light, 1973a). Elevated amylase levels resulting from esophageal rupture or malignancy differ from those found in pancreatitis in that the salivary isoform is also increased (Sherr, 1972; Kramer, 1989). Isoenzyme evaluation may therefore help in diagnosing effusions with elevated amylase levels of unknown origin.

LD levels in pleural fluid rise in proportion to the degree of pleural inflammation. In addition to the use of LD in separating exudates from transudates, declining LD levels during the course of an effusion indicate that the inflammatory process is resolving, whereas increasing levels indicate a worsening condition requiring aggressive workup or treatment. LD isoenzyme analysis may rarely be helpful in diagnosing problematic exudates (Vergnon, 1984) but is not recommended for routine use.

pH. The pH of normal pleural fluid is 7.64 (Good, 1980). A parapneumonic exudate with a pH of more than 7.20 to 7.30 generally resolves completely with medical therapy alone. A combination of low pH (<7.30) and low glucose (<60 mg/dL or 3.33 mmol/L) indicates (1) a complicated parapneumonic effusion (loculated or associated with empyema) that requires surgical drainage; (2) rheumatoid pleuritis; or (3) a malignant effusion with a poorer prognosis and response to pleurodesis (Potts, 1978; Good, 1980; Rodriquez-Panadero, 1989). A pH value of below 6.0 is characteristic of esophageal rupture, although severe empyema is sometimes also this low (Good, 1980).

Urinothorax, a collection of urine presumably produced by lymphatic drainage of perirenal accumulations into the pleural cavity, is also associated with a pleural fluid pH of less than 7.30. These effusions are transudative because of their low protein content, and they have a creatinine level greater than that of simultaneously drawn serum (Miller, 1988).

LIPIDS. Lipid measurements are helpful in identifying chylous effusions. Pleural fluid triglyceride levels above 110 mg/dL indicate a chylous effusion. Values of between 60 and 110 mg/dL (0.68 to 1.24 mmol/L) are less certain and require lipoprotein electrophoresis for chylomicrons to confirm a chylothorax (Staats, 1980). Nonchylous and pseudochylous effusions generally have triglyceride levels of under 50 mg/dL (0.56 mmol/L) and no chylomicrons.

Cholesterol measurements are useful in separating transudates from exudates, as described earlier. Elevated levels and the presence of cholesterol crystals are seen rarely in association with long-standing pleural effusions, usually of several years duration.

TUMOR MARKERS. *Carcinoembryonic antigen* (CEA) is the most useful fluid marker for malignancy, but reported cut-off values vary considerably. Sensitivity for malignant effusions is about 40% to 50% overall and 60% to 70% for lung or breast carcinoma using a cut-off value of 5 ng/mL (Mezger, 1988; Tamura, 1988).

Immunologic Studies

Approximately 5% of patients with RA and 50% of those with systemic lupus erythematosus develop pleural effusions at some time during the course of their disease.

RF is commonly present in pleural effusions associated with seropositive RA. Although a pleural fluid titer of 1:320 or greater in a patient with known RA is reasonable evidence of rheumatic pleuritis (Halla, 1980), elevated RF titers (up to 1:1280) have been identified in 41% of patients with bacterial pneumonia, 20% of patients with malignant effusions, and 14% of patients with tuberculosis, making a routine test for RF of little value (Levine, 1968).

ANA titers may be useful in the diagnosis of effusions due to lupus pleuritis because they have a sensitivity of about 85% using a cut-off titer of 1:160 (Good, 1983). Specificity is not high, however, because elevated ANA titers also occur in other conditions.

Decreased *complement levels* (CH_{50} below 10 U/mL or C4 levels below 10×10^{-5} U/g protein) are seen in most patients with rheumatoid or lupus pleuritis (Hunder, 1972; Halla, 1980). These measurements are not highly specific, however, and are of little value for routine diagnosis. They are sometimes helpful in the diagnosis of otherwise enigmatic effusions.

3

Microbiologic Examination

Bacteria most commonly associated with parapneumonic effusions are *Staphylococcus aureus* and certain gram-negative bacilli. Anaerobic bacteria are isolated in a significant proportion of cases, so both anaerobic and aerobic cultures should be performed in patients with parapneumonic effusions (Bartlett, 1974).

The sensitivity of Gram's stain is not well documented in pleural fluid, but, as in other body fluids, it rarely exceeds 70% (Kjeldsberg, 1993). Screening specimens stained with acridine orange can increase sensitivity by 20% (Hanes, 1988). This stain is recommended for laboratories with fluorescent microscopy capability.

Direct staining of tuberculous effusions for acid-fast bacteria has a sensitivity of about 10%, and cultures are positive in only about 30% of cases (Kumar, 1981). *Pleural biopsy* yields the highest culture sensitivity (50% to 75%) and may provide a rapid presumptive diagnosis of tuberculosis by histopathologic demonstration of granulomas. The combination of culture and acid-fast stains with pleural biopsy can increase the sensitivity up to 95% (Jay, 1986). Analysis for *adenosine deaminase* or *interferon-gamma*, if available, can provide rapid chemical evidence of tuberculous effusions in immunocompetent hosts (Ribera, 1988; Hsu, 1993).

PERICARDIAL FLUID

From 10 to 50 mL of fluid is normally present in the pericardial space, produced by a transudative process similar to pleural fluid. Pericardial effusion may be produced by inflammatory, malignant, or hemorrhagic processes; common causes are summarized in Table 19–20. Many of the recommended laboratory tests described for pleural fluid (see Table 19–17) also pertain to pericardial effusions. The value of separating pericardial fluid accumulations into transudates and exudates is not established, however.

Table 19–20. CAUSES OF PERICARDIAL EFFUSIONS

Infection
Bacterial pericarditis
Tuberculosis
Fungal pericarditis
Viral or mycoplasma pericarditis
AIDS-related
Neoplasm
Metastatic carcinoma
Lymphoma
Myocardial infarct
Hemorrhage
Trauma
Anticoagulant therapy
Leakage of aortic aneurysm
Metabolic
Uremia
Myxedema
Rheumatoid disease
Systemic lupus erythematosus

Specimen Collection and Gross Examination

Pericardial effusions of unknown cause or large effusions generally require laboratory examination. Fluid is obtained either by pericardiotomy following limited thoracotomy or by pericardiocentesis, the sterile aspiration of fluid by needle. Normal pericardial fluid is pale yellow and clear. Large effusions (> 350 mL) are most often caused by malignancy or uremia or are idiopathic (Colombo, 1988; Corey, 1993). AIDS is becoming an increasingly common cause of large pericardial effusions (Reynolds, 1992).

Infection or malignancy typically produces turbid effusions, whereas effusions due to uremia are usually clear and straw-colored. These and several other conditions may also produce hemorrhagic effusions.

Bloodlike fluid obtained by pericardiocentesis may represent hemorrhagic effusion or inadvertent aspiration of blood from the heart. Blood obtained from a heart chamber has a hematocrit comparable to that of peripheral blood, and blood gas analysis yields results similar to those obtained with venous or arterial blood. In contrast, the hematocrit of a hemorrhagic effusion is usually lower than that of the peripheral blood. Blood gas analysis shows a pH and Po_2 that are lower and a Pco_2 that is higher than those of venous or arterial blood (Mann, 1978). Blood from a cardiac puncture clots, whereas a hemorrhagic effusion usually does not.

A milky appearance suggests the presence of a true chylous or pseudochylous effusion. Identification and differentiation of these are discussed in the earlier section, Pleural Fluids, Gross Examination (page 17).

Microscopic Examination

Hematocrit and red cell counts document the presence of a hemorrhagic effusion but are of limited value for differential diagnosis.

Total leukocyte counts of over 10,000 cells/μL suggest bacterial, tuberculous, or malignant pericarditis. However, low counts are also encountered in these conditions, limiting the value of this measurement (Agner, 1979). Formal leukocyte differentials add little diagnostic information, but a stained smear should always be examined.

Cytologic identification of malignant cells is usually not difficult. Metastatic carcinoma of the lung and breast are most frequently observed in malignant pericardial effusions and are virtually never the initial presentation (Yazdi, 1980; Monte, 1987). Cytology has a sensitivity of 87%, a specificity of 100%, and a diagnostic accuracy of 94% (Meyers, 1989).

Chemical Analysis

PROTEIN. Protein determination is of little diagnostic value in the differential diagnosis of pericardial effusions.

GLUCOSE. Pericardial glucose levels may be decreased to less than 40 mg/dL (< 2.22 mmol/L) in bacterial, tuberculous, rheumatic, or malignant effusions. Glucose determination has little practical value in differential diagnosis, however.

pH. Pericardial fluid pH may be markedly decreased (< 7.10) in rheumatic or purulent conditions. Malignancy, uremia, tuberculosis, and idiopathic disorders may have moderate decreases in the range of 7.20 to 7.40 (Kindig, 1983). The value of pH measurements in diagnosis requires further evaluation.

LIPIDS. Separation of true chylous and pseudochylous effusions may be facilitated by triglyceride and cholesterol measurements as well as by lipoprotein electrophoresis for chylomicrons.

ENZYMES. *Adenosine deaminase* activity is a useful adjunctive test for tuberculous pericarditis in cases with negative stains in which tuberculosis is suspected. Sensitivity has been reported to be 93% and specificity 97% using a cut-off value of 40 U/L (Koh, 1994).

Immunologic Studies

High titers of antinuclear antibody have been described in effusions associated with lupus erythematosus but are not specific for that condition (Leventhal, 1990).

Microbiologic Examination

The sensitivity of Gram's stain and culture of pericardial fluid for bacterial pericarditis is about 50% to 80%, respectively, similar to results in other body fluids.

Diagnosis of a specific etiologic agent in viral pericarditis is generally unnecessary because morbidity is low, and pericardial fluid viral cultures usually do not grow an organism (Bellinger, 1987).

Sensitivity of acid-fast stains and culture for tuberculous pericarditis is about 50% (Agner, 1979). Sensitivity may be increased to as high as 90% if a pericardiectomy tissue specimen is also provided.

PERITONEAL FLUID

Up to 50 mL of fluid is normally present in the mesothelium-lined potential space that represents the peritoneal cavity. Like pleural and pericardial fluid, peritoneal fluid is produced as an ultrafiltrate of plasma that is dependent on vascular permeability and hydrostatic and oncotic Starling forces. A patient with a peritoneal effusion is said to have *ascites*, and the fluid is known as *ascitic fluid*.

Transudates and Exudates

Some common causes of peritoneal effusions are listed in Table 19–21. Laboratory criteria for dividing ascitic fluid into transudates and exudates are not as well defined as they are for pleural fluid. For example, infected or malignancy-related samples are not uncommonly reported with protein concentrations in the transudate range, and many patients with cirrhotic ascites or heart failure have protein values in the exudative range (Runyon, 1992).

The *serum-ascites albumin gradient*, defined as the serum albumin concentration minus the ascitic fluid albumin concentration, is considered a more physiologically appropriate test. Ascites caused by portal hypertension has a gradient of at least 1.1 g/dL (≥ 11 g/L), whereas ascites produced by other causes has a gradient of < 1.1 g/dL (Runyon, 1992). Like every other criterion used to separate transudates from exudates, the serum-ascites albumin gradient is an imperfect discriminator. Patients with "mixed" ascites, for example, hepatic cirrhosis with ascites and peritoneal tuberculosis, tend to have wide gradients.

Specimen Collection

PARACENTESIS. Diagnostic paracentesis is performed in most patients with new ascites or if there is a change in the clinical picture of a patient with existing ascites such as rapid fluid accumulation or development of fever. A minimum of 30 mL is needed for complete evaluation. If possible, at least 100 mL should be provided for cytologic examination. Samples for cell counts should be placed in a lavender top (EDTA) tube (Becton Dickinson, Rutherford, NJ). Culture specimens should include blood culture bottles that have been inoculated at the bedside with ascitic fluid (Marshall, 1988).

DIAGNOSTIC PERITONEAL LAVAGE (DPL). This procedure is useful in the triage of patients with blunt or penetrating trauma to the abdominal area who have equivocal clinical signs of internal injury or are otherwise unresponsive to examination. A peritoneal dialysis catheter is inserted through a small incision into the abdominal cavity. If less than 15 mL of gross blood can be aspirated, DPL is performed by infusing 1 liter of saline or Ringer's lactate (20 mg/kg in children) and retrieving the fluid by gravity drainage. At least 600 mL should be recovered to ensure reliable results (Feied, 1989). The catheter is sometimes left in place so that DPL can be repeated in 2 to 3 hours if the initial results are negative or indeterminate.

Commonly accepted criteria for interpretation of DPL after trauma are shown in Table 19–22. Positive results have a sensitivity of 96%, a specificity of 99%, and an overall accuracy of about 98% for blunt abdominal trauma (Gomez, 1987). The positive predictive value is reported to be only 23% for an isolated (no other abnormal criteria) leukocyte count of 500/L or greater, however (Soyka, 1990). Sensitivity and specificity are somewhat less with penetrating trauma.

Other applications of DPL include the evaluation of patients with suspected acute peritonitis or pancreatitis (Robert, 1986; Larson, 1992).

PERITONEAL DIALYSIS. Dialysate fluid from patients with renal disease undergoing chronic ambulatory peritoneal dialysis is examined for evidence of infection.

PERITONEAL WASHINGS. The peritoneal cavity is flooded with saline solution and "washed" intraoperatively to document early intra-abdominal spread of ovarian and endometrial carcinomas. Samples are generally sent for cytologic examination only.

Recommended Tests

The most useful tests for the evaluation of peritoneal fluid are listed in Table 19–23. Relative importance varies depending on the type of sample and the clinical indications. RBC and leukocyte counts, for example, are more important than cytology or the serum-ascites albumin gradient in the

Table 19–21. CAUSES OF PERITONEAL EFFUSIONS

Transudates (increased hydrostatic pressure or decreased plasma oncotic pressure)
Congestive heart failure
Hepatic cirrhosis
Hypoproteinemia (e.g., nephrotic syndrome)
Exudates (increased capillary permeability or decreased lymphatic resorption)
Infections
Tuberculosis
Primary bacterial peritonitis
Secondary bacterial peritonitis (e.g., appendicitis)
Neoplasms
Hepatoma
Metastatic carcinoma
Lymphoma
Mesothelioma
Trauma
Pancreatitis
Bile peritonitis (e.g., ruptured gallbladder)
Chylous effusion
Damage or obstruction to thoracic duct (e.g., trauma, lymphoma, carcinoma, tuberculosis, parasitic infestation)

Table 19–22. STANDARD CRITERIA FOR EVALUATION OF PERITONEAL LAVAGE

Positive result
Aspiration of >15 mL gross blood on catheter placement
Grossly bloody lavage fluid
RBC > 100,000/µL after blunt trauma
RBC > 50,000/µL after penetrating trauma
WBC > 500/µL
Indeterminate
Small amount of gross blood on catheter placement
RBC 50,000–100,000/µL after blunt trauma
RBC 1000–50,000/µL after penetrating trauma
WBC 100–500/µL
Negative
RBC < 50,000/µL after blunt trauma
RBC < 1000/µL after penetrating trauma
WBC < 100/µL

Modified from Feied CF: Diagnostic peritoneal lavage. Postgrad Med 1989; 85(4):40.

3

Table 19–23. RECOMMENDED TESTS IN PERITONEAL EFFUSION

Useful in most patients
Gross examination
Cytology
Stains and culture for organisms
Serum-ascites albumin concentration gradient
Useful in certain circumstances
Leukocyte count and differential count
RBC count (lavage)
Alkaline phosphatase
Cholesterol (malignancy-related ascites)
Amylase
Tumor markers
Immunology-flow cytometry
Lactate dehydrogenase

Modified from Kjeldsberg CR, Knight JA: Body Fluids: Laboratory Examination of Amniotic, Cerebrospinal, Seminal, Serous and Synovial Fluids, 3rd ed. © American Society of Clinical Pathologists, Chicago, 1993.

evaluation of trauma. Gross examination provides immediate information that is useful in clinical and laboratory triage.

Gross Examination

Transudates are usually pale yellow and clear. Exudates are cloudy or turbid due to accumulation of leukocytes, tumor cells, or protein. The presence of food particles, foreign material, or green bile staining in a DPL specimen indicates perforation of the gastrointestinal tract or biliary tract. Acute pancreatitis and cholecystitis may also cause green discoloration.

Blood-tinged or grossly bloody fluid must be distinguished from traumatic tap, in which the blood usually clears with continued paracentesis. As little as 15 mL of blood turns a liter of fluid bright red and opaque, so that newsprint cannot be read through the lavage tubing. This corresponds to an RBC count of 100,000/μL and provides immediate feedback to the surgeon performing the DPL. Bloody ascites not related to traumatic tap is also seen in malignancy and tuberculosis.

Milky fluid that does not clear with centrifugation suggests a chylous or pseudochylous effusion. True chylous effusions are rare. They are caused by disruption or blockage of lymphatic flow by trauma, lymphoma, carcinoma, tuberculosis, hepatic cirrhosis, adhesions, or parasitic infestation (Lesser, 1970). Differentiation of true chylous and pseudochylous effusions is discussed in the earlier section Pleural Fluid, Gross Examination (page 17).

Microscopic Examination

The total leukocyte count is useful in distinguishing ascites due to uncomplicated cirrhosis from spontaneous bacterial peritonitis (SBP), which is caused by migration of bacteria from the intestine into the ascitic fluid (Plate 19–12). Approximately 90% of patients with SBP have leukocyte counts of greater than 500 cells/μL, over 50% of which are neutrophils (Runyon, 1984; Stewart, 1986).

Ascitic fluid absolute neutrophil counts have become the preferred method for the diagnosis of SBP. Cut-off values of 250 and 500 neutrophils/μL have been used; diagnostic accuracy is about 94% for 500 cells/μL and about 90% for 250 cells/μL (Stassen, 1986; Albillos, 1990).

Cell counts and protein and albumin gradient values vary with fluid shifts associated with ascites formation and resolution. Diuresis, for example, can cause the WBC to increase from 300 cells/μL to 1000/μL or more. When obtained by DPL, a leukocyte count of 200 cells/μL or more is reported to be associated with a 99% probability of acute peritonitis (Alverdy, 1988; Larson, 1992).

Eosinophilia (> 10%) is most commonly associated with chronic peritoneal dialysis but has also been reported with congestive heart failure, vasculitis, lymphoma, and ruptured hydatid cyst (Adams, 1977).

Cytology has an overall sensitivity of 40% to 60% for malignant ascites. However, peritoneal carcinomatosis accounts only for about two-thirds of malignant effusions; cytology has a sensitivity of more than 95% when confined to these cases (Runyon, 1988). Immunocytochemical stains are useful in characterizing atypical cells in equivocal cases (Kjeldsberg, 1993). DNA ploidy studies by flow cytometry are too insensitive for routine use but may identify an aneuploid peak in selected cases in which cytology is equivocal or negative (Weisman, 1987; Zarbo, 1991).

Chemical Analysis

PROTEIN. As discussed previously, the serum-ascites albumin gradient is superior to the total protein content in differentiating cirrhosis from other forms of peritoneal effusion (Runyon, 1992). Spontaneous bacterial peritonitis is often associated with a low protein level and a high gradient, however, making protein measurements of little value in this disorder. Extracellular fluid shifts associated with ascites formation and resorption also cause variations in protein content.

GLUCOSE. Peritoneal fluid glucose levels are reportedly decreased in 30% to 60% of cases of tuberculous peritonitis and in approximately 50% of patients with abdominal carcinomatosis (Polak, 1973; Brown, 1976). However, sensitivity and specificity are generally too low to be of practical value.

ENZYMES. *Amylase* activity in normal peritoneal fluid is similar to blood levels. An ascites level of more than three times the serum value is good evidence of a pancreatic origin, such as acute pancreatitis, pancreatic pseudocyst, or trauma (Runyon, 1987a). Gastroduodenal perforation, acute mesenteric vein thrombosis, or intestinal strangulation or necrosis may also produce elevated amylase levels. Various nonpancreatic malignancies may rarely produce elevations of ascites amylase. Isoenzyme evaluation usually shows the salivary isoform in these cases (Kosches, 1989). Routine amylase measurement is not cost-effective in the evaluation of trauma (Alyono, 1981). It is not recommended in the routine evaluation of ascites because the prevalence of pancreatic ascites is low. Retrospective amylase measurement on a stored specimen is indicated, however, if initial studies are not diagnostic.

Elevated *alkaline phosphatase* levels (> 10 IU/L) have some value in predicting bowel injury in patients with indeterminate diagnostic peritoneal lavage who would otherwise not undergo laparotomy (Jaffin, 1993).

LD activity is often increased in patients with malignant effusions (Gerbes, 1991). An ascitic fluid/serum LD ratio of greater than 0.6 has a reported sensitivity of 80% (Boyer, 1978). Combined measurement of ascitic fluid LD and cholesterol is purported to achieve total discrimination of peritoneal carcinomatosis from cirrhosis and hepatocarcinoma-related ascites (Castaldo, 1994). Additional studies are necessary to confirm the value of this combination. LD has also been used for the early diagnosis of spontaneous bacterial peritonitis, in which it has a diagnostic accuracy of about 74% using an ascitic fluid/serum ratio cut-off point of 0.4 (Lee, 1987).

LACTATE. Ascitic fluid lactate has been used with pH measurements to differentiate SBP from uncomplicated ascites. Sensitivity and specificity are approximately 90% using a cut-off value of 40 mg/dL (4.44 mmol/L), with a positive predictive value of 62% (Stassen, 1986). Although not as accurate as leukocyte counts, the high specificity of lactate in hepatic ascites suggests that it has some value in the diagnosis of SBP in otherwise equivocal cases. Malignant and tuberculous ascites are also associated with elevated lactate.

Patients with hollow viscus perforation, gangrenous intestine, peritonitis, or intra-abdominal abscess have a peritoneal fluid minus plasma lactate level of at least 1.5 mmol/L (13.5 mg/dL), which reportedly separates these patients completely from those with other conditions producing acute conditions of the abdomen (DeLaurier, 1994). Additional studies are necessary to determine the use of lactate measurement in surgical decision making.

CREATININE AND UREA. Measurement of creatinine and urea nitrogen is sometimes useful to differentiate peritoneal fluid from urine. Elevated peritoneal urea nitrogen and creatinine associated with elevated serum urea but normal creatinine (due to back-diffusion of urea) suggests bladder rupture (Kjeldsberg, 1993).

AMMONIA. Levels significantly greater than the accompanying blood values (twice the upper limit of normal for plasma) have been associated with perforated peptic ulcer, ruptured appendix, bowel strangulation, and ruptured bladder with extravasation of urine (Mansberger, 1967). The clinical value of this measurement has yet to be established.

BILIRUBIN. Ascitic fluid bilirubin greater than 6.0 mg/dL (103 μmol/L) and an ascitic fluid/serum bilirubin ratio of over 1.0 suggests choleperitoneum from a ruptured gallbladder (Runyon, 1987b).

pH. Ascitic fluid pH may be helpful in the diagnosis of SBP in patients with cirrhotic ascites, especially if it is used in conjunction with leukocyte counts (Attali, 1986; Stassen, 1986). A pH of less than 7.32 or a blood-ascitic fluid pH difference of more than 0.1 have a reported sensitivity and specificity of about 90% for SBP, the pH differential being slightly more accurate. Patients with an ascitic fluid pH of less than 7.15 have a poor prognosis (Attali, 1986). Low pH is also found in patients with malignant and pancreatic ascites and tuberculous peritonitis (Attali, 1986; Stassen, 1986; Albillos, 1990).

LIPIDS. Ascitic fluid cholesterol is moderately useful in separating malignant ascites from cirrhotic ascites (Mortensen, 1988; Castaldo, 1994). Sensitivity and specificity average about 90% using a cut-off value of 45 to 48 mg/dL (1.2 mmol/L).

TUMOR MARKERS. These tests are seldom necessary for the diagnosis of carcinoma in the presence of a good cytologic examination but have some practical value in following the patient's response to therapy. CEA has a sensitivity of only 40% to 50% and a specificity of about 90% using a cut-off point of 3 ng/mL (Mezger, 1988).

Ascitic fluid CA-125 is elevated to some degree in a variety of nonmalignant conditions. Extremely high levels are more likely to be caused by epithelial carcinomas of the ovary, fallopian tubes, or endometrium, however. Using a cut-off point of 3652 U/mL, the sensitivity of CA-125 for müllerian epithelial carcinomas is about 70%, with a specificity of nearly 100% (Pinto, 1992).

Microbiologic Examination

In SPB Gram's stain has a sensitivity of only 25% (Lee, 1987), and routine cultures are positive in only about 50% of cases (Castellote, 1990). Inoculation of blood culture bottles at the bedside and concentration of large volumes of fluid can improve sensitivity, but up to 35% of infected patients may still have negative ascitic fluid cultures (Marshall, 1988).

The sensitivity of acid-fast stains for tuberculosis is no more than 20% to 30%. Cultures have a sensitivity of 50% to 70% (Reimer, 1985). Laparoscopic examination with biopsy may be helpful in cases in which tuberculosis is suspected. Adenosine deaminase activity in ascitic fluid is elevated in nearly all cases of tuberculous peritonitis studied (Voigt, 1989; Dwivedi, 1990).

3

Cerebrospinal Fluid

Abramson JS, Hampton KD, Babu S, et al: The use of C-reactive protein from cerebrospinal fluid for differentiating meningitis from other central nervous system diseases. J Infect Dis 1985; 151:854.

Albright RE, Christenson RH, Emlet JL, et al: Issues in cerebrospinal fluid management. CSF Venereal Disease Research Laboratory testing. Am J Clin Pathol 1991; 95:397.

Albright RE, Christenson RH, Habig RL, et al: Cerebrospinal fluid (CSF) TRAP: A method to improve CSF laboratory efficiency. Am J Clin Pathol 1988; 90:707.

American College of Physicians: The diagnostic spinal tap. Ann Intern Med 1986; 104:880.

Bailey EM, Domenico P, Cunha BA: Bacterial or viral meningitis? Measuring lactate in CSF can help you know quickly. Postgrad Med 1990; 88:217.

Benjamin DR, Opheim KE, Brewer L: Is C-reactive protein useful in the management of children with suspected bacterial meningitis? Am J Clin Pathol 1984; 81:779.

Benson RL, Ansbacher L, Hutchison RE, et al: Cerebrospinal fluid centrifuge analysis in primary amebic meningoencephalitis due to *Naegleria fowleri*. Arch Pathol Lab Med 1985; 109:668.

Bigner SH: Cerebrospinal fluid (CSF) cytology: Current status and diagnostic applications. J Neuropathol Exp Neurol 1992; 51:235.

Blake J, Berman P: The use of adenosine deaminase in the diagnosis of tuberculosis. S Afr Med J 1982; 62:19.

Bonadio WA, Smith DS, Goddard S, et al: Distinguishing cerebrospinal fluid abnormalities in children with bacterial meningitis and traumatic lumbar puncture. J Infect Dis 1990; 162:251.

Bouza E, Dreyer JS, Hewitt WL, et al: Coccidioidal meningitis: An analysis of thirty-one cases and review of the literature. Medicine 1981; 60:139.

Britton C, Hultman E, Murray V, et al: The diagnostic accuracy of CSF analyses in stroke. Acta Med Scand 1983; 214:3.

Cameron PD, Boyce JM, Ansari BM: Cerebrospinal fluid lactate in meningitis and meningococcaemia. J Infect 1993; 26:245.

Centers for Disease Control and Prevention: Diagnosis of tuberculosis by nucleic acid amplification methods applied to clinical specimens. MMWR, 1993; 42:686.

Chalmers AC, Aprill BS, Shephard H: Cerebrospinal fluid and human immunodeficiency virus: Findings in healthy, asymptomatic, seropositive men. Arch Intern Med 1990; 150:1538.

College of American Pathologists (CAP): Chemistry Survey Set M-B, 1991.

Davis LE, Schmitt JW: Clinical significance of cerebrospinal fluid tests for neurosyphilis. Ann Neurol 1989; 25:50.

DeSalles AAF, Kontos HA, Becker DP, et al: Prognostic significance of ventricular CSF lactic acidosis in severe head injury. J Neurosurg 1986; 65:615.

Donald PR, Malan C: Cerebrospinal fluid lactate and lactate dehydrogenase activity in the rapid diagnosis of bacterial meningitis. S Afr Med J 1986; 69:39.

dos Santos JGN: Fatal primary amebic meningoencephalitis: A retrospective study in Richmond, Virginia. Am J Clin Pathol 1970; 54:737.

Dyson D, Cassaday G: Use of limulus lysate for detecting gram-negative neonatal meningitis. Pediatrics 1976; 58:105.

Edberg SC: Conventional and molecular techniques for the laboratory diagnosis of infections of the central nervous system. Neurol Clin 1986; 4:13.

Engelke S, Bridgers S, Saldanha RL, et al: Cerebrospinal fluid lactate dehydrogenase in neonatal intracranial hemorrhage. Am J Med Sci 1986; 291:391.

Fishman RA: Cerebrospinal Fluid in Diseases of the Nervous System, 2nd ed. Philadelphia, W. B. Saunders, 1992.

Gerbaut L, Macart M: Is standardization more important than methodology for assay of total protein in cerebrospinal fluid? Clin Chem 1986; 32:353.

Graves M: Cerebrospinal fluid infections. *In* Herndon RM, Brumback RA (eds): The Cerebrospinal Fluid. Boston, Kluwer Academic Publishers, 1989, p 143.

Greenlee JE: Approach to diagnosis of meningitis. Cerebrospinal fluid examination. Infect Dis Clin N Am 1990; 4:583.

Hall CD, Snyder CR, Robertson KR, et al: Cerebrospinal fluid analysis in human immunodeficiency virus infection. Ann Clin Lab Sci 1992; 22:139.

Hayward RA, Oye RK: Are polymorphonuclear leukocytes an abnormal finding in cerebrospinal fluid? Results from 225 normal cerebrospinal fluid specimens. Arch Intern Med 1988; 148:1623.

Hayward RA, Shapiro MF, Oye RK: Laboratory testing on cerebrospinal fluid: A reappraisal. Lancet 1987; 8523:1.

Herndon RM, Brumback RA (eds): The Cerebrospinal Fluid. Boston, Kluwer Academic Publishers, 1989.

Hische EAH, Tutuarima JA, Wolters EC, et al: Cerebrospinal fluid IgG and IgM indexes as indicators of active neurosyphilis. Clin Chem 1988; 34:665.

Jeffrey GM, Frampton CM, Legge HM, et al: Cerebrospinal fluid b2-microglobulin levels in meningeal involvement by malignancy. Pathology 1990; 22:20.

Jones HD, Urquhart N, Mathias RG, et al: An evaluation of oligoclonal banding and CSF IgG index in the diagnosis of neurosyphilis. Sex Transm Dis 1990; 17:75.

Kärkelä J, Pasanen M, Kaukinen S, et al: Evaluation of hypoxic brain injury with spinal fluid enzymes, lactate, and pyruvate. Crit Care Med 1992; 20:378.

Kasper LM, Moorehead WR, Oel TO, et al: An alternative method assaying cerebrospinal fluid protein in the presence of methotrexate. Clin Chem 1988; 34:2091.

Kaufman L: Serodiagnosis of fungal disease. *In* Rose NR, Friedman H (eds): Manual of Clinical Immunology. Washington, DC, American Society for Microbiology, 1976, p 371.

Kjeldsberg CR, Knight JA: Body Fluids, 3rd ed. Chicago, American Society of Clinical Pathologists Press, 1993.

Klee GG, Tallman RD, Goellner JR, et al: Elevation of carcinoembryonic antigen in cerebrospinal fluid among patients with meningeal carcinomatosis. Mayo Clin Proc 1986; 61:9.

Knight JA, Dudek SM, Haymond RE: Early (chemical) diagnosis of bacterial meningitis-cerebrospinal fluid glucose, lactate, and lactate dehydrogenase compared. Clin Chem 1981; 27:1431.

Kuberski T: Eosinophils in cerebrospinal fluid: Criteria for eosinophilic meningitis. Hawaii Med J 1981; 40:97.

Lang DT, Berberian LB, Lee S, et al: Rapid differentiation of subarachnoid hemorrhage from traumatic lumbar puncture using the D-dimer assay. Am J Clin Pathol 1990; 93:403.

Lefvert AK, Link H: IgG production within the central nervous system: A critical review of proposed formulae. Ann Neurol 1985; 17:13.

Lolli F, Siracusa G, Amato MP, et al: Intrathecal synthesis of free immunoglobulin light chains and IgM in initial multiple sclerosis. Acta Neurol Scand 1991; 83:239.

Lott JA, Warren P: Estimation of reference intervals for total protein in cerebrospinal fluid. Clin Chem 1989; 35:1766.

Luxton RW, Patel P, Keir G, et al: A micro-method for measuring total protein in cerebrospinal fluid by using benzethonium chloride in microtiter plate wells. Clin Chem 1989; 35:(8)1731.

Marton KI, Gean AD: The spinal tap: A new look at an old test. Ann Intern Med 1986; 104:840.

Mayefsky JH, Roughmann KJ: Determination of leukocytosis in traumatic spinal tap specimens. Am J Med 1987; 82:1175.

McGuinness GA, Weisz SC, Bell WE: CSF lactate levels in neonates. Am J Dis Child 1983; 137:48.

Medley S: Acridine orange: Method for diagnosis of amoebic meningitis? Med J Aust 1980; 2:635.

Mizock BA, Rackow EC, Burke GS: Elevated cerebrospinal fluid glutamine in septic encephalopathy. J Clin Gastroenterol 1989; 11:362.

Muller F, Moskophidis M: Estimation of the local production of antibodies to *Treponema pallidum* in the central nervous system of patients with neurosyphilis. Br J Vener Dis 1983; 59:80.

Novak RW: Lack of validity of standard corrections for white blood cell counts of blood-contaminated cerebrospinal fluid in infants. Am J Clin Pathol 1984; 82:95.

Oda K, Egawa H, Okuhara T, et al: Meningeal involvement in Bence Jones multiple myeloma. Cancer 1991; 67:1900.

Odom LF, Wilson H, Cullen J, et al: Significance of blasts in low-cell count cerebrospinal fluid specimens from children with acute lymphoblastic leukemia. Cancer 1990; 66:1748.

Pappu ID, Purolit DM, Levkoff AH: CSF cytology in the neonate. Am J Dis Child 1982; 136:297.

Peacock JEJ, McGinnis MR, Cohen MS: Persistent neutrophilic meningitis: Report of four cases and review of the literature. Medicine 1984; 63:379.

Powers W: Cerebrospinal fluid lymphocytosis in acute bacterial meningitis. Am J Med 1985; 79:216.

Rabinovitch A, Cornbleet PJ: Body fluid microscopy in US laboratories. Data from two College of American Pathologists surveys, with practice recommendations. Arch Pathol Lab Med 1994; 118:13.

Radhakrishnan VV, Annamma M, Shobha S: Correlation between culture of *Mycobacterium tuberculosis* and IgG antibody to *Mycobacterium tuberculosis* antigen-5 in the cerebrospinal fluid of patients with tuberculous meningitis. J Infect 1990; 21:271.

Ragland SA, Arsura E, Ismail Y, et al: Eosinophilic pleocytosis in coccidioidal meningitis: Frequency and significance. Am J Med 1993; 95:254.

Rajantie J, Koskiniemi M, Siimes MA, et al: CSF fibronectin concentration in Burkitt's lymphoma: An early marker for CNS involvement. Eur J Haematol 1989; 42:313.

Rudick RA, French CA, Breton D, et al: Relative diagnostic value of cerebrospinal fluid kappa chains in MS, comparison with other immunoglobulin tests. Neurology 1989; 39:964.

Ryall RG, Peacock MK, Simpson DA: Usefulness of beta 2-transferrin assay in the detection of cerebrospinal fluid leaks following head injury. J Neurosurg 1992; 77:737.

Sarff LD, Platt LH, McCracken GH: Cerebrospinal fluid evaluation in neonates: Composition in high-risk infants with and without meningitis. J Pediatr 1976; 88:473.

Schriever H, Gambino SR: Protein turbidity produced by trichloroacetic acid and sulfosalicylic acid at varying temperatures and varying ratios of albumin and globulin. Am J Clin Pathol 1965; 44:667.

Shephard MD, Whiting MJ: Nephelometric determination of total protein in cerebrospinal fluid and urine using benzalkonium chloride as precipitation reagent. Ann Clin Biochem 1992; 29:411.

Shibata D, Nichols P, Sherrod A, et al: Detection of occult CNS involvement of follicular small cleaved lymphoma by the polymerase chain reaction. Modern Pathol 1990; 3:71.

Silverman LM, Christenson RH: Amino acids and proteins. *In* Burtis CA, Ashwood ER (eds): Tietz Textbook of Clinical Chemistry, 2nd ed. Philadelphia, W. B. Saunders, 1994, p 625.

Simon RP, Abele JS: Spinal-fluid pleocytosis estimated by the Tyndall effect. Ann Intern Med 1978; 89:75.

Sloman AJ, Kelly RH: Transferrin allelic variants may cause false positives in the detection of cerebrospinal fluid fistulae. Clin Chem 1993; 39:1444.

Souverijn JHM, Smit WG, Peet R, et al: Intrathecal Ig synthesis: Its detection by isoelectric focusing and IgG index. J Neurol Sci 1989; 93:211.

Spanos A, Harrell FEJ, Durack DT: Differential diagnosis of acute meningitis: An analysis of the predictive value of initial observations. JAMA 1989; 262:2700.

Steele RW, Marmer DJ, O'Brien MD, et al: Leukocyte survival in cerebrospinal fluid. J Clin Microbiol 1986; 23:965.

Talstad I: Electronic counting of spinal fluid cells. Am J Clin Pathol 1984; 81:506.

Torre D, Zeroii C, Issi M, et al: Cerebrospinal fluid concentration of fibronectin in meningitis. J Clin Pathol 1991; 44:783.

Tourtellotte WW, Staugaitis SM, Walsh MJ, et al: The basis of intra-blood-brain barrier IgG synthesis. Ann Neurol 1985; 17:21.

Trotter JL, Rust RS: Human cerebrospinal fluid immunology. *In* Herndon RM, Brumback RA (eds): The Cerebrospinal Fluid. Boston, Kluwer Academic Publishers, 1989, p 179.

Tubergen DG, Cullen JW, Boyett JM, et al: Blasts in CSF with a normal cell count do not justify alteration of therapy for acute lymphoblastic leukemia in remission: A Childrens Cancer Group study. J Clin Oncol 1994; 12:273.

Twijnstra A, Nooyen WJ, van Zanten AP, et al: Cerebrospinal fluid carci-

noembryonic antigen in patients with metastatic and nonmetastatic neurological diseases. Arch Neurol 1986, 43:269.
Walts AE: Cerebrospinal fluid cytology: Selected issues. Diagn Cytopathol 1992; 8:394.
Ward E, Gushurst CA: Uses and techniques of pediatric lumbar puncture. Am J Dis Child 1992; 146:1160.
Weller M, Sommer N, Stevens A, et al: Increased intrathecal synthesis of fibronectin in bacterial and carcinomatous meningitis. Acta Neurol Scand 1990; 82:138.
Weller M, Stevens A, Sommer N, et al: Humoral CSF parameters in the differential diagnosis of hematologic CNS neoplasia. Acta Neurol Scand 1992; 86:129.
Wenger JD, Hightower AW, Broome CV, et al: Bacterial meningitis in the United States: Report of a multistate surveillance study, 1986. J Infect Dis 1990; 162:1316.
Woods GL: Tuberculosis. Role of the clinical laboratory in providing rapid diagnosis and assessment of disease activity. Am J Clin Pathol 1994; 101:679.
Zandman-Goddard G, Matzner Y, Konijn AM, et al: Cerebrospinal fluid ferritin in malignant CNS involvement. Cancer 1986; 58:1146.

Synovial Fluid

Amor B, Dougados M, Carlioz R, et al: Lymphocyte arthritis. Rev Rheum 1984; 31:733.
Baker DG: Chemistry, serology, and immunology. *In* Gatter RA, Schumacher HR (eds): A Practical Handbook of Joint Fluid Analysis, 2nd ed. Philadelphia, Lea and Febiger, 1991, p 70.
Borenstein DG: Stains, cultures, and other tests for infection. *In* Gatter RA, Schumacher HR (eds): A Practical Handbook of Joint Fluid Analysis, 2nd ed. Philadelphia, Lea and Febiger, 1991, p 63.
Borenstein DG, Gibbs CA, Jacobs RP: Gas-liquid chromatographic analysis of synovial fluid. Arthritis Rheum 1982; 25:947.
Centers for Disease Control and Prevention: Diagnosis of tuberculosis by nucleic acid amplification methods applied to clinical specimens. MMWR, 1993; 42:686.
Clayburne G, Baker DG, Schumacher HR: Estimated synovial fluid leukocyte numbers on wet drop preparations as a potential substitute for actual leukocyte counts. J Rheumatol 1992; 19:60.
Cohen AS, Goldenberg D: Synovial fluid. *In* Laboratory Diagnostic Procedures in the Rheumatic Diseases, 3rd ed. New York, Grune and Stratton, 1985.
Curtis GDW, Newman RJ, Slack MPE: Synovial fluid lactate and the diagnosis of septic arthritis. J Infect 1983; 6:239.
Ettlinger RE, Hunder GC: Synovial effusions containing cholesterol crystals. Mayo Clin Proc 1979; 54:366.
Gatter RA, Schumacher HR: A Practical Handbook of Joint Fluid Analysis, 2nd ed. Philadelphia, Lea and Febiger, 1991.
Goldenberg DL, Reed JI: Bacterial arthritis. N Engl J Med 1985; 312:764.
Golightly MG: Laboratory considerations in the diagnosis and management of Lyme borreliosis. Am J Clin Pathol 1993; 99:168.
Hasselbacher P: Variation in synovial fluid analysis by hospital laboratories. Arthritis Rheum 1987; 30:637.
Jones AC, Chuck AJ, Arie EA, et al: Diseases associated with calcium pyrophosphate deposition disease. Semin Arthritis Rheum 1992; 22:188.
Kay J, Eichenfield AH, Athreya BH, et al: Synovial fluid eosinophilia in Lyme disease. Arthritis Rheum 1988; 31:1384.
Kjeldsberg CR, Knight JA: Body fluids, 3rd ed. Chicago, American Society of Clinical Pathologists Press, 1993.
Lazcano O, Li CY, Pierre RV, et al: Clinical utility of the alizarin red s stain on permanent preparations to detect calcium-containing compounds in synovial fluid. Am J Clin Pathol 1993; 99:90.
Luukkainen R, Kaarela K, Huhtala H, et al: Prognostic significance of synovial fluid analysis in rheumatoid arthritis. Ann Med 1989; 21:269.
McCarty DJ: Crystal identification in human synovial fluids. Rheum Dis Clin North Am 1988; 14:253.
Nocton JJ, Dressler F, Rutledge BJ, et al: Detection of *Borrelia burgdorferi* DNA by polymerase chain reaction in synovial fluid from patients with Lyme arthritis. N Engl J Med 1994; 330:229.
Podell TE, Ault M, Sullam P, et al: Synovial fluid eosinophilia. Arthritis Rheum 1980; 23:1060.
Rabinovitch A, Cornbleet PJ: Body fluid microscopy in US laboratories. Data from two College of American Pathologists surveys, with practice recommendations. Arch Pathol Lab Med 1994; 118:13.
Rosenthal A, Ryan LM, McCarty DJ: Arthritis associated with calcium oxalate crystals in an anephric patient treated with peritoneal dialysis. JAMA 1988; 260:1280.
Rosett W, Hodges GR: Antimicrobial activity of heparin. J Clin Microbiol 1980; 11:30.
Shmerling RH: Synovial fluid analysis. A critical reappraisal. Rheum Dis Clin North Am 1994; 20:503.
Shmerling RH, Delbanco TL, Tosteson ANA, et al: Synovial fluid tests. What should be ordered? JAMA 1990; 264:1009.
Sledge CB: Biology of the Joint. *In* Kelley WN, Harris ED, Ruddy S, Sledge CB (eds): Textbook of Rheumatology, 3rd ed. Philadelphia, W. B. Saunders, 1989, p 1.
Weinberger A, Simkin PA: Plasma proteins in synovial fluids of normal human joints. Semin Arthritis Rheum 1989; 19:66.
Wise CM, White RE, Agudelo CA: Synovial fluid lipid abnormalities in various disease states: Review and classification. Semin Arthritis Rheum 1987; 16:222.
Wolf AW, Benson DR, Shoji H, et al: Current concepts in synovial fluid analysis. Clin Orthop 1978; 134:261.

Pleural Fluid

Adelman M, Albelda S, Gottlieb J, et al: Diagnostic utility of pleural fluid eosinophilia. Am J Med 1984; 77:915.
American College of Physicians: Diagnostic thoracentesis and pleural biopsy in pleural effusions. Ann Intern Med 1985; 103:799.
American Thoracic Society: Guidelines for thoracentesis and needle biopsy of the pleura. Am Rev Respir Dis 1989; 140:257.
Bartlett JG, Thadepalli H, Gorback SL, et al: Bacteriology of empyema. Lancet 1974; 1:338.
Brook I: Measurement of lactic acid in pleural fluid. Respiration 1980; 40:344.
Cheson BD: Clinical utility of body fluid analyses. Clin Lab Med 1985; 5:195.
Dines DE, Pierre KV, Franzen SJ: The value of cells in the pleural fluid in the differential diagnosis. Mayo Clin Proc 1975; 50:571.
Gästrin B, Lövestad A: Diagnostic significance of pleural fluid lactate concentration in pleural and pulmonary disease. Scand J Infect Dis 1988; 20:85.
Good JT, King TE, Antony VB, et al: Lupus pleuritis. Chest 1983; 84:714.
Good JT, Taryle DA, Maulitz RM, et al: The diagnostic value of pleural fluid pH. Chest 1980; 78:55.
Halla JT, Schrohenloher RE, Volankis JE: Immune complexes and other laboratory features of pleural effusions. Ann Intern Med 1980; 92:748.
Hamm H, Brohan U, Bohmer R, et al: Cholesterol in pleural effusions. A diagnostic aid. Chest 1987; 92:296.
Hanes VE, Lucia HL: Acridine orange as a screen for organisms in clinical specimens and comparison with Gram's stain. Arch Pathol Lab Med 1988; 112:529.
Hsu WH, Chiang CD, Huang PL: Diagnostic value of pleural adenosine deaminase in tuberculous effusions of immunocompromised hosts. J Formos Med Assoc 1993; 92:668.
Hunder GG, McDuffie FC, Hepper NGG: Pleural fluid complement activity in systemic lupus erythematosus and rheumatoid arthritis. Ann Intern Med 1972; 76:357.
Ibrahim RE, Teich D, Smith BR, et al: Flow cytometric surface light chain analysis of lymphocyte-rich effusions. Cancer 1989; 63:2024.
Jay SJ: Pleural effusions. II: Definitive evaluation of the exudate. Postgrad Med 1986; 80:181.
Jonasson JG, Ducatman BS, Wang HH: The cell block for body cavity fluids: Do the results justify the cost? Mod Pathol 1990; 3:667.
Katz RL, Raval P, Manning JT, et al: A morphologic, immunologic, and cytometric approach to the classification of non-Hodgkin's lymphoma in effusions. Diagn Cytopathol 1987; 3:91.
Kjeldsberg CR, Knight JA: Body Fluids, 3rd ed. Chicago, American Society of Clinical Pathologists Press, 1993.
Kramer MR, Saldana MJ, Cepero RJ, et al: High amylase levels in neoplasm-related pleural effusion. Ann Intern Med 1989; 110:567.
Kumar S, Seshadri MS, Koshi G, et al: Diagnosing tuberculous pleural effusion: Comparative sensitivity of mycobacterial culture and histopathology. Br Med J 1981; 283:(6283)20.
Levine H, Szanto M, Grieble HG, et al: Rheumatoid factor in nonrheumatoid pleural effusions. Ann Intern Med 1968, 69:487.
Light RW: Pleural Diseases, 2nd ed. Philadelphia, Lea and Febiger, 1990.
Light RW, Ball WC Jr: Glucose and amylase in pleural effusions. JAMA 1973a; 225:257.
Light RW, Erozan YS, Ball WC Jr: Cells in pleural fluid: Their value in differential diagnosis. Arch Intern Med 1973b; 132:854.
Light RW, MacGregor MI, Luchsinger PC, et al: Pleural effusions: The diagnostic separation of transudates and exudates. Ann Intern Med 1972; 77:507.
Meisel S, Shamiss A, Thaler M, et al: Pleural fluid to serum bilirubin concentration ratio for the separation of transudates from exudates. Chest 1990; 98:141.

Mezger J, Permanetter W, Gerbes AL, et al: Tumour associated antigens in diagnosis of serous effusions. J Clin Pathol 1988; 41:633.
Miller KS, Wooten S, Sahn SA: Urinothorax: A cause of low pH transudative pleural effusions. Am J Med 1988; 85:448.
Naylor B: Cytological aspects of pleural, peritoneal and pericardial fluids from patients with systemic lupus erythematosus. Cytopathology 1992; 3:1.
Potts DE, Taryle DA, Sahn SA: The glucose-pH relationship in parapneumonic effusions. Arch Intern Med 1978; 138:1378.
Ribera E, Ocana I, Martinez-Vasquez JM, et al: High level of interferon gamma in tuberculous pleural effusion. Chest 1988; 93:308.
Rodriquez-Panadero F, Mejias JL: Low glucose and pH levels in malignant pleural effusions. Am Rev Respir Dis 1989; 139:663.
Romero S, Candela A, Martín C, et al: Evaluation of different criteria for the separation of pleural transudates from exudates. Chest 1993; 104:399.
Sahn SA: The differential diagnosis of pleural effusions. West J Med 1982; 137:99.
Sahn SA, Good JT: In defense of low glucose levels in pleural fluid. Chest 1980; 77:242.
Sherr HP, Light RW, Merson MH, et al: Origin of pleural fluid amylase in esophageal rupture. Ann Intern Med 1972; 76:985.
Staats BA, Ellefson RD, Budahn LL, et al: The lipoprotein profile of chylous and non-chylous pleural effusions. Mayo Clin Proc 1980; 55:700.
Tamura S, Nishigaki T, Moriwaki Y, et al: Tumor markers in pleural effusion diagnosis. Cancer 1988; 61:298.
Valdés L, Pose A, Suàrez J, et al: Cholesterol: A useful parameter for distinguishing between pleural exudates and transudates. Chest 1991; 99:1097.
Venrick MG, Sidaway MK: Cytologic examination of serous effusions. Processing techniques and optimal number of smears for routine preparation. Am J Clin Pathol 1993; 99:182.
Vergnon JM, Guidollet J, Gateau O, et al: Lactic dehydrogenase isoenzyme electrophoretic patterns in the diagnosis of pleural effusion. Cancer 1984; 54:507.

Pericardial Fluid

Agner RC, Gallis HA: Pericarditis. Differential diagnosis considerations. Arch Intern Med 1979; 139:407.
Bellinger RL, Vacek JL: A review of pericarditis. 2. Specific pericardial disorders. Postgrad Med 1987; 82:105.
Colombo A, Olson HG, Egan J, et al: Etiology and prognostic implications of a large pericardial effusion in men. Clin Cardiol 1988; 11:389.
Corey GR, Campbell PT, Van-Trigt P, et al: Etiology of large pericardial effusions. Am J Med 1993; 95:209.
Kindig JR, Goodman MR: Clinical utility of pericardial fluid pH determination. Am J Med 1983; 75:1077.
Koh KK, Kim EJ, Cho CH, et al: Adenosine deaminase and carcinoembryonic antigen in pericardial effusion diagnosis, especially in suspected tuberculous pericarditis. Circulation 1994; 89:2728.
Leventhal LJ, DeMarco DM, Zurier RB: Antinuclear antibody in pericardial fluid from a patient with primary cardiac lymphoma. Arch Intern Med 1990; 150:1113.
Mann W, Millen JE, Glauser FL: Bloody pericardial fluid. The value of blood gas measurements. JAMA 1978; 239:2151.
Meyers DG, Bouska DJ: Diagnostic usefulness of pericardial fluid cytology. Chest 1989; 95:1142.
Monte SA, Ehya H, Lang WR: Positive effusion cytology as the initial presentation of malignancy. Acta Cytol 1987; 31:448.
Reynolds MM, Hecht SR, Berger M, et al: Large pericardial effusions in the acquired immunodeficiency syndrome. Chest 1992; 102:1746.
Yazdi HM, Hajdu SI, Melamed MR: Cytopathology of pericardial effusions. Acta Cytol 1980; 24:401.

Peritoneal Fluid

Adams HW, Mainz DI: Eosinophilic ascites. Am J Digest Dis 1977; 22:40.
Albillos A, Cuervas-Mons V, Millán I, et al: Ascitic fluid polymorphonuclear cell count and serum to ascites albumin gradient in the diagnosis of bacterial peritonitis. Gastroenterology 1990; 98:134.
Alverdy JC, Saunders J, Chamberlin WH, et al: Diagnostic peritoneal lavage in intra-abdominal sepsis. Am Surg 1988; 54:456.
Alyono D, Perry JFJ: Value of quantitative cell count and amylase activity of peritoneal lavage fluid. J Trauma 1981; 21:345.
Attali P, Turner K, Pelleteir G, et al: pH of ascitic fluid: Diagnostic and prognostic value in cirrhotic and noncirrhotic patients. Gastroenterology 1986; 90:1255.
Boyer TD, Kahn AM, Telfer BR: Diagnostic value of ascitic fluid lactic dehydrogenase, protein, and WBC levels. Arch Intern Med 1978; 138:1103.
Brown JD, An ND: Tuberculous peritonitis. Am J Gastroenterol 1976; 66:277.
Castaldo G, Oriani G, Cimino L, et al: Total discrimination of peritoneal malignant ascites from cirrhosis and hepatocarcinoma-associated ascites by assays of ascitic cholesterol and lactate dehydrogenase. Clin Chem 1994; 40:478.
Castellote J, Xiol X, Verdaguer R, et al: Comparison of two ascitic fluid culture methods in cirrhotic patients with spontaneous bacterial peritonitis. Am J Gastroenterol 1990; 85:1605.
DeLaurier GA, Ivey RK, Johnson RH: Peritoneal fluid lactate acid and diagnostic dilemmas in acute abdominal disease. Am J Surg 1994; 167:302.
Dwivedi M, Misra SP, Misra V, et al: Value of adenosine deaminase estimation in the diagnosis of tuberculous ascites. Am J Gastroenterol 1990; 85:1123.
Feied CF: Diagnostic peritoneal lavage. Questions and answers. Postgrad Med 1989; 85:40.
Gerbes AL, Jungst D, Xie Y, et al: Ascitic fluid analysis for the differentiation of malignancy-related and nonmalignant ascites. Cancer 1991; 68:1808.
Gomez GA, Alvarez R, Plasencia G, et al: Diagnostic peritoneal lavage in the management of blunt abdominal trauma: A reassessment. J Trauma 1987; 27:1.
Jaffin JH, Ochsner MG, Cole FJ, et al: Alkaline phosphatase levels in diagnostic peritoneal lavage as a predictor of hollow visceral injury. J Trauma 1993; 34:829.
Kjeldsberg CR, Knight JA: Body Fluids, 3rd ed. Chicago, American Society of Clinical Pathologists Press, 1993.
Kosches DS, Sosnowik D, Lendvai S, et al: Unusual anodic migrating isoamylase differentiates selected malignant from nonmalignant ascites. J Clin Gastroenterol 1989; 11:43.
Larson FA, Haller CC, Delcore R, et al: Diagnostic peritoneal lavage in acute peritonitis. Am J Surg 1992; 164:449.
Lee HH, Carlson RW, Bull DM: Early diagnosis of spontaneous bacterial peritonitis: Values of ascitic fluid variables. Infection 1987; 15:232.
Lesser GT, Bruno MS, Enselberg K: Chylous ascites. Arch Intern Med 1970; 125:1073.
Mansberger AR: Peritoneal ammonia levels in acute intra-abdominal disease: A reappraisal. Am J Surg 1967; 113:37.
Marshall JB: Finding the cause of ascites. The importance of accurate fluid analysis. Postgrad Med 1988; 83:189.
Mezger J, Permanetter W, Gerbes AL, et al: Tumour associated antigens in diagnosis of serous effusions. J Clin Pathol 1988; 41:633.
Mortenson PB, Kristensen SD, Bloch A, et al: Diagnostic value of ascitic fluid cholesterol levels in the prediction of malignancy. Scand J Gastroenterol 1988; 23:1085.
Pinto MM, Bernstein LH, Rudolph RA, et al: Diagnostic efficiency of carcinoembryonic antigen and CA125 in the cytologic evaluation of effusions. Arch Pathol Lab Med 1992; 116:626.
Polak M, Torres Da Costa AC: Diagnostic value of the estimation of glucose in ascitic fluid. Digestion 1973; 8:347.
Reimer LG: Approach to the analysis of body fluids for the detection of infection. Clin Lab Med 1985; 5:209.
Robert JH, Meyer P, Rohner A: Can serum and peritoneal amylase and lipase determinations help in the early prognosis of acute pancreatitis? Ann Surg 1986; 203:163.
Runyon BA: Amylase levels in ascitic fluid. J Clin Gastroenterol 1987a; 9:172.
Runyon BA: Ascitic fluid bilirubin concentration as a key to choleperitoneum. J Clin Gastroenterol 1987b; 9:543.
Runyon BA, Hoefs JC: Ascitic fluid analysis in the differentiation of spontaneous bacterial peritonitis from gastrointestinal tract perforation into ascitic fluid. Hepatology 1984; 4:447.
Runyon BA, Hoefs JC, Morgan TR: Ascitic fluid analysis in malignancy-related ascites. Hepatology 1988; 8:1104.
Runyon BA, Montano AA, Akriviadis EA, et al: The serum-ascites albumin gradient is superior to the exudate-transudate concept in the differential diagnosis of ascites. Ann Intern Med 1992; 117:215.
Soyka JM, Martin M, Sloan EP, et al: Diagnostic peritoneal lavage: Is an isolated WBC count $\geq 500/mm^3$ predictive of intra-abdominal injury requiring celiotomy in blunt trauma patients? J Trauma 1990; 30:874.
Stassen WN, McCullough AJ, Bacon BR, et al: Immediate diagnostic criteria for bacterial infection of ascitic fluid. Gastroenterol 1986; 90:1247.
Stewart RJ, Gupta RK, Purdie GI, et al: Fine catheter aspiration cytology of peritoneal cavity improves decision-making about difficult cases of acute abdominal pain. Lancet 1986; 2:1414.
Voigt MD, Trey C, Lombard C, et al: Diagnostic value of ascites adenosine deaminase in tuberculous peritonitis. Lancet 1989; 1:751.
Weisman GS, McKinley MJ, Budman DR, et al: Flow cytometry. A technique in the diagnosis of malignant ascites. J Clin Gastroenterol 1987; 9:599.
Zarbo RJ: Flow cytometric DNA analysis of effusions. A new test seeking validation. Am J Clin Pathol 1991; 95:2.

Chapter 20

Clinical Application of Human Chorionic Gonadotropin

Stuart D. Flynn, M.D.
David B. Seifer, M.D.

3

Within the past 15 years, there has been an explosion of information and technology related to the role of human chorionic gonadotropin (hCG) in obstetrics and gynecology. What was initially offered as a pregnancy test has evolved into a sophisticated diagnostic tool aiding clinicians in the differential diagnosis of a broad spectrum of diseases. This chapter discusses much of this new information and technology and the related clinical applications.

HUMAN CHORIONIC GONADOTROPIN

hCG is a glycoprotein composed of two dissimilar subunits—an α-polypeptide subunit (92 amino acids, molecular weight 14,500) and a β-polypeptide subunit (145 amino acids, molecular weight 22,200). This heterodimer is very closely related to two other gonadotropins—follicle-stimulating hormone (FSH) and luteinizing hormone (LH)—as well as to thyroid-stimulating hormone (TSH), all three of which are pituitary glycoprotein hormones. The α-subunits of all four of these hormones are nearly identical, consisting of 92 amino acids in the same sequence (Hussa, 1981). The unique immunologic and biological properties of each of these are conveyed by the differences in the β-subunit amino acid sequence. However, there still is significant homology among the β-subunits of the four hormones, such as between hCG and LH or hCG and TSH, resulting in some overlap in biological activity (Hussa, 1981; Fradkin, 1989). The separated subunits manifest no biological activity, whereas the biological activity of hybrid molecules (i.e., the α-subunit from one molecule combined with the β-subunit from another) is determined by the β-subunit (Gray, 1988). Evidence also suggests that the biological activity is dependent on reversible tertiary or quaternary structural configuration of subunits in the intact molecule (Ross, 1977).

Although a prohormone hypothesis for hCG biosynthesis had been considered, it is now favored that the α- and β-subunits are synthesized individually and subsequently bound noncovalently. The subunits are linked to carbohydrate side chains that include sialic acid, fucose, galactose, and mannose (Ross, 1977). The carbohydrate structure may be essential to glycoprotein hormone-target cell interaction, although there is disagreement about whether the role of the carbohydrate is in subunit-subunit interaction, hormone-receptor interaction, or subsequent activation of adenylate cyclase in the target tissue (Hussa, 1981). *In vivo* hCG activity is decreased by progressive removal of sialic acid, whereas the *in vitro* activity is not affected (Ross, 1977). This decrease of *in vivo* activity with desialylation corresponds to a decrease in hCG plasma half-life.

Serum hCG levels rise rapidly in early gestation. The hCG level doubles every two days below the concentration of 1200 mIU/mL, every three days between the concentrations of 1200 and 6000 mIU/mL, and every four days above the concentration of 6000 mIU/mL (Speroff, 1994). Peak levels are attained in the latter part of the first trimester of pregnancy (Hussa, 1981). The hCG activity can be measured by five general methods: bioassay, agglutination immunoassay, radioimmunoassay (RIA), radioreceptor assay (RRA), and immunometric assay.

Bioassay

The first clinically useful bioassay was introduced by Ascheim (1927) and by Zondek (1931) and was characterized by enlargement and luteinization of the corpus luteum of the immature mouse after injection of urine from normally pregnant women. Zondek (1931) noted similar results when the urine from women with choriocarcinoma or ovarian cancer or from men with testicular neoplasms was used. These assays were followed by Friedman's test (1931) and the *Xenopus laevis* test (Shapiro, 1934), using urine from pregnant women, with the end point being ovulation in the rabbit and South African toad, respectively. Two subsequent tests reported in 1948—the *Rana pipiens* frog test (Wiltberger, 1948) and the Galli-Mainini toad test (1948)—measured the release of spermatozoa from the male frog and toad, respectively, two to four hours after injection of urine from pregnant women. Although these last two tests were relatively rapid, they were not very sensitive.

Bioassays have several associated problems that significantly limit their usefulness as routine pregnancy tests. These include the need to have relatively strict standardization of the test animals, including constant environmental and dietary regimens; technical difficulties; relative high cost; and interference from LH. Thus, various immunoassays have replaced bioassays for routine testing, although bioassays are still used in some research laboratories.

Immunoassay

Bioassays have largely been replaced by immunoassays, with the first of these reported in 1960 (Wide). The concentration of hCG may be expressed as

IU/mL urine or serum
ng/mL urine or serum

The relationship between IU/mL and ng/mL is expressed as

$$1 \text{ ng/mL} = 9 \text{ to } 11 \text{ mIU/mL}$$

The International Unit (IU) is based on bioassays (Storring, 1980), with the standard being the gonadotropin activity of a powdered urinary gonadotropin maintained at the World Health Organization in London.

Immunoassays are rapid, inexpensive, and relatively reliable tests for pregnancy. However, they lack sensitivity and do not lend themselves to easy measurement of the amount of hCG in the specimen. In addition, differences in recognition of nicked hCG, free β, and other hCG variants cause discordant results among different immunoassays (Cole, 1992, 1993). Six basic types of immunoassays have been described: complement fixation, sol particle immunoassay, hemagglutination inhibition (HAI), latex particle agglutination inhibition (LAI), direct agglutination, and enzyme immunoassay. The latter four of these assays are discussed in this chapter because they represent commonly used pregnancy tests.

In the HAI assay, erythrocytes coated with hCG are incubated with anti-hCG serum and the patient's urine. In pregnancy, the hCG in the urine neutralizes the hCG antibody, and thus no agglutination occurs when the hCG-coated erythrocytes are added. This assay is performed in test tubes, with a positive result (hCG in the urine) characterized by a sharply demarcated ring or doughnut at the bottom of the tube. Agglutination occurs in the absence of hCG in the urine (a negative test result), resulting in a uniform film at the bottom of the tube (Fig. 20–1). The assay time for HAI is approximately two hours.

LAI is similar in principle to HAI, with the substitution of hCG-coated latex particles for the hCG-coated erythrocytes.

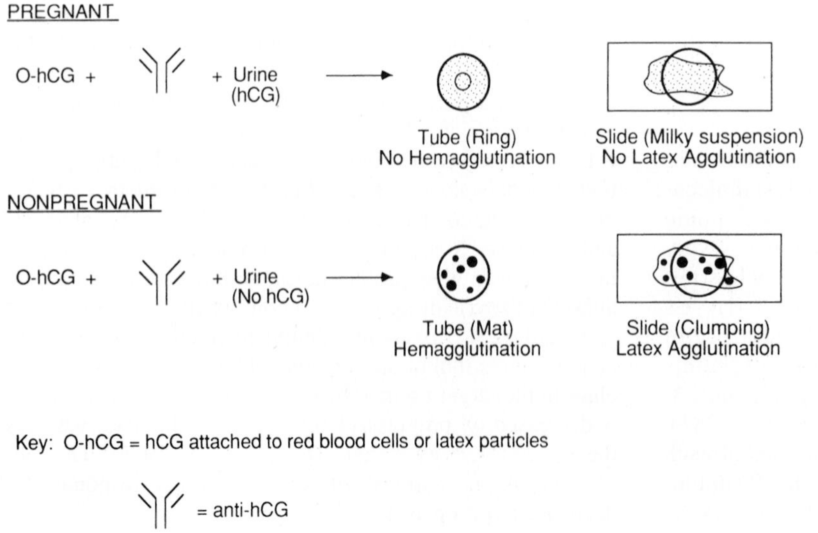

Figure 20–1. Agglutination inhibition immunoassay tests for hCG.

Most LAI tests are performed on glass slides and require only a few minutes to complete. In pregnancy, the hCG in the urine neutralizes the antiserum, resulting in no agglutination and a milky suspension on the slide. The absence of hCG in the urine allows the anti-hCG present in the test kit to agglutinate the hCG-coated latex particles, resulting in clumping of the particles on the slide.

In the direct agglutination test, antibody to hCG is coated on erythrocytes or latex particles. Thus, the results are opposite those seen in HAI or LAI tests, because agglutination occurs in the presence of hCG (pregnancy).

Slide LAI tests have a stated sensitivity ranging from 500 to 3500 mIU/mL, whereas most HAI tests are sensitive, with a detected range stated to be between 150 and 4000 mIU/mL (Hussa, 1987).

Home pregnancy tests use some of the preceding immunoassays and represent a significant commercial endeavor. Unfortunately, it has been demonstrated that laypersons have more difficulties performing and interpreting these tests than experienced technologists, although the manufacturers of the home kits claim 90% accuracy (Hicks, 1989). Differences in recognition of different hCG molecules by immunoassays have now been acknowledged as potential sources of discordant results between home pregnancy tests (Cole, 1993).

Radioimmunoassay

Radioimmunoassays (RIAs) are competitive-binding assays in which both the hCG in the test serum and a radiolabeled hCG compete for binding with an anti-hCG antibody. Thus, an inverse correlation exists between the number of radioactive counts in the antibody complex and the amount of hCG in the patient's serum. Quantitative measurements of hCG may be obtained by RIA. The RIA using antibodies against both the α- and β-subunits exhibits significant cross-reaction with both LH and FSH. Antisera against the β-subunit result in an RIA that is much more specific for hCG. However, even these assays, such as the SB6 RIA, using rabbit antisera generated against the β-subunit, have some cross-reaction with LH that may result in aberrant low-level hCG values (Vaitukaitis, 1972).

Rapid RIAs have decreased the time of the assay from days to several hours. These have taken advantage of chemical precipitants such as dioxane or polyethylene glycol. However, rapid RIAs are not as precise as the longer, conventional RIAs.

Radioreceptor Assay

Radioreceptor assays (RRAs) use gonadotropin target tissue such as rat or pig testes, ovaries from superovulating rats, and corpora lutea from ovaries of pregnant cows (Hussa, 1987). The receptors on the plasma membrane preparations from these organs are the source of binding for hCG instead of the anti-hCG antibodies used in RIAs. The RRA can be more rapid (one hour) but less specific than the β-subunit RIA because of cross-reactions with LH, such as in the menstrual midcycle peak or in the postmenopausal state. RRAs are performed with serum and have a stated sensitivity of approximately 20 to 50 mIU/mL.

3

Immunometric Assay

Immunometric assays are solid-phase immunoassays and include immunoradiometric assay (IRMA), immunoenzymatic assay (IEMA), immunofiltration (Rapak, 1993) and enzyme-linked immunosorbent assay (ELISA). Unlike competitive-binding assays, in these tests both the capture antibody attached to the solid phase and the detection antibody are added in large excess (Hussa, 1987). In addition, these assays use labeled antibody rather than labeled antigen, and the antigen-antibody binding is directly proportional to the amount of antigen present. The monoclonal antibody attached to the solid state is directed toward an epitope of the α-subunit, whereas the second monoclonal antibody, labeled with a radioisotope or an enzyme (e.g., alkaline phosphatase), is directed at an epitope on the β-subunit (Fig. 20–2). The

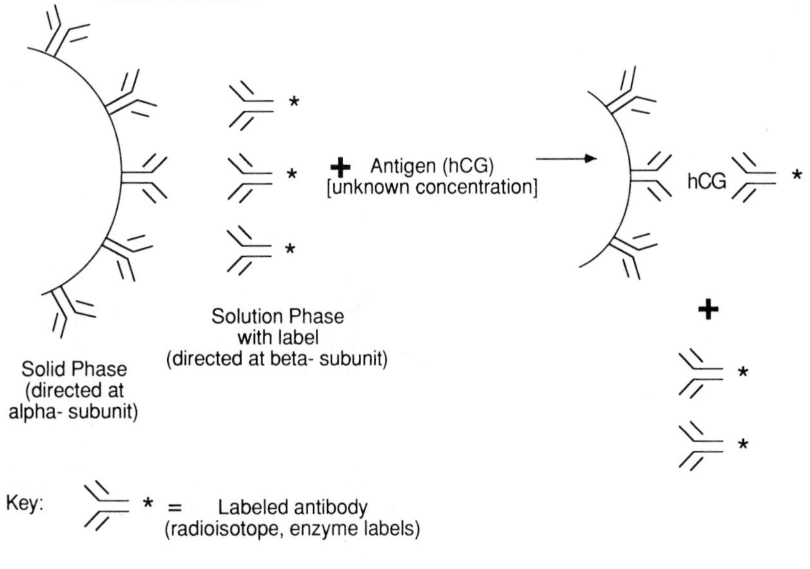

Figure 20–2. Immunometric assay for hCG. (From Robert O. Hussa, The Clinical Marker hCG. Praeger Publishers, New York, a division of Greenwood Press, Inc., 1987, p. 28, © 1987 by Praeger Publishers. Reprinted with permission.)

ELISA has the advantage of not using a radioisotope and is a relatively quick assay (one hour) with a stated sensitivity of 50 mIU/mL. One solid-phase immunoassay, immunoconcentration (Tandem ICON II hCG, Hybritech, Inc., San Diego, CA), uses antibody-coated surfaces with a higher ratio of surface area to sample volume (Valkirs, 1985). ICON minimizes the kinetic problems associated with other solid-phase immunoassays, requires no instrumentation, is easy and fast to perform (minutes), and has a stated sensitivity of 25 to 50 mIU/mL. The determination of a serum quantitative hCG range compares well with the standard quantitative serum hCG immunoassays (Kooi, 1992; Norman, 1992).

Examples of pregnancy kits used in laboratory, office, and home are shown in Table 20–1. Owing to such factors as low sensitivity, long performance time, need for animal facilities, and high cost, bioassays have been replaced by other tests. Until the past few years, urine and slide agglutination tests were popular because they are rapid and inexpensive. The slide tests can be interpreted quickly (minutes), but both the slide and the tube tests have relatively low sensitivity, with a 5% to 10% false-negative rate even when hCG is at its maximum level ([60 to 80 days] Derman, 1979). Causes of false-positive results include error in test performance, inaccurate reading of test results, testing too soon after pregnancy termination, proteinuria in excess of 1 g per 24 hours, drugs (methadone and antipsychotics), and hematuria.

The development of solid-phase IEMAs has resulted in a more sensitive and reliable visual pregnancy test than the agglutination tests (Hussa, 1987). However, the advent of ICON seems to make it the method of choice for physicians' offices, the emergency room, and the clinical laboratory, given its simplicity, speed (minutes), and sensitivity (25 to 50 mIU/mL) (Norman, 1992). Automated immunoassay systems (Baxter-Dade Stratus II, Abbott IMx intact hCG and total β-hCG) also offer highly accurate and precise results in about one fourth of the time required for a Hybritech batch run (Witherspoon, 1992).

Diagnosis of Normal Pregnancy

During a normal nonpregnant menstrual cycle, the corpus luteum remains viable for 14 days until it is no longer sensitive to support provided by LH. Without a pregnancy to produce hCG, the corpus luteum regresses, becoming a corpus albicans, and loses its ability to produce its principal secretory product, progesterone. As a result, endometrial desquamation occurs as clinically demonstrated by menses. However, if conception does occur, the syncytiotrophoblast produces hCG, which is responsible for rescuing and maintaining the corpus luteum beyond its normal 14-day lifespan. Therefore, hCG rescues the corpus luteum from luteolysis and is thus referred to as a luteotropic hormone. Progesterone produced by the corpus luteum is essential in supporting the viability of a pregnancy until approximately 7 to 10 weeks' gestation. At that time, the developing placenta may produce sufficient amounts of progesterone initially to supplement and eventually to replace the production of progesterone by the corpus luteum.

In a normal pregnancy, the syncytiotrophoblast secretes a

Table 20–1. PREGNANCY TEST KITS USED IN LABORATORY, OFFICE AND HOME SITES

Type of Test	Testing Site	Manufacturer	Trade Name	Type of Assay
Serum	Laboratory	Hybritech	Tandem-R	Immunoradiometric assay
Serum	Laboratory	Abbott Laboratories	IMX HCG	Microparticle fluorimetric assay
Serum or urine	Laboratory	Wallace	Delfia HCG	Time-resolve fluorescence assay
Serum	Laboratory	PB Diagnostics	Opus hCG	Enzyme-linked fluorimetric assay
Serum	Laboratory	Biomerica	IRMA-HCG	Immunoradiometric assay
Serum	Laboratory	Baxter Diagnostics	Stratus HCG	Enzyme-linked fluorimetric assay
Serum or urine	Laboratory	Scrono Diagnostics	MAIAclone	Immunoradiometric assay
Serum or urine	Laboratory	Organon Teknika	NMI	Immunoradiometric assay
Serum	Laboratory	Abbott Laboratories	β-HCG 15/15	Enzyme-linked immunosorbent assay
Serum	Laboratory	Ciba Corning	AC5180	Chemiluminescence assay
Serum	Laboratory	Baxter Diagnostics	Stratus βHCG	Enzyme-linked fluorimetric assay
Serum	Laboratory	Abbott Laboratories	IMX β-HCG	Microparticle fluorimetric assay
Serum	Laboratory	Immunonuclear (INC)	Gammadab βHCG	RIA
Serum	Laboratory	ICN	HCGβ RIA	RIA
Serum or urine	Laboratory	Amersham	Amerlex-M	RIA
Serum or urine	Laboratory	Diagnostics Products	HCG	RIA
Urine	Office	Hybritech	Tandem-ICON	Immunoconcentration assay
Urine	Office	Abbott Laboratories	TestPack Combo	Dye-based sandwich assay
Urine	Office	Quidel	RAMP	Enzyme-linked immunosorbent assay
Urine	Office	Becton Dickinson	Precise	Dye-based sandwich assay
Urine	Office	Wampole	UCG-BETA Stat	Hemagglutination
Urine	Office	Organon Teknika	Pregnosticon	Dye-based single site assay
Urine	Office	Roche Diagnostics	Pregnosis	Latex agglutination
Urine	Office	Stanbio	Quicktell	Latex competitive assay
Urine	Home	Leeco Diagnostics	Preview	Dye-based sandwich assay
Urine	Home	Whitehall Laboratories	Clear Blue Easy	Dye-based sandwich assay
Urine	Home	Becton Dickinson	Q-test	Dye-based sandwich assay
Urine	Home	Parke-Davis	E.P.T.	Dye-based twin antibody assay
Urine	Home	Carter Wallace	First Response	Dye-based single site assay

Modified from Cole LA, Seifer DB, Kardana A, Braunstein GD: Selecting human chorionic gonadotropin immunoassays: Consideration of cross-reacting molecules in first-trimester pregnancy serum and urine. Am J Obstet Gynecol 1993; 168(5):1580–1586.

detectable amount of hCG almost immediately on implantation, which is six to eight days after conception (Braunstein, 1976). Levels of hCG rise rapidly, with a doubling time of 1.4 to 3.5 days, until reaching a peak of approximately 100,000 mIU/mL of serum after 60 to 80 days (Fritz, 1987) (Fig. 20–3). hCG levels decline from their peak to a plateau of 10,000 to 20,000 mIU/mL at 15 to 16 weeks, a level that is maintained for the remainder of the pregnancy. The presence of free β-hCG in early and free α-hCG in late pregnancy, when codetermined with total hCG, may aid in the general evaluation of placental function and in the diagnosis of threatened abortion and ectopic pregnancy (Cole, 1988a). After delivery of a term pregnancy, hCG regresses to nondetectable levels within approximately two weeks (Steier, 1984).

Indications for qualitative β-hCG testing include any suspicion of a possible pregnancy, as in the case of a missed period, abnormal vaginal bleeding, or galactorrhea. Physicians, before prescribing birth control pills, steroids, or particular antibiotics (i.e., tetracycline or chloramphenicol), may be prudent to rule out pregnancy to prevent inadvertent teratogenic effects. Similar reasons would motivate a clinician to rule out pregnancy before ordering/obtaining x-ray studies, chemotherapy, or radiotherapy.

Diagnosis of Ectopic Pregnancy

The incidence of ectopic pregnancy has increased sixfold in the United States since 1970. Ectopic pregnancy represents a guarded prognosis with respect to a woman's survival as well as her future reproductive potential. Approximately 10% of all maternal mortality is the result of ectopic pregnancy. Only one third of women who have sustained an ectopic pregnancy will subsequently go on to deliver a liveborn infant. The reported recurrence risk of sustaining an ectopic pregnancy ranges from 4% to 27% (Marchbanks, 1988).

The increased incidence of ectopic pregnancies may be attributed to several factors, including an increased rate of pelvic inflammatory disease, the introduction of microsurgical techniques for the treatment of fallopian tube disease, a larger number of elective sterilizations being performed, the increased use of ovulation induction medications, and the increased popularity of assisted reproductive technology (i.e., *in vitro* fertilization, gamete intrafallopian tube transfer). The greatest clinical challenge with respect to ectopic pregnancy is in making a diagnosis as early as possible and delivering prompt intervention to avoid rupture, hemorrhage, and destruction of the fallopian tube. Diagnostic techniques include high-resolution ultrasonography and, most importantly, assays using monoclonal antibodies for the β-subunit of hCG.

As discussed previously, quantitative β-hCG doubles its concentration approximately every two days until approximately 10 weeks' gestation. If this doubling time does not occur, an abnormal pregnancy is suspected. More specifically, serum β-hCG level that does not rise at least 66% in 48 hours is consistent with a nonviable pregnancy approximately 80% of the time (Kadar, 1981, 1988). The differential diagnosis would include a possible ectopic gestation if an intrauterine pregnancy could not be clearly demonstrated by ultrasonography. Transabdominal ultrasonography has been the most useful technique for identifying an intrauterine pregnancy as early as 42 days from the last menstrual period. A corresponding hCG titer at 42 days' gestation is 6500 mIU/mL. The absence of a gestational sac when the serum hCG concentration was reported to be greater than 6500 mIU/mL had been shown to be associated with an ectopic pregnancy in 87% of cases (Romero, 1985). Thus, the hCG discriminatory zone for differentiating an ectopic pregnancy from an intrauterine pregnancy was initially determined to be 6500 mIU/mL. However, the clinical utility of this criterion had been limited to the 40% of women with suspected ectopic pregnancies who presented with an hCG titer exceeding 6500 mIU/mL (Romero, 1985). RIAs have proved to be a very sensitive means by which to measure hCG, with a sensitivity of 5 to 10 mIU/mL. This has resulted in a false-negative rate of less than 1% for ectopic pregnancies, and results may be available within three hours (DeCherney, 1989). Two thirds of patients with ectopic pregnancies exhibit a decrease, a plateau, or an inability to achieve the predicted slope for increasing hCG production with serial measurements (DeCherney, 1989). As mentioned, ultrasonography is critical in making the diagnosis in the remaining one third of patients.

β-Core fragment (β-core), a small degraded molecule, is the main hCG/β-subunit–related molecule in pregnancy urine. In preliminary studies comparing the results from two types of β-core test, three types of hCG, and one free β-subunit test, the two β-core tests gave values for tubal preg-

3

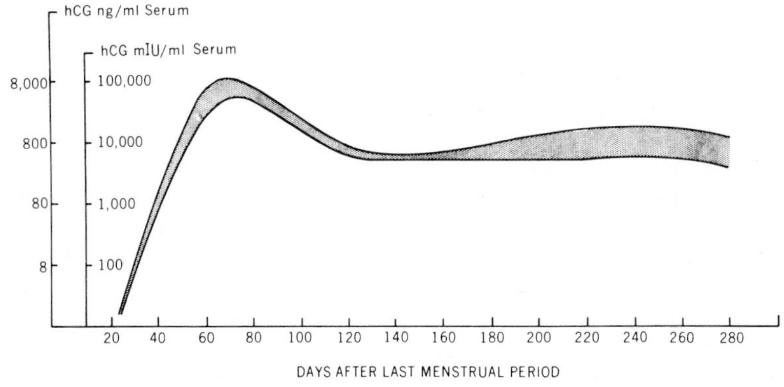

Figure 20–3. Serum hCG levels during normal pregnancy. (Adapted from Lau, HL: Testing for pregnancy. *In* Practice of Medicine, Vol. II. Hagerstown, Md., Harper & Row, 1975, Chap. 29; and Braunstein GD, Rasor J, Adler D, Danzer H, Wade ME: Am J Obstet Gynecol 1976; 126:678.)

nancy threefold more different from normal pregnancy than all other tests (Cole, 1994a). At a selected cut-off level, the β-core test had a very high predictive value (>98%), higher than that indicated with ectopic pregnancy for ultrasonography, serum hCG, or culdocentesis.

In an effort to improve the predictive value of the combined use of ultrasonography and quantitative serum hCG determination, transvaginal ultrasonography has been used. An hCG discriminatory zone of approximately 1400 mIU/mL has been noted to correspond to a visualized gestational sac by transvaginal ultrasonography approximately 35 days from the last menstrual period (Fossum, 1988). At present, the diagnosis of a very early ectopic pregnancy before five weeks from the last menstrual period remains a particular clinical challenge.

After surgical removal of an ectopic pregnancy, the time necessary for disappearance of hCG from the blood has been noted to range from 1 to 31 days, with a median of 8.5 days (Steier, 1984). It has been recommended that patients having undergone conservative surgery for ectopic pregnancy (i.e., salpingostomy) be monitored with serial serum β-hCG determinations until titers return to nonpregnant levels in order to preclude undetected persistent ectopic trophoblastic tissue (Seifer, 1990, 1991, 1993, 1994).

It is important to note that quantitative β-hCG values mentioned in this discussion are derived from the International Reference Preparation (IRP). Another reference standard established by the World Health Organization is the Second International Standard of hCG (2nd IS hCG). hCG concentrations are calibrated approximately twice as high when using the IRP as compared with the 2nd IS hCG. An excellent discussion of the history and further relevance of these standards may be found in the text by Hussa (1987).

Evaluation of Abortion

The incidence of early loss of pregnancy has been documented to be as high as 31% (Wilcox, 1988). This relatively common event of the human reproductive cycle may present in various different clinical situations. In a premenopausal woman with uterine bleeding accompanied by a positive pregnancy test result within 20 weeks from her last menses, the differential diagnosis includes threatened, missed, inevitable, incomplete, or complete abortion. Each type of abortion is clinically defined by the status of the internal os of the cervix (open versus closed) and whether or not products of conception have been passed from the uterine cavity. A clinician must often include the possibility of an ectopic pregnancy, a hydatidiform mole, or choriocarcinoma in the differential diagnosis. A combination of the patient's history, results of a physical examination, pelvic ultrasonography, and serial quantitative β-hCG titers provide information needed for effective management.

Serial quantitative titers of β-hCG indicative of an abnormal pregnancy are suggested by a plateauing or a decrease from the expectant doubling time displayed by a normal intrauterine pregnancy. After spontaneous abortion, serum β-hCG becomes nondetectable within 9 to 35 days, with a median of 19 days. This is in contrast to induced abortion, in which titers become nondetectable within 16 to 60 days, with a median of 30 days. Investigators attribute this difference in rate of regression of β-hCG to the amount of residual vital trophoblastic tissue remaining after evacuation of the uterus (Steier, 1984). An IEMA for the detection of urinary hCG based on the same antibodies used for the standard IRMA can serve as an efficient screening assay for the detection of early fetal loss (O'Connor, 1992).

Diagnosis and Evaluation of Down Syndrome

In Down syndrome pregnancies, β-hCG measured in maternal serum in the second trimester is on average two times the unaffected median value. When combined with maternal serum α-fetoprotein (AFP) and unconjugated estriol, these analytes constitute a triple marker screen in common use today in the United States (Canick, 1993).

Diagnosis and Evaluation of Gestational Trophoblastic Disease

Gestational trophoblastic disease (GTD) occurs in approximately 1 in 1000 pregnancies, with approximately 3500 new cases of hydatidiform mole diagnosed each year in the United States (Atrash, 1986). Prognosis for survival is excellent if the diagnosis is made early and treatment is initiated in a timely manner. In the United States, 82% of hydatidiform moles completely resolve after uterine evacuation, whereas 15% progress to chorioadenoma destruens and 3% to choriocarcinoma.

Clinical presentation may include vaginal bleeding after a missed period, discrepancy between uterine size and gestational age, nausea, vomiting, pre-eclampsia, thyrotoxicosis, neurologic symptoms, and in 25% of cases bilateral theca-lutein cysts. A classic example of GTD is noted in a woman with an enlarged uterus and positive β-hCG, without a fetal heartbeat, and with a characteristic snowstorm pattern noted on pelvic sonogram.

Women with GTD typically produce concentrations of hCG equal to or exceeding levels produced in normal pregnancy for similar gestational age. When hCG levels are monitored before treatment, levels fail to plateau at the end of the first trimester and continue to rise in proportion to the increase in trophoblast cell mass. After evacuation of the uterus, quantitative β-hCG titers must be measured weekly until nondetectable levels are noted for three weeks, followed by monthly titers for one year. During this follow-up period, the regression of hCG should be plotted and compared with a standard regression curve (Morrow, 1977). The majority of patients whose regression curves deviate during follow-up from the standard postevacuation regression curve may be identified within three weeks, and 87% can be identified by six weeks (Schlaerth, 1981). If hCG titers plateau or rise, indicating persistent GTD, further clinical workup is necessary to rule out metastatic disease.

Reports now indicate that the ratio of serum free β-subunit of hCG to total hCG may be valuable in the evaluation of GTD (Khazaeli, 1986; Fan, 1987; Ozturk, 1988). Free β-subunit is present in normal pregnancy and averages less than 4% of the total hCG up to the time of the hCG peak (Cole, 1988a). The free β-hCG/hCG ratio is higher in GTD and correlates strongly with the type of GTD. The ratio has been shown to be lowest in patients with hydatidiform mole, intermediate in invasive mole, and highest in choriocarcinoma, correlating with the degree of immaturity, or differentiation of the trophoblastic cell (Fan, 1987). This ratio may also be of value in predicting those patients with hydatidiform mole who will experience spontaneous remission (lower ratio) versus persistent disease (higher ratio [Khazaeli, 1986]). Also, a highly specific IRMA result may predict very early tumor recurrence in patients with gestational choriocarcinoma (Ozturk, 1988).

Pregnancy serum samples contain predominantly intact hCG, whereas trophoblastic disease serum samples are more heterogeneous, containing a varying mixture of intact hCG and uncombined and degraded molecules. All multiple antibody sandwich assays detect intact hCG, and most do not detect one or all of the degraded molecules. Thus, it is important to understand the utility of each assay and the potential limitation of each in monitoring trophoblastic disease (Cole, 1994b).

Based on the metatastic workup, prognosis can be determined. Factors associated with poor prognosis include serum hCG titers greater than 40,000 mIU/mL, greater than four months from last pregnancy, failure of previous chemotherapy, brain or liver metastases, and antecedent term pregnancy (McDonald, 1983). Patients without metastatic disease or those belonging to the metastatic disease group with a favorable prognosis may receive single-agent methotrexate or actinomycin D. Patients belonging to the group with a poor prognosis receive multiagent chemotherapy for treatment.

Five-year survival for those with nonmetastatic disease or those belonging to the group with metastatic disease with a favorable prognosis is 100%, as compared with a range of survival of 66% to 90% for those belonging to the metastatic disease group with a poor prognosis. After successful treatment, patients are requested to avoid pregnancy for one year. The risk of developing a trophoblastic tumor in the second year of follow-up is less than 1 in 1000 (Bagshawe, 1984).

Surveillance of Ovarian Germ Cell Tumors

Serial quantitative β-hCG concentrations can be helpful in monitoring patients for evidence of persistence or recurrence of ovarian germ cell tumors after initial chemotherapy or surgery. Absolute levels of β-hCG are probably of less practical value than rates of increase or decrease from initial baseline levels, which are obtained before therapy. β-hCG can serve as a tumor marker for various ovarian germ cell tumors, which include choriocarcinoma, endodermal sinus tumor, embryonal carcinoma, and dysgerminoma.

Administration of Human Chorionic Gonadotropin for Induction of Ovulation During *In Vitro* Fertilization

Administration of hCG is an integral part of the induction and timing of ovulation for *in vitro* fertilization. After selected fertility medications are administered to foster the development of multiple follicles, 10,000 IU of hCG is given. hCG simulates the spontaneous LH surge that normally occurs during a natural cycle and thus triggers a resumption of meiosis. The oocyte originally arrested in prophase of the first meiotic division may then proceed to develop to metaphase II of the second meiotic division and thus become receptive to fertilization. Ovulation predictably occurs 36 to 38 hours after the administration of hCG, at which time oocyte retrieval can be initiated (Seibel, 1988).

Evaluation of Testicular Tumors

β-hCG titers are extremely useful in both diagnosis and treatment of testicular tumors. They have contributed greatly to the diagnosis, immunohistochemical classification, staging, and follow-up surveillance of these tumors. Germ cell tumors account for more than 90% of testicular tumors and are classified histologically as either seminomas (40%) or nonseminomas (60%). Greater than 40% of men with testicular tumors have been shown to have serum hCG present. Furthermore, when hCG is assayed in conjunction with AFP, as many as 50% to 90% of men with nonseminomatous testicular tumors have been noted to have elevated levels (Hussa, 1987).

Radical orchiectomy followed by radiotherapy has traditionally been the preferred treatment for low-stage seminoma of the testis. Five-year survival rates for patients with seminoma range from 80% to 97%. Nonseminoma germ cell tumors are less radiosensitive and thus more difficult to treat. Although it is becoming somewhat controversial because of the success of salvage chemotherapy, retroperitoneal lymphadenectomy after radical orchiectomy is still used in most patients. Adjuvant chemotherapy is given to patients with higher-stage disease. The treatment of testicular germ cell neoplasms has been thoroughly reviewed by Loehrer (1988).

The titer of hCG may be a factor in influencing recommended treatment. Patients with seminoma and elevated β-hCG may have a less favorable prognosis than those with seminoma with normal titers. Therefore, it has been suggested that these tumors be approached in a more aggressive manner, including retroperitoneal lymphadenectomy with chemotherapy after pathologic staging (Pritchett, 1985).

After chemotherapy for advanced germ cell neoplasms, the magnitude of decline in hCG titers has been noted to be prognostic for long-term response (Picozzi, 1984).

Ectopic Human Chorionic Gonadotropin Production in Nontrophoblastic Tumors

Various nontrophoblastic tumors and even non-neoplastic tissue have been reported to be associated with the presence of hCG-like immunoreactivity in the serum and tissue extracts of patients. Many of the studies using RIA for the detection of hCG have been summarized by Hussa (1981). Nontrophoblastic tumors producing hCG-like immunoreactivity, in order of decreasing frequency, include breast, ovarian, pancreatic, cervical, gastric, and hepatic cancers. Immunoreactive hCG may also be present in ascites of patients with malignant tumors (Hoermann, 1992).

The initial enthusiasm about the possibility of the use of hCG as a nontrophoblastic tumor marker has not been realized. The low percentage with detectable levels of hCG and the associated low titers (1 to 10 mIU/mL) have severely limited the use of hCG in detecting and monitoring the therapy of patients with the previously mentioned neoplasms. In addition, no substantial evidence shows that the trend in hCG titers correlates with clinical treatment of these particular tumors. Thus, hCG may serve as a marker only for the diagnosis of nontrophoblastic cancers and at present offers very little as far as follow-up surveillance after initial treatment is concerned.

There is a great deal of enthusiasm about the recent observation that in the urine from patients who are pregnant and from some cancer patients there is a small form of β-subunit hCG (urinary gonadotropin fragment [UGF] or urinary gonadotropin peptide) that may represent both a specific and a sensitive marker for tumor detection. UGF has a molecular weight of 10,000 and is composed of two disulfide-linked polypeptide chains. In the placenta, UGF is directly secreted by the trophoblasts and does not represent a degradation product (Cole, 1988b). Immunohistochemical studies using an antibody to UGF revealed staining of some normal tissues (placenta, gastric mucosa, breast ductal epithelium) and carcinomas (lung, ovary, cervix, breast [Kardana, 1988]). A rapid, simple radioimmunometric assay has been developed to measure UGF as well as hCG and the β-subunit of hCG (O'Connor, 1988). With this assay, 80% of positively tested individuals actually had some form of gynecologic malignancy (O'Connor, 1988). Cole (1988c) noted that 72 of 112 (64%) women with active gynecologic cancer had urine UGF levels exceeding the cut-off value. Detectable UGF levels were noted in 70% of patients with cervical cancer, 73% with ovarian cancer, and 77% with endometrial cancer (Cole, 1988d). Another study revealed elevated UGF levels in 24 of 28 women with gynecologic cancers, and a correlation was observed between UGF levels and changing clinical status during therapy in 23 of these 24 patients (Wang, 1988). Thus, preliminary studies suggest that UGF levels may be valuable in the monitoring of therapy in patients with gynecologic cancers.

Ascheim S, Zondek B: Das hormon des hypophysenvorderlappens: Testobjeckt zum nachweis des hormons. Klin Wochenschr 1927; 6:248.

Atrash HK, Hogue CJR, Grimes DA: Epidemiology of hydatidiform mole during early gestation. Am J Obstet Gynecol 1986; 154:906.

Bagshawe KD: Clinical applications of hCG. Adv Exp Med Biol 1984; 176:313.

Braunstein GD, Rasor J, Adler D, et al: Serum human chorionic gonadotropin levels throughout normal pregnancy. Am J Obstet Gynecol 1976; 126:678.

Canick JA, Saller DN: Maternal serum screening for aneuploidy and open fetal defects. Obstet Gynecol Clin North Am 1993; 20:443.

Cole LA: Occurrence and properties of glycoprotein hormone free subunits. *In* Kell B, Grotjan H (eds): Microheterogeneity of Glycoprotein Hormones. New York, CRC Press, 1988a.

Cole LA, Birken S: Origin and occurrence of human chorionic gonadotropin beta-subunit core fragment. Mol Endocrinol 1988b; 2:825.

Cole LA, Kardana A: Discordant results in human chorionic gonadotropin assays. Clin Chem 1992; 38:263.

Cole LA, Kardana A, Seifer DB, Bohler HCL Jr: Urine hCG β-subunit core fragment, a sensitive test for ectopic pregnancy. J Clin Endocrinol Metab 1994a; 78:497.

Cole LA, Kohorn EI, Kim GS: Detecting and monitoring trophoblastic disease: New perspectives on measuring human chorionic gonadotropin levels. J Reprod Med 1994b; 39:193.

Cole LA, Schwartz PE, Wang Y: Urinary gonadotropin fragments (UGF) in cancers of the female reproductive system. Gynecol Oncol 1988c; 31:82.

Cole LA, Seifer DB, Kardana A, Braunstein GD: Selecting human chorionic gonadotropin immunoassays: Consideration of cross-reacting molecules in first-trimester pregnancy serum and urine. Am J Obstet Gynecol 1993; 168:1580.

Cole LA, Wang Y, Elliott M, et al: Urinary human chorionic gonadotropin free beta-subunit and beta-core fragment: A new marker of gynecologic cancers. Cancer Res 1988d; 48:1356.

DeCherney AH: Ectopic pregnancy. ACOG American College of Obstetricians and Gynecologists Technical Bulletin 1989; 126.

Derman R, Edelman DA, Berger GS: Current status of immunologic pregnancy tests. Int J Gynaecol Obstet 1979; 17:190.

Fan C, Goto S, Furuhashi Y, Tomoda Y: Radioimmunoassay of the serum free beta-subunit of human chorionic gonadotropin in trophoblastic disease. J Clin Endocrinol Metab 1987; 64:313.

Fossum GT, Davajan V, Kletzky OA: Early detection of pregnancy with transvaginal ultrasound. Fertil Steril 1988; 49:788.

Fradkin JE, Eastman RC, Lesniak MA, Roth J: Specificity spillover at the hormone receptor—exploring its role in human disease. N Engl J Med 1989; 320:640.

Friedman MH, Lapham ME: A simple rapid procedure for the laboratory diagnosis of early pregnancies. Am J Obstet Gynecol 1931; 21: 405.

Fritz MA, Guo S: Doubling time of human chorionic gonadotropin (hCG) in early normal pregnancy: Relationship to hCG concentration and gestational age. Fertil Steril 1987; 47:584.

Galli-Mainini CD: Pregnancy test using the male batrachia. JAMA 1948; 138:121.

Gray CJ: Glycoprotein gonadotropins. Structure and synthesis. Acta Endocrinol 1988; 288:20.

Hicks JM, Iosefsohn M: Reliability of home pregnancy-test kits in the hands of laypersons. N Engl J Med 1989; 320:320.

Hoermann R, Gerbes AL, Spoettl G, et al: Immunoreactive human chorionic gonadotropin and its free beta subunit in serum and ascites of patients with malignant tumors. Cancer Res 1992; 52:1520.

Hussa RO: Human chorionic gonadotropin, a clinical marker: Review of its biosynthesis. Ligand Rev 1981; 3:1.

Hussa RO: The Clinical Marker hCG. New York, Praeger, 1987.

Kadar N, Caldwell BU, Romero R: A method of screening for ectopic pregnancy and its indications. Obstet Gynecol 1981; 58:162.

Kadar N, Romero R: Serial human chorionic gonadotropin measurements in ectopic pregnancy. Am J Obstet Gynecol 1988; 158:1239.

Kardana A, Taylor ME, Southall PJ, et al: Urinary gonadotropin peptide—isolation and purification, and its immunohistochemical distribution in normal and neoplastic tissues. Br J Cancer 1988; 58:281.

Khazaeli MB, Hedayat MM, Hatch KD, et al: Radioimmunoassay of free beta-subunit of human chorionic gonadotropin as a prognostic test for persistent trophoblastic disease in molar pregnancy. Am J Obstet Gynecol 1986; 155:320.

Kooi S, Kock HCLV: An office semiquantitative serum human chorionic gonadotropin determination. Fertil Steril 1992; 58:522.

Loehrer PJ, Williams SD, Einhorn LH: Testicular cancer: The quest continues. J Natl Cancer Inst 1988; 80:1373.

Marchbanks PA, Annegers JF, Coulam CB, et al: Risk factors for ectopic pregnancy: A population-based study. JAMA 1988; 259:1823.

McDonald TW, Ruffolo EH: Modern management of gestational trophoblastic disease. Obstet Gynecol Surv 1983; 38:67.

Morrow CP, Kletzky, OA, Disaia PJ, et al: Clinical and laboratory correlates of molar pregnancy and trophoblastic disease. Am J Obstet Gynecol 1977; 128:424.

Norman RJ, Gilmore TA, McLoughlin JW: Simple quantitative measurement of serum choriogonadotropin compared with immunoradiometric, immunoenzymometric, and chemiluminescent assays. Clin Chem 1992; 38:144.

O'Connor JF, Hanson FW, Lasley BL: Prospective assessment of early fetal loss using an immunoenzymometric screening assay for detection of urinary human chorionic gonadotropin. Fertil Steril 1992; 57: 1220.

O'Connor JF, Schlatterer JP, Birken S, et al: Development of highly sensitive immunoassays to measure human chorionic gonadotropin, its beta-subunit, and beta core fragment in the urine: Application to malignancies. Cancer Res 1988; 48:1361.

Ozturk M, Berkowitz R, Goldstein D, et al: Differential production of human chorionic gonadotropin and free subunits in gestational trophoblastic disease. Am J Obstet Gynecol 1988; 158:193.

Picozzi VJ, Freiha FS, Hannigan JF, Torti FM: Prognostic significance of a decline in serum human chorionic gonadotropin after initial chemotherapy for advanced germ-cell carcinoma. Ann Intern Med 1984; 100:183.

Pritchett TR, Skinner TG, Selser SF, Kern WH: Seminoma with elevated human chorionic gonadotropin: The case for retroperitoneal lymph node dissection. Urology 1985; 25:344.

Rapak A, Szewczuk A: Semiquantitative assay of human chorionic go-

nadotropin by a simple and fast immunofiltration technique. Eur J Clin Chem Clin Biochem 1993; 31:153.
Romero R, Kadar N, Jeanty P, et al: Diagnosis of ectopic pregnancy: Value of the discriminatory human chorionic gonadotropin zone. Obstet Gynecol 1985; 66:357.
Ross GT: Clinical relevance of research on the structure of human chorionic gonadotropin. Am J Obstet Gynecol 1977; 129:795.
Schlaerth JB, Morrow CP, Kletzky OA, et al: Prognostic characteristics of serum human chorionic gonadotropin titer regression curve following molar pregnancy. Obstet Gynecol 1981; 58:478.
Seibel MM: A new era in reproductive technology. N Engl J Med 1988; 318:828.
Seifer DB, Gutmann JN, Doyle MB, et al: Persistent ectopic pregnancy following laparoscopic linear salpingostomy. Obstet Gynecol 1990; 76: 1121.
Seifer DB, Diamond MP, DeCherney AH: Persistent ectopic pregnancy. Obstet Gynecol Clin North Am 1991; 18:153.
Seifer DB, Gutmann JN, Grant WD, et al: Comparison of persistent ectopic pregnancy after laparoscopic salpingostomy versus salpingostomy at laparotomy for ectopic pregnancy. Obstet Gynecol 1993; 81:378.
Seifer DB, Silva PD, Grainger DA, et al: Reproductive potential after treatment for persistent ectopic pregnancy. Fertil Steril 1994; 62:194.
Shapiro HA, Zwarenstein HA: A rapid test for pregnancy on *Xenopus laevis*. Nature 1934; 133:762.
Speroff L, Glass RH, Kase NG: Clinical Gynecologic Endocrinology and Infertility, 5th ed. Baltimore, Williams and Wilkins, 1994.
Steier JA, Bergsjo P, Myking O: Human chorionic gonadotropin in maternal plasma after induced abortion, spontaneous abortion, and removed ectopic pregnancy. Obstet Gynecol 1984; 64:391.
Storring PO, Gaines-Das RE, Bangham DR: International reference preparation of human chorionic gonadotropin for immunoassay: Potency estimates in various bioassay and protein binding assay systems; and international reference preparations of the alpha and beta subunits of human chorionic gonadotropin for immunoassay. J Endocrinol 1980; 84:295.
Vaitukaitis JL, Braunstein GD, Ross GT: A radioimmunoassay which specifically measures human chorionic gonadotropin in the presence of human luteinizing hormone. Am J Obstet Gynecol 1972; 113:751.
Valkirs G, Chisum D, Barton R: Qualitative two-side IEMA for serum hCG using immunoconcentration technology. Clin Chem 1985; 31:960.
Wang Y, Schwartz PE, Chambers JT, Cole LA: Urinary gonadotropin fragments (UGF) in cancers of the female reproductive system. Gynecol Oncol 1988; 31:91.
Wide L, Gemzell CA: An immunological pregnancy test. Acta Endocrinol 1960; 35:261.
Wilcox AJ, Weinberg CR, O'Connor JF, et al: Incidence of early loss of pregnancy. N Engl J Med 1988; 319:189.
Wiltberger PD, Miller DF: The male frog, *Rana pipiens*, as a new test animal for early pregnancy. Science 1948; 107:198.
Witherspoon LR, Shuler SE, Joseph GF, et al: Immunoassays for quantifying choriogonadotropin compared for assay performance and clinical application. Clin Chem 1992; 38:887.
Zondek B: Die hormone des ovariums und des hypophysenvorderlappens. Berlin, Springer, 1931.

Chapter 21

Examination of Amniotic Fluid

Robert E. Wenk, M.D., M.S.
Jerald M. Rosenbaum, M.D.

HISTORICAL PERSPECTIVE

Amniocentesis was initially carried out as treatment for polyhydramnios in the 1870s. Diagnostic amniocentesis, however, was first used to predict erythroblastosis only in the early 1950s. The range of laboratory examinations of amniotic fluid (AF) has been widening since its initial use in predicting severity of hemolytic disease. Advances in prenatal diagnosis of hereditary, teratologic, and infectious disorders suggest continuing interest in AF as an informative specimen source (Weaver, 1989). A subjective historical summary of progress in diagnostic testing of AF is given in Table 21–1.

Generally, second- and third-trimester amniocentesis is a safe procedure. It is complicated only infrequently (0.5%) by bleeding, infection, fetoplacental trauma, fluid leak, and alloimmunization of the mother to fetal antigens. Nevertheless, newer antenatal diagnostic approaches that are under development promise more direct, earlier, or more accurate means of fetal diagnosis (Table 21–2). In the interest of brevity, this chapter does not deal with the general topic of prenatal diagnosis but focuses on the conditions that warrant AF studies, current methods, and future use of AF in clinical and laboratory medicine.

Before diagnostic amniocentesis is attempted, its goals, limitations, and follow-up options should be understood. There is a growing need to ensure that an informed couple has consented to undergo prenatal tests that may raise difficult medical questions and impose difficult family and interventional decisions (Elias, 1994). Parents have a legal right to decide whether or not to undergo AF testing. Physicians, on the other hand, must be informed about an increasing number of tests for a bewildering number of genetic and acquired fetal diseases. Test results may suggest examination of the partners or family members in follow-up. All the options must be offered (e.g., pregnancy termination, preparations for a handicapped child, medical and surgical treatments, and so on), and counselors and support agencies must be contacted. Laboratory staff should ensure the documentation of informed consent and be ready to participate in consultations with physicians, geneticists, and counselors. A team approach is appropriate.

EMBRYOLOGY AND FLUID PHYSIOLOGY

The amniotic sac arises entirely from embryonic structures during the first week of gestation. It consists of an outer mesodermal layer, which initially separates it from an extraembryonic coelomic space, and an inner ectodermal layer. During growth, the amniotic cavity expands, reflects over the embryo and its umbilical cord, and fills with aqueous fluid, suspending both living and nonviable cells. Amniocentesis can be carried out after 10 weeks, but this early sampling is technically difficult, cell culture is slow because few viable cells are retrieved, the procedure is risky because fetal mortality may be higher, and talipes deformity may be increased (Nicolaides, 1994). Most amniocenteses are now carried out during the second trimester for diagnosis of genetic disease and during the third trimester to assess fetal

Table 21–1. ADVANCES IN AMNIOTIC FLUID EXAMINATION

Year	Diagnostic Value and Test Method
1952	Prediction of hemolytic disease of newborns (HDN)
1955	Microscopic determination of fetal sex by Barr body study
1961	Management of Rho HDN by spectrophotometry
1966	Amniotic cell culture and karyotyping
1968	Galactosemia diagnosis by Gal-1-P uridyl transferase activity
1971	Respiratory distress syndrome assessment by surfactant analysis
1972	Neural tube defects (NTD) associated with increased α-fetoprotein
1975	Diagnostic DNA analysis (homozygous ß-thalassemia)
1981	Acetylcholinesterase test reduces false-positive tests for NTD
1984	Screening for endemic fetal infections (rubella, *Toxoplasma*)
1987	Steroidal analysis for congenital adrenal hyperplasia
1993	Induced amniotic fluid cells of patients with muscular dystrophy lack dystrophin
1994	Fetal DNA for Rho allele predicts HDN from amniotic fluid cells

pulmonary maturity and the severity of alloimmune fetal hemolytic disease.

In the first trimester, AF is primarily maternal in origin, but the suspended cells are entirely fetal, unless maternal ones were accidentally introduced during amniocentesis. Fetal urine is the major source of AF after the first trimester, but the umbilical cord, amniotic membrane, and fetal gastrointestinal and pulmonary tracts make contributions.

Normal AF volume at term is 0.5 to 1.5 L. Increased AF volume, associated with rapidly developing fetal edema, is termed acute hydramnios. Recipient twin transfusion syndrome, hydrops fetalis of various causes, and fetal heart failure are notable etiologies. (In twin-twin transfusion syndrome, there is acute shunting of blood from a donor twin to a growth-retarded recipient of the same sex. Vascular anastomoses are present in a monochorionic diamniotic placenta and may partly account for the phenomenon, which can reverse direction. Before 28 weeks of gestation, therapeutic amniocentesis can be lifesaving; otherwise, the death rate of one or both twins is about 50% [Saunders, 1992].) Chronic hydramnios is associated with fetal disorders characterized by poor fetal swallowing, with maternal diabetes, and with toxemia of pregnancy. Oligohydramnios ($<$300 mL AF volume) may accompany chronic fetal illness or distress and may indicate the need for measurements of fetal well-being, such as fetal capillary or cord blood pH or maternal urinary estriol. Oligohydramnios also occurs in placental insufficiency, donor-twin transfusion syndrome, and malformations of the fetal urinary tract.

FETAL GENETIC DIAGNOSIS

Cytogenetics

Cytogenetic examinations of cells from second- or third-trimester AF require several simultaneous cell cultures for 5 to 10 days because only one third of harvested cells are capable of survival and division. Indications for cytogenetic analysis are tabulated (Table 21–3). Advanced maternal age accounts for most AF cytogenetic assessment. Pitfalls of amniotic cell culture and karyotyping include accidental culture of maternal cells (1%) and pseudomosaicism (5%). The latter is an *in vitro* artifact consisting of a chromosomal abnormality in cells of only one primary culture (Moertel, 1992).

Amniotic cytogenetic studies may have advantages over those carried out on other fetal specimens (Bell, 1987; Meade, 1991). Failure to obtain samples occurs 60% less often after amniocentesis than chorionic villus sampling (CVS). Amniocentesis poses a slightly lower risk of fetal loss (0.5%) and fewer major complications than CVS (risk: 1% to 2%), cordocentesis, or fetal biopsy. Because the AF karyotype is performed on fetal cells, there are significantly fewer false-positive numerical abnormalities and mosaicisms, which are found in about 5% of CVS cultures. It has been suggested that because CVS is carried out earlier in pregnancy, a number of the detected chromosomally abnormal fetuses would have aborted spontaneously. Thus, the rate and cost of interventions and pregnancy terminations are increased with CVS. Whether early CVS may be a cause of some limb reduction anomalies is controversial (Firth, 1994).

Amniotic cytogenetics requires 7 to 12 days between sampling and reporting results because of the need for long-term culture of the few viable amniotic cells collected. Faster procedures have therefore been proposed, including fluorescence *in situ* hybridization (FISH), a procedure for probing

Table 21–2. COMPARISON OF FLUIDS IN FETAL CELL SAMPLING

Site	Earliest Gestational Sampling Time	Advantages	Disadvantages
Amniotic fluid	10 weeks	Safety (if carried out after 14 weeks) Direct DNA tests	Maternal cells mistaken for fetal Few cells, slow growth Fetal loss, lung hypoplasia if <12 weeks
Coelocentesis	6–10 weeks	Early Direct DNA tests	Cell cultures fail Experimental
Cordocentesis	18 weeks	Direct tests of fetal cells, plasma, serum etc. Most accurate karyotype	Higher fetal losses Availability limited Late
Maternal blood	10 weeks	Noninvasive Early	Fetal cells rare Experimental
Chorionic villus sample	8–12 weeks	Early Rapid karyotype	Higher fetal losses Limb, jaw defects Maternal cells recovered in error Detects mosaicism confined to placenta

Table 21–3. INDICATIONS FOR CYTOGENETIC AMNIOCENTESIS

Maternal age older than 35 years associated with increased risk of a child with a chromosome abnormality
Screening test (e.g., triple marker) suggests trisomy 21, 18, other chromosome disorder
Ultrasound examination suggests chromosomal abnormality because of anomalies
Previous child with trisomic disorder if the trisomy is the result of parental translocation
Known parental balanced translocation, inversion, or aneuploidy
Familial breakage syndromes (Bloom's syndrome, Fanconi's anemia, etc.)
Mother exposed to significant irradiation (e.g., radiotherapy)
Familial disorder for which fetal cytogenetic diagnosis is possible

chromosomes in mitotic metaphase or in cells that are not dividing (interphase). The procedure is currently considered adjunctive but is capable of microscopically demonstrating common aneuploidies of chromosomes 13, 18, 21, X, and Y, thus detecting many cytogenetic disorders that fail to cause spontaneous abortion (Ward, 1993). Results are available within 1 to 2 days, labor expense is low, cell culture is unnecessary, and more than 70% of all aneuploidies are detected. Unfortunately, other numerical and structural chromosomal anomalies are not identified by interphase FISH. Errors (failures to hybridize probe to target) have been reported in assessing sex and autosomal chromosomes. Therefore, given the present state of the art, standard cytogenetic evaluation must be carried out to provide the most complete information to physicians and patients.

More experimental than FISH are chemical molecular methods for the trisomies (e.g., 47,+21). Polymerase chain reaction (PCR) amplification of short tandem repeat sequences of DNA, known to be carried on the trisomic chromosome, can be distinguished from one another (they are allelic) and qualified to determine whether two or three copies of the alleles are present (Fig. 21–1). Advantages of this technology are rapidity and the ability to analyze few cells (Pertl, 1994). It also has limitations: Parents must be heterozygous for a marker allele, and nondisjunction at meiosis II may be indistinguishable from uniparental disomy.

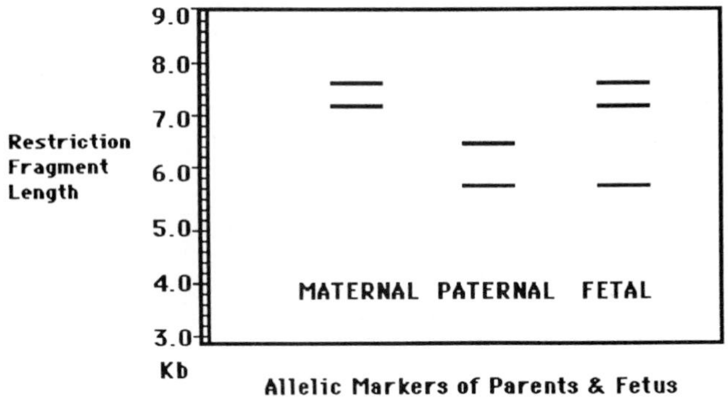

Figure 21–1. A Down syndrome fetus's chromosome 21 DNA at a hypothetical polymorphic locus near the centromere. Each parent is heterozygous; each band represents a DNA fragment derived from a parental chromosome 21. As in 70% of DS cases, the trisomy 21 fetus shows both maternal alleles and one paternal band. This indicates a nondisjunction in meiosis I during maternal oogenesis, followed by fertilization by a sperm cell containing a single chromosome 21. The bands are obtained by digestion of DNA with a specific endonuclease, amplification using PCR, electrophoresis on a sizing gel, and a detection method (e.g., ethidium bromide stain).

Down Syndrome Screening

Screening programs have been initiated for the intrauterine detection of Down syndrome (DS), the most common numerical autosomal disease of live-born infants. Advanced maternal age is associated with an increased risk of a DS pregnancy. Before the advent of maternal serum screening tests, women older than 35 years, whose age-specific risk of delivering a child with DS was 1:270, were offered amniotic cytogenetic analysis to detect a DS fetus. (At age 35, the risk of pregnancy loss secondary to amniocentesis equals the risk of delivering a live-born infant with a chromosomal abnormality.) As a result of this, it was found that most live-born children with DS (75%) were born to women younger than 35 years. Maternal serum screening became an appropriate assay for younger women. The first maternal serum test quantified α-fetoprotein (AFP) concentration, but this was neither specific (Table 21–4) nor sufficiently sensitive.

Current AFP testing provides a determination of risk of DS pregnancy and has been shown to detect about 60% of the cases. Increased accuracy is achieved by combining the information given by advanced maternal age and three laboratory markers in maternal serum sampled at 14 to 22 weeks' gestation. Maternal serum AFP (MSAFP) level tends to be decreased if the fetus has DS, human chorionic gonadotropin (hCG) level tends to be increased, and unconjugated estriol (UE3) tends to be decreased (Haddow, 1992). The triple-marker screening protocol effectively detects a majority (~80%) of DS. It has also been shown to detect Edwards' syndrome (47,+18), a disorder associated with decreased hCG, AFP, and UE3 (Fig. 21–2). Turner's syndrome (45,X) may also be detected. Proper interpretation of the data requires accurate assessment of gestational age and knowledge of other critical factors such as maternal weight, multiple gestation, and so on. Confirmation can be obtained by AF cytogenetic study.

Triple-marker screening was later extended to women older than 35 years in order to avoid unnecessary first-trimester diagnostic amniocenteses with their associated risk of miscarriage (0.3% to 0.5%) (Haddow, 1994). Because the serum markers are independent of maternal age, they can offset advanced age as a sole indicator of DS risk. Test sensitivity, however, is about 90% in this group, and thus some children with DS will be borne by those older women who do not benefit from cytogenetic analysis because of the protocol. In summary, cytogenetic amniocentesis can be offered when risk of DS is 1:190 or greater (the risk of miscarriage from the procedure) in pregnant women of any age. An algorithm for screening for DS during pregnancy is shown in Figure 21–3.

Table 21–4. CONDITIONS ASSOCIATED WITH DECREASED MATERNAL SERUM α-FETOPROTEIN

Some normal pregnancies	Gestational age overestimated
Fetal death (late)	Spontaneous, missed abortion
Molar pregnancy	Choriocarcinoma
Down syndrome	Edwards' syndrome (trisomy 18)

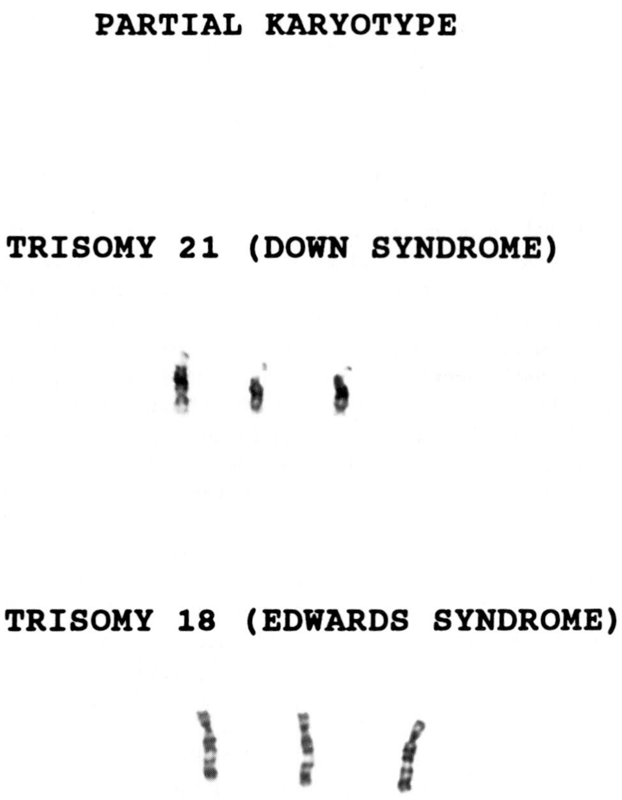

Figure 21–2. Partial karyotypes of trisomies 21 and 18, associated with Down and Edwards' syndromes, respectively. Trisomy may be the result of meiotic nondisjunction (NDJ) of the entire chromosome as depicted, mitotic NDJ, robertsonian translocation, or inheritance of three copies of only the critical region of the involved chromosome following a structural duplication.

The method of DS screening outlined earlier has been confirmed as highly effective (Goodburn, 1994). Better means may become available, however, including examination of maternal serum for free β-hCG and pregnancy-associated plasma protein A (PAPP-A) as early as 10 to 12 weeks of gestation (McIntosh, 1994). Effectiveness of these experimental screening protocols requires confirmation.

Other Reasons for Amniotic Cytogenetic Analysis

Obstetric ultrasound examination sometimes demonstrates anomalies that suggest the possibility of a chromosome disorder. Multisystem malformations are associated with abnormal amniotic karyotypes (trisomies 13, 18, 21, triploidy, Turner's syndrome, and unbalanced structural disorders) in more than 25% of cases (Nicolaides, 1992). High recurrence risk (associated with some parental structural chromosomal rearrangements encountered in a previous pregnancy, such as t[14;21]), may also indicate study.

Rarely, a familial chromosomal instability syndrome is encountered. Instability is related to hereditary defects in deoxyribonucleic acid (DNA) replication and repair. Syndromes include Fanconi's anemia, Bloom's syndrome, ataxia-telangiectasia, xeroderma pigmentosa, progeria, Wiskott-Aldrich syndrome, and others (Schroeder, 1982).

Single-Gene Disorders

More detailed information about the general topic of prenatal diagnostic methods, in addition to AF genetic tests, may be found elsewhere (Weaver, 1989; Grabowski, 1990;

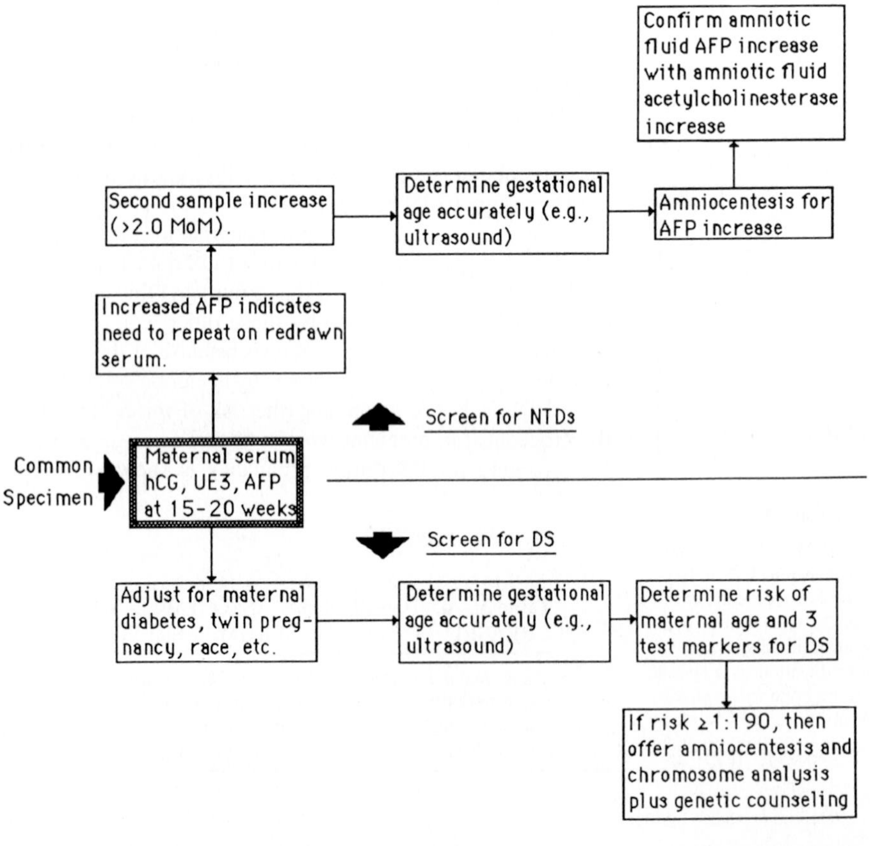

Figure 21–3. An algorithm for simultaneous screening for Down syndrome fetuses and open neural tube defects. Positive screening may be followed by amniotic fluid analyses.

Grebner, 1993). Selected topics related to AF are presented later.

Both hereditary and nongenetic fetal disorders may be detected from amniotic samples. Examples of nongenetic diseases include congenital hypothyroidism (in which AF thyroid-stimulating hormone [TSH] is increased) and fetal hydantoin syndrome (in which the amniocyte epoxide hydrolase level is low).

Purely hereditary (single-gene) diseases can be evaluated by study of metabolites of uncultured amniotic cells, cultured AF cells, and supernatant fluid. Two interesting examples are described next: X-linked muscular dystrophy and autosomal recessive congenital adrenal hyperplasia. In addition, amniotic cells can be used as sources of DNA for directly evaluating other single-locus diseases, including the hemoglobinopathies, cystic fibrosis, fragile X syndrome, α-1-antitrypsin deficiency, phenylketonuria, and the hemophilias. Aspects of fragile X syndrome and cystic fibrosis are described as examples. Rho alloimmune hemolytic disease and alloimmune thrombocytopenia have both genetic and immunologic components that may be evaluated by AF tests. Each of these alloimmune disorders is described.

It should be noted that AF contamination by maternal cells (cultured and uncultured) can cause error in molecular analyses as well as in cytogenetics. Maternal DNA analysis can be used to demonstrate contamination error, which may occur in nearly one in five cases (Rebello, 1994).

X-linked Muscular Dystrophies

Two clinical variants of X-linked muscular dystrophy (Duchenne's and Becker's) are usually caused by one of various mutations in the single gene encoding for the protein dystrophin (chromosome Xp21.2). In approximately two thirds of affected males or carrier females, the deleterious mutation (usually a deletion) can be identified by molecular methods. Point mutations and some deletions are not detected. Dystrophin is limited in its tissue distribution; therefore, biopsy samples of skeletal muscle stained with a fluorescein-labeled antibody to dystrophin demonstrate the abnormality when the molecular methods fail. Fetal muscle biopsy, however, is both difficult and risky as a prenatal diagnostic method.

Although dystrophin is normally absent from amniocytes, its manufacture may be initiated by retroviral transfection of amniotic cells with *MYOD*, a human gene that induces amniocyte myogenesis if the dystrophin gene is functional. Failure to demonstrate dystrophin by immunofluorescence cytology after *MYOD* transfection is evidence of some form of muscular dystrophy in a male fetus. Test sensitivity appears to be 100% for Duchenne's dystrophy (absent dystrophin, severe disease), and specificity appears to be 98% in this currently experimental test. Patients with the milder Becker's form of dystrophy often manufacture a truncated protein or a small amount of dystrophin. These cases may require Western blot or enzyme-linked immunosorbent assay (ELISA) methods, rather than immunofluorescence, to demonstrate abnormal protein (Sancho, 1993).

Congenital Adrenal Hyperplasia

Congenital adrenal hyperplasia (CAH) consists of a group of autosomal recessive clinical disorders caused by deficiency of one of several enzymes in the biosynthetic pathway to cortisol. The most frequent (95%) is 21-hydroxylase deficiency caused by mutations in both parental alleles at a locus on chromosome 6p21.3. Each known variant allele is in linkage disequilibrium with a specific HLA haplotype, is frequent within defined populations, and is associated with one of several specific clinical syndromes termed salt-wasting, simple-virilizing, late-onset, cryptic, and null. Virilization of affected females occurs between 9 and 13 weeks' gestation. In families at risk, first-trimester prenatal diagnosis is sometimes possible by determining the HLA haplotype marker of the defective 21-hydroxylase alleles or by DNA probes of targeted intragenic base sequences in first-trimester chorionic villus cells. Amniotic cells are sufficient for DNA diagnosis in the second trimester, but earlier diagnosis and treatment (with dexamethasone) are desirable to avoid later surgery in severely virilized girls.

Amniotic supernate may be used in the second trimester (16 weeks) to evaluate the adequacy of treatment by analyzing for increased concentrations of 17-hydroxyprogesterone (17HP) in the salt-wasting variant or androstenedione (d4A) in salt-wasting and simple-virilizing CAH. 17HP is a precursor of both cortisol and aldosterone, whereas d4A is an androgen produced by metabolic shunting. Increases in 17HP and d4A are evidence of inadequate treatment (Dorr, 1993). Chemical analyses of AF supernate may be useful in confirming diagnosis of congenital adrenal hyperplasia (after a five-day suspension of treatment) as well as for determining the efficacy of maternal dexamethasone administration from the fifth gestational week (Pang, 1990).

Fragile X Syndrome

Fragile X syndrome is the most common familial type of mental retardation (frequency: 1/2500 females, 1/1500 males). The fragile X chromosome is named for its folate-sensitive site at Xq27.3. Microscopically, the chromosome appears as if it is about to fragment in cytogenetic preparations using specific cell culture conditions in which folate is depleted. Diagnosis from amniotic (or CVS) cytogenetics poses a problem because of variable expression and difficulty in inducing the chromosomal appearance. Molecular methods that have been developed provide more reliable detection of disease and are now the methods of choice. Southern blots are used to determine the size and state of hypermethylation of DNA. PCR is used to determine the length of CGG trinucleotide repeat sequences, which are markedly increased (>200 repeats) in overt disease (mutation) and somewhat increased (>52 repeats) in family members who carry the defect (premutation). Although early prenatal diagnosis is feasible (e.g., from chorionic DNA), a cautious approach is warranted and confirmation by amniocyte DNA analysis may be required to resolve ambiguous results (Marchese, 1994).

Cystic Fibrosis

Cystic fibrosis (CF) is a very frequent autosomal recessive disease of Caucasians, affecting about 1/2500, but disease is not limited to specific populations. Many different mutations in the CF transmembrane regulator (*CFTR*) gene cause variant disease phenotypes. DNA probe analyses must be able to detect dozens of different CF variants. Thus, when variant alleles have been identified in a specific family, carrier detection and diagnosis of disease are possible, but genetic heterogeneity precludes simple universal screening and counselling. Current recommendations are that couples known to be at risk and contemplating pregnancy should be made aware of DNA tests for CF (Harrington, 1992). If already pregnant, a woman may elect to have fetal DNA analysis.

Direct diagnosis of fetal CF has been described, using single-strand conformation polymorphism (SSCP) analysis (Desgeorges, 1993). PCR is used to amplify short regions of the gene's DNA coding sequence, denaturing the amplified DNA into two strands, performing gel electrophoresis of the single strands, hybridizing with labeled probes, and observing for abnormally shifted bands on autoradiograms. SSCP may provide a means of prenatal diagnosis when mutation analysis and restriction fragment polymorphisms are uninformative or not possible.

Table 21–5. CONDITIONS ASSOCIATED WITH INCREASED MATERNAL SERUM α-FETOPROTEIN

Gestational age underestimated	Open neural tube defects
Multiple pregnancy	Intrauterine death (early)
Growth retardation	Maternal α-fetoprotein–producing neoplasm
Fetal distress	Hydrocephaly
Gastroschisis	Tetralogy of Fallot
Omphalocele	Hydrops fetalis (any cause)
Congenital nephropathies (various)	Turner's syndrome without hygroma
Sacrococcygeal teratoma	Cystic hygroma
Congenital neoplasms	Placental defects
Duodenal atresia	Microcephaly
Esophageal atresia	Cyclopia
Abdominal pregnancy	

MULTIFACTORIAL FETAL DISORDERS

Multifactorial fetal disorders often involve multigenic and environmental factors in their pathogenesis. Examples include erythroblastosis fetalis and many congenital anomalies.

Major physical anomalies are observed in as many as 3% of births but cannot be easily ascribed to simple interactions of heredity and environment. Depending on their pathogenesis, the critical time in gestation when they arise, and the tissues affected, they can be generally classified as *malformations*, intrinsically abnormal developmental processes (e.g., neural tube defects arise early); *disruptions*, breakdowns or interference with originally normal developmental processes (e.g., limb defects related to amniotic bands arise later); and *deformations*, changes in form or position of a body part caused by nondisruptive mechanical forces (e.g., oligohydramniotic facial compression arises very late in gestation).

Neural Tube Defects

Neural tube defects (NTDs) arise between 17 and 30 days' gestation and develop in as many as 1% of some Caucasian populations (e.g., in Ireland), although less frequently in other groups. Most cases are sporadic, the recurrence risk in families with one affected individual ranges from 0.3% to 43% (average 5%), depending on the number and degree of affected relatives. NTDs are a leading cause of stillbirth and death in early infancy, with two thirds of affected live-born infants being female. Folate supplementation (4 to 5 mg/day) has been associated with a 70% decrease in the risk of recurrence after the birth of an affected child (Czeizel, 1992). Open NTDs can occur at either caudal (neural tube fusion site 5) or cephalic sites (sites 2 and 4) and result in meningomyelocele or anencephaly. Each of these open defects occurs in 0.1% of births in the United States.

Maternal Serum α-Fetoprotein Screening

A pregnant woman's serum AFP is increased in concentration when her unborn child possesses an open NTD. AFP concentration in fetal serum is 300 mg/dL (maximal at 12 to 15 weeks), and AFP diffuses into AF (maximal at 15 to 16 weeks) and maternal serum (maximal at 32 weeks). Maternal serum α-fetoprotein increase was established as an indicator of fetal NTDs before maternal serum AFP decrease became a marker of fetal DS. The two screening algorithms for NTD and DS can be initiated simultaneously (see Fig. 21–3). MSAFP increases are not specific for NTDs: AFP is increased in a number of fetal anomalies, twin pregnancies, and other conditions (Table 21–5).

Serum AFP examination is carried out at 14 to 22 weeks' gestation (16 to 18 weeks is optimal). Gestational age is usually estimated by simple dating in whole weeks (rounding downward) from the last menstrual period. AFP concentrations are adjusted for maternal weight, race, and presence of insulin-dependent diabetes mellitus. If concentrations exceed 2.0 multiples of the fiftieth percentile (median) of the frequency distribution of normal values for a given week of pregnancy, a second serum specimen is collected one week after the first (see Fig. 21–3). A second abnormal serum increase is followed up by high-resolution ultrasonography to detect a gross NTD or other anomaly and to detect a multiple pregnancy but, most importantly, to detect an underestimation of gestational age.

Amniotic Fluid α-Fetoprotein

After the finding of an abnormal MSAFP, if gestational age is correct, amniocentesis may be carried out, depending on clinical indications and circumstances. AFP analyses on AF samples are also carried out concurrently with cytogenetic studies, if either parent was born with an NTD, or in a mother who previously delivered a child with an open NTD, or whose sister delivered a child with an open NTD. Concentrations of AFP in AF (AF AFP) are expressed in multiples of the median (MoM) of normal values of the data collected in a given laboratory:

MoM = average of patient's duplicate results ÷ median of the reference interval for a given gestational age in weeks

AF AFP concentrations are a thousandfold greater than maternal serum concentrations. Unlike serum, AF AFP concentration declines between 16 and 22 weeks.

Acetylcholinesterase

If AF AFP is increased, amniotic acetylcholinesterase (AChE) activity is determined. AChE, like AFP, is increased with open fetal NTDs, but the enzyme determination presents the diagnostic advantage that AChE is independent of gestational age. Although their results are less affected by fetal blood than AFP, AChE tests should be avoided in grossly bloody AF. Follow-up of a bloody tap includes ultrasound examination and repeated AF studies when blood has cleared (in two weeks) (see Traumatic [Bloody] Amniocentesis).

AChE appears to be as sensitive as and more specific than AF AFP in detecting NTDs. It produces half as many false-positive results. Unfortunately, until recently, the test was labor intensive, expensive, subjective, and prone to interference when enzyme activity was measured. Therefore, it was not considered useful in screening. Because AF AChE testing is unnecessary in 95% of cases but is invaluable when AFP results are high (>2.0 MoM), optimal screening results are currently achieved when AF AFP and AChE tests are used in tandem (Wald, 1989).

Monoclonal antibody immunoassays for AChE between 16 and 24 weeks may replace kinetic enzyme or electrophoretic methods in the future because they are more objective, more specific, and less labor intensive, and they avoid interference with the enzyme activity measurements (Loft, 1990). AChE determination can be carried out using maternal serum or AF. In AF, AChE may be less elevated in fetal abdominal wall defects and other anomalies than in NTDs, suggesting differential diagnostic value (Loft, 1993). If automated, AChE determinations could replace AFP tests (Hangaard, 1991).

Erythroblastosis Fetalis

Developments such as cordocentesis, nucleic acid probes for target sequences of the Rh factor (Rho,D), and changes in clinical methods are modifying laboratory participation in the management of alloimmune hemolytic disease. Older methods, however, have not been discarded and may be used when the new ones are not available.

Alloimmune Fetal Hemolytic Disease

Maternal alloimmunization to red blood cell antigens may follow transfusion or fetomaternal hemorrhage. When maternal IgG alloantibodies cross the placenta, they may bind to fetal erythrocyte antigens that were paternally inherited. Sensitized fetal red blood cells may have decreased survival, and the rate of hemolysis may increase with advancing gestation. Severe disease in a fetus is marked by anemia, congestive heart failure (hydrops), and intrauterine death.

A fetus does not develop jaundice after a fetal hemolytic anemia. Catabolism of released hemoglobin to unconjugated bilirubin is not problematic because the placenta ordinarily excretes the pigment. Also, stress induction of fetal hepatocytes to produce glucuronyl transferase may increase nontoxic conjugated bilirubin (which accounts for as much as 50% of AF bilirubin).

Maternal Alloimmunization

Decline in the frequency of cases of Rho(D) alloimmune hemolytic disease is related primarily to a decrease in family size and secondarily to preventive passive immunization by administration of Rho immune globulin (RhIg). Severe Rho(D) disease after pregnancy immunization is related to failures of prophylaxis against immunizing events: fetomaternal hemorrhage in late pregnancy, parturition, intragestational trauma, amniocentesis, spontaneous abortion, undertreatment, and emergency obstetric transfusion.

Severe non-Rho(D) alloimmune hemolytic disease is occasionally encountered. Although many alloimmune causes are possible, Kell (K1), hr′(c), and A(BO) hemolytic disease are fairly frequent. Therefore, all women should be screened for atypical antibodies twice during pregnancy, if possible, once at the first prenatal visit and again after 28 weeks. Further screening may be indicated by gestational trauma, antepartum bleeding (e.g., threatened abortion), and medical interventions such as amniocentesis, CVS, external version, and intrauterine transfusion. Notably, new maternal alloantibodies against red blood cells have been induced by intrauterine transfusion in about one quarter of cases. These antibodies are usually directed against fetal antigens, but they are specific for donor cell antigens in about 20% (Vietor, 1994). Kleihauer's stain of maternal blood films may demonstrate fetomaternal hemorrhage, which, if sufficient in volume, may explain fetal compromise or indicate need for repeated or higher doses of RhIg.

Management of the Rho Alloimmunized Pregnancy

3

Although the most elegant methods have been developed for treating Rho(D) disease, all hemolytic disease is managed in a similar way. When active immunization against the Rho(D) antigen is discovered by maternal serum antibody screening during the first trimester, the presence of alloantibody alone is cause for a four-step follow-up.

First, one must ascertain by history that active immunization to Rho(D) has occurred—that is, no prophylactic RhIg was administered before serologic screening of an Rho(D)-negative gravida. Prophylactic intramuscular RhIg is administered after all invasive procedures, after trauma, at 28 weeks of gestation, and immediately postpartum. Preventive administration of RhIg does not usually raise titers to greater than about 8 (equivalent to about 0.25 IU/mL). The problem of a false-positive screen for irregular antibodies arises fairly often, and either the obstetrician or the patient herself must be called to obtain the clinical history.

Second, it is important to know if the fetus in the current, actively immunized pregnancy possesses the Rho(D) antigen. Because the alloimmunized mother is homozygous for absence of D (i.e., she is dd), the fetus can be either Dd or dd, depending on the paternal genotype. Ideally, simple red blood cell phenotyping of the male partner should allow determination of the chances of fetal inheritance of the reacting D antigen. That is, it might be determined first if he is one of 16% of Rho-negative (dd) Caucasian men, approximately 48% of heterozygous (Dd) men, or 36% of homozygous (DD) men. Second, if he carries the D antigen, the probability of his heterozygosity for D could be calculated from his CcDEe phenotype and known population haplotype frequencies. Study of the male partner's red blood cell phenotype, however, may not be informative because the partner may not be the father of the unborn child, paternal phenotype may not correctly specify the genotype after probability calculations, and even a known heterozygous father would sire an Rho(D)-negative child half the time. Therefore, it is better to determine the fetal type directly to achieve greater certainty.

Fetal red blood cell phenotyping is possible using cells obtained by CVS at 9 to 11 weeks or from cordocentesis samples. Small samples require extraordinary laboratory methods. CVS also can serve as a source of DNA for analysis, as described subsequently. However, early CVS appears to be associated with increases in fetal mortality, late complications, fetal limb and jaw anomalies, and fetomaternal hemorrhage, which can result in an anamnestic antibody response, increased fetal hemolysis, and worsened anemia.

A less invasive evaluation is possible by probing amniocytic DNA for the genomic RhD sequences (Bennett, 1993; Simsek, 1994). One or 2 mL of AF is sampled in the first or second trimester. DNA is extracted from fetal cells, and RhD locus–specific exonic sequences (chromosome 1p34-36) are amplified using selected primers and the PCR. Nonspecific sequences found in both the RHD gene and the adjacent RHCE gene may be amplified simultaneously (multiplex PCR) as an internal control for possible sample-specific failure of the PCR reaction. Within a few hours, the amplified products can be electrophoresed and visualized on an agarose gel using ethidium bromide staining. An RHD-positive fetus demonstrates a characteristic band size on the gel, whereas an RHD-negative fetus produces only the band representing the nonspecific sequence. (Without the use of the nonspecific sequence, PCR failure could result in mistyping an RHD-positive fetus as RHD negative. RHD-positive and -negative samples are also analyzed to control reagents and procedures.)

The PCR method may produce false RHD-positive results. Because DNA is examined only when a mother is at risk for Rho(D) alloimmunization (she is RHD negative), there is no possibility of her cells causing false-positive results. Precautions are necessary, however, to avoid extraneous sources of DNA contamination. Furthermore, present techniques allow for nonspecificity of oligonucleotide primers if there is low hybridization stringency or if weak D serologic variants (with similar RHD DNA target sequences) are encountered. False RHD negatives may be caused by omitting a primer or by primer failing to hybridize during initial PCR cycles. Use of more than one set of target sequences in the RHD gene may be useful in avoiding some errors. To date, fetal genotyping of only the RHD gene has been carried out as a means of predicting the presence of the antigen causing the hemolytic disease, and the procedure for RHD gene analysis is not widely available.

Third, if the mother demonstrates alloantibody to an antigen determined with certainty (from DNA) or greater than 90% probability (from paternal phenotype) to be present in the fetus, or if paternal antigens cannot be determined, severity and progress of hemolysis should be established. In some centers, titration of maternal antibodies is considered irrelevant and ultrasonography may be performed to assess for hydrops. In the absence of fetal edema, severity of fetal hemolytic disease may be determined by the severity of jaundice in AF. In other centers, a critical titer is established (usually ≥ 16 or ≥ 32 or a two-tube or fourfold rise) before attempting amniocentesis (Welch, 1993). Critical titer is one below which severe disease is not supposed to occur (based on past experience). An argument against using maternal titers as indicators of severity is that moderate hemolytic disease (requiring exchange transfusion) and severe disease (deaths) actually do occur in as many as 10% of newborns with titers considered less than critical.

Although Liley's graphic method for predicting severity from AF spectrophotometry cannot be extrapolated into the second trimester, AF collected at 18 to 20 weeks still may be used to detect and manage pregnancies at high risk for severe alloimmunization (Queenan, 1993). Fetal blood sampling and hemoglobin determination, however, provide a more accurate assessment of (hemolytic) anemia than AF examination before 26 weeks. Notably, about two thirds of cases of severe anemia (hemoglobin <6 g/dL) are undetectable by single AF spectrophotometric examinations. Some severely affected fetuses without hydrops cannot be detected by any means other than direct blood sampling (Nicolaides, 1986). Absence of fetal anemia indicates follow-up by amniotic pigment study and ultrasound examination. Fetal blood sampling is repeated with the detection of hydrops or when AF absorbance exceeds the midpoint of the midzone on Liley's prediction graph (Fig. 21–4). Otherwise, AF pigment is simply monitored (e.g., at one- or two-week intervals) until fetal pulmonary maturity is identified and delivery is possible (see Procedure for Liley's Test and Surfactant Analysis: Fetal Pulmonary Maturity).

Fetal blood sampling (cordocentesis) is not universally available, involves greater risks of fetal mortality and maternal complications, may be clinically unsuitable in some cases, and is refused by patients in others. In the third trimester, amniocentesis provides about 95% accuracy in determining severity of anemia (Steyn, 1992). Empirically, both historical and recent series of cases have shown sufficient correlation between newborn hemoglobin concentrations and net AF absorbance measurements at 450 nm for case management in the third trimester.

Fourth, once severe disease is certain, obstetric management depends on various clinical factors including the gestational age, fetal and maternal complications (e.g., hydrops), fetal pulmonary maturity, resources of available health care institutions, and the skills of obstetricians and neonatologists. Clinical pathology and transfusion medicine services provide important data and blood components for treatment of patients, including surfactant analysis; the positive identification of fetal blood in a cordocentesis sample (by absence of plasma hCG, increased red blood cell volume, and red blood cell immunophenotyping); provision of irradiated, filtered, CMV-negative, compatible red blood cell suspensions; and so on.

Procedure for Liley's Test

Bilirubin imparts a yellow color to AF, but it should be noted that the AF pigment can be either maternal or fetal in origin. (Maternal hemolytic or sickle disorders can increase bilirubin in AF.) In erythroblastosis, severity of hemolysis correlates with the net absorbance of light at a 450-nm wavelength. Because bilirubin is bound to albumin, its concentration is dependent on protein turnover, and its concentration in AF does not change rapidly. If a previous erythroblastotic pregnancy's outcome was fetal death, AF of the current gestation is first sampled 10 weeks before the gestational week of the death. Analyses are most accurate after 26 to 28 weeks.

A specimen of AF is collected, centrifuged or filtered, and examined with a recording spectrophotometer. If the light absorbance of the fluid is plotted continuously between wavelengths of 350 and 700 nm, the resulting curve can be used to determine whether or not the AF contains bilirubin or other

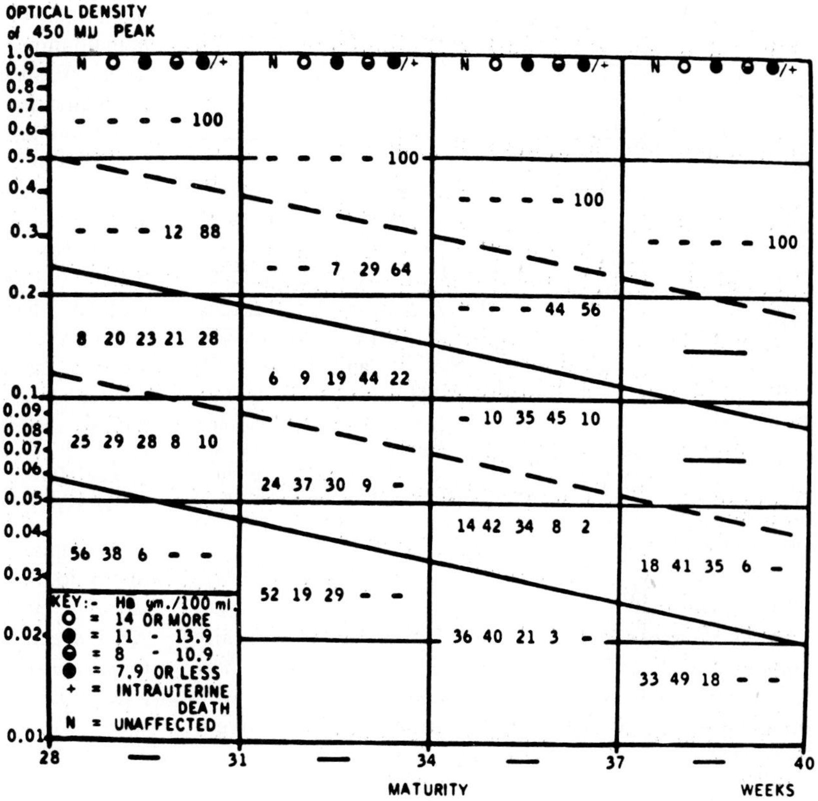

Figure 21–4. Liley's correlative graph for predicting the severity of hemolytic disease as determined from cord blood hemoglobin concentrations of newborns delivered several days after amniotic pigment analysis. (Liley AW: Am J Obstet Gynecol 1963; 86:485.)

pigmented products of hemolysis and to quantify the bilirubin pigment that is present.

Net absorbance at 450 nm is the difference between the observed and the expected (background) absorbance of the AF lacking bilirubin. Background AF absorbance decreases as the duration of an unaffected pregnancy increases after 28 weeks but not before 26 weeks, when it is constant. The decrease is the effect of dilution, and it is depicted as negatively sloped lines that demarcate Liley's lower, mid-, and upper prediction zones for mild, moderate, and severe hemolysis, respectively. The greater the net absorbance at 450 nm, the greater is the hemolysis and the lower is the umbilical cord hemoglobin at any given age of gestation.

Five to 10 mL of AF is usually collected. The specimen should not be exposed to light because bilirubin is photosensitive. After centrifugation or filtration to remove cells and large particulates, the supernatant fluid is examined. A spectral absorbance curve is obtained (Fig. 21–5) to determine the net absorbance (optical density, OD) at 450 nm. An alternative approach involves analysis of bilirubin by a sensitive diazotization method (Gambino, 1966).

The initial curve may plot wavelength (abscissa) against total absorbance (ordinate) on linear scales. The curvilinear plot can be transferred to a semilog ordinate scale to convert it to a straight line by selecting the two absorbance values observed at 365 and 550 nm (Fig. 21–6). The two points are above and below the 450-nm absorbance peak of bilirubin pigment, and thus the straight line represents the background absorbance of the fluid itself. The actual absorbance at 450 nm is recorded from the original (linear) plot. The expected absorbance at 450 nm (if no pigment was present) is recorded from the transfer (log) plot. The difference between actual and expected absorbance (OD) values is the net absorbance (OD) at 450 nm.

The calculated net absorbance is transferred to the Liley graph, which denotes weeks of gestation on the linear abscissa and net absorbance on the logscale ordinate. Interpretation is made from the point or points plotted on the Liley graph. Serial testing is common practice and allows for trending sequential net absorbances. High and increasing net absorbances may indicate need for more frequent AF analyses, early delivery, or more invasive tests and treatment.

Trends are usually unidirectional, either paralleling the negatively sloped lines on Liley's graph or showing a positive slope. The slopes of trend lines may change in some cases, sometimes dramatically (Fig. 21–7). This is more likely to occur when early net absorbance values are in the midzone.

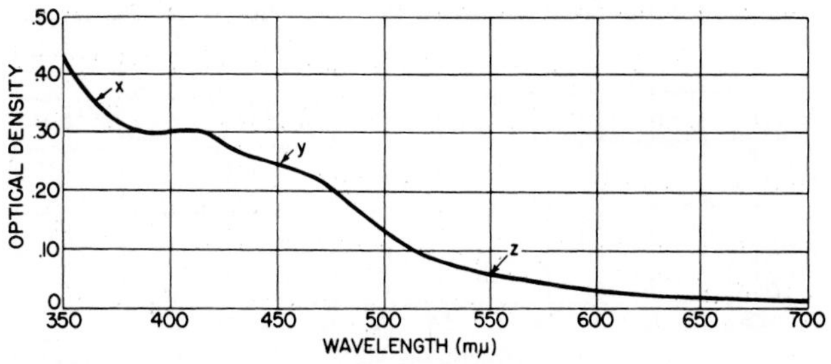

Figure 21–5. Spectrophotometric record of the absolute absorbance (optical density, O.D.) of light between 350 and 700 nm determined in an amniotic fluid sample from a case of hemolytic disease (containing bilirubin pigment). A water blank was used. (Redrawn from original scan.)

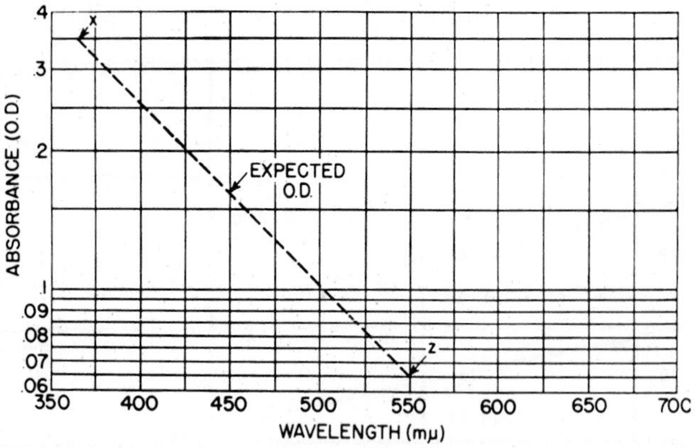

Figure 21–6. Semilog transfer of the 365- and 550-nm datapoints recorded in Figure 21–5. The curvilinear plot of the background AF is now represented by a straight line. The expected absorbance (A) at 450 nm is determined from the line and subtracted from the observed A at 450 nm to produce the net A. Net A (net O.D.) is a measure of bilirubin concentration and empirically correlates with severity of fetal hemolytic disease.

After 30 weeks' gestation, the Liley test result is usually combined with an assessment of fetal lung maturity. The combination of pigment and surfactant analyses assists with the clinical decision about whether or not to induce delivery (see Surfactant Analysis: Fetal Pulmonary Maturity).

Pitfalls in Interpreting Amniotic Fluid Pigment Analyses

Tracings must be interpreted by a knowledgeable person because it is important to recognize pitfalls, obtain the clinical history and blood bank information, and study other laboratory data before writing an interpretive report. Pigments

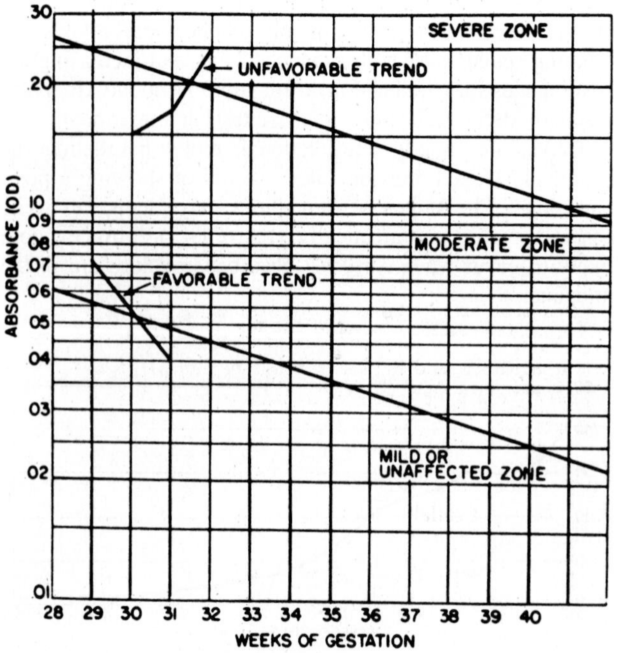

Figure 21–7. Sequential net absorbance values of AF showing an increasing severity of hemolysis in one case (upper curve) and a favorable trend in another case (lower curve). Trended data yield more accurate assessments of disease severity and progression than single measurements.

other than bilirubin may affect results. Hemoglobin, methemalbumin, meconium, and fetal acidosis produce characteristic spectrophotometric effects. Blood contamination is frequently encountered. Maternal jaundice or hemolysis can also cause misinterpretation. The presence of fetal cells indicates worsening of anemia by blood loss, may explain rise in maternal antibody (anamnestic response), and may be associated with an unexpected increase in net absorbance at 450 nm. The last effect is the result of bilirubin in fetal plasma (which is increased in even mild disease) admixing with AF. Meconium staining of AF is a sign of fetal distress. Exposure of AF to light, fetal acidosis, maternal use of steroids, markedly increased hemoglobin, and poor calibration all may cause inaccurate net absorbance measurements.

Laboratory Identification of Amniotic Fluid

Attempts at amniocentesis occasionally result in aspirate that is not the AF expected. Fetal ascites, AF of a twin, amniotic cyst contents, and maternal urine may be submitted as AF. A spectrophotometric tracing of maternal urine is similar to normal AF, but the curve is of greater negative slope. Maternal urine is the most frequent specimen mistaken for AF. It contains urea nitrogen in a concentration of about 300 mg/dL and creatinine exceeding 10 mg/dL, whereas AF urea nitrogen concentration is usually about 30 mg/dL and creatinine is less than 3.5 mg/dL. Precautionary creatinine or urea nitrogen measurements of AF should be carried out routinely. Use of dipsticks to detect protein and glucose in AF are less useful because these two materials may be present in the urine of pregnant women.

The identification of AF with certainty is currently problematic. Aside from the erroneous sampling of maternal urine after attempted amniocentesis, there are other reasons for identifying whether fluid is truly amniotic. For example, the presence of vaginal AF can indicate premature rupture of membranes (PROM). Clinically, AF is identified nonspecifically as vaginal pooled fluid with an alkaline pH and a ferning pattern when dried on a glass surface. Unfortunately, cervical mucus also causes ferning, and the test is not specific.

One potentially specific laboratory marker is a unique Western blot pattern of fibronectin and tenascin isoforms (Linnala, 1994). The fetal domain of fibronectin can be detected in cervicovaginal fluid by a monoclonal antibody in 94% of women with PROM and 50% of those with preterm contractions without rupture. The antigen is found in less than 5% of vaginal fluids of women who have uncomplicated pregnancies and who deliver at term (Lockwood, 1991). Thus, this experimental test for fetal fibronectin appears to herald preterm labor but does not differentiate ruptured and unruptured membranes.

Traumatic (Bloody) Amniocentesis

Blood is visually evident even when diluted by AF a thousandfold (v/v). Bloody taps occur in 2% to 3% of early amniocentesis aspirates and 20% of late ones. The blood is sometimes of fetal origin, raising the possibilities of fetomaternal hemorrhage (with potential for primary or anamnestic alloimmunization).

Kleihauer's staining of AF red blood cells prepared on a

glass slide allows for discrimination among pure fetal, pure adult, and mixed red blood cell populations. Fetal cells contain hemoglobin F, which resists alkaline buffer elution. Fetal cells appear as red, refractile, large cells on an eosin-stained Kleihauer preparation. Maternal cells appear as uncolored ghosts or dull red, poorly stained intermediate cells (indicating increased maternal erythropoiesis). Kleihauer's stains are difficult to control technically, and alternate methods have been developed (immunofluorescence staining of hemoglobin F, electrophoresis or isofocusing of hemoglobin F, flow cytometry). Notably, ordinary cell counters can be used in very bloody specimens of AF to ascertain that fetal blood was sampled. Counters can also determine the proportions of fetal cells in mixed populations because fetal cells have mean corpuscular volumes of 140 fL, whereas adult cells are usually less than 100 fL.

Alloimmune Thrombocytopenia

Maternal IgG alloantibodies to paternally inherited fetal platelet antigens can give rise to passive alloimmune fetal and newborn thrombocytopenia. (The pathogenesis of alloimmune thrombocytopenia is similar to that of erythroblastosis.) The frequency of newborn alloimmune thrombocytopenia is 1/5000 births. Affected infants are at risk for gastrointestinal or central nervous system bleeding. Intracranial hemorrhage can produce neurologic damage or death. Unlike red blood cell alloimmunization, the disease arises frequently (50%) in primiparous patients.

Because antibodies bind to platelets that are quickly removed from circulation, laboratory diagnosis may or may not be possible, depending on the concentrations of platelet alloantibodies in maternal serum. That is, it may not be possible to detect low-titer antibody, to determine its specificity, or to ascertain incompatibility of maternal antibody and paternal platelets. Diagnosis sometimes depends on a history of a previously affected child. A low maternal platelet count is occasionally encountered and alerts a physician. Although this is usually evidence of maternal autoimmune disease, workup may reveal alloimmune fetal thrombocytopenia. (Possibly, decrease in maternal platelets is caused by an "innocent bystander" mechanism similar to post-transfusion purpura.)

Once fetal disease has been diagnosed, percutaneous umbilical blood sample (PUBS) and capillary blood of the presenting part (at delivery) can be used to determine fetal and newborn platelet counts. Intravenous immunoglobulin can be given to the mother to protect the passively immunized thrombocytopenic fetus, if PUBS platelet counts exceed 50,000/μL. Lower counts may indicate intrauterine transfusion or cesarean section. After delivery, washed, irradiated, serologically screened maternal platelets can be used for transfusion of the newborn.

The maternal antibodies in passive alloimmune thrombocytopenia are usually directed against platelet-specific antigens, but HLA antigens may occasionally be involved. Half of all cases are caused by HPA1 (PI^{A1}) antibodies directed against an antigen lacking in 2% of the population.

Recurrence of disease is very high. Whether a subsequent fetus or newborn is affected depends, in part, on the platelet type and zygosity of the father of that subsequent offspring.

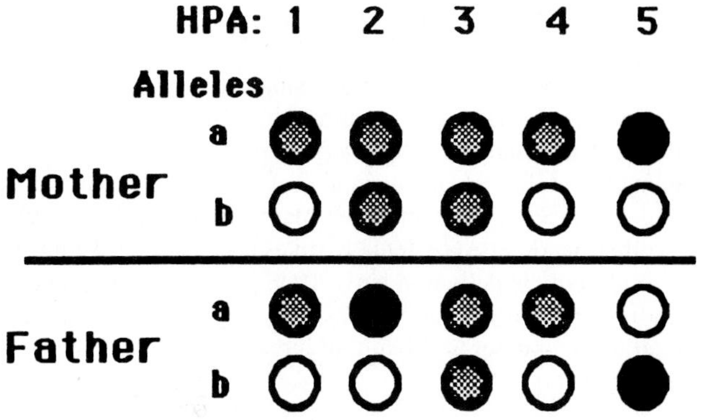

Figure 21-8. A DNA dotblot of the parents of a newborn severely affected by alloimmune thrombocytopenia. The DNA encoding five diallelic platelet antigen polymorphisms was evaluated with allele specific oligonucleotides. In the HPA5 system, the mother appears to be homozygous for an antigen (5a) lacking in her apparently homozygous (5b) partner. This allowed her to manufacture alloantibody to the fetopaternal 5b antigen. All future offspring of the couple are at risk. (Redrawn from original.)

It is now possible to genotype fetal platelets for specific antigens (e.g., HPA1) by evaluating amniocyte DNA sequences (using PCR) encoding platelet glycoprotein IIIa (Bennett, 1994). A dotblot of DNA from a couple with a severely affected firstborn is shown in Figure 21-8. Other methods of DNA analysis are possible and may be simpler than dotblots (Skogen, 1994).

SURFACTANT ANALYSIS: FETAL PULMONARY MATURITY

Lung Maturation

Of fetal organs, the lungs mature quite late. Maturation is marked by production of a detergent-like material, surfactant, which forms a film on the alveolar surfaces. Type II alveolar pneumocytes produce surfactant, which is secreted in aggregated lamellar bodies that range in size from 2 to 5 μm in diameter. Lamellar bodies diffuse out of the lungs and bronchial tree into AF. They impart a turbid appearance to the fluid. After delivery, the presence of surfactant reduces surface tension at the tissue-air interface. Surfactant decreases the work of breathing in air by reducing resistance to lung expansion during inspiration and preventing collapse during expiration. Deficiency of surfactant produces respiratory distress syndrome (RDS), a disorder that results in hypoxia, acidosis, and escape of blood proteins into alveolar air spaces (hyaline membrane disease).

Mechanical ventilators assist newborns with RDS but can overinflate the lungs to cause alveolar rupture, interstitial emphysema, and bronchopulmonary dysplasia. Exogenous surfactant is available as a therapeutic option in RDS but is not yet in prophylactic use.

Before delivery, respiration causes surfactant to diffuse from the unexpanded lungs through the bronchial tree, into the AF. AF surfactant can be measured after third-trimester amniocentesis. Surfactant analysis is important in managing disorders predisposing to RDS: preterm labor, PROM, maternal diabetes, chronic maternal hypertension, fetal growth retardation, alloimmune hemolytic disease, and cesarean section.

Classifying the Small Fetus

A small fetus may be either small for gestational age (SGA) or appropriate for gestational age (AGA). An SGA fetus can die *in utero* or at delivery. It produces adequate surfactant but suffers from placental insufficiency. Clinical treatment of an SGA fetus involves planned early delivery. On the other hand, an AGA fetus is small because it is young. If an AGA fetus is delivered early, RDS is frequent. If prevention of premature labor is unsuccessful, steroids may be given to the mother to attempt to induce fetal surfactant production.

Amniotic Fluid Surfactant

Pulmonary surfactant is a mixture of lipids, carbohydrates, and proteins (Hawgood, 1990). Current clinical tests, however, determine lipid properties of surfactant. The majority of the lipid is phospholipid, with lecithin as the major component. Between 50% and 85% of molecular lecithin is saturated with fatty acids at both its α and β positions. Approximately 62% is disaturated phosphatidylcholine (DSPC) (Brown, 1982). Other phospholipids present are phosphatidylgycerol (PG) (10%), phosphatidylinositol, phosphatidylserine, and phosphatidylethanolamine. Sphingomyelin, composing about 2% of surfactant, appears to have little independent surface active properties, but its concentration in AF remains constant during the third trimester. Therefore, it can be used as an internal standard against which lecithin can be compared. (The reference method for pulmonary maturation is the lecithin : sphingomyelin [L/S] ratio test; see Chemical Methods.)

Surfactant may be measured by either physical or chemical means. The great number of procedures available suggests that none is ideal in predicting RDS or its absence. Physical methods do not measure phospholipids individually but test some nonchemical property of surfactant. A method's usefulness is related to clinical accuracy, low cost, simplicity, and speed.

Physical Methods

OD measurements determine the turbidity of mature AF, an effect of surfactant-containing lamellar bodies. Indeed, experienced obstetricians can often predict lung maturity by gross inspection of AF. OD is a simple and rapid measurement, but it is affected by pigments (bilirubin, heme, porphyrins), cell debris, and methods of removing debris. Hydramnios causes dilution and falsely immature results.

Microviscosity of AF correlates with the reference L/S ratio test results in clinical trials. In this method, a fluorescent probe (1,6-diphenyl-1,3,5-hexatriene) polarizes incident light at 365 nm and emits light at wavelengths greater than 418 nm. In AF, the probe partitions between albumin and surfactant. The greater the concentration of surfactant is, relative to a constant concentration of albumin, the lower is the viscosity. Fluorescence depolarization is related to the hydrophobic matrix of surfactant and its decreased viscosity. The method is unaffected by dilution but may overestimate maturity in concentrated specimens (e.g., in fetal urinary tract obstruction). Samples are prepared by filtration to avoid loss of surfactant by centrifuge precipitation. Effects of the methods for AF preparation have not been evaluated. Because blood and meconium lipids increase microviscosity, specimens with visible pigmentation should not be analyzed. Bilirubin pigment slightly increases results.

An automated fluorescence polarization assay using the Abbott TDx instrument (Abbott Laboratories, Irving, TX) is widely used. This rapid determination appears accurate in most clinical situations (Bayer-Zwirello, 1993; Bender, 1994).

Foam stability assays depend on the longevity of bubbles under standard conditions. Proteins, free fatty acids, and other biological materials can form relatively stable bubbles when air is mixed with water. Ethanol, however, can serve as an antifoaming agent. When surfactant is added to a standard mixture of 47.4% ethanol and water (v/v) which produces surface tension of 29 dynes/cm, the surface tension is lowered, the ethanol effect is overcome, and the bubbles are stable. There are several other variants of bubble stability tests (simple shake test, manual foam stability index). Control of some procedures is difficult, and the presence of blood causes interference.

Amniotic particle counting determines the concentration of lamellar bodies suspended in AF. This technique uses the platelet channel of an automated hematology cell counter. Particles measured vary in size from 2 to 20 fL. The assay is simple and rapid. Counts greater than 32,000 particles per microliter correlate with fetal maturity (Dubin, 1988; Fakhoury, 1994).

Chemical Methods

Before 35 weeks' gestation, the major component of surfactant is α-palmatic β-myristic lecithin. After that time, dipalmitic lecithin predominates, and PG appears about a week later. PG increases to term and maintains alveolar stability. Concentration of phosphatidylinositol increases in AF and parallels the increase in the L/S ratio until 36 weeks, when PG appears.

The lung maturation process, as observed chemically, occurs rapidly (1 to 2 days). Because sphingomyelin content in AF is constant during the third trimester, it serves as a reference material against which surfactant lecithin can be compared. The L/S ratio avoids problems associated with variability in chemical extraction and inaccuracy in estimates of absolute concentration per AF volume.

The L/S test was the first practical chemical test to assess fetal pulmonary status (Gluck, 1971). It continues to be the standard test against which other tests are compared, unless a new test is compared directly with clinical outcomes. A commercial kit (Fetal-Tek 200, Helena Laboratories, Beaumont, TX) is available.

After extraction and purification with solvents, AF surfactant phospholipids are chromatographed on thin-layer silica. The phospholipids are made visible by heat charring or staining. Densitometric quantification determines the L/S ratio. Acetone-precipitated L/S ratios greater than 2.0 usually indicate maturity; those of 1.5 indicate borderline maturity. When mothers are not diabetic, AF L/S ratios of 2.0 or greater predict absence of severe RDS with probability of 95% (specificity). L/S ratios of 2.0 or less predict RDS with probability of 25% (sensitivity). Some believe that the L/S ratio test is unsatisfactory in diabetic women (Dubin, 1992), in whose neonates RDS can be noted when L/S ratios are greater than 2.0.

The L/S test method is slow, expensive, method variable, and sometimes inaccurate. Preanalytical variables affect accuracy. One variable is dilution by secretions, if AF is recovered vaginally. Analytical error results from overcentrifugation (speed and time), blood contamination (hemolysis), and imprecision of thin-layer chromatography. Meconium can prevent clear separation of lecithin and sphingomyelin.

Phospholipid Profile and Phosphatidylglycerol

In addition to an L/S ratio of 2.0 or greater, the presence of PG on the thin-layer chromatogram of the L/S test indicates fetal pulmonary maturity with virtual certainty (Higuchi, 1990). Because chromatography is cumbersome and often unavailable when needed (nights, weekends), more rapid tests for PG have been used. A rapid, slide, lipid agglutination method for PG is available and can screen for pulmonary maturity (Amnio-Stat-FLM, Irvine Scientific, Santa Ana, CA). If immature or equivocal results are observed, the chromatographic method is indicated (Ashwood, 1992). PG may be enzymatically determined, but glycerol may interfere (Jones, 1994).

AMNIOTIC FLUID AND INTRAUTERINE INFECTIONS

About 5% of fetal deaths are caused by several maternal, fetal, and membranous infections (Table 21–6). Exposure to infectious agents during pregnancy or at delivery is associated with a 20% perinatal death rate or retardation, congenital anomalies, and lifelong disabilities. Various serologic, culture, and molecular methods have been used to detect prevalent or likely fetal infections. Availability of DNA probe procedures is still limited, but rapid PCR amplification of toxoplasmosis DNA in amniocytes has been cited as at least diagnostically equivalent to the accepted and effective culture, mouse inoculation, and serologic methods (Dupouy-Camet, 1992; Hohlfeld, 1994). Similarly, PCR shows promise for prenatal cytomegalovirus diagnosis (Hogge, 1993). AF may be useful in several suspected infectious diseases, as shown in Table 21–7.

A fraction of women undergo PROM. Amniocentesis has been advocated for those cases with fetal tachycardia or nonreactive stress test results. One third of patients with PROM produce positive AF Gram's stains and cultures and should be delivered on the basis of the demonstrated bacterial infection (Asrat, 1990).

Table 21–6. CONGENITAL INFECTIONS

Viral	Bacterial	Other
Cytomegalovirus	*Listeria*	*Chlamydia*
Rubella	Syphilis	*Candida*
Hepatitis B	Tuberculosis	Malaria
Herpes	*Salmonella*	Trypanosomes
Rubeola	*Streptococcus* group B	*Toxoplasma*
Vaccinia	*Brucella*	
Varicella	Tularemia	
Coxsackie B	*Staphylococcus*	
Western equine encephalitis	Anthrax	
Human immunodeficiency virus		

Table 21–7. PERINATAL INFECTIONS DETECTABLE IN AMNIOTIC FLUID

Agents	Possible Methods of Diagnosis
Listeria	Culture, Gram's stain
Mycobacteria	Acid-fast stain, culture
Neisseria	Culture, Gram's stain
Mycoplasma hominis	Culture
Treponema pallidum	Direct immunofluorescence, darkfield microscopy
Cytomegalovirus	Culture, polymerase chain reaction
Rubella	Culture
Toxoplasma	Mouse inoculation, polymerase chain reaction
Candida	Culture
Chlamydia	Polymerase chain reaction

AMNIOTIC FLUID EMBOLUS

When AF enters the maternal circulation (e.g., at delivery), it may embolize systemically and cause severe pulmonary symptoms, circulatory failure, and disseminated intravascular coagulopathy. Historically, pathologic diagnosis was possible by sampling (usually postmortem) maternal blood from the right side of the heart or the inferior vena cava. A third layer was often visible grossly above the red blood cell and leukocyte layers. Microscopically, the third layer contained mucus and fetal squames. Antemortem diagnosis of AF embolus may now be possible using maternal serum tests for increases of either zinc coproporphyrin I or Tn antigen (NeuAc alpha 2-GalNAc alpha 1-0-Ser/Thr) (Kanayama, 1992; Kobayashi, 1993).

Ashwood E: Evaluating health and maturation of the unborn: The role of the clinical laboratory. Clin Chem 1992; 38:1523.

Asrat T, Nageotte MP, Garite TJ, et al: Gram stain results from amniocentesis in patients with preterm premature rupture of membranes—comparison of maternal and fetal characteristics. Am J Obstet Gynecol 1990; 163:887.

Bayer-Zwirello L, Jetson J, Rosenbaum J, et al: Amniotic fluid surfactant-albumin ratio as a screening test for fetal lung maturity: Two years clinical experience. J Perinatol 1993; 13:354.

Bell JA, Pearn HJ, Smith A: Prenatal cytogenetic diagnosis: Amniotic cell culture versus chorionic villus sampling. Med J Austral 1987; 146:27.

Bender TM, Stone LR, Amenta JS: Diagnostic power of lecithin/sphingomyelin ratio and fluorescence polarization assays for respiratory distress syndrome compared by relative operating characteristic curves. Clin Chem 1994; 40:541.

Bennett PR, Le Van Kim C, Colin Y, et al: Prenatal determination of fetal RhD type by DNA amplification. N Engl J Med 1993; 329:607.

Bennett PR, Warwick R, Vaughan J, et al: Prenatal determination of human platelet antigen type using DNA amplification following amniocentesis. Br J Obstet Gynaecol 1994; 101:246.

Brown LM, Duck-Chong CG: Methods of fetal lung maturity. Crit Rev Clin Lab Sci 1982; 16:85.

Czeizel AE, Dudas I: Prevention of the first occurrence of neural tube defects by periconceptional vitamin supplementation. N Engl J Med 1992; 327:1832.

Desgeorges M, Boulot P, Kjellberg P, et al: Prenatal diagnosis for cystic fibrosis using SSCP analysis. Prenat Diagn 1993; 13:147.

Dorr HG, Sippell WG: Prenatal dexamethasone treatment in pregnancies at risk for congenital adrenal hyperplasia due to 21-hydroxylase deficiency: Effect on midgestational amniotic fluid steroid levels. J Clin Endocrinol Metab 1993; 76:117.

3

Dubin S: Determination of lamellar body size, number, density and concentration by differential light scattering from amniotic fluid: Physical significance of A650. Clin Chem 1988; 34:938.

Dubin S: Assessment of fetal lung maturity by laboratory methods. Clin Lab Med 1992; 12:603.

Dupouy-Camet J, Bougnoux ME, Lavareda de Souza S, et al: Comparative value of polymerase chain reaction and conventional biologic tests for the prenatal diagnosis of congenital toxoplasmosis. Ann Biol Clin (Paris) 1992; 50:315.

Elias SE, Annas GJ: Generic consent for genetic screening. N Engl J Med 1994; 330:1611.

Fakhoury G, Daikoku NH, Benser J, et al: Lamellar body concentrations and the prediction of fetal pulmonary maturity. Am J Obstet Gynecol 1994; 170:72.

Firth HV, Boyd PA, Chamberlain PF, et al: Analysis of limb reduction defects in babies exposed to chorionic villus sampling. Lancet 1994; 343:1069.

Gambino SR, Freda VJ: The measurement of amniotic fluid bilirubin by the method of Jendrassik and Grof: Its correlation with spectrophotometric analysis. Am J Clin Pathol 1966; 46:198.

Gluck L, Kulovich MV, Borer R, et al: Diagnosis of the respiratory distress syndrome by amniocentesis. Am J Obstet Gynecol 1971; 109:440.

Goodburn SF, Yates JRW, Raggatt PR, et al: Second trimester maternal serum screening using alpha-fetoprotein, human chorionic gonadotrophin, and unconjugated oestriol: Experience of a regional program. Prenat Diagn 1994; 14:391.

Grabowski, GA, Desnick RJ: Antenatal metabolic diagnosis: A compendium. *In* Filkins K, Russo JF (eds): Human Prenatal Diagnosis. New York, Marcel Dekker, 1990, pp 99–146.

Grebner EE: Basic concepts in biochemical antenatal diagnosis. Obstet Gynecol Clin North Am 1993; 20:421.

Haddow JE, Palomaki GE, Knight GJ, et al: Prenatal screening for Down's syndrome with use of maternal serum markers. N Engl J Med 1992; 327:588.

Haddow JE, Palomaki GE, Knight GJ, et al: Reducing the need for amniocentesis in women 35 years of age or older with serum markers for screening. N Engl J Med 1994; 330:1114.

Hangaard J, Whittaker M, Loft AGR, et al: Quantification and phenotyping of serum cholinesterase by enzyme antigen immunoassay: Methodological aspects and clinical applicability. Scand J Clin Lab Invest 1991; 51:349.

Hawgood S, Clements JA: Pulmonary surfactant and its apoproteins. J Clin Invest 1990; 86:1.

Higuchi M, Hirano H, Gotoh K, et al: Comparison of amniotic fluid disaturated phosphatidylcholine, phosphatidylglycerol and lecithin/sphingomyelin ratio in predicting the risk of developing neonatal respiratory distress syndrome. Gynecol Obstet Invest 1990; 29:92.

Hogge WA, Buffone GJ, Hogge JS: Prenatal diagnosis of cytomegalovirus (CMV) infection: A preliminary report. Prenat Diagn 1993; 13:131.

Hohlfeld P, Daffos F, Costa J-M, et al: Prenatal diagnosis of congenital toxoplasmosis with a polymerase chain reaction test on amniotic fluid. N Engl J Med 1994; 331:695.

Jones GW, Ashwood ER: Enzymatic measurement of phosphatidylglycerol in amniotic fluid. Clin Chem 1994; 40:518.

Kanayama N, Yamazaki T, Naruse H, et al: Determining zinc coproporphyrin in maternal plasma—a new method for diagnosing amniotic fluid embolism. Clin Chem 1992; 38:526.

Kobayashi H, Ohi H, Terao T: A simple noninvasive, sensitive method for diagnosis of amniotic fluid embolism by monoclonal antibody TKH-2 that recognizes NeuAc alpha 2-6GalNAc. Am J Obstet Gynecol 1993; 168:848.

Linnala A, von Kosull H, Virtanen I: Isoforms of cellular fibronectin and tenascin in amniotic fluid. FEBS Letters 1994; 337:167.

Lockwood CJ, Senyei AE, Dische R, et al: Isoforms of fibronectin in cervical and vaginal secretions as a predictor of preterm delivery. N Engl J Med 1991; 325:669.

Loft AGR: Determination of amniotic fluid acetylcholinesterase activity in the antenatal diagnosis of foetal malformations: The first ten years. Clin Chem Clin Biochem 1990; 28:893.

Loft AGR, Hogdall E, Larsen S, et al: A comparison of amniotic fluid alpha-fetoprotein and acetylcholinesterase in the prenatal diagnosis of open neural tube defects and anterior abdominal wall defects. Prenat Diagn 1993; 13:93.

Marchese S, Thomas J: Fragile X syndrome and its relationship to mental retardation. Genetics in Practice (Allegheny Health, Education, and Research Foundation Center for Medical Genetics. A Newsletter for Health Professionals) 1994; 1(2):5.

McIntosh MCM, Iles R, Teisner B, et al: Maternal serum human chorionic gonadotropin and pregnancy-associated plasma protein A markers for fetal Down syndrome at 8–14 weeks. Prenat Diagn 1994; 14:203.

Meade TW, Ammala P, Aynsley-Green M, et al: Medical research council European trial of chorion villus sampling. Lancet 1991; 337:1491.

Moertel CA, Stupca PJ, Dewald GW: Pseudomosaicism, true mosaicism and maternal cell contamination in amniotic fluid processed with *in situ* culture and robotic harvesting. Prenat Diagn 1992; 12:671.

Nicolaides K, Brizot MDL, Patel F, et al: Comparison of chorionic villus sampling and amniocentesis for fetal karyotyping at 10–13 weeks gestation. Lancet 1994; 344:435.

Nicolaides KH, Rodek CH, Mibashan RS, et al: Have Liley charts outlived their usefulness? Am J Obstet Gynecol 1986; 155:90.

Nicolaides KH, Snijders RJM, Gosden CM, et al: Ultrasonographically detectable markers of fetal chromosomal abnormalities. Lancet 1992; 340:704.

Pang S, Pollack MS, Marshall RN, et al: Prenatal treatment of congenital adrenal hyperplasia due to 21-hydroxylase deficiency. N Engl J Med 1990; 322:111.

Pertl B, Shu CY, Sherlock J, et al: Rapid molecular method for prenatal detection of Down's syndrome. Lancet 1994; 343:1197.

Queenan J, Tomai TP, Ural SH, et al: Deviation in amniotic fluid optical density at a wavelength of 450 nm in Rh-immunized pregnancies from 14–40 weeks gestation: A proposal for clinical management. Am J Obstet Gynecol 1993; 168:1370.

Rebello MT, Abas A, Nicolaides K, et al: Maternal contamination of amniotic fluid demonstrated by DNA analysis. Prenat Diagn 1994; 14:109.

Sancho S, Mongini T, Tanji K, et al: Analysis of dystrophin expression after activation of myogenesis in amniocytes, chorionic-villus cells, and fibroblasts. N Engl J Med 1993; 329:915.

Saunders NJ, Snijders RJM, Nicolaides KH: Therapeutic amniocentesis in twin-twin transfusion syndrome appearing in the second trimester of pregnancy. Am J Obstet Gynecol 1992; 166:820.

Schroeder TM: Genetically determined chromosomal instability syndromes. Cytogenet Cell Genet 1982; 33:119.

Simsek S, Bleeker PMM, Von Dem Borne AEG: Prenatal determination of fetal RhD type. (Letter.) N Engl J Med 1994; 330:795.

Skogen B, Bellissimo DB, Hessner MJ, et al: Rapid determination of platelet alloantigen genotypes by polymerase chain reaction using allele-specific primers. Transfusion 1994; 34:955.

Steyn DW, Pattinson RC, Odendaal HJ: Amniocentesis—still important in the management of severe rhesus incompatibility. S Afr Med J 1992; 82:321.

Vietor HE, Kanhai HHH, Brand A: Induction of additional red cell alloantibodies after intrauterine transfusions. Transfusion 1994; 34:970.

Wald N, Cuckle H, Nanchahal K: Amniotic fluid acetylcholinesterase measurement in the prenatal diagnosis of open neural tube defects: Second report of the collaborative acetylcholinesterase study. Prenat Diagn 1989; 9:813.

Wald NJ, Cuckle HS, Densem JW, et al: Maternal serum screening for Down's syndrome in early pregnancy. Br Med J 1988; 297:883.

Ward BE, Gersen SL, Carelli MP, et al: Rapid prenatal diagnosis of chromosomal aneuploides by fluorescence in situ hybridization: Clinical experience with 4,500 specimens. Am J Hum Genet 1993; 52:854.

Weaver DD: Catalog of Prenatally Diagnosed Conditions, 2nd ed. Baltimore, Johns Hopkins University Press, 1989.

Welch CR, Makepeace PA, Walkinshaw SA: Management of pregnancies complicated by rhesus (D) antibodies. Br J Hosp Med 1993; 49:1993.

Chapter 22

Andrology Laboratory and Fertility Assessment

Siddhartha Sarkar, Ph.D.
John Bernard Henry, M.D.

3

AN OVERVIEW

Andrology laboratory service provides various measurements and examinations that offer results to assist clinicians in arriving at a correct conclusion about the fertility of a patient. The determinations are primarily directed toward analysis of semen or its major constituent, spermatozoa (sperm), including concentration, motility, and morphology. Ten to 20% of American couples, numbering two to four million, have impaired fertility and spend about a billion dollars annually in medical care (U.S. Congress OTA Report, 1988). Physicians in infertility practice use semen analysis results to counsel couples about the outlook for future fertility, to select donors for therapeutic insemination, and to select among the assisted reproductive technologies (ART) of *in vitro* fertilization (IVF) including gamete or embryo transfer (Cohen, 1992). Various medical and surgical therapies for male infertility are evaluated by preoperative and postoperative semen analysis. Semen analysis is also used to screen for exposure to reproductive toxicants and to set their regulatory levels (Lamb, 1994).

The principal practice of andrology laboratories was formerly based on spermatozoa (sperm) and testicular physiology, and the routine activity was limited compared with laboratories of today. Not long ago, semen analysis was used in suspected rape cases or in the establishment or denial of paternity on grounds of sterility. In contrast, forensic analysis is currently carried out by detecting polymorphic semen antigens with monoclonal antibodies or by deoxyribonucleic acid (DNA) fingerprinting and DNA typing (Jeffreys, 1993). Since the landmark decisions of *Skinner* v. *Oklahoma* in 1942, which is notable for its explicit mention of a "right to have offspring," and *Roe* v. *Wade* in 1973, permitting women to choose to discontinue a pregnancy, reproduction has become the converging point of conflict in ethical issues (McCullough, 1994). The introduction of IVF technique in 1978 with the birth of Louise Brown (Brinsden, 1992) opened a new era that has challenged and changed our concepts of family life. Sperm selection for offspring's sex (Fletcher, 1983), being carried out in some andrology laboratories, is another such ethical issue (Billings, 1992).

Conception and establishment of pregnancy require a series of successful events: ovulation and endometrial preparation for implantation, sperm production and transport in the male, sperm and oocyte transport in the female, and finally, fertilization and embryonic development (Taylor, 1992). Sperm and ova production to fertilization and embryo formation are shown in Figures 22–1 and 22–2 (Amann, 1994; Blasco, 1984); reproductive failure would be the consequence if any of these events did not follow its normal course. As new methods are developed to identify the weak gaps, new therapeutic procedures are used to compensate for them and the defining conditions of unexplained infertility change. The commonly used diagnostic steps for unexplained infertility are semen analysis, endometrial biopsy, serum progesterone estimation, laparoscopy, hysterosalpingogram, postcoital test (PCT), and the detection of sperm antibody. A schedule for workup of isolated abnormalities in semen parameters (Sigman, 1991) is shown in Figure 22–3. Not included in the standard semen analysis is a group of procedures commonly known as sperm function tests (Mortimer, 1994), which include sperm movement characteristics in semen, sperm-cervical mucus interaction, detection of capacitation, acrosome reaction, zona binding, and penetration

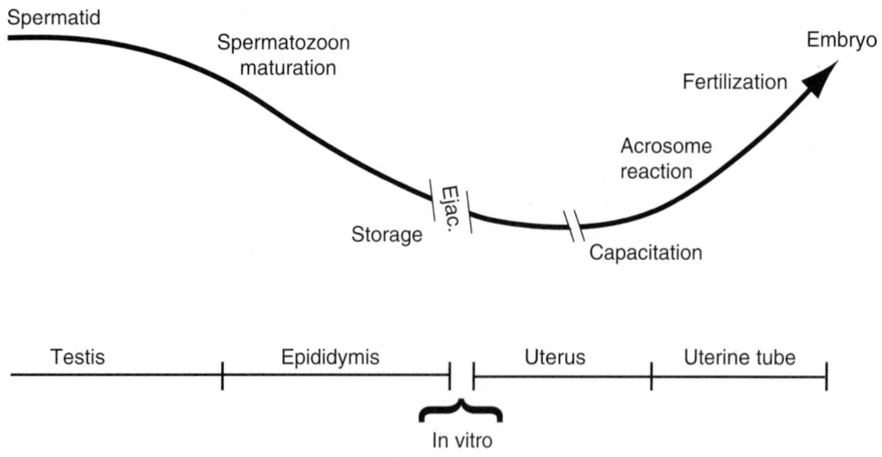

Figure 22–1. Pathway from sperm production to fertilization and embryo formation. (With permission of Amann RP, Hammerstedt RH: *In vitro* evaluation of sperm quality: An opinion. J Androl 1994; 14:397–408.)

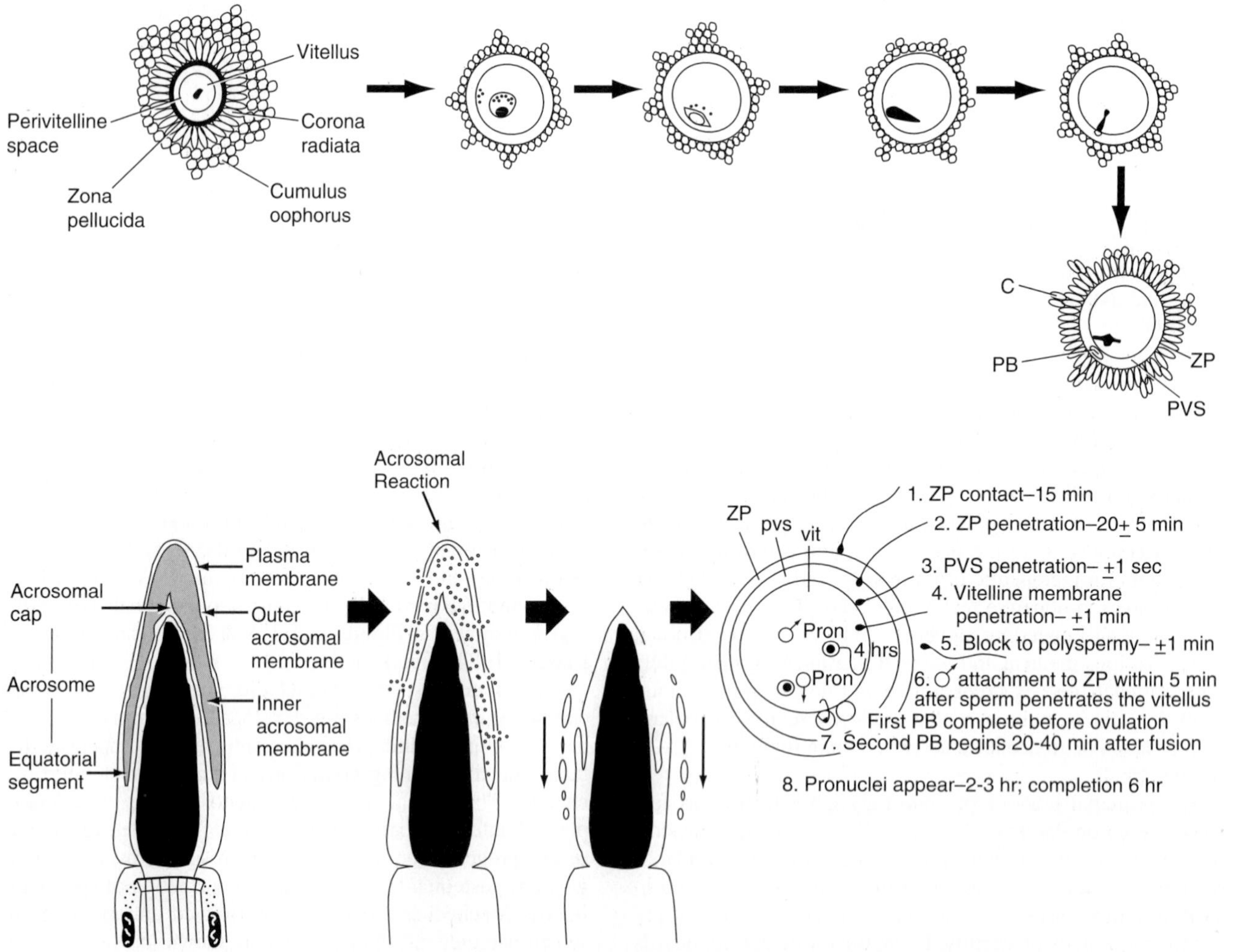

Figure 22–2. Preovulatory maturation of the egg from the germinal vesicle stage to the secondary oocyte surrounded by the perivitelline space (PVS), zona pellucida (ZP), and first polar body (PB). The lower part of the figure shows sperm with central condensed nucleus surrounded by an inner and outer membrane undergoing the acrosomal reaction with release of proteolytic enzymes necessary for the capacitation of sperm: contact of sperm with ZP (15 minutes), penetration of the ZP (20 minutes), penetration of PVS and vitelline membrane, and consequent block of polyspermy. Fusion of male and female pronuclei and formation of the second PB occur 20 to 40 minutes after fusion. (With permission of Blasco L: Clinical tests for fertilizing ability. Fertil Steril 1984; 41:177–192. Reproduced with the permission of the publisher, The American Fertility Society.)

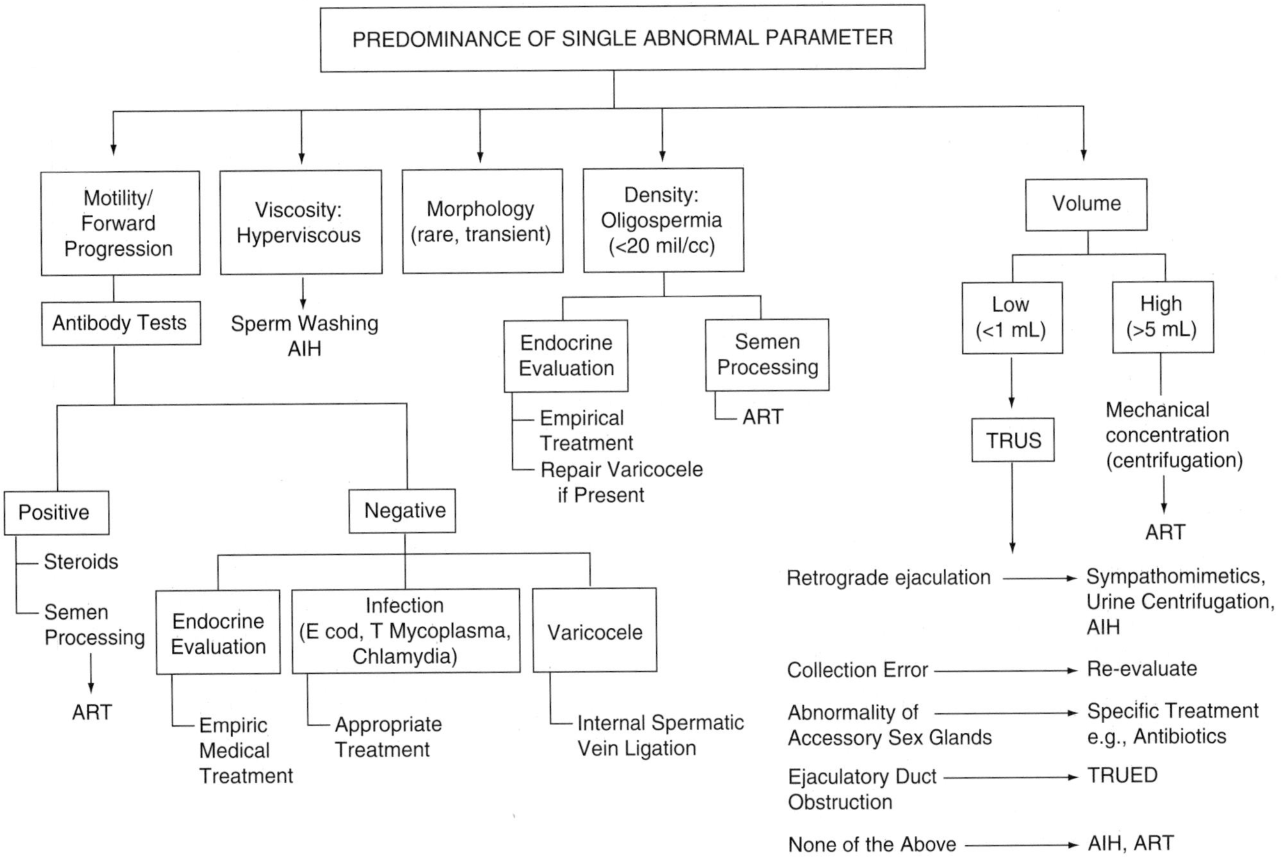

Figure 22–3. Algorithm for the workup of isolated abnormalities in semen parameters. (With permission of Sigman M, Lipschulz LI, Howards SS: Evaluation of the subfertile male. *In* Lipschulz I, Howards SS [eds]: Infertility in the Male. Mosby–Year Book, 1991, pages 179–210.)

3

and fusion with vitelline membrane, followed by the formation of sperm pronucleus. These assays cover a span of sperm's life cycle from its production to fertilization, and the results are particularly useful when sperm autoantibodies are present in semen and in cases of unexplained infertility. A report summarizing the observations from various clinics stated that the relative frequencies of defects diagnosed among infertile couples were ovulation defects 30%, semen abnormality 22%, tubal defect 17%, other disorders 12%, and endometriosis in the remaining 5% of the cases (Taylor, 1992).

Preoperative and postoperative semen analysis after varicocelectomy is performed within three to four months of the surgical procedure to determine improvements in sperm morphology and motility. Although 15% to 20% of the normal male population can be found to have scrotal varices, this number approaches 40% in subfertile men, and varicocele is the most common surgically removable abnormality. A varicocele occurs predominantly on the left side, but an additional right-sided varicocele may occur in 50% of the patients. Ligation of a varicocele may help oligospermia with poor sperm motility and poor sperm morphology in the presence of normal levels of gonadotropin. A varicocele may alter convective transport through testicular capillaries owing to an increase in venous pressure, which may enhance the exchange of interstitial fluid and the production of testicular lymph. Local concentrations of substrates within the interstitial compartment could change dramatically as a result. Deterioration of the functioning of endothelial cells present in distinct vascular segments such as the arterioles, capillaries, and venules may explain the pathogenesis of fertility impairment in patients with a varicocele, because in testes, the bulk of the secreted tissue products reach the systemic blood by the venous effluent (Gilbert, 1994).

In an azoospermic or low-volume severely oligospermic patient, one must discriminate between low sperm production and impaired sperm delivery or a combination. Although testicular biopsy is the definitive test for sperm production, a significantly elevated follicle-stimulating hormone (FSH) level is a strong indication of abnormal seminiferous epithelium. An ultrasonographic scan of the vas, seminal vesicles, and ejaculatory ducts may reveal the specific defect responsible for problems with delivery of sperm—namely, vasal agenesis, seminal vesicle agenesis or atresia, fullness of the seminal vesicles caused by obstruction, and prostatic cysts or calculi causing ejaculatory duct blockage. Bilateral absence of the vasa deferentia (found in 1% of infertile males) in patients with cystic fibrosis results from the defect in the cystic fibrosis gene and is probably a primary rather than an indirect secondary effect of the defective gene (Oates, 1994). Transrectal ultrasonography may be used to identify similar abnormalities in the male genital system, some of which are treatable.

Deterioration of semen quality and reduction in sperm count, often attributed to environmental toxins, have been observed in the past few decades (Gray, 1992). Toxins enter our system presumably through drinking water contaminated by runoff from agricultural use. About 60,000 chemicals are in commercial use, and 500 new chemicals are coming into use each year. Information from surveys about the potential harmful effects of many of those chemicals, particularly the halogen-containing reproductive toxicant, glycol and glycol ethers, metals and estrogenic substances, appears alarming (Lamb, 1994). A toxin may cause infertility in males by several different mechanisms, either adversely affecting the differentiation of fetal testis, or directly by damaging the seminiferous tubules and stem cells, or inhibiting the sperm maturation process in the adult testis. A toxin may also act indirectly, inducing changes in the function of the hypothalamus and pituitary. Although animal studies may not be comparable in each case for an understanding of the human ailment, they bring into focus some insidious ways in which the metabolites of a seemingly innocuous agent can be utterly specific in choosing targets to produce the toxic effect (Gray, 1992). An example of such reproductive toxins is Vinclozolin, a fungicide, registered for use on several fruits and vegetables, ornamental plants, and turfgrass (Kelce, 1994). Vinclozolin competes weakly with androgen for binding to the androgen receptor (Ki > 700 μM), but two of its degradative products, 2-[[(3,5-dichlorophenyl)-carbamoyl]oxyl]-2-methyl-3-butanoic acid (M1) and 3′,5′- dichloro-2-hydroxy-2-methylbut-3-enanilide (M2), are effective antagonists of androgen binding (Ki = 92 and 9.7 μM, respectively). Leydig's cell tumors, as well as atrophic ventral prostate and seminal vesicle, resulted from chronic exposure in adult male rats. Dams exposed from gestational day 14 to postnatal day 3 produced male pups with several reproductive abnormalities, reduced anogenital distance, nipple development, cleft phallus with hypospadias, suprainguinal ectopic testis, vaginal pouch, epididymal and testicular granulomas, atrophic seminal vesicles, and ventral prostate glands. All are indications of the antiandrogenic activity of the fungicide. Interestingly, neither Vinclozolin nor its degradation products inhibits 5 α-reductase activity, which converts testosterone to the more potent androgen 5 α-dihydrotestosterone.

A spinoff from the *in vitro* and genetic cytotechnologies is sperm micromanipulation and its various applications (Cohen, 1992). One of its many uses is enhancing sperm penetration for oligospermic or asthenospermic donors by introducing a few sperm through drilled zona into the perivitelline space (subzonal sperm insertion, SUZI) or directly in the cytoplasm (intracytoplasmic sperm injection, ICSI). Another use of ICSI is fertilizing the egg with a small number of sorted X or Y sperm for sex selection of the offspring, a technique (Sarkar, 1974) that has been successful in animal trials (Johnson, 1993). The technique should be specially applicable to carriers of sex chromosome–linked gene defects. Sperm selection against defective genes linked to autosomal chromosomes may be possible with the use of other cell separation techniques (Sarkar, 1984).

The general concern over the infectivity of tissue fluids that may contain human immunodeficiency virus (World Health Organization [WHO], 1992), particularly for cryopreserved specimens acquired for artificial insemination by donor (American Fertility Society, 1990), has added a separate dimension to the safety procedures of the andrology laboratory. Additional technical training may be required of the staff who are already prepared for handling infected material from patients with sexually transmitted diseases. Perhaps because of these concerns and the Clinical Laboratory Improvement Amendments (1992), standardization of laboratory procedures and quality control and its assessment are gaining acceptance internationally (see Chaps. 1 and 6). The detailed knowledge of fertilization and intensive exploration of the human genome (Griffin, 1992) have greatly enlivened the manipulative possibilities of sperm acting as a vector in endowing parental genes to the embryo (Liu, 1994).

DIAGNOSTIC PROCEDURES

Semen Analysis

Semen analysis can be recommended as a cost-effective procedure for couples who have failed to conceive after six months of unprotected intercourse. The basic examination of semen consists of determining sperm concentration, percent motility, and morphology according to the guidelines described in the World Health Organization (WHO) laboratory manual for the examination of semen and semen–cervical mucus interaction (WHO, 1992). A more descriptive book, *Practical Laboratory Andrology* (Mortimer, 1994), may also be useful as a reference and guide in interpreting the results of semen analysis. The principal issues of semen analysis and male fertility evaluation have been described succinctly in two reviews (Gilbert, 1992, 1994).

The patient should be instructed to collect semen after three days and no longer than five days of sexual abstinence, and his name, date and time of collection, length of abstinence, and the interval between collection and analysis should be recorded on the semen analysis report form. Longer periods of abstinence usually result in a higher semen volume but reduced sperm motility. A second semen specimen aliquot may be collected in another two hours if a long period of abstinence is suspected. The man should evacuate his bladder before ejaculation. A preweighed sterile plastic (polypropylene) container with a screw top should be provided by the laboratory for semen collection, and the semen specimen should be delivered to the laboratory within one hour of collection while being kept close to the body to maintain body temperature during the transit interval. A sample of postejaculate urine may be collected at this time. Two specimens collected within two- to three-week intervals should be used for evaluation, and if they are markedly different, additional specimens should be collected. Semen specimens should ideally be collected in the privacy of a room adjacent to the laboratory, because for some samples, sperm should be separated from seminal plasma as soon as possible. Semen should be obtained by masturbation, and if circumstances preclude such collection, special Silastic condoms should be made available for semen collection with intercourse. Incomplete semen specimens should not be analyzed.

An initial macroscopic examination of semen specimen is performed after liquefaction, which usually occurs in less than 60 minutes at room temperature. Failure to liquefy may indicate inadequate prostate secretion, and proteolytic enzymes such as bromelin, plasmin, or chymotrypsin may have to be added. It is important that the semen specimen be thoroughly mixed before subsequent examination, and the viscosity of the semen sample recorded. The volume of ejaculate can be measured by the difference of weights of the collection cup before and after specimen collection. The appearance of a yellowish hue in a semen specimen is associated with pyospermia, and a rust color with small bleeding in the seminal vesicle. The pH ranges from 7.2 to 7.8 but may be 8.0 or greater owing to acute infection in the prostate, seminal vesicle, or epididymis. The pH may be 7.0 or lower if there is an obstruction in the ejaculatory ducts or when the specimen consists of mainly prostatic fluid.

Initial microscopic examination is performed to obtain estimates of sperm concentration, motility, and agglutination. Other cellular elements such as polygonal cells of the urethral tract, as well as round cells such as the spermatogenic cells and leukocytes, can also be observed when sperm are counted in a hemocytometer (see Chap. 24). Because sperm motility and velocity are highly dependent on temperature, assessment of motility is performed on a microscope with a warm stage. A fixed volume of 8 μL under a 22 × 22-mm glass coverslip produces a 16.5-mm depth in the wet preparation. A hemocytometer or any of the chambers available must be used for enumeration of spermatozoa (sperm) count. At least four different fields in each of the two specimen aliquots from a well-mixed semen collection should be counted, and the mean of the eight separate readings recorded. Total sperm count is then calculated by multiplying the concentration (normal concentration 20 to 50 million/mL) of the sample times its volume (normal range 2 to 5 mL). Motility (normal range 50% or greater) is expressed as the percent of sperm that have movements, and the forward progression (normal range 2, and a maximum of 4 if excellent) is noted. Spermatozoa moving rapidly in a straight line with little yaw and lateral movement are graded as 4, and they are graded as 3 when the motion is slower. Sperm motility graded as 2 is still slower, with substantial yaw, and grade 1 has no forward progression. Zero progression denotes absence of any motility. If motility is less than 50%, a viability stain of eosin Y with nigrosin as a counterstain is performed. In brightfield microscopy, red dye appears to be accumulated in the head of nonmotile sperm.

Agglutination of spermatozoa is noted when motile spermatozoa stick to each other in various orientations such as head to head, tail to tail, midpiece to midpiece, or other mixed ways depending on the specificity of sperm antibodies directed against these sperm structures. Clumping of spermatozoa to debris or because of bacterial infection may be differentiated from agglutination due to the presence of sperm-specific antibodies. Agglutination is suggestive of an immunologic cause of infertility, and a description of the type of agglutination should be recorded.

Round cells should be differentiated into two classes, immature germ cells with a single or double highly condensed nucleus with a relatively larger area of surrounding cytoplasm; and the polymorphonuclear leukocytes, which are smaller than the germ cells and have an increased nuclear-to-cytoplasmic ratio. Peroxidase staining specifically identifies the polymorphonuclear leukocytes in the presence of all other cells in semen including lymphocytes. In addition, bacterial contamination and the presence or absence of epithelial cells should be noted. If no sperm are seen in association with a low semen volume, a fructose test should be performed to confirm the presence of fluid from the seminal vesicle, and the same test should be performed on postejaculate urine to rule out retrograde ejaculation.

The analysis of morphologic characteristics of spermatozoa has gained importance in recent years for its predictive value as a fertility determinant. Morphologically abnormal spermatozoa usually have multiple defects, and the average number of defects per spermatozoa, designated as teratozoospermic index, is a significant predictor of sperm function both *in vivo* and *in vitro*. Any sperm with an acrosomal cap less than one third of the head surface, retaining a cytoplasmic droplet of more than half of the head size, and with a tail less than 45 μm long is considered abnormal. Strict criteria proposed by Kruger (1988) consider all borderline forms as abnormal. Of particular note is the direct relationship between acrosome size and the frequency of both pregnancy and fertilization. Diff-Quik stain (Baxter Healthcare Corporation, McGraw Park, IL) is usually the method of choice for spermatozoa, and the traditional feathering technique is used for a thin slide preparation of semen.

Immunologic Assays

The presence of sperm antibody binding to head or tail antigens is considered specific for immunologic infertility. The antibodies are usually of the IgA or IgG and rarely of IgM class; IgA antibodies are considered to have the most clinical significance. Two current methods of detecting sperm-bound antibodies are the mixed agglutination reaction assay (MAR tests for IgG and IgA) and the immunobead assay (Fertility Technologies, Inc., Natick, MA), which detect all classes. Both tests require motile sperm. The direct MAR test can be performed on fresh whole semen, and the result can be read within a few minutes with a light microscope. This test is performed by mixing semen with latex beads coated with human IgG. To this mixture, monospecific antisera to human IgG is added. The formation of mixed agglutinates between beads and motile spermatozoa indicates the presence of sperm antibody. Under light microscopy, the localized binding of the beads to specific sperm structures identifies the antibody as being specific to head, tail, or any other region of the sperm structure. An indirect test can also be performed with this reagent to detect the presence of sperm antibody in semen, cervical mucus, or serum.

The immunobead assay can detect all three immunoglobulin classes of sperm antibody when beads are coated with monospecific antisera to each class; therefore, sperm are washed to remove all free immunoglobulin before the beads are added. An indirect assay can also be designed with this reagent. The test is best read under phase microscopy. Increased risk of the presence of sperm antibody in men is expected as a result of vasectomy, repeat infections, obstruction of the ducts, cryptorchidism, varicocele, testicular biopsy, trauma, torsion, cancer, and genetic predisposition (Gilbert, 1992). The origin of sperm antibody in women is usually associated with intense mucosal inflammation of the genital tract.

Microbiologic Assays

Genital tract infections may have significant adverse effects on male and female fertility. For example, *Escherichia coli* can cause sperm agglutination and immobilization, and the adherence of *E. coli* to sperm is mediated by mannose and mannose-binding cell surface structures present on both cell types (Wolff, 1993; Sarkar, 1974). Special precaution should be taken in collecting semen specimen for bacteria or yeast detection, in order to eliminate the possibilities of external sources of contamination. The culture of seminal plasma to assess the presence of both aerobic and anaerobic organisms may help in the diagnosis of male accessory gland infection, particularly of the prostate. If the concentration of bacteria exceeds 1000 colony-forming units per milliliter, the colonies should be identified and tested for antibiotic sensitivity. Genital infections often require the involvement of a specialized microbiology laboratory service.

Biochemical Assays

The functioning of the accessory glands, especially the seminal vesicle, prostate, and epididymis, can be tested by examining the presence and amounts of specific tissue constituent products. Content of zinc and citric acid in semen, as well as its pH and acid phosphatase activity, is a reliable measure of prostate gland secretion. Fructose in semen reflects the secretory function of the seminal vesicles. In case of azoospermia caused by the congenital absence of vasa deferentia, a low fructose level may indicate an associated dysgenesis of the seminal vesicles. Ejaculatory duct obstruction or agenesis of the vasa deferentia and seminal vesicles may result in the production of semen with low volume, low pH, no coagulation, and no characteristic semen odor. Neutral α-glucosidase originates solely from the epididymis, and its measurement is of diagnostic value for distal ductal obstruction when considered with hormonal and testicular parameters.

Fertilizing Functions or Sperm Function Tests

Defective sperm function may affect various fertilizing activities such as the transport of sperm in the male and female reproductive tracts and events directly related to fertilization such as specific zona binding, penetration, and formation of the male pronucleus. Many factors may be responsible for defective sperm function. Evidence indicates that peroxidase damage, induced by the excessive generation of reactive oxygen species, may be one. Abnormally high activity levels of creatine phosphokinase and a low ratio of muscle (CK − M) to the combined activities of muscle and brain isoforms (CK − M + B), may be indicative of abnormal activities of the midpiece. Creatine kinase (CK) is a key enzyme in the energy generation and transport of spermatozoa; it catalyzes the regeneration of adenosine triphosphate to support the tubulin-dynein interaction during the motility cycle. Sperm function tests specifically include the (1) sperm penetration assay (SPA), (2) hemizona assay, (3) acrosin assay, (4) hypo-osmotic swelling (HOS) test, and (5) cervical mucus penetration assay.

1. The SPA uses zona-denuded golden hamster eggs as hosts for the penetration of human spermatozoa, thus testing sperm for fertilizing capacity. A spermatozoon must complete many of its preceding functions in order to be successful in penetrating the egg. Thus, the SPA test measures sperm capacitation, the acrosome reaction, sperm-oolemma fusion, sperm incorporation in the ooplasm, and decondensation of the sperm chromatin. A positive SPA test result, however, does not include the steps of sperm binding and passing through the zona and falls short of guaranteeing normal embryo development. A negative SPA test result can be a false indication because the acrosome reaction as a specific result of interaction with zona is not tested in this procedure.
2. The hemizona assay uses unfertilized oocytes obtained through donation; they are bisected, and the number of sperm tightly bound to the outer surface is counted. The two halves of the hemizona are presumably functionally equivalent, thus providing controlled comparison for binding. The results of this test show good correlation with strict criteria morphology and IVF rates.
3. The acrosin assay measures acrosin, a trypsin-like serine proteinase specific to sperm acrosome, and it is responsible for the penetration of the zona pellucida, after the binding of sperm to zona triggers its release.
4. The HOS test measures the membrane integrity of sperm. Sperm membrane is a highly differentiated structure, and each separate area of the membrane is metabolically distinct in its ability to transport molecules selectively. When viable sperm are exposed to hypo-osmotic conditions, water enters the cell, resulting in swelling and curling of the tail, which can be visualized under phase microscopy. Results of the HOS test correlate highly with those of the SPA test in normal ejaculates.
5. Cervical mucus penetration assay measures the relative ability of motile sperm to penetrate cervical mucus at midcycle, compared with a standard mucus sample. Spermatozoa are susceptible to the pH changes of the cervical mucus. Acid mucus immobilizes, whereas alkaline mucus enhances sperm motility. The optimum pH range is 7 to 8.5, which is the normal range for cervical mucus in midcycle. Estrogen-prepared mucus favors penetration; however, the ideal time window for maximum penetration may vary from cycle to cycle. The assay quantitates penetration by counting the number of motile sperm at different travel distances from the point of entry. Because the water (and calcium ion) content of the mucus is highest during the estrogen surge, a larger number of sperm can penetrate and have higher swimming velocity compared with the time of progesterone control when the water content is 10% lower. The PCT performed at this time also indicates greater penetrability of sperm at this time. Human or

bovine cervical mucus is used to test the penetration of motile sperm and can be correlated with the PCT results.

Automated Analysis of Semen

Routine evaluation of semen is often carried out by an automated technology system that uses the sperm head movement to derive the magnitudes of various swimming parameters. There is yet another automated system for morphologic analysis. Automation seeks to establish a standard of accuracy of measurements of various parameters and promote interlaboratory comparisons. Because human sperm are heterogeneous in morphology and motility parameters, one important limitation common to automated systems is to set a common standard against which each specimen can be compared. Hence, semen evaluation by manual methods performed by trained technical staff remains the standard practice of andrology laboratories.

THERAPEUTIC PROCEDURES

Sperm Wash

Preparing spermatozoa for insemination is becoming a major activity for andrology laboratories. Spermatozoa for clinical procedures such as IVF, gamete intrafallopian tube transfer (GIFT), intrauterine insemination, and others require that a motile sperm population be removed from seminal plasma within one hour of ejaculation, because of inhibitory effects of seminal plasma on fertilization. Contaminating seminal plasma can be effectively removed by diluting semen with nutrient medium and repeat centrifugation (Mortimer, 1994). However, pelleting live sperm along with dead sperm and other cellular and tissue debris impairs sperm functions, presumably because of the production of reactive oxygen species. Therefore, sedimentation through a Percoll gradient as a selective technique for live spermatozoa is commonly used for wash preparations for assisted reproductive techniques. Other therapeutic uses of sperm wash are retrograde ejaculation in which sperm is recovered from urine, isolating free motile sperm from semen containing sperm antibody, or intrauterine insemination of women with toxic factors or sperm antibody in cervical mucus.

Semen Cryopreservation

Semen cryopreservation or sperm banking is recommended for men to preserve their reproductive potential before they begin cancer therapy, before surgical sterilization by vasectomy, to ensure the availability of sperm at the precise moment as in assisted reproduction, or for men who are in unique life-threatening situations as in military service. It is also recommended for donors who have low sperm counts but good cryosurvival, because it provides the opportunity to pool stored ejaculates for insemination. Donor semen for therapeutic procedures is cryopreserved, because it allows sufficient time to test the specimen aliquot for the presence of viruses or other infectious agents before insemination. Cryopreservation also ensures the ready availability of a wide variety of genotypes (and donor phenotypes) for selection and multiple inseminations.

QUALITY CONTROL AND LABORATORY SAFETY

Each aspect of the testing process should be established by the procedures of quality control and the diagnostic utility, and the user's satisfaction should be monitored by the process of quality assurance. Patient confidentiality should be highlighted as an integral part of the training routine. Maintaining standards in the performance of laboratory procedures is best accomplished by determining intratechnician and intertechnician variability at regular intervals and keeping an eye on the potential for discrepancy between the measurements (see Chaps. 1 and 6). Predetermined methods should be used to train laboratory personnel, and a reference method should be available for calibration of each procedure. A comprehensive review of semen analysis assesses the technical caliber and quality of testing (Baker, 1994).

Amann RP, Hammerstedt RH: *In vitro* evaluation of sperm quality: An opinion. J Androl 1994; 14:397–408.

American Fertility Society: New guidelines for the use of semen donor insemination. Fertil Steril 1990; 53(Suppl 1):1S–13S.

Baker DJ, Paterson MA, Klaassen JM, et al: Semen evaluations in the clinical laboratory—how well are they being performed? Lab Med 1994; 25:509–514.

Billings PR: DNA on Trial, Genetic Identification and Criminal Justice. Cold Spring Harbor, NY, Cold Spring Harbor Laboratory Press, 1992.

Blasco L: Clinical tests for fertilizing ability. Fertil Steril 1984; 41:177–192.

Brinsden PR, Rainsbury PA: A Textbook of *In Vitro* Fertilization and Assisted Reproduction. Park Ridge, NJ, Parthenon Publishing, 1992.

Clinical Laboratory Improvement Amendments (CLIA): Garden Grove, CA, Medcom, 1992.

Cohen J, Malter HE, Talensky BE: Microsurgical Fertilization. *In* Brisden A, Rainsbury PA (eds): A Textbook of *In Vitro* Fertilization and Assisted Reproduction. Park Ridge, NJ, Parthenon Publishing, 1992, pp 205–226.

Fletcher JC: Ethics and Public Policy: Should Sex Selection Be Discouraged? *In* Bennett NG (ed): Sex Selection of Children. New York, Academic Press, 1983, pp 213–252.

Gilbert BR, Cooper GW, Goldstein M: Semen analysis in the evaluation of male factor subfertility. AUA Update Series 1992; 11:250–255.

Gilbert BR, Schlegel PN, Goldstein M: Office evaluation of the infertile male. AUA Update Series 1994; 13:70–75.

Gray LE Jr: Chemically induced alteration in sexual and functional development. *In* Colborn T, Clement C (eds): The Wildlife/Human Connection. Princeton, NJ, Princeton Scientific, 1992.

Griffin JE: Androgen resistance—the clinical and molecular spectrum. N Engl J Med 1992; 326:611–618.

Jeffreys AJ, Pena SDJ: Brief introduction to human DNA fingerprinting. Experientia 1993; 67(Suppl):1–20.

Johnson LA, Welch GR, Keyvan K, et al: Gender preselection in humans? Flow cytometric separation of X and Y spermatozoa for the prevention of X-linked diseases. Hum Reprod 1993; 8:1733–1739.

Kelce WR, Monosson E, Gamscik MP, et al: Environmental hormone disruptors: Evidence that vinclozolin developmental toxicity is mediated by antiandrogenic metabolites. Toxicol Appl Pharmacol 1994; 126: 276–285.

Kruger T, Acosta A, Simmons K, et al: Predictive value of sperm morphology in *in vitro* fertilization. Fertil Steril 1988; 49:112–117.

Lamb EJ, Bennett S: Epidemiologic studies of male factors in infertility. Ann NY Acad Sci 1994; 709:165–178.

Liu J, Lissens W, Silber SJ, et al: Birth after preimplantation diagnosis of the cystic fibrosis ΔF508 mutation by polymerase chain reaction in human embryos resulting from intracytoplasmic sperm injection with epididymal sperm. JAMA 1994; 272:1858–1860.

McCullough LB, Chervenak FA: Ethics in Obstetrics and Gynecology. New York, Oxford University Press, 1994.

Mortimer D: Practical Laboratory Andrology. New York, Oxford University Press, 1994.

Oates RD, Amos JA: The genetic basis of congenital bilateral absence of the vas deferens and cystic fibrosis. J Androl 1994; 15:1–8.

Sarkar S: Carbohydrate antigens of human sperm and autoimmune induction of infertility. J Reprod Med 1974; 13:93–99.

Sarkar S, Jolly DJ, Friedmann T, et al: Swimming behavior of X and Y human sperm. Differentiation 1984; 27:120–125.

Sarkar S, Jones OW, Shioura N: Constancy in human sperm DNA content. Proc Natl Acad Sci USA 1974; 71:3512–3516.

Sigman M, Lipschulz LI, Howards SS: Evaluation of the subfertile male. *In* Lipschulz I, Howards SS (eds): Infertility in the Male. St. Louis, Mosby–Year Book, 1991, pp 179–210.

Taylor PJ, Collins JA: Unexplained Infertility. New York, Oxford University Press, 1992.

U.S. Congress, Office of Technology Assessment, Infertility: Medical and Social Choices, OTA-BA-358. Washington, D.C., U.S. Government Printing Office, May 1988.

Wolff H, Panhans A, Stolz W, et al: Adherence of *Escherichia coli* to sperm: A mannose mediated phenomenon leading to agglutination of sperm and *E. coli*. Fertil Steril 1993; 60:154–158.

World Health Organization: WHO Laboratory Manual for the Examination of Human Semen and Sperm–Cervical Mucus Interaction. London, Cambridge University Press, 1992.

Chapter 23

Laboratory Diagnosis of Gastrointestinal Tract and Exocrine Pancreatic Disorders

Yuan S. Kao, M.D., FCAP
Frank Ju-Feng Liu, M.D., FCAP
Daniel R. Alexander, M.D.

3

EXAMINATION OF GASTRIC CONTENTS

Analysis of gastric secretion, like most other laboratory tests, is seldom itself of pathologic significance but must be interpreted in light of the patient's history and the results of other *in vivo* and *in vitro* tests. Furthermore, there are no sharply delineated normal ranges in gastric analysis, such as the reference intervals commonly used in many laboratory determinations in chemistry or hematology. It is indeed only at the extremes of gastric secretion that one can say with certainty that an underlying disease exists. The situation is further complicated by the usage of old terminology and the introduction of newer determinations. Because of its limitations and its value, gastric analysis is performed infrequently at the present time. Gastroscopy, roentgenography, and gastric cytology are far more useful in establishing the diagnosis of gastric pathology than is gastric analysis.

A properly performed gastric analysis requires a relatively large investment of time by the physician, who must perform the intubation and supervise the collection of specimen. Although the procedure is a benign experience, intubation is apt to be unpleasant and sometimes traumatic for the patient. In view of these facts and the inherent limitations of the information gained through gastric analysis, a definite indication for such tests is essential. In general, gastric analysis is performed for the following reasons:

1. To determine whether the patient can secrete any gastric acid. The finding of anacidity is of major importance in the patient with pernicious anemia, the patient

in whom pernicious anemia is suspected and who has been treated with vitamin B_{12} before the diagnosis has been unequivocally established, and the patient in whom an ulcerative lesion of the stomach is suspected.
2. To measure the amount of acid produced by a patient with symptoms of peptic ulcer, or with a suspected duodenal ulcer, or with a postoperative marginal ulcer that shows no demonstrable lesion on roentgenography.
3. To support the diagnosis of a hypersecretory state characteristic of Zollinger-Ellison syndrome.
4. To determine the completeness of vagotomy.
5. To aid in the differential diagnosis of gastric ulcer from duodenal ulcer.

Composition of Gastric Secretion

Gastric secretion is a complex solution, the synthesis of which is not completely understood. Although the cells that secrete hydrochloric acid, pepsin, and mucus have been clearly identified, the varying concentrations of inorganic ions in particular remain the object of speculation.

HYDROCHLORIC ACID. Hydrochloric acid is secreted by the parietal cells located in the isthmus and neck of the gastric glands of the fundus and body of the stomach but not those at the narrow rim of the cardia or the pylorus and antrum. The stomach secretes hydrochloric acid at a concentration of more than one million times the plasma concentration (about 160 mEq/L prior to dilution with other secretory components). The major role of hydrochloric acid in digestion is to provide the high acidity necessary to activate pepsin from pepsinogen but also, to a limited extent, to hydrolyze polypeptides and disaccharides directly. Because of the ease of measurement and relatively good correlation with disease states, determination of hydrochloric acidity is the most commonly used clinical index of gastric secretory activity.

ELECTROLYTES. Gastric secretion contains all the electrolytes found in other body fluids in a combined osmolar concentration equal to or slightly greater than plasma. The individual electrolytes vary widely in concentration, and, with the exception of hydrogen ion, such variations have no known clinical significance.

MUCUS. Gastric mucus is a complex mixture of mucoproteins and mucopolysaccharides. Physiologically, it acts as a barrier to protect the gastric mucosa from acid autodigestion. Mucus is secreted by specialized cells of the gland necks in the fundus and body of the stomach, by cells of the surface epithelium, and by the acinar cells of the cardia, antrum, and pylorus.

DIGESTIVE ENZYMES AND NONDIGESTIVE ENZYMES. Pepsin, the major digestive enzyme of gastric secretion, is secreted by chief cells (peptic cells) located at the base of the gastric glands of the body and fundus. Pepsin is secreted as pepsinogen I (A) and pepsinogen II (C) according to electrophoretically separated isozymogens. These two proenzymes are activated by gastric acid at an optimal pH of 1.6 to 2.4. Pepsin catalyzes the degradation of proteins to proteoses and peptones but does not liberate free amino acids. A small amount of pepsinogen enters the blood, presumably by direct absorption from the peptic cells, and is secreted in the urine as uropepsinogen. Gastrin also has a proteolytic activity at a higher pH optimum (pH 3.2) than pepsin. Gastric lipase plays an important role in the digestion of dietary fat, especially when pancreatic function is not well developed, as in the neonate, or is compromised, as in cystic fibrosis. Gastric lipase has a pH optimum of between 4.5 (against tricaprylin) and 5.5 (against triolein). Various nondigestive enzymes such as lactate dehydrogenase, aspartate aminotransferase, isocitrate dehydrogenase, alkaline phosphatase, alanine aminotransferase, and ribonuclease have been described. Except perhaps for ribonuclease, the role of these enzymes in digestion is not known.

MISCELLANEOUS SUBSTANCES. Small amounts of serum albumin and γ-globulin are normally present in gastric secretion. Albumin is frequently increased in gastric secretion in patients with giant hypertrophic gastritis or Ménétrier's disease, in carcinoma, and in benign peptic ulcer. Intrinsic factor, a glycoprotein, is elaborated by parietal cells. It promotes vitamin B_{12} absorption in the ileum. Blood group-specific substances (ABH, Lewis) are present in the gastric secretion in approximately 80% of individuals (i.e., those possessing the dominant secretor gene in either a homozygous or heterozygous state). Gastrointestinal peptide hormones may or may not be present in gastric secretion.

Nomenclature of Gastric Secretion

Various terms have been employed to describe qualitatively the results of gastric secretion tests. Most of these terms originated from translation of the older concepts of gastric acid and therefore must be redefined or discarded. The old terms, such as free acid, combined acid, total acid, achlorhydria, hypochlorhydria, hypersecretion, and hyposecretion, should be avoided entirely. Achlorhydria and hypochlorhydria, however, continue to appear in the literature. Gastric secretion can best be measured objectively according to volume, titratable acidity, and pH of each specimen aliquot of gastric secretion.

1. *Volume* is expressed in milliliters. The total volume is the sum of the individual specimen sample values.
2. *Titratable acidity* is expressed in milliequivalents per liter (mEq/L). This is determined by titration of a suitable aliquot of gastric secretion with 0.1 N NaOH to neutrality (pH of 7.0, or 7.4 as preferred by some). The end point should be measured electrometrically with a suitable pH meter, or it can be determined calorimetrically with phenol red (color change of yellow to red in the pH range 6.8 to 8.4).
3. *pH* is measured electrometrically.

Acid output is expressed in milliequivalents. The acid output of each sample can be calculated by multiplying its volume in milliliters by the titratable acidity and dividing by 1000. The *total acid output* is the sum of the individual acid output values. The *basal acid output* (BAO) in milliequivalents per hour is based on a one-hour collection of gastric secretion, which generally consists of four individually segregated 15-minute specimen collection samples. The *maximal acid output* (MAO) is defined as the sum of milliequivalents of acid secreted in one hour (four 15-minute samples) following injection of histamine, pentagastrin, or betazole (Histalog). This is not to be confused with the *maximal histamine response*, which is defined by Kay (1953) as the output of acid in milliequivalents in the period from 15 to 45 minutes after injection of histamine. The term *peak acid output* (PAO) is defined as the greatest acid output in any two successive 15-minute periods in the augmented histamine test. *Anacidity* is defined as a failure of the pH to fall below either 6.0 or 7.0 in the augmented histamine, pentagastrin, or Histalog test. This definition of anacidity represents the most reasonable compromise between clinical usefulness and strict physicochemical definition.

Gastric Intubation and Collection of Gastric Secretion

Prior to gastric intubation, the patient should be informed in detail about the procedure to obtain the fullest possible cooperation and to avoid undue apprehension. Towels or a large apron should be provided to protect clothing. The best recovery of gastric secretion is obtained with the patient in a sitting position. The bedfast patient should lie on his left side with his head elevated approximately 45 degrees. For intubation, a Levin tube or an equivalent can be passed through the nose, or a Rehfuss or similar tube can be passed through the mouth. Whether to use oral or nasal intubation depends on the preference of the individual examiner. It is likely that less difficulty will be encountered with nasal intubation. It is essential that the tube have a radiopaque tip so that it can be adjusted fluoroscopically. The tube may or may not be chilled with ice prior to intubation.

For oral intubation, the patient is instructed to open the mouth and project the chin slightly forward and upward. The tip of the tube is placed on the superior aspect of the posterior portion of the tongue, and the tube is then pushed gently to the posterior pharynx. The tube should avoid contact with the uvula as much as possible. After the patient has closed his mouth gently on the tube he should be encouraged to alternate swallowing and deep oral breathing while the tube is pushed intermittently to its destination as the patient swallows.

It is common for gastric tubes to be calibrated with several measurements, one of which is 55 cm; this corresponds to the approximate distance from the mouth to the antrum. It is imperative, however, that the tip lie in the most dependent portion of the stomach, which will usually be the antrum if the patient is sitting, or in the middle of the greater curvature if the patient is lying on the left side. Placement of the gastric tube is extremely important. Inappropriate placement of the tube leads to inadequate aspiration of gastric secretion. Following correct positioning, the tube should be directed lateral to the third molar tooth and maintained in position by taping it to the patient's face.

The principles of nasal intubation are similar to those of oral intubation. With the patient's chin elevated, the moistened tube is directed slightly upward and then pushed gently posteriorly into the nasopharynx and esophagus. Spraying of local anesthetic prior to intubation should rarely be necessary. A water recovery test for positioning of the nasogastric tube during gastric secretory study may be necessary.

If gastric secretion is to be collected over a period of time, as in the basal 1-hour secretion test, continuous aspiration should be employed because intermittent withdrawal of secretion has been shown to result in significantly lower recovery volumes. Continuous aspiration can be performed either with a syringe or by mechanical means; however, a significantly greater recovery is achieved with a syringe than with a suction apparatus. It is important to caution the patient to expectorate all saliva and upper respiratory secretions while aspiration is in progress.

Gastric intubation for secretory studies is contraindicated for patients with esophageal varices, diverticula, stenosis, malignant neoplasms, aortic aneurysm, recent severe gastric hemorrhage, congestive heart failure, or pregnancy.

Physical Examination of Gastric Contents

Normal fasting gastric secretion is a pale gray, translucent, slightly viscous fluid with a faintly pungent odor. The fasting volume varies up to about 50 mL. Following a 12-hour fast, the presence of food particles is distinctly abnormal and indicates delayed gastric emptying, often the result of pyloric obstruction.

BILE. Yellow to green coloration is the result of bile, which is occasionally regurgitated in the normal stomach and frequently accompanies excessive gagging during intubation. A large amount of bile, however, is an abnormal finding and usually indicates obstructing lesions of the small intestine distal to the ampulla of Vater.

MUCUS. Mucus is normally present in the gastric secretion. It may result from swallowed saliva and upper respiratory secretions and to a minor degree from the reflux of duodenal contents. The latter is identified by its staining property. Saliva is identified by its frothy flocculent nature, which causes it to float on the surface of the gastric secretion. Upper respiratory secretions are highly tenacious and may contain dust particles.

BLOOD. Flecks or streaks of blood are commonly seen as a result of minor trauma during intubation. Blood of a greater amount and longer duration in the acid-secreting stomach is brown and granular, the so-called coffee-ground appearance. Blood can arise from gastric lesions such as gastritis, ulcer, or carcinoma or from lesions in the mouth, nasopharynx, and respiratory tract. The presence of blood should be confirmed by an orthotoluidine or guaiac test. When testing the specimen using Hemoccult II (SmithKline Diagnostics, San Jose, CA), one may encounter a false-negative result if the pH of the gastric secretion is below 4.0. Gastroccult (SmithKline Diagnostics, San Jose, CA), a guaiac-based slide test, is specifically designed for detecting occult blood in gastric secretion (Hovsepian, 1986). Likewise, the Apt test, a qualitative test originally designed to detect fetal hemoglobin (HbF) in grossly bloody stools, has also been used to identify HbF in hematemesis of the newborn. The test, based on the fact that HbF is more resistant to alkali denaturation than adult hemoglobin, has a relatively low sensitivity, and the result must be interpreted with caution (McRury, 1994).

pH. pH should be measured electrometrically with a reliable pH meter.

Microscopic Examination of Gastric Contents

A variety of structures can be recognized on microscopic examination. Components such as erythrocytes, leukocytes, epithelial cells, yeast, bacteria, and particles of mucus can be found in the normal stomach. Cellular elements are usually in various stages of autolysis or digestion; thus their specific identity may be difficult to determine.

The presence of small numbers of erythrocytes is of no consequence. Leukocytes may be of gastric origin or from swallowed secretions. Increased numbers of leukocytes may result from inflammation of the gastric mucosa, mouth, or upper respiratory tract. Less commonly, they may come from the pancreas, biliary tract, or duodenum. Epithelial cells are found in small numbers as a result of desquamation from various mucosae. Squamous cells can be dislodged from the mouth, nose, pharynx, or esophagus. Gastritis often results in a significant increase in columnar epithelial cells, but this is usually not of pathognomonic significance.

The normal stomach does not have an established microbiologic flora. Although bacteria and yeasts can be regularly cultured from gastric secretion, these usually reflect the flora of the mouth and upper respiratory tract. Mycobacterial species may be recovered from the gastric secretion in patients with pulmonary tuberculosis. Strong associations between *Helicobacter pylori* and chronic superficial gastritis as well as antral gastritis are well established. A causal relationship between peptic ulcer disease and *H. pylori* is more difficult to establish. However, nearly all patients with duodenal ulcer have *H. pylori* gastritis. The association between *H. pylori* infection and gastric ulcer is only slightly less strong (NIH Consensus Development Conference, 1994). The microorganism *H. pylori* is characteristically found in or under the mucus layer on the enterocytes. Thus, the bacteria can be demonstrated in the biopsy specimen by staining with Giemsa's or Warthin-Starry stain. Both histologic demonstration of the organism and direct detection of urease activity in the tissue specimen have a sensitivity and specificity of greater than 90%. Culture of the organism is the least sensitive diagnostic test; it is positive in approximately 70% to 80% of cases. Noninvasive tests such as serologic tests for IgG antibody to *H. pylori* antigens and breath tests for urease activity have a sensitivity and specificity of greater than 95% (Hazell, 1987; NIH Consensus Development Conference, 1994). Direct morphologic identification of the bacteria from the gastric secretion has not been successful.

Yeasts are often present in large numbers in retained gastric contents, such as in patients with pyloric obstruction. Protozoan and metazoan parasites occur rarely and then usually in patients with reflux of duodenal contents. *Giardia lamblia* trophozoites or cysts, *Strongyloides* larvae, or *Ascaris* or hookworm ova can also be found.

Tests for Evaluation of Gastric Function

BASAL GASTRIC SECRETION. In basal gastric secretion, the acid is secreted in the absence of an external stimulus. It represents the response of the stomach to endogenous stimuli, which are continually present in the interdigestive or fasting state. Endogenous stimuli include psychoneurogenic influences, mediated by the vagus nerves, and hormonal stimuli, such as gastrin and perhaps adrenocorticosteroids. For clinical validity it is essential that basal physiologic and environmental conditions be maintained as much as possible during collection of the secretion. Minimum requirements include the following: (1) The patient must be in the fasting state and free from the sight or odor of food. (2) All medications influencing gastric secretion must be withheld for 24 hours. These include antacids, antisecretory drugs, and secretory stimulants. (3) The patient should be removed from environmental situations provoking untoward psychological reactions such as fear, anger, or depression.

The one-hour morning aspiration is now the standard method of measuring basal secretion. The basal acid output, like the stimulated acid output, varies considerably among individuals and is higher in men than in women (Feldman, 1983). The mean basal acid output reported for normal males ranges from 1.3 to 4.0 mEq/h in various series. This variation among series is a reflection in part of different collection techniques and methods of measuring titratable acid. Although low values had been observed in older individuals, a recent study indicated that gastric acid secretion increases with age in an otherwise healthy population (Katelaries, 1993). Somewhat lower than normal values are reported in most large series in patients with gastric carcinoma and benign gastric ulcer. Higher than normal values are observed in those with duodenal ulcer or marginal ulcer following partial gastrectomy with gastrojejunostomy (Table 23–1). An extremely high acid output is present in patients with the Zollinger-Ellison syndrome. A high ratio of basal acid output to maximal acid output is of even greater significance, however, in the diagnosis of the Zollinger-Ellison syndrome. It is important to emphasize that no pathognomonic range exists for any of the disease states listed, with the possible exception of the very high acid output in patients with the Zollinger-Ellison syndrome.

Technique—Basal Acid Output

1. Following a 12-hour overnight fast, the patient is intubated. Water may be taken until 8 hours prior to intubation.
2. Residual gastric secretion is aspirated, measured, and qualitatively examined.

Table 23–1. GASTRIC ACID OUTPUT IN VARIOUS CONDITIONS

Condition	Basal Acid Output (mEq H^+/h)	Maximal Acid Output (mEq H^+/h)
Control	0–5	5–20
Achlorhydria	0	0
Gastric carcinoma	0–5	0–10
Gastric ulcer	0–5	0.2–15
Duodenal ulcer	0–5	5–30
Zollinger-Ellison syndrome	5–70	10–100

Modified from Craig RM: Alimentary tract and exocrine pancreas. *In* Noe DA, Rock RC (eds): Laboratory Medicine. Baltimore, Williams & Wilkins, 1994, pp 383–400.

3. Continuous aspiration is begun, preferably manually with a syringe. The aspirate should be segregated into 15-minute samples. Usually the first one or two samples are discarded to allow for adjustment of the patient to the intubation procedure. Subsequent to this adjustment period, four 15-minute samples are collected.
4. For each 15-minute sample, the volume, pH, and titratable acidity are measured and the acid output is calculated. The sum of the acid outputs in the four samples, expressed in milliequivalents, represents the one-hour basal acid output.

MAXIMAL STIMULATION TESTS. Maximal stimulation tests are tests that result in an output of hydrochloric acid that cannot be increased substantially with additional stimulation. In these tests, a dose of histamine acid phosphate, an analogue of histamine (Histalog), or the synthetic pentapeptide pentagastrin (Peptavlon) is injected, and the gastric secretion is collected for analysis. Because histamine acid phosphate and Histalog induce untoward systemic effects of histamine, they have now largely been replaced by pentagastrin. The maximum rate of acid secretion is characteristically attained within 15 minutes after injection of pentagastrin and is maintained for approximately 30 minutes. By 60 minutes, acid secretion usually has fallen to basal levels. The maximum acid output, representing the sum of the acid outputs for the four 15-minute specimens, is the most generally accepted expression of gastric acid secretion. Values for various conditions are listed in Table 23–1.

According to Marks (1962), the range for maximal acid output in normal males is 4.9 to 38.9 mEq/h. A maximal acid output of greater than 40 mEq/h is found in about 40% of males with duodenal ulcer but only rarely in normal individuals. In addition to marked hypersecretion, the patient with Zollinger-Ellison syndrome has a high ratio of basal to maximal acid output. Ratios greater than 60% are strongly indicative of this disorder, whereas ratios between 40% and 60% are suggestive. Maximal acid output is not of great help in distinguishing benign gastric ulcer from gastric carcinoma unless anacidity is found, in which case benign peptic ulceration can be excluded.

Anacidity in the maximal secretory test is most commonly found in adults with pernicious anemia, chronic atrophic gastritis, Ménétrier's disease, gastric carcinoma, gastric ulcer, vitiligo, rheumatoid arthritis, thyrotoxicosis, or iatrogenic causes (postvagotomy, postgastric resection), and in those taking certain medications (e.g., H-receptor antagonists) (Wolfe, 1988). Pernicious anemia in adults is virtually always accompanied by anacidity, but this does not hold true in the rare cases of juvenile pernicious anemia, in which normal acid secretion may be present. Abnormally high acid secretion rates have been observed in Zollinger-Ellison syndrome, hypertrophic hypersecretory gastropathy, duodenal ulcer, small intestinal resection, and, rarely, systemic mastocytosis (Wolfe, 1988). Contamination of refluxed gastric juice with bile acids may predispose the patient to the development of strictures and Barrett's esophagus (Stein, 1994).

Technique—Maximal Acid Output (Kay, 1953; Baron, 1979)

1. At the conclusion of the basal secretion study, pentagastrin is administered subcutaneously at a dose of 6 μg/kg body weight (see Physicians' Desk Reference).
2. Proceed with the collection of gastric secretion in four 15-minute specimens for 1 hour.
3. Record the volume, pH, and titratable acidity for each specimen as previously described. The maximal acid output is calculated as the sum of the four 15-minute specimens.

INSULIN HYPOGLYCEMIA TEST. Hypoglycemia, resulting from the administration of insulin, is a potent stimulus of gastric acid secretion. The major component of this stimulus is transmitted by the vagus nerves, and the stimulation can be abolished by vagotomy. The hypoglycemic response is complex, however, and probably consists of three phases. For about 30 minutes after insulin injection there is a slight depression of gastric secretion, presumably owing to the secretion of antral somatostatin. The predominant effect during the remainder of the first two hours consists of marked enhancement of gastric secretion. It is believed that this results from cephalic-vagal stimulation of the parietal cells. Vagal stimulation also enhances the release of gastrin in the antrum. The final effect, which is manifested after two hours, also stimulates gastric secretion, presumably by a humoral mechanism.

The insulin test is valid only if the blood glucose level falls below 50 mg/dL at some point in the test, which usually occurs 30 minutes after insulin administration. The test is further valid only if the stomach has been shown to be capable of secreting hydrochloric acid. Therefore, if no acid is present in either the basal or the postinsulin period, it is necessary to perform a maximal stimulation test in an attempt to evoke acid secretion. If the stomach is truly anacid, no conclusion can be drawn about the completeness of vagotomy, but the possibility of simple peptic ulceration is then excluded. The assessment of gastric function following vagotomy has been reviewed (Read, 1974). No clear delineation of normal or abnormal gastric function results from the insulin test. Nevertheless, several generalizations can be made. Vagotomy can be considered to be complete if the larger acid output in the two postinsulin hours is less than the larger acid output of the two basal hours. Incomplete vagotomy is likely if the acid output in the two-hour postinsulin period exceeds that of the two-hour basal period by more than 0.5 mEq (Stempien, 1962). Incomplete vagotomy is also suggested by an acid output of greater than 2 mEq in either basal hour. The time of increased acid output in the insulin test appears to be of some prognostic significance in incompletely vagotomized patients. Bell (1965) reported on 42 patients who were shown to have incomplete vagotomy by the insulin test. Of 28 patients who had an elevated acid output in the first postinsulin hour, 10 eventually developed recurrent peptic ulceration. In contrast, peptic ulceration recurred in only one of the remaining 14 patients who showed an elevated acid output in the second postinsulin hour.

Technique (Modified from Hollander, 1948)

1. After a 12-hour overnight fast, the patient is intubated. A two-hour basal secretion test is performed by collecting eight 15-minute samples.
2. Blood samples for glucose determinations are obtained on completion of the basal secretion study and at 30, 60, and 90 minutes after insulin injection.

3. Insulin is administered intravenously either at a fixed dosage of 15 or 20 units or at a calculated dosage of 0.20 U/kg body weight. It is essential that a 50-mL syringe filled with 50% (w/v) glucose solution be readily available for intravenous injection to counteract any serious hypoglycemic episodes.
4. Gastric secretion is collected in 15-minute specimen samples for two hours after insulin injection.
5. For each basal and postinsulin gastric sample, the volume and titratable acidity are determined, and the acid output is calculated.

SHAM FEEDING. Testing for completeness of vagotomy by inducing hypoglycemia with insulin has occasionally resulted in serious complications. Sham feeding has been used as a safer alternative for testing vagal stimulation of gastric acid secretion. The procedure for sham feeding also requires gastric intubation; however, instead of administering insulin, patients are given a sandwich to chew and spit out. The gastric contents are first suctioned at 15-minute intervals for one hour to determine the basal gastric acid output; sham feeding follows, and then poststimulation gastric content suctioning is done at 15-minute intervals for another hour. This procedure has been shown to be as accurate as the insulin test without risking potential hypoglycemic complications (Kronborg, 1980; Athow, 1986).

URINE ACID OUTPUT TEST. More recently, a noninvasive test for assessing the completeness of vagotomy has been developed as a modification of sham feeding that does not require gastric intubation. This test relies on the postprandial alkaline tide produced by release of bicarbonate from the stomach parietal cells into the bloodstream following gastric acid secretion. Thus, when basal acid secretion is constant, the urine acid output also remains constant. Following increased gastric acid secretion, an alkaline tide into the bloodstream is detected by a decrease in the urine acid output. With this technique, gastric acid output following sham feeding was found to have a strong inverse correlation to urine acid output (Thomas, 1993). Because gastric intubation is not necessary for this test, patients may be permitted to swallow the food. When a test meal was substituted for sham feeding, postprandial urine acid output was better able to differentiate between vagotomized patients without recurrent duodenal ulcer and those with recurrent ulcer (Johnson, 1990). Thus, if vagotomy is complete, the two- and three-hour postprandial urine acid output does not decrease.

Miscellaneous Tests

MYCOBACTERIAL CULTURE. Aspiration of gastric contents for mycobacterial culture is indicated in patients in whom pulmonary tuberculosis is suspected but who are unable to produce adequate sputum samples. This procedure is particularly indicated for young children who cannot effectively expectorate pulmonary secretions. It is essential that the gastric content be collected in the early morning prior to eating or drinking and preferably immediately on awakening before increased motor activity of the stomach has emptied its contents. Because gastric acidity is inimical to the survival of mycobacterial bacilli as well as to most other bacteria, it is important to submit specimens immediately for decontamination and culture. Acid-fast stains on gastric contents are unreliable because saprophytic acid-fast microorganisms are frequently present in the mouth.

EXFOLIATIVE CYTOLOGY OF THE STOMACH. As mentioned previously, gastric cytology, gastroscopy, and roentgenography are at present the most useful procedures for the investigation of benign or malignant lesions of the stomach. To a large extent these three procedures complement each other, but in the final analysis the most discriminating information is provided by exfoliative cytology or biopsy. Multiple techniques are available for obtaining specimens, including sample aspiration of gastric content, the use of abrasive balloons or brushes, and gastric lavage with saline, buffered salt solutions, or solutions of papain or chymotrypsin. Accuracy rates of more than 90% have been reported for exfoliative cytology in the diagnosis of gastric carcinoma.

DETERMINATION OF INTRINSIC FACTOR. The gastric secretion used for routine gastric analysis is satisfactory for the assay of intrinsic factor. Failure to secrete intrinsic factor is commonly seen in atrophic gastritis in patients with loss of the parietal cell population or the presence of antibodies to intrinsic factor. Failure to secrete intrinsic factor can be determined either by *in vitro* assay using blocking or binding antibodies or by measuring the absorption of radiolabeled vitamin B_{12} *in vivo* (Schilling's test) with and without the addition of intrinsic factor.

DETERMINATION OF TUMOR MARKERS IN GASTRIC SECRETION. Because of methodologic variation, variation due to gastric pH, and nonstandardization of sampling collection, conflicting results of efforts to detect tumor markers in the gastric juice have been reported in patients with benign and malignant gastric diseases (Gion, 1988) (see Chap. 45).

SUCROSE PERMEABILITY TEST FOR SCREENING GASTRIC DAMAGE. This test is based on the principle that the healthy gastrointestinal mucosa is relatively impermeable to disaccharides. However, in the presence of gastrointestinal damage, sucrose is absorbed and an increased amount of sucrose is excreted in urine after an oral load of sucrose is administered (Sutherland, 1994).

DETERMINATION OF PLASMA GASTRIN. Although not an integral part of gastric analysis per se, radioimmunoassay of plasma or serum gastrin is a valuable adjunct in the diagnosis of the Zollinger-Ellison syndrome and pernicious anemia, both of which are associated with marked elevation of gastrin. The two diseases are readily distinguished on the basis of concomitant gastric acid secretion studies and by the fact that intragastric instillation of dilute hydrochloric acid results in a precipitous decrease in plasma gastrin in pernicious anemia, whereas no appreciable change in gastrin concentration occurs in the Zollinger-Ellison syndrome. Fasting plasma gastrin concentrations in duodenal ulcer patients do not differ from those in normal individuals but may be persistently elevated in the postprandial state. Small increases in plasma gastrin are associated with gastric ulcer and with aging (Trudeau, 1971).

Gastrin is a polypeptide hormone produced by the G cells of the antral mucosa of the stomach, the proximal duodenum, and, to a lesser extent, the pancreas, where most gastrinomas occur. Gastrin is produced in three forms: as a 34-amino acid polypeptide, G-34 (big gastrin); a 17-amino acid form, G-17 (little gastrin); and G-14 (minigastrin). G-34 is usually produced in larger amounts and has a longer half-life but lower biologic activity than G-17. G-17 can be produced physiologically by trypsinization of G-34 or is secreted directly by the antral mucosal G cells. G-14 is a minor form accounting for only about 5% of total gastrin. In each of these forms, a tetrapeptide at the carboxyterminal end is essential for biologic activity. Pentagastrin, marketed as Peptavalon (Ayerst), is a synthetic form of the C-terminal end used diagnostically as a potent parietal cell secretagogue. The radioimmunoassay for gastrin uses an antibody specific for the C-terminal end common to all forms. In this assay, ^{125}I-labeled G-17 competes with a mixture of gastrin forms in the patient sample for a limited number of C-terminal antibody binding sites. Antibody-bound radioactivity is inversely proportional to the gastrin level, which in normal fasting patients is less than 100 ng/L but may be increased physiologically to more than 300 ng/L. Aberrant gastrin-like peptides lacking the C-terminal end may be produced by tumor cells; however, they lack biologic activity and are not detectable by routine gastrin assay.

Conditions associated with increased serum gastrin levels include (1) hypersecretion by G cells that are unresponsive to physiologic negative feedback signals, as in Zollinger-Ellison syndrome, or are hyporesponsive, as in duodenal ulcer disease; (2) conditions associated with end organ unresponsiveness to gastrin stimulation, such as following gastrectomy, pernicious anemia, atrophic gastritis, gastric carcinoma involving the body of the stomach, gastric ulcer disease, and omeprazole therapy; (3) compensatory gastrin hypersecretory states following loss of other acid secretagogues such as after vagotomy and in patients on long-term H_2-blocker therapy.

An autonomous gastrinoma (Zollinger-Ellison syndrome) can be distinguished by hyperacidity that is unresponsive to negative feedback inhibition following intragastric acid instillation and also by a paradoxical rise in gastrin levels following intravenous secretin injection.

EXAMINATION OF DUODENAL CONTENTS AND PANCREATIC EXOCRINE SECRETION

Examination of Duodenal Contents

Composition of Duodenal Contents

The duodenal contents are composed of exocrine pancreatic secretion, bile, intestinal secretion mixed with gastric secretion, and possibly partially digested food particles. Clinical examination is usually performed with the patient in the fasting state, and specimen samples are collected in such a manner that gastric secretion is effectively excluded.

Pancreatic exocrine secretion probably exceeds 1500 mL/day in the normal adult and is thus the major contributor to the duodenal contents. It is a colorless, clear, nonviscid, alkaline solution with a pH of approximately 8.0. The secretion consists of 1% to 2% organic material, mostly enzymes or their precursors, including trypsinogen, chymotrypsinogen, amylase, lipase, lecithinase, elastase, collagenase, leucine aminopeptidase, and various esterases. It also contains about 1% inorganic material, with sodium the major cation and bicarbonate the major anion. Compared with serum, sodium and potassium are present in about the same concentrations, whereas calcium and magnesium are present in lower concentrations. The bicarbonate concentration varies directly with the rate of pancreatic secretion and ranges from 25 to 150 mEq/L, whereas chloride varies inversely with the rate of secretion, so that the sum of these two ions remains approximately constant.

Pancreatic exocrine secretion occurs in response to both vagal and gastric stimuli. The vagal component is relatively slight and results in a small volume of secretion that is rich in enzymes. Two hormones, secretin and cholecystokinin, which are elaborated by the duodenal mucosa, are potent stimuli of pancreatic secretion. They are released into the blood following the entry of peptone, amino acid, or fluid into the duodenum. Acid by itself can apparently stimulate the release of secretin. Secretin results in a copious flow of pancreatic secretion that is low in enzyme content and high in bicarbonate. Cholecystokinin, on the other hand, stimulates the pancreas to secrete enzymes and consequently results in degranulation of the acinar cells. Clinical tests using these two enzymes have been established. Gastrin, although a weak stimulus, may provoke pancreatic exocrine secretion. The gastrin is released by food in the stomach or perhaps through vagal stimulation.

3

The daily volume of duodenal secretion (succus entericus) is not known. As with the pancreatic exocrine secretion, the succus entericus contains a variety of digestive enzymes that are capable of breaking down ingested foods. However, the enzymatic activities are considered relatively weak.

Approximately 500 to 1000 mL of bile enters the duodenum daily. Bile is yellow to brown or green in color and usually alkaline, with a pH of 7.0 to 8.5. In addition to bile salts, chiefly sodium glycocholate and taurocholate, bile contains bilirubin pigment, cholesterol, phospholipids, and various inorganic salts. Alkaline phosphatase, the only enzyme present in a significant amount in bile, has no function in digestion.

Duodenal Intubation and Collection of the Fluid

Duodenal intubation can be performed by using various types of tubes including a double-lumen tube, such as the Diamond or Dreiling tube, or a three-lumen tube, and certain types of instruments for small bowel biopsies (Linscheer, 1976). It is essential that the tube have a radiopaque tip so that its position can be verified fluoroscopically.

For intubation, the technique described by Raskin (1958) is recommended: Following an overnight fast, a sedative dose of a benzodiazepine is administered parenterally. A double-lumen Diamond tube is inserted into the mouth and passed about 45 cm, which brings the tip approximately to the cardia. The patient is then placed in the left lateral decubitus position on a table, the cephalic end of which is elevated 16 inches. The tube is then slowly swallowed for another 15 cm, which brings the tip to a position along the greater curvature. The patient then sits on the edge of the examining table with the body bent forward at the waist as far as possible. Several deep inspirations will assist in allowing the tube to enter the antrum. Peristalsis will move the tube into the duodenum if the patient lies in the right lateral decubitus position with the face elevated for about 5 minutes. Finally, the patient lies on his back for another 5 minutes while the tube is slowly advanced another 10 to 15 cm. The tube is adjusted with fluoroscopic visualization so that its tip is located in the middle of the third portion of the duodenum. Proper location of the tube can be maintained by taping it to the patient's face. This entire procedure can usually be completed in about 15 minutes.

Secretions are collected with continuous suction by a vacuum pump or suitable apparatus that can obtain a pressure of at least 25 mm Hg. During aspiration, the patient may lie on either the back or the right side. The duodenal aspirate can be collected in suitable containers, such as centrifuge test tubes, which can be placed as a trap in the suction line. This facilitates the frequent changing of containers that is required. The character of the aspirate can be monitored continuously by placing a section of glass tubing in the duodenal tube just before the collection container. The gastric aspirate is discarded.

In addition to the conditions that are contraindications to gastric intubation, duodenal intubations should not be performed as a general rule in patients with acute cholecystitis or acute pancreatitis.

Macroscopic and Microscopic Examination of Duodenal Contents

In the fasting state the residual content of the duodenum varies by up to 20 mL. The fluid is transparent or slightly translucent, pearly gray, and moderately viscid unless it is mixed with gastric secretion, in which case a slight turbidity is observed. Bile staining is usually absent, but its presence is of no significance. Slight blood streaking can result from the intubation procedure. A large amount of blood may suggest a neoplasm, usually involving the ampulla of Vater. The presence of food particles is distinctly abnormal and usually indicates either intestinal obstruction or a duodenal diverticulosis. Sediment or flocculent debris can be seen in patients with inflammation of the duodenal mucosa, pancreas, or biliary tract.

For microscopic examination of cellular elements, the duodenal contents should be collected in containers chilled in an ice bath and should be examined as soon as possible. Following centrifugation, the cellular elements may be examined unstained. A few leukocytes or epithelial cells are normal. Increased numbers of polymorphonuclear leukocytes and exfoliated epithelial cells enmeshed in mucus, with or without masses of bacteria, can be found in patients with inflammation of the duodenum, bile ducts, or pancreas. The presence of bile staining may prove of some help in differentiating inflammatory conditions of the biliary tract. Rarely, parasites such as larvae of *Strongyloides stercoralis*, cysts or trophozoites of *Giardia lamblia* or *Entamoeba histolytica*, or the ova of *Necator*, *Ancylostoma*, or *Ascaris* can be found.

Chemical Examination of Duodenal Contents

The most important electrolyte in duodenal contents is bicarbonate, but its measurement is indicated only in tests of pancreatic function such as the secretin test. Determination of chloride, bilirubin, and urobilinogen provides no useful information.

Determination of amylase, lipase, or trypsin activity in the pancreatic secretion following secretin or pancreozymin stimulation is an important index of pancreatic exocrine function. Variations in these three enzyme levels usually parallel one another, so only one of the three determinations is indicated. Amylase is most commonly measured and is the most stable. Determination of lipase and trypsin in addition to amylase is occasionally helpful in infants in whom cystic fibrosis is suspected or who have diarrhea or steatorrhea of unknown cause. Methods of determining either serum amylase or lipase can be easily adapted to the duodenal contents. Trypsin activity can be determined by testing for digestion of gelatin coating on x-ray film as is done for fecal trypsin.

Examination of Stimulated Bile

Because bile flow into the duodenum is intermittent in the fasting state, it is usually necessary to induce bile flow with a suitable stimulant if examination of bile is indicated. Although secretin is a potent choleretic agent, the increased volume of bile produced by the liver is stored in the gallbladder if the cystic duct is patent. In the presence of normal gallbladder function, secretin can result in a decrease in or even cessation of bile flow into the duodenum. Pancreozymin, on the other hand, usually results in abundant bile flow. Magnesium sulfate functions as an active cholagogue when applied topically to the duodenal mucosa but not when administered orally. Olive oil is probably an even more potent cholagogue but has the disadvantage of interfering with subsequent microscopic examination of the bile.

To obtain stimulated bile, duodenal intubation is performed, and the position of the tube is confirmed fluoroscopically. Following aspiration of residual duodenal contents through the duodenal tube, 50 to 100 mL of a sterile 25% saturated solution of magnesium sulfate is slowly introduced. A minute or so later, the magnesium sulfate and duodenal content are aspirated. The collected fluid is pooled and discarded until yellow bile first appears in quantity. Three fractions of bile are subsequently collected in separate containers. The first of these to appear, the A bile, is light yellow and watery; it usually amounts to 5 to 20 mL and originates in the common duct. The B bile is viscid and deep yellow-brown and appears abruptly 1 to 3 minutes after the A fraction. The B bile, which normally amounts to 30 to 75 mL, originates in the gallbladder. After the B bile appears, the bile again becomes pale yellow and watery; this C bile presumably comes from the hepatic ducts and intrahepatic radicles. The absence of B bile is associated with advanced cholecystitis, cholelithiasis with obstructed cystic duct, or recent cholecystectomy. However, absence of B bile is not proof of gallbladder disease, and this finding should be confirmed by other diagnostic procedures.

Microscopic Examination of Duodenal Bile

It has been suggested that detection of cholesterol or bilirubinate crystals in duodenal bile could be used to distinguish between patients with or without gallstones. Cholesterol crystals are transparent and rectangular or rhomboidal. Calcium bilirubinate crystals are amorphous yellow to orange. The finding of bile sand, often in deep red-brown bile, is highly suggestive of cholelithiasis or calculus elsewhere in the biliary tract. Bockus (1931) found that the presence of either or both of these crystals was associated with calculi in approximately 90% of patients. Ramond (1988) analyzed gallbladder bile obtained by direct puncture and aspiration before cholangiography and found that the presence of cholesterol crystals in the gallbladder bile had an 87% sensitivity, 97% specificity, and positive predictive value of 97%. Bilirubinate crystals, when present alone, had a 71% sensitivity, 93% specificity, and positive predictive value of 88%. Inflammation of the biliary tract is often accompanied by flocculent debris, which often consists of bile-stained epithelial cells, leukocytes, and clumps of bacteria. Culture of stimulated bile is occasionally informative. However, interpretation is frequently difficult and depends on quantitative as well as qualitative evaluation of cultures.

Screening for Pancreatic Disorders

Determination of amylase and lipase activity in body fluids has for years been the cornerstone of the laboratory approach to the diagnosis of acute and chronic relapsing pancreatitis, in which release of these substances into blood and urine is increased. Except for the diagnosis of pancreatic carcinoma and chronic pancreatitis, examination of stimulated pancreatic fluid through duodenal aspiration has been until recently the only reliable means of assessing pancreatic secretory function. These tests are not suitable for screening for the pancreatic disease-prone individual or patients with the predisease state. However, they are useful for screening for predisposing conditions. For example, because alcoholism or gallstone disease is present in over 80% of patients with pancreatitis, biochemical tests sensitive to liver damage, such as serum aspartate aminotransferase or γ-glutamyl transpeptidase, may be useful. In alcoholics, hypertriglyceridemia may trigger pancreatitis; therefore, serum triglyceride determinations may also be useful. Serum calcium measurements may be indicated because patients with hyperparathyroidism should be screened. Steroids, thiazides, sulfonamides, azathioprine, and birth control pills have also been implicated as causes of pancreatitis, although not commonly.

Pancreatic carcinoma is one of the leading causes of cancer deaths in the United States, and unfortunately there is no established effective screening test for its early diagnosis. Although pancreatic function tests, abdominal ultrasound, computed tomography (CT), endoscopic retrograde cholangiopancreatography, galactosyltransferase isoenzyme II, carcinoembryonic antigen, α-fetoprotein, CA 19-9, and pancreatic oncofetal antigen tests have been used, no single test has proved to have both high sensitivity and specificity.

Cystic fibrosis is a common cause of pancreatic insufficiency in the pediatric population. In these patients, secretion of bicarbonate from the pancreas into the duodenum is impaired, resulting in persistent acidification of duodenal and jejunal contents. Protein and fat malabsorption syndromes are the main clinical findings with pancreatic insufficiency secondary to cystic fibrosis. This disease is an autosomal recessive genetic disorder caused by mutation in the cystic fibrosis transmembrane conductance regulator (*CFTR*) gene, which codes for a cyclic AMP–regulated chloride channel (Anderson, 1991; Bear, 1992). A single mutation in the *CFTR* gene causing cystic fibrosis involves a specific deletion of three base pairs coding for phenylalanine at amino acid position ΔF508 (delta-F508). This mutation has been detected in approximately 70% of cystic fibrosis patients (Kerem, 1989, 1990; Riordan, 1989). A strong correlation has been shown between ΔF508 and pancreatic insufficiency (Kristidis, 1992). The ability to detect this common genetic mutation causing cystic fibrosis provides a powerful tool for the prenatal diagnosis of the disease, improved methods of identifying spouses of cystic fibrosis carriers, and population-based screening programs for carriers of the cystic fibrosis gene (Lemna, 1990; Colton, 1990). However, more than 300 other sequence alterations in the *CFTR* gene have been identified since 1989 (Tsui, 1992). The relationship between mutations in *CFTR* (genotype) and disease presentation (phenotype) is not straightforward (Kiesewetter, 1993). For example, Highsmith and colleagues (1994) identified a group of patients with pulmonary disease similar to that seen in cystic fibrosis, normal sweat chloride concentration, and no common mutation in the *CFTR* gene with conventional genetic analysis of genomic DNA but a point mutation in intron 19 of *CFTR* identified using direct sequencing of messenger RNA transcripts. Most of the patients in this group, however, did not have phenotypic evidence of pancreatic insufficiency. Up to 95% of all cystic fibrosis patients have *CFTR* mutation genotypes known to be associated with pancreatic insufficiency.

Amylase (α-1,4-Glucan-4-Glucanohydrolase, E.C. 3.2.1.1)

Biochemistry and Physiology

Amylases are enzymes that catalyze the hydrolysis of amylopectin, amylose, glycogen, and their partially hydrolyzed products. α-Amylase occurs in animal tissue and fluids. It splits α-1,4-glucosidic linkages in polysaccharides containing three or more α-1,4-linked D-glucose units in random fashion. On hydrolysis by α-amylase, amylose gives rise to a mixture of maltose and glucose, whereas amylopectin yields a mixture of branched and unbranched oligosaccharides. Because α-1,6-glucosidic linkages are not hydrolyzed by the enzyme, the polysaccharides that remain after hydrolysis are limit dextrins. α-Amylase rapidly decreases the ability of amylose and starch to stain blue with iodine and decreases the viscosity of starch solutions. Other amylases include β-amylase, found in both animals and plants; an exoenzyme, α-1,4-glucanomaltohydrolase, E.C. 3.2.1.2); and γ-amylase, α-1,4-glucanoglucohydrolase, E.C. 3.2.1.3), found in numerous fungi. Of these three amylases, only α-amylase is of clinical interest.

Isoamylases

The α-amylase present in blood and urine of normal individuals is predominantly of pancreatic and salivary origin. α-Amylase of pancreatic and salivary origin is abbreviated to P-type and S-type amylase (isoenzyme, isoamylase), respectively, whenever such a distinction is needed. These two types of amylase are closely related enzymes but also have organ-specific variations. They have the same amino acid composition and yield similar but not identical peptide maps. Each appears to consist of a single polypeptide chain without subunits. Pancreatic amylase has a molecular weight of 54,000. Higher molecular weights have been reported for salivary amylase. Both amylases contain sulfhydryl groups. Pancreatic amylase is believed to have five binding sites for substrates (Wermus, 1979). Amylases are metalloenzymes containing at least one atom of calcium per molecule; they require this metal for their catalytic activities. The pH for optimal activity ranges from 6.9 to 7.0. The pH optimum for salivary amylase varies with the anion used as activator, of which chloride is the most important. Optimal chloride concentration is 10 mmol/L, and the activation is allosteric. Bromide and iodide ions also activate amylase. The isoelectric points (pI) have been reported to be 7.6 and 7.2 for P-type and 6.4 and 5.8 for S-type isoamylases. Other pI values have also been documented (Scully, 1981; Bossuyt, 1981).

Human pancreatic amylase and salivary amylase are controlled by independent genes. At neutral pH, both amylases exhibit the same action pattern, although there are differences in molecular weight, carbohydrate content, and amide groups. At both high and low temperature extremes, pancreatic amylase is more labile than salivary amylase. Pancreatic amylase, P-type, is synthesized by the acinar cells of the pancreas and is tissue specific. Salivary amylase, S-type, is present in and believed to be synthesized by parotid, sweat, and lactating mammary glands, lung, fallopian tube, and possibly, liver. After electrophoresis of human serum on agar gel, Kamaryt (1965) observed two bands with amylolytic activity, both of which appeared in the γ-globulin region. The mobility of the less anodic isoenzyme corresponded to that of the amylase band obtained from pancreas, and the more anodic one corresponded to the band of amylase from salivary gland. A minimum of three and a maximum of five serum amylases were found by De la Lande (1969) using polyacrylamide gel electrophoresis. These isoenzymes were designed as AmySE-1, -2, -3, -4, and -5, respectively, according to their mobilities. It was concluded that AmySE-1 and SE-2 were probably of pancreatic origin, and SE-2 and SE-3 were the most active isoenzymes in normal human serum. In his study of 1000 blood donors, Vacikova (1969) reported the presence of four amylase monomers and five possible combinations of isoenzymes designated as SP, sSP, SPp, sSpP, and P.

With refinement of separation techniques, it was found (Spiekerman, 1974) that human amylase of pancreatic origin contained one or two major and one or more minor isoenzymes, whereas salivary amylase generally yielded one or two major and three to six minor amylolytic bands. In normal individuals and in patients with mumps, pancreatitis, pancreatectomy, and chronic relapsing pancreatitis, Otsuki (1976) determined isoamylases in serum and urine as well as in saliva, pancreatic juice, and the homogenates of human pancreas. He found that as many as seven amylase isoenzymes were separated from these specimens. He concluded that essentially all the isoenzymes in human serum and urine were derived from the pancreas and salivary gland, and that the isoenzymes of 98% of normal individuals consisted of two major and two to three minor isoamylases.

Assigning amylase-1 to the isoenzyme with the slowest mobility, Otsuki (1976) found that it also was the major isoenzyme among four pancreatic isoamylases and that amylase-3 was the major isoenzyme among three salivary isoamylases. This finding is in agreement with the findings of Spiekerman (1974) that, as a group, human pancreatic isoenzymes migrate more slowly in the electric field toward the anode than do salivary isoamylases.

The assignment of number 1 to the slowest migrating isoamylase and number 7 to the fastest migrating isoamylase is contrary to the commonly accepted isoenzyme numbering practice, in which the fastest migrating isoenzyme is given the subscript 1, such as LD_1. Isoamylase nomenclature is further complicated by other reports (Aw, 1966; Legaz, 1976) in which isoamylases were named either S or P to indicate their origin, followed by a subscript number to indicate their electrophoretic mobility—for example, S_1 being the slowest migrating salivary isoamylase.

Using a DEAE-Sephadex column for the separation, Fridhandler (1972) reported that in normal serum the P-type isoamylase constituted 28% to 49% of the total amylase activity, but in the corresponding urine the percentage of pancreatic amylase was significantly higher. When QAE-Sephadex A-50, a better ion exchanger for the separation of P-type and S-type isoamylases, was used, it was found that in serum the percentage of total amylase activity contributing to P-type isoamylase ranged from 12.7% to 76.3%, with most of the values falling below 50%; for S-type isoamylase, it averaged 57.6% (Heffernon, 1977). As for the corresponding urine samples, 62.3% (range, 30.5% to 94%) of amylase was P-type isoamylase and 37.6% was S-type isoamylase. However, according to Gillard (1979), based on polyacrylamide disk–gel electrophoresis, only 43% of total serum amylase was of pancreatic origin. When a selective inhibitor for S-type isoamylase was employed, an average of 48% (range, 27% to 70%) of pancreatic isoenzyme was found in normal individuals (Huang, 1982). Conversely, Otsuki (1976) found that in normal adult serum the activity of P-type amylase averaged 52.3% of the total, and P-type activity was higher than that of S-type in almost all normal adults. Bossuyt (1981) reported that the serum isoamylase pattern was clearly related to age. Using thin-layer gel isoelectric focusing techniques, it was found that the contribution of P-type isoenzymes increased from an average of 25% and peaked at 42% of the total amylase activity at age 40, after which the contribution of P-type decreased rather rapidly to less than 20% after age 70. All these reports agreed that there was no significant difference in results between normal males and females.

Macroamylasemia

Macroamylasemia was first discovered by Wilding (1964) and was later so named by Berk and coworkers (1979) to describe a condition of persistently elevated serum amylase activity with no apparent clinical symptoms of a pancreatic disorder. It was attributed to the presence of an amylase-globulin complex whose larger size precluded its excretion into urine even though renal function was unimpaired. Macroamylase is a circulating complex of normal amylase linked to an immunoglobulin in most cases and to a polysaccharide in others. The immunoglobulins involved are IgA and IgG. The composition of macroamylases is heterogeneous. Analysis of the complex after acid dissociation re-

Table 23–2. DIFFERENTIAL DIAGNOSIS OF HYPERAMYLASEMIA AND MACROAMYLASEMIA

Condition	Serum Amylase	Serum Lipase	Urinary Amylase	Cam : Ccr	Serum Macroamylase
Pancreatic hyperamylasemia	High	High	High	High	Absent
Salivary hyperamylasemia	High	Normal	Low or normal	Low or normal	Absent
Macroamylasemia type 1	High	Normal	Low	Very low	High
Macroamylasemia type 2	High	Normal	Low or normal	Low	Moderate
Macroamylasemia type 3	Normal	Normal	Normal	Low or normal	Trace

Cam : Ccr (amylase clearance : creatinine clearance ratio) = (urinary amylase/serum amylase) × (serum creatinine/urinary creatinine)
Modified from Kleinman DS, O'Brien JF: Macroamylase. Mayo Clin Proc 1986; 61:669.

vealed that P-type and S-type isoamylases were present in variable proportions. The molecular weight has been estimated at 150,000 to more than one million. Macroamylasemia may also occur in hyperamylasemic patients with undiminished urine amylase and in patients with normal serum and urine amylase activity. Serum lipase may also form a complex with circulating immunoglobulins, resulting in macrolipasemia (Zaman, 1984). Table 23–2 shows the features of different types of macroamylasemia.

Amylase, unlike most serum enzymes, is filtered by the renal glomeruli and partially reabsorbed in the renal tubules. Little is known about the normal mechanism of the entrance of pancreatic enzymes, such as amylase, into blood, where normally the pancreatic enzyme appears to account for less than 50% of serum amylase activity. Increased serum activity in acute pancreatitis presumably results from the escape of enzyme into the interstitial tissue and peritoneal cavity, leading to increased absorption through the lymphatics and veins. The renal clearance of amylase has been estimated to be 1 to 3 mL/min and appears to be constant over a wide range of urine flow rates; therefore, increased release into the blood is followed by increased excretion in the urine owing to reduced tubular reabsorption of amylase.

Both the salivary and pancreatic amylases clear very rapidly from the blood; their half-lives are approximately two hours. Salivary and pancreatic amylases catalyze the hydrolysis of glucosidase bonds of glycogen, starch, and breakdown products of these in the digestive tract; however, in serum, urine, or tissue, amylase has no known function. During the first year of life, little or no pancreatic amylase is produced. In neonates, the source of amylase is apparently the salivary glands (Hadorn, 1968).

In humans, α-amylase is normally present in pancreas (approximately 200 mg/kg), salivary glands, liver, muscle, adipose tissue, saliva, blood, urine, feces, milk, semen, kidney, brain, lung, fallopian tube, intestine, spleen, and heart. There is very little quantitative information in the literature comparing the amylase concentrations per gram of tissue in the various organs.

Reference ranges for serum amylase differ greatly owing to the assays used to measure the enzyme. Serum amylase levels in neonates are normally close to zero. Amylase is first detectable between the ages of two and three months and reaches low normal adult levels by one year of age. The adult amylase value is usually reached by the age of five years. The pancreatic amylase rises with age to a peak of about 40% of the total serum amylase level at age 50 years and decreases thereafter (O'Donnell, 1980; Bossuyt, 1981). Serum amylase reference ranges are the same for both men and women and are not affected by food intake or time of day. There is a broad range of values for the urine amylase level: the 24-hour excretions of amylase range from 271 to 3671 units (Lott, 1970).

Analytical Methods

TOTAL SERUM OR URINE AMYLASE. α-Amylase is one of the most stable enzymes; in serum and urine it is stable for one week at room temperature and for at least six months under refrigeration in well-sealed containers. It may be kept in the frozen state much longer without appreciable loss of activity. Plasma specimens that have been anticoagulated with citrate or oxalate should be avoided for amylase determination because amylase is a calcium-containing enzyme and falsely low enzyme activities are obtained from such specimens (Young, 1975). Heparinized plasma specimens do not interfere with the amylase assay.

Since the first method for amylase determination was described in 1831, more than 200 different methods, based on different principles and substrates, have been developed. In an interlaboratory study of amylase methodologies (College of American Pathologists [CAP] Chemistry Survey, 1994), 4828 laboratories that participated in the survey used 43 commercially available amylase methods. The mean amylase values for specimen C-06 in the survey were reported to range from 37.2 to 86.2 IU/L, for specimen C-07 from 166.7 to 372.5 IU/L, for specimen C-08 from 64.8 to 152.5 IU/L, for specimen C-09 from 208.2 to 506.2 IU/L, and for specimen C-10 from 210.6 to 506.7 IU/L, depending on the methods used. Enzyme activities, of course, vary depending on the specific substrate used and on conditions such as pH and temperature, as discussed in Chapter 13.

One of the most disturbing problems in the determination of amylase activity by different methods is the interconvertibility of the results (Sax, 1972). Although the use of international units has been recommended, they are seldom used by the manufacturers of the amylase reagent. Different methods use different expressions of unit based on the manufacturer's definition. The interconversion among different units is extremely difficult, and sometimes impossible, because many of the substrates used either are ill defined or are not the natural substrate for amylase; in some cases, the substrates are the partial breakdown products of starch, the natural substrate for amylase. Some methods use a pH that is not optimal for amylase. Therefore, the attempt to interconvert the different units for amylase among different methods is not recommended. As a result, different methods have different "expected reference ranges" (Marshall, 1980). The analytical methods for total amylase concentration may be classified into six broad categories: saccharogenic methods, amyloclastic and iodometric methods, chromogenic (chromolytic, dyed-starch) methods, coupled-enzymatic (kinetic) methods, turbidimetric and nephelometric methods, and viscometric methods. With the great number of different methodologies for determining amylase concentration available today, each with its merits and drawbacks, one must choose a method based on accuracy, precision, ease of operation, and other requirements such as equipment availability and caliber of laboratory personnel. Regardless of the method chosen, caution must be exercised to avoid contamination of specimens with saliva because its amylase content is approximately 700 times that of serum. Red cells contain no amylase, so hemolysis generally presents no problem with most of the methods except those coupled-enzyme methods in which the released peroxide is determined by a coupled peroxidase reaction. It may not be the same for urine amylase. A recent interlaboratory proficiency test showed that the coefficient of variation of serum amylase ranged from 1.9% to 11.9% by a variety of methods (CAP Enzyme Chemistry Surveys Set C-1 through 7-B, 1994), whereas the coefficient of variation of urine amylase ranged from 19% to 68.1% (CAP Urine Chemistry Series 1 Set U-C, 1993). Improvement of the urine amylase assay, therefore, is urgently needed.

ISOAMYLASE. The fractionation of amylase in serum, urine, or other body fluids may be achieved by physical means, such as electrophoresis, chromatography, and isoelectric focusing, and each isoenzyme is then quantitated either by direct densitometry or by amyloclastic or saccharogenic techniques. A simplified, readily adaptable chromatographic method has been described by Fridhandler (1980). A chemical inhibition assay employing a salivary amylase–specific protein inhibitor is also being used for isoenzyme determinations (Huang, 1982) and is commercially available (Tietz, 1984). The chemical inhibition isoamylase determination is simple, fast, and suitable for emergency situations; thus, any clinical laboratory can perform isoamylase determinations. An immunoinhibition method using a monoclonal antibody to inhibit the salivary amylase and subsequently quantitate the remaining pancreatic amylase has been reported (Mifflin, 1985). Because of its simplicity, acceptable analytical precision, and good correlation with the isoamylase electrophoretic method, this method should be further investigated for clinical application.

MACROAMYLASE DETECTION METHOD. Several methods are available to detect macroamylase. Direct identification of macroamylase requires ultracentrifugation or chromatography. Indirect methods that rely on dissociating amylase from other proteins such as the temperature-sensitive amylase assay have also been used. A chromatographic screening procedure has been developed by Fridhandler (1971).

Interpretation

SERUM AND URINE TOTAL AMYLASE. Elevations of serum and urine amylase are observed in a wide variety of disorders. Most of the elevations of serum amylase are due to increased rates of amylase entry into the bloodstream, decreased rates of clearance, or both.

Determinations of serum and urine amylase activity, although not specific indices, have been used most extensively in the laboratory diagnosis of acute pancreatitis for the past 50 years. Reported diagnostic sensitivity and specificity of serum amylase for the diagnosis of acute pancreatitis vary greatly. This great variation is, of course, affected by methodologic differences, diagnostic criteria, and reference intervals. The diagnostic sensitivity and specificity of serum amylase in acute pancreatitis have been reported to be 70% to 98% and 70% to 76%, respectively; sensitivity and specificity of urine amylase are 80% to 98% and 80% to 90%, respectively (Lente, 1982).

Serum amylase activity rises within 6 to 48 hours of onset of acute pancreatitis in about 80% of patients but not proportionally to the severity of the disease. Values of over 600 Somogyi units/dL, or over four times the upper limit of normal, are highly suggestive of the diagnosis. Activity usually returns to normal in three to five days in patients with the milder edematous forms of the disease. Elevated values persisting longer than this suggest continuing necrosis or possible pseudocyst formation. The levels of serum amylase elevation are not necessarily correlated with the severity of acute pancreatitis (Ventrucci, 1989). The urine amylase activity rises promptly, often within several hours of the rise in serum activity, and may remain elevated after the serum activity has returned to the normal range. Values of over 1000 Somogyi units/h are seen almost exclusively in patients with acute pancreatitis. False-negative results are often seen when the urine specimen is taken too soon or too late or in patients with fulminating necrosis in which the production of amylase is decreased or has ceased. In a majority of patients with acute pancreatitis, serum amylase activity is elevated and there is a concomitant increase in urine amylase activity. There may be instances, however, in which the elevated urine amylase is not accompanied by a concomitant increase in serum amylase.

As may be surmised, increased renal clearance of amylase accounts for the greater diagnostic value of the urine amylase determination in the diagnosis of acute and relapsing pancreatitis, and the ratio of amylase clearance to creatinine clearance expressed as a percentage has been used diagnostically. This ratio (Cam/Ccr) can be calculated by the following formula:

$$\text{Clearance ratio (percent)} = \frac{\text{urine amylase activity}}{\text{serum amylase activity}} \times \frac{\text{serum creatinine concentration}}{\text{urine creatinine concentration}} \times 100$$

The normal ratio averages 1% to 4%, whereas that for patients with pancreatitis usually exceeds 4% and is often in the range of 7% to 15%. Unfortunately, about one third of patients with pancreatitis have normal ratios, and elevated ratios may be found in patients with burns, ketoacidosis, renal insufficiency, heart disease, and duodenal perforation, as well as following thoracic surgery. Thus, the ratio adds little to the diagnostic armamentarium.

Approximately 20% of patients with pancreatitis have normal or near-normal amylase activity. In hyperlipemic patients with pancreatitis, normal serum and urine amylase levels are frequently encountered. The spuriously normal levels are believed to be the result of suppression of amylase activity by triglyceride or by a circulating inhibitor in serum (Warshaw, 1975).

Lower than normal serum amylase activity may be found in patients with chronic pancreatitis and has also been reported in such diverse and unexpected conditions as congestive heart failure, pregnancy (during the second and third trimesters), gastrointestinal cancer, bone fractures, and pleurisy.

Serum amylase may be elevated in patients with pancreatic carcinoma but too late to be diagnostically useful. It is also elevated frequently (in over 60% of cases) in patients with diabetic ketoacidosis. Polyacrylamide gel electrophoresis has demonstrated that in this condition it is usually salivary rather than pancreatic amylase that is elevated. Serum amylase activity may also be elevated in patients with cholecystitis or peptic ulcer, or following gastric resection, renal transplant, viral hepatitis, or ruptured ectopic pregnancy; very high activity has been reported in patients with carcinoma of the lung. Fewer hyperamylasemic patients may be found to have intestinal obstruction, mesenteric thrombosis, and peritonitis. In some of these patients, pancreatic secretions find their way into the peritoneal cavity and are absorbed into the bloodstream; in others, there may be inflammation involving the pancreas.

Increased ascites fluid amylase levels have been seen in patients with pancreatitis, a leaking pancreatic pseudocyst, pancreatic duct rupture, pancreatic cancer, abdominal tumors that secrete amylase, and perforation of a hollow viscus (Wendt, 1984).

ISOAMYLASE. Whether or not the isoenzyme determination of amylase is of diagnostic value is controversial. It certainly adds little additional information to the differential diagnosis of pancreatitis and parotitis because the clinical symptoms are quite different and easily differentiated. However, in clinically unexplained hyperamylasemia, information obtained from isoamylase determination may be of value in distinguishing acute pancreatitis from other intra-abdominal catastrophes associated with elevated amylase activities.

A great number of reports have supported the finding that in acute pancreatitis P-type amylase is invariably elevated in both serum and urine (Otsuki, 1976; Bossuyt, 1981; Huang, 1982). The S-type isoenzyme, however, is decreased to zero to 15% of the total activity of serum hyperamylasemia in patients with acute pancreatitis, to 12% to 25% in those with chronic relapsing pancreatitis, and to zero in those with carcinoma of the head of the pancreas. The P-type isoenzyme is also elevated in chronic relapsing pancreatitis, hypoparathyroidism, and glomerulonephritis. S-type amylase has been found to be increased in the serum of patients with chronic pancreatitis, mumps, pancreatic insufficiency, Sjögren's syndrome, cholelithiasis, common duct narrowing, alcohol ingestion, acute gastroenteritis, acute respiratory insufficiency, chronic renal failure, and lung cancer and with other cancer-associated hyperamylasemias. Isoenzyme studies on serum, urine, and duodenal fluid from patients with cystic fibrosis revealed that two thirds of the patients had no or little pancreatic amylase (Taussig, 1974).

The relative activity of P-type isoamylase may be highly useful as a diagnostic index of pancreatic pseudocyst (Warshaw, 1980). The P_1 isoamylase (the slowest migrating or least anodic) normally accounts for 80% to 90% of total amylase activity; P_2 and P_3 account for 0% to 4% in both serum and pancreatic juice. The mean ratios of P_2/P_1 and P_3/P_1 in fresh pancreatic juice, normal serum, acute pancreatitis serum, chronic pancreatitis serum, and pancreatic cancer serum were always less than 0.25 and less than 0.04, respectively. The ratio was elevated after incubation of the specimens at 37°C in about 90% of sera from patients with proven pseudocysts but not from others. In several cases, this isoamylase analysis ruled out a pseudocyst correctly, whereas ultrasound or computed tomography (CT) scan erroneously indicated the presence of a pseudocyst.

The clinical usefulness of isoamylase determination may still be somewhat limited, especially in patients with pancreatic disorders with concomitant renal insufficiency, which alone may increase the P-type isoenzyme to as much as three times the upper limit of normal (Berk, 1979). However, with the availability of a simpler and more reliable isoamylase method, a better defined normal isoamylase pattern, and more clinical information on isoamylase changes in relation to different disease states, the analysis of isoenzymes can provide a new dimension in the differential diagnosis of pancreatic diseases (Huang, 1982; Tietz, 1984; Massey, 1985). Serum pancreatic isoamylase determinations provide a much higher diagnostic sensitivity and specificity than the total serum amylase for the diagnosis of acute pancreatitis (Massey, 1985; Ventrucci, 1989).

MACROAMYLASE. More than 200 cases of macroamylasemia have been reported, with a frequency of 1.05% in randomly selected patients, 2.56% among persons with hyperamylasemia, and 0.98% in persons with normal serum amylase (Klonoff, 1980). Macroamylasemia per se is not a disease entity because no clinical symptoms consistently accompany it. It is an acquired and benign condition that may occur in apparently healthy individuals and is found more frequently in males than in females. The age at the time of discovery in most patients is in the fifth through seventh decades. The occurrence of macroamylasemia may be an early sign of disease, either as a marker or as a nonspecific disease-induced dysproteinemia with amylase-binding capability, and it may be regarded as one of the immunoglobulin-complexed enzyme disorders.

Clinically, it is important to differentiate macroamylasemia from other conditions associated with hyperamylasemia. Any patient with hyperamylasemia, a very low (less than 1%) amylase/creatinine clearance ratio, and normal renal function should be considered for the possibility of having macroamylasemia. Definitive identification of macroamylasemia, however, requires direct demonstration of the existence of macroamylase molecules by ulracentrifugation, chromatography, or other physical techniques. A detection method using chromatography has been in use for many years (Fridhandler, 1971). A rapid and simple assay based on selective precipitation of macroamylase in a polyethylene glycol solution has also been reported (Levitt, 1982).

Lipase (Triacylglycerol Acylhydrolase, E.C. 3.1.1.3)

Biochemistry and Physiology

The pancreas is the major and primary source of serum lipase. Human pancreatic lipase is a glycoprotein with a molecular weight of 45,000 daltons. In contrast to amylase, which is present in both the pancreas and the salivary glands, lipase is not present in the salivary glands. Lipases are defined as enzymes that hydrolyze preferentially glycerol esters of long chain fatty acids at the carbon 1 and 3 ester bonds, producing two moles of fatty acid and one mole of β-monoglyceride per mole of triglyceride. After isomerization, the third fatty acid can be split off at a slower rate. Lipolysis increases in proportion to the surface area of the lipid droplets, and the absence of bile salts in duodenal fluid with a resultant lack of emulsification renders lipase ineffective.

The presence of colipase and bile salt is required for full catalytic activity and the greatest specificity of the pancreatic lipase. Serum lipase is inhibited by proteins, bile acids, and phospholipids; colipase acts to reverse this inhibition. Both lipase and colipase are secreted by the pancreas and are, therefore, present in the serum. Colipase is present in the blood of patients with pancreatitis but in variable concentrations and usually below normal and below the amount needed to activate pancreatic lipase fully. To determine accurately and fully the pancreatic lipase activity in patients with pancreatitis it is essential to add colipase to the reagent pack (Lott, 1986).

Pancreatic lipase must be differentiated from lipoprotein lipase, aliesterase, and arylester hydrolase, which are related but different enzymes. These enzymes' activities may be included in the measurement of lipase activity unless the suitable assay conditions for "pancreatic" lipase are adapted. Lipase is also present in liver, stomach, intestine, white blood cells, fat cells, and milk.

Calcium is necessary for maximal lipase activity, but at a concentration higher than 5×10^{-3} M, it has an inhibitory effect. It is speculated that the inhibitory effect is due to its interference with the action of bile salts at the water-substrate interface. Like serum albumin, bile salts prevent the denaturation of lipase at the interface. Heavy metals and quinine inhibit lipase activity.

Lipase is filtered by the glomeruli owing to its low molecular weight; it is normally completely reabsorbed by the proximal tubules and is absent from normal urine. In patients with failure of renal tubular reabsorption caused by renal disorders, lipase is found in the urine. Urine lipase activity is inversely related to the creatinine clearance (Lott, 1986).

Analytical Methods

Serum lipase is stable up to one week at room temperature and may be kept stable longer if it is refrigerated or frozen. The optimal reaction temperature is about 40°C. The optimal pH is 8.8, but other values ranging from 7.0 to 9.0 have been reported. This difference probably is due to the effect of the difference in types of substrate, buffer, incubation temperature, and concentrations of reagents used. Serum is the specimen of choice for blood lipase assays. Icterus, lipemia, and hemolysis do not interfere with turbidimetric lipase assays.

The classic method is that of Cherry (1932), in which olive oil is used as a substrate, avoiding inclusion of nonspecific esterase activity in the assay result. Oleic acid released after a 16- to 18-hour incubation period at 37°C is titrated with standard alkali, and the results are expressed as milliliters 0.05 N NaOH (corrected for blank). This procedure is too slow to be useful. Therefore, modifications have been developed, largely aimed at speeding up the test and improving substrate sensitivity and reproducibility. One of the more successful of these is the Tietz-Fiereck (1972) modification. The newer titrimetric methods are still labor intensive, making them unsuitable for routine use, although they can be completed in the same day.

Three serum lipase assays that can be performed in a few minutes are commercially available. A modification of the Shihabi and Bishop turbidimetric method is available on the Automated Chemistry Analyzer (ACA) (DuPont Clinical Systems, Wilmington, DE), and a similar method, requiring only spectrophotometry and amenable to automation, is available from Boehringer-Mannheim Diagnostics (BMD), Indianapolis, IN. An automated thin-film procedure has been developed for the Ektachem (EK) Analyzers (Eastman Kodak, Rochester, NY).

Evaluations of these three new lipase assays in comparison with the titrimetric lipase revealed that the DuPont ACA lipase reagents do not contain colipase and both the BMD lipase and the EK lipase methods do have colipase. The BMD and EK lipase methods had better agreement with the titrimetric method and had greater analytical sensitivity than did the DuPont ACA procedure, probably owing to the presence of colipase in the BMD and EK reagents. All three lipase methods are simple and rapid and have acceptable analytical precision. The precision of the ACA, BMD, and titrimetric lipase methods was similar, whereas the EK procedure showed significantly better precision at all concentrations of lipase activity. The upper reference limit (URL) ranges of serum lipase concentrations for adults by the ACA, BMD, and EK lipase procedures are 140, 140, and 200 U/L, respectively (Lott, 1986).

Interpretation

In acute pancreatitis serum lipase activity tends to become elevated at about the same time as, if not earlier than, the elevation of serum amylase, and it remains elevated for a much longer period of time, about 7 to 10 days. Increased lipase activity rarely lasts longer than 14 days, and prolonged increases suggest a poor prognosis or the presence of a cyst (Tietz, 1993).

Serum lipase is much more sensitive and specific than serum amylase in diagnosing acute pancreatitis when the serum lipase reagent is added with colipase (Lott, 1986; Ventrucci, 1989; Tietz, 1993). Lott (1986) reported a diagnostic sensitivity of 100% and a specificity of 56% by the EK lipase method; a sensitivity of 86% and specificity of 61% by the BMD lipase method; a sensitivity of 82% and specificity of 62% by the DuPont ACA lipase procedure; and a sensitivity of 94% and specificity of 50% by the titrimetric lipase method. In comparison, he found a diagnostic sensitivity of 75% and specificity of 33% by the EK amylase assay and a sensitivity of 96% and specificity of 34% by the DuPont ACA amylase assay for acute pancreatitis. However, serum lipase measured by the EK method is often elevated in patients with nonpancreatic abdominal diseases, particularly the gastrointestinal and hepatobiliary disorders, because the substrate in this technique is more likely to be hydrolyzed by intestinal lipase than by pancreatic lipase. Therefore, patients with an acute condition of the abdomen who have an increased serum EK lipase and a normal or low serum amylase are more likely to have gastrointestinal or hepatobiliary disorders. The combined use of serum lipase and serum amylase is effective in ruling out acute pancreatitis. Although determination of serum lipase has diagnostic advantages over serum amylase for acute pancreatitis, it is not specific for acute pancreatitis. Serum lipase may also be elevated in patients with chronic pancreatitis, obstruction of the pancreatic duct, and nonpancreatic conditions including renal diseases, various abdominal diseases such as acute cholecystitis, intestinal obstruction or infarction, duodenal ulcer, and liver disease, as well as alcoholism, and diabetic ketoacidosis, and in patients who have undergone endoscopic retrograde cholangiopancreatography (Lott, 1986; Tietz, 1993). Patients with trauma to the abdomen uniformly have increases in both serum amylase and lipase, whereas those with primarily head injury or manipulation of the parotid gland during surgery have a significant increase in serum amylase only (Lott, 1986). Elevation of serum lipase activity in patients with mumps strongly suggests significant pancreatic as well as salivary gland involvement by the disease.

In view of the improved performance of currently available lipase assays and their amenability to automation, serum lipase and amylase tests have been and continue to be widely used in the diagnosis of acute pancreatitis. Both serum amylase and serum lipase are elevated in many patients who have inflammatory or other disorders of organs in the abdominal cavity but no evidence of pancreatitis. It is concluded that the pancreas is exquisitely sensitive to inflammatory or metabolic disturbances in the peritoneum and nearby organs (Lott, 1986; Tietz, 1991).

Serum Elastase-1

Elastase (E.C. 3.4.21.36) is produced in the acinar portion of the pancreas and appears in the exocrine pancreatic secretion as a zymogen precursor, proelastase, which is activated by trypsin. Elastase is present in pancreatic juice and to a small extent in the serum. Elastase is a pancreatic proteolytic enzyme that hydrolyzes the yellow scleroprotein that is the basic ingredient of yellow elastic connective tissue. There are two types of elastase: elastase-1, which is anionic and has a molecular weight of 30,000, and elastase-2, which is cationic and has a molecular weight of 25,000. Until recently, attempts to assay elastase activity had not been successful owing to the lack of sufficient sensitivity of the methods used and the presence of inhibitors in blood.

A sensitive and specific radioimmunoassay (RIA) of serum elastase-1 has become available in clinical practice (Satake, 1982). Gullo (1987) evaluated the diagnostic value of serum elastase-1 concentrations by RIA and compared its diagnostic sensitivity and specificity with those of serum total amylase and pancreatic isoamylase in patients with pancreatic diseases. Serum elastase-1 concentrations were markedly elevated in all 29 patients (100%) with acute pancreatitis. Total serum amylase was increased in 26 (89%) patients, and abnormal pancreatic isoamylase levels were seen in 28 (97%). Serial measurements of all three enzymes in acute pancreatitis showed that elastase-1 remained abnormally elevated longer than amylase and pancreatic isoamylase. Of 21 chronic pancreatitis patients with a painful relapse, 16 (76%) patients had an elastase-1 concentration above the upper normal limit; 11 (52%) showed elevated serum amylase, and 13 (62%) had increased serum pancreatic isoamylase. Diagnostic specificities of serum elastase, amylase, and pancreatic isoamylase for acute pancreatitis obtained by studying 46 control patients with nonpancreatic abnormal pain were 95.7%, 84.8%, and 82.6%, respectively.

Serum concentrations of amylase, pancreatic isoamylase, lipase, trypsinogen, and elastase-1 were studied in 145 patients with pancreatic disease and in 66 patients with abdominal pain of nonpancreatic origin for the purpose of evaluating the diagnostic efficiency of these five enzyme assays (Ventrucci, 1989). For the diagnosis of acute pancreatitis, the elastase-1 assay showed the highest sensitivity (100%) and specificity (98.5%) followed in order by lipase, P-isoamylase, amylase, and trypsinogen. In patients with chronic pancreatitis, the studied enzymes demonstrated a significant diagnostic sensitivity only in those who had either a painful relapse of the disease or pancreatic cysts. In both conditions, elastase-1 was the enzyme most frequently elevated, indicating that elastase-1 is the best marker for chronic pancreatitis in relapse or its cystic complication. In the remission of chronic pancreatitis, the behavior of serum pancreatic enzymes was highly variable; consequently, enzyme assays were of little diagnostic value in this period.

Serum pancreatic enzymes have poor diagnostic sensitivity and specificity for pancreatic cancer. It is concluded that serum pancreatic enzyme assays are useful in the diagnosis of acute pancreatitis, acute relapse of chronic pancreatitis, and cystic complications of chronic pancreatitis. For routine initial diagnosis of acute pancreatitis, a serum lipase determination is the recommended test because it is simple, rapid, and readily available in all clinical laboratories. However, it is advisable to measure both amylase and lipase in the diagnosis of acute pancreatitis. Serum elastase-1 assay would be the method of choice in the later stages of acute pancreatitis and in patients with relapse or cystic complications of chronic pancreatitis. Future refinements and simplification of the serum elastase-1 assay, particularly a nonradioisotopic method, will make this test the best laboratory method for the diagnosis of pancreatic disorders.

Other Pancreatic Enzymes

Proteolytic enzymes such as trypsin, chymotrypsin, and carboxypeptidases in pancreatic juices may, in patients with acute pancreatitis, leak into the interstitial fluid and eventually reach the plasma. Attempts to assay trypsin in the blood of patients with acute pancreatitis by means of conventional enzyme methods have not generally been very successful because trypsin activity is inhibited by trypsin inhibitors such as α-antitrypsin, inter-α-antitrypsin, and α_2-macroglobulin in the serum. More recently, however, radioimmunoassay techniques have been developed to measure circulating trypsins in plasma. It has been found that the measurement of immunoreactive trypsin is a specific and reliable diagnostic test of exocrine pancreatic function. The concentration of immunoreactive trypsin is grossly elevated in patients with acute pancreatitis and chronic relapsing pancreatitis without any overlap with normal controls (Masoero, 1980). Serial determinations of immunoreactive trypsin activity showed that the degree and duration of elevation followed the same pattern as that characteristic of serum amylase. However, patients with a two- to fivefold increase in serum amylase without evidence of pancreatic damage have been found to have normal immunoreactive trypsin activity. Therefore, this test can supplement tests used to discriminate between pancreatic and nonpancreatic lesions. Serum immunoreactive trypsin levels were very low in patients with chronic pancreatitis and normal in those with mild or moderate pancreatic insufficiency or mumps (Gullo, 1980). It has been suggested that normal ranges of immunoreactive trypsin levels be established according to age groups (Koehn, 1981).

Trypsin and chymotrypsin are nearly always present in grossly measurable quantities in the stools of normal young children. Frequently much less activity is detectable, however, in the adult stool, except in conditions causing rapid transit through the gastrointestinal tract. The enzymes are apparently partially destroyed by bacteria within the gastrointestinal tract, and activity is seldom detectable at all by the cruder tests in the presence of constipation. The simpler tests are therefore not very useful for adults. On the other hand, many bacteria produce proteolytic enzymes that may give positive results in the absence of pancreatic enzymes. For this reason, results must be interpreted with caution in children also (Ammann, 1968).

A number of methods have been devised for detecting and measuring proteolytic enzyme activity in stools and duodenal fluid. These include tests based on the ability of stool solutions to digest such substrates as serum proteins, hemoglobin, casein, and gelatin. The methods lack specificity and precision; however, one has been widely used as a screening test for cystic fibrosis of the pancreas. It depends on the ability of a stool suspension to digest the gelatin emulsion of x-ray film by the following procedure: Serial dilutions are made of stool with a barbital buffer, pH 8. Strips of x-ray film are partially immersed in them and are incubated for one hour at 37°C. Proteolytic activity is indicated by digestion and removal of the opaque emulsion from the film. Methods for the determination of fecal trypsin may be reviewed in a prior edition (16th) of this text (pp. 753–756).

Secretin Test

The exocrine secretory capacity of the pancreas can be assessed by intubating the duodenum and subjecting the pancreas to stimulation with a test meal, secretin, and pancreozymin. However, such testing is now slipping from favor because intubation is so unpopular with patients; in addition, pancreatic disease is usually advanced before exocrine function is appreciably reduced. Therefore, the test is of little help in distinguishing between chronic pancreatitis and carcinoma. In the secretin test, bicarbonate secretory capacity is best expressed in terms of output (secretory rate). The distribution of bicarbonate output of normal subjects is apparently very skewed, with a sharp cut-off at the lower end of the reference interval. Subjects with normal pancreatic function generally secrete more than 15 mmol HCO_3 in 30 minutes. Wormsley (1970) has shown that diagnostic discrimination between normal and chronic pancreatitis may be improved by considering bicarbonate concentration and volume together or by calculating bicarbonate output. He recommended that bicarbonate concentration always be assessed in conjunction with the secretory rate.

Dreiling (1950) has published the most extensive study of the secretin test. Using his criteria for the lower limit of normal for volume, bicarbonate concentration, and enzyme output, false-positive results were found in 5.1% of 2723 patients without pancreatic disease and false-negative results were detected in 5.2% of 1725 patients with proven pancreatic disease.

Augmented Secretin Test

The standard test is adequate for the diagnosis of well-established pancreatic lesions causing gross destruction of the exocrine pancreas. The augmented test (4.0 to 5.0 secretin U/kg) is particularly valuable if the response to 1.0 U/kg is equivocal because augmented stimulation enhances secretory deficiencies found in patients with inflammation and cancer (Bordalo, 1975). See Table 23–3 for patterns of normal and abnormal findings.

Until recently, attention has been directed largely toward the pattern of secretory deficiency. Discordant secretion is a pattern of increased flow after secretin stimulation, with lesser increases in bicarbonate secretion. This condition is present in some patients with the Zollinger-Ellison syndrome, hemochromatosis, and alcoholic and nonalcoholic cirrhosis. Preliminary findings of the secretory patterns in these patients show that (1) biliary cirrhotics and nonalcoholic cirrhotics had elevated volumes and high normal bicarbonate secretion and (2) patients with the Zollinger-Ellison syndrome, hemochromatosis, and alcoholic cirrhosis had a marked increase in volume and a lesser increase in bicarbonate secretion above the upper limit of normal. Methods for performing and interpreting the secretin test and the augmented secretin test are described in the 16th edition of this text (pp. 753–756).

Miscellaneous Tests

Leukocytosis is usually present in patients with acute pancreatitis, in whom white blood cell counts sometimes reach 30,000/mm^3. There may also be signs of hemoconcentration. A falling serum calcium level points to the more serious form of pancreatitis, as does turbidity of the serum. The falling calcium value presumably results from formation of calcium soaps from fatty acids plus glycerol liberated by the action of

Table 23–3. PATTERNS OF SECRETION OBSERVED FOLLOWING THE AUGMENTED SECRETIN TEST

		HCO_3^-		
	Volume	*Concentration*	*Output*	**Amylase**
Normal	↑↑	↑	↑↑	↑↑
Chronic pancreatitis	↑	= or ↓	↑	↑
Pancreatic cancer	= or ↓	↑	↑	↑

Modified from Bordalo O, Noronha M, Lamy J, Dreiling DA: Standard and augmented secretin testing in chronic pancreatic disease. Am J Gastroenterol 1975; 64:125. © by Williams & Wilkins, 1975.

pancreatic lipase. Hyperbilirubinemia occurs in many patients, not only those with gallstones but also those in whom pancreatitis appears to be related to alcoholism. The reason is not well understood. Results of other liver function tests may also be abnormal. Transient hyperglycemia may also occur.

Malabsorption, discussed later in this chapter, may be caused by an inadequate pancreatic secretion and may result from chronic pancreatitis or pancreatic carcinoma. Various tests for malabsorption, such as the serum carotenoid level, the glucose tolerance test, the ^{14}C-labeled triglyceride breath test, the starch tolerance test, and the three-day fecal fat determination, may be useful diagnostically, as may gross and microscopic examinations of stool. Only about one third of patients with pancreatic carcinoma are reported to have abnormal results in the starch tolerance test. A larger percentage may have a "flat" glucose tolerance curve, but this is very nonspecific diagnostically. The D-xylose test, discussed later in this chapter in the section on malabsorption, is a very useful test for distinguishing malabsorption caused by pancreatic disease from that caused by intestinal disorders. The following tests have been reported to provide a better indicator of pancreatic function than malabsorption tests as well as a diagnosis of pancreatic carcinoma: (1) Lactoferrin, a protein secreted by the pancreas, is higher in the pancreatic juice of patients with chronic pancreatitis than in that of normal controls or patients with pancreatic carcinoma (Fedail, 1979; Multigner, 1981). (2) A tubeless technique employs oral administration of a synthetic peptide, *N*-benzol-L-tyrosyl-*p*-aminobenzoic acid (BT-PABA). This substrate is broken down in the intestine by pancreatic chymotrypsin, and the released PABA is absorbed and excreted in urine. The variation in gastric emptying, absorption, and hepatic metabolism of PABA is then corrected by simultaneous administration of ^{14}C-PABA (Tetlow, 1981). (3) Galactosyltransferase isoenzyme II has been found to be raised in patients with pancreatic carcinoma, so it can be used in an attempt to distinguish between pancreatic carcinoma and chronic pancreatitis. However, this enzyme is not specific; it may be elevated in the presence of other gastrointestinal carcinomas (Podolsky, 1981).

Sweat Test

Principle

Pilocarpine is introduced into the skin by iontophoresis to stimulate locally increased sweat gland secretion (Gibson, 1959). The resulting sweat is absorbed by filter paper or gauze, weighed, diluted with water, and analyzed for sodium and chloride concentrations. The method is painless and reliable if performed properly. Total body sweating in patients with cystic fibrosis is hazardous, and a number of deaths from the procedure have been recorded.

When performed properly in duplicate, the Gibson-Cooke test has a sensitivity of 90% to 99%. However, a study performed at a cystic fibrosis center and studies by others revealed that up to 43% of the tests originally performed on patients referred to the center were incorrect (Rosenstein, 1978; Shwachman, 1979). The unacceptably high rates of incorrect results have been attributed to problems associated with sweat specimen sample collection and test analysis. Methodologic unreliability, technical errors, inadequate and inappropriate collection of sweat, inexperience of laboratory workers, lack of appropriate quality controls, and misinterpretation of test results were found to be sources of errors (LeGrys, 1994). To provide the best possible quality of sweat testing, laboratories are referred to the document Sweat Testing: Sample Collection and Qualitative Analysis: Proposed Guidelines (document C34-P, 1993), developed by the National Committee for Clinical Laboratory Standards (NCCLS) (Villanova, PA) to improve the performance of the sweat test for the diagnosis of cystic fibrosis (LeGrys, 1994). This NCCLS document includes a discussion of sweat stimulation, qualitative measurements of sweat chloride and sodium, and quality control issues. The College of American Pathologists (CAP) and the Cystic Fibrosis Foundation have jointly developed the External Proficiency Testing Survey for Sweat Test Analysis (Set SW) for laboratories to further improve the quality of the sweat test. The Cystic Fibrosis Foundation recommends that laboratories that perform few sweat tests per year should refer patients to a cystic fibrosis center (LeGrys, 1994).

3

Other than iontophoresis, sweat collection may be accomplished without pilocarpine stimulation by placing a weighed gauze pad on the patient's back overnight. The pad is sealed tightly to prevent evaporation and removed in the morning. The pad is then weighed, diluted with water, and analyzed for sodium and chloride. The analytical method for determination of sweat electrolytes is described in Chapter 7.

Interpretation

Cystic fibrosis (mucoviscidosis) of the pancreas is an autosomal recessive disease with an incidence of 1:1600 white births and 1:17,000 black births in the United States. Approximately one in every 20 Caucasians is a carrier. Cystic fibrosis is characterized by abnormal secretion from the various exocrine glands of the body, including the pancreas, salivary glands, peritracheal, peribronchial, and peribronchiolar glands, lacrimal glands, sweat glands, mucosal glands of the small bowel, and even the bile ducts. Involvement of the intestinal glands may result in the presence of meconium ileus at birth. Chronic lung disease and malabsorption resulting from pancreatic involvement are the major clinical problems of those who survive beyond infancy.

Laboratory diagnosis depends largely on the demonstration of increased sodium and chloride in the sweat. Unfortunately, unless the sweat test is correctly performed, it probably is the least reliable test and has a high proportion of false-positive and false-negative results. Several modifications have been made to render the test more reproducible and the results more definitive (Hammond, 1982). In children, chloride concentrations of over 60 mmol/L of sweat on at least two occasions are diagnostic. Levels of between 50 and 60 mmol/L are suggestive in the absence of adrenal insufficiency. Patients in whom cystic fibrosis is suspected on the basis of indeterminate sweat electrolyte results may undergo confirmatory testing by having the sweat electrolytes test repeated following administration of a mineralocorticoid such as fludrocortisone. In these patients, the electrolyte values would remain unchanged, whereas normal controls would show a decrease in sweat electrolytes. Sodium concentrations in sweat tend to be slightly lower than those of chloride in patients with cystic fibrosis, but the reverse is true in normal subjects (Shwachman, 1981). Sweat chloride concentrations of more than 60 mmol/L may be found in some patients with malnutrition, hyperhidrotic ectodermal dysplasia, nephrogenic diabetes insipidus, renal insufficiency, glucose-6-phosphatase deficiency, hypothyroidism, mucopolysaccharidosis, and fucosidosis. These disorders are usually easily differentiated from cystic fibrosis by their clinical symptoms. False-negative sweat test results (nonelevated electrolyte concentrations) have been reported in patients with cystic fibrosis in the presence of hypoproteinemic edema (MacLean, 1973).

Sweat electrolytes in about half of a group of premenopausal adult women were shown to undergo cyclic fluctuation, reaching a peak chloride concentration most commonly 5 to 10 days prior to the onset of menses. Peak values were slightly under 65 mmol/L. Men showed random fluctuations up to and just under 70 mEq/L. For this reason, interpretation of sweat electrolyte values in adults must be approached with caution. In Chapter 59 of Part VII, Molecular Pathology, a genetic diagnostic approach is presented.

Serum Tumor Markers for Pancreatic Cancer

(see also Chaps. 14, 15, and 45)

Despite the continuous and intense research effort by many investigators to find sensitive and specific serum tumor markers for pancreatic cancer that may help in the early diagnosis of this cancer at a stage when it can be resected and cured, none of the currently available tumor markers is sensitive and specific enough to be used routinely in cancer screening or diagnosis. Oncofetal antigens including carcinoembryonic antigen (CEA), α-fetoprotein (AFP), pancreatic oncofetal antigen (POA), basic fetoprotein, and α-CAP 1 have been evaluated. CEA, the most widely used marker, has not been shown to be useful as a diagnostic aid in pancreatic cancer. Although 85% of patients with cancer of the pancreas have elevated CEA, 65% of patients with other cancers and 46% of those with benign diseases also have elevated CEA values. AFP and POA are not clinically useful for pancreatic cancer. Tumor antigens including non–cross-reacting antigen (NCA), α_2-glycoprotein, β_2-microglobulin, CA 19-9, and DU-Pan-2 monoclonal antibodies have been or are being evaluated for the diagnosis and clinical management of pancreatic cancer, but thus far none has proved to be useful (DiMagno, 1988).

Combined uses of five pancreatic enzymes, including serum amylase, P-isoamylase, lipase, trypsinogen, and elastase-1, have been evaluated for the diagnosis of pancreatic cancer. None of the enzymes investigated had enough sensitivity to be clinically useful, nor was a specific pattern of serum pancreatic enzymes for pancreatic cancer determined. Among the five enzymes evaluated, elastase-1 was most frequently seen to be abnormal, showing positive results in 47% of patients with pancreatic cancer who were studied. However, because elastase-1 was also elevated in all patients with acute pancreatitis who were studied and in a significant number of those with chronic pancreatitis with acute relapse and cystic complication, this test has a rather limited role and specificity in the diagnosis of pancreatic cancer (Ventrucci, 1989).

Because pancreatic cancer has a high mortality rate when it is diagnosed and no effective salvage therapy is available, the use of tumor markers to monitor patient response to therapies does not result in extension of patient survival time. Therefore, the effort in developing tumor marker testing for pancreatic cancer should be directed toward the development of marker tests that can be used to diagnose the disease at the earliest stage when the tumor is resectable and curable and can be treated effectively.

Some tumors of the pancreas secrete neuroendocrine products and thus may produce clinical manifestations before they become large enough to cause obstruction or before widespread invasion occurs. Gastrinomas, as previously discussed, occur most often in the pancreas. Other hormone-secreting tumors of the pancreas include those that produce vasoactive intestinal peptide (VIP), pancreatic polypeptide (PP), and other islet cell tumors that produce insulin, glucagon, and somatostatin. VIPomas cause a complex of symptoms, including profuse watery diarrhea, hypotension, cutaneous vasodilation, hypokalemia, and achlorhydria, known as the Verner-Morrison syndrome. PPomas are not known to produce any specific clinical syndrome but do produce excess amounts of peptide hormone that, like VIP, can be quantified by RIA for diagnosis and post-treatment follow-up. RIA may also be used to diagnose pancreatic islet cell tumors that produce excess insulin, glucagon, or somatostatin, all of which may have clinical manifestations related to disturbances in glucose metabolism.

DIARRHEA, MALABSORPTION, AND EXAMINATION OF FECES

Diarrhea

The large intestine receives about 500 to 1500 mL of fluid from the ileum daily, but only about 150 mL is normally lost in the stool each day. The large intestine normally absorbs water, chloride, and sodium but excretes bicarbonate and potassium. Under normal conditions, the large intestine of an adult can absorb about double the amount of fluid coming from the ileum daily. If the amount of fluid entering or secreted into the large intestine exceeds the capacity for absorption, diarrhea results. Table 23–4 outlines the pathophysiologic causes of diarrhea. In general, watery diarrheas can be divided into secretory and osmotic (nonsecretory) types and combinations of both. The differential diagnosis of secretory diarrhea and osmotic diarrhea can be made by determination of fecal osmolality. In general, in secretory diarrhea, fecal osmolality is about twice the sum of the fecal sodium and potassium levels, whereas in osmotic diarrhea, fecal osmolality is greater than twice the sum of fecal sodium and potassium values (Binder, 1984).

When performing a work-up of a patient for the differential diagnosis of diarrhea, the history is most important. Additionally, establishing the presence or absence of fecal polymorphonuclear or mononuclear leukocytes is very useful. Fecal leukocytes are usually present in bacterial infection of the intestines by such organisms as *Salmonella*, *Shigella*, *Yersinia*, and invasive *Escherichia coli* as well as in nonbac-

Table 23–4. CLASSIFICATION OF DIARRHEA*

Inflammatory/Exudative—Immune-mediated injury of GI mucosa

Inflammatory bowel disease
- Crohn's disease, ulcerative colitis

Infectious
- *Salmonella, Shigella, Campylobacter*, enteroinvasive *E. coli, Yersinia enterocolitica*, HIV enteropathy, opportunistic infections, *Entamoeba histolytica*

Other
- Ischemic colitis, protein-losing enteropathy, graft vs. host disease, radiation enteritis, eosinophilic gastroenteritis

Secretory—Increased secretion of water and electrolytes into the GI tract lumen

Enteric infections
- *Salmonella, Shigella*, enterotoxigenic *E. coli, V. cholera*, staphylococci, *Clostridia*, protozoa, rotavirus, Norwalk virus, enteric adenovirus

Hormone-mediated
- Carcinoid syndrome, Zollinger-Ellison syndrome, VIPoma, hyperthyroidism, systemic mastocytosis

Other
- Villous adenoma of rectum or sigmoid colon, bile acid malabsorption

Osmotic—Nonabsorbed substances retain water in the GI tract lumen

Maldigestion—Incomplete breakdown of protein, lipid, and/or carbohydrates

Pancreatic insufficiency
- Chronic pancreatitis, cystic fibrosis, obstruction at ampulla of Vater, pancreatic adenocarcinoma, somatostatinoma

Carbohydrate intolerance
- Lactase deficiency, isomaltase-sucrase deficiency, trehalase deficiency

Other
- Biliary obstruction, resection of ileum, chronic intestinal ischemia

Malabsorption—Incomplete absorption of substances across the GI mucosa

Short bowel syndrome, Whipple's disease, celiac disease, tropical sprue, bacterial overgrowth, abetalipoproteinemia, GI lymphoma, glucose-galactose malabsorption, congenital chloridorrhea, hypogammaglobulinemia, parasitic infections

Osmotically active dietary products
- Psyllium fiber, magnesium citrate, sorbitol

Altered motility—Increased peristalsis reduces transit time down GI tract

Irritable bowel syndrome, hyperthyroidism, fecal impaction, neurologic diseases, diabetes, hypocalcemia, systemic sclerosis, GI bleeding, post-vagotomy

Increased filtration—GI capillary hydrostatic/oncotic pressure imbalance

Portal hypertension, severe hypoalbuminemia, partial small bowel obstruction

Iatrogenic—Medical treatment side effect

GI surgery

Abdominal radiation therapy

Medications
- Magnesium citrate, laxatives, antibiotics, cardiac medications, chemotherapeutic drugs, metoclopramide, cisapride, lactulose, theophyllin, others

Factitious—Self-induced

Surreptitious laxative abuse associated with psychiatric disorders

*Pathophysiologic subdivisions are not mutually exclusive.

terial inflammatory processes, such as ulcerative colitis, and occasionally in antibiotic-associated colitis. Fecal leukocytes are usually not present in the stools of patients with diarrhea secondary to viruses, toxigenic bacteria (*Staphylococcus, E. coli, Clostridium perfringens, Vibrio cholerae*), and parasites (*Giardia, Entamoeba*). Laboratory tests used in the differential diagnosis of diarrhea are listed in Table 23–5. The selection of tests should be guided by the clinical history, physical examination findings, and initial screening test results.

Carcinoid Tumors and the Carcinoid Syndrome

Carcinoid tumors are neuroendocrine neoplasms of enterochromaffin cells belonging to the amine precursor uptake and decarboxylation (APUD) system. Many of these enterochromaffin cells are also known as argentaffin cells for their ability to take up silver stain in histologic sections. These cells are widely distributed throughout many organs, transforming into carcinoid tumors most commonly in the appendix, terminal ileum, rectum, and bronchus and less often in the jejunum, duodenum, stomach, liver, pancreas, and gonads. They are often detected as incidental findings at autopsy or appendectomy, reflecting their indolent behavior, for which they are dubbed "carcinoid." They become symptomatic late in the course of the disease. Carcinoid tumors reach a peak incidence in the sixth decade of life, causing mechanical small bowel obstruction or paraneoplastic manifestations of the carcinoid syndrome.

The carcinoid syndrome is caused by endocrine factors released from the tumor resulting in episodic skin flushing, abdominal cramps, nausea, vomiting, diarrhea, hypotension, bronchoconstriction, cyanosis, and cardiac lesions characterized by endocardial and valvular thickening and fibrosis, predominantly involving the right ventricle. These symptoms

Table 23–5. LABORATORY TESTS IN THE DIFFERENTIAL DIAGNOSIS OF DIARRHEA

Test	Method	Use
Initial screening tests		
Fecal leukocytes	Wright's stain or methylene blue	Identify inflammatory diarrhea
Hemoccult test	Peroxidase reaction for hemoglobin	Identify hemorrhagic diarrhea
Fecal osmotic gap	FOG = Fecal osmolality − (2 × [fecal Na+K])	Distinguish secretory vs. osmotic diarrhea
Stool alkalinization	Color change after adding NaOH to stool	Phenolphthalein laxative ingestion
24-hour stool volume	Timed collection and volume measurement	Quantify volume of diarrhea
Infectious causes		
Stool bacterial culture	Routine culture and sensitivity	Identify *Shigella, Salmonella, Campylobacter*
Stool special culture	Specialized culture and serotyping	Identify *E. coli* 0157:H7, *Yersinia, Vibrio*
Stool *C. difficile* toxin assay	Tissue culture cytotoxicity	Pseudomembranous colitis
HIV serology	ELISA	HIV enteritis
Stool rotavirus screen	Antigen enzyme immunoassay	Rotavirus enteritis
Stool ova and parasites	Wet mount	Enteric parasitic infection
Stool mycobacteria	Acid-fast stain and culture, PCR	M. tuberculosis, MAI
Stool protozoans	Iodine or modified acid fast stain	*Cryptosporidium, Isospora belli*, etc.
E. histolytica Ab titers	Serology	*Entamoeba histolytica*
Stool *Giardia* antigen	Enzyme immunoassay	*Giardia lamblia*
Endocrine causes		
Urine 5-HIAA	HPLC	Carcinoid syndrome
Blood serotonin	HPLC	Carcinoid syndrome
Serum VIP	RIA	VIPoma
Serum TSH, free T_4	Immunoassay	Hyperthyroidism
Serum gastrin	RIA	Zollinger-Ellison syndrome
Serum calcitonin	RIA	Hypocalcemia-related diarrhea
Serum somatostatin	RIA	Somatostatinoma
Maldigestion		
Lactose tolerance test	See text	Lactase deficiency
Secretin test	See text	Pancreatic insufficiency
Bentiromide test	See text	Pancreatic insufficiency
Sweat chloride	See text	Pancreatic insufficiency (cystic fibrosis)
Stool reducing sugars	Clinitest tablets	Carbohydrate intolerance
Malabsorption		
D-Xylose absorption test	See text	Evaluate surface area of intestinal mucosa
72-hour fecal fat content	Saponification and titration	Lipid malabsorption
Fecal fat stain	Sudan stain	Lipid malabsorption
Serum carotene	Spectrophotometry	Lipid malabsorption
^{14}C-xylose breath test	See text	Lipid malabsorption
Antiendomysial antibody	Serology	Celiac disease
Antigliadin antibody	Serology	Celiac disease
H_2 breath test	Expired H_2 by gas chromatography	Carbohydrate malabsorption
Bacterial colony count	Small bowel aspirate quant. culture	Bacterial overgrowth
Other and miscellaneous		
Serum ionized calcium	Ion-specific electrode	Hypocalcemia-related diarrhea
Serum protein and albumin	Biuret reaction, anionic dyes	IBD, protein-losing enteropathy
Stool α_1-antitrypsin	See text	Protein-losing enteropathy
Quantitative immunoglobulins	Nephelometry	Agammaglobulinemia
Colon biopsy	Endoscopic biopsy	Neoplasia, lymphocytic colitis, collagenous colitis
Intestinal biopsy	Endoscopic or open biopsy	Whipple's disease, MAI, abetalipoproteinemia, lymphoma, amyloidosis, eosinophilic gastroenteritis, agammaglobulinemia, intestinal lymphangiectasia, Crohn's disease, tuberculosis, graft versus host disease, giardia and other parasitic infections

PCR = polymerase chain reaction; HPLC = high-pressure liquid chromatography; RIA = radioimmunoassay; IBD = inflammatory bowel disease; MAI = mycobacterium avium-intracellulare; HIV = human immunodeficiency virus; ELISA = enzyme-linked immunosorbent assay; 5-HIAA = 5-hydroxyindoleacetic acid.

are most often associated with increased release of serotonin from the tumor cells, although other neurotransmitter hormones including kallikrein, bradykinin, histamine, prostaglandins, and tachykinins including neuropeptide K and substance P have also been implicated. In addition, carcinoids may synthesize and release other hormones including gastrin, adrenocorticotropic hormone (ACTH), insulin, glucagon, somatostatin, human chorionic gonadotropin (hCG) subunits, VIP, PP, motilin, and calcitonin. These other hormones are often detectable only by immunohistochemical analysis of the excised carcinoid tumor, although they may occasionally be secreted in sufficient quantity to produce a clinically recognizable syndrome.

Enterochromaffin cells of carcinoid tumors produce serotonin from the amino acid tryptophan by the following pathway:

$$\text{Tryptophan} \xrightarrow{\text{tryptophan hydroxylase}} \text{5-HTP} \xrightarrow{\text{dopa decarboxylase}}$$

$$\text{5-HT} \xrightarrow[\text{aldehyde dehydrogenase}]{\text{monoamine oxidase,}} \text{5-HIAA}$$

where 5-HTP = 5-hydroxytryptophan, 5-HT = 5-hydroxytryptamine (serotonin), and 5-HIAA = 5-hydroxyindoleacetic acid.

The most common laboratory method used for the diagnosis of carcinoid syndrome is measurement of the metabolite 5-HIAA from urine collected over a 24-hour period. The urine should be acidified to a pH of 2 to 3 with approximately 10 ml of 6 N HCl to prevent oxidation. Many methods of assaying 5-HIAA have been developed including colorimetry, fluorometry, gas chromatography, radioimmunoassay, and fluorescence polarization immunoassay. However high-pressure liquid chromatography (HPLC) is now the preferred assay method because of its technical convenience and high sensitivity and specificity. The range of normal values for urinary 5-HIAA is between 2 and 8 mg/24 h, which may vary slightly among reference laboratories. False-positive increases in urinary 5-HIAA may occur in patients consuming foods rich in serotonin such as bananas, plantains, tomatoes, eggplant, pineapple, kiwi fruit, walnuts, hickory nuts, pecans, and avocados. Drugs including acetaminophen and guaifenesin may also produce false-positive results. False-negative results may occur in patients taking reserpine, salicylates, monoamine oxidase (MAO) inhibitors, phenothiazines, and L-dopa.

For patients with indeterminate urinary 5-HIAA levels, serotonin (5-HT) in blood can also be assayed. Blood for serotonin levels should be collected in an ethylenediamine tetraacetic acid (EDTA) tube containing ascorbic acid as a preservative. Most of the serotonin in blood is taken up and stored in platelets. Thus, either whole blood or platelet-rich plasma may be used to assay serotonin levels, with HPLC again being the preferred technique. The reference interval for whole blood serotonin is 50 to 200 ng/ml, or 125 to 500 ng/10^9 platelets when platelet-rich plasma is used. One recent study of patients with carcinoid tumors reported that platelet serotonin was a more sensitive test than urinary 5-HIAA and also more specific in that diets containing serotonin-rich foods did not cause false-positive results (DeVries, 1993). Finally, atypical carcinoid tumor variants deficient in dopa decarboxylase have been described that may secrete large quantities of 5-HTP, with blood serotonin and urinary 5-HIAA in the normal ranges.

Malabsorption Syndromes

Classification

The malabsorption syndromes result from impaired digestion or assimilation of foodstuffs by the small bowel. Maldigestion usually results from pancreatic disease such as chronic pancreatitis, carcinoma of the pancreas, or cystic fibrosis of the pancreas. Generally, there is associated creatorrhea, evidenced by the presence of undigested meat fibers in the feces, and steatorrhea due to an increase in fat, largely triglycerides.

Hepatic maldigestion results from interference with bile flow. Loss of bile salts interferes with fat emulsification, diminishing the surface area available for lipolytic action. In addition, bile salt activation of lipase activity is lost. Patients are usually jaundiced, pass dark urine, and have other signs of liver disease. Hepatic steatorrhea may coexist with pancreatic steatorrhea, as in patients with a neoplasm obstructing the ampulla of Vater.

Enteric malabsorption comprises a variety of conditions that have in common normal digestion but inadequate net assimilation of foodstuffs. This may result from competition by bacteria or altered bacterial flora, as in the blind loop syndrome or diverticulosis of the small bowel; from obstruction to the flow of lymph, as in Whipple's disease and lymphoma; from diseases affecting the small bowel mucosa, as in amyloidosis, inflammation following irradiation, and other types of small bowel inflammation; from a diminished mucosal surface area, as in gastroileostomy or small bowel resection; or from alterations in small bowel mucosal function, as in atrophy secondary to wheat protein sensitivity, gluten or gliadin sensitivity in celiac disease, or relative vitamin B_6 or B_{12} deficiency. Malassimilation also occurs in patients with vasculitis, diabetes mellitus, carcinoid syndrome, and hypogammaglobulinemia. In some of these situations, malabsorption may result from rapid transit of small bowel contents, because diarrheal syndromes may be associated with malabsorption.

These conditions all cause general malabsorption, of which steatorrhea is a major sign. Steatorrhea may be defined as the presence of more than 5 g of lipid (measured as fatty acids) in feces per 24 hours. Normal individuals with a normal fat intake excrete up to 5 g of lipid daily. Although the source of fecal lipid is largely dietary, gastrointestinal excretions, cellular desquamation, and bacterial metabolism also contribute. Lipids are normally present as soaps and triglycerides. In addition, lipoids are present, including higher alcohols, paraffins, and vegetable carotenoids. Although diet has some effect on it, the pattern of lipids excreted may be very different from the lipids ingested in the diet, and the quantity of fat ingested by a normal individual has a relatively small effect on the total output of fat. According to one study, fecal lipid is equal to a constant (2.93 g) plus 2.1% of the dietary fat intake. On a fat-free diet, the output of fat normally varies from 1 to 4 g/day. In severe cases of steatorrhea, stools are generally fluid, semi-fluid, or soft and pasty, bulky, pale, and foul-smelling. They may be foamy and may tend to float on water. Floating stools contain gas, which may also appear in stools from healthy people, so the sign is not specific.

Patients with malabsorption are liable to develop deficiencies of fat-soluble vitamins (A, D, E, and K). Primary and secondary alterations of the bowel mucosa may also result in deficiencies of water-soluble vitamins. In addition, these patients are liable to weight loss because of large caloric loss and are likely to have other evidence of nutritional deficiencies, such as hypoprothrombinemia, glossitis, anemia, edema, ascites, and osteomalacia. Malabsorption may involve a single foodstuff or vitamin or only a small group of substances. For example, pernicious anemia results from failure to absorb vitamin B_{12} owing to a deficiency of intrinsic factor. Then, too, different foodstuffs are absorbed primarily in different locations, so that a lesion of regional enteritis localized to the distal ileum may affect only vitamin B_{12} and bile salt absorption. Lactose intolerance caused by lactase deficiency is an example of a specific malabsorption syndrome.

Differentiating Causes

When a diagnosis of malabsorption has been established, the differential diagnosis becomes important for distinguishing pancreatic from enteric malabsorption. In children the definitive test for cystic fibrosis, the main cause of pancreatic malabsorption in children, is the sweat electrolyte determination. This test should be used whenever clinical evidence warrants it, although screening tests based on absent stool trypsin and on semiquantitative demonstrations of increased sweat chloride have been applied. One of the most valuable differential diagnostic tests, especially in adults, is the

D-xylose absorption test (Santiago-Borrero, 1971). In this procedure, a 25-g dose of pentose sugar in water is administered orally, and the amount excreted in the urine over a five-hour period is determined. If the amount excreted in the urine is less than 3 g, the diagnosis is most likely enteric malabsorption because pancreatic enzymes are not required for absorption of D-xylose. Poor kidney function may also result in low excretion; thus the test is difficult to interpret in patients with renal disease. If the test is performed in these circumstances, blood values should also be assayed. High blood values coupled with low urine values are expected in renal disease. Because reference values in this situation are not available, the test is better avoided in patients with renal disease.

Alternatively, the cellobiose-mannitol sugar permeability test (Strobel, 1983) and lactulose-mannitol test (Juby, 1989) have been shown to be useful in the diagnosis of celiac disease. The principle of the tests is based on the observation that patients with celiac disease underabsorb small molecules, such as mannitol, but paradoxically absorb larger molecules, such as cellobiose and lactulose, to a greater degree than controls. The value of the cellobiose-mannitol test in patients with known abnormal histopathology on jejunal biopsy has been confirmed (Strobel, 1984). However, the test has several drawbacks; it is time-consuming and difficult to perform. The lactulose-mannitol test using an enzymatic determination is simple to perform; thus, it can be used as a screening test (Juby, 1989).

Other tests may be used as alternatives to the D-xylose test, although isotopic techniques and the starch tolerance test have been used by some workers for this purpose (Althausen, 1961). Quantitative specific fecal trypsin and chymotrypsin assays may be helpful, as may the Schilling test for vitamin B_{12} absorption, which tends to be abnormal in patients with enteric steatorrhea and in which the abnormality is not correctable with intrinsic factor. Probably the best alternative laboratory diagnostic aid is duodenal intubation and jejunal biopsy.

Intestinal Disaccharidase Deficiency

Many of the previously listed conditions causing malabsorption may also be associated with intolerance to disaccharides. Disaccharide absorption is diminished either from primary disaccharidase deficiencies such as sucrase-isomaltase deficiency, lactase deficiency, primary alactasia, primary trehalase deficiency, or secondary disaccharidase deficiencies due to celiac disease, tropical sprue, acute viral gastroenteritis, or drugs such as orally administered neomycin, kanamycin, and methotrexate. These secondary disaccharidase deficiencies are usually transient and involve more than one enzyme. Although the incidence of lactose intolerance due to congenital lactase deficiency is low, the prevalence of lactose intolerance in adults is quite high; about 10% of whites and 70% to 80% of American blacks and an even greater percentage of Asians manifest some degree of lactose intolerance even though they were able to digest lactose well as infants. In these disorders, unhydrolyzed and unabsorbed carbohydrates are fermented by intestinal bacteria, producing gas, lactic acid, or other organic acids. Normally, absorption of digested carbohydrates is rapid and fairly complete in the proximal small intestine. Unhydrolyzed disaccharides or unabsorbed monosaccharides due to deficiencies in transport are osmotically active and hence cause secretion of water and electrolytes into the small and large intestines. This often results in protracted diarrhea as well as complaints of bloating and flatulence.

Screening tests for disaccharidase deficiencies include oral challenge of suspected disaccharides to reproduce the abdominal symptomatology followed by stool analysis. The stools are usually watery, acid, explosive, and fermentative. Stool pH of less than 5.5 is suggestive, but the measurement of pH is not valid if the patient is taking oral antibiotics. High pH does not exclude the diagnosis. Abnormally high stool pH is common in normal infants between three and seven days of age. Stools can be analyzed for sugars by chromatography or by one of the semiquantitative nonspecific tests for urinary sugar adapted for stool analysis. The Clinitest tablet (Ames Company, Elkhart, IN) is suitable for this purpose. The presence of 0.5 g/dL or greater of reducing substances is considered abnormal. In patients with intolerance to sugar, the amount of total reducing substances in the stool usually exceeds 250 mg/dL feces. Children in whom intolerance to sugar has been proved can excrete more than 1 g/dL of total reducing substances when fed an offending sugar (Kerry, 1964).

An oral tolerance test using a specific sugar such as lactose or sucrose can be used to establish a specific carbohydrate intolerance. Although the oral tolerance test is fairly specific and sensitive, in some instances, 23% to 30% false-positive results were noted following administration of lactose—i.e., a flat tolerance curve and less than a 20 mg/dL (1.1 mmol/L) increase in blood sugar (Krasilnikoff, 1975). Delayed gastric emptying appears to be the cause of the false-positive result because duodenal instillation of lactose eliminates the flat tolerance curve.

Definitive diagnosis of disaccharidase deficiencies depends on the demonstration of low specific enzyme activity in the mucosae of small intestinal biopsy material. An assay for disaccharidase has been published (Dahlquist, 1968).

Glucose-Galactose Malabsorption

Primary glucose-galactose malabsorption is a rare hereditary disorder of active absorption of glucose and galactose from the small intestine. It is inherited as an autosomal recessive trait. Symptoms and signs are similar to those seen in patients with disaccharide malabsorption, diarrhea being the main problem. Stools are watery and always contain several grams of glucose and galactose per 100 mL.

LABORATORY TESTS. Diagnostic laboratory tests for this disorder include identification of glucose and galactose in the stools using glucose oxidase, galactose oxidase, or chromatography, and oral glucose and oral galactose tolerance tests, in which a flat curve is expected. A flat glucose tolerance curve alone does not, of course, indicate the presence of this disorder. Many variables affect blood glucose levels. Flat glucose tolerance curves are normal in newborn babies. Furthermore, blood glucose levels are affected by oral fructose loading (Meeuwisse, 1970). If oral sugar tolerance tests yield equivocal results, intubation and perfusion of a segment of the small intestine may be indicated to establish the diagnosis.

Protein-Losing Enteropathy

Many gastrointestinal disorders such as Ménétrier's disease, gastric cancer, chronic gastritis, benign or malignant tumors, Crohn's disease, celiac disease, tropical sprue, ulcerative colitis, intestinal lymphatic obstruction (intestinal lymphangiectasia), graft-versus-host disease of the intestine, bacterial overgrowth (Whipple's disease), and infectious enteritis (viral, bacterial, and parasitic) may result in a mild to severe degree of protein malabsorption and excessive transmucosal loss of serum protein. The hypoproteinemia may or may not be associated with edema. The laboratory test commonly employed in the diagnosis of protein-losing enteropathy has been based on the measurement of fecal radioactive chromium after intravenous injection of radioactive chromium–labeled albumin. This technique, however, is cumbersome and has been replaced by determination of fecal α_1-antitrypsin as an endogenous marker of intestinal protein loss. α_1-Antitrypsin is a serum protease inhibitor that is resistant to intestinal proteolysis and is not reabsorbed. Furthermore, the α_1-antitrypsin clearance, calculated by multiplying the number of grams of stool collected in 24 hours by the ratio of fecal to serum α_1-antitrypsin concentrations, has been well correlated with chromium-51–labeled albumin as a measure of mucosal protein exudation. In this method, both fecal and blood α_1-antitrypsin levels are measured by radial immunodiffusion, and the results are expressed either as milligrams per gram of stool or as clearance (Florent, 1981; Weisdorf, 1983). The test is not reliable in patients with α_1-antitrypsin deficiency. Moreover, α_1-antitrypsin is broken down by an acidic environment that may persist in the gastrointestinal tract distal to the stomach, yielding false-negative results. False-positive results may occur in patients with gastrointestinal bleeding.

Collection of Feces

Uninstructed patients sometimes exhibit considerable ingenuity in collecting stool specimens, but a few simple instructions are likely to produce more satisfactory specimens. A scoured, well-rinsed bedpan is a convenient collection container. If the patient does not own one, a carefully cleaned, rinsed, and boiled glass jar of suitable size is a satisfactory alternative. Patients should be warned against passing urine at the same time into the bedpan or container because, among other things, urine has a harmful effect on protozoa. Tongue depressors or pieces of cardboard are reasonably convenient instruments for transferring the stool from bedpan to transport vessel, for which plastic, cardboard, and glass containers are available. We prefer 2-ounce ointment jars with screw caps for small stool samples because they are odor-free, leakproof, and easy to transport. Patients should be instructed not to contaminate the outside of the container and not to overfill the container. Gas, which frequently accumulates, should be released gradually by carefully loosening of the cap. Failure to observe this simple precaution, especially in the case of an overfilled container, can result in an explosive release of contents.

Fecal matter left on the physician's gloved finger at the time of a rectal examination may be transferred to a piece of filter paper for inspection and testing for occult blood. Because of wide variation in bowel habits, intestinal transit time, and bulk of stool, special consideration must be given to methods of timed stool collection. For collection of timed urine specimens, the urinary bladder can be emptied before and at the end of the collection period; the gastrointestinal tract, however, cannot be emptied completely at will. Therefore, the amount of stool collected in a 24-hour period usually correlates very poorly with the amount of food ingested during a similar period of time. For determining the 24-hour fecal excretion of any substance, stool should be collected over a period of at least three days, and calculations should be based on the entire specimen divided by the number of days of collection. The accuracy of this method can be enhanced somewhat by having the patient ingest carmine dye (0.3 g) at the beginning and charcoal (1 g) at the end of a collecting period, collecting the stools from the beginning of the appearance of the dye to the beginning of the appearance of the charcoal. However, *Salmonella cubana* outbreaks in Massachusetts and California were traced to carmine dye. Another method of signaling the collection period involves the use of inert, nonabsorbable stool markers. These are taken in divided uniform doses for several days prior to the beginning of the collection, continuing through the collection period. The concentration of the material found in the stool specimen is then used to determine the quantity of stool containing one day's ingestion of the material as an indication of the 24-hour output. For this purpose, chromium sesquioxide (Cr_2O_3) has been used, and its concentration in the feces is determined chemically. The substitution of radioactive chromium or zirconium isotope has made it possible to determine concentration by measuring the radioactivity of the stool, but these methods, as currently used, are too time-consuming for routine determinations.

Fecal specimen sample collection at home is by no means simple and easy unless the patient has been instructed properly. Hoffman (1973) has described a collection method that has the advantages of ease of transportation and storage, absence of requirements for special equipment, and acceptability to patients and laboratory staff.

A pediatric method described by Jelliffe (1973) includes the use of a thick-walled glass tube, which is lubricated by dipping into water and then inserted into the young child's rectum. In about two thirds of cases, a core of feces can be obtained, which can be poked out with an applicator stick into the container.

Examination of Feces

Macroscopic Examination of Feces

Inspection of the feces is important because it may lead to a diagnosis of parasitic infestation, obstructive jaundice, diarrhea, malabsorption, rectosigmoidal obstruction, dysentery, ulcerative colitis, or gastrointestinal tract bleeding.

The quantity, form, consistency, and color of the stool should be noted. Normally, 100 to 200 g of stool is passed per day. When diarrhea is present the stool is watery. Passage of large amounts of mushy, foul-smelling, gray stool that floats on the water is characteristic of steatorrhea. Constipation may be associated with passage of small, firm, spherical masses of stool (scybala). Constipation most often results from the irritable colon syndrome in patients with anxiety or from overuse of laxatives. In such patients, repeated tests for occult (hidden) blood are called for to detect more serious organic problems such as carcinoma, which may also, of course, afflict those patients.

A narrow, ribbon-like stool suggests the possibility of spastic bowel or rectal narrowing or stricture. Clay color suggests diminution or absence of bile or the presence of barium sulfate. Blood, especially blood originating from the lower gut, may cause the stool to be red; beets in the diet may mimic this. Bleeding from the upper gastrointestinal tract is more likely to cause the stool to be black and have a tarry consistency. Bismuth, iron, and charcoal may also cause a black color. Stool that is allowed to stand in the air for a time may darken on the surface. Green stools may result from ingestion of spinach and other green vegetables or calomel, or it may result from the presence of biliverdin, seen in patients taking antibiotics orally. It is not unusual to see seeds and vegetable skins. Parasites are considered in Chapter 53.

MUCUS. The presence of recognizable mucus in a stool specimen is abnormal and should be reported. Translucent gelatinous mucus clinging to the surface of the formed stool suggests spastic constipation or mucous colitis. It is seen in stools of emotionally disturbed patients and may result from excessive straining. Bloody mucus clinging to the fecal mass suggests neoplasm or inflammatory processes of the rectal canal. Mucus associated with pus and blood is found in stools of patients with ulcerative colitis, bacillary dysentery, ulcerating diverticulitis, and intestinal tuberculosis. Patients with villous adenoma of the colon may pass copious quantities of mucus, amounting to 3 or 4 L in 24 hours. They frequently develop severe dehydration and electrolyte disturbances, especially hypokalemia.

PUS. Patients with chronic ulcerative colitis and chronic bacillary dysentery frequently pass large quantities of pus with the stool, the recognition of which requires microscopic examination. This also occurs in patients with localized abscesses or fistulas communicating with the sigmoid colon, rectum, or anus. Large amounts of pus seldom accompany the stools of patients with amebic colitis; therefore, its presence is evidence against this diagnosis. No inflammatory exudate is seen in the watery stools of patients with viral gastroenteritis.

Microscopic Examination of Feces

FAT (Drummey, 1961). The crudest technique is microscopic examination using Sudan III, Sudan IV, or Oil Red O stain. The procedure has been widely employed for screening because of its simplicity. In our experience, results have correlated well with quantitative measurements when aliquots of the same homogenized stool have been analyzed. For this purpose, a small aliquot of stool suspension is placed on a slide and mixed with two drops of 95% ethanol and then by two drops of saturated ethanolic solution of Sudan III, with further mixing. A coverslip is then applied. Under these conditions fatty acids are present as lightly stained flakes or as needle-like crystals that do not stain and therefore may be missed. Soaps also do not stain but appear as well-defined amorphous flakes or as rounded masses or coarse crystals. Neutral fats, however, appear as large orange or red droplets. When 60 or more stained droplets of neutral fats per high-power field are seen, one may be reasonably certain that the patient has steatorrhea. Caution is advisable in interpretation, however, because mineral oil or castor oil may mimic neutral fat. The procedure is then repeated, adding several drops of 36% (v/v) acetic acid to the stool mixture and warming the slide several times over a flame until slight boiling occurs. This converts neutral fats and soaps to fatty acids and melts the fatty acids, causing them to form droplets that stain strongly with Sudan III. The slide is then examined while warm. After this procedure, the presence of up to 100 stained droplets per high-power field is considered normal. Patients with steatorrhea of pancreatic origin are likely to have greater increases in fatty acids and soaps. Use of Oil Red O has been advocated by some because it permits substitution of isopropanol for ethanol.

MEAT FIBER (Moore, 1971). The technique for sampling is identical to that used for Sudan preparations for detection of fecal fat. The stool is mixed thoroughly on a slide with a 10% alcohol solution of eosin, allowed to stain for three minutes, and then examined for muscle fibers. The entire area under the coverslip is examined, and only rectangular fibers with clearly evident cross-striation are counted. It appears that examination for meat fibers yields results that correlate well with chemical determination of fat excretion.

LEUKOCYTES (Harris, 1972). A small fleck of mucus or a drop of liquid stool is placed on a glass microscopic slide with a wooden applicator stick. Two drops of Löffler methylene blue are added and mixed thoroughly and carefully. A coverslip is placed on the mixture, which is allowed to stand for two to three minutes for good nuclear staining. Using low-power scanning, rough quantitative counts are made by approximating the average number of leukocytes and erythrocytes. All differential counts should be made under high power, counting 200 cells when possible. Only those cells clearly identified as either mononuclear or polymorphonuclear are included in the differential count. Macrophages and epithelial cells that cannot be clearly identified are ignored. The initial cell counts should be performed at the time of presentation of the specimen.

Other Tests

Latex agglutination assays of the stool specimens to detect rotavirus and adenovirus gastroenteritis are now commercially available. The tests for rotavirus have been shown to have high sensitivity, specificity, positive predictive values, and negative predictive values. However, for primary adenovirus screening, a low sensitivity was observed in one product. In general, latex agglutination tests offer a good alternative to electron microscopic examination or culture confirmation for viral gastroenteritis (Thomas, 1994).

Fecal Blood

General Considerations

Bleeding into the gastrointestinal tract of any degree is always alarming and should never be ignored, although often it results from minor pathology, such as hemorrhoids and anal fissures. Bleeding from the jejunum and ileum is very rare.

Drugs, particularly salicylates, steroids, rauwolfia derivatives, phenylbutazone, and indomethacin, have been associated with increased gastrointestinal blood loss in normal subjects and even more pronounced blood loss in patients with gastrointestinal tract pathology. This effect may follow even parenteral administration of the drugs. Apparent fecal peroxidase activity has been shown to increase with the use of carmine as a stool marker and occasionally with massive iron therapy. The latter, however, may result from actual bleeding secondary to gastrointestinal irritation produced by some iron compounds. Loss of more than 50 to 75 mL of blood from the upper gastrointestinal tract generally imparts a dark red to black color and a tarry consistency to the stool ("tarry stool"). Persistence of a tarry appearance for two or three days suggests loss of at least 1000 mL of blood. Following this amount of bleeding, occult blood may persist for 5 to 12 days. Somewhat smaller quantities of blood entering the lower gastrointestinal tract may produce similar-appearing stools or may appear as bright red blood. Such stools should be considered grossly bloody only after the blood has been verified by chemical tests to avoid confusion with coloring from dietary substances or medications. Smaller increases in blood content may not alter the appearance of the stool. Such stools are said to contain "occult blood," detection of which can be most useful in uncovering or localizing disease. This is especially important because early diagnosis and treatment of patients with colonic cancer result in a relatively good prognosis for survival (Greegor, 1971).

The Hemoccult test (SmithKline Diagnostics, San Jose, CA), when used to screen for colorectal cancer, has a low rate of positivity overall (1% to 3.5%) but a high positive predictive value for neoplastic lesions (44% to 50%), most being resectable Dukes Stage A and B carcinomas as well as adenomatous polyps (Winawer, 1980). A study of positive occult blood findings in stools by Couglin (1987) showed that roughly one third are caused by bleeding from the anal canal, one third from some type of colorectal inflammation, and one third from cancer and polyps.

Tests for Fecal Occult Blood

The most commonly employed screening tests for the detection of occult blood depend on determination of the peroxidase and pseudoperoxidase activity of red blood cells including hemoglobin. The indicators used in the test system include guaiac, orthotoluidine, orthodinisidine, and benzidine. In the presence of peroxidase or pseudoperoxidase in the fecal specimen and with the addition of hydrogen peroxide in the test, the indicator is oxidized to a blue quinone compound (in the case of guaiac) or other color compound, depending on the reagent used. The intensity of the color reaction depends on the enzyme activity of hemoglobin or other peroxidase, the presence of other coloring matter, the presence (or absence) of inhibitors, and the sensitivity of the test material. Reagents differ chiefly in sensitivity. Of the reagents used in the test, guaiac is the least sensitive. However, the more sensitive reagents can be adapted to provide a less sensitive test by varying the amount and purity. Because the normal individual loses 2.0 to 2.5 mL of blood into the gastrointestinal tract daily, it is reasonable to use a test that begins to turn positive with a blood loss of more than 5 to 10 mL per day. This corresponds to 5 to 10 mg of hemoglobin/g stool, assuming a blood hemoglobin level of 15 g/dL and an average stool volume of 150 g.

There are at least eight commercially available guaiac-based tests. Hemoccult II (SmithKline Diagnostics, San Jose, CA) is currently the most widely used commercial guaiac test (Knight, 1989). It seems to have the lowest percentage of false-positive results, approximately 1% to 12%. The range of false-positive results reported for other guaiac-based preparations is 6% to 76% (Morris, 1976). Hemoccult detected 37% of stools containing 2.0 to 5.0 mg hemoglobin/g stool, 60% of stools containing 5.0 to 20.0 mg hemoglobin/g stool, and 95% of stools with more than 20.0 mg hemoglobin/g stool, which corresponds to a blood loss of more than 20 mL a day. However, the ratio of volume of blood loss to stool volume as well as the amount of blood loss was an important factor in obtaining a positive result. Two thirds of the stools were positive for occult blood with Hemoccult when the calculated volume of blood loss was 10% of stool volume, and nearly all specimens were positive when the volume of blood loss was 30% of stool volume (Stroehlein, 1976).

The sensitivity of occult blood tests for detecting asymptomatic colorectal carcinomas and adenomas is difficult to estimate. Between 50% and 87% of tests in patients with known colorectal carcinoma have been reported to yield positive results with Hemoccult (Knight, 1989). Because the pseudoperoxidase activity of hemoglobin tends to be altered as it passes through the gastrointestinal tract, bleeding from the upper gastrointestinal tract is less likely to produce a positive result than is lower gastrointestinal tract bleeding. Ebaugh (1958) has shown that there is an 80- to 120-fold decrease in the peroxidase activity of blood passing through the gastrointestinal tract compared to blood added directly to the feces. The specificity of Hemoccult II administered according to American Cancer Society guidelines has been estimated at about 98% (Eddy, 1987). The positive predictive value of the test in two controlled trials was reported to be 10% for carcinoma and 30% for adenomas for the initial screening test (Winawer, 1980; Gilbertson, 1980). However, a study by Alquist and colleagues (1993) showed that in their screening tests, fecal blood tests appear to be a poor marker for colorectal neoplasia.

Certain dietary constituents may cause guaiac-based fecal occult blood tests to be positive in the absence of blood loss. These include myoglobin and hemoglobin of ingested meat and fish, which have peroxidase activity. Aspirin-containing preparations and iron compounds are known to increase gastrointestinal tract bleeding. Bacteria in the intestines as well as digested vegetables and fruits, such as horseradish and turnips, bananas, black grapes, pears, and plums, also contain peroxidase and can falsely elevate fecal peroxidase activity (for a detailed listing of these substances, see Gnauck, 1984). Modification of the tests intended to destroy plant and bacterial peroxidases by heating the fecal suspension may also denature some of the peroxidase activity of hemoglobin and is therefore not recommended. Vitamin C and other antioxidants can suppress peroxidase activity and may give a false-negative result. Thus, appropriate dietary restriction is necessary to minimize false-positive results.

HemoQuant (SmithKline Diagnostics, San Jose, CA) test is based on the conversion of heme to fluorescent porphyrin. The test is not affected by dietary peroxidase, vitamin C, specimen storage, or hydration and offers the advantage of a quantitative estimation of bleeding. Although the test was initially reported to have a high sensitivity for colorectal cancer, later reports indicated that it was not suitable for screening for colorectal neoplasias (St. John, 1993).

Several immunologic tests employing antisera to human hemoglobin to detect fecal occult blood have been described, including radial immunodiffusion, enzyme-linked immunoassay, latex agglutination, and hemagglutination. This type of approach overcomes some of the false-positive and false-negative results of guaiac-impregnated slide tests and offers a great chemical specificity for human blood. However, the test detects a very low concentration of fecal hemoglobin, resulting in too many false-positive results (Armitage, 1985). Recent studies have indicated that an immunologic test (HemeSelect, SmithKline Diagnostics, San Jose, CA) is more sensitive and specific for symptomatic colorectal cancer than are guaiac-based methods and thus appears to be a potential screening test for colorectal neoplasia (St. John, 1993).

Quantitative methods have been developed to study gastrointestinal bleeding using radioactive chromium-51 (Fall, 1971). These methods have greater specificity than peroxidase tests. Furthermore, they can be combined with other techniques to determine the location of bleeding, when present. Because they involve considerable time, effort, and expense, their use should be reserved for patients presenting special diagnostic problems. The procedures are based on the ability of radioactive chromium to bind to red blood cells and on the fact that radioactive chromium is not reabsorbed from the gastrointestinal tract but is excreted in the feces, where it can be measured by γ-ray spectrometry (Markisz, 1982).

Finally, techniques for measuring peroxidase activity are subject to considerable experimental error, particularly when large numbers of stool specimens must be screened by mass production methods. Specimens show marked variability in consistency and in the tendency to disperse in suspensions. This leads to inconsistencies in the amount of aliquot used and in the portion of aliquot actually available to react in suspension. The reproducibility of filter paper techniques is limited by the tendency of liquid stools to be absorbed into the substance of the paper. Further errors result from inaccurate measurement of reagents, inaccurate timing of the reaction, and varying interpretations of the color developed. Inconsistencies may also arise from sampling by patients or incomplete mixing of blood with the stool. Blood arising in the upper gastrointestinal tract is mixed relatively uniformly throughout the specimen, but blood from the lower gastrointestinal tract is likely to be segmental in distribution within the stool, or it may only coat the surface. Anorectal blood frequently produces red streaking of the surface. The presence of such focally distributed blood should be reported after chemical verification. In routine testing for occult blood, an attempt is made to use an aliquot from the center of the formed stool.

In patients with severe gastrointestinal hemorrhage, the diagnostic problems are not such as to necessitate a very sensitive test to detect blood in feces. The real benefit of these tests is as a screening procedure for hemorrhage that may bleed intermittently. To be valid, the test employed must be repeated at least three and preferably six times with the patient on a diet free of exogenous sources of peroxidase activity. In addition, the patient should be requested to include liberal amounts of high-residue foods in the diet such as prunes, bran, raw vegetables, corn, and peanuts. This regimen is usually unacceptable to the patient, so positive results of tests on a normal diet must be repeated following a three- or four-day period of abstinence from meats, fish, and vegetable sources of peroxidase activity. Only after this regimen can a positive series of test results be considered an indication for further evaluation of the patient.

HEMOCCULT II SLIDE TEST FOR OCCULT BLOOD
(SmithKline Diagnostics, San Jose, CA)

PROCEDURE. A very small stool specimen is collected on the tip of a wooden applicator. A thin smear of specimen is applied inside the circle. The cover is closed and the applicator discarded. The specimen is allowed to dry (it is important that the specimen dry completely). Next, the perforated window in the back of the slide is opened, and two or three drops of developing solution are applied to the slide opposite the specimen. The results are read after 30 seconds.

RESULTS

Positive. Reactions that produce a blue color, regardless of whether the reaction is weak or strong, are positive.

Negative. No detectable blue anywhere on the slide indicates a negative result for occult blood. Reactions that do not produce a blue color should be considered not trace but negative.

Note. The sensitivity of slides can be increased by rehydrating them prior to adding developing solution (Castiglione, 1993), but this results in a high false-positive rate. Macrae (1982) suggested that the high false-positive rate resulting from rehydration of slides can be reduced if the patient maintains a low-peroxidase diet. According to Thomas (1992), Hemoccult II was shown to be significantly more sensitive for carcinoma of the sigmoid and descending colon than for rectal or right-sided cancers. HemoccultSENSA (SmithKline Diagnostics, San Jose, CA), employing rehydration, is a more sensitive guaiac test than Hemoccult (sensitivity of 94% and 89%, respectively) (St. John, 1993).

The American Cancer Society has made the following recommendations for using the Hemoccult II test (Gnauck, 1984):

1. Subjects should avoid ingesting red meat and high-peroxidase foods for three days before and during testing.
2. Use of vitamin C, iron tablets, and nonsteroidal anti-inflammatory drugs should be avoided.
3. Two samples of each of three consecutive stools should be tested.
4. The delay between preparation and laboratory testing should not exceed six days.
5. Slides should not be dehydrated.
6. A single positive smear should be considered a positive test result, even in the absence of dietary restriction.

HemeSelect TEST FOR OCCULT BLOOD
(SmithKline Diagnostics, San Jose, CA)

This test is based on the principle of reverse passive hemagglutination. The assay uses formalin-fixed chicken erythrocytes coated with antihuman hemoglobin antibody. The punched-out filter paper of the fecal smears is then used to obtain a diluted fecal solution to which the coated chicken erythrocytes are added. Hemagglutination occurs in the presence of hemoglobin in the fecal solution. Because the test does not cross-react with animal hemoglobins or dietary peroxidases no diet restrictions are required.

Tests for Steatorrhea

Screening Tests

Screening tests for detection of steatorrhea include microscopic examination of feces for fat globules and determination of serum carotenoid. Carotenoids are a group of compounds that are the major precursors of vitamin A in humans. Absorption of carotenoid in the intestines depends on the presence of dietary fat and its normal absorption. Because carotenoids are not stored in the body to any appreciable degree, lack of carotenoids in the diet or disturbances in absorption of lipids from the intestine can result in decreasing levels of serum carotenoid. This is a simple and useful screening test for steatorrhea. In addition to steatorrhea and poor dietary intake, low levels of serum carotenoid may also be caused by liver diseases and high fever. Elevated serum carotenoid levels are seen in patients with hypothyroidism, diabetes, hyperlipidemia, and excessive intake of carotene. The principle of the test is based on the normal transport of carotenoid in serum as a complex with lipoprotein. These carotenoid bonds are broken with ethanol, and the pigments are extracted with petroleum ether. After absorbance is determined, the concentration is calculated by reference to a standard curve (Levinson, 1969).

Definitive Test for Steatorrhea

The definitive test for steatorrhea is the fecal fat determination. The amount of fat in feces may be determined and expressed as a percentage by weight of wet stool, a percentage by weight of dry stool, a percentage of ingested fat retained (absorbed), or a chemically determined amount of fat per 24-hour stool collection. Because of wide variations in water content of stool, wet weight concentration is the least informative. Dry weight concentration is only slightly less variable because of the effect of diet on bulk. Total output of fat per 24 hours, based on chemical analysis of at least a three-day stool collection, is the most reliable measurement. For this purpose, the patient is placed on a standard diet containing 100 g fat/day. In infants and children, for whom the standard 100-g diet cannot be used, "percent coefficient of fat retention" is a more useful expression. This is the difference between fecal fat and ingested fat expressed as a percentage of the ingested fat:

$$\text{Coefficient of fat retention} = \left(\frac{\text{dietary fat} - \text{fecal fat}}{\text{dietary fat}}\right) \times 100$$

The coefficient of fat retention in normal children and adults is 95% or higher, although in premature infants it may be much lower than this. A low value otherwise is indicative of steatorrhea.

Laboratory Tests for Fat Malabsorption

The normal fat content of feces consists primarily of fatty acids, fatty acid salts (soaps), and neutral fats, with higher alcohols, paraffins, sterols, and vegetable carotenoids present in significantly smaller amounts. Fractionation of total lipids into free fatty acids and neutral fats was thought formerly to aid in assessment of the exocrine functions of the pancreas. However, owing to the presence of bacterial lipase and the spontaneous hydrolysis of neutral fats, fractionation of total lipids provides no additional information about the cause of steatorrhea.

Several laboratory procedures are available for the evaluation of fat malabsorption. Titrimetric methods quantitate various chemical forms of fatty acids, whereas gravimetric and microscopic procedures evaluate total fecal fat. The titrimetric method of Van de Kamer has been the most widely used procedure for the quantitation of fecal fats (Van de Kamer, 1949). Breath tests represent a more recent approach to the diagnosis of fat malabsorption. In these tests the specific radioactivity of $^{14}CO_2$ is measured after the ingestion of a test meal containing ^{14}C-labeled triglycerides.

TITRIMETRIC METHOD. The titrimetric method of Van de Kamer (1949) serves as the laboratory procedure for the definitive diagnosis of steatorrhea. In this method fats and fatty acids are converted to soap (saponified) by boiling feces with alcoholic potassium hydroxide, yielding a solution that contains soaps derived from neutral fats and fatty acids and soaps originally present in the stool. After cooling, excess hydrochloric acid is added to convert soaps to fatty acids. These are extracted with petroleum ether. An aliquot is evaporated, taken up in neutral alcohol, and titrated with sodium hydroxide. Fats are calculated as fatty acids.

In some cases of malabsorption, the coefficient of fat retention can be improved by substituting medium-chain fatty acids for long chain fatty acids in the diet. The Van de Kamer method does not quantitatively recover medium-chain fatty acids. Braddock (1968) has improved recovery of medium-chain fatty acids from feces by slightly modifying the Van de Kamer procedure. He reduced the amount of water used during saponification and distilled the excess alcohol prior to extraction, resulting in complete recovery of medium-chain and long-chain fatty acids.

BREATH TEST. The test is based on the measurement of $^{14}CO_2$ in expired air following the ingestion of various ^{14}C-labeled triglycerides (triolein, tripalmitin, and trioctanoin) (Meeker, 1980). Steatorrhea from either pancreatic insufficiency or other causes results in a decreased absorption of triglycerides by the digestive system. This in turn results in a decrease in expired CO_2 derived from metabolism of triglyceride fatty acids.

Procedure. After an overnight fast the patient consumes a ^{14}C-labeled triglyceride. Periodically, breath CO_2 is collected in a trapping solution containing an indicator that changes color when a predetermined amount of CO_2 is in solution. The radioactivity of the $^{14}CO_2$ is then measured in a liquid scintillation counter, and the results are reported as a percentage of the dose of $^{14}CO_2$ excreted per hour.

Comment. To distinguish pancreatic insufficiency from other causes of steatorrhea some investigators have developed a two-stage breath test (Goff, 1982). In the first stage of the test the patient consumes a ^{14}C-labeled triglyceride, and the $^{14}CO_2$ is measured as previously described. The second stage of the test is performed five to seven days later and is the same as the first stage except that the patient is given an oral dose of pancreatic enzymes along with the dose of ^{14}C-labeled triglyceride. In patients with steatorrhea due to pancreatic insufficiency the amount of $^{14}CO_2$ expired should increase relative to the amount of $^{14}CO_2$ expired in the first stage of the test. Patients with steatorrhea from other causes should show no significant change in the amount of $^{14}CO_2$ expired following the oral administration of pancreatic enzymes.

Celiac Disease

Celiac disease is perhaps the most common cause of malabsorption in developed countries. It is characterized by the presence of severe mucosal lesions in the proximal small intestine following exposure to gluten. The noninvasive D-xylose test has been used for the differential diagnosis of this disorder. Other tests used in screening for this disease before invasive biopsy include immunologic tests for antigliadin (AGA) and antiendomysial (EmA) antibodies, and the cellobiose-mannitol permeability test. In one study, the combination of AGA and EmA used to diagnose celiac disease had a sensitivity and specificity of 100% (Carroccio, 1993). Similar diagnostic accuracy was obtained by combining AGA serology with the cellobiose-mannitol permeability test (Troncone, 1992).

D-Xylose Test

The D-xylose absorption test is a valuable test for the differential diagnosis of malabsorption. In this procedure a 25-g dose of pentose sugar in water is administered orally, and the amount excreted over a five-hour period in the urine is determined. If the amount excreted is less than 3 g, the diagnosis is mostly likely enterogenous malabsorption because pancreatic enzymes are not required for absorption of D-xylose. D-Xylose is passively absorbed in the small intestine and is not metabolized by the liver, although a portion of an orally or intravenously administered dose is destroyed. The accuracy of the method depends not only on the rate of absorption of D-xylose but also on the rate of excretion by the kidneys. It is therefore advisable in patients with renal disease to collect a blood sample for xylose quantitation two hours after the administration of xylose.

METHOD (Reiner, 1965)

PRINCIPLE. D-Xylose (25 g) is administered orally. Blood level is determined two hours later; urine excretion over a five-hour postadministration period is also determined. Chemical determination depends on dehydration of pentose to furfural in the presence of acid, followed by condensation of furfural with *p*-bromoaniline to form a colored compound. At 70°C about 9% of the available pentose is converted to furfural, but at this temperature very little furfural is formed from other precursors. *p*-Bromoaniline is used because it does not form any appreciable color with other substances; and thiourea, which is an antioxidant, also helps to prevent the formation of interfering colored compounds.

SAMPLE COLLECTION

1. Allow patient nothing by mouth after midnight on the day of the test.
2. Between 8:00 and 9:00 A.M. patient voids. Discard urine.
3. Immediately after patient voids, give orally 25 g of D-xylose dissolved in 250 mL (8 oz) of tap water, followed immediately by an additional 250 mL of tap water. Note time. In children, administer 0.5 g D-xylose/kg body weight up to 25 g, adjusting the amount of water accordingly.
4. Exactly two hours (one hour for children) after administration of D-xylose, draw 4 mL of venous blood. This should be sent to the laboratory immediately.
5. Allow patient no further fluid or food and keep him or her on bed rest or in a chair until the test is completed. Patient may experience mild diarrhea later in the day from the D-xylose.
6. Save all urine voided during the test. Five hours after the start of the test have the patient void. Add this urine to the rest. Send pooled urine to the laboratory immediately.

REAGENTS

1. Somogyi deproteinizing reagents: (a) zinc sulfate; dissolve 5 g of $ZnSO_4 \cdot 7\ H_2O$ in deionized water and dilute to 100 mL with deionized water; (b) barium hydroxide, 0.3 N; dissolve 25 g of $Ba(OH)_2 \cdot 8\ H_2O$ in deionized water and dilute to 500 mL with deionized water.
2. Saturated thiourea: Add about 4 g of thiourea to 100 mL of glacial acetic acid. Shake and decant the supernatant.
3. D-Xylose color reagent: Make fresh before each use. Add 4 g *p*-bromoaniline to 200 mL of the saturated solution of thiourea in glacial acetic acid.
4. Stock D-xylose standard (2.0 mg/mL). Dissolve 0.20 g D-xylose in 0.3% (w/v) benzoic acid in a 100-mL volumetric flask and dilute to volume with 0.3% benzoic acid.
5. Working D-xylose standard (0.040 mg/mL). Dilute 2.0 mL of the stock D-xylose standard to volume in a 100-mL volumetric flask with 0.3% (w/v) benzoic acid.
6. Working D-xylose standard (0.10 mg/mL). Dilute 5.0 mL of the stock D-xylose standard to volume in a 100-mL volumetric flask with 0.3% (w/v) benzoic acid.
7. Working D-xylose standard (0.20 mg/mL). Dilute 10 mL of the D-xylose stock standard to volume in a 100-mL volumetric flask with 0.3% (w/v) benzoic acid.

PROCEDURE

1. Prepare an appropriate quantity of D-xylose color reagent.
2. Prepare a protein-free supernatant 1:10 solution as follows: Mix one volume of serum, seven volumes of deionized water, one volume of zinc sulfate, and one volume of 0.3 N barium hydroxide. Mix after the addition of each solution. Centrifuge the solution and collect the supernatant for D-xylose determination.
3. Measure the volume of urine and prepare 1:50, 1:100, and 1:250 dilutions with deionized water.
4. Pipette 0.5 mL of water, standards, serum filtrate, and urine dilutions in a series of duplicate tubes.
5. Add 2.5 mL of *p*-bromoaniline reagent to all tubes.

6. Incubate one of the duplicate tubes in a water bath at 70°C ± 2°C for 10 minutes. Cool tubes in running water to room temperature. Use the unheated set of tubes as blanks.
7. Place the heated and unheated tubes in a dark place for 70 minutes.
8. Read each set of tubes in a spectrophotometer at 520 nm. The unheated tube serves as a blank for each corresponding heated tube. Read within 30 minutes.
9. Construct a standard curve by plotting corrected absorbance versus D-xylose concentration in milligrams per milliliter for the three xylose standards. The standard curve should be linear and pass through the origin.

CALCULATIONS

Concentration

$$\text{mg D-xylose/dL} = \text{mg/mL} \times 10 \times 100$$

where mg/mL is obtained from the standard curve using the corrected absorbance, 10 is the correction for the dilution used in preparing the protein-free filtrate, and 100 converts mg/mL to mg/dL.

Urine Concentration

Read the concentration of D-xylose in milligrams per milliliter corresponding to the corrected absorbance for the diluted urine from the standard curve.

For the 1 : 50 dilution:

$$\text{g D-Xylose excreted in 5 h} = (\text{mg/mL D-xylose}) \times (50:1) \times (\text{urine volume in liters})$$

For the 1 : 100 dilution:

$$\text{g D-Xylose excreted in 5 h} = (\text{mg/mL D-xylose}) \times (100:1) \times (\text{urine volume in liters})$$

For the 1 : 250 dilution:

$$\text{g D-Xylose excreted in 5 h} = (\text{mg/mL D-xylose}) \times (250:1) \times (\text{urine volume in liters})$$

NORMAL VALUES. With a 25-g dose of D-xylose, adults should excrete at least 4 g xylose in the five-hour urine specimen. The blood concentration should be 36 ± 16 mg/dL (2.4 ± 1.07 mmol/L). Children should normally excrete 16% to 33% of the dose in the five-hour urine sample, and the blood concentration should be greater than 30 mg/dL (2.01 mmol/L).

Tests for Reducing Substances in Feces

(Kerry, 1964)

PROCEDURE. Add one volume of stool to two volumes of distilled water and mix thoroughly. Transfer 15 drops of this suspension to a clean test tube and add a Clinitest tablet. The reaction and interpretation of results are described in Chapter 18.

INTERPRETATION. The presence of 0.25 g/dL reducing substances or less is considered normal; from 0.25 g/dL to 0.5 g/dL is regarded as suspicious; more than 0.5 g/dL is interpreted as an abnormal amount of sugar. Sucrose, of course, is not a reducing sugar and will not react in this test. However, in patients with sucrose intolerance, little sucrose but large amounts of glucose and fructose are found in the stool, presumably due to hydrolysis of sucrose by intestinal bacteria, so that the test is positive nonetheless.

Oral Lactose Tolerance Test

(Gudmand-Hoyer, 1977)

Following an overnight fast, administer orally 50 g of lactose dissolved in 400 mL of water. Draw fasting blood and blood samples at 30, 60, and 120 minutes after ingestion as for a glucose tolerance test. Also collect a five-hour stool specimen, examining and recording the appearance, consistency, and pH.

Patients with lactase deficiency exhibit a peak rise of less than 20 mg/dL in reducing substances expressed as glucose. In all persons with flat tolerance curves, the test should be repeated within two days and the less abnormal of the two curves used for interpretation. A control test may be performed, using 25 g glucose and 25 g galactose if the lactose test indicates malabsorption. Some investigators use a 100-g dose, which has been reported by some to yield more definitive results. It may cause symptoms in patients with mild lactase deficiency. In children, the dose of lactose or other sugars is 2 g/kg body weight.

3

Alquist DA, McGill DB, Schwartz S, et al: Fecal blood levels in health and disease: A study using HemoQuant. N Engl J Med 1985; 312:1422.

Alquist DA, Wieand HS, Moertel CG, et al: Accuracy of fecal occult blood screening for colorectal neoplasia. A prospective study using Hemoccult and Hemoquant. JAMA 1993; 269:1262.

Althausen TL, Uyeyama K: Further experience with the starch tolerance test for pancreatic insufficiency. Gastroenterology 1961; 40:470.

Ammann RW, Tagwercher E, Kashiwagi H, et al: Diagnostic value of fecal chymotrypsin and trypsin assessment for detection of pancreatic disease. Am J Dig Dis 1968; 13:123.

Anderson MP, Rich DP, Gregory RJ, et al: Generation of cAMP-activated chloride currents by expression of CFTR. Science 1991; 251:679.

Armitage N, Hardcastle JD, Amar SS, et al: A comparison of an immunological fecal occult blood test Fecatwin sensitive/FECA EIA with Hemoccult in population screening for colorectal cancer. Br J Cancer 1985; 51:799.

Athow AC, Lewin MR, Sewerniak AT, et al: Gastric secretory responses to modified sham feeding and insulin after vagotomy. Br J Surg 1986; 73:132.

Aw SE, Hobbs JR: Human isoamylases. Biochem J 1966; 99:16P.

Baron JH: Clinical Tests of Gastric Secretion. History, Methodology, and Interpretation. New York, Oxford University Press, 1979.

Bear CE, Li CH, Kartner N, et al: Purification and functional reconstruction of the cystic fibrosis transmembrane conductance regulator (CFTR). Cell 1992; 68:809.

Bell PRF, Checketts RG, Johnston D, et al: Augmented histamine response after incomplete vagotomy. Lancet 1965; 2:978.

Berk JE, Fridhandler L, Neuw RL: Amylase and isoamylase activities in renal insufficiency. Ann Intern Med 1079; 90:351.

Binder HJ: The pathophysiology of diarrhea. Hosp Prac 1984; 19:107.

Bockus HL, Shay H, Willard JH, et al: Comparison of biliary drainage and cholecystography in gallstone diagnosis with especial reference to bile microscopy. JAMA 1931; 96:311.

Bordalo O, Noronha M, Lamy J, et al: Standard and augmented secretin testing in chronic pancreatic disease. Am J Gastroenterol 1975; 64:125.

Bossuyt PJ, Bogaert RV, Scharpe SL, et al: Relation of age to isoenzyme pattern and total activity of amylase in serum. Clin Chem 1981; 27:451.

Braddock LI, Fleisher DR, Barbero GJ: A physical chemical study of the Van de Kamer method for fecal fat analysis. Gastroenterology 1968; 55:165.

Carroccio A, Iacono G, Montalto G, et al: Immunologic and absorption tests in celiac disease: Can they replace intestinal biopsies? Scand J Gastroenterol 1993; 28:673.

Castiglione G, Biagini M, Barchielli A, et al: The effect of rehydration on guaiac-based faecal occult blood testing in colorectal cancer screening. Br J Cancer 1993; 67:1142.

Cherry IS, Crandall LA Jr: The specificity of pancreatic lipase: Its appearance in the blood after pancreatic injury. Am J Physiol 1932; 100:266.

Colton HR: Screening for cystic fibrosis—public policy and personal choices. N Engl J Med 1990; 322:328.

Corrao G, Corazza GR, Andreani ML: Serological screening of celiac disease: Choosing the optimal procedure according to various prevalence value. Gut 1994; 35:771.

Coughlin RJ, Friend WG: Dietary restriction and fecal occult blood testing. Am Fam Phys 1987; 35:118.

Dahlquist A: Assay of intestinal disaccharidases. Anal Biochem 1968; 22:99.

De la Lande FA, Boettcher B: Electrophoretic examination of human serum amylase isoenzyme. Enzymologia 1969; 37:355.

DeVries EGE, Kema IP, Sloof MJ, et al: Recent developments in diagnosis and treatment of metastatic carcinoid tumors. Scand J Gastroenterol 1993; 28(S200):87.

DiMagno EP: Early diagnosis of chronic pancreatitis and pancreatic cancer. Med Clin North Am 1988; 72(5):797.

Dreiling DA, Hollander F.: Studies in pancreatic function. II. A statistical study of pancreatic secretion following secretin in patients without pancreatic disease. Gastroenterol 1950; 115:620.

Drummey GD, Benson JA, Jones GM: Microscopical examination of the stool for steatorrhea. N Engl J Med 1961; 264:85.

Ebaugh FG Jr, Clements T Jr, Rodan G, et al: Quantitative measurement of gastrointestinal blood loss. Am J Med 1958; 25:169.

Eddy MD, Nugent FW, Eddy JF, et al: Screening for colorectal cancer in a high risk population: Results of a mathematical mode. Gastroenterology 1987; 92:682.

Fall DJ, Kupier DH, Pollard HM: Use of isotopes for various tests for occult blood in feces. Cancer 1971; 28:135.

Fedail S, Harvey R, Salmon P, et al: Trypsin and lactoferrin levels in pure pancreatic juice in patients with pancreatic disease. Gut 1979; 20:983.

Feldman M, Richardson CT, Walsh JH: Sex-related differences in gastric release and parietal cell sensitivity in healthy human beings. J Clin Invest 1983; 71:715.

Florent C, L'Hirondell C, Dasmazures C, et al: Intestinal clearance of alpha-1-antitrypsin: A sensitive method for the detection of protein-losing enteropathy. Gastroenterology 1981; 81:777.

Fridhandler L, Berk JE: Macroamylasemia. Adv Clin Chem 1978; 20:267.

Fridhandler L, Berk, JE: Simplified chromatographic method for isoamylase analysis. Clin Chem Acta 1980; 101:135.

Fridhandler L, Berk JE, Ueda M: Macroamylasemia: Rapid detection method. Clin Chem 1971; 17:423.

Fridhandler L, Berk JE, Ueda M: Isolation and measurement of pancreatic amylase in human serum and urine. Clin Chem 1972; 18:1493.

Gibson LE, Cook RE: A test for concentration of electrolytes in sweat in cystic fibrosis of the pancreas utilizing pilocarpine by iontophoresis. Pediatrics 1959; 23:545.

Gilbertson VA, McHugh RB, Schuman LM, et al: The early detection of colorectal cancers: Preliminary report of results of the occult blood study. Cancer 1980; 45:2899.

Gillard BK: Quantitative gel-electrophoretic determination of serum amylase isoenzyme distributions. Clin Chem 1979; 25:1919.

Gion M, Dittadi R, Munegato G, et al: Tumor marker radioimmunoassay in gastric juice. Methodologic drawbacks due to pH variations. Gastroenterology 1988; 94:1271.

Gnauck R, Macrae FA, Fleisher M: How to perform the fecal occult blood test. CA 1984; 34:134.

Goff JS: Two-stage triolein breath test differentiates pancreatic insufficiency from other causes of malabsorption. Gastroenterology 1982; 83:44.

Greegor DH: Occult blood testing for detection of asymptomatic colon cancer. Cancer 1971; 28:131.

Gudmand-Hoyer E, Simony KO: Individual sensitivity of lactose in lactose malabsorption. Am J Dig Dis 1977; 22:177.

Gullo L, Ventrucci M, Pezzilli R, et al: Diagnostic value of serum elastase I in pancreatic disease. Br J Surg 1987; 74:44.

Hadorn B, Zoppi G, Schmerling DH, et al: Quantitative assessment of exocrine function in infants and children. J Pediatr 1968; 73:39.

Hammond KB, Johnston BJ: Sweat test for cystic fibrosis. *In* Faulkner WR, Meites S (eds): Selected Methods for the Small Clinical Chemistry Laboratory, Vol. 9. Washington, DC, American Association of Clinical Chemistry, 1982.

Harris JC, Dupont HL, Hornick RB: Fecal leukocytes in diarrhea illness. Ann Intern Med 1972; 76:697.

Hazell SL, Borody TL, Gal A, et al: *Campylobacter pylori* gastritis I. Detection of urease as a marker of antral colonization and gastritis. Am J Gastroenterol 1987; 82:292.

Heffernon JJ, Fridhandler L, Berk JE, et al: Assay of amylase and isoamylase activities in serum and urine. Am J Gastroenterol 1977; 67:473

Highsmith WE, Burch LH, Zhou Z, et al: A novel mutation in the cystic fibrosis gene in patients with pulmonary disease but normal sweat chloride concentrations. N Engl J Med 1994; 331:974.

Hoffman NE, LaRusso NF, Hoffman AF: An improved method for fecal collection: The field-kit. Lancet 1973; 1:1422.

Hollander F: Laboratory procedures, in the study of vagotomy (with particular reference to the insulin test). Gastroenterology 1984; 11:419.

Hovsepian MD, Linskey ME, Fedorak R: Failing to detect occult blood. Ann Intern Med 1986; 105:471.

Huang WY, Tietz NW: Determination of amylase isoenzymes in serum by use of a selective inhibitor. Clin Chem 1982; 28:1525.

Jelliffe DB, Jelliffe EFD: Collection of stool sample. Lancet 1973; 2:618.

Johnson CD, Rai AS: Urine acid output as a test of completeness of vagotomy. Br J Surg 1990; 77:417.

Juby LD, Rothwell J, Axon ATR: Lactulose/mannitol test: An ideal screen for celiac disease. Gastroenterology 1989; 96:79.

Kamaryt J, Laxova R: Amylase heterogeneity, some genetic and clinical aspects. Humangenetik 1965; 1:579.

Katelaris PH, Lin SF, Napoli J: Effect of *H. pylori* infection and gastritis with atrophy on serum gastrin and gastric acid secretion. Gut 1993; 34:1032.

Kay AW: Effect of large doses of histamine on gastric secretion of HCl, an augmented histamine test. BMJ 1963; 2:77.

Kerem B, Rommens JM, Buchannan JA, et al: Identification of the cystic fibrosis gene: genetic analysis. Science 1989; 245:1073.

Kerem E, Corey M, Kerem BS, et al: The relation between genotype and phenotype in cystic fibrosis—analysis of the most common mutation (delta F508). N Engl J Med 1990; 323:1517.

Kerry KR, Anderson CM: A ward test for sugar in feces. Lancet 1964; 1:981.

Kiesewetter S, Macek M Jr, Davis C, et al: A mutation in cystic fibrosis transmembrane conductance regulator produces different phenotype depending on chromosomal background. Nat Genet 1993; 5:274.

Klonoff DC: Macroamylasemia and other immunoglobulin-complexes enzyme disorders. West J Med 1980; 133:339.

Knight KK, Fielding JE, Battista RN: Occult blood screening for colorectal cancer. JAMA 1989; 261:587.

Koehn HD, Mostbeck A: Age-dependence of immunoreactive trypsin concentration in serum. Clin Chem 1981; 27:502.

Krasilnikoff PA, Gudmand-Hover E, Moltke HH: Diagnostic value of disaccharide tolerance tests on children. Acta Paediatr Scand 1975; 64:693.

Kristidis P, Bozon D, Corey M, et al: Genetic determination of exocrine pancreatic function in cystic fibrosis. Am J Hum Genet 1992; 50:1178.

Kronborg O, Andersson D: Acid response to sham feeding as a test for completeness of vagotomy. Scand J Gastroenterol 1980; 15:119.

Layne EA, Mellow MH, Lipman TO: Insensitivity of guaiac slide tests for detection of blood in gastric juice. Ann Intern Med 1981; 94:774.

Legaz ME, Kenny MA: Electrophoretic amylase fractionation as an aid in diagnosis of pancreatic disease. Clin Chem 1976; 22:57.

LeGrys VA, Burnett RW: Current status of sweat testing in North America: Results of the College of American Pathologists Needs Assessment Survey. Arch Pathol Lab Med 1994; 118:865.

Lemna WK, Feldman GL, Kerem B, et al: Mutation analysis for heterozygote detection and the prenatal diagnosis of cystic fibrosis. N Engl J Med 1990; 322:291.

Lente FV: Diagnosing acute pancreatitis the enzyme way. Diagnostic Med 1982; 5:50.

Levinson SA, McFate RR: Clinical Laboratory Diagnosis. Philadelphia, Lea and Febiger, 1969, p 402.

Levitt MD, Ellis C: A rapid and simple assay to determine if macroamylase is the cause of hyperamylasemia. Gastroenterology 1982; 83:378.

Linscheer WG, Abele JE: A new directable small bowel biopsy device. Gastroenterology 1976, 71:575.

Lott JA, Mercier JE: A semi-automated method for determining amylase activity in serum and urine. Clin Chem 1970; 16:390.

Lott JA, Patel ST, Sawney AK, et al: Assays of serum lipase: Analytical and clinical considerations. Clin Chem 1986; 37:1290.

MacLean WC Jr, Tripp RW: Cystic fibrosis with edema and falsely negative sweat test. J Pediatr 1973; 83:86.

Macrae F, St. John DJB, Caligiore P, et al: Optimal dietary conditions for Hemoccult testing. Gastroenterology, 1982; 82:899.

Markisz JA, Front D, Royal HD, et al: An evaluation of ^{99m}Tc-labelled red blood cell scintigraphy for the detection of localization of gastrointestinal bleeding site. Gastroenterology 1982; 83:394.

Marks IN, Bank S, Louw JH, et al: The augmented histamine test, an analysis of 672 consecutive tests. S Afr Med J 1962; 36:807.

Marshall JJ: Concerning the measurement of alpha-amylase activity in international units. Clin Biochem 1980; 13:4.

Masoero G, Andriulli A, Recchia S, et al: Trypsin-like immunoreactivity in the diagnosis of acute pancreatitis. Scand J Gastroenterol 1980; 15 (Suppl. 62):21.

Massey TH: Efficiency in the diagnosis of acute pancreatitis increased by improved electrophoresis of amylase isoenzyme P3 on cellulose acetate. Clin Chem 1985; 31:70.

McRury JM, Barry RC: A modified Apt test: A new look at an old test. Pediatr Emerg Care 1994; 10:189.

Meeker HE, Chen IW, Connell AM, et al: Clinical experience in ^{14}C-palmitin breath test for malabsorption. Am J Gastroenterol 1980; 73:277.

Meeuwisse GW, Linquist B: Glucose-galactose malabsorption: Study on the intermediate carbohydrate metabolism. Acta Paediatr Scand 1970; 59:74.

Mifflin TE, Benjamin DC, Bruns DE: Rapid quantitative, specific measurement of pancreatic amylase with use of a monoclonal antibody. Clin Chem 1985; 31:1283.

Moore JG, Engler E Jr, Bigler AH, et al: Simple fecal test of absorption: A prospective study and critique. Am J Dig Dis 1971; 16:97.

Morris DW, Hansell JR, Ostrow JD et al: Reliability of chemical test for fecal occult blood in hospitalized patients. Am J Dig Dis 1976; 21:845.

Multigner L, Figarella C, Sarles H: Diagnosis of chronic pancreatitis by measurement of lactoferrin in duodenal juice. Gut 1981; 22:350.

Newcomer AD, Hofmann AF, DiMagno EP, et al: Tridenin breath test. Gastroenterology 1979; 76:6.

NIH Consensus Development Conference: *Helicobacter pylori* in peptic ulcer disease. JAMA 1994; 272:65.

O'Donnell MD, Miller NJ: Plasma pancreatic and salivary-type amylase and immunoreactive trypsin concentrations: Variations with age and reference ranges for children. Clin Chem Acta 1980; 104:265.

Otsuki M, Saeki S, Yuu H, et al: Electrophoretic pattern of amylase isoenzymes in serum and urine of normal person. Clin Chem 1976; 22:439.

Podolsky D, McPhee M, Alpert E, et al: Galactosyl transferase isoenzyme II in the detection of pancreatic cancer: Comparison with radiologic, endoscopic and serologic tests. N Engl J Med 1981; 304:1313.

Ramond MJ, Dumont M, Belghiti J, et al: Sensitivity and specificity of macroscopic examination of gallbladder bile for gallstone recognition and identification. Gastroenterology 1988; 95:1339.

Raskin HF, Wenger J, Sklar M, et al: The diagnosis of cancer of the pancreas, biliary tract, and duodenum by combined cytologic and secretory methods. Gastroenterology 1958; 34:996.

Read RC, Hall WH: Objective assessment of gastric function after vagotomy. Curr Probl Surg 1994, 1:July.

Reiner M, Cheung HL: Xylose. *In* Meites S (ed): Standard Methods of Clinical Chemistry, Vol. 5. New York, Academic Press, 1965, p 257.

Riordan JR, Rommens JM, Kerem B, et al: Identification of the cystic fibrosis gene: Cloning and characterization of complementary DNA. Science 1989; 245:1066.

Robinson MHE, Marks CG, Farrands PA, et al: Population screening for colorectal cancer: Comparison between guaiac and immunological fecal occult blood tests. Br J Surg 1994; 81:448.

Rommens JM, Iannuzzi MC, Kerem B, et al: Identification of the cystic fibrosis gene: Chromosome walking and jumping. Science 1989; 245:1059.

Rosenstein BJ, Langbaum TS, Gordes E, et al: Cystic fibrosis: Problems encountered with sweat testing. JAMA 1978; 240:1987.

Rosenthal P, Thompson J, Singh M: Detection of occult blood in gastric juice. J Clin Gastroenterol 1984; 6:119.

St. John DJB, Young GP, McHutchinson JG, et al: Comparison of the specificity and sensitivity of Hemoccult and Hemoquant in screening for colorectal neoplasia. Ann Intern Med 1992; 117:376.

St. John DJB, Young GP, Alexeyeff MA, et al: Evaluation of new occult blood tests for detection of colorectal neoplasia. Gastroenterology 1993; 104:1661.

Santiago-Borrero PJ, Santini R, Maldonado N: The xylose excretion test in normal children and in pediatric patients with tropical sprue. Pediatrics 1971; 48:59.

Satake K, Chung YS, Umeyma K: Serum elastase I levels in pancreatic disease. Am J Surg 1982; 144:239.

Sax SM: Interconversion of Enzyme Units. Santa Monica, Clinton Laboratories, 1972.

Scully C, Eckersal PD, Emond RTD, et al: Serum alpha-amylase isoenzymes in mumps: Estimation of salivary and pancreatic isoenzymes by isoelectric focusing. Clin Chim Acta 1981; 113:281.

Shwachman H, Mahmoodian A: Quality of sweat test performance in the diagnosis of cystic fibrosis. Clin Chem 1979; 25:158.

Shwachman H, Mahmoodian A, Neff RK: The sweat test: Sodium and chloride values. J Pediatr 1981; 98:576.

Somogyi M: Modification of two methods for the assay of amylase. Clin Chem 1960; 6:23.

Songster CL, Barrows GH, Jarrett DD: Immunochemical detection of fecal occult blood—the fecal smear punch-disc test: A new non-invasive screening test for colorectal cancer. Cancer 1980; 45:1099.

Spiekerman AM, Perry P, Hightower NC, et al: Chromogenic substrate method for demonstrating multiple forms of alpha-amylase after electrophoresis. Clin Chem 1974; 20:324.

Stein HJ, Feussner H, Kauer W, et al: Alkaline gastroesophageal reflux: Assessment by ambulatory esophageal aspiration and pH monitoring. Am J Surg 1994; 167(1):163.

Stempien SJ: Insulin gastric analysis: Technic and interpretations. Am J Dig Dis 1962; 7:138.

Strobel S, Brydon WG, Ferguson A: Cellobiose/mannitol sugar permeability test complements biopsy histopathology in clinical investigation of the jejunum. Gut 1984; 25:1241.

Stroehlein JR, Farrbanks UF, McGill DB, et al: Hemoccult detection of fecal occult blood quantitated by radioassay. Am J Dig Dis 1976; 21:841.

Sutherland LR, Verhoef M, Wallace JL, et al: A simple, non-invasive marker of gastric damage: Sucrose permeability. Lancet 1994; 343:998.

Taussig LM, Wolf RO, Woods RE et al: Use of serum amylase isoenzyme in evaluation of pancreatic function. Pediatrics 1974; 54:229.

Tetlow VA, Herman H, Kay GH et al: Diagnostic accuracy of the PABA excretion index (using C-PABA). Gut 1981; 22:A4441.

Thomas EE, Roscoe, DL, Book L, et al: The utility of latex agglutination assays in the diagnosis of pediatric viral gastroenteritis. Am J Clin Pathol 1994; 101:742.

Thomas JE, Eastham, EJ, Weaver LT: New non-invasive test of gastric acid secretion for use in children. Gut 1993; 34:738.

Thomas WM, Hardcastle JD, Jackson J, et al: Chemical and immunological testing for fecal occult blood: A comparison of two tests in symptomatic patients. Br J Cancer 1992; 65:618.

Tietz NW, Fiereck EA: Measurement of lipase in serum. *In* Cooper GR (ed): Standard Methods of Clinical Chemistry, Vol. 7. New York, Academic Press, 1972, pp 19–31.

Tietz NW, Shuey DF: A commercially available S-type amylase isoenzyme in serum. Clin Chem 1984; 30:1227.

Tietz NW, Shuey DF: Lipase in serum—The elusive enzyme: An overview. Clin Chem 1993; 39:746.

Troncone R, Starita A, Coletta S, et al: Anti-gliadin antibodies, D-xylose, and cellobinose/mannitol permeability test as indicators of mucosal damage in children with celiac disease. Scand J Gastroenterol 1992; 27:703.

Trudeau WL, McGuigan JE: Relations between serum gastrin levels and rates of gastric hydrochloric acid secretion. N Engl J Med 1971; 284:408.

Tsui LC: The spectrum of cystic fibrosis mutations. Trends Genet 1992; 8:392.

Vacikova A, Blochova RW: Isoamylase in blood donors. Humangenetik 1969; 8:162.

Van de Kamer JH, Ten Bokel Huinink H, Weyers HW: Rapid method for the determination of fat in feces. J Biol Chem 1949; 177:347.

Ventrucci M, Pezzilli R, Gullo L, et al: Role of serum pancreatic enzyme assays in diagnosis of pancreatic diseases. Dig Dis Sci 1989; 27:39.

Warshaw AL, Bellini CA, Lesser PB: Inhibition of serum and urine amylase activity in pancreatitis with hyperlipemia. Ann Surg 1975; 182:72.

Warshaw AL, Lee KH: Aging changes of pancreatic isoamylases and the appearance of "old amylase" in the serum of patients with pancreatic pseudocysts. Gastroenterology 1980; 79:1246.

Weisdorf SA, Salati LM, Judy S, et al: Graft-versus-host disease of the intestine: A protein-losing enteropathy characterized by fecal alpha-1-antitrypsin. Gastroenterology 1983; 85:1076.

Weller D, Thomas D, Hiller J, et al: Screening for colorectal cancer using an immunochemical test for fecal occult blood: Results of the first 2 years of a South Australian programme. Aust NZ J Surg 1994; 64:464.

Wendt P, Fritsch A, Schulz F, et al: Proteinases and inhibitors in plasma and peritoneal exudate in acute pancreatitis. Hepatogastroenterology 1984; 31:277.

Wermus G, Adams T, Menson R: A stoichiometric method for the determination of serum amylase. *In* Lorentz K: Alpha-amylase assay: Current state and future development. J Clin Biochem 1979; 17:499.

Wilding P, Cooke WT, Nicholson GI: Globulin-bound amylase: A cause of persistently elevated levels in serum. Ann Intern Med 1964; 60: 1053.

Winawer SJ: Screening for colorectal cancer: An overview. Cancer 1980; 45:1093.

Wolfe MM, Soll AH: The physiology of gastric acid secretion. N Engl J Med 1988; 319:1707.

Wormsley KG: Test of pancreatic function. Proc R Soc Med 1970; 63:431.

Young DS, Pestaner LC, Gibberman V: The effect of drugs on clinical laboratory tests. Clin Chem 1975; 21:255D.

Zaman Z, Van Orshoven A, Marien G, et al: Simultaneous macroamylasemia and macrolipasemia. Clin Chem 1994; 40:939.

Part 4

HEMATOLOGY, COAGULATION, AND TRANSFUSION MEDICINE

Edited by
Frederick R. Davey, M.D.
John Bernard Henry, M.D.

Chapter 24

Basic Examination of Blood

Michael W. Morris, M.S., DLM(ASCP)SH
Frederick R. Davey, M.D.

Hematology encompasses the study of blood cells and coagulation. It includes analyses of the concentration, structure, and function of cells in blood; their precursors in the bone marrow; chemical constituents of plasma or serum intimately linked with blood cell structure and function; and function of platelets and proteins involved in blood coagulation. Increasingly, molecular biological techniques enable the detection of genetic mutations underlying the altered structure and function of cells and proteins that result in hematologic disease.

HEMOGLOBIN (Hb)

Hemoglobin (Hb), the main component of the red blood cell, is a conjugated protein that serves as the vehicle for the transportation of oxygen and carbon dioxide. When fully saturated, each gram of hemoglobin holds 1.34 mL of oxygen. The red cell mass of the adult contains approximately 600 g of hemoglobin, capable of carrying 800 mL of oxygen. The terminology, symbols, and absorption maxima are given in Table 24–1.

A molecule of hemoglobin consists of two pairs of polypeptide chains ("globin") and four prosthetic heme groups, each containing one atom of ferrous iron. Each heme group is precisely located in a pocket or fold of one of the polypeptide chains. Located near the surface of the molecule, the heme reversibly combines with one molecule of oxygen or carbon dioxide.

The main function of hemoglobin is to transport oxygen from the lungs, where oxygen tension is high, to the tissues, where it is low. At an oxygen tension of 100 mm Hg in the pulmonary capillaries, 95% to 98% of the hemoglobin is combined with oxygen. In the tissues, where the oxygen tension may be as low as 20 mm Hg, the oxygen readily dissociates from hemoglobin; in this instance, less than 30% of the oxygen would remain combined with hemoglobin.

Reduced hemoglobin (Hb) is hemoglobin with iron unassociated with oxygen. When each heme group is associated with one molecule of oxygen, the hemoglobin is called oxyhemoglobin (HbO_2). In both Hb and HbO_2, iron remains in the ferrous state. When iron is oxidized to the ferric state, methemoglobin (hemiglobin; Hi) is formed, and the molecule loses its capacity to carry oxygen or carbon dioxide.

Anemia, a decrease to below normal of the hemoglobin concentration, erythrocyte count, or hematocrit, is a common condition and is frequently a complication of other diseases. Clinical diagnosis of anemia or of high hemoglobin based on estimation of the color of the skin and of visible mucous

Table 24–1. NOMENCLATURE AND ABSORPTION MAXIMA OF HEMOGLOBINS

Term	Symbol	Absorption Peak 1 λ (ε)	Absorption Peak 2 λ (ε)	Absorption Peak 3 λ (ε)
Hemoglobin	Hb	431 (140)	555 (13.04)	
Oxyhemoglobin	HbO_2	415 (131)	542 (14.37)	577 (15.37)
Carboxyhemoglobin	HbCO	420 (192)	539 (14.36)	568.5 (14.31)
Hemiglobin (methemoglobin)	Hi	406 (162)	500 (9.04)	630 (3.70)
Hemiglobincyanide (cyanmet Hb)	HiCN	421 (122.5)	540 (10.99)	

The wavelength (λ) in nanometers for each maximum is followed by the extinction coefficient (ε) placed in parentheses.

Modified from van Assendelft OW: Spectrophotometry of Haemoglobin Derivatives. Assen, The Netherlands, Royal Van Gorcum Ltd., 1970.

membranes is highly unreliable. The correct estimation of hemoglobin is important and is routinely performed on practically every patient.

Determining the Concentration of Hemoglobin

The cyanmethemoglobin (hemiglobincyanide; HiCN) method has the advantage of convenience and a readily available, stable standard solution. The oxyhemoglobin method and chemical method (iron content) are no longer routinely employed in the clinical laboratory (van Assendelft, 1970).

Hemiglobincyanide (HiCN) Method

PRINCIPLE

Blood is diluted in a solution of potassium ferricyanide and potassium cyanide. The potassium ferricyanide oxidizes hemoglobins to hemiglobin (Hi; methemoglobin), and potassium cyanide provides cyanide ions (CN^-) to form hemiglobincyanide (HiCN), which has a broad absorption maximum at a wavelength of 540 nm (Fig. 24–1; see Table 24–1). The absorbance of the solution is measured in a spectrophotometer at 540 nm and compared with that of a standard HiCN solution.

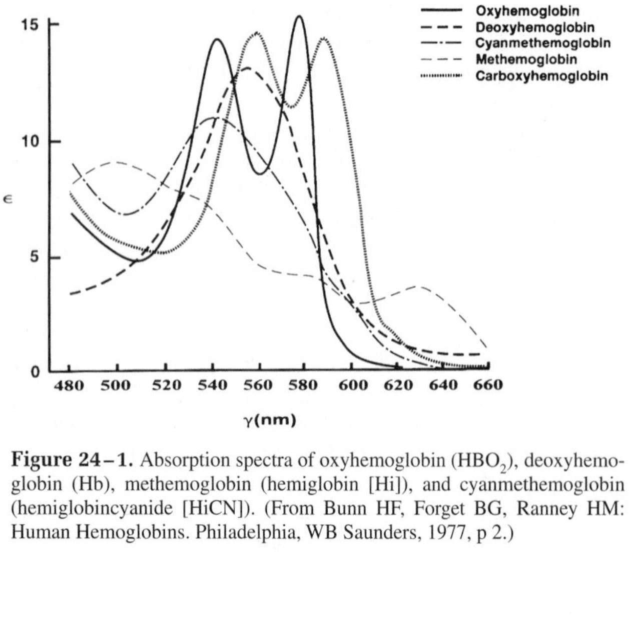

Figure 24–1. Absorption spectra of oxyhemoglobin (HBO_2), deoxyhemoglobin (Hb), methemoglobin (hemiglobin [Hi]), and cyanmethemoglobin (hemiglobincyanide [HiCN]). (From Bunn HF, Forget BG, Ranney HM: Human Hemoglobins. Philadelphia, WB Saunders, 1977, p 2.)

REAGENT

The diluent is detergent-modified Drabkin's reagent:

Potassium ferricyanide, $K_3Fe(CN)_6$	0.20 g
Potassium cyanide, KCN	0.05 g
Dihydrogen potassium phosphate (anhydrous) KH_2PO_4	0.14 g
Nonionic detergent—e.g., Sterox S.E. (Harleco) or Triton X-100 (Rohm and Haas)	0.5 mL 1.0 mL
Distilled water to	1000 mL

The solution should be clear and pale yellow, have a pH of 7.0 to 7.4, and give a reading of zero when measured in the photometer at 540 nm against a water blank.

Substituting dihydrogen potassium phosphate, KH_2PO_4, in this reagent for sodium bicarbonate, $NaHCO_3$, in the original Drabkin reagent shortens the time needed for complete conversion of Hb to HiCN from 10 minutes to 3 minutes. The detergent enhances lysis of erythrocytes and decreases turbidity from protein precipitation.

KCN must be handled carefully in the preparation of the Drabkin solution, because salts or solutions of cyanide are poisonous. The diluent itself contains only 50 mg KCN per liter, less than the lethal dose for a 70-kg person. However, because HCN is released by acidification, exposure of the diluent to acid must be avoided. Reagents and samples should be disposed of in running water in the sink. The diluent keeps well in a dark bottle at room temperature but should be prepared fresh once a month.

METHOD

Twenty microliters of blood is added to 5.0 mL of diluent (1:251), mixed well, and allowed to stand at room temperature for at least three minutes (Dacie, 1991). The absorbance is measured, against the reagent blank, in the photoelectric colorimeter at 540 nm or with an appropriate filter. A vial of HiCN standard is then opened and the absorbance measured, at room temperature, in the same instrument in a similar fashion. The test sample must be analyzed within a few hours of dilution. The standard must be kept in the dark when not in use and discarded at the end of the day.

$$\text{Hb (g/dL)} = \frac{A^{540}\ \text{test sample}}{A^{540}\ \text{standard}} \times \frac{\text{concentration of standard (mg/dL)}}{100\ \text{mg/g}} \times 251 \qquad (24\text{-}1)$$

It is usually convenient to calibrate the photometer to be used for hemoglobinometry by preparing a standard curve or table that will relate absorbance to Hb concentration in g/dL.

The absorbance of fresh HiCN standard is measured against a reagent blank. Absorbance readings are made of fresh HiCN standard and of dilutions of this standard in the reagent (1 in 2, 1 in 3, 1 in 4) against a reagent blank. Hb values (in g/dL) are calculated for each solution as described previously. When the absorbance readings are plotted on a linear graph as the ordinates against Hb concentration as the abscissae, the points should describe a straight line that passes through the origin.

An advantage of the HiCN method is that most forms of hemoglobin (Hb, HbO_2, Hi, and HbCO, but not SHb) are measured. The test sample can be directly compared with the HiCN standard, and the readings can be made at the convenience of the operator because of the stability of the diluted samples.

Increased absorbance not due to hemoglobin may be caused by turbidity due to abnormal plasma proteins, hyperlipemia, large numbers of leukocytes (counts greater than 30×10^9/L), or fatty droplets, any of which may lead to increased light scattering and apparent absorbance.

Errors in Hemoglobinometry

The sources of error may be those of the sample, the method, the equipment, or the operator.

ERRORS INHERENT IN THE SAMPLE

Improper venipuncture technique may introduce hemoconcentration, which will make hemoglobin concentration and cell counts too high. Improper technique in fingerstick or capillary sampling can produce errors in either direction.

ERRORS INHERENT IN THE METHOD

The HiCN method is the method of choice. The use of HiCN standard for calibration of the instrument and for the test itself eliminates a major source of error. The broad absorption band of HiCN in the region of 540 nm makes it convenient to use both in filter-type photometers and in narrow-band spectrophotometers. With the exception of SHb, all varieties of hemoglobin are converted to HiCN.

ERRORS INHERENT IN THE EQUIPMENT

Equipment is not uniformly accurate. A good grade of pipette with a guaranteed accuracy exceeding 99% is desirable. Calibration of pipettes will lessen errors. Unmatched cuvettes can introduce significant error; therefore, flow-through cuvettes are preferred.

The wavelength settings, the filters, and the meter readings require checking. The photometer must be calibrated in the laboratory before its initial use and must be rechecked frequently to reduce the method's error to 2% ($\pm$CV).

OPERATOR'S ERRORS

Human errors can be reduced by good training, understanding the clinical significance of the test and the necessity for a dependable method, adherence to oral and written instructions, and familiarity with the equipment and with the sources of error. Errors increase with fatigue and tend to increase near the end of the day. A technologist who is patient and critical by nature and by training and who is interested in the work is less prone to make errors.

The preceding discussion applies to manual techniques of hemoglobinometry. Automated equipment is widely used and eliminates most errors.

Hemoglobin Derivatives

The two physiologic hemoglobins, oxyhemoglobin and reduced hemoglobin, are readily converted into a series of compounds through the action of acids, alkalies, oxidizing and reducing substances, heat, and other agents.

Hemiglobin (Methemoglobin [Hi])

Hi is a derivative of hemoglobin in which the ferrous iron is *oxidized* to the ferric state, resulting in the inability of Hi to combine reversibly with oxygen. The polypeptide chains are not altered.

Up to 1.5% of the hemoglobin is Hi in the normal person. Increases of Hi will cause cyanosis and functional anemia if high enough and will cause cyanosis at lower concentrations. Cyanosis becomes obvious at a concentration of about 1.5 g Hi/dL—that is, 10% of hemoglobin. Comparable degrees of cyanosis will be caused by 5 g Hb/dL blood, 1.5 g Hi/dL blood, and 0.5 g SHb/dL blood. The degree of cyanosis, however, does not necessarily correlate with the concentration of Hi.

A small amount of Hi is always being formed but is reduced by enzyme systems within the erythrocyte. The most important is the NADH-dependent methemoglobin reductase system (NADH-cytochrome b5 reductase). Others, which may function mainly as reserve systems, are ascorbic acid, reduced glutathione, and NADPH-methemoglobin reductase. The latter requires a natural cofactor or an auto-oxidizable dye such as methylene blue for activity (see Fig. 26–14).

Methemoglobinemia, an increased amount of Hi in the erythrocytes, results from either an increased production of Hi or decreased NADH-cytochrome b5 reductase activity and may be hereditary or acquired (Jaffe, 1989). The hereditary form is divided into two major categories.

In the first, methemoglobinemia is due to a decrease in the capacity of the erythrocyte to reduce the Hi that is constantly being formed back to Hb. This is most often due to *NADH-cytochrome b5 reductase deficiency,* which is inherited as an autosomal recessive characteristic. The homozygote has methemoglobin levels of 10% to 50% and is cyanotic. Polycythemia is present as a compensating mechanism only occasionally. Hemiglobin concentrations of 10% to 25% may give no apparent symptoms; levels of 35% to 50% result in mild symptoms, such as exertional dyspnea and headaches; and levels exceeding 70% are probably lethal. Therapy with ascorbic acid or methylene blue in this form of hereditary methemoglobinemia will reduce the level of Hi, the latter apparently by activation of the NADPH-methemoglobin reductase system. Heterozygotes have intermediate levels of NADH-cytochrome b5 reductase activity and normal blood levels of Hi. They may become cyanotic because of methemoglobinemia after exposure to oxidizing chemicals or drugs in amounts that will not affect normal persons.

In the second major category of hereditary methemoglobinemia, the reducing systems within the erythrocyte are intact, but the structure of the hemoglobin molecule itself is abnormal. A genetically determined alteration in the amino acid composition of either α- or β-globin chains may form a hemoglobin molecule with an increased tendency toward oxidation and a decreased susceptibility of the methemoglobin formed to reduce back to hemoglobin. Five abnormal hemoglobins have been identified, whose principal consequence is asymptomatic cyanosis as a result of methemoglobinemia; they are designated as various forms of *hemoglobin M (HbM).* The HbM defects are inherited as autosomal dominant traits (Bunn, 1986). Methylene blue therapy in such persons is without effect.

Most cases of methemoglobinemia are classified as secondary or acquired, due mainly to exposure to drugs and chemicals that cause increased formation of hemiglobin. Chemicals or drugs that directly oxidize HbO_2 to Hi include nitrites, nitrates, chlorates, and quinones. Other substances—aromatic amino and nitro compounds—probably act indirectly through a metabolite, because they do not cause Hi formation *in vitro.* These substances include acetanilid, phenacetin, sulfonamides, and aniline dyes. Very large doses of ferrous sulfate may produce methemoglobinemia. Levels of drugs or chemicals that would not cause significant methemoglobinemia in a normal person may do so in someone with a mild reduction in NADH-cytochrome b5 reductase activity who ordinarily is not cyanotic (newborn infants and persons heterozygous for NADH-cytochrome b5 reductase deficiency) (Bunn, 1986).

Hemiglobin is reduced back to Hb by the erythrocyte enzyme systems. It can also be reduced (slowly) by the administration of reducing agents, such as ascorbic acid or sulfhydryl compounds (glutathione, cysteine); these agents, as well as methylene blue, are of value in cases of hereditary NADH-cytochrome b5 reductase deficiency. In cases of acquired or toxic methemoglobinemia, methylene blue is of great value; its rapid action is not based on its own reduction capacity but on its acceleration of the normally slow NADPH-methemoglobin reductase pathway.

Hemiglobin can combine reversibly with various chemicals (e.g., cyanides, sulfides, peroxides, fluorides, and azides). Because of the strong affinity of Hi for cyanide, the therapy of cyanide poisoning is to administer nitrites to form Hi, which then combines with the cyanide. Thus, the free cyanide (which is extremely poisonous to the cellular respiratory enzymes) becomes less toxic when changed to HiCN.

Hemiglobin and sulfhemoglobin are quantitated by spectrophotometry. If Hi is elevated, drugs or toxic substances must first be eliminated as a cause. Congenital methemoglobinemia due to NADH-cytochrome b5 reductase deficiency is determined by assay of the enzyme. An abnormal hemoglobin (HbM; see Chap. 26) may also be responsible for methemoglobinemia noted at birth or in the first few months of life.

Sulfhemoglobin

Sulfhemoglobin is a mixture of oxidized, partially denatured forms of hemoglobin that form during oxidative hemolysis (Jandl, 1987). During oxidation of hemoglobin, sulfur (from some source, which may vary) is incorporated into heme rings of hemoglobin, resulting in a green hemochrome. Further oxidation usually results in the denaturation and precipitation of hemoglobin as Heinz bodies (Fig. 24–2).

Sulfhemoglobin cannot transport oxygen, but it can combine with CO to form carboxysulfhemoglobin. Unlike methemoglobin, sulfhemoglobin cannot be reduced back to hemoglobin, and it remains in the cells until they break down.

$$\text{Hb} \underset{\text{tissues}}{\overset{\text{lungs}}{\rightleftharpoons}} \text{HbO}_2 \underset{\text{NADH-cytochrome 5b reductase}}{\overset{\text{Oxidation}}{\rightleftharpoons}} \text{Hi} \longrightarrow \text{SHb} \longrightarrow \begin{array}{c}\text{Denatured}\\ \text{hemoglobin}\\ \text{(Heinz bodies)}\end{array}$$

Figure 24–2. Simplified concept of oxidation of hemoglobin (Hb) as proposed by Jandl (1960). Reversible binding and release of oxygen occur in lungs and tissues: oxidation of ferrous ions and formation of hemoglobin are reversible in the red cell to a limited extent: continued oxidation leads to irreversible conformational changes and sulfhemoglobin: still further oxidation results in denaturation of the hemoglobin and precipitation within the erythrocyte as Heinz bodies.

Sulfhemoglobin has been reported in patients receiving treatment with sulfonamides or aromatic amine drugs (phenacetin, acetanilid), as well as in patients with severe constipation, in cases of bacteremia due to *Clostridium perfringens,* and in a condition known as enterogenous cyanosis. The normal concentration of sulfhemoglobin *in vivo* is less than 1% and in these conditions seldom exceeds 10% of the total hemoglobin. It results in cyanosis and is usually asymptomatic. The reason some patients develop methemoglobinemia, some sulfhemoglobinemia, and others Heinz bodies and hemolysis is not well understood.

Carboxyhemoglobin (HbCO)

Endogenous carbon monoxide (CO) produced in the degradation of heme to bilirubin normally accounts for about 0.5% of carboxyhemoglobin in the blood and is increased in hemolytic anemia. Hemoglobin can combine with carbon monoxide with an affinity 210 times greater than that for oxygen. Carbon monoxide will bind with hemoglobin even if its concentration in the air is extremely low (e.g., 0.02% to 0.04%). In such cases, HbCO will build up until typical symptoms of poisoning appear (Goldsmith, 1968).

HbCO cannot bind to and carry oxygen. Furthermore, increasing concentrations of HbCO shift the Hb-oxygen dissociation curve increasingly to the left, thus adding to the anoxia. If a patient poisoned with carbon monoxide receives pure oxygen, the conversion of HbCO to HbO_2 is greatly enhanced. HbCO is light sensitive and has a typical, brilliant, cherry red color.

Acute carbon monoxide poisoning is well known and is further discussed in Chapter 17. Chronic poisoning, a result of prolonged exposure to small amounts of carbon monoxide, is less well recognized but is of increasing importance. The chief sources of the gas are gasoline motors, illuminating gas, gas heaters, defective stoves, and the smoking of tobacco. Exposure to carbon monoxide is thus one of the hazards of modern civilization. Enough of the gas has even been found in the air of busy streets of large cities to cause mild symptoms in persons such as traffic police officers who are exposed to it over long periods of time. Chronic exposure through tobacco smoking may lead to chronic elevation of HbCO and an associated left shift in the oxygen dissociation curve; smokers tend to have higher hematocrits than nonsmokers and may have polycythemia (Smith, 1978).

Healthy persons exposed to various concentrations of the gas for an hour do not experience definite symptoms (headache, dizziness, muscular weakness, and nausea) unless the concentration of the gas in the blood reaches 20% to 30% of saturation; however, it appears that in chronic poisoning, especially in children, serious symptoms may occur with lower concentrations.

HbCO may be quantitated by differential spectrophotometry or by gas chromatography.

Tests for Hemoglobin Derivatives

Naked eye examination of the blood specimen can yield some information. The normal appearance of the serum or plasma identifies the red cells as the site of the pigment.

Shaking of normal whole blood in the air for 15 minutes imparts to it a bright red color as the Hb is converted to HbO_2. The blood is cherry red when the pigment is HbCO in carbon monoxide poisoning. The color is chocolate brown in methemoglobinemia and mauve-lavender in sulfhemoglobinemia.

SPECTROPHOTOMETRIC IDENTIFICATION OF HEMOGLOBINS

The various hemoglobins have characteristic absorption spectra, which can be determined easily with a spectrophotometer. The useful absorbance maxima are given in Table 24–1. The maxima for Hi vary considerably with pH. The maxima given in the two right-hand columns are useful for distinguishing among these forms of hemoglobin. The absorbance between 405 and 435 nm (the Soret band) is considerably greater and may be used when small concentrations of hemoglobin are to be measured.

HEMATOCRIT (PACKED CELL VOLUME)

Before taking a sample from a tube of venous blood for a hematologic determination, it is important to mix the blood thoroughly. If the tube has been standing, this requires at least 60 inversions of the tube, or two minutes on a mechanical rotator; less mixing reduces precision unacceptably (Fairbanks, 1971).

The hematocrit of a sample of blood is the ratio of the volume of erythrocytes to that of the whole blood. It is expressed as a percentage or as a decimal fraction. The units (L/L) are implied. The venous hematocrit agrees closely with the hematocrit obtained from a skin puncture; both are greater than the total body hematocrit. Dried heparin and ethylenediaminetetraacetic acid (EDTA) are satisfactory anticoagulants. The hematocrit may be measured directly by centrifugation with macromethods or micromethods, or indirectly as the product of the mean corpuscular volume (MCV) × red cell count in automated instruments. In blood kept at room temperature, swelling of erythrocytes between 6 and 24 hours raises the hematocrit and MCV. Cell counts and indices are stable for 24 hours at 4°C (Brittin, 1969b).

The Wintrobe macromethod hematocrit employs centrifugation of blood in a thick-walled glass tube with a uniform internal bore and a flattened bottom. It is no longer used.

Micromethod

Equipment

A capillary hematocrit tube about 7 cm long with a uniform bore of about 1 mm is used. For blood collection directly from a skin puncture, heparinized capillary tubes are available.

Procedure

The microhematocrit tube is filled by capillary attraction, from either a free-flowing puncture wound or a well-mixed venous sample. The capillary tube should be filled to at least 5 cm. The empty end is sealed with modeling clay. The filled tube is placed in the radial grooves of the microhematocrit centrifuge head with the sealed end away from the center. The bottom of the tube is placed against the rubber gasket to prevent breakage. Centrifugation for five minutes at 10,000 to 12,000 g is satisfactory unless the hematocrit exceeds 50%; in that case, centrifugation should be continued for five additional minutes to ensure minimal plasma trapping.

The capillary tubes are not graduated. The length of the blood column, including the plasma, and of the red cell column alone must be measured in each case with a millimeter rule and a magnifying lens or with one of several commercially available measuring devices. The instructions of the manufacturer must be followed.

Interpretation of Results

Typical reference values for adult males are 0.41 to 0.51; for females, 0.36 to 0.45. A value below an individual's normal or below the reference interval for age and sex indicates anemia, and a higher value indicates polycythemia. The hematocrit reflects the concentration of red cells, not the total red cell mass. The hematocrit is low in hydremia of pregnancy, but the total number of circulating red cells is not reduced. The hematocrit may be normal or even high in shock accompanied by hemoconcentration, though the total red cell mass may be considerably decreased owing to blood loss. The hematocrit is unreliable as an estimate of anemia immediately after a loss of blood or immediately following transfusions.

Sources of Error

CENTRIFUGATION

Adequate duration and speed of centrifugation are essential for a correct hematocrit. The red cells must be packed so that additional centrifugation does not further reduce the packed cell volume.

In the course of centrifugation, a small proportion of the leukocytes, platelets, and plasma are trapped between the red cells. The error resulting from the former is, as a rule, insignificant. The amount of trapped plasma is larger in high hematocrits than in low hematocrits. Trapped plasma accounts for about 1% to 3% of the red cell column in normal blood (about 0.014 in a hematocrit of 0.47), slightly more in macrocytic anemias, spherocytosis, and hypochromic anemias (Dacie, 1991). Even greater amounts of plasma are trapped in the hematocrits of patients with sickle cell anemia and vary with the degree of sickling and consequent rigidity of the cells. In using the microhematocrit as a reference method for calibrating automated instruments, correction for trapped plasma is recommended (ICSH, 1980).

SAMPLE

Posture, muscular activity, and prolonged tourniquet-stasis can cause the same order of changes in hematocrit and cell concentrations as it does for nonfilterable soluble constituents (see Chap. 1). Unique to the hematocrit is the error due to excess EDTA (inadequate blood for a fixed amount of EDTA): The hematocrit will be falsely low as a result of cell shrinkage, but the hemoglobin and cell counts will not be affected.

OTHER ERRORS

Technical errors include failure to mix the blood adequately before sampling, improper reading of the level of cells and plasma, and inclusion of the buffy coat as part of the erythrocyte volume.

With good technique the precision of the hematocrit, expressed as ± 2 CV (coefficient of variation), is ± 1%. With low hematocrit values, the CV is greater because of reading error.

Macroscopic Examination

When the hematocrit determination is performed by centrifugation, inspection of the specimen after spinning may furnish valuable information. The relative heights of the red cell column, buffy coat, and plasma column should be noted.

The buffy coat is the red-gray layer between the red cells and plasma; it includes platelets and leukocytes.

An orange or green color of the plasma suggests increased bilirubin, and pink or red suggests hemoglobinemia. Poor technique in collecting the blood specimen is the most frequent cause of hemolysis. If the specimens are not obtained within an hour or two after a fat-rich meal, cloudy plasma may point to nephrosis or certain abnormal hyperglobulinemias, especially cryoglobulinemia.

BLOOD CELL COUNTING

Counts of erythrocytes, leukocytes, and platelets are each expressed as concentrations—cells per unit volume of blood. The unit of volume was expressed as cubic millimeters (mm^3) because of the linear dimensions of the hemacytometer (cell counting) chamber: 1 mm^3 = 1.00003 μL. The International Committee for Standardization in Hematology recommends that the unit of volume be the liter as on the right in the following examples:

Erythrocytes:

$5.00 \times 10^6/mm^3 = 5.00 \times 10^6/\mu L = 5.00 \times 10^{12}/L$

Leukocytes:

$7.0 \times 10^3/mm^3 = 7.0 \times 10^3/\mu L = 7.0 \times 10^9/L$

Platelets:

$300 \times 10^3/mm^3 = 300 \times 10^3/\mu L = 300 \times 10^9/L$

Except for some platelet counts and low leukocyte counts, the hemacytometer is no longer used for routine blood cell counting. Yet it is still necessary for the technologist to be able to use this method effectively and to know its limitations.

Any cell counting procedure includes three steps: dilution of the blood, sampling the diluted suspension into a measured volume, and counting the cells in that volume.

Erythrocyte Counts

Dilutors

Semiautomatic dilution of the blood for hemoglobin or for cell counts is more rapid and accurate than manual dilution.

SEMIAUTOMATED METHODS

Instruments are available for precise and convenient diluting, which both aspirate the sample and wash it out with the diluent. The dilutor should perform a 1:250 or 1:500 dilution with a CV of less than 1%.

MANUAL

Manual RBC counts are almost never performed.

Combining a microcapillary tube with a plastic vial containing a premeasured volume of diluent, the Unopette (Becton-Dickinson, Franklin Lakes, NJ) is a valuable system for manual dilutions. After the capillary tube is filled, it is pushed into the container, and the sample is washed out by squeezing the soft plastic vial. This system is especially convenient for microsampling. Unopettes are available with diluents for counts of red cells, white cells, platelets, eosinophils, and reticulocytes, as well as for hemoglobin and osmotic fragility determinations.

Electronic Counting Methods (Brittin and Brecher, 1971)

ELECTRICAL IMPEDANCE

Cells passing through an aperture through which a current is flowing cause changes in electrical resistance that are counted as voltage pulses. This principle, illustrated in Figure 24–3, is used in instruments marketed by Coulter (Coulter Electronics, Inc., Hialeah, FL 33010: S-Plus series, STKR, MAXM, STKS, etc.), TOA (TOA Medical Electronics, Los Alamitos, CA 90720: Sysmex CC-800, E-5000, NE-8000, SE-9000, etc.), Abbott (Abbott Diagnostics, Abbott Park, IL 60064: Cell-Dyn 1400, 1600cs, 3000, 3500, etc.), Serono-Baker (Serono-Baker Diagnostics, Allentown, PA 18103-9562: System 9000, etc.), Nova (Nova Biomedical, Waltham, MA 02254-9141: Celltrak series), Roche (Roche Diagnostic Systems, Inc., Montclair, NJ 07042-5199: COBAS ARGOS), and others. An accurately diluted suspension of blood (CS) is made in an isotonic conductive solution (such as Isoton) that preserves the cell shape. The instrument has a glass cylinder (GC) that can be filled with the conducting fluid and has within it an electrode (E_2) and an aperture

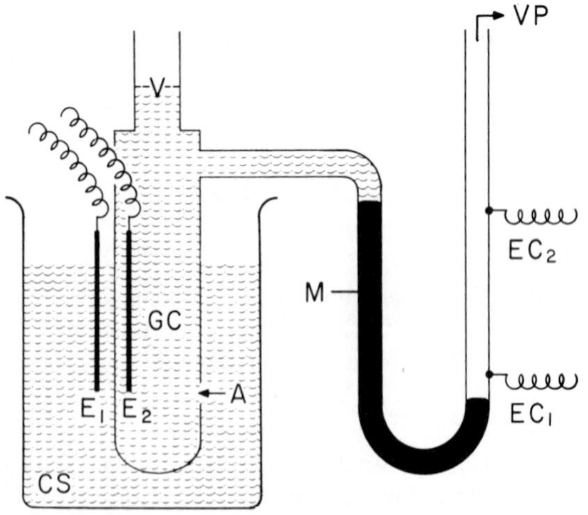

Figure 24–3. Schematic diagram of particle counter in which changes in electrical resistance are counted as voltage pulses. CS = cell suspension, GC = glass cylinder, A = aperture, E_1 and E_2 = platinum electrodes, V = valve, M = mercury column, EC_1 and EC_2 = electrical contacts, VP = vacuum pump. (Diagram adapted from Ackermann, 1972.)

(A) of 100 μm diameter in its wall. Just outside the glass cylinder is another electrode (E_1). The cylinder is connected to a U-shaped glass tube that is partly filled with mercury (M) and that has two electrical contacts (EC_1 and EC_2). The glass cylinder is immersed in the suspension of cells to be counted (CS) and is filled with conductive solution and closed by a valve (V). A current now flows through the aperture between E_1 and E_2. As mercury moves up the tube, the cell suspension is drawn through the aperture into the cylinder. Each cell that passes through the aperture displaces an equal volume of conductive fluid, increasing the electrical resistance and creating a voltage pulse, because its resistance is much greater than that of the conductive solution. The pulses, which are proportional in height to the volume of the cells, are counted. This is the "Coulter principle."

In the simplest system, the counting mechanism is started when the mercury contacts EC_1 and stopped when it contacts EC_2; during this time, the cells are counted in a volume of suspension exactly equal to the volume of the glass tubing between contact wires EC_1 and EC_2.

If two or more cells enter the aperture simultaneously, they will be counted as one pulse; this produces a coincidence error that must be corrected. The size of the coincidence error can be diminished by decreasing the concentration of cells and decreasing the size of the aperture. However, decreasing the cell concentration increases the effect of errors in dilution, increases the inherent counting error, and makes more critical the error due to the background "noise" of contaminating particles. With decreased aperture size, partial or complete plugging of the aperture with debris becomes a problem. Therefore, a balance is struck, and for a given count above a critical number, a coincidence correction is made by referring to a chart supplied by the manufacturer (for older-style semiautomated instruments) or is performed internally by new instruments.

A threshold setting or pulse discriminator allows the exclusion of pulses below an adjustable height on the certain counters. On others, a second threshold also excludes the counting of pulses *above* a certain height. One therefore counts only the cells in the "window" between the two settings. Systematically changing each threshold by given increments, one can determine a frequency distribution of relative cell volumes. Such cell size distributions can be automatically plotted and are valuable in the study of red cells, white cells, or platelets when two or more changing populations of cells are present. Blood cell histograms are based on this principle and are now routinely produced by the multichannel hematology analyzers.

Instruments that handle the data from the changes in electrical resistance digitally (e.g., the Coulter Counter) are stable and infrequently require calibration. Therefore, properly maintained, they can be relied on as primary reference machines to give a correct red cell count if the specimens are properly mixed and diluted (Brittin, 1971).

Before counting, one checks the adjustment of the threshold by counting the diluted suspension of red cells at successively increasing increments. To ensure that smaller particles (background "noise") are excluded from the count, the adjustment should be in the middle of the plateau. Larger foreign particles in the diluent are quantitated in a background or blank count that may be subtracted from the cell count. The final cell dilution should allow a particle count of at least 5000, which should be at least 20 times the blank count.

In the Coulter Counter, the dilution for the red cell count is 1:50,000, usually made in two steps: first, 20 μL of blood in 10 mL (1:500), followed by 100 μL of the first dilution in 10 mL of diluent (1:100). Because 0.5 mL of the cell suspension is counted, 50,000 cells (after correction for coincidence) will be counted for a normal red cell count of 5×10^{12}/L.

For a normal red cell count, therefore, the Poisson error will be about 0.5% $\left(CV = \frac{\sqrt{n}}{n}\right)$ and, for a very low count, closer to 1%. The actual precision of red cell counting is about twice this, or 1% to 2% (CV), and errors of dilution bring the precision achieved in practice to 2% to 4% (Brittin, 1971).

4

LIGHT SCATTERING

In the electro-optical analyzers (Fig. 24–4), a light-sensitive detector measures light scattering. All major multichannel analyzers now employ the optical method, at least to some extent. The size of the pulse detected is proportional to the size of the particle (WBC, RBC, or platelet). These instruments are discussed in more detail in the later section Multichannel Instruments. The precision of the instruments employing the optical method is equivalent to that of systems utilizing electrical impedance.

Erythrocyte Indices

Wintrobe introduced calculations for determining the size, content, and Hb concentration of red cells; these erythrocyte indices have been useful in the morphologic characterization

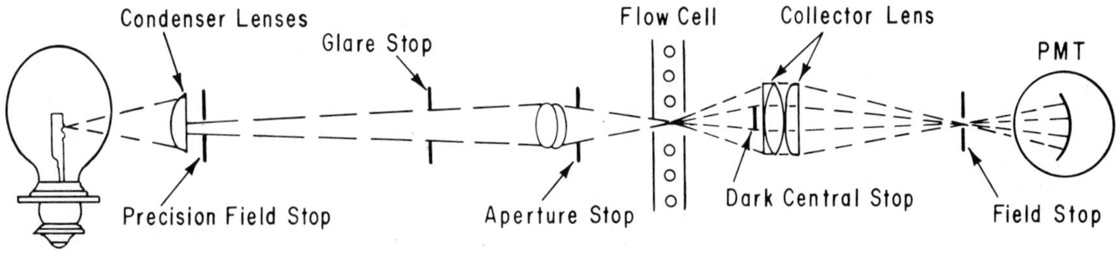

Figure 24–4. Schematic diagram of the electro-optical cell counter. Light is focused on the flow cell. Only light scattered by a cell reaches the photomultiplier tube (PMT), which converts it to an electrical pulse. (From Mansberg HP: Advanc Automated Anal 1970; 1:213. Reprinted courtesy of Technicon Instrument Corporation, Tarrytown, NY.)

of anemias. They may be calculated from the red cell count, hemoglobin concentration, and hematocrit.

Mean Cell Volume (MCV)

The MCV is the volume of the average red cell and is calculated from the hematocrit and the red cell count. MCV = Hct × 1000/RBC (in millions per μL), expressed in femtoliters or cubic micrometers. If the hematocrit = 0.45 and the red cell count = 5×10^{12}/L, 1 L will contain 5×10^{12} red cells, which occupy a volume of 0.45 L.

$$\text{MCV} = \frac{0.45\ \text{L}}{5 \times 10^{12}} = 90 \times 10^{-15}\ \text{L} \qquad (24\text{-}2)$$

One femtoliter (fL) = 10^{-15} L = 1 cubic micrometer (μm^3).

Mean Cell Hemoglobin (MCH)

The MCH is the content (weight) of Hb of the average red cell; it is calculated from the Hb concentration and the red cell count.

$$\text{MCH} = \frac{\text{Hb (in g/L)}}{\text{RBC (in millions per } \mu\text{L)}} \qquad (24\text{-}3)$$

The value is expressed in picograms. If the Hb = 15 g/dL and the red cell count is 5×10^{12}/L, 1 L contains 150 g of Hb distributed in 5×10^{12} cells.

$$\text{MCH} = \frac{150\ \text{g}}{5 \times 10^{12}} = 30 \times 10^{-12}\ \text{g (pg)} \qquad (24\text{-}4)$$

One picogram (pg) = 10^{-12} g = 1 micromicrogram ($\mu\mu$g)

Mean Cell Hemoglobin Concentration (MCHC)

The MCHC is the average concentration of Hb in a given volume of packed red cells. It is calculated from the Hb concentration and the hematocrit.

$$\text{MCHC} = \frac{\text{Hb (in g/dL)}}{\text{Hct}}, \text{ expressed in g/dL} \qquad (24\text{-}5)$$

If the Hb = 15 g/dL and the Hct = 0.45, the

$$\text{MCHC} = \frac{15\ \text{g/dL}}{0.45} = 33.3\ \text{g/dL} \qquad (24\text{-}6)$$

Discussion

Indices are determined in the electrical impedance instruments somewhat differently. The MCV is derived from the mean height of the voltage pulses formed during the red cell count, and the Hb is measured by optical density of HiCN. The other three values are calculated as follows: Hct = MCV × RBC;

$$\text{MCH} = \frac{\text{Hb}}{\text{RBC}};\ \text{MCHC} = \frac{\text{Hb}}{\text{Hct}} \qquad (24\text{-}7)$$

The reference values for the indices will depend on whether they are determined from the centrifuged hematocrit or from the cell counters. The values in normal persons will be similar if both are corrected for trapped plasma. However, because of increased trapped plasma in hypochromic anemias and sickle cell anemia, the MCHC calculated from the microhematocrit will be significantly lower than the MCHC derived from the electrical impedance counters.

With the Coulter Model S Plus IV, 95% reference intervals for normal adults are as follows: MCV = 80 to 96 fL; MCH = 27 to 33 pg; and MCHC = 33 to 36 g/dL (Williams, 1995). In a healthy person, variation is slight, no more than ± 1 unit in any of the indices. Deviations from the reference value for an individual or outside the reference intervals for normal persons are useful, particularly in characterizing morphologic types of anemia.

In *microcytic anemias,* the indices may be as low as an MCV of 50 fL, an MCH of 15 pg, and an MCHC of 22 g/dL; rarely do any become lower.

In *macrocytic anemias,* the values may be as high as an MCV of 150 fL and an MCH of 50 pg, but the MCHC is normal or decreased (Dacie, 1991). The MCHC typically increases only in spherocytosis, and rarely is over 38 g/dL.

Leukocyte Counts

In the total leukocyte count, no distinction is made among the six normal cell types (neutrophils and bands, lymphocytes, monocytes, eosinophils, and basophils). Although each cell type has its particular function in defending the body against foreign threats, in this discussion we are concerned with the total leukocyte concentration in the blood. The reference interval for adults is 4.5 to 11.0 × 10^9/L.

Sample

Heparin is unsatisfactory as an anticoagulant; EDTA should be used.

Hemacytometer Method

Although this method is only occasionally used in leukocyte counting, the technologist should be able to perform it (1) as a check on the validity of electronic methods for calibration, (2) as a check on the validity of electronic counts in patients with profound leukopenia or thrombocytopenia, (3) for blood specimens with platelet counting interference (i.e., very microcytic RBC), and (4) as a back-up method. It is also commonly used as a method for counting cells in cerebro-spinal fluid.

COUNTING CHAMBER

The hemacytometer is a thick glass slide with inscribed platforms of known area and precisely controlled depth under the coverslip.

Counting chambers and coverglasses should be rinsed in lukewarm water immediately after use; wiped with a clean, lint-free cloth; and allowed to air dry. The surfaces must not be touched with gauze or linen because these materials may scratch the ruled areas.

DILUTING FLUID

The diluting fluid lyses the erythrocytes so that they will not obscure the leukocytes. The fluid must be refrigerated and filtered frequently to remove yeasts and molds.

PROCEDURE

1. Well-mixed blood is diluted 1:20 in diluting fluid, and the vial is rotated for about five minutes. The chamber is loaded with just enough fluid to fill the space beneath the coverglass.

2. The cells are permitted to settle for several minutes, and the chamber is surveyed with the low-power objective to verify uniform cell distribution.
3. Counting is performed. The condenser diaphragm of the microscope is partially closed to make the leukocytes stand out clearly under a low-power (10×) objective lens. The leukocytes are counted in each of the four large (1 mm^2) corner squares (A, B, C, and D in Fig. 24–5). A total of eight large corner squares from two sides of a chamber are counted.
4. Each large square encloses a volume of 1/10 mm^3, and the dilution is 1:20. A general formula is as follows:

$$\text{Leukocyte count (cells/mm}^3) = \frac{cc}{lsc} \times d \times 10 \qquad (24\text{-}8)$$

where cc is the total number of cells counted, d is the dilution factor, 10 is the factor transforming value over one large square (1/10 mm^3) to the volume in mm^3, and lsc is the number of large squares counted.
In leukopenia, with a total count below 2500, the blood is diluted 1:10. In leukocytosis, the dilution may be 1:100 or even 1:200.

SOURCES OF ERROR

Errors may be due to the nature of the sample, to the operator's technique, and to inaccurate equipment. Errors that are inherent in the distribution of cells in the counting volume are called "field" errors and can be minimized only by counting more cells. Hemacytometer leukocyte counts yield a CV of about 6.5% for normal and increased counts and about 15% in leukopenic blood. Electronic counters, on the other hand, result in CVs of approximately 1% to 3%.

ERRORS DUE TO THE NATURE OF THE SAMPLE. Partial coagulation of the venous blood introduces errors by changes in the distribution of the cells or decrease of their number.

Failure to mix the blood thoroughly and immediately before dilution introduces an error, which depends on the degree of sedimentation.

OPERATOR ERRORS. Errors caused by faulty technique may occur during dilution, when the chamber is loaded, and when the cells are counted.

ERRORS DUE TO EQUIPMENT. Equipment errors can be diminished by using pipettes and hemacytometers certified by the U.S. Bureau of Standards.

INHERENT OR FIELD ERRORS. Even in a perfectly mixed sample, variation occurs in the number of suspended cells that are distributed in a given volume (i.e., come to rest over a given square). This "error of the field" is the minimal error. Another error is the "error of the chamber," which includes variations in separate fillings of a given chamber and in sizes of different chambers. Still another is the "error of the pipette," which includes variations in filling a given pipette and in the sizes of different pipettes.

In performing a WBC count, if 200 cells are counted using two chambers and one pipette, the CV = 9.1%, corresponding to 95% confidence limits of ±18.2% (twice the CV). Using four chambers and two pipettes and counting twice as many cells reduces the 95% confidence limits to ±12.8%. This relatively large percentage of error is of little practical consequence because of the physiologic variation of the leukocyte count.

NUCLEATED RED CELLS. Nucleated red cells will be counted and cannot be distinguished from leukocytes with the magnification used. If their number is high, as seen on the stained smear, a correction should be made according to the following formula:

$$\text{True leukocyte count} = \frac{\text{total count} \times 100}{100 + \text{No. of NRBC}} \qquad (24\text{-}9)$$

where No. of NRBC = the number of nucleated red cells that are counted during the enumeration of 100 leukocytes in the differential count.

EXAMPLE. The blood smear shows 25 nucleated red cells per 100 leukocytes. The total nucleated cell count is 10,000.

$$\text{True leukocyte count} = \frac{10{,}000 \times 100}{125} = 8000/\mu L\ (8.0 \times 10^9/L)$$
(24-10)

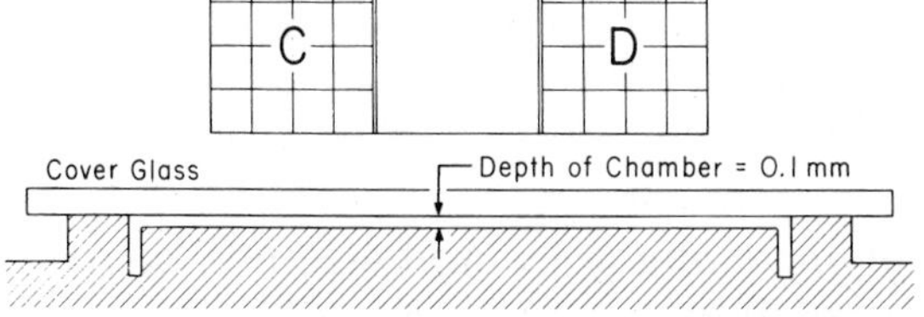

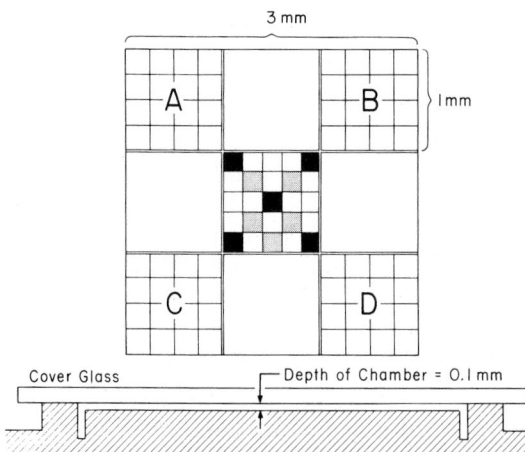

Figure 24–5. The upper figure is a diagram of the improved Neubauer ruling; this is etched on the surface of each side of the hemacytometer. The large corner squares, A, B, C, and D, are used for leukocyte counts. The five black squares in the center are used for red cell counts or for platelet counts, and the 10 black plus shaded squares for platelet counts. Actually, each of the 25 squares within the central sq mm has within it 16 smaller squares for convenience in counting.

The lower figure is a side view of the chamber with the coverglass in place.

Electronic Counting of Leukocytes (Brittin, 1971)

The principle is the same as that for red cells, except that in either electro-optical or impedance counting, the red cells are lysed before counting. This discussion is confined to the small semiautomated impedance instruments. Larger instruments are discussed later under Multichannel Instruments.

DILUENT SOLUTION

1. Physiologic saline, Isoton, or one of the other commercially available diluting fluids is used—10 mL for 20 μL of blood. (a) To this are added two drops of a 3% saponin solution (or one of the commercially available reagents—e.g., Zaponin) for lysis of the red cells. Five minutes are required to ensure complete stromatolysis. (b) Alternatively, one can use a commercially available reagent that both lyses red cells and converts Hb to HiCN (e.g., Zapoglobin); this allows the hemoglobin concentration and the leukocyte count to be determined from the same dilution.

4

2. Cetrimide-citrate-saline has advantages over saponin in that stromatolysis and dilution occur with one procedure, and the leukocytes are stable for several hours (Cartwright, 1968). A 1:500 dilution is achieved by diluting 20 μL of blood directly in 10 mL of cetrimide-citrate-saline.

THRESHOLD (PULSE DISCRIMINATOR) SETTING

Prior to counting with any new instrument, diluent, or lysing agent, it may be necessary to construct a threshold curve. This is done by performing multiple leukocyte counts on a normal blood sample at threshold settings differing by small increments from zero to a point at which the cells are no longer being counted. They may have to be done at different aperture current settings in order to select one that yields a good plateau. The threshold setting is selected so that baseline noise and small particles are not included in the count. The height of the plateau should be checked by several replicate hemacytometer leukocyte counts.

PROCEDURE

Details of operation and coincidence correction charts are supplied by the instrument manufacturer. Background counts greater than 100 should be corrected for coincidence and subtracted from the corrected leukocyte count; if less than 100, background counts can be ignored.

SOURCES OF ERROR

With small single-channel analyzers, about 0.5 mL of the 1:500 dilution of blood is counted, so that 10,000 cells are actually counted for a white cell count of 10,000 per μL. If two counts are made from one dilution and averaged, the error (±2 CV) is approximately ±10% in the normal range. If two dilutions of blood are made with an automatic dilutor and triplicate counts are done on each and averaged, the error (±2 CV) is ±4.6% in the normal range. Gagon (1966) showed that the leukocyte concentration in blood anticoagulated with EDTA is stable for 24 hours at 8°C or 25°C. Counts with heparinized blood may be either higher or lower than those with other anticoagulants and were not reproducible.

Speed of performance, elimination of visual fatigue of the technician, and improved precision are decisive advantages of the electronic cell counter over the hemacytometer.

Platelet Counts

Platelets are thin disks, 2 to 4 μm in diameter and 5 to 7 fL in volume (in citrated blood). They function in hemostasis, in maintaining vascular integrity, and in the process of blood coagulation. Reference values for platelet counts are 150 to 450×10^9/L.

In EDTA-blood, the mean platelet volume (MPV) increases with time up to one hour *in vitro*, is relatively stable between one and three hours, and then increases further with time. Change from a discoid to a spherical shape accounts for this increase in apparent volume in EDTA compared with citrate (Rowan, 1982). For reproducible results, platelet volume should be measured with multichannel instruments between one and three hours after the blood is drawn. The

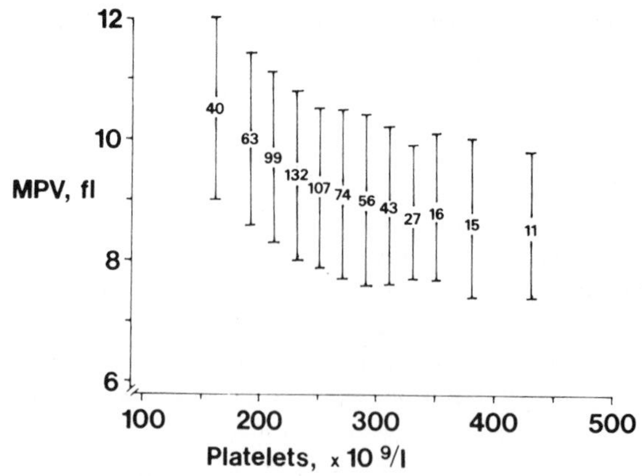

Figure 24–6. Mean platelet volume related to platelet count in 683 normal subjects. Each group is shown as mean (number) 2 S.D. (bar) of subjects grouped by platelet counts of 128–179, 180–199, 200–219, 220–239, 240–259, 260–279, 280–299, 300–319, 320–339, 340–359, 361–403, 406–462 × 10^9/L. The number of the mean position is the number of subjects in the group. (From Bessman JD, Williams LJ, Gilmer PR Jr: Am J Clin Pathol 1981; 76:289.

frequency distribution of platelet volumes in a person is log normal. The reference values for MPV are approximately 6.5 to 12 fL in adults. There is, however, a nonlinear, inverse relationship between the MPV and the platelet count within normal individuals (Fig. 24–6). Therefore, reference values for the MPV appear to vary with the platelet count (Bessman, 1981). The MPV is generally increased in hyperthyroidism (Ford, 1988) and myeloproliferative disease (Small, 1981).

Platelets are more difficult to count, because they are small and must be distinguished from debris. Another source of difficulty is their tendency to adhere to glass, to any foreign body, and particularly to one another. It is often possible to recognize a significant decrease in the number of platelets by a careful inspection of stained films. With capillary blood, films must be made evenly and quickly after the blood is obtained in order to avoid clumping and to minimize the decrease due to adhesion of platelets to the margins of the injured vessels. The estimate can be improved by examining stained films made from venous blood with EDTA as an anticoagulant (EDTA-blood), in which platelets are evenly distributed and clumping normally does not occur. Their morphology on films is described in the section Platelets, under Blood Film Examination.

The visual method of choice employs the phase-contrast microscope. This is the reference method. Laboratories performing over five platelet counts per day can justify electronic platelet counting; both the voltage pulse counting and the electro-optical counting systems are satisfactory.

Hemacytometer Method—Phase-Contrast Microscope

SPECIMEN

Venous blood is collected with EDTA as the anticoagulant. Blood from skin puncture wounds produces more variation but is satisfactory if the blood is flowing freely and if only the first few drops are used.

DILUENT SOLUTION

One percent ammonium oxalate is mixed in distilled water. A stock bottle is kept in the refrigerator. The amount needed for the day is filtered before use, and the unused portion is discarded at the end of the day.

PROCEDURE

1. Well-mixed blood is diluted 1:100 in diluting fluid, and the vial containing the suspension is rotated on a mechanical mixer for 10 to 15 minutes.
2. The hemacytometer is filled in the usual fashion, using a separate capillary tube for each side.
3. The chamber is covered with a Petri dish for 15 minutes to allow the platelets to settle in one optical plane. A piece of wet cotton or filter paper is left beneath the dish to prevent evaporation.
4. The platelets appear round or oval and frequently have one or more dendritic processes. Their internal granular structure and a purple sheen allow the platelets to be distinguished from debris, which is often refractile. Ghosts of the red cells that have been lysed by the ammonium oxalate are seen in the background.
5. Platelets are counted in 10 small squares (the black squares in Fig. 24–5), five on each side of the chamber. If the total number of platelets counted is less than 100, more small squares are counted until at least 100 platelets have been recorded—10 squares per side (black plus checked squares, Fig. 24–5) or all 25 squares in the large central square on each side of the hemacytometer, if necessary. If the total number of platelets in all 50 of these small squares is less than 50, the count should be repeated with 1:20 or 1:10 dilutions of blood.

CALCULATION

Because each of the 25 small squares defines a volume of 1/250 μL (1/25 mm^2 area × 1/10 mm depth), the platelet count (per μL) $= \dfrac{\text{No. cells counted}}{\text{No. squares counted}} \times \text{dilution} \times 250.$

By adjusting the number of squares so that at least 100 platelets are counted, the field error (the statistical error due to counting a limited number of platelets in the chamber) can be kept in the same range for low platelet counts as for high platelet counts. It has been shown that the CV due to combined field, pipette, and chamber errors is about 11% when at least 100 platelets are counted and 15% when 40 platelets are counted.

SOURCES OF ERROR

Most of the sources of error are the same as those discussed previously for the red cell and white cell counts. Blood in EDTA is satisfactory for five hours after collection at 20°C and for 24 hours at 4°C, provided that no difficulty was encountered in collection. Platelet clumps in the chamber imply a maldistribution and negate the reliability of the count; a new sample of blood must be collected. The causes of platelet clumping are likely to be initiation of platelet aggregation and clotting before the blood reaches the anticoagulant; imperfect venipuncture; delay in the anticoagulant contacting the blood; or, in skin puncture technique, delay in sampling. Capillary blood gives similar mean values, but errors are about twice those with venous blood, probably because the platelet level varies in successive drops of blood from the skin puncture wound.

Electronic Counting—Electrical Impedance

Because even relatively inexpensive whole blood counters now incorporate platelet counting capabilities, stand-alone platelet counters are not often used.

Sources of Error

Careful technique is especially important at all steps in platelet counting: collection of blood, having a particle-free diluent, microtechnique in diluting, and cleanliness in glassware and in the aperture of the counter.

With instruments using platelet-rich plasma, excessive numbers of red cells in the plasma will give falsely low counts, because platelets entering the aperture at the same time as red cells will not be detected. High leukocyte counts will also produce a falsely low platelet count, because white cells erratically filter out platelets when aspirating into the microcapillary tube. Platelets as large as red cells will be screened out by the upper threshold, also giving a falsely low count. On the other hand, if the sample is hemolyzed or if red cell fragments or very microcytic RBCs are in the blood, the platelet count is apt to be falsely high.

Whenever the platelet count is in question (e.g., very low or high count, or any type of instrument "flag" or distribution abnormality) the blood film must be examined before the count can be reported. This is to check for concordance of the apparent numbers on the film with those from the machine and to detect abnormalities such as those just mentioned that are prone to produce erroneous counts.

At times, the blood film (prepared from EDTA-blood) must be checked to corroborate the count and to detect abnormalities in platelets or other blood elements that may give a false value. Fragments of leukocyte cytoplasm that are sometimes numerous in leukemias may falsely elevate the count. The phase-contrast hemocytometer method must be employed in these cases. Counts are falsely low when platelets adhere to neutrophils (platelet satellitism) (Ahmed, 1978) or when platelets clump because of agglutinins (Lombarts, 1988), spontaneous aggregation, or incipient clotting due to faulty blood collection. The first two of these phenomena appear to depend on EDTA (Dacie, 1991).

Platelet counts tend to be the least reproducible of the blood cell counts, and the technologist must be vigilant to ensure their accuracy. This includes a readiness to confirm suspicious or abnormal results with a freshly drawn sample.

LIGHT SCATTERING

The Technicon analyzers (H-6000 and H*1, H*2, H*3) utilize light-scatter techniques for platelet counting. The H-6000 employs a sensitive photodiode to enumerate platelets (Kaplow, 1983). The H*1 uses a laser light source and high-angle detector to count platelets in the presence of erythrocytes (Bollinger, 1987). Both instruments generate a histogram showing the relative number of platelets versus platelet size (0 to 20 fL).

Multichannel Instruments

Coulter Hematology Systems

COULTER COUNTER MODEL S-PLUS SERIES

Coulter Electronics produces a large array of electrical impedance hematology analyzers. The compact semiautomated systems provide only the basic WBC, RBC, Hgb, Hct, and indices and are designed for small laboratories performing only a few tests per day (Nixon, 1986). At the other end of the spectrum, the Coulter MAXM, ONYX, STKR, and STKS provide for walk-away operation using a positive identification bar code system and closed-vial sampling. Eighteen to 20 parameters are provided, including WBC, RBC, Hgb, Hct, MCV, MCH, MCHC, Plat, RDW (red cell distribution width), and MPV (mean platelet volume), plus the histogram differential leukocyte count (absolute and relative lymphocytes, granulocytes, mononuclear cells). The "Interpretive Report" notes the presence of suspected eosinophilia, basophilia, blasts, atypical lymphocytes, immature granulocytes, NRBCs, and other abnormalities such as RBC flags for anisocytosis, microcytosis, and macrocytosis (Schoentag, 1988).

Coulter analyzers utilize the electrical impedance principle that they developed and began marketing in the early 1960s. Figure 24–7 shows the flow diagram from the Model S, an early whole-blood analyzer. In most instruments, about 125 to 250 μL of whole blood is aspirated directly and mechanically diluted in Isoton that maintains the size of the cells and conducts electricity. Throughput is up to 135 samples per hour with less than 1% carry-over. One dilution (about 1:6250; 1.6 μL whole blood plus 10 mL Isoton) is used to determine the erythrocyte and platelet measurements. In another dilution (about 1:251; 42.9 μL whole blood plus 6 mL Isoton plus 1.0 mL Lyse S III diff), the erythrocytes are lysed and the hemoglobin is converted to hemiglobincyanide. From this suspension, the hemoglobin concentration is measured colorimetrically at about 530 nm and the leukocyte parameters determined. Red and white blood cell counts are performed in triplicate and are based on the principle employed in Figure 24–3. An average of the three aperture determinations is reported, unless one result disagrees with the other two by more than a predetermined amount, in which case the discordant result is discarded and the mean of the other two is printed out. If all three results disagree, none is accepted (a "vote out"), and no value is printed. The mean cell volume (MCV) and red cell distribution width (RDW) are derived from the RBC histogram (RDW and histograms are discussed later in this chapter). The hematocrit is calculated by multiplying the MCV by the red cell count. The other indices (MCH, MCHC) are calculated.

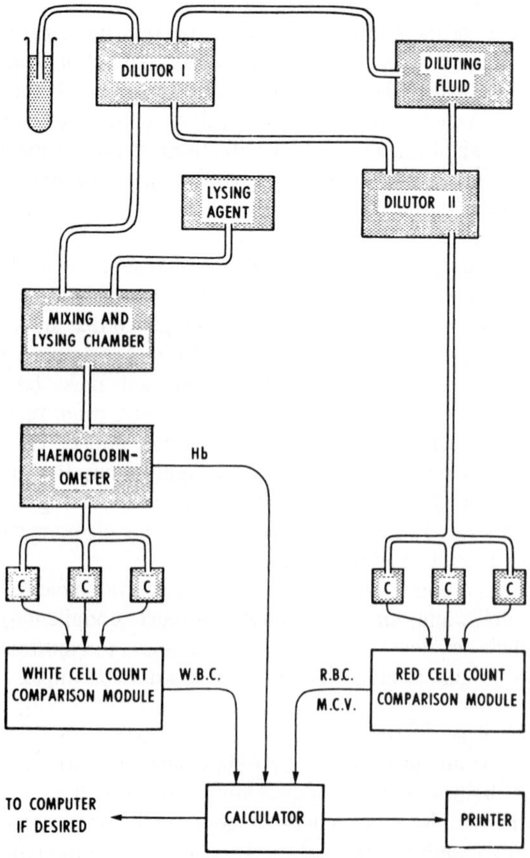

Figure 24–7. Flow diagram of the Coulter Model S. The blood sample is presented manually to the instrument, as indicated by the tube, upper left. (From Pinkerton PH, et al: J Clin Pathol 1970; 23:68.)

PLATELET COUNTING AND MPV. Except for the lower line instruments, most hematology analyzers now perform an automated whole blood platelet count as a part of the complete blood count. In the Coulter S-Plus series, platelets are enumerated in triplicate simultaneously with the erythrocyte count. Particles in the range of 2 to 20 fL are counted as platelets. Platelet count and distribution are determined using a 64-channel pulse-height analyzer (Channelyzer). By least square fitting, an algorithm based on the log normal size distribution of platelets extrapolates a curve in the range of 0 to 70 fL, provided that counting statistics are valid. The mean platelet volume (MPV) is determined from the arithmetic mean of the extrapolated histogram. MPV reference values are about 6.5 to 12 fL, but platelet size normally varies inversely with platelet count (Bessman, 1981) (see Fig. 24–6). Even for abnormal platelet counts, this reverse relationship holds true when marrow function remains normal; for example, MPV tends to be high in idiopathic thrombocytopenia purpura and low in reactive thrombocytosis. However, with an improperly functioning marrow, as occurs in folate deficiency or aplastic anemia, the MPV may be low despite thrombocytopenia (Schoentag, 1988). Platelet volume increases approximately 20% in EDTA during the first two hours, owing at least partly to the discocyte-to-echinocyte transformation (Threatte, 1993). The utility of the MPV is compromised by its variability, which is due to the lack of standard conditions for determining this value (Threatte, 1993).

RED CELL DISTRIBUTION WIDTH (RDW). The red cell distribution width (RDW) is an estimate of erythrocyte anisocytosis. A 256-channel pulse height discriminator is used to enumerate erythrocytes in the three RBC/PLT apertures as particles from 36 to 360 fL (μm^3). The RDW is the CV of the distribution of individual red cell volumes. In the Coulter instruments, it is derived from the central area of the RBC histogram. The RDW reference value (University Hospital, SUNY—Health Science Center at Syracuse) is 13.1% ± 1.5% (11.6% to 14.6%).

Bessman (1983) has proposed a system of classification of anemias based on the RDW and the MCV. This scheme has been used to help discriminate between uncomplicated heterozygous thalassemia (with a normal RDW and low MCV) and iron deficiency (high RDW and normal to low MCV). Of all the red cell measurements performed by multichannel instruments, the RDW appears to be the first to become abnormal in iron deficiency anemia due to chronic blood loss (McClure, 1985). Morgan (1988) also showed that an increased RDW is a sensitive but nonspecific indicator of iron deficiency in chronic hemodialysis patients. The RDW, therefore, can be a helpful adjunct in the classification and management of disorders involving the erythrocyte. Red cell histograms (discussed later) can be valuable in the diagnosis and treatment of such patients.

BLOOD CELL HISTOGRAMS. The Coulter Models S-Plus II through V, JS, ST, STKR, and STKS provide size distributions (cell volume in fL) versus relative number or frequency of cells for WBCs, RBCs, and platelets. Figure 24–8*A* shows typical normal distributions for all the cell types. The distributions are displayed along with the numerical data on the cathode ray tube of the data terminal and can be printed on a matrix printer-plotter. Figure 24–8 illustrates analyses from the same normal blood sample on (*A*) the Coulter STKS compared with (*B*) the Sysmex NE-8000 and (*C*) the Miles (Technicon) H*1. Figure 24–9 shows the results from an acute leukemia specimen run on the same respective analyzers.

The erythrocyte and platelet histograms depict the native size of the cells (x-axis) versus their frequency (y-axis). In the WBC impedance channel, the diluent lyses the RBCs and alters the WBCs. The lysing reagent punctures the leukocyte cytoplasmic membrane and causes it to collapse around the shrunken nucleus and granules. These altered leukocytes are drawn by vacuum through the three $100 \times 75-\mu m$ apertures and are counted and sized according to their impedance. Particles larger than 35 fL are considered leukocytes, and a 256-channel analyzer stores the information regarding the number of different-sized leukocytes. A Coulter proprietary computerized algorithm is used to classify the cells into three categories. Both percentage and absolute counts are determined. The percentage for each cell type is multiplied by the total leukocyte count (WBC) to obtain the absolute number of cells. Particles between 35 and about 90 fL are considered lymphocytes, those between 90 and approximately 160 fL are "mononuclear" (normally primarily monocytes), and those from 160 to 450 fL are granulocytes. There is some degree of automatic adjustment of these thresholds to compensate for individual variation in the location of the peaks and valleys. A spectrum of flags is used to indicate problems with a sample concerning linearity, lack of agreement among the apertures, or region flags due to unacceptable distribution caused by unusual cell populations that interfere with the typical valleys between the cell types (Cox, 1985). Table 24–2 (Schoentag, 1988) lists the regional areas of interference and possible causes of R flags on the Coulter analyzers. The laboratory staff (especially those reporting the "three-part differential") must be able to interpret properly all three histograms and know how they are affected by different conditions.

Experience reported in the literature has been generally favorable regarding the utility of these instruments in performance of a screening leukocyte differential count. Agreement between manual counts and instruments has been especially good for lymphocyte and granulocyte counts, with correlation coefficients of 0.85 or greater (Cox, 1985; Miers, 1987). The "mononuclear" count has been less satisfactory, with an r value of about 0.5. Monocytes are typically the major cell types in the mononuclear region; because of their lower numbers in the blood, they show decreased precision in the reference manual differential leukocyte count compared with automated results. Many other less frequent or unusual cell types (eosinophils, basophils, atypical lymphocytes, plasma cells, blast cells, and immature granulocytes) also appear in the mononuclear or granulocyte region and affect the correlation between the two methods. Application of the three-part differential count depends in part on the types of patients in the institution. Flagged or incomplete three-part differential counts are generally less frequent (about 16%) in nontertiary care hospitals (Duncan, 1987; Kalish, 1986) compared with tertiary care institutions (Miers, 1987; Ross, 1985b). Missed abnormalities (false-negative reports) from use of the instrument differential appear to be equal (9%—Kalish, 1986) or less frequent (6%—Griswold, 1985, 4%—Pierre, 1987) when compared with the manual/visual procedure using the National Committee for Clinical Laboratory Standards (NCCLS) reference method (Pierre, 1987). Most laboratories using instrument differential counts have action limits based on the CBC and leukocyte differential results that determine whether the counts can be accepted or require verification by scanning the blood film or performing a manual differential count (Koepke, 1985; Payne, 1986).

COULTER STKR

On the STKR, Coulter has enhanced the three-part differential by use of computer algorithms to produce a "complete differential with interpretive report." The blood cell histograms are analyzed to permit some degree of automatic interpretation. Eosinophils are normally reported as less than 0.7 ($\times 10^9$/L) and basophils as less than 0.2 ($\times 10^9$/L). If the histogram indicates that this threshold may be exceeded, no result prints out for the affected cell type, either eosinophil or basophil. The interpretive report also includes flags for the suspected presence of atypical lymphocytes or blasts (determined from interference at about 90 fL, between the lymphocytes and mononuclear), eosinophilia or immature granulocytes, and nucleated red blood cells or platelet clumps (determined from a lack of return of the WBC histogram to baseline to the left of the lymphocytes at about 35 fL). The instrument can also be user-programmed to flag absolute increases or decreases of lymphocytes or granulocytes. The RBC histogram is examined for normal distribution, anisocytosis (determined from the RDW), microcytosis, and macrocytosis (based on the MCV). Analysis of the platelet histogram is based on the normal nomogram derived from the inverse relationship between platelet count and MPV. Flag-

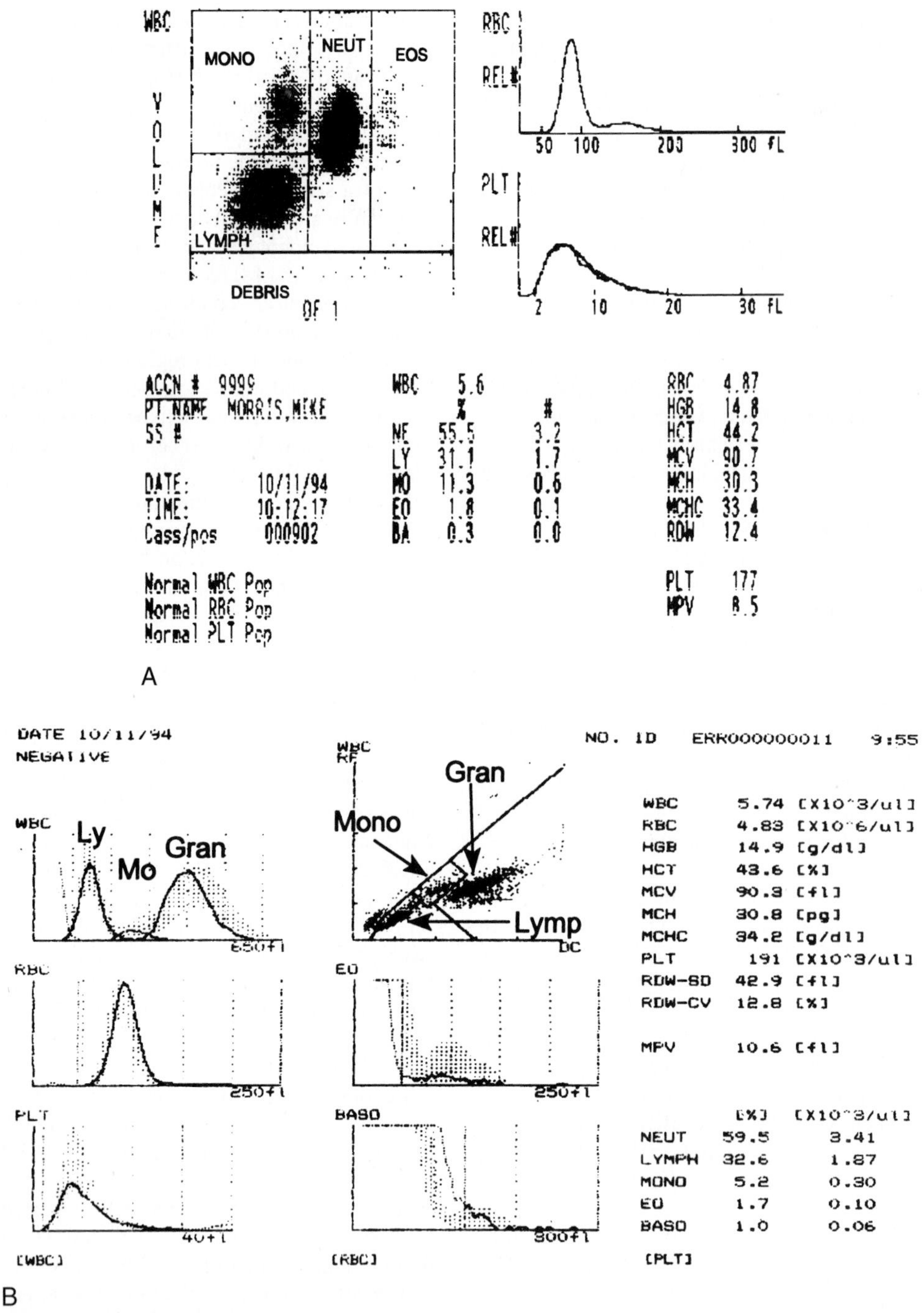

Figure 24–8. *A*, Normal blood on Coulter STKS. The red blood cell (RBC) and platelet histograms plot cell frequency (REL #, or relative number) on the Y axis versus cell volume on the X axis. In the RBC plot, particles sized 36 to 360 fL are considered to be erythrocytes. This is the typical narrow bell-shaped curve, the tail to the right is due to coincidence—more than one cell passing through the aperture at once and being sensed as a single larger cell. The red cell distribution width (RDW) is normal at 12.4 (reference interval 11.5% to 14.5%). The platelet histogram (*lower right*) is from particles sized 2 to 20 fL, showing the typical log normal distribution, skewed to the right.

The white blood cell (WBC) scattergram plots leukocyte volume (determined by impedance) versus laser light scatter (DF1) on the X axis. The cell population's designated regions have been added. Relative counts (%) and absolute counts (#, $\times 10^3/\mu L$) are given for the 5 WBC types and interpretations for the WBC, RBC, and platelet populations. Manual (400 cells counted) differential: 55.5% neutrophils, 0.5 band, 29.5 lymphocytes, 4.0 atypical lymphocytes, 9.0 monocytes, 1.0 eosinophil, and 0.5 basophil.

B, Sysmex NE-8000 results from same blood specimen as 24–8*A*. On the left side of the figure, histograms for WBC (trimodal WBC histogram), RBC and platelets (PLT) show relative number on Y axis versus impedance determined size on X axis. The shaded (*dotted*) areas represent the normal distribution. On the right are the three WBC plots, which are used to determine the five leukocyte types. In the upper right is the scatterplot of radiofrequency (RF) on the Y axis versus DC impedance sizing on the X axis. The computer analyzes the distributions and places thresholds to segregate cell populations. Designations have been added for the cell types. The right middle and lower histograms (volume versus frequency) are derived from use of temperature regulation and cell-specific lysing reagents that shrink other leukocytes and leave eosinophils and basophils intact and, therefore, larger in size.

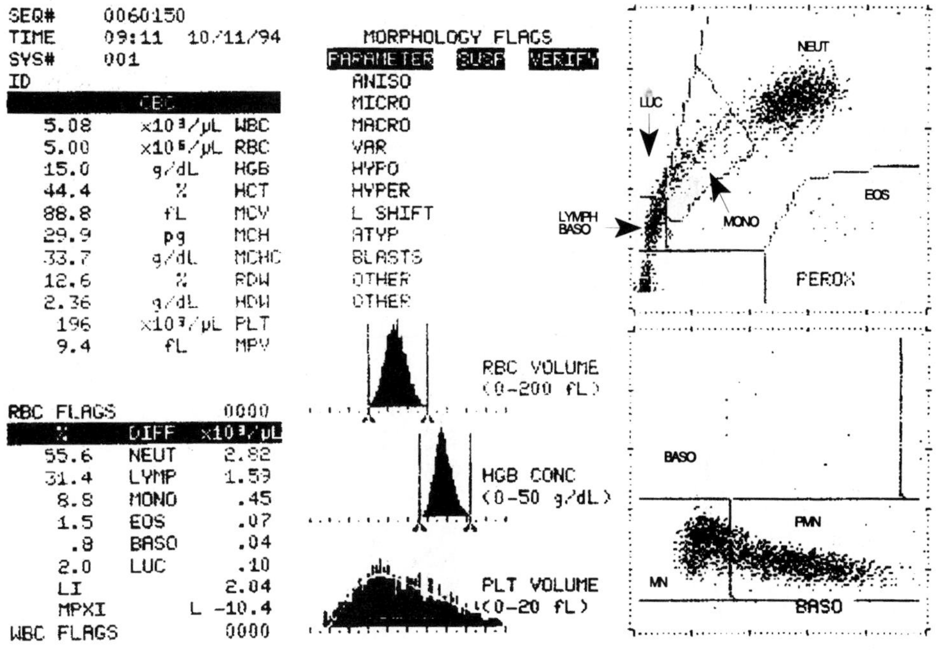

C

Figure 24–8 *Continued.* *C,* Miles H*1 results of same normal blood specimen as in *A* and *B.* In the peroxidase plot of size (light scatter, Y axis) versus peroxidase staining intensity (X axis), cell region designations are added. The analyzer computer performs cluster analysis and segregates the various cell types. Large unstained cells (LUCs) correspond to atypical (larger) lymphocytes. The basophil/lobularity plot shows basophils with intact cytoplasm above; below and to the left are mononuclear cells (lymphocytes, monocytes) with granulocytes (bands, eosinophils and neutrophils) to the right.
RBC volume, hemoglobin concentration, and platelet histograms are normal, reflected also in the RBC indices and platelet count.

4

ging occurs if MPV, PLT, or the relationship between them is abnormal. Figure 24–10 shows an abnormal sample as analyzed on the Coulter STKR with interpretive report.

COULTER STKS

Coulter's latest top-of-the-line analyzer is the STKS. This flow cytometer–based model incorporates the VCS technology combining simultaneous volumetric impedance measurements (V), cell conductivity (C) determined by high-frequency electromagnetic probing of the cell, and scatter (S) from a laser light source. WBCs are analyzed in their near native state in an electro-optical flow cell. Typically, over 8000 WBCs are analyzed, or 20 seconds counting, whichever comes first. Cell volume is determined using the traditional Coulter principle of impedance. Conductivity is determined using a high-frequency electromagnetic probe, which provides information on the cells' internal constituents (chemical composition, nuclear characteristics, and granular constituents). Conductivity especially helps in differentiating between cells of the like size such as small lymphocytes and basophils. Forward angle scatter of a helium-neon laser–generated monochromatic light is determined by cell surface characteristics, morphology, and granulation. Laser light scatter (DF1) is particularly important in recognition of granular cells such as eosinophils. By plotting each cell according to its VCS measurements, each cell is placed in a characteristic leukocyte cluster on a three-dimensional grid. Scatterplots are displayed on a CRT with color coding for different population densities. Figure 24–8*A* shows results from a normal sample on the STKS. Figure 24–9*A* depicts the STKS results from a patient with acute monocytic leukemia FAB AML, M5a and approximately 85% blasts.

The STKS has been extensively evaluated in the literature, either individually against the manual differential count (Cornbleet, 1993; Verheul, 1993; Warner, 1991) or more frequently against the manual count and other automated analyzers such as the Technicon H*1 (Robertson, 1992); Abbott Cell-Dyn 3000 (Stroop, 1994); STKS or S-Plus IV and Sysmex NE-8000 and Technicon H*1 (Burns, 1992; Warner, 1990) or against the Technicon H*1 (or H*2) and Sysmex NE-8000 and Cell-Dyn 3000 (Bentley, 1993; Buttarello, 1992, 1993). Studies show the STKS's acceptability as a routine hematology analyzer with very high correlation coefficients compared with manual and other instruments for neutrophils and lymphocytes and satisfactory to good coefficients for eosinophils and monocytes. Basophils continue to be less precise, largely because of their usual low frequency, but this rarely would be a clinically significant problem. Continuous updating of instrument software versions complicates interpretation of comparative studies but typically leads to improved accuracy of instrument results. Overall, WBC differential screening for abnormals has been acceptable, with considerable variability depending on the author and the particular WBC flag. Warner (1991) showed 6% false-negative results overall and 3% false-positive results, whereas Stroop (1994) reported 25% false-negative results and 6.2% false-positive results. Robertson's studies (1992) revealed false-positive rates of 5%, 2%, and 31% for blasts, variant lymphocytes, and immature granulocytes/bands, respectively, with respective false-negative rates of 0%, 0.4%, and 2%.

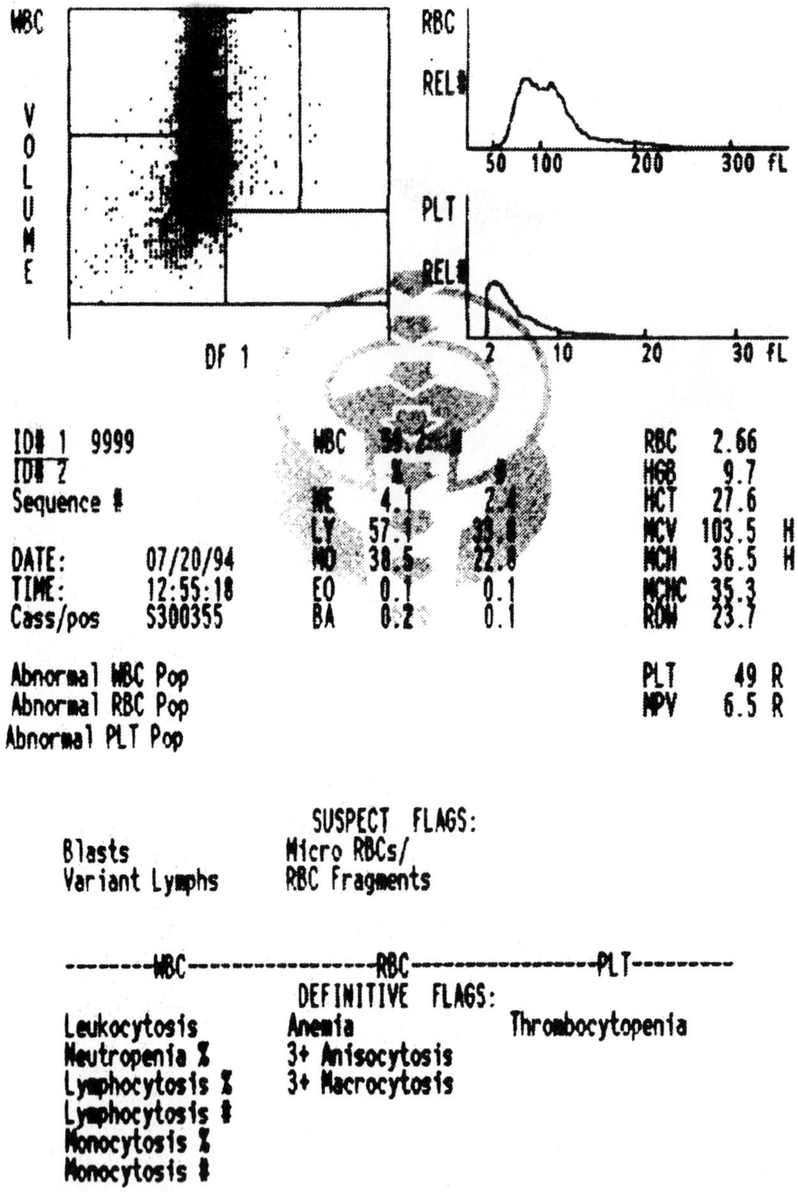

A

Figure 24–9. *A,* Coulter STKS. Acute monocytic leukemia (FAB, M5a) with 85% blasts that lie in the lymphocyte and monocyte areas but correctly produce a blast suspect flag. Patient's high MCV and RDW result in 3+ definitive flags for macrocytosis and anisocytosis. Platelet count of 49 leads to thrombocytopenia flag. Manual differential count: 85% monoblast, 0.5 myelocytes, 1.0 bands, 1.0 neutrophils, 11.5 lymphocytes, 0.5 atypical lymphocytes, 0.5 monocytes, and rare NRBC. Blasts are Sudan Black B, myeloperoxidase, and chloroacetate esterase negative; 50% are alpha naphthyl butyrate positive. Cytogenetic studies show rearrangements between chromosomes 10 and 11, which has been reported in AML, M5a.

Germain (1994) reported that 8% of specimens from HIV-positive patients had a falsely elevated basophil count (values of from 11% to 29% basophils). About 90% of the time, incubation of the sample at 37°C returned the basophil count to normal. Cohen (1993) found the STKS to be less accurate than the S-Plus IV in analyzing HIV-infected populations. On the STKS, about 20% of patients were falsely deemed granulocytopenic, especially those who were macrocytic. In HIV patients, macrocytosis is usually caused by zidovudine therapy.

Although Verheul (1993) was able to reduce the overall laboratory differential load by 70%, the STKS was unsuitable for screening neonates because of a 75% suspect flag rate.

TOA Systems

SYSMEX CC-800

The Sysmex CC-800 is an eight-parameter cell counter that employs the impedance principle of detection (Carlson, 1986). Precision is claimed to equal that of the Coulter Model S-Plus II. Up to 100 samples on a turntable are analyzed at 80 per hour using 0.5 mL whole blood. A quality-control program stores control values, calculates moving mean, and plots Levey-Jennings charts on a cathode ray tube. A microprocessor monitors and provides alerts for abnormal patient values, manometer performance, reagent supply, aperture clogging, diluent temperature, and electronics. The instrument provides histograms of WBC, RBC, and platelets and enumerates subpopulations of each based on size.

SYSMEX E-5000

The TOA Sysmex E-5000 also uses the impedance principle to classify cells. Three population percentages are routinely determined: *lymphocytes* (formerly called small cell ratio [SCR]); *mixed* (formerly middle cell ratio [MCR],

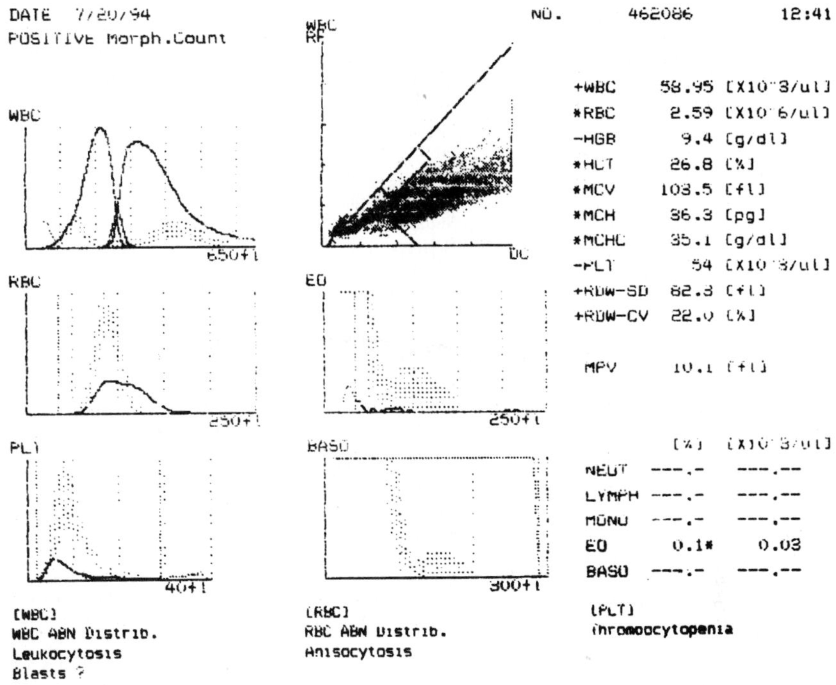
DATE 7/20/94
POSITIVE Morph.Count
NO. 462086 12:41
WBC
RBC
PLT
EO
BASO
+WBC 58.95 [X10^3/ul]
*RBC 2.59 [X10^6/ul]
-HGB 9.4 [g/dl]
*HCT 26.8 [%]
*MCV 103.5 [fl]
*MCH 36.3 [pg]
*MCHC 35.1 [g/dl]
-PLT 54 [X10^3/ul]
+RDW-SD 82.3 [fl]
+RDW-CV 22.0 [%]
MPV 10.1 [fl]
NEUT
LYMPH
MONO
EO 0.1* 0.03
BASO
[WBC]
WBC ABN Distrib.
Leukocytosis
Blasts ?
[RBC]
RBC ABN Distrib.
Anisocytosis
[PLT]
Thromobocytopenia

B

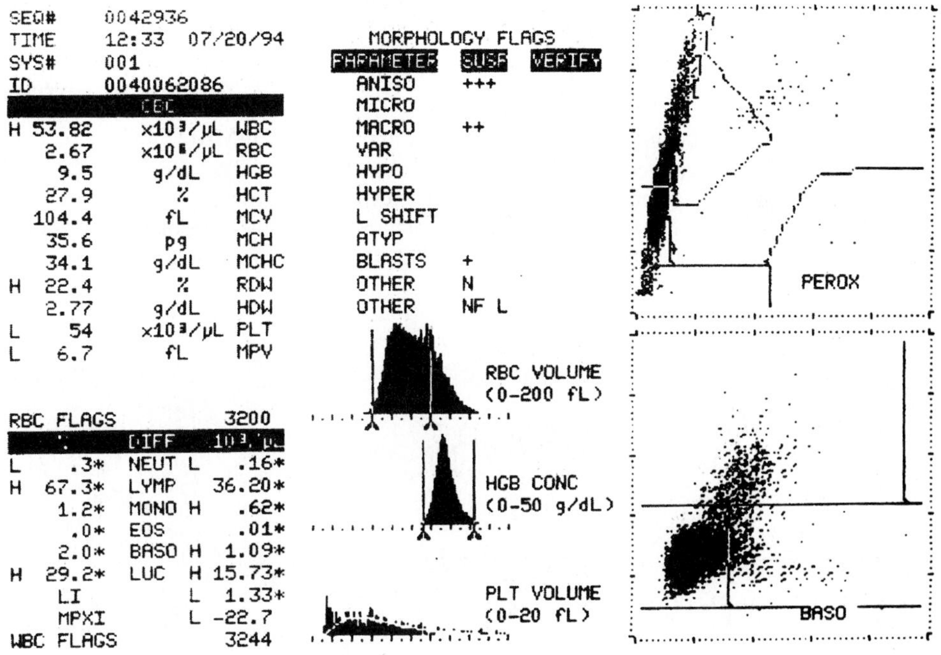
SEQ# 0042936
TIME 12:33 07/20/94
SYS# 001
ID 0040062086
CBC
H 53.82 x10³/µL WBC
2.67 x10⁶/µL RBC
9.5 g/dL HGB
27.9 % HCT
104.4 fL MCV
35.6 pg MCH
34.1 g/dL MCHC
H 22.4 % RDW
2.77 g/dL HDW
L 54 x10³/µL PLT
L 6.7 fL MPV
RBC FLAGS 3200
DIFF
L .3* NEUT L .16*
H 67.3* LYMP 36.20*
1.2* MONO H .62*
.0* EOS .01*
2.0* BASO H 1.09*
H 29.2* LUC H 15.73*
LI L 1.33*
MPXI L -22.7
WBC FLAGS 3244
MORPHOLOGY FLAGS
PARAMETER SUSP VERIFY
ANISO +++
MICRO
MACRO ++
VAR
HYPO
HYPER
L SHIFT
ATYP
BLASTS +
OTHER N
OTHER NF L
RBC VOLUME (0-200 fL)
HGB CONC (0-50 g/dL)
PLT VOLUME (0-20 fL)
PEROX
BASO

C

Figure 24–9 *Continued.* *B*, The same specimen as shown in *A*. Sysmex NE-8000. The trimodal WBC histogram shows two major cell populations with high absolute numbers (far above the normal shaded curve areas). The size versus radiofrequency (RF) shows a population extending up and to the right from the lymphocyte area and another below the granulocyte area. Although the differential count is suppressed, an appropriate blast flag is generated.

C, The same specimen as shown in Figure 24–9*A* and *B*. The Miles H*1 reports mostly lymphocytes and a high (29.2%) large unstained cell (LUC) population for those cells in the peroxidase plot above the lymphocytes, resulting in a blast flag. Note also the predominance of cells (blasts) to the far left in the mononuclear area of the basophil/lobularity plot. Anisocytosis and macrocytosis flags are appropriate, the hemoglobin (HGB) concentration histogram shows that individual erythrocytes are normochromic.

which includes monocytes, atypical lymphocytes, blasts, myelocytes, eosinophils, basophils, and others); and *neutrophils* (formerly large cell ratio [LCR], which includes neutrophils, bands, myelocytes, and metamyelocytes). The absolute cell counts are also calculated. Figure 24–11 shows the WBC, RBC, and PLT histograms from the E-5000. Data show this instrument to be an acceptable screening instrument (Payne, 1987; Pierre, 1987).

The E-5000 also determines a platelet large cell ratio (P-LCR), which represents the proportion of large platelets (platelets between 12 fL and the upper discriminator level, divided by total platelet count). This may be useful for detecting platelet clumping, giant platelets, and cell fragments or for monitoring hematopoietic function. The manufacturer's reference interval for P-LCR is approximately 13% to 43%. For the TOA Sysmex E-5000 Analyzer, the RDW is the width of the histogram (in femtoliters) at 20% of the height of the histogram from the base to the highest peak. For this

Table 24–2. FLAGS ON COULTER ANALYZERS

	Region	Possible Causes
R1	Left of lymphocytes (~35 fL)	Nucleated RBCs Platelet clumps Fibrin strands Cold agglutinins Cryoglobulins Malaria Heinz bodies
R2	Lymphocyte/mononuclear (~90 fL)	Atypical lymphocytes Plasma cells Blasts Monocytosis Eosinophilia Basophilia Hairy cells Sézary cells
R3	Mononuclear/granulocyte (~160 fL)	Immature granulocytes Eosinophilia Basophilia Monocytosis
R4	Right of granulocytes (~450 fL)	High granulocyte count
RM	Multiple R flags	Multiple causes

From Schoentag RA: Hematology analyzers. Clin Lab Med 1988; 8:653.

RDW, the TOA's reference interval is 37 to 54 fL. Instead, or in addition, the more traditional RDW as a CV may be chosen on the E-5000.

SYSMEX NE-8000

The Sysmex NE-8000 uses a hydrodynamically focused flow cytometer with direct current electrical impedance (referred to as DC on the scattergram) and radio frequency conductivity (RF) to place white blood cells into the granulocyte, lymphocyte, and monocyte categories (Bentley, 1993; Burns, 1992). Eosinophils and basophils are selectively counted in two separate channels using impedance sizing measurement after proprietary lysis or shrinkage of the other cell types. Neutrophils are calculated by subtracting the sum of the separately measured eosinophils plus basophils from the total granulocyte number. Figure 24–8*B* shows the NE-8000 results and cytograms from a normal blood sample. Figure 24–9*B* shows an acute monocytic leukemia patient from the same blood specimen as Figure 24–9*A* on the Coulter STKS and Figure 24–9C on the Technicon H*1.

The NE-8000 also provides an acceptable five-cell population differential count (Warner, 1990) and was judged safe and effective for diagnostic use (Bentley, 1993). Correlation coefficients compared with the manual differential counts were excellent for neutrophils and lymphocytes and acceptable for other cell types (Buttarello, 1992; Warner, 1990). However, several authors (Bentley, 1993; Buttarello, 1992; Warner, 1990) found considerable variation in the monocyte counts.

SYSMEX SE-9000

The latest top-of-the-line TOA analyzer, the Sysmex SE-9000 has added an Immature Cell Channel to provide additional information on blasts and immature myeloid cells. This should improve the specificity and accuracy of the WBC flags. The analyzer also permits a quantitative review of the degree of flagging.

Technicon Instruments (Miles, Inc.)

HEMALOG D

The *Hemalog D* (Technicon Instruments Corp., Tarrytown, NY) automatically samples blood from a turntable at the rate of 90 per hour. Erythrocytes are lysed, leukocytes are separated into three channels and fixed, and reagents are

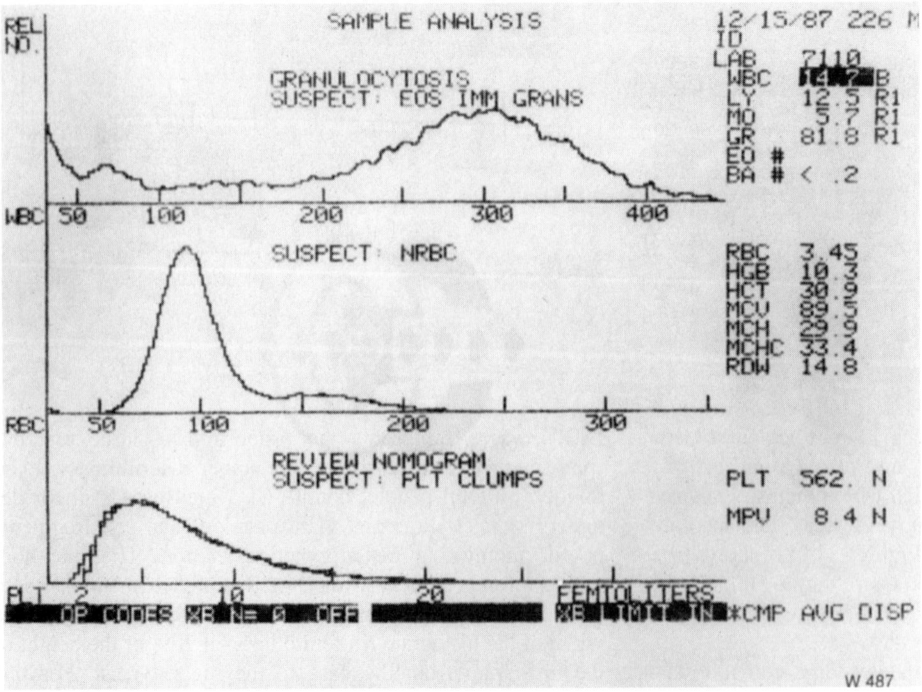

Figure 24–10. Coulter STKR report from a patient with clumped platelets and thrombocytosis. The total WBC count (14.7) is backlit to warn that something is elevating the baseline at about 35 fL, also causing a R1 flag. In this case, clumped platelets are interfering at the left side of the lymphocyte population. This has also resulted in a "SUSPECT: PLT CLUMPS" in the platelet histogram and "SUSPECT: NRBC" in the RBC histogram, because either is a possible cause of the "high take-off" on the WBC histogram. The WBC histogram also gives a true positive result for granulocytosis (at operator-defined limits) but a false-positive result for eosinophilia (note no EO# printed) and/or immature granulocytes. Although platelet clumps are sometimes seen on the right side of the platelet histogram, they are not seen in this case. Manual leukocyte differential count: 74 neutrophils, 11 n bands, 9 lymphocytes, 6 monocytes.

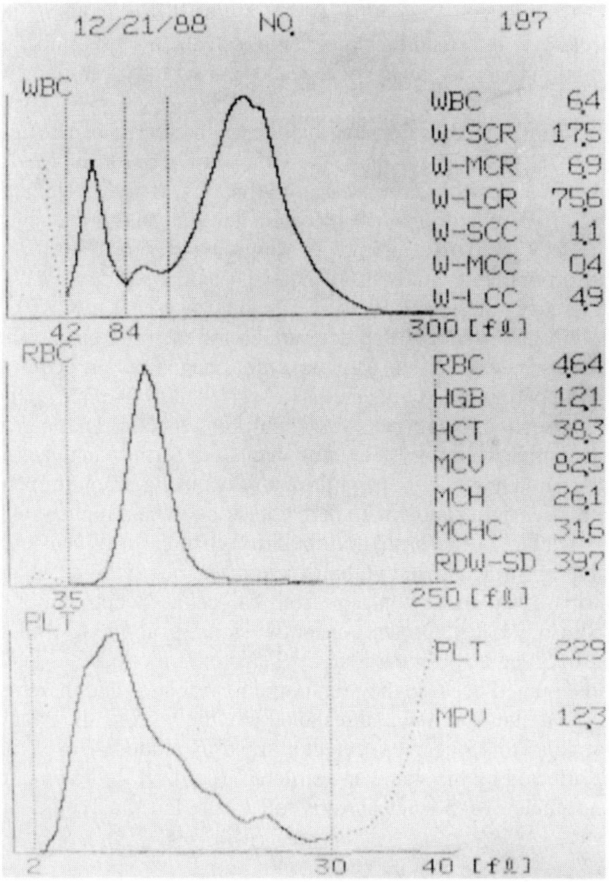

Figure 24–11. Report from TOA Sysmex E-5000. Normal sample, but slightly low MCHC. Small (SCR), medium (MCR), and large (LCR) cell ratios are now being termed lymphocyte, mixed, and neutrophil percentages, respectively, to increase acceptance and decrease confusion. Absolute counts are also calculated. The instrument gives the fL cut-off points (thresholds) between the cell types: these can also be adjusted by the operator on any particular sample. The RDW selected here is the fL spread at 20% of the height to the highest RBC peak. The reference interval for this RDW is 37 to 54 fL. The threshold to the right between the platelets and RBCs is also specified and the RBCs (dotted continuation of line) cause the curve to the right to rise, in this case at 30 fL. Printing of the platelet large cell ratio (P-LCR, percentage > 12 fL) is suppressed. Manual leukocyte differential count: 72 neutrophils, 19 lymphocytes, 9 monocytes.

introduced for cytochemical reactions (Mansberg, 1974). In a photo-optical system, size (using a darkfield detector sensitive to light scatter) and light absorption (using a brightfield detector sensitive to stain density) are measured as each cell passes through the flow cell. In the *peroxidase channel,* immature neutrophils, neutrophils, and eosinophils (which contain peroxidase) absorb light. A pH of 3.2 is used; eosinophils stain more deeply than neutrophils and are distinguished from them by greater absorption and less scatter. Immature and toxic neutrophils have greater peroxidase activity than mature neutrophils and are designated "high peroxidase cells" (HPX cells); they are separated by greater absorption and equal or greater scatter. Although it has been generally assumed that an increase in HPX cells is due to increased bands and immature neutrophils, it is likely that an increased HPX count is often due to toxic granulation in the neutrophils (Peacock, 1982). Lymphocytes are distinguished by low scatter and low absorption. "Large unstained cells" (LUCs) have high scatter and low absorption and include atypical lymphocytes and blasts. A higher than expected LUC count after initial chemotherapy in acute myelogenous leukemia may be an early means of detecting patients in whom remission with subsequent therapy is unlikely (Winkle, 1982). The cells are counted and instantaneously plotted (scatter versus absorption) on a scattergram, which is electronically displayed and may be photographed (Fig. 24–12). Platelets and erythrocyte stroma are excluded by a lower threshold. In the *lipase channel,* monocytes are stained by α-naphthyl butyrate esterase activity and counted; they are separable from other cells by high scatter and high absorption. In the third channel, basophils are counted as their granular heparin stains with alcian blue. Heparinized blood, therefore, cannot be used.

Ten thousand leukocytes are counted in each channel; the results are expressed both as percentages and as absolute concentrations. The total leukocyte count is determined in the peroxidase channel. An optional addition is an automatic slide maker (Autoslide) that makes and stains blood films on a roll of plastic tape, mounts the blood films on glass slides, and identifies them by accession number for reference or examination if needed. The reference intervals achieved with the Hemalog D are similar to those achieved with the manual technique (Simmons, 1974).

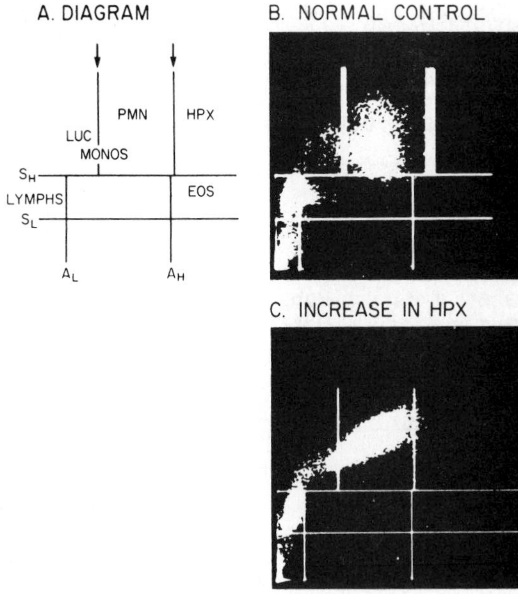

Figure 24–12. The appearance of HPX cells in the peroxidase channel of the Hemalog D. As shown in the line drawing (*A*), fixed thresholds are set on the horizontal axis for light scatter (S_H = high scatter; S_L = low scatter), and on the vertical axis for light absorbance (A_H = high absorbance; A_L = low absorbance). The neutrophil (PMN) population is identified by size and peroxidase staining; vertical thresholds set to identify PMNs are designated with arrows. Other distinct populations include large unstained cells (LUC), monocytes (MONO), lymphocytes (LYMPH), and eosinophils (EOS). Cells that have the same size (light scatter) as PMNs but fall above the designated absorption threshold are termed high peroxidase cells (HPX). A photograph of the cell distribution from a normal volunteer (*B*) is compared with a donor with an increase (>4%) in HPX cells (*C*). (From Peacock JE, Ross DW, Cohen MS: Am J Clin Pathol 1982; 78:445.)

H-6000

The Technicon H-6000 incorporates the eight-parameter CBC and platelet count with the cytochemical differential principle of the earlier Hemalog D. Stirred whole blood is aspirated and drawn into three manifolds: basophil and alkaline peroxidase for WBC and leukocyte differential count, and an RBC/platelet/hemoglobin manifold for CBC and platelets. Hemoglobin is determined using the HiCN reaction. The RBC/PLT optics assembly has two detection channels. A photodiode enumerates RBCs, and the light scatter signals are integrated to determine hematocrit. A more sensitive photomultiplier tube senses scatter from platelets. The differential portion is similar to that of the Hemalog D except that monocytes are measured in the peroxidase manifold rather than in a separate esterase channel. The H601 printer provides a copy of the CBC and differential, RBC, platelet histograms, and scatter versus absorption display of the leukocytes in the peroxidase channel (Fig. 24–13).

H*1

The H*1 was introduced in 1985. It produces all of the results of the H-6000 and has a number of additional useful features. The instrument is a fairly small single-sample analyzer with separate components for the benchtop analyzer, floor level electronic/pneumatic power supply, and CRT with interactive menu-driven keyboard with dual printers and optional dot matrix printer-plotter. Using 100 μL of whole blood per sample, the instrument cycles at 80 samples per hour for CBC and platelet count or 60 samples per hour, including the leukocyte differential count. Single-specimen closed-tube aspiration or walk-away automated closed-tube sampling is optional.

The H*1 uses a tungsten halogen light source and cytometer for peroxidase analysis. Time required for this cytochemical reaction is decreased by heating to 75°C. The analyzer's computer also performs cluster analysis of the segregated cell types instead of applying rigid scatter and absorption thresholds. The mean peroxidase index (MPXI, reference interval −10 to +10), a measure of neutrophil-staining intensity, is also determined for each specimen. This enables detection of patients with congenital or acquired myeloperoxidase deficiency (Ross, 1985a). The top right-hand section of Figure 24–8*C* shows a typical normal peroxidase plot from the H*1. Leukocytes are further analyzed in a separate channel (basophil/lobularity) using a helium-neon red laser light source with detectors at a low and higher angle of scatter. In the basophil/lobularity channel, a diluent containing surfactant and phthalic acid lyses the erythrocytes and strips away the cytoplasm from all cells except basophils (Simson, 1986). On the y-axis, the signal from the low-angle (2 to 3 degrees) forward scatter detector is plotted. Basophils are counted because they retain their cytoplasm and therefore exceed the horizontal threshold. On the x-axis, the higher angle (5 to 15 degrees) detector signal is plotted. This signal is affected by the shape and structure (density) of the remaining nuclei. Mononuclear cells fall to the left, and cells with

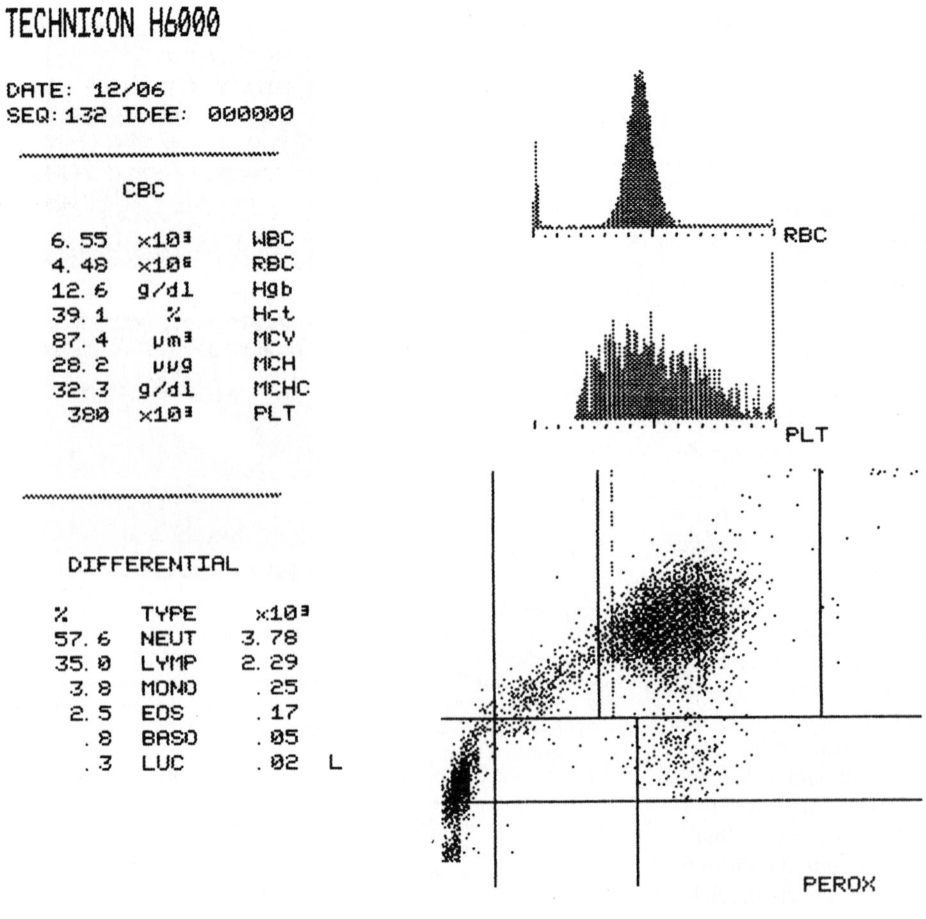
TECHNICON H6000
DATE: 12/06
SEQ: 132 IDEE: 000000
CBC
6. 55 x10³ WBC
4. 48 x10⁶ RBC
12. 6 g/dl Hgb
39. 1 % Hct
87. 4 µm³ MCV
28. 2 µµg MCH
32. 3 g/dl MCHC
380 x10³ PLT
DIFFERENTIAL
% TYPE x10³
57. 6 NEUT 3. 78
35. 0 LYMP 2. 29
3. 8 MONO . 25
2. 5 EOS . 17
. 8 BASO . 05
. 3 LUC . 02 L
RBC
PLT
PEROX

Figure 24–13. Printout from the Technicon H-6000 includes the six RBC measurements and the WBC and platelet counts; the size distributions of the RBCs and platelets; the differential leukocyte count listed as percentage and as absolute counts (cells × $10^3/\mu$L); and the scatter versus absorption display of leukocytes in the peroxidase channel. In the latter display (which provides most of the information for classifying the leukocytes), the horizontal lines represent low and high thresholds for light scatter and the vertical lines represent thresholds for light absorbance. See Figure 24–12 for further details.

successively more structured or lobulated nuclei fall to the right, separated by a vertical threshold. Blasts are usually shifted farthest to the left, followed as one moves to the right on the x-axis by lymphocytes and monocytes (immature granulocytes, if present, are also in the mononuclear area), bands, eosinophils, neutrophils, and nucleated red blood cells. The lower right-hand side of Figure 24–8*B* shows a basophil/lobularity plot from a normal person. Comparison and integration of the results from the peroxidase and basophil/lobularity channels enable specific flags for blasts, atypical lymphocytes, immature granulocytes, left shift, and NRBC (Bollinger, 1987; Schoentag, 1988).

The Coulter STKS and the Sysmex NE-8000 have been compared with the H*1 (Burns, 1992; Warner, 1990). Buttarello (1992, 1993) also adds the Abbott Cell Dyn 3000. All find the H*1 instrument to be acceptable as a CBC and leukocyte differential analyzer. The H*1 performed well in recognition of basophils (Burns, 1992; Warner, 1990). It also showed good correlation with the manual method for neutrophils, lymphocytes, monocytes, and eosinophils (Burns, 1992; Buttarello, 1992; Warner, 1990). The Technicon H*2 had a very low WBC differential rejection rate (1%) on the instrument (Bentley, 1992), mandating a rigorous review of results before reporting.

Clinical reports are favorable regarding the H*1's usefulness in detecting blasts in acute leukemia (Ialongo, 1993; Kline, 1989) and in distinguishing acute myeloblastic from acute lymphoblastic leukemias (Krause, 1988; Penchansky, 1991; Tsakona, 1992). Lanza (1992) showed that the large unstained cells (LUCs) and blasts in chronic B-lymphocytic leukemia correlated with survival and prognostic factors such as lymphoid subtypes. The H*1 may also help characterize myelodysplastic syndromes (Watson, 1987) and aid in the detection of infectious or inflammatory disease (Bentley, 1987; Wenz, 1987). In general, the instrument surpasses the screening capabilities of the routine manual eye count differential, especially when combined with other review criteria.

Total leukocytes also are counted in the basophil/lobularity channel as a check on the WBC count from the peroxidase channel. In cases of discrepancy between the two WBC counts (as can occur with incomplete RBC lysis in the peroxidase channel), the count from the basophil/lobularity channel is reported. Lack of complete erythrocyte lysis in the H-6000 peroxidase channel and therefore interference with the instrument total and differential leukocyte counts sometimes permit detection of abnormal hemoglobins, such as Hb C, S, E, and D.

RBC/platelet data are also derived using the laser-based optical system of the basophil/lobularity channel. The erythrocytes are converted into spheres (without change of volume) and lightly fixed with glutaraldehyde. This is necessary because laser light scatter is affected by shape. Once RBCs are spherical, low-angle scatter is a function of RBC size; from this, MCV and RDW as well as anisocytosis, microcytosis, and macrocytosis flags can be determined. High-angle scatter is primarily determined by the RBC density (hemoglobin concentration per cell). This permits flags for variation (VAR) in chromasia (anisochromia), hypochromia, and hyperchromia. Histograms of cell volume versus frequency and hemoglobin concentration versus frequency can therefore be produced. These histograms allow detection of abnormal erythroid populations that are present in small proportions. The RBC histograms are shown in the center of Figures 24–8*C* and 24–9C. The H*1 also calculates a hemoglobin distribution width (HDW) from the hemoglobin concentration data. With further clinical experience, this may prove to be a helpful parameter. Mohandas (1986) showed that anisochromia (increased HDW) occurs in sickle cell anemia, and Ballas (1988) showed that some erythrocytes in patients with Hb SC disease are hyperchromic and microcytic. Robertson (1992) showed that the H*1 erythrogram pattern is useful in screening for thalassemia. Gulley (1990) reports that high neutrophil myeloperoxidase activity (MPXI) on the H*1 is a simple and useful indicator of megaloblastic anemia, particularly when the MCV is below 100 fL. Ialongo (1989) reports that the hemoglobin concentration histogram is good at revealing the presence of a high percentage of hyperchromic microcytic red cells in hereditary spherocytosis; patients who have not undergone splenectomy showed the increase even more dramatically.

The (Miles) Technicon H*2 is faster, with a throughput of 100 CBCs and differentials per hour, and it allows one to choose either a cassette system or continuous feed for walk-away operation. Technicon claims accurate results for blood samples as old as 48 hours. The H*3 also adds automated reticulocyte analysis at 100 per hour and full-color workstation displays.

Platelets are enumerated in the RBC/PLT channel using a higher gain setting on the high-angle scatter detector. A platelet histogram from 0 to 20 fL is produced.

Abbott Diagnostics

CELL-DYN 3000

The Cell-Dyn 3000 is a multiparameter hematology analyzer that uses technology called Multi-Angle Polarized Scatter Separation (MAPSS) to perform the leukocyte differential count (Stroop, 1994). A laser beam is shaped into a wide profile and focused on a quartz flow cell. This beam shape makes laser alignment less critical than with other flow cytometers. Blood is diluted in a solution maintaining WBCs in a near native state but rendering RBCs transparent to the laser. Four simultaneous light scattering measurements are made on each white cell. Zero-degree forward angle is primarily determined by cell *size*. Ten-degree light scatter is an indicator of cell structure or *complexity* and is especially helpful to resolve basophils and separate all cell populations. Ninety-degree light scatter separates granulated cells and is called *lobularity*. Depolarized 90-degree light scattering resolves eosinophils because of their large crystalline *granularity*. Abnormal cells can have distinctive locations in the size-versus-complexity scatterplot and help to determine WBC suspect flags (Cornbleet, 1992) such as for blasts, variant lymphs, bands, and immature granulocytes. Figure 24–14 is a Cell-Dyn 3500 report from a patient with severe enteritis and a left shift including blasts.

The Cell-Dyn 3000 has been evaluated against the manual differential count (Cornbleet, 1992; van Leeuwen, 1991) and against the STKS, NE-8000, and H*1 and H*2 (Bentley, 1993; Buttarello, 1992, 1993). Van Leeuwen's (1991) evaluation shows good accuracy and reproducibility, with high sensitivity and fair specificity permitting a 70% decrease in leukocyte differential workload. Cornbleet (1992) showed 83% specificity for WBC flags and 82% sensitivity to detec-

4

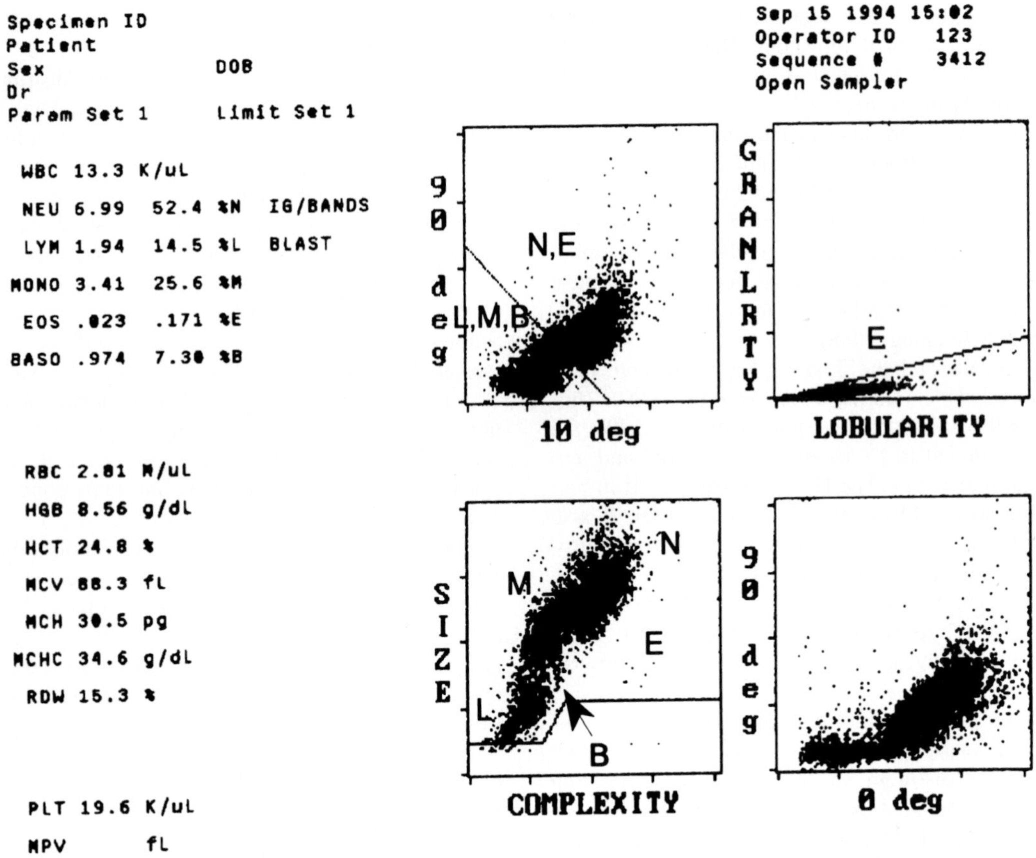

Figure 24–14. Abbott Cell-Dyn 3500. Patient with severe enteritis and left shift as far as blasts. Cell populations are labeled (N = neutrophil, E = eosinophil, L = lymphocyte, B = basophil, M = monocyte). Scatterplot of 90 degrees (lobularity) laser light scatter versus 10 degrees (complexity) separates neutrophils and eosinophils from other cells. Granularity (90 degrees depolarized) versus lobularity separates eosinophils. Size (10 degrees) versus complexity shows best spread of all cell types. Blasts, immature granulocytes and monocytosis were well reported; basophils were over called. Manual differential count: 4 blasts, 1 NRBC, 4 myelocytes, 1 metamyelocyte, 4 bands, 34 neutrophils, 21 lymphocytes, 27 monocytes, 1 eosinophil.

tion of more than 5% abnormal cells. Correlation coefficients for all cell types except basophils were good. The device's primary deficiency was in detecting less than 5% NRBCs, lymphoblasts, or hairy cells and more than 5% reactive lymphocytes. Flagging was also poor for bands with many false-positive and false-negative results. The Cell-Dyn 3000 had very low levels of WBC differential reject rates—0% in Bentley's (1993) study. Clinical sensitivity and ability to identify quantitative abnormalities was similar to those of the H*2, NE-8000, and STKS (Bentley, 1993). Buttarello (1993) showed a high morphologic false-positive rate (16%) for the instrument.

The latest in the series is the Cell-Dyn 3500. The unit is small and quiet. A confirmatory WBC count is based on aperture impedance analysis. It also has an automated sampler and enhanced database capabilities and a choice of four definable parameter sets for CRT display.

Calibration

A number of commercial calibrants (Baker, Coulter, Dade, Fisher, R + D) are available for calibrating hematology analyzers. The target values are assigned from instruments that are calibrated frequently with whole blood using reference procedures. These blood cell suspensions are generally suitable for calibration, provided that the manufacturer's instructions are rigorously followed. The success of the calibration process should be verified by running three level controls, checking the instrument results against reference procedures for a few specimens, and, if possible, closely monitoring $\bar{x}$B moving averages for the RBC indices (Bull, 1974). Calibration using the commercially available calibrants is much easier and faster than performing a complete whole blood calibration by replicate reference methods and in most laboratories probably yields a better end result.

If a commercial calibrant is not available, or if there is doubt about its validity, a whole blood calibration may be necessary. Details for one method of doing so follow.

Fresh normal blood should be used for calibration, as emphasized by Brittin (1969a) and Gilmer (1977). Hemoglobin is determined by the HiCN method, using a certified standard and photometer. Hematocrit is measured by the microhematocrit technique. Red cell counts and white cell counts are performed with single-channel analyzers. For RBCs, a 1:50,000 dilution is made in a single step to reduce error. A 2 μL ± 0.25% Microcap pipette is used to deliver the blood into 100 mL (±0.08) of Isoton in a volumetric flask. (Alternatively, 5 μL, 10 μL, or 20 μL pipettes of similar accuracy may be used to deliver blood into 250, 500, or 1000 mL of diluent, respectively.) The blood for the white cell count is diluted 1:500, again with a Microcap, 20 μL ± 0.25% of blood in 10 mL of Isoton.

Each of the preceding steps is performed in triplicate (each dilution is read in duplicate) on fresh blood from 10 to 20 normal persons. If desired, the hematocrit can be corrected by subtracting the average proportion of trapped plasma found in the hematocrits of normal persons (ICSH, 1980). This has been estimated to be between 1.5% and 3% (Dacie, 1991). If a 3% correction factor is used, for a hematocrit of 0.44, then 0.44 − 0.013 = 0.427. The red cell indices are then calculated. The white cell count is checked by performing duplicate hemacytometer or analyzer counts. The normal blood specimens are run in triplicate on the instrument, and the results are averaged. The difference between the values from the reference procedure and the hematology analyzer is determined for each specimen so that the percentage difference can be calculated. A normal specimen is then run on the analyzer, and the values are reset in the instrument by multiplying by the proper correction factor. For example, if the instrumental hemoglobin values were on the average 5% lower than the cyanmethemoglobin reference values, the instrumental hemoglobin would be multiplied by 1.05, and this value would be used to set the instrument. It is important that this calibration not be changed until a "drift" away from these values has been statistically demonstrated by quality control procedures. At that time, after any necessary maintenance work has been done, the instrument is recalibrated in the same fashion. The calibration settings should not be changed on the basis of a single determination of a control suspension of cells. Recent analyzers are stable; recalibration is usually unnecessary more often than every few months.

The method of calibration described gives values for red cell indices from the cell counters comparable with those calculated from the individual methods, except that the reference values reflect the slight difference due to correction of the hematocrit for trapped plasma. It is clear that in disorders in which trapped plasma is considerably increased (in the microhematocrit) owing to rigidity or shape of red cells, such as iron deficiency anemia and sickle-cell disease, the hematocrit and MCV are lower and the MCHC slightly higher with electronic analyzers than with conventional methods. The instrument probably gives the more correct values.

Quality Control

Commercially available blood cell control specimens may be used and charted every morning and at intervals during the day, but this is expensive and, alone, not entirely satisfactory. Brittin (1971) discussed this problem in his excellent review of instrumentation, and Brittin (1969b) presented a useful method for using patient blood samples in quality control. He demonstrated that all seven values (WBC, RBC, Hb, Hct, and indices) are stable in blood collected in EDTA for at least 24 hours at 4°C. At least 5 and preferably 10 specimens with hematologic values in the normal range are selected on day one, kept in the refrigerator, and re-analyzed on day two. A significant change in any channel between the two days can be detected statistically using the Student-t test for paired samples:

$$t_n = \frac{\bar{d}}{S_d}\sqrt{n}, \text{ with } n - 1 \text{ degrees of freedom} \qquad (24\text{-}11)$$

n = number of pairs of observations
$\bar{d}$ = mean of the differences (from day to day)
S_d = standard deviation of the differences

$$\text{or } = \sqrt{\frac{\Sigma(d^2) - \frac{(\Sigma d)^2}{n}}{n-1}} \qquad (24\text{-}12)$$

The t value is calculated for each parameter. If the calculated t value exceeds that critical value for the 95% limits found in a statistical table of t values, the difference is significant at the 5% level. For n = 5, the critical t value is 2.78. For example, if the t score calculated from the five pairs of white cell counts exceeds 2.78, one can be 95% confident that there is a significant difference between the two days. A significant t value should alert one to possible trouble, and persistently significant t scores in the same channel indicate the need for action. Often, simple inspection of the values will reveal whether the mean difference from one day to the next differs significantly from zero. The calculations can be easily programmed for a desktop computer, and it is helpful to chart the t values.

The tendency for drift throughout the day can be monitored by repeating this procedure twice a day or more simply by running two or three specimens from the first morning batch at intervals throughout the day.

This method will detect a developing loss of calibration, such as may be due to electronic drift. However, a significant loss of calibration that occurs more abruptly, owing to mechanical or electronic breakdown, may not be detected until the following day. Bull (1974, 1983) has shown that calculation of a moving average for the MCV, MCH, and MCHC of each successive 20 samples run on the analyzer throughout the day provides an effective, rapidly available indicator of loss of calibration. This indicator is based on the demonstrated constancy of the mean values for these indices in medium-sized to large hospitals from day to day and week to week. If the moving average changes by 3%, the calibration must be checked at once. Variations of this method, of increasing complexity, may be performed on a hand calculator or a programmable calculator or may be programmed into the laboratory computer system.

The quality control programs in the larger-volume multichannel hematology analyzers are comprehensive; patient and control values (including blood cell histograms) are stored in libraries. Moving averages of red cell indices are calculated every 20 samples and flagged when laboratory-defined limits are exceeded. This permits better and more frequent monitoring of instrumental function than day-to-day comparisons allow. Also helpful are delta checks (comparison with previous results for the same patient) and interlaboratory comparisons.

Sources of Error

Modern analyzers have carry-over of 1% or less, virtually eliminating this problem.

Increased white cell counts, over 30×10^9/L, usually produce a slight but significant false elevation of the hemoglobin as a result of turbidity. A very high white count can also elevate the hematocrit and the MCV because the white cells are counted and sized with the red cells.

England and colleagues (1976b) reviewed errors that influence the MCV determined by voltage pulse analysis. From their studies, it appears that if the MCV is calibrated in the normal range only, microcytic MCVs will be overestimated when compared with those determined by microhematocrits corrected for plasma trapping. They suggest that the MCV be calibrated with both small cells and normal-sized cells. High glucose concentrations (above 400 mg/dL) and hyperosmolality due to other causes may cause a spuriously high MCV and hematocrit but may cause low MCHC as measured on the Coulter Counters (Holt, 1982). Examples are diabetes, hypernatremia, and blood drawn distal to an intravenous glucose line. The probable mechanism is that when diluted in Isoton, the RBCs swell because Isoton is relatively hypotonic to the hypertonic blood sample. Incubating a 1:224 dilution (44.7 L blood plus 10 mL Isoton) for 10 minutes before analysis will correct the problem.

Cold agglutinins in high titer tend to give spurious macrocytosis and low red cell counts with impossibly high MCHCs (Hattersley, 1971). Warming the blood or the diluent eliminates this problem.

In some patients with leukemia, the white cells appear to be fragile and escape being counted, giving a falsely low count. Erroneously low white counts also occur in uremia or in some patients receiving immunosuppressive drugs (Luke, 1971). Hemacytometer counts should be used to check the white counts of such patients. Taft (1973) reported pseudoleukocytosis due to IgG or IgM paraprotein. Whenever the instrument leukocyte count is at odds with an estimate on the blood film, a hemacytometer count should be performed.

Very high lipid levels cause plasma turbidity, which falsely elevates the hemoglobin, MHC, and MCHC (Nosanchuk, 1974). Cyanmethemoglobin must be determined manually, using an appropriate volume of patient plasma in the blank to zero the spectrophotometer. To calculate the appropriate amount of Drabkin diluent to add to 20 μL of patient plasma to prepare a blank, use the following formula:

$$N = \frac{5\ \text{mL}}{(1 - \text{Hct})} \qquad (24\text{-}13)$$

where N = mL of Drabkin to be added to 20 μL of patient plasma. For example, if the patient has a hematocrit of 0.45,

$$N = \frac{5}{(1 - 0.45)} = \frac{5}{0.55} = 9.1\ \text{mL Drabkin} \qquad (24\text{-}14)$$

As an alternative, a hemoglobin reading can be determined on the patient's plasma, multiplied by the plasmacrit, and subtracted from the whole blood hemoglobin result.

Cornbleet (1983) summarizes many of the causes of spurious results from automated hematology cell analyzers (Table 24–3).

Reticulocyte Counts

Principle

Reticulocytes are immature non-nucleated red cells that contain ribonucleic acid (RNA) and continue to synthesize hemoglobin after loss of the nucleus. When blood is briefly incubated in a solution of new methylene blue or brilliant cresyl blue, the RNA is precipitated as a dye-ribonucleoprotein complex. Microscopically, the complex appears as a dark blue network (reticulum) or dark blue granules that allow reticulocytes to be identified and enumerated.

REAGENT

One percent new methylene blue in a diluent of citrate-saline (one part 30 g/L sodium citrate plus four parts 9 g/L sodium chloride).

Procedure

Three drops each of reagent and blood are mixed in a test tube, incubated 15 minutes at room temperature, and remixed.

Two wedge films are made on glass slides and air dried.

Viewed microscopically with an oil-immersion lens, reticulocytes are pale blue and contain dark blue reticular or granular material (Fig. 24–15), and red cells stain pale blue or blue-green.

The percentage of reticulocytes is determined in at least 1000 red cells. A Miller disc inserted in the eyepiece allows rapid estimation of large numbers of red cells by imposing two squares (one square is nine times the area of the other square) onto the field of view (Brecher, 1950). Reticulocytes are counted in the large square and red cells in the small square in successive microscopic fields until at least 300 red cells are counted. This process estimates reticulocytes among at least 2700 red cells, as follows:

$$\text{Reticulocytes (percent)} = \frac{\text{No. reticulocytes in large square}}{\text{No. red cells in small square} \times 9} \times 100 \qquad (24\text{-}15)$$

The absolute reticulocyte count is determined by multiplying the reticulocyte percentage by the red cell count.

Reference Values

Normal adults have a reticulocyte count of 0.5% to 1.5% or 24 to 84×10^9/L. In newborn infants, the percentage is 2.5% to 6.5%; this falls to the adult range by the end of the second week of life.

Interpretation

Because reticulocytes are immature red cells that lose their RNA a day or so after reaching the blood from the marrow, a reticulocyte estimates the rate of red cell production. An absolute reticulocyte count or reticulocyte production index is more helpful than the percentage (see Chap. 25).

Sources of Variation

Because such a small number of actual reticulocytes are counted, the sampling error in the reticulocyte count is relatively large. The 95% confidence limits may be expressed as follows:

$$R \pm 2\sqrt{\frac{R(100 - R)}{N}} \qquad (24\text{-}16)$$

where R is the reticulocyte count in percent and N is the number of erythrocytes examined. This means that if only 1000 erythrocytes are evaluated, the 95% confidence limits

Table 24–3. POTENTIAL CAUSES OF ERRONEOUS RESULTS WITH AUTOMATED CELL COUNTERS

Parameter	Causes of Spurious Increase	Causes of Spurious Decrease
WBC	Cryoglobulin, cryofibrinogen Heparin Monoclonal proteins Nucleated red cells Platelet clumping Unlysed red cells	Clotting Smudge cells Uremia plus immunosuppressants
RBC	Cryoglobulin, cryofibrinogen Giant platelets High WBC (>50,000/μL)	Autoagglutination Clotting Hemolysis (*in vitro*) Microcytic red cells
Hemoglobin	Carboxyhemoglobin (>10%) Cryoglobulin, cryofibrinogen Hemolysis (*in vitro*) Heparin High WBC (>50,000/μL) Hyperbilirubinemia Lipemia Monoclonal proteins	Clotting Sulfhemoglobin (?)
Hematocrit (automated)	Cryoglobulin, cryofibrinogen Giant platelets High WBC (>50,000/μL) Hyperglycemia (>600 mg/dL)	Autoagglutination Clotting Hemolysis (*in vitro*) Microcytic red cells
Hematocrit (Microhematocrit)	Hyponatremia Plasma trapping	Excess EDTA Hemolysis (*in vitro*) Hypernatremia
MCV	Autoagglutination High WBC (>50,000/μL) Hyperglycemia Reduced red cell deformability	Cryoglobulin, cryofibrinogen Giant platelets Hemolysis (*in vitro*) Microcytic red cells Swollen red cells
MCH	High WBC (>50,000/μL) Spuriously high Hgb Spuriously low RBC	Spuriously low Hgb Spuriously high RBC
MCHC	Autoagglutination Clotting Hemolysis (*in vitro*) Hemolysis (*in vivo*) Spuriously high Hgb Spuriously low Hct	High WBC (>50,000/μL) Spuriously low Hgb Spuriously high Hct
Platelets	Cryoglobulin, cryofibrinogen Hemolysis (*in vitro* and *in vivo*) Microcytic red cells Red cell inclusions White cell fragments	Clotting Giant platelets Heparin Platelet clumping Platelet satellitosis

From Cornbleet J: Spurious results from automated hematology cell analyzers. Lab Med 1983; 14:509.

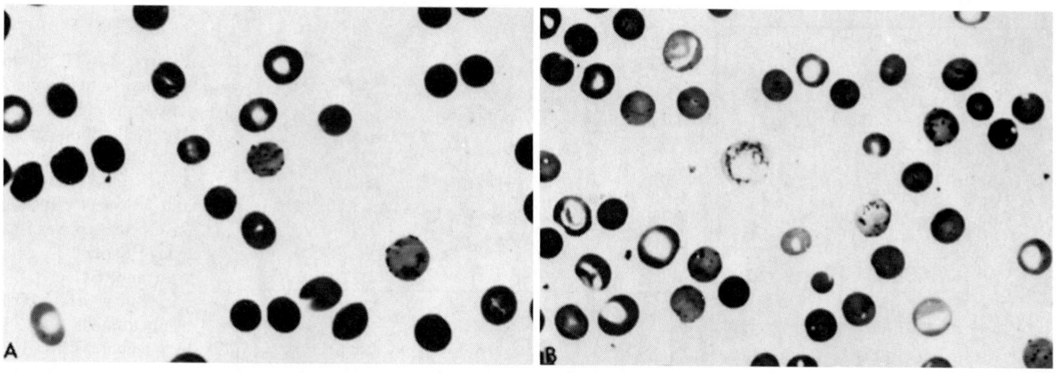

Figure 24–15. Reticulocytes; on air-dried film made after vital staining of blood with new methylene blue dye. RNA precipitates with the dye and appears as blue granules, which are sometimes connected into a network of reticulum.

4

for a 1% count are 0.4% to 1.6%; for a 5% count, 3.6% to 6.4%; and for a 10% count, 8.1% to 11.9%.

Flow cytometric counting of reticulocytes is now practical when instrumentation is available. Fluorescent dyes such as acridine orange or thioflavin T bind to the RNA and allow detection of reticulocytes; large numbers of cells counted result in enhanced precision and increased accuracy in routine practice (Metzger, 1987).

Thiazole orange fluorescent dye can be used to bind to RNA in reticulocytes, and 10,000 to 50,000 cells can be simply and quickly counted on the Beckton-Dickinson FACScan (Pappas, 1992). Results normally correlate well with those of the manual procedure, with a similar reference interval but much better precision. With this instrument and technique, however, results may be falsely high in the presence of Howell-Jolly bodies, NRBCs, sickled cells, or giant platelets (Lofsness, 1994; Pappas, 1992). TOA markets a stand-alone automated reticulocyte analyzer, the Sysmex R-1000, with 5 to 10 times improved precision (Batjer, 1994; Tichelli, 1990). The Sysmex R-1000 uses auramine-O and provides automated aspiration, dilution, incubation, and measurement. TOA claims that a high-level fluorescent discriminator eliminates interference by the inclusions above. Using laser light, the instrument measures and plots fluorescent intensity (staining) versus forward scatter intensity (size)—see Figure 24–16. Reticulocytes are grouped into low, middle, and high fluorescent ratio (LFR, MFR, HFR). Precise flow cytometer reticulocyte counts permit earlier detection of recovery or engraftment after bone marrow transplant (Batjer, 1994; Lazarus, 1992). The Sysmex R-3000 provides automated, closed-container walk-away reticulocyte determination at 80 samples per hour.

The Miles (Technicon) H*3 analyzes blood stained off-line (15-minute to 90-minute incubation) with oxazine 750 dye. For each RBC and reticulocyte, the cytometer determines volume, hemoglobin content, hemoglobin concentration, and fluorescent staining by simultaneous measurement of low-angle scatter, high-angle scatter, and absorption (Fig. 24–17). Brugnara (1994a) showed that measurement of reticulocyte cell hemoglobin content can be a useful early indicator of iron-deficient erythropoiesis and of response to iron therapy (Brugnara, 1994b).

BLOOD FILM EXAMINATION

Making and Staining Blood Films

Examination of the blood film is an important part of the hematologic evaluation. The reliability of the information obtained depends heavily on systematic examination of well-made and well-stained films. Blood films should be prepared immediately if possible.

Three methods of making films are described here: the two-slide or wedge method, the coverglass method, and the spinner method.

Wedge Method

Place a drop of blood 2 to 3 mm in diameter about 1 cm from the end of a clean, dust-free slide that is on a flat surface. With the thumb and forefinger of the right hand, hold the end of a second (spreader) slide against the surface of the first slide at an angle of 30 to 45 degrees and draw it back to contact the drop of blood. Allow the blood to spread and film the angle between the two slides. Push the spreader slide at a moderate speed forward until all the blood has been spread into a moderately thin film. The spreader slide should be clean, dry, and slightly narrower than the first slide so that the edges can be easily examined with the microscope.

The slides should be rapidly air dried by waving the slides or with an electric fan. The thickness of the film can be adjusted by changing the angle of the spreader slide or the speed of spreading or by using a smaller or larger drop of blood. At a given speed, increasing the angle of the spreader slide will increase the thickness of the film. At a given angle, increasing the speed with which the spreader slide is pushed will also increase the thickness of the film. The film should not cover the entire surface of the slide. In a good film, there is a thick portion and a thin portion and a gradual transition from one to the other. The film should have a smooth, even appearance and be free from ridges, waves, or holes. The edge of the spreader must be absolutely smooth. If it is rough, the film has ragged tails containing many leukocytes.

In films of optimal thickness, there is some overlap of red cells in much of the film but even distribution and separation of red cells toward the thin tail. The faster the film is air dried,

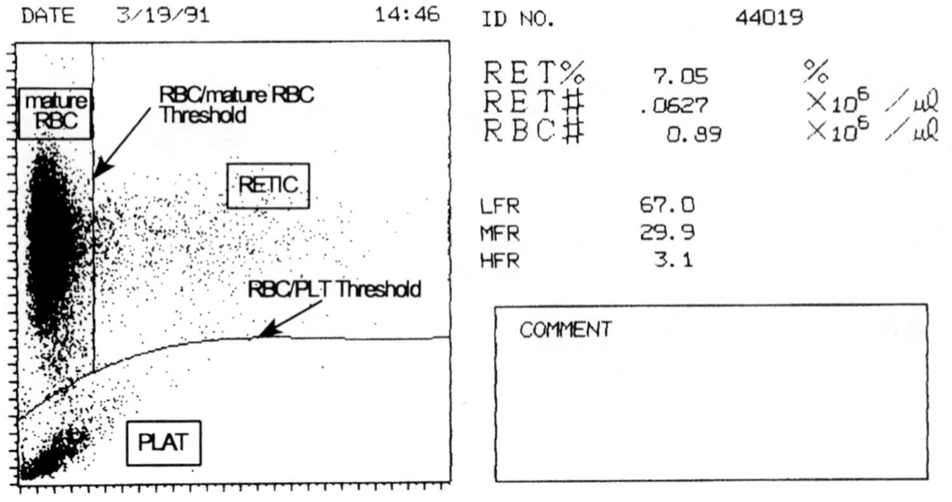

Figure 24–16. Sysmex R-1000 automated Reticulocyte Analyzer. Scattergram using auramine-o fluorescent dye. Cell volume as a function of forward angle laser light intensity on the Y axis and fluorescence on the X axis. Note thresholds separating RBCs and platelets from reticulocytes. Patient is extremely anemic with an RBC of $0.89 \times 10^6/\mu L$, but the patient has 7.05% reticulocytes by instrument, was 7.9% determined by manual Miller disc method with new methylene blue N.

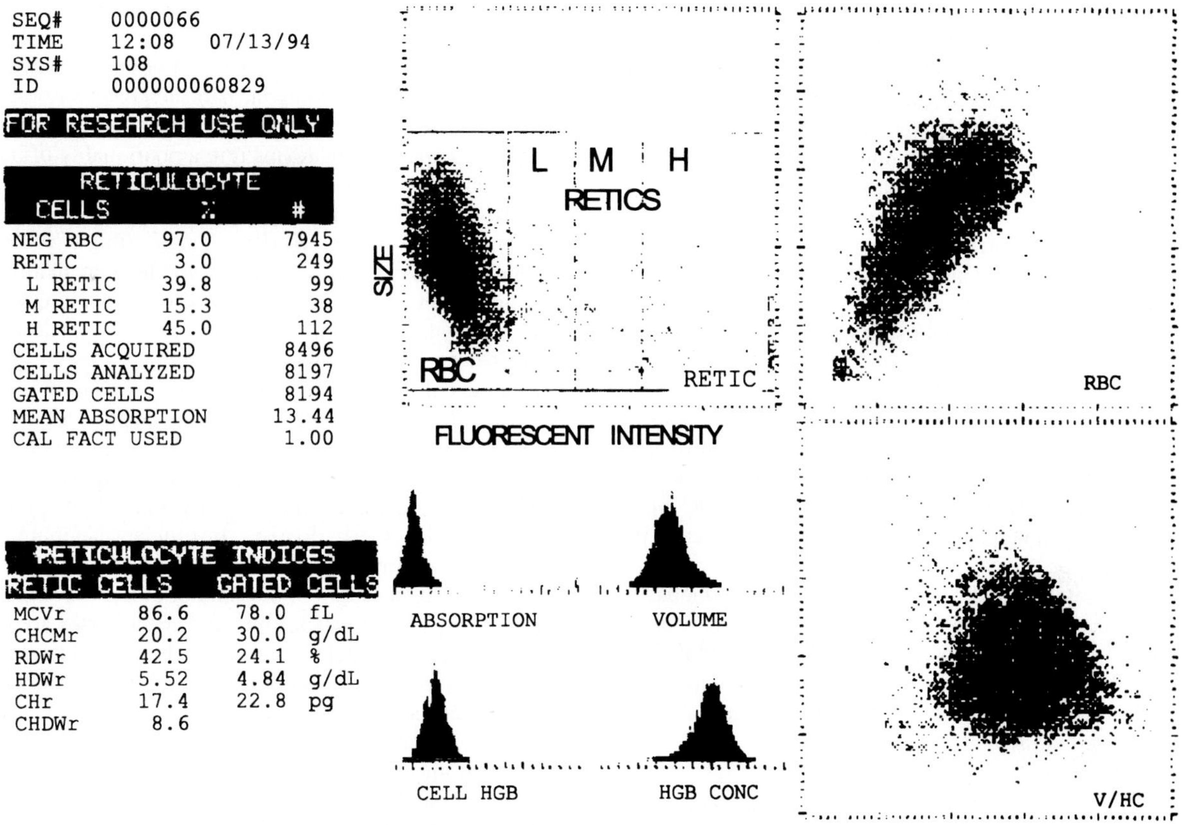

Figure 24–17. Miles H*3 reticulocyte analysis using off-line incubation of 3 μL whole blood added to a prepackaged single-test vial containing Oxazine 750 dye. The reticulocyte mode on the H*3 is called up and the incubated sample aspirated through the probe. Size on Y axis and fluorescence on X axis. Instrument printout shows percent and absolute reticulocyte count and low, medium, and high fluorescence intensity populations of reticulocytes. H*3 also shows MCV, hemoglobin concentration per cell and RDW for mature RBCs and reticulocytes.

the better the spreading of the individual cells on the slide. Slow drying (in humid weather, for example) results in contraction artifacts of the cells.

The slide may be labeled with a lead pencil on the frosted end or directly on the thicker end of the blood film.

Coverglass Method

No. 1 or 1½ coverglasses, 22 mm square, are recommended.

Touch a coverglass to the top of a small drop of blood without touching the skin and place it, blood side down, crosswise on another coverglass so that the corners appear as an eight-pointed star. If the drop is not too large and if the coverglasses are perfectly clean, the blood will spread out evenly and quickly in a thin layer between the two surfaces. Just as it stops spreading, pull the coverglasses quickly but firmly apart on a plane parallel to their surfaces. The blood usually is much more evenly spread on one of the coverglasses than it is on the other. Coverglasses should be placed film side up on clean paper and allowed to dry in the air, or they may be inserted back to back in slits made in a cardboard box.

Films from venous blood may be prepared similarly by placing a drop of blood on a coverslip and proceeding as described.

Spinner Method

Blood films that combine the advantages of easy handling of the wedge slide and uniform distribution of cells of the coverglass preparation may be made with special types of centrifuges known as spinners (Rogers, 1973).

The spinner slide produces a uniform blood film, in which all cells are separated (a monolayer) and randomly distributed. White cells can be easily identified at any spot in the film. A wedge smear has a disproportion of monocytes at the tip of the feather edge, of neutrophils just in from the feather edge, and of both at the lateral edges of the film (Rogers, 1973). This is of little practical significance, but it does result in slightly lower monocyte counts in wedge films.

Blood Stains

The aniline dyes used in blood work are of two general classes: basic dyes, such as methylene blue, and acid dyes, such as eosin. Nuclei and certain other structures in the blood are stained by the basic dyes and, hence, are called basophilic. Structures that take up only acid dyes are called acidophilic or eosinophilic. Other structures stained by a combination of the two are called neutrophilic.

Polychrome methylene blue and eosin stains are the outgrowth of the original time-consuming Romanowsky method and are widely used. They differentially stain most normal and abnormal structures in the blood.

The thiazine's basic components consist of methylene blue (tetramethylthionine) and, in varying proportions, its analogues produced by oxidative demethylation: azure B (trimethylthionine); azure A (asymmetric dimethylthionine); symmetric dimethylthionine; and azure C (monomethylthionine) (Lillie, 1977). The acidic component, eosin, is derived from a xanthene skeleton.

Most Romanowsky stains are dissolved in methyl alcohol and combine fixation with staining. Among the best known methods are Giemsa and Wright stains.

WRIGHT STAIN

This is a methyl alcoholic solution of eosin and a complex mixture of thiazines, including methylene blue (usually 50% to 75%), azure B (10% to 25%), and other derivatives (Lubrano, 1977). Wright stain certified by the Biological Stain Commission is commercially available as a solution ready for use or as a powder.

The buffer solution (pH 6.4) contains primary (monobasic) potassium phosphate (KH_2PO_4), anhydrous 6.63 g; secondary (dibasic) sodium phosphate (Na_2HPO_4), anhydrous 2.56 g; and distilled water to make 1 L. A more alkaline buffer (pH 6.7) may be prepared by using 5.13 g of the potassium salt and 4.12 g of the sodium salt.

PROCEDURE

1. To prevent the plasma background of the film from staining blue, blood films should be stained within a few hours of preparation or fixed if they must be kept without staining.
2. Fixation and staining may be accomplished by immersing the slides in reagent-filled jars or by covering horizontally supported slides or coverslips with the reagents. In the latter method, covering the film with copious stain avoids evaporation, which leads to precipitation.
3. Fixation is for one to two minutes with absolute methanol.
4. The slide is next exposed to undiluted stain solution for two minutes. Then, without removing the stain from the horizontal slide, an equal amount of buffer is carefully added and mixed by blowing gently.
5. The stain is flushed from the horizontal slide with water. Washing for more than 30 seconds reduces the blue staining. The back of the slide is cleaned with gauze.
6. The slide is allowed to air-dry in a tilted position.
7. Coverglasses are mounted film side down on a slide with Canada balsam or other mounting medium.

Films stained well with Wright stain have a pink color when viewed with the naked eye. Under low power, the cells should be evenly distributed. The red cells are pink, not lemon yellow or red. There should be a minimum of precipitate. The color of the film should be uniform. The blood cells should be free from artifacts, such as vacuoles. The nuclei of leukocytes are purple, the chromatin and parachromatin clearly differentiated, and the cytoplasmic neutrophilic granules tan in color. The eosinophilic granules are red-orange and each is distinctly discernible.

The basophil has dark purple granules. Platelets have dark lilac granules. Bacteria (if present) are blue. The cytoplasm of lymphocytes is generally light blue; that of the monocytes has a faint blue-gray tinge. Malarial parasites have sky-blue cytoplasm and red-purple chromatin. The colors are prone to fade if the preparation is mounted in a poor quality of balsam or exposed to the light.

STAINING PROBLEMS

Excessively Blue Stain. Thick films, prolonged staining time, inadequate washing, or too high an alkalinity of stain or diluent tends to cause excessive basophilia. In such films, the erythrocytes appear blue or green, the nuclear chromatin is deep blue to black, and the granules of the neutrophils are deeply overstained and appear large and prominent. The granules of the eosinophils are blue or gray. Staining for less time or using less stain and more diluent may correct the problem. If these steps are ineffective, the buffer may be too alkaline, and a new one with a lower pH should be prepared.

Excessively Pink Stain. Insufficient staining, prolonged washing time, mounting the coverslips before they are dry, or too high an acidity of the stain or buffer may cause excessive acidophilia. In such films, the erythrocytes are bright red or orange, the nuclear chromatin is pale blue, and the granules of the eosinophils are sparkling brilliant red. One of the causes of the increased acidity is exposure of the stain or buffer to acid fumes. The problem may be a low pH of the buffer, or it may be the methyl alcohol, which is prone to develop formic acid as a result of oxidation on standing.

Other Staining Problems. Inadequately stained red cells, nuclei, or eosinophilic granules may be due to understaining or excessive washing. Prolonging the staining or reducing the washing may solve the problem.

Precipitate on the film may be due to unclean slides; drying during the period of staining; inadequate washing of the slide at the end of the staining period, especially failure to hold the slide horizontally during initial washing; inadequate filtration of the stain; or dust settled on the slide or smear.

OTHER STAINS

Besides Wright stain, Romanowsky-type stains include a number of others: Giemsa, Leishman, Jenner, May-Grünwald, MacNeal, and various combinations. Some have been particularly recommended for certain purposes, such as Giemsa stain for excellence in staining malarial parasites and protozoa.

REFERENCE METHOD

Studies have demonstrated the ability of the combination of just two dyes—azure B and eosin Y—to give the full range of colors provided by ideal Romanowsky staining of blood and marrow cells. This is the reference method for Romanowsky staining (ICSH, 1984).

Erythrocytes

In the blood from a healthy person, the erythrocytes, when not crowded together, appear as circular, homogeneous discs of nearly uniform size, ranging from 6 to 8 μm in diameter (Fig. 24–18). However, even in normal blood, individual cells may be as small as 5.5 μm and as large as 9.5 μm. The

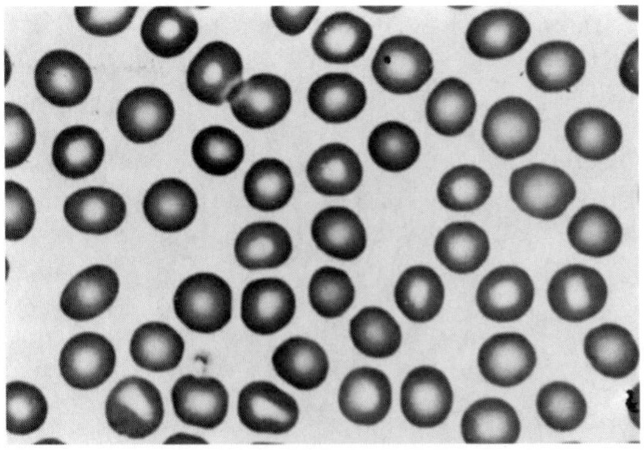

Figure 24–18. Normal blood film (×875).

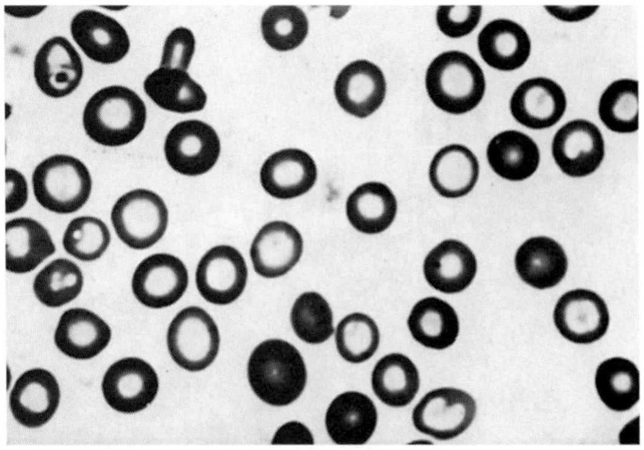

Figure 24–20. Iron-deficiency anemia. Most of the cells are hypochromic and microcytic. Note elliptical cells. Anisocytosis is slight in degree (×875).

center of each is somewhat paler than the periphery. In disease, erythrocytes vary in their hemoglobin content, size, shape, staining properties, and structure.

Color

HEMOGLOBIN CONTENT

The depth of staining furnishes a rough guide to the amount of hemoglobin in red cells, and the terms normochromic, hypochromic, and hyperchromic are used to describe this feature of red cells. *Normochromic* refers to normal intensity of staining (Figs. 24–18 and 24–19). When the amount of hemoglobin is diminished, the central pale area becomes larger and paler. This is known as *hypochromia.* The MCH and MCHC are usually decreased (Fig. 24–20). In megaloblastic anemia, because the red cells are larger and hence thicker, many stain deeply and have less central pallor (Figs. 24–21 and 24–22). These cells are *hyperchromic* because they have an increased hemoglobin content (MCH), but the hemoglobin concentration (MCHC) is normal. In hereditary spherocytosis, the cells are also hyperchromic (Fig. 24–23); though the hemoglobin content (MCH) is normal, the hemoglobin concentration (MCHC) is usually increased because of a reduced surface/volume ratio.

The presence of hypochromic cells and normochromic cells in the same film is called *anisochromia* or, sometimes, dimorphic anemia (Fig. 24–24). This is characteristic of sideroblastic anemias but also is found some weeks after iron therapy for iron-deficiency anemia or in a hypochromic anemia after transfusion with normal cells.

POLYCHROMATOPHILIA

A blue-gray tint to the red cells (polychromatophilia or polychromasia) is a combination of the affinity of hemoglobin for acid stains and the affinity of RNA for basic stains. The presence of residual RNA in the red cell indicates that it is a young red cell that has been in the blood for one to two days. These cells are larger than the mature red cells and may lack the central pallor (Fig. 24–25). Young cells with residual RNA are polychromatophilic red cells on air-dried films stained with Wright stain but are reticulocytes when stained supravitally with brilliant cresyl blue. Therefore, increased polychromasia implies reticulocytosis; it is most marked in hemolysis and in acute blood loss.

Size

The red cells may be abnormally small, or *microcytes* (see Figs. 24–20, 24–22, and 24–26); they may be abnormally large, or *macrocytes* (see Figs. 24–21, 24–22, and 24–24);

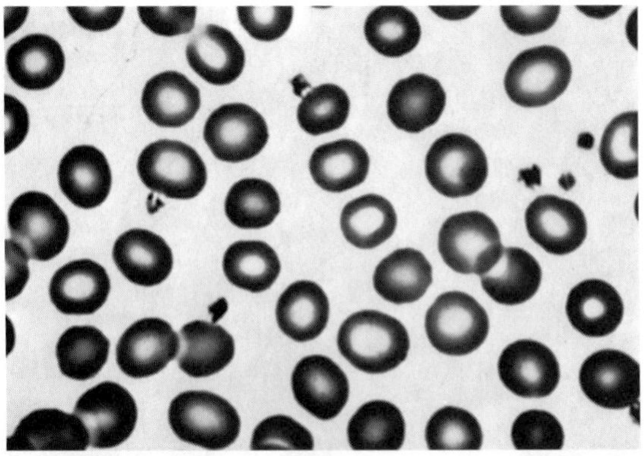

Figure 24–19. This blood film shows a small number of slightly hypochromic red cells; most are normochromic. Cell diameters are normal. MCV and MCHC are normal. The irregular bodies 2 to 3 μm in diameter are normal blood platelets (×875).

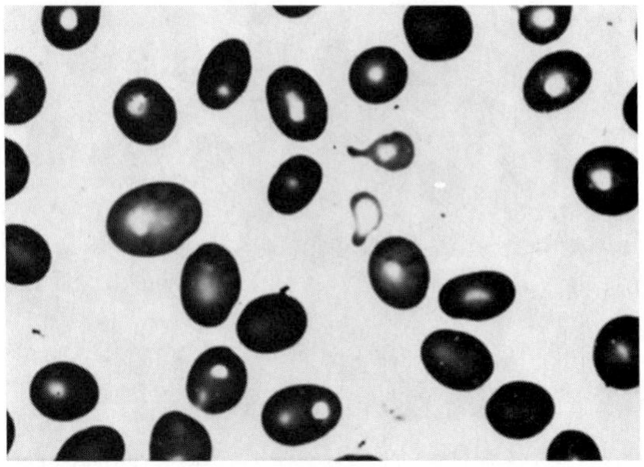

Figure 24–21. Megaloblastic anemia. Macrocytosis. Marked anisocytosis. Note elliptical cells and teardrop-shaped cells (×875).

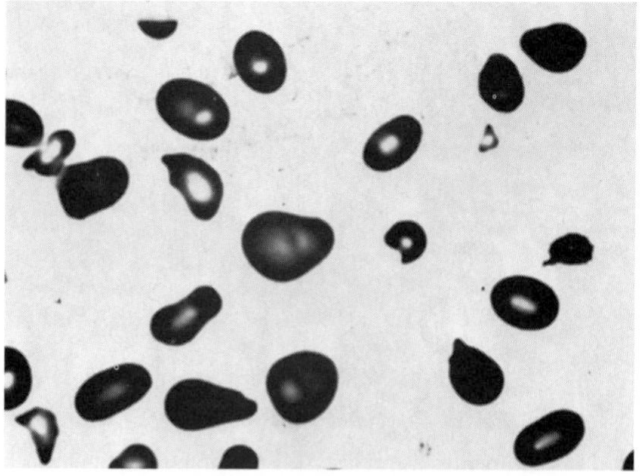

Figure 24–22. Megaloblastic anemia, macrocytosis, marked anisocytosis (×875).

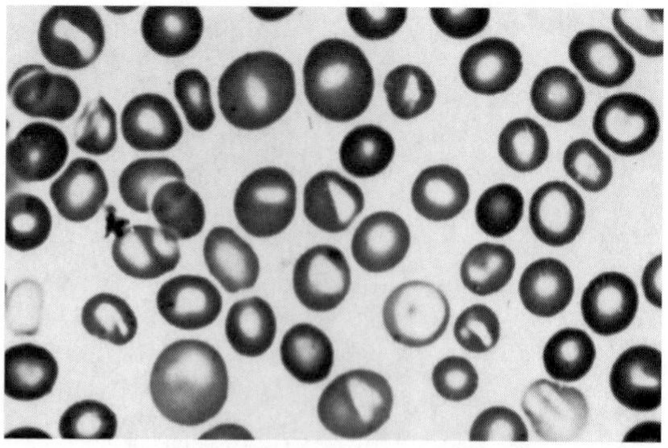

Figure 24–24. Sideroblastic anemia. Dimorphic populations of hypochromic cells and normochromic cells, some of which are macrocytic. Moderate anisocytosis (×875).

or they may show abnormal variation in size *(anisocytosis)* (see Figs. 24–20 through 24–26). Anisocytosis is a feature of most anemias; when it is marked in degree, both macrocytes and microcytes are usually present (see Figs. 24–21 and 24–22). In analyzing causes of anemia, the terms *microcytic* and *macrocytic* have most meaning when considered in terms of cell volume rather than cell diameter. The mean cell volume is measured directly on a multichannel analyzer. We perceive the diameter directly from the blood film and infer volume (and the hemoglobin content) from it. Thus, the red cells in Figure 24–20 are microcytic; because they are hypochromic, they are thinner than normal and the diameter is not decreased proportionately to the volume. Also, the mean cell volume in the blood of the patient with spherocytosis (see Fig. 24–25) is in the normal range; though many of the cells have a small diameter, their volume is not decreased because they are thicker than normal.

Shape

Variation in shape is called *poikilocytosis.* Any abnormally shaped cell is a poikilocyte. Oval, pear-shaped, teardrop-shaped, saddle-shaped, helmet-shaped, and irregularly shaped cells may be seen in a single case of anemia such as megaloblastic anemia (see Figs. 24–21 and 24–22).

Elliptocytes are most abundant in hereditary elliptocytosis

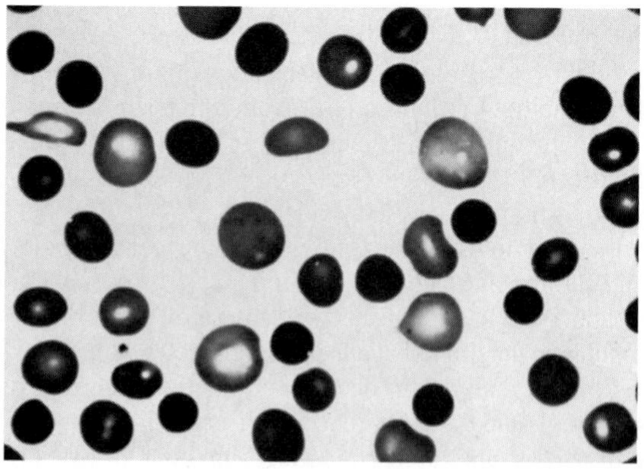

Figure 24–25. Autoimmune hemolytic anemia. The paler, large cells are polychromatic macrocytes (i.e., young reticulocytes.) The small, dense cells are spherocytes. Moderate anisocytosis (×875).

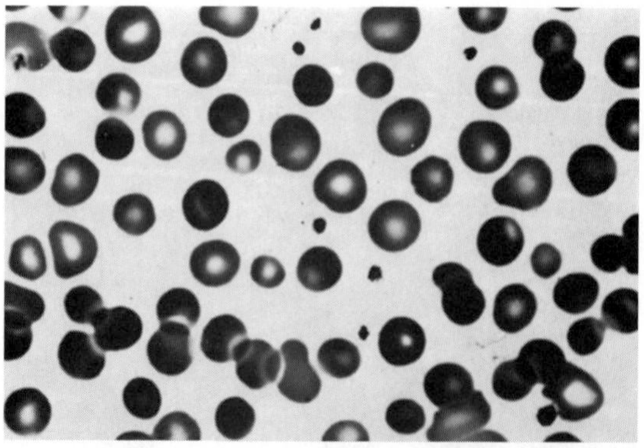

Figure 24–23. Hereditary spherocytosis. The denser cells are more spherocytic. Note that they have minimal and eccentric pallor, moderate anisocytosis. Although the cell diameter is reduced, the MCV is within the normal range (×875).

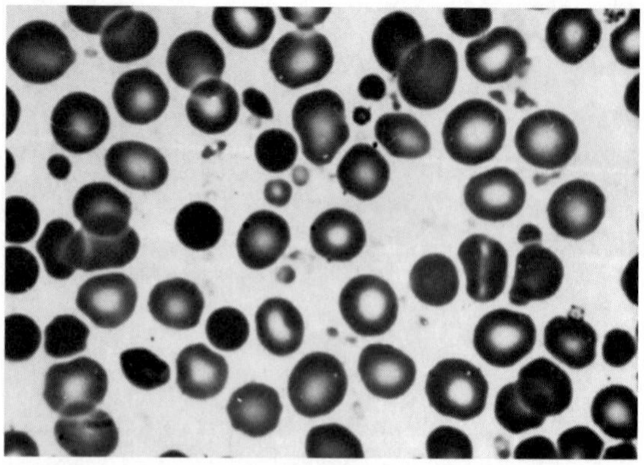

Figure 24–26. Blood film from a patient who has just suffered extensive body burns. Note the many tiny red cell fragments that have budded off the red cells as a result of the heat, leaving spherocytes. Marked anisocytosis (×875).

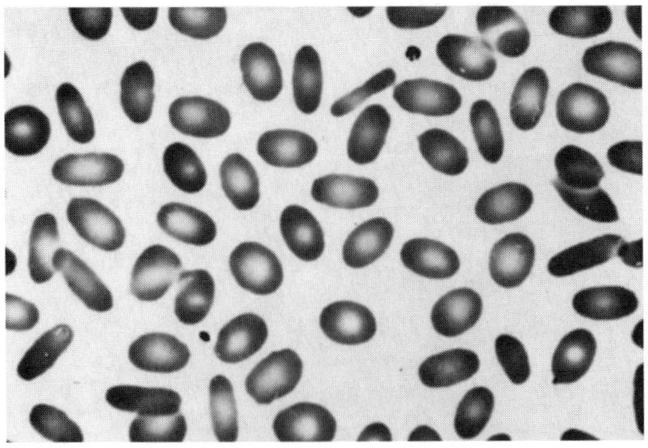

Figure 24–27. Hereditary elliptocytosis. Incidental finding, no anemia (×875).

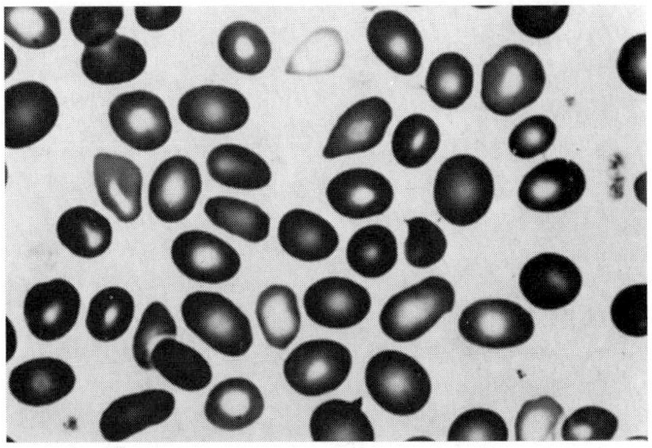

Figure 24–29. Same specimen as shown in Figure 24–28. A few hypochromic microcytic cells are present also (×875).

(Fig. 24–27), in which most of the cells are elliptical; this is a dominant condition that is only occasionally associated with hemolytic anemia. Elliptocytes are seen in normal persons' blood but account for less than 10% of the cells. They are more common, however, in iron-deficiency anemia, myelofibrosis with myeloid metaplasia (Figs. 24–28 and 24–29), megaloblastic anemias (see Figs. 24–21 and 24–22), and sickle cell anemia.

Spherocytes are nearly spherical erythrocytes in contradistinction to normal biconcave discs. Their diameter is smaller than normal. They lack the central pale area or have a smaller, often eccentric, pale area (because the cell is thicker and can come to rest somewhat tilted instead of perfectly flattened on the slide). They are found in hereditary spherocytosis (HS, see Fig. 24–23), in some cases of autoimmune hemolytic anemia (AHA, see Fig. 24–25), and in some conditions in which there has been a direct physical or chemical injury to the cells, such as heat (see Fig. 24–26). In each of these three instances, tiny bits of membrane (in excess of hemoglobin) are removed from the adult red cells, leaving the cell with a decreased surface/volume ratio. In HS and AHA, this occurs in the reticuloendothelial system; in other instances (e.g., the patient with body burns), this may occur intravascularly.

Target cells are erythrocytes that are thinner than normal (leptocytes) and when stained show a peripheral rim of hemoglobin with a dark, central, hemoglobin-containing area. They are found in obstructive jaundice (Fig. 24–30), in which there appears to be an augmentation of the cell surface membrane; following splenectomy, when there is a lack of normal reduction of surface membrane as the cell ages; in any hypochromic anemia, especially thalassemia; and in hemoglobin C disease.

Schistocytes (cell fragments) indicate the presence of hemolysis, whether in megaloblastic anemia (see Fig. 24–22), severe burns (see Fig. 24–26), or microangiopathic hemolytic anemia (Fig. 24– 31). The latter process is associated with either small blood vessel disease or fibrin in small blood vessels and results in intravascular fragmentation; particularly characteristic are helmet cells and triangularly shaped cells. Burr cells are irregularly contracted red cells with prominent spicules and are seen in the same process; however, this term is used differently by different hematologists and therefore leads to confusion.

Acanthocytes are irregularly spiculated red cells in which the ends of the spicules are bulbous and rounded (Fig. 24–32); they are seen in abetalipoproteinemia, hereditary or acquired, and in certain cases of liver disease. *Crenated cells,* or echinocytes (Fig. 24–33), are regularly contracted cells that commonly occur as an artifact during preparation of films or that may be due to hyperosmolarity or to the discocyte-echinocyte transformation. *In vivo,* the latter may be associated with decreased red cell ATP as a result of any of several causes.

Artifacts resembling crenated cells consisting of tiny pits

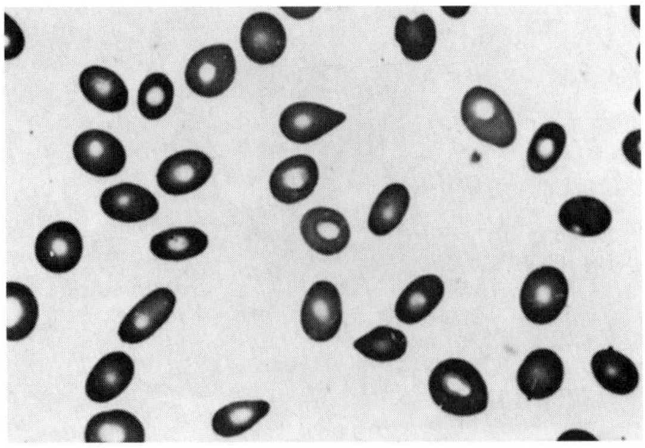

Figure 24–28. Blood film from patient with myelofibrosis with myeloid metaplasia. Numerous elliptocytes. Teardrop-shaped cells (×875).

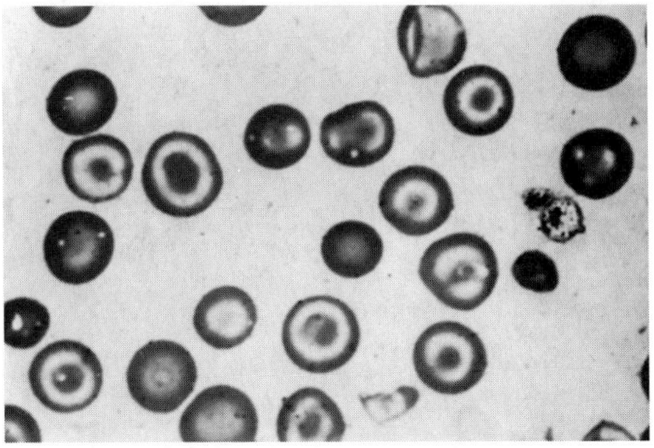

Figure 24–30. Target cells that have an increased cell diameter. Blood film from a patient with obstructive jaundice (×875).

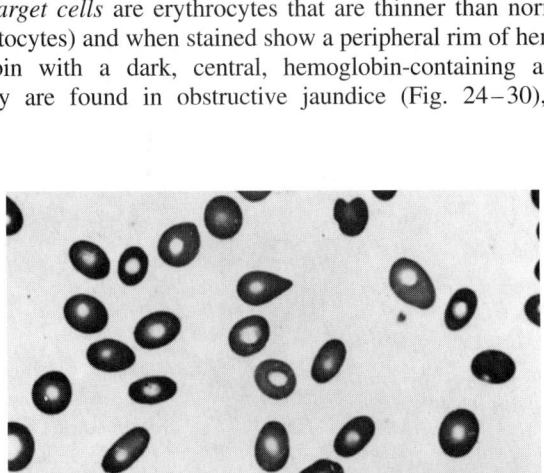

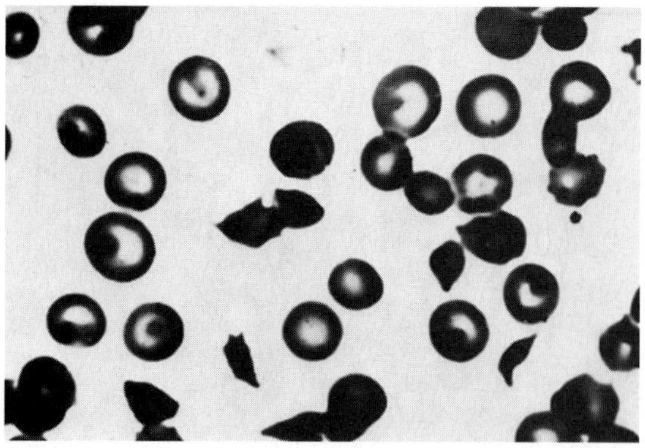

Figure 24–31. Microangiopathic hemolytic anemia; hemolytic-uremic syndrome. Note irregularly contracted cells, schistocytes, a few crenated cells. One nucleated red cell is present (× 875).

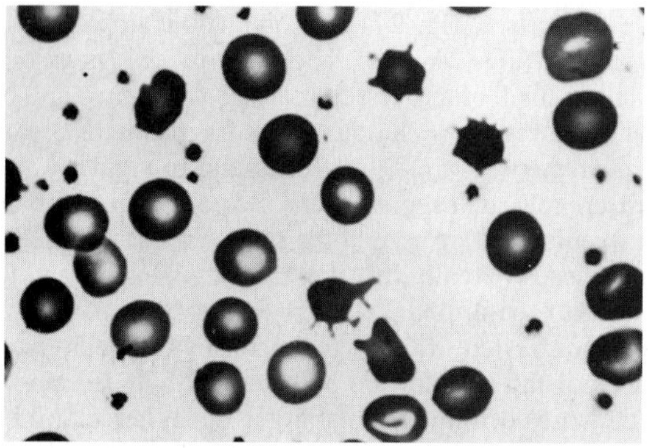

Figure 24–32. Acanthocytes. Note the long spicules, which tend to have bulbous ends (× 875).

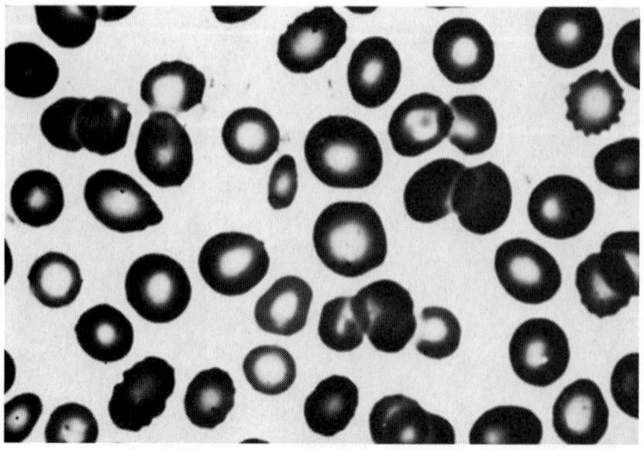

Figure 24–33. Megaloblastic anemia. A few crenated cells are present (× 875).

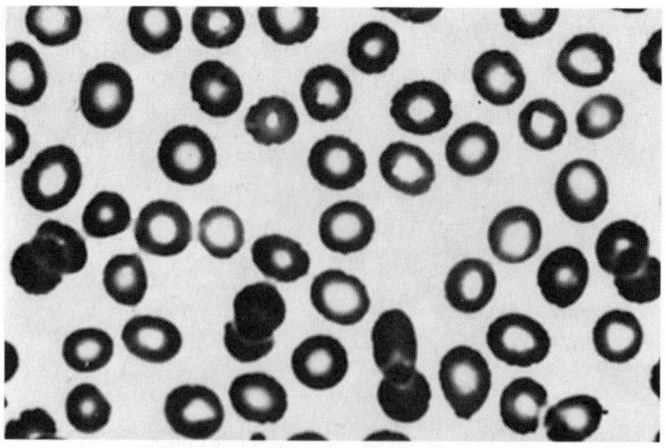

Figure 24–34. Artifact due to water in the methyl alcohol fixative. If bubbles are small in size (as shown here), they cause an indented appearance that may be confused with crenation (× 875).

or bubbles indenting the red cells (Fig. 24–34) may be caused by a small amount of water contaminating the Wright stain (or absolute methanol, if this is used first as a fixative).

Structure

BASOPHILIC STIPPLING (PUNCTATE BASOPHILIA)

Basophilic stippling is characterized by the presence, within the erythrocyte, of irregular basophilic granules, which vary from fine to coarse (Fig. 24–35). These granules stain deep blue with Wright stain. The erythrocyte containing them may stain normally in other respects, or it may exhibit polychromatophilia. Fine stippling is common when there is increased polychromatophilia, and, therefore, with increased production of red cells. Coarse stippling may be seen in lead poisoning or other diseases with impaired hemoglobin synthesis, in megaloblastic anemia, and in other forms of severe anemia; it is attributed to an abnormal instability of the RNA in the young cell.

Red cells with inorganic iron-containing granules (as demonstrated by stains for iron) are called *siderocytes*. Sometimes these granules stain with Wright stain; if so, they are called *Pappenheimer bodies*. In contrast with basophilic stippling, Pappenheimer bodies are few in a given red cell and are rare in the peripheral blood except after splenectomy.

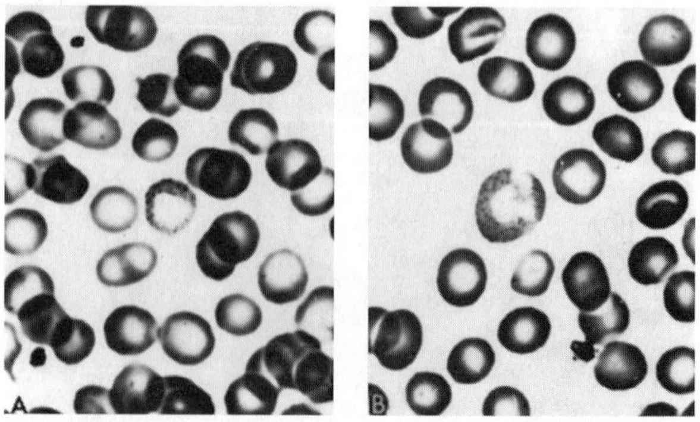

Figure 24–35. Basophilic stippling. One stippled red cell in the center of each field. *A*, Thalassemia minor; *B*, lead poisoning (× 875).

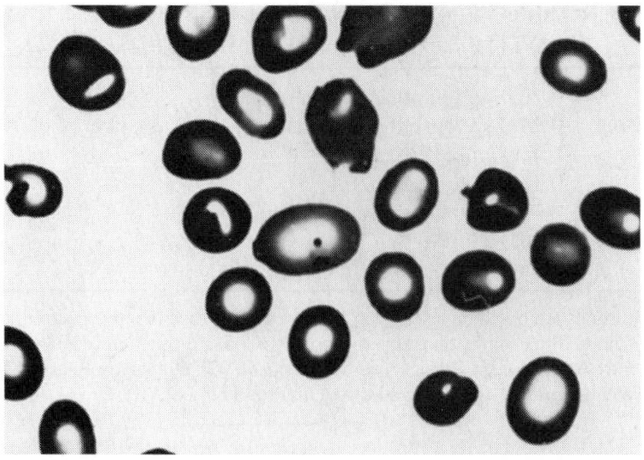

Figure 24–36. Megaloblastic anemia. The central oval macrocyte has four Howell-Jolly bodies; the lower three are touching one another (× 875).

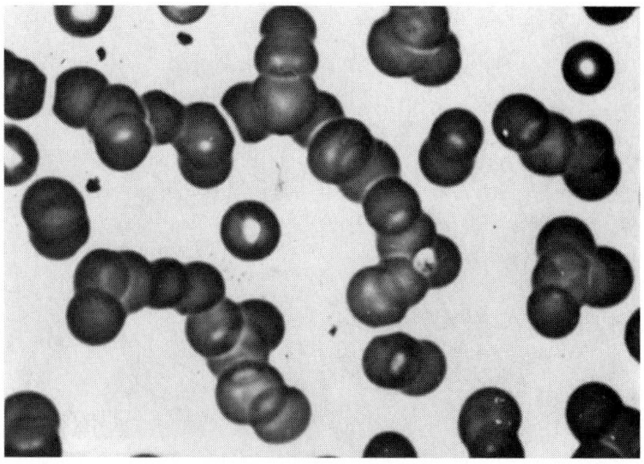

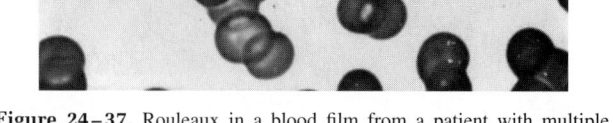

Figure 24–37. Rouleaux in a blood film from a patient with multiple myeloma (× 875).

HOWELL-JOLLY BODIES

Howell-Jolly bodies are smooth, round remnants of nuclear chromatin. Single Howell-Jolly bodies may be seen in megaloblastic anemia, in hemolytic anemia, and after splenectomy. Multiple Howell-Jolly bodies in a single cell (Fig. 24–36) usually indicate megaloblastic anemia or some other form of abnormal erythropoiesis.

CABOT RINGS

Cabot rings are ring-shaped, figure-of-eight, or loop-shaped structures. Occasionally they are formed by double or several concentric lines. They are observed rarely in erythrocytes in pernicious anemia, lead poisoning, and certain other disorders of erythropoiesis. They stain red or reddish purple with Wright stain and have no internal structure. The rings are probably microtubules remaining from a mitotic spindle (Bessis, 1977). They are interpreted as evidence of abnormal erythropoiesis.

MALARIAL STIPPLING

Fine granules may appear in erythrocytes that harbor *Plasmodium vivax.* With Wright stain, the minute granules, "Schüffner's granules," stain purplish red. They are sometimes so numerous that they almost hide the parasites. These red cells usually are larger than normal.

ROULEAU FORMATION

Rouleau formation is the alignment of red cells on one another so that they resemble stacks of coins. On air-dried films, rouleaux appear as in Figure 24–37. Elevated plasma fibrinogen or globulins cause rouleaux to form and also promote an increase in the erythrocyte sedimentation rate. Rouleau formation is especially marked in paraproteinemia (monoclonal gammopathy). *Agglutination,* or clumping, of red cells is more surely separated from rouleaux in wet preparations, and on air-dried films (Fig. 24–38) tends to show more irregular and round clumps than the linear rouleaux do. Cold agglutinins are responsible for this appearance.

Nucleated Red Cells

In contrast with erythrocytes of lower vertebrates and with most mammalian cells, the mammalian erythrocyte lacks a nucleus.

Nucleated red cells *(normoblasts)* are precursors of the non-nucleated mature red cells in the blood. In the human, normoblasts are normally present only in the bone marrow (Fig. 24–39). The stages in their production (Plate 24–1), from the earliest to the latest are the pronormoblast, basophilic normoblast, polychromatophilic normoblast, and orthochromatic normoblast.

In general, nucleated red cells that might appear in the blood in disease are polychromatic normoblasts. Sometimes, however, the cytoplasm is so basophilic that it is difficult to recognize the cell as erythroid except by the character of the nucleus, intensely staining chromatin, and sharp separation of chromatin from parachromatin. Such erythroid cells are often mistaken for lymphocytes, an error that usually can be prevented by careful observation of the nucleus. The *megaloblast* (Fig. 24–40) is a distinct, nucleated erythroid cell, not merely a larger normoblast. It is characterized by large size and an abnormal "open" nuclear chromatin pattern. Cells of this series are not found in normal marrow but are characteristically present in the marrow and sometimes the blood of patients with pernicious anemia or other megaloblastic anemias (see Chap. 26).

SIGNIFICANCE

Normoblasts are present normally only in the blood of the fetus and of very young infants. In the healthy adult, they are confined to the bone marrow and appear in the circulating

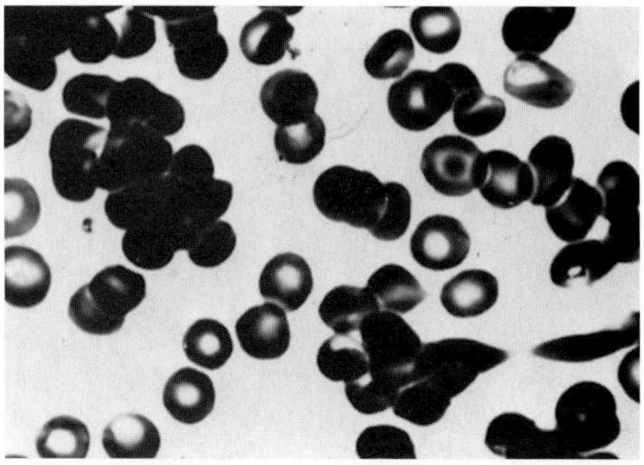

Figure 24–38. Blood film from a patient with a high titer of cold agglutinins. Red cells aggregate in clumps. Separation of cells during making the film may distort the cells (*lower right*) (× 875).

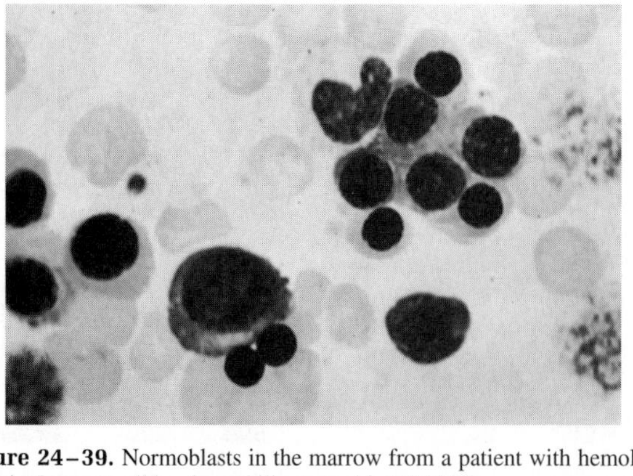

Figure 24–39. Normoblasts in the marrow from a patient with hemolytic anemia. Largest cell is a basophilic normoblast (×875).

Table 24–4. CONDITIONS ASSOCIATED WITH LEUKOERYTHROBLASTOSIS

0.63	0.26 Solid tumors and lymphomas
	0.24 Myeloproliferative disorders, including chronic myeloid leukemia (CML)
	0.13 Acute leukemias
0.37	0.03 Benign hematologic conditions
	0.08 Hemolysis
	0.26 Miscellaneous, including blood loss

Proportions are based on a series of 215 cases discovered in a prospective study of 50,277 blood film examinations in a six-month period, a proportion of 0.004.

Data are from Weick JK, Hagedorn AB, Linman JW: Leukoerythroblastosis: Diagnostic and prognostic significance. Mayo Clin Proc 1974; 49:110.

blood only in disease, in which their presence usually denotes an extreme demand made on the marrow, extramedullary hematopoiesis, or marrow replacement. Large numbers of circulating nucleated red cells are particularly found in hemolytic disease of the newborn (erythroblastosis fetalis; see Chap. 26) and thalassemia major (see Chap. 26).

LEUKOERYTHROBLASTOTIC REACTION

The presence of normoblasts and immature cells of the neutrophilic series in the blood is known as a *leukoerythroblastotic reaction.* This often indicates space-occupying disturbances of the marrow, such as myelofibrosis with myeloid metaplasia, metastatic carcinoma, leukemias, multiple myeloma, Gaucher's disease, and others. Nonetheless, in the study of Weick (1974), over a third of the patients with a leukoerythroblastotic reaction did not have malignant or potentially malignant disease (Table 24–4). In patients with metastatic malignancy, a leukoerythroblastotic reaction is good evidence for marrow involvement by tumor.

Leukocytes

Differential Leukocyte Count

Before evaluating leukocytes on the Romanowsky-stained blood film, one should first determine that the film is well made, the distribution of the cells is uniform, and the staining of cells is satisfactory. Learning to identify normal cells with low power (100× magnification) as well as with the oil immersion lens (1000×) enables one to find abnormal cells readily when they are present.

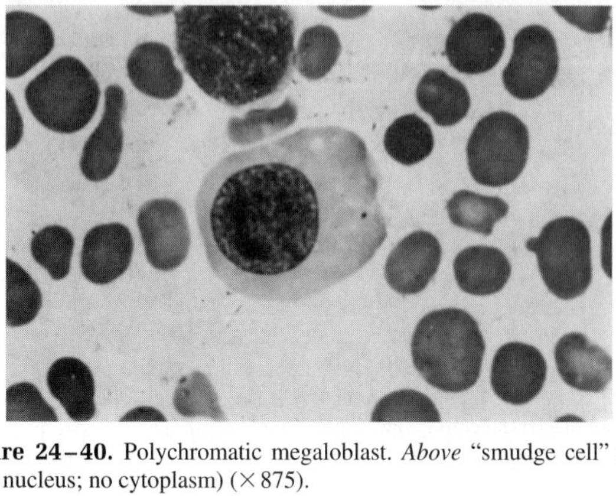

Figure 24–40. Polychromatic megaloblast. *Above* "smudge cell" (damaged nucleus; no cytoplasm) (×875).

One first scans the counting area of the slide and, in wedge films, the lateral and feather edges, where monocytes, neutrophils, and large abnormal cells (if present) tend to be disproportionately represented. Suspicious cells are detected at 100× magnification and confirmed at high power. Because nucleated red cells, macrophages, immature granulocytes, immature lymphoid cells, megakaryocytes, and abnormal cells are not normally found in blood, they should be recorded if present.

While scanning under low power, one should estimate the leukocyte count from the film. Even though it is a crude approximation, it sometimes enables one to detect errors in total count. One then proceeds to determine the percentage of distribution of the different types of leukocytes, which is known as the differential leukocyte count. In the crenellation technique of counting, the field of view is moved from side to side across the width of the slide in the counting area, just behind the feather edge, where the red cells are separated from one another and are free of artifacts. As each leukocyte is encountered, it is classified until 100, 200, 500, or 1000 leukocytes have been counted. The greater the number of cells counted, the greater the precision (Table 24–5), but for practical reasons 100 cells are usually counted.

The count may be recorded with a mechanical or electronic tabulator. Leukocytes that cannot be classified should be placed together in an unidentified group. In some conditions, notably leukemia, there may be many of these unidentified leukocytes. During the differential leukocyte counting procedure, the morphology of erythrocytes and platelets is examined and the number of platelets is estimated.

The absolute concentration of each variety of leukocyte is its percentage times the total leukocyte count. An increase in absolute concentration is an *absolute increase;* an increase in percentage only is a *relative increase.* With a low total leukocyte count, for example, the neutrophil count may be relatively normal (normal percentage) but absolutely decreased. Reference intervals are more useful if given as absolute concentrations rather than as percentages (Table 24–6).

Leukocytes Normally Present in the Blood

NEUTROPHIL (POLYMORPHONUCLEAR NEUTROPHILIC LEUKOCYTE; SEGMENTED NEUTROPHILIC GRANULOCYTE)

Neutrophils average 12 μm in diameter; they are smaller than monocytes and eosinophils and slightly larger than basophils. The nucleus stains deeply; it is irregular and often

Table 24–5. NINETY-FIVE PERCENT CONFIDENCE LIMITS FOR VARIOUS PERCENTAGES OF BLOOD CELLS OF A GIVEN TYPE AS DETERMINED BY DIFFERENTIAL COUNTS

a	n = 100	n = 200	n = 500	n = 1000	n = 10,000
0	0.0–3.6	0.0–1.8	0.0–0.7	0.0–0.4	0.0–0.1
1	0.0–5.4	0.1–3.6	0.3–2.3	0.5–1.8	0.8–1.3
2	0.0–7.0	0.6–5.0	1.0–3.6	1.2–3.1	1.7–2.3
3	0.6–8.5	1.1–6.4	1.7–4.9	2.0–4.3	2.6–3.4
4	1.1–9.9	1.7–7.7	2.5–6.1	2.9–5.4	3.6–4.5
5	1.6–11.3	2.4–9.0	3.3–7.3	3.7–6.5	4.5–5.5
6	2.2–12.6	3.1–10.2	4.1–8.5	4.6–7.7	5.5–6.5
7	2.9–13.9	3.9–11.5	4.9–9.6	5.5–8.8	6.5–7.6
8	3.5–15.2	4.6–12.7	5.8–10.7	6.4–9.9	7.4–8.6
9	4.2–16.4	5.4–13.9	6.6–11.9	7.3–10.9	8.4–9.6
10	4.9–17.6	6.2–15.0	7.5–13.0	8.2–12.0	9.4–10.7
15	8.6–23.5	10.4–20.7	12.0–18.4	12.8–17.4	14.3–15.8
20	12.7–29.2	14.7–26.2	16.6–23.8	17.6–22.6	19.2–20.8
25	16.9–34.7	19.2–31.6	21.3–29.0	22.3–27.8	24.1–25.9
30	21.2–40.0	23.7–36.9	26.0–34.2	27.2–32.9	29.1–31.0
35	25.7–45.2	28.4–42.0	30.8–39.4	32.0–38.0	34.0–36.0
40	30.3–50.3	33.2–47.1	35.7–44.4	36.9–43.1	39.0–41.0
45	35.0–55.3	38.0–52.2	40.6–49.5	41.9–48.1	44.0–46.0
50	39.8–60.2	42.9–57.1	45.5–54.5	46.9–53.1	49.0–51.0
55	44.7–65.0	47.8–62.0	50.5–59.4	51.9–58.1	54.0–56.0
60	49.7–69.7	52.9–66.8	55.6–64.3	56.9–63.1	59.0–61.0
65	54.8–74.3	58.0–71.6	60.6–69.2	62.0–68.0	64.0–66.0
70	60.0–78.8	63.1–76.3	65.8–74.0	67.1–72.8	69.0–70.9
75	65.3–83.1	68.4–80.8	71.0–78.7	72.2–77.7	74.1–75.9
80	70.8–87.3	73.8–85.3	76.2–83.4	77.4–82.4	79.2–80.8
85	76.5–91.4	79.3–89.6	81.6–88.0	82.6–87.2	84.2–85.7
90	82.4–95.1	85.0–93.8	87.0–92.5	88.0–91.8	89.3–90.6
91	83.6–95.8	86.1–94.6	88.1–93.4	89.1–92.7	90.4–91.6
92	84.8–96.5	87.3–95.4	89.3–94.2	90.1–93.6	91.4–92.6
93	86.1–97.1	88.5–96.1	90.4–95.1	91.2–94.5	92.4–93.5
94	87.4–97.8	89.8–96.9	91.5–95.9	92.3–95.4	93.5–94.5
95	88.7–98.4	91.0–97.6	92.7–96.7	93.5–96.3	94.5–95.5
96	90.1–98.9	92.3–98.3	93.9–97.5	94.6–97.1	95.5–96.4
97	91.5–99.4	93.6–98.9	95.1–98.3	95.7–98.0	96.6–97.4
98	93.0–99.8	95.0–99.4	96.4–99.0	96.9–98.8	97.7–98.3
99	94.6–99.9	96.4–99.9	97.7–99.7	98.2–99.5	98.7–99.2
100	96.4–100.0	98.2–100.0	99.3–100.0	99.6–100.0	99.9–100.0

n is the number of cells counted; a, the observed percentage of cells of the given type. The limits for n = 100, 200, 500, and 1000 are exact; for n = 10,000, they have been determined with Freeman and Tukey's approximation as described in the Geigy tables.

Courtesy of Prof. C. L. Rümke.

Table 24–6. NORMAL LEUKOCYTE COUNT, DIFFERENTIAL COUNT, AND HEMOGLOBIN CONCENTRATION AT VARIOUS AGES

	Leukocytes								
Age	***Total Leukocytes***	***Total Neutrophils***	***Band Neutrophils***	***Segmented Neutrophils***	***Eosinophils***	***Basophils***	***Lymphocytes***	***Monocytes***	**Hemoglobin (g/dL Blood)**
12 mo	11.4 (6.0–17.5)	3.5 (1.5–8.5)	0.35	3.2 (1.0–8.5)	0.30 (0.05–0.70)	0.05 (0–0.20)	7.0 (4.0–10.5)	0.55 (0.05–1.1)	12.6 (11.1–14.1)
		31	*3.1*	*28*	*2.6*	*0.4*	*61*	*4.8*	
4 yr	9.1 (5.5–15.5)	3.8 (1.5–8.5)	0.27 (0–1.0)	3.5 (1.5–7.5)	0.25 (0.02–0.65)	0.05 (0–0.2)	4.5 (2.0–8.0)	0.45 (0–0.8)	12.7 (11.2–14.3)
		42	*3.0*	*39*	*2.8*	*0.6*	*50*	*5.0*	
6 yr	8.5 (5.0–14.5)	4.3 (1.5–8.0)	0.25 (0–1.0)	4.0 (1.5–7.0)	0.23 (0–0.65)	0.05 (0–0.2)	3.5 (1.50–7.0)	0.40 (0–0.8)	13.0 (11.4–14.5)
		51	*3.0*	*48*	*2.7*	*0.6*	*42*	*4.7*	
10 yr	8.1 (4.5–13.5)	4.4 (1.8–8.0)	0.24 (0–1.0)	4.2 (1.8–7.0)	0.20 (0–0.60)	0.04 (0–0.2)	3.1 (1.5–6.5)	0.35 (0–0.8)	13.4 (11.8–15.0)
		54	*3.0*	*51*	*2.4*	*0.5*	*38*	*4.3*	
21 yr	7.4 (4.5–11.0)	4.4 (1.8–7.7)	0.22 (0–0.7)	4.2 (1.8–7.0)	0.20 (0–0.45)	0.04 (0–0.2)	2.5 (1.0–4.8)	0.30 (0–0.8)	15.5 (13.5–17.5)
		59	*3.0*	*56*	*2.7*	*0.5*	*34*	*4.0*	13.8 (12.0–15.6)

Note: Values are expressed as mean (95% reference) values. For leukocytes and differential count cell types, the units are cells × $10^9/\mu L$; the numbers in italic type are mean percentages.

Source: For leukocyte and differential count. Altman PL, Dittmer DS (eds): Blood and Other Body Fluids. Washington, DC, Federation of American Societies for Experimental Biology, 1961; for hemoglobin concentrations. Dalman PR: Developmental changes in red blood cell production and function. *In* Rudolph AM, Hoffman JIE (eds): Pediatrics, 18th ed. Norwalk, CT, Appleton & Lange, 1987, pp 1011 and 1012.

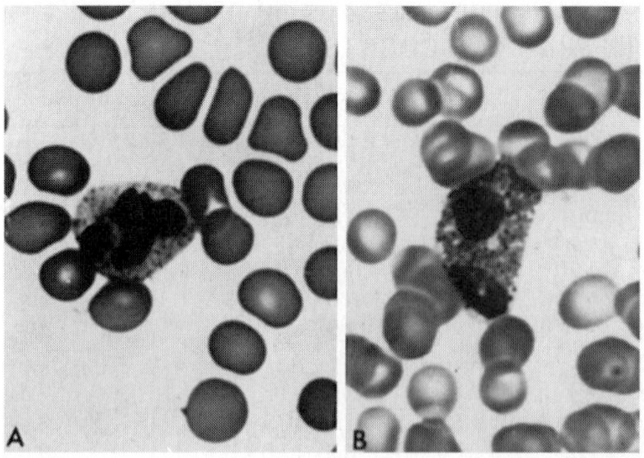

Figure 24–41. *A*, Neutrophil. The cytoplasm is filled with tiny granules, some of which stain more deeply than others (toxic granulation). Note that most of the red cells lack central pallor, an artifact seen near the feather edge of the film. *B*, Eosinophil. Typically this cell has fewer nuclear lobes and larger cytoplasmic granules than the neutrophil (×875).

assumes shapes comparable to such letters as E, Z, and S. What appear to be separate nuclei normally are segments of nuclear material connected by delicate filaments.

A filament has length but no breadth as one focuses up and down. A *segmented neutrophil* has at least two of its lobes separated by a filament. A *band neutrophil* has either a strand of nuclear material thicker than a filament connecting the lobes, or a U-shaped nucleus of uniform thickness. The nucleus in both types of neutrophils has coarse blocks of chromatin and rather sharply defined parachromatin spaces. If, because of overlapping of nuclear material, one cannot be certain as to whether a filament is present, the cell should be placed in the segmented category (Mathy, 1974). The number of lobes in normal neutrophils ranges from two to five, with a median of three.

The cytoplasm, itself colorless, is packed full of tiny granules (0.2 to 0.3 μm) that stain tan to pink with Wright stain (Fig. 24–41*A* and Plate 24–1). About two thirds of these are specific granules and one third azurophil granules. The intensity of the red-blue or purple staining of the azurophil granules in the more immature neutrophils (see Chap. 25) has diminished; with light microscopy, the two types of granules often cannot be distinguished in the mature cell.

Segmented neutrophils average 56% of leukocytes; reference intervals are 1.8 to 7.0×10^9/L in white adults but have a lower limit of about 1.1×10^9/L in blacks. Band neutrophils average 3% of leukocytes; the upper reference value is about 0.7×10^9/L in whites and slightly lower in blacks (using the preceding definition and counting 100 cells in the differential, see Table 24–6).

Normally about 10% to 30% of the segmented neutrophils have two lobes, 40% to 50% have three lobes, 10% to 20% four, and no more than 5% have five lobes. A shift to the left occurs when there are increased bands and less mature neutrophils in the blood, as well as a lower average number of lobes in segmented cells.

Neutrophil production and physiology are discussed in Chapter 25. Neutrophilia or neutrophilic leukocytosis is an increase in the absolute count, and neutropenia is a decrease; they are discussed in Chapter 27.

EOSINOPHIL (EOSINOPHILIC GRANULOCYTE)

Eosinophils average 13 μm in diameter. The structure of these cells is similar to that of the polymorphonuclear neutrophils, with the striking difference that, instead of the neutrophilic granules, their cytoplasm contains larger round or oval granules with a strong affinity for acid stains (see Fig. 24–41*B* and Plate 24–1*F* and *G*). Eosinophils are easily recognized by the size and color of the granules, which stain bright red with eosin. The cytoplasm is colorless. The nucleus stains somewhat less deeply than that of the neutrophils and usually has two connected segments (lobes), rarely more than three.

Eosinophils average 3% of the leukocytes in adults, and the upper reference value is 0.6×10^9/L when calculated from the differential count. If allergic persons are excluded, the upper limit is probably 0.35×10^9/L or 350/μL. The lower reference value is probably 40/μL; a decrease in eosinophils (eosinopenia) can be detected only by counting large numbers of cells as in direct hemacytometer counts (Dacie, 1991) or with a flow cytometer automated differential counter.

Eosinophilia, an increase in eosinophils, and eosinopenia are discussed in Chapter 27.

BASOPHIL (BASOPHILIC GRANULOCYTE)

In general, basophils resemble neutrophils, except that the nucleus is less segmented (usually merely indented or partially lobulated), and granules are larger and have a strong affinity for basic stains (Fig. 24–42 and Plate 24–1*H* and *I*). In some basophils, most of the granules may be missing because they are soluble in water, leaving vacuoles or openings in the cytoplasm. The granules then are a mauve color. In a well-stained film, the granules are deep purple, and the nucleus is somewhat paler and is often nearly hidden by the granules, so that its form is difficult to distinguish. Unevenly stained granules of basophils may be ring shaped and resemble *Histoplasma capsulatum* or protozoa.

Basophils are the least numerous of the leukocytes in normal blood and average 0.5%. The 95% reference values for adults are 0 to 0.2×10^9/L when derived from the differential count. Direct hemacytometer counts employing Alcian blue (Gilbert, 1975) or automated differential counts on the H-6000 or H*1 allow a narrower reference interval.

Basophilia (basophilic leukocytosis) and basopenia (de-

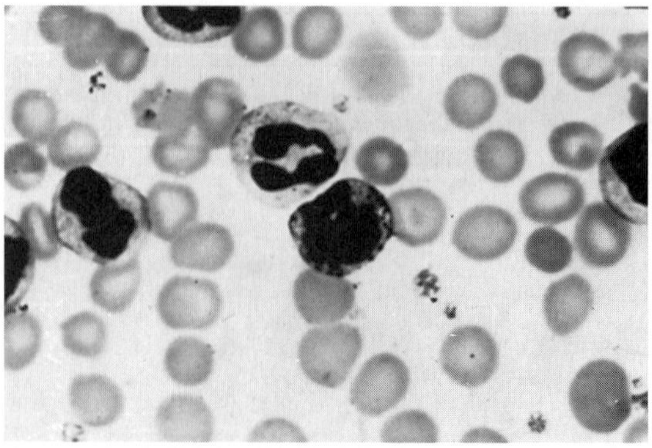

Figure 24–42. Neutrophil (above) and basophil (below). The basophil is smaller and has large, deeply basophilic granules that often can be partially washed out, leaving vacuoles (×875).

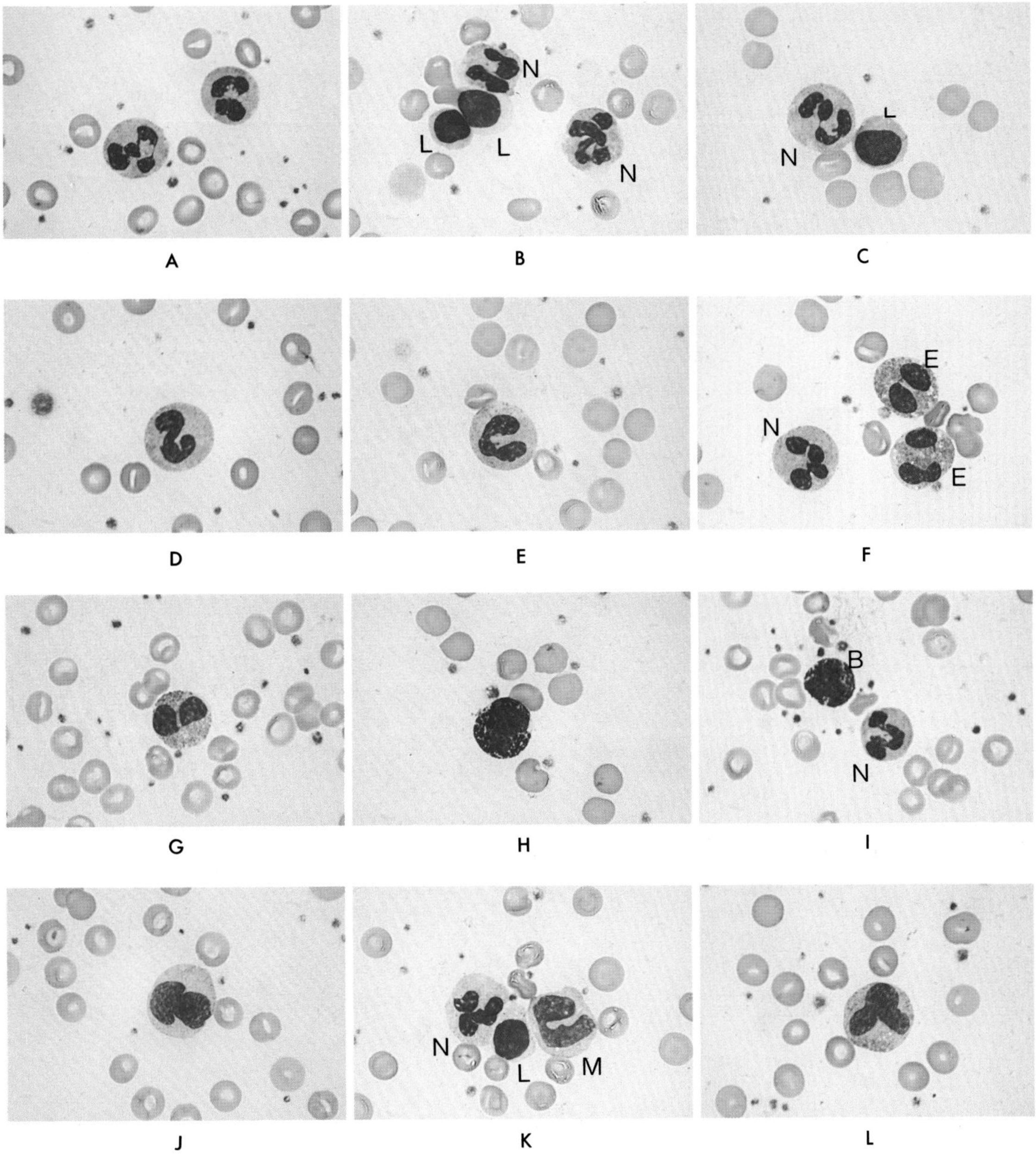

Plate 24–1. These photomicrographs are from buffy coat preparations of blood from a normal individual. Therefore, the number of leukocytes and platelets per field is greater than in blood films made directly. *A*, Neutrophils. The cell on the right has a few nuclear spicules or extensions. These rather pointed spicules are directed toward the centrosomal region of the cell. Such nuclear extensions may be found in normal individuals but are more frequent in those with chronic illnesses (Bessis, 1977). They should be distinguished from the sex chromatin appendages, which have a drumstick appearance. *B*, Lymphocytes (L) of slightly different size and chromatin condensation, and neutrophils (N). *C*, Neutrophil (N) and lymphocyte (L). *D* and *E*, Band neutrophils. In *E*, note the incomplete segmentation. *F*, Neutrophil (N) and eosinophils (E). Eosinophils have larger granules and, on the average, fewer lobes than do neutrophils. *G*, Eosinophil. *H*, Basophil. *I*, Basophil (B); neutrophil (N). *J*, Monocyte. *K*, Neutrophil (N); lymphocyte (L); monocyte (M). The monocyte has more delicately staining chromatin than the other cells; this usually can be appreciated at low magnification. *L*, Monocyte.

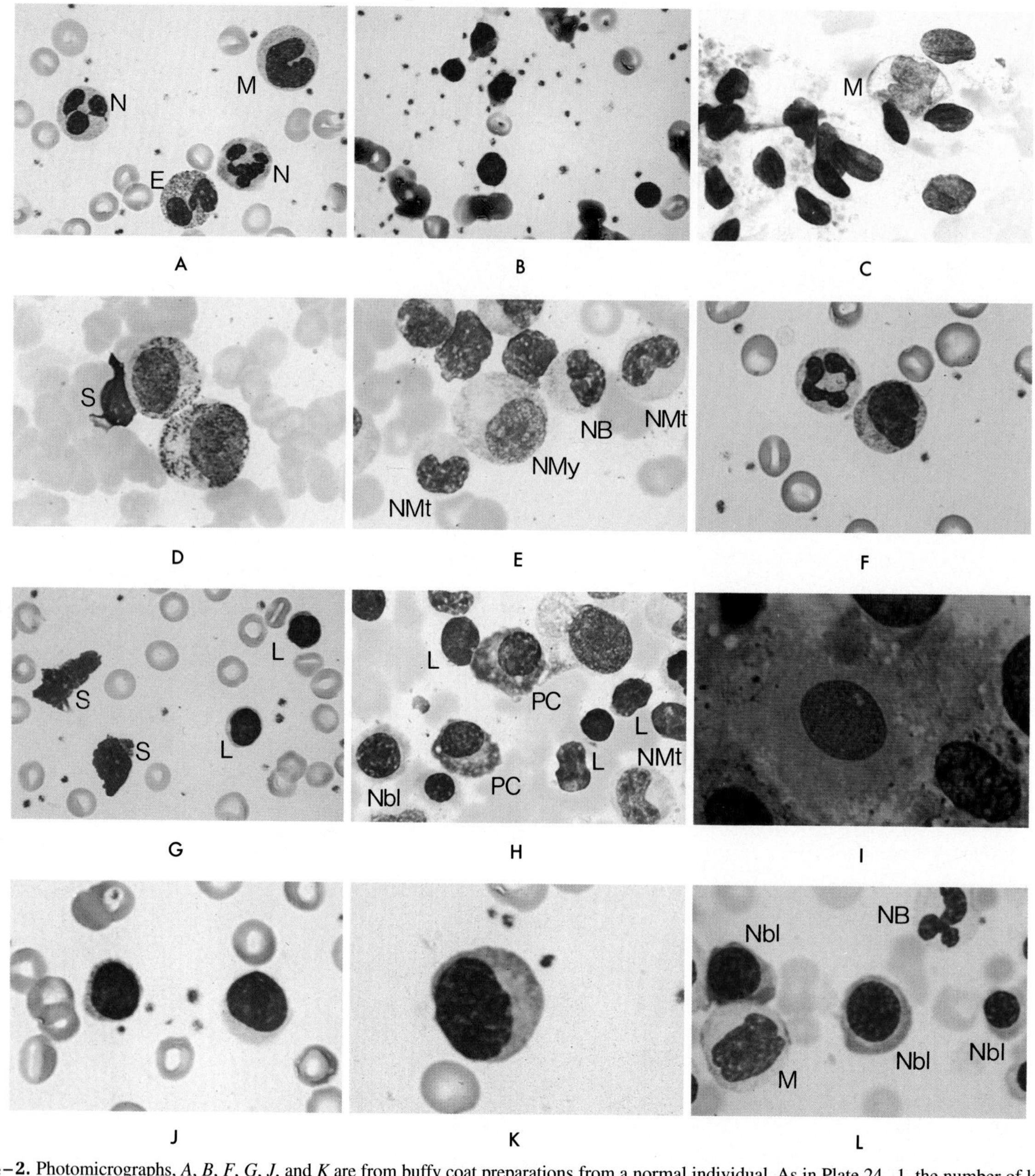

Plate 24–2. Photomicrographs, *A*, *B*, *F*, *G*, *J*, and *K* are from buffy coat preparations from a normal individual. As in Plate 24–1, the number of leukocytes and platelets per field is greater than in blood films made directly. *A*, Neutrophils (N), eosinophil (E), and monocyte (M) are easily identifiable in this thin, well-spread area of film. *B*, Thick area of same film as *A*, same magnification. Slow drying and shrinkage have made cell identification much less certain. *C*, Endothelial cells and a monocyte (M) at the feather edge of a normal blood film. Endothelial cells have an oval nucleus that is folded or "creased" and abundant, ill-defined cytoplasm. *D*, Two neutrophil myelocytes and the nucleus of a broken or smudged cell (S). Normal marrow. *E*, Neutrophil myelocytes (NMy), neutrophil metamyelocytes (NMt), and neutrophil band form (NB), Normal marrow. *F*, Monocyte (*right*) and neutrophil (*left*). *G*, Lymphocytes (L) and broken, smudged nuclei (S). *H*, Plasma cells (PC), normoblast (Nbl), lymphocytes (L), neutrophil metamyelocyte (NMt). Normal marrow. *I*, Macrophage. These cells have reticular nuclei and abundant cytoplasm containing scattered pigment granules. Bone marrow. *J*, Lymphocytes. *K*, Atypical lymphocyte. Increased cytoplasmic basophilia and more distinct separation of chromatin from parachromatin distinguish this "activated lymphocyte" from resting normal lymphocytes (*J*). *L*, Normoblasts (Nbl), monocyte (M), and neutrophil band (NB). Normal marrow.

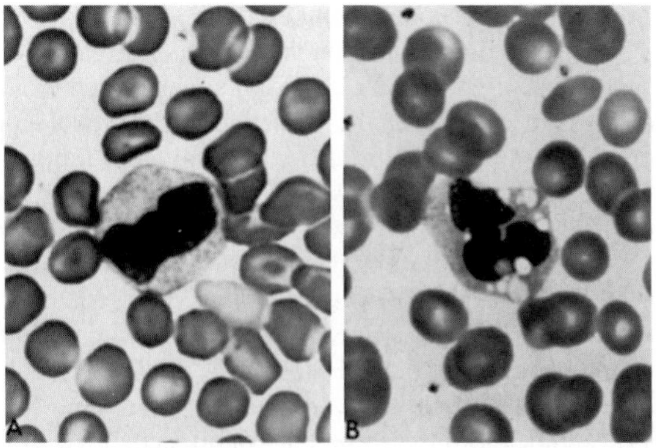

Figure 24–43. *A* and *B*, Monocytes. Of the normal blood cells, the monocyte is the largest and has the most delicate chromatin pattern; it has a propensity to form cytoplasmic vacuoles (*B*), which usually indicate phagocytosis (× 875).

creased absolute basophil count) are discussed in Chapter 27.

MONOCYTE

The monocyte is the largest cell of normal blood (Fig. 24–43 and Plate 24–1*J*, *K*, and *L*). Its diameter generally is about two to three times that of an erythrocyte (14 to 20 μm), although they sometimes are smaller. The monocyte contains a single nucleus, which is partially lobulated, deeply indented, or horseshoe shaped. The nucleus of a monocyte sometimes appears round or oval.

The cytoplasm is abundant. The nuclear chromatin often appears to be in fine, parallel strands separated by sharply defined parachromatin. The nucleus stains less densely than that of other leukocytes. The cytoplasm is blue-gray and has a ground-glass appearance and often contains fine red to purple granules that are less distinct and smaller than the granules of neutrophils. Blue granules sometimes are seen.

When the monocyte transforms into a macrophage, it becomes larger (20 to 40 μm); the nucleus may become oval and the chromatin more reticular or dispersed, so that nucleoli may be visible (Plate 24–2*I*). A perinuclear clear zone (Golgi) may be evident. The fine red or azurophil granules vary in number or may have disappeared. The more abundant cytoplasm tends to be irregular at the cell margins and to contain vacuoles. These are phagocytic vacuoles, which may contain ingested red cells, debris, pigment, or bacteria. Evidence of phagocytosis in monocytes or the presence of macrophages in directly made blood films is pathologic and often indicates active infection.

Monocytes average 4% of leukocytes, and the reference interval for adults is approximately 0 to 0.8×10^9/L, depending on the method of performing the differential count (see Table 24–6).

Monocyte production is discussed in Chapter 25. An increase in monocytes (monocytosis) and a decrease (monocytopenia) are discussed in Chapter 27.

LYMPHOCYTE

Lymphocytes are mononuclear cells without specific cytoplasmic granules. Small lymphocytes are about the size of an erythrocyte or slightly larger (6 to 10 μm) (Plates 24–1*B* and *C*, and 24–2*G* and *J*). The typical lymphocyte has a single, sharply defined nucleus containing heavy blocks of chromatin. The chromatin stains dark blue with Wright stain, whereas the parachromatin stands out as lighter-stained streaks; at the periphery of the nucleus, the chromatin is condensed. Characteristically, there is a gradual transition or "smudging" between the chromatin and the parachromatin. The nucleus is generally round but is sometimes indented at one side. The cytoplasm stains pale blue except for a clear perinuclear zone.

Larger lymphocytes, 12 to 15 μm in diameter, with less densely staining nuclei and more abundant cytoplasm, are common, especially in the blood of children, and they may be difficult to distinguish from monocytes. The misshapen, indented cytoplasmic margins of lymphocytes are due to the pressure of neighboring cells. The cytoplasm of about one third of the large lymphocytes contains a few round, red-purple granules. They are larger than the granules of neutrophilic leukocytes (Fig. 24–44*B*). There is a continuous spectrum of sizes between small and large lymphocytes, and, indeed, there can be a transition from small to large to blast forms as well as the reverse (see Plate 24–2*J* and *K*). It is not meaningful to classify small lymphocytes and large lymphocytes separately. A significant proportion of atypical lymphocytes and blast forms (nonleukemic lymphoblast, reticular lymphocytes) must be noted; these indicate transformation of lymphoid cells as a response to antigenic stimulation (see Chap. 25).

Plasma cells have abundant blue cytoplasm, often with light streaks or vacuoles, an eccentric round nucleus, and a well-defined clear (Golgi) zone adjacent to the nucleus (see Plate 24–2*H*). The nucleus of the plasma cell has heavily clumped chromatin, which is sharply defined from the parachromatin, and often arranged in a radial or "wheel-like" pattern. Plasma cells are not present normally in blood.

Lymphocytes average 34% of all leukocytes and range from 1.5 to 4×10^9/L in adults.

The lymphocytes and their derivatives, the plasma cells, operate in the immune defenses of the body. Lymphocytosis and plasmacytosis are discussed in Chapter 27.

Artifacts

BROKEN CELLS

Damaged or broken leukocytes constitute a small proportion of the nucleated cells in normal blood. Bare nuclei from

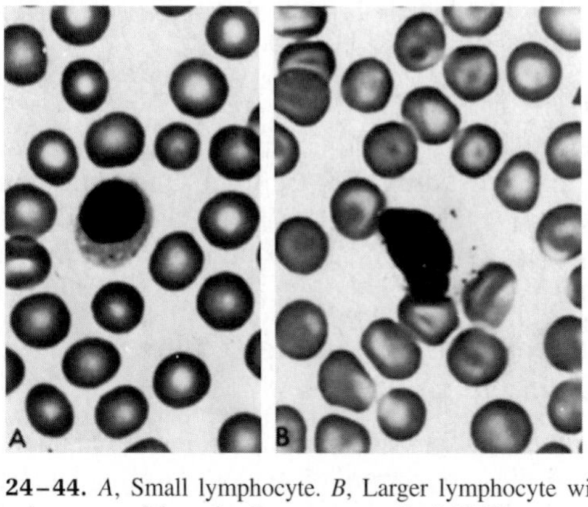

Figure 24–44. *A*, Small lymphocyte. *B*, Larger lymphocyte with granules: note that many of the red cells are target cells (× 875).

4

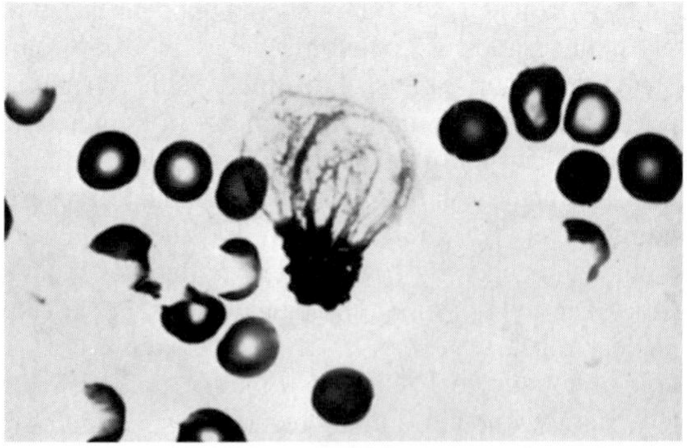

Figure 24–45. Basket cell. This is a nuclear remnant from a damaged or broken white blood cell (×875).

ruptured cells vary from fairly well-preserved nuclei without cytoplasm to smudged nuclear material (see Plate 24–2*G*), sometimes with strands arranged in a coarse network, the so-called basket cells (Fig. 24–45). They probably represent fragile cells, usually lymphocytes, that have been broken in preparing the film. They are apt to be numerous in the case of atypical lymphocytosis (see Chap. 27), chronic lymphocytic leukemia, and acute leukemias.

DEGENERATIVE CHANGES

As EDTA-blood ages in the test tube, leukocyte morphology begins to change (Sacker, 1975). The degree of change varies among cells and in different persons. Within a half hour, the nuclei of neutrophils may begin to swell, with some loss of chromatin structure. Cytoplasmic vacuoles appear, especially in monocytes and neutrophils. Nuclear lobulation appears in mononuclear cells; deep clefts may cause the nucleus to resemble a clover leaf (radial segmentation of the nuclei; Rieder cells). Finally, loss of the cytoplasm and a smudged nucleus may be all that remains of the cell.

Degenerative changes occur more rapidly in oxalated blood than in EDTA-blood. They arise more rapidly with increasing concentrations of EDTA, such as occur when evacuated blood collection tubes are incompletely filled.

CONTRACTED CELLS

In the thicker part of wedge films, drying is slow. Obvious changes in the film are rouleaux of the erythrocytes and shrinkage of the leukocytes. Because the leukocytes are contracted and heavily stained, mononuclear cells are difficult to distinguish. Optimal cell identification is usually impossible in these areas (see Plate 24–2*B*).

ENDOTHELIAL CELLS

Endothelial cells from the lining of the blood vessel may appear in the first drop of blood from a fingerstick specimen, or, rarely, in venous blood (see Plate 24–2*C*). They have an immature reticular chromatin pattern and may be mistaken for histiocytes or for tumor cells.

Sources of Error in the Differential Leukocyte Count

Even in perfectly made blood films, the differential count is subject to the same errors of random distribution. For interpretation of day-to-day or slide-to-slide differences in the same patient, it is helpful to know how much of the variation is ascribable to chance alone (Rümke, 1985). Table 24–5 gives 95% confidence limits for different percentages of cells in differential counts performed, classifying a total of 100 to 10,000 leukocytes. In comparing the percentages from two separate counts, if one number lies outside the confidence limits of the other, the difference probably is significant (i.e., not due to chance). Thus, on the basis of a 100-cell differential count, if the monocytes were 5% one day and 10% the next, the difference probably is due solely to sampling error. Although the difference *could be* real, one cannot be sure because of the small number of cells counted. If, on the other hand, the differential count totaled 500 cells, the difference between 5% and 10% is significant; one can be reasonably certain (with a 5% chance of being wrong) that the difference is real and not due to chance alone. Of course, this is a minimal estimate of the error involved in differential counts, because it does not include mechanical errors (due to variations in collecting the blood samples, inadequate mixing, irregularities in distribution depending on the type and quality of the blood films, and poor staining) or errors in cell identification, which depend on the judgment and experience of the observer. Meticulous technique as well as accurate and consistent cell classification are therefore required. The physician who interprets the results must be aware of the possible sources of error, especially the error due to chance in the distribution of cells.

Table 24–6 shows the distribution of the various types of leukocytes in the blood of normal persons. Absolute concentrations are given, because these are much more significant than percentages alone.

Automated Differential Leukocyte Counting

Because the differential leukocyte count is nonspecific, imprecise, error-prone, usually labor intensive, expensive to perform, and of limited clinical significance as a screening test, some investigators have suggested that it may be prudent to discontinue use of the differential count as an inpatient screening test for adults (Connelly, 1982). For example, Moyer (1990) reports that of 387 asymptomatic and clinically well children, 75% had an abnormality in at least one of the relative (percentage) or absolute (total) differential count numbers, yet no new or unsuspected illness was discovered in this group. Not only is there the expense of the original WBC differential count, but it may lead to an unnecessary expensive workup. Nevertheless, it continues to be among the widely used procedures.

Automation of the differential count eliminates some of the detractions. Ideally, requirements for the automated differential leukocyte counting system should include the following: (1) the distribution of cells analyzed should be identical with that in the blood, (2) all leukocytes usually found in blood diseases should be accurately identified, or detected and flagged in some way, (3) the speed of the process should enable a large number of cells to be counted in order to minimize statistical error, and (4) the instrument should be cost effective (Bentley, 1977).

The impedance counters and flow cytometer systems and their differential counts are discussed in the section Blood Cell Histograms. The electro-optical/cytochemical systems have the advantage of rapidly analyzing larger numbers of cells, significantly reducing the statistical error of counting. They can be more fully automated than the digital image processors. The disadvantage is that the categories of cells are not completely consonant with those with which we are familiar on Romanowsky-stained films. An "unclassified" category is difficult to interpret. When a result is abnormal, a film must be made and examined. Yet this kind of precision in differential leukocyte counting was not previously available. Analytical variation in the H*1 is small enough that physiologic variations previously undetected become apparent, and an individual's own baseline reference values become meaningful (Statland, 1978).

Of the major multiparameter hematology analyzers studied (Coulter STKS, Technicon H*1, Sysmex NE-8000, Cell-Dyn 3000), none was found to be clearly superior (Bentley, 1993). Likewise, none of the instruments permits doing away with the microscope (Burns, 1992). Because of concern regarding the instrument flags, each laboratory should devise a policy for blood film examination and visual counting when indicated. Camden (1993) provides guiding questions to be asked in selecting a new hematology analyzer for your laboratory. The International Committee for Standardization in Haematology (1984) also published a protocol for evaluation of automated blood cell counters.

The other principle employed in the systems was digital image processing, which uses computer identification of cells on stained blood films.

DIGITAL IMAGE PROCESSING

A uniformly made and stained blood film is placed on a motor-driven microscope stage. A computer controls scanning the slide and stopping it when leukocytes are in the field. The optical details (e.g., nuclear and cytoplasmic size, density, shape, and color) are recorded by a television camera, analyzed by computer, and converted to digital form; these characteristics are compared with a memory bank of such characteristics for the different cell types. If the pattern "fits" that of a normal cell type, it is identified as such; otherwise, it is classified as "other" or unknown. The coordinates of the unknown cells are kept by the instrument and relocated at the end of the count so that the technologist can classify them. Because computerized classifiers can tolerate only limited variation in staining, manufacturers significantly improved blood stain composition, stability, and reproducibility (Lapen, 1982).

Four such systems were available commercially and clinically evaluated: the LARC (Leukocyte Automatic Recognition Computer), the Hematrak, the "diff-3 system," and the ADC-500. The last of these digital image processing differential counters (Hematrak) was marketed in 1986. Because some systems are still used and because the principle is notable, a brief discussion is given.

The Hematrak (Dutcher, 1974) uses Romanowsky-stained wedge films and classifies 100 leukocytes in about 40 seconds. Erythrocyte morphology is determined and platelet estimates are made before or after the count and entered on the console. Programs are available for automated reticulocytes, automated platelet estimates, and automated red cell measurements. The identification of leukocytes, including band neutrophil counts, and the detection of abnormal cells have been reported to be satisfactory (Egan, 1974). Later Hematrak models, such as the 480, 450, 450 QP, and 590, have slide cassettes permitting walk-away performance of leukocyte differentials, including erythrocyte morphology and platelet estimates. With the Hematrak 590, up to 100 label-identified blood films are processed per batch in about an hour and a half. Unlike the other pattern recognition instruments, the Hematrak accommodated either spun or wedge smears.

Intelligent Medical Imaging (IMI), Inc. (Palm Beach Gardens, FL 33410) has marketed the Micro 21, an automated, walk-away microscope, since 1994. Thus far, only WBC differentials have FDA approval; other microscopic procedures (reticulocyte count, body fluids, AFBs, DNA probes) are planned. "Neural Vision" is IMI's proprietary neural networking and image processing employed to mimic visual artificial intelligence. Cell features measured or derived appear analogous to those of previous pattern recognition methods.

Platelets

In films made from EDTA-blood and stained with Romanowsky stains, platelets are round or oval, 2 to 4 μm in diameter, and separated from one another (see Plate 24–1). The platelet count may be estimated from such films. On the average, if the platelet count is normal, about one platelet is found per 10 to 30 red cells. At 1000 × magnification, this is equivalent to about 7 to 20 platelets per oil immersion field in the areas of optimal red cell morphology.

Platelets contain fine purple granules that usually fill the cytoplasm. Occasionally, granules are concentrated in the center (the "granulomere") and surrounded by a pale cytoplasm (the "hyalomere"); these are probably activated platelets, the appearance resulting from contraction of the microtubular band (see Chap. 28). A few platelets may have a decreased concentration of granules (hypogranular platelets).

In EDTA-blood from normal persons, the fraction of platelets that exceed 3 μm in diameter and the fraction of platelets that are hypogranular are both less than 5% if the films are made at 10 minutes or 60 minutes after the blood is drawn. If films are made immediately or at three hours after blood drawing, the fraction of large platelets and the fraction of hypogranular or activated platelets are increased (Zeigler, 1978). These artifacts make it necessary to standardize time of film preparation when evaluating platelet size from films.

In patients with immune thrombocytopenia, large platelets are increased in number. They are also increased in patients with the rare Bernard-Soulier syndrome (see Chap. 28) and in patients with myelophthisis or myeloproliferative syndromes; in the latter, the platelets are frequently hypogranular or have a distinct granulomere and hyalomere.

In blood films made from skin puncture wounds, platelets assume irregular shapes with sharp projections and tend to clump together.

4

PHYSIOLOGIC VARIATION

Physiologic Variation in Erythrocytes

Changes in red cell values are greatest during the first few weeks of life (Fig. 24–46). At birth, as much as 100 to 125 mL of placental blood may be added to the newborn if tying the cord is postponed until its pulsation ceases. In a study of newborns whose cords had been clamped late, the average capillary red cell counts were 0.4×10^{12}/L higher 1 hour after and 0.8×10^{12}/L higher 24 hours after birth compared with newborns whose cords had been clamped early.

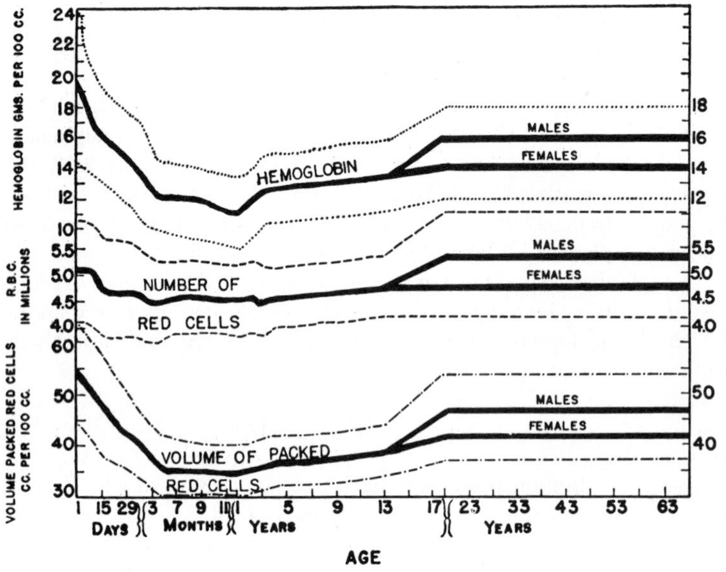

Figure 24–46. Values for hemoglobin, hematocrit (volume of packed red cells), and red cell counts from birth to old age. Mean values are heavy lines. Reference interval for hemoglobin is indicated by dotted lines, for red cell counts by interrupted lines, and for hematocrit by dotted interrupted lines. The scales on the ordinate are similar so that relative changes in hemoglobin, red cell count, and hematocrit are apparent on inspection. The scale for age, however, is progressively altered. (From Wintrobe MM: Clinical Hematology, 7th ed. Philadelphia, Lea & Febiger, 1974.)

Capillary blood (obtained by skin puncture) gives higher RBC and Hb values than venous blood (cord). The differences may amount to about 0.5×10^{12} RBC/L and 3 g Hb/dL. The slowing of capillary circulation and the resulting loss of fluid may be responsible. Examination of venous blood furnishes more consistent results than examination of capillary blood.

In the full-term infant, *nucleated red cells* average about 0.5×10^9/L. The normoblast count declines to about 200/μL at 24 hours, 25/μL at 48 hours, and less than 5/μL at 72 hours. By seven days, it is rare to find circulating normoblasts (Nathan, 1993).

The normal *reticulocyte count* at birth ranges from 3% to 7% during the first 48 hours, during which time it rises slightly. After the second day, it falls rather rapidly to 1% to 3% by the seventh day of life.

Hemoglobin concentration in capillary blood during the first day of life averages 19.0 g/dL, with 95% of normal values falling between 14.6 and 23.4 g/dL. In cord blood, the average is 16.8 g/dL, with 95% of normals between 13.5 and 20 g/dL (Nathan, 1993). The hemoglobin level of venous blood frequently increases initially at the end of 24 hours compared with that of cord blood. At the end of the first week, the level is about the same as in cord blood, and it does not begin to fall until after the second week. During the first two weeks, the lower limit of normal is 14.5 g/dL for capillary blood and 13.0 g/dL for venous blood.

The hematocrit in capillary blood on the first day of life averages 0.61, with 95% of normal values between 0.46 and 0.76. In cord blood, the average is 0.53. The changes during the first few weeks parallel the hemoglobin concentration.

The Hb and Hct are highest at birth but fall rather steeply in the first days and weeks of life to a minimum at two months of age, when the lower limit of the 95% reference values and the mean value for the Hb are 9.4 and 11.2 g/dL, respectively, and for the Hct are 0.28 and 0.35, respectively. After the age of four months, the lower limit for the Hb is 11.2 g/dL and the Hct is 0.32; the values rise gradually until about age 5 years and somewhat more steeply in boys than in girls thereafter (Dallman, 1991).

The normal MCV at birth ranges from 104 to 118 fL, compared with the adult reference interval of 80 to 96 fL. Because the RBC does not fall as much as the Hb and Hct do, the MCV decreases abruptly, then gradually, during the first few months of life. The lowest value is reached at about 1 year. In studies in which iron deficiency and thalassemia are excluded, the lower reference limit (95% reference values) for the MCV gradually rises between the ages of 1 year and 15 years—in boys from 70 to 76 fL, and in girls from 70 to 78 fL (Dallman, 1991).

Reference intervals for red blood cell values in sexually mature adults are given in Table 24–7. The indices are similar in males and females, but the Hb is 1 to 2 g/dL higher in males, with commensurate increments in Hct and RBC (see Fig. 24–46). This difference is believed to be mainly the effects of androgen in stimulating erythropoietic production and its effect on the marrow. Estrogen probably has a slight suppressing effect on red cell production (Erslev, 1990).

In older men, the Hb tends to fall; in older women, the Hb tends to fall to a lesser degree (in some studies) or even rise slightly (in other studies). In older persons, therefore, the sex difference is less than 1 g Hb/dL (Dacie, 1991).

Posture and muscular activity change the concentration of the formed elements. The Hb, Hct, and RBC increase by several percent when a person stands from a recumbent position (Mollison, 1979); strenuous muscular activity causes a further increase, presumably owing primarily to loss of plasma water.

Diurnal variation that is not related to exercise or to analytical variation also occurs. The Hb is highest in the morning, falls during the day, and is lowest in the evening, with a mean difference of 8% to 9% (Dacie, 1991).

In persons living at a higher altitude, the Hb, Hct, and RBC are elevated over what they would be at sea level. The difference is about 1 g Hb/dL at 2 kilometers altitude and 2 g Hb/dL at 3 km. Increased erythropoiesis is secondary to anoxic stimulation of erythropoietin production. Smokers also tend to have mild erythrocytosis (see Chap. 26).

Table 24–7. TYPICAL BLOOD CELL VALUES IN A NORMAL POPULATION OF YOUNG ADULTS

	Men		Women
White cell count (× 10^9/L blood)		7.8 (4.4–11.3)	
Red cell count (× 10^{12}/L blood)	5.21 (4.52–5.90)		4.60 (4.10–5.10)
Hemoglobin (g/dL blood)	15.7 (14.0–17.5)		13.8 (12.3–15.3)
Hematocrit (percent)	46 (41.5–50.4)		40.2 (35.9–44.6)
Mean cell volume (fL/red cell)		88.0 (80.0–96.1)	
Mean cell hemoglobin (pg/red cell)		30.4 (27.5–33.2)	
Mean cell hemoglobin concentration (g/dL RBC)		34.4 (33.4–35.5)	
Red cell distribution width (CV, percent)		13.1 (11.6–14.6)	
Platelet count (× 10^9/L blood)		311 (172–450)	

The mean and reference internal (normal range) are given. Because the distribution curves may be non-gaussian, the reference interval is the nonparametric central 95% confidence interval. Results are based on 426 normal adult men and 212 normal adult women. Studies were performed on the Coulter model S-Plus IV. (Nelson and Morris, SUNY-Health Science Center at Syracuse).

Physiologic Variation in Leukocytes

The total white cell count at birth and during the first 24 hours of life varies within wide limits. Neutrophils are the predominant cell, varying from 6 to 28 × 10^9/L; about 15% of these are band forms (Altman, 1974), and a few myelocytes are present. Neutrophils drop to about 5 × 10^9/L during the first week of life and remain at about the same level thereafter. Lymphocytes are about 5.5 × 10^9/L at birth and change little during the first week. They become the predominant cell, on the average, after the first week of life and remain so until about age seven, when neutrophils again predominate. The upper limit of the 95% reference interval for lymphocytes at age 6 months is 13.5, at 1 year 10.5, at 2 years 9.5, at 6 years 7.0, and at 12 years 6.0 × 10^9/L. For neutrophils at the same ages, the values are 8.5, 8.5, 8.5, 8.0, and 8.0 × 10^9/L, respectively, all somewhat higher than those for adults (see Table 24–6).

Diurnal variation has been recognized in the neutrophil count, with highest levels in the afternoon and lowest levels in the morning at rest. However, Statland (1978) has shown, using precise methods (Hemalog D), that diurnal variation in neutrophils and in total WBC varies from subject to subject; some persons show little diurnal variation, but the pattern is consistent for the individual.

Exercise produces leukocytosis, which includes an increased neutrophil concentration as a result of a shift of cells from marginal to circulating granulocyte pool (see Chap. 25); increased lymphocyte drainage into blood also appears to contribute to the total increase.

Both the average and the lower reference value for neutrophil concentration in the black population are lower than in the white; this difference must be considered in assessing neutropenia.

Cigarette smokers have higher average leukocyte counts than nonsmokers. The increase is greatest (about 30%) in heavy smokers who inhale and affects neutrophils, lymphocytes, and monocytes (Corre, 1971).

There appear to be mild changes during the menstrual cycle (England, 1976a). Neutrophils and monocytes fall and eosinophils tend to rise during menstruation. Basophils have been reported to fall during ovulation (Mettler, 1974).

The availability of precise automated leukocyte analyzers provides the potential for investigating physiologic sources of variation that have been obscured by the statistical error in traditional microscopic differential counts (Statland, 1978).

Physiologic Variation in Platelets

The average platelet count is slightly lower at birth than in older children and adults and may vary from 84 × 10^9/L to 478 × 10^9/L (Nathan, 1993). After the first week of life, the reference intervals are those of the adult. No sex difference is clearly established. In women, the platelet count may fall at the time of menstruation.

ERYTHROCYTE SEDIMENTATION RATE

Principle

When well-mixed venous blood is placed in a vertical tube, erythrocytes tend to fall toward the bottom. The length of fall of the top of the column of erythrocytes in a given interval is called the erythrocyte sedimentation rate (ESR). Several factors are involved.

Plasma Factors

An accelerated ESR is favored by elevated levels of fibrinogen and, to a lesser extent, α_2-, β-, and γ-globulins. These asymmetric protein molecules have a greater effect than other proteins in decreasing the negative charge of erythrocytes (zeta potential) that tends to keep them apart. The decreased zeta potential promotes the formation of rouleaux, which sediment more rapidly than single cells. Removal of fibrinogen by defibrination lowers the ESR.

The ESR does not correlate absolutely with any of the plasma protein fractions. Albumin and lecithin retard sedimentation, and cholesterol accelerates the ESR.

Red Cell Factors

Anemia increases the ESR, because the change in the erythrocyte/plasma ratio favors rouleau formation, independent of changes in the concentration of the plasma proteins. By any method of measurement, the ESR is most sensitive to altered plasma proteins in the hematocrit range of 0.30 to 0.40 (Bull, 1975).

The sedimentation rate is directly proportional to the weight of the cell aggregate and inversely proportional to the surface area. Microcytes sediment slower than macrocytes, which have decreased ratios of surface area to volume. Rouleaux also have a decreased ratio of surface area to volume and accelerate the ESR. Red cells with an abnormal or irregular shape, such as sickle cells or spherocytes, hinder rouleau formation and lower the ESR.

Stages in the Erythrocyte Sedimentation Rate

Three stages can be observed: (1) In the initial 10 minutes, there is little sedimentation as rouleaux form. (2) For about 40 minutes, settling occurs at a constant rate. (3) Sedimentation slows in the final 10 minutes as cells pack at the bottom of the tube.

Methods

WESTERGREN METHOD

Because of its simplicity, the Westergren method is widely used. The National Committee for Clinical Laboratory Standards has recommended it as the standard method.

EQUIPMENT. The Westergren tube is a straight pipette 30 cm long, 2.5 mm in internal diameter, and calibrated in millimeters from 0 to 200. It holds about 1 mL. The Westergren rack is also used.

REAGENT. A 0.105 molar solution of sodium citrate is used as the anticoagulant-diluent solution (31 g of $Na_3C_6H_5O_7 \cdot H_2O$ added to 1 L of distilled water in a sterile glass bottle). This is filtered and kept refrigerated without preservatives.

PROCEDURE

1. Four mL of whole blood is added to 1.0 mL of sodium citrate and mixed by inversion.
2. A Westergren pipette is filled to the 0 mark and placed exactly vertical in the rack at room temperature without vibration or exposure to direct sunlight.
3. After exactly 60 minutes, the distance from the 0 mark to the top of the column of red cells is recorded in millimeters as the ESR value. If the demarcation between plasma and red cell column is hazy, the level is taken where the full density is first apparent.

MODIFIED WESTERGREN METHOD

A modification of the Westergren method produces the same results but employs blood anticoagulated with EDTA rather than with citrate. This is more convenient, because it allows the ESR to be determined from the same tube of blood as is used for other hematologic studies. Two milliliters of well-mixed EDTA-blood is diluted either with 0.5 mL of 3.8% sodium citrate or with 0.5 mL of 0.85% sodium chloride. Precision is poor with undiluted blood anticoagulated with EDTA (ICSH, 1977).

The ESR gradually increases with age. Westergren's original upper limits of normal (10 mm/hour for men and 20 mm/hour for women) appear to be too low. According to studies of Böttiger (1967) and Zauber (1987), upper limits of reference values for the Westergren method should be as follows:

	Men	*Women*
Below age 50 years	15 mm/h	20 mm/h
Above age 50 years	20	30
Above age 85 years	30	42

SOURCES OF ERROR

If the concentration of the anticoagulant is higher than recommended, the ESR may be elevated. Sodium citrate or EDTA does not affect the rate of sedimentation if used in the proper concentration. Heparin, however, alters the membrane zeta potential and cannot be used as an anticoagulant.

Bubbles left in the tube when it is filled will affect the ESR. Hemolysis may modify the sedimentation. The cleanliness of the tube is important.

Tilting the tube accelerates the ESR. The red cells aggregate along the lower side while the plasma rises along the upper side. Consequently, the retarding influence of the rising plasma is less effective. An angle of even 3 degrees from the vertical may accelerate the ESR by as much as 30%.

Temperature should be within the range of 20°C to 25°C. Lower or higher temperatures sometimes alter the ESR. If the blood has been kept refrigerated, it should be permitted to reach room temperature before the test is performed.

The test should be set up within two hours after the blood sample is obtained (or 12 hours if EDTA is used as the anticoagulant and the blood is kept at 4°C); otherwise, some samples with elevated ESRs will be falsely low (Morris, 1975). On standing, erythrocytes tend to become spherical and less readily form rouleaux.

There is no effective method for correcting for anemia in the Westergren method.

ZETA SEDIMENTATION RATIO

A centrifugal device (the Zetafuge) spins capillary tubes in a vertical position in four 45-second cycles (Bull, 1972). This results in controlled compaction and dispersion of erythrocytes, allowing rouleaux to form and sediment in three minutes. The capillary tube is then read like a microhematocrit, giving a value referred to as a zetacrit. The true hematocrit is divided by the zetacrit, and the result, expressed as a percentage, is the zeta sedimentation ratio (ZSR). It is not affected by anemia, which makes it easier to interpret. Its sensitivity to moderate elevation of the ESR by fibrinogen is the same as that of the Westergren method. The ZSR requires only a 100-μL sample and is considerably faster. The adult reference interval is 41% to 54% for both sexes.

A few clinical trials (Morris, 1977) showed the ZSR to be a satisfactory alternative to the ESR, but the Zetafuge is no longer produced.

The *Diesse Ves-matic* (Diesse Diagnostica Senese, Milano, Italy) instrument provides automated mixing and infrared end-point determination after 20 minutes of sedimentation. Samples showed good correlation with ICSH values and offer a safer, quicker, and more standardized ESR (Caswell, 1991).

MICRO-ESR METHOD

Barrett (1980) described a micro-ESR method using 0.2 mL of blood to fill a plastic disposable tube 230 mm long with a 1-mm internal bore. Capillary blood values correlated well with venous blood micro-ESR and Westergren ESR values. This method has more utility in pediatric patients.

Interpretation

The ESR is one of the oldest laboratory tests still in use. Its usefulness has decreased as more specific methods of evaluating disease (such as C-reactive protein) have been developed (Zlonis, 1993).

In pregnancy, the ESR increases moderately, beginning at the tenth to twelfth weeks, and returns to normal about one month post partum.

The ESR tends to be markedly elevated in monoclonal blood protein disorders such as multiple myeloma or macroglobulinemia, in severe polyclonal hyperglobulinemia due to inflammatory disease, and in hyperfibrinogenemia.

Moderate elevations are common in active inflammatory disease such as rheumatoid arthritis, chronic infections, collagen disease, and neoplastic disease. The ESR has little diagnostic value in these disorders, but it can be useful in monitoring disease activity. It is simpler than measurement of serum proteins, which has tended to replace the ESR. Because the test results often are normal in patients with neoplasms, connective tissue disease, and infections, a normal ESR does not exclude these diagnostic possibilities (Sox, 1986).

The ESR is of little value in screening asymptomatic patients for disease; history and physical examination will usually disclose the cause of an elevated ESR (Sox, 1986).

The ESR is useful and is indicated in establishing the diagnosis and in monitoring temporal arteritis and polymyalgia rheumatica (Zlonis, 1993).

In Hodgkin's disease, the ESR may be a useful prognostic blood measurement in the absence of systemic ("B") symptoms (fever, weight loss, night sweats). In one study (Vaughan Hudson, 1987), one third of asymptomatic patients had both an ESR of less than 10 mm/hour and an excellent survival rate regardless of age, stage, or histopathology. The survival rate of asymptomatic patients with an ESR of at least 60 mm/hour was as poor as that for patients with systemic symptoms.

Ahmed P, Minnich V, Michael JM: Platelet satellitosis with spurious thrombocytopenia and neutropenia. Am J Clin Pathol 1978; 69:473.

Altman PL, Dittmer DS: Biology Data Book. Bethesda, Federation of American Societies for Experimental Biology, 1974.

Ballas SK, Kocher W: Erythrocytes in HbSC disease are microcytic and hyperchromic. Am J Hematol 1988; 28:37.

Barrett BA, Hill PI: A micromethod for the erythrocyte sedimentation rate suitable for use on venous or capillary blood. J Clin Pathol 1980; 33:1118.

Batjer JD, Riddell K, Fritsma GA: Predicting bone marrow transplant engraftment by automated flow cytometric reticulocyte analysis. Lab Med 1994; 25:22.

Bentley SA, Lewis SM: Automated differential leukocyte counting: The present state of the art. Br J Haematol 1977; 35:481.

Bentley SA, Johnson A, Bishop CA: A parallel evaluation of four automated hematology analyzers. Am J Clin Pathol 1993; 100:626.

Bentley SA, Pegram MD, Ross DW: Diagnosis of infective and inflammatory disorders by flow cytometric analysis of blood neutrophils. Am J Clin Pathol 1987; 88:177.

Berkson J, Magath TB, Hurn M: The error of estimate of the blood cell count as made with the hemocytometer. Am J Physiol 1940; 128:309.

Bessis M: Blood Smears Reinterpreted, translated by G Brecher. New York, Springer-Verlag, 1977.

Bessman JD, Williams LJ, Gardner FH: Improved classification of anemias by MCV and RDW. Am J Clin Pathol 1983; 80:322.

Bessman JD, Williams LJ, Gilmer PR Jr: Mean platelet volume—the inverse relation of platelet size and count in normal subjects, and an artifact of other particles. Am J Clin Pathol 1981; 76:289.

Bollinger PB, Drewinko B, Brailas CD, et al: The Technicon H-1—an automated hematology analyzer for today and tomorrow. Am J Clin Pathol 1987; 87:71.

Böttiger LE, Svedberg CA: Normal erythrocyte sedimentation rate and age. Br Med J 1967; 2:85.

Brecher G, Schneiderman M: A time-saving device for the counting of reticulocytes. Am J Clin Pathol 1950; 20:1079.

Brittin GM, Brecher G: Instrumentation and automation in clinical hematology. Prog Hematol 1971; 7:299.

Brittin GM, Brecher G, Johnson CA: Evaluation of the Coulter Counter Model S. Am J Clin Pathol 1969a; 52:679.

Brittin GM, Brecher G, Johnson CA, et al: Stability of blood in commonly used anticoagulants—use of refrigerated blood for quality control of the Coulter Counter Model S. Am J Clin Pathol 1969b; 52:690.

Brugnara C, Colella GM, Cremins J, et al: Effects of subcutaneous recombinant human erythropoietin in normal subjects: Development of decreased reticulocyte hemoglobin content and iron-deficient erythropoiesis. J Clin Lab Med 1994a; 123:660.

Brugnara C, Laufer MR, Friedman AJ, et al: Reticulocyte hemoglobin content (CHr): Early indicator of iron deficiency and response to therapy. Blood 1994b; 83:3100.

Bull BS: Is a standard ESR possible? Lab Med 1975; 6:31.

Bull BS, Brailsford JD: The zeta sedimentation ratio. Blood 1972; 40:550.

Bull BS, Korpman RA: Autocalibration of hematology analyzers. J Clin Lab Auto 1983; 3:111.

Bull BS, Elashoff RM, Heilbron DC, et al: A study of various estimators for the derivative of quality control procedures from patient erythrocyte indices. Am J Clin Pathol 1974; 61:473.

Bunn HF, Forget BG, Ranney HM: Human Hemoglobins. Philadelphia, W.B. Saunders Company, 1977.

Bunn HF, Forget BG: Hemoglobin: Molecular, Genetic and Clinical Aspects. Philadelphia, W.B. Saunders Company, 1986.

Burns ER, Lampasso J, Kowatch N, et al: Performance characteristics of state-of-the-art hematology analyzers. Clin Lab Sci 1992; 5:181.

Buttarello M, Gadotti M, Lorenz C, et al: Evaluation of four automated hematology analyzers: A comparative study of differential counts (imprecision and inaccuracy). Am J Clin Pathol 1992; 97:345.

Buttarello M, Lorenz C, Gadotti M, et al: Diagnostic performance: A comparative study of the leukocyte differential count on four automated haematology analysers. Eur J Clin Chem Clin Biochem 1993; 31:251.

Camden TL: How to select the ideal hematology analyzer. Med Lab Obs 1993; (Feb):29.

Carlson DA, Io RK, Statland BE: Evaluation of the Sysmex CC-800: An automated eight parameter hematology instrument. Am J Clin Pathol 1986; 86:55.

Cartwright GE: Diagnostic Laboratory Hematology, 4th edition, New York, Grune & Stratton, 1968.

Caswell M, Stuart J: Assessment of Diesse Ves-matic automated system for measuring erythrocyte sedimentation rate. J Clin Pathol 1991; 44:946 (erratum J Clin Pathol 1992; 45:184).

Cohen AJ, Peerschke EI, Steigbigel RT: A comparison of the Coulter STKS, Coulter S+IV, and manual analysis of white blood cell differential counts in a human immunodeficiency virus-infected population. Am J Clin Pathol 1993; 100:611.

Connelly DP, McClain MP, Crowson TW, et al: The use of the differential leukocyte count for inpatient case finding. Hum Pathol 1982; 13:294.

Cornbleet J: Spurious results from automated hematology cell analyzers. Lab Med 1983; 14:509.

Cornbleet PJ, Myrick D, Judkins S, et al: Evaluation of the Cell-Dyn 3000 differential. Am J Clin Pathol 1992; 98:603.

Cornbleet PJ, Myrick D, Levy R: Evaluation of the Coulter STKS five-part differential. Am J Clin Pathol 1993; 99:72.

Corre F, Lellouch J, Schwarz D: Smoking and leukocyte counts—results of an epidemiological survey. Lancet 1971; 2:632.

Cox CJ, Haberman TM, Payne BA: Evaluation of the Coulter Counter Model S-Plus IV. Am J Clin Pathol 1985; 84:297.

Dacie JV, Lewis SM: Practical Haematology, 7th edition. Edinburgh, Churchill Livingstone, 1991.

Dallman PR: Blood and blood-forming tissues. *In* Rudolph AM, Hoffman JI (eds): Pediatrics, 19th ed. Norwalk, CT, and Los Altos, CA, Appleton & Lange, 1991.

Duncan KL, Gottfried EL: Utility of the three-part leukocyte differential count. Am J Clin Pathol 1987; 88:308.

Dutcher TF, Benzel JE, Egan JJ, et al: Evaluation of an automated differential leukocyte counting system: I. Instrument description and reproducibility studies. Am J Clin Pathol 1974; 62:525.

Egan JJ, Benzel JF, Hart DJ, et al: Evaluation of an automated differential leukocyte counting system: III. Detection of abnormal cells. Am J Clin Pathol 1974; 62:537.

England JM, Bain BJ: Total and differential leucocyte count. Br J Haematol 1976a; 33:1.

England JM, Down MC: Measurement of the mean cell volume using electronic particle counters. Br J Haematol 1976b; 32:403.

Erslev AJ: Anemia of endocrine disorders. *In* Beutler E, Lichtman MA, Coller BS, et al (eds): Williams Hematology, 5th edition. New York, McGraw-Hill, 1995, p 462.

Fairbanks VF, Fahey JL, Beutler E: Clinical Disorders of Iron Metabolism, 2nd edition. New York, Grune & Stratton, 1971.

Ford HC, Toomath RJ, Carter JM, et al: Mean platelet volume is increased in hyperthyroidism. Am J Hematol 1988; 27:190.
Germain PR, Lammers DB: False basophil counts on the Coulter STKS hematology analyzer. A study of specimens from patients infected with the Human Immunodeficiency Virus. Lab Med 1994; 25(6):376.
Gilbert HS, Ornstein L: Basophil counting with a new staining method using Alcian blue. Blood 1975; 46:279.
Gilmer PR Jr, Williams LJ, Koepke JA, et al: Calibration methods for automated hematology instruments. Am J Clin Pathol 1977; 68:185.
Goldsmith JR, Landow SA: Carbon monoxide and human health. Science 1968; 162:1352.
Griswold DJ, Champagne VD: Evaluation of the Coulter S-Plus IV three-part differential in an acute care hospital. Am J Clin Pathol 1985; 84:49.
Gulley ML, Bentley SA, Ross DW: Neutrophil myeloperoxidase measurement uncovers masked megaloblastic anemia. Blood 1990; 76:1004.
Hattersley PG, Gerard PW, Caggiano V, et al: Erroneous values on the Model S Coulter due to high titer cold agglutinins. Am J Clin Pathol 1971; 55:442.
Holt JT, De Wandler MJ, Arvan DA: Spurious elevation of the electronically determined mean corpuscular volume and hematocrit caused by hyperglycemia. Am J Clin Pathol 1982; 77:561.
Ialongo P, Lubrano MC, Fenu S, et al: Haematological monitoring of acute lymphoblastic leukemia by automated flow cytochemistry Bayer Technicon H*1. Haematol 1993; 78:89.
Ialongo P, Vignetti M, Cigliano G, et al: Flow cytometric measurement (H*1 Technicon) of microcytic and hyperchromic red cell populations in pediatric patients affected by hereditary spherocytosis. Haematology 1989; 74:547.
International Committee for Standardization in Haematology (ICSH): Recommendation for measurement of erythrocyte sedimentation rate of human blood. Am J Clin Pathol 1977; 68:505.
International Committee for Standardization in Haematology (ICSH): Expert Panel on Blood Cell Sizing: Recommendation for reference method for determination of packed cell volume of blood. J Clin Pathol 1980; 33:1.
International Committee for Standardization in Haematology (ICSH): ICSH reference method for staining of blood and bone marrow films by azure B and eosin Y (Romanowsky stain). Br J Haematol 1984; 57:707.
International Committee for Standardization in Haematology (ICSH): Protocol for evaluation of automated blood cell counters. Clin Lab Haematol 1984; 6:69.
Jaffe, ER, Hultquist DE: Cytochrome b5 reductase deficiency and enzymopenic hereditary methemoglobinemia. *In* Scriver CR, Beaudet AL, Sly WS, et al (eds): The Metabolic Basis of Inherited Disease. New York, McGraw-Hill, 1989, p 2267.
Jandl JH: Blood: Textbook of Hematology. Boston, Little Brown, 1987.
Kalish RJ, Becker K: Evaluation of the Coulter S-Plus V three-part differential in a community hospital, including criteria for its use. Am J Clin Pathol 1986; 86:751.
Kaplow L, Orlowski L, Vaznelis ME: Evaluation of the Technicon H6000 hematology system. J Clin Lab Autom 1983; 3:167.
Kline A, Bird A, Adams L, et al: Identification of blast cells in the peripheral blood of patients with acute leukemia using the Technicon H*1. Clin Lab Haematol 1989; 11:111.
Koepke JA, Dotson MA, Shifman MA: A critical evaluation of the manual/visual differential leukocyte counting method. Blood Cells 1985; 11:173.
Krause JR, Costello RT, Krause J, et al: Use of the Technicon H-1 in the characterization of leukemias. Arch Path Lab Med 1988; 112:889.
Lampasso JA: Error in hematocrit value produced by excessive ethylenediamine-tetraacetate. Am J Clin Pathol 1965; 44:109.
Lanza F, Moretti S, Latorraca S, et al: Flow cytochemical analysis of peripheral lymphocytes in chronic B lymphocytic leukemia and its correlation with morphologic features. Leuk Res 1992; 16:639.
Lapen D: A standardized differential stain for hematology. Cytometry 1982; 2:309.
Lazarus HM, Chahine A, Lacerna K, et al: Kinetics of erythrogenesis after bone marrow transplantation. Am J Clin Pathol 1992; 97:574.
Lillie RD (ed): H.J. Conn's Biological Stains, 9th edition. Baltimore, Williams & Wilkins, 1977.
Lofsness KG, Kohnke ML, Geier NA: Evaluation of automated reticulocyte counts and their reliability in the presence of Howell-Jolly bodies. Am J Clin Pathol 1994; 101(1):85.
Lombarts AJ, deKieviet W: Recognition and prevention of pseudothrombocytopenia and concomitant pseudoleukocytosis. Am J Clin Pathol 1988; 89:634.
Lubrano GJ, Dean WW, Heinsohn HG, et al: The analysis of some commercial dyes and Romanowsky stains by high-performance liquid chromatography. Stain Technol 1977; 52:13.
Luke RG, Koepke JA, Siegel RR: The effects of immunosuppressive drugs and uremia on automated leukocyte counts. Am J Clin Pathol 1971; 56:503.
Mansberg HP, Saunders AM, Groner W: The Hemalog D white cell differential system. J Histochem Cytochem 1974; 22:711.
Mathy KA, Koepke JA: The clinical usefulness of segmented vs. stab neutrophil criteria for differential leukocyte counts. Am J Clin Pathol 1974; 61:947.
McClure S, Custer E, Bessman JD: Improved detection of early iron deficiency in nonanemic subjects. JAMA 1985; 253:1021.
Mettler L, Shirwani D: Direct basophil count for timing ovulation. Fertil Steril 1974; 25:718.
Metzger DK, Charache S: Flow cytometric reticulocyte counting with thioflavin T in a clinical hematology laboratory. Arch Pathol Lab Med 1987; 111:540.
Miers MK, Fogo AB, Federspiel CF, et al: Evaluation of the Coulter S-Plus IV three-part differential as a screening tool in a tertiary care hospital. Am J Clin Pathol 1987; 87:745.
Mohandas N, Kum YR, Tycko DH: Accurate and independent measurement of volume and hemoglobin concentration of individual red cells by laser light scattering. Blood 1986; 68:506.
Mollison PL: Blood Transfusion in Clinical Medicine. Oxford, Blackwell Scientific Publications, 1979, p 128.
Morgan DL, Peck SD: The use of red cell distribution width in the detection of iron deficiency in chronic hemodialysis patients. Am J Clin Pathol 1988; 89:513.
Morris MW, Pinals RS, Nelson DA: The zeta sedimentation ratio (ZSR) and activity of disease in rheumatoid arthritis. Am J Clin Pathol 1977; 68:760.
Morris MW, Skrodzki Z, Nelson DA: Zeta sedimentation ratio (ZSR), a replacement for the erythrocyte sedimentation rate (ESR). Am J Clin Pathol 1975; 64:254.
Moyer VA, Grimes R: Total and differential leukocyte counts in clinically well children. Am J Dis Child 1990; 144:1200.
Nathan DG, Oski, FA: Hematology of Infancy and Childhood, 4th ed. Philadelphia, W.B. Saunders Company, 1993.
Nixon GA, Mentrup P: Automated office hematology instruments. Prim Care 1986; 13:727.
Nosanchuk JS, Roark MF, Wanser C: Anemia masked by triglyceridemia. Am J Clin Pathol 1974; 62:838.
Pappas AA, Owens RB, Flick JT: Reticulocyte counting by flow cytometry—a comparison with manual methods. Ann Clin Lab Sci 1992; 22(2):125.
Payne BA, Pierre RV: Using the three-part differential: Part 2. Implementation of the system. Lab Med 1986; 17:517.
Payne BA, Pierre RV, Lee WK: Evaluation of the TOA E-5000 automated hematology analyzer. Am J Clin Pathol 1987; 88:51.
Peacock JE, Ross DW, Cohen MS: Automated cytochemical staining and inflammation, further assessment of the "left shift." Am J Clin Pathol 1982; 78:445.
Penchansky L, Krause JR: Flow cytochemical study of acute leukemia of childhood with the Technicon H*1. Lab Med 1991; 22(3):184.
Pierre RV, Payne BA, Lee WK, et al: Comparison of four leukocyte differential methods with the National Committee for Clinical Laboratory Standards (NCCLS) reference method. Am J Clin Pathol 1987; 87:201.
Robertson EP, Lai HW, Wei DC: An evaluation of leucocyte analysis on the Coulter STKS. Clin Lab Haemat 1992; 14:53.
Robertson EP, Pollock A, Yau KS: Use of Technicon H*1 technology in routine thalassemia screening. Med Lab Sci 1992; 49:259.
Rogers, C.H.: Blood sample preparation for automated differential systems. Am J Med Technol 1973; 39:435.
Ross DW, Kaplow LS: Myeloperoxidase deficiency: Increased sensitivity for immunocytochemical compared to cytochemical detection of enzyme. Arch Path Lab Med 1985a; 109:1005.
Ross DW, Watson JJ, David PH, et al: Evaluation of the Coulter three-part differential screen. Am J Clin Pathol 1985b; 84:481.
Rowan RM, Fraser C: Platelet size distribution analysis. *In* van Assendelft OW, England JM (eds): Advances in Hematological Methods: The Blood Count. Boca Raton, FL, CRC Press, 1982, p 125.
Rümke CL: The imprecision of the ratio of two percentages observed in differential white blood cell counts: A warning. Blood Cells 1985; 11:137.
Sacker LS: Specimen collection. *In* Lewis SM, Coster JF (eds): Quality Control in Haematology. New York, Academic Press, 1975, p 211.
Schoentag RA: Hematology analyzers. Clin Lab Med 1988; 8:653.
Simmons A, Leaverton P, Elbert G: Normal laboratory values for differential white cell counts established by manual and automated cytochemical methods (Hemalog D). J Clin Pathol 1974; 27:55.
Simson E (ed): Proceedings of the Technicon H*1 Hematology Symposium. Tarrytown, NY, Technicon Instruments Inc, 1986.
Small BM, Bettigole RE: Diagnosis of myeloproliferative disease by analysis of platelet volume distribution. Am J Clin Pathol 1981; 76:685.
Smith JR, Landaw SA: Smoker's polycythemia. N Engl J Med 1978; 298:6.
Sox HC Jr, Liang MH: The erythrocyte sedimentation rate—guidelines for rational use. Ann Intern Med 1986; 104:515.
Statland BE, Winkel P, Harris SC, et al: Evaluation of biologic sources of variation of leukocyte counts and other hematologic quantities using very precise automated analyzers. Am J Clin Pathol 1978; 69:48.
Stroop DM, Triplett RC, Perrotta G, et al: Comparison of the Abbott Cell

DYN 3000 SL and the Coulter STKS Hematology Analyzers. Ann Clin Lab Sci 1994; 24(3):250.
Taft EG: Pseudoleukocytosis due to cryoprotein crystals. Am J Clin Pathol 1973; 60:669.
Threatte GA: Usefulness of the mean platelet volume. Clin Lab Med 1993; 13(4):937.
Tichelli A, Gratwohl A, Driessen A, et al: Evaluation of the Sysmex R-1000: An automated reticulocyte analyzer. Am J Clin Pathol 1990; 93:70.
Tsakona CP, Kinsey SE, Goldston, AH: Use of flow cytochemistry via the H*1 in FAB identification of acute leukaemias. Acta Haematol 1992; 88:72.
van Assendelft OW: Spectrophotometry of Haemoglobin derivatives. Assen, The Netherlands, Royal Van Gorcum Ltd, 1970.
van Leeuwen I, Eggels PH, Bullen JA: A short evaluation of a new haematological cell counter—the Cell-Dyn 3000 following a modified tentative NCCLS-procedure. Eur J Clin Chem Clin Biochem 1991, 29:105.
Vaughan Hudson B, Maclennan KA, Bennett MH, et al: Systemic disturbance in Hodgkin's disease and its relation to histopathology and prognosis. Clin Radiol 1987; 38:257.
Verheul FE, Spitters JM, Bergmans CH: Evaluation and performance of the Coulter STKS. Eur J Clin Chem Clin Biochem 1993; 31(3):179.
Warner BA, Reardon DM: A field evaluation of the Coulter STKS. Am J Clin Pathol 1991; 95(2):207.
Warner BA, Reardon DM, Marshall DP: Automated haematology analysers: A four-way comparison. Med Lab Sci 1990; 47:285.
Watson JS, Ross DW: Characterization of myelodysplastic syndromes by flow cytochemistry with the Technicon H*1. Med Tech 1987; 4:18.
Weick JK, Hagedorn AB, Linman JW: Leukoerythroblastosis: Diagnostic and prognostic significance. Mayo Clin Proc 1974; 49:110.
Wenz B, Ramirez MA, Burns ER: The H*1 Hematology Analyzer: Its performance characteristics and value in the diagnosis of infectious disease. Arch Pathol Lab Med 1987; 111:521.
Williams WJ, Morris MW, Nelson DA: Examination of the blood. *In* Beutler E, Lichtman MA, Coller BS, et al (eds): Williams Hematology, 5th ed. New York, McGraw-Hill, 1995, p 8.
Winkel P, Olesen T, Nissen NI: Automated cytochemistry in the prediction of remission following chemotherapy of patients with de novo acute myeloblastic leukemia. Am J Clin Pathol 1982; 77:50.
Zauber NP, Zauber AG: Hematologic data of healthy very old people. JAMA 1987; 257:2181.
Zeigler Z, Murphy S, Gardner FH: Microscopic platelet size and morphology in various hematologic disorders. Blood 1978 51:479.
Zlonis M: The mystique of the erythrocyte sedimentation rate—a reappraisal of one of the oldest laboratory tests still in use. Clin Lab Med 1993; 13:787.

Chapter 25

Hematopoiesis

Robert E. Hutchison, M.D.
Frederick R. Davey, M.D.

STEM CELLS

In postnatal life in humans, erythrocytes, granulocytes, monocytes, and platelets are normally produced only in the bone marrow. Lymphocytes are produced in the secondary lymphoid organs as well as in the bone marrow and thymus gland. Most bone marrow cells are morphologically recognizable precursors of granulocytes or erythrocytes; there are smaller numbers of platelet precursors (megakaryocytes), lymphocytes, monocytes, macrophages, stromal cells (endothelial cells, fibroblasts, osteoblasts and osteoclasts), eosinophils, plasma cells, basophils, mast cells, and blasts. The last group includes stem cells, both hematopoietic progenitor cells, which are capable of self-renewal and differentiation, and committed progenitor cells, which differentiate along a specific pathway.

Hematopoietic Stem Cells

A pluripotential or multipotential stem cell is present in the marrow and gives rise to two major progenitors—the lymphoid stem cell and the myeloid or hematopoietic stem cell. The latter is a common precursor cell for granulocytes and monocytes, erythrocytes, and megakaryocytes. Evidence of this in animal models was demonstrated experimentally by Till (1961), who injected isologous bone marrow cells into irradiated mice. Seven to ten days later spleen colonies formed that contained erythroid cells, granulocytes, megakaryocytes, or a mixture of cell types. It was shown that all the differentiating cells in a single colony were derivatives of a single stem cell, and after retransplanting cells from a single colony with only one differentiated cell type, multipotential stem cells were still present in the individual colonies. These multipotential stem cells were operationally designed colony-forming units spleen (CFU-S).

Evidence in the human of a multipotential hematopoietic stem cell was derived from myeloproliferative disorders (polycythemia vera, myelofibrosis with myeloid metaplasia, chronic myelogenous leukemia). In these disorders it was shown that one precursor cell gives rise to the abnormal erythrocytes, granulocytes, and megakaryocytes but not to marrow fibroblasts, and in most cases not to lymphocytes. These are, therefore, monoclonal disorders.

Hematopoietic precursor cells can be detected immunologically using monoclonal antibodies against the CD34 antigen, a glycoprotein associated with hematopoietic precursors that is encoded on chromosome 1q (Molgaard, 1989). These cells comprise approximately 1% to 4% of bone marrow cells and have the morphology of blasts. They also occur in small numbers in the peripheral blood and increase with administration of growth factors or some chemotherapeutic agents, allowing the use of peripheral blood as well as bone marrow to obtain stem cells for bone marrow transplantation (Siena, 1989).

The pluripotent or multipotential stem cell gives rise to committed stem cells, which in turn proliferate or differentiate and mature, resulting in maintenance of a hematopoietic system that is consistent yet highly responsive to changing needs for oxygenation, defense, and hemostasis. The control of hematopoiesis involves varying gene expressions, stimulatory factors, and feedback mechanisms about which we are currently learning a great deal.

Committed Progenitor Cells

Committed progenitor cells (committed stem cells) are characterized by their ability to form colonies *in vitro* in response to a soluble factor. Bradley (1966) and Ichikawa (1966) described *in vitro* culture systems in which granulocytic differentiation occurred from normal mouse hemopoietic cells; the technique was later adapted for human cells by Pike (1970). The cultures consist of two layers of cells in agar: an upper layer of blood or bone marrow contains "target" stem cells (colony-forming cells [CFC] or colony-forming units in culture [CFU-C]); a lower layer of blood cells (feeder layer) contains a diffusible substance (colony-stimulating activity [CSA]) necessary to stimulate the CFC to proliferate and differentiate into colonies. After a period of 7 to 14 days, colonies become visible in the upper layer; these are composed of neutrophils, monocytes (macrophages), a mixture of these two cell types, or eosinophils. The CSA necessary in the feeder layer is produced by monocytes or activated T lymphocytes. It was shown that each colony was derived from a single progenitor (stem) cell. Because both neutrophils and monocytes were found in the same colony, it became clear that neutrophils (granulocytes) and monocytes were both derived from a single committed progenitor cell (CFU-GM) in response to a soluble substance—granulocyte-monocyte colony-stimulating factor (GM-CSF).

Commitment of a pluripotent stem cell along an increasingly specific path is the first requirement for differentiated hematopoiesis. This is currently thought to be, at least initially, a stochastic or random event, in which a proportion of stem cells express limited portions of their genetic repertoire and are either positively or negatively selected (Trinchieri, 1993). Differentiation of embryonic stem (ES) cells in culture involves interaction with stromal cells and growth factors. This is demonstrated by the finding that ES cells differentiate *in vitro* into the variety of blood cell precursors when cocultured with a stromal cell line lacking production of macrophage-stimulating factor (M-CSF), which inhibits production of blood cells except macrophages. Manipulation of culture conditions with other growth factors encourages differentiation along other blood cell lines (Nakono, 1994).

The earliest bone marrow cell that is a progenitor of stromal cells as well as hematopoietic cells is recognizable immunologically by its expression of CD34 with lack of the major histocompatibility complex (MHC) Class II antigen HLA-DR (Deeg, 1993). The earliest hematopoietic cell is CD34+, HLA-DR+, and CD38− (Deeg, 1993; Terstappen, 1991). Lineage commitment can be recognized by additional expression of CD38 antigen along with other antigens such as CD71 for erythroid, CD33 for myeloid, CD10 for B-lymphoid, and CD7/CD5 for T-lymphoid differentiation (Terstappen, 1991). Selection and differentiation with progressively narrower lineage restrictions are influenced by local effects in the bone marrow microenvironment and humoral factors (Trinchieri, 1993) and probably involve MHC Class II molecule interactions (Deeg, 1993).

Hematopoietic Growth Factors

Soluble or membrane-bound biochemical factors contributing to control of hematopoiesis are referred to as hematopoietic growth factors or interleukins (IL). They consist of acidic glycoproteins that are functionally diverse but structurally conserved (Kaushansky, 1993). Elucidation of these factors is occurring rapidly in a fashion very different from that characteristic of other biochemical systems in the past. Genes associated with hematopoietic growth factors are identified, cloned, and sequenced, and the products are generated by recombinant DNA methods. Molecular structures are frequently predicted using computer models from sequence data as well as analyzed directly by crystallography and magnetic resonance spectroscopy. Pure molecules are used experimentally and several are now used therapeutically as drugs. The rapid growth in knowledge of hematopoietic growth factors and the complexity of their activities defy simple summation. The factors noted here along with their primary known functions are listed in an order designed to facilitate reference rather than strictly according to importance.

Erythropoietin (EPO) stimulates proliferation, growth, and differentiation of erythroid precursors, resulting in increased erythrocyte counts, and may have a minor effect on megakaryocytes. EPO, an 18-kDa protein (34 to 39 kDa when glycosylated) encoded on the long arm of chromosome 7, is primarily produced in the kidney in adult life and is induced by hypoxia (Bagby, 1991). Recombinant EPO is used clinically to treat anemia, particularly that associated with renal failure, chemotherapy, or bone marrow infiltration by cancer (Mertelsmann, 1994).

Granulocyte-monocyte colony-stimulating factor (GM-

CSF) is a pan-myeloid growth factor that stimulates erythroid, granulocyte, monocyte, megakaryocyte, and eosinophil progenitors (Bagby, 1991), resulting primarily in increases of neutrophils, monocytes, and eosinophils and in activation of phagocytic function (Mertelsmann, 1994). It is a 14- to 35-kDa glycoprotein encoded on the long arm of chromosome 5. GM-CSF is used clinically to combat neutropenia in patients receiving chemotherapy and those undergoing bone marrow transplantation (Mertelsmann, 1994). Myeloid hyperplasia may result in the bone marrow in these patients.

Granulocyte colony-stimulating factor (G-CSF) stimulates granulocyte production and functional activation. It is an 18-kDa protein encoded on the long arm of chromosome 17 (Bagby, 1991). G-CSF is used to treat neutropenia (Mertelsmann, 1994).

Monocyte-macrophage colony-stimulating factor (M-CSF) stimulates monocyte-macrophage production and activity. It consists of two species of glycoprotein (40- to 50- and 70- to 90-kDa) that are encoded on the long arm of chromosome 5 (Bagby, 1991).

Thrombopoietin is a newly characterized growth factor that is the primary regulator of platelet production. It is homologous with erythropoietin and may act on the same stem cells. Thrombopoietin and erythropoietin appear to act in competition for a common precursor cell (Wendling, 1994; Kaushansky, 1994; Lok, 1994; de Sauvage, 1994; Metcalf, 1994; McDonald, 1993).

Interleukin 1 (IL1) is a broadly active cytokine produced by monocytes, fibroblasts, endothelial cells, and, to some extent, almost all cells. It exists as two 31-kDa protein forms encoded by different genes on chromosome 2. IL1 is induced by inflammation and results in production of other cytokines (IL1, IL6, GM-CSF, and G-CSF) by leukocytes, stromal and epithelial cells (Bagby, 1991). It is thus a modulator of inflammation.

Interleukin 2 (IL2) stimulates growth and activation of T lymphocytes, B lymphocytes, and natural killer (NK) cells. It is a 23-kDa product encoded on the long arm of chromosome 4 and is produced by activated T cells (Bagby, 1991). It has been a subject of intense interest owing to its role as an autocrine factor in T-cell malignancies and its experimental use as a modulator of therapeutic antitumor immune activity. IL2 is a good example of the intricacies of growth factor ligand and receptor interactions. Serum IL2 (ligand) attaches to IL2 receptors on T cells, resulting in activation and further IL2 production as well as up-regulation (increased expression) of IL2 receptors in a positive feedback (autocrine) loop. This loop is inhibited by the presence of soluble IL2 receptors in the serum that bind to available IL2 ligand.

Interleukin 3 (IL3) is a multipotential colony-stimulating factor that has activity analogous to that of GM-CSF but at an earlier level. The 14- to 28-kDA protein is encoded near the GM-CSF gene on the long arm of chromosome 5. It is produced by T cells and mast cells and probably imparts its activities indirectly by stimulating other cytokines (Bagby, 1991).

Interleukin 4 (IL4) is an 18-kDa protein produced by activated T cells and has multiple activities including stimulation of activated B cells, T cells, macrophages, and mast cells. It induces isotype switching from IgG to IgE in B cells, induces IL2 receptor expression on T cells, and induces G-CSF and M-CSF in monocytes (Bagby, 1991).

Interleukin 5 (IL5) activates cytotoxic T cells, induces immunoglobulin secretion, and stimulates eosinophils. It is a 50- to 60-kDa product of the long arm of chromosome 5 that is produced by activated T cells (Bagby, 1991).

Interleukin 6 (IL6) is a broadly active factor that appears to exert its influence indirectly through synergy with other factors. It functions along with IL3 to increase replication of myeloid precursors, synergizes with IL2 and IL4, and stimulates platelet production. It is a 26-kDa product of the short arm of chromosome 7 (Bagby, 1991).

Interleukin 7 (IL7) is a less well described growth factor that stimulates production of immature lymphoid (pre-B and pre-T) cells (Bagby, 1991).

Interleukin 8 (IL8) is a chemotactic factor for neutrophils and T cells. It is an 8- to 10-kDa protein produced by activated T cells (Herbert, 1993).

Interleukin 9 (IL9) is a T-cell growth factor and mast cell-activating factor that also has effects in stimulating erythroid and myeloid proliferation. It is a 30- to 40-kDa glycoprotein encoded on chromosome 5 (Quesniaux, 1994).

Interleukin 10 (IL10) is a lymphocyte regulatory cytokine that acts in a complex fashion largely by inhibiting the Th1 subset of T-helper cells. It thus inhibits IL2, IL3, tumor necrosis factor (TNF), interferon γ, and GM-CSF. It also stimulates thymocytes and mast cells. A homologous product of Epstein-Barr virus (BCRF1) is thought to have resulted from viral capture of human host genetic information and has effects thought to promote virus survival (Quesniaux, 1994).

Interleukin 11 (IL11) promotes formation of antigen-specific Ig-secreting B cells and synergizes with IL3 to stimulate megakaryocyte production and pluripotential stem cell proliferation. It is a 23-kDa glycoprotein encoded on the long arm of chromosome 19 (Quesniaux, 1994).

Interleukin 12 (IL12) is a stimulatory factor for natural killer (NK) cells and both CD4+ and CD8+ T cells. It is a 70-kDa glycoprotein (Quesniaux, 1994).

Interleukin 13 (IL13) is a 10-kDa protein produced by activated T cells and shows activity similar to that of IL4, including anti-inflammatory effects on macrophages and regulation of B-cell functions. It does not, however, stimulate T cells (Zurawski, 1994).

Interleukin 14 (IL14), also called high-molecular-weight B-cell growth factor, has effects on B-cell maturation. It induces B-cell proliferation, inhibits immunoglobulin secretion, and induces selective expansion of B-cell populations. It is a 53-kDa protein produced by T cells and some malignant B cells (Ambrus, 1993).

Interleukin 15 (IL15) is a T-cell growth factor produced by a variety of tissues. It shares activities with IL2, shows partial antigenic similarity, and appears to use components of the IL2 receptor (Grabstein, 1994).

Kit ligand (KL) is the ligand for the tyrosine kinase receptor *c-kit* and has been referred to as stem cell factor or steel factor. It synergizes with most other growth factors including

GM-CSF and IL3 to stimulate myeloid, erythroid, and lymphoid progenitors (Quesniaux, 1994).

Cytoadhesion Molecules in Hematopoiesis

Cytoadhesion molecules are required to modulate many interactions between hematopoietic cells and growth factors, stromal cells, endothelium and extracellular matrix. These cell surface molecules influence induction, differentiation, and function of hematopoietic cells and often have multiple functions. Several major families of adhesion molecules exist. These include the adhesion molecules of the immunoglobulin supergene family, the integrins and the selectins (Long, 1992; Inghirami, 1993).

The immunoglobulin supergene family includes T-cell receptors and immunoglobulins, which are specialized for antigen detection. It also includes lymphocyte functional antigens LFA2 (CD2) and LFA3 (CD58) and intercellular cytoadhesion molecules (ICAM1 and ICAM2). LFA2 and LFA3 are involved in antigen-independent cell attachment of T lymphocytes. ICAM1, present on some erythroid and granulocytic progenitors as well as macrophages, appears to have a role in progenitor cell cytoadhesion.

Integrins are receptors for cells and also proteins of the extracellular matrix. They are each composed of two membrane-spanning α and β chains and their function appears to be β-chain dependent. The β1 integrins include six proteins identified on activated T cells and referred to as very late antigens (VLA). VLA2 binds collagen and laminin, and VLA3 binds collagen and fibronectin. The β2 integrin LFA1 (CD11a/CD18) is the counterreceptor for ICAM1 and is restricted to blood cells. It and other so-called leukocyte integrins MAC1 ([R3] [CD11b/CD18]) and gp 150, 95 (CD11c/CD18) are necessary for migration during inflammation. LFA1 is also involved in T-cell and NK cell cytotoxicity and, in association with other molecules including CD44, functions in lymphoid and myeloid cell ontogenesis and lymphocyte migration.

The selectin LEC-CAM family molecules have a lectin-binding domain, an endothelial growth factor receptor domain, and an area homologous with complement-binding proteins—thus the acronym LEC. These molecules include a lymphocyte homing receptor (MEL14), which interacts with a ligand on the endothelium of lymph node high endothelial venules (HEV), resulting in entry of lymphocytes into the lymph node. A similar molecule, ELAM1, is involved in neutrophil-endothelial cell interaction during inflammation. Another selectin, GP140 (CD62), is also involved in leukocyte-endothelial cell interaction. It is found in platelet granules and endothelial cells, is mobilized during coagulation, and is inducible on neutrophils and monocytes.

Many extracellular matrix components interact with receptors on hematopoietic cells. These include fibronectin, thrombospondin, hyaluronic acid, homonectin, and heparan sulfate. Receptors for some of these are known. CD44, receptor for hyaluronic acid, is an antigenically related group of inducible cell surface proteins variably expressed on all leukocytes. It is required for early granulopoiesis as well as trafficking of mature lymphocytes. Additional cytoadhesion molecules that have effects on hematopoiesis are known (Long, 1992), and undoubtedly many more remain to be described.

HEMATOPOIETIC TISSUES

Embryonic and Fetal Hematopoiesis

Beginning in the first month of prenatal life, the first blood cells arise outside the embryo in the mesenchyme of the yolk sac as *blood islands*. The cells are predominantly *primitive erythroblasts*, which are large and megaloblastic, are formed intravascularly, and retain their nuclei. At the sixth week, hematopoiesis begins in the liver, and this becomes the major hematopoietic organ of early and midfetal life. *Definitive erythroblasts,* which become non-nucleated red cells, are formed extravascularly in the liver, and granulopoiesis and megakaryocytes are present to a lesser degree. In midfetal life, the spleen and to a lesser extent lymph nodes play a minor role in hematopoiesis, but the liver continues to dominate. In the latter half of fetal life, the bone marrow becomes progressively more important as a site of blood cell production, and the liver's role diminishes.

Postnatal Hematopoiesis

4

Shortly after birth, hematopoiesis in the liver ceases, and the marrow is the only site of production of erythrocytes, granulocytes, and platelets. Hematopoietic stem cells and committed progenitor cells are maintained in the marrow. Lymphocytes (of the B-cell type) continue to be produced in the marrow as well as in the secondary lymphoid organs, whereas T lymphocytes are produced in the thymus and also in the secondary lymphoid organs (see later section in this chapter under Lymphocytes).

At birth, the total marrow space is occupied by active hematopoietic (red) marrow. As body growth progresses and marrow space increases during infancy, only part of that space is needed for hematopoiesis; the remaining space is occupied by fat cells. Later in childhood, only the flat bones (the skull, vertebrae, thoracic cage, shoulder, and pelvis) and the proximal parts of the long bones (femora and humeri) are sites of blood formation. The remaining marrow space is fatty or yellow marrow that can be replaced by hematopoietic cells if continuous, intensive stimulation exists.

The marrow circulation is closed—that is, arterioles deriving from central longitudinal arteries (i.e., in long bones) connect directly with broad venous sinuses that anastomose and eventually empty into central longitudinal veins. The flattened endothelium of the sinuses is partially covered by adventitial reticular cells, a form of fibroblast that elaborates argentophilic reticulin fibers. These reticular cells and fibers form the supporting meshwork of the marrow stroma, where the hematopoietic cells reside. The reticular cells are but minimally phagocytic; they may swell and take up water, may become fat cells, and possibly may induce hematopoietic stem cells to become committed progenitor cells. After proliferation and maturation have occurred in the marrow stroma, blood cells gain entrance to the blood through or between the endothelial cells of the sinus wall. This requires displacement of adventitial cells.

ERYTHROCYTE PRODUCTION

The erythrocyte is a vehicle for the transport of hemoglobin, which is produced in precursor cells of the erythrocytes, the normoblasts. The function of hemoglobin is the transport of oxygen and carbon dioxide. The erythrocyte is also metabolically capable of keeping hemoglobin in a functional state.

Normoblastic Maturation

(Plate 25–1)

The earliest recognizable erythroid precursor is the *pronormoblast* (Fig. 25–1 and Plate 25–1*A* and *I*). At about 20 μm diameter, it is the largest of the erythroid precursors. The nucleus has a fine, uniform chromatin pattern that is somewhat more distinct and more intensely staining than that of the myeloblast. The nuclear membrane is prominent. One or more prominent nucleoli are present. The cytoplasm has a heterogeneous quality and is moderate in amount and moderately basophilic; no granules are present. The pronormoblast undergoes mitosis and forms two basophilic normoblasts.

The *basophilic normoblast* (Plate 25–1*B, C, J,* and *K*) is somewhat smaller and has slightly coarser chromatin that stains intensely; the chromatin may be partially clumped and the pattern may suggest a wheel with broad spokes. The parachromatin (the nonchromatin part of the nucleus) is distinct and stains pink. Nucleoli are present but not often visible. The nuclear/cytoplasmic (N/C) ratio is moderate; about one fourth of the total cell area appears to be cytoplasm. The cytoplasm is deeply basophilic owing to the abundance of RNA; much of this is evident as polyribosomes in electron micrographs. The cell borders of early normoblasts frequently are made irregular by pseudopodia.

After mitosis of the basophilic normoblast, evidence of continuing hemoglobin production becomes visible in the cytoplasm of the two daughter cells as polychromasia—i.e.,

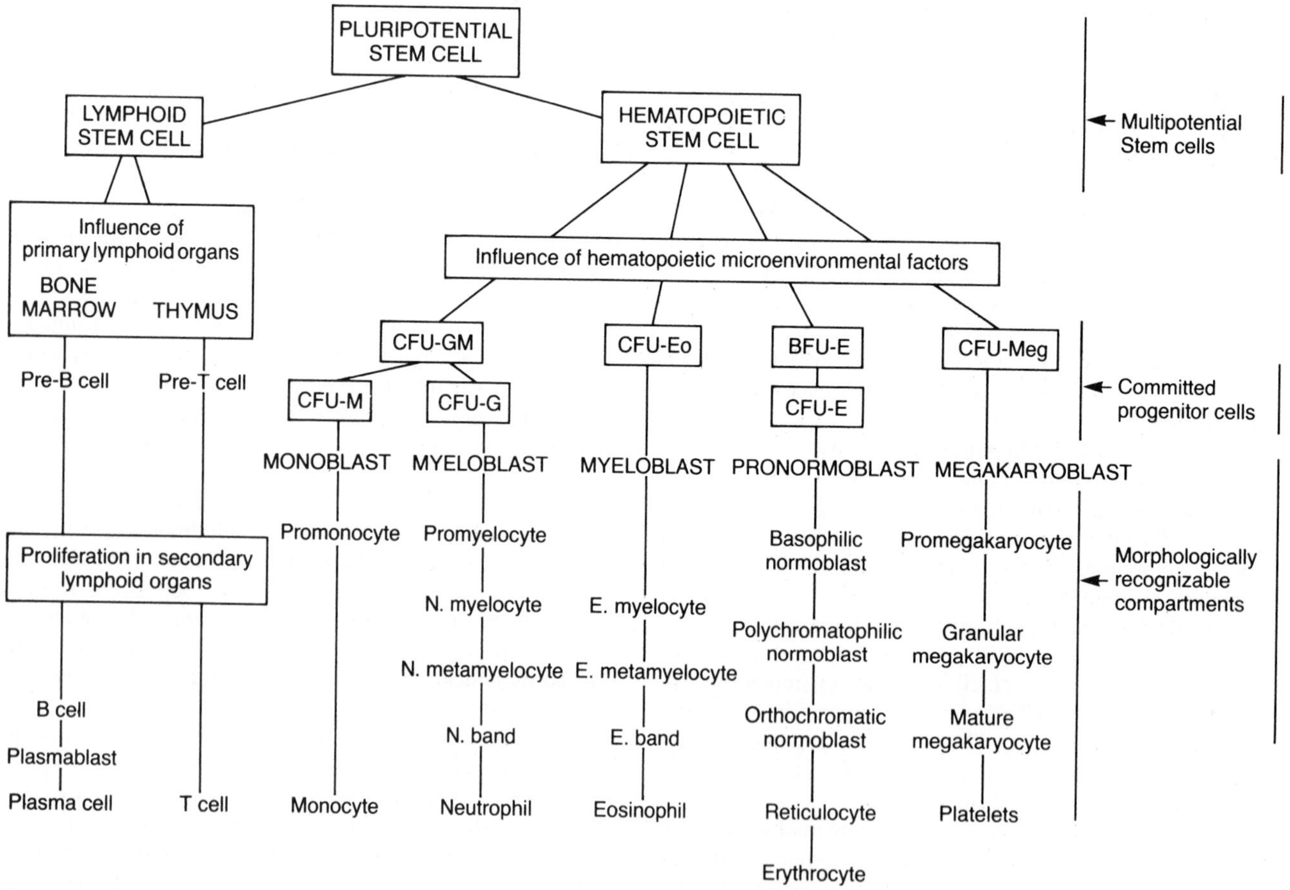

Figure 25–1. Hypothetical scheme of hematopoiesis.
CFU-GM = Colony-forming unit (cell)—granulocyte/monocyte
CFU-M = Colony-forming unit (cell)—monocyte
CFU-G = Colony-forming unit (cell)—granulocyte
CFU-Eo = Colony-forming unit (cell)—eosinophil
BFU-E = Burst-forming unit (cell)—erythroid
CFU-E = Colony-forming unit (cell)—erythroid
CFU-Meg = Colony-forming unit (cell)—megakaryocyte

mixtures of the red-staining of hemoglobin with the blue of RNA in varying shades of gray. This cell is the *polychromatophilic normoblast* (see Fig. 24–37 and Plate 25–1*C, J, K, L,* and *M*), which is slightly smaller than the basophilic normoblast. The nucleus occupies about half of the area of the cell, stains intensely, and has moderately condensed chromatin that is sharply distinct from the pink parachromatin. The polychromatophilic normoblast undergoes one or two mitotic divisions.

After the last mitosis, the nucleus becomes small and dense (pyknotic), and the *orthochromatic normoblast* stage is reached (see Fig. 24–37 and Plate 25–1*D*). Mitosis is no longer possible. The cell is smaller than the polychromatophilic normoblast and has a lower N/C ratio. The cytoplasm contains more abundant hemoglobin and fewer polyribosomes and remains slightly polychromatophilic.

Finally, accompanied by cytoplasmic contractions and undulations, the nucleus and a small rim of cytoplasm are ejected from the orthochromatic normoblast, forming the *reticulocyte.* On air-dried films with Romanowsky's stains, the reticulocyte is polychromatophilic as a result of the retention of RNA.

In the marrow, developing erythroid cells are usually in contact with macrophages in what are termed "erythroblastic islands" (Plate 25–1*N*). These erythroblastic islands are usually broken up when aspirated marrow is spread on slides, but fragments of macrophage cytoplasm are sometimes seen attached to the separated normoblasts, especially on Prussian blue-stained films.

During proliferation and maturation, iron is transferred from plasma transferrin into the cells in the normoblastic series. The pronormoblast and basophilic normoblast have the highest content of RNA, which begins to decline in the polychromatophilic normoblasts as hemoglobin increases in amount. Synthesis of RNA gradually decreases in each stage through the orthochromatic normoblasts. Of course, when the nucleus is no longer present (in the reticulocyte), RNA synthesis ceases, yet the RNA already present remains for a few days, and protein and heme synthesis continue in the reticulocyte until the cell loses its RNA and mitochondria.

During this maturation process, three or four mitotic divisions occur in a period of three days, resulting in the potential production of 16 reticulocytes from each pronormoblast. The reticulocytes are larger than mature red cells and are sticky. They remain in the marrow stroma for one to two days before they are released into the blood.

In the marrow the number of reticulocytes is about equal to that of nucleated erythrocytes and slightly higher than the number of reticulocytes in the circulating blood. If sufficiently severe hypoxia is present, this marrow pool of reticulocytes can be released, approximately doubling the number of circulating reticulocytes.

Normally, reticulocytes remain as such, slowly synthesizing hemoglobin for two to three days in the marrow and one day in the blood. Residual ribosomes, mitochondria, and other organelles are then removed, and the mature erythrocytes circulate for about 120 days. During this time they gradually age, certain enzymatic activities diminish, and they are finally destroyed by phagocytic cells of the reticuloendothelial system.

Megaloblastic Maturation

(Plate 25–1)

The abnormal maturation of erythroid precursors that occurs in vitamin B_{12} deficiency or folic acid deficiency (see Chap. 26) is known as megaloblastic maturation, and the abnormal erythroid cells are called *megaloblasts.* Because of the impaired ability of the cells to synthesize DNA, the intermitotic and mitotic phases are prolonged. This results in enlarged cells in which nuclear maturation lags behind cytoplasmic maturation (nuclear cytoplasmic dissociation). The nuclear chromatin pattern is more delicate and more "open," and parachromatin is prominent. Karyorrhexis, or breaking up of the nucleus, and Howell-Jolly bodies are frequently noted. Megaloblastic development parallels normoblastic maturation; the stages of promegaloblast, basophilic megaloblast, polychromatophilic megaloblast, and orthochromatic megaloblast may be recognized (Plate 25–1*E* to *H*).

Regulation of Erythrocyte Production

The number of erythrocytes in the blood may be regulated by changing the rate of production. The rate of erythrocyte destruction does not vary appreciably in normal individuals. Increased production of erythrocytes occurs when oxygen transport to the tissues is impaired, as in anemia, in cardiac or pulmonary disorders, and in the low oxygen tension of high altitudes. On the other hand, production of erythrocytes is decreased when an individual is hypertransfused or exposed to high oxygen tension.

Oxygen affinity of hemoglobin is modulated by the concentration of phosphates, in particular 2,3-diphosphoglycerate (2,3-DPG), in the red cell. These phosphates combine with the β chains of reduced hemoglobin and diminish its affinity for oxygen (Fig. 25–2). In areas of tissue hypoxia, as oxygen moves from hemoglobin into the tissues, the amount of reduced hemoglobin in the red cells increases, binding more 2,3-DPG, further reducing its oxygen affinity so that more oxygen can be delivered to the tissues. If hypoxia persists, depletion of free 2,3-DPG leads to increased glycolysis, production of more 2,3-DPG, and a persistently lower oxygen affinity of the hemoglobin.

Tissue hypoxia induces formation of erythropoietin, a hormone that travels in the plasma to the marrow, where it effects the production of more red cells. It acts by inducing committed progenitor cells (CFU-E and BFU-E) in the marrow to proliferate and differentiate into pronormoblasts, by shortening the generation time of normoblasts, and by promoting early release of reticulocytes into the blood. The result is increased numbers of marrow normoblasts in a normal ratio of cell types, a condition known as normoblastic hyperplasia.

Measurement of erythropoietin may be accomplished by bioassay using mice or by *in vitro* immunologic methods. Elevated levels are detected in patients with erythroid hyperplasia and aplastic anemia. Decreased levels below the normal range are found in normal individuals after transfusion and in patients with polycythemia vera.

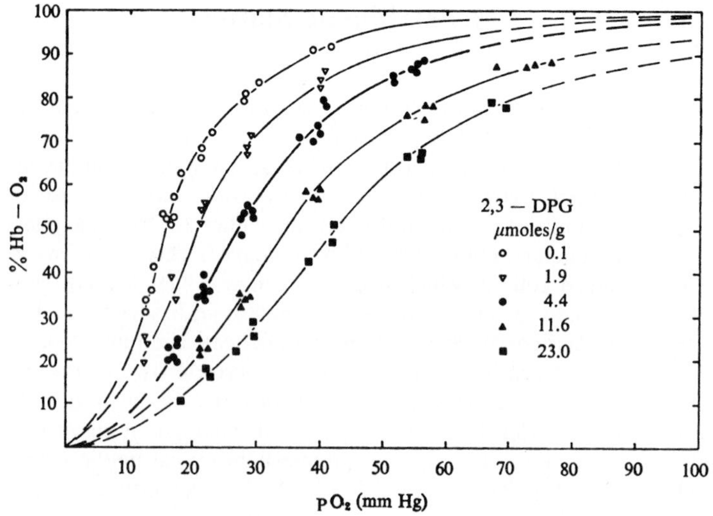

Figure 25–2. Oxygen dissociation curves of hemoglobin at different concentrations of 2,3-diphosphoglycerate (DPG). The curve is sigmoidal and shifts to the right with increasing concentrations of 2,3-DPG; this results in decreased affinity of hemoglobin for oxygen and increased delivery of oxygen to the tissues. (From Duhm J: *In* Rorth M, Astrup P [eds]: Oxygen Affinity of Hemoglobin and Red Cell Acid Base Status [Alfred Benzon Symposium IV]. Copenhagen. Munksgaard International Publishers, 1972, p 583.)

Synthesis of Hemoglobin

HEME SYNTHESIS. Heme synthesis occurs in most cells of the body except mature erythrocytes but is most abundant in the erythroid precursors. Succinylcoenzyme A condenses with glycine to form the unstable intermediate α-amino β-ketoadipic acid, which is readily decarboxylated to δ-aminolevulinic acid (ALA) (Fig. 25–3). This condensation requires pyridoxal phosphate (vitamin B_6) and occurs in mitochondria.

ALA is excreted normally in small amounts in the urine, but in certain abnormalities of heme synthesis (e.g., lead poisoning) excretion is increased. Two molecules of ALA condense to form the monopyrrole porphobilinogen, which is catalyzed by the enzyme ALA-dehydrase. Porphobilinogen is also normally excreted in small amounts in the urine. Markedly elevated amounts appear in the urine in acute intermittent porphyria and are easily detected by a color reaction with Ehrlich's aldehyde reagent.

Four molecules of porphobilinogen react to form uroporphyrinogen III or I (Fig. 25–4). The Type III isomer is converted, by way of coproporphyrinogen III and protoporphyrinogen, to protoporphyrin. In certain diseases when this pathway is partially blocked, Type I isomers of uropor-

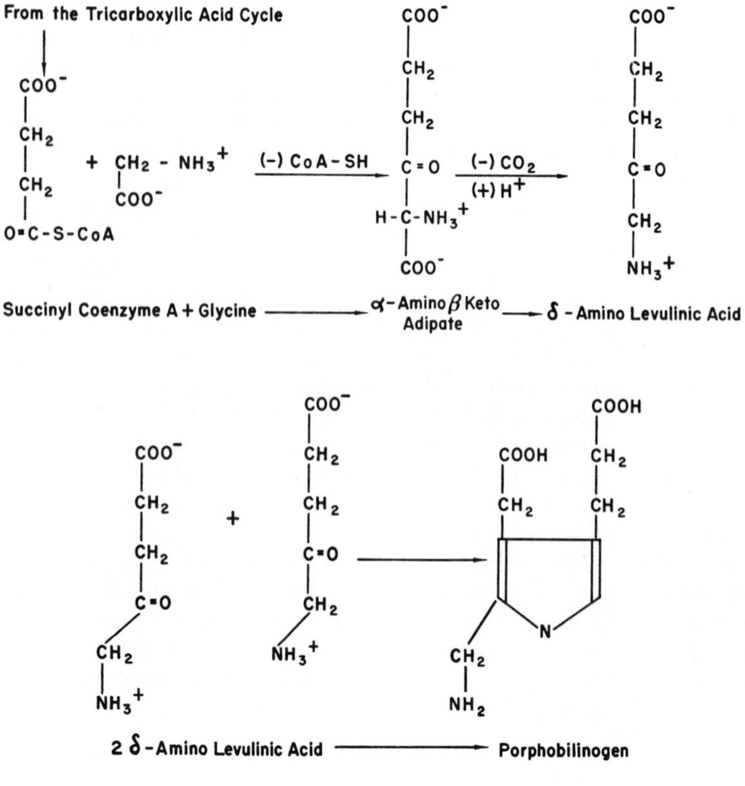

Figure 25–3. Formation of porphobilinogen from succinylcoenzyme A and glycine. (From Leavell BS: Fundamentals of Clinical Hematology, 4th ed. Philadelphia, W.B. Saunders Company, 1976.)

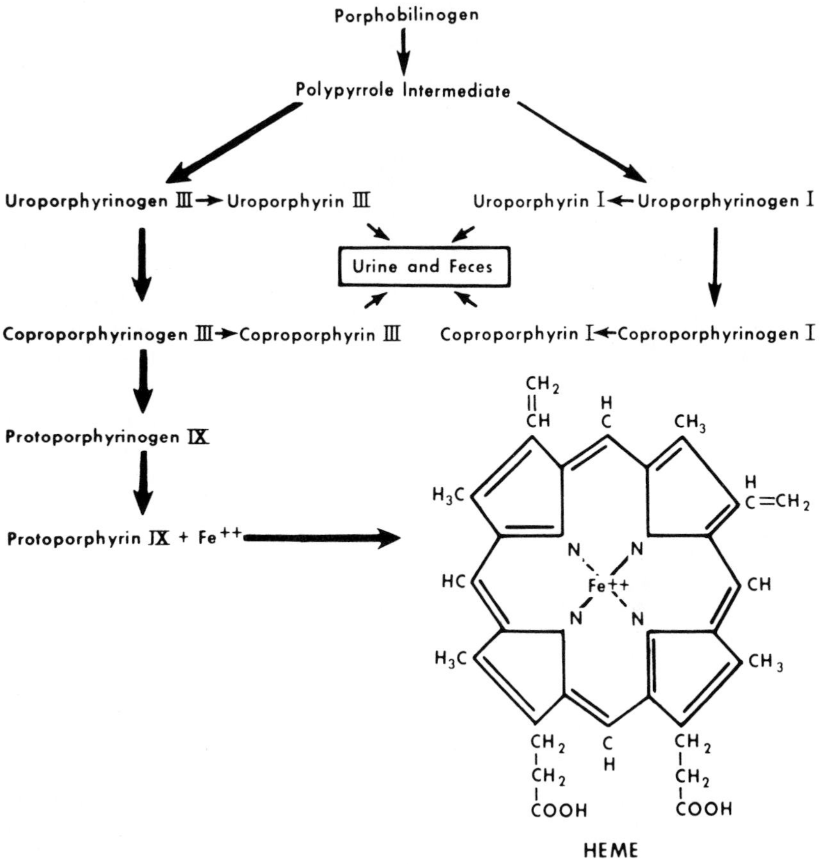

Figure 25–4. Formation of heme from porphobilinogen. (From Leavell BS: Fundamentals of Clinical Hematology, 4th ed. Philadelphia, W.B. Saunders Company, 1976.)

4

phyrinogen and coproporphyrinogen are formed, and their oxidized excretion products, uroporphyrin I and coproporphyrin I, are increased in amount.

Protoporphyrin is normally found in mature erythrocytes. In patients with lead poisoning or iron deficiency, levels of free erythrocyte protoporphyrin are increased.

Iron is inserted into protoporphyrin by the mitochondrial enzyme ferrochetalase to form the finished heme moiety.

GLOBIN SYNTHESIS. Globin synthesis occurs in the cytoplasm of normoblasts and reticulocytes. The polypeptide chains are manufactured on the ribosomes. Specific small soluble RNA (sRNA) molecules determine the placement of each amino acid according to the code in the messenger RNA (mRNA). Progressive growth of the polypeptide chain begins at the amino end. This process of protein synthesis occurs on ribosomes clustered into polyribosomes, which are held together by mRNA. Because the reticulocyte can synthesize hemoglobin for at least two days after loss of its nucleus, the mRNA for hemoglobin is apparently quite stable. The polypeptide chains released from the ribosomes are folded into their three-dimensional configurations spontaneously.

Control of hemoglobin synthesis is exerted primarily through the action of heme. Increased heme inhibits further heme synthesis by inhibiting the activity and synthesis of ALA synthase. Heme also promotes globin synthesis, mainly at the site of chain initiation, the interaction of ribosomes with mRNA.

Structure and Function of Hemoglobin (Bunn, 1986)

In each hemoglobin molecule, one heme group is inserted into a hydrophobic pocket of one folded polypeptide chain. Normal adult hemoglobin A consists of four heme groups and four polypeptide chains (two α chains and two β chains), which form a roughly globular hemoglobin molecule (Fig. 25–5). The ferrous iron atoms have six coordination bonds—four to the pyrrole nitrogens of heme, one to the imidazole nitrogen of histidine of the globin chain (87-α or 92-β), and one that is reversibly bound to oxygen. As the oxygen partial pressure increases, the four heme groups sequentially bind one molecule of oxygen each. In the process, a change in the overall configuration of the hemoglobin molecule occurs, and this altered configuration favors the additional binding of oxygen.

The sigmoid-shaped oxygen dissociation curve of hemoglobin reflects this increasing affinity for oxygen with an increasing partial pressure of oxygen in the lungs (see Fig. 25–2). In the tissues, the conversion of HbO_2 to Hb, the decreasing pH and increasing temperature produced by metabolic processes, and the binding of more 2,3-DPG to Hb result in a shift of the Hb-oxygen dissociation curve to the right, which favors the release of oxygen from hemoglobin.

Carbon dioxide is transported in erythrocytes as well as in plasma. A small part of red cell carbon dioxide is dissolved and a small part is bound to amino groups of hemoglobin as

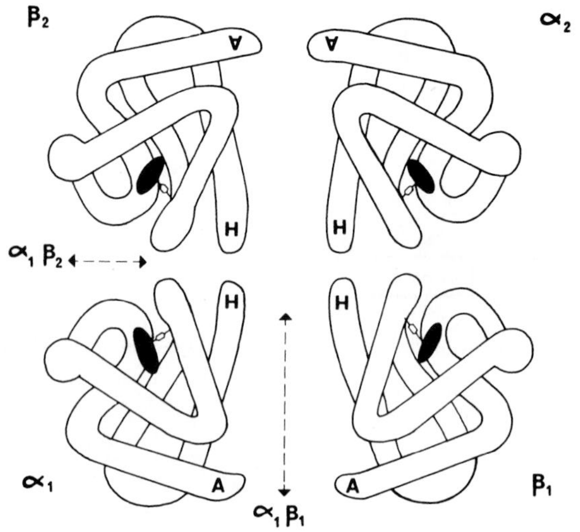

Figure 25–5. The hemoglobin molecule (tetramer, molecular weight 64,500 daltons). The heme group for each monomeric polypeptide chain is depicted as a black disc, connected to an imidazole group of histidine, and located near the surface of the molecule in a "pocket" formed by the polypeptide chain. The letters A and H designate alphahelic segments of each polypeptide chain: A is the N-terminal segment, and H is the C-terminal segment. The four monomers are separated in this drawing, but actually make contact along a relatively large area ($\alpha_1\beta_1$), which is thought to be the relatively fixed or stabilizing contact area, and a smaller ($\alpha_1\beta_2$) area thought to be the functional contact area, where movement occurs during oxygenation and deoxygenation, changing the molecular configuration. (From White JM, Dacie JV: Prog Hematol 1971; 7:69. Orlando, FL, Grune & Stratton Inc, by permission.)

carbamino carbon dioxide, but most is in the bicarbonate form. The enzyme carbonic anhydrase catalyzes the transformation of carbon dioxide to bicarbonate in red cells in the tissue capillary bed and catalyzes the reverse reaction (the release of carbon dioxide from bicarbonate) in the erythrocytes in the capillary bed of the lungs.

ERYTHROCYTE DESTRUCTION

The erythrocyte gradually undergoes metabolic changes during the course of its 120-day lifespan, at which time the less viable senescent cell is removed from the circulation. Certain glycolytic enzymes diminish in activity as the cell ages. Older red cells have a smaller surface area and an increased mean cell hemoglobin concentration (MCHC) compared with younger cells. Furthermore, aged red cells lose sialic acid from their membranes, exposing an asialoglycophorin. This senescent antigen is recognized and an autoantibody is synthesized by the host. After the binding of the autoantibody, the senescent cell is removed from the circulation by the reticuloendothelial system. About three million cells are normally removed from the blood per second without any demonstrable histologic evidence of erythrophagocytosis.

In some pathologic states, the reticuloendothelial system removes younger sensitized or abnormal red cells at a rapid rate. Subsequently, erythrophagocytosis is often evident. In autoimmune hemolytic anemia, the reticuloendothelial system removes red cells following the binding of autoantibodies or complement to reticulocytes and young red cells. In other pathologic states, red cells are removed because of structural defects that interfere with their normal passage through the microcirculation of the reticuloendothelial system.

Degradation of Hemoglobin

After removal of the red cell from the circulation, hemoglobin is broken down with the macrophages of the reticuloendothelial system into its three constituents—iron, protoporphyrin, and globin. The iron goes into storage and may be completely reused. The globin may be degraded and returned to the amino acid pool of the body. In contrast, the protoporphyrin ring is split, converted to bilirubin, and excreted from the body.

In the macrophage, the protoporphyrin ring is cleaved by a heme oxidase enzyme at the α-methene bridge, yielding one mole of carbon monoxide (CO) and one mole of biliverdin. The carbon monoxide appears in the blood as HbCO and is eventually exhaled. Biliverdin is reduced to bilirubin in the macrophage, and bilirubin is transported to the liver by plasma albumin (see Chap. 12). It is removed from the plasma by the liver cell, conjugated mainly with glucuronide, and excreted in the bile. In the intestine, reduction by bacteria occurs, and bilirubin is transformed into urobilinogen, mesobilirubinogen, and stercobilinogen, compounds that are collectively designated urobilinogens.

Estimations of exhaled carbon monoxide, hemoglobin carbon monoxide, or fecal urobilinogen can be used as measures of hemoglobin breakdown. When production of red cells is diminished and the level of circulating hemoglobin is low, as in aplastic anemia, urobilinogen excretion is reduced. When destruction of erythrocytes is increased, as in hemolytic anemia, all three substances are increased in amount.

In normal humans, about 80% to 90% of the excreted bile pigment measured as fecal urobilinogen is derived from the breakdown of senescent erythrocytes that have lived 100 to 120 days. However, about 10% to 20% of the pigment is excreted within the first few days. This early labeled bile pigment comes from nonhemoglobin heme formed in the liver as well as from the breakdown of newly formed hemoglobin in the bone marrow. Much of the latter may represent hemoglobin from the nucleus and pieces of cytoplasm of the orthochromatic normoblast that are lost during the process of nuclear extrusion.

In certain hematologic diseases, notably thalassemia, megaloblastic anemia, refractory normoblastic anemia, and erythropoietic porphyria, this early labeled bile pigment fraction may be markedly increased. This intramedullary destruction of hemoglobin, which never appears in circulating erythrocytes, is known as ineffective erythropoiesis.

ERYTHROKINETICS

The balance between delivery of erythrocytes to the blood and removal of erythrocytes from the blood results in a relatively constant hemoglobin mass in the circulation. Anemia occurs when the removal of erythrocytes from the blood is increased and cannot be compensated by increased production, or when the delivery of erythrocytes to the blood is decreased, or when both processes exist together.

When anemia develops, tissue hypoxia leads to elevated levels of erythropoietin in the plasma. The resultant normoblastic hyperplasia produces more erythrocytes for delivery to the circulation. The marrow in a normal individual is capable of six to eight times the normal output of erythrocytes with extreme stimulation. This capacity must be compared with the output actually attained when one is evaluating the marrow response of a given patient.

Measurements that assess *effective erythropoiesis* (production and delivery of erythrocytes to the circulation), *ineffective erythropoiesis,* and destruction of erythrocytes may be necessary to determine the mechanism and the cause of anemia.

Measurements of Total Production of Erythrocytes or Hemoglobin

The *total mass of erythropoietic cells* in the body cannot be easily measured. An estimate is made by examining a sample of bone marrow from a normally active site and determining the cellularity and the percentage of total nucleated cells that are erythropoietic (see later section, Bone Marrow Examination). When marrow activity increases, usually the additional hematopoietic cells replace the fat in the red marrow sites before extension occurs into the yellow marrow of the long bones. One assumes that the sample is representative of the marrow as a whole, an assumption that is usually valid.

The *plasma iron turnover* is calculated from the serum iron level and the rate of removal of injected radioactive iron from the plasma. About 25% to 30% of the iron is not used in erythropoiesis and is primarily taken up by the liver. The remaining 70% to 75% is taken up by erythropoietic cells and is therefore a measure of total erythropoiesis, both effective and ineffective.

Measurements of Total Destruction of Erythrocytes or Hemoglobin

Determination of *fecal urobilinogen* provides an estimate of the total excretion of bile pigments—the breakdown products of heme. This measurement includes pigment derived from hemoglobin formed and destroyed in the marrow without ever reaching the circulating erythrocytes. Limitations of this measurement include the possibility of diminished conversion of bilirubin to urobilinogen because of oral administration of broad-spectrum antibiotics, and failure of pigment to reach the intestine in patients with obstructive jaundice. In severe liver disease, less reabsorbed urobilinogen is excreted in the bile and more is excreted in the urine. The urine urobilinogen is not as good a measure of urobilinogen excretion for two reasons: Removal by the kidney is usually a minor component of the total excretion, and with a normally functioning liver, clearance of reabsorbed urobilinogen in the plasma is so effective that considerable increases in the circulating blood may result in little or no elevation of the urine urobilinogen.

Measurements of Effective Production of Erythrocytes

RETICULOCYTE COUNT. Because the RNA of the reticulocyte disappears about a day after its entry into the blood, enumeration of reticulocytes is a measure of the number of cells being delivered by the marrow to the blood each day—that is, a measure of effective erythropoiesis. The absolute reticulocyte count is calculated by multiplying the reticulocyte percentage by the erythrocyte count. To give a meaningful expression of erythropoiesis, the absolute reticulocyte count, or some estimate of it, and not simply the percentage must be used. The normal absolute reticulocyte count is approximately 50×10^9/L, or 1% of circulating erythrocytes. Because the normal maturation time for reticulocytes in the blood is one day, production is 50×10^9 reticulocytes per liter per day.

A second consideration is the need for an adjustment for increased maturation time of reticulocytes in the blood owing to accelerated release from the marrow, an effect of erythropoietin. The need for this is recognized by the presence of large polychromatic cells or nucleated red cells in the blood film, indicating a shift of excessively immature reticulocytes from the marrow into the blood. To avoid an overestimate of the daily erythrocyte production, a correction factor is used based on the estimated maturation time of reticulocytes in the blood. This varies inversely with hematocrit as follows (Hillman, 1992):

Hematocrit (%)	Reticulocyte Maturation Time (days)
45	1.0
35	1.5
25	2.0
15	2.5

If a patient has a hematocrit of 0.25, a red cell count of 2.89 $\times 10^{12}$/L, and a reticulocyte count of 7%, he will have an absolute reticulocyte count of 202×10^9/L. Because the average normal absolute reticulocyte count is 50×10^9/L, he has

$$\frac{202 \times 10^9/\text{L}}{50 \times 10^9/\text{L}}$$

or four times as many reticulocytes as normal. However, this result must be corrected for increased maturation time (shift): $4 \times \frac{1}{2} = 2$. Therefore, two times as many reticulocytes are entering the blood per day as in a normal individual—that is, the red cell production is two times normal.

If only the hematocrit is available, the same correction can be made as follows:

Correction for anemia:

$$\frac{\text{Patient's reticulocyte count (7\%)}}{\text{Normal reticulocyte count (1\%)}} \times \frac{\text{Patient's Hct (0.25)}}{\text{Normal Hct (0.45)}} = 4$$

Correction for shift:

$$\text{Corrected reticulocyte index (4)} \times \frac{1}{\text{maturation time (2)}} = 2$$

4

These corrections are necessary to assess the degree of red cell production in response to anemia.

A normal individual with a normal supply of iron can increase red cell production by two times normal within a week if the hematocrit drops to 0.35, or to three times normal if the hematocrit drops to 0.25. Only if there is a parenteral supply of iron (such as in hemolysis) can the maximal red cell production of six to eight times normal be achieved. If an appropriate marrow response to anemia has not been reached in one to two weeks, some impairment of red cell production exists.

The *erythrocyte utilization of iron* is a measure of the amount of an injected dose of iron that appears in the hemoglobin of circulating erythrocytes. It is derived from the plasma iron turnover and the percentage of radioactive iron that has been injected and that appears in the circulating erythrocytes after two weeks, assuming that none of the newly formed cells have been destroyed in that time interval. This, too, is a measure of effective erythropoiesis.

Measurements of Effective Survival of Erythrocytes in Blood

The *erythrocyte survival* can be determined by removing a sample of blood, labeling the erythrocytes with ^{51}Cr, inactivating the excess ^{51}Cr remaining in the plasma, and reinjecting the labeled erythrocytes into the patient. The ^{51}Cr is bound to the β chain of the hemoglobin molecule and for the most part is not released until the red cell is removed from the circulation and the hemoglobin is degraded. Measurements of radioactivity in red cells are made at 2 hours or 24 hours (the zero time, or 100% level) and at one- to three-day intervals until more than 50% of the activity has disappeared. The results are usually expressed as the ^{51}Cr half-survival time. The normal range is 28 to 38 days. (The reason it is not 60 days is that ^{51}Cr is eluted from the hemoglobin at the rate of about 1% per day.) If the production of erythrocytes equals their destruction (i.e., if a steady state exists), the erythrocyte survival is also a measure of the effective production of erythrocytes.

SUMMARY. Total erythropoiesis refers to the total production of hemoglobin or red cells; effective erythropoiesis refers to production of hemoglobin or red cells that reach the circulation; and ineffective erythropoiesis refers to production of hemoglobin or red cells that never reach the circulating blood. These concepts of the *erythrokinetic* approach to the study of anemia are useful, especially in anemias that defy easy classification.

NEUTROPHILS

(Plate 25–2)

The common progenitor cell for neutrophils and monocytes (CFU-GM) divides and gives rise to the progenitor cells for granulocytes (CFU-G) and for monocytes (CFU-M). CFU-G and CFU-M give rise to myeloblasts and monoblasts, respectively, with stimulation by colony-stimulating factors for granulocytes and monocytes (see Fig. 25–1 and Table 25–1).

Table 25–1. RECOMBINANT HUMAN HEMATOPOIETIC COLONY-STIMULATING FACTORS

Name	Protein Size (kDa)	Sources	Hematopoietic Lineages
G-CSF	18–22	Monocytes Fibroblasts	n
GM-CSF	14–35	T cells Endothelial cells Fibroblasts	n.m.e.E.M.
Interleukin-3	14–28	T cells	n.m.e.b.E.M.
M-CSF	35–45 (×2) 18–26 (×2)	Monocytes Fibroblasts Endothelial cells	m
Erythropoietin	34–39	Kidney	E

The M-CSF proteins are homodimers of the indicated sizes. The hematopoietic lineages that result from the action of the factors on the stem cells and progenitor cells are as follows: n = neutrophils; m = monocytes; e = eosinophils; b = basophils; E = erythroid cells; and M = megakaryocytes.

Modified from Clark SC, Kamen R: Science 1987; 236:1229–1237. Copyright 1987 by the AAAS; and Nathan DG, Sieff CA: Prog Hematol 1987; 15:1.

Morphology of Neutrophil Precursors

The *myeloblast* (see Plate 25–2*A*) is a cell about 15 μm in diameter with a moderately high N/C ratio; a large oval to quadrangular nucleus; a very fine, uniform chromatin pattern; a delicate nuclear membrane; and two to five nucleoli. The cytoplasm is pale, clear blue, and without granules. The appearance of azurophil granules (~0.5 μm diameter) heralds the earliest promyelocyte (see Plate 25–2*B*) and indicates that the cell is to be a neutrophil. The *promyelocyte* stage encompasses the entire period of production of azurophil granules. The promyelocyte is slightly larger than the myeloblast. The nuclear chromatin begins to condense a bit, and the nucleoli are less obvious. The cytoplasm is basophilic and is filled by more and more azurophil granules (Plate 25–2*C*). The *neutrophil myelocyte* stage begins with the appearance of specific neutrophil granules, at first only in the Golgi region; as more specific granules develop, they spread throughout the cytoplasm (Plate 25–2*D* to *H*). With successive mitoses, the number of azurophil granules (which have ceased production at the end of the promyelocyte stage) is diminished. The early neutrophil myelocyte, therefore, has a rather fine, dispersed nuclear chromatin pattern, many azurophil granules, and few specific granules. The late neutrophil myelocyte has a somewhat more condensed chromatin pattern, a cytoplasm well filled with specific granules, and rather few azurophil granules. The myelocyte is the latest stage capable of cell division. Next is the *neutrophil metamyelocyte*, which is distinguished by an indented, kidney-shaped nucleus with more condensed chromatin (Plate 25–2*F* and *G*). From this stage on, changes in the cytoplasm are insignificant. In the *band neutrophil* (stab form), the nucleus has more condensed chromatin and a rather uniform elongated shape. Partial constriction of the nucleus occurs in the band stage, until a fine filament (length but no breadth) is formed between two of the lobes, at which point the cell is classified as a *segmented neutrophil.*

The mature human neutrophil has twice as many specific

granules as azurophil granules. The azurophil granules (formed in the promyelocyte stage) contain lysosomal enzymes (acid hydrolases—acid phosphatase, β-glucuronidase, and so on), peroxidase, muramidase, and cationic antibacterial proteins, along with other enzymes and proteins. The specific granules (formed in the myelocyte stage) contain lactoferrin, collagenase, and muramidase, as well as other enzymes and proteins. Tertiary granules, similar in size to the specific granules, contain gelatinase. Alkaline phosphatase is located in yet another type of granule lighter in density than specific granules (Boxer, 1988).

Distribution and Kinetics

The distribution of this cell series in the body is depicted in Figure 25–6. For each neutrophil in the blood vessels, about 16 precursors are present in the marrow. From the time of differentiation into a myeloblast through about five mitotic divisions (three of which occur at the myelocyte stage), it takes about 14 days until the progeny of that cell reach the blood. The last eight days are spent in the maturation and storage pool. When a neutrophil enters the blood, it moves readily between a circulating granulocyte pool (CGP), which is sampled in the leukocyte count, and a marginal granulocyte pool (MGP), which is not, but is either marginated along vessel walls or sequestered in capillary beds. In less than a day after it arrives, the neutrophil emigrates from the circulation in a random manner and enters the tissues. From there, if not used in an inflammatory exudate, neutrophils leave the body within a few days via secretions in bronchi, saliva, gastrointestinal tract, and urine, or they are destroyed by the reticuloendothelial system.

Function

Neutrophils are able to move in a zigzag manner, but their motion changes to a straight-line path if a chemotactic attractant (e.g., a bacterium coated with certain components of complement) is within a certain distance. Neutrophils have receptors for the Fc portion of IgG as well as for complement (C3) and bind and phagocytize the coated particle. Phagocytosis occurs, with the formation of a phagocytic vacuole that contains the ingested particle; accompanying this process is an increase in metabolic activity and energy production. Specific granules, followed shortly by azurophil granules, empty their contents into the phagocytic vacuoles, a process known as degranulation. Bactericidal activity occurs within the vacuole, mediated by H_2O_2, peroxidase, and a halide ion generating the free halogen, or by other enzymatic activity.

Neutrophils are thus important in defense against infectious disease (see Chap. 27). If their enzymes are activated and released outside the cell, neutrophils can cause tissue necrosis, tissue injury, and inflammation.

EOSINOPHILS

Eosinophils are produced in the bone marrow. It seems likely from *in vitro* culture studies that there is a separate eosinophilic committed progenitor cell (CFU-Eo) in the marrow that is distinct from the CFU-GM, CFU-G, and CFU-M. The colony-stimulating factor that induces the CFU-Eo to proliferate and differentiate into eosinophil colonies (CSF-Eo; interleukin-5) is produced by T lymphocytes (Campbell, 1987).

Morphology of Eosinophil Precursors

The cell that is the precursor for the earliest recognizable eosinophil, the eosinophil myelocyte, is presumably a distinctive myeloblast. However, it is morphologically indistinguishable from the myeloblasts that give rise to neutrophils and monocytes or to basophils (see Fig. 25–1 and Plate 25–2). In the early eosinophil myelocyte, the granules are large and take the basophilic stain (Plate 25–2*H*). As the cell matures, the granules appear olive-green (Plate 25–2*I*) and finally assume the characteristic red-orange color (Plates 25–2*I* and 24–1*F* and *G*). Nuclear maturation is similar to that of the neutrophil. Eosinophils are slightly larger than neutrophils and have fewer nuclear lobes.

Electron micrographs of eosinophils show characteristic granules that have a dense crystalloid core in a less dense matrix. Immature granules appearing in the myelocyte at first

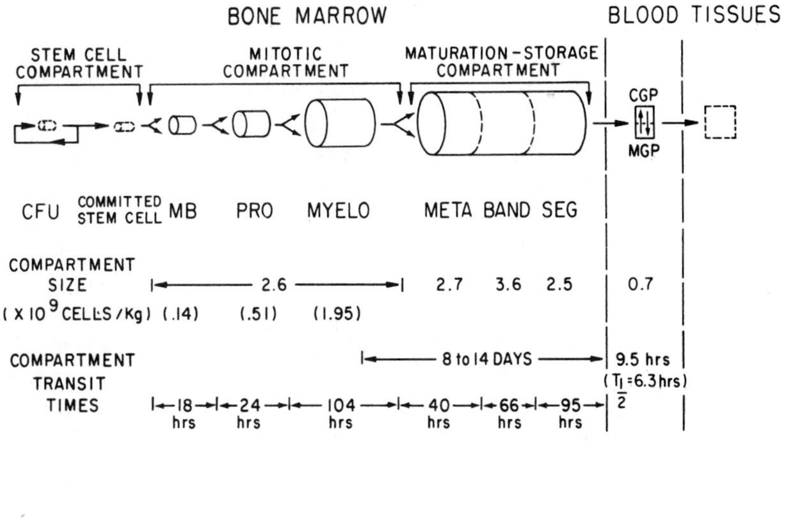

Figure 25–6. Neutrophil production, distribution, and kinetics. CFU = Multipotential stem cell; MB = myeloblast; PRO = promyelocyte; MYELO = myelocyte; META = metamyelocytes; SEG = segmented neutrophil; CGP = circulating granulocyte pool; MGP = marginal granulocyte pool. The cylinders representing the various compartments are drawn proportional to their sizes. The compartment transit times on the next to last line are from $DF^{32}P$ studies; those on the last line are from tritiated thymidine studies. (From Wintrobe MM et al: Clinical Hematology, 7th ed. Philadelphia, Lea & Febiger, 1974.)

have no crystalloids but develop them as maturation proceeds. Mature granules are of two types: the larger granule (0.5 to 1.5 μm in largest diameter) has a dense crystalloid, and the smaller granule (0.1 to 0.5 μm in diameter) has no crystalloid. The smaller granules appear later during maturation, after the myelocyte stage.

Eosinophil-specific granules contain major basic protein (MBP) in the crystalloid core; MBP is toxic to parasites and cells, neutralizes heparin, and induces histamine release from basophils. Granule constituents in the matrix include acid hydrolases, peroxidase, phospholipase, and cathepsin. The specific granules also contain eosinophil cationic protein (ECP), eosinophil-derived neurotoxin (EDN), and eosinophil protein X (EPX). ECP shortens coagulation time and alters fibrinolysis; it also inhibits lymphocyte proliferation and is a potent neurotoxin. EDN and EPX are strong neurotoxins (Gleich, 1986). The smaller granules contain arylsulfatase; both granule types contain peroxidase and acid phosphatase. Eosinophil peroxidase is different from the type of peroxidase present in neutrophils and monocytes; also, eosinophils contain no alkaline phosphatase or muramidase.

Distribution and Kinetics

The kinetics of eosinophils are similar to those of neutrophils. They spend less than eight hours in the blood and do not re-enter the circulation once they leave it. Eosinophils are considerably less numerous in blood and marrow than are neutrophils. Eosinophils in the tissues, however, are at least 100 times as numerous as the total eosinophils in the blood; they are located primarily in skin, lung, and gastrointestinal tract—i.e., the epithelial barriers to the outside world.

Function

The function of eosinophils is not completely understood. Eosinophils leave the blood when adrenal corticosteroid hormones increase. Eosinophils proliferate in response to immunologic stimuli; this proliferative response is mediated, at least with some antigens, by T lymphocytes, monocytes, and mast cells. Eosinophils destroy helminths by generating potent oxidants and releasing cationic proteins. Eosinophils participate in some inflammatory conditions, particularly allergic reactions, asthma, and certain myocardial diseases (Gleich, 1986). Although eosinophils phagocytose foreign particles and antigen-antibody complexes, this may not be their main function. There is evidence that eosinophils modulate reactions that occur when tissue mast cells and basophils degranulate. Among the chemotactic factors that attract eosinophils, eosinophil chemotactic factor of anaphylaxis (ECFA) is present in basophils and mast cells; also, eosinophils contain substances that inactivate factors released by mast cells and basophils, such as histamine, slow-reacting substances of anaphylaxis, and platelet-activating factor.

BASOPHILS AND MAST CELLS

There is no evidence of basophil development in the *in vitro* colonies containing neutrophils and monocytes or eosinophils, and it is probable that basophils develop from a separate committed progenitor cell that has been derived from the hematopoietic stem cell.

Morphology

Basophils probably develop from a cell resembling a myeloblast. The first recognizable stage is a *basophil myelocyte*, which has the appearance of the specific basophil granules. These granules (about 0.2 to 1 μm in diameter) are larger than the azurophil granules of the promyelocyte and often are irregular in shape. As the cell matures, the granules become more metachromatic (red-purple) owing to the increasing acid mucopolysaccharide (heparin) content. During maturation, cytoplasmic RNA decreases, and the nucleus partially segments. Because of incomplete nuclear segmentation, stages analogous to the neutrophil are not readily identified. In mature basophils, the nucleus has condensed but smudged chromatin, and the background cytoplasm lacks basophilia (residual RNA) (Plate 25–2*K* and *L*).

In contrast, *tissue mast cells* are connective tissue cells of mesenchymal origin that contain metachromatic cytoplasmic granules. They are widely distributed throughout the organism, including bone marrow, thymus, and spleen, but they do not normally appear in blood. On Romanowsky-stained films (Plate 25–2*M*) they are usually larger than basophils and have a low N/C ratio and a round or oval reticular nucleus that is usually obscured by abundant red-purple granules. The granules are smaller, more round and regular, and less soluble than basophil granules. The cytoplasmic granules are often spindle-shaped rather than round.

Kinetics

Because basophils are the least numerous of the leukocytes, their kinetics have been more difficult to uncover. Production appears to be similar to that of the neutrophil and the eosinophil. The basophil's time in the marrow is approximately seven days; it circulates in the blood; and it is not normally found in tissues, in contrast to mast cells (Curnutte, 1987).

Function

With regard to circulating numbers, basophils respond to adrenal corticosteroids in a fashion similar to that of eosinophils.

Basophil granules contain histamine, heparin, and peroxidase. Basophils synthesize and store histamine and ECFA. They synthesize and release slow-reacting substance of anaphylaxis (SRSA) and probably platelet-activating factor (PAF) at the time of stimulation but do not store them. Basophils lack hydrolytic enzymes such as alkaline and acid phosphatase, at least in cytochemically demonstrable amounts. Glycogen is abundant outside the granules. Although ultrastructurally different, mast cells have similar cytochemical characteristics except for the presence of proteolytic enzymes and serotonin, which basophils lack. In tissues, the two cell types appear to function in a similar manner.

Basophils (as well as mast cells) appear to be involved in

immediate hypersensitivity reactions, such as allergic asthma. Immunoglobulin E (reagin) binds readily to basophil and mast cell membranes. When specific antigen reacts with the membrane-bound IgE, degranulation occurs with the release of mediators of immediate hypersensitivity—e.g., histamine, SRSA, PAF, heparin, and ECFA. The last substance leads to the accumulation of eosinophils, which contain substances that tend to counteract these mediators. Basophils are also involved in some delayed hypersensitivity reactions, "cutaneous basophil hypersensitivity," such as contact allergies, in which they appear to undergo a different type of degranulation response.

MONOCYTES AND MACROPHAGES

Monocytes share the same committed progenitor cell as neutrophils, the CFU-GM (see Fig. 25–1).

Morphology

In normal marrow it is not possible morphologically to distinguish the "monoblast" from the myeloblast. The earliest recognizable cell in this series is the *promonocyte,* which is 15 to 20 μm in diameter, somewhat larger than the myeloblast. The N/C ratio is moderate, and the nucleus may be oval or indented with a fine uniform or slightly streaked chromatin pattern and two to five nucleoli. The cytoplasm is basophilic with a ground-glass appearance and a variable number of fine azurophilic granules (Plate 25–3*A*). The *monocyte*, which is present in both blood and marrow, is only slightly smaller; it has a moderate to low N/C ratio and an indented or lobed nucleus with a fine streaked, only slightly condensed, delicate chromatin pattern. Nucleoli are indistinct or obscured. The cytoplasm is opaque, more gray than blue, and contains an abundance of fine azurophilic granules (Plate 25–3*B*).

In the promonocyte stage, the granules contain acid hydrolase, arylsulfatase, and peroxidase; they represent primary lysosomes. There may be more than one type of granule. As the cell matures, peroxidase activity diminishes, and acid phosphatase and arylsulfatase activity increase. The enzyme activity occurs in the rough endoplasmic reticulum (RER), Golgi zone, coated vesicles, and digestive vacuoles, suggesting that in the macrophage the coated vesicles are a second form of primary lysosome that shuttles hydrolytic enzymes from the Golgi to the digestive vacuoles.

Kinetics

After promonocytes are formed, they undergo two or three mitotic divisions in a period of about 50 to 60 hours before being released into the blood. Under conditions of increased demand, the cycle time can shorten, leading to earlier release of more immature cells into the blood. Blood monocytes are distributed in a circulating monocyte pool and a marginal monocyte pool in a ratio of 1 : 3.5. Once monocytes enter the blood, they leave randomly with a half-time of 8.4 hours; this time period is shortened in patients with splenomegaly or acute infection, and may be prolonged in monocytosis. After monocytes leave the blood, they spend several months, perhaps longer, in the tissue phase.

Function

The monocyte is formed in the marrow, transported by the blood, and migrates into the tissues, where it is transformed into a histiocyte or macrophage (see Plate 24–2*I*), in which form it spends the majority of its lifespan. The blood monocytes and tissue macrophages make up a mononuclear phagocyte system (reticuloendothelial system).

The mononuclear phagocyte system has an important role in defense against microorganisms, including mycobacteria, fungi, bacteria, protozoa, and viruses. The cells are motile and respond to chemotactic factors (complement components as well as lymphokines and γ-interferon from activated T lymphocytes); they become immobilized by migration-inhibition factor (MI) from activated lymphocytes. They engage in phagocytosis, a process that is enhanced if the particle is coated by IgG or complement, for which the macrophages have membrane receptors. After phagocytosis, they kill ingested microorganisms.

These mononuclear phagocytes are an integral part of both humoral and cell-mediated immunity. They handle or process antigens, providing contact of the antigen (or antigenic information) with lymphocytes. They also respond to various lymphokines and act as effector (e.g., cytotoxic) cells in the cell-mediated immune response. They have the ability to kill a variety of malignant cells (Mavier, 1984).

Macrophages remove and process senescent cells and debris through phagocytosis and digestion: for example, erythrocytes, leukocytes, and megakaryocyte nuclei by macrophages in the marrow; inhaled particulate material by alveolar macrophages in the lungs.

Macrophages may be "activated" by either specific factors (e.g., cytophilic antibody) or nonspecific factors (e.g., in response to phagocytized material). Activation results in enlargement of the cell and enhanced metabolism, phagocytosis, microbicidal activity, cytotoxicity, and so on.

Macrophages synthesize and secrete a large number of biologically active molecules, including certain complement components, transferrin, muramidase, IL1, tumor necrosis factor, certain colony-stimulating factors, and interferon.

This system, therefore, has multiple functions that include host defense, control of hematopoiesis, and policing of the environment within the body (Johnston, 1988).

MEGAKARYOCYTES

Platelets originate from polyploid megakaryocytes, the largest of all hematopoietic cells, which number less than 1% of the total nucleated marrow cells. Megakaryocytes arise from the multipotential hematopoietic stem cell and then from a committed progenitor cell, the CFU-Meg (see Fig. 25–1). Based on *in vitro* and *in vivo* studies, it is likely that megakaryocyte proliferation is regulated by at least two humoral factors: a factor (Meg-CSF) that induces the CFU-Megs to proliferate, and a thrombopoietin-like factor that promotes differentiation and maturation of megakaryocytes (Mazur, 1987).

Table 25–2. CYTOLOGIC CHARACTERISTICS OF STAGES OF MEGAKARYOCYTIC MATURATION: DIAGRAMS OF NUCLEAR CONFIGURATIONS AND NUCLEAR/CYTOPLASMIC RATIOS AT EACH STAGE ARE IN THE FIRST COLUMN

	Stage	Nuclear Morphology	Cytoplasmic Staining (Wright-Giemsa)	Approximate Size Range	Demarcation Membranes	Granules	Suggested Name
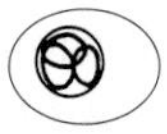	I	Compact (lobed)	Basophilic	6–24 μm	Present by electron microscopy	Few present by electron microscopy	Megakaryoblast
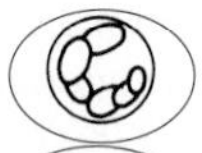	II	Horseshoe	Pink center	14–30 μm	Proliferating to center of cell	Starting to increase	Promegakaryocyte
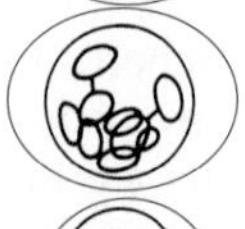	III	Multilobed	Increasingly more pink than blue	16–56 μm	Extensive but asymmetric	Great numbers	Granular megakaryocyte
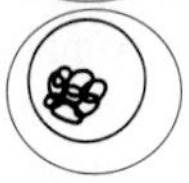	IV	Compact but highly lobulated	Wholly eosinophilic	20–50 μm	Evenly distributed	Organized into "platelet fields"	Mature megakaryocyte

From Williams N, Levine RF: The origin, development and regulation of megakaryocytes. Br J Haematol 1982; 52:173–180.

Morphology

Committed progenitor cells are not morphologically distinguishable from lymphocytes. The different maturation stages of megakaryocytes are illustrated in Table 25–2. Megakaryocyte development is characterized by *endomitosis*, nuclear division without cytoplasmic division, which results in ploidies varying from 2N to 64N. Most are 8N and 16N, with smaller numbers on either side. Nuclear lobes do not correlate precisely with ploidy. Nuclear chromatin is intensely staining, rather dispersed early, more compact and dense later. Nucleoli are small at all stages of megakaryocyte development.

The earliest recognizable *megakaryoblast* has overlapping nuclear lobes and a small amount of basophilic cytoplasm. In the *promegakaryocyte* nuclear lobes increase and spread out, and red-pink granules become visible, first in the center of the cell. The *granular megakaryocyte* is characterized by spreading of the red-pink granules diffusely through most of the cytoplasm and further increases and spreading of the nuclear lobes. In the *mature megakaryocyte* the nucleus is more compact, basophilia have disappeared, and the granules are clustered into small aggregates. At an ultrastructural level this appearance is produced by invaginated surface membranes (demarcation membranes) that separate the cytoplasm into individual platelets. Platelets are ultimately shed as cytoplasmic fragments by fusion of the demarcation membranes. In the marrow, megakaryocytes are adjacent to sinus walls, and platelets are released into the lumen.

Megakaryocytes in Blood

Whole megakaryocytes or fragments are occasionally found in normal blood films. In buffy coat films they are present consistently. Megakaryocytes are frequently found in the capillaries of the lungs. Kaufman (1965) presented experimental data suggesting that pulmonary megakaryocytes do not originate in the lungs but are carried there in venous blood. There is evidence suggesting that at least some platelets are released from megakaryocytes in the pulmonary circulation (Mazur, 1987).

Megakaryocyte fragments in blood films may be as small as lymphocytes and are recognized by the deeply stained chromatin (which has a sharper chromatin-parachromatin separation than that of lymphocytes) and by fragments of attached megakaryocyte cytoplasm (Plate 25–3*G*). They are found more frequently than normal in patients with myelophthisic processes, myeloproliferative disorders, or stress or injury to the marrow.

Dwarf or micromegakaryocytes (Plate 25–3*H*), on the other hand, show evidence of abnormal megakaryopoiesis: agranular cytoplasm with hyaloplasmic zones or pseudopods, and association with large atypical platelets that have similar cytoplasmic characteristics. These abnormal dwarf megakaryocytes are rarely found in any condition except myeloproliferative or myelodysplastic disorders.

Kinetics

The maturation time for megakaryocytes in the marrow is about five days in humans. Platelets are released into the marrow sinuses over a period of several hours, and the megakaryocyte nuclei undergo phagocytosis by macrophages. Newly released platelets appear larger, more active metabolically, and more effective hemostatically. Platelets circulate at a stable concentration that averages 275×10^9/L. At any one time, about two thirds of the total platelets are present in the circulation, and about one third are present in the spleen. In asplenic individuals, all platelets are circulating; on the other hand, in patients with diseases characterized by splenic enlargement, 80% to 90% of platelets may be sequestered in the spleen, resulting in a decreased concentration of circulating platelets (thrombocytopenia) on the basis of this altered distribution.

Platelets survive 8 to 11 days in the circulation. Some platelets are probably used in maintaining vascular integrity and in plugging small vascular injuries (random loss), and others are probably removed by the mononuclear phagocytic system when they become senescent.

Function

Platelets normally (1) maintain the integrity (leak-free state) of the blood vessels, and (2) form hemostatic plugs to stop blood loss from injured vessels and, in the process, promote coagulation of plasma factors (see Chap. 28).

LYMPHOCYTES

Primary Lymphoid Tissue

During fetal life, lymphocyte precursors originate in the bone marrow and undergo antigen-independent lineage commitment. Maturation and selection of T cells occur primarily in the thymus, and that of B cells occurs in the marrow and peripheral lymphoid organs (Denning, 1988; Bertoli, 1988).

B-CELL DEVELOPMENT: BONE MARROW. A distinct organ, the bursa of Fabricius, is present in birds and serves as the primary site of B-cell development. In the human, a bursal equivalent exists in the liver during the eighth or ninth week of gestation and later is found in the bone marrow after the hematopoietic stem cells have populated that organ. During adult life, generation of B cells occurs in the bone marrow.

B-cell differentiation can be divided conveniently into two stages (Cooper, 1987). The initial stage of B-cell differentiation involves the antigen-independent generation of diversity. The second stage is regulated by antigen triggering, T-cell interaction, macrophages, and various growth factors (Fig. 25–7). This stage occurs predominantly in the secondary lymphoid organs.

A stem cell gives rise to the first recognizable B cell in humans and mammals. This cell, known as the pre-B cell, is characterized by the presence of intracytoplasmic μ heavy chain without any surface-bound immunoglobulin ($SIg^{-}\mu^{+}$). Humoral proteins influence pre-B cell differentiation.

In becoming a pre-B cell, a lymphoid stem cell undergoes *DJ* and *VDJ* gene segment rearrangement to form a functional *V* gene for the μ heavy chain (Fig. 25–8). A productive heavy chain gene rearrangement is then followed by a rearrangement of the *VJ* gene segment of the light chain. In a B cell one of four light chain genes can be rearranged. The controls exerted during pre-B cell development allow only one productive *VH* and *VL* gene to emerge, limiting each B cell to one unique antibody structure (Bertoli, 1988). Isotype switching (changing from IgM/IgD to IgG1, and so on) and constant heavy (*CH*) gene deletions occur in pre-B cells and more differentiated B cells. The switching of μ cells to $\gamma 1$ or $\alpha 2$ cells occurs by the formation of a DNA loop in which all intervening *CH* genes are deleted (Fig. 25–9). A different mechanism regulates IgD expression. Because there is no switch region for $C\delta$, the IgD and IgM are usually expressed together.

Pre-B cells give rise to B cells that characteristically possess surface-bound immunoglobulins. In the peripheral blood, approximately 6% to 15% of B cells express surface-bound IgM (90% of these coexpress IgD), 1% to 3% express IgG, and 0.5% to 2% express IgA. Mature B cells also express receptors for Fc portions of Ig isotypes, C3b and C3d fragments of complement, interferon, and B cell–stimulating factor (IL4). A subset of mature B cells binds to mouse rosettes and possesses CD5 (LEU1) antigen.

In the second stage of differentiation, B cells interact with antigen in the presence of T cells and macrophages and

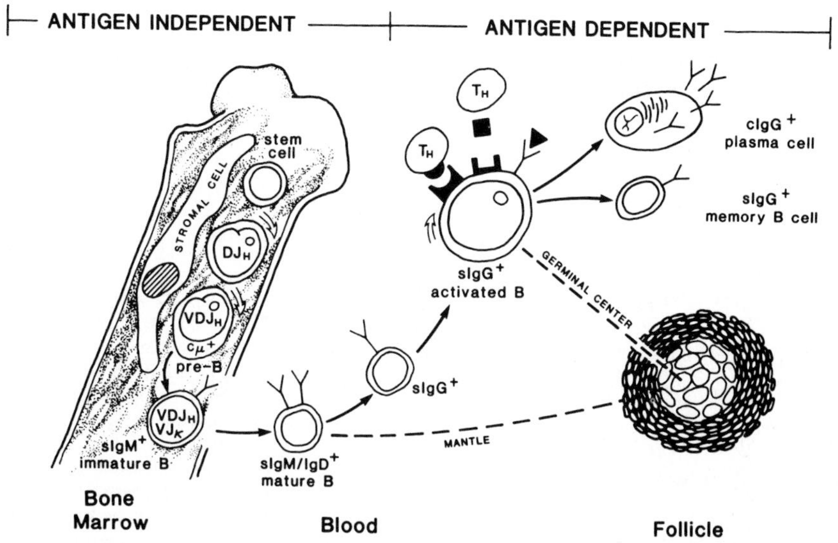

Figure 25–7. Differentiation of pre-B cells into B cells occurs independently of antigen, whereas the proliferation and terminal differentiation of B cells are antigen driven. Hematopoietic stem cells with stromal cell help give rise to pre-B cells. These proliferate (*open arrow* denotes cell cycling), rearrange DJ and VDJ gene segments, then express μ chains in cytoplasm ($c\mu^{+}$). A small, resting pre-B cell (not shown) with rearranged VJK gene assembles a complete IgM_k molecule, becoming an immature B cell and leaving the bone marrow expression of SIgD, marks entry of the cell into the mature, resting phase (G_0) characteristic of most blood and mantle zone B cells. Switching an alternative isotype (IgG in this case) may occur before encounter with antigen or afterward. Antigen triggers the resting B cell to enlarge (G_1) and present processed antigen and DR to the antigen-specific T cell receptor–T_3 complex. T-helper cells (T_H) secrete growth factors that bind to newly expressed receptor, further enhancing proliferation (S and M phases) in germline centers. The activated B cell can be induced to differentiate into plasma cells, which secrete their abundant cytoplasmic IgG. Alternatively, it can become a memory B cell with refined specificity poised to deliver an anamnestic immune response on its next encounter antigen. (Reproduced from Bertoli LF, Burrows PD: Normal B-lineage cells: Their differentiation and identification. Clin Lab Med 1988; 8:15, with permission.)

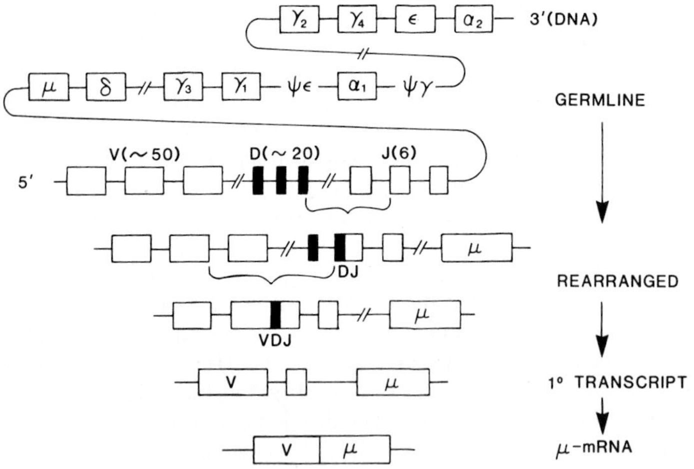

Figure 25–8. Generation of a functional Ig gene requires DNA rearrangement. In the germline and in somatic nonlymphoid cells, V, D, and J gene segments are widely separated in the DNA of chromosome 14. A cell committed to the B lineage first undergoes D to J rearrangement, juxtaposing the D and J segments, and deleting intervening DNA sequences. This is followed by V to DJ rearrangement, generating a complete VDJ exon. The primary RNA transcript is processed to yield a contiguous V (VDJ) μ mRNA. (Reproduced from Bertoli LF, Burrows PD: Normal B-lineage cells: Their differentiation and identification. Clin Lab Med 1988; 8:15, with permission.)

transform into plasma cells. In this process, an internal message is sent following the activation of membrane phospholipase C, which, along with calcium and phosphatidyl serine, activate protein kinase C. As a result, certain genes are activated, and the B cell is put into a proliferative mode. During this process, B cells develop receptors for B-cell differentiation factor (BCDF, IL6) as well as transferrin and other growth factors. B cells present antigen to T-helper cells through major histocompatibility complex II (MHCII) molecules on the B-cell membrane. This interaction activates T-helper cells to release IL4 and IL6, which bind to receptors on the B cell, promoting B-cell proliferation, differentiation, and plasma cell formation.

Plasma cells are characterized by abundant cytoplasmic immunoglobulin reflecting the immunoglobulin commitment of the activated B cell. At this stage, Fc and C3 receptors, HLA-DR antigen, and surface-bound immunoglobulin are greatly reduced, but PCA-1 and PCA-2 antigens are preserved (Bertoli, 1988). Thus, the lymphocytes bearing SIg give rise to cells committed to the synthesis of IgM, IgG, and IgA.

T-CELL DEVELOPMENT: THYMUS GLAND. The human thymus has two parts—the cortex and the medulla. The cortex is subdivided into two portions, the subcapsular cortex and the inner cortex, and is populated predominantly by small lymphocytes with a few scattered epithelial cells. Fibrous septa extend from the capsule to the medullary region. The medulla is composed mostly of epithelial cells with a small component of lymphocytes. In the medulla, Hassall's corpuscles, small islands of partially hyalinized epithelial cells, are present.

The microenvironment of the thymus is necessary for the differentiation of T cells (Denning, 1988). Prothymocytes migrate from the bone marrow or fetal liver to the thymus gland, where they are processed into functionally mature T cells for circulation in the blood to the peripheral or secondary lymphoid tissues. As thymic cells mature, they acquire and lose certain membrane determinants that can be recognized by various monoclonal antibodies. Three maturational stages have been recognized in the ontogeny of T cells. In the first stage, the CD7, CD2, and CD45 antigens are expressed. In the second stage, CD1, CD3, CD4, CD5, CD8,

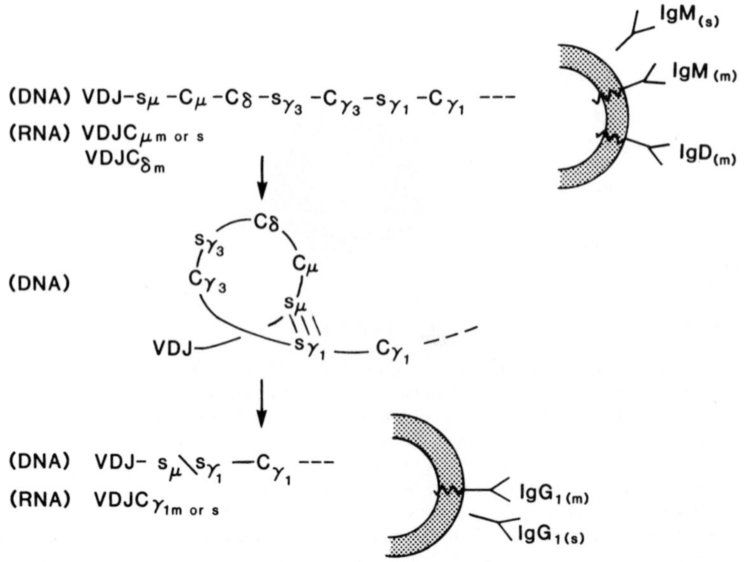

Figure 25–9. Alternate strategies for expression of non-IgM isotypes. IgD can be coexpressed with IgM by alternative processing of a primary RNA transcript of VDJ-Cμ-cδ to yield μ membrane (m), μ secretory (s), and δ_m RNAs. The production of IgG, IgA, or IgE isotypes involves DNA rearrangement. During the switch from IgM to IgG, for example, intrachromosomal recombination between homologous switch (s) regions results in deletions of C_μ, C_δ, and $C_{\gamma 3}$ so that $C_{\gamma 1}$ is now the first C gene 3′ of the VDJ exon. Thus, the same variable region is expressed with a different constant region. (Reproduced from Bertoli LF, Burrows PD: Normal B-lineage cells: Their differentiation and identification. Clin Lab Med 1988; 8:15, with permission.)

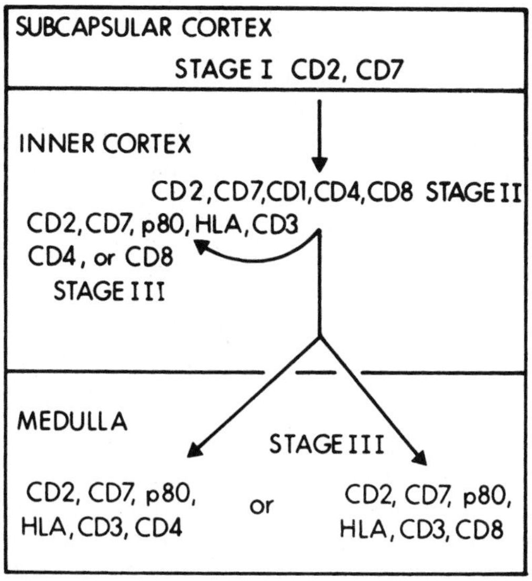

Figure 25–10. Human intrathymic T-cell maturation. (Adapted from Haynes BF: The role of the thymic microenvironment in promotion of early stages of human T-cell maturation. Clin Res 1986; 34:422–431. Reproduced from Denning SM, Haynes BF: Differentiation of human T cells. Clin Lab Med 1988; 8:1, with permission.)

and HLA antigens are observed on thymic cells. During the end of this stage, thymic cells begin to segregate into CD4+ and CD8+ populations. In the third stage, this segregation becomes complete and two separate mature T-cell populations are formed—CD4+ (helper-inducer) cells and CD8+ (suppressor-cytotoxic) cells (Fig. 25–10). As thymic cells differentiate, they migrate from the subcapsular cortex to the inner cortex, the medulla, and finally the peripheral blood and secondary lymphoid tissues. Prothymocytes and essentially all thymocytes possess terminal deoxynucleotidyl transferase (TdT). However, as thymocytes mature, this enzyme is reduced and is not expressed in peripheral blood T cells.

The T-cell receptor (TCR/CD3) for antigen interaction is necessary for antigen-specific T-cell activation (Denning, 1988). T-cell specific genes encode for polypeptide chains for the T-cell receptor (Royer, 1987). TCRA and TCRB genes encode for chains that form the T-cell receptor on mature T cells, whereas the TCRG and TCRD genes code for chains expressed on immature thymocytes and NK cells. The T-cell receptor genes undergo rearrangement in a manner similar to the rearrangement of immunoglobulin genes (Fig. 25–11). The TCRG gene rearranges in the thymus prior to the rearrangement of the TCRB gene. If TCRG gene rearrangement is successful, this cell may mature into an NK cell or a cell responsible for antibody-dependent cell-mediated cytotoxicity (Cossman, 1988). The rearrangement of the TCRA gene follows the rearrangement of the TCRB gene that occurs in the first stage of T-cell differentiation (Denning, 1988). In addition to the heterodimeric glycoproteins (α/β or γ/δ), the TCR/CD3 complex also consists of additional subunits: CD3-Σ, -ζ, and -η (Blumberg, 1990).

Activation of T cells occurs by two separate pathways. The T-cell antigen-independent pathway occurs through the binding of CD2 molecules and results in the release of IL1 and IL2, and the proliferation and differentiation of immature T cells in the thymus. The T-cell antigen-dependent pathway occurs through the binding of the T-cell receptor by antigen with appropriate MHC II antigen interaction on macrophages and/or B cells. This results in the release of IL1 by the activated macrophages, which in turn leads to the formation of IL2 receptors on T cells and the subsequent synthesis and release of IL2 by these activated T cells. These events result in the activation and maturation of T-helper cells, T-suppressor cells, T-cytotoxic cells, and other immunoregulatory cells (Denning, 1988).

Secondary Lymphoid Tissue

In late fetal and postnatal life, lymphocytes are produced in the secondary lymphoid tissue: spleen, lymph nodes, and intestine-associated lymphoid tissue. Lymphocytes of the secondary lymphoid organs are progeny from stem cells that have been influenced by primary lymphoid organs. The secondary lymphoid organs are thus composed of a mixture of B cells and T cells. Lymphopoiesis in secondary lymphoid organs depends solely on antigenic stimulation. B cells and

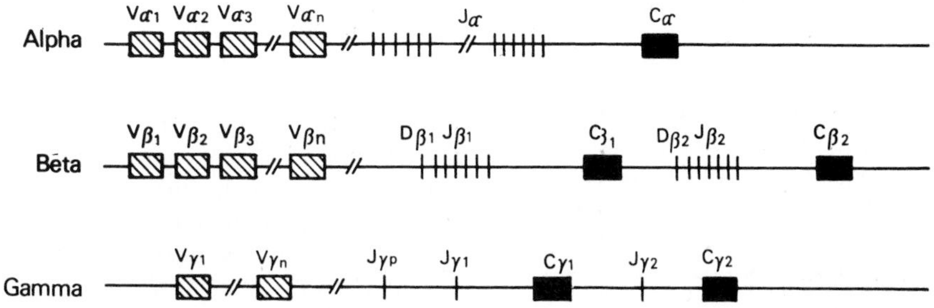

Figure 25–11. T-cell receptor gene family. The unrearranged α, β, and γ genes share an overall configuration that is similar to that of the evolutionary related immunoglobulin genes. For each locus, a series of variable region (V) genes lies upstream or the diversity (D, in the case of β) and joining (J) segments. The rearrangement process directly joins a V gene to either a J gene or a joined DJ (for β) to produce a continuous V gene and an altered restriction fragment size that is detectable by Southern blot hybridization. The α gene includes more than 50 J_α segments spanning as much as 100 kb, thus limiting evaluation or rearrangement of the α gene. β gene rearrangements can be readily detected with either J_β or C_β probes. Likewise, γ gene rearrangements are identified with either J_γ or C_γ probes. The γ gene is unusual in that it contains only a few (8 to 10) rearranging V genes. The δ gene is located between V_α and J_α. (Reproduced from Cossman J, Uppenkamp M: T-cell gene rearrangements and the diagnosis of T-cell neoplasms. Clin Lab Med 1988; 8:31, with permission.)

T cells tend to localize in anatomically distinct parts of the lymphoid tissues, where proliferation can take place.

Lymphocyte Function and Physiology

T cells and their progeny function in cell-mediated immunity, which includes delayed hypersensitivity, graft rejection, graft-versus-host reactions, defense against intracellular organisms (such as tubercle bacillus and brucella), and probably defense against neoplasms. B cells and their progeny perform in humoral immunity, or the production of antibodies, either as lymphocytes or after transformation into plasma cells.

The majority of the circulating lymphocytes are T cells, which have a lifespan of months to years. The B cells are a minor population (10% to 20% of the lymphocytes), probably have a short lifespan measured in days, and are distinguished by the presence of considerable immunoglobulin on their surface membrane.

Lymphocytes, especially T cells, recirculate from blood to lymph; in the postcapillary venule in lymphoid tissue the lymphocyte travels from the blood through the endothelium and into the lymphoid tissue, where it may stay or percolate through and return to the blood via the thoracic duct lymph. Small lymphocytes (Plate 25–3*J*) have little cytoplasm and, in electron micrographs, few organelles and relatively little RNA. After antigenic stimulation, small lymphocytes (B cells or T cells, depending on the nature of the antigen) become activated, increase their RNA synthesis, and undergo blast transformation. On Wright's-stained films, these blasts are large (15 to 25 μm) cells with abundant, rather deep blue cytoplasm, a large reticular nucleus with uniform chromatin, and prominent nucleoli (Plate 25–3*J* and *K*). This is the cell that is called the *reticular lymphocyte* (nonleukemic lymphoblast, "immunoblast"). If the blasts are derived from B cells, the new lymphocytes function in the production of antibodies (B cells, plasma cells); if the blasts are derived from T cells, the progeny act in the cellular immune response. The latter is mediated by several soluble factors produced by the activated T cell, including IL2, which induces the proliferation of T cells; IL3, which is a multipotential colony-stimulating factor; IL4, which promotes the proliferation of B cells; IL5, which enhances the proliferation of eosinophils as well as B cells; IL6, which promotes differentiation of B cells; lymphotoxin, which is directly toxic to cells; and migratory inhibitory factor, which promotes adherence of macrophages and keeps them at the site.

Plasma cells have abundant blue cytoplasm, often with light streaks or vacuoles, an eccentric round nucleus, and a well-defined clear (Golgi) zone adjacent to the nucleus. The nucleus of the plasma cell has heavily clumped chromatin, which is sharply defined from the parachromatin and often arranged in a radial or wheel-like pattern (see Plates 24–2*H* and 25–3*L*).

BONE MARROW EXAMINATION

Marrow aspiration biopsy can be carried out as an office procedure on ambulatory patients with minimal risk. It compares favorably with ordinary venipuncture and is less traumatizing than a lumbar puncture. As for any other special procedure, however, the indications for marrow examination should be clear. In each instance the physician should have in mind some reasonable prediction of its result and consequent benefit to the patient. Without exception, the peripheral blood should be examined carefully first. It is a relatively uncommon circumstance to find hematologic disease in the bone marrow without evidence of it in the peripheral blood.

It is estimated that the weight of the marrow in the adult is 1300 to 1500 g. The marrow can undergo complete transformation in a few days and occasionally even in a few hours. As a rule, this rapid transformation involves the whole organ, as evidenced by the fact that a small sample represented by a biopsy or aspiration is usually fairly representative of the whole marrow. This conclusion is in accord with results of studies of biopsy samples removed simultaneously from several sites. According to these observations, the various sites chosen for removal of marrow for studies are in most instances equally good. Consequently, the difficulty of access, the risks involved, the ease of obtaining a good biopsy specimen, and the discomfort of the patient are the main factors involved in selecting a particular site in a particular patient. Occasionally, failure to obtain quantitatively or qualitatively adequate material in one site may be followed by success in another location. Also, the need for repeated aspirations or biopsies may indicate the use of several different sites. We regard the posterior iliac crest as the preferred site. The large marrow space allows both aspiration and biopsy to be performed with ease at one time. The techniques of marrow aspiration and biopsy have been adequately reviewed (Hyun, 1988).

Preparation of the Aspirate for Examination

Two commonly used preparations are marrow films and histologic sections.

MARROW FILMS. Delay, no matter how brief, is undesirable. Films can be made in the same way as for ordinary blood counts. Gray particles of marrow are visible with the naked eye. They are the best material for the preparation of good films and serve as landmarks for the microscopic examination of stained smears.

Direct Films. A drop of marrow is placed on a slide a short distance from one end. A film 3 to 5 cm long is made with a spreader, not wider than 2 cm, dragging the particles behind but not squashing them. A trail of cells is left behind each particle.

Imprints. Marrow particles can also be used for preparation of imprints. One or more visible particles are picked up with a capillary pipette, the broken end of a wooden applicator, or a toothpick and transferred immediately to a slide and made to stick to it by a gentle smearing motion. The slide is air-dried rapidly by waving it and then is stained.

Crush Preparations. Marrow particles in a small drop of aspirate may be placed on a slide near one end. Another slide is carefully placed over the first. Slight pressure is exerted to crush the particles, and the slides are separated by pulling them apart in a direction parallel to their surfaces.

All films should be dried rapidly by whipping them through the air or by exposing them to a fan.

As the aspirated material is being spread, the appearance of fat as irregular holes in the films gives assurance that marrow and not just blood has been obtained.

HISTOLOGIC SECTIONS. The needle biopsy and the clotted marrow particles (fragments) are fixed in Zenker's acetic solution (5% glacial acetic acid; 95% Zenker) for 6 to 18 hours, or in B-5 fixative for 1 to 2 hours (Hyun, 1988). Excessive time in either fixative makes the tissue brittle. The tissue is processed routinely for embedding in paraffin, cut at 4 μm, and stained routinely with hematoxylin and eosin. Giemsa and periodic acid–Schiff stains are frequently useful. Embedding the tissue in plastic material allows examination of thinner sections and better survival of protein structure so that enzyme histochemistry and immunocytochemistry are practical for identification of cell lineages.

Sections provide the best estimate of cellularity and a picture of marrow architecture but are somewhat inferior for the study of cytologic details. Another disadvantage of clot sections is that particles adequate for histologic sections are not always obtained, especially in conditions in which the diagnosis depends on marrow evidence—e.g., myelofibrosis or metastatic cancer. Biopsy sections generally overcome this disadvantage.

Staining Marrow Preparations

ROMANOWSKY'S STAIN. Marrow films should be stained with a Romanowsky's stain (e.g., Wright-Giemsa) in a manner similar to that used for blood films (see Chap. 24). A longer staining time may be necessary for marrows with greater cellularity.

PERLS' TEST FOR IRON

Procedure. One film containing marrow particles is fixed for 10 minutes in formalin vapor, immersed for 10 minutes in a freshly prepared solution that contains 0.5% potassium ferrocyanide and 0.75% hydrochloric acid, rinsed, dried, and counterstained with Nuclear Fast Red (Chroma-Gesellschaft, distributed by Roboz Surgical Instrument Co., Inc., Washington, DC 20036).

Interpretation. The Prussian blue reaction is produced when hemosiderin or ferritin is present; iron in hemoglobin is not stained. It is reported as negative or 1+ to 5+. Storage iron, which is contained in macrophages, can be evaluated only in the marrow particles on the film. In adults, 2+ is normal, 3+ slightly increased, 4+ moderately increased, and 5+ markedly increased.

Storage iron in the marrow is located in macrophages. Normally a small number of blue granules are seen. In iron deficiency, blue-staining granules are absent or extremely rare. Storage iron is increased in most other anemias, infections, hemochromatosis, hemosiderosis, hepatic cirrhosis, uremia, and cancer, and after repeated transfusions (see Plate 26–1*D* and *E*).

Sideroblasts are normoblasts that contain one or more particles of stainable iron. Normally, from 20% to 60% of the late normoblasts are sideroblasts; in the remainder, no blue granules can be detected. The percentage of sideroblasts is decreased in iron deficiency anemia (in which storage iron is decreased) and also in the common anemias associated with infection, rheumatoid arthritis, and neoplastic disease (in which storage iron is normal or increased). The number of sideroblasts is increased when erythropoiesis is impaired for other reasons; it is roughly proportional to the degree of saturation of transferrin. The Prussian blue reaction can also be performed on slides previously stained with a Romanowsky's stain to identify sideroblasts or to determine whether iron is present in other cells of interest.

Sections. Routine hematoxylin and eosin stains are satisfactory for most purposes. Romanowsky's stains can be used to good advantage with Zenker-fixed or B-5–fixed material.

Iron stains are best performed on films that contain particulate marrow tissue. They are less sensitive in sections of marrow because some iron is lost in processing and a lesser thickness of tissue is examined in sections.

Examination of Marrow

It is desirable to establish a routine procedure to obtain the maximum information from examination of the marrow.

PERIPHERAL BLOOD. The complete blood cell count, including platelet count and reticulocyte count, should be performed on the day of the marrow study and the results incorporated into the report. The pathologist or hematologist who examines the marrow should also carefully examine the blood film as previously described (see Chap. 24) and incorporate the observations into the marrow report.

CELLULARITY OF THE MARROW. Marrow cellularity is expressed as the ratio of the volume of hematopoietic cells to the total volume of the marrow space (cells plus fat and other stromal elements). Cellularity varies with the age of the subject and the site. For example, at age 50 years, the average cellularity in the vertebrae is 75%; sternum, 60%; iliac crest, 50%; and rib, 30%. Normal cellularity of the iliac bone at different ages has been well defined by Hartsock (1965), as summarized in Figure 25–12. If the percentage is increased for the patient's age, the marrow is hypercellular, or hyperplastic; if decreased, the marrow is hypocellular, or hypoplastic.

Marrow cellularity is best judged by histologic sections of biopsy or aspirated particles (Fig. 25–13) but should also be estimated from the particles that are present in marrow films.

4

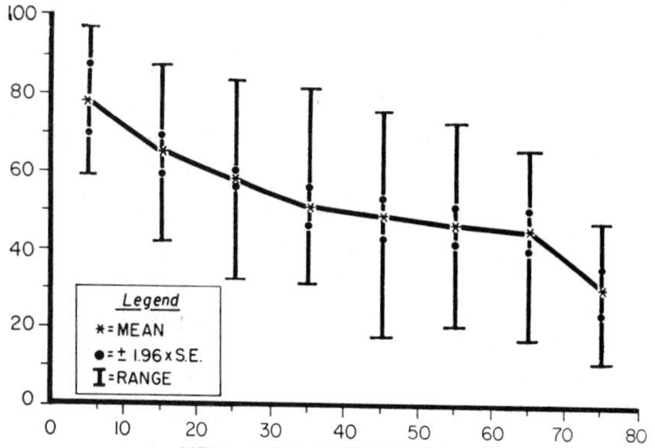

Figure 25–12. Marrow cellularity in hematologically normal individuals. Percent cellularity on the ordinate, versus age, grouped by decade, on the abscissa. (From Hartsock RJ, Smith EB, Petty CS: Am J Clin Pathol 1965; 43:326.)

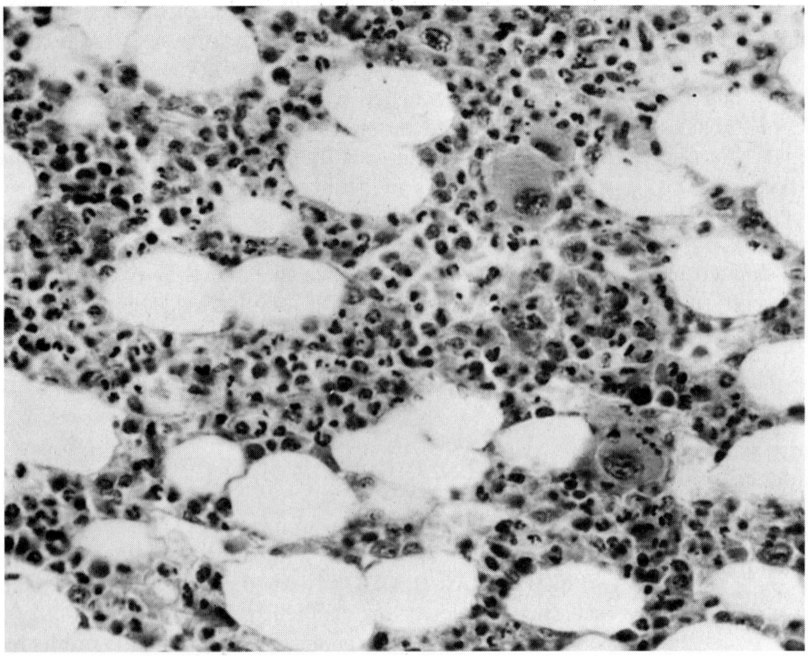

Figure 25–13. Marrow biopsy (× 1470). Cellularity here is between 60% and 70%, which is normal for an adult. Three megakaryocytes are present, which is normal for this size field. Granulocytic maturation appears normal with all stages present. Very few normoblasts are noted. (Normoblasts have intensely staining nuclei and tend to occur in clusters.) The myeloid:erythroid (M:E) ratio is higher than 4:1, indicating erythroid hypoplasia. No other abnormalities are noted.

This is done by comparing the areas occupied by fat spaces and nucleated cells in the particles as well as the density of nucleated cells in the "tail" or fallout of the particles. Comparison of films and sections on each marrow specimen enables the observer to estimate cellularity reasonably well from films, a skill that is useful when sectioned material is unavailable.

DISTRIBUTION OF CELLS. The distribution of the various cell types can be ascertained in two ways. First, several slides are scanned under low and then high magnification, and then, on the basis of previous experience, the observer estimates the number and distribution of cells. Second, an actual differential count of 300 to 1000 cells is made and the percentage of each type of cell is calculated. A combination of both methods is preferred. The second of these methods, careful differential counting, is an essential part of training in this work without which accuracy in the first method may be difficult to achieve. The differential count also affords an objective record from which future changes may be measured.

One first scans the marrow films under low power (100 × or 200 × magnification), looking for irregularities in cell distribution, the number of megakaryocytes, and the presence of abnormal cells. Then one selects areas on the films where marrow cells are both undiluted with blood cells and separated and spread out sufficiently to allow optimal identification. These areas are usually just behind marrow particles on the direct films or near the particles on the crushed films. The differential count is performed at 400 × or 1000 × magnification. Examples of reference intervals for differential counts of the marrow at selected different ages are given in Table 25–3.

Changes in the marrow cell distribution are most dramatic in the first month of life, during which a predominance of granulocytic cells at birth changes to a predominance of lymphocytes. This predominance of lymphocytes characterizes the bone marrow during infancy. A small proportion of "immature" or transitional lymphoid cells (fine nuclear chromatin, high N/C ratio, small to intermediate cell size) is normally present; it may be that these cells include stem cells and progenitor cells. These cells probably include cells designated as "hematogones"; they may be increased in patients with iron deficiency anemia, immune thrombocytopenic purpura, and other disorders, especially in infancy (Muehleck, 1983). Normoblasts fall after birth, rise to a maximum level at two months, and then fall to a stable, relatively low level by four months and remain there during most of infancy.

The myeloid:erythroid (M:E) ratio is the ratio of total granulocytes to total normoblasts. In newborns and infancy, it is somewhat higher than in later childhood or adult life (see Table 25–3). In adults, the range is broad, varying from about 1.2 to 1 to 5 to 1.

Both the differential count and the M:E ratio are relative values and must be interpreted with respect to the cellularity or to other evidence that one of the systems is normal.

An *increased* M:E ratio (e.g., 6 to 1) may be found in patients with infection, chronic myelogenous leukemia, or erythroid hypoplasia. A *decreased* M:E ratio (i.e., less than 1.2 to 1) may indicate a depression of leukopoiesis or a normoblastic hyperplasia, depending on the marrow cellularity.

The number of megakaryocytes is estimated more reliably in sections than in marrow films. In scanning areas of films with good cellularity under low power (100 ×), an average of one to three megakaryocytes should be found in each field in normal marrow.

MATURATION. While examining the cells during the differential count, one should evaluate whether maturation is normal—that is, whether nuclear and cytoplasmic development is in balance. Impaired cytoplasmic maturation in normoblasts, for example, occurs when hemoglobin synthesis is impaired; impaired nuclear maturation occurs in megaloblastic anemias. Bizarre or dysplastic maturation occurs as a result of certain drugs, in some leukemias, and in dysmyelopoietic syndromes.

PRESENCE OF RARE CELL TYPES OR ABNORMAL CELLS. In scanning the marrow, one looks for the presence of rare or unexpected cell types.

Table 25–3. DIFFERENTIAL CELL COUNTS OF BONE MARROW IN PERCENT OF TOTAL NUCLEATED CELLS

	Rosse (1977)			Mauer (1969)	Jandl (1987)
Cell Types	**Birth (Mean, S.D.)**	**1 Month (Mean, S.D.)**	**18 Months (Mean, S.D.)**	**Childhood (Mean, Range)**	**Adult (Mean, Range)**
Normoblasts, total	14.48 ± 7.24	8.04 ± 5.00	8.21 ± 3.71	23.1	21.5 (14.2 − 30.4)
Pronormoblasts	0.02 ± 0.06	0.10 ± 0.14	0.08 ± 0.13	0.5 (0.0 − 1.5)	0.6 (0.2 − 1.4)
Basophilic n.	0.24 ± 0.25	0.34 ± 0.33	0.50 ± 0.34	1.7 (0.2 − 4.8)	2.0 (0.7 − 3.7)
Polychromatophilic n.	13.06 ± 6.78	6.90 ± 4.45	6.97 ± 3.56	18.2 (4.8 − 34.0)	12.4 (12.2 − 24.2)
Orthochromatic n.	0.69 ± 0.73	0.54 ± 1.88	0.44 ± 0.49	2.7 (0.0 − 7.8)	6.5 (2.0 − 22.7)
Neutrophils, total	60.37 ± 8.66	32.35 ± 7.68	36.06 ± 7.40	57.1	56.0 (45.1 − 66.5)
Myeloblasts	0.31 ± 0.31	0.62 ± 0.50	0.06 ± 0.08	1.2 (0.0 − 3.2)	1.0 (0.5 − 1.8)
Promyelocytes	0.79 ± 0.91	0.76 ± 0.65	0.64 ± 0.59	1.4 (0.0 − 4.0)	3.4 (2.6 − 4.6)
Myelocytes	3.95 ± 2.93	2.50 ± 1.48	2.49 ± 1.39	18.3 (8.5 − 29.7)	11.9 (8.1 − 16.9)
Metamyelocytes	19.37 ± 4.84	11.30 ± 3.59	12.42 ± 4.15	23.3 (14.0 − 34.2)	18.0 (9.8 − 25.3)
Bands	28.89 ± 7.56	14.10 ± 4.63	14.20 ± 5.23		11.0 (8.5 − 20.8)
Segmented	7.37 ± 4.64	3.64 ± 2.97	6.31 ± 3.91	12.9 (4.5 − 29.0)	10.7 (8.0 − 16.0)
Eosinophils	2.70 ± 1.27	2.61 ± 1.40	2.70 ± 2.16	3.6 (1.0 − 9.0)	3.2 (1.2 − 6.2)
Basophils	0.12 ± 0.20	0.07 ± 0.16	0.10 ± 0.12	0.06 (0.0 − 0.8)	<0.1 (0.0 − 0.2)
Lymphocytes, total	15.6	49.0	45.5	16.0 (4.8 − 35.8)	15.8 (10.8 − 22.7)
Transitional	1.18 ± 1.13	1.95 ± 0.94	1.99 ± 1.00		
Small	14.42 ± 5.54	47.05 ± 9.24	43.55 ± 8.56		
Plasma cells	0.00 ± 0.02	0.02 ± 0.06	0.06 ± 0.08	0.4 (0.2 − 0.6)	1.8 (0.2 − 2.2)
Monocytes	0.88 ± 0.85	1.01 ± 0.89	2.12 ± 1.59		1.8 (0.2 − 2.8)
Megakaryocytes	0.06 ± 0.15	0.05 ± 0.09	0.07 ± 0.12		<0.1 (0.0 − 0.2)
Reticulum cells					0.3 (0.0 − 0.5)
M:E ratio	4.2	4.0	4.4	2.9 (1.2 − 5.2)	2.5 (1.2 − 5.0)

Data are from Rosse C, et al: J Lab Clin Med 1977; 89:1225; Mauer AM: Pediatric Hematology. New York, McGraw-Hill, 1969; and Jandl JH: Blood: Textbook of Hematology. Boston, Little, Brown and Co, 1987.

Tissue mast cells (Plate 25–2*M*) are normally very infrequent. They are increased in number in aplastic or refractory anemias and in lymphoproliferative disorders.

Osteoblasts (Plate 25–3*I*) are cells that synthesize the collagen matrix of bone. *Osteoclasts* (Plate 25–3*C*) are cells that resorb bone and are thought to result from the fusion of histiocytes. Both cell types are normally present in small numbers in the aspirates of infants and children. They are uncommonly seen in adult marrow except when bone destruction or repair is occurring, as in hyperparathyroidism, Paget's disease, metastatic tumor, or a recent biopsy at the same site.

Osteoblasts are large cells with a single eccentric nucleus that has reticular chromatin and a prominent nucleolus. The cytoplasm is moderately basophilic; a large pale Golgi's zone is separated from the nucleus rather than abutting it as in plasma cells. Osteoblasts are often present in clusters and may be confused with immature plasma cells or myeloma cells.

Osteoclasts are large multinucleated cells up to 100 μm diameter that may be mistaken for megakaryocytes. They have multiple nuclei that are separate (not joined as in megakaryocytes). The chromatin is reticular, and a prominent nucleolus is usually present. The cytoplasm may be basophilic but usually has pink-purple granules that resemble megakaryocytic granules. Coarse fragments of purple-staining material are often present.

Clusters of *metastatic neoplastic cells* may be found in one or more marrow films of patients with metastatic tumor in the bone sampled, or they may be found in biopsy sections and not films, in both, or, less commonly, in one or more films and not the biopsy. Some metastatic neoplastic cells resemble myeloblasts or other primitive blasts. The clue to recognition is that they almost always appear in clusters or clumps of cells; this is not true of hematopoietic blast cells.

EVALUATION OF THE BIOPSY SPECIMEN. Histologic sections allow better estimates of marrow cellularity and the number of megakaryocytes than do marrow films (see Fig. 25–13). In good histologic preparations, cell distribution and maturation abnormalities can be determined quite reliably. In addition to allowing more reliable detection of lymphomas or metastatic tumors, the histologic pattern is often useful in diagnosing the type of neoplasm. Other focal lesions not found in films include granulomas, abscesses, and vascular lesions.

In some conditions, such as myelofibrosis and leukemic reticuloendotheliosis (hairy cell leukemia), the bone marrow cannot be aspirated, and biopsy is necessary to establish a diagnosis.

Trabeculae should always be examined to detect bone abnormalities. Osteosclerosis with thickened bone trabeculae may accompany myelofibrosis or may be congenital. In osteoporosis the bone trabeculae are thin. Osteomalacia is characterized by a recognizable osteoid seam. Osteitis fibrosa occurs in hyperparathyroidism and is characterized by irregular osteoclastic bone resorption, endosteal fibrosis, and some osteoblastic activity in areas of bone regeneration. Irregularly widened trabeculae with a "mosaic" pattern are typical findings in Paget's disease of bone.

INTERPRETATION. The *summary* of the marrow report includes an estimate of cellularity, an estimate of the number of megakaryocytes, the M:E ratio, statements about any cytologic or maturation abnormalities, an estimate of the storage iron and proportion of sideroblasts, and statements about any other abnormal findings. The abnormalities in the blood cell counts and morphology are also summarized.

Then an *interpretation* of the observed findings is made, which of course includes a diagnosis if this is possible. In making such an interpretation, one should combine the marrow and blood observations with clinical findings and other laboratory data.

Alterations in blood and marrow cells are discussed with reference to the diseases and disorders considered in subsequent chapters.

Indications for Marrow Study

In patients with microcytic anemias, evaluation of the iron stores and sideroblasts allows categorization of the anemia—i.e., iron deficiency, anemia of chronic disease, or sideroblastic.

In macrocytic anemias, marrow examination confirms whether the process is megaloblastic or not; in some cases the changes in the blood are minimal, yet the marrow is megalobastic.

In normocytic anemias (or macrocytic anemias) with no increased reticulocyte production index, the marrow is evaluated for quantitative or qualitative abnormalities in erythropoiesis—e.g., pure red cell aplasia or myelodysplasia.

In neutropenia, thrombocytopenia, or pancytopenia, marrow study is helpful in assessing the presence and normality of the precursor cells in each series. This enables one to assess the probabilities of decreased production, impaired maturation, or increased destruction as the mechanism of the disorder. In patients with cytopenias, marrow examination sometimes reveals the presence of leukemia or other hematologic neoplasia.

In immunoglobulin abnormalities, the diagnosis of plasma cell myeloma or macroglobulinemia may be confirmed if infiltrations of abnormal plasma cells or lymphocytes are present.

Marrow examination is essential for the diagnosis and classification of acute leukemia. It is frequently performed to assist in the diagnosis and staging of other neoplasms including lymphomas and metastatic tumors and to assess the response to therapy of hematologic disorders.

If the marrow cannot be aspirated ("dry tap"), biopsy is essential. Marrow biopsy should also be performed if there are blood changes suggesting myelofibrosis with myeloid metaplasia or if granulomatous disease or metastatic tumor is suspected.

Ambrus JL Jr, Pippin J, Joseph A, et al: Identification of a cDNA for a human high-molecular-weight B-cell growth factor. Proc Natl Acad Sci USA 1993; 90:6330.

Bagby GC, Segal GM: Growth factors and control of hematopoiesis. *In* Hoffman R, Berry EJ, Shattil SJ, et al (eds): Hematology, Basic Principles and Practice. New York, Churchill Livingstone, 1991.

Bertoli LF, Burrows PD: Normal B-lineage cells: Their differentiation and identification. Clin Lab Med 1988; 8:15.

Blumberg RS, Ley S, Sancho J, et al: Structure of the T-cell antigen receptor: Evidence for two CD3 epsilon subunits in the T-cell receptor-CD3 complex. Proc Natl Acad Sci USA 1990; 87:7220.

Boxer LA, Smolen JE: Neutrophil granule constituents and their release in health and disease. Hematol Oncol Clin North Am 1988; 2:101.

Bradley TR, Metcalf D: The growth of mouse bone marrow cells in vitro. Aust J Exp Biol Med Sci 1966; 44:287.

Bunn HF, Forget BG: Hemoglobin: Molecular, Genetic and Clinical Aspects. Philadelphia, W.B. Saunders Company, 1986.

Campbell HD, Tucker WQJ, Hort Y, et al: Molecular cloning, nucleotide sequence, and expression of the gene encoding eosinophil differentiation factor (interleukin 5). Proc Natl Acad Sci USA 1987; 84:6629.

Cooper MD: B lymphocytes: Normal development and function. N Engl J Med 1987; 317:1452.

Cossman J, Uppenkamp M: T-cell gene rearrangements and the diagnosis of T-cell neoplasms. Clin Lab Med 1988; 8:31.

Curnutte JT: Disorders of granulocyte function and granulopoiesis. *In* Nathan DG, Oski FA (eds): Hematology of Infancy and Childhood, 4th ed. Philadelphia, W.B. Saunders Company, 1993.

de Sauvage FJ, Hass PE, Spencer SD, et al: Stimulation of megakaryocytopoiesis and thrombopoiesis by the c-Mpl ligand. Nature 1994; 369:533.

Deeg HF, Huss R: Major histocompatibility complex class II molecules, hemopoiesis and the marrow microenvironment. Bone Marrow Transplant 1993; 12:425.

Denning SM, Haynes BF: Differentiation of human T cells. Clin Lab Med 1988; 8:1.

Gleich GJ, Adolphson CR: The eosinophilic leukocyte: Structure and function. Adv Immunol 1986; 39:177.

Grabstein KH, Eisenman J, Shanebeck K, et al: Cloning of a T cell growth factor that interacts with the beta chain of the interleukin-2 receptor. Science 1994; 264:965.

Hartsock RJ, Smith EB, Petty CS: Normal variations with aging of the amount of hematopoietic tissue in bone marrow from the anterior iliac crest. Am J Clin Pathol 1965; 43:326.

Herbert CA, Baker JB: Interleukin-8: A review. Cancer Invest 1993; 11 (6):743.

Hillman RS, Finch CA: Red Cell Manual, 6th ed. Philadelphia, F. A. Davis, 1992.

Hyun BH, Gulati GL, Ashton JK: Bone marrow examination: Techniques and interpretation. Hematol Oncol Clin North Am 1988; 2:513.

Ichikawa Y, Pluznik DH, Sachs L: *In vitro* control of the development of macrophages and granulocyte colonies. Proc Natl Acad Sci USA 1966; 56:488.

Inghirami G, Knowles DM: The immune system: Structure and function. *In* Knowles D (ed): Neoplastic Hematopathology. Baltimore, Williams and Wilkins, 1993.

Johnston RB Jr: Current concepts: Immunology. Monocytes and macrophages. N Engl J Med 1988; 318:747.

Kaufman RM, Airo R, Pollack S, et al: Origin of pulmonary megakaryocytes. Blood 1965; 25:767.

Kaushansky K, Karplus PA: Hematopoietic growth factors: Understanding functional diversity in structural terms. Blood 1993; 82:3229.

Kaushansky K, Lok S, Holly RD, et al: Promotion of megakaryocyte progenitor expansion and differentiation by the c-Mpl ligand thrombopoietin. Nature 1994; 369:568.

Lok S, Kaushansky K, Holly RD, et al: Cloning and expression of murine thrombopoietin cDNA and stimulation of platelet production in vivo. Nature 1994; 369:565.

Long MW: Blood cell cytoadhesion molecules. Exp Hematol 1992; 20:289.

Mavier P, Edgington TS: Human monocyte-mediated tumor cytotoxicity. I. Demonstration of an oxygen-dependent myeloperoxidase-independent mechanism. J Immunol 1984; 132:1980.

Mazur EM: Megakaryocytopoiesis and platelet production: A review. Exp Hematol 1987; 15:340.

McDonald TP, Sullivan PS: Megakaryocytic and erythrocytic cell lines share a common precursor cell. Exp Hematol 1993; 21:1316.

Mertelsmann R: Hematopoietic cytokines: From biology and pathophysiology to clinical application. Leukemia 1994; 7(Suppl 2):5168–5177.

Metcalf D: Blood thrombopoietin—at last. Nature 1994; 369:519.

Molgaard HV, Spurr ND, Greaves MF: The hemopoietic stem cell antigen, CD34, is encoded by a gene located on chromosome 1. Leukemia 1989; 3(11):773.

Muehleck SD, McKenna RW, Gale PF, et al: Terminal deoxynucleotidyl transferase (TdT)—positive cells in bone marrow in the absence of hematologic malignancy. Am J Clin Pathol 1983; 79:277.

Nakono T, Kodama H, Honjo T: Generation of lymphohematopoietic cells from embryonic stem cells in culture. Science 1994; 265:1098.

Pike BL, Robinson WA: Human bone marrow colony growth in agar-gel. J Cell Physiol 1970; 76:77.

Quesniaux VFJ: Interleukins 9, 10, 11, and 12 and kit ligand: A brief overview. Res Immunol 1994; 143:385.

Royer HD, Reinherz EL: T lymphocytes: Ontogeny, function, and relevance to clinical disorders. N Engl J Med 1987; 317:1136.

Siena S, Bregni M, Brando B, et al: Circulation of CD34+ hematopoietic stem cells in the peripheral blood of high-dose cyclophosphamide-treated patients: Enhancement by intravenous recombinant human granulocyte-macrophage colony-stimulating factor. Blood 1989; 74(6):1905.

Terstappen LW, Huang S, Safford M, et al: Sequential generations of hematopoietic colonies derived from single nonlineage-committed CD34 + CD38- progenitor cells. Blood 1991; 77(6):1218.

Till JE, McCulloch EA: A direct measurement of the radiation sensitivity of normal mouse bone marrow cells. Rad Res 1961; 14:213.

Trinchieri G: The hematopoietic system and hematopoiesis. *In* Knowles D (ed): Neoplastic Hematopathology. Baltimore, Williams and Wilkins, 1993.

Wendling F, Maraskovsky E, Debili N, et al: cMpl ligand is a humoral regulator of megakaryocytopoiesis. Nature 1994; 369:571.

Zurawski G, de Vries JE: Interleukin-13 elicits a subset of the activities of its close relative interleukin-4. Stem Cells 1994; 12:169.

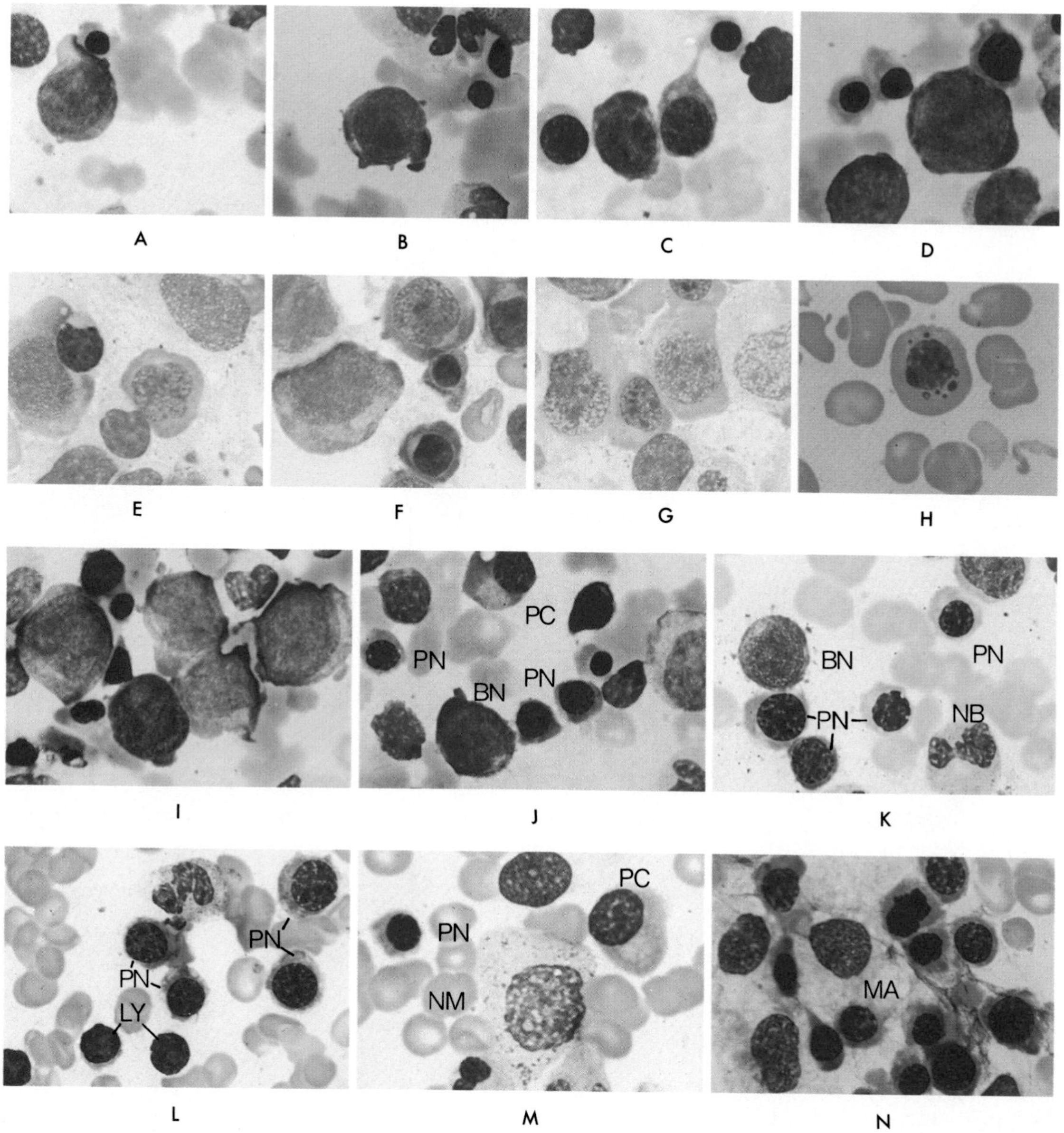

Plate 25–1. Normoblastic series. *A* to *D*, Megaloblastic series. *E* to *H*, Same magnification. *A*, Pronormoblast, normal marrow. A small orthochromatic normoblast is in contact with the pronormoblast. A broken nucleus of an unidentifiable cell is partly in the field. *B*, Basophilic normoblast, normal marrow. Note the intense cytoplasmic basophilia and irregular cytoplasmic protrusions, which are common. *C*, Basophilic normoblast, *center*: polychromatophilic normoblasts (PN) on either side. The PN on the left is more mature, having more condensed nuclear chromatin and more cytoplasmic hemoglobin than the PN on the right. *D*, Orthochromatic normoblasts; *left*, normal marrow. Note the pyknotic nuclei. Cytoplasm retains RNA and is polychromatophilic. A basophilic normoblast and a polychromatophilic normoblast are in the field. *E*, Promegaloblast; *left*, overlying its edge is a small cell with intensely staining nuclear chromatin, probably part of a late polychromatophilic megaloblast. In the center an earlier polychromatophilic megaloblast is in contact with a lymphocyte. *F*, Basophilic megaloblast; *left*, polychromatophilic megaloblasts; *center*. *G*, Polychromatophilic megaloblasts. Note, in addition to the large size (compared with C), the prominent parachromatin; this is an "open" nuclear chromatin pattern. *H*, Orthochromatic megaloblast with karyorrhexis and multiple Howell-Jolly bodies. *I*, A group of four pronormoblasts. One basophilic normoblast, and a few later forms, from a marrow aspirate showing normoblastic hyperplasia. *J*, Contrast the basophilic normoblast (BN) and the polychromatophilic normoblasts (PN) with the plasma cell (PC); these cells are sometimes confused. *K*, Basophilic normoblast (BN) with several "pseudopods," four polychromatophilic normoblasts (PN), and a neutrophil band form (NB). *L*, Contrast the lymphocytes (LY) with smudged nuclear chromatin, and the polychromatophilic normoblasts (PN), which are sometimes confused. Here, the PNs have delayed cytoplasmic maturation (less hemoglobin than expected for the degree of nuclear development). The normoblasts have sharper separation of nuclear chromatin and parachromatin than the lymphocytes. *M*, Small polychromatophilic normoblast (PN) damaged early neutrophil myelocyte (NM), and plasma cell (PC). *N*, Erythroblastic island. The macrophage in the center (MA) has abundant partially vacuolated cytoplasm, which is in contact with several normoblasts; one of the latter is in mitosis.

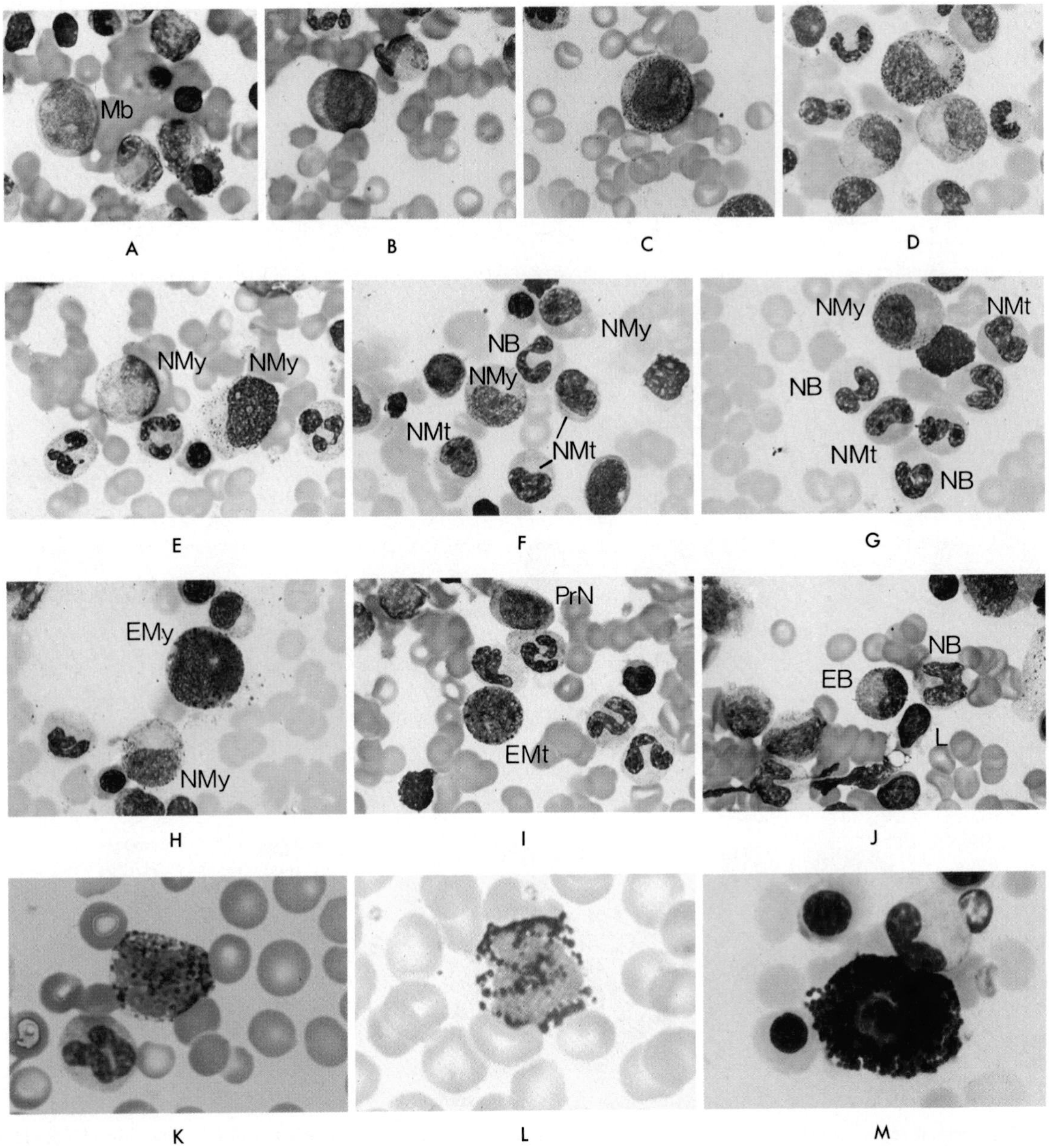

Plate 25–2. *A*, Myeloblast (Mb). *B*, Early promyelocyte has more basophilic cytoplasm than the myeloblast. A few azurophilic granules are in the vicinity of the Golgi zone. *C*, Promyelocyte. Later state has more numerous azurophilic granules. *D*, Neutrophil myelocytes. Newly formed specific granules have appeared in the Golgi zone adjacent to the nucleus. The azurophilic granules, which were formed in the promyelocyte stage, are best seen in the upper cell. As maturation proceeds, the azurophilic staining quality is lost. *E*, Neutrophil myelocytes (NMy), a late polychromatophilic normoblast, and three neutrophils. In the NMy on the left, opaque granules overlying the nucleus give it a pale or "motheaten" appearance. *F*, N. myelocytes (NMy), N. metamyelocytes (NMt), and N. band form (NB) NMt and monocytes are frequently confused with one another. *G*, N. myelocyte (NMy), N. metamyelocytes (NMt), N. band forms (NB), and a broken or smudged cell. *H*, Eosinophil myelocyte (EMy), contrasted with a neutrophil myelocyte (NMy), is larger and has larger granules. The eosinophil granules that appear early in development have a basophilic staining reaction; as the cell matures, they become olive-green, then eosinophilic in their staining characteristics. *I*, Eosinophil metamyelocyte (EMt). Neutrophils and a pronormoblast (PrN) are present. *J*, Eosinophil band form (EB), neutrophil band form (NB), and lymphocyte (L). The granules in the EB have the staining reaction characteristic of the mature cell. *K*, Basophil and neutrophil. *L*, Mature basophil. The nuclei in basophils do not normally segment. Immature basophils have cytoplasmic basophilia (outside the granules), which this cell lacks. *M*, Tissue mast cell; *center*, bone marrow. Mast cell granules are smaller, rounder, less water soluble and more abundant than basophil granules; they usually obscure the nucleus.

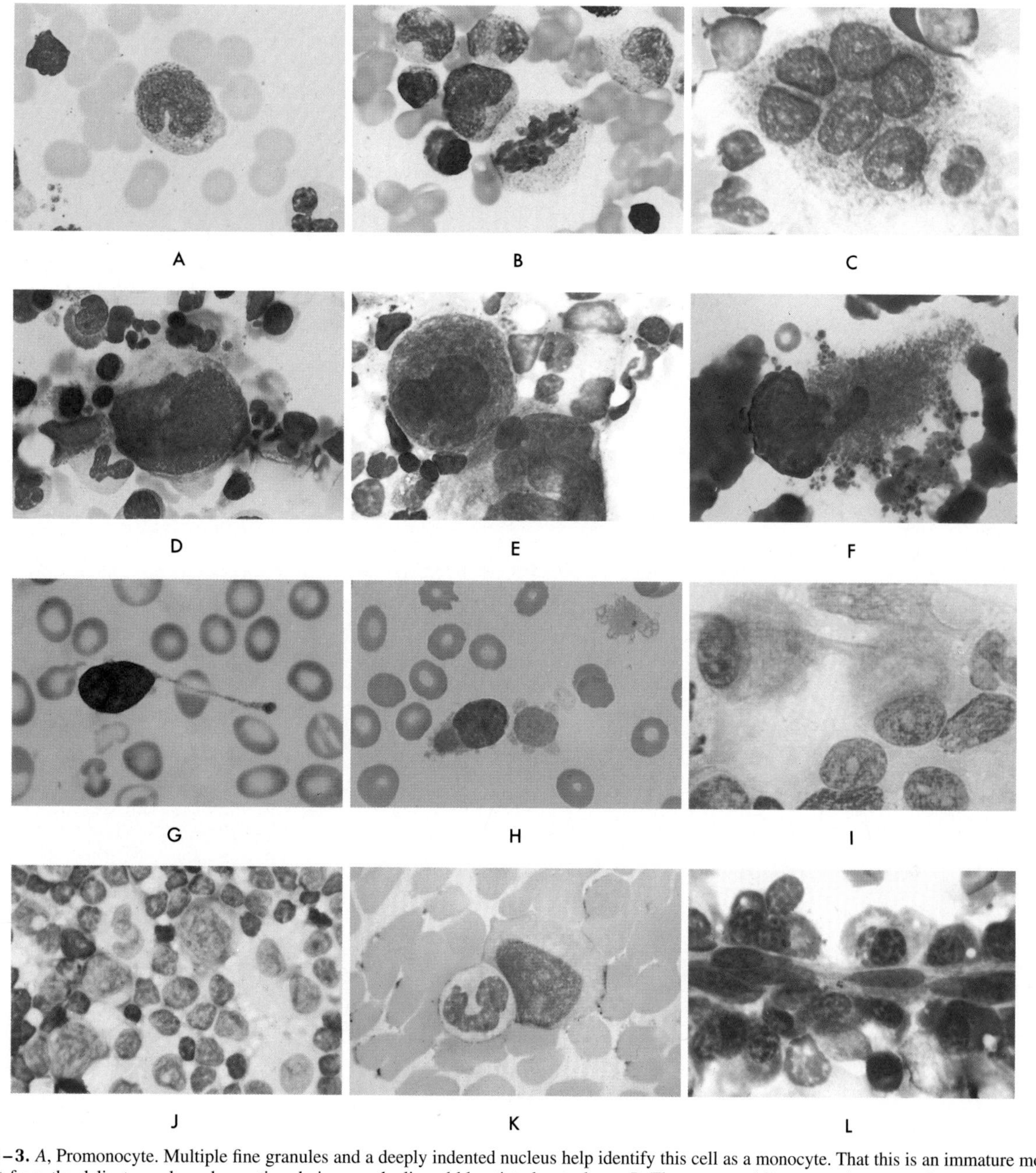

Plate 25–3. *A*, Promonocyte. Multiple fine granules and a deeply indented nucleus help identify this cell as a monocyte. That this is an immature monocyte is evident from the delicate nuclear chromatin, obvious nucleoli, and blue-tinted cytoplasm. *B*, Three neutrophil metamyelocytes at the top, a monocyte in the center of the group of cells, a small plasma cell, and a neutrophil myelocyte in mitosis. *C*, Osteoclast. Separate nuclei with relatively large nucleoli are the major features that distinguish this cell from a megakaryocyte. *D*, Megakaryoblast. *E*, Early megakaryocyte (bottom); the later megakaryocyte at the top has more compact nuclear material and clustering of granules. *F*, Megakaryocyte, releasing platelets. *G*, Megakaryocyte nuclear fragment with long strand of cytoplasmic material. *H*, Dwarf megakaryocyte and two atypical platelets from the blood of a patient with myelofibrosis with myeloid metaplasia. The atypical platelets are large, lack the normal number of granules, and have pseudopods. *I*, Osteoblasts. The eccentric nucleus, reticular chromatin pattern, large nucleolus, basophilic cytoplasm, and large pale Golgi zone separated from the nucleus are characteristic. *J*, Lymph node imprint from a patient with reactive lymph node hyperplasia. Note four or five histiocytes with abundant cytoplasm; numerous small lymphocytes; and stages in blast transformation, including three large reticular lymphocytes (nonleukemic lymphoblasts). *K*, Reticular lymphocyte (nonleukemic lymphoblast) in the blood of a patient with atypical pneumonitis and increased cold agglutinins. Note the large nucleoli; reticular nuclear chromatin; and moderately abundant, opaque, basophilic cytoplasm. *L*, Plasma cells lining sinusoidal endothelium in a marrow film from a patient with rheumatoid arthritis. In reactive plasmacytosis in marrow, plasma cells are frequently oriented in this manner. The chromatin in coarse blocks and the pale Golgi zone immediately adjacent to the nucleus are in contrast to the appearance of osteoblasts.

Chapter 26

Erythrocytic Disorders

M. Tarek Elghetany, M.D.
Frederick R. Davey, M.D.

ANEMIAS

General Manifestations

Anemia is considered to be present if the hemoglobin concentration or the hematocrit is below the lower limit of the 95% reference interval for the individual's age, sex, and geographic location (altitude) (see Fig. 24–47; Table 26–1). This means that 2.5% of normal individuals will be classified as anemic. Conversely, an individual whose hemoglobin falls within the reference intervals for his or her age and sex yet significantly below his or her own reference values should be considered anemic.

Causes of anemia fall into three major pathophysiologic categories: impaired red cell production, blood loss, or accelerated red cell destruction (hemolysis) in excess of the ability of the marrow to replace these losses. The presence of anemia may be a sign of an underlying disorder whose cause should be identified, because correction may be very important to the individual. Dilutional anemia with normal or increased total red cell mass may occur with pregnancy, macroglobulinemia, and splenomegaly.

Anemia also may be classified by red cell morphology as macrocytic, normocytic, or microcytic, an approach that is useful in differential diagnosis (see Laboratory Diagnosis of Anemia). Both the pathophysiologic and morphologic classifications should be understood. Some anemias have more than one pathogenetic mechanism and go through more than one morphologic stage, such as blood loss anemia.

Clinical Signs of Anemia

Clinical signs and symptoms result from the diminished delivery of oxygen to the tissues and, therefore, are related to the lowered hemoglobin concentration and blood volume, and are dependent on the rate of these changes. Modifying factors are compensatory adjustments in the cardiac output, the respiratory rate, and the oxygen affinity of hemoglobin. When anemia develops slowly in a patient who is not otherwise severely ill, hemoglobin concentrations as low as 6 g/dL may develop without producing any discomfort or physical signs as long as the patient is at rest.

In general, the anemic patient complains of easy fatigability and dyspnea on exertion, and often of faintness, vertigo, palpitation, and headache. The more common physical findings are pallor, a rapid bounding pulse, low blood pressure, slight fever, some dependent edema, and systolic murmurs. In addition to these general signs and symptoms, certain clinical findings are characteristic of the specific type of anemia.

Blood Loss Anemia

Acute Posthemorrhagic Anemia

Blood may be lost from the circulation externally, into the gastrointestinal tract, or into a tissue space or a body cavity. If blood is lost over a short period of time in amounts sufficient to cause anemia, *acute posthemorrhagic anemia* occurs.

After a single episode of bleeding, the major manifestations are those due to depletion of blood volume (hypovolemia). After a day or so, blood volume returns to previous levels by movement of fluid into the circulation, and anemia becomes evident.

The earliest hematologic change is a transient fall in the platelet count, which may rise to elevated levels within an hour. The next development is a moderate neutrophilic leukocytosis with a shift to the left; a maximum leukocyte count

Table 26–1. REFERENCE VALUES BELOW WHICH ANEMIA IS CONSIDERED TO EXIST AT SEA LEVEL

Age (Years)	Hb (g/dL)	Hct (Liter/Liter)
0.6 to 4	11	0.33
5 to 9	11.5	0.345
10 to 14	12	0.36
Adults—men	14	0.42
Adults—women	12	0.36
Pregnant women	11	0.33

From Committee on Iron Deficiency: Iron deficiency in the United States. JAMA 1968; 203:407. Copyright 1968. American Medical Assocation.

of 10 to 35 × 10^9/L may occur in two to five hours. The hemoglobin (Hb) and hematocrit (Hct) do not fall immediately but slowly as tissue fluids move into the circulation to compensate for the lost blood volume. The fall in Hb and Hct may not reveal the full extent of the red cell loss until two or three days after the hemorrhage.

The anemia that develops at first is normochromic and normocytic, with a normal mean cell volume (MCV) and mean cell hemoglobin concentration (MCHC) and only minimal anisocytosis and poikilocytosis. Increased erythropoietin (EPO) secretion stimulates erythroid proliferation in the marrow, and reticulocytes begin to reach the circulation in three to five days, reaching a maximum by 10 days or so. During this period, transient macrocytosis (increased MCV), increased polychromasia, and normoblasts may appear in the blood. It takes about two to four days after the blood loss for the leukocyte count to return to normal, and about two weeks for the morphologic changes to disappear. Return of red cell values is slower.

Chronic Posthemorrhagic Anemia

If blood is lost in small amounts over an extended period of time, both the clinical and hematologic features that characterize acute posthemorrhagic anemia are lacking. Regeneration of red cells occurs at a slower rate.

The reticulocyte count may be normal or slightly increased. Significant anemia does not usually develop until after storage iron is depleted; the anemia, therefore, is one of iron deficiency (q.v.). The anemia is at first normochromic and normocytic, and gradually the newly formed red cells become microcytic, then hypochromic. The leukocyte count is normal or slightly decreased, owing to neutropenia. Platelets are commonly increased, and only later, in severe iron deficiency, are they likely to be decreased.

The cause of blood loss must be identified, because it is toward this that definitive treatment must be directed.

Impaired Production—Iron Deficiency

Iron Metabolism

Iron is an essential component of hemoglobin, of myoglobin (in muscle cells), and of certain enzymes (in most body cells) (Fairbanks, 1995). The major pools of iron in the body are illustrated in Figure 26–1. Two thirds or more of the body's total iron is in the erythron (normoblasts and erythrocytes); each milliliter of red cells contains about 1 mg of iron. Storage iron is present in macrophages of the reticuloendothelial system in two forms: ferritin and hemosiderin. Ferritin is a water-soluble complex of ferric salt and a protein, apoferritin. Apoferritin has a molecular weight of approximately 450,000 daltons and consists of 24 subunits with a variable ratio of H (heavy) and L (light) types. Apoferritin forms a shell around a crystalline core of predominately ferric oxyhydroxide (FeOOH). Hemosiderin is water-insoluble and consists mostly of aggregates of FeOOH core crystals with partially or completely degraded protein shell. Most of the iron used in hemoglobin synthesis is that recently released from degraded Hb in macrophages and transported to the normoblasts by plasma transferrin (β-globulin, molecular weight 80,000 daltons). Transferrin binds to transferrin receptors on the cell membrane of erythroid precursors, reticulocytes, and most body cells. The transferrin-transferrin receptor complex is rapidly internalized, iron is released, and apotransferrin returns to the circulation and binds more iron.

Very little iron is lost from the body, and this mainly from loss of cells in the gastrointestinal tract and to a lesser extent from the skin and in the urine. The iron excreted in women averages more than that in men as a result of menstrual blood loss. Iron balance is maintained by control of absorption. In the United States, dietary iron averages 15 mg/day with 6% absorption in men, and 11 mg/day with 12% absorption in women. Absorption can be increased in iron deficiency but only to about 20% of ingested iron in meat-containing diets and less in vegetarian diets. Absorption takes place largely in the small intestine, most efficiently in the duodenum.

In plasma, the total iron averages 110 μg/dL (1.1 mg/L or 19.7 μmol/L). The great majority of this iron is bound to the transferrin, which has a capacity to bind 330 μg of iron/dL (or 59.1 μmol/L) and therefore is about one third saturated. A very small amount of iron in plasma is in ferritin. Plasma (or serum) ferritin averages about 100 μg/L in men (less in women: about 50 μg/L).

Iron Deficiency Anemia

When iron loss exceeds iron intake for a time long enough to deplete the body's iron stores, insufficient iron is available for normal hemoglobin production. When well developed, iron deficiency is characterized by a hypochromic microcytic anemia.

Iron deficiency results only when there is an increased need for iron (e.g., during rapid growth in infancy and childhood or during pregnancy) or when excessive loss of blood has reduced the body's reserves of iron (e.g., following repeated hemorrhages, excessive menstruation, or multiple pregnancies).

Iron deficiency is probably the most common cause of anemia between the ages of 6 and 24 months. It is caused by insufficient dietary iron to meet the needs of rapid growth. After the first four to six months of life, the iron stores present from birth have been exhausted, and the infant depends on dietary iron. An infant maintained on milk and carbohydrates without supplements of iron-containing foods is likely to develop an iron deficiency anemia, the so-called milk anemia of infancy. Defective absorption of iron and eventual iron deficiency anemia occur after total gastrectomy or even subtotal

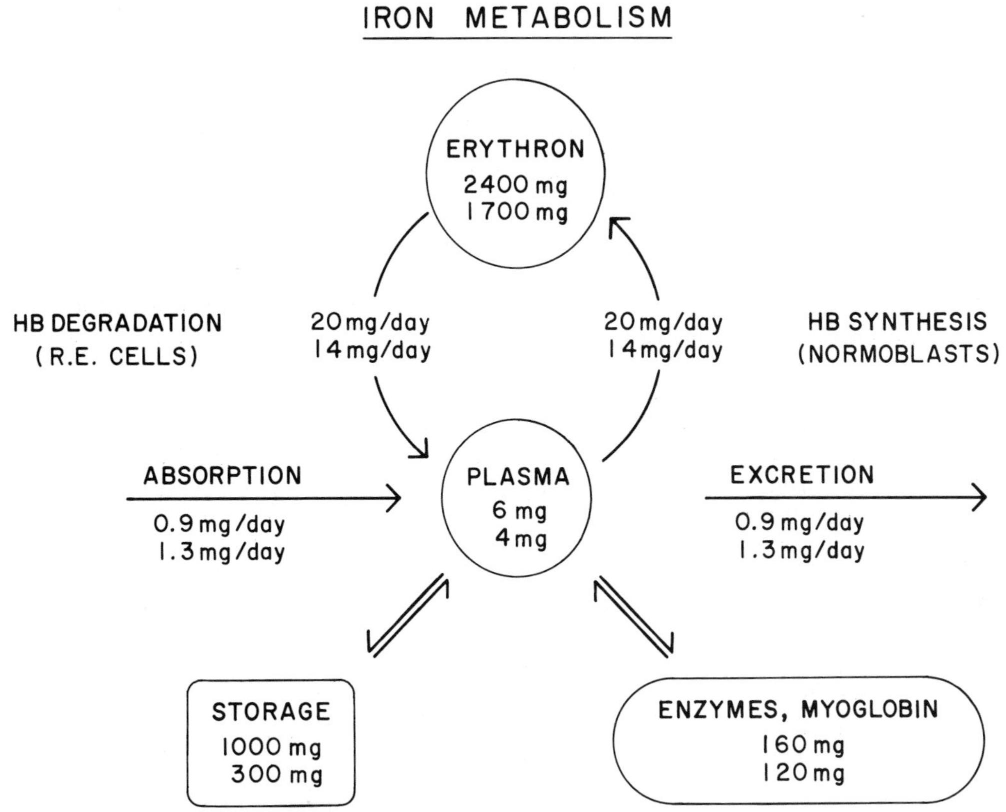

Figure 26–1. Scheme of iron metabolism. The upper figure in each position is average for an 80-kg man; the lower figure is for a 65-kg woman. (Data from Hillman and Finch, 1974.) The plasma iron, bound largely to transferrin, is central in one scheme. It completely turns over several times a day in supplying iron for heme synthesis.

Each day, about 1/120 of the total circulating red cells are destroyed and the same number of new red cells are delivered to the blood. That proportion of the total erythron iron enters the plasma from the site of Hb degradation, the macrophages of the reticuloendothelial (RE) system, and travels (bound to transferrin) to the normoblasts in the marrow. Storage iron largely resides also in the macrophages of the RE system. Absorbed iron enters the plasma pool, bound to transferrin. Excreted iron is largely from loss of cells.

4

gastrectomy. Except for the sprue syndrome, other causes of malabsorption of iron are extremely rare.

If an adult male had absolutely no iron intake or absorption (which would be extremely unlikely), his body iron stores of 1000 mg would last for three to four years before he would even begin to become iron deficient. Therefore, almost all cases of iron deficiency anemia in adult males are due to chronic blood loss.

The sequence of events in developing iron deficiency anemia is usually as follows (Hillman, 1985): When blood loss exceeds absorption, a negative iron balance exists. Iron is mobilized from stores, storage iron decreases, plasma ferritin decreases, iron absorption increases, and plasma iron-binding capacity (transferrin) increases. This stage is known as *iron depletion.* After iron stores are depleted, the plasma iron concentration falls, saturation of transferrin falls below 15%, and the percentage of sideroblasts decreases in the marrow. As a result of lack of iron for heme synthesis, red cell protoporphyrin increases. This second stage is *iron deficient erythropoiesis;* anemia may not yet be present. The third stage is *iron deficiency anemia;* in addition to the above-mentioned abnormalities, anemia is detectable. The anemia is at first normochromic and normocytic, gradually becomes microcytic, and finally microcytic and hypochromic.

CLINICAL FEATURES. Clinical findings may be due to the underlying cause of the blood loss itself, to the general manifestations of anemia (see previous discussion), or to iron deficiency. Those that are probably attributable to lack of tissue iron include paresthesias, such as numbness and tingling; atrophy of the epithelium of the tongue with burning or soreness; fissures or ulcers at the corners of the mouth (angular stomatitis); chronic gastritis, which leads to decreased gastric secretions but few symptoms; pica, which is the craving to eat unusual substances such as dirt or ice; concave or spoon-shaped nails (koilonychia); and difficulty swallowing owing to webs of tissue or partial strictures at the junction of the esophagus and hypopharynx. Koilonychia and strictures of the esophagus and hypopharynx are relatively uncommon. Splenomegaly may occur but is uncommon.

LABORATORY FEATURES

Blood. In early iron deficiency anemia, the stained blood film often shows normochromic normocytic erythrocytes (Fairbanks, 1971). In later stages, the picture is one of microcytosis, anisocytosis, poikilocytosis (including elliptical and elongated cells), and varying degrees of hypochromia. Reticulocytes are usually decreased in absolute numbers except following iron therapy. The MCV is low, and the Hb and Hct are relatively lower than the erythrocyte count. Osmotic fragility may be decreased because the red cells are thinner than normal (see Fig. 24–20; Plate 26–1*J*).

The leukocyte count is normal or slightly lowered. Granulocytopenia and a small number of hypersegmented neutrophils may be present. Megaloblastic changes in severe iron deficiency may be related to decreased activity of the enzyme ribonucleotide reductase, which contains an essential nonheme iron atom (Beck, 1991). However, the detection of hypersegmented neutrophils should raise suspicion about the presence of mild folate deficiency, which may become more overt after iron therapy (Dallman, 1993). Platelets may be increased, whether the iron lack is due to blood loss or dietary deficiency, but tend to be decreased in severe anemia.

Marrow. Normoblastic hyperplasia occurs early, but in later stages, the limiting effect of severe iron deficiency restricts erythropoiesis to the basal level. The normoblasts are smaller than normal, deficient in the amount of hemoglobin in the cytoplasm, and irregular in shape with frayed margins (see Plate 26–1*G*). Giant neutrophil bands or metamyelocytes, if present, are rarely due to iron deficiency per se; usually they indicate an associated cobalamin or folate deficiency (see the section entitled Megaloblastic Anemia). Iron stains should be performed routinely (see Chap. 25 and Plates 26–1*D* and *E*). *Storage iron* is absent, unless iron has recently been administered in some form. The proportion of normoblasts that are *sideroblasts* is decreased (less than 20%); this proportion is usually about the same as the percent saturation of transferrin (or total iron-binding capacity [TIBC]) and is a measure of iron delivery to the normoblasts.

Serum Iron. The reference interval is 50 to 160 μg/dL (9 to 29 μmol/L) in adults. The level is lower in iron deficiency but also in infections and the anemia of chronic disease.

Serum Iron-Binding Capacity. The reference interval for adults is 250 to 400 μg/dL (45 to 72 μmol/L). In iron deficiency anemia, the serum TIBC is increased. It is normal or decreased in the anemia of chronic disease. If chronic infection coexists with chronic blood loss, the TIBC may not be increased, even though the patient is iron deficient.

Percent Saturation of TIBC. The ratio of serum iron to TIBC is the percent saturation of the TIBC. Normally, this is 20% to 55%; values below 15% indicate iron-deficient erythropoiesis.

There is normally a marked diurnal variation in serum iron, with highest values in the morning and lowest values late in the day. Consequently, fasting morning blood specimens are preferred for the diagnosis of iron deficiency.

Somewhat lower reference intervals for serum iron are normal in iron sufficient infants from the second month through the twelfth month. Saarinen (1977) studied infants in whom iron deficiency was excluded by normal hemoglobin, MCV, and serum ferritin values. The TIBC gradually rose during the first year of life. After the first four months of life, through the first year, the lower reference value for percent saturation in normal infants was 10% rather than 20% as in adults. Thereafter, values slowly rise to adult levels at about the age of two years (Jacobs, 1974).

Serum Ferritin. In adults, the reference values are 12 to 300 μg/L, with higher values in men than in women. Serum ferritin appears to be in equilibrium with tissue ferritin and is a good reflection of storage iron in normal subjects and in most disorders. The equivalence of 1 μg/L of serum ferritin with 8 to 10 mg storage iron has been suggested. In patients with some hepatocellular diseases, malignancies, and inflammatory diseases, serum ferritin is a disproportionately high estimate of storage iron because serum ferritin is an acute phase reactant. In such disorders, iron deficiency anemia may exist with a normal serum ferritin concentration. In the presence of inflammation, persons with a serum ferritin level of less than 50 to 60 μg/L are likely to respond to iron therapy (Finch, 1986). A *low* value, however, below 12 μg/L, indicates low iron stores; falsely low values mimicking iron deficiency have not been found.

In infancy and childhood, between the ages of 6 months and 15 years, the reference interval for serum ferritin is 7 to 142 μg/L (Siimes, 1974), somewhat lower than early infancy or adult life. In men, serum ferritin gradually rises between the ages of 18 and 30 years, whereas in women it does not (Finch, 1977); representative geometric mean values of the skewed distribution of reference values were 127 μg/L for men and 46 μg/L for women.

Erythrocyte Porphyrins. Because heme is formed by insertion of iron into protoporphyrin IX, the latter is increased in iron deficient erythropoiesis, whether owing to iron deficiency or anemia of chronic disease. It is also increased in lead poisoning and in some cases of sideroblastic anemia but is normal in thalassemia. A relatively simple micromethod measuring free erythrocyte porphyrins (FEP) in whole blood (Piomelli, 1973) has been shown to be useful in distinguishing microcytosis due to iron deficiency from that due to β-thalassemia minor (Stockman, 1975). The normal reference interval was 10 to 99 μg/dL of erythrocytes; in iron deficiency, the erythrocyte porphyrins became elevated when the saturation of the TIBC was less than 15%.

DIFFERENTIAL DIAGNOSIS. Anemia due to iron deficiency usually must be distinguished from other microcytic or hypochromic anemias. These include the thalassemia traits, long-standing anemia of chronic disease, and the sideroblastic anemias (see later discussions of these entities). Bone marrow storage iron and serum ferritin is decreased in iron deficiency and normal or elevated in all others. In *thalassemia trait,* the FEP is normal, serum iron is normal, and the condition is present in family members. In β-thalassemia trait, the Hb A_2 and often the Hb F are increased. Indeed, the Hb A_2 is often decreased in iron deficiency. In *anemia of chronic disorders* (chronic infection, rheumatoid arthritis, or neoplastic disease), although the serum iron is low, as in iron deficiency, the TIBC is low or normal. In the *sideroblastic anemias,* which include chronic lead poisoning, the serum iron and percent TIBC saturation are increased, and pathologic ring sideroblasts are present in the marrow.

MANAGEMENT. The first principle in therapy is that the underlying cause be identified and corrected. Ferrous iron is given orally, about 200 mg/day, in three doses between meals. This regimen provides 20 to 40 mg of absorbed iron per day, which, with the iron produced by turnover of senescent red cells, is sufficient to increase production to two or three times normal (Hillman, 1985). The reticulocyte count will reach a maximum at 5 to 10 days then gradually decrease toward normal. Monitoring the hemoglobin is best; Hb should increase by 0.1 to 0.2 g/dL/day after the fifth day and by at least 2 g/dL each three weeks. After the hemoglobin has returned to normal, iron therapy should be continued for at least two months in order to replenish storage iron.

Impaired Production—Megaloblastic Anemia

Macrocytosis with Normoblastic Marrow

Macrocytic anemias that are not megaloblastic may be due to early release of erythrocytes from the marrow, as in response to acute blood loss or hemolysis; this is a shift macrocytosis, because it results from a premature release of reticulocytes from the marrow (Hillman, 1985). Macrocytosis not due to reticulocytosis is found commonly in hypothyroidism and in individuals with an excessive alcohol intake, as well as in some cases of aplastic or refractory anemias and of nonalcoholic liver disease (Chanarin, 1976).

Megaloblastic Anemia

BLOOD. Macrocytic anemias associated with megaloblastosis differ from nonmegaloblastic macrocytic anemia in that macro-ovalocytes and giant hypersegmented neutrophils are present in the blood (Figs. 24–21, 24–22, 24–33, 24–36, 24–40, and 26–2; see Plate 26–1*K*). Pancytopenia is the rule. The anemia is macrocytic with an elevated MCV and is characterized by macro-ovalocytes and often extreme degrees of anisocytosis and poikilocytosis. Microcytes and dacrocytes are common. Basophilic stippling, multiple Howell-Jolly bodies, nucleated red cells with karyorrhexis, and even megaloblasts may be seen. Leukopenia is present. Granulocytes have increased numbers of lobes, presumably a result of abnormal nuclear maturation. Five lobes in more than 5% of the neutrophils constitute hypersegmentation (Herbert, 1985), as do any neutrophils with six or more lobes. Thrombocytopenia usually is encountered and, on rare occasions, is sufficiently severe to be responsible for bleeding. It is worth noting that significant morphologic changes may occur in the blood in the absence of anemia and also that neurologic symptoms may be present in the absence of anemia.

MARROW. Megaloblastic anemia is characterized by enlargement of all rapidly proliferating cells of the body, including marrow cells (Plate 25–1*E* to *H*; Plate 26–1*B* and *H*). The major abnormality is the diminished capacity for DNA synthesis. The cells have both a prolonged intermitotic resting phase and a block early in mitosis. The number of mitotic figures is increased. RNA synthesis is less impeded than is DNA synthesis; hence, cytoplasmic maturation and growth continue, accounting for enlargement of the cells. The delicate chromatin and the prominent parachromatin result in a distinctly more open chromatin pattern than is seen in the normoblastic series. The nuclei undergo karyorrhexis readily, and multiple Howell-Jolly bodies may be present. There usually are more cells analogous to the pronormoblast and basophilic normoblast (e.g., the promegaloblast and basophilic megaloblast) than are seen in normal erythropoiesis. This has sometimes been termed maturation arrest, or nuclear-cytoplasmic asynchrony. Giant polychromatic megaloblasts are especially distinctive. The same general features are seen in the other cell lines. In the granulocytic series, the cells are larger, with retarded nuclear maturation and large cytoplasmic mass; often, the specific granules themselves are distinctly larger. The chromatin pattern is less condensed (more open), and as a result, the nucleus appears to stain poorly. Abnormally contorted nuclear configurations are common. The giant metamyelocyte is the most characteristic of the abnormal granulocytes. Megakaryocytes, too, are large and have separated nuclear lobes or nuclear fragments.

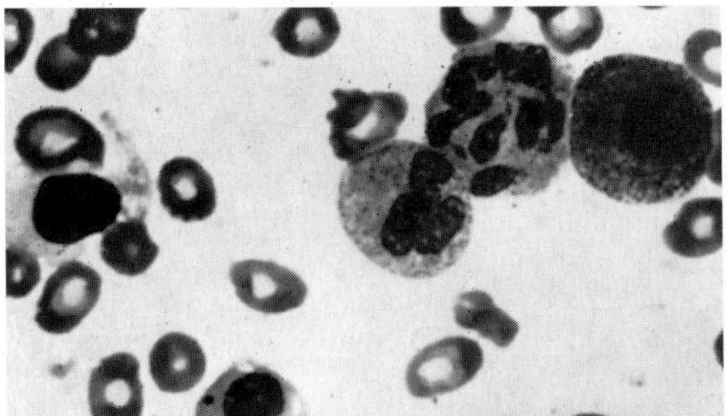

Figure 26–2. Megaloblastic anemia. *Below*, Orthochromatic megaloblast with four Howell-Jolly bodies. *Above, right*, Two giant neutrophils (one of which has nine nuclear lobes and could be called a macropolycyte) and an eosinophil with poor nuclear maturation. (× 875.)

The bone marrow is hyperplastic. The fat is replaced, and red marrow extends into the long bones. The number of erythroid precursors (megaloblasts) is increased, and the myeloid/erythroid ratio is decreased. If the megaloblastic process is incompletely developed or if the patient has been inadequately treated, the findings may be only partial. Because they persist longer, the granulocytic alterations are especially helpful in assessing recently treated megaloblastic anemia. The marrow findings result from the effects of impaired nucleic acid synthesis, leading to megaloblastosis, and hypoxic stress, giving rise to increased numbers of erythroid cells. If the patient is transfused with packed red cells, the number of erythroid precursors diminishes but the cytologic abnormalities persist.

ERYTHROKINETICS. In megaloblastic anemias, the mass of erythroid tissue is increased, plasma iron turnover is rapid, and urine and fecal urobilinogen are increased. These measures indicate an *increase of total erythropoiesis* that may be up to three times normal. Decreased rate of appearance of iron in the Hb of circulating erythrocytes and reticulocytopenia indicate *ineffective erythropoiesis.* In addition to increased destruction of the defective erythroid precursors in the marrow, survival of circulating erythrocytes is short, indicating hemolysis. Indirect serum bilirubin is increased, serum iron is increased, endogenous carbon monoxide production is increased, and serum lactate dehydrogenase (LD) usually is greatly elevated. Serum muramidase may be elevated, implying ineffective granulocytopoiesis.

Megaloblastic anemia is nearly always due to cobalamin or folic acid deficiency. The findings described are similar for either.

Cobalamin (Vitamin B_{12}) Metabolism

Vitamin B_{12} (cyanocobalamin) has a molecular weight of 1355 daltons. The molecule's two major parts are (1) a planar group (the corrin nucleus), a ring structure surrounding a cobalt atom; and (2) a nucleotide group, which consists of the base, 5,6-dimethylbenzimidazole, and a phosphorylated ribose esterified with 1-amino, 2-propanol. A cyanide group is in coordinate linkage with the trivalent cobalt. Different

4

forms of vitamin B_{12} result from replacement of the cyanide by hydroxy, adenosyl, or methyl groups; generically, these are termed *cobalamins.*

Cobalamin is the only vitamin exclusively synthesized by microorganisms. It is found in practically all animal tissues. It is stored primarily in the liver in the form of adenosylcobalamin. The human liver contains approximately 1 μg per gram of liver. Cobalamin is released by digestion of proteins of animal origin and then is bound by gastric intrinsic factor (IF), a 44-kDa glycoprotein produced in the parietal cells of the stomach. This cobalamin-IF complex then adheres to specific receptor sites on the epithelial cells of the ileum, at which site the cobalamin is absorbed. Several hours are required for absorption. The IF itself is not absorbed from the gut and is lost without recycling (Cooper, 1993).

Once absorbed, cobalamin is transported in the plasma as methylcobalamin, bound to a group of proteins named transcobalamin I (TC I), transcobalamin II (TC II), and transcobalamin III (TC III). Ninety percent of newly absorbed cobalamin is bound to TC II, which serves as the chief transport protein, rapidly delivering the vitamin to the liver, hematopoietic cells, and other dividing cells. Some cobalamin binds to TC I, which prevents its loss from the plasma; this cobalamin is a passive reservoir in equilibrium with body stores in the liver. The reference values for plasma cobalamin depend on the method of assay but commonly are 200 to 900 ng/L (150 to 670 pmol/L). One third of the binding sites on transcobalamins are normally occupied. TC I is 70% to 90% saturated and binds most of the plasma cobalamin; this is very slowly cleared from the plasma. TC II is only about 5% saturated; much of newly absorbed cobalamin bound to TC II is removed from the plasma during the first few hours, but a small fraction remains bound for several weeks (Hall, 1975).

The relative importance of the transcobalamins is illustrated by the effects of congenital deficiency (Cooper, 1993). Lack of TC II results in severe megaloblastic anemia in infancy; yet the serum cobalamin level is normal. Lack of TC I is not accompanied by anemia or megaloblastosis; yet the serum cobalamin level is decreased.

TC I and III are R-type proteins (rapidly moving on electrophoresis). TC III is probably an isoprotein of TC I, unsaturated with cobalamin and thus less charged. Much of the serum TC III is released from granulocytes during blood clotting *in vitro;* TC III does not appear to bind significant amounts of plasma cobalamin under normal conditions. TC I may arise from granulocytes as well as from other tissues. Elevation of TC I and III accounts for the elevation of total cobalamin-binding proteins in myeloproliferative diseases. TC I is synthesized by granulocytes whereas TC II is produced by the liver, macrophages, and ileum. TC III is produced by various cells in the body such as fibroblasts, macrophages, enterocytes, renal cells, hepatocytes, gastric mucosa and endothelium (Cooper, 1993).

The daily requirement for cobalamin is in the range of 2 to 5 μg/day. The body's stores of 2 to 5 mg will last for several years if intake is cut off, as is the case if total gastrectomy is performed (Beck, 1991).

Cobalamin Deficiency

Cobalamin deficiency is produced by any of several mechanisms.

INADEQUATE INTAKE. A dietary deficiency is an *extremely rare* cause of megaloblastic anemia in the United States and is seen only in persons who completely abstain from animal food, including milk and eggs. Only strict vegetarians are known to develop this form of cobalamin deficiency.

DEFECTIVE PRODUCTION OF INTRINSIC FACTOR. This is the most common cause of cobalamin deficiency.

PERNICIOUS ANEMIA. Pernicious anemia (PA) is a conditioned nutritional deficiency of cobalamin that is caused by a failure of the gastric mucosa to secrete IF. This abnormality is genetically determined but usually is not manifested until late in life; less than 10% of cases occur in persons under the age of 40.

Clinical Features. The disorder is equally common in males and females. Symptoms of anemia and the combination of skin pallor and jaundice giving a lemon-yellow tone to the skin are often present. The tongue may be sore, smooth, and pale (atrophic glossitis) or red and raw (acute glossitis). *Gastrointestinal symptoms* may be prominent and include episodic abdominal pain, constipation, and diarrhea. Diffuse and irregular degeneration of the white matter of the *central nervous system* characteristically involves the posterior and lateral columns of the spinal cord (subacute combined degeneration) and sometimes other sites. Symmetric sensations of pins and needles of the distal extremities, numbness and tingling, loss of position sensation (difficulty with balance and gait), and loss of vibratory sensation (perhaps the most constant sign) are indicative of posterior column lesions. Lateral column involvement gives rise to weakness, spasticity, and increased deep tendon reflexes. Sometimes the brain may be affected, and the patient shows irritability, emotional instability, or a change in personality. Neuropsychiatric disorders may be associated with cobalamin deficiency even without accompanying hematologic manifestations (Lindenbaum, 1988).

Gastric Findings. Atrophic gastritis of varying degree is found in most adults with PA, and gastric atrophy involving all coats of the wall in the remainder. IF and HCl are secreted by gastric parietal cells in the human; in adult PA, IF secretion is absent and almost always there is histamine-refractory achylia and achlorhydria—a decreased volume of gastric juice and lack of HCl secretion.

Immune Abnormalities. Autoantibodies have been found in the serum of patients with PA (Babior, 1995; Jandl, 1987). *Antiparietal cell antibodies* react with gastric parietal cells and are present in over 90% of patients. These parietal cell antibodies are also present in patients with chronic gastritis, such as that associated with iron deficiency, and in some patients with thyroiditis and myxedema; they are also present in 4% to 5% of age-matched healthy individuals.

Another type of autoantibody is directed against IF. *Anti-IF antibodies* occur in the serum, saliva, and gastric juice of about 75% of patients with PA. Two types of anti-IF antibodies occur. Blocking antibodies prevent the binding of cobalamin by IF, and binding antibodies bind to the cobalamin-IF complex and prevent the complex from binding to receptors in the ileum. Although these antibodies can cause some functional impairment *in vivo,* it is not clear whether the antibodies are the cause or an effect of the disease. IF antibodies in the absence of PA occur in a small percentage of individuals with hyperthyroidism (Graves' disease) and similarly in persons with insulin-dependent diabetes.

Family studies in patients with PA have shown an increased incidence of the disease in relatives, and many relatives have achlorhydria and partial defects of cobalamin absorption. Relatives of patients with PA also have a higher incidence of gastric parietal cell antibodies and thyroid antibodies than normal individuals.

It is possible that adult PA is a genetically determined autoimmune gastritis. However, the relationship of the gastric lesion to the antibodies remains unclear.

Pernicious Anemia in Children. Two forms of PA in children exist. *Congenital PA* occurs in the first few years of life. IF secretion is lacking, but acid secretion and the appearance of the gastric mucosa are normal. Antibodies to parietal cells and to IF are absent. *Juvenile PA* occurs usually in older children and is like that of adults, with gastric atrophy, achlorhydria, and serum antibody to IF; antibody to parietal cells, however, is usually absent (Babior, 1995).

GASTRECTOMY. Surgical removal of the stomach (total or even subtotal occasionally) removes the source of IF. Gastrectomy leads to megaloblastic anemia after the body's stores of cobalamin have been exhausted, in three to six years, if cobalamin therapy has not been given. Frequently, the anemia is in part due to iron deficiency.

DEFECTIVE ABSORPTION OF COBALAMIN

Malabsorption Syndromes. Celiac disease, tropical sprue, resection of the small bowel, or inflammatory disease of the small bowel may be associated with multiple defects of absorption, including other vitamins. Folic acid deficiency (absorbed principally in the upper small bowel) is more commonly seen than cobalamin deficiency (absorbed principally in the lower small bowel) in diseases leading to malabsorption. The reason for this is probably the lesser amount of time necessary for depletion of body stores of folic acid.

The Imerslund-Gräsbeck syndrome is an autosomally recessive inherited defect in the intestinal absorption of cobalamin, in the presence of normal IF (Babior, 1995).

Lack of Availability of Cobalamin. In certain countries, infestation with the fish tapeworm *(Diphyllobothrium latum)* is common enough that cobalamin deficiency may occur occasionally when it is present. The worm successfully competes with the host for the ingested cobalamin. The condition is most common in Finland but is rarely seen in the United States.

Bacteria in a blind loop of intestine may also preferentially use ingested cobalamin to the detriment of the host.

DIAGNOSIS OF COBALAMIN DEFICIENCY. Recognition of megaloblastic anemia indicates the likelihood of cobalamin deficiency or folic acid deficiency. In addition, evidence of neurologic involvement favors cobalamin deficiency. This diagnosis can be established by one of four methods: therapeutic trial, serum cobalamin assay, methylmalonic acid and homocysteine assays, and the deoxyuridine suppression test.

Therapeutic Trial. With the patient on a diet low in cobalamin and folate, a parenteral physiologic dose of cobalamin (10 μg/day) is given. Optimal hematologic response indicates deficiency, and consists of reticulocytosis beginning on the third or fourth day and reaching a peak on the seventh day. Erythropoiesis becomes normoblastic by two days, and leukopoiesis becomes normal by 12 to 14 days (Cooper, 1993). Within a week, leukocyte and platelet counts have returned to normal and the hemoglobin concentration begins to rise.

Serum Cobalamin Assay. This is the usual method of detecting a cobalamin deficient state. Microbiological assay of serum cobalamin employs an organism (e.g., *Euglena gracilis*) that requires cobalamin for growth. Radioisotopic dilution assays are more rapid and widely used and give results comparable with those of the *Euglena* assay, provided that the binding protein is specific for biologically active cobalamin; a standardized IF preparation is most satisfactory.

Reference values are 200 to 900 ng/L. In megaloblastic anemia due to cobalamin deficiency, serum cobalamin is usually less than 100 ng/L. Individuals with folate deficiency and mild cobalamin deficiency and who are pregnant have borderline values between 100 and 200 ng/L. Measurement of TC II–bound cobalamin may provide additional information because it may indicate early deficiency.

Methylmalonic Acid and Homocysteine Assays. Because a cobalamin coenzyme is essential for the isomerization of methylmalonate to succinate, excretion of increased amounts of methymalonate is found in cobalamin deficiency. Provided that the rare inborn error of metabolism methylmalonic aciduria is not present, this is a sensitive test for cobalamin deficiency, but it is not usually necessary for the diagnosis. In addition, plasma levels of methylmalonic acid and homocysteine are increased as well. Following several weeks of therapy, their plasma concentration returns to normal.

4

Deoxyuridine Suppression Test. The deoxyuridine suppression test measures the ability of marrow cells *in vitro* to use deoxyuridine in DNA synthesis. Normally, in marrow cells the major source of thymidine for DNA is by *de novo* synthesis from deoxyuridine, which requires intact cobalamin and folate enzymes; therefore, less than 10% of added tritium-labeled thymidine (^{3}H-Tdr) is incorporated into DNA. In megaloblastic marrows due to cobalamin or folate deficiency, deoxyuridine cannot be efficiently converted to thymidine, and more ^{3}H-Tdr is taken up into DNA. An abnormal deoxyuridine suppression test indicates either cobalamin or folate deficiency (Chanarin, 1976). A lymphocyte microdeoxyuridine suppression test (Herbert, 1985) requires only 1 mL of blood, making this diagnostic modality available for infants and children.

DETECTING THE CAUSE OF COBALAMIN DEFICIENCY. Clinical history is useful in suggesting whether cobalamin or folate deficiency is the cause of megaloblastic anemia. Clinical associations of PA include a family history of PA in one third of patients, certain endocrine deficiencies (thyroid disease, diabetes mellitus, hypothyroidism, Addison's disease), and certain immune disorders (immune thrombocytopenic purpura, autoimmune hemolytic anemia [AHIA], and acquired hypogammaglobulinemia). Cobalamin deficiency is likely in strict vegetarians, and in patients with paresthesias, neuropathy, or a previous gastrectomy (Chanarin, 1976).

In cobalamin-deficient patients, it is important to demonstrate a lack of IF. To do so, the ability of the patient to absorb an oral dose of radioactive cobalamin may be measured. The usual method is the Schilling test, which measures radioactivity in a 24-hour sample of urine. Two hours after oral administration of 0.5 to 2.0 μg of radioactive cobalamin, a large flushing dose of nonlabeled cobalamin is given parenterally. Normal individuals excrete over 7% of a 1-μg dose of ingested cobalamin in the urine in 24 hours, whereas patients lacking IF excrete less. If the excretion is low, the test must be repeated using the same procedure except that hog IF is given orally along with the labeled cobalamin. If the 24-hour excretion is normal, the low value in the first part was due to IF deficiency. If the excretion remains abnormal in the second part of the procedure, an explanation for malabsorption of cobalamin on the basis of intestinal disease must be sought. The validity of the results depends on good renal function and an accurate urine collection. The Schilling test is abnormal in PA even after the patient is treated with cobalamin and is in remission. Some patients may absorb vitamin B_{12} in water (as given in the original Schilling test) but fail to absorb vitamin B_{12} bound to protein in food. A modification of the Schilling test is being introduced to include protein-bound B_{12} using egg yolk or chicken serum (Cooper, 1993).

Other tests that establish the diagnosis of PA are direct assay of IF, demonstrating it to be deficient in gastric juice. The combination of megaloblastic anemia, decreased serum cobalamin, and serum antibodies to IF is essentially diagnostic of PA, obviating the need for the Schilling test (Lindenbaum, 1983).

Folic Acid Metabolism

Folic acid or pteroyl monoglutamic acid contains three parts: pteridine, para-aminobenzoate, and L-glutamic acid (Beck, 1991). In nature, folic acid occurs mainly as less soluble polyglutamates, with multiple glutamic acid residues attached to one another. Folic acid is present in a wide variety of foods, such as eggs, milk, leafy vegetables, yeast, liver, and fruits, and it also is formed by intestinal bacteria.

Conjugase enzymes in bile and intestine hydrolyze the polyglutamates prior to absorption, which is rapid and occurs in the proximal jejunum. Folate is rapidly removed from plasma to cells and tissues for utilization. The principal form of folate in serum, erythrocytes, and liver is 5-methyltetrahydrofolate (5-methyl-FH_4); the liver is the chief storage site. The minimal daily requirement is about 50 μg of pteroyl monoglutamate or 400 μg of total folate; a typical reference interval for serum folate is 5 to 21 μg/L (11 to 48 nmol/L) and for red cell folate 150 to 600 μg/L (340 to 1360 nmol/L) of red blood cells.

Folic Acid Deficiency

INADEQUATE INTAKE OF FOLATE

Evolution of Laboratory Abnormalities. Herbert delineated the sequence of events in the onset of folate-deficient megaloblastic anemia. After a folate-deficient diet was initiated, the various abnormalities were established as follows: three weeks, low serum folate; five weeks, hypersegmented neutrophils in bone marrow; seven weeks, hypersegmented neutrophils in peripheral blood, with bone marrow showing increased and abnormal mitoses and basophilic intermediate megaloblasts; 10 weeks, bone marrow showing some large metamyelocytes and polychromatophilic intermediate megaloblasts; 13 weeks, high excretion of formiminoglutamic acid (FIGLU) in urine; 17 weeks, low erythrocyte folate; 18 weeks, macro-ovalocytosis of erythrocytes with many large metamyelocytes in bone marrow; 19 weeks, overtly megaloblastic bone marrow; 20 weeks, anemia (Herbert, 1985).

At this time, changes in the intestinal epithelium had not yet appeared. Therefore, in humans with no dietary intake of folic acid, anemia will appear in three to six months. The peripheral blood and bone marrow features of megaloblastic anemia due to folic acid deficiency are similar to those of cobalamin deficiency; however, leukopenia and thrombocytopenia are less constant. Folic acid deficiency usually has been found in association with some complicating factor.

Nutritional Folate Deficiency. Megaloblastic anemia due to lack of folate is most commonly associated with insufficient dietary intake. The usual diet does not contain much above the minimal requirements, and body stores in the adult are sufficient for only about three months' needs. Dietary folate deficiency is especially common in the tropics and in India, and even in those locations it is usually associated with increased demand for folate in pregnancy, rapid growth in infancy, infection, or hemolytic anemia.

Folate deficiency in infancy is uncommon in the United States. Human milk or fresh cow's milk contains sufficient folate, but heated milk, powdered milk, and goat's milk do not. If the infant's milk lacks folate, if the diet is low in ascorbic acid, or if infection or diarrhea is a problem, megaloblastic anemia may occur (Mauer, 1969).

Megaloblastic anemia in pregnancy is not uncommon because of the fetal requirements for folate. The mother's plasma folate level gradually falls during pregnancy, and at birth, the plasma level in the newborn averages five times that of the mother. Megaloblastic anemia is more frequent in multiparous women, may be precipitated by infection, and is usually due to folate deficiency rather than cobalamin deficiency. Pregnant women should receive, in addition to iron, folic acid supplements.

Elderly persons on inadequate diets in the United States may develop folate-deficient megaloblastic anemia.

Liver Disease. Liver disease associated with alcoholism may lead to folate-deficient megaloblastic anemia because of the grossly inadequate diet of the alcoholic. With an adequate dietary folic acid intake, however, the anemia that is found with liver disease is macrocytic and normoblastic, not megaloblastic.

DEFECTIVE ABSORPTION OF FOLATE. Defective absorption of folic acid occurs in association with malabsorption syndromes discussed previously and in the blind loop syndrome, in which bacteria preferentially use folate.

Nontropical sprue, or adult celiac disease, is an important cause of malabsorption in adults or children that is related to dietary gluten (wheat protein). Included among the signs of malabsorption may be megaloblastic anemia due to folic acid deficiency (Beck, 1991). Jejunal biopsy shows villous atrophy. The folate deficiency as well as the malabsorption responds to a gluten-free diet. Folic acid therapy (parenteral) corrects the folate deficiency but not the general malabsorption.

Tropical sprue is a poorly understood malabsorptive disorder that is common in the Caribbean, India, and Southeast Asia. Evidence of malabsorption includes megaloblastic anemia due to folate deficiency. Treatment with folic acid brings considerable improvement in the general malabsorption as well as the anemia, but antimicrobial treatment is recommended in addition.

Megaloblastic anemia or decreased serum and red cell folate without anemia has been associated with the long-term use of anticonvulsant drugs, phenytoin, phenobarbital, and primidone. The problem appears to be a drug-induced malabsorption of pteroylpolyglutamate. Oral contraceptives cause malabsorption of folate in a small proportion of women, owing to impaired deconjugation of pteroylpolyglutamate (Beck, 1991).

INCREASED REQUIREMENT FOR FOLATE. The increased need in infants and pregnant women (multiple births) has been mentioned. Increased cell turnover that occurs in neoplasia and in the markedly stimulated hematopoiesis of hemolytic anemias may result in megaloblastic erythropoiesis. The basis for this problem is increased need for a marginal supply of folate.

INADEQUATE USE OF FOLATE. Inadequate use of folic acid is relatively rare.

Folic acid antagonists, such as methotrexate, block folic acid metabolism and, because of this action, are used in therapy of some malignant neoplasms. In addition to inhibiting the growth of the tumor, they also induce megaloblastic hematopoiesis.

In addition to the previously mentioned nutritional problem in alcoholics, *alcohol* may exert a direct effect in suppressing hematopoiesis by blocking metabolism of folate.

DIAGNOSIS OF FOLATE DEFICIENCY. Folic acid deficiency or cobalamin deficiency is suspected when the blood and bone marrow show findings characteristic of megaloblastic anemia; usually serum folate and cobalamin levels are then determined.

Serum and Red Cell Folate. A microbiological assay for folic acid activity employing *Lactobacillus casei* is a reliable method for the definitive diagnosis (Beck, 1991). Radioisotopic methods employing different folate binders are widely used because of rapidity and greater convenience. Although the correlation with the microbiological assay is generally good, discrepancies seem to be frequent and, on the basis of other data, tend to be resolved in favor of the microbiological assay.

The serum folate level is decreased (<3 μg/L) in megaloblastic anemia due to folate deficiency but is usually normal or increased in cobalamin deficiency. A low serum folate level precedes the decrease of red cell or tissue folate; it indicates a negative folate balance but does not by itself indicate tissue folate deficiency. In cobalamin deficiency, serum folate is decreased in 10% of cases, increased in 20%, and normal in the remainder (Tietz, 1990).

The red cell folate is a better test of body folate stores and is decreased in megaloblastic anemia due to folate deficiency. In cobalamin deficiency, however, red cell folate is low in almost two thirds of cases, so this needs to be excluded before regarding a low red cell folate as proof of severe folate deficiency. Therefore, three measurements are often useful in distinguishing between deficiencies of folic acid and cobalamin (Table 26–2).

Urinary Formiminoglutamic Acid. Folic acid coenzymes are required for the conversion of FIGLU to glutamic acid in the catabolism of histidine. When oral histidine is given, FIGLU appears in increased amounts in the urine if folate deficiency is present. The test is useful in patients with megaloblastic anemia due to antifolate drugs; these patients have normal serum folate levels but greatly decreased tissue coenzyme levels (Beck, 1991).

Therapeutic Trial. The therapeutic trial remains an excellent way to discriminate between folic acid and vitamin B_{12} deficiency. Physiologic doses of folic acid (parenteral, 50 to 200 μg/day) allow an adequate reticulocyte response in patients with folic acid deficiency but not in those with cobalamin deficiency.

On the other hand, the usual therapeutic doses of folic acid (5 to 15 mg/day) or larger doses of cobalamin (500 to 1000 μg) may induce a partial response in a patient with megaloblastic anemia due to the other deficiency.

Deoxyuridine Suppression Test. See earlier discussion.

Plasma Homocysteine Assay. As with cobalamin deficiency, total plasma homocysteine is increased in 80% to 90% of patients with folate deficiency. The level of methymalonic acid is normal (Cooper, 1993).

Therapy for Megaloblastic Anemia

Although it may be necessary to treat severely anemic patients with both vitamins, it is usually possible to determine which is the cause and treat only with that particular vitamin.

The maximal reticulocyte response occurs in five to seven days. Within four to six hours after the initial therapy (if parenteral), the marrow shows decreased early megaloblasts and the appearance of pronormoblasts. Within two to four days, the marrow is predominantly normoblastic. Granulocytic abnormalities return to normal more slowly, and hypersegmented neutrophils disappear from the blood only after 12 to 14 days.

PA is treated parenterally with 1000 μg of hydroxycobala-

Table 26–2. CORRELATION OF VITAMIN B_{12} AND FOLATE LEVELS WITH CLINICAL STATUS: THREE LABORATORY TESTS NEEDED TO SEPARATE FOUR CLINICAL SITUATIONS

Clinical Situation	Serum Vitamin B_{12} (pg/mL)	Serum Folate (ng/mL)	Red Cell Folate (ng/mL)
Normal*	Normal (200–900)	Normal (5–16), indeterminate (3–5), or low (<3)	Normal (>150)
Vitamin B_{12} deficiency	Low (<100)	Normal (5–16) or high (>16)	Low (<150)
Folic acid deficiency	Normal	Low	Low
Deficiency of both	Low	Low	Low

*Normal includes transient states of negative folate balance.

From Herbert V: Biology of disease. Megaloblastic anemias. Lab Invest 1985; 52:3. © by U.S. and Canadian Academy of Pathology, Inc.

min daily for two weeks, then twice weekly until the anemia is corrected, then monthly for the lifetime of the patient (Allen, 1992). Oral cobalamin therapy can be used only in patients with nutritional deficiency.

In folate deficiency, oral therapy is generally used at a dosage of 1 to 2 mg/day. Cobalamin deficiency must be excluded and corrected if present to avoid the occurrence of neuropathies of cobalamin deficiency.

Other Defects of Nucleoprotein Synthesis

Other defects of nucleoprotein synthesis may lead to megaloblastic anemias that do not respond to cobalamin or folic acid.

CONGENITAL DEFECTS. Oroticaciduria is a very rare autosomal recessive condition in which certain enzymes required for pyrimidine synthesis are absent. The findings are excessive urinary excretion of orotic acid, failure of normal growth and development, and megaloblastic anemia that is refractory to cobalamin and folate but that responds to uridine.

Inborn defects in enzymes involved in folate metabolism have also been described.

SYNTHETIC INHIBITORS. Synthetic inhibitors of purine synthesis (6-mercaptopurine, thioguanine, azathioprine), of pyrimidine synthesis (5-fluorouracil), or of deoxyribonucleotide synthesis (cytosine arabinoside or hydroxyurea) are used in chemotherapy for neoplasia and concomitantly may produce megaloblastosis.

REFRACTORY ANEMIAS. Anemias that are megaloblastic and that fail to respond to cobalamin or folic acid are considered with the myelodysplastic syndromes (see Chap. 27). The megaloblastic changes usually are atypical and do not include the characteristic granulocytic features, but other dysplastic changes are present.

Impaired Production—Other

Anemia of Chronic Disorders

The anemia most commonly seen in chronic infections, rheumatoid arthritis, and neoplastic disease is usually mild and is overshadowed by the basic disease (Means, 1992). Usually, the anemia does not progress in severity and has characteristic morphologic, biochemical, and kinetic disturbances (Cartwright, 1971).

The erythrocytes usually are normocytic and normochromic, and occasionally are microcytic and hypochromic. Anisocytosis and poikilocytosis are slight. The reticulocyte count usually is not elevated. Leukocytes and platelets are not distinctively altered, except by the causative disease.

The marrow is normocellular or minimally hypocellular or hypercellular, and the cell distribution is not greatly disturbed. The normoblasts may have frayed hypochromic cytoplasm, and the appearance of hemoglobin in the cells may be delayed (as in iron deficiency anemia). Sideroblasts are decreased, but storage iron is normal or increased.

The serum iron concentration is characteristically decreased, the TIBC is decreased or normal (in contrast to iron deficiency anemia, in which the TIBC is elevated), and the percent saturation is decreased. Erythrocyte protoporphyrin and serum ferritin are elevated.

The anemia seems to be the result of several factors. However, the most important pathogenetic mechanisms include inhibition of erythropoiesis by cytokines and an altered iron metabolism. Tumor necrosis factor-α (TNF) plays a significant role in inflammation and immune response. TNF levels are increased in patients with cancer, rheumatoid arthritis, infections and AIDS. *In vitro* inhibition of human erythroid colony formation (BFU-E and CFU-E) by TNF has been reported. Similarly, an inhibitory action of interleukin-1 (IL-1) and γ-interferon (γ-IFN) on erythropoiesis has been implicated.

EPO levels, although above normal, have been disproportionate to the degree of anemia indicating relative EPO deficiency in anemia of chronic disease. Inhibitory effects of cytokines on EPO synthesis sites such as renal and liver cells have been suggested. Increased apoferritin production by some cytokines, especially IL-1, may play a role in altered iron metabolism because it may facilitate the retention of iron as ferritin in the reticuloendothelial system (Rapaport, 1987).

The anemia usually fails to respond to iron therapy. However, patients treated with EPO have shown improvement.

Anemia of Renal Insufficiency

The correlation between the severity of the anemia and the degree of elevation of the blood urea nitrogen is positive but not strictly linear. When the blood urea nitrogen (BUN) exceeds 100 mg/dL (36 nmol/L), the hematocrit is usually below 0.30 (Erslev, 1995a).

Several factors are often involved in the anemia of chronic renal failure. Decreased production of EPO by the damaged kidney is probably the important factor in most cases in which the BUN exceeds 100 mg/dL. Both ineffective erythropoiesis and impaired ability of the marrow to respond to EPO appear to be present in some degree.

Inhibitors of erythropoiesis have been demonstrated in the plasma of patients with chronic renal failure (Hockings, 1987). The nature of these inhibitory factors is not known; however, parathyroid hormone and spermine have been implicated as inhibitors of erythropoiesis.

Hemolysis is a significant feature in many cases of chronic renal failure. There appears to be an extracorpuscular factor in uremic plasma that has a detrimental effect on red cell metabolism and results in morphologically deformed cells (echinocytes and spiculated red cells). Numerous irregularly contracted and fragmented cells are seen in the hemolytic-uremic syndrome and in malignant hypertension as a result of traumatic damage incurred by the red blood cells in traversing the damaged small blood vessels. Changes in red cell membrane ATPase and transketolase may render the red cells more sensitive to oxidant drugs or chemicals.

In addition, bleeding is a common problem in chronic renal disease, probably owing either to thrombocytopenia, in some patients, or to platelet functional defects, which are present in most patients. Anemia due to iron deficiency from blood loss should always be suspected. Folic acid deficiency may be a problem in patients in a dialysis program, because folic acid is readily moved into the dialysis bath.

Anemia in Liver Disease

Chronic posthemorrhagic anemia; hypoplastic anemia secondary to viral-induced marrow suppression; folate-deficient megaloblastic anemia due to poor nutrition in alcoholic cirrhosis; and acquired hemolytic anemias associated with either Coombs-positive red blood cells, congestive splenomegaly, or lipid disturbances may occur in liver disease (Phillips, 1987).

In addition to these types, there is an anemia associated with liver disease that is characterized by shortened red blood cell survival and relatively inadequate red cell production. It is exaggerated by an increased blood volume that appears to correlate with the degree of portal hypertension. The red blood cells are normocytic or macrocytic (thin macrocytes). Frequently, target cells are present, especially in obstructive jaundice (Fig. 24–30); these cells have an increased surface membrane with increased cholesterol and lecithin content. However, the phospholipid/cholesterol ratio is normal. Reticulocytes may be slightly increased, and platelets may be normal or decreased. The bone marrow may be slightly hypercellular, and erythropoiesis is macronormoblastic rather than megaloblastic. Changes in leukocytes, such as are present in megaloblastic anemias, are not seen, and this type of anemia does not respond to cobalamin (vitamin B_{12}) or folic acid. The anemia is of unknown origin.

A small proportion of patients with severe cirrhosis have a hemolytic anemia associated with spur cells, which are red blood cells with thorny projections similar to acanthocytes. As with target cells, the spur cells are secondary to lipid abnormalities in the plasma; they have increased surface membrane with increased cholesterol but normal phospholipid content in the membrane. These irregular cells have decreased deformability and tend to be trapped in the spleen and destroyed (Beck, 1991).

Anemia in Endocrine Disease

Uncomplicated anemia in hypothyroidism is mild to moderate; it is normochromic and normocytic without reticulocytosis and with normal red blood cell survival. It reflects a decreased marrow production due to a smaller tissue oxygen requirement and subsequent reduced EPO secretion. Because plasma volume is decreased in hypothyroidism, the apparent degree of anemia may not be proportional to the decrease in red cell mass. Hypothyroidism may, of course, be complicated by iron deficiency or folic acid or vitamin B_{12} deficiency (Orwoll, 1987).

In adrenal cortical hormone deficiency, there is a mild normochromic normocytic anemia. The etiology is unclear, but it is corrected by hormone replacement.

Deficient testosterone secretion in men results in a decrease in red cell production of 1 to 2 g Hb/dL (to a value comparable with that of the woman); this appears to be due to the effect of androgens on EPO secretion.

Pituitary deficiency tends to result in a greater depression of hemoglobin concentration because of the effect on multiple endocrine glands and possibly the loss of growth hormone effect.

A small number of patients with hyperparathyroidism have a normocytic, normochromic anemia. Earlier studies suggested that the parathyroid hormone may suppress normal erythropoiesis. More recent studies failed to support this theory. The anemia of hyperparathyroidism is likely related to marrow fibrosis or decreased EPO secretion secondary to renal calcification (Erslev, 1995b).

Anemia Associated with Bone Marrow Infiltration (Myelophthisic Anemia)

This anemia is associated with marrow replacement by (or involvement with) metastatic carcinoma, multiple myeloma, leukemia, lymphoma, lipidoses or storage disease, and certain other conditions.

The characteristic finding in the blood is the presence of varying number of normoblasts and immature neutrophils; these are responsible for the descriptive terms *leukoerythroblastotic reaction, leukoerythroblastic anemia,* and *leukoerythroblastosis* (see Table 24–5).

Normochromic and normocytic (occasionally macrocytic) anemia of varying severity is present. Reticulocytes are often increased, and the number of normoblasts usually is out of proportion to the severity of the anemia. The leukocyte count is normal or reduced (occasionally elevated), and immature neutrophils and even myeloblasts may be found. Platelets are normal or decreased, and bizarre, atypical platelets can sometimes be seen.

Examination of the marrow usually reveals the condition responsible for this reaction. Mechanical crowding out of the hematopoietic tissue by the pathologic process has been assumed but not proved and probably is not the usual cause. Often, the amount of erythropoietic tissue in the marrow as determined by morphologic and kinetic studies is normal or increased. The mechanism described in the section on anemia of chronic disorders may often play a role, but the reason for the outpouring of immature cells into the blood is not clear.

In addition to myelophthisic anemias, circulating normoblasts and immature neutrophils can also be seen in hemolytic anemias, severe anemias due to other causes, severe infections, and congestive heart failure, but usually, the normoblasts are not as numerous.

The *leukoerythroblastotic reaction* associated with myelophthisic anemias cannot always be distinguished from the blood picture of myelosclerosis with myeloid metaplasia (MMM), which is one of the myeloproliferative disorders. In MMM, enlargement of the spleen and liver is almost always found. In the blood film, more severe red blood cell abnormalities, leukocytosis, myeloblasts and immature granulocytes of all varieties (not just neutrophils), increased basophils, more atypical platelets, more numerous megakaryocyte fragments, and dwarf megakaryocytes are all findings more characteristic of MMM than of a leukoerythroblastotic reaction of some other cause. Examination of the bone marrow by a needle biopsy or surgical biopsy is necessary to differentiate MMM from myelophthisic anemias.

Aplastic Anemia

The term aplastic anemia usually refers to pancytopenia associated with a severe reduction in the amount of hematopoietic tissue that results in deficient production of blood cells. The marrow, although hypocellular, may have patchy areas of normocellularity or even hypercellularity. The diagnosis of severe aplastic anemia is made in pancytopenic patients when at least two of the following three peripheral blood values—granulocytes less than 0.5×10^9/L, platelets less than 20×10^9/L, or reticulocytes less than 1% (corrected for hematocrit)—are present and the bone marrow is either markedly hypocellular or moderately hypocellular with less than 30% of residual hematopoietic cells (Camitta, 1982).

CLINICAL FEATURES. The clinical course may be acute and fulminating, with profound pancytopenia and a rapid progression to death, or the disorder may have an insidious onset and a chronic course. The symptoms and signs depend on the degree of the deficiencies: bleeding from thrombocytopenia, infection from neutropenia, and signs and symptoms of anemia. As a rule, splenomegaly and lymphadenopathy are absent.

Etiology. Aplastic anemias are of diverse etiology. Since 1980, in approximately 70% of cases, no specific etiologic agent could be correlated with the disease; such cases are considered idiopathic. Drug-related and chemical-related aplastic anemias account for 11% to 20%, and those associated with infectious hepatitis account for 6% of cases (Alter, 1993).

PATHOGENESIS. Hematopoietic failure may occur at any level in the differentiation of bone marrow precursor cells. There may be insufficient or defective pluripotent stem cells (CFU-S) or committed stem cells (CFU-C). The microenvironment may be unable to provide for the normal development of hematopoietic cells. The appropriate humoral and cellular stimulators for hematopoiesis may be absent. In addition, bone marrow failure could result from excessive suppression of hematopoiesis by T lymphocytes or macrophages. Finally, stem cells could interact among themselves, with one clone inhibiting the growth of another (Alter, 1978).

In most cases of aplastic anemia, it is likely that damage to the hematopoietic stem cell by a known or unknown agent in some way alters the ability of the cell to proliferate or differentiate. The committed granulocyte-monocyte precursor cells (CFU-GM) are decreased in blood and marrow in most patients with aplastic anemia (Kern, 1977). In a small proportion of cases, it may be that the defect is in the hematopoietic microenvironment, which fails to support stem cell growth; this may be the case when bone marrow transplants repeatedly will not engraft. Also, inhibition of stem cell growth may be mediated by blood or bone marrow lymphocytes in some cases of aplastic anemia (Good, 1977). In addition, immunologic mechanisms may suppress hematopoiesis, as is likely in some pure red cell aplasias. An excellent review of the pathogenesis of aplastic anemia is provided by Alter (1993).

PROGNOSIS. Complications are due to infection, bleeding, and problems of iron overload from repeated transfusions. The prognosis appears to depend upon the severity of marrow damage. In a series of 101 patients treated by conventional methods (Williams, 1978), 25% of patients died within four months of the onset of symptoms, 50% died within 12 months, and 71% died within five years. Those who died within four months had significantly lower reticulocyte, neutrophil, and platelet counts; a lower percentage of myeloid cells in the marrow; and a shorter interval between onset of symptoms and visit to the physician (Lynch, 1975). Other factors that correlated with a poor prognosis included male gender but not the age of the patient or etiology of the aplasia (Williams, 1978). In some survivors, partial recovery is common. With the introduction of modern treatment protocols by immunosuppressive therapy and bone marrow transplantation, long-term survival rates of more than 60% are reported. The survivors have much higher risk of developing myelodysplastic syndrome, paroxysmal nocturnal hemoglobinuria, and acute leukemia (Narayanan, 1994).

Because of the high mortality rate, it is important to identify early those patients who have a poor prognosis for bone marrow transplantation.

MANAGEMENT. Treatment includes bone marrow transplantation for patients younger than 50 years of age if there is a human leukocyte antigen (HLA)–matched donor. Antilymphocyte globulin and corticosteroids are useful in some patients. Androgens appear to be least helpful in the stimulation of any residual marrow. Supportive care must be used with caution. Certainly, appropriate antibiotics should be used to combat infections; however, the risk for sensitization should be considered with the administration of blood products. Single donor platelets or platelets from HLA-matched donors are preferred (Alter, 1993).

IDIOPATHIC APLASTIC ANEMIA. In patients with pancytopenia and a hypocellular marrow, a search should be made for evidence of significant exposure to radiation, drugs, and chemicals of known or possible propensity to injure the marrow so that further exposure can be eliminated. Nevertheless, in approximately 70% of the cases of aplastic anemia, no suspected causal relationship to toxic agents can be found, and these are the cases that are designated as idiopathic.

The symptoms and signs do not differ, but the onset is commonly more insidious than in toxic or hypersensitive aplastic anemias.

BLOOD. The red blood cells usually are normal in size and shape, although in some cases, there may be varying degrees of anisocytosis and poikilocytosis or macrocytosis. In a nontransfused patient, the red blood cell distribution width (RDW) is normal. However, following transfusion, there is an increase in the RDW and, in some cases, the emergence of a bimodal population of red cells (Bessman, 1983). Polychromasia, stippling, and normoblasts are most often conspicuously absent. Leukopenia with marked decrease in granulocytes and a relative lymphocytosis are observed. In severe leukopenia, there is often also an absolute lymphocytopenia. Neutrophil granules may be larger than normal and may stain dark red (unlike the so-called toxic granules found in infections), and the neutrophil alkaline phosphatase may be elevated. Thombocytopenia is part of the picture. The serum iron usually is increased. The serum cobalamin and folate levels usually are normal. Although an occasional patient is hypogammaglobulinemic, most patients have normal levels of serum immunoglobulins.

BONE MARROW. In most cases, the aspirate consists of red cells, lymphocytes, some plasma cells, and fatty particles. Marrow sections show fatty tissue with inconspicuous fibrosis and islands of lymphocytes and plasma cells (see Plate 26–1*C*). Though focal areas of normocellularity or hypercellularity sometimes may be present, the overall cellularity is decreased. Storage iron is increased.

Erythrokinetics. The increased serum iron concentration is a valuable early sign of erythroid hypoplasia and reflects the decreased plasma iron turnover. In addition, the erythrocyte use of iron is decreased. Both effective and total erythropoiesis, therefore, are decreased in aplastic anemia.

APLASTIC ANEMIA ASSOCIATED WITH CHEMICAL OR PHYSICAL AGENTS

Toxic Aplastic Anemias. A number of physical and chemical agents produce marrow damage in all humans and animals exposed to a sufficient dose. Examples are ionizing radiation; mustard compounds; benzene; and antineoplastic agents such as busulfan, urethane, and antimetabolites.

Ionizing Radiation. The effects depend on the radiosensitivity of the cells and the capacity of the cells to regenerate, as well as the survival rate of the cells in the blood. Erythroid cells are most sensitive, granulocytes have intermediate sensitivity, and the megakaryocytes are the least sensitive of the three. Stromal cells are relatively insensitive.

After acute exposure to radiation, the reticulocyte count falls, but the red blood cells decline slowly because of their long survival. Within the first few hours, there is a neutrophilic leukocytosis due to a shift from marginal and probably marrow storage pools. A fall in lymphocytes occurs after the first day and is responsible for the early leukopenia. After five days or so, granulocytes begin to fall. The platelets decrease later. Platelets are often the last to return to normal in the recovery phase.

Hypersensitive Aplastic Anemias. A large number of drugs produce marrow damage in some individuals after single or repeated exposures. Effects are not dose related as they are in toxic aplasia. Agents include antimicrobial drugs (e.g., salvarsan, chloramphenicol, sulfonamides, chlortetracycline, streptomycin), anticonvulsants (e.g., mephenytoin, trimethadione), analgesics (e.g., phenylbutazone), antithyroid drugs (e.g., carbimazole), antihistaminics (e.g., tripelennamine), insecticides (e.g., DDT), and other chemicals—some known (e.g., gold compounds, quinacrine, chlorpromazine, hair dyes, bismuth, mercury) and others unknown.

Chloramphenicol is an important drug in this category. Reactions of the marrow to chloramphenicol are of two types, which are possibly unrelated (Yunis, 1964).

In about half the patients who receive chloramphenicol, increased serum iron, reticulocytopenia with anemia, neutropenia, and thrombocytopenia are found. The marrow may show decreased erythroid cells and vacuolization of primitive erythroid and granulocyte precursors. These changes are dose related, time dependent, and reversible.

In a very small proportion of persons receiving chloramphenicol, an irreversible aplastic anemia develops that may be fatal. No relationship has been established between the reversible erythropoietic lesion and the development of aplastic anemia; it may be that individual susceptibility is responsible for the latter. For this reason, it is essential that restraint be employed in using the drug, because monitoring its administration with blood cell counts is not an effective preventive measure.

APLASTIC ANEMIA ASSOCIATED WITH OTHER DISEASE

Infection. Marrow aplasia has been described as an infrequent sequela to infectious hepatitis, occurring a few months after onset when the hepatitis is resolving. Most cases are non-A, non-B hepatitis, with only rare cases of A or B types. These patients usually are males and younger than age 20; the prognosis usually is grave. Parvovirus has been associated with transient erythroid aplastic crisis in patients with chronic hemolytic disorders (Young, 1984). Human immunodeficiency virus and Epstein-Barr virus may also cause hematopoietic depression. The mechanism of virus-induced bone marrow failure may be related to direct cytotoxicity, immune-mediated mechanisms or stromal injury (Alter, 1993).

Paroxysmal Nocturnal Hemoglobinuria. This rare hemolytic process (see later discussion) may be followed by aplastic anemia. Usually in paroxysmal nocturnal hemoglobinuria (PNH), a variable degree of marrow hypofunction coexists. Curiously, in some patients who present with aplastic anemia, the red blood cell defect of PNH may be present or may appear during the course of the disease. According to Lewis (1967), about 15% of patients with aplastic anemia have a demonstrable PNH red blood cell defect, with or without clinical hemolysis.

Pregnancy. Pregnancy occurring in a patient with acquired aplastic anemia may make the pancytopenia more severe. Occasionally, however, aplastic anemia occurs during pregnancy and remits following delivery. In some such cases, aplasia recurs during a second pregnancy. The infants may be anemic, thrombocytopenic, or leukopenic (Fleming, 1973).

Thymoma. Although thymomas usually are associated with pure red blood cell aplasias, other bone marrow elements may also become depressed. Pancytopenia, often with hypoplastic bone marrow, occurs in 10% to 15% of cases with thymoma. Thymectomy results in a good remission in one third of the patients. Most of the patients are women older than 50 years of age (Hirst, 1967).

CONSTITUTIONAL APLASTIC ANEMIA. The term constitutional aplastic anemia designates individuals with a congenital or genetic predisposition to bone marrow failure. In a study of 40 patients with constitutional aplastic anemia, 26 patients had Fanconi's anemia, 10 patients had familial aplastic anemia without classic signs of Fanconi's anemia, and 4 patients presented with amegakaryocytic thrombocytopenia that later developed into complete aplasia (Alter, 1978).

Fanconi's Anemia. In Fanconi's anemia, the pancytopenia becomes obvious after infancy and usually is significant by the eighth year of life. Often, more than one member of a family is affected. The anemia usually is normochromic and may be macrocytic; the marrow generally is hypocellular. Developmental anomalies are present and may include hyperpigmentation, short stature, hypogonadism, malformations of the extremities (e.g., aplasia of the radius and abnormalities of the thumbs), microcephaly, and malformation of other organs (e.g., heart and kidneys). Chromosomal defects consisting of random breaks and rearrangements characteristically are present in blood lymphocytes as well as in marrow cells. The chromosomal breakage becomes more evident when the cultured cells are challenged with alkylating and DNA cross-linking agents such as mitomycin C and diepoxybutane. Patients with Fanconi's anemia are at a higher risk of developing leukemia and nonhematologic tumors, particularly in the liver (Alter, 1993).

Familial Aplastic Anemia. In a subset of Fanconi's anemia, patients may have pancytopenia and a hypocellular marrow without major developmental anomalies. In some cases, there may be skin hyperpigmentation, a narrow palpebral fissure, or stunted growth. Sometimes, the patient with aplastic anemia may have a relative with classic Fanconi's anemia (O'Gorman Hughes, 1974).

However, aplastic anemia may occur in members of a family without the stigmata of Fanconi's syndrome. In this group, males are more likely to be affected than females. The age at diagnosis varies from younger than 1 year to 77 years.

A few children present with bleeding manifestations secondary to amegakaryocytic thrombocytopenia. As their disease progresses, they develop a pancytopenia and a hypocellular marrow. In some cases, the patients have the developmental abnormalities associated with Fanconi's anemia, whereas in other cases, no anomalies are identified.

Pancytopenia and hypoplastic anemia may develop in a subset of patients with other familial disorders. Some patients with dyskeratosis congenita, Shwachman-Diamond syndrome, and amegakaryocytic thrombocytopenia have been reported to develop aplastic anemia (Alter, 1993).

Pure Red Cell Aplasia

TRANSITORY ARREST OF ERYTHROPOIESIS. This condition may occur during the course of a hemolytic anemia (often preceded by an infection), and the combination of aplasia and hemolysis becomes a life-threatening situation. Red blood cell production may occasionally cease during or following rather minor infections in normal children or adults, at which time the marrow will show absence of all but a few of the most immature erythroid precursors. Aplastic episodes in chronic hemolytic anemias often appear to be due to parvovirus infection. This virus inhibits erythropoiesis by infecting mature erythroid progenitor cells (CFU-E). The aplastic crises resulting from parvovirus infection are transient, with erythroid marrow recovery in one to two weeks after onset (Young, 1984).

TRANSIENT ERYTHROBLASTOPENIA OF CHILDHOOD. Transient erythroblastopenia of childhood (TEC) occurs in previously healthy children, usually younger than eight years of age, with most cases occurring between one and three years of age. It is characterized by a moderate to severe normocytic anemia and severe reticulocytopenia. A history of a viral infection within the past three months is frequently elicited. The bone marrow generally is normocellular and shows virtual absence of erythroid precursors, except for a few early forms. The patients recover within one or two months without therapy. The pathogenesis appears to involve humoral inhibition of erythropoiesis or decreased stem cells in many of the patients who have been studied, but parvovirus is not the cause of TEC (Alter, 1993).

CONGENITAL RED CELL APLASIA (DIAMOND-BLACKFAN ANEMIA; CONGENITAL HYPOPLASTIC ANEMIA). This is a rare, constitutional red blood cell aplasia that usually becomes obvious during the first year of life but may occur as late as six years of age. The severe anemia is normochromic and slightly macrocytic; reticulocyte level is low; leukocytes are normal or slightly decreased; platelets are normal or increased; and the marrow usually shows a reduction in all developing erythroid cells but normal granulocytic and megakaryocytic cell lines. In a small number of cases, residual erythroid precursors are detected. These precursors are mostly pronormoblasts. Fetal hemoglobin (Hb F) is elevated (5% to 25%) to a degree not expected for the patient's age, and the antigen i is often present. These findings contrast with those of transient arrest of erythropoiesis (transient erythroblastopenia of childhood). In transient erythroblastopenia of childhood, the red blood cells are normocytic, the Hb F is normal, the antigen i is absent, and red blood cell enzymes are at a lower level (characteristic of an older cell population) (Alter, 1993).

The defect appears to be in the erythroid-committed progenitor cells. CFU-Es and BFU-Es are decreased in the marrow, and BFU-Es, which normally circulate, are absent or decreased in the blood. In addition, these progenitor cells fail to respond in *in vitro* culture systems to normal T cells and to usual levels of EPO, suggesting a qualitative defect.

About 75% of patients respond at least partially to corticosteroids, and the overall long-term survival rate is about 65%, although many patients require long-time steroid use (Alter, 1993).

ACQUIRED PURE RED CELL APLASIA. In middle-aged adults, selective failure of red blood cell production occurs rarely. Reticulocytopenia and a cellular marrow devoid of all but the most primitive erythroid precursors are characteristic. Leukocyte and platelet production are normal. About half of the reported cases have been associated with thymoma, usually a noninvasive spindle cell type. However, only 5% to 10% of patients with thymoma have the anemia. Remission of the anemia occurs in about one fourth of the cases following surgical removal of the thymoma. Chronic acquired red blood cell aplasia has also been associated with other conditions, such as drugs, collagen vascular disorders, lymphoproliferative disorders of granular lymphocytes, or other disorders with immunologic aberrations. Most of these anemias appear to be part of a spectrum of autoimmune cytopenias in which the target cells are either erythroid stem cells or normoblasts. In some patients, antibodies that react with these cells have been identified. Corticosteroids and immunosuppressive drugs have been used as therapy, but less than half the patients achieve satisfactory remission (Alter, 1993).

Sideroblastic Anemia

Sideroblastic anemia is characterized by hypochromic, often microcytic, red cells in the blood usually mixed with normochromic cells, so that the appearance is dimorphic (see Fig. 24–24). The serum iron concentration is increased, the TIBC is decreased, and the percent saturation of the iron-binding protein is greatly elevated. The marrow shows markedly increased storage iron, erythroid hyperplasia with evidence of defective hemoglobinization, and increased numbers of sideroblasts. In addition, there are increased numbers of siderotic granules per cell, and granules surround the nucleus (at least two thirds of the circumference) forming ring sideroblasts (see Plate 26–1*E* and *F*). In the latter, iron loading of mitochondria is seen by electron microscopy. These findings are associated with defective synthesis of heme, which may be due to any of several possible enzyme defects (Pasanen, 1986). Occasionally, megaloblast-like changes are seen in the erythroid cells, but changes typical of cobalamin or folate deficiency are not seen in granulocytes unless folate deficiency coexists.

HEREDITARY SIDEROBLASTIC ANEMIAS

Hereditary Sex-Linked Anemia. This condition occurs in males and may not appear until adolescence. It is rare, but a few well-documented family studies exist. In contrast to acquired sideroblastic anemia, the ring sideroblast abnormality is usually found in late, nondividing erythroblasts (Bottomley, 1982).

Inheritance Undetermined. In a few cases, severe sideroblastic anemia has been found in female children but not in family members. The clinical and hematologic features are similar to those described in males with the sex-linked type. The type of inheritance remains unclear in these patients (Bottomley, 1982).

ACQUIRED SIDEROBLASTIC ANEMIAS

Primary (Idiopathic) Sideroblastic Anemia. When other causes of sideroblastic anemia cannot be identified, the term primary or idiopathic is applied. Idiopathic sideroblastic anemia (ISA) is more common, has its onset in later adult life, and is seen in either sex. The dimorphic anemia has both hypochromic-microcytic and macrocytic red blood cells, and the MCV is usually high (see Plate 26–1*I*). At least 40% of erythroblasts (early and late forms) in bone marrow are ring sideroblasts. In addition to the marrow findings described previously, megaloblastic alterations are observed in over 50% of the cases, and they usually remain after therapy with cobalamin and folic acid. Many patients have mild leukopenia or thrombocytopenia, or both.

The etiology of ISA is not understood. A subgroup of patients who respond distinctly but incompletely to pyridoxine therapy (so-called pyridoxine-responsive anemia) appears to have a primary abnormality in δ-aminolevulinic acid (ALA) synthetase itself. The activities of both ALA synthetase and the mitochondrial enzyme heme synthetase are decreased in erythroblasts, leading to impairment of heme synthesis (Pasanen, 1986).

The exact relationship between ISA and hematologic malignancies is not clear. In one study using G6PD isoenzyme analysis of peripheral blood cells from a patient with ISA, all blood cell lines including B and T lymphocytes were shown to be clonal (Prchal, 1978). This suggests that, at least in some cases, ISA is the result of a clonal abnormality of a pluripotential stem cell.

ISA is generally considered to constitute a subgroup of the myelodysplastic syndromes (refractory anemia with ring sideroblasts [RARS]) (Bennett, 1982; see also Chap. 27). About ten percent of patients with ISA develop acute leukemia; in those who have pancytopenia, dysplastic changes involving other cell lines, and (especially) increased blast cells, the probability of evolution into acute leukemia is higher (Jandl, 1987).

SECONDARY (DRUG-INDUCED OR TOXIN-INDUCED) SIDEROBLASTIC ANEMIA. This form of sideroblastic anemia is secondary to some agent that interferes with heme synthesis; recognition is important because hematologic improvement occurs if the agent is removed.

The *antituberculosis drugs* isoniazid, cycloserine, and pyrazinamide cause sideroblastic abnormalities in some patients on long-term therapy.

Lead poisoning is an important member of this group because environmental exposure to lead usually is unrecognized and needs to be detected. Lead interferes with heme synthesis by blocking the enzymes ALA synthetase, ALA dehydrase, and heme synthetase. These blocks are only partial and of different degree; ALA and coproporphyrin are increased in the urine. *Chloramphenicol* also results in ring sideroblast formation, probably by inhibiting mitochondrial protein synthesis.

Ethanol-induced anemia is perhaps the most common of the reversible sideroblastic anemias. Folate deficiency, hypomagnesemia, and hypokalemia are concomitant findings. After withdrawal of alcohol intake, the abnormal sideroblasts usually disappear within a few days.

A small number of patients with a variety of inflammatory or neoplastic diseases such as rheumatoid arthritis, malignant lymphoma and multiple myeloma may also manifest sideroblastic anemia.

Refractory Anemia

There is an ill-defined group of chronic anemias usually occurring in individuals older than 50 years of age. Normocytic or macrocytic anemia, reticulocytopenia, often pancytopenia, and a hypercellular marrow showing erythroid hyperplasia with a variable degree of dyserythropoiesis are present. Often, the patient has been treated with cobalamin, folic acid, and iron without response. The process is usually unremitting and, in a small proportion of cases, develops additional dysplastic changes in marrow cells and increased blast cells and evolves into an acute leukemia. Refractory anemias, therefore, are considered one of the myelodysplastic syndromes (see Chap. 27).

Congenital Dyserythropoietic Anemias

Several forms of apparently hereditary anemias characterized by abnormal erythropoiesis with ineffective erythropoiesis and splenomegaly have been identified. In general, they tend to be more benign than β-thalassemia major, which forms another group of hereditary anemias with ineffective erythropoiesis.

At least three types have thus far been separated on the basis of marrow and serologic findings (Lewis, 1973). Congenital dyserythropoietic anemias (CDA)-I has megaloblastic changes with some binuclearity, internuclear chromatin bridges, and a macrocytic anemia. CDA-II is more common than the others and shows binuclearity and multinuclearity of erythroid precursors with pluripolar mitoses and karyorrhexis. The anemia is normocytic. CDA-II is distinguished from the others because it has a positive acidified serum test (with some, but not all normal sera) and a negative sucrose hemolysis test. It is known as hereditary erythroblastic multinuclearity with positive acidified serum test (HEMPAS). The red blood cells have an antigen not present on normal or PNH cells, and about one third of normal sera contain the corresponding antibody. CDA-III has giant erythroid precursors, with more pronounced multinuclearity and a macrocytic anemia. In contrast to CDA-I and CDA-II, which are autosomal recessive, CDA-III has autosomal dominant inheritance (Jandl, 1987).

Hemolysis—General

Anemias that are due primarily to increased red blood cell destruction are *hemolytic anemias.* A shortened red blood cell survival time, therefore, proves that hemolysis is present; this measurement usually is unnecessary in practice.

Hemolytic anemias may be due to a defect of the red blood

cell itself, an *intrinsic hemolytic anemia:* these types usually are hereditary and are commonly grouped as *membrane, metabolic,* or *hemoglobin* defects. Alternatively, the hemolysis may be due to a factor outside the red blood cell and acting on it, an *extrinsic hemolytic anemia:* these types are almost always acquired. The terms *intravascular hemolysis* and *extravascular hemolysis* refer to the *site* of the destruction of the red blood cell: within the circulating blood or outside it, respectively.

ERYTHROCYTE SURVIVAL STUDIES. A shortened red blood cell survival time defines hemolysis. If the hemolytic process is moderate or severe, the following studies suffice to show that hemolysis is present. If the hemolytic process is mild or obscure, red blood cell survival studies may be necessary.

Radioactive chromium (^{51}Cr) is convenient and widely used. Labeled chromate is added to a blood sample *in vitro* and binds to β-chains of hemoglobin. The chromated red blood cells are injected intravenously, and their disappearance is measured by counting blood, which is sampled every one to two days for 10 to 14 days. Residual activity is an index of the intravascular lifespan of the labeled red cells. Because ^{51}Cr emits γ-rays, external scanning can detect sites of red cell destruction.

The erythrocyte lifespan is usually expressed as the period during which one half of the radioactivity remains in the blood (the $T_{1/2}$ ^{51}Cr; Fig. 26–3). Chromium normally elutes from the red blood cells at a rate of 1% per day. Thus, the half-life of the ^{51}Cr-labeled erythrocytes in normal individuals is 25 to 32 days instead of 60 days. Blood loss, change in hematocrit, and recent blood transfusions significantly complicate the interpretation of survival data; therefore, a steady state is necessary for usable results.

In AHIAs, the slope of red blood cell survival produces a straight line when plotted on semilogarithmic paper (see Fig. 26–3). In other hemolytic anemias, two cell populations may exist. In these situations, the survival curve may be composed of an initial steep slope, followed by a flatter component (Fig. 26–4). This type of curve has been seen in hereditary enzyme-deficiency hemolytic anemias, sickle cell anemia, and PNH (Dacie, 1991).

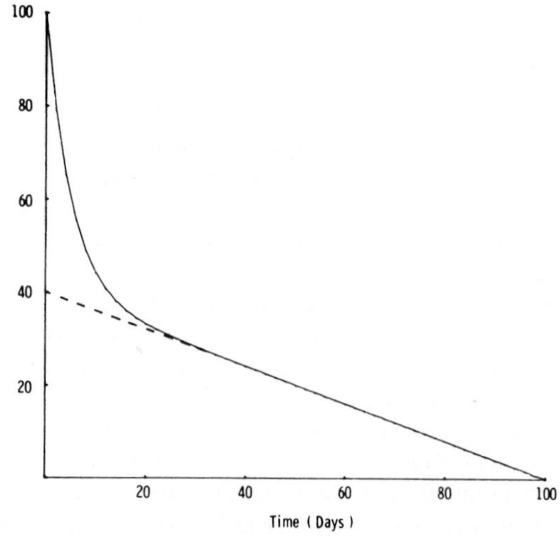

Figure 26–4. Results of ^{51}Cr erythrocyte survival curve in a patient with hemolytic anemia containing two cell populations. The percent survival is on the ordinate. By extrapolating the flatter curve to time 0, it can be estimated that 40% of the cells have a mean lifespan of 100 days. Sixty percent of cells have a mean lifespan of five days. (From Bentley SA: Clin Haematol 1977;6:601.)

Hemoglobin Destruction

Laboratory findings differ, depending on the site of blood destruction, the amount of destroyed blood, and the rate of destruction. If the destruction is *intravascular* and the quantity of destroyed blood is large, free hemoglobin and methemalbumin is present in the plasma (hemoglobinemia and methemalbuminemia). The urine may contain free hemoglobin and also hemosiderin.

Free hemoglobin readily dissociates into $\alpha\beta$ dimers $\alpha_2\beta_2$—$2\alpha\beta$, which are bound to haptoglobin, an α_2-globulin, and the hemoglobin-haptoglobin complex is rapidly removed from the circulation and catabolized by the liver parenchymal cells. This process prevents hemoglobin from appearing in the urine. However, when the plasma hemoglobin level exceeds 50 to 200 mg/dL (8 to 31 μmol/L), which is the capacity of haptoglobin to bind hemoglobin, the free $\alpha\beta$ dimers

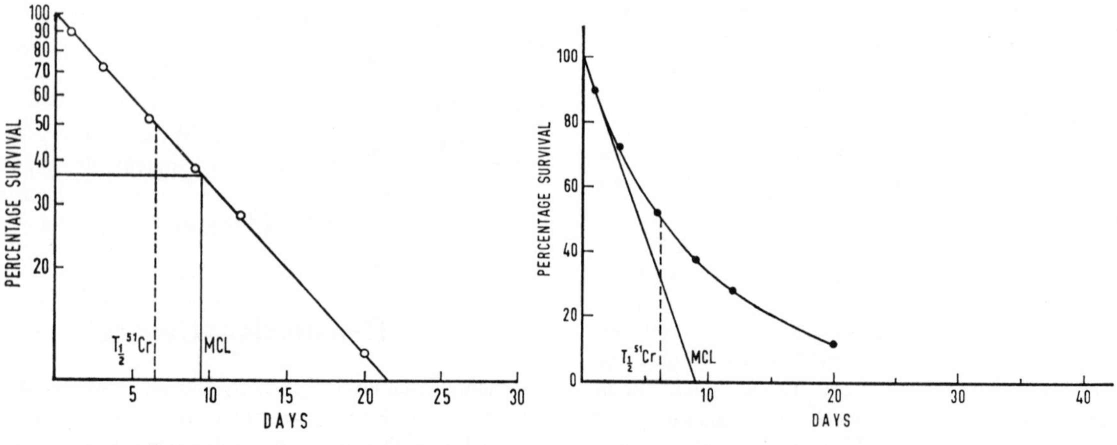

Figure 26–3. Results of ^{51}Cr erythrocyte survival curve in patients with autoimmune hemolytic anemia. The results are plotted on semilogarithmic graph paper. The mean cell lifespan (MCL) was 9 to 10 days and is recorded at a period when 37% of cells were still circulating. The time of 50% survival ($T_{1/2}Cr$) was 6 to 7 days. (From Dacie JV, Lewis SM: Practical Hematology, 5th ed. Edinburgh, Churchill Livingstone, 1975.)

of hemoglobin readily pass through the glomerulus of the kidney. Part of the hemoglobin is then absorbed by the proximal tubular cells, where the hemoglobin iron is converted to hemosiderin. When these tubular cells are later shed into the urine, *hemosiderinuria* results. If the amount of hemoglobin in the tubular lumen exceeds the capacity of the tubular cell to absorb it, it reaches the urine *(hemoglobinuria).* In the process, it may be oxidized to methemoglobin (hemiglobin). Plasma hemoglobin not bound to haptoglobin nor removed by the kidney is oxidized to hemiglobin. The oxidized heme groups (hemin) are bound to *hemopexin,* a β-globulin, and the complex is rapidly cleared by the hepatic parenchymal cells. If hemopexin is depleted, hemin groups bind to albumin, forming methemalbumin. Once hemopexin again becomes available, it removes the hemin groups from albumin for hepatic clearance (Hillman, 1985).

LD is released from red blood cells and is increased in serum in hemolysis, especially in intravascular hemolysis; it is cleared more slowly than is hemoglobin. If the upper reference value is 207 IU/L, the LD in hemolytic anemia may be increased as much as 800 IU/L. In megaloblastic anemia, for reasons that are unclear, the LD is greatly increased to several thousand units. Serum LD is also increased in other forms of cellular injury (see Chap. 13).

The normal plasma hemoglobin level is 0.5 to 5 mg/dL (0.08 to 0.78 μmol/L). A rise to 10 mg/dL imparts to the plasma a yellow to orange color. With further increase, the color becomes pink. Levels up to 25 to 30 mg/dL are common in hemolytic anemia. Higher levels usually indicate intravascular hemolysis and are seen in hemolytic transfusion reactions and in paroxysmal cold and nocturnal hemoglobinurias.

If hemolysis is primarily *extravascular,* no hemoglobinemia, hemoglobinuria, or hemosiderinuria is present. Hemolysis is detected by measuring an increase in one of the products of heme catabolism (see Chap. 25).

1. An increase in CO expired (a research technique), or in the blood carboxyhemoglobin level.
2. An increase in indirect-reacting serum bilirubin; because this is bound to albumin, it will not appear in the urine.
3. An increase in urine urobilinogen or, more consistently, in fecal urobilinogen.

The normal urobilinogen in a 24-hour specimen is 0.5 to 4 mg (0.8 to 6.75 μmol) in urine and 40 to 280 mg (0.068 to 0.470 mmol) in the stool. Following excessive hemolysis, it may increase to 5 to 200 mg in the urine and to 300 to 400 mg in the stool. The examination of feces is more dependable than examination of the urine because it may show an increase when the urine shows none. It may show an increase even when the serum bilirubin concentration is not raised because the normal liver can remove large amounts of (indirectly reacting) bilirubin and of reabsorbed urobilinogen from the blood.

Hemolytic anemia is characterized also by increased red blood cell production. Because of the availability of maximal amounts of iron for hemoglobin formation, red blood cell production reaches the maximal degree possible (about eight times normal) in severe chronic hemolytic anemia, if complicating factors such as folate deficiency do not intervene. If red blood cell destruction exceeds the capacity of the marrow to replace red blood cells at the same rate, hemolytic anemia occurs. With less severe hemolysis, the marrow may be able to produce enough red cells so that anemia does not occur; this is called compensated hemolysis.

BLOOD FILM. The anemia is normocytic or macrocytic. Macrocytosis is due to the presence of immature red blood cells, which are larger than normocytes. Polychromasia usually is prominent; it may be excessively basophilic and normoblasts may be present, both of which indicate a shift of marrow reticulocytes into the blood.

Other red blood cell abnormalities may give a clue to the nature of the hemolytic process. Spherocytes suggest hereditary spherocytosis or autoimmune hemolysis (see Figs. 24–23 and 24–25); schistocytes imply traumatic hemolytic anemia (see Fig. 24–31); sickle cells, target cells, and crystals suggest a hemoglobinopathy (Plate 26–2). When hemolytic anemia is acute, increased numbers and younger forms of leukocytes and platelets often are released from the marrow together with erythrocytes. The result is leukocytosis with a shift to the left and thrombocytosis with both normal and giant platelets.

BONE MARROW. Normoblastic hyperplasia is present and may be striking in degree. Storage iron usually is increased and sideroblasts are normal or increased in number, reflecting the abundance of available iron for hemoglobin synthesis.

Sudden worsening of the degree of anemia may occur in chronic hemolytic anemias and may be due to either of two basic mechanisms. Occasionally, episodes of bone marrow failure (transient arrest of erythropoiesis; see earlier discussion) characterized by erythroid hypoplasia and reticulocytopenia may upset the equilibrium between production and destruction of red blood cells. In most instances, these *aplastic crises* are probably due to parvoviral infection (Young, 1984). On the other hand, an increased rate of red blood cell destruction may occur, associated with infection or other illness that increases splenic size. This condition is not associated with erythroid aplasia, and is called a *hemolytic crisis.*

Hemolysis—Membrane Disorders

HEREDITARY SPHEROCYTOSIS. Hereditary spherocytosis (HS) affects 1 in 5000 of the population, occurring predominantly in those of Northern European ancestry. It is characterized by spherocytic red blood cells that are intrinsically defective, splenomegaly, and familial occurrence (most often autosomal dominant). In about 15% to 30% of cases, however, neither parent is affected. The hemolytic process is variable in severity and is corrected by splenectomy, although the spherocytosis remains.

The laboratory findings are those of a chronic extravascular hemolytic process: evidence of increased pigment catabolism, erythroid hyperplasia, and reticulocytosis. The direct antiglobulin test is negative. The red blood cells characteristically have increased osmotic fragility. On the blood film, spherocytes have a smaller diameter and are more intensely stained than normal cells. They have decreased or absent central pallor; if present, the pallor may be eccentric (Fig. 24–23; Plate 26–2*J*). The MCV is normal and the MCHC is often increased, reflecting a decrease in cell surface.

Osmotic Fragility Test. Red blood cells are suspended in a series of tubes containing hypotonic solutions of NaCl varying from 0.9% to 0.0%, incubated at room temperature for 30 minutes, and centrifuged. The percent hemolysis in the supernatant solutions is measured and plotted for each NaCl concentration. Cells that are more spherical, with a decreased surface/volume ratio, have a limited capacity to expand in hypotonic solutions and lyse at a higher concentration of NaCl than do normal biconcave red blood cells. They are said to have increased osmotic fragility. Conversely, cells that are hypochromic and flatter have a greater capacity to expand in hypotonic solutions, lyse at a lower concentration than do normal cells, and are said to have decreased osmotic fragility (Fig. 26–5).

The osmotic fragility of freshly drawn blood usually is increased in HS, but may be normal in mildly affected patients. In blood that is incubated at 37°C for 24 hours before performing the test, the osmotic fragility is almost always increased (Fig. 26–6).

The increased osmotic fragility of freshly drawn blood is characteristic but not specific; it may occur in acquired spherocytic anemias. A greater difference in median fragility (after incubation from before incubation) occurs in HS cells than in control normal cells; this is an important diagnostic feature in HS.

Autohemolysis Test. Sterile, defibrinated blood is incubated at 37°C for 48 hours (Dacie, 1991). During this time, red blood cells undergo a complex series of changes, lose membrane, and become more spherocytic. In normal blood, without added glucose, the amount of autohemolysis at 48 hours is 0.2% to 2.0%. In normal blood, incubated with added glucose, the amount of autohemolysis is less—0% to 0.9%.

In HS, autohemolysis is virtually always increased; with glucose, the lysis is diminished to a variable extent. Rarely, patients with strong clinical and laboratory evidence for HS have normal incubated osmotic fragility. In these patients, the abnormal autohemolysis test is useful in confirming a diagnosis of HS (Fukagawa, 1979).

The erythrocytes are abnormally permeable to sodium, and there is no defect in energy metabolism, which is, in fact, increased. The increased metabolic activity has been explained as an attempt to compensate for a membrane defect that leaks cations, with degenerative changes and the loss of cell membrane accelerated by the metabolic and physical stress of passage through the spleen (Jandl, 1987).

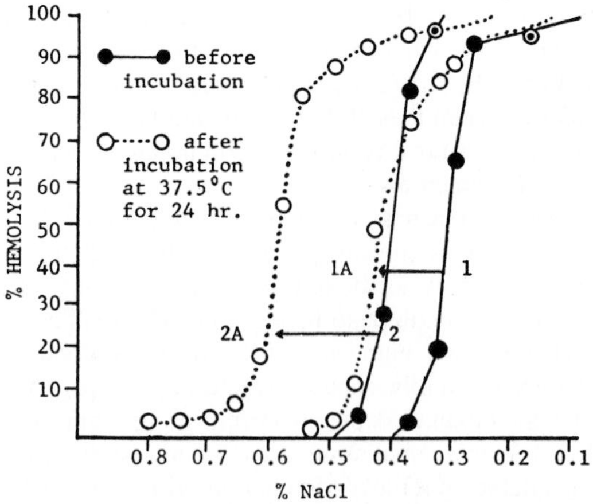

Figure 26–6. The effect of incubation on erythrocyte osmotic fragility. The change in the osmotic fragility curve from "before incubation" to "after incubation" is illustrated for normal blood (1 → 1A) and for blood from a patient with hereditary spherocytosis (2 → 2A). Blood in hereditary spherocytosis characteristically shows a greater increase in fragility with incubation than does normal blood or even blood of acquired spherocytosis (e.g., autoimmune hemolytic anemia).

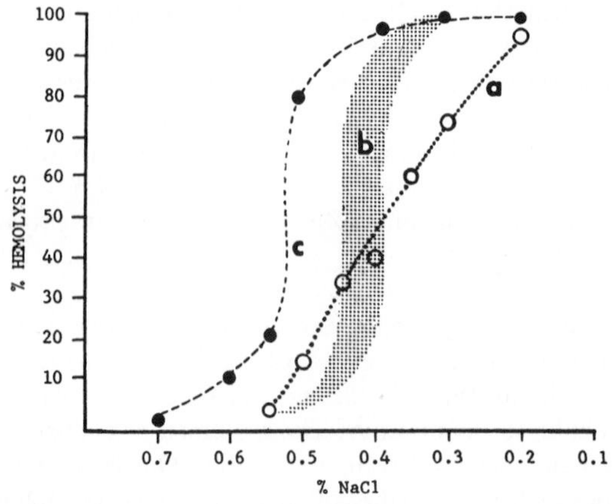

Figure 26–5. Erythrocyte osmotic fragility. *a*, Thalassemia, showing a small fraction of cells with increased fragility (*lower left*) and a larger fraction of cells with decreased fragility (*upper right*). *b*, Normal curves fall in shaded area. *c*, Hereditary spherocytosis, showing increased osmotic fragility.

The genetic defects in HS are heterogeneous but affect the skeletal proteins of the red blood cell membrane. Probably all affected individuals have mutations that lead to a quantitative decrease in spectrin. The loss of surface area in HS is probably related to separation and loss of membrane lipid bilayer from the skeleton. Recent studies suggest that normal spectrin density is required for normal cohesion between the lipid bilayer and membrane skeleton (Mohandas, 1993). The degree of spectrin deficiency as measured by radioimmunoassay appears to correlate with the degree of spherocytosis and the clinical severity (Agre, 1986).

HEREDITARY ELLIPTOCYTOSIS. Hereditary elliptocytosis (HE) is an autosomal dominant condition that probably includes more than one genetic variant. All cases of HE are associated with weakening of the membrane skeleton and defective association of proteins that hold the skeleton together (Becker, 1993). The most common defined abnormality appears to be a defect in spectrin resulting in impaired association of spectrin dimers into spectrin tetramers and spectrin oligomers. (This defect is also found in hereditary pyropoikilocytosis [HPP]). Other abnormalities include a defect in spectrin causing impaired binding of spectrin to ankyrin, a defective band 3 protein, and a deficiency of protein 4.1. Nonhypochromic elliptocytes are abundant in the blood film, numbering over 25% (see Fig. 24–27), whereas in normal individuals, less than 15% of the red blood cells are elliptical. The deformity is increased in sealed, moist preparations.

Most persons with the common form of HE (about 90% of cases) are nonanemic; a minority of this group (perhaps 10% to 20%) have mild hemolysis. In a subgroup of common HE, especially in black families, affected neonates transiently have moderate poikilocytosis, red blood cell fragmentation, and budding, with hemolytic anemia; during the first year of life, hemolysis declines and typical HE emerges (Becker, 1993).

Hemolytic HE accounts for 10% of cases. Mild to moderate hemolytic anemia and splenomegaly are present, with both elliptocytes and spherocytes, and abnormal osmotic fragility and autohemolysis tests.

Southeast Asian ovalocytosis occurs with high frequencies (20% to 30%) in certain populations of the Far East, particularly Malaysia. Hemolysis usually is absent or mild. The erythrocytes are less elongated, and some have the appearance of stomatocytic ovalocytes. This condition is associated with increased resistance to malaria. The underlying defect is related to a mutation in band 3 (Becker, 1993; Mohandas, 1993).

HEREDITARY PYROPOIKILOCYTOSIS. HPP is a rare, moderately severe congenital hemolytic anemia that is characterized by microcytosis, striking micropoikilocytosis and fragmentation, and autosomal recessive inheritance. It occurs primarily in blacks. In contrast to normal red blood cells, which show budding and fragmentation when heated to 49°C, HPP red blood cells fragment at 45° to 46°C. As in some cases of HE, the membrane abnormality involves defective spectrin function. Recent studies suggest that the HPP phenotype is a severe form of HE (Mohandas, 1993).

HEREDITARY STOMATOCYTOSIS (HEREDITARY HYDROCYTOSIS). This is a rare, autosomally transmitted disorder. Heterozygotic individuals have no anemia and 1% to 25% stomatocytes in the blood film. In presumed homozygotic individuals, about one third of the red cells are stomatocytes, and there is a mild to moderate hemolytic anemia. The membrane abnormality results in increased permeability of the membrane to Na^+ and K^+ (and therefore water), resulting in hydrated, macrocytic red blood cells. The MCV may be as high as 150 fL. The osmotic fragility and autohemolysis are increased. Although the exact membrane defect is not known, several reports indicate the absence of a membrane protein located in the band 7 region called stomatin (Becker, 1993).

PAROXYSMAL NOCTURNAL HEMOGLOBINURIA. PNH is an acquired stem cell disorder characterized by the production of abnormal erythrocytes, granulocytes, and platelets (Beutler, 1995; Rosse, 1993). The red blood cell defect renders them more susceptible to complement-mediated intravascular lysis. Three types of erythrocytes have been described according to their in vitro sensitivity: type I with normal sensitivity, type II with medium sensitivity (3 to 5 times the normal level), and type III with extreme sensitivity (15 to 25 times the normal level). Several complement defense proteins are decreased or absent in PNH. These proteins include decay accelerating factor (DAF, CD55), membrane inhibitor of reactive lysis (MIRL, CD59), and C8 binding protein (homologous restriction factor). DAF is a glycoprotein which antagonizes the convertase complexes of complement. MIRL is a protein that controls the membrane attack complex, C5b-9. Other proteins that are deficient in PNH include CD58 (leukocyte function antigen 3), CD14 (endotoxin-binding protein receptor), CD24 and CD16 (Fcγ receptor). Membrane-associated enzymes such as acetyl cholinesterase and leukocyte alkaline phosphatase may be deficient as well. Recent work indicates that deficient proteins and enzymes are attached to the cell membrane by a common glycolipid anchor called glycosylphosphatidyl inositol (GPI). Deficiency of GPI results in secondary deficiency of the attached proteins. Therefore, PNH can be redefined as partial or complete lack of GPI-linked proteins on a population of cells of the hematopoietic system (Rosse, 1993).

Clinically, PNH usually occurs in young adults and is characterized by chronic intravascular hemolysis with or without obvious hemoglobinuria. Hemosiderinuria is, however, almost constantly present. Typical nocturnal or sleep-related hemoglobinuria is present in less than 25% of patients. Bouts of hemolysis could be initiated by infection, surgery, whole blood transfusion, injection of contrast dyes, and even intense exercise.

The blood usually shows a normocytic anemia with a reticulocytosis that is often less than expected for the degree of anemia. Hypochromic microcytic anemia is not uncommon, however, and is due to loss of iron in the urine. Neutropenia occurs in three fifths and thrombocytopenia in two thirds of patients at some time during the course of disease, so that pancytopenia is common. The direct antiglobulin test usually is negative.

The marrow is usually hypercellular with normoblastic hyperplasia, but it may be hypocellular. In some patients, marrow failure may occur during the course of PNH; in others, aplastic anemia is the initial diagnosis, with signs of PNH later manifesting themselves. An abnormal line of cells probably develops in an aplastic or regenerating marrow (Lewis, 1967).

Thrombotic complications are common. The disease may undergo partial remissions and exacerbations. In over half of patients, both the proportion of abnormal cells and the clinical severity decrease with time.

Sucrose Hemolysis Test. This test should be performed whenever the diagnosis of PNH is considered, also in hypoplastic anemias, and in any hemolytic anemia of obscure origin (Hartmann, 1970). The principle of the test is that sucrose provides a medium of low ionic strength that promotes the binding of complement to the red blood cells. In PNH, a proportion of the red blood cells is abnormally sensitive to complement-mediated lysis.

The patient's washed red blood cells are mixed with ABO-compatible normal serum (fresh or properly stored) and isotonic (10%) sucrose. The tube is incubated at room temperature for 30 minutes and then centrifuged, and the percent hemolysis in the supernatant is determined. Two control tubes eliminate the serum, and the cells should be negative. Less than 5% hemolysis in the test specimen is negative, 5% to 10% is suspicious, and over 10% is positive and virtually diagnostic for PNH. Suspicious results can be seen in some other hematologic diseases, especially megaloblastic anemia and AHIA. False-negative results occur if the serum lacks complement activity.

Acidified Serum Test (Ham Test). Definitive diagnosis of PNH depends on a positive acidified serum test (Dacie, 1991; Ham, 1939). In acidifed serum, complement is activated by the alternate pathway, binds to red blood cells, and lyses the abnormal PNH cells that are unusually susceptible to complement. The patient's washed red blood cells are mixed with ABO-compatible normal serum (fresh or properly stored) and acid; after an hour's incubation at 37°C, the PNH cells are lysed, as indicated in Table 26–3. The patient's own serum may or may not result in lysis, de-

4

Table 26–3. ACIDIFIED SERUM TEST

	1	2	3	4	5	6	7
Fresh normal serum	0.5	0.5			0.5	0.5	
Patient's serum			0.5				
Heat-inactivated normal serum				0.5			0.5
0.2 N HCl		0.05	0.05	0.05		0.05	0.05
50% patient's red cells	0.05	0.05	0.05	0.05			
50% normal red cells					0.05	0.05	0.05
Pattern of lysis in positive test	Trace	+++	+	−	−	−	−

Modified from Dacie JV, Lewis SM: Practical Haematology, 4th ed. New York, Grune & Stratton, 1968.

pending on residual complement, and the other tubes provide controls.

In PNH, usually 10% to 50% of the cells are lysed. If lysis also occurs with heat-inactivated serum, the test is not positive, because spherocytic or antibody-sensitized cells may be responsible.

A positive acidified serum test occurs in congenital dyserythropoietic anemia, type II (CDA-II) or HEM-PAS (see earlier discussion). In this situation, however, lysis does not occur with the patient's own serum, and only with about 30% of normal sera. Also, the sucrose hemolysis test is negative in CDA-II. The hemolysis is probably due to a naturally occurring antibody directed against an as yet undefined antigen.

Flow cytometry using immunofluorescent staining of red blood cells with a monoclonal antibody against deficient proteins such as CD55, 58, and 59 may be useful in the diagnosis and study of PNH (Hillmen, 1992).

Hemolysis—Hemoglobin Disorders

In 1949, Pauling and his associates described an electrophoretically abnormal hemoglobin type in patients with sickle cell anemia. Their studies initiated the concept of molecular disease—that is, a molecular variation in a single protein can be responsible for the entire spectrum of clinical, laboratory, and pathologic manifestations that characterize a disease. The subsequent finding that the abnormality was due to the substitution of a single amino acid in a polypeptide chain of hemoglobin inaugurated the field of biochemical genetics.

At present, nearly 500 hemoglobin variants with known structure have been described. The great majority of these variants have been characterized as a single amino acid substitution in one of the polypeptide chains (α, β, γ or δ), which can be explained by a single base substitution in the corresponding triplet codon of the gene. In a small number of abnormal hemoglobins, the polypeptide chain is abnormally long or short as a result of termination errors, frame-shift mutations, crossover in phase, deletion of codons, or fused or hybrid chains (Bunn, 1986).

Normal Hemoglobins

The heme group is identical in all variants of human hemoglobin. The protein part of the molecule (globin) consists of four polypeptide chains. At least three distinct hemoglobin types are found postnatally in normal individuals, and the structure of each has been determined.

Hb A ($\alpha_2\beta_2$). Hemoglobin A is the major normal adult hemoglobin. The polypeptide chains of the globin part of the molecules are of two types: two identical α-chains, each with 141 amino acids; and two identical β-chains, with 146 amino acids each. Each chain is linked with one heme group. The molecule is ellipsoidal, with the four heme groups at the surface of the molecule, where they function by combining reversibly with oxygen (see Fig. 25–5).

Hb F ($\alpha_2\gamma_2$). Hemoglobin F is the major hemoglobin of the fetus and the newborn infant. The increased affinity for oxygen of fetal blood over adult blood is not due to the hemoglobin itself but probably to the environment in the red blood cell. The two α-chains are identical to those of Hb A; and two γ-chains, with 146 amino acid residues, differ from β-chains. In normal individuals, Hb F has two types of γ-chains, which differ in one amino acid, having either alanine (Aγ) or glycine (Gγ) at position 136. The ratio of Gγ to Aγ chains changes from 3:1 at birth to 2:3 by age 12 months (Weatherall, 1981).

During fetal life, Hb F predominates, because α-chain production and γ-chain production are high (Fig. 26–7). β-chain production begins before the twentieth week of prenatal life, so that Hb A is 10% of the total between 20 and 35 weeks and 15% to 40% at the time of birth. After birth, smaller amounts of Hb F are produced; by 6 months Hb F usually is less than 8% and by 12 months it is less than 5% in about 90% of infants. Between 12 and 24 months of age, Hb F usually is less than 3%, but varies from 3% to 10% in about 20% of infants. After two years of age, Hb F is normally less than 2% in children. Only traces of Hb F ($<$ 1.0%) are found in adults. During fetal life, all red blood cells produce and contain Hb F, whereas in adults, only 0.2% to 7% do so (Weatherall, 1981). The Hb F–containing cells (F cells) may increase in number when reactivation of Hb F synthesis occurs in normal pregnancy and in some disorders of erythropoiesis. The total Hb F rarely exceeds 20% in these conditions. In newborns, approximately 10% of total hemoglobin is a negatively charged variant of Hb F, designated Hb F_1, owing to acetylation of the N terminal ends of the γ-chains. Hb F_1 is found in all stages of fetal development and in patients with elevated Hb F levels. Both Gγ and Aγ chains are equally acetylated (Bunn, 1986).

Hb A2 ($\alpha_2\delta_2$). Hemoglobin A_2 accounts for 1.5% to 3.5% of normal adult hemoglobin. Its two α-chains are the same as in Hb A and Hb F; its two δ-chains differ from β-chains in only eight of their 146 amino acids.

δ-chain synthesis begins late in fetal life and occurs only in normoblasts (not reticulocytes). The level of Hb A_2 gradually increases during the first year of life, at which time the adult level is reached. Hb A_2 is increased in some β-thalassemias. Iron deficiency causes decreased Hb A_2 synthesis.

EMBRYONIC HEMOGLOBINS. The zeta (ζ) chain is the

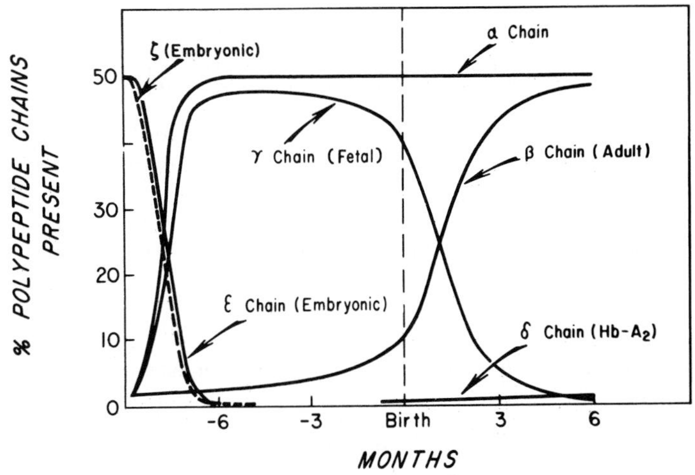

Figure 26–7. Relative proportions of polypeptide chains of hemoglobin present during fetal and neonatal life. (From Bunn HF, Forget BG, Ranney HM: Human Hemoglobins. Philadelphia, W.B. Saunders Company, 1977.)

embryonic analogue of the α-chain and may combine with epsilon (ϵ) chains to form Hb Gower-1 ($\zeta_2\epsilon_2$) or with γ-chains to form Hb Portland-1 ($\zeta_2\gamma_2$). The ϵ-chain is the embryonic counterpart of the γ-, β-, and δ-chains and combines with α-chains to form Hb Gower-2 ($\alpha_2\epsilon_2$). Hb Gower-1, Hb Portland-1, and Hb Gower-2 are the embryonic hemoglobins and are found in normal human embryos and fetuses with a gestational age of less than three months (see Figs. 26–7 and 26–8).

Genetics. Analysis of pedigrees has shown that the α and non-α-genes are on different chromosomes, and that two functioning α-genes are on a haploid chromosome (balanced by only one β-gene). DNA technology, cloning of specific human DNA fragments, and restriction endonuclease mapping have elucidated detailed globin gene arrangements (Bunn, 1986). Two ζ-genes and the two α-genes are on chromosome 16. Genes for the ϵ-chain, the two γ-chains, the δ- and β-chains are located on chromosome 11 (Fig. 26–9). As in other genes, the coding sequences (exons) of the globin genes are interrupted by noncoding DNA sequences (introns). Introns are transcribed into RNA but are removed from the premessenger RNA by precise splicing reactions before the resultant mRNA is translated into protein.

GLYCOSYLATED HEMOGLOBINS. Approximately 5% of Hb A undergoes post-translational glycosylation, resulting in linkage of sugars to serine, asparagine, and hydroxylysine residues. The glycosylated hemoglobins have been designated Hb A_{Ia} (<1%), Hb A_{Ib} (<2%), and Hb A_{Ic} (3%). Glycosylation of hemoglobin increases linearly over the 120-day lifespan of the red blood cell. Hb A_{Ic} is elevated twofold to threefold in patients with diabetes mellitus. The measurement of Hb A_{Ic} has been used as an index of metabolic con-

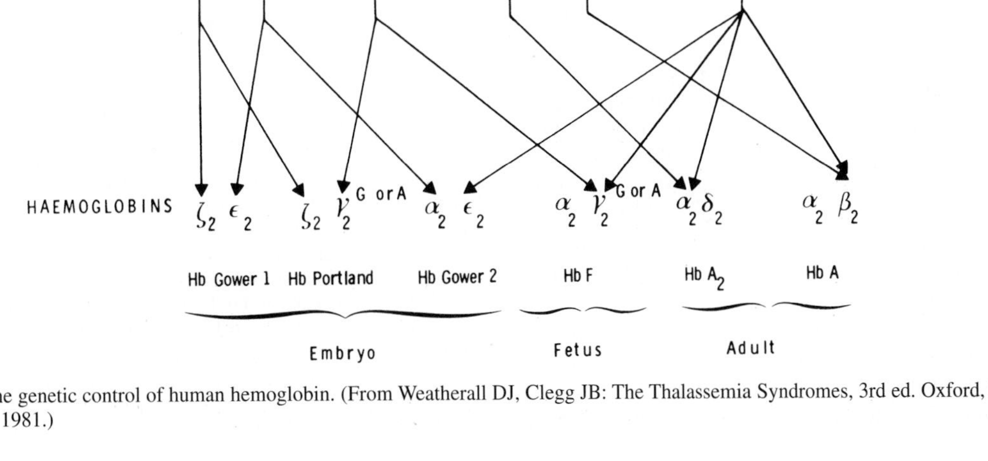

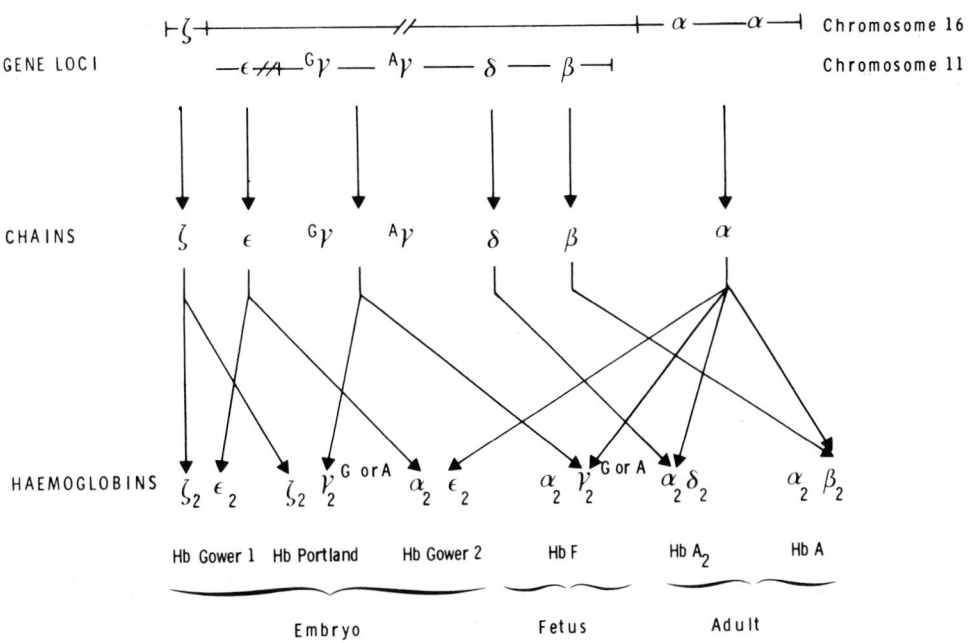

Figure 26–8. The genetic control of human hemoglobin. (From Weatherall DJ, Clegg JB: The Thalassemia Syndromes, 3rd ed. Oxford, Blackwell Scientific Publications, 1981.)

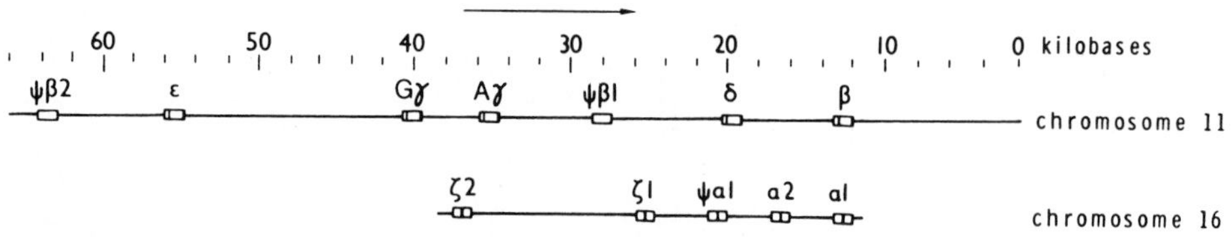

Figure 26–9. The physical arrangement of globin genes on chromosomes 11 and 16. Chromosome 11 has five functional β-like globin genes and two β-like nonfunctional pseudogenes ($\psi\beta_2$ and $\psi\beta_1$). Chromosome 16 has four functional α-like genes and one non-functional α pseudogene ($\psi\alpha_1$). The arrow indicates the direction of transcription of the two clusters of globin genes. (From Weatherall DJ, Clegg JB: The Thalassaemia Syndromes, 3rd ed. Oxford, Blackwell Scientific Publications, 1981.)

trol of diabetes during the preceding two to three months (Bunn, 1994).

Abnormal Hemoglobins and Nomenclature

Normal adult hemoglobin is designated Hb A; fetal hemoglobin, Hb F; that found in sickle cell anemia, Hb S; and those associated with methemoglobinemia, Hb M. Other hemoglobins were assigned letters of the alphabet, then geographic names, or both—usually to distinguish different Hbs with similar characteristics, such as electrophoretic mobilities. There are several variants of Hb D, G, J, and M, for example.

The polypeptide chain on which the abnormality is present can be indicated as a superscript—such as Hb S = $\alpha_2{}^A\beta_2{}^S$, Hb I = $\alpha_2{}^I\beta_2{}^A$. The common designation is the number of the amino acid residue in the superscript along with the substituted amino acid—such as Hb S = $\alpha_2\beta_2{}^{6Val}$; Hb I = $\alpha_2{}^{16Asp}\beta_2$ (Fig. 26–10). Amino acid substitutions in some of the known hemoglobin variants are listed and classified by functional characteristics in Table 26–4.

HEMOGLOBIN ELECTROPHORESIS. Hemoglobin molecules in an alkaline solution have a net negative charge and move toward the anode in an electrophoretic system. Those with an electrophoretic mobility greater than that of Hb A at pH 8.6 are known as the fast hemoglobins; these include Hb Bart's and the two fastest, Hb H and Hb I. Hb C is the slowest of the common hemoglobins. A few in order of increasing mobility are Hbs A_2, E = O = C, G = D = S, F, A, K, J, Bart's, N = I, H (Fig. 26–11).

Different media and different buffers vary in efficiency of separation. None is both practical and adequate for *all* separations and for screening purposes.

A practical method for routine hemoglobin electrophoresis is cellulose acetate at alkaline pH (Briere, 1965). It is rapid and reproducible and separates hemoglobins S, F, C, A, and A_2. Quantification of the major bands is easily accomplished. If an S band is present, a solubility test or sickling test must be performed. Citrate agar electrophoresis at an acid pH (Milner, 1975) provides ready separation of hemoglobins that migrate together on cellulose acetate: S from D and G, and C from E and O (see Fig. 26–11; Schmidt, 1973). When these two methods are combined with electrophoresis of globin chains in 6M urea, most hemoglobin variants can be identified presumptively. As an alternative, isoelectric focusing on polyacrylamide gel provides sharp separation of most hemoglobin variants (Bunn, 1986).

Final characterization of abnormal hemoglobins is beyond the scope of the clinical laboratory. It consists of purification of the abnormal hemoglobin with starch-block electrophoresis, hybridization experiments to determine whether the abnormality lies in the α- or β-chain, and so-called fingerprinting. In the latter procedure, the polypeptide chains are split by enzymatic digestion into peptides that are separated by performing horizontal paper electrophoresis and vertical chromatography in sequence. This peptide map, or fingerprint, is compared with that prepared from normal hemoglobin, and the peptide in which the abnormality occurs can be located. The abnormal peptide is then eluted and its amino acid content determined. Amino acid sequencing has been automated. With the use of molecular genetic techniques, determining the primary structure or amino acid sequence of

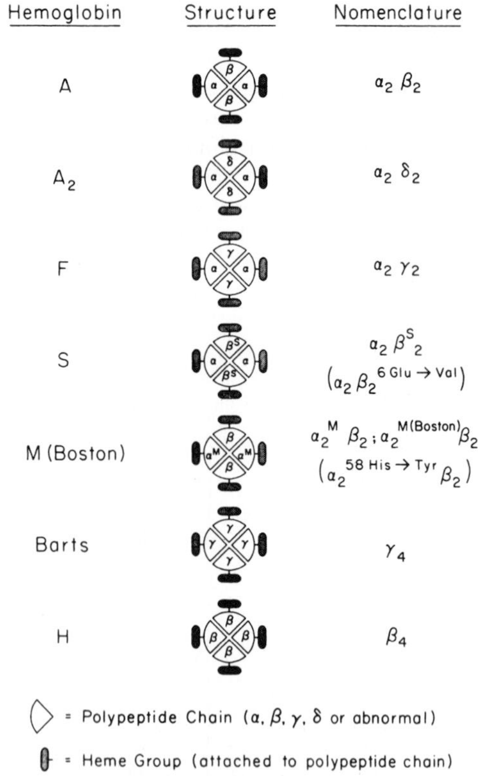

Figure 26–10. Configuration and nomenclature of normal and abnormal hemoglobins. Each triangle represents one folded polypeptide chain; the bar attached to its external surface represents a heme group. The drawing is schematic. Each heme group is near the surface of the molecule, located in a pocket formed by folds of its polypeptide chain and attached to that chain by an imidazole group. In most hemoglobinopathies (e.g., Hb S, Hb G Philadelphia), the affected polypeptide chains differ from normal in only one amino acid. In Hb S, the designation could also be written as $\alpha_2\beta_2{}^{6Val}$, and in Hb G Philadelphia, $\alpha_2{}^{68Lys}\beta_2$, indicating the site of the substitution and the amino acid that replaces the one usually present. (After Krieg, 1967.)

Table 26–4. FUNCTIONAL CLASSIFICATION OF HEMOGLOBIN VARIANTS

I. Homozygous: Hemoglobin polymorphisms: the variants that are most common

Hb S	$\alpha_2\beta_2^{6Val}$	Severe hemolytic anemia; sickling
Hb C	$\alpha_2\beta_2^{6Lys}$	Mild hemolytic anemia
Hb D Punjab	$\alpha_2\beta_2^{121Gln}$	No anemia
Hb E	$\alpha_2\beta_2^{26Lys}$	Mild microcytic anemia

II. Heterozygous: Hemoglobin variants causing functional aberrations or hemolytic anemia in the heterozygous state

A. Hemoglobins associated with methemoglobinemia and cyanosis

1. Hb M Boston	$\alpha_2^{58Tyr}\beta_2$	4. Hb M Milwaukee	$\alpha_2\beta_2^{67Glu}$	7. Hb FM Fort Ripley	$\alpha_2\gamma_2^{92Tyr}$
2. Hb M Iwate	$\alpha_2^{87Tyr}\beta_2$	5. Hb M Hyde Park	$\alpha_2\beta_2^{92Tyr}$		
3. Hb M Saskatoon	$\alpha_2\beta_2^{63Tyr}$	6. Hb FM Osaka	$\alpha_2\gamma_2^{63Tyr}$		

B. Hemoglobins associated with altered oxygen affinity

1. Increased affinity and polycythemia
   - a. Hb Chesapeake $\alpha_2^{92Leu}\beta_2$
   - b. Hb J Capetown $\alpha_2^{92Gln}\beta_2$
   - c. Hb Malmo $\alpha_2\beta_2^{97Gln}$
   - d. Hb Yakima $\alpha_2\beta_2^{99His}$
   - e. Hb Kempsey $\alpha_2\beta_2^{99Asn}$
   - f. Hb Y psi (Ypsilanti) $\alpha_2\beta_2^{99Tyr}$
   - g. Hb Hiroshima $\alpha_2\beta_2^{146Asp}$
   - h. Hb Rainier $\alpha_2\beta_2^{145Cys}$
   - i. Hb Bethesda $\alpha_2\beta_2^{145His}$
2. Decreased affinity—may have mild anemia or cyanosis
   - a. Hb Kansas $\alpha_2\beta_2^{102Thr}$
   - b. Hb Titusville $\alpha_2^{94Asn}\beta_2$
   - c. Hb Providence $\alpha_2\beta_2^{82Asn}$
   - d. Hb Agenogi $\alpha_2\beta_2^{90Lys}$
   - e. Hb Beth Israel $\alpha_2\beta_2^{102Ser}$
   - f. Hb Yoshizuka $\alpha_2\beta_2^{108Asp}$

C. Unstable hemoglobins

1. Hb may precipitate as Heinz bodies after splenectomy; "congenital Heinz body anemia"
   - a. Severe hemolysis; no improvement after splenectomy
     - Hb Bibba $\alpha_2^{136Pro}\beta_2$
     - Hb Hammersmith $\alpha_2\beta_2^{42Ser}$
     - Hb Bristol $\alpha_2\beta_2^{67Asp}$
     - Hb Olmsted $\alpha_2\beta_2^{141Arg}$
   - b. Severe hemolysis; improvement after splenectomy
     - Hb Torino $\alpha_2^{43Val}\beta_2$
     - Hb Ann Arbor $\alpha_2^{80Arg}\beta_2$
     - Hb Genova $\alpha_2\beta_2^{28Pro}$
     - Hb Shepherd's Bush $\alpha_2\beta_2^{74Asp}$
     - Hb Koln $\alpha_2\beta_2^{98Met}$
     - Hb Wein $\alpha_2\beta_2^{130Asp}$
   - c. Mild hemolysis; intermittent exacerbations
     - Hb L-Ferrara $\alpha_2^{47Gly}\beta_2$
     - Hb Hasharon $\alpha_2^{47His}\beta_2$
     - Hb Leiden $\alpha_2\beta_2^{6or7}$ (Glu deleted)
     - Hb Freiburg $\alpha_2\beta^{23}$ (Val deleted)
     - Hb Seattle $\alpha_2\beta_2^{70Asp}$
     - Hb Louisville $\alpha_2\beta_2^{42Leu}$
     - Hb Zurich $\alpha_2\beta_2^{63Arg}$
     - Hb Gun Hill $\alpha_2\beta^{91-97}$ (5 a. a. deleted)
   - d. No disease
     - Hb Etobicoke $\alpha_2^{84Arg}\beta_2$
     - Hb Dakar $\alpha_2^{112Gln}\beta_2$
     - Hb Sogn $\alpha_2\beta_2^{14Arg}$
     - Hb Tacoma $\alpha_2\beta_2^{30Ser}$
2. Tetramers of normal chains; appear in thalassemias
   - Hb Bart's γ_4
   - HbH β_4
   - Hb α_4

Modified, in part, from Winslow RM, Anderson WF: The hemoglobinopathies. *In* Stanbury JB, Wyngaarden JB, Fredrickson DS, Goldstein JL, Brown MS (eds.): The Metabolic Basis of Inherited Disease, 5th ed. New York, McGraw-Hill, 1983, pp 2281–2317.

4

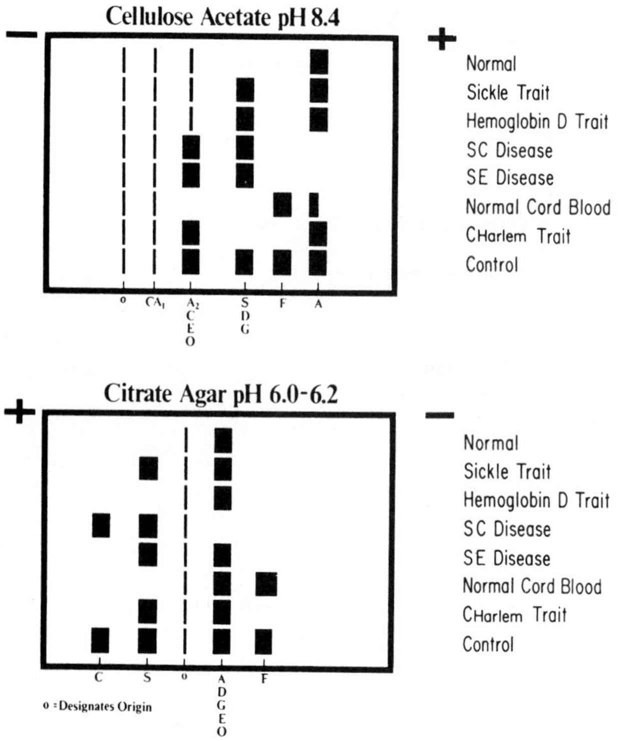

Figure 26–11. Hemoglobin electrophoresis. Comparison of various hemoglobin samples on cellulose acetate and citrate agar, showing relative mobilities. The control is a composite sample. The relative amounts of hemoglobin are not necessarily proportional to the size of the band; for example, in sickle trait (Hb AS), Hb A always exceeds Hb S in amount. (From Schmidt, 1976.)

globin chains can now be performed by determining the base sequence of the mRNA or DNA for the globin chains. This type of analysis is less laborious than classic amino acid sequencing and just as reliable (Bunn, 1986). Discussion of techniques for the identification of hemoglobins is provided by Huisman (1977, 1986).

Hb A_2 QUANTITATION. Estimating Hb A_2 visually or by densitometry from cellulose acetate membranes is unreliable (Schmidt, 1975). Satisfactory methods that can be readily performed in a clinical laboratory are cellulose acetate electrophoresis followed by elution of the Hb A_2 band and measuring this spectrophotometrically as a percentage of the total (Marengo-Rowe, 1965). More convenient for large numbers of samples is microchromatography using DEAE-cellulose and inexpensive glassware (Efremov, 1974; Huisman, 1975).

Reference intervals for Hb A_2 are 1.5% to 3.5% of total hemoglobin.

Hb A_2 estimation is useful in identifying individuals with β-thalassemia trait, in whom it is elevated up to 7%. Hb A_2 values from normal individuals do not overlap with those of individuals with β-thalassemia trait when performed by microchromatography; however, there is some overlap with the cellulose acetate electrophoresis method (Huisman, 1986). Hb A_2 is also occasionally increased in megaloblastic anemia, and it may be decreased in iron deficiency anemia. If an individual with β-thalassemia trait has concomitant severe iron deficiency, the usually elevated Hb A_2 may be in the normal range; in this instance, retesting should be performed after the iron deficiency is corrected.

ALKALI DENATURATION TEST FOR Hb F. Fetal hemoglobin resists alkali denaturation; adult hemoglobin does not (Singer, 1951). A hemolysate is alkalinized and then neutralized, and the denatured adult hemoglobin is precipitated by ammonium sulfate. A filtrate then contains only alkali-resistant hemoglobin, which is measured and expressed as a percentage of the total.

The modification of Betke (1959) gives reference intervals of 0.2% to 1.0% for adults.

Elevated Hb F is found in some hemoglobinopathies, in β-thalassemias, and in hereditary persistence of fetal hemoglobin (HPFH).

In certain acquired hematopoietic disorders, the Hb F level may be elevated. These include megaloblastic anemia, myelofibrosis, aplastic anemia, leukemias, erythroleukemia, refractory anemias, and PNH. It is also increased in pregnancy.

ACID ELUTION SLIDE TEST FOR Hb F. The modification of the original method of Kleihauer and Betke by Shepard (1962) is useful for analyzing the distribution of Hb F among red blood cells. Hemoglobins other than Hb F are eluted from the red blood cells on an air-dried blood film by a citric acid–phosphate buffer (pH 3.3). Only Hb F remains in the fixed red blood cells, and the distribution can be determined after staining.

In normal adults, almost all red blood cells appear as ghosts; 1% to 5% of red blood cells contain residual hemoglobin (Hb F). If increased Hb F is due to most types of HPFH, the Hb F is distributed evenly among red blood cells. If the cause is thalassemia or hemoglobinopathy, the distribution of the Hb F is heterogeneous among red blood cells.

Abnormal Hemoglobin Syndromes

In *hemoglobinopathies,* the structure of one of the four types of polypeptide chains formed is abnormal; this is usually due to substitution of a single amino acid. A large number of hemoglobin variants that do not cause disease have been discovered in surveys. In clinically significant disease, either the β-chain or the α-chain is affected. Involvement of the γ-chain and δ-chain occurs, but because of the small amount of hemoglobin involved, they are less often detected and rarely of any clinical significance. Depending on the type of amino acid and the site involved, the hemoglobin may be functionally abnormal and have altered chemical and physical properties.

In *thalassemias,* globin chains, usually of normal structure, are produced at a decreased rate. β-Thalassemia refers to decreased production of β-chains; therefore, HbF $(\alpha_2\gamma_2)$ or HbA_2 $(\alpha_2\delta_2)$ is often increased with respect to Hb A $(\alpha_2\beta_2)$. α-Thalassemia refers to decreased production of α-chains: Hb A $(\alpha_2\beta_2)$, Hb A_2 $(\alpha_2\delta_2)$ and Hb F $(\alpha_2\gamma_2)$ are decreased proportionally.

In *homozygous β-hemoglobinopathies,* both allelic genes for the abnormal β-chains are present, so that no normal β-chains (hence, no Hb A) are produced. Examples are sickle cell disease (Hb SS) and hemoglobin C disease (Hb CC). Because α-, γ-, and δ-genes (and chain production) are normal, the Hb F and Hb A_2 formed are structurally normal, although they may be increased in amount.

Homozygous α-hemoglobinopathies have not been described.

In *heterozygous β-hemoglobinopathies,* the abnormal hemoglobin is present in addition to Hb A; Hb F and Hb A_2 are structurally normal. Examples are sickle cell trait (Hb AS) and hemoglobin C trait (Hb AC). The normal Hb A quantitatively exceeds the abnormal hemoglobin present because of slower production of abnormal β-chains than of normal β-chains, selective early destruction of the red cells with higher concentrations of the abnormal hemoglobin, or selective removal of the abnormal hemoglobin from the cell.

In *heterozygous α-hemoglobinopathies,* the abnormality in the α-chain affects all three hemoglobin types. Therefore, six different hemoglobin types are found—the three normal hemoglobins and the three abnormal forms. Examples are Hb D Baltimore, Hb Ann Arbor, and Hb M Boston.

Combinations of abnormalities exist. *Double heterozygotes for two β-chain abnormalities* produce two different abnormal β-chains; therefore, there are two abnormal hemoglobins and no hemoglobin A. An example of this is Hb SC disease. Double heterozygotes for β- and δ-chain abnormalities and for α- and β-chain abnormalities are rare but have provided important information. The latter have four major hemoglobin types on electrophoresis: $\alpha_2^A\beta_2^A$; $\alpha_2^X\beta_2^A$; $\alpha_2^A\beta_2^Y$; and $\alpha_2^X\beta_2^Y$.

Double heterozygotes for β-hemoglobinopathy and β-thalassemia are well known. Here, the quantity of abnormal hemoglobin exceeds the normal hemoglobin, in contrast to the heterozygous β-hemoglobinopathies, in which the reverse is true. Examples are Hb S thalassemia and Hb E thalassemia.

β-HEMOGLOBINOPATHIES

Hemoglobins S, C, D, and E are believed to be polymorphisms because their frequency is greater than can be explained by mutation alone (Lehmann, 1977). They occur in homozygous as well as heterozygous form and involve the β-chain.

SICKLE CELL DISEASE. Homozygous Hb S disease is a serious chronic hemolytic anemia, first manifested in early childhood and often fatal before the age of 30 years. With modern medical care, however, many patients live longer. Hemoglobin S is found almost exclusively in the black population; 0.1% to 0.2% of the blacks born in the United States have sickle cell anemia (Schneider, 1976).

In hemoglobin S, the glutamic acid in the sixth position on the β-chain is replaced by valine. This substitution is on the surface of the molecule and changes its charge and, hence, its electrophoretic mobility. Hemoglobin S is freely soluble when fully oxygenated; when oxygen is removed from Hb S, polymerization of the abnormal hemoglobin occurs, forming tactoids (fluid crystals) that are rigid and deform the cell into the shape that gave the cell its name. In homozygous Hb S disease, sickling occurs at physiologic oxygen tensions and the rigidity of the red cells is responsible for the hemolysis as well as for most of the complications. These irreversibly sickled cells result from membrane reorganization during repeated episodes of sickling and unsickling, in addition to cell dehydration, which markedly reduces cellular deformability (Mohandas, 1993). The rigid cells are more vulnerable to trauma and are readily trapped by the reticuloendothelial system, especially the spleen, accounting for the hemolysis. As a result of the hemolysis, severe continued marrow hyperplasia during childhood produces bone changes: expansion of the marrow space, thinning of the cortex, and radial striations seen in the skull on x-ray study. Leg ulcers are common.

Complications. In early childhood, bilateral painful swelling of the dorsa of the hands or feet occurs as a result of sickling and capillary stasis; this is known as the *hand-foot syndrome* or sickle cell dactylitis. It lasts about two weeks; is accompanied by changes of periostitis, as observed by x-ray study; and does not occur after the age of four years.

The spleen is central to three complications: A *sequestration crisis* refers to sudden pooling of blood and rapid enlargement of the spleen, resulting in hypovolemic shock. This may occur in early childhood, when splenomegaly is present. *Functional asplenia* (Pearson, 1969) consists of inadequate antibody responses under some conditions and an impaired ability of the reticuloendothelial system to clear bacteria and particulate material from the blood, probably owing to reticuloendothelial blockade. This may partly explain the increased risk of infection in children with the disease. Salmonellal and pneumococcal infections are unusually prevalent in children with sickle cell anemia. Vaso-occlusive episodes result in progressive infarction, fibrosis, and contraction of the spleen, so-called *autosplenectomy.* Although splenomegaly is present in childhood, a small fibrotic remnant is the rule in the adult.

From early childhood, patients cannot produce a concentrated urine, apparently as a result of anoxic damage in the medullae of the kidneys. Hematuria as a result of papillary necrosis is common.

Vaso-occlusive crises are debilitating episodes of abdominal and bone or joint pain, accompanied by fever, which are probably due to plugging of small blood vessels by masses of sickled cells. Bone necrosis occurs and may be a focus for salmonellal osteomyelitis. Aseptic necrosis of the femoral head is occasionally a complication. The various complications that result from recurring vaso-occlusive crises involve many systems (Diggs, 1965).

Aplastic crises can occasionally afflict any patient with chronic hemolytic anemia. A temporary failure of red blood cell production that would not be noticed in a person with a normal red blood cell lifespan will cause a serious fall in hemoglobin concentration in hemolytic anemia. This may be a result of infection, exposure to toxic drugs, or folic acid deficiency; sometimes no cause can be found. *Hemolytic crises* due to a further increase in hemolysis are rare. Other causes for an increase in jaundice (e.g., gallstones, hepatitis) should be sought.

Blood. The anemia is normochromic and normocytic; polychromasia is increased; and normoblasts are present. Target cells are numerous, and Howell-Jolly bodies are regularly seen in older children and adults as a result of asplenia. Sickle cells are often found in the stained smear (Fig. 26–12; see Plate 26–2*A*). The microhematocrit as an estimate of degree of anemia is unreliable because of excessive plasma trapping. Osmotic fragility usually is decreased, and mechanical fragility is increased. Neutrophilia and thrombocytosis are usual. The marrow shows normoblastic hyperplasia and increased storage iron.

Sickling Test—Metabisulfite. Adding sodium metabisulfite, a reducing substance, to blood enhances deoxygenation of Hb and sickling of Hb S (see Plate 26–2*D*). The test does not distinguish sickle cell anemia from sickle trait or

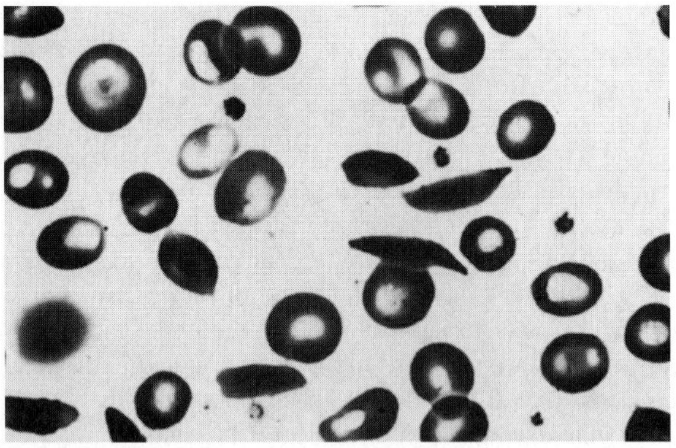

Figure 26–12. Sickle cell anemia. Note that the elongated pointed cells have greater density in the center than near the edges, in contrast to elliptocytes. Linked molecules of reduced Hb S, forming tactoids, distort the cells. (× 875.)

other Hb S syndromes because all red blood cells sickle; however, sickling occurs more rapidly with greater amounts of Hb S in the cells. Positive tests may occur with other rare abnormal hemoglobins (e.g., Hb C–Harlem and Hb I) and Hb Bart's. False-negative tests may occur if Hb S concentration is less than 10% (as in very young infants) or if deoxygenation is inadequate (e.g., deterioration of reagent).

Solubility Test—Dithionite. Red blood cells are lysed, Hb S is reduced by dithionite (sodium hydrosulfite), and the reduced Hb S is insoluble in concentrated inorganic buffers. The polymers of deoxy Hb S obstruct light rays and produce opacity. The test is useful in screening large numbers of people for the presence of Hb S or other sickling hemoglobins. Positive reactions (turbid solution) occur also in the presence of many Heinz bodies, as in unstable hemoglobin disorders after splenectomy, and in blood protein disorders due to precipitation of plasma proteins. Negative reactions (clear solution) occur with normal and most abnormal Hbs, and also if the amount of Hb S is too small, as in severe anemia, or if the reagent has deteriorated.

Hb Electrophoresis. In cellulose acetate electrophoresis at pH 8.6, no Hb A will be found if the patient has not been transfused recently; over 80% of the hemoglobin will be Hb S, 1% to 20% Hb F, and 2% to 4.5% Hb A_2 (Wrightstone, 1974). The fetal hemoglobin is distributed unevenly among the red blood cells. Hb S, Hb D, and Hb G–Philadelphia have the same electrophoretic mobility at alkaline pH, but of these, only Hb S produces a positive sickling test. In agar gel electrophoresis at pH 6.0, Hb D and Hb G migrate with Hb A, differently from Hb S (see Fig. 26–11).

SICKLE CELL TRAIT (Hb AS). Sickle cell trait is the most common hemoglobinopathy in the United States. This heterozygous condition is present in about 9% of American blacks (Schneider, 1976). Under normal circumstances, no clinical signs of disease or hematologic abnormalities are present. However, acidosis or hypoxia due to aircraft flight, respiratory infection, anesthesia, or congestive heart failure may cause sickling and vascular complications with visceral infarcts, including hematuria. Impaired ability to concentrate urine is found in adults with the trait. Sickle cell trait confers protection on children from the lethal effects of *Plasmodium falciparum* malaria, which may account for the major distribution of Hb S in central Africa.

The stained blood film appears normal, except perhaps for a few target cells. Blood cell counts are normal. The sickle cell preparation is positive, and almost all the red blood cells eventually sickle. The solubility test is positive.

Electrophoresis. The findings are Hb A, 50% to 65%; Hb S, 35% to 45%; Hb F, normal; Hb A_2, normal to slightly increased, up to 4.5%. Less than 35% Hb S often indicates the coexistence of one or more α-thalassemia genes (Weatherall, 1981), which is also associated with microcytosis.

HEMOGLOBIN C DISEASE. Homozygous hemoglobin C disease is a mild hemolytic anemia with splenomegaly that is often asymptomatic but occasionally results in jaundice and abdominal discomfort. In the United States, 0.02% of blacks have Hb C disease (Schneider, 1976).

Blood. Slight normochromic, normocytic to microcytic anemia with an admixture of microcytes and spherocytes; a minimal increase in reticulocytes; and numerous target cells are seen in the blood. Osmotic fragility is biphasic, with both increased and decreased fragility. Hexagonal or rod-shaped crystals may be seen in erythrocytes in the stained smear, especially after splenectomy or after slow drying of the smear (Fig. 26–13; see Plate 26–2*B* and *C*). The red blood cells are dehydrated, owing to loss of cations and water as a result of interaction of the abnormal hemoglobin with the red blood cell membrane. As a consequence, the cells are more rigid and less deformable than normal, increasing their likelihood of being trapped and destroyed in the spleen. The MCV is normal or decreased, and the MCHC is normal or increased. Reticulocytosis is less than expected, probably because of a shift to the right in the oxyhemoglobin dissociation curve (Bunn, 1986).

Electrophoresis. The findings are no Hb A; over 90% Hb C; less than 7% Hb F. Hb E and Hb O-Arab have the same migration as Hb C on alkaline electrophoresis. They can be separated on agar gel at an acid pH (see Fig. 26–11).

HEMOGLOBIN C TRAIT (Hb AC). Hemoglobin C is prevalent in West Africans and in about 2% to 3% of American blacks. The heterozygous state is asymptomatic, without anemia, and mild hypochromia and target cells (up to 40%) may be present.

Electrophoresis. The findings are Hb A, 50% to 60%; Hb C, 30% to 40%. Lower proportions of Hb C and mi-

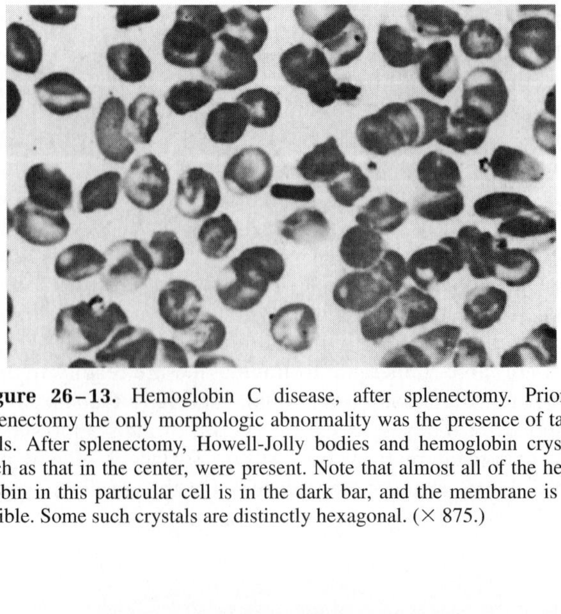

Figure 26–13. Hemoglobin C disease, after splenectomy. Prior to splenectomy the only morphologic abnormality was the presence of target cells. After splenectomy, Howell-Jolly bodies and hemoglobin crystals, such as that in the center, were present. Note that almost all of the hemoglobin in this particular cell is in the dark bar, and the membrane is still visible. Some such crystals are distinctly hexagonal. (× 875.)

crocytosis usually are associated with coexistence of α-thalassemia.

HEMOGLOBINS D AND G. Hemoglobin G–Philadelphia is the most common G-variant in American blacks. Hb D–Punjab and Hb D–Los Angeles are the same ($\alpha_2\beta_2^{121\ Gln}$) and constitute the most common D-variant in American blacks (<0.02%). Hb G is somewhat more frequent than Hb D in American blacks (Schneider, 1976). Homozygosity and heterozygosity for either Hb D or Hb G exhibit no clinical or hematologic abnormalities, except a few target cells on the blood film of individuals who are homozygous for Hb D. Homozygotes for Hb D are found in India, and homozygotes for Hb G are found in Ghana (Bunn, 1986).

Electrophoresis. Hb D and Hb G–Philadelphia ($\alpha_2^{68\ Lys}\beta_2$) have mobilities on alkaline electrophoresis identical to that of Hb S but have negative solubility and sickling tests. Hb D and Hb G migrate differently from Hb S on agar gel at an acid pH. Because α-chains are affected, Hb G shows a double Hb A_2 band on alkaline electrophoresis. As stated previously, Hb G is somewhat more frequent than Hb D in American blacks (Schneider, 1976).

In the homozygous state, Hb D accounts for about 95% of the total hemoglobin, and Hb A_2 is normal. In the heterozygote, Hb D accounts for less than half of the hemoglobin.

HEMOGLOBIN E DISEASE AND TRAIT. Hb E (β26 Glu→Lys) is the second most prevalent abnormal hemoglobin worldwide and the third in the United States, behind S and C. It is found primarily in Southeast Asia, and especially in people of Thai and Burmese extraction, but is also found in blacks and whites. Hb E trait (Hb AE) is asymptomatic, with microcytosis (average MCV = 73) and no anemia. Hemoglobin E disease is also asymptomatic; it resembles thalassemia trait, with microcytosis (average MCV = 67), erythrocytosis, and slight, if any, anemia. Target cells are numerous on the blood film. Hb E β-Thalassemia is a more severe disease than Hb E disease, and resembles β-thalassemia major; Hb A is reduced or absent.

Hb E is associated with a β-thalassemia phenotype *as well as with* a structurally abnormal globin chain because the base substitution causing the amino acid substitution also causes alternative splicing of precursor β-mRNA molecules. This is because of the location of the base substitution in exon 1, near the 5′ end of IVS-1 (Bunn, 1986).

In the laboratory, Hb E can be demonstrated to be unstable; it precipitates abnormally in the heat denaturation test and with isopropanol. Yet this has no *in vivo* significance; the red blood cell survival is normal in Hb E disease.

Electrophoresis. Hb E migrates similarly to Hb A_2, Hb C, and Hb O–Arab on alkaline electrophoresis. On agar gel at acid pH, Hb E migrates with Hb A, Hb O–Arab tends to separate from A, and Hb C is distinct. In the homozygote, Hb E accounts for over 90% of the hemoglobin, with Hb F from 1% to 10%, no Hb A, and normal Hb A_2. In the heterozygote, Hb A is 65% to 70% of the total hemoglobin, and Hb E is 30% to 35%. If one or more α-thalassemia genes is also present, the proportion of Hb E decreases and the MCV is also lower.

DOUBLY HETEROZYGOUS STATES (β-HEMOGLOBIN)

A different abnormal β-chain inherited from each parent may result in interaction of Hb C, D, or E with Hb S to produce hemolytic anemia of variable severity.

HEMOGLOBIN SC DISEASE. The frequency of Hb SC disease is about the same as that of Hb SS disease in American blacks. The severity is intermediate between sickle cell trait and sickle cell disease, with almost all the manifestations of sickle cell anemia appearing but with less frequency. The onset is usually early in childhood, but real difficulties do not occur until the teens or later. Fatigue, dyspnea on effort, frequent upper respiratory infections, attacks of mild jaundice, and arthralgias are seen. Crises usually are rare and mild. Painful crisis occurs more often in joints and muscles than in the abdomen. Constant hip and low back pain may be present with aseptic necrosis of the head of the femur on x-ray study. Hematuria and splenic infarcts have been described. Leg ulcers occur only occasionally. In pregnancy, there is a tendency toward increased frequency of crisis—both clinical and hematologic. Painful crises are related to infarction, and sudden death may occur following childbirth. In contrast to sickle cell anemia, splenomegaly usually is present. The body habitus is normal or stocky in contrast to the asthenic features in sickle cell anemia.

Blood. Anemia varies from moderate to very mild and is normochromic-normocytic. Anisocytosis and poikilocytosis are mild to severe, and target cells are numerous—up to 85% of the erythrocytes. Plump and angulated sickled cells are often present on the film. The sickling test is positive.

Electrophoresis. Hb C and Hb S occur in about equal amounts. Hb F ranges from normal to 7%. Because no normal β-chains can be produced, Hb A is absent.

HEMOGLOBIN SD DISEASE. SD disease simulates but is less severe than sickle cell anemia, and thus may also resemble SC disease. The sickling test is positive.

4

Electrophoresis. The pattern is indistinguishable from sickle cell anemia because Hb S and Hb D cannot be separated on routine (alkaline) electrophoresis. Agar gel electrophoresis at pH 6.2 separates Hb S and Hb D; solubility studies (Hb D is more soluble than Hb S) and family studies help reveal the true nature of the condition. One parent is likely to have a negative sickling test and an abnormal hemoglobin with the mobility of Hb S.

Other doubly heterozygous β-hemoglobinopathies occur but are even less common.

HETEROZYGOUS HEMOGLOBINOPATHIES

A number of amino acid substitutions occur in the heme pocket, where they either increase the stability of the methemoglobin form (Hb M) or alter the affinity of the heme for oxygen; the latter usually alters the stability of the molecule as well.

Other substitutions affect the αβ contact sites; these also can change stability and oxygen affinity of the molecule (Perutz, 1968).

These functionally significant hemoglobinopathies are heterozygous; usually the concentration of the abnormal hemoglobin is less than 50%. Generally, the hemoglobins with abnormal α-chains form a smaller proportion of the total (10% to 25%) than do those with abnormal β-chains (35% to 50%).

HEMOGLOBINS ASSOCIATED WITH METHEMOGLOBINEMIA AND CYANOSIS

Hemoglobin M. Seven abnormal hemoglobins are associated with clinical methemoglobinemia and cyanosis that do not respond to methylene blue (see Table 26–4). The common feature is that all have an amino acid substitution at or near the heme group, so that methemoglobin is unusually stable, and reduction to ferrous heme and hence reversible binding of oxygen are prevented.

Cyanosis from birth is seen in hemoglobin M disease with α-chain abnormalities and in fetal Hb M (Hb FM–Osaka). In fetal Hb M, cyanosis disappears after the γ-chains have been replaced by β-chains by six months of age. Cyanosis does not appear until nearly six months of age in Hb M variants with β-chain abnormalities for the same reason (Bunn, 1986). The cyanosis is, of course, not associated with enzyme abnormalities in the red blood cell, toxic drugs, or cyanotic heart disease, conditions that must be considered in the differential diagnosis.

All Hb M disorders thus far discovered have been in heterozygotes, probably because homozygosity is lethal. Some types of Hb M do not separate from Hb A on alkaline electrophoresis. If the hemolysate is first converted to methemoglobin, the Hb M will migrate differently from normal methemoglobin at pH 7.1. The absorption spectra of the eluted Hb M, which may be distinctive, can be compared with that of normal methemoglobin (Bunn, 1986). Amino acid analysis of peptide maps of tryptic digests of the abnormal hemoglobin enables identification of the Hb M. This may be performed at a reference laboratory.

HEMOGLOBINS ASSOCIATED WITH ALTERED OXYGEN AFFINITY

Increased Affinity and Polycythemia. Over 50 abnormal hemoglobins with high oxygen affinity that are associated with familial erythrocytosis have been described (Bunn, 1993). Some are listed in Table 26–4. The oxygen dissociation curve is shifted to the left. The P_{50}, the partial pressure of oxygen at which hemoglobin is 50% saturated, is decreased. Under physiologic conditions, the normal P_{50} of whole blood is 26 mm Hg; in this disorder, it has ranged from 5 to 23 mm Hg. Because the hemoglobin has high affinity for oxygen, the tissues are relatively hypoxic at any given PO_2, resulting in increased EPO production and polycythemia. Because the amino acid substitution is inside the molecule, usually the abnormal hemoglobin is indistinguishable from Hb A on electrophoresis (Stamatoyannopoulos, 1971).

Hemoglobin Chesapeake. An α-chain abnormality associated with mild asymptomatic polycythemia in a white family was the first described (Charache, 1966). The features were similar to those of benign familial polycythemia. The abnormal hemoglobin, accounting for about 30% of the total, had an increased affinity for oxygen that resulted in significantly elevated hematocrit levels. The abnormal hemoglobin could be detected by starch block or starch gel electrophoresis.

These disorders are autosomal dominant; only heterozygotes have been described. The hemoglobin concentration has ranged from 15 to 23.8 g/dL. Only about half of these abnormal hemoglobins can be separated from Hb A by starch gel or cellulose acetate electrophoresis at pH 8.6. Measurement of oxygen affinity is required to establish the diagnosis (Bunn, 1986).

Decreased Affinity and Cyanosis. Fifteen abnormal hemoglobins are stable and have decreased oxygen affinity (see Table 26–4; Bunn, 1986). Individuals with this condition have mild anemia and a hemoglobin-oxygen dissociation curve that is shifted to the right (increased P_{50}). Three of these variants are associated with cyanosis. The hemoglobin level may be somewhat low on the basis of the high P_{50}.

Hemoglobin Kansas. This low-affinity hemoglobin, described in a white boy, had just the opposite property from Hb Chesapeake. The clinical features were cyanosis since infancy, normal arterial oxygen tension, and reduced oxygen saturation. Electrophoresis after conversion to methemoglobin allowed separation from Hb A (Reissman, 1961).

UNSTABLE HEMOGLOBINS

Over 100 hemoglobin variants have been described in which the hemoglobin precipitates within the red blood cell as Heinz bodies (Bunn, 1993). Some are listed in Table 26–4. Most of the abnormalities are β-chain; some are α-chain. Rare unstable hemoglobins such as Hb F–Poole are related to an unstable γ-chain variant. Amino acid substitution or deletion renders the Hb molecule unstable. Precipitated Hb attaches to the cell membrane and shortens its survival; the cells are inflexible; Heinz bodies are removed by the spleen; the further damaged cells have a shortened survival. The oxygen affinity usually is abnormal and may be increased or decreased. Some of these unstable hemoglobins cause so-called congenital Heinz body hemolytic anemias.

All patients have been heterozygous. The clinical features have shown considerable variation, from severe hemolytic anemia in the first year of life (e.g., Hb Hammersmith, Hb Bristol) to a very mild chronic hemolytic anemia (e.g., Hb Louisville, Hb Hasharon) that may be exacerbated by drugs (e.g., Hb Zurich). A few unstable hemoglobins have been discovered incidentally in clinically normal individuals (e.g., Hb Tacoma, Hb Sogn).

Jaundice and splenomegaly are common, as in other hemolytic anemias. More distinctive in some cases is the excretion of darkly pigmented urine (only during hemolytic crises in mild variants). The urine pigment appears to be dipyrrole, probably a breakdown product of denatured hemoglobin. Cyanosis is present in some patients and is due to methemoglobinuria and sulfhemoglobinemia or to low oxygen affinity.

The anemia is normocytic and normochromic to hypochromic, the latter because of the removal of precipitated hemoglobin from aging red blood cells by the macrophages of the spleen and other reticuloendothelial organs. Prominent basophilic stippling probably related to excessive clumping of ribosomes is a common feature. Patients with relatively high hemoglobin concentrations in the steady state usually have hemoglobin variants with a high oxygen affinity and an unexpectedly high reticulocyte count (e.g., Hb Köln, Hb Gun Hill). On the other hand, patients with rather low hemoglobin concentrations may be relatively asymptomatic if their hemoglobin has a low oxygen affinity; their reticulocyte counts are unexpectedly low for the hemoglobin concentration (e.g., Hb Hammersmith). Heinz bodies are rarely seen in circulating red blood cells before splenectomy, although sometimes they may be generated by incubating the red blood cells with brilliant cresyl blue or new methylene blue. After splenectomy, Heinz bodies are readily demonstrable in a large proportion of cells; the blood film shows irregularly contracted cells and basophilic stippling that may be pronounced.

In splenectomized patients, the Heinz bodies may interfere with hemoglobin determinations and with electronic platelet and white blood cell counts. Before measuring the absorbance of the hemolysate, it should be centrifuged to remove the Heinz bodies. Platelet and leukocyte counts should be performed by visual methods.

Hemoglobin electrophoresis is normal in about one fourth of patients. Hb A_2 may be elevated in β-chain variants because of the loss of the abnormal hemoglobin from the cells. Hb F may be increased to a level of 10% to 15%. The key laboratory determinations are the heat instability and isopropanol precipitation tests.

HEAT INSTABILITY TEST. Most unstable hemoglobins precipitate more rapidly than normal hemoglobins when incubated at 50°C (Dacie, 1991). Both normal and unstable hemoglobins precipitate more rapidly in Tris-buffer than in phosphate buffers. In a hemolysate in Tris-buffer, an easily visible precipitate forms within an hour if an unstable hemoglobin is present; the control sample is clear or slightly cloudy. Slight precipitation is equivocal; the test should be repeated and the isopropanol precipitation test performed as well. Precipitates accounting for 10% to 40% of the total Hb are found in unstable hemoglobin disorders.

ISOPROPANOL PRECIPITATION TEST. A relatively nonpolar solvent weakens the internal bonds of hemoglobin and decreases its stability (Carrell, 1972). An unstable hemoglobin precipitates within 20 minutes in the nonpolar solvent isopropanol, whereas a normal hemolysate remains clear for 30 to 40 minutes. False-positive results occur with high levels of Hb F.

Thalassemias

Thalassemias comprise a heterogeneous group of hereditary disorders of hemoglobin synthesis that occur predominantly in persons of Mediterranean, African, and Asian ancestry.

The common characteristic of these disorders is impaired production of polypeptide chains of hemoglobin—that is, the *rate* of synthesis is diminished but the chain formed is, in most cases, structurally normal. In β-thalassemias, β-chain production is decreased. α-Thalassemia, $\delta\beta$-, δ-, and $\sigma\delta\beta$-thalassemias have decreased synthesis of the respective polypeptide chains. These various conditions constitute the so-called thalassemia syndromes. Weatherall (1994) and Bunn (1986) have summarized evidence for the genetic defects in these syndromes, which in the majority of cases, result in a quantitative deficiency of messenger RNA (mRNA).

Molecular Defects

In the β-thalassemias, there is considerable heterogeneity in the molecular defects. Most are single-base substitutions that produce defects in transcription, RNA splicing, or translation (via frameshifts or nonsense codons), resulting in decreased mRNA or unstable mRNA. In rare variants, the production of highly unstable β-globin chains results in β-thalassemia (Kazazian, 1988).

In β°-thalassemia, β-chain synthesis is absent. The β-globin genes are intact; only very rarely is the gene deleted. In some cases, mRNA is absent; in other cases mRNA is present but nonfunctional. There is considerable heterogeneity in the molecular defects.

In β^{+} thalassemia, β-globin chains are present but reduced in quantity, because the molecular defects have resulted in the production of decreased amounts of mRNA or unstable mRNA (Table 26–5).

In $\delta\beta$-thalassemias, different deletions involving both the δ- and the β-genes have been described. In $\gamma\delta\beta$-thalassemia, a long deletion including the γ-genes and the δ-gene stops short of the β-gene, but the output of the latter is greatly reduced. Lepore hemoglobins have normal α-chains and abnormal $\delta\beta$-chains. Abnormal $\delta\beta$-chains are produced by $\delta\beta$-fusion genes that are the result of unequal crossover between δ- and β-globin genes during meiosis.

The α-thalassemias generally are due to gene deletion of various lengths. The α°-thalassemia determinant (α-thalassemia 1) results from deletion of both α-globin genes on the chromosome, which therefore directs no α-chain synthesis. The α^{+} thalassemia determinant (α-thalassemia 2) is due to either various-sized *deletions* that result in the absence of one of the two α-globin genes on chromosome 16 or *nondeletion defects* that reduce the output of mRNA.

Hb Constant Spring is due to an abnormal termination codon in an α-globin gene that results in an elongated α-chain with 31 extra amino acids. For unknown reasons, the chain synthesis is slow, resulting in the clinical findings of α-thalassemia.

β-Thalassemia

The clinical and hemoglobin findings in the β-thalassemias are summarized in Table 26–6. The disorders are very heterogeneous, phenotypically as well as at the level of the

Table 26–5. MAJOR CATEGORIES OF β-THALASSEMIA SYNDROMES AND THEIR ASSOCIATED BIOCHEMICAL AND MOLECULAR DEFECTS

			Hb F (γ-Chain) Synthesis				
	Hb A (β-Chain)	**Hb A_2 (δ-Chain)**	***Amount***	***Cellular Distribution***	**α: Non-α-Globin Chain Imbalance**	**β-Globin mRNA**	**β-Globin Gene DNA**
β^{+}-Thalassemia	↓	+	+	Heterogeneous	++++	↓	+
β^{0}-Thalassemia	0	+	+	Heterogeneous	++++	0	+
						↓	+
$\delta\beta$-Thalassemia	0	0	++/+++	Heterogeneous	++/+++	0	0
Hereditary persistence of fetal hemoglobin	0	0	++++	Uniform	+	0	0

From Forget BG: Molecular studies of genetic disorders affecting the expression of the human β-globin gene: A model system for the analysis of inborn errors of metabolism. Recent Progr Horm Res 1982; 38:257.

Table 26–6. β-THALASSEMIAS

Syndrome	Genotype	Clinical Features	Hemoglobin Pattern
Homozygous states:			
β^+ thalassemia	β^+/β^+	Thalassemia major: or thalassemia intermedia	↓ Hb A. ↑ Hb F, variable Hb A_2
β^0 thalassemia	β^0/β^0	Thalassemia major	0 Hb A, variable Hb A_2, residual Hb F
$\delta\beta^0$/thalassemia	$\delta\beta^0/\delta\beta^0$	Thalassemia intermedia	0 Hb A and Hb A_2, 100% Hb F
Hb Lepore	Lepore/Lepore	Thalassemia major	0 Hb A, Hb A_2; 75% Hb F, 25% Hb Lepore
Heterozygous states:			
β^+ thalassemia	β^+/β	Thalassemia minor	↑ Hb A_2, slight ↑ Hb F
β^0 thalassemia	β^0/β	Thalassemia minor	↑ Hb A_2, slight ↑ Hb F
$\delta\beta^0$ thalassemia	$\delta\beta^0/\delta\beta$	Thalassemia minor	5–20% Hb F
Hb Lepore	Hb Lepore/β	Thalassemia minor	↑ Hb F, ↓ Hb A_2, 5–15% Hb Lepore

Modified from Orkin SH, Nathan DG: Reprinted, by permission of the New England Journal of Medicine, 1976; 295:710.

molecular defects. The terms *thalassemia major, thalassemia intermedia,* and *thalassemia minor* refer to clinical severity and are not genetic designations.

HOMOZYGOUS β-THALASSEMIA (THALASSEMIA MAJOR; COOLEY'S ANEMIA). With an absence (β°) or a marked decrease (β^+) in β-chain production, γ-chain production remains high (Hb F is elevated), and there is an excess of α-chains. Aggregates of α-chains (α_4) are unstable and precipitate in the normoblast or red cell and damage the cells. Precipitates and cells are removed, causing ineffective erythropoiesis and a severe hemolytic anemia.

Clinical findings include jaundice and splenomegaly, which become evident early in childhood. Prominent frontal bones, cheek bones, and jaws impart a mongoloid appearance. These changes and the roentgenographic findings of thinned cortex of the long and flat bones and thickening of the skull with osteoporosis (hair-on-end appearance) reflect the extreme bone marrow hyperplasia in response to the hemolytic process. Growth is stunted, and puberty is delayed. Most patients require regular transfusions and develop problems due to iron loading. Hemochromatosis commonly develops, and the major cause of death is cardiac failure due to myocardial siderosis by the end of the third decade.

Blood. Unlike most hemolytic diseases, the anemia is hypochromic and microcytic. This is probably due to the defect in hemoglobin synthesis. Extreme poikilocytosis with bizarre shapes, target cells, ovalocytosis, Cabot rings, Howell-Jolly bodies, nuclear fragments, siderocytes, anisochromia, anisocytosis, and often extreme normoblastosis are present. Poikilocytosis is more striking in patients with intact spleens; normoblastosis is more severe after splenectomy. Normoblasts have hypochromic cytoplasm and, especially after splenectomy, aggregates of densely staining hemoglobin (see Plate 26–2*F*), which probably represent precipitated α-chains (with heme attached). Incubation of the blood with methyl violet (as for Heinz bodies) stains these precipitates in both red blood cells and normoblasts. The reticulocyte count is less elevated than expected for the degree of anemia because of destruction of erythroid precursors in the marrow. Osmotic resistance of the red cells, serum iron, and indirect-reacting bilirubin are increased.

Marrow. Marked normoblastic hyperplasia is present. Many late normoblasts show inclusion bodies as in the blood. Intramedullary destruction of hemoglobin (ineffective erythropoiesis) is markedly increased in thalassemia major. Storage iron and sideroblasts are increased.

Hemoglobin Studies. In β°-thalassemia, Hb A is absent, Hb F is as high as 98%, and Hb A_2 is about 2%. In β^+-thalassemias (Mediterranean), Hb F is 60% to 95%, with Hb A present. Although Hb A_2 may or may not be increased, the ratio of A_2 to A is always increased. In blacks with β^+-thalassemia, the clinical features are less severe (so-called thalassemia intermedia) and transfusion usually is unnecessary; Hb F is 20% to 40%, Hb A_2 is 2% to 5%, and Hb A levels are higher.

HETEROZYGOUS β-THALASSEMIA (THALASSEMIA MINOR; COOLEY'S TRAIT). Clinical findings are as follows: The features in heterozygous β-thalassemia vary from moderately severe anemia (thalassemia intermedia) to completely normal clinical findings. The severe intermediate forms of heterozygous thalassemia are rare and are found in Mediterranean individuals but not in blacks; in the latter, heterozygous thalassemia is uniformly mild. In many persons, there is a mild hypochromic, microcytic anemia with slight hemolytic jaundice and splenomegaly. Most individuals with thalassemia minor, however, have no symptoms or abnormal physical signs.

Blood. Usually, there is no anemia. Characteristically, the red blood cell count is elevated and the hemoglobin and hematocrit are reduced. The mean cell hemoglobin (MCH) is low, usually less than 22 pg; and MCV is low, between 50 and 70 fL. The MCHC is sometimes low but often normal. On stained films, the cells have a moderate degree of microcytosis and poikilocytosis; target cells and basophilic stippling are often present (see Plate 26–2E). Osmotic fragility is decreased. The serum iron concentration is normal or high, and the serum ferritin level is normal.

Marrow. Normoblastic hyperplasia and elevated storage iron may be found.

Hemoglobin Studies. Hb A_2 is elevated in the 3.5% to 7% range. Hb F is slightly elevated in about half of the cases. If the Hb F exceeds 5%, it is likely that a gene for HPFH is also present.

In some cases of heterozygous β-thalassemia, the Hb A_2 is normal. One form, designated *Type 1 normal Hb A_2 β-thalassemia,* has a normal hemoglobin pattern and minimal hematologic changes (the so-called silent β-thalassemia gene). The other, *Type 2 normal Hb A_2* β-thalassemia, has typical thalassemic red blood cell changes. Globin synthesis studies are necessary to identify Type 1 and to distinguish Type 2 from α-thalassemia minor (Weatherall, 1983).

δβ-THALASSEMIAS. In the homozygous state, these

forms are characterized by thalassemia intermedia and absence of both Hb A and Hb A_2. Heterozygotes have thalassemia minor, with 5% to 20% Hb F and normal Hb A_2.

HEMOGLOBIN LEPORE SYNDROMES. Hb Lepore is an abnormal hemoglobin that has a normal α-chain combined with a composite $\delta\beta$-chain (Weatherall, 1994). It probably occurs as a result of chromosome misalignment with crossing-over and fusion of genetic material at the $\delta\beta$-gene complex. Different Hb Lepores have been described, depending on the point of fusion. Because the composite $\delta\beta$-chain is synthesized at a slow rate, it results in a hypochromic microcytic red cell morphology resembling the thalassemias (see Table 26–6). Lepore migrates similarly to Hb S on alkaline electrophoresis.

Double Heterozygosity for β-Thalassemia and β-Hemoglobinopathy

Patients doubly heterozygous for β-thalassemia and a β-chain hemoglobin variant have levels of Hb A that are *less* than the level of the variant hemoglobin. In the simple sickle cell trait, for example, the level of Hb A always exceeds that of Hb S.

SICKLE CELL THALASSEMIA (HB S/β-THALASSEMIA). Hb S/β°-thalassemia is more severe than Hb S/β^+-thalassemia. The anemia and clinical findings vary from slight to severe, with manifestations similar to those in sickle cell anemia (Hb SS). In contrast to Hb SS, the spleen in Hb S/β-thalassemia remains enlarged after childhood and into adult life.

Blood. Pronounced microcytosis, variable hypochromia, and many target cells are present. Sickled cells are uncommon. The MCV and MCH are low.

Hemoglobin Studies. The solubility test and sickling test, of course, are positive. In Hb S/β^+-thalassemia, Hb A is 15% to 30%; Hb S is over 50%; Hb F is 1% to 20%; and Hb A_2 is increased, usually over 4.5%. Although these individuals clinically may resemble those with sickle trait (Hb AS), in S/β^+-thalassemia the amount of Hb S always exceeds Hb A; in Hb AS, Hb A always exceeds Hb S.

In Hb S/β°-thalassemia, Hb A is absent; Hb S is 75% to 90%; Hb F is 5% to 20%; and Hb A_2 is usually increased, over 4.5%. This disorder clinically and hematologically resembles sickle cell disease. The main difference is that in Hb S/β°-thalassemia, the MCV and MCH are lower and the Hb A_2 is increased. Family study is often necessary for a clear distinction (Lehmann, 1977; Wrightstone, 1974).

HEMOGLOBIN C THALASSEMIA (HB C/β-THALASSEMIA). This condition occurs mainly in blacks, in whom it tends to result in little disability. Patients of Mediterranean extraction usually have moderately severe hemolytic anemia.

Blood. The MCH and MCV are reduced. On the blood film are hypochromic target cells, fragmented red cells, and microspherocytes, many of which have a folded appearance.

Hemoglobin Studies. In Hb C/β°-thalassemia, Hb C is 90% to 95%, Hb F is 5% to 10%, and Hb A is absent. In Hb C/β^+-thalassemia, Hb A is 20% to 30% and Hb C 70% to 80%. Hb A_2 levels cannot be studied when Hb C is present, because there are no satisfactory methods for separating the two.

HEMOGLOBIN E THALASSEMIA (HB E/β-THALASSEMIA). This disorder is manifested by a severe anemia, with a clinical and hematologic features similar to that of thalassemia major.

Hemoglobin Studies. Hb E is 15% to 95%, Hb F is 5% to 85%. It is of interest that Hb A is nearly always absent. This emphasizes the fact that absence of Hb A cannot be taken as proof of homozygosity; it must be supported by family studies.

α-Thalassemias

Whereas there is one β-globin gene per haploid genotype, there are two α-globin genes. The normal haplotype is designated $\alpha\alpha$/. The mild α-thalassemia determinant (-α/) is α^+-thalassemia, also called α-thalassemia 2, a deletion of one gene. The severe α-thalassemia determinant (–/) is α°-thalassemia, also called α-thalassemia 1, a deletion of two genes. The main forms of α-thalassemias are outlined in Table 26–7.

HYDROPS FETALIS WITH HB BART'S. Complete absence of α-chains is incompatible with life. Infants are stillborn with severe edema, marked anemia, and marked hepatosplenomegaly. The blood shows marked anisocytosis, poikilocytosis, microcytosis, and erythroblastosis. ABO or Rh incompatibility is absent. Because of the absence of α-chains, no Hb A ($\alpha_2\beta_2$) or Hb F ($\alpha_2\gamma_2$) is present. Large quantities of Hb Bart's (γ_4) and some Hb H (β_4) are present; both of these types migrate faster than Hb A on alkaline electrophoresis.

HEMOGLOBIN H DISEASE. Three of the four α-genes are

4

Table 26–7. α-THALASSEMIAS

			Hemoglobin Pattern	
Syndrome	**Genotype**	**Clinical Features**	*Newborn*	*After First Year*
Hydrops fetalis	– –/– –	Fetal or neonatal death with severe anemia	Hb Bart's > 80% Hb H. Hb Portland	—
Hb H disease	– –/– α (– –/$\alpha\alpha^{CS}$)	Chronic hemolytic anemia	Hb Bart's 20–40% (Hb CS present)	Hb H 5–30% Hb Bart's ± trace (Hb CS 2–3%)
Thalassemia minor	– –/$\alpha\alpha$ –α/–α $\alpha\boxed{\alpha}/\alpha\boxed{\alpha}$	Little or no anemia: thalassemic RBC	Hb Bart's 2–20%	None
Silent carrier	–α/$\alpha\alpha$ ($\alpha\alpha$/$\alpha\alpha^{CS}$)	No clinical or hematologic abnormality	Hb Bart's 1–2% (Hb CS present)	None (Hb CS 1%)
Normal	$\alpha\alpha$/$\alpha\alpha$	No clinical or hematologic abnormality	Hb Bart's 0-trace	None

α^{CS} = α-structural gene for HB Constant Spring: $\boxed{\alpha}$ = non-deletion α-thalassemia gene.
Modified from Wintrobe MM, Lee GR, Boggs DR, et al: Clinical Hematology, 8th ed. Philadelphia, Lea and Febiger, 1981.

absent. A chronic anemia with the clinical picture of thalassemia intermedia is usual, although the severity varies. Hb H disease has been described in almost all racial groups, especially those in Southeast Asia, Greece, and parts of the Middle East; it is very rare, however, in blacks.

Blood. MCV and MCH are decreased. The blood film shows hypochromia, target cells, and anisopoikilocytosis (see Plate 26–2*G*). Reticulocytes are usually 4% to 5%. Vital staining of the blood with an oxidizing dye such as brilliant cresyl blue induces pale blue inclusion bodies (Hb H precipitates) in many of the red cells, which contrast with the deep blue precipitates of RNA in reticulocytes (see Plate 26–2*H*). After splenectomy, single large Heinz bodies are seen.

Hemoglobin Studies. Hemoglobin electrophoresis shows a rapidly migrating band of Hb H (β_4), accounting for 4% to 30% of the hemoglobin, and traces of the slightly less rapidly migrating Hb Bart's (γ_4). Hb H can be precipitated *in vitro* and lost from the hemolysate by careless handling or prolonged storage. Hb Bart's is alkali resistant and may be measured with Hb F (which is not increased in Hb H disease). The percentage of Hb Bart's is 20% to 40% at birth; it gradually falls thereafter, but the level in adults in variable.

Hemoglobin H Preparation. During incubation of two parts of blood in one part of 1% brilliant cresyl blue stain, the unstable Hb H (β_4) gradually precipitates as multiple small pale blue inclusions uniformly distributed on the red cell membrane (see Plate 26–2*H* and *I*) (Jones, 1981). Hb H inclusions must be distinguished from (1) the granules and reticular networks in reticulocytes, which are darker blue in color; and (2) preformed Heinz bodies, which are larger, also darker blue, and often attached to the membrane. After 10 to 20 minutes of incubation at room temperature, Hb H inclusions are present in at least half of the red blood cells in Hb H disease and in a very rare red blood cell in α-thalassemia minor. The larger Heinz bodies may be found after splenectomy in Hb H disease.

THALASSEMIA MINOR (HETEROZYGOUS α°-THALASSEMIA OR HOMOZYGOUS α^{+}-THALASSEMIA). Absence of two α-genes results in clinical features similar to β-thalassemia minor, with very mild anemia, microcytosis, a normal serum iron, normal serum ferritin, and normal red blood cell protoporphyrin.

Hemoglobin Studies. Diagnosis is best made by finding 5% to 6% Hb Bart's in cord blood; normally, only trace amounts (<0.5%) are found. In adults, Hb H inclusion bodies in some cases can be found in a very small percentage of red blood cells (perhaps 1 in 10^5), if *exhaustively sought after* (Wasi, 1974) and if the sample is enriched for Hb H–containing red blood cells (Jones, 1981). Otherwise, no evidence of hemoglobin imbalance is detectable by standard techniques, and the diagnosis is one of excluding iron deficiency and β-thalassemia or demonstrating a decreased α-chain/β-chain synthesis ratio (~0.6).

SILENT CARRIER OF α-THALASSEMIA (HETEROZYGOUS α^{+}-THALASSEMIA). One of four α-globin genes is absent. No hematologic abnormality is detectable in adults; MCV, blood film, and hemoglobin studies are normal. In infants, Hb Bart's accounts for 1% to 2% of the cord blood hemoglobin. The diagnosis cannot be made reliably in the adult with these techniques.

Hemoglobin Constant Spring. Hb Constant Spring (Hb $\overline{CS}$) is an α-chain variant with 31 extra amino acids. It is synthesized slowly and results in a thalassemia-like picture. The homozygous state appears as a mild thalassemia with microcytosis and 5% to 8% Hb $\overline{CS}$, normal Hb A_2, trace amounts of Hb Bart's, and the rest Hb A (Weatherall, 1994). The heterozygous state shows no hematologic abnormality: normal Hb A and A_2, and about 1% Hb $\overline{CS}$. The abnormal Hb migrates more slowly than Hb A_2 at alkaline pH and is easily missed. The gene behaves similarly to that in a silent carrier (α^{+}-thalassemia trait) and is found in about 40% of cases of Hb H disease in Southeast Asia (see Table 26–7).

Hereditary Persistence of Fetal Hemoglobin

A group of conditions with Hb F production persisting beyond infancy without significant hematologic abnormalities is known as HPFH. It is found in about 0.1% of American blacks; there are also a Greek form and other variants (Weatherall, 1994).

In blacks, the homozygote has slightly microcytic, hypochromic red blood cells without anemia. Hb F is 100%; no Hb A or Hb A_2 is present. This lack of β and δ-chain synthesis has been shown to be due to deletion of the $\delta\beta$-gene complex (Weatherall, 1994).

In the heterozygote, no hematologic abnormalities are found. Hb F is 20% to 30%, and Hb A_2 is 1% to 2.1%, with the remainder Hb A. With the acid elution technique, the Hb F is homogeneously distributed among the red cells in the form found in blacks or the *pancellular* type of HPFH. This is in contrast to β-thalassemia, in which the distribution is heterogeneous.

The most common *heterocellular* HPFH is the Swiss type. There are no hematologic changes and 1% to 3% Hb F, which is heterogeneously distributed among the red cells. It is difficult to define because it overlaps the normal. When it is inherited with a β-thalassemia gene, the result is a higher Hb F than is found in a heterozygous β-thalassemia alone (Weatherall, 1981).

Prenatal Diagnosis of Hemoglobin Disorders

In populations in which there is a significant incidence of severe forms of thalassemia or sickle cell anemia, women should be screened early in pregnancy for thalassemia and the sickle cell trait (Alter, 1988; Weatherall, 1985, 1994). If both parents are carriers, prevention of severe disease is possible through genetic counselling and offering prenatal diagnosis with the option of therapeutic abortion.

Fetal blood analysis has been employed since 1974 for the diagnosis of thalassemia major using samples obtained by placental aspiration or direct vision fetoscopy at 18 to 20 weeks' gestation. Washed red blood cells are incubated with labeled amino acids, and synthetic rates of α-, β-, and γ-globin chains are determined. A β/γ ratio of less than 0.035 indicates homozygous β-thalassemia; the normal β/γ ratio is 0.10 to 0.12 at this age. Although the fetal mortality rate for the procedure is 5% to 10%, this procedure has been well accepted in several populations and has led to major decreases in the incidence of new cases of β-thalassemia major in these areas.

Fetal DNA analysis can be performed on samples of fetal cells obtained by amniocentesis at 16 to 18 weeks' gestation

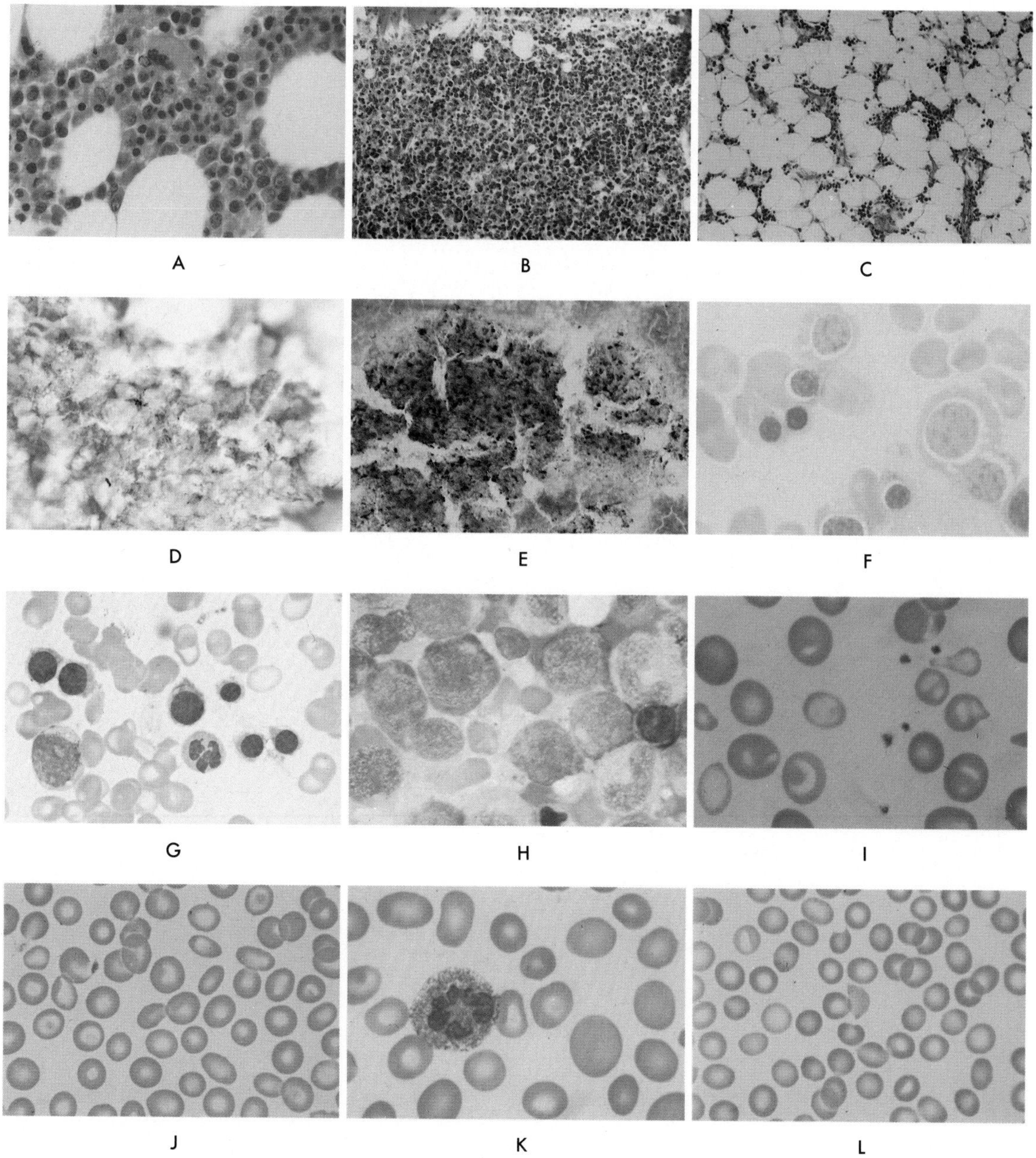

Plate 26–1. *A*, Section of normal marrow. The cellularity (i.e., the ratio of the space occupied by cells to the total) is about 0.5 to 0.6. The erythroid/granulocytic (E/G) ratio is normal, about ⅓. A megakaryocyte is in the upper center. *B*, Section of hyperplastic marrow, megaloblastic anemia. The cellularity is over 0.95. *C*, Section of hypocellular marrow, aplastic anemia. The cellularity is about 0.10 or less. Although they are not discernible at this magnification, most of the cells are lymphocytes and plasma cells. *D*, Marrow film, Prussian blue reaction, no counterstain, normal marrow. Storage iron stains blue-green and is within macrophages. On a scale of 0 to 5+, the amount of storage iron here is judged as 1+, which is in the normal range for a woman, probably somewhat low for a man. In iron deficiency anemia, no blue-green staining iron is visible. *E*, Marrow film, Prussian blue reaction, no counterstain, sideroblastic anemia. On a scale of 0 to 5+, the amount of storage iron is judged at 5+, which is markedly increased. *F*, Marrow film, Prussian blue reaction, counterstained with nuclear fast red, sideroblastic anemia. The normoblasts in the field contain multiple siderotic granules. Two ring sideroblasts are left of the center. The wide perinuclear space in some cells is an artifact. *G*, Marrow film, iron deficiency anemia. The six normoblasts have irregular margins and irregular clear spaces, reflecting lack of hemoglobin synthesis, i.e., defective cytoplasmic maturation. Also in the field are a neutrophil and an immature monocyte. *H*, Marrow film, megaloblastic anemia. Basophilic and polychromatophilic megaloblasts predominate in this field; two giant-band neutrophils are present. The "open," non-condensed chromatin pattern and large cell size are characteristic of defective nuclear maturation. *I*, Blood film, primary acquired sideroblastic anemia. Dimorphic red cell populations normocytic to macrocytic and normochromic, microcytic, and hypochromic. *J*, Blood film, iron deficiency anemia, same patient as in *G*. The red cells are microcytic; some are also hypochromic; a few target cells and an increased proportion of elliptocytes are present. *K*, Blood film, megaloblastic anemia. The oval macrocytes and hypersegmented neutrophil are presumptive evidence of megaloblastosis. Note the prominent large neutrophil granules. *L*, Blood film, lead poisoning. The red cells are slightly microcytic with some hypochromic cells. The poikilocyte in the center contains basophilic stippling.

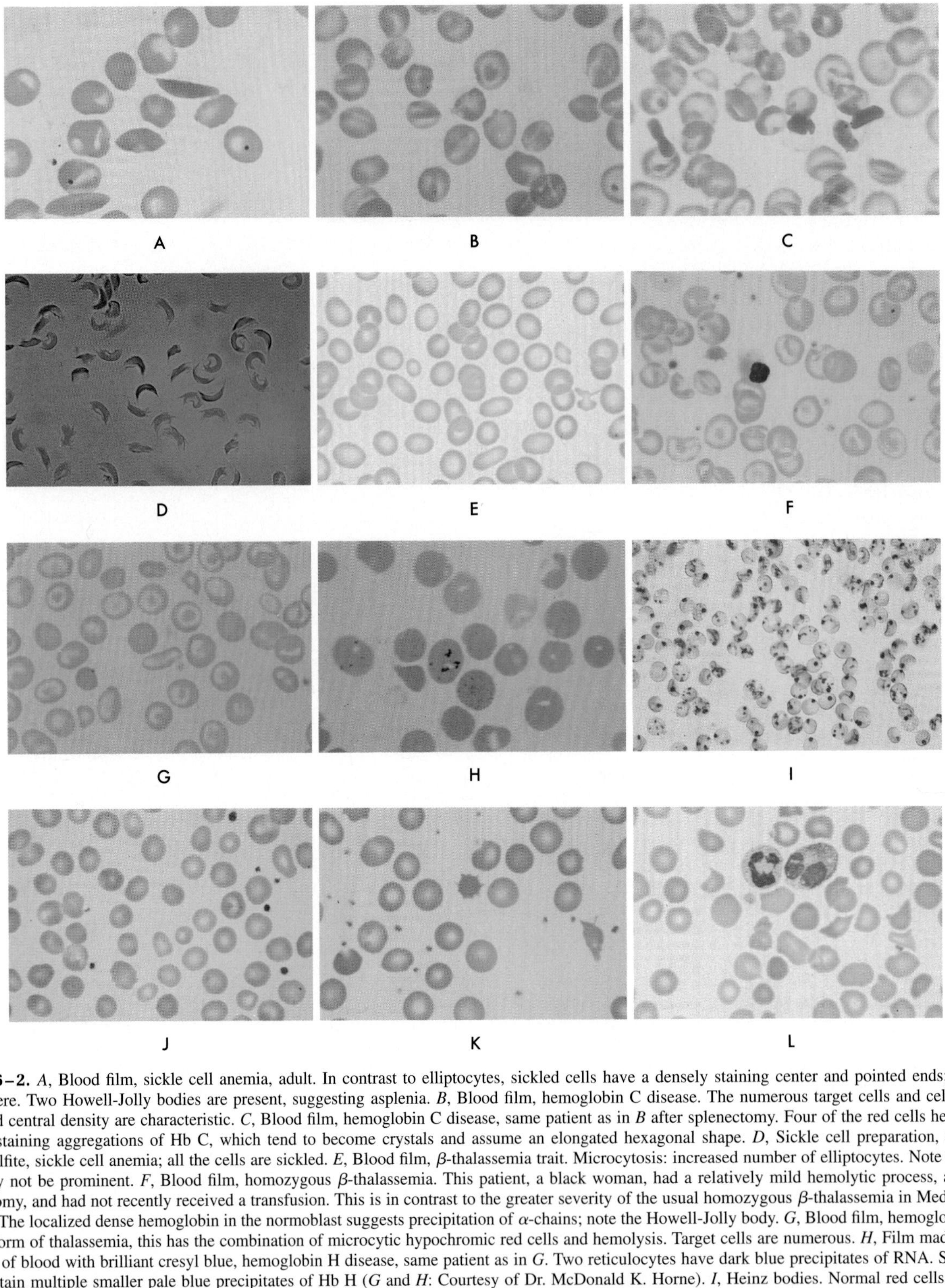

Plate 26–2. *A*, Blood film, sickle cell anemia, adult. In contrast to elliptocytes, sickled cells have a densely staining center and pointed ends; three are shown here. Two Howell-Jolly bodies are present, suggesting asplenia. *B*, Blood film, hemoglobin C disease. The numerous target cells and cells with an elongated central density are characteristic. *C*, Blood film, hemoglobin C disease, same patient as in *B* after splenectomy. Four of the red cells here contain densely staining aggregations of Hb C, which tend to become crystals and assume an elongated hexagonal shape. *D*, Sickle cell preparation, in sodium metabisulfite, sickle cell anemia; all the cells are sickled. *E*, Blood film, β-thalassemia trait. Microcytosis: increased number of elliptocytes. Note that target cells may not be prominent. *F*, Blood film, homozygous β-thalassemia. This patient, a black woman, had a relatively mild hemolytic process, a previous splenectomy, and had not recently received a transfusion. This is in contrast to the greater severity of the usual homozygous β-thalassemia in Mediterranean peoples. The localized dense hemoglobin in the normoblast suggests precipitation of α-chains; note the Howell-Jolly body. *G*, Blood film, hemoglobin H disease. A form of thalassemia, this has the combination of microcytic hypochromic red cells and hemolysis. Target cells are numerous. *H*, Film made after incubation of blood with brilliant cresyl blue, hemoglobin H disease, same patient as in *G*. Two reticulocytes have dark blue precipitates of RNA. Several red cells contain multiple smaller pale blue precipitates of Hb H (*G* and *H*: Courtesy of Dr. McDonald K. Horne). *I*, Heinz bodies. Normal red cells incubated with an oxidant drug, acetyl-phenyldrazine, and stained while in suspension by methyl violet; finally, an air-dried film was made and stained with Wright stain. Purple-staining Heinz bodies are precipitates of denatured hemoglobin that tend to be attached to the cell membrane. *J*, Blood film, hereditary spherocytosis. In milder cases, the morphologic clues are a decreased red cell diameter and a decreased amount of central pallor that tends often to be eccentric. *K*, Blood film, pyruvate kinase deficiency, after splenectomy. The contracted, deformed cells were not present prior to splenectomy; they probably represent the most ATP-depleted cells. *L*, Blood film, hemolytic-uremic syndrome. Note the irregularly shaped schistocytes, including helmet cells.

or by chorionic villus sampling (CVS) at 8 to 12 weeks' gestation. The latter is preferable in that it allows therapeutic abortion to take place in the first trimester. However, a recent study indicates that CVS is associated with six-fold increase in limb anomalies (Olney, 1995).

Restriction endonucleases are enzymes that cut DNA into fragments at specific sites depending on base sequences. The fragments are separated by gel electrophoresis, then immobilized on nitrocellulose. Radioactively labeled gene probes then hybridize with the fragments that contain the gene and are detected by autoradiography.

Direct identification of gene mutations may be made by using restriction enzymes and appropriate DNA probes (Table 26–8). In this way, *deletions* may be detected in α-thalassemias or in the rare forms of β-thalassemias due to deletions.

Sickle cell disease provides an example of a variant that is due to a *mutation affecting a restriction site.* Certain restriction endonucleases (Dde I, Mst II) cleave normal DNA at the $\beta^{5,6,7}$-globin gene site, and the sickle mutation at β^6 abolishes the cleavage site. The resulting patterns of DNA fragments that contain the β-globin gene allow clear distinction among normal DNA, heterozygous β^s-DNA, and homozygous β^s-DNA (Chang, 1982; Orkin, 1982).

Restriction fragment length polymorphism (RFLP) linkage analysis depends on harmless single-base changes in DNA that are inherited and either remove existing restriction enzyme sites or produce new ones. If such a site is close to a globin gene, it can be used as a linkage marker for that gene. This approach requires studying a family with multiple restriction enzymes to determine whether a RFLP can be found to be used as a marker for the thalassemia gene (for example) in that family.

Oligonucleotide probes are short synthetized DNA segments that hybridize to homologous sequences in the gene but not if even one base is different. Probes both for the normal segment of DNA and for the same segment of DNA containing a known mutation are used. This technique can define a person's genotype with respect to a given mutation.

In addition, techniques have employed the polymerase chain reaction that amplifies DNA and minimizes the amount required for analysis, and also have substituted nonradioactive for radioactive probes. Rapid analysis of fetal DNA, allowing the detection of sickle cell anemia and of thalassemia major, in many cases is now possible, even in a heterogenous population (Kazazian, 1988; Saiki, 1988; Weatherall, 1994).

Table 26–8. SOME HEMOGLOBIN DISORDERS THAT CAN BE IDENTIFIED DIRECTLY BY FETAL DNA ANALYSIS*

Structural Hemoglobin variants
Hemoglobin S (*Dde* I, *Mst* II, *Mnl* 1)
Hemoglobin O Arab (*Eco* RI)
Hemoglobin Lepore
Thalassemias
α^0 thalassemia
a^+ thalassemia (deletion)
a^+ thalassemia (non-deletion)
5 base-pair deletion IVS I (*Hph* I)
T → C initiation codon (*Nco* I)
β^0 thalassemia (deletion)
β^0 thalassemia
IVS 2 splice junction (*Hph* I)
IVS I (−25 base-pair) (*Fnu* 4H, *Mst* II)
Codon 6 (−16 base-pair) (*Mst* II)
Codon 39, chain termination (*Mae* I)
β^+ thalassemia
IVS 2 745 (*Rsa* I, *Kpn* I)
−87 C → G (*Avr* II)

*Appropriate restruction enzymes are shown in parentheses.
From Weatherall DJ: Prenatal diagnosis of inherited blood diseases. Clin Haematol 1985; 14:747.

Hemolysis—Metabolic Disorders

Deficient enzyme activity in the erythrocyte may result in abnormalities that lead to premature destruction and hemolytic anemia; these disorders usually are inherited. However, interference with or oxidative stress on erythrocyte metabolism sometimes can result in hemolysis in individuals who have normal erythrocytes.

ERYTHROCYTE METABOLISM. The mature red blood cell lacks mitochondria and, therefore, oxidative phosphorylation and Krebs cycle activity. Energy production is mainly glycolytic, 90% of which occurs through the Embden-Meyerhof pathway, as glucose is metabolized to lactic acid with the net production of two moles of adenosine triphosphate (ATP) (Fig. 26–14). ATP is needed for the energy-requiring reactions in the cell: for active cation transport across the membrane, for maintaining membrane deformability, and for preserving the cell's biconcave shape. Most of the hemiglobin (methemoglobin) produced in the normal cell (about 3% of the total per day) is reduced by nicotinamide adenine dinucleotide (NAD)-linked Met Hb reductase. The pentose phosphate pathway (hexose monophosphate shunt) generates nicotinamide adenine dinucleotide phosphate (NADPH) in the first two steps, through the enzymes glucose-6-phosphate dehydrogenase (G6PD) and 6-phosphogluconate. NADPH production is linked to glutathione reduction and, through this mechanism, to preservation of vital enzymes and hemoglobin from oxidation. Small amounts of oxidized hemoglobin (methemoglobin) are reduced by glutathione (GSH). Activity of the pentose phosphate pathway increases when the cell is exposed to an oxidant drug, probably as a result of increased NADP production. If an enzyme in this pathway lacks activity, GSH cannot be produced and hemoglobin will be oxidized by the oxidant stress. Oxidation in the red blood cells is mediated by high-energy derivatives of oxygen referred to collectively as activated oxygen (Carrell, 1975). Oxidized Hb denatures and precipitates as Heinz bodies, which adhere to the membrane, inducing rigidity and a tendency to lysis. Moderate enzyme deficiencies in this pathway (e.g., in G6PD) may not be associated with anemia under normal conditions; however, an acute hemolytic episode occurs if the cells are challenged by oxidant stress (e.g., drugs, infection).

Deficiencies in the Embden-Meyerhof pathway result in impaired ATP generation and a chronic hemolytic anemia. The mechanism of the red blood cell destruction here is less clear. Heinz bodies are not formed. It appears that lack of cell

4

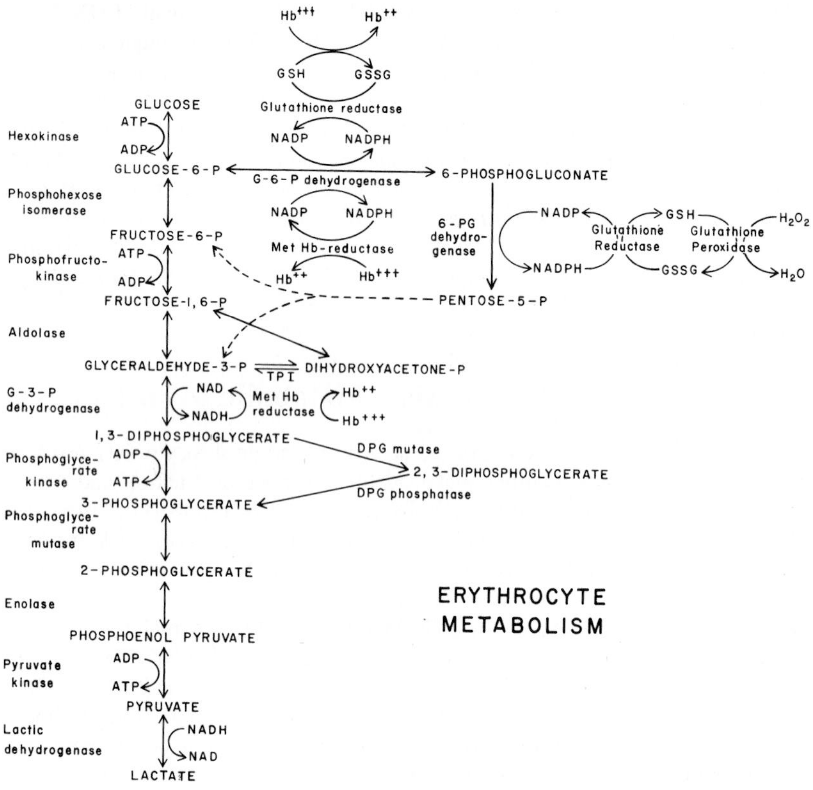

Figure 26–14. Erythrocyte metabolism is discussed in the text. Normally, most hemiglobin (methemoglobin, Hb^{+++}) is reduced to hemoglobin (Hb^{++}) by nicotinamide adenine dinucleotide–linked methemoglobin reductase (NAD, Met Hb reductase). NADP-linked methemoglobin reductase requires methylene blue for activation and is more effective in drug-induced methemoglobinemia than the normal cell mechanism. GSH = reduced glutathione; GSSG = oxidized glutathione.

deformability and impaired cation pumping may be important in the hemolytic process (LaCelle, 1971).

The Rapoport-Luebering shunt provides for the conversion of 1,3-diphosphoglycerate (1,3-DPG) to 2,3-diphosphoglycerate (2,3-DPG) instead of directly to 3-phosphoglycerate (3-PG) (see Fig. 26–14). If this shunt is operating, generation of two moles of ATP (per mole of glucose) is bypassed; the result is no net energy production in glycolysis. However, 2,3-DPG combines with the β-chain of hemoglobin and decreases the affinity of hemoglobin for oxygen. At a given partial pressure of oxygen, therefore, increased 2,3-DPG allows more oxygen to leave hemoglobin and go to the tissues; the oxygen dissociation curve is shifted to the right (see Fig. 25–2). Increased activity of this shunt is apparently stimulated by hypoxia.

GLUCOSE-6-PHOSPHATE DEHYDROGENASE DEFICIENCY. About 10% of male American blacks who were given the antimalarial drug primaquine during the Korean War developed a self-limited, acute hemolytic anemia (Beutler, 1978, 1994). Only the older red blood cells were destroyed, and it was eventually determined that the deficiency in the susceptible red blood cells was in G6PD.

It has since been found that G6PD deficiency is widespread throughout the world. Among whites, the highest incidence is in Kurdish Jews; the deficiency is also found in blacks and in Asians.

Because G6PD is determined by a gene on the X chromosome, full expression of the deficiency is found in the male hemizygote. Partial expression may be found in the heterozygous female who has two populations of red blood cells, one normal and one deficient. The deficiency of G6PD limits the regeneration of NADPH, which renders the cell vulnerable to oxidative denaturation of hemoglobin. Because, normally, G6PD is highest in young cells and decreases as the cell ages, in persons with G6PD deficiency, the older cells are preferentially destroyed.

Hemolytic susceptibility in affected persons can increase greatly during intercurrent illness or on exposure to various drugs that have oxidant properties (Table 26–9).

The genetic heterogeneity is great and is expressed as variation in the stability and the electrophoretic and catalytic properties of the enzymes, in the degree of deficiency, in the types of cells in the body affected, in the types of drugs that will produce hemolysis, and in the susceptibility to chronic hemolysis or to neonatal jaundice. The most common (normal) G6PD isoenzyme in all population groups is designated as B. In blacks, an electrophoretically more rapid variant A is prevalent and has almost the same activity; 20% of black males have this variant. Eleven percent of black males have the A- type of G6PD, which has only 5% to 15% of the nor-

Table 26–9. DRUGS AND CHEMICALS THAT HAVE CLEARLY BEEN SHOWN TO CAUSE CLINICALLY SIGNIFICANT HEMOLYTIC ANEMIA IN G6PD DEFICIENCY

Acetanilid	Primaquine
Methylene blue	Sulfacetamide
Nalidixic acid (Negram)	Sulfanilamide
Naphthalene	Sulfamethoxazole (Gantanol)
Niridazole (Ambilhar)	Sulfapyridine
Nitrofurantoin (Furadantin)	Thiazolesulfone
Pamaquine	Toluidine blue
Pentaquine	Trinitrotoluene (TNT)
Phenylhydrazine	

From Beutler E: Hemolytic Anemia in Disorders of Red Cell Metabolism. New York, Plenum Medical Book Company, 1978.

mal enzyme activity; it is these individuals who are susceptible to hemolysis after ingesting oxidant drugs or during infection. The most common variant in whites is G6PD-Mediterranean, found in Mediterranean populations; the level of enzyme activity in affected males is low, often less than 1%. These individuals usually are not anemic but may have somewhat more severe and non–self-limited hemolytic anemia with infections, and with a wider variety of drugs than the black variant (Beutler, 1978). In a subgroup of G6PD-deficient subjects, severe hemolysis may occur within hours after eating fava beans (called favism). Although the vast majority of G6PD-deficient subjects worldwide are not anemic, a small proportion of persons with G6PD-Mediterranean (and persons with some rarer variants) have a chronic nonspherocytic hemolytic anemia.

The laboratory findings during active hemolysis are those of hemolytic anemia in general. In the blood film, one finds poikilocytes, some spherocytes, and irregularly contracted cells that stain densely and have contraction of Hb from a part of the cell membrane. These probably are cells from which Heinz bodies have been removed by the spleen. After supravital staining with methyl violet, Heinz bodies may be present early in an acute hemolytic episode. G6PD deficiency may be detected by one of the screening tests: the dye reduction test, the ascorbate cyanide test, or a fluorescent spot test. Confirmation is made with a quantitative assay.

Heinz Bodies. When hemoglobin denatures, it forms precipitates that are known as Heinz bodies (Dacie, 1991). These precipitates cannot be detected in Romanowsky-stained, air-dried blood films, but after vital staining with methyl violet or crystal violet, Heinz bodies stain deep purple. They vary from 1 to 4 μm in diameter and often attach to the red blood cell membrane. They also stain, but less intensely, as pale blue inclusions in reticulocyte stains—such as new methylene blue.

The presence of Heinz bodies in freshly drawn blood indicates that (1) an oxidizing drug or chemical (e.g., phenylhydrazine, chlorate, naphthalene, or dapsone) has been ingested in sufficient amount to overwhelm the normal protective mechanisms of the red blood cell and denature hemoglobin; (2) a drug such as primaquine (see Table 26–9) has been ingested by an individual with G6PD deficiency (or another defect resulting in a deficiency of reduced glutathione) so that hemoglobin is not protected from oxidative denaturation; or (3) the subject has an unstable hemoglobin or thalassemia.

Ascorbate Cyanide Test. When blood is incubated with a solution of sodium cyanide and sodium ascorbate, hydrogen peroxide is generated from the coupled oxidation of ascorbate and hemoglobin (Jacob, 1966). Cyanide inhibits catalase, hydrogen peroxide is available to oxidize hemoglobin, and the brown color of methemoglobin is discernible. This occurs more rapidly in G6PD-deficient cells than in normal cells.

The ascorbate cyanide test is not specific, in that pyruvate kinase (PK) deficiency, PNH, and unstable hemoglobins give a positive result. It is the most sensitive of the screening tests, in that it uses intact cells and will detect the deficiency in black males during hemolytic episodes and in heterozygotes (Fairbanks, 1969).

Fluorescent Spot Test. Whole blood is added to a mixture of glucose-6-phosphate (G6P), NADP, saponin, and buffer, and a spot of this mixture is placed on filter paper and observed for fluorescence with ultraviolet light. If G6PD is present, NADP is converted to NADPH. Because phosphogluconate dehydrogenase is present in most hemolysates, further NADP is converted to NADPH (see Fig. 26–14). NADPH fluoresces, but NADP does not. The normal control sample fluoresces brightly, and lack of fluorescence indicates G6PD deficiency. By reoxidizing any small amounts of NADPH formed, oxidized glutathione (GSSG) enhances the ability of the test to detect mild G6PD deficiency. This is the recommended screening test for G6PD deficiency (Beutler, 1979b).

Quantitative Assay of G6PD. For G6PD, most assays are based on the rate of reduction of NADP to NADPH, measured spectrometrically at 340 nm, when a hemolysate is incubated with G6P (Beutler, 1984).

In heterozygotes or in acute hemolysis in black subjects with G6PD deficiency, the diagnosis may be obscured even with the assay because of the increased level of G6PD in reticulocytes and younger erythrocytes. Usually, however, the ascorbate cyanide screening test is positive in these instances.

PYRUVATE KINASE DEFICIENCY. The most common red blood cell enzyme deficiency involving the Embden-Meyerhof glycolytic pathway, PK deficiency results in a mild to moderately severe hemolytic anemia with splenomegaly (Tanaka, 1962). The anemia may be detected in infancy, or not until adult life in milder cases. Patients tolerate the anemia well because of high levels of 2,3-DPG, which occur as a result of the block in glycolysis. The blood film may show no notable red blood cell abnormalities until after splenectomy, when echinocytes, irregularly contracted cells, and crenated red blood cells may be prominent. Reticulocyte counts are elevated and increase further after splenectomy.

Inheritance is autosomal recessive, but this is probably true only in consanguineous families. PK mutants are numerous and are not detected in phenotypically normal heterozygotes who have one half the normal PK activity. Most individuals with PK-deficient hemolytic anemias are therefore probably double heterozygotes for two mutant genes (Valentine, 1979). Acquired PK deficiency occurs occasionally in myelodysplastic disorders and leukemias (Miwa, 1981; Valentine, 1979).

The autohemolysis test gives variable results. Some patients show only a mild increase in autohemolysis that is partially prevented by glucose (Type I), and others have a greater increase that is not prevented by glucose (Type II). Heinz bodies are not found. The diagnosis is made by a specific screening test or enzyme assay.

Splenectomy is indicated in cases requiring transfusions. After splenectomy, the hemoglobin concentration usually increases by 1 to 2 g/dL and the reticulocytes increase sharply, although hemolysis persists (Miwa, 1981).

Fluorescent Spot Test. PK catalyzes the phosphorylation of ADP to ATP by phosphoenolpyruvate (PEP) with the formation of pyruvate (Beutler, 1984). Pyruvate then reduces any NADH present to NAD with the formation of lactate (see Fig. 26–14). Loss of fluorescence of NADH under ultraviolet light is observed as evidence of the presence of PK.

Leukocytes must be removed from the sample because normally they contain about 300 times as much PK as do red blood cells, and in PK deficiency, the red blood cells but not the leukocytes are deficient.

Quantitative Assay of PK. The same principle is employed as in the screening test, but the rate of decrease of absorbance at 340 nm is measured. A negative screening test or a normal PK assay (using the standard high substrate [PEP] concentrations) does not rule out PK-deficient hemolytic anemia. Because mutant PK enzymes may have normal activity at high PEP concentrations and decreased activity at low PEP concentrations, it is necessary to perform the assay in both ways (Beutler, 1984).

OTHER GLYCOLYTIC ENZYME DEFICIENCIES. Other enzyme deficiencies in the *Embden-Meyerhof pathway* are rarer (Keitt, 1981; Valentine, 1989). When severe, they produce hemolytic anemias, with two exceptions: (1) LD deficiency has no clinical manifestations. (2) Deficiencies of 2,3-DPG mutase and 2,3-DPG phosphatase activities occur together and result in erythrocytosis as a result of lack of 2,3-DPG, shifting the oxygen dissociation curve of Hb to the left.

Other enzyme deficiencies in the *hexose monophosphate shunt* are rare. They include the two enzymes involved in glutathione synthesis: γ-glutamyl cysteine synthetase and glutathione synthetase. As in G6PD deficiency, hemolysis increases with oxidant drug exposure or infection.

There is no good evidence, however, for the causation of chronic hemolytic anemia by 6-phosphogluconate deficiency, glutathione reductase (GR) deficiency, or glutathione peroxidase (GP_x) deficiency (Beutler, 1979a). GR contains flavine-adenine dinucleotide and is often partially deficient because of dietary riboflavin deficiency. GP_x is one half normal in about 30% of the Jewish population as a result of homozygosity for a gene for low GP_x activity; in addition, GPx activity is dependent on selenium intake in the diet. In neither case is there an association with a hematologic disorder.

PYRIMIDINE-5'-NUCLEOTIDASE (PN) DEFICIENCY. When RNA is degraded in the reticulocyte, pyrimidine nucleotides must be dephosphorylated by pyrimidine-5'-nucleotidase (PN) in order to cross the red cell membrane (Paglia, 1981). Autosomal recessive PN deficiency results in accumulation of pyrimidines, and the impaired degradation of RNA results in pronounced basophilic stippling in red blood cells on the blood film. This is probably one of the more common enzyme deficiencies responsible for hereditary hemolytic anemia (Beutler, 1979a).

The disorder is characterized by mild to moderate chronic hemolysis, reticulocytosis (~10%), marked basophilic stippling, and splenomegaly without notable improvement after splenectomy. A screening test compares the ultraviolet absorption of deproteinized extracts of red blood cells at 260 nm with that at 280 nm. In PN deficiency, the major aborption peak is shifted from the normal 260 nm to 280 nm, which is the maximum for the pyrimidines uridine diphosphate and cytidine diphosphate. Confirmation requires an assay showing decreased nucleotidase activity (Beutler, 1984).

Acquired PN deficiency occurs in lead poisoning and is probably responsible for the basophilic stippling in that condition.

Hemolysis—Acquired; Extrinsic

Chemical Agents

AGENTS HEMOLYTIC TO NORMAL CELLS. The action of chemical agents depends on the dose and on other factors, many of which are known only vaguely. They range from simple substances, such as water, to some that are highly complex.

When used as irrigating fluid, distilled water was found responsible for acute hemolytic anemia as a result of entry into venous channels during transurethral resection.

In addition to anemia, some chemicals produce methemoglobinemia, and some are responsible for cyanosis (toluene, trinitrotoluene, nitrobenzene, acetanilid, and phenacetin). Some may lead to aplastic anemia (toluene and trinitrotoluene). Promin, a sulfone derivative, makes blood turn chocolate brown.

Lead toxicity may produce progressive anemia, with basophilic stippling, reticulocytosis, normoblastemia, Cabot rings, Howell-Jolly bodies, and leukocytosis. Lead not only causes damage to the red cell and hemolysis but also produces defects in the heme synthetic pathway. In cases of chronic exposure to lead, basophilic stippling, more in the marrow than in the peripheral blood, and coproporphyrinuria are the characteristic findings. These changes produce defective erythrocytes, which are removed by the spleen.

AGENTS HEMOLYTIC TO ABNORMAL CELLS. Certain drugs and chemicals that have oxidizing activity (see Table 26–9) may produce hemolytic anemia in individuals with G6PD deficiency or other defects resulting in glutathione deficiency. In addition, unstable hemoglobins such as Hb Zürich have a propensity for drug-induced hemolytic anemia. Premature infants, although they have high levels of G6PD, have glutathione instability and low levels of glutathione and may develop hemolytic anemia when given large doses of synthetic water-soluble analogues of vitamin K.

It must be remembered that, if the exposure to these oxidant substances is great enough, acute hemolytic anemia may be produced in normal individuals.

During the acute hemolytic episode, Heinz bodies can frequently be demonstrated by direct vital staining of blood with methyl violet. Red blood cells with Heinz bodies are removed from the circulation by the spleen, or the Heinz bodies are extracted from the red blood cells by splenic action. Therefore, Heinz bodies may not be found in the blood if the spleen is effectively removing them or after the acute hemolytic process has abated.

Tests for G6PD deficiency, the most common underlying cause of drug-sensitive hemolytic anemia, are described earlier in this chapter.

Physical Agents

HEAT. Extensive burns produce hemolytic anemia, probably because of direct damage to red blood cells. The blood film may show remarkable morphologic abnormalities of the red blood cells, including budding fragmentation of the membrane and microspherocytosis. The most severe abnormalities are often found immediately after extensive burns, before a reticulocyte response has had time to develop (see Fig. 24–26). The badly damaged cells are rapidly removed from the circulation.

TRAUMATIC HEMOLYSIS. Hemolytic anemia, characterized by striking morphologic abnormalities of the red blood cells, which include fragments (schistocytes) and irregularly contracted cells (triangular cells, helmet cells), has been attributed to physical trauma to the red blood cells (see Fig. 24–31; Plate 26–2*L*). The basis of the hemolytic process is probably damage to the red blood cells in their contact with loose fibrin meshworks (intravascular coagulation) or with pathologic vascular lesions. Fragmentation of the cells results with or without intravascular lysis. Two general categories are recognized in this group of disorders, aptly termed the "red cell fragmentation syndrome."

Cardiac Valvular Disease and Prostheses. Chronic intravascular hemolysis associated with low serum haptoglobin, hemosiderinuria, reticulocytosis, and red blood cell abnormalities (e.g., schistocytes and irregularly contracted cells) may occur after surgical replacement of a diseased heart valve with a prosthesis or after surgical repair of a septal defect with a plastic patch (Marsh, 1969). This has been attributed to mechanical damage of red blood cells in the turbulent environment of a leaky valve or of a roughened surface uncovered by endothelial cells. Repair of the valve or coverage of the patch by endothelium has improved the hemolytic process. Other studies have shown that some patients with cardiac valvular disease have a hemolytic process that may be altered by surgery. The chronic intravascular hemolysis may lead to iron deficiency as a result of loss of hemoglobin in the urine.

Microangiopathic Hemolytic Anemia. Hemolytic anemia with red blood cell fragmentation (e.g., schistocytes and irregularly contracted cells) has been described in malignant hypertension, thrombotic thrombocytopenic purpura, and disseminated carcinoma, in which a common factor was the presence of pathologic lesions involving small blood vessels. The hypothesis was advanced that the hemolytic anemia in these conditions may be an expression of mechanical or perhaps chemical effects of the vascular lesions on the red blood cells, and the process was designated microangiopathic. The role of disseminated or local intravascular coagulation has been recognized as an important factor (although not necessarily the inciting factor) in the pathogenesis of microangiopathy and the resultant hemolysis (Brain, 1972).

A rather distinct clinical state that probably belongs in the latter group as far as the hemolytic mechanism is concerned is the *hemolytic-uremic syndrome (HUS).* It occurs most commonly in infants younger than two years of age and is often preceded by an infection associated with diarrhea. It is likely that some of these cases are due to one of several 0 serotypes of *Escherichia coli* that produce a verotoxin. *E. coli* 0157:H7, for example, produces a verotoxin that probably is cytotoxic to vascular endothelium as well as to intestinal epithelium (Griffin, 1988) and has been incriminated in outbreaks of hemorrhagic colitis associated with HUS. Other etiologic agents (chemicals, viruses) have been implicated as well. Hemolytic anemia with schistocytes (owing to interaction of red cells with microvascular thrombotic lesions), variable thrombocytopenia, and uremia are the cardinal features. Death formerly occurred in almost half of the cases; the renal pathology has included acute glomerulonephritis and thrombotic and necrotic vascular lesions associated with patchy, bilateral renal cortical necrosis. With supportive therapy, including transfusions and dialysis, some investigators have reported that the mortality rate has been reduced to 5% to 15%. Nonetheless, about 15% of patients develop chronic and end-stage renal failure.

HUS appears to be related in some way to *thrombotic thrombocytopenic purpura (TTP).* TTP may occur at any age, but the median age at diagnosis is 35 years; it occurs more often in females than in males. The triad of clinical manifestations present in most patients includes hemolytic anemia, thrombocytopenia, and neurologic symptoms; in addition, fever and renal diseases are often present. Pathologically, microvascular occlusive lesions with hyaline thrombi and endothelial proliferation are widespread throughout the body. The etiology is unknown; different pathologic mechanisms and probably different etiologies are implicated (Lian, 1987). Endothelial injury with release of large von Willebrand factor multimers into the plasma, impaired prostacyclin production by endothelium, formation of microvascular platelet thrombi, and impaired local fibrinolytic activity appear to be involved in the pathogenesis. The disease is acute and, until the 1980s, was fatal in well over half of the cases. With the therapy of plasma exchange by plasmapheresis and plasma transfusions (in addition to platelet inhibitors), the remission rate has improved from about 30% to over 80% (Shepard, 1987). Preeclampsia and eclampsia are microangiopathic disorders occurring with pregnancy and sharing some features of HUS or TTP. Approximately 4% to 12% of patients with severe eclampsia develop HELLP syndrome: *H*emolysis, *E*levated *L*iver enzymes and *L*ow *P*latelet count. Most patients recover within a few days after delivery. A small subset of patients develop severe persistent multisystem disease that requires plasma exchange (Martin, 1991).

Infectious Agents

Destruction of erythrocytes by plasmodia is responsible for the anemia in malaria. This is supported by the observation that the osmotic and mechanical fragility of parasitized erythrocytes is increased. Inhibition of marrow activity may be an additional factor. Fulminant hemoglobinuria (blackwater fever) is a complication of *P. falciparum* malaria.

Oroya fever, a frequently fatal disease that occurs in Peru, is characterized by a hemolytic anemia and leukocytosis. *Bartonella bacilliformis* is the responsible agent.

Babesiosis, a protozoan infection transmitted by ticks from rodents or cattle, is associated with hemolysis; parasites may be seen in red blood cells in Romanowsky-stained blood films.

Hemolytic anemia with cold agglutinins may complicate mycoplasmal pneumonia and infectious mononucleosis. This is due to the effect of antibody on the red blood cells.

Hemolytic anemia of varying severity is frequent in some bacterial infections. A notable example is *Clostridium perfringens* septicemia following septic abortion or biliary tract surgery, which may be accompanied by a dramatic and life-threatening hemolytic crisis.

Immune Hemolytic Anemias

Immune hemolytic anemias are disorders in which erythrocyte survival is reduced because of the deposition of immunoglobulin or complement, or both, on the red blood cell membrane. The immune hemolytic anemias can be grouped according to the presence of autoantibodies, isoantibodies, or drug-related antibodies (Table 26–10).

AUTOIMMUNE HEMOLYTIC ANEMIA. The AIHAs are due to an altered immune response resulting in the production of antibody against the host's own erythrocytes, with subsequent hemolysis. The AIHAs can be classified according to

4

Table 26–10. CLASSIFICATION OF IMMUNE HEMOLYTIC ANEMIAS

Autoimmune hemolytic anemias
Associated with warm antibodies
Associated with cold antibodies
Combined warm and cold antibodies
Isoimmune hemolytic anemias
Hemolytic disease of newborn
Rh incompatibility
ABO incompatibility
Drug-induced hemolytic anemia
Adsorption of immune complexes to red cell membrane
Adsorption of drug to red cell membrane
Induction of autoantibody by drugs
Nonimmunologic adsorption of immunoglobin to red blood cell membrane

serologic or clinical characteristics (Table 26–11). Some AIHAs are mediated by antibodies with maximum binding affinity at 37°C, and other AIHAs are mediated by antibodies with their maximum binding affinity at 4°C. In addition, AIHAs could be viewed according to their association with other disorders. In a study of 1834 patients, approximately 40% of cases of AIHA have been associated with an underlying disease, while the remainder are idiopathic (Sokol, 1992).

Etiology and Pathophysiology. The cause of the production of autoantibody in patients with AIHA is unknown. However, several mechanisms have been suggested. Autoimmune antibodies are sometimes produced following an infection. This is typically seen with the elaboration of anti-I in patients with *Mycoplasma pneumoniae* infections. It has been hypothesized that the autoantibody may be a response to sensitization from a breakdown component of the *M. pneumoniae* organism. In infectious mononucleosis, anti-i antibody is present in the serum of patients and it occasionally results in AIHA. Because the i-antigen is normally on the lymphocyte membrane, perhaps in this disorder the production of anti-i is part of an effort to remove host-infected B cells.

The development of AIHA in patients with lymphoproliferative disorders or with autoimmune disorders may relate to some abnormality with B cells, T cells, macrophages, or the interaction among these cells. Perhaps loss of T-cell suppressor function could result in unrestrained production of red blood cell antibody by B cells. This hypothesis is strengthened by the observation that methyldopa, a drug known to cause the development of anti-red cell antibodies, inhibits the activation of suppressor T lymphocytes (Kirtland, 1980).

In AIHA associated with warm-type antibody, there is IgG coating of erythrocytes with or without complement fixation. Clearance of red blood cells occurs mostly in the spleen. In the absence of complement fixation, it appears that the Fc portion of the red blood cell–bound IgG immunoglobulin interacts with the Fc receptor present on the membrane of splenic macrophages located along the cords of Billroth. Thus, sensitized erythrocytes are retained, phagocytosed, or fragmented by splenic macrophages during their passage through the spleen.

In AIHA associated with the production of cold-type autoantibody, the erythrocytes are usually coated with IgM immunoglobulin. Under these circumstances, the fixation of complement frequently occurs. In paroxysmal cold hemoglobinuria, the offending antibody is an IgG immunoglobulin that fixes complement. If the entire complement sequence is activated, there may be intravascular hemolysis. This phenomenon may occur in cases of cold hemagglutinin disease as well as in paroxysmal cold hemoglobinuria. If complement activation fails to proceed to completion but is halted at an intermediate stage, intravascular lysis of the erythrocytes may not occur. However, extravascular hemolysis can still

Table 26–11. AUTOIMMUNE HEMOLYTIC ANEMIA (AIHA)

		Cold AIHA		
Condition	**Warm AIHA**	***CHAD***	***PCH***	**Mixed AIHA**
Idiopathic	282 (23)	194 (16)	5 (<1)	47 (4)
Drug-induced disorders	184 (15)	0	0	2 (<1)
Neoplasia	165 (14)	81 (7)	0 (0)	26 (2)
Non-Hodgkin's lymphoma	27	25	0	8
Chronic lymphocytic leukemia	65	4	0	8
Hodgkin's lymphoma	11	7	0	5
Carcinomas	37	30	0	4
Miscellaneous	25	15	0	1
Infections	9 (<1)	76 (6)	14 (1)	2 (<1)
Pneumonia-mycoplasma	0	21	0	0
Viral pneumonia	2	19	0	0
Infectious mononucleosis	0	11	1	0
Miscellaneous	7	25	13	2
Collagen diseases	30 (2)	15 (1)	0 (0)	20 (2)
Systemic lupus erythematosus	7	4	0	16
Rheumatoid arthritis	21	6	0	4
Others	2	5	0	0
Miscellaneous disorders	45 (4)	20 (2)	0	6 (<1)
Totals	715 (58)	386 (32)	19 (2)	103 (8)

Note: Numbers in parentheses are percentages. CHAD = cold hemagglutinin disease; PCH = paroxysmal cold hemoglobinuria.

Modified and reprinted with permission from Sokol RJ, Hewitt S: CRC Critical Reviews in Oncology-Hematology, 1985; 4:125. Copyright CRC Press, Inc., Boca Raton, FL.

continue. In this situation, sensitized cells with C3b on the membrane are bound in the liver by the interaction of C3b and its receptors on Kupffer cells. Erythrocytes may be phagocytosed entirely, or portions of the cells may be removed, resulting in fragmentation and spherocyte formation.

Approximately 7% of patients with AIHA satisfy diagnostic criteria for both warm and cold autoantibodies (Sokol, 1992). In these cases, IgG and C3d sensitize the erythrocytes. The serum contains IgM cold autohemagglutinins (optimally reactive at 4°C, but with a high thermal amplitude to 37°C) and IgG warm autoantibodies.

AIHA Associated with Warm Antibody. The warm antibody type of AIHA is slightly more frequent in females than in males and is most likely to occur in individuals 40 years of age or older. The clinical signs and symptoms frequently are those of an underlying disorder. However, in individuals with idiopathic AIHA, the patient may have noted the presence of a mild upper respiratory tract infection just prior to the onset of hemolysis. As the disorder progresses, there may be weakness, dizziness, and fever. Jaundice can be a presenting complaint.

Laboratory findings include the presence of a moderate to severe anemia. The neutrophil count may be increased. In a small proportion of cases, thrombocytopenia can exist. The peripheral film frequently shows spherocytosis, red blood cell fragmentation, polychromasia, and a few normoblasts (see Fig. 24–25). Reticulocyte percentage is high in approximately 50% of patients. The lack of reticulocytosis should not keep one from making a diagnosis of AIHA. The bone marrow exhibits normoblastic erythroid hyperplasia, sometimes with mild megaloblastic changes.

There is usually a decrease in serum haptoglobin and an increase in unconjugated bilirubin. The osmotic fragility and autohemolysis test can be either normal or abnormal.

The direct and indirect antiglobulin tests indicate the presence of erythrocyte antibodies. The specificity of the autoantibody is usually directed against antigens of the Rh system. However, activity against U, LW, Kell, jk^a, and Fy^a antigens may also occur. The warm antibody is most likely an IgG immunoglobulin with subclass IgG1 and less frequently with IgG3. When either IgG2 or IgG4 is present on the red blood cells alone, there is no associated hemolytic reaction (Petz, 1980). Occasionally, the antibody may be an IgA immunoglobulin and rarely an IgM immunoglobulin. Complement may be detected on the erythrocyte membrane in slightly over half of the cases.

In some cases, sensitized red blood cells contain less immunoglobulin than can be detected using commercially prepared antiglobulins, which are normally sensitive to 250 to 500 molecules of IgG per red blood cell (Gilliland, 1976). Under these circumstances, the autoantibody can at times be detected with an antiglobulin consumption test.

The clinical course of AIHA associated with warm antibody is characterized by periods of remissions and relapse. In secondary AIHA, the course and prognosis are related to the nature of the underlying disorder. In idiopathic AIHA, the complications of the hemolytic disorder may be severe and lead to the demise of the patient.

AIHA Associated with Cold Antibody. AIHA associated with cold antibody can be mediated by an IgM immunoglobulin and less frequently by an IgG immunoglobulin. The IgM autoantibody is associated with a syndrome known as cold hemagglutinin disease, whereas the IgG autoantibody is seen with paroxysmal cold hemoglobinuria.

Cold Hemagglutinin Disease. Cold hemagglutinin disease occurs in individuals usually older than 50 years of age and in females more often than in males. In some cases, cold hemagglutinin disease is associated with a lymphoreticular malignancy or autoimmune disorder. Other cases appear as a complication of infection (especially with *M. pneumoniae*). Cases unassociated with an underlying disorder are listed as idiopathic.

Symptoms and signs vary widely. Some individuals may complain of acrocyanosis or Raynaud's phenomenon. Others have episodes of hemolysis following exposure to cold.

The laboratory findings usually indicate anemia. Spherocytes and polychromatophilic erythrocytes are present to a variable degree in the blood film. There may be marked red blood cell agglutination, which should be differentiated from rouleau formation (see Figs. 24–37 and 24–38). A mild leukocytosis can exist.

The cold antibody is usually an IgM immunoglobulin with anti-I, or less frequently anti-i, specificity. Rarely do other specificities exist. In the chronic idiopathic form of cold hemagglutinin disease, the antibody tends to be monoclonal IgM, κ with anti-I specificity or IgM, λ with anti-i specificity (Petz, 1980). The autoantibody is also capable of fixing complement. When the titer of cold antibody is very high, the thermal range of antibody activity may extend up to 37°C. The direct antiglobulin test is positive only if the reagents contain anti-complement activity. Thus, one usually observes a positive antiglobulin reaction with the broad spectrum and non-γ reagents but no agglutination with only the γ reagent.

4

Paroxysmal Cold Hemoglobinuria. Paroxysmal cold hemoglobinuria is a very rare disorder that can occur in an individual of any age. Females are as frequently involved as males. Patients have symptoms of acute hemolysis following exposure to the cold. There are chills, fever, pain in the back and legs, and hemoglobinuria. The acute form may follow an acute viral illness, but the chronic form is associated with congenital syphilis.

The laboratory features consist of anemia, elevated reticulocyte count, increased concentration of indirect bilirubin, and the presence of hemoglobin in the urine.

The serum contains a cold hemolysin with biphasic activity. This antibody, first described by Donath and Landsteiner (1904), is an IgG immunoglobulin that fixes the first components of complement (C1 to C4) in the cold (4°C). As the temperature rises to 25° to 37°C, the remainder of the complement proteins are activated and erythrocyte lysis results. The specificity of the antibody is directed against the P antigen. In general, the prognosis is good.

AIHA Associated with Warm and Cold Antibodies. AIHA associated with both warm and cold autoantibodies is mediated by IgG warm antibodies and complement as well as IgM cold hemagglutinins. Females are more likely to have this condition than are males. There appears to be an association between the combined warm and cold antibody AIHA and systemic lupus erythematosus (SLE) in that 15% to 42% of these patients have SLE (Shulman, 1985; Sokol, 1985). In one study (Shulman, 1985), 6 of 12 patients (50%) had idiopathic AIHA and 4 of these (33%) had concomitant thrombocytopenia (Evans' syndrome); all 12 patients had severe hemolysis that responded dramatically to corticosteroid therapy.

ISOIMMUNE HEMOLYTIC ANEMIA. Isoimmune hemolytic anemia usually occurs in newborns following the transplacental passage of maternal antifetal red blood cell antibody. Isoimmune hemolytic disease of the newborn most frequently results from incompatibility in Rh and ABO erythrocyte antigens between the mother and the fetus. In rare cases, some other red blood cell antigen may be responsible for this disorder (see Chap. 38).

In isoimmune hemolytic disease of the newborn due to *Rh incompatibility,* prior sensitization is necessary to initiate the disease process. This sensitization usually occurs during pregnancy when Rh(D) fetal red blood cells cross the placenta and enter the circulation of a mother with Rh negative cells. Maternal sensitization can also occur by a previous incompatible transfusion. Under either of these circumstances, maternal IgG antibodies are produced against the fetal cells. If a subsequent pregnancy occurs in a sensitized mother, fetal erythrocytes again reach the maternal circulation and restimulate an antibody response, resulting in transfer of anti-Rh(D) antibody across the placenta and reduced fetal red blood cell survival.

In the *ABO system,* anti-A or anti-B antibodies of the IgG class may arise spontaneously in the mother; their presence does not require prior transfusion or pregnancy. As a result, first-born children may suffer from isoimmune hemolytic disease when ABO incompatibility exists.

The clinical features of *isoimmune hemolytic disease of the newborn due to Rh incompatibility* vary greatly. Some newborns experience only mild jaundice. Others initially appear markedly pale and then develop jaundice. They can have prominent hepatosplenomegaly. The disease may be complicated by a bleeding diathesis, marked acid-base abnormalities, and kernicterus. In very severe cases, patients can present with hydrops fetalis.

Early examination of the blood usually reveals an increase in nucleated erythrocytes, which may include forms as immature as pronormoblasts. Although this finding gave the disease its name, *erythroblastosis fetalis,* erythroblastosis is not always present, especially if the examination is not performed immediately after birth.

Up to 2.0×10^9 nucleated red cells/L in term infants and up to 5.0×10^9/L in premature infants are commonly seen in this disorder. Normally, nucleated red cells average 0.5×10^9/L in term infants and 1.0 to 1.5×10^9/L in premature infants. Blood from the umbilical vein for early examination is more reliable than peripheral (capillary) blood because the erythrocyte count and the hemoglobin may be significantly altered between birth and ligation of the cord.

Generally, there is a macrocytic anemia of varying severity and an increase in reticulocytes. Occasionally, anemia may develop suddenly on the second or third day. The leukocyte count is frequently elevated, with immature leukocytes. There is pronounced normoblastic hyperplasia of the marrow.

In severely affected infants, there may be thrombocytopenia, depression of the prothrombin complex procoagulants, or diffuse intravascular coagulation.

A direct antiglobulin test on fetal erythrocytes indicates the presence of an IgG antibody. When the maternal serum and an eluate from the fetal erythrocytes are incubated separately with a panel of O cells, one usually can demonstrate the presence of antibody with Rh(D) specificity. In Rh negative pregnant women known to be sensitized to Rh(D), the titer of anti-Rh(D) antibody is measured periodically during pregnancy to serve as a guide for performing amniocentesis (see Chap. 31).

Isoimmune hemolytic disease of the newborn associated with ABO incompatibility is less severe than that observed with Rh incompatibility. Occasionally, the diagnosis is suggested by the presence of unexplained hyperbilirubinemia in a group A or B newborn infant from a group O mother.

Laboratory findings usually show a mild anemia and modest reticulocytosis. In contrast to Rh isoimmune disease, spherocytosis in ABO isoimmune disease may be prominent. However, there may be no anemia. The fetal cells are usually weakly positive with the antiglobulin reagents. Serum from the newborn and eluates from the cells should contain anti-A or anti-B antibody. In addition, the maternal serum should contain high titers of anti-A or anti-B antibodies of the IgG subclass.

DRUG-INDUCED IMMUNE HEMOLYTIC ANEMIA. Immune hemolytic anemia may occur following the administration of drugs. Four mechanisms appear to mediate the immune hemolysis (Petz, 1980).

Adsorption of Immune Complexes to Red Blood Cell Membrane. Numerous drugs are known to provoke an antibody response with subsequent adsorption of immune complexes to the erythrocyte membrane (Table 26–12). The drug-induced antibody is usually IgM and tends to fix complement, resulting in lysis of cells.

Patients present with acute intravascular hemolysis, hemoglobinemia, and hemoglobinuria. The direct antiglobulin reaction is positive if the reagents contain anticomplement activity. The reaction usually is negative with the γ-reagent because it contains little anti-IgM or complement specificity.

The diagnosis can be determined by incubating the patient's serum with the offending drug in the presence of target erythrocytes, and observing agglutination, lysis, or sensitization of the erythrocytes.

Table 26–12. DRUGS ACCEPTED AS CAUSING IMMUNE HEMOLYTIC ANEMIA BY THE ADSORPTION OF IMMUNE COMPLEXES TO RED CELLS

Stibophen
Quinidine
Para-aminosalicylic acid
Quinine
Phenacetin
Chlorinated hydrocarbon-containing insecticides
Antihistamines
Sulfonamides
Isonicotinic acid hydrazine
Chlorpromazine
Aminopyrine
Dipyrone
Melphalan
Mefenamic acid
Sulfonylureas
Insulin
Rifampin

Modified from Petz LD, Garratty G. Clin Haematol 1975; 4:181.

Adsorption of Drug to the Red Blood Cell Membrane. Penicillin and cephalosporin combine with protein normally present on the erythrocyte membrane. These drugs, once bound to the red blood cell membrane, form haptenic groups and provoke an immune response. Both IgM and IgG antibodies are made, but only the IgG antibodies are associated with the immune hemolysis. Complement is not involved. The erythrocytes, coated with IgG antibody, are presumably removed via the Fc receptors on macrophages in the spleen.

The direct antiglobulin test is strongly positive. Antibody eluted from patients' erythrocytes react only with red blood cells previously treated with penicillin or cephalosporins.

Induction of Autoantibody by Drugs. In approximately 15% of patients using the antihypertensive drug methyldopa, a positive direct antiglobulin reaction is present. The antibody is of the IgG class and, in some studies, appears to have Rh specificity (Croft, 1968). However, other studies indicate that there may be nonspecific erythrocyte adsorption of γ-globulin altered by exposure to methyldopa (Gottlieb, 1974). Kirtland (1980) demonstrated that methyldopa caused an elevation of intracellular lymphocyte cyclic AMP and an inhibition of T-lymphocyte suppressor activity. The investigators postulated that these effects may lead to unregulated autoantibody production by B cells in some patients.

The development of the positive antiglobulin reaction is dose dependent. Thirty-six percent of patients have a positive antiglobulin reaction when consuming 2 g or more of methyldopa per day, and 11% have a positive reaction when taking only 1 g daily. An immune hemolytic anemia occurs in less than 1% of patients. Methyldopa also decreases mononuclear phagocytic activity, which may explain the rarity of hemolytic anemia despite the common presence of autoantibodies (Sokol, 1992). L-Dopa, procainamide, and mefenamic acid are additional drugs that have been reported to cause an AHIA in a fashion similar to methyldopa.

Nonimmunologic Adsorption of Immunoglobulins to the Red Blood Cell Membrane. Cephalosporins appear to alter the erythrocyte membrane, resulting in the nonspecific adsorption of plasma proteins to its surface. As a result, IgG and IgM immunoglobulin may be loosely bound to the red blood cell membrane. This phenomenon can then cause a positive direct antiglobulin reaction (Petz, 1980).

Laboratory Diagnosis of Anemia

The diagnosis and study of anemia require the proper use and interpretation of laboratory measurements. The prerequisites for the efficient use of the laboratory are a careful history and physical examination, both of which lead to the initial laboratory measurements and provide important guidance in determining the nature of the anemia.

Whether the patient is anemic can be ascertained by determining whether the hemoglobin, hematocrit, or erythrocyte count lies below (1) the reference intervals for age and sex, or (2) the patient's previous values, even though these are within the reference intervals. Then the task is to define the underlying cause or mechanism for the anemia.

Usually, the complete blood count (white blood cells, red blood cells, Hb, Hct, MCV, MCH, MCHC) and examination of a Wright-stained film are parts of the routine examination of the blood. It is possible that all these values could be normal in the presence of a mild macrocytic anemia, in which the red blood cell count does not fall below the normal range, and the macrocytes present (and detectable on the blood film) do not elevate the MCV above the normal range.

Once anemia is discovered, the basic examination of the blood should include the following: (1) hemoglobin, hematocrit, red blood cell count, and erythrocyte indices; (2) blood film examination; (3) leukocyte count; (4) platelet count; and (5) reticulocyte count.

With current multichannel instruments, all red blood cell values and the indices have comparable precision. Indices are *mean* values, however, and do not detect different populations of cells that balance each other. For example, combined deficiencies of folate and iron may give rise to populations of macrocytic and hypochromic microcytic cells, which could yield normal indices. Careful examination of the blood film is essential, and cell volume distribution curves are very useful in defining this type of abnormality (see Chap. 24).

The size of the erythrocytes, determined by the MCV and examination of the blood film, determines the morphologic type of anemia. In addition, certain findings on the blood film suggest mechanisms that are involved.

Increased numbers of *polychromatic* macrocytes, with or without normoblasts, suggest increased erythropoiesis, and in the untreated patient, this usually is due to hemorrhage or hemolysis. In this situation, the history (of blood loss) or physical examination (jaundice or splenomegaly) will help in arriving at the appropriate diagnosis.

Findings suggestive of hemolysis are *poikilocytes* (abnormally shaped red blood cells), *sickle cells, irregularly contracted forms* (including red blood cell fragments or schistocytes), and *spherocytes.* Sometimes it is difficult to detect spherocytes in hereditary spherocytosis because of minimal anisocytosis. The two findings in the red blood cells that are helpful in this situation are the presence of a low mean cell diameter (MCD) between 6.0 and 6.5 m (normal = 7.0 to 7.4) and red blood cells with eccentric pallor.

Target cells may be found in hemoglobinopathies, especially in the presence of Hb C, Hb D, and Hb E, and in the thalassemias. They may be present in any *hypochromic* anemia, although usually in smaller numbers. Target cells without microcytosis are also found in liver disease and in the absence of the spleen or of splenic function.

Fine *basophilic stippling* (which is due to precipitation of RNA) may be found in polychromatic red blood cells associated with a significant increase in the generation of erythrocytes, as in response to hemorrhage or hemolysis. *Coarse basophilic stippling* suggests an abnormality in hemoglobin synthesis. It is found in megaloblastic anemias, thalassemias, refractory anemias, and lead poisoning. In particular, hypochromasia or microcytosis with stippling excludes the diagnosis of iron deficiency anemia and is more suggestive of thalassemia or lead poisoning.

The combination of *oval macrocytes* (especially egg-shaped macrocytes) and *hypersegmented neutrophils* indicates the very likely existence of megaloblastic anemia.

Finally, examination of the blood film allows the evaluation of *qualitative abnormalities in leukocytes and platelets,* as well as an estimate of their numbers. Blood diseases that may be first suspected or detected in this manner are many and include chronic lymphocytic leukemia; compensated hemolytic anemia; early megaloblastic anemia; and anomalies of red blood cells, such as HE, or of leukocytes, such as myelodysplasia or the Pelger-Hüet anomaly.

After the basic studies just mentioned, the choice of further procedures depends on the morphologic type of the anemia, as determined by the indices and the blood film.

Macrocytic Anemia (Increased Mean Cell Volume)

The macrocytic anemias are normochromic, as determined by appearance on the film and by the MCHC. The first step is to ascertain whether the anemia is megaloblastic. The clues from the film have been mentioned. A *bone marrow aspiration* should be performed to confirm the presence of megaloblastosis.

MEGALOBLASTIC MARROW. If the marrow is *megaloblastic,* with characteristic changes in both red blood cell and white blood cell precursors, in all likelihood, the anemia is due to folate or cobalamin deficiency.

See the sections on diagnosis of cobalamin deficiency and of folate deficiency. Once the *type* of deficiency is defined, the *cause* must be determined.

NONMEGALOBLASTIC MARROW. If the marrow is *not megaloblastic,* conditions that can be associated with macrocytosis should be investigated. These include liver disease; hemolytic anemias; hypothyroidism; excessive alcohol intake; hypoplastic anemias; and refractory anemias with hyperplastic bone marrow, which include the myelodysplastic syndromes. Anemias associated with these disorders, although they *may* be macrocytic, are more usually normocytic and thus are considered with the normocytic anemias.

Microcytic and Hypochromic Anemias (Decreased Mean Cell Volume and Mean Cell Hemoglobin)

If the counts are performed on a multichannel instrument, the MCHC is likely to be in the normal range, with slight to moderate degrees of hypochromia. Consequently, the MCV has assumed the leading role in the detection of microcytic hypochromic anemias.

These anemias reflect a quantitative defect in hemoglobin synthesis:

1. *Iron deficiency anemias* are due to increased requirement or blood loss not balanced by intake.
2. *Anemia of chronic disorders* is associated with infection, neoplasia, or collagen disease. This anemia may be normochromic and normocytic but in long-standing disease is often hypochromic and microcytic.
3. *Thalassemia* is a genetically determined impairment in the rate of globin synthesis.
4 *Sideroblastic anemia* is that group of refractory anemias with erythroid hyperplasia of the marrow in which a defect in hemoglobin synthesis creates a population of hypochromic microcytic cells. The blood film is dimorphic, and macrocytes may prevail, making the MCV normal or high.

Because *iron deficiency* is the most common anemia, the first step is to determine whether the body lacks iron.

When blood loss cannot be documented, serum ferritin, serum iron and iron-binding capacity, or bone marrow study for iron should be performed. These studies usually discriminate between the two most common anemias in this category, iron deficiency and simple chronic anemia associated with some other disease—frequently chronic infection or cancer. In both, the serum iron concentration is low, but in iron deficiency, the total iron-binding capacity is elevated, whereas in simple chronic anemia it is normal or decreased. Storage iron in the marrow is depleted in iron deficiency but is normal or elevated in simple chronic anemia. Iron deficiency anemia in an adult male almost always means chronic blood loss; the source must be found and corrected, if necessary.

Hypochromic anemias (or erythrocytoses) with basophilic stippling and normal or increased serum iron are most likely *thalassemias,* and the next examinations to perform are hemoglobin electrophoresis and determination of Hb A_2 and Hb F. Family studies often are necessary.

Sideroblastic anemias include idiopathic refractory sideroblastic anemias, which are part of the myelodysplastic syndromes (see Chap. 27), as well as anemias that occur after therapy with certain drugs (e.g., isoniazid) or in chronic lead poisoning. Coarse basophilic stippling is common in this group of anemias.

Table 26–13 summarizes some laboratory distinctions within the microcytic anemias.

Normocytic and Normochromic Anemias (Normal Mean Cell Volume)

This large group of anemias has many causes. A useful approach is evaluation of the erythrokinetics in a given patient (see Chap. 25). Often, the reticulocyte production index (RPI) and examination of the bone marrow suffice. The RPI is the simplest measure of effective erythropoiesis.

OPTIMAL MARROW RESPONSE: RETICULOCYTE PRODUCTION INDEX GREATER THAN TWO. If the output of reticulocytes has exceeded two times normal, as determined by the absolute reticulocyte count or RPI, it can be assumed that the marrow has reached an optimal response. The cause for the anemia is then either *acute blood loss* or *hemolysis.* If blood loss cannot be proved, evidence that hemolysis is in fact present must be sought.

Erythroid hyperplasia of the marrow, serum bilirubin, and urine or fecal urobilinogen indicate whether erythropoietic activity and destruction are increased. Red blood cell survival determination may be needed to prove hemolysis in some cases. Low serum haptoglobin points to hemolysis, but a normal level does not exclude it. None of these measurements specify whether hemolysis is intravascular or extravascular, but elevated plasma hemoglobin, hemoglobinuria, and hemosiderinuria indicate intravascular hemolysis.

Once it is determined that excessive hemolysis is occurring, the type of hemolytic mechanism must be ascertained.

The *direct antiglobulin (Coombs') test* is a useful guide to further study.

If the direct antiglobulin reaction is *positive* using broad-spectrum reagents, tests to determine the presence of IgG, IgM, or complement on the red blood cells should be undertaken. If immunoglobulin is present on the red blood cells, tests for antibody specificity, cold agglutinins, Donath-Landsteiner antibody, and serum protein electrophoresis may help define the process.

Table 26–13. LABORATORY FEATURES IN MICROCYTIC HYPOCHROMIC ANEMIAS

	Serum Iron	Serum TIBC	% Saturation	Marrow: % *Sideroblasts*	Marrow: *Iron Stores*	Serum Ferritin	FEP	Hb A_2	Hb F
Iron deficiency	↓	↑	↓	↓	↓	↓	↑	N-↓	N
β-Thalassemia trait	N (↑)	N	N	N	N-↑	N-↑	N	↑	N-↑
Anemia of chronic disease	↓	N-↓	↓	↓	N-↑	N-↑	↑	N	N
Sideroblastic anemia	↑	↓	↑	↑	↑	↑	↑ (↓)	N	N-↑

TIBC = total iron-binding capacity; FEP = free erythrocyte porphyrins; ↓ = decreased; N = normal; ↑ = increased.

If the direct antiglobulin reaction is *negative,* the examinations performed next depend on the clinical findings and the results of the measurements already made.

If hereditary spherocytosis is suspected, osmotic fragility before and after 24-hour incubation at 37°C and family studies will be necessary.

If a nonspherocytic congenital hemolytic anemia is suspected, screening for G6PD and PK deficiencies, hemoglobin electrophoresis, and a sickle cell test are helpful. If these tests are negative, the heat instability, isopropanol solubility, and autohemolysis tests should be considered.

If thalassemia seems likely, determinations of HbA_2 and Hb F and perhaps a search for Hb H inclusions are appropriate. Thalassemias usually are microcytic and hypochromic anemias; β-thalassemia major, β-thalassemia intermedia, and hemoglobin H disease are hemolytic disorders and may have an increased RPI.

If drug-induced hemolysis is suspected, a test for Heinz bodies, screening test for G6PD, and if possible, tests for a drug-dependent autoantibody are indicated.

If the nature of the hemolytic anemia is obscure, a sucrose hemolysis test for paroxysmal nocturnal hemoglobinuria should be performed.

INADEQUATE MARROW RESPONSE: RETICULOCYTE PRODUCTION INDEX LESS THAN TWO. The mechanism of the anemia may be ineffective erythropoiesis. Conditions with the greatest degree of ineffective erythropoiesis appear in other categories (e.g., megaloblastic anemia and thalassemia), but some idiopathic refractory anemias have a hyperplastic bone marrow and impaired delivery of the cells to the blood. In some of these anemias, abnormalities in erythroid precursors suggestive of megaloblastic change may be present, but the granulocytic and megakaryocytic changes usually seen in megaloblastic anemia are lacking.

A low reticulocyte count may indicate decreased production caused by inadequate stimulation of the marrow. Chronic renal disease may result in impaired production of EPO. Certain endocrinopathies, such as hypopituitarism or hypothyroidism, may result in regulation of hemoglobin production at a lower level as a result of decreased tissue need for oxygen.

A large group of normochromic anemias associated with various chronic diseases form a heterogeneous group characterized by failure of the marrow to meet the need caused by a slightly decreased red blood cell survival. Some of these types are anemia of chronic disorders associated with infection, cancer, or rheumatoid arthritis and have the defect in iron metabolism noted previously under the hypochromic microcytic anemias.

Inability of the marrow to respond to EPO may be due to damage to the marrow by drugs or toxic chemicals, to unknown causes, or to infiltration of the marrow by neoplastic cells or fibrous tissue.

In those conditions with low reticulocyte counts in which the marrow is not effectively producing erythrocytes, it usually is helpful to examine the bone marrow. Other studies to determine the underlying disease process can then proceed according to the marrow picture, the assessment of erythrokinetics, and the clinical findings.

4

POLYCYTHEMIA

Polycythemia (erythrocytosis) is classically defined as an elevated hematocrit level above the normal range rather than an increased hemoglobin concentration or red blood cell count (Landaw, 1990).

Absolute polycythemia refers to an increase in the total red blood cell mass in the body; in *relative polycythemia,* the total red blood cell mass is normal, but the hematocrit is elevated because the plasma volume is decreased. Polycythemia may be classified as in Table 26–14.

Table 26–14. CLASSIFICATION OF POLYCYTHEMIA

Relative polycythemia

1. Diminished plasma volume: dehydration; shock
2. Spurious polycythemia (stress polycythemia; Gaisböck's syndrome)

Absolute polycythemia

1. Secondary polycythemia (increased erythropoietin)
    a. Appropriate erythropoietin production; hypoxia
        1. Arterial oxygen unsaturation: high altitude; pulmonary disease; cyanotic heart disease; smoker's polycythemia; methemoglobinemia; Hb M
        2. High oxygen affinity hemoglobinopathy
    b. Inappropriate erythropoietin production
        1. Neoplasms: renal carcinoma; cerebellar hemangioma; hepatoma; uterine fibroids; adrenal cortical neoplasms
        2. Renal pathology: cysts; hydronephrosis; transplantation
    c. Familial polycythemia
2. Polycythemia vera

Modified from Berlin NI: Semin Hematol, 1975; 12:339.

Relative Polycythemia

Relative polycythemia refers to an increase in hematocrit or red blood cell count as a result of decreased plasma volume; the total red blood cell mass is not increased. This occurs in acute dehydration, such as occurs in severe diarrhea or burns, and in patients on diuretic therapy.

In *spurious polycythemia* (Gaisböck's syndrome), the red blood cell mass is often high normal and the plasma volume is low normal; patients with this condition have been regarded as an extreme of the normal physiologic state. Almost all are men, have a high incidence of tobacco smoking, and tend to be obese and to have hypertension. Weinreb (1975) compared a group of these patients with a second group, which was similar except that the elevated hematocrit was due primarily to decreased plasma volume. The latter group had a greater tendency toward hypertension and hypercholesterolemia, and had a poorer rate of survival.

Smoking as a cause of polycythemia has been stressed (Smith, 1978); it is likely that smoking is an important factor in some cases of spurious polycythemia.

Absolute Polycythemia

Appropriate Erythropoietin Production Due to Hypoxia

ARTERIAL OXYGEN UNSATURATION. Lack of oxygen reaching the blood for whatever reason results in arterial unsaturation, impaired oxygen delivery to the tissues, increased production of EPO, erythroid hyperplasia in the marrow, and resultant erythrocytosis. The red blood cell mass is increased. As a response to the hypoxia, the red blood cell 2,3-DPG and the P_{50} are increased. In contrast to polycythemia vera, there usually is no leukocytosis or thrombocytosis, and the neutrophil alkaline phosphatase is normal. Arterial oxygen unsaturation may be the cause of polycythemia in persons living at high altitudes; in patients with chronic pulmonary disease and a block in diffusion of oxygen into the blood; in cyanotic heart disease in which there is right to left shunt; in cigarette smokers (Smith, 1978); and in methemoglobinemia whether due to enzyme deficiency (see Chap. 24), chronic drug effect, or a structurally abnormal hemoglobin (Hb M). (See the section entititled Hemoglobin M.)

HIGH OXYGEN AFFINITY HEMOGLOBINOPATHY. Another cause of tissue hypoxia is the presence of a structurally abnormal hemoglobin that has a high affinity for oxygen (Adamson, 1975). (See the section entitled Hemoglobins Associated with Altered Oxygen Affinity.) As in other functional hemoglobinopathies, the disorder occurs in the heterozygote. The abnormal hemoglobin releases less oxygen to the tissues than does normal hemoglobin at the same PO_2; the oxygen dissociation curve is shifted to the left, and the P_{50} is decreased. The red blood cell 2,3-DPG is not increased. As in arterial oxygen unsaturation, there is increased EPO production and erythrocytosis. It must be emphasized that routine hemoglobin electrophoresis often does not detect these hemoglobin variants because the amino acid substitution is at one of the $\alpha\beta$ contact sites or near the heme pocket. A low P_{50}, therefore, is presumptive evidence for a hemoglobinopathy. Some high-affinity hemoglobins associated with polycythemia are unstable; in these instances, the heat instability test is positive. Carbon monoxide poisoning causes hypoxia by two mechanisms: direct reduction of oxygen saturation and interference with oxygen release from hemoglobin (Landaw, 1990).

Inappropriate Erythropoietin Production

NEOPLASMS. Neoplasms, either benign or malignant, have been associated with polycythemia. Renal neoplasms account for the majority. In almost all cases, erythrocytosis has disappeared after resection of the tumor. The mechanism is not clear. Some of these neoplasms have been shown to contain, and presumably produce, EPO (e.g., cerebellar hemangioma, hypernephroma, some hepatomas).

RENAL DISORDERS. In other neoplasms or growths (e.g., renal cysts, hydronephrosis, ovarian carcinoma, some hepatomas), it appears that the mass impinging on the kidney induces increased renal production of EPO as a result of increased pressure or local hypoxia within the kidney. In most patients who have erythrocytosis following renal transplantation, the native kidneys have been left in place. Renal ischemia due to arterial narrowing is the probable mechanism for increased EPO production and erythrocytosis in these cases (Jandl, 1987).

FAMILIAL POLYCYTHEMIA. The most common familial polycythemia is due to the presence of a *high oxygen affinity hemoglobin,* which is inherited as an autosomal dominant trait (see earlier discussion). Autonomous or unexplained excessive production of EPO that results in polycythemia may be inherited as an autosomal dominant trait (Distelhorst, 1981) or as an autosomal recessive characteristic (Adamson, 1975). Both suggest a *defective regulation of EPO* production as the cause of polycythemia. Individuals with the recessive type have involvement earlier in life, have higher Hb and Hct levels, and more often have splenomegaly than do persons with polycythemia due to high oxygen affinity hemoglobinopathy.

Marked decrease in red blood cell 2,3-DPG associated with *deficiency of 2,3-DPG mutase and 2,3-DPG phosphatase* activities results in polycythemia and appears to be inherited as an autosomal recessive condition.

In other families, there is a genetically determined *expansion of the pool of EPO-responsive erythroid progenitor cells* (Prchal, 1985).

Polycythemia Vera

Polycythemia vera is a panmyelosis—that is, a condition in which excessive proliferation occurs in megakaryocytes and granulocytes, as well as in erythrocytes. It is manifested by erythrocytosis, leukocytosis, and thrombocytosis of varying degrees. The etiology is unknown. Polycythemia vera is discussed with the myeloproliferative disorders (see Chap. 27).

Measurement of Erythrocyte and Plasma Volume

The diagnosis of absolute polycythemia depends on reliable measurements of erythrocyte and plasma volumes. The erythrocyte and plasma volumes are measured by the use of

Table 26–15. CLINICAL EFFECT OF VARIABLE RELATIONSHIP BETWEEN RED CELL VOLUME AND PLASMA VOLUME

Red Cell Volume	Plasma Volume	Cause	Effect
Normal	High	Pregnancy Cirrhosis Nephritis Congestive cardiac failure	Pseudoanemia
Normal	Low	Stress Peripheral circulatory failure Dehydration Edema Prolonged bed rest	Pseudopolycythemia
Low	Normal	Anemia	Accurate reflection of degree of anemia
Low	High	Anemia	Anemia less severe than indicated by blood count
Low	Low	Hemorrhage Severe anemia (when hematocrit below 0.2)	Anemia more severe than indicated by blood count
High	Normal to low	Polycythemia	Accurate reflection of polycythemia or polycythemia less severe than apparent
High	High	Polycythemia (when hematocrit >0.5)	Polycythemia more severe than apparent
Normal or even high	High	Marked splenomegaly	Pseudoanemia

From Dacie JV, Lewis SM: Practical Haematology, 5th ed. Edinburgh, Churchill Livingstone, 1975.

radioactive isotopic tracers and the dilution principle. The most commonly employed tracers are ^{51}Cr in the form of sodium chromate bound to erythrocytes for measurement of erythrocyte volume. Iodine-125 or iodine-131 is bound to albumin and can be used to measure plasma volume.

For detailed description of measurement of red blood cell and plasma volume, see the report of the International Committee for Standardization in Hematology (1980).

ERYTHROCYTE VOLUME. In brief, blood is collected from the patient and the erythrocytes are labeled with ^{51}Cr. The chromated erythrocytes are washed in saline. An aliquot of the ^{51}Cr erythrocytes diluted in saline is injected intravenously into the patient. After a period of equilibration, usually 10 to 20 minutes, a sample of blood is withdrawn from the opposite arm. In cases in which the equilibration time is likely to be prolonged (as in splenomegaly, heart failure, or shock), another sample should be withdrawn 60 minutes after injection.

Radioactivity of each sample is recorded by a scintillation counter. The erythrocyte volume (EV) is calculated using the formula

$$\text{EV (mL)} = \frac{\text{I(cpm)}}{\text{C(cpm/mL)}}$$

where I = total injected radioactivity (counts per minute)

C = radioactivity in erythrocytes after mixing is complete (counts per minute per milliliter of erythrocytes).

PLASMA VOLUME. Approximately 20 mL of blood is withdrawn from a patient. After centrifugation, the plasma is removed and radioiodine-labeled albumin is added. After mixing, the labeled plasma is injected intravenously into the patient. At 10, 20, and 30 minutes following the injection, 5 mL of blood is removed and the radioactivity is counted in a well-type scintillation counter. The radioactivity at zero time (P_0) is determined by plotting the three points on semilogarithmic graph paper and extrapolating to zero time. A standard is prepared by diluting an aliquot of the radioiodine-labeled albumin with saline containing a small amount of detergent.

The plasma volume (PV) is calculated using the formula

$$\text{PV (mL)} = \frac{\text{S(cpm/mL)} \times \text{D} \times \text{V(mL)}}{\text{P}_0\text{(cpm/mL)}}$$

where S = counting rate of standard (counts per minute/mL)

D = dilution of diluted standard solution

V = volume of radioiodine-labeled albumin solution injected

P_0 = counting rate of plasma sample corrected to zero time (counts/minute/mL).

INTERPRETATION. The normal erythrocyte volume for men is 20 to 36 mL/kg, and for women, it is 19 to 31 mL/kg. The plasma volume for men is 25 to 43 mL/kg, and for women, it is is 28 to 45 mL/kg. In newborns and premature infants, the red blood cell volume and plasma volume in mL/kg are higher than in adults.

Patients with polycythemia have red blood cell volumes exceeding 36 mL/kg for men and 32 mL/kg for women. Changes in erythrocyte volume and plasma volume in a variety of conditions are recorded in Table 26–15.

Adamson JW: Familial polycythemia. Semin Hematol 1975; 12:383.
Agre P, Asimos A, Casella JF, et al: Inheritance pattern and clinical response to splenectomy as a reflection of erythrocyte spectrin deficiency in hereditary spherocytosis. N Engl J Med 1986; 315:1579.
Allen RH: Megaloblastic anemias. *In* Wyngaarden JB, Smith LH Jr, Bennett JC (eds): Cecil Textbook of Medicine, 19th ed. Philadelphia, W.B. Saunders Company, 1992, p 847.
Alter BP, Young NS: The bone marrow failure syndromes. *In* Nathan DG and Oski FA (eds): Hematology of Infancy and Childhood, 4th ed. Philadelphia, W.B. Saunders Company, 1993, p 216.
Alter BP: Prenatal diagnosis: General introduction, methodology, and review. Hemoglobin 1988; 12:763.
Alter BP, Potter NU, Li FP: Classification and aetiology of the aplastic anemias. Clin Haematol 1978; 7:431.
Babior BM: The megaloblastic anemias. *In* Beutler E, Lichtman MA, Coller BS, Kipps TJ (eds): Williams Hematology, 5th ed. New York, McGraw-Hill, 1995, p 471.
Beck WS (ed): Hematology, 5th ed. Cambridge, MA, The MIT Press, 1991.
Becker PS, Lux SE: Disorders of the red cell membrane. *In* Nathan DG, Oski FA (eds): Hematology of Infancy and Childhood, 4th edition, p 529. Philadelphia, W.B. Saunders Company, 1993.

Bennett JM, Catovsky D, Daniel MT, et al: Proposals for the classification of the myelodysplastic syndromes. Br J Haematol 1982; 51:189.

Bessman JD, Gilmer PR, Gardner FH: Improved classification of anemias by MCV and RDW. Am J Clin Pathol 1983; 30:322.

Betke K, Marti HR, Schlict I: Estimation of small percentages of foetal haemoglobin. Nature 1959; 184:1877.

Beutler E: Hemolytic Anemia. *In* Beutler E (ed): Disorders of Red Cell Metabolism. New York, Plenum Medical Book Company, 1978.

Beutler E: Red cell enzyme defects as nondiseases and as diseases. Blood 1979a; 54:1.

Beutler E, Glumbe, KG, Kaplan JC, et al: International Committee for Standardization in Haematology: Recommended screening test for glucose-6-phosphate dehydrogenase (G-6-PD) deficiency. Br J Haematol 1979b; 43:469.

Beutler E: Red Cell Metabolism: A Manual of Biochemical Methods, 3rd ed. Orlando, Grune & Stratton, 1984.

Beutler E: Paroxysmal nocturnal hemoglobinuria. *In* Beutler E, Lichtman MA, Coller BS, Kipps TJ (eds): Williams Hematology, 5th ed. New York, McGraw-Hill, 1995, p 252.

Beutler E: The molecular biology of enzymes and erythrocyte metabolisms. *In* Stamatoyannopoulos G, Nienhuis AW, Majerus PW, Varmus H (eds): The Molecular Basis of Blood Diseases, 2nd ed. Philadelphia, W.B. Saunders Company, 1994, p 331.

Bottomley S: Sideroblastic anemia. Clin Haematol 1982; 11:389.

Brain MC: Microangiopathic haemolytic anaemia (MHA). Br J Haematol 1972; 23 (Suppl):45.

Briere R, Golias T, Batsakis JG: Rapid qualitative and quantitative hemoglobin fractionation, cellulose acetate electrophoresis. Am J Clin Pathol 1965; 44:695.

Bunn HF: Sickle hemoglobin and other hemoglobin mutants. *In* Stamatoyannopoulos G, Nienhuis AW, Majerus PW, Varmus H (eds): The Molecular Basis of Blood Diseases, 2nd ed. Philadelphia, W.B. Saunders Company, 1994, p 207.

Bunn HF, Forget BG: Hemoglobin: Molecular, Genetic and Clinical Aspects. Philadelphia, W.B. Saunders Company, 1986.

Bunn HF: Human hemoglobins; normal and abnormal; methemoglobinemia. *In* Nathan DG, Oski FA (eds): Hematology of Infancy and Childhood, 4th ed. Philadelphia, W.B. Saunders Company, 1993, p 698.

Camitta BM, Strob R, Thomas ED: Aplastic anemia: Pathogenesis, diagnosis, treatment and prognosis. N Engl J Med 1982; 306:645, 712.

Carrell RW, Kay R: A simple method for the detection of unstable hemoglobins. Br J Haematol 1972; 23:615.

Carrell RW, Winterbourn CC, Rachmilewitz EA: Activated oxygen and hemolysis. Br J Haematol 1975; 30:259.

Cartwright GE, Lee GR: The anemia of chronic disorders. Br J Haematol 1971; 21:147.

Chanarin I: Investigation and management of megaloblastic anaemia. Clin Haematol 1976; 5:747.

Chang JC, Kan YW: A sensitive new prenatal test for sickle-cell anemia. N Engl J Med 1982; 307:30.

Charache S, Weatherall DJ, Clegg JB: Polycythemia associated with a hemoglobinopathy. J Clin Invest 1966; 45:813.

Cooper BA, Rosenblatt DS, Whitehead VM: Megaloblastic anemia. *In* Nathan DG, Oski FA (eds): Hematology of Infancy and Childhood, 4th ed. Philadelphia, W.B. Saunders Company, 1993, p 698.

Croft JD Jr, Swisher SN, Gilliland BC, et al: Coombs' test positivity induced by drugs: Mechanisms of immunologic reactions and red cell destruction. Ann Intern Med 1968; 68:176.

Dacie JV, Lewis SM: Practical Haematology, 7th ed. Edinburgh, Churchill Livingstone, 1991.

Dallman PR, Yip R, Oski FA: Iron deficiency and related nutritional anemias. *In* Nathan DG, Oski FA (eds): Hematology of Infancy and Childhood, 4th ed. Philadelphia, W.B. Saunders Company, 1993, p 413.

Diggs LW: Sickle cell crises. Am J Clin Path 1965; 44:1.

Distelhorst CW, Wagner DS, Goldwasser E, et al: Autosomal dominant familial erythrocytosis due to autonomous erythropoietin production. Blood 1981; 58:1155.

Donath J, Landsteiner K: Uber paroxysmale Haemoglobinurie. Munch Med Wschr 1904; 51:1590.

Efremov CD, Huisman THJ, Bowman K, et al: Microchromatography of hemoglobins. II. A rapid method for determination of hemoglobin A_2. J Lab Clin Med 1974; 83:657.

Erslev AJ: Anemia of chronic renal failure. *In* Beutler E, Lichtman MA, Coller BS, Kipps TJ (eds): Williams Hematology, 5th ed. New York, McGraw-Hill, 1995a, p 456.

Erslev AJ: Anemia of endocrine disorders. *In* Beutler E, Lichtman MA, Coller BS, Kipps TJ (eds): Williams Hematology, 5th ed. New York, McGraw-Hill, 1995b, p 462.

Fairbanks VF, Beutler E: Iron metabolism. *In* Beutler E, Lichtman MA, Coller BS, Kipps TJ (eds): Williams Hematology, 5th ed. New York, McGraw-Hill, 1995, p 369.

Fairbanks VF, Fahey JL, Beutler E: Clinical Disorders of Iron Metabolism, 2nd ed. New York, Grune & Stratton, 1971.

Fairbanks VF, Fernandez MN: The identification of metabolic errors associated with hemolytic anemia. JAMA 1969; 208:316.

Finch CA, Bellotti V, Stray S, et al: Plasma ferritin determination as a diagnostic tool. West J Med 1986; 145:657.

Finch CA, Cook JD, Labbe RF, et al: Effect of blood donation on iron stores as evaluated by serum ferritin. Blood 1977; 50:441.

Fleming AF: Hypoplastic anaemia of pregnancy. Clin Haematol 1973; 2:477.

Fukagawa N, Friedman S, Gill FM, et al: Hereditary spherocytosis with normal osmotic fragility after incubation. Is the autohemolysis test really obsolete? JAMA 1979; 242:63.

Gilliland BC: Coombs-negative immune hemolytic anemia. Semin Hematol 1976; 13:267.

Good RA: Aplastic anemia—suppressor lymphocytes and hematopoiesis. N Engl J Med 1977; 296:41.

Gottlieb AJ, Wurzel HA: Protein-quinone interaction: In vitro induction of indirect antiglobulin reactions with methyldopa. Blood 1974; 43:85.

Griffin PM, Ostroff SM, Tauxe RV, et al: Illnesses associated with *Escherichia coli* 0157:H7 infections: A broad clinical spectrum. Ann Intern Med 1988; 109:705.

Hall CA: Transcobalamins I and II as natural transport proteins of vitamin B_{12}. J Clin Invest 1975; 56:1125.

Ham TH: Studies on the destruction of red blood cells. I. Chronic hemolytic anemia with paroxysmal nocturnal hemoglobinuria: An investigation of the mechanism of hemolysis, with observations on five cases. Arch Intern Med 1939; 64:1271.

Hartmann RC, Jenkins DE Jr, Arnold AB: Diagnostic specificity of sucrose hemolysis test for paroxysmal nocturnal hemoglobinuria. Blood 1970; 35:462.

Herbert V: Biology of disease: Megaloblastic anemias. Lab Invest 1985; 52:3.

Hillman RS, Finch CA: Red Cell Manual, 5th ed. Philadelphia, F.A. Davis, 1985.

Hillmen P, Hows JM, Luzzatto L: Two distinct patterns of glycosyl phosphatidylinositol (GPI) linked protein deficiency in the red cells of patients with paroxysmal nocturnal haemoglobinuria. Br J Haematol 1992; 80:339.

Hirst E, Robertson TI: The syndrome of thymoma and erythroblastopenia anemia. Medicine 1967; 46:225.

Hockings WG: Hematologic abnormalities in patients with renal disease. Hematol Oncol Clin North Am 1987; 1:229.

Huisman THJ: The Hemoglobinopathies. Methods in Hematology, Vol 15. Edinburgh, Churchill Livingstone, 1986.

Huisman THJ, Jonxis JHP: The Hemoglobinopathies. Techniques of Identification. New York, Marcel Dekker, Inc, 1977.

Huisman THJ, Schroeder WA, Brodie AN, et al: Microchromatography of hemoglobins. III. A simplified procedure for the determination of hemoglobin A2. J Lab Clin Med 1975; 86:700.

International Committee for Standardization in Haematology: Recommended methods for measurement of red-cell and plasma volume. J Nucl Med 1980; 21:793.

Jacob HS, Jandl JH: A simple visual screening test for glucose-6-phosphate dehydrogenase deficiency employing ascorbate and cyanide. N Engl J Med 1966; 274:1162.

Jacobs A: Erythropoiesis and iron deficiency anemia. *In* Jacobs A, Worwood M: Iron in Biochemistry and Medicine. New York, Academic Press, 1974, p 405.

Jandl JH: Blood: Textbook of Hematology. Boston, Little, Brown, and Co. 1987.

Jones JA, Broszeit HK, LeCrone CN, et al: An improved method for detection of red cell hemoglobin H inclusions. Am J Med Technol 1981; 47:94.

Kazazian HH Jr, Boehm CD: Molecular basis and prenatal diagnosis of beta-thalassemia. Blood 1988; 72:1107.

Keitt AS: Diagnostic strategy in a suspected red cell enzymopathy. Clin Haematol 1981; 10:3.

Kern P, Heimpel H, Heit W, et al: Granulocytic progenitor cells in aplastic anaemia. Br J Haematol 1977; 35:613.

Kirtland HH, Mohler DN, Horwitz DA: Methyldopa inhibition of suppressor-lymphocyte function. A proposed cause of autoimmune hemolytic anemia. N Engl J Med 1980; 302:825.

LaCelle PL, Weed RI: The contribution of normal and pathologic erythrocytes to blood rheology. Prog Hematol 1971; 7:1.

Landaw SA: Polycythemia vera and other polycythemia states. Clin Lab Med 1990; 10:857.

Lehmann H, Huntsman RG, Casey R, et al: Erythrocyte disorders, anemias related to abnormal globin. *In* Williams WJ, Beutler E, Erslev AJ, Rundles, RW (eds): Hematology, 2nd ed. New York, McGraw-Hill, 1977, p 494.

Lewis SM, Dacie JV: The aplastic anaemia—paroxysmal nocturnal haemoglobinuria syndrome. Br J Haematol 1967; 13:236.

Lewis SM, Verwilghen RL: Dyserythropoiesis and dyserythropoietic anemias. Prog Hematol 1973; 8:99.

Lian EC-Y: Pathogenesis of thrombotic thrombocytopenic purpura. Semin Hematol 1987; 24:82.

Lindenbaum J: Status of laboratory testing in the diagnosis of megaloblastic anemia. Blood 1983; 61:624.
Lindenbaum J, Healton EB, Savage DG, et al: Neuropsychiatric disorders caused by cobalamin deficiency in the absence of anemia or macrocytosis. N Engl J Med 1988; 318:1720.
Lynch RE, Williams DM, Reading JC, et al: The prognosis in aplastic anaemia. Blood 1975; 45:517.
Marengo-Rowe AJ: Rapid electrophoresis and quantitation of haemoglobins on cellulose acetate. J Clin Pathol 1965; 18:790.
Marsh GW, Lewis SM: Cardiac haemolytic anaemia. Semin Hematol 1969; 6:133.
Martin JN Jr, Blake PG, Perry KG, et al: The natural history of HELLP syndrome: Patterns of disease progression and regression. Am J Obstet Gynecol 1991; 164:1500.
Mauer AM: Pediatric Hematology. New York, McGraw-Hill, 1969.
Means RT Jr, Krantz SB: Progress in understanding the pathogenesis of the anemia of chronic disease. Blood 1992; 80:1639.
Milner PF, Gooden H: Rapid citrate-agar electrophoresis in routine screening for hemoglobinopathies using a simple hemolysate. Am J Clin Pathol 1975; 64:58.
Miwa S: Pyruvate kinase deficiency and other enzymopathies of the Embden-Meyerhof pathway. Clin Haematol 1981; 10:57.
Mohandas N, Chasis JA: Red blood cell deformability, membrane material properties and shape: Regulation by transmembrane, skeletal and cytosolic proteins and lipids. Semin Hematol 1993; 30:171.
Narayanan HN, Geary CG, Freemont AJ, Kendra JR: Long-term follow-up of aplastic anemia. Br J Haematol 1994; 86:837.
O'Gorman Hughes DW: Aplastic anemia in childhood. III. Constitutional aplastic anemia and related cytopenias. Med J Aust 1974; 2:519.
Olney RS, Khoury MJ, Alo CJ, et al: Increased risk of transverse digital deficiency after chorionic villus sampling: Results of the United States multistate case-control study, 1988–1992. Teratology 1995; 51:20.
Orkin SH, Little PFR, Kazazian HH Jr, et al: Improved detection of the sickle mutation by DNA analysis. Application to prenatal diagnosis. N Engl J Med 1982; 307:32.
Orwoll ES, Orwoll RL: Hematologic abnormalities in patients with endocrine and metabolic disorders. Hematol Oncol Clin North Am 1987; 1:261.
Paglia DE, Valentine WN: Haemolytic anaemia associated with disorders of the purine and pyrimidine salvage pathways. Clin Haematol 1981; 10:81.
Pasanen A, Tenhunen R: Heme synthesis in sideroblastic anaemias. Scand J Haematol 1986; 36; 45(Suppl):60.
Pauling L, Itano HA, Signer SJ, et al: Sickle cell anemia. A molecular disease. Science 1949; 110:543.
Pearson HA, Spencer RP, Cornelius EA: Functional asplenia in sickle cell anemia. N Engl J Med 1969; 281:923.
Perutz MF, Lehmann H: Molecular pathology of human hemoglobin. Nature (London) 1968; 219:902.
Petz LD, Garratty G: Acquired Immune Hemolytic Anemias. New York, Churchill Livingstone, 1980.
Phillips DL, Keefe EB: Hematologic manifestations of gastrointestinal disease. Hematol Oncol Clin North Am 1987; 1:207.
Piomelli S: A micromethod for free erythrocyte porphyrins: The FEP test. J Lab Clin Med 1973; 81:932.
Prchal JT, Crist WM, Goldwasser E, et al: Autosomal dominant polycythemia. Blood 1985; 66:1208.
Prchal JT, Throckmorton DW, Carroll AJ III, et al: A common progenitor for human myeloid and lymphoid cells. Nature 1978; 274:590.
Rapaport SI: Introduction to Hematology, 2nd ed. Philadelphia, J.B. Lippincott, 1987.
Reissman KR, Ruth WE, Nomura TA: A human hemoglobin with lowered oxygen affinity and impaired heme-heme interactions. J Clin Invest 1961; 40:1826.
Rosse WF: The glycolipid anchor of membrane surface proteins. Semin Hematol 1993; 30:219.
Saarinen UM, Siimes MA: Developmental changes in serum iron, total iron-binding capacity, and transferrin saturation in infancy. J Pediatr 1977; 91:875.
Saiki RK, Chang CA, Levenson CH, et al: Diagnosis of sickle cell anemia and beta-thalassemia with enzymatically amplified DNA and nonradioactive allele-specific oligonucleotide probes. N Engl J Med 1988; 319:537.
Schmidt RM: Laboratory diagnosis of hemoglobinopathies. JAMA 1973; 224:1276.
Schmidt RM, Rucknagel, DL, Necheles TF: Comparison of methodologies for thalassemia screening by HbA_2 quantitation. J Lab Clin Med 1975; 86:873.
Schneider RG, Hightower B, Hosty TS, et al: Abnormal hemoglobins in a quarter million people. Blood 1976; 48:629.
Shepard KV, Bukowski RM: The treatment of thrombotic thrombocytopenic purpura with exchange transfusions, plasma infusions, and plasma exchange. Semin Hematol 1987; 24:178.
Shepard MK, Weatherall DJ, Conley CL: Semiquantitative estimation of the distribution of fetal hemoglobin in red cell populations. Bull Johns Hopkins Hosp 1962; 110:293.
Shulman IA, Branch DR, Nelson JM, et al: Autoimmune hemolytic anemia with both cold and warm autoantibodies. JAMA 1985; 253:1746.
Siimes MA, Addiego JE, Dallman PR: Ferritin in serum: Diagnosis of iron deficiency and iron overload in infants and children. Blood 1974; 43:581.
Singer K, Chernoff AI, Singer L: Studies on abnormal hemoglobins. I. Their demonstration in sickle cell anemia and other hematologic disorders by means of alkali denaturation. Blood 1951; 6:413.
Smith JR, Landaw SA: Smoker's polycythemia. N Engl J Med 1978; 298:6.
Sokol RJ, Hewitt S: Autoimmune hemolysis: A critical review. CRC Critical Rev Oncol Hematol 1985; 4:125.
Sokol RJ, Booker DJ, Stamps R: The pathology of autoimmune hemolytic anemia. J Clin Pathol 1992; 45:1047.
Stamatoyannopoulos G, Bellingham AJ, Lenfant C, et al: Abnormal hemoglobins with high and low oxygen affinity. Ann Rev Med 1971; 22:221.
Stockman JA, Weiner LS, Simon GE, et al: The measurement of free erythrocyte porphyrin (FEP) as a simple means of distinguishing iron deficiency from beta-thalassemia trait in subjects with microcytosis. J Lab Clin Med 1975; 85:113.
Tanaka KR, Valentine WN, Miwa S: Pyruvate kinase (PK) deficiency hereditary non-spherocytic hemolytic anemia. Blood 1962; 19:267.
Tietz NW (ed): Clinical Guide to Laboratory Tests, 3rd edition. Philadelphia, W.B. Saunders Company, 1995.
Valentine WN: Hemolytic anemia and inborn errors of metabolism. Blood 1979; 54:549.
Valentine WN, Tanaka KR, Paglia DE: Pyruvate kinase and other enzyme deficiency disorders of the erythrocyte. *In* Scriver CR, Beaudet AL, Sly WS, et al (eds): The Metabolic Basis of Inherited Disease, 6th ed. New York, McGraw-Hill, 1989, p 2341.
Wasi P, Na-Nakorn S, Pootrakul S-N: The alpha-thalassemias. Clin Haematol, 1974; 3:383.
Weatherall DJ: The diagnostic features of the different forms of thalassaemia. *In* Weatherall DJ (ed): Methods in Hematology. Edinburgh, Churchill Livingstone, 1983, p 1.
Weatherall DJ: Prenatal diagnosis of inherited blood diseases. Clin Haematol 1985; 14:747.
Weatherall DJ, Clegg JB: The Thalassaemia Syndromes, 3rd ed. Oxford, Blackwell Scientific Publications, 1981.
Weatherall DJ: The thalassemias. *In* Stamatoyannopoulos G, Niehuis AW, Majerus PW, Varmus H (eds). The Molecular Basis of Blood Disease, 2nd ed. Philadelphia, W.B. Saunders Company, 1994, p 157.
Weinreb NJ, Shih C-F: Spurious polycythemia. Semin Hematol 1975; 12:397.
Williams DM, Lynch RE, Cartwright GE: Prognostic factors in aplastic anemia. Clin Haematol 1978; 12:467.
Wrightstone RN, Huisman THJ: On the levels of hemoglobins F and A_2 in sickle-cell anemia and related disorders. Am J Clin Pathol 1974; 61:375.
Young N, Mortimer P: Viruses and bone marrow failure. Blood 1984; 63:729.
Yunis AA, Bloomberg GR: Chloramphenicol toxicity: Clinical features and pathogenesis. Prog Hematol 1964; 4:138.

Chapter 27

Leukocytic Disorders

Frederick R. Davey, M.D.
Robert E. Hutchison, M.D.

NON-NEOPLASTIC DISORDERS

Quantitative study of leukocytes includes measuring the concentration of all the white blood cells, the total leukocyte count (white blood cell count; WBC), and the relative and absolute concentrations of the various forms of white blood cells. The term *leukocytosis* refers to an increase in the total WBC above the upper limit of normal for an individual's age and sex. *Leukopenia* is a total WBC below normal. Although all leukocytes act in defending the body, their functions differ and it is best to regard them as separate systems. An increase or decrease in the absolute concentration of cells in each series is termed *neutrophilia* (neutrophilic leukocytosis) and *neutropenia, eosinophilia* (eosinophilic leukocytosis) and *eosinopenia; basophilia* (basophilic leukocytosis) and *basopenia, lymphocytosis* and *lymphocytopenia,* and *monocytosis* and *monocytopenia.* Qualitative study of leukocytes includes evaluation for structural abnormalities in the cytoplasm and nucleus and for functional abnormalities as well.

One purpose of the study of leukocytes is to help in establishing a diagnosis. Occasionally, the examination alone may furnish a specific diagnosis—for example, in leukemia. More frequently, it may be diagnostically helpful together with other clinical and laboratory data—for example, in acute appendicitis or infectious mononucleosis. Another purpose is to help in establishing a prognosis. For example, leukopenia in acute appendicitis or pneumonia is considered prognostically unfavorable.

Finally, study of the leukocytes is helpful in following the course of disease. For example, toxic effects of radiotherapy and chemotherapy may be recognized, and recovery monitored, by examination of leukocytes.

For these reasons, the leukocyte count is performed for almost every patient admitted to the hospital regardless of disease.

Granulocytic and Monocytic Disorders

Neutrophilia

Neutrophilic leukocytosis or neutrophilia refers to an absolute concentration of neutrophils in the blood above normal levels for age. Reference intervals are given in Table 24–6; age variations are discussed in Chapter 24.

MECHANISMS. The primary factors influencing the neutrophil count are (1) the rate of inflow of cells from the bone marrow, (2) the proportion of neutrophils in the marginal granulocyte pool (MGP) and the circulating granulocyte pool (CGP), and (3) the rate of outflow of neutrophils from the blood.

Physiologic leukocytosis is produced by factors or situations that do not involve tissue damage. Severe exercise, hypoxia, stress, or the injection of epinephrine results in a decrease in the MGP and a corresponding increase in the CGP, resulting in a pseudoneutrophilia. This simple redistribution of cells between the CGP and MGP may be the result of epinephrine-induced activation of β-receptors on endothelial cells, releasing cyclic adenosine monophosphate (cAMP), which alters the adhesive properties of neutrophils and increases the release of neutrophils into circulation (Boxer, 1980).

Stress of greater severity or injection of endotoxin, corticosteroids, or etiocholanolone results in an increased inflow of cells to the blood from the marrow storage pool. As a result, the maturation and storage pool in the marrow is diminished, and both MGP and CGP are enlarged. A greater neutrophilia is possible in this situation because of the much larger size of the storage pool than the CGP and MGP. Band neutrophils and metamyelocytes are likely to be present.

In both of the preceding situations, acute neutrophilia occurs as a result of redistribution of cells, without input from increased production. Chronic neutrophilia may be produced by corticosteroids, which decrease the egress of neutrophils from the blood and result in increased CGP and MGP without necessarily increasing the production of neutrophils.

In contrast to the preceding discussion, *pathologic leukocytosis* is an increased WBC that occurs as a result of disease, and usually is a response to tissue damage (Table 27–1). This leukocytosis is most often a form of neutrophilia.

In addition to the random loss of neutrophils from the circulation in various body secretions, neutrophils leave the blood by ameboid movement when attracted to a focus of inflammation in tissues, presumably by chemotactic substances. It is from the MGP that the neutrophils leave the blood, pass between capillary endothelial cells, and reach the tissues.

In acute infection, increased margination of neutrophils and outflow from blood to tissues would lead to neutropenia were there not a flow of neutrophils from the marrow storage compartment into the blood. Because the latter overcompensates, the result is neutrophilia. Usually, production and storage compartments then increase in the marrow and are able to sustain the increased CGP (neutrophilia) and MGP in the face of the increased flow of neutrophils from the blood into the inflammatory site. In these instances, the marrow shows granulocytic hyperplasia (decreased erythrocytic precursor cell/granulocytic precursor cell [E/G] ratio and increased cellularity), with maturation intact.

If the demand for neutrophils is extremely great, as in severe infection, there may be depletion of the marrow storage pool and a decreased CGP (neutropenia) and MGP, because the supply of cells is insufficient for the demand. In these instances, the marrow shows increased numbers of early neutrophil precursors, through the myelocyte stage, but decreased numbers of metamyelocytes, bands, and neutrophils.

CAUSES

Infection. Systemic infections due to various bacteria, fungi, spirochetes, and viruses may cause neutrophilia. In some, neutrophilia may be preceded by a transient neutropenia, especially if the infection is severe. Some bacterial infections, such as typhoid fever, paratyphoid fever, and brucellosis, result in persistent neutropenia. Whether this is due to the mechanism cited previously for severe infection or to a toxic depression of the marrow, or to a combination of causes, is not clear.

Appendicitis, salpingitis, otitis media, and other localized infections caused by pyogenic organisms usually result in neutrophilia.

A characteristic pattern of response to infection includes progressive neutrophilic leukocytosis, an increase of young forms (shift to the left), and a fall in eosinophils. When the infection begins to subside and the fever drops, a gradual transformation in the blood picture occurs: The total number of leukocytes goes down, and the number of monocytes increases. This monocytic phase is gradually replaced by a relative or slight absolute lymphocytosis and eosinophilia as recovery proceeds.

Other disorders associated with neutrophilia are presented in the following section. In some of them, one or more of the mechanisms described previously are operating; in others, the mechanism is unclear.

Toxic

Metabolic. Uremia, eclampsia, gout, diabetic acidosis.

Drugs and Chemicals. Lead, mercury, potassium chlorate, digitalis, epinephrine, corticosteroids, turpentine, ethylene glycol, benzene, and myeloid growth factors.

Physical and Emotional Stimuli. Heat, cold, muscular activity, anoxia, pain, fear, anger.

Tissue Destruction or Necrosis. Myocardial infarc-

Table 27–1. PATHOLOGIC LEUKOCYTOSIS

Cause	Cell Type
Allergy	Eosinophil
Brucellosis	Lymphocyte, monocyte
Convulsions	Neutrophil or lymphocyte
Drugs and poisons	
ACTH	Neutrophil
Epinephrine	
Camphor	Neutrophil and eosinophil
Copper sulfate, phosphorus	Eosinophil
Tetrachlorethane, epinephrine	Monocyte, neutrophil, and lymphocyte
Other (acetanilid, arsenicals, benzene, CO, digitalis, lead, phenacetin, turpentine, venoms)	Neutrophil
Myeloid growth factors (G-CSF, GM-CSF, M-CSF)	Neutrophil, monocyte
Hemolysis	Neutrophil
Hemorrhage	Neutrophil
Hodgkin's disease	Neutrophil, eosinophil, and monocyte
Infectious lymphocytosis	Lymphocyte
Infectious mononucleosis	Lymphocyte, atypical changes
Leukemia	Granulocyte, lymphocyte, or monocyte
Loeffler's syndrome, periarteritis nodosa, pernicious anemia	Eosinophil
Polycythemia vera	Neutrophil, eosinophil, basophil
Toxemias: diabetic acidosis, eclampsia, gout, uremia	Neutrophil
Tuberculosis	Neutrophil, eosinophil, lymphocyte, monocyte
Tumors involving	
Marrow and serous cavities	Neutrophil and eosinophil
Ovary	Eosinophil
GI tract and liver	Neutrophil
Typhoid fever	Lymphocyte

tion, burns, surgical operations, crush injuries, fractures, neoplastic disease (especially with extensive necrosis).

Hemorrhage. Especially if bleeding has occurred within a serous cavity (peritoneal, pleural, joint, subdural).

Hemolysis. Especially with rapid hemolysis, as in hemolytic crises or hemolytic transfusion reactions.

Hematologic Disorders. Myeloproliferative disorders, myelogenous leukemia, postsplenectomy state.

SOLID TUMORS. Neutrophilia is occasionally seen in patients with solid tumors, particularly large-cell carcinomas of the lung. The neutrophilia is secondary to several factors including response to tissue necrosis and underlying infection as well as to the production of myeloid growth factors (Peterson, 1993).

Determinants. Certain host factors modify the degree of neutrophilic response. Children respond more intensely than adults. The degree of neutrophilia produced may be impaired by the same factors that impair erythrocyte production (iron, folate or cobalamin deficiency) or by marrow failure due to other causes. Imperfectly defined factors that enable the body to localize an infection may play a role: The more localized the process, the more pronounced the neutrophilia.

Other factors modifying the neutrophilic response are due more to the microorganism than to the host. Pyogenic bacteria, especially, induce neutrophilia. Within limits, the more virulent the agent, the higher the neutrophil count. When the infection is overwhelming, however, there is apt to be a neutropenia and greater shift to the left as a result of the mechanism described previously.

Treatment of infections with antibiotic agents may modify the leukocytic response to infection. Steroid therapy, although causing neutrophilia, tends to impair the host response to infection, probably because of diminished movement of neutrophils into the tissues and increased lysosomal stability.

Neutropenia

Neutropenia is a reduction of the absolute neutrophil count below 2×10^9/L for whites and below 1.3×10^9/L for blacks. The term *agranulocytosis* has been used for severe neutropenia; this is almost always associated with depletion of eosinophils and basophils as well. If the neutrophil count is less than 1×10^9/L, the risk of infection is considerably increased over normal, and if there are less than 0.5×10^9 neutrophils per liter, the risk of infection is greater still.

The mechanisms by which neutropenia occurs include (1) decreased flow of neutrophils from marrow into blood as a result of either lack of production or ineffective production, (2) increased removal of neutrophils from the blood, (3) altered distribution between the CGP and the MGP, or (4) combinations of these. Neutropenias are not so neatly classified as anemias. A sound approach has been made using data from radioisotopic measurements of proliferative activity, maturation time, survival in the circulation, and measurement of MGP and CGP, in addition to the usual bone marrow and peripheral blood studies. A classification is given in Table 27–2. It should be noted that drugs induce neutropenia through several mechanisms and are a very important consideration in any differential diagnosis of leukopenia.

Table 27–2. CLASSIFICATION OF NEUTROPENIA

I. *Myeloid hypoplasia*
   A. Infantile genetic agranulocytosis (Kostmann); familial neutropenia; cyclic neutropenia; chronic (hypoplastic) neutropenia; neutropenias associated with lymphocytic disorders, myelophthisic neutropenia
   B. Drug induced
      1. Cytolytic
         a. Alkylating agents (nitrogen mustard, cyclophosphamide, chlorambucil, busulfan)
         b. Ionizing radiation
         c. Mitosis inhibitors (colchicine, vinblastine, vincristine)
         d. DNA depolymerization (procarbazine)
      2. Metabolic interference with DNA synthesis
         a. Purine and pyrimidine antagonists (cytosine arabinoside,* methotrexate,* 6-mercaptopurine, azathioprine, hydroxyurea)
         b. Phenothiazine type (phenothiazines, benzodiazepines, antithyroid compounds,* sulfonamides,* antibiotics, anticonvulsants)
         c. Others (chloramphenicol,* benzene*)
      3. Idiosyncratic
         a. Acute, days to weeks (quinine, quinidine, indomethacin, procainamide, thiazides, sulfonamides,* phenylbutazone,* antithyroids*)
         b. Chronic, months to years (chloramphenicol,* phenylbutazone,* benzene,* gold salts*)

II. *Marrow hyperplasia with ineffective granulocytopoiesis*
   A. Chédiak-Higashi syndrome; megaloblastic anemia; myeloproliferative disorders (these may belong in IV)
   B. Drug induced
      1. Impaired nucleic acid synthesis (cytosine arabinoside,* methotrexate,* phenytoin)
      2. Others (alcohol, chloramphenicol*)

III. *Decreased survival in circulation* due to increased utilization or increased destruction
   A. Bacterial infections; viral infections; protozoal infections; chronic benign neutropenia of childhood; chronic idiopathic neutropenia in adults; splenic neutropenia; neonatal isoimmunization neutropenia; acquired immunoneutropenia
   B. Drug induced (immunologic mechanism)
      Aminopyrine, amidopyrine, phenylbutazone,* sulfapyridines*

IV. *Combination of impaired production (I or II) and decreased survival (III)*
   A. Megaloblastic anemia; severe bacterial infections; mycobacterial infections; chronic idiopathic myelokathexis
   B. Drug induced (very likely)
      Alcohol, purine and pyrimidine inhibitors, aminopyrine

V. *Pseudoneutropenia (shift from circulating granulocyte pool [CGP] to marginal granulocyte pool [MGP]*
   A. Endotoxin
   B. Drug induced: anesthetic agents, ether, pentobarbital

*Drugs cited for more than one mechanism.

Adapted from Finch SC: *In* Williams WJ, Beutler E, Erslev AJ, and Lichtman MA (eds): Hematology, 3rd ed. New York, McGraw-Hill, 1983.

MYELOID HYPOPLASIA. Kostmann's infantile genetic agranulocytosis is a rare autosomal recessive condition appearing in early infancy. The marrow usually shows increased early granulocytes but few maturing forms, and the neutrophil survival is normal. An intrinsic defect in myeloid precursor cells with dysmyelopoiesis appears to be present (Athens, 1993).

Chronic familial neutropenia and cyclic neutropenia appear to be autosomal dominant conditions. Cyclic neutropenia usually has a periodicity of about 21 days, and appears to be due to periodic stem cell failure. Neutrophil precursors disappear prior to the fall in circulating neutrophils and reappear during the neutropenic phase. Other congenital and familial neutropenias have been described (Athens, 1993).

Patients with dysfunctional lymphocytes frequently exhibit some degree of neutropenia. Males with X-linked agammaglobulinemia often are neutropenic.

Isolated neutropenia or agranulocytosis is uncommon in adults. When the marrow is damaged by a myelophthisic process such as metastatic carcinoma or Gaucher's disease replacing the marrow or by drugs, usually the damage is not limited to granulopoiesis but affects normoblasts and megakaryocytes as well. Because of the short lifespan of granulocytes, however, neutropenia is the earliest recognizable effect in the blood. It takes weeks before damage to the erythropoietic tissue becomes manifest because of the long lifespan of erythrocytes. Platelets have a rather short lifespan but, on the other hand, megakaryocytes are more resistant to damage.

Drugs are an important cause of neutropenia and, as outlined in Table 27–2, may act in different ways. Drugs that have the effect of destroying or interfering with mitosis of the proliferating cells are frequently used in the therapy of malignant disease. Important and limiting side effects of such chemotherapy are severe neutropenia with its risk of infection and severe thrombocytopenia with risk of bleeding; anemia is more readily controlled with transfusion.

Idiosyncratic drug effects refer to those in which host susceptibility factors predominate—that is, there is little relationship with dose and duration of drug therapy.

INEFFECTIVE GRANULOCYTOPOIESIS. Neutropenia due to ineffective granulocytopoiesis occurs in megaloblastic anemias, with drugs that have an antifolate effect, and in starvation. In these conditions, there usually is an associated anemia and thrombocytopenia. Anemia is usually present if therapy is prolonged, and often thrombocytopenia is present as well. The marrow usually is hyperplastic. In addition to increased destruction of cells in the marrow, there is some evidence that circulating neutrophils have a shortened survival. Indirect evidence for increased granulocyte turnover in this group of neutropenias with hypercellular marrow is an increased serum muramidase (lysozyme).

DECREASED SURVIVAL. Transient neutropenia may occur early in some infections, followed by leukocytosis once the marrow production catches up with the demand. As previously noted, in severe, extensive bacterial infection, neutropenia with a shift to the left may be due to inability of marrow production to keep up with the peripheral utilization. Some bacterial infections, notably brucellosis and *Salmonella* infections, are prone to be associated with neutropenia; they may have some depressing effect on the marrow as well. Patients with viral infections such as measles and rubella have neutropenia for several days after appearance of the rash; this is probably due in part to increased utilization. Lymphocytosis is present and persists after the neutropenia subsides.

The neutropenia of hypersplenism has been attributed to selective removal of neutrophils by the spleen. It is associated with neutrophilic hyperplasia of the marrow and is corrected by splenectomy. Splenomegaly due to many causes may result in a shortened neutrophil survival and neutropenia; these include congestive splenomegaly, Felty's syndrome, Gaucher's disease, and lymphoma. In some cases of Felty's syndrome (neutropenia and splenomegaly in rheumatoid arthritis), there may be a neutrophil-specific antibody involved.

Evidence has been accumulating that there are antibodies capable of clumping leukocytes of all varieties under proper experimental conditions (leukoagglutinins). Leukopenia in the newborn may be produced by leukoagglutinins from the mother. Studies have demonstrated that autoantibodies also may be responsible for immune neutropenia or immune panleukopenia. Several antibodies with agglutinating or cytotoxic activity against specific neutrophilic antigens have been considered responsible for neutropenia. An autoantibody with cytotoxic activity against mature granulocytes, monocytes, and lymphocytes as well as primitive myeloid cells has been shown to result in episodic autoimmune panleukopenia.

Drug-induced neutropenia due to immune mechanisms has been well described for aminopyrine. In about 1% of persons, 7 to 10 days after first taking the drug, chills, headache, fever, and neutropenia with a shift to the left occur. Slight granulocytic hyperplasia is noted in the marrow. If the drug is continued, mucosal ulceration and sepsis may occur, and granulocytic precursors may disappear from the marrow. If, on the other hand, the drug is discontinued, the neutrophil count returns to normal levels in a week. An antibody develops in these patients that, in the presence of the drug, causes enhanced destruction of neutrophils. The antibody probably is directed against a drug–plasma protein complex; the resulting antigen-antibody complex nonspecifically adsorbs on the cells and leads to their destruction.

COMBINATIONS. As indicated, some of the conditions discussed previously are probably combinations of increased destruction and impaired effective production.

PSEUDONEUTROPENIA. Small doses of endotoxin cause a shift of neutrophils into the MGP from the CGP, giving an apparent neutropenia, prior to causing a leukocytosis. In animals, anesthetic agents such as ether cause the same kind of pseudoneutropenia.

Morphologic Alterations in Neutrophils

In addition to quantitative changes, qualitative morphologic alterations also occur in neutrophils. Some of these alterations, such as toxic granules or cytoplasmic vacuoles, are acquired and disappear after the stimulus that provoked them is gone. Others are hereditary and persist through life, with or without functional impairment. These are well illustrated and reviewed by Brunning (1970).

It should be noted that disorders of leukocyte function may exist without any structural abnormality detectable with the usual modes of morphologic examination.

TOXIC GRANULATION. Toxic granules are dark blue to purple cytoplasmic granules in the metamyelocyte, band, or neutrophil stage. They are peroxidase positive and may be nu-

4

merous or few in number; there may be less peroxidase activity in toxic than in normal neutrophils. Toxic granulation is found in severe infections or other toxic conditions (Plate 27–1*A*).

Normally, neutrophil granules are tan to pink in color in neutrophil metamyelocytes, bands, and mature forms. Even the nonspecific or azurophil granules that are dark blue in the promyelocyte stage normally lose their basophilia in the mature neutrophil, where they constitute about one third of the granules in the human. Toxic granules are azurophil granules that have retained their basophilic staining reaction by lack of maturation or that have developed increased basophilia in the mature neutrophil. In addition, perhaps skipped divisions during the development of the neutrophil may result in a greater proportion of the granules being of the azurophil type. Increased basophilia of azurophil granules simulating toxic granules may occur in normal cells with prolonged staining time or decreased pH of the staining reaction.

Irregular basophilia of the cytoplasm is also common in toxic conditions and appears to reflect impaired cytoplasmic maturation. If discrete, this focal basophilia is known as a Döhle inclusion body (see later).

Cytoplasmic vacuoles are also signs of toxic change if the possibility of degeneration artifacts can be eliminated by making films from fresh blood free of anticoagulant. Vacuoles or irregular depletion of granules implies that phagocytosis has occurred (Plate 27–1*B*).

Another toxic change in the neutrophil is the occasional appearance of several sharp or blunt spicules extending out from the nucleus (see Plate 24–1*A*).

DÖHLE INCLUSION BODIES. Döhle inclusion bodies are small, oval inclusions in the peripheral cytoplasm of polymorphonuclear neutrophils that stain pale blue with Wright's stain. They are remnants of free ribosomes or rough endoplasmic reticulum persisting from an earlier stage of development. Originally, Döhle bodies were described as being especially prominent in scarlet fever, but they are seen in many other infectious diseases, in burns, in aplastic anemia, and following administration of toxic agents. They frequently accompany toxic granulation in the neutrophil. With the light microscope, Döhle bodies resemble the inclusions seen in the May-Hegglin anomaly (Plate 27–1*C*).

MAY-HEGGLIN ANOMALY. May-Hegglin anomaly is a rare autosomal dominant condition characterized by the presence of pale blue inclusions resembling Döhle bodies in neutrophils, giant platelets, and in some persons, by thrombocytopenia. The inclusions are larger and more prominent than the Döhle bodies found in patients with infections (Plate 27–1*C*). They have been described in eosinophils, basophils, and monocytes, as well as in neutrophils (Brunning, 1970). The blue staining of the inclusions can be abolished by prior treatment of the cells with ribonuclease. With electron microscopy, the appearance of the inclusions differs from that of Döhle bodies, suggesting structural alterations in RNA.

ALDER-REILLY ANOMALY. Dense azurophilic granulation in all white blood cells was described by Alder in 1939 (Plate 27–1*D*). In neutrophils, it may resemble toxic granulation, but it is unrelated to infection and is not transient. In 1941, Reilly described similar granulocytes in some but not all patients with gargoylism (Hurler's syndrome or, more generally, the genetic mucopolysaccharidoses). Other observations have shown that the heavy granulation in neutrophils can occur either as a feature of the genetic mucopolysaccharidoses or independently in otherwise healthy persons (Brunning, 1970).

Occurring more often than the Alder-Reilly anomaly in the genetic mucopolysaccharidoses is a metachromatic inclusion in the lymphocytes surrounded by a clear space (Plate 27–1*E*). Macrophages in the marrow frequently contain similar granulation (Plate 27–1*F*). This group of disorders is inherited and is characterized by deficiencies or derangement in various lysosomal enzymes required for degrading mucopolysaccharides. The result is abnormal deposition and storage of mucopolysaccharides in multiple organs. Skeletal abnormalities are prominent.

PELGER-HUËT ANOMALY. This hereditary, autosomal dominant condition involves failure of normal segmentation of granulocytic nuclei. Most nuclei are band shaped to have two segments but no more (Plate 27–1*G*). The chromatin is coarse, and these are not normal young band forms. When a large number of band neutrophils appear in the differential count in a patient without infection or other cause, careful analysis of the blood films of the patient and of family members occasionally establishes the presence of the Pelger-Huët anomaly. The cells are functionally normal.

A similar appearing, acquired disorder of nuclear segmentation in granulocytes may occasionally be found in cases of granulocytic leukemia, myeloproliferative disorders, some infections, and after exposure to certain drugs (Brunning, 1970); this is sometimes called the pseudo–Pelger-Huët anomaly. In addition to the band forms and neutrophils with only two segments, mature cells with round, nonsegmented nuclei and coarse chromatin are common, in contrast to the congenital Pelger-Huët anomaly.

CHÉDIAK-HIGASHI SYNDROME. This rare, autosomal recessive disorder is characterized by partial albinism, photophobia, abnormally large granules in leukocytes and other granule-containing cells, and frequent pyogenic infections. An accelerated lymphoma-like phase occurs, with lymphadenopathy, hepatosplenomegaly, and pancytopenia; lymphoid infiltrates are widespread, and death ensues at an early age. Granulocytes, monocytes, and lymphocytes contain giant granules (Plate 27–1*H* and *I*), which appear to be abnormal lysosomes. Leukocyte functional abnormalities exist. The pathogenesis of this disorder is linked to a cellular abnormality causing increased fusion of cytoplasmic granules (Jandl, 1987).

Functional Disorders of Neutrophils

Inherited and acquired disorders affecting leukocytes may result in abnormal function and consequent susceptibility to infections (Boxer, 1995). Often, the leukocytes are normal in number and in morphologic appearance.

Deficiencies of humoral factors (i.e., antibodies or components of complement) may result in defective chemotaxis or opsonization. Cellular abnormalities (i.e., contractile protein dysfunction or enzyme deficiencies) may result in defects in motility, phagocytosis, or microbial killing.

Eosinophilia

Eosinophilia exists if blood eosinophils exceed $0.35 \times 10^9/L$ when large numbers of cells are counted, as with automated instruments or direct chamber counts, or $0.5 \times 10^9/L$

when the count is calculated from the 100- or 200-cell differential and the total leukocyte count. The major function of eosinophils is to release granule contents or reactive oxygen species generated by the cell membrane to damage the target organism or offending cell (Shurin, 1988).

ALLERGIC DISEASES. Allergic and atopic conditions such as bronchial asthma and seasonal rhinitis (hay fever) are characterized by eosinophilia. These immune reactions are mediated by IgE, which results in mast cell and basophil degranulation with the release of a chemotactic factor for eosinophils. Eosinophils are found in the blood, marrow, and sputum (in bronchial asthma), and in nasal and conjunctival discharges (in hay fever). Blood eosinophilia usually is only mild or moderate (0.4 to 1.0×10^9/L).

Absolute eosinophil counts have been useful in the management of asthma because in that disorder, the level of eosinophils positively correlates with pulmonary performance, indicates the adequacy of steroid therapy, and may indicate the presence of complicating infections.

SKIN DISORDERS. Atopic dermatitis and eczema are often accompanied by blood eosinophilia, especially in children. In pemphigus, eosinophilia is characteristic. Eosinophilia is frequently associated with acute urticarial reactions but is uncommon in chronic urticaria.

PARASITIC INFESTATIONS. Eosinophilia is more pronounced if tissues are invaded (for example, trichinosis) than when parasites are inhabiting the lumen of a viscus (for example, tapeworm). Eosinophilia disappears in some forms of infestation when encystment occurs (for example, cysticercosis).

In trichinosis, eosinophil levels begin to rise in the blood within days after infection. The peak of the eosinophilia is during the third or fourth week. Eosinophilia may be absent, however, in severe infestation with trichinae.

Leukocytosis and eosinophilia extending over months are seen in visceral larva migrans (dog and cat roundworm) infestation. In this condition, pulmonary lesions (Loeffler's syndrome) may be present.

Another parasitic infestation with eosinophilia is creeping eruption caused by larvae of the dog or cat hookworm.

INFECTIOUS DISEASES. Eosinophilia of various degrees is seen in some infectious diseases. In scarlet fever, eosinophilia is commonly associated with the cutaneous rash, which is probably allergic in nature. Chorea may be associated with eosinophilia, but other forms of rheumatic fever are not.

In conditions characterized by neutrophilia, eosinophilia is uncommon; often, this may be due to increased adrenal corticosteroid secretion in disease. For example, when a lesion that is responsible for eosinophilia (such as an *Echinococcus* cyst) becomes infected and suppurates, neutrophilia replaces eosinophilia. The same phenomenon is also observed in acute infections (for example, *Pneumococcus* pneumonia).

PULMONARY EOSINOPHILIAS. Loeffler's syndrome is characterized by repeated, transient pulmonary exudates accompanied by cough, often producing sputum that contains eosinophils. The syndrome resolves in a few weeks. It may be caused by certain drugs, inhaled antigens, or helminth (roundworm) infestation during periods of dissemination when the parasites pass from the blood into the alveoli of the lung.

The *PIE* syndrome (pulmonary infiltration with eosinophilia) refers to a more severe disorder characterized by a chronic and relapsing fever, cough, dyspnea, and other symptoms. The etiology may be bacterial, viral, or fungal infection; an allergic reaction to drugs; or parasitic infestations. The difference between the PIE syndrome and Loeffler's syndrome appears to be one of severity (Lee, 1993).

Tropical pulmonary eosinophilia is a syndrome of paroxysmal cough and bronchospasm associated with marked eosinophilia. It is found mainly in India, Southeast Asia, and the South Pacific. There is a predilection for males and for Indians among racial groups living in an endemic area. Serum IgE levels are very high. Interestingly, epinephrine induces a rise instead of a fall in blood eosinophils. The disease is probably a hyperimmune reaction caused by microfilariae, which may be found occasionally in lung or lymph node biopsy specimens but not in blood. The patients have a high titer of filarial complement-fixing antibodies in the blood. Response to the antifilarial drug diethylcarbamazine is curative.

HYPEREOSINOPHILIC SYNDROME. Persistent high levels of eosinophils for long periods of time, no evidence of known causes of eosinophilia, and signs and symptoms of organ involvement are criteria for inclusion of patients in this syndrome. The organ most consistently affected is the heart, with mural thrombi and endocardial and myocardial fibrosis. Hepatosplenomegaly is common. Most patients have a hypersensitivity reaction of some type; it is an open question whether some patients have a form of eosinophilic leukemia. Regardless of cause, large numbers of circulating eosinophils appear to damage the heart by some unknown mechanism.

Reactive eosinophilia can often be differentiated from an eosinophilic leukemia by the use of cytochemical stains. Eosinophilic leukemias usually have an increased proportion of myeloblasts and eosinophilic myelocytes. In addition, the presence of an abnormal karyotype in a patient with eosinophilia may suggest the appearance of a leukemic clone.

BLOOD DISEASES. In chronic myelogenous leukemia (CML), some cases of acute myelomonocytic leukemia, and to a lesser extent, other myeloproliferative disorders, eosinophilia is present. Mild eosinophilia may be found in marrow and blood in pernicious anemia.

OTHER CONDITIONS. Splenectomy is frequently followed by eosinophilia and lymphocytosis. This may last for several months.

There is no satisfactory explanation for occasional instances of moderate and even severe eosinophilia, general or local, in patients with various neoplasms and a variety of other conditions (for example, ovarian cysts). Eosinophilia is seen more frequently in neoplasms involving serous surfaces and bone and in those with necrosis. Eosinophilia associated with malignant tumors often persists until the primary neoplasm is removed or significantly reduced in size. The eosinophils may be hypogranular and vacuolated. In addition, the eosinophil count may exceed 100×10^9/L. In Hodgkin's disease, the majority of patients do not have blood eosinophilia, although when present it is sometimes marked in degree.

Various drugs have been reported to be responsible for eosinophilia: pilocarpine, physostigmine, digitalis, para-aminosalicylic acid, sulfonamides, and others. On the other hand, atropine is supposed to depress the eosinophils.

Hereditary eosinophilia occurs rarely in the absence of other recognized causes of eosinophilia (Naiman, 1964).

Eosinopenia

Eosinopenia is a decreased level of circulating eosinophils, below the lowest reference value of 0.04×10^9/L. In order to be detected, large numbers of cells must be counted, using direct hemacytometer counts or automated counts with an instrument such as the Technicon H-6000 or H1.

Eosinopenia occurs in any situation that results in acute stress, owing to adrenal glucocorticoid and epinephrine secretion (either causes eosinopenia), and also in acute inflammatory states. A rapid decrease in circulating eosinophils occurs as a result of margination or migration into inflammatory sites. Release of eosinophils from the marrow is temporarily inhibited, and later eosinophil production is inhibited. Once the acute process subsides, immune stimulation of eosinophil production may occur; this process is mediated by T lymphocytes. Eosinopenia of 0 to 0.03×10^9/L also may occur in Cushing's syndrome or following the administration of corticosteroids.

Basophilia

Basophilia is an increase of basophils in the blood to a level above 0.2×10^9/L, if calculated from the differential count and the total leukocyte count, and above 0.08×10^9/L, if counted directly in a hemacytometer chamber or with automated instruments (Gilbert, 1975b).

Basophilia is seen most frequently in allergic reactions, chronic myeloid leukemia, myeloid metaplasia (extramedullary myelopoiesis), polycythemia vera (PCV), and acute basophilic leukemia. Relative basophilia may be transient following irradiation. Basophilia may be present in hypothyroidism and chronic hemolytic anemia and following splenectomy.

Basopenia

A decreased basophil count (less than 0.01×10^9/L) can be detected only when large numbers of basophils are counted directly. With direct basophil counting, it has been determined that basophils, like eosinophils, show diurnal variation. The level is lowest in the morning and highest during the night. Sustained treatment with adrenal glucocorticoids induces a basopenia. Acute infection or stress results in a fall in basophils. About half of patients with hyperthyroidism have a basopenia (Gilbert, 1975b).

Monocytosis

Monocytosis is an increase of monocytes above the upper reference value, usually 1.0×10^9/L (see Table 24–7).

Monocytosis is present during the recovery stage from acute infections and from agranulocytosis, in which it is considered a favorable sign. In contrast, an increase of monocytes in tuberculosis is a poor prognostic sign.

Monocytosis may be present in subacute bacterial endocarditis. In this condition, monocytes may show phagocytosis of other blood cells, red blood cells, and leukocytes. It may be present in mycotic, rickettsial, protozoal, and viral infections.

Infectious disease, however, is an uncommon cause of monocytosis. In a study of 160 successive cases of absolute monocytosis (Maldonado, 1965), over half (85) were associated with *hematologic disease*. Twenty had monocytic or granulocytic leukemia; 20 had lymphoma (Hodgkin's disease was most frequent); 7 had multiple myeloma; 6 had myeloproliferative disorders; and in 18, the cause was indeterminate. *Other malignant diseases* accounted for 13 cases; *connective tissue disorders,* 16; *infectious disease,* 9; *fever of unknown origin,* 7; *ulcerative colitis,* 4; *regional enteritis,* 4; *nontropical sprue,* 2; and *cirrhosis,* 3 cases. *Miscellaneous* and *indeterminate causes* made up the remaining 17 cases. Among hematopoietic dysplasias, an unexplained monocytosis occasionally seems to precede the development of leukemia by months or years (see the section entitled Myelodysplastic Syndromes).

Monocytopenia

A decrease in circulating monocytes below the lower reference value of 0.2×10^9/L is monocytopenia. Few studies have dealt with monocytopenia. During therapy with prednisone, monocytes fall during the first few hours after the first dose but return to above original levels by 12 hours. Monocytopenia has also been observed in hairy cell leukemia (HCL).

Lymphocytic and Plasmacytic Disorders

Lymphocytes in Normal Individuals

In normal individuals, the absolute numbers of lymphocytes and T cells are highest at birth (Fig. 27–1). At that time, lymphocytes represent approximately 90% of all leukocytes. During the first three to seven days of life, there is a slight decrease in the number of lymphocytes. However, during the second week of life, the lymphocyte count returns to the level observed at birth. Cellular immune function in the newborn is comparable with that in normal adults.

During the first decade of life, the absolute lymphocyte count and the absolute number of T cells decrease but remain higher than observed in the adult. By the time of adolescence, the absolute lymphocyte count and the absolute number of T cells have leveled off at values observed throughout adulthood. The absolute number of B lymphocytes remains stable during all stages of life (Davey, 1977). In adolescence and adulthood, lymphocytes constitute about 20% to 40% of all leukocytes or 1.5 to 4.0×10^9 cells per liter.

There is some disagreement regarding the absolute number of lymphocytes and number of T cells in aged individuals. Although some studies (Diaz-Jouanen, 1975) indicate that there is a decrease in total lymphocyte count and T-cell numbers, other investigators find no significant change in total lymphocytes or T cells in aged individuals (Davey, 1977; Weksler, 1974). The distribution of lymphocyte subsets in adults is given in Table 27–3. The CD4:CD8 (T-helper/T-suppressor) cell ratio is usually 2, with a range of 1.5 to 3.0. Conflicting results are found concerning the T-lymphocyte subsets in the neonate. In comparison with adult blood, the number of total T cells and CD8-positive T cells may be identical or decreased, whereas CD4-positive T cells may be identical or increased (De Waele, 1988).

Lymphocytosis

Lymphocytosis is an increase in the number of lymphocytes in the peripheral blood; the reference intervals are 1.5 to

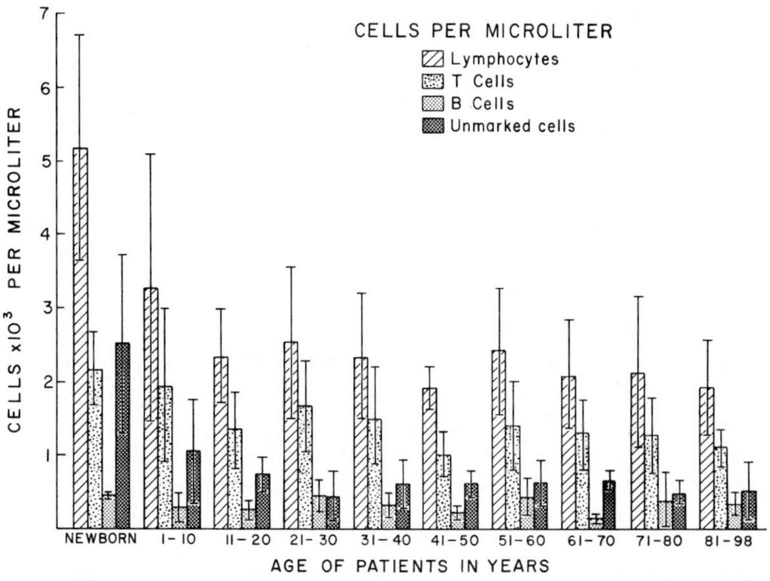

Figure 27-1. Absolute counts of total lymphocytes. T cells, B cells, and unmarked cells (non-T, non-B) in normal individuals at different ages, by decade. (From Davey FR, Huntington S: Age-related variation in lymphocyte subpopulations. Gerontology 1977; 23:381. Basel S. Karger AG. Used by permission.)

4.0 × 10^9/L in the adult and 1.5 to 8.8 × 10^9/L in the child. Relative lymphocytosis (an increase in the percentage of lymphocytes) is present in various conditions and is especially prominent in disorders with neutropenia.

INFECTIOUS LYMPHOCYTOSIS. This disorder is characterized by lymphocytosis associated with viral infection and occurs mainly in children. The incubation period is 12 to 21 days.

Antibody and viral studies have indicated that a relationship exists between infectious lymphocytosis and coxsackievirus A, coxsackievirus B6, echoviruses, and adenovirus type 12. No association has been noted with Epstein-Barr virus (EBV), cytomegalovirus, or herpesvirus. Although the disease usually has no systemic manifestations, sometimes vomiting, fever, abdominal discomfort, signs suggesting involvement of the nervous system, cutaneous rashes, upper respiratory infections, or diarrhea occur. Leukocytosis (20 to 50 × 10^9/L, occasionally over 100 × 10^9/L) precedes the clinical manifestations. From 60% to 95% of blood leukocytes are small mature lymphocytes and are probably of T-cell origin (Cassuto, 1977). In contrast to infectious mononucleosis, atypical lymphocytes (see the section entitled Lymphocytosis) are uncommon. There usually is an associated eosinophilia. The lymphocytosis usually lasts three to five weeks, or sometimes longer. Other blood changes are unusual. The marrow has no characteristic changes; an increased percentage of lymphocytes has been observed but is probably an artifact as a result of admixture of peripheral blood. Lymph node enlargement is rare and minimal when present. The spleen and liver are rarely, if ever, enlarged. Lymph node biopsy may show reactive follicular hyperplasia but no characteristic changes.

The tests for infectious mononucleosis (see later discussion) are negative. In some cases, there has been an increase of white blood cells in the cerebrospinal fluid, with about 40% lymphocytes. The course is benign.

Another form of infectious lymphocytosis in children has a chronic course. The leukocyte count is 10 to 25 × 10^9/L, with 60% to 80% lymphocytes of normal appearance. Slight eosinophilia, monocytosis, and plasmacytosis are also present. As a rule, the children have enlargement of the tonsils, lymph nodes, and spleen and a history of re-

4

Table 27-3. LYMPHOCYTE SUBSETS IN PERIPHERAL BLOOD OF NORMAL ADULT

Cluster Designation	Representative Monoclonal Antibodies	Expression on Normal Cells	Median Percent Positive	Range (Percent)
CD1	Na 1/34, Leu-6	Thymocytes	5	1–15
CD2	9.6, Leu-5	Pan-T cell	76	34–91
CD3	T3, Leu-4	Pan-T cell	63	28–77
CD4	OKT4, Leu-3	Helper/inducer T cell	50	32–62
CD5	UCHT2, Leu-1	Pan-T cell	77	42–84
CD7	3A1, Leu-9	Pan-T cell	64	38–88
CD8	Leu-2	Cytotoxic/suppressor T cell	28	2–36
CD10	J5	Restricted B cell	4	1–11
CD16	Leu-11	Natural killer cell	11	5–19
CD19	B4, Leu-12	Pan-B cell	8	3–14
CD20	B1	Pan-B cell	8	3–15
CD24	BA1	Pan-B cell	30	24–32

Constructed from data presented in McMichael AJ (ed): Leukocyte Typing III. White Cell Differentiation Antigens. Oxford University Press, 1987.

current upper respiratory infections. The marrow shows no abnormalities.

PERTUSSIS. Whooping cough (pertussis) occurs during childhood, especially in unimmunized children. The etiologic agent is *Bordetella pertussis (Haemophilus pertussis),* which produces an inflammatory reaction in the entire respiratory tract.

The incubation period is approximately two weeks, and the first symptoms are those of a head cold. Later, the patient develops paroxysms of coughing productive of thick sputum. There is frequently pain over the trachea and bronchi.

Patients frequently develop significant lymphocytosis with counts higher than 30×10^9/L recorded. The lymphocyte count is highest during the first three weeks of the illness, then decreases during the fourth and subsequent weeks (Lagergren, 1963). The lymphocytes are small and mature, and are increased due to the release of lymphocytosis-promoting factor (LPF) released from the organism. Each of these factors causes a transient increased mobilization of lymphocytes from lymphoid organs, followed by inhibition of recirculation of lymphocytes from blood into the lymphatic system. Thus, the lymphocytosis is due to a redistribution of lymphocytes into the peripheral circulation without increased lymphopoiesis (Rai, 1971; Spangrude, 1985).

CHRONIC LYMPHOCYTOSIS. A persistent peripheral blood chronic lymphocytosis is an uncommon event in adults. In most cases in which this abnormality has been discovered, the diagnosis of chronic lymphocytic leukemia is made subsequently. However, in a few cases, the lymphocytosis waxed and waned over months to years and may have spontaneously disappeared (Chanarin, 1984). The peripheral blood lymphocytes from these patients often possess a mature T-cell or natural killer cell immunophenotype (Bassan, 1988). The patients usually have no significant clinical symptoms or physical findings. However, patients with a suppressor cell (CD8) phenotype often exhibit a variety of rheumatic symptoms and some patients have even shown classic Felty's syndrome (Newland, 1984). The lymphocytes from some of these patients have been shown to result from a clonal expansion of T cells. Persistent polyclonal lymphocytosis has been reported in adults as an infrequent event in smokers and in the postsplenectomy state (Hutchison, 1988).

HUMAN T-LYMPHOTROPIC VIRUS-TYPE I–ASSOCIATED TRANSIENT T-CELL LYMPHOCYTOSIS. Human T-lymphotropic virus-type 1 (HTLV-1) is a retrovirus associated with adult T-cell leukemia, particularly in endemic areas of Japan, the Caribbean basin, and the southeastern United States. Several cases have now been reported of a transient T-cell lymphocytosis in patients infected with this virus (Kinoshita, 1985; Ehrlich, 1988). In most patients, the disorder is characterized by few clinical symptoms consisting of fever, limited lymphadenopathy, and occasional skin rash. The peripheral blood lymphocyte count usually is less than 20×10^9/L; however, 10% to 40% of these lymphocytes are immature forms. In most of these cases, the lymphocytosis is the result of monoclonal proliferation of T cells. Although some patients with this infection progress to adult T-cell leukemia, almost 90% of patients with antibodies against HTLV-1 are symptom free. Although most individuals exhibit only a virus-like syndrome, others manifest a chronic progressive leukemia, and still others develop tropical spastic paraparesis (Davey, 1991).

INFECTIOUS MONONUCLEOSIS. Infectious mononucleosis (IM) usually is a self-limited infectious disease of the reticuloendothelial tissue, with characteristic clinical, hematologic, and pathologic features, as well as specific serologic alterations.

Etiology and Pathophysiology. IM is a disorder secondary to an infection with the EBV. When the primary infection occurs during early childhood, the disease often goes unnoticed. However, when the infection involves adolescent individuals or adults, the resultant disorder is the IM syndrome. In most cases, the virus gains entry into the body through the oropharyngeal epithelial and lymphoid tissues, and the virus appears to infect both tissues. The virus attaches to C3d complement receptors (CD21) on B-lymphoid cells and is absorbed into the cells. The EBV then stimulates DNA synthesis in these B cells and induces the formation of several new antigens, including the viral capsid antigen (VCA); the membrane antigen (MA); early antigen (EA), both diffuse (EA-D) and the restricted (EA-R) subtypes; Epstein-Barr nuclear antigens (EBNA); and the lymphocyte-detected membrane antigen (LYDMA) (Harrington, 1988). Thus, the earliest phase of this disease is characterized by an infection of B cells that proliferate, develop neoantigens, circulate, stimulate an immune response, and synthesize immunoglobulin (Sixbey, 1984).

The humoral immune response is characterized by the rise in titer of viral capsid antibodies IgM and IgG during the incubation and early prodrome period. The titer of IgM capsid antibody starts to fall during the second and third weeks of illness and then diminishes to undetectable levels within the following several months (Fig. 27–2). The IgG viral capsid antibody decreases during convalescence but remains detectable for life. Approximately two to three weeks after the onset of illness, the EBV antibodies against the early antigens appear and then decline over the succeeding two months. The titer of the EBV nuclear antigen antibodies rises during the later portion of convalescence and is apparently detectable throughout life.

The cellular immune response in IM is characterized by a proliferation and activation of T cells usually during the second week of illness in response to the EBV-induced B-cell infection and activation. Because these activated T cells are mostly from the cytotoxic and suppressor cell subpopulation, there is a marked suppression and destruction of EBV-infected B cells. Indeed, most of the atypical lymphocytes observed in the peripheral blood of patients with IM during the second week of illness possess the CD8 antigen. These cytotoxic and suppressor T cells kill infected B cells and diminish the polyclonal antibody production induced by the EBV. In addition to the cytotoxic T cells, the activity of natural killer cells has a profound effect on limiting the proliferation of the EBV-infected B cells in patients with IM (Purtilo, 1983). It is also likely that EBV-infected B cells are destroyed, at least in part, through the mechanism of antibody-dependent cellular cytotoxicity, a process requiring the presence of both cytotoxic cells and antibody. This process of B-cell proliferation followed by the inhibitory and destructive effects of EBV-directed antibody production, as well as T-cell and natural killer cell cytotoxic effects, occurs

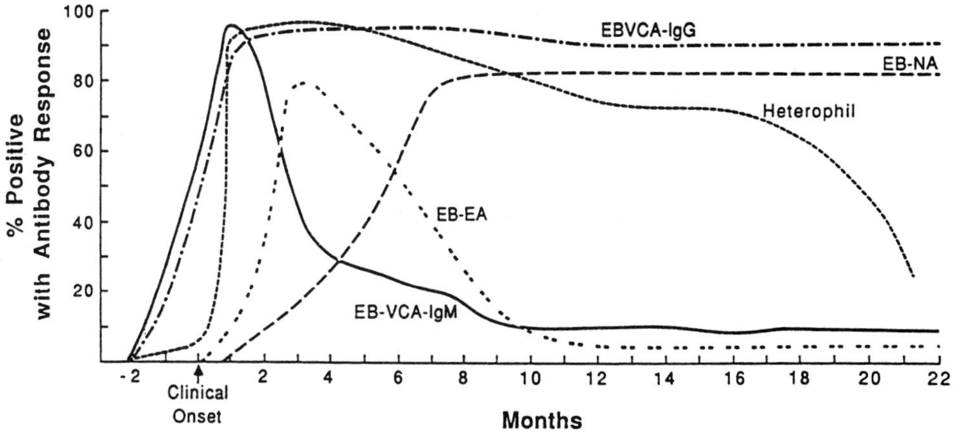

Figure 27–2. Percentage of individuals with antibody responses at different time intervals. (Reproduced with permission: Davey FR, Kurec AS: Infectious Mononucleosis. ASCP Hematology Check Sample, vol 30: H88-10[H-201]. Chicago, American Society of Clinical Pathologists, 1988.)

within the patient's peripheral blood, bone marrow, lymphoid tissues, and perhaps to a limited degree, all tissues of the body.

Clinical Features. The disease has been observed in patients from three months to 70 years of age but is most common in adolescents and young adults. The onset is vague, indefinite, and similar to the onset of other infectious diseases. Patients usually have fever, sore throat, and lymphadenopathy (Table 27–4).

Complications. Of the rare anemias associated with IM, hemolytic anemia is the most common, occurring in 1% to 3% of cases. The cause now appears to be related to the anti-i antibody produced frequently in this disease.

Mild thrombocytopenia occurs in about half the cases, but the platelet count is not often less than 100×10^9/L. Thrombocytopenic purpura with hemorrhagic complications is exceedingly rare.

Abnormal liver function tests indicative of hepatitis occur in 85% to 100% of patients. Clinical jaundice is rare, but cases have been reported in which jaundice and acute pharyngitis were the only clinical manifestations of IM, with positive hematologic and serologic findings.

Approximately one third of patients with IM carry β-hemolytic streptococci in the pharynx. Thus, one should give attention to strict clinical, hematologic, and serologic criteria in distinguishing IM from streptococcal pharyngitis.

Hematologic Features. Leukocytes are increased, usually ranging from 12 to 25×10^9/L. Rarely, counts as high as 80×10^9/L have been recorded. The leukocytosis usually is due to lymphocytosis (60% to 90%) composed of a variety of atypical lymphocytes. The total leukocyte count, as a rule, returns to normal within three weeks. The atypical lymphocytes have nuclear alterations and an increase in the amount and basophilia of cytoplasm.

Nuclei may have so-called open chromatin and deep indentations (leukocytoid lymphocytes, Downey type I; Plate 27–2*E*). The cytoplasm shows basophilia, an increase of azurophilic granules, and frequently, vacuoles. Some cells resemble plasma cells; some resemble monocytes. Cells that have a relatively smooth but still mature nucleus and abundant smooth cytoplasm with patchy peripheral and radial basophilia have been called stress lymphocytes or Downey type II (see Plates 27–2*A* to *D,* 27–7*I*). They are often the most numerous. Occasionally, lymphocytes have transformed into blastlike cells, presumably in response to the viral stimulation. These immature lymphocytes, usually representing only a small percentage of the total lymphocyte count, are large reticular lymphocytes (nonleukemic lymphoblasts) with a coarsely reticular nucleus and abundant, deeply basophilic cytoplasm (Downey type III; see Plates 27–2*C* and *G,* 27–7*H,* 25–3*J* and *K*). In contrast, lymphoblasts of acute lymphocytic leukemia are usually smaller, with a very fine chro-

Table 27–4. CLINICAL FINDINGS IN 106 CASES OF INFECTIOUS MONONUCLEOSIS

	No. Cases	Percent		No. Cases	Percent
Lymphadenopathy	101	95.3	Skin rash	5	4.7
Fever	93	87.7	Epistaxis	3	2.8
Pharyngitis	64	60.4	Icterus	3	2.8
Without membrane	50	47.2	Loss of weight	2	1.9
With membrane	14	13.2	Diarrhea	2	1.9
Splenomegaly	51	48.1	Arthritic pains	2	1.9
Headache	26	24.5	Purpura	2	1.9
Hepatomegaly	24	22.6	Gingivitis	2	1.9
Prostration	11	10.4	Convulsions	1	0.9
Emesis	10	9.4	Toothache	1	0.9
Pain in abdomen	8	7.6	Albuminuria	14	13.2
Upper abdomen	6	5.7	Positive test for syphilis	3	2.8
Lower abdomen	2	1.9	Relapses (17 days to 2 months)	7	6.5
Stiffness or pain in neck	6	5.7	Recurrence (1 year)	1	0.9

Table 27–5. CAUSES OF LYMPHOCYTOSIS

Lymphocytosis Associated with Atypical Lymphocytes			**Lymphocytosis Associated with Small Mature Lymphocytes**
Percent of White Cells That Are Atypical Lymphocytes *>20*	*<20*	*Uncommon Causes*	
Infectious mononucleosis Infectious hepatitis Post-transfusion syndrome Cytomegalovirus infection *p*-Aminosalicylic acid (PAS) hypersensitivity Phenytoin (Dilantin) and mephenytoin (Mesantoin) hypersensitivity	(a) Infections Mumps,* varicella,* rubeola, rubella, atypical pneumonia, herpes simplex, herpes zoster, roseola infantum, influenza,* other viral illnesses, tuberculosis,* rickettsialpox, brucellosis,* toxoplasmosis* (b) Radiation (c) Other Letterer-Siwe disease Agranulocytosis Lead intoxication Stress Leukemia and lymphoma*	Tertiary syphilis* Congenital syphilis* Smallpox Tetrachlorethane poisoning Trinitrotoluene poisoning Organic arsenical hypersensitivity Severe dermatitis herpetiformis	Infectious lymphocytosis Pertussis

*Higher counts of atypical lymphocytes are occasionally found.
Modified from Wood TA, Frenkel EP: The atypical lymphocyte. Am J Med 1967; 42:923.

matin pattern and very little cytoplasm (Plates 27–1*L*, 27–2*H*, 27–4*G*).

Often the number of monocytes rises transiently. The term mononucleosis refers to an increase of lymphocytes and not monocytes.

The cytologic alterations are not pathognomonic of IM. Similar cells are found in a variety of disorders, including cytomegalovirus mononucleosis, toxoplasmosis, and infectious hepatitis, and usually to a lesser extent in viral pneumonia, varicella, mumps, and viral exanthemas of children (Table 27–5).

Neutrophils are relatively and absolutely decreased in most cases during the first week of illness. During this time, there may be a shift to the left, with an increase of band cells and metamyelocytes. Toxic granules and Döhle bodies may be seen. The eosinophils are within normal limits.

The bone marrow from patients with IM usually shows an increased cellularity. There is an increased number of lymphocytes, macrophages, plasma cells, megakaryocytes, and erythroid cells. The neutrophilic series appears decreased. About half of the cases may have collections of mononuclear cells forming loose granulomas.

Serologic Findings

Heterophil Antibody. Paul (1932) first described the presence of sheep cell agglutinins in the sera of patients with IM. Unfortunately, the presence of sheep cell agglutinins is not a specific finding for IM and can be present in other disorders.

Davidsohn (1937) demonstrated that the heterophil antibodies in patients with IM are absorbed by beef erythrocytes, in contrast to heterophil antibodies present in other disorders. The heterophil antibodies in other disorders are absorbed by the Forssman antigen, such as that found in guinea pig kidney. The differential absorption test (Paul-Bunnell-Davidsohn test) is highly specific for IM (Davidsohn, 1969).

The spot test for IM (Lee, 1968) is based on the principle that horse erythrocytes are more sensitive than sheep erythrocytes in testing for IM. Serum is mixed with a suspension of finely ground guinea pig kidney on one part of the slide, with a suspension of beef erythrocyte stroma on another. Horse erythrocytes are added to each spot and mixed. A positive test for IM shows agglutination of horse erythrocytes of serum absorbed with guinea pig kidney but not by serum absorbed with beef erythrocyte stroma. The spot test has proved to be a simple, rapid, highly specific, and sensitive test for the heterophil antibodies of IM. False-positive tests occur but are very rare. False-negative tests occur, particularly in young children, who produce heterophil antibodies (IgM) in limited amounts. In heterophil negative IM, the diagnosis may be substantiated by assay for antibody to EBV.

As previously mentioned, several antibodies are produced by the host in response to a variety of EBV antigens (see Fig. 27–2). Antibody to the VCA arises within the first two weeks of the onset. This antibody is measured by an immunofluorescent method and is probably the most widely used assay for determining exposure to EBV. Assaying for the presence of EBV antibody usually is limited to the few cases of heterophil negative IM.

In addition to heterophil and EBV antibodies, patients with IM frequently produce antibodies to a wide variety of antigens. Antibodies against human erythrocytes, leukocytes, and platelets have been described. Patients with IM have an increased frequency of cold agglutinins. Positive tests to rheumatoid factor and antinuclear factor have been reported.

Differential Diagnosis. The clinical, hematologic, and serologic features of IM permit an accurate diagnosis to be made in over 90% of the cases. When the heterophil (monospot) test is negative, one must consider several possibilities. The patient could still have EBV antibody-positive but heterophil-negative IM. However, cytomegalovirus infection is the most common cause of heterophil-negative mononucleosis. Other possibilities include toxoplasmosis, infectious hepatitis, and ingestion of drugs (*p*-aminosalicylic acid, phenytoin [Dilantin], and diaminodiphenylsulfone).

Course. IM is a benign disorder, and complications occur in less than 5% of patients. The disorder usually resolves in three to four weeks. Fatalities are extremely rare, but tend to occur in members of the same family (Purtilo, 1979). Further studies indicate that the affected individuals frequently suffered from sex-linked lymphoproliferative syndrome.

CYTOMEGALOVIRUS INFECTION. Some individuals infected with cytomegalovirus develop a syndrome similar to infectious mononucleosis. This disorder can occur following massive blood transfusions (post-transfusion mononucleosis) or spontaneously in previously healthy individuals (cytomegalovirus mononucleosis). The patient has fever, chills, profound malaise, and myalgia. There may be a sore throat (but not exudative pharyngitis) and lymphadenopathy. Occasionally, splenomegaly is found, but hepatomegaly does not occur.

Leukocytosis is characteristic with absolute lymphocytosis. Usually, 20% or more of the leukocytes are atypical lymphocytes. Bone marrow aspirates have shown an increased number of normal lymphocytes and atypical lymphocytes. Hepatic enzymes are frequently abnormal. In a small percentage of patients, there may be an increased titer of cold agglutinins, rheumatoid factor, and antinuclear antibodies. There is no rise in heterophil, EBV, or *Toxoplasma* antibodies. The diagnosis usually is made by isolating the cytomegalovirus from urine or by demonstrating a rise in antibody by the complement fixation of indirect hemagglutination techniques (Jordan, 1973).

TOXOPLASMOSIS. In children and adults, toxoplasmosis can produce a disorder similar to infectious mononucleosis. Patients have fever, lymphadenopathy, and an increased number of atypical lymphocytes in the peripheral blood. Rarely is there splenomegaly. Pharyngitis and upper respiratory tract infection are usually absent.

The histopathology of lymph nodes usually is distinctive and correlates closely with elevated *Toxoplasma* antibody titers (Dorfman, 1973). Bone marrow biopsy specimens have no specific pathologic lesion.

The diagnosis is established by demonstrating an elevation of *Toxoplasma* antibodies by fluorescent-antibody, or hemagglutination techniques.

MISCELLANEOUS CAUSES OF LYMPHOCYTOSIS. Numerous disorders have been associated with lymphocytosis. A partial listing of illnesses associated with relative or absolute lymphocytosis is provided in Table 27–5.

Lymphocytopenia

Lymphocytopenia is present when the absolute lymphocyte count is below 1.5×10^9/L in adults and below 3.0×10^9/L in children. A number of immunologic deficiency disorders that are genetically determined have lymphocytopenia along with various other immunologic defects of either humoral or cell-mediated immunity. Lymphocytopenia in these disorders is due to impaired lymphopoiesis. Increased levels of adrenocortical hormones, the administration of chemotherapeutic drugs, or irradiation results in lymphocytopenia. Impaired drainage of the intestinal lymphatics with loss of lymphocytes into the intestines owing to a number of causes has been implicated as a mechanism for lymphocytopenia. In advanced cases of non-Hodgkin's and Hodgkin's lymphomas, as well as in terminal cases of carcinoma, lymphocytopenia often is observed.

ACQUIRED IMMUNODEFICIENCY SYNDROME. Acquired immunodeficiency syndrome (AIDS) usually is a progressively fatal infectious disorder with characteristic clinical, hematologic, and serologic abnormalities.

Etiology. AIDS is a disorder secondary to an infection with the human immunodeficiency viruses 1 (HIV-1) and 2 (HIV-2), RNA retroviruses that are cytotropic for $CD4^+$ T cells and for macrophages. The infection is spread by contamination with secretions, excretions, blood, and tissues that contain the virus. Because of the cytotropic effect of the AIDS viruses for $CD4^+$ cells, there is marked decrease in the number of T-helper cells and an imbalance in T-suppressor and cytotoxic cells in the blood and the lymphoid tissues of the body. As a result, a profound cellular immune depression occurs, which is characterized by infections with a variety of opportunistic organisms (Jandl, 1987). Initially, B cells are not involved and immunoglobulin levels are normal or increased. However, as the disease progresses, there is an increased frequency of non-Hodgkin's lymphoma (NHL), most often of B-cell lineage (Egerter, 1988). In addition, the function of monocytes and natural killer cells is abnormal.

Hematologic Features. The most common hematologic abnormality in patients with AIDS is anemia of chronic disease and lymphopenia (80% to 85% of cases), particularly of the T-helper and inducer (CD4) subset. Thrombocytopenia occurs in approximately 30% of cases, and neutropenia occurs in 40%, often with a shift to the left; the former often is immune mediated.

The peripheral blood film usually displays atypical lymphocytes that have a plasmacytoid appearance. Monocytes are often large with a fine nuclear chromatin and cytoplasmic vacuoles. Immune-mediated anemia, thrombocytopenia and neutropenia also have been described in AIDS.

The bone marrow usually is normocellular to hypercellular. There often is an increased number of immature myeloid precursor cells, macrophages laden with iron, and plasma cells. There are defects in bone marrow progenitor cells such as colony forming unit–granulocyte, monocyte (CFU-GM), colony forming unit–granulocyte, erythrocyte, monocyte, megakaryocyte, pluripotential stem cell (CFU-GEMM), colony forming unit–megakaryocyte (CFU-MK), and burst forming unit–erythrocyte (BFU-E). Frequent dysplastic features provide evidence of ineffective hematopoiesis (Hoxie, 1995). Many drugs used to treat AIDS and its infectious complications also are myelosuppressive.

Functional Disorders of Lymphocytes

Functional disorders of lymphocytes can be inherited or acquired. The immune deficiency may be due to a disorder in monocytes, B cells, T cells, stem cells, suppressor cells, or a combination. Acquired functional abnormalities of lymphocytes are most frequently observed in lymphoid malignancies. Decreased B-cell function is observed in chronic lymphocytic leukemia, in which two thirds of the patients have hypogammaglobulinemia. In multiple myeloma, there is a diminished synthesis of normal immunoglobulin in the presence of high levels of paraprotein.

Diminished T-cell activity has been described in patients with Hodgkin's disease, sarcoidosis, and leprosy. In Hodgkin's disease, the diminished T-cell activity may be the result

4

of the suppressive effects of monocytes. In autoimmune diseases, a loss of suppressor T cells has been observed.

In severe malnutrition and in patients with terminal malignancies, there is diminished humoral and cell-mediated immunity.

The diagnosis of functional disorders of lymphocytes requires the use of skin tests, enumeration of B and T cells and their subsets, measurement of serum immunoglobulin and antibodies, and a variety of *in vitro* lymphocyte assays that record their response to mitogens and antigens.

Plasmacytosis

Plasma cells are not normally present in circulating blood. They are increased in a variety of chronic infections, in allergic states, in the presence of neoplasms, and in other conditions in which the serum γ-globulin concentration is elevated. Plasma cells have also been recorded in the blood of patients with viral disorders, including rubella, measles, chickenpox, and mumps. They are moderately increased in cutaneous exanthemas, infectious mononucleosis, syphilis, subacute bacterial endocarditis, sarcoidosis, and collagen diseases. Their increase usually is linked with an increase in lymphocytes, monocytes, and eosinophils.

In the marrow, an average of 1% to 2% of plasma cells are present in adults. An increase beyond 4% is significant; lower values are found in children (see Table 25–3). Increases of up to 20% of plasma cells may be found in a variety of conditions other than multiple myeloma, including metastatic carcinoma, chronic granulomatous infections, conditions linked with hypersensitivity, and following the administration of cytotoxic drugs. They are often increased in aplastic anemia, but this is probably just a relative increase. On the other hand, they are decreased or absent in agammaglobulinemia.

Leukemoid Reactions

A leukemoid reaction is an excessive leukocytic response. It includes leukocytosis of 50×10^9/L or higher with a shift to the left; lower counts, even below normal, with considerable numbers of immature granulocytes; and similar quantitative or qualitative changes in lymphocytes or monocytes. Depending on the predominant cell, leukemoid reactions may be neutrophilic, eosinophilic, lymphocytic, or monocytic. No clear explanation for these apparent temporary aberrations in normal regulatory control mechanisms is yet available. The reactions are irregular in degree, even when associated with the same inciting agent.

NEUTROPHILIC LEUKEMOID REACTIONS. Excessive neutrophilia may occur in many situations, including hemolysis, hemorrhage, malignancy with bone involvement, Hodgkin's disease, myelofibrosis, infections (especially tuberculosis), severe burns, eclampsia, and certain intoxications.

Examination of the blood usually is more helpful than marrow examination. Leukemoid reactions lack the characteristic differential count that is seen in chronic myelogenous leukemia, including the so-called myelocyte peak, eosinophilia, and basophilia. Also, the leukemic hiatus so characteristic of acute leukemia is absent.

EOSINOPHILIC LEUKEMOID REACTIONS. Cells as immature as eosinophilic myelocytes rarely appear in the blood in reactive eosinophilia, in which the leukocyte count may exceed 50×10^9/L. Eosinophilic leukemoid reactions usually occur in children and usually are caused by parasitic infections. The idiopathic hypereosinophilic syndrome in adults is leukemoid (Fauci, 1982).

ERYTHROBLASTOSIS. In patients with or without anemia, circulating normoblasts frequently are accompanied by a neutrophilic leukemoid reaction; this, then, is a *leukoerythroblastotic reaction*. Moderate anemia with normoblasts in the peripheral blood is fairly common in metastatic carcinoma involving bone marrow.

LYMPHOCYTIC LEUKEMOID REACTIONS. Extremely high counts of normal-appearing lymphocytes may occur in infectious lymphocytosis and in pertussis. When atypical lymphocytes are strikingly increased or immature (which may occur in conditions such as infectious mononucleosis), the distinction from leukemia may be difficult. Tuberculosis may be associated with either type of lymphocytosis.

Examination of the marrow often is useful, because lymphocytes are minimally increased, if at all, in most leukemoid reactions in contrast to leukemia.

NEOPLASTIC AND RELATED DISORDERS PRIMARILY INVOLVING LEUKOCYTES

Definition and Classification of Leukemias

Leukemia is a generalized neoplastic proliferation or accumulation of leukopoietic cells with or without involvement of the peripheral blood. Leukocytosis, abnormal circulating cells, and infiltration of nonhematopoietic tissues are frequently but not invariably present.

The *acute leukemias,* if no remission is induced, usually are fatal within three months. The bone marrow usually is packed with primitive cells of the series involved with very little evidence of differentiation. Patients with *chronic leukemias* usually survive more than one year after the onset of symptoms if no remission occurs. The cell type is more differentiated.

The leukemias are also classified according to cytologic characteristics. There are two major cytologic categories—myeloid and lymphoid—which are further divided depending on the level of differentiation of the predominant cell type. The proliferation in acute myeloid leukemia (AML) consists predominantly of myeloblasts, whereas in CML it consists mostly of more differentiated cells (myelocytes, metamyelocytes, neutrophils) and relatively few myeloblasts. In acute lymphoblastic leukemia, the proliferation is of lymphoblasts. In contrast, in chronic lymphocytic leukemia, it is composed of small mature lymphocytes.

Myeloid Disorders

The myeloid disorders comprise a group of closely related syndromes characterized by self-perpetuating proliferation of one or more type of bone marrow cells: erythroid precursors, granulocytes and monocytes, and megakaryocytes. The proliferation is abnormal, and the causes are incompletely understood. Marrow, spleen, liver, and lymph nodes may be involved; these are the organs that normally participate in hematopoiesis. All cell lines may be committed to the proliferative process (panmyelosis), or a single cell line may predominate.

The *AMLs* include the myeloblastic with minimal differentiation, myeloblastic without maturation, myeloblastic with maturation, promyelocytic, myelomonocytic, monoblastic, monocytic, erythroleukemic, and megakaryocytic leukemias. The *chronic myeloproliferative disorders* include CML, PCV, myelofibrosis with myeloid metaplasia, and essential thrombocythemia (ET). An additional group of disorders are the *myelodysplastic syndromes (MDS).* They include refractory anemia, refractory anemia with ringed sideroblasts, refractory anemia with excess blasts, chronic myelomonocytic leukemia, and refractory anemia with excess blasts in transformation.

AML, the chronic myeloproliferative disorders, and many of the MDS are clonal proliferative diseases that involve erythroid, granulocytic, monocytic, and megakaryocytic cell lines, all derived from a common hematopoietic stem cell line. The leukemic cells from patients with AML and MDS have been shown to be clonal proliferations with characteristic chromosomal and oncogene translocations (Jandl, 1987). Studies in individuals with a chronic myeloproliferative disorder who were heterozygous for glucose-6-phosphate dehydrogenase (G6PD) isoenzymes have indicated that only one isoenzyme was present in erythrocytes, granulocytes, monocytes, and platelets, whereas both isoenzymes were found in other tissues of these patients. This has been demonstrated in CML (Fialkow, 1977), in PCV (Adamson, 1976), in myelofibrosis with myeloid metaplasia, and in ET (Fialkow, 1981). Such evidence strongly supports the concept that the chronic myeloproliferative disorders are also clonal in nature (and by implication, neoplastic), having arisen from a single pluripotential hematopoietic stem cell. However, the fibrosis that may occur in the marrow in these conditions is not monoclonal and hence is likely to be reactive. The new clone of cells seems to have a proliferative advantage over normal cells that it gradually replaces and then often results in bone marrow failure with anemia, neutropenia, and thrombocytopenia.

Acute Myeloid Leukemia

CLINICAL FEATURES. AML is the most common form of acute leukemia during the first few months of life. During childhood and adolescence, it is relatively rare. However, during the middle and later years of life it becomes the most frequently observed form of acute leukemia.

The onset of AML often resembles an acute infection or even a septic condition. Changes include signs of granulocytic insufficiency, with ulcerations of mucous membranes (especially of the mouth and throat) and fever. Enlargement of lymph nodes, spleen, and liver usually is not pronounced. Marked prostration and general malaise may be present. In untreated cases, the course is rapidly progressive.

FAB CLASSIFICATION. The French-American-British (FAB) Cooperative Group has published criteria for the classification of acute leukemias (Bennett, 1976, 1985a, 1985b, 1991) and for the MDS, or preleukemias (Bennett, 1982). The FAB classification is based on morphology of cells in Romanowsky-stained blood and marrow films and certain supplemental cytochemical reactions or serum lysozyme levels (Tables 27–6 and 27–7). It requires the need for excellent technical preparations of blood and marrow films and stresses the need for caution before diagnosing leukemia from hypocellular marrow specimens.

The FAB classification proposes that the initial assessment of a bone marrow specimen suspected of AML or myelodysplastic syndrome be based on a 500-cell count. First, it is necessary to calculate the percentage of erythroid precursor cells. With the exception of the erythroleukemias (M6), the diagnosis of AML is established when 30% or more of the nucleated cells of the bone marrow are blasts and/or leukemic cells (abnormal promyelocytes or promonocytes). The diagnosis of erythroleukemia is established when more than 50% of the bone marrow cells are erythroid precursor cells and when myeloblasts represent more than 30% of the remaining nonerythroid cells (NECs). The diagnosis of myelodysplastic syndrome is suggested when less than 30% of the NECs are myeloblasts, and dysplastic alterations are present in cells of the myeloid, erythroid, and/or megakaryocytic series. Once the diagnosis of AML has been made, only NECs should be considered in the differential count for the further assignment of the subtypes (M1 to M5, M7).

The FAB group recognizes three types of blast cells: All have central nuclei with fine, uncondensed chromatin and prominent nucleoli (usually three to five) (Plate 27–1*J* and *K*). Type I blasts lack cytoplasmic granules, but Type II blasts have a small number (<20) of primary (azurophilic) granules. Type III blasts are similar to Type II blasts with the exception of more abundant azurophilic granules. Neutrophilic promyelocytes are larger, have lower nuclear/cytoplasmic ratios and more dense nuclear chromatin than Type III blasts and show concentration of granules in the Golgi zone.

A helpful finding in the diagnosis of AML is the presence of Auer rods. With Romanowsky stains, Auer rods are linear or spindle-shaped, red-purple inclusions in the cytoplasm of myeloblasts or promyelocytes (see Plate 27–4*I*). Less commonly, they may be seen in more mature neutrophils. Auer rods are derivatives of azurophilic granules and stain positively for Sudan black B, myeloperoxidase, ASD chloroacetate esterase, and acid phosphatase. Auer rods can be found in any of the subtypes of AML, but they are especially associated with M1 to M3. Their presence ensures the diagnosis of AML or, at least, refractory anemia with excess blasts in transformation.

Acute Myeloblastic Leukemia with Minimal Differentiation (MO). In acute myeloblastic leukemia with minimal differentiation (MO), myeloblasts (Type I) display less than 3% positivity with Sudan black B, myeloperoxidase, or ASD chloroacetate esterase (Bennett, 1991) (Plate 27–3*A*). However, when examined for myeloid and lymphoid markers using either flow cytometry or immunocytochemistry, at least 20% of the blasts exhibit myeloid-associated antigens (CD13, CD33, or CD14) without specific lymphoid antigens.

Acute Myeloblastic Leukemia Without Maturation (M1). In acute myeloblastic leukemia without maturation (M1), myeloblasts (Type I and II) must represent at least 90% of the NECs in the bone marrow (Bennett, 1985a, 1985b) (Plate 27–4*A*). Because M1 can be confused with acute lym-

4

Table 27–6. CYTOCHEMICAL REACTIONS IN NORMAL BLOOD CELLS AND BLAST CELLS OF ACUTE LEUKEMIA

		Esterases				
	Peroxidase Sudan Black B	***α-Naphthyl Acetate***	***α-Naphthyl Butyrate***	***Naphthol ASD Chloroacetate***	**PAS**	**Acid Phosphatase**
Promyelocyte	+/++	−/±	−	+/++	±/+	+/++
Neutrophil	++	−/±	−	+/++	+++	+
Monocyte	−/±	+++	++/+++	−/±	±	++
Lymphocyte	−	−/±[a]	−/±[a]	−	−/+	−/++
Erythroblast	−	−/±[b]	−	−	−	±/−
Megakaryocyte	−	+++	±	−	++	++
ALL	−	−/+[c]	−	−	+/++[d]	−/+[c]
AML (M0)	−	−	−	−	−	−
AML (M1)	+	−	−	+	+	−
AML (M2)	++	−/+	−/+	++	+	+
APL (M3)	+++	−/++	−	+++	±/++	++
AMML (M4)	++	++/+++	++	++	−/++	++
AMoL (M5)	−/±	+++	+++	−/±	++	+
EL (M6)	−	++	+	−	++	−
MegL (M7)	−	+	−/±	−	++	+
AUL	−	−	−	−	−	−

− = negative
± = weak or few positive cells
+ = moderate
++ = moderately strong
+++ = strongly positive (most cells)
ALL = acute lymphoblastic leukemia
AML (M0) = acute myeloblastic leukemia with minimal differentiation
AML (M1) = acute myeloblastic leukemia without maturation
AML (M2) = acute myeloblastic leukemia with maturation
APL (M3) = acute promyelocytic leukemia
AMML (M4) = acute myelomonocytic leukemia
AMoL (M5) = acute monocytic leukemia
EL (M6) = acute erythroleukemia
MegL (M7) = acute megakaryoblastic leukemia
AUL = acute undifferentiated leukemia
PAS = periodic acid–Schiff stain
[a] positivity is focal, not diffuse
[b] in erythroleukemia and in some erythroid maturation defects, positivity is strong
[c] focal cytoplasmic positivity in a small proportion of ALL
[d] coarse blocks are typical
In M1 through M5, the cytochemical reactions for the esterases apply to all of the mononuclear nonerythroid, nonlymphoid cells.
In M6, the cytochemical reactions cited in the table apply to the erythroblasts, not the myeloblasts, which are also present and which are likely to be Sudan black B or peroxidase positive.
Modified with permission from Nelson DA, Davey FR: Leukocyte esterase. *In* Beutler E, Lichtman MA, Coller BS, Kipps TJ (eds): Williams Hematology, 5th ed. New York, McGraw-Hill, 1995.

phoblastic leukemia, particularly the L2 subtype, cytochemical staining reactions are essential in making the correct diagnosis. At least 3% of the blasts must stain for either myeloperoxidase or Sudan black B. Positive staining for ASD chloroacetate esterase can also be used in the diagnosis of M1; however, the ASD chloroacetate esterase tends to be less sensitive than the former two staining methods.

Acute Myeloblastic Leukemia with Maturation (M2). In acute myeloblastic leukemia with maturation, myeloblasts represent 30% to 89% of the total marrow cells, granulocytes from promyelocytes to neutrophils are greater than 10% of the NECs, and monocytes and their precursor cells are less than 20% of the NECs. Dysplastic changes are present in at least one cell lineage, and Type III blasts are observed. In this subtype, the majority of the blasts (usually more than 85%) stain with myeloperoxidase, Sudan black B, and ASD chloroacetate esterase (Plate 27–4*C* and Plate 27–1*J*). In addition, less than 20% of the blasts stain diffusely and strongly with α-naphthyl acetate esterase or α-naphthyl butyrate esterase. Serum levels of lysozyme are within normal limits.

Acute Promyelocytic Leukemia (M3). Promyelocytes instead of myeloblasts predominate in the marrow in hypergranular promyelocytic leukemia (M3) (McKenna, 1982). Azurophilic granules are abundant and intensely stained. Auer rods are found in almost all cases, and frequently are multiple (10 or more) in a given cell (Plate 27–4*I*). The disorder is characterized by bleeding that is more severe than would be expected from the degree of thrombocytopenia. This is attributed to intravascular coagulation that is apparently initiated by the procoagulant material from the granules of the abnormal cells.

A variant of M3 is hypogranular or microgranular promyelocytic leukemia (M3V), in which cytoplasmic granules appear sparse with light microscopy and numerous, but smaller, with electron microscopy (Bennett, 1980; Golomb, 1980). The cytochemical staining reactions are a little less positive than in the hypergranular M3. In microgranular M3V, cells with Auer rods and hypergranular promyelocytes are found only in small numbers. Nuclei of most leukemic cells are bilobed or reniform, and confusion with an atypical monocytic leukemia is frequent.

In acute promyelocytic leukemia, over 85% of the leukemic cells stain for myeloperoxidase, Sudan black B, and ASD

Table 27–7. FRENCH-AMERICAN-BRITISH (FAB) CLASSIFICATION OF THE ACUTE MYELOID LEUKEMIAS

Subtype	Criteria	Approximate Percentage of Cases
M0: Myeloblastic with minimal differentiation	≥30% of ANC are Type I blast <3% of blasts are Px/SBB positive ≥20% of blasts are positive for myeloid associated antigens while negative for lymphoid antigens	—
M1: Myeloblastic without maturation	≥30% of ANC are Type I and Type II blasts ≥90% of NEC are blasts ≥3% of blasts are Px/SBB positive	20
M2: Myeloblastic with maturation	≥30% of ANC are Type I and Type II blasts <90% of NEC are blasts ≥10% of NEC are promyelocytes or more mature granulocytes <20% of NEC are of monocytic lineage Usually >85% of blasts are positive for SBB/Px/CAE	30
M3: Promyelocytic, hypergranular	≥30% blasts and abnormal hypergranular promyelocytes Auer rods and multiple Auer rods Usually >85% of leukemic cells are positive for SBB/Px/CAE	12
M3V: Promyelocytic, microgranular	≥30% blasts and abnormal microgranular promyelocytes Rare hypergranular promyelocytes Rare Auer rods and multiple Auer rods Usually >85% of leukemic cells are positive for SBB/Px/CAE	4
M4: Myelomonocytic	≥30% of ANC are Type I and Type II blasts Percentage of myeloblasts, promyelocytes, myelocytes, and later granulocytes is ≥30% <80% NEC are monoblasts, promonocytes, or monocytes >20% of blasts are positive for SBB/Px/CAE >20% of blasts are positive for αNAE, αNBE	12
M4E: Myelomonocytic with eosinophilia	Same as M4 plus abnormal eosinophilia Eosinophils with large abnormal basophilic granules; eosinophilic granules are often PAS positive, eosinophils are often CAE positive	4
M5A: Monocytic, poorly differentiated	≥30% of ANC are blasts ≥80% of NEC are monoblasts, promonocytes, or monocytes ≥80% of monocytic cells are monoblasts <20% of leukemic cells are CAE positive ≥80% of leukemic cells are αNAE, αNBE positive	
M5B: Monocytic, differentiated	≥30% of ANC are blasts ≥80% of NEC are monoblasts, promonocytes, or monocytes <80% of monocytic cells are monoblasts <20% of leukemic cells are CAE positive ≥80% of leukemic cells are αNAE, αNBE positive	12
M6: Erythroleukemia	≥50% ANC are erythroblasts ≥30% NEC are blasts Many erythroid precursor cells are PAS positive	3
M7: Megakaryoblastic	≥30% of ANC are megakaryoblasts or leukemic cells Leukemic cells are platelet peroxidase positive on electron microscopy or positive for glycoproteins Ib or IIb/IIIa as demonstrated by immunocytochemical methods	<1

ANC = all nucleated cells; NEC = nonerythroid cells; SBB = Sudan black B; Px = myeloperoxidase; CAE = ASD chloracetate esterase; αNAE = α-naphthyl acetate esterase; αNBE = α-naphthyl butyrate esterase; PAS = periodic acid–Schiff.

From Bennett JB, Catovsky D, Daniel M, Flandrin G, Galton DAG, Gralnick HR, Sultan C: Criteria for the diagnosis of acute leukemia of megakaryocyte lineage (M7). Ann Intern Med 1985; 103:460; and proposed revised criteria for the classification of acute myeloid leukemia. Ann Intern Med 1985; 103:620.

chloroacetate. In approximately 25% of the cases, more than 20% of the leukemic cells stain strongly and diffusely for α-naphthyl acetate esterase. However, these leukemic cells do not exhibit any immunophenotypic characteristics of monocytes, and clinically these cases behave similarly to other cases of acute promyelocytic leukemia.

Acute Myelomonocytic Leukemia (M4). In the bone marrow of patients with acute myelomonocytic leukemia (M4), myeloblasts constitute more than 30% of the total marrow cells (Plate 27–1*K* and Plate 27–4*D, E, F*). The sum of the monoblasts, promonocytes, and monocytes is more than 20% but is less than 80% of the NECs. The cells of the granulocytic series (myeloblasts, promyelocytes, myelocytes, and other more mature forms) represent 30% to 80% of the NECs. If these bone marrow findings are accompanied by a peripheral blood monocytosis (5×10^9/L or more), a diagnosis of M4 is ensured. However, if the monocyte count is less than 5×10^9/L, additional laboratory measurements are needed (i.e., serum lysozyme greater than three times normal, or 20% or more of the blasts staining for either α-naphthyl acetate esterase or α-naphthyl butyrate esterase) (Bennett, 1985a).

In myelomonocytic leukemia (M4), there is variable staining of the leukemic cells with myeloperoxidase, Sudan black B, ASD chloroacetate esterase, and periodic acid–Schiff (PAS). However, in most cases, leukemic cells exhibit a diffuse and intense stain with α-naphthyl acetate esterase or α-naphthyl butyrate esterase. In rare cases, these nonspecific esterases cannot be demonstrated and the diagnosis must be made on the Romanowsky stains alone. Immunocytochemical staining for lysozyme may be helpful in these cases to confirm a monocytic component.

In a small percentage of cases of M4 AML, there is a slight to moderate eosinophilia (1% to 33%) (Bitter, 1984). This variant is called acute myelomonocytic leukemia with eosinophilia (M4EO) (Plate 27–3*B*). In rare cases, the eosinophilia may be very pronounced, but in most cases, it represents approximately 5% of the NECs. Many of these eosinophils have abnormally large basophilic granules admixed with normal eosinophilic granules. When stained with PAS, the eosinophilic granules themselves are positive, whereas normal eosinophils demonstrate only intergranular staining. Another distinguishing characteristic is the positive staining of these abnormal eosinophils with ASD chloroacetate esterase, a feature not present in normal eosinophils. Counterstaining with chlorazol fast pink is often useful in identifying all of the eosinophils.

Acute Monocytic Leukemia (M5). The diagnosis of acute monocytic leukemia (M5) depends on the identification of 80% or more of the marrow NECs as monoblasts, promonocytes, or monocytes. Two subtypes of M5 AML are recognized: M5 without differentiation (monoblastic, M5A) is characterized by large blasts accounting for 80% or more of the marrow monocytic cells (Plate 27–3*C*), whereas M5 with differentiation (M5B) has fewer monoblasts (<80% of the marrow monocytic cells) and more promonocytes and monocytes (see Plates 27–1*K* and 27–3*D*) (Bennett, 1985a). Promonocytes differ from mature monocytes by less chromatin condensation and convoluted nuclei. The α-naphthyl acetate esterase and the α-naphthyl butyrate esterase stain the leukemic cells diffusely and intensely (80% or more of the leukemic cells). Occasionally, the leukemic cells fail to stain with the nonspecific esterase and the diagnosis must be made by the Romanowsky stains or immunophenotypic techniques. This is particularly the case with the monoblastic (M5A) leukemias.

Erythroleukemia (M6). The diagnosis of erythroleukemia (M6) is made when more than 50% of the nucleated cells of the bone marrow are erythroblasts and 30% or more of the NECs are myeloblasts. Morphologic abnormalities of the erythroblasts are often pronounced, with atypical megaloblastic features, bizarre nuclear shapes, and multinucleated giant forms. The cytoplasm may contain pseudopods or vacuoles, particularly in the pro- and basophilic erythroblasts.

Very rarely, there is virtually no granulocytic involvement in the neoplastic process and primitive erythroblasts predominate, in which case the condition has been called *erythemic myelosis.* In most cases, there is a mixture of variable proportions of erythroid precursors and myeloblasts (sometimes abnormal monocytic and megakaryocytic elements are present as well) and, in the past, the term erythroleukemia has been employed to connote this subtype. At present, the term erythroleukemia (M6) includes both subtypes.

Occasionally, one sees progression from an initial erythemic myelosis to erythroleukemia to a final termination in a subtype of acute myeloblastic leukemia (FAB M2 or M4) in a single patient. This group of disorders has been designated the *Di Guglielmo syndrome*. However, with the widespread use of the FAB classification, this term is rarely used and is primarily of historic interest.

In some cases of M6, the erythroid cells may show strong cytoplasmic PAS positively. This is granular in early erythroid precursors and diffuse in later stages (Plate 27–4*K*). Erythroid precursors are PAS negative in normal individuals and in most diseases, including nutritional megaloblastic anemia. They are sometimes positive, however, in iron deficiency anemia, thalassemia, and refractory anemia with ring sideroblasts (Hayhoe, 1984). In erythroleukemia, myeloblasts usually stain for Sudan black B, myeloperoxidase, and ASD chloroacetate esterase. A nonspecific esterase-positive monocytic component is often evident (Plate 27–4*L*). Neoplastic erythroid precursors also are sometimes positive for the α-naphthyl acetate and α-naphthyl butyrate esterases (Hayhoe, 1984).

Acute Megakaryoblastic Leukemia (M7). The diagnosis of acute megakaryoblastic leukemia, like other forms of AML, depends on identification of an infiltrate of blast cells representing 30% or more of the nucleated cells of the bone marrow, and at least 30% of the blasts must be megakaryoblasts (Bennett, 1985b). The blast cells are demonstrated to be of megakaryoblastic lineage either by the platelet peroxidase technique (Breton-Gorius, 1973) or by immunophenotyping methods using monoclonal antibodies against platelet glycoproteins Ib or IIb/IIIa (Erber, 1987) (Plate 27–3*E*).

The blasts in acute megakaryoblastic leukemia (M7) are often listed as undifferentiated using the FAB classification as a guide. Megakaryoblasts are very polymorphic; some blasts simulate lymphoblasts, both L1 and L2 forms. Other blasts are larger and have pseudopods or stringy cytoplasmic projections. The cytoplasm usually is light blue and may or may not possess granules. The nuclei often have one to three nucleoli.

In the peripheral blood, there usually is pancytopenia with marked leukopenia and anemia. Megakaryocytic fragments are sometimes present in the blood. The bone marrow shows pronounced myelofibrosis, often resulting in futile attempts at obtaining marrow aspirate films.

Megakaryoblasts do not stain with Sudan black B, myeloperoxidase, ASD chloroacetate esterase, or α-naphthyl butyrate esterase. α-Naphthyl acetate esterase may be positive. The PAS reaction shows diffuse and peripheral granular (often in large blocks) staining.

COURSE. Table 27–7 shows the approximate distribution of cases according to the FAB classification. Current data suggest that a small proportion of patients with M4 and M5 variants enter a complete remission. Patients with erythroleukemia may have a very poor prognosis (Roggli, 1981). However, patients with M2, M3, and M4E tend to have a higher response rate and longer survival than patients with other FAB subtypes of AML (Griffin, 1986). Prognostic features of AML are recorded in Table 27–8.

Other Forms of Acute Nonlymphoid Leukemia

ACUTE UNDIFFERENTIATED (STEM CELL) LEUKEMIA. This is a variety of acute leukemia in which the predominant cells are blast forms that cannot be classified using morphologic, cytochemical, ultrastructural, immunologic, or

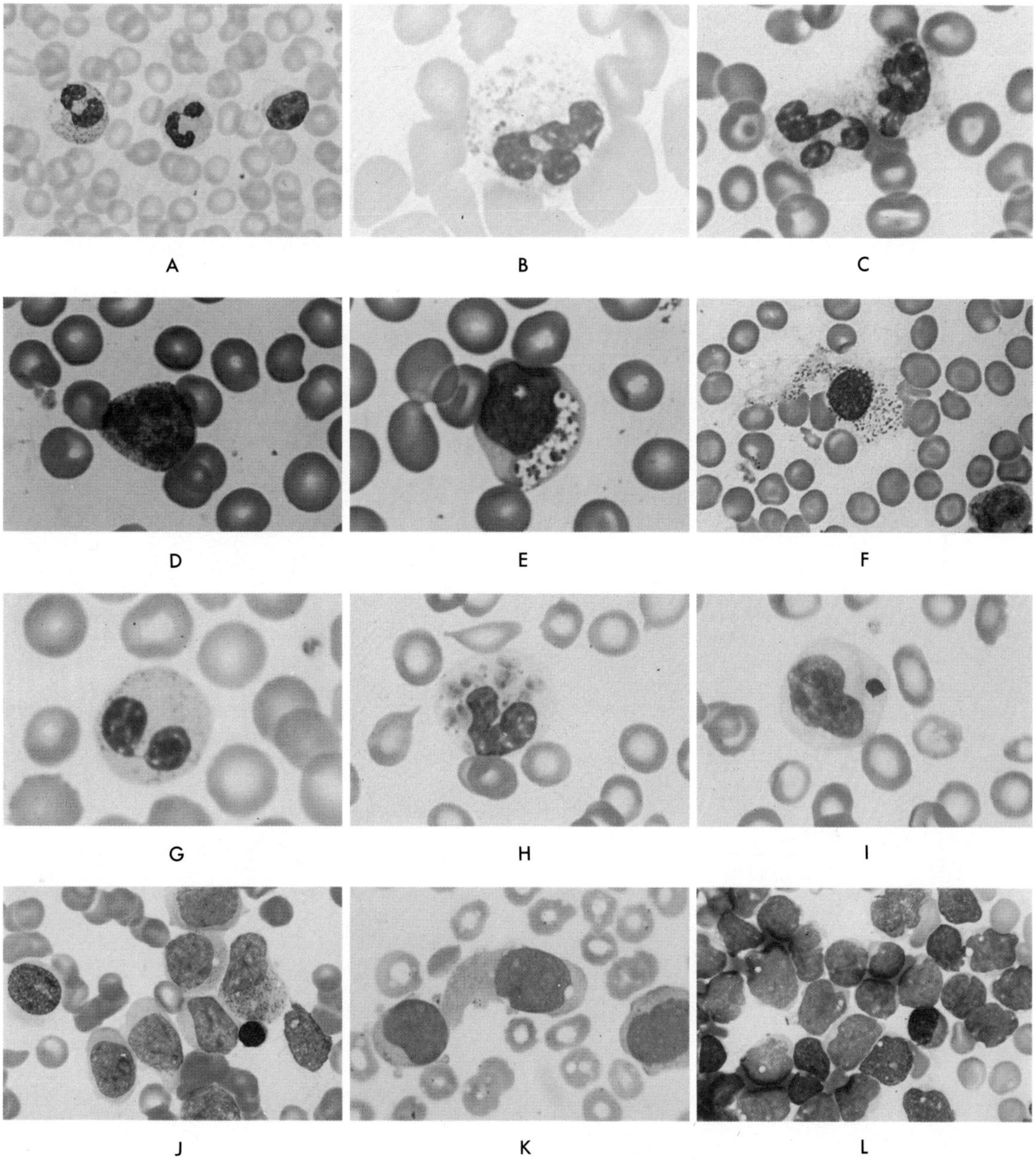

Plate 27–1. *A,* Toxic neutrophil, *left,* with cytoplasmic vacuoles and heavy azurophilic granules. Normal neutrophil, *center.* Lymphocyte, *right. B,* Toxic neutrophil. Partial degranulation, fusion of granules, vacuoles, and phagocytized diplococcus. Blood film from a patient with meningococcemia. *C,* May-Hegglin anomaly. Note the large, pale blue inclusions at the outer margins of each neutrophil. *D,* Alder-Reilly anomaly, Hurler's syndrome. Deeply staining azurophilic granules almost obscure the nucleus of the neutrophil. The Alder-Reilly anomaly may be found in some cases of mucopolysaccharidosis (in which case the granules are usually metachromatic), or it may be found as a hereditary anomaly in apparently healthy persons. These cells resemble neutrophils with intense toxic granulation. *E,* Lymphocyte with basophilic inclusions surrounded by halos, characteristic of mucopolysaccharidosis. These inclusions are metachromatic. Peripheral blood film, Hurler's syndrome. *F,* Histiocyte or macrophage with numerous basophilic inclusions, which are surrounded by clear spaces or halos. These granules are metachromatic and characteristic of mucopolysaccharidosis. Bone marrow film, Hurler's syndrome. *G,* Pelger-Huët anomaly, neutrophil. *H,* Chédiak-Higashi anomaly, band neutrophil. Neutrophil granules have fused into irregular masses that stain gray rather than tan. *I,* Chédiak-Higashi anomaly, lymphocyte. Azurophilic inclusions are much larger than azurophilic granules in lymphocytes of normal persons. *J,* Acute myelogenous leukemia. Several myeloblasts and one abnormal neutrophil myelocyte. *K,* Acute myelomonocytic leukemia. Blast, *left*; immature monocytes, *center* and *right. L,* Acute lymphoblastic leukemia. The lymphoblasts have more nuclear irregularity and a higher nuclear to cytoplasmic ratio than myeloblasts.

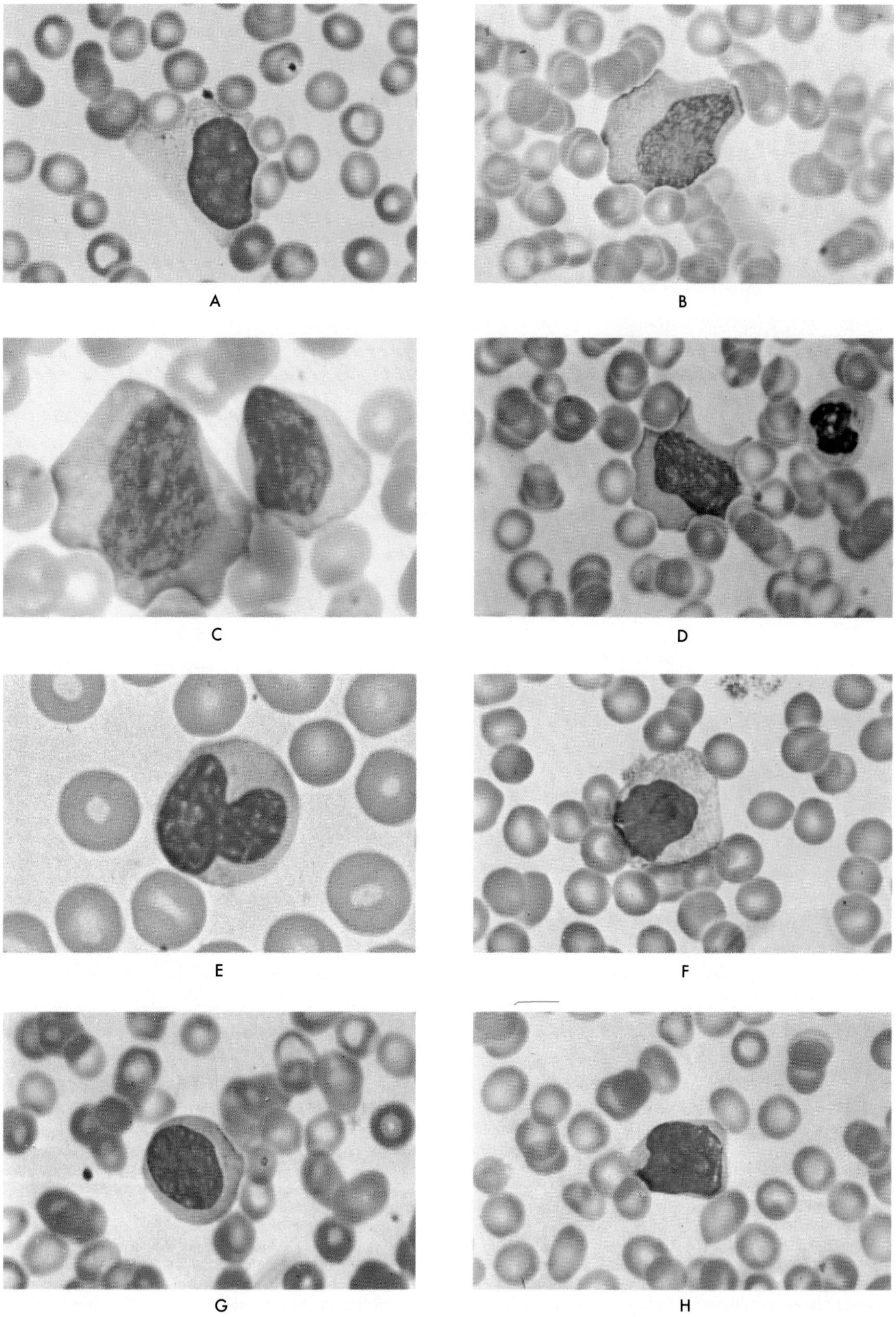

Plate 27–2. *A*, Infectious mononucleosis. All the photographs of the lymphocytes of infectious mononucleosis are from patients with characteristic clinical findings and with positive differential tests. The lymphocyte is larger than any normal so-called large lymphocyte. The cytoplasm is abundant, clear, and moderately basophilic, especially close to the edges of the cell; red azure granules are accumulated along the upper periphery. The cytoplasm is delicate, and the surrounding red cells leave an indentation in the cytoplasm, giving it a scalloped appearance. The nucleus is oval, and the chromatin is delicate and less dense than in normal large lymphocytes. Three nucleoli are seen clearly. The two red cells adjacent on the right made indentations, even in the nucleus, suggesting that it is plastic. There is a light perinuclear zone. The characteristic lymphocytes in infectious mononucleosis are called atypical lymphocytes. *B*, Atypical lymphocyte, infectious mononucleosis. Notice sharp separation of nuclear chromatin and parachromatin, and basophilic cytoplasm. *C*, Reticular lymphocyte (nonleukemic lymphoblast), *left;* atypical lymphocyte with greater nuclear maturity, *right*. Infectious mononucleosis. *D*, Atypical lymphocyte, *center*; normal lymphocyte, *right*. Infectious mononucleosis. *E*, Atypical lymphocyte with "leukocytoid" nucleus. Infectious mononucleosis. *F*, Normal monocyte. *G*, Reticular lymphocyte (nonleukemic lymphoblast); infectious mononucleosis. The nuclear chromatin is uniform and granular (or reticular). Nucleoli are conspicuous. The cytoplasm is deeply basophilic. Note the difference between this cell and the lymphoblast of acute leukemia (*H*). *H*, Lymphoblast, acute lymphoblastic leukemia.

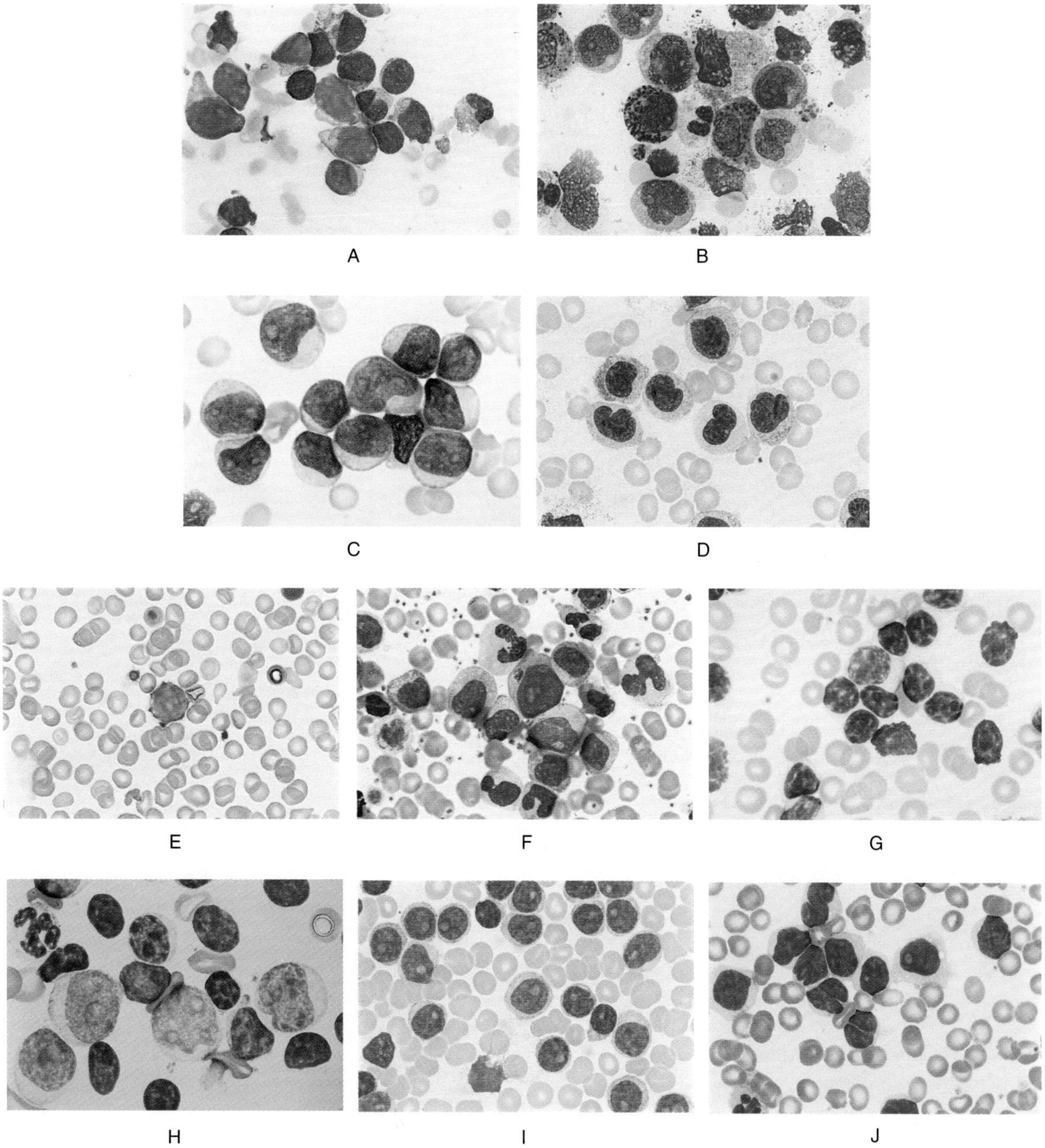

Plate 27–3. *A*, Acute myeloblastic leukemia with minimal differentiation (AML-MO), Wright-Giemsa stain of bone marrow. No maturation is evident, Sudan black and myeloperoxidase reactions are negative, but flow cytometric studies demonstrate blasts to possess CD13 and CD33 antigens. *B*, Acute myelomonocytic leukemia with esoinophilia (AML-M4EO), Wright-Giemsa stain of bone marrow. Maturation is evident and there is a moderate eosinophilia. Many eosinophils have large basophilic granules. *C*, Acute monoblastic leukemia (AML-M5A), Wright-Giemsa stain of bone marrow. More than 80% of the cells are monoblasts. *D*, Acute monocytic leukemia (AML-M5B), Wright-Giemsa stain of blood. Leukemia cells show maturation to promonocytes and monocytes. *E*, Acute megakaryoblastic leukemia, (AML-M7), alkaline phosphatase antialkaline phosphatase (APAALP) against CD41 (GPIIb/IIIa). *F*, Chronic myelogenous leukemia (CML), Wright-Giemsa stain of blood. There is a leukocytosis with a spectrum of granulocytic cells, *G*, Chronic lymphocytic leukemia (CLL), Wright-Giemsa stain of the blood. Ninety percent or more of the cells are small lymphocytes. *H*, Chronic lymphocytic leukemia, mixed cell type (CLL/PLL), Wright-Giemsa stain of the blood. Prolymphocytes represent more than 10% and less than 55% of blood lymphocytes. *I*, Prolymphocytic leukemia (PLL), Wright-Giemsa stain of the blood. Prolymphocytes represent more than 55% of the blood lymphocytes. *J*, Leukemic phase of intermediate NHL, Wright-Giemsa stain of blood. Leukemic cells possess condensed nuclear chromatin and slight nuclear indentations or clefts.

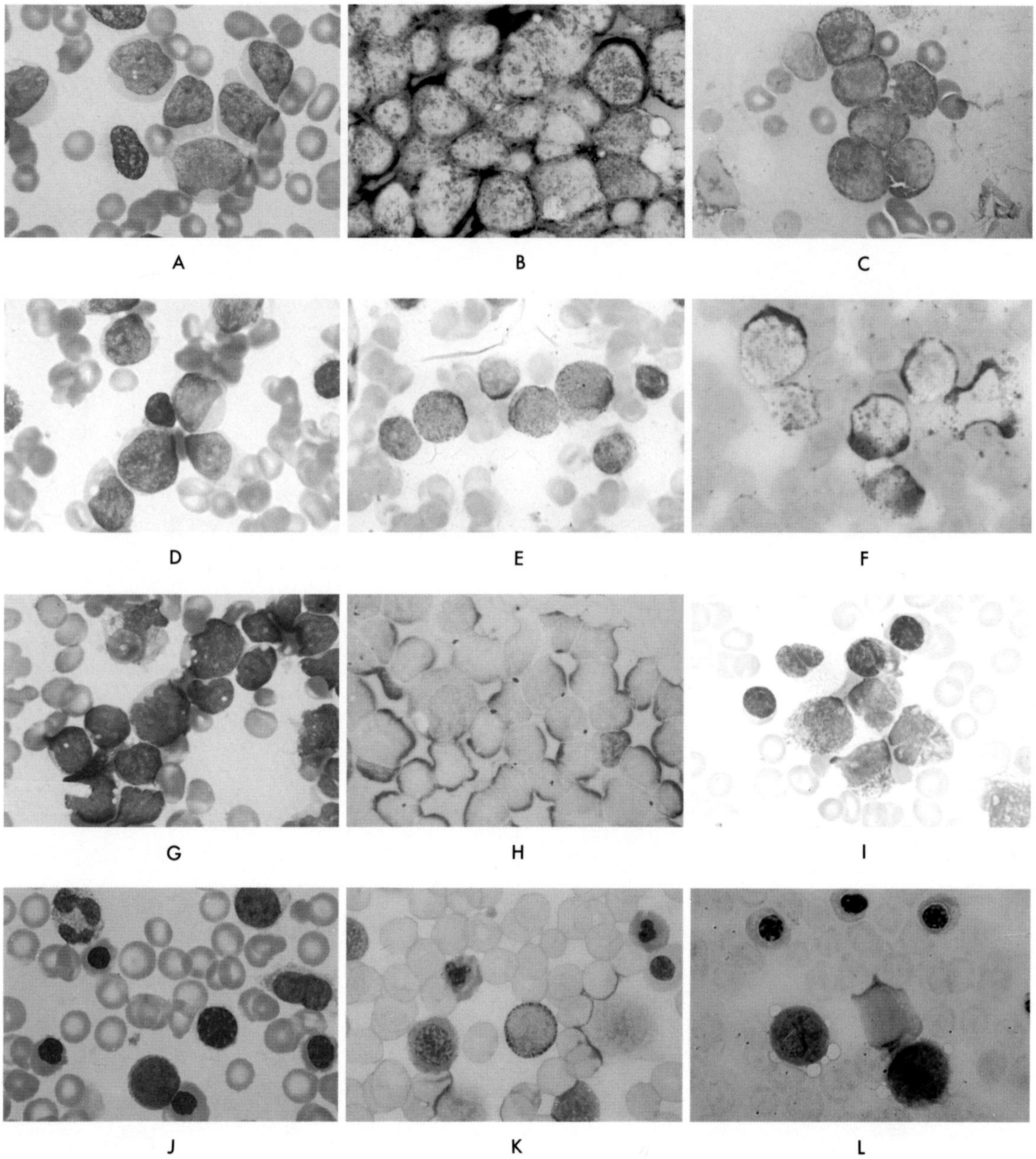

Plate 27–4. *A*, Acute myeloblastic leukemia (AML), Wright-Giemsa stain. No maturation is evident. This corresponds to the M1 category of the French-American-British (FAB) classification (see Table 27–7). *B*, AML, Sudan black B reaction. Same case as in *A*. Although granules are not visible with the Wright-Giemsa stain, all of the blasts contain sudanophilic material (brown granules). The peroxidase reaction was similarly positive. *C*, Acute myeloblastic leukemia with partial maturation (M2). Naphthol ASD chloroacetate esterase reaction. All stages of developing neutrophils have a positive reaction. *D*, Acute myelomonocytic leukemia (AMML), Wright-Giemsa stain. No cytoplasmic maturation is evident. This stain alone does not allow a definitive diagnosis. *E*, AMML, Sudan black B reaction. Same case as *D*. A moderate proportion of the blasts contains sudanophilic material. *F*, AMML, α-naphthyl acetate esterase reaction. Same case as *D*. Most of the blasts contain nonspecific esterase (which is fluoride sensitive). Cytochemical reactions, therefore, lead to the diagnosis of myelomonocytic leukemia. *G*, Acute lymphoblastic leukemia (ALL), Wright-Giemsa stain. Most of the blasts are small and the cytoplasm is scanty. This corresponds to the L1 category of the FAB classification (see Table 27–8). *H*, ALL, periodic acid–Schiff (PAS) reaction. Same case as *G*. A moderate proportion of the blasts contains one or more large granules or "blocks" of PAS-positive material. *I*, Acute promyelocytic leukemia, Wright-Giemsa stain. The majority of cells have abundant azurophil granules, often large. Usually, some cells contain multiple Auer rods, as in the cell at the right. The nuclei are irregularly shaped or indented (Reider forms). This is the hypergranular promyelocytic category M3 of the FAB classification. *J*, Erythroleukemia, Wright-Giemsa stain. One primitive blast *(lower center),* one abnormal monocyte *(upper right),* one neutrophil, and five nucleated erythroid cells are present. Most of the latter are abnormal. *K*, Erythroleukemia, PAS reaction. Same case as *J*. Of the six nucleated erythroid cells in this field, five are PAS positive: in the most immature, the reactive material is granular *(lower center);* in the others, it is diffuse. A monocyte and a blast are PAS negative; a neutrophil is PAS positive. *L*, Erythroleukemia, α-naphthyl butyrate reaction. Same case as *J*. Monocytes are strongly positive for this nonspecific esterase reaction; they were increased in number and morphologically abnormal and part of the leukemic process. Erythroid, granulocytic, and monocytic cell lines are demonstrably involved in this case.

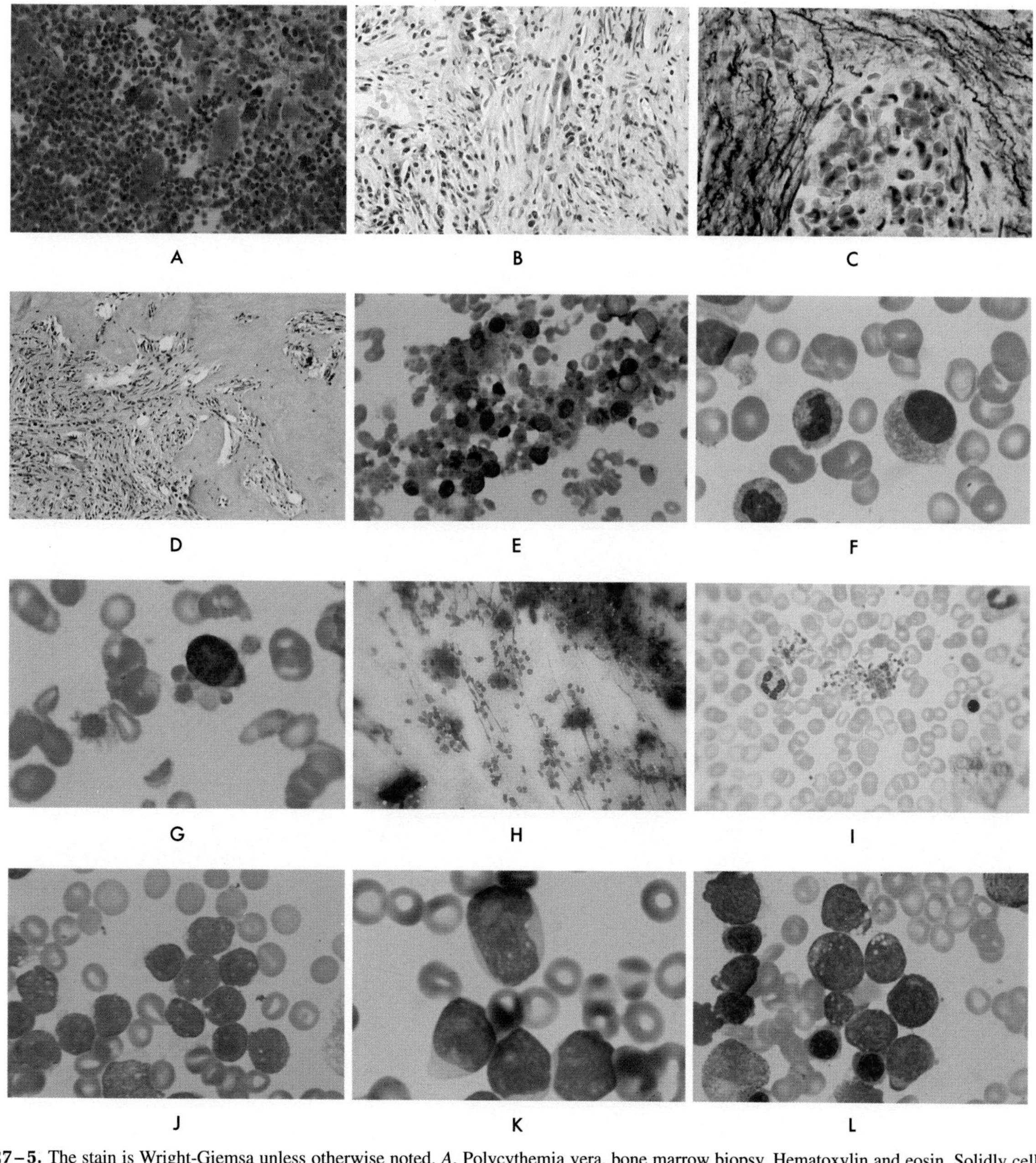

Plate 27–5. The stain is Wright-Giemsa unless otherwise noted. *A*, Polycythemia vera, bone marrow biopsy. Hematoxylin and eosin. Solidly cellular marrow with panmyelosis, i.e., the hypercellularity is due to increased erythroid, granulocytic, and megakaryocytic proliferation. *B*, Myelofibrosis with myeloid metaplasia (MMM), bone marrow biopsy, H & E. Reticulin and collagen fibrosis accounts for the increased intercellular material; note the distortion of the megakaryocytes *(right center).* This marrow is considerably less cellular than in *A. C*, MMM, bone marrow biopsy, reticulin stain. Reticulin fibers are coated with silver in this reaction and appear dark. They are the major component of the myelofibrosis in the early phases of MMM: only later does the collagen staining reaction appear. Note the large vascular space; these are often present in the marrow in MMM. *D*, MMM with osteosclerosis, bone marrow biopsy, H & E stain. Note the irregular new bone formation and apparent continuity of fibers from the marrow with those in the bone *(upper center). E*, MMM, touch preparation of marrow biopsy. A mass of abnormal platelets, most with diminished granules, and many separate, small megakaryocytic nuclei (each the size of a small lymphocyte). These abnormal micromegakaryocytes and masses of atypical platelets can often be found on touch preparations of marrow biopsies in MMM. Usually aspiration of marrow tissue is impossible. *F*, MMM, blood film. To the right of the neutrophil near the center is a micromegakaryocyte; note the intensely staining nuclear chromatin and fine azure granules in the cytoplasm. Often the cytoplasm is less abundant in these cells. *G*, MMM, blood film. The nucleated cell is a micromegakaryoblast. Cells such as this are frequently mistaken for lymphocytes. Adjacent to it are three large poorly granular platelets; another is seen to the left in the field. *H*, Thrombocythemia, bone marrow film, low power. An abundance of megakaryocytes dominate the marrow films from most aspirations in thrombocythemia. *I*, Thrombocythemia, blood film. Individual platelets usually appear normal, except that they are frequently large. The features of the blood film are considerably increased numbers of platelets, neutrophilia, and often hypochromic microcytic red cells as a result of chronic blood loss. *J*, ALL, FAB-L1, marrow film. The blasts are small and have nuclear/cytoplasmic (N/C) ratios, inconspicuous nucleoli, and regular nuclear outline (×400). *K*, ALL, FAB-L2, blood film. The blasts are large and have lower N/C ratios, prominent nucleoli, and often irregular nuclear outlines (×800). *L*, ALL, FAB-L3, marrow film. The blasts are moderately large and uniform in size and have a moderate amount of intensely basophilic cytoplasm, which often contains vacuoles (×400).

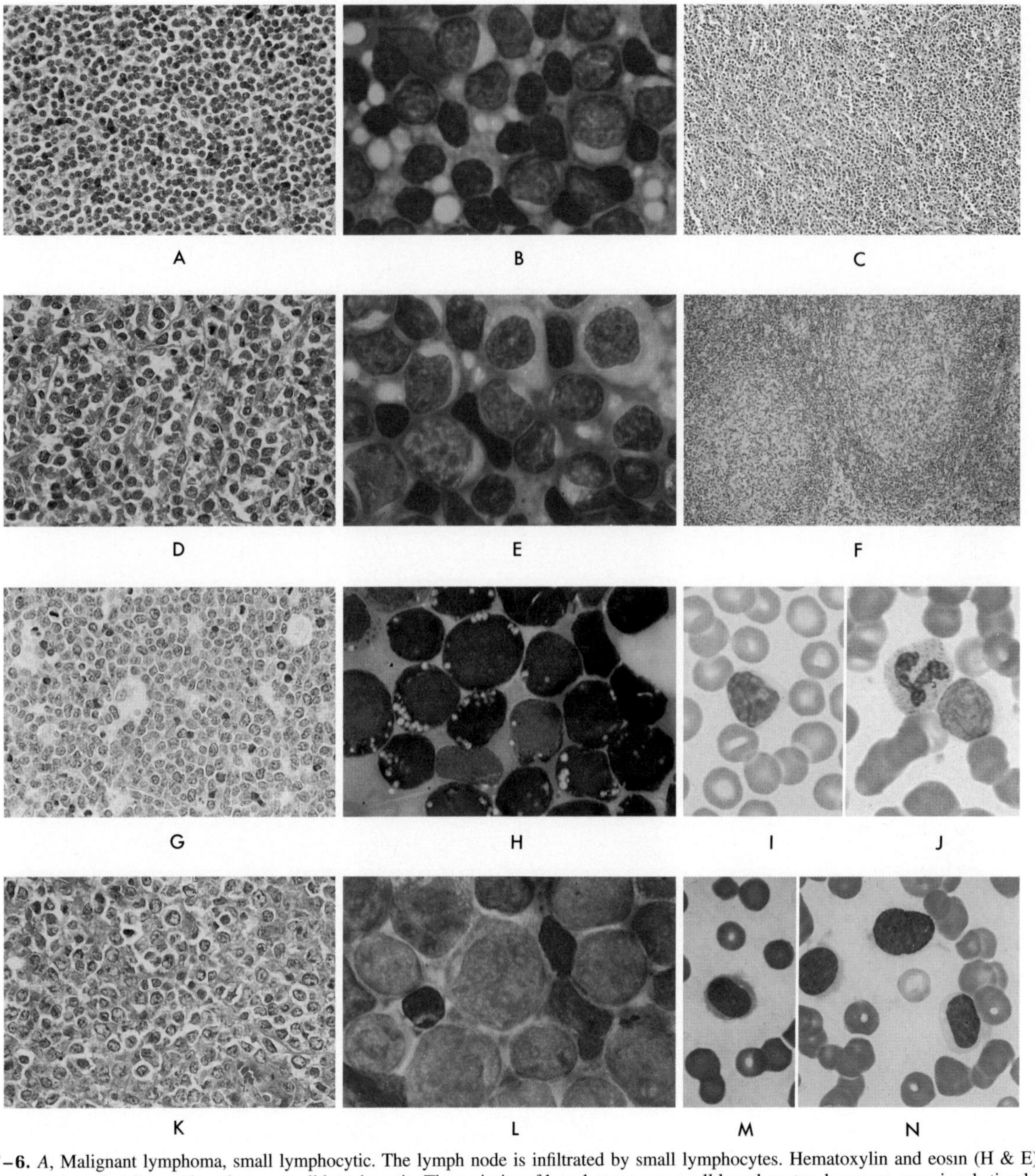

Plate 27–6. *A*, Malignant lymphoma, small lymphocytic. The lymph node is infiltrated by small lymphocytes. Hematoxylin and eosin (H & E), ×400. *B*, Touch preparation of malignant lymphoma, small lymphocytic. The majority of lymphocytes are small lymphocytes; however, occasional stimulated lymphocytes are present. Wright-Giemsa, ×900. *C*, Non-Hodgkin's lymphoma with diffuse pattern. Compare with *F*. H & E, × 100. *D*, Malignant lymphoma, follicular, small cleaved cell. Note the presence of lymphoid cells with angulated and clefted nuclei, occasional nucleoli, and scant cytoplasm. Mitotic figures are more frequent than in *A*. H & E, ×400. *E*, Touch preparation of malignant lymphoma, small cleaved cell. The majority of cells are stimulated lymphocytes with occasional mature lymphocytes. Wright-Giemsa, ×900. *F*, Non-Hodgkin's lymphoma with follicular pattern. Compare with *C*. H & E, × 100. *G*, Malignant lymphoma, small noncleaved cell (Burkitt's lymphoma). Primitive lymphoid cells are positioned around tissue macrophages. H & E, ×400. *H*, Touch preparation of Burkitt's lymphoma. Neoplastic cells contain fine reticular chromatin. Cytoplasm is intensely basophilic and frequently contains multiple vacuoles. Wright-Giemsa, ×900. *I, J*, Sezary cells, blood film, from a patient with mycosis fungoides. Wright-Giemsa stain, ×400. These are mononuclear cells with scanty cytoplasm and a deeply indented or convoluted nucleus. The cell on the left has more chromatin condensation than the cell adjacent to the neutrophil on the right. *K*, Malignant lymphoma, diffuse large cell. Large lymphoid cells with prominent nuclei, thickened nuclear membrane, conspicuous nucleoli, and more abundant cytoplasm. H & E, ×400. *L*, Touch preparation of malignant lymphoma, diffuse large cell. Neoplastic cells are large, measuring approximately 20 μm in diameter. The nuclear chromatin is fine and reticular; nucleoli are prominent. Wright-Giemsa, ×900. *M, N,* Hairy cell leukemia, blood film, Wright-Giemsa stain, ×400. The two left-most cells are "hairy cells." They have less condensed but more intensely staining chromatin and more irregular cytoplasmic margins than normal lymphocytes (cell at farthest right).

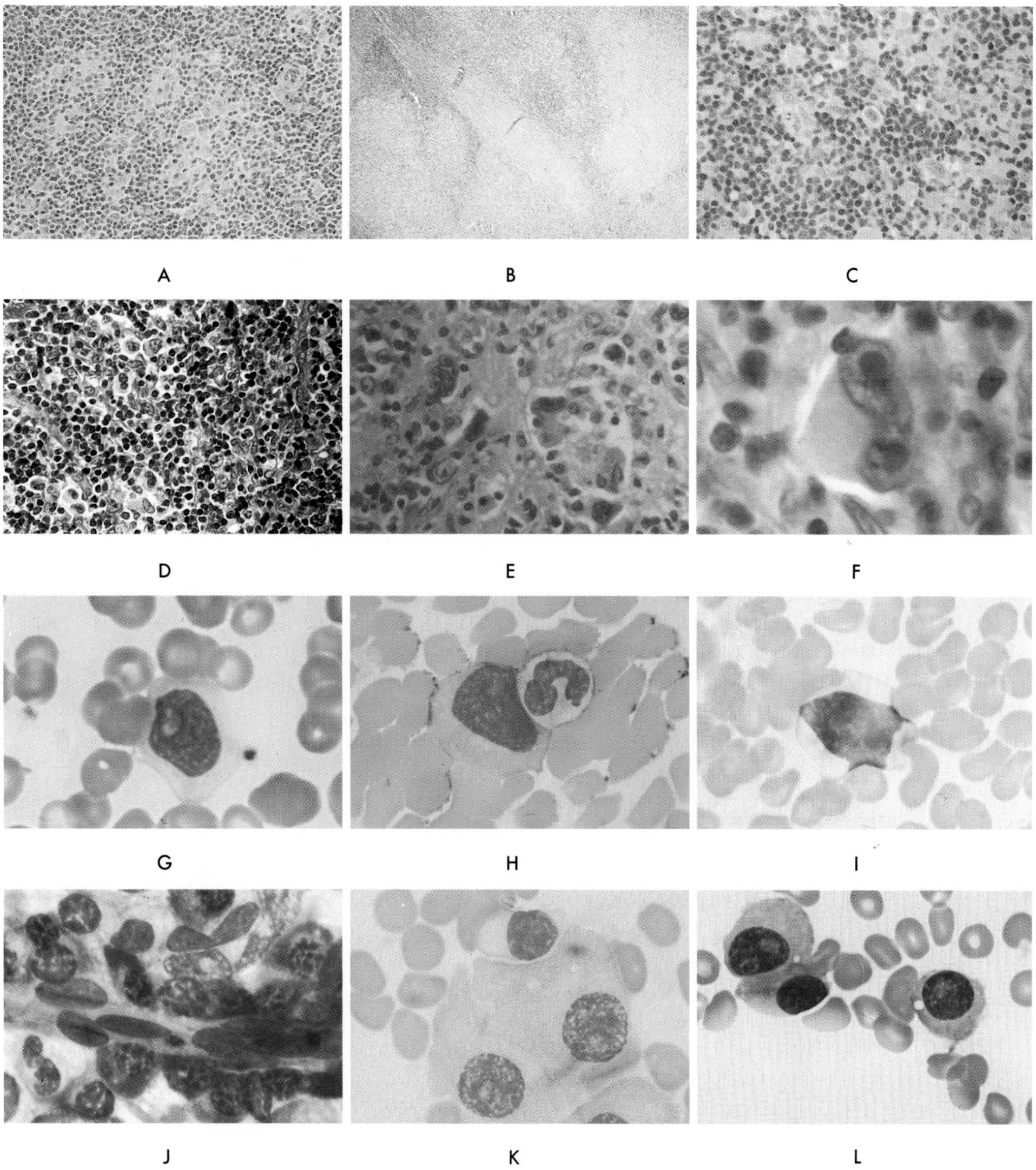

Plate 27–7. *A*, Hodgkin's disease, lymphocyte predominance type. The mature lymphocyte is the most common cell. Histiocytes are frequently present. Reed-Sternberg cells are rare. Eosinophils and plasma cells are infrequent. Hematoxylin and eosin (H & E), ×250. *B*, Hodgkin's disease, nodular sclerosis type. Broad bands of collagen course through the lymph node, forming nodules of lymphoid tissue. H & E, ×100. *C*, Hodgkin's disease, nodular sclerosis type. Note presence of "lacunar" Reed-Sternberg cells with multinuclei and pale cytoplasm. H & E, ×400. *D*, Hodgkin's disease, mixed type. There are numerous Reed-Sternberg cells and histiocytes. Eosinophils and plasma cells are characteristically present. H & E, ×400. *E*, Hodgkin's disease, lymphocyte depletion type. There are several multinucleated Reed-Sternberg cells and many abnormal mononuclear cells. Lymphocytes are less prominent. There is a background of proteinaceous material and disorderly fibrosis, H & E ×400. *F*, Reed-Sternberg cell, in Hodgkin's disease, mixed type. *G*, Malignant lymphoma, small cleaved cell, leukemic phase. Blasts, such as this cell, and cells with more chromatin condensation and notched nuclei (as in Plate 27–6*E*) are found in the blood in a minority of patients with small cleaved cell lymphoma, usually late in the disease. *H*, Lymphocytic reaction. This reticular lymphocyte in the blood of a patient with a viral infection resembles the malignant blast in *G*. This type of reactive blast form ("non-leukemic lymphoblast") usually has more deeply basophilic cytoplasm and is associated with numerous characteristic atypical lymphocytes, as in *I*. *I*, Atypical lymphocyte, blood film. *J*, Plasma cells adjacent to the endothelial cells lining a blood vessel in bone marrow film from a patient with rheumatoid arthritis. In mature plasma cells, the nuclear chromatin is coarsely clumped and the cytoplasm is deeply basophilic. *K*, Multiple myeloma, bone marrow film. The abnormal plasma cells have abundant cytoplasm and eccentric nuclei. In contrast to normal plasma cells, however, the cytoplasm is less deeply basophilic, the chromatin is not coarsely clumped, and nucleoli are prominent. *L*, Multiple myeloma, bone marrow film. The dissociation between advanced cytoplasmic maturation (abundant, usually basophilic cytoplasm with a prominent Golgi zone) and delayed nuclear maturation (prominent nucleolus, less chromatin condensation) is the most useful feature in distinguishing the abnormal plasma cells in myeloma from normal plasma cells.

Table 27–8. PROGNOSTIC FACTORS IN ACUTE MYELOID LEUKEMIA

Factors	Favorable	Unfavorable
Age	<45 years	<2 years, >60 years
Leukocytosis	<25 × 10^9/L	>100 × 10^9/L
CNS involvement	Absent	Present
Response to therapy	Rapid	Delayed/incomplete
Auer rods	Present	Absent
FAB type	M2, M3, M4EO	M5, M6, M7
Cell markers	CD2 or CD19	CD13, CD14, CD33
Cytogenetics	t(15;17), t(8;21) inv (16)/del (16q)	−7; del (7q), −5; del (5q), 11q23 abnormalities, 3q21 and 3q26 abnormalities, complex karyotypic abnormalities

Modified from Lee GR, Bithell TC, Foerster J, Athens JW, Lukens JN (ed): Wintrobe's Clinical Hematology, 9th ed. Philadelphia, Lea and Febiger, 1993.

DNA analytical methods. This entity is rare. The use of electron microscopy, immunophenotypic methods, and DNA analytical techniques has demonstrated the lineage of neoplastic cells from several cases of acute leukemia that were considered to be undifferentiated by standard morphologic and cytochemical procedures (Raghavachar, 1986; Sobol, 1987).

ACUTE MIXED-LINEAGE LEUKEMIA. In this disorder, patients with acute leukemia have two separate populations of neoplastic cells with different lineage expression or one population of leukemic cells with multiple lineage expression. Cases of acute mixed myeloid/lymphoid leukemia and cases of acute mixed B-cell/T-cell leukemia have been identified in both pediatric and adult patients (Sobol, 1987; Stass, 1986). Using standard morphologic and cytochemical techniques, these cases can be confused with subtypes of acute lymphoid leukemia. As a result, immunophenotypic or DNA analytical techniques are required to confirm the diagnosis of acute mixed-lineage leukemia.

GRANULOCYTIC SARCOMA. This neoplasm has also been called myeloblastic sarcoma, extramedullary myeloid cell tumor, and chloroma. It represents a localized tumor of myeloblasts or monoblasts infiltrating extramedullary sites. These tumors have been reported to occur in the skin, lymph nodes, nasopharyngeal and upper respiratory tract tissues, breast, ovary, bone, perineural and epidural structures, the eye and other orbital structures, and a variety of soft tissues (Neiman, 1981). Granulocytic sarcomas have been reported in 3% to 8% of autopsied cases of CML and may precede the occurrence of AML in 0.6% of cases (Muss, 1973).

Patients with reported granulocytic sarcomas range in age from 2 to 81 years. Three clinical settings are found: (1) no known disease, (2) a known myeloproliferative disorder, and (3) AML (Neiman, 1981). The diagnosis depends on recognizing the nature of the primitive cells that can often be mistaken for NHLs, amelanotic melanomas, or undifferentiated carcinoma. The diagnosis can be facilitated by making touch imprint preparations of cut sections of the tumor and staining them with Romanowsky stains and by cytochemical reactions. In formalin-fixed, embedded tissue, the naphthol ASD chloroacetate esterase reaction and the use of immunocytochemical methods employing polyclonal and monoclonal antibodies against determinants found in myeloid and monocytic cells may be very helpful (Davey, 1988). In addition, ultrastructural examination of these tissues to demonstrate myeloid granules may be crucial.

ACUTE BASOPHILIC LEUKEMIA. Acute basophilic leukemia is a rare form of AML in which the blastic cells differentiate along the basophil lineage. The peripheral blood usually demonstrates anemia and thrombocytopenia with leukocytosis. The bone marrow is infiltrated by blastic cells simulating lymphoblasts or myeloblasts. Blasts are generally negative for Sudan black B and myeloperoxidase. There may be an increase in mature basophils or in blasts staining with toluidine blue. The diagnosis often rests on the identification of blasts with basophilic granules by ultrastructural methods (Brunning, 1994).

Chronic Myeloproliferative Disorders

The chronic myeloproliferative disorders are composed of CML, PCV, myelofibrosis with myeloid metaplasia (MMM), and ET. These four disorders are grouped together because they share several clinical and laboratory characteristics. They are clonal proliferations of a pluripotential stem cell that can differentiate along granulocytic, erythroid, and megakaryocytic lines. In addition, these four disorders have a chronic course that often terminates as acute leukemia, myelofibrosis, or a coagulopathy.

4

Chronic Myelogenous Leukemia

CLINICAL FEATURES. CML occurs in young and middle-aged adults. However, the age-specific incidence increases markedly after 50 years of age. The onset is insidious, and the disorder may be discovered accidentally on a routine blood test. The patient may have symptoms of anemia and weight loss or simply may complain of malaise. The spleen enlarges progressively, and the patient begins to lose weight and have fever and night sweats associated with increased metabolism as a result of granulocyte turnover. The discomfort associated with an enlarged spleen may bring the patient to the doctor. Infarcts in the spleen may produce left upper quadrant pain. Excessive bleeding or bruising may occur in the later stages of the disease. Lymphadenopathy, although often present, is rarely prominent.

LABORATORY FEATURES

Blood. The leukocyte count usually is over 50×10^9/L and may exceed 300×10^9/L. The differential count is characteristic. There is a complete spectrum of granulocytic cells, from a few myeloblasts to mature neutrophils (Plate 27–3*F*). Myeloblasts are less than 10% of the cells. Myelocytes and neutrophils both exceed the other cell types. This bimodal distribution helps exclude other myeloproliferative disorders and reactive leukocytoses. The relative percentage of neutrophil myelocytes increases as the total leukocyte count increases. Basophilia is consistently present. Eosinophilia is almost always noted, along with the presence of eosinophil myelocytes. Monocytes are also absolutely increased in most patients.

Anemia is present in the majority of patients at the time of diagnosis. In others, it appears during the course of the disease as a result of decreased RBC production. Erythrocytes are normochromic and normocytic. A few normoblasts can usually be found.

Thrombocytosis is present at the time of diagnosis in over half of patients. Less than 15% of patients have thrombocytopenia.

Marrow. The marrow is markedly hypercellular primarily as a result of granulocytic proliferation, with all stages represented. Eosinophil and basophil precursors are often increased. Normoblasts tend to be decreased. Frequently the marrow cannot be aspirated because of the density of cells packed together or (especially later in the disease) because of increased reticulin, which can be demonstrated on marrow biopsy. In a minority of patients, macrophages are found laden with blue pigment (sea-blue histiocytes) or appearing indistinguishable from Gaucher cells (pseudo-Gaucher cells). These are likely due to phagocytosis of cellular debris resulting from increased cell turnover.

It is well to remember that even a typical bone marrow is not diagnostic of CML. On the other hand, the diagnosis can be made from the peripheral blood film in most cases.

Neutrophil Alkaline Phosphatase. The neutrophil alkaline phosphatase (NAP) is greatly reduced or absent in over 90% of patients with CML. It is greatly elevated in PCV; elevated, normal, or low in myelofibrosis with myeloid metaplasia; and normal or elevated in leukemoid reactions. During remission of CML with a normal-appearing blood picture, in most cases, the NAP continues to be low; in about one third of patients, it returns to normal. The NAP increases in the accelerated and blastic phases of the disease. It may also increase in response to infection, as it does in normal individuals.

Cytogenetic Abnormalities. In over 95% of patients with typical CML, cultured cells from the blood or bone marrow possess the t(9;22)(q34; q11). The abnormally small chromosome formed by this translocation is called the Philadelphia (Ph^1) chromosome (Nowell, 1960). It appears that the Ph^1 chromosome is present in precursors of granulocytes, normoblasts, megakaryocytes, and B lymphocytes but not in skin cells. The normal *ABL1* gene is located on the long arm of chromosome 9, whereas the *BCR* gene is on the long arm of chromosome 22. In CML, a reciprocal exchange of DNA results in *BCR* sequences moving to chromosome 9 and *ABL1* sequences to chromosome 22. This translocation results in a *BCR-ABL1* gene fusion that forms a novel RNA transcript and, subsequently, a protein growth factor that possesses tyrosine kinase activity. This protein has a higher tyrosine kinase activity than does the normal protein 145 coded for by *ABL1*. Morphologic and clinical reassessment of patients with CML who lack the Ph^1 chromosome has revealed that nearly all of these patients have either an atypical myeloproliferative disorder other than CML or chronic myelomonocytic leukemia (a myelodysplastic syndrome) (Jandl, 1987; Kaye, 1984). Some patients with the typical hematologic findings of CML but who lack the Ph^1 chromosome on karyotypic analysis have been found to have the *ABL1-BCR* gene fusion by molecular probe analysis (Morris, 1986).

Other Findings. Serum cobalamin and transcobalamins usually are increased considerably, as a result of increased transcobalamin I, and are thought to reflect the size of the total blood granulocyte pool. The serum muramidase is also increased.

Course. After a median period of about three years, the disease changes into a more aggressive or accelerated phase. This is characterized by one or more features of progressive myeloproliferation: basophilia, thrombocytosis, leukocytosis, increasing splenomegaly, anemia, and reticulin myelofibrosis. These features become refractory to chemotherapy. Preceding these changes, new clones of cells with cytogenetic abnormalities may be demonstrated, and frequently, a change occurs in the *in vitro* growth characteristics of the committed progenitor cells in soft agar cultures.

In about one third of cases, the accelerated phase is characterized by a progressive increase in blasts (10% to 30%) and promyelocytes; when blasts exceed 30% of cells in blood or marrow, it is regarded as the blastic phase of the disease. In the majority of cases, the blastic phase follows the accelerated phase by a few months; in a small proportion of cases, the blastic phase may be the first presentation of the disease (Peterson, 1976). These patients usually have the Ph^1 chromosome, with or without morphologic evidence of CML, such as basophilia. The NAP becomes normal or high in most patients in the blastic phase.

The morphologic patterns in the blastic phase of CML resemble acute myeloblastic leukemia in the majority of cases, although Auer rods are rarely found. In approximately one third of cases, however, the appearance is that of acute lymphoblastic leukemia (ALL) (Rosenthal, 1977). In these latter cases, the blasts are positive for terminal deoxynucleotidyl transferase (Marks, 1978). The distinction is useful because the latter (ALL) may respond to ALL-oriented therapy but the former (AML) do not (Peterson, 1976). Median survival after onset of the blastic phase of CML is about 2 months overall and about 10 months in patients who respond by going into remission.

Treatment with either busulfan or hydroxyurea usually controls the disease in the chronic phase, but without hematologic bone marrow remission or clearing of the Ph^1 chromosome. Treatment with interferon (IFN) has produced complete hematologic remission in approximately 70% of patients with CML, and over half of the responders show suppression of the Ph^1 chromosomes. In some patients, there has been complete disappearance of the *BCR-ABL1* fusion gene (Yoffe, 1987). The long-term usefulness of IFN is presently being studied.

Polycythemia Vera (Erythremia, Primary Polycythemia)

PCV is characterized by excessive proliferation of erythroid, granulocytic, and megakaryocytic elements in the marrow (panmyelosis). This is reflected in the blood in an absolute increase in the red blood cell mass, leukocytosis, and thrombocytosis. Erythropoietin excretion in the urine is decreased. The production of erythrocytes appears to be autonomous, but it does respond to erythropoietin when the patient has become anemic through blood loss. The cause of this panmyelosis and pancytosis is unknown.

CLINICAL FEATURES. The disease is slightly more frequent in men than in women. It usually begins in middle age. Affected patients exhibit ruddy cyanosis. Splenomegaly is present in two thirds of patients. Thrombotic or hemorrhagic phenomena occur in about half of the patients. Myocardial infarction, cerebral thrombosis, splenic infarction, pulmonary infarcts, and thrombophlebitis account for the most frequent thrombotic episodes; upper gastrointestinal bleeding, often from peptic ulcer, is the most common bleeding problem. Pruritus, especially after bathing, is common.

BLOOD. The erythrocytes number 6 to 12×10^{12}/L, and the hemoglobin is 18 to 24 g/dL. The mean cell volume (MCV), mean cell hemoglobin (MCH), and mean cell hemoglobin concentration (MCHC) are normal or low. The erythrocytes are hypochromic and microcytic if chronic blood loss has occurred. Macrocytes, polychromatic cells, and normoblasts may be found but are not a prominent feature of the disease. Red blood cell production is increased. Red blood cell destruction is normal during the period of erythrocytosis; later in the disease, as splenomegaly develops, red blood cell survival diminishes. The total blood volume is increased, primarily because of the increased red blood cell mass, although the plasma volume also may be elevated to a lesser degree. Blood viscosity is high, and it may be difficult to prepare good blood films. The erythrocyte sedimentation rate (ESR) is reduced.

The platelet count is increased in about two thirds of patients, often to levels exceeding 1000×10^9/L. In 80% of untreated patients, functional platelet abnormalities can be detected by platelet aggregation studies (Gilbert, 1975a). Decreased aggregation in response to epinephrine is most common but may be found in response to other reagents as well. No consistent clotting defect has been found in PCV.

Moderate neutrophilic leukocytosis in the range of 10 to 30 $\times 10^9$/L is common. Immature granulocytes are seen in about one half of cases, and basophils often are absolutely increased. The NAP is markedly elevated in 80% of patients. Serum transcobalamins and serum muramidase usually are elevated.

The arterial oxygen saturation is normal. Hyperuricemia appears in many patients with PCV as a result of the increased nucleic acid metabolism, and in some patients, secondary gout or renal uric acid stones occur.

Soft agar culture of blood cells reveals normal to increased numbers of colonies. The colony-stimulating activity (granulocyte-monocyte colony stimulating factor [GM-CSF]) in the blood usually is increased.

MARROW. The marrow characteristically is hypercellular, with all the elements (erythroid, granulocytic, and megakaryocytic) sharing the hyperplasia; fat is decreased (Plate 27–5*A*). In a study of patients of the Polycythemia Vera Study Group (PVSG), 90% had moderate or marked hypercellularity; only 6% were normocellular and none hypocellular. Increased reticulin is often present and correlates positively with the cellularity. Storage iron is decreased or absent in 95% of cases.

In vitro culture of marrow cells results in the growth of substantial numbers of erythroid colonies without added erythropoietin; this suggests that the clone is erythropoietin independent or abnormally sensitive to erythropoietin.

DIAGNOSIS. Criteria of the PVSG for the diagnosis of PCV are as follows:

1. Increased total erythrocyte volume (male, $\geq$36 mL/kg; female, $\geq$32 mL/kg).
2. Normal arterial oxygen saturation ($\geq$92%).
3. Either splenomegaly, or two of the following: (a) thrombocytosis ($>400 \times 10^9$/L), (b) leukocytosis ($>12 \times 10^9$/L), (c) increased NAP, (d) increased serum vitamin B_{12} ($>$900 μg/L) or unsaturated B_{12}-binding capacity ($>$2200 μg/L).

If doubt remains about the diagnosis of PCV, a search for other causes of polycythemia should be made.

COURSE. PCV is a chronic disease; patients usually live 10 to 20 years under good control. Phlebotomy, chlorambucil, radioactive phosphorus (^{32}P), and hydroxyurea have been used to control the manifestations of the disease. Because of the high incidence of complications in untreated cases, surgery should not be undertaken unless the hematocrit has been reduced to normal levels.

In about 20% to 40% of patients, progressive anemia, gradual splenic enlargement, and further elevation of the leukocyte count, with more immature granulocytes and more circulating nucleated red cells, may occur. Many erythrocytes become oval, teardrop-shaped cells (dacrocytes) become prominent, and poikilocytic red blood cells increase in number. Bone marrow aspiration becomes impossible because of myelofibrosis, and splenomegaly increases, owing to extramedullary hematopoiesis. The manifestations at this stage of the disease are indistinguishable from myelofibrosis with myeloid metaplasia (Plate 27–5*B* to *G*).

Another late complication of PCV is acute leukemia (Landaw, 1975). An increased risk of developing acute leukemia is associated with PCV itself (phlebotomy treatment alone). To this is added the leukemogenic potential contributed by the effective myelosuppressive agents; of these, the risk with chlorambucil exceeds that with ^{32}P. It does appear, however, that treatment with phlebotomy alone results in shorter survival than treatment with myelosuppressive agents.

Myelofibrosis with Myeloid Metaplasia

Synonyms for what is probably the same basic disease process include agnogenic myeloid metaplasia, myelosclerosis with myeloid metaplasia, myeloid megakaryocytic hepatosplenomegaly, aleukemic myelosis, and many others.

DEFINITION. This is a chronic, progressive panmyelosis characterized by a triad of findings: varying degrees of fibrosis of the marrow, massive splenomegaly due to extramedullary hematopoiesis, and a leukoerythroblastic anemia with marked red blood cell abnormalities, circulating normoblasts, immature granulocytes, and atypical platelets. Myelofibrosis with myeloid metaplasia is an uncommon disease with an incidence one third that of CML (Jandl, 1987).

CLINICAL FEATURES. The disorder occurs typically in persons over the age of 50 and has an insidious onset, with weight loss, anemia, and abdominal discomfort due to the large spleen. Often, the liver is enlarged as well, and the patient may be slightly jaundiced. On x-ray study, diffuse or patchy osteosclerosis may appear in one third to one half of patients; osteoporosis may be seen also.

BLOOD. A moderate normochromic, normocytic anemia (frequently with some hypochromic cells and basophilic stippling), moderate anisocytosis, and marked poikilocytosis, including prominent teardrop forms (dacrocytes) and elliptocytes, are characteristic. Normoblasts are often present in numbers out of proportion to the degree of anemia, and a slight reticulocytosis is frequently found. The anemia may have a complicated origin, with components of marrow failure, ineffective erythropoiesis, and hemolysis. The leukocyte count is normal or, more commonly, moderately increased; immature neutrophils and occasionally even myeloblasts are present. The NAP is most often elevated, but occasionally may be normal or decreased. Chromosomal studies have not shown the presence of the Ph^1 chromosome, which is so characteristic of CML. However, 80% of patients acquire nonspecific chromosomal alterations, and their appearance frequently reflects a conversion to AML or CML. Basophils are often increased in number. Platelets are normal or decreased in number (rarely increased) and often are atypical, with distinct zones: a clear hyaloplasm and a central pale chromomere that lacks the usual concentration of azurophilic granules (Plate 27–5*E* to *G*). Micromegakaryocytes the size of lymphocytes with both nucleus and cytoplasm or small megakaryoblasts usually may be found if searched for; on rare occasions, they are present in considerable numbers (Plate 27–5*E* to *G*; see also Plate 25–4*H*).

In vitro culture studies of blood cells have generally shown considerably increased colonies (CFU-GM) and clusters, which are similar to the pattern in CML. The serum colony-stimulating activity (GM-CSF) appears to be very high.

Serum uric acid is frequently increased. Serum cobalamin and unsaturated transcobalamin are normal or elevated.

MARROW. It usually is impossible to aspirate marrow, and a needle biopsy or a surgical biopsy is necessary; this is especially true later in the course of the disease. Early in the disease, the marrow may be hypercellular, with panmyelosis and prominently increased megakaryocytes that are frequently abnormal. On histologic sections, there is a diffuse increase in reticulin fibers, which is demonstrable with silver stains (Rappaport, 1966); patchy fibrosis may be present.

Later, the marrow becomes more fibrotic, with residual islands of atypical megakaryocytes, erythroid, and granulocytic precursors. The fibrosis is of loose connective tissue with scanty collagen, but reticulin fibers are abundant. Foci of osteoid may be found, and the bony trabeculae are sometimes irregularly thickened (myelosclerosis). The marrow may show a mixture of hyperplasia and fibrosis in one sample, or it may vary in different sites of the body (Plate 27–5*B* to *D*).

COURSE. A significant proportion of cases of myelofibrosis with myeloid metaplasia represent a late stage, after many years' progression, of typical PCV. The usual course of myelofibrosis with myeloid metaplasia is one of progressive anemia and enlargement of the spleen; hemolysis frequently becomes an increasing element in the anemia. Infections may be a serious problem. Portal hypertension occurs in 10% to 20% of cases and may result in bleeding esophageal varices. It may be due to portal vein thrombosis or intrahepatic obstruction as a result of myeloid metaplasia coupled with increased portal blood flow.

The median survival is about five years, slightly longer than that of chronic granulocytic leukemia, but considerably less than that of PCV; however, patients occasionally may live as long as 10 to 15 years. In patients with longer survival, frequently the terminal event is acute leukemia.

Thrombocythemia

As distinguished from *thrombocytosis,* the term *thrombocythemia* should probably be confined to situations in which the platelet count is persistently elevated to levels at least three times normal. Thrombocythemia, thus defined, usually is part of the general picture of other myeloproliferative disorders: PCV, CML, and rarely, myelofibrosis with myeloid metaplasia.

Occasionally, however, thrombocythemia may be the predominant feature of the hematologic picture, and in these cases, it is commonly associated with bleeding problems. Evidence suggests that thrombocythemia is a clonal disorder similar to PCV and CML.

CLINICAL FEATURES. Characteristic features are recurrent, spontaneous hemorrhages, which are most commonly gastrointestinal. Hemorrhages occasionally are preceded or accompanied by thrombosis in superficial or deep veins. Purpura has not been described. Slight splenomegaly as measured with radioisotopic techniques occurs in 50% of cases.

BLOOD. The most striking feature is the marked increase in platelets (usually greater than 1000×10^9/L), often with abnormal and giant forms and usually accompanied by fragments of megakaryocytes (Plate 27–5*I*). Neutrophilic leukocytosis is almost always present, and the NAP usually is normal. Hypochromic microcytic anemia due to chronic blood loss is present in many cases; at other times, erythrocytosis may be evident. Platelet function defects in thrombocythemia are frequently demonstrable. The most typical finding is decreased aggregation in response to epinephrine.

MARROW. The marrow shows a panmyelosis with increased megakaryocytes (Plate 27–5*H*). Megakaryocyte clusters usually are present. Splenic extramedullary hematopoiesis may be present.

DIAGNOSIS. Revised criteria of the PVSG for the diagnosis of thrombocythemia are as follows (Murphy, 1986):

1. Platelet count exceeding 600×10^9/L
2. Hemoglobin <13 g/dL or normal red blood cell mass
3. Stainable iron in marrow or failure of one month of iron therapy to raise hemoglobin by 1 g/dL
4. No Ph^1 chromosome
5. Collagen fibrosis of marrow is absent, or less than one third of biopsy specimen without both splenomegaly and leukoerythroblastic reaction
6. No known cause for thrombocytosis present (such as malignancy, chronic inflammatory disease, or history of splenectomy)

COURSE. Most cases are stable for many years, but a small proportion may merge into other chronic myeloproliferative disorders or, rarely, develop into acute leukemia.

Myelodysplastic Syndromes

MDS occur primarily in persons over age 50 and usually present as an anemia refractory to hematinics, with or without neutropenia and thrombocytopenia. Liver, spleen, or lymph nodes usually are not enlarged. The marrow is hypercellular and maturation is abnormal in one or more of the three hematopoietic cell lines, and blast cells often are increased. This group of disorders has been called preleukemias or dysmyelopoietic syndromes because of the high proportion of cases that ultimately progress to overt acute leukemia. The FAB Cooperative Group (Bennett, 1976, 1982) has described and classified these disorders.

TYPES OF ABNORMAL CELLULAR MATURATION. *Dyserythropoiesis* includes nuclear fragmentation or karyorrhexis, multinuclearity, irregularly staining cytoplasm, basophilic stippling, and ring sideroblasts (Bennett, 1986). Erythroid cells may be decreased or increased in number. Erythrocytic abnormalities in the blood film include oval macrocytes, anisochromia, basophilic stippling, dacrocytes, and reticulocytopenia.

Dysgranulopoiesis included retarded nuclear maturation and distorted cytoplasmic maturation, with azurophilic granules either unstained or abnormally large and decreased numbers of specific granules. In the blood film, one may see nuclear hyposegmentation (pseudo–Pelger-Huët anomaly) or bizarre hypersegmentation, and irregular retention of cytoplasmic basophilia or lack of cytoplasmic granules.

Dysmegakaryocytopoiesis includes large megakaryocytes with unsegmented nuclei, micromegakaryocytes, and megakaryocytes with two or more small unconnected nuclei. Megakaryocytes may be decreased in number. In the blood film, giant hypogranular platelets are frequent and micromegakaryocytes are seen rarely.

BLOOD AND MARROW FINDINGS. Five types of myelodysplastic syndromes have been defined by the FAB Cooperative Group (Bennett, 1982). However, some observers have expanded the classification of MDS to include chronic myelomonocytic leukemia in transformation and myelodysplastic syndrome, unclassified (Brunning, 1994).

Refractory Anemia. Anemia with reticulocytopenia and abnormal erythrocytes are the presenting findings of refractory anemia (RF). Abnormal granulocytes are rare, and blasts are less than 1 percent in the blood. The marrow is normocellular to hypercellular with erythroid hyperplasia and/or dyserythropoiesis and fewer than 5 percent blasts.

Refractory Anemia with Ring Sideroblasts. In refractory anemia with ring sideroblasts (RARS), in addition to the findings of RA, ring sideroblasts are present and exceed 15% of all marrow cells. Defective cytoplasmic maturation and anisochromic erythrocytes are associated abnormalities.

Refractory Anemia with Excess Blasts. In refractory anemia with excess blasts (RAEB), the blood shows cytopenia in two or three of the cell lines, and less than 5% circulating blasts. The marrow is hypercellular, with variable erythroid or granulocytic hyperplasia. Dyspoietic changes are present in all three cell lines, and 5% to 20% of the marrow cells are blasts.

Chronic Myelomonocytic Leukemia. In chronic myelomonocytic leukemia (CMML), the blood shows a persistent monocytosis ($>1 \times 10^9$/L), frequently neutrophilia with morphologic abnormalities, and less than 5% blasts. The marrow is similar to that in RAEB but often has increased promonocytes. These may be distinguished from the abnormal myelocytes by nonspecific esterase staining.

RAEB in Transformation. In RAEB in transformation (RAEB-T), the findings are similar to those in RAEB, with the addition of any of the following: (1) greater than 5% blasts in the blood, (2) 20% to 30% blasts in the marrow, or (3) the presence of Auer rods. In this group are patients with cytopenias and symptoms of short duration that do not fit into the other categories of MDS or of AML. (A minimum of 30% blasts in the blood or bone marrow is required for the diagnosis of AML.)

Chronic Myelomonocytic Leukemia in Transformation (CMML-T). CMML in transformation (CMML-T) is a term used for cases in which the features of CMML exist plus the finding of Auer rods or the presence of 20% to 29% blasts in the bone marrow or 5% to 29% blasts in the blood.

Myelodysplastic Syndrome, Unclassified. The myelodysplastic syndrome, unclassified, category is used when the clinical and hematologic findings of myelodysplasia exist, but without specific features to allow placement in one of the other six categories. Patients often have cytopenias with panhyperplasia of the bone marrow. There usually are less than 5% blasts in the bone marrow, but it possesses a degree of myelodysplasia greater than that seen in refractory anemia or ringed sideroblasts are less than required for the diagnosis of RARS.

COURSE. The course of MDS ranges from slowly progressive forms (RA, RARS) to more aggressive conditions (RAEB, RAEB-T). The median survival of the more aggressive forms is approximately 3 to 22 months, whereas that of the slowly progressive conditions is 16 to 52 months (Mufti, 1986).

Lymphoid Disorders

The lymphoid disorders represent a group of neoplastic conditions originating from cells of the lymphoreticular system. When neoplastic cells involve predominantly the blood and bone marrow, the condition is called leukemia. However, when the condition is predominantly limited to lymph nodes and/or organs, the disorder usually is called lymphoma. Some types of lymphomas, in their natural course, typically develop into leukemia; for example, a diffuse, small lymphocytic lymphoma may in time involve the blood and thus be indistinguishable from chronic lymphocytic leukemia. Blood involvement also occurs with lymphoblastic and Burkitt types of lymphomas and occasionally with follicular lymphomas.

Acute Lymphoblastic Leukemia

CLINICAL FEATURES. This disorder occurs in all age groups, with a peak occurrence in children between 2 and 10 years of age. A second peak in the frequency of ALL occurs in middle-aged and elderly adults. Individuals with this disorder often present with symptoms of fatigue, fever, and bleeding. Generalized lymphadenopathy, splenomegaly, and hepatomegaly are common findings. Because the leukemic cells infiltrate many tissues of the body, other symptoms may occur. Leg pain can be associated with periosteal infiltrates; and headaches, nausea, and vomiting with meningeal leukemia. A rapid onset of unconsciousness usually indicates subarachnoid hemorrhage.

BLOOD. Anemia is present if clinical manifestations are fully developed. It is usually normocytic. Frequently, nucleated red cells are present. Thrombocytopenia of moderate to marked degree is the rule. The leukocyte count occasionally is very high (over 100×10^9/L), often is slightly elevated but is perhaps most frequently normal or decreased. The pre-

Table 27–9. FRENCH-AMERICAN-BRITISH (FAB) CLASSIFICATION OF THE ACUTE LYMPHOBLASTIC LEUKEMIAS (L)

Cytology	L1	L2	L3
Size	Small	Large	Large and homogeneous
Chromatin	Homogeneous	Variable	Finely stippled
Shape	Regular	Irregular	Oval to round
Nucleoli	Rare	Present	1–3
Cytoplasm	Scanty	Moderate	Moderate
Basophilia	Moderate	Variable	Intense

From Bennett JM, et al: Br J Haematol 1976; 33:451. Blackwell Scientific Publications, Ltd., Oxford.

Table 27–10. FAB SCORING SYSTEM FOR L1 AND L2 VARIANTS

Criteria*	Score
High N/C ratio ≥ 75% of cells	+
Low N/C ratio ≥ 25% of cells	−
Nucleoli: 0–1 (small) ≥ 75% of cells	+
Nucleoli: 1 or more (prominent) ≥ 25% of cells	−
Irregular nuclear membrane ≥ 25% of cells	−
Large cells > 50% of cells	−

*Criteria that are not met (or intermediate results) result in no score. The possible total score for a case ranges from −4 to +2. A score of 0 to +2 results in a diagnosis of L1, and a score of −1 to −4 in a diagnosis of L2. N/C ratio = nuclear/cytoplasmic ratio.

From Bennett JM, et al: Br J Haematol 1981; 47:553. Blackwell Scientific Publications, Ltd., Oxford.

dominant cell is the lymphoblast or immature lymphocyte (see Plate 27–1*L* and Plate 27–2*H*).

MARROW. By the time the patient is symptomatic, the hematopoietic cells and fat usually are replaced by diffuse infiltration of lymphoblasts.

In the L1 type according to the FAB classification (Table 27–9), the lymphoblast has a high nuclear/cytoplasmic ratio. The nuclei are regular and not indented or twisted. The chromatin pattern is fine and uniform. Usually only one or two nucleoli are present. The cytoplasm is scanty in amount, pale blue, and homogeneous, usually without granules (see Plates 27–1*L*, 27–4*G*, and 27–5*J*). The L1 type is homogeneous in these characteristics and is the type of leukemia that is common in children. In L2, a larger cell type prevails (Plates 27–2*H* and 27–5*K*) and usually there is more variation in cytologic features within and between cases. It is less common in children and is the usual adult type of ALL. L3 represents the Burkitt type of ALL (see Plates 27–5*L* and 27–6*H*). The cells are large and uniform; they have a round or oval nucleus with prominent nucleoli and deeply basophilic cytoplasm that usually contains vacuoles.

The precision of the diagnosis of the L1 and L2 variants has been improved by employing a scoring method (Bennett, 1981; Table 27–10). In this system, the nuclear/cytoplasmic ratio, number and prominence of nucleoli, nuclear shape, and cell size are the features that distinguish between L1 and L2 variants.

Approximately 71% of cases of childhood ALL are L1, 27% are L2, and 2% are L3 variants. In adult patients with ALL, however, L2 is the most commonly observed cytologic variant. In addition, it appears that more children with the L1 variant remain in hematologic remission at one year than children with L2 morphology. The prognostic significance of the FAB classification in adults is not yet clear, but more patients with L1 morphology may obtain a complete remission than patients with the L2 variant.

CYTOCHEMISTRY. (see Table 27–6). The blasts are negative for Sudan black B, peroxidase, and naphthol ASD chloroacetate esterase. The diagnosis of ALL cannot be made with certainty until the Sudan black B or peroxidase reaction has been performed to show that the blasts are negative. In a few cases of L2, azurophilic granules may be present, but they are Sudan black B and peroxidase negative. The acid phosphatase reaction is moderately or strongly positive in the blasts in about 20% of cases of ALL. Most of these appear to be T-cell leukemias. The PAS stain usually shows coarse blocks of material in at least some lymphoblasts (Plate 27–4*H*).

IMMUNOLOGIC CELL MARKERS. ALL can be divided into four subtypes, depending on the reaction of blasts with lymphocyte cell marker assays (Table 27–11). T-cell leukemias, which account for 10% to 20% of cases of ALL, occur predominantly in boys, who tend to be slightly older than children with early pre–B-cell ALL (common ALL) (see later). Patients with T-cell ALL usually have a high leukocyte count and a widening of the mediastinum as seen on x-ray study.

The most frequent form of ALL in children is the early pre-B cell. The diagnosis can be made only when antisera specific for Tdt and for the CD10, CD19, CD24, and HLA-DR antigens react with the patient's blasts. The diagnosis of pre–B-cell ALL rests on the demonstration of μ heavy chain, within the cytoplasm of the blasts. Patients with early pre–

Table 27–11. IMMUNOPHENOTYPIC CLASSIFICATION OF ACUTE LYMPHOBLASTIC LEUKEMIA (ALL)

Subsets of ALL	Immunophenotype										Approximate Percentage of Population
	Tdt	*DR*	*CD2*	*CD5*	*CD10*	*CD19*	*CD20*	*CD24*	*SIg*	*CIg*	
T cell	+	−	+	+	−	−	−	−	−	−	10–20
Early pre-B	+	+	−	−	+	+	−	+	−	−	60–70
Pre-B	+	+	−	−	+	+	+	+	−	+	15–20
B cell	−	+	−	−	−	+	+	+	+	−	1–3

Tdt = terminal deoxynucleotidyl transferase
DR = HLA-DR histocompatibility antigen
CD = cluster designation: CD2 and CD5, pan–T cell; CD10, common ALL; CD19, CD20, CD24, pan–B cell
SIg = surface immunoglobulin
CIg = cytoplasmic immunoglobulin

B-cell ALL and pre–B-cell ALL have similar laboratory and clinical features as well as a relatively good prognosis.

In the B-cell type of ALL, lymphoblasts have surface immunoglobulin restricted to one light chain and usually correspond to the L3 variant of the FAB classification. In contrast, the other immunologic subtypes of ALL show no distinctive correlation with the FAB classification. The B-cell type is the rarest subgroup of ALL and has a less favorable prognosis, although recent therapeutic results in children are encouraging (Crist, 1991). It likely represents a more advanced phase of sporadic Burkitt's lymphoma.

Chronic B- and T-Lymphoid Leukemias (Small Lymphocytic Leukemias)

For many years, the variability of the clinical course and the heterogeneity of the neoplastic cells from patients with chronic lymphocytic leukemia was accepted as part of the disease spectrum. However, with studies involving the correlation of clinical course with the morphologic appearance and immunophenotype of neoplastic cells an enhanced recognition of several neoplastic disorders of small mature lymphocytes has emerged. The FAB (Bennett, 1989) presented a classification of chronic (mature) B- and T-lymphoid leukemias and Brunning and McKenna (1994) offered a similar classification of small lymphocytic leukemias.

Chronic Lymphoid Leukemias of B-Cell Type

CHRONIC LYMPHOCYTIC LEUKEMIA (CLL) OF B CELL TYPE

CLINICAL FEATURES. CLL is rare under the age of 40; most cases occur over the age of 60. It is more than twice as common in men as in women. The onset is insidious, and the disease is commonly discovered by chance during the investigation of another problem. Lymphadenopathy, asymptomatic or associated with symptoms such as weakness, fatigue, anorexia, and weight loss, may cause the patient to come to the physician. Enlarged lymph nodes usually are evident, and frequently hepatosplenomegaly is also found (Table 27–12).

BLOOD. The leukocyte count usually is between 30 and 200×10^9/L, although lower counts may be present in early disease. In the typical type of CLL, 90% or more of the cells are small lymphocytes that are monotonously similar in appearance and usually look normal (Plate 27–3*G*). Nuclear chromatin may be coarsely condensed and more sharply separated by parachromatin than in normal lymphocytes, or in some cases, the chromatin is less condensed than normal. Sometimes nucleoli are evident in many of the lymphocytes. Size variation is minimal. Cytoplasm is of small to moderate amount. Less than 10% of lymphocytes are prolymphocytes or reticular lymphocytes (transformed lymphocytes).

Often there is neither anemia nor thrombocytopenia at the time of diagnosis. Anemia due to impaired production does develop as the marrow is replaced by leukemic cells. In addition, erythrocyte lifespan in some patients with CLL may be reduced. This is especially true when there is marked splenomegaly. Autoimmune hemolytic anemia develops in about 10% of patients. Thrombocytopenia often is slight and occasionally becomes severe as the disease progresses, so that hemorrhagic manifestations appear. Thrombocytopenia usually is due to hypoproliferation but may also be secondary to an immune process or splenic sequestration. A staging classification of cases of CLL has been offered by a National Cancer Institute sponsored working group (Cheson, 1988). The prognosis of patients with CLL correlates with the size of the total body lymphocyte pool and the presence of anemia or thrombocytopenia. The median survival for patients with CLL is about six years.

MARROW. The usual early finding is the presence of slight to moderate lymphocytosis. Because the lymphocytes are morphologically normal, examination of marrow films may be equivocal. Histologic sections of aspirated particles or biopsy material are very helpful. Small to medium-sized areas of lymphocytes are present and have indistinct margins; lymphocytes are infiltrating into adjacent hematopoietic tissue. The degree of lymphocyte infiltration correlates with the survival of the patient. Patchy, nodular, or interstitial involvement of the bone marrow by neoplastic lymphocytes is associated with a relatively good outcome. However, a diffuse infiltrate of the bone marrow usually correlates with a poor prognosis (Bartl, 1982a; Montserrat, 1987).

4

CHRONIC LYMPHOCYTIC LEUKEMIA, MIXED CELL TYPES

Two subtypes exist. The first, *mixed cell type of CLL*, is composed of both large and small lymphocytes in the blood.

Table 27–12. COMPARISON OF CHRONIC LYMPHOCYTIC LEUKEMIA (CLL), PROLYMPHOCYTIC LEUKEMIA (PL), NON-HODGKIN'S LYMPHOMA (NHL), AND HAIRY CELL LEUKEMIA (HCL)

	CLL	PL	NHL	HCL
Mean age	55	65	60	50
Male/female ratio	2:1	6.5:1	2.5:1	4:1
Initial mean lymphocytic count ($\times 10^9$/L)	90	350	40	Usually pancytopenia
Lymphadenopathy	Moderate	Mild	Moderate	Mild
Splenomegaly	Moderate	Frequently massive	Moderate	Frequently massive
Hepatomegaly	Moderate	Moderate to massive	Moderate	Mild
Morphology of neoplastic cell	Small lymphocyte (T-cell variant clover leaf nuclei)	Prolymphocyte	Small cleaved	Hairy cell
Lineage of neoplastic cells	≈95% B cell ≈ 5% T cell	≈95% B cell ≈ 5% T cell	Virtually all B cell	Virtually all B cell
Response to therapy	Good	Poor	Fair	Good
Mean survival (years)	6–7	1	4–5	5–6

Adapted from Galton DAG, Goldman JM, Wiltshaw E, Catovsky D, Henry K, Goldenberg GJ: Br J Haematol 1974; 27:7. Oxford, Blackwell Scientific Publications.

The larger lymphocytes have more abundant basophilic cytoplasm with lower nuclear/cytoplasmic ratio. The nuclear chromatin is clumped, and nucleoli are variably present. Less than 10% of the cells are prolymphocytes. There is no evidence at this time that the clinical course of mixed cell type CLL differs from the typical type of CLL. The second, *chronic lymphocytic leukemia/prolymphocytic leukemia (CLL/PLL)*, is composed of a dimorphic population of prolymphocytes (>10% and less than 55%) and small lymphocytes in the blood (see Plate 27–3*H*). The bone marrow sections may contain foci of transformed cells or mixtures of small lymphocytes and prolymphocytes. The clinical course is between CLL and prolymphocytic leukemia (PLL).

PROLYMPHOCYTIC LEUKEMIA

PLL was originally described as a variant of CLL (Galton, 1974). The male/female ratio is 6.5:1 and the mean age is 65 years. PLL is characterized by a very marked lymphocytosis (usually $> 100 \times 10^9$/L; mean 355×10^9/L), massive splenomegaly, moderate hepatomegaly, and inconspicuous lymphadenopathy. The malignant lymphoid cells have a large vesicular nucleolus, condensed nuclear chromatin, and moderate amount of cytoplasm. More than 55% of blood leukemic cells are prolymphocytes (see Plate 27–3*I*). PLL usually is less responsive to treatment than CLL in general and has a poorer prognosis.

LEUKEMIC MANIFESTATIONS OF NON-HODGKIN'S LYMPHOMA

In the past, the term lymphosarcoma cell leukemia was used to connote the appearance of neoplastic cells, often in large numbers (mean 40×10^9/L), in the blood of patients with NHL. The cells have variably condensed nuclear chromatin and oval or notched nuclei in more than 30% of the cells. Occasional large blastlike cells may be present (Plate 27–7*G*). Bone marrow involvement is common and typically shows a paratrabecular localization of lymphocytic infiltration. Because this type of cell usually is associated with a follicular lymphoma, the term *leukemic phase of follicular lymphoma* is most often used.

The *leukemic phase of intermediate NHL or mantle zone lymphoma* is characterized by the presence of medium size cells with condensed nuclear chromatin and inconspicuous nucleoli with slight nuclear indentations and clefts (see Plate 27–3*J*). However, the clefts are not as pronounced as in follicular lymphoma. In a few cases, there are large cells with abundant, slightly basophilic cytoplasm similar to those of CLL of mixed cell type.

HAIRY CELL LEUKEMIA

Bouroncle (1958) described HCL, which is clinically variable in its manifestations. It occurs more frequently in males than in females. The mean age of afflicted patients is 50 years. It has an insidious onset and is characterized by proliferation of the abnormal cells in the reticuloendothelial organs and blood. Splenomegaly is the predominant physical finding (see Table 27–12).

Pancytopenia or depression of only two cell lines is the usual finding, with variable numbers of hairy cells. In the majority of cases, bone marrow aspiration is difficult. Marrow biopsy shows a marrow that varies in cellularity, often having both hypocellular and hypercellular areas and reticulin fibrosis. Hairy cells usually are present in large numbers.

Morphologically, the cells are medium sized (10 to 20 μm diameter), with round to oval nuclei, although many are notched or dumbbell shaped. The chromatin pattern is usually uniformly reticular similar to that of a monocyte, and nucleoli are small and inconspicuous. In some cells, chromatin is more condensed, resembling that of a lymphocyte. The cytoplasm is moderate in amount, often has numerous hairlike projections and frayed borders, and stains gray with Wright's stain (Plate 27–6*M* and *N*).

Cytochemically, these cells contain acid phosphatase, which is resistant to inhibition by tartrate; this is in contrast to the isoenzymes of acid phosphatase present in other hemic cells (Yam, 1971a). The cells are usually subtypes of B lymphocytes. The clinical course is usually chronic, but may be acute or subacute. The median survival is between five and six years. Traditionally, splenectomy has offered significant benefit to many patients. However, treatment with either α-interferon or $2'$-deoxycoformycin has been reported to induce remission.

SPLENIC LYMPHOMA WITH VILLOUS LYMPHOCYTES

Splenic lymphoma with villous lymphocytes (SLVL) is a disorder with many clinical, laboratory, and morphologic features that are similar to HCL. The disease is more common in men than women. Patients are often in their seventh decade of life and present with splenomegaly. In contrast to HCL, the leukocyte count is elevated (25×10^9/L and approximately one half of the patients possess a monoclonal gammopathy, usually IgM. The neoplastic cells are medium sized with clumped chromatin, moderately basophilic cytoplasm, and short cytoplasmic villi, often with a polar distribution. The bone marrow may demonstrate patchy infiltrates or massive involvement. In the spleen, the neoplastic infiltrate expands from the white pulp into the red pulp. The TRAP stain usually is negative, although positive reactions have been recorded. This may represent a leukemic phase of splenic marginal zone lymphoma (Harris, 1994).

IMMUNOLOGIC MARKERS

Most cases of CLL, follicular lymphoma, HCL, and PLL possess immunologic cell markers that help identify the disorder (Table 27–13). With the exception of HCL, neoplastic cells from these disorders contain surface-bound immunoglobulin usually restricted to IgM and IgD and to a single light chain, supporting the clonal origin of the leukemic cells. HCL cells usually exhibit only IgG surface bound immunoglobulin. Neoplastic cells from cases of NHL may possess surface IgG in addition to IgM and IgD. NHL and PLL cells usually have greater concentrations of membrane-bound IgM than cells from patients with CLL.

In virtually all cases of B-cell CLL, 25% to 90% of neoplastic cells form spontaneous rosettes with mouse erythrocytes. In approximately 40% of cases of HCL, neoplastic cells also form rosettes with mouse erythrocytes. However, leukemic cells from other B-cell malignancies rarely form rosettes with mouse erythrocytes. This useful marker for CLL has generally fallen into disuse, however, due to the need for fresh mouse red blood cells and the lack of a monoclonal antibody against the receptor. Characteristic anomalous labeling of B-cell CLL for the T-cell marker CD5 has largely supplanted the mouse rosette assay. The diagnosis of CLL is

Table 27–13. IMMUNOPHENOTYPIC CLASSIFICATION OF CHRONIC LYMPHOID LEUKEMIAS OF THE B-CELL TYPE

Subsets	SIg	MR	DR	CD5	CD11c	CD19	CD22	CD23	CD24	CD25	FMC7
CLL	+	+	+	+	−/+	+	−/+	+	+	−/+	−
PLL	++	−	+	−	−	+	+	−	+	−	+
ICL (MCL)	++	−	+	+	−	+	+	−/+	+	−	+
FL	++	−	+	−	−	++	+	+	+	−	+
HCL	++	−	+	−	+	+	+	−	−/+	+	+

Immunophenotypes

SIg	Surface immunoglobulins
MR	Receptor for mouse rosettes
DR	HLA-DR
CD5	Pan–T-cell antigen and subset of B cells
CD11c	B2 subfamily of integrin receptor molecules
CD19	Pan–B-cell antigen
CD22	Pan–B-cell antigen
CD23	Subset of B cells
CD24	Pan–B-cell antigen and some granulocytes
CD25	TAC (receptor for interleukin-2)
FMC7	Receptor for subset of B cells

CLL = chronic lymphocytic leukemia; PLL = prolymphocytic leukemia; ICL (MCL) = intermediate cell lymphoma (mantle zone cell lymphoma); FL = follicular lymphoma; HCL = hairy cell leukemia.

strongly suggested when neoplastic cells show low-intensity monoclonal surface-bound immunoglobulin, mouse rosette receptors, coexpression of CD5 with CD19, CD20, CD22 and other B-cell antigens but are negative for FMC7 antigen. In contrast, neoplastic cells from patients with HCL are characteristically CD5 negative but are CD11c, CD19, and CD25 positive. PLL cells are strongly positive for monoclonal surface-bound immunoglobulin, negative for mouse rosettes and CD11c, but positive for CD19, CD20, CD22, CD23, and CD24 antigens. PLL also typically labels with antibody FMC7.

T-Cell Lymphoid Leukemias

The immunologic phenotyping of neoplastic cells from patients with chronic lymphoid leukemia has indicated that a small percentage of cases are derived from T-cell lineage (Table 27–14) (Kadin, 1988).

Large Granulated Lymphocyte (LGL) Leukemia

The median age of these patients is 63 years. It is unusual to see pediatric patients with this disease. Patients are often asymptomatic; however, symptoms related to rheumatoid arthritis or Felty's syndrome, or both, are present in approximately 30% of patients. In approximately one half of the patients, there is splenomegaly and neutropenia. Anemia and thrombocytopenia can be seen alone or associated with neutropenia. Lymphocytosis is a constant feature. Large granulated lymphocytes are of moderate size with abundant light blue cytoplasm, eccentrically placed nuclei with a condensed chromatin pattern. Azurophilic cytoplasmic granules vary in number and size. The bone marrow exhibits a moderate infiltrate of granulated lymphocytes. All other marrow elements are present and show full maturation. Immunophenotypically there are two subtypes of large granulated lymphocytic leukemia. The most common is positive for CD3 and CD8 antigens, show variable expression for CD16 and CD57 antigens, and lack natural killer cell function. The second type are negative for CD3 and CD8 antigens, but positive for CD56 antigen and natural killer cell function (Brunning, 1994). This disorder usually has a chronic course, with the major complication relating to increased infections as a result of neutropenia. An additional type, with expression of CD3 and CD56, has been reported to present with high large granulated lymphocyte counts and follow an aggressive course (Gentile, 1994).

Table 27–14. IMMUNOPHENOTYPIC CLASSIFICATION OF CHRONIC LYMPHOID LEUKEMIAS OF THE T-CELL TYPE

	Immunophenotype					
Subset	*TdT*	*CD2*	*CD3*	*CD4*	*CD8*	*CD25*
Large granulated lymphocyte leukemia	−	++	++	−	+	
Adult T-cell leukemia-lymphoma	−	++	++	++	−	++
T-prolymphocytic leukemia	−	++	+	+	−/+	−/+
Sezary's syndrome and mycosis fungoides	−	++	++	+	−	−

Tdt = terminal deoxynucleotidyl transferase
CD2 = pan–T-cell antigen
CD3 = pan–T-cell antigen
CD4 = T-helper cell antigen
CD8 = T-suppressor cell antigen
CD25 = activated T cells, activated B cells, activated macrophages

Adult T-Cell Leukemia-Lymphoma

Adult T-cell leukemia-lymphoma (ATLL) is endemic in southwestern Japan, the Caribbean basin, the southeastern United States, and central Africa. The etiologic agent in this malignancy is the HTLV-1 (Poiesz, 1980). Transmission of HTLV-1 may occur from mother to child, or through intravenous drug abuse, sexual contact, or blood transfusion. Only a minority of individuals infected with HTLV-1 develop ATLL. Some individuals exhibit only a flulike syndrome, others develop a progressive leukemia, and still others manifest an aggressive lymphoproliferative disorder often involving lymph nodes, skin, liver, spleen, bone marrow, and blood (Davey, 1991).

Laboratory findings indicate moderate anemia, thrombocytopenia, and lymphocytosis. The blood film demonstrates the presence of moderately large blastic cells. The nuclear outline is characteristically convoluted or clover leafed with condensed chromatin. Nucleoli are small or absent, and the cytoplasm is agranular and basophilic. In the chronic form, 10% to 50% of the peripheral blood cells are abnormal cells, whereas in the acute form, greater than 50% of the cells exhibit characteristic morphology. The bone marrow may demonstrate minimal to marked involvement in 50% to 60% of patients. Patients may show variable involvement of the spleen, lymph nodes, liver, and bones. In the chronic form, the life expectancy is one to two years, whereas in the acute form survival is less than one year.

T-Prolymphocytic Leukemia

T-prolymphocytic leukemia is an uncommon disorder with a median age of 69 years, and the disease is slightly more frequent in males than in females. Patients present with a marked lymphocytosis (200×10^9/L), anemia, and thrombocytopenia. In most cases, the neoplastic cell is a prolymphocyte; however, in approximately 20% of patients the lymphocytes lack distinctive features and do not possess a prominent nucleolus. T-prolymphocytic leukemia is a rapidly progressive malignancy, with a survival time usually of less than one year.

Mycosis Fungoides and Sézary's Syndrome

Mycosis fungoides is a lymphoreticular neoplasm primarily involving the skin. As the disorder evolves, neoplastic cells infiltrate the lymph nodes and other visceral organs.

Mycosis fungoides occurs twice as frequently in men as in women. It usually affects individuals in their middle to late years.

The disorder first appears as an eczematoid, psoriaform, or nonspecific exfoliative dermatitis. The lesions tend to form plaques and then tumors that often ulcerate. Some patients develop generalized erythroderma.

Biopsies of the skin reveal lymphocytic and mononuclear cell infiltrates in the dermis. Neoplastic cells and normal-appearing lymphocytes infiltrate the epidermis and form clusters known as Pautrier's abscesses. These abscesses usually are accompanied by parakeratosis, acanthosis, spongiosis, and elongation of rete pegs. The nuclei of the neoplastic cells frequently have a cerebriform appearance.

In advanced stages of the disease, neoplastic cells infiltrate the lymph nodes, liver, spleen, and other organs.

Occasionally, atypical mononuclear cells with cerebriform nuclei are present in the peripheral blood (Plate 27–6*I* and *J*). In addition, when lymphocytosis exists (especially in the erythremic patient), the disorder is called *Sézary's syndrome.* Neoplastic cells from patients with mycosis fungoides and Sézary's syndrome appear to be T lymphocytes; in almost all cases, the cells demonstrate helper activity.

The disorder may follow a prolonged chronic course. However, following lymph node infiltration, the disease becomes more progressive, and death, usually due to infection, occurs within two years.

Malignant Lymphoma

Malignant lymphoma is a clonal neoplastic proliferation of lymphoid cells involving principally lymphoid organs rather than blood. Often, lymphoma begins in and involves lymph nodes predominantly, although other sites such as the spleen and the gastrointestinal tract are frequent areas of origin as well. As the disease progresses, proliferation spreads to lymphoid tissue beyond the site of origin. In advanced disease, infiltrations of neoplastic cells are found in many organs throughout the body and may eventually involve the blood.

NON-HODGKIN'S LYMPHOMAS

Classification. Following the introduction of the widely accepted Rappaport classification of NHL in 1966, a number of different classification schemes were proposed to better describe the diversity of NHL histology and to categorize immunologic subtypes. The subsequent simultaneous use of multiple classifications led to confusion among oncologists. To remedy this confusion, the United States National Cancer Institute initiated a multi-institutional study including a panel of expert hematopathologists to review over 1000 cases of NHLs. This study analyzed clinical outcome as well as histologic features and resulted in a scheme for translating between classifications known as the "Working Formulation of Non-Hodgkin's Lymphoma for Clinical Usage" (Non-Hodgkin's Lymphoma Pathologic Classification Project, 1982) (Table 27–15).

Since the publication of the Working Formulation, the importance of B-cell and T-cell derivation in the classification of lymphomas became universally recognized. Additionally, new entities have been identified. Because the Working Formulation is commonly used in the United States by most centers involved in clinical trials funded by the National Cancer Institute, it should be maintained for now as a basis for classification of NHLs. Recent comprehensive reviews of the classification of NHLs are available (Jaffe, 1995; Knowles, 1992). In addition, an excellent review of current concepts in this field and a new proposed comprehensive classification for the non-Hodgkin's and Hodgkin's lymphomas, as well as other lymphoproliferative disorders, has been offered (Harris, 1994) but has not been as yet widely accepted.

The Working Formulation stratifies histologic types of NHL into grades based on the clinical outcome of the 1175 patients who were studied. Among other findings, it demonstrated the significance of differentiating the follicular from the diffuse pattern of cases with similar cytology. Independent of cell type, the follicular pattern has a more favorable survival.

WORKING FORMULATION OF NON-HODGKIN'S LYMPHOMAS

Low-Grade Malignancy

Malignant Lymphoma, Small Lymphocytic (SL). (Plate 27–6*A* to *C*). In this condition, the cell type is the small lymphocyte, with clumped chromatin indistinguishable

Table 27–15. CLINICAL CHARACTERISTICS OF 1014 PATIENTS IN THE TEN SUBTYPES OF THE WORKING FORMULATION OF NON-HODGKIN'S LYMPHOMAS FOR CLINICAL USAGE*

Prognostic Group	Low Grade			Intermediate Grade				High Grade		
Subtype	SL	FSC	FM	FL	DSC	DM	DL	IBL	LBL	SNC
Percent	3.6	22.5	7.7	3.8	6.9	6.7	19.7	7.9	4.2	5.0
Age range (years)	26–79	3–87	26–99	16–82	10–91	22–90	10–88	10–81	11–90	3–90
Median age	60.5	54.3	56.1	55.4	57.9	58.0	56.8	51.3	16.9	29.8
Sex ratio (M:F)	1.2	1.3	0.8	1.8	2.0	1.1	1.0	1.5	1.9	2.6
Pathologic stage (%)										
I	3	8	15	15	9	19	16	23	7	13
II	8	10	12	12	19	26	30	29	20	21
III	8	16	28	15	12	13	10	16	2	9
IV	81	66	46	58	60	42	44	33	72	57
Bone marrow involved†	71	51	30	34	32	14	10	12	50	14
Survival										
Median (years)	5.8	7.2	5.1	3.0	3.4	2.7	1.5	1.3	2.0	0.7
5-year (%)	59.0	70.0	50.0	45.0	33.0	38.0	35.0	32.0	26.0	23.0
Complete remission (%)	61	73	65	61	56	69	59	53	69	48
Median time to relapse (years)	>5.4	5.0	5.2	>8.0	2.1	4.3	>8.4	3.5	1.1	>7.7

*Non-Hodgkin's lymphoma pathologic classification project. Writing Committee, National Cancer Institute-sponsored study of classifications of non-Hodgkin's lymphomas. Summary and description of a working formulation for clinical use. Cancer 1982; 49:2112.

†At initial evaluation.

from the normal lymphocyte. Mitoses are rarely seen. The pattern of node and marrow involvement is characteristically diffuse. Although it may begin in lymph nodes, the accumulative process involves the bone marrow early in its course, and the blood lymphocyte count is then elevated. The resulting diagnosis, therefore, is often chronic lymphocytic leukemia rather than lymphoma. It is essentially the same disease.

Plasmacytoid lymphocytes may be prominent in patients with gammopathies, although plasma cells may be numerous without evidence of a paraproteinemia.

Malignant Lymphoma, Follicular, Predominantly Small Cleaved Cell (FSC). (Plate 27–6*D* to *F*). There is predominantly a follicular pattern. The proliferating cell is a lymphocyte with a nucleus that has less condensation of chromatin than the normal circulating lymphocyte; an irregular, clefted or indented nuclear shape; and small, inconspicuous nucleoli. The cytoplasm is scant in amount.

Malignant Lymphoma, Follicular, Mixed Small Cleaved and Large Cell (FM). The pattern is follicular, and the lymphoma is composed of both large and small cleaved lymphocytes. Large noncleaved cells are also present and contain multiple prominent nucleoli.

Intermediate-Grade Malignancy

Malignant Lymphoma, Follicular, Predominantly Large Cell (FL). Large cleaved and noncleaved cells are observed in a follicular pattern. The large cleaved cells usually are more numerous. Many mitotic figures are present within the tumor.

Malignant Lymphoma, Diffuse Small Cleaved Cell (DSC). This tumor is composed of small lymphocytes with scanty cytoplasm. The nuclear membrane is irregular, angulated, and often cleaved. There is no evidence of a nodular pattern. A small number of large cleaved cells may be present. Diffuse mantle zone lymphoma (see Miscellaneous) may be included in this category.

Malignant Lymphoma, Diffuse, Mixed Small and Large Cell (DM). Some of these lymphomas represent the diffuse counterpart of follicular mixed lymphomas. However, some may be composed of lymphocytes containing irregular and lobated nuclei and represent a T-cell neoplasm.

Malignant Lymphoma, Diffuse, Large Cell (DL). (Plate 27–6*K* and *L*). The tumor is composed predominantly of large cleaved and noncleaved cells. The nucleus has reticular chromatin and usually a multiple nucleoli, some of which are attached to the nuclear membrane. The cytoplasm is moderately abundant. Small lymphocytes occasionally are present. There is no evidence of a follicular pattern.

High-Grade Malignancy

Malignant Lymphoma, Large Cell, Immunoblastic (IBL). This lymphoma is composed of large cells with oval vesicular nuclei and one or more prominent nucleoli. In the plasmacytoid subtype, the nuclei appear to be eccentrically placed with abundant cytoplasm suggesting plasmacytic differentiation. In the clear cell subtype, the nuclei are placed centrally and the cytoplasm has a clear appearance. The polymorphous subtype contains a mixture of small lymphocytes with twisted nuclei and larger lymphocytes with clear cytoplasm. Many cases of anaplastic large cell lymphoma may be placed in this category. These large cells may have hyperlobated nuclei simulating Reed-Sternberg cells. Immunoblastic lymphomas may be of T-cell or B-cell immunophenotype.

Malignant Lymphoma, Lymphoblastic (LBL). These tumors typically have a diffuse pattern. The neoplastic cells have fine chromatin and scanty cytoplasm. In approximately 50% of the cases, the nuclear contour is convoluted. In the remaining cases, the nuclei are round. Mitoses are numerous. On touch preparations, the cells simulate lymphoblasts of ALL. These tumors are usually of the T-cell type and are closely related to T-cell ALL, to which they often evolve.

Malignant Lymphoma, Small Noncleaved Cell (SNC). (Plate 27–6*G* and *H*). The cells are homogeneous with round to oval nuclei, approximately the size of a histiocyte nucleus; reticular chromatin; multiple small nucleoli; and slight to moderate amounts of amphophilic cytoplasm. The mitotic rate is high, and macrophages with abundant cytoplasm interspersed among the tumor cells give a starry sky histologic appearance. Touch preparations reveal cells similar to the morphology of L3 ALL. These are almost all of B-cell lineage.

Miscellaneous. This group includes composite lymphoma, mycosis fungoides, true histiocytic lymphoma, anaplastic large cell lymphoma, extramedullary plasmacytoma, mantle cell lymphoma, monocytoid B-cell lymphoma, low-grade lymphoma of mucosa-associated lymphoid tissue (MALT), mantle zone lymphoma, T-cell–rich B-cell lymphoma, angiotropic large cell lymphoma (Lukes, 1992) and otherwise unclassifiable lymphomas. The majority of these are discussed by Harris (1994).

A summary of the major clinical features of the subtypes of the working formulation of NHLs can be found in Table 27–15.

Immunologic Classification of Non-Hodgkin's Lymphomas. Using a variety of immunologic techniques, one can categorize a malignant lymphoid proliferation according to cells of origin and level of differentiation (Harris, 1994). It now appears that the lymphoproliferative disorders are neoplastic tumors that are blocked at certain stages of differentiation. Thus, most cases of ALL represent a proliferation of cells at the earliest stage of B-cell differentiation, whereas CLL and poorly differentiated lymphocytic lymphoma are blocked at the early to middle stages of differentiation. Multiple myeloma represents a B-cell neoplasm that can fully differentiate. The majority of low-grade and intermediate-grade lymphomas, as well as small non-cleaved cell lymphoma, are of B-cell derivation. Most lymphoblastic lymphomas are of the T-cell precursor phenotype. Diffuse mixed, diffuse large cell and immunoblastic lymphomas are a mixture of B-cell and peripheral T-cell types.

HODGKIN'S DISEASE. The current classification of Hodgkin's disease is that of the Rye conference (Lukes, 1966). Hodgkin's disease is generally regarded as a malignant lymphoma, but has a different histologic appearance in that the cells reacting to the neoplasm usually predominate rather than the neoplastic cells themselves. The hallmark of Hodgkin's disease is the Reed-Sternberg (RS) cell (Plate 27–7*F*), which is a large binucleated or multinucleated cell, with each nucleus bearing a very large nucleolus.

Hodgkin's disease may occur at any time from early childhood to old age. Increased frequency is noted between 15 and 35 years of age and after age 50. Males predominate, especially in childhood; disease in females under age 30 usually is of the nodular sclerosis type.

Classification. Diagnosis is made histologically, usually from a lymph node biopsy (Table 27–16).

The *lymphocytic predominance* group shows numerous lymphocytes with a variable degree of histiocytic proliferation without necrosis or fibrosis and few Reed-Sternberg cells (Plate 27–7*A*). Moderately large cells with convoluted nuclei and moderately prominent nucleoli, so-called lymphocytic/histiocytic (L/H), are present in variable numbers. Prognosis is best in this group, which tends to be localized to the cervical nodes and occurs most frequently in young males.

Nodular sclerosis is characterized by broad bands of collagen extending from the capsule and separating nodules of lymphoid tissue and the presence of lacunar cells, which are large atypical histiocyte-like cells with abundant pale cytoplasm. Classic Reed-Sternberg cells may be difficult to find, but multinucleated variants usually are readily found (Plate 27–7*B* and *C*). This variety of Hodgkin's disease is common and often is first discovered as a mediastinal mass in a young woman.

The *mixed cellularity type* contains a diffuse infiltrate of a variety of cell types: lymphocytes, plasma cells, eosinophils, histiocytes, and Reed-Sternberg cells, which are often numerous. Mummified cells (densely staining pyknotic RS cells) usually are present. Necrosis and disorderly fibrosis may be present (Plate 27–7*D*).

The rare *lymphocyte depletion* type (Plate 27–7*E*) contains numerous RS cells and variants with a paucity of background lymphocytes. It may be confused with immunoblastic NHL, undifferentiated carcinoma, or melanoma. It frequently contains variable amounts of diffuse fibrosis. It is sometimes associated with an acute febrile illness accompanied by pancytopenia and lymphocytopenia. There may be a paucity of peripheral lymphadenopathy, although some patients have a generalized enlargement of lymph nodes. The lack of leukocytosis and thrombocytosis and more frequent involvement of the bone marrow contrast with other forms of Hodgkin's disease (Neiman, 1973).

The identification of the lineage of Reed-Sternberg cells has been a difficult and often controversial subject. The concept that Hodgkin's disease is a heterogeneous entity has emerged (Haluska, 1994). There is now evidence that the Reed-Sternberg cell is an activated lymphocyte (either T cell or B cell). In most cases of Hodgkin's disease (excluding lymphocyte predominance), Reed-Sternberg cells exhibit CD15 and CD30 antigens but not CD45 (leukocyte common antigen—LCA) or T-cell or B-cell antigens (Harris, 1994). However, in the nodular subtype of lymphocyte predominance, the neoplastic cells appear to be of B-cell lineage (Pinkus, 1985).

Blood. Normocytic, sometimes severe, anemia is seen in about 50% of cases.

The leukocyte count may be elevated, normal, or reduced. The differential count shows neutrophilia, lymphocytopenia, monocytosis, and eosinophilia. Either all or any combination of these may be present.

Neutrophilic leukocytosis is seen, especially when lymph nodes are involved; and neutropenia is seen when bone marrow is involved. The blood changes seem to depend on the stage of the disease and on some poorly understood mechanisms. The NAP is elevated during activity of the disease; it returns to normal during remissions.

Table 27–16. HISTOLOGIC CLASSIFICATION OF HODGKIN'S DISEASE

Subtype	Major Morphologic Alteration	Percentage of Cases
Lymphocyte predominance	Usually diffuse, sometimes vaguely nodular pattern, abundant lymphocytes, few Reed-Sternberg cells, no fibrosis	7
Nodular sclerosis	Nodular pattern formed by birefringent collagen bands; moderate number of lymphocytes, eosinophils, plasma cells; lacunar variant of Reed-Sternberg cells	68
Mixed cellularity	Diffuse involvement; numerous Reed-Sternberg cells; moderate number of lymphocytes, eosinophils, plasma cells	23
Lymphocyte depletion	Diffuse involvement; decreased cellularity; occasionally numerous, bizarre-shaped Reed-Sternberg cells	2

The most frequent finding is a moderate leukocytosis, with WBCs ranging from 12 to 25 $\times$ 10^9/L and a relative and even absolute lymphopenia. A slight shift to the left may be present in the neutrophils. As a rule, lymphopenia is prognostically a poor omen.

Monocytosis is frequent. Eosinophilia has been described in about 20% of patients and may be extreme. The platelet count may be increased, normal, or decreased, the latter especially with marrow involvement.

Both the histologic changes noted and the blood and marrow findings appear to be manifestations of different host responses to the disease.

Marrow. The incidence of bone marrow involvement in untreated cases of Hodgkin's disease is approximately 10% (Bartl, 1982b). Positive bone marrow biopsies vary with stage of disease (Stage I, 1%; II, 2%; III, 25%; and IV, 45%) and with histologic pattern (lymphocyte predominance, 8%; nodular sclerosis, 4%; mixed cellularity, 9%; lymphocyte depletion, 22%).

In 80% of uninvolved bone marrow biopsy specimens, there are a variety of nonspecific reactions. Frequently, there is granulocytic hyperplasia, slight monocytosis, and eosinophilia. In some cases, there is marrow hypoplasia, and in others, there are epithelial cell granulomas and lymphoid nodules. The latter features often are associated with a favorable prognosis (Bartl, 1982b).

Clinical Staging. Clinical staging presently is employed to determine the extent of the disease at the time of diagnosis. Besides history and physical examination, extensive radiographic studies, radioisotope scans, CBC, platelet count, bone marrow biopsy, liver function studies, urinalysis, and skin tests for delayed hypersensitivity are performed. *Stage I disease* is limited to lymph nodes in one anatomic region or two contiguous regions on one side of the diaphragm. *Stage II disease* involves more than two contiguous regions or two noncontiguous regions on one side of the diaphragm. *Stage III disease* is present on both sides of the diaphragm but is confined to lymphoid tissue. *Stage IV disease* involves bone marrow or any other organ, in addition to lymphoid tissue. All stages are additionally classified as A if systemic symptoms are absent and B if they are present. This extensive diagnostic approach is to define areas of involvement and facilitate radiation therapy, which is combined with chemotherapy. It is part of the current aggressive approach to the management of Hodgkin's disease, which is resulting in longer survival and apparent cure in many patients.

Immunologic studies in Hodgkin's disease have shown that cell-mediated immunity is defective when extensive disease is present.

Plasma Cell Dyscrasias and Lymphoreticular Malignancies Associated with Abnormal Immunoglobulin Synthesis

Polyclonal gammopathy refers to an increase in the serum of several different immunoglobulins that are the products of many different clones of plasma cells. This is usually a response to antigenic stimulation.

Monoclonal gammopathy refers to an increase in the serum of one specific class, subclass, and type of immunoglobulin molecule (or fragment thereof); this is the product of plasma cells or lymphocytes that originated from a single cell or clone. Monoclonal gammopathy is found in multiple myeloma, some lymphomas (including Waldenström's macroglobulinemia and heavy chain diseases), some patients with primary amyloidosis, a few patients with carcinoma, and some individuals with no known underlying disease *(benign monoclonal gammopathy).* The last group may constitute up to one third of all monoclonal gammopathies; it includes primarily elderly individuals who have a lower concentration of the homogeneous immunoglobulin (less than 2 g/dL) that does not change for long periods of time.

Multiple Myeloma

Multiple myeloma is a neoplastic proliferation of plasma cells or morphologically abnormal plasma cells (myeloma cells), primarily occurring in the bone marrow either in nodules or diffusely. Although plasma cells also proliferate in lymph nodes and spleen, these organs are rarely enlarged.

CLINICAL FEATURES. Multiple myeloma is rare in patients younger than age 40. The mean age at the time of diagnosis is 62 years. The incidence of this disease is equal in men and women. Bone pain is the most common symptom, and pathologic fractures are frequent. Neurologic symptoms may be prominent from encroachment of tumor that has broken through the bony cortex on spinal nerves or spinal cord. Bone destruction leads to calcium mobilization, with an increase of calcium in the serum and metastatic calcification. The growth of myeloma cells in the marrow produces multiple tumors, which appear on x-ray study as multiple punched-out osteoporotic lesions; occasionally, the growth is diffuse and appears as diffuse osteoporosis. An unusual propensity to infection is common because of impaired production of antibodies.

Blood. There usually is a normochromic normocytic anemia; normoblasts may be present in the blood. The leukocyte count is slightly decreased, normal, or slightly increased. Occasionally, young neutrophils or even myeloblasts may be found. The platelet count usually is normal but may be decreased. The most striking feature of the blood film is the marked degree of rouleau formation, which may make cell counting difficult.

Marrow. The bone marrow shows the presence of plasma cells or myeloma cells, varying from less than 1% to over 90%, depending on the degree of involvement in the site of the marrow aspirated. A diagnosis usually relies on the presence of at least 10% of the bone marrow nucleated cells being plasma cells. Cytologically, the cells may be indistinguishable from normal plasma cells (Plate 27–7*J*), but they usually show abnormal chromatin, such as less clumping of nuclear chromatin, large nucleoli, lack of perinuclear clear zone, lighter blue cytoplasm, or varying degrees of anaplasia (Plate 27–7*K* and *L*). The dissociation of nuclear and cytoplasmic maturation is a distinctive feature of the myeloma cells. Plasma cell maturity and extent of infiltration of plasma cells into the biopsy specimen correlate significantly with patient survival (Bartl, 1982c). Patients with mostly immature plasma cells and heavy infiltration of the marrow have a poor prognosis, whereas those with mature plasma cells and patchy infiltrates have better survival.

Immunoglobulins. Serum globulin usually is increased, often strikingly so. This increase is responsible for the tendency toward rouleau formation and an elevated ESR. Serum protein electrophoresis usually shows an M-spot, a homogeneous band in the γ- or β-region; less commonly, there is hypogammaglobulinemia (when only light chains are produced by the neoplastic plasma cells). Immunoelectrophoresis indicates that the monoclonal protein is IgG in over half the cases of multiple myeloma, IgA in about one fifth, IgD in less than 1 percent, and IgE very rarely. In each of these groups of myeloma, some patients secrete light chains (kappa or lambda) in addition to the whole immunoglobulin molecule. In about one quarter of patients with multiple myeloma, only light chains (Bence Jones protein) are produced by the abnormal plasma cells. Hypogammaglobulinemia is found in the latter group because light chains are filtered through the renal glomerulus, leaving little or none in the serum, in addition to the fact that immunoglobulin production by the nonmalignant plasma cells is greatly reduced in all patients with multiple myeloma.

Roughly 5% of myeloma proteins are cryoglobulins—that is, proteins that precipitate from cooled serum and redissolve on warming.

Proteinuria is frequently present in multiple myeloma. In somewhat over 50% of patients, light chains of immunoglobulin are detected by electrophoresis of a concentrate of urine on which they migrate as a narrow band in the γ-globulin region. If renal damage has occurred, albumin and whole immunoglobulin molecules are also found in the urine. Excretion of light chains of immunoglobulin sometimes results in obstruction and loss of nephrons, and the so-called myeloma kidney. Renal insufficiency is common and is the presenting feature of multiple myeloma in some cases.

Amyloidosis, which is present in about 10% to 15% of cases of multiple myeloma, may be a factor in the renal failure. Amyloid fibrils in cases of myeloma appear to have as their major protein component the light chains of immunoglobulin molecules.

The diagnosis of multiple myeloma is secure if the marrow contains large numbers of morphologically bizarre, malignant-appearing plasma cells. If large numbers of normal-appearing plasma cells and plasma-cell precursors are present in the marrow, the diagnosis is not established unless punched-out, lytic bone lesions are demonstrated on x-ray study, or light chain proteinuria or a monoclonal gammopathy is also present. Clonality can be confirmed by immunohistochemical demonstration of a monoclonal cytoplasmic immunoglobulin.

The prognostic importance of several different laboratory measurements and clinical features has been demonstrated. These clinicopathologic features have been correlated with the total body tumor cell mass and used as a basis for a clinical staging system (Table 27–17) (Durie, 1975). Serum levels of β_2-microglobulin also correlate with stage of disease and survival at diagnosis (Bataille, 1984). Measurements of serum β_2-microglobulin can be very useful in evaluating response to treatment, particularly in patients with light chain disease.

Median length of survival after diagnosis is approximately three years. In almost 5% of patients, acute leukemia develops (usually myelomonocytic). This may be preceded by sideroblastic anemia.

Table 27–17. MYELOMA CLINICAL STAGING SYSTEM

			Median Survival
Stage I		Low myeloma cell mass ($<0.6 \times 10^{12}$ cells/M^2)	
	Criteria:	All of the following	
		Hb $>$ 100 g/L	
		Serum calcium $<$3.0 mmol/L	
		X-ray: normal bone structure or one lesion only	
		M-component production rates	64 mo
		IgG value $<$50 g/L	
		IgA value $<$30 g/L	
		Urine light chain excretion $<$4 g/24 h	
Stage II		Intermediate myeloma cell mass ($0.6–1.2 \times 10^{12}$ cells/M^2)	
	Criteria:	Fitting neither Stage I nor Stage III	32 mo
Stage III		High myeloma cell mass ($>1.2 \times 10^{12}$ cells/M^2)	
	Criteria:	Any of the following	
		Hb $<$ 85 g/L	
		Serum calcium $>$3.0 mmol/L	
		Advanced lytic bone lesions	
		M-component production rates	6 mo
		IgG value $>$70 g/L	
		IgA value $>$50 g/L	
		Urine light chain excretion $>$12 g/24 h	
Subclassification			
	A = Serum creatinine value $<$20 mg/L		
	B = Serum creatinine value $>$20 mg/L		

From Durie BG, Salmon SE: Cancer 1975; 36:842.

Plasma Cell Leukemia

Often in multiple myeloma, a few plasma cells are found in the peripheral blood. Only in the rare instances of myeloma in which large numbers of plasma cells circulate (either $>$20% of blood leukocytes or $> 2 \times 10^9$/L) is the term plasma cell leukemia used (Woodruff, 1978). Patients with plasma cell leukemia tend to have tissue infiltration, advanced stage disease, and poor survival.

Waldenström's Macroglobulinemia

Macroglobulins (IgM immunoglobulins) constitute 3% to 10% of serum proteins. They have a high molecular weight (10^6 daltons), a sedimentation constant of 18 to 20 Svedberg units, and a high carbohydrate content and are characterized by a heavy chain and either kappa or lambda light chains. Increases of serum macroglobulins that are polyclonal may be seen in chronic infections or in collagen diseases. Monoclonal macroglobulinemia is found in a few individuals without detectable disease, in some patients with malignant lymphoma, and in patients with chronic lymphocytic leukemia. It appears that Waldenström's macroglobulinemia is a variant of well-differentiated lymphocytic lymphoma or CLL in which there is a greater degree of maturation of the B lymphocytes into plasma cells.

CLINICAL FEATURES. Waldenström's macroglobulinemia is found in individuals older than age 40, with a peak incidence between ages 60 and 70. It is characterized by a general proliferation of lymphocytes (and plasma cells) and the presence of at least 1 g/dL of monoclonal IgM in the serum, amounting to at least 15% of the total serum protein.

The clinical features of the disease are effects of the increased levels of serum macroglobulins, which commonly cause symptoms due to increased viscosity; and the cell proliferation itself, which accounts for hepatosplenomegaly and some degree of lymphadenopathy. In contrast to multiple myeloma, bone pain and osteolytic lesions on x-ray study are rare. Hyperviscosity and sludging of blood may lead to visual disturbances, neurologic symptoms, impaired kidney function, and right-sided congestive heart failure. Hemorrhagic phenomena may be caused by the macroglobulins adhering to platelets, which interferes with their function, and forming complexes with plasma-clotting factors, which impairs their activity. Cryoglobulinemia occurs somewhat more frequently than with myeloma and may be responsible for sensitivity to cold and Raynaud's phenomenon.

BLOOD. Normochromic, normocytic anemia is sometimes associated with thrombocytopenia or pancytopenia. Relative or slight absolute lymphocytosis usually is found. Marked rouleau formation is present on the blood film, and the sedimentation rate usually is extremely rapid, although it may be low if macrocryoglobulins are present and the test is carried out at a lower temperature. The anemia is occasionally hemolytic, with a positive Coombs' test.

MARROW. Often, the marrow cannot be aspirated readily. Lymphoid cells are increased in number. These usually resemble normal small lymphocytes, but sometimes plasmacytoid cells are present and plasma cells may be increased in number. PAS-positive inclusions often are seen in the cytoplasm and nucleus of the lymphoid cells. Tissue mast cells are increased in number.

IMMUNOGLOBULINS. Serum globulin usually is markedly increased.

The *relative serum viscosity* may be simply measured using an Ostwald viscometer. The average time for descent of the serum at room temperature is expressed as a ratio to that of distilled water. The normal range is 1.4 to 1.8. It is considerably elevated in most patients with macroglobulinemia. Symptoms of hyperviscosity appear in most patients when the relative serum viscosity is between 6 and 8, although the threshold varies among patients.

The identification of the paraprotein is achieved by *immunoelectrophoresis.* Together with the μ heavy chains, only one type of light chain is found. The total monoclonal IgM often exceeds 10 mg/mL (1 g/dL).

Light chain proteinuria occurs in about 10% of patients.

Heavy Chain Disease

A small number of patients produce and excrete heavy chain fragments without associated light chains. Some of these proteins show structural mutations.

GAMMA HEAVY CHAIN DISEASE. Gamma heavy chain disease (γ-HCD) clinically resembles malignant lymphoma rather than myeloma, with lymphadenopathy, hepatosplenomegaly, fever, and propensity to infections. Anemia is constantly present, often with leukopenia and thrombocytopenia. Atypical lymphocytes or plasma cells are frequently present in the blood, and a few cases have terminated in plasma cell leukemia. The marrow usually is abnormal, with increased plasma cells and lymphocytes and eosinophils, but is not diagnostic. Usually, but not always, the histologic appearance of lymphoid tissue indicates a malignant lymphoproliferative disease. A rather broad serum protein spike has been found in the β-γ region in most patients, accompanied by hypogammaglobulinemia. The diagnosis is made by showing that the protein reacts on immunoelectrophoresis with antisera to γ-chains but not to light chains. The protein is also found in the urine in varying amounts, although concentration techniques may be necessary to demonstrate it.

ALPHA HEAVY CHAIN DISEASE. Alpha heavy chain disease (α-HCD) appears to be more common than γ-HCD, and involves a younger age group. The uniform clinical pattern in most patients is malabsorption and diarrhea accompanying a massive lymphoplasmacytic infiltration of intestinal mucosa, or a histiocytic lymphoma of the intestine. In a few patients, the respiratory tract has been involved instead. Bone marrow and other lymphoid organs have not been involved. Usually, routine protein electrophoresis is negative, but small amounts of α-chain may be detected in the serum and sometimes in the urine with immunoelectrophoresis. The abnormal protein does not contain light chains.

MU HEAVY CHAIN DISEASE. The few patients who have been described as having mu heavy chain disease (μ-HCD) have had chronic lymphocytic leukemia with vacuolated plasma cells in the marrow. Routine serum electrophoresis showed only hypogammaglobulinemia. The mu heavy chain was detected by serum immunoelectrophoresis; it was not found in the urine. In most patients, however, the urine contained light chains in large amounts (Franklin, 1975).

Laboratory Assays Useful in the Diagnosis of Hematologic Malignancies

4

The diagnosis and classification of many hematologic malignancies have been considerably advanced by the application of cytochemical, immunocytochemical, cytogenetic, and DNA analytical techniques. The use of cytochemical and immunocytochemical procedures has aided in identifying the lineage and stage of maturation of both normal and neoplastic hemic cells. The employment of cytogenetic and DNA analytical techniques has greatly facilitated the recognition of certain chromosomal and genetic abnormalities in specific hematologic malignancies and has provided a new insight into the etiology and pathogenesis of these disorders.

Cytochemical Assays

It is often difficult to differentiate the leukemic blasts of acute lymphoblastic leukemia from those of AML (particularly acute myeloblastic leukemia without maturation, M1; acute monoblastic leukemia, M5A; and acute megakaryoblastic leukemia, M7) using Romanowsky-stained films alone. Several cytochemical staining procedures are helpful in making this distinction. When the results of appropriate cytochemical reactions are used together with the morphologic appearance of Wright-Giemsa–stained films, a precise diagnosis can be made in most cases. The following cytochemical reactions have proved helpful in the diagnosis and classification of several hematologic malignancies.

SUDAN BLACK B STAIN AND PEROXIDASE (MYELOPEROXIDASE). Sudan black B stains phospholipids and sterols. It appears to stain both azurophilic and specific granules in neutrophils, whereas the peroxidase is found only in azurophilic granules (Sheehan, 1947). Cytoplasmic granules stain faintly in neutrophil precursors and strongly in mature neutrophils with Sudan black B. Eosinophilic granules are also positive but often show a central pallor. Monocytes may be unstained or may contain a few positive granules. Lymphocytes and lymphoblasts are negative, but at least some myeloblasts contain Sudan black–positive granules (see Plate 27–4*B* and *E*).

The peroxidase reaction is based on the principle that in the presence of hydrogen peroxide, myeloperoxidase in leukocyte granules oxidizes benzidine dihydrochloride from a colorless form to a blue or brown derivative that is localized at the site of the enzyme (Kaplow, 1965, 1975). Myeloperoxidase activity is present at all stages of neutrophil development and is localized in the azurophilic (nonspecific) granules. Eosinophils show an intense reaction. Lymphocytes, mature basophils, and erythroid forms do not stain. Monocytes stain less intensely than do neutrophils, and the granular precipitates are smaller. Using 3,3′-diaminobenzidine-HCl (DAB) as a substrate for the peroxidase reaction instead of benzidine-HCl results in a greater proportion of positive blast cells in AML (Cardullo, 1981). DAB demonstrates catalase as well as myeloperoxidase, and the cytochemical reaction has been called hydroperoxidase.

The Sudan black B and the peroxidase reactions show roughly similar patterns in the various cell types (see Table 27–6) (Hayhoe, 1984). The Sudan black B and the hydroperoxidase reactions are somewhat more sensitive than the myeloperoxidase reaction in our experience. These techniques are most useful in distinguishing subtypes of AML from acute lymphoblastic leukemia.

Peroxidase activity may be absent in some toxic neutrophils from patients with infection, AML, and the rare congenital myeloperoxidase deficiency.

ESTERASES. The leukocyte esterases hydrolyze an ester that is a derivative of naphthalene (Li, 1973; Yam, 1971b). A naphthol (or naphthyl) compound is liberated and rapidly couples with a diazonium salt present in the mixture, resulting in a brightly colored precipitate at or near the site of the enzyme activity.

The cytochemical reactions for esterases are positive in many cell types. The chloroacetate esterase reaction, using naphthol ASD chloroacetate as a substrate, is positive in neutrophils and precursors and weak or negative in monocytes and precursors and in other blood cells (see Plate 27–4*C*). The reactions of chloroacetate esterase are similar to those of Sudan black B and peroxidase in the acute leukemias, but they are more specific for the neutrophil series. Whereas chloroacetate esterase is more consistently negative in monocytes than Sudan black B or peroxidase, it is also less sensitive than the latter two staining reactions in the cells of the granulocytic series.

The nonspecific esterases, using α-naphthyl acetate or α-naphthyl butyrate as substrates, are strongly positive in monocytes but weak or negative in granulocytes (see Plate 27–4*F* and *L*). Megakaryocytes are positive for α-naphthyl acetate esterase but negative for α-naphthyl butyrate esterase. Macrophages are positive for both. α-Naphthyl acetate esterase also is positive in basophils and plasma cells, focally positive in resting T lymphocytes, and weakly positive in the normoblasts of some normal individuals. Sodium fluoride inhibits the reaction in monocytes, megakaryocytes, platelets, and plasma cells but not that in neutrophils or lymphocytes (Li, 1973). When the reaction is performed at a pH of 8, α-naphthyl butyrate esterase can be used to differentiate subpopulations of T lymphocytes, B lymphocytes, null cells, and monocytes.

α-Naphthyl acetate esterase and α-naphthyl butyrate esterase are useful in distinguishing neutrophil precursors from monocytes and precursors in the acute leukemias (see Table 27–6). The α-naphthyl acetate esterase reaction is focally positive in the blasts of a small proportion of patients with acute lymphoblastic leukemia. In some cases, this focal activity is associated with neoplastic T lymphocytes. In addition, a positive reaction may be also observed in the leukemic cells of megakaryocytic, eosinophilic, and basophilic leukemias, and in the erythroblasts of erythroleukemia.

PERIODIC ACID–SCHIFF (PAS) REACTION. The PAS reaction is based on the principle that periodic acid (HIO_4) is an oxidizing agent that converts hydroxy groups on adjacent carbon atoms to aldehydes. The resulting dialdehydes are combined with Schiff's reagent to give a red-colored product. A positive reaction therefore is seen with polysaccharides, mucopolysaccharides, and glycoproteins.

In blood cells, a positive PAS reaction usually indicates the presence of glycogen. This is demonstrated by digestion with amylase and consequent loss of staining. Neutrophils react at all stages of development, most strongly in the mature stage. The same is true of eosinophils. The glycogen is not in the granules, but in background cytoplasm. Myeloblasts contain a few small PAS positive granules. Monocytes have a faint staining reaction in the form of fine granules. Lymphocytes may contain a few small or large granules. Normoblasts are normally PAS negative.

In erythroleukemia (see Plate 27–4*K*) and in thalassemia, some of the erythroid precursors are PAS positive. This is true to a lesser extent in iron deficiency anemia and sideroblastic anemias. In acute lymphoblastic leukemia, the lymphoblasts often contain large, coarse clumps of PAS positive material (see Plate 27–4*H*). In chronic lymphocytic leukemia and NHLs as well as in infectious mononucleosis, the lymphocytes may have increased numbers of PAS-positive granules.

ACID PHOSPHATASE. Acid phosphatase in the cells hydrolyzes the substrate, naphthol AS-BI phosphoric acid (Katayama, 1977). The naphthol released is insoluble and couples with so-called hexazotized pararosaniline. The colored precipitate in the cytoplasm of the cells indicates acid phosphatase activity. If L(+) tartaric acid is in the solution, it inhibits the isoenzymes of acid phosphatase that are present in most cells but not those of the cells of HCL.

Red granules in the cytoplasm indicate acid phosphatase activity. The reaction is positive to varying degrees in most normal (and abnormal) leukocytes. Monocytes stain more intensely than neutrophils and precursors. Lymphocytes normally contain little activity; T cells appear to react positively; B cells usually are negative.

The acid phosphatase reaction is useful in two areas. First, one of the elements in confirming a diagnosis of *HCL* (see earlier discussion) is the presence of tartrate-resistant acid phosphatase in the abnormal cells. It must be realized, however, that a small fraction of cases of HCL do not show this reaction (Katayama, 1977). Second, in the subclassification of *acute lymphoblastic leukemia,* definite focal positivity for acid phosphatase in the blasts is evidence in favor of T-cell origin. A diffusely positive reaction product is not specific for T lymphocytes.

NEUTROPHIL ALKALINE PHOSPHATASE. The enzyme is located in neutrophils from the metamyelocyte to the segmented stage, probably in a tertiary granular fraction. It can be detected by exposure to the substrate (a naphthol phosphate) in the presence of a diazonium salt (fast blue or fast violet) at an alkaline pH 9.5 (Kaplow, 1963). The substrate is hydrolyzed by the enzyme, releasing a phosphate and an arylnaphtholamide. The arylnaphtholamide is immediately coupled to the diazonium salt, forming an azo dye. After counterstaining, 100 mature neutrophils are scored (0 to 4) according to the intensity of the staining reaction, from negative to the most intense. Adding the scores for the 100 neutrophils gives a total score with a possible range of 0 to 400. Reference values must be determined for each laboratory and usually are about 20 to 100.

Increased activity occurs in infections, PCV, Hodgkin's disease, and in some cases of myelofibrosis with myeloid metaplasia. Decreased activity is found in CML, AMLs, paroxysmal nocturnal hemoglobinuria, aplastic anemia, hereditary hypophosphatasia, and some viral infections, especially infectious mononucleosis.

Immunologic Assays

Leukocyte antigen-specific monoclonal antibodies applied in either immunofluorescence or immunoenzymatic assays are powerful tools for the identification of lineage and stage of maturation of both lymphoid and myeloid cells. As a result, these methods have been widely employed in the diagnosis and classification of hematologic malignancies. It generally is recognized that the immunofluorescence flow cytometric procedure is more sensitive and more reliable in labeling weak surface antigens than immunocytochemical methods (Sobol, 1988). However, the latter techniques allow for a more detailed cytologic examination of the neoplastic cells as well as identification of cytoplasmic constituents. Furthermore, immunocytochemical assays do not require specialized equipment and can be performed in routine hematology laboratories (Kurec, 1988).

IMMUNOFLUORESCENCE ASSAYS. Lineage-specific, fluorescence-conjugated monoclonal antibodies against various determinants on lymphoid or myeloid cells are incubated with mononuclear cell suspensions. In cases of leukemia, immunophenotyping studies are best performed on specimens from bone marrow, where there is usually a higher percentage of blast cells. In lymphoma, portions of lymph nodes need to be teased into a cellular suspension for immunophenotypic evaluation. Following incubation, the labeled cells are enumerated by flow cytometry. Cell preparations may be stained with two or more fluorochromes. For example, one monoclonal antibody is conjugated with fluorescein isothiocyanate and a second monoclonal antibody with phycoerythrin. This procedure permits the identification of antigens on one or two cell populations (Keren, 1989).

IMMUNOENZYMATIC CYTOCHEMICAL METHODS. A variety of enzymatic immunocytochemical assays may be used. For example, in the alkaline phosphatase antialkaline phosphatase method, a primary mouse monoclonal antibody is used to identify cellular or membranous antigens. A rabbit antimouse immunoglobulin acts as an antibody bridge connecting the primary mouse monoclonal antibody with the alkaline phosphatase antialkaline phosphatase complexes (mouse monoclonal antialkaline phosphatase bound to calf intestinal alkaline phosphatase). The alkaline phosphatase with the complexes hydrolyses the substrate naphthol AS-BI phosphate or naphthol AS-MX phosphate, to phosphate and arylnaphtholamide, which is coupled to the diazonium dye fast red, forming an insoluble precipitate (Kurec, 1988). Endogenous alkaline phosphatase is blocked by the use of levamisole. A bright red precipitate forms at the antigen-antibody sites. Membrane antigens exhibit a linear stain, and cytoplasmic antigens demonstrate a focal or diffuse cellular stain (Cordell, 1984). Other similar methods use the binding of the small molecule biotin to avidin or streptavidin. Biotin-labeled secondary antibodies bind avidin or streptavidin conjugated with alkaline phosphatase or horseradish peroxidase to hydrolyze a substrate and develop the color reaction. A variety of substrates can be used to produce red, brown, blue or other colors. Biotin can also be used to label nucleic acid probes for *in situ* hybridization. Immunocytochemical techniques are now partially automated in many large laboratories using a variety of commercial equipment, and reliable commercial kits are available for small laboratories.

A partial list of monoclonal antibodies that have proved useful in the diagnosis and classification of hematologic malignancies is presented in Table 27–18.

Chromosomal Abnormalities

Chromosomal analyses are useful in the diagnosis and classification of hematologic malignancies (Yunis, 1986). In many of the MDS, leukemias, and NHLs, a specific chromosomal alteration is present. The most common types of cytogenetic abnormalities are balanced translocations, chromosomal deletions, and cytogenetic manifestations of gene amplification (extrachromosomal double minute chromatin bodies and chromosomally integrated, homogeneously stained regions) (Brodeur, 1986). Associated with these structural alterations is the activation of oncogenes either as a result of translocation of proto-oncogenes to more active chromosomal sites or owing to a loss of suppressor, regulator, or differentiation genes (Brodeur, 1986). A listing of the most common chromosomal abnormalities associated with hematologic malignancies is provided in Table 27–19.

DNA Analytical Assays

The diagnosis and classification of many hematologic malignancies can be made at the molecular level. In these situations, DNA from neoplastic cells is incubated with restriction endonucleases that recognize certain nucleotide sequences and cleave DNA at specific sites. The resultant DNA fragments are separated by electrophoresis on agarose gels and are identified after transfer to nitrocellulose paper after hybridization with a radioactive DNA probe (Southern, 1975).

With this technique, malignancies of B cells and T cells can be determined. Genes for the light and heavy chains of immunoglobulin and the genes for the $\alpha\beta\gamma\delta$-chains of the T-cell receptor are rearranged from the germ line to an active configuration during the differentiation of uncommitted lymphoid cells to committed B or T cells. When a monoclonal population of lymphoid cells is present, digested fragments of DNA of uniform size that hybridize with radiolabeled or enzyme-labeled probes are identified as discrete bands on electrophoretic gels. Clonal rearrangement of immunoglobulin genes (particularly light chain genes) is strong evidence in support of a B-cell malignancy (Pugh, 1988). Likewise, the recognition of T-cell receptor gene (particu-

Table 27–18. MONOCLONAL ANTIBODIES USEFUL FOR IMMUNOPHENOTYPING LYMPHOID AND MYELOID NEOPLASTIC DISORDERS

Antibody	CD No.	Antigen Expression on Normal Cells	Source of Antibody*
OKT6	1a	Thymocytes	1
T-11	2	Pan-T cells	2
Leu-4	3	Pan-T cells	3
Leu-3	4	T helper/inducer	3
Leu-1	5	Pan-T cells, subsets of B cells	3
Leu-9	7	Pan-T cells	3
Leu-2	8	T cytotoxic/suppressor	3
J5	10	Pre-B cells (common ALL† antigen)	2
OKM1	11b	Granulocytes, monocytes, natural killer cells	1
p 159/95	11c	Monocytes/histiocytes	4
My7	13	Granulocytes/monocytes	2
My4	14	Monocytes/granulocytes	2
Leu M1	15	Granulocytes, Reed-Sternberg cells	3
Leu 11c	16	Natural killer cells, granulocytes, macrophages	3
B4	19	Pan-B cells	2
B1	20	Pan-B cells	2
B2	21	B cell subset	2
Leu-14	22	Pan-B cells	3
B6	23	B cell subset	2
BA-1	24	B cells; granulocytes	5
ACT-1	25	Activated T-cells, activated B-cells, activated macrophages	4
Ber-H2	30	Activated T-cells, activated B-cells, Reed-Sternberg cells	4
My9	33	Granulocytes/monocytes	2
DAKO-MPO	—	Myeloperoxidase	4
Platelet glycoprotein IIb/IIIa	42a	Platelets	4
Leukocyte (ZD1)	45	Leukocytes	3
Y1/82A	68	Monocytes/macrophages	4
Ret-40	—	Glycophorin A; erythroid precursor cells and red blood cells	4
Y2/51	61	Platelet glycoprotein IIIa; megakaryocytes and platelets	4
C17	41	Platelet glycoprotein IIb/IIIa; megakaryocytes and platelets	4
HLA-DR	—	HLA-DR major histocompatibility antigen, B cells, stem cells, activated T cells	3

*1 = Ortho Diagnostics; 2 = Coulter Immunology; 3 = Becton Dickinson; 4 = DAKO Corporation; 5 = Boehringer Mannheim Biochemical.
†ALL = acute lymphoblastic leukemia.

Table 27–19. CHROMOSOMAL ABNORMALITIES ASSOCIATED WITH HEMATOLOGIC MALIGNANCIES

Type of Malignancy	Chromosomal Abnormality	Involved Genes	Approximated Frequency (%)
AML (M2)	t(8;21) (q22;q22)	AML-1	20
AML (M3)	t(15;17) (q22;q21)	Retinoic acid receptor gene	100
AML (M4E)	inv(16) (p13;q22)	Not known	20
CML	t(9;22) (q34;q11)	c-ABL1	100
ALL (L3) and Burkitt's lymphoma	t(8;14) (q24;q32)	c-MYC	100
	t(2;8) (p13;q24)	Ig heavy chain	
	t(8;22) (q24;q11)	Kappa light chain	
		Lambda light chain	
Follicular lymphoma	t(14;18) (q32;q21)	BCL-2	85
T-cell neoplasms	t(8;14) (q24;q11)	c-MYC (8q24)	
		T-cell receptor α-chain	
	t(7;14) (q35;q11)	TCL-1	
		T-cell receptor β-chain	
	T(11;14) (p13;q11)	TCL-2	
		T-cell receptor α-chain	
AML-M4/AML-M5	t(9;11) (p22;q23)		
	del (11) (q23)		
	t(10–11) (p11–p15;q23)	Multiple	35
	t(11;17) (q23;q25)		
	t(11;19) (q23;p13)		
	t(11q)		
AML-M6	-5/del (5q), -7/del (7q)		33
	complex defects		
AML-M7	t(1;22) (p13;p13)		
	multiple defects		
MDS	-5/del (5q)		
	-7/del (7q)		
ALL (L1 and L2)	t(9;22) (q34;q11)	c-ABL1	20–25 (adults)
ALL (L1 and L2)	t(1;19) (q23;p13)	PBX1,E2A	5–6 (children)

AML = acute myeloid leukemia; CML = chronic myelogenous leukemia; ALL = acute lymphoblastic leukemia. See text for description of subtypes.

larly β-chain) rearrangement is very suggestive of a T-cell malignancy (Crossman, 1988). Using the Southern DNA analytical technique and similar methods to measure RNA transcripts, it is also possible to demonstrate translocated oncogenes (e.g., *MYC* in Burkitt's lymphoma) (Croce, 1985), as well as to detect the formation of fusion genes (e.g., *BCR-ABL1* in CML) (Champlin, 1985). Amplification of targeted gene segments by polymerase chain reaction is useful in identification of small populations of neoplastic cells. When these methods become simplified and further automated for general laboratory usage, they will be increasingly helpful in the early diagnosis and classification of hematologic malignancies. Similarly, *in situ* hybridization can be used to demonstrate neoplastic cells, or viral nucleic acid segments or oncogenes in cells present in tissue sections.

Adamson JW, Fialkow PJ, Murphy S, et al: Polycythemia vera: Stem-cell and probable clonal origin of the disease. N Engl J Med 1976; 295:913.

Alder A: Über konstitutionell bedingte Granulationsveränderungen der Leukocyten. Deutsch Arch Klin Med 1939; 183:372.

Athens JW: Neutropenia. *In* Lee GR, Bithell TC, Foerster J, et al (eds): Wintrobe's Clinical Hematology, 9th ed. Philadelphia, Lea and Febiger, 1993, p 1589.

Bartl R, Frisch B, Burkhardt R, et al: Assessment of marrow trephine in relation to staging in chronic lymphocytic leukemia. Br J Haematol 1982a; 51:1.

Bartl R, Frisch B, Burkhardt R, et al: Assessment of bone marrow histology in Hodgkin's disease: Correlation with clinical features. Br J Haematol 1982b; 51:345.

Bartl R, Frisch B, Burkhardt R, et al: Bone marrow histology in myeloma: Its importance in diagnosis, prognosis, classification and staging. Br J Haematol 1982c; 51:361.

Bassan R, Buzzetti M, Marini B, et al: Investigation of chronic lymphocytosis in adults. Am J Clin Path 1988; 89:783.

Bataille R, Grenier J, Sang J: Beta-2-microglobulin in myeloma: Optimal use for staging, prognosis, and treatment—a prospective study of 160 patients. Blood 1984; 63:468.

Bennett JM: Classification of the myelodysplastic syndromes. Clin Haematol 1986; 15:909.

Bennett JM, Catovsky D, Daniel M-Th, et al: Proposals for the classification of the acute leukaemias. French-American-British (FAB) Co-operative Group. Br J Haematol 1976; 33:451.

Bennett JM, Catovsky D, Daniel M-Th, et al: A variant form of hypergranular promyelocytic leukemia (M3). Br J Haematol 1980; 44:169.

Bennett JM, Catovsky D, Daniel M-Th, et al: The French-American-British (FAB) Co-operative Group: The morphological classification of acute lymphoblastic leukaemia: Concordance among observers and clinical correlations. Br J Haematol 1981; 47:553.

Bennett JM, Catovsky D, Daniel M-Th, et al: The French-American-British (FAB) Co-operative Group: Proposals for the classification of the myelodysplastic syndromes. Br J Haematol 1982; 51:189.

Bennett JM, Catovsky D, Daniel M-Th, et al: Proposed revised criteria for the classification of acute myeloid leukemia. A report of the French-American-British cooperative group. Ann Intern Med 1985a; 103:620.

Bennett JM, Catovsky D, Daniel M-Th, et al: Criteria for the diagnosis of acute leukemia of megakaryocytic lineage (M7). A report of the French-American-British cooperative group. Ann Intern Med 1985b; 103:460.

Bennett JM, Catovsky D, Daniel M-T, et al: The French-American-British (FAB) Cooperative Group. Proposal for the classification of chronic (mature) B and T lymphoid leukemias. J Clin Pathol 1989; 42:567.

Bennett JM, Catovsky D, Daniel M-T, et al: Proposal for the recognition of minimally differentated acute myeloid leukemias (AML-M0). Br J Haematol 1991; 78:325.

Bitter MA, LeBeau MM, Larson RA, et al: A morphologic and cytochemical study of acute myelomonocytic leukemia with abnormal marrow eosinophils associated with inv(16) (p13q22). Am J Clin Pathol 1984; 81(6):733.

Bouroncle BA, Wiseman BK, Doan CA: Leukemic reticuloendotheliosis. Blood 1958; 13:609.

Boxer LA: Neutrophil disorders: qualitative abnormalities of the neutrophil. *In* Beutler E, Lichtman MA, Coller BS, Kipps TJ (eds): Williams Hematology, 5th ed. New York, McGraw-Hill, 1995, p 828.

Boxer LA, Allen JM, Baehner RL: Diminished polymorphonuclear leukocyte adherence. Function dependent on release of cyclic AMP by endothelial cells after stimulation of B-receptors by epinephrine. J Clin Invest 1980; 66:268.

Breton-Gorius J, Daniel MT, Flandrin G, et al: Peroxidase activity of circulating micromegakaryoblasts and platelets in a case of acute myelofibrosis. Br J Haematol 1973; 25:331.

Brodeur GM: Molecular correlates of cytogenetic abnormalities in human cancer cells: Implications for oncogene activation. Prog Hematol 1986; 14:229.

Brunning RD: Morphologic alterations in nucleated blood and marrow cells in genetic disorders. Hum Pathol 1970; 1:99.

Brunning RD, McKenna RW: Atlas of Tumor Pathology. Tumors of the Bone Marrow. Washington, D.C., Armed Forces Institute of Pathology, 3rd series, Fascicle 9. 1994.

Cardullo LD, Morilla R, Catovsky D: Significance of Phi bodies in acute leukemia. J Clin Pathol 1981; 34:153.

Cassuto JP, Schneider M, Bourg M, et al: Acute infectious lymphocytosis as a T-cell lymphoproliferative syndrome. BMJ 1977; ii:1331.

Champlin RE, Golde DW: Chronic myelogenous leukemia: Recent advances. Blood 1985; 65:1039.

Chanarin I, Harrisingh D, Tidmarsh E, et al: Significance of lymphocytosis in adults. Lancet 1984; 2:897.

Cheson BD, Bennett JM, Rai KR, et al: Guidelines for clinical protocols for chronic lymphocytic leukemia: Recommendations of the National Cancer Institute–Sponsored Working Group. Am J Hematol 1988; 29:152.

Cordell JL, Falini B, Erber WN, et al: Immunoenzymatic labeling of monoclonal antibodies using immune complexes of alkaline phosphatase and monoclonal anti-alkaline phosphatase (APAAP complexes). J Histochem Cytochem 1984; 32:219.

Crist, WM, Pullen DJ, Rivera GK: Acute lymphoid leukemia. *In* Ferbach DJ, Vietti TJ (eds): Clinical Pediatric Oncology, 4th ed. St. Louis, Mosby–Year Book, 1991.

Croce CM, Nowell PC: Molecular basis of human B cell neoplasia. Blood 1985; 65:1.

Crossman J, Uppenkamp M: T-cell gene rearrangements and the diagnosis of T-cell neoplasms. Clin Lab Med 1988; 8:31.

Davey FR, Huntington S: Age-related variation in lymphocyte subpopulations. Gerontology 1977; 23:381.

Davey FR, Hutchison RE: Pathology and immunology of adult T-cell leukemia/lymphoma. Current Opinion in Oncology 1991: 3:13.

Davey FR, Olson S, Kurec AS, et al: The immunophenotyping of extramedullary myeloid cell tumors in paraffin-embedded tissue sections. Am J Surg Pathol 1988; 12:699.

Davidsohn I: Serologic diagnosis of infectious mononucleosis. JAMA 1937; 108:289.

Davidsohn I, Lee CL: The clinical serology of infectious mononucleosis. *In* Carter RL, Penman HG (eds): Infectious Mononucleosis. Oxford, Blackwell Scientific Publications, 1969.

De Waele M, Foulon W, Renmans W, et al: Hematologic values and lymphocyte subsets in fetal blood. Am J Clin Pathol 1988; 89:742.

Diaz-Jouanen E, Strickland RG, Williams RC: Studies of human lymphocytes in the newborn and the aged. Am J Med 1975; 58:620.

Dorfman RF, Remington JS: Value of lymph-node biopsy in the diagnosis of acute acquired toxoplasmosis. N Engl J Med 1973; 289:878.

Durie BGM, Salmon SE: A clinical staging system for multiple myeloma: Correlation of measured myeloma cell mass with presenting clinical features, response to treatment and survival. Cancer 1975; 36:842.

Egerter DA, Beckstead JH: Malignant lymphomas in the acquired immunodeficiency syndrome. Arch Pathol Lab Med 1988; 112:602.

Ehrlich GD, Han T, Bettigole R, et al: Human T-lymphotropic virus type I–associated benign transient immature T-cell lymphocytosis. Am J Hematol 1988; 27:49.

Erber WN, Breton-Gorius J, Villeval JL, et al: Detection of cells of megakaryocyte lineage in haematological malignancies by immuno-alkaline phosphatase labelling cell smears with a panel of monoclonal antibodies. Br J Haematol 1987; 65(1):87.

Fauci AS, Harley JB, Roberts WC, et al: The idiopathic hypereosinophilic syndrome. Clinical, pathophysiologic, and therapeutic considerations. Ann Intern Med 1982; 97:78.

Fialkow PJ, Faguet GB, Jacobson RJ, et al: Evidence that essential thrombocythemia is a clonal disorder with origin in a multipotent stem cell. Blood 1981; 58:916.

Fialkow PJ, Jacobson RJ, Papayannopoulou T: Chronic myelocytic leukemia: Clonal origin in a stem cell common to the granulocyte, erythrocyte, platelet and monocyte/macrophage. Am J Med 1977; 63:125.

Franklin EC: μ-Chain disease. Arch Intern Med 1975; 135:7.

Galton DAG, Goldman JM, Wiltshaw E, et al: Prolymphocytic leukaemia. Br J Haematol 1974; 27:7.

Gentile TC, Uner AH, Hutchison RE, et al: CD3+ CD56+ Aggressive variant of large granular lymphocyte leukemia. Blood 1994; 84:2315.

Gilbert HS: Definition, clinical features and diagnosis of polycythaemia vera. Clin Haematol 1975a; 4:263.

Gilbert HS, Ornstein L: Basophil counting with a new staining method using Alcian blue. Blood 1975b; 46:279.

Golomb HM, Rowley JD, Vardiman JW, et al: "Microgranular" acute promyelocytic leukemia: A distinct clinical, ultrastructural, and cytogenetic entity. Blood 1980; 55:253.

Griffin JD, Davis R, Nelson DA, et al: Use of surface marker analysis to predict outcome of adult myeloblastic leukemia. Blood 1986; 68:1232.

Haluska FG, Brufsky AM, Canellos GP: The cellular biology of the Reed-Sternberg cell. Blood 1994; 84:1005.

Harrington DS, Weisenburger DD, Purtilo DT: Epstein-Barr virus–associated lymphoproliferative lesions. Clin Lab Med 1988; 8:97.

Harris NL, Jaffe ES, Stein H, et al: A revised European-American classification of lymphoid neoplasms: A proposal from the International Lymphoma Study Group. Blood 1994; 84:1361.

Hayhoe FGJ: Cytochemistry of acute leukemias. Histochem J 1984; 16:1051.

Hoxie JA: Hematologic manifestations of AIDS. *In* Hoffman R, Benz EJ, Shattil SJ, et al (eds): Hematology. Basic Principles and Practice, 2nd ed. New York, Churchill Livingstone, 1995.

Hutchison RE, Kurec AS, Davey FR: Lymphocytic surface markers in lymphoid leukemoid reactions. Clin Lab Med 1988; 8:237.

Jaffe ES (ed): Surgical Pathology of the Lymph Nodes and Related Organs. Philadelphia, W.B. Saunders Company, 1995.

Jandl JH: Blood, Textbook in Hematology. Boston, Little, Brown and Co., 1987.

Jordan MC, Rousseau WE, Stewart JA, et al: Spontaneous cytomegalovirus mononucleosis: Clinical and laboratory observations in nine cases. Ann Intern Med 1973; 79:153.

Kadin ME, Said J: T-cell lymphomas and leukemias of post-thymic differentiation. Clin Lab Med 1988; 8:135.

Kaplow LS: Cytochemistry of leukocyte alkaline phosphatase. Am J Clin Pathol 1963; 39:439.

Kaplow LS: Simplified myeloperoxidase stain using benzidine dihydrochloride. Blood 1965; 26:215.

Kaplow LS: Substitute for benzidine in myeloperoxidase stains. Am J Clin Pathol 1975; 63:451.

Katayama I, Yang JPS: Reassessment of a cytochemical test for differential diagnosis of leukemic reticuloendotheliosis. Am J Clin Pathol 1977; 68:268.

Kaye FJ, Najfeld V, Singer J, et al: Confirming evidence for the clonal development and stem cell origin of Philadelphia chromosome–negative chronic myelogenous leukemia. Am J Hematol 1984; 17:93.

Keren DF: Flow cytometry in Clinical Diagnosis. Chicago, American Society of Clinical Pathologists, 1989.

Kinoshita K, Amagasaki T, Ikeda S, et al: Preleukemic state of adult T cell leukemia: Abnormal T lymphocytosis induced by human adult T cell leukemia-lymphoma virus. Blood 1985; 66:120.

Knowles DM: Neoplastic Hematopathology. Baltimore, Williams & Wilkins, 1992.

Kurec AS, Baltrucki L, Mason DY, et al: Use of APAAP method in the classification and diagnosis of hematologic disorders. Clin Lab Med 1988; 8:223.

Lagergren J: The white blood cell count and the erythrocyte sedimentation rate in pertussis. Acta Paediatr 1963; 52:405.

Landaw SA: Acute leukemia in polycythemia vera. Semin Hematol 1975; 13:33.

Lee CL, Davidsohn I, Panczyszyn O: Horse agglutinins in infectious mononucleosis. II. The spot test. Am J Clin Pathol 1968; 49:12.

Lee GR, Bithell TC, Foester J, et al: Wintrobe's Clinical Hematology, 9th ed. Philadelphia. Lea and Febiger, 1993.

Li CY, Lam KW, Yam LT: Esterases in human leukocytes. J Histochem Cytochem 1973; 21:1.

Lukes RJ, Craver LL, Hall TC, et al: Hodgkin's disease, report of Nomenclature Committee. Cancer Res 1966; 26:1311.

Lukes RJ, Collins RD: Tumors of the hematopoietic system. *In* Atlas of Tumor Pathology. Washington, D.C., Armed Forces Institute of Pathology, Second Series, Fascicle 28, 1992.

Maldonado JE, Hanlon DG: Monocytosis: A current appraisal. Mayo Clin Proc 1965; 40:248.

Marks SM, Baltimore D, McCaffrey R: Terminal transferase as a predictor of initial responsiveness to vincristine and prednisone in blastic chronic myelogenous leukemia. N Engl J Med 1978; 298:812.

McKenna RW, Parkin J, Bloomfield CD, et al: Acute promyelocytic leukaemia: A study of 39 cases with identification of hyperbasophilic microgranular variant. Br J Haematol 1982; 50:201.

Montserrat E, Rozman C: Bone marrow biopsy in chronic lymphocytic leukemia: A review of its prognostic importance. Blood Cells 1987; 12:315.

Morris CM, Reeve AE, Fitzgerald PH, et al: Genomic diversity correlates with clinical variation in Ph1 negative chronic myeloid leukemia. Nature 1986; 320:281.

Mufti GJ, Galton DAG: Myelodysplastic syndromes: Natural history and features of prognostic importance. Clin Haematol 1986; 15:953.

Murphy S, Iland H, Rosenthal D, et al: Essential thrombocythemia: An interim report from the Polycythemia Vera Study Group. Semin Hematol 1986; 23:177.

Muss HB, Moloney WC: Chloroma and other myeloblastic tumors. Blood 1973; 42:721.

Naiman JL, Oski FA, Allen FH, et al: Hereditary eosinophilia: Report of a family and review of the literature. Am J Hum Genet 1964; 16:195.

Neiman RS, Barcos M, Berard C, et al: Granulocytic sarcoma: A clinicopathologic study of 61 biopsied cases. Cancer 1981; 48:1426.

Neiman RS, Rosen PJ, Lukes RJ: Lymphocyte-depletion Hodgkin's disease. N Engl J Med 1973; 288:751.

Newland AC, Catovsky D, Linch D, et al: Chronic T cell lymphocytosis: A review of 21 cases. Br J Haematol 1984; 58:433.

Non-Hodgkin's Lymphoma Pathologic Classification Project: National Cancer Institute–sponsored study of classifications of non-Hodgkin's lymphoma. Cancer 1982; 49:2112.

Nowell PC, Hungerford DA: A minute chromosome in human chronic granulocytic leukemia. Science 1960; 132:1497.

Paul JR, Bunnell WW: The presence of heterophile antibodies in infectious mononucleosis. Am J Med Sci 1932; 183:90.

Peterson L, Hrisinko MA: Benign lymphocytosis and reactive neutrophilia. Laboratory features provide diagnostic clues. Clin Lab Med 1993; 13:863.

Peterson LC, Bloomfield CD, Brunning RD: Blast crisis as an initial or terminal manifestation of chronic myeloid leukemia. A study of 28 patients. Am J Med 1976; 60:209.

Pinkus GS, Said JW: Hodgkin's disease, lymphocyte predominance type, nodular—a distinct entity? Unique staining profile for L & H variants of Reed-Sternberg cells defined by monoclonal antibodies to leukocyte common antigen, granulocyte-specific antigen, and B-cell specific antigen. Am J Pathol 1985; 118:1.

Poiesz BG, Ruscetti FW, Gordon AF, et al: Detection and isolation of type C retrovirus particles from fresh and cultured lymphocytes of patients with cutaneous T-cell lymphoma. Proc Natl Acad Sci U S A 1980; 77:7415.

Pugh WC, Stass SA: Immunoglobulin gene rearrangement and its implications for the study of B-cell neoplasia. Clin Lab Med 1988; 8:45.

Purtilo D, Paquin L, DeFlorio D, et al: Immunodiagnosis and immunopathogenesis of the X-linked recessive lymphoproliferative syndrome. Semin Hematol 1979; 16:309.

Purtilo DT: Immunopathology of X-linked lymphoproliferative syndrome. Immunol Today 1983; 4:291.

Raghavachar A, Bartram CR, Ganser A, et al: Acute undifferentiated leukemia: Implications for cellular origin and clonality suggested by analysis of surface markers and immunoglobulin gene rearrangement. Blood 1986; 68:658.

Rai KR, Chanana AW, Cronkite EP, et al: Studies on lymphocytes. XVIII. Mechanisms of lymphocytosis induced by supernatant fluids of *Bordetella pertussis* cultures. Blood 1971; 38:49.

Rappaport H: Tumors of the hematopoietic system. *In* Atlas of Tumor Pathology. Washington, D.C., Armed Forces Institute of Pathology, Section III, Fascicle 1966, p 88.

Reilly WA: The granules in the leukocytes in gargoylism. Am J Dis Child 1941; 62:489.

Roggli VL, Surback J, Saleem A: Prognostic factors and treatment effects on survival in erythroleukemia: A retrospective study of 134 cases. Cancer 1981; 48:1101.

Rosenthal S, Canellos GP, DeVita VT Jr, et al: Characteristics of blast crisis in chronic granulocytic leukemia. Blood 1977; 49:705.

Sheehan HL, Storey GW: An improved method of staining leukocyte granules with Sudan black B. J Pathol Bacteriol 1947; 59:336.

Shurin SB: Pathologic states associated with activation of eosinophils and with eosinophilia. Hematol Oncol Clin North Am 1988; 2:171.

Sixbey JW, Nedrud JG, Raab-Traub N, Hanes RA, et al: Epstein-Barr virus replication in oropharyngeal epithelial cells. N Engl J Med 1984; 310:1225.

Sobol RE, Bloomfield CD, Royston I: Immunophenotyping in the diagnosis and classification of acute lymphoblastic leukemia. Clin Lab Med 1988; 8:151.

Sobol RE, Mick R, Royston I, et al: Clinical importance of myeloid antigen expression in adult acute lymphoblastic leukemia. N Engl J Med 1987; 316:1111.

Southern EM: Detection of specific sequences among DNA fragments separated by gel electrophoresis. J Mol Biol 1975; 98:503.

Spangrude GJ, Sacchi F, Hill HR, et al: Inhibition of lymphocyte and neutrophil chemotaxis by pertussis toxin. J Immunol 1985; 135:4135.

Stass SA, Mirro J: Lineage heterogeneity in acute leukaemia: Acute mixed-lineage leukemia and lineage switch. Clin Haematol 1986; 15:811.

Weksler ME, Hütteroth TH: Impaired lymphocyte function in aged humans. J Clin Invest 1974; 53:99.

Woodruff RK, Malpas JS, Paxton AM, et al: Plasma cell leukemia (PCL): A report on 15 patients. Blood 1978; 52:839.

Yam LT, Li CY, Lam KW: Tartrate-resistant acid phosphatase isoenzyme in the reticulum cells of leukemic reticuloendotheliosis. N Engl J Med 1971a; 284:357.

Yam LT, Li CY, Crosby WH: Cytochemical identification of monocytes and granulocytes. Am J Clin Pathol 1971b; 55:283.

Yoffe G, et al: Molecular analysis of interferon-induced suppression of Philadelphia chromosome in patients with chronic myeloid leukemia. Blood 1987; 69:961.

Yunis JJ, Brunning RD: Prognostic significance of chromosomal abnormalities in acute leukemias and myelodysplastic syndromes. Clin Haematol 1986; 15:597.

Chapter 28

Blood Platelets

Jonathan L. Miller, M.D., Ph.D.

PLATELET FUNCTIONAL ANATOMY

A well-prepared peripheral blood film (see Plate 24–1) offers an opportunity to evaluate platelet numbers, size, distribution, and light microscopic structure. Although subtle abnormalities of platelet structure usually require electron microscopic analysis, gross absence or asymmetry of granulation and grossly aberrant platelet surfaces may be evident. In films from nonanticoagulated fingerstick specimens, some platelet clumping is an expected feature. In instances of observed abnormalities, artifacts resulting from improper specimen collection or handling should always be considered, and a repeat specimen obtained if a satisfactory explanation for the abnormality is not apparent.

In cases of suspected platelet structural abnormalities, electron microscopy allows much more precise characterization of the defect. Optimal preparation methods for the study of platelet ultrastructure have been described (Gerrard, 1979), and it is essential that meticulous care be taken in the collection and processing of such specimens.

Normal features of the platelet that may be visualized ultrastructurally are shown in Figure 28–1. The outer surface of the platelet, the *glycocalyx*, is rich in glycoproteins, both those integral to the platelet membrane and those adsorbed from the plasma. A submembranous band of *microtubules*, composed of the protein tubulin, provides structural support for the normally discoid cell. Contractile *microfilaments*, may also be seen. These are composed principally of platelet actin and platelet myosin. An extensive *open canalicular system* within the platelet has been demonstrated by a variety of methods to be in direct communication with the extracellular environment. Often seen in close proximity to the open canalicular system is the *dense tubular system*. This system, apparently derived from the smooth endoplasmic reticulum, shows positive staining for platelet peroxidase activity (Breton-Gorius, 1972), in accord with its role as a site of arachidonic acid metabolism within the platelet. The dense tubular system is also believed to function as a calcium-sequestering pump, providing low levels of cytoplasmic calcium in the resting platelet (Statland, 1969). Immunocytochemical studies (Herbener, 1988) have now demonstrated Ca^{+2}-ATPase activity in the open canalicular system and possibly also the dense tubular system.

A variety of inclusions can be recognized within the platelet cytoplasm. Both *mitochondria* and *glycogen* can be identified. Lighter staining *α granules*, less frequent *dense core* (or "bull's eye") *granules, lysosomes,* and *peroxisomes* may also be seen. The α granules contain a number of different proteins, including platelet fibrinogen, the platelet-derived growth factor (PDGF), von Willebrand factor (vWF), the Factor V binding protein multimerin (Hayward, 1991; Hayward, 1993), the lectin-like molecule P-selectin (Stenberg, 1985; Berman, 1986), β-thromboglobulin (βTG), and the heparin-neutralizing platelet factor 4 (PF4). The dense core granules are known to be the locus of stored nonmetabolic pools of adenosine diphosphate (ADP), adenosine triphosphate (ATP), 5-hydroxytryptamine (5-HT), and calcium.

In recent years detailed study of the platelet *membrane glycoproteins* has led to an improved understanding of platelet function. Through radioactive labeling and, more recently, chemical labeling with nonradioactive biotin (Fabris, 1992a) of surface glycoprotein amino acid or

4

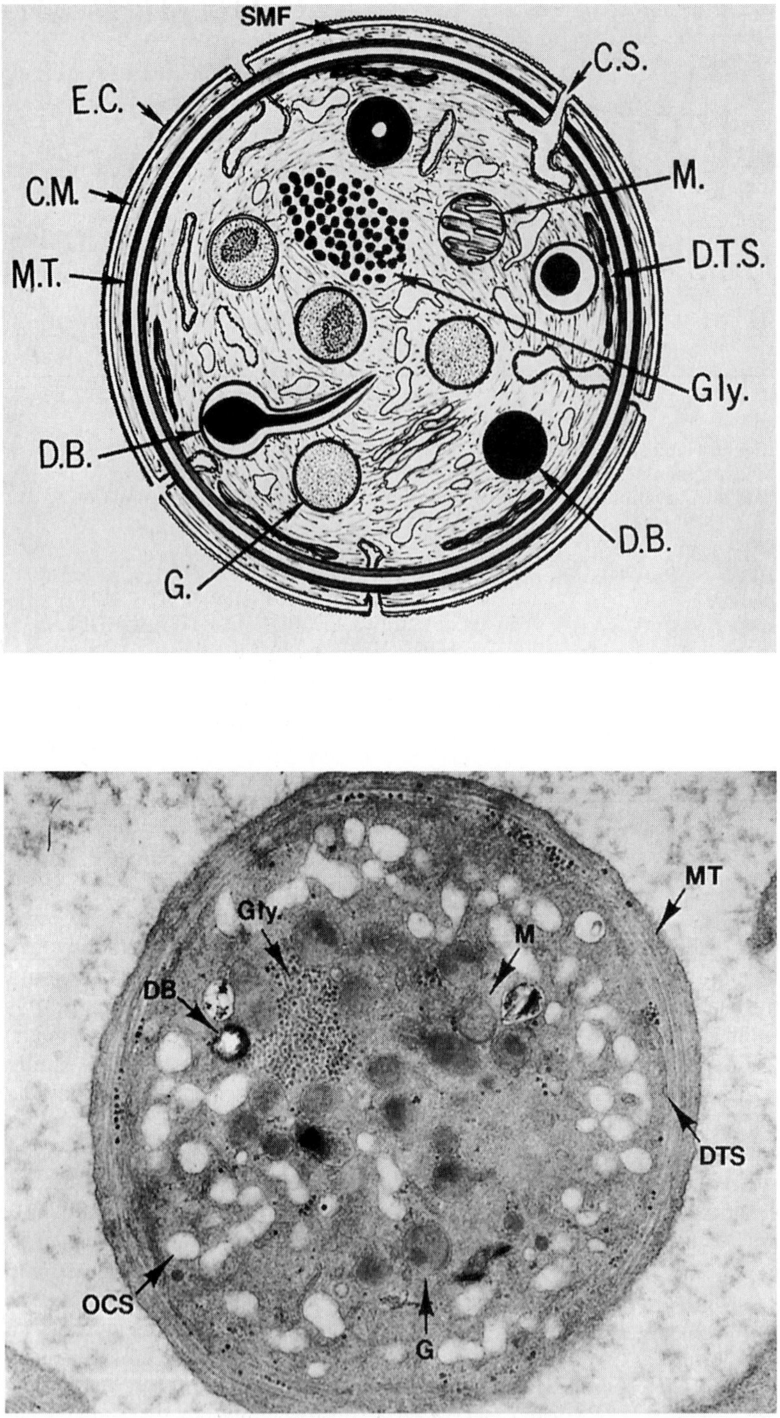

Figure 28–1. Discoid platelets. The diagram summarizes ultrastructural features observed in thin sections of discoid platelets cut in the equatorial plane. Components of the peripheral zone include the exterior coat (EC), trilaminar unit membrane (CM), and submembrane area containing specialized filaments (SMF) that form the wall of the platelet and line channels of the surface connected canalicular system (CS). The matrix of the platelet interior is the sol-gel zone containing actin microfilaments, structural filaments, the circumferential band of microtubules (MT), and glycogen (Gly). Formed elements embedded in the sol-gel zone include mitochondria (M), granules (G), and dense bodies (DB). Collectively they constitute the organelle zone. The membrane systems include the surface connected canalicular system (CS) and the dense tubular system (DTS), which serve as the platelet sarcoplasmic reticulum. The electron micrograph shows a platelet sectioned in the equatorial plane (30,000), which reveals most of the structures indicated on the diagram. (From White JG: *In* Bloom AL, Forbes CD, Thomas DP, Tuddenham EGD [eds.]: Haemostasis and Thrombosis. New York, Churchill Livingstone, 1994.)

sugar residues, solubilization of the platelet membranes, electrophoretic separation of the solubilized proteins on polyacrylamide gels, and autoradiography of the gels, the different platelet membrane glycoproteins can be identified (Nurden, 1986). The appearance of the major platelet membrane glycoprotein bands is illustrated in Figure 28–2.

Platelet Activities in Hemostasis and Their Laboratory Measurements

Following vascular injury, blood platelets rapidly *adhere* to the exposed subendothelium (Fig. 28–3), with plasma vWF serving as a glue connecting subendothelial collagen to

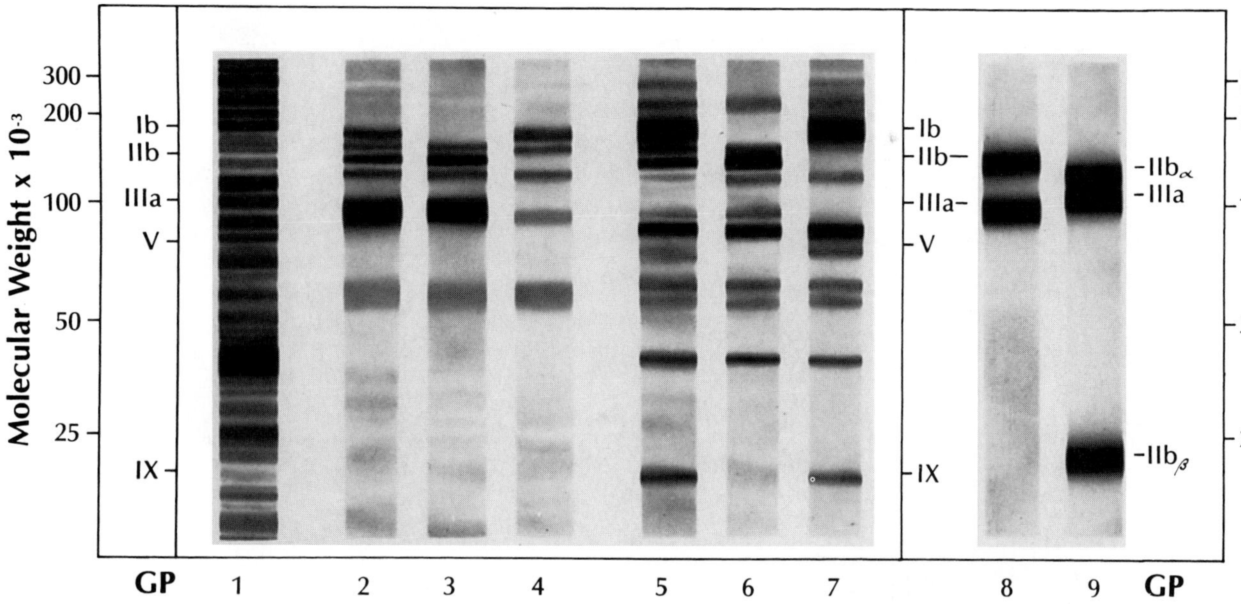

Figure 28–2. Analysis of platelet proteins and antiplatelet antibodies by SDS–polyacrylamide gel electrophoresis and immunoblotting. This figure is an artist's rendering of the original material to allow a clearer, more consistent presentation of typical analyses. Solubilized platelet proteins were separated by electrophoresis through a slab gel containing a 7% to 12% exponential gradient of polyacrylamide. All samples are unreduced, except for lane 9, in which the proteins are reduced with 5% β-mercaptoethanol. The ordinates mark the position of the major platelet membrane glycoproteins in the unreduced form; therefore, these notations are not applicable to lane 9. Lane 1 represents a Coomassie brilliant blue protein stain of normal whole platelets. Among the major membrane glycoproteins, only GP IIb is separated from other polypeptides and is present as a distinct band. Lanes 2 to 4 represent autoradiographs of platelet cell surface proteins labeled by lactoperoxidase-catalyzed radioiodination, and lanes 5 to 7 represent fluorographs of platelets labeled by sequential treatment with neuraminidase, galactose oxidase, and sodium [^{3}H]borohydride (to label cell surface carbohydrate). Lanes 2 and 5 represent normal platelets. Lanes 3 and 6 represent platelets from a patient with Bernard-Soulier syndrome. The lack of GP Ib can be seen with both techniques, whereas the apparent absence of GP V, GP IX, and a high molecular weight band that may contain complexes of GP Ib can only be seen in lane 6. Lanes 4 and 7 represent platelets from a patient with Glanzmann's thrombasthenia, demonstrating their deficiency of GP IIb and GP IIIa. Lanes 8 and 9 are Western blots of unreduced (lane 8) and reduced (lane 9) platelet proteins using a mixture of polyclonal rabbit anti-GP IIb and anti-GP IIIa antisera as the primary antibody. Disulfide bond reduction causes the dissociation of GP IIb into two subunits: GP IIb_α, with a slightly faster migration than GP IIb, and GP IIb_β, which can be seen at the position of $M_r = 22{,}000$. Glycoprotein IIIa is apparently rich in intramolecular disulfide bonds and assumes a larger size and slower electrophoretic migration after reduction. (From Nurden AT, George JN, Phillips DR: Platelet membrane glycoproteins: Their structure, function, and modification in disease. *In* Phillips DR, Shuman MA [eds]: Biochemistry of Platelets. Orlando, FL, Academic Press, Inc, 1986.)

the platelet through the platelet's glycoprotein Ib/IX receptor complex (Clemetson, 1989; Roth, 1991; Ruggeri, 1994). In patients with von Willebrand's disease, the initial adhesive event may not occur (Turitto, 1983). Subsequent spreading of platelets that have adhered to subendothelium may be dependent on platelet-collagen interactions mediated by platelet membrane glycoprotein Ia (Nieuwenhuis, 1986). In pathologically narrowed arterioles or small arteries, where platelets may flow at high velocities, conformational changes in the platelet glycoprotein Ib/IX complex may be induced by high shear forces, resulting in the binding of vWF to the platelet (Roth, 1991; Chow, 1992). Additionally, at high shear rates, the platelet membrane glycoprotein IIb/IIIa complex may also be involved in adhesion to subendothelium, with vWF mediating this process (Weiss, 1989; Peterson, 1987; Ikeda, 1991). Although a number of *in vitro* laboratory tests have been used to assess the adhesion properties of platelets, most have now been abandoned owing to poor reproducibility or predictive value. It has been suggested (Turitto, 1994) that to achieve physiologically meaningful results, a test of platelet adhesion should be performed under direct visual observation on whole blood (preferably not anticoagulated), using a vascular or well-characterized collagen surface, with controlled-flow conditions simulating a particular area of the vascular system. Several *ex vivo* experimental systems in which blood flows at controlled shear rates through devices with carefully defined surfaces may in the near future permit a much closer approximation to the *in vivo* environment than is possible in the clinical laboratory today (Weiss, 1986; Sakariassen, 1986; Moake, 1988; Ikeda, 1991; Sakariassen, 1983; Johnson, 1992; Barstad, 1994).

Through activation of the coagulation system (see Chap. 29) thrombin is produced and serves as another very potent stimulus for platelet activation. On stimulation by thrombin, collagen, or various other agents, platelets change in shape from discoid to spherical, extend pseudopods, undergo internal contraction resulting in centralization of their α granules and dense core granules, and ultimately release from the cell the contents of these granules. Depending on the strength of the stimulus, the contents of the α granules, dense core granules, or even lysosomal granules may be released (Fig. 28–4). As a result of platelet activation, conformational changes in the glycoprotein IIb/IIIa complex occur (Sims, 1991; Phillips, 1991; Frelinger, 1991), resulting in the formation of receptors capable of binding several plasma proteins, most notably fibrinogen (Bennett, 1979). Through bridging provided by fibrinogen in the presence of calcium, platelets now show a stickiness toward each other, resulting in *platelet aggregation. In vivo,* aggregates of platelets reinforced by fibrin are termed *thrombi.*

The initial laboratory evaluation of platelets includes a

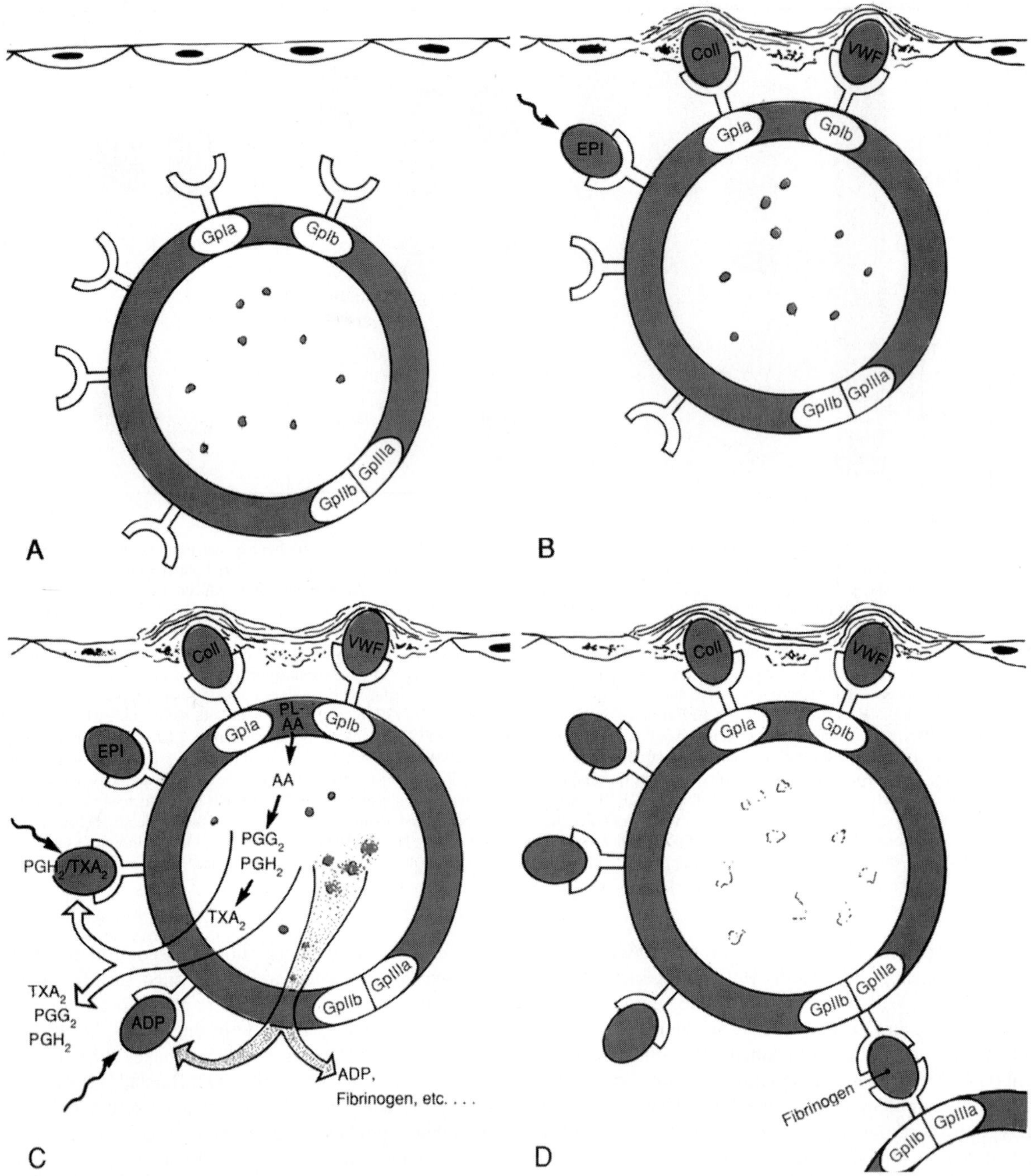

Figure 28–3. General scheme of platelet-vessel wall interactions and platelet activation. *A*, The thromboresistant properties of intact vascular endothelial cells promote blood fluidity and prevent the activation of circulating platelets. *B*, Focal vascular injury exposes subendothelial connective tissue. Platelet adhesion (platelet-vessel wall interaction) is mediated by collagen (Coll) binding directly to platelet receptors localized to membrane GPIa (at lower shear rates) or by vWF bridging of connective tissue to platelet membrane vWF receptors localized to GPIb (at high shear rates). Other agonists, such as epinephrine (EPI), may also bind to specific platelet-surface receptors to initiate or amplify platelet activation. *C*, Adherent platelets undergo the release reaction, during which prepackaged storage granule constituents (eg, ADP) are secreted, and arachidonic acid (AA) is hydrolyzed from phospholipid (PL) pools and metabolized to biologically active eicosanoids (e.g., PGG_2, PGH_2, TXA_2). Released ADP, PGH_2, and TXA_2 are platelet stimulants than bind to specific platelet receptors to amplify the activation process and to activate neighboring platelets. *D*, The process of platelet aggregation (platelet-platelet interaction) is mediated by fibrinogen binding to specific receptors that are exposed on the platelet surface with the formation of the Ca^{2+}-dependent GPIIb/IIIa heterodimer complex. Fibrinogen links aggregating platelets by binding to GPIIb/IIIa on opposing membranes of neighboring platelets. At high shear levels, vWF substitutes for fibrinogen as the ligand mediating platelet aggregation. This scheme does not illustrate various other platelet receptors that are exposed during the process of platelet activation, such as the binding sites for coagulation factor Xa, which confer procaoagulant properties on the platelet surface, or receptors for inhibitors (e.g., prostaglandins) that tend to offset activating signals. (From Schafer AI: The platelet life cycle: Normal function and qualitative disorders. *In* Handin RI, Lux SE, Stossel TP [eds] Blood: Principles and Practice of Hematology. Philadelphia, J.B. Lippincott, 1995, p 1098.)

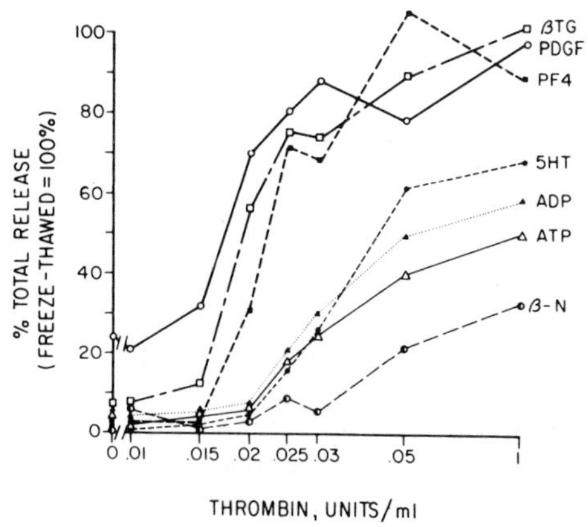

Figure 28–4. Platelet release reaction as a function of stimulus strength. With increasing thrombin concentrations, constituents of the α granules (platelet factor 4, PF4; platelet-derived growth factor, PDGF; *β*-thromboglobulin, *β*TG), dense granules (ATP; ADP; serotonin, 5HT), and lysosomal granules (*β-N*-acetylglycosaminidase, *β-N*) are released. (From Witte LD, et al: Studies of the release from human platelets of the growth factor for cultured human arterial smooth muscle cells. Circ Res 1978; 42:402. By permission of the American Heart Association, Inc.)

platelet count. This measurement has now become a routine component of the complete blood count (CBC) in an era of electronic particle counting instrumentation. Many instruments additionally provide a value for *mean platelet volume* (MPV) or may even display a histogram of platelet volumes. In healthy individuals the MPV varies inversely with platelet count, so that interpretation of MPV values as abnormally low or high is best done by referring to the patient's platelet count (Bessman, 1981, 1986). Evaluation of the peripheral blood film should permit at least a rough corroboration of the measured count and platelet size distribution. Because platelets may undergo variable degrees of activation and subsequent spreading in the preparation of the blood film, the apparent size distribution of platelets in the blood film may, in some cases, deviate significantly from actual volume distributions. In cases of severe thrombocytopenia, or whenever cellular fragments may be spuriously affecting the automated count, a manual phase contrast count with a hemocytometer chamber should be performed (Brecher, 1950). The reference interval for the platelet count is approximately 150 to 400 × 10^9/L.

No currently available laboratory test faithfully reflects the platelets' ability to accomplish their enormously complex series of functions in a manner consistent with normal hemostasis. For many years the template *bleeding time* test has been used by many laboratories as a sort of "global" test for the adequacy of primary hemostasis. In this procedure a disposable device is used that consists of either a spring-loaded blade that descends vertically into the epidermis (described in detail by Hoyer, 1982) or a blade that cuts the epidermis as it makes a rotary arc (Buchanan, 1989). In these tests a blood pressure cuff is placed around the upper arm and inflated to maintain a constant pressure of 40 mm Hg. A standardized cut is then made on the volar surface of the forearm, a timer is started, and at 30-second intervals the resulting drops of blood are blotted with filter paper (taking care that the paper does not directly touch the wound edge itself). When blood no longer stains the filter paper, the timer is stopped. At platelet counts of more than 100 × 10^9/L, bleeding times should fall within the laboratory's established reference interval (Thompson, 1983). Prolonged bleeding times in such cases are most frequently associated with prior ingestion of drugs that have an antiplatelet action (e.g., aspirin), von Willebrand's disease, congenital platelet abnormalities, or acquired disorders of platelet function (e.g., uremia).

Whereas a carefully performed bleeding time test may provide useful information during the evaluation of a patient who presents with a history of increased bleeding, the usefulness of the bleeding time test is less clear in the frequently encountered context of preoperative hemostatic screening of asymptomatic patients. In an extensive review of published papers reporting the extent of clinical bleeding in a wide variety of settings, Rodgers (1990) concluded that the available data did not provide convincing evidence that the relationship between platelet count and bleeding time is predictively useful in the individual patient typically encountered in clinical practice. They also concluded that the degree of bleeding from a standardized template cut in the skin cannot be relied on in an individual patient to predict the risk of bleeding elsewhere in the body, such as at operative sites. A recent prospective study of 40 patients with negative bleeding histories and no recent intake of nonsteroidal anti-inflammatory drugs who underwent coronary artery bypass surgery found no predictive relationship between the preoperative bleeding time test and either perioperative or postoperative bleeding (De Caterina, 1994). Although there are clearly limitations to the usefulness of the bleeding time test, particularly for a normal or only slightly prolonged bleeding time in the context of a generally asymptomatic patient, judicious use of the bleeding time test remains valuable, and a dramatically prolonged bleeding time in the absence of technical artifact provides strong suspicion for an underlying disorder of primary hemostasis.

Further evaluation of a suspected defect of platelet function can be obtained through laboratory study of *platelet aggregation and secretion* in response to a battery of platelet-stimulating agents. When citrated platelet-rich plasma is continuously stirred in a *platelet aggregometer* and a light beam is passed through the suspension, platelet aggregation in response to an added chemical stimulus can be monitored by changes in light transmittance (Born, 1962; Zucker, 1989). A discoid to spheroidal shape change is seen as an initial decrease in transmittance, whereas the subsequent formation of platelet clumps allows more light to pass through the suspension to the photodetector and is recorded as an increase in light transmittance. In instruments equipped with a second channel for monitoring secretion, the release of ATP from platelet dense granules is simultaneously measured. This is accomplished by adding the firefly luminescence substrate and enzyme, luciferin and luciferase, to the platelet-rich plasma; released ATP then functions as a cofactor in the light-producing luciferin-luciferase reaction, and light emission is recorded with a second photodetector. Because of separation of wavelengths, the aggregation and release channels can be monitored independently (Fig. 28–5). The release of ATP in most cases may be assumed to reflect the release of the other constituents of dense granules, which are less easily measured (i.e., ADP, serotonin, calcium). Direct measurement of serotonin may also be performed (Holmsen, 1989). A variety of reagents are commonly used to induce platelet aggregation, including collagen, epinephrine, ADP, ristocetin, and the calcium ionophore A23187 (Fig. 28–6). Arachidonic acid or cryoprecipitate may also serve as useful stimuli in appropriate

4

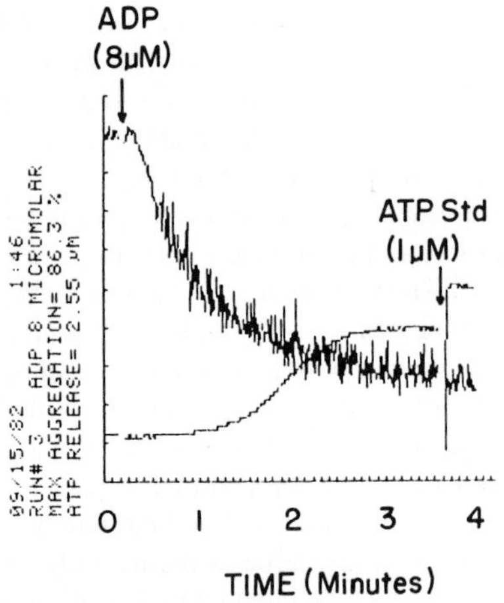

Figure 28–5. Simultaneously measured platelet aggregation and secretion of ATP. *Upper trace*: Platelet aggregation. Increasing aggregation shown as downward deflection, with platelet-rich plasma initially set at 90% full vertical scale and platelet-poor plasma at 10%. *Lower trace*: Platelet secretion. Increasing secretion of ATP shown as upward deflection. As indicated by right arrow, ATP was added following the secretory response as an internal calibration standard. Data corresponding to the measurements are indicated to the left of the traces. (From Miller JL: Am J Clin Pathol 1984; 81:471.)

circumstances. Although clearly of paramount importance as a platelet stimulus *in vivo*, thrombin is difficult to employ with platelet-rich plasma owing to interference from the formation of fibrin. The partially trypsinized γ-thrombin, however, retains platelet-stimulating activity but largely lacks clotting activity and may prove useful (Charo, 1977). An approach to the simultaneous testing of platelet aggregation and ATP secretion is found in Miller (1984).

By means of impedance measurement, the aggregation of platelets not only in platelet-rich plasma but also in whole blood may be evaluated (Cardinal, 1980). Following the addition of a platelet agonist to the stirred sample, conductance between two electrodes falls as platelets aggregate on the electrode surfaces. The resulting curves of electrical impedance versus time share many similarities to those of light transmittance versus time, although characteristic differences between these two approaches are observed (Ingerman-Wojenski, 1984; Joseph, 1987). When impedance aggregometry is combined with ATP secretion measurement on whole blood samples (Ingerman-Wojenski, 1984), relatively rapid evaluation of platelet function, requiring only a small volume of blood, may be performed.

The contractile abilities of activated platelets also result in

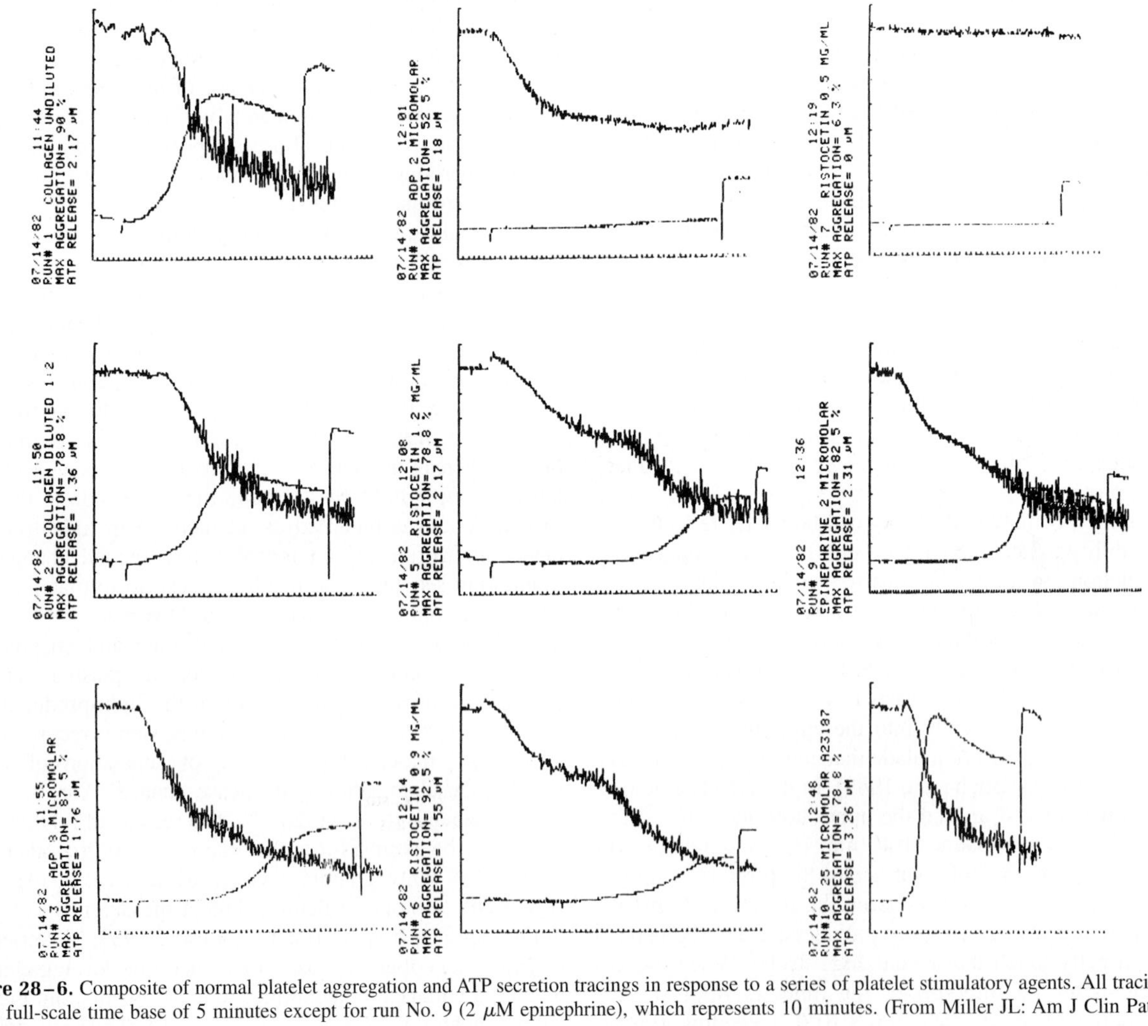

Figure 28–6. Composite of normal platelet aggregation and ATP secretion tracings in response to a series of platelet stimulatory agents. All tracings represent a full-scale time base of 5 minutes except for run No. 9 (2 μM epinephrine), which represents 10 minutes. (From Miller JL: Am J Clin Pathol 1984; 81:471.)

contraction (or "retraction") of formed clots. In the test tube, *clot retraction* can be quantitatively assessed (Owen, 1969). In thrombocytopenia or in Glanzmann's thrombasthenia, clot retraction is delayed or incomplete.

Platelets serve as the key mediators not only of primary hemostasis but also of a number of activation steps of coagulation factors. Platelets have been shown to play a role in the activation of "contact factors" XII and XI (Walsh, 1972; Ogston, 1981). Moreover, following the simultaneous exposure of platelets to collagen and thrombin, or to calcium ionophore A23187, platelet membrane phospholipids (particularly phosphatidylserine) undergo a "flip-flop" translocation from the internal to the external surface of the membrane (Hemker, 1983; Bevers, 1985), resulting in the availability of highly ordered phospholipoprotein surfaces for the activation of Factors IX and X and prothrombin (see Table 29–2). Platelets additionally contain endogenous Factor V, which appears to play a key role in the formation of a receptor on the platelet surface for activated Factor X (Miletich, 1978). Study of these various procoagulant activities of platelets is not currently standard in most laboratories but may be indicated in individual situations.

Pathways of Platelet Activation by Platelet Stimuli

Despite a great amount of research on platelet physiology and pharmacology, a clear understanding of the actual sequence of reactions following initial platelet stimulation has not yet been achieved. The mobilization of arachidonic acid from membrane phospholipids and its metabolism through the cyclo-oxygenase pathway to the potent proaggregatory agent thromboxane A_2 (see Fig. 28–3) is an intermediary mechanism occurring in response to a variety of platelet stimuli that has now been well defined. However, even after potent cyclo-oxygenase-inhibiting agents such as acetylsalicylic acid (aspirin) have fully blocked this pathway, strong stimuli such as thrombin, high concentrations of collagen, and calcium ionophore A23187 remain capable of producing full aggregatory responses.

Except in cases of simple cell agglutination, such as that induced by ristocetin, all platelet aggregating agents require the presence of free calcium ions. The roles of calcium in platelet function appear to be multiple and include promotion of platelet contractile and secretory phenomena and the formation (or unmasking) of membrane receptors. Agents that interfere with intraplatelet calcium fluxes (e.g., local anesthetics), calcium-binding proteins (e.g., phenothiazines), or extracellular free calcium (e.g., chelating agents) may accordingly be expected to produce inhibitory results when platelet function is tested (Feinstein, 1981). Although a full picture of the pathways of platelet activation remains incomplete, it is now clear that platelet activation involves a highly ordered interplay between membrane receptors for platelet stimuli, guanine nucleotide-binding proteins ("G proteins"), phospholipases C and A_2, calcium, protein kinase C, and membrane receptors for adhesive ligands. A schema integrating much of what is currently known about these interrelationships is shown in Figure 28–7.

4

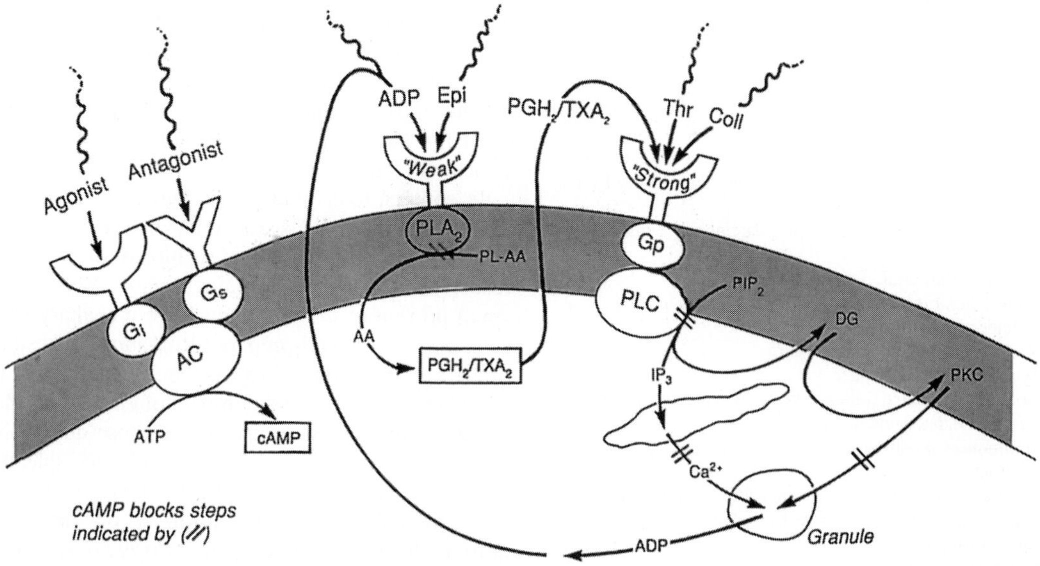

Figure 28–7. Outline of signal-response coupling in platelets. Weak agonists (e.g., ADP, epinephrine) stimulate phospholipase A_2 (PLA_2) mediated hydrolysis of free arachidonic acid (AA) from membrane phospholipid (PL) pools. AA is converted by means of the cyclo-oxygenase pathway to endoperoxides PGG_2 and PGH_2 and to thromboxane A_2 (TXA_2). PGG_2, PGH_2, TXA_2, and other strong agonists (e.g., thrombin, collagen) stimulate phospholipase C (PLC) through a G protein (Gp). PLC cleaves phosphatidylinositol 4,5-bis-phosphate (PIP_2) to generate two second messengers: diacylglycerol (DG), which activates protein kinase C (PKC) and inositol 1,4,5-triphosphate (IP_3), which translocates Ca^{2+} from intracellular storage sites to activate PLA_2. PKC activation and Ca^{2+} mobilization act synergistically to induce secretion; ADP released from storage granules during secretion amplifies functional platelet responses by acting as a weak agonist. These activation pathways are modulated by cAMP, the major inhibitory second messenger in platelets. cAMP is generated from ATP by adenylyl cyclase (AC), which is under dual control by an inhibitory G protein (Gi) that is linked to agonists and a stimulatory G protein (Gs) that is linked to antagonists (e.g., PGI_2). cAMP, directly or indirectly, inhibits a number of processes in platelet activation, including PLA_2, PLC, PKC, and Ca^{2+} mobilization. cGMP (not shown) is also an inhibitory second messenger in platelets. (From Schafer AI: The platelet life cycle: Normal function and qualitative disorders. *In* Handin RI, Lux SE, Stossel TP [eds]: Blood: Principles and Practice of Hematology. Philadelphia, J.B. Lippincott, 1995, p 1100.)

QUANTITATIVE PLATELET DISORDERS

Thrombocytopenia

Decreased numbers of circulating platelets can result from a wide variety of causes (Table 28–1), and the resulting bleeding tendency may be the first sign of an underlying disease process. Usually the clinical history will permit differentiation between an acquired and a congenital process, although some congenital thrombocytopenias (e.g., those associated with Fanconi's anemia) are typically delayed 3 to 10 years in onset.

Acquired aplastic anemias involving the erythroid and granulocytic lines as well as the megakaryocytic line are seen more commonly than are pure megakaryocytic aplasias.

Table 28–1. MECHANISMS UNDERLYING THROMBOCYTOPENIA

A. Disorders of production
  1. Decreased megakaryocytopoiesis
    a. Congenital disorders (Fanconi's anemia, TAR syndrome, intrauterine drugs or infection, etc.)
    b. Acquired hypoplasia (radiation, chemicals, alcohol, insecticides, drugs such as thiazides, chloramphenicol, or cancer chemotherapy, infections, lupus erythematosus, idiopathic, etc.)
  2. Ineffective platelet production
    a. Hereditary thrombocytopenia (autosomal dominant, May-Hegglin anomaly, Wiskott-Aldrich syndrome, etc.)
    b. Vitamin B_{12} or folate deficiency
    c. Other (myelodysplastic syndrome, paroxysmal nocturnal hemoglobinuria, etc.)

B. Disorders of distribution and dilution
  1. Splenic pooling (congestive infiltrative, inflammatory, infectious, hyperplastic, neoplastic etc.)
  2. Hypothermia
  3. Dilution by transfused stored blood

C. Disorders of destruction
  1. Combined consumption
    a. Snake venoms
    b. Tissue injury (surgical, trauma, anoxia, toxic necrosis, etc.)
    c. Obstetric complications (abruptio placentae, retained dead fetus, amniotic fluid embolism, toxemia, etc.)
    d. Neoplasms (promyelocytic leukemia, carcinoma, hemangioma, etc.)
    e. Infection (bacterial, viral, rickettsial, etc.)
    f. Intravascular hemolysis
  2. Isolated platelet consumption
    a. Thrombotic thrombocytopenic purpura
    b. Hemolytic-uremic syndrome
    c. Vasculitis (disseminated lupus erythrematosus, other collagen vascular disease, bacteremia, etc.)
    d. Cardiopulmonary prostheses
  3. Immune destruction
    a. Autoimmune (acute, chronic, transplacental, secondary, etc.)
    b. Acquired immunodeficiency disorder (AIDS)
    c. Post-transfusion purpura
    d. Isoimmune neonatal purpura
    e. Drug-induced antibodies (gold, quinine, quinidine, sulfonamide derivatives, etc.)
    f. Others

D. Combination thrombocytopenia
  1. Alcoholic liver disease
  2. Lymphoproliferative disorders
  3. Cardiopulmonary bypass
  4. Others (malignancies, infection, etc.)

Modified from Burstein SA, Harker LA: *In* Bloom AL, Thomas DP (eds): Haemostasis and Thrombosis. Edinburgh, Churchill Livingstone, 1981.

Table 28–2. CLINICAL FEATURES OF IMMUNOLOGIC THROMBOCYTOPENIC PURPURA

	Children	Adults
Occurrence		
Peak age (years)	2–4	15–40
Sex (F:M)	Equal	2.6:1
Presentation		
Onset	Acute (most with symptoms < 1 week)	Insidious (most with symptoms > 2 months)
Symptoms	Purpura (<10% with severe bleeding)	Purpura (typically bleeding not severe)
Platelet count	Most <20,000/μL	Most <20,000/μL
Course		
Spontaneous remission	83%	2%
Chronic disease	24%	43%
Response to splenectomy	71%	66%
Eventual complete recovery	89%	64%
Morbidity and mortality		
Cerebral hemorrhage	<1%	3%
Hemorrhagic death	<1%	4%
Mortality of chronic, refractory disease	2%	5%

Modified from George JN, El-Harake MA, Aster RH. *In* Beutler E, Lichtman MA, Coller BS, Kipps TJ (eds): Williams Hematology, 5th ed. New York, McGraw-Hill, 1995, p 1316. Reproduced with permission of McGraw-Hill.

Toxic chemical exposures, viral illnesses, and, frequently, unexplained causes may underlie the aplasia.

Study of the bone marrow is usually required to assess whether the thrombocytopenia is due at least in part to a failure of platelet production. Bone marrow aspirates are often less reliable than bone marrow biopsies for ascertaining the actual numbers of megakaryocytes present. In some instances abnormalities in megakaryocyte structure may be found, although the mere presence of an increased proportion of the more immature, basophilic megakaryocytic forms must not be taken as evidence of a qualitative megakaryocytic disorder.

In contrast to estimations of megakaryocyte numbers, it is usually difficult to assess abnormalities in megakaryocyte size or lobulation pattern from biopsy or clot sections. This results from the fact that one section may sample only a small portion of the relatively large megakaryocyte cell. For such purposes a well-prepared Romanowsky's stain on an aspirate smear or on a biopsy touch preparation is typically most helpful. Decreased numbers of circulating platelets may be seen with *splenomegaly* of any cause due to the resulting increase in *sequestration of platelets* by the spleen.

One of the most important and frequently encountered forms of enhanced consumption of platelets is in the acquired disorder *immunologic thrombocytopenic purpura* (ITP). The clinical history is usually most helpful in arriving at a tentative diagnosis, and particularly in distinguishing between the acute and chronic forms of ITP (Table 28–2). The study of platelet-associated immunoglobulins in patients in whom ITP is suspected has been widely used in an effort to identify immune-mediated processes. However, the predictive value of positive findings in such cases is questionable because immunoglobulins not influencing platelet survival or function may be associated with platelets in a wide variety of clinical settings (Kelton, 1982). Although high sensitivity for the detection of platelet-associated immunoglobulins can now be achieved by a variety of techniques (e.g., von dem Borne, 1980; Shaw, 1984; Kelton, 1985; Court, 1987; Tijhuis, 1991), including flow cytometry (Rosenfeld, 1986, 1987; Kunicki, 1987, 1989), positive results must be interpreted with caution owing to the low specificity of all of these tests for ITP (Kelton, 1989). Such problems in interpretation would probably not apply, however, to the demonstration of antiplatelet antibodies in patient serum that can be demonstrated to bind to platelets only in the presence of specific drugs (e.g., quinidine). A recent approach offering considerable diagnostic power measures antiplatelet antibodies bound to specific glycoprotein complexes (most frequently glycoproteins IIb/IIIa and Ib/IX) either on the patient's own platelets or following incubation of patient serum with normal platelets, by solubilizing the complexes in detergent, "capturing" them with monoclonal antibodies directed against epitopes within the complexes, and then quantifying the amount of human antibody bound to the complex with heterologous antihuman immunoglobulin (Kiefel, 1991, 1987; McMillan, 1987). Other approaches in which patient serum is reacted against normal platelet glycoprotein complexes that have been captured on beads, immobilized on nitrocellulose, or isolated by other means have proved useful in many instances but may give false-negative results for antibodies that recognize specific conformational states of the glycoprotein molecules present only in the native platelet (Fabris, 1992b; Pfueller, 1988; Nieminen, 1992; Fujisawa, 1993).

In patients with suspected heparin-induced thrombocytopenia, study of serotonin release from platelets preincubated with radioactive serotonin appears to be of diagnostic value provided that the platelets are challenged with optimally chosen concentrations of heparin (Sheridan, 1986). Studies employing this technique suggest that the thrombocytopenia observed in affected patients may be caused by heparin-IgG immune complexes binding to platelet Fc receptors (Kelton, 1988) and to platelet factor 4 (Visentin, 1994). It has recently been suggested that platelet microparticles with procoagulant activity may subsequently be produced in some patients with heparin-induced thrombocytopenia, leading to the development of thrombotic complications or disseminated intravascular coagulation (Warkentin, 1994).

Definitive assessment of platelet survival may be accomplished by labeling either the patient's own or heterologous platelets with a radioactive isotope and following the survival of the reinfused platelets. The ^{51}Cr and diisopropyl fluorophosphate ($DF^{32}P$) labels used in the past provide a number of methodologic problems and have been increasingly supplanted by ^{111}In (Heaton, 1979, 1989). Successful measurement of platelet lifespan using the nonradioactive label biotin has recently been reported in dogs (Heilmann, 1993). Until concerns about biotin's potential for toxicity and immunogenicity are fully addressed, however, this method is not applicable in humans. Nonisotopic methods based on the recovery of malondialdehyde formation in platelets newly released from the marrow following aspirin ingestion (Stuart, 1975) and the cleavage of the extracellular portion of glycoprotein Ib (Beer, 1994) have also been reported.

It must be emphasized that other routine studies may provide very helpful correlative data for elucidating the cause of thrombocytopenia. The blood film frequently reveals fragmented erythrocytes in *thrombotic thrombocytopenic purpura* (TTP) or the *hemolytic-uremic syndrome* (HUS). In the acute phase of *disseminated intravascular coagulation* (DIC) there is often an associated hypofibrinogenemia and an increase in fibrin(ogen) degradation products (see Chap. 29). Isoimmune neonatal thrombocytopenia should be suspected when thrombocytopenia occurs in the newborn period.

Thrombocytosis

Increased platelets counts, or thrombocytosis, may be seen both as a benign reactive process and as a manifestation of a myeloproliferative disorder (Table 28–3; see also Chap. 27). The blood film should confirm an electronic cell count, showing that the increased particles in fact correspond to platelets and not to cell fragments or other entities. The smear also affords an opportunity to assess deviations in platelet size, morphologic appearance, and clumping tenden-

Table 28–3. CONDITIONS IN WHICH ELEVATED PLATELET COUNTS MAY BE FOUND

Myeloproliferative disorders
Essential (primary) thrombocythemia
Polycythemia vera
Chronic myelogenous leukemia
Idiopathic myelofibrosis
Secondary thrombocytosis
Malignant diseases, including hematologic malignancies
Chronic inflammatory diseases, including hematologic malignancies
Connective tissue disorders
Inflammatory bowel disease
Tuberculosis
Hepatic cirrhosis
Chronic pancreatitis
Temporal arteritis
Chronic pneumonitis
Acute inflammatory disease
Infection
Mucocutaneous lymph node syndrome
Acute blood loss
Iron deficiency
Hemolytic anemia
Surgery
Splenectomy
Other surgical procedures
Response to drugs
Vincristine
Epinephrine
Interleukin-1β
Response to exercise
Recovery from thrombocytopenia ("rebound")
Withdrawal of myelosuppressive drugs, including alcohol
Therapy for vitamin B_{12} deficiency
Prematurity
Vitamin E deficiency in infants
Miscellaneous*
Osteoporosis, cardiac disease, renal transplant, diabetes mellitus, dry gangrene, renal failure, nephrotic syndrome, pregnancy, seizures, multicentric angiofollicular lymph node hyperplasia, familial

*Thrombocytosis has been infrequently or inconsistently reported in a variety of conditions, many of which are included here for completeness.

Modified from Williams WJ:. *In* Beutler E, Lichtman MA, Coller BS, Kipps TJ (eds): Williams Hematology, 5th ed. New York, McGraw-Hill, 1995, p 1361. Reproduced with permission of McGraw-Hill.

4

cies. In autonomous thrombocytoses that are part of myeloproliferative syndromes, large hypogranular platelets are sometimes seen.

It has been stated that reactive processes typically do not produce platelet counts of over 1000×10^9/L but that myeloproliferative processes frequently do; nonetheless, this criterion is reliable neither for diagnosis nor for the decision about whether to institute antiplatelet therapy. Particularly in patients with myeloproliferative syndromes, the individual patient may be asymptomatic, have a tendency to bleed, or have a tendency to form thromboses; at present, the most appropriate clinical approach appears to be to respond to such tendencies once they become evident. In documented cases of myeloproliferative syndromes there have been reports of abnormalities in platelet and megakaryocyte structure, platelet surface membrane receptors, platelet aggregation patterns, platelet coagulant activity, and arachidonic acid metabolism. Despite statistically significant abnormalities in comparisons of populations of patients with myeloproliferative disorders or reactive thrombocytosis, in the individual patient platelet-sizing parameters and platelet function studies are unlikely to be capable of differentiating between these disorders (Sehayek, 1988).

INHERITED DISORDERS OF PLATELET FUNCTION

(Table 28–4)

Surface Membrane Abnormalities

Our understanding of qualitative platelet disorders in molecular terms has made the greatest advance in disorders involving abnormalities of the surface membrane glycoprotein complexes IIb/IIIa and Ib/IX. Laboratory evaluation of these disorders is correspondingly well developed.

In nonanticoagulated blood films prepared from patients with *Glanzmann's thrombasthenia*, platelets typically are present in normal numbers and are individually normal in appearance but show a characteristic tendency to remain isolated, without the platelet-platelet clumping characteristic of normal blood films. In the aggregometer, platelets show a striking failure to aggregate in response to all aggregating agents. Ristocetin does induce an initial agglutination and a normal degree of release, but disagglutination then follows rather than a secondary wave corresponding to true aggregation. The platelet release reaction also usually proceeds normally with strong stimuli such as calcium ionophore or thrombin but may be diminished with collagen or the weaker stimuli ADP and epinephrine. Clot retraction is decreased mildly to severely.

A rather wide variety of additional cellular abnormalities were described in the earlier literature on Glanzmann's thrombasthenia. However, a unifying concept of this disease emerged from studies by Nurden and Caen (1974) and by Phillips and coworkers (1975, 1977) showing that patients with Glanzmann's thrombasthenia shared a decrease in content of surface membrane glycoproteins IIb and IIIa. Because the platelet antigen $P1^{A1}$ is associated with glycoprotein IIIa, this antigen is typically decreased in patients with Glanzmann's thrombasthenia (Kunicki, 1978a; van Leeuwen, 1981). Relative estimation of platelet glycoprotein IIb/IIIa molecules through binding of specific monoclonal antibodies permits diagnosis of Glanzmann's thrombasthenia by flow cytometry requiring only small volumes of blood for the assay (Montgomery, 1983; Kempfer, 1991). Actual quantitation of the platelet receptor molecules present is accomplished most accurately by study of the binding of radiolabeled monoclonal antibodies to platelet glycoproteins (Scudder, 1992). Platelet glycoprotein analyses showing loss of the IIb/IIIa complex provide definitive diagnoses of these patients (see Fig. 28–2).

As a consequence of the abnormality of glycoproteins IIb and IIIa, platelets from patients with Glanzmann's thrombasthenia fail to bind ^{125}I-fibrinogen following stimulation with ADP or epinephrine (Bennett, 1979; Mustard, 1979). This lack of the normally inducible fibrinogen-binding sites appears to be the dominant pathologic lesion in Glanzmann's thrombasthenia. A growing number of specific deletions and point mutations in the DNA coding for glycoproteins IIb and IIIa have been reported (for review see Coller, 1995). Clinical symptomatology results from either homozygous or doubly heterozygous expression of such defects, with singly heterozygous individuals usually free of bleeding manifestations.

The blood film from a patient with *Bernard-Soulier's disease* may resemble that from some patients with immunologic thrombocytopenic purpura (ITP) in that the platelets tend to be larger than normal, and there is a mild to moderate thrombocytopenia. Findings in the aggregometer are almost the reciprocal of those in Glanzmann's thrombasthenia: aggregation and release are normal with all agents *except* ristocetin. In addition, the release reaction induced by thrombin may be decreased.

Unlike von Willebrand's disease (vWD), in which there is also diminished platelet agglutination in response to ristocetin, in Bernard-Soulier's disease the addition of exogenous vWF (present in plasma cryoprecipitate fractions) does not restore ristocetin-induced agglutination of platelets. This important difference is attributable to the finding that whereas in vWD there is a deficiency in plasma vWF, in Bernard-Soulier's disease the deficiency is in the platelet membrane receptor to which the vWF must bind for normal hemostasis.

When platelet surface membrane glycoproteins from patients with Bernard-Soulier's disease are analyzed, a striking decrease in glycoprotein Ib is seen (Nurden, 1975). When very sensitive techniques for detection of this glycoprotein are employed, residual amounts of Ib may, however, be detected (Drouin, 1988; Finch 1990). Restriction fragment length polymorphism studies of one family with Bernard-Soulier's disease in fact demonstrated that the underlying molecular defect in Bernard-Soulier's disease may not be due to the gene encoding the glycoprotein Ib α chain (Finch, 1990). Although glycoprotein Ib is believed to contain the actual site for the ristocetin-dependent binding of vWF, glycoprotein IX is known to be complexed in a 1:1 ratio with glycoprotein Ib (Berndt, 1985a) and to be markedly deficient in patients with Bernard-Soulier's disease (Clemetson, 1982; Drouin, 1988). Additionally, the platelets of patients with Bernard-Soulier's disease have been reported to be deficient in glycoprotein V (Berndt, 1983; Stricker, 1986). Mutations have now been described both in glycoprotein Ib α chain

Table 28–4. DIAGNOSTIC CRITERIA FOR INHERITED DISORDERS OF PLATELET FUNCTION

Major Categories	Aggregation Pattern in Platelet-Rich Plasma	Release of ATP and Serotonin	Inheritance	Other Characteristic Abnormalities
I. Surface membrane defects				
Glanzmann's thrombasthenia	Markedly decreased with all agents except ristocetin (which may show a reversible single wave)	May be decreased with collagen, ADP, and epinephrine; normal with thrombin and calcium ionophore	Autosomal recessive	Glycoproteins IIb and/or IIIa decreased, absent, or functionally abnormal; platelet fibrinogen may be decreased; decreased clot retraction; decreased platelet clumping on blood film
Bernard-Soulier's disease	Markedly decreased with ristocetin, without correction by von Willebrand factor; may be decreased with thrombin; normal response to other agents	Decreased with ristocetin (or with the snake venom botrocetin)	Usually autosomal recessive; rare variant autosomal dominant	Platelets appear large on blood film and are frequently decreased in number; glycoproteins Ib and/or IX decreased, absent, or functionally abnormal; decreased adhesiveness to subendothelium or to glass beads; decreased receptor for quinidine-dependent antibodies
Platelet-type von Willebrand's disease	Increased with low ristocetin concentrations; uniquely agglutinated by asialo-von Willebrand factor; normal responses to other agents	Cryoprecipitate by itself produces release; normal with other agents	Autosomal dominant	Borderline thrombocytopenia; selective decrease of higher molecular weight von Willebrand factor multimers in plasma; increased platelet binding of normal von Willebrand factor
Collagen receptor defect	Markedly decreased or absent with collagen; normal response to other agents	Decreased with collagen		Decreased adherence to collagen both at low and high shear rates; may be associated with deficiency of platelet thrombospondin; may revert to normal at menopause
II. Granule defects				
Dense granule deficiencies (Hermansky-Pudlak, Chédiak-Higashi, and Wiskott-Aldrich syndromes and thrombocytopenia with absent radii syndromes) or as an isolated abnormality	Decreased aggregation, particularly of second phase, with weak agents; usually normal response to arachidonic acid, calcium ionophore, and high concentration of weaker agents	Decreased	Autosomal (except for Wiskott-Aldrich syndrome, which is sex-linked)	Decreased dense granule content of ADP, ATP, 5-HT, and calcium; increased total platelet ATP/ADP ratio; oculocutaneous albinism and reticuloendothelial ceroid deposition in Hermansky-Pudlak syndrome; thrombocytopenia associated with Chédiak-Higashi and Wiskott-Aldrich syndromes, and thrombocytopenia with absent radii; decreased autologous platelet survival and an increase in platelet-associated IgG is seen in Wiskott-Aldrich syndrome
α granule deficiencies (gray platelet syndrome)	Decreased with all agents	Decreased with all agents	Autosomal	Large, pale-appearing platelets on blood film, accompanied by thrombocytopenia; decreased α granules by electron microscopy; decreased cellular content of platelet fibrinogen, platelet factor 4, and platelet-derived growth factor; possible marrow fibrosis

(Table continued on next page)

4

Table 28–4. DIAGNOSTIC CRITERIA FOR INHERITED DISORDERS OF PLATELET FUNCTION *Continued*

Major Categories	Aggregation Pattern in Platelet-Rich Plasma	Release of ATP and Serotonin	Inheritance	Other Characteristic Abnormalities
Combined dense and α granule deficiencies	Decreased	Decreased		Heterogeneity of granule deficiencies reported
III. Defects in signal transduction				
Defects in calcium mobilization	Decreased with ADP, epinephrine; normal response to collagen, thrombin, or other strong agonists	Decreased with ADP, epinephrine; normal response to collagen, thrombin, or other strong agonists		Exact molecular mechanisms underlying defects still unknown
Defects in arachidonic acid mobilization	Decreased with ADP, epinephrine, collagen; normal response to arachidonic acid	Decreased with ADP, epinephrine, collagen; normal response to arachidonic acid		Normal dense granule content of ADP and ATP
Defects in arachidonic acid metabolism	Decreased with weak agents; unresponsive to arachidonic acid but normal response to platelet endoperoxides	Decreased with weak agents; normal response to platelet endoperoxides		Formation of lipoxygenase products from exogenous ^{14}C-arachidonic acid appears to be normal
IV. Miscellaneous				
Isolated disorders of aggregation and release as a concomitant finding in a variety of pathologic states including Epstein syndrome, the May-Hegglin anomaly, Down syndrome, inherited connective tissue disorders, and congenital heart disease	Variable	Variable		Heterogeneity of defects

(Ware, 1990; Simsek, 1994; Kunishima, 1994) and in glycoprotein IX (Clemetson, 1994; Wright, 1993) that, when present in homozygous or doubly heterozygous fashion result in a classic Bernard-Soulier's phenotype. A point mutation in the leucine-rich region of the glycoprotein Ib α chain may also produce a Bernard-Soulier's phenotype even when it is expressed only by a single allele (Miller, 1992; Ware, 1993).

It is interesting that whereas virtually all normal platelets possess a binding site for antiplatelet antibodies arising in patients with a hypersensitivity to quinidine or quinine, platelets from patients with Bernard-Soulier's disease do not appear to have this receptor (Kunicki, 1978b). Berndt (1985b) has provided evidence that such antibodies may be binding to glycoprotein IX, to the beta (β) subunit of glycoprotein Ib, or to a region defined by the association of glycoproteins Ib and IX. It has been suggested by Pfueller (1988), however, that quinine- and quinidine-induced thrombocytopenia may result from antibodies that are quite heterogeneous among patients, recognizing neoantigens composed either of various epitopes on the platelet surface and the drug, or of new conformations of platelet glycoproteins induced by the drug. Additionally, in some patients quinidine-dependent antibodies may also be directed against epitopes present within the glycoprotein IIb/IIIa complex (Pfueller, 1988; Chong, 1991; Visentin, 1991; Nieminen, 1992).

In the autosomal dominant bleeding disorder termed *platelet-type von Willebrand's disease* (Miller, 1982; Weiss, 1982) patients characteristically have low-normal platelet counts, normal Factor VIII coagulant activity and vWF antigen, and decreased ristocetin cofactor activity (see discussion of vWD in Chap. 29). On agarose gel electrophoresis of plasma there is a selective decrease of the higher molecular weight multimers, similar to that seen in Type 2 vWD. However, unlike platelets from patients with Type 2 vWD, platelets from patients with platelet-type vWD show an increased ability to bind normal vWF (Miller, 1983). In the diagnostic laboratory this increased binding is reflected by the ability of unusually low concentrations of ristocetin (0.3 to 0.5 mg/mL) to produce strong aggregation of platelets in this disorder, a finding also observed in Type 2B vWD (Ruggeri, 1980). Cryoprecipitate, however, when added to platelet-type vWD platelets without additional aggregating agents, is capable of inducing aggregation; cryoprecipitate added to normal or to Type 2B vWD platelets, in contrast, does not produce aggregation. Platelets from patients with platelet-type vWD also show unique agglutination reactions with desialylated vWF (asialo vWF) (Miller, 1987). The molecular basis of platelet-type vWD was recently shown to be due to a single base mutation resulting in the replacement of a glycine by valine at amino acid residue 233 of the glycoprotein Ib α chain (Miller, 1991). A substitution of valine for methionine just six amino acids away at residue 239 has subsequently been reported in two additional kindreds (Russell, 1993; Takahashi, 1995). These mutations are believed to produce conformational changes in the receptor leading to abnormally heightened vWF binding (Pincus, 1991; Pincus, 1994).

Nieuwenhuis (1985, 1986) reported the absence of the high-molecular-weight (168,000 daltons) glycoprotein Ia in a 33-year-old woman with a mild bleeding disorder whose platelets showed no response to collagen. Kehrel (1988) identified a second female patient with similar findings but whose platelets additionally had a lack of intact thrombospondin. Most interestingly, not only the bleeding tendency but also the structural and functional platelet abnormalities disappeared at the onset of menopause in this patient.

Storage Granule Abnormalities

A variety of platelet disorders have been described in which the primary abnormality is a deficiency of one or more types of storage granules. Several syndromes involving the dense storage granules in particular are now recognized, all of which are associated with additional clinical abnormalities distinct from those of the platelets themselves (Nichols, 1981).

In the *Hermansky-Pudlak* syndrome (Hermansky, 1959) patients have a deficiency of dense granules. They characteristically manifest an oculocutaneous albinism, and macrophages of their reticuloendothelial system contain ceroid-like deposits. Patients with the Chédiak-Higashi syndrome may also be partially albino and appear prone to frequent infections. As in granulocytes from patients with this disorder, giant inclusion granules may be found in the platelet cytoplasm. Patients with the *Chédiak-Higashi* syndrome as well as those with the *Wiskott-Aldrich syndrome* (Grottum, 1969) and the *thrombocytopenia with absent radii (TAR)* syndrome (Day, 1972) have a decreased platelet count in addition to deficiencies in dense granule content. Unlike the other syndromes, which show autosomal recessive patterns of inheritance, the Wiskott-Aldrich syndrome is sex-linked.

Disorders involving the dense granules have been characterized as showing diminished platelet aggregation, particularly of the second phase, with the weaker agents (ADP, epinephrine, low concentrations of collagen). However, arachidonic acid and higher concentrations of the weaker agents as well as the stronger agents (calcium ionophore, thrombin) may produce a relatively normal degree of aggregation. The release of dense granule materials (ADP, ATP, serotonin, calcium) is typically decreased in such patients. In storage granule abnormalities, assay of the *total* cellular content of ATP and ADP reveals a characteristic increase in the ratio of ATP to ADP, reflecting decreased nucleotides in the dense granular storage pool. This is due to the lower ATP/ADP ratio (2:3) in the storage pool compared to a much higher ration (8:1 to 10:1) in the cytoplasmic metabolic pool (Weiss, 1994). It should be emphasized that in patients in whom a platelet storage pool deficiency is suspected, normal platelet aggregation responses do not *exclude* this diagnosis, as demonstrated in a study comprising 106 patients with prolonged bleeding times and biochemically established decreases in the level of platelet serotonin and ADP (Nieuwenhuis, 1987).

Patients possessing an absence of the α *granules* have also been described. Because of the pale color of these large platelets on Romanowsky-stained blood films, this disorder has been named the *gray platelet* syndrome (Raccuglia, 1971). On electron microscopy there appears to be a selective decrease of α granules (White, 1979), and biochemical analyses have confirmed associated decreases in cellular content of platelet fibrinogen, platelet factor 4, β-thromboglobulin, and platelet-derived growth factor. Both aggregation and the platelet release reaction have been reported to be characteristically decreased in these patients. In addition to patients showing a selective decrease of either α or dense granules, rare patients may also present with platelets that exhibit a combined deficiency of α and dense granules.

Abnormalities in Signal Transduction

A number of patients with varying degrees of clinical bleeding appear to have a normal complement of storage granules, but secretion by their platelets is somehow impaired. The mechanisms for such impairment potentially include a lesion anywhere in the sequence of reactions subserving signal transduction (see Fig. 28–7). Several patients have in fact been reported in whom an underlying abnormality appears to involve impaired calcium mobilization (Lages, 1981; Hardisty, 1983; Rao, 1989).

An abnormality in the mobilization of arachidonic acid from membrane phospholipids may be suspected in patients whose platelets fail to aggregate well in response to agonists such as ADP, epinephrine, and collagen, yet respond quite normally to the direct addition of arachidonic acid (Rao, 1984). In contrast, when platelets fail to respond to arachidonic acid but show a normal aggregation and release pattern in response to the endoperoxide prostaglandin G_2, *and the possibility of drug ingestion can be absolutely eliminated*, a deficiency of the enzyme cyclo-oxygenase should be considered (Nichols, 1981). A deficiency of thromboxane synthetase has also been encountered in several patients (Defreyn, 1981; Wu, 1981; Mestel, 1980).

ACQUIRED DISORDERS OF PLATELET FUNCTION

Patients with previously normal hemostasis may acquire a variety of disorders of platelet function. The most frequent cause is ingestion of drugs that have inhibitory effects upon platelets (see later discussion), but a number of other disease states may also adversely affect platelet function.

Patients with *myeloproliferative disorders* may present not only with abnormalities of platelet numbers (see earlier section, Quantitative Platelet Disorders) but also with qualitative platelet abnormalities. These abnormalities may be at the level of platelet membrane glycoproteins (Bolin, 1977), membrane receptors for platelet agonists or antagonists (Kaywin, 1978; Ganguly, 1978; Cooper, 1978), platelet coagulant activity (Walsh, 1977), platelet α granule thrombospondin (Booth, 1984), adenine nucleotide content (Cowan, 1975; Rendu, 1979), or prostaglandin synthesis (Keenan, 1977; Schafer, 1982; Jubelirer, 1980; Pareti, 1982). Studies of platelet aggregation may be helpful, most frequently revealing decreased responsiveness to epinephrine (Spaet, 1969; Schafer, 1984) or to other platelet stimuli. Structural abnormalities have been identified not only in the platelets (Maldonado, 1974b) but also in the megakaryocytes (Maldonado, 1974a) in a number of patients with myeloproliferative disorders. Demonstration of platelet peroxidase activity through ultrastructural cytochemistry may permit the identification of megakaryocytic lineage in blast crises of CML (Breton-Gorius, 1978), acute megakaryoblastic leukemia (see Chap. 27), or in other hematologic neoplasms. The availability of monoclonal antibodies specific for platelet glycoproteins has facilitated the identification of megakaryocytic-platelet lineage in both acute and chronic leukemias. There appears to be excellent agreement between the immunologic and platelet peroxidase techniques (Tabilio, 1984).

Patients with myeloma or lymphoproliferative disorders associated with *paraproteins* frequently have been observed to have prolonged bleeding times and abnormal platelet function (Perkins, 1970; Penny, 1971; Lackner, 1973). It has been proposed that coating of the platelet by immunoglobulin may be responsible for impaired aggregation (Bang, 1972), but other mechanisms may also be involved. Patients with lymphoproliferative disorders may occasionally develop antibodies against specific platelet antigens.

Open heart surgery using *cardiopulmonary bypass* is typically associated both with a decrease in the number of circulating platelets and with the development of platelet functional defects (McKenna, 1975). Depletion of platelet α granules (Harker, 1980) following bypass has been reported. The infusion of prostacyclin during bypass surgery in experimental animals at doses too low to prevent the release of granule proteins did, nevertheless, prevent prolongation of bleeding times (Malpass, 1981). This finding underscores the complexities involved in elucidating mechanisms underlying hemostatic impairment in such procedures (Bick, 1985; Mammen, 1985). Additionally, activation of both the coagulation and fibrinolytic systems, anticoagulation with heparin, and neutralization of heparin with protamine—events that typically accompany open heart surgery—clearly may contribute to the development of a hemostatic imbalance (Bick, 1985; Mammen, 1985). The antiprotease aprotinin may afford some protection to platelets in patients undergoing cardiopulmonary bypass (Orchard, 1993).

Acquired storage pool deficiency has been reported in patients with systemic lupus erythematosus and other autoimmune disorders (Regan, 1974; Zahavi, 1974; Weiss, 1980), chronic ITP (Clancy, 1972), DIC (Pareti, 1976), and a variety of other hematologic or nonhematologic disorders. The mechanisms leading to deficiencies appear to be varied. Deficiencies of platelet dense granules have been demonstrated in isolated platelets both by means of an altered ATP/ADP ratio (see earlier) and by abnormalities of serotonin uptake (Pareti, 1980).

Patients with *uremia* have long been known to suffer impairment of primary hemostasis. The increased blood levels of guanidinosuccinic acid (Horowitz, 1970) and phenolic acids (Rabiner, 1970) that may be found in uremic patients have been shown to be capable of inducing dysfunction of normal platelets *in vitro*. Additionally, increased vascular prostacyclin production (Remuzzi, 1977) and decreased platelet thromboxane production (Smith, 1981) have been reported in uremic patients, both of which alterations would be expected to contribute to impaired hemostasis.

Platelet function is inhibited both *in vivo* and *in vitro* by a great number of *drugs*. Some of the major drugs known to impair platelet function are listed according to their mechanism of action on platelets in Table 28–5. Interpretation of bleeding times or of platelet function tests is complicated considerably when the patient has recently taken one or more such agents. Considerable variation exists among drugs in the duration of their antiplatelet effects. In the case of the nonsteroidal anti-inflammatory agent ibuprofen, platelet function has been shown to return to normal within 24 hours of the last oral administration (McIntyre, 1978; Cronberg, 1984). In contrast, in the case of aspirin, which irreversibly

Table 28–5. DRUGS THAT AFFECT PLATELET FUNCTION

1. Drugs that affect prostanoid synthesis or action
   - Cyclo-oxygenase inhibitors
     - Aspirin
     - Nonsteroidal anti-inflammatory agents
       - Indomethacin, phenylbutazone, ibuprofen, sulfinpyrazone, sulindac, meclofenamic acid, etc.
   - Thromboxane synthetase inhibitors
     - Dazoxiben, OKY-1581
   - Thromboxane receptor antagonists
   - SQ 28668, AH 23848
2. Drugs that increase platelet cyclic AMP
   - Adenylate cyclase activators
     - Prostaglandins I_2, D_2, E_1
   - Phosphodiesterase inhibitors
     - Dipyridamole
     - Methyl xanthines
       - Caffeine, theophylline, aminophylline
3. Antimicrobials
   - Penicillins
   - Cephalosporins
   - Nitrofurantoin
   - Hydroxychloroquine
4. Cardiovascular drugs
   - β-Adrenergic blockers (propranolol)
   - Vasodilators (nitroprusside, nitroglycerin)
   - Diuretics (furosemide)
   - Calcium channel blockers
   - Quinidine
5. Anticoagulants
   - Heparin, coumadin
6. Thrombolytic agents
   - Streptokinase, tissue plasminogen activator, urokinase
7. Psychotropics and anesthetics
   - Tricyclic antidepressants
     - Imipramine, amitryptyline, nortriptyline
   - Phenothiazines
     - Chlorpromazine, promethazine, trifluoperazine
   - Local anesthetics
   - General anesthesia (halothane)
8. Chemotherapeutic agents
   - Mithramycin
   - BCNU
   - Daunorubicin
9. Miscellaneous agents
   - Dextrans
   - Ticlopidine
   - Lipid lowering agents (clofibrate, halofenate)
   - Quinidine
   - ε-Aminocaproic acid
   - Antihistaminics
   - Ethanol
   - Vitamin E
   - Radiographic contrast agents
   - Food items (onions, garlic, ginger)

From Rao AK, Carvalho ACA: Acquired qualitative platelet defects. *In* Colman RW, Hirsh J, Marder VJ, Salzman EW (eds): Hemostasis and Thrombosis, 3rd ed. Philadelphia, J.B. Lippincott, 1994, p 694.

acetylates the platelet's cyclo-oxygenase enzyme, up to 10 days must elapse before the affected circulating platelets are fully replaced by new platelets. Elective studies of platelet function should be planned to minimize recent drug exposure to the extent that abstinence from medications would be unlikely to compromise significantly the health or well-being of the patient.

Table 28-6. EVALUATION OF PATIENTS WITH SUSPECTED PLATELET DISORDERS

History and physical examination
Detailed evaluation of bleeding tendencies—onset, frequency, duration and severity, transfusion requirement, and characteristic sites of involvement
Bleeding associated with surgery or trauma—tonsillectomy, tooth extractions, and circumcision
Drug history—including multi-ingredient formulations that may contain aspirin or other antiplatelet agents
Family history—inheritance pattern and severity of bleeding
Complete physical examination—including signs of recent bleeding (petechiae, ecchymoses, purpura, etc.), restricted joint mobility, and findings associated with particular congenital abnormalities (absent radii, albinism, teleangiectasia, and inherited connective tissue disorders)
Coagulation and fibrinolytic system testing
Screening (and, if indicated, more definitive) tests to detect abnormalities not related to platelets
Basic laboratory evaluation of platelets
CBC including platelet count (and possibly platelet volume data) by electronic cell counter
Peripheral blood smear evaluation of platelets—platelet numbers, size, appearance, and clumping tendency
Bleeding time
Usually omitted in the absence of clinical history suggesting a disorder of primary hemostasis or in the presence of significant thrombocytopenia; may help in the diagnosis of von Willebrand's disease and functional platelet disorders
Evaluation of plasma von Willebrand factor
von Willebrand factor antigen
von Willebrand factor functional activity, most frequently measured as ristocetin cofactor activity
Platelet function studies
Platelet aggregation (and simultaneous ATP release when firefly luciferin-luciferase reaction utilized) on platelet-rich plasma or whole blood in response to agonists such as ADP, epinephrine, collagen, ristocetin, thrombin
Clot retraction—of limited usefulness, although may be impaired in Glanzmann's thrombasthenia
Specialized studies relating to platelet function
Quantitation of platelet receptors for adhesive ligands by assay of monoclonal antibody or ligand binding to glycoprotein complexes, most notably IIb/IIIa or Ib/IX
SDS-polyacrylamide gel electrophoresis or Western blot evaluation of platelet membrane glycoproteins
Platelet adhesion to defined surfaces in *ex vivo* flow systems
Shear-induced platelet aggregation studies
Studies of uptake and release of radioactive serotonin
Specialized studies relating to decreased platelet numbers
Antiplatelet antibody studies by platelet suspension immunofluorescence test, flow cytometry, platelet membrane glycoprotein antigen capture techniques, etc.
Drug-dependent antiplatelet antibodies studied by above methods
Heparin-induced thrombocytopenia evaluated with respect to the ability of patient serum to stimulate active responses by normal platelets (serotonin secretion, microparticle formation, etc.) as a function of varying heparin concentrations
Measurement of platelet lifespan by radioactive or nonradioactive methods
Electron microscopic examination of platelet ultrastructure
Analysis of constituents of intracellular granules—α granules, dense granules, and lysosomal granules
Evaluation of platelet coagulant activities

EVALUATION OF PATIENTS WITH SUSPECTED PLATELET DISORDERS

Evaluation of patients with a clinical history or symptoms suggesting a bleeding tendency involves consideration of the coagulation and fibrinolytic systems (see Chap. 29) as well as of the blood platelets. An approach to such evaluation is outlined in Table 28-6. A carefully conducted history can be the single most important factor leading to a diagnosis in many patients. Determination of whether the disorder is likely to be congenital or acquired is most important. A platelet count in conjunction with a prolonged bleeding time will help to determine whether the bleeding tendency is explainable by decreased platelet numbers alone or whether another abnormality is present. Because vWD is far more common than congenital disorders of platelet function, an evaluation of disordered primary hemostasis frequently necessitates analysis of the Factor VIII/vWF complex, as discussed in Chapter 29. Finally, although many patients are adequately diagnosed through the application of basic studies, some require one or more of the specialized studies indicated in Table 28-6 to allow a definitive diagnosis to be reached.

Bang NU, Heidenreich RO, Trygstad, CW: Plasma protein requirements for human platelet aggregation. Ann NY Acad Sci 1972; 201:280.

Barstad RM, Roald HE, Cui Y, et al: A perfusion chamber developed to investigate thrombus formation and shear profiled in flowing native human blood at the apex of well-defined stenoses. Arterioscler Thromb 1994; 14:1984.

Beer JH, Büchi L, Steiner B: Glycocalicin: A new assay—The normal plasma levels and its potential usefulness in selected diseases. Blood 1994; 83:691.

Bennett JS, Vilaire G: Exposure of platelet fibrinogen receptors by ADP and epinephrine. J Clin Invest 1979; 64:1393.

Berman CL, Yeo EL, Wencel-Drake JD, et al: A platelet alpha granule membrane protein that is associated with the plasma membrane after activation. Characterization and subcellular localization of platelet activation-dependent granule-external membrane protein. J Clin Invest 1986; 78:130.

Berndt MC, Gregory C, Chong BH, et al: Additional glycoprotein defects in Bernard-Soulier's syndrome: Confirmation of genetic basis by parental analysis. Blood 1983; 62:800.

Berndt MC, Gregory C, Kabral A, et al: Purification and preliminary characterization of the glycoprotein Ib complex in the human platelet membrane. Eur J Biochem 1985a; 151:637.

Berndt MC, Chong BH, Bull HA, et al: Molecular characterization of quinine/quinidine drug-dependent antibody platelet interaction using monoclonal antibodies. Blood 1985b; 66:1292.

Bessman JD, Williams LJ, Gilmer PR: Mean platelet volume. Am J Clin Pathol 1981; 76:289.

Bessman JD: Automated Blood Counts and Differentials. A Practical Guide. Baltimore, The Johns Hopkins University Press, 1986.

Bevers EM, Rosing J, Zwaal RF: Development of procoagulant binding sites on the platelet surface. Adv Exp Med Biol 1985; 192:359.

Bick RL: Hemostasis defects associated with cardiac surgery, prosthetic devices, and other extracorporeal circuits. Semin Thromb Hemost 1985; 11:249.

Bolin RB, Ikumura T, Jamieson GA: Changes in distribution of platelet membrane glycoproteins in patients with myeloproliferative disorders. Am J Hematol 1977; 3:63.

Booth WJ, Berndt MC, Castaldi PA: An altered platelet granule glycoprotein in patients with essential thrombocythemia. J Clin Invest 1984; 73:291.

Born GVR: Aggregation of blood platelets by adenosine diphosphate and its reversal. Nature 1962; 194:927.

Brecher G, Cronkite EP: Morphology and enumeration of human blood platelets. J Appl Physiol 1950; 3:365.

4

Breton-Gorius J, Guichard J: Ultrastructural localization of peroxidase activity in human platelets and megakaryocytes. Am J Pathol 1972; 66:277.

Breton-Gorius J, Reyes F, Vernant JP, et al: The blast crisis of chronic granulocytic leukaemia: Megakaryoblastic nature of cells as revealed by the presence of platelet peroxidase: A cytochemical ultrastructural study. Br J Haematol 1978; 39:295.

Buchanan GR, Holtkamp CA: A comparative study of variables affecting the bleeding time using two disposable devices. Am J Clin Pathol 1989; 91:45.

Burstein SA, Harker LA: Quantitative platelet disorders. *In* Bloom AL, Thomas DP (eds): Haemostasis and Thrombosis. Edinburgh, Churchill Livingstone, 1981, pp 279–300.

Cardinal DC, Flower RJ: The electronic aggregometer: A novel device for assessing platelet behavior in blood. J Pharmacol Methods 1980; 3:135.

Charo IF, Feinman RD, Detwiler TC: Interrelations of platelet aggregation and secretion. J Clin Invest 1977; 60:866.

Chong BH, Du X, Berndt MC, et al: Characterization of the binding domains on platelet glycoproteins Ib-IX and IIb/IIIa complexes for the quinine/quinidine-dependent antibodies. Blood 1991; 77:2190.

Chow TW, Hellums JD, Moake JL, et al: Shear stress-induced von Willebrand factor binding to platelet glycoprotein Ib initiates calcium influx associated with aggregation. Blood 1992; 80:113.

Clancy R, Jenkins E, Firkin B: Qualitative platelet abnormalities in idiopathic thrombocytopenic purpura. N Engl J Med, 1972; 286:622.

Clemetson KJ: Biochemistry of platelet membrane glycoproteins. Prog Clin Biol Res 1989; 283:33.

Clemetson JM, Kyrle PA, Brenner B, et al: Variant Bernard-Soulier syndrome associated with a homozygous mutation in the leucine-rich domain of glycoprotein IX. Blood 1994; 84:1124.

Clemetson K, McGregor JL, James E, et al: Characterization of the platelet membrane glycoprotein abnormalities in Bernard-Soulier syndrome and comparison with normal by surface-labeling techniques and high-resolution two-dimensional gel electrophoresis. J Clin Invest 1982; 70:304.

Coller BS: Hereditary qualitative platelet disorders. *In* Beutler E, Lichtman MA, Coller BS, et al (eds): Williams Hematology, 5th ed. New York, Mcgraw-Hill, 1995, pp 1364–1385.

Cooper B, Schafter AI, Puchalsky D, Handin RI: Platelet resistance to prostaglandin D_2 in patients with myeloproliferative disorders. Blood 1978; 52:618.

Court WS, Bozeman JM, Soong SJ, et al: Platelet surface-bound IgG in patients with immune and nonimmune thrombocytopenia. Blood 1987; 69:278.

Cowan DH, Graham RC, Jr, Baunach D: The platelet defect in leukemia: Platelet ultrastructure, adenine nucleotide metabolism, and the release reaction. J Clin Invest 1975; 56:188.

Cronberg S, Wallmark E, Soderberg I: Effect on platelet aggregation of oral administration of 10 non-steroidal analgesics to humans. Scand J Haematol 1984; 33:155.

Day HJ, Holmsen H: Platelet adenine nucleotide "storage pool deficiency" in thrombocytopenic absent radii syndrome. JAMA 1972; 221:1053.

De Caterina R, Lanza M, Manca G, et al: Bleeding time and bleeding: An analysis of the relationship of the bleeding time test with parameters of surgical bleeding. Blood 1994; 84:3363.

Defreyn G, Machin SJ, Carreras LO, et al: Familial bleeding tendency with partial platelet thromboxane synthetase deficiency: Reorientation of cyclic endoperoxide metabolism. Br J Haematol 1981; 49:29.

Drouin J, McGregor JL, Parmentier S, et al: Residual amounts of glycoprotein Ib concomitant with near-absence of glycoprotein IX in platelets of Bernard-Soulier patients. Blood 1988; 72:1086.

Fabris F, Cordiano I, Mazzuccato M, et al: Labeling of platelet surface glycoproteins with biotin derivatives. Thromb Res 1992a; 66:409.

Fabris F, Cordiano I, Steffan A, et al: Identification of anti-platelet autoantibodies by Western blot in 45 patients with idiopathic thrombocytopenic purpura (ITP). Haematologica 1992b; 77:122.

Feinstein MB, Rodan GA, Cutler LS: Cyclic AMP and calcium in platelet function. *In* Gordon JL (ed): Platelets in Biology and Pathology—2. New York, Elsevier/North-Holland Biomedical Press, 1981, pp 437–472.

Finch CN, Miller JL, Lyle VA, Handin RI: Evidence that an abnormality in the glycoprotein Ib alpha gene is not the cause of abnormal platelet function in a family with classic Bernard-Soulier disease. Blood 1990; 75:2357.

Frelinger AL III, Du X, Plow EF, et al: Monoclonal antibodies to ligand-occupied conformers of integrin $\alpha_{IIb}\beta_3$ (glycoprotein IIb-IIIa) alter receptor affinity, specificity, and function. J Biol Chem 1991; 266:17106.

Fujisawa K, Tani P, McMillan R: Platelet-associated antibody to glycoprotein IIb/IIIa from chronic immune thrombocytopenic purpura patients often binds to divalent cation-dependent antigens. Blood 1993; 81:1284.

Ganguly P, Sutherland SB, Bradford HR: Defective binding of thrombin to platelets in myeloid leukemia. Br J Haematol 1978; 39:599.

George JN, El-Harake MA, Aster RH: Thrombocytopenia due to enhanced platelet destruction by immunologic mechanisms. *In* Beutler E, Lichtman MA, Coller BS, Kipps TJ (eds): Williams Hematology, 5th ed. New York, McGraw-Hill, 1995, p 1316.

Gerrard JM, Kindom SE, Peterson DA, et al: Lysophosphatidic acids: Influence on platelet aggregation and intracellular calcium flux. Am J Pathol 1979; 96:423.

Grottum KA, Hovig T, Holmsen H, et al: Wiskott-Aldrich syndrome: Qualitative platelet defects and short platelet survival. Br J Haematol 1969; 17:373.

Hardisty RM, Machin SJ, Nokes TJC, et al: A new congenital defect of platelet secretion: Impaired responsiveness of the platelets to cytoplasmic free calcium. Br J Haematol 1983; 53:543.

Harker LA, Malpass TW, Branson HE, et al: Mechanism of abnormal bleeding in patients undergoing cardiopulmonary bypass: Acquired transient platelet dysfunction associated with selective alpha granule release. Blood 1980; 56:824.

Hayward CP, Bainton DF, Smith JW, et al: Multimerin is found in the alpha-granules of resting platelets and is synthesized by a megakaryocytic cell line. J Clin Invest 1993; 91:2630.

Hayward CPM, Warkentin TE, Horsewood P, et al: Multimerin: A series of large disulfide-linked multimeric proteins within platelets. Blood 1991; 77:2556.

Heaton WA, Heyns ADP, Joist JH: Measurement of in vivo platelet turnover and organ distribution using ^{111}In labeled platelets. Methods Enzymol 1989; 169:172.

Heaton WA, Davis HH, Melch MJ, et al: Indium-111: A new radionuclide label for studying human platelet kinetics. Br J Haematol 1979; 42:613.

Heilmann E, Friese P, Anderson S, et al: Biotinylated platelets: A new approach to the measurement of platelet life span. Br J Haematol 1993; 85:729.

Hemker HC, van Rijn JLML, Rosing J, et al: Platelet membrane involvement in blood coagulation. Blood Cells 1983; 9:303.

Herbener GH, Dean WL: Immunocytochemical localization of the Ca^{2+}-ATPase polypeptide in human platelets. Biochem Biophys Res Commun 1988; 153:848.

Hermansky F, Pudlak P: Albinism associated with hemorrhagic diathesis and unusual pigmented reticular cells in the bone marrow: Report of two cases with histochemical studies. Blood 1959; 14:162.

Holmsen H, Dangelmaier CA: Measurement of secretion of serotonin. Methods Enzymol 1989; 169:205.

Horowitz HI, Stein IM, Cohen BD, White JG: Further studies on the platelet inhibitor effect of guanidinosuccinic acid: Its role in uremic bleeding. Am J Med 1970; 49:336.

Hoyer LW: The assessment of von Willebrand's disease. *In* Bloom AL (ed): Methods of Hematology, Vol. 5. The Hemophilias. New York, Churchill-Livingstone, 1982, pp 106–121.

Ikeda Y, Handa M, Kawano K, et al: The role of von Willebrand factor and fibrinogen in platelet aggregation under varying shear stress. J Clin Invest 1991; 87:1234.

Ingerman-Wojenski CM, Silver MJ: A quick method for screening platelet dysfunctions using the whole blood lumi-aggregometer. Thromb Haemost 1984; 51:154.

Johnson PC, Sheppeck RA, Bercell SA, et al: Customized neonatal incubator for measurement of platelet-artificial microvascular graft interactions under controlled flow, temperature, and transmural pressure. J Appl Biomater 1992; 3:1.

Joseph R, Welch KMA, D'Andrea G, Levine SR: Epinephrine does not induce platelet aggregation in citrated whole blood. Thromb Res 1987; 45:871.

Jubelirer SJ, Russell F, Vaillancourt R, Deykin D: Platelet arachidonic acid metabolism and platelet function in ten patients with chronic myelogenous leukemia. Blood 1980; 56:728.

Kaywin P, McDonough M, Insel PA, Shattil SJ: Platelet function in essential thrombocythemia: Decreased epinephrine responsiveness associated with a deficiency of platelet α-adrenergic receptor. N Engl J Med, 1978; 299:505.

Keenan JP, Wharton J, Shepherd AJN, Bellingham AJ: Defective platelet lipid peroxidation in myeloproliferative disorders: A possible defect of prostaglandin synthesis. Br J Haematol 1977; 35:275.

Kehrel B, Balleisen L, Kokott R, et al: Deficiency of intact thrombospondin and membrane glycoprotein Ia in platelets with defective collagen-inducted aggregation and spontaneous loss of disorder. Blood 1988; 71:1074.

Kelton JG, Powers PJ, Carter CJ: A prospective study of the usefulness of the measurement of platelet-associated IgG for the diagnosis of idiopathic thrombocytopenic purpura. Blood 1982; 60:1050.

Kelton JG, Murphy WG, Lucarelli A, et al: A prospective comparison of four techniques for measuring platelet-associated IgG. Br J Haematol 1989; 71:97.

Kelton JG, Denomme G, Lucarelli A, et al: Comparison of the measurement of surface or total platelet-associated IgG in the diagnosis of immune thrombocytopenia. Am J Hematol 1985; 18:1.

Kelton JG, Sheridan D, Santos A, et al: Heparin-induced thrombocytopenia: Laboratory studies. Blood 1988; 72:925.

Kempfer AC, Frontroth JP, Lazzari MA: Visualization of platelet glycoproteins Ib and IIIa by immunoenzymatic stain using avidin-biotin peroxidase complex. Thromb Res 1991; 64:395.

Kiefel V, Santoso S, Weisheit M, et al: Monoclonal antibody-specific immunobilization of platelet antigens (MAIPA): A new tool for the identification of platelet-reactive antibodies. Blood 1987; 70:1722.

Kiefel V, Santoso S, Kaufmann E, et al: Autoantibodies against platelet glycoprotein Ib/IX: A frequent finding in autoimmune thrombocytopenic purpura. Br J Haematol 1991; 79:256.

Kunicki TJ, Aster RH: Deletion of the platelet-specific alloantigen Pl^{A1} from platelets in Glanzmann's thrombasthenia. J Clin Invest 1978a; 61:1225.

Kunicki TJ, Johnson MM, Aster RH: Absence of the platelet receptor for drug-dependent antibodies in the Bernard-Soulier syndrome. J Clin Invest 1978b; 62:716.

Kunicki TJ, Furihata K, Bull B, Nugent DJ: The immunogenicity of platelet membrane glycoproteins. Trans Med Rev 1987; 1:21.

Kunicki TJ, Beardsley DS: The alloimmune thrombocytopenias: Neonatal alloimmune thrombocytopenic purpura and post-transfusion purpura. *In* Coller BS (ed): Progress in Hemostasis and Thrombosis, Vol. 9. Philadelphia, W.B. Saunders, 1989, pp 203–232.

Kunishima S, Miura H, Fukutani H, et al: Bernard-Soulier syndrome Kagoshima: Ser 444 —> stop mutation of glycoprotein (GP) Ibα resulting in circulating truncated GPIbα and surface expression of GPIbβ and GPIX. Blood 1994; 84:3356.

Lackner H: Hemostatic abnormalities associated with dysproteinemias. Semin Hematol 1973; 10:125.

Lages B, Malmsten C, Weiss HJ, et al: Impaired platelet response to thromboxane-A2 and defective calcium mobilization in a patient with a bleeding disorder. Blood 1981; 57:545.

Maldonado J: Dysplastic platelets and circulating megakaryocytes in chronic myeloproliferative disease. Blood 1974a; 43:811.

Maldonado JE, Pintado T, Pierre RV: Dysplastic platelets and circulating megakaryocytes in chronic myeloproliferative disease. I. The platelets: Ultrastructure and peroxidase reaction. Blood 1974b; 43:797.

Malpass TW, Hanson SR, Savage B, et al: Prevention of acquired transient defect in platelet plug formation by infused prostacyclin. Blood 1981; 57:736.

Mammen EF, Koets MH, Washington BC, et al: Hemostasis changes during cardiopulmonary bypass surgery. Semin Thromb Hemost 1985; 11:281.

McIntyre BA, Philp RB, Inwood MJ: Effect of ibuprofen on platelet function in normal subjects and hemophiliac patients. Clin Pharmacol Ther 1978; 24:616.

McKenna R, Bachmann F, Whittaker B, et al: The hemostatic mechanism after open-heart surgery. II. Frequency of abnormal platelet functions during and after extracorporeal circulation. J Thorac Cardiovasc Surg 1975; 70:298.

McMillan R, Tani P, Millard F, et al: Platelet-associated and plasma anti-glycoprotein autoantibodies in chronic ITP. Blood 1987; 70:1040.

Mestel F, Oetliker O, Beck E, et al: Severe bleeding associated with defective thromboxane synthetase [letter]. Lancet 1980; 1:157.

Miletich JP, Jackson CM, Majerus PW: Properties of the factor Xa binding site on human platelets. J Biol Chem 1978; 253:6908.

Miller JL: Platelet function testing: An improved approach utilizing lumi-aggregation and an interactive computer system. Am J Clin Pathol 1984; 81:471.

Miller JL, Castella A: Platelet-type von Willebrand's disease. Characterization of a new bleeding disorder. Blood 1982; 60:790.

Miller JL, Kupinski MJ, Castella A, Ruggeri ZM: von Willebrand factor binds to platelets and induces aggregation in platelet-type but not Type IIB von Willebrand disease. J Clin Invest, 1983; 72:1532.

Miller JL, Cunningham D, Lyle VA, et al: Mutation in the gene encoding platelet glycoprotein Ibα in platelet-type von Willebrand disease. Proc Natl Acad Sci USA 1991; 88:4761.

Miller JL, Lyle VA, Cunningham D: Mutation of leucine-57 to phenylalanine in a platelet glycoprotein Ib alpha leucine tandem repeat occurring in patients with an autosomal dominant variant of Bernard-Soulier disease. Blood 1992; 79:439.

Miller JL, Ruggeri ZM, Lyle VA: Unique interactions of asialo von Willebrand factor with platelets in platelet-type von Willebrand disese. Blood 1987; 70:1804.

Moake JL, Turner NA, Stathopoulos NA, et al: Shear-induced platelet aggregation can be mediated by vWF released from platelets, as well as by exogenous large or unusually large vWF multimers, requires adenosine diphosphate, and is resistant to aspirin. Blood 1988; 71:1366.

Montgomery RR, Kunicki TJ, Taves C, et al: Diagnosis of Bernard-Soulier syndrome and Glanzmann's thrombasthenia with a monoclonal assay on whole blood. J Clin Invest 1983; 71:385.

Mustard JF, Kinlough-Rathbone RL, Packham MA, et al: Comparison of fibrinogen associaton with normal and thrombasthenic platelets on exposure to ADP or chymotrypsin. Blood 1979; 54:987.

Nichols WL, Didisheim P, Gerrard JM: Qualitative platelet disorders. *In* Pollar L (ed): Recent Advances in Blood Coagulation—3. New York, Churchill Livingstone, 1981, pp 41–80.

Nieminen U, Kekomaki R: Quinidine-induced thrombocytopenic purpura: Clinical presentation in relation to drug-dependent and drug-independent platelet antibodies. Br J Haematol 1992; 80:77.

Nieuwenhuis HK, Akkerman JW, Houdijk WP, Sixma JJ: Human blood platelets showing no response to collagen fail to express surface glycoprotein Ia. Nature 1985; 318:470.

Nieuwenhuis HK, Akkerman J-WN, Sixma JJ: Patients with a prolonged bleeding time and normal aggregation tests may have storage pool deficiency: Studies on one hundred six patients. Blood 1987; 70:620.

Nieuwenhuis HK, Sakariassen KS, Houdijk PM, et al: Deficiency of platelet membrane glycoprotein Ia associated with a decreased platelet adhesion to subendothelium: A defect in platelet spreading. Blood 1986: 68:692.

Nurden AT, Caen JP: An abnormal platelet glycoprotein pattern in three cases of Glanzmann's thrombasthenia. Br J Haematol 1974; 28:253.

Nurden AT, Caen JP: Specific roles for platelet surface glycoproteins in platelet function. Nature 1975; 255:720.

Nurden AT, George JN, Phillips DR: Platelet membrane glycoproteins: Their structure, function, and modification in disease. *In* Phillips DR, Shuman MA (eds): Biochemistry of Platelets. Orlando, FL, Academic Press, 1986, pp 159–224.

Ogston D: Contact activation of blood coagulation. *In* Poller L (ed): Recent Advances in Blood Coagulation—3. New York, Churchill Livingstone, 1981, pp 109–123.

Orchard MA, Goodchild CS, Prentice CRM, et al: Aprotinin reduces cardiopulmonary bypass-induced blood loss and inhibits fibrinolysis without influencing platelets. Br J Haematol 1993; 85:533.

Owen CA, Jr, Bowie EJW, Didisheim P, Thompson JH: The Diagnosis of Bleeding Disorders. Boston, Little, Brown and Co., 1969.

Pareti FI, Capitanio A, Mannucci PM: Acquired storage pool disease in platelets during disseminated intravascular coagulation. Blood 1976; 48:511.

Pareti FI, Capitanio A, Mannucci L, et al: Acquired dysfunction due to the circulation of "exhausted" platelets. Am J Med 1980; 69:235.

Pareti FI, Gugliotta L, Mannucci L, et al: Biochemical and metabolic aspects of platelet dysfunction in myeloproliferative disorders. Thromb Haemost 1982; 47:84.

Penny R, Castaldi PA, Whitsed HM: Inflammation and haemostasis in paraproteinaemias. Br J Haematol 1971; 20:35.

Perkins HA, McKenzie MR, Fudenberg HH: Hemostatic defects in dysproteinemias. Blood 1970; 35:695.

Peterson DM, Strathopoulos NA, Giorgio TD, et al: Shear-induced platelet aggregation requires von Willebrand factor and platelet membrane glycoproteins Ib and IIb-IIIa. Blood 1987; 69:625.

Pfueller SL, Bilston RA, Logan D, et al: Heterogeneity of drug-dependent platelet antigens and their antibodies in quinine- and quinidine-induced thrombocytopenia: Involvement of glycoproteins Ib, IIb, IIIa, and IX. Blood 1988; 72:1155.

Phillips DR, Agin PP: Platelet membrane defects in Glanzmann's thrombasthenia. Evidence for decreased amounts of two major glycoproteins. J Clin Invest 1977; 60:535.

Phillips DR, Charo IF, Scarborough RM: GPIIb-IIIa: The responsive integrin. Cell 1991; 65:359.

Phillips DR, Jenkins CSP, Lüscher EF, Larrieu MJ: Molecular differences of exposed surface proteins on thrombasthenic platelet plasma membranes. Nature 1975; 257:599.

Pincus MR, Carty RP, Miller JL: Structural implications of the substitution of Val for Met at residue 239 in the alpha chain of human platelet glycoprotein Ib. J Protein Chem 1994; 13:629.

Pincus MR, Dykes DC, Carty RP, et al: Conformational energy analysis of the substitution of Val for Gly 233 in a functional region of platelet GPIbα in platelet-type von Willebrand disease. Biochim Biophys Acta 1991; 1097:133.

Rabiner SF, Molinas F: The role of phenol and phenolic acids on the thrombocytopathy and defective platelet aggregation of patients with renal failure. Am J Med 1970; 49:346.

Raccuglia G: Gray platelet syndrome: A variety of qualitative platelet disorder. Am J Med 1971; 51:818.

Rao AK, Carvalho ACA: Acquired qualitative platelet defects. *In* Colman RW, Hirsh J, Marder VJ, Salzman EW (eds): Hemostasis and Thrombosis, 3rd ed. Philadelphia, J.B. Lippincott, 1994, p 694.

Rao AK, Koike K, Willis J: Platelet secretion defect associated with impaired liberation of arachidonic acid and normal myosin light chain phosphorylation. Blood 1984; 64:914.

Rao AK, Kowalska MA, Disa J: Impaired cytoplasmic ionized calcium mobilization in inherited platelet secretion defects. Blood 1989; 74:664.

Regan MG, Lackner H, Karparkin S: Platelet function and coagulation profile in lupus erythematosus. Ann Intern Med 1974; 81:462.

Remuzzi G, Cavenaghi AE, Mecca G, et al: Prostacyclin-like activity and bleeding in renal failure. Lancet 1977; 2:1195.

Rendu R, Lebret M, Nurden A, Caen JP: Detection of an acquired platelet storage pool disease in three patients with a myeloproliferative disorder. Thromb Haemost 1979; 42:794.

Rodgers RPC, Levin J: A critical reappraisal of the bleeding time. Semin Thromb Hemost 1990; 16:1.

Rosenfeld CS, Bodensteiner DC: Detection of platelet alloantibodies by flow cytometry. Am J Clin Pathol 1986; 85:207.

4

Rosenfeld CS, Nichols G, Bodensteiner DC: Flow cytometric measurement of antiplatelet antibodies. Am J Clin Pathol 1987; 87:518.

Roth GJ: Developing relationships: Arterial platelet adhesion, glycoprotein Ib, and leucine-rich glycoproteins. Blood 1991; 77:5.

Ruggeri ZM, Pareti FI, Mannucci PM, et al: Heightened interaction between platelets and factor VIII/von Willebrand factor in a new subtype of von Willebrand's disease. N Engl J Med 1980; 302:1047.

Ruggeri ZM: Glycoprotein Ib and von Willebrand factor in the process of thrombus formation. Ann NY Acad Sci 1994; 714:200.

Russell SD, Roth GJ: Pseudo-von Willebrand disease: A mutation in the platelet glycoprotein Ibα gene associated with a hyperactive surface receptor. Blood 1993; 81:1787.

Sakariassen KS, Aarts PAMM, de Groot PHG, et al: A perfusion chamber developed to investigate platelet interaction in flowing blood with human vessel wall cells, their extracellular matrix and purified components. J Lab Clin Med, 1983; 102:522.

Sakariassen KS, Nievelstein PF, Coller BS, et al: The role of platelet membrane glycoproteins Ib and IIb-IIIa in platelet adherence to human artery subendothelium. Br J Haematol 1986; 63:681.

Schafer AI: Deficiency of platelet lipoxygenase activity in myeloproliferative disorders. N Engl J Med, 1982; 306:381.

Schafer AI: Bleeding and thrombosis in the myeloproliferative disorders. Blood 1984; 64:1.

Schafer AI: The platelet life cycle: Normal function and qualitative disorders. *In* Handin RI, Lux SE, Stossel TP (eds): Blood: Principles and Practice of Hematology. Philadlephia, J.B. Lippincott, 1995, p 1100.

Scudder LE, Kalomiris EL, Coller BS: Preparation and functional characterization of monoclonal antibodies against glycoprotein Ib. Methods Enzymol 1992; 215:295.

Sehayek E, Ben-Yosef N, Modan M, et al: Platelet parameters and aggregation in essential and reactive thrombocytosis. Am J Clin Pathol 1988; 90:431.

Shaw GM, Axelson J, Maglott JG, LoBuglio AF: Quantification of platelet-bound IgG by ^{125}I-staphylococcal protein A in immune thrombocytopenic purpura and other thrombocytopenic disorders. Blood 1984; 63:154.

Sheridan D, Carter C, Kelton JG: A diagnostic test for heparin-induced thrombocytopenia. Blood 1986; 62:27.

Sims PJ, Ginsberg MH, Plow EF, et al: Effect of platelet activation on the conformation of the plasma membrane glycoprotein IIb-IIIa complex. J Biol Chem 1991; 266:7345.

Simsek S, Admiraal LG, Modderman PW, et al: Identification of a homozygous single base pair deletion in the gene coding for the human platelet glycoprotein Ibα causing Bernard-Soulier syndrome. Thromb Haemost 1994; 72:444.

Smith MC, Dunn M: Impaired thromboxane production in renal failure. Nephron 1981; 29:133.

Spaet TH, Lejnieks F, Gaynor E, Goldstein ML: Defective platelets in essential thrombocythemia. Arch Itern Med 1969; 124:135.

Statland BE, Heagan BM, White JG: Uptake of calcium by platelet relaxing factor. Nature 1969; 223:521.

Stenberg PE, McEver RP, Shuman MA, et al: A platelet alpha-granule membrane protein (GMP-140) is expressed on the plasma membrane after activation. J Cell Biol 1985; 101:880.

Stricker RB, Shuman MA: Quinidine purpura: Evidence that glycoprotein V is a target platelet antigen. Blood 1986; 67:1377.

Stuart MJ, Murphy S, Oski FA: A simple nonradioisotope technic for the determination of platelet life-span. N Engl J Med, 1975; 292:1310.

Tabilio A, Vainchenker W, Van Haecke D, et al: Immunological characterization of the leukemic megakaryocytic line at light and electron microscopic levels. Leuk Res 1984; 8:769.

Takahashi H, Murata M, Moriki T, et al: Substitution of Val for Met at residue 239 of platelet glycoprotein Ib alpha in Japanese patients with platelet-type von Willebrand disease. Blood 1995; 85:727.

Thompson AR, Harker LA: Manual of Hemostasis and Thrombosis, 3rd ed. Philadelphia, F.A. Davis, 1983.

Tijhuis GJ, Klaassen RJL, Modderman PW, et al: Quantification of platelet-bound immunoglobulins of different class and subclass using radiolabelled monoclonal antibodies: Assay conditions and clinical application. Br J Haematol 1991; 77:93.

Turitto VT, Baumgartner HR: Initial deposition of platelets and fibrin on vascular surfaces in flowing blood. *In* Colman RW, Hirsh J, Marder, VJ, Salzman EW (eds): Hemostasis and Thrombosis, 3rd ed. Philadelphia, J.B. Lippincott, 1994, p 805.

Turitto VT, Weiss HJ, Baumgartner HR: Decreased platelet adhesion on vessel segments in von Willebrand's disease: A defect in initial platelet attachment. J Lab Clin Med 1983; 102:551.

van Leeuwen EF, von dem Borne AEG, Jr, von Riesz LE, et al: Absence of platelet-specific alloantigens in Glanzmann's thrombasthenia. Blood 1981; 57:49.

Visentin GP, Ford SE, Scott JP, et al: Antibodies from patients with heparin-induced thrombocytopenia/thrombosis are specific for platelet factor 4 complexed with heparin or bound to endothelial cells. J Clin Invest 1994; 93:81.

Visentin GP, Newman PJ, Aster RH: Characteristics of quinine- and quinidine-induced antibodies specific for platelet glycoproteins IIb and IIIa. Blood 1991; 77:2668.

von dem Borne AEG, Helmerhorst FM, van Leeuwen EF, et al: Autoimmune thrombocytopenia: Detection of platelet autoantibodies with the suspension immunofluorescence test. Br J Haematol 1980; 45:319.

Walsh PN, Murphy S, Barry WE: The role of platelets in the pathogenesis of thrombosis and hemorrhage in patients with thrombocytosis. Thromb Haemost 1977; 38:1085.

Walsh PN: The role of platelets in the contact phase of blood coagulation. Br J Haematol 1972; 22:237.

Ware J, Russell SR, Marchese P, et al: Point mutation in a leucine-rich repeat of platelet glycoprotein Ib alpha resulting in the Bernard-Soulier syndrome. J Clin Invest 1993; 92:1213.

Ware J, Russell SR, Vicente V, et al: Nonsense mutation in the glycoprotein Ib alpha coding sequence associated with Bernard-Soulier syndrome. Proc Natl Acad Sci USA 1990; 87:2026.

Warkentin TE, Hayward CPM, Boshkov LK, et al: Sera from patients with heparin-induced thrombocytopenia generate platelet-derived microparticles with procoagulant activity: An explanation for the thrombotic complications of heparin-induced thrombocytopenia. Blood 1994; 84:3691.

Weiss HJ: Inherited abnormalities of platelet granules and signal transduction. *In* Colman RW, Hirsh J, Marder VJ, Salzman EW (eds): Hemostasis and Thrombosis, 3rd ed. Philadelphia, J.B. Lippincott, 1994, pp 741–749.

Weiss HJ, Meyer D, Rabinowitz R, et al: Pseudo von Willebrand's disease: An intrinsic platelet defect with aggregation by unmodified human factor VIII/von Willebrand factor and enhanced adsorption of its high-molecular-weight multimers. N Engl J Med 1982; 306:326.

Weiss HJ, Rosove HM, Lages BA, Kaplan KL: Acquired storage pool deficiency with increased platelet-associated IgG. Report of five cases. Am J Med 1980; 69:711.

Weiss HJ, Turitto VT, Baumgartner HR: Role of shear rate and platelets in promoting fibrin formation on rabbit subendothelium. Studies utilizing patients with quantitative and qualitative platelet defects. J Clin Invest 1986; 78:1072.

Weiss HJ, Hawiger J, Ruggeri ZM, et al: Fibrinogen-independent platelet adhesion and thrombus formation on subendothelium mediated by glycoprotein IIb-IIIa complex at high shear rate. J Clin Invest 1989; 83:288.

White JG: Ultrastructural studies of the gray platelet syndrome. Am J Pathol 1979; 95:445.

White JG: *In* Bloom AL, Forbes CD, Thomas DP, Tuddenham EGD (eds): Haemostasis and Thrombosis. New York, Churchill Livingstone, 1994.

Williams WJ: Secondary thrombocytosis. *In* Beutler E, Lichtman MA, Coller BS, Kipps TJ (eds): Williams Hematology, Ed. 5. New York, McGraw-Hill, 1995, p 1361.

Witte LD, Kaplan KL, Nossel HL, et al: Studies of the release from human platelets of the growth factor for cultured human arterial smooth muscle cells. Circ Res 1978; 42:402.

Wright SD, Michaelides K, Johnson DJD, et al: Double heterozygosity for mutations in the platelet glycoprotein IX gene in three siblings with Bernard-Soulier syndrome. Blood 1993; 81:2339.

Wu KK, Minkoff IM, Rossi EC, et al: Hereditary bleeding disorder due to a primary defect in platelet release reaction. Br J Haematol 1981; 47:241.

Zahavi J, Marder VJ: Acquired "storage pool disease" of platelets associated with circulating anti-platelet antibodies. Am J Med, 1974; 56:883.

Zucker MB: Platelet aggregation measured by the photometric method. Methods Enzymol 1989; 169:117.

Chapter 29

Blood Coagulation and Fibrinolysis

Jonathan L. Miller, M.D., Ph.D.

NORMAL COAGULATION MECHANISMS

The arrest of bleeding depends on primary platelet plug formation in conjunction with elaboration of a stable fibrin clot. The formation of this clot involves the sequential interaction of a series of plasma proteins in a highly ordered and complex fashion as well as the interaction of these complexes both with blood platelets and with materials released from tissues. In recent years there has been intensive investigation of all aspects of the blood coagulation system. With the increased availability of purified coagulation factors for research, it has been possible to study the interactions (and conditions for interactions) among individual factors directly. In many cases, this has led to a deeper understanding of interactions that had been defined in previous decades by means of "experiments of nature," in which patients with bleeding disorders were found to be deficient in a specific factor. In other instances, however, new interactions have now been established, including apparent "cross-over reactions" connecting the classically formulated "intrinsic" and "extrinsic" systems, as well as important positive and negative feedback loops occurring at multiple levels of the cascade. Moreover, in recent years cDNAs for the coagulation factors have been cloned and sequenced, with the result that the primary amino acid structures of the corresponding proteins have now been determined.

Of major conceptual importance is the method of approaching and understanding the many chemical reactions that subserve hemostasis from the initial bleeding stimulus to final formation of a stable clot. To accomplish this task, it is necessary to understand first the normal series of reactions and then how to localize an abnormality to the specific factor or factors responsible. An examination of the factors that participate in the normal hemostatic mechanism is presented first (Table 29–1 and Fig. 29–1). Laboratory methods of localizing hemostatic abnormalities are considered next. In the latter process, portions of the normal coagulation cascade are artificially broken up into smaller incomplete segments that lend themselves to laboratory localization of factor defects. It must be emphasized, however, that tests (see later under Laboratory Screening Tests of Coagulation) such as the activated partial thromboplastin time (PTT), prothrombin time (PT), or thrombin time (TT) are merely convenient laboratory aids to diagnosis. The "intrinsic pathway," "extrinsic pathway," and other segments that these tests appear to define should accordingly not be thought of as actual physiologic pathways of hemostasis.

Overview of the *In Vivo* Coagulation Cascade

The flow of the reactions believed to underlie hemostasis *in vivo* is depicted by bold print and thick arrows in Figure 29–1. Tissue injury promotes the association of "tissue fac-

Table 29–1. MOLECULAR PROPERTIES OF COAGULATION PROTEINS

	Synonyms	Site of Synthesis	Molecular Mass (kDa)	Function	Protein Characteristics	Plasma Concentration	Chromosomal Location	Gene Organization
Factor XII	Hageman factor	Hepatocyte	80	Protease zymogen		30 μg/ml	5	14 exons
Factor XI		Hepatocyte	160	Protease zymogen	Homodimeric	5 μg/ml	4	15 exons
Factor IX	Christmas factor	Hepatocyte	56	Protease zymogen	Vitamin K–dependent	5 μg/ml	X	8 exons
Factor VIII	Antihemophilic factor	Liver	330	Cofactor	Cofactor to Factor IXa	0.1 μg/ml	X	26 exons
Factor VII		Hepatocyte	50	Protease zymogen	Vitamin K–dependent	0.5 μg/ml	13	9 exons; adjacent to Factor X gene
Tissue factor	Tissue thromboplastin	Many cell types	37	Cofactor	Transmembrane protein	0	1	6 exons
Factor X	Stuart factor	Hepatocyte	56	Protease zymogen	Vitamin K–dependent	10 μg/ml	13	8 exons; adjacent to Factor VII gene
Factor V	Proaccelerin	Hepatocyte, megakaryocyte	330	Cofactor	Cofactor to Factor Xa	10 μg/ml	1	Similar to Factor VIII
Prothrombin (Factor II)		Hepatocyte	72	Protease zymogen	Vitamin K–dependent	100 μg/ml	11	14 exons
Fibrinogen (Factor I)		Hepatocyte	340	Structural	Dimeric, with each monomer having three subchains	200–400 mg/dl	4	Separate genes for α, β, and γ chains (5, 8, and 9 exons, respectively)
Factor XIII	Fibrin-stabilizing factor; Laki-Lorand factor	Hepatocyte	320	Transamidation	Tetrameric (a_2b_2)	10 μg/ml	1 (b) 6 (a)	a and b genes on different chromosomes
von Willebrand factor		Endothelial cell, megakaryocyte	220 (multimers up to 20×10^6)	Platelet adhesion	Carries Factor VIII in plasma	10 μg/ml	12	52 exons; pseudogene on chromosome 22
Protein C		Hepatocyte	62	Regulatory (protease zymogen)	Vitamin K–dependent	5 μg/ml	2	8 exons
Protein S		Hepatocyte	80	Regulatory	Vitamin K–dependent	25 μg/ml	3	15 exons; pseudogene on chromosome 3
Thrombomodulin		Endothelial cell	75–105	Regulatory	Expressed on endothelial surface	0	20	No introns
Antithrombin III		Hepatocyte	60	Regulatory	Forms complex with heparin	150 μg/ml	1	6 exons
Tissue factor pathway inhibitor	Lipoprotein-associated coagulation inhibitor; extrinsic pathway inhibitor	Endothelial cell	33	Regulatory	Circulates in plasma; disulfide-linked to apolipoprotein A-II	115 μg/ml	2	9 exons

Modified from Schafer AI: Coagulation cascade: An overview. *In* Loscalzo J, Schafer AI (eds): Thrombosis and Hemorrhage. Boston, Blackwell Scientific Publishers, 1994, p 4. Reprinted by permission of Blackwell Science, Inc.

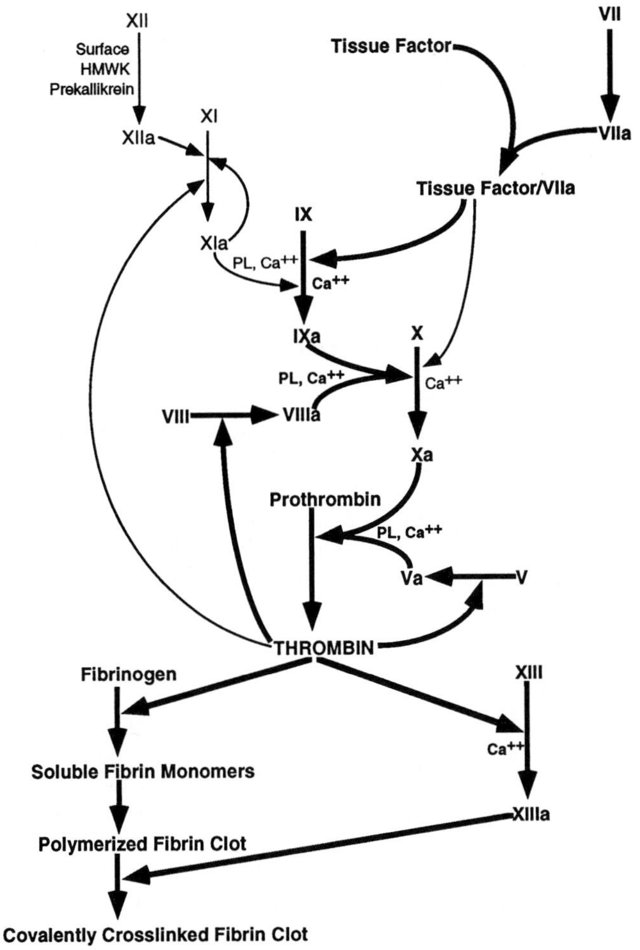

Figure 29–1. Coagulation pathway. Proteins indicated in bold type and connected by thick arrows are believed to comprise the predominant *in vivo* pathway following tissue injury. If the injury is severe enough, activation of Factor XI and the subsequent activation of Factor IX by Factor XIa may occur. Required cofactors are indicated along the arrows of the individual activation reactions. (PL represents phospholipid, which is present on the surface membranes of platelets *in vivo*.)

tor," a 263-amino acid transmembrane glycoprotein (Ruf, 1994) together with an activated form of Factor VII (Factor VIIa) to initiate the coagulation cascade *in vivo*. Factor VIIa, a serine protease, cleaves Factor IX to produce Factor IXa, another serine protease, which in turn, in the presence of activated Factor VIII (Factor VIIIa), activates Factor X to Factor Xa. The Factor VIIa–tissue factor complex under certain conditions can activate Factor X directly—for example, under the standard conditions established for the *in vitro* PT test (see Fig. 29–4).

Factor Xa, in the presence of activated Factor V (Factor Va), then activates prothrombin (Factor II) to thrombin. Thrombin has many roles in hemostasis, but clearly a central role is its ability to cleave bonds in the fibrinogen molecule to produce monomeric fibrin—the building block of the actual clot. Fibrin monomers subsequently polymerize to form a fibrin clot, which is subsequently stabilized through covalent cross-linking by Factor XIIIa. A deficiency of any of the factors involved in this complex sequence of reactions results in a clinically significant bleeding tendency.

Further Considerations of the Coagulation Cascade

It had been thought for many years that the coagulation cascade could be initiated through activation of the "contact" factors, which include Factor XII (Hageman factor), prekallikrein, high-molecular-weight kininogen, and Factor XI. Yet, with the exception of Factor XI, it is now widely accepted that deficiencies of the contact factors do not result in any increased bleeding tendency. Reconciliation of these clinical observations with the classic intrinsic pathway (which was believed to be initiated by activation of the contact factors) is thus difficult. An emerging alternative view that is increasingly gaining acceptance is the following: Normal *in vivo* hemostasis probably does not involve the participation of Factor XII, prekallikrein, or high-molecular-weight kininogen, despite the requirement for their presence in the *in vitro* clotting test, the PTT (see Fig. 29–4). The usual starting point for the coagulation cascade would thus be Factor VII, not Factor XII. Not explained by this schema, however, is the clinical observation that deficiencies of Factor XI may be associated with significant bleeding. A possible explanation of this paradox is that the critical *in vivo* activation of Factor XI occurs not through the proteolytic action of Factor XIIa but rather through direct proteolytic attack by thrombin or by another serine protease (Rapaport, 1992; Gailani, 1993; Naito, 1991). In this view, thrombin initially produced through the Factor VIIa–tissue factor pathway cleaves Factor XI to produce Factor XIa, thereby providing an additional means of activating Factor IX to Factor IXa. Although thrombin has been shown to be capable of activating Factor XI using purified reagents under carefully defined conditions, it is still unclear whether or not similar events occur *in vivo* (Scott, 1992). Because, following an initiating injury, the Factor VIIa-tissue factor pathway is believed to operate for only a limited time before natural inhibitors effectively turn it off (see later discussion), in the presence of a substantial injury, the pathway requiring activation of Factor IX by Factor XIa would become critical (Rapaport, 1992).

An additional puzzle presented by our current understanding of the coagulation cascade is how Factor VII actually becomes activated. Laboratory studies indicate that Factor VII can be transformed to its active enzymatic form following proteolytic attack by Factors XIIa, Xa, IXa, or thrombin (Broze, 1994) or by autoactivation in the presence of tissue factor (Yamamoto, 1992). Which, if any, of these potential activators is primarily responsible for achieving activation of Factor VII *in vivo* is presently unknown.

Activation of Factor IX by Factor XIa does not require the presence of tissue factor, but it does require negatively charged phospholipids as well as ionized calcium. *In vivo*, blood platelets are presumed to be the primary source of these phospholipids. In the resting state a limited amount of phospholipid is present on the platelet surface, but during platelet activation in the course of hemostasis (see Chap. 28) there appears to be a "flip-flop" of phosphatidylserine and phosphatidylethanolamine from the cytoplasmic surface to the outer surface of the platelet membrane (Bevers, 1982; Hemker, 1983). This shift of phospholipids probably is instrumental in providing an optimal surface for facilitating co-

4

agulant activation reactions. In the laboratory, phospholipid extracts ("partial thromboplastins") added to platelet-free plasma replace platelet phospholipid in supporting the activation of Factor IX by Factor XIa as well as in the subsequent steps shown in Figure 29–1 where platelets are indicated as cofactors.

Following the activation of Factor IX by Factor VIIa-tissue factor, Factor IXa forms a complex with phospholipid and activated Factor VIII that, in the presence of calcium, activates Factor X. Factor VIII is a critical molecule in hemostasis, and its hereditary absence constitutes the disorder known as hemophilia A (see later discussion). Thrombin cleaves peptide bonds within Factor VIII to produce the activated form of this cofactor. Schematic representation of the Factor VIII gene and gene product is shown in Figure 29–2. Thrombin similarly cleaves peptide bonds within Factor V to produce the active form of this analogous cofactor.

Once formed, Factor Xa in turn becomes the activator of the zymogen prothrombin. *In vivo*, this reaction is thought to proceed on the surface of platelets, where activated Factor V (of plasma or platelet origin) in the presence of calcium forms a receptor for Factor Xa, and the potent "prothrombinase" thereby formed catalyzes the conversion of prothrombin to the active enzyme thrombin. The importance of each of these cofactors to the production of thrombin, as well as the dramatic contrast of reaction rates when simple phospholipids are substituted for platelets in this process, is evident in Table 29–2. The interactions of prothrombin, Factor Xa, Factor Va, and Factor VIIIa with the platelet surface have been extensively studied (Rosenberg, 1987; Sims, 1989; Nesheim, 1991).

Table 29–2. EFFECTS OF COFACTORS UPON RATE OF THROMBIN FORMATION FROM PROTHROMBIN

Cofactors	Relative Rate
Factor Xa, Ca^{2+}	1
Factor Xa, phospholipid, Ca^{2+}	50
Factor Xa, phospholipid, Factor Va, Ca^{2+}	20,000
Factor Xa, platelets, Ca^{2+}	300,000

From Miletich JP, et al: J Biol Chem 253:6908, 1978.

Clot Formation

Thrombin formation marks a critical event in the hemostatic process. Thrombin directly cleaves peptide fragments from the α and β chains of fibrinogen (fibrinopeptides A and B, respectively) to create fibrin monomers that subsequently assemble into a highly ordered, polymeric fibrin clot. Thrombin also functions as an extremely potent physiologic stimulus of platelet activation (see Chap. 28). As mentioned previously, thrombin proteolysis of native Factors VIII and V produces activated forms of these molecules (see Fig. 29–1), providing amplification for the activation of Factor X and prothrombin, respectively.

Formation of fibrin polymer is the end point detected in the major clotting time tests of the coagulation system (PT, PTT, and TT). This clot, however, is still rather loose, being held together principally by electrostatic interactions between neighboring molecules of fibrin monomer. Final stabilization of the clot is achieved by the formation of covalent lysine to glutamine linkages between γ chains of adjacent

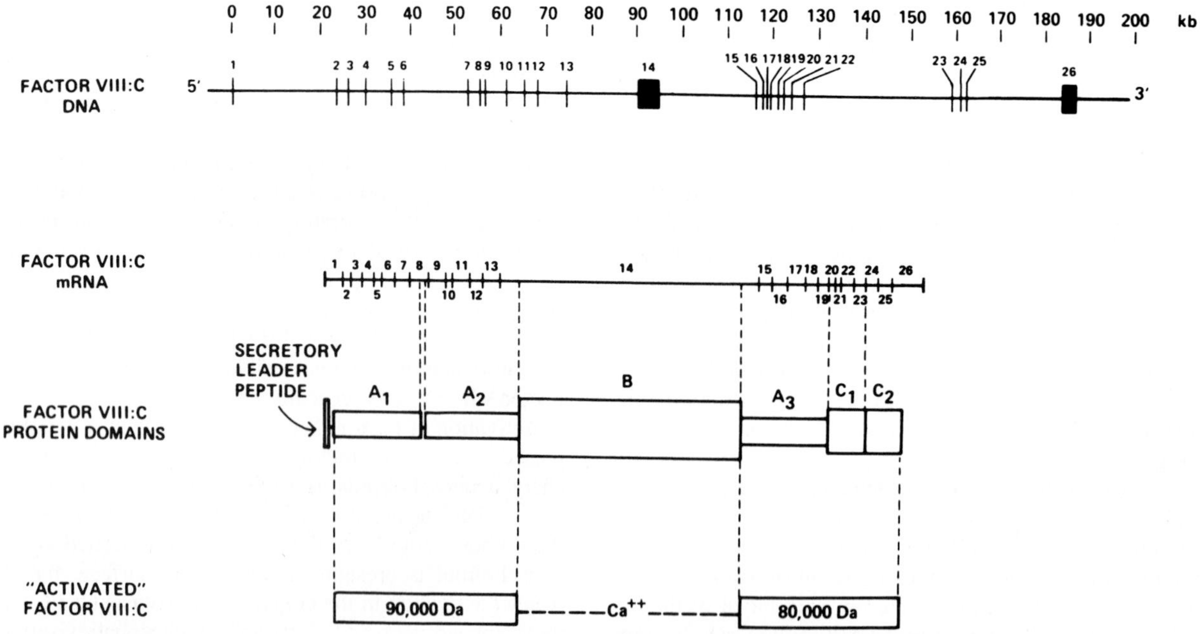

Figure 29–2. Schematic representation of Factor VIII gene, mRNA, protein domains, and "activated" form. The arrangement of secretory leader peptide, A_1, A_2, B, A_3, C_1, and C_2 domains of the Factor VIII protein is shown, and the relationship with the coding sequences of the mRNA is depicted. The activated form of Factor VIII consists of two polypeptide chains: a heavy, 90-kilodalton (kDa) chain and a light, 80 kDa chain, which contain A_1A_2 and $A_3C_1C_2$ domains, respectively. (From Antonarakis SE: The molecular genetics of hemophilia A and B in man: Factor VIII and Factor IX deficiency. Adv Hum Genet 1988; 17:27.)

fibrin molecules as well as between adjacent α chains through the activity of *Factor XIIIa (fibrin-stabilizing factor)*. This transglutaminase enzyme is formed from its inactive zymogen (Factor XIII) by the proteolytic action of thrombin. Not only is calcium required for Factor XIII activation, but fibrinogen itself may serve as a cofactor in this reaction. Factor XIIIa additionally covalently cross-links the physiologic inhibitor of fibrinolysis, α_2-antiplasmin inhibitor, to the fibrin clot, making the clot less susceptible to lysis by plasmin.

When platelets are present during clot formation, there is eventual contraction of the formed clot, which is thought to be mediated by the platelet contractile protein, thrombosthenin. The precise *in vivo* correlate of this "clot retraction" observable in the test tube is not fully understood.

Natural Inhibitors of Coagulation

A variety of natural inhibitors serve to put "brakes" on a cascade that, if left unchecked, might extend the mere cessation of a bleed into a massive thrombosis of the circulatory system. The system of checks and balances is complex, involving both a number of molecules termed natural anticoagulants (Fig. 29–3) and an entire fibrinolytic system that is poised to dissolve formed clots once they are formed (see later on).

Initiation of the Factor VIIa-tissue factor pathway of blood coagulation soon results in formation of Factor Xa (see earlier). The tissue factor pathway inhibitor (TFPI), a 34-kDa protein, is a complex molecule that binds both Factor Xa and the Factor VIIa–tissue factor complex (Girard, 1990;

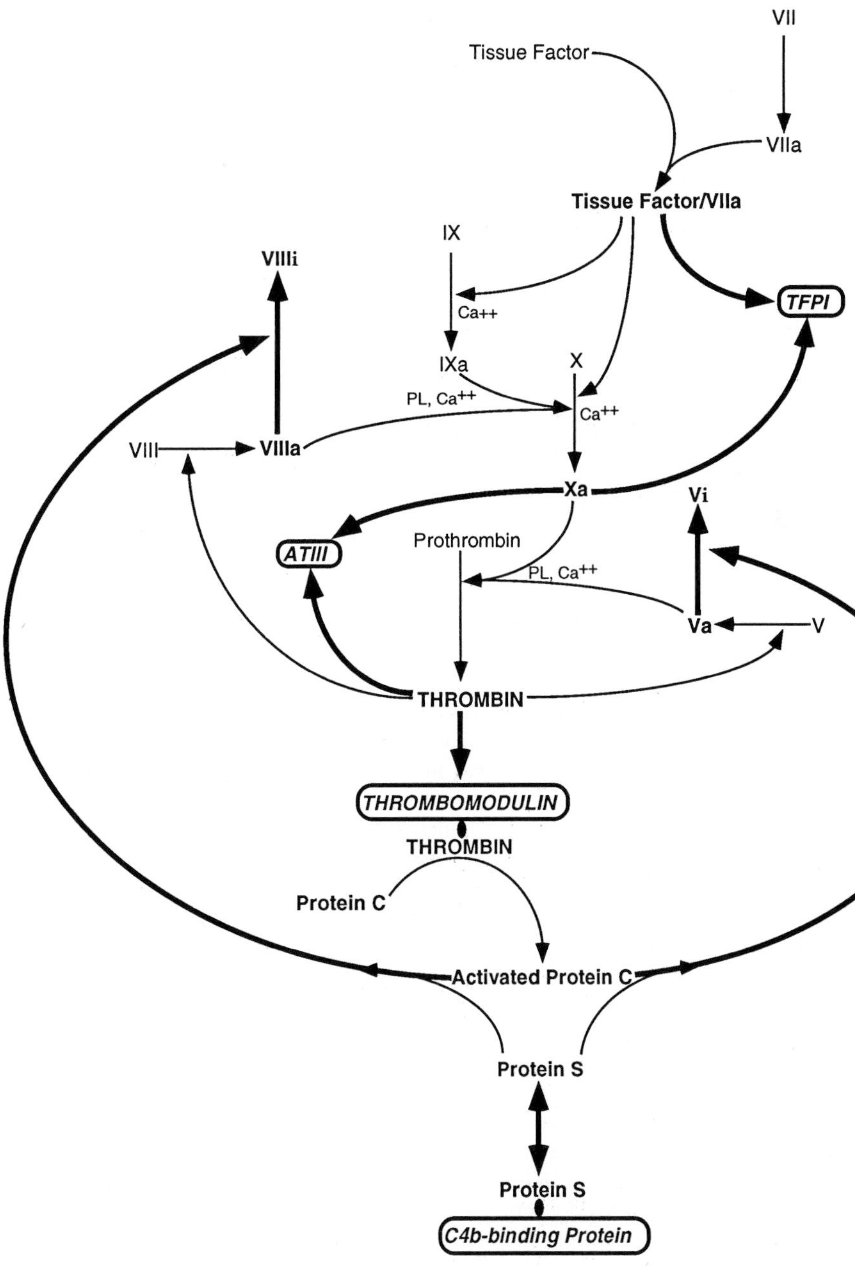

Figure 29–3. Natural inhibitors of coagulation. Reactions represented by thick arrows indicate the major mechanisms by which enzymes and cofactors of the coagulation pathway are inhibited. (ATIII = antithrombin III; TFPI = tissue factor pathway inhibitor.) Proteins that exert an inhibitory effect by binding components of the coagulation system are shown in italics.

Rapaport, 1992). As a result, TFPI down-regulates the Factor VII–tissue factor pathway. In the presence of substantial injury, though, thrombin molecules that have been formed from the zymogen prothrombin may sustain the clotting cascade through thrombin activation of Factor XI, Factor VIII, and Factor V.

A key target for natural anticoagulants is thrombin itself. There are in fact several different ways in which thrombin activity is regulated. Antithrombin III is a member of the "serpin" superfamily of *ser*ine *p*roteinase *in*hibitors (Carrell, 1985), which also includes α_1-antitrypsin, α_2-antiplasmin, heparin cofactor II, and plasminogen activator inhibitor. Antithrombin III is the principal physiologic inhibitor of thrombin and of Factor Xa. It has also been shown to possess inhibitor activity against Factors XIIa, XIa, and IXa. Antithrombin III and thrombin appear to form a 1 : 1 complex that is enzymatically inactive and can be detected by specific antibodies raised against the complex. Monitoring the titer of this antigenic complex is one means of assessing the extent of *in vivo* coagulation. In the presence of heparin, the anticoagulant activity of antithrombin III is greatly enhanced, and this enhancement is in fact believed to constitute the primary mechanism of heparin's anticoagulant effects. For example, the rate constant for the reaction between thrombin and antithrombin III is increased more than 2000 times in the presence of heparin (Barrowcliffe, 1994). *Heparin cofactor II* is an additional, although comparatively minor, inhibitor of thrombin (Tollefsen, 1982). The hereditary deficiency of heparin cofactor II may be associated with a tendency toward thrombosis (Sie, 1986; Tran, 1986). Thrombin activity is also inhibited by the glycoprotein α_2-*macroglobulin* (molecular weight 725,000 daltons). With the exception of kallikrein, none of the other coagulant enzymes is significantly inhibited by α_2-macroglobulin. Thrombin interacts with α_2-macroglobulin in such a fashion that although the thrombin–α_2-macroglobulin complex still retains enzymatic activity against small synthetic substrates, its actions on large natural substrates are effectively inhibited, most likely owing to steric hindrance.

Thrombin activity is additionally modulated in a rather different manner. A transmembrane glycoprotein on endothelial cells termed *thrombomodulin* (Esmon, 1981) serves as a sort of sink for circulating thrombin molecules. Once bound to the thrombomodulin, thrombin undergoes a change in conformation that dramatically alters its substrate preference. The ability of thrombin to cleave procoagulant molecules or activate platelets is greatly diminished in conjunction with the acquisition of a new substrate preference—the natural anticoagulant zymogen precursor protein C (Kisiel, 1977). Activated protein C (APC) in turn serves as an important modulator both of coagulation and of fibrinolysis.

Protein C is a 62-kDa protein whose synthesis depends on vitamin K. Following activation of the zymogen by thrombin, APC proteolytically cleaves Factors Va and VIIIa to inactive forms (Factors Vi and VIIIi, respectively) of these important coagulant factors.

APC injected into dogs also appears to lead to the release into the circulation of plasminogen activator (Comp, 1981), although subsequent studies performed in a primate model were unable to establish such a relationship between protein C and the fibrinolytic system (Colucci, 1984). An additional vitamin K–dependent natural anticoagulant, termed *protein S*, appears to function as a cofactor for the inactivation of clotting factors by activated protein C. Thus, protein S bound to phospholipid greatly accelerates the inactivation of Factor Va by APC; similar interactions occurring *in vivo* may be localized to the surface of platelets, peripheral blood cells, or endothelial cells (Rosenberg, 1987).

Since the description by Griffin (1981) of familial thrombotic disease associated with decreased levels of protein C, many additional kindreds have been reported. Heterozygotes for protein C deficiency that have approximately 50% of normal protein C levels may experience thrombotic events, typically in adulthood. It must be emphasized, however, that there is great variability in the expression of clinical symptoms among heterozygotes. Thus, the heterozygous parents of homozygous infants with purpura fulminans and venous thrombosis may themselves be entirely asymptomatic. The apparent lack of concordance between a thrombotic tendency and protein C levels consistent with heterozygous deficiency in a study of the general population (Miletich, 1987) has added further complexity to this important issue, raising the possibility that those patients with protein C deficiency who actually become symptomatic might have an additional abnormality.

Protein C antigen levels may be measured by Laurell electroimmunoassay or other immunologic methods in essentially the same manner as von Willebrand factor (see later). Functional assay of protein C initially proved more difficult to standardize but is being used with increasing frequency in clinical laboratory evaluation and may be helpful in identifying patients who have a *qualitative* abnormality of protein C. In patients on warfarin therapy, it is difficult to interpret the results of protein C assays. In this instance it is sometimes helpful to assay another vitamin K–dependent factor (e.g., Factor II or Factor X) in parallel with the protein C assay to be able to make at least a rough estimate about the degree to which vitamin K antagonism may be reducing the assayed levels of these factors.

Hereditary venous thrombosis may also be associated with heterozygous protein S deficiency (i.e., levels of protein S approximately 50% of normal). Because circulating protein S loses its functional activity on becoming complexed with C4b-binding protein, measurement of the distribution of protein S between free and bound forms is helpful in the laboratory evaluation of protein S deficiency (Comp, 1986).

In 1993 Dahlbäck reported a kindred with a strong family history of recurrent thromboses in whom there appeared to be APC "resistance" (Dahlbäck, 1993). Through a series of studies in several laboratories it has recently become apparent that a mutation in the Factor V molecule (most typically a point mutation at amino acid residue 506) (Dahlbäck, 1994; Greengard, 1994; Bertina, 1994) that prevents effective proteolysis by APC at this site constitutes a major cause of this resistance. Additional causes of APC resistance also must be considered, including autoantibodies that may arise in association with lupus anticoagulants (Bokarewa, 1994). Based on studies available to date, APC resistance as an underlying cause of thrombosis may be more prevalent than deficiencies of antithrombin III, protein C, and protein S together (Svensson, 1994; Bauer, 1994). Assay of APC resistance is performed by assessing the ability of exogenously added APC to impede the time needed for clot formation in a standard clotting assay, most typically a modification of the PTT (Dahlbäck, 1993).

Laboratory Screening Tests of Coagulation (Fig. 29–4)

All coagulation testing is critically dependent on the quality of the plasma specimen obtained. A clean venipuncture with a minimum of trauma to tissues is required. Often a two-syringe technique is used, in which a few milliliters of blood obtained in the first syringe either is used for purposes other than coagulation testing or is discarded. Citrate is the anticoagulant routinely used for coagulation screening tests as well as for many of the more specialized coagulation tests. Citrated plasma essentially free of platelets is prepared by standard centrifugation procedures.

The prothrombin time (PT) is performed by adding a source of tissue factor and phospholipid (typically an extract from brain or lung) to citrated plasma, adding an excess of calcium, and measuring the time to clot formation. Recombinant tissue factor has also recently been employed (Tripodi 1993, Bader 1994, Roussi 1994). Prolongations of the PT may be associated with deficiencies of factors comprising the classic extrinsic pathway—Factors VII, X, V, II, and fibrinogen, a combination of these factors, or the presence of an inhibitor. It must be emphasized that the *in vitro* PT test differs in an important way from the actual cascade believed to occur *in vivo*. Under the conditions established for the PT test, Factor VIIa in the presence of tissue factor effectively activates Factor X to Factor Xa. Thus, despite the crucial involvement of Factor IX in the Factor VIIa–tissue factor pathway that occurs *in vivo, the level of Factor IX in the patient plasma does not affect the result of the PT determination.*

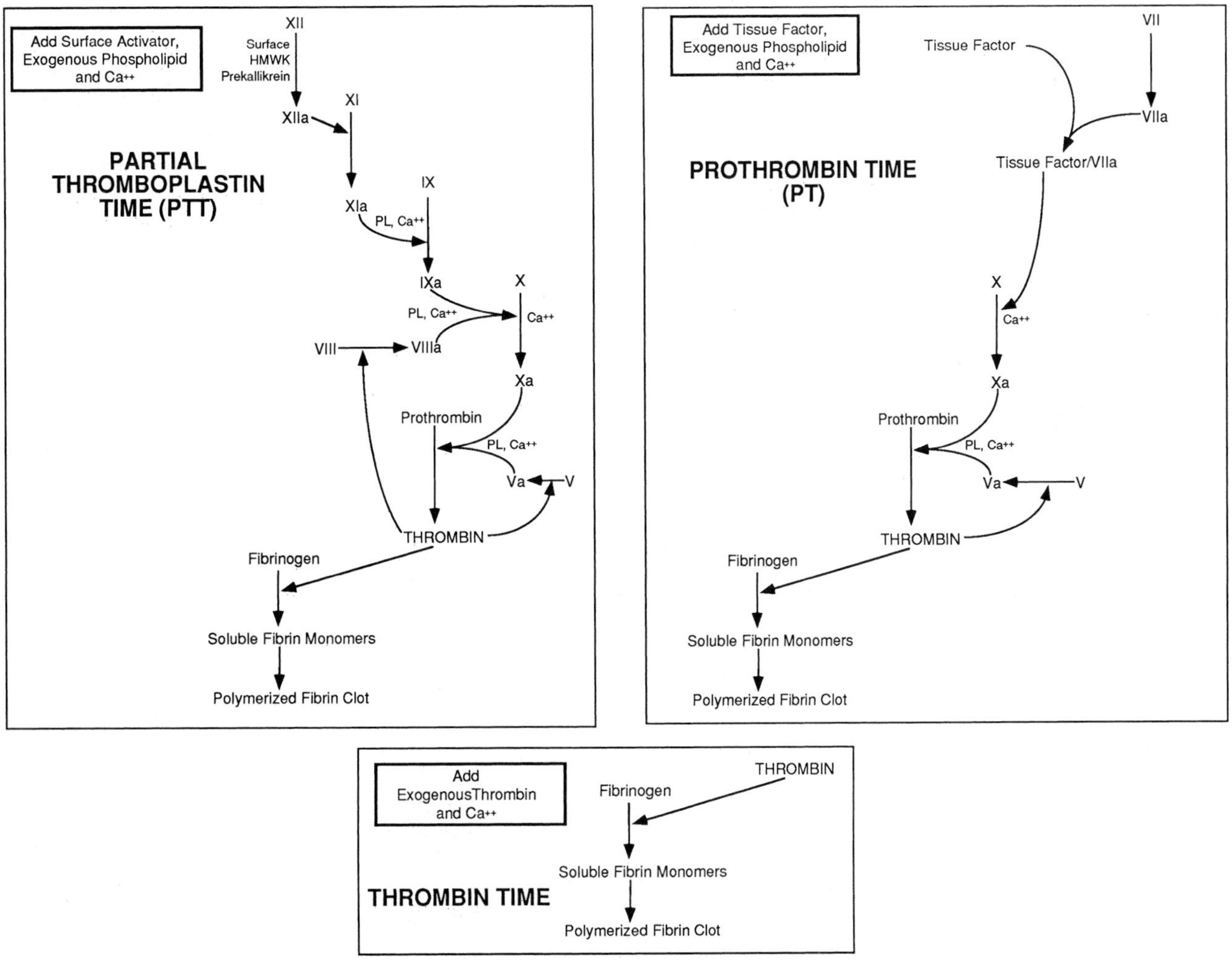

Figure 29–4. Coagulation screening tests. The end point in each of these tests is the number of seconds until the detection of a clot, following addition of the indicated reagents to citrated platelet-free patient plasma. Required cofactors are indicated along the arrows of the individual activation reactions. Although these tests follow the general flow of the *in vivo* coagulation system illustrated in Figure 29–1, the screening tests have been optimized so as to identify specific factors that may be abnormal in quantity or function. Although a deficiency of a single factor may lead to a prolongation of a screening test, occasionally a deficiency of one factor may be masked by an increase in the level of one or more other factors, such as a greatly elevated level of Factor VIII. Note that in the prothrombin time (PT) test, the tissue factor/VIIa complex directly activates Factor X, without the need for Factor IX. (PL represents exogenously added phospholipid.)

The *activated partial thromboplastin time* (aPTT, or simply PTT) is performed on citrated plasma by activating the contact factors (e.g., with kaolin, ellagic acid, or celite), adding a standardized phospholipid preparation as a platelet substitute, and then measuring the time to clot formation following the addition of an excess of calcium. The PTT is prolonged by a deficiency of factors comprising the classic intrinsic pathway—prekallikrein, high-molecular-weight kininogen, Factors XII, XI, IX, VIII, X, V, II, and fibrinogen, or by inhibitors directed against the involved factors or complexes. Shortening of the PTT may be seen in conjunction with an activated coagulation system, for instance, in a patient with a compensated, low-grade consumptive coagulopathy.

The thrombin time (TT) is performed by adding exogenous thrombin to citrated plasma and measuring the time to clot formation. A deficiency (or abnormality) of fibrinogen and the presence of heparin or fibrin(ogen) degradation products are the most common causes of a prolonged TT.

NORMAL FIBRINOLYSIS

Clot formation interrupts blood loss from damaged vessels, but ultimately the clot must be removed if blood flow is to resume. This latter condition is achieved through dissolution of the clot by the *fibrinolytic system* (Table 29–3). The enzyme *plasmin* sequentially cleaves a series of bonds in the fibrin molecules, releasing peptidic *fibrin degradation products* (FDP), and producing clot lysis.

Several mechanisms leading to the formation of active plasmin have been elucidated (Fig. 29–5). Activation of the contact factors of coagulation is associated with conversion of the inactive zymogen, *plasminogen*, to the active enzyme plasmin.

Table 29–3. MOLECULAR COMPONENTS OF THE PLASMA FIBRINOLYTIC SYSTEM AND THEIR CHARACTERISTICS

Name	Molecular Form(s) M_r	Molecular Form(s) Chains	Plasma Concentration	Plasma Half-Life	Selected Functional Properties
Plasminogen	88,000 (Glu1) 83,000 (Lys77)	Single	2.4 μmol/L (210 mg/L)	2.2 days 0.8 days	Zymogen; lysine binding sites for fibrin on the kringle portions; activator-sensitive site at Arg560–Val
Plasmin	88,000 (Glu1) 83,000 (Lys77) 38,000 (Val442)	Two	0	0.1	Serine protease; active site on the light chain (M_r 26,000); variable heavy chain containing kringle structures
Plasminogen activators					
Endogenous					
Tissue plasminogen activator (t-PA)	72,000	One or two	2 μg/L	5 min	Single-chain form rapidly converted to two-chain form by plasmin or in the presence of fibrin, high fibrin affinity and increased activity in the presence of fibrin
Single-chain urokinase-like plasminogen activator (scu-PA) (pro-urokinase)	54,000	Single	6.5 pmol/L (4 μg/L)	Stable	Low intrinsic activity; plasmin converts to a two-chain active enzyme (UK)
Two-chain urokinase	54,000 33,000	Two		10 min	Serine protease; normally present in urine
Exogenous					
Streptokinase (SK)	48,000	Single		30 min	Inactive by itself; forms active equimolar complex with plasminogen
Acyl-plasminogen streptokinase activator complex (APSAC)	131,000	Complex		70 min	Lys-plasminogen complexed to SK, made chemically inert by acyl attachment, binds to fibrin, active upon spontaneous deacylation
Inhibitors					
α_2-Plasmin inhibitor	69,000	Single	1 μmol/L (69 mg/L)	2.6 days	Inhibits plasmin by forming an irreversible complex with the catalytic site; prevents plasmin binding to fibrin and is itself bound to fibrin by Factor XIII_a
Plasminogen activator inhibitor-1 (PAI-1)	50,000	Single	2 nmol/L (25 μg/L)		Interacts with the catalytic site of UK or t-PA to form an inactive complex; occurs in both active and latent forms

From Francis CW, Marder VJ: Physiologic regulation and pathologic disorders of fibrinolysis. *In* Colman RW, Hirsh J, Marder VJ, Salzman EW (eds): Hemostasis and Thrombosis: Basic Principles and Clinical Practice, 3rd ed. Philadelphia, JB Lippincott, 1994, p 1077.

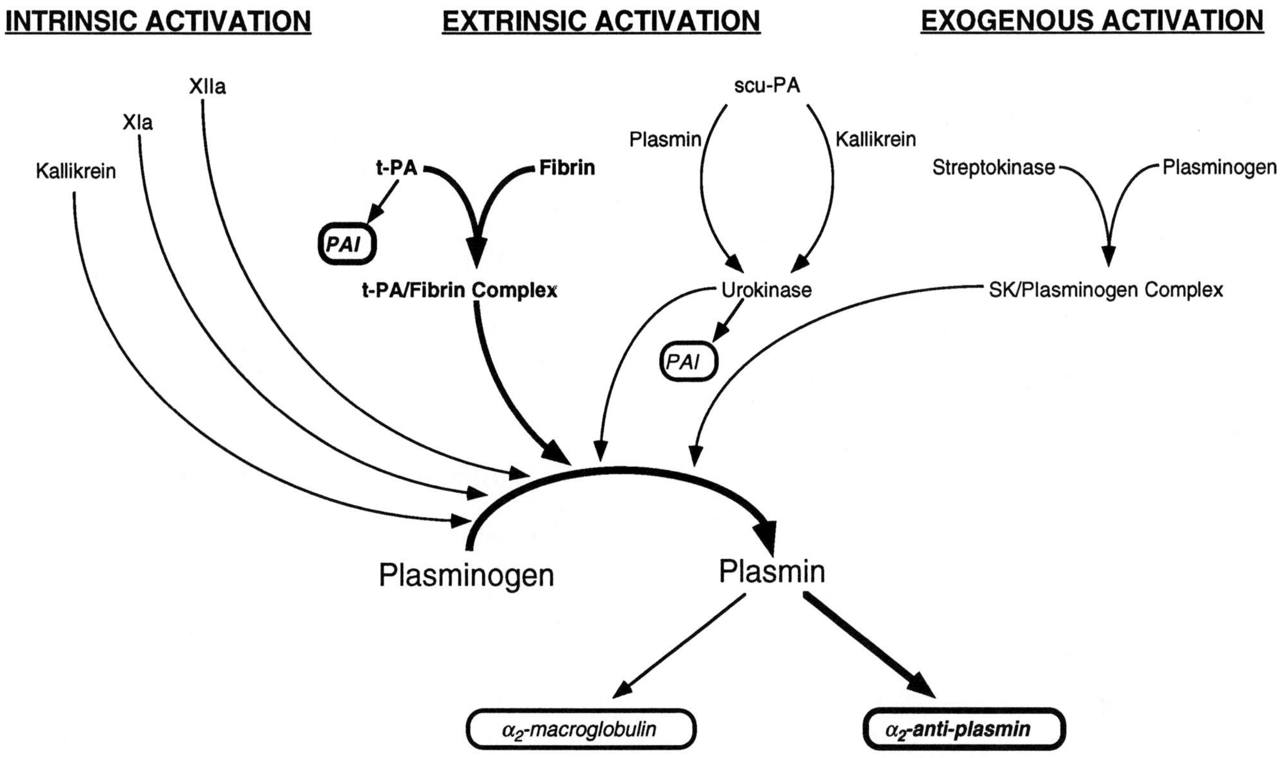

Figure 29–5. Activation and inhibition of the fibrinolytic system. Inhibitors of plasminogen activator or of plasmin are shown in italics. (t-PA = tissue plasminogen activator; scu-PA = single-chain urokinase precursor; PAI = tissue plasminogen activator inhibitor.)

Factor XIIa, kallikrein, and high-molecular-weight kininogen all appear to play roles in this process. Native plasminogen, which has a molecular weight of 88,000 daltons and an amino-terminal glutamic acid ("glu-plasminogen"), undergoes limited proteolytic cleavage of the amino-terminal region, resulting in "lys-plasminogen." Lysplasminogen then undergoes cleavage of a single arginine-valine bond, resulting in active plasmin ("lys-plasmin"). Activation of plasminogen by the other pathways (see later discussion) proceeds via cleavage of the same arginine-valine bond. Although glu-plasminogen can also undergo this arginine-valine bond cleavage, activation proceeds at a much faster rate if glu-plasminogen is first converted to lys-plasminogen.

Tissue plasminogen activator (t-PA) is a 70,000-dalton enzyme produced in vascular and other tissues. Binding of t-PA to fibrin greatly enhances its activity. In recent years, recombinant human t-PA has been approved as a thrombolytic agent. Because it requires fibrin (as is present in the target thrombi) to work effectively as a plasminogen activator, t-PA produces relatively little lysis of circulating fibrinogen. Plasminogen activator inhibitor-1 (PAI-1) and PAI-2 are natural inhibitors that serve to check plasminogen activation.

Urokinase and its single-chain precursor scu-PA (see Table 29–3), are potent plasminogen activators found in human urine and are also produced by kidney cell cultures. Purified urokinase has been used clinically in thrombolytic therapy.

The bacterial protein *streptokinase* also possesses plasminogen activator activity and is used in thrombolytic therapy. Streptokinase differs from the previously described plasminogen activators in that it is not an enzyme. Instead, streptokinase binds to plasminogen (or to plasmin), whereupon the streptokinase-plasmin(ogen) complex then develops plasminogen activator activity. Antigenicity of streptokinase has been a limiting feature, and work is currently in progress to try to identify functional portions of the streptokinase molecule that may possess much lower antigenic activity.

From a clinical standpoint, the various pathways used for the activation of plasminogen (see Fig. 29–5) offer advantages and disadvantages in terms of efficiency of clot lysis and concomitant fibrinogenolysis. By means of highly innovative genetic engineering, hybrid molecules possessing the desired regions of the different plasminogen activators have in fact now been produced (Haber, 1989; Lijnen, 1992). To date, the clinical laboratory has had a relatively small role in monitoring the course of antifibrinolytic therapy. A coagulation rate assay for fibrinogen (Clauss technique) has been suggested for monitoring thrombolytic therapy (Garabedian, 1988). Bell (1995) has also recommended monitoring prolongation of the TT to manage fibrinolytic therapy.

Plasmin, once formed, is capable not only of degrading fibrin clots (*fibrinolysis*) but also, as mentioned earlier, of degrading native fibrinogen (*fibrinogenolysis*). The sequence of proteolytic steps by which this latter process occurs has been intensively studied, and an increasingly complex nomenclature of degradation products has resulted. A simplified schematic diagram of these steps is presented in Figure 29–6. The earliest proteolytic activity results in the still-clottable X fragment, which is subsequently degraded to the unclottable Y and D fragments. The Y fragment, consisting of D plus E portions, is then itself split into these components. Small peptides are also produced at a number of the proteolytic cleavages.

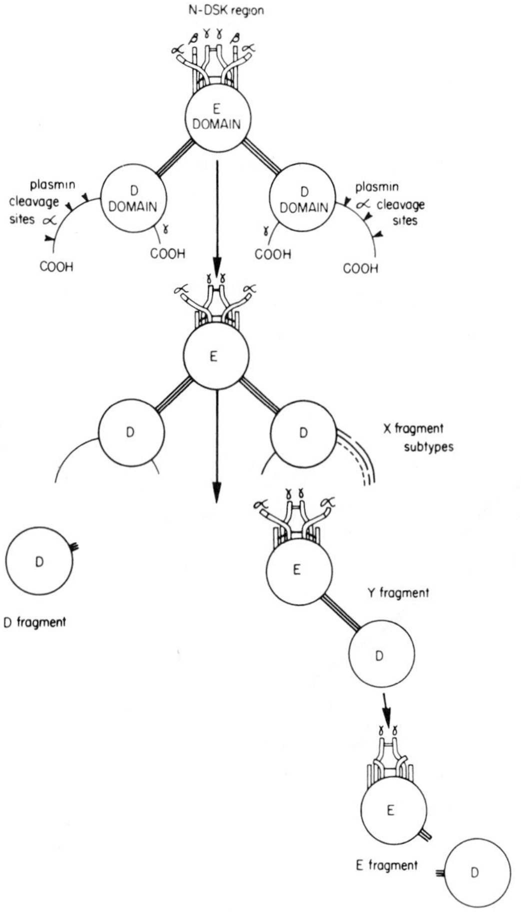

Figure 29–6. Degradation of fibrinogen by plasmin. (From Rosenberg RD: Hemorrhagic disorders I. Protein interactions in the clotting mechanism. *In* Beck WS [ed]: Hematology, 5th ed. Cambridge, MA, MIT Press, 1991, p 531.)

When a normally cross-linked fibrin clot is dissolved by plasmin, isolated D and E fragments are not the characteristic end-stage fragments. Rather, a variety of complexes are found, most characteristically one composed of two D and one E moieties (D_2E fragment), which is called a *D-dimer.* The degradation of cross-linked fibrin is shown schematically in Figure 29–7.

By rendering fibrinogen unclottable and lysing fibrin clots, plasmin directly counterbalances the tendency toward coagulation. Direct effects of plasmin against the aggregation of platelets induced by thrombin have also been demonstrated (Miller, 1975; Adelman, 1986; Michelson, 1990; Lu, 1993). Plasmin additionally exerts proteolytic attack on activated Factors VIIIa and Va, hastening their inactivation. FDP produced in fibrinolysis themselves possess anticoagulant effects, inhibiting fibrin polymerization and enzymatic activity of some coagulant enzymes, most notably thrombin.

The primary inactivator of plasmin is a protein of 70 kDa known as α_2-antiplasmin. α_2-Antiplasmin quickly forms a 1:1 stoichiometric complex with plasmin, and the assay of this complex may serve as a useful indicator of *in vivo* fibrinolysis (Collen, 1980; Suffredini, 1989). α_2-Macroglobulin can also be shown to have antiplasmin activity, but it is slower acting and probably of only minor importance in normal hemostasis.

Except in instances such as disseminated intravascular coagulation or therapeutic thrombolysis, it is unusual for actual fibrinogenolysis to occur *in vivo*. Even in the rare patient with a congenital absence of α_2-antiplasmin, significant fibrinogenolysis is not observed. Within the gel-phase of a clot, however, conditions are quite different. Despite the presence of α_2-antiplasmin cross-linked to polymerizing fibrin by Factor XIIIa, plasmin present within the clot is nevertheless able to bring about eventual fibrin dissolution. The precise mechanisms whereby fibrinolytic activators and inactivators actually reach a balance favoring or hindering fibrinolysis are complex and are still being elucidated.

Laboratory Tests of Fibrinolysis

FDP produced during fibrinolysis *in vivo* may bind to fibrinogen or remain freely circulating. Because only the latter fraction is measured when patient serum is assayed for FDP, false-negative values constitute a potential problem for this test. In the tanned red cell hemagglutination inhibition immunoassay, FDP present in the patient's serum neutralize antifibrinogen antiserum, thereby preventing the antiserum from agglutinating fibrinogen-coated erythrocytes. A more rapid, semi-quantitative method assesses the ability of FDP present in patient serum directly to agglutinate latex beads coated with antifibrinogen antibody. If the antibody used in this assay recognizes only neoantigens created by the proteolytic action of thrombin on fibrinogen, then patient plasma may be substituted for patient serum in the assay. Similarly, immunoassays specific for the cross-linked D-dimer fragment of fibrin can be performed directly on patient plasma, thus avoiding the potential problem that FDP recovered in the serum fraction of clots prepared *in vitro* may not faithfully reflect circulating FDP levels. D-dimer levels generally rise together with the appearance of thrombin-antithrombin III (TAT) complexes and of the prothrombin fragment 1.2 that results from activation of prothrombin to thrombin, although in individual patients actual rises in the levels of these markers may vary considerably (Boisclair, 1990; Velasco, 1992; Wada, 1993; Vaziri, 1994).

The *whole blood clot lysis time* is a simple screening test in which a tube of whole blood is allowed to clot, and dissolution of the clot is subsequently examined. In normal individuals the clot remains undissolved even 24 hours after clot formation. In the absence of normal antiplasmin activity and in some fibrinolytic states, lysis may be observed after several hours. Plasma can also be admixed with dilute acid to precipitate a fraction relatively rich in plasminogen activator, plasminogen, and fibrinogen but relatively poor in antiplasmins. This "euglobulin" fraction can subsequently be redissolved in buffer and clotted by recalcification, and the time for clot lysis then measured. Such *euglobulin clot lysis* is normally complete in two to four hours but may be shortened with increased fibrinolysis, particularly in association with increased plasminogen activator activity.

Both *plasminogen* and *α_2-antiplasmin* may be measured antigenically in patient plasma. Functional plasminogen and antiplasmin assays that use synthetic substrates in either

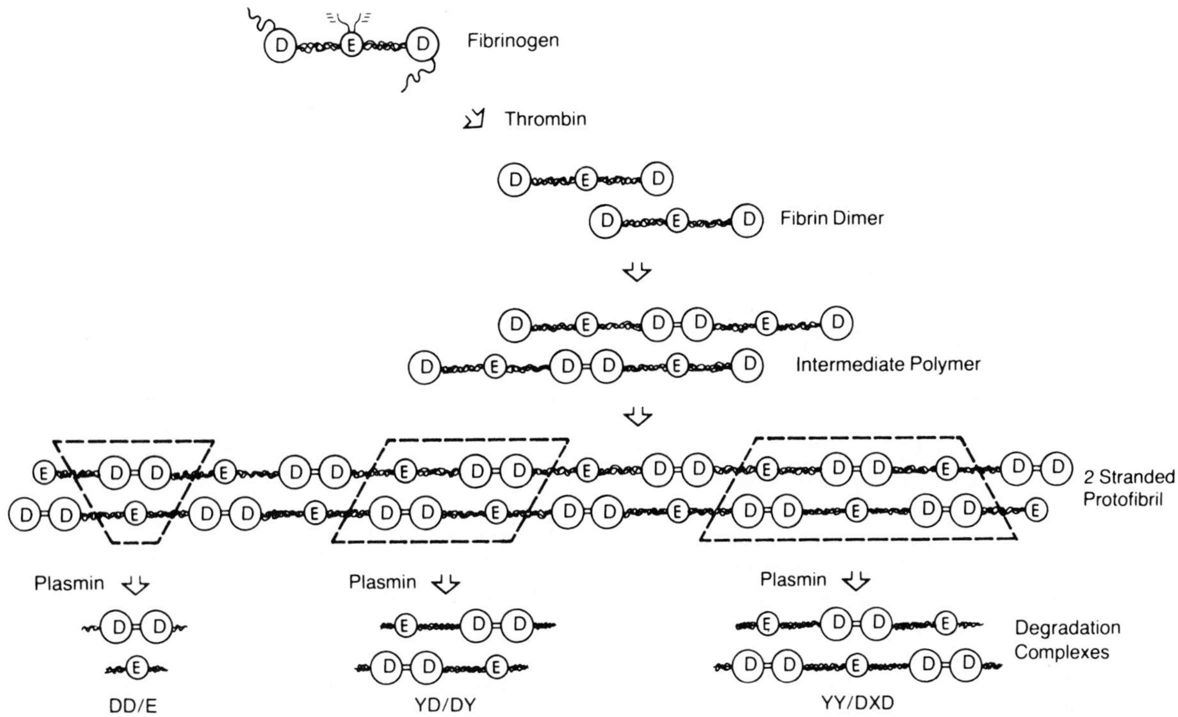

Figure 29–7. Plasmic degradation of cross-linked fibrin. Plasmic degradation of the two-stranded protofibril results in a series of noncovalently bound complexes, the smallest of which is DD/E. Each complex consists of fragments derived from each strand of the protofibril, attached noncovalently to complementary regions. For convenience, the α-chain extensions are not shown. (From Francis CW, Marder VJ: Mechanisms of fibrinolysis. *In* Beutler E, Lichtman MA, Coller BS, Kipps TJ [eds]: Williams Hematology, 5th ed. New York, McGraw-Hill, 1995, p 1258.)

spectrophotometric or fluorometric measuring systems have recently become available. Assay of PAI-1 levels is currently under investigation in a number of clinical situations, including malignancy (Foekens, 1994; Landau, 1994; Bouchet, 1994) and pre-eclampsia (Halligan, 1994).

CONGENITAL DEFICIENCIES OF HEMOSTATIC FACTORS

Hemophilia A

Hemophilia A is the most common congenital disorder of the coagulation factors. Its incidence is usually cited as 1 in 10,000 males, although Brettler (1994), has suggested that the true incidence may actually be twice this figure. This deficiency of normal Factor VIII is caused by a defect on the X chromosome, with the result that hemizygous males are primarily affected. Although female carriers ordinarily do not have a bleeding diathesis, there are a number of conditions in which females may also experience clinical Factor VIII deficiency (Bloom, 1987; Ingerslev, 1989; Mannucci, 1978). These genetic abnormalities in phenotypic females include a single functional X chromosome bearing the hemophilia gene, extreme lyonization in a heterozygote, and true homozygosity for the hemophilia gene. In kindreds for which apparent hemophilia is manifested in autosomal rather than sex-linked inheritance patterns, the possibility of the Normandy variant of von Willebrand's disease should be considered (see later discussion). In approximately one third of newly diagnosed cases of hemophilia, no antecedent family history of bleeding can be obtained, suggesting the presence of either several generations of silent carriers or a recent mutation.

"Spontaneous" hemorrhages are seen frequently in patients having less than 1 U/dL of Factor VIII. (Factor activities are expressed as arbitrary units [U] per deciliter, where 100 U/dL corresponds to the activity present in a normal plasma pool.) Patients with such levels are considered *severe* hemophiliacs. Levels of Factor VIII up to 5 U/dL are usually associated with *moderate* clinical severity, and patients with values above 5 U/dL are considered *mild* hemophiliacs and typically bleed excessively only in situations involving trauma or surgical procedures.

Bleeding histories in patients with hemophilia typically indicate bleeding into joints or muscles, excessive postoperative hemorrhage, and generally easy bruising. Bleeding at mucous membrane or skin sites is not as pronounced as in patients with von Willebrand's disease or platelet disorders. Intracranial hemorrhage remains a major cause of death in hemophiliacs.

Although the bleeding time in patients with newly diagnosed hemophilia is frequently normal, studies by Buchanan (1980) and Eyster (1981) indicate that some patients with hemophilia may in fact show a prolongation of the template bleeding time (see Chap. 28). The PT and the TT are characteristically normal. Tests that screen for the "intrinsic pathway" will be abnormal if they are of adequate sensitivity. The PTT will be prolonged if Factor VIII levels are below 40 U/dL, and this has proved to be an acceptable screening test in most cases. It is important to emphasize, however, that when a hemophiliac is being treated, particularly postoperatively, the PTT is not an acceptable substitute for specific Factor VIII assays. Both overestimation and underestimation of actual Factor VIII levels may result from attempts to interpret PTT values in patients undergoing Factor VIII replacement therapy and may lead to inappropriate subsequent therapy.

Although some laboratories employ a two-stage technique based on the thromboplastin generation test (Denson, 1976), most laboratories now assay Factor VIII clotting activity in a one-stage technique based on the PTT (Hardisty, 1962; Cinotti, 1991). Patient plasma is accordingly assessed for its ability to shorten the time to clot formation of plasma devoid of Factor VIII activity (such as plasma from a severe hemophiliac). When pooled normal plasma is diluted serially with buffer so that its content of Factor VIII progressively declines, a plot of the resulting clotting times versus the logarithm of the corresponding plasma dilutions should be linear. If the patient plasma is taken through a similar series of dilutions, a line drawn through the corresponding patient points should be parallel to a line drawn through the normal points, with the degree of displacement above or below the normal line providing a quantitative measure of the decrease or increase, respectively, of the Factor VIII level of the patient plasma. Concern about the validity of the assay arises if these two lines are not parallel. In particular, when the clotting times corresponding to the greater patient dilutions define a line parallel to that of normal plasma, but the clotting times corresponding to the least diluted patient plasma fail to shorten sufficiently to fall on that line, the presence of an inhibitor must be suspected. In the general population such an inhibitor most frequently turns out to be a lupus anticoagulant (see later), although in a hemophiliac patient the possibility of a specific inhibitor directed against Factor VIII is of major concern. An alternative to assessing the actual parallelism of patient and normal dilutions is to use computational algorithms based on the clotting times of a series of dilutions of patient plasma, and this approach appears to be particularly suited to automated instrumentation for clotting assays. A somewhat different approach to Factor VIII measurement that entirely avoids using clotting as an end point is the chromogenic assay, in which cleavage of a synthetic substrate results in a measurable color change (Cinotti, 1991). Chromogenic assays may be particularly useful in the context of a lupus-like anticoagulant because they appear to be relatively unaffected by the presence of such inhibitors.

Human alloantibodies to the Factor VIII coagulant moiety are produced in 10% to 25% of patients with severe hemophilia who receive Factor VIII replacement therapy (see later). These antibodies typically do not produce precipitin reactions. Used earlier in antibody neutralization studies, these alloantibodies identified "cross-reacting material" in the plasma of some patients with mild to moderate hemophilia (so-called CRM + patients). Quantitative, more reproducible studies have used such antibodies in immunoradiometric assays of Factor VIII coagulant antigen (VIII:Ag) (Lazarchick, 1978). In normal individuals the correlation between plasma Factor VIII (activity) and VIII:Ag is excellent. Although Factor VIII activity is not found in *serum*, VIII:Ag remains detectable in serum, usually at 60% to 85% of the plasma level (Hoyer, 1982). Levels of VIII:Ag are very low or undetectable in most patients with severe hemophilia. In patients with mild to moderate hemophilia, VIII:Ag levels usually are equal to or slightly greater than Factor VIII coagulant activity. In those few hemophiliacs in whom VIII:Ag levels remain normal, there is likely to be a qualitative abnormality of the Factor VIII molecules. Reaction of CRM+ Factor VIII with a panel of well-defined monoclonal antibodies may be potentially useful in the genotypic and phenotypic analysis of such patients (Tanaka, 1992).

On the average, maternal carriers have 50 U/dL of Factor VIII activity, yet the individual variation in levels is too great to allow detection of carriers from Factor VIII assays alone in individual women. Predictive value of such assays is increased, however, if in addition to Factor VIII values, measurement is also made of von Willebrand factor antigen (vWF:Ag). vWF:Ag is commonly assayed by the Laurell electroimmunoassay technique, in which electrophoresis of patient plasma through agarose containing rabbit antiserum against human vWF is performed (Zimmerman, 1971). The height of the resulting immunoprecipitin lines (resembling rockets) is proportional to the concentration of vWF present in the plasma (Fig. 29–8). In normal individuals the ratio of vWF:Ag to Factor VIII approaches unity. Like Factor VIII, vWF appears to have characteristics of an acute phase reactant, so that transient elevations in Factor VIII are generally accompanied by similar elevations in vWF. In carriers of hemophilia A, vWF levels are normal, and Factor VIII levels are frequently one half or less as great, resulting in characteristically decreased Factor VIII/vWF:Ag ratios. As Graham (1979) has emphasized, however, carrier identification based solely on a comparison between patient ratios and those

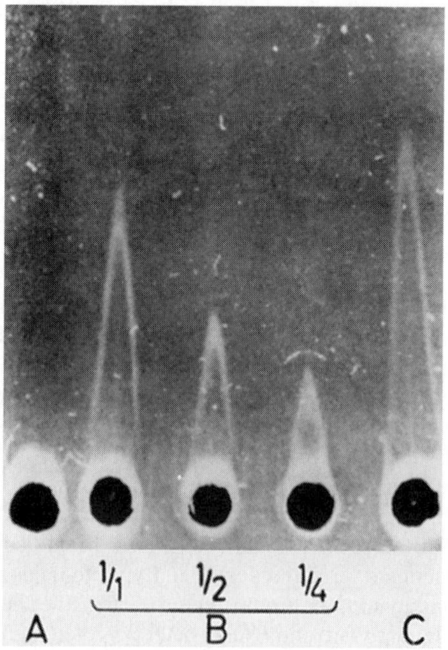

Figure 29–8. Laurell immunoelectrophoresis assay of von Willebrand factor. *A*, Plasma from patient with von Willebrand's disease. *B*, Doubling dilutions of normal plasma, *C*, Plasma from a patient with hemophilia A. (From Rizza CR: von Willebrand's disease. *In* Biggs R [ed]: The Treatment of Haemophilia A and B and von Willebrand's Disease. Oxford, Blackwell Scientific Publications, 1978.)

obtained in normal individuals may lead to serious errors. Graham has proposed that laboratories establish a discriminant analysis based on pools of both obligate carriers and normal individuals, and that the resulting patient discriminant value be combined with pedigree analysis of the patient's family to obtain a final estimate of carrier likelihood. A stepwise procedure for calculating the probability of carriership, using a universal linear discriminant that allows for the effects of both age and ABO blood type, has been published (Green, 1986).

The prenatal diagnosis of hemophilia was advanced by the development of VIII:Ag assays (Firshein, 1979). Samples of blood obtained from unaffected fetuses at 18 to 20 weeks of gestation could be assessed for the presence of detectable levels of VIII:Ag as well as ratios of VIII:Ag to vWF appropriate for fetal age. However, this approach has tended to be confined to specialized centers.

In recent years, the virtual explosion of knowledge in molecular biology has had a significant impact on the detection of carriers and the prenatal diagnosis of hemophilia. The most widely practiced approach uses restriction length polymorphism (RFLP) analysis of either intragenic or very closely linked extragenic polymorphisms (see, for example, Antonarakis, 1988) to determine the segregation of Factor VIII alleles identified with an affected hemophilic male within a kindred (Schwaab, 1993). By combining information gained from the DNA analyses with conventional assays of Factor VIII (and von Willebrand factor) activity and careful pedigree analysis, correct assignment of carriership status may be increased still further (Poon, 1992). In 1991 a directory of known deletions, point mutations, and other mutations affecting Factor VIII expression was published (Tuddenham, 1991) in the anticipation that periodic updates would follow. However, until recently there has appeared to be a significant limitation in the molecular characterization of hemophilia because in approximately 50% of cases of severe hemophilia A, the underlying mutations could not be found even with quite thorough evaluation of the coding regions and splice junctions of the Factor VIII gene (Higuchi, 1991). However, recent reports (Goodeve, 1994; Lakich, 1993) have now focused on intron 22 as a source of up to 40% to 50% of the mutations seen in hemophilia. Using probes spanning the coding region, intron-exon splice junctions, and regions of intron 22, Naylor and colleagues (Naylor, 1991, 1992, 1993) have reported a successful method of rapidly identifying virtually all mutations in the hemophiliac patients they have studied. Their approach takes advantage of the expression of detectable mRNA for Factor VIII in circulating leukocytes, which is reverse transcribed to cDNA. Then both amplified cDNA and genomic DNA from the patient's leukocytes are hybridized with a variety of probes, following which single nucleotide mismatches between patient and probe DNA are detected and localized by the hydroxylamine-osmium tetroxide-piperidine chemical approach (Cotton, 1988; Smooker, 1993), and the localized region of the amplified patient DNA is then directly sequenced for precise identification of the mutation. There is little doubt that molecular biologic techniques will continue to be refined and will dominate the detection of carriers and prenatal diagnosis during the coming years.

Hemophilia is treated principally by Factor VIII replacement therapy, either as Factor VIII concentrates purified from human plasma or as a recombinant product. The incidence of development of inhibitor antibodies to the transfused Factor VIII has varied widely over a range of 18% to 52% in more recent reports (Feinstein, 1995), appearing to exceed the earlier reported incidence of only 10% to 15%. Because the degree of anamnestic response and the antibody titer greatly affect the therapeutic approach in individual patients, it is important that laboratories be able to provide reproducible inhibitor level measurements. Although inhibitor assays based on the PTT have been found useful (Lossing, 1977; Ewing, 1982), the two-hour "Bethesda" method (Kasper, 1975, 1982) has achieved wide acceptance, and inhibitors are generally expressed in Bethesda units. One Bethesda unit corresponds to the ability of patient plasma to inactivate 50% of the Factor VIII activity of an equal volume of normal plasma following a two-hour incubation at 37°C. For patients receiving porcine Factor VIII replacement therapy, or for whom studies are needed to determine whether an established anti-Factor VIII inhibitor may cross-react with porcine Factor VIII, a modification of the Bethesda assay may be performed in which porcine Factor VIII rather than human Factor VIII is used as substrate.

Current modes of therapy for patients with inhibitors include the use of higher doses of Factor VIII replacement therapy in patients with low-titers of inhibitors. In some patients in whom adequate levels of Factor VIII cannot be achieved with human Factor VIII concentrate, porcine Factor VIII concentrate may prove successful, although antibodies to the porcine Factor VIII may be produced subsequently. In patients with high titers of inhibitors, nonactivated or activated Factor IX concentrates may be used in an attempt to "bypass" the Factor VIII inhibitory activity. There is currently no accepted laboratory test for monitoring such bypass therapy; the response must be assessed clinically. Factor VIIa has also been used successfully on an experimental basis in several patients with inhibitors to Factor VIII (Stein, 1993; Bell, 1993). Pharmacodynamic studies suggest that PT determinations may be potentially useful for monitoring the level of Factor VIIa in such patients (Lindley, 1994).

Hemophilia B

Congenital deficiency of Factor IX, or hemophilia B, is also an X chromosome-linked disorder and occurs approximately one fifth as frequently as hemophilia A. The clinical manifestations of hemophilia B are virtually indistinguishable from those of hemophilia A. Because replacement therapy is entirely different, consisting primarily of plasma fractions enriched by Factor IX rather than Factor VIII, it is the responsibility of the laboratory to differentiate these two disorders.

As in hemophilia A, patients with hemophilia B typically have a prolonged PTT, a normal TT, and a normal bleeding time. Although most also have a normal PT, one subgroup of patients (the B_m variant) has a prolonged PT when ox brain thromboplastin is employed, presumably owing to inhibition of thromboplastin by the abnormal Factor IX (Kidd, 1963; Hougie, 1967). In rare kindreds, the Factor IX level appears to increase as the individual matures (Leyden variant) (Veltkamp, 1970; Briet, 1982; Coyle, 1994).

With a clinical suspicion of hemophilia, a prolonged PTT, and a normal Factor VIII level, a specific assay for Factor IX activity should be performed. As with Factor VIII assays, either a one-stage or a two-stage clotting assay or a chromogenic assay may be performed, using substrates severely deficient in Factor IX (Brandt, 1990; Wagenvoord, 1990). Levels of circulating Factor IX activity usually correlate with clinical severity, as described previously for Factor VIII.

A number of variants of hemophilia B have been described; they appear to reflect different functional abnormalities of altered Factor IX molecules and are reviewed by Roberts (1993). Carrier detection of hemophilia B by conventional methodology has proved to be more complicated than that of hemophilia A, with varying opinions about the role of determinations of Factor IX antigenic levels in the different variants (Graham, 1979; Kasper, 1977; Pechet, 1978; Thompson, 1977). However, molecular approaches to carrier detection and prenatal diagnosis have paralleled the advances previously described for hemophilia A and are capable of providing a high level of information (Aguilar-Martinez, 1994; Martinez, 1994; Montandon, 1990).

Inhibitors to Factor IX develop in about 3% of hemophilia B patients overall and in approximately 7% to 10% of those with severe disease (Shapiro, 1979). These inhibitors are usually immediately acting antibodies as opposed to the time-dependent antibodies characteristic of hemophilia A, and titers tend to fall more rapidly on the termination of Factor IX exposure than usually seen with inhibitors to Factor VIII.

Von Willebrand's Disease

Although hemophilia A has traditionally been considered the most frequently occurring congenital bleeding disorder, increasing identification of patients with milder forms of von Willebrand's disease (vWD) suggests that the overall incidence of vWD is equal to or even greater than that of hemophilia A. Transmission of vWD is usually autosomal dominant. A small number of cases have been described, however, in which transmission appears to be autosomal recessive.

Patients with vWD characteristically bleed from mucous membranes and cutaneous sites. Easy bruising, epistaxis, gastrointestinal bleeding, and excessive bleeding following tonsillectomy or dental extractions may be prominent. Menorrhagia may be pronounced. Hemarthroses and deep muscle hematomas, in contrast, are not usually characteristic of vWD except in the most severe cases in which there is a concomitant severe decrease of Factor VIII (see earlier under Hemophilia A).

vWF circulating in the blood is synthesized by endothelial cells (Jaffe, 1974). The only other cell known to synthesize vWF is the megakaryocyte (Nachman, 1977), and vWF synthesized by megakaryocytes is stored in the α granules of platelets (Cramer, 1985). The biosynthesis of vWF by cultured endothelial cells has been reviewed (Handin, 1989). The vWF gene is quite large, spanning approximately 175 kb of genomic DNA, and is located on the short arm of chromosome 12 (Ginsburg, 1985). When mature vWF is subjected to chemical reduction, a single band of 220 to 225×10^3 daltons is seen by SDS-polyacrylamide gel electrophoresis (SDS-PAGE). This band in fact corresponds to a heavily glycosylated, monomeric subunit of 2050 amino acids. Dimers of this subunit form a series of vWF *multimers*, which may be best appreciated by the technique called *multimeric analysis*. By this technique, plasma (or the lysate from endothelial cells, megakaryocytes, or platelets) is electrophoresed on agarose (Ruggeri, 1981; Ciavarella, 1985), and a labeled anti-vWF antibody is incubated with the gel (or with a blot transfer from the gel). The gel (or blot) is then washed free of unbound antibody, and autoradiography or enzyme-linked color development is performed to detect regions to which the vWF has migrated. Protein migrations on the agarose gel are strongly dependent on molecular size. Depending on the type and concentration of the agarose, separation of protein bands in the highest molecular weight or lower molecular weight regions of the gel may be optimized. Examples of the same plasma samples analyzed at different agarose concentrations are shown in Figure 29–9. Normal plasma possesses an extremely wide range of these multimers, ranging from 400,000 to over 20 million daltons. Even higher molecular weight multimers are found in extracts of endothelial cells or megakaryocytes (Moake, 1982; Kupinski, 1985). Although resolution of the individual multimeric bands decreases as the molecular weight of the band increases, in the lower molecular weight region of the gel, it is possible to discern a pattern of an intense central band, sandwiched by two (or, depending on resolution of the gel, up to four or more) "satellite" bands. These satellite bands may represent the presence of pro-vWF fragments that have not been cleaved from the molecule during the process of vWF synthesis (Lynch, 1986; Dent, 1991; Fischer, 1994). Crossed immunoelectrophoresis (CIE) affords similar qualitative information but lacks resolution of the multimeric bands.

Circulating vWF is complexed with Factor VIII coagulant protein and serves as a carrier for Factor VIII, stabilizing it from proteolytic destruction and helping to increase its concentration at sites of vascular injury. vWF appears to play a central role in the adhesion of platelets to subendothelial surfaces following vessel injury. Demonstration of prolonged template bleeding times (see Chap. 28) in patients with vWD is accordingly of diagnostic importance. Additionally, the PTT in some patients is prolonged if there is a sufficiently decreased Factor VIII activity. The PT and TT are normal. Although tests of platelet adhesiveness in glass bead columns show decreased adhesiveness in patients with vWD, difficulties in reproducibility have prompted the abandonment of this test in most laboratories.

Measurement of the different component activities of the Factor VIII-vWF complex is necessary for a more specific diagnosis. The Laurell "rocket" immunoelectrophoresis technique (see Fig. 29–8) is a commonly used quantitative method of detecting total vWF antigenically. For quantitation of vWF:Ag, immunoradiometric (IRMA) and enzyme-linked immunosorbent (ELISA) assays are also available (Goodall, 1985; McCraw, 1987; Chand, 1986) and may be used either in conjunction with or as an alternative to the Laurell assay. The ability of vWF to interact with platelets may be assayed as the vWF's *ristocetin cofactor* activity. This test is performed by quantitating the ability of patient plasma (the source of vWF's ristocetin cofactor activity) to support ristocetin-induced agglutination of either freshly washed (Weiss, 1973) or formalin-fixed (Macfarlane, 1975) normal platelets

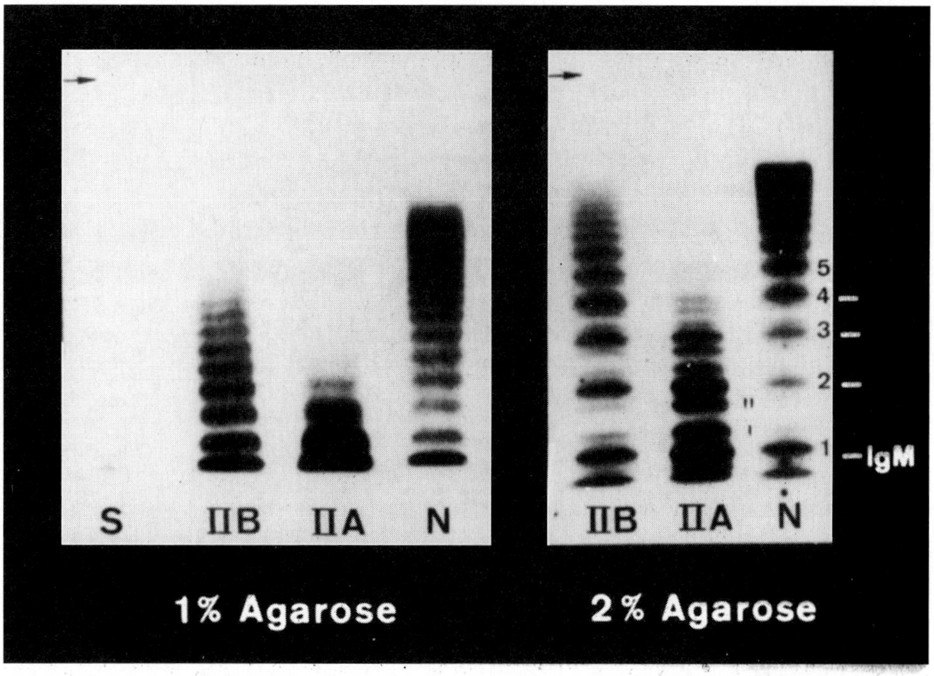

Figure 29–9. SDS electrophoresis in 1% (*left*) and 2% (*right*) agarose gels of normal plasma (N): plasma from a patient with vWD type IIA (IIA), a patient with vWD type IIB (IIB), and a patient with severe vWD (S). The arrow indicates the interface between stacking and running gel. The cathode was at the top and the anode at the bottom of the gel. Numbers from 1 to 5 indicate the smallest major bands in normal plasma, whereas the intervening bands are indicated by primes. The position of IgM and its cross-linked oligomers is shown by white marks. (From Ruggeri ZM, Zimmerman TS: The complex multimeric composition of Factor VIII/von Willebrand factor. Blood 1981; 57:1140.)

by the antibiotic ristocetin. This test is generally considered a more sensitive assay of decreases in vWF functional activity than aggregation studies based on the direct addition of ristocetin to the patient's own platelet-rich plasma. Although not generally available in clinical laboratories, instruments permitting study of platelet aggregation under conditions of defined shear stress may better assess the functional interaction of vWF with platelets (Peterson, 1987; Ikeda, 1991; Chow, 1992). Measurement of Factor VIII activity is performed as described earlier in the evaluation of hemophilia A.

vWD comprises a quite heterogeneous group of quantitative and qualitative disorders affecting the vWF molecule. In keeping with recent recommendations of a subcommittee of the International Society on Thrombosis and Haemostasis (Sadler, 1994a, 1994b), the classification of inherited vWD subtypes included in Table 29–4 employs both primary (Types 1, 2, and 3) and secondary (A, B, M, N) levels that produce a total of six diagnostic entities. The primary levels distinguish partial (Type 1) and virtually full (Type 3) quantitative deficiencies of an apparently normal molecule from qualitative disorders of the vWF molecule (Type 2). vWF mutations leading to decreased platelet-dependent function are considered to produce examples of Type 2A vWD if the vWF lacks high-molecular-weight multimers; Type 2M vWD exists if high-molecular-weight vWF multimers are present. Thus, in Type 2M disorders, the mutations alter vWF function by some means other than simply reducing the amount of high-molecular-weight vWF multimers. Mutations of vWF leading to heightened interaction with platelet glycoprotein Ib are considered to produce examples of Type 2B vWD whether or not there is a decrease in the high-molecular-weight multimers. vWF mutations that impair the ability of the vWF molecule to bind Factor VIII comprise the Type 2N category. It should be noted that although a series of diagnostic tests are used to reach as specific a diagnosis as possible, the classification system itself is intended to reflect phenotypes rather than to be assay dependent.

Clinical expression in Type 1 disease may be highly variable. In fact, in milder cases vWF may be within normal limits at the time of the initial study, necessitating repeated studies to reach a diagnosis (Zimmerman, 1983). Discrimination between normal individuals and those with mild Type I vWD may also be further complicated by the effect of ABO blood type. As discussed by Gill (1987), in some blood group AB individuals with a genetic defect of vWF this diagnosis may be overlooked because plasma vWF levels tend to be elevated in persons with this blood type. Additionally, in some patients a decreased level of vWF is attributable to their blood group O status rather than to an inherited abnormality of the vWF gene itself.

The Type 2A and 2B forms of vWD are recognized by a selective absence of the higher molecular-weight multimers of vWF. In *Type 2A*, concentrations of ristocetin that are more than adequate to promote platelet aggregation in platelet-rich plasma (PRP) from normal individuals (1.5 to 2.0 mg/mL) are unable to produce significant aggregation in patient PRP. Conversely, in *Type 2B*, not only do intermediate concentrations of ristocetin (0.9 to 1.2 mg/mL) produce aggregation, but aggregation is typically produced by ristocetin concentrations even lower than those required to produce aggregation in normal PRP (0.3 to 0.5 mg/mL).

In recent years great progress has been made in establishing the pathophysiology of the qualitative vWD disorders. Most Type 2A and 2B mutations have been found to occur within a relatively small region of the gene (Fig. 29–10). Moreover, *in vitro* expression studies have now been able to reproduce the key 2A and 2B phenotypes seen *in vivo* (Sadler, 1994c).

An additional disorder showing selective absence of the higher molecular-weight multimers of plasma vWF has been

Table 29–4. DISORDERS INVOLVING VON WILLEBRAND FACTOR AND FACTOR VIII

	Inherited von Willebrand's Disease Subtypes									
		Qualitative vWF Abnormality								
	1	*2A*	*2B*	*2M*	*2N*	*3*	**Hemophilia A**	**Platelet-type (Pseudo) vWD**	**Acquired vWD**	**Acquired Factor VIII Inhibitors**
Defining attribute	vWF partial quantitative deficiency	↓ HMW multimers, ↓function	↓ HMW multimers, ↑function	Despite all multimers, ↓function	↓ vWF affinity for Factor VIII	vWF full quantitative deficiency	Factor VIII mutations	Platelet glycoprotein Ibα mutations	Autoantibodies develop against vWF	Autoantibodies develop against Factor VIII
Commonest genetics	Autosomal dominant	Autosomal dominant	Autosomal dominant	Autosomal dominant	Autosomal dominant	Autosomal recessive	Sex-linked	Autosomal dominant	Acquired	Acquired
Bleeding time	Often increased	Usually increased	Usually increased	Often increased	Usually normal	Markedly increased	Usually normal	Usually increased	Often increased	Normal
Platelet count	Normal	Normal	Decreased	Normal	Normal	Normal	Normal	Decreased	Usually normal	Normal
Factor VIII	Often decreased	May be decreased	May be decreased	May be decreased	Markedly decreased	Markedly decreased	Markedly decreased	May be decreased	May be decreased	Markedly decreased
vWF antigen	Usually decreased	Usually decreased	Often decreased	Usually decreased	Usually normal	Markedly decreased	Normal	Often decreased	Usually decreased	Normal
Ristocetin cofactor	Usually decreased	Decreased	Decreased	Usually decreased	Usually normal	Markedly decreased	Normal	Decreased	Usually decreased	Normal
vWF binding to platelets	Decreased	Decreased	Increased due to abnormal vWF	Decreased	Usually normal	Markedly decreased	Normal	Increased due to abnormal platelet glycoprotein Ibα	Usually normal but rarely increased	Normal
vWF multimer pattern	Normal	HMW multimers absent	HMW multimers may be absent	Abnormal structure, but all HMW multimers present	Normal	All multimers markedly decreased	Normal	HMW multimers absent	HMW multimers may be absent	Normal
vWF binding to Factor VIII	Normal	Normal	Normal	Usually normal	Markedly decreased	Presumably normal	Usually normal	Normal	May be decreased	May be decreased

HMW = High molecular weight

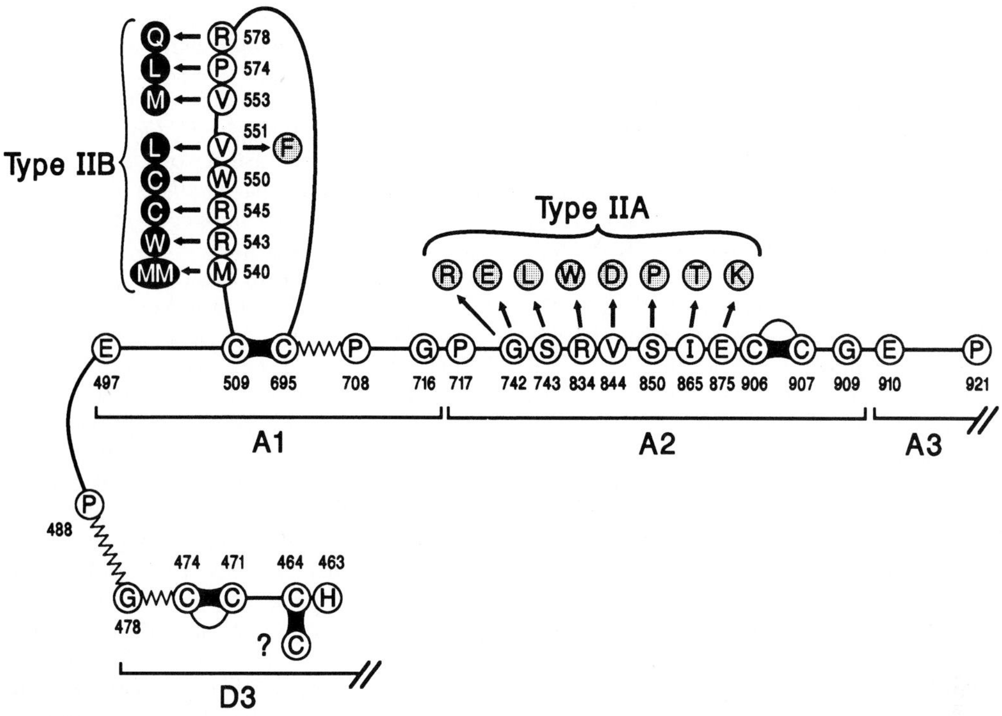

Figure 29–10. Mutations in vWF exon 28 that cause vWD Type 2A and Type 2B. The segment of mature vWF shown is encoded by exon 28 and includes amino acid residues 463 to 921. The positions of repeated domains D3, A1, A2, and A3 are indicated. The zigzag segments from Cys 474 to Pro 488 and Cys 695 to Pro 708 indicate regions proposed to interact directly with platelet GPIb. Mutations reported to cause vWD Type 2A (*shaded circles*) and Type 2B (*black circles*) are indicated by brackets; one proposed type IIA mutation, Val 551 to Phe 551, occurs in the region of the type IIB mutations. (From Sadler JE, Davie EW: Hemophilia A, hemophilia B, and von Willebrand disease. *In* Stamatoyannopoulos G, Nienhuis AW, Majerus PW, Varmus H [eds]: The Molecular Basis of Blood Diseases, 2nd ed. Philadelphia: W. B. Saunders Company, 1994, p 683. As adapted from Sadler, JE: Von Willebrand factor. J Biol Chem 1991; 266:22777; with permission of the American Society for Biochemistry and Molecular Biology.)

termed *platelet-type* (or *pseudo*) *vWD* (Miller, 1982; Weiss, 1982). Although this is a primary disorder of platelets (see Chap. 28) rather than of the vWF molecule, it is typically considered in the diagnostic evaluation of patients who show heightened interaction between their platelets and circulating vWF; in these patients low concentrations (0.3 to 0.5 mg/mL) of ristocetin added to patient PRP induce aggregation. Typically a borderline thrombocytopenia, bleeding times near the upper limit of normal, and an abnormally enhanced ability of patient *platelets* to bind circulating vWF are seen. The ability of cryoprecipitate with no added ristocetin to produce aggregation in PRP provides a quite simple method of distinguishing platelet-type vWD from Type 2B vWD (Miller, 1983; see also Chap. 28). Additionally, platelet-type vWD platelets have a unique ability to be agglutinated by desialylated human vWF (asialo-vWF) (Miller, 1987). When the plasma from Type 2B but not platelet-type vWD patients is incubated with normal platelets, a "neutral" monoclonal antibody directed against vWF that does not interfere with the binding of vWF to platelet glycoprotein Ib/IX will detect heightened binding induced by low concentrations of ristocetin (Scott, 1991; Miller, 1991).

The most severely affected patients with vWD typically have an autosomal recessive disorder that has been termed *Type 3* vWD. Inheritance patterns are either truly homozygous or doubly heterozygous. vWF antigen is nearly undetectable, ristocetin cofactor activity markedly reduced or absent, and Factor VIII activity moderately to severely reduced.

Other Congenital Deficiencies

In comparison with hemophilia A and B (and vWD), congenital deficiencies of the other coagulation factors are quite rare. Additionally, inheritance of these latter disorders is autosomal and in most instances recessive as well.

Deficiencies of Factor XII, high-molecular-weight kininogen, or prekallikrein are not associated with clinical bleeding tendencies. In *Factor XI deficiency* (of which the highest incidence appears to be in Ashkenazi Jews) the degree of bleeding is quite variable (Bolton-Maggs, 1988; Saito, 1985). The application of molecular genetic techniques to the study of Factor XI deficiency has led to the identification of several mutations, two of which appear to account for the great majority of cases in the Ashkenazic Jewish population (Hancock, 1991; Asakai, 1991; Seligsohn, 1993).

Patients with a deficiency of one of the above "contact" factors typically have a prolonged PTT and normal PT and TT. If the PTT is corrected when patient plasma is mixed with an equal volume of normal plasma, and assays of Factors VIII and IX are within normal limits, the abnormality may be presumed to be localized to the contact factors. Normalization of the PTT following prolonged incubation of plasma with the activating agent (e.g., kaolin) suggests that the deficiency may be in prekallikrein. Substrate plasmas deficient in Factors XI, XII, high-molecular-weight kininogen, or prekallikrein are commercially available for the performance of specific assays.

Factor VII deficiency may be associated with serious bleeding tendencies. Levels of 3 to 10 U/dL of Factor VII are frequently adequate to prevent serious bleeding, but the presence of only trace levels has been associated with major hemorrhages (Rapaport, 1981). The onset of hemorrhagic symptoms may occur early in life or may be delayed until adolescence or even later (Bloom, 1987). Laboratory studies in these patients show a prolonged PT but a normal PTT and TT. In this setting a Russell's viper venom time (RVVT), in which the snake venom directly activates Factor X, may be useful. A normal RVVT suggests a deficiency of Factor VII activity, and a specific assay for Factor VII should be employed to confirm this diagnosis. Dysfunctional Factor VII variants resulting from missense mutations that impair the ability of Factor VII to bind to tissue factor, to undergo activation to Factor VIIa, or to bind to substrate have recently been reported (Chaing, 1994; Takamiya, 1993; Bernardi, 1994).

Deficiency of Factor X activity appears to derive from a variety of qualitative as well as quantitative abnormalities of the Factor X molecule and is variable in its clinical severity. In most (but not all) cases both the PTT and the PT are prolonged. Although in the originally reported kindreds the RVVT was abnormal, variants with a normal or only slightly prolonged RVVT have been reported (Roberts, 1981). Molecular genetic analyses of Factor X deficiency have shown the presence of gene deletions, germline mosaicism, and several point mutations (Watzke, 1990; Wieland, 1991; Odom, 1994).

Congenital deficiency of Factor V is quite rare. Moreover, the level of plasma Factor V is not well correlated with clinical severity. Studies of patients with congenital Factor V deficiency have suggested a correlation between severity of bleeding and an inability of patient platelets to bind Factor Xa and increase the rate of thrombin formation at the platelet surface (Miletich, 1978). Because the platelet surface may serve as a key site for the activation of the coagulation proteins *in vivo*, this explanation is appealing and might even apply to deficiencies of other factors. Additionally, about one third of patients with Factor V deficiency have experienced a prolonged bleeding time, again possibly attributable to an abnormality in platelet-associated Factor V (Bloom, 1987). Detection of decreased plasma levels of Factor V is based on a prolonged PTT and PT but a normal TT in the absence of an inhibitor; specific assay of Factor V may then be performed by using a modified PT test, using as substrate normal plasma that has been depleted of Factor V. Although point mutations in the Factor V gene have recently been identified that destroy proteolytic sites for activated protein C (see earlier section on APC resistance), the resulting structural modifications of the Factor V molecule do not appear to impair Factor V coagulant activity significantly.

Although quite rare, *hereditary prothrombin disorders* representing a variety of qualitative abnormalities (dysprothrombinemias) have been reported, as have true hypoprothrombinemias. The PT and usually also the PTT are prolonged, and Factors VII, X, V, and fibrinogen are usually normal. Clinical, laboratory, and genetic aspects of prothrombin disorders have recently been reviewed by Roberts (1994).

Inherited disorders of fibrin formation and stabilization (Table 29–5) comprise both quantitative deficiencies and qualitative abnormalities of fibrinogen and also deficiencies of the fibrin cross-linking enzyme, Factor XIII. Structural defects in the fibrinogen molecule, in particular, may predispose the patient to bleeding or thrombosis. Routine laboratory testing—particularly the *thrombin time*—may provide the first clue to the existence of a fibrinogen abnormality. Additionally, an abnormal *reptilase time* may signal the presence of an abnormal fibrinogen molecule; this test can be particularly useful if there is any question about whether a prolonged TT is due to heparin in the patient sample because the reptilase time is not prolonged by heparin. Discrepancies in fibrinogen assayed by antigenic versus functional methodologies may further raise the suspicion of a dysfibrinogenemia. Measurement of total clottable protein by the method of Ratnoff and Menzie (1951) is widely used as a reference method. However, in cases of dysfibrinogenemia, measurement of fibrinogen using the *rate* of clot formation by the method of Clauss (1957) or one of the several variations of this method may prove significantly more sensitive in detecting the abnormality (Beck, 1979, 1982). Immunologic measurement of fibrinogen typically agrees fairly closely with functional assays in patients with true hypofibrinogenemias but may produce significantly higher values in patients with dysfibrinogenemias. More sophisticated studies, however, are usually required to characterize specific functional defects of the fibrinogen molecule such as defects of fibrinopeptide A release, fibrinopeptide B release, fibrin polymerization, fibrin stabilization, potentiation of plasminogen activation, and susceptibility to lysis by plasmin (Gralnick, 1995).

Because any test involving coagulation of the patient's own plasma is dependent on the level of functional fibrinogen present, the PTT and the PT, in addition to the TT, may be prolonged in patients with fibrinogen disorders. In contrast, these tests are normal in patients with Factor XIII deficiency. Solubility of a formed clot in 5-molar urea reflects the lack of covalent fibrin-fibrin cross-linkages in severe Factor XIII deficiency. In less severe deficiencies of Factor XIII, diagnosis of the abnormality may require demonstration of a decreased ability of patient plasma to catalyze incorporation into casein of the fluorescent probe monodansylcadaverine (Lorand, 1969) or of the radioactive probe ^{14}C-putrescine (Dvilansky, 1970).

ACQUIRED DISORDERS OF COAGULATION

Factor VIII

Inhibitors in patients with congenital deficiencies of Factor VIII have been discussed previously. Inhibitors to Factor VIII arise rarely in previously healthy individuals, most notably in women subsequent to childbirth. Although variable in severity, most inhibitors eventually disappear over a period of months, but occasionally they disappear only after several years. Unlike inhibitors that develop in some patients with hemophilia A, these inhibitors characteristically do not show an anamnestic response following Factor VIII therapy. In addition, the antibody may react with the Factor VIII coagulant moiety in such a way that the inhibitor–Factor VIII

Table 29–5. FUNCTIONAL CLASSIFICATION OF CONGENITAL DYSFIBRINOGENEMIAS WITH KNOWN STRUCTURAL DEFECTS CAUSING BLEEDING ALONE OR BLEEDING COMBINED WITH THROMBOSIS

Name	Defect/Mutation	Age/Sex	Major Symptoms	Possible Mechanism
Fibrinogen A Release Defects				
Mitaka II	Aα(11) Glu→Gly	14/F	Easy bruising	Defective thrombin binding to fibrinogen
Rouen I	Aα(12) Gly→Val	—/—	—	Altered Asp(7)-Arg(16) sequence impairs interaction with thrombin
Louisville I	Aα(16) Arg→His	54/M	Easy bruising/postoperative bleeding	—
Adelaide I	"Aα chain"	16/F	Postoperative/postpartum bleeding	—
Fibrinopeptide B Release Defects				
Christchurch II	Bβ(14) Arg→Cys	—/—	Recurrent epistaxis	Bβ thrombin reactive site affected; new disulfide bond formation
Baltimore II	Bβ(448) Arg→Lys A→G	—/—	Postpartum bleeding	Identified defect may be a normal polymorphism only
Fibrinopeptide A and B Release Defects				
Birmingham I	Aα(16) Arg→His	23/M	Mucosal bleeding; hematomas causing neurological compression	Intermittent reduction of high-molecular-weight multimers present
Sheffield I	Aα(16) Arg→His	—/F	Postdental extraction/postpartum bleeding	—
Magdeburg II	"Bβ chain"	—/—	Mild bleeding	—
Fibrinopeptide A Release and Polymerization Defects				
Frankfurt II	Aα(16) Arg→CYS	—/—	Mild bleeding	—
Frankfurt III	Aα(16) Arg→Cys	—/—	Mild bleeding	—
Frankfurt XIII	Aα(16) Arg→Cys C→T	—/—	Postdental bleeding	—
Metz I	Aα(16) Arg→Cys	—/F	Antenatal and postpartum hemorrhage	—
Giessen I	Aα(16) Arg→His	22/F	Antenatal and postpartum hemorrhage	—
Milan VI	Aα(16) Arg→His	18/F	Gastrointestinal bleeding	—
New Britain I	Aα(16) Arg→His	—/—	Postoperative bleeding	—
Stony Brook II	Aα(16) Arg→His	28/M	Recurrent hemarthroses	—
Munich I	Aα(19) Arg→Asn	—	Antenatal/mucosal hemorrhage	—
Mannheim I	Aα(19) Arg→Gly	—/F	Menorrhagia/postpartum bleeding	—
Detroit I	Aα(19) Arg→Ser	17F	Menorrhagia	—
Valhalla I	"Bβ chain"	34/F	Posttrauma bleeding/poor wound healing	—
Fibrinopeptide A and B Release and Polymerization Defects				
Homburg III	Aα(16) Arg→Cys	61/F	Recurrent minor bleeding	—
Ledyard I	Aα(16) Arg→Cys	10/M	Minor bleeding	Altered thrombin binding site due to a new disulfide bond formation at Cys(16)
Barcelona II	Aα(16) Arg→His	50/M	Postdental bleeding	—
Chapel Hill II	Aα(16) Arg→His	61/F	Minor bleeding	Retarded alpha polymer formation
White Marsh I	Aα(16) Arg→His	19/F	Postpartum bleeding	—
Polymerization Defects Alone				
Kyoto II	Aα(18) Pro→Leu CCA→CTA codon	27/F	Postpartum bleeding	—
Lima I	Aα(141) Arg→Ser	16/F	Hematuria	Extra oligosaccharide at Aα(139); Asn causes impaired lateral association of fibrils
Marburg I	Aα(461) Lys→610 A→T	20/F	Postpartum bleeding and recurrent thromboembolic events	Abnormal fibrinogen albumin complexes formed
Chapel Hill I	"Aα chain"	12/F	Postdental extraction bleeding	Alteration of sites involved in fibrin gel network branching
Saga I	γ(275) Arg→His	16/F	Hematuria	Abnormal fragment D present
Polymerization and Stabilization Defects				
Baltimore I	γ(292) Gly→Val G→T	20/F	Recurrent thromboembolic events; minor bleeding	
Asahi I	γ(310) Met→Thr T→C codon	33/M	Posttrauma bleeding	Delayed dimerization due to conformational change in γ chain
Frankfurt VII	γ(310) Met→Thr	—/—	Postmenopausal bleeding	Impaired platelet aggregation support by fibrinogen
Fibrinogen A and B Release Defects				
Naples I/Milan II	Bβ(68) Ala→Thr G→A	26/M	Recurrent thromboembolic events; arterial thrombosis (C.V.A.)	Reduced thrombin binding to fibrin
Fibrinopeptide A Release and Polymerization Defects				
Hershey II	Aα(16) Arg→Cys G→A	78/F	Arterial thrombosis	—

Table continued on following page

Table 29–5. FUNCTIONAL CLASSIFICATION OF CONGENITAL DYSFIBRINOGENEMIAS WITH KNOWN STRUCTURAL DEFECTS CAUSING BLEEDING ALONE OR BLEEDING COMBINED WITH THROMBOSIS *(Continued)*

Name	Defect/Mutation	Age/Sex	Major Symptoms	Possible Mechanism
Fibrinopeptide A and B Release and Polymerization Defects				
Aarhus I	Aα(19) Arg→Gly	31/F	Transient ischemic attacks postpartum	Reduced association between factor XIII and fibrinogen
New York I	Bα(9-72) deletion Exon 2 deletion	31/F	Severe recurrent thromboembolic disease	Abnormal thrombin and plasminogen binding to fibrin
Polymerization Defects Alone				
Dusard I/Paris V	Aα(554) Arg→Cys	37/M	Recurrent thromboembolic disease	Reduced fibrin enhancement of tissue plasminogen activator (t-PA activation); abnormal fibrin-albumin complexes formed
Milan III	Aα chain defect	13/F	Recurrent thrombophlebitis	—
Ijmuiden I	Bβ(44) Arg→Cys C→T	—/—	—	Reduced rate of t-PA activation; abnormal fibrin-albumin complex formed
Nijmegen I	Bβ(44) Arg→Cys C→T	49/F	Recurrent thromboembolic disease; arterial thrombosis	Reduced t-PA binding to fibrin; abnormal fibrin-albumin complexes formed
Oslo I	Bα chain defect	32/F	Recurrent thromboembolic disease during pregnancy	Increased fibrinogen binding affinity for platelets
Bergamo II	γ(275) Arg→His	—/F	Recurrent thromboembolic disease during pregnancy; arterial thrombosis (C.V.A.)	—
Haifa I	γ(275) Arg→His	30/F	Arterial occlusion	Fibrinogen not protected by calcium against plasmin digestion
Vlissingen I/Frankfurt IV	γ(319–320) deletion A→G deletion	23/F	Pulmonary embolism	Reduced calcium binding to fibrinogen
Richfield I	γ chain defect	28/M	Deep vein thrombosis; myocardial infarction	Fibrin clot was plasmin-resistant

From Gralnick H, Connaghan DG: Hereditary abnormalities of fibrinogen. *In* Beutler E, Lichtman MA, Coller BS, et al (eds): Williams Hematology, 5th ed. New York, McGraw-Hill, 1995, pp 1443–1444.

complex retains significant Factor VIII activity (Biggs, 1972; Gawyrl, 1982).

Von Willebrand Factor

A number of cases of acquired vWD have been seen in patients with autoimmune disease or with lymphoproliferative or, rarely, other neoplastic disorders (Miller, 1990; Coppes, 1992). The resulting bleeding diathesis results from antibody interference with one or more of the functions normally subserved by vWF (Mannucci, 1984; Van Genderen, 1994). In some cases it is possible that the neoplastic cells may act by binding vWF (Richard, 1990), in particular, the high-molecular-weight vWF multimers (Joist, 1978).

Factor IX

Inhibitors arising in patients with congenital deficiencies of Factor IX have been discussed earlier. Inhibitors in nonhemophiliacs are very rare but have occurred in a small number of women postpartum and in a small number of patients with autoimmune disorders or the nephrotic syndrome (Shapiro, 1979).

Other Coagulation Factors

Isolated inhibitors of these factors are quite rare, and few generalizations can be made. Occasional patients with autoimmune or neoplastic disorders produce antibodies that appear specific for individual factors. Development of inhibitors to Factor XIII has occurred following drug ingestion, most notably isoniazid. Inhibitors to Factor V have also been attributed to antibiotic therapy in rare patients, or have appeared to commence following major surgery. Finally, deficiencies of Factor X occasionally arise in association with amyloidosis, most likely due to binding of the Factor X by amyloid (Furie, 1981).

Lupus-like Anticoagulant

About 5% to 10% of patients with systemic lupus erythematosus, a significant number of patients on phenothiazine therapy, patients taking a variety of other drugs, occasional patients with lymphoproliferative disorders, and occasional patients in whom neither an underlying disease nor a drug can be identified develop inhibitors known as lupus-like anticoagulants. These inhibitors are heterogeneous but have in common the quality of being IgG or IgM antibodies that appear to be directed at phospholipid or phospholipoprotein components involved in the activation of coagulation factors. The outstanding feature of these anticoagulants is that, unless an additional hemostatic abnormality is present (most often thrombocytopenia, for example, in the case of systemic lupus), *the presence of a lupus-like anticoagulant is not associated with a clinical bleeding tendency.*

A lupus-like anticoagulant usually comes to attention first by a prolonged PTT. The PT is either normal or mildly prolonged, and the TT is normal. Because the need to diagnose a lupus-like anticoagulant is often part of a preoperative patient workup, further testing is usually required to eliminate the possibility of a clinically significant coagulation inhibitor. Unfortunately, currently no single test is specific for identification of a lupus-like anticoagulant (Shapiro, 1982). The following criteria have been suggested by Mueh (1980):

1. For patients whose PTT is at least five seconds above the upper limit of the normal range, one part of patient plasma is mixed with one part of normal plasma, and a PTT is then performed (i.e., without prior incubation of the plasma mixture). The PTT of the mixture remains prolonged at least five seconds longer than that of the same normal plasma run in parallel.
2. At least two specific one-stage assays for factors of the intrinsic system (i.e., Factors VIII, IX, XI, or XII) reveal apparent factor deficiencies of less than 50% of normal.
3. As the patient plasma is increasingly *diluted* in these assays (i.e., beyond the 1:5 or 1:10 dilution normally used in a factor assay), the measured activity of one or more of these factors appears to increase.
4. No other apparent causes of the abnormal coagulation studies can be identified.

Similar criteria have been recommended in an international cooperative study (Green, 1983).

The tissue thromboplastin inhibition test (Schleider, 1976) has been used to identify a lupus-like anticoagulant. In this test the thromboplastin source used in prothrombin determinations is diluted to increase its sensitivity to inhibitors. Despite its sensitivity, this test should not be considered specific for lupus-like inhibitors.

The substitution of resting or activated platelets for exogenous phospholipid in the PTT or dilute RVVT tests has been shown to correct the abnormality associated with a lupus-like anticoagulant (Thiagarajan, 1980; Shapiro, 1981). Such assays have now received wide acceptance in the evaluation of patients with suspected lupus-like anticoagulants. Subsequently, Rauch (1990) reported that mice immunized with phosphatidylethanolamine in the hexagonal II phase, but not in the bilayer phase, produced antiphospholipid antibodies that had lupus-like anticoagulant activity. Hexagonal II phase phospholipid has in fact now been used in a neutralization assay for the diagnosis of lupus-like anticoagulants (Triplett, 1993). Stevenson (1994), however, has pointed out that a sensitive dilute RVVT can be constructed for the detection of lupus-like anticoagulants without a specific requirement either for platelets or for hexagonal II phase phospholipids. Rather, Stevenson (1994) simply used a rabbit brain extract in a diluted form for the detection of lupus-like anticoagulants and in a concentrated form as a correcting reagent.

Occasionally a lupus-like anticoagulant may be present in a patient for whom assay of a specific intrinsic system coagulation factor is required. When available, chromogenic assays are generally preferred in these situations. If a PTT-based clotting system is used for assay of a factor, it is important to perform multiple dilutions of the patient sample and, when interpretating the resulting clotting times, to rely most heavily on dilutions that in a logarithmic plot are approximately parallel to a line drawn through the corresponding points of the standard plasma (Fig. 29–11). Alternatively, a two-stage

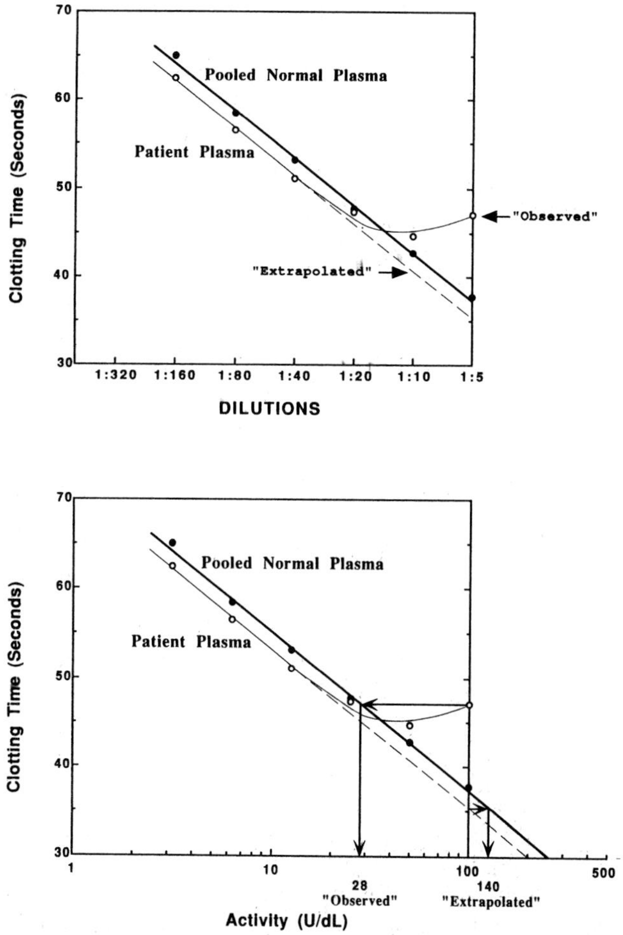

Figure 29–11. Coagulation factor assays in the presence of a lupus-like anticoagulant. *Upper panel:* The clotting times for serial dilutions of pooled normal plasma were plotted (*closed circles*) together with the best-fit logarithmic regression line (standard curve). Clotting times for serial dilutions of patient plasma were then plotted on the same graph (*open circles*). A straight line providing the best fit to the patient values at greater dilutions was then generated, with the requirement that this line remain parallel to the standard curve. Extrapolation of this line beyond these patient values is also indicated (*dashed line*). *Lower panel:* From the observed patient value at the 1:5 dilution and from the extrapolated patient value at the 1:5 dilution, horizontal lines were drawn to intersect the standard curve. Vertical lines were then dropped from these intersections to the X-axis (which was then relabeled as factor activity in U/dL, with the 1:5 dilution of pooled normal plasma arbitrarily defined as 100 U/dL). These intersections then defined the clearly underestimated "Observed" and the more accurate "Extrapolated" activities, as shown.

clotting assay may be considered because the lupus-like anticoagulant appears to have less effect on these assays (Green, 1983).

Liver Disease

Hemostasis in liver disease is complex owing to the many different roles of the liver in the synthesis of coagulation and fibrinolysis factors, the breakdown or removal of factor complexes, and our poor understanding of the influence of liver disease on platelet production and function. Decreases in the vitamin K–dependent factors (Factors II, VII, IX, X) are the earliest changes usually encountered in liver disease; they result in a prolonged PT and possibly also PTT. Fibrinogen levels may be decreased or increased depending on the type of liver disease present. Even in patients with chronic liver disease accompanied by high fibrinogen levels, however, the TT may be prolonged; in at least some cases this appears to be attributable to disordered fibrinogen synthesis resulting in functionally abnormal fibrinogen molecules.

Factor VIII, vWF antigen, and ristocetin cofactor activities are frequently elevated in patients with acute hepatic failure or chronic liver disease. Such elevations would not be inconsistent with severe hepatocellular damage on the basis of our current knowledge that vWF is synthesized by endothelial cells and megakaryocytes and that Factor VIII produced from hepatic synthesis may be derived from hepatic reticuloendothelial cells rather than from hepatocytes themselves.

Patterns of screening tests and specific assay results typically found in different types of liver disease are shown in Table 29–6. An assessment of bleeding risk in patients with liver disease can, in most instances, be based on the results of the routine coagulation screening tests and the platelet count.

Vitamin K Deficiency

Inadequate vitamin K levels lead to an impairment in the synthesis of coagulation Factors VII, IX, and X and prothrombin. This fat-soluble vitamin promotes the postribosomal addition of a second carboxyl group to glutamic acid in the zymogen molecules, producing γ-carboxyglutamic acid (or Gla) forms of these molecules. The highly negatively charged Gla regions are thought to be responsible for binding the molecules to negatively charged phospholipids (e.g., at the surfaces of activated platelets) in a complex process mediated by calcium ions (Jackson, 1994).

In vitamin K deficiency the PT typically is prolonged, and the PTT may also be prolonged. Because fibrinogen synthesis is not vitamin K dependent, the TT remains normal. The inhibitory coagulation factor protein C is also vitamin K dependent, and its functions may be impaired during vitamin K deficiency.

Vitamin K is normally obtained through both dietary intake of vitamin K_1 produced by plants and the production of vitamin K_2 by intestinal bacteria. Inadequate diet, biliary obstruction, intestinal malabsorption, and gut sterilization by antibiotics are among the contributing causes of clinical vitamin K deficiency. Vitamin K deficiency in the neonatal period may also predispose the infant to hemorrhagic disease of the newborn. Parenteral administration of vitamin K_1 will correct the associated coagulation abnormalities within 6 to 24 hours.

Intentional induction of a vitamin K deficiency–like state forms the basis of therapeutic anticoagulation induced by *warfarin* or its derivatives. These pharmacologic antagonists of vitamin K can be taken orally and result in the development of a full anticoagulant effect in several days. Technical variations among testing laboratories can result in significantly different levels of clinical anticoagulation despite seemingly comparable PT ratios. Sustained cooperation among a number of laboratories in different countries has resulted in development of the International Sensitivity Index (ISI) and the International Normalized Ratio (INR), which have been designed to allow standardization of PT reporting worldwide. In brief, when the logarithms of plasma PTs obtained in a prescribed series of normal patients and patients taking warfarin using the primary International Reference Thromboplastin are plotted against the logarithms of PTs obtained using an individual thromboplastin reagent, the resulting slope is the ISI for that thromboplastin reagent. If the PT ratio performed using the individual thromboplastin reagent is raised to the power of the ISI, the result is the INR—i.e., the PT ratio that would have been obtained if the International Reference Thromboplastin had actually been used for the patient testing. As demonstrated by Ng (1993) and by Cunningham (1994), however, attainment of a truly assay-independent INR may be very difficult in practice.

With thromboplastin reagents of increasing ISI, not only do the resulting limits between underdosage and overdosage become narrower, but the discrimination from normal also diminishes. In choosing thromboplastin reagents, accordingly, the laboratory must consider not only the sensitivities of the individual reagents for use in detecting individual factor deficiencies (for which a low ISI reagent might actually prove too sensitive), but also their ability to provide good monitoring of oral anticoagulation.

A quite different approach to monitoring oral anticoagulant therapy avoids PT testing altogether. Instead, an anti-

Table 29–6. HEMOSTATIC ABNORMALITIES IN LIVER DISEASE AND VITAMIN K DEFICIENCY

Condition	Platelets	APTT	PT	Factor V	Factor VII	TT	Fibrinogen Clauss Assay	Serum FDPs D-dimer	Clot Lysis Time
Acute hepatitis									
Without liver failure	N	N	N or ↑	N or ↓	N or ↓	N or ↑	N or ↑	N	N
With liver failure	N or ↓	↑	↑↑	↓↓	↓↓	↑↑	↓↓	N or ↑	↓
Liver cirrhosis (stable)	N or ↓	N or ↑	↑	↓ or N	↓	↑ or N	N or ↓	N or ↑	N or ↓
Liver cirrhosis (decomp)	↓	↑ or N	↑↑	↓	↓↓	↑ or N	↓ or N	N or ↑	↓ or N
Biliary cirrhosis	N or ↓	↑	↑↑	↓ or N	↓↓	↑ or N	↑ or N	N or ↑	↓ or N
Obstructive jaundice	N	↑ or N	↑↑	N or ↑	↓↓	N or ↑	↑ or N	N	N
Vitamin K deficiency	N	↑ or N	↑↑	N	↓↓	N	N	N	N

APTT = Activated partial thromboplastin time; PT = prothrombin time; TT = thrombin time; FDPs = fibrinogen/fibrin degradation products; N = normal; ↑ = increased; ↓ = decreased; decomp = decompensated

From Joist JH: Hemostatic abnormalities in liver disease. *In* Colman RW, Hirsh J, Marder VJ, Salzman EW (eds): Hemostasis and Thrombosis: Basic Principles and Clinical Practice, 3rd ed. Philadelphia, J. B. Lippincott, 1994, p 913.

body is employed in an immunoassay that recognizes only the normal (or "native") form of prothrombin and not those molecules lacking γ-carboxylation of glutamic acids, which are produced as a consequence of warfarin therapy (Furie, 1984). This approach has the potential advantage of being less dependent on specimen handling than a functional assay. Moreover, early clinical studies suggest that use of this approach to guide oral anticoagulant dose administration may result in a lower incidence of bleeding or thrombotic episodes (Furie, 1990).

Heparin

Heparin is a sulfated mucopolysaccharide that is capable of binding to antithrombin III, thereby greatly increasing the anticoagulant activity of the antithrombin III molecule (Barrowcliffe, 1994). Administration of heparin provides a potent form of anticoagulation that rapidly inhibits the activities of thrombin, Factor Xa, and the other serine protease coagulation factors (see Table 29–1). The PTT is the test most commonly employed for monitoring heparin therapy. It should be emphasized that standardization of PTT reagents in the individual laboratory for heparin monitoring is of considerable importance in the development of a PTT therapeutic range (Thomson, 1982; Ingram, 1982). Amidolytic anti-Factor Xa and anti-Factor IIa assays offer an alternative approach to monitoring heparin therapy (van den Besselaar, 1990). Anti-Factor Xa assays also provide a means of monitoring therapy with low-molecular-weight heparin fractions that do not produce the characteristic prolongations of the PTT observed with unfractionated heparin preparations.

Plasma samples obtained for coagulation testing occasionally show striking prolongations in the TT, together with variable prolongations of the PTT, and occasionally also of the PT. When no other cause is apparent, the presence of heparin arising in the patient, in an infusion line, or in the blood processing itself must be considered. In particular, whenever all three of these tests are prolonged more than 90 seconds, the possibility of the presence of heparin should be considered first. Commercially available ecteola (epichlorohydrin triethanolamine) cellulose anion-exchange resins now allow rapid removal of even full therapeutic doses of heparin from plasma; following this, most coagulation tests approach preheparin values. Enzymatic removal of heparin with heparinase has also been reported (van den Besselaar, 1993). Alternatively, the presence of heparin can be established if the addition of protamine sulfate or polybrene normalizes the test values (Hoffman, 1980). These positively charged substances neutralize the negatively charged heparin molecule.

Consumptive Thrombohemorrhagic Disorders

A wide variety of systemic and localized pathologic processes may lead to activation of the coagulation or fibrinolytic systems or both (Fig. 29–12). Depending on the balance struck between these two systems in the individual case, the immediate clinical result may be thrombosis, bleeding, or even a combination of the two.

The release of thromboplastic material into the circulation triggers the coagulation system, which subsequently activates the fibrinolytic system. Such an event has been termed *consumptive coagulopathy*, or *disseminated intravascular coagulation* (DIC). A wide variety of underlying causes may predispose to DIC, and it is imperative to detect the underlying condition so that therapy specific for the disorder can be instituted. Clinically suspected acute DIC can be verified by laboratory testing. Typically, the patient's platelet count drops, and the PTT, PT, and TT are prolonged. FDP are elevated, and the patient's fibrinogen level is decreased from its previous value. Increased thrombin formation may be monitored by assaying the F1-2 fragment of prothrombin that remains after cleavage of prothrombin by the Xa complex. Radioimmunoassay for *fibrinopeptide A* released from fi-

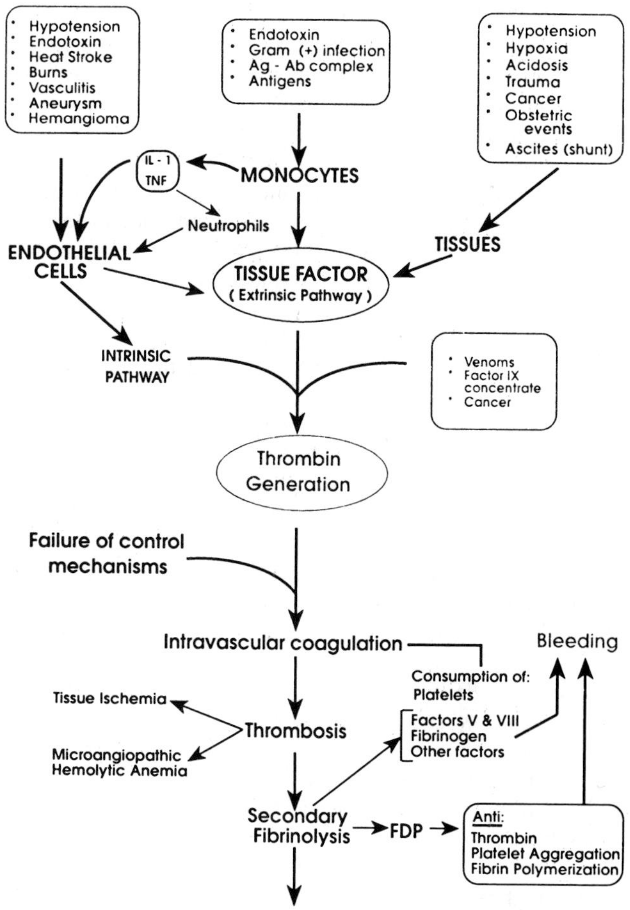

Figure 29–12. Main initiation pathways of DIC and its consequences. Triggers can activate (1) the extrinsic coagulation system by tissue factor expressed on cell surfaces; (2) the intrinsic coagulation system by causing injury to endothelial cells; and (3) coagulation factors, e.g., Factor X by cancer cells, Factor II by snake venoms. All of these elements lead to thrombin generation that in the presence of failure of the control mechanisms results in intravascular coagulation. This, in turn, can lead to thrombosis (that may be minimized by triggering secondary fibrinolysis) and to consumption of platelets, fibrinogen, and other coagulation factors. Bleeding can be caused by depletion of these essential hemostatic components; by the anticoagulant effects of fibrinogen/fibrin degradation products; and by further depletion of fibrinogen, Factor V, and Factor VIII by plasmin if generated in excess by the secondary fibrinolysis or if uninhibited due to diminished antiplasmin levels. (From Seligsohn U: Disseminated intravascular coagulation. *In* Beutler E, Lichtman MA, Coller BS, Kipps TJ [eds]: Williams Hematology, 5th ed. New York, McGraw-Hill, 1995, p 1499.)

brinogen by thrombin reflects *in vivo* thrombin activity and is nearly always increased (Nossel, 1974). Paracoagulation tests for circulating fibrin monomers such as the *ethanol gelation test* or the *serial dilution protamine sulfate test* (Niewiarowski, 1971) may also be positive.

Should the initiating process persist, DIC may progress from an acute to a more chronic form. Chronic DIC may be encountered, for example, in patients with malignancies or autoimmune disorders (Marder, 1994). In some instances in which the rate of consumption of individual hemostatic components is not excessive, a compensatory increase in production may lead to a normalization, or even an increase, in their circulating levels.

The initiation of *systemic hyperfibrinolysis* without a prominent accompanying DIC is a decidedly less common occurrence. Among disorders in which it may be encountered occasionally are liver disease and certain tumors that appear to produce plasminogen activators (Donati, 1981). Thrombolytic therapy (see previously) also may lead to a systemic hyperfibrinolytic state. Decreased fibrinogen (due to active plasmin in the circulation), increased FDP, and shortened whole blood or euglobulin clot lysis times are typical findings. In the rare instance of fibrinolysis unaccompanied by coagulation, the plasma D-dimer test for cross-linked fibrin D_2E fragments should be negative despite an increased serum FDP (as long as the detecting antibody recognizes determinants on fibrinogen rather than only on fibrin).

Localized renal thrombi or multiorgan thrombus formation is associated with the *hemolytic-uremic syndrome* (HUS) and *thrombotic thrombocytopenic purpura* (TTP), respectively. The pathophysiology of this family of disorders, which remains controversial, has been reviewed (Moake, 1994). Laboratory findings typically include thrombocytopenia and microangiopathic hemolytic anemia. Although the TT may be prolonged and the level of FDP increased, convincing evidence of DIC is usually not present in most cases. When laboratory evidence of DIC is found, it is thought to be secondary to the severe hemolysis and subsequent release of red cell fragments that may occur in HUS and TTP (Bukowski, 1982).

APPROACH TO THE PATIENT

Hemostatic evaluation in the individual patient begins first with a thorough clinical history and physical examination. It is critical to determine whether the degree of bleeding appears disproportionate to the inciting incident(s). Tracing the onset of an apparent bleeding tendency can help to determine whether the abnormality is inherited or acquired. A careful systems review and questions about previous surgery, dental procedures, trauma, and blood transfusions may reveal important clues to a disorder or may reinforce a clinical impression of hemostatic normality. A detailed family history may provide important information about the mode of transmission of inherited disorders or may reinforce the impression that a particular disorder is acquired.

The pattern of bleeding in primary hemostatic (platelet or vWF) disorders tends to be different from that in secondary hemostatic (coagulation) disorders (Table 29–7), although some degree of overlap of these features is to be expected. In disorders of primary hemostasis, the bleeding time typically is prolonged. If the platelet count is normal and there is no history of ingestion of drugs that could have a detrimental effect on platelet function, the possibility of vWD should be considered. Measurement of vWF antigen and ristocetin cofactor activity should be performed and, if the levels are decreased, further characterization by means of multimeric analysis of vWF may be undertaken. Normal values of vWF antigen and ristocetin cofactor activity raise the possibility of a qualitative platelet defect, either congenital or acquired. Platelet aggregation (or lumi-aggregation), together with evaluation of platelet morphology on a peripheral blood smear, may suggest a recognizable platelet defect. More specialized platelet studies (see Table 28–6) may be of additional help in reaching a diagnosis. Repeated studies of the patient, together with studies of members of the patient's family, may be necessary before a definitive diagnosis can be reached in some cases.

Table 29–7. PATTERNS OF CLINICAL BLEEDING IN DISORDERS OF HEMOSTASIS

	Disorders of Primary Hemostasis (Platelet-Vascular Problem)	Disorders of Secondary Hemostasis (Coagulation Factor Problem)
Onset of bleeding	Spontaneous or immediately after trauma	Delayed after trauma
Sites of bleeding	Superficial surfaces	Deep tissues
Skin	Petechiae, ecchymoses	Hematomas
Mucous membranes	Common (nasal, oral, gastrointestinal, genitourinary)	Rare
Other sites	Rare	Common (joint muscle, retroperitoneal)
Clinical examples	Thrombocytopenia, functional platelet defect, vascular fragility	Congenital coagulation factor deficiency, acquired inhibitor, anticoagulation
	Disseminated intravascular coagulation, liver failure	Disseminated intravascular coagulation, liver failure

From Schafer AI: Approach to bleeding. *In* Loscalzo J, Schafer AI (eds): Thrombosis and Hemorrhage. Boston, Blackwell Scientific Publishers, 1994, p 409. Reprinted by permission of Blackwell Science, Inc.

Disorders of secondary hemostasis usually do not present with a prolonged bleeding time. The whole blood clot lysis test or a variant thereof can serve as a screening test (albeit not very sensitive) for enhanced fibrinolysis. Should an abnormality in fibrinolysis be suspected, measurement of serum FDP or plasma D-dimer, euglobulin clot lysis time, or more specialized tests may be undertaken.

Routine use of the PT, PTT, and TT offer great help in narrowing the diagnostic possibilities in most patients with secondary hemostatic disorders. Although there is no one single approach to such patients, some form of progression from the simpler screening types of tests to specific assays for only a small number of different factors is necessary. Figure 29–13 represents such an approach to the diagnosis of both inherited and acquired disorders of secondary hemostasis.

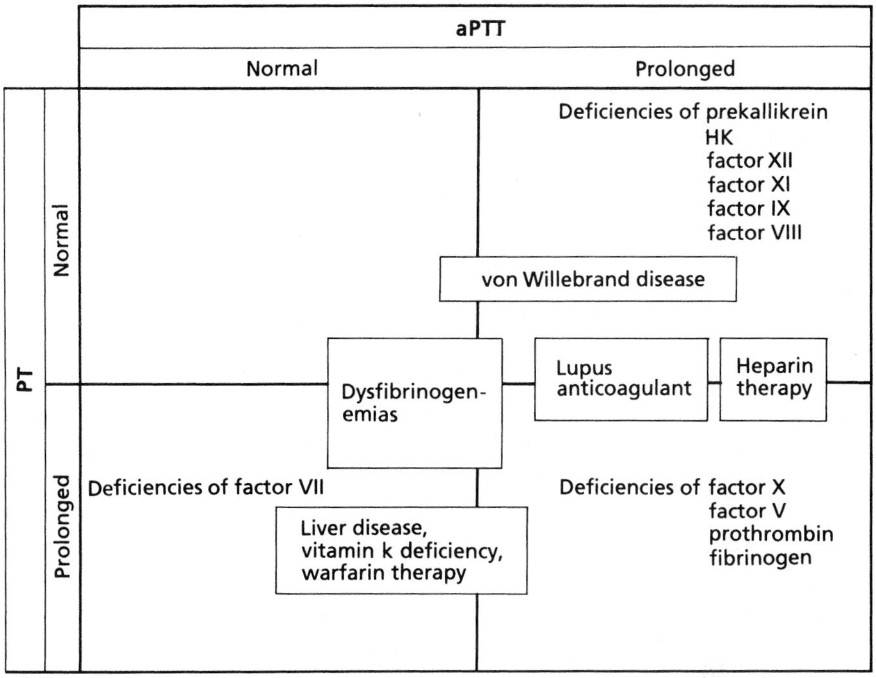

Figure 29–13. Matrix of diagnostic possibilities with abnormalities of the prothrombin time (PT) and/or the activated partial thromboplastin time (aPTT). Patients with disorders indicated as boxed insets may exhibit different patterns of abnormalities of the PT or aPTT. For example, in von Willebrand's disease, the PT is normal but the aPTT may be either prolonged or normal. In the lupus anticoagulant or in patients receiving heparin, the usual pattern is a prolonged aPTT and a normal PT; however, in some cases, the PT may also be prolonged. In patients with liver disease, vitamin K deficiency, or on warfarin therapy, the usual pattern is a prolonged PT and a normal aPTT; however, in more severe cases, the aPTT may also be prolonged. Any combination of results of the PT and aPTT may be seen in dysfibrinogenemias. (From Schafer AI: Approach to bleeding. *In* Loscalzo J, Schafer AL [eds]: Thrombosis and Hemorrhage. Boston, Blackwell Scientific Publications, 1994, p 418. Reprinted by permission of Blackwell Science, Inc.)

Adelman B, Michelson AD, Loscalzo J, et al: Plasmin effect on platelet glycoprotein Ib-von Willebrand factor interactions. Blood 1986; 65:32.

Aguilar-Martinez P, Romey MC, Schved JF, et al: Factor IX gene mutations causing haemophilia B: Comparison of SSC screening versus systematic DNA sequencing and diagnostic applications. Hum Genet 1994; 94:287.

Antonarakis SE: The molecular genetics of hemophilia A and B in man: Factor VIII and factor IX deficiency. Adv Hum Genet 1988; 17:27.

Asakai R, Chung DW, Davie EW, et al: Factor XI deficiency in Ashkenazi Jews in Israel. N Engl J Med 1991; 325:153.

Bader R, Mannucci PMM, Tripadi A, et al: Multicentric evaluation of a new PT reagent based on recombinant human tissue factor and synthetic phospholipids. Thromb Haemost 1994; 71:292.

Barrowcliffe TW, Thomas DP: Heparin and low molecular weight heparin. *In* Bloom AL, Forbes CD, Thomas DP, Tuddenham EGD (eds): Haemostasis and Thrombosis, 3rd ed. New York, Churchill Livingstone, 1994, p 1417.

Bauer KA: Hypercoagulability—A new cofactor in the Protein C anticoagulant pathway. N Engl J Med 1994; 330:566.

Beck EA: Congenital abnormalities of fibrinogen. Clin Haematol 1979; 8:169.

Beck EA: Congenital disorders of fibrin formation and stabilization. *In* Colman RW, Hirsh J, Marder VJ, Salzman EW (eds): Hemostasis and Thrombosis. Philadelphia, J. B. Lippincott, 1982, p 185.

Bell BA, Birch K, Glazer S: Experience with recombinant factor VIIA in an infant hemophiliac with inhibitors to FVIII:C undergoing emergency central line placement. A case report. Am J Pediatr Hematol Oncol 1993; 15:77.

Bell WR: Fibrinolytic therapy: Indications and management. *In* Hoffman R, Benz EJ Jr, Shattil SJ, et al (eds): Hematology: Basic Principles and Practice, 2nd ed. New York, Churchill Livingstone, 1995, p 1814.

Bernardi F, Liney DL, Patracchini P, et al: Molecular defects in CRM+ factor VII deficiencies: Modelling of missense mutations in the catalytic domain of FVII. Br J Haematol 1994; 86:610.

Bertina RM, Koeleman BP, Koster T, et al: Mutation in blood coagulation factor V associated with resistance to activated protein C. Nature 1994; 369:64.

Bevers EM, Comfurius P, van Rijn JL, et al: Generation of prothrombin-converting activity and the exposure of phosphatidylserine at the outer surface of platelets. Eur J Biochem 1982; 122:429.

Biggs R, Austen DEG, Denson KWE, et al: The mode of action of antibodies which destroy factor VIII. II. Antibodies which give complex concentration graphs. Br J Haematol 1972; 23:137.

Bloom AL: Inherited disorders of blood coagulation. *In* Bloom AL, Thomas DP (eds): Haemostasis and Thrombosis, 2nd ed. New York, Churchill Livingstone, 1987, p 436.

Boisclair MD, Lane DA, Wilde JT, et al: A comparative evaluation of assays for markers of activated coagulation and/or fibrinolysis: Thrombin-antithrombin complex, D-dimer and fibrinogen/fibrin fragment E antigen. Br J Haematol 1990; 74:471.

Bokarewa MI, Blomback M, Egberg N, et al: A new variant of interaction between phospholipid antibodies and the protein C system. Blood Coag Fibrinol 1994; 5:37.

Bolton-Maggs PHB, Wan-Yin BY, McCraw AH, et al: Inheritance and bleeding in factor XI deficiency. Br J Haematol 1988; 69:521.

Bouchet C, Spyratos F, Martin PM, et al: Prognostic value of urokinase-type plasminogen activator (uPA) and plasminogen activator inhibitors PAI-1 and PAI-2 in breast carcinomas. Br J Cancer 1994; 69:398.

Brandt JT, Arkin CF, Bovill EG, et al: Evaluation of APTT reagent sensitivity to factor IX and factor IX assay performance. Results from the College of American Pathologists Survey Program. Arch Pathol Lab Med 1990; 114:135.

Brettler DB, Levine PH: Clinical manifestations and therapy of inherited coagulation factor deficiencies. *In* Colman RW, Hirsh J, Marder VJ, et al (eds): Hemostasis and Thrombosis: Basic Principles and Clinical Practice, 3rd ed. Philadelphia, J. B. Lippincott, 1994, p 169.

Briet E, Bertina RM, Van Tilburg NH, et al: Hemophilia B Leyden. A sex-linked hereditary disorder that improves after puberty. N Engl J Med 1982; 306:788.

Broze GJ Jr: The tissue factor pathway of coagulation: Factor VII, tissue factor, and tissue factor pathway inhibitor. *In* Bloom AL, Forbes CD, Thomas DP, Tuddenham EGD (eds): Haemostasis and Thrombosis, 3rd ed. New York, Churchill Livingstone, 1994, p 349.

Buchanan GP, Holtkamp CA: Prolonged bleeding time in children and young adults with hemophilia. Pediatrics 1980; 66:951.

Bukowski RM: Thrombotic thrombocytopenic purpura: A review. *In* Spaet TH (ed): Progress in Hemostasis and Thrombosis, Vol. 6. New York, Grune & Stratton, 1982, p 287.

Carrell R, Travis J: Alpha-1 antitrypsin and the serpins: Variation and countervariation. Trends Biochem Sci 1985; 10:20.

Chaing S, Clarke B, Sridhara S, et al: Severe factor VII deficiency caused by mutations abolishing the cleavage site for activation and altering binding to tissue factor. Blood 1994; 83:3524.

Chand S, McCraw A, Hutton R, et al: A two-site, monoclonal antibody-based immunoassay for von Willebrand factor: Demonstration that vWF function resides in a conformational epitope. Thromb Haemost 1986; 55:318.

Chow TW, Hellums JD, Moake JL, et al: Shear stress-induced von Willebrand factor binding to platelet glycoprotein Ib initiates calcium influx associated with aggregation. Blood 1992; 80:113.

Ciavarella G, Ciavarella N, Antoncecchi S, et al: High-resolution analysis of von Willebrand factor multimeric composition defines a new variant of Type I von Willebrand disease with aberrant structure but presence of all size multimers (Type IC). Blood 1985; 66:1423.

Cinotti S, Longo G, Messori A, et al: Reproducibility of one-stage, two-stage and chromogenic assays of factor VIII activity: A multi-center study. Thromb Res 1991; 61:385.

Clauss A: Gerinnungsphyiologische Schnellmethode zur Bestimmung des Fibrinogens. Acta Haematol 1957; 17:237.

Collen D: On the regulation and control of fibrinolysis. Thromb Haemost 1980; 43:77.

Colucci M, Stassen JM, Collen D: Influence of protein C activation on blood coagulation and fibrinolysis in squirrel monkeys. J Clin Invest 1984; 74:200.

Comp PC, Doray D, Patton D, et al: An abnormal plasma distribution of protein S occurs in functional protein S deficiency. Blood 1986; 67:504.

Comp PC, Esmon CT: Generation of fibrinolytic activity by infusion of activated protein C into dogs. J Clin Invest 1981; 68:1221.

Coppes MJ, Zandvoort SW, Sparling CR, et al: Acquired von Willebrand disease in Wilms' tumor patients. J Clin Oncol 1992; 10:422.

Cotton RG, Rodrigues NR, Campbell RD: Reactivity of cytosine and thymine in single-base-pair mismatches with hydroxylamine and osmium tetroxide and its application to the study of mutations. Proc Natl Acad Sci USA 1988; 85:4397.

Cowan JF, Khan MB, Vargo J, Joist JH: An improved method for evaluation of blood coagulation in heparinized blood. Am J Clin Pathol 1981; 75:60.

Coyle TE, Spicer T, Michalovic D, et al: Moderate hemophilia B Leyden: Identification by polymerase chain reaction, sequencing, and oligomer restriction. Am J Hematol 1994; 46:234.

Cramer EM, Vainchenker W, Vinci G, et al: Gray platelet syndrome: Immunoelectron microscopic localization of fibrinogen and von Willebrand factor in platelets and megakaryocytes. Blood 1985; 66:1309.

Cunningham MT, Johnson GF, Pennell BJ, et al: The reliability of manufacturer-determined, instrument-specific international sensitivity index values for calculating the international normalized ratio. Am J Clin Pathol 1994; 102:128.

Dahlbäck B, Carlsson M, Svensson PJ: Familial thrombophilia due to a previously unrecognized mechanism characterized by poor anticoagulant response to activated protein C: Prediction of a cofactor to activated protein C. Proc Natl Acad Sci USA 1993; 90:1004.

Dahlbäck B, Hildebrand B: Inherited resistance to activated protein C is corrected by anticoagulant cofactor activity found to be a property of factor V. Proc Natl Acad Sci USA 1994; 91:1396.

Denson WE: The simplified two-stage assay for factor VIII. *In* Biggs R (ed): Human Blood Coagulation, Haemostasis and Thrombosis, 2nd ed. Oxford, Blackwell Scientific Publishers, 1976, p 688.

Dent JA, Galbusera M, Ruggeri ZM: Heterogeneity of plasma von Willebrand factor multimers resulting from proteolysis of the constituent subunit. J Clin Invest 1991; 88:774.

Donati MB, Poggi A, Semeraro N: Coagulation and malignancy. *In* Poller L (ed): Recent Advances in Blood Coagulation. New York, Churchill Livingstone, 1981, p 227.

Drake TA, Morrissey JH, Edgington TS: Selective cellular expression of tissue factor in human tissues. Am J Pathol 1989; 135:1087.

Dvilansky A, Britten AHF, Loewy AG: Factor XIII assay by an isotope method. I. Factor XIII (transamidase) in plasma, serum leukocytes, erythrocytes and platelets and evaluation of screening tests of clot solubility. Br J Haematol 1970; 18:339.

Edson JR: Discussion of the control of heparin therapy by the activated partial thromboplastin time: Sensitivity of various thromboplastins to heparin. *In* Triplett DA (ed): Standardization of Coagulation Assays: An Overview. Skokie, IL, College of American Pathologists, 1982, p 204.

Esmon CT, Owen WG: Identification of an endothelial cell cofactor for thrombin-catalyzed activation of protein C. Proc Natl Acad Sci USA 1981; 78:2249.

Ewing NP, Kasper CK: In vitro detection of mild inhibitors to factor VIII in hemophilia. Am J Clin Pathol 1982; 77:749.

Eyster ME, Gordon RA, Ballard JO: The bleeding time is longer than normal in hemophilia. Blood 1981; 58:719.

Feinstein DI: Inhibitors in hemophilia. *In* Hoffman R, Benz EJ Jr, Shattil SJ, et al (eds): Hematology: Basic Principles and Practice, 2nd ed. New York, Churchill Livingstone, 1995, p 1686.

Firshein SI, Hoyer LW, Lazarchick J, et al: Prenatal diagnosis of classic haemophilia. N Engl J Med 1979; 300:937.

Fischer B, Mitterer A, Schlokat U, et al: Structural analysis of recombinant von Willebrand factor: Identification of hetero- and homo-dimers. FEBS Lett 1994; 351:345.

Foekens JA, Schmitt M, van Putten WL, et al: Plasminogen activator inhibitor-1 and prognosis in primary breast cancer. J Clin Oncol 1994; 12:1648.

Francis CW, Marder VJ: Physiologic regulation and pathologic disorders of fibrinolysis. *In* Colman RW, Hirsh J, Marder VJ, Salzman EW (eds): Hemostasis and Thrombosis, 3rd ed. Philadelphia, J. B. Lippincott, 1994, p 1076.

Francis CW, Marder VJ: Mechanisms of fibrinolysis. *In* Beutler E, Lichtman MA, Coller BS, Kipps TJ (eds): Williams Hematology, 5th ed. New York, McGraw-Hill, 1995, p 1258.

Furie B, Diuguid CF, Jacobs M, et al: Randomized prospective trial comparing the native prothrombin antigen with the prothrombin time for monitoring oral anticoagulant therapy. Blood 1990; 75:344.

Furie B, Furie BC: The molecular basis of blood coagulation. Cell 1988; 53:505.

Furie B, Liebman HA, Blanchard RA, et al: Comparison of the native prothrombin antigen and the prothrombin time for monitoring oral anticoagulant therapy. Blood 1984; 64:445.

Furie B, Voo L, McAdam KPWJ, et al: Mechanism of factor X deficiency in systemic amyloidosis. N Engl J Med 1981; 304:827.

Gailani D, Broze GJ Jr: Factor XI activation by thrombin and factor XIa. Semin Thromb Hemost 1993; 19:396.

Garabedian HD, Gold HK, Leinbach RC, et al: Laboratory monitoring of hemostasis during thrombolytic therapy with recombinant human tissue-type plasminogen activator. Thromb Res 1988; 50:121.

Gawyrl MS, Hoyer LW: Inactivation of factor VIII coagulant activity by two different types of human antibodies. Blood 1982; 60:1103.

Gill JC, Endres-Brooks J, Bauer PJ, et al: The effect of ABO blood group on the diagnosis of von Willebrand disease. Blood 1987; 69:1691.

Ginsburg D, Handin RI, Bonthron DT, et al: Human von Willebrand factor (vWF): Isolation of complementary DNA (cDNA) clones and chromosomal localization. Science 1985; 228:1401.

Girard TJ, MacPhail LA, Likert KM, et al: Inhibition of factor VIIa-tissue factor coagulation activity by a hybrid protein. Science 1990; 248:1421.

Gitschier J, Kogan S, Levinson B, et al: Mutations of factor VIII cleavage sites in hemophilia A. Blood 1988; 72:1022.

Goodall AH, Jarvis J, Chand S, et al: An immunoradiometric assay for human factor VIII/von Willebrand factor (VIII:vWF) using a monoclonal antibody that defines a functional epitope. Br J Haematol 1985; 59:565.

Goodeve AC, Preston FE, Peake IR: Factor VIII gene rearrangements in patients with severe haemophilia A. Lancet 1994; 43:329.

Graham JB: Genotype assignment (carrier detection) in the haemophilias. Clin Haematol 1979; 8:115.

Gralnick H, Connaghan DG: Hereditary abnormalities of fibrinogen. *In* Beutler E, Lichtman MA, Coller BS, et al (eds): Williams Hematology, 5th ed. New York, McGraw-Hill, 1995, p 1439.

Green D, Hougie C, Kazmier FJ, et al: Report of the working party on acquired inhibitors of coagulation: Studies of the "lupus" anticoagulant. Thromb Haemost 1983; 49:144.

Green PP, Mannucci PM, Briët E, et al: Carrier detection in hemophilia A: A cooperative international study. II. The efficacy of a universal discriminant. Blood 1986; 67:1560.

Greenfield C, Hiles I, Waterfield MD, et al: Epidermal growth factor binding induces a conformational change in the external domain of its receptor. EMBO J 1989; 8:4115.

Greengard JS, Eichinger S, Griffin JH, et al: Brief report: Variability of thrombosis among homozygous siblings with resistance to activated protein C due to an Arg to Gln mutation in the gene for factor V. N Engl J Med 1994; 331:1559.

Griffin JH, Evatt B, Zimmerman TS, et al: Deficiency of protein C in congenital thrombotic disease. J Clin Invest 1981; 68:1370.

Haber E, Quertermous T, Matsueda GR, et al: Innovative approaches to plasminogen activator therapy. Science 1989; 243:51.

Halligan A, Bonnar J, Sheppard B, et al: Haemostatic, fibrinolytic and endothelial variables in normal pregnancies and pre-eclampsia. Br J Obstet Gynaecol 1994; 101:488.

Hancock JF, Wieland K, Pugh RE, et al: A molecular genetic study of factor XI deficiency. Blood 1991; 77:1942.

Handin RI, Wagner DD: Molecular and cellular biology of von Willebrand factor. *In* Coller BS (ed): Progress in Hemostasis and Thrombosis, Vol. 9. Philadelphia, W. B. Saunders, 1989, p 233.

Hardisty RM, Macphorson JC: A one-stage factor VIII (anti-haemophilic globulin) assay and its use on venous and capillary plasma. Thromb Diath Haemorrh 1962; 7:215.

Hemker HC, van Rijn JLML, Rosing J, et al: Platelet membrane involvement in blood coagulation. Blood Cells 1983; 9:303.

Higuchi M, Kazazian HH Jr, Kasch L, et al: Molecular characterization of severe hemophilia A suggests that about half the mutations are not within the coding regions and splice junctions of the factor VIII gene. Proc Natl Acad Sci USA 1991; 88:7405.

Hoffman JJML, Meulendijk PN: Evaluation of a heparin neutralizer. Thromb Res 1980; 18:897.

Hougie C, Twomey JJ: Haemophilia B_M: A new type of factor IX deficiency. Lancet 1967; 1:698.

Hoyer LW: Biochemistry of factor VIII. *In* Colman RW, Hirsh J, Marder VJ, Salzman EW (eds): Hemostasis and Thrombosis. Philadelphia, J. B. Lippincott, 1982, p 39.

Ikeda Y, Handa M, Kawano K, et al: The role of von Willebrand factor and fibrinogen in platelet aggregation under varying shear stress. J Clin Invest 1991; 87:1234.

Ingerslev J, Schwartz M, Lamm LU, et al: Female haemophilia A in a fam-

ily with seeming extreme bidirectional lyonization tendency: Abnormal premature X-chromosome inactivation? Clin Genet 1989; 35:41.
Ingram GIC, Brozovic M, Slater NGP: Bleeding Disorders: Investigation and Management, 2nd ed. Oxford, Blackwell Scientific Publishers, 1982, p 326.
Jackson CM: Physiology and biochemistry of prothrombin activation. *In* Bloom AL, Forbes CD, Thomas DP, Tuddenham EGD (eds): Haemostasis and Thrombosis, 3rd ed. New York, Churchill Livingstone, 1994, p 397.
Jaffe EA, Hoyer LW, Nachman RL: Synthesis of von Willebrand factor by cultured human endothelial cells. Proc Natl Acad Sci USA 1974; 71:1906.
Joist JH, Cowan JF, Zimmerman TS: Acquired von Willebrand's disease. Evidence for a quantitative and qualitative factor VIII disorder. N Engl J Med 1978; 298:988.
Joist JH: Hemostatic abnormalities in liver disease. *In* Colman RW, Hirsh J, Marder VJ, Salzman EW (eds): Hemostasis and Thrombosis: Basic Principles and Clinical Practice, 3rd ed. Philadelphia, J. B. Lippincott, 1994, p 913.
Kasper CK, Aledort LM, Counts RB, et al: A more uniform measurement of factor VIII inhibitors. Thromb Diath Haemorrh 1975; 34:869.
Kasper CK, Ewing NP: Measurement of inhibitor to factor VIII C (and IX C). *In* Bloom AL (ed): The Hemophilias. New York, Churchill Livingstone, 1982, p 39.
Kasper CK, Osterud B, Minami JY, et al: Hemophilia B: Characterization of genetic variants and detection of carriers. Blood 1977; 50:351.
Kidd P, Denson KWE, Biggs R: The thrombotest reagent and Christmas disease. Lancet 1963; 2:522.
Kisiel W, Canfield W, Errison L, et al: Anticoagulant properties of bovine plasma protein C following activation by thrombin. Biochemistry 1977; 16:5824.
Kogan SC, Doherty M, Gitschier J: An improved method for prenatal diagnosis of genetic diseases by analysis of amplified DNA sequences. Application to hemophilia A. N Engl J Med 1987; 317:985.
Kupinski JM, Miller JL: Multimeric analysis of von Willebrand factor in megakaryocytes. Thromb Res 1985; 38:603.
Lakich D, Kazazian HH Jr, Antonarakis SE, et al: Inversions disrupting the factor VIII gene are a common cause of severe haemophilia A. Nature Gen 1993; 5:236.
Landau BJ, Kwaan HC, Verrusio EN, et al: Elevated levels of urokinase-type plasminogen activator and plasminogen activator inhibitor type-1 in malignant human brain tumors. Canc Res 1994; 54:1105.
Lazarchick J, Hoyer LW: Immunoradiometric measurement of the factor VIII procoagulant antigen. J Clin Invest 1978; 55:1048.
Lijnen HR, Collen D: Remaining perspectives of mutant and chimeric plasminogen activators. Ann NY Acad Sci 1992; 667:357.
Lindley CM, Sawyer WT, Macik BG, et al: Pharmacokinetics and pharmacodynamics of recombinant factor VIIa. Clin Pharmacol Ther 1994; 55:638.
Lorand L, Urayama T, de Kiewiet JWC, Nossel HL: Diagnostic and genetic studies of fibrin-stabilizing factor with a new assay based on amine incorporation. J Clin Invest 1969; 48:1054.
Lossing TS, Kasper CK, Feinstein DI: Detection of factor VIII inhibitors with the partial thromboplastin time. Blood 1977; 49:793.
Lu H, Soria C, Soria J, et al: Reversible translocation of glycoprotein Ib in plasmin-treated platelets: Consequences for platelet function. Eur J Clin Invest 1993; 23:785.
Lynch DC, Zimmerman TS, Ling EH, et al: An explanation for minor multimer species in endothelial cell-synthesized von Willebrand factor. J Clin Invest 1986; 77:2048.
Macfarlane DE, Stibbe J, Kirby EP, et al: A method for assaying von Willebrand factor (ristocetin cofactor). Thromb Diath Haemorrh 1975; 34:306.
Mannucci PM, Coppola R, Lombardi R, et al: Direct proof of extreme lyonization as a cause of low factor VIII levels in females. Thromb Haemost 1978; 39:544.
Mannucci PM, Lombardi R, Bader R, et al: Studies of the pathophysiology of acquired von Willebrand's disease in seven patients with lymphoproliferative disorders or benign monoclonal gammopathies. Blood 1984; 64:614.
Mannucci PM, Lombardi R, Pareti FI, et al: A variant of von Willebrand's disease characterized by recessive inheritance and missing triplet structure of von Willebrand factor multimers. Blood 1983; 62:1000.
Marder VJ, Feinstein DI, Francis CW, et al: Consumptive thrombohemorrhagic disorders. *In* Colman RW, Hirsh J, Marder VJ, Salzman EW (eds): Hemostasis and Thrombosis, 3rd ed. Philadelphia, J. B. Lippincott, 1994, p 1023.
Martinez PA, Romey MC, Schved JF, et al: Direct carrier testing of haemophilia B by SSCP. Clin Lab Haematol 1994; 6:15.
McCraw A, Chand S, Tuddenham EG, et al: A monoclonal antibody based immunoradiometric assay for von Willebrand factor: Survey of a large patient group. Thromb Res 1987; 45:101.
Menache D: Congenital abnormal fibrinogens. *In* Menache D, Surgenor DM, Anderson H (eds): Hemophilia and hemostasis. New York, Alan R. Liss, 1981, p 205.
Michelson AD, Gore JM, Rybak ME, et al: Effect of *in vivo* infusion of recombinant tissue-type plasminogen activator on platelet glycoprotein Ib. Thromb Res 1990; 60:421.
Miletich JP, Majerus DW, Majerus PW: Patients with congenital factor V deficiency have decreased factor Xa binding sites on their platelets. J Clin Invest 1978; 62:824.
Miletich JP, Jackson CM, Majerus PW: Properties of the factor Xa binding site on human platelets. J Biol Chem 1978; 253:6908.
Miletich J, Sherman L, Broze G Jr: Absence of thrombosis in subjects with heterozygous protein C deficiency. N Engl J Med 1987; 317:991.
Miller JL, Katz AJ, Feinstein MB: Plasmin inhibition of thrombin-induced platelet aggregation. Thromb Diath Haemorrh 1975; 33:286.
Miller JL: Sorting out heightened interactions between platelets and von Willebrand factor: "IIB or not IIB?" is becoming an increasingly answerable question in the molecular era. Am J Clin Pathol 1991; 96:681.
Miller JL: von Willebrand disease. Hematol Oncol Clin North Am 1990; 4:107.
Miller JL, Castella A: Platelet-type von Willebrand's disease: Characterization of a new bleeding disorder. Blood 1982; 60:790.
Miller JL, Kupinski JM, Castella A, et al: von Willebrand factor binds to platelets and induces aggregation in platelet-type but not type IIB von Willebrand disease. J Clin Invest 1983; 72:1532.
Miller JL, Ruggeri ZM, Lyle VA: Unique interactions of asialo von Willebrand factor with platelets in platelet-type von Willebrand disease. Blood 1987; 70:1804.
Moake JL, Rudy CK, Troll JH, et al: Unusually large plasma factor VIII: von Willebrand factor multimers in chronic relapsing thrombotic thrombocytopenia purpura. N Engl J Med 1982; 307:1432.
Montandon AJ, Green PM, Bentley DR, et al: Two factor IX mutations in the family of an isolated haemophilia B patient: Direct carrier diagnosis by amplification mismatch detection (AMD). Hum Genet 1990; 85:200.
Morrissey JH, Fakhrai H, Edgington TS: Molecular cloning of the cDNA for tissue factor, the cellular receptor for the initiation of the coagulation protease cascade. Cell 1987; 50:129.
Mosher DE: Disorders of blood coagulation. *In* Wyngaarden JB, Smith LH Jr (eds): Textbook of Medicine, 18th ed. Philadelphia, W. B. Saunders, 1988, p 1060.
Mueh JR, Herbst KD, Rapaport SI: Thrombosis in patients with the lupus anticoagulant. Ann Intern Med 1980; 92:156.
Nachman R, Levine R, Jaffe EA: Synthesis of factor VIII antigen by cultured guinea pig megakaryocytes. J Clin Invest 1977; 60:914.
Naito K, Fujikawa K: Activation of human blood coagulation factor XI independent of factor XII. Factor XI is activated by thrombin and factor XIa in the presence of negatively charged surfaces. J Biol Chem 1991; 266:7353.
Naylor JA, Green PM, Montandon AJ, et al: Detection of three novel mutations in two haemophilia A patients by rapid screening of whole essential region of factor VIII gene. Lancet 1991; 337:635.
Naylor JA, Green PM, Rizza CR, et al: Analysis of factor VIII mRNA reveals defects in everyone of 28 haemophilia A patients. Hum Mol Genet 1993; 2:11.
Naylor JA, Green PM, Rizza CR, et al: Factor VIII gene explains all cases of haemophilia A. Lancet 1992; 340:1066.
Nemerson Y, Zur M: Is hemophilia a disease of the tissue factor pathway of coagulation? *In* Menache D, Surgenor DM, Anderson H (eds): Hemophilia and Hemostasis. New York, Alan R Liss, 1981, p 77.
Nesheim M, Pittman DD, Giles AR, et al: The effect of plasma von Willebrand factor on the binding of human Factor VIII to thrombin-activated human platelets. J Biol Chem 1991; 266:17815.
Ng VL, Levin J, Corash L, et al: Failure of the International Normalized Ratio to generate consistent results within a local medical community. Am J Clin Pathol 1993; 99:689.
Niewiarowski S, Gurewick V: Laboratory identification of intravascular coagulation: The serial dilution protamine sulfate test for the detection of fibrin monomer and fibrin degradation products. J Lab Clin Med 1971; 77:665.
Nossel HL, Yudelman I, Canfield RE, et al: Measurement of fibrinopeptide A in human blood. J Clin Invest 1974; 54:43.
Odom MW, Leone G, De Stefano V, et al: Five novel point mutations: Two causing haemophilia B and three causing factor X deficiency. Mol Cell Probes 1994; 8:63.
Pechet L, Tarks CY, Stevens J, et al: Relationship of factor IX antigen and coagulant in hemophilia B patients and carriers. Thromb Haemost 1978; 40:465.
Pecorara M, Casarino L, Mori PG, et al: Hemophilia A: Carrier detection and prenatal diagnosis by DNA analysis. Blood 1987; 70:531.
Peterson DM, Strathopoulos NA, Giorgio TD, et al: Shear-induced platelet aggregation requires von Willebrand factor and platelet membrane glycoproteins Ib and IIb-IIIa. Blood 1987; 69:625.
Poon MC, Hoar DI, Low S, et al: Hemophilia A carrier detection by restriction fragment length polymorphism analysis and discriminant analysis based on ELISA of factor VIII and vWf. J Lab Clin Med 1992; 119:751.
Rapaport SI: The activation of factor IX by the tissue factor pathway. *In*

4

Menache D, Surgenor DM, Anderson H (eds): Hemophilia and Hemostasis. New York, Alan R. Liss, 1981, p 57.

Rapaport SI, Rao VM: Initiation and regulation of tissue factor-dependent blood coagulation. Arterioscler Thromb 1992; 12:1111.

Ratnoff OD, Menzie C: A new method for the determination of fibrinogen in small samples on plasma. J Lab Clin Med 1951; 37:316.

Rauch J, Janoff AS: Phospholipid in the hexagonal II phase is immunogenic: Evidence for immunorecognition of nonbilayer lipid phases in vivo. Proc Natl Acad Sci USA 1990; 87:4112.

Richard C, Cuadrado MA, Prieto M, et al: Acquired von Willebrand disease in multiple myeloma secondary to absorption of von Willebrand factor by plasma cells. Am J Hematol 1990; 35:114.

Rizza CR: von Willebrand's disease. *In* Biggs R (ed): The Treatment of Haemophilia A and B and von Willebrand's Disease. Oxford, Blackwell Scientific Publishers, 1978.

Roberts HR: Molecular biology of hemophilia B [review]. Thromb Haemostas 1993; 70:1.

Roberts HR, Griffith MJ, Braunstein KM, et al: Structural abnormalities of the vitamin K-dependent clotting factors. *In* Menache D, Surgenor DM, Anderson H (eds): Hemophilia and Hemostasis. New York, Alan R. Liss, 1981, p 85.

Roberts HR, Lefkowitz JB: Inherited disorders of prothrombin conversion. *In* Colman RW, Hirsh J, Marder VJ, Salzman EW (eds): Hemostasis and Thrombosis: Basic Principles and Clinical Practice, 3rd ed. Philadelphia, J. B. Lippincott, 1994, p 200.

Rosenberg RD, Bauer KA: Thrombosis in inherited deficiencies of antithrombin, Protein C and Protein S. Hum Pathol 1987; 18:253.

Rosenberg RD: Hemorrhagic disorders I. Protein interactions in the clotting mechanism. *In* Beck WS (eds): Hematology, 5th ed. Cambridge, MIT Press, 1991, p 531.

Roussi J, Drouet L, Samama M, et al: French multicentric evaluation of recombinant tissue factor (recombiplastin) for determination of prothrombin time. Thromb Haemost 1994; 72:698.

Ruf W, Edgington TS: Structural biology of tissue factor, the initiator of thrombogenesis in vivo. FASEB J 1994; 8:385.

Ruggeri ZM, Lombardi R, Gatti L, et al: Type IIB von Willebrand's disease: Differential clearance of endogenous versus transfused large multimer von Willebrand factor. Blood 1982a; 60:1453.

Ruggeri ZM, Nilsson IM, Lombardi R, et al: Aberrant structure of von Willebrand factor in a new variant of von Willebrand's disease (Type IIC). J Clin Invest 1982b; 70:1124.

Ruggeri ZM, Pareti FI, Mannucci PM, et al: Heightened interaction between platelets and factor VIII/von Willebrand factor in a new subtype of von Willebrand's disease. N Engl J Med 1980; 302:1047.

Ruggeri ZM, Zimmerman TS: von Willebrand factor and von Willebrand disease. Blood 1987; 70:895.

Ruggeri ZM, Zimmerman TS: The complex multimeric composition of factor VIII/von Willebrand factor. Blood 1981; 57:1140.

Sadler JE: A revised classification of von Willebrand disease. For the subcommittee on von Willebrand factor of the scientific and standardization committee of the International Society on Thrombosis and Haemostasis. Thromb Haemost 1994b; 71:520.

Sadler JE, Davie EW: Hemophilia A, Hemophilia B, and von Willebrand disease. *In* Stamatoyannopoulos G, Nienhuis AW, Majerus PW, Varmus H (eds): The Molecular Basis of Blood Diseases, 2nd ed. Philadelphia, W. B. Saunders, 1994c, p 683.

Sadler JE, Gralnick HR: A new classification for von Willebrand disease. Blood 1994a; 84:676.

Saito, Ratnoff OD, Bouma BN, et al: Failure to detect variant (CRM+) plasma thromboplastin antecedent (factor XI) molecules in hereditary plasma thromboplastin antecedent deficiency: A study of 125 patients of several ethnic backgrounds. J Lab Clin Med 1985; 106:718.

Schafer AI: Approach to bleeding. *In* Loscalzo J, Schafer AL (eds): Thrombosis and Hemorrhage. Oxford, Blackwell Scientific Publishers, 1994, p 418.

Schleider MA, Nachman RL, Jaffe EA, et al: A clinical study of the lupus anticoagulant. Blood 1976; 48:499.

Schwaab R, Oldenburg J, Tuddenham EG, et al: Mutations in haemophilia A. Br J Haematol 1993; 83:450.

Scott CF, Colman RW: Fibrinogen blocks the autoactivation and thrombin-mediated activation of factor XI on dextran sulfate. Proc Natl Acad Sci USA 1992; 89:11189.

Scott JP, Montgomery RR: The rapid differentiation of type IIb von Willebrand's disease from platelet-type (pseudo-) von Willebrand's disease by the "neutral" monoclonal antibody binding assay. Am J Clin Pathol 1991; 96:723.

Seligsohn U: Factor XI deficiency. Thromb Haemost 1993; 70:68.

Seligsohn U: Disseminated intravascular coagulation. *In* Beutler E, Lichtman MA, Coller BS, Kipps TJ (eds): Williams Hematology, 5th ed. New York, McGraw-Hill, 1995, p 1499.

Shapiro SS: Antibodies to blood coagulation factors. Clin Haematol 1979; 8:207.

Shapiro SS, Thiagarajan P, De Marco L: Mechanism of action of the lupus anticoagulant. Ann NY Acad Sci 1981; 370:359.

Shapiro SS, Thiagarajan P: Lupus anticoagulants. *In* Spaet TH (ed): Progress in Hemostasis and Thrombosis, Vol. 6. New York, Grune & Stratton, 1982, p 263.

Sie P, Dupouy D, Pichon J, et al: Constitutional heparin co-factor II deficiency associated with thrombosis. Lancet 1986; 2:413.

Sims PJ, Wiedmer T, Esmon CT, et al: Assembly of the platelet prothrombinase complex is linked to vesiculation of the platelet plasma membrane. Studies in Scott syndrome: An isolated defect in platelet procoagulant activity. J Biol Chem 1989; 264:17049.

Smooker PM, Cotton RG: The use of chemical reagents in the detection of DNA mutations. Mutation Res 1993; 288:65.

Solum NO, Rigollot C, Budzynski AZ, et al: A qualitative evaluation of the inhibition of platelet aggregation by low molecular weight degradation products of fibrinogen. Br J Haematol 1983; 24:419.

Spicer EK, Horton R, Bloem L, et al: Isolation of cDNA clones coding for human tissue factor: Primary structure of the protein and cDNA. Proc Natl Acad Sci USA 1987; 84:5148.

Stein J, Ratnoff OD: An inhibitor of antihemophilic factor (factor VIII) in an 18-month-old nonhemophilic child. Am J Pediatr Hematol Oncol 1993; 15:346.

Stevenson KJ, Seddon JM: The role of lipids in the detection of lupus anticoagulant by the dilute Russell viper venom test: Are platelets or reagents containing hexagonal HII phases necessary? Br J Haematol 1994; 86:583.

Suffredini AF, Harpel PC, Parrillo JE: Promotion and subsequent inhibition of plasminogen activation after administration of intravenous endotoxin to normal subjects. N Engl J Med 1989; 320:1165.

Suzuki K: Activated protein C inhibitor. Semin Thromb Hemost 1984; 10:154.

Svensson PJ, Dahlbäck B: Resistance to activated protein C as a basis for venous thrombosis. N Engl J Med 1994; 330:517.

Takamiya O, Kemball-Cook G, Martin DM, et al: Detection of missense mutations by single-strand conformational polymorphism (SSCP) analysis in five dysfunctional variants of coagulation factor VII. Hum Mol Genet 1993; 2:1355.

Tanaka I, Kasper CK, Fulcher CA: Enzyme-linked immunoassays for CRM positive hemophilia A using monoclonal antibodies with defined epitopes. Thromb Res 1992; 67:491.

Thiagarajan P, Shapiro SS, De Marco L: Monoclonal immunoglobulin M lambda coagulation inhibitor with phospholipid specificity. Mechanism of a lupus anticoagulant. J Clin Invest 1980; 66:397.

Thompson AR: Factor IX antigen by radioimmunoassay in heterozygotes for hemophilia B. Thromb Res 1977; 11:193.

Thomson JM: The control of heparin therapy by the activated partial thromboplastin time: Sensitivity of various thromboplastins to heparin. *In* Triplett DA (ed): Standardization of Coagulation Assays: An Overview. Skokie, IL, College of American Pathologists, 1982, p 195.

Tollefsen DM, Majerus DW, Blank MK: Heparin cofactor II: Purification and properties of a heparin-dependent inhibitor of thrombin in human plasma. J Biol Chem 1982; 257:2162.

Tran TH, Marbet GA, Duckert F: Association of hereditary heparin co-factor II deficiency with thrombosis. Lancet 1986; 2:413.

Triplett DA, Barna LK, Unger GA: A hexagonal (II) phase phospholipid neutralization assay for lupus anticoagulant identification. Thromb Haemost 1993; 70:787.

Tripodi A, Arbini A, Chantarangkul V, et al: Recombinant tissue factor as substitute for conventional thromboplastin in the prothrombin time test. Thromb Haemost, 1992; 67:42.

Tuddenham EG, Cooper DN, Gitschier J, et al: Haemophilia A: Database of nucleotide substitutions, deletions, insertions and rearrangements of the factor VIII gene. Nuc Acids Res 1991; 19:4821.

van den Besselaar AM, Meeuwisse-Braun J, Bertina RM: Monitoring heparin therapy: Relationships between the activated partial thromboplastin time and heparin assays based on ex-vivo heparin samples. Thromb Haemost 1990; 63:16.

van den Besselaar AM, Meeuwisse-Braun J: Enzymatic elimination of heparin from plasma for activated partial thromboplastin time and prothrombin time testing. Blood Coagul Fibrinolysis 1993; 4:635.

Van Genderen PJJ, Vink T, Michiels JJ, et al: Acquired von Willebrand disease caused by an autoantibody selectively inhibiting the binding of von Willebrand factor to collagen. Blood 1994; 84:3378.

Vaziri ND, Gonzales EC, Shayestehfar B, et al: Plasma levels and urinary excretion of fibrinolytic and protease inhibitory proteins in nephrotic syndrome. J Lab Clin Med 1994; 124:118.

Velasco F, Torres A, Rojas R, et al: Increase in the D-dimer levels during treatment in patients with acute myelogenous leukemia. Haemostasis 1992; 2:117.

Veltkamp JJ, Meilof J, Remmelts HG, et al: Another genetic variant of haemophilia B: Haemophilia B Leyden. Scand J Haematol 1970; 7:82.

Wada H, Minamikawa K, Wakita Y, et al: Increased vascular endothelial cell markers in patients with disseminated intravascular coagulation. Am J Hematol 1993; 44:85.

Wagenvoord R, Hendrix H, Tran T, et al: Development of a sensitive and rapid chromogenic factor IX assay for clinical use. Haemostasis 1990; 20:276.

Warwick RM, Vaughan J, Murray N, et al: *In vitro* culture of colony forming unit-megakaryocyte (CFU-MK) in fetal alloimmune thrombocytopenia. Br J Haematol 1994; 88:874.

Watzke HH, Lechner K, Roberts HR, et al: Molecular defect ($Gla^{+14} \rightarrow$ Lys) and its functional consequences in a hereditary factor X deficiency (factor X "Vorarlberg"). J Biol Chem 1990; 265:11982.

Weiss HJ, Meyer D, Rabinowitz R, et al: Pseudo–von Willebrand's disease. An intrinsic platelet defect with aggregation by unmodified human factor VIII/von Willebrand factor and enhanced adsorption of its high-molecular-weight multimers. N Engl J Med 1982; 306:326.

Weiss HJ, Hoyer LW, Rickles FR, et al: Quantitative assay of a plasma factor deficient in von Willebrand's disease that is necessary for platelet aggregation. Relationship to factor VIII procoagulant activity and antigen content. J Clin Invest 1973; 52:2708.

Wieland K, Millar DS, Grundy CB, et al: Molecular genetic analysis of factor X deficiency: Gene deletion and germline mosaicism. Hum Genet 1991; 86:273.

Wilde JT, Kitchen SK, Greaves M, Preston FE: Plasma D-dimer levels and their relationship to serum fibrinogen/fibrin degradation products in hypercoagulable states. Br J Haematol 1989; 71:65.

Yamamoto M, Nakagaki T, Kisiel W: Tissue factor–dependent autoactivation of human blood coagulation factor VII. J Biol Chem 1992; 267: 19089.

Zimmerman TS, Abildgaard CF, Meyer D: The factor VIII abnormality in severe von Willebrand's disease. N Engl J Med 1979; 301:1307.

Zimmerman TS, Ratnoff OD, Powell AE: Immunologic differentiation of classic hemophilia (factor VIII deficiency) and von Willebrand's disease, with observations on combined deficiencies of antihemophilic factor and proaccelerin (factor V) and on an acquired circulating anticoagulant against antihemophilic factor. J Clin Invest 1971; 50:244.

Zimmerman TS, Ruggeri ZM: von Willebrand's disease. Clin Haematol 1983; 12:175.

Chapter 30

Immunohematology

John Bernard Henry, M.D.
Wendy V. Beadling, M.S., MT(ASCP)SBB

BASIC IMMUNOHEMATOLOGY

The term *immunohematology* defines the immunologic properties and reactions of all blood components and constituents. Immunohematology is intimately related to *transfusion medicine*, which represents a section of clinical pathology that involves the transfusion of blood, its components, and its derivatives. Furthermore, immunohematology encompasses the performance of laboratory examinations, evaluation of results and reactions, and additional procedures as required for the study of the pathogenesis, diagnosis, prevention, and management of immunization (sensitization) associated with transfusion, pregnancy, and organ transplantation. Immunohematologic resolution of parentage problems may also be included. Investigators in this field also have made important contributions to human genetics, anthropology, and criminology and forensics.

Blood Group Antigens

The term *blood group* refers not only to erythrocyte antigen systems but also to the immunologic diversity expressed by other blood constituents including leukocytes, platelets, and plasma. Blood constituent antigens that are produced by alleles at a single gene locus or by a group of closely linked loci make up a blood group antigen *system*. Most blood group genes, with a few exceptions, are located on the autosomal chromosomes and are inherited following Mendelian rules of inheritance, leading to their application as useful genetic markers. Most blood group alleles demonstrate codominance as well, meaning that genetic heterozygotes at a particular locus will express both gene products.

Many membrane-associated structures of blood cells and constituents of plasma may be defined as *antigens* because they can react with a complementary antibody or cell receptor. Most of these antigens are also *immunogens*, because they can elicit an antibody-mediated immunologic response if introduced as a foreign substance into a responsive host. Each antigen may have a variety of different epitopes or specific antigenic determinants. Epitopes are discrete, immunologically active regions of the antigen, whose molecular configuration confers the ability to interact with specific lymphocyte membrane receptors or secreted complementary antibody. In the process of antigenic stimulation, many cells are involved with recognition of the various epitopes contained within a complex antigen (see Chaps. 32 and 35).

Immunogenicity

The ability of an antigen to elicit an immune response is known as its immunogenicity. The immunogenicity of an antigen is determined not only by certain innate characteristics of the antigen itself but also by the host's genetically determined immune responsiveness. Characteristics of antigens that determine their immunogenicity include the degree of foreignness; molecular size and configuration, which may change with temperature, pH, and ionic environment; and antigenic complexity as measured by the number of available epitopes or antigenic determinants.

Blood group antigens vary greatly in their ability to elicit an immune response. The A, B, and D (Rh_o) antigens are certainly the most immunogenic, and thus all blood transfused must be matched for these antigens between the blood donor and the recipient. Approximately 50% to 75% of D-negative persons would produce anti-D if transfused with only one unit of D-positive blood. After the D antigen, K is the next most immunogenic, with Fy^a and other antigens within the

Table 30–1. RELATIVE IMMUNOGENICITY OF SELECTED CLINICALLY IMPORTANT BLOOD GROUP ANTIGENS*

Antigen	Relative Potency	Antigen	Relative Potency
D	0.70	K	0.10
c	0.041	E	0.0338
k	0.030	e	0.0112
Fy^a	0.0046	C	0.0022
Jk^a	0.0014	S	0.0008
Jk^b	0.0006	s	0.0006

*These figures represent the approximate percentage of persons negative for a specific antigen who, if transfused with one unit of corresponding antigen-positive blood, would develop antibodies to that specific antigen. When relative potency of K antigen is 0.1 as estimated by Kornstad (1957), the relative potency of other blood groups can be estimated as shown by Mollison (1993).

Rh system, such as C, c, E, and e, also classified as fairly immunogenic based on the frequency with which their corresponding antibodies are encountered. Using the same criteria, one finds that the other common blood group antigens, such as Fy^b, Jk^a, Jk^b, and s, are much less immunogenic. The relative immunogenicity of some clinically important red cell antigens is listed in Table 30–1.

Chemical Composition

The chemical composition of an antigen determines most of its physical and biological properties, including immunogenicity. As a general rule, purified carbohydrate and simple monosaccharides are not immunogenic except in certain species, such as humans and mice (Goodman, 1994a). Also, pure lipid or nucleic acids are not immunogenic, but they can be antigenic because they may serve as haptens. Haptens are well-defined chemical groupings that are too small to be immunogenic by themselves but can react with specific antibody induced when the hapten is attached to a carrier protein.

Although pure protein may be immunogenic, the most potent immunogens usually are complex macromolecular glycoproteins or lipoproteins. Thus, it is not surprising that red cell antigens for which the chemical composition has been determined are usually glycoproteins, lipoproteins, or glycolipids. Experiments with peptide chain polymers have shown that the inclusion in proteins of aromatic amino acids such as tyrosine and phenylalanine greatly contributes to increased immunogenicity (Kuby, 1991). In glycoproteins, immunogenicity may also be influenced by the extent of branching in the polysaccharide side chains. Whereas the immunogenicity of an antigen relates to the total complex molecular structure, the areas in which antigen combines with specific antibody (i.e., the epitopes) are usually limited to one or a few simple structures such as terminal sugars or amino or fatty acid residues. These are often referred to as the immunodominant structures because they determine the specificity of the antigen-antibody interaction.

Antigen Density

The number of antigenic sites on a foreign substance, whether a complex molecule or a cell, will obviously contribute to the strength and end result of an immunologic response. Studies of blood group antigens have demonstrated that antigen density contributes to the efficiency of antibody binding and to the extent of complement activation, thus determining the likelihood of red cell hemolysis.

Various techniques have been used to determine the number of copies of certain blood group antigens on the red cell membrane. In the past, radioimmunoassay (Hughes-Jones, 1971) or enzyme-linked immunosorbent assay (Caren, 1982) using specific polyclonal or monoclonal antibody labeled with a radioactive isotope, such as ^{125}I, or with an enzyme have been used to indirectly calculate the number of antigen sites by measuring the number of attached, labeled antibodies. Another method uses ferritin-labeled anti-IgG against red cells sensitized with various IgG blood group antibodies to count antigen sites by electron microscopy (Masouredis, 1980). More recently, automated flow cytometry using antibodies labeled with fluorescein isothiocyanate (FITC) has been used to quantitate and analyze red cell antigen distribution for a number of blood group systems (Nance, 1988). Table 30–2 lists some of the estimated antigenic sites on each erythrocyte.

Table 30–2. NUMBER OF MEMBRANE SITES FOR SELECTED NATIVE ERYTHROCYTE ANTIGENS ESTIMATED BY RADIOIMMUNOASSAY*

Antigen	Phenotype	Number of Antigenic Sites	Antigen	Phenotype	Number of Antigenic Sites
A	A_1 adult	$810–1170 \times 10^3$	D	DCce	$9.9–14.6 \times 10^3$
	newborn	$250–370 \times 10^3$		Dce	$12–20 \times 10^3$
	A_2 adult	$240–290 \times 10^3$		DcEe	$14–16.6 \times 10^3$
	newborn	140×10^3		DCe	$14.5–19.3 \times 10^3$
	A_1B adult	$460–850 \times 10^3$		DcE	$15.5–33.3 \times 10^3$
	newborn	220×10^3		DCcEe	$23–21 \times 10^3$
	A_2B adult	140×10^3		D−−	$110–202 \times 10^3$
B	B adult	750×10^3		weak D (D^u)	$0.8–3 \times 10^3$
	A_1B adult	430×10^3	c	c+C−	$70–85 \times 10^3$
I	I+	500×10^3		c+C+	$37–53 \times 10^3$
K	K+k−	6.1×10^3	e	e+E−	$18.2–24.4 \times 10^3$
	K+k+	3.5×10^3		e+E+	$13.4–14.5 \times 10^3$
			E	e−E+	$0.45–25.6 \times 10^3$

*Figures taken from Mollison (1993).

Red Cell Membrane Structure and Biochemistry

Experimental research on human erythrocyte membranes has provided a better understanding of other cell membrane systems, particularly in the area of membrane composition and membrane-cytoskeletal associations. Like other cells, erythrocytes are enclosed by a lipid bilayer, 4 to 5 nm in thickness, primarily composed of phospholipids, cholesterol, and some glycolipids. There is also a variety of membrane proteins that may be classified either as peripheral proteins, which can be easily dissociated in intact form by simple detergent extraction of erythrocyte ghosts, or as integral or transmembrane proteins, which can be dissociated only after harsher extraction techniques.

The peripheral membrane proteins that compose the membrane skeleton include spectrin, ankyrin, protein 4.1, actin, and tropomyosin and are located just adjacent to the cytoplasmic surface of the phospholipid bilayer (Mohandas, 1993). These proteins form a meshwork that provides support and stability to the lipid envelope (Fig. 30–1).

The integral or transmembrane proteins span the phospholipid bilayer and are anchored to the peripheral protein meshwork at specific points. One of the most abundant integral membrane proteins composes protein band 3, so named because of its mobility on sodium dodecyl sulfate–polyacrylamide gel electrophoresis (SDS-PAGE). Band 3 molecules exist in dimer or tetramer form in the cell membrane and are made up of two distinct domains: (1) the intracytoplasmic domain that serves as an attachment point for spectrin via ankyrin and (2) the membrane-associated domain that carries out anion exchange functions (Jennings, 1989).

The other predominant group of transmembrane proteins consists of the glycophorins A, B, C, and D. These glycoproteins are glycosylated at various points on the external membrane surface with tetrasaccharides containing a high content of sialic acid residues that confer the net negative charge to the red cell membrane. Glycophorin C is associated with peripheral protein 4.1 and probably serves a role in maintenance of membrane shape and mechanical properties. The glycophorins may also serve as red cell receptors for certain bacterial, viral, or parasitic organisms (Cartron, 1993b).

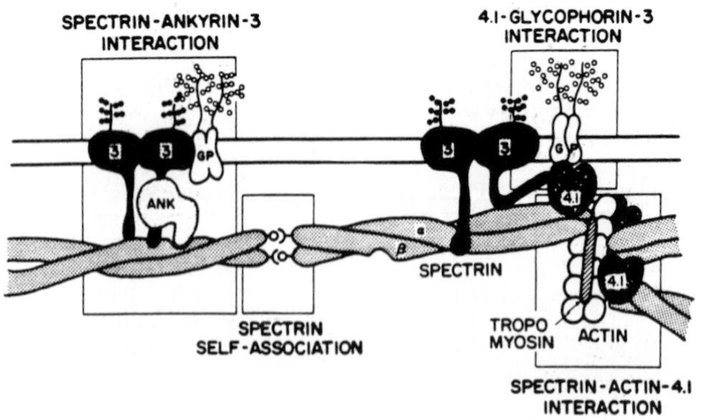

Figure 30–1. Red cell membrane structure, showing the membrane skeleton (spectrin, ankyrin [ANK], protein 4.1, actin, and tropomyosin) on the cytoplasmic side of the phospholipid bilayer. Certain structures, band 3 proteins (3) and glycophorin (GP), are anchored to the cytoskeleton and traverse the phospholipid bilayer. (From Lux SE: Disorders of the red cell membrane. *In* Nathan DG, Oski FA [eds]: Hematology of Infancy and Childhood, 3rd ed. Philadelphia, W.B. Saunders Company, 1987.)

Another important integral membrane glycoprotein, with about half as many copies per erythrocyte as band 3 and glycophorin A, is protein band 4.5, or the glucose transporter. This 55,000-dalton transmembrane protein is proposed to consist of 12 membrane-spanning loops with exposed cytoplasmic portions, one of which is glycosylated with a single, highly branched N-linked oligosaccharide (Muekler, 1985).

Location of Red Cell Membrane Blood Group Antigens

Extensive studies of secretions and red cell membrane extracts, as well as more recent techniques involving cloning of blood group genes and the study of their products, have yielded information as to the biochemistry and location of some of the blood group antigens on certain well-defined structures of the erythrocyte membrane (Table 30–3).

CARBOHYDRATE ANTIGENS

A number of common carbohydrate blood group antigens, including H, A, B, P_1, P, I, and i, are located on oligosaccharide chains attached directly to membrane glycosphingolipids or to the membrane-associated domains of integral protein bands 3 and 4.5 (Anstee, 1990). There is also some evidence of carbohydrate activity associated with the glycophorins. All of these carbohydrate antigens have a common precursor consisting of lactosylceramide or ceramide dihexose (CDH). P antigen is produced by the addition of N-acetyl galactosamine (GalNAc) to CDH to form globoside, the most abundant glycosphingolipid in the red cell membrane. Addition of GalNAc, followed by D-galactose, to CDH results in the formation of *para*globoside. Specific transferase enzymes coded for by the ABO, P, and Ii blood group genes then add specific sugars to paragloboside to form the H, A, B, P_1, and i antigens. The antigen specificities of H, A, B, and P_1 are determined by a terminal molecular configuration that includes a single immunodominant sugar. The i antigen specificity is determined by a minimum of two repeating units of D-galactose and GalNAc in linear formation, whereas I antigen is present when these repeating units are incorporated in a more complex branching structure.

The relationship between the common precursor paragloboside and some of the integral carbohydrate red cell antigens is summarized in Figure 30–2. The biochemistry of these antigens is discussed in more detail in the later section, Erythrocyte Antigens and Antibodies.

PROTEIN ANTIGENS

SIALOGLYCOPROTEINS. The red cell membrane glycophorins are made up of four different types of polypeptide chains designated α, β, γ, and δ. Glycophorins A and B are known to contain antigens of the MNSs blood group system. The α chains make up glycophorin A (GPA) and contain the M and N antigens, whereas δ chains make up glycophorin B (GPB) and contain the S, s, and U antigens. The β and γ chains make up glycophorins C and D, respectively, and contain a group of high-incidence antigens belonging to the Gerbich blood group system (Cartron, 1993b).

Antigenic activity of GPA and GPB resides at the amino terminus of the polypeptide backbone that extends into the

Table 30–3. SOME BIOCHEMICALLY DEFINED PROTEIN BLOOD GROUP ANTIGENS

Blood Group	Protein Characteristic	Function or Significance	cDNA Cloned
Rh	30- to 32-kDa integral membrane protein	Unknown: possibly related to lipid transport	Yes
LW	37- to 47-kDa glycoprotein	Has homology to ICAM-2	Yes
Duffy	35- to 43-kDa glycoprotein	Chemokine receptor	Yes
Kell	93-kDa glycoprotein	Structurally part of zinc-binding metalloproteinase family	Yes
Kx	32 kDa	Unknown	No
Kidd	50 kDa	Possibly urea transporter	No
MN	43-kDa integral membrane protein	Glycophorin A	Yes
Ss	25-kDa integral membrane protein	Glycophorin B	Yes
Lutheran	78 kDa, 85 kDa	Unknown; Ig superfamily	Yes
Xg^a	22- to 29-kDa	Unknown	No
Gerbich	39 kDa	Glycophorins C and D	Yes
Chido-Rogers	200-kDa glycoprotein	Complement component 4 (C4)	Yes
Knops-McCoy	Variably sized glycoprotein (170–220 kDa)	Complement C3b/C4b receptor Type 1 (CR1)	Yes
JMH	76-kDa, PI-linked glycoprotein	CDw108	No
Diego	95–105 kDa	Band 3 (anion transporter)	Yes
Cartwright	160-kDa, PI-linked homodimer	Acetylcholinesterase	Yes
Scianna	60 kDa	Unknown	No
Dombrock	47- to 58-kDa, PI-linked glycoprotein	Unknown	No
Colton	28-kDa integral membrane protein	Aquaporin (water channel)	Yes
Cromer	70-kDa, PI-linked glycoprotein	Decay-accelerating factor (CD55)	Yes

PI = phosphatidylinositol.
Modified with permission from Telen MJ, Rao N: Recent advances in immunohematology. Curr Opin Hematol 1994; 1:143–150.

extracellular environment. Antigenic specificity depends on amino acid sequence differences and, apparently for some M and N antigens, on the presence of attached tetrasaccharide chains containing N-acetyl neuraminic acid.

OTHER MEMBRANE PROTEINS

Rh. The Rh system antigens have been isolated to three highly homologous but distinct membrane proteins that are necessary for maintaining normal membrane integrity, because absence of these proteins in Rh_{null} cells results in abnormal erythrocyte morphology and survival. Evidence suggests that most of the structure of the approximately 30-kDa proteins is highly hydrophobic and is embedded in the phospholipid bilayer with five or six extracellular hydrophilic loops (Cartron, 1993a). Antigenic properties may reside on these loops, and evidence indicates that antigenicity depends on membrane phospholipids for proper orientation of the polypeptide loops.

Kell. The Kell blood group system antigens have been isolated to a single 93-kDa protein that migrates at the same rate as protein band 3 on SDS-PAGE. However, various ana-

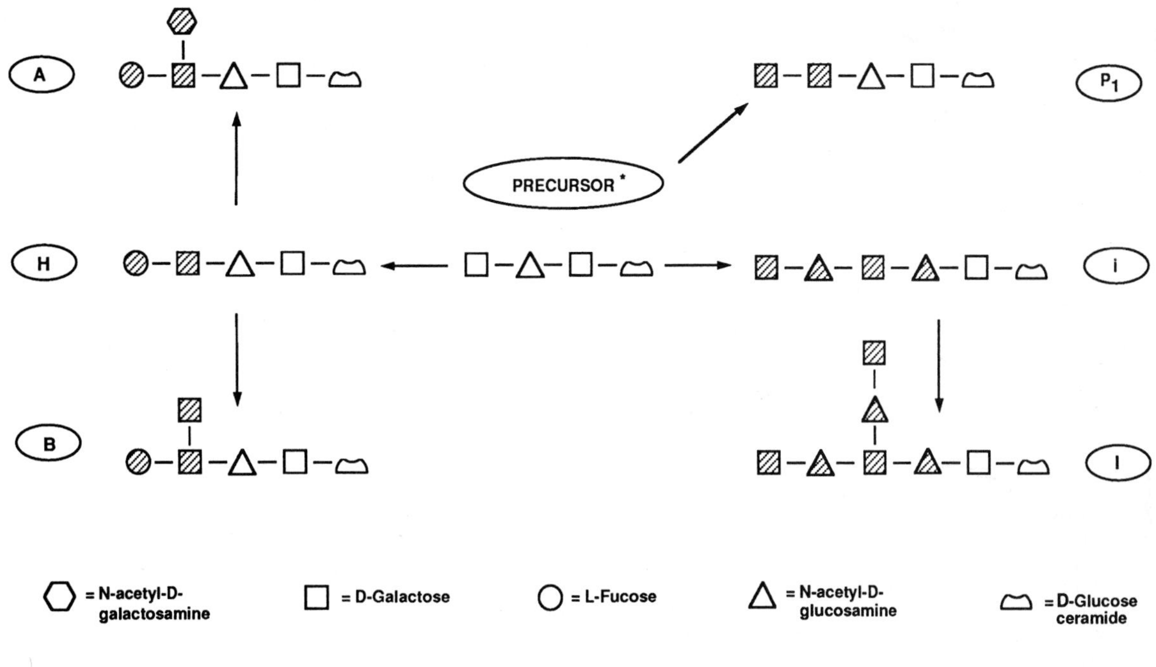

* Precursor = paragloboside
(Shading = immunodominant structures)

Figure 30–2. Some known erythrocyte antigenic determinants.

lytical techniques have shown they are not the same proteins. Most of the Kell protein is extracellular and probably exhibits a folded configuration linked by intrachain disulfide bonds. The extracellular domain is also glycosylated with five to six oligosaccharide chains (Redman, 1993). Differences in antigen specificity may depend on differences in both amino acid sequence and carbohydrate composition. Evidence indicates that the Kell structure is a transmembrane protein, because the cytoplasmic domain is complexed with several red cell membrane skeletal proteins.

Blood Group Antibodies

Immunoglobulins and Antigen-Binding Sites

Immunoglobulins are naturally occurring proteins having antibody-like structure and activity. Although immunoglobulins in general are normal plasma components, specific antibody activity develops only in response to antigenic stimulation. To understand antibodies, one must first be familiar with immunoglobulin structure and function, which are reviewed in Chapters 32 and 35. Properties of immunoglobulins that are relevant to blood banking are summarized in Tables 30–4, 30–5, and 30–6.

The specificity of an antibody is related to the hypervariable regions of an immunoglobulin. There are three hypervariable regions each in the light and heavy chains (Goodman, 1994b), as shown in Fig. 35–1. Amino acid sequence heterogeneity in the hypervariable regions, which allows for variation in the configuration of the peptide chains in the variable loops, determines the combining specificity for each antibody. The combining site of an antibody, where it is in physical contact with an antigenic determinant or epitope, is called the *paratope*. In the case of a globular protein, as many as 20 amino acids of the antibody-combining site may be in contact with the antigen, although the overall binding energy of the reaction suggests that only a proportion of those amino acids actively contribute to the force of attraction between antigen and antibody (Roitt, 1991).

Because one basic molecular unit of immunoglobulin contains two Fab or antigen-binding portions, all antibodies of all classes are at least bivalent, with polymers such as IgM and IgA having a valency that is some multiple of 2, as shown in Table 30–4.

Blood Group Alloantibodies and Autoantibodies

Most clinically significant blood group antibodies fall into the IgG or IgM immunoglobulin classes, with occasional IgA forms found among autoantibodies and against antigens in certain blood group systems. Blood group antibodies are usually classified as (1) alloantibody, which reacts with a foreign antigen not present on the patient's own erythrocytes, or as (2) autoantibody, which reacts with an antigen on the patient's own cells and with that same antigen on the cells of other persons. Erythrocyte autoantibodies are discussed later.

Some alloantibodies to erythrocyte antigens are called naturally occurring—that is, the antigenic stimulus is unknown. Naturally occurring antibodies may appear regularly in the serum of persons who lack the corresponding antigen, such as in the ABO blood group system. Other naturally occurring antibodies seem to appear only in a certain percentage of the population who lack the respective antigen.

Many blood group alloantibodies are produced as the result of immunization to foreign erythrocyte antigens either by exposure through transfusion of blood components or through pregnancy, usually at the time of delivery. It is the presence of such alloantibodies to erythrocyte or other blood cell antigens that necessitates the selection of specific antigen-negative components for transfusion. Identification of alloantibodies with selection or preparation of compatible blood components currently remains one of the primary functions of a transfusion medicine service.

Complement and Blood Banking

Complement is important to blood banking because of its involvement in the sensitization and destruction of either transfused red cells by alloantibody or destruction of autologous red cells in the case of an autoantibody. It is also important to some serologic testing in the detection of *in vivo* or *in vitro* antigen-antibody reactions. Because a detailed description of complement components, their detection and quanti-

Table 30–4. IMPORTANT PROPERTIES OF FIVE CLASSES OF HUMAN IMMUNOGLOBULIN (Ig)

	IgG	IgM	IgA	IgD	IgE
Heavy chain class	γ	μ	α	δ	ε
Light chains	κ or λ	κ or λ	κ or λ	κ or λ	κ or λ
Special chains		J	J, SC		
No. of 4 peptide units	1	5	1–3	1	1
Valency (Ag binding)	2	10	2–4	2	2
Development in immune response	Late secondary	Early primary			
Half-life *in vivo* (days)	22	5	6	3	2.5
Serum concentration (mg/mL)	8–16	0.5–2	1.4–4	0–0.04	Trace
Percentage of total serum Ig	80	6	13	1	
Extravascular distribution	Tissue fluids		Secretions		Secretions
Inactivated by sulfhydryl reagents	−	++++	+/−		
Crosses placenta	Yes	No	No	No	No
Induces agglutination	+	++++	++		
Fixes complement	+	++++	+	+	+
(Pathway)	Classic, alternative?	Classic	Alternative possible	Alternative possible	Alternative possible

Modified from Roitt I: Essential Immunology, 7th ed. Oxford, Blackwell Scientific Publications, 1991.

Table 30–5. SOME KNOWN PROPERTIES OF THE FOUR IMMUNOGLOBULIN G SUBCLASSES

Subclasses of IgG	IgG1	IgG2	IgG3	IgG4
Heavy chain subclass	$\gamma 1$	$\gamma 2$	$\gamma 3$	$\gamma 4$
Allotypic markers	a, x, f, z	n	b0, b1, b3, b4, b5 c3, c5, g, s, t, u, v	4a, 4b (isoallotypes)
Half-life *in vivo* (days)	21	21	7	21
Relative serum concentration	64–70%	23–28%	4–7%	3–4%
Placental transfer	++	+/−	++	++
Complement fixation	+++	++	++++	+/−
Macrophage binding	+++	+	+++	+/−
Binding to staph protein A	Yes	Yes	No	Yes
Antibodies showing subclass restriction	IgG anti-A/B Anti-Rh	Anti-dextrans	Anti-Rh	Anti-AHF

Modified from Roitt I: Essential Immunology, 7th ed. Oxford, Blackwell Scientific Publications, 1991.

tation, and their changes in various diseases is presented in Chapter 36, a brief outline of the complement system as it applies to blood banking will be discussed.

Role of Complement in Erythrocyte Destruction

Alloantibodies or autoantibodies that combine with erythrocyte antigens are the most common reason for complement activation on the erythrocyte surface *in vivo.* Complement may also be activated on erythrocytes via a carrier/hapten reaction with antibody such as that seen with penicillin-erythrocyte complexes reacting with antipenicillin antibodies. Components of the complement cascade may also be attached to the membrane via a nonspecific mechanism as seen with certain drugs or when erythrocytes are "innocent bystanders" in another immune reaction.

Erythrocyte-antibody complexes usually activate complement by the classic pathway. However, the mode of destruction and extent of hemolysis of erythrocytes involved in complement activation depends primarily on the class of immunoglobulin involved and the activity of a person's reticuloendothelial (RE) system.

Intravascular Hemolysis

Intravascular hemolysis of erythrocytes is usually caused by antibodies directed against the ABO erythrocyte antigens. Other IgM antibodies that exhibit a broad thermal range, as well as some IgG antibodies that are potent activators of complement (e.g., antibodies of the Kidd blood group system), can also induce intravascular hemolysis. Intravascular lysis occurs when the complement cascade is activated completely through to the membrane attack complex, and the cells are destroyed by osmotic swelling.

Extravascular Hemolysis

IgG antibodies cause most extravascular hemolysis as a result of activity of the RE system. As shown in Table 30–7, phagocytic cells such as macrophages and monocytes have receptors for the C3b and C4b complement fragments. Thus, for those IgG antibodies that can activate complement, erythrocytes that have C3b or C4b attached may be immobilized and engulfed by cells with these receptors and are thus removed by phagocytosis.

Some erythrocytes that have been involved in complement activation may escape extravascular destruction by the action of inactivator proteins that help down-regulate the complement cascade. After the activation of C3, with splitting of the molecule into C3a and C3b, erythrocyte-bound C3b may be further split into C3c and C3d by C3b inactivator protein. C3d remains attached to the erythrocyte, and because it has no enzymatic or opsonic properties, erythrocytes coated with C3d may subsequently be released back into the peripheral circulation (Fig. 30–3) as spherocytes.

Erythrocytes sensitized by IgG antibodies that fail to acti-

Table 30–6. VARIANTS OF HUMAN IMMUNOGLOBULINS (Ig)

Variation	Meaning	Variant	Determined Location	Examples
Isotypic	Ig determinants present in all normal humans	Classes	C_H	IgG, IgM, IgA, IgD, IgE
		Subclasses	C_H	IgG1, IgG2, IgG3, IgG4 IgA1, IgA2
		Types	C_L	κ, λ
Allotypic	Genetic markers present in some individuals but not in others	Allotypes	C_H	G1m(a), (x), (f), (z) G2m(n), G2m(−n) G3m(b), (c), (g), etc.
			C_L (κ chains only)	Km(1), (2), (3)
Idiotypic	Sum of variable domain determinants unique to a specific immunoglobulin molecule	Idiotypes	V_H or V_L	Determinant of individual myeloma protein (monoclonal Ig molecule)

Modified from Roitt I: Essential Immunology, 7th ed. Oxford, Blackwell Scientific Publications, 1991.

Table 30–7. COMPLEMENT RECEPTORS ON HUMAN CELLS

	Complement Receptors	
Human Cells	*C3b, C4b*	*C3d*
Macrophages/monocytes	+	–
Granulocytes	+	–
Erythrocytes	+	–
B lymphocytes	+	+

vate complement may also be removed by the RE system, because phagocytic cells also have receptors for the Fc portion of IgG. Although phagocytosis is not complement dependent, Mollison (1989) has demonstrated that erythrocytes coated with IgG and complement tend to show accelerated removal by the liver, whereas erythrocytes coated only with IgG tend to be destroyed more slowly in the spleen.

Role of Complement in Serologic Testing

HEMOLYSIS

Occasionally, serum alloantibodies or autoantibodies may be detected in serologic tests by virtue of *in vitro* hemolysis during the testing process. Hemolysis is considered a positive reaction when present in a test designed to detect erythrocyte antibodies. Blood group antibodies that have been reported to demonstrate *in vitro* hemolysis include immune forms of anti-A and anti-B; anti-P_1, anti-P, and anti-PP_1P^k; anti-Jk^a and anti-Jk^b; anti-Le^a and anti-Le^b; and anti-Vel.

Certain procedures, such as the Donath-Landsteiner test, are purposely designed to detect specific blood group hemolysins in serum. This test requires a fresh blood sample to ensure an adequate supply of complement, because complement is relatively unstable and deteriorates during storage. It is also important not to draw such a sample into anticoagulant such as EDTA or citrate, because chelation of calcium ions by the anticoagulant would prevent complement activation.

DIRECT ANTIGLOBULIN TESTING (DAT)

For serologic detection of complement fixation *in vivo* caused by autoantibodies or alloantibodies, broad-spectrum antihuman globulin (AHG) serum must be used for direct antiglobulin testing (see the later section, Antihuman Globulin Test). At minimum, broad-spectrum AHG must contain anti-IgG and anti-C3d reactivity, but it usually also contains anti-C3b reactivity. Some broad-spectrum reagents may have anti-C4b or anti-C4d reactivity as well; occasionally, there is reactivity against the κ and λ light chains of IgM or IgA.

C4 complement components are common on autologous cells when complement has been activated *in vitro* by cold agglutinins in the patient's serum after the blood sample has been drawn. Consequently, for valid interpretation of DAT results, it is recommended that a sample drawn in EDTA be used for detection of complement components attached *in vivo*.

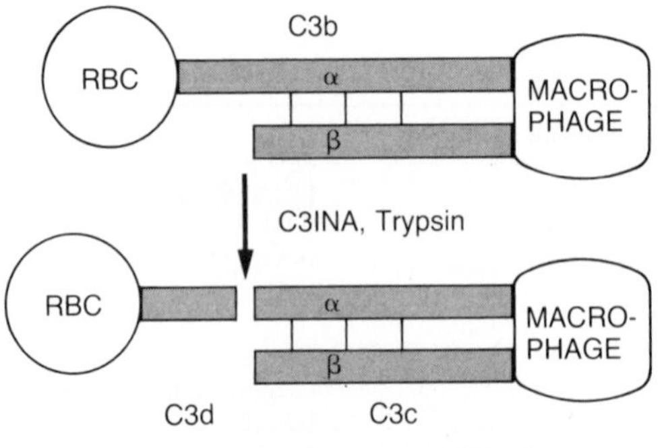

Figure 30–3. When C3 is activated, C3a and C3b are formed. C3b has red blood cell (RBC) receptor on one end and macrophage receptor on the other end to facilitate erythrophagocytosis. When C3b is cleaved by C3INA *in vivo* or by trypsin *in vitro*, C3c and C3d are formed. C3d remains on the RBC and may be detected by anti-C3d.

INDIRECT ANTIGLOBULIN TESTING (IAT)

It is unclear whether anticomplement reactivity is needed in antihuman globulin reagents used for serum antibody detection by indirect antiglobulin testing (see later section, Antihuman Globulin Test). There have been reports of antibodies that could only be detected by their ability to bind complement, but these have been extremely rare (Walker, 1993). There is a slight risk, however, that one might miss clinically significant examples of complement-dependent antibodies by using an AHG reagent that lacks anticomplement activity. Another advantage of using broad-spectrum AHG containing anticomplement activity is that the reactions in indirect antiglobulin tests often are stronger than those seen with monospecific anti-IgG alone (Wright, 1979). However, many laboratories have opted to use anti-IgG in antibody detection and identification tests and in crossmatch procedures, because use of the reagent will avoid detection of complement activation by clinically insignificant cold-reactive autoantibodies or alloantibodies.

ERYTHROCYTE ANTIGENS AND ANTIBODIES

ABO System

In 1900, Karl Landsteiner discovered the A and B antigens of the ABO blood group system and their corresponding antibodies by observing that the serum of certain individuals agglutinated the erythrocytes of others. This finding demonstrated one of the unique characteristics of the ABO system, which is that the serum of normal persons almost always contains potent hemagglutinins against the antigens they lack, a feature not associated with other blood group antigen systems.

Human Antigen Distribution and Development

Although ABO antigens have been detected on erythrocytes in a six-week-old fetus, they do not reach full adult expression on erythrocytes until three years of age (Mollison, 1993). The ABO antigens are found ubiquitously throughout the body, both as part of epithelial and endothelial cell membranes and as soluble substances in secretions and biological fluids. Because the ABO antigens are found on most tissues of the body, they are often referred to as "histo-blood group" antigens. This wide antigen distribution combined with the presence of preformed potent antibodies makes the ABO system of paramount importance in blood transfusion and organ transplantation.

As mentioned previously, extensive immunologic and biochemical studies show that the ABO antigens are found predominantly on erythrocyte membrane protein bands 3 and 4.5, membrane glycophorin, and structural glycolipids. Platelets have also been shown to possess ABO antigens, both intrinsic to the platelet membrane and acquired by passive absorption of plasma ABO glycolipids. Studies using monoclonal antibody–specific immobilization have pinpointed the location of the intrinsic platelet ABO antigens on specific membrane glycoproteins (Santoso, 1991). ABO antigens can also be detected on lymphocytes, although it is currently believed that the antigens are acquired from the plasma, and debate continues in the literature as to whether granulocytes express ABO antigens at all.

Common Phenotypes

Common ABO phenotypes include A, B, O, and AB and are distributed variably among various racial groups. Table 30–8 shows the serologic reactions of erythrocytes and serum for the four common phenotypes as well as the phenotype frequencies in several United States population groups.

ABO Subgroups

The A and B phenotypes are divided into subgroups classified serologically according to their reactions with anti-A, anti-B, and anti-H, and to which soluble antigens are present in the saliva of secretors (Table 30–9). Subgroups of A and B differ from the common phenotypes quantitatively, because there are fewer numbers of antigen sites on the erythrocyte membrane of the subgroups, and perhaps qualitatively, because the serum of subgroups may sometimes contain weakly reactive antibodies that react with normal A or B antigens.

The major subdivisions of the A phenotype are A_1 and A_2, which occur in 80% and 20% of the group A population, respectively. The much rarer A subgroups, such as A_3, A_x, and A_m, and the B subgroups are only seen occasionally, and identification is usually of little practical importance with regard to transfusion.

Subgroups of A are distinguished by their lack of agglutination with anti-A_1 lectin prepared from *Dolichos biflorus* or with anti-A_1 reagent derived from serum of group O or B persons that has been absorbed with A_2 cells. Table 30–10 lists some of the differentiating characteristics of A_1 and the commonly encountered A_2 erythrocyte subgroup.

Genetics and Biochemistry

Several independent sets of genes control expression of the ABO blood group antigens: (1) the *ABO* genes themselves, which include the four common alleles—A_1, A_2, *B,* and *O,* (2) the *H* locus, and (3) the *SE* locus. The *ABO* locus has been mapped to the long arm of chromosome 9, whereas both the *H* and *SE* loci are currently assigned to chromosome 19.

Production of ABO antigens depends on the sequential action of specific transferases coded for by the *H* and *ABO* genes. These enzymes transfer a specific sugar from a donor nucleotide derivative to the carbohydrate chains of a precursor molecule (see Fig. 30–2). In the three-locus model of ABO production, the *H* gene produces fucosyl transferase that acts first to attach L-fucose to the second carbon of the terminal galactose of precursor Type 1 or 2 oligosaccharide chains. Erythrocytes have only Type 2 chains, whereas Type 1 chains predominate in the secretory glands.

The function of the *H* structural gene is controlled by one of two regulatory systems: (1) the *SE* system in the secretory glands or (2) the proposed *Z* system on the erythrocyte membrane (Pittiglio, 1986). This model is summarized diagrammatically in Figure 30–4. In 80% of the population, possession of a dominant *SE* gene allows expression of *H* in the secretory glands. These persons are called secretors because soluble H, A, or B substance may be detected in their saliva and other secretory fluids. Individuals who are genotypically *se/se* are known as nonsecretors and account for the other 20% of the population. The *Z* gene, which appears to be a high-frequency allele, allows expression of *H* on the erythrocyte membrane. Persons who are genotypically *z/z* at the erythrocyte regulatory locus are exceedingly rare.

After H antigen is produced on the erythrocytes or in the secretions, the *A*-encoded or *B*-encoded transferases act to attach *N*-acetyl-D-galactosamine or D-galactose, respectively, to the third carbon of the terminal galactose on H-active chains. Studies using DNA cloning and sequencing techniques clearly show the allelic nature of the *A* and *B* genes, which have large sections of identical nucleotide sequence but also demonstrate four consistent nucleotide substitutions (Yamamoto, 1990). These, in turn, result in four amino acid substitutions that account for the difference in specificity of the two enzymes produced by the *A* and *B* alleles.

The *O* allele is similar in sequence to the *A* and *B* genes

4

Table 30–8. ROUTINE ABO GROUPING RESULTS AND PHENOTYPE FREQUENCIES

Cells Against Known Antisera		Serum Against Red Cells of Known Phenotype			Frequencies (%) in U.S. Population			
Anti-A	*Anti-B*	*A*	*B*	Interpretation	*White*	*Black*	*Native American*	*Asian*
−	−	+	+	O	45	49	79	40
+	−	−	+	A	40	27	16	28
−	+	+	−	B	11	20	4	27
+	+	−	−	AB	4	4	<1	5

Composite figures calculated from Mourant (1976).

Table 30–9. SEROLOGIC DIFFERENTIATION OF THE ABO GROUPS

	Red Cells with Anti-					Serum with Red Cells			Substances in Saliva of Secretors	Level of Transferase in Serum	Antigen Sites per RBC × 10^3
Phenotype	***A***	***A_1***	***B***	***A, B***	***H***	***A_1***	***B***	***O***			
A_1	++++	++++	0	++++	0/+	0	++++	0	A, H	Normal (optimal activity at pH 6.0)	810–1170
A_{int}	++++	++	0	++++	++	0	++++	0	A, H		
A_2	++++	0	0	++++	+++	§	++++	0	A, H	Decreased (optimal activity at pH 7.0)	240–290
A_3	$++^{mf}$	0	0	$++^{mf}$	+++	§	++++	0	A, H	Low	30
A_x	0/±	0	0	++	++++	+*	++++	0	H	Very low	4
A_m	0‡	0	0	0	++++	0	++++	0	A, H	Low (A_1 or A_2 enzyme may be present)	0.2–1.9
B	0	0	++++	++++	++	++++	0	0	B, H	Normal	750
B_3	0	0	$++^{mf}$	$++^{mf}$	+++	++++	0	0	B, H	Low	
O	0	0	0	0	++++	++++	++++	0	H	Normal	1700
O_h	0	0	0	0	0	++++	++++	++++	None† (classic Bombay)	Normal	

mf = mixed field (minor population of agglutinates).
*A_x subgroups usually have anti-A_1 but not always.
†Bombay secretors (presumably H_z) have been reported.
‡A antigen specificity demonstrated only after adsorption/elution procedures.
§May have anti-A_1 in serum.

but possesses a single nucleotide deletion at position 258. This produces a shift in the reading frame during translation that results in an enzymatically inactive protein (Yamamoto, 1990). Thus, these studies confirm that the *O* allele is indeed a silent gene or amorph. Similarly, molecular techniques have been used to identify the genetic polymorphisms leading to the A_2 subgroup and other rare phenotypes such as A_3, A_x, and cis-AB (Yamamoto, 1994).

There is some evidence to support a two-locus model for ABO production in which *H* and *SE* are two closely linked structural genes that both produce an H enzyme (Oriol, 1981). The *H* gene would produce a fucosyl transferase acting preferentially on Type 2 precursor chains to produce Type 2 H antigen, whereas *SE* would produce a slightly different enzyme acting preferentially on Type 1 precursor chains to form soluble Type 1 H antigen. Biochemical evidence for two distinct H enzymes has yet to be demonstrated, however, so at present the three-locus model is generally accepted.

In either model, absence of the *H* gene (designated as *hh*) leads to the Bombay erythrocyte phenotype denoted as O_h. In the classic Bombay phenotype, precursor substance can not be converted to H, and therefore a person's inherited *ABO* genes can not be expressed on the erythrocytes or in the secretions. Another form of Bombay phenotype, designated as H_z, results from inheritance of the very rare *z/z* genotype at the erythrocyte regulatory locus as described previously. These persons may express A, B, or H substances in their secretions, depending on the *SE* and *ABO* genes they have inherited.

ABO Antibodies

Human ABO antibodies have historically been called naturally occurring, although it is known that production of these antibodies is triggered soon after birth by exposure through ingestion or inhalation of antigenic substances in nature such as bacterial polysaccharides and plant pollen. This has been

Table 30–10. DIFFERENTIATING CHARACTERISTICS OF THE A_1 AND A_2 SUBGROUPS

Group	A_1	A_2
Quantitative Differences		
Reaction with diluted anti-A	++++	++
No. of antigen sites: Adult	1,000,000	250,000
Newborn	310,000	140,000
Qualitative Differences		
Reaction with *Dolichos biflorus* (Anti-A_1) lectin	++++	0
Anti-A_1 in serum	No	1–8%
Glycolipid erythrocyte variants containing antigens	A^a, A^b, A^c, A^d (linear and complex branched chains)	A^a, A^b (linear chains only)
N-acetyl-galactosaminyl transferase activity	Normal activity Optimal at pH 6	Decreased activity Optimal at pH 7

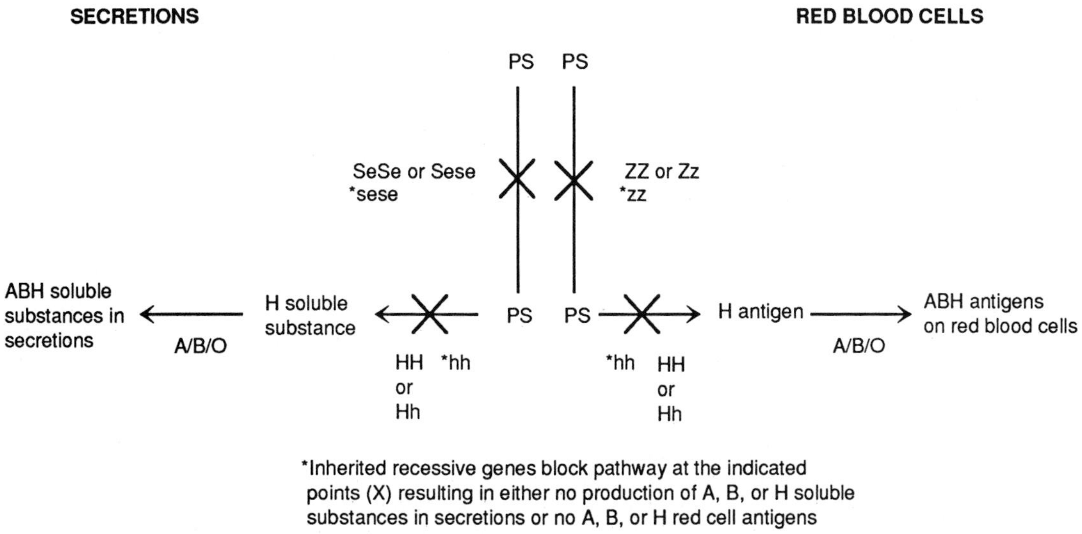

Figure 30–4. Proposed genetic pathway for biosynthesis of the A, B, and H antigens. (Modified with permission from Harmening DM: Modern Blood Banking and Transfusion Practices, 3rd ed. Philadelphia, FA Davis, 1994, p 93.)

proven by experiments with animals kept in germ-free environments from birth that fail to develop the expected ABO agglutinins. Detectable levels of ABO agglutinins in humans usually develop by about 3 to 6 months of age. Some of the characteristics of various ABO antibodies are summarized in Table 30–11.

COMMON ABO ANTIBODIES

The common ABO antibodies include anti-A, anti-B, and anti-A,B. Anti-A,B is an antibody produced exclusively by group O persons that appears to react with a structure common to both the A and B antigens. Anti-A,B is useful in differentiating the A_x and B_x subgroups, because these cells are agglutinated by anti-A,B but not by anti-A or anti-B.

Studies have shown that naturally occurring ABO agglutinins are distributed among the IgG, IgM, and IgA classes and usually show an optimal temperature of reactivity of 4°C. Immune forms of ABO antibodies, on the other hand, seem to be primarily IgG and react equally well at 37°C as at 4°C. These forms result from an identifiable immune stimulus such as an ABO incompatible pregnancy, deliberate injection of blood group substance for the purpose of reagent antiserum production, or accidental infusion of ABO-incompatible red cells. Immune antibodies are generally of higher titer and less readily neutralized by soluble blood group substances than are the naturally occurring forms.

LESS COMMON ABO ANTIBODIES

ANTI-A_1. Anti-A_1 is usually detected in the serum of some A subgroups (see Table 30–9) as a naturally occurring antibody that is generally considered clinically insignificant. However, there have been isolated reports of increased de-

Table 30–11. ABO ANTIBODIES

Specificity	Serum			Other Sources
	Group	*Incidence*	*Characteristics*	
Anti-A	B	All	Titer 1:32–2048 Average 1:256 Primarily IgM	Colostrum (IgA) Saliva (IgA) Tears
Anti-B	A	All	Titer 1:8–512 Average 1:64 Primarily IgM	Ascitic fluid Anti-A found in several snail species Anti-B found in salmon roe and the fungus, *Fomes fomentarius*
Anti-A, B	O, O_h	All	May have higher titer in pregnancy because of immune stimulation Reacts with A_x and B_x red cells	
Anti-A_1	A_2 A_x A_2B	1–8% Most 22–35%	Usually clinically insignificant Rare transfusion reactions are reported	Human group O or B sera absorbed with A_2 cells *Dolichos biflorus* lectin
Anti-H	O_h A_1, A_1B nonsecretors	All Some	Usually benign cold autoagglutinin except in O_h phenotype	*Ulex europaeus* lectin Several eel species Immunized chicken

struction of transfused A_1 erythrocytes demonstrated by anti-A_1 reactive at 37°C (Mollison, 1993). Anti-A_1 may also be prepared as a lectin from *Dolichos biflorus* and is useful in testing for A subgroups, as described previously.

ANTI-H. Anti-H is usually a benign cold autoagglutinin found most frequently in group A_1 and A_1B nonsecretors. Auto–anti-H shows varying activity with cells of different ABO groups, because group O cells contain the greatest amount of H antigen activity followed by A_2, A_2B, B, A_1, and A_1B. However, in persons of the O_h phenotype, anti-H acts as a potent erythrocyte agglutinin or hemolysin of high titer and broad thermal range and thus causes considerable difficulty in finding compatible blood for transfusion, because all normal erythrocytes contain the H antigen to some degree.

Anti-H lectin prepared from *Ulex europaeus* provides an excellent reagent for determining secretor status and detecting H antigen on erythrocytes. Although it is stronger than human anti-H, the lectin may be weakly to nonreactive with A_1 or A_1B erythrocytes.

ABO GROUPING PROCEDURES

Antisera and reagent erythrocytes for the performance of ABO grouping are well standardized and readily available commercially. ABO grouping is carried out at room temperature with only an immediate-spin centrifugation step required to promote a macroscopic agglutination reaction. Components of the initial protocol for determination of ABO grouping include (1) *forward* grouping, in which one drop of a 3% to 5% erythrocyte suspension is tested with one drop each of commercially prepared anti-A and anti-B, and (2) *reverse* grouping, in which two drops of patient or donor serum are tested against one drop of reagent erythrocytes of known A_1 and B phenotype. These are the minimal reagents required for routine ABO testing of recipients, and the results of the forward and reverse grouping should agree with each other (see Table 30–8) before any results are reported or blood is transfused. In contrast with forward grouping, in which reactions are usually strong and clear cut, the reactions of serum grouping may vary greatly in strength. An extended period of incubation at room temperature or incubation at 4°C may be required to demonstrate the presence of weak serum agglutinins.

Some blood banks routinely include the use of anti-A,B in the forward grouping procedure. However, this reagent does not usually yield any additional useful information except for the detection of the A_x or B_x subgroups, as previously mentioned. Anti-A,B is also used as a convenient reagent in quick confirmation ABO testing such as that performed on group O donor units received by a transfusion service from a donor center or in repeat testing to confirm patient ABO results.

Anti-A_1 also may sometimes be used in forward testing to confirm a suspected A subgroup, as previously described. If anti-A_1 is suspected in the serum of such a subgroup, A_2 and O cells may be additionally tested in the reverse grouping to confirm the presence of anti-A_1. Group O cells are also used in reverse testing to confirm the suspected presence of an unexpected room-temperature reactive alloantibody.

ABO GROUPING DISCREPANCIES

Interpretation of ABO blood grouping results is generally straightforward. However, for some of the weaker subgroups or rare phenotypes, careful observation of forward grouping reactions for mixed field reactions (minor population of agglutinates) or special techniques, such as absorption/elution, secretor studies, or tests for serum A, B, or H transferases, may be necessary to confirm the true ABO status of an individual.

If the results of forward and reverse grouping do not agree, the testing should always first be repeated to rule out any clerical or technical error. If results are unchanged, a discrepancy is present that may be due to problems with either the patient's serum or the patient's cells. Table 30–12 lists some of the many reasons for ABO discrepancies. These problems and the protocols for resolution are reviewed more completely by Walker (1993) and Harmening (1994).

If a blood transfusion is urgently needed and a discrepancy occurs that cannot be resolved in a timely manner, group O packed red blood cells, AB fresh frozen plasma, or both may be given in an emergency. However, it is important to obtain enough of a pretransfusion blood specimen from the patient that the workup may be continued later or an aliquot of the specimen may be sent to a reference laboratory for further evaluation.

Table 30–12. SOME CAUSES OF ABO GROUPING DISCREPANCIES

	Forward Typing Problems	Reverse Typing Problems
Unexpected positive reactions	Acquired B antigen associated with colon and gastric cancers, intestinal obstructions Cord cells contaminated with Wharton's jelly Autoagglutination caused by cold autoantibodies Cells heavily coated with warm autoantibody Polyagglutination Acriflavine antibody (against dye used in anti-B) Genetic chimerism* Bone marrow transplants* Transfusion reactions due to administration of red cells outside ABO group*	Rouleaux-forming proteins present, e.g., plasma expanders, monoclonal gamma globulins Room-temperature alloantibody present, e.g., anti-M, N, P_1 Cold autoagglutinin present, e.g., anti-I, IH Passively acquired ABO antibodies Subgroup of A with anti-A_1 in serum *cis*-AB with weak anti-B in serum
Unexpected negative reactions	A or B subgroups Antigen depression due to leukemia or other disease state High levels of soluble blood group substances associated with pseudomucinous ovarian cyst	Age of patient (elderly, newborn) Hypogammaglobulinemia Immunosuppression Genetic chimerism

*Look for mixed field appearance of reactions with reagent antisera.

Rh System

Background

The first and most clinically important characterization of the Rh system antigens came when Landsteiner and Wiener (1940) published studies of animal experiments involving the immunization of guinea pigs and rabbits with rhesus monkey erythrocytes. The antiserum produced agglutinated 85% of human erythrocytes, and the antigen defined was called the Rh factor. Anti-Rh was later reported to have the same specificity as antibodies studied earlier by Levine and Stetson (1939) that were responsible for hemolytic disease of the newborn.

Today, the Rh system is probably the most complex erythrocyte antigen system in humans, encompassing some 50 antigens, many phenotypic variants, and complex serologic relationships. Hence, the following review is basic and includes some of the most current information. For a detailed, historical review of the Rh system, readers should consult Race and Sanger (1975), Issitt (1985), and Mollison and coworkers (1993).

Rh System Genetics

THEORIES OF INHERITANCE

Using five basic antisera, anti-D, anti-C, anti-E, anti-c, and anti-e, Wiener identified five different factors or antigens (Table 30–13) that, from population and family studies, appeared to be inherited as two complexes of up to three factors each. There were eight possible combinations of three-factor complexes if one included "d" as designating the lack of D, because no anti-d had ever been demonstrated. Wiener did not use the DCE nomenclature, which was formulated later by Fisher and Race, in his studies or publications; instead, he used a system based on his theory of inheritance of the Rh antigens.

Wiener proposed a single-locus inheritance system with eight alternate common alleles coding for membrane structures that he called *agglutinogens*. Each individual would therefore produce two agglutinogens, one derived from the paternal and one inherited from the maternal gene, and each agglutinogen expressed up to three different antigenic determinants or factors. Wiener's nomenclature for the eight different genes and the allelic frequencies in the U.S. population are listed in Table 30–14.

Fisher and Race later proposed a different inheritance theory and nomenclature system based on genetic evidence of the antithetical nature of the C and c and the E and e antigens (Race, 1948); *antithetical* describes antigens produced by allelic genes at a single locus. Because cross-over in the Rh system has never been well documented, these investigators proposed a system of three closely linked loci or subloci on each chromosome inherited as a block of genes, which is called a haplotype—that is, the genetic contribution of one member of a chromosome pair (Fig. 30–5). They also introduced the *DCE* nomenclature to name the alleles, including the use of "d" to designate the lack of *D* (see Table 30–14). Although many find the Fisher-Race nomenclature easier to remember and understand, both Fisher-Race and Wiener notations are still commonly used in blood banking, and thus one must be conversant in both "languages," particularly when reading literature relating to the Rh system.

Table 30–13. COMPARISON OF WIENER, FISHER-RACE, AND ROSENFIELD NOMENCLATURES FOR ANTIGENS OF THE Rh BLOOD GROUP SYSTEM

Wiener	Fisher-Race	Rosenfield
Rh_o	D	Rh1
rh′	C	Rh2
rh″	E	Rh3
hr′	c	Rh4
hr″	e	Rh5

Table 30–14. COMPARISON BETWEEN WIENER AND FISHER-RACE NOMENCLATURES FOR THE Rh HAPLOTYPES AND THEIR POPULATION FREQUENCIES*

		Frequencies in U.S. Population			
Wiener	**Fisher-Race**†	***White***	***Black***	***Native American***	***Asian***
R^o	*Dce*	0.04	0.44	0.02	0.03
R^1	*DCe*	0.42	0.17	0.44	0.70
R^2	*DcE*	0.14	0.11	0.34	0.21
R^z	*DCE*	0.00	0.00	0.06	0.01
r	*dce*	0.37	0.26	0.11	0.03
r′	*dCe*	0.02	0.02	0.02	0.02
r″	*dcE*	0.01	0.00	0.01	0.00
r^y	*dCE*	0.00	0.00	0.00	0.00

*Composite figures calculated from Mourant (1976).
†In Fisher-Race nomenclature, "d" indicates the lack of D antigen.

Rosenfield proposed a numerical system of naming the antigens in 1962, because the ever increasing number of Rh antigens rendered an alphabetic notation impractical (see Table 30–13). It was also appreciated that this nomenclature contained no inferences as to the genetic inheritance of the antigens.

MOLECULAR GENETICS RESEARCH

As it turns out, neither Wiener nor Fisher and Race were completely correct about the inheritance of the Rh system genes. New evidence from studies utilizing DNA cloning and nucleotide sequencing, along with amino acid analysis of the gene products, show that the Rh system antigens are controlled by a set of two closely linked genes per haploid genome mapped to chromosome 1 (Cartron, 1993a). In D-positive persons, the *D* gene produces a membrane protein containing the D antigen, whereas a second *CE* gene apparently produces two highly related, but separate, proteins containing the Cc and Ee antigens. Southern blot analysis of genomic DNA of D-negative persons showed that one of the Rh system genes is completely lacking (Fig. 30–6), indicating that this is the gene that produces the D antigen. Sequence homology between the *D* and *CE* genes and their predicted gene products suggests the two genes may have developed from a common ancestor gene by duplication (Cartron, 1993a).

Biochemistry

As mentioned previously, the Rh polypeptides have been shown to reside on fatty-acylated erythrocyte membrane pro-

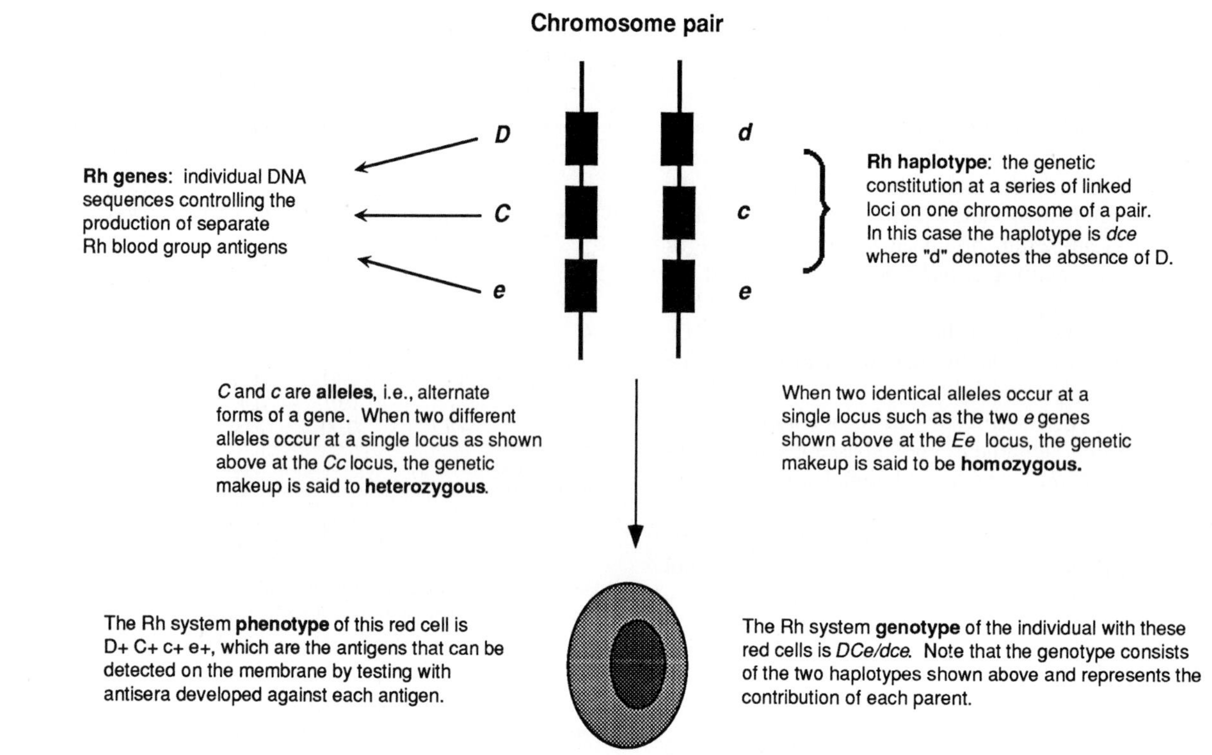

Figure 30–5. Fisher's theory of Rh system inheritance with definitions of genetic terms relevant to immunohematology.

teins that are necessary for structural membrane integrity. These proteins migrate from 28 to 33 kDa on SDS-PAGE. Immunoprecipitation experiments using Rh antibodies have also coprecipitated glycosylated proteins of higher molecular weight. It is believed that these so-called "Rh-related" proteins may be associated with the Rh polypeptides in the erythrocyte membrane to form a functional complex and that interaction of both the Rh polypeptides and the Rh-related glycoproteins may contribute to antigenic specificity.

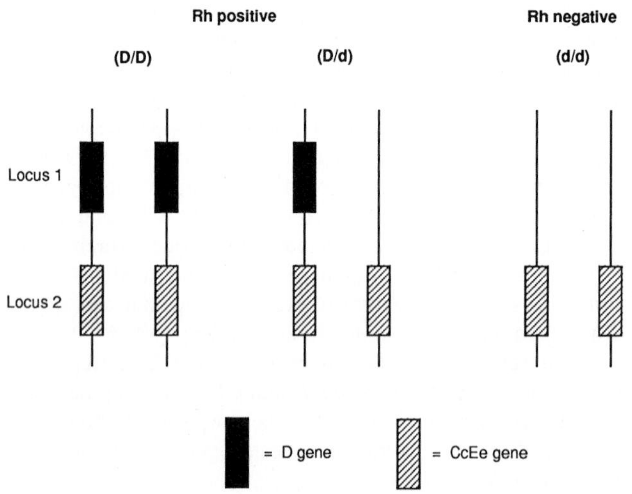

Figure 30–6. The Rh locus structure based on Southern Blot analysis. (Based on data from Colin Y, Cherif-Zahar B, Le Van Kim C, et al: Genetic basis of the RhD-positive and RhD-negative blood group polymorphism as determined by Southern analysis. Blood 1991; 78:2747.)

Rh Antigens

D (Rh_o) ANTIGEN

The D antigen is, after the A and B erythrocyte antigens, the second most immunogenic and, therefore, clinically significant blood group antigen. Until about the mid-1960s, the D antigen, or Rh_o antigen as it is most frequently called, was responsible for most cases of severe hemolytic disease of the newborn (HDN). Studies with monoclonal antibodies have identified at least eight D-protein epitopes that are probably determined by the folding and assembly of the cytoplasmic loops and transmembrane portions of the protein. Erythrocytes of the common Rh phenotypes have a range of about 10 to 33×10^3 D antigen sites per cell on the erythrocyte membrane (see Table 30–2).

Most tests for the D antigen with today's monoclonally derived or modified polyclonal antisera give clear-cut positive or negative reactions using room temperature techniques. However, some D-positive persons react weakly or not at all with anti-D by routine testing and can be detected only by using the AGT. Historically, the phenotype of these persons was called D^u, but because a variety of different mechanisms lead to this weak reactivity, the term weak D is now preferred because it does not imply a single definable phenotype.

Some weak D phenotypes are apparently the result of a quantitative reduction in the number of D antigen sites. This may be due to a *trans* effect of the *C* gene in a *dCe* or *dCE* complex that suppresses expression of *D* on the other chromosome. Other types of weak D may be the result of an alternative allele at the *D* locus that codes for weaker antigen expression. This seems to be common in the black population as part of a *Dce* or R^o gene complex.

Another type of weak D is due to a qualitative variation in the D protein that is produced. As mentioned previously, the D antigen has at least eight separate epitopes identifiable by monoclonal antibodies, and it has often been referred to as the D antigen mosaic. Persons who lack one or more of these epitopes are called D variants or D mosaics, and they may produce antibody against the parts of the mosaic that they lack.

OTHER Rh ANTIGENS

ANTIGENS C AND c, E AND e. The C, c, E, and e antigens are the four other common Rh system antigens, in addition to D, that account for most common Rh phenotypes. Some variant forms of these antigens do exist and are often restricted in frequency to a particular racial group.

The C^w antigen (Rh8) is found in approximately 2% of the white population and is most frequently, but not always, associated with a *DCe* (R^1) gene complex. Thus, virtually all erythrocytes that are C^w positive are also C positive. Although C^w was originally considered the product of an alternative allele at the *C* locus, more recent studies of rare genotypes that produce C^w in combination with the *c* gene suggest that C^w may be a low-incidence marker antigen produced on variant forms of the Cc protein (Issitt, 1985).

The antigen VS or e^s (Rh20) is rare in whites, but it is found in about 25% of the black population as part of Dce^s, dce^s, or dCe^s gene complexes. In many blacks, unusual phenotypes with variant e antigens, as well as the existence of a number of reports of e-like antibodies made by e-positive persons, have led some to conclude that the e antigen is a mosaic structure much like the D protein.

Many other unusual variants of Rh gene complexes producing enhanced or weakened expressions of the five common antigens, as well as rare low-incidence markers, have also been described. These are reviewed in more detail in Race and Sanger (1975) and Issitt (1985).

G ANTIGEN AND ANTI-G. The G antigen was described in 1958 by Allen and Tippet with the report of a serum, anti-CD, that reacted with cells that were positive for neither C nor D antigen (Case, 1987). These investigators theorized the existence of the G antigen and proposed that many anti-CD antigens contained an anti-G component. Their studies showed that the G antigen was produced by virtually all gene complexes containing either a *D* or a *C* gene, but that rare complexes such as r^G found in their original discovery could produce G without C or D. The discovery of G finally explained earlier case reports in which exposure to erythrocytes that were D − C + (G +) or D + C − (G +) gave rise to antibodies with apparent anti-CD specificity.

COMPOUND Rh ANTIGENS AND THEIR CORRESPONDING ANTIBODIES. Some Rh antibodies were eventually discovered that would agglutinate only those cells possessing two common Rh antigens produced by genes in the *cis* position (Table 30–15). These have come to be defined as antibodies directed against compound antigens and include anti-ce (f or Rh6), anti-Ce (Rh7), anti-cE (Rh27), and anti-CE (Rh22). Anti-Ce is a common component of most human anti-C produced by D-positive recipients, because the C-positive immunizing cells most likely had at least one *DCe* gene complex based on the frequency of R^1 in the general population. Anti-cE may also less frequently be a component of some anti-E antisera produced by D-positive persons, because the E-positive immunizing cells in that case would likely have had at least one *DcE* (R^2) gene complex. The existence of antibodies such as anti-ce, which are not just simple mixtures of two separate antibodies, suggests a certain spatial proximity of the Cc and Ee proteins on the erythrocyte membrane giving rise to these compound antigenic determinants.

Table 30–15. REACTIONS OF ANTIBODIES TO FOUR COMPOUND Rh ANTIGENS WITH THE EIGHT Rh HAPLOTYPES

Antibody	Haplotypes Giving Positive Reactivity
CE	R^z (DCE) r^y (dCE)
Ce	R^1 (DCe) r′ (dCe)
cE	R^2 (DcE) r″ (dcE)
ce (f)	R^o (Dce) r (dce)

Deletion Phenotypes

The first example of erythrocytes lacking any expression of Cc or Ee antigens was described in 1950 and was notated as D− − (Tippett, 1987). This rare occurrence was called a deleted phenotype and, in addition to *C* and *E* locus antigens, was shown to lack all high-frequency Rh antigens with the exception of Rh29 or "total Rh." This phenotype does, however, demonstrate exalted D antigen expression, with a range of 100,000 to 200,000 antigen sites per cell. Partial deletion phenotypes such as Dc− and DC^w− have also been found.

Rh_{null} Syndrome

The first example of erythrocytes lacking all Rh expression was found in an Australian aboriginal woman in an anthropologic survey (Tippett, 1987). The designation Rh_{null} was adopted to denote this rare phenotype, which has been documented in only a small number of families world-wide. There appear to be two genetic mechanisms by which the Rh_{null} phenotype arises.

In one pathway, an individual apparently is homozygous for an amorph or silent allele (designated $\overline{\overline{r}}$ in Wiener notation) at the Rh complex locus. Parents and siblings of the propositus will be heterozygotes for one $\overline{\overline{r}}$ gene and one normal haplotype. DNA analysis of one individual of the amorph type of Rh_{null} has shown absence of the *D* gene but presence of a *CE* gene, a pattern identical to that found in normal D-negative controls. Nucleotide sequence analysis of *CE* transcripts from the Rh_{null} amorph individual and D-negative normal controls showed no differences that indicate mutation in the coding region. Thus, the molecular basis for the so-called amorph type of Rh_{null} has yet to be explained (Cherif-Zahar, 1993).

The second pathway was proposed by Levine, who discovered a second family in which suppression of normal Rh gene expression was the apparent mechanism for the Rh_{null} phenotype (Race, 1975). Levine hypothesized a regulatory locus, calling the normal allele X^1r and the suppressor allele $X^\circ r$. In

4

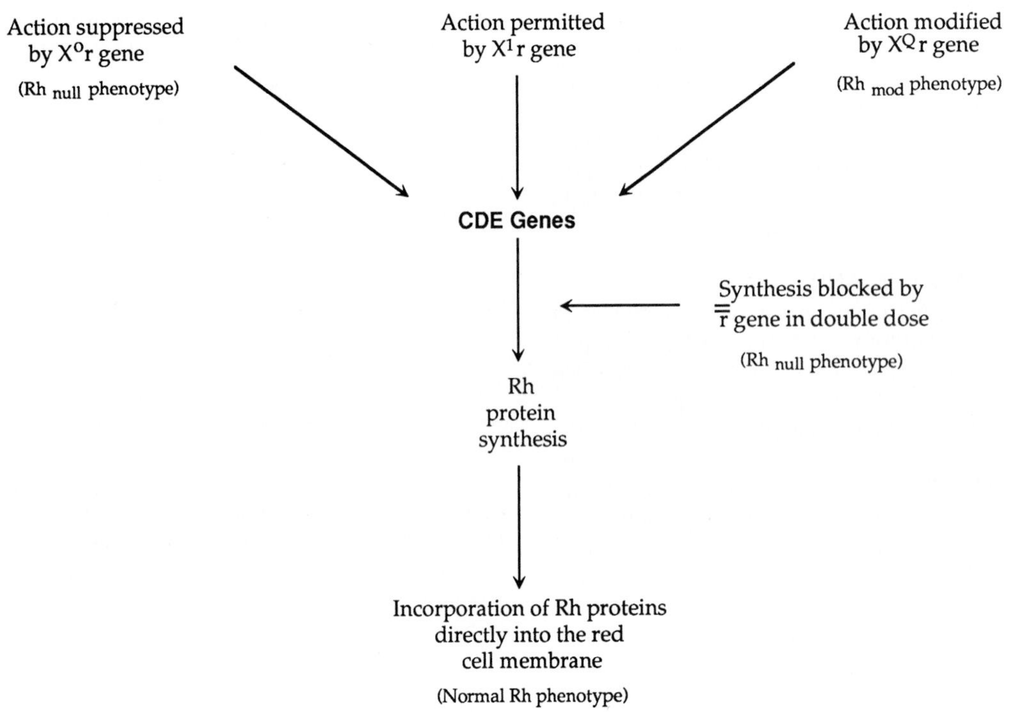

Figure 30–7. Possible genetic pathways in the biosynthesis of the Rh antigens. (Modified with permission from Issitt PD: Applied Blood Group Serology, 3rd ed. Miami, Montgomery Scientific Publications, 1985, p 263.)

this pathway, the Rh_{null} individual is able to pass a normal Rh haplotype to offspring, who will then express those genes inherited. Figure 30–7 summarizes the proposed mechanism for biosynthesis of the Rh proteins and production of the Rh_{null} phenotype.

Persons of the Rh_{null} phenotype have abnormally depressed expression of the S, s, and U antigens and lack the high-frequency antigen Fy^5, the LW protein, and the Rh-related glycoproteins. These multiple abnormalities suggest that the Rh proteins are necessary for correct expression of certain membrane glycoproteins. On the other hand, expression of M, N, En^a, Dombrock, and Kidd antigens tends to be enhanced on Rh_{null} cells. All Rh_{null} propositi studied presented with a compensated hemolytic anemia associated with abnormal erythrocyte morphology (stomatocytosis) and increased osmotic fragility, consistent with the hypothesis concerning the Rh protein's role in maintaining membrane integrity and proper cell volume. The serum of immunized Rh_{null} persons may contain a multitude of anti-Rh specificities including anti-Rh29, which reacts with all except other Rh_{null} cells, thus posing a difficult transfusion problem if these antibodies are present in a recipient.

Rh Antibodies

Antibodies directed against the common Rh antigens that are routinely encountered by blood bankers are, with few exceptions, immune in origin and are usually of the IgG_1 and IgG_3 subclasses, although rare IgM and IgA forms also occur. Naturally occurring forms of anti-C^w and anti-E are not infrequently seen. Many Rh system antibodies are commonly first detected in screening tests after the 37°C incubation phase with albumin, and almost all will be detected by the antihuman globulin technique. Serologic reactivity is enhanced by enzyme-treated erythrocytes. All Rh system antibodies have been associated with hemolytic transfusion reactions (HTRs). However, because Rh antibodies generally do not fix complement, incompatible erythrocytes are almost always cleared through extravascular destruction (Mollison, 1993).

Anti-D antibodies may develop after fetal-maternal hemorrhage (FMH) or rarely as a result of transfusion, because recipient and donor are usually matched for Rh type. Once a person is immunized, detectable anti-D may last in the circulation throughout a lifetime, and secondary exposure will cause a prompt and vigorous anamnestic response.

Human IgG anti-D is used in the preparation of Rh_0 immune globulin, which is used to prevent sensitization to the D antigen, primarily in Rh_0-negative women after delivery of an Rh_0-positive baby. Rh_0 immune globulin may also be used when an Rh_0-negative woman of childbearing age has accidentally received a transfusion with Rh_0-positive erythrocytes or has received a large number of erythrocyte-contaminated platelets from Rh_0-positive donors. Administration of one vial containing 300 μg of IgG anti-D is recommended for every 15 mL of D-positive erythrocytes (not whole blood) introduced through either FMH or transfusion. Rh_0 immune globulin must be given within 72 hours of exposure in order to prevent active immunization.

Rh Typing Procedures

Routine Rh system typing for blood donors and recipients includes only tests for the D (Rh_0) antigen. Testing by the collection facility for weak D (D^u) in donors yielding negative results by room temperature methods is required as stated in the American Association of Blood Banks' *Standards for Blood Banks and Transfusion Services* (Klein, 1994). If either routine or weak D testing yields positive results, the unit label shall read "Rh POSITIVE." Testing for weak D in recipients is optional, although blood banks who do prenatal and postnatal testing should perform the test for weak D at least once prior to delivery in all pregnant women who initially test as D negative. Tests for the C, c, E, and e antigens may be done to determine the most probable genotype in the evaluation of antibody problems or in the performance of paternity studies. Table 30–16 lists the phenotypes that can be determined by extended testing with the five basic Rh system–typing sera and indicates the most common genotypes within a given phenotype.

Several types of antisera are available for detection of the Rh antigens. These include modified tube reagents that contain a high-molecular-weight protein additive, chemically modified IgG sera in which the antibody molecules have been treated with a reducing reagent, saline reactive antisera prepared from human IgM antibody, and most recently, monoclonal/polyclonal blended reagents. Because of the possibility of false-positive reactions due to reagent additives or diluents, particularly with the modified tube antisera, manufacturers of Rh typing sera recommend always running a parallel diluent control or an albumin or saline negative control, depending on the medium in which the reagent is suspended. Typing for the D antigen is carried out at room temperature using one drop of a 3% to 5% erythrocyte suspension and one drop each of commercial anti-D and the appropriate negative control reagent in an immediate spin technique.

LW System

LW is almost always discussed in conjunction with the Rh system because historically they were thought to be one and the same. However, data accumulated throughout the years finally showed that the anti-Rh sera raised initially in rabbits by Landsteiner and Wiener were not reacting with the human D antigen at all but with a separate, high-frequency antigen subsequently named LW in honor of its discoverers. Although two separate antigens, D and LW are nevertheless strongly associated phenotypically, because all D-positive cells are strongly LW positive, whereas D-negative cells type only weakly LW positive; also, as previously mentioned, Rh_{null} cells lack the LW protein completely.

Evidence that led to the conclusion that Rh_o and LW were truly two different antigens included the following: (1) human D-negative or D-positive erythrocytes could stimulate the "anti-Rh" antisera in guinea pigs, and the antibody could be adsorbed onto human D-negative cells, (2) if human "incomplete" anti-D was incubated with D-positive erythrocytes, the cells could still react with the animal-derived "anti-Rh" agglutinating antibody, and (3) although human anti-D could be used to differentiate between D-positive and D-negative cord red blood cells, the animal anti-Rh would strongly agglutinate all cord cells regardless of D status. Family studies of propositi who had made anti-LW confirmed the genetic independence of the two systems (Issitt, 1985).

Serologic studies show that LW antigen expression is heterogeneous and demonstrates a spectrum of antigen strength. LW phenotypes were originally classified according to the amount of LW antigen present on the erythrocytes as measured by strength of agglutination with selected examples of anti-LW (Table 30–17). Although LW3 and LW4 erythrocytes appear to be LW negative by routine techniques, the cells of these phenotypes actually possess small amounts of LW antigen as shown by serologic studies and by animal immunization experiments. It is possible that only Rh_{null} cells are truly LW negative (Storry, 1992). In typing for the LW antigen, one must give special attention to the source of the antiserum used, because antibodies produced by different LW-negative phenotypes also seem to react heterogeneously with the LW antigen.

The nomenclature of the LW system was changed with the discovery of a new low-frequency antigen, Ne^a, that was

4

Table 30–16. FREQUENCIES OF COMMON Rh PHENOTYPES*

Reaction with Anti-†					Phenotype		Genotype		Frequencies‡			
D	*C*	*c*	*E*	*e*	*Rh*	*DCE*	*Rh*	*DCE*	*White*	*Black*	*Native American*	*Asian*
+	+	+	+	+	Rh_1Rh_2	DCcEe	R^1R^2	*DCe/DcE*	0.1176 (89%)	0.0374 (100%)	0.2992 (89%)	0.294 (97%)
							R^1r''	*DCe/dcE*	0.0084 (6%)		0.0088 (3%)	
							r^1R^2	*dCe/DcE*	0.0056 (5%)		0.0135 (4%)	0.0084 (2.8%)
							rR^z	*dce/DCE*			0.0132 (4%)	0.0006 (0.2%)
+	+	+	−	+	Rh_1rh	DCce	R^1R^0	*DCe/Dce*	0.0168 (5%)	0.1495 (63%)	0.0176 (15%)	0.042 (50%)
							R^1r	*DCe/dce*	0.3108 (95%)	0.0884 (37%)	0.0968 (85%)	0.042 (50%)
+	−	+	+	+	Rh_2rh	DcEe	R^2R^0	*DcE/Dce*	0.0112 (10%)	0.0968 (63%)	0.0136 (15%)	0.0126 (50%)
							R^2r	*DcE/dce*	0.1035 (90%)	0.0572 (37%)	0.0748 (85%)	0.0126 (50%)
+	+	−	−	+	Rh_1Rh_1	DCe	R^1R^1	*DCe/DCe*	0.176 (91%)	0.029 (81%)	0.194 (92%)	0.490 (93%)
							R^1r'	*DCe/dCe*	0.017 (9%)	0.007 (19%)	0.017 (8%)	0.028 (7%)
+	+	−	+	+	Rh_1Rh_z	DCEe	R^1R^z	*DCe/DCE*			0.053 (100%)	
+	−	+	+	−	Rh_2Rh_2	DcE	R^2R^2	*DcE/DcE*	0.02 (88%)	0.012 (100%)	0.116 (94%)	0.044 (100%)
							R^2r''	*DcE/dcE*	0.003 (12%)		0.007 (6%)	
+	+	+	+	−	Rh_2Rh_z	DCcE	R^2R^z	*DcE/DCE*			0.041 (100%)	
+	−	+	−	+	Rh_0Rh_0	Dce	R^0R^0	*Dce/Dce*	0.0016 (5%)	0.1936 (46%)	0.0004 (8%)	0.0009 (33%)
							R^0r	*Dce/dce*	0.0296 (95%)	0.2286 (54%)	0.0044 (92%)	0.0018 (67%)
−	−	+	−	+	rhrh	dce	*rr*	*dce/dce*	0.1369 (100%)	0.0676 (100%)	0.0121 (100%)	0.0009 (100%)
−	+	+	−	+	rh′rh	dCce	*rr′*	*dce/dCe*	0.0055 (100%)	0.0014 (100%)	0.0044 (100%)	0.0012 (100%)
−	−	+	+	+	rh″rh	dcEe	*rr″*	*dce/dcE*	0.0028 (100%)		0.0022 (100%)	

*Estimated from haplotype frequencies (p,q from Table 30–14) using p^2 for homozygotes and 2pq for heterozygotes.
†+ = positive; − = negative.
‡(%) = percentage of genotypes within a given phenotype.

Table 30–17. RELATIONSHIP OF OLD AND NEW NOMENCLATURES FOR THE LW SYSTEM

Old Phenotype Designation	Amount of LW[a] Antigen on Red Cell	New Phenotype Designation*	Possible Genotypes
LW1	Greatest	LW (a+b−) or LW (a+b+)	LW^aLW^a, LW^aLW^b, LW^aLW
LW2	↓	LW (a+b−) or LW (a+b+)	LW^aLW^a, LW^aLW^b, LW^aLW
LW3	↓	LW (a−b+)	LW^bLW^b, LW^bLW
LW4	Least	LW (a−b−)	*LWLW*

*Determined by routine agglutination methods.

present in persons of the LW3 phenotype (Sistonen, 1982). The Ne[a] antigen came to be known as LW[b], the partner of the high-frequency antigen LW[a], previously designated LW. The old LW classification is compared with the newly designated LW phenotypes in Table 30–17. The LW (a−b−) phenotype results from homozygotes for the silent allele *LW*.

Despite being weakly phenotypically positive for LW (actually LW[a]) antigen, as described earlier, persons of both the LW3 and the LW4 phenotypes can make anti-LW. The antibody produced by those of the LW4 phenotype acts as anti-LW[ab]. Studies of LW in relation to disease indicate that loss of LW antigens along with transient anti-LW production has been associated with changes in immunologic state, including pregnancy, Hodgkin's disease, and autoimmune thrombocytopenic purpura (Storry, 1992).

The phenotypic relationship between LW and Rh remains unclear. Studies on Rh_{null} erythrocytes show that proper expression of LW depends on normal production of the Rh polypeptides. One early suggestion was that the LW antigens resulted from glycosylation of the Rh proteins, because biochemical studies showed the LW antigens to be present on a glycosylated protein integrally associated with the erythrocyte cytoskeleton (Storey, 1992). Later studies, however, demonstrate that Rh and LW have no precursor relationship (Cartron, 1993a); an alternative hypothesis will have to be proposed for simultaneous absence of these two proteins in the Rh_{null} syndrome.

Other Erythrocyte Antigens and Antibodies

Literally hundreds of erythrocyte antigens (over 600) have been reported in the literature and have been organized so far into 22 blood group systems (Table 30–18). Some of these antigens are of high frequency and are found on nearly all erythrocytes ("public" antigens); others are rarely present ("private" antigens) and are of relatively little practical importance in most routine transfusion cases. The antigens and the antibodies produced against them that blood bankers most often detect are described in the sections to follow. Table 30–19 may be used as a convenient reference that lists the more commonly encountered antibodies according to their immunoglobulin class, serologic phase of detection, clinical significance, and statistics on finding compatible blood.

Lewis System

LEWIS ANTIGENS

The Lewis system of antigens is produced from the same Type I precursor chains on which soluble ABO substances are built. However, unlike the ABO antigens, Lewis system antigens cannot be synthesized directly on erythrocyte membrane structures. These antigens are produced in cells that have yet to be identified from which the antigens are secreted into the saliva and other body fluids. In the plasma, Lewis antigens are attached to glycosphingolipid and are carried by lipoproteins that are secondarily adsorbed onto the erythrocyte membrane in a reversible process. Like the ABO antigens, Lewis antigens are distributed widely in body fluids and tissues and can be important clinically in relation to transfusion and solid organ transplantation. Lewis antigens are not well developed on the erythrocyte at birth, so cord erythrocytes will type as Le(a−b−). The frequency of the common adult Lewis phenotypes is shown in Table 30–20.

GENETICS AND BIOCHEMISTRY

The Lewis genetic locus has been assigned to chromosome 19 with the alleles *LE* and *le* occurring at the locus. The *LE* gene codes for the enzyme, α-4-L fucosyl transferase, which adds fucose at the fourth carbon of N-acetylglucosamine (GNAc), which is the subterminal sugar of Type I precursor chain. This addition results in the formation of Le[a] antigen.

Production of Le[b] antigen depends on the genetic interaction among the *LE*, *SE*, and *H* genes. The three-gene model of ABO antigen production (see Fig. 30–4) reminds us that *SE* regulates expression of the *H* gene in secretory cells, and if one inherits *SE*, Type I H substance will be produced. The enzyme encoded by *LE* also can add fucose to Type I H substance at the fourth carbon of GNAc to form Le[b] antigen. Because H substance is the precursor for Le[b], one must be a secretor to form Le[b]. Consequently, all nonsecretors can

Table 30–18. HUMAN ERYTHROCYTE BLOOD GROUP SYSTEMS CLASSIFIED ACCORDING TO 1993 ISBT* REPORT

Name	System No.	Name	System No.
ABO	001	Xg	012
MNS	002	Scianna	013
P	003	Dombrock	014
Rh	004	Colton	015
Lutheran	005	Landsteiner-Wiener	016
Kell	006	Chido-Rogers	017
Lewis	007	Hh	018
Duffy	008	Kx	019
Kidd	009	Gerbich	020
Diego	010	Cromer	021
Yt (Cartwright)	011	Knops	022

*Data from Daniels GL, et al: International Society of Blood Transfusion Working Party on Terminology for Red Cell Surface Antigens, São Paulo Report. Vox Sang 1993; 65:77.

Table 30–19. SEROLOGIC CHARACTERISTICS AND CLINICAL SIGNIFICANCE OF RED CELL ALLOANTIBODIES

		Most Common Phase of Reactivity			Clinical Significance		Approximate % of Compatible Donors	
Antibody	**Usual Ig Class**	***Sal***	***Alb***	***AGT***	***HTR***	***HDN***	***White***	***Black***
D	IgG	Few	X	X	Yes	Yes	15	8
C	IgG		X	X	Yes	Yes	30	68
E	IgG	Few	X	X	Yes	Yes	70	98
c	IgG		X	X	Yes	Yes	20	1
e	IgG		X	X	Yes	Yes	2	2
C[w]	IgG/IgM	Some	X	X	Yes	Yes	98	100
K	IgG	Rare		X	Yes	Yes	91	97
k	IgG			X	Yes	Yes	0.2	0.1
Kp[a]	IgG	Rare		X	Yes	Yes	98	99.9
Kp[b]	IgG			X	Yes	Yes	<0.1	0.1
Js[a]	IgG			X	Yes	Yes	>99.9	81
Js[b]	IgG			X	Yes	Yes	<0.1	1
Fy[a]	IgG			X	Yes	Yes	34	90
Fy[b]	IgG			X	Yes	Yes	17	77
Jk[a]	IgG			X	Yes	Yes	23	9
Jk[b]	IgG			X	Yes	Yes	28	5
M‡	IgM	X			Few	Yes	22	30
N	IgM	X			Rare	Rare	28	26
S	IgG/IgM		Some	X	Yes	Yes	45	69
s	IgG			X	Yes	Yes	11	3
U	IgG			X	Yes	Yes	0	1
Lu[a]*	IgM	X			?	Yes	92	96
Lu[b]*	IgG			X	Yes	Mild	<0.1	<0.1
P_1†	IgM	X	Some		Rare	No	21	6
P	IgM	X	Some	Some	Probable	Yes	<0.1	0.1
PP_1P^k†	IgG/IgM	X	Some	Some	Probable	Yes	<0.1	0.1
Le[a]†	IgM	X	Some		Yes	No	78	77
Le[b]†	IgM	X			Yes	No	28	45
I	IgM	X	Few		Rare	No	<0.1	<0.1
i	IgM	X	Few		?	No	<0.1	<0.1

*Exhibits characteristic mixed field agglutination pattern.
†May occasionally show *in vitro* hemolysis.
‡Most examples of anti-M also have a small but significant IgG component.

produce only Le[a] from Type I precursor, and thus their erythrocyte phenotype after adsorption of antigen is Le(a + b −).

In secretors, the *H*-specified and *LE*-specified fucosyl transferases compete for Type I precursor chains. Many more H chains are made than Le[a] chains, and those H chains may then go on to be converted to Le[b] as previously described. Probably because of the higher plasma Le[b] concentration, Le[b] is the antigen primarily adsorbed by erythrocytes; therefore, the erythrocyte phenotype in secretors is Le(a − b +) by routine agglutination methods. Secretor saliva, however, contains both Le[a] and Le[b] antigens in readily detectable concentrations. Figure 30–8 depicts the interaction between the *H*, *SE*, and *LE* genes and the resulting antigens expressed on the erythrocytes and in the saliva.

Table 30–20. PHENOTYPES OF THE LEWIS SYSTEM

	Reactions with Anti-		Frequencies (%) of U.S. Adults	
Phenotypes	***Le[a]***	***Le[b]***	***White***	***Black***
Le(a+b−)	+	−	22	23
Le(a−b+)	−	+	72	55
Le(a−b−)	−	−	6	22
Le(a+b+)*	+	+		

*Encountered occasionally in infants or young children who subsequently become Le(a−b+).

Persons who are homozygous for the *le* allele do not produce Le[a] or Le[b] antigens, and their erythrocyte phenotype is Le(a − b −). The discovery of two antibodies in the early 1970s that reacted with Le(a − b −) erythrocytes from secretors (anti-Le[d]) and nonsecretors (anti-Le[c]) led to the hypothesis that the *le* gene was actually not an amorph but coded for a separate α-3-L fucosyl transferase that could add fucose to Type II precursor or Type II H antigen on erythrocytes, resulting in the formation of Le[c] and Le[d] antigens, respectively. However, this hypothesis was effectively refuted by phenotypic family studies on *LE/le* heterozygotes (Issitt, 1985). Subsequently, it was shown that Le[c] is most likely unconverted Type I precursor and that Le[d] is simply Type I H substance, either of which may be adsorbed onto the erythrocyte membrane. Anti-Le[c] and anti-Le[d] have thus far been produced primarily as the result of animal immunization experiments, and no clinical significance in humans has been documented.

Adult Le(a − b −) cells also lack the antigen Le[x], which may be a common determinant of Le[a] and Le[b]. For all practical purposes serologically, anti-Le[x] acts as an inseparable mixture of anti-Le[a] and anti-Le[b], because the antibody reacts with all but other Le(a − b −) cells. Because anti-Le[x] also ag-

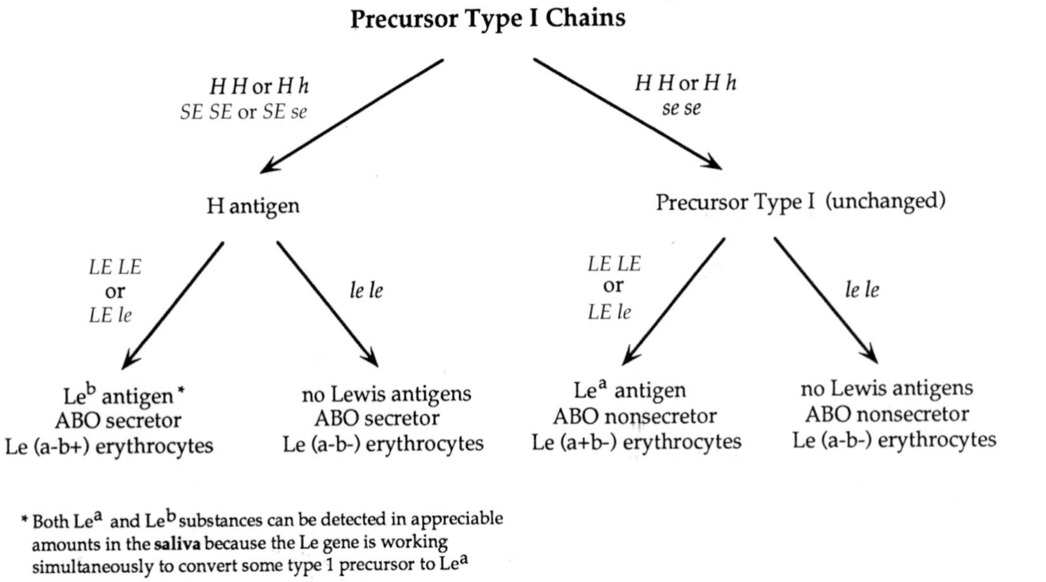

Figure 30–8. Interaction of *LE/SE/H* genes in the production of Lewis and ABO blood group antigens in the secretory cells.

glutinates 90% of all cord bloods in whites (Pittiglio, 1986) initially typing as Le(a − b −), Le^x may be a determinant in the early formation of Le^a and Le^b antigens.

LEWIS ANTIBODIES

Both anti-Le^a and anti-Le^b are usually naturally occurring antibodies of the IgM class. Although their optimal temperature of reactivity is room temperature or lower, many of these antibodies, particularly anti-Le^a, react well at temperatures up to 37°C. Both antibodies are most commonly detected as agglutinins after the 37°C incubation phase of the indirect antiglobulin antibody screen or crossmatch. Reactivity is enhanced by use of enzyme-treated cells. Because the antibodies readily activate complement, they may be reactive in the antihuman globulin (AHG) of testing if polyspecific AHG is used. Also, *in vitro* hemolysis sometimes occurs with anti-Le^a and more rarely with anti-Le^b.

Hemolytic transfusion reactions due to anti-Le^a have been reported, but none due to anti-Le^b has been reported. For most sera containing Lewis antibodies detected as agglutinins after 37°C incubation, studies have shown that selection of blood compatible by crossmatch using the indirect antiglobulin technique is appropriate and that screening for antigen-negative units with commercial antisera is unnecessary. Any example of anti-Le^a or anti-Le^b that is hemolytic *in vitro* or shows strong reactivity in the AHG phase of testing should be treated as clinically significant, and antigen-negative blood should be transfused. When antigen-negative blood could not be found for a patient who demonstrates clinically significant Lewis antibodies, plasma containing soluble Lewis antigen corresponding to the patient's antibody or antibodies has been infused prior to erythrocyte transfusion in order to neutralize or inhibit the patient's antibody (Mollison, 1993).

Lewis antibodies have not been implicated in HDN because the vast majority of anti-Le^a and anti-Le^b are IgM, and the corresponding antigens are poorly developed on the erythrocytes at birth.

I and i Antigens

Like the A, B, H, and Lewis antigens, the I and i blood group antigens are derived from complex glycosphingolipids or glycoproteins. Because I and i are not discrete antithetical antigens produced by allelic genes, they cannot correctly be classified as a blood group "system." Experiments with removal of ABH sugars from erythrocytes and on cells from persons of the O_h phenotypes show that the Ii antigens are defined by a series of repeating carbohydrate structures on oligosaccharide chains more proximal to the erythrocyte membrane than is the case with the ABO antigens (Harmening, 1994). The activity of i antigen is associated with linear H_2 structures, whereas I antigen activity occurs on the more complex branched H_3 chains. It is hypothesized that an *I* gene codes for an enzyme responsible for branching of the H chains to produce I antigen.

At birth, cord cells for all practical purposes are I − i +. From birth to 18 months of age, the i antigen expression gradually decreases as I antigen increases to the adult erythrocyte phenotype of I + i −. The changing expression of the Ii antigens from linear to branched chains most likely reflects the ontogenic development of fetal to adult erythrocytes (Hakomori, 1981). Rare individuals do not develop the I + i − adult phenotype and remain i + I −, which is called the i_{adult} phenotype. This appears to be the result of a recessive inheritance pattern. Table 30–21 shows the transformation in Ii pheno-

Table 30–21. THE I AND i ANTIGENS

Phenotype	Relative Antigen Strength *I*	Relative Antigen Strength *i*	Incidence
i_{adult}	Weakest	Strongest	Rare
i_{cord}	Weak	Strong	All newborns
I_{int}	Strong	Weak	Rare adults
I	Strongest	Weakest	Almost all adults

type from birth to adulthood. In addition to being an erythrocyte antigen, the I antigen is also found on leukocytes and platelets and in soluble form in many body fluids.

Anti-I can be an autoantibody or an alloantibody. Because the frequency of I-negative adults is very low, alloanti-I is relatively rare and is found in persons of the i_{adult} phenotype as a naturally occurring antibody. Alloanti-I may be IgM or IgG. Conversely, autoanti-I is a common, low-titered, benign, IgM, cold agglutinin found in many normal persons, but it can also be a pathologic antibody in those with acquired cold autoimmune hemolytic anemia. High-titered anti-I is usually associated with *Mycoplasma pneumoniae* infection (see Erythrocyte Autoantibodies).

Anti-i is relatively uncommon, but potent examples of autoanti-i have been most frequently reported in the serum of patients with infectious mononucleosis or in persons with alcoholic cirrhosis. Anti-i has never been described as an alloantibody (Mollison, 1993). Both anti-I and anti-i reactivities are optimal at temperatures below 22°C and are enhanced by enzyme treatment of erythrocytes.

Because of the biochemical relationship and spatial proximity of I antigen to the ABH and Lewis antigens on the erythrocyte membrane, antibodies against compound antigens such as anti-IH, anti-IA, anti-IB, anti-iH, and anti-ILe^{bH} have been described. Such antibodies only react optimally with cells that possess both antigens.

P System

Although the three antigens P_1, P, and P^k are not all produced by allelic genes, they will be referred to collectively as the P system. These antigens are biochemically related to the ABH antigens such as Lewis and Ii as previously described. The P, P_1, and P^k antigens are found on erythrocytes, platelets, leukocytes, and tissue fibroblasts; P and P^k have also been found in plasma.

Biochemically, the P^k, P, and P_1 antigens are produced via separate biosynthetic pathways in which specific transferases add immunodominant sugars to the erythrocyte precursor, ceramide dihexose (CDH). CDH also carries the type 2 chains on which A, B, H, and I antigens are made, but because the P system genes act first, their gene products (antigens) are situated closer to the erythrocyte membrane (Harmening, 1994). The genetics controlling these biosynthetic pathways are still not clear, although it is apparent that production of the three antigens is controlled by two independent genetic systems (Mollison, 1993).

Although P is a high-frequency antigen found on almost all cells, only 79% of whites and 94% of blacks are positive for the P_1 antigen. Table 30–22 shows the frequency of the various phenotypes within the P system and the antigens that are produced. The degree of antigen expression varies among persons who are P_1 positive. *In vitro*, the P_1 antigen deteriorates rapidly during erythrocyte storage at 1°C to 6°C.

Table 30–22. PHENOTYPE FREQUENCIES AND ASSOCIATED ANTIGENS IN THE P SYSTEM

Phenotypes	Phenotype Frequencies (%) — *White*	*Black*	Antigens Produced
P_1	79	94	P_1, P
P_2	21	6	P
P_1^k	Very rare	Very rare	—
P_2^k	Very rare	Very rare	P_1, P^k
p	Very rare	Very rare	P^k

Anti-P_1 produced by P_2-positive persons is the most commonly encountered P system antibody and is usually a naturally occurring, weak, IgM agglutinin reactive at temperatures below 22°C. Because the antibody binds complement effectively, however, anti-P_1 is often detected by laboratories using polyspecific AHG sera.

Most anti-P_1 may be inhibited by a commercially available soluble P_1 substance derived from pigeon egg protein or prevented from reacting by prewarming techniques. If the antibody is truly reactive by prewarmed antiglobulin methods or is hemolytic *in vitro*, antigen-negative units should be provided for transfusion because anti-P_1 has been associated with both delayed and immediate hemolytic transfusion reactions. For anti-P_1 reactive only at room temperature or below, blood compatible by the antihuman globulin crossmatch (unscreened for P_1 antigen) is appropriate. Anti-P_1 has not been associated with HDN, probably because the antigen is poorly developed at birth, and because most antibody is IgM.

Anti-P may be found as a naturally occurring IgM alloantibody in the serum of all persons of the P^k and p phenotypes and is a potent hemolysin of all cells containing the P antigen. Fortunately, it is a rare antibody. Anti-P specificity is also associated with an IgG biphasic hemolysin produced in paroxysmal cold hemoglobinuria, or PCH (see Erythrocyte Autoantibodies).

Anti-PP_1P^k (formerly called anti-Tj^a) is present as a naturally occurring mixture of separable specificities in all people with the p phenotype (P_{null}). This mixture may be IgM only or IgM plus IgG and is potentially very hemolytic. The anti-P portion of anti-PP_1P^k is usually IgG and has been associated with habitual early abortion. Anti-P^k may be prepared by selective adsorption of anti-PP_1P^k with globoside (P antigen).

MNSs System

The MNSs system antigens are glycoprotein antigens determined by two closely linked genes that have been assigned to chromosome 4. M and N are found on glycophorin A and S and s on glycophorin B, two integral membrane sialoglycoproteins. The M and N determinants of glycophorin A, which is 131 amino acids in length and glycosylated with numerous tetrasaccharide units, are specified by two amino acid substitutions at positions one and five of the polypeptide chain (Fig. 30–9). Results of inhibition studies of anti-M and anti-N using octapeptides containing the first eight amino acids of the M and N sialoglycoproteins suggest that the first amino acid substitution at position one is the critical antigenic determinant for the M or N antigens (Pedersen, 1990). The portion of glycophorin A that carries the M and N antigens is cleaved from the membrane by proteolytic enzymes so that reactivity with the corresponding antibodies is usually abolished.

The S and s determinants of glycophorin B, which is 72 amino acids in length and glycosylated similarly to glycophorin A, are specified by a single amino acid substitution at position 29 in the polypeptide chain. Glycophorin B also carries the high-frequency antigen U at a location closer to the membrane than S or s (see Fig. 30–9). Approximately 1% of blacks lack the U antigen as well as the S and s antigens and

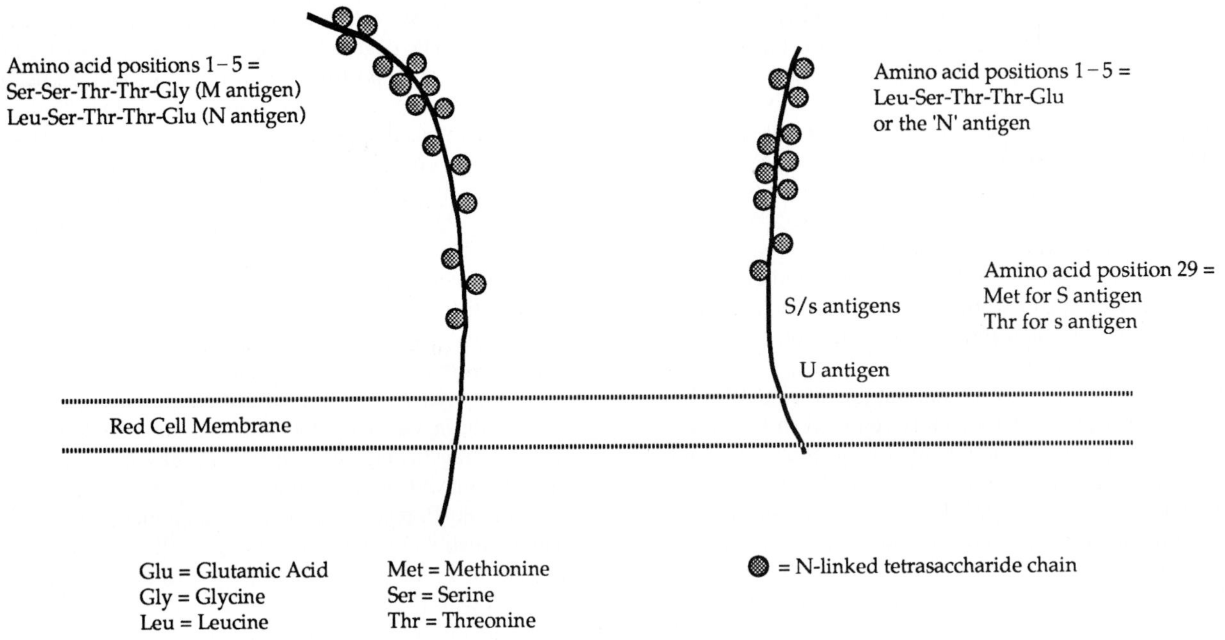

Figure 30–9. The MN and Ss sialoglycoproteins in the red cell membrane.

have been shown to totally lack glycophorin B or to possess only between 2% and 5% of the glycophorin B found in normal cells (Issitt, 1985). The rare allele at the *S* locus responsible for the S−s−U− or S−s−U+^{w} phenotype in blacks has been designated S^{u}. Table 30–23 shows the phenotypes and frequencies within the MNSs system. Issitt (1985) has extensively reviewed the biochemistry and serology of this blood group system.

Anti-M is a commonly encountered, naturally occurring agglutinin usually reactive at temperatures below 22°C. Reactivity of some anti-M may be enhanced by acidification of the serum to pH 6.5. Although predominantly IgM, anti-M can have an IgG component and as such has been occasionally implicated in cases of HDN, some of which have been severe.

Anti-N is a rare antibody found as a naturally occurring IgM agglutinin. Only persons of the rare S−s− phenotype are truly N antigen negative, because the first 26 amino acids at the NH_2 terminus of the Ss glycoprotein, designated 'N,' are identical to the N determinant (see Fig. 30–9), which probably accounts for the scarcity of human anti-N. A lectin with anti-N specificity can be made from the seeds of *Vicia graminea* and is commercially available for phenotyping purposes. Most anti-M and anti-N are clinically insignificant, but both have been reported as rare causes of hemolytic transfusion reactions.

Table 30–23. PHENOTYPES OF THE MNSs SYSTEM

Reactions with Anti-						Phenotype Frequencies (%)	
M	*N*	*S*	*s*	*U*	Phenotype	*White*	*Black*
+	−				M+N−	28	26
+	+				M+N+	50	44
−	+				M−N+	22	30
		+	−	+	S+s−U+	11	3
		+	+	+	S+s+U+	44	28
		−	+	+	S−s+U+	45	69
		−	−	−	S−s−U−	0	<1
		−	−	+	S−s−U+	0	Rare

Anti-S, anti-s, and anti-U usually result from immune stimulation, and most are IgG reactive at 37°C. Most are detectable only by the antihuman globulin technique. Enzyme treatment of erythrocytes may decrease the reactivity of anti-S, but anti-s and anti-U are unaffected. All three of these antibodies have been associated with hemolytic transfusion reactions and HDN.

Many examples of anti-M, anti-N, anti-S, and anti-s exhibit the dosage phenomenon *in vitro*. Commercially prepared anti-M and anti-N sera usually differentiate heterozygotes from homozygotes if a titer and scoring technique is used for phenotyping. Phenotyping in the MNSs antigen system often yields much useful information in paternity testing.

Lutheran System

The first two antigens of the Lutheran system, Lu^{a} and Lu^{b}, were discovered in 1946 and 1956, respectively; until the 1970s, the system was thought to be a simple two-allele system assigned to chromosome 19. Since then, three more pairs of alleles closely linked to Lu^{a} and Lu^{b} have been described, the most recent inclusion being that of the genes coding for the previously described antigens Au^{a} and Au^{b} (Daniels, 1991). The system currently consists of eight established Lutheran system antigens (Table 30–24) and a number of "para-Lutheran" antigens.

Various studies show that the Lutheran system antigens are carried on glycoproteins and that intact disulfide bonds probably contribute to the conformation of the antigenic determinants (Poole, 1992). Lu^{a} and Lu^{b} seem to be unaffected or only mildly affected by the commonly used blood bank enzymes such as ficin and papain, but these antigens are destroyed by treatment with trypsin or chymotrypsin. The biochemistry of the Lutheran system is well reviewed by Daniels (1988).

Table 30–24. ANTIGENS AND PHENOTYPES OF THE LUTHERAN SYSTEM

Antithetical Antigens	Approximate Frequency (%)	Common Lutheran Phenotypes	Frequency (%) in U.S. Population	
			White	*Black*
Lu1 (Lu^a)	8	Lu (a+b−)	0.1	0.1
Lu2 (Lu^b)	>99			
Lu6	>99	Lu (a+b+)	6.7	5.2
Lu9	2			
Lu8	>99	Lu (a−b+)	93.2	94.7
Lu14	2.4			
Lu18 (Au^a)	80	Lu (a−b−)	Very rare	
Lu19 (Au^b)	50			

Anti-Lu^a and anti-Lu^b are uncommon antibodies that are only rarely associated with hemolytic transfusion reactions or hemolytic disease of the newborn. Anti-Lu^a may be stimulated by incompatible transfusion, but it is usually transient and weak. Anti-Lu^b is rare because of the high frequency of the antigen in the population. Although both antibodies may be mixtures of IgG, IgM, or IgA, anti-Lu^b is almost always at least partly IgG. Most examples of anti-Lu^a and some of anti-Lu^b act as saline agglutinins reactive at room temperature, but anti-Lu^b is also commonly detected by the antihuman globulin technique. A distinctive pattern of agglutination is characteristic of Lutheran antibodies, which consists of a minor population of small agglutinates against a background of unagglutinated cells known as mixed field agglutination.

Another Lutheran system antibody, anti-Lu^3, is made by those with the rare recessive Lutheran (a−b−) phenotype. The Lu(a−b−) phenotype is unusual in that it may be the result of three alternative genetic mechanisms. The most common of these is a dominant inheritance pattern determined by a gene named *In(Lu)* that suppresses normal expression of Lutheran system antigens. *In(Lu)* also suppresses expression of antigens unrelated to Lutheran, including the P_1 and i antigens.

Kell System

The Kell blood group system was the first new erythrocyte antigen system to be discovered with the newly developed antiglobulin technique in the investigation of a case of HDN. The antibody responsible was directed against what is now known as the K antigen, but which at the time was christened Kell after the original propositus. The K antigen ranks second in immunogenicity only to the D antigen, if A and B antigens are excluded from consideration.

Today, the Kell blood group is a complex system of 23 antigens. Production of Kell system antigens is presumably controlled by a series of closely linked loci that have been assigned to chromosome 7 (Redman, 1993). Kell system antigens can basically be divided into groups of high-frequency and low-frequency antigens, with only K and Js^a falling in between. Table 30–25 shows the frequency of the Kell system phenotypes in the general population.

The Kell system antigens are found only in erythroid tissues and seem to be associated with a single transmembrane glycoprotein (Redman, 1993). They are unaffected by proteolytic enzymes but are denatured by reducing reagents such as dithiothreitol (DTT) and 2-aminoethylisothiouronium bromide (AET), indicating that disulfide bonds are important in the antigenic configuration. The biosynthesis of these antigens is still not clearly understood, but it has been hypothesized that the basic precursor substance is the K_x erythrocyte membrane protein (Rouger, 1990). This hypothesis is supported by indirect evidence—the rare Kell null (K_o) phenotype, in which no Kell system antigens are expressed, and the McLeod phenotype, discussed subsequently. K_o cells possess approximately twice as much K_x as is found on cells of normal Kell phenotypes. However, no biochemical evidence supports this hypothesis.

Production of K_x is controlled by an X-linked gene at the locus, *XK*. Possession of an alternative recessive allele at the *XK* locus results in absence of the K_x protein associated with weak expression of the Kell system antigens and with an abnormal erythrocyte morphology. This is called the McLeod phenotype. Some males with the McLeod phenotype also have chronic granulomatous disease (CGD). For a number of years, early absorption studies with anti-K_x and both normal and CGD neutrophils led to the hypothesis that neutrophils also possess K_x membrane protein and that lack of neutrophil K_x was responsible for the neutrophil biochemical defect seen in CGD. Branch and colleagues (1986), however, showed by flow cytometric analysis that K_x is absent from even normal neutrophils, so K_x is not directly related to CGD. Thus, the clinical association sometimes observed between CGD and the McLeod phenotype is probably due to the fact that the genes controlling both syndromes are contiguous on the X chromosome (Redman, 1993).

Of the antibodies to Kell system antigens, anti-K is the most frequently encountered; other antibodies, such as anti-Kp^a and anti-Js^a, are much more rare. Most Kell system antibodies are IgG and reactive at 37°C, although there have been a few examples of naturally occurring IgM forms of anti-K. Most Kell system antibodies are detectable only by the antihuman globulin technique. All have been implicated in cases of hemolytic transfusion reactions and hemolytic disease of the newborn.

Duffy System

The Duffy system currently consists of five known Duffy-controlled antigens, two of which, Fy^a and Fy^b, are controlled by allelic genes at a locus mapped to chromosome 1. Fy^a and Fy^b antigens are known to be cleaved from the erythrocyte membrane by proteolytic enzymes, whereas Fy3, Fy4, and

Table 30–25. PHENOTYPE FREQUENCIES IN THE KELL SYSTEM

Reactions with Anti-						Phenotype	Frequency (%) in U.S. Population	
K	*k*	*Kp^a*	*Kp^b*	*Js^a*	*Js^b*		*White*	*Black*
+	0					K+k−	0.2	Rare
+	+					K+k+	8.8	2
0	+					K−k+	91	98
		+	0			Kp(a+b−)	Rare	0
		+	+			Kp(a+b+)	2.3	Rare
		0	+			Kp(a−b+)	97.7	100
				+	0	Js(a+b−)	0	1
				+	+	Js(a+b+)	Rare	19
				0	+	Js(a−b+)	100	80
0	0	0	0	0	0	K_o	Exceedingly rare	

4

Table 30–26. PHENOTYPE FREQUENCIES IN THE DUFFY SYSTEM

	Frequency (%) in U.S. Population		Probable Genotype	
Phenotype	*White*	*Black*	*White*	*Black*
Fy(a+b−)	17	9	Fy^aFy^a	Fy^aFy^4
Fy(a+b+)	49	1	Fy^aFy^b	Fy^aFy^b
Fy(a−b+)	34	22	Fy^bFy^b	Fy^bFy^4
Fy(a−b−)	Extremely rare	68	*FyFy*	Fy^4Fy^4

Fy5 are protease-resistant. The Duffy antigens are carried on a transmembrane erythrocyte glycoprotein containing one or more N-linked oligosaccharides (Riwom, 1994), which was recently definitively identified as the erythrocyte chemokine receptor (Neote, 1994).

The incidence of the Fy^a and Fy^b antigens differs markedly in the white and black populations, as shown in Table 30–26. Originally, Fy(a−b−) status, which was found as the major phenotype in blacks, was thought to be the result of a silent *Fy* allele. However, cells from most blacks with this phenotype were later found to react with an antibody characterized in 1973 and called anti-Fy^4, suggesting the existence of an Fy^4 allele common to blacks (Issitt, 1985). Cells of the Fy(a−b−) phenotype have been shown to be resistant to infection with the malarial organism, *Plasmodium vivax.* Evidence suggests that the Fy^a and Fy^b antigens are located at the parasite's site of the entry into the erythrocyte (Miller, 1975).

Anti-Fy^a is the most commonly encountered antibody to Duffy system antigens. Anti-Fy^b occurs less frequently and is usually found with other specificities in the serum of immunologic responders. Both are usually immune-stimulated, IgG antibodies and are detected only by use of the antihuman globulin technique. Both anti-Fy^a and anti-Fy^b have been associated with hemolytic transfusion reactions and hemolytic disease of the newborn. Issitt (1985) provides a detailed review of the serologic activity of anti-Fy^3, anti-Fy^4, and anti-Fy^5.

Kidd System

Unlike some of the other blood groups previously described, since the discovery of the Kidd system Jk^a and Jk^b antigens in the 1950s, no other antigens have been added to this system (Table 30–27). The two antigens are coded for by allelic genes, but no consensus has been reached as to which chromosome contains the Kidd locus. A $Kidd_{null}$ or Jk(a−b−) phenotype was described soon after the characterization of the antigens; the frequency of this phenotype reaches almost 1% in the Polynesian population, but otherwise is rare. The Jk(a−b−) phenotype sometimes results from inheritance of the recessive allele, *Jk*, in double dose or from a dominant suppressor gene at a locus separate from Kidd.

Knowledge of the biochemistry of the Kidd antigens still is relatively limited. However, they are probably protein in nature and appear to be restricted to erythrocytes. The weak reactivity of the Kidd antibodies with antigen-positive erythrocytes led to the early inference that there were only a small number of membrane antigen sites. However, studies on antigen density showed that the weak reactions were not due to decreased binding sites (Mougey, 1990). It is now hypothesized that the Kidd antigens are clustered on the membrane and thus not very accessible to antibody.

The protein on which the Kidd antigens are situated functions, in a manner yet to be elucidated, in urea or water transport across the erythrocyte membrane (Edwards-Moulds, 1988). This was discovered when it was noticed that cells of the Jk(a−b−) phenotype resist lysis by 2M urea, which is a lytic agent used in some automated hematology analyzers. Undoubtedly, further study of this phenomenon by membrane biologists in addition to attempts to clone the Kidd genes will answer many questions concerning the genetics and biochemistry of the system.

Anti-Jk^a and anti-Jk^b are both immune-stimulated, IgG antibodies detectable only by the antihuman globulin technique (AGT). Studies have shown that they are almost always of the subclass IgG_1 or IgG_3 (Mougey, 1988). The reactivity of both antibodies is enhanced by use of enzymes and by the presence of complement. Some blood bankers will not use monospecific anti-IgG in their indirect antiglobulin tests (IAT) tests because of the possibility of missing a complement-dependent Kidd antibody, as discussed previously in the section Complement and Blood Banking.

Anti-Jk^a and anti-Jk^b are usually low in titer and weak in avidity, and in most cases they disappear rapidly from the patient's system after immunization. The antibodies also classically demonstrate the dosage phenomenon *in vitro.* This combination of attributes may render detection or identification of Kidd antibodies difficult. Undoubtedly, this is one of the reasons that Kidd antibodies are associated with about one quarter of delayed transfusion reactions in which antibody is detected only as the result of an anamnestic response. In addition, the *in vivo* activity of Kidd antibodies also explains why they are responsible for over 75% of severe delayed reactions involving true hemolytic sequelae (Ness, 1990). Because the Kidd antibodies are effective activators of complement, *in vivo* hemolysis may be extensive, because the cell-bound antibody and complement act synergistically to cause rapid hepatic clearance of incompatible cells. The Kidd antibodies have also both been implicated in hemolytic disease of the newborn.

Other Systems

Two groups of antibodies, the high titer/low avidity (HTLA) and Bg antibodies, as well as anti-Sd^a, are commonly detected by the antibody screen or crossmatch utilizing the antihuman globulin technique. They have limited clinical significance but are a considerable nuisance, because they must be investigated just as any other blood group antibody. All of the antigens against which these antibodies are directed, with the exception of Bg, are present in abundant soluble form in plasma or other body fluid. They are summarized in Table 30–28. Table 30–29 summarizes a few other

Table 30–27. PHENOTYPES OF THE KIDD SYSTEM

	Reactions with Anti-			Frequencies (%) in U.S.	
Phenotype	Jk^a	Jk^b	$Jk^{ab}(3)$	*Caucasian*	*Black*
Jk(a+b−)	+	−	+	28	57
Jk(a+b+)	+	+	+	49	34
Jk(a−b+)	−	+	+	23	9
Jk(a−b−)	−	−	−	Very rare	

Table 30–28. HIGH TITER, LOW AVIDITY (HTLA), Bg, AND SID ANTIBODIES

Blood Group System or Antigen Collection	Comments	Incidence in Whites (%)
HTLA Antibodies		
Chido/Rodgers	Ch^a, Rg^a, and JMH are determinants of the C4 complement component coded for at the HLA locus, abundant in plasma	98 (Ch^a); 97 (Rg^a)
John Milton Hagen		98 (JMH)
Knops	Kn^a and McC^a are determinants of erythrocyte complement receptor 1	99 (Kn^a)
McCoy		99 (McC^a)
York	Yk^a and Cs^a are white cell determinants expressed on erythrocytes and in plasma	92 (Yk^a)
Cost-Sterling		98 (Cs^a)
Bg Antibodies	Bg antibodies react with HLA antigen remnants on the mature erythrocyte membrane Bg^a = HLA-B7 Bg^b = HLA-Bw17 Bg^c = HLA-A28	
SID Antibodies	Sd^a antigen is abundant in urine; rare "super-Sid" erythrocytes with very strong expression of the Sd^a antigen exist, also known as the Cad+ phenotype. Transfusion of these cells to a recipient with anti-Sd^a was implicated in one transfusion reaction. Anti-Sd^a shows a unique mixed field agglutination pattern of tightly packed, refractile agglutinates.	96 (Sd^a)

miscellaneous well studied blood group systems consisting of two antithetical antigens (usually one "public" and one "private").

Erythrocyte Autoantibodies

Although blood bank technologists spend much of their time detecting and identifying serum alloantibodies, serologic evaluation for the presence of erythrocyte autoantibodies is also an important, though less frequent, endeavor. Autoantibodies, in general, are produced by an individual's immune system against "self" or an antigen that is present in that same person. Although produced against self-antigens, these antibodies will also usually react with the same antigen found in other normal persons. If the antibodies produced are against blood cell constituents, the pathologic result could be hemolytic anemia, thrombocytopenia, or leukopenia, but often the autoantibodies cause no demonstrable clinical symptoms.

The direct antiglobulin test (DAT) contributes directly to the diagnosis of autoimmune hemolytic anemia (AIHA), because it can confirm the presence of antibody that has attached *in vivo* to the patient's own erythrocytes. The test thus can help differentiate AIHA from anemias caused by a congenital abnormality in the patient's erythrocyte structure, enzymes, or hemoglobin. The DAT may be positive because of IgG or complement components, depending on the class or subclass of autoantibody involved. A positive DAT by itself, however, does not mean a person has AIHA, because one study showed that up to 8% of hospitalized patients have positive DATs without any signs of hemolysis (Petz, 1993).

The serum of a patient with suspected AIHA may also be screened for the presence of free autoantibody by the indirect antiglobulin technique. By this testing, autoantibodies are frequently categorized according to the temperature of *in vitro*

4

Table 30–29. OTHER BLOOD GROUP SYSTEMS CONSISTING OF TWO KNOWN ANTITHETICAL ANTIGENS

System	Phenotype	Frequency (%) in Whites*	Optimal Reaction Phase	Implicated in: *Hemolytic Transfusion Reaction*	Implicated in: *Hemolytic Disease of the Newborn*
Diego†	Di(a+b−)	0	AGT	Yes	Mild
	Di(a+b+)	Very rare			
	Di(a−b+)	100			
Cartwright	Yt(a+b−)	91.9	AGT	Possible	No
	Yt(a+b+)	7.9			
	Yt(a−b+)	0.2			
Dombrock	Do(a+b−)	17.2	AGT with enzymes	Yes	Mild
	Do(a+b+)	49.5			
	Do(a−b+)	33.3			
Colton	Co(a+b−)	89.3	AGT with enzymes	Yes	Mild
	Co(a+b+)	10.4			
	Co(a−b+)	0.3			
	Co(a−b−)	Very rare			
Scianna	Sc:1,−2	99.7	Most AGT; some saline	No	No
	Sc:1, 2	0.3			
	Sc:−1, 2	Very rare			
	Sc:−1, −2	Very rare			

AGT = antiglobulin test.
*Insufficient data for reliable calculation of frequencies in blacks.
†Di^a antigen has a much higher frequency in Asians and Native Americans.
Modified from Walker RH (ed): Technical Manual, 11th ed. Bethesda, MD, American Association of Blood Banks, 1993.

reactivity as cold (usually IgM) or warm (usually IgG). The causative antibodies of these categories of anemias are described here; however, Chapter 26 reviews the etiology and pathophysiology of AIHA.

Warm Reactive Autoantibodies

Persons with warm reactive autoantibodies account for approximately 80% of the cases of AIHA each year, AIHA having a total incidence of about 1:80,000 (Prasad, 1993). Warm autoimmune hemolytic anemia (WAIHA) may be classified either as primary or idiopathic (of unknown etiology) or as secondary—that is, associated with some other disease state, such as another autoimmune process (frequently systemic lupus erythematosus), lymphoproliferative disorders, or certain viral infections. With the advent of improved diagnostic procedures, the percentage of WAIHA classified as idiopathic has dropped to about 30% of cases. Patients with warm autoantibodies and a positive DAT will not all present with symptomatic anemia but may exist in a chronic compensated state for some time before their condition progresses to overt anemia.

Causative antibodies of WAIHA are usually IgG and polyclonal in nature, showing optimal *in vitro* reactivity at 37°C. The vast majority of warm autoantibodies that are in the serum and recovered in eluates from the patients' erythrocytes can only be demonstrated by use of the indirect antiglobulin technique.

Warm autoantibodies will be demonstrated on the patient's erythrocytes in about 80% of cases of WAIHA. The DAT profiles show that about 30% to 40% are due to IgG only, 40% to 50% are due to IgG and complement, and about 10% are due to complement only (Prasad, 1993). When the DAT is negative, other studies have reported that more sensitive techniques such as radioisotope-labeled or enzyme-labeled direct antiglobulin testing can demonstrate low levels of IgG or, less frequently, IgM or IgA on the erythrocytes (Engelfriet, 1992).

Immunoglobulin subclass studies in cases of WAIHA have showed the causative antibodies to be predominantly IgG_1 and/or IgG_3 (see Table 30–5). Despite the ability of these subclasses to activate complement, immune destruction of the patient's autologous cells occurs largely through the spleen and liver via extravascular pathways. Patients whose erythrocytes are coated with IgG_3, however, are more likely to have overt anemia, apparently because of the greater capacity of IgG_3 for binding to Fc receptors on macrophages (Engelfriet, 1992). Some erythrocytes may also be destroyed via cytotoxic killing by other cells with Fc receptors.

Specificity of the causative antibodies of WAIHA is generally broad, with reactivity against all normal human erythrocytes. However, many of these broadly reactive antibodies do show specificity for some unidentified high-frequency antigen within the Rh system, because the autoantibodies will not react with Rh_{null} cells or cells with Rh deletion phenotypes. Some autoantibodies will demonstrate a single Rh specificity such as anti-e (most frequently) or anti-c. Warm autoantibody specificities have also been reported to include those in the Kell, Kidd, MNSs, and ABO blood group systems, as well as anti-Vel and anti-LW. However, only about 4% of persons with WAIHA will show a single simple specificity (Issitt, 1985).

Occasionally, the autoantibody mimics a single alloantibody specificity, but further testing shows that the antibody can be absorbed to exhaustion with either antigen-positive or antigen-negative erythrocytes. These mimicking antibodies can occur in patients with or without the corresponding antigen, and the autoantibody may or may not be reactive, at least *in vitro,* with the patient's own cells. It is these cases that provide a challenge for the blood bank technologist who must employ special techniques (e.g., antibody adsorption) to decide if a simple alloantibody or a mimicking autoantibody is present.

Although transfusion is usually avoided for as long as possible in patients with WAIHA, the use of least incompatible blood (as determined by comparison to an autocontrol) for transfusion of patients with an autoantibody of unknown specificity is generally accepted. However, before such a decision is made, one must exclude the possibility of the simultaneous presence of other serum alloantibodies by further serologic investigation, including warm autoadsorption followed by antibody detection on the absorbed serum. Autoadsorption can only be performed on patients who have not recently undergone transfusion, however.

Cold Reactive Autoantibodies

Cold autoantibodies may be detected in the serum of many normal persons if they are tested under the right conditions. However, most of these antibodies are benign cold agglutinins that show optimal reactivity at 4°C and little or no reactivity at 37°C. Cold agglutinins are usually a nuisance that may interfere with ABO typing procedures or with antibody detection and crossmatching techniques using polyspecific antihuman globulin if complement is activated *in vitro*. Although usually ignored as clinically insignificant, cold agglutinins may become important, depending on their thermal range, during procedures in which the patient's core temperature will be decreased to as low as 28°C, as in cardiopulmonary bypass surgery. When cold agglutinins are detected, one of the following antibodies can often be identified.

ANTI-H

Anti-H is usually seen as a benign cold agglutinin (with the exception of Bombays) in A_1 or A_1B nonsecretors with optimal reactivity at 4°C. Detectable anti-H will normally react well with group O or A_2 cells and weakly or not at all with A_1 or A_1B cells, leading to a situation in which anti-H may cause a positive antibody screening test while all crossmatches appear compatible. Anti-H can be avoided by prewarming or by inhibition with secretor saliva as a source of soluble antigen, which is the basis for testing of secretor status (see Hemagglutination Inhibition).

ANTI-I

Anti-I is normally found as a low-titer, IgM cold agglutinin in most adult sera. However, anti-I is also one of the most common specificities associated with cold autoimmune hemolytic anemia (CAIHA), also sometimes referred to as cold hemagglutinins disease (CHD). CAIHA accounts for about 20% of total cases of AIHA. As with warm AIHA, CAIHA may be idiopathic or secondarily associated with a disease state, particularly after infections with certain bacteria or viruses. Anti-I is the most frequent causative antibody of idiopathic CAIHA and is also the cause of secondary CAIHA with acute onset following infection with *Mycoplasma pneu-*

moniae. In secondary CAIHA, it is believed that the *Mycoplasma* organism somehow alters the erythrocyte such that the I antigen is no longer recognized as "self." The autoanti-I formed is truly against erythrocyte antigen and can not be absorbed out by a preparation of the infectious agent or organism (Issitt, 1985).

In contrast with the low-titer anti-I agglutinins found in normal sera, anti-I in CAIHA usually develops at very high titers in a range of at least 1:10,000 up to as high as 1:1,000,000. The antibody also has a wider thermal amplitude than benign anti-I and may be monoclonal or polyclonal (Prasad, 1993). The mechanism of hemolysis appears to be that the antibody reacts with erythrocytes at around 32°C or lower in the peripheral vessels of the extremities, and complement is activated. Hemolysis of erythrocytes, however, is rarely intravascular, but instead occurs via extravascular pathways involving cells of the liver with receptors for C3b. Hemolysis may be chronic or episodic, depending on the thermal range of the antibody, and may be triggered by exposure to cold temperatures. DATs on erythrocytes from patients with CHD, if positive, are due to C3 components, usually C3d.

Because of the broad reactivity of anti-I in CAIHA with nearly all adult erythrocytes, the antibody may cause great difficulty in compatibility testing. As with warm autoantibodies, one of the primary concerns is to detect and identify underlying IgG alloantibodies, if present. Techniques to circumvent the autoanti-I in serum testing include prewarming, cold autoadsorption, adsorption with rabbit erythrocyte stroma (REST), or treatment of the serum with sulfhydryl reagents, such as dithiothreitol (DTT) and 2-mercaptoethanol (2-ME). Information regarding all of these procedures may be found in the American Association of Blood Banks' *Technical Manual* (American Association of Blood Banks, 8101 Glenbrook Road, Bethesda, Maryland 20814–2749) (Walker, 1993).

ANTI-i

Anti-i usually is detected as an IgM, cold autoantibody in patients with infectious mononucleosis or with certain lymphoproliferative disorders. The latter group may have monoclonal forms of anti-i. Perhaps 10% to 20% of patients with infectious mononucleosis have significant cold agglutinin titers, but few go on to actually develop CAIHA (Prasad, 1993).

ANTI-Pr

Anti-Pr antibodies (originally called anti-Sp) are an infrequent cause of CAIHA. Anti-Pr specificities may initially react as anti-I does but may be differentiated by their equally strong reactions with cord cells and with adult cells (cord cells are I antigen–negative); by the fact that anti-Pr is nonreactive with enzyme-treated erythrocytes, whereas anti-I is enhanced by enzyme treatment; and by the fact that anti-Pr is nonreactive in an alkaline (pH 9) test system, whereas anti-I is only mildly affected. Anti-Pr in patients with CAIHA is usually monoclonal and may be IgG, IgM, or IgA.

Table 30–30 shows the serologic differentiation of various, usually benign, cold agglutinating autoantibodies.

ANTI-P

Anti-P is observed primarily in patients with PCH, which is a syndrome often seen in children following infection by mumps, chickenpox, measles, and other viruses. Historically, PCH was also seen in syphilitic patients. In PCH, anti-P is known as the Donath-Landsteiner (DL) antibody. It is an IgG, biphasic autohemolysin that can bind to erythrocytes at cold temperatures and cause intravascular hemolysis of erythrocytes at body temperature. This characteristic can be demonstrated *in vitro* in the Donath-Landsteiner test to help diagnose PCH. Erythrocytes sensitized by the DL antibody usually yield a positive result on the direct antiglobulin test because of C3 components during or right after an episode of hemolysis (Prasad, 1993) but may yield completely negative results between attacks. Because the antibody elutes from erythrocytes relatively easily during the washing steps of a routine direct antiglobulin test, the test is usually negative with anti-IgG.

Positive Direct Antiglobulin Tests and Hemolytic Anemia Induced by Medication

Many drugs are known to induce positive results on a direct antiglobulin test (DAT) and sometimes cause acquired hemolytic anemia. Traditionally, four mechanisms have been proposed to explain sensitization of autologous erythrocytes with immunoglobulin, complement, or other serum proteins that is induced by drugs as illustrated in Figure 30–10. For a more complete discussion of this topic, see Garraty (1994) and Walker (1993).

STIMULATION OF ERYTHROCYTE AUTOANTIBODY PRODUCTION

About 20% of hypertensive patients who receive methyldopa (Aldomet) for three to six months or longer eventually demonstrate a positive DAT, but only approximately 0.8% of them develop hemolytic anemia (Petz, 1993). The DAT gradually becomes negative after the termination of methyldopa treatment, taking from a few months up to two years. Serologically, antibodies eluted from erythrocytes or free in the

Table 30–30. DIFFERENTIATION OF COLD AGGLUTINATING ANTIBODIES

	Antigens Present			Cold Antibody				
Test Erythrocytes	***H***	***I***	***i***	***Anti-H****	***Anti-I†***	***Anti-i‡***	***Anti-IH***	***Anti-Pr§***
O adult	+	+	−	3+	3+	0	3+	3+
O cord	+	−	+	3+	0 to +	3+	1+	3+
A_1 adult	−	+	−	1+	3+	0	1+	3+
A_2 adult	+	+	−	2+	3+	0	2+	3+

*May be neutralized by soluble H substance found in secretor saliva.
†Associated with *Mycoplasma pneumoniae* infection; reactivity enhanced by proteases.
‡Associated with infectious mononucleosis and other forms of reticulosis.
§Pr receptors on red blood cells destroyed by proteases.

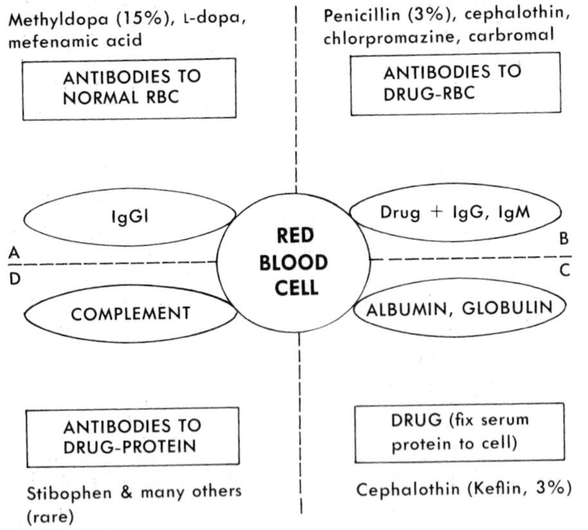

Figure 30–10. Four possible mechanisms for drug-induced positive direct antiglobulin test. Reactive agents on erythrocytes are in ovals; reactive agents in serum are in rectangles. Examples of drugs in each category are given.

serum are indistinguishable from autoantibodies found in patients with idiopathic warm autoimmune hemolytic anemia. The antibodies are usually of the IgG class with both κ and λ light chains, and many show Rh specificity. About 10% of patients with Parkinson's disease receiving levodopa, which is closely related to methyldopa, also develop erythrocyte autoantibodies, but these autoantibodies rarely result in overt hemolysis. Several hypotheses have been proposed for the development of autoantibodies induced by methyldopa and levodopa, including erythrocyte membrane alteration or an increase in responsiveness to self-antigen, but neither has been proven. Other drugs that have been reported to result in autoantibody production and hemolytic anemia are procainamide, chlorpromazine, nomifensine, and mefenamic acid (Petz, 1993).

DRUG ADSORPTION MECHANISM

About 3% of patients receiving large doses of penicillin intravenously ($> 10 \times 10^6$ IU/day) develop a positive DAT, although only a few of these patients will have hemolytic anemia (Garraty, 1993). Breakdown products of benzyl penicillin can bind firmly to erythrocytes, which results in the formation of haptenic benzylpenicilloyl (BPO) determinants. Patients may make antibodies to BPO that then attach to the drug/erythrocyte complex, yielding a positive DAT due to IgG. These antibodies may also be demonstrated in the serum when penicillin-coated erythrocytes are used as test cells in combination with the patient's serum. The DAT becomes negative again within several days to several weeks after the penicillin is discontinued.

Penicillin antibodies may be IgM or IgG. IgM antibodies are common if a sensitive method is used for detection. Antibodies associated with immune hemolytic anemia are of the IgG type. Hemolysis is usually through extravascular destruction mediated by cells with Fc receptors, although rare cases of complement-mediated intravascular lysis have been reported. Several cases of acquired hemolytic anemia have also been reported in association with the first-generation cephalosporin, cephalothin, in a mechanism similar to that of penicillin.

NONIMMUNOLOGIC ADSORPTION OF SERUM PROTEINS

Studies of patients taking from 6 to 14 g/day of cephalothin for prolonged periods have been reported to develop a positive DAT with a frequency ranging widely from 3% to 81% (Garraty, 1993). Subsequently, it was shown that erythrocytes exposed to cephalothin can adsorb plasma or serum proteins (albumin, immunoglobulins, complement) nonimmunologically. These proteins may be detected by broad-spectrum AHG sera in the DAT. It has been hypothesized that the adsorption is due to a change in erythrocyte membrane properties by the drug. Other drugs within the cephalosporin family may also have this effect; however, hemolysis has never been associated with this phenomenon.

IMMUNE COMPLEX THEORY

A wide variety of drugs may cause hemolytic anemia via the so-called immune complex mechanism. The theory is that the drug complexes with a carrier protein in the serum, producing haptenic determinants that stimulate antibody formation. The formation of a carrier/drug/antibody complex may then be followed by nonspecific attachment to the erythrocyte membrane, resulting in complement activation. The DAT is usually positive because of C3d only. Drugs acting by this mechanism most often are associated with episodes of acute intravascular hemolysis that may prove fatal. The antibodies involved can be detected only in test systems in which serum or eluate, test erythrocytes, and free drug are all present simultaneously. Some drugs that have been reported to cause hemolytic anemia by this mechanism include stibophen, rifampin, quinine, quinidine, streptomycin, tetracycline, sulfonylurea derivatives, insecticides, isoniazid, chlorpromazine, antihistamines, and the second-generation and third-generation cephalosporins.

The immune complex theory has been criticized for a number of reasons: (1) the antibodies involved in this mechanism bind to cells via their Fab, not Fc, domains, (2) no one has ever actually demonstrated immune complexes on platelets, erythrocytes, or neutrophils involved in these reactions, and (3) some of the antibodies show specificity for well characterized erythrocyte or platelet antigens (Garraty, 1994).

UNIFIED MODEL OF DRUG-INDUCED HEMOLYTIC ANEMIA

There have been suggestions that one unifying model explains three of the previously described mechanisms—drug adsorption, immune complex, and autoantibody formation—for drug-induced erythrocyte sensitization (Salama, 1992). The hypothesis suggests that the immune process involved is always initiated by a primary interaction between erythrocytes and the drug or its metabolites, even though the drug may be only loosely bound to the erythrocyte *in vivo*. This provides the composite determinants (or neoantigen) necessary for production of drug-dependent antibodies, as in the drug adsorption and immune complex mechanisms, or drug-independent autoantibodies by virtue of subtle alteration of the erythrocyte membrane. Because none of the other mechanisms has been disproved, however, the question of how drug antibodies are formed and why they display certain serologic reactivity and clinical manifestations is still open to further research.

IMMUNOHEMATOLOGY TESTS AND PROCEDURES

Specific hemagglutination is the single most important reaction in blood banking because it is the end point of almost all test systems designed to detect erythrocyte antigens and antibodies. The hemagglutination process actually occurs in two stages. The first stage is simply the combination of paratope and epitope in a reversible reaction that follows the law of mass action and has an associated equilibrium constant. Antigen and antibody are held together by noncovalent attractions. In stage two, multiple erythrocytes with bound antibody form a stable latticework through antigen/antibody bridges formed between adjacent erythrocytes. This latticework is the basis of all visible agglutination reactions. A number of factors influence either the first or second stages of the agglutination reaction.

Factors Affecting Hemagglutination

First Stage

EFFECT OF TEMPERATURE

This may affect both the equilibrium constant and the rate of reaction. For IgM antibodies, both of these parameters may be increased by decreasing the temperature of the reaction environment to 24°C or 4°C. IgG antibodies, on the other hand, react slowly at cold temperatures and thus are tested for at 37°C.

EFFECT OF pH

The pH affects the equilibrium constant. At a pH range of 6.5 to 7.0, the ionic forces of attraction between oppositely charged chemical groups on antibody and antigen are optimal for most blood group antibodies. However, certain antibodies, such as anti-M and anti-Pr, react better at a more acidic pH.

ENHANCEMENT MEDIA

LOW IONIC STRENGTH SOLUTIONS. The rate of combination of antigen and antibody is increased in a low ionic strength environment. In an isotonic saline medium, sodium cations accumulate around negatively charged sialic acid residues on the erythrocyte membrane, while chloride anions accumulate around positive charges on the antibody molecule. This acts to neutralize the attractive forces between antigen and antibody. Addition of a low ionic strength solution (LISS) into the reaction system reduces the neutralization of opposite charges, thus increasing the rate of reaction and the amount of antibody attached to the erythrocytes.

POLYETHYLENE GLYCOL. The addition of the linear polymer, polyethylene glycol (PEG), to the test system also accelerates the rate and amount of antibody combination with antigen. This is attributed to the increase in relative concentration of reactants (antigen and antibody) with respect to each other by the addition of large space-occupying molecules (Wenz, 1990). Because PEG also tends to induce nonspecific aggregation of the erythrocytes, examination for agglutination can be performed only at the final step of the AGT after all serum and PEG has been washed away. IgM antibody-induced agglutination could be missed by using this reagent; therefore, when using PEG in an AGT crossmatch protocol, one must perform an immediate-spin test of the donor cells and patient's serum before adding PEG in order to detect ABO incompatibility as soon as possible.

TIME OF INCUBATION

Different antigen/antibody reactions reach equilibrium over different periods of time. Blood group antibodies are usually detectable using incubations of between 15 and 60 minutes. These times may be varied within the limitations of a specific procedure or application. For example, incubation time may be increased from 30 to 45 minutes if one is trying to strengthen the reactions of a weakly reactive antibody.

Second Stage

Formation of the latticework during the second stage of hemagglutination is naturally impeded by the fact that erythrocytes in solution normally repel each other. This is due to the net negative charge of the erythrocytes produced by the high sialic acid content of the erythrocyte membrane. As previously mentioned, if erythrocytes are suspended in an ionic medium such as saline, cations arrange themselves around the erythrocytes to form an "ionic cloud." Cations closest to the erythrocyte are firmly bound and move with the erythrocyte, whereas the outer cations move freely. The difference in charge at the surface between the inner and outer cation layers, called the surface of shear, creates an electrical potential named the zeta potential (Fig. 30–11). The zeta potential keeps erythrocytes in solution about 25 nm apart (Harmening, 1994). Another factor that may be important in keeping erythrocytes apart is the water of hydration. Proponents of this theory suggest that the hydrophilic polar heads of lipid molecules making up the erythrocyte membrane bilayer attract water molecules. The water thus creates a surface tension that helps to keep the erythrocytes apart.

IgM antibodies usually can facilitate the second stage of hemagglutination because of their diameter of approximately 35 nm, which allows them to span the distance between two adjacent erythrocytes. Most IgG antibodies, on the other hand, usually cannot induce agglutination on their own. However, hemagglutination can be induced in two ways, either by reducing the distance between the erythrocytes or by providing bridges between two antibodies that cannot attach to two erythrocytes because of the distance between the erythrocytes (Fig. 30–12).

ANTIGEN DENSITY AND ACCESSIBILITY

The importance of the type, number, and location of antigens in the ability of a given antibody to cause agglutination of adjacent erythrocytes is illustrated by the ABO and Rh antigens. The number of ABO antigen sites may be close to one million per cell, and they are considered to be extramembranous; thus, erythrocytes are easily agglutinated by appropriate antibodies. On the other hand, Rh antigens are expressed in about 10,000 to 30,000 sites per cell and are considered to be intramembranous; thus, they are less easily agglutinated by appropriate antibodies. Also, erythrocytes that are ho-

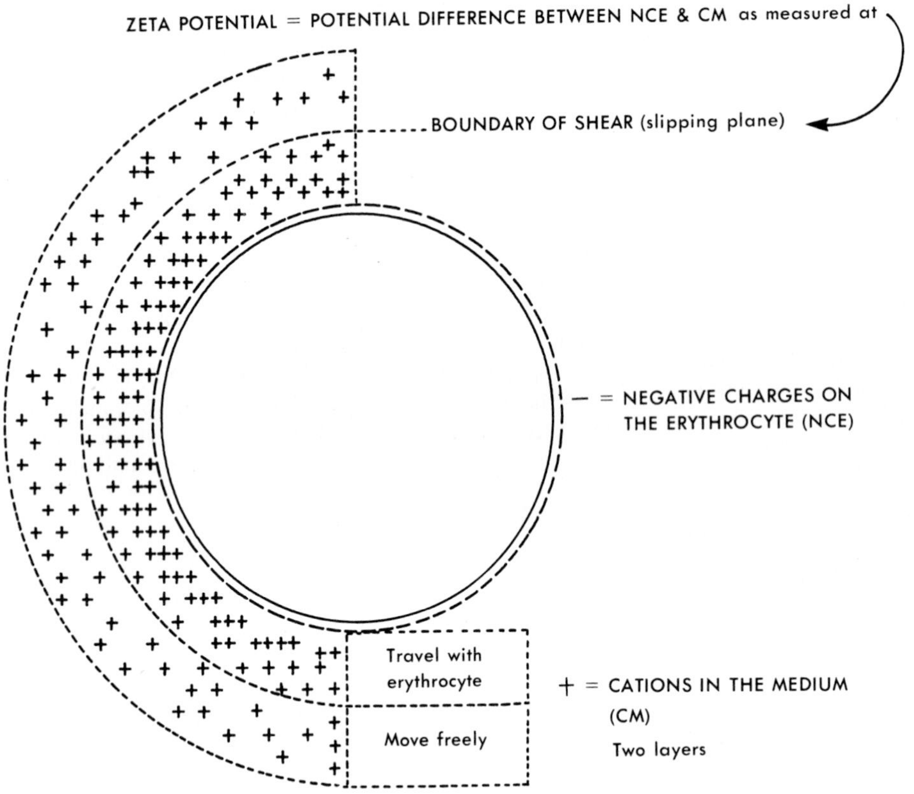

Figure 30–11. The measurement of zeta potential of erythrocytes.

mozygous for a particular erythrocyte antigen will often react more strongly with the corresponding antibody than erythrocytes that are heterozygous because there are twice as many copies, or a double dose, of the antigen per cell. This is often referred to as dosage.

ANTIBODY CONCENTRATION

The ability of a particular antibody to cause agglutination depends on a minimum number of antibody molecules attached per erythrocyte. Increasing the serum to cell ratio may induce agglutination by certain antibodies (usually IgM).

CENTRIFUGATION

Agglutination is enhanced by centrifugation as the antibody-sensitized erythrocytes physically are brought closer together.

USE OF ENHANCEMENT REAGENTS

PROTEOLYTIC ENZYMES. Treatment of erythrocytes with proteolytic enzymes, such as neuraminidase, trypsin, papain, bromelin, or ficin, irreversibly reduces the sialic acid content and lowers the zeta potential values. Because sialic acid is known to contain the determinants for M and N antigens, enzyme treatment of erythrocytes usually destroys these antigens along with several antigens belonging to other blood groups (e.g., Fy^a, Fy^b). Enzymatic cleavage of these glycoproteins, however, better exposes other antigens, thereby inducing direct hemagglutination by certain IgG antibodies such as those directed against Rh system antigens.

ALBUMIN. Addition of albumin to the test system will sometimes cause antibodies that do not normally agglutinate erythrocytes in saline to become direct agglutinins, particularly the Rh antibodies. The exact mechanism of albumin enhancement is not yet known. One theory is that albumin reduces zeta potential by increasing the dielectrical constant of the medium, which is the ability of a solution to dissipate a charge. Others believe that albumin replaces the water of hydration surrounding the erythrocyte. Either way, the cells are allowed to approach each other more closely for production of the latticework formation.

POLYCATIONS. Polybrene and protamine, which may be used with both automated and manual test systems, provide an excess number of cations that neutralize the negative charges on the erythrocyte and produce nonspecific aggregation of the erythrocytes. Specific antibodies then can attach to the corresponding antigens on more than one cell and produce antibody-mediated latticework formation. The final addition of certain electrolytes counteracts the effects of Polybrene or protamine and disperses the nonspecific aggregation, whereas antibody-induced agglutination remains.

ANTIHUMAN GLOBULIN REAGENTS

Even with use of enhancement reagents, such as albumin, enzymes, or polycations, and the final step of centrifugation, many IgG antibodies still cannot produce detectable hemagglutination. To visualize reactions by these antibodies (historically called "incomplete" antibodies), antihuman globulin sera must be utilized. The antibodies to human globulin or complement components in these reagents act as bridges between erythrocytes already sensitized with antibody or complement (Fig. 30–13). This is the basis of the antiglobulin test or AGT described subsequently in further detail.

NONSPECIFIC AGGREGATION

In addition to the nonspecific aggregates formed by Polybrene and protamine, many other chemicals may induce non-

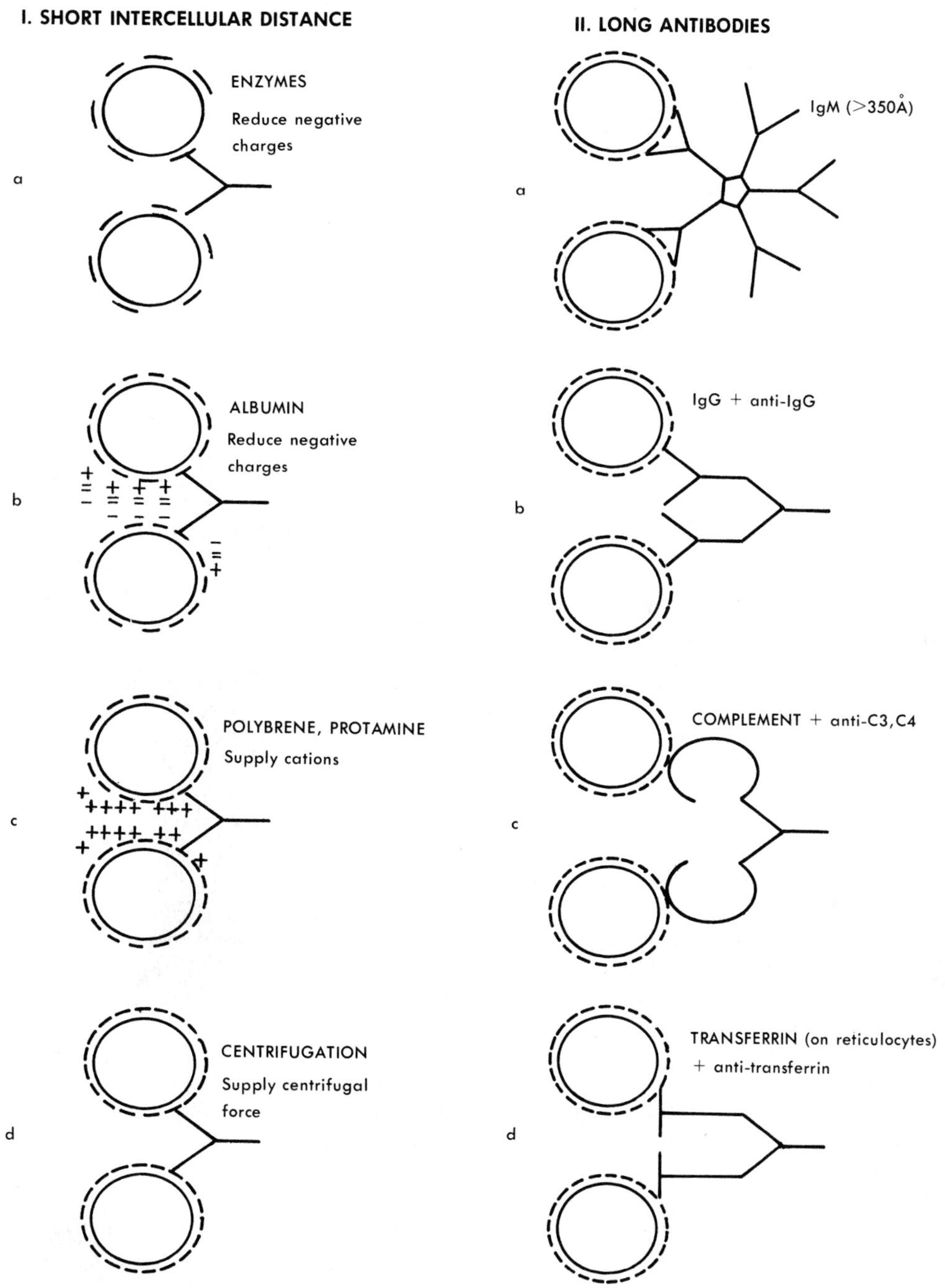

Figure 30–12. Two basic mechanisms of inducing hemagglutination.

specific hemagglutination. One such phenomenon is rouleaux formation. Patients with multiple myeloma, Waldenstrom's macroglobulinemia, or hyperviscosity syndromes will have high concentrations of abnormal serum proteins that may change the net surface charge on the erythrocyte membrane. The erythrocytes thus cluster together and may resemble macroscopic hemagglutination. Plasma expanders, such as dextran and hydroxyethyl starch, and some intravenous x-ray contrast materials may also cause rouleaux formation. Rouleaux can be differentiated from true agglutination by microscopic examination for the classic "stacked-coin" formation and by dispersion on the replacement of serum with saline. Nonspecific agglutination may also be found in cord blood contaminated with Wharton's jelly. The presence of hyaluronic acid, together with albumin, has been shown to be responsible and is usually solved by the addition of hyaluronidase.

Antihuman Globulin Test

The AGT is also commonly called the Coombs' test in honor of one of the investigators who developed the test for laboratory use (Coombs, 1945), although the principle was actually described much earlier in 1908 by Moreschi (Harmening, 1994). As described previously, the AGT is based on

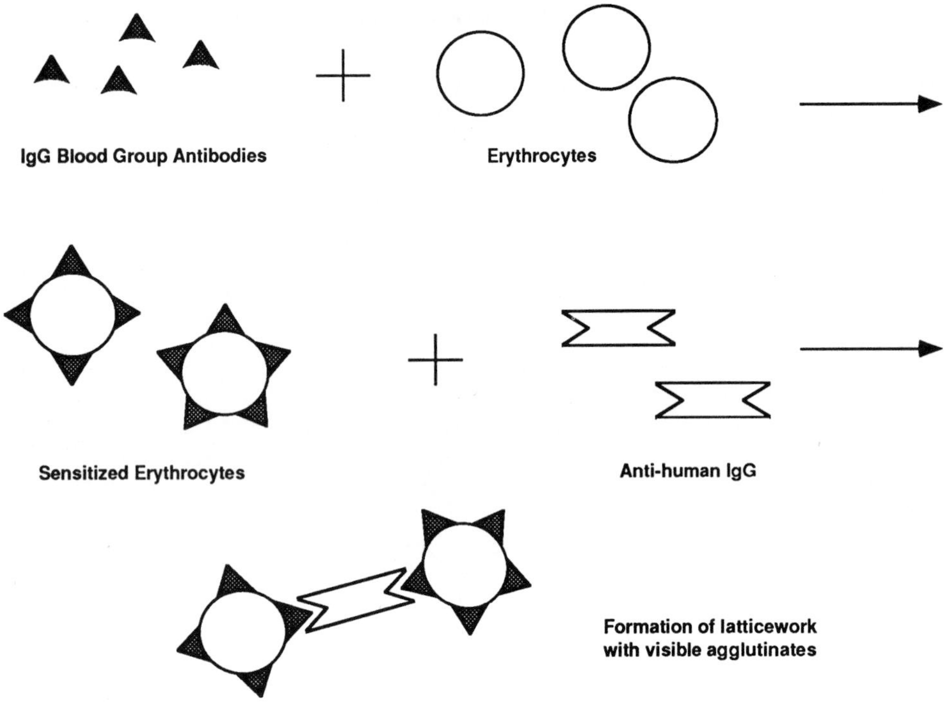

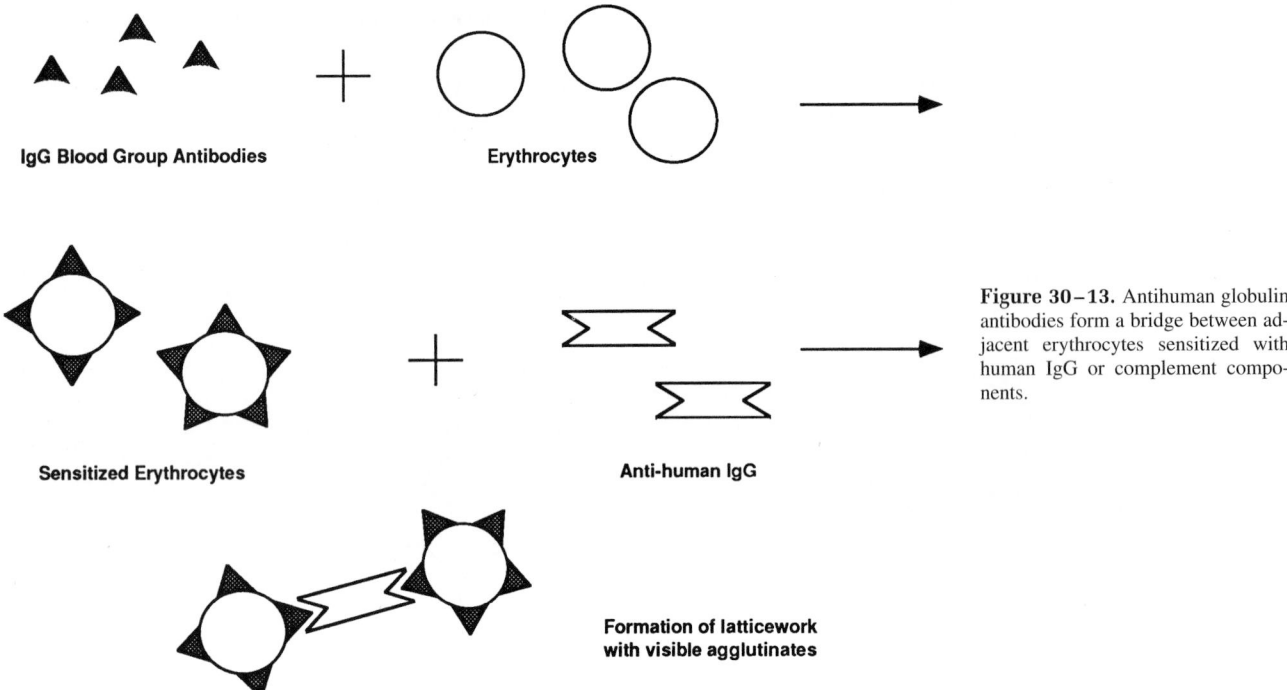

Figure 30–13. Antihuman globulin antibodies form a bridge between adjacent erythrocytes sensitized with human IgG or complement components.

the principle that specific antihuman globulin antibodies act as a bridge that induces agglutination of erythrocytes coated with human immunoglobulin or complement (see Fig. 30–13). The AGT has become a powerful tool in testing for antigens or antibodies undetectable by other techniques. When the AGT is used to detect antibodies bound to erythrocytes *in vivo,* it is called the direct antiglobulin test (DAT). When the AGT is used to detect the reaction of antibody and erythrocytes *in vitro* after an appropriate incubation phase, it is called the indirect antiglobulin test (IAT).

Antihuman Globulin Sera

Antihuman globulin (AHG) sera may be produced by hyperimmunizing animals, usually rabbits, with purified immunoglobulin or complement to produce high-titered, high-avidity, IgG antibodies. For a given batch of reagent, the animal sera is harvested, pooled, absorbed to remove heterophile agglutinins, and then titered to ascertain the dilution necessary for optimal reactivity in routine use. Polyspecific or broad-spectrum AHG contains IgG antibodies to both human immunoglobulin (primarily IgG) and the C3 complement components C3b and C3d. Today's polyspecific reagents are usually a blend of polyclonal IgG antibodies against the spectrum of human IgG subclasses and monoclonal antibodies against C3b and C3d complement components. The monoclonal anticomplement activity may consist of either IgG or IgM antibodies. The activity of the two components will vary somewhat among different manufacturers and between lots produced by the same manufacturer, but all AHG sera must contain levels of anti-IgG and anti-C3d activity that meet or exceed the reference standards of the Food and Drug Administration (FDA) (21 CFR 600.52). Most manufacturers absorb out any anti-C4 activity from their polyspecific AHG reagents, because it has been shown that *in vitro* complement activation by clinically insignificant cold agglutinins results in much more binding of C4d than of C3d (Mollison, 1993). Excluding anti-C4 activity thus reduces the number of false-positive results in both DAT and IAT testing.

Monospecific anti-IgG, anti-IgM, and anti-IgA, as well as anti-C3 and anti-C4, anti-C3b and anti-C3d, anti-C4b, and anti-C4d reagents are also commercially available. Because immunization against IgG may also produce anti–light chain antibodies in a polyclonal response, one should remember that polyclonal, monospecific anti-IgG sera may cross-react with the light chains of IgM or IgA molecules unless the manufacturer specifies that the reagent is heavy chain–specific. Many of the anticomplement sera are now monoclonal in origin. Currently, at least one commercial reagent company (Gamma Biologicals, Houston, Texas) is marketing a monoclonal, monospecific anti-IgG reagent as well.

Sensitivity of the Antihuman Globulin Test

Although the AGT is extremely sensitive, a negative test result by no means excludes the presence of antibodies on erythrocytes. It is estimated that 100 to 500 IgG or C3 molecules bound per erythrocyte are required for detection by antiglobulin antibodies (Harmening, 1994); a smaller number of molecules bound per erythrocyte would give a negative reaction. Also, AHG sera may possess greater activity against some subclasses of IgG than against others; consequently, certain antihuman globulin sera may produce negative results with erythrocytes coated by a particular IgG subclass.

Quality Control of the Antihuman Globulin Test

In order to standardize antiglobulin sera and to confirm true negative antiglobulin reactions, two types of quality control cells are normally used: those coated with IgG and those coated with C3b or C3d. To sensitize erythrocytes with

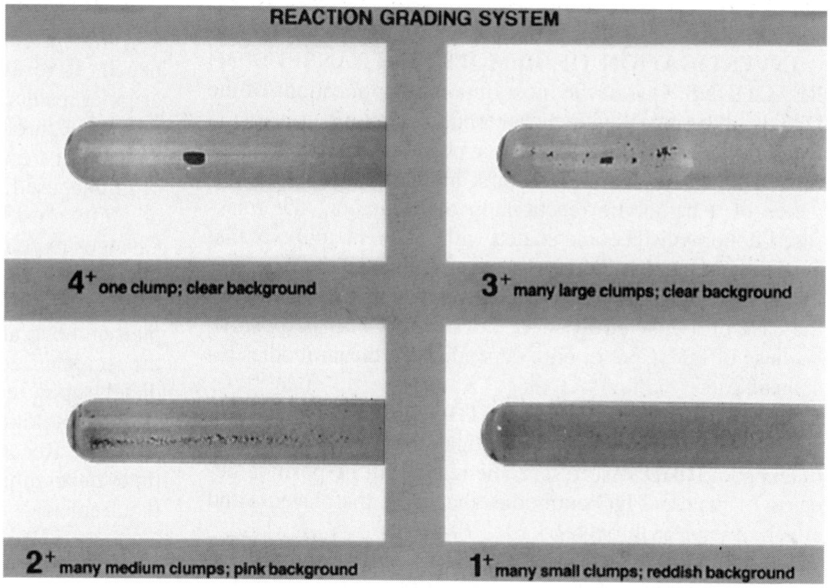

Figure 30–14. Agglutination grading system showing macroscopic hemagglutination reactions.

IgG, Rh antibodies are usually used. C3b-coated erythrocytes can be prepared by incubation of whole blood in a low-ionic-strength sucrose medium or by incubation of erythrocytes with human anti-Le[a] or anti-I. Additional incubation of cells prepared by both of these methods with fresh serum or trypsin will split C3b, leaving the cells coated with only C3d. IgG or complement-coated control cells should give about a 2+ reaction (Fig. 30–14) when tested with anti-IgG or anti-C3b and C3d.

Quality control cells for the AGT are often referred to as check cells, Coombs' control cells, or sensitized cells. In a true-negative AGT, free antiglobulin reagent should remain in the test system in an active state. False-negative reactions may occur if the antiglobulin reagent is inactivated by residual serum globulins because of incomplete washing or contamination of the reagent prior to testing, or if the reagent was mistakenly not added. Thus, control cells sensitized with IgG must be added to either a negative direct or indirect AGT and centrifuged. Observance of agglutination of the control cells confirms the reactivity of the anti-IgG component of the specific antiglobulin reagent added. If the control cells fail to agglutinate in any tube, the tests must be repeated because they are invalid and may have yielded false-negative results.

Procedures

For the direct antiglobulin test (DAT), blood samples should be drawn in EDTA to prevent sensitization of cells with complement *in vitro* through the activation of complement beyond C1q. A 3% to 5% saline suspension of patient erythrocytes is prepared for testing. One drop of this cell suspension is subsequently washed at least four times with saline, and then polyspecific AHG containing anti-IgG and anti-C3d must be added so that *in vivo* sensitization with either IgG or complement may be detected (see Role of Complement in Serologic Testing).

For the various applications of the indirect antiglobulin technique (IAT), patient, donor, or reagent erythrocytes are incubated with appropriate serum or commercially prepared antisera, usually at 37°C, for the time period indicated in the standard operating procedure (SOP) for the particular assay being performed. Depending on the procedure, tubes may be centrifuged after incubation and then examined for hemolysis or agglutination. Whether this step is performed or not, the next step should be thorough washing of the erythrocytes at least four times to remove all unbound free serum globulins or extraneous protein. Failure to completely remove unbound proteins will result in neutralization of the antiglobulin reagent when it is added to the test, giving a false-negative reaction. After washing, either polyspecific antihuman globulin or monospecific anti-IgG is added to all tubes to detect *in vitro* sensitization of the test cells by antibody or complement.

In grading and interpretation of results for both DAT and IAT techniques, the protocol may include optional microscopic examination to confirm macroscopically negative tests. However, all laboratories are required to confirm any negative antiglobulin test by use of quality control cells as previously described. Table 30–31 lists common causes for false-negative and false-positive results in using the AGT.

Table 30–31. REASONS FOR FALSE-POSITIVE OR FALSE-NEGATIVE REACTIONS IN ANTIGLOBULIN TESTING

False-Positive Reactions	False-Negative Reactions
Contamination of reagents	Reagent failure*
Overcentrifugation	Improper washing*
Direct agglutination by strong cold agglutinins	Failure to add antiglobulin reagents*
Overincubation with enzyme-treated cells	Improper centrifugation
Improper use of enhancement reagents	Serum/cell ratio too low
Saline stored in glass or metal containers	Delayed washing (elution of weakly attached antibody)
Dirty glassware	

*Will be detected by use of Coombs' control cells.

Applications of the Direct Antiglobulin Test

INVESTIGATION OF HEMOLYTIC TRANSFUSION REACTIONS. One of the most important applications of the DAT is in the investigation of potential hemolytic transfusion reactions. The development of a positive DAT soon after transfusion of red cells is the first immunohematologic evidence of a hemolytic reaction. In this situation, the transfused donor cells become coated with recipient antibody that was already present, in the case of an immediate reaction, or that is increasing in titer as part of an anamnestic response, in the case of a delayed reaction. DAT results may be positive because of IgG, C3d, or both depending on the antibodies responsible.

HEMOLYTIC DISEASE OF THE NEWBORN (HDN). A positive DAT result in the investigation of possible HDN is diagnostic. If HDN is present, the result will be positive because of maternal IgG antibodies that cross the placenta and attach to fetal erythrocytes.

INVESTIGATION OF AUTOANTIBODIES. A positive DAT result in the investigation of possible autoimmune hemolytic anemia is also diagnostic. Most warm autoantibodies cause a positive DAT result because of IgG and rarely because of both IgG and C3d. Cold autoagglutinins often cause a positive DAT result because of C3d only, although the responsible antibody may rarely be detected by anti-IgM, if available.

ANTIBODIES INDUCED BY MEDICATION. Antibodies induced by medication cause a positive DAT result because of IgG or C3d, or both, depending on the mechanism involved (see Erythrocyte Autoantibodies).

Applications of the Indirect Antiglobulin Technique

DETECTION AND IDENTIFICATION OF ERYTHROCYTE ANTIBODIES IN SERA. Reagent red blood cells of known phenotype are incubated with the patient's serum. To detect patient antibodies that have bound to the reagent red blood cells, either polyspecific antiglobulin reagent or monospecific anti-IgG may be used.

TYPING OF ERYTHROCYTE ANTIGENS. The detection of many erythrocyte antigens requires incubation at 37°C with specific antisera followed by conversion to an antiglobulin test. To detect specific binding of antisera to erythrocytes possessing the corresponding antigens, polyspecific antiglobulin reagent or monospecific anti-IgG may be used.

CROSSMATCHING. Donor erythrocytes are incubated with patient serum at 37°C followed by conversion to an antiglobulin test in order to detect antibodies that may have been missed by the antibody screen because of absence of the corresponding antigen or diminished antigen concentration (dosage/zygosity) on the screening cells. To detect recipient antibodies bound to the donor erythrocytes, polyspecific antiglobulin reagent or monospecific anti-IgG may be used.

Compatibility Testing

General Considerations

DOCUMENTATION

All blood banks must have a manual or computerized system of record keeping. Records must be complete and retrievable within a reasonable time frame. In a manual record-keeping system, all forms should be filled out with ink, not pencil. If results must be changed on manual worksheets, original results are not to be obliterated; a single line should be placed through them and the new results initialed by the technologist making the change. A continuously updated list of initials used by all personnel working in the blood bank on all shifts must be part of the permanent blood bank records. Changes to computerized results must be appropriately documented in the computer.

Recipient information, including such items as name, hospital number, and results of all testing, should be entered into the computer or recorded on the appropriate worksheet immediately upon testing; the date, time of testing, and initials of the technologist performing the work should also be recorded. Records must be maintained for different periods of time depending on federal, state, and accrediting agency requirements.

LABORATORY SAFETY

All safety precautions for a clinical laboratory should be observed, including the currently recommended protocols for barrier protection (see Chap. 1). Pipetting of blood components by mouth is not acceptable; a mechanical device should be used instead. All blood components, even if screening test results for infectious agents were completely negative, are potential transmitters of hepatitis B or C, HIV, HTLV-I, or other pathogens and should be handled according to the guidelines for Universal Blood and Body Fluid Precautions. Discarded blood components and patient specimens should be autoclaved before final disposal or placed in a puncture-resistant container for eventual incineration. Needles, scalpels, or any other sharp objects such as broken glass should be placed into a sharps container immediately after use.

METHODS

EQUIPMENT. Testing for erythrocyte antigens or antibodies may be performed using slides, test tubes, capillary tubes, microtiter plates, or gel or column agglutination techniques once these technologies have been approved for use in the United States by the FDA. These procedures may be semiautomated or fully automated, particularly in facilities that perform large-volume testing, such as blood collection centers. Currently, methods employing test tubes are the most widely used in hospital blood banks. Batch testing using microtiter plates is becoming increasingly popular, whereas slide testing has become almost obsolete, at least in the Unites States. Unless otherwise specified, procedures referred to in this chapter employ tube testing. Because each type of test has many variations, one should use the technique that has been evaluated and has proven its reliability for the desired application. The American Association of Blood Banks' *Technical Manual* (Walker, 1993), *Methods in Immunohematology* (Judd, 1994), and *Immunohematology Methods* (Mallory, 1993) are excellent general references for most common procedures as well as for more specialized techniques.

INCUBATION. Many tests require a period of incubation to allow the antigen-antibody reaction to occur. ABO and Rh testing is routinely carried out at room temperature with a minimal incubation time. Most indirect antiglobulin tests use 37°C incubation, and incubation times vary with the type of enhancement medium used in testing, if any. Generally incubation times range from 15 minutes with albumin to 60 minutes without the use of any enhancement medium. Use of low-ionic-strength solutions can decrease incubation times by 5 to 10 minutes. When a short incubation period is used, the tubes should be placed in a dry bath or water bath to speed up equilibration to the desired temperature, because the heat conductivity of air is poor. Low-ionic-Polybrene procedures require only one minute of incubation prior to addition of Polybrene.

CENTRIFUGATION. In most tests, centrifugation is the final step required to enhance agglutination and to facilitate the reading of results. The time of centrifugation required for each phase or type of testing should be determined for each centrifuge by yearly functional calibration using the appropriate controls and test media. Centrifuge speeds at each setting should be checked quarterly with a stroboscope to confirm that they fall within manufacturer specifications.

GRADING OF REACTIONS. Agglutination is observed and graded according to the strength of the reaction. The presence of hemolysis usually indicates a potent antibody capable of fixing complement *in vitro*. After incubation of tests applying the indirect antiglobulin technique or in ABO reverse grouping, the serum should be observed for evidence of hemolysis prior to resuspending the cell button. When one is reading for agglutination, the tube should be shaken, using a gentle wrist action, until all cells are dislodged. This is most easily accomplished by holding the tube at a sharp angle so that the fluid "cuts" across the cell button such that the cells can be easily resuspended. When cells no longer adhere to the tube, it should be tilted back and forth gently until an even suspension of cells (or agglutination) is observed. Proper illumination with a concave mirror is an invaluable aid for macroscopic reading. By placing the tube about 2.5 inches above a 3-inch concave mirror, one can easily differentiate aggregates from the free cells by looking at the mirror, not at the tube. The strength of the reaction can be graded or scored as follows:

Grade	Meaning	Score
H	Hemolysis, presence of free hemoglobin	10
4+	One solid aggregate	10
3+	Several medium to large aggregates	8
2+	Many small to medium aggregates with a clear background	5
1+	Many small aggregates with a turbid background	3
±	Few small aggregates, many unagglutinated erythrocytes	2
0	Absence of aggregates	0

All negative reactions, when required by the procedure, should be read under a microscope and recorded as follows:

Grade	Meaning	Score
±m	Presence of microscopic aggregates	1
0	Absence of aggregates	0
mf	Presence of minor population of aggregates (also known as mixed field agglutination)	
R	Rouleaux, appearing like a stack of coins; disappears with addition of saline	

Figure 30–14 shows the appearance of some of the different grades of agglutination. Although the grade of agglutination gives an approximate idea regarding the potency or strength of a particular antibody, the scoring method is much more useful in semiquantitation, particularly when used in conjunction with titers to compare the relative antibody strengths of two different sera.

Required Compatibility Test Procedures

The term compatibility testing has historically been used synonymously with the crossmatch. In its broader meaning, however, compatibility testing is a process composed of many procedures designed to provide the safest blood product possible for the recipient of a transfusion. These steps include proper record keeping, accurate donor and recipient identification, and the actual serologic testing of the recipient specimen prior to transfusion. The steps required in compatibility testing are outlined in the following sections.

RECIPIENT IDENTIFICATION

Proper identification of patient blood specimens and donor units is absolutely essential in blood banking. Recipient blood specimens should be labeled by the phlebotomist at the bedside directly from information on the patient's wristband. If the patient's wristband is not attached for any reason, signed confirmation of the patient's identity must be obtained before the blood is drawn. The recipient's blood specimen label should include at least the patient's full name, hospital identification number, and specimen collection date and time, and it should be securely attached to the specimen tube when it is accepted by blood bank personnel. Unlabeled or improperly labeled blood specimens are unacceptable. During testing, all test tubes or other types of aliquot or reaction containers must also be accurately identified.

CHECK OF PREVIOUS RECORDS

Manual or computerized records should always be checked for previous results on a given patient. ABO and Rh tests on the current specimen should be checked against previous results, if available, to help verify that the specimen was collected from the correct person. Information on any unexpected antibodies identified previously is also extremely important because the titer of an antibody may fall to levels that cannot be detected by antibody screening procedures. If a clinically significant antibody was previously identified, the patient must receive erythrocytes negative for the corresponding antigen even if current test results for antibody detection are negative.

ABO TESTING

DONORS. Before transfusion of any red blood cell component, the transfusion service doing the crossmatch must reconfirm the ABO group of all units and Rh type of those red blood cell units labeled Rh NEGATIVE to detect any labeling errors. Repeat testing by the transfusion service for weak D is not required by the American Association of Blood Banks (Klein, 1994), although some state regulations still mandate this testing.

RECIPIENTS. Every patient blood specimen accompanied by an appropriately completed requisition for transfusion of a blood component must also be tested for ABO group and Rh type. The test for weak D is not required on recipients. The patient blood specimen to be used for compatibility testing must not be older than 72 hours if the recipient has undergone transfusion or has been pregnant within three months prior to the scheduled transfusion.

Antibody Detection

All specimens submitted for pretransfusion testing must be tested by methods that demonstrate clinically significant antibodies. These methods must include incubation at physiologic or body temperature (37°C) followed by conversion to the antiglobulin test. This is commonly called the antibody screen and is an application of the indirect antiglobulin technique, as previously described.

REAGENT RED BLOOD CELLS

The reagent red blood cells or screening cells for detection of antibodies in a patient's serum are usually obtained from commercial manufacturers. The American Association of Blood Banks' *Standards for Blood Banks and Transfusion Services* (Klein, 1994) requires that antibody detection in recipients be performed using reagent cells that are not pooled, so two or three group O cells from different donors are used for the procedure. Sets of screening cells are selected so that all antigens corresponding to most commonly encountered erythrocyte antibodies are represented. When possible, cells that are homozygous for selected antigens are used, which increases the likelihood of detecting weak or dosing antibodies. Each lot of screening red blood cells is accompanied by an "antigram" that lists the antigenic makeup of each cell (Fig. 30–15).

ANTIBODY DETECTION PROTOCOLS

A large number of different antibody detection protocols are in use today that vary with regard to incubation time, incubation temperature, and enhancement media. Currently, none of the available techniques can detect all erythrocyte antibodies; it is unlikely that there will be such a technique in the future. Because the purpose of the antibody screen is to detect clinically significant antibodies, which typically react at body temperature, most laboratories omit room temperature incubation completely because antibodies that react below 37°C are not considered clinically significant. In the most common protocol, tubes containing one volume of 3% to 5% screening reagent cells and two volumes of patient serum (giving an average serum/cell ratio of approximately 50:1) are incubated at 37°C with an enhancement medium for the time specified by the manufacturer of the enhancement reagent used, centrifuged, and read for hemolysis or agglutination. The screening cells are then washed four times with saline, and antihuman globulin serum is added.

Because different blood group antibodies commonly show characteristic reaction patterns by the indirect antiglobulin technique (see Table 30–19), close examination of the results of the antibody screening test may yield helpful information when the screen is positive.

Direct agglutination of the cells in albumin after 37°C incubation usually indicates the presence of an Rh antibody.

IgM antibodies of a wide thermal range may also show reactions in albumin such as anti-I, anti-P_1, and the Lewis antibodies. However, these reactions generally become much weaker after conversion to the antiglobulin test.

With rare exception, the presence of *in vitro* hemolysis of the reagent cells after 37°C indicates the presence of Lewis, Kidd, Ii, P, PP_1P^k, or Vel antibodies.

The vast majority of IgG antibodies, with the exception of Rh, will not be detected until after washing and conversion to the AGT.

Reactions of the different screening cells in multiple phases or with varying strengths usually indicates that more than one antibody is present.

If an antibody screen result is positive, the antibody must be identified (see Antibody Identification).

CROSSMATCHING

MAJOR CROSSMATCH. A major crossmatch testing donor cells against recipient serum is usually required before administration of erythrocyte components. A 3% to 5% saline suspension of donor erythrocytes is prepared from an integral segment taken from the selected donor unit. Cells are usually washed once to remove any anticoagulant or plasma protein that could interfere with the testing. For many years, the major crossmatch was required to include 37°C incubation followed by conversion to the antiglobulin test, just as in the antibody screen. However, in 1984, this requirement was eliminated by the American Association of Blood Banks' *Standards for Blood Banks and Transfusion Services* as long as the antibody screen on the patient is completely negative and there is no known history of previous clinically significant antibodies. Instead, only a crossmatch procedure designed to detect ABO incompatibility need be used. This usually consists of testing the donor cells and patient serum at room temperature for agglutination or hemolysis by immediate spin or by centrifugation following a five-minute room temperature incubation (Walker, 1993). This procedure has come to be known as the abbreviated crossmatch.

Ironically, this was nearly the same standard of testing in place some 20 years before, as endorsed by Grove-Rasmussen (1964). His study on the safety of the antibody screen utilizing 37°C incubation and conversion to the antiglobulin test, as well as later reports on the efficacy of the antibody screen (Boral, 1977; Cordle, 1990; Heddle, 1992; Mintz,

LOT NO: 000456
EXPIRES: 00/00/00

SCREENING CELL MASTER LIST

VIAL		Rh								MNSs				P	Lewis		Luth-eran		Kell				Duffy		Kidd		Sex Linked
	Donor	D	C	E	c	e	f	C^w	V	M	N	S	s	P_1	Le^a	Le^b	Lu^a	Lu^b	K	k	Kp^a	Js^a	Fy^a	Fy^b	Jk^a	Jk^b	Xg^a
I	R_1R_1	+	+	0	+	+	0	0	0	+	0	+	0	+	+	0	0	+	0	+	0	0	+	+	+	0	+
II	R_2R_2	+	0	+	+	0	0	0	0	+	+	+	+	+	0	+	0	+	+	+	0	0	0	+	+	+	+

Figure 30–15. The "antigram" accompanying each lot of reagent screening red blood cells.

1982), show that at least 99% of commonly encountered antibodies will be detected by the antibody screen if at least two separate reagent red blood cells containing the common blood group antigens, including K, are used. When the frequency of occurrence of the common antibodies is multiplied by the actual antigen frequencies in the population to give a theoretical calculated rate of incompatibility, it can be seen that the antibody screen is probably greater than 99% effective in preventing incompatible transfusions (Boral, 1977). Therefore, only rarely will the crossmatch be expected to pick up a clinically significant antibody missed by the antibody screen. This might occur, for instance, if the recipient had an antibody to a low-frequency antigen not present on the screening cells, such as anti-Kp^a or anti-Wr^a.

Use of the abbreviated crossmatch procedure in clinical settings has shown it to be a safe and cost-effective alternative to the full crossmatch (Cordle, 1990; Shulman, 1985, 1990), though there are a few reports of this technique failing to detect ABO incompatibility when the recipient ABO antibodies are of low titer or the donor cells belong to an ABO subgroup with weaker than normal antigen expression (Berry-Dortch, 1985; Shulman, 1987). This procedure has also been reported to give false-negative results regarding ABO incompatibility in the rare presence of a prozone effect (Judd, 1988) and because of a delay in centrifugation, which is apparently attributable to steric hindrance of agglutination by fixation of the C1 complement component to the membrane of the incompatible erythrocytes prior to centrifugation (Shulman, 1990). Suspension of donor cells in EDTA-saline eliminates this latter problem. In addition to false-negative results, the immediate-spin crossmatch can cause false-positive results due to rouleaux, cold-reactive antibodies, or fibrin, all of which may result in delay of issuing the blood for transfusion (Meyer, 1989).

The abbreviated crossmatch has not been universally accepted for the reasons stated and because the antibody screen might fail to detect clinically significant antibodies because of human error (Napier, 1991), the presence of a dosing antibody, or deterioration of antigen from the reagent cells during storage. Laboratories that prefer to retain the antiglobulin phase of the crossmatch argue that the savings in labor and expense do not outweigh the additional, though slight, risk of transfusing an incompatible unit to a patient that could have been avoided through use of the full antiglobulin crossmatch procedure. However, reports in the literature surveying the experience of various institutions who have adopted the abbreviated crossmatch show the actual incidence of missing a *clinically significant* antibody is low, less than 0.05% (Cordle, 1990; Mintz, 1982). In addition, a multicenter study involving 1.3 million abbreviated crossmatches demonstrated an observed risk of acute hemolytic reaction of only 0.0004% following transfusion of these units (Shulman, 1990). In the rare instances in which patients did receive incompatible blood for transfusion because of the elimination of the AHG crossmatch, none resulted in death or long-term adverse clinical effects.

The obvious reported advantages of the abbreviated crossmatch include the streamlining of testing allowing for increased workloads without increased staffing, cost-savings resulting from decreased technologist time and decreased crossmatch to transfusion (C/T) ratios, and, just as important, increased efficiency and speed in releasing blood in emergency situations in which the elimination of needless delay may actually save lives. Thus, in weighing the level of acceptable risk versus the benefits to patient care derived from the abbreviated crossmatch, the available data have prompted our own and many other transfusion services to replace the full antihuman globulin crossmatch procedure with the abbreviated crossmatch for all eligible patients.

One source of debate in eliminating the antihuman globulin crossmatch has been the question of whether to use a set of three, rather than two, reagent screening cells in order to theoretically increase the sensitivity of the antibody screen and thus decrease the likelihood of not detecting, for instance, a dosing antibody. A three-cell screening panel ensures homozygosity for more antigens such as Jk^a, Jk^b, Fy^a, Fy^b, S, and s, against which the corresponding antibodies are likely to exhibit dosage, but it is also more expensive to buy and use. However, in one study of 3380 serum samples (Cordle, 1990), the authors concluded that there was no statistically significant difference in the incidence of irregular antibodies detected by either the two-cell or the three-cell screening panels. A more recent study of 159,262 separate patients (Hoeltge, 1995) used a three-cell screen for all pretransfusion testing but looked at the actual number of *clinically significant* antibodies detected that would be expected to exhibit dosage. Only 0.3% of all antibodies found included those with the aforementioned characteristics detected as single specificities; the rest of such antibodies were found in a mixture of specificities that would almost always cause a positive antibody detection test result anyway. Thus, the authors proposed that knowledge of the prevalence of such antibodies allows one to perform an informed cost-benefit analysis of utilizing the more expensive three-cell screening panel.

Going one step beyond the abbreviated crossmatch, one institution proposed a standard operating procedure that would replace the abbreviated serologic crossmatch with a computer or "electronic" crossmatch (Butch, 1992). This has been advocated for some time by those who argue that the immediate-spin serologic crossmatch will continue to fail occasionally in its ultimate purpose to identify ABO incompatibilities between a recipient and an incompatible donor who might be chosen erroneously for crossmatch. Proponents of the electronic crossmatch believe that the best way to ensure compatibility is to reduce the human error factor that would allow the wrong units to be crossmatched in the first place by assigning final verification of ABO compatibility between donor and recipient to a computer system (Judd, 1991). This would also eliminate time-consuming investigation of false-positive serologic reactions. According to the current *Standards for Blood Banks and Transfusion Services* (Klein, 1994), the "electronic crossmatch" is permissible as long as the blood bank information system has been validated on site to prevent the release of ABO-incompatible blood and components and at least two separate determinations of the recipient's blood group have been made, including one on the current specimen being used for compatibility testing. In addition, the same rules apply to use of the computer crossmatch as apply to use of the abbreviated crossmatch regarding any past or current history of clinically significant antibodies in the recipient.

PREOPERATIVE CROSSMATCH PROTOCOLS. Because of the reported efficacy of a well-controlled antibody screening procedure in detecting clinically significant antibodies, a type and screen protocol for many routine surgical procedures that do not require transfusion was advocated by Mintz and coworkers (1976), Henry and colleagues (1977), and Boral and Henry (1977). The type and screen protocol, when used in conjunction with preoperative blood ordering guidelines (Henry, 1977; Mintz, 1976), also referred to as the "maximum surgical blood order schedule" (Friedman, 1976), allows for much more efficient blood inventory management and reduction in the C/T ratio. For elective surgical procedures that do not routinely require transfusion, only a type and antibody screen is ordered. Blood orders for elective surgical procedures requiring transfusion are set at a level that reflects actual use according to the utilization patterns of surgeons for the same operative procedure at individual hospitals. For blood ordering guidelines to be successful, they should come under periodic review and revision based on the surgeon's experiences as new surgical procedures are adopted and techniques are refined. (Refer to the back inside book cover for suggested preoperative blood ordering guidelines.)

The preoperative type and screen protocol requires no further serologic work as long as the patient's antibody screen is negative and there is no known history of clinically significant antibodies. If a patient unexpectedly requires transfusion, ABO-compatible and Rh-compatible units are selected, and an abbreviated crossmatch is performed. If no agglutination or hemolysis is seen, the blood can be safely released to the operating room with a minimal turnaround time.

If the preoperative type and screen results in a positive antibody screen, the antibody must be identified. Two antigen-negative units are then held for use by the patient during surgery and must be crossmatched with the patient's serum using a full antiglobulin crossmatch procedure prior to transfusion. This same rule applies to patients with known histories of clinically significant antibodies, even if the screen is not positive at the time of elective surgery.

COMPATIBILITY TESTING IN EMERGENCIES

In urgent situations, blood may have to be released for transfusion prior to completion of compatibility tests or even before a patient blood specimen is available. If the ABO and Rh type of the patient are not known, group O negative packed red blood cells are released. If a blood specimen is available and there is time to perform ABO and Rh typing, type-specific blood may be released. All units are conspicuously labeled to indicate that they are uncrossmatched and that the patient's serum has not been screened for irregular antibodies. In these situations, the patient's physician signs a release form stating that the clinical situation warrants the release of uncrossmatched blood. In such cases, the antibody screen is promptly completed, and crossmatches are performed using the laboratory's protocol. In the event of a positive screen or incompatible crossmatch, the physician is notified of any antibodies or incompatibility detected.

COMPATIBILITY TESTING IN MASSIVE TRANSFUSION

If a patient receives a volume of blood equal to or exceeding his or her blood volume, the patient is considered to be massively transfused. Under these circumstances, laboratories still employing the full antiglobulin crossmatch may safely switch to the abbreviated crossmatch to detect any ABO incompatibility. If the patient has a known, clinically significant erythrocyte antibody, however, antigen-negative units must be used for transfusion even though the antibody may be diluted and undetectable because of the large volume of blood and fluids transfused. Transfusion of antigen-positive units could result in an increase of antibody titer and lead to a delayed hemolytic transfusion reaction. Most protocols for massive transfusion return to the use of the routine crossmatch procedure on the day following the emergency.

Antibody Identification

USING A PANEL OF RED BLOOD CELLS

As mentioned previously, a positive antibody screen or antihuman globulin crossmatch mandates identification of the causative antibody so that antigen-negative blood can be provided for transfusion. This is accomplished by testing an extended panel of reagent red blood cells against the recipient's serum using the indirect antiglobulin technique. The pattern of positive and negative serum reactions is then compared with the phenotype pattern on the accompanying antigram to find a "match." Following is a greatly simplified example:

Cells in a panel	**Known antigenic composition**					**Test serum**	
	D	**C**	**c**	**E**	**e**	**Y**	**Z**
No. 1	+	+	+	−	−	+	−
No. 2	+	+	−	+	+	+	+
No. 3	+	−	+	−	+	+	−
No. 4	−	−	+	−	+	−	−
No. 5	−	+	−	−	+	−	−
No. 6	−	−	+	+	+	−	+

Panel 1

In Panel 1, serum Y reacts with cells number 1 through 3, which are positive for the D antigen, but does not react with cells number 4 through 6, which are negative for the D antigen; thus, the pattern of positive and negative serum reactions matches the phenotype of the panel for the D antigen, and therefore serum Y appears to contain anti-D. Similarly, the pattern of reactivity for serum Z matches the phenotype of the panel for the E antigen, and thus serum Z appears to contain anti-E. However, before such an identification can be conclusively stated, one must evaluate the chance that serum Z is reacting by coincidence with an antigen other than E that is present on the two E-positive cells and is absent from the four E-negative cells, leading to an erroneous conclusion. The same possibility must be considered for the probable anti-D in serum Y. In antibody identification, therefore, one must be sure that enough cells of differing antigenic composition are tested to definitively identify a single antibody or combination of antibodies in a given serum.

The minimum number of cells positive for each antigenic determinant that is required for a desired level of confidence can be estimated by Fisher's exact method for a 2×2 table (Race, 1975), as follows:

Total number of cells in a panel	**Probability of coincidence with number of cell samples that react positively**				
	1	**2**	**3**	**4**	**5**
6	1:6	1:15	1:20		
7	1:7	1:21	1:35		
8	1:8	1:28	1:56	1:70	
9	1:9	1:36	1:84	1:126	
10	1:10	1:45	1:120	1:210	1:252

2 × 2 table

Statistically, a chance of coincidence of 1 in 20, or 5% (i.e., the 95% confidence interval), is acceptable, although use of the 99% confidence interval with a chance of coincidence of 1% or less is generally recommended (Mollison, 1993). From the 2 × 2 table shown, it may be determined that a panel of seven cells with a minimum of two representing each antigen would be required to achieve the 95% confidence interval. To reduce the chance of erroneous conclusions to less than 1%, one would need a panel of nine cells with a minimum of four for each antigen. Most manufacturers supply reagent cell panels with 10 or 11 cells in order to reach the 99% confidence interval for identification of many of the commonly encountered antibodies. However, because it is difficult to ensure that at least three cells represent each antigen, additional cells may have to be tested from other panels for definitive identification of certain antibodies, particularly those directed against low-frequency or high-frequency antigens.

The following simplified example is used to illustrate the identification of a single antibody:

Cells in a panel	**Known antigenic composition**									**Serum reaction**	
	D	C	c	E	e	K	k	Fy^a	Fy^b	37°C	AGT
No. 1	+	+	+	−	+	−	+	+	+	−	+
No. 2	+	+	−	−	+	−	+	+	−	−	+
No. 3	+	−	+	+	+	+	+	−	+	−	−
No. 4	−	+	+	−	+	+	+	−	+	−	−
No. 5	−	−	+	−	+	−	+	+	−	−	+
No. 6	−	−	+	+	−	−	+	−	+	−	−
No. 7	−	+	+	−	+	−	+	+	+	−	+
No. 8	−	−	+	−	+	−	+	−	+	−	−

Panel 2

One of the first steps that is performed by many technologists in evaluating antibody identification results is to rule out those antibodies for which the serum has failed to react with a cell known to carry the corresponding antigen. It is best to rule out antibodies based on cells demonstrating the homozygous form of an antigen so as not to erroneously rule out weakly reactive or dosing antibodies. Panel 2 shows that there is no reaction of the serum with cells No. 3, 4, 6, or 8. Thus, anti-D, anti-c, and anti-Fy^b may be ruled out with cell No. 3. Anti-e may be ruled out with cell No. 4. Anti-E and anti-k may be ruled out using cell No. 6, but nothing additional may be ruled out using cell No. 8. Thus, after the ruling out process, anti-C, anti-K, and anti-Fy^a remain as possibilities. However, Fy^a is the only antigen phenotype pattern that matches the pattern of serum reactivity, so that anti-Fy^a may be tentatively identified in the serum with a chance of coincidence of 1:70, or 1.5%. To complete this identification, one must test cells homozygous for the C and K antigens that are *negative* for the Fy^a antigen against the serum to rule out those antibodies, and an additional Fy^a-positive cell should be tested to achieve a less than 1% chance of coincidence.

Figure 30–16 shows an actual antibody identification. Several conclusions can be drawn from the results:

- Because the auto control is negative, the serum reactivity appears to be due to alloantibodies.
- Using the homozygous "rule of thumb" for ruling out antibodies, cells No. 3, 5, 6, and 7 may be used to rule out antibodies directed against D, C, c, e, f, V, M, N, s, P_1, Le^a, Le^b, Lu^b, k, Fy^b, Jk^a, Jk^b, and Xg^a.
- Because of reactions seen in different phases and demonstrating different agglutination strengths, at least two antibodies are likely present in the serum.
- Cells No. 4 and 10 show direct agglutination in the 37°C phase followed by stronger agglutination in the antihuman globulin (AHG) phase, which is typical of Rh system antibodies. These are the only two cells on the panel positive for the E antigen, which has not been crossed out. Thus, it is likely that anti-E is one of the antibodies involved.
- Cells No. 2 and 8 show strong agglutination in the AHG phase only. Looking at the antigens across the top of the panel that have not been crossed out, one sees that the phenotype of the panel cells for the K antigen fits the serum reactivity of these two cells. Thus, anti-K probably is a second antibody involved.
- The remaining serum reactions with cells No. 1, 9, and 11 cannot be explained by either anti-E or anti-K, but could be explained by anti-Fy^a, because all three of these cells are positive for the Fy^a antigen, and anti-Fy^a has not been ruled out.
- Because the panel in Figure 30–16 contains more than 10 cells of various phenotypes, the 2×2 table shows that the 99% confidence interval may be achieved by having three separate cells positive for each antigenic determinant reacting with the serum. Thus, anti-Fy^a can be identified with confidence; however, two more cells positive for K antigen only and one more cell positive for E antigen only must be tested with the serum to conclusively identify the presence of anti-K and anti-E.
- Anti-C^w and anti-S should be ruled out by testing another cell (or cells) positive for C^w and positive in the homozygous state for S that at the same time are negative for the Fy^a, K, and E antigens. Anti-Lu^a, anti-Kp^a, and anti-Js^a may be ruled out by testing appropriate cells positive for these antigens. If necessary, heterozygous cells can be used, because it is so difficult to find cells homozygous for these antigens, especially if the blood bank laboratory has limited resources in terms of other reagent red cell panels.

If an antibody identification workup is being performed for the first time on a particular patient, once all other antibodies have been ruled out by testing additional cells, patient erythrocytes should be tested for the antigens to which he or she has developed antibodies as a confirmation of the identification. The patient's erythrocytes should lack the antigens corresponding to the antibodies present.

Finally, and most important, red blood cell units for transfusion should be tested with known commercial antisera (see Testing for Erythrocyte Antigens), if available, to prove the lack of all antigens to which the patient has clinically significant serum antibodies, and all units for transfusion, even if already screened for antigens, *must* be crossmatched with the patient's serum utilizing 37°C incubation followed by conversion to the antiglobulin test. As previously described, the abbreviated crossmatch protocol is *not* permitted when the patient currently has demonstrable clinically significant antibodies or any history of the same.

SPECIAL TECHNIQUES USED IN ANTIBODY IDENTIFICATION

Patients who have undergone multiple transfusions may respond by forming multiple irregular erythrocyte antibod-

Name John Doe
Hospital Number 000123456
ABO O Rh Pos
DAT: Neg ; IgG ______ ; C3________

Date Drawn ____________
Date Tested ____________
Interpretation ____________
____
Technologist ____________

		Rh								MNSs				P	Lewis		Luth-eran		Kell				Duffy		Kidd		Sex Linked	Vial			
Rh Phenotype		D	C	E	c	e	f	C^w	V	M	N	S	s	P_1	Le^a	Le^b	Lu^a	Lu^b	K	k	Kp^a	Js^a	Fy^a	Fy^b	Jk^a	Jk^b	Xg^a		37°C	AHG	CC
1	rr	0	0	0	+	+	+	0	0	+	0	+	0	+	+	0	0	+	0	+	0	0	+	+	+	0	+	1	0	1	
2	rr	0	0	0	+	+	+	0	0	+	+	0	+	+	0	+	0	+	+	+	0	0	0	+	0	+	+	2	0	3	
3	r'r	0	+	0	+	+	+	0	0	+	0	+	+	+	0	+	0	+	0	+	0	0	0	+	0	+	0	3	0	0	2
4	r"r	0	0	+	+	+	+	0	0	+	+	+	+	0	0	+	+	+	0	+	0	0	0	+	0	+	0	4	1	2	
5	rr	0	0	0	+	+	+	0	0	0	+	+	+	+	0	+	0	+	0	+	0	0	0	+	0	+	+	5	0	0	2
6	R_or	+	0	0	+	+	+	0	+	+	+	0	+	+	0	0	0	+	0	+	0	0	0	0	+	0	0	6	0	0	2
7	R_1R_1	+	+	0	0	+	+	0	0	+	0	+	+	0	+	0	0	+	0	+	0	0	0	+	+	+	0	7	0	0	2
8	R_1R_1	+	+	0	0	+	+	0	0	+	+	+	+	+	0	+	0	+	+	+	0	0	+	0	0	+	+	8	0	3	
9	$R_1R_1^w$	+	+	0	0	+	+	+	0	+	+	0	+	+	0	+	0	+	0	+	0	0	+	+	+	+	+	9	0	1	
10	R_2R_2	+	0	+	+	0	+	0	0	+	+	0	+	+	+	0	0	+	0	+	0	+	0	0	+	+	+	10	1	2	
11	rr	0	0	0	+	+	+	0	0	0	+	0	+	+	0	+	+	+	0	+	+	0	+	+	+	0	0	11	0	1	
																												Auto	0	0	2
																												Cord			
																												SCI			
																												SCII			
																												A_1 Cell			
																												B Cell			

CC = Coombs' control cells

Figure 30–16. An example of antibody identification.

ies. Autoantibodies can often mask the presence of alloantibodies and will react with all cells tested including all reagent red blood cells for antibody identification and all donor units crossmatched. When complicated problems such as these are encountered, special techniques are required to resolve the problem and find compatible units for transfusion. Some of these techniques are described subsequently.

HEMAGGLUTINATION INHIBITION. One application of hemagglutination inhibition is to neutralize a specific antibody with its corresponding soluble substance in antibody identification tests. Certain blood group antigens are found in abundant soluble form either in human saliva, serum, or other body fluids, as well as in substances in nature, and include such antigens as ABH, Le^a, Le^b, I, P_1, Sd^a, Rg^a, and Ch^a.

Table 30–32 lists sources of soluble substances for hemagglutination inhibition procedures. These soluble substances share the same antigenic specificity as those found on the erythrocytes and can neutralize the corresponding specific antibody in a given serum. Serum containing antibody that can be neutralized with a specific soluble substance will no longer agglutinate erythrocytes possessing that particular antigen after addition of the neutralizing substance. This technique can be used to confirm the specificity of a suspected antibody, and it can be useful when working with a serum specimen containing multiple specificities. If one antibody can be neutralized with a source of soluble antigen, the remaining antibodies will be easier to identify. This is particularly helpful when the inhibited antibody previously reacted with a large percentage of cells tested.

Table 30–32. SOURCES OF SOLUBLE ANTIGENS FOR HEMAGGLUTINATION INHIBITION PROCEDURES

Soluble Substance	Source
Le^a, Le^b	Secretor saliva
P_1	Hydatid cyst fluid, pigeon eggs
Sd^a	Urine, guinea pig urine
Ch^a, Rg^a	Plasma
I	Mother's milk
H	Saliva

Hemagglutination inhibition is also used to determine the secretor status of persons by detection of H substance in saliva, or it can be used to identify weak ABO subgroups by detection of A or B substance in the saliva when the erythrocytes fail to produce expected agglutination with corresponding antisera. Saliva is mixed with antibody of known specificity and then subsequently tested with indicator cells possessing the corresponding antigen. The absence of agglutination in hemagglutination inhibition indicates a positive test result and signifies the presence of a specific soluble antigen in the fluid tested. The strength of the antibody used in the test must be adjusted to yield a reaction of 2+ or less (see Fig. 30–14) with the indicator cells. If the antibody concentration is too high, insufficient neutralizing substance may lead to only partial neutralization of the antibody, and a false-negative result will be obtained.

ADSORPTION. Adsorption is a process used to remove antibodies from sera. The adsorption procedure may be performed using washed, enzyme-treated, or formalinized erythrocytes or erythrocyte stromata. The type of antigenic material chosen depends on the specific application for which adsorption is being used. The incubation temperature and times to be used in the adsorption process depend on the immunoglobulin class and thermal range of the antibodies being adsorbed. In general, using a low ratio of antibody to antigen will increase the efficiency of the adsorption. Also, periodic mixing of the serum and cells during the adsorption period is helpful, because this maximizes the amount of contact between antigen and antibody. Adsorption has the following applications:

Removal of Cold or Warm Autoantibodies. This is necessary to detect the presence of any underlying antibodies that may be masked by the autoantibodies. Autologous erythrocytes are typically used for the adsorption, provided the patient has received no transfusions in the last three to four months. For most autoantibodies, enzyme treatment of the adsorbing cells prior to adsorption increases the amount of autoantibody that can be removed from the serum.

Removal of a Single Alloantibody. This is useful when attempting to identify multiple antibodies in a single serum, especially if one of the antibodies is directed against an antigen of high frequency. Adsorption is performed using cells with the appropriate antigen that will remove the desired antibody, which will then simplify the identification of the antibodies remaining in the adsorbed serum.

Purposeful Sensitization of Erythrocytes. This is usually done and then combined with subsequent elution studies. One example of the use of adsorption-elution studies is in the classification of rare ABO subgroups in which the antigen expression is so weak that the erythrocytes are not agglutinated by their corresponding antisera. By adsorbing a specific antibody, such as anti-A, onto erythrocytes suspected of being positive for the A antigen, and then eluting and identifying the antibody as anti-A by appropriate tests, one can indirectly prove the presence of the antigen on the erythrocytes.

Removal of Unwanted ABO Agglutinins. This may be done in the preparation of raw antisera for antigen screening purposes. When a rare antibody is found in the plasma of a donor or in a patient specimen, it can be used to screen donor units for the corresponding antigen as long as interfering ABO hemagglutinins are first removed. Antigen-negative units are then retyped using licensed antisera, if available. Stromata or formalinized cells may be useful for adsorption in this application in order to avoid hemolysis that might be induced by the ABO antibodies during the adsorption procedure.

ELUTION. When a direct antiglobulin test first yields a positive result, the antibody generally must be removed from the patient's erythrocytes so that it may be identified. Elution is the process used to remove antibodies bound to erythrocytes. Because one desires to examine only antibody removed from the erythrocytes themselves, the technologist first washes the cells to be eluted numerous times prior to elution with large volumes of saline in order to remove any serum containing unbound antibody. To ensure the complete removal of serum antibody, the saline from the last wash must be tested against appropriate cells to detect any residual unbound antibody. The last wash control should show absence of antibody reactivity before the elution procedure is performed. Eluates are often prepared in a saline medium and should therefore be tested on the same day. When storage is anticipated, the eluate should be prepared in group AB serum or 6% albumin and kept at −20°C or lower.

Elution of red blood cells may be accomplished by a variety of methods that alter or reverse the forces of attraction that hold the antigen and antibody together. The Landsteiner-Miller heat elution dissociates antibody from erythrocyte antigens by heating at 56°C to 60°C for 10 minutes with frequent agitation. This procedure is actually effective only in the removal of IgM antibodies such as ABO. ABO antibodies may also be removed by a method called the freeze-thaw elution, which changes the conformation of the red cell membrane to cause antibody dissociation. This procedure is useful when only a small amount of specimen is available, such as in evaluating newborns for the possibility of hemolytic disease due to ABO incompatibility between mother and baby.

Organic solvents may also be used as an effective elution method that typically gives good yields of IgG antibody. Organic solvents such as ether, ethanol, chloroform, xylene, and methylene chloride have all been used, although ether elution has been one of the most frequently used methods by many laboratories in the past. The organic solvent procedures are generally no longer employed as a routine method of elution because of the carcinogenic, toxic, or explosive properties of the chemicals used. However, organic solvent elutions may still be used when a highly effective method that gives an excellent yield of antibody is necessary—for instance, when *in vivo* erythrocyte sensitization is highly suspected but the direct antiglobulin test result is negative.

Another method of elution involves the alteration of pH such that the attractive forces produced by oppositely charged chemical structures on antigen and antibody are neutralized. One example of such a method is the digitonin-acid elution. The acid elution has been adapted into kit form by a number of manufacturers to render the elution procedure safe, efficient, and easy to perform. This method is generally suitable for most applications in which elution is needed.

Sonication is another method of elution that has been described in which high-frequency sound waves are used to dissociate antibody from the erythrocyte membrane. For a comprehensive review of elution procedures, see Mallory (1993).

Elution has the following applications:

- To determine the specificity of antibodies bound to patient erythrocytes *in vivo*, such as in cases of acute or delayed hemolytic transfusion reactions, hemolytic disease of the newborn, autoimmune hemolytic anemia, and antibodies induced by medication.
- To confirm the presence of a single antibody in a mixture of several serum antibodies. The antibody is first adsorbed onto a carefully selected source of antigen-positive cells and then eluted from the cells and identified using a panel of reagent red blood cells.
- To demonstrate the identity of a weak subgroup of A

such as A_x, A_m, and A_{el}. Erythrocytes of these phenotypes may not be agglutinated by anti-A or anti-A,B, but they will adsorb enough anti-A added to the cells that it can then be eluted. The eluted antibody is tested against appropriate cells to identify it as anti-A, which confirms the presence of A antigen on these cells.

- To prepare a small amount of monospecific antisera for typing purposes by separation from other unwanted antibodies, such as anti-A, anti-B, or other irregular antibodies, which would interfere with the monospecific antibody in erythrocyte typing.

ENZYME TREATMENT. Bromelin, papain, trypsin, and ficin are widely used to treat erythrocytes in order to enhance certain antibody reactivity or to provide more effective adsorption of antibody in autoadsorption procedures. Bromelin (0.5% at pH 5.5) or cysteine papain (0.1% at pH 6.5) can be mixed together with serum and reagent red blood cells in a one-stage enzyme technique. In the two-stage technique, a 0.1% solution of papain, trypsin, or ficin at pH 7.3 is used to pretreat reagent red blood cells. The cells are then washed, resuspended, and tested with the appropriate serum. The two-stage test is much more sensitive than the one-stage test; consequently, improper performance of the test may yield a high incidence of false-positive reactions, especially when the test is followed by an antiglobulin test.

Enzyme treatment is usually used in antibody identification in one of two ways. If a weak antibody that is not easily identified is found in a patient serum, enzyme treatment of the reagent cells followed by retesting may enhance the reactivity of the antibody. This may aid in its identification by allowing the antibody to react with all antigen-positive cells on a panel, thus enabling recognition of a definitive reaction pattern. Enhancement of antibody reactivity with enzyme-treated cells is demonstrated in the Rh, Kidd, Lewis, Ii, and P systems. In fact, rare examples of Rh and Kidd antibodies can be detected only with enzyme-treated cells.

On the other hand, enzyme treatment reduces or destroys reactivity of the M, N, Fy^a, Fy^b, Xg^a, Pr, Yt^a, Ch^a, Rg^a, and sometimes S antigens. This can be used to eliminate the reactivity of one or more antibodies in a serum allowing detection of underlying antibodies. In another application, an antibody that has so far eluded identification may be tested with enzyme-treated cells. If the antibody fails to react by the enzyme technique, its specificity can be assigned to one of the antigens that are sensitive to enzyme treatment. This can aid in the identification of an antibody.

ANTIBODY TITRATION. Antibody titration is a method used to semiquantitatively determine the amount of antibody present in a given serum. Serial twofold dilutions of the serum are prepared and then tested with erythrocytes possessing the corresponding antigen. Each dilution is read for macroscopic agglutination, and the titer of the antibody is expressed as the reciprocal of the highest serum dilution that gives macroscopic agglutination. Antibody titration has several applications. In prenatal studies, clinically significant IgG alloantibodies that can cause hemolytic disease of the newborn are titered periodically in the maternal serum during pregnancy. An increasing titer usually indicates that fetal cells possess the corresponding antigen and are stimulating the mother to produce more antibody, thus providing valuable information to the physician regarding how the pregnancy should be managed. Antibody titration is also used in the classification of high-titer, low-avidity (HTLA) antibodies. Most antibodies (excluding HTLA) that initially give weak ($\pm$ or $\pm^m$) reactions in indirect antiglobulin tests will react to at most the 1:2 dilution if a titration is performed. However, HTLA antibodies characteristically give weak ($\pm$ or $\pm^m$) reactions, yet will usually react to a dilution equal to or greater than 1:64 when the serum is titered. If such an antibody is suspected, a titer is performed to demonstrate that the weakly reactive antibody is still reactive at a high dilution, thus allowing its classification as an HTLA. These antibodies include anti-Ch^a, anti-Rg^a, anti-Yk^a and others (see Table 30–28).

Testing for Erythrocyte Antigens

A variety of circumstances necessitate the typing of erythrocytes for selected blood group antigens. To select blood for transfusion, one must determine the patient's ABO group and Rh type. When one is resolving a complicated antibody problem, it may be useful to test the patient's erythrocytes for the other common blood group antigens to determine which antigens the patient lacks, thus providing information as to which red cell antibodies the patient could form.

When a patient has a known antibody, donor units must be tested to demonstrate lack of the corresponding antigen. Because some antigens have differing frequencies among various ethnic groups, valuable time may be saved if screening is conducted within selected donor populations. In larger blood centers, a percentage of all group O units may be screened for selected high-incidence antigens or other antigens (e.g., E, Fy^a, Jk^a, K) as requested. Units lacking certain antigens are frozen and saved for later use with other patients who may have the corresponding antibody or antibodies.

Erythrocyte antigens also are typed in the resolution of paternity cases and in the determination of zygosity for D in the husband of a D-negative woman when there is the potential for Rh hemolytic disease of the newborn.

GENERAL CONSIDERATIONS

ERYTHROCYTE SUSPENSION. With the possible exception of ABO and Rh typing (depending on the technique used), a 3% to 5% saline suspension of erythrocytes is usually prepared for all procedures. One drop of the 3% to 5% suspension is used for each test. For typings of ABO, Lewis, Chido, Bg, Yt^a, and Sd^a, washed erythrocytes are preferable, because the presence of soluble antigen in the plasma could neutralize antibodies in the typing serum.

REAGENTS. Whenever possible, licensed reagents or those of equivalent quality should be used for erythrocyte typing. Positive and negative controls should be performed on a daily basis. Reagents should be stored according to manufacturers' instructions, which is most commonly at 2°C to 4°C. In addition, the method of testing recommended by the manufacturer must be carefully followed; the use of an antiglobulin test or microscopic examination when it is not recommended may result in the detection of contaminating antibodies, giving a false-positive result.

Sources of Reagents. The most common source of antisera is plasma collected from blood donors who are found to have been sensitized to an antigen or antigens via transfusion or pregnancy. The specificity of the antibody is identified, and other unwanted antibodies, such as ABO antibodies, are absorbed from the serum. The antiserum is then tested for specificity, avidity, and titer according to the FDA guidelines. Antisera for most common red cell antigens are available commercially.

Monoclonal Antibodies. Monoclonal antibodies are synthesized by lymphocyte hybridomas, which are produced by the fusion of antibody-producing cells from immunized animals (often mice) and neoplastic myeloma cells. Some of the hybridoma cells can grow continuously in a selective culture medium and will secrete the same antibody produced by the original fused B lymphocyte (Mollison, 1993). Hybridomas producing a desirable antibody are isolated and subcultured indefinitely to provide a continuous source of antibodies with identical specificity. These hybridoma cells can also be maintained in a frozen state or reinjected into mice to produce ascites tumors with very high concentrations of monoclonal antibodies in the fluid. Human monoclonal antibodies with specificity for blood group antigens have also been produced by transformation of human B lymphocytes with Epstein-Barr virus into lymphoblastoid cells that can grow in culture and secrete antibody (Mollison, 1993).

Monoclonal antibodies differ from conventional antibodies in three aspects: (1) *specificity*—they react with just one instead of multiple antigenic determinants; (2) *purity*—all, not just a fraction, of the serum protein content is immunoglobulin; and (3) *reproducibility*—the same specificity and affinity is expected from every subculture of a single clone. When using monoclonal antibodies for erythrocyte typing, however, one must be familiar with their characteristics. Monoclonal antibodies may show unexpected crossreactivities because of their high potency and affinity. Because of their narrow specificity, some monoclonal antibodies may not react with all examples of an antigen. For instance, many human monoclonal anti-D reagents will not react with weak D variants. Thus, the anti-D reagent marketed for routine use is usually a blend of monoclonal and polyclonal antibody because of this problem.

Currently, erythrocyte typing reagents derived from murine monoclonal antibodies that are available commercially in the United States include anti-A, anti-B, anti-M, anti-N, anti-Le^a, anti-Le^b, and anti-C3d. Human monoclonal anti-D, anti-E, anti-c, anti-Jk^a, and anti-Jk^b have also been produced and are now available. In the near future, monoclonal reagents will be available for human leukocyte antigen (HLA) typing as well. The combination of monoclonal antibodies and flow cytometry holds promise for development of new automated methods of erythrocyte and leukocyte typing for immunohematologic investigation. (See Part V for a review of use of monoclonal antibodies as reagents.) In addition to clinical uses, monoclonal antibodies are being used extensively in research into the biochemical and functional properties of the erythrocyte membrane blood group proteins.

Lectins. Lectins are specific receptor proteins present in plant seeds and in some invertebrate animals and lower vertebrates. Although many lectins have been reported, only a few have been found useful in blood banking (Bird, 1988), and these are listed in Table 30–33.

Anti-H lectin prepared from *Ulex europaeus* strongly agglutinates group O erythrocytes. It reacts weakly with A_2 cells and very weakly with A_1 or B cells. Most anti-H lectin preparations are readily inhibited by the immunodominant sugar of H substance, L-fucose, and some are also inhibited by N-acetyl-D-glucosamine. Because the potency of the lectin may vary with the preparation, each lot should be standardized before use. Anti-H lectin is most useful in the determination of secretor status and in the classification of weak A subgroups.

Table 30–33. LECTINS USEFUL IN BLOOD BANKING

Lectin	Activity Inhibited by	Serologic Specificity
Ulex europaeus	L-fucose N-acetyl-D-glucosamine	Anti-H
Lotus tetragonolobus	L-fucose	Anti-H
Vicia graminea	β-D-galactose	Anti-N
Arachis hypogaea	β-D-galactose	Anti-T, anti-Tk
Dolichos biflorus	α-N-acetyl-D-galactosamine	Anti-A, anti-Tn, anti-Cad
Salvia sclarea	α-N-acetyl-D-galactosamine	Anti-Tn
Salvia horminum	α-N-acetyl-D-galactosamine	Anti-Tn, anti-Cad (separable)
Bandeiraea simplicifolia	α-D-galactose (BS-I) N-acetyl-D-glucosamine (BS-II)	Anti-B Anti-Tk
Helix pomatia	α- or β-N-acetyl-D-galactosamine	Anti-A, -TN, -Cad
Glycine soja	N-acetyl-D-galactosamine	Anti-T, -Tn, -Cad

Anti-A_1 lectin prepared from *Dolichos biflorus* agglutinates A_1 erythrocytes, an activity that can be inhibited by A substance or N-acetyl-D-galactosamine. Anti-A_1 lectin is most commonly used to distinguish A_1 phenotypes from phenotypes of the A subgroups.

Anti-N lectin prepared from *Vicia graminea* agglutinates erythrocytes possessing the N antigen, and its activity is inhibited by D-galactose. In addition to typing erythrocytes, anti-N lectin has been useful in elucidating the chemical composition of the M and N antigens.

Anti-T lectin prepared from *Arachis hypogaea* (peanut), anti-Tn lectin from *Salvia sclarea,* and separable anti-Tn + anti-Cad lectin from *Salvia horminum* are useful in the study of erythrocyte polyagglutination.

TYPING OF ERYTHROCYTES WITH A POSITIVE DIRECT ANTIGLOBULIN TEST (DAT) RESULT. Many antisera used for typing of erythrocyte antigens require use of the indirect antiglobulin technique. If the erythrocytes being tested yield a positive DAT result, these reagents cannot be used because a false-positive reaction will result from the positive DAT result. Most elution methods that remove blood group antibodies from the surface of erythrocytes destroy either the cells or the antigens. However, treatment of antibody-coated erythrocytes with chloroquine diphosphate dissociates antibody while leaving the antigens intact. Chloroquine-treated erythrocytes can then be typed for antigens that require the use of antihuman globulin reactive antisera. Care should be exercised when interpreting results of typing for Rh system antigens with chloroquine-treated cells, because these antigens may be weakened and could give false-negative reactions with certain antisera.

New Technologies and Automation in Blood Bank Testing

Throughout the history of immunohematology as a clinical laboratory discipline, manual agglutination tests have been the most popular methods employed for the various procedures described in this chapter. In general, blood banks have lagged behind other areas of the clinical laboratory in automation of manual methods. The conventional manual agglutination method was first automated in large blood centers for the performance of ABO and Rh donor grouping. The instrumentation used adapted the continuous flow technology previously developed for clinical chemistry. Instruments employing continuous flow technology such as the AutoAnalyzer (Technicon, Tarrytown, New York) were some of the earliest automated systems adapted to blood banking and may still be in use by some facilities today. Another early automated batch-processing system used for donor grouping, introduced in 1969, was the Groupamatic (Kontron Instruments, Everett, Massachusetts).

Since the late 1980s, many blood centers worldwide have implemented the PK7100 Automated Pretransfusion Blood Testing System (Olympus Corporation, Lake Success, New York) for large-volume donor processing. The system is fully automated with bar-coded donor specimen identification and consists of a microprocessor, analyzer unit, photometer, and printer. Agglutination is still the final end point for the Olympus method, but the PK7100 uses microplates with a patented terraced-well design (Gibbons, 1986). Agglutinated erythrocytes settle out onto the terraced steps of the wells, while unagglutinated cells roll to the bottom of the well to form a compact, distinct button that is not disturbed by automated handling, resulting in more definite positive and negative readings by the photometric scanning unit. The PK7100 can perform up to 12 different tests on each specimen with a throughput of 240 specimens per hour. Besides ABO and Rh testing, the Olympus system is FDA-approved for cytomegalovirus and syphilis screening as well, and it can also be used for rare antigen screening (e.g., c, e, k) if desired. Outside of the United States, Olympus systems are also used for infectious disease screening for hepatitis B, hepatitis C, HIV, and HTLV-I.

In the 1980s, solid-phase test systems were developed as an alternative to agglutination tests for ABO and Rh testing (Plapp, 1992). For these procedures, microplate wells are coated with the appropriate antibodies. Test cells are added, and after incubation and centrifugation, the wells are read manually or with an automated reading device. For positive reactions, the erythrocytes adhere to the entire bottom surface of the antibody-coated well, whereas for negative reactions, a tightly packed cell button is formed in the bottom of the well.

This same principle was used to develop a solid-phase, red cell adherence method for antibody detection and identification, which until recently have proved to be the greatest challenge for automation. For these tests, reagent red cells are bound to the microplate wells. Serum and an enhancement reagent are added and incubated, allowing for antibody to bind to the solid phase. After washing to remove unbound serum components, antiglobulin-coated red cells are added and centrifuged. If a reaction has occurred, the bottom surface of the well will be covered by adherent antiglobulin-coated cells, whereas a discrete button in the bottom of the well indicates a negative reaction. Immucor (Atlanta, Georgia) currently markets several solid-phase kits including Capture-R, Capture-R Ready Screen, and Capture-R Ready ID kits for antibody detection and identification, as well as Capture-P and Capture-P Ready Screen kits for use in platelet crossmatching and detection of antiplatelet antibodies (Plapp, 1992). With these kits, the microplate methods can be combined with automated pipetting devices, plate readers, and printers to produce semiautomated systems for ABO and Rh testing and antibody screening.

Among the newest technologies developed for pretransfusion donor and recipient testing is the gel test, developed and patented by Lapierre and colleagues and released for European use by Diamed AG in 1988 (Lapierre, 1990). A different concept utilizing a similar principle is column agglutination technology (CAT), which is currently marketed in Europe by Ortho Diagnostics under the name of BioVue (Reis, 1993). Both of these products utilize the differential centrifugation of erythrocytes through a small column filled with either a dextran acrylamide gel (Diamed) or glass bead microparticles in a density gradient diluent (Ortho). Diamed's gel test can be used for ABO and Rh typing, antibody detection and identification, and crossmatching. Ortho's system at present is adapted only for direct or indirect antiglobulin testing (AGT).

In the application of this technology for AGT, antiglobulin reagents are incorporated into the gel or glass bead column matrix. After incubation of precisely measured volumes of reagent red blood cells, serum, and enhancement reagent in the reaction chamber above the column matrix (or simply the addition of patient cells in the direct test), the plastic card or cassette containing six microcolumns is centrifuged under carefully controlled conditions in a specially designed centrifuge. Erythrocytes that have been sensitized by IgG antibodies or complement agglutinate as they come into contact with the antiglobulin reagent in the matrix and are trapped, depending on the size of the agglutinates, either near the top of the column or throughout the matrix. Cells that have not been sensitized do not agglutinate and thus form a pellet at the bottom of the microtube. The reactions can be graded from negative to 4+ according to the pattern seen, with the strongest reaction being an intact band of agglutinated cells near the top of the matrix, as depicted in Figure 30–17.

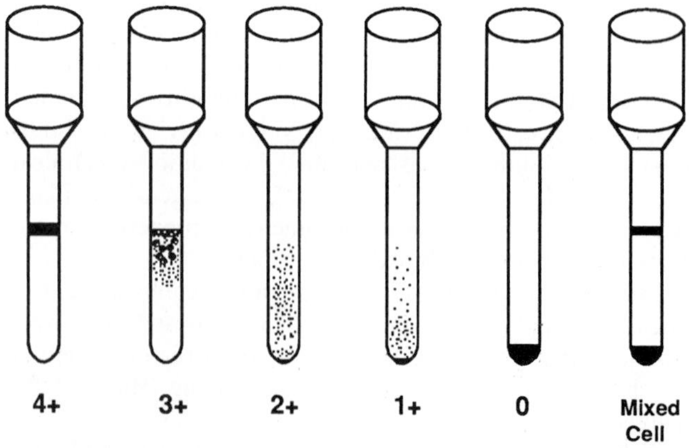

Figure 30–17. Appearance of reaction patterns and grading for the gel test or column agglutination system.

An important aspect of this technology, as applied to AGT, is the elimination of the need for a washing step, because the serum does not travel down through the matrix during centrifugation, and thus there is no danger of neutralization of the antiglobulin reagent. Another interesting aspect is that the reactions are stable in either the gel test or the CAT for at least 30 minutes. These two characteristics made possible the introduction, in Europe in 1992, of the first instrument to perform completely automated antiglobulin testing by the gel technique. An updated version of the automated gel testing system is currently available in Europe from Diamed using a system called the ID-Matic II. Tests that are available include blood grouping, direct antiglobulin testing, antibody detection and identification, crossmatching, sickle cell testing, and infectious disease screening, with a maximum throughput of 288 cards per hour (Malyska, 1995).

FDA approval for use of these technologies in the United States is still pending, but obviously the eventual availability of automated antiglobulin testing, in addition to ABO and Rh typing already available, will increase the attractiveness of this technology for large-volume testing performed at blood collection centers. As the technology becomes more commonplace and cost-effective, large transfusion services may decide to employ automation as well.

Anstee DJ: Blood group–active surface molecules of the human red blood cell. Vox Sang 1990; 58:1.

Berry-Dortch S, Woodside CH, Boral LI: Limitations of the immediate spin crossmatch when used for detecting ABO incompatibility. Transfusion 1985; 25:176.

Bird GWG: Lectins: A hundred years. Immunohematology 1988; 4:45.

Boral LI, Henry JB: The type and screen: A safe alternative and supplement in selected surgical procedures. Transfusion 1977; 17:163.

Branch DR, Gaidulis L, Lazar GS: Human granulocytes lack red cell K_x antigen. Br J Haematol 1986; 62:747.

Butch SH, Judd WJ, Steiner EA, et al: The computer crossmatch. Transfusion 1992; 32(Suppl):5s.

Caren LD, Bellavance R, Grumet FC: Demonstration of gene dosage effects on antigens in the Duffy, Ss and Rh systems using an enzyme-linked immunosorbent assay. Transfusion 1982; 22:475.

Cartron JP, Agre P: Rh blood group antigens: Protein and gene structure. Semin Hematol 1993a; 30:193.

Cartron JP, Le Van Kim C, Colin Y: Glycophorin C and related glycoproteins: Structure, function, and regulation. Semin Hematol 1993b; 30: 152.

Case J: Compound and complex Rh antigens. *In* Vengelen-Tyler V, Pierce S (eds): Blood Group Systems: Rh. Arlington, Virginia, American Association of Blood Banks, 1987, p 55.

Cherif-Zahar B, Raynal V, Le Van Kim C, et al: Structure and expression of the Rh locus in the Rh-deficiency syndrome. Blood 1993; 82:656.

Code of Federal Regulations. Title 21—Food and Drugs, Part 660, Subpart F—Anti-human globulin. Washington, DC, US Government Printing Office, 1993.

Colin Y, Cherif-Zahar B, Le Van Kim C, et al: Genetic basis of the RhD-positive and RhD-negative blood group polymorphism as determined by Southern analysis. Blood 1991; 78:2747.

Coombs RRA, Mourant AF, Race RR: A new test for the detection of weak and "incomplete" Rh agglutinins. Br J Exp Pathol 1945; 26:225.

Cordle DG, Strauss RG, Snyder EI, et al: Safety and cost containment data that advocate abbreviated pretransfusion testing. Am J Clin Pathol 1990; 94:428.

Daniels G: The Lutheran blood group system: Monoclonal antibodies, biochemistry and the effect of In(Lu). *In* Pierce SR, Macpherson C (eds): Blood Group Systems: Duffy, Kidd, and Lutheran. Arlington, Virginia, American Association of Blood Banks, 1988, p 119.

Daniels GL, Le Pennec PY, Rouger P, et al: The red cell antigens Au^a and Au^b belong to the Lutheran system. Vox Sang 1991; 60:191.

Edwards-Moulds J: The Kidd blood group system: drug-related antibodies and biochemistry. *In* Pierce SR, Macpherson CR (eds): Blood Group Systems: Duffy, Kidd, and Lutheran. Arlington, Virginia, American Association of Blood Banks, 1988, p 73.

Engelfriet CP, Overbeeke MA, von dem Borne AE: Autoimmune hemolytic anemia. Semin Hematol 1992; 29:3.

Friedman BA, Oberman HA, Chadwick AR, et al: The maximum surgical blood order schedule and surgical blood use in the United States. Transfusion 1976; 16:380.

Garraty G: Immune cytopenia associated with antibiotics. Transfus Med Rev 1993; 7:255.

Garraty G: Review: Immune hemolytic anemia and/or positive direct antiglobulin tests caused by drugs. Immunohematology 1994; 10:41.

Gibbons DS, Kano T, Edelmann M: A terraced microplate system for automated ABO and Rh grouping. American Clinical Products Review, Nov 1986.

Goodman JW: Immunogens and antigens. *In* Stites DP, Terr AI, Parslow TG, (eds): Basic and Clinical Immunology, 8th ed. Norwalk, Connecticut, Appleton & Lange, 1994a, p 50.

Goodman JW: Immunoglobulin proteins. *In* Stites DP, Terr AI, Parslow TG, (eds): Basic and Clinical Immunology, 8th ed. Norwalk, Connecticut, Appleton & Lange, 1994b, p 66.

Grove-Rasmussen M: Routine compatibility testing standards of the AABB as applied to compatibility tests. Transfusion 1964; 4:200.

Hakomori S: Blood group ABH and Ii antigens of human erythrocytes: Chemistry, polymorphism, and their developmental change. Semin Hematol 1981; 18:39.

Harmening DM: Modern Blood Banking and Transfusion Practices, 3rd ed. Philadelphia, FA Davis, 1994.

Heddle NM, O'Hoski P, Singer J, et al: A prospective study to determine the safety of omitting the antiglobulin crossmatch from pretransfusion testing. Br J Haematol 1992; 81:579.

Henry JB, Mintz PD, Webb W: Optimal blood ordering for elective surgery. JAMA 1977; 237:451.

Hoeltge GA, Domen RE, Rybicki LA, et al: Multiple red cell transfusions and alloimmunization. Arch Pathol Lab Med 1995; 119:42.

Hughes-Jones NC, Gardner B, Lincoln P: Observations of the number of available c, D, e, and E antigen sites on red cells. Vox Sang 1971; 21:210.

Issitt PD: Applied Blood Group Serology, 3rd ed. Miami, Montgomery Scientific Publications, 1985.

Jennings ML: Structure and function of the red blood cell anion transport protein. Annu Rev Biophys Chem 1989; 18:397.

Judd WJ: Are there better ways than the crossmatch to demonstrate ABO incompatibility? Transfusion 1991; 31:192.

Judd WJ: Methods in Immunohematology, 2nd ed. Durham, North Carolina, Montgomery Scientific Publications, 1994.

Judd WJ, Steiner EA, O'Donnell DB, et al: Discrepancies in reverse ABO typing due to prozone: How safe is the immediate-spin crossmatch? Transfusion 1988; 28:334.

Klein HG: Standards for Blood Banks and Transfusion Services, 16th ed. Bethesda, Maryland, American Association of Blood Banks, 1994.

Kornstad L, Heisto H: The frequency of formation of Kell antibodies in recipients of Kell-positive blood. *In* Proceedings of the 6th Congress of the European Society of Haematology, Copenhagen, 1957, p 754.

Kuby J: Immunology, 2nd ed. New York, WH Freeman and Company, 1991.

Landsteiner K, Wiener AS: An agglutinable factor in human blood recognized by immune sera for rhesus blood. Proc Soc Exp Biol Med 1940; 43:223.

Lapierre Y, Rigal D, Adam J, et al: The gel test: A new way to detect red cell antigen-antibody reactions. Transfusion 1990; 30:109.

Levine P, Stetson RE: An unusual case of intragroup agglutination. JAMA 1939; 113:126.

Mallory D (ed): Immunohematology Methods, 1st ed. Rockville, Maryland, American National Red Cross, 1993.

Malyska H: Personal communication, 1995.

Masouredis SP, Sudora E, Mahan L, et al: Quantitative immunoferritin microassay of Fy^a, Fy^b, Jk^a, V and Di^b antigen site numbers on human red cells. Blood 1980; 56:969.

Meyer EA, Shulman IA: The sensitivity and specificity of the immediate-spin crossmatch. Transfusion 1989; 29:99.

Miller LH, Mason SJ, Dvorak JA, et al: Erythrocyte receptors for (*Plasmodium knowlesi*) malaria: Duffy blood determinants. Science 1975; 189:561.

Mintz PD, Haines AL, Sullivan MF: Incompatible crossmatch following nonreactive antibody detection test: Frequency and cause. Transfusion 1982; 22:107.

Mintz PD, Nordine RB, Henry JB, et al: Expected hemotherapy in elective surgery. N Y J Med 1976; 76:532.

Mohandas N, Chasis JA: Red blood cell deformability, membrane material properties and shape: Regulation by transmembrane, skeletal, and cytosolic proteins and lipids. Semin Hematol 1993; 30:171.

Mollison PL: Further observations on the patterns of clearance of incompatible red cells. Transfusion 1989; 39:347.

Mollison PL, Engelfriet CP, Contreras M: Blood Transfusion in Clinical Medicine, 9th ed. Oxford, Blackwell Scientific Publications, 1993.

Mougey R: A review: The Kidd system. Immunohematology 1990; 6:1.

Muekler M, Caruso C, Baldwin SA et al: Sequence and structure of a human glucose transporter. Science 1985; 229:941.

Nance ST: Applications of flow cytometry in blood transfusion science. *In* Moore SB (ed): Progress in Immunohematology. Arlington, Virginia, American Association of Blood Banks, 1988, p 1.

Napier JA: The crossmatch. Br J Haematol 1991; 78:1.

Neote K, Mak JY, Kolakowski LF, et al: Functional and biochemical analysis of the cloned Duffy antigen: Identity with the red blood cell chemokine receptor. Blood 1994; 84:44.

Ness PM, Shirey RS, Thoman SK, et al: The differentiation of delayed serologic and delayed hemolytic transfusion reactions: Incidence, long-term serologic findings, and clinical significance. Transfusion 1990; 30:688.

Oriol R, Danilovs J, Hawkins BR: A new genetic model proposing that the *Se* gene is a structural gene closely linked to the *H* gene. Am J Hum Genet 1981; 33:421.

Pedersen JT, Kaplan H, Wedock L, et al: Octapeptide segments from the amino terminus of glycophorin A contain the antigenic determinants of the M and N blood group systems. J Lab Clin Med 1990; 116:527.

Petz LD: Drug-induced autoimmune hemolytic anemia. Transfus Med Rev 1993; 8:242.

Pittiglio DH: Genetics and biochemistry of A, B, H, and Lewis antigens. *In* Wallace ME, Gibbs FL (eds): Blood Group Systems: ABH and Lewis. Arlington, Virginia, American Association of Blood Banks, 1986, p 1.

Plapp FV, Rachel JM: Automation in blood banking: Machines for clumping, sticking, and gelling. Am J Clin Pathol 1992; 98(Suppl 1):S-17.

Poole J: Review: The Lutheran blood group system—1991. Immunohematology 1992; 8:1.

Prasad AS: Acquired hemolytic anemias. *In* Bick RL (ed): Hematology: Clinical and Laboratory Practice, 1st ed, Vol I. St. Louis, CV Mosby, 1993, p 391.

Race RR: The Rh genotypes and Fisher's theory. Blood 1948; 3:27.

Race RR, Sanger R: Blood Groups in Man, 6th ed. Oxford, Blackwell Scientific Publications, 1975.

Redman CR, Marsh WL: The Kell blood group system and the McLeod phenotype. Semin Hematol 1993; 30:209.

Reis KJ: Column agglutination technology: The antiglobulin test. Transfusion 1993; 33:639.

Riwom S, Janvier D, Navenot JM, et al: Production of a new murine monoclonal antibody with Fy6 specificity and characterization of the immunopurified N-glycosylated Duffy-active molecule. Vox Sang 1994; 66:61.

Roitt I: Essential Immunology, 7th ed. Oxford, Blackwell Scientific Publications, 1991.

Rouger P: Defects of McLeod red blood cells and association with disease. *In* Laird-Fryer B, Levitt J, Daniels G (eds): Blood Group Systems: Kell. Arlington, Virginia, American Association of Blood Banks, 1990, p 79.

Salama A, Mueller-Eckhardt C: Immune-mediated blood cell dyscrasias related to drugs. Semin Hematol 1992; 29:54.

Santoso S, Kiefel V, Mueller-Eckhardt C: Blood group A and B determinants are expressed on platelet glycoproteins IIa, IIIa, and Ib. Thromb Haemost 1991; 65:196.

Shulman IA: The risk of an overt hemolytic transfusion reaction following the use of an immediate spin crossmatch. Arch Pathol Lab Med 1990; 114:412.

Shulman IA, Nelson J, Kent D, et al: Experience with a cost effective crossmatch protocol. JAMA 1985; 254:93.

Shulman IA, Nelson JM, Lam HT, et al: Additional limitations of the immediate spin crossmatch to detect ABO incompatibility. Am J Clin Pathol 1987; 87:677.

Sistonen P, Tippett P: A "new" allele giving further insight into the LW blood group system. Vox Sang 1982; 42:252.

Storry JR: Review: The LW blood group system. Immunohematology 1992; 8:87.

Tippett P: Rh blood group system: The D antigen and high- and low-frequency Rh antigens. *In* Vengelen-Tyler V, Pierce S (eds): Blood Group Systems: Rh. Arlington, Virginia, American Association of Blood Banks, 1987, p 25.

Walker RH (ed): Technical Manual, 11th ed. Bethesda, Maryland, American Association of Blood Banks, 1993.

Wenz B, Apuzzo J, Shah DP: Evaluation of the polyethylene glycol–potentiated indirect antiglobulin test. Transfusion 1990; 30:318.

Wright MS, Issitt PD: Anticomplement and the indirect antiglobulin test. Transfusion 1979; 19:688.

Yamamoto F, Clausen H, White T, et al: Molecular genetic basis of the histo-blood group ABO system. Nature 1990; 345:229.

Yamamoto F-I: Review: Recent progress in the molecular genetic study of the histo-blood group ABO system. Immunohematology 1994; 10:1.

Chapter 31

Transfusion Medicine

Leonard I. Boral, M.D., M.B.A.
John Bernard Henry, M.D.

with a section on Stem Cells by
Bruce E. Kloster, M.D.

Transfusion medicine is a multidisciplinary specialty concerned with the proper selection and utilization of blood components as well as the removal of blood or blood components in the treatment or prevention of disease. The term blood banking is being replaced by the term transfusion medicine in order to stress the increasing role of patient care and evaluation of clinical results in this specialty (Klein, 1987). The blood components—red cells, platelets, granulocytes, fresh frozen plasma, and cryoprecipitate—are made directly from a unit of whole blood, using different methods of physical separation (i.e., centrifugation and freezing). Blood derivatives—albumin, plasma protein fraction, immune serum globulin, coagulation factor concentrates—are produced by the pharmaceutical industry and are usually made from plasma pools of thousands of donor units, using modifications of the Cohn ethanol fractionation technique. The basic principle of this method is that different proteins can be precipitated from plasma, without denaturation, by adjusting the amount of ethanol added (Rock, 1986).

When considering transfusion therapy, the physician must weigh the expected benefits against the potential dangers (NIH Consensus Conference, 1988). The risks of transfusion include the possible development of transfusion-transmitted diseases, immunization or sensitization, and transfusion reactions. The following are several helpful recommendations for using transfusion therapy.

The safest blood a person can receive is his or her own. Consequently, presurgical autologous deposit should be considered for all elective surgeries when the patient is relatively healthy and has a good chance of needing blood during or directly after surgery. Intraoperative and postoperative blood salvage as well as normotensive hemodilution should also be contemplated in selected surgical cases. These procedures are discussed in more detail later in this chapter.

Blood products (components and derivatives) must only be transfused when definitely indicated. The physician should reflect on each patient's needs before ordering blood. The decision to transfuse a patient (the transfusion trigger) should not be based on a number (such as the old 10 g of hemoglobin/30% hematocrit rule) but should be based on the patient's complete evaluation: (1) the patient's age as related to his or her health (patients over 70 often have poorer cardiovascular status than younger persons, who will tolerate hypoxemia and hypotension better), (2) the severity of the anemia, (3) the natural history of the cause of the anemia, (4) the rapidity of the onset of anemia, (5) the estimated blood loss, if applicable, (6) the degree of atherosclerosis affecting the coronary or cerebral arteries, (7) the degree of cardiac or pulmonary disease, and (8) types of current medications.

Additionally, the type of blood product that should be ordered will require some knowledge of the patient's future blood component needs as well as his or her current and future immune status. Should the patient receive leukoreduced blood, CMV-negative units, irradiated components, or some combination of these?

For those who need a number as a guide, the National Institutes of Health (NIH, 1988) Consensus Conference suggested a hematocrit of 21. Others have suggested even lower numbers—that is, a hematocrit of about 15% (McDonald, 1994; Rock, 1995, Viele, 1994). However, this is for younger patients who have an excellent cardiopulmonary reserve, with minimal chance of compromising cardiac output, and who have excellent pulmonary oxygen exchange. For those who want additional information when deciding how low to go before initiating the transfusion of blood, invasive monitoring for deriving oxygen extraction ratios has been suggested (Levine, 1990).

Take, for example, two different patients whose hemoglobin is 8 g/dL. A 20-year-old man who is in stable medical condition after a car accident that caused several fractures of his leg bones probably does not need red blood cells, because he will be inactive, in casts, for the next several weeks and his body will have time to produce enough red cells before he becomes physically active again. On the other hand, an 80-year-old man with angina and a decreased hemoglobin of 8 g/dL from blood loss due to a car accident would probably need increased numbers of red blood cells from a transfusion to enhance the blood's oxygen-carrying capacity, especially to his heart.

When a transfusion is indicated, always use a filter. Use as few of the products as possible, because the incidence of transfusion-transmitted diseases increases with the number of exposures to donors. Some derivatives, such as albumin, plasma protein fraction, immune serum globulin, and Rh immune globulin, are considered relatively safe products because the method of production virtually eliminates hepatitis and acquired immune deficiency syndrome (AIDS) viruses. However, in 1994, hepatitis C virus was reported to have been transmitted by intravenous immune serum globulin (CDC, July 21, 1994). The manufacturer involved has now added a solvent-detergent treatment in the manufacturing process to further inactivate contaminating viruses. Until recently, coagulation factor concentrates, made from thousands of pooled plasma units, posed a high risk for the transmission of hepatitis and AIDS, but newer methods of production have decreased this risk to below that of cryoprecipitate, as discussed later.

Before describing further how to use blood components and derivatives, the blood collection process should first be explained.

BLOOD COLLECTION

The collection and subsequent transfusion of blood comes under the watchful eye of several government regulatory agencies—the Food and Drug Administration (FDA), the Health Care Financing Administration (HCFA), the Occupational Safety and Health Administration (OSHA), and the State Department of Health. Inspections are performed by these agencies to assure regulatory compliance. Additionally, the American Association of Blood Banks (AABB), a professional association, provides the scientific leadership and mechanisms to deal with progress and change by providing the AABB Standards. The AABB, the College of American Pathologists (CAP), and the Joint Commission on Accreditation of Hospital Organizations (JCAHO) all make available voluntary inspections by peers, and each has its own written standards.

About 5% of the general population donates blood with an average of 1.7 donations per donor per year to provide the 13 million red cell products that are transfused annually to over four million patients. Almost all donations are from volunteers, but some places in the United States still pay for donor blood, and according to FDA regulations these units must be labeled "Paid Donor." Twenty-five years ago, more paid donor blood was used, but blood from paid donations has carried a four to eight times greater risk for hepatitis transmission (Kahn, 1981). Consequently, the use of paid donor blood has almost been and should be eliminated.

Donor Registration

The first step in the donation process, registration, makes a record of the donor identification so that the donor can be contacted in the future, if necessary. The information requested includes full name, date of birth, social security number, or other appropriate means of identification (driver's license number), date of donation, address, telephone number, and sex. Additionally, race may be asked in order to allow the reference laboratory to more easily identify donors of specific compatible types for patients with antibody problems. The donors must also sign a consent form giving permission to draw the unit and perform required laboratory testing (e.g., for human immunodeficiency virus [HIV]).

Donor Selection

The decision on whether to accept or defer a donor is based on two broad questions. Might the procedure be harmful to the donor? Might the donor's blood be a risk to the recipient? The FDA (U.S. Department of Health and Human Services, 21 CFR), the American Association of Blood Banks (AABB) (Jones, 1994; Klein, 1994; Walker, 1993), the American Red Cross, and the College of American Pathologists all have medical guidelines and requirements to help make this determination. Most blood centers have a medical deferral rate of less than 12% (Tomasulo, 1980b).

Medical History and Miniphysical

The following is an abbreviated summary based on the AABB donor criteria (Jones, 1994; Klein, 1994; Walker, 1993). The medical history and limited physical examination are performed on the day of donation. This interview must be conducted in an area that permits adequate privacy so that other persons nearby cannot hear the answers to the questions.

Basic Qualifications of the Potential Blood Donor

1. Appears to be in good health.
2. Age: at least 18 years old (age of majority) or, if state law permits, 17 years old. Persons younger than 17 may donate with written permission from their legal guardian. In the past, the upper age limit for blood donation was 66 without the blood bank medical director's approval. However, so many successful homologous and autologous donations have taken place in donors over 75 years of age that the upper age limit for blood donation is no longer defined.
3. Body weight: 110 lb (50kg) or more to remove 450 (±45) mL of blood collected in 63 mL of citrate phosphate dextrose (CPD) or citrate phosphate dextrose adenine (CPDA-1) anticoagulant plus up to 30 mL of additional blood used for testing. Donors under 110 lb may be drawn if the volume of blood donated is decreased in proportion to their weight and if the anticoagulant is decreased accordingly (Walker, 1993, pp. 11–12). Unexplained weight loss of more than 10 lb is a reason for deferral.
4. Temperature: not to exceed 37.5°C or 99.5°F.
5. Pulse: shall reveal no pathologic cardiac abnormalities; should be regular, 50 to 100 beats per minute; a lower pulse rate is acceptable for athletes.
6. Blood pressure: systolic pressure no higher than 180 mm Hg; diastolic pressure not higher than 100 mm Hg; exceptions may be made by the blood bank physician.
7. Minimum hemoglobin:

By fingerstick, by venipuncture, or by ear lobe puncture:

For both males and females—specific gravity by copper sulfate > 1.053, 12.5 g/dL hemoglobin (Hb), 38% hematocrit (HCT).

Deferral

1. Permanent: high-risk history for AIDS, which includes (a) men who have had sex with another man any time since 1977, (b) hemophiliacs, (c) intravenous drug abusers, either past or present, or (d) persons who have engaged in sex for money or drugs any time since 1977; confirmed positive laboratory test for AIDS; symptoms of AIDS; history of viral hepatitis after age 11; the only donor implicated in a post-transfusion hepatitis or AIDS case; confirmed positive test for hepatitis B surface antigen (HBsAg); positive tests for hepatitis B core antibody (anti-HBc); confirmed positive test for hepatitis C antibody (HCAb); confirmed positive test for human T-cell lymphotropic virus (HTLV)-1/2; malignant solid tumors, except for basal cell carcinoma of the skin and carcinoma in situ of the cervix; hematologic malignancies; chemotherapeutic agents administered for malignancy; chronic cardiopulmonary, liver, or renal disease; serious abnormal bleeding tendencies; and those who have ever taken the drug etretinate (Tegison) for the treatment of psoriasis.

The two items listed above stating "since 1977" are under review for blood donors and may be changed to read "in the preceding 5 years," as per Centers for Disease Control and Prevention (CDC) guidelines published for tissue banks (CDC, May 20, 1994).

In December 1987, the FDA asked blood centers to permanently defer donors who received pituitary-derived human growth hormone (FDA memorandum November 25, 1987). The NIH reported that some persons who received this pituitary-derived hormone contracted Creutzfeldt-Jacob disease many years later (NIDDK Fact Sheet, 1987). It should be noted that recombinant human growth hormone, which is not associated with Creutzfeldt-Jacob disease, became available for use in 1985. Additionally, persons who have received a tissue transplant of cornea or dura mater must be permanently deferred because of the risk of transmission of the Creutzfeldt-Jacob agent.

2. Temporary: active disease under treatment such as cold, flu, tuberculosis, syphilis, infections; curable dis-

4

eases of the heart, lung, kidney, liver, and gastrointestinal (GI) tract; and treatment with antibiotics.
3. For three years: an immigrant or refugee coming from an area considered endemic for malaria, three years after departure, or those who have had a diagnosis of malaria, three years after becoming asymptomatic.
4. For one year: after hepatitis B immune globulin administration, after therapeutic rabies vaccination (after bite from an animal), rape victims, healthcare workers with percutaneous exposure to blood or body fluids, close contact with viral hepatitis, tattoo, sexual contact with a prostitute or other persons in a high-risk group for AIDS; incarceration in a jail for more than 72 consecutive hours, transfusion of blood components, travel to areas endemic for malaria (with or without prophylactic therapy). Note that alanine aminotransferase (ALT) testing is no longer required for the donor selection process.
5. For two months: recent blood donation.
6. For six weeks: following delivery of a baby.
7. For one month: German measles (rubella) vaccination and after cessation of the drug isotretinoin (Accutane) for acne treatment or after the cessation of the drug finasteride (Proscar) for the treatment of benign prostatic hyperplasia.
8. For two weeks: after vaccination with oral polio, measles (rubeola), mumps or yellow fever, or for two weeks after the immune reaction to smallpox vaccination.
9. For 48 hours: whole blood donation deferred after hemapheresis.

In addition, the donor, in many instances, is able to confidentially self-exclude his or her unit so that he or she may indicate that it should be tested but not used for transfusion. Many blood centers accomplish this task by using a non-eye-readable, barcoded label applied to the donor registration form or the blood bag that denotes whether or not the unit may be used for transfusion.

Phlebotomy

The donor is placed in the supine position, either on a flat bed or in a specially designed donor chair. The donor blood bag, sample tubes, and donor record should be properly identified and labeled before blood is drawn. The venipuncture site should be free of skin lesions. Both antecubital fossae must be inspected for needle marks, a sign of drug addiction.

A tourniquet is applied to the upper arm above the antecubital venipuncture site. The prospective area is palpated by the phlebotomist to evaluate and determine the best vein. The tourniquet is released, and then the skin overlying the chosen vein is prepared using an aseptic technique. A soap scrub is performed followed by application of a germicidal solution, which is usually an iodine derivative. Blood is removed via a sterile, closed container system and a single venipuncture. If more than one skin puncture is necessary, another sterile closed system container with another attached sterile needle must be used. Because multiple blood components are made from a single blood donor, the closed system chosen usually has a main plastic bag with additionally attached satellite bags.

Four hundred fifty milliliters ±10% (405 to 495 mL) of blood are withdrawn over a period of 7 to 10 minutes and mixed with 63 mL of citrate phosphate dextrose adenine-1 (CPDA-1) or citrate phosphate dextrose (CPD) anticoagulant. Additionally, a maximum of 30 mL are drawn into pilot tubes for testing for a theoretical total maximum of 525 mL of whole blood drawn. During the phlebotomy procedure, the blood and anticoagulant are mixed at least one to two times per minute. At the end of the procedure, the tubing is clamped near the needle, and the needle is removed from the donor's arm. The blood in the tubing is then stripped into the bag for purposes of anticoagulation, and then the blood is allowed to run back into the tubing. The tubing is then sealed to provide segments for future testing and crossmatching.

After the blood is collected, it is stored between 1°C and 6°C, unless it is to be used as a source of platelets. If used for platelet production, it should be stored at room temperature (20°C to 24°C) until the platelets are removed. The platelets must be separated from the blood within eight hours of collection.

Donor Reactions

One of the most common adverse responses to blood donation is the vasovagal reaction. Its major manifestation is a slow heart rate (sometimes less than 60 beats per minute) as opposed to hypovolemic shock, wherein the heart rate is often greater than 100 beats per minute. In both the vasovagal reaction and hypovolemia, additional signs and symptoms include dizziness, diaphoresis, pallor, nausea, vomiting, and even fainting. Vasovagal reactions may be caused by pain (at the time of needle insertion), apprehension, or the sight of blood. Symptoms of hypovolemia can occur during blood donation in someone who is already partially dehydrated or on a hot day, and, therefore, occurs more frequently in the summer.

Sometimes apprehension can cause hyperventilation leading to respiratory alkalosis, which may induce tonic-clonic movements similar to a convulsion. If a convulsion-type reaction does occur, administration of oxygen with appropriate intervention to prevent airway obstruction should ensue. Hyperventilation can be corrected by having the donor breathe into a paper bag.

Hematomas occur when the integrity of the vein is compromised by the needle. The arm should be elevated, and compression should be applied to the site. Cold compresses should be used at the venipuncture site several times during the first 24 to 48 hours to help stop the bleeding and ease the pain. The cold compresses are then discontinued, and warm compresses may be employed several times daily to ameliorate pain. The donor should be told to refrain from exercising that arm for a few days. Tylenol and not aspirin should be used for pain, because aspirin may cause further bleeding because of its antiplatelet activity.

For the more severe reaction in which hypotension is suspected, it is best to stop the phlebotomy by removing the needle and elevate the legs by placing pillows under the feet, legs, and thighs so that the legs are above the head. This will cause blood to flow into the brain and, it is hoped, alleviate the symptoms of hypotension. If the donor is conscious, fluids should be administered orally. If hypotension is prolonged (longer than 45 minutes) so that the donor cannot stand up, it may be necessary to administer intravenous fluids to the donor in order to stabilize the blood pressure.

BLOOD PROCESSING TESTS

ABO and Rh Typing (see Chap. 30)

The ABO group is tested on the red cells by "forward typing" the donor cells using known anti-A and anti-B reagents. The "reverse typing" examines the donor sera for expected antibodies and is performed using known A and B reagent red blood cells. Any discrepancies between forward and reverse typings must be resolved before the donor unit can be released (see Chap. 30).

Direct typing for the Rh_0 (D) antigen is performed using an anti-D reagent and the appropriate control. Persons typing D-negative on initial testing must be examined by the antihuman globulin (AHG) test for the detection of the D^u variant (weak D). All ABO types and Rh_0 (D) negative units must be confirmed by the hospital transfusion service prior to transfusion.

Antibody Screen

About 4 in 1000 blood donations demonstrate unexpected antibodies. It is the usual practice to pool four donor sera and then test for unexpected antibodies using screening reagent red blood cells. Pooling dilutes any antibodies present but will still detect any moderately strong antibodies. Any weak antibodies not detected will be greatly diluted when the unit is transfused, causing no untoward effect in the recipient.

Syphilis

The wisdom of testing blood donors for syphilis has been questioned for many years, but such testing continues to be required. If the donor has spirochetemia, serologic tests are usually negative, whereas, in the presence of antispirochete antibodies, the donor blood is not infectious. Additionally, spirochetes cannot survive in blood stored for 96 hours at 1°C to 6°C (Chambers, 1969). However, the FDA and the AABB require that syphilis testing be performed as a surrogate marker for detecting donors who might be at a high risk for transmitting transfusion-related diseases.

Hepatitis (see Chap. 12)

Blood testing for hepatitis B began in the early 1970s. Scientists soon found that most post-transfusion hepatitis cases did not have the characteristics of either hepatitis A or B, and the term non-A, non-B hepatitis was coined for these residual cases. With the discovery of the etiologic agent for non-A, non-B hepatitis in the late 1980s, now referred to as hepatitis C, it was further possible to define another non-A, non-B hepatitis entity called hepatitis E. Hepatitis E is an epidemic infection contracted from contaminated water and not associated with blood transfusions.

Eighty to ninety percent of post-transfusion hepatitis is caused by hepatitis C (non-A, non-B hepatitis), 10% by hepatitis B virus, and a small percentage by cytomegalovirus, Epstein-Barr virus, and hepatitis A virus. Hepatitis B and hepatitis C are initially relatively mild diseases in most cases, but both can go on to become chronic hepatitis and cirrhosis. The chronic complications of hepatitis occur much more frequently with hepatitis C than with hepatitis B. Hepatitis A often is a mild disease that has no serious long-term effects, because recovery provides lasting immunity with no known associated chronic viral carrier state. Hepatitis A has only rarely been implicated in transfusion-transmitted hepatitis (Noble, 1984; Sheretz, 1984). Consequently, blood intended for transfusion is only tested for hepatitis B and hepatitis C.

Each unit of donated blood is tested for hepatitis B surface antigen (HBsAg) by enzyme immunoassay (EIA) or radioimmunoassay (RIA) third-generation methods. Because false-positive results for HBsAg occur, the FDA has developed a donor re-entry algorithm, as shown in Figure 31–1, to be used to re-enter donors into the system when initial testing for HBsAg is positive (FDA memorandum, December 2, 1987). A third-generation, FDA-licensed HBsAg test and an FDA-licensed confirmatory test (neutralization) for HBsAg must be used in order for this re-entry algorithm to apply. For complete details on FDA compliance with this protocol, or any future protocol, see the original document.

ALT and hepatitis B core antibody (anti-HB_c) tests have been performed as surrogate tests for the detection of hepatitis C (non-A, non-B hepatitis) to prevent as much as 58% of transfusion-transmitted hepatitis (Menitove, 1988). During the summer of 1986, the AABB required that the ALT test be implemented and did the same for the anti-HBc test during the fall of 1987. Even with the implementation of the original hepatitis C antibody testing in May of 1990, these two surrogate tests were retained to provide the safest units of blood possible. With the increased sensitivity of the upgraded hepatitis C antibody test, there was no advantage to continuing ALT testing, so the AABB dropped the requirement to perform ALT testing on blood donors in June of 1995. ALT testing was never a requirement of the FDA. Many blood banks continue to use ALT testing in order to meet the requirements of the European pharmaceutical industry. The European ALT cutoff is usually twice the upper limit of normal. All blood components from units testing above the cutoff should be discarded and the donor notified of the abnormal result.

Units found to be positive for anti-HBc are discarded. Because there is some question as to the reproducibility of positive test results for anti-HBc, the donors are notified and indefinitely excluded if (1) any two donations show a positive anti-HBc test or (2) a positive anti-HBc is confirmed by another method (EIA versus RIA) or by another company's reagents or by showing that there is also a positive anti-HBs. Even though anti-HBc positive donors are excluded as whole blood donors, their plasma may be included in plasma fractionation pools used to make derivatives. It is believed that anti-HBc plasma units, which often also contain anti-HBs, should be included in these pools to neutralize any small amounts of HBsAg not detected by current testing methods (Menitove, 1988).

On May 2, 1990, the FDA licensed a first-generation test

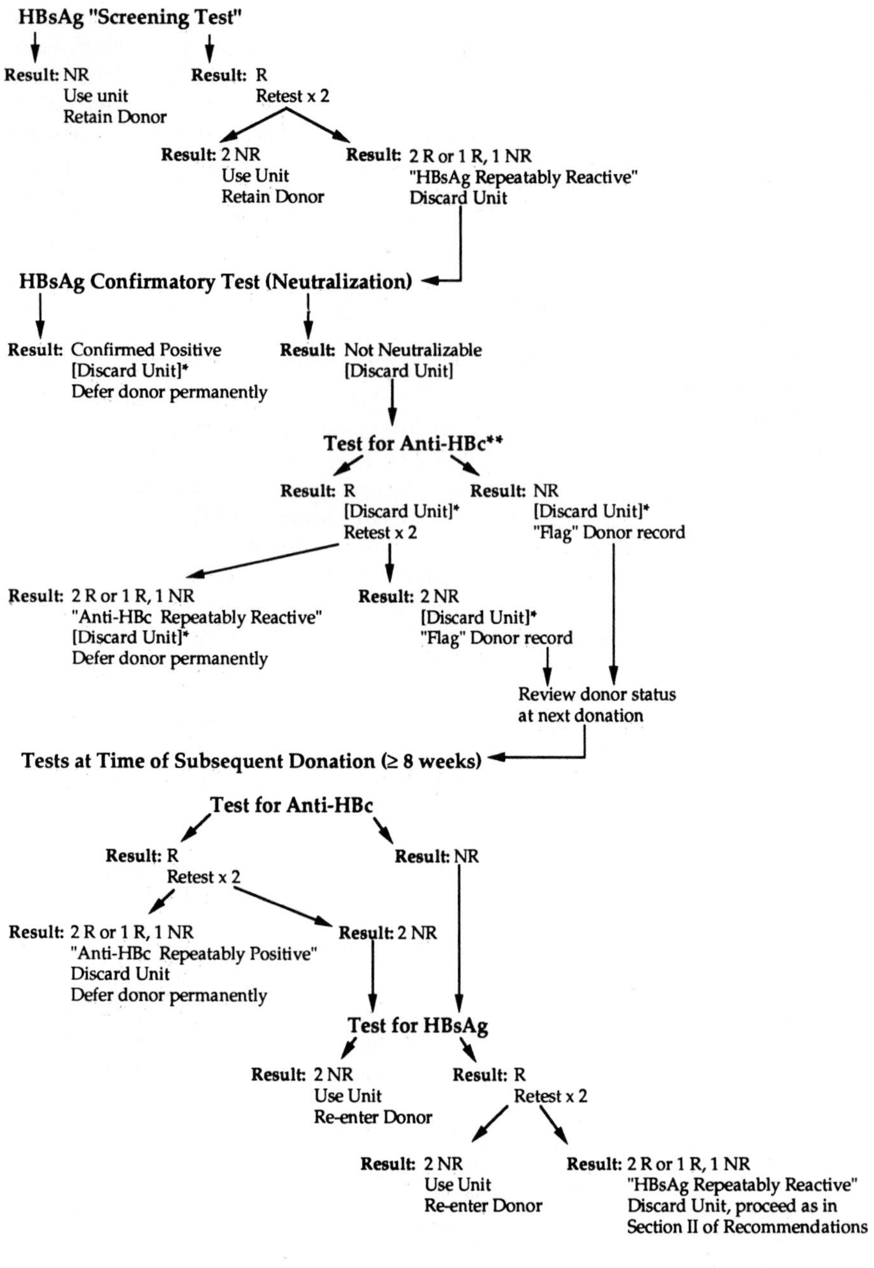

Figure 31–1. Flow chart for hepatitis B surface antigen testing in donors. NR = nonreactive; R = reactive. (Figure modified from FDA memorandum, December 2, 1987. For complete details on FDA compliance with this protocol or any future protocol, see original document.)

for detecting antibodies to hepatitis C virus (HCV). This test primarily detected antibodies to the c100-3 antigen (nonstructural region), a single recombinant antigen. On March 13, 1992, the FDA licensed the second-generation EIA test, referred to as the multi-antigen test because it detects antibodies to HCV using several recombinant antigens—the composite antigen c200 (includes two antigens from the nonstructural region, c100-3 and c33c) and the nucleocapsid protein c22-3. Even this more sensitive second-generation test will not detect about 10% of persons infected with HCV (Alter, 1994).

Two FDA-licensed supplemental tests are available to determine further specificity of those persons testing repeatedly reactive by the screening EIA test for HCV. Both of these tests use the recombinant immunoblot assay (RIBA). Specimens are classified as (1) positive if at least two of the four commercial recombinant HCV antigens show reactivity, (2) indeterminate if (a) only one antigen shows reactivity or (b) only one antigen shows reactivity and there is reactivity to superoxide dismutase, and (3) negative if (a) there is no reactivity or (b) there is only reactivity to superoxide dismutase.

Although these supplemental tests for HCV antibody are positive in the vast majority of those from the high-risk population (intravenous drug abusers, homosexuals), they are confirmed as positive in only about 50% of the low-risk donor population (Alter, 1994).

Donors testing repeatedly reactive for anti-HCV by EIA testing on initial presentation may be considered for re-entry as donors after a minimum waiting period of 6 months (FDA memo, August 5, 1993). To be re-entered, a donor must test nonreactive in both a licensed multi-antigen EIA screening test and a licensed multi-antigen supplemental test for antibodies to HCV.

Donors should be permanently deferred (1) if they test reactive more than once by an FDA-licensed EIA multi-antigen screening test for anti-HCV or (2) if they test repeatedly reactive on an initial FDA-licensed multi-antigen test and the result is confirmed on an FDA-licensed supplemental test. Donors placed in either of these two categories may not be considered for re-entry. Blood products that are repeatedly reactive to anti-HCV on testing are discarded. Currently, lookback for anti-HCV is not required. The concepts of donor re-entry and lookback are defined in detail in the next topic, AIDS.

AIDS

As knowledge concerning AIDS evolved, the blood banking community took steps to attempt to stop transfusion-transmitted AIDS. In March 1983, the FDA issued guidelines for self-deferral of donors at risk for AIDS: male homosexuals or bisexuals with multiple male partners, intravenous drug abusers, immigrants from Haiti or Central Africa after 1977, hemophiliacs, persons showing symptoms of AIDS (night sweats, prolonged episodes of fever or diarrhea, lymphadenopathy, significant unexplained weight loss, thrush, or evidence of Kaposi's sarcoma), and sexual partners of these groups. In December 1984, the FDA redefined risk behavior for "multiple" homosexual partners as more than one; in September 1985, the definition became even more stringent when the FDA announced that even one homosexual encounter since 1977 was to be considered high-risk behavior. Human immunodeficiency virus (HIV) antibody testing began in March 1985, and soon thereafter, there was concern that high-risk persons might use the blood center to obtain a free test in those areas without alternative test sites. Consequently, the FDA asked blood centers to provide a system whereby donors could not only expect their blood to be fully tested but confidentially exclude their unit from being transfused. In October 1986, sexual contact with a prostitute during the previous six months was recognized as high-risk behavior by the FDA. The FDA added sub-Saharan Africa to the high-risk category in April 1988 because of the risk of HIV-2.

Because of the availability of an HIV-2 test and a combined HIV-1/2 test as well as other technical and scientific advances, the FDA modified the donor selection and deferral procedures as published in a memorandum dated April 23, 1992:

1. Deferral is 12 months instead of a lifetime for the sexual partners of persons demonstrating high-risk behavior.
2. Voluntary, instead of recommended, use of the confidential unit exclusion.
3. Place or country of origin would no longer be used as a reason for deferral.
4. Not only written, but now oral communications are required by appropriately trained personnel who would directly ask each donor whether he or she has engaged in any high-risk behaviors for HIV and who would present educational materials describing the clinical signs and symptoms of AIDS; the records of unsuitable donors would not need to include the answers to each of the direct questions about risk behavior but could indicate that the deferral was based on high-risk behavior.
5. Deferral is 12 months for persons treated for syphilis or gonorrhea.

HIV Antibody Testing

Donor blood HIV screening is performed using one of the commercially available, FDA-licensed combination HIV-1,2 tests performed by EIA. A solid-phase EIA method employing denatured viral antigen coated on beads or microtiter wells is used today. Serum is added to the denatured viral antigen. If anti-HIV-1 or anti-HIV-2 is present in the donor's serum, it will bind to the viral antigen. The HIV antibody (Ab) is detected using antihuman globulin (AHG)-tagged reagents. Initially negative tests are negative. Initially reactive tests are usually repeated twice. If these two repeat tests are negative, the unit is considered negative and used for transfusion. If on total testing, the unit is reactive two of three or three of three times, it is considered repeatedly reactive and all components made from this unit are destroyed. To ensure appropriate counseling of the donor, this repeatedly reactive specimen must undergo a series of supplemental tests to see if it is confirmed positive for either HIV-1 or HIV-2 antibodies, as shown in Figure 31–2. First, the supplementary tests for HIV-1 Ab are performed. If these HIV-1 tests are negative, HIV-2 Ab tests must be performed to rule out the possibility

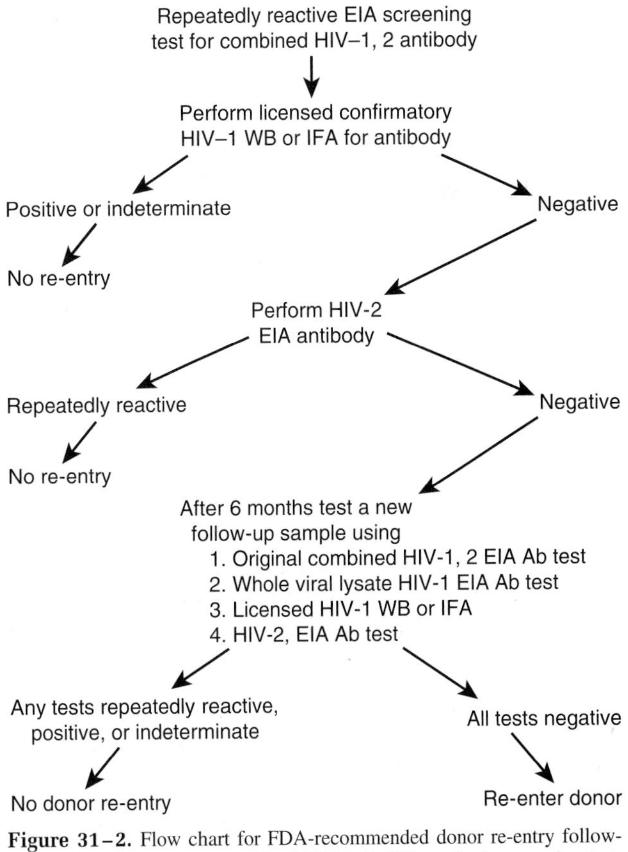

Figure 31–2. Flow chart for FDA-recommended donor re-entry following a repeatedly reactive combined HIV-1, 2, EIA antibody screening test. (Figure modified from FDA memorandum, April 23, 1992. For complete details on FDA compliance with this protocol, see original document.) It is assumed that the HIV-1 antigen test will be part of the HIV Ab re-entry program when it becomes available for use.

4

of HIV-2 infection. The confirmatory tests for HIV-1 include the FDA-licensed HIV-1 Western blot (WB) tests or the FDA-licensed HIV-1 immunofluorescence assay (IFA). For HIV-2, there is an FDA-licensed, EIA Ab test that detects serum HIV-2 Ab directed against HIV-2 antigens.

The WB test (Cyrus, 1988) is simply an antigen-antibody detection procedure in its final step. The difficulty arises in separating the denatured viral antigens into their various purified protein bands. First, the denatured virus is disrupted and electrophoresed on polyacrylamide gel (PAGE), where the viral proteins are separated according to size. This gel is then blotted (transferred) onto nitrocellulose paper by sending a current through the PAGE at 90 degrees to its surface. The separated viral protein bands (antigens) are then exposed to the donor's serum. If HIV-1 Ab is truly present in the serum, specific protein bands will appear after the addition of antihuman globulin (AHG) and will be tagged with an enzyme substrate system, such as biotin-avidin. The specific bands that may appear include (1) protein (p) 18, p24, and p55, which correspond to the group-specific antigen (GAG)/viral core gene products; (2) p31, p51, and p66, which correspond to the polymerase (POL) gene products; and (3) glycoprotein (gp) 41, gp120, and gp160, which correspond to the envelope (ENV) gene products of HIV-1 (CDC, 1989). Several systems for HIV-1 WB interpretation evolved over time:

1. FDA-licensed DuPont test, now referred to as the Cambridge Biotech (Worcester, Massachusetts) test: p24 (GAG), plus p31 (POL), plus gp41 (ENV), or gp120/gp160 (ENV). Note that this original criterion has changed, as explained later.
2. American Red Cross: similar to Cambridge Biotech in that three bands, one corresponding to each of the structural genes—GAG, POL, and ENV—are required, but no specific bands within each category are needed to call a specimen positive. Note that this original criterion has changed, as explained subsequently.
3. Association of State and Territorial Public Health Laboratory Directors (ASTPHLD)/CDC: any two of the following: p24 (GAG), gp41 (ENV), and gp120/gp160 (ENV); note that p31 (POL) is not required.
4. Consortium of Retrovirus Serology Standardization (CRSS): two bands, one from each of the following two categories: (a) p24 (GAG) or p31 (POL), (b) gp41 (ENV) or gp120/gp160 (ENV).

The CDC compared these four methods of interpreting HIV-1 antibody confirmatory testing by Western blot and concluded that the three-gene-product (GAG, POL, and ENV) approach to define a positive Western blot was not sensitive enough for public health or clinical practice because it provided indeterminate, rather than positive, Western blot results in several known AIDS patients (CDC, 1989). It should be noted that the Cambridge Biotech and the Red Cross criteria were originally developed to meet the needs of the low-risk blood donor centers, whereas the criteria of the ASTPHLD/CDC and the CRSS were developed to meet the needs of those patients being seen in clinics serving many high-risk persons. In April of 1992, the Cambridge Biotech package insert changed such that only two of the following three bands are required for confirmation: p24, gp41, and gp120/160, as recommended by the CDC (CDC, 1991). It was apparently felt that the POL gene product, p31, was too low in sensitivity to be required for confirmation. The Red Cross has also changed their requirements from three bands to two bands, consistent with the ASTPHLD/CDC criteria.

An indeterminate HIV-1 Western blot result is reported in the presence of any band or groups of bands that do not meet the criteria for a positive result as noted earlier. These bands may exist in HIV-1 or non-HIV-1 zones. A negative WB pattern is the complete absence of any bands.

For example, a serum specimen is received for HIV-1 Western blot confirmation after having been found repeatedly reactive on the EIA HIV-1,2 antibody screen. If bands were seen on the HIV-1 Western blot in p24 and gp41, all of the current criteria would define this specimen as positive. On the other hand, if bands were noted in p24 and p38 (non-HIV), the specimen would be considered indeterminate. If no bands were seen, the specimen would be negative.

A donor who is HIV-1 Western blot indeterminate still has a chance of developing an HIV-1 antibody diagnostic pattern in the future, but most indeterminates in the donor population either lose their WB reactivity or do not progress over the next six months if they have not been exposed to HIV-1. These indeterminates may be showing some cross-reactivity with a retrovirus other than HIV-1 and cannot be used for transfusion.

High-risk persons who are early seroconverters and show an indeterminate HIV-1 WB pattern will progress to a diagnostic HIV-1 Ab pattern within six months (CDC, 1989).

Because these are antibody identification tests and it takes several weeks to develop antibodies after exposure, it is theoretically possible to have HIV viremia and be able to transmit the virus from donor to recipient while the HIV antibody test is negative. This time frame is called the "window-phase" and was estimated to be 45 days for the blood donor population (Petersen, 1994) in 1992, but 22 to 25 days in 1995 (CCBC Newsletter, Aug. 11, 1995).

In the late 1980s, investigators using polymerase chain reaction (PCR) technology published data implying that the window phase of HIV could be as long as one year. However, this work could not be repeated, and the false results are now thought to have occurred because of PCR "carryover" (Busch, 1992). Because of these original studies, the waiting period for blood donors involved in HIV-related exposure activities was prolonged from six months to one year.

The HIV-1 antigen test was not originally required for blood donor screening because, after review of the available data on March 23, 1989, the FDA Blood Products Advisory Committee concluded that this test would provide no additional blood donor screening information. However, the committee did recommend that the HIV-1 p24 antigen test be licensed for diagnostic and prognostic indicators in patients. The FDA changed its policy on HIV-1 antigen (Ag) screening of blood donors in August of 1995 because there were documented incidents of HIV-1 transmission through blood transfusion from donors who were HIV-1 Ab negative but who were later found in retrospective studies to be HIV-1 Ag positive. It is anticipated that with the addition of the HIV-1 Ag test, the window phase will decrease by about six days to somewhere between 16 and 19 days and that 5 to 10 transfusion-transmitted HIV-1 cases will be prevented (CCBC Newsletter, 1995). When HIV-1 Ag testing starts, all repeatedly reactive HIV-1 Ag tests will require a neutralization test for confirmation. Those donors confirming positive on the neutralization test will be permanently deferred, and their donation will be discarded. Donors who are negative on neutralization testing will (1) have their current donation discarded; (2) be deferred, and (3) should be retested on a newly drawn specimen at least 8 weeks later, at which time they could be automatically reinstated if all new donor screening tests, including the HIV-1 Ag, are found to be negative and the donors meet all other suitability criteria. Those donors who are repeatedly HIV-1 Ag reactive on any subsequent evaluation must be permanently deferred, regardless of the results of the neutralization test.

The April 23, 1992, FDA memorandum also permitted the use of an alternative HIV-1 confirmatory technology, the licensed immunofluorescence assay, Fluorognost HIV-1 IFA (Waldheim Pharmazeutika, GmbH, Vienna, Austria). In this IFA, T cells that express HIV-1 antigen (the virus) are fixed to wells on a glass slide. Separate wells containing fixed T cells negative for HIV-1 antigen (uninfected) are provided as a negative control. HIV-1 antibodies, if present in the serum, will bind to the fixed infected T cells. These bound antibodies are detected with AHG conjugated to fluorescein, which emits fluorescent light in the presence of ultraviolet light. The fluorescent light emission is evaluated microscopically and reported as positive, negative, or indeterminate (FDA, April 23, 1992).

In those specimens repeatedly reactive by the combined HIV-1,2 EIA Ab test, in which supplemental HIV-1 Ab testing is negative or indeterminate, the FDA-licensed HIV-2 EIA Ab test must be performed to rule out the presence of HIV-2 Ab. If this HIV-2 EIA Ab test is repeatedly reactive, other investigational, supplemental tests may further delineate the nature of this repeatedly reactive HIV-2 Ab test for the purpose of counseling the donor (FDA memorandum, April 23, 1992):

1. An HIV-2 WB test is considered positive if band gp105 (ENV) alone, or with gp34 (ENV), plus either bands (1) p26 (GAG) or (2) p31 (POL, endonuclease) or p68/58/55 complex (POL, reverse transcriptase) are present (CBC, HIV-2 WB kit, package insert, Cambridge Biotech Corp., Worcester, Massachusetts); the indeterminate and negative WB categories are defined as for the HIV-1 WB test.
2. A radioimmunoprecipitation HIV-2 assay.
3. A recombinant HIV-2 EIA Ab test.

Shortly after the introduction of HIV antibody testing of blood donors, the ethical issue of whether to tell past recipients that they had received blood from a currently HIV antibody positive donor arose. In June 1986, the national blood banking organizations suggested notifying these recipients and referred to the process as "lookback." Currently, in the blood banking community, there is some discussion on the necessity of a universal lookback (CCBC Newsletter, Sept. 2, 1994). In universal lookback, an attempt is made to perform the standard tests for transfusion-transmitted diseases on every blood recipient, about 6 months after a transfusion, as a proactive effort to search for infected individuals and their associated blood donors.

In the volunteer blood donor population, approximately 0.12% of donors are repeatedly reactive using the combination HIV-1,2 screening EIA test, as shown in Table 31–1. Only about 14% of those in whom the test is repeatedly reactive will be confirmed as positive by the FDA-licensed Western blot test for HIV-1, the FDA-licensed IFA for HIV-1, and the FDA-licensed recombinant EIA antibody test for HIV-2. Consequently, the vast majority of the combined HIV-1,2 screening EIA Ab tests in the low-risk donor population that are repeatedly reactive give a biologically false-positive reaction. This false-positive reaction could be due to (1) technical problems in performing the test, such as improper washing or conducting the test at improper reaction temperatures, and (2) biological causes, such as reactivity between HLA-DR antibodies in the donor's serum, which react with HLA-DR antigens present on the cell line used to produce the viral antigen or serum containing high IgG levels or serum from those who have recently been vaccinated against flu. Because of this high rate of biological false-positive reactivity, the FDA has provided a blood donor re-entry algorithm (FDA memorandum, April 23, 1992), as shown in Figure 31–2, the important aspects of which include:

1. A 6-month interval between donor specimen collections to rule out viral incubation in the window phase.
2. Negative reactions by a licensed supplemental HIV-1 Ab test—the HIV-1 WB or the HIV-1 IFA.
3. Negative reactions by a licensed HIV-1 EIA Ab test made from a whole viral lysate.
4. Negative reactions by a second, different, licensed HIV-2 Ab test.

For complete details concerning FDA compliance with

4

Table 31–1. REPEATEDLY REACTIVE AND CONFIRMATORY TESTING FOR TRANSFUSION-TRANSMITTED DISEASES

	ALT							
	1–2× NML	*>2× NML*	**HBsAG**	**Anti HIV-1,2**	**Anti HTLV-1,2**	**Anti-HCV**	**Anti-HBC**	**STS**
1992–93*	1.32%	0.194%	0.055% RR	0.115% RR	0.058% RR	0.394% RR	1.39%	0.28%
% confirmatory of those RR*	—	—	70%	14%	9%	67%	—	—
Risk of disease from transfusion†	—	—	1/200,000 donors	1/225,000	1/70,000	1/3,300		

NML = normal; RR = repeatedly reactive; STS = serologic test for syphilis

*Data from Sandler GS, Smith J: Preface to the 1994 Overview. *In* Brubaker DB, Lamberson H, Dock N (eds): Technical and Public Health Aspects of Disease Testing. Bethesda, Maryland, American Association of Blood Banks, 1994.

†Dodd RY: Adverse consequences of blood transfusion: Qualitative risk estimates. *In* Nance ST (ed): Blood Supply: Risks, Perceptions and Prospects for the Future. Bethesda, Maryland, American Association of Blood Banks, 1994, pp 1–24.

this and any other FDA algorithm, please see the original document.

HTLV-1

In December 1988, blood centers were required by the FDA to perform human T-cell lymphotropic virus type 1 (HTLV-1) antibody testing on each unit of blood collected (CDC, 1988; FDA memorandum, November 29, 1988). Because the virus has been transmitted only by cellular blood products, the FDA has not required source plasma donations, intended for use in further manufacturing, to be tested. The screening test is an HTLV-1 EIA Ab detection method similar in principle to that performed for HIV antibody. Those units repeatedly reactive (two of three or three of three elevations) for HTLV-1 antibody are destroyed, and nonlicensed supplemental tests are used to confirm the specificity of the EIA Ab test:

1. The HTLV-1 WB test best determines antibodies to the group specific antigen [GAG] core proteins, p19, p24, and p28; the envelope proteins gp46 and gp61/68 complex are only variably present.
2. The radioimmunoprecipitation assay (RIPA) best determines antibodies to the envelope proteins gp46 and gp61/68 complex.
3. A recombinant WB that contains the usual Western blot antigens as well as recombinant p21e and recombinant gp46 antigen bands.

Whatever systems are used for confirmation, to be considered positive, the HTLV-1 confirmatory tests must demonstrate antibodies to the p24 GAG core protein plus antibodies to at least one ENV glycoprotein band—gp46 or the gp61/68 complex (CDC, 1988; FDA memorandum, November 29, 1988). Some investigators are determining the usefulness of the recombinant p21e antigen (Ness, 1994) in the confirmatory scheme. Because of the antigenic and structural similarities between HTLV-1 and HTLV-2, routinely available testing methods cannot distinguish between these two retroviral antibodies. However, testing with PCR and with recombinant HTLV-2 antigens may be useful in counseling patients thought to be positive for HTLV-2.

Donors whose previous HTLV-1 antibody test results were repeatedly reactive on EIA, but who were not confirmed may donate again at a later time. If the test results on that next donation are nonreactive on EIA, the unit can be used for transfusion (Walker, 1993, p. 103). However, if the test results on this second donation are HTLV-1 repeatedly reactive by EIA, whether confirmed or not, the donor is notified and indefinitely deferred (CDC, 1988; FDA memorandum, November 29, 1988).

A lookback program for HTLV-1 has also been recommended, but it must be realized that it may take years to decades for the virus to manifest itself as either adult T cell leukemia/lymphoma or as tropical spastic paraparesis, also known as the HTLV-1-associated myelopathy (Fridley, 1989). Apparently, the vast majority of persons who are HTLV-1 antibody positive never demonstrate symptoms (CDC, 1988; FDA memorandum, November 29, 1988). HTLV-2 virus may be associated with hairy cell leukemia (CDC, 1988; FDA memorandum, November 29, 1988) or chronic neurodegenerative diseases (Ness, 1994). Neither HTLV-1 nor HTLV-2 causes AIDS.

Further information on transfusion-transmitted diseases, such as cytomegalovirus (CMV) and parvovirus B19, may be found later in this chapter in the section entitled Diseases Transmitted Through Blood Transfusion.

Table 31–1 shows that the positive results of many donors are not confirmed after they test repeatedly reactive by the screening test. These viral screening tests are highly sensitive but not specific, so this finding is not unexpected. Table 31–1, under "risk of disease from transfusion," essentially shows the window phase for each of the viruses listed. The risk of transfusion-transmitted hepatitis C is 1 in 3300 using the first-generation hepatitis C test and is expected to be much lower with third-generation testing.

BLOOD PRESERVATION

Anticoagulants and Red Blood Cell Additives

Citrate was first used as a blood anticoagulant in 1914 (Hustin). It binds calcium and therefore prevents the activation of the coagulation cascade. Dextrose was added to citrate in 1916 (Rous) to provide an energy source for the red blood cells, but because of the alkaline pH, caramelization took place during heat sterilization. Consequently, the citrate and dextrose had to be separately sterilized and mixed together just prior to the blood collection. In the early 1940s, the pH of this citrate dextrose mixture was decreased by adding citric acid (Loutit, 1943). This new solution, acid citrate dextrose (ACD), with a lowered pH, could be heat sterilized without caramelization and became the standard blood anticoagulant.

During the 1950s, citrate phosphate dextrose (CPD) was developed (Gibson, 1957). CPD was prepared by adding inorganic phosphate buffer to ACD to increase adenosine triphosphate (ATP) production and therefore increase red blood cell viability. CPD requires less citric acid than ACD does. Consequently, the pH is higher, so that 2,3-diphosphoglycerate (2,3-DPG) is better maintained during red blood cell storage and is not depleted for two weeks. 2,3-DPG promotes the release of oxygen, from hemoglobin in the red blood cells, to the tissues.

Adenine was shown to improve the survival of stored, anticoagulated, donor red blood cells (Simon, 1962). The addition of adenine to CPD, CPDA-1, by commercial blood bag manufacturers during the 1970s increased the maximum shelf-life of blood from 21 days (ACD, CPD) to 35 days at 1°C to 6°C storage. Adenine provides a substrate for red blood cells to maximize ATP synthesis and thereby increases red blood cell viability.

The shelf-life of blood was increased to 42 days with the commercial introduction of red blood cell additives (Roberts, 1986) during the 1980s. First, blood is collected in CPD or citrate phosphate double dextrose (CP2D). Then the plasma is removed, and the red blood cell additive (e.g., Adsol [Fenwal]) is added from an integrally attached bag. The additive solution consists of saline, adenine, and a high concentration of dextrose. Mannitol, a red blood cell membrane stabilizing agent, may also be part of the additive system.

Table 31–2. CHARACTERISTICS OF WHOLE BLOOD STORED FOR 35 DAYS IN CPDA-1 (N = 10)*

	Storage Time (Days)				
	0	*7*	*14*	*21*	*35*
Plasma dextrose (mg/dL)	432	374	357	324	282
Plasma sodium (mEq/L)	169	162	159	157	153
Plasma potassium (mEq/L)	3.3	12.3	17.6	21.7	17.2
Plasma chloride (mEq/L)	84	81	79	77	79
Plasma bicarbonate (mEq/L)	12.0	17.0	12.5	12.2	8.0
Whole-blood pH	7.16	6.94	6.93	6.87	6.73
Whole-blood lactate (mg/dL)	19	62	91	130	202
Plasma LD (units)	296	1002	1222	1457	1816
Whole-blood ammonia (μg/dL)	82	280	423	521	703
Plasma hemoglobin (mg/dL)	0.5	13.1	24.7	24.7	45.6
WBC ($\times 10^3/\mu$L)	7.2	4.0	3.0	2.8	2.4
Hematocrit (%)	35	36	35	36	36
RBC hemoglobin (g/dL)	12	12	12	12	12
RBC ($\times 10^6/\mu$L)	4.0	4.0	3.9	3.9	3.9
Red blood cell 2,3-DPG (μmol/gHb)†	13.2	—	—	—	0.7
Red blood cell ATP (μmol/gHb)	4.18	—	—	—	2.40

*Data from Latham JT, Bove JR, Weirich FL: Chemical and hematologic changes in stored CPDA-1 blood. Transfusion, 1982; 22:158.

†Moore GL, Peck CC, Sohmer PR, Zuck TF: Some properties of blood stored in anticoagulant CPDA-1 solution. Transfusion, 1981; 21:135.

From Snyder EL (ed.): Blood Transfusion Therapy, A Physician's Handbook. Arlington, Virginia, American Association of Blood Banks, 1987, p 7.

Biochemical Changes During Liquid Storage

For all the anticoagulant preservative solutions mentioned above, biochemical changes occur during red blood cell storage. Comparison of the first day of CPDA-1 storage to the last day of shelf-life shows that the pH drops from about 7.2 to 6.7; ATP drops considerably; 2,3-DPG decreases from 100% to less than 10%; plasma potassium rises; plasma sodium decreases; and plasma hemoglobin increases (Table 31–2). These alterations are of greatest concern during massive and neonatal transfusions.

Storage of Frozen Red Blood Cells

Three methods are used to freeze red blood cells: high glycerol (40% w/v final concentration), agglomeration, and low glycerol (20% w/v final concentration) (Dawson, 1977). This section discusses only the high glycerol method because it is the procedure used by the vast majority of laboratories in the United States (see Frozen Red Blood Cells). Glycerol is a cryoprotective agent that enters the cell, alters its tonicity, and therefore changes its freezing rate.

Freezing should take place using red blood cells less than six days old to maintain high levels of 2,3-DPG. However, red blood cells of any acceptable storage time might be considered for freezing.

Glycerolization takes place at room temperature using red blood cells from which almost all of the plasma has been removed. The slow addition of the glycerol, the constant agitation of the red blood cells, and time for equilibration avoid a sudden change of osmotic pressure that could otherwise contribute to hemolysis during the thawing procedure. A special polyolefin freezing bag is usually used to reduce hemolysis and to provide a container that better withstands the cold temperatures. Because these plastic bags can easily be cracked by handling, they are placed into metal or cardboard canisters for protection. The canister, with its enclosed glycerolized red blood cell product, is then placed in an electric freezer that can maintain temperatures colder than −65°C. Frozen red blood cells processed by acceptable techniques can be stored for up to 10 years.

The frozen red blood cells may be thawed by placing them with their protective canister in a 37°C waterbath or dry warmer. Thawing takes about 10 minutes. The glycerol must be removed gradually from the red blood cells to avoid *in vitro* or *in vivo* hemolysis. Because the intracellular red cell environment of frozen red blood cells is hypertonic (compared with plasma) owing to the glycerol, decreasing concentrations of hypertonic solutions must be used to allow the glycerol to exit from the cells. This is best accomplished with commercially available cell washers. Special procedures must be used for donors with sickle cells or the cells will form a jelly-like mass and hemolyze during deglycerolization (Meryman, 1976).

Following deglycerolization, the shelf-life of the red blood cell product is 24 hours at 1°C to 6°C storage, because the bag has been entered.

PREPARATION AND SELECTION OF BLOOD COMPONENTS AND DERIVATIVES

Preparation of Blood Components

Blood components are prepared from whole blood by using large refrigerated centrifuges. The high-gravity forces developed in these machines cause the blood to separate into liquid plasma and its different cellular elements. Table 31–3 is a chart of common blood components and derivatives

Table 31-3. COMMON BLOOD COMPONENTS AND DERIVATIVES USED IN HEMOTHERAPY

Blood Component or Derivative	Characteristics	Approximate Volume	Shelf-Life	Indications and Comments
Whole blood	RBC and plasma; WBC and platelets not viable after 24 hr storage. Labile clotting factors significantly decreased after 2 days of storage. Hct 35% (dilution by anticoagulant). Blood 450 mL. CPD or CPDA-1 anticoagulant 63 mL.	520 mL	ACD, CPD—21 days at 1–6°C. CPDA—1–35 days at 1–6°C.	Most useful for massive transfusion where both red cell mass and plasma volume are required; active, brisk bleeding. The flow characteristics are rapid.
Packed red blood cells	Packed RBC with reduced plasma volume; WBC, platelets, and coagulation factors as for whole blood. Hct 69%.	260 mL	As whole blood.	Most useful for increasing red cell mass when symptomatic anemia is present; chronic anemia. Hct is high so flow characteristics are viscous and slow. Can be used with colloids or crystalloids to increase rate of flow for active, brisk bleeding or massive transfusion.
Red blood cells with additive solution (adenine-saline)	RBC with reduced plasma volume and an additional 100 mL of additive solution. Hct 53%.	340 mL	42 days at 1–6°C.	Can be used like whole blood or packed red blood cells. Hct is at a slightly elevated level but rapid flow rates can be achieved.
Washed red blood cells	RBC, no plasma, minimal platelets. 70–80% WBC removed if manual wash. 90% WBC removed if automated wash. Hct adjustment as per amount of saline added. 5% loss of red cells due to wash procedure.	250 mL	24 hr at 1–6°C after wash.	Increased red cell mass as for packed red cells. Most useful for preventing febrile and allergic reactions due to leukocytes or plasma proteins and for preventing anaphylactic reaction in IgA-deficient recipients.
Frozen deglycerolized red blood cells	RBC, no plasma, no platelets, removal of 95% of WBC. Hct adjustment as per amount of saline added. Up to 20% of red cells lost due to procedure.	250 mL	10 years at −65°C or colder. 24 hr at 1–6°C after wash.	Most useful for supply of rare blood, inventory control, and autotransfusion. Also, as per washed red blood cells.
Random-donor platelet concentrate	Platelets (5.5×10^{10}); some WBC (i.e., lymphocytes), 50 mL of plasma, few RBC (less than 0.5% Hct).	50 mL	5 days, room temperature (20–24°C) constant, gentle agitation.	Used for quantitative or qualitative platelet disorders. May be used when bleeding (slow ooze) due to severe thrombocytopenia or for prophylactic therapy. 6–10 units raises platelet count about 50,000 per microliter in an adult.
Single-donor platelet concentrate by apheresis	Platelets (3.0×10^{11}); some WBC (i.e., lymphocytes), 250 mL plasma, few RBCs (less than 0.5% Hct).	250 to 300 mL	5 days at room temperature, constant, gentle agitation. 1 day if open system.	Indications as per random-donor platelets. Used as supplement to inventory when there are not enough random-donor platelets. Most useful in immunologically refractory patient when given as HLA match with recipient. Fewer donor exposures.
Single-donor granulocyte concentrate by apheresis	Granulocytes (1.0×10^{10}) and other WBC, 250 mL plasma, minimal platelets, RBC about 10% Hct.	300 mL	12–24 hr at room temperature, no agitation.	Most useful for septic, severely granulocytopenic patient unresponsive to 48 hr of antibiotic therapy. Potential for aggregated WBC to plug pulmonary capillaries. Perform RBC crossmatch because of quantity of RBC present.
Fresh frozen plasma	Plasma proteins, all coagulation factors, complement.	200 to 260 mL	1 year at −18°C, or colder.	Most useful in the bleeding patient with multiple coagulation deficiency problems secondary to liver disease, disseminated intravascular coagulopathy (DIC), or dilutional changes from massive transfusions. Also useful for the treatment of Factor V or Factor XI deficiency. Should not be used as volume expander or source of protein nutrition because of risk of transfusion-transmitted disease.

Table 31–3. COMMON BLOOD COMPONENTS AND DERIVATIVES USED IN HEMOTHERAPY *Continued*

Blood Component or Derivative	Characteristics	Approximate Volume	Shelf-Life	Indications and Comments
Cryoprecipitate	80 units of Factor VIII, other plasma proteins, von Willebrand factor, Factor XIII, fibrinogen (200 mg), fibronectin.	10 to 15 mL	1 year at −18°C or colder.	Most useful for von Willebrand disease, Factor XIII deficiency, or hypofibrinogenemia. See text for exception in von Willebrand variant and for use of DDAVP. Cryoprecipitate should not be used for a newly diagnosed hemophilia A case, because there are factor concentrates available that have been modified to eliminate the AIDS virus and possibly hepatitis.
Factor VIII concentrate	Quantity of Factor VIII units are marked on lyophilized bottle.	25 mL, as per manufacturer's instructions for reconstitution with sterile diluent.	2 yr at 2–8°C storage.	Used for hemophilia A (Factor VIII deficiency). Lacks high molecular weight von Willebrand factor. See text for use of DDAVP.
Factor IX concentrate	Contains Factors II, VII, IX, and X.	25 mL, as per manufacturer's instructions for reconstitution with sterile diluent.	2 yr at 2–8°C storage.	Most useful for patients with hereditary deficiency of Factors II, VII, IX, or X. Sometimes used in patients with high Factor VIII antibodies because product contains activated coagulation factors. May cause DIC if severe liver disease present.
Albumin	5 g/100 mL	250 to 500 mL	3 yr below 30°C.	Most useful for hypovolemic shock or hypoproteinemia.
	25 g/100 mL	50 to 100 mL		Hypertonic (25 g/100mL) albumin solution rapidly increases intravascular oncotic pressure, but draws water from tissues into the intravascular space. Therefore, it is a good idea to monitor arterial and central venous pressure when using this product.
Plasma protein fraction	5 g/100 mL. Contains primarily albumin and some α- and β-globulins.	250 to 500 mL	3 yr below 30°C.	Same as for albumin.
Immune serum globulin	Mostly IgG antibodies, and some IgA and IgM antibodies.	10 mL	3 yr below 30°C.	Treatment or prophylaxis of hypogammaglobulinemia. Prevents and modifies hepatitis A and hepatitis C.
Rh immune globulin	IgG anti-D(Rh_O).	1 mL	1½ yr at 2–8°C.	Prevents hemolytic disease of the newborn in Rh negative women exposed to Rh positive red cells.

showing their characteristics, quantity, shelf-life, and indications. Table 31–4 lists various conditions and the recommended therapy for using specific blood components or derivatives.

Centrifugation

The outcome of centrifugation depends on two factors: the relative centrifugal force (RCF) and the duration of centrifugation. The RCF, or g force, is the product of $1.118 \times 10^{-5} \times r \times N^2$, where r is the radius of the rotor in centimeters and N is the number of revolutions per minute. Because different rotors have different radii, different speeds are used to achieve the same RCF in different centrifuges. The following RCF-per-minute combinations are useful in the preparation of blood components: 5000 g for 5 minutes for preparation of packed RBC or platelet concentrate; 5000 g for 7 minutes for preparation of cryoprecipitate, or cell-free plasma. These combinations are referred to as a "heavy spin," as opposed to 2000 g for 3 minutes, known as a "light spin," which is used to produce platelet-rich plasma.

For preparation of a platelet concentrate, centrifugation is performed at room temperature (20°C to 24°C); for all other blood components, centrifugation is carried out between 1°C and 6°C. Balancing the material in opposite sides of the centrifuge head is important and can be easily done with rubber disks of different weights. A protective plastic bag placed around the blood is useful because of the potential for breakage. The ports and tubings attached to the bag should be protected from breakage. Manual braking of the centrifuge disturbs the contents of the blood bag and should be avoided. All safety precautions should be observed.

Because platelets are in such great demand at most regional blood centers, the following protocol is the most prevalent for producing blood components. The whole blood unit, with its two attached satellite bags, is first centrifuged using a light spin, yielding platelet-rich plasma (PRP) in the upper portion

Table 31–4. BLOOD COMPONENTS AND DERIVATIVES RECOMMENDED FOR VARIOUS CLINICAL CONDITIONS

Clinical Conditions	Preparations Recommended and Comments
Active bleeding	Whole blood or packed red blood cells (RBC), less than 7 days old, if possible, for massive bleeding. Platelets and FFP on occasion for massive bleeding
Anemia: transient	Packed RBC of any acceptable shelf-life
Anemia: aplastic	Washed RBC less than 7 days old (to reduce frequency of transfusion and exogenous iron) and/or leukoreduced RBC to decrease HLA exposure
Routine surgery	Whole blood, packed RBC, of any acceptable shelf-life
Cardiopulmonary bypass	RBC and crystalloid or colloid solutions. Platelets sometimes necessary when off bypass equipment. Fresh frozen plasma (FFP) needed occasionally
Repeated febrile reactions	Leukoreduced RBC and platelets
Repeated allergic reactions	Washed RBC; washed or plasma reduced platelets
Intrauterine transfusion	CMV-negative group O Rh-negative RBC. Irradiation of RBC should be considered to prevent graft versus host disease if fetus <1200 gm or if relative is a directed donor
Exchange transfusion for newborn	CMV-negative whole blood, if available. Packed group O Rh-negative RBC or mother's type less than 7 days old plus 5% albumin. FFP instead of albumin, if coagulation factors are required. Possible irradiation of RBC as for intrauterine transfusion
Immunosuppressed (T-cell)	Leukoreduced, irradiated packed RBC and platelet concentrates and irradiated granulocyte concentrates.
Hemodialysis, renal or hepatic failure	Packed RBC
Anti-IgA requiring transfusion	Washed RBC or blood from IgA-deficient donors
Thrombocytopenia with hemorrhage or impending hemorrhage	Random-donor platelet concentrate. HLA-compatible single-donor apheresed platelets in immunologically refractory patients
Agammaglobulinemia or prevention of hepatitis A, hepatitis B, or hepatitis C	Immune serum globulin, recommended for accidental needle sticks (specific hepatitis A and B immunization is available)
Hemophilia or von Willebrand's disease	DDAVP, if mild to moderate disease: Factor VIII concentrate (pasteurized or equivalent safety measures) for severe hemophilia A. DDAVP or cryoprecipitate for von Willebrand's disease (see text for exceptions in certain variants)
Afibrinogenemia, dysfibrinogenemia, or hypofibrinogenemia	Cryoprecipitate, FFP, no commercial concentrate available
Other coagulopathy	FFP
Shock without hemorrhage	Albumin, other colloids, or crystalloid solutions
Cerebral edema	25% albumin (pulls fluid from tissues into intravascular space) with diuretic therapy
Prevention of Rh sensitization	Rh immune globulin for RH_O(D) negative women to prevent hemolytic disease of the newborn or for inadvertent transfusion of several milliliters of Rh_O(D) positive RBC contained in RH_O(D) positive blood components such as platelets
Uremia-induced platelet dysfunction	Cryoprecipitate and/or DDAVP
Directed donor—blood relative	Irradiated whole blood or packed RBC

and red blood cells (RBC) in the lower portion. The PRP, about 250 mL, is expressed into an attached satellite bag, leaving the RBC in the primary bag. The three attached bags are recentrifuged using a heavy spin to produce an aggregated platelet button from the PRP. Approximately 200 mL of platelet-poor plasma is removed, leaving 50 mL of platelet-poor plasma with the platelet button. The 200 mL of plasma may be placed into the second satellite bag to make recovered plasma or fresh frozen plasma (FFP), or it is returned to the RBC to make modified whole blood. Meanwhile, the bag containing the platelet button and 50 mL of plasma is separated from the primary bag containing the red cells and allowed to rest undisturbed for an hour at room temperature to enhance platelet disaggregation. The platelets are then placed on a mechanical rotator to gently resuspend the platelet button. Most of the platelets from the whole blood unit are present in the platelet concentrate. The platelet concentrate must be agitated continuously at controlled room temperature to maintain optimal platelet function.

Selection of Blood Components

Whole Blood

Whole blood is a product in which all of the red cells and most of the plasma from the original unit remain. The shelf life, at 1°C to 6°C storage, is 35 days for units drawn in CPDA-1 anticoagulant and 21 days for units drawn in CPD or ACD. A whole blood unit could be whole blood, modified by the removal of 50 mL of plasma in the preparation of platelets or 10 to 15 mL of plasma in the preparation of cryoprecipitate. The platelets and white blood cells (WBC) in whole blood are not active because they require separation from whole blood and special storage conditions to maintain their viability and function. There is no scientific justification for the use of "fresh blood" stored for less than 24 hours. The major indication for whole blood is volume replacement in trauma cases in which there is more than a one-third loss of blood volume and impending hemorrhagic shock. This product provides both volume and the oxygen-carrying capacity of red blood cells.

Whole blood should not be considered for those patients with chronic anemia and normal blood volume. The chronic anemia patient needs the oxygen-carrying capacity of the red blood cells and not the volume. Too much volume may cause the patient to go into pulmonary edema. The immediate effect of a one-unit whole blood transfusion in an adult is to increase the hematocrit by about 1% to 3%.

Red Blood Cells

Red blood cells (RBC), also known as packed red blood cells or packed cells, may be prepared from whole blood by overnight sedimentation (during refrigerated storage), or by the more popular refrigerated centrifugation using a heavy spin, anytime during the 21-day or 35-day storage period. Two hundred to 250 mL of plasma will be extracted, leaving the RBC with a hematocrit of approximately 70% to 80%. Quality control is needed to ensure that stored packed RBC have a hematocrit of less than 80% so that there is adequate plasma glucose for RBC metabolism and enough citrate to maintain the pH at acceptable levels (close to 7.0) during the storage period. The immediate effect of transfusing one unit of packed red cells into an adult is to increase the hematocrit by about 3%.

When removing the maximum amount of plasma, leaving a 90% hematocrit for packed RBC, a red blood cell additive system must be used for long term RBC storage. Two major RBC additive systems exist commercially—one in which the original RBC anticoagulant is CPD and the other in which the anticoagulant is CP2D, which contains additional glucose. In both cases, the RBC are packed, and the plasma is removed and replaced with 100 mL of the additive solution present in an integrally attached satellite bag. This solution (Roberts, 1986) consists of saline with (1) adenine, to provide improved RBC viability because of enhanced ATP synthesis, (2) extra glucose, to provide energy for the cells, and in some cases (3) mannitol, which acts as a RBC stabilizing agent. The expiration date of these RBC in additive solutions is extended to 42 days from the date of collection. The increase in acellular fluid of these cells containing 100 mL of additive solution (lower hematocrit), as compared with the usual packed blood cells with only 50 mL of plasma, permits more rapid infusion of blood.

The major indication for packed RBC is to increase the oxygen-carrying capacity of blood in persons with chronic anemia.

Leukocyte-Reduced Red Blood Cells

Packed RBC contain 2×10^9 to 5×10^9 leukocytes per unit; random donor platelet concentrates contain 0.5×10^8 to 2.5×10^8 leukocytes per unit; apheresed platelets by older techniques contained 10^9 WBC, but apheresed platelets with current leukoreduced protocols contain only 10^6 WBC (Lane, 1994).

Several methods are available to prepare leukocyte-reduced RBC. All methods of preparation for use in preventing febrile nonhemolytic transfusion reactions must reduce the leukocyte count to less than 5×10^8 in the final component and retain at least 80% of the original RBC, whereas to prevent HLA sensitization, the WBC content must be less than 5×10^6 (Klein, 1994, p. 12).

For all practical purposes, the newer, easy to use, 3-log (99.9%) leukoreduction filters, which provide final blood components with less than 5×10^6 WBC (Klein, 1994, p. 12), are used not only for their intended purposes of preventing HLA sensitization but also for preventing febrile nonhemolytic transfusion reactions and, in selected cases, for decreasing the chances of viral transmission (i.e., cytomegalovirus), graft versus host disease (GVHD), and immunosuppression (Bordin, 1994). Consequently, the following discussion on the less than 1-log (90%) leukoreduction techniques is historical.

In one method, the bag containing whole blood is inverted and centrifuged. Most of the RBC are then removed through the bottom of the bag, leaving the uppermost layer of RBC, the buffy coat (WBC and platelets), and plasma. Another procedure is to prepare packed cells and wash these RBC twice with several hundred milliliters of normal saline, using centrifugation and removal of the buffy coat.

In the spin-cool filter technique (Parravicini, 1984), blood older than four days is recentrifuged to aggregate WBC-platelet-fibrin plugs and allowed to stand overnight so that the fibrin plug can mature, making disaggregation unlikely. The blood is then put through a microfilter to remove these fibrin plugs during the transfusion. This method had the advantage of retaining the original shelf-life because the unit is entered only at the time of transfusion.

Thus far, the methods discussed remove less than 90% (1 log) of the WBC. If an automated cell washer is used, about 90% of the WBC can be removed. If blood is glycerolized, frozen, and washed, about 95% of the WBC may be removed. Many of these methods require entering the bag and therefore cause the shelf-life to be limited to 24 hours from preparation. For a further discussion of leukocyte-reduced blood products, see the section on Filters and the section on Inflammatory Cytokines Involved in Immune-Mediated Hemolysis later in this chapter.

Neocytes

Neocytes (younger RBC) can be prepared by differential centrifugation, taking into account that the younger cells are larger and more buoyant than the smaller, more dense, older cells.

Neocytes are useful in the treatment of young patients with severe chronic anemia (e.g., thalassemia patients) who require repeated transfusions (Propper, 1980). Each milliliter of RBC contains about 1 mg of iron, which theoretically can be deposited in tissues and cause hemosiderosis. If neocytes, with an average 90-day life span, are transfused instead of conventional RBC, with an average 60-day life span, RBC transfusion requirements and the chance of inducing hemosiderosis may be reduced.

Frozen Red Blood Cells

There are three methods of freezing RBC (Dawson, 1977). The predominant technique used in this country is the high-glycerol (40% w/v final concentration) procedure in which the blood is stored for up to 10 years at −65°C or colder. Another method, the low-glycerol (14% to 17.5% w/v final concentration) technique employs liquid nitrogen storage at −120°C to −196°C for up to 10 years. Both procedures use a thawing and washing step that removes most of the glycerol prior to transfusion of the RBC. Because these are open systems, the red cells become outdated 24 hours after deglycerolization. The third method, agglomeration, employs a deglycerolization technique in which, in the presence of a low-ionic-strength solution, the cells "agglomerate," forming large clumps that sink to the bottom of the bag. The supernatant can be removed, and a wash procedure can be instituted. See the earlier section, Storage of Frozen Red Blood Cells, for more information.

The use of frozen, deglycerolized RBC has decreased since the late 1970s because it has been shown that the hepatitis virus cannot be "washed" out of blood (Alter, 1978; Haugen, 1979) and because deglycerolized RBC are used less in potential kidney transplant recipients who have now been shown to have better kidney graft survival if they are exposed to the HLA material in the buffy coat (Opelz, 1980). Although 95% of the WBC are removed in the freeze-thaw process, some viable lymphocytes remain (Kurtz, 1978) and could theoretically produce GVHD. Consequently, even frozen, deglycerolized RBC should be irradiated prior to transfusion in the severely immunocompromised patient.

Rejuvenation of Liquid Stored Erythrocytes

RBC, in the liquid state, show many changes with storage (see Table 31–2). Their 2,3-DPG level decreases markedly after 10 days, and their post-transfusion survival is reduced to below 80% at the end of their shelf-life. Both can be restored by incubation with media containing pyruvate, inosine, glucose, and phosphate with or without adenine (Valeri, 1972). The RBC can be frozen in the presence of glycerol and stored until needed. The same process can be applied to fresh RBC to increase the 2,3-DPG level to about 160% of normal; thus, two units of such modified blood can have the functional effect of three conventional units. Such a rejuvenation solution is commercially available in the United States.

The rejuvenation procedure may be performed up to three days after RBC expiration if the units are continuously stored at appropriate refrigerated temperatures. After rejuvenation, the unit may be washed and transfused within 24 hours or may be frozen using glycerolization and stored for future use.

Platelet Concentrates

Random-donor platelets are produced from whole blood within eight hours of collection (depending on the bag manufacturer and type of anticoagulant used) by centrifugation using a light spin to produce platelet-rich plasma. The platelet-rich plasma is transferred into a satellite bag, and then the plasma is given a hard spin to form an aggregated platelet button and platelet-poor plasma. All but about 50 mL of the plasma is removed to produce platelet concentrate. The 200 mL of platelet-poor plasma that is left can be placed back on the RBC to make modified whole blood, frozen to make FFP, or used as recovered plasma for further manufacturing.

This platelet concentrate is left undisturbed for one hour to allow gentle disaggregation of the platelet button. The platelets are next subjected to continuous gentle agitation at room temperature (20°C to 24°C) for up to five days of storage. It is important to ensure that the pH of all the platelets is maintained at 6.0 or above so that they remain functional and that at least 75% of the units tested have a minimal dose of 5.5×10^{10} platelets.

Bleeding from severe thrombocytopenia (less than 20,000 per μL) is characterized by slow diffuse oozing from venipuncture and surgical sites, petechiae, ecchymosis, gingival bleeding, conjunctival hemorrhage, hematuria, and melena. Hemostasis from platelets usually is adequate if the bleeding time does not exceed twice the upper limit of normal (12 to 15 minutes). Risk factors for thrombocytopenic hemorrhage must also be considered as shown later in Table 31–5.

Platelets are transfused (1) to prophylactically correct severe thrombocytopenia to prevent catastrophic hemorrhage in the central nervous system or other vital organs, especially in leukemia and lymphoma patients undergoing high-dose chemotherapy, (2) to bleeding patients in surgery or trauma cases with platelet counts of 75,000 or less, and (3) to bleeding patients with thrombocytopathy (qualitative abnormal platelet dysfunction), who may have normal platelet counts.

Table 31–5. INCREASED RISK FACTORS FOR THROMBOCYTOPENIC BLEEDING

Rapid onset of thrombocytopenia-disseminated intravascular coagulation, septicemia
Fever
Coagulation factor deficiency
Poor vascular integrity
Uremia
Intracranial or gastrointestinal sites of malignancy
Medications—aspirin, piroxicam (Feldene), ticlopodine, heparin, sodium warfarin (Coumadin), chemotherapy
Mucosal injury from chemotherapy
Protracted vomiting
Rapid tumor lysis

Platelet therapy is probably not effective for persons with conditions causing rapid platelet consumption, such as disseminated intravascular coagulation (DIC), idiopathic thrombocytopenic purpura (ITP), gram-negative septic shock, and severe hypersplenism (NIH Consensus Conference, 1987).

Rh antigens are not found on platelets, but because platelet concentrates contain some red cells (about 0.5% hematocrit), efforts should be made to give Rh-negative platelets to Rh-negative females of child-bearing age or younger. This is often not possible, so Rh immune globulin (RhIG) therapy should be considered to prevent immunization and the potential for hemolytic disease of the newborn subsequently.

ABO-incompatible platelets may be administered to adults with only a minor decrease in the expected increment in platelet count, because platelets demonstrate weak ABO antigenicity. When using this procedure, a volume reduction step should be considered to decrease the amount of incompatible plasma, which could otherwise result in a strongly positive direct antiglobulin test (DAT) on the RBC. Because of their much smaller blood volumes, pediatric patients should receive platelets containing ABO-compatible plasma. This sometimes is accomplished by removal of ABO-incompatible plasma, with replacement using 5% albumin or AB plasma.

The Platelet Immunologic Refractory State

The transfusion of multiple platelet concentrates often creates an immunologic, antibody-mediated, refractory state in which further random-donor platelet infusions fail to bring about any increment in the recipient's one-hour post-transfusion count. This state occurs in 40% to 70% of patients receiving repeated platelet transfusions for hematologic malignancies (Howard, 1978; Schiffer, 1982a, 1982b). It may become evident as early as three weeks after the start of therapy. Only 10% of persons with solid tumors become refractory (Schiffer, 1982a). In cases of aplastic anemia, the refractory state may occur in 75% of patients (Silvergleid, 1980). It is thought that the reason that aplastic anemia patients have a higher rate of the immunologic platelet refractory state than do those with malignancies is that patients with malignancies receive chemotherapy, which makes them immunosuppressed.

A patient who becomes immunologically refractory to

random-donor platelets has usually developed an HLA antibody that reacts directly with the transfused platelets. Platelets express varying amounts of HLA-A and HLA-B antigens but demonstrate no significant amounts of HLA-C, D, or DR antigens (Silvergleid, 1980). Platelet transfusions from donors mismatched for cross-reactive HLA antigens provide hemostasis and platelet survival equivalent to those of perfectly matched platelets (Schiffer, 1980). The use of selective mismatching for cross-reactive HLA antigens allows for adequate numbers of donors to be found from a pool of 1500 rather than a pool of 10,000, which is needed if only perfect HLA matches are required (Tomasulo, 1980a). HLA-B8, B12, Bw4, and Bw6 are variably expressed on platelets but are readily detectable on lymphocytes, the cells that are used for HLA lymphocytotoxicity testing. A donor with these antigens on his or her lymphocytes could have decreased expression of them on his or her platelets and therefore could be used as a donor for recipients in whom these antigens would otherwise be regarded as a mismatch. Persons negative for HLA-A2 antigen have a better response to single-donor platelets with major mismatches than do those who possess the HLA-A2 antigen (Tomasulo, 1980a). Perhaps the HLA-A2 negative person is not as good a responder as the HLA-A2 positive person. Selective mismatching of platelets may not be successful in all patients.

Most apheresis programs base donor choice on the recipient's HLA typing and match the recipient with appropriate, previously typed donors. Because the expression of the HLA antigens are more prominent than the ABO system on the platelet surface (ABO is very weak), HLA-matched donors are often selected without regard to the ABO system. Donor selection procedures may include a crossmatch, which uses patient serum against donor lymphocytes. The lymphocyte crossmatch procedure is not always a good predictor of platelet survival and ranges in accuracy from 30% to 75% (Silvergleid, 1980; Slichter, 1980).

In addition to HLA typing, some programs perform a percent reactive antibody (PRA), as is done in solid organ transplantation (see Chap. 38). The PRA is a lymphocytotoxicity (HLA) test measuring the degree of antibody reactivity that a patient's serum has against a panel of lymphocytes, representing various HLA antigens from the general population. Those whose antibodies react to more than 90% of the panel cells are unlikely to respond well to single-donor, HLA-matched platelets unless the match is perfect.

Thrombocytopenic patients who continue to receive single-donor, HLA-matched platelets can become refractory even to these products. The antibody that then develops is probably directed against platelet-specific antigens. A compatible unit can be found only by using a crossmatch that employs platelets. Consider how few donors would be available who offered a specific HLA type in addition to being negative for Pl^{A1}: less than 2% of the population. Theoretically, it seems that it would be better to perform crossmatches using platelets rather than lymphocytes to predict platelet survival. Many direct platelet antibody and platelet crossmatch tests have been developed that employ EIA, RIA, and immunofluorescence tagged anti-IgG techniques (Sinor, 1988), but further study is needed to determine the tests' interlaboratory reproducibility and ability to predict the survival of single-donor transfused platelets. A commercially available, solid-phase red cell adherence, platelet antibody detection assay is becoming increasingly popular.

Once the thrombocytopenic patient no longer responds to HLA-matched, single-donor platelets, little can be done to raise the platelet count unless autologous cryopreserved platelets are available. Autologous DMSO-cryopreserved platelets obtained from the patient during remission can provide adequate hemostasis and may be stored up to three years in the vapor phase of liquid nitrogen.

Prevention of the Platelet Immunologic Refractory State

Historically, European investigators (Eernisse, 1981) showed that the removal of most of the lymphocytes that contaminate platelet concentrates will significantly decrease alloimmunization, but many platelets were also removed in these older techniques. Others (Gmur, 1983) began using single-donor apheresed platelet support for severe thrombocytopenia to decrease the number of donor exposures and subsequent potential sensitization, rather than using multiple donors through the usual random-donor platelet transfusions. To decrease leukocyte contamination of platelets, many blood bankers empirically employed centrifugation using the special Leukotrap bag (Cutter Biologicals, Emeryville, California). Many are starting to use the new selective adsorption filters that remove 99.9% of leukocytes, as discussed later in this chapter under Filters, to delay HLA alloimmunization to transfused platelet products.

Additionally, ultraviolet irradiation of platelet concentrates has been shown to nullify the lymphoproliferative response and the ability of lymphocytes to act as stimulator cells without affecting platelet function (Bordin, 1994; Kahn, 1985b).

The widespread, exclusive use of single-donor platelets would limit the donors available to persons in the refractory state, because most apheresis centers have only a small number of donors, usually less than 1500. However, many blood centers are enlarging their apheresis donor pools in order to provide increasing numbers of single-donor apheresis products to lessen recipient exposure to multiple platelet concentrates.

An animal model (Bordin, 1993) has shown some interesting, but yet not totally clarified, phenomena:

1. 30% of rabbits become immunologically refractory to leukoreduced platelet transfusions with no significant advantage of 3-log over 2-log reduction filters.
2. Platelet refractoriness can be reduced by combining plasma removal with 3-log leukoreduction.

Perhaps alloimmunization in this animal model is caused not only by the number of intact WBC in the blood component but by the presence of HLA or other major histocompatibility antigens in either soluble or microparticle form, such that they escape the leukofiltration process.

Leukocytes disintegrate, leaving nonfilterable WBC fragments that increase with time of storage. These WBC fragments have been found to be immunogenic in animal experiments (Bordin, 1993). Consequently, prestorage WBC filtration and minimizing plasma infusion would probably be the best way to decrease HLA sensitization and the subsequent platelet refractory state.

Granulocyte Concentrate

Granulocytes are prepared by apheresis from a single donor. To obtain at least 1.0×10^{10} granulocytes, donors are administered steroids several hours prior to the procedure to raise the peripheral blood granulocyte count. Steroids make the granulocytes in the marginating pool go to the circulating pool. In addition, donors are exposed to hydroxyethyl starch (HES), a RBC-sedimenting agent, during the procedure. Although unproven clinically, "buffy coat," prepared from a single unit of fresh whole blood, has also been used as a source of granulocytes (about 0.7×10^9) in the treatment of the septic neutropenic neonate (Baley, 1987; Cairo, 1987).

Granulocyte concentrates, prepared by apheresis, with a total volume of 250 to 300 mL, contain other WBC, platelets (equivalent to a unit of apheresis platelets), enough RBC (10% Hct) to require RBC crossmatch, and about 250 mL of plasma. They are stored without agitation at room temperature and must be administered within 24 hours, but bacterial killing function rapidly decreases soon after production of this blood component.

Granulocytes are transfused once daily for four to five days when neutropenia of less than 500/μL has resulted in a bacterial infection unresponsive to therapy with the appropriate third-generation broad-spectrum antibiotic for 48 hours (Strauss, 1987). Because these newer antibiotics are so effective and because of the use of G-CSF and GM-CSF to reduce the period of severe neutropenia after high-dose chemotherapy, the need for granulocytes has decreased substantially over the years. Also, some severe complications such as acute pulmonary insufficiency are associated with granulocyte therapy. Amphotericin B, an antifungal agent, should not be infused shortly before or after a granulocyte transfusion because of the association of acute respiratory distress syndrome, probably caused by granulocyte agglutinates plugging the pulmonary capillaries. These appear as pulmonary infiltrates ("white lung") on chest radiographs. Furthermore, there is some question as to whether granulocytes are effective in eliminating systemic fungal infections.

The monitoring of a successful granulocyte transfusion is difficult because of the short half-life of six to eight hours and because functional granulocytes will go to the site of infection and will not circulate. The easiest way to check the efficacy of the granulocyte transfusion is to look for resolution of the symptoms of septicemia. Granulocytes may also be labeled with indium-111; after transfusion, a nuclear scan is performed to see if there is activity at the clinical site of infection (McCullough, 1981). There is no effective pretransfusion compatibility test for granulocytes, but because this component contains so many RBC, a major RBC crossmatch should be performed.

Fresh Frozen Plasma

Fresh frozen plasma (FFP) is prepared by centrifuging whole blood and separating 200 to 260 mL of the upper liquid plasma. The plasma must be frozen at −18°C or colder within eight hours of collection in order to maintain the labile coagulation factors, Factors V and VIII. Its frozen shelf-life is one year. FFP is composed of over 90% water, 6% to 8% protein, and a small percentage of carbohydrates and lipids. One milliliter of FFP contains 100% or one unit of coagulation activity. FFP should be thawed at 37°C with constant agitation and transfused within 24 hours when stored at 1°C to 6°C.

Although FFP has been used in the past for volume expansion, this indication is no longer recognized because of the risk of transfusion-transmitted disease and the availability of other, safer products such as 5% albumin or normal saline. However, a solvent/detergent (S/D) treated pooled FFP product is currently being evaluated for clinical use. This S/D treatment eliminates lipid-coated viruses (HIV-1, HIV-2, HTLV-1, HTLV-2, hepatitis B, hepatitis C, CMV) but not hepatitis A virus or parvovirus B19. FFP should also not be used as a source of protein nutrition, because other commercial preparations not made from blood are available (NIH Consensus Conference, 1985). The primary use of FFP is in the bleeding patient with multiple coagulation deficiency problems secondary to liver disease, DIC, or dilutional changes from massive transfusions. Because a large volume of FFP that could cause fluid overload is normally required to correct bleeding episodes in factor-deficient patients, commercially available concentrates are the first treatment of choice. However, FFP is employed to stop bleeding episodes in Factor V or XI deficiencies, because no concentrate is available.

Cryoprecipitate

Cryoprecipitate, prepared from one unit of whole blood, contains at least 80 units of Factor VIII, about 50% of the von Willebrand factor (vWF) in the original unit, at least 200 mg of fibrinogen, and about 25% of the Factor XIII present in the original unit, as well as considerable fibronectin activity.

Cryoprecipitate is produced by slowly thawing (overnight) a unit of FFP at 1°C to 6°C, leaving a small amount of white precipitate (cryoprecipitate). The material is centrifuged, and all but 10 to 15 mL of the supernatant plasma is removed. The cryoprecipitate is then refrozen at − 18°C or colder and may be stored frozen for one year. It is thawed at 37°C and stored at 1°C to 6°C up to six hours prior to use.

Until recently, cryoprecipitate was the product of choice for bleeding, severe hemophiliacs, but because of the newer methods (Prodouz, 1994) of inactivating viruses used in the pooled concentrates, commercial Factor VIII is the product of choice. The major use of cryoprecipitate is for the treatment of severe von Willebrand's disease, because commercial Factor VIII concentrate has minimal, if any, functional high-molecular-weight vWF. (See the later section, Factor VIII Concentrate, and Chap. 28 for further discussion of von Willebrand's disease.) Standard doses of cryoprecipitate have caused thrombocytopenia in patients with the platelet-type variant of von Willebrand's disease (Montgomery, 1994). Low-dose cryoprecipitate may be useful in these cases (Montgomery, 1994).

Since fibrinogen concentrates are no longer available because of their high risk of hepatitis, cryoprecipitate may be used for hypofibrinogenemia. Cryoprecipitate is also a source of concentrated fibronectin. This protein acts as an opsonin because it is thought to coat bacteria so that they are more easily cleared by the phagocytes of the body. Fibronectin is greatly diminished in both burn and traumatic shock patients. Consequently, replacement therapy, using cryoprecipitate for fibronectin-deficient patients, may help to reverse septicemia in these patients (Saba, 1982).

Selection of Blood Derivatives

Blood derivatives are made by the pharmaceutical industry from pools of thousands of units of plasma using the principles of Cohn ethanol fractionation (Rock, 1986). Albumin and plasma protein fractions have been relatively safe products for years because they have been subjected to pasteurization. However, effective viricidal techniques were not widely available for factor concentration until the 1980s, and consequently, many of those who received these factor concentrates in the early 1980s contracted AIDS or hepatitis, or both. Today, blood derivatives are relatively safe products.

Factor VIII Concentrate

Factor VIII concentrate is a lyophilized product made from pooled plasma using the Cohn ethanol fractionation method. In 1984, some manufacturers began heat treating the lyophilized (dry state) Factor VIII products at 60°C for over 24 hours. Although this procedure was probably enough to inactivate the HIV virus, it did not completely inactivate the hepatitis B or hepatitis C viruses. Other methods of viral inactivation have been found to be more effective against these two viruses, but they considerably reduce the Factor VIII yield: wetted, intermediate-phase, lyophilized product exposed to pressurized steam; pasteurization, in which liquid Factor VIII is exposed to 60°C for 10 hours; and monoclonal Factor VIII antibody affinity columns used to isolate Factor VIII followed by washing and further viral inactivation steps. The most promising method of viricidal treatment is solvent/detergent exposure in which the solvent, tri-n-butyl phosphate, and any one detergent—cholate, Tween 80, or Triton X-100—is used to inactivate viruses with lipid coats such as HIV-1,2, hepatitis B, hepatitis C, HTLV-1,2, EBV, and CMV. However, nonlipid envelope viruses such as hepatitis A and parvovirus B19 are not destroyed in this process (Prodouz, 1994).

Factor VIII concentrate is transfused intravenously into patients with moderate to severe congenital Factor VIII deficiency (hemophilia A) when bleeding occurs. 1-Deamino-8-D-arginine vasopressin (desmopressin acetate, DDAVP), a pharmacologic agent, should first be used in mild to moderate hemophilia A to stimulate a twofold or threefold increase in Factor VIII production and release from endothelial cells (Lusher, 1984).

Patients with von Willebrand's disease have a combined plasma deficiency of Factor VIII and vWF (which leads to platelet aggregation dysfunction). Usually, bleeding episodes in mild to moderate von Willebrand's disease are best treated with DDAVP because desmopressin induces significant increments in both Factor VIII and the vWF (Mannucci, 1988). However, DDAVP has caused thrombocytopenia in Type II B and the platelet-type von Willebrand variants (Montgomery, 1994). For bleeding episodes in severe von Willebrand's disease, cryoprecipitate has been the treatment of first choice because DDAVP can seldom raise the deficient factors to hemostatic levels in patients with severely depressed levels and because commercial Factor VIII concentrate has not contained much functional, high-molecular-weight vWF. It is known, however, that some intermediate-purity Factor VIII concentrates do have variable amounts of high-molecular-weight vWF. The lack of, or lower than expected amounts of, high-molecular-weight vWF in commercial Factor VIII concentrates is most likely due to proteolysis of this factor by proteases released from lysed excess numbers of WBC and platelets. One investigator found that the use of protease inhibitors in the production of Factor VIII concentrate diminished the loss of high-molecular-weight vWF (Mannucci, 1994). Perhaps in the future, manufacturers will either better separate the WBC from the plasma or employ protease inhibitors so that Factor VIII concentrates will have reasonable and standard amounts of vWF. The French are investigating the use of a specific vWF concentrate that contains only minimal amounts of Factor VIII concentrate (Montgomery, 1994).

In newly diagnosed severe hemophilia, whether due to Factor VIII or Factor IX deficiency, hepatitis B vaccine should be given as soon as possible. This vaccine usually will prevent hepatitis B infection.

When significant Factor VIII inhibitors (antibodies) are present, bleeding episodes can be stopped using alternative methods: porcine Factor VIII, Factor IX concentrate (contains some activated coagulation factors), anti-inhibitor coagulation complex (activated coagulation factors), or plasma exchange with high-dose Factor VIII administration.

Factor IX Concentrate

Factor IX concentrate is a lyophilized product made from pooled plasma using the Cohn ethanol fractionation method. Besides Factor IX, it usually contains Factors II, VII, and X. It is transfused intravenously when treating bleeding episodes in patients with Factor IX congenital deficiency (hemophilia B, Christmas disease), but it is also useful for those with congenital Factor VII or X deficiencies. As mentioned earlier, Factor IX concentrate may be administered to Factor VIII–deficient patients with significant inhibitor activity, because Factor IX concentrate often contains activated coagulation factors.

Heat treatment of the lyophilized (dry) product was begun in 1984, which probably resulted in inactivation of HIV but not hepatitis virus. Methods of viral inactivation similar to those noted for Factor VIII are currently in place (Prodouz, 1994).

Because Factor IX concentrate may contain activated coagulation factors, it may cause DIC in patients with severe liver disease in whom antithrombin production is inadequate.

Anti-Inhibitor Coagulation Complex

Anti-inhibitor coagulation complex, also known as Factor VIII inhibitor bypass activity (feiba), is a lyophilized product made from pooled plasma using the Cohn ethanol fractionation method. It contains activated vitamin K–dependent coagulation factors (II, VII, IX, X) and their precursors, as well as kinin-generating proteins. Viricidal techniques have been used to reduce the risk of HIV and hepatitis transmission such that no transfusion-transmitted diseases have been reported with this product.

Anti-inhibitor coagulation complex is used to stop bleeding episodes in patients with high levels of Factor VIII inhibitor. Because of the amount of activated coagulation factors in this product, Factor VIII is bypassed so that coagulation can occur.

This product should be used with caution in liver disease and the hyperthrombotic state.

Plasma Protein Fraction and Albumin

Plasma protein fraction (PPF) and albumin are plasma colloid derivatives made from pools of plasma using the Cohn ethanol fractionation process (Rock, 1986). After separation from plasma, they are pasteurized by heating to 60°C for 10 hours to inactivate viruses such as hepatitis and HIV. Fifty percent sucrose and 2M glycine are added as stabilizers to prevent excessive protein denaturation (Prodouz, 1994). The heating process inactivates all of the coagulation factors. PPF contains about 83% albumin and 17% α and β globulins. Albumin is a more refined product, containing 96% albumin and 4% α-globulins. Because neither product has γ-globulins, there are no ABO blood group antibodies present and, consequently, compatibility testing is not required prior to infusion. The 5% PPF and albumin products are osmotically equivalent to plasma, whereas the 25% (25 g of protein per 100 mL) albumin solution is very hyperosmotic compared with plasma and will draw tissue fluid into the intravascular space.

Albumin and PPF 5% solutions are indicated as plasma expanders for the treatment of hypovolemia and shock. Per milliliter, they are the most expensive volume expanders, and therefore crystalloids (normal saline and Ringer's lactate) should be considered first. The rapid infusion of PPF is contraindicated in cardiopulmonary bypass. The product contains bradykinin precursors that cannot be broken down when activated because the pulmonary capillaries are bypassed. The end result is hypotension. Albumin does not contain bradykinin precursors, so this restriction does not apply. These two colloids are useful to raise blood pressure in therapeutic plasma exchange, dialysis, shock, and other potentially hypotensive situations. Albumin may also be useful in hemolytic disease of the newborn to bind indirect bilirubin. These products are unjustified as a source of nutrition (because enteric and parenteral alimentation and hyperalimentation fluids are available) and are of questionable use in the general management of hypoalbuminemia due to liver disease, protein-losing enteropathy, and protein-losing nephropathy.

Immune Serum Globulin

Immune serum globulin (ISG) is a solution or a lyophilized preparation containing many of the antibodies present in human blood. It is prepared from large pools of plasma using the Cohn ethanol fractionation process (Sacher, 1988), and it is commercially available in the intramuscular (IM) or intravenous (IV) form. The manufacturing process apparently inactivates hepatitis B, hepatitis C, and HIV viruses. However, in 1994, hepatitis C was found to be transmitted in IV ISG (CDC, 1994); since then, manufacturers have added a solvent/detergent step.

At least 90% of either the IV or the IM product is IgG. However, IgA, IgM, and other plasma proteins are also present in small quantities. The half-life of pharmacologically produced ISG in the bloodstream ranges between 18 and 32 days, depending on the preparation (Berkman, 1988). ISG for IM use may not be administered intravenously, because the aggregated IgG molecules can activate complement and produce anaphylactic shock.

ISG is used for the replacement of γ-globulins in those immunodeficiency states in which antibody formation is severely impaired, leaving the patient subject to frequent infections. These conditions include congenital agammaglobulinemia, common variable immunodeficiency, Wiskott-Aldrich syndrome, and severe combined immunodeficiency. The IV solution is administered to those patients who do not tolerate IM injections well because of bleeding tendencies or small muscle mass. The IV preparation has also been used to create a blockade of the reticuloendothelial system (RES), also known as the mononuclear phagocyte system, in order to increase the platelet count in patients with autoimmune thrombocytopenic purpura (Bussel, 1988a) and has been similarly used to improve the condition of other autoimmune diseases. The IM ISG solution has been used to provide passive immunity to persons exposed to either hepatitis A or hepatitis C.

The IV preparation should be infused over several hours (Berkman, 1988). Rapid infusion may cause flushing, tachycardia, and hypotension, but slowing the infusion rate usually stops this adverse reaction. Because of the presence of IgA in the product, anaphylaxis may occur in those patients with antibodies directed against IgA.

Specific hyperimmune IM ISG is available to provide passive immunity in specific situations: hepatitis B (HBIG), tetanus, varicella zoster, measles, and Rh immune globulin.

SPECIAL SITUATIONS

Hemapheresis

Hemapheresis is a procedure in which whole blood is removed from a person, anticoagulated, and separated into components. The desired components are retained, and the unwanted portions remaining are returned to the donor. This procedure can be used to obtain components intended for transfusion (platelets, granulocytes, plasma) or to remove pathologic elements, cells, or dissolved plasma factors circulating in the blood.

There are cell/plasma separators that separate components by centrifugal force, and there are also plasmapheresis machines, using special membrane technology, that allow plasma but not cellular elements to pass through the membrane (Pineda, 1987). Only the cell/plasma separators will be covered in this section.

Historical Perspective

Duke, in 1910, was first to show that the bleeding thrombocytopenic patient greatly benefited from the infusion of functional platelets derived from fresh whole blood. During the 1950s and early 1960s, the major cause of death associated with hematologic malignancies was hemorrhage due to marrow replacement with tumor cells or, more likely, due to marrow suppression by chemotherapy. In 1951, Dillard developed a method to separate and concentrate platelets from whole blood, and investigators in the early 1950s began to experimentally transfuse platelets to patients with thrombocytopenic hemorrhage (Gardner, 1954).

Platelet concentrates were not used routinely until the late 1960s, when plastic bags with multiple satellite containers became readily available. Once hemorrhagic problems were somewhat overcome, the major cause of death in hematologic malignancies became infection. This led to the development of apheresis equipment in the late 1960s and early 1970s to provide granulocytes for the treatment of iatrogenically induced neutropenia. These machines also could provide single-donor platelets, which were eventually found useful for patients who were immunologically refractory to random-donor platelet concentrates. Several cytapheresis machines became commercially available in the early 1970s.

The Aminco (no longer manufactured), the Cobe/IBM 2997 (no longer manufactured), the Cobe Spectra, and the Fenwal CS-3000 are continuous flow machines requiring two venipuncture sites. The Aminco machine had a large bowl whose walls were perpendicular to the bottom of the bowl. Centrifugation of citrated whole blood in the Aminco bowl separated blood so that the lightest blood element in density, plasma, was closest to the inside wall, while platelets, being the lightest in density of the cellular elements, were closest to the plasma layer. This was followed by lymphocytes, granulocytes, and lastly red cells (the heaviest in density of the blood elements), which were found against the outside wall. Various blood elements could be collected by evacuation channels placed in specific blood layers. The desired element was saved, and the unwanted portions were returned to the donor in a continuous flow fashion. The Aminco bowl was reusable and could be autoclaved.

The Cobe/IBM 2997 was similar in principal to the Aminco equipment but used donut-shaped disposable plastic equipment. The apheresis division of IBM was sold to the Cobe Company, which provides the 2997 technology today. In 1988, Cobe began to market a new device called the Spectra. It has many of the characteristics of the Cobe/IBM 2997 but is a more automated and computerized version and produces platelet apheresis products with minimal WBC contamination. The Spectra is also mobile and thus can be moved to a patient's room to perform therapeutic apheresis procedures.

The CS-3000, produced by Fenwal, became commercially available in the early 1980s. It is a continuous flow apparatus that comprises two specially configured rotating chambers. In one chamber, platelet-rich plasma is separated from anticoagulated whole blood. The platelet-rich plasma is evacuated from this separation chamber and pumped to the other chamber, where the platelets are separated from plasma. The platelets may then be collected. Granulocytes are produced, using a similar mechanism but a differently configured chamber. Plasma may be separately collected using either the platelet or the granulocyte procedure.

Both the Cobe Spectra and the Fenwal CS3000 can be used to harvest stem cells from bone marrow or peripheral blood.

The Haemonetics Company produces an intermittent flow cell separator based on the Latham bowl. This bowl has sides that are at an acute angle to the bottom of the bowl. Because of the bowl configuration, when citrated whole blood enters the bowl, RBC go to the bottom and outside of the bowl and allow for packing of RBC and the pushing up of the lighter plasma and cell elements outside through the top of the bowl. Thus, blood elements may be sequentially collected into different bags. When the RBC fill the bowl and all of the rest of the blood elements have been displaced from the bowl, the procedure is stopped; the RBC are then evacuated, and the procedure is started again. The desired components are retained, and those not wanted are returned to the donor. Each procedure is called a "pass"; six to eight passes are needed to collect enough platelets or granulocytes to provide appropriate therapy to thrombocytopenic or granulocytopenic recipients. A surge protocol for platelet production has been developed that briefly increases the flow rate from about 80 to 200 mL/min, using plasma separated during the initial phase of the apheresis procedure, and allows for platelet collection relatively free of WBC and RBC contamination. The extracorporeal volume is much greater (more than 500 mL) using this equipment than the continuous flow (about 200 mL extracorporeal volume). However, a single needle technique may be employed, making intermittent flow techniques an advantage in those donors and patients in whom venous access is poor. In addition, the intermittent flow equipment is more easily mobile, because it weighs much less than the continuous flow machines.

Apheresis Donations

The plateletpheresis procedure requires about two hours. Apheresis donors must undergo additional testing beyond what is necessary for normal blood donors.

The AABB standards require that 75% of apheresed platelets contain at least 3.0×10^{11} platelets and that all units have a pH greater than 6.0 at the maximum storage time. The apheresis donor loses more platelets but about the same amount of plasma (i.e., 250 mL) as a whole blood donor. Because the continuous flow apheresis donor loses only about 3 mL of RBC, the limiting factor for frequency of platelet donations becomes donor platelet production. After an apheresis platelet donation, the platelet count may drop as much as 50%. Consequently, donors with counts of less than 150,000/μL are usually not accepted. The count ordinarily returns to pre-apheresis levels within 24 hours. The AABB standards recommend that the interval between plateletpheresis donations be at least 48 hours. Other guidelines, which also must be considered, permit no more than 1000 mL (1200 mL for a donor weighing over 80 kg) of plasma to be removed in seven days and no more than 25 mL of RBC per week. For frequent plateletpheresis donors, quantatitive IgM and IgG levels or serum protein electrophoresis must be performed every four months, as for plasma donors.

The loss of RBC becomes a limiting factor when certain intermittent flow apheresis equipment is used. Such machines permit 20 to 30 mL of RBC to be lost per procedure. Still other types of equipment may cause the donor to lose as much as 3×10^8 lymphocytes. Theoretically, immunologic memory cells may be present in these lost cells; no long-term adverse immunologic deficiencies have been reported from plateletpheresis, however. The FDA has suggested that plateletpheresis procedures be performed no more than every 48 hours, twice a week, and 24 times a year (FDA memorandum, October 7, 1988).

Furthermore, the AABB standards do not allow a donor who will be the sole source of a platelet preparation (i.e., random-donor platelet concentrate for neonates or plateletpheresis donor for adults) to have ingested aspirin, piroxicam (Feldene), or other platelet aggregation inhibitors within three days of donation or ticlopodine within 14 days of donation.

The granulocytapheresis procedure takes about 2.5 hours to perform. To achieve a minimum yield of 1.0×10^{10}, the donor is given corticosteroids several hours prior to the procedure to raise the peripheral granulocyte count to between 8,000 and 15,000/μL. Therefore, donors with hypertension, diabetes mellitus, active stomach ulcers, or a history of tuberculosis should not donate granulocytes. Granulocytapheresis donors are also exposed to hydroxyethyl starch (HES), an agent used to sediment the RBC during centrifugation, to improve granulocyte separation. The half-life of granulocytes in the bloodstream is only 7.5 hours, and turnover is rapid. However, because of the considerable plasma (250 mL) that is lost, there should still be a 48-hour interval between procedures.

The apheresis donor is subject to all the reactions of a normal blood donor but additionally could develop the following:

1. Chills, caused by the rapid reinfusion of room-temperature blood components or volume expanders; treatment is to slow the infusion, use blankets on the donor or patient, or a blood warmer.
2. Citrate toxicity from the rapid reinfusion of citrated plasma resulting in hypocalcemia, with symptoms of paresthesias, carpopedal spasm, or tetany; treatment may include administering Tums (calcium-containing medication) by mouth or calcium gluconate intravenously.
3. Allergic reactions to HES; treatment may include administering antihistamines.

Therapeutic Hemapheresis

Therapeutic hemapheresis is the removal of harmful cellular or plasma factors from a person's circulation.

During continuous plasma exchange, the removal of one plasma volume (about 2500 mL in adults) with the replacement of an equivalent amount of fluid will result in about a 65% removal of the pathologic substance, but a two-volume plasma exchange will remove only about 85% of the material (Klein, 1985). The replacement fluid is usually 5% albumin or a combination of 5% albumin and normal saline (Guidelines, 1992). Neither of these solutions contains coagulation factors, so coagulation and fibrinogen studies should be performed after several days of treatment as well as potassium and calcium levels (Westphal, 1987). The AABB standards caution that patients taking angiotensin-converting enzyme (ACE) inhibitors who need plasma exchange utilizing albumin or PPF as the replacement fluid should have their drug therapy withheld for 24 hours, if the drug half-life is less than six hours, or 48 hours, if the drug half life is over six hours, because of the potential risk of anaphylactoid reaction. This is especially true when staph protein A columns are being used. Apparently, excess bradykinin is generated when albumin or PPF are exposed to artificial membranes. The bradykinin is inhibited from breaking down by the presence of ACE inhibitors, resulting in urticaria, wheezing, and hypotension. The use of FFP should be avoided because of potential disease transmission. Most protocols (Clinical, 1993; Guidelines, 1992) require a one-volume plasma exchange a few days a week and usually do not require the use of FFP except in thrombotic thrombocytopenic purpura (TTP). Plasma exchange will more effectively remove IgM, which is predominantly intravascular, than will IgG, which is found intravascularly as well as extravascularly. Abnormal IgM accumulates relatively slowly. When excess quantities of abnormal IgG are rapidly removed from the intravascular space, IgG is pulled from the tissues into the intravascular space. The removal of IgG also causes a "rebound" effect (i.e., increased IgG synthesis). Therefore, chemotherapeutic drugs should be considered in these instances to diminish the excess IgG production.

The AABB (Guidelines, 1992) and the American Society for Apheresis have categorized diseases by their response to therapeutic apheresis:

1. Category I—Indicated as standard, primary therapy
2. Category II—Indicated as suggestive of efficacy and on a second-line, adjunctive basis
3. Category III—Indicated as uncertain with inconclusive evidence for efficacy
4. Category IV—Not indicated; therapeutic trials have shown a lack of efficacy

Table 31–6 lists a number of diseases treated by apheresis, their therapeutic category, and the most likely reason why therapeutic hemapheresis can ameliorate the patient's symptoms.

Hyperviscosity syndrome, usually caused by increased IgM (i.e., Waldenstrom's macroglobulinemia) and sometimes caused by IgG or IgA elevations (i.e., multiple myeloma) can induce decreased mentation because of sluggish brain circulation and vascular insufficiency. One to two days of plasma exchange will acutely lower the total protein levels so that cognitive functions return. When chemotherapy or immunosuppression is not sufficient to improve the status of patients with autoimmune diseases and they are compromised by a life-threatening process, plasmapheresis can help ameliorate the condition. Plasma exchange is especially helpful as ancillary treatment (Guidelines, 1992) in myasthenia gravis (autoantibody directed against the acetylcholine receptor of the motor endplates), Eaton-Lambert syndrome (a myasthenia gravis-like syndrome often associated with small cell carcinoma of the lung), Goodpasture syndrome (autoantibody directed against the basement membrane of the kidney and lungs), and immune complex disorders. Plasmapheresis has also been found useful in the following antibody-related problems: post-transfusion purpura (PL^{A1} antibody), acute (Guillain-Barré syndrome) and chronic inflammatory demyelinating polyneuropathy, and hemophilia A refractory to Factor VIII concentrate because of high-titer Factor VIII antibodies. Therapeutic cytapheresis is used to acutely lower cellular elements when they are much more abundant than normal. When myeloblasts are elevated above 100,000/μL, in acute myeloblastic leukemia or the blast phase of chronic myelogenous leukemia, leukostasis may occur, leading to fatal pulmonary or cerebral vascular insufficiency. This leukostasis phenomenon is thought to be further aggravated when chemotherapy is started, so cytoreduction using apheresis is employed first.

When chemotherapy seems to have little effect on the rising leukocyte counts of some chronic lymphocytic leukemia patients, lymphapheresis may be used to acutely decrease the tumor load and allow the chemotherapeutic agents to work

Table 31–6. RATIONALE FOR THERAPEUTIC HEMAPHERESIS

Disease	Category*	Abnormal Substance Removed
Plasmapheresis		
Hyperviscosity syndrome	I	Abnormal proteins
Myasthenia gravis	I	Autoantibody to acetylcholine receptor
Eaton-Lambert syndrome	I	Autoantibody to myoneural junction
Goodpasture syndrome	I	Autoantibody to basement membrane of glomeruli and lungs
Post-transfusion purpura	I	Platelet-specific antibody
Thrombotic thrombocytopenic purpura	I	Platelet-aggregating toxic factor
Acute Guillain-Barré	I	Probable autoantibody
Chronic inflammatory demyelinating polyneuropathy	II	Probable autoantibody
Multiple sclerosis	III	Possible autoantibody
Systemic vasculitis from autoimmune disease	II	Immune complexes
Rapidly progressive glomerulonephritis	II	Immune complexes
Rh isoimmunization	III	Rh_O (D) antibodies
Autoimmune thrombocytopenic purpura	III	Autoantibody to platelets
Autoimmune hemolytic anemia	III	Autoantibody to RBC
Factor VIII inhibitors	I	Factor VIII antibodies
Hyperlipidemia	I	Excess lipids and abnormal lipoproteins
Protein-bound toxins (mushroom poisoning)	II	Toxin bound to plasma proteins
Renal transplant rejection	III	Combined removal of antibody and cytotoxic lymphocytes
Cytapheresis		
Hyperleukemic leukostasis in AML or CML (blasts) greater than 100,000/μL	I	Excess myeloid blasts
Thrombocytosis	I	Excess platelets
Chronic lymphocytic leukemia	II	Abnormal lymphocytes
Sickle cell crisis	I	Sickled erythrocytes

AML = acute myeloid leukemia; CML = chronic myeloid leukemia.
*Categories taken from Guidelines for Therapeutic Apheresis, AABB Extracorporeal Therapy Committee, American Association of Blood Banks, Bethesda, Maryland, May, 1992. See text for definition of categories.

better. Thrombocytapheresis is used in symptomatic patients with essential thrombocytosis or myelofibrosis whose platelet counts are greater than one million per microliter. Symptoms include headache and both thrombotic and bleeding episodes.

Red blood cell exchange has been used as an effective treatment in sickle cell crisis (category I) and as prophylaxis in pregnancy for sickle cell disease patients (category III) in order to decrease the risks of obstetric complications and to improve the chances of the fetus reaching term (Rock, 1995).

Some conditions in which therapeutic hemapheresis has been shown not to be helpful (category IV) include fulminant hepatic failure, amyotrophic lateral sclerosis, and schizophrenia (Guidelines, 1992).

Autologous Transfusions

The safest blood a recipient can receive is his or her own; this procedure is called an autologous donation or transfusion. The advantages (Gilcher, 1987a) of autologous transfusion to the patient or donor include the prevention of transfusion-transmitted infectious diseases, the elimination of alloimmunization to the cellular elements and plasma proteins, the elimination of graft versus host disease, and the erythropoietic stimulation caused by repeated preoperative phlebotomy. The anemia produced with autologous donation may even be beneficial, because it is thought to improve capillary blood flow.

Presurgical Blood Donation

All patients who can medically tolerate phlebotomy should attempt to donate blood for themselves, if they meet criteria and are expected to need blood for anticipated surgery. Even patients expecting to undergo elective coronary artery bypass surgery are participating in autologous donation programs (Barnes, 1989; Owings, 1989). If several units are required within a few weeks, iron supplementation of 320 mg ferrous sulfate or ferrous gluconate, given three times daily, should be considered (Gilcher, 1987b). Recombinant erythropoietin administration can be useful in the autologous donation process by stimulating donor red cell production so that more units could be donated in less time. Units of blood may be donated as often as every 72 hours, and AABB standards recommend that the last donation take place up to 72 hours prior to surgery. Additional standards recommend that the donor's hemoglobin be at least 11 g/dL and that the donor not have bacteremia at the time of donation. Presurgical blood donation is especially important to patients with rare blood types or blood compatible with only a small percentage of the population. The crossing over of unused autologous units to the general blood supply is frowned on because the reason for the original donation is to help oneself and not others. Therefore, the answers to the donor questionnaire may be suspect. Additionally, autologous donations have been shown to have a higher incidence of disease markers than heterologous volunteer donations. Assuming that the autologous donor has met all the donor suitability criteria intended to protect the recipient, including the confidential self-exclusion, there is still some doubt as to how truthful the donor will be in answering the medical history questions pertaining to high-risk activities if the donor is donating for himself or herself. In fact, reports show an increased chance of an autologous donor unit being positive for anti-HBc as compared with the general donor pool (Starkey, 1989).

The FDA has required that a permanent, nonremovable

autologous label be placed on all autologous blood donations and that if an autologous unit is shipped outside of the collecting facility, it must tested at least for the required FDA tests—anti-HIV-1/2, HBsAg, and syphilis (FDA memoranda of February 12, 1990). Those units crossed-over to the general blood inventory need to be fully tested and must meet all the usual donor suitability criteria, including the confidential unit exclusion.

Intraoperative Salvage

Intraoperative salvage is a system whereby blood is aspirated from the operative field and then transfused to the patient. In some cases, the transfusion is done directly, using a filter, whereas in other cases the blood is first washed to remove surgical debris, phospholipids, activated complement, and tissue activators of the coagulation system (Popovsky, 1987; Stehling, 1989). This type of procedure should not be used if the operative site is grossly contaminated with bacteria or malignant tumor cells.

Normovolemic hemodilution is a technique involving phlebotomy of up to several units during induction of anesthesia with the concomitant volume replacement of crystalloid (3:1, crystalloids to whole blood). The hematocrit can be decreased to as low as 20%; therefore, each milliliter of blood loss depletes the total RBC volume much less than usual (Popovsky, 1987; Stehling, 1989).

Another surgical blood-saving technique is induced hypotension, which is used primarily in younger adults for orthopedic (especially spinal) or intracranial vascular procedures. The systolic blood pressure is reduced by about 20 mm Hg; consequently, this method should not be used in anyone who could have poor coronary or cerebral artery circulation (Popovsky, 1987; Stehling, 1989).

By combining presurgical autologous blood donations with intraoperative salvage, it has been estimated that 40% to 50% (Gilcher, 1987a) of all surgical procedures can be handled using autologous transfusions.

Directed Transfusions

With the public's concern about AIDS, a growing number of patients are requesting directed donations (Pura, 1987). For this kind of donation, the patient directly solicits blood from family and friends. The entire process is based on the false assumption that blood donated by family and friends is safer than that from the regular volunteer donor population. First of all, the directed donor is under more pressure to donate than the anonymous donor. If the potential directed donor does not donate, the recipient may learn of his or her unsuitability and possible high-risk behavior. Also, the extra paperwork and logistic problems contribute to increased probability of clerical errors. Some feel that support for directed donations will decrease the nation's blood supply, because regular donors might withhold their routine donations until asked by a specific recipient. Another disadvantage is the possibility of litigation directly against the donor, because the donor's identity is known by the recipient. Confidentiality has been surrendered in this system. The American Association of Blood Banks, the American Red Cross, and the Council of Community Blood Centers originally tried to discourage directed donations because of legal problems, ethical issues, and the lack of evidence that the process is any safer than the existing system. Current AABB guidelines recommend that directed donations from blood relatives be irradiated because of reports of graft versus host disease in immunocompetent blood recipients who have received directed transfusions from relatives. A more detailed discussion concerning this issue may be found later in this chapter under Transfusion-Associated Graft versus Host Disease.

Many hospitals perceive directed donations as advantageous and, because of public pressure, perform this procedure routinely. One main advantage is the positive psychological benefit to patients and donors. In this competitive health care environment, the hospitals that provide directed donations use it as a marketing tool. Many feel that directed donations will increase the blood supply by stimulating more first-time donors who then can be recalled to make future blood donations to the general community.

To accommodate the dedicated directed donor, AABB standards have been changed to allow whole-blood donations more frequently than every eight weeks (Klein, 1994, p. 3). This special donation procedure must be requested by the recipient's physician, must be approved by the blood bank physician, and must have the informed consent of the donor. Blood donations, in this situation, may be made as often as every three days as long as the donor meets all the usual criteria, including minimum hemoglobin. Additionally, the FDA requires that a donor donating whole blood more often than every eight weeks be examined by a physician who certifies that the donor is in good health at the time of donation (U.S. Dept. of Health and Human Services, 21 CFR).

Massive Blood Transfusions

Transfusions are considered massive when the amount of infusion equals the patient's blood volume within 24 hours. Because a one-blood-volume exchange should leave only 35% of the originally circulating blood and plasma elements, it used to be routine to give 10 units of platelets and 2 units of FFP with each 10 units of RBC transfused. This automatic trigger formula must be more closely examined in the era of AIDS.

A prospective study (Counts, 1979) of 27 massively transfused patients showed that major causes of microvascular bleeding were dilutional thrombocytopenia (less than 100,000 platelets per microliter) in five patients and DIC in three. In these eight patients who developed abnormal bleeding, it took a mean of 35 units of blood for coagulopathy to develop. Factor V levels remained above the 5% to 10% level necessary for coagulation. Factor VIII levels remained above the 30% minimum needed for adequate coagulation in all but two patients who developed DIC. Consequently, it is believed that there must be a large reserve of Factor VIII. This theory should not be surprising, because Factor VIII is an acute phase reactant that significantly rises with stress.

Six of the eight patients with abnormal bleeding and platelet counts below 100,000/μL responded well to platelet transfusions. Dilutional thrombocytopenia did not occur as often as expected, probably because platelets were released into the circulation from the sequestered splenic platelet pool. Because this study showed that the platelet count did not fall below 100,000/μL until more than 18 units of blood were transfused, the current recommendations in massively transfused adult patients are to get a platelet count, as a baseline, after 15 units of blood are transfused (1.5 blood volumes) and then wait for the signs of thrombocytopenia (slow diffuse oozing in the operative field) before infusing the platelets.

It once was the practice to administer sodium bicarbonate to combat the acidosis of hemorrhagic shock and to overcome the acid load of banked blood. This is no longer the case. We now know that a patient in hemorrhagic shock who has rapid restoration of blood volume, and therefore reperfusion of organs and tissues, will quickly restore buffering capacity, dissipating the organic acids produced as intermediary metabolites during shock (Collins, 1982). Furthermore, in the post-transfusion period, many of these patients who undergo massive transfusion become alkalotic because they metabolize the sodium citrate contained in the anticoagulated banked blood.

For very rapid infusion of whole blood, calcium gluconate infusion might be considered to overcome citrate toxicity. Additionally, a blood warmer should be used whenever there is rapid transfusion of blood components recently removed from the refrigerator.

Transfusion in Cardiopulmonary Bypass

Cardiopulmonary bypass is an essential system for open heart surgery (Milam, 1983). The patient's heparinized venous blood is drained into a 37°C chamber where the partial pressure of oxygen is restored to the level of arterial blood and the excess oxygen and carbon dioxide are removed. Then the blood is pumped back to the patient. A cardiotomy aspiration system is also used to pump blood salvaged from the chest cavity back to the oxygenation chamber to be reused. With the bypass system, a significant extracorporeal blood space, about (10 mL/lb body weight of patient), is created and can be compensated for by using crystalloid solutions. This hemodilution has the advantages of conserving blood and reducing the complications of blood transfusion. To partially overcome the substantial anemia that occurs by the end of the procedure, RBC remaining in the pump system can be centrifuged, washed, and reinfused to the patient.

Systems are also available to reinfuse shed blood safely in the early postoperative period. Preoperative donations of autologous blood are now becoming more common in the patient undergoing open heart surgery (Chambers, 1991). Because of these various methods, postoperative transfusion of homologous blood in open heart surgery has decreased markedly.

Coagulation parameters in the early postoperative period require careful attention. Protamine titration to overcome the heparin effect at the end of the procedure, and administration of FFP generally correct most coagulation abnormalities.

Transient thrombocytopenia or thrombocytopathy is often associated with cardiopulmonary bypass because of the exposure to foreign surfaces. The decision to transfuse platelets should be based on whether the slow diffuse oozing of thrombocytopenia is present. If the decision is to transfuse, platelets should be administered after the patient comes off bypass. Otherwise, the newly infused platelets are likely to be damaged because they will come in contact with the foreign material of the extracorporeal equipment.

Cardiovascular surgery has some predisposing medical conditions as well as technical processes that make bleeding episodes more probable than in other types of surgery. Prior to open heart surgery, patients may be taking aspirin or Coumadin or may have just undergone a percutaneous transluminal coronary angioplasty procedure and have received plasminogen activators. Additionally, platelets and coagulation factors may be diminished because of hemodilution and because of contact with the thrombogenic surfaces of the cardiopulmonary bypass equipment.

Protease release is probably the main culprit involved in consuming coagulation factors and making platelets dysfunctional. It is, therefore, not surprising that aprotinin, a serine protease inhibitor that both inhibits plasmin and kallikrein activity and preserves platelet adhesiveness works to significantly reduce blood loss and blood component use during open heart surgery (Chambers, 1991). Additionally, Desmopressin, which induces an increase in circulating high-molecular-weight von Willebrand factor and probably makes platelets more adhesive, has variably been shown to decrease bleeding in open heart surgery (Chambers, 1991). Prostacyclin, although it preserves platelets, has not been effective in decreasing blood loss in cardiovascular surgery.

Neonatal Hemotherapy

The neonatal period extends to the fourth month of life. The blood volume of a full-term newborn is 85 mL/kg, whereas that of a premature baby (less than 1200 g) can be higher than 100 mL/kg (Walker, 1993, p. 437). Sick neonates are subjected to multiple blood laboratory determinations. Even with microsampling techniques, iatrogenic blood loss can exceed 10 mL/day. In a 1-kg premature infant, this could be 10% of the blood volume and would necessitate multiple small-volume blood transfusions for replacement.

Newborns do not adjust or compensate as rapidly as adults when subjected to hypovolemia or hypoxia. With these conditions, the left ventricular stroke volume is decreased in the neonate, and peripheral vascular resistance increases instead of the heart rate (Walker, 1993, p. 437). Therefore, the blood transfused should be less than seven days old in order to maximize 2,3-DPG levels so that oxygen is optimally released to the tissues.

Blood for large neonatal intensive care units is usually provided as O-negative units drawn into four integrally attached blood packs. Consequently, one fourth of the total unit, 125 mL, can be used daily for all the patients in the neonatal care area. Multiple blood bags can also be attached to a blood unit via a sterile docking device. The blood is kept refrigerated and entered in a sterile fashion multiple times during a 24-hour period. The blood is usually drawn in a syringe, through a filter, and allowed to come to room temperature (about 20 minutes) prior to slow infusion.

Because premature infants have an immature immune system and are at increased risk for the severe complications of CMV, either frozen deglycerolized RBC (CMV is nonviable after freezing) or CMV antibody negative RBC should be infused. Alternatively, a three-log leukoreduction filter may be used to remove WBC containing possible CMV from the RBC product. One must also consider irradiating either cellular blood products given to low-birth-weight, premature neonates or blood coming from blood relatives who are directed donors in order to avoid graft versus host disease. Because sick neonates have a great chance of being hypoxic or acidotic, it is best to make sure that the RBC infused are negative for hemoglobin S.

Hemolytic Disease of the Newborn

Fetal blood elements are composed of antigens inherited from both the mother and the father. Any antigens lacking in the mother, yet present on the baby's cells, may cause an immune response by the mother directed against the baby's cells, if transplacental fetomaternal hemorrhage (TPH) has occurred. Maternal IgG can cross the placenta and if directed against the baby's cells may cause hemolytic disease of the newborn (HDN), isoimmune neonatal neutropenia, or isoimmune neonatal thrombocytopenia. The most common of these conditions is HDN due to anti-D produced in an Rh_0 (D) negative mother and directed against the baby's Rh_0 (D) positive red cells. Before the introduction of Rh immune globulin (RhIG), HDN due to Rh_0 (D) accounted for almost 50% of deaths in the perinatal period (Sacher, 1987, p. 24). The dose of RBC causing sensitization can be as low as 0.1 mL (Walker, 1993, p. 441) but usually requires more. However, 20% of Rh_0-negative individuals exposed to the Rh_0 (D) antigen will not respond at all (Mollison, 1993, pp. 228–234).

Any IgG red cell antibody can cause HDN. These IgG antibodies include the Rh (D, C, c, E, e), Duffy (Fy^a, Fy^b), Kidd (Jk^a, Jk^b), and Kell (K, k) systems. Interestingly, many of the antibodies directed against high-incidence antigens were first discovered because they caused HDN. Anti-Rh_0 (D) is the most common cause of HDN because the D antigen is so immunogenic. Because the ABO system is naturally occurring and has not only IgM but also IgG antibodies, it too may cause HDN, but such disease is seldom severe. IgM antibodies of the Lewis, I, and P systems do not cause HDN because they cannot cross the placenta. Additionally, Lewis and I antigens are not well developed on neonatal RBC.

The transplacental passage of maternal IgG directed against fetal RBC induces immune hemolysis and fetal anemia of varying degrees. In severe cases typical of the Rh system, the fetus may develop anasarca, ascites, and heart failure in association with anemia, hypoxia, and depressed serum proteins because of poor liver function. This condition is known as hydrops fetalis and often results in death *in utero*. The peripheral blood smear from the extreme extravascular hemolysis and anemia shows large numbers of nucleated red cells and reticulocytes. Consequently, this condition is also known as erythroblastosis fetalis. On the other hand, HDN due to ABO incompatibility shows spherocytosis on the peripheral blood smear, a much less severe anemia, and usually a mild clinical course.

Prevention of HDN

Once a mother is sensitized and produces antibodies directed against the baby's RBC, the condition cannot be reversed. Therefore, HDN must be prevented when possible. During the early 1960s, Rh immune globulin [RhIG] was developed (Freda, 1964). RhIG is given to unsensitized Rh_0 (D) negative mothers in the antenatal and immediate postnatal period to remove any Rh_0-positive fetal red cells that may have entered the maternal circulation. This early removal of Rh_0 (D) positive fetal red cells from the circulation of an Rh_0 (D) negative mother prevents maternal anti-Rh_0 (D) production and thereby prevents possible HDN in the next pregnancy. HDN due to ABO antibodies can occur with the first pregnancy because these antibodies occur naturally. HDN due to all other IgG antibody systems usually arises with the second pregnancy. It takes weeks to months to produce IgG RBC antibodies after exposure. Because transplacental hemorrhage (TPH) usually does not occur until the third trimester or at delivery, severe HDN does not ordinarily occur with the first baby but during the second and subsequent pregnancies.

Prior to immunoprophylaxis with RhIG, 7% to 8% of Rh-negative women having Rh-positive, ABO-compatible infants developed anti-Rh_0 (D) within six months of delivery, whereas only 1% of Rh_0-negative mothers delivering ABO-incompatible babies were immunized (Sacher, 1987, p. 25). This shows the sparing effect of rapid removal of Rh-positive, ABO-incompatible fetal cells from the mother's circulation.

The use of postpartum RhIG therapy in unsensitized Rh-negative mothers with an ABO-compatible fetus has decreased the incidence of HDN from 8% to 1.8% (Sacher, 1987, p. 25). HDN has been further reduced to only 0.1% to 0.2% of Rh-negative mothers by administering antenatal RhIG routinely at 28 to 30 weeks of gestation and after amniocentesis, spontaneous or induced abortions, ectopic pregnancy, hydatidiform mole, chorionic villus sampling, percutaneous umbilical blood sampling (PUBS), or abdominal trauma. The additional use of antenatal RhIG should theoretically decrease HDN, because fetal cells have been observed in the maternal circulation of 7% of pregnant women during the first trimester, 16% during the second trimester, 29% during the third trimester, and 40% at term (Sacher, 1987, p. 28).

A 300-μg dose of RhIG is sufficient to remove 15 mL of Rh_0 (D) positive packed red cells or the Rh_0 (D) positive RBC from 30 mL of whole blood. This 300-μg dose should be administered to unimmunized, Rh_0 (D) negative mothers at 28 to 30 weeks of gestation and again to these mothers within 72 hours after delivery of an Rh-positive infant. The timing of these two doses is based on the assumption that the RhIG will offer protection for about 12 weeks (Sacher, 1987, p. 32). For events with potential for TPH prior to 12 weeks gestation, a 50-μg RhIG dose is recommended for unimmunized Rh-negative women (Sacher, 1987, p. 28). Afterward, the regular 300-μg dose is suggested.

The administration of RhIG has no effect on the mother. Little of the RhIG crosses the placenta. RhIG sometimes causes a positive direct antiglobulin test in Rh_0 (D) positive babies, but they do not have erythroblastosis fetalis.

It has been estimated that only 0.3% of TPH will be greater than 30 mL (Walker, 1993, p. 464). Therefore, Rh_0 (D) negative women at risk for developing HDN in the future should be checked to make sure that the 300-μg, RhIG dose given within 72 hours of delivery was sufficient enough to remove all the Rh-positive fetal red cells. This should be done about three days after RhIG administration.

Microscopic examination of the D^u test once was used to detect TPH but has been proven to be a relatively insensitive method in that it will not always detect TPH of 30 mL. The erythrocyte rosetting test will apparently detect TPH of 10 mL (Walker, 1993, pp. 464, 681). This test is performed by adding maternal red cells to reagent anti-D. The mixture is washed, and reagent D-positive cells are added. If Rh_0 (D) positive fetal cells from the mother's blood specimen are present, RBC rosetting in a mixed field environment will be seen microscopically. To quantitate the amount of TPH, a Kleihauer-Betke acid elution is necessary. The basis of this test is that fetal hemoglobin is resistant to acid, whereas adult hemoglobin will dissolve when exposed to acid (Walker, 1993, pp. 465, 682). In the presence of acid, adult cells appear as depigmented "ghost cells" with intact RBC membranes, whereas fetal cells with hemoglobin F maintain the normal RBC staining characteristics. Additionally, one may search for residual anti-D. If anti-D is present after RhIG administration, it is in excess and has probably taken care of any Rh-positive fetal red cells. The titer of anti-D is important, because if it is due to RhIG it will be 1:4 or less. Titers of anti-D greater than 1:4 probably indicate an anamnestic response in the mother to the presence of Rh_0 (D) positive fetal red cells.

Immunized (Sensitized) Rh_o (D)–Negative Mothers

Maternal serum anti-D titers up to 1:16 are usually not associated with a high percentage of fetal deaths. Anti-D titers should be performed every two to three weeks; if they show an increase, amniocentesis for bilirubin pigment studies should be considered. Bilirubin pigment, found in amniotic fluid, is a hemoglobin breakdown product and is a reflection of fetal hemolysis and HDN severity (see Chap. 20). When appropriate, amniocentesis is initially performed at about 28 weeks' gestation but may be done earlier if a prior pregnancy demonstrated severe HDN or if the anti-D titers are high. Diagnosis of fetal immune hemolytic anemia using fetal RBC obtained by the relatively new percutaneous umbilical blood sampling technique might also be considered and will be explained in more detail later.

Amniotic fluid is normally straw-colored early in pregnancy, colorless later in pregnancy, and bright yellow if severe HDN is present (see Chap. 21). Once collected, amniotic fluid should be protected from light to prevent breakdown of the bilirubin pigment. Centrifugation and filtering of the amniotic fluid are performed to remove particulate matter. Continuous spectrophotometric analysis between 350 and 700 nm is then conducted. The presence of bilirubin pigment leads to an abnormal elevation of the optical density (O.D.) at 450 nm. The change in O.D. at 450 nm between the estimated baseline (a straight line drawn between the points at 375 and 525 nm on the amniotic fluid curve to approximate the position of a normal amniotic fluid curve) and the top of the amniotic fluid curve at 450 nm is known as the ΔO.D. at 450 nm. (O.D. may also be referred to as absorbance [A].) The ΔO.D. at 450 nm is 0.23, as shown in Figure 31–3, and is calculated by subtracting the actual reading at 450 nm (0.39) from the estimated baseline at 450 nm (0.16). If RBC are present, they may lyse prior to removal and cause an oxyhemoglobin peak at 410 nm (Tietz, 1994). If the oxyhemoglobin peak is substantial, 5% of the ΔO.D. at 410 nm, $0.17 \times 5\% = 0.01$, should be subtracted from the ΔO.D. at 450 nm, $0.23 - 0.01 = 0.22$, because of the effect of the oxyhemoglobin contamination on the optical density read at 450 nm. Meconium staining of the amniotic fluid will contribute, in addition to bilirubin pigment, to the elevation at 450 nm, but there is no way to quantitatively compensate for meconium contamination (Tietz, 1994). Meconium has a broad elevation with a variable peak from 400 to 415 nm, as shown in Figure 31–4. Both meconium and oxyhemoglobin take about three weeks to clear.

After the ΔO.D. at 450 nm is calculated, it is placed on the Liley curve shown in Figure 31–5 and compared with past readings, if available, to see if the trend is increasing or decreasing. With increasing gestational age, the ΔO.D. is expected to decrease, if no further problems occur, because of the dilutional effect of the increase in amniotic fluid with fetal age.

4

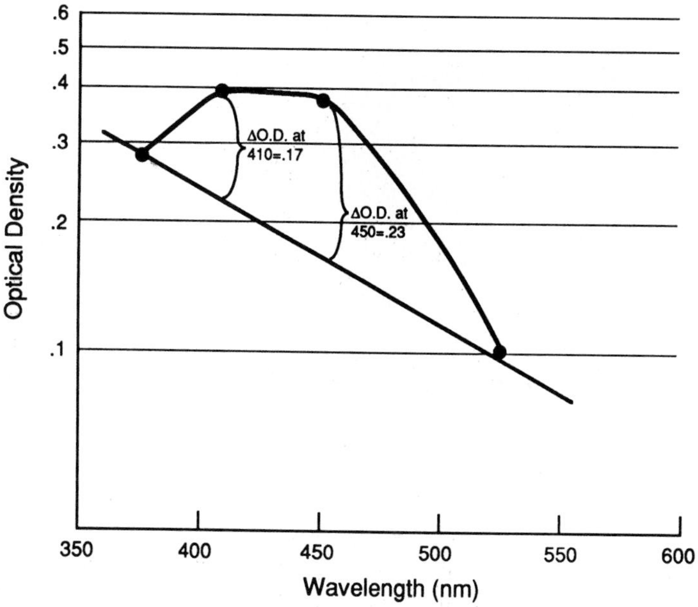

Figure 31–3. Amniotic fluid analysis. Baseline drawn between 375 and 525 nm on the actual curve to approximate the linearity of a normal curve. Bilirubin ΔO.D. at 450 nm = 0.23. Oxyhemoglobin ΔO.D. at 410 nm = 0.17. 0.23 − 5% (0.17) = 0.22 = ΔO.D. at 450 nm due to bilirubin. ΔO.D. = change in optical density. (Modified from Tietz NW: Fundamentals of Clinical Chemistry, 3rd ed. Philadelphia, W.B. Saunders Company, 1987, p 918.)

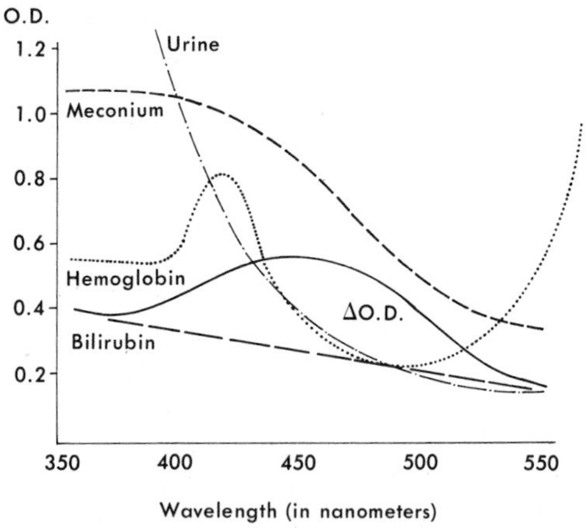

Figure 31–4. Differentiation of pigments commonly found in amniotic fluid by spectrophotometric scan.

The upper zone (high ΔO.D. at 450 nm) on the Liley curve correlates with the severe manifestations of HDN and fetal death; the middle zone correlates with moderately affected fetuses; and the lower zone (low ΔO.D. at 450 nm) correlates with mildly affected or unaffected fetuses.

Once the amniotic fluid is analyzed and the trend observed, there are three alternatives: allow the pregnancy to continue to term, perform intrauterine transfusion, or induce early labor. The maturity of the fetus must be considered in this decision, because if the fetus is less than 32 weeks old, its chances of viability after birth are diminished. Fetal age is determined by the date of the last menstrual period, by the size of the uterus, and by ultrasound measurements of both the length of the femur and the biparietal diameter. If the decision is to induce early labor, it is wise to determine the lecithin-sphingomyelin (L/S) ratio of the amniotic fluid to see if the surfactant activity of the fetal lung is sufficient. About 98% of babies with an L/S ratio of greater then 2.0 will not develop respiratory distress syndrome (RDS) if delivered within 24 hours of the test, whereas about 50% of the babies with an L/S ratio of 1.5 to 2.0 will develop RDS (Tietz, 1994). If the L/S ratio is less than 1.5, severe RDS should be anticipated.

Intrauterine transfusion (Sacher, 1987, p. 36) is performed by injecting hyperpacked (90% hematocrit) O-negative, CMV-negative (when appropriate) irradiated red cells into the fetal peritoneal cavity. About 80% of these RBC enter the fetal circulation via the lymphatics. Intrauterine transfusions are repeated every 10 to 21 days until delivery. Fetal transfusions using the relatively new percutaneous umbilical vein technique might also be considered and will be discussed more fully.

Plasmapheresis of the mother has been attempted with the intent of lowering the maternal IgG Rh_o (D) level so that the effect on the fetus will be diminished, but its efficacy is questionable, so it is listed in Category III in Table 31–6.

Percutaneous Umbilical Blood Sampling

Percutaneous umbilical blood sampling (PUBS), also known as cordocentesis, is becoming an important tool in fetal/maternal medicine. The technique allows for both diagnosis, through fetal blood aspiration, and therapy through direct access to the fetal circulation.

The PUBS procedure uses a long ultrasound-guided needle, 20 to 25 gauge, which ideally punctures the umbilical cord within 1 to 2 cm of its placental insertion, a point where the cord is well anchored and the risk of maternal blood contamination from the placenta is minimal (King, 1989). Most physicians prefer using the umbilical vein over the artery, because the vein is larger, is straighter in its course, and has a thinner wall. Furthermore, the incidence of inducing fetal bradycardia may be increased if the umbilical artery is entered (Nicolaides, 1988). A small blood sample may be aspi-

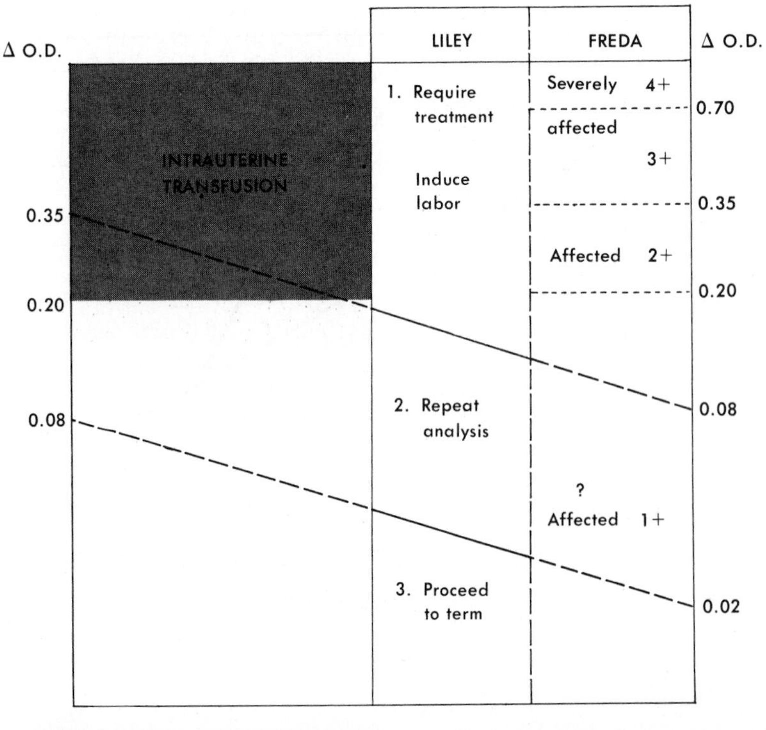

Figure 31–5. Methods of Liley and of Freda on the assessment of fetal prognosis by the values of ΔO.D. at 450 nm of bilirubin pigment in amniotic fluid. (Modified from WR Dito: Amniotic Fluid Analysis in Pregnancy at Risk. © 1975 by the American Society of Clinical Pathologists, Chicago. Also see Freda [1984].)

rated and sent for the desired studies, which should include a Kleihauer-Betke test and a mean corpuscular RBC volume (much higher in the fetus than in the adult) to assure that the specimen is from the fetus and not the mother.

After withdrawal of the needle, the fetus is monitored by using ultrasound to detect any significant blood leakage and by observing the fetal heart rate to discover any bradycardia related to fetal distress.

The major complications from the use of PUBS are blood extravasation from the puncture site, fetal bradycardia, and chorioamnionitis; the rate of procedure-related fetal loss is between 1% and 2% (Ludomirski, 1988; Nicolaides, 1988). This is lower than the fetal loss rate of 2% to 5% noted with fetoscopy (Ludomirski, 1988). To diminish the chance of developing chorioamnionitis, one investigator (Ludomirski, 1988) routinely administers broad-spectrum antibiotics to the mother after the procedure.

Indications

PUBS can be performed after the seventeenth week of gestation (Ludomirski, 1988; Nicolaides, 1988). It is useful in the prenatal diagnosis of the following:

1. Inherited and acquired blood disorders, including hemoglobinopathies, coagulopathies, autoimmune and alloimmune thrombocytopenia, and inherited immunodeficiency syndromes
2. Infections including rubella, toxoplasmosis, and cytomegalovirus
3. Inherited metabolic disorders
4. Hypoxia or acid base imbalance found in conditions related to fetal distress

Amniocentesis followed by two to three weeks of culture usually provides enough cells for biochemical and cytogenetic analysis. Karyotyping of fetal blood lymphocytes can be available within three days (King, 1989) so that PUBS would be useful when the patient's first presentation comes later than usual in the pregnancy or when the previous culture has failed. However, even more rapid is the moderately safe technique of chorionic villus sampling. This is a type of placental biopsy that yields 15 to 30 mg of tissue, which usually is sufficient material with which to perform direct biochemical and cytogenetic analysis, which can be available in several hours (Wapner, 1988).

Because of the higher risks of fetoscopy to both the mother and the fetus, PUBS will probably replace fetoscopy in most situations. Additionally, because amniocentesis for HDN is not reliable until the third trimester of pregnancy (Ludomirski, 1988; Nicolaides, 1988) and gives only indirect evidence of fetal hemolysis, PUBS will probably be used increasingly for HDN because it provides direct access to fetal RBC to permit a hematocrit/hemoglobin and direct antiglobulin test.

In the past, fetal RBC transfusions for HDN were performed, usually after the twenty-fifth week of gestation, by injecting the cells into the fetus intraperitoneally. Intravascular absorption of the RBC from the peritoneum could be hampered if ascites were present. The ability to conduct direct intravascular transfusions in the fetus, using PUBS, allows the transfusion therapy to begin several weeks earlier and provides for a better and more rapid therapeutic response. Platelets can also be transfused directly into the fetal circulation using PUBS when thrombocytopenia in the fetus is severe (King, 1989).

Exchange Transfusion

Once the fetus with HDN is delivered, there are further problems that may necessitate neonatal exchange transfusion. Excess bilirubin in the fetus derived from extravascular hemolysis is handled by release to the mother's circulation, where it is bound to maternal albumin, conjugated in the mother's liver, and then excreted into the bile. In the newborn with HDN, the glucuronyl transferase levels in the immature liver are low, and the amount of serum albumin is limited. Therefore, the excess unconjugated (free) bilirubin increases in the neonatal circulation. The blood-brain barrier is poorly developed in the neonate, so the unconjugated (free) bilirubin passes into the brain, as shown in Figure 31–6. Because bilirubin has an affinity for the basal ganglia, it accumulates there. The term kernicterus is used to describe this phenomenon. Clinically, kernicterus first results in lethargy and opisthotonos but eventually goes on to respiratory failure and death. In milder cases, the infant may appear normal but later exhibits mental retardation. To prevent kernicterus, exchange transfusions are performed when the unconjugated serum bilirubin reaches 6 to 9 mg/dL in premature infants, when the bilirubin rises to 18 mg/dL in the full-term infant, or when there is a rapid rise in the bilirubin, exceeding 8.6 μmol/L/hour (Walker, 1993, p. 456). The exchange transfusion should take place earlier if acidosis or anoxia is present.

Besides increasing hyperbilirubinemia, several other laboratory evaluations indicate HDN. Anemia (less than 15 g/dL) is present, and the peripheral smear shows nucleated red cells (erythroblastosis) and reticulocytes if the condition is due to warm reacting IgG antibodies (Rh, Kell, Duffy systems) or spherocytes if the condition is due to ABO incompatibility. ABO incompatibility only rarely causes HDN severe enough to require exchange transfusion; when it occurs, it is in a type-O mother who has a type A, B, or AB baby. The direct antiglobulin test (DAT) will be positive because the mother's IgG antibodies will be coating the fetal cells. However, the strength of the DAT does not correlate with the severity of the HDN.

Exchange transfusion removes unbound IgG antibody, excess bilirubin, and antibody-coated RBC. It also corrects the anemia and replaces fetal RBC with adult RBC, which have better release of oxygen to the tissues. Besides hyperbilirubinemia, exchange transfusion is used for sepsis, disseminated intravascular coagulation, polycythemia, respiratory distress syndrome, hyperammonemia, and toxin removal (Seibel, 1987).

The blood used for the exchange transfusion should be ABO compatible, less than one week old to provide maximum 2,3-DPG levels, and close to body temperature. In the premature infant who weighs less than 1200 g and who is potentially immunocompromised, blood irradiated with 25 Gy is used to prevent graft versus host disease. CMV-negative blood should be provided if the mother is CMV negative. The administration of 1 mL of 10% calcium gluconate solution for every 100 mL of citrated blood infused might also be considered, because the immature liver may handle the cit-

4

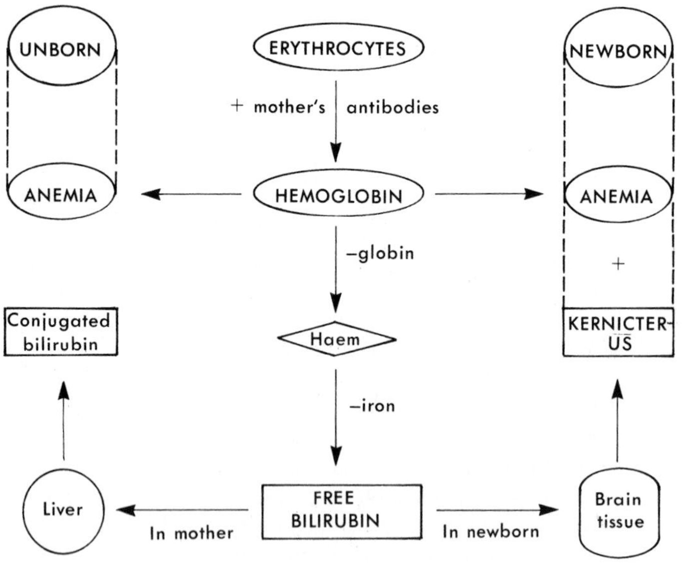

Figure 31–6. The effect of immune hemolysis in the unborn (anemia only) and in the newborn (anemia and kernicterus). This difference is due to the fact that the newborn's liver has insufficient glucuronidase to conjugate free bilirubin, which has a high affinity for brain tissue, thus producing kernicterus.

rate poorly. If calcium is employed, a different IV line should be used so that the calcium administered will not overcome the citrate anticoagulant in the transfused blood, thereby causing the blood to clot in the IV line.

The red cell crossmatch in the newborn or fetus is usually performed using the mother's serum. However, if the mother and baby are not of the same ABO blood groups, group O blood should be transfused. If the mother's serum is not available, the baby's serum and the eluate of the baby's cells (if the DAT is positive) can be used for crossmatching.

When the mother has an antibody to a high-incidence antigen on her baby's RBC, the best chance of finding a compatible unit is to test the mother's RBC for compatibility. If compatible, the mother's blood donation can be used after the antibody has been removed by washing the blood. Additionally, the mother's blood should be irradiated prior to the infusion to prevent graft versus host disease.

Similarly, in the case of isoimmune thrombocytopenia of the newborn, in which the mother produces an IgG antibody against a high-incidence platelet antigen, usually $P1^{A1}$, on the baby's platelets, the best platelet product to give the baby in order to correct the thrombocytopenia is the mother's washed, irradiated platelets. The mother's platelets should be negative for the antigen to which she is producing the antibody. Immune serum globulin has been administered to mothers in subsequent pregnancies when they have had a previous child born with isoimmune thrombocytopenia. Maternal ISG treatment has successfully raised the platelet count of the fetus in utero (Bussel, 1988b).

Cytokines as Therapeutic Agents and Their Effect on Blood Banking

Hematopoietic Growth Factors

Cytokines are hormone-like substances, secreted by cells, that influence other cells by either stimulating or inhibiting them. They are usually named by their cellular source or their biological activity on the target cells. One class of cytokine is the hematopoietic growth factors, also known as colony-stimulating factors (CSF). These factors are polypeptides released by B and T lymphocytes, monocytes, macrophages, fibroblasts, endothelial cells, various epithelial cells, some tumor cells, and in the case of erythropoietin (EPO), renal cortical interstitial cells (Zanjani, 1989). As their name suggests, CSF cause single hematopoietic progenitor cells to form colonies *in vitro*—hence the term colony-forming units (CFU). The term cytokine includes interferons, interleukins, tumor necrosis factors, colony-stimulating factors, and transforming growth factors.

Erythropoietin

EPO, one type of CSF, promotes RBC production by stimulating erythroid precursors to proliferate, differentiate, and mature. Its primary site of production is the kidney, but small quantities are also produced by the liver. EPO is increased during hypoxemia and is suppressed with hyperoxemia or bilateral nephrectomy.

Recombinant EPO has been shown to either eliminate or significantly reduce the RBC transfusion requirements of end stage renal disease and to correct the uremic hemostatic abnormalities in these patients. Complications of EPO therapy include hypertension, headache, clotting of vascular access devices, and aching in the long bones.

Additionally, EPO has been used to significantly ameliorate the anemia found in (1) HIV patients receiving zidovudine therapy, (2) malignancy, (3) autoimmune disease, and (4) the premature newborn (Goodnough, 1994).

EPO can also be used to facilitate the aggressive withdrawal of units of autologous blood over several weeks. Note that the effects of EPO are not immediate; several weeks of therapy are needed before there is a recognizable response manifested as an increase in the hematocrit.

Similar to the case with EPO, the recent discovery of thrombopoietin (Metcalf, 1994) assuredly will greatly reduce the need for platelet transfusions in many thrombocytopenic conditions once the recombinant form is commercially produced, tested, and approved for use.

Other Colony-Stimulating Factors

Recombinant granulocyte-macrophage colony-stimulating factor (GM-CSF) has been shown to stimulate the proliferation and differentiation of peripheral blood phagocytes (granulocytes and monocytes), activate mature phagocytes, increase peripheral leukocyte counts, shorten the period of neutropenia after intensive chemotherapy, and accelerate myeloid recovery after bone marrow transplantation. Similarly, recombinant granulocyte colony-stimulating factor (G-CSF) has been shown to reduce periods of neutropenia after intensive chemotherapy by stimulating marrow production of granulocyte precursors and enhancing the release of granulocytes and their precursors into the peripheral blood. G-CSF has induced substantial improvement in neutrophil counts in patients with congenital idiopathic neutropenia, cyclic neutropenia, and acquired chronic neutropenia. GM-CSF has been much less effective in this last group of conditions (Goodnough, 1994).

Interleukins

Another class of cytokine, the interleukins, comprise a group of soluble proteins secreted by lymphocytes and macrophages in response to foreign antigenic stimuli. Interleukins are helpful in coordinating activities involved with mounting both a cellular and a humoral immune response, but they also contribute to hematopoietic stimulation. For example, interleukin-1 (IL-1), which is released by activated macrophages and participates in T-cell activation, has also been shown to promote growth of primitive hematopoietic stem cells.

Of all the interleukins, IL-2 has received the most publicity because of its use in adoptive immunotherapy for cancer. IL-2 mediates the expansion of cytotoxic lymphocytes after they are activated. Lymphokine-activated killer (LAK) cells are produced by incubating peripheral blood lymphocytes, taken from a cancer patient, with recombinant IL-2. These reactive cytotoxic lymphocytes are induced to proliferate when put in culture for several weeks with IL-2. The LAK cells are then reinfused into the same cancer patient along with high doses of IL-2. LAK cell therapy has caused tumor regression in renal cell cancer, melanoma, colorectal cancer, and non-Hodgkin's lymphoma, but the response rate is only about 20% (Rosenberg, 1988). The treatment has proven to be moderately toxic and usually requires several days of intensive care after therapy is instituted. The toxicity is thought to be caused by the required high doses of IL-2, which induces capillary permeability and hypotension, leading to fluid retention and organ dysfunction.

A modification of LAK cell therapy, called tumor infiltrating lymphocytes (TILs), is currently being evaluated for its antineoplastic capabilities in patients with advanced cancers who have not responded to standard forms of treatment (Topalian, 1988). TILs are derived from surgically removed solid tumor specimens by enzymatically digesting the tumor tissue and selectively expanding the subset of lymphocytes responsive to recombinant IL-2 by placing the specimens in culture for several weeks. TILs and recombinant IL-2 are administered after pretreatment of the patient with cyclophosphamide. TILs have been found to be cytotoxic T lymphocytes that are apparently much more effective against tumor cells and more tumor specific than LAK cells (Topalian, 1988).

Unlike LAK cell therapy, for TILs to be effective against the tumor, cyclophosphamide must be administered to the patient, prior to the TILs infusion, to make the patient immunosuppressed in an attempt to eliminate suppressor T cells (Klein, 1989). LAK cells and TILs are the first of a new generation of blood cell components grown outside the body and then used to modify the immune response.

PRETRANSFUSION TESTING

Pretransfusion testing provides the basis for selecting the most appropriate blood component for the recipient so that the blood product survives adequately and so that no harm or poor interaction occurs when the product is transfused. The general steps in the process include:

1. Proper identification of the recipient and the blood specimen collected from the recipient
2. Review of any previous records of the recipient and comparison with the current results
3. Determination of the ABO/Rh type and testing for unexpected antibodies
4. Selection of the appropriate ABO/Rh-compatible blood component for the recipient
5. Performing tests to look for incompatibility between the recipient's serum and donor cells

General Considerations

The transfusion request form must have the patient's first and last name as well as a unique hospital identification number. If any of the required information is missing or the writing is illegible, the form cannot be accepted.

The phlebotomist must confirm the identity of the patient by comparing the information on the patient's wristband to that on the transfusion request form. The specimen should be labeled at the bedside and include the first and last name of the patient, the unique hospital number of the patient, the date of collection, and the initials of the phlebotomist. In an emergency in which the patient is unconscious and unknown, an emergency identity bracelet should be placed on the patient prior to obtaining the specimen.

If the blood specimen is obtained from an intravenous line, the line should be flushed with normal saline and the first 5 mL of blood drawn should be discarded to prevent residual fluid from interfering with the testing. Serum is preferred to plasma (1) because in plasma, small clots sometimes develop, making it difficult to distinguish from an agglutination reaction, and (2) because plasma, if anticoagulated with citrate or EDTA, binds calcium so that complement activation and subsequent cell lysis is prevented. Plasma can be converted to serum by treating it with thrombin, protamine, or glass beads, depending on the anticoagulant. Hemolyzed specimens should not be used, because antibody-induced hemolysis cannot be detected.

If the patient has been pregnant or has undergone transfusion in the past three months (Klein, 1994, p. 25), the blood sample should be less than three days old, because detectable antibody can occur at any time up to three months after exposure. The choice of three days by the AABB standards is somewhat arbitrary but accommodates preadmission testing on Friday for Monday morning surgery.

Neonatal patients can be treated differently. If the initial tests demonstrate no unexpected antibodies and the infant has received no blood transfusions, it is not necessary to perform further testing during the four-month neonatal period. After the initial ABO/Rh typing, repeat testing can be omitted for the remainder of the neonatal period if the infant has (1) received its own ABO type or group O cells and (2) received its own Rh type or Rh-negative cells (Klein, 1994, p. 28).

The information on the transfusion request form and the specimen label must be identical. Illegible or incomplete labels should be reasons not to accept the specimen. The blood specimens from the recipient and donor must be sealed or stoppered and stored at 1°C to 6°C for seven days after the transfusion (Klein, 1994, p. 30). This post-transfusion storage time has been selected so that, in the event of a delayed hemolytic transfusion reaction, a pretransfusion specimen will be available for re-evaluation.

The prior transfusion history records of the recipient should be compared with current testing results to make sure that there are no discrepancies. If there was a clinically significant antibody in the past that is not currently demonstrable, the patient should still receive blood negative for the corresponding antigen. If blood containing the previous red cell antigen is transfused, a more rapid secondary immune (anamnestic) response may be induced in the recipient.

Every recipient should undergo serologic testing before blood is issued. The tests should include ABO/Rh typing and a screen for unexpected antibodies. If ABO/Rh discrepancies occur, give O-negative and crossmatch-compatible units until the problem is resolved.

The hospital transfusion service must confirm the ABO type on each donor unit and repeat the Rh type on Rh-negative units. If a discrepancy is detected between the tests performed at the hospital transfusion service and those performed at the blood center, the unit should be isolated and returned to the blood center for resolution of the problem. All donor unit serologic testing should be done using an integrally attached segment, rather than the test tube, because the segments are the true representation of the blood in the bag. The donor cells should be washed before testing in order to eliminate interference from plasma and from fibrin clots.

Antibody Screen

Antibody detection or screening is much more important in patients than in donors because the adult patient has 2 to 3 liters of plasma, a much greater amount than is found in a unit of blood (250 mL of plasma). Furthermore, weak-reacting antibodies can become stronger owing to a secondary immune (anamnestic) response after appropriate antigen stimulation from an incompatible blood transfusion. Antibody screening is done with at least two screening cells, tested separately, to detect the commonly encountered clinically significant antibodies (Boral, 1977). The antiglobulin phase must be included routinely for this test. IgG, antibody-coated RBC (check cells) should be used with any negative antiglobulin test to eliminate the possibility of a falsely negative test. A negative antibody screen does not exclude the presence of unexpected antibodies in the patient's serum. Antibodies to low-incidence antigens may be rarely detected only during the crossmatch and not on the antibody screen. Unexpected antibodies are those other than in the ABO system. The antibodies of the ABO system (anti-A, anti-B, anti-A,B) are naturally occurring and expected. Clinically significant antibodies are those that are known to cause transfusion reactions or decreased RBC survival. Usually, antibodies detected at 37°C (body temperature) are clinically significant, whereas those reacting only at room temperature or below are probably insignificant and inactive at body temperatures (Giblett, 1977). Some antibodies cannot be detected by heterozygous cells and need a homozygous cell to cause agglutination. This is called the dosage effect and occurs in the Rh, Kell, Duffy, and Kidd systems. Commercial companies attempt to provide reagent screening cells that are homozygous for these systems. Those providing three-cell reagent screens can usually guarantee homozygosity for these systems.

ABO/Rh typing with an antibody screen (type and screen) may be ordered without a crossmatch for patients undergoing surgical procedures that normally do not require blood. The results of the type and antibody screen procedure make available to the surgeon and anesthesiologist the ABO/Rh type of the patient and the knowledge that no unexpected antibodies are present. If antibodies are found, two crossmatch-compatible, antigen-negative units should be placed on hold in case significant bleeding occurs. A list of elective surgery procedures acceptable for the type and screen category is provided in Table 31–7.

The Crossmatch

The major crossmatch consists of testing the patient's serum against the donor's RBC. The crossmatch is expected to detect ABO incompatibility and clinically significant unexpected antibodies. If the antibody screen, taken through the antiglobulin phase, showed no clinically significant antibodies and there is no previous record of such antibodies, the antiglobulin phase of the crossmatch can be omitted and only testing methods that detect ABO incompatibility are required (Klein, 1994, p. 26). This last step may be satisfied by performing only an immediate-spin crossmatch or by performing a computer system verification when the computer has

Table 31–7. PROCEDURES FOR WHICH BLOOD IS USUALLY CROSSMATCHED BUT FOR WHICH TYPE AND SCREEN WOULD APPEAR ADEQUATE

Type of Surgery	Procedure
General	Cholecystectomy; exploratory laparotomy; thyroidectomy; parathyroidectomy; parotidectomy; colostomy; vein stripping
Gynecologic	Hysterectomy; uterine suspension; tuboplasty; ovarian wedge resection
Neurosurgery	Laminectomy; ventriculoperitoneal shunt
Orthopedic	Total knee; medial meniscectomy; leg amputation; arthroscopy; removal of hip pin
Otolaryngology	Transantral ethmoidectomy; Caldwell-Luc
Plastic	Reduction mammoplasty; skin flap; skin graft
Urologic	Transurethral resection of the prostate; pyelolithotomy; ureterolithotomy; cystotomy; transurethral resection of bladder tumor; fulguration of bleeding bladder tumor, orchiectomy; orchiopexy; ureteral reimplantation

Reprinted by permission from the *New York State Journal of Medicine*, copyright by the Medical Society of the State of New York. From Mintz PD, Nordine RB, Henry JB, Webb WR: Expected hemotherapy in elective surgery. NY State J Med 1976; 76:532.

been appropriately validated to prevent the release of ABO-incompatible blood components (Klein, 1994, p. 26). It should be noted that the immediate-spin crossmatch does not always detect ABO incompatibility (Berry-Dortch, 1985; Lamberson, 1986). If, at any time, a clinically significant antibody is found, the antiglobulin phase of the crossmatch is required.

It is no longer necessary to perform a minor crossmatch (a mixture of patient cells with donor plasma), because donor units are screened for unexpected antibodies.

Some laboratories routinely include an autocontrol, but this test is probably useful only if the patient has recently undergone transfusion (Judd, 1980).

Blood ordering schedules that list the number of crossmatches to be ordered or the category of type and screen for many different elective surgery procedures have been published (Boral, 1979; Friedman, 1976; Mintz, 1976) and can be tailored to a specific hospital through examination of previous records of blood utilization. Implementing such a guideline can reduce the number of unnecessary crossmatches and can help in identifying potential problem cases by further investigation when too many units are ordered.

Selection of Units

If the patient cannot receive an RBC component of his or her own ABO group, an alternative ABO group may be used (Table 31–8). Group O is considered the universal RBC donor because the expected antibodies of the ABO system—anti-A, anti-B, and anti-A,B—will not react with group O red cells. Group AB patients are the universal red cell recipient because their serum contains no expected ABO antibodies. Consequently, group AB patients can receive packed or washed RBC (removed antibodies) from group A, B, AB, or O donors.

If the component to be transfused contains 5 mL or more of RBC, the donor's RBC must be ABO-compatible with the recipient's serum. If large amounts of incompatible plasma are transfused, the patient may develop a positive direct antiglobulin test with possible damage and decreased survival of the patient's own RBC.

Rh_0 (D) positive blood should be transfused to Rh_0 (D) positive patients. Rh_0 (D) negative blood is acceptable for Rh_0 (D) positive patients, but because the Rh_0 (D) negative blood accounts for only 15% of the donor population, it should be reserved for Rh_0 (D) negative patients.

Table 31–8. ABO AND RH_0 (D) COMPATIBILITY IN BLOOD TRANSFUSION

Blood Type of Recipient	Blood Type of Donor					
	O	*A*	*B*	*AB*	*D−*	*D+*
O	Yes	No	No	No		
A	S	Yes	No	No		
B	S	No	Yes	No		
AB	S	S	S	Yes		
D−					Yes	E
D+					Yes	Yes

S = substitute as packed red blood cells or wash to eliminate antibodies; E = only under extreme emergency conditions, especially if the recipient is a young female.

Rh_0 (D) negative patients should receive Rh_0 (D) negative blood. Sometimes ABO-compatible, Rh_0 (D) negative blood is not readily available. At these times, Rh_0 (D) negative blood should be reserved for Rh_0 (D) negative females of child-bearing age (under 45 years old) or younger to avoid the formation of anti-Rh_0 (D). If exposed to Rh_0 (D) positive RBC, these women may develop HDN with future pregnancies. Additionally, Rh_0 (D) negative blood should be reserved for those Rh_0 (D) negative patients who have already exhibited anti-Rh_0 (D). In times of Rh_0 (D) negative blood shortages, it is permissible to transfuse Rh_0 (D) positive blood to Rh_0 (D) negative patients who are men or older women if they do not already have an anti-Rh_0 (D) antibody. However, it must be realized that many of these persons may subsequently develop an anti-Rh_0 (D) antibody about three months later. Therefore, if an Rh_0 (D) negative person is expected to undergo chronic transfusion, that person should probably not be sensitized, if possible.

Sometimes it is necessary for a patient who has received many units of group O blood to receive blood from his or her original blood group—A, B, or AB. This may be done when compatibility tests no longer demonstrate incompatible ABO antibodies. If tests show incompatibility, it is best to remain with group O transfusions.

Only ABO and Rh_0 (D) antigens are routinely tested on blood units. If an antibody is detected in the patient's serum, the units must be tested appropriately, and only corresponding antigen-negative RBC should be transfused.

It is anticipated that all ABO donor units soon will be converted to group O (the universal donor type). Exoglycosidase α-galactosidase has been used to remove B antigen (terminal α-linked galactose), leaving behind the group O structure (Lenny, 1994). There have been no adverse effects, but the titer of anti-B has increased significantly in the recipient. A similar enzymatic process has been used to remove A antigen from A_2 blood, but the complete removal of A antigen from the more complex A_1 blood has not yet been perfected. Once all types of donor units can be converted to group O, there will be much fewer blood supply problems and much fewer incidents of acute immune intravascular hemolytic transfusion reactions. Imagine what blood banking will be like when and if we can remove Rh, Kell, Duffy, and Kidd antigens from red cells.

Interpretation of Compatibility Testing

Compatibility testing includes the ABO/Rh testing of the donor and recipient, antibody screen on the recipient specimen, and the major crossmatch.

Ninety-five percent of specimens demonstrate a negative antibody screen and a negative crossmatch. Given these conditions, the transfusion can be conducted relatively safely.

If the antibody screen is positive and the crossmatch is positive, the unit should not be used for transfusion unless the blood bank physician has been consulted about the risks of transfusing incompatible blood. First, the antibody should be identified by performing an RBC antigen panel. After antibody identification, donor units should be screened to provide the appropriate antigen-negative units. The screen can be conducted using reagent antibody or serum from the patient. If the antibody detected is directed against a high-incidence antigen, it may be necessary to contact the Rare Donor File (Berry-Dortch, 1983) to provide compatible blood.

If the RBC panel detects a specific antibody and the autocontrol is positive, examine the autocontrol under the microscope for mixed field agglutination. If the patient has undergone transfusion within the past three months, the antibody might be reacting with the transfused cells remaining in the circulation, resulting in a mixed field reaction. This would indicate a delayed transfusion reaction. An elution should be done to identify the antibody on the RBC. Additionally, mixed field agglutination could occur if donor antibodies are transfused and react with the recipient's cells.

Autoantibodies may create many problems in serologic testing. The cause of the autoantibody production may be disease associated, drug induced, or idiopathic. Cold autoantibodies can interfere with ABO/Rh testing, the antibody screen, and the crossmatch. When cold antibodies (i.e., anti-I) have a high thermal range, they can bind complement so that the antiglobulin phase of the antibody screen or crossmatch will be positive. Such antibodies are also often positive on the immediate spin phase of these tests. To prevent interference from cold autoantibodies in ABO/Rh testing, the RBC must be separated from the plasma while the blood specimen is maintained at 37°C from the time of the phlebotomy. The cells should then be washed in saline at 37°C. Serum can be obtained from the clotted specimen, which is kept at room temperature. Additionally, the specimen should be prewarmed (Walker, 1993, p. 642) for the antibody screen and crossmatch when a cold autoantibody interferes in routine testing. Autoadsorption of the cold autoantibody at 4°C may be necessary.

Aldomet (methyldopa) is a common cause of warm autoantibody production. Autoimmune disease can also cause this phenomenon. The presence of a warm autoantibody can interfere with Rh_o (D) typing if the anti-Rh_o (D) reagent contains significant amounts of potentiators. Chemically modified anti-Rh_o (D) is helpful for Rh_o (D) typing in these situations. If the patient has not undergone transfusion in the past three months, the serum can be autoadsorbed at 37°C in an attempt to remove all the autoantibody, allowing a search for specific alloantibodies. Additionally, an eluate can be performed to detect specific antibodies.

Warm autoadsorbed serum may be used to find serologically compatible units. Should the patient have autoantibodies without alloantibodies, transfusion of least incompatible units (reacting less strongly than the autocontrol) may be attempted. Patients can usually tolerate such transfusions unless an underlying alloantibody has been missed.

The *in vivo* compatibility test may be attempted under special conditions, when patients require blood in the presence of an incompatible crossmatch, and the nature of the incompatibility has not been elucidated or compatible blood cannot be found. For this test, RBC survival studies, using small samples of RBC tagged with radioactive indium or technetium, have been performed (Davey, 1987; Marcus, 1987).

The antibody screen sometimes is negative and the crossmatch positive. This condition may indicate the presence of an antibody directed against low-frequency antigens. An RBC antigen panel should be performed to identify the antibody. Incompatibility will also occur if the donor RBC yield a positive direct antiglobulin test (DAT). The DAT is not routinely performed on donor units, and it is estimated that between 1 in 1000 and 1 in 13,000 healthy donors produce a positive DAT (Garratty, 1988). In this case, the donor cells will be incompatible with the serum of all potential recipients, and therefore the unit should be discarded. Another reason for this condition is that the donor cells could be in a polyagglutinable state from T activation (T, Tn, Tk). Last, and most important, this condition could result from ABO incompatibility. ABO antibodies would react with incompatible cells in the crossmatch but would not react with the screening RBC, which are always group O.

If the RBC antibody screen (group O cells) is positive, but the crossmatch is negative, anti-Le^{bH} might be suspected. This antibody is produced by A_1, B, or A_1B phenotypes and reacts with cells that have the H (O or A_2) as well as the Le^b antigens (Walker, 1993, p. 221).

Table 31–9 shows the time it takes to conduct the tests required for preparing for a blood transfusion. Table 31–10 is interesting because it summarizes the cumulative probability of safe blood transfusion as different serologic tests are added. If random blood, taken off the shelf without any testing, were to be used, almost two thirds of these transfusions would be compatible. When ABO groups are matched, over 99% are compatible. Matching for Rh_o (D) improves the odds by 0.4%, whereas antibody screening increases the odds only 0.14%. The crossmatch increases the safety only 0.01%. Recently, there has been less emphasis on the crossmatch, and many hospitals are only using the immediate-spin or abbreviated crossmatch after completing an antibody screen taken through the antiglobulin phase (see Chap. 30).

INFUSION OF BLOOD COMPONENTS

Proper Identification

Most fatal transfusion reactions are due to clerical errors resulting in an ABO-incompatible transfusion (Myhre, 1980). Therefore, ABO typing from the correct specimen is vital.

Table 31–9. APPROXIMATE TIME REQUIRED FOR PREPARING FOR A BLOOD TRANSFUSION*

Procedures	Time in Minutes
1. Collecting the blood	10
2. ABO and Rh typing	10
3. ABO and Rh typing plus antibody screening	45
4. Typing, antibody screening, and crossmatching	60
5. Antibody identification, additional	60+ (up to several days)
6. Fresh-frozen plasma thawing	40
7. Cryoprecipitate thawing	20
8. Washing erythrocytes	45
9. Thawing and washing of frozen erythrocytes	60

*Excluding pick-up and delivery.

Table 31–10. PROBABILITY OF SAFE BLOOD TRANSFUSION

Procedure	Compatibility Individual (%)	Compatibility Cumulative (%)
None	64.4	64.4
ABO grouping	35.0	99.4
Rh typing	0.4	99.8
Antibody screening	0.14	99.94
Crossmatching	0.01	99.95
Autotransfusion	100	100

Modified from Walker RH: On the safety of the abbreviated crossmatch. *In* Polesky HF, Walker RH (eds): Safety in Transfusion Practices. Skokie, Illinois, College of American Pathologists, 1982, pp 71–106.

Correct identification of the recipient is probably the most crucial activity in the blood transfusion process. There are two times when the patient must be properly identified, once at the time of the specimen collection, and again at the initiation of the blood transfusion. During specimen collection, the transfusion request form and specimen label must be compared with the patient's wristband to assure identity of the first and last names as well as the unique hospital number. Similarly, before a blood component can be started, the blood product label, the attached compatibility tag, and the patient's wristband must be compared to assure that the first and last names as well as the unique hospital numbers are the same and that ABO/Rh types of the product and recipient are compatible.

Emergency situations, in the Emergency Room, operating room, or intensive care units, are the times when identification errors most often occur. Therefore, personnel from these areas who are involved in collecting specimens and starting blood transfusions must be particularly cautious during emergencies.

Conditions Affecting the Infusion of Blood Components

Intravenous Fluid

Normal (0.9%) saline is usually employed to start an IV line prior to instituting a blood transfusion. Five percent dextrose in water (D5W) is hypotonic and may cause RBC aggregation and hemolysis, whereas Ringer's lactate may cause clotting because of its calcium content. Packed RBC may be diluted with normal saline or rarely with ABO-compatible plasma or 5% albumin to decrease the viscosity and allow for increased rates of infusion.

Medications should not be added to or administered in the same line with blood components. The excessively high or low pH of some drugs may induce hemolysis if they are added to RBC. Additionally, if medication were added to a unit of blood and the unit were discontinued because of a transfusion reaction, the full dose of the medication would not be given. Lastly, if a transfusion reaction occurs, it would be difficult to discern whether the reaction was due to the drug or to the blood.

RBC should be stored in a monitored blood bank refrigerator until immediately before transfusion. Therefore, a blood component should not be requested until an intravenous line has been started.

Filters

Blood components and derivatives must be transfused through a filter to remove fibrin clots and other particulate debris. Most standard blood and platelet transfusion sets contain first-generation filters with a pore size of approximately 170 μm. The surface area of the filters varies widely, as does the arrangement of the filter and drip chamber. Under normal conditions, one filter can be used for two to four units of blood. However, the condition of the filter and the total time (less than four hours) of infusion must be considered and the filter changed accordingly.

Microaggregates consist of platelets, degenerating WBC, cell fragments, nuclei, and fibrin. They form progressively in whole blood or packed RBC after about 5 days of refrigerated storage. These microaggregates can be as large as 100 μm in diameter. Second-generation microaggregate filters, with pore sizes between 20 and 40 μm, are composed principally of plastic wool fibers. They are available as either screen filters, which remove microaggregates by direct interception, or depth filters, which are made of several layers of mesh or of foam. They are probably most useful to prevent the infusion of large numbers of microaggregates, which might occur during the massive transfusions used in cardiopulmonary bypass, or to prevent microaggregate-induced hypoxia in patients with previously compromised pulmonary function who have undergone transfusion. Microaggregate filters do not remove individual WBC. Microaggregate filters should not be used with either platelet or granulocyte concentrates, because a large percentage of these viable cellular elements are retained by these filters.

The spin-cool-filter method was discussed earlier, in the section entitled Leukocyte-Reduced Red Cells. It was a popular, relatively inexpensive method, using microaggregate filters to remove less than 85% of the leukocytes.

Third-generation leukoreduction filters are available that selectively remove 99.9% (3 logs) of WBC from RBC (Kickler, 1989) and platelet (Wenz, 1989) products, leaving fewer than 5×10^6 WBC in their respective blood components. The potential applications of these 3-log selective adsorption filters include the prevention of HLA sensitization, febrile nonhemolytic transfusion reactions, viral transmission (i.e., CMV, HTLV-1), transfusion-associated immune suppression,

4

and graft versus host disease (Bordin, 1994). However, because 3-log WBC filtration is not assured under all conditions—that is, slow flow (Ledent, 1994)—it is best to use other proven techniques wherever possible: CMV serologically negative units or frozen-thawed blood components to prevent CMV infection and the irradiation of blood components to prevent GVHD. 3-Log leukoreduction filtration should be saved for when no better method exists—such as prevention of HLA sensitization—or when time does not permit use of an assured alternative method. Techniques to further reduce white cell contamination of blood components are currently under investigation: (1) a newly developed filter that removes 6 logs of WBC (Sadoff, 1992) and (2) filtration directly after platelet rich plasma production but before the hard spin to produce platelet concentrates (Dzik, 1992).

Blood Warmers

Rapid infusion of large volumes of cold blood may precipitate ventricular arrhythmia and even death. A blood warmer is recommended for patients receiving many units of cold blood in a short time, in massive transfusion, in exchange transfusions, in transfusion of premature infants, and in patients with strong cold autoagglutinins. The temperature of the blood warmer should be maintained at about 37°C. No hemolysis or increase in plasma potassium level will result at this temperature; however, hemolysis is possible when the blood temperature exceeds 42°C (Klein, 1994, p. 32). Warming the patient with cold agglutinin disease during the transfusion is recommended.

Speed of Infusion

In most administration sets, 15 drops equal 1 mL. At a rate of 60 drops/min, $60/15 \times 60 = 240$ mL of blood can be transfused in one hour. The duration of the transfusion can thus be estimated by the rate of infusion. Under normal conditions for an average adult without cardiopulmonary dysfunction, one unit of blood should be infused within one or two hours. If the unit of blood needs to be infused slowly, the transfusion should be completed within four hours. Blood transfusion should not be used to keep intravenous lines open, and extended time for infusions should be avoided. Blood is an ideal culture medium, and when it warms up over several hours at room temperature it allows growth of bacteria that may enter the system during blood collection or infusion.

In massive bleeding, the rate of infusion can be accelerated via large needles at more than one site. In patients with severe anemia or heart failure, the rate of infusion should be reduced, and concurrent use of diuretics, digitalis, or both may be helpful. It may be necessary to transfuse only half of one unit at one time. The remaining half should be stored in a blood bank refrigerator and used later but within 24 hours. As a rule, during the first 15 minutes of transfusion, the rate of infusion should be slow to allow observation of any patient reaction, especially when a least incompatible unit is being transfused or when previous transfusion reactions have been reported.

Monitoring the Patient

Transfusion is a serious and potentially hazardous treatment. Reactions can be fatal if proper precautions are not observed. In the United States, any fatal transfusion reaction must be reported within 24 hours to the FDA. Most transfusion reactions develop within 30 minutes of transfusion. If the patient is being monitored carefully by medical or nursing personnel, most fatal transfusion reactions can be avoided by prompt, early, and appropriate action. A patient's vital signs should be taken and recorded shortly before the transfusion to serve as a baseline, then every 15 minutes after the beginning of the transfusion and again at the end of the transfusion.

TRANSFUSION REACTIONS

Nonhemolytic Transfusion Reactions

At least 3% of all transfusions result in either a febrile nonhemolytic transfusion reaction or an allergic reaction.

Febrile Nonhemolytic Transfusion Reactions

The febrile nonhemolytic transfusion reaction (FNHTR) is defined as a temperature increase of greater than a 1°C during or shortly after a transfusion of blood or one of its components. This reaction may be accompanied by chills. FNHTRs are seen in 1% to 3% of RBC transfusions and up to 30% in platelet transfusions. FNHTRs occur more frequently in patients who have undergone transfusion repeatedly or who have had multiple pregnancies.

The traditional mechanism for FNHTR has been attributed to the interaction of recipient plasma antibodies directed against HLA antigens on donor WBC and platelets or rarely the reverse, in which donor plasma antibodies react with HLA antigens on recipient WBC and platelets. It is known that the transfusion of single-donor apheresed platelets leads to much fewer FNHTRs than random-donor platelets do, and that the transfusion of leukoreduced RBC (1 log or greater) leads to much fewer FNHTRs than do nonleukoreduced RBC. Today, most physicians use 3 log leukoreduction whenever a recipient is expected to receive multiple transfusions of cellular products over time, in order to prevent or decrease the possibility of HLA sensitization. However, other mechanisms must be in place, because FFP and plasma from platelet concentrates can cause FNHTRs. In fact, the reactions from the plasma portion of the platelets are more severe than those from the cellular components (Heddle, 1994). Moreover, FNHTRs occur in males who have no history of prior transfusions. Antigen-antibody reactions are, therefore, not the only mechanisms that induce FNHTRs.

Bioreactive substances generated by leukocytes during storage of cellular blood components are now thought to play a major role in causing transfusion reactions. Tumor necrosis factor (TNF), interleukin (IL)-1B, and IL-6 are endogenous pyrogens that have been found to progressively increase during storage of platelets containing more than 3×10^9 WBC, especially after 3 days of storage (Muylle, 1993). Prestorage leukoreduction by 3-log WBC filtration has significantly reduced the level of these three cytokines and IL-8 during storage of platelet concentrates (Bordin, 1994; Stack, 1994) and thereby decreased the incidence of FNHTRs. IL-8 recruits WBC from the bone marrow into the blood stream and is probably responsible for creating leukocytosis.

Fever may also be the first sign of either a hemolytic transfusion reaction or a bacterially contaminated unit; consequently, FNHTR requires a more extensive transfusion reaction workup. The fever of FNHTR will respond to antipyretics. If severe chills occur, meperidine should be considered. Leukocyte-poor blood products are usually prescribed only after the second FNHTR, because repeat febrile transfusion reactions in the same patient are uncommon (Menitove, 1982). The FNHTR can sometimes be prevented by administering antipyretics prior to the transfusion of the blood components.

Allergic Reactions

Allergic reactions caused by transfusion are manifested by hives and itching but may progress to a more systemic response with wheezing and stridor. They are usually IgE mediated.

Tissue mast cells and circulating basophils store histamine. Released histamine causes respiratory and gastrointestinal smooth muscle to contract and capillaries to dilate. The clinical response to generalized histamine release is headache, facial flushing, hypotension, dyspnea and wheezing, vomiting, and diarrhea.

Histamine content in platelet concentrates rises progressively, in some units as high as 22 mg/mL; if these high-content histamine units are rapidly infused, bronchospasm and wheezing might occur (Muylle, 1988). Other associated hypotensive substances that may be found in platelet concentrates include (1) serotonin, present in dense granules of the platelets and (2) platelet activating factor, generated by granulocytes and monocytes. Enough serotonin (Wiggins, 1988), platelet activating factor (Yamanaka, 1992), or both can be released into the plasma to cause hypotension.

Patients having an allergic reaction should be treated with antihistamines. If the urticaria remain relatively localized and do not progress, and if the antihistamines have provided symptomatic relief, the transfusion (which should have been stopped when the reaction was noted) from the same unit may be reinstituted. The same unit should not be restarted if there are widespread urticaria or a generalized rash or wheezing. Prevention of allergic reactions can be accomplished by (1) administering antihistamine prior to the transfusion or (2) by using washed RBC. Because allergic reactions are not one of the symptoms of an acute hemolytic transfusion reaction, extensive laboratory investigations are not necessary.

Anaphylactic Reactions

Anaphylactic reactions occur suddenly after transfusion of only a few milliliters of blood and are characterized by acute respiratory distress, laryngeal edema, and coughing due to bronchospasm. Other accompanying symptoms may include flushing of the skin, nausea, vomiting, and diarrhea. This type of reaction may occur in IgA-deficient patients who demonstrate potent IgG anti-IgA and who are exposed to IgA-containing plasma products (Mollison, 1993, pp. 690–694). Treatment includes epinephrine and steroids. Prevention of future episodes requires the use of washed RBC products or the use of blood components from IgA-deficient donors.

Bacterial Contamination

Bacterial contamination of blood components is rare and in red cells is usually due to cold-growing, gram-negative, endotoxin-producing bacteria such as *Pseudomonas, Citrobacter freundii, Escherichia coli,* and *Yersinia enterocolitica*; in platelets, the contaminating organisms can be either gram positive or gram negative. From 1976 to 1990, several fatalities were reported to the FDA from either contaminated RBC or platelets and included the following: eight from *Yersinia enterocolitica,* seven from *Staphylococcus aureus,* six from *Staphylococcus epidermidis,* and five from *Klebsiella* species (Sazama, 1994). The reaction to the transfusion of heavily contaminated blood is characterized by bright red malar (facial) flushing, high fever, a subjective feeling of heat, abdominal cramps, vomiting, diarrhea, and shock (Mollison, 1993, p. 698). Sometimes DIC also occurs. Treatment consists of antibiotics and steroids.

Bacterial contamination of blood can be prevented by paying careful attention to preparation of the venipuncture site during blood donations, following AABB guidelines once the unit is entered, and transfusing blood products within four hours. Extra care should be taken to avoid inducing micropunctures of the blood bag, during clamping and during component preparation and from sharp edges—likely items include the centrifuge bucket, plasma expressors, and platelet rotators. When thawing FFP or cryoprecipitate, it is best to enclose the component in an additional plastic bag so as not to expose the component bag directly to microbes possibly growing in the 37°C water bath. Donors should be carefully questioned to see if they have had any mucosal trauma that might cause bacteremia for a few days (e.g., dental procedure, colonoscopy or sigmoidoscopy, manipulation of the genitourinary tract).

The blood bank technologist must look for signs of visible contamination before the unit is released for transfusion—purplish discoloration of the blood, the presence of clots or clumping, dark color of the plasma due to hemolysis, or the presence of gas in the unit (Weisz-Carrington, 1986, p. 342). One group (Kim, 1992), found that blood in contaminated bags darkens because of hemolysis and the drop in Po_2 as compared with a brighter color in the segments.

Circulatory Overload

Circulatory overload from transfusions is most common in patients with compromised cardiac or pulmonary disease or with normovolemic chronic anemia. Symptoms include dyspnea and coughing from pulmonary edema and a sudden increase in systolic blood pressure. The treatment is diuretics and oxygen but may even include phlebotomy in severe cases. Digitalis may also be helpful. Patients at high risk for developing a hypervolemic transfusion reaction should undergo transfusion slowly and be given packed RBC rather than whole blood.

Noncardiogenic Pulmonary Edema

Transfusion-associated noncardiogenic pulmonary edema, also known as transfusion-related acute lung injury (TRALI), is rare and is characterized by bilateral pulmonary edema in the absence of heart failure. Acute respiratory distress occurs, and pulmonary infiltrates are seen on chest x-ray. It is caused by either (1) leukoagglutinins (granulocyte-specific antibodies) or HLA antibodies that react with WBC to produce WBC aggregates that are trapped in the pulmonary capillaries or (2) activation of the complement components C3a or C5a, which subsequently release histamine and serotonin from tissue basophils and platelets. These substances can directly aggregate granulocytes that lodge in the pulmonary microvascular circulation (Walker, 1993, p. 483). Treatment includes high-dose steroids and general respiratory support.

Post-Transfusion Purpura

Post-transfusion purpura is a condition characterized by severe thrombocytopenia occurring about a week after a blood transfusion. This situation is usually caused by antibodies to the platelet-specific antigen, $P1^{A1}$, but may be caused by other platelet-specific antibodies as well (Aster, 1993). The mechanism is not clearly understood, but somehow the anti-$P1^{A1}$ not only attacks the transfused $P1^{A1}$-positive platelets but also involves the patient's $P1^{A1}$-negative platelets. The cause may be (1) an innocent bystander condition, in which an antigen-antibody reaction induces extensive platelet aggregation, or (2) soluble $P1^{A1}$ substance in the transfused plasma, which might be absorbed onto the patient's platelets and directly react with the patient's anti-$P1^{A1}$. The treatment is plasmapheresis.

Hemosiderosis

Hemosiderosis is a condition caused by iron deposition in vital organs, such as the liver and heart, with their subsequent malfunctions. It occurs in patients who need chronic transfusions such as thalassemics. Each unit of blood contains about 200 mg of iron (Walker, 1993, p. 486); after 100 red cell transfusions, total body iron deposition can be significant. Consequently, measures must be taken in these patients to reduce iron overload. One such method is to infuse neocytes when transfusions are required, so that fewer transfusions are necessary (Propper, 1980). Treatment with desferrioxamine, an iron chelating agent, is also important in lowering the body iron stores in patients with thalassemia.

Graft versus Host Disease (GVHD)

When immunologically competent allogeneic T lymphocytes are transfused into a person who is severely immunocompromised because of lymphocyte deficiency or malfunction, transplanted T lymphocytes may engraft in the host's lymphoid or hematopoietic tissue and become functional. These engrafted allogeneic T lymphocytes recognize the antigens on the host's cells as foreign and mount a cellular or humoral immune response against the host, creating the syndrome of GVHD.

ACUTE GVHD

Acute GVHD is primarily a cellular, cytotoxic response against the host that occurs in severely immunosuppressed patients within three months of exposure to foreign transplanted T lymphocytes. It occurs in up to 70% of allogeneic bone marrow transplant recipients and often responds to immunosuppressive therapy; however, as many as 20% of patients with this syndrome will die from its effects (Leitman, 1985). The first sign of acute GVHD is usually fever followed by a generalized maculopapular rash that may progress to bullae formation and desquamation. Other clinical manifestations include profuse watery diarrhea and hepatomegaly with elevated liver transaminases and hyperbilirubinemia.

The diagnosis of acute GVHD is suspected because of the clinical manifestations and may be confirmed by skin biopsy. When the clinical signs are primarily epidermal, the major differential diagnoses are drug reaction and viral infection. The skin biopsy is pathognomonic for GVHD if it shows in the lower third of the epidermis, the presence of single, epidermal cell necrosis (apoptosis) in association with a "satellite" lymphocyte (Brubaker, 1994).

CHRONIC GVHD

Chronic GVHD presents more than three months after exposure to foreign transplanted T lymphocytes, which are involved in generating both a cellular and a humoral immune response against the host. It occurs in up to 40% of long-term survivors of allogeneic bone marrow transplantation (Conlon, 1984). The clinical manifestations of chronic GVHD resemble those of the autoimmune diseases scleroderma and Sjögren's syndrome. The signs and symptoms include an erythematous rash, most prominent in the malar and palmar areas, which may progress to cutaneous atrophy and sclerosis; the sicca syndrome; esophageal fibrosis; elevated liver aminotransferases (AST/ALT); restrictive and obstructive pulmonary disease; autoantibody formation; chronic anemia, leukopenia, or thrombocytopenia; arthritis; and myositis. When chronic GVHD is limited to skin and hepatic manifestations, the prognosis is good, but when the symptoms are extensive and not responsive to immunosuppressive therapy, the prognosis is poor (Conlon, 1984).

TRANSFUSION-ASSOCIATED GVHD

A more aggressive form of acute GVHD is seen when severely immunosuppressed patients receive regular blood components. These persons present rapidly with acute GVHD in less than 30 days from the time they are exposed to transplanted lymphocytes. In addition to the usual symptoms of acute GVHD, they exhibit prominent pancytopenia. The pancytopenia occurs because donor cytotoxic T lymphocytes react against the host's bone marrow cells. This is in contradistinction to acute GVHD seen in allogeneic bone marrow transplant recipients, in which the host marrow comprises donor hematopoietic elements so that the bone marrow is not a site for the graft versus host reaction. Ninety percent of transfusion-associated GVHD results in death, primarily due to infections but also to hemorrhagic complications secondary to pancytopenia (Brubaker, 1994). Transfusion-associated GVHD can be confirmed by examining the patient's blood and finding a chimeric situation, using cytogenetic or HLA studies, that show the transfused cell phenotype.

Post-transfusion GVHD can theoretically be prevented in susceptible recipients by either (1) inactivating the lymphocytes through irradiation so that they cannot respond to foreign antigenic stimulation or (2) limiting the number of lymphocytes transfused to fewer than those required to produce GVHD, somewhere below 1×10^7 lymphocytes per kilogram of body weight (Leitman, 1985).

Cellular blood components contain significant numbers of lymphocytes: whole blood about 100×10^7 per unit; washed RBC, 25×10^7 per unit; random-donor platelet concentrate, 4×10^7 per unit; single-donor apheresed platelets, 30×10^7 per unit; and granulocytes, about 500×10^7 per unit (Leitman, 1985). Transfusion-associated GVHD can occur if these products are infused into a severely immunocompromised patient. Transfusion-associated GVHD has occurred after the use of 3-log leukoreduction filters and even after the infusion of nonfrozen fresh plasma, with an estimated infusion dose of 8×10^4 WBC (Akahoshi, 1992). Consequently, irradiation is used to inactivate lymphocytes in cellular blood components. A 25-Gy (2500 rads) exposure to a cesium-137 or cobalt-60 source is adequate to prevent GVHD without significantly altering RBC, platelet, or granulocyte functions or their *in vivo* survival (Brubaker, 1994). At 5 Gy, the proliferative response of lymphocytes to foreign Class II antigens (the mixed lymphocyte culture test) is ablated, and at 15 Gy, there is a 90% decrease in the lymphocyte response to mitogens (Leitman, 1985).

Although lymphocyte functions are not totally eliminated at 15 Gy, until recently it was thought that a 15-Gy dose provided enough lymphocyte inactivation to prevent GVHD. However, the FDA mandated a minimum dose of 25 Gy (FDA, 1993) after there was a case of transfusion-associated GVHD subsequent to using blood products irradiated at 15 Gy (Lowenthal, 1993) and after *in vitro* studies did not show a complete lack of growth of T cells until 25 Gy was used (Moroff, 1992). 25-Gy irradiation has some minimal adverse effects on RBC, including reduced 24-hour post-transfusion survival time after 28 days of storage. Consequently, the maximum storage time for irradiated RBC products is 28 days. Other abnormalities include increased plasma potassium, increased plasma hemoglobin, and decreased RBC ATP. 25-Gy irradiation causes no significant damage to platelets or granulocytes. Its main effect is on lymphocytes, the reproductive capacity of which is eliminated.

Those who should receive irradiated blood products include autologous and allogeneic bone marrow transplant recipients, patients with congenital immunodeficiency syndromes such as severe combined immunodeficiency syndrome and Wiskott-Aldrich syndrome, fetuses, low-birthweight premature neonates, those with hematologic malignancies, those undergoing high-dose chemotherapy for solid tumors, and those receiving transfusion from blood relatives. Because theoretically there are few, if any, lymphocytes in FFP or cryoprecipitate, it is probably unnecessary to irradiate these frozen noncellular plasma products. However, frozen, deglycerolized RBC should probably be irradiated because of the occasional mitotically active lymphocyte found in this product (Kurtz, 1978).

Conditions demonstrating only humoral immunodeficiency, such as agammaglobulinemia, or nonlymphoid cellular abnormalities, such as chronic granulomatous disease, probably do not require irradiated blood products. Similarly, aplastic anemia patients, whose stem cell defect is not in the lymphoid line, demonstrate normal cellular immune function and are therefore not thought to be at increased risk for post-transfusion GVHD. However, if a patient with aplastic anemia receives regular transfusions in close proximity to therapy with anti-thymocyte globulin, GVHD could be a problem.

Because of the extreme suppression of cellular immunity in AIDS, there is a theoretical risk of transfusion-associated GVHD. However, because no cases of transfusion-associated GVHD have been reported in AIDS, it is not necessary to provide AIDS patients with irradiated blood products. Full-term infants also do not need irradiated blood.

Some recent evidence has emerged that blood recipients who are not immunocompromised can develop transfusion-associated GVHD if they share HLA determinants on blood donated by family members. Reports have discussed the use of "fresh blood" from first-degree relatives utilized in open heart surgery, which resulted in transfusion-transmitted GVHD. Apparently, these studies revealed that the engraftment usually occurred with donor lymphocytes in which one of the two HLA haplotypes was the same as that of the recipient (Vogelsang, 1990). The AABB at first recommended, in November of 1989, that blood from first-degree relatives (parents, children, siblings) be irradiated, but then extended this recommendation to include all genetically related blood donors in May of 1993.

Hemolytic Transfusion Reactions

Acute Nonimmune Hemolysis

Although antibody-mediated activation of the complement system is the most notable cause of intravascular hemolysis, nonimmunologic causes can damage donor RBC before infusion. For example, hemolysis can occur if a unit of blood is overheated in an improperly functioning blood warmer or frozen after being placed in an unmonitored refrigerator or placed on a windowsill during winter.

Hemolysis can take place also when packed RBC are diluted with a hypotonic solution such as 5% dextrose in water, or when packed RBC are transfused through a small-bore needle (i.e., 21 gauge) using a blood pressure cuff. Calcium, found in Ringer's lactate, can overcome the citrate anticoagulant and cause clotting with subsequent hemolysis (Ryden, 1975). The only fluids that might be considered for mixing with blood are 0.9% saline (normal saline), 5% (not 25%) albumin, and ABO-compatible plasma. Bacterial contamination of a donor unit can result in the transfusion of hemolyzed blood and endotoxic shock. Less commonly, if a patient on quinine receives blood from a donor deficient in glucose-6-phosphate dehydrogenase (G6PD), the donor RBC will be hemolyzed.

The transfused RBC, however, may not be the cells being destroyed. If the patient is G6PD deficient and receiving quinine, it is the patient's RBC, rather than those of the donor, that are hemolyzed. Likewise, a patient with paroxysmal nocturnal hemoglobinuria (PNH) may hemolyze autologous RBC, especially when receiving a blood product containing complement. A patient in sickle cell crisis, in which hypoxia occurs in tissues, also may hemolyze autologous RBC. Distilled water may enter the blood circulation as a result of bladder irrigation during prostate surgery and thereby hemolyze patient RBC intravascularly. Patient RBC may also be hemolyzed by certain toxins such as those resulting from *Clostridium welchii* infection.

If hemolysis is demonstrated and if examination of residual blood from the transfused units reveals no hemolysis, antibody-mediated hemolysis may be suspected.

Acute Immune Hemolysis

The most severe, life-threatening, acute hemolytic transfusion reaction is almost always due to the transfusion of ABO-incompatible blood into a recipient after an identification error or some other clerical mistake (Myhre, 1980). This

ABO incompatibility causes intravascular hemolysis, shock, DIC, and subsequent renal failure. The initial signs and symptoms include pain at the infusion site, fever, chills, chest pain, hypotension, shock, nausea, vomiting, flushing of the skin, dyspnea, hemoglobinuria, oliguria, back pain, and generalized bleeding from the severe thrombocytopenia due to DIC. In the anesthetized, unconscious patient, the first signs will be hypotension and generalized bleeding at the venipuncture and surgical incision sites (Brown, 1986).

Because severe acute hemolytic transfusion reactions are almost always due to a clerical error (Myrhe, 1980), the transfusion reaction investigation should begin with an immediate comparison of the donor unit paperwork with the identifying information on the patient's wrist band. It is important to try to prevent a second such reaction in another patient, if it is found that the blood units were inadvertently switched.

Treatment of acute, immune intravascular hemolytic transfusion reactions centers on overcoming the DIC. Intravenous fluids will ameliorate the hypotension and promote renal blood flow. Diuretics are also administered in an attempt to promote renal blood flow. Platelet transfusions should be considered if life-threatening bleeding occurs from severe thrombocytopenia.

Acute extravascular hemolysis can occur with incompatible transfusion due to the non-ABO red cell systems. These can be serious but are not as severe as for the ABO system, because DIC and complement activation usually do not occur. Extravascular hemolysis is seen with IgG antibodies in the Rh, Kell, Kidd, and Duffy systems. Fever, anemia, increased bilirubin, and a positive DAT are the usual signs and symptoms. Treatment is supportive.

Delayed hemolytic transfusion reactions result from an anamnestic response to renewed antigen exposure. A previously developed antibody may disappear; re-exposure to the antigen causes a rapid antibody response, usually within two weeks of transfusion. These IgG antibodies are from the same antigenic systems as mentioned for extravascular hemolysis and produce the same symptoms, but the sole manifestation of a delayed hemolytic transfusion reaction may only be a drop in hematocrit or hemoglobin (Pineda, 1978).

Pathologic Physiology of Immune Hemolysis *In Vivo*

Hemolytic reactions due to antigen-antibody reactions are designated immune hemolysis. Immune hemolysis *in vivo* is divided into two basic types (Fig. 31–7), intravascular and extravascular. Antibodies, such as anti-A and anti-B, which can activate complement, may cause intravascular hemolysis if sufficiently active *in vivo* at body temperature (i.e., wide thermal range). Symptoms such as flushing of the skin, pain at injection site, shock, and hypotension may be related to activation of complement and the subsequent release of histamine, serotonin, or kinins. Hemoglobin released from the lysed erythrocytes combines with haptoglobin and usually deposits in the liver, where it is subsequently split into iron and bilirubin. Because the amount of haptoglobin in blood is limited, hemoglobin can also be handled in alternative ways. The heme released can combine with albumin to form methemalbumin or combine with hemopexin. It is then processed in the liver into bilirubin and free iron. In the laboratory, the following can be demonstrated: free plasma hemoglobin; a decrease in (1) haptoglobin, (2) hemopexin, and (3) albumin-binding capacity; and an increase in (1) lactate dehydrogenase, (2) hemoglobinuria, and (3) hemosiderinuria. A positive DAT with mixed field agglutination is also noted. Serum bilirubin may be increased four to six hours after the initiating event (Fig. 31–8).

Most IgG antibody-coated red cells are destroyed extravascularly, mainly through phagocytosis by the reticuloendothelial system, also known as the mononuclear phagocyte

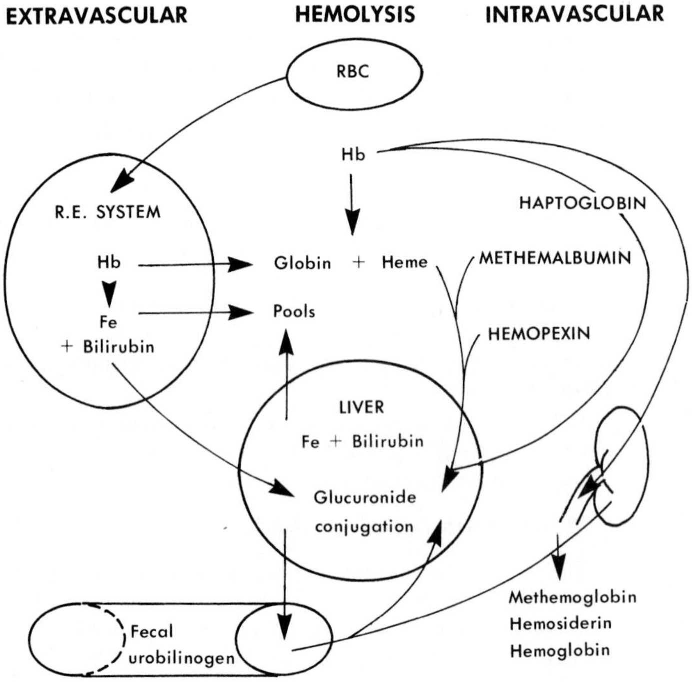

Figure 31–7. Two types of hemolysis *in vivo*.

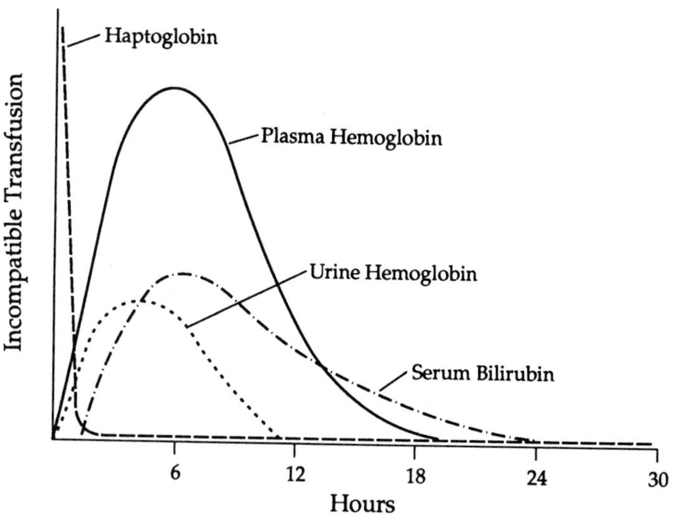

Figure 31–8. Laboratory findings in intravascular hemolysis. Positive direct antiglobulin test and presence of minor population of agglutinates are not listed. (Modified from Huestis DW, Bove JR, Case J: Practical Blood Transfusion, 4th ed. Boston, Little, Brown & Co., 1988.)

system, of the spleen (Mollison, 1993, pp. 439–497). Complement-coated erythrocytes are similarly destroyed predominantly in the liver. Some IgG antibodies may activate complement *in vivo,* such as anti-K, anti-Fy[a], and anti-Jk[a], and cause the complement and IgG-coated RBC to be destroyed primarily in the liver. IgG-coated erythrocytes can be destroyed by lymphocytes with Fc receptors.

Inflammatory Cytokines Involved in Immune-Mediated Hemolysis

Inflammatory cytokines are now thought to play an active role in the development of fever and DIC due to immune hemolysis. Both pyrogens IL-1B and tumor necrosis factor (TNF), when injected alone into animals in high doses, produce hypotension, shock, and death. However, IL-1B and TNF work synergistically so that shock and pulmonary hemorrhage occur at one tenth the original high dose as compared with when each is given alone (Okusawa, 1988).

Washed ABO-incompatible RBC incubated at 37°C with heparinized whole blood have been shown to result in rapid TNF production by peripheral blood phagocytes. This TNF production peaks with a concentration of greater than 1 ng/mL at 2 to 4 hours and returns to the baseline by 24 hours (Davenport, 1994). The amount of TNF produced is proportional to the degree of hemolysis. Both hemolysis and TNF production require the presence of a heat-labile protein, probably complement. This increase in TNF induces fever and is thought to initiate DIC by causing leukocyte adhesion onto endothelial surfaces, which may lead to WBC trapping and tissue ischemia. Additionally, both IL-1B and TNF can decrease thrombomodulin and induce tissue factor production by endothelial cells, thereby favoring thrombosis. TNF has been found to be increased in a clinical acute immune hemolysis episode due to ABO incompatibility (Butler, 1991). Additionally, IL-8 increases in the above *in vitro* model, but this increase starts at 4 hours and peaks at 24 hours. IL-8 recruits WBC from the bone marrow and is probably responsible for the leukocytosis seen clinically in acute immune intravascular hemolysis.

Similar studies using IgG-coated RBC incubated at 37°C with human monocytes in tissue culture show low-level (100 pg/mL) IL-1B, IL-6, and TNF production within 24 hours. Compared with ABO incompatibility mentioned earlier, this response is much less and delayed. IL-8 is elevated at high levels (1 ng/mL within 24 hours), a condition similar to that described for ABO incompatibility.

From these *in vitro* models, it has been suggested (Davenport, 1994) that the clinical response difference between immune acute intravascular hemolysis and extravascular hemolysis reactions is due to the higher amounts of and earlier formation of TNF, which leads to the systemic response of generalized DIC, hypotension, and shock in intravascular hemolysis. It is further postulated that the lower-level response rates of inflammatory cytokines in the IgG antibody-coated model are probably analogous to the local phenomenon seen in the reticuloendothelial system of the spleen and liver that occurs with extravascular hemolysis. Additionally, it is felt that the elevation at 24 hours of IL-1B and IL-6 seen in the IgG-coated RBC model may simulate the mechanism, producing immune-delayed hemolytic reaction *in vivo,* because both IL-1B and IL-6 promote growth and differentiation of B cells, which lead to antibody production.

4

Transfusion Reaction Investigation

Most transfusion reaction investigations are conducted to make sure that the reaction is not due to acute intravascular immune hemolysis from an ABO-incompatible transfusion. Because almost any unusual sign or symptom occurring during a transfusion can be the initial event of a serious reaction, *the transfusion must be stopped for any reaction. The IV line must be kept open* with crystalloids in case immediate treatment is necessary to overcome hypotension. *The attending physician and the blood bank must be notified* as soon as possible.

Additionally, the following investigations should be performed if acute, immune intravascular hemolysis is suspected (Brown, 1986; Walker, 1993, pp. 471–479):

1. A clerical check of the compatibility tag on the blood bag, the blood bag label, and the patient identification (wristband) for discrepancies.

2. Examination of the pretransfusion clotted blood specimen, an EDTA anticoagulated post-transfusion blood specimen, and the blood bag.

a. Look for hemolysis in the post-transfusion specimen. If pink or red serum is present, compare with the pre-transfusion specimen. More measurements may be indicated from the process described in Figures 31–7 and 31–8.

b. Perform a DAT on the post-transfusion EDTA specimen. A mixed field reaction is strongly suspicious of an antibody-mediated transfusion reaction. If the DAT is negative and hemolysis has occurred but ABO incompatibility has been ruled out, several non-immune mechanisms, mentioned earlier, should be considered as the cause of the intravascular hemolysis.

The initial portion of the transfusion reaction investigation should include (1) stopping the transfusion, (2) notifying the attending physician and blood bank, (3) checking the clerical work, (4) inspecting the post-transfusion serum for hemolysis, and (5) performing a DAT on the post-transfusion specimen (Klein, 1994, p. 35). Further workup is not necessary unless there is evidence for hemolysis. Allergic and circulatory overload reactions require medical attention, but no blood bank technical evaluation is necessary.

3. Perform a Gram's stain on the blood in the bag and a culture, if necessary, to determine the presence of bacterial contamination, if indicated; i.e. symptoms/signs of gram negative sepsis.
4. Repeat the ABO/Rh typing, antibody screen, and the crossmatch to see if a patient antibody is directed against donor cells. If an antibody is suspected, a RBC panel should be performed for identification of the antibody.
5. Examination of the post-transfusion urine.

a. Look for a dark color and, if present, test for hemoglobinuria.

b. Perform other measurements of constituents shown in Figures 31–7 and 31–8.

6. Determination, on a post-transfusion anticoagulated specimen, of prothrombin time (PT), partial thromboplastin time (PTT), platelet count, fibrinogen, and fibrin split products, if DIC is suggested.
7. Measurement of Hct/Hb at frequent intervals if hemolysis is observed.

Diseases Transmitted Through Blood Transfusion

Blood is tested for the HIV-1,2 antibody and HIV-1 antigen to prevent the transmission of AIDS; for the HTLV-1 antibody to prevent tropical spastic paraparesis and adult T-cell leukemia; for hepatitis B surface antigen and hepatitis B core antibody to prevent hepatitis B; and for hepatitis C antibody to prevent hepatitis C. Blood is subjected to VDRL or the RPR card test to screen blood for syphilis.

Cytomegalovirus (CMV) is an obligate intracellular organism found within leukocytes. It sometimes lies dormant within these cells, so it may be difficult to determine whether an active CMV infection in a transfused patient is the direct result of the transfusion itself or the reactivation of a latent CMV infection. In healthy persons, CMV infections are often asymptomatic but can produce a mild, self-limiting, flu-like illness. However, in the severely immunosuppressed patient, CMV can be devastating and causes multiorgan problems including pneumonia, hepatitis, and cytopenias. Therefore, CMV-seronegative (antibody-negative) cellular blood products should be considered for CMV-seronegative patients who are severely immunosuppressed, such as premature, low-birthweight infants; patients undergoing solid organ or bone marrow transplantation who receive a seronegative transplant; those with congenital immunodeficiency; or those with AIDS (Tegtmeier, 1989). Additionally, CMV-seronegative blood products should be considered for the CMV-seronegative pregnant woman because of the vulnerability of the fetus. Because almost all of the WBC, and therefore active CMV, is removed in the freeze-thaw-wash process, frozen, deglycerolized RBC can be used as an alternative to CMV-seronegative blood. CMV infectivity is determined by performing an antibody test on the serum. Similar to the case with HIV, a positive CMV antibody test means that the patient has been exposed to the virus and may be infectious. It does not mean that the person is immune from having the disease. Use of the 3-log leukoreduction filter has also been shown to prevent CMV transmission. However, this filter does not remove 3 logs of WBC under all conditions (Ledent, 1994), as mentioned earlier.

Parvovirus B19 is a nonlipid, enveloped virus, which can withstand the usual viricidal treatments including heat and solvent/detergent techniques. It is not cell associated, so 3-log leukoreduction filters would not be expected to decrease infectivity. It has been found in Factor VIII and Factor IX concentrates (Luban, 1994). It is usually a mild, self-limiting disease and, in children, is the cause of erythema infectiosum, also known as fifth disease.

In susceptible persons, parvovirus B19 infects proliferating hematopoietic cells by attaching onto its P antigen RBC receptor. In patients with chronic hemolytic anemias, such as sickle cell disease, sickle C disease, and hereditary spherocytosis, an acute aplastic crisis can occur. This virus can be devastating to the fetus, in which it may cause anemia and hydrops fetalis. It infects not only dividing fetal hematopoietic cells but also fetal myocardial cells (Luban, 1994). Additionally, parvovirus B19 can cause chronic cytopenias with associated generalized symptoms of fever, malaise, and joint pain in immunocompromised patients.

The incidence of parvovirus B19 IgG seropositivity ranges from about 10% in children under 5 to 60% in adults over 20 years of age (Luban, 1994). IgG antibody gives lifetime immunity. The major route of transmission is respiratory, but blood transfusion can also transmit this disease. Persons whose RBC are P antigen negative show natural resistance to this virus (Brown, 1994).

Few cases of malaria are transmitted because of the donor standards excluding those likely to transmit this disease. Other parasites (Shulman, 1994; Weisz-Carrington, 1986, pp. 343–344) causing babesiosis, Chagas' disease, trypanosomiasis, kala-azar, filariasis, and toxoplasmosis are rarely, if ever, transmitted by blood in the United States. Lyme disease, a tick-borne spirochete (*Borrelia burgdorferi*), also can be transmitted by blood (Aoki, 1989; Badon, 1989).

Transfusion-Induced Immunosuppression

It is postulated that blood transfusions cause a generalized down-regulation of the immune system by reducing the capacity of T cells to secrete IL-2 (Blumberg, 1994), perhaps by macrophage secretion of prostaglandin E_2. Both natural killer cells and lymphokine activated killer cells are IL-2 dependent and, therefore, would play a diminished role in organ transplant rejection, in attacking and killing tumor cells, and in protecting against bacterial and viral infection in those receiving blood transfusions.

Animal studies (Blumberg, 1994) have shown that blood transfusions reduce the mixed lymphocyte response to foreign antigens; decrease helper T cell, natural killer cell, and cell-mediated lymphocytotoxicity activity; and increase suppressor T cells.

Interestingly, it is known that patients who have undergone multiple transfusions have significantly less chance of rejecting a transplanted organ (i.e., kidney) than do those who have never undergone transfusion. The picture isn't as clear for malignant tumors. Studies (Blumberg, 1994; Bordin, 1994; Lane, 1994) show conflicting results—that transfusions may either impair host defenses, leading to increased rate of tumor recurrence and metastasis, or that they may show no effect. Many other immunosuppressive factors are often not accounted for in patient studies: extent and duration of surgical dissection, length of anesthesia, drugs, the type of malignancy, and prior transfusions or pregnancies. One group (Blumberg, 1994) has speculated from a review of the literature that the postoperative bacterial infection rate is not significantly different when comparing patients with one unit allogeneic and one unit autologous transfusions to those receiving no transfusions—all are at about 5%. However, the postoperative infection rate for those receiving two units of allogeneic transfusions is 25% and for three units is 40%, as compared with those receiving two and three units of autologous blood, for whom the rate is 5% and 10%, respectively (Blumberg, 1994). Another group's (Bordin, 1994) review of clinical studies estimates that the bacterial infection rate with allogenic transfusions is 20% to 30% as compared with either no transfusions or autologous transfusions, which have between 5% and 10% infection rates. At this time, no other investigators feel that this relationship between allogeneic transfusions and increased bacterial infections has been definitely proved because (1) these observations were not derived from randomized, controlled, prospective studies or (2) the definition of infection has varied from the specific culture proven to the broad "fever present."

Through all this, there has been one large (475 patients evaluated), prospective, randomized, controlled trial assessing the effect of allogeneic and autologous transfusions versus no transfusion in patients with colorectal cancer (Busch, 1993). The conclusions were that there was no difference in the tumor recurrence rates for those receiving either allogeneic (41% at 4 years) or autologous (38% at 4 years) transfusions, but the recurrence rate for those not receiving blood was definitely lower (27% at 4 years). This study indicates that the act of receiving a transfusion establishes a subgroup with poorer prognosis than that of those who do not receive blood at all. Interestingly, there was also no difference in the postoperative infection rate for those receiving transfusions—25% for allogeneic, 27% for autologous.

STEM CELLS

The 1990 Nobel Prize for Medicine was awarded to E. Donnall Thomas for his contributions to the field of stem cell transplantation in animal models and humans (Thomas, 1977). The number of autologous or allogeneic stem cell transplants has increased dramatically over the past several years, and over 10,000 procedures are performed worldwide each year (Bortin, 1992). Despite its increasing popularity, stem cell transplantation is successful for only a minority of patients. Post-transplant relapse and graft versus host disease (GVHD) are significant hurdles to even greater use of stem cell transplantation. Numerous studies on modifying the collection, processing, and storage of stem cells are underway to resolve these problems.

The bone marrow and blood cells of greatest interest include totipotential stem cells, committed hematopoietic progenitor cells, and lymphoid cells (see Chap. 25). All blood cells arise from the rare totipotential stem cells, and thus long-term repopulation of the marrow depends on transplantation of these cells. Assurance of rapid hematologic recovery may depend on transplantation of sufficient numbers of committed hematopoietic progenitor cells. Both totipotential stem cells and committed progenitor cells have been reported as necessary for rapid, long-term engraftment in mice (Jones, 1990) and are suspected to be necessary in humans (Juttner, 1985). Lymphoid cells play a role in enhancement of engraftment and prevention of relapse; however, lymphoid cells are also responsible for the development of GVHD.

The progenitor cell assays most often used to predict the engraftment time after stem cell transplantation include colony-forming units–granulocyte/monocyte (macrophage) (CFU-GM), burst-forming units–erythroid (BFU-E), and colony-forming units–granulocyte/erythrocyte/macrophage/megakaryocyte (CFU-GEMM) (Table 31–11). Recipients of marrows with higher progenitor cell assay results generally have shorter periods of aplasia (Emminger, 1989). Unfortunately, the two weeks required for progenitor cell assays delay receipt of the most vital information regarding a stem cell collection's adequacy. Thus, at the time of collec-

Table 31–11. COMMON TERMS

Progenitor Cell Assays	
Colony-forming units—granulocyte/monocyte (macrophage)	CFU-GM
Colony-forming units—granulocyte/erythrocyte/macrophage/megakaryocyte	CFU-GEMM
Burst-forming units—erythroid	BFU-E
Cytokines	
Granulocyte-colony stimulating factor	G-CSF
Granulocyte/monocyte-colony stimulating factor	GM-CSF
Erythropoietin	EPO
Steel factor*	SLF

*Also known as stem cell factor or kit ligand

tion, the total nucleated or mononuclear cell counts are generally used to determine the adequacy of an individual stem cell harvest (Kessinger, 1987). The numbers of total nucleated or mononuclear cells in the product are only indirect measures of the quantity of totipotential stem cells, committed progenitor cells, and lymphoid cells necessary for optimal engraftment. The subpopulation of cells that express the CD34 antigen contain the early hematopoietic progenitor cells and the totipotential stem cells. If problems with interlaboratory standardization can be resolved, CD34 cell counts may offer more rapid estimates of a stem cell collection's adequacy, because flow cytometric cell phenotyping can be performed in a few hours (Siena, 1991).

Bone Marrow Stem Cells

For bone marrow transplantation (BMT), adequate quantities of marrow cells can be obtained from the posterior iliac crest using the techniques described by Thomas (1970). The quantity of marrow cells needed for successful engraftment is not known and, at the time of bone marrow harvesting, estimates of adequacy are generally based on total nucleated bone marrow cells (Torres, 1985). Most centers obtain at least 2 to 4×10^8 total nucleated bone marrow cells per kilogram of recipient body weight.

The risks to the bone marrow donor are usually minimal. Because general or regional anesthesia is administered, the possibility of reaction to the anesthetic must be considered. Other donor complications such as infection at the skin puncture sites, systemic infections, hematomas, and neuralgias are also risks. Anemia as a result of the 750 to 1500 mL of blood lost during bone marrow harvest can be adequately handled by pretransplant autologous blood storage. Some centers also salvage RBC from autologous bone marrow grafts during processing. In addition to HLA matching, allogeneic donors should be evaluated using the standard criteria applied to blood donors. The potential for transmission of not only hepatitis, HIV, HTLV, and syphilis but also CMV should be considered.

Peripheral Blood Stem Cells

In mice, (Micklem, 1975) and in dogs (Storb, 1968), peripheral blood stem cells (PBSC) have effectively repopulated aplastic bone marrow. Human trials of autologous peripheral blood stem cell transplantation with numerous malignancies have been reported, including leukemia (Goldman, 1980), lymphoma (Kessinger, 1991), multiple myeloma (Ventura, 1990), breast carcinoma (Kessinger, 1988), small cell carcinoma of the lung (Stiff, 1987a), neuroblastoma (Lasky, 1989), and soft tissue sarcoma (Williams, 1990). A review by Reiffers (1991) concludes that for patients with acute leukemia, the risk of disease reoccurrence is similar for PBSC and autologous bone marrow transplantation (ABMT). The largest series of patients with non-Hodgkins intermediate and high-grade lymphomas who underwent PBSC transplantation included 41 patients (Kessinger, 1990). Each of these patients had a bone marrow abnormality (either tumor involvement of the marrow or marrow hypocellularity) that made ABMT unsuitable. The event-free survival rate at 5 years was 28%, which is comparable with the outcome reported for patients with non-Hodgkins lymphoma who were treated with ABMT (Philip, 1987). Thus, patients whose bone marrow is unsuitable for autologous BMT can benefit from autologous PBSC transplantation. Some centers add the collection of PBSC to ABMT to enhance hematologic recovery. Use of mobilized PBSC and ABMT results in earlier engraftment than does ABMT alone, with a resultant decrease in the morbidity associated with pancytopenia (Peters, 1991).

In all animal species tested and in humans, peripheral blood has significantly lower numbers of hematopoietic progenitor cells than bone marrow does (McCarthy, 1984). In humans, 1 of every 1000 mononuclear cells (MNC) in the bone marrow is a CFU-GM, whereas only 1 of every 100,000 mononuclear cells in the peripheral blood is a CFU-GM (Table 31–12) (McCarthy, 1984). For this reason, large volumes (45 to 60 liters) of autologous whole blood are processed using cytapheresis (leukapheresis)/apheresis technology during 3 to 5 days of collection to yield at least 6.5×10^8 mononuclear cells (MNC) per kilogram of recipient weight (Kessinger, 1991). In addition, most PBSC collection protocols use chemotherapy-induced mobilization (To, 1990) or cytokine-induced (G-CSF or GM-CSF) mobilization to increase the number of hematopoietic progenitor cells in the blood (Molineux, 1990). The minimum number of MNC needed for a successful transplant is not known and is likely affected by donor variability. The most accurate predictor of engraftment is the CFU-GM, which requires 2 weeks to complete testing. Thus, as with a bone marrow harvest, one must estimate when a sufficient number of cells have been collected.

The rarity of early hematopoietic progenitor cells in peripheral blood leads to the use of mobilization techniques in most autologous PBSC collection protocols. Most experience has been gained using chemotherapy-induced aplasia, which gives a resultant rebound of CFU-GM to levels 10-fold to 100-fold higher than the baseline levels of CFU-GM in peripheral blood (To, 1984). The rebound typically occurs 12 to 16 days post chemotherapy; timing of the collection is crucial because the optimal period for collection often lasts only 4 to 5 days (To, 1984). The various criteria used to determine when to initiate collection include the time a specific number of neutrophils return to the circulation (Korbling, 1990), the time the absolute number of MNC reaches a specific value (Ventura, 1990), the time the percentage of monocytes reaches a certain value (Stiff, 1987a), and the time of recovery of platelet counts (To, 1990). Not surprisingly, the optimal timing varies from patient to patient.

Table 31–12. COMPARISON OF BONE MARROW (BM), PERIPHERAL BLOOD (PB), AND CORD BLOOD (CB) AS SOURCES FOR STEM CELLS

	CFU-GM* Frequency	Volume Processed	Currently Used for
BM	1/1000	0.75–1.0 L	Autologous Allogeneic
PB	1/100,000	45–60 L	Autologous
CB	1/1000	0.075–0.28 L	Autologous Allogeneic

*Approximate values as ratio of CFU-GM to mononuclear cells.

Recent work suggests that cytokine-induced mobilization of autologous PBSC may be more predictable (Haas, 1990; Molineux, 1990). Either G-CSF or GM-CSF is administered daily, beginning three to four days before PBSC collection and continuing throughout the collection, to mobilize early hematopoietic progenitor cells. In addition, simultaneous use of chemotherapy-induced and cytokine-induced mobilization techniques suggest an additive effect (Siena, 1989). Patients with a history of extensive therapy for their malignancies or metastatic involvement of the bone marrow may be the most suitable candidates for cytokine-induced mobilization (To, 1990). It is not yet clear whether tumor cells are equally mobilized by cytokines.

The potential for allogeneic PBSC transplantation has been demonstrated in animal models. Mice (Goodman, 1962) and dogs (Korbling, 1979) have received successful allogeneic transplantations following marrow ablative irradiation. Chromosomal markers have been used to establish the origin of donor versus recipient hematopoietic progenitor cells. The recipients were found to have donor blood cells over a period of one third of their expected life spans.

The inability to specifically identify the totipotential stem cell in humans has markedly limited the experience of allogeneic PBSC transplantation in humans. The fact that autologous PBSC transplants are successfully performed does not prove that totipotential stem cells have been transplanted. The possibility exists of stem cells surviving the marrow ablative regimen and eventually repopulating the marrow, with the PBSC merely supporting the recipient during what would have been a long period of aplasia. Supporting evidence that recipient stem cells can survive a marrow ablative regimen comes from allogeneic BMT recipients who have eventually developed permanent populations of both donor and recipient marrow cells (Branch, 1982). Until marker studies can prove the transplantation of totipotential peripheral blood stem cells, the use of allogeneic PBSC transplantation is likely to remain limited. Another substantial hurdle to allogeneic PBSC transplantation is the enhanced risk of GVHD from the large number of T lymphocytes found in peripheral blood compared with bone marrow. It is possible that T-cell depletion will resolve this complication.

Cord Blood Stem Cells

Umbilical cord blood has been found to contain a high concentration of hematopoietic progenitor cells and is proving to be an interesting source of stem cells for transplantation (Broxmeyer, 1989). Ontologically, the totipotential stem cells and committed hematopoietic progenitors are first found in the yolk sac, then the fetal liver and spleen, and eventually in fetal bone marrow (Johnson, 1975; Tavassoli, 1991). The migration of these primitive cells is not completely understood, but the presence of early hematopoietic progenitors in murine and human umbilical cord blood is well documented (Broxmeyer, 1989). Although the volume of blood recovered from the umbilical cord and placenta is roughly 75 to 280 mL, the concentration of CFU-GM in cord blood may be up to 30 to 1200 times that found in adult blood (Knudtzon, 1974; Ueno, 1981). By day one after birth, the concentration of circulating CFU-GM is reduced to 22% to 49% of that found in cord blood (Broxmeyer, 1992). During the first month of life, the level of CFU-GM remains approximately five times higher than in adult peripheral blood (Geissler, 1986).

Gluckman, Broxmeyer, and colleagues (1989) first reported successful transplantation of human cord blood; the case involved a patient with Fanconi's anemia whose HLA-identical sibling's cord blood was collected, frozen, and later infused. Engraftment of the donor cells was documented by cytogenetics, ABO typing, and DNA polymorphism assays. After one year, the lymphoid system was 98% donor origin. To date, more than 50 cord blood transplants have been reported with donor cell engraftment in 39 of 44 evaluable patients (Wagner, 1994).

A critical question is whether enough totipotential stem cells and committed hematopoietic progenitor cells are present in a typical cord blood collection for transplantation into adults. Of interest are the findings of Broxmeyer and colleagues of increased capacity of cord blood CFU-GEMM cells to be replated *in vitro* and still form colonies, which suggests a more immature subpopulation of cells than is seen in adult bone marrow (Carow, 1991). In a modified CFU-GM assay, which studied CFU-GM responsive to GM-CSF plus steel factor (SLF) in culture, comparison of the number of CFU-GM between cord blood specimens and bone marrow specimens used in ABMT showed higher total numbers of progenitors in all of the cord blood specimens than in the successfully engrafting bone marrow specimens with the lowest number of these cells (Broxmeyer, 1992). The data suggest that, despite the small volume obtained, cord blood may contain a more immature population of cells and thus may suffice for effective transplantation of adults. In addition, recipients of cord blood transplants have had little graft versus host disease (GVHD), possibly as the result of the relative immaturity of cord blood stem cells or lymphoid cells (Wagner, 1994).

Cord blood can be collected during either vaginal delivery or cesarean section. Differing techniques include milking of blood from the clamped, cut umbilical cord and needle and syringe aspiration of the umbilical and placental veins. The anticoagulated specimens vary considerably in volume, and the greatest volume is associated with early cord clamping (Bertolini, 1993). Careful cleansing of the cord to avoid contamination by either bacteria or maternal blood is recommended. Maternal lymphocytes pose the theoretical risk of GVHD in the recipients, although the number of cells needed for this complication is uncertain.

Stem Cell Processing

Totipotential stem cells, committed hematopoietic progenitors, and lymphocytes are all contained in the buffy coat of the bone marrow and peripheral blood stem cell collections. Processing of these two stem cell collections with either automated or manual centrifugation equipment can decrease the volume of the harvest, the hematocrit, the number of granulocytes, and, in bone marrow, the amount of fat in the product. RBC do not survive the freezing process; therefore, decreasing the hematocrit can minimize the amount of free hemoglobin reinfused. Similarly, decreasing the number of granulocytes, which release DNA and clump when lysed, can decrease the possibility of respiratory dysfunction, occasionally seen on reinfusion. Depending on the apheresis machine used, PBSC products may not need processing. Attempts to remove RBC and granulocytes from cord blood have resulted in large losses of hematopoietic progenitor cells (Broxmeyer, 1989). Thus, no processing of cord blood is recommended. Record keeping is crucial and includes the volume of product collected, cell counts (total nucleated and mononuclear), lot numbers of reagents, unit numbers, and product location. In addition, results of bacteriologic cultures and quantitation of a progenitor assay, usually CFU-GM, are recorded. We have developed and use a database (File Maker Pro) that provides rapid retrieval of product characteristics and locations.

ABO-Mismatched Transplantation

Major ABO-mismatched BMT poses the risk of a hemolytic transfusion reaction, given the significant number of RBC in the bone marrow harvest. Approximately 70% of the RBC in the harvest are removed during automated processing to minimize the RBC contaminant. The transition from recipient to donor blood type occurs over several weeks and can be monitored. During this time, transfusion of group O packed red cells minimizes the risk of transfusion-related hemolysis. The persistence of recipient antibody to donor RBC delays the hematologic recovery of RBC, but not WBC or platelets (Hows, 1983).

Minor ABO-mismatched BMT may result in low-grade hemolysis from donor antibodies to recipient RBC. Volume reduction during processing can help avoid this complication. The presence of donor lymphocytes in the bone marrow product will occasionally lead to the production of isohemagglutinins and a transient delayed hemolytic reaction beginning one to two weeks post transplant (Hows, 1986). Neither major nor minor ABO-mismatched BMT appear to be associated with graft failure or graft versus host disease (Braine, 1982; Gale, 1977).

T-Cell Depletion of Allogeneic Bone Marrow

Graft versus host disease (GVHD) is the major complication of allogeneic bone marrow transplantation, as the result of T lymphocytes in the transplant. The incidence of severe acute GVHD in HLA-identical sibling transplants may reach 35% and even higher in HLA-identical, nonrelated transplants (Deeg, 1984; Storb, 1985). Numerous studies have focused on reducing the risk of GVHD by depletion of T cells from the bone marrow. Techniques to achieve removal of 99% to 99.9% of the T lymphocytes from the bone marrow product include counterflow elutriation centrifugation (Wagner, 1990), adherence to sheep erythrocytes (Fischer, 1986) or soybean lectin agglutinin (Reisner, 1983), complement-mediated lysis (Mitsuyasy, 1986), immunotoxin-mediated cell destruction (Filipovich, 1984), and physical separation with immunomagnetic beads (Gee, 1987).

These studies have met with some success in reducing severe acute GVHD at the expense of increased rates of graft failure and increased risk of relapse. A graft versus leukemia (GVL) effect has been associated with GVHD, and it has been noted that depletion of T cells increases the risk of relapse, especially in chronic myelogenous leukemia (Goldman, 1988). Use of anti-T cell antibodies and complement in one study lowered the incidence of GVHD but did not provide the recipients with a survival advantage because of increased engraftment failure and relapse (Mitsuyasy, 1986). T-cell depletion also carries the potential risk of B-cell neoplasms and infections. Efforts are underway to estimate the number of T cells to add back to T-lymphocyte-depleted bone marrow to resolve these complications.

Purging of Tumor Cells from Autologous Marrow

Autologous BMT is a possibility for patients who have chemotherapy dose-responsive malignancies and who lack HLA-matched sibling donors. Often their malignancies involve the marrow either as the primary location (e.g., acute leukemias) or as a secondary location, as in metastatic breast carcinomas or some lymphomas. Not surprisingly, residual tumor cells have been demonstrated in autologous bone marrow harvests from patients with these diseases (Peters, 1990; Vaughan, 1987). Efforts to purge marrow by immunologic techniques are frequently directed at tumor specific antigens using monoclonal antibodies and complement-mediated lysis (Ramsay, 1985), monoclonal antibody-toxin conjugates (Uckun, 1990), or binding to monoclonal antibody-coated magnetic beads (Anderson, 1989). This negative selection approach offers the potential of little or no toxicity to hematopoietic progenitors. However, difficulties with antigenic heterogeneity have yet to be resolved (Gee, 1987).

Techniques employing chemotherapy purging most often use the active derivative of cyclophosphamide, 4-hydroperoxycyclophosphamide (4-HC). The efficacy of autologous BMT with 4-HC purged marrow was first shown in a rat model of leukemia in which sufficiently high concentrations led to cure of the rat (Sharkis, 1980). Phase I and Phase II trials of *ex vivo* 4-HC purging have demonstrated the feasibility of this technique in humans (Kaizer, 1985; Rosenfeld, 1989; Yeager, 1986). Toxicity to hematopoietic progenitor cells during *ex vivo* 4-HC purging can lead to a delay in hematopoietic recovery (defined as 500 granulocytes per mL) of 19 days in patients with non-Hodgkins lymphoma and 39 days in patients with acute myelogenous leukemia (Rowley, 1991). The potential for delay in or failure of engraftment leads many centers to store an unpurged "backup" marrow to be used if the transplant fails to engraft.

Positive selection, by isolation of CD34-positive cells, is an indirect method of reducing the number of contaminating tumor cells in the marrow product. Approximately 1.5% of nucleated bone marrow cells express the CD34 antigen, and this subpopulation contains essentially all totipotential stem cells and most of the committed progenitor cells (Civin, 1984). A study in nonhuman primates reported successful transplantation with marrow enriched for CD34-positive cells (Berenson, 1988). Experience with humans has been limited, but one study of 10 patients being treated for breast carcinoma describes engraftment of all evaluable patients (Berenson, 1991).

Expansion of Stem Cells

The ability to expand both totipotential stem cells and committed hematopoietic progenitors *in vitro* would be a major advance in technology, especially for the use of cord blood in adult transplantation. Currently, expansion of committed progenitors has been demonstrated in short-term suspension culture, and CFU-GM from cord blood can be increased more than 12 times with combinations of cytokines such as GM-CSF and steel factor (SLF) (Broxmeyer, 1992). It is not clear whether totipotential stem cells can be expanded *in vitro.* This would require self-renewal—that is, replication without differentiation—and is the subject of intense study. Because the totipotential stem cell has not yet been identified, the measurement of these cells and documentation of their self-renewal can only be extrapolated. An alternative to *in vitro* expansion of totipotential stem cells is the expansion of stem cells *in vivo,* either prior to collection or post transplant, through the use of cytokines. Because interactions between stem cells and stromal cells appears crucial to self-renewal, *in vivo* expansion and self-renewal may be more feasible than the *in vitro* approach (Broxmeyer, 1989, 1991).

Cryopreservation

Although allogeneic bone marrow can be processed and infused immediately, autologous bone marrow or autologous peripheral blood stem cell transplantation requires storage of the product during the period of chemotherapy induction. The most commonly used cryopreservative technique involves the intracellular cryoprotectant dimethylsulfoxide (DMSO) with either autologous plasma or human albumin. A final concentration of 10% DMSO with 20% autologous plasma and 1×10^8 to 2×10^8 nucleated cells per mL is optimal. The final volume of cells and cryopreservative solution is approximately 100 to 800 mL and may have a hematocrit of 5% to 15%. The product is frozen at a controlled rate of 1°C to 3°C per minute to approximately −85°C and then stored in liquid nitrogen in either the vapor or the liquid phase. Measurements of cryopreservation efficacy as estimated by CFU-GM survival rates are complicated by the osmolar shock experienced by marrow cells as they are introduced to the culture media. One study in humans reported that poor cell survival (less than 50% CFU-GM survival) was predictive for delayed or failed engraftment. Cryopreserved human stem cell products are directly infused to the recipient and thus may experience similar osmolar shock (Gorin, 1986).

Recent efforts to place processed stem cell collections directly into −80°C freezers without controlled rate freezing have used a combination of 5% DMSO and 6% hydroxyethyl starch (HES) (Stiff, 1987b). The mechanism of HES cryopreservation is not completely understood but is probably related to the formation, in 20% solutions of HES, of a reversible glass at approximately −20°C (Takahashi, 1988). Marrows stored with DMSO and HES have been reported to retain 82% ± 39% of the CFU-GM when stored at −80°C for 1 to 4 months (Takahashi, 1988). A lesser concentration of DMSO may diminish the patient's symptoms on infusion.

Stem Cell Infusion

Unfiltered infusion of processed bone marrow, peripheral blood stem cells, or cord blood through a central venous line is generally accomplished with only minor complications. If cryopreserved, the aliquots of product are rapidly thawed in a 37°C water bath, and the aliquots are infused over 4 hours (Kessinger, 1988). The entire 100-mL to 800-mL product may require two days of infusion. The DMSO used can stimulate histamine release with resultant dyspnea, hypotension, nausea, diarrhea, and skin rash (Davis, 1990). Pretreatment with antihistamines can minimize these side effects. Other potential complications of stem cell infusions include volume overload and, in bone marrow transplants, pulmonary embolism of fat or particulates and effects of anticoagulation. Hemoglobinuria from lysed RBC is common but resolves without therapy (Kessinger, 1994). In addition to these reactions, allogeneic stem cell infusions pose the risk of allergic reactions to blood components, acute or delayed hemolytic reactions from ABO incompatibilities, and GVHD. Plasma, fat, RBC, or granulocytes can be reduced during processing. On rare occasions, anaphylaxis and cardiac arrest have been reported with the infusion of DMSO cryopreserved marrow (Davis, 1990; Vriesendorp, 1984).

ARTIFICIAL BLOOD

There is no substitute for blood. However, in this time of concern for transfusion-transmitted diseases, many companies (Dracker, 1994) have joined the research efforts to find a RBC substitute to carry oxygen to the tissues.

Perfluorocarbons

Perfluorocarbons (PFC) are relatively large organic molecules that are chemically inert, nonimmunogenic, and not metabolized. They can dissolve 40% to 70% oxygen per unit volume (Allen, 1986), which is more than blood can. The amount of oxygen in the PFC depends on the external environment's oxygen concentration. Addition of surfactant, such as egg white lecithin or the synthetic polymer Pluronic F-68 (Green Cross Corp., Osaka, Japan), causes the PFC to emulsify and thereby become miscible with blood. Because they do not carry carbon monoxide, PFC may be useful in carrying oxygen to the tissues during cases of carbon monoxide poisoning. Because of their small size, 1/70 that of an RBC, PFC can be used to deliver oxygen distal to a partial vascular occlusion such as in an acute myocardial infarct, a stroke, or sickle cell crisis. PFC are also used to deliver oxygen to the interior of a tumor to enhance subsequent treatment with ionizing irradiation (Allen, 1986). The FDA has approved the use of PFC for percutaneous transluminal coronary angioplasty.

The disadvantages of PFC are (1) the lack of affinity for oxygen (oxygen simply dissolves in the material), (2) the necessity for the patient therefore to be in a high-oxygen environment with the possible development of oxygen toxicity to the lungs, and (3) the potential for blockade of the reticuloendothelial system (RES) (clearing mechanism for PFC) and subsequent diminished clearing of pathogens.

For several years, Fluosol-DA was permitted for investigational human use in emergency situations. However, the FDA (1983) questioned its use because of lack of convincing evidence that PFC were more efficient in carrying oxygen than existing IV solutions and because of concern over possible toxicity to macrophages, neutrophils, monocytes, lungs, and platelets (Kahn, 1985a). Furthermore, it was concluded by Gould (1986) that Fluosol-DA is ineffective in overcoming the effects of anemia.

Hemoglobin Solutions

When a crude extract of hemoglobin is transfused, the red cell stroma infused acts as an antigen that can combine with the recipient's antibodies and cause DIC with kidney failure. When the red cell stroma is removed, the hemoglobin solution becomes a relatively nontoxic product.

The half-life of stroma-free hemoglobin is short. Free hemoglobin remains in the circulation only two to four hours (Allen, 1986). Outside the RBC, the hemoglobin tetramer readily dissociates to dimers and monomers that are rapidly cleared by the kidney. Hemoglobin is also bound by plasma proteins such as haptoglobin and cleared by the RES (see Fig. 31–7).

Two methods are used to stabilize the hemoglobin molecule in solution. One is to use intramolecular cross-links, which stabilize the tetramer, and the other is to employ intermolecular cross-links, which produce a high-molecular-weight polymer of hemoglobin (Allen, 1986). These processes can increase the intravascular half-life of hemoglobin to 15 to 30 hours, but the oxygen affinity remains high so that oxygen is poorly released to the tissues.

Pyridoxylated hemoglobin is treated with pyridoxal-5-phosphate, an analogue of 2,3-DPG, to reduce the oxygen affinity for the hemoglobin so that it more closely approximates that seen in RBC. Therefore, this product can better release oxygen to the tissues.

Because of the relatively short time free hemoglobin remains in the circulation, its usefulness may be limited only to emergency situations.

Human trials of the hemoglobin preparations have all revealed several adverse clinical effects—nausea, vomiting, fever, generalized discomfort, vasoconstriction, increased vascular pressure, and increased blood pressure (Goodrich, 1994). The vasoconstriction is thought to be due to free hemoglobin irreversibly binding endothelial nitrous oxide when the hemoglobin leaks out from the vascular spaces.

Encapsulated Hemoglobin

Encapsulated hemoglobin can be made by surrounding hemoglobin molecules with liposomes comprising either nonimmunogenic phospholipids or phospholipids and neutral fats (Allen, 1986). These liposomes are closed, spherical vesicles with an internal aqueous environment and a cell membrane-like outer layer consisting of lipids. When 2,3-DPG is included in the internal compartment with the hemoglobin, the oxygen affinity is decreased to those levels seen with hemoglobin in the RBC.

Within a few hours of intravenous administration, 50% of the liposomes are cleared from the circulation, primarily by the RES of the liver and some by the RES of the spleen. Additional clearing mechanisms include irreversible binding to tissues and lysis by plasma lipoproteins (Allen, 1986). There is concern about this rapid encapsulated hemoglobin clearance by the RES and its blockade by the liposomes, which might result in decreased immunity to pathogens.

Liposome technology has also been used to produce artificial platelets that can bind fibrinogen and agglutinate along with activated platelets (Allen, 1986).

Akahoshi M, Takanashi M, Masuda M, et al: A case of transfusion associated GVHD not prevented by white cell-reduction filters. Transfusion 1992; 32:169–172.

Allen RW, Kahn RA, Baldassare JJ: Advances in the production of blood cell substitutes with alternate technologies. *In* Wallas CH, McCarthy LJ (eds): New Frontiers in Blood Banking. Arlington, Virginia, American Association of Blood Banks, 1986, pp 21–49.

Alter HJ, Tabor E, Meryman HT, et al: Transmission of hepatitis B virus infection by transfusion of frozen-deglycerolized RBC. N Engl J Med 1978; 294:637.

Alter M: Review of the serologic testing for hepatitis C virus infection and risk of post-transfusion hepatitis. Arch Pathol Lab Med 1994; 118:342–345.

Anderson IC, Shpall EJ, Leslie DS, et al: Elimination of malignant clonogenic breast cancer cells from human bone marrow. Cancer Res 1989; 49:4659.

Aoki SK, Holland PV: Lyme disease—another transfusion risk? Transfusion 1989; 29:646.

Aster RH: Platelet-specific alloantigen systems: History clinical significance, and molecular biology. *In* Nance ST (ed): Alloimmunity: 1993 and Beyond. Bethesda, Maryland, American Association of Blood Banks, 1993, pp 83–116.

Badon SJ, Fister RD, Cable RG: Survival of *Borrelia burgdorferi* in blood products. Transfusion 1989; 29:581.

Baley JE, Stork EK, Warkentin PI, et al: Buffy coat transfusions in neutropenic neonates with presumed sepsis: A prospective, randomized trial. Pediatrics 1987; 80:712.

Barnes A, Pachciarz J: Current strategies in preoperative autologous donation. *In* Carlson KB, Golub AH (eds): Limiting Homologous Exposure: Alternative Strategies. Arlington, Virginia, American Association of Blood Banks, 1989, pp 25–40.

Berenson RJ, Andrews RG, Bensinger WI, et al: Antigen CD34+ marrow cells engraft lethally irradiated baboons. J Clin Invest 1988; 81:951.

Berenson RJ, Bensinger WI, Hill RS, et al: Engraftment after infusion of CD34+ marrow cells in patients with breast cancer or neuroblastoma. Blood 1991; 77:1717.

Berkman SA, Lee ML, Gale RP: Clinical uses of intravenous immunoglobulins. Semin Hematol 1988; 25:140.

Berry-Dortch S, Boral LI: Where to get blood for patients with antibodies to high frequency antigens: Problems and solutions. Chicago, American Society of Clinical Pathologists, Immunohematology Check Sample IH 6, 1983.

Berry-Dortch S, Woodside CH, Boral LI: Limitations of the immediate spin crossmatch when used for detecting ABO incompatibility. Transfusion 1985; 25:176.

Bertolini F, Lazzari L, Corsini C, et al: Cord blood banking for stem cell transplant. International Journal of Artificial Organs 1993; 16(Suppl 5):111.

Blumberg N, Heal JM: Transfusion associated immunomodulation. *In* Anderson KC, Ness PM (eds). Scientific Basis of Transfusion Medicine. Philadelphia, WB Saunders Co., 1994, pp 580–597.

Boral LI, Cornell TA, Danemiller FJ, et al: A guideline for anticipated blood usage during elective surgery. Am J Clin Pathol 1979; 71:680.

Boral LI, Henry JB: The type and screen: A safe alternative and supplement in selected surgical procedures. Transfusion 1977; 17:163.

Bordin JO, Bardossy, L, Blajchman MA: Experimental animal model of refractioness to donor platelets: The effects of plasma removal and the extent of WBC reduction in allogeneic alloimmunization. Transfusion 1993; 33:798.

Bordin JO, Heddle NM, Blajchman MA: Biologic effects of leukocytes present in transfused cellular blood products. Blood 1994; 84:1703–1721.

Bortin MM, Horowitz MM, Rimm AA: Increasing utilization of allogeneic bone marrow transplantation. Results of the 1988–1990 survey. Ann Intern Med 1992; 116:505.

Branch DR, Gallagher MT, Forman SJ, et al: Endogenous stem cell repopulation resulting in mixed hematopoietic chimerism following total body irradiation and marrow transplantation for acute leukemia. Transplantation 1982; 34:226.

Brown KE, Hibbs JR, Gallinella G, et al: Resistance to parvovirus B19 due to lack of virus receptor (erythrocyte P antigen). N Engl J Med 1994; 330:1192–1196.

Brown SL, Boral LI: Detection of mixed field agglutination in a surgical patient receiving blood transfusions. Chicago, American Society of Clinical Pathologists, Immunohematology Check Sample IH 5, 1986.

Broxmeyer HE, Douglas GW, Hangoc G, et al: Human umbilical cord blood as a potential source of transplantable hematopoietic stem/progenitor cells. Proc Natl Acad Sci U S A 1989; 86:3828.

Broxmeyer HE, Hangoc G, Cooper S, et al: Growth characteristics and expansion of human umbilical cord blood and estimation of its potential for transplantation of adults. Proc Natl Acad Sci U S A 1992; 89:4109.

Brubaker DB: Transfusion associated GVHD. *In* Anderson KC, Ness PM (eds): Scientific Basis of Transfusion Medicine, Implications for Clinical Practice. Philadelphia, WB Saunders Co., 1994, pp 544–579.

Busch MP: Retrovirus and blood transfusions: The lessons learned and the challenges yet ahead. *In* Nance SJ (ed): Blood Safety: Current Challenges, Bethesda, Maryland, American Association of Blood Banks, 1992, pp 1–44.
Busch ORC, Hop WCJ, Hoynk van Papendrecht MAW, et al: Blood transfusions and prognosis in colorectal cancer. N Engl J Med 1993; 328:1372–1376.
Bussel JB: Intravenous immunoglobulin therapy of immune hematological disease. *In* Garner RJ, Sacher RA (eds): Intravenous Gammaglobulin Therapy. Arlington, Virginia, American Association of Blood Banks, 1988a, pp 99–112.
Bussel JB, Berkowitz RL, McFarland JG, Lynch L, Chitkara U: Antenatal treatment of neonatal alloimmune thrombocytopenia. N Engl J Med 1988b; 319:1374.
Butler J, Parker D, Pillai R, et al: Systemic release of neutrophil elastase and tumor necrosis factor alpha following ABO incompatible blood transfusion. Br J Haematol 1991; 79:525–526.
Cairo MS: Granulocyte transfusions in neonates with presumed sepsis. Pediatrics 1987; 80:738.
Carow CE, Hangoc G, Cooper SH, et al: Mast cell growth factor (c-kit ligand) supports the growth of human multipotential (CFU-GEMM) progenitor cells with a high replating potential. Blood 1991; 78:2216.
Centers for Disease Control (CDC): Public Health Service Working Group: Licensure of screening test for antibody to human T-lymphotropic virus type 1. MMWR 1988; 37(48):736.
Centers for Disease Control (CDC): Guidelines for preventing transmission of HIV through transplantation of human tissues and organs. MMWR 43 (RR-8), May 20, 1994, p 12.
Centers for Disease Control (CDC): Outbreak of hepatitis C associated with intravenous immunoglobulin administration—U.S., Oct. 1993–June 1994. MMWR 43 1994; (28):505–509.
Centers for Disease Control (CDC): Interpretive criteria used to report Western blot results for HIV-1-antibody testing—U.S. MMWR 40 1991; (40):692–695.
Centers for Disease Control (CDC): Interpretation and use of the Western blot assay for serodiagnosis of human immunodeficiency virus type 1 infections. MMWR 1989; 38(S-7):1.
Chambers LA, Kruskall MS: Strategies to limit homologous blood use in cardiac surgery. *In* Baldwin ML, Kurtz SR (eds): Transfusion Practice in Cardiac Surgery. Arlington, Virginia, American Association of Blood Banks, 1991, pp 13–31.
Chambers RW, Foley HT, Schmidt PJ: Transmission of syphilis by fresh blood components. Transfusion 1969; 9:32.
Civin CI, Strauss LC, Brovall C, et al: Antigenic analysis III: A hematopoietic progenitor cell surface antigen defined by a monoclonal antibody raised against KG-1a cells. J Immunol 1984; 133:157.
Collins JA: The pathophysiology of hemorrhagic shock. *In* Collins JA, Murawski K, Shafer AW (eds): Massive Transfusion in Surgery and Trauma. New York, Alan R. Liss, 1982, pp 5–29.
Council of Community Blood Centers Newsletter, September 2, 1994, Washington DC.
Council of Community Blood Centers Newsletter, Aug. 11, 1995, Washington, DC.
Counts RB, Haisch C, Simon TL, Maxwell NG, et al: Hemostasis in massively transfused trauma patients. Ann Surg 1979; 190:91.
Cyrus S: Western blot, radioimmunoprecipitation and immunofluorescence assays. *In* Vengelen-Tyler V, Baldwin ML (eds): Understanding Technology New to the Blood Bank. Arlington, Virginia, American Association of Blood Banks, 1988, pp 31–45.
Davenport R: Cytokines and erythrocyte incompatibility. Curr Opin Hematol 1994; 1:452–456.
Davey RJ: Red cell radiolabeling in transfusion medicine. *In* Davey RJ, Wallace ME (eds): Diagnostic and Investigational Uses of Radiolabeled Blood Elements. Arlington, Virginia, American Association of Blood Banks, 1987, pp 39–66.
Davis JM, Rowley SD, Braine HG, et al: Clinical toxicity of cryopreserved bone marrow graft infusion. Blood 1990; 75:781.
Dawson RB, Barnes A Jr (eds): Clinical and Practical Aspects of the Use of Frozen Blood. Washington DC, American Association of Blood Banks, 1977.
Deeg HJ, Thomas ED, Flournoy N, et al: Cyclosporine A prophylaxis for graft-versus-host disease: A randomized study in patients undergoing marrow transplantation for acute nonlymphoblastic leukemia. Blood 1984; 65:1325.
Dillard GHL, Brecher G, Cronkite CP: Separation, concentration and transfusion of platelets. Proc R Soc Exp Biol Med 1951; 78:796.
Dito WR, Patrick CW, Shelly J: Clinical Pathological Correlations in Amniotic Fluid. Chicago, American Society of Clinical Pathologists, 1975.
Dracker RA, Beadling W, Lauenstein K: The search for a clinically useful blood substitute. Lab Med 1994; 25:718—723.
Duke WW: The relationship of blood platelets to hemorrhagic disease. Description of a method for determining the bleeding time and coagulation time and report of three cases of hemorrhagic disease relieved by transfusion. JAMA 1910; 55:1185.
Dzik WH, Cusack WF, Sherburne B, Kickler T: The effect of prestorage white cell reduction on the function and viability of stored platelet concentrates. Transfusion 1992; 32:334–339.
Eernisse JG, Brand A: Prevention of platelet refractoriness due to HLA antibodies by administration of leukocyte-poor blood components. Exp Hematol 1981; 9:77.
Emminger W, Emminger-Schmidmeier W, Hocker P, et al: Myeloid progenitor cells (CFU-GM) predict engraftment kinetics in autologous transplantation in children. Bone Marrow Transplant 1989; 4:415.
Filipovich AH, Vallera DA, Youle RJ, et al: Ex-vivo treatment of donor bone marrow with anti-T-cell immunotoxins for prevention of graft-versus-host disease. Lancet 1984; 1:469.
Fischer A, Durandy A, de Villartay JP, et al: HLA-haploidentical bone marrow transplantation for severe combined immunodeficiency using E rosette fractionation and cyclosporine. Blood 1986; 67:444.
Food and Drug Administration (Center for Biologics Evaluation and Research): Autologous Blood Collection and Processing Procedures. Communication to all registered blood establishments. Bethesda, Maryland, February 12, 1990.
Food and Drug Administration (Center for Biologics Evaluation and Research): HCV clarification of the use of unlicensed anti-HCV supplemental test results in regard to donor notification. Communications sent to all registered blood establishments. Bethesda, Maryland, August 19, 1993.
Food and Drug Administration (Center for Biologics Evaluation and Research): HTLV-1 antibody testing. Communication to all registered blood establishments. Bethesda, Maryland, November 29, 1988.
Food and Drug Administration (Center for Biologics Evaluation and Research): Recommendations regarding license amendments and procedures for gamma irradiation of blood products. Communications sent to all registered blood establishments. Bethesda, Maryland, July 22, 1993.
Food and Drug Administration (Center for Biologics Evaluation and Research): Revised recommendations for the prevention of HIV transmission by blood and blood products. Communications sent to all registered blood establishments. Bethesda, Maryland, April 23, 1992.
Food and Drug Administration (Office of Biologics and Research Review): Deferral of donors who have received human pituitary-derived growth hormone. Communications to all registered blood establishments. Bethesda, Maryland, November 25, 1987.
Food and Drug Administration (Office of Biologics Research and Review): Recommendations for the management of donors and units that are initially reactive for hepatitis B surface antigen (HBsAG). Communication to all registered blood establishments, December 2, 1987.
Freda VJ: The antepartum management of Rh disease. *In* Garratty G (ed): Hemolytic Disease of the Newborn. Arlington, Virginia, American Association of Blood Banks, 1984, pp 33–51.
Freda VJ, Gorman JG, Pollack W: Successful prevention of experimental Rh sensitization in man with an anti-Rh gamma-globulin antibody preparation: A preliminary report. Transfusion 1964; 4:26.
Fridley JL, Ellis K: Human T-cell lymphotropic virus, type 1 (HTLV-1) disease manifestations and implications for transfusion therapy. Chicago, American Society of Clinical Pathologists, Transfusion Medicine Check Sample TM 1, 1989.
Friedman BA, Oberman HA, Chadwick AR, Kingdom KI: The maximum blood order schedule and surgical blood use in the United States. Transfusion 1976; 16:380.
Gale RP, Feig S, Ho W, et al: ABO blood group system and bone marrow transplantation. Blood 1977; 50:185.
Gardner FH, Howell D, Hirsch ED: Platelet transfusion utilizing platelet equipment. J Lab Clin Med 1954; 43:196.
Garratty G: The clinical significance (and insignificance) of red-cell-bound IgG and complement. *In* Wallace ME, Levitt JS (eds): Current Applications and Interpretation of the Directed Antiglobulin Test. Arlington, Virginia, American Association of Blood Banks, 1988, pp 1–24.
Gee AP, Bruce KM, van Hilten J, et al: Selective loss of expression of a tumor-associated antigen on a human leukemia cell line induced by treatment with monoclonal antibody and complement. J Natl Cancer Inst 1987; 78:29.
Geissler K, Geissler W, Hinterberger W, et al: Circulating committed and pluripotential haemopoietic progenitor cells in infants. Acta Haematol 1986; 75:18.
Giblett ER: Blood group antibodies: An assessment of some laboratory practices. Transfusion 1977; 17:299.
Gibson JG: A citrate-phosphate-dextrose solution for preservation of human blood. Am J Clin Pathol 1957; 28:569.
Gilcher RO, Belcher L: Autologous blood. *In* Garner RJ, Silvergleid AJ (eds): Autologous and Directed Blood Programs. Arlington, Virginia, American Association of Blood Banks, 1987a, pp 1–13.
Gilcher RO, Belcher L: Preoperative autologous blood donation programs. *In* Garner RJ, Silvergleid AJ (eds): Autologous and Directed Blood Programs. Arlington, Virginia, American Association of Blood Banks, 1987b, pp 15–29.
Gluckman E, Broxmeyer HE, Auerback AD, et al: Hematopoietic reconstitution in a patient with Fanconi's anemia by means of umbilical-cord blood from an HLA-identical sibling. N Engl J Med 1989; 321:1174.

Gmur J, von Felton A, Osterwalder B, et al: Delayed alloimmunization using random single donor platelet transfusion: A prospective study in thrombocytopenic patients with acute leukemia. Blood 1983; 62:473.

Goldman JM, Gale RP, Horowitz MM, et al: Bone marrow transplantation for chronic myelogenous leukemia in chronic phase: Increased risk for relapse associated with T-cell depletion. Ann Intern Med 1988; 108:806.

Goldman JM, Johnson SM, Islam A, et al: Haematological reconstitution after autografting for chromic granulocytic leukaemia in transformation: The influence of previous splenectomy. Br J Haematol 1980; 45:223.

Goodman JW, Hodgson GS: Evidence for stem cells in the peripheral blood of mice. Blood 1962; 19:702.

Goodnough LT: Role of hematopoietic growth factors in transfusion medicine. Curr Opin Hematol 1994; 1:462–470.

Goodrich RP, Sowemino-Coker SO, Weinstein R: Advances in erythrocyte preservation and hemoglobin substitutes. Curr Opin Hematol 1994; 1:162–169.

Gorin NC: Collection, manipulation and freezing of haemopoietic stem cells. *In* Gladstone AH (ed): Clinics in Haematology. London, WB Saunders, 1986, p 19.

Gould SA, Rosen AL, Sehgal LR, Sehgal HL, et al: Fluosol-DA as a red-cell substitute in acute anemia. N Engl J Med 1986; 26:1653.

Guidelines for therapeutic hemapheresis. American Association of Blood Banks Extracorporeal Therapy Committee, American Association of Blood Banks, Bethesda, Maryland, May, 1992.

Haas R, Ho AD, Bredthauer U, et al: Successful autologous transplantation of blood stem cells mobilized with recombinant human granulocyte-macrophage colony-stimulating factor. Exp Hematol 1990; 18:94.

Haugen RK: Hepatitis after the transfusion of frozen red cells and washed red cells. N Engl J Med 1979; 301:393.

Heddle NM, Klama L, Singer J, et al: The role of the plasma from platelet concentrates in transfusion reactions. N Engl J Med 1994; 331:625–628.

Howard JE, Perkins HA: The natural history of alloimmunization to platelets. Transfusion 1978; 18:496.

Hows J, Beddow K, Gordon-Smith E, et al: Donor-derived RBC antibodies and immune hemolysis after allogeneic bone marrow transplantation. Blood 1986; 67:177.

Hows JM, Chipping PM, Palmer S, et al: Regeneration of peripheral blood cells following ABO incompatible allogeneic bone marrow transplantation for severe aplastic anaemia. Br J Haematol 1983; 53:145.

Huestis DW, Bove JR, Caser J: Practical Blood Transfusion, 4th ed. Boston, Little Brown, 1988.

Hustin A: Principe d'une nouvelle methode de transfusion mucuese. J Med Brux 1914; 2:436.

Johnson GR, Moore MAS: Role of stem cell migration in initiation of mouse fetal liver haematopoiesis. Nature 1975; 258:726.

Jones FS (ed): Accreditation Requirements Manual of the American Association of Blood Banks, 5th ed. Bethesda, Maryland, American Association of Blood Banks, 1994.

Jones RJ, Wagner JE, Celano P, et al: Separation of pluripotent haematopoietic stem cells from spleen colony-forming cells. Nature 1990; 347:188.

Judd WJ, Butch SH, Oberman HA, et al: The evaluation of a positive direct antiglobulin test in pretransfusion testing. Transfusion 1980; 20:17.

Juttner CA, To LB, Haylock DN, et al: Circulating autologous stem cells collected in very early remission from acute non-lymphoblastic leukaemia produce prompt but incomplete haemopoietic reconstitution after high dose melphalan or supralethal chemoradiotherapy. Br J Haematol 1985; 61:739.

Kahn RA: Donor screening to prevent posttransfusion hepatitis. *In* Keating LJ, Silvergleid AJ (eds): Hepatitis, A Technical Workshop. Washington DC, American Association of Blood Banks, 1981, pp 99–125.

Kahn RA, Allen RW, Baldassare J: Alternate sources and substitutes for therapeutic blood components. Blood 1985a; 66:1.

Kahn RA, Duffy BF, Rodey GE: Ultraviolet irradiation of platelet concentrate abrogates lymphocyte activation without affecting platelet function *in vitro*. Transfusion 1985b; 25:547.

Kaizer H, Stuart RK, Brookmeyer R, et al: Autologous bone marrow transplantation in acute leukemia: A phase I study of in vitro treatment of marrow with 4-hydroperoxycyclophosphamide to purge tumor cells. Blood 1985; 65:1504.

Kessinger A, Armitage JO: Harvesting marrow for autologous transplantation from patients with malignancies. Bone Marrow Transplant 1987; 2:15.

Kessinger A, Armitage JO, Landmark JD, et al: Autologous peripheral hematopoietic stem cell transplantation restores hematopoietic function following marrow ablative therapy. Blood 1988; 71:723.

Kessinger A, Bierman PJ, Vose JM, et al: High-dose cyclophosphamide, carmustine, and etoposide followed by autologous peripheral stem cell transplantation for patients with relapsed Hodgkin's disease. Blood 1991; 77:2322.

Kessinger A, Nademanee A, Forman SJ, et al: Autologous bone marrow transplantation for Hodgkin's and non-Hodgkin's lymphoma. Hematol Oncol Clin North Am 1990; 4:577.

Kessinger A: Peripheral blood stem cells. *In* Anderson KC, Ness PM (eds): Scientific Basis of Transfusion Medicine. Philadelphia, WB Saunders Co, 1994, p 489.

Kickler TS, Bell W, Ness PM, Pall D: Depletion of white cells from platelet concentrates using a new adsorption filter. Transfusion 1989; 29:411.

Kim DM, Brecher ME, Bland LA, et al: Visual identification of bacterially contaminated red cells. Transfusion 1992; 32:221–225.

King JC, Sacher RA: Percutaneous umbilical cord sampling. *In* Sacher RA, Strauss R (eds): Contemporary Issues in Pediatric Transfusion Medicine. Arlington, Virginia, American Association of Blood Banks, 1989, pp 33–53.

Klein HG (ed): Standards for Blood Banks and Transfusion Services, 16th ed. Bethesda, Maryland, American Association of Blood Banks, 1994.

Klein HG: Effect of plasma exchange on plasma constituents: Choice of replacement solutions and kinetics of exchange. *In* MacPherson JL, Kasprisin DO (eds): Therapeutic Hemapheresis, Vol II. Boca Raton, Florida, CRC Press, 1985, pp 3–14.

Klein HG: Transfusion medicine: The evolution of a new discipline. JAMA 1987; 258:2108.

Klein HG, Leitman SF: Adoptive immunotherapy in the treatment of malignant disease. Transfusion 1989; 29:170.

Knudtzon S: In vitro growth of granulocyte colonies from circulating cells in human cord blood. Blood 1974; 43:357.

Korbling M, Fliedner TM, Calvo W, et al: Albumin density gradient purification of canine hemopoietic blood stem cells: Long-term allogeneic engraftment without GVH-reaction. Exp Hematol 1979; 7:277.

Korbling M, Holle R, Haas R, et al: Autologous blood stem-cell transplantation in patients with advanced Hodgkin's disease and prior radiation to the pelvic site. J Clin Oncol 1990; 8:978.

Kurtz SR, VanDeinse WH, Valeri CR: The immunocompetence of residual leukocytes at various stages of red cell cryopreservation with 40% w/v glycerol in an ionic medium at −80° C. Transfusion 1978; 18:441.

Lamberson RD, Boral LI, Berry-Dortch S: Limitations of the crossmatch for detection of incompatibility between A B RBC and B patient sera. Am J Clin Pathol 1986; 86:511.

Lane TA: Leukocyte reduction of cellular blood components. Arch Pathol Lab Med 1994; 118:392–404.

Lasky LC, Bostrom B, Smith J, et al: Clinical collection and use of peripheral blood stem cells in pediatric patients. Transplantation 1989; 47:613.

Ledent E, Berlin G: Inadequate white cell reduction by bedside filtration of red cell concentrates. Transfusion 1994; 34:765–768.

Leitman SF, Holland PV: Irradiation of blood products, indications and guidelines. Transfusion 1985; 25:293.

Lenny LL, Hurst R, Goldstein J, Galbraith RA: Transfusion to group O subjects of 2 units of red cells enzymatically converted from group B to group O. Transfusion 1994; 34:209–214.

Levine E, Rosen A, Sehgal L, et al: Physiologic effects of acute anemia: Implications for a reduced transfusion trigger. Transfusion 1990; 30:11–14.

Loutit JF, Mollison PL, Young IM: Citric acid–sodium citrate–glucose mixtures for blood storage. J Exp Physiol 1943; 32:183.

Lowenthal RM, Chalis DR, Griffiths RA, et al: Transfusion associated GVHD: Report of an occurrence following the administration of irradiated blood. Transfusion 1993; 33:524–529.

Luban NLC: Human parvovirus: Implications for transfusion medicine. Transfusion 1994; 34:821–26.

Ludomirski A, Weiner S: Percutaneous fetal umbilical blood sampling. Clin Obstet Gynecol 1988; 31:19.

Lusher JM: Desmopressin acetate (DDAVP): Its use in disorders of hemostasis. Chicago, American Society of Clinical Pathologists, Thrombosis and Hemostasis Check Sample TH 5, 1984.

Mannucci PM: Desmopressin: A nontransfusional form of treatment for congenital and acquired bleeding disorders. Blood 1988; 72:1449.

Mannucci PM: Lattuada A Ruggin ZM: Proteolysis of von Willebrand factor in therapeutic plasma concentrates. Blood 1994; 83:3018–3027.

Marcus CS, Myhre BA, Angulo MC, Salk RD, et al: Radiolabeled red cell viability II. 99mTc and 111-In for measuring the viability of heterologous red cells in vivo. Transfusion 1987; 27:420.

McCarthy DM, Goldman JM: Transfusion of circulating stem cells. CRC Crit Rev Clin Lab Sci 1984; 20:1.

McCullough J, Weiblen BJ, Clay ME, Forstrom L: Effect of leukocyte antibodies on the fate in vivo of Indium-III-labeled granulocytes. Blood 1981; 58:164.

McDonald TB, Berkowitz RA: Massive transfusion in children. *In* Jeffries LC, Brecher ME (eds): Massive Transfusion. Bethesda, Maryland, American Association of Blood Banks, 1994, pp 97–123.

Menitove JE: Rationale for surrogate testing to detect non-A, non-B hepatitis. Transfusion Med Rev 1988; 2:65.

Menitove JE, McElligott MC, Aster RH: Febrile transfusion reaction: What blood component should be given next? Vox Sang 1982; 42:318.

Meryman HT, Hornblower M: Freezing and deglycerolizing sickle trait RBC. Transfusion, 16:627, 1976.

Metcalf D: Thrombopoietin: At last. Nature 369:519–520, 1994.

Micklem HS, Anderson N, Ross E: Limited potential of circulating haemopoietic stem cells. Nature 1975; 256:41.

Milam JD: Blood transfusion in heart surgery. Surg Clin North Am 1983; 63:1127.

Mintz PD, Nordine RB, Henry JB, Webb WR: Expected hemotherapy in elective surgery. N Y State J Med 1976; 76:532.

Mitsuyasy RT, Champlin RE, Gale RP, et al: Treatment of donor bone marrow with monoclonal anti-T-cell antibody and complement for the prevention of graft-versus-host disease. A prospective, randomized, double-blind trial. Ann Intern Med 1986; 105:20.

Molineux G, Podjda Z, Hampson IN, et al: Transplantation potential of peripheral blood stem cells induced by granulocyte colony-stimulating factor. Blood 1990; 76:2153.

Mollison PL, Engelfriet CP, Contreras M: Blood Transfusion in Clinical Medicine, 9th ed. Oxford, Blackwell Scientific Publications, 1993.

Montgomery RB, Coller BS: von Willebrand disease. *In* Colman RW, Hirsh J, Marder VJ, Salzman EW (eds): Hemostasis and Thrombosis, 3rd ed. Philadelphia, JB Lippincott, 1994, pp 134–168.

Moroff G, Luban NLC: Prevention of transfusion associated GVHD. Transfusion 1992; 32:102–103.

Morstyn G, Campbell L, Souza LM, Alton KL, et al: Effect of granulocyte colony stimulating factor on neutropenia induced by cytotoxic chemotherapy. Lancet 1988; 2:667.

Murkin JM, Lux J, Shannon NA, et al: Aprotinin significantly decreases bleeding and transfusion requirements in patients receiving aspirin and undergoing cardiac operations. J Thorac Cardiovasc Surg 1994; 107:554–561.

Muylle L, Laekeman G, Herman AG, Peetermans ME: Histamine levels in stored platelet concentrate. Relationship to white cell content. Transfusion 1988; 28:226–228.

Muylle L, Joos M, Wouters R, et al: Increased TNFa, IL-1 and IL-6 levels in the plasma of stored platelet concentrates: Relationships between TNFa and IL-6 levels and febrile transfusion reactions. Transfusion 1993; 33:195–199.

Myhre B: Fatalities from blood transfusions. JAMA 1980; 244:1333.

Ness PM, Nass CC: Blood donor testing for HIVI/II and HTLVI/II. Arch Pathol Lab Med 1994; ll8:337–341.

Nicolaides KH: Cordocentesis. Clin Obstet Gynecol 1988; 31:123.

NIDDK Fact Sheet: Human growth hormone and Creutzfeldt-Jacob disease. U.S. Department of Health and Human Services. NIH Publication No. 88-2793, December 1987.

N.I.H. Consensus Conference: Fresh frozen plasma. Indications and risks. JAMA 1985; 253:551.

N.I.H. Consensus Conference: Platelet transfusion therapy. JAMA 1987; 257:1777.

N.I.H. Consensus Conference: Perioperative RBC transfusion. JAMA 1988; 260:2700.

Noble RC, Kane MA, Reeves SA, Roeckel I: Posttransfusion hepatitis A in a neonatal intensive care unit. JAMA 1984; 252:2711.

Okusawa S, Gelfand JA, Ikejima T, et al: Interleukin-1 induces a shock-like state in rabbits. Synergism with TNF and the effect on cyclooxygenase inhibition. J Clin Invest 1988; 81:1162–1172.

Omaha NE: The University of Nebraska Medical Center, 1991.

Opelz G, Terasaki PI: Dominant effect of transfusions on kidney graft survival. Transplantation 1980; 29:153.

Owings DV, Kruskall MS, Thurer RL, Donovan LM: Autologous blood donations prior to elective cardiac surgery. Safety and effect on subsequent blood use. JAMA 1989; 262:1963.

Parravicini A, Rebulla P, Apuzzo J, Wenz B, Sirchia G: The preparation of leucocyte-poor red cells for transfusion by a simple cost-effective technique. Transfusion 1984; 24:508.

Peters WP, Rosner G: A bottom-line analysis of the financial impact of hematopoietic colony-stimulating factors and CSF-primed peripheral blood progenitor cells. Blood 1991; 78(Suppl 1):6a.

Peters WP, Shpall EJ, Jones RB, et al: High-dose combination cyclophosphamide (CPA), cisplatin (cDDP) and carmustine (BCNU) with bone marrow support as initial treatment for metastatic breast cancer: Three- to six-year follow-up. Proc Am Soc Clin Oncol 1990; 9:31.

Petersen LR, Satten GA, Dodd R, et al: Duration of time from the onset of HIV-1 infectiousness to development of detectable antibody. Transfusion 1994; 34:283–289.

Philip T, Armitage JO, Spitzer G, et al: High-dose therapy and autologous bone marrow transplantation after failure of conventional chemotherapy in adults with intermediate-grade or high-grade non-Hodgkin's lymphoma. N Engl J Med 1987; 316:1493.

Pineda AA: New apheresis technologies. *In* Westphal RG, Kasprisin DO (eds): Current Status of Hemapheresis: Indications, Technology and Complications. Arlington, Virginia, American Association of Blood Banks, 1987, pp 71–86.

Pineda AA, Taswell HE, Brzica SM Jr: Delayed hemolytic transfusion reaction. An immunologic hazard of blood transfusion. Transfusion 1978; 18:1.

Popovsky MA: The role of autologous transfusion in surgery and the emergency room. *In* Garner RJ, Silvergleid AJ (eds): Autologous and Directed Blood Programs. Arlington, Virginia, American Association of Blood Banks, 1987, pp 47–63.

Prodouz KN, Fratantoni JC: Viral inactivation of blood products. *In* Anderson KC, Ness PM (eds): Scientific Basis of Transfusion Medicine, Implications for Clinical Practice. Philadelphia, WB Saunders Co., 1994, pp 852–873.

Propper RD, Button LN, Nathan DG: New approaches to the transfusion management of thalassemia. Blood 1980; 55:55.

Pura LS, Smith LE, Goldfinger D: Establishment of a directed donor blood program in a hospital-based blood bank. *In* Garner RJ, Silvergleid AJ (eds): Autologous and Directed Blood Programs. Arlington, Virginia, American Association of Blood Banks, 1987, pp 31–45.

Ramsay N, LeBien TW, Nesbit M, et al: Autologous bone marrow transplantation for patients with acute lymphoblastic leukemia in second or subsequent remission: Results of bone marrow treated with monoclonal antibodies BA-1, BA-2, BA-3 plus complement. Blood 1985; 66:508.

Reiffers J, Marit G, Rice A, et al: Peripheral blood stem cell transplantation in patients with acute myeloid leukemia. *In* Dicke KA, Armitage JO, Dicke-Evinger MJ (eds): Autologous Bone Marrow Transplantation. Proceedings of the Fifth International Symposium, pp 823.

Reisner Y, Kapoor N, Kirkpatrick D, et al: Transplantation for severe combined immunodeficiency with HLA-A, B, D, DR incompatible parental marrow cells fractionated by soybean agglutinin and sheep RBC. Blood 1983; 61:341.

Roberts SC, Snyder EL: Preservation solutions for blood component storage: Current status and future trends. Chicago, American Society of Clinical Pathologists, Immunohematology Check Sample IH 1, 1986.

Rock G: Production of plasma products and derivatives. *In* Wallas CH, McCarthy LJ (eds): New Frontiers in Blood Banking. Arlington, Virginia, American Association of Blood Banks, 1986, pp 51–87.

Rock WA Jr, Boral LI: Blood product replacement in obstetrics and gynecology. *In* Rock JA (ed): Advances in Obstetrics and Gynecology, vol 2. St Louis, MO, Mosby–Year Book, Inc., 1995, pp 71–89.

Rosenberg SA, Lotze MT, Mule JJ: New approaches to immunotherapy of cancer using interleukin-2. Ann Intern Med 1988; 108:853.

Rosenfeld S, Shadduck RK, Przepiorka D, et al: Autologous bone marrow transplantation with 4-hydroperoxycyclophosphamide purged marrows for acute nonlymphocytic leukemia in late remission or early relapse. Blood 1989; 74:1159.

Rous P, Turner JP: Preservation of living red blood corpuscles *in vitro*: II. The transfusion of kept cells. J Exp Med 1916; 23:219.

Rowley SD, Piantadosi S, Marcellus DC, et al: Analysis of factors predicting speed of hematologic recovery after transplantation with 4-hydroperoxycyclo-phosphamide-purged autologous bone marrow grafts. Bone Marrow Transplant 1991; 7:183.

Ryden SE, Oberman HA: Compatibility of common intravenous solutions with CPD blood. Transfusion 1975; 15:250.

Saba TM: Reversal of plasma fibronectin deficiency in septic-injured patients by cryoprecipitate infusion. *In* Collins JA, Murawski K, Shafer AW (eds): Massive Transfusion in Surgery and Trauma. New York, Alan R. Liss, 1982, pp 129–150.

Sacher RA: Intravenous gammaglobulin products: Development, pharmacology and precautions. *In* Garner RJ, Sacher RA (eds): Intravenous Gammaglobulin Therapy. Arlington, Virginia, American Association of Blood Banks, 1988, pp 1–30.

Sadoff BJ, Stromberg RR, Miller K, et al: Experimental 6 log white cell-reduction filters for red cells. Transfusion 1992; 32:129:33.

Sacher RA, Queenan JT: Hemolytic disease of the newborn: Antenatal and prophylactic management. *In* Kasprisin DO, Luban NLC (eds): Pediatric Transfusion Medicine, Vol 1. Boca Raton, Florida, CRC Press, 1987, pp 23–41.

Salzman EW, Weinstein MJ, Weintraub RM, et al: Treatment with desmopressin acetate to reduce blood loss after cardiac surgery: A double blind randomized trial. N Engl J Med 1986; 314:1402.

Sazama K: Bacteria in blood for transfusion. Arch Pathol Lab Med 1994; 118:350–365.

Schiffer CA: Introduction: Future research in platelet transfusion. *In* Schiffer CA (ed): Platelet Physiology and Transfusion. Washington DC, American Association of Blood Banks, 1980, pp 1–6.

Schiffer CA, Dutcher JP, Hogge DE, et al: Histocompatible platelet transfusion for patients with leukemia. Plasma Ther Trans Technol 1982a; 3:273.

Schiffer CA, Slichter SJ: Platelet transfusion from single donors. N Engl J Med 1982b; 307:245.

Seibel M, Gross S: Exchange transfusion in the neonate. *In* Kasprisin DO, Luban NLC (eds): Pediatric Transfusion Medicine, Vol 1. Boca Raton, Florida, CRC Press, 1987, pp 43–52.

Sharkis SJ, Santos GW, Colvin OM: Elimination of acute myelogenous leukemic cells from marrow and tumor suspensions in the rate with 4-hydroperoxy-cyclophosphamide. Blood 1980; 55:521.

Sherertz RJ, Russell BA, Reuman PD: Transmission of hepatitis A by transfusion of blood products. Arch Intern Med 1984; 144:1579.

Shulman IA: Parasitic infections and their impact on blood donor selection and testing. Arch Pathol Lab Med 1994; 118:366–370.

Siena S, Bregni M, Brando B, et al: Circulation of CD34+ hematopoietic stem cells in the peripheral blood of high-dose cyclophosphamide treated patients: Enhancement by intravenous recombinant human granulocyte-macrophage colony-stimulating factor. Blood 1989; 74:1905.

Siena S, Bregni M, Brando B, et al: Flow cytometry for clinical estimation of circulating hematopoietic progenitors for autologous transplantation in cancer patients. Blood 1991; 77:400.

Silvergleid AJ: Clinical platelet transfusions. *In* Silver H (ed): Blood, Blood Components and Derivatives in Transfusion Therapy. Washington DC, American Association of Blood Banks, 1980, pp 45–88.

Simon ER, Chapman RG, Finch CA: Adenine in red cell preservation. J Clin Invest 1962; 41:351.

Slichter SJ: Selection of compatible platelet donors. *In* Schiffer CA (ed): Platelet Physiology and Transfusion. Washington DC, American Association of Blood Banks, 1980, pp 83–92.

Stack G, Snyder EL: Cytokine generation in stored platelet concentrates. Transfusion 1994; 34:20–25.

Starkey JM, MacPherson JL, Bolgiano DC, et al: Markers for transfusion-transmitted disease in different groups of blood donors. JAMA 1989; 262:3452.

Stehling L: Surgery without transfusion: The anesthesiologist's view. *In* Carlson KB, Golub AH (eds): Limiting Homologous Exposure: Alternative Strategies. Arlington, Virginia, American Association of Blood Banks, 1989, pp 87–106.

Stiff PJ, Koester AR, Eagleton LE, et al: Autologous stem cell transplantation using peripheral blood stem cells. Transplantation 1987a; 44:585.

Stiff PJ, Koester AR, Weidner MK, et al: Autologous bone marrow transplantation using unfractionated cells cryopreserved in dimethylsulfoxide and hydroxyethyl starch without controlled-rate freezing. Blood 1987b; 70:974.

Storb R, Deeg HJ, Thomas ED, et al: Marrow transplantation for chronic myelocytic leukemia: A controlled trial of cyclosporine versus methotrexate for prophylaxis of graft-versus-host disease. Blood 1985; 66: 698.

Storb R, Epstein RB, Thomas ED: Marrow repopulating ability of peripheral blood cells compared to thoracic duct cells. Blood 1968; 32:662.

Strauss RG: Granulocyte transfusions: Uses, abuses, and indications. *In* Kolins J, McCarthy LJ (eds): Contemporary Transfusion Practice. Arlington, Virginia, American Association of Blood Banks, 1987, pp 65–83.

Takahashi T, Hirsch A, Erbe E, Williams RI: Mechanism of cryoprotection by extracellular polymeric solutes. Biophys J 1988; 54:509.

Tavassoli M: Embryonic and fetal hematopoiesis: An overview. Blood Cell 1991; 17:269.

Tegtmeier GE: Posttransfusion cytomegalovirus infections. Arch Path Lab Med 1989; 113:236.

Thomas ED, Storb R: Technique for human marrow grafting. Blood 1970; 36:507.

Thomas ED, Lochte HL Jr, Cannon JH, et al: Supralethal whole body irradiation and isologous marrow transplantation in man. J Clin Invest 1959; 38:1709–1716.

Tietz NW: Fundamentals of Clinical Chemistry, 3rd ed. Philadelphia, WB Saunders Co., 1994, pp 917–927.

To LB, Haylock DN, Kimber RJ, et al: High levels of circulating haemopoietic stem cells in very early remission from acute non-lymphoblastic leukaemia and their collection and cryopreservation. Br J Haematol 1984; 58:399.

To LB, Shepperd KM, Haylock DN, et al: Single high doses of cyclophosphamide enable the collection of high numbers of hemopoietic stem cells from the peripheral blood. Exp Hematol 1990; 18:442.

Tomasulo PA: Management of the alloimmunized patient with HLA-matched platelets. *In* Schiffer CA (ed): Platelet Physiology and Transfusion. Washington DC, American Association of Blood Banks, 1980a, pp 69–81.

Tomasulo PA, Anderson AJ, Paluso MB, et al: A study of criteria for blood donor deferral. Transfusion 1980b; 20:511.

Topalian SL, Solomon D, Avis FP, et al: Immunotherapy of patients with advanced cancer using tumor-infiltrating lymphocytes and recombinant interleukin-2: A pilot study. J Clin Oncol 1988; 6:839.

Torres A, Alonso MC, Gomez-Villagran JLG, et al: No influence of number of donor CFU-GM on granulocyte recovery in bone marrow transplantation for acute leukemia. Blut 1985; 50:89.

Uckun FM, Kersey JH, Vallera DA, et al: Autologous bone marrow transplantation in high-risk remission T-lineage acute lymphoblastic leukemia using immunotoxins plus 4-hydroperoxy-cylophosphamide for marrow purging. Blood 1990; 76:1723.

Ueno Y, Koizumi S, Yamagami M, et al: Characterization of hemopoietic stem cells (CFU-C) in cord blood. Exp Hematol 1981; 9:717.

U.S. Department of Health and Human Services, Food and Drug Administration: The code of federal regulations, 21 CFR, Parts 600, 606, 607, 610, and 640, current edition. Washington DC, US Government Printing Office.

Valeri CR, Zaroulis CG: Rejuvenation and freezing of outdated stored human red cells. N Engl J Med 1972; 187:1307.

Vaughan WP, Weisenburger DD, Sanger W, et al: Early leukemic recurrence of non-Hodgkin lymphoma after high-dose anti-neoplastic therapy with autologous marrow rescue. Bone Marrow Transplant 1987; 1:373.

Ventura GJ, Barlogie B, Hester JP, et al: High dose cyclophosphamide, BCNU and VP-16 with autologous blood stem cell support for refractory multiple myeloma. Bone Marrow Transplant 1990; 5:265.

Viele MK, Weiskopf, RB: What can we learn about the need for transfusion from patients who refuse blood? The experience with Jehovah's Witnesses. Transfusion 1994; 34:396–401.

Vogelsang GB: Transfusion-associated graft-versus-host disease in immunocompromised hosts. Transfusion 1990; 30:101.

Vriesendorp R, Aalders JG, Sleijfer DT, et al: Effective high-dose chemotherapy with autologous bone marrow infusion in resistant ovarian cancer. Gynecol Oncol 1984; 17:271.

Wagner JE, Santos GW, Noga SJ, et al: Bone marrow graft engineering by counterflow centrifugal elutriation: Results of a phase I-II clinical trial. Blood 1990; 75:1370.

Wagner JE, Kernan NA, Broxmeyer HE et al: Transplantation of umbilical cord blood in 50 patients: Analysis of the registry data. (Abstract 1564.) Blood 1994; 84(10 Suppl 1): 395a.

Walker RH: On the safety of the abbreviated crossmatch. *In* Polesky HF, Walker RH (eds): Safety in Transfusion Practices. Skokie, Illinois, College of American Pathologists, 1982, pp 71–106.

Walker RH (ed): Technical Manual, 11th ed. Bethesda, Maryland, American Association of Blood Banks, 1993.

Wapner RJ, Jackson L: Chorionic villus sampling. Clin Obstet Gynecol 31:328, 1988.

Weisz-Carrington P: Principles of Clinical Immunohematology. Chicago, Year Book Medical Publishers, 1986.

Wenz B: Leukocyte-free red cells: The evolution of a safer blood product. *In* McCarthy LJ, Baldwin ML (eds): Controversies of Leukocyte-Poor Blood and Components. Arlington, Virginia, American Association of Blood Banks, 1989, pp 27–48.

Westphal RG: Complications of hemapheresis. *In* Westphal RG, Kasprisin DO (eds): Current Status of Hemapheresis: Indications, Technology and Complications. Arlington, Virginia, American Association of Blood Banks, 1987, pp 87–104.

Wiggins RC, Glatfelter A, Campbell AM, et al: Acute hypotension due to platelet serotonin induced hemoreflexes after intravenous injection of dextransulfate in the rabbit. Circ Res 1985; 57:262–277.

Williams SF, Bitran JD, Richards JM, et al: Peripheral blood-derived stem cell collections for use in autologous transplantation after high dose chemotherapy: An alternative approach. Bone Marrow Transplant 1990; 5:129.

Yamanaka S, Miura K, Yukimura T, et al: Putative mechanism of hypotensive action of platelet activating factor in dogs. Circ Res 1992; 70:893–890.

Yeager AM, Kaizer H, Santos GW, et al: Autologous bone marrow transplantation in patients with acute nonlymphocytic leukemia, using *ex vivo* marrow treatment with 4-hydroperoxycyclophosphamide. N Engl J Med 1986; 315:141.

Zanjani ED, Ascensao JI: Erythropoietin. Transfusion 1989; 29:56.

Part 5

IMMUNOLOGY AND IMMUNOPATHOLOGY

Edited by

Robert M. Nakamura, M.D.
David J. Bylund, M.D.
Howard S. Fox, M.D., Ph.D.
John Bernard Henry, M.D.

Chapter 32

Overview of the Immune System

Howard S. Fox, M.D., Ph.D.

The immune system consists of multiple defenses designed to protect the body from infectious agents and to maintain internal homeostasis by removing damaged cells. The skin and mucosal surfaces function as barriers, a very important first line of defense, but once breached, they give way to immune mechanisms that are activated sequentially to protect the host. A number of specific and nonspecific mechanisms serve to shield the body and attack invading organisms. In this overview, the basic components of immunity are described: the cells, their mediators, and some of the processes necessary to drive immune responses. References are provided to recent, more extensive discussions of the basic mechanisms involved in immune system function.

DEVELOPMENT OF CELLS OF THE IMMUNE SYSTEM

The immune system comprises organized lymphoid tissue, such as the lymph nodes, spleen, and mucosa-associated lymphoid tissues, as well as circulating cells. Immune cells derive from multipotent hematopoietic progenitor cells (Weissman, 1994). During physiologic development, hematopoiesis begins in the yolk sac, moves to the liver in the fetus, and continues in the bone marrow from infancy to death. The first differentiation step is a division into lymphoid and myeloid precursors. Lymphoid precursors give rise to the B and T lymphocytes and natural killer (NK) cells, whereas the myeloid precursors eventually form red blood cells, platelets, monocytes and macrophages, dendritic cells, neutrophils, basophils, and eosinophils.

T-lymphocyte differentiation occurs in the thymus. The thymus gland, which is organized into an inner medulla and outer cortex, contains numerous epithelial cells that nurse and provide the correct milieu for T-cell development. Cells originating in the bone marrow pass into the thymus and from its cortex to the medulla, during which time the T cell acquires its specificities. The majority of these cells die within the thymus, but through a series of steps involving negative selection against self-reactive cells and positive selection of cells that can see antigen in the context of self–major histocompatibility complex (MHC) molecules, T cells emerge (von Boehmer, 1994; Nossal, 1994). Such cells then have the characteristics of mature T cells, expressing either the CD4 or CD8 cell surface molecule. Genes that produce antigen receptors on T cells rearrange early during these cells' stay in the thymus. That is, rearrangements of the variable (V), diversity (D, not present in α or γ chains), and joining (J) regions with respect to the constant (C) region result in cells expressing the T-cell antigen receptor heterodimer, ready to encounter antigen (Fig. 32–1). The majority of circulating cells and those in lymphoid tissue express the $\alpha\beta$-chains, but some, largely in the skin and gut, express the $\gamma\delta$-chains.

B-lymphocyte differentiation occurs within the bone marrow. B cells also undergo the processes of positive and negative selection, which can occur both in the bone marrow and peripherally (von Boehmer, 1994; Nossal, 1994). Just as the thymic epithelium nurtures T cells, stromal reticular cells contribute to B-cell development. Within the bone marrow, immunoglobulin gene rearrangements occur, with the heavy chain V-D-J segments joining the μ C region, followed by V-J rearrangement of the light chain (light chains lack D segments) joining to κ λ C segments (see Fig. 32–1). In addition to IgM expression dictated by these rearrangements, alternative splicing allows the expression of IgD. This creates the functional B cell, ready to encounter antigen.

Immune cells of the myeloid lineage—mast cells, baso-

5

	Variable			Constant
TcR α chain	$V\alpha_n$		$J\alpha_n$	$C\alpha$
TcR β chain	$V\beta_n$	$D\beta_{1,2}$	$J\beta_n$	$C\beta_{1,2}$
Ig heavy chain	Vh_n	Dh_n	Jh_n	$C\mu, \delta, \gamma_{1\text{-}4}, \varepsilon, \alpha_{1,2}$
Ig light chain	$V\kappa_n, \lambda_n$		$J\kappa_n, \lambda_n$	$C\kappa, \lambda$

Figure 32–1. Organization of T cell receptor and immunoglobulin genes. Both the TcR and Ig molecules are heterodimeric, with the individual genes encoded on different chromosomes. Both the TcR and Ig have variable regions, made up of numerous segments encoding variable (V), diversity (D, not found in the TcR α chain or the Ig light chain), and joining (J) segments, which undergo genomic rearrangements within T and B cells, respectively, to form a functional gene. The rearranged variable region is then joined by RNA splicing to the constant region to form the mature mRNA transcript. Furthermore, in the case of the Ig heavy chain, class switching can occur by genomic rearrangement, for example, in changing from B-cell secretion of IgM ($C\mu$) to IgG_2 ($C\gamma_2$).

phils, eosinophils, neutrophils, dendritic cells, and monocytes—all develop in the bone marrow. Both dendritic cells and monocytes then migrate to lymphoid organs and tissues. Subsequently, the blood-borne monocytes differentiate into mature macrophages. In particular organs, they are known by such specialized names as Kupffer cells of the liver, osteoclasts of the bone, and microglia of the brain.

ANTIGEN RECOGNITION AND CELL ACTIVATION

For a specific immune response to occur, the immune system must first recognize a stimulus and become activated by it (Fig. 32–2) (Janeway, 1994; Weiss, 1994). B cells use a form of IgM or IgD, or both, on their exterior membrane to

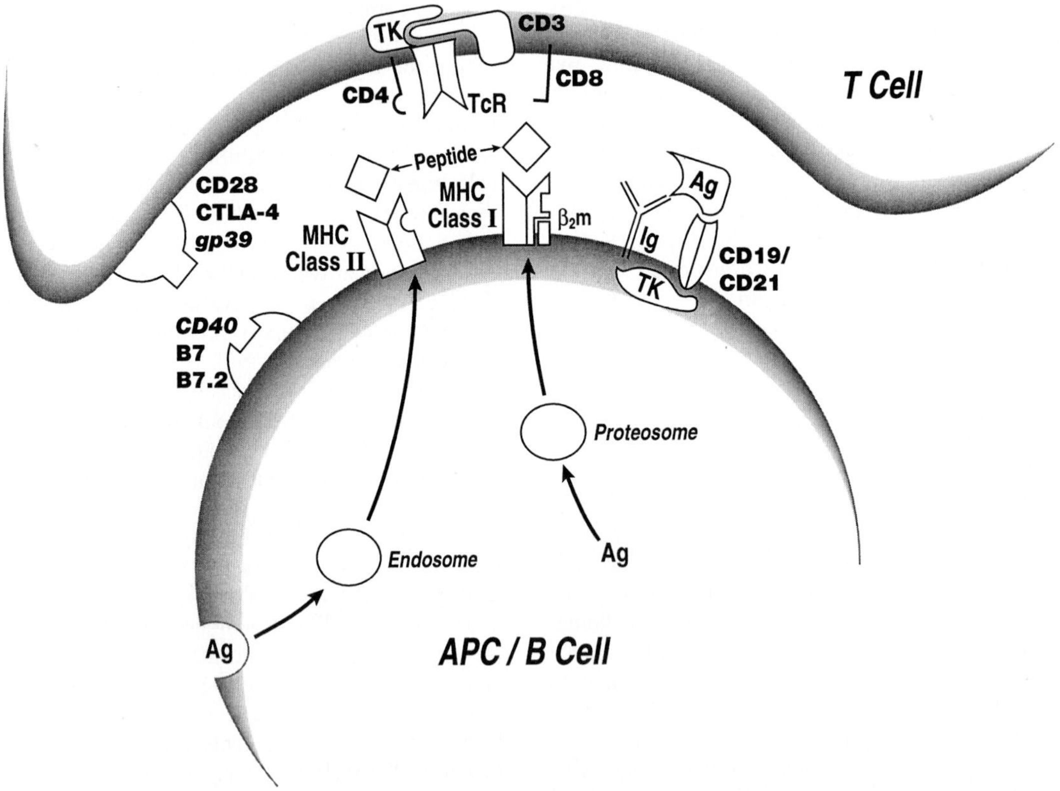

Figure 32–2. Cellular interactions in the immune system. Antigen-presenting cells (APC) process external or internal antigens (Ag) and present antigen peptide fragments, in association with an MHC molecule, to T cells. On the T cell, a specific TcR, along with the coreceptor CD4 or CD8 molecule, recognizes the antigen/MHC complex. Cellular activation proceeds through the CD3 complex and activation of tyrosine kinases (TK). The B-cell receptor is composed of membrane-bound Ig complexed to associated membrane proteins, and the CD19/CD21 coreceptor. On antigen recognition, cellular TK are also activated. Costimulatory activation of T cells or B cells is provided by cellular receptors binding their ligands (the ligands B7 or B7.2 for T-cell costimulation through CD28 and CTLA-4 molecules, and the gp39 ligand for the B cell CD40 molecule). (Adapted from Paul W, Seder R: Lymphocyte responses and cytokines. Cell 1994; 76:229; and Weiss A, Littman D: Signal transduction by lymphocyte antigen receptors. Cell 1994; 76:263.)

recognize a specific antigen. These cell surface molecules cannot transmit a signal to carry the immune response forward but instead do so through associated cellular transmembrane glycoproteins and intracellular tyrosine kinases such as Lyn, Fyn, and Syk. The T-cell receptor transmits signals through association with the CD3 complex of proteins, consisting of δ-, ϵ-, γ-, ζ-, and η-chains. T-cell signaling also is associated with the activation of tyrosine kinases, in this case Fyn, Lck, and ZAP-70.

In contrast to B cells, however, the T-cell receptor cannot directly recognize an antigen. For the T-cell receptor to see an antigen, the antigen must be processed into a small peptide and presented in the groove of an MHC molecule (Germain, 1994). Two types of MHC molecules exist: (1) Class I glycoproteins, which associate with the β_2-microglobulin invariant chain, and (2) Class II glycoproteins, which are present on the cell surface as an $\alpha\beta$ heterodimer.

Intracellularly produced antigens, such as viral proteins, can be degraded by a proteasome complex, thereby breaking the larger protein into peptides. These peptides are then transported to the endoplasmic reticulum, where they complex with MHC Class I molecules and β_2-microglobulin, and then travel through the Golgi complex to the cell surface. Extracellular as well as some intracellular antigen molecules can be presented to T cells by a second pathway, in which their peptides, which have been degraded by endosomes, fuse with vacuoles containing the MHC Class II molecules in addition to an invariant chain. The peptides can replace the invariant chain, and this complex is transported to the cell surface. Through these processes, fragments of protein antigens are presented to T cells in the context of host MHC molecules. Individual subsets of T cells specifically recognize distinct MHC classes owing to binding of these cells' coreceptor molecule (CD4 or CD8) to the particular MHC molecule (Class II or Class I, respectively). Thus, the $CD4^+$ T cells, generally defined as helper and inducer cells, see antigen presented by MHC Class II molecules, whereas the $CD8^+$ T cells, which are cytotoxic T cells, recognize antigen in the context of MHC Class I molecules.

The $CD4^+$ subset of T cells serves an important role as helper and effector cells in immune interactions, highlighted by the immunodeficiency associated with their depletion in patients with acquired immunodeficiency syndrome (AIDS). Although T cell–independent immune responses can occur under certain conditions, in general, $CD4^+$ T-cell help is required for adequate defense against antigenic attack. But an intermediary must bring an antigen to the attention of these T cells. It is macrophages, dendritic cells, and B cells that are capable of processing an antigen and presenting it to T cells. Additionally, macrophages and dendritic cells can process all available antigens, whereas B cells can internalize a specific antigen bound to the surface immunoglobulin, process it, and present it to T cells. The antigen presented by the MHC class II molecules to the given T-cell receptor thus provides the specificity to instigate $CD4^+$ T-cell help.

However, two signals are needed for the initial activation of T cells: the first is provided by the T cells' recognition of an antigen, and the second by the presence of antigen-nonspecific costimulatory molecules (Janeway, 1994). This latter system uses the CD28 molecule on naive T cells (those never exposed to an antigen), and CTLA-4 on cells that have previously encountered antigen, as well as B7 or B7.2 molecules on the antigen-presenting cell. A second system may also be used, consisting of the heat-stable antigen (HSA) on antigen-presenting cells and its yet uncharacterized ligand on T cells. Both $CD4^+$ and $CD8^+$ T cells can be costimulated by these systems.

B cells have similar mechanisms to allow activation (Janeway, 1994). A coreceptor exists, consisting of the CD19/CD21 complex, but is not as well characterized as the CD4 or CD8 T-cell coreceptors. Costimulatory molecules are also present to induce B-cell activation. In this case, the CD40 molecule on B cells must interact with its ligand (known as gp39, the tumor necrosis factor [TNF]–related activation protein, or simply the CD40 ligand) to allow $CD4^+$ T-cell help. As with many basic biological mechanisms, the function of this system is best illustrated in a disease state. X-linked immunodeficiency with an excess of IgM is a relatively rare form of primary immunodeficiency in which B cells fail to switch from IgM to IgG or another Ig class and fail to form memory B cells. T cells from individuals with this disorder were recently found to be defective in CD40 ligand expression, owing to defects in the CD40 ligand gene (Allen, 1993; Korthauer, 1993; DiSanto, 1993). The failure of this system resulted in faulty T-B cell cooperation and immunodeficiency, showing the necessity of T-cell help for B-cell function.

B-CELL AND T-CELL MEMORY

B cells play an important role in the primary immune response through the production of antibody. Re-exposure to a previously experienced antigen induces a secondary response of greater magnitude than the first one. This response is also of heightened specificity owing to affinity maturation, in which selection of high-affinity B-cell clones occurs. Somatic mutation of the immunoglobulin genes in B cells additionally can modulate the specificity of the antibody they make, with the higher affinity clones selected for expansion. Immunoglobulin class switching from IgM to IgG also occurs, owing primarily to T-cell help and production of cytokines such as interleukin 4 (IL-4) and interferon-γ (IFNγ) by distinct T-helper cell classes (Paul, 1994). Although the highly differentiated plasma cells produce and secrete antibody, these cells are relatively short lived. Memory B cells, which persist for long periods of time after initial exposure to an antigen, also go through processes of affinity maturation and class switching but appear to have a separate lineage from the cells mediating primary immune responses. Memory B cells are distinguishable by their low expression of HSA and higher expression of CD44, compared with naive cells (Sprent, 1994).

The majority of T cells also die following a primary immune response, but the remaining memory cells likely come from the same lineage as those effective in the primary response. Although somatic mutation does not cause affinity maturation in the T-cell receptor genes, high affinity clones of T cells may be selected to persist and become memory cells. Memory T cells are characterized by low expression of CD45R and CD62L (the leukocyte-endothelial cell adhe-

5

sion molecule LECAM-1) and high levels of CD44; the opposite pattern of expression is found on naive cells (Sprent 1994).

EFFECTOR MECHANISMS OF THE IMMUNE RESPONSE

Immune cells must recognize foreign invaders and destroy them, and do so in both antigen-specific and nonspecific manners (Roitt, 1994). Extracellular organisms, such as bacteria or parasites, can bind to and activate neutrophils and macrophages, which can then phagocytose the organism. The subsequent release of the neutrophils' granular contents (including myeloperixodase, lysozyme, defensins, and lactoferrin) and production of reactive oxygen and nitrogen intermediates lead to death of the invader. Eosinophils also contain specific protein granules, such as the major basic protein and cationic proteins, which are active against parasites. Furthermore, microorganisms can activate the alternative complement pathway, which may unleash phagocytosis, chemotaxis of immune cells, production and release of immune mediators from mast cells (including IL-3 through IL-6, chemotactic factors, histamines, leukotrienes, prostaglandins, and thromboxanes) and direct lysis of the organism. Extracellular organisms can also confront specific antibodies produced by B cells. Binding of such antibodies to the organisms' antigens activates the classic pathway of the complement cascade, ultimately neutralizing the organism or marking it for uptake by phagocytes.

Intracellular organisms, such as mycobacteria or viruses, are killed by a number of mechanisms. For example, infection of cells by viruses induces the production of IFN, making surrounding cells resistant to infection. NK cells can recognize a virally infected cell, then release their granule contents, including perforin, granzymes, and lymphotoxin (known as LTα or TNFβ), thereby killing the infected cell. Moreover, NK cells, which have receptors for the Fc region of antibody, use these receptors to participate in antigen-specific immunity. To do so, B-cell–produced specific antiviral antibodies mark viral antigen on the surfaces of infected cells, leading to antibody-dependent cell-mediated cytotoxicity by NK cells. Specific immunity is also achieved by T cells. Cytotoxic T lymphocytes, generally CD8$^+$ cells, have T-cell receptors that specifically recognize viral proteins produced in the infected cell in association with host MHC class I molecules. Recognition of the virus-MHC duo triggers killing of the infected cells, again, through the release of perforin, granzymes, and TNFβ. Additionally, IFNγ production protects surrounding cells from infection.

Intracellular microbes within antigen-presenting cells such as macrophages can also be killed through specific T-helper (CD4$^+$) cells. When infected cells present antigens from the organism on their surfaces in association with host MHC class II molecules, recognition of the antigen-MHC unit by a T-cell specific receptor incites the release of cytokines, including IFNγ, that activate macrophages and their antimicrobial function.

HYPERSENSITIVITY REACTIONS

Although it is intended to protect the host, the immune system can also cause tissue damage through mechanisms known as hypersensitivity reactions (Roitt, 1994). Immediate, or Type I, hypersensitivity occurs through the interaction of antigen (allergen) with mast cell IgE. The result can be dramatic anaphylaxis as well as atopic reactions through the release of molecules such as histamine and leukotrienes. Type II hypersensitivity consists of antibody-dependent reactions in which antibodies bind to cellular components, engendering destruction of the cell via complement or phagocytes, or altering cellular functions. Transfusion reactions, autoimmune hemolytic anemia, and Graves' disease are examples of pathologies induced by antibodies. Immune complex–mediated, or Type III, hypersensitivity arises owing to the local or systemic deposition of antigen-antibody complexes secondary to persistent production of both antigen and antibody. Serum sickness, systemic lupus erythematosus, and extrinsic allergic alveolitis exemplify diseases that can result when immune complexes induce complement fixation and stimulation of mast cells as well as neutrophils. Finally, Type IV hypersensitivity occurs through memory T-cell–mediated processes and is known as delayed-type hypersensitivity. Following antigen-specific stimulation, an excessive immune response may occur. Subsequent cytokine production and proliferation of additional lymphocytes and macrophages, and sometimes eosinophils and neutrophils, yields an inflammatory infiltrate with the potential to cause extensive tissue damage. Contact dermatitis, allograft rejection, and tuberculosis all arise from such cell-mediated responses.

PERSPECTIVES

The immune system is made up of a complex series of cells and their products, whose interactions serve to protect the host. Yet, deficiencies in or inappropriate activation of such components can harm the host. The mechanisms by which these derangements occur and the methods for testing components of the immune system to obtain diagnostic information are illuminated in the following chapters.

Allen R, Armitage R, Conley M, et al: CD40 ligand gene defects responsible for X-linked hyper-IgM syndrome. Science 1993; 259:990.

DiSanto J, Bonnefoy J, Gauchat J, et al: CD40 ligand mutations in x-linked immunodeficiency with hyper-IgM. Nature 1993; 361:541.

Germain R: MHC-dependent antigen processing and peptide presentation: Providing ligands for T lymphocyte activation. Cell 1994; 76:287.

Janeway C, Bottomly K: Signals and signs for lymphocyte responses. Cell 1994; 76:275.

Korthauer U, Graf D, Mages H, et al: Defective expression of T-cell CD40 ligand causes X-linked immunodeficiency with hyper-IgM. Nature 1993; 361:539.

Nossal G: Negative selection of lymphocytes. Cell 1994; 76:229.

Paul W, Seder R: Lymphocyte responses and cytokines. Cell 1994; 76:241.

Roitt IM: Essential Immunology. Oxford, Blackwell Scientific Publications, 1994.

Sprent J: T and B memory cells. Cell 1994; 76:315.

von Boehmer H: Positive selection of lymphocytes. Cell 1994; 76:219.

Weiss A, Littman D: Signal transduction by lymphocyte antigen receptors. Cell 1994; 76:263.

Weissman I: Developmental switches in the immune system. Cell 1994; 76:207.

Chapter 33

Immunoassays and Immunochemistry

Yasushi Kasahara, Ph.D., D.M.Sc.
Robert M. Nakamura, M.D.

IMMUNOASSAYS AND IMMUNOCHEMISTRY

General Characteristics of Antigen-Antibody Reaction

Biological ligands (commonly referred to as a key and corresponding keyhole), based on the affinity between molecules, such as enzyme and substrate, hormone and receptor, antigen and antibody, and others, play an important role in living organisms. Based on specific recognition characteristics, immunoassays (antigen-antibody reactions) have become widely used as analytical tools, despite the wide range of methodologies available in clinical laboratory testing. Relying on antigen-antibody specificity, immunoassays can be credited for the elimination of tedious pretreatment processes of specimens, such as blood containing thousands of molecules.

Immunoassays can be used for the detection of either antigens or antibodies. For antigen detection, the corresponding specific antibody should be prepared as one of the reagents. The reverse is true for antibody detection. The sensitivity of immunoassays has been enhanced through the development of new types of signal detection systems and solid-phase technology. Immunoassays have been optimized to detect less than 0.1 pg/mL of antigen present in blood. They can be applied to the detection of haptens as small molecules, proteins and protein complexes as macromolecules, as well as of any antibody to allergens, infectious agents, and autologous antigens.

Characteristics of Antigens

Antigens can be defined as any substance that can represent antigenic sites (epitopes) to produce corresponding antibodies, from small molecules such as haptens and hormones, to macromolecules such as proteins, glycoproteins, glycolipids, and other natural products. Artificial chemical compounds can also be antigens acting as haptens. Antigens should have at least one epitope. Epitopes that can be recognized by antibodies include amino acid sequences of peptides in proteins and high-dimensional protein structures such as neoantigenic sites.

Characteristics of Antibodies

Immunoglobulin, an important plasma protein, refers to antibodies in the context of the biological functions of immunoglobulin specific to antigens. Antibodies, therefore, are produced in response to antigenic stimulations. Antibodies are formed of both functional and heterogeneous molecules that bind antigens via the antigen-combining site. There are five classes (isotypes) of immunoglobulin: IgG, IgM, IgA, IgD, and IgE. IgG immunoglobulins are further divided into four subclasses, and both IgA and IgM have two subgroups. All known antibody molecules have a heavy chain with either a κ or a λ light chain. The molecular structure of antibodies is composed of variable regions and constant regions. The hypervariable domain (epitope-binding spot), located in a part of the variable region, can be assembled to interact with a wide variety of epitopes (antigen determinants). In laboratory medicine, two categories of antibodies can be distinguished: antibodies as reactants and antibodies as analytes. Antibodies as analytes are often classified by IgG, IgM, IgA subtypes. Antibodies as reactants are prepared from antiserum obtained through animal immunization with purified antigen.

Polyclonal Antibodies

A polyclonal antibody can be obtained through immunization with an antigen, which presents various epitopes. In other words, the antibody is specific against each epitope. The avidity of a polyclonal antibody to a complex antigen is usually stronger than a single monoclonal antibody. Carrier proteins may be needed for the immunization of rather small molecules, such as haptens or hormones, as a way to compensate for the weak antigenicity of the antigens.

Monoclonal Antibodies

Monoclonal antibodies (Koehler and Milstein, 1975) have been developed using the following current biotechnologies: somatic cell infusion, selection of the resulting hybridoma, and limiting dilution to obtain monoclonals. They are defined as uniform homogeneous antibodies directed to epitopes, not to whole antigen molecules. An established cell line allows for the secretion of all reactive immunoglobulin specific to single epitopes. Monoclonal antibodies have made it possible to analyze molecules on an epitope-to-epitope basis because of their narrow specificity, which differentiates a single amino-acid mutation on peptides. Yet monoclonal antibodies do not have the ability to recognize entire molecules that polyclonal antibodies have. For monoclonal antibodies, different antigens with a common epitope appear to be the same antigen. CA 19-9 antibody as a tumor marker can detect the size and shape of different molecules that have common carbohydrate epitopes. Monoclonal antibodies enable the identification of isoenzymes, subtypes, isotypes of protein, and conformational changes of molecules, and so on, because they can discern the slightest differences in molecules.

Monoclonal antibodies are cross-reactive with epitopes; this cross-reactivity can be explained by the probable existence of the same amino-acid sequence, carbohydrates, or lipids on different molecules. Monoclonal antibody technology has allowed for the development of extremely useful and nearly ideal immunoassay systems for clinical laboratory testing.

The production methods and applications of monoclonal antibodies have been extensively reviewed (Nakamura, 1983; Zola, 1987). The advantages of monoclonal antibodies are as follows:

1. Monoclonal antibodies provide a well-defined reagent.
2. Monoclonal antibody production can yield an unlimited quantity of homogeneous reagent with highly consistent affinity and specificity.
3. Monoclonal antibodies can be prepared through immunization with a nonpurified antigen.

Monoclonal antibodies have certain limitations in their use, as follows:

1. Insufficient reactivity in precipitation or agglutination because of weak network formation in the immunocomplex occurs when single monoclonal antibodies are applied.
2. Antigens with multiple heterogeneous epitopes are more difficult to characterize immunochemically.

Antibody Production by Recombinant Technology

A new technology called phage display has emerged for the production of antibodies (Winter, 1994). In this method, antibody fragments of predetermined binding specificity are constructed from a repertoire of antibody V genes, thereby eliminating the need for immunization and hybridoma technology. The V genes can be assembled *in vitro*. The phage selected from the repertoire by binding to antigen and antibody fragments is expressed in infected bacteria. Furthermore, the binding affinity of the antibodies is improved through the mutation. In the near future this technology will allow for the use of specific antibodies with high avidity.

Kinetics of Antigen-Antibody Reaction

Certain aspects of equilibrium or the law of mass action in chemistry can be applied to the antigen-antibody reaction. The kinetics of the reversible Ag-Ab reaction is as follows (Steward, 1986):

$$\mathrm{Ag+Ab} \underset{K^2}{\overset{K^1}{\rightleftarrows}} \mathrm{AgAb},$$

where Ag represents free antigen; Ab represents free antibody sites, AgAb represents the antigen-antibody complex concentration, K^1 and K^2 are the association and disassociation rate constants, respectively. The rate of formation of the antigen-antibody complex is represented as follows:

$$\frac{dt\,[AgAb]}{dt} = K^1\,[Ag]\,[Ab] - K^2\,[AgAb],$$

and at equilibrium the net rate is zero. Therefore,

$$\frac{K^1}{K^2} = \frac{[AgAb]}{[Ag]\,[Ab]} = K^a \text{ (association equilibrium constant or affinity).}$$

K^a is the parameter limited to site-to-site reactions, although antigens and antibodies often have multiple binding sites on the molecule. The apparent association constant for multiple antigen and antibody reactions may be referred to as *avidity* instead of affinity. The K^a value may be obtained from the following equations and experimental data:

$$Ab = Abt - (AgAb).$$

Ab is the antibody concentration at equilibrium, Abt represents the total original antibody concentration, F is free antigen or analyte, and B is bound antigen or analyte.

$$K^a = \frac{B}{(Abt - B)\,F},$$

or

$$\frac{B}{F} = K^a\,(Abt - B).$$

A Scatchard plot is produced when the amount of antigen bound (B) is plotted on the X axis and the B/F ratio of analytes is plotted on the Y axis. Two parameters that can be determined from the Scatchard plot are the association or affinity constant from the slope of the line and the concentration of antibody-binding sites from the X intercept (Scatchard, 1949).

OVERVIEW OF GENERAL PRINCIPLES OF IMMUNOASSAYS

Classes of Immunoassays

A brief classification and list of features of various immunoassays appears in Table 33–1. Precipitation immunoassays provide the most simple method by which antigens and antibodies react with each other without involving the detection of any labels. The resulting antigen-antibody complex in gel or liquid phase may be observed qualitatively as a precipitant by the naked eye and quantitatively with a detector.

The particle agglutination immunoassay (Kasahara, 1992b) uses inert particles as labels, as opposed to direct precipitation of the antigen-antibody complexes. Antigens or antibodies attached to particles such as erythrocytes, latex, or metal sol react with the analyte in the specimen. As a result of this immune reaction, the large particles show significant agglutination patterns that may be seen by the naked eye.

Yalow and Berson (1959) reported on the development of a radioimmunoassay (RIA) using radioisotopes as labels. This breakthrough allowed for the quantitative detection of a trace level of analytes and contributed to the advancement of basic research and clinical medicine. Insulin, for example, was quantified by RIA, which subsequently replaced the insulin bioassay. RIA may be formatted in a solid-phase procedure for easy separation of bound and free labels. Since the development of RIAs, the search for alternative labels to hazardous radioisotopes has intensified, with the aim of developing nonisotopic immunoassays using enzymes, fluorescent labels, and other reporter groups.

The enzyme immunoassay (EIA), using enzymes as labels, was developed in the early 1970s (Engvall, 1971; Van Weeman, 1971) and rapidly gained wide popularity. Enzymes can amplify signals depending upon the turnover of enzyme catalytic activity. Efforts to improve substrates and to increase sensitivity have led to the introduction of chromophore, fluorophore, and later chemiluminescent compounds. Depending on the substrate chosen, the assay method can be defined as a fluorescent enzyme immunoassay or a chemiluminescent enzyme immunoassay. Fluorescent immunoassays (FIA) use fluorophores as labels. Fluorophores require optimal wavelength light energy for their excitation to produce detectable emission light. FIA sensitivity is likely to decrease because of the background fluorescence present in biological specimens. Fluorophores that have a delayed fluorescence emission of 100 nanoseconds are suitable for application on time-resolved FIA. The introduction of various fluorophores resulted in improvements such as the elimination of background noise and the introduction of sophisticated instrumentation that can detect low concentrations (10^{-15} M) of analytes.

Table 33–1. CLASSIFICATION OF VARIOUS IMMUNOASSAYS AND THEIR CHARACTERISTICS

	Labels (Reporter Groups)	B/F Separation*	Signal Detection	Sensitivity
Precipitation immunoassays		Not required	Naked eye, turbidity, nephrometry	~10 μg/ml‡
Particle immunoassays	Blood cells, artificial particles (gelatin, particles, latex, etc.)	Not required	Naked eye, pattern analyzer, spectrophotometry, particle counting	~5 ng/ml§
Radioimmunoassays	Radioisotopes (^{125}I, ^{3}H)	Required	Photon counting	~5 pg/ml‖
Enzyme immunoassays	Enzymes	Required	Naked eye, spectrophotometry, photon counting	~0.1 mg/ml (CL-EIA)¶
Fluorescent immunoassays	Fluorophores	Required†	Photon counting	~5 pg/ml‖
Chemiluminescent immunoassays	Chemiluminescent compounds	Required†	Photon counting	~5 pg/ml‖

*Washing step for separation of bound labels in immunocomplex from free labels.
†Homogeneous assays included are not required for B/F separation.
Data sources: ‡Ritchie (1978); §Haux (1988); ‖ Sgoutas 1989); ¶ Isomura (1994).

Chemiluminescent immunoassays use chemiluminescent compounds as labels. Chemiluminescent compounds include chemically synthesized molecules as well as natural products such as aequorin. Unlike fluorophores, most chemiluminescent compounds require chemical rather than light energy to generate emission light. The reduction-oxidation reaction is a process common to all chemiluminescent assays. Signal amplification is not expected of chemiluminescent labels because chemiluminescent molecules generate just one photon through molecular decomposition. Recently a series of improved compounds for electrochemiluminescence have proved suitable for application on immunoassays. Metal chelate with tri-biphenyls emits light through a continuous reduction-oxidation reaction on the surface of electrodes.

In the various types of assays mentioned earlier, the main factors affecting assay sensitivity are the association constant (affinity or avidity) of the reactant, the signal intensity of the labels, and the signal-to-noise ratio of the detection signal caused by either background from the signals themselves or by a nonspecific reaction. When the material reactant and labels are fixed, the reduction of background noise becomes crucial to increase sensitivity.

^{125}I isotopes require about 7 million molecules to generate 1 photon/sec based on half-life calculations of radioisotopes (Bounaud, 1987). Chemiluminescent substrates to enzymes can increase events by an order of magnitude six times greater than that of ^{125}I. This is attributable to the catalytic amplification capacity of enzymes.

Conjugation Chemistry

Depending on the assay chosen, the method of conjugation that couples one molecule to others, enzymes (or cofactors) to antigens (or antibodies), or antigens (or antibodies) to solid phase also varies. The coupling reaction applied should be performed under conditions that avoid the reduction of any of the biological activities of the protein. In the glutaraldehyde method (Avrameas, 1978), glutaraldehyde, with two (or possibly more) aldehyde groups as a coupling reagent, has been used for conjugation of protein amino groups. This method is based on mixed reactions, including aldol condensation at high pH (the pKa of the NH_2 residue is 8.6 to 10.8). In this method shown in Figure 33–1, the resulting conjugate has different forms because of the existence of multiple active sites for coupling. The periodate oxidation method (Nakane, 1966) for the conjugation of antibodies uses horseradish peroxidase, which contains carbohydrates in its molecules. The methods mentioned earlier are not suitable for regulation of site-specific reactions, such as when configurational stereospecificity of conjugates is required.

As shown in Figure 33–2, new coupling methods (Kato, 1975; Kitagawa, 1978) have been developed using a sophisticated coupling reagent, m-maleimidobenzyl-N-hydroxysuccinimide ester (MBS). The MBS reagent has an activated ester and maleimide within one molecule, and will react with an NH_2 group and SH group, respectively. The carboxy group can also be used as specific site for conjugating with the NH_2 or proteins using N-hydroxysuccinimide (NHS) as the coupling reagent. The NHS coupling reagent extends to conjugate protein or the carboxyl group introduced on the solid phase.

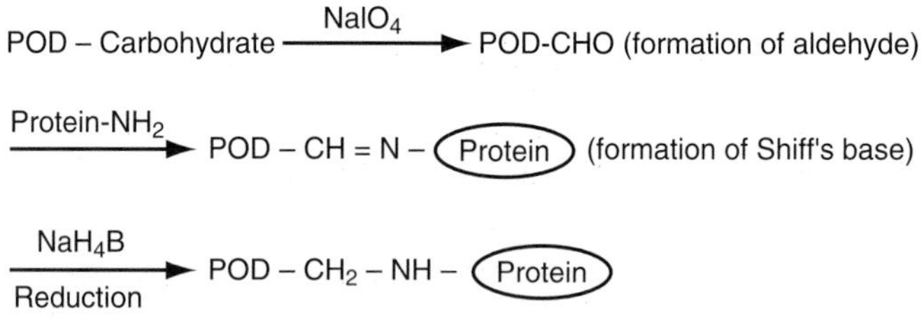

Figure 33–1. Coupling scheme for conjugation of protein with horseradish peroxidase (POD) based on Nakane method.

Characteristics of the Solid Phase

All heterogeneous immunoassays using conjugate with labels, including radioisotopes, require at least one separation step to distinguish the reacted immunocomplex (bound) from unreacted materials (free). Solid-phase immobilization of antigens or antibodies is obtained by covalent binding or physical adsorption through noncovalent interactions. Gel particles made of agarose, polyacrylamide, and plastic beads, such as polystyrene, have been used as the solid phase, as well as particles coated with iron oxide that can be separated by a magnetic field.

The inner wall of a tube, a microtiter well, and a plastic bead and disk are commonly used as solid phases. With these relatively large solid phases, shaking of the reaction mixture may be needed to shorten the time needed for the immune reaction to take place. The prozone phenomenon or hook effect caused by high concentrations of an analyte is likely to be observed when limited quantities of solid-phase antibody are present. Microtiter or strip-type plates may cause an "edge effect." This effect can be explained by the different kinetics of the immune reaction or enzyme activity with variations in temperature. A difference in temperature may be present between the wells located at the edge of the microtiter plate and the center of the plate. A difference of about 2°C may be observed with an infrared thermometer between the edge and center of wells at ambient temperature. The size and shape of the solid phase are critical factors affecting the capturing capacity of solid-phase antibody or antigen, and the kinetics of

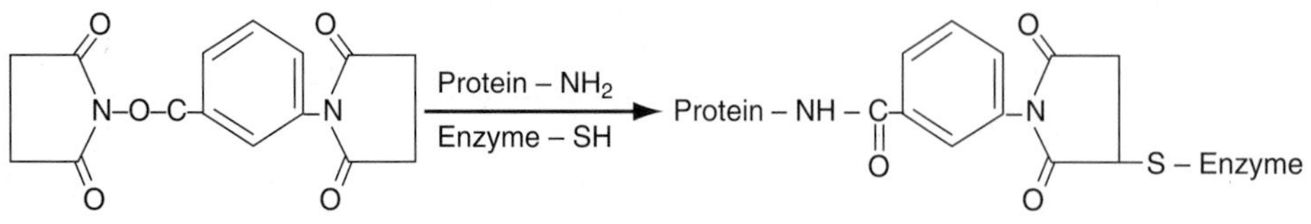

Figure 33–2. Preparation of enzyme-protein conjugate using heterobifunctional coupling reagent.

Table 33–2. PARTICLES USED AS LABELS FOR PARTICLE AGGLUTINATION/IMMUNOASSAY

	Supply	Supply
Human erythrocyte	Direct hemagglutination (Landsteiner)	ABO blood type
	Erythrocyte antibody hemagglutination: titer plate/slide	Human immunodeficiency virus (HIV) antibody
Avian erythrocyte	Direct hemagglutination	Human influenza virus
Fixed animal erythrocyte	Passive hemagglutination: titer plate	*T. pallidum* antibody
	Reverse passive hemagglutination: titer plate	Hepatitis B virus (HBV) surface antigen
Latex	Reverse passive agglutination: slide	Chorionic gonadotropin
	Reverse passive agglutination: turbidimetry	IgE
	Reverse passive agglutination	Ferritin
Latex (color)	Immunochromatography	Human chorionic gonadotropin (hCG)
Microcapsule	Passive agglutination: titer plate	*T. pallidum* antibody
Gelatin particle	Passive agglutination: titer plate	HIV, *T. pallidum* antibody
	Reverse passive agglutination: TV camera	Human hemoglobin (hHb)
Polypeptide particle	Passive and reverse agglutination	*T. pallidum* antibody, HBs
Silicate particle	Passive agglutination: titer plate/TV camera	*T. pallidum* antibody
Gold particle	Reverse agglutination enhancement photometry	Total estrogen
Metal sols	Reverse agglutination	hCG, hHb

From Kasahara (1992b). Reproduced with permission.

the immune reaction. Ferrite or latex particles 3000 Å in diameter provide a larger total surface area for immunoabsorbency than usually obtained with other solid phases. The larger total surface area helps shorten the immunologic reaction time.

The particles used for the particle agglutination assay are listed in Table 33–2. The phenomenon particle agglutination (direct agglutination) caused by an immune reaction was first observed in tests after incubation with infected patient serum. The agglutination of erythrocytes after incubation with serum led to the discovery of ABO blood types. Particle immunoassays are based on the agglutination principle and use the reactant of either an antibody or an antigen attached to the inert particle as a label, as opposed to direct precipitation of an antigen-antibody immune complex. As a label, the particle can significantly increase the immunoassay sensitivity regardless of whether the resulting agglutination is detected by the naked eye or with spectrophotometric instruments for quantification.

Erythrocytes, gelatin particles, liposomes, metal sols, and various kinds of latex particles, including latex modified with iron oxide or dyes, are all suitable solid phases. The diameter of these particles used for agglutition reactions varies from 7 to 0.01 μm. No single theory can explain the kinetics of agglutination (Kasahara, 1992b) because of the wide variety of particle sizes used as labels. For particles larger than 3 to 5 μm in diameter, Brownian motion of dispersed particles acting in accordance with the diffusion coefficient is not observed at room temperature. However, the theory of potential energy of interaction between particles, or the theory of colloidal coagulation reaction, can apply to small particles such as latex microparticles. The IgM antibody, being multivalent, is estimated to be 750 times more efficient than the bivalent IgG antibody in an agglutination reaction. The distance between particles in flocculation should be less than or equal to 120 Å because of the molecular length of the antibody. In summary, the important factors to consider in an immunoreaction are the surface properties of particles, such as the charge and hydrophobicity, and the stability of dispersion.

PRECIPITIN AND NEPHELOMETRIC IMMUNOASSAYS

Background and Principles of Precipitin Reaction

The precipitate that forms when large complexes of antigen and antibody combine to form an insoluble lattice has been widely used to identify and quantitate immunoprecipitin reactions. The modes of application of precipitin techniques have the advantages of sensitivity, specificity, and simplicity. The sensitivity limitation of these assays is a major consideration. Even under the best conditions of enhanced sensitivity afforded by the newer light-scattering techniques, the accuracy and sensitivity of immunoprecipitin assays remain below the range of 0.1 to 0.5 mg/dL. This range limits certain applications of immunoprecipitin assays, but precipitin techniques appear to be quite sufficient for the quantification of many major serum proteins. The precipitin reaction forms the basis for many quantitative and qualitative immunochemical techniques now used in the clinical laboratory (Kabat, 1961).

Factors affecting the precipitin reaction were extensively investigated by Heidelberg in 1935, who found that the relative proportions of reactants; conditions of temperature, pH, and ionic strength of the medium; and the antibody characteristics of avidity and affinity were all equally important in the formation of the immune precipitate. An illustration of the pattern of precipitin formation when there is sequential addition of increasing quantities of antigen to a fixed quantity of antiserum is shown in Figure 33–3. It can be noted that there is a point at which precipitation is maximum or optimal, designated as the *point of equivalence.* Continued addition of antigen once the point of equivalence has been reached produces a solubilizing effect on the precipitate. The dynamic range suitable for the determination of analytes should be up to the zone of equivalence. Optimization of the antibody concentration as a reactant is necessary, in addition

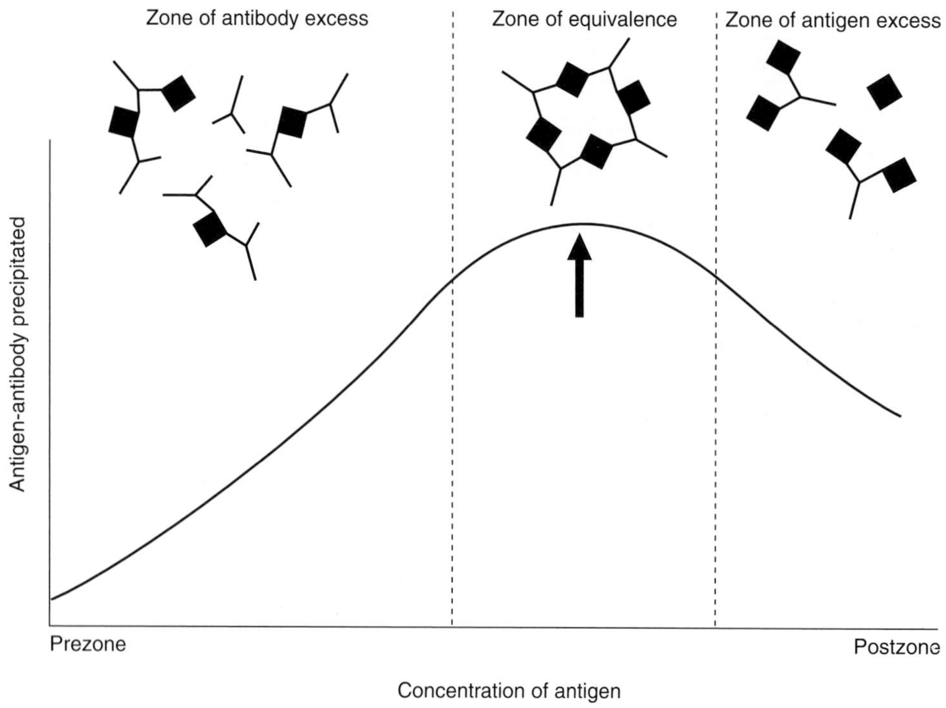

Figure 33–3. Quantitative precipitin curve. Immune complex as precipitin increases up to equivalence point which is optimal ratio of antigen to antibody.

to optimization of buffer solutions. Typical precipitant reaction methods are as follows:

Qualitative precipitant assay methods

Single immunodiffusion (Williams, 1970)
Double immunodiffusion (Garvey, 1977)
Double immunodiffusion in two dimensions (Williams, 1970)
Electroimmunodiffusion reaction (Ritzmann, 1975)
Immunoelectrophoresis (Rose, 1973)

Semiquantitative precipitant assay methods

Single radial immunodiffusion (Mancini, 1965, Lahey, 1965)
Single dimension electroimmunodiffusion (Axelsen, 1975) ("rocket" electrophoresis)

Nephelometric Immunoassays

A number of techniques for immunoprecipitin analysis have been developed that use light-scattering devices (Ritchie, 1978). The occurrence of immune complex formation has been related to the amount of such light scattering and has been used as a basis for antigen quantitation. Sophisticated instruments have been designed to rapidly measure light scattering. Measurements of scattered light are generally referred to as *turbidimetry* or *nephelometry*.

PARTICLE IMMUNOASSAY

Principle of Particle Agglutination

The agglutination reaction may be used to detect antibodies in specimens with specific antigens sensitized to a particle (passive or direct agglutination) (Fig. 33–4*B*). Reverse agglutination using a corresponding antibody sensitized to particles can be employed to detect soluble antigens in the specimen (Fig. 33–4*A*). A hapten unit single-binding site (for drugs, hormones, or small particles) does not form a cross-linking structure, and hence does not become agglutinated unless it is immobilized on the solid phase. As shown in Figure 33–5*A* and *B*, when a particle or carrier sensitized with a hapten is used as a reactant, an agglutination inhibition reaction must occur for the detection of the hapten to occur. This assay is based on a competitive-type principle in which agglutination of hapten particles with a limited amount of antibody, whether free or sensitized on particles, is inhibited by the hapten present in the specimen. Also, labeled particles can react with reactants fixed on the solid phase of the membrane. After immunologic reaction, particles within the immunocomplex begin to show color development on part of the membrane. This type of assay is gaining popularity as a simple device for the detection of human chorionic gonadotropin (hCG) and other analytes.

Hemagglutination

Hemagglutination tests (Boyden, 1951) are simple to perform and do not require special equipment. For this reason, advanced and developing countries have adopted a variety of hemagglutination tests. A popular worldwide hemagglutination test is used for the detection of antibody to *Treponema pallidum*, marketed as Serodia-TP, by Fujirebio, Inc. (Tokyo, Japan). In the United States, the hemagglutination test for *Treponema pallidum* was approved in 1981 by the Centers for Disease Control. It was also recommended by the World Health Organization because of its superiority over other tests in terms of specificity and sensitivity (Kasahara, 1992b).

In the *Treponema pallidum* agglutination test, the reagent consists of sensitized and unsensitized sheep red cells, and a serum diluent solution for the reconstitution of lyophilized sensitized cells as a positive control. Both qualitative and semiquantitative tests can be carried out using the following serum dilution protocol, using a titer plate as a reaction con-

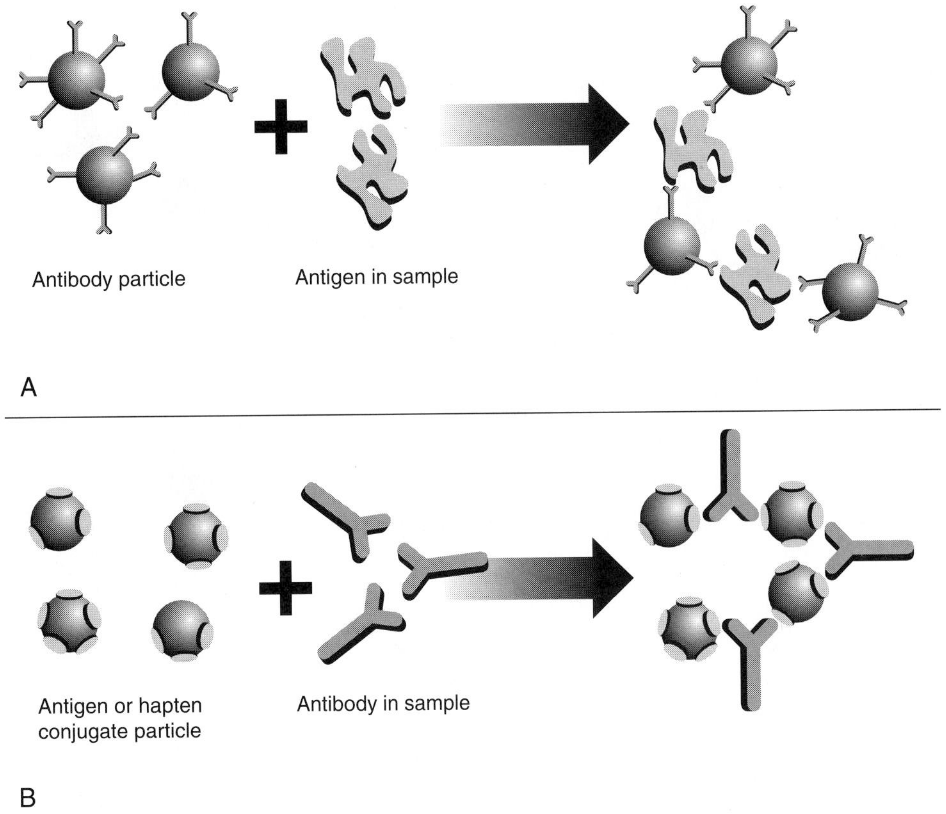

Figure 33–4. Principles of passive particle agglutination immunoassay for detection of antigen with multiple epitopes (A) or antibodies (B). (From Nakamura RM, Kasahara Y, Rechnitz GA (eds): Immunochemical Assays and Biosensor Technology for the 1990s. Washington, D.C.: American Society for Microbiology, ASM Press, 1992.)

tainer as follows: Using a 25 mL pipette dropper, place four drops of serum diluent in well 1 (Fig. 33–6) and one drop in wells 2 to 4 for the qualitative assay (wells 4 to 8 are for the semiquantitative assay). The resulting agglutination patterns are shown in Figure 33–7. Negative patterns, indicating that immunoreaction has not taken place, show condensed flocculation particles with a cross-packing structure at the bottom of the microtiter well. On the other hand, positive patterns, indicating that immunoreaction has occurred, show an expanded agglutination pattern of particles. Agglutinated particles cannot be sedimented any further to obtain condensation as negative patterns because their global shape is lost on account of the agglutination of particles. In the first and second rows, serum and unsensitized cells (negative control) were used, respectively. Specimens 1 and 2 show negative results. Specimens 3 to 8 show either negative or positive results, depending on the specimen dilution. Positive results are observed for both specimens 7 and 8, up to 1:2560 (rows 3 to 8).

Hemagglutination kits are now available for the detection of antibodies to hepatitis type B (HBV), hepatitis type C (HCV), human immunodeficiency virus (HIV) 1/2, thyroid, globulin, thyroid microsome, and other substances. Reverse hemagglutination tests are used for the detection of HBV surface antigen, α-fetoprotein, human hemoglobin using stools as specimens (occult blood test), and so on. The sensitivity of these tests is about 50 ng/mL for antigen (analyte) detection. Recently, Kemp (1988) developed a new hemagglutination assay that uses a mouse monoclonal antibody specific to the surface antigen of human erythrocytes. The antibody can recognize an epitope common to different types of red cells or to abnormal cells, such as those found in sickle cell anemia. As shown schematically in Figure 33–8, blood cells in the specimens are used as the solid-phase particles, and the resulting agglutination can be observed by the naked eye. Bivalent antibodies are conjugated chemically so that one antibody specifically reacts with the surface epitopes of the blood cell, and the other is specific to the target antigen or analyte. This assay can be applied for the detection of antibody to HIV as well as for the detection of various antigens. Unlike conventional agglutination formats, it does not require the separation of plasma or serum. This assay is simple and saves time and also has safety advantages, because it eliminates the need for serum separation for hazardous HIV- or HBV-positive specimens.

5

Gelatin Particle Agglutination

The development of a special gelatin particle with a highly hydrophilic surface able to prevent nonspecific binding of materials present in a specimen has provided an alternative to erythrocytes (Ikeda, 1984). The particle is made by phase separation and three-dimensional cross-linkage at 40°C at optimum pH. The resulting particle is fixed with formaldehyde or glutaraldehyde, and its diameter is about 3 μm. The physical properties of gelatin particles in comparison with those of erythrocytes are shown in Figure 33–9. A gelatin particle has no antigenicity and is therefore free from problems associated with heterophile antibodies when erythrocytes are used as particles. This type of artificial particle requires much less serum dilution to avoid nonspecific binding and guarantees more sensitive detection compared with blood cells. Other synthetic particles (Hirayama, 1991) made from block copolymer composed of L-glutamic acid and derivatives have been developed by Hirayama (1991) as alternatives to gel particles. These synthetic particles can be stained with any color of dye because the particles themselves are colorless, as are gelatin particles.

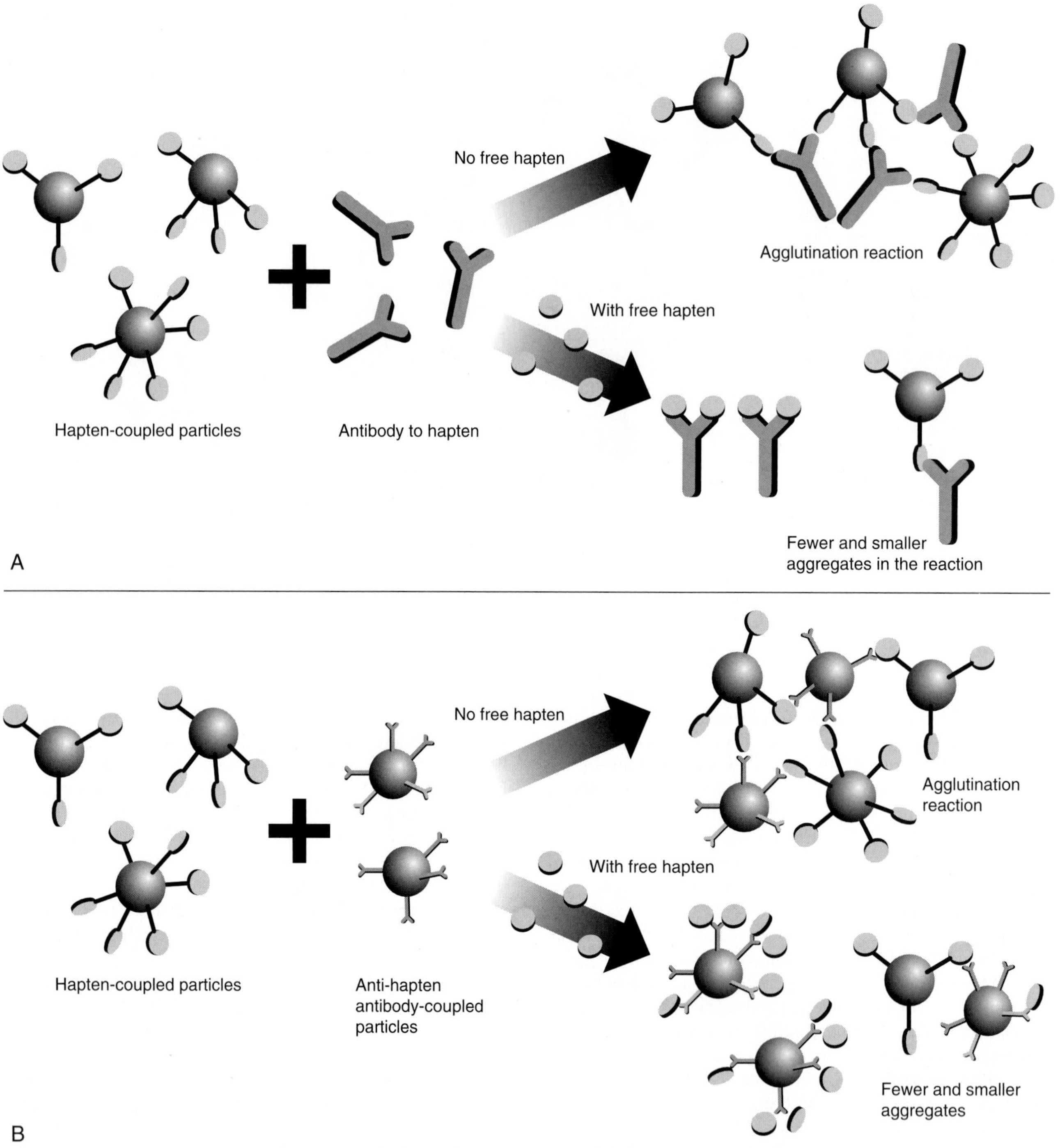

Figure 33–5. Principles of particle inhibition immunoassay for detection of antigen with single epitope (hapten), using antigen particles with free (A) or fixed (B) antibody. (From Nakamura RM, Kasahara Y, Rechnitz GA [eds]: Immunochemical Assays and Biosensor Technology for the 1990s. Washington, D.C.: American Society for Microbiology, ASM Press, 1992.)

The gelatin particle agglutination test was initially applied to the detection of antibodies to human T-cell lymphotropic virus (HTLV-1), which was first discovered as a retrovirus in humans. This agglutination test (Ikeda, 1984) soon became particularly popular for blood screening for HIV, HBV, and HCV because of its high sensitivity and specificity, its simplicity, and the fact that strict temperature control is not required to perform the tests. Gelatin particle agglutination can replace any assay based on hemagglutination, with the exception of assays using red cells as particles in specimens.

Latex Agglutination

Latex agglutination (Galvin, 1984), using latex as particles, has been used for the detection of various analytes, such as human chorionic gonadotropin for qualitative pregnancy tests, and for the quantitative detection of other plasma pro-

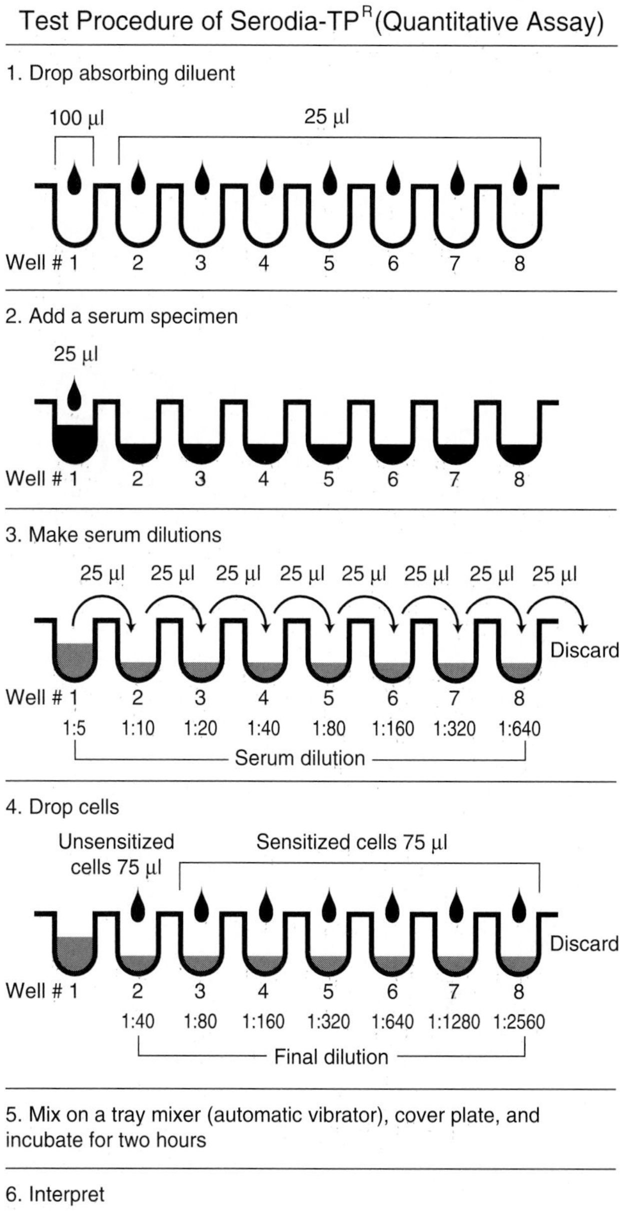

Figure 33–6. Hemagglutination assay for detection of *T. palladium* antigen (Serodia-TP, Fujirebio, Inc., Tokyo, Japan) based on semiquantitative test protocols. (From Nakamura RM, Kasahara Y, Rechnitz GA (eds): Immunochemical Assays and Biosensor Technology for the 1990's. Washington, D.C.: American Society for Microbiology, ASM Press, 1992.)

5

teins with or without instrumentation. The format of this qualitative assay is simple. For example, one might only have to mix a couple of drops of latex sensitized with reactant and specimen using a stick on a black slide. Two to three minutes later, phase inversion agglutination resulting from the immunoreaction can be observed by the naked eye. Latex agglutination was adapted for quantification assays using light detection methods based on either turbidimetry (light absorption) or nephelometry (light scattering). With these techniques, latex agglutination achieves an enhanced sensitivity of subnanograms per milliliter, while the sensitivity of the assay measuring intact precipitation of the antigen-antibody complex is less than 0.5 μg/mL.

Latex Turbidimetric Assay

Apparent light adsorption (light loss by scattering on the surface of a particle) is proportional to the diameter of the particle up to the limit of detection, which depends on the wavelength of light used. Most latex reagents commercially available use latex with a diameter of less than 1 μm and are applied in automated chemistry analyzers using photometric measuring principles. To further improve sensitivity, efforts were made to upgrade reagents and instrumentation, and to work with the optimum particle size, the most appropriate wavelength, and the most suitable computer software. There are now automated systems that use latex particles and can perform about 200 tests per hour at a subnanogram-per-milliliter sensitivity.

Particle-Counting Immunoassay

The particle-counting immunoassay (PACIA) (Masson, 1986) uses optical cell counting to assess the decrease in the number of unagglutinated particles after an immune reaction. In the PACIA format, either the rate assay, that is, the rate of

Agglutination Patterns of Serodia-TP*

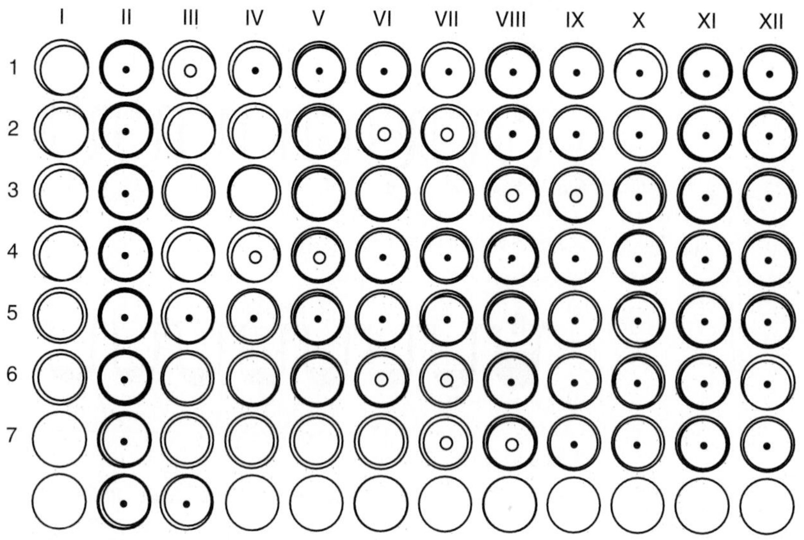

A

Interpretation

Row No.	II	III	IV	V	VI	VII	VIII	IX	X	XI	
Type of cells added	Unsensitized cells	Sensitized cells									Result
Final dilution of serum specimen	1:40	1:80	1:160	1:320	1:640	1:1280	1:2560	1:5120	1:10240	1:20480	Titer
Serum specimen											
No. 1	—	±	—	—	—	—	—	—	—	—	Inconclusive
No. 2	—	++	++	+	+	—	—	—	—	—	1:640
No. 3	—	++	++	++	++	++	+	—	—	—	1:2560
No. 4	—	+	+	—	—	—	—	—	—	—	1:160
No. 5	—	—	—	—	—	—	—	—	—	—	Negative
No. 6	—	++	++	++	+	—	—	—	—	—	1:640
No. 7	—	++	++	++	++	+	—	—	—	—	1:1280
Medium control	—	—									

B *Trade mark for agglutination test for *T. pallidum* antibody, Fujirebio, Inc., Tokyo, Japan

Figure 33–7. Hemagglutination patterns for detection of anti–*T. palladum* antibody (A) and interpretation as positive or negative at final serum dilution. (From Nakamura RM, Kasahara Y, Rechnitz GA (eds): Immunochemical Assays and Biosensor Technology for the 1990's. Washington, D.C.: American Society for Microbiology, ASM Press, 1992.)

decrease in the number of unagglutinated particles, or the end-point assay can be applied. The end-point assay guarantees a sensitivity at the nanogram-per-milliliter level, but incubation for a longer period of time is required for immunologic reactions.

Other Particle Immunoassays

Quasi-elastic scattering immunoassays were developed using a measurement of the change in response to particle size distribution. This technique uses a laser light beam to measure the reduction in the mean diffusion coefficient of particles as a result of immunoreaction. Other methods measure the change in angular anisotropy of scattered light with the increasing average size of the particle. Particles with diameters about equal to the size of a wavelength achieve a size-dependent angular variation of scattered light.

Summary

Indirect hemagglutination and gelatin particle agglutination tests using microtiter plates are the most popular procedures for qualitative and semiquantitative testing of various analytes. These tests do not require additional instrumentation or strict temperature control. Most importantly, these tests guarantee a sensitivity equal to or higher than conven-

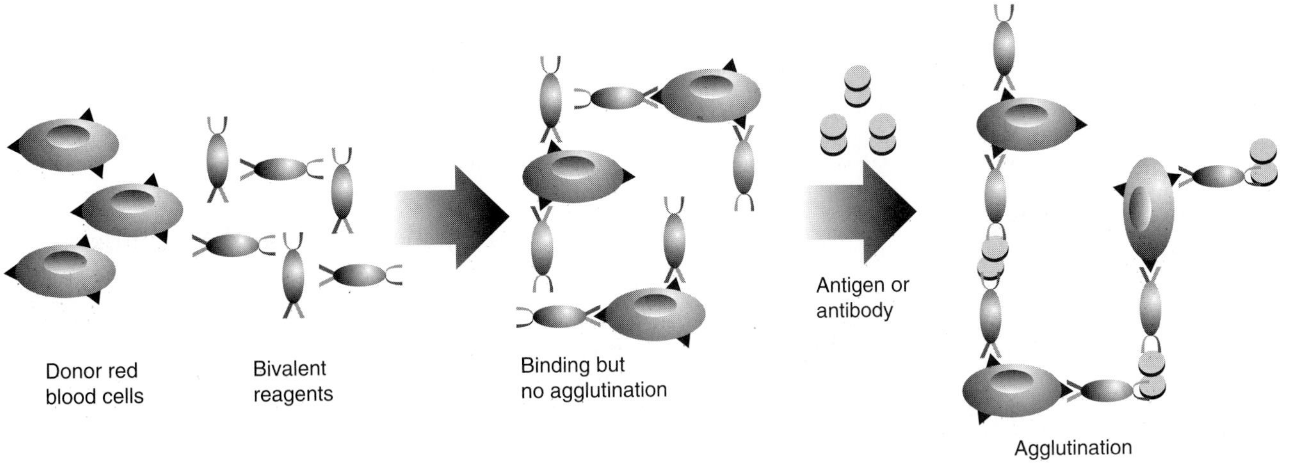

Figure 33–8. Schematic presentation of an assay based on autologous erythrocyte agglutination, using erythrocytes in the specimen as particles. (From Nakamura RM, Kasahara Y, Rechnitz GA (eds): Immunochemical Assays and Biosensor Technology for the 1990's. Washington, D.C.: American Society for Microbiology, ASM Press, 1992.)

tional enzyme immunoassays when applied to antibody detection of infectious agents. Latex as a solid phase provides great kinetic advantages, such as a shorter immunoreaction time as a result of its behavior in the colloidal dimension. For this reason, it was possible to adapt latex for use in existing or sophisticated instruments by applying different principles resulting in an assay sensitivity of about three orders of magnitude greater than immunoprecipitation. Latex is susceptible to interferences from unknown factors present in specimens. To eliminate this problem, various absorbents have to be used in both the reagent and the incubation medium. The great advantage of particle immunoassay is its simplicity, because it does not require separation of bound and free reactants. This should be emphasized when comparing it with other heterogeneous assay methods.

RADIOIMMUNOASSAY

Background

Since RIA technology, using radioisotopes as labels, was first developed by Yalow and Berson (1959), it has improved dramatically in sensitivity and precision. Numerous variations in the method have been introduced into the clinical

5

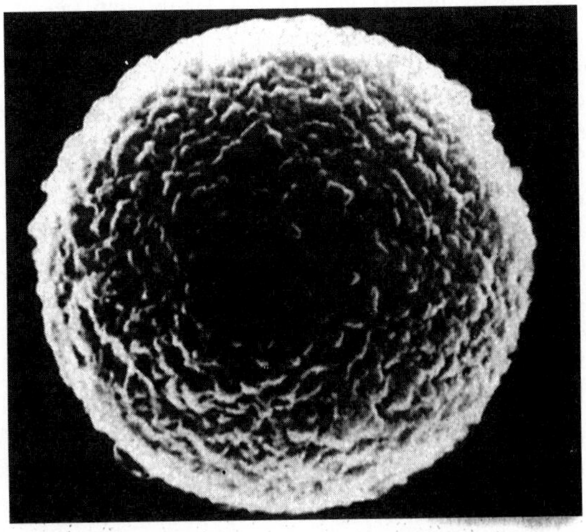

Figure 33–9. Electron micrograph (×25000) and physical properties of gelatin particles in comparison with sheep erythrocytes. (From Nakamura RM: Fluorescence immunoassays. *In* Nakamura RM, Kasahara Y, Rechnitz GA (eds): Immunochemical Assays and Biosensor Technology for the 1990s. Washington, D.C.: American Society for Microbiology, ASM Press, 1992, pp 149–167.)

physical properties	carrier	
	gelatin particles	sheep erythrocytes
diameter ; μm	2 ~ 6	6
specific gravity	1.05 ~ 1.10	1.10
electrophoretic mobility ; μm/sec/V/cm	-0.75 ~ -1.85	-1.15

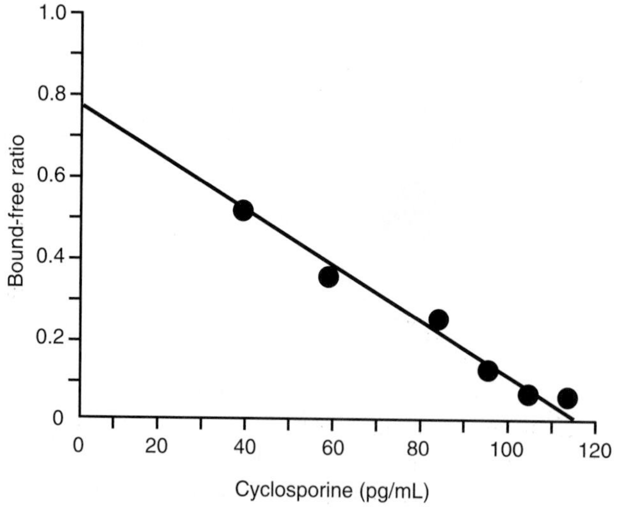

Figure 33–10. Scatchard plot of cyclosporine antibody binding characteristics (Ka = 8.1×10^9 L/M, Kd = 1.2×10^{-10} M/L).

laboratory. There are two main RIA techniques, competitive and noncompetitive heterogeneous formats, which require washing steps to separate bound and free labels (conjugates). The competitive assay follows the law of mass action, which specifies the reaction between analytes and binding proteins, receptors, and antibody. The key factor in assay optimization is the binding capability of the antibody. The Scatchard plot of the ratio of bound to free antibody to analyte concentration is commonly used to evaluate antibody performance. Figure 33–10 shows the Scatchard plot for cyclosporin determination. As described earlier, this plot gives the affinity (association constant K^a) for a particular antibody. Radioactive emissions, such as gamma rays of ^{125}I labels, can be measured in terms of counts per minute (CPM) using a gamma scintillation counter. Typical radioisotopes used as labels and their properties are shown in Table 33–3. The choice of label affects the assay protocol considerably. For example, the most popular label, ^{125}I, requires a rather short time for signal counting but has a limited shelf life because of its short half-life. On the other hand, ^{3}H label requires a longer time for counting thereby increasing the total assay time. Most RIAs now use ^{125}I as labels to expedite the conjugation process and to retain the biological activity of the reactants. A commonly used method for conjugation of ^{125}I with proteins is the chloramine-T method (Hunter, 1962). Tyrosine, in particular, has more reactivity with iodate because of its hydroxy group at the para-position on the aromatic ring. The signal can be measured in terms of CPM as gamma ray emissions. Unlike enzymes, isotopes as labels with a small Stoke's radius are not likely to disrupt antigenic activity because of steric hindrance when isotopes are conjugated with small antigens (haptens).

Table 33–3. PROPERTIES OF RADIOISOTOPES USED AS LABELS FOR RADIOIMMUNOASSAYS

Isotope	Half-Life	Type of Decay	Specific Activity (mCi/μmol)
^{125}I	60 days	γ	2200
^{131}I	8.1 days	$\beta-/\gamma$	16,100
^{3}H	12.3 years	$\beta-$	29
^{14}C	5760 years	$\beta-$	6062
^{32}P	14.3 days	$\beta-$	9120

Assay Principles and Methods

Various competitive methods (antigen excess) based on the competitive binding reaction (Ekins, 1960) to antibodies between labeled antigens and nonlabeled antigens (analytes present in the specimen) have been developed for a wide range of analytes. A widely used competitive method is shown in Figure 33–11. At first, a certain amount of labeled antigen and antigen in the specimen react competitively with a certain amount of antibody coated on a solid phase, such as sepharose beads or the inner wall of plastic tubes. After incubation for a period of time, the immune reaction reaches equilibrium, and then the mixture is washed to separate the immune complex fixed on the solid phase from unreacted conjugates and antigens. The washing step is referred to as B/F (bound over free) separation. Using the competitive principle, the plot of bound percentage against log concentration of analyte provides the standard curve shown in Figure 33–11. The CPM plot on the standard curve yields the concentration of analytes.

In the second antibody method shown in Figure 33–12, the antibody specific to a particular antigen (analyte) first competitively reacts with the conjugate and the antigen. Then the immune complex is captured by the second antibody, which is specific to the first antibody on the solid phase. When the second antibody is used on a fine solid phase, the resulting immune complex produced by the second reaction can be separated as a precipitant from the unreacted molecules. For antibody determination, the labeled antibody and the antibody in the specimen react with the antigen (analyte) on the solid phase, in a competitive manner. The steep portion of the slope of the standard curve provides more precise data, and the discrepancy between duplicate values gives a quick estimate of assay precision. Competitive methods require smaller amounts of antibody or antigen (analyte) as the reagent compared with the sandwich-type assays to be discussed.

Noncompetitive assays, initially proposed by Miles (1968), have gained popularity in recent years. The immunoradiometric assays (IRMA) or sandwich assays, shown in Figure 33–13, have a different analyte-antibody relationship. While the classic competitive assay is titered to achieve a response with a minimum amount of antibody, the sandwich assay uses an excessive amount of antibody. Monoclonal antibody technology has made it possible to manufacture large amounts of specific antibodies at moderate costs, thereby allowing the sandwich assay to be exploited.

The sandwich assay utilizes a stoichiometric excess of reagent antibody and is more sensitive than the competitive assay. When background noise is omitted, the ultimate sensitivity of the sandwich assay is one molecule of analyte, which is theoretically possible when the amount of antibody used in the assay system approaches infinity. As shown in Figure 33–13, the antibody on the solid phase first captures

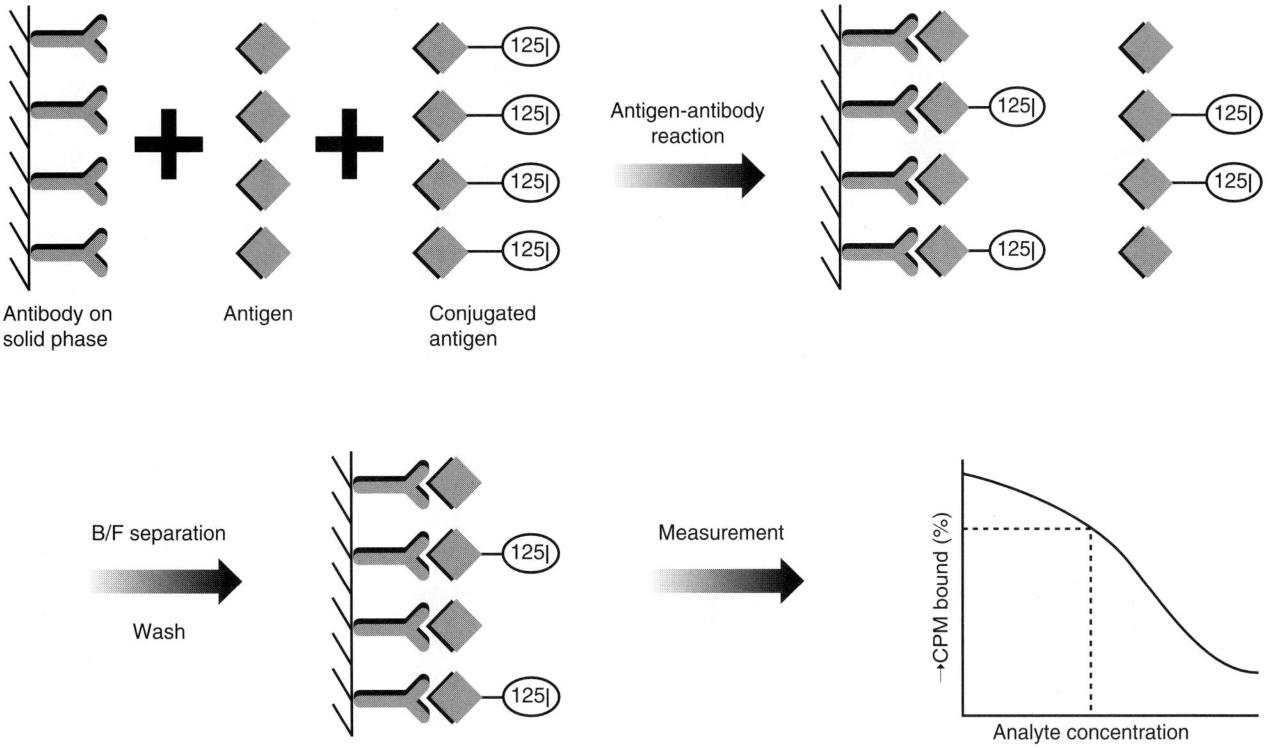

Figure 33–11. Assay principle of competitive RIA using first antibody as solid phase.

the antigen (analyte) in the specimen. Following B/F separation, the conjugate reacts with the antigen (analyte) fixed on the solid phase, and the signal can then be counted after the elimination of free conjugates through a washing step. This assay requires antigens with more than two antigenic sites. When different antibodies, that is a solid-phase antibody specific to one antigenic site and a conjugate antibody specific to another antigenic site, are used, the assay protocol can be simplified and a one-step sandwich assay can be performed. Thus the solid phase, the antigen in the specimen, and the conjugate can mix together simultaneously. Interference does not occur because the antibodies on both the solid phase and the conjugate are capable of recognizing different antigenic sites. In this assay the signal generated is proportional to the analyte concentration present in the specimen, as in the two-step sandwich assay. This assay method can be applied to antibody detection with assay formats using either antigen as the solid phase and labeled antigen, or antigen as the solid phase and labeled antibody specific to the target antibody. Using the sandwich format, assay sensitivity (Espinosa, 1987) is high. An example is IRMA for the determination of the peptide hormone TSH. The level of assay sensitivity is below 0.07 μU/mL of TSH with IRMA, as compared with about 0.7 μU/mL with conventional competitive antigen-labeled assay.

Summary

Compared with other immunoassays, RIAs are advantageous for a number of reasons: (1) precision and high sensitivity, (2) ease of isotope conjugation, (3) signal detection without optimization, and (4) stability against interference from the assay environment, among others. Disadvantages of RIAs are the short shelf life of the reagents and the need to protect against hazardous radioactivity. Furthermore, RIAs may not be applied to homogeneous immunoassays because signals from isotopes cannot modulate antigen-antibody reactions. A shift from RIAs to nonisotopic assays will eventually take place. Still, RIA assays may be preferred when new analytes are discovered and only small amounts of the purified reagent are available for assay development.

5

ENZYME IMMUNOASSAY

Background and Classification

Quantitative immunoassays using enzymes as labels were developed as an alternative to radioisotopes, (Engvall, 1971; Van Weeman, 1971; Avrameas, 1971). The most widely used are the enzyme-linked immunoabsorbent assay (ELISA), the enzyme immunoassay (EIA), and the enzyme-multiplied immunoassay technique (EMIT), which is a registered tradename of SYVA Co. (Rubenstein, 1972). Essentially, heterogeneous EIAs are quite similar to RIAs, except that they use enzymes as labels. Enzymes make it possible to develop homogeneous EIAs, eliminating the otherwise necessary washing steps for B/F separation. Table 33–4 compares the features of heterogeneous and homogeneous EIAs with RIAs. Improvements in EIAs have provided many innovative formats with different degrees of speed, sensitivity, simplicity, and precision. The advantages and disadvantages of EIAs are listed in Table 33–5 (Nakamura, 1992b).

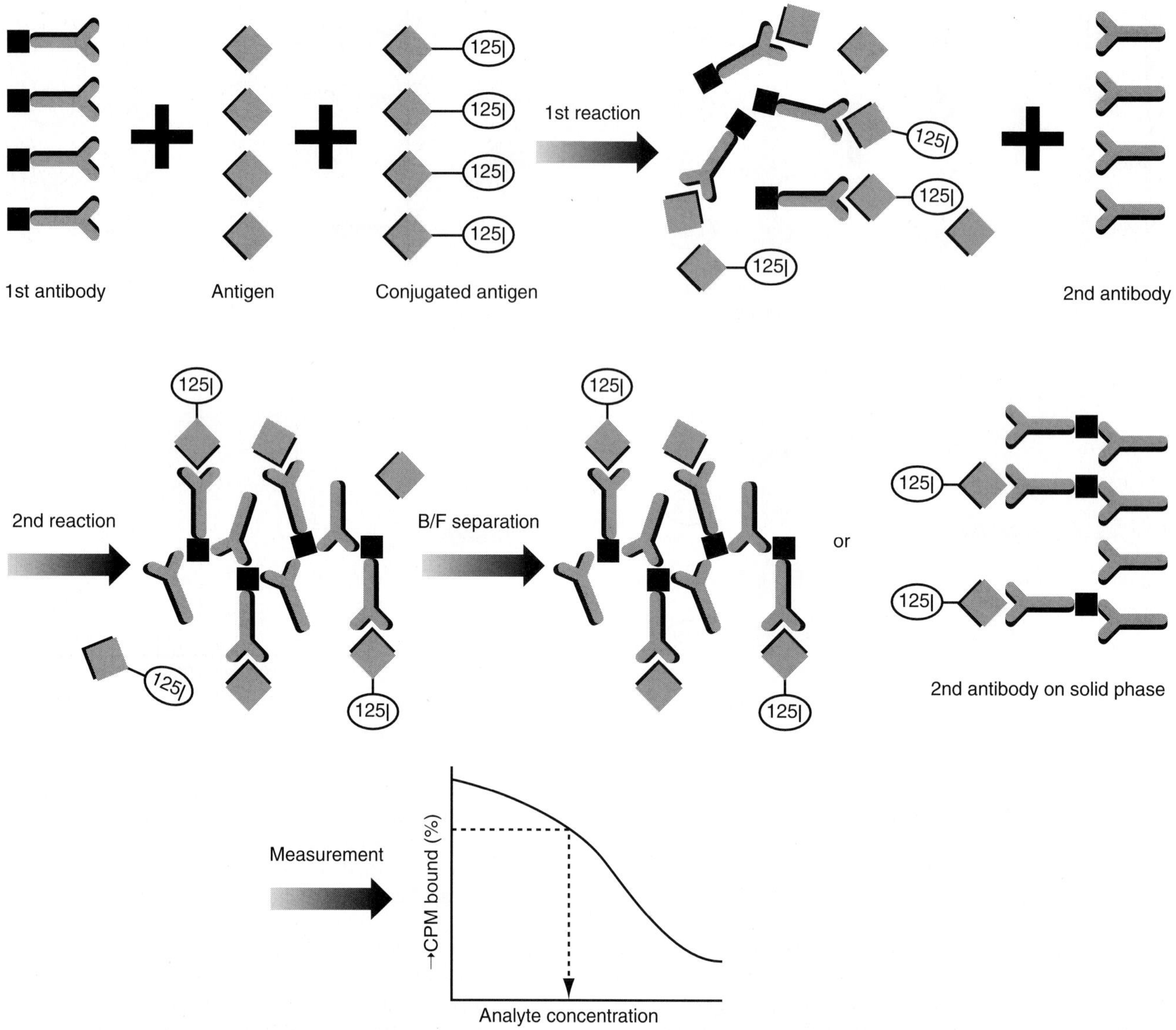

Figure 33–12. Assay principle of competitive RIA using second antibody for B/F (bound/free) separation.

Heterogeneous Enzyme Immunoassays

The assay principle of heterogeneous EIAs is similar to that of RIAs, except that enzyme activity, not radioactivity, is measured. EIAs require a secondary process to obtain signals through the catalytic reaction of enzymes and optimization of enzyme activity. The solid phase for the separation of bound and free conjugates can be microtiter plate wells, plastic beads, plastic tubes, magnetic particles, etc. The use of small magnetic particles allows shortening of the immunoreaction time, thereby reducing the total assay time. The development of substrates to be cleaved by enzymes was marked by the introduction of colorimetric and fluorometric substances, and later chemiluminescent substances, which increased sensitivity. The enzymes commonly used in various heterogeneous EIAs are horseradish peroxidase, alkaline phosphatase, β-galactosidase, glucose oxidase, urease, and catalase. Listed in Table 33–6 are horseradish peroxidase, β-galactosidase, and alkaline phosphatase, which are the most widely used enzymes. The characteristics of these enzymes are shown in Table 33–6.

The assay format of heterogeneous EIAs, like RIAs, can be divided into competitive and noncompetitive assays, as shown in Figure 33–14. Competitive assays (analyte excess) use antigen-enzyme conjugates (Fig. 33–14, 1a), while noncompetitive assays (reactant excess) include two-site immunometric sandwich assays and indirect assays to measure antibodies (Fig. 33–14, 2a, 2b). Immunometric sandwich assays have now gained much popularity for the determination of antigen hormones, tumor markers, plasma proteins, and infectious agents. Indirect assays for antibody measurement (Fig. 33–14, 2b) have been adopted for the detection of antibodies to infectious agents (HIV, HBV, HCV, etc.) and to autoantibodies.

Heterogeneous EIA consists of the following steps:

1. The solid phase attached by reactants is used for the separation of bound or free conjugates, regardless of

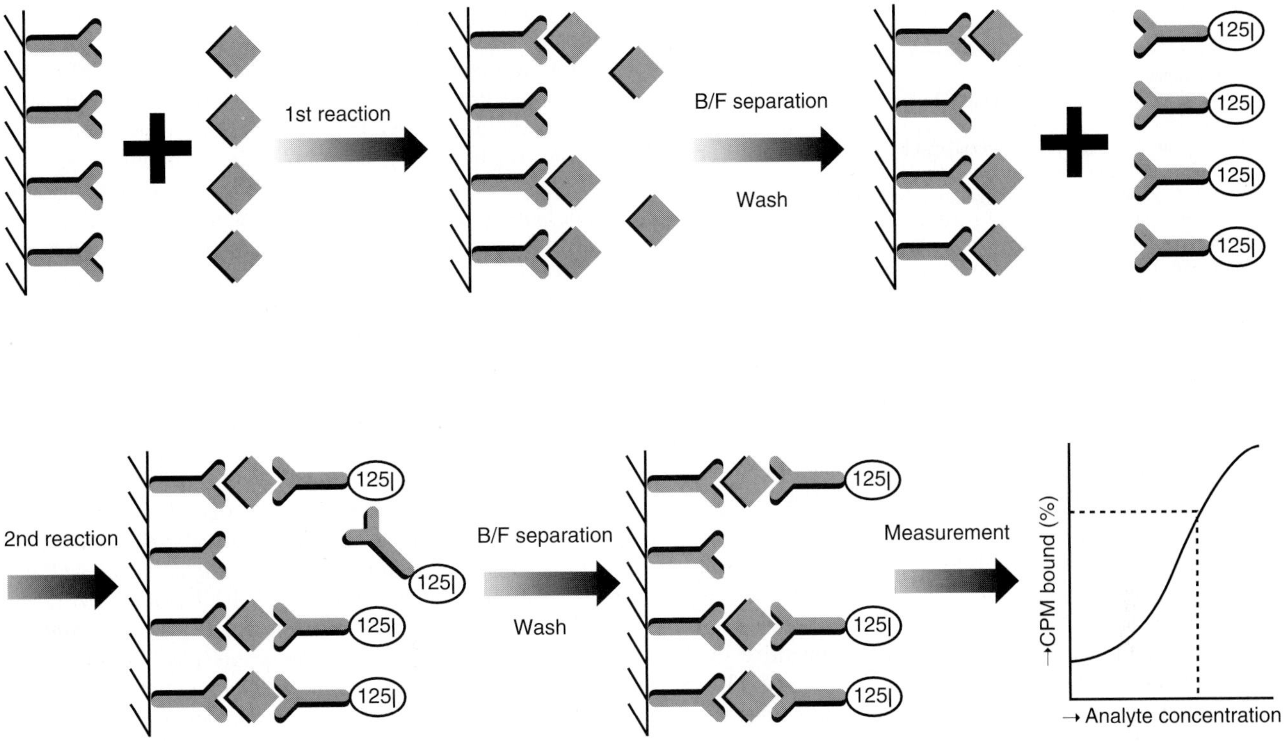

Figure 33–13. Assay principle of competitive RIA sandwich method using solid phase, also referred to as immunoradiometric assay (IRMA).

Table 33–4. COMPARISON OF RADIOIMMUNOASSAY, HETEROGENEOUS ENZYME IMMUNOASSAY, AND HOMOGENEOUS ENZYME IMMUNOASSAY

Assay	Immunological Reaction Steps	Enzyme Reaction Steps	Signal Detection Steps
Radioimmunoassay Sample + (labeled analyte or Ab) — ^{125}I	Immunologic reaction with washing steps for separation	—	Radioactive decay (γ ray)
Heterogeneous Enzyme Immunoassay Sample + (labeled analyte or Ab) — E	Immunologic reaction with washing steps for separation	Enzyme reaction with additional reagent	Optical density fluorescence luminescence
Homogeneous Enzyme Immunoassay Sample + (labeled analyte or Ab) — X	Immunologic and/or systemic reaction is carried out in one solution, which includes reagent for signal development of enzyme	Immunologic and/or systemic reaction is carried out in one solution, which includes reagent for signal development of enzyme	Optical density fluorescence luminescence

X, enzyme or cofactors.

Table 33–5. ADVANTAGES AND DISADVANTAGES OF ENZYME IMMUNOASSAY

A. Advantages

1. Sensitive assays can be developed by the amplification effect of enzymes.
2. Reagents are relatively cheap and can have a long shelf-life.
3. Multiple simultaneous assays can be developed.
4. A wide variety of assay configurations can be developed.
5. Equipment can be inexpensive and is widely available.
6. No radiation hazards occur during labeling or disposal of wastes.
7. Rapid simple EIA adaptable to automation can be developed.
8. Homogeneous EIA can be developed for haptens and proteins.

B. Disadvantages

1. Measurement of enzyme activity can be more complex than measurement of the activity of some types of radioisotopes.
2. Enzyme activity may be affected by plasma constituents.
3. Homogeneous assays at the present time have the sensitivity of 10^{-9} M and are not as sensitive as radioimmunoassays.
4. Homogeneous EIAs for large protein molecules have been developed but require complex immunochemical reagents.

EIA, enzyme immunoassay.
From Nakamura (1992b). Reproduced with permission.

whether the assay is based on the competitive or the noncompetitive format (see Figs. 33–11 and 33–13).

2. Following the addition of conjugate and incubation, there is a wash with a buffer solution containing a wetting agent, one or two steps after the immune reaction. The immune reaction should reach certain yields to obtain a stable and precise assay.
3. The solid phase, with the immune complex containing either enzyme-labeled antigen or antibody, is incubated at constant temperature with the enzyme-substrate solution.
4. The enzyme reaction is stopped (rate assay is not needed), and the substrate reaction product is measured with various detectors depending on the substrate used.

Colorimetric Enzyme Immunoassay

This assay uses substrates to develop a color by prime catalytic reaction with the enzyme reaction of ABTS [diammonium salt of 2,2′-azino-di (3-ethyl-benzothiazoline sulphonate-6)]. ABTS with H_2O_2 to peroxidase and the p-nitrophenylphosphate reaction with alkaline phosphatase are commonly used procedures. A spectrophotometer is used to measure the optical density of the resulting chromogen. There are many instruments, for the measurement of optical density in tubes or microtiter plates ranging from a fully automated system that performs sample pipetting and data printout to more simple manual devices. When the EIA reaction is performed on nitrocellulose (Western blotting) or other membranes, substrates that generate insoluble dyes are utilized. An hCG pregnancy test with an immunoassay format that is sold as an over-the-counter test commonly uses either benzidine derivatives to react with peroxidase or phosphate derivatives to react with alkaline phosphatase to generate insoluble dyes. The dye accumulating on the solid phase through enzyme reaction can be read by the naked eye. Theoretically, the measurement of optical density is limited from 0 to 2.0. Therefore, the determination of optical density for analytes that require the determination of a wide dynamic range can be problematic, even when an excess amount of conjugate and solid phase with sufficient capturing capacity are used with a sandwich-type assay.

Efforts to improve EIAs, the milestone of nonisotopic immunoassays, brought to light several disadvantages of RIAs, such as hazardous isotopic waste, radiolysis of labeled analytes, and the short half-life of ^{125}I. Ishikawa (1989) developed an ultrasensitive EIA that is able to detect 3 fmol of specific IgG antibody. To achieve this level of sensitivity, several tedious steps are required, such as immune complex transfer from a first solid phase to another solid phase to reduce background signals. Colorimetric EIAs are now the most popular immunochemical assays. However, more sensitive assays, such as chemiluminescent EIAs, may gradually replace the colorimetric EIAs.

Fluorescent Enzyme Immunoassay

Fluorescent EIAs are identical to other EIAs except that they use fluorescent substrates. In the fluorescent EIA, a fluorophore is generated by an enzyme reaction. Following excitation of the fluorophore at its optimal light excitation wavelength, wavelengths of light are emitted that produce maximum fluorescence. Instruments such as a fluorometer require both a supplier of the excitation light source and a photon multiplier as a detector of the emission fluorescence. There may be substances that emit fluorescent light present in the specimen. These substances may increase the background signal, which may interfere with the assay's sensitivity. Thus, close attention should be paid to the selection of substrates for EIAs to avoid interfering factors. Compared with colorimetric EIAs, fluorescent assays generate a signal intensity that is at least one order of magnitude greater.

Table 33–6. CHARACTERISTICS OF TYPICAL ENZYMES USED AS LABELS FOR ENZYME IMMUNOASSAY

Characteristics	Peroxidase (EC1.11.1.7)	Enzyme β-Galactosidase (EC3.2.1.23)	Alkaline Phosphatase (EC3.1.3.1)
Source	Horseradish	*E. coli*	Bovine intestine
Molecular weight (daltons)	ca. 40,000	ca. 530,000	ca. 100,000
Specific activity	250 U/mg	600 U/mg	2500 U/mg
Turnover rate*	10,000	318,000	250,000
Measurement of enzyme	Colorimetry, fluorometry, luminometry	Colorimetry, fluorometry	Colorimetry, fluorometry
Highly sensitive measurement	Luminometry	Fluorometry	Fluorometry
Method for enzyme labeling	Periodate oxidation (Nakane method)	Dimaleimide method, cross-linking reagent†	Glutaraldehyde method

*Number of substrate molecules produced by a molecule of enzyme for one-minute reaction; molecule number/min.
†The reagent contains chemically reactive groups, such as maleimide and succinimide.

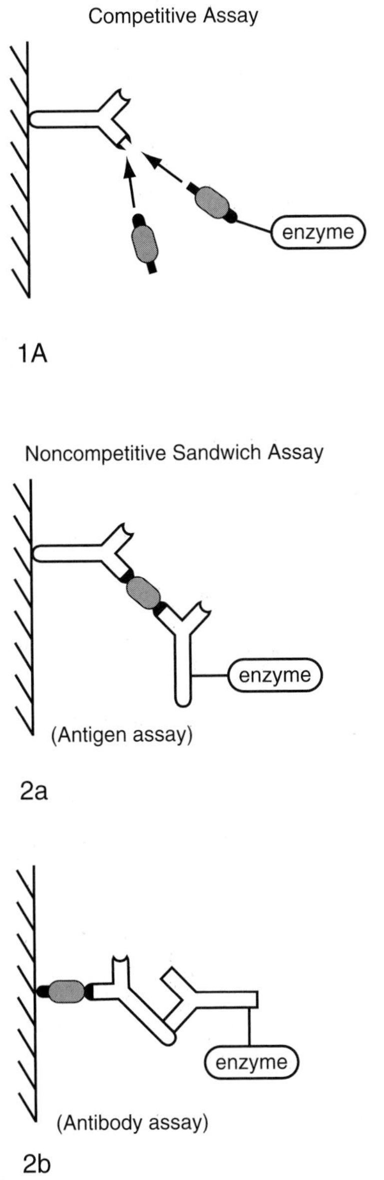

Figure 33–14. Assay principles of heterogeneous enzyme immunoassay (EIA) using solid phase; (1a) competitive assay and (2a and b) noncompetitive sandwich assay.

Chemiluminescent Enzyme Immunoassay

Chemiluminescent enzyme immunoassays (CL-EIA) use chemiluminescent substrates that react with various enzymes employed as labels. The chemiluminescent enzymatic reaction generates light, similar to bioluminescence, which involves the use of natural substrates such as luciferin. Over the past 20 years, much attention has been paid to the application of chemiluminescence in immunoassays, and a variety of systems consisting of substrates with enzymes have been developed. Current systems using either luminol derivatives to peroxidase with an enhancer or dioxetane derivatives to alkaline phosphatase achieve highly sensitive immunoassays. These assays are effective tools in practical diagnosis. The enzymatic oxidation reaction of luminol analogs has long been used for CL-EIA. Using peroxidase with H_2O_2 is a common method that is interchangeable with an alternative coupling enzyme producing H_2O_2, such as glucose oxidase or uricase. The discovery of enhancers (Kricka, 1991) for luminol-based chemiluminescence remarkably improved the assay's sensitivity. Enhancers include phenol derivatives and aromatic compounds. For example, luminol-peroxidase with p-iodophenol as an enhancer achieves a light emission increase of up to 2800-fold in the optimized reaction mixture. This assay is able to detect TSH at 0.04 μU/mL using serum as the specimen. However, oxidative reactions, such as for luminol, are likely to be interfered with by multiple factors that cause increased nonspecific background signals (noise).

Bronstein (1990) developed a chemiluminescent substrate for alkaline phosphatase that differs considerably from other compounds. This new substrate is known as AMPPD (admantyl 1,2-dioxetane phosphate), an admantyl dioxetane derivative. It requires no additional molecules for the emission of chemiluminescent light, unlike luminol, which needs oxidative compounds from outside the luminol molecules. AMPPD is a novel molecule that is a complete substrate because it is composed of the admantyl group as a stabilizer of the entire substrate, the dioxetane bond as an energy source and cleavage site of the enzyme, and a phenyl group for chemiluminescence, all assembled within one molecule. The structure of the molecule and the reaction process for light generation are shown in Figure 33–15. Phosphate cleavage by alkaline phosphatase triggers chemically initiated electron exchange luminescence (CIEEL) decomposition of AMPPD by releasing electron-rich dioxetane. A chemiluminescent with a maximum wavelength of 477 nm can be detected within a couple of minutes to a few hours, depending on substrate concentration. The alkaline phosphatase with AMPPD assay system has a sensitivity of 10^{-20} mol or less (Bronstein 1989, 1991).

CL-EIA uses AMPPD as a substrate to react with alkaline phosphatase, which is used as the enzyme label. CL-EIA can be performed on a fully automated instrument that can process 120 tests per hour with a random access mode containing 12 parameters. In the CL-EIA instrument, a reagent with 0.3-μm diameter ferrite particles is employed to shorten the immunoreaction time and to provide a larger surface area for the immunoabsorbent. For each test, the solid phase and conjugate are provided packed in plastic cartridges. The total assay time from sampling to data output is fixed at 30 minutes for all analytes, regardless of whether they have different assay formats, that is, the competitive or sandwich methods. The relationship between the chemiluminescent signal and the concentration of analytes is linear up to about seven orders of dynamic range. The sensitivity of CL-EIA (Nishizono, 1991) was 10-fold greater than standard RIAs when α-fetoprotein was assayed; α-fetoprotein was detected at a level of 30 pg/mL with an assay time of 30 minutes. Thus the new chemiluminescent EIA systems are a definite improvement over RIAs in terms of sensitivity, time efficiency, procedural simplicity and are gaining increasing popularity in the market.

5

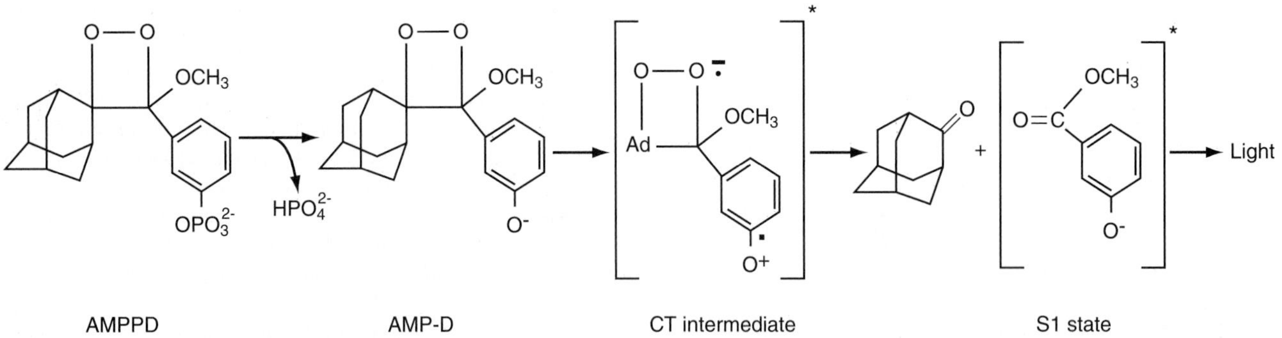

Figure 33–15. Admantyl 1,2-dioxetane phosphate (AMPPD); a chemiluminescent substrate for alkaline phosphatase (ALP) detection. Hydrolytic phosphate cleavage by ALP initiates chemically initiated electron exchange luminescence (CIEEL) decomposition of AMPPD by releasing the electron-rich dioxetane phenolate 2 (AMP-D). Charge transfer from the phenolate to the dioxetane ring takes place forming the charge transfer (CT) intermediate and subsequent breakdown of the cyclic peroxide. There is a release of energy with light emission.

Homogeneous Enzyme Immunoassays

Background

Two options are available to eliminate tedious assay procedures. One is to design fully automated instruments to access heterogeneous types of reagents, and the other is to develop innovative reagents that do not require complicated washing steps, such as those needed for heterogeneous EIAs. Enzymes and their cofactors are advantageous labels in homogeneous EIAs because enzyme activity can be modulated easily by changing factors in the microenvironment of the Ag-Ab reaction. This is not the case when using radioisotope decay as the signal. At present, homogeneous EIAs are generally less sensitive than their heterogeneous counterparts. Conventional heterogeneous EIAs have equal sensitivity as RIAs in many applications, whereas homogeneous EIAs (Nakamura, 1988) remain one or two orders of magnitude less sensitive than RIAs. Homogeneous EIAs may require complex immunochemical reagents, but the assay systems are rapid and simple, and are adaptable to conventional instruments. There are various types of homogeneous EIAs. In each of these assays the antigen-antibody interaction modulates the activity of the enzyme or enzyme label in the presence of the substrate. Modulation of the enzyme activity reflects the degree of the immunochemical reaction. Table 33–7 lists the characteristics of typical homogeneous EIAs. Homogeneous EIAs can be classified as competitive and noncompetitive binding assays. Competitive assays usually consist of enzyme-labeled antigens; however, the antigen (analyte) may be conjugated to the substrate or a prosthetic group of the enzyme in other assay formats. In contrast, noncompetitive binding assays use a conjugate of antibody labeled with enzyme. Among the various methods reported, five homogeneous EIAs deserve our attention.

Enzyme-Multiplied Immunoassay Technique

The enzyme-multiplied immunoassay technique (EMIT), the first homogeneous EIA, was developed by Rubinstein (1972). The EMIT system is diagrammed in Figure 33–16. In EMIT, the conjugation of enzymes to haptens does not disrupt enzyme activity; however, the binding of hapten-specific antibodies to haptens results in the inhibition of enzyme activity. Free haptens in the standard or sample relieve this inhibition by competing for antibodies. Thus, in the presence of antibodies enzyme activity is proportional to the concentration of free haptens. As a general rule, the antibody inhibits the enzyme by inducing or preventing confirmational changes necessary for enzyme activity (Rowley, 1975).

Table 33–7. CLASSIFICATION AND CHARACTERISTICS OF TYPICAL HOMOGENEOUS ENZYME IMMUNOASSAYS

Name and Assay Type	Conjugate	Manner of Modulation
Competitive		
EMIT	Antigen with lysozyme, G6PD*	Steric hindrance
SLFIA	Antigen with substrate	Steric hindrance
ARIS	Antigen with prosthetic group	Steric hindrance
Enzyme-channeling immunoassay	Antigen with G6PDH and hexokinase	Enhancement by proximity
Biotin-enzyme avidin immunoassay	Antigen with avidin	Steric hindrance
CEDIA	Antigen with fragments of β-galactosidase	Steric hindrance
Noncompetitive		
Hybrid antibody immunoassay	Hybrid antibodies specific to antigen and to inhibitor	Steric hindrance
Proximal linkage immunoassay	Antibody with G6PDH and hexokinase	
EIHIA	Antibody with amylase	Steric hindrance

*G6PD, glucose-6-phosphate dehydrogenase.
Bold indicates the enzyme name is spelled out and the enzyme is discussed in detail in the text.
From Kasahara (1992a). Reproduced with permission.

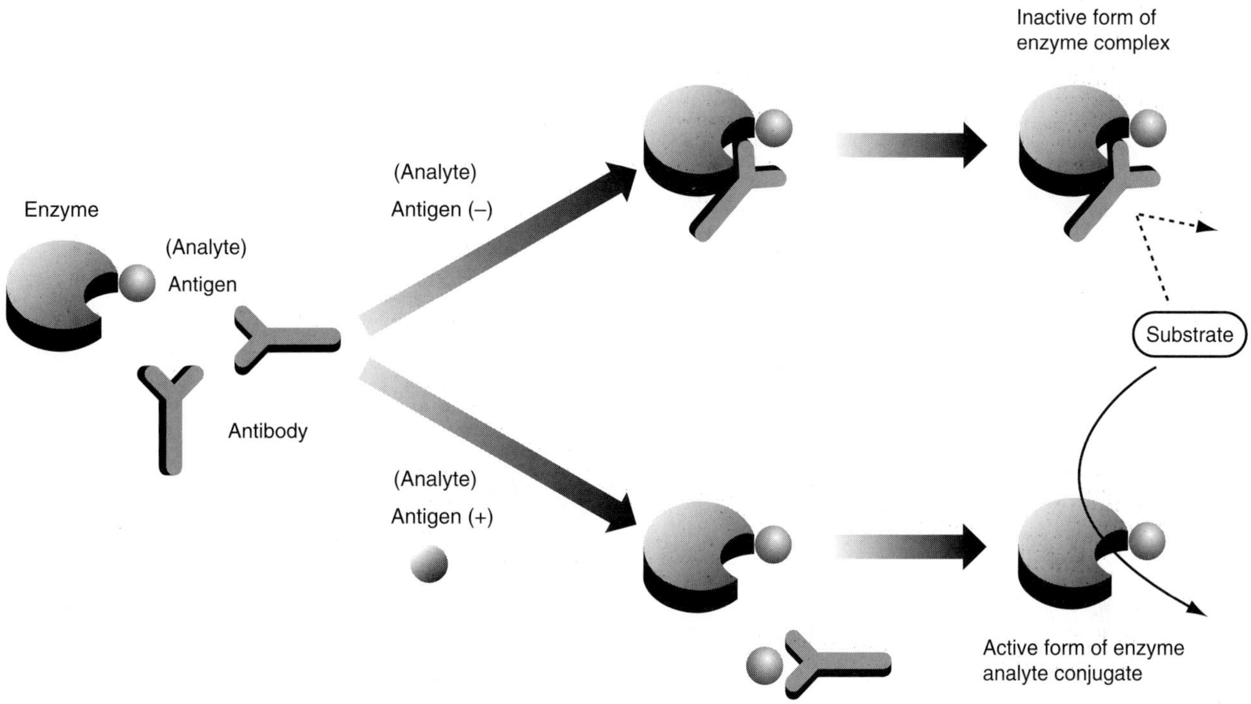

Figure 33–16. Enzyme-multiplied immunoassay technique (EMIT) system diagram: The activity of an enzyme as a label is inhibited by the binding of antibody to the antigen (analyte) conjugated with enzyme. The analyte is usually a hapten. Glucose-6-phosphate dehydrogenase (G6PD) and lysozome are usually used as enzymes. In the assay, enzyme activity is proportional to concentration of analyte. (From Nakamura RM, Kasahara Y, Rechnitz GA (eds): Immunochemical Assays and Biosensor Technology for the 1990's. Washington, D.C.: American Society for Microbiology, ASM Press, 1992.)

The exception to the inhibition mechanism is the EMIT thyroxine assay, which uses malate dehydrogenase. In this assay, the thyroxine-malate dehydrogenase conjugate is enzymatically inactive, but it becomes activated when it is bound by thyroxine antibody (Ullman, 1975). It is believed that conjugated thyroxine inhibits the enzyme by binding to the active site, thus increasing the "apparent" Km of the substrate. The antibody reactivates the enzyme by "pulling" the thyroxine out of the active site. In the EMIT assay system, malate dehydrogenase and glucose-6-phosphate dehydrogenase have been found to be most useful because they are less likely to be affected by serum constituents. These assays generally measure drug at a concentration of milligrams per liter. However, the digoxin assay has a much lower limit of sensitivity, in the range of 1 μg/L.

Substrate-Labeled Fluorescent Immunoassay

The substrate-labeled fluorescent immunoassay (SLFIA) (Burd, 1977) uses a characteristic fluorogenic substrate, umbelliferyl β-galactoside, attached to the antigen (analyte) as a conjugate. Umbelliferone is the fluorescent product produced when the substrate is cleaved with β-galactosidase. The enzyme β-galactosidase cannot cleave the substrate-antigen complex when it is reacted with the specific antibody. The free antigen (analyte) in the specimen solution competes with the antigen conjugated with the substrate to form the immunocomplex (Figure 33–17). Antigen concentration in the sample is proportional to the fluorescent intensity of the cleaved fluorescent product. SLFIA can be used to assay drugs and haptens, as well as protein ligands such as IgG and IgM. A disadvantage of this method is that the amplification properties of the enzyme are not utilized, and thus the assay system has limited sensitivity in the range of 10^{-9} to 10^{-10} molar concentration of the analyte.

Apoenzyme Reactivation Immunoassay

The apoenzyme reactivation immunoassay (ARIS) is a homogeneous assay developed by Morris (1981) using the prosthetic group consisting of flavin adenine dinucleotide (FAD)-conjugated antigen (analyte) and glucose oxidase apoenzyme. As shown in Figure 33–18, the antigen (analyte) and a constant amount of analyte-FAD conjugate compete for a limited amount of specific antibody. At equilibrium, the level of free conjugate is proportional to the amount of antigen (analyte) in the specimen. The apoenzyme combines with the free but not the antibody-bound form of conjugate to reactivate glucose oxidase activity in proportion to the amount of free conjugate in the mixture. The active enzyme is generated in the procedure, and an amplification mechanism is also built into this assay. ARIS has been used to assay for theophylline and IgG (Bogulaski, 1984). This FAD-labeled conjugate assay is readily adapted to the measurement of other haptens, drugs, and hormones as well as large molecular weight proteins (Burd, 1977).

Enzyme Inhibitory Homogeneous Immunoassay

The enzyme inhibitory homogeneous immunoassay (EIHIA), developed by Ashihara (1987, 1991), consists of anti-

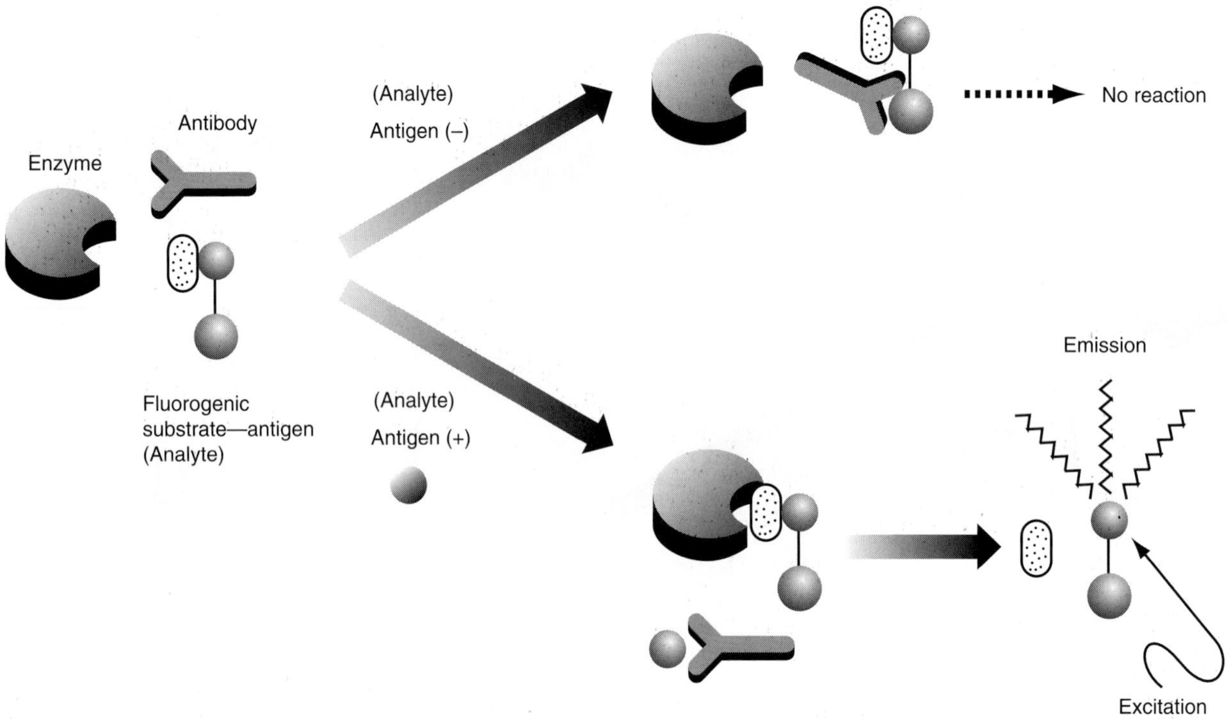

Figure 33–17. Substrate-labeled fluorescent immunoassay (SLFIA). The substrate β-galactosylumbelliferone is conjugated with the antigen (analyte) and forms a nonfluorescent substrate. The substrate can be cleaved by an enzyme β-galactosidase to form a fluorescent product. However, when the substrate-antigen conjugate is allowed to react with specific antibody to the antigen, there is no cleavage of the substrate complex with the β-galactosidase enzyme. In this assay, the concentration of the antigen (analyte) is directly proportional to the fluorescent intensity measured. (From Nakamura RM, Kasahara Y, Rechnitz GA (eds): Immunochemical Assays and Biosensor Technology for the 1990's. Washington, D.C.: American Society for Microbiology, ASM Press, 1992.)

body conjugated with enzyme and insoluble substrate. This assay is most suitable for the determination of large antigens (analytes). Because the immunocomplex of conjugate with large antigen increases the steric hindrance of the enzyme to substrates (Fig. 33–19), α-amylase has been used as an enzyme for the assay of ferritin. EIHIA based on a noncompetitive binding assay requires a significant time period for incubation to achieve a sensitive detection level. Using this method, the measuring range of ferritin in serum is 15 to 650 ng/mL. EIHIA has also been applied on a simple dry-film format. The dry film consists of three major layers, each containing a developing zone for immunologic and enzymatic reaction, a barrier zone, and a color-developing zone. An inhibitor specific to human amylase present in serum is used to prevent serum background. The assay is completed in only six minutes by simply placing the specimen on the slide using dry chemistry instrumentation (Fuji Film Co.). Nevertheless, the sensitivity of the system remains inadequate for application to analytes such as tumor markers.

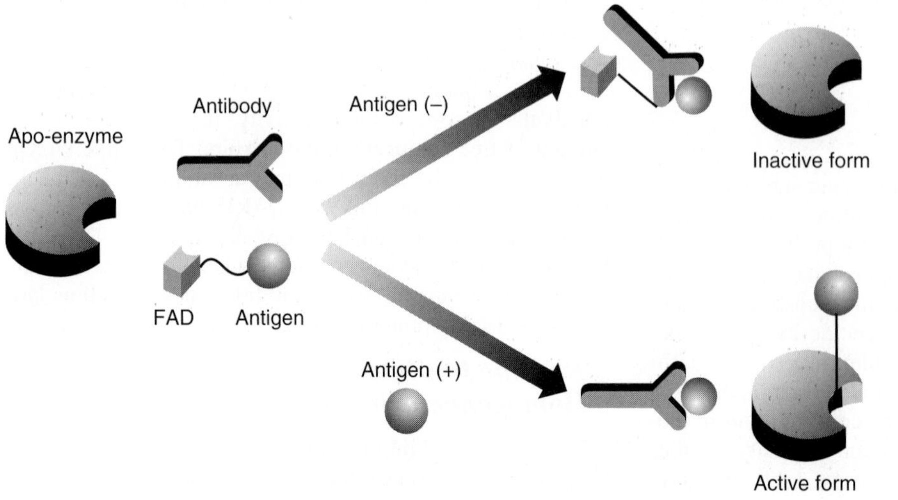

Figure 33–18. Apoenzyme reactivation immunoassay (ARIS). Flavin adenine dinucleotide (FAD) attached to the antigen is used. The apoenzyme is apoglucose oxidase which requires FAD cofactor for activity. In the assay, concentration of antigen (analyte) is proportional to enzyme activity generated. (From Nakamura RM, Kasahara Y, Rechnitz GA (eds): Immunochemical Assays and Biosensor Technology for the 1990's. Washington, D.C.: American Society for Microbiology, ASM Press, 1992.)

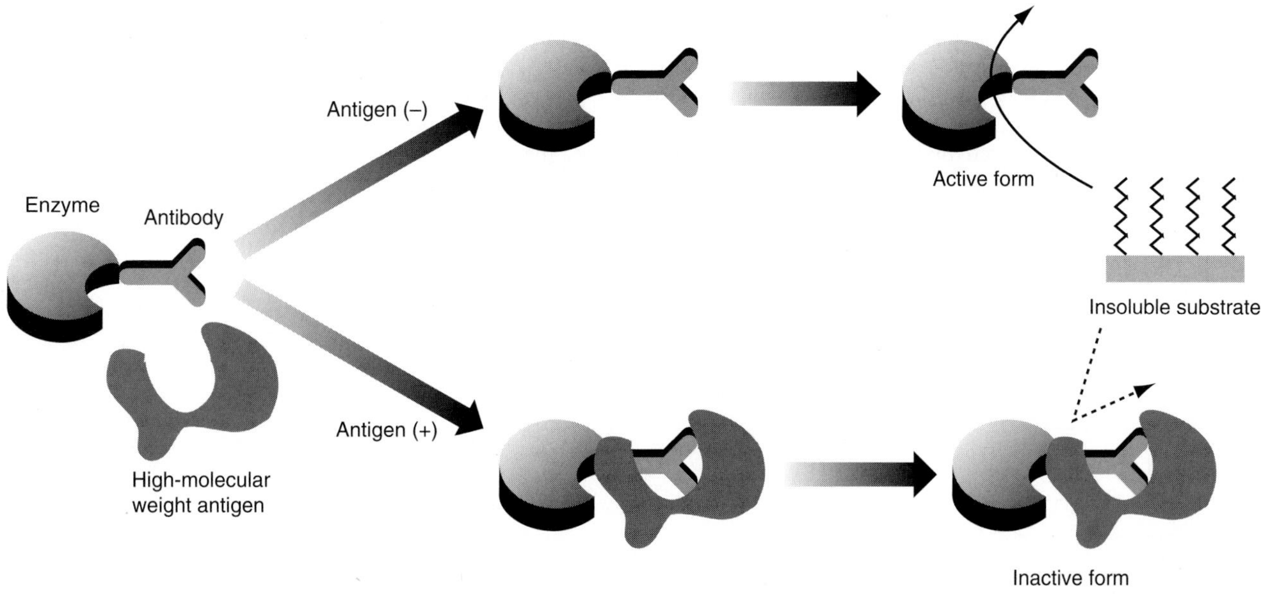

Figure 33–19. Enzyme inhibitory homogeneous immunoassay (EIHIA). The enzyme is α-amylase from *Bacillus subtilis* or dextranase from *Chaetomium gracile* and is conjugated to the specific antibody to the high molecular weight antigen. The high-molecular-weight antigen can be ferritin or α-fetoprotein. The α-amylase enzyme is inactive when the enzyme antibody conjugate is reacted with specific antibody. The active enzyme form can react with the starch insoluble substrate. The antigen concentration is directly proportional to the enzyme activity of assay reaction. (From Nakamura RM, Kasahara Y, Rechnitz GA (eds): Immunochemical Assays and Biosensor Technology for the 1990's. Washington, D.C.: American Society for Microbiology, ASM Press, 1992.)

Cloned Enzyme Donor Immunoassay

The cloned enzyme donor immunoassay (CEDIA) was first achieved through the application of recombinant DNA technology to homogeneous immunoassays by Henderson (1986). Microgenics Corp. (Concord, CA) was able to engineer β-galactosidase protein into a large polypeptide (an enzyme acceptor, EA) and a small polypeptide (an enzyme donor, ED). EAs and EDs reconstruct to form enzymatically active tetramers. In the assay (Fig. 33–20), a hapten antigen

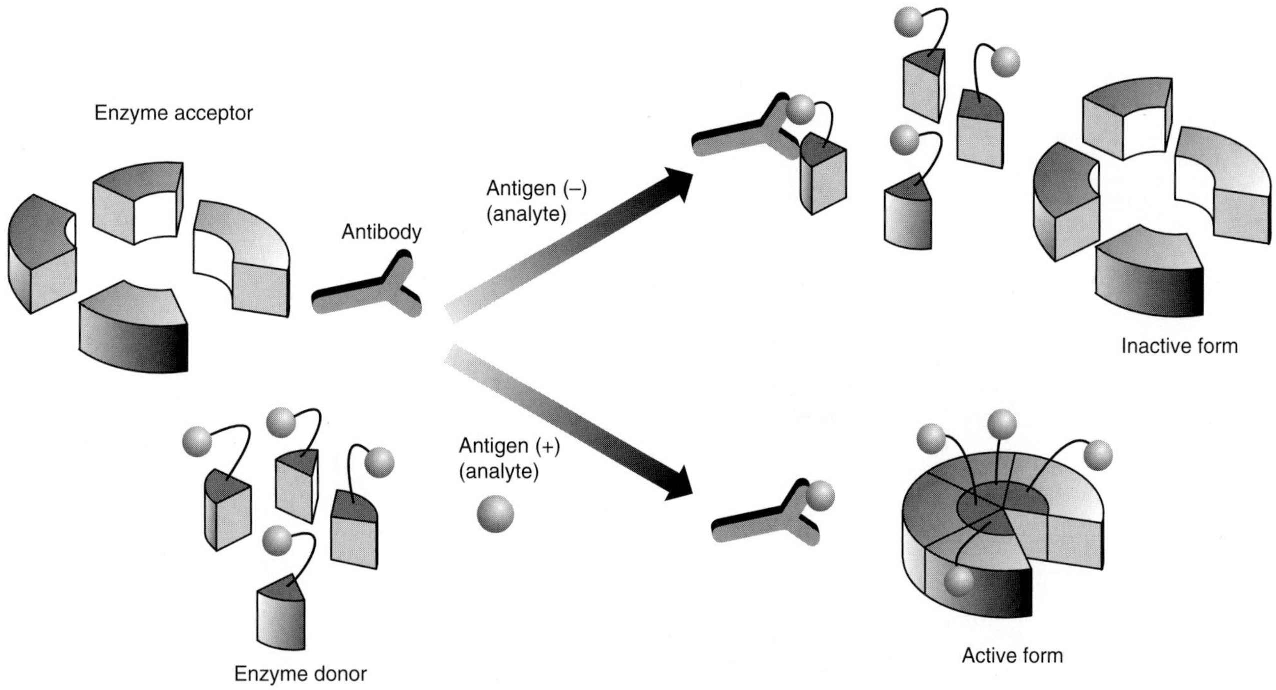

Figure 33–20. Cloned enzyme donor immunoassay (CEDIA). Enzyme acceptors associate with enzyme donors to form an active β-galactosidase tetramer. The antibody inhibits the association of enzyme acceptor with enzyme donor-antigen conjugate. (From Nakamura RM, Kasahara Y, Rechnitz GA (eds): Immunochemical Assays and Biosensor Technology for the 1990's. Washington, D.C.: American Society for Microbiology, ASM Press, 1992.)

(analyte) is attached to an ED, and an analyte-specific antibody is used to inhibit the spontaneous assembly of the active enzyme. The antigens (analytes) in patient serum compete with the analytes in the analyte-ED conjugate for antibody, modulating the amount of active β-galactosidase formed. The signal generated by enzyme substrates is directly proportional to the analyte concentration in the patient serum. The test for digoxin is a 5- to 15-minute colorimetric assay that requires no serum pretreatment or predilutions. The assay system is suitable for use with automated chemistry analyzers.

Instrumentation Enzyme Immunoassay

The demand for instrumentation that can perform large volumes of tests with random access capability has emphasized the need to improve reagents and to avoid tediousness in performing heterogeneous EIAs. Individual cartridges of prepacked reagent were thus designed for simple application on a fully automated assay system. A schematic presentation of this system is shown in Figure 33–21. Operating the system is relatively straightforward. The operator selects the

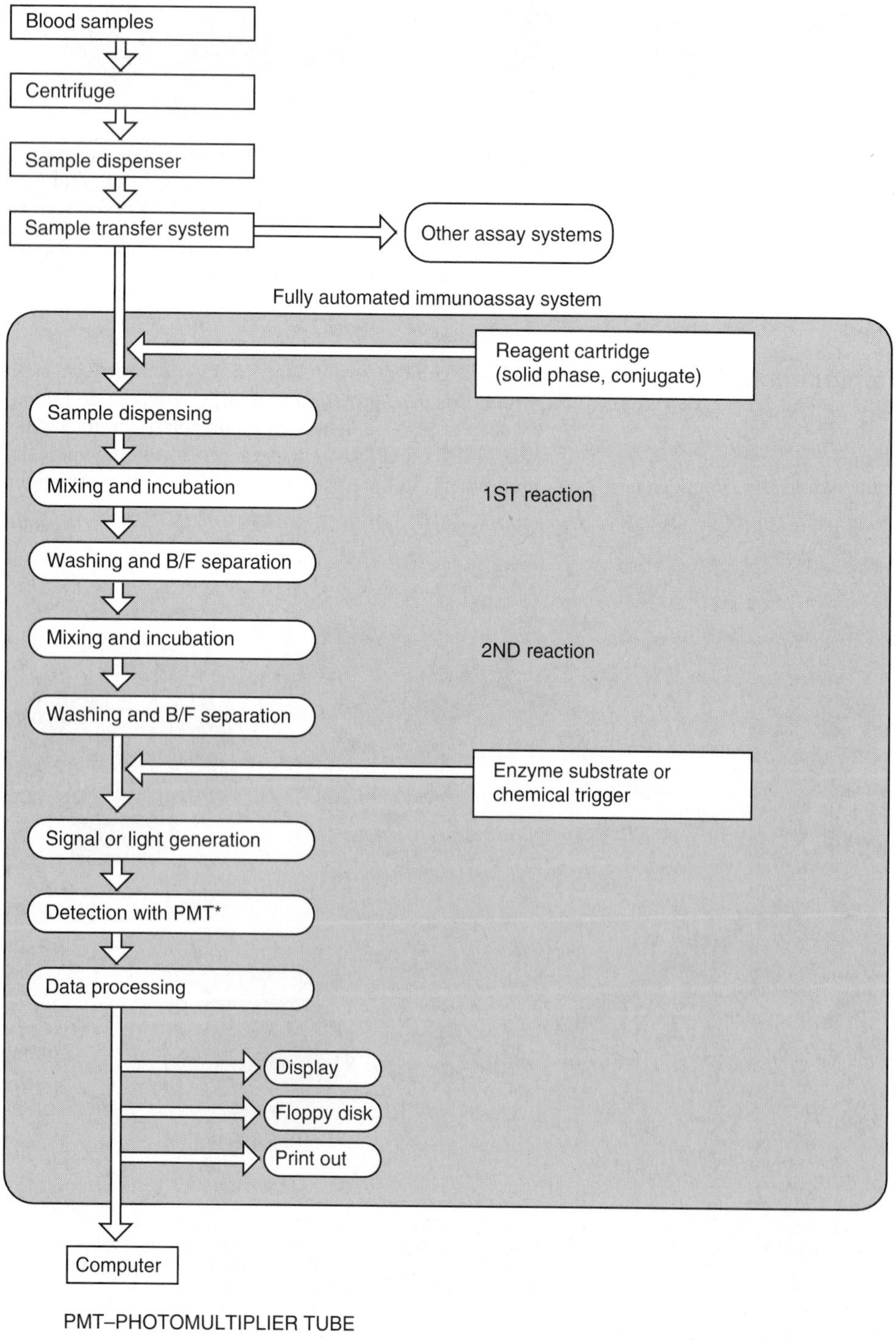

Figure 33–21. Brief diagram of fully automated immunoassay system in clinical laboratory automation.

desired test cartridges for each specimen. Test results are printed out within 30 minutes and sent automatically on-line to the mainframe. The instrument picks up the cartridge for a particular analyte and dispenses the sample from the sample tube; all subsequent steps of the assay are performed sequentially on the reaction line. Finally, the resulting signals are measured by detectors, depending on the signal generated. This system can perform about 100 to 150 tests/hr, with each sample specimen processing 10 to 20 analytes with the random-access procedure. The concentration of analytes can be calculated from the standard data curve automatically.

Summary

EIAs can be applied to all antigen-antibody systems, including those involving serum protein, hormones, drugs, and other antigens and the antibodies directed against pathogens. Heterogeneous EIAs using chromogenic substrates have a sensitivity comparable with that of RIAs, and they have gained wide acceptance for application in various immunoassays. Heterogeneous EIAs using sophisticated substrates that generate chemiluminescent light and small particles as the solid phase are sensitive enough to detect less than 1 pg/mL of analytes. Their sensitivity is thus much higher than that of RIAs. In addition, the assay procedure is greatly simplified by fully automated instruments. Compared with heterogeneous EIAs, homogeneous EIAs have certain limitations in sensitivity, dynamic range, and large analyte application. Also, high background signals and noise are inevitable because of the elimination of washing steps for the separation of bound and free conjugates. The homogeneous EIAs are advantageous because they are based on a simple assay format and can be adapted to existing automatic instrumentation. At this time, heterogeneous EIA with fully automated instruments remains the best choice in terms of sensitivity and simplicity, as well as for safety reasons, because they do not require the use of radioisotopes.

FLUORESCENT IMMUNOASSAY

Background and Classification

Coons (1941) first introduced the use of fluorescent compounds as immunochemical labels to detect antigens in tissue sections. Immunofluorescence assays on tissue sections are currently very well established in the clinical laboratory. Over the past several years, many fluorescent immunoassay (FIA) procedures have been developed to detect the concentration of drugs, hormones, and a wide variety of proteins and polypeptides (Nakamura, 1992a). In the initial stages of development, analytic fluorescent immunoasssays were hindered by a decrease in sensitivity because of background fluorescence of biological samples. Gradually, the sensitivity of fluorimetric methods improved, and the detection of analytes at concentrations of 10^{-15} M became possible. Further advancements were achieved through improvements in instrumentation and the introduction of unique substrates with various immunochemical and enzymatic reactions.

Selection of the fluorochrome label is important. The label should be stable and should demonstrate high absorptivity and quantum yield. It should also emit at appropriate wavelengths and should not interfere with ligand-antibody reactions. Most fluorophores or fluorescent compounds are organic compounds with a ring structure. When these molecules are irradiated with light at appropriate wavelengths, electrons within the molecules are excited and change to a higher energy state. As the excited electron returns to the ground state, energy is released in the form of a photon of lower energy (longer wavelength) than the exciting light. The fluorescence spectrum reveals a wavelength of maximal excitation and maximal emission, characteristic of a particular fluorescent compound. The time between excitation and emission is also characteristic of a specific fluorophore. The standard label, fluorescein isothiocyanate (FITC), has an absorption-emission time interval of less than 1 nanosecond, whereas other compounds exhibit delayed fluorescence with an interval of several hundred nanoseconds.

The various FIAs may be classified as follows: (1) heterogeneous and homogeneous, (2) ligand or antibody labeled, (3) competitive or noncompetitive, and (4) solid or nonsolid phase. The most common methods will be discussed.

Heterogeneous Fluorescent Immunoassay

Heterogeneous FIA procedures include a washing step to separate bound from free fluorescent labels. The assay procedure is similar to that of heterogeneous enzyme immunoassays and radioimmunoassays. Most of the commercially available assays use a solid-phase antigen or antibody system. The assay can be either competitive or noncompetitive, a property RIAs and EIAs also share.

Fluoroimmunometric Method

The analyte reacts with excess labeled antibodies in the solution. Residual labeled antibodies bind to excess solid-phase bound antigens. The solid-phase matrix is washed and the fluorescence intensity is inversely related to the analyte concentration. This method is adaptable for the assay of haptens and complex proteins. Solid-phase FIA procedures were developed for the serologic assay of antibodies to rubella, toxoplasmosis, viral antigens, and antinuclear antibodies. Heterogeneous FIA methods for antigen determination were developed for serum proteins and hormones, including immunoglobulins, cortisol, progesterone, and thyroxin. The major advantage of heterogeneous FIAs is the significant reduction in interference by naturally fluorescent substances in patient samples, because of physical removal of interference factors during the separation step.

Radial Partition Immunofluorometric Assay

In radial partition immunoassays, radial chromatography is used and the assay is carried out on glass-fiber filter papers (Giegel, 1982). The procedure has been automated for the assay of hCG and several other analytes in serum (Rogers, 1986).

Time-Resolved Fluoroimmunoassay

This methodology makes use of special instrumentation and special fluorescent labels to increase assay sensitivity. It involves the use of fluorescent labels exhibiting delayed fluorescence with a time period of 100 nanoseconds or more between excitation and emission. Because most substances responsible for background fluorescence have a short decay period, the measurement of the delayed fluorescence signal will significantly reduce the effects of background fluorescence. This is accomplished with the time-resolved fluorometer, a special instrument that produces a fast light pulse that excites the fluorophore. Fluorescence is measured a little while after excitation. Thus, the effect of nonspecific background, which generally decays in less than 10 nanoseconds, can be removed (Halonen, 1973; Soini, 1983). The fluorophores exhibiting delayed fluorescence that have been used in these assays include (Soini, 1979) the following:

1. Pyrene derivatives with a decay time of almost 100 nanoseconds.
2. Rare earth metal chelate labels that have a very long decay time of almost 50 to 100 microseconds. These include europium (Eu^{3+}), samarium (Sm^{3+}), and terbium (Tb^{3+}).

Time-resolved fluoroimmunoassays have been developed to measure many analytes, including hCG, IgG, cortisol, insulin, and others.

Homogeneous Fluorescent Immunoassay

By definition, these immunoassays are performed on homogeneous specimen samples: They do not require the separation of bound from free conjugates and are usually not sensitive to background interference in the samples. Homogeneous FIAs also have the advantage of being quick to perform. However, when compared with heterogeneous assays, they show certain disadvantages. Homogeneous FIAs have a limited sensitivity near 10^{-10} mol/L with standard instrumentation. Labeled impurities in the sample may increase background interference. The assays require relatively pure labeled antigen or specific antibody, as well as special instrumentation to achieve a higher sensitivity.

Fluorescence Polarization Assay

A polarizing lens or prism can resolve light into rays in a single plane. When viewed at right angles to exciting beams of vertically polarized or natural light, fluorescent solutions emit partially polarized fluorescence. The fluorescence polarization principle was first applied to immunoassay procedures by Dandliker (1970, 1973). The fluorescence polarization of small fluorescent-labeled molecules tumbling freely in the solution is very low. When the labeled molecule is complexed with antibody, molecular motion is slowed and fluorescence polarization is increased. These modulating changes in fluorescence polarization may be measured to distinguish between free and antibody-bound fluorescent-labeled antigens. Studies with labeled antibody or antibody fragments showed no change in polarization upon mixing antigen and labeled antibody, even though other evidence indicated that a reaction had occurred. This method is most useful for the measurement of small antigens and haptens, which produce the greatest change in polarized fluorescence with antibody binding of labeled antigen (Jolley, 1981). Abbott Laboratories (Lake Bluff, IL) has adapted this system for the assay of many therapeutic drugs (Abbott TDX).

Fluorescence Excitation Transfer Immunoassay

The fluorescence excitation transfer (FETI) method (Ullman, 1976) uses two labels, fluorescein as the donor fluorescent label and rhodamine as the acceptor or quencher. Fluorescein isothiocyanate has a maximum emission of 525 nm, and tetraethylrhodamine has a strong absorption peak at 525 nm. Therefore, when FITC-labeled antigen and rhodamine-labeled antibody bind, there is a *quenching* of FITC fluorescence. This phenomenon involves an energy transfer from an electronically excited fluorescent dye to an acceptor dye. The rate of energy transfer is inversely proportional to the sixth power of the distance between the donor and acceptor molecules. For adequate reduction of fluorescence with quenching, the donor-acceptor distance between the labels should be about 50 to 70 Å. This method is useful for the assay of antigen with multivalent antigenic determinants. Separate portions of specific antibody are labeled with fluorescein and rhodamine. The admixture of differently labeled fluorescein-tagged antibody and rhodamine-labeled antibody reduces the intensity of the fluorescein label by adjusting the ratio and amount of donor and acceptor so that they can react in close proximity to permit energy transfer.

Fluorescent Protection Immunoassay

In this assay (Nargessi, 1979), the protein antigen is labeled with fluorescein and then is reacted with specific antibody to the antigen. The antigen-specific antibody will sterically inhibit the reaction of a second antibody specific to fluorescein, which, in turn, will quench the fluorescence of fluorescein when it binds to the fluorophore. The specific antifluorescein antibody may increase in size, but its ability to interact with fluorescein coupled to the surface of the antigen within a small space will decrease. The procedure may be used to assay either for antibody concentration or for antigen (analyte) concentration in a homogeneous system.

CHEMILUMINESCENT IMMUNOASSAY

Background

Chemiluminescent immunoassays use chemiluminescence-generating molecules as labels, such as luminol derivatives, acridinium esters, or nitrophenyl oxalate derivatives and ruthenium tri-bipridyl [$Ru(bpy)^{+2}_{3}$] with trypropylamine (TPH) for electrochemiluminescence. Basically, the assay method does not differ from that of heterogeneous im-

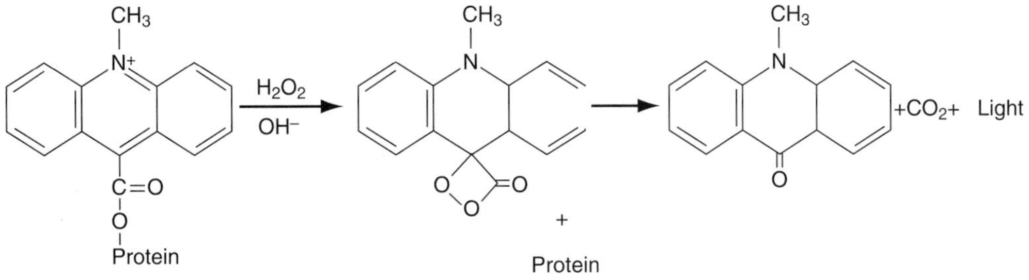

Acridinium ester

Figure 33–22. Chemiluminescent immunoassay mechanism with acridinium ester based on oxidative decomposition.

munoassays, RIAs, and FIAs. Light generation of luminol derivatives requires OH^- and H_2O_2 as a chemical trigger or H_2O_2 with peroxidase as enhanced chemiluminescent triggers. Acridinium esters chemically triggered with OH^-/H_2O_2 display a relatively high chemiluminescent quantum yield for light emission compared with luminol. Other chemiluminescent molecules, including, for example, aequorin, a natural compound, will be applied to this assay in the near future. Labels of chemiluminescent compounds produce light electrochemically on the surface of electrodes and can be applied to homogeneous assay formats. Both CLIAs using acridinium esters and electro CLIAs are applicable for practical testing in diagnostics. A description of their characteristics follows.

Chemiluminescent Immunoassay Using Acridinium Ester as Labels

In this method (Weeks, 1983), acridinium esters (Fig. 33–22) are directly conjugated with protein molecules. Acridinium esters can oxidatively react with H_2O_2 under low pH conditions to produce high-energy intermediates that decompose to the excited fragment, generating light. The rate of light emission of acridinium esters is extremely fast, within 5 to 10 seconds after the initiation of the oxidation reaction. Flash-type chemiluminescence, as this process is referred to, has a much steeper spectrum of light emission to reactive time than glow-type chemiluminescence triggered by enzymes. The sensitivity of this assay is higher than that of RIA, and testing is less time consuming. The solubility of acridinium esters and the stability of conjugates with proteins in storage periods have been improved through modification of the molecule and conjugation chemistry. This technology is likely to bring improvements in the assay of haptens, such as hormones.

Electrochemiluminescent Immunoassay (ECLIA)

ECLIA uses electrochemical compounds that generate light electrochemically linked with the reaction of the oxidative-reduction type of cycles as labels instead of conventional molecules. With the optimization of conditioning solutions, the selection of appropriate conjugation method, and the development of suitable compounds such as $RU(bpy)_3^{2+}$ [ruthenium (II) tri (bipyridyl)] and tripropylamine (TPA), it became possible to apply electrochemiluminescent technology to immunoassays (Blackburn, 1991). $RU(bpy)_3^{2+}$ has a reaction site for the conjugation of analytes using a heterobifunctional coupling reagent such as NHS. $RU(bpy)_3^{2+}$ conjugated with antibodies can apply to sandwich-type assays for large molecules of analyte. The conjugate generates light on the surface of gold electrodes. $RU(bpy)_3^{2+}$ on solid phase and TPA are oxidized on the surface of electrodes to form $RU(bpy)_3^{3+}$ and TPA+*, respectively. TPA+* spontaneously loses electrons. $RU(bpy)^{+3}_3$ can generate light of emission wavelength at 620 nm when it returns to $RU(bpy)_3^{2+}$ as a ground state through reduction with TPA*.

The efficiency of light generation (quantum yield) depends on the proximity between the electrode and conjugate, and thereby on the diffusion mobility of the conjugate. Free conjugates can generate more light than conjugates fixed on the solid phase as a result of immunoreaction. This allows easy access to the homogeneous assay format, but background noise interferes with assay sensitivity, as it does in other homogeneous assays. The assay protocol for the determination of proteins is the same as that of 46 heterogeneous assays, namely, magnetic microparticles coated with antibody as the solid phase and sample mix together for immunoreaction. After washing for bound and free conjugates by magnetic separation according to the assay format, the solid-phase suspension is introduced into the detector with the electrode to measure chemiluminescence. The detection limit of ECLIAs has been reported as 0.2 to 0.4 ng/mL for the determination of carcinoembryonic antigen and 0.4 ng/mL for α-fetoprotein. This assay does not require complicated instruments. A further advantage is that ECLIAs have a short signal time detection, like FIAs and other CLIAs.

Ashihara Y, Hishizono I, Miyagama E, Kasahara Y: Homogeneous enzyme immunoassay for macromolecular antigens using biotin enzyme. J Clin Lab Anal 1987; 1:80–82.

Ashihara et al: Immunoassay for determining low and high molecular antigens with a dry multilayer film. Clin Chem 1991; 37:1525–1526.

Avrameas S, Guilbert B: Dosage enzymoimmunologique de proteines a l'aide d'immunoabsorbants et d'antigenes marques aux enzymes. CR Acad Sci 1971; 273:205–2707.

Avrameas S, Ternynck T, Guesdon JL: Coupling of enzymes to antibodies and antigens. Scand J Immunol 1978; 7 (Suppl):7–23.

Axelsen NH (ed): Quantitative immunoelectrophoresis: New developments and applications. Scand J Immunol 1975; (Suppl. 2):1–230.

Blackburn GF, Shah HP, Kenten JH, et al: Electrochemiluminescence detection for development of immunoassay and DNA probe assays for clinical diagnostics. Clin Chem, 1991; 37:1534.

Bogulaski RC, Maggio ET, Nakamura RM: Clinical Immunochemistry: Principles of Methods and Applications. Little, Brown & Co., Boston, 1984.

Bounaud MP, Bounara JY, Bouin-Pineau MH, et al: Chemiluminescence immunoassay of thyrotropin with acridinium-ester-labeled antibody evaluated and compared with two other immunoassays. Clin Chem 1987; 33:2096.

Boyden SV: The absorption of protein on erythrocytes treated with tannic acid and subsequent hemagglutination by antiprotein sera. J Exp Med 1951; 93:107–120.

Bronstein I, Edwards B, Voyta JC: 1.2-dioxetanes: Novel chemiluminescent enzyme substrates. J Biol Chem 1990; 4:99.

Bronstein I, Juo RR, Voyta JC: Novel chemiluminescent adamantyl 1, 2 dioxetane enzyme substrate. *In* Stanley P, Kricka LJ (eds): Bioluminescence and Chemiluminescence. Chichester, England, John Wiley & Son, 1991, pp 74–82.

Bronstein I, Voyta J, Thorpe G, et al: Chemiluminescent assay of alkaline phosphatase applied in an ultra-sensitive enzyme immunoassay of thyrotropin. Clin Chem, 1989; 35:1441.

Burd JF, Wong RC, Feeney JE, et al: Homogeneous reactant-labeled fluorescent immunoassay for therapeutic drugs exemplified by gentamicin determination in human serum. Clin Chem 1977; 23:1402–1408.

Coons AH, Creech JH, Jones RN: Immunologic properties of an antibody containing a fluorescent group. Prop Soc Exp Biol Med 1941; 47:200.

Dandliker WB, de Saussure, VA: Fluorescence polarization in immunochemistry. Immunochemistry 1970; 7:799.

Dandliker WB, Kelly RJ, Dandliker J, et al: Fluorescence polarization immunoassay. Theory and experimental method. Immunochemistry 1973; 10:219.

Ekins RP: The estimation of thyroxine in human plasma by an electrophoretic technique. Clin Chem Acta 1960; 5:453.

Engvall E, Perlmann O: Enzyme linked immunosorbent assay (ELISA). Quantitative assay of immunoglobulin G. Immunochemistry 1971; 8:871.

Espinosa RJ, Brugues MJ, Lianos OJ, et al: Technical and clinical performances of six sensitive immunoradiometric assays of thyrotropin in serum. Clin Chem 1987; 33:1439.

Fahey JL, McKelvey EM: Quantification determination of serum immunoglobulins in antibody-agar plates. J Immunol 1965; 94:84–90.

Galvin JP: Particle enhanced immunoassays—a review, diagnostic immunology. *In* Rippey JH, Nakamura RM (eds): Technology Assessment. Skokie, Illinois, College of American Pathologists, 1984, pp 18–30.

Garvey JS, Cremer NE, Sussdorf DH: Methods in Immunology, 3rd ed. Reading, MA, WA Benjamin, 1977, pp 273–327.

Giegel JL, Brotherton MM, Cronen P, et al: Radial partition immunoassay. Clin Chem 1982; 28:1894.

Halonen P, Meurman O, Lovgren T, et al: Detection of viral antigens by time resolved fluoroimmunoassay. *In* Bachman PA (ed): Current Topics in Microbiology and Immunology. New York, Springer-Verlag, 1973, pp 133–146.

Haux P, Dybois H, McGovern M, et al: Evaluation of the TIna-quant® ferritin assay on the Boehringer Mannheim/Hitachi 704 system. Clin Chem 1988; 34:1174 (Abstr).

Heidelberg M, Kendall FE: The precipitin reaction between type III pneumococcus polysaccharide and homologous antibody. J Exp Med 1935; 61:563–591.

Henderson DR, Freidman SB, Harris JD, et al: CE-DIA, a new homogeneous immunoassay system. Clin Chem 1986; 32:1637.

Hirayama C, Ihara H, Shibata M, et al: Polypeptide artificial carrier particles for use in passive agglutination immunoassay. Polymer J 1991; 23:161.

Hunter WH, Greenwood FC: Preparation of iodine-131 labeled human growth hormone of high specific activity. Nature 1962; 194:495–496.

Ikeda M: New agglutination test for serum antibodies to adult T-cell leukemia virus. Gann 1984; 75:845–848.

Ishikawa E, Kohono T: Development and application of sensitive enzyme immunoassay for antibodies. J Clin Lab Anal 1989; 3:252.

Isomura M, Veno M, Shimada K, et al: Highly sensitive chemiluminescent enzyme immunoassay with gelatin-coated ferrite solid phase. Clin Chem 1994; 40:1830.

Jolley ME: Fluorescence polarization immunoassay for the determination of therapeutic drug levels in human plasma. J Anal Toxicol 1981; 5:236.

Kabat EA: Kabat and Meyer's Experimental Immunochemistry, 2nd ed. Springfield, Illinois, Charles C Thomas, 1961.

Kasahara Y: Homogeneous enzyme immunoassays. *In* Nakamura RM, Kasahara Y, Rechnitz GA (eds): Immunological Assays and Biosensors for the 1990s. American Society for Microbiology, Washington, DC, 1992a, pp 169–182.

Kasahara Y: Principles and applications of particle immunoassay. *In* Nakamura RM, Kasahara Y, Rechnitz GA (eds): Immunological Assays and Biosensors for the 1990s. Washington DC, American Society for Microbiology, 1992b, pp 127–147.

Kato K, Hamaguchi Y, Fukui H, Ishikawa E: Enzyme-linked immunoassay, a simple method for synthesis of the rabbit antibody-β-D-galactosidase complex and its general applicability. J Biochem 1975; 78:423–425.

Kemp BE, Rylatt DB, Bundesen PG, et al: Autologous red cell agglutination assay for HIV-1 antibodies: Simplified test with whole blood. Science 1988; 241:1352–1354.

Kitagawa T, Fujitake T, Taniyama H, Aikawa T: Enzyme immunoassay of viomycin, new cross-linking reagent for enzyme-labelling and a preparation method for antiserum of viomycin. J Biochem 1978; 83:1493–1501.

Koehler G, Milstein C: Continuous cultures of fused cells secreting antibody of predefined specificity. Nature 1975; 256:495.

Kricka LJ: Chemiluminescent and bioluminescent techniques. Clin Chem 1991; 37:1439.

Mancini G, Carbonara AO, Hereman JF: Immunochemical quantitation of antigens by single radial immunodiffusion. Immunochemistry 1965; 2:235.

Masson PL, Holy HW: Immunoassay by particle counting. *In* Rose NR, Friedman H, Fahey JL (eds): Manual of Clinical Laboratory Immunology, 3rd ed. Washington DC, American Society for Microbiology, 1986, pp 43–48.

Miles LEM, Hales CM: Labelled antibodies and immunological assay systems. Nature 1968; 219:186.

Morris DL, Ellis PB, Carrico FJ, et al: Flavin adenine dinucleotide as label in homogeneous colorimetric immunoassays. Anal Chem 1981; 53:658.

Nakane PK, Pierce GB: Enzyme-labeled antibodies: Preparation and application for localization of antigens. J Histochem Cytochem 1966; 14:929–931.

Nakamura RM: Monoclonal antibodies: Methods and clinical applications. Clin Physiol Biochem 1983; 1:160.

Nakamura RM: Fluorescence immunoassays. *In* Nakamura RM, Kasahara Y, Rechnitz GA (eds): Immunological Assays and Biosensors for the 1990s. Washington DC, American Society for Microbiology, 1992a, pp 205–227.

Nakamura RM, Kasahara Y: Heterogeneous enzyme immunoassays. *In* Nakamura RM, Kasahara Y, Rechnitz GA (eds): Immunological Assays and Biosensors for the 1990s, Washington DC, American Society for Microbiology, 1992b, pp 149–167.

Nakamura RM, Voller A, Bidwell DE: Enzyme immunoassays: Heterogeneous and homogeneous systems. *In* Weir M (ed): Handbook of Experimental Immunology, Vol 1, 4th ed. London, Blackwell Scientific Publications, 1986, p 271.

Nakamura RM, Robbins BA: Current status of homogeneous enzyme immunoassays. J Clin Lab Anal 1988; 2:51.

Nargessi RD, Landon J, Smith DS: Use of antibodies against the label in non-separation non-isotopic immunoassay; "Indirect quenching" fluoroimmunoassay of protein. J Immunol Methods 1979; 26:307.

Nishizono I, Iida S, Suzuki N, et al: Rapid and sensitive chemiluminescent enzyme immunoassay for measuring tumor markers. Clin Chem 1991; 37:1639.

Ritchie R: Automated Immunoanalysis, Part I and Part II. New York, Marcel Decker, 1978.

Ritzmann SE, Daniels JC (eds): Serum Protein Abnormalities—diagnostic and Clinical Aspects. Boston, Little, Brown and Co., 1975.

Rogers LC, Kahn SE, Oeser TH, Bermes EW: The stratus immunofluorometric assay system evaluated for quantifying human chorionic gonadotropin in serum. Clin Chem 1986; 32:1402.

Rose NR, Bigazzi PE (eds): Methods in Immunodiagnosis. New York, John Wiley and Sons, 1973, pp 1–30.

Rowley GL, Rubenstein JE, Huisjen J, Ullman EF: Mechanism by which antibodies inhibit hapten-malate dehydrogenase conjugates. J Biol Chem 1975; 250:3759.

Rubenstein KE, Schneider RS, Ullman EF: Homogeneous enzyme immunoassay. A new immunological technique. Biochim Biophys Res Commun 1972; 47:846.

Scatchard G: The attractions of proteins for small molecules and ions. Ann NY Acad Sci 1949; 51:660.

Sgoutas DS, Baron EG, Hammarstrom M, et al: Four sensitive thyrotropin assays critically evaluated and compared. Clin Chem 1989; 25:1785.

Soini E, Hemmila I: Fluoroimmunoassay: Present status and key problems. Clin Chem 1979; 25:353.

Soini E, Kojola H: Time resolved fluorometer for lanthanide chelates: A new generation of nonisotopic immunoassays. Clin Chem 1983; 29:65.

Steward MW: Overview: Introduction to methods used to study the affinity and kinetics of antibody-antigen reactions. *In* Weir M (ed): Handbook of Experimental Immunology, Vol I: Immunochemistry, 4th ed. London, Blackwell Scientific Publications, 1986, p 25.

Ullman EF, Blakemore J, Leute RK, et al: Homogeneous enzyme immunoassay for thyroxine. Clin Chem 1975; 21:1011.

Ullman EF, Schwartzberg M, Rubenstein KD: Fluorescent excitation transfer assay: A general method for determination of antigen. J Biol Chem 1976; 251:4172.

Van Weeman BD, Schuurs, AHWM: Immunoassay using antigen enzyme conjugates. FEBS Lett 1971; 15:232.

Weeks I, Beheshti I, McCapra, et al: Acridinium esters as high specific activity labels in an immunoassay. Clin Chem 1983; 29:1474.

Williams CA, Chase MW (eds): Methods in Immunology and Immunochemistry, Vol III. New York, Academic Press, 1970.

Winter G, Griffiths AD, Hawkins RE, Hoogenboom HR: Making antibodies by phage display technology. Annu Rev Immunol 1994; 12:433–455.

Yalow RS, Berson SA: Assay of plasma insulin in human subjects by immunological methods. Nature 1959; 184:1648.

Zola H: Monoclonal Antibodies: A Manual of Techniques. Boca Raton, Florida, CRC Press, 1987.

Chapter 34

Laboratory Evaluation of the Cellular Immune System

Helene Paxton, M.S., MT(ASCP)
Susanna Cunningham-Rundles, Ph.D.
Maurice R.G. O'Gorman, M.S.C., Ph.D., D(ABMLI)

5

Laboratory evaluation of the cellular immune system has developed gradually out of research studies during the past 20 years and is currently undergoing a process of standardization that may lead to broader and more effective use of this versatile approach to diagnosis and treatment of immune disorders.

Until comparatively recently, basic study of the human cellular immune system has been focused mainly on two areas: (1) primary immunodeficiency, which reveals the impact of congenital immune defects on host defense, and (2) autoimmune diseases, in which the effect of excessive or inappropriate immune activity is evident. In addition, cellular immune aspects of certain diseases with immune dysfunctional features, such as chronic viral infection, cancer, malnutrition, or traumatic injury, have been studied.

The concept of immune surveillance, introduced by Burnet in 1970, postulated that the immune system would eliminate dangerous mutant cells in healthy, immunocompetent persons. This theory led to an attempt to find general or common immune defects in patients with cancer and suggested that it might be possible to develop a kind of universal yardstick of immune parameters that could effectively quantify immune competence for virtually any person. This ultimately resulted in the development of standardized microtiter plate testing of human immune response (Cunningham-Rundles, 1976).

Much has been learned from bone marrow transplantation, which began in the mid-1970s with the reconstitution of the human immune system in primary immunodeficiency, specifically severe combined immune deficiency (SCID) disorders (Reisner, 1983; Pollack, 1983). Basic principles of immune recognition, including identification of the major histocompatibility complex (MHC), were obtained in the struggle to overcome graft rejection, graft-versus-host disease, and viral reactivation in bone marrow recipients (Meuwissen, 1969; Kersey, 1971; Sullivan, 1978).

Although many of the early studies were based on a simpler view of immune response and used complicated, specialized tests that were sometimes difficult to interpret, these efforts served as the basis for current work. Research laboratory assays designed to test lymphocyte and monocyte function found major application in clinical evaluation of immunodeficiencies such as bare lymphocyte syndrome, leukocyte adhesion deficiency disorder (LAD), and immunodeficiency associated with chronic granulomatous disease (CGD) (Touraine, 1979; Springer, 1984; Barnes, 1970).

Until recently, however, relatively few of the immune assays used in research laboratories were in widespread use in clinical immunology laboratories. In fact, among general medical practitioners, the concept of immunity has generally been equated with humoral immunity, the presence of potentially protective antibodies to an infectious agent introduced by natural infection or by immunization.

This limited approach to immune assessment occurred partly because immunology is a very young science. Immunology has been called the last science (Moulin, 1989, 1991), existing in its current form only since the 1960s. In addition, cellular immune function is fundamentally complex and not easy to measure. Basic humoral immune tests measure the specific antibody product of a response formed in the past *in vivo* to a specific virus or microbe. In contrast, cellular immune assays measure current response *in vitro* by elicitation of a functional response at the time of the test.

Because peripheral blood lymphocytes are resting cells, the cellular immune reaction must be generated freshly in the test system. The system must be capable of triggering the response, supporting the reaction by accurately providing all needed elements available *in vivo*, and having a measurable end point. The choice of test signal is very important. If the test signal is nonspecific—for example, mitogens, which directly trigger response, or allogeneic cells, which express MHC Class II antigens recognized as foreign—a relatively large fraction of isolated mononuclear cells from all healthy persons will be capable of reacting in an appropriately designed system. If the test signal is an antigen previously encountered *in vivo*, then a smaller proportion of the cells from the donor will react. This latter type of reaction, the classic delayed-type hypersensitivity Type IV reaction (Kirkpatrick, 1988), is a secondary response comparable to a humoral immune response to a booster immunization.

However, unlike the booster-type reaction, which occurs *in vivo*, the cellular immune response *in vitro* is not based on a preformed product and so requires an assay with sufficient specificity and sensitivity to elicit response in the present. In its most powerful form, cellular immune testing mirrors past reaction, demonstrates current function or immunocompetence, and predicts future ability.

Events during the early 1980s dramatically changed the field of cellular immunology. The development of monoclonal antibodies directed against human immune cell surface determinants provided a more accurate and ultimately quantifiable way to define lymphocyte subpopulations (Reinherz, 1980; Platt, 1983; Lanier, 1986). The burgeoning field of cytokine research made possible the identification of the signaling system at the level of secreted product, receptor, and finally gene activation (Gillis, 1977; Gearing, 1988; Davis, 1988; Shaw, 1987). The appearance of the human immunodeficiency virus (HIV) occurred virtually in parallel with the potential to identify $CD4^+$ T cells (see page 886, Methodology: Measurement of Lymphocyte Activation and Proliferation in the Evaluation of Cellular Immunodeficiency). The first analyses of cellular immune functional deficiency in the new syndrome were based on analysis of lymphocyte proliferative response (Siegal, 1981; Masur, 1981). These studies provided strong evidence that destruction of T lymphocytes was sufficient to produce mortal immunodeficiency resulting in susceptibility to opportunistic infections, the hallmark of underlying immunodeficiency.

As knowledge about the interaction of HIV with host cells has developed, it has become increasingly apparent that cellular immune function is not directly related to cellular number (Leibovits, 1990; Bonagura, 1992). In acquired immunodeficiency syndrome (AIDS) in particular and in clinical cellular immunology in general, investigators are searching for tests of lymphocyte function that accurately reflect the nature and extent of human immune alteration and can ultimately predict host defense *in vivo*.

This chapter presents current cellular immunologic tests in light of future trends. Cellular immune assessment is moving away from single assays and single-number fixed end points toward an integrated analysis of cell function at several levels that reflect cellular interactions as a moving process.

CLINICAL CRITERIA FOR EVALUATION OF CELLULAR IMMUNITY: IMPLICATIONS FOR INTERPRETATION

Decision to Test

Although in theory the interpretation of immune tests develops out of a careful differential approach to screening, in practical terms, patients' immune response is studied in the context of clinical presentation or history. However, immune tests may be expensive and time consuming, and thus the choice of test is often guided by clinical suspicion. Because few, if any, cellular immune tests are totally and specifically diagnostic, interpretation should be approached with caution. A major responsibility for the clinical immunology laboratory is to establish a sufficient range of tests, perform sufficient retesting to determine the nature and extent of the immune alteration, and consider alternative potential causes.

The decision to test immune response in a patient who presents for treatment usually arises for one of the reasons described in Table 34–1. Increased or unexplained susceptibility to infection, increased severity of common infections, and unusual reaction to immunization are common reasons for immune evaluation. Potential HIV infection has now replaced possible primary immunodeficiency as the leading presumptive diagnosis. However, as discussed subsequently, primary immunodeficiency disease may thus be underdiagnosed.

Unusual infections, especially opportunistic agents or se-

Table 34–1. PRESENTATION OF POSSIBLE IMMUNODEFICIENCY

Frequent bacterial infection
Unusually severe systemic reaction to a virus
Development of infection with an unusual organism such as fungus or protozoan
Systemic reaction following live virus vaccination
Family history of recurrent infections
Exposure to the human immunodeficiency virus

vere infections unresponsive to treatment and certain allergic or atopic states, may prompt immune testing. Lingering viral illnesses such as mononucleosis and chronic fatigue syndrome following Epstein-Barr virus infection, as well as other microbial related illnesses such as Kawasaki's disease, toxic shock, and Lyme disease, may lead to cellular immune testing.

Immune changes may accompany many clinical entities, including malignancies and treatment of malignancies, hematologic diseases such as Fanconi's anemia, immune thrombocytopenia, lymphoproliferative disorders such as histiocytosis, and the hemoglobinopathies such as hemophilia, sickle-cell anemia, and thalassemia, as well as a fairly wide range of chromosomal abnormalities such as Down syndrome, Bloom's syndrome, Williams' congenital dyskeratosis, epidermolysis bullosa, and Duncan's syndrome (X-linked lymphoproliferative disorder). Autoimmune diseases such as the rheumatic diseases, mixed connective tissue disease, systemic lupus erythematosus, amyotrophic lateral sclerosis, multiple sclerosis, and myasthenia gravis may be associated with cellular immune changes and are discussed further in Chapters 41 and 43.

Primary Versus Secondary Immunodeficiency

The principal features of primary immunodeficiency or suspected acquired immunodeficiency due to HIV infection must be distinguished from immune changes associated with other clinical conditions described earlier, for example traumatic injury such as burns or accidents resulting in major blood loss or organ damage, which often produce a period of vulnerability to infections. In addition, other conditions such as underlying premalignancy or undiagnosed infectious diseases may produce immune changes that could appear phenotypically identical to primary immunodeficiency.

Although HIV infection can be diagnosed by direct testing, the clinical immunology laboratory is frequently used as a proving ground before approaching the patient or guardian for informed consent for HIV testing. This is based on the observation that at least among HIV-positive adults, inverted CD4/CD8 ratio is virtually always found. Thus, as a result of the current AIDS epidemic, inverted CD4/CD8 ratio has become identified as a marker of HIV infection.

In fact, a number of diseases involving the immune system, in addition to HIV infection, can actually produce inverted CD4/CD8 ratio or extremely low CD4 cell numbers. These include but are not limited to DiGeorge's syndrome, benign thymoma, thalassemia, Kawasaki's disease, protein-calorie malnutrition, and malignancy. In addition, sequestration of cells can drain T cells from the peripheral blood during certain types of traumatic injury. Some examples of non–HIV-related inverted CD4/CD8 ratio and low CD4 numbers are shown in Table 34–2. The infant described as case 3 presented with multiple septic abscesses at the gastrointestinal (GI) tract and was thought to have a primary immunodeficiency disorder. However, this evaluation occurred after a near-drowning episode in a bathtub later found to contain traces of drain cleaner. Caustic damage to the GI tract produced the unusual lesion and the peripheral T-cell subset, imbalance, which resolved rapidly. This case also illustrates the need to conduct confirmatory testing as soon as possible when a patient is stable.

Primary immunodeficiency disorders nearly always present in the context of infection or hematologic changes. Immunodeficiency disorders are discussed in detail in Chapter 40. Laboratory evaluation usually requires a stepwise approach not only to minimize blood drawing but in order to choose wisely among available tests for the purpose of differential diagnosis. Some presumptive diagnosis may appear

5

Table 34–2. INVERTED CD4/CD8 RATIO, LOW CD4 IN NON-HIV IMMUNODEFICIENCY

		Lymphocyte Subsets				
Case Study	**Age**	*%CD3*	*%CD4*	*%CD8*	**ABS #**	**Diagnosis**
1. Initial	3 years	56	26	29	209	Idiopathic CD4 deficiency
2. Initial	6 years	73	18	24	330	Dyskeratosis
3. Initial	3 months	29	15	10	762	Congenital R/O immunodeficiency
1 week	—	43	25	15	2846	Caustic gastrointestinal trauma
4. Initial	6 years	89	62	32	874	Red blood cell aplasia
3 years	—	93	36	57	272	Red blood cell aplasia
5. Initial	3 months	83	51	31	2734	Noonan's syndrome
5 months	—	76	18	48	96	—
6. Initial	4 months	36	25	7	304	Williams' syndrome
1 year	—	51	42	12	2794	—
7. Initial	1 week	0	0	24	0	DiGeorge's syndrome
8. Initial	12 years	64	20	33	ND	Thalassemia
9. Initial	8 years	65	26	47	ND	Immune neutropenia
10. Initial	50 years	74	18	51	ND	Uveal melanoma
1 day	—	72	45	35	ND	Post hyperthermia

ABS # = Absolute number of CD4 T lymphocytes.

to be too frequently suspected—for example, Wiskott-Aldrich syndrome, which may be ruled out in cases of unexplained thrombocytopenia. However, Wiskott-Aldrich syndrome may be missed if response to mitogens alone rather than to antigens as well is not tested, and the immune defect may become more marked with time.

Clinical Significance of Tests of Immunodeficiency

An issue that frequently confronts clinical laboratory directors is how to evaluate the potential clinical significance of impaired immune response *in vitro*. Studies of even relatively well-defined disorders have shown very significant differences in clinical impact. However, the use of newer testing strategies can be helpful in subclassifying patients by level and extent of defect.

For example, studies of DiGeorge's syndrome (DiGeorge, 1974)—classically a triad of thymic and parathyroid aplasia and conotruncal defects—showed marked differences in the severity of infections associated with a relatively similar immunology laboratory picture of reduced numbers of mature T cells and poor response to mitogen caused by thymic hypoplasia. A very high degree of fatality was initially associated with this syndrome, but with improved surgical and anesthesia methods, it became clear that a significant number of infants appeared to develop normally (Bastian, 1989) without severe infections. Some infants did, however develop intractable and ultimately fatal infections, and there was no clear way to predict outcome. It is now possible to use more exact lymphocyte phenotype analysis and to analyze the levels of immune defects in DiGeorge's syndrome. Using longitudinal testing for several months and a multiple parametric approach, it now seems that severity may be predictable from consistently low $CD4^+$ T-cell numbers, inverted CD4/CD8 ratio, and reduced lymphokine interleukin-2 (IL2) production (Cunningham-Rundles, 1994b).

As noted earlier, T-cell function may be as important or more important in HIV infection than loss of $CD4^+$ T cells, although loss or rate of loss is predictive of survival. In some virus-associated illnesses, there is considerable uncertainty about how to close the link is between immune deficit detected *ex vivo* and immune function *in vivo*, as for example in the chronic fatigue syndrome. Even in this complex setting, however, there is a suggestion that patients can be staged to some degree using a panel approach to lymphocyte functional and immunophenotyping methods (Landay, 1991; Lloyd, 1992).

The Effect of Age on Immune Response

Current studies demonstrate that the immune system changes as part of the aging process (Gillis, 1981; Inkeles, 1977; Bogdan, 1994). Although there is considerable variation in this change and controversy about the cause, it is essential that the clinical laboratory use age-matched controls.

Study of pediatric patients presents particular issues for the laboratory diagnosis of immunodeficiency. The development of a child's immune system is not complete at birth, and in addition, children have not been exposed to a wide variety of abnormal environmental agents and may have vulnerability to infections. Congenital viral exposure or prematurity alone may be associated with immune abnormalities. Key differences in pediatric immune response include marked lymphocytosis at birth, elevation of B cells, increased $CD4^+/CD8^+$ T-cell ratio, and few natural killer (NK) cells (Fletcher, 1992; Yabuhara, 1990; Cunningham-Rundles, 1993). These differences are reflected in marked variations in the normal range of lymphocyte subsets and must be taken into account in evaluation of results (Denny, 1992). Also observed in pediatric patients are marked differences in response to various activators as compared with adults. The neonatal response of premature infants to certain microbial activators may be stronger than that of adults or full-term infants because of rapid changes in immune regulation (Veber, 1991).

Malnutrition and Immune Response

Although it is generally thought to be relatively rare in this country, malnutrition is frequently associated with immunodeficiency and causes significant vulnerability to infections (Chandra, 1993). For example, zinc deficiency can present as a profound immunodeficiency that may be related to the primary lack of zinc uptake at the GI tract, acrodermatitis enteropathica, or lack of adequate zinc in the diet (Moynahan, 1974; Prasad, 1963). Persons with hypogammaglobulinemia and associated malabsorption affecting zinc levels may show poor proliferative response *in vitro* and infections that resolve with zinc repletion (Cunningham-Rundles, 1981). This is associated with the fact that zinc is required for the biological activity of thymic hormone, needed for the production of functionally mature T cells (Dardenne, 1982). Many of the infections associated with protein-calorie malnutrition—specifically tuberculosis, herpes, *Pneumocystis carinii* pneumonia, and measles—are intracellular pathogens, suggesting that the cellular immune system has been critically affected (Bonagura, 1989).

In many clinical settings, malnutrition is associated with impairment of immune function, infectious complications, and inability to produce relevant immune response (e.g., trauma, renal disease, hepatic disease) (Shronts, 1993; Beisel, 1993). Patients with cancer, as discussed later, have particular disturbances in the interaction between nutrition and immunity.

Cancer

In cancer, immunodeficiency or alteration may occur in association with the development of malignancy or metastasis or may be caused by chemotherapy or radiation therapy. Loss of immune response has been found to be almost universal with advanced disease and is associated with development of opportunistic infections, often the proximate cause of death. It is now recognized that primary immunodeficiency is associated with an increased incidence of cancer (Cunningham-Rundles, 1987) and that certain tumors develop in association with HIV infection (Krown, 1983; Davis, 1984).

Inverted CD4/CD8 ratio and increased suppressor cell activity are often observed in patients with untreated cancer (Livingston, 1987). In general, chemotherapy produces transient suppression of immune response that resolves within a short time, whereas radiation may have long-term effects on immune response (Katz, 1993). The lingering immunodeficiency associated with Hodgkin's disease is well known and appears to be associated with etiology (Andreesen, 1984; Shulof, 1980).

METHODOLOGIC APPROACH TO CELLULAR IMMUNE TESTING

Human studies have been based on observation of peripheral blood immune cells because the peripheral compartment is most accessible and readily measured, but this approach may not reflect regional events (Cunningham-Rundles, 1994a). Knowledge of the differences between systemic and mucosal immune response may ultimately explain many current paradoxes arising when immune response measured *in vitro* or *ex vivo* is compared with host defense *in vivo* (Xu-Amano, 1993).

Systemic cellular immune function appears to be regulated through functionally distinct T-helper–type cytokine patterns, such that when T-helper Type 1, Th-1 cytokines, IL2, interferon-γ (IFNG) are produced, cellular immune host defense is favored and that when T-helper Type 2, Th-2, cytokines IL4, IL5, IL6, and IL10 are produced, B-cell response is induced (Barnes, 1993; Yamamura, 1991).

In contrast to systemic immunity, the primary activity of mucosal immune response is to protect the mucosa by blocking microbial, toxin, and antigen entry through secretion and transport of IgA to the lumen of the gut, a process mediated by a special type of memory T cells with reduced proliferative capacity capable of providing B-cell help (Kagnoff, 1993; Marsh, 1993). Both lamina propria T lymphocytes and intraepithelial T lymphocytes develop in relative independence of the thymus, and they function differently from peripheral blood T cells in using the CD2 signal transduction pathway rather than the T-cell receptor/CD3 pathway. Studies suggest that normal mucosa may down-regulate mucosal T-cell reactivities (Quiao, 1993). Triggering of these cells, however, can produce an inflammatory response. New studies show that genes for inflammatory cytokines, including tumor necrosis factor-α (TNFA) exist in lymphoid cells of the human GI tract (Pang, 1993) and that recombinant IL1 can induce intraepithelial lymphocyte proliferation (Mowat, 1993).

At present, tests of mucosal immunity are usually not performed in the clinical immunology laboratory and with rare exceptions the immune cells under study are from the peripheral blood compartment. For this reason, the use of *in vivo* skin testing and examination of humoral immune response to previously encountered vaccines is useful to cellular immunologists because these provide another level of assessment. *De novo* immunization can be helpful, although this is an experimental procedure. When lymph node, bone marrow, spleen, or tonsillar tissue is available, the clinical immunology laboratory may be able to construct a dimensional picture of immune system function for an individual patient. In all cases, the use of a stepwise approach and repeat testing is highly informative.

Stages of Study: The Scanning Stage

Evaluation of immune function in a patient with possible immunodeficiency is normally achieved in a series of stages. The first stage is a *scanning analysis* of possible areas of deficiency and is outlined in Table 34–3. These scanning studies should be accomplished by appropriate flow cytometric analysis of lymphocytes subpopulations and in children must include use of a B-cell marker to assess possible B-cell shifts, which may occur transiently in neonates and be reflected in low T-cell populations. The use of an NK marker is also strongly recommended even in young children, although this population may be reduced or absent at birth (Zola, 1983).

The scanning stage includes a panel approach to assess mitogenic and antigenic proliferative response. The proliferative response of lymphocytes to a range of activators continues to be one of the most sensitive tools to assess normal function and, when this includes an appropriate T-cell and B-cell activator, can be specifically useful in defining areas of defect. Although this is not always done, the use of multiple concentrations of each activator is strongly recommended.

Because of the frequent limitation of blood that can be drawn for such studies, it is essential that the first evaluation include parallel studies including a complete blood count, hematologic analysis of hemoglobin, hematocrit, and so forth on the same specimen of blood. It is essential that the differential be carried out (this is frequently canceled automatically in the hematology laboratory when the white blood cell count is in a normal range).

Functional studies need to be carried out on fresh anticoagulated blood whenever possible (or blood stored at room temperature in the dark for less than 24 hours) before mononuclear cells are isolated. When blood is being sent by air or transport to a distant laboratory, it is extremely important to include a control specimen drawn in parallel from a healthy person to serve as an internal standard for the shipping process.

In addition, the type of tube chosen to draw the blood is important. The use of lithium heparin or EDTA-containing tubes is not recommended for any lymphocyte functional studies. Sodium heparin (preservative free) or acid citrate dextrose tubes must be used. Blood collected in heparinized tubes can also be used for flow cytometric analysis, although timing for specimen preparation and analysis is critical (Nicholson, 1993).

Table 34–3. BASIC SCANNING IMMUNOLOGY STUDIES

Complete blood count/differential
Lymphocyte subpopulation analysis (numbers and percentages of T and B cells) by flow cytometry
Lymphocyte activation *in vitro* to mitogens and microbial activators
Serum immunoglobulins, including immunoglobulin subclasses if evidence of clinical infections with encapsulated bacteria. In some cases, immunoglobulin levels are normal but heterogeneous nonbinding antibodies are produced; thus, additional studies are needed

5

The question of when the blood should be drawn is important. In general, most data have been obtained with blood drawn in the morning, and circadian effects may influence results. When this cannot be done, it is helpful to continue to maintain a uniformity of drawing time for an individual patient. This is most critical when measuring absolute numbers of T-cell subsets in the monitoring of HIV disease or as part of a clinical trial (Malone, 1990).

Stages of Study: The Confirming Stage

General Aspects

Once the screening of a single individual has been achieved and evidence of potential gaps has been observed, these tests should be confirmed by repeat tests of aspects of the first series. Minimally, a positive and a negative (normal range and abnormal range) test should be carried out. Additional tests may sometimes be added to the panel to provide the beginning phase of analytical studies, as discussed subsequently.

It is important to make appropriate arrangements to draw blood when a patient is in the most clinically stable state. This usually does not occur at the first evaluation but can sometimes be achieved at the succeeding one. Double baseline studies are recommended before intervention is undertaken, and these can encompass the confirming phase. Some cases of apparent immunodeficiency may be marked by sequestration of immune cells, which is reflected in low percentages of T cells in the peripheral compartment (see Table 34–2, case 3). T cells are more subject to stress depletion. This is usually accompanied by reduced response *in vitro* even when a system using a standardized number of isolated mononuclear cells, because the transit of cells out of the peripheral compartment is not usually an even process. This reduced response may resolve when the underlying conditions have changed. This stage should also include a careful reevaluation of a patient's medical history and a patient's family history. Studies that may be used at this confirming stage are shown in Table 34–4.

Thymic Presence

The x-ray test for thymic shadow may be inadequate because the thymus is highly prone to stress depletion (Clarke, 1986). As described later in Methodology: Flow and Image Cytometry, expression of normal maturation antigens acquired during thymic development suffices to identify the presence of a working thymus.

Table 34–4. CONFIRMING AND FIRST-STAGE ANALYTICAL STUDIES

Radiograph for thymic shadow
Skin test
Natural killer cell activity (if child is 6 months or older)
Cytokine production in response to activation T-helper 1, T-helper 2 (IL-2, interferon-γ, IL-4, and so on)
Mixed lymphocyte culture reaction with patient as stimulator and patient as responder
Response to immunization
Test for presence of age-appropriate specific antibodies
Naturally occurring antibody response to isohemagglutinins (anti-A and B blood group substances) if patient has A, B, or O blood type
Test for adenosine deaminase and purine nucleoside phosphorylase enzyme deficiency

Table 34–5. CAUSES OF SKIN TEST ANERGY

Lack of appropriate antigenic history when panel does not include ubiquitous activators
Primary immunodeficiency
Viral infections
Malnutrition
Granulomatous diseases
Neoplasia

The Skin Test

The use a skin test panel can be important at this point. This approach to cellular immune assessment originally served as the departure point for the development of the cellular immune functional tests and measures delayed-type hypersensitivity directly *in vivo*. Experience with the delayed-type hypersensitivity skin test during previous decades has shown good overall correlation between lack of reactivity, termed anergy, and immunodeficiency but has not been useful as an analytical tool to distinguish the reason for lack of response. The skin test is not very quantifiable. The use of the purified protein derivative skin test to assess possible presence of *Mycobacterium tuberculosis* is an exception, although of course anergic individuals do not respond and false-positive results occur in persons who have been vaccinated with bacille Calmette Guérin.

Reasons for lack of skin test response are shown in Table 34–5. Some studies have been based on a *de novo* immunization skin test using dinitronitrofluorobenzene. Although this was once used rather extensively, this approach is no longer considered useful because of ambiguities in the underlying mechanism of reaction, which has some features of producing contact sensitivity, and because of lingering alteration in skin. The introduction of the skin window test may ultimately provide a more quantitative and informative measure of *in vivo* immune response because the reaction can be used to test autologous tumor response (Black, 1988) and the types of cells entering the region can be studied.

Despite some reservations, however, the importance of the skin test as a convincing demonstration that immune defects noted *in vitro* may have prognostic significance *in vivo* should not be underestimated. The measure of cell-mediated immunity (CMI) using Multitest (Merieux, France) is particularly recommended (Kniker, 1979) because it provides a broad range of test antigens as well as positive and negative controls.

Stages of Study: Analytical Immune Studies

Analytical studies are generally outlined in Table 34–6. Although a complete description of these approaches is beyond the scope of this discussion, these studies in general are aimed at defining the underlying mechanism of immune defect and proceed through a series of steps. Although there are different possible ways of doing this, one good way is to assess the general level of defect by following the general plan

Table 34-6. ANALYTICAL AND IMMUNOREGULATORY STUDIES

Development of activation antigens during response to stimulation, such as Tac antigen, transferrin receptor, up-regulation for MHC Class II on T cells, soluble receptors, and so on
Early activation response, e.g., calcium channels
Immunoregulation
Response to IL-1, IL-2, interferons
Development of effector functions
Immunoglobulin synthesis *in vitro*
Cytotoxic T-cell activity
Suppressor cell/factor analysis
Gene activation, cell cycle analysis
Response to immunization: *de novo* immunization

of assessing the presence of cell types and relative proportions of each in light of areas of diminished general function and then to perform studies of effector function.

Differential Immune Function

The two main immune cell types (Haynes, 1990; Paul, 1993) are T lymphocytes (T cells) and B lymphocytes (B cells). T cells are defined by expression of the T-cell receptor, which binds to antigen and CD3, a surface determinant associated with the T-cell receptor that is essential for activation. T cells have different, clonally variable receptors for a large range of antigens, require thymic maturation for normal function, and mediate cellular immunity. B cells are identified by surface immunoglobulin (detected by monoclonal antibodies such as CD19, CD20) and on appropriate activation develop into plasma cells secreting specific antibody and thus mediate humoral immunity. Loss of the normal thymus compromises T-cell function and affects T-dependent B-cell activation. Failure at the bone marrow level can affect both T-cell and B-cell immune response, although specific lineages may be involved. This is described in more detail later in Methodology: Measurement of Lymphocyte Activation and Proliferation in the Evaluation of Cellular Immunodeficiency.

The distinction between specific and nonspecific immune response is a fundamental necessity in immune response because the system must be able to distinguish between self and nonself. In general, this is accomplished by the incorporation of the molecular complex MHC self-antigen system into the antigen recognition phase. Antigen must be processed and presented in the context of self-MHC to be recognized and lead to response and the development of immune memory. The antigen-processing function is carried out by antigen-presenting cells, the best studied of which is the monocyte. This response triggers lymphocyte activation and proliferation and may include production of effector cells and triggering of B cells to produce antibody. This kind of immunity, often termed adaptive immunity, is retained as memory and is typically elicited after immunization or natural infection (Owen, 1993; Schuurman, 1979). Lack of expression of MHC Class II antigen can be detected on lymphocytes by flow cytometry by using HLA-DR or HLA-DQ monoclonals and is a hallmark of one form of a congenital immunodeficiency (bare lymphocyte syndrome) (Schuurman, 1979) (Table 34-7).

A second fundamental type of immunity, described as innate immunity, does not have memory and is not improved by repeated contact. This immunity is mediated by phagocytic cells, some of which, like the monocyte, can also process and present antigen. Innate immunity is also mediated by certain cytokines, such as interferons (Cohen, 1994; Germain, 1993), which confer nonspecific protection. NK cells are an integral component of the nonadaptive, innate immune system. Unlike phagocytic cells, NK cells are not functionally developed at birth, probably because the key cytokine, IFNG which is needed for development and maturation of this system, is also down-regulated at birth.

This third arm, represented by the NK (natural killer) cell, which is neither B-cell nor exactly T-cell-like in having neither surface immunoglobulin nor a rearranged T-cell receptor, can be defined. This cell, once called the K cell, null cell, or third population, has eluded conventional classification by cell lineage analysis. CD56 is currently considered the most definitive marker of the NK cell (Trinchieri, 1992). However, NK cells are best known as cells that can kill nonspecifically (naturally) virus-infected cells and bacteria and prevent tumor cell metastasis. If activated by a key cytokine IL-2, which triggers NK cell differentiation into the lymphokine-activated killer cells (Ortaldo, 1988), these cells can kill many tumor cell types. The NK system is constitutively active and does not have to be primed by antigen to kill. When armed with specific antibody, however, these cells can kill specifically. Functional evaluation of this cell population can be readily achieved using a short-term chromium release assay (known as an NK cytotoxicity assay using K-562 cells as targets) and is a valuable tool in assessing immune response.

Development of Immune Response

If cell populations have been determined to be essentially intact in the absence of activation, the issue of intrinsic failure may be studied by many different approaches, including the use of expanded lymphocyte surface marker analysis, framework determinants to the T-cell receptor, and activation antigens such as CD25, CD38, and HLA-DR, (see Table 34-7). Absence of MHC Class II up-regulation in response to IFNG is one example. Although cell populations may express a reference normal differentiation antigen, they may also coexpress other inappropriately, and this may be a key

5

Table 34-7. IMMUNOPHENOTYPING LYMPHOCYTE SUBPOPULATIONS

Basic peripheral blood panel (Whole blood, lysed red blood cells*)
CD45/CD14
Isotype mouse immunoglobulin controls
CD3/CD19
CD3/CD4
CD3/CD8
CD3-/CD56 and 16
Isolated mononuclear cells, activation panel†
CD45/CD14
Isotype mouse immunoglobulin controls
CD3/CD25 (IL-2R)
CD3/HLA-DR

*If low CD3, then repeat and add CD2. Further, monoclonals against T-cell receptor paired with CD3 may be added. Monocyte markers may also be evaluated. These may also be perfomed using three or four-color reagents using CD45 gating.

†After 2 days of culture, remove cells and wash before staining with monoclonal antibodies listed; analyze control cells containing no activator, then analyze activated cells. Activators may include mitogen, IL-2, and/or interferon-γ.

to functional abnormality. For example, $CD8^+$ T cells coexpressing CD38 are not functionally the same as CD8 cells that do not express this marker and are expanded in HIV disease (Giorgi, 1989). In some primary immunodeficiency syndromes, up-regulation of the IL2 receptor in response to IL2 may be abnormal. Receptors may not be translocated normally, or receptors may be shed prematurely (Cunningham-Rundles, 1990).

The development of response may be kinetically abnormal, because of delayed secondary recruitment during the amplification phase. This should be tested by performing time course studies. In some cases, cytokines may not be made or may be functionally altered. Effector functions may be missing or impaired. Evaluation of this may require a detailed approach. Attempts to restore response by cytokine addition may be useful, although this may circumvent by compensation rather than fill in the actual deficiency. When suppressor cell mechanisms are suspected, removal of cells by magnetic or flow cytometric approaches may be useful. Monitoring population characteristics in these cases is critical. Study of response of subpopulations also requires careful evaluation of normal cells in parallel, because immune response is to a large degree under negative control.

The cellular immunology laboratory is advised to choose basic analytical studies, which are normally performed on an online basis to provide a strongly developed basis for comparison. The establishment of laboratory normal ranges and maintenance of reagent quality control, especially for certain variable elements such as serum, are essential for accuracy and sensitivity of these tests.

LYMPHOCYTE PROLIFERATION AS AN IN VITRO METHOD OF ASSESSING CELLULAR IMMUNITY

Cellular Immunology: Lymphocyte Activation and Proliferation

As discussed earlier, the immune system has been divided into the humoral and cellular components. This separation is in no way absolute because there is considerable interdependence between B and T cells. The production of specific antibodies requires functional T cells, and alternatively, specific T-cell responses to antigens require processing and presentation of antigenic peptides and costimulatory molecules by B lymphocytes. For example, hyper-IgM syndrome, characterized by significant reduction of all classes of immunoglobulin other than IgM, is due to the abnormal expression of a T-cell surface marker. This marker, gp39, binds to CD40 on B lymphocytes and induces proliferation, differentiation, and immunoglobulin class switching.

Measurement of lymphocyte activation/proliferation has evolved substantially since the late 1950s and early 1960s, when cell division was determined by counting lymphocytes that had transformed into blasts. The latter method was largely replaced by quantitation of incorporated radiolabeled nucleic acid precursors into newly synthesized deoxyribonucleic acid (DNA). Many clinical laboratories still measure lymphocyte proliferation with this method. More recently, the measurement of proliferation-associated markers, estimates of the percentages of cells in specific phases of the cell cycle, quantitation of secreted cytokines/cytokine receptors, and determinations of the number of cell division following stimulation have been developed to assess cellular immune responses. This section reviews the events involved in T-lymphocyte activation/proliferation and introduces new methods that have been developed to assess the latter.

Unraveling the Biochemical Pathways of Lymphocyte Activation

After the specific interaction of mitogen or antigen with a lymphocyte, several cellular processes occur, culminating ultimately in the synthesis of DNA and the division of one parent cell into two daughter cells. Ongoing investigations are unraveling the molecular and biochemical events involved in antigen processing/presentation, antigen recognition, signal transduction, gene transcription, and ultimately DNA synthesis and lymphocyte proliferation. Specific abnormalities underlying many immunodeficiency diseases may occur at any point in the lymphocyte activation pathway. Unfortunately, abnormalities in bulk proliferation assays indicate only that there is limited or no cell division. These assays provide no information about the underlying abnormality in lymphocyte activation. More sophisticated assays are required to investigate the underlying T-cell abnormalities.

Antigen-Induced Activation of T Lymphocytes

Antigen-induced activation of T lymphocytes is a very complex process. Antigen is processed by B cells or monocytes, leading to the assembly of immunogenic peptides into the Class I or Class II products of the MHC genes. The peptide/MHC complex is presented to T cells bearing the appropriate T-cell receptor, and the signal is transduced to the nucleus. Several genes are transcribed, including *IL2* and *IL2* receptor genes. T cells expressing the *IL2* receptor respond to IL2 (originally described as T-cell growth factor), resulting in a rapid increase in the production of ribonucleic acid (RNA), proteins, and lipids, followed by DNA synthesis and ultimately cell division.

T-Cell Recognition, Activation, and Signal Transduction

The T-cell receptor responsible for specific recognition of antigen is linked to other molecules that are ultimately responsible for the transduction of signals to the nucleus.

The response that a T lymphocyte undergoes on the ligation of its receptor is very complex. Proliferation, differentiation, or anergy in response to a specific stimulus depends on many factors, including but not limited to the genetic background, costimulatory molecules on the antigen-presenting cell, coreceptors on the T cells, dose of antigen, and the cytokines present in the extracellular milieu.

The T-cell receptor complex is composed of both a heterodimeric antigen recognition structure (i.e., the T-cell receptor) and a transducing complex referred to as CD3. The antigen-binding components of this complex cannot be expressed on the cell surface without CD3 (Weiss, 1991). The antigen recognition structure is composed of structurally divergent alpha and beta chains (or less frequently the gamma and delta chains), and the CD3-transducing complex is composed of five invariant polypeptide chains, alpha, beta, epsilon and a zeta chain dimer. The zeta chain dimer (a zeta homodimer, or zeta with an eta or with an Fc epsilon RI gamma chain (Weiss, 1994), contains specific amino acid sequences known as antigen recognition activation motifs (ARAM). Originally described by Reth (1989), these motifs have an essential role in the early events following T-cell activation (Irving, 1991). CD4 and CD8 molecules on the surface of T cells are noncovalently attached to the T-cell receptor complex and bind to HLA Class II and Class I molecules, respectively, on the antigen-presenting cell. Processed antigen is presented to T cells in the context of the MHC antigens. In general, $CD4^+$ T cells responds to exogenously processed antigens presented in the context of MHC Class II, and $CD8^+$ T cells respond to endogenously processed antigens presented in the context of MCH Class I. Both CD4 and CD8 are associated with tyrosine kinase involved in the early events following T-cell activation. Other molecules on both the antigen-presenting cell and the responding T cell bind to each other and serve to increase the avidity of the binding. These molecules are referred to as adhesion molecules. Abnormal expression of a specific group of these molecules, the B2 leukocyte integrins, leads to a profound immunodeficiency state (Anderson, 1987).

In addition to the MHC-Ag-TCR/CD3/CD4 or CD8 interaction and the adhesion molecule cointeractions, activation of naive T cells requires costimulatory signals. Much information on the role of costimulatory molecules in T-cell activation has been derived from experiments using cells transfected with the TCR/CD3 complex but lacking costimulatory molecules. The latter, identified on antigen-presenting cells, include B7 (CD80) (Linsley, 1991a), B7.2 (Azuma, 1993), and heat-stable antigen (Liu, 1992). On T cells, CD28 binds B7 and the CTLA4 receptor binds both B7 and B7.2 (Linsley, 1991b). The receptor on T cells for heat stable antigen has not been identified. Antigen presentation in the presence of reagents that block the binding of the costimulating molecules leads to specific cellular anergy or tolerance to that antigen but does not affect the responses to other antigens (Tan, 1993) (i.e., leads to the specific induction of tolerance to that antigen). The ability to make nonimmunogenic transplantable tumors immunogenic by transfecting them with the B7 gene (Townsend, 1993; Chen, 1992; Baskar, 1993; Janeway, 1993) suggests that costimulatory molecules have a role in T-cell activation *in vivo*.

Signal Transduction Following Antigen-Specific Stimulation

The presentation of antigen to T cells leads to aggregation of the T-cell receptor complexes. The T-cell receptor itself has a small cytoplasmic tail with no known transducing activity. It is the associated zeta chains containing the ARAM motifs that have been shown to coprecipitate protein tyrosine kinase activity. Two well-known classes of cytoplasmic protein tyrosine kinases are involved in the very early events following T-cell activation, SRC and SYK/ZAP-70. Of the SRC family, three members are generally expressed in T cells, LCK, FYN, and YES, whereas ZAP-70 is exclusively expressed in T cells and NK cells. The nature of the interaction of these cytoplasmic kinases with the ARAM motifs of the TCR/CD3 complex is fairly well understood (Weiss, 1994). Activation of the TCR-association tyrosine kinases leads to activation of phospholipase C (Imboden, 1985), which hydrolyzes phosphatidylinositol and leads to the generation of the second messengers diacylglycerol (DAG) and inositol triphosphate. DAG activates protein kinase C, and IP3 leads to rapid and sustained increase in cytoplasmic calcium. These events lead to the induction of DNA-binding proteins and the transcription of numerous genes including those encoding IL2 and IC2 receptor. For a detailed review of the molecular transduction pathways leading to IL2 transcription following T-cell receptor activation, please refer to Weiss (1994).

T-Cell Responses

The designation of Type I versus Type II responses has been preferred for those T-cell responses that lead to cytokine secretion patterns known to be involved in cellular immunity versus cytokine secretion patterns observed in humoral immunity, respectively. Type I responses are characterized by the secretion of cytokines known to induce the activation and proliferation of T cells and monocytes, namely IL2, IFNG, and IL12. Type II responses are characterized by the secretion of cytokines that stimulate B cells to divide and differentiate into immunoglobulin-secreting cells, (i.e., interleukins 4, 5, 10, and 13). Evidence suggests that the secretion of Type I cytokines regulates the secretion of Type II cytokines and vice versa (Paul, 1994). For example, in the presence of IL4, both in vivo (Chatelain, 1992) and in vitro (Seder, 1992, 1993), T cells do not develop into IFNG–secreting cells (i.e., this environment favors the development of a humoral immune response). It has been suggested that the relative amounts of IL4 and IL12 that are present during the stimulation of naive T cells shift the response one way or the other (Paul, 1994).

Several factors are involved in regulating the type of T-cell response that ensues after antigenic stimulation. In addition to the cytokine environment, evidence suggests that the dose of antigen influences the type of response (Bretscher, 1992; Madrenas, 1995). The predominant response that develops after T-cell activation has significant clinical implications. It has been postulated that the development of a Type I response to HIV infection may lead to protective immunity (Clerici, 1994). Clearly, a Type II response is not protective, because most infected persons seroconvert and eventually succumb to a profound immunosuppression. Clerici and Shearer argue that repeated exposure to low-dose HIV-1 may lead to protective Type I cellular immunity (reviewed in Clerici, 1993). The latter laboratory has developed a method to measure cytokine secretion patterns in response to HIV-1 antigen exposure *in vitro*. Their results indicate that between 39% and 75% of HIV-1–seronegative and polymerase chain reaction (PCR)–negative high-risk individuals' peripheral blood mononuclear cell (gay men, intravenous drug users, and infants born to HIV-1–positive mothers) secreted IL2 in response to the env protein *in vitro*. These scientists propose that these seronegative high-risk individuals have developed protective cell-mediated immunity as a result of low-dose immunization or infection.

In animal models, the generation of a Type I or a Type II

5

response may lead to protection or lack of protection in response to infection. For example, some strains of mice develop a prominent cellular response to specific infectious agents, whereas other strains develop a prominent humoral response. Development of a cellular immune response against intracellular organisms appears to be protective, whereas development of a Type II response against these organisms leads to enhanced disease. This concept was reviewed by Paul (1994). Identical infections leading to disparate outcomes in different mouse strains suggest that the genetic background of the mice is also involved in the regulation of a Type I versus a Type II response.

T-cell abnormalities are most commonly designated as acquired or innate. As more of the underlying abnormalities leading to T-cell immunodeficiency are being discovered, Gelfand (1993) has proposed that the disorders should be classified using a comprehensive system that would identify the disorders according to abnormalities in differentiation, maturation, or function. These designations would begin to focus on the actual physiologic or biochemical defect and may ultimately provide new options for therapy. For a review of specific molecular abnormalities leading to abnormal T-cell activation/proliferation, please refer to Amaiz-Villena (1992) and Gelfand (1993).

Methodology: Measurement of Lymphocyte Activation and Proliferation in the Evaluation of Cellular Immunodeficiency

Developmental defects, inherited genetic abnormalities, and acquired infections may cause profound immunodeficiency states. Similarly, trauma and therapeutic intervention may also lead to immunodeficiency. Bulk assays used to ascertain whether or not an individual has a decreased T-cell proliferative response have been available for some time. The rapid development of immunologic reagents including monoclonal antibodies to a multitude of cell surface markers, specific cytokine assays, and novel and simplified molecular methods has led to an increased understanding of the mechanisms involved in T-cell activation and proliferation in both health and disease.

Procedures Used to Assess T-Cell Activation and Proliferation

Lymphocytes are unique in that they express surface receptors able to identify virtually any molecule or foreign substance (antigen). Structural diversity within these receptors is created by the differential rearrangement of the T-cell receptor genes. In general, only a limited number of circulating lymphocytes are able to recognize any one antigen. *In vivo*, when a lymphocyte recognizes a foreign antigen, the cells proliferate rapidly in a clonal manner in order to generate a large number of both effector and memory cells. This process is usually referred to as acquired immunity.

During the past several years, new methods have been developed to measure different cellular events known to occur along the pathway to cell division. *It must be emphasized that many methods measure early events in T-lymphocyte activation, which may or may not correlate with cell division.*

Tritiated Thymidine Incorporation Assay ^3H(TdR Assay)

The most common *in vivo* procedure used to test for cellular immunity is a simple skin test. A positive skin test result for the detection of a delayed-type hypersensitivity response implies intact cellular immunity as well as intact monocyte chemotaxis (Borut, 1980). Although skin testing is easily performed, negative results are difficult to interpret in young children, and skin testing is not as sensitive as *in vitro* lymphocyte stimulation assays (Borut, 1980). Other *in vivo* correlates of cell-mediated immunity include contact sensitivity, granuloma formation, and allograft rejection.

Most laboratories assess the proliferative capacity of lymphocytes by measuring the amount of newly synthesized DNA that is formed after stimulation with mitogen or antigens. In general, only a limited number of T cells respond to any one antigen *in vitro*; therefore, cells must be cultured from 6 to 10 days in order to detect a response. Mitogens, on the other hand induce the rapid proliferation of up to 100% of the T cells. For this reason, proliferation can be detected in two to four days and thus provides an effective screening tool. *In vitro* lymphocyte transformation in response to a mitogen was first reported by Nowell in 1960. Mitogens in general are the most potent stimuli because they activate the largest proportion of lymphocytes relative to alloantigens and then antigens.

Flow Cytometry in the Evaluation of Lymphocyte Activation/Proliferation

Bulk assays, in addition to their inherent technical problems, provide no information on the specific cell subsets that are responding. Flow cytometry with inherent multiparameter potential has become the instrument of choice in analytical cellular immunology. Figure 34–1 illustrates some of the cellular events occurring along the T-cell activation/prolifera-

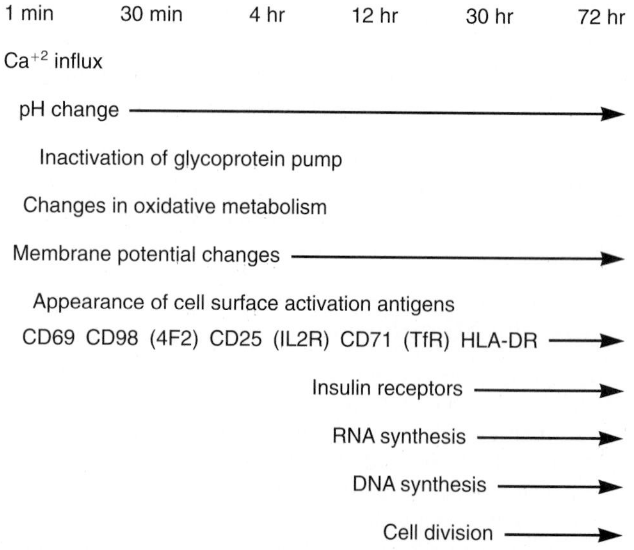

Figure 34–1. The time course of events involved in T-lymphocyte activation, which can be detected by flow cytometry. (Modified from Shapiro HM: Practical Flow Cytometry, 3rd ed. New York, Wiley-Liss, 1995, p 397. Copyright © Wiley-Liss, 1995. Reprinted by permission of Wiley-Liss, Inc., a subsidiary of John Wiley & Sons, Inc.)

tion pathway that can be measured in a flow cytometer. For a comprehensive review of flow cytometry and methods used to assess lymphocyte activation and proliferation, please refer to Bauer (1993) and Shapiro (1995) and see the later section Methodology: Flow and Image Cytometry.

Clearly, one of the earliest events that occurs after T-cell activation is the rapid increase in intracellular free calcium. This is followed by a change in pH and changes in the membrane potential. All of the effects can be measured flow cytometrically using functional probes. Unfortunately, these assays have not been sufficiently reliable to be used routinely in clinical settings. More easily and reproducibly measured is the increase in the expression of cell surface molecules that occurs after lymphocyte activation. After T-cell activation via CD3/TCR or via CD2 (the alternate T-cell activation pathway), the first measurable surface marker induced is CD69. This marker is a disulfide-linked homodimer that is present on 20% to 30% of normal thymocytes but that is not expressed on resting peripheral blood T cells. After T-cell activation, CD69 transcripts are detected within 30 minutes (Lopez-Cabrera, 1993) and cell surface expression can be detected within 2 to 3 hours (Testi, 1989). CD69 reaches peak levels in 18 to 24 hours and declines with a half-life of approximately 24 hours if the stimulus is removed. CD69 induction correlates with the extent of CD3 cross-linking and requires sustained levels of intracellular calcium (Testi, 1989). It appears that the key event responsible for CD69 induction in lymphocytes is the activation of the *RAS* ongogene (D'Ambrosio, 1994). CD69 is itself able to generate intracellular signals (Testi, 1994); however, its ligand has not been identified. With multiparametric flow cytometry, it is possible to measure the increase in CD69 expression on specific lymphocyte subsets. The development of commercial kits will standardize measurements and ensure some reproducibility (Becton Dickinson, Mountain View, CA). The relationship of CD69 induction pathway and the pathway leading to cell division is not clear. For example, we have observed strong induction of CD69 with anti-CD3 at four hours without subsequent cell proliferation as measured by ^{3}HTdR, at three days incorporation (Fig. 34–2). Although CD69 measurements can be performed in whole blood, the utility and significance of such measurements in a clinical setting remain to be established. Other cell surface markers appear on activated T cells at variable times after activation, including CD25 (the alpha chain of the IL-2 receptor), CD71 (both of the latter within 24 to 48 hours), and HLA-DR (after 48 hours).

Another flow cytometry–based method that has attained significant use in clinical laboratories is the measurement of lymphocytes in the various phases of the cell cycle (see page 886, Methodology: Flow and Image Cytometry, DNA Analysis the later section for review). In general, cell cycle analyses are performed by measuring the level of fluorescence intensity emitted by DNA staining dyes. The most common dye used is propidium iodide (PI), which intercalates stoichiometrically into DNA (i.e., the amount or intensity of fluorescence is proportional to the amount of DNA in a cell). Using complex mathematical formulas, it is possible to measure the percentage of cells with a DNA content between 2N and 4N, which correlates with the percentage of cells in the S-phase of the cell cycle. Peripheral blood lymphocytes

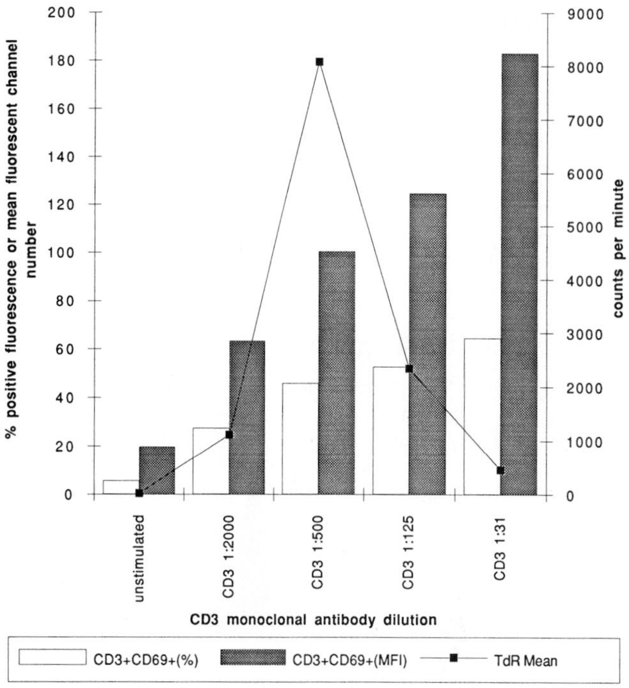

Figure 34–2. The relationship between the level of expression of CD69 on T cells after four hours and the proliferative response after three days in whole blood cultures stimulated with the same concentrations of anti-CD3. The high level of CD69 expression without significant incorporation of tritiated thymidine (i.e., no proliferation at high concentrations of anti-CD3 lymphocytes) was consistently observed in whole blood obtained from healthy adults as well as HIV-1–infected adults.

are in general in the resting phase of the cell cycle, with less than 5% of the cells in the S-phase.

Some laboratories have replaced the tritiated thymidine incorporation assays with a combination of cell surface marker induction assays and a measurement of the percentage of cells in various phases of the cell cycle after activation (Cost, 1993).

Dyes that have been developed can stably integrate into the membranes of live lymphocytes (Fig. 34–3). After excess dye is washed away, the lymphocytes are stimulated to divide. With each successive division, the amount of dye per cell is decreased. The fluorescence emitted from the cells after culture can be modeled, and the number of cell divisions can be estimated. This method has been standardized into a kit that includes both the software required for analyses and the tracking dye (Sigma Immunochemicals, St. Louis, MO). This assay may provide the most accurate assessment of the actual proliferative response in *in vitro* culture systems, with the substantial advantage over standard bulk assays of allowing the measurement of specific lymphocyte subsets. The use of multiparametric flow cytometry combined with tracking dyes allow the assessment of the proliferative responses within specific lymphocyte subsets. Kits for measuring lymphocyte proliferation using the tracking dyes have not only recently been developed and have not yet been widely tested in a clinical setting.

New assays are being developed to measure different events involved in T-cell activation. New technologies that have been developed allow measurement of the earliest phosphoryla-

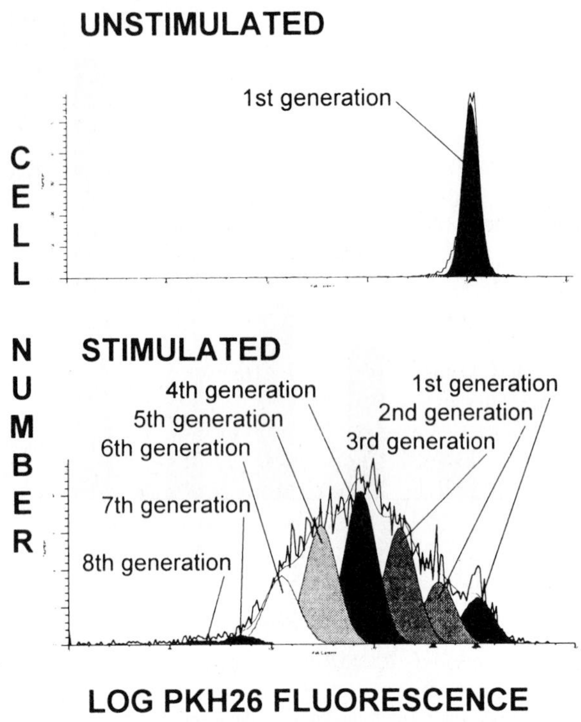

Figure 34–3. Use of tracking dye PKH26 in mitogen stimulated and unstimulated peripheral lymphocytes after five days in culture. Cell proliferation is indicated by the dilution of the fluorescence intensity with each succeeding generation. (Modified from Shapiro, HM: Practical Flow Cytometry, 3rd ed. New York, Wiley-Liss, 1995, p 313. Copyright © Wiley-Liss, 1995. Reprinted by permission of Wiley-Liss, Inc., a subsidiary of John Wiley & Sons, Inc.)

tion/dephosphorylation events, through signal transduction, gene transcription, and cell division. As these methods are adapted for routine clinical use, a veritable armamentarium of methods to assess many of the specific steps involved in lymphocyte activation and proliferation, will become available. Although many of these new technologies are still within the domain of research laboratories, some of the methods have been simplified and adapted for use in clinical laboratories. Within the next few years, the clinical applicability of the CD69 assays and the tracking dye assays should be appreciated. Correlation of these methods to standard and historical methods remains to be performed and validated. Clearly, the lack of achievable standardization and the continued lack of inter-laboratory reproducibility with the historical methods make new approaches to measurements attractive to both the clinical and research laboratory.

GRANULOCYTE FUNCTION IN CELL-MEDIATED IMMUNITY

Both monocytes and granulocytes are derived from a common parental precursor. Granulocytes are extremely important in the early inflammatory response, and abnormalities in their functions lead to profound deficiencies in cellular immunity. Abnormalities occur at any point in a series of processes required for granulocytes function, including difficulty in leaving the vasculature (diapedesis), movement toward the offending agent (chemotaxis, chemokinesis), engulfment of the offending agent (phagocytosis), and killing via the generation of toxic oxygen radicals.

Since the original observation by Metchnikoff that phagocytosis is part of host defense, numerous procedures have been developed to assess granulocyte functions. A thorough review of these methods is clearly beyond the scope of this text. For reviews of the conventional methods as well as flow cytometric methods, refer to Metcalf (1986) and Robinson (1993), respectively. Highlighted here are some of the recent developments in granulocyte function assays that have increased their adaptation for use in a clinical setting. The development of whole blood assays simplifies the procedures, limits the amount of blood required, and helps to standardize methods both within and between laboratories. Two diagnostic whole blood assays are used for the detection of CGD and LAD Type I (O'Gorman, 1993, 1995).

The diagnosis of LAD can be ascertained by the level of expression of B2 leukocyte integrins expressed on the surface of both resting and activated granulocytes. Patients with LAD express significantly reduced levels of each of the B2 leukocyte integrins (i.e., CD11a, CD11b, and CD11c on both resting and activated granulocytes). The reduced expression of each of these alpha chains had been associated with a mutation in the CD18 beta chain.

Patients with CGD sustain repeated infections because of an inability of their granulocytes to kill phagocytosed pathogens. Mutations in NADPH oxidase, an enzyme system involved in the generation of toxic oxygen radicals, prevents their granulocytes from generating an oxidative burst. The latter can be assessed rapidly in a flow cytometric assay—for example, nonfluorescent laser-sensitive dye is loaded into granulocytes in whole blood. The latter are stimulated to generate an oxidative burst that oxidizes the dye and renders it brightly fluorescent. Many variations of this assay have been published and are currently performed routinely in specialized clinical laboratories. Mutations have been reported in each of the four known components of the NADPH oxidase system. By measuring the cell surface expression of the p22 phox subunit simultaneously with an assessment of the oxidative burst potential, Emmendorfer (1994) claims that additional information about the specific subunits affected in patients with CGD can be obtained. Granulocyte function is only briefly reviewed here, and these tests are still primarily performed in clinically oriented research laboratories. (Please refer to the previous citations for excellent and comprehensive reviews.)

METHODOLOGY: FLOW AND IMAGE CYTOMETRY

The use of flow cytometry (laser-based cell analysis) has become the standard of laboratory clinical practice in the study of the cellular immune response, as previously indicated (Kamientsky, 1969; Hertzenberg, 1976). The measures of immunocompetence and the immune modulation of specific surface markers and receptors, the lineage characterization by the immunophenotyping of lymphomas and leukemias, the definition of malignancy using specific chromosome probes, as well as the study of tumor heterogeneity by multiparameter DNA measures are commonly performed analyses in many laboratories, as discussed in previous sections, and are detailed in Keren (1989) and Keren (1989a) as well as in many other references mentioned throughout this text. The classification of cell types by these means enables the definition of biological and effector function on a molecular basis and allows the relationship of these measures to relate to disease process and definition. These are but a few of the applications that are possible using laser-based technologies. Two major technologies are used. The first is characterized as flow-through, in which the particles being counted and their physical and chemical characteristics are measured by the particles passing in a fluid stream in a single-cell suspension. In the second, known as static analysis, the particles are stationary and the stage or the laser moves as in image analysis (Martin-Reay, 1994). Image analysis technology is slowly making its mark in the laboratory in the evaluation of touch preparations or cytospins, chromosome preparations, and tissue sections for certain applications. Advances in the availability of fluorescent probes for use in fluorescence *in situ* hybridization (FISH) and chromosome painting will make analysis a more relevant and useful tool in the clinical laboratory (Weinberg, 1993). Instrumentation development combining the strengths of flow cytometry and the static advantages of image analysis has been introduced. These instruments, known as scanning cytometers, make the traditional flow cytometry measures of forward scatter, side scatter, and fluorescence on cells in suspension or fixed on to a glass slide. Experience with these systems will determine if this approach offers measurement advantages not available with the current flow cytometric and image system configurations (Martin-Reay, 1994) (Fig. 34–4). Image analysis is not further considered in this chapter.

The combined advances in electronic pulse processing, optics, and data storage with advances in computer technology and software have allowed the flow cytometry technology to become routine in the laboratory. Further, the wide availability of workshop clustered monoclonal antibodies (Shaw, 1993) labeled in multicolor, directly conjugated, and in premixed formats has allowed the simultaneous detection of multiple surface antigens as well as cytoplasmic and nuclear constituents. *The ability to perform multiparameter analysis is the greatest strength of flow cytometry.* The major manufacturers have made the art of flow cytometry into a routine laboratory measurement—a "black box" science, much to the dismay of many. As already described, this "black box" approach phenomenon is largely the result of the use of flow cytometry in the phenotyping of T-cell subsets for the monitoring of patients with HIV (Shapiro, 1993; Centers for Disease Control, 1992; Calvelli, 1993). Before the onset of the HIV epidemic, flow cytometry use in the laboratory was primarily for the characterization of leukemias and other hematologic malignancies and for DNA analysis of tumors for synthesis phase (S-phase) and DNA index (DI). Although flow cytometry technology may be more black box, the HIV epidemic has brought the power of the flow cytometer to a much larger number of institutions and laboratories (College of American Pathology [CAP], 1990–1995). This has allowed the technology to be an integral part of many diagnoses and an important adjunct in treatment of patients. Despite its simplification, many issues with regard to Food and Drug Administration regulation, proficiency testing, data management, and reproducibility of data remain. This is particularly true in the area of DNA analysis (CAP, 1990–1995). It is not the purview of this chapter to describe all the nuances of a flow cytometer or image cytometer. Current flow cytometers all can adequately perform routine phenotyping and DNA analysis. Most laboratory problems lie in the nonavailability of standard quality control reagents and calibrators and the lack of reliable, rapid methods for data transfer and storage compatible with laboratory information systems. Readers are urged to review the many references for the appropriate selection of a flow cytometer or image cytometer with details of their many configurations and capabilities (Shapiro, 1993, 1995). More important for clinicians is the understanding of the technology, the strengths, and the pitfalls in quality control and quality assurance, specimen preparation, and data interpretation.

The Light Source and Signal Processing

Today's clinical flow cytometer is used primarily for immunophenotyping and for DNA analysis and some functional assays such as calcium. It rarely has the capability to perform sorting, and this property remains with research instruments in the highly specialized laboratory. The clinical flow cytometer now uses helium-neon and argon ion air-cooled lasers or a single air-cooled argon ion emitting at 488 nm as compared with the not-so-distant, large, water-cooled, argon ion laser, which necessitated dedicated power and special plumbing (Bogh, 1993). Today's laser has a low-milliwatt output between 10 and 20 mW and lasts for more than 6000 hours. These lasers, as compared with their predecessors, are easy to maintain and much cheaper to replace. If a laboratory is interested in performing five or more colors of analyses using Hoescht's ultraviolet-stimulated probes, it is then necessary to use the larger water-cooled 5-W lasers in combination with the air-cooled lasers. Most multifaceted clinical flow cytometers use a single argon ion-air cooled laser with a minimum of four photomultiplier tubes. The most common instrument configurations include the Becton-Dickinson FACScan, the Coulter Profile II, the Ortho Cytoron, and most recently the Coulter XL. The introduction of the XL brings forth the latest technology in flow cytometry with the use of digital signal pulse processing (Coulter, 1994; Shapiro, 1995) with high-resolution analog digital converters (ADCs), negating the use of logarithmic amplifiers (log amps). The log values are now simply read from a mathematical table (Coulter, 1994). This is an important development because it removes the issues of linearity and low-end sensitivity (threshold) in the measurement of fluorescence intensity. In the traditional flow cytometer, the fluorescence measurements are made on a linear scale but have to be converted to log in order to fit on a reasonable scale (to fit all the peaks of interest). This process in the nondigital instruments is done with the use of ACDs with log amps. Unfortunately, this conversion of linear signal through the ADC to the log amps al-

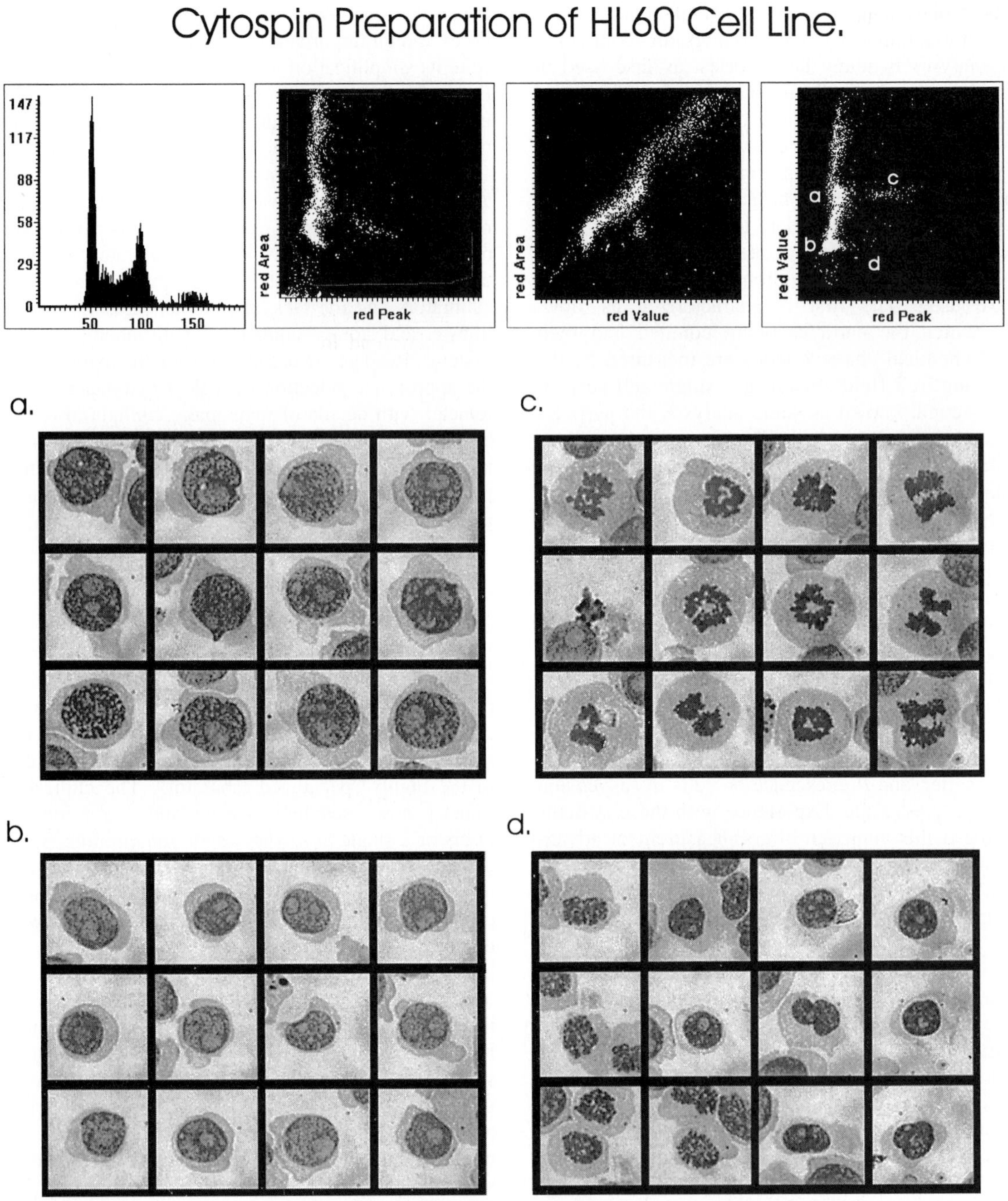

Figure 34–4. Use of the laser scanning cytometer (LSC) produces data that are comparable to flow cytometric data; however, because the machine is slide based, it has several key differences.

Unlike flow cytometry, in which all of the information for each cell is contained in single electronic pulse for each parameter, the LSC uses hundreds of measurements to calculate and extract parameters for each cell. It also is possible to derive subparameters. The cell value is the total amount of fluorescence per cell, but subparameters such as cell area and peak value are also important. The figure shows data from a cytospin preparation of HL-60 cells that were stained with propidium iodine (PI). The single parameter histogram of the red value is shown, as well as the three possible combinations of the red subparameters. Of particular interest is the cluster of cells located below the letter c.

The slide was restained with eosin/hematoxylin, and cells from the lettered areas (see earlier) were relocated. The digital snapshots of the first 20 cells relocated in each region are shown. Cells in region c are mitotic, whereas the cells in region d, b, and a are consistent with cells progressing through stages G_1a, G_1b, and G_2m of the cell cycle. (Courtesy of CompuCyte, Cambridge, Massachusetts.)

lows a lot of noise, causing increased signal processing coefficients of variation (CVs) with increased fluorescence signal. This makes each measurement decade different in sensitivity because the CVs of the signal conversion increase with higher channel numbers (Shapiro, 1995a). Although average technologists using a clinical flow cytometer do not really understand the cause of the variable sensitivity of the log amps in their instruments, they are confronted with the results or the lack of response in certain regions of their logarithmic scale. Linearity is particularly important in the measurement of DNA content (because DNA measurements are made in linear scale, the log amp problems are avoided but other, similar electronic factors enter in) because the DI value is dependent on its accuracy. Further, linearity is becoming increasingly important in the measurement of quantitative fluorescence measurements of proliferation and activation (Auer, 1994; Shapiro, 1995). The laboratory must institute measures of linearity, sensitivity and resolution, and quality control before performing clinical work. Daily quality control steps are defined later in this chapter. Readers are again urged to review appropriate references for more detail (Bauer, 1993; Shapiro, 1995).

The Flow Cell

Two common flow cells are in use in the clinical laboratory, but because most clinical instruments are used in the measurement of CD4 cells in the monitoring of HIV disease, most clinical systems used a closed system as a biohazard precaution. The first, known as a stream-in-air or flow-in-air flow cells, allows the optical measurement point to fall outside the chamber. This type of cell minimizes the distance between the flow chamber and the sample injector tip and thus minimizes carry-over between specimens and the sample wash time necessary between samples. This chamber allows greater sample flow rate variability than a closed system (Shapiro, 1993; Bogh, 1993). Other advantages of the stream-in-air tips are important in cell sorting and are not considered here. In the closed system, often referred to as a quartz tip, the focal point is within the chamber. Disadvantages of these quartz systems are the thickness of the quartz and thus the diffraction of the laser beam or the scattering of the signal. Additionally, the relatively large surface area (200 microns) makes the flow rate more difficult to control. The success of these quartz tips in the clinical system depends on the illumination and the collection optics. The major manufacturers have made many advances in these systems to provide both the safety and maximum sensitivity with the use of low-power, laser-based systems (Bogh, 1993). It is often difficult for clinical operators to understand how the fluidic system drives the sample through, to allow the precise alignment of the particles or cells through the sheath fluid. Confounding are all the terms used in the definition of these systems, which include the flow rate, the sheath pressure, the core size, the resulting particle velocity, the resulting CVs, and so forth. The most important factor for a laboratory worker to understand is that in DNA analysis, the cells are analyzed at a slow flow rate to increase the time a particle spends in the beam, allowing greater sensitivity and better CVs. In immunophenotyping, sensitivity is typically not an issue, and the particle flow rate can be increased. Sensitivity in immunophenotyping may become problematic as activation measurements necessitating quantitative measurements performed by flow cytometry take on greater clinical significance (Shapiro, 1993; Weinberg, 1993). Most clinical systems are compromises to accommodate the two most common applications of immunophenotyping and DNA analysis (Shapiro, 1993, 1995a; Goetzman, 1993). Research flow cytometers have much greater flexibility and operator control for controlling the sample flow rate, differential pressure, and time.

Colors and More Colors: Applications of Fluorochromes

Most laboratories are still using the most common fluorochromes, fluorescein isothiocyanate (FITC, 530 nm emission) and phycoerythrin (PE, 575 nm emission) for immunophenotyping and PI (625 nm emission) in the measures of DNA (Shapiro, 1995b). These fluorescent dyes are directly conjugated by the antibody of interest and simultaneously added to a patient's sample. The use of a secondary antibody such as a goat anti-mouse (GAM) IgG labeled with fluorescein is no longer necessary for extra sensitivity, and therefore the background fluorescence is minimized. Most clinically used antibodies in the study of HIV are premixed and prediluted for use in whole blood technologies. PI can be used simultaneously with FITC in multiparameter DNA analysis, although this requires preservation of the cell membrane (Clevenger, 1993).

New dyes that have become available to the clinical laboratory allow the simultaneous measurement of four colors with directly labeled monoclonal antibodies and excited with a single 488-nm laser. This availability will revolutionize the current performance of flow cytometry in laboratory practice. These dyes with a red and far red emission include PE Texas Red tandems (625 nm emission), PE-Cy-5 tandem (675 emission), and allophycocyanin (675 emission), to name a few (Fig. 34–5). The early tandems were problematic because of excess free PE in solution, leading to excess background fluorescence and issues with compensation. New technologies for the synthesis of these dyes are exploding, solving most of the technical issues, and new dyes are constantly being added for use in the clinical laboratory (Clevenger, 1993). With the availability of the red and far red dyes, an HIV subset analysis can be performed in a single tube with greater surety. A single tube with 100 μl of whole blood is simultaneously stained with CD45 PE-Cy-5, CD3 PE-Texas Red, CD8 FITC, and CD4 PE. With the new digitized signal processing, compensation (discussed later) is easily performed, and the analysis is performed using the CD45 as a gating agent with side scatter (SSC) and the simultaneous analysis of CD3, CD4, and CD8 (Fig. 34–6*A* and *B*). Another interesting phenomenon is that these new dyes have allowed the use of fluorescence as a trigger in place of the usual forward light scatter parameter. This is possible because the far red dye spectra are not found in components of most cells or they do not have much autofluorescence competition in nature as found with FITC. Further, they can be excited at wavelengths that minimize the autofluorescence from cell constituents such as riboflavin. Therefore, when performing a rare event (cells present at less than 0.1% of total population) analysis using a fluorescent trigger, many cells can be analyzed very rapidly. This method is also used to label leukocytes in unlysed blood using fluorescence as a trigger. A dye that marks the leukocytes' nuclei or cytoplasm and not the erythrocytes' is used. Rare event evaluation methods for the clinical laboratory are really in their infancy. Several approaches are being tried and evaluated. In the evaluation of minimal residual disease (MDR), they include polymerase chain reaction (PCR), flow cytometry combined with nuclear probes, flow cytometry with use of multiple markers defining the leukemic phenotype, and various

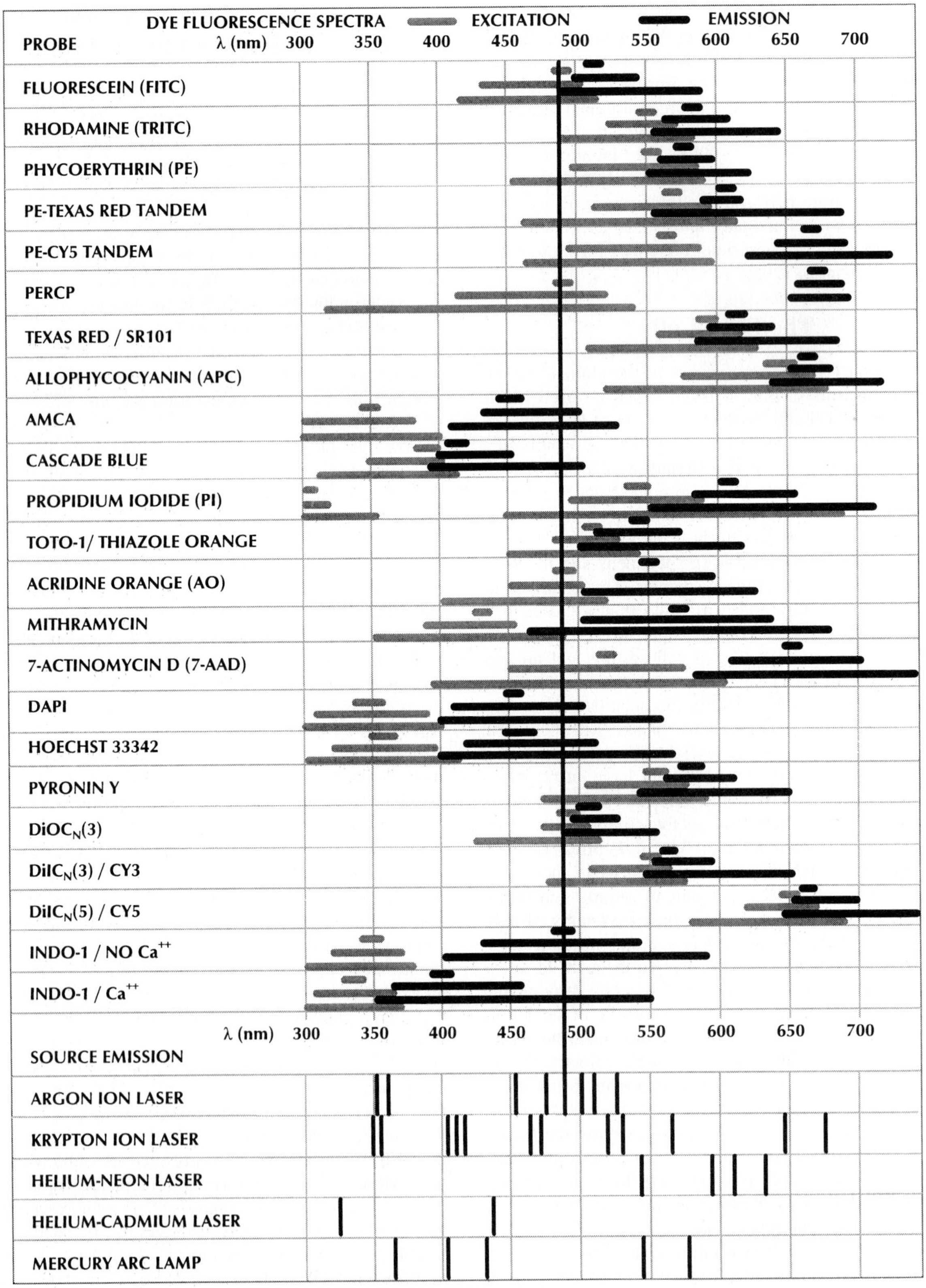

Figure 34–5. Common fluorescence dyes used in multicolor, multiparameter flow cytometry. (From Shapiro, HM: Practical Flow Cytometry, 3rd, ed. New York, Wiley-Liss, 1995, p 245. Copyright © Wiley-Liss, 1995. Reprinted by permission of Wiley-Liss, Inc., a subsidiary of John Wiley & Sons, Inc.)

applications of FISH. Data suggest that true bone marrow remission in myelogenous leukemia really never occurs as far as flow cytometry analysis is concerned; it is simply a matter of level of sensitivity and event detection (Campana, 1995). This obviously has great implications when correlating flow cytometry results versus morphologic criteria of remission and prediction of relapse. How this will affect treatment strategies in various hematologic malignancies continues to be evaluated. The use of multicolor fluorescence has allowed the concept of multiparameter analysis to become a reality in most laboratories. The parameters can evaluate different functional subsets of a particular cell population using an intracellular fluorescent probe, use of several colors to identify small clusters of otherwise unidentifiable events (as in MDR), activation status of cells in a particular disease stage—for example, use of HLA-DR and CD38 on CD4 and CD8s in HIV staging using an anchor gate approach, as well as looking at cell surface expression and the DI or S-phase of a particular cell population as in defining the CD19 S-phase in an acute leukemia. Obviously, the possible combinations are nearly infinite, and their sophistication enhanced by the specific dyes and DNA/RNA probes available (Fig. 34–7). A discussion of some of these approaches and techniques follows.

Gating and Analysis

Immunophenotyping: T-Gates and Anchor Gates

The analysis of cell populations with the flow cytometer uses a combination of parameters that, when applied, define a specific cell population. Flow cytometry uses similar parameters to those that have been used for many years in hematology, including size (forward light scatter), cytoplasmic granularity (side scatter), affinities for specific dyes, and so forth and combine them with the immunologic tools already mentioned. These include multiple fluorescent dyes bound to antibodies or probes, DNA measurements as measured using either PI or 4′6-diamidino-2-phenylindole (DAPI), and other nuclear markers. The key is the simultaneous detection of these parameters in today's analytical systems. For many years, the clinical laboratory flow cytometer could only use three simultaneous measurements including forward angle light scatter (FALS) versus SSC versus FITC or PE. Staining of cell populations was limited by the unavailability of directly conjugated monoclonal antibodies, necessitating the use of a secondary GAM reagent or the use of biotin-labeled antibodies. Definition of positive and negative populations in high-background cases made it necessary to use a subtraction channel-by-channel algorithm to define positive from negative (Bagwell, 1993). In cases in which the cell population had a defined boundary between negative and positive, a cursor was set so that no more than 2% of the events considered negative fell to the right of the cursor, defining the positive events when using a matched isotypic control. Although this approach seemed reasonable at the time (Lewis, 1993) and worked well with bright cell clusters, it has become quite cumbersome when identifying leukemic cells or performing analyses of cell activation markers. Leukemic cells were particularly problematic, because each leukemia has its own "relative" fluorescent intensity and isotype controls may have little relevance. Applying hard-and-fast rules to cursor settings led to the underestimation of positive clusters. The failure of this approach is especially dramatic in the analysis of monoclonality by kappa and lambda light chain expression. Small but significant differences are often lost. Use of isotype controls in certain situations has been challenged on many fronts, both from technical aberrations associated with their use and from the added cost to the laboratory. Routine software algorithms do not yet have the capability of making intensity measurements and defining clusters based on population means intensities, although these will soon be available. Clearly, the need to remember what we are measuring and understanding the biology of the population of interest need to be considered when designing an analysis protocol. Fortunately, some sophisticated software approaches and better reagents have allowed us to use multiparameter gating to define populations, rather than trying to make estimates of fluorescence expression using cursor values. Many investigators have used the multiparameter approach in defining cluster and other populations of interest (Shapiro, 1995c; Loken, 1987; Terstappen, 1988; Terstappen, 1990; Verwer, 1993). These approaches take many forms, and a few are reviewed here.

With the coming of multicolor fluorescence came the need to analyze the number of cells expressing one or more colors at the same time on a particular cell population defined by FALS and SSC regions. When this method was first developed, scientists were basically thinking about the mathematics and the accounting of all cells and the number of these cells expressing one or more colors. A binary approach to this analysis was developed, known as prism (Coulter, Hialeah, FL). These analysis regions were hardgated and set into the instrument by the operator. These regions could not be redefined at a later time using list mode analysis, which caused a lot of frustration. This approach was later modified to allow some regating, and other manufacturers as well third-party software made this prism binary approach on a postanalysis basis. Loken then defined bone marrow populations using CD45 versus SSC gating a unique approach to defining the heterogeneous populations found in bone marrow (Figs. 34–7 to 34–9). They and others (Borowitz, 1992) developed the concept of patterns defining specific leukemic states. Shapiro used a ginger root to define the evolution of this concept (Shapiro, 1995c). Loken further promoted the use of CD45 and CD14 dual-parameter analysis gated on the lymphocyte region of FALS versus SSC for peripheral blood (Loken, 1990). Many agencies embraced and promoted this approach for most of the HIV flow cytometry panels in order to minimize the effect of contaminating monocytes in the lymphocyte population because they might interfere with a true CD4 lymphocyte count as monocytes have CD4 receptors on their surface (Passlick, 1989). Agencies promoting this type of analysis included Centers for Disease Control and Prevention (CDC, 1992), National Institute of Allergy and Infectious Disease, Division of AIDS (NIH, DAIDS) (Calvelli, 1993), New York State, National Committee for Clinical Standards (NCCLS, 1992), and the CAP (1990–1995). Unfortunately, even though this approach solved a lot of problems, it did not ensure that each tube in the panel had the same contents as the tube containing the CD45 and

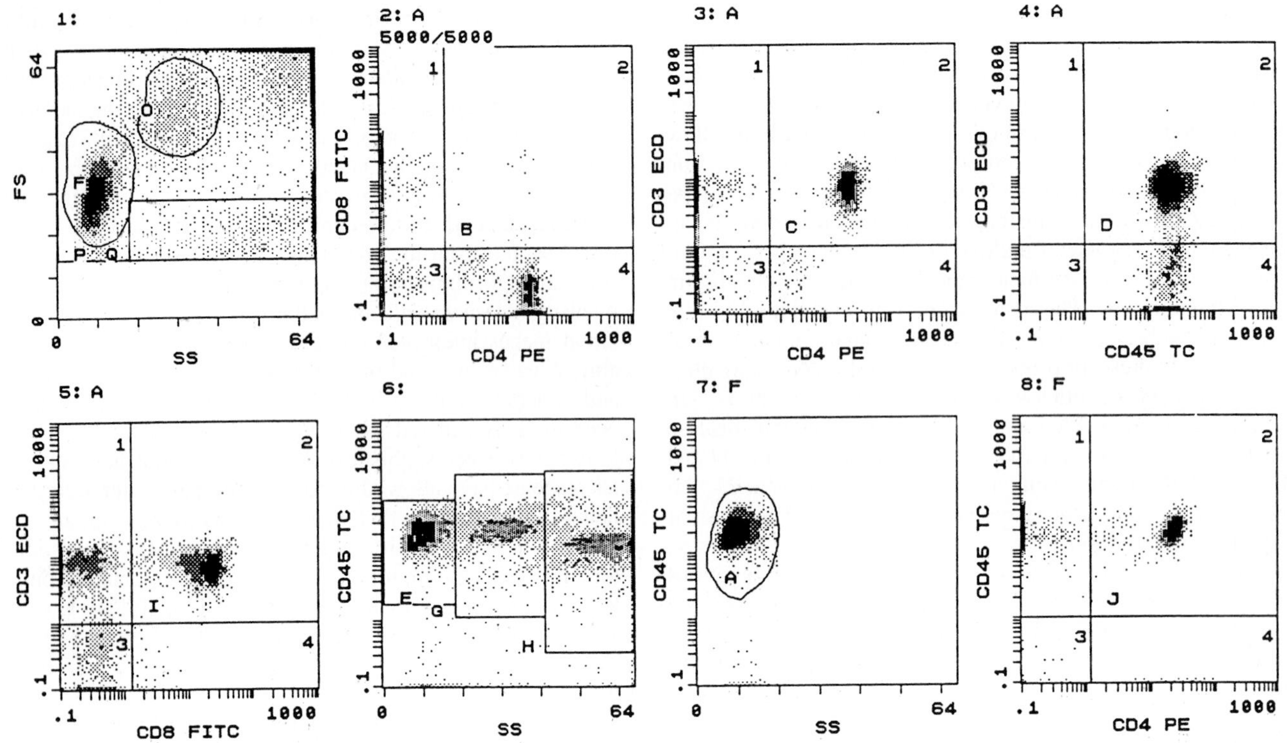

4 COLOR CD45/4/3/8

Hist #	Region	%	Count
1	F F	31.3	4845
	O O	7.8	1209
	P P	99.9	15448
	Q Q	6.1	939
2	B1 B	47.2	2362
	B2 B	0.5	27
	B3 B	15.4	768
	B4 B	36.9	1843
3	C1 C	51.8	2591
	C2 C	34.7	1737
	C3 C	10.9	544
	C4 C	2.6	128
4	D1 D	0.0	0
	D2 D	86.6	4328
	D3 D	0.0	0
	D4 D	13.4	672
5	I1 I	39.9	1997
	I2 I	46.6	2331
	I3 I	12.7	636
	I4 I	0.7	36
6	E lymphs	31.8	4915
	G monos	11.4	1769
	H grans	55.5	8583
7	A A	98.8	4785
8	J1 J	62.4	3021
	J2 J	36.5	1770
	J3 J	0.7	33
	J4 J	0.4	21

A

Figure 34–6. *A*, Use of four-color flow cytometry in the performance of HIV monitoring panel. Method demonstrates the use of CD45 as gating strategy and use of CD45 and light scatter in the performance of three-part differential (H-6). Use of four-color flow cytometry allows performance of T-cell subsets to be measured in same tube and all cells to be accounted for. Histogram 7 is gated on region F contained in histogram 1, FALS vs SSC. In histogram 1, use of Q-region defines debris. Debris greater than 15% of total events usually results in specimen being unacceptable. This gating and staining approach allows all parameters to be checked against each other. (Directly conjugated monoclonal antibodies were either Coulter or Becton Dickinson clones for FITC and PE clones, Coulter for ECD, and Caltag Corporation for Cy-5 CD45.)

CD14, and the required purity correction might be overestimated, leading to incorrect values for CD4. These issues were reviewed during a conference held by the CDC, a year after the HIV guidelines for the performance of CD4 counts were published (Stelzer, 1993; CDC, 1993). Other analyses of this approach have been performed by the ACTG Flow Advisory Committee in the DAIDS Proficiency CD4/CD8 program (CDC, 1993; Kagan, 1993) and by the CAP in their proficiency testing program (Homberger, 1993). A new approach to gating was evaluated in HIV panels that followed from Loken's original approach to bone marrow definition of clusters (Loken, 1990). Use of a CD45 as a gating parameter

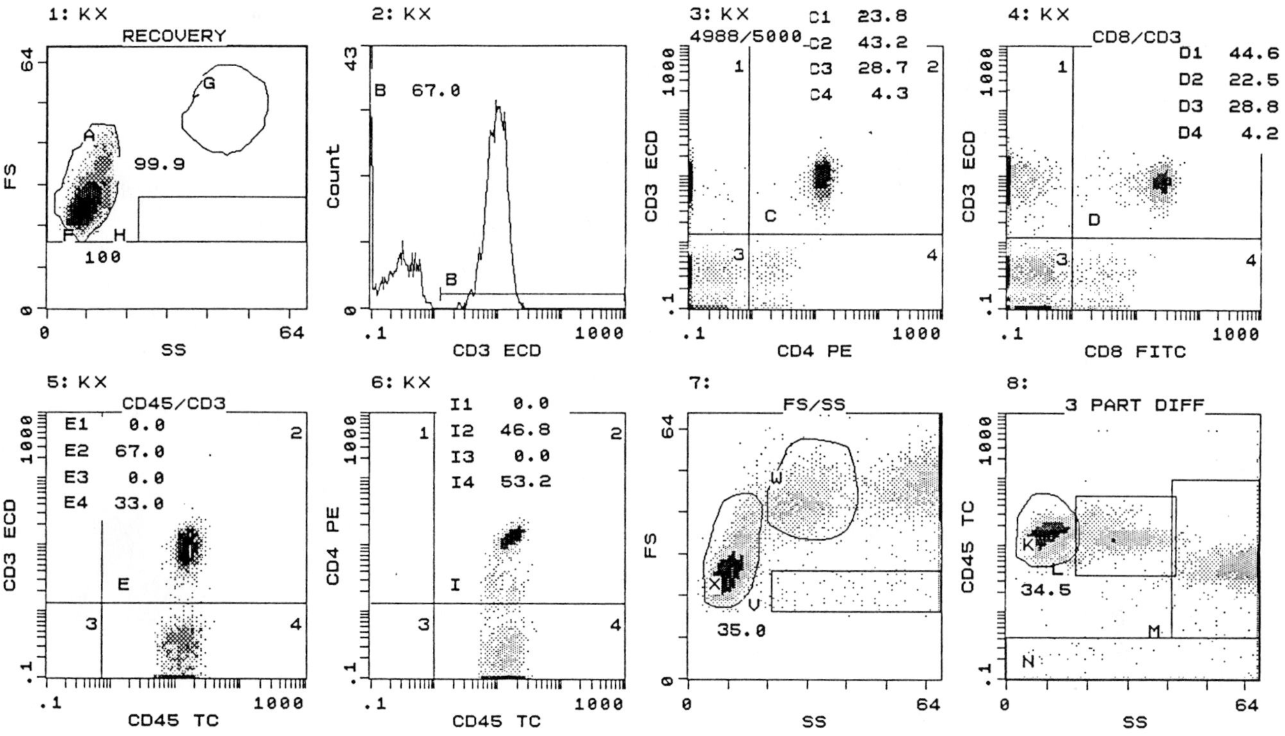

B

Figure 34–6 *Continued B*, HIV monitoring panel as in *A*, except that in this case, the panels incorporate the use of a lymphocyte recovery parameter calculated on FALS vs SSC and CD45 vs SSC. Additionally, the use of a T-gate is demonstrated in H: 2. These gating strategies allow multiple values of CD3 to be calculated and checked against each other.

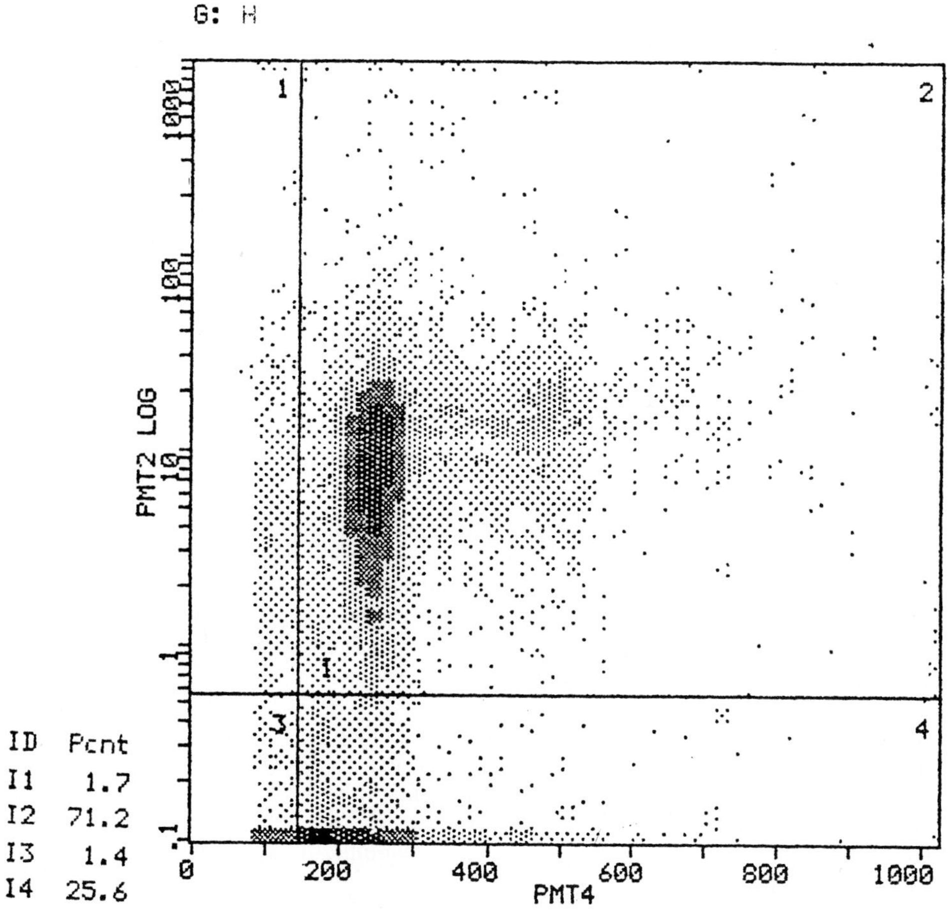

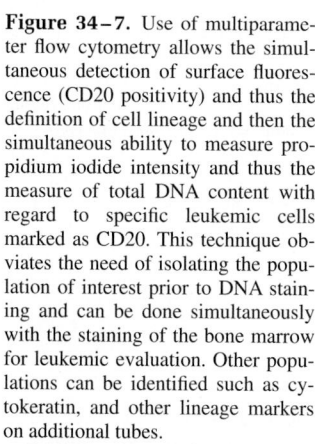

Figure 34–7. Use of multiparameter flow cytometry allows the simultaneous detection of surface fluorescence (CD20 positivity) and thus the definition of cell lineage and then the simultaneous ability to measure propidium iodide intensity and thus the measure of total DNA content with regard to specific leukemic cells marked as CD20. This technique obviates the need of isolating the population of interest prior to DNA staining and can be done simultaneously with the staining of the bone marrow for leukemic evaluation. Other populations can be identified such as cytokeratin, and other lineage markers on additional tubes.

Bone marrow sample was stained with CD20 FITC (Coulter, Miami, FL) and then fixed using methanol, permeabilized using 0.1% Triton X, and stained with standard RNAse, propidium iodide (PI) solution. Peripheral blood lymphocytes were used as normal, noncycling control (data not shown).

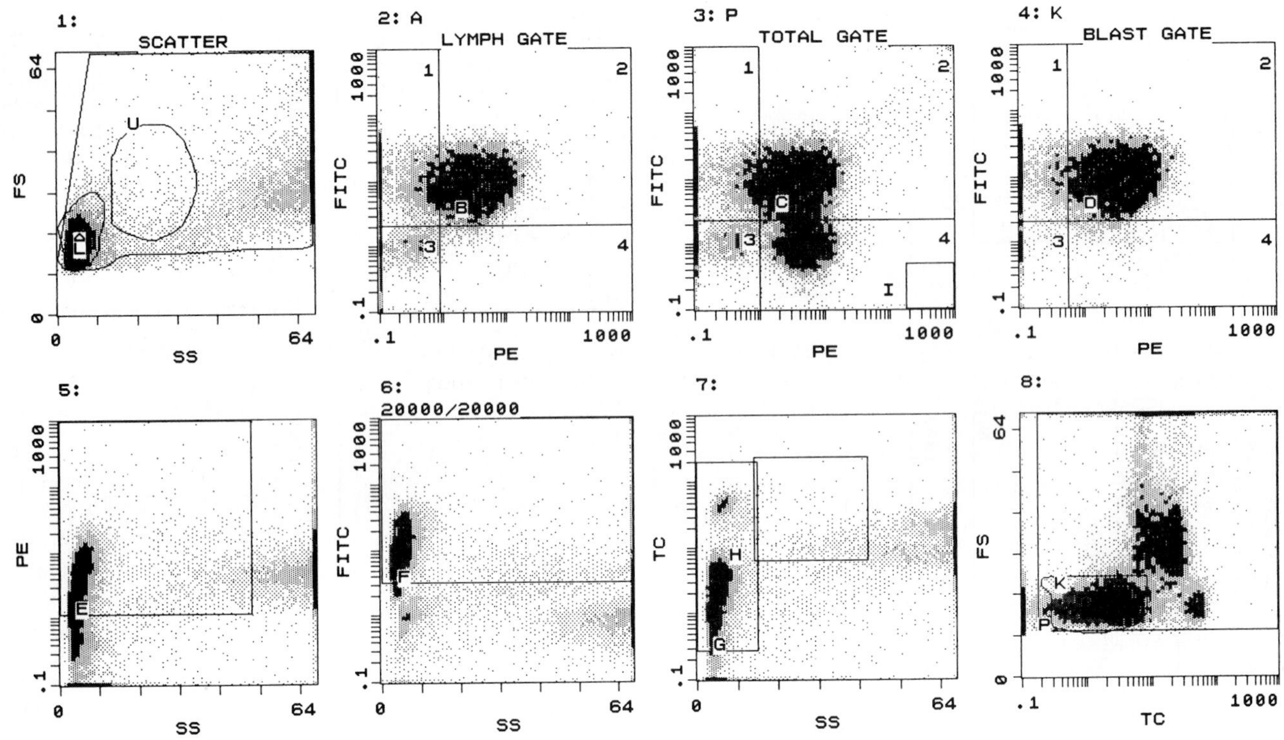

BONE MARROW 45 GATE
CD34/CD33/CD45

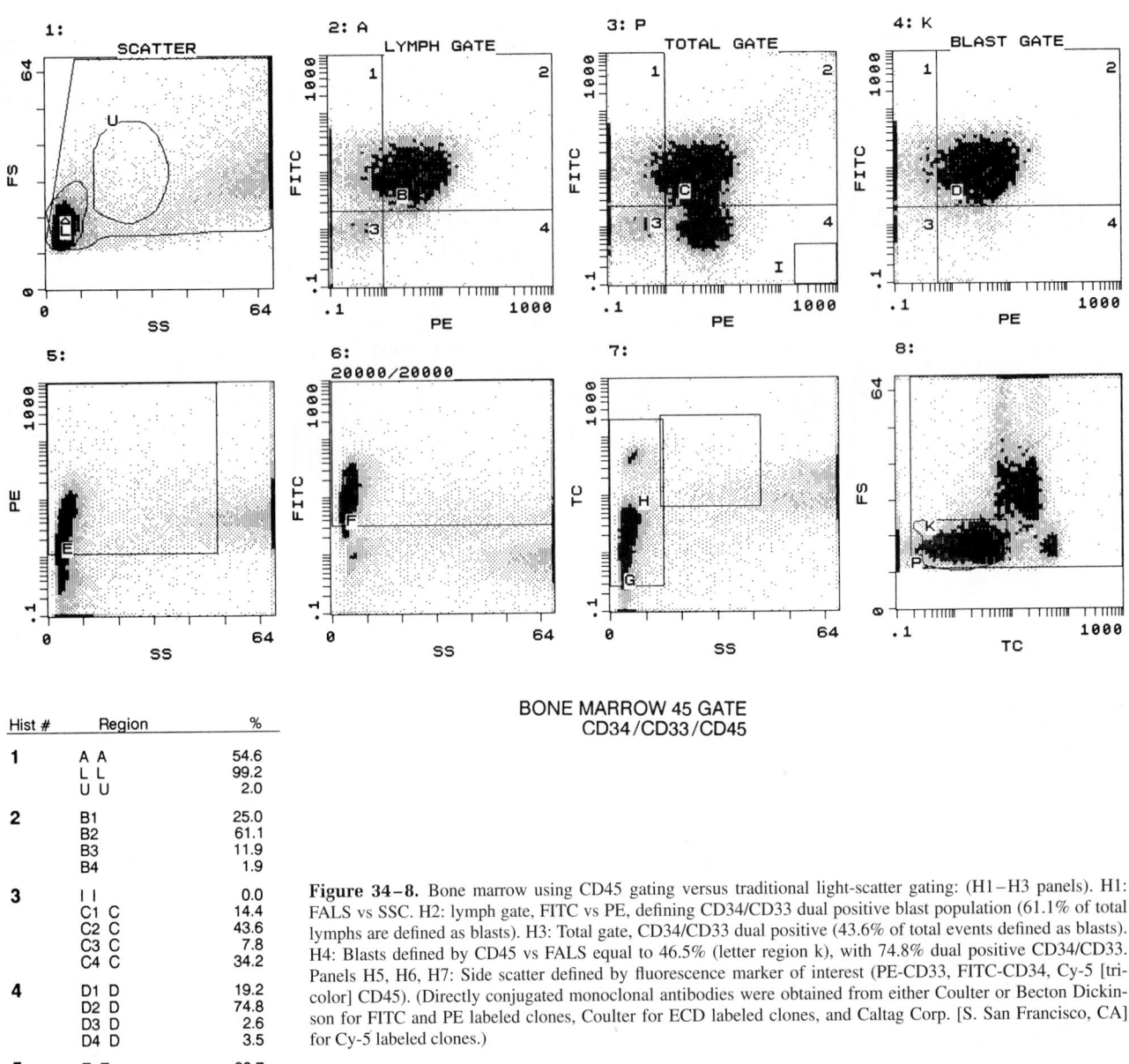

Hist #	Region	%
1	A A	54.6
	L L	99.2
	U U	2.0
2	B1	25.0
	B2	61.1
	B3	11.9
	B4	1.9
3	I I	0.0
	C1 C	14.4
	C2 C	43.6
	C3 C	7.8
	C4 C	34.2
4	D1 D	19.2
	D2 D	74.8
	D3 D	2.6
	D4 D	3.5
5	E E	38.7
6	F F	54.1
7	G G	51.3
	H H	2.8
8	K K	46.5
	P P	94.8

Figure 34–8. Bone marrow using CD45 gating versus traditional light-scatter gating: (H1–H3 panels). H1: FALS vs SSC. H2: lymph gate, FITC vs PE, defining CD34/CD33 dual positive blast population (61.1% of total lymphs are defined as blasts). H3: Total gate, CD34/CD33 dual positive (43.6% of total events defined as blasts). H4: Blasts defined by CD45 vs FALS equal to 46.5% (letter region k), with 74.8% dual positive CD34/CD33. Panels H5, H6, H7: Side scatter defined by fluorescence marker of interest (PE-CD33, FITC-CD34, Cy-5 [tri-color] CD45). (Directly conjugated monoclonal antibodies were obtained from either Coulter or Becton Dickinson for FITC and PE labeled clones, Coulter for ECD labeled clones, and Caltag Corp. [S. San Francisco, CA] for Cy-5 labeled clones.)

has simplified the analysis of bone marrow, leukemias, and HIV panels. In bone marrow and leukemia workups, the CD45 is usually set as the third or fourth color and is paired either with forward light scatter or side scatter; this allows the definition of a potential blast (malignant) population. The blast population is then defined using a panel of monoclonals using the three color parameters available (see Figs. 34–8 and 34–9*A* and *B*). In the HIV, one-tube, four-color method, CD45 allows the definition of a large lymphocyte-gated region, which is secondarily gated for CD45. This can also be done without the use of the light scatter parameters, as previously described. (This can also be done using a two-tube, three-color panel.)

Another gating strategy is the use of two- or three-color definition of a particular subset of interest. This approach, commonly now referred to as an anchor gate, uses the particular properties of some cells to investigate another set of parameters. When applied specifically to T cells, it is referred to as a T-gate (Mandy, 1992). Use of an anchor gate (Paxton, 1994) is especially useful when looking at activation markers, as in the HIV subsets of CD3/CD8 expressing CD38 and HLA-DR or looking at the expression of CD45Ra and CD45Ro against either CD3/CD4 or CD3/CD8. The advantage of this method is that it is intuitive and each color acts as a quality control check for the other subset (Figs. 34–10 to 34–13). Further, we have the choice to define the expression of biologically relevant markers in relation to functional or biologically relevant populations. This approach lends itself well to quantitative fluorescence (see histograms 2 and 3, respectively). Although the concept of quantitative fluorescence is not new, the techniques to measure fluorescence equivalents or fluorescence thresholds or other similar designations are. Quantitative fluorescent measurements will be described after DNA gating and analysis. Another approach to anchor gating is in CD34 harvesting, which uses CD34 staining and PI in the identification of CD34 progenitor cells. This method has great utility in bone marrow transplantation protocols in which progenitor cells are harvested from cord blood or peripheral blood (Bender, 1991; O'Gorman, 1995) (Fig. 34–14*A* to *E*).

DNA Analysis

Conceptually, the performance of DNA analysis should be more simple than immunophenotyping analysis, but the review of published data and its prognostic capabilities as well as performance by laboratories on proficiency tests indicates otherwise (Nicholson, 1993; Coon, 1994). A DNA consensus conference was held and the proceedings published in *Cytometry* (Shankey, 1993). This report reviewed major tumor types and the clinical value of the performance of ploidy by DI and the value of S-phase. These parameters were analyzed in terms of their effectiveness as prognostic markers. The 1994 CAP conference #26 looked at the previous markers and some additional potential tumor surrogates. In each case, the DI and S-phase were less predictable as prognostic markers than hoped. This was largely attributed to the variability in the performance and analysis of these assays and in the definition of tumor heterogeneity and therefore the appropriate sampling of the tumor. Specific recommendations were made in each tumor type for the appropriate quality control measurements that should be performed and the proper deconvolution of the histograms.

Sample Preparation

DNA preparative methods are reasonably simple and inexpensive to perform. Many references for the original methods exist, as well as many modifications. The most common methods are those used on fresh and frozen tissues developed by Krishan, Vindelov, Crissman, Steinkamp, and others (Rabinovitch, 1993; Vindelov, 1994) and those used on paraffin blocks with preparations of Hedley (1983). In each case, whether the cells are enucleated or the cell membrane is preserved, the DNA dye PI is the most commonly used in most clinical laboratories and has already been described. PI staining is straightforward as long as timing, saturation, and removal of RNA parameters are followed. Measures of the gross karyotic abnormalities are made by comparing the peak (fluorescence intensity, PI uptake) of the tumor versus a diploid calibrator. Factors affecting this measurement include the CV of the peaks for both the calibrator and suspected tumor, the G2/G1 ratio, or the linearity of the instrument and percent of tumor present (sampling) in the sample. It is not unusual to find laboratories reporting out a diploid tumor result on a sample containing "no" tumor. Tumors with near diploid values need stringent rules of interpretation, as does the definition of tetraploidy. Further problems occur in the definition of aggregates, doublets, debris, treatment of sliced and cut nuclei, and S-phase population. The descriptive and semi-quantitative acronym BAD is used by the software analysis packages to model the effects of background, aggregates, and doublets (Rabinovitch, 1993, 1994) (Figs. 34–15*A* to *C* and 34–16*A* and *B*).

The resulting S-phase and DI measurements using a single-parameter mode of analysis (PI only) is subject to these deconvolution algorithms, leading to great interlaboratory variability (Coon, 1994). These deconvolution algorithms for DNA have been extensively studied (Coon, 1994; Rabinovitch, 1993, 1994; Wheeless, 1991; Shankey, 1993), but many models used for analysis need further study. The DNA consensus document makes specific recommendations applicable to certain tumor types and suggests that laboratories perform their analyses accordingly, but even with these guidelines there remains a level of ambiguity in the interpretation and performance for the clinical laboratory. These ambiguities contribute to the discordance of results in comparative studies as well as in proficiency tests (Coon, 1988, 1994; Wheeless, 1991). The difficulty in achieving consensus makes the interpretation of results more difficult for the novice laboratory as well as for clinicians who are trying to compare their laboratory results with the recent literature in the treatment of their patients. This is especially true in the classification of S-phase values. S-phase measures are subject to the effects of debris and aggregate modeling as described by Rabinovitch (1993, 1994), Bagwell (1993), Shankey (1993), Coon (1988), Wheeless (1991), and others. The area between 2C and 4C is subject to artifactual interference. Further, it is critical that the decisions made with regard to which mathematical model is used for a particular tumor be kept constant and that the list mode data be retained without modeling in case further analysis is necessary.

The issue of binning the S-phase data as low, medium, and high or the use of tertiles (Shankey, 1993; Rabinovitch, 1994) further confuses the interpretation of results. Because of the difficulties in DNA histogram analysis, it has been suggested by some that DNA measurements should be performed only by expert laboratories. The Food and Drug Administration to date has not cleared any methods and still considers this a research test. Unfortunately, the standard of medical practice suggests otherwise. A standard or guideline such as an NCCLS document does not exist for laboratories, except as previously indicated. Therefore, stringent quality control parameters need to be followed to allow meaningful DNA measures.

Other approaches using DNA and RNA probes such as thymidine derivatives, bromodeoxyuridine (BrdU), variously abbreviated, and so (Fig. 34–17) and acridine orange (RNA) are used to improve the quality of the models in the estimation of proliferative and kinetic properties of a specific tumor. It is important to remember that proliferation measures are not the same as measures of S-phase quantitation, which are a static model or a picture in time of all the cells being analyzed. The integration of the area for the number of cells between 2C and 4C in a DNA histogram is not capable of giving any information with regard to cells "stuck" in S_0 (cells actually stop DNA synthesis) or measure the number of infiltrating normal cells that also might be proliferating.

Text continues on page 905

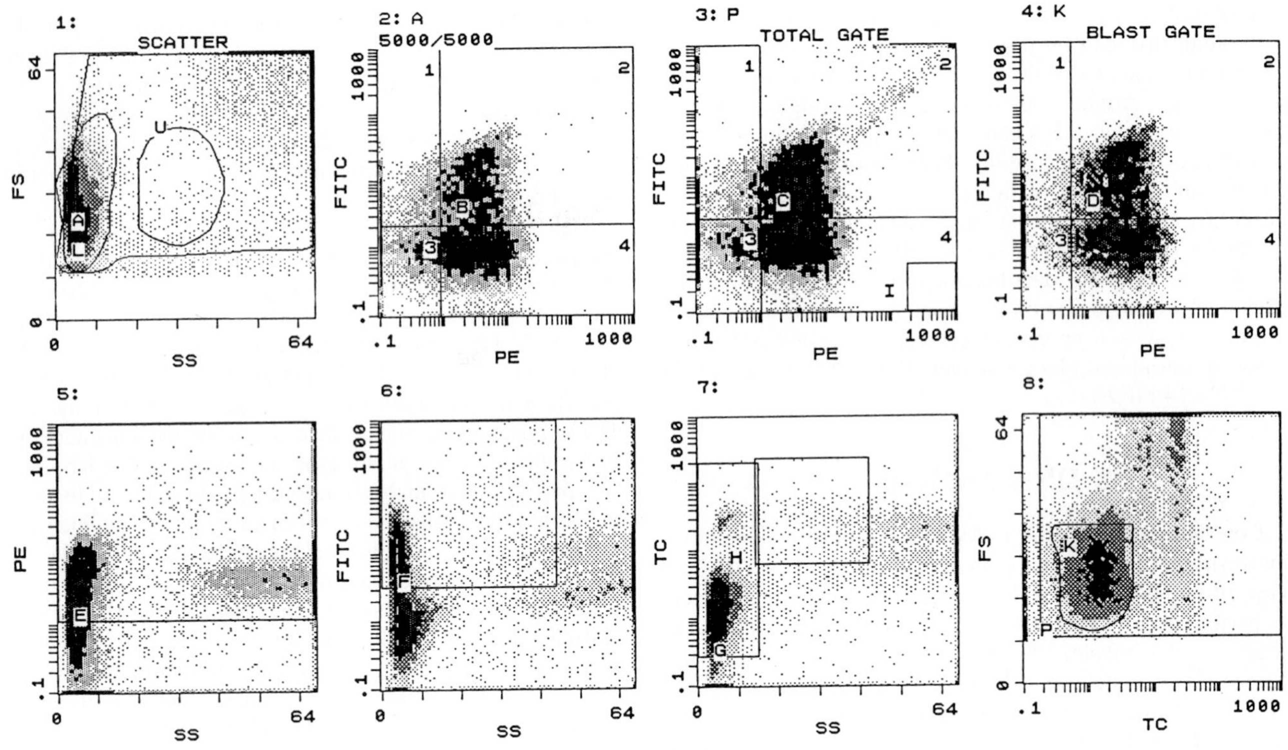

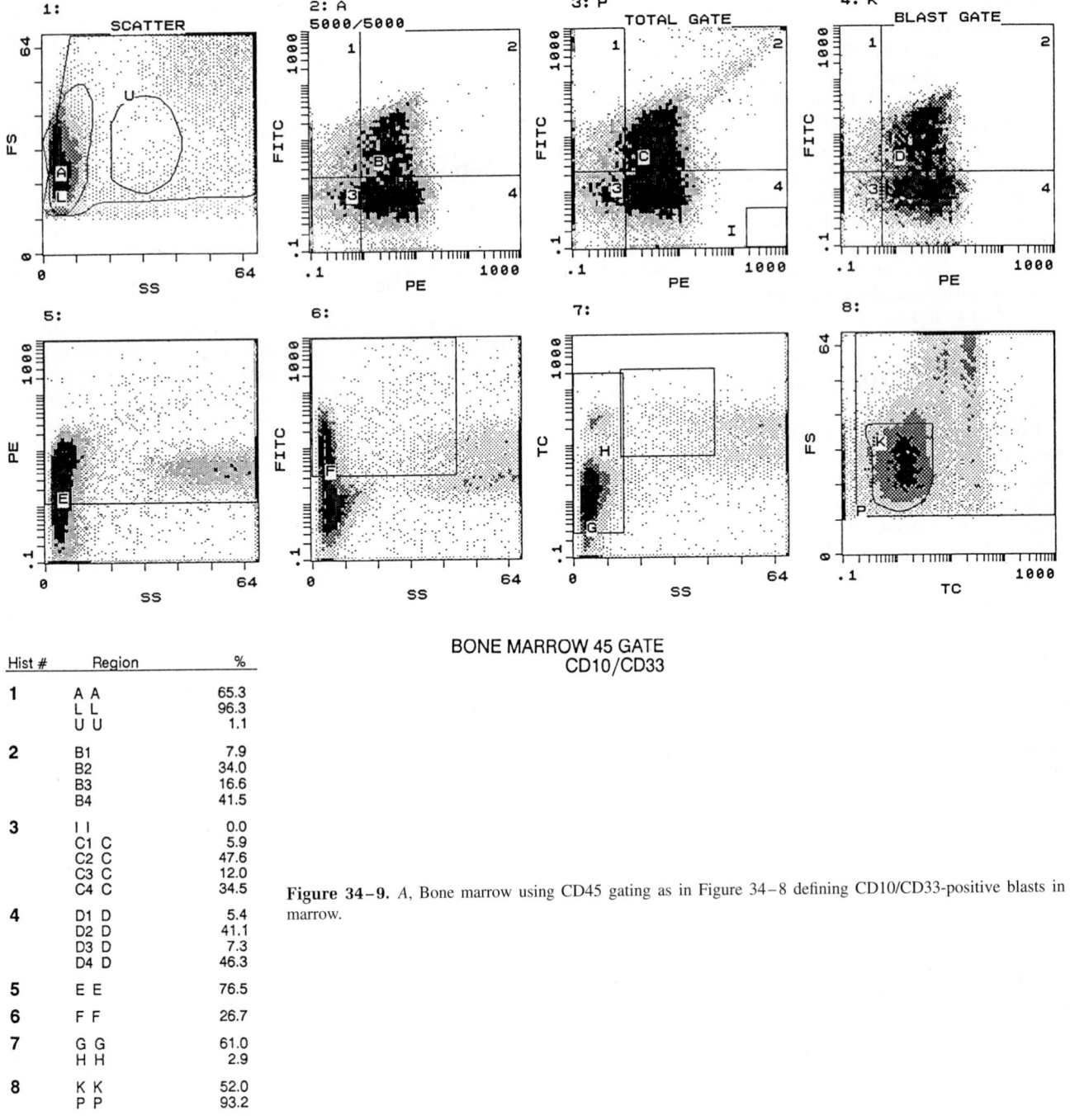

BONE MARROW 45 GATE
CD10/CD33

Hist #	Region	%
1	A A	65.3
	L L	96.3
	U U	1.1
2	B1	7.9
	B2	34.0
	B3	16.6
	B4	41.5
3	I I	0.0
	C1 C	5.9
	C2 C	47.6
	C3 C	12.0
	C4 C	34.5
4	D1 D	5.4
	D2 D	41.1
	D3 D	7.3
	D4 D	46.3
5	E E	76.5
6	F F	26.7
7	G G	61.0
	H H	2.9
8	K K	52.0
	P P	93.2

A

Figure 34–9. *A*, Bone marrow using CD45 gating as in Figure 34–8 defining CD10/CD33-positive blasts in marrow.

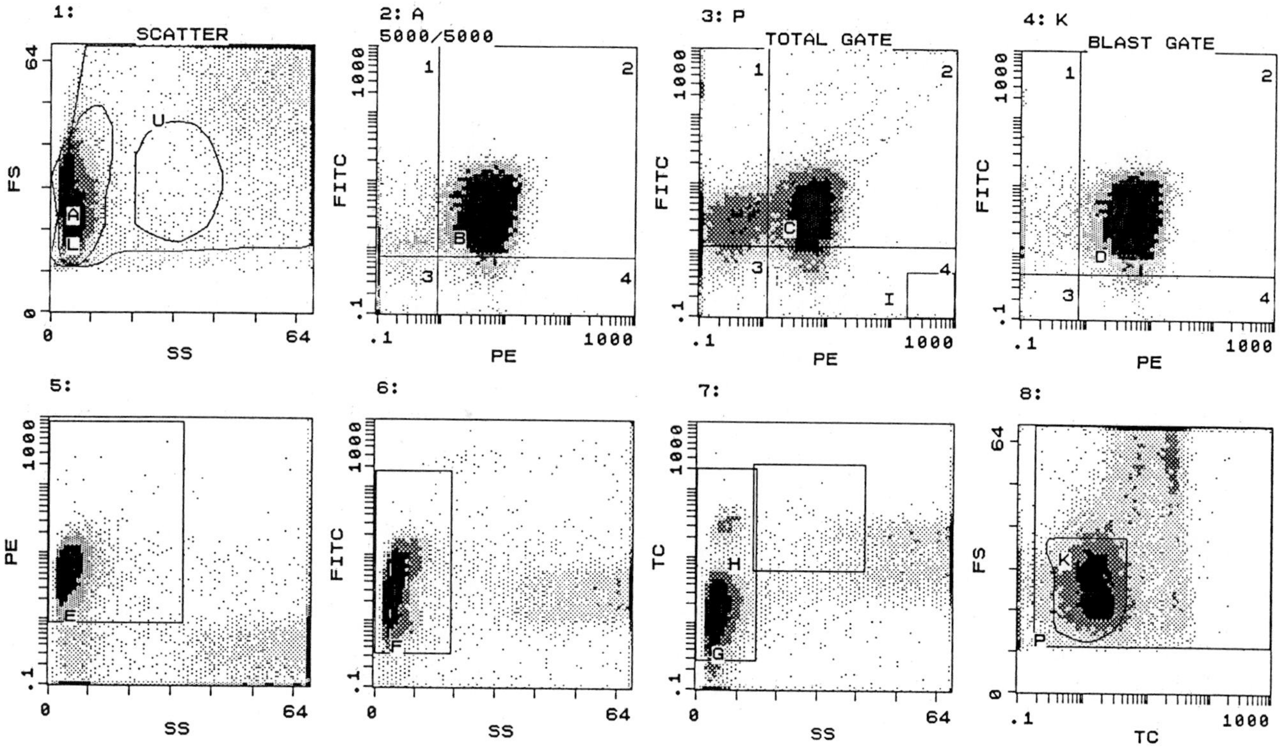

BONE MARROW 45 GATE
CD19/CD22

Hist #	Region	%
1	A A	67.9
	L L	97.3
	U U	0.9
2	B1	5.7
	B2	86.6
	B3	4.3
	B4	3.5
3	I I	0.0
	C1 C	28.3
	C2 C	59.3
	C3 C	6.1
	C4 C	6.3
4	D1 D	3.6
	D2 D	94.9
	D3 D	0.3
	D4 D	1.2
5	E E	63.6
6	F F	69.7
7	G G	65.6
	H H	2.3
8	K K	55.2
	P P	96.1

B

Figure 34–9 *Continued B*, Bone marrow using CD45 gating as in Figure 34–8 defining CD19/CD22-positive blast sin marrow.

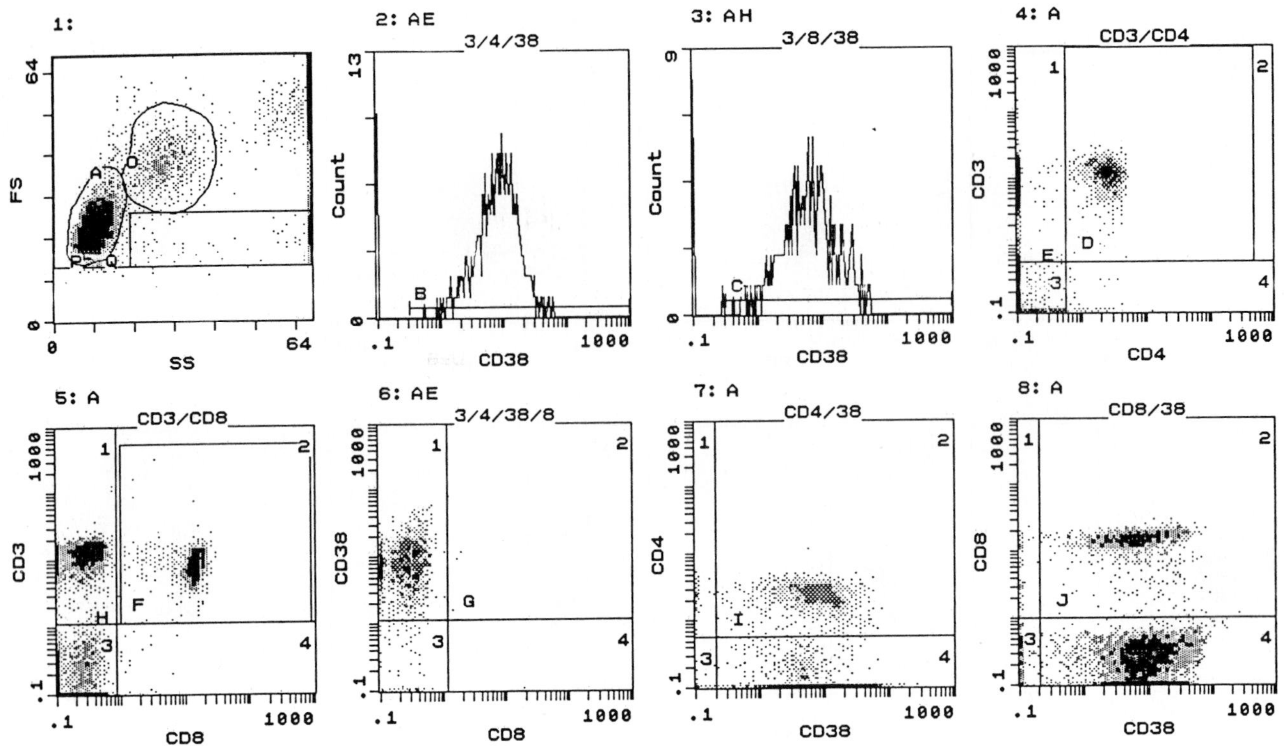

CD8/CD38/CD3/CD4

Hist #	Region	%	Count
1	A A	62.0	5000
	O O	10.4	835
	P P	99.8	8045
	Q Q	3.3	268
2	B I	96.0	1434
3	C C	95.4	1124
4	E E	29.9	1494
	D1 D	31.9	1593
	D2 D	29.9	1494
	D3 D	37.0	1850
	D4 D	1.3	63
5	H H	23.6	1178
	F1 F	34.7	1735
	F2 F	23.7	1187
	F3 F	41.1	2053
	F4 F	0.5	25
6	G1 G	93.0	1389
	G2 G	0.4	6
	G3 G	6.5	97
	G4 G	0.1	2
7	I1 I	1.1	57
	I2 I	30.0	1500
	I3 I	2.3	115
	I4 I	66.6	3328
8	J1 J	0.9	46
	J2 J	23.0	1152
	J3 J	2.5	126
	J4 J	73.5	3676

Figure 34–10. Use of four-color flow cytometry in the performance of activation studies with the use of so-called anchor gating (Paxton, 1994). In histogram 4 and 5, anchor gates defined by CD3/CD4 (letter region E) and CD3/CD8 (letter region H) are used to measure CD38. CD38 value for CD3/CD4 is in panel 2 and 4 gated on lymph region A and anchor gate E. CD38 value for CD3/CD8 is in panel 3 and 5 gated on lymph region A and anchor gate H. Histograms makes measures of CD38 against CD4 and CD8 on open gate A without defining $CD3^{+}$ cells with anchor. Panel 6, looks for four-color events defining cells as positive for CD3, CD4, CD8 and CD38. Note that there should be few events in quadrant 4 and serves as quality control for nonspecific staining. (Directly conjugated monoclonal antibodies used in these histograms were usually obtained from either Coulter or Becton Dickinson for PE and FITC, Coulter for ECD and Caltag Corp. for Cy-5 CD45. Whole blood lysing was performed using a Coulter Q-prep using standard manufacturer's protocol.)

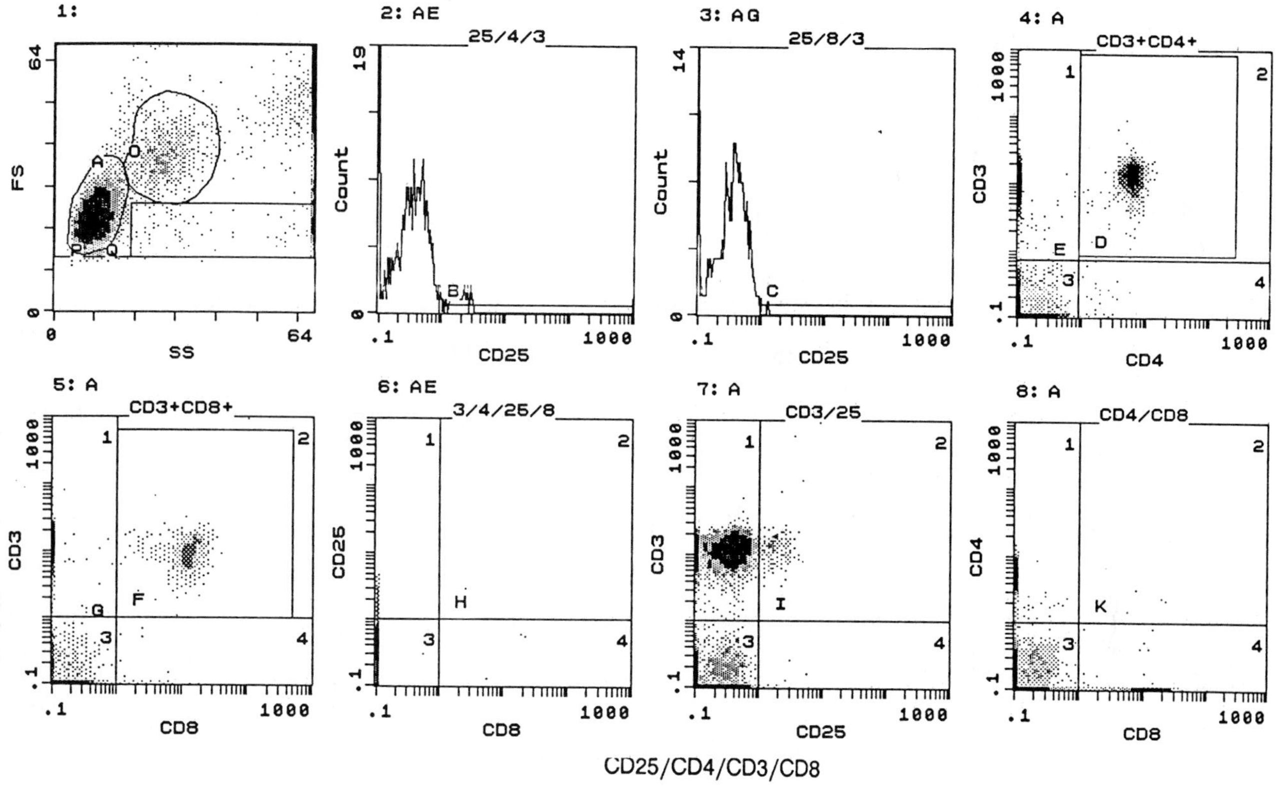

Hist #	Region	%	Count
1	A A	61.2	5000
	O O	10.7	872
	P P	99.8	8151
	Q Q	3.2	261
2	B B	8.3	133
3	C C	1.3	14
4	E E	31.9	1593
	D1 D	27.0	1352
	D2 D	31.9	1595
	D3 D	40.4	2019
	D4 D	0.7	34
5	G G	22.1	1104
	F1 F	36.6	1832
	F2 F	22.1	1105
	F3 F	40.5	2026
	F4 F	0.7	37
6	H1 H	8.7	138
	H2 H	0.1	2
	H3 H	91.0	1450
	H4 H	0.2	3
7	I1 I	54.8	2740
	I2 I	3.9	197
	I3 I	41.0	2049
	I4 I	0.3	14
8	K1 K	32.4	1620
	K2 K	0.1	5
	K3 K	44.8	2238
	K4 K	22.7	1137

Figure 34–11. Use of four-color flow cytometry in the performance of activation studies with the use of so-called anchor gating as in Figure 34–10. In this case, CD25 up-regulation is being measured on CD3/CD4 and CD3/CD8 anchor gates. Use of single parameter histograms (2, 3) allows the quantitative measurements of fluorescence intensity. Use of digital pulse processing allows the linear measurement and therefore a more accurate and reproducible representation of signal (Auer, 1994).

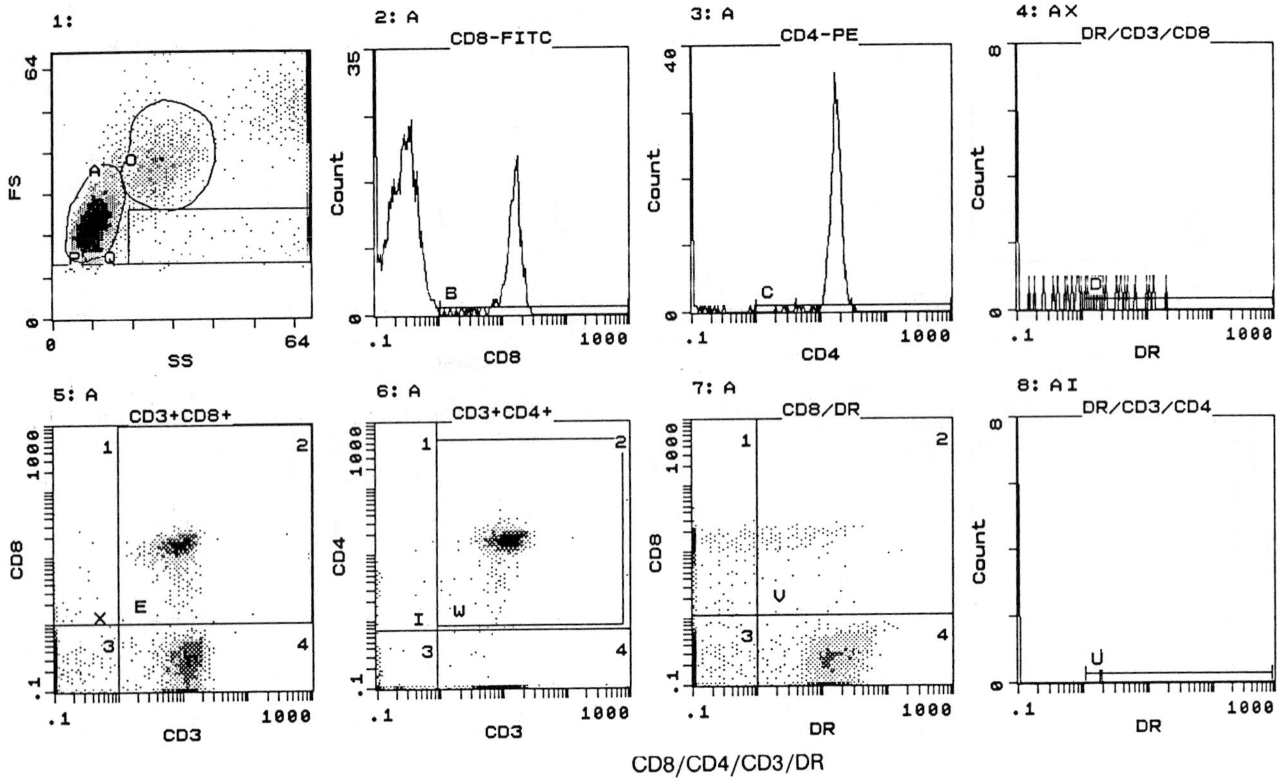

Hist #	Region	%	Count
1	A A	60.9	5000
	O O	11.3	932
	P P	99.7	8189
	Q Q	3.2	261
2	B B	24.8	1241
3	C C	33.9	1696
4	D D	11.0	132
5	X F	24.0	1201
	E1 E	0.8	40
	E2 E	24.0	1201
	E3 E	38.7	1937
	E4 E	36.4	1822
6	I I	33.3	1665
	W1 H	0.6	32
	W2 H	33.4	1672
	W3 H	38.8	1941
	W4 H	27.1	1355
7	V1 H	22.0	1100
	V2 H	2.8	138
	V3 H	38.3	1913
	V4 H	37.0	1849
8	U G	1.9	32

Figure 34–12. Use of four-color flow cytometry in the performance of activation studies with the use of anchor gating as in Figures 34–10 and 34–11. In this case, HLA-DR is used in place of CD25.

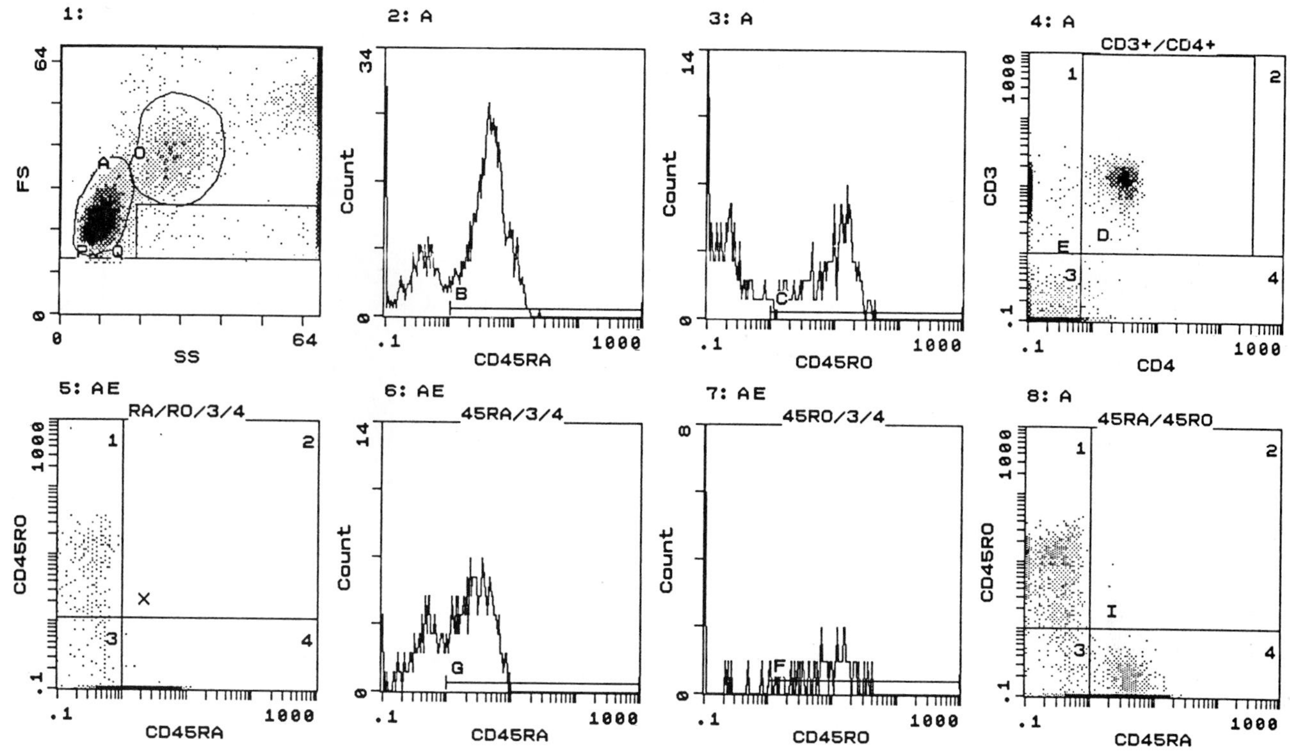

Hist #	Region	%	Count
1	A A	61.8	5000
	O O	10.5	849
	P P	99.7	8069
	Q Q	3.1	254
2	B B	72.6	3630
3	C C	18.5	923
4	E E	30.7	1534
	D1 D	28.0	1402
	D2 D	30.7	1534
	D3 D	39.0	1949
	D4 D	2.3	115
5	X1 F	16.1	247
	X2 F	0.0	0
	X3 F	17.1	263
	X4 F	66.8	1024
6	G G	66.9	1027
7	F F	16.6	254
8	I1 I	18.4	918
	I2 I	0.0	2
	I3 I	8.6	431
	I4 I	73.0	3649

Figure 34–13. Four-color flow cytometry in the performance of functional studies allows the study of reciprocal cell populations as in the study of CD45Ro (defined as memory) and CD45Ra (defined as functionally naive) on a particular T-cell subset. This figure demonstrates the definition of an anchor (Paxton, 1994) of CD3/CD4 (region E) evaluated in histograms 5, 6, and 7 for expression of RA/RO expression. Histograms 2, 3, and 8 measure RA/RO on non-CD4 cells. This can be used as a comparative measure to the CD3/CD4 without going to a second tube. Five-color fluorescence would allow the simultaneous use of CD8, which would be measured and compared with CD4. Note again the clear, absence of nonspecific staining now available using directly conjugated clones. Use of digital pulse processing allows the direct quantitation of these markers in fluorescence equivalents and comparison from time point to time point in a longitudinal study using single parameter histograms, as in histograms 2, 3, 6, and 7. (Directly conjugated monoclonal antibodies for CD45Ra and CD45Ro were obtained from either Coulter or Becton Dickinson. All assays were performed using standard whole blood lysing methods.)

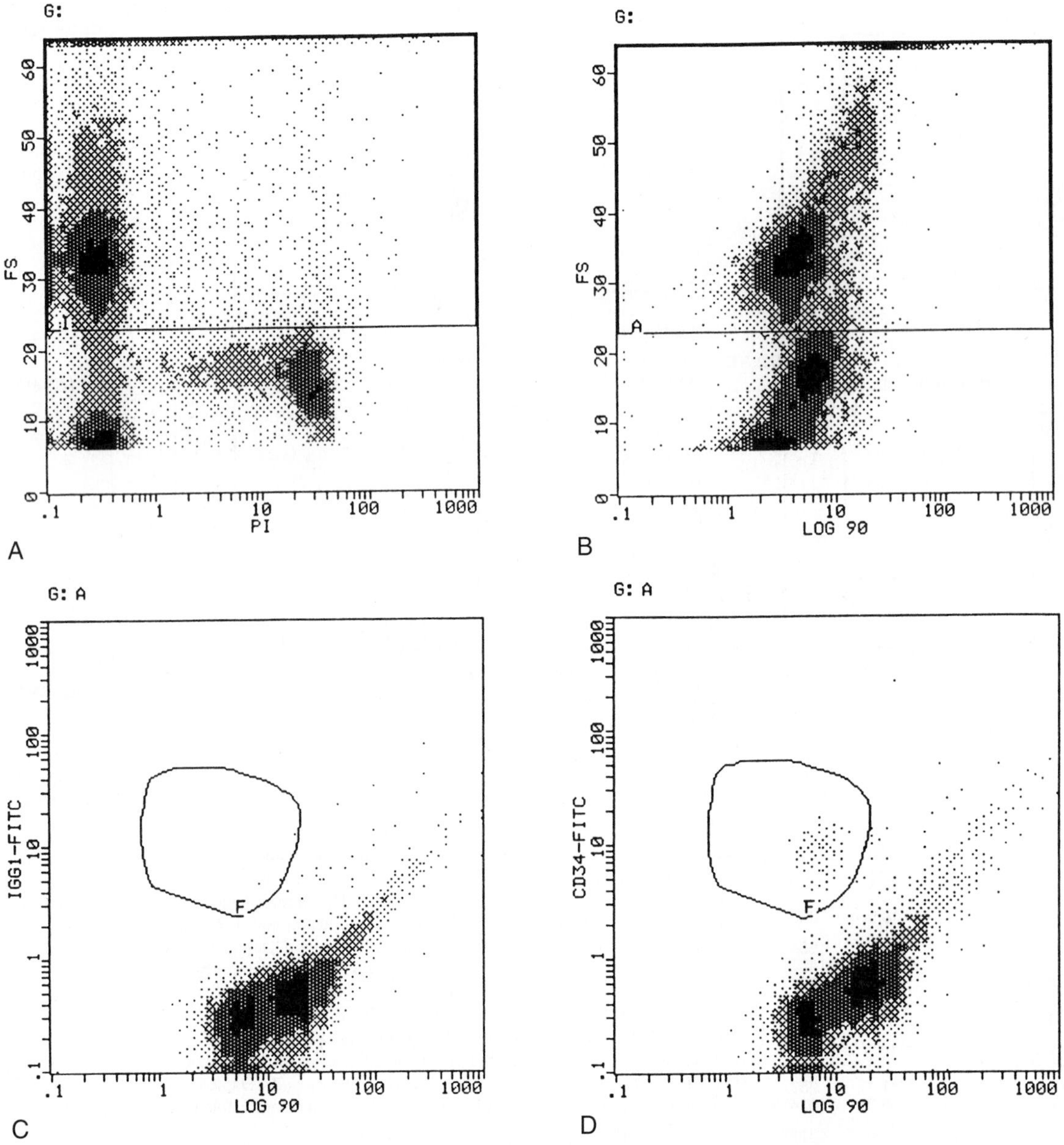

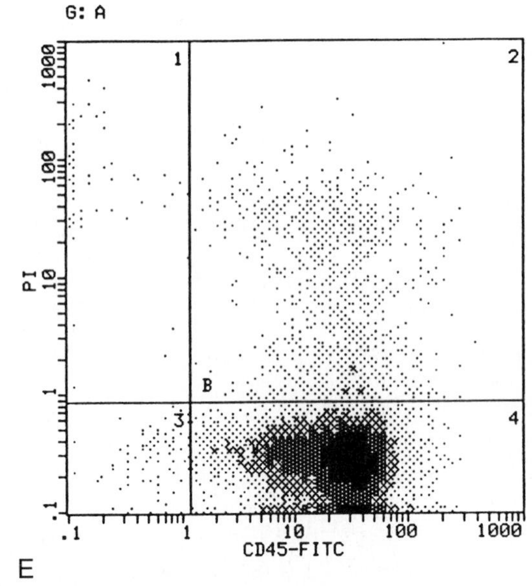

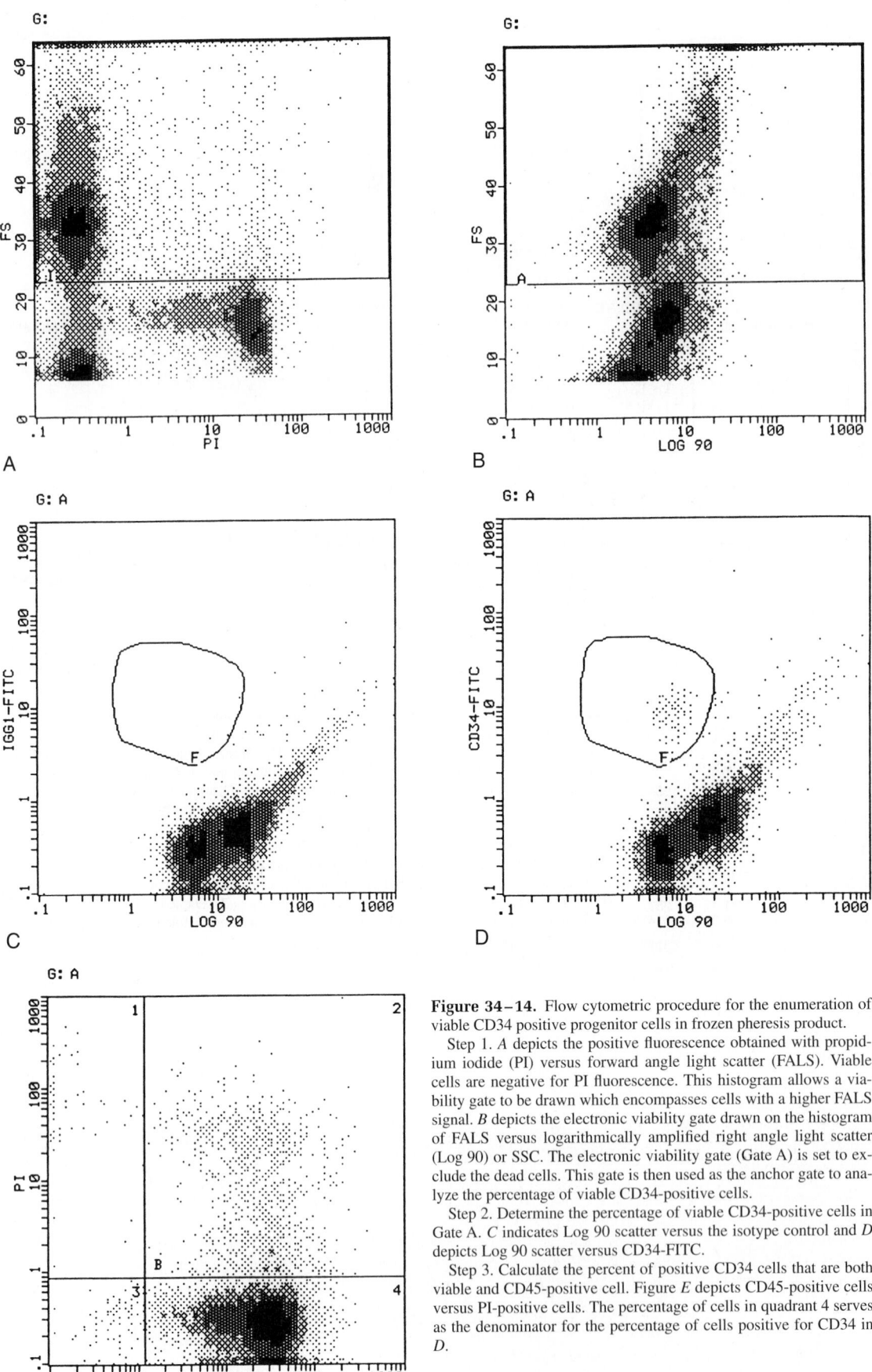

Figure 34–14. Flow cytometric procedure for the enumeration of viable CD34 positive progenitor cells in frozen pheresis product.

Step 1. *A* depicts the positive fluorescence obtained with propidium iodide (PI) versus forward angle light scatter (FALS). Viable cells are negative for PI fluorescence. This histogram allows a viability gate to be drawn which encompasses cells with a higher FALS signal. *B* depicts the electronic viability gate drawn on the histogram of FALS versus logarithmically amplified right angle light scatter (Log 90) or SSC. The electronic viability gate (Gate A) is set to exclude the dead cells. This gate is then used as the anchor gate to analyze the percentage of viable CD34-positive cells.

Step 2. Determine the percentage of viable CD34-positive cells in Gate A. *C* indicates Log 90 scatter versus the isotype control and *D* depicts Log 90 scatter versus CD34-FITC.

Step 3. Calculate the percent of positive CD34 cells that are both viable and CD45-positive cell. Figure *E* depicts CD45-positive cells versus PI-positive cells. The percentage of cells in quadrant 4 serves as the denominator for the percentage of cells positive for CD34 in *D*.

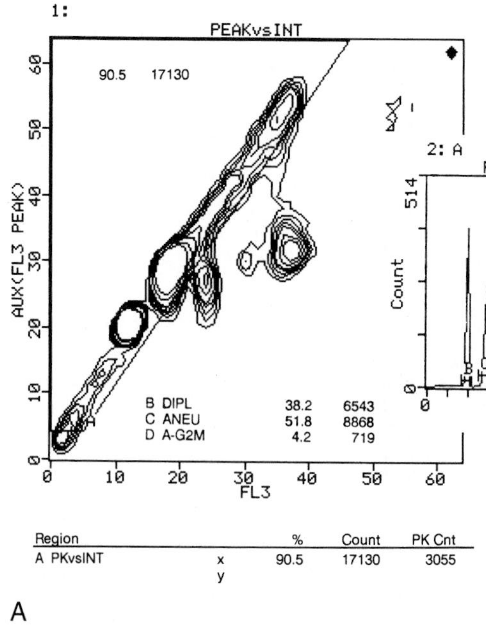

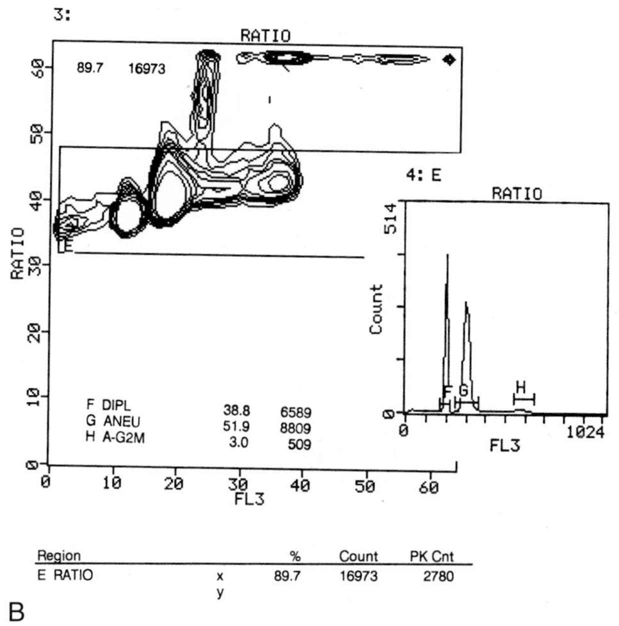

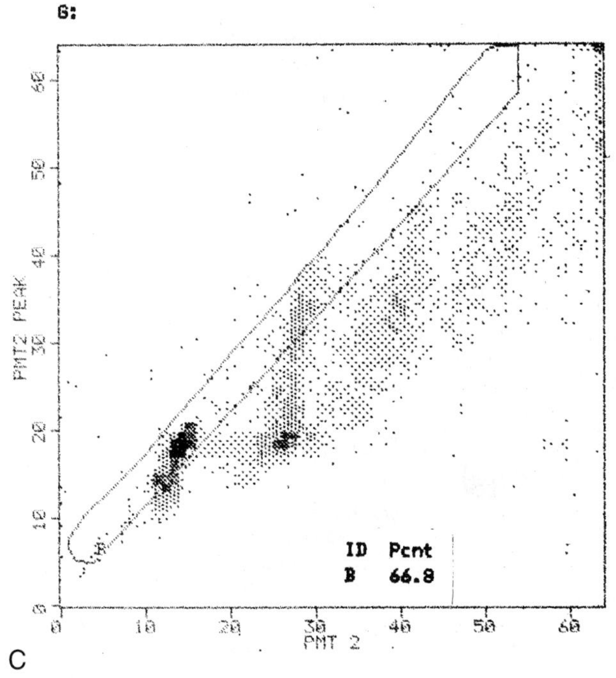

Figure 34–15. Use of different approaches to gating for DNA analysis. *A* demonstrates traditional peak versus integral with corresponding exclusion of doublets. Single-parameter histogram (insert) demonstrates linear propidium iodide (PI) intensity demonstrating diploid peak (2N) and aneuploid G_0/G_1 peak with corresponding G_2M. *B* demonstrates new method of gating (Bauer, personal communications [1994]) using the ratio of peak versus integral measurement versus FL3 (area). This method is being evaluated for greater consistency in the evaluation of S-phase values. *C* Peak versus integral demonstrating that 66.8% of the events are falling within the gated population (peak versus integral, gate b).

5

The S-phase value may often be higher than the actual proliferative capacity owing to artifacts of tumor heterogeneity. The single-parameter histogram yields reasonable results when dealing with an asynchronous, relatively homogeneous cell population. Pulse labeling is most commonly used in larger academic settings and is most often used to measure the effectiveness of radiation and chemotherapy by obtaining true measures of the $G_0/G1$ cells as well as $G2 + M$ compartments, which are not possible using single-parameter measures of S-phase.

Other approaches using nuclear and cytoplasmic probes as well as surface markers can be used to separate a population of interest from a mixture of cell types. This type of multiparameter analysis is especially useful in the measure of S-phase in hematologic malignancies (see Fig. 34–7). Specific blast populations can be identified by FITC fluorescence and FALS, and those events analyzed for DNA content and S-phase using PI. Staining methods are altered to preserve cell surface properties or nuclear properties (Clevenger, 1993; Ramaekers, 1993; Carothers, 1994; Bauer, 1994). These methods usually involve staining the surface marker of interest with the monoclonal antibody, fixing in an alcohol, then treating with a detergent to allow penetration of PI or other nuclear dye. Staining methods are selectively modified to preserve specific membrane and nuclear properties specific to the probe of interest (Bauer, 1994).

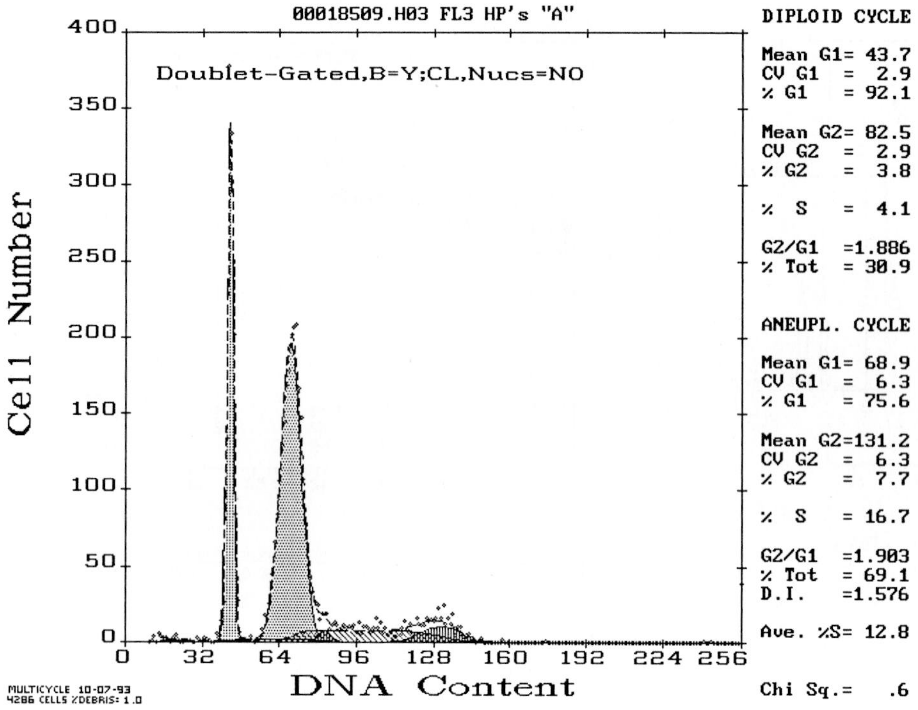

A

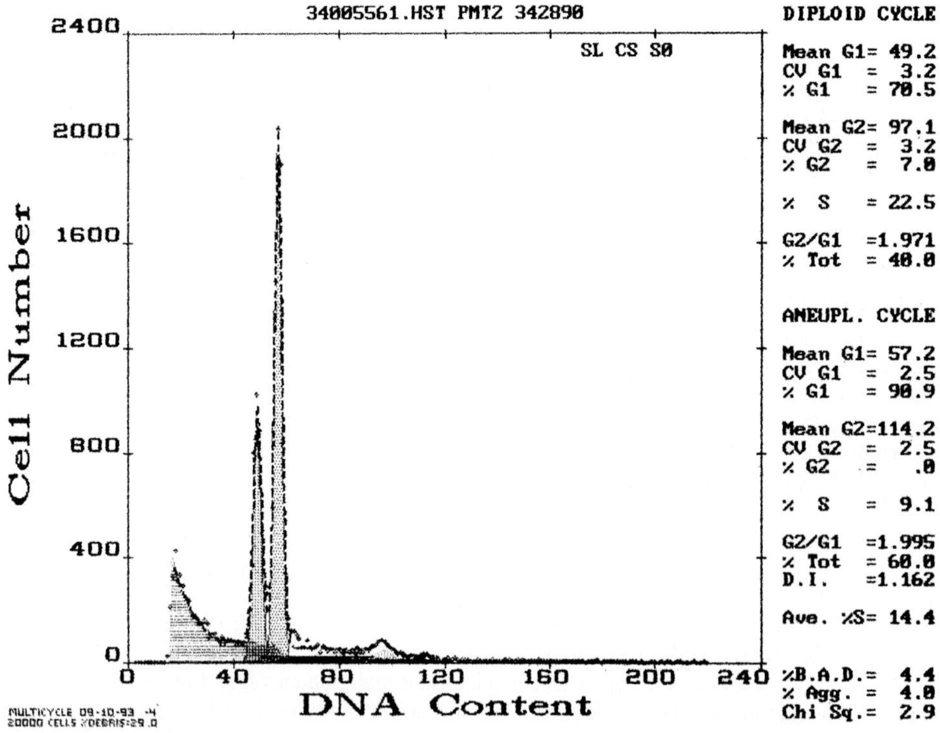

B

Figure 34–16. *A* and *B* demonstrate the use of a computer-modeling approach on two different sample types. In *A*, a fixed cell line preparation is demonstrated. This sample shows little debris and good recovery of aneuploid population. Both populations demonstrate good CVs. S-phase value is consistent for a cell line specimen. In *B*, a paraffin section sample is demonstrated with the presence of debris and a near-diploid aneuploid peak. CVs are good, and debris is minimum. Sample demonstrates an S-phase of 9%. (Multicycle Software, Phoenix Flow System, San Diego, CA.)

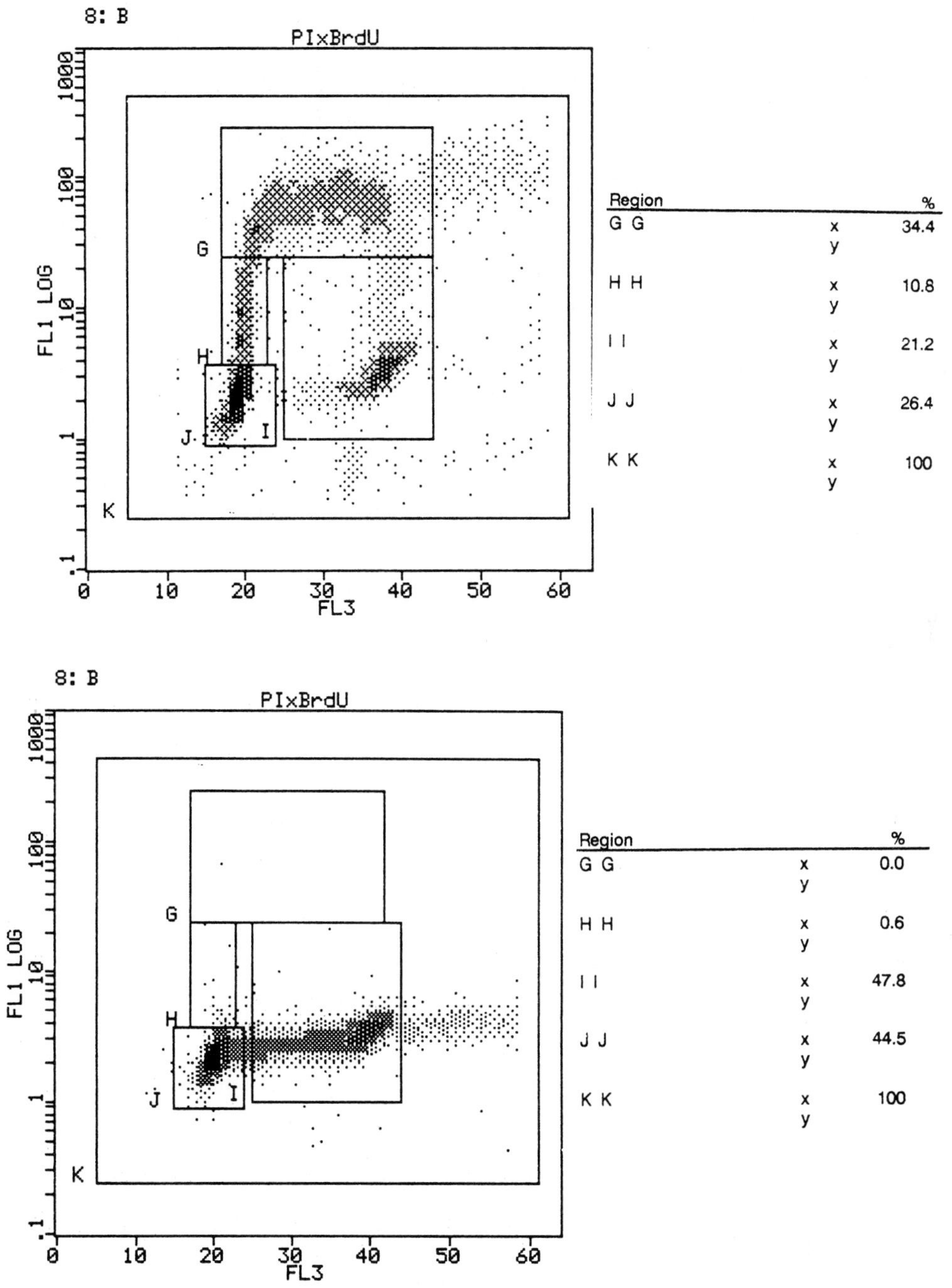

Figure 34–17. These histograms demonstrate the use of multiparameter DNA analysis using BrdU as a nuclear probe. This was performed using an exponentially growing CEM cell line that was pulsed with BrdU and then labeled with an anti-BrdU FITC antibody and stained for DNA content with propidium iodide (PI). The lower figure demonstrates a negative control (noncycling cell line or peripheral blood lymphocytes [PBLs]) used to validate the BrdU staining. Negative controls are mandatory in the successful interpretation of these analyses. These studies give a better understanding of the cells in cycle and which phase of the cell cycle they are in.

Quantitative Fluorescence Measurements

The definition of cell types in immunologic terms such as effector cells implies the property of these cells to regulate, whether up or down, specific molecular functions through surface receptors. Known as immunologic phenotypes (Poncelet, 1993), these cells need other measurable properties to define their biological roles in maturation and in disease processes. One of the observed phenomena is the differential expression of cell surface antigens (CDs) in relative terms and in absolute quantitative terms. Before the availability of absolute measures, descriptive terms such as bright or dim, bimodal, and so forth were used in the literature to describe a visual phenomenon of antigen density differences. Although descriptive, these terms are hard to define and to standardize between laboratories and between patients. They also lack precision in defining an event and cannot be objectively used to monitor patients' treatment or call definition (cell type) by measures of CD expression and their overlapping expression. Evidence suggests that quantitative differences in antigen expression in chronic lymphocytic leukemia and other leukemias may be important in determining the prognosis (Poncelet, 1986). These measures are also used in the definition of residual disease and in the investigation of a viral effect or activation in HIV disease (Tamalet, 1991). The percent of a specific cell present often does not give the true clinical picture. This is particularly true in leukopenic cases and when the blast population is a relatively small percentage of total cells present.

Investigators (Poncelet, 1985, 1986; Schwartz, 1994; Vogt, 1991) have described the use of polystyrene beads or cell lines coated with saturating amounts of antibody to determine the absolute number of receptors or antigenic sites per cell, also referred to as antigen density (Poncelet, 1993). It is important to point out that variations in immunophenotyping percentages occur if staining antibodies are not used at saturating concentrations, resulting in incorrect results. Although this phenomenon is well known and has been extensively documented and described, monoclonal antibody users, in trying to be cost conscious by diluting commercial clones, often fall into this trap, as demonstrated in proficiency surveys (Homberger, 1993). The use of fluorescence intensity measurements should give the user a means to avoid this situation.

The use of cell lines or microbeads to build a standard curve follows certain assumptions (modified from Poncelet, 1986):

1. Antibodies at saturating conditions should bind to cell surface through monovalent interaction.
2. The number of antigenic sites per cell can be inferred from the amount of bound antibody.
3. Fluorescence intensity can be related by using a calibration curve with cells of different antigen expression or with beads coated with different amounts of mouse immunoglobulin at saturating antibody concentrations. These measures are subject to variation of binding capacity of specific monoclonal antibodies to the mouse immunoglobulin as well as the polystyrene interactions with specific clones. These measures may not be able to be transferred from laboratory to laboratory and may not be the same for different manufacturers' monoclonals of the same specificity (Schwartz, 1994; Paxton, 1995).
4. Mean channel fluorescence intensity of these particles as measured by flow cytometry can then be used to estimate the molecule of equivalent soluble fluorochrome of a particular cell.
5. These measures, if performed by an indirect measure using a constant source of goat anti-mouse immunoglobulin, are independent of subclass of antibody used to define the antigen.
6. These measures can also be performed using directly conjugated monoclonals at saturation using appropriate bead standards. More care has to be taken to avoid spatial problems relative to the size of fluorochrome molecule and fluorescein/protein ratios.

These models are still novel to most laboratories, and technical issues remain, but these approaches help define malignant and biologically relevant cell types based on quantitative antigen expression. The differential expression of specific antigens helps define normal from aberrant populations and mature from immature. These measurements can also be used to establish clonality and surface immunoglobulin expression in a more quantitative manner.

Although early in its development, quantitative phenotypes will help us define cluster analysis software programs for cell quantification and identification by establishing mean channel fluorescence intensity as a means of separating cells of different functional phenotypes.

QUALITY CONTROL AND QUALITY ASSURANCE IN THE CELLULAR LABORATORY

Throughout this chapter we have tried to point out areas where the clinician as well as the laboratory must pay particular attention to the methods used and the interpretations made in the evaluation of the cellular response. Quality assurance and quality control parameters are not well defined in this area of the laboratory, and few absolute standards exist as compared with chemistry analytes or humoral antibody measures. The success of the cellular laboratory rests in its approach to the problem and the longitudinal assessment of the condition being diagnosed. It was clearly pointed out that baseline studies need to be repeated if the original evaluation is performed at a time of immunologic stress.

Basic parameters of diurnal variations in lymphocyte subsets are obvious but are often forgotten or overlooked. Malone (1990) pointed out that the variability in the CD4 measures of absolute counts is 50% due to biology and the other 50% due to other technical issues. Factors affecting the longitudinal evaluation of CD4 absolute counts in a clinical trial setting have been reviewed in Fei (1993). Further, Fahey (1990) reviewed the prognostic value of both humoral and cellular assays in HIV. In other clinical cellular assays, variability is inherent in the assay owing to lack of standard formats and methods as well as reagents. Further, instrument calibration and sensitivity are not well monitored. Cytotoxic T-lymphocyte assays are particularly hard to standardize. Historic assays such as mitogen proliferation are also fraught with variability between laboratories. Therefore, laboratories offering these immunologic tests must have an extensive database by which they can interpret an individual patient's result. Cellular laboratories must establish normal ranges for their assays and be aware that adult normal ranges are not applicable to pediatric assays. This is particularly problematic because pediatric normal ranges are difficult to determine owing to lack of available subjects in the first year of life, and correct interpretation of laboratory results depends on these. Comparisons of data between laboratories (inter) should be undertaken carefully.

When available, a cellular immunology laboratory must use the available standards in the performance of flow cytometry and DNA analysis and should be aware of the state and federal regulations with regard to the laboratory including the Human Health and Services Clinical Laboratory Improvement Act of 1988. Further, they should participate in proficiency testing, when available, and be involved in continuing education seminars including competency evaluations for all personnel involved in testing. All assays performed in the laboratory must include a normal control and, when possible, in-process controls to establish the validity of the assay. Shipped samples must be carefully monitored for exposure to heat and cold and time since patient procurement. A clinical history should accompany the samples for particular studies being undertaken so that the laboratory director can take the correct approach to testing.

Many books have been written about quality control and the proper performance of specific assays and have been referred to many times in this chapter. Readers are urged to remember that the cellular laboratory is faced with a more difficult job of interpretation because the data are not easily standardized. Further, quality assurance of the sample and evaluation being performed depends on careful documentation of the biological and logistical parameters that may influence the results.

The future of tests used in the evaluation of the cellular component of the immune response resides in the development of new methods that may lend themselves to better standardization, as reviewed in this chapter.

Amaiz-Villena A, Timon M, Rodriguez-Gallego C, et al: Human T-cell activation deficiencies. Immunol Today 1992; 13:259–265.

Anderson DC, and Springer TA: Leukocyte adhesion deficiency: An inherited defect in the MAC-1, LFA-1 and p150,95 glycoproteins. Annu Rev Med 1987; 138:175–194.

Andreesen JO, Osterholz J, Lohr GW, et al: A Hodgkin cell specific antigen is expressed on a subset of auto and alloactivated T (helper) lymphoblasts. Blood 1984; 63:1299–1302.

Auer RE: From counting to quantitative measures: Realizing the potential of flow cytometry. (Abstract 365a.) ISAC Cytometry 1994; (Suppl 7): 68.

Azuma M, Daisuke I, Yagita H, et al: B70 antigen is a second ligand for CTLA-4 and CD28. Nature 1993; 366:76–79.

Bagwell BC: Theoretical aspects of flow cytometry data analysis: *In* Bauer D, Duque RE, Shankey TV (eds): Clinical Flow Cytometry: Principles and Applications. Baltimore, Williams and Wilkins, 1993, pp 41–61.

Barnes, PF, Shuzhuang L, Abrams JS, et al: Defining protective responses to pathogens: Cytokine profiles in leprosy lesions. Science 1993; 254:277–279.

Barnes RD, Bishnun NP, Holliday J: Impaired lymphocyte transformation and chromosomal abnormalities in fatal granulomatous disease in childhood. Acta Paediatr Scand 1970; 59:403–416.

Baskar S, Ostrand-Rosenberg S, Nabavi N, et al: Constitutive expression of B7 restores immunogenicity of tumor cells expressing truncated MHC class II molecules. Proc Natl Acad Sci USA 1993; 90:5687–5690.

Bastian J, Law S, Vogler L, et al: Prediction of persistent immunodeficiency in the DiGeorge anomaly. J Pediatr 1989; 115:391.

Bauer KD, Duque RE, Shankey TV: Flow cytometric analysis of granulocytes. *In* Bauer KD, Duque RE, Shankey TV (eds): Clinical Flow Cytometry: Principles and Applications. Baltimore, Williams and Wilkins, 1993, pp 405–434.

Bauer KD, Jacobberger JW: Analysis of intracellular proteins. Methods Cell Biol 1994; 41:351–376.

Beisel WR: Impact of infectious disease on the interaction between nutrition and immunity. *In* Cunninghan-Rundles S (ed): Nutrient Modulation of Immune Response. New York, Marcel Dekker, 1993, pp 475–480.

Bender JG, Unverzagt KL, Walker DE, et al: Identification and comparison of CD34-positive cells and their subpopulations for normal peripheral blood and bone marrow using multicolor flow cytometry. Blood 1991; 77:1591–1596.

Black MM, Zachrau RE, Ashikari RH, et al: Skin window reactivity to autologous breast cancer: An index of prognostically significant cell mediated immunity. Cancer 1988; 62:72–83.

Bogdan JD, Bendich A, Kemp FW, et al: Daily micronutrient supplements enhance delayed hypersensitivity skin test responses in older people. Am J Clin Nutr 1994; 60:437–447.

Bogh LD, Duling TA: Flow cytometry instrumentation in research and clinical laboratories. Clin Lab Sci 1993; 6:167–173.

Bonagura VR, Cunningham-Rundles S, Edwards BL, et al: Common variable hypogammaglobulinemia in recurrent *Pneumocystis carinii* on intravenous y-globulin therapy, and natural killer deficiency. Clin Immunol Immunopathol 1989; 51:216–231.

Bonagura VR, Cunningham-Rundles S, Shuval S: Dysfunction of natural killer cells in HIV+ children with *Pneumocystic carinii* pneumonia. J Pediatr 1992; 121:195–201.

Borowitz MJ: Acute lymphoblastic leukemia. *In* Knowles DM (ed): Neoplastic Hematopathology. Baltimore, Williams and Wilkins, 1992, pp 1295–1314.

Borut TC, Ank BJ, Gard BS, et al: Tetanus toxoid skin test in children: Correlation with in vitro lymphocyte stimulation and monocyte chemotaxis. J Pediatr 1980; 94:567–573.

Bretscher P, Wei G, Menon JN, Bielefeldt-Ohmann H: Establishment of stable cell mediated immunity that makes "susceptible" mice resistant to *Leishmania major*. Science 1992; 257:539–542.

Burnet FM: Immunological Surveillance. Oxford, England, Pergamon Press, 1970.

Calvelli TC, Denny TN, Paxton H, et al: Guideline for flow cytometric immunophenotyping: A report from the National Institute of Allergy and Infectious Diseases, Division of AIDS. Cytometry 1993; 14:702–715.

Campana D, Pui CH: Detection of minimal residual disease. Blood 1995; 85:1416–1434.

Carothers AD: Counting, measuring, and mapping in FISH-labelled cells: Sample size consideration and implications for automation. Cytometry 1994; 16:298–304.

Centers for Disease Control: Guidelines for the performance of CD4+ T-cell determinations in persons with human immunodeficiency virus infection. MMWR 1992; 41:1–17.

Centers for Disease Control: CD4 Conference, Atlanta, Georgia, June 23–24, 1993.

Chandra RK: Nutrition and the immune system. Proc Nutr Soc 1993; 52:77–84.

Chatelaine R, Varekila K Coffman RL: IL-4 induces a T_h2 response in *Leishmania major*-infected mice. J Immunol 1992; 148:1182–1187.

Chen L, Ashe S, Bradu WA, et al: Costimulation of antitumor immunity by the B7 counterreceptor for the T lymphocyte molecules CD28 and CTLA-4. Cell 1992; 71:1093–1102.

Clarke AG, MacLennan KA: The many facets of thymic involution. Immunol Today 1986; 7:204–205.

Clerici M, Shearer GM: The T_h1-T_h2 hypothesis of HIV infection: New insights. Immunol Today 1994; 15:575–581.

Clerici M, Shearer GM: A T_H1 T_H2 switch is a critical step in the etiology of HIV infection. Immunol Today 1993; 14:107–111.

Clevenger CV, Shankey TV: Cytochemistry II: Immunofluorescence measurement of intracellular antigens. *In* Bauer KD, Duque RE, Shankey TV (eds): Clinical Flow Cytometry: Principles and Applications. Baltimore, Williams and Wilkins, 1993; pp 157–175.

Cohen JJ: Cells involved in host defense: The new immunology. J Nutr Immunol 1994; 2(4):73–85.

College of American Pathology: Conference #26: Clinical relevance of prognostic markers in solid tumors. Park City, Utah, June 23–25, 1994.

College of American Pathology Flow Cytometry Proficiency Survey Summary Reports FL series, 1990–1995.

Compucyte Corp: Personal communications. Cambridge, Massachusetts, 1995.

Coon JS, Deitch AD, deVere White RW, et al: Interinstitutional variability in DNA flow cytometric analysis of tumors: The National Cancer Institute's Flow Cytometry Network (NCI-FCN) experience. Cancer 1988; 61:126–130.

Coon JS, Paxton H, Lucy L, Homberger H: Interlaboratory variation in DNA flow cytometry. Results of the College of American Pathologists' survey. Arch Pathol Lab Med 1994; 118:681–685.

Cost KM, Fineman D, Steger S: A flow cytometry-based screening assay for lymphocyte proliferation. Clin Immunol Newsletter 1993; 13:82–85.

Coulter XL: Procedure Manual. Coulter Corp., Miami, FL, 1994.

Cunningham-Rundles C, Cunningham-Rundles S, Iwata T, et al: Zinc deficiency depressed thymic hormones and T lymphocyte dysfunction in patients with hypogammaglobulinemia. Clin Immunol Exp Pathol 1981; 21:387–396.

Cunningham-Rundles C, Siegal FD, Cunningham-Rundles S, et al: Incidence of cancer in 98 patients with common varied immunodeficiency in the United States. J Clin Immunol 1987; 7:294–303.

Cummingham-Rundles S: Malnutrition and gut immune function. Curr Opin Gastroenterol 1994a; 10:664–670.

Cunningham-Rundles S, Chen C(X), Bussel JB, et al: Human immune development: Implications for congenital HIV infection. Ann NY Acad Sci 1993; 693:20–34.

Cunningham-Rundles S, Hansen JA, Dupont B: Lymphocyte transformation to antigens and mitogens. Clin Immunobiol 1976;3:151–194.

Cunningham-Rundles S, Harbison M, Guirguis S, et al: New perspectives on use of thymic factors in immune deficiency. Ann NY Acad Sci 1994b; 730:20–27.

Cunningham-Rundles S, Yeger-Arbitman, Nachman R, et al: New variant of MHC class II deficiency with interleukin-2 abnormality. Clin Immunol Immunopathol 1990; 56:116–123.

D'Ambrosio D, Cantrell DA, Frati L, et al: Involvement of p21ras activation in CD69 expression in T cells. Eur J Immunol 1994; 24:616–620.

Dardenne M, Pleau JM, Nabarra B, et al: Contribution of zinc and other metals to the biological activity of the serum thymic factor. Proc Natl Acad Sci USA 1982; 79:5370–5373.

Davis JM, Mouradian JM, Fernandez RD, et al: Acquired immunodeficiency syndrome. Arch Surg 1984; 119:90–95.

Davis MM, Bjorkman PJ: T cell antigen receptor genes and T cell recognition. Nature 1988; 334:395–402.

Denny TR, Yogeu R, Gelman R, et al: Lymphocyte subsets in healthy children during the first 5 years of life. JAMA 1992; 267:1484.

DiGeorge AM: Congenital absence of the thymus and its immunologic consequences: Concurrence with congenital hypothyroidism. *In* Bergsma D (ed): Birth Defects Immunologic Deficiency Disease in Man, Vol 4(1). White Plains, New York, The National Foundation-March of Dimes, 1974, p 116.

Emmendorffer A, Nakamura M, Rothe G, et al: Evaluation of flow cytometric methods for diagnosis of chronic granulomatous disease variant under routine laboratory conditions. Cytometry 1994; 18:147–155.

Fahey JL, Taylor JMG, Detels R, et al: The prognostic value of cellular and serologic markers in infection with human immunodeficiency virus type 1. N Engl J Med 1990; 322:166–172.

Fei DTW, Paxton H, Chen B: Difficulties in precise quantitation of CD4+ T lymphocytes for clinical trials. A review. Biologicals 1993; 21:221–231.

Fletcher MA, Moseley JE, Hassett J, et al: Effect of age on human immunodeficiency virus type-1 induced changes in lymphocyte populations among patients with congenital clotting disorders. Blood 1992; 80:831.

Gearing AJH, Thorpe R: The international standard for human interleukin-2: Calibration by international collaborative study. J Immunol Methods 1988; 334:3–15.

Gelfand EW: Abnormalities of signal transduction and T cell immunodeficiency. *In* Gupta S, Griscelli C (eds): New Concepts in Immunodeficiency Disease. New York, Wiley and Sons, 1993, pp 231–248.

Germain RN, Margulies DH: The biochemistry and cell biology of antigen processing and presentation. Annu Rev Immunol 1993; 11:403–450.

Gillis SR, Kosak R, Durante M, et al: Immunologic studies of aging: Decreased production pf and response to T cell growth factor by lymphocytes from aged humans. J Clin Invest 1981; 67:937.

Gillis SR, Smith KA: Long term culture of tumour specific cytotoxic T cell. Nature 1977; 268:154–158.

Giorgi JV, Detels RT: T-cell subsets alterations in HIV-infected homosexual men: NIAID Multicenter AIDS Cohort Study. Clin Immunol Immunopathol 1989; 52:10–18.

Goetzman EA: Flow cytometry: Basic concept and clinical applications in immunodiagnostics. Clin Lab Sci 1993; 6:177–182.

Haynes BF, Denning SM, Le PT, Singer KH: Human intrathymic T cell differentiation. Semin Immunol 1990; 2:67–77.

Hedley DW, Friedlander ML, Taylor IW, et al: Method for analysis of cellular DNA content of paraffin-embedded pathological material using flow cytometry, J Histochem Cytochem 1983; 31:1333–1335.

Hertzenberg LA, Sweet RG, Herzenberg LA, et al: Fluorescence activated cell sorting. Sci Am 1976; 234:108.

Homberger HA, Rosebstock W, Paxton H, et al: Assessment of interlaboratory variability of immunophenotyping: Results of the College of American Pathologist Flow Cytometry Survey. Ann NY Acad Sci 1993; 677:43–49.

Imboden JB, Stobo JD: Transmembrane signaling by the T cell antigen receptor: Perturbation of the T3-antigen receptor complex generated inositol phosphates and releases calcium ions from intracellular stores. J Exp Med 1985; 161:446–456.

Inkeles B, Innes JB, Kuntz MM, et al: Immunologic studies of aging III. Cytokinetic basis for the impaired response from aged humans to plant lectins. J Exp Med 1977; 145:1176.

Irving BA, Weiss A: The cytoplasmic domain of the T cell receptor zeta chain is sufficient to couple to receptor associated signal transduction pathways. Cell 1991; 64:890–901.

Janeway CA, Bottomly K: Signals and signs for lymphocyte response. Cell 1993; 76:275–285.

Kagan J, Gelman R, Waxdal M, et al: NIAID Div. of AIDS, flow cytometry quality assessment program. Ann NY Acad Sci 1993; 677:50–52.

Kagnoff MF: Immunology of the intestinal tract. (Review.) Gastroenterology 1993; 105:1275–1280.

Kamentsky LA, Melamed MR: Instrumentation for automated examination of cellular specimens. Proc IEEE 1969; 57:2007.

Katz P, Fauci AS: Immunosuppressives and immunoadjuvants. *In* Samter M, Talmage DW, Frank MM, et al (eds): Immunological Diseases, 4th ed. Boston, Little, Brown and Co., 1993, pp 675–698.

Keren DF: Surface marker assays in immunodeficiency diseases. *In* Keren DF (ed): Flow Cytometry in Clinical Diagnosis. Chicago, ASCP Press, 1989a, pp 213–247.

Keren DF (ed): Flow Cytometry in Clinical Diagnosis. Chicago, ASCP Press, 1989.

Kersey JH, Meuwissen HJ, Good RA: Graft-versus-host reactions following transplantation of allogeneic hematopoietic cells. Hum Pathol 1971; 2:389.

Kirkpatrick CH: Delayed hypersensitivity. *In* Sampter M, Talmage DW, Frank MM, et al (eds): Immunological Diseases. Boston, Little Brown and Co., 1988, pp 261–277.

Kniker WT, Anderson CT, Roumiantzeff M: The MULTITEST system: A standardized approach to evaluation of delayed type hypersensitivity and cell mediated immunity. Ann Allergy 1979; 43:73–79.

Krown SE, Real FX, Cunningham-Rundles S, et al: Preliminary observation on the effect of recombinant leukocyte A interferon in homosexual men with Kaposi's sarcoma. N Eng J Med 1983; 308:1071–1076.

Landay AL, Jessop C, Lennette ET, et al: Chronic fatigue syndrome: Clinical condition associated with immune activation. Lancet 1991; 338:707–712.

Lanier L, Philips JH, Hackett J, et al: Natural killer cells: Definition of a cell type rather than a function. J Immunol 1986; 137:2735–2741.

Leibovitz E, Riguad M, Pollack H, et al: *Pneumocystis carinii* pneumonia in infants infected with the human immunodeficiency virus with more than 450 CD_4+ T cells. N Engl J Med 1990; 323:531–533.

Lewis DE, Cytochemistry I: Cell surface immunofluorescence. *In* Bauer KD, Duque RE, Shankey TV (eds): Clinical Flow Cytometry: Principles and Applications. Baltimore, Williams and Wilkins, 1993; pp 143–156.

Linsley PS, Brady W, Grosmaire L, et al: Binding of the B cell antigen B7 to CD28 costimulates T cell proliferation and interleukin-2 mRNA accumulation. J Exp Med 1991a; 173:721–730.

Linsley PS, Brady W, Urnes M, et al: CTLA-4 is a second receptor for the B cell activation antigen B7. J Exp Med 1991b; 174:561–569.

Liu Y, Jones B, Aruffo A, et al: Heat stable antigen is a costimulatory molecule for CD4 T cell growth. J Exp Med 1992; 175:437–445.

Livingston PE, Cunningham-Rundles S, Marfleet G, et al: Inhibition of suppressor cell activity in melanoma patients by cyclophosphamide. J Biol Res Mod 1987; 6:392–493.

Lloyd A, Hickie I, Hickie C, et al: Cell-mediated immunity in patients with chronic fatigue syndrome, healthy control subjects and patients with major depression. Clin Exp Immunol 1992; 87:76–79.

Loken MR, Brosman JM, Back BA, et al: Establishing optimal lymphocyte gates for immunophenotyping by flow cytometry. Cytometry 1990; 11:453–459.

Loken MR, Shah VO, Dattilio KL, et al: Flow cytometric analysis of human bone marrow II. Normal B lymphocyte development. Blood 1987; 70:1316–1324.

Lopez-Cabrera M, Santis AG, Fernandez-Ruis E, et al: Molecular cloning, expression, and chromosomal localization of the human earliest lymphocyte activation antigen AIM/CD69, a new member of the C-type animal lectin superfamily of signal transmitting receptors. J Exp Med 1993; 178:537–547.

Madrenas J, Wange RL, Wang JL, et al: Zeta phosphorylation without ZAP-70 activation induced by TCR antagonists or partial agonists. Science 1995; 267:515–518.

Malone JL, Simms TE, Wagner KF, et al: Sources of variability in repeated T-helper lymphocyte counts from human immunodeficiency virus type1-infection patients: Total lymphocyte count fluctuations and diurnal cycle are important. J Acquir Immun Defic Syndr 1990; 3:144–151.

Mandy F, Bergeron M, Recktenwald D, et al: A simultaneous three-color T-cell subset analysis with single laser flow cytometers using T-cell gating protocol. Comparison with conventional two-color immunophenotyping method. J Immunol Methods 1992; 156:151–162.

Marsh MN, Cummins AG: The interactive role of mucosal T lymphocytes in intestinal growth, development and enteropathy. J Gastroenterol Hepatol 1993; 8:270–278.

Martin-Reay DG, Kamenstsky LA, Weinberg DS, et al: Evaluation of a new slide-based laser scanning cytometer for DNA analysis of tumors: Comparison with flow cytometry and image analysis. Am J Clin Pathol 1994; 102:432–438.

Masur H, Michelis MA, Greene JB, et al: A community acquired outbreak of *Pneumocystis carinii* pneumonia: Initial manifestation of cellular immune dysfunction. N Engl J Med 1981; 305:1431–1438.

Metcalf JA, Gallin JI, Nauseef WM, et al: Laboratory manual of neutrophil function. New York, Raven Press, 1986.

Meuwissen HJ, Gatti RA, Terasaki PI, et al: Treatment of lymphopenic hypogammaglobulemia and bone marrow aplasia by transplantation of allogeneic marrow. Crucial role of histocompatibility matching. N Engl J Med 1969; 281:691.

Moulin AM: Immunology old and new: The beginning and the end. *In* Paulin MH (ed): Essays on the History of Immunology. Toronto, Wall and Thompson, 1989, pp 292–298.

Moulin AM: Le demier language de la medecine; histoire de l'immunologie de Pasteur au SIDA. Paris, Presses Universitaires de France, 1991.

Mowat AM, Hutton AK, Garside P, et al: A role for interleukin-1 alpha in immunologically mediated intestinal pathology. Immunology 1993; 80:110–115.

Moynahan EM: Acrodermatitis enteropathica: A lethal inherited human zinc deficiency disorder. Lancet 1974; 2:399–400.

National Committee for Clinical Laboratory Standards: Clinical applications of flow cytometry: Quality assurance and immunophenotyping of peripheral blood lymphocytes; NCCLS Document H42-T (ISBN 1-56238-155-5). Villanova, Pennsylvania, 1992.

Nicholson JKA, Green TA, Collaborating Laboratories: Selection of anticoagulants for lymphocyte immunophenotyping: Effect of specimen age on results. J Immunol Methods 1993; 165:31–35.

Nicholson KA, Jones BM, Hubbard M: CD4 T-Lymphocyte determinations on whole blood specimens using a single-tube three color assay. Cytometry 1993; 14:685–689.

Nowell PC: Phytohemagglutinin: An initiator of mitosis in cultures of humaneukocytes. Cancer Res 1960; 20:462–466.

O'Gorman M: Laboratory protocol, personal communication, 1995.

O'Gorman MRG, and Corrochano V: Rapid whole-blood flow cytometry assay for diagnosis of chronic granulomatous disease. Clin Diagn Lab Immunol, 1995; 2:227–232.

O'Gorman MRG, McNally AC, Anderson DC, et al: A rapid whole blood lysis technique for the diagnosis of moderate or severe leukocyte adhesion deficiency (LAD). Ann NY Acad Sci 1993; 667:427–430.

Ortaldo JR, Longo DL: Human natural lymphocyte effector cells: Definition, analysis of activity, and clinical effectiveness. J Natl Cancer Inst 1988; 80:999–1010.

Owen MJ, Jenkinson E: Ontogeny of the immune response. *In* Lachman PJ, Peters DK, Rosen FS, et al (eds): Clinical Aspects of Immunology. London, Blackwell Scientific, 1993, pp 3–12.

Pang G, Buret A, Batey RT, et al: Morphological, phenotypic and functional characteristics of a pure population of CD56+ CD16- CD3- large granular lymphocytes generated from human duodenal mucosa. Immunology 1993; 79:498–505.

Passlick B, Flieger D, Ziegler-Heitbrock W: Identification and characterization of a novel monocyte sub-population in human peripheral blood. Blood 1989; 74:2527–2534.

Paul WE: Fundamental Immunology, 3rd ed. New York, Bauer Press, 1993.

Paul WE, Seder RA: Lymphocyte responses to cytokines. Cell 1994; 76:241–251.

Paxton H: Unpublished laboratory data presented in symposiums during '94 and '95 as part of Coulter Corp. countdowns held in 15 U.S. cities and Canada.

Paxton H, Pins M, Denton G, et al: Comparison of CD4 cell count by a simple enzyme-linked immunosorbent assay using the Trax CD4 test kit and by flow cytometry and hematology. Clin Diagn Lab Immunol 1995; 2:104–114.

Platt JL, Grant BW, Eddy AA: Immune cell populations in cutaneous delayed hypersensitivity. J Exp Med 1983; 158:1227–1230.

Pollack MS, Kirkpatrick DV, Kapoor N, et al: The use of HLA typing to monitor engraftment following transplantations of lectin-fractionated histo-incompatible marrow in patients with immunodeficiency and leukemia. Transplant Proc 1983; 343:21–34.

Poncelet P, Carayon P: Cytofluorometric quantification of cell-surface antigens by indirect immunofluoresence using monoclonal antibodies. J Immunol Methods 1985; 85:65–74.

Poncelet P, George F, Lavabre-Bertrand T: Immunological detection of membrane bound antigens and receptors. Cells and Tissues Methods of Immunological Analysis 1993; 3:389–417.

Poncelet P, Lavabre-Bertrand T, Caryon P: Quantitative phenotypes of B chronic lymphocytic leukemia B cells established with monoclonals antibodies from the B cell protocol. *In* Reinherz EL, Haynes BF, Nadler LM, et al (eds): Leukocyte Typing II, Vol 2. New York, Springer-Verlag, 1986; pp 229–343.

Prasad AS, Miale A Jr, Farid Z, et al: Zinc metabolism in patients with the syndrome of iron deficiency anemia, hepatosplenomegaly, dwarfism and hypogonadism. J Lab Clin Med 1963; 61:537–549.

Quiao L, Schumann G, Autschbach F, et al: Human intestinal mucosa alters T-cell reactivities. Gastroenterology 1993; 105:814–819.

Rabinovitch PS: Practical considerations for DNA content and cell cycle analysis. *In* Bauer KD, Duque RE, Shankey TV (eds): Clinical Flow Cytometry: Principles and Applications. Baltimore, Williams and Wilkins, 1993, pp 143–156.

Rabinovitch PS: DNA content histogram and cell-cycle analysis. Methods Cell Biol 1994; 41:263–295.

Ramaekers FC, Hopman AH: Detection of generic aberrations in bladder cancer using in situ hybridization. Ann NY Acad Sci 1993; 677: 199–213.

Reinherz EL, Schlossman SF: The differentiation and function of human T lymphocytes. Cell 1980; 19:821–827.

Reisner Y, Kapoor N, Kirkpatrick D, et al: Transplantation for severe combined deficiency with HLA-A, B, D, DR incompatible parental marrow cells fractionated with soybean agglutinin and sheep red blood cells. Blood 1983; 61:341–348.

Reth M: Antigen receptor tail clue. Nature 1989; 338:383–384.

Robinson JP, Carter WO: Flow cytometric analysis of granulocytes. *In* Bauer KD, Duque RE, Shankey TV (eds): Clinical Flow Cytometry. Principles and Applications. Baltimore, Williams and Wilkins, 1993, pp 405–434.

Schuurman RKB, Van Rood JJ, Vossen JM, et al: Failure of lymphocyte membrane expression in two siblings with combined immunodeficiency. Clin Immunol Immunopath 1979; 14:18–24.

Schwartz A: Product brochure. San Juan, Puerto Rico, Flow Cytometry Standards Corp., 1994.

Seder RA, Gazzinelli R, Sher A, et al: IL-12 acts directly on CD4 T cells to enhance priming for IFN-gamma production and diminishes IL-4 inhibition of such priming. Proc Natl Acad Sci USA 1993; 90:10188–10192.

Seder RA, Paul WE, Davis MM, et al: The presence of interleukin-4 during in vitro priming determines the lymphokine-producing potential of CD4+T cells from T cell receptor transgenic mice. J Exp Med 1992; 176:1091–1098.

Shankey TV, Rabinovitch PS, Bagwell CB, et al: Guidelines for implementation of clinical DNA cytometry. Cytometry 1993; 14:472–477.

Shapiro HM: Trends and developments in flow cytometry instrumentation. Ann NY Acad Sci 1993; 677:155–166.

Shapiro HM: Practical Flow Cytometry, 3rd ed. New York, Wiley-Liss, 1995.

Shapiro HM: Parameters and probes. *In* Shapiro HM (ed): Practical Flow Cytometry, 3rd ed. New York, Wiley-Liss, 1995b, pp 129–348.

Shapiro HM: Using flow cytometers. *In* Shapiro HM (ed): Practical Flow Cytometry, 3rd ed. New York, Wiley-Liss, 1995c, pp 376–377.

Shapiro HM: How flow cytometers work. *In* Shapiro HM (ed): Practical Flow Cytometry, 3rd ed. New York, Wiley-Liss, 1995a, pp 75–178.

Shaw J, Meerovich K, Elliott JF: Induction, suppression and superinduction of lymphokine IL-2 mRNA in T lymphocytes. Mol Immunol 1987; 24:409.

Shaw S: Leukocyte differentiation antigen database. NIH and 5th International Workshop on Leukocyte Differentiation Antigens (Version 1.1) 1993. Nov 3–7, Boston, MA, USA.

Shront EP: Basic concepts of immunology and its application to clinical nutrition. Nutr Clin Pract 1993; 8(4):177–183.

Shulof RS, Bockmna RS, Garofalo JA, et al: Multivariate analysis of T-cell functional defects and circulating serum factors in adult Hodgkin's disease. Cancer 1980; 48:964–973.

Siegal FP, Lopez C, Hammer GS, et al: Severe acquired immunodeficiency in male homosexuals manifested by chronic perianal ulcerative herpes simplex lesions. N Engl J Med 1981; 305:1439–1444.

Springer TA, Thompson WS, Miller LJ, et al: Inherited deficiency of the Mac-1, LFA-1, p150,95 glycoprotein family and its molecular basis. J Exp Med 1984; 160:1901–1918.

Stelzer GT, Shults KE, Loken MR: CD45 gating for routine flow cytometric analysis of human bone marrow specimens. Ann NY Acad Sci 1993; 677:265–280.

Sullivan JL, Wallen WC, Johnson FL: Epstein Barr virus infection following bone marrow transplantation. Int J Cancer 1978; 22:132–140.

Tamalet JC, Chermann F, Kourilsky F, et al: Surface CD4 density remains constant on lymphocytes of HIV-infected patients in the progression of disease. Res Immunol 1991; 142:291–298.

Tan P, Anasetti C, Hansen JA, et al: Induction of alloantigen-specific hyperresponsiveness in human T lymphocytes by blocking interactions of CD28 with its natural ligand B7/BB1. J Exp Med 1993; 177:165–173.

Terstappen LWMM, Loken MR: Five-dimensional flow cytometry as a new approach to blood and bone marrow differentials. Cytometry 1988; 9:548–556.

Terstappen LW, Loken MR: Myeloid cell differentiation in normal bone marrow and acute myeloid leukemia assessed by multi-dimensional flow cytometry. Anal Cell Pathol 1990; 2:220–240.

Testi, R, D'Ambrosio D, De Maria R, Santoni A: The CD69 receptor: A multipurpose cell-surface trigger for hematopoietic cells. Immunol Today 1994; 15:479–483.

Testi R, Phillips JH, Lanier LL: Leu 23 induction as an early marker of functional CD3/T cell antigen receptor triggering: Requirement for receptor cross-linking, prolonged elevation of intracellular [Ca++] and stimulation of protein kinase. J Immunol 1989; 142:1854–1860.

Touraine JL, Betuel H, Suillet MG, et al: Combined immunodeficiency disease associated with absence of cell surface HLA A and B antigens. J Pediatr 1979; 93:47–59.

Townsend SE, Allison JP: Tumor rejection after direct costimulation of CD8+ T cells by B7-transfected melanoma cells. Science 1993; 259:368–370.

Trinchieri G: The hematopoietic system and hematopoiesis. *In* Knowles DM (ed): Neoplastic Hematopathology. Baltimore, Williams & Wilkins, 1992, pp 1–25.

Veber MB, Cunningham-Rundles S, Schulman M, et al: Acute shift in immune response to microbial activators in very low birthweight infants. Clin Exp Immunol 1991; 83:391–395.

Verwer BJH, Terstappen LWMM: Automatic linear assignment of acute leukemias by flow cytometry. Cytometry 1993; 14:649–659.

Vindelov LL, Christensen I: Detergent and proteolytic enzyme-based techniques for nuclear isolation and DNA content analysis. Methods Cell Biol 1995; 219–229.

Vogt RF, Cross GD, Philips DL, et al: Inter-laboratory study of cellular fluorescence intensity measurements with fluorescein labeled microbead standards. Cytometry 1991; 12:6.

Weinberg DS: Relative applicability of image analysis and flow cytometry in clinical medicine. *In* Bauer KD, Duque RE, Shankey TV (eds): Clinical Flow Cytometry: Principles and Applications. Baltimore, Williams and Wilkins, 1993; pp 359–371.

Weiss A: Molecular and genetic insights into T cell antigen receptor structure and function. Annu Rev Genet 1991; 25:487–510.

Weiss A, Littman DR: Signal transduction by lymphocyte antigen receptors. Cell 1994; 76:263–274.

Wheeless LL, Coon JS, Cox C, et al: Precision of DNA flow cytometry in interinstitutional analyses. Cytometry 1991; 12:405–412.

Xu-Amano J, Kiyono H, Jackson RJ, et al: Helper T-cell subsets for immunoglobulin A responses: Oral immunization with tetanus toxoid and cholera toxins as adjuvants selectively induces T_h2 cells in mucosa associated tissues. J Exp Med 1993; 178:1309–1321.

Yabuhara A, Kawai H Kamiyame A: Development of natural killer cytotoxicity during childhood: Marked increases in number of natural killer cells with adequate cytotoxic abilities during infancy to early childhood. Pediatr Res 1990; 28:316.

Yamamura MK, Uyemura RJ, Deans K, et al: Defining protective responses to pathogens: Cytokin profiles in leprosy lesions. Science 1991; 254:277–279.

Zola H, Moore HA, Bradley J, et al: Lymphocyte subpopulations in human cord blood: Analysis with monoclonal antibodies. J Reprod Immunol 1983; 5:311.

Chapter 35

Laboratory Evaluation of Immunoglobulin Function and Humoral Immunity

Nimrat Bawa, M.D.
Russell H. Tomar, M.D.

Antibodies are the effector molecules of humoral (B-cell–mediated) immunity. They are immunoglobulins that react specifically and bind with the antigen that stimulated their production. Immunoglobulins comprise about 20% of plasma proteins. Antibody activity is associated with the slowest migrating proteins on electrophoresis, the γ globulins. The focus of this chapter is to discuss the general structural and functional properties of immunoglobulins, their laboratory evaluation, and their clinical significance.

STRUCTURAL PROPERTIES OF ANTIBODIES

Antibody Molecules

Much work has been done and published on the structural properties of antibodies (Padlan, 1991; Poljak, 1991; Tedford, 1991). An immunoglobulin molecule is a Y-shaped glycoprotein. It has two identical antigen-binding sites at the tips of the Y (Fab region) and binding sites for complement components and/or various cell surface receptors on the tail of the Y (Fc region). Each immunoglobulin molecule is composed of two identical heavy (H) chains and two identical light (L) chains. These polypeptide chains are held together by noncovalent interactions that are stabilized by disulfide bonds. Parts of both the H and L chains form the antigen-binding sites. Each immunoglobulin L and H chain consists of a variable region of about 110 amino acid residues at its amino-terminal end (the tips of the Y), which forms the antigen-binding site, followed by a constant region. The H constant region is three or four times larger than that of the L chain. Each chain is composed of repeating, similarly folded domains: an L chain has one variable region (V_L) and one constant region (C_L) domain, whereas the H chain has one variable region (V_H) and three or four constant region (C_H) domains (Fig. 35–1). The amino acid sequence variation in the variable regions of both L and H chains is for the most part confined to three small hypervariable regions which come together at the amino-terminal end of the molecule to form the antigen-binding site. Each antigen-binding site is only large enough to bind an antigenic determinant the size of five or six sugar residues.

There are five different heavy chain isotypes (γ, α, μ, δ, and ϵ) and two light chain isotypes (κ and λ), with some of the isotypes having further subtypes. For example, γ has subtypes $\gamma1$, $\gamma2$, $\gamma3$, and $\gamma4$. The isotypes are formed as a result of variations in the constant region of the heavy and

5

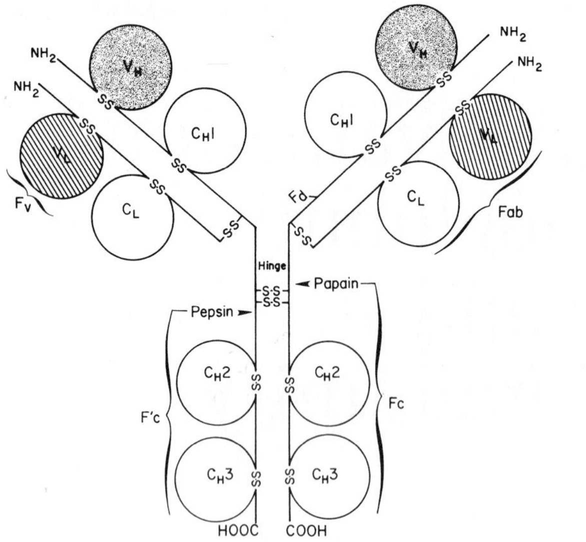

Figure 35–1. Schematic representation of immunoglobulin G molecule. The relative positions of the *interchain* disulfide bonds and the *intrachain* disulfide bonds that form the loop regions are shown. Each of the loops delineates the domain of the light and heavy chain labeled accordingly. The probable sites of enzymatic cleavage in the "hinge" region by papain or pepsin are indicated. The papain fragments are designated Fab and Fc. The pepsin fragments are Fc′ and Fab′2 (two Fab fragments disulfide linked). Digestion of Fab with pepsin under the proper conditions yields the fragment Fv (V_H and V_L noncovalently associated). The part of the heavy chain that contributes to the Fab fragment is designated Fd.

light chains. These isotypic designations are the basis for the nomenclature of antibodies. Because the heavy chain alone determines effector functions, immunoglobulins are conveniently referred to by their heavy chain isotype (class) using an English letter terminology (IgG, IgA, IgM, IgD, IgE).

Antibodies have two identical antigen-binding sites. An antigen-binding site is made up of amino acids from one H chain class and one L chain class. Thus, the four-chain Y monomer molecules (see Fig. 35–1) possess two identical antigen-combining sites and are said to be *bivalent*. Such antibody molecules can cross-link antigen molecules into a large lattice if the antigen molecules each have three or more antigenic determinants. Once the lattice reaches a certain size, it precipitates out of solution (Davies, 1983). This cross-linking is of physiologic importance because it enhances the engulfment of antigen, such as that expressed by bacteria, and by phagocytic leukocytes. It is also involved in activation of the complement system. In addition, cross-linking may be required for the triggering of antibody-producing cells (B lymphocytes) by antigen. The efficiency of antigen-binding and cross-linking reactions by antibodies is greatly increased by a flexible hinge region where the arms of the Y join the tail, allowing the distance between the two antigen-binding sites to vary.

Multivalence affects the avidity with which an antibody can bind certain types of antigens. A particulate antigen (such as a bacterium or virus) has repeating antigenic determinants on its surface. An antibody molecule may interact with a single particle in such a manner that both of its antigen-combining sites are bound to antigenic determinants on that particle rather than to antigenic determinants on two adjacent particles. When this type of binding occurs, the effective energy of interaction or avidity is greatly increased compared with that associated with monovalent attachments to two particles. This mechanism has been shown to be physiologically important in the neutralization of viruses by antibodies of relatively low binding affinity.

The protective effect of immunoglobulins is not due simply to their ability to bind antigen. They engage in a variety of biological activities mediated by the tail of the Y, the Fc region of the molecule. This part of the antibody molecule determines what will happen to the antigen once it is bound. Immunoglobulins with the same antigen-binding capacity can have a variety of different Fc regions and therefore different functional properties, such as activating the complement system and attaching to Fc receptors on macrophages, thereby aiding phagocytosis of antigens.

Because of its exposed location and loosely folded structure, the *hinge region* is readily attacked by various proteolytic enzymes. As the name suggests, the hinge region confers a certain amount of flexibility on the molecule, allowing it to assume the Y-shaped structure. This permits an antibody to become attached to a single particle (e.g., a bacterium) through both of its antigen-combining sites or, alternatively, to stretch out to its full length to join two particles. The unique properties conferred by the hinge region on Ig molecules are related to its rich content of proline and hydrophilic amino acid residues. The inter-H-chain disulfide bonds of IgG, IgA, and IgD molecules are located in the hinge region (see Fig. 35–1).

The proteolytic enzymes papain and pepsin cleave antibody molecules into different characteristic fragments that lead to an understanding of the structure-function relationship of the protein. Papain cleavage produces two separate and identical Fab (fragment antigen-binding) fragments, each with one antigen-binding site, and one Fc fragment (so-called because in nonhuman primates it readily crystallizes). On the other hand, pepsin cleavage produces one $F(ab')_2$ fragment, so-called because it consists of two covalently linked F(ab′) fragments (each slightly larger than a Fab fragment); the rest of the molecule is broken down into smaller fragments of various sizes (see Fig. 35–1). Because $F(ab')_2$ fragments are bivalent, they can still cross-link antigens and form precipitates. This is not true of the univalent Fab fragments. However, neither of these fragments (subunits of antibodies) has the other biological properties of intact antibody molecules because they lack the tail, the Fc region, that mediates these properties.

Each B-cell clone makes antibody molecules with a unique antigen-binding site. Initially, the molecules are inserted into the plasma membrane, where they serve as cell surface receptors for antigen. When antigen binds to the membrane-bound antibodies, B cells are activated to multiply, differentiate to a plasma cell, and synthesize a large amount of soluble antibody with the same antigen-binding site, which is secreted into the blood. Humoral antibodies defend humans and animals against infection by inactivating viruses and bacterial toxins via its V_H/V_L domains, and by recruiting complement and various cells to kill and ingest invading microorganisms via its C_L domains in the Fc region of the molecule. The biological properties of the various immunoglobulin domains are summarized in Table 35–1.

Table 35-1. BIOLOGICAL PROPERTIES OF IMMUNOGLOBULIN DOMAINS (IgG)

Domain	Known or Probable Function
C_H3	1. Cytotrophic reactions involving: (a) Macrophages and monocytes (b) Heterologous mast cells (c) Cytotoxic killer (K) cells (d) B cells 2. Noncovalent assembly of heavy and light chains
C_H2	1. Binding of complement (Clq) 2. Control of catabolic rate
C_H1/C_L	1. Noncovalent assembly of heavy and light chains 2. Covalent assembly of heavy and light chains 3. Spacers between interdomain interactions involving antigen binding and effector functions
V_H/V_L	1. Antigen binding 2. Noncovalent bonding of heavy and light chains

From Dorrington KJ, Painter RH: Biological activities of the constant region of immunoglobulin G. *In* Mandel TE, et al (eds): Progress in Immunology III. Canberra City, Australian Academy of Science, 1977.

Antibody-Antigen Interaction

The binding of an antigen to antibody is reversible. The affinity and the number of binding sites contribute to the strength of an antibody-antigen interaction. This reversible binding is a result of many relatively weak noncovalent forces, including hydrophobic and hydrogen bonds, van der Waals forces, and ionic interactions. These weak forces are effective only when the antigen molecule is close enough to allow some of its atoms to fit into complementary recesses (regions) on the antibody surface. The complementary regions of a four-chain antibody unit are its two identical antigen-binding sites, whereas the corresponding region on the antigen is an antigenic determinant. Most antigenic macromolecules have many different antigenic determinants; if two or more of them are identical, the antigen is said to be multivalent.

The *affinity* of an antibody molecule reflects the tightness of the fit of an antigenic determinant to a single antigen-binding site, and it is independent of the number of antigenic sites. However, the total *avidity* of an antibody for a multivalent antigen, such as a polymer with repeating subunits, is defined as the total binding strength of all of its binding sites together. A typical IgG molecule binds at least 10,000 times more strongly to a multivalent antigen if both antigen-binding sites are engaged than if only one site is involved.

For the same reason, if the affinity of the antigen-binding sites in an IgG and an IgM molecule is the same, the IgM molecule (because it is a pentamer and thus has 10 binding sites) will have a very much greater avidity for a multivalent antigen than an IgG molecule (which has two binding sites). This difference in avidity is important in view of the fact that antibodies produced early in an immune response usually have much lower affinities than those produced later. The increase in the average affinity of antibodies produced as time passes after immunization is called *affinity maturation*. This occurs because the antibody response to an antigen is heterogeneous—that is, antibodies with different antigen-combining sites are elicited against the antigen by the responding clones of B lymphocytes. Because of its high total avidity, IgM, the major Ig class produced early in immune responses, can function even when each of its binding sites has only a low affinity.

The size of the antigen-antibody complex is determined by the valence of the antigen and the relative concentrations of the antigen and the antibody. The antigen-antibody precipitation reaction is based on the cross-linking of multivalent antigens by bivalent antibodies. If only one species of antibody (a monoclonal response) is present, molecules with only one antigenic determinant cannot be cross-linked. If an antigen is bivalent, it can form small cyclic complexes or linear chains with antibody, whereas an antigen with three or more antigenic determinants can form large three-dimensional lattices that readily precipitate. However, the majority of antisera elicited against an antigen contain a variety of different antibodies (a polyclonal response) that react with different determinants on the antigen and can cooperate in cross-linking the antigen. By contrast, homogeneous (monoclonal) antibodies can precipitate molecules only with repeating identical antigenic determinants.

Given valence conditions that allow the formation of large aggregates, the size of the antigen-antibody complexes that form depends critically on the relative molar concentrations of the two reactants. If there is an excess of either antigen or antibody, large complexes are unlikely to form (Fig. 35-2).

The size and composition of antibody-antigen complexes are not only important in influencing precipitation reactions *in vitro*, they are crucial in determining the fate of the complexes in the body. Complexes formed at equivalence or in antibody excess have multiple protruding Fc regions and therefore bind strongly to Fc receptors in macrophages, which ingest and degrade them. Small complexes, formed in antigen excess, have only one Fc region per complex. Therefore, they bind poorly to Fc receptors on macrophages and are less efficiently destroyed. Instead they may be deposited in small blood vessels in the skin, kidneys, joints, and brain, where they may activate the complement system, causing inflammation and the destruction of tissue.

Although it appears that antigen-antibody complexes have a rigid "lock and key" appearance, antibodies are dynamic entities and undergo structural fluctuations (Karplus, 1983; Wilson, 1991). Conformational changes may even be required for the binding. These adjustments include side chain shifts of up to 2 to 3 Å, aromatic ring rotations, conformational changes, and even small rotations between V_H and V_L domains (Bhat, 1990; Stanfield, 1990; Herron 1991).

5

THE GENETIC BASIS OF ANTIBODY DIVERSITY

It is estimated that a human is able to make at least 10^6 to 10^9 different antibody molecules. Special genetic mechanisms have evolved to produce the very large number of immunoglobulin molecules that develop in response to antigen stimulation without the need for an excessive number of genes (Edward, 1993).

Immunoglobulin molecules are produced by three separate gene pools encoding the κ, λ, and H chains, respectively. The gene pools for light and heavy chains reside on different chromosomes. In each pool, separate gene segments that encode for different parts of the variable regions of light and heavy chains can be brought together by site-specific recombination events during B-cell differentiation. The light chain gene pools contain one or more constant (C) genes and sets

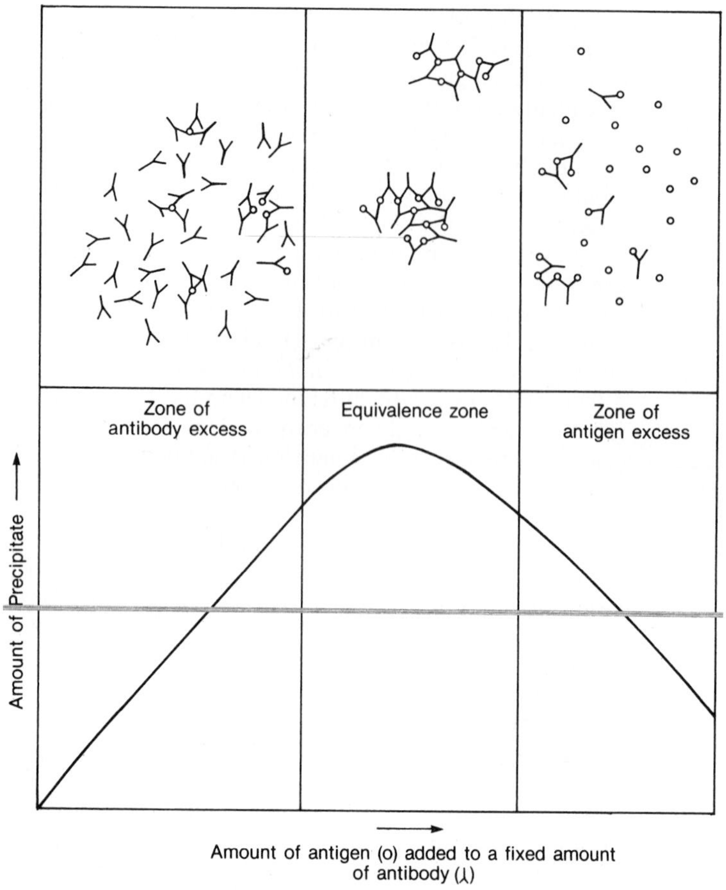

Figure 35–2. Antibody and antigen concentrations influence the size of antigen-antibody complexes formed. The largest complexes form when both molecules are present at approximately the same molar concentration (zone of equivalence), whereas the smallest complexes form when the antigen is present in great excess. Note that the small complexes formed in antigen excess have only a few antibody molecules per complex; for this reason, they are inefficiently cleared from the extracellular fluids by macrophages.

of variable (V) and joining (J) gene segments. The H-chain gene pool contains a set of C genes and sets of V, diversity (D), and J gene segments. To make an antibody molecule, a V_L gene segment is recombined with a J_L gene segment to produce a V gene for the light chain; and a V_H gene segment is recombined with a D and J_H segment to produce a V gene for the heavy chain (Fig. 35–3). Each of the assembled gene segments is then cotranscribed with the appropriate constant region sequence to produce a messenger RNA molecule that encodes for the complete polypeptide chain. By variously combining inherited gene segments encoding for V_L and V_H regions, vertebrates can make thousands of different light chains and thousands of different H chains that can associate to form millions of different antibody molecules.

The baseline repertoire of antibody molecules can be expanded still further by somatic hypermutation, which seems to be activated by exposure to antigen. Thus, the selective role of antigen in the presence of somatic mutation appears to lead to a fine tuning of the immune response and to a virtually unlimited diversity of antibody molecules. Somatic point mutations in immunoglobulin genes occur in B cells (not germ cells) during the lifetime of the animal or of humans (Tonegawa, 1983). The somatic hypermutations are largely confined to the H-chain and L-chain variable region genes and the introns immediately surrounding them. It is estimated that close to one mutation will occur in either the H- or L-chain V region of an individual cell with each cell division. This not only increases antibody diversity but may also cause a change in the affinity with which the antibody binds its ligand. Those B cells that emerge that can bind the antigen more avidly have an advantage over other B cells that do not bind the antigen as avidly. As the concentration of antigen falls, those B cells that have more avid receptors dominate the population of responding cells. This results in a greater affinity of the antibodies being produced on rechallenge than in the initial response. Thus this process of somatic hypermutation can result in the presence in immunized individuals of high-affinity antibodies that are much more effective on a weight basis.

All B cells initially make IgM antibodies. Some later switch to make antibodies of other classes (isotypes) that have the same antigen-binding site (idiotype) as the original IgM antibodies *(allelic exclusion)* (Fig. 35–4, Table 35–2). Such class switching in combination with allelic exclusion allows the same antigen-binding sites (same V_H and light chain) to be distributed among antibodies with many different biological properties (secondary effector functions).

Thus the gene organization mechanism permits the assembly of immunoglobulin molecules with a variety of specificities. Antibody diversity depends on the presence of multiple gene segments, their rearrangement into different sequences, the combination of different light and heavy chains in the assembly of immunoglobulin molecules, and somatic mutations.

GENERAL PROPERTIES OF IMMUNOGLOBULINS

(Spielgelberg, 1974; Carayannopoulos, 1993)

The various classes of human immunoglobulins and their properties are summarized in Tables 35–3 and 35–4.

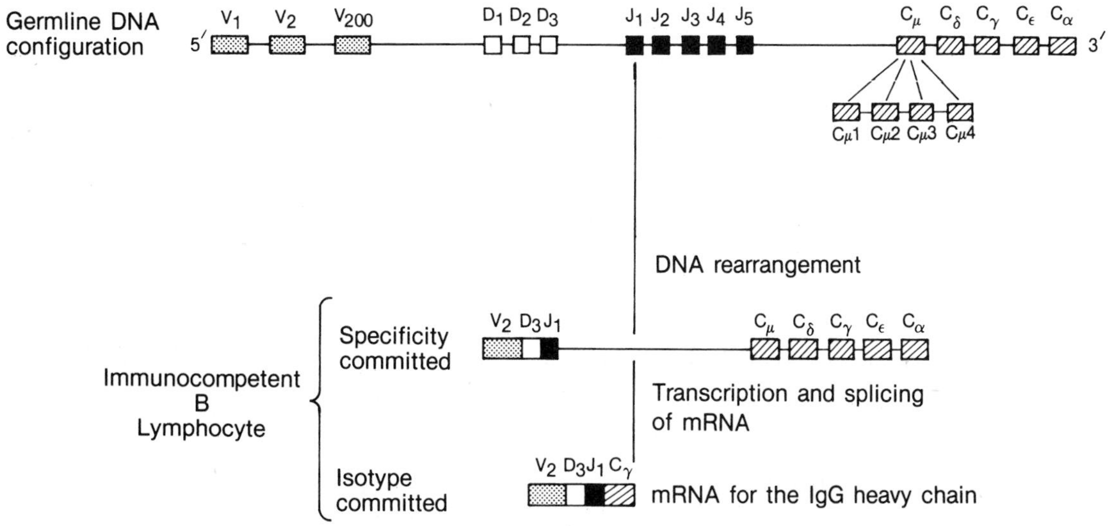

Figure 35–3. Organization and rearrangement of the heavy chain Ig genes (exons) on the mouse 12 chromosome. Each V_H gene also has a leader sequence, which is not shown. The constant region genes are identified by the heavy chain isotype, and more than one gene exists for the C_γ and C_α isotypes. Unlike C_α and C_λ genes, C_H genes are composed of multiple exons, as illustrated for the C_μ gene ($C_{\mu 1}-C_{\mu 4}$ domains). The switch sites are located at the 5′ end of each of the C_H genes and are also not shown. The solid line represents the intervening sequences (introns) between the genes or gene segments. Each heavy chain is encoded by four distinct gene segments, V, D, J, and C. (Redrawn from Marcu KB: Immunoglobulin heavy-chain constant-region genes. Cell 1982; 29:719. © by Cell Press.)

Immunoglobulin M

This glycoprotein is the major class of antibody secreted into the blood in the early stages of a *primary* antibody response. Normally, the secreted form of IgM is a pentamer composed of five four-chain units, a macroglobulin with a 19S sedimentation rate and a molecular weight of 900,000. However, in human autoimmune disorders, such as systemic lupus erythematosus (SLE), the monomeric 7S form may be detected in appreciable amounts in serum. Selective IgM deficiency is a rare disorder associated with the absence of IgM and normal levels of other immunoglobulin classes. The cause of this disorder is unknown.

Because pentameric IgM has a total of 10 antigen-binding sites, it is more efficient than 7S monomeric IgM or IgG molecules in cross-linking antigen and in activating the complement system when bound to antigen. Thus, this high efficiency in binding and activating complement, coupled with its early appearance during the course of infection, makes IgM a particularly potent agent in combating microbial invasions.

Each IgM pentamer contains one copy of another polypeptide chain, called a *J (joining) chain*, which has a molecular weight of 15 kDa. This accessory polypeptide is produced by IgM-secreting cells. It is an acidic glycoprotein with a high content of cysteine residues and thus is disulfide linked between two adjacent IgM monomeric Fc regions at the carboxyl-terminal end. Presumably, oligomerization is initiated at this site.

IgM is also the first class of antibody to be produced by developing B cells. The immediate precursors of B cells, called pre-B cells, make μ chains but not light chains, which accumulate in the cells. Pre-B cells then begin to synthesize light chains that combine with μ chains to form four-chain monomer IgM molecules. The two μ-chain and two light-chain component is inserted into the plasma membrane, where it functions as a receptor for antigen. At this point, the cells have become B lymphocytes and can respond to antigen.

Perhaps because of its large size, secreted pentamer IgM is not found to any significant extent in tissue spaces; it is confined to the blood circulation and does not cross the placenta. IgM is a minor component of secretory immunoglobulins at mucosal surfaces and in breast milk.

IgM is phylogenetically the most primitive of the immunoglobulins, and most variants of the genes from the μ chain appear to have evolved into heavy-chain genes for the other immunoglobulin classes. Additional physical and biological properties of IgM as well as the other classes of immunoglobulin are given in Tables 35–3 and 35–4.

Figure 35–4. The structure of the light and heavy chains showing the positions and lengths of the hypervariable regions in the V_L domain (designated Lv1, Lv2, Lv3) and V_H domain (designated Hv1, Hv2, Hv3). The amino acid residues are numbered starting from the N-terminal. In some heavy chains, an additional (?) hypervariable region (N84–N91) has been observed. The diagram also illustrates the region(s) where the major immunoglobulin variants may be found. The idiotypic determinants are found exclusively in the V_L and V_H domains and the isotypic marker in the constant regions of both chains. The allotypic markers can occur throughout the entire length of both chains.

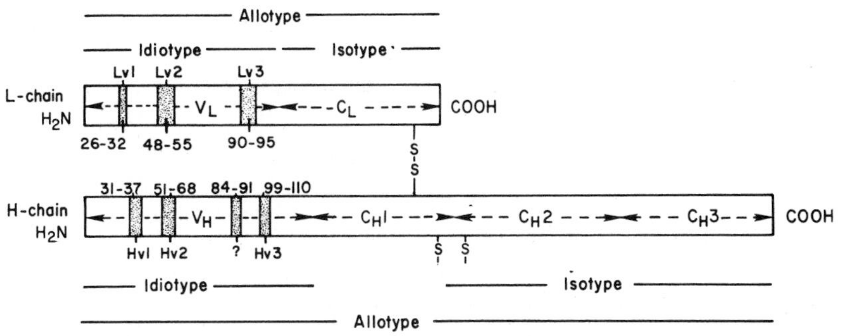

Table 35–2. SUMMARY OF IMMUNOGLOBULIN VARIANTS

Type of Variation	Distribution	Variant	Location	Examples
Isotypic	All variants present in serum of a normal individual	Classes	C_H	IgM, IgE
		Subclasses	C_H	IgA_1, IgA_2
		Types	C_L	κ, λ
		Subtypes	C_L	λOz^+, λOz^-
		Subgroups	V_L, V_H	$V_{\kappa I}$, $V_{\kappa II}$, V_{HI}, V_{HII}
Allotypic	Allelic forms not present in all individuals	Allotypes	Mainly C_H/C_L Occasionally V_H/V_L	Gm group (human γ chain; e.g., IgG1, G1m3, and G1m17) b_4, b_5, b_6, b_9 (rabbit light chain)
Idiotypic	Antigenic individuality specific to each Ig molecule	Idiotypes	V_H/V_L	Determinant identified by antibody specific to an individual immunoglobulin

Immunoglobulin G

IgG is the most well studied isotype at both the structural and functional levels (Burton, 1985). Antibodies of this class constitute the major immunoglobulin in the blood. They are copiously produced during *secondary* immune response. The Fc region of IgG molecules binds to specific receptors on phagocytic cells, such as macrophages and polymorphonuclear leukocytes, thereby increasing the efficiency with which the phagocytic cells can ingest and destroy infecting microorganisms that have become coated with IgG antibodies in response to the infection. The best known function of IgG is complement activation via the classic cascade. The Fc region of IgG can bind to and thereby activate the first component of the complement system, which unleashes a biochemical attack that kills the microorganism. At least two molecules of IgG are required for complement activation compared to one molecule of IgM, which has more than two Fc regions.

IgG molecules are the only antibodies that can pass from mother to fetus. Cells of the placenta that are in contact with maternal blood have receptors that bind the Fc region of IgG molecules and mediate their passage to the fetus. The antibodies are first ingested by receptor-mediated endocytosis and then transported across the cell and released by exocytosis into the fetal blood. Other classes of antibodies do not bind to these receptors and therefore cannot pass across the placenta. The ability of IgG to cross the placenta provides a major line of defense against infection for the first weeks of an infant's life. Normally, the human fetus begins to receive significant quantities of maternal IgG transplacentally at around 12 weeks' gestation. The quantity increases steadily until, at birth, cord serum contains a concentration of IgG comparable to that of maternal serum. Barring any immunologic disorders, adult levels of IgG are reached by the seventh year of life and remain relatively constant thereafter.

IgG antibodies have a high diffusion coefficient, which enables them to diffuse into the extravascular body spaces more readily than other Ig classes. IgG, being the predominant immunoglobulin in these spaces, carries the major burden of neutralizing bacterial toxins and of binding microorganisms to enhance their phagocytosis. Furthermore, only IgG anti-

Table 35–3. PHYSICAL PROPERTIES OF HUMAN IMMUNOGLOBULINS

WHO Designation	IgM	IgG	IgA	IgD	IgE
Heavy chains	μ	γ	α	δ	ϵ
Heavy chain subclasses	μ_1, μ_2	γ_1, γ_2, γ_3, γ_4	α_1, α_2	—	—
Light chains	κ or λ	κ or λ	κ or λ	κ or λ	κ or λ
Molecular formula	$IgM(\kappa)\ (2\mu 2\kappa)_5$ $IgM(\lambda)\ (2\mu 2\lambda)_5$	$IgG(\kappa)\ 2\gamma 2\kappa$ $IgG(\lambda)\ 2\gamma 2\lambda$	$IgA(\kappa)\ (2\alpha 2\kappa)_{1-3}$ $IgA(\lambda)\ (1\alpha 2\lambda)_{1-3}$ $IgA(\kappa)\ (2\alpha 2\kappa)_2S$† $IgA(\lambda)\ (2\alpha 2\lambda)_2S$	$IgD(\kappa)\ 2\delta 2\kappa$ $IgD(\lambda)\ 2\delta 2\lambda$	$IgE(\kappa)\ 2\epsilon 3\kappa$ $IgE(\lambda)\ 2\epsilon 2\lambda$
Number of four-chain units per molecule	5	1	1–3	1	1
Heavy chain molecular weight, daltons	70,000	50,000–60,000	55,000	62,000	70,000
Light chain molecular weight, daltons	23,000	23,000	23,000	23,000	23,000
Sedimentation coefficient, S_{20W}	18.0–19.0	6.7–7.0	6.6–14.0	6.9–7.0	7.9–8.0
Molecular weight, daltons	900,000	143,000–160,000	159,000–447,000	177,000–185,000	187,000–200,000
Electrophoretic mobility	$\gamma^1-\beta^1$	$\gamma^2-\alpha^1$	$\gamma^2-\beta^2$	γ^1	γ^1
Carbohydrate content, percent	7–14	2.2–3.5	7.5–9.0	12–13	11–12
Heavy chain allotypes	—	Gm	Am	—	—
Light chain allotypes	Km(κ)*	Km(κ)*	Km(κ)*	Km(κ)*	Km(K)
Valency for antigen binding	5(10)	2	2.4 (? polymeric forms)	2	2
Number of domains on the heavy chains	5	4	4	4	5

*Formerly designated Inv marker.
†Dimer in external secretions carries secretory component -S.

Table 35–4. PROPERTIES OF HUMAN IMMUNOGLOBULINS

	IgM	IgG	IgA	IgD	IgE
A. Physiologic					
Normal adult serum concentration mg/mL	1.2–4.0	8.0–16.0	0.4–2.2	0.03	17–450 ng/mL
International units/mL	69–322	92–207	54–268	—	<100
Percent total immunoglobulin	13	80	6	1	0.002
Intravascular distribution, percent	41	48	76	75	51
Synthetic rate, mg/kg/d	2.2	35	24	0.4	0.003
Catabolic rate in serum, percent/d	10.6	6	24	37	90
(or half-life, d)	(5–6)	(18–23)	(5–6.5)	(2.8)	(2.3)
B. Biological					
Agglutinating capacity	+4	±	+2	—	—
Complement-fixing capacity via classic pathway	+4	+	—	—	—
Homologous anaphylactic hypersensitivity	—	—	—	—	+4
Heterologous guinea pig anaphylaxis	—	+	—	—	—
Fixation to homologous mast cells and basophils	—	±	—	—	+4
Cytophilic binding to macrophages	—	+	±	—	—
Placental transport to fetus	—	+	—	—	—
Rheumatoid factor-binding activity	—	+	—	—	—
Present in external secretions	±	+	+4	—	+2
Other characteristic properties:					
IgM—Produced early in immune response, first effective defense against bacteremia					
IgG—Combats microorganisms and their toxins in extravascular fluids					
IgA—Defends external body surfaces					
IgD—Present on lymphocyte surface of immunocompetent cells, important for B-cell activation and/or immunoregulation					

bodies coating target cells, such as tumor cells, can sensitize them for extracellular killing by the process called antibody-dependent cell cytotoxicity (ADCC). The ADCC killer (K) cells also possess Fc receptors for IgG.

There are four subclasses of human IgG, 1 through 4. The four subclasses reflect the existence of four antigenetically distinct H chains ($\gamma 1$ through $\gamma 4$), which are similar but not identical in amino acid sequence and general properties. For example, IgG1 is the dominant subclass in adult humans. IgG3 is the most effective binder of complement, followed by IgG1 and IgG2. IgG4 in most cases fails completely to bind complement by the classic pathway. All of the subclasses except IgG2 have been demonstrated to cross the placenta. A summary of the physical and biological properties of IgG is given in Tables 35–3 and 35–4 and for the subclasses in Table 35–5.

Immunoglobulin A

Antibodies of this class comprise the major class of antibody in secretions (milk, saliva, tears, and respiratory and intestinal secretions). It exists as a four-chain monomer (like IgG) or as a dimer of two such monomer units. IgA molecules

Table 35–5. PROPERTIES OF HUMAN IMMUNOGLOBULINS G SUBCLASSES

	IgG1	IgG2	IgG3	IgG4
A. Physiologic				
Percent distribution of total normal serum IgG	66 ± 8	23 ± 8	7.3 ± 3.8	4.2 ± 2.6
Synthetic rate, mg/kg/d, in serum	25	?	3.4	?
Fraction catabolic rate, percent/d	8	6.9	16.8	6.9
(half-life, d)	(23)	(23)	(7)	(23)
Ratio of $\kappa:\lambda$	1.4–2.4	1.0–1.1	1.1–1.3	5.0–7.0
Allotypic markers (Gm types)	a,z,f,x	n	bo,bi,bz g,st,etc.	?
B. Biological				
Complement-fixing capacity via classic pathway	+2	±	+3	−
Heterologous skin-binding capacity	+	−	+	+
Placental transport to fetus	+	±	+	+
Macrophage receptor	+	−	+	−
Reaction with protein A	+	+	−	+
Dominant antibody activitites:				
Antitetanus toxoid	+2	+	+	±
Antidiphtheria toxoid	+2	+	+	±
Antithyroglobulin	+2	+	+	±
Anti-DNA	+2	+2	±	±
Anti-Rh	+2	−	−	±
Anti-Factor VIII	−	−	−	+
Antidextran	−	+	−	−
Antilevan	−	+	−	−
Antiteichoic acid	−	+	−	−
Number of interheavy chain disulfide bonds in hinge region	2	4	5	2
Position of light-heavy chain disulfide bond on the heavy chain	N214	N131	N131	N131

5

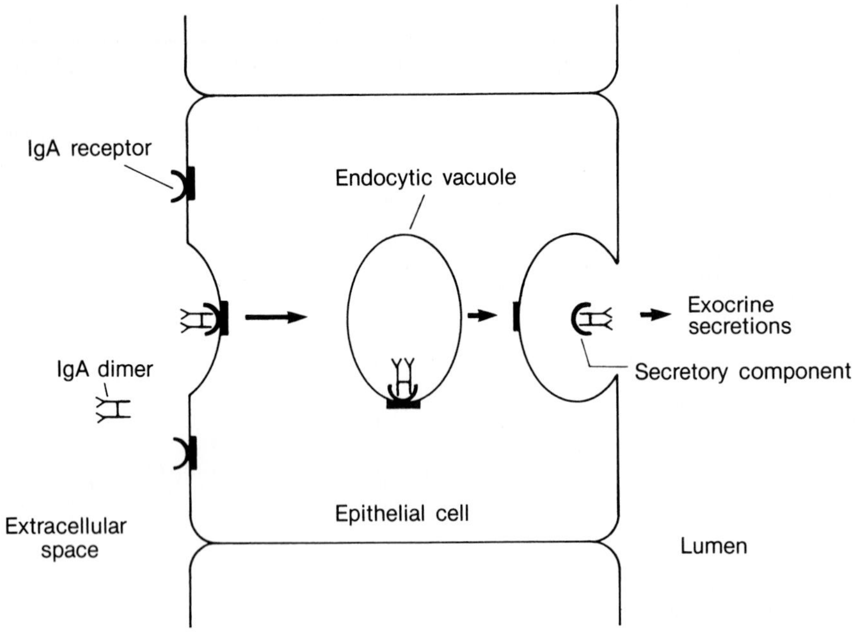

Figure 35–5. The mechanism by which the secretory component mediates the transport of a dimeric IgA molecule across an epithelial cell. The entire complex is transported from the extracellular fluid into the lumen of the epithelial tube. The secretory component is synthesized by the epithelial cell as a transmembrane glycoprotein and serves as a receptor on its basolateral surface for binding the IgA dimer. The receptor-IgA complex enters the cell in an endocytotic vesicle, which crosses the cell and is exocytosed at the apical surface. Cleavage of the receptor frees the dimer IgA for discharge at the exterior surface (lumen side). The portion of the receptor that remains attached to the IgA dimer is called the secretory component. This transport mechanism is responsible for depositing IgA in the various exocrine secretions (e.g., saliva, milk, bile, tears, and sweat), as well as in the mucous layer that protects the inner lining of the nasopharyngeal passages, intestine, and genitourinary tract.

in secretions are dimers that carry a single J chain, similar to the one associated with pentameric IgM, and an additional glycopolypeptide chain called *secretory component* (SC) of 70,000 daltons. IgA dimers pick up SC from the surface of the epithelial cells lining the intestine, bronchi, or the milk, salivary, or tear ducts. Secretory component is synthesized by the epithelial cells and is initially exposed on the nonluminal (external) surface of these cells, where it serves as a receptor for binding dimer IgA. The resulting dimer IgA-receptor complexes are ingested by receptor-mediated endocytosis, transferred across the epithelial cell cytoplasm in the form of a membrane vesicle, which fuses with the plasma membrane on the luminal side of the epithelial cell. The extramembranal portion of the IgA receptor is then enzymatically cleaved and released as part of the secretory IgA molecule ($[\alpha_2L_2]_2$-Jα) into the lumen. The amino-terminus of the dimer IgA receptor remaining attached to dimer IgA is the SC (Fig. 35–5). Thus, the fully assembled dimeric secretory IgA molecule is the synthetic product of two distinct types of cells, plasma cells and epithelial cells. In addition to this transport role, SC may also protect the dimer IgA molecules from being digested by proteolytic enzymes in secretions.

In humans it has been possible to classify IgA antibodies into two subclasses, IgA1 and IgA2, based on differences in antigenic structure and variation in the arrangement of interchain disulfide bridges. Whereas IgA2 is a minor component of serum IgA, this subclass is the dominant form in secretions. Furthermore, secretory IgA reaches adult levels sooner than serum IgA. The IgA system in the intestinal tract of humans, for example, may be fully developed by two years of age, whereas serum IgA levels do not normally reach adult concentrations until 12 years of age.

Because of its presence near external membranes, secretory IgA constitutes a first line of defense against microorganisms in the external environment. It has been postulated that IgA inhibits the adherence of microorganisms to the surface of mucosal cells, thereby preventing their entry into body tissues. One property of secretory IgA that is important in this respect is its multivalence, which is associated with high avidity of binding to antigens; this may be especially relevant in the neutralization of viruses. Antiviral activity by IgA antibodies has been demonstrated in individuals given either of the polio vaccines. Secretory IgA may also combine with certain antigens in food, preventing their absorption into the bloodstream and thus reducing the incidence of allergic reactions. For example, IgA immunodeficiencies can lead to increased levels and incidence of humoral antibodies directed against antigens derived from food and intestinal organisms.

IgA possesses the following effective properties: it fixes complement through the alternative pathway; through a specific Fc receptor on macrophages it can serve as an opsonin for phagocytosis; and it can induce eosinophil degranulation through a specific receptor, which has implicated IgA in antiparasitic responses. The physical and biological properties of IgA are listed in Tables 35–3 and 35–4.

Immunoglobulin D

Although only a minor component of the serum, IgD is a major membrane immunoglobulin found on the surface of a high proportion of B lymphocytes, especially in newborns. During the course of B cell differentiation, these cells synthesize and display IgD molecules as well as IgM molecules. Whereas this appears to contradict the one-cell–one-immunoglobulin rule, the antigen-binding sites (idiotype) of the two types of molecules and their light chains are identical. Only their C_H regions differ. The membrane-bound IgD may serve as one of the receptors with which B cells bind antigen and are stimulated to undergo clonal proliferation. There is some evidence to suggest that IgM-bearing B cells can respond to certain T-independent antigens and that the acquisition of IgD is needed for B cells (IgM- and IgD-bearing) to respond to T-cell help required for T-dependent antigen responsiveness.

Furthermore, if IgD molecules are selectively removed from IgM- and IgD-bearing B cells by taking advantage of the much greater sensitivity of δ chain to papain, the cells are rendered susceptible to becoming tolerant. The precise role played by surface IgD in an immune response remains unknown, but the generally held view is that it turns on, turns off, or modulates (controls) B cell division or differentiation.

IgD usually is detected in serum at about six months of age, and its concentration throughout life is always very low. In disease states, however, IgD concentration can vary greatly. In chronic infections, IgD serum levels increase, as do those of the other immunoglobulins. To date, no specific increase of IgD has been associated with a particular disease. Patients with allergies and autoimmune diseases do not show an abnormal IgD concentration. IgD is usually absent in hypogammaglobulinemic individuals.

To date, IgD has not been assigned a specific biological role as a humoral antibody. IgD activity against a number of antigens has been reported on occasion. Surface IgD, which has proteins like those of surface IgM, is a marker for mature B cells, and its role as a receptor is generally accepted even though the nature and purpose of the signal it transmits remain controversial (Carsetti, 1993; Roes, 1993). IgD does not bind complement, does not cross the placenta, and does not bind to cells through its Fc region. The secreted form of IgD as well as that of the other immunoglobulins lacks the carboxyl-terminal transmembrane peptide that anchors it to the surface of B cells. Tables 35–3 and 35–4 list additional properties of IgD.

Immunoglobulin E

Of the various classes of immunoglobulins, IgE is present at the lowest serum concentration (see Table 35–4). It has the ability to attach to human skin (homocytotropic antibody) and to initiate aspects of the allergic reaction (reaginic antibody). The biological activity of IgE is accounted for by its property of binding through the Fc region to basophils and to their tissue equivalent, mast cells. IgE may also be important in the humoral immune response to parasitic disease because it is often found at high levels in the serum of patients with helminthic infection. IgE may play a part in allowing white blood cells, antibodies, and complement components to enter sites of inflammation leading to an immediate hypersensitivity reaction. IgE antibodies provide a striking example of the *bifunctional* nature of antibody molecules. The Fc portion of the molecule binds to the target cells, whereas the Fab portion binds the allergen (see Chap. 44 for the role of IgE in allergic diseases and related assays). Serum IgE levels in selected conditions are shown in Table 35–6.

Like IgA, IgE is produced mainly in the linings of the respiratory and intestinal tracts and is part of the external secretory system of antibody. A deficiency of IgE has been inconsistently associated with deficiency of IgA in individuals with impaired immunity who present with undue susceptibility to infection. IgE does not cross the placenta, and IgE-antigen complexes do not bind complement by the classic pathway (see Table 35–4).

Summary

There are five different classes of antibodies (IgM, IgG, IgA, IgD, and IgE), four subclasses of IgG antibodies (IgG1, IgG2, IgG3, and IgG4), and two subclasses of IgA antibodies (IgA1 and IgA2) in humans. Each of these antibody isotypes possesses a distinct H chain (μ, γ, α, δ, ϵ; $\gamma 1$, $\gamma 2$, $\gamma 3$, $\gamma 4$; and $\alpha 1$, $\alpha 2$, respectively). The H chains contain the Fc region of the antibody, which determines what other proteins will bind to the antibody and therefore the biological properties of the class and subclass. Either type of L chain (κ or λ) can be associated with any class of H chain.

The structural differences among the five classes of immunoglobulins correspond to functional differences in their sites of production and action, their relative levels of production in primary and secondary immune responses, and their roles as physiologic effectors. For example, IgG is prevalent in both blood and tissue fluids, whereas IgM is chiefly confined to the blood, and secretory IgA is found primarily on epithelial surfaces. IgD and IgE are principally bound to cells, IgD to B cells, and IgE to basophils and mast cells.

Table 35–6. SERUM IgE LEVELS IN SELECTED CONDITIONS

Elevated
Atopic dermatitis
IgE myeloma
Hyper-IgE and recurrent infections
Wiskott-Aldrich syndrome
Hodgkin's disease (especially late stages)
Bronchopulmonary aspergillosis
Pemphigoid
Parasites (such as ascariasis)
Leprosy
AIDS
Elevated to normal
Allergic rhinitis
Allergic asthma
Extrinsic allergic alveolitis
Cystic fibrosis
Aspergilloma
Drug allergies
Severe liver disease
Allergic urticaria
Kawasaki disease
Periarteritis nodosa
Normal
Intestinal lymphangiectasia
Bronchiolitis
Pemphigus
Thyroiditis
Chronic renal failure
Normal to decreased
Leukemias
Multiple myeloma
Isolated IgA deficiency
Decreased
Ataxia-telangiectasia
Sex-linked hypogammaglobulinemia
Congenital hypogammaglobulinemia
Acquired hypogammaglobulinemia
IgE deficiency

Modified from Waldmann TA, Strober W, Polmar SH, Terry WD: *In* Ishizaka K, Dayton DH, Jr (eds): The Biological Role of the Immunoglobulin E System. Washington, D.C., U.S. Government Printing Office, 1975; and Arbesman CA: *In* Ishizaka K, Dayton DH, Jr (eds): The Biological Role of the Immunoglobulin E System, Washington, D.C., U.S. Government Printing Office, 1975.

5

CLINICAL SIGNIFICANCE OF IMMUNOGLOBULINS

Immunoglobulins play important roles in disease pathogenesis, diagnosis, prevention, and therapy.

Disease Pathogenesis

Hyperimmunoglobulinemia is a prominent feature of multiple myeloma and Waldenström's macroglobulinemia. Antibodies against native antigens may result in autoimmune diseases, as discussed in Chapters 41 and 43. Hypo- or agammaglobulinemia is often the prime characteristic of some immunodeficiency disorders (see Chap. 40).

Hyperimmunoglobulinemia

SERUM IMMUNOGLOBULIN LEVELS

Valid interpretation of serum immunoglobulin levels requires recognition of biological variations that exist throughout the lifespan of the individuals. The most important of these variables are age, sex, and race.

Studies on a large unselected group of healthy white subjects (3213) from a single community (Tecumseh, Michigan) showed that the mean concentrations of IgG and IgA increased with age, with slight but significant differences between the sexes. Females had higher serum levels of IgG and lower levels of IgA (Tables 35–7 and 35–8). Although these sex differences for IgG and IgA are statistically significant, their biological meaning is not apparent. IgM levels in these subjects remained relatively constant with age. However, females had higher mean levels of IgM (1.06 mg/mL) than males (0.77 mg/mL).

Several studies have reported that immunoglobulin levels are higher in persons with pigmented skins. Table 35–8 presents the results obtained in a healthy biracial population in Evans County, Georgia. Blacks had higher levels of the three major immunoglobulins (IgM, IgG, and IgA) than did whites. The most prominent difference was in IgG. No urban-rural difference in immunoglobulin levels was noted in this study. White subjects in Rochester, New York, had serum levels of IgM and IgG similar to those of white subjects in rural Georgia. A triracial study in Durban, Natal, South Africa, showed that Bantu male adults had significantly higher levels of IgM (32% more), IgG (40% more), and IgA (32% more) in their sera than comparable whites in this community who were born in the same year and had the same ABO blood group. Healthy Asiatic male adults had about 20% more IgG, 23% more IgA, and 7% more IgM than comparable whites. A study of subjects in the Washington, D.C., metropolitan area revealed that blacks had significantly higher IgG levels than whites but similar IgA and IgM levels (Tollerud, 1995). Control groups used in these studies were matched for age, sex, and race as well as for several environmental factors (Cassidy, 1974; Lichtman, 1967). Increases in γ globulin are often first noted after serum protein electrophoresis, a measurement of total protein, or measurements of albumin and γ-globulin fractions. Reference values for the different immunoglobulins vary with age, sex, and race (see Tables 35–7 and 35–8).

Table 35–7. SERUM IMMUNOGLOBULIN CONCENTRATIONS

Age (Years)	Mean IgG (mg/mL)		Mean IgA (mg/mL)	
	White Male	*White Female*	*White Male*	*White Female*
5–9	10.28	11.05	1.09	1.10
10–14	10.41	11.13	1.16	1.15
15–19	10.55	11.20	1.23	1.21
20–24	10.69	11.28	1.32	1.28
25–29	10.83	11.35	1.40	1.35
30–34	10.98	11.43	1.50	1.42
35–39	11.12	11.50	1.59	1.49
40–44	11.27	11.58	1.70	1.57
45–49	11.42	11.66	1.81	1.65
50–54	11.57	11.74	1.93	1.74
55–59	11.72	11.81	2.06	1.83
60–64	11.88	11.89	2.20	1.93
65–69	12.04	11.97	2.34	2.03
70–74	12.20	12.05	2.49	2.14
75+	12.36	12.13	2.66	2.26

The data were derived from 3213 serum samples collected from an unselected group of subjects from a single healthy community (Tecumseh, Michigan) (Cassidy, 1974).

Increases in immunoglobulins are referred to as monoclonal or polyclonal. Monoclonal immunoglobulins from any one individual are structurally identical and are believed to result from the clonal expansion of a single immunoglobulin-producing lymphoid cell, and hence are specific for a particular antigen. Polyclonal immunoglobulins in the same individual are structurally different from each other in one or more important ways—by class, as polyclonal IgG, IgA, or IgM; by light chain; or by antigen specificity. Polyclonal immunoglobulins arise from the expansion of several to many different immunoglobulin-producing lymphoid cells.

POLYCLONAL IMMUNOGLOBULINS

Polyclonal increases in immunoglobulins have been associated with many disease states (Table 35–9) (Buckley, 1977; Cushman, 1973). Serum protein electrophoresis is often sufficient to establish this condition. Immunoelectrophoresis, immunofixation, and determination of individual immunoglobulins or immunoglobulin light chains may be helpful at times to confirm a polyclonal distribution or an increased concentration in one or more immunoglobulin classes. Increases in serum immunoglobulins may result from decreased catabo-

Table 35–8. SERUM IgG CONCENTRATION IN A BIRACIAL POPULATION

Sex	Age (Years)	No. Samples Tested	Whites Mean (± SE) (mg/mL)	No. Samples Tested	Blacks Mean (± SE) (mg/mL)
	15–34	17	11.2 (7.3)	21	13.4 (6.5)
Men	35–54	17	10.8 (5.9)	19	13.5 (9.0)
	55–74	20	10.9 (7.4)	20	13.3 (5.8)
	15–34	19	10.6 (6.3)	18	15.6 (8.0)
Women	35–54	19	12.3 (3.4)	15	15.4 (6.4)
	55–74	20	10.9 (6.1)	16	14.2 (9.6)

The data are representative of subjects living in Evans County, Georgia (Lichtman, 1967).

Table 35–9. POLYCLONAL HYPERIMMUNOGLOBULINEMIAS: SOME ASSOCIATED DISEASE STATES

Condition	Immunoglobulin Classes
Immunodeficiency diseases	
Hyperimmunoglobulin E and recurrent infections	IgE
Wiskott-Aldrich syndrome	IgA, IgE
"Dysgammaglobulinemia Type I"	IgM
Hyperimmunoglobulin A and recurrent infections	IgA
AIDS	All classes
Infections	
Congenital infections (syphilis, toxoplasmosis, rubella, cytomegalovirus)	IgM
Infectious mononucleosis	IgM or all
Trypanosomiasis	IgM or all
Intestinal parasitism	All classes
Several helminthic infections	IgE
Visceral larva migrans	All classes
Chronic granulomatous disease of childhood	All classes
Leprosy	All classes
Chronic infection in general	All classes, with a preference for IgG
Liver diseases	
Chronic active hepatitis	IgG predominates
Acute hepatitis	IgG predominates
Biliary cirrhosis	IgM predominates
Lupoid hepatitis	All classes
Pulmonary disorders	
Pulmonary hypersensitivity syndrome	All classes
Sarcoidosis	All classes
Berylliosis	All classes
"Autoimmune" disorders	
Systemic lupus erythematosus	All classes
Rheumatoid arthritis	IgA or all
Many "autoimmune" states such as thyroiditis	All classes
Scleroderma	All classes
Cold agglutinin disease	IgM
Anaphylactoid purpura	IgA
Miscellaneous	
Down syndrome	All classes
Amyloidosis	All classes
Narcotic addiction	IgM
Renal tubular disease	All classes

lism and increased synthesis. The control mechanisms for these events are not well understood. The implications of elevated immunoglobulins are unknown. Most immunoglobulins appear not to be directed toward a definable, specific, or set of specific antigenic determinants. It should also be noted that most autoantibodies are not monoclonal but polyclonal. In general, persistent polyclonal increases in γ globulin are thought to be related to antigenic stimulation of a chronic nature or a loss of immunoglobulin regulation.

MONOCLONAL IMMUNOGLOBULINS

Monoclonal immunoglobulins or fragments of immunoglobulins have been associated with a number of disease conditions (Table 35–10) (Atkinson, 1977; Benbassat, 1976; Schafer, 1978; Wells, 1974; Kelly, 1985). These immunoglobulins have also been referred to as immunoglobulins with restricted heterogeneity.

The incidence of monoclonal immunoglobulins (M components) in unselected population studies is estimated to be 0.9% (Bachman, 1965; Axelsson, 1968; Cohen, 1985). Of course, a much higher percentage of positive results is found

Table 35–10. SELECTED CONDITIONS ASSOCIATED WITH MONOCLONAL IMMUNOGLOBULINS

Multiple myeloma
Macroglobulinemia of Waldenström
Chronic lymphocytic leukemia
Other leukemias
Lymphomas
"Benign" monoclonal gammopathy
Systemic capillary leak syndrome
Amyloidosis
Chronic liver disease such as chronic active hepatitis, primary biliary cirrhosis
Autoimmune disorders, including rheumatoid arthritis, systemic lupus erythematosus, thyroiditis, pernicious anemia, polyarteritis nodosa, Sjögren's syndrome
Gaucher's disease
Malignancies of various types
Hereditary spherocytosis
HIV infection including AIDS

in clinical laboratories where the sera to be tested are preselected. Multiple myeloma, Waldenström's macroglobulinemia, and B-cell neoplasms are some of the diseases that are associated with an elevated level of monoclonal immunoglobulins. It was earlier believed that monoclonal gammopathies were rare in cases of chronic lymphocytic leukemia or well-differentiated lymphocytic lymphoma. It has now been shown that when high-resolution electrophoresis and immunofixation are combined to study samples from these patients, the majority are found to have a monoclonal gammopathy (Keren, 1988). Monoclonal gammopathies have also been demonstrated in patients with Burkitt's lymphoma and B-cell acute lymphocytic leukemia.

The term monoclonal gammopathy of undetermined significance (MGUS) was coined by Kyle to categorize individuals in whom a monoclonal component is demonstrated in the serum but who lack other key features for diagnosing a malignant condition (Kyle, 1982). Subjects with MGUS may have as many as 10% plasma cells in the bone marrow. This is considerably less than the bone marrow plasmacytosis associated with multiple myeloma. About 20% of individuals with MGUS will develop a malignant B-cell lymphoproliferative disorder, most commonly multiple myeloma, over a 10-year period. Some of the other cases develop into chronic lymphocytic leukemia, amyloidosis, well-differentiated lymphocytic lymphoma, and other B-cell proliferative diseases. The majority of cases of MGUS do not progress to any other overt clinical disease. Subjects with MGUS have quantities of M component ranging from 300 mg/dL to greater than 3000 mg/dL and usually do not have Bence Jones protein in the urine. It is recommended that such patients be followed with serum protein electrophoresis every 6 to 12 months to determine whether the process is progressing or regressing.

Disease Diagnosis

Laboratory evaluation of immunoglobulin levels and functions may be helpful in the diagnosis and management of diseases. The use of complement fixation tests, hemagglutination assays, and other immunoassays can detect an increased or changing titer of antibodies against specific antigens such as those present on microorganisms.

Requests to examine sera for the presence of a monoclonal

protein are usually generated by a physician who recognizes that a patient has clinical symptoms and signs of such a disorder, or by the laboratory examination of a serum protein electrophoresis that suggests a monoclonal protein. If there is indeed an M component in a serum protein electrophoresis, a quantitative measurement of immunoglobulins by radial immunodiffusion, nephelometry, or another suitable technique can identify the specific immunoglobulin if only one of the major three classes is increased. Of course, this neither determines the light chain of a monoclonal immunoglobulin nor detects light chain myelomas. Biclonal gammopathies may be confusing.

Quantitative immunoglobulins are useful in monitoring the course of the disease and its treatment and may be helpful in separating a benign from a malignant condition. Monoclonal IgG levels of 2 g/100 mL or IgA levels of 1 g/100 mL (Isobe, 1971) or greater suggest a malignant condition. In many malignant immunocytopathies, the concentration of nonmonoclonal immunoglobulins is reduced. Thus, a deficiency of polyclonal immunoglobulins is suggestive of malignancy. Paradoxically, the patient with a malignant immunocytopathy is immunodeficient even though he possesses large amounts of a "nonsense" immunoglobulin produced by a poorly controlled clone of lymphoid cells.

Immunoelectrophoresis

Immunoelectrophoresis (IEP) or immunofixation (IEF) are useful in detecting specific monoclonal proteins. Thus, in patients with suspicious signs, symptoms, or especially hematopathologic findings in the peripheral blood, bone marrow, or lymph node, an IEP may be diagnostic. Whether or not serum protein electrophoresis should precede IEP or IEF depends on the relative availability of these techniques and the sophistication of each in a laboratory. For example, agarose serum protein electrophoresis detects most M components. However, electrophoresis on paper or cellulose acetate is not as sensitive. Another way of selecting sera for IEP or IEF is by reviewing serum protein electrophoresis determinations.

In an alternative approach suggested by Keren and his associates (Keren, 1988), serum values and the ratio of κ/λ are determined in conjunction with high-resolution electrophoresis. Serum immunofixation is performed if electrophoresis shows no abnormality, polyclonal hypergammaglobulinemia, or hypogammaglobulinemia, and the κ/λ ratio is not within reference limits. Serum immunofixation is also recommended in instances in which the κ/λ ratio is "normal" but an unusual band is seen on electrophoresis.

IEP is a sensitive, relatively uncomplicated procedure used to detect M components and their heavy and light chain components. IEP allows one to semi-quantitate the concentration of the immunoglobulins. Patients' sera should be compared with "normal" sera or a "normal" pool. For example, from a pool of 100 to 200 mL of blood from healthy individuals, 1-mL aliquots are quick-frozen with dry ice and acetone and stored at −70°C. The unused control serum is not refrozen but is discarded after retaining it for three days at 4°C.

The following types of antisera are recommended: anti-whole human sera; anti-IgG (γ chains), anti-IgM (μ); anti-IgA (α), anti-κ, and anti-λ (Fig. 35–6). It is important to realize that not all antisera are alike in strength and specificity and it is possible that the M component may not be detected with one of the antisera yet may be found with a second. Thus, each lot of antisera should be compared for titer, such as by gel diffusion against control sera, and specificity against whole human serum in an IEP. Interpretation of an IEP may take considerable experience, but generally one is searching for a disruption of a normally smooth line—that is, by bowing, thickening, or changed mobility. Examples of IEP are shown in Figure 35–6. IEP is a useful technique but has limitations. It may identify the presence of heavy and light chains but does not ensure that one indeed has an entire immunoglobulin molecule composed of two heavy chains and two light chains.

It is also possible, but unusual, for monoclonal immunoglobulins to be present in amounts below the level of detection of the system used. The lower level of detection can be estimated by diluting a known monoclonal immunoglobulin and testing it by IEP. Because monoclonal proteins of IgM, IgA, IgD, and IgE may be present in relatively small quantities compared with IgG, the light chain portion of the whole non-IgG immunoglobulin may not be detected by IEP. The inability to detect light chains of immunoglobulins in lesser concentrations in the presence of IgG of greater concentration is referred to as an umbrella effect. Therefore, other procedures may be required to rule out heavy chain or Franklin's disease. It is possible that the serum being tested and the antibody being used are not in the proper concentrations and that the M component may be missed. Finally, it is possible that the antisera being used will not detect the available determinants on a particular M component. If one has a high index of suspicion, it may be useful to use a second antiserum from another source.

Immunofixation

IEF is rapidly replacing IEP in the clinical laboratory because of its speed, sensitivity, and ease of interpretation. Comparative studies performed in our laboratory indicate that the two procedures are of comparable sensitivity. IEF also has the advantage of a more rapid read-out because diffusion through gel is not required. Replicate samples of patient serum are subjected to electrophoresis through high-resolution gel before monospecific antisera are applied directly to the separated serum proteins. The gel is washed, and the protein-antibody conjugates are stained and read directly (Fig. 35–7).

Either technique may be applied to other body fluids, most commonly urine. Monoclonal light chains in the urine, Bence Jones protein, may be detected in more than half of patients with multiple myeloma (Isobe, 1971; Wells, 1974). Polyclonal light chains may be detected in patients with other disorders, usually as part of complete immunoglobulin molecules. Detection of Bence Jones protein by heat is reviewed in Chapter 18. IEP/IEF of urine is more specific and more sensitive than the older Bence Jones assay. IEP/IEF may be performed on urine samples with sufficient protein or subsequent to concentration by lyophilization or selective membranes (Minicon, Amicon). Measurement of serum viscosity is discussed in Chapter 27.

Disease Prevention and Therapy

Administration of preformed antibodies obtained from another individual of the same species (homologous γ globu-

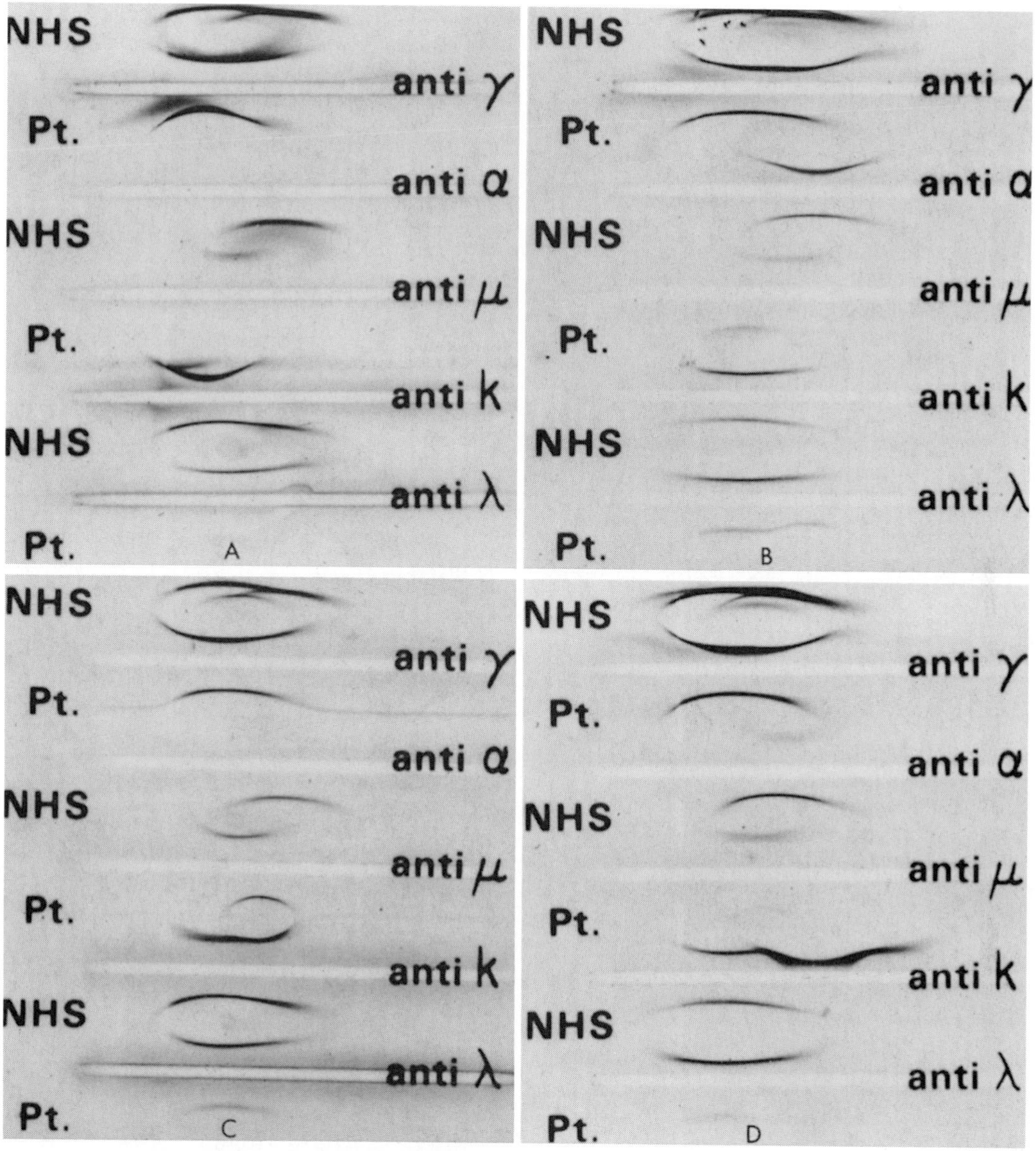

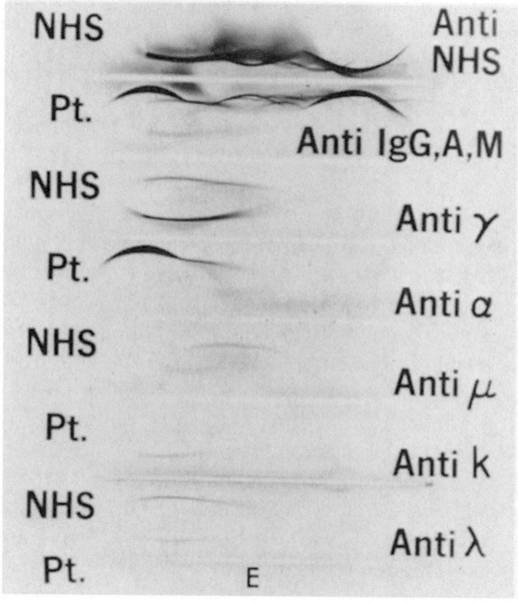

Figure 35–6. Monoclonal immunoglobulins demonstrated by serum immunoelectrophoresis. Aliquots of patient serum and a pool of normal human serum were subjected to electrophoresis on polyacrylamide at pH 8.6 (Poly-E-Film, Pfizer). The separated proteins were reacted overnight with antisera to (1) whole human serum; (2) a combination of IgG, IgA, and IgM; (3) γ-; (4) α-; (5) μ-; (6) κ; and (7) λ-chains, respectively. The membranes were washed and stained with Amido Black B. *A*, IgG-κ M component. *B*, IgA-λ M component. *C*, IgM-κ M component. *D*, κ-Light chain M component. *E*, γ-Heavy chain M component.

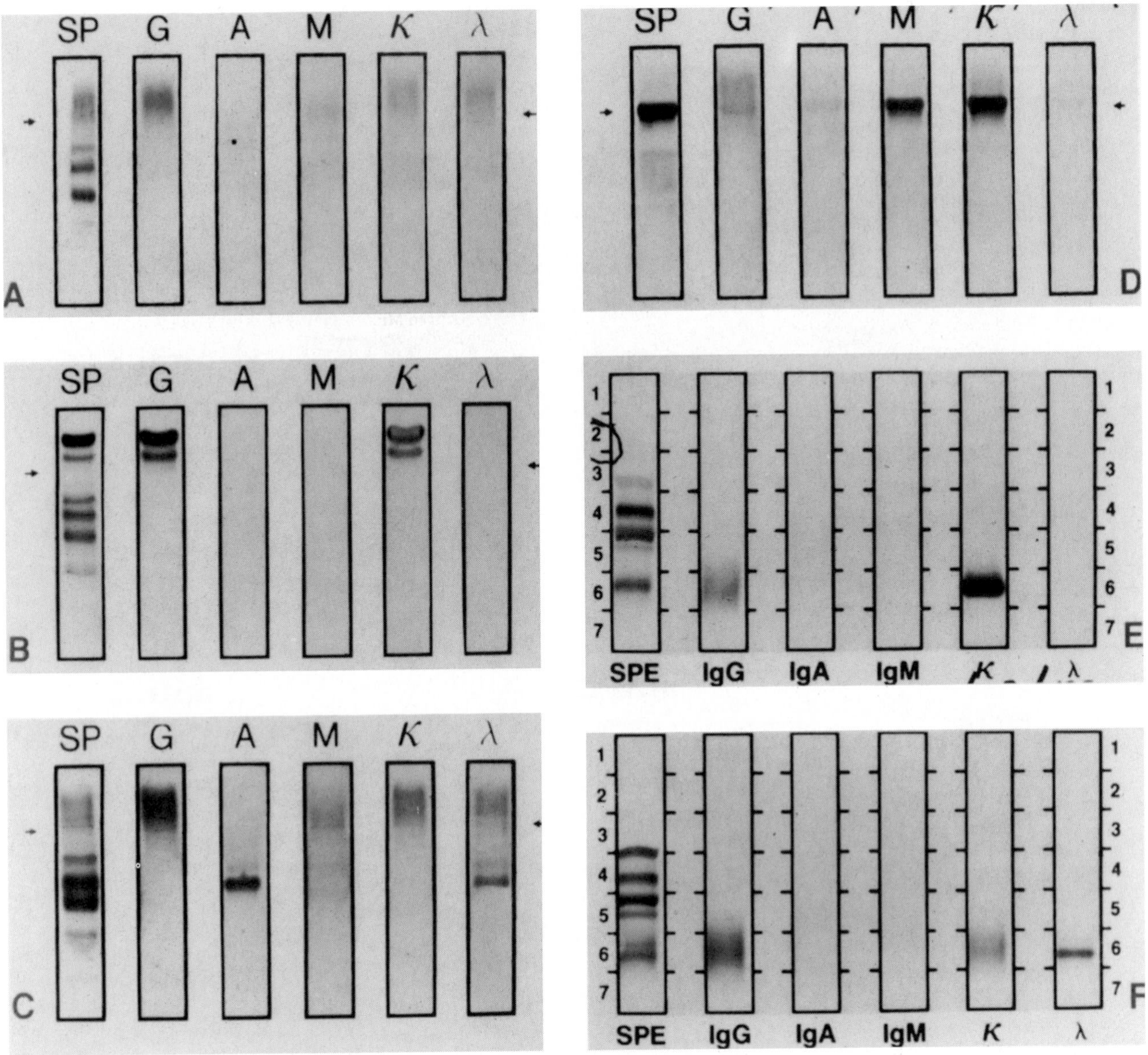

Figure 35–7. Monoclonal immunoglobulins demonstrated by serum immunofixation. Replicate samples of patient serum are subjected to electrophoresis through agarose at pH 8.6. The separated proteins are allowed to react with monospecific antisera, the gels washed, fixed, and stained. SP or SPE = sample not washed nor reacted with antisera (serum electrophoresis); G or IgG = sample reacted with anti-IgG; A or anti-IgA = sample reacted with anti-IgA; M or anti-IgM = sample reacted with anti-IgM; K or anti-kappa = sample reacted with anti-κ; L or anti-lambda = sample reacted with anti-λ. *A*, "normal." *B*, IgG-K M components (2). *C*, IgA-lambda M component. *D*, IgM-kappa M component. *E*, κ-chain M component. *F*, λ-chain M component.

lins) or a different species (heterologous γ globulins) results in immediate protection against infection. The immunity is short lived and decays as the antibodies are used and catabolized. Passive protection in neonatal life is based on transfer of maternal antibodies across the placenta or through colostrum (Pennington, 1991).

Pooled human γ globulin is useful for temporary protection against several viral and bacterial infections (Berkman, 1990; Hammarstrom, 1990; Desai, 1991). Depending on the dose used and the time of administration, the disease may be modified to a mild form or entirely prevented. The effect is more complete and more predictable if one uses hyperimmune preparations made from the plasma of individuals who are either convalescing from the disease in question or have been recently immunized against it. Such preparations contain a higher concentration of specific antibodies. Antibodies may also be produced in animals, such as horses, and in the past these found widespread use. However, prior sensitization to foreign proteins may lead to clinical reactions such as anaphylaxis, serum sickness, pyrexia, and local Arthus reactions.

Monoclonal antibodies have revolutionized many areas of medicine, including research, diagnostics, and therapy. Murine, human, and humanized monoclonal antibodies have all been developed (Lefrano, 1990; Mountain, 1992; Morrison, 1992; Ward, 1992; Shin, 1993). Many monoclonal antibodies, often replacing polyclonal antisera, are used for diagnostic purposes (see Chap. 33). Perhaps the most important therapeutic applications of monoclonals are seen in the fields of transplantation and oncology (Neame, 1994; Stevenson, 1990; Vitetta, 1993). OKT3, a murine monoclonal antibody against the CD3 receptor on lymphocytes, is often used as an antirejection therapy to block the activity of cytotoxic T lymphocytes in renal transplant recipients (Ortho Multicenter Transplant Study Group, 1985). Many potential clinical applications of monoclonal antibodies are being evaluated. Monoclonal antibodies against a variety of bacteria or their products are potentially useful in patients with gram-positive and gram-negative shock (Chmel, 1990; Peake, 1993; Fink, 1993); anticytokine and antineutrophil adhesion molecule monoclonal antibodies may be effective in conditions associated with acute inflammation and cytokine release, e.g., acid aspiration, ischemia or reperfusion injury (myocardial infarction, hemorrhagic shock, aortic aneurysm repair); and antibodies inhibiting neutrophil adhesion may be effective in asthma, pulmonary fibrosis, meningitis, and cerebral malaria. Clinical research will determine the extent of the role of monoclonal antibodies in disease prevention and therapy.

Atkinson JP, Waldmann TA, Stein SF, et al: Systemic capillary leak syndrome and monoclonal IgG gammopathy. Medicine 1977; 56:225.

Axelsson N, Hellen J: Frequency of M components in 6995 sera from an adult population. Br J Haematol 1968; 15:417.

Bachman R: The diagnostic significance of the serum concentration of pathological proteins. Acta Med Scand 1965; 178:801.

Benbassat J, Fluman N, Zlotnick A: Monoclonal immunoglobulin disorders: A report of 154 cases. Am J Med Sci 1976; 27:325.

Berkman SA, Lee ML, Gale RP: Clinical uses of intravenous immunoglobulins. Ann Intern Med 1990; 112:278.

Bhat TN, Bentley GA, Fischmann TO, et al: Small rearrangements in structures of Fv and Fab fragments of antibody D1.3 upon antigen binding. Nature 1990; 347:483.

Buckley RH: *In* Altman PL, Katz DD (eds): Human Health and Disease. Bethesda, MD, FASEB, 1977.

Burton DR: Immunoglobulin G: Functional sites. Mol Immunol 1985; 22:161.

Carayannopoulos L, Capra JD: Immunoglobulins structure and function. *In* Paul WE (ed): Fundamental Immunology. New York, Raven Press, 1993, p 283.

Carsetti R, Kohler G, Lamers MC: A role for immunoglobulin D: Interference with tolerance induction. Eur J Immunol 1993; 23:168.

Cassidy JT, Nordby GL, Dodge HJ: Biologic variation of human serum immunoglobulin concentrations: Sex-age specific effects. J Chronic Dis 1974; 27:507.

Chmel H: Role of monoclonal antibody therapy in the treatment of infectious disease. Am J Hosp Pharm 1990; 47:S11.

Cohen HJ: Multiple myeloma in the elderly. Clin Geriatr Med 1985; 1:827.

Cushman P, Grieco MH: Hyperimmunoglobulinemia associated with narcotic addiction. Am J Med 1973; 54:320.

Davies DR, Metzer H: Structural basis of antibody function. Ann Rev Immunol 1983; 1:87.

Desai RG: Recent advances in intravenous immunoglobulin therapy: Concluding remarks. Current trends and future directions. Cancer 1991; 68:1460.

Edward EM: Immunoglobulins—molecular genetics. *In* Paul WE (ed): Fundamental Immunology. New York, Raven Press, 1993, p 315.

Fink MP: Adoptive immunotherapy of gram-negative sepsis: Use of monoclonal antibodies to lipopolysaccharide. Crit Care Med 1993; 21:S32.

Hammarstrom L, Smith CI: New and old aspects of immunoglobulin application. The use of intravenous IgG as prophylaxis and for treatment of infections. Infection 1990; 18:314.

Herron JN, He XM, Ballard DW: An antibody to single-stranded DNA: Comparison of the three-dimensional structures of the unliganded Fab and a deoxynucleotide-Fab complex. Proteins 1991; 11:159.

Isobe T, Osserman EF: Pathologic conditions associated with plasma cell dyscrasias: A study of 806 cases. Ann NY Acad Sci 1971; 190:507.

Karplus M, McCammon JA: Dynamics of proteins: Elements and function. Annu Rev BioChem 1983; 53:263.

Kelly RH, Tardy TJ, Shah PM: Benign monoclonal gammopathy: A reassessment of the problem. Immunol Invest 1985; 14:193.

Keren DF, Warren JS, Lowe JB: Strategy to diagnose monoclonal gammopathies in serum: High-resolution electrophoresis, immunofixation and kappa/lambda quantification. Clin Chem 1988; 34:2196.

Kyle RA: Monoclonal gammopathy of undetermined significance (MGUS): A review. Clin Haematol 1982; 11:123.

Lefrano G, Lefrano MP: Antibody engineering and perspectives in therapy. Biochemie 1990; 72:639.

Lichtman MA, Vaughan JH, Hames CG: The distribution of serum immunoglobulins, anti-γ-G globulins and antinuclear antibodies in White and Negro subjects in Evans County, Georgia. Arthritis Rheum 1967; 10:204.

Morrison SL: In vitro antibodies: Strategies for production and application. Ann Rev Immunol 1992; 10:239.

Mountain A, Adair JR: Engineering antibodies for therapy. Biotechnol Genet Eng Rev 1992; 10:1.

Neame PB, Soamboonsrup P, Quigley JG, et al: The use of monoclonal antibodies and immune markers in the diagnosis, prognosis, and therapy of acute leukemia. Transfusion Med Rev 1994; 8:59.

Ortho Multicenter Transplant Study Group: A randomized clinical trial of OKT3 monoclonal antibody for acute rejection of cadaveric renal transplants. N Engl J Med 1985; 313:337.

Padlan EA: Anatomy of the antibody molecule. Mol Immunol 1991; 31(3):169.

Peake S: Monoclonal antibodies—immunotherapy for the critically ill. Anaesth Intens Care 1993; 21:739.

Pennington JE: Immunoglobulin therapy in infectious disease. Cleve J Med 1991; 58:309.

Poljak RJ: Structure of antibodies and their complexes with antigens. Mol Immunol 1991; 28(12):1341.

Roes J, Rajewski K: Immunoglobulin D (IgD)—deficient mice reveal an auxiliary receptor function for IgD in antigen-mediated recruitment of B-cells. J Exp Med 1993; 177:45.

Schafer AI, Miller JB, Lester EP, et al: Monoclonal gammopathy in hereditary spherocytosis: A possible pathogenetic relation. Ann Intern Med 1978; 88:45.

Shin SU, Wright A, Morrison SL: Hybrid antibodies. Int Rev Immunol 1993; 10:177.

Spielgelberg HL: Biological activities of immunoglobulins of different classes and subclasses. Adv Immunol 1974; 19:259.

Standfield RL, Fieser TM, Lerner RA, et al: Crystal structures of an antibody to a peptide and its complex with peptide antigen at 2.8 Å. Science 1990; 248:712.

Stevenson FK, George AJ, Glennie MJ: Anti-idiotypic therapy of leukemias and lymphomas. Chem Immunol 1990; 48:126.

Tedford MC, Stimson WH: Molecular recognition in antibodies and its application. Experientia 1991; 47:1129.

Tollerud DJ, Brown LM, Blattner WA, et al: Racial differences in serum immunoglobulin levels: Relationship to cigarette smoking, T-cell subsets, and soluble interleukin-2 receptors. J Clin Lab Anal 1995; 9:37.

Tonegawa S: Somatic generation of antibody-diversity. Nature 1983; 302:575.

Vitetta ES, Thorpe PE, Uhr JW: Immunotoxins: Magic bullets or misguided missiles? Trends Pharmacol Sci 1993; 14:148.

Ward ES: Antibody engineering: The use of *Escherichia coli* as an expression host. FASEB J 1992; 6:2122.

Wells JV, Fudenberg HH: Paraproteinemias. DM 1:45, 1974.

Wilson IA, Stanfield RL, Rini JM, et al: Structural aspects of antibodies and antibody-antigen complexes. Ciba Foundation Symposium 1991; 159:13.

Wright A, Shin SU, Morrison SL: Genetically engineered antibodies: Progress and prospects. Crit Rev Immunol 1992; 12:125.

5

Chapter 36

Complement and Kinins: Mediators of Inflammation

Wasiuddin Ahmed Khan, Ph.D.
Delbert R. Wigfall, M.D.
Michael M. Frank, M.D.

STRUCTURAL AND FUNCTIONAL RELATIONSHIPS

The complement system is composed of a series of circulating blood proteins that serve as mediators of the inflammatory response. In addition, the complement proteins are important in the opsonization of foreign particulate matter, including a variety of microorganisms, and in cytolytic reactions against certain susceptible cells (prokaryotic or eukaryotic cells) and enveloped viruses. Thus, the complement system has evolved as a complex, interacting series of over 30 proteins designed to mediate host defense reactions and to protect against infections. There are very few individuals deficient in any one of these proteins. In sharp contrast to inherited defects in the coagulation cascade, the absence of a component is not often overtly responsible for manifestation of a disease state. In certain diseases the complement system is functioning normally but is being activated under abnormal circumstances. For example, circulating immune complexes may be deposited in the kidneys of patients with systemic lupus erythematosus, and these circulating complexes may activate complement in a perfectly normal fashion. This normal activation process may lead to renal inflammation and glomerular damage. In this case, the complement system is functioning normally but nevertheless is intimately associated with the development of disease.

Complement proteins circulate as inactive precursors in serum and are activated in a very precise order of biochemical reactions (Table 36–1). With each of the earlier acting components, activation of the protein is associated with cleavage of the protein component. The larger fragment produced by the protein cleavage is usually responsible for continuation of the complement sequence. The smaller fragment often has the function of promoting the inflammatory response. There are a number of ways in which complement proteins can be activated. For example, proteolytic enzymes, such as those released from certain bacteria, may cleave a complement protein, leading to the uncovering of an active site and the propagation of the complement sequence. More often, antigen-antibody complexes on microbial or viral surfaces are the inciting agents.

Table 36–1. PLASMA COMPLEMENT PROTEINS

Proteins	Molecular Weight (kDa)	Chromosomal Localization	Concentration (mg/mL)
C1	750		
C1q	410	$1p^{34-36}$	70
C1r	85	$12p^{13}$	35
C1s	85	$12p^{13}$	35
C1 Inh	105	$11p^{11}$	200
C4	~200	$6p^{21.3}$	450–750
C2	105	$6p^{21.3}$	20
C3	~190	19	1000–1600
C5	190	$9q^{32}$	75
C6	115	5q	50–70
C7	115	5q	50–70
C8	100	$1p^{34}$	55
C9	71	$5p^{13}$	60
Factor B	~90	$6p^{21.3}$	200
Factor D	~24	unknown	~1
Properdin	~53	$Xp^{11.3}$	~25
Factor 1	~88	$4q^{24}$	35
Factor H	~150	1q	500
C4 binding protein	~570	1q	300
SP-40	80	unknown	~75
S protein (vitronectin)	80	unknown	500

Complement Nomenclature

There are two major pathways of complement activation in serum; they are referred to as the classic and the alternative pathways. Figure 36–1 illustrates the general sequence of reactions of each of these pathways. The nine proteins of the classic pathway are designated by an upper case letter C followed by a number. The numbers generally follow the order of action of the components with the exception of C4, which acts before C2 and C3. Components reacting solely in the alternative pathway are designated by upper case letters. Regulatory proteins are referred to by a descriptive title or a letter (such as C4 binding protein and Factor H). Single component or multicomponent complexes that have enzymatic activity are designated by a bar over the component(s), such as $\overline{C1r2}$. Fragments or subunits of the various components are designated by a lower case letter suffix, such as C3b. Components or fragments that have lost activity through chemical denaturation of the action of control proteins are usually designated by a prefix lower-case i, such as iC3 or iC3b.

Classic Pathway

The classic pathway, which was described around the turn of the century, was the first of the two complement pathways to be discovered. Much of our understanding of the mechanism of complement action is derived from studies of this pathway, which is responsible for the lysis of most antibody-sensitized cells. Nine proteins or components comprise the classic pathway. The functional activity of the various components has been well elucidated, and more recent work has focused on the physiochemical basis for their activity (Hammer, 1988). Under most conditions, initiation of complement activation by the classic pathway requires the interaction of antigen with C1-fixing antibody. Not all classes of immunoglobulin activate the classic pathway. IgM and IgG subclass IgG1, IgG2, and IgG3 bind and activate C1. This reaction has been studied in detail in several model systems. The precise molecular nature of the antigen-antibody C1 interaction is not clear, but it is known that C1 binds to the Fc fragment of antibody in the antigen-antibody complex by a noncovalent, easily reversed ionic linkage with the immunoglobulin CH2 domain. Recent data suggest that multiple points of interaction with antibody are required for C1 activation. C1 itself is a 740,000 dalton macromolecular protein complex that contains a single C1q molecule complexed of two C1r and two C1s chains that are held together in the presence of calcium ions. The portion of the C1 molecule that interacts with immunoglobulin is the C1q subcomponent. Electron microscopic studies show that C1q is a structure consisting of six globular heads (sites of immunoglobulin attachment) attached by collagen-like fibrillar stalks to a central subunit (Fries, 1987). The ability of C1q to interact with aggregated immunoglobulin has provided the basis for a number of tests designed to detect the presence of soluble immune complexes in patient blood samples. Radiolabeled C1q is added to the serum or plasma sample, and one of a number of techniques is used to differentiate free C1q from that bound to protein components of serum. The binding of C1q suggests the presence of immunoglobulin complexes in the serum or plasma sample (Zubler, 1976).

The binding of C1 to antibody in turn leads to its activation. It appears that a single molecule of most IgM antibodies bound by multiple antibody sites to an antigen can "fix" or bind and activate one molecule of C1. Although C1 binding by a single IgG molecule has been described, C1 binding requires an IgG doublet, two molecules side by side, in most of the experimental models studied (Borsos, 1965). The fact that the binding of C1 by IgG requires cooperative interaction of several IgG molecules has consequences of clinical importance. Because IgG molecules bind to a cell surface in a random fashion, the attachment of hundreds or thousands of IgG molecules to an antigen may be required to generate a C1-fixing site. This is thought to be the explanation for the fact that anti-Rh antibodies of the complement-fixing subclasses generally do not provide a site for complement fixation when they bind to human erythrocytes. The appropriate Rh antigens are sparsely scattered on the erythrocyte surface, and this is thought to preclude the formation of antibody doublets and subsequent complement fixation. Interestingly, binding of ^{125}I-C1q to IgG anti-Rh0(D)-coated cells has been reported with binding at affinities high enough to suggest multivalent attachment and hence the presence of IgG at least in doublets (Hughes-Jones, 1981). Nevertheless, complement activation is not noted in most anti-Rh-mediated hemolytic states, whereas it is noted in hemolytic states mediated by cold agglutinins and anti-A and anti-B blood group substance antibodies.

The activation of C1 leads to the generation of an enzymatic site that in model systems has esterase activity. This activation is associated with cleavage of each of the two C1r chains producing an enzymatically active site on each of the two generated C1r light chains, which then cleave the two C1s chains to form $\overline{C1s2}$. $\overline{C1s2}$ is capable of interacting with

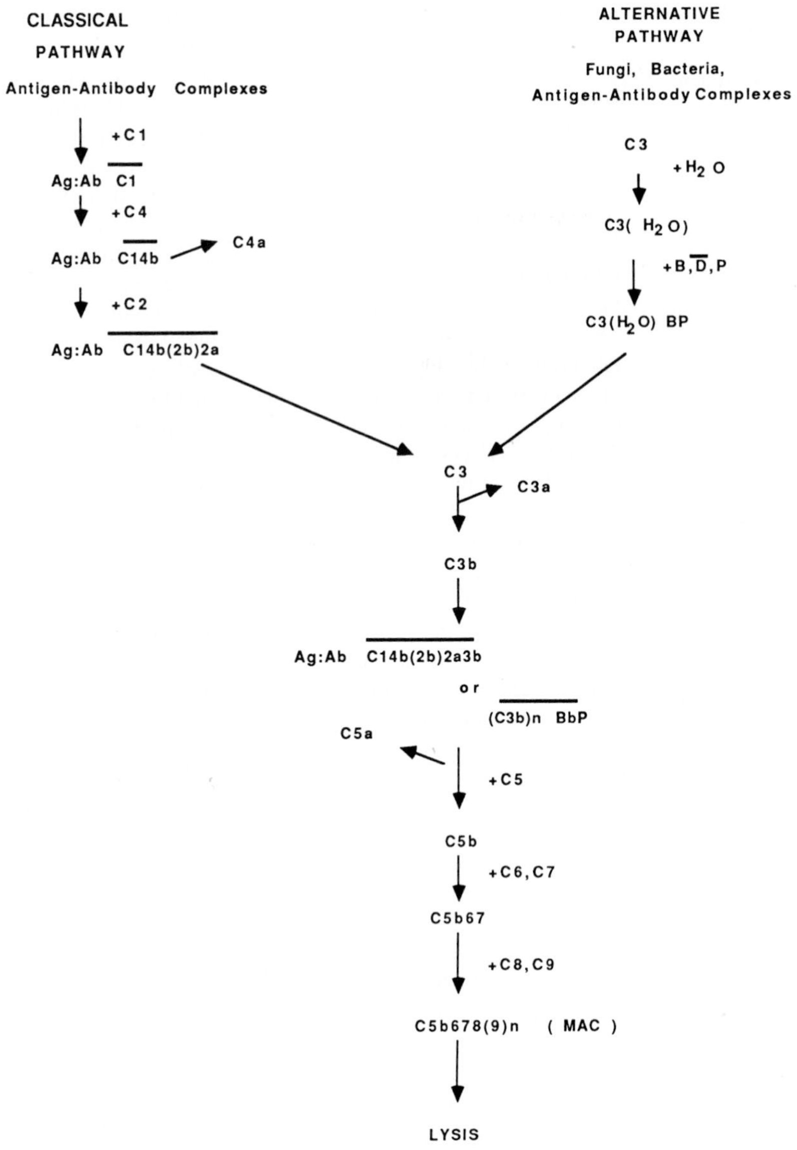

Figure 36–1. The components of the classic (classical) and alternative pathways, which converge to form a convertase that cleaves C3. In the classic pathway, antigen-antibody complexes sequentially bind and activate C1, C4, and C2. In the alternative pathway, C3 undergoes hydrolysis of its thioester bond, which induces a change in conformation. It then binds factor B (B), which is cleaved by factor D (D) to form a convertase that is stabilized by properdin (P). C3b, the cleavage product of C3, also has a cleaved thioester bond and is capable of activating the alternative pathway. The C3b-containing convertase of both pathways continues sequential binding of the late-acting components until the sequence of activation is complete. MAC denotes the membrane attack complex.

the next component in the complement sequence, C4. C4 is cleaved by C1s2 acting as an enzyme, and two cleavage fragments are formed (C4a and C4b). The larger fragment (C4b) is highly reactive for a few moments after its formation and appears to covalently bind to any suitable receptor in the microenvironment. Covalent binding involves formation of an amide or ester bond with an appropriate substrate following cleavage of an internal thioester within the C4 (Fries, 1987).

Two genes for C4 exist, and two types of C4 are often produced, C4A and C4B (O'Neill, 1978a; Awdeh, 1980). Multiple alleles for each gene exist, and individuals with a deletion of one of these genes are fairly common. These two gene products differ in hemolytic efficiency and in their tendency to form amide as opposed to ester bonds. It has been found that the Chido and Rodgers blood group antigens arise from degradation fragments of C4B and C4A, respectively bound to red cells (O'Neill, 1978b). On activation, some of the activated C4 molecules bind to the erythrocyte cell membrane as a cluster around the antigen-antibody-C1 site. Therefore, one antibody site can lead to the deposition of many C4b molecules (Borsos, 1970).

In the presence of magnesium ions, C4b acts as a site for the binding and subsequent cleavage of the next component in the sequence, C2. $\overline{\text{C1s2}}$ in association with C4b cleaves C2 into two fragments, C2a and C2b, leading to formation of the unstable enzymatic complex, $\overline{\text{C1s24b(2b)2a}}$. The complex of C4b bound to cleaved C2, referred to as the classic pathway C3 convertase, functions to cleave C3, a pivotal component that functions in both pathways. The C2a molecule in this complex is thought to serve as the enzyme in the cleavage of C3 as well as C5 later in the sequence. C2a, however, does not cleave C3 in the absence of C4b, which is required for C3 binding. C3b, the major cleavage fragment of C3, is covalently bound at the activating site, and, again, amplification is an important part of the reaction in that hundreds of C3b molecules may be deposited at each complement fixing site. C3a, the smaller fragment that is released, has no apparent further role in the cytolytic cascade (see Fig.

36–2 for C3 binding and degradation). If C3 is not present, the C1s24b(2b)2a complex decays to C1s24b, releasing inactivated fragments of C2. Many of the remaining reactions in the complement sequence follow this general formulation. The C4b(2b)2a3b complex can bind and then cleave C5 into two fragments, C5a and C5b. Again, C5b associates with the cell membrane to continue the hemolytic sequence, and the C5a fragment is released. This general pattern is continued for C6, C7, C8, and C9; however, the reactions differ in detail. Activation of these components does not appear to be accompanied by cleavage. When all of the complement components have reacted with a site on the cell surface, the cell membrane may be damaged in such a way that the cell lysis occurs (Fries, 1987).

Alternative Pathway

The existence of a second pathway of complement activation was first suggested by Pillemer (1954). This pathway, currently referred to as the alternative pathway, is important in the control of microbial infection. Because this pathway does not have an absolute requirement for antibody and does not use C1, C4, or C2, it is of particular importance before the appearance of antibody during the course of an infection.

Critical to an understanding of the function of this pathway is an understanding of the function of C3 (Fig. 36–2). C3 is a two-chain molecule that is held in a strained configuration by the presence of a thioester linkage between a cysteine in position 338 and glutamic acid in position 341 (De Bruijn, 1985). This highly reactive group is buried in a hydrophobic pocket within the molecule. On removal of the C3a peptide from the α chain of C3, the pocket is exposed, and the thioester reacts either with an antigenic surface nearby to form an ester or amide linkage or with water to be hydrolyzed (Tack, 1983). With the opening of this thioester, the C3 molecule undergoes a marked alteration in configuration. If Mg^{2+} is available, it can now react with Factor B of the alternative pathway. In the presence of Factor D, Factor B is cleaved, forming a complex of the altered C3 (C3b) with the cleavage fragments of bound Factor B ($\overline{C3bBb}$). This complex of two protein fragments can bind a fresh molecule of C3 and cleave it to form more C3b. The newly formed C3b can, in turn, continue alternative pathway activation. Thus, the pathway has an intrinsic feedback capability and can act on C3 to provide further amplification (Gotze, 1977).

In plasma, native C3 is not completely stable. Water can slowly penetrate the hydrophobic pocket even when C3a is

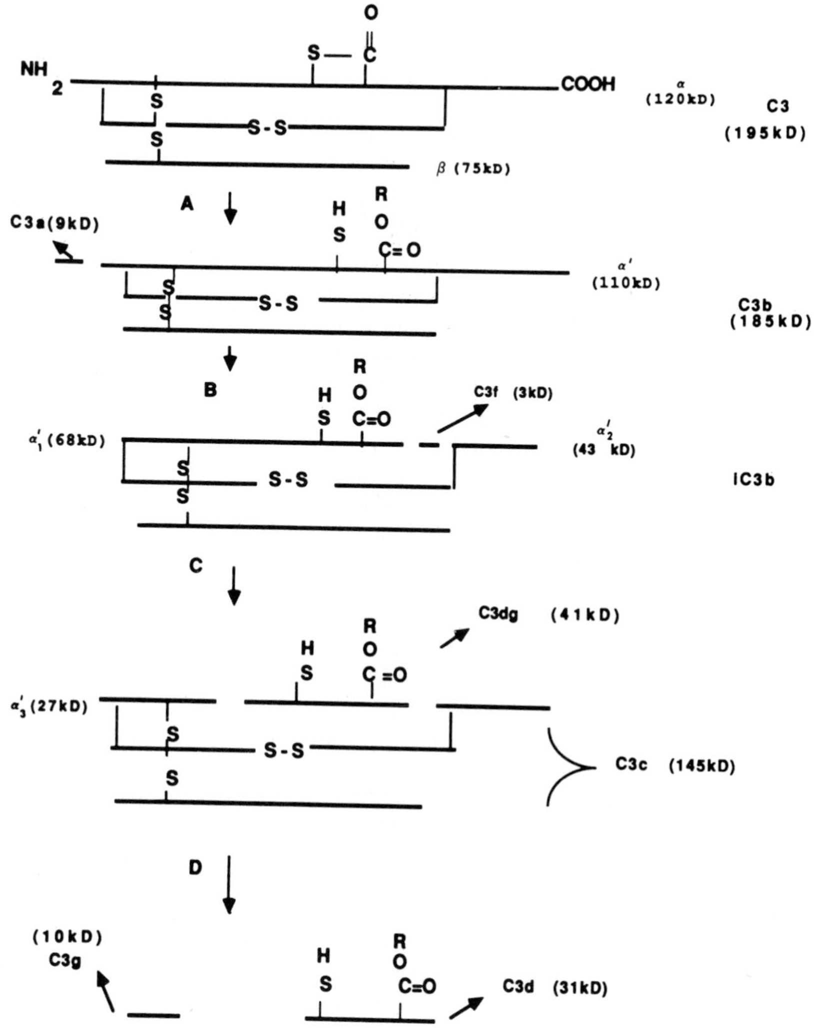

Figure 36–2. C3 cleavage and the C3b inactivation sequence. The approximate molecular weight of each chain or fragment is given in kilodaltons. Enzymes and cofactors believed responsible for each cleavage (designated by capital letters) are A, C3 convertase; B, factor H or CR1 + Factor I; C, CR1 + Factor I; and D, trypsin, elastase, or plasmin.

not cleaved from the molecule (Pangburn, 1981). Again, the thioester is hydrolyzed, and the molecule undergoes a conformational change. It can accept Factor B in the presence of Mg^{2+}, and Factor D can cleave the C3 bound B to generate a C3 cleaving enzyme complex. Spontaneous activation of the alternative pathway could lead to unregulated complement-mediated damage. For this reason, the activity of C3 with a cleaved thioester is under rigid control (see Regulation of Activation subsequently).

In both the alternative and classic pathways, the C3 cleaving convertase tends to decay. The decay is rapid in the case of the alternative pathway convertase and is stabilized by properdin (Gotze, 1977). Properdin is found in normal serum in an inactive state and becomes activated on binding to $\overline{\text{C3bBb}}$. Binding of properdin increases the half-life of the C3 convertase more than threefold. Properdin mediates this effect primarily by impeding the decay of the Bb. Interestingly, in some individuals with glomerulonephritis with very low C3, the alternative pathway C3 convertase is stabilized by another protein, C3Nef (C3 nephritic factor) (Gotze, 1977), a protein that binds to the convertase and prevents its decay. C3Nef interacts with the C3 convertase to form a fluid phase complex, $\overline{\text{C3bBb}}$(C3Nef), that has a 10-fold longer half-life than $\overline{\text{C3bBb}}$. C3Nef also apparently protects the alternative pathway C3 convertase from decay association by Factor H (Fearon, 1980) (see later under Regulation of Complement Activation). Analysis of C3Nef has demonstrated that the protein is an autoantibody formed against the C3 convertase. C3Nef appears to be responsible for the very low C3 level present in these patients but is not thought at present to play a central role in the development of nephritis.

The Mechanism of Cell Lysis

The biomechanical basis of the terminal events involved in complement-mediated lysis has been greatly clarified in the last decade; however, a number of aspects of the process remain unresolved. It is believed that the membrane lytic sequence is initiated when C5b interacts with C6. With the binding of C7, the complex becomes more hydrophobic, and, if formed near a cell, it will insert itself into the cell membrane lipid. This newly formed complex, C5b67, can bind C8 and one or more molecules of C9. The binding of C8 alone can lead to the formation of a small transmembrane pore and slow lysis of erythrocytes. Electron microscopy shows the formation of a hollow cylinder-like structure formed by the assembly of these components in the presence of excess C9. This complex, referred to as the membrane attack complex (MAC), is thought to have a lipid-associated external surface and a hydrophilic center through which ions pass freely. Thus, the insertion of the MAC disrupts the osmotic and chemical equilibrium of the cell (Mayer, 1984; Shin, 1988). On certain cells, such as erythrocytes, one lesion can cause cell lysis; however, on other cells with more complex metabolism, a lesion may be internalized and destroyed, thereby providing some protection from complement lysis.

Recent studies have revealed that C9 has a strong tendency to polymerize, leading to a re-evaluation of the terminal events in cell lysis. It has been shown that polymerized C9 (polyC9) alone may produce cell lesions under some circumstances. When C9 undergoes polymerization, its surface hydrophobicity increases, and a neoantigen that is absent from native C9 is expressed. Interestingly, antibodies against the polyC9 neoantigen react strongly with detergent-extracted MAC. Moreover, the ultrastructure of polyC9 is similar to that of the MAC complex. According to one proposed theory, the C5b-8 complex serves to bind C9 and to initiate its polymerization. PolyC9 is responsible for the cylinder-like lesion seen on electron microscopy, and C5b-8 does not have a central role in forming the visualized transmembrane channel leading to cell lysis. This alternative theory on the mechanism of cell lysis remains an area of active investigation (Zalman, 1990).

Biological Functions Associated with Activation

As discussed, the complement system subserves many functions in addition to inducing cell lysis. Many of the features of the inflammatory response are promoted by complement fragments, and complement plays a key role in opsonization. Table 36–2 lists the most widely accepted biological functions of complement components and complement fragments (Fries, 1987; Joiner, 1984; Frank, 1994).

The anaphylatoxins C3a, C4a, and C5a are biologically active, low-molecular-weight peptides that are generated by the enzymatic cleavage of their parent molecules during complement activation (Goldstein, 1988). In general, anaphylatoxins are defined by their biological effects on smooth muscle, mast cells, small blood vessels, and peripheral blood leukocytes. The specific effects mediated by these peptides include degranulation of mast cells and basophils with subsequent release of various mediators in the absence of cytotoxicity; the induction of human neutrophil aggregation; smooth muscle contraction; enhanced vascular permeability; induction of serotonin release from guinea pig platelets and thromboxane release from guinea pig macrophages; and stimulation of mucus release from goblet cells (Marom, 1985). One important effect of the reaction of the anaphylatoxins with basophils is to cause vessel dilation, leading to increased blood flow to an inflammatory site. The function of C4a is generally similar to that of C3a; however, C4a is far less effective in its biological effects on a molar basis. C5a is by far the most potent of the human anaphylatoxins. For instance, the effect of C5a is 200-fold greater than that of C3a and 3000-fold greater than that of C4a in causing smooth muscle contraction of guinea pig ileum. It should be noted, however, that the relative effectiveness of these peptides is both tissue and species specific. C3a and C4a are both cationic polypeptides that have a similar structure and molecular weight (9000 daltons). Apparently C3a and C4a bind to the same cell surface receptors; however, quantitative studies of the receptors for C3a and C4a have not yet been published. Notably, the receptors that recognize C3a and C4a are distinct from those that bind C5a. Cell surface receptors that recognize these peptides exist on neutrophils, mast cells, monocytes, eosinophils, and platelets. Many of the responses mediated by the anaphylatoxins involve receptor-ligand interactions; however, other, more complex mechanisms are thought to be involved in the wide range of biological effects elicited by these peptides. In addition to its role as an anaphylatoxin, C5a has many other important biological properties that appear to be mediated by

Table 36–2. INHERITED DEFICIENCIES IN COMPLEMENT AND COMPLEMENT-RELATED PROTEINS

Deficient Component or Subcomponent	Clinical Pattern of Inheritance	Reported Major Clinical Correlates*
C1q	Autosomal recessive	Glomerulonephritis, systemic lupus erythematosus (SLE)
C1r	Probably autosomal recessive	Syndrome resembling SLE
C1s	Found in combination with C1r deficiency	SLE
C4	Probably autosomal recessive (two separate loci, C4A and C4B)†	Syndrome resembling SLE
C2	Autosomal recessive, HLA-linked	SLE, discoid lupus erythematosus, juvenile rheumatoid arthritis, glomerulonephritis
C3	Autosomal recessive	Recurrent pyogenic infections, glomerulonephritis
C5	Autosomal recessive	Recurrent disseminated neisserial infections, SLE
C6	Autosomal recessive	Recurrent disseminated neisserial infections
C7	Autosomal recessive	Recurrent disseminated neisserial infections, Raynaud's phenomenon
C8 β chain or C8 α-γ chains	Autosomal recessive	Recurrent disseminated neisserial infections
C9	Autosomal recessive	None identified
Properdin	X-linked recessive	Recurrent pyogenic infections, fulminant meningococcemia
Factor D	Autosomal recessive	Recurrent pyogenic infections
C1 inhibitor	Autosomal dominant	Hereditary angioedema (HAE), increased incidence of several autoimmune diseases‡
Factor H	Autosomal recessive	Glomerulonephritis
Factor I	Autosomal recessive	Recurrent pyogenic infections
CR1	Autosomal recessive§	Association between low numbers of erythrocyte CR1 and SLE
CR3	Autosomal recessive¶	Leukocytosis, recurrent pyogenic infections, delayed umbilical-cord separation
DAF	?	Paroxysmal nocturnal hemoglobinuria (PNH)
HRF	?	PNH

*Note that many people with complement deficiencies, especially of C2 and the terminal components, are clinically well. A substantial number of patients with defects in C5 through C9 have had autoimmune disease. Deficiencies of C1-9 are associated with CH_{50} of 0. Deficiencies of C1, C4, and C2 associated with SLE often have negative LE preps. Deficiencies of C3-9 are associated with the absence of bactericidal activity of serum. Deficiency of C3 or C5 is associated with absent or diminished chemotactic activity of serum and may be associated with absent leukocyte response to infection. The genes for C2, C4, and Factor B are clearly linked to HLA.

†The deficiency in persons lacking C4A or C4B is referred to as "q0", for quantity zero. Thus, such a deficiency can be designated C4Aq0 or C4Bq0. Persons with such deficiencies are reported to have a higher than normal incidence of autoimmune diseases. Similarly, heterozygous C-2 deficient persons are reported to have an increased incidence of autoimmune disease.

‡Approximately 85% of cases involve silent alleles, and 15% involve alleles encoding for acquired dysfunctional variant C1-inhibitor protein. In HAE, C1 is normal or depressed, C3 is always normal, C4 is depressed. In the acquired disease, C1 and C4 are depressed, antigenic C1-inhibitor is normal or high, functional C1-inhibitor is zero.

§Homozygosity for a low (not absent) numerical expression of CR1 on erythrocytes is detectable *in vitro* and appears to be associated with SLE. An acquired defect in the number of CR1 receptors may also be operative.

¶Low, but not absent, levels of leukocyte CR3 are detectable in both parents of most CR3-deficient children.

interaction with specific high-affinity cellular receptors. The binding of C5a to neutrophils produces a profound response, including an increase in adhesion, aggregation, and induction of an oxidative response, and the release of lysosomal enzymes. Moreover, C5a is strongly chemotactic for monocytes and neutrophils, inducing the migration of the cells toward the source of complement activation. Thus, a local complement-activating inflammatory reaction can thereby induce increased blood flow to tissue, the adherence of neutrophils to local endothelium, and directed migration of phagocytes to inflammatory sites. Neutrophils aggregated by C5a can embolize to the lung, causing changes in pulmonary gas exchange and even death (Davitz, 1987). This may occur in patients undergoing cardiopulmonary bypass or renal dialysis.

The opsonic properties of the complement proteins depend on the presence of specific receptors for these proteins on the surface of phagocytic cells (see later section, Complement Receptors). Foreign materials with opsonically active fragments bound to their surfaces interact with these receptors, leading first to adherence to the cell membrane of the phagocyte and a second to phagocytosis. C3b and its inactivated form, iC3b, are the most important opsonic fragments in the complement system. C3d (and presumably C3dg) fragment has also been shown to have a role in monocyte phagocytosis (Gaither, 1987). There is also evidence that C1q, via specific C1q receptors, promotes phagocytosis by macrophages (Bobak, 1987). Further details on complement receptor function in the phagocytic process are reviewed subsequently in the section Complement Receptors.

5

Regulation of Complement Activation

Regulation of activation occurs at multiple steps in the complement sequence. Thus, generation of the biologically active complement fragments is controlled by specific plasma protein inhibitors or by cell membrane-associated inhibitory proteins (Fries, 1987). The classic pathway components C1, C2, C4, and C3, are each under some form of regulation once they are activated. Regulation of C5b67 complex and of the terminal components C8 and C9 is also described.

The enzymatic activity of activated C1 is destroyed by the C1 inhibitor (C1-Inh) (Schapira, 1986). The C1-Inh binds in a stoichiometric 1:1 complex with each of the enzymatically active fragments, C1r and C1s, to block their enzymatic activity. Thus, four molecules of the 105,000-dalton C1-Inh interact with one molecule of macromolecular-activated C1 containing two C1r light chains and two C1s light chains to destroy its activity. In binding, the C1 inhibitor dissociates C1 into its subunits, leaving C1q bound to the antigen-antibody complex. C1r and C1a are released into the fluid phase in the form of two ($\overline{C1r}$-$\overline{C1s}$) C1-Inh$_2$ complexes. This complex is highly stable and resists dissociation.

C1-Inh also inhibits activated Hageman factor and its fragments, clotting Factor XI, plasmin, and kallikrein (Ratnoff, 1969). Patients with hereditary angioedema have low functional levels of C1-Inh (described subsequently under Diagnosis or Assessment of Clinical Activity) (Oltvai, 1991; Davis, 1988).

The activity of C4b is regulated by Factor I (the C3b/C4b inactivator (Fries, 1987). Factor I cleaves C4b in several steps, leading to generation of several small fragments. One of these, C4d, derived from the α chain, which contains the site of the covalent bond between C4b and the activating surface, remains cell bound. The proteolysis of surface-bound C4b by Factor I is enhanced by a serum protein, the C4b binding protein (C4BP), which, in addition, is required for Factor I cleavage of fluid phase C4b. C4BP also binds to fluid-phase and particle-bound C4b, displacing C2a and destroying convertase activity (Gigli, 1979).

The activity of C3b is also under rigid control (Fig. 36–2) (Fries, 1987). The inactivation of C3b is physiologically relevant because functionally active C3b interacts with the late components of the classic pathway to cause membrane damage and recruits alternative pathway factors as well. As with C4b, Factor I degrades C3b enzymatically. The C4BP and more importantly another serum protein, Factor H, act as cofactors to enhance its cleavage. The cell membrane receptor for C3b, termed CR1, also acts as a cofactor to facilitate the cleavage of bound C3b by Factor I (Table 36–3). CR1, which is present on human erythrocytes and many types of leukocytes, is of major importance in control of C3b degradation. In addition, because of its ability to bind C3b, it aids in the transport of C3b-coated immune complexes to sites of degradation in Kupffer cells within the liver (Cornacoff, 1983). Factor I cleavage of C3b in the presence of Factor H produces an inactive form of the molecule iC3b, which is incapable of engaging C5 or Factor B; however, iC3b remains covalently attached to the activating site and is capable of interacting with specific receptors (CR3) on phagocytic cells to promote phagocytosis. In the presence of CR1, Factor I proceeds further to mediate the formation of a smaller C3 fragment, C3dg. Under physiologic conditions, CR1 is very efficient in promoting Factor I cleavage of iC3b, whereas Factor H is not. The cleavage product formed by CR1 plus Factor I, C3dg, may be cleaved further to C3d by serum enzymes such as elastase, trypsin, and plasmin (Ross, 1982; Davis, 1984). The low-molecular-weight fragments, C3dg and C3d, contain the antigen-binding site of C3b, which allows them to remain attached to the activating surface. The larger fragments of iC3b, C3c, is released from the activating surface. C3dg and C3d also bind to specific receptors for these fragments (CR2 and CR4). The biological effects of these fragments (described subsequently) continue to be examined (Frade, 1992).

There is evidence that other leukocyte cell surface glycoproteins may play a role in C3b regulation. One such glycoprotein, referred to as membrane control protein (MCP), is reported to act as a cofactor in Factor I–mediated cleavage of C4b (Liszewski MK, 1992) and of C3b (Cole, 1985; Seya, 1986). Complement receptor 2 (CR2) is reported to have a similar role in Factor I cleavage of iC3b (Mitomo, 1987). In addition to their roles as cofactors for Factor I–mediated cleavage of C3b and iC3b, Factor H and CR1 regulate complement activation by another mechanism as well. Both Factor H and CR1 have been shown to accelerate the functional decay of the unstable C3 convertase of the alternative pathway, thus reducing amplification at the C3 step. Factor H accelerates the decay of the alternative pathway by promoting the dissociation of Bb from the complex. It also inhibits C5 activation in the classic pathway by binding directly to C3b (Fries, 1987). Interestingly, CR1 functions to accelerate the decay of the surface bound alternative pathway C3 convertase C3bBb much more efficiently than it does the classic pathway convertase $\overline{C1s24b(2b)2a}$ (Nicholson-Weller, 1982). This may be due to different binding affinities of CR1 for C3b and C4b. As we will discuss later, a different membrane protein (DAF) is more efficient in regulating surface-bound classic pathway activation at this step (see Table 36–3).

On some surfaces, like those of normal human cells, the control proteins interact with C3b, leading to its rapid degradation as just described. On other surfaces, like those of many microorganisms, C3b resists degradation (protected site) and continues to bind Factor B to activate the alternative pathway and induce destruction. The chemical nature of the protected site that confers resistance to Factors H and I is not yet defined. In a number of systems, the presence of sialic acid on a surface augments the susceptibility of C3b to degradation (Fearon, 1978). Conversely, the repeating polysaccharide subunits present on many bacteria inhibit the binding of the regulatory proteins.

Table 36–3. CELL MEMBRANE PROTEINS WITH COMPLEMENT-INHIBITORY ACTIVITY

Common Name	CD Nomenclature	Molecular Weight (kDa)	Target	Mechanism of Action
Decay-accelerating factor (DAF)	CD55	70	C3bBb, C4b2a	Dissociation of C3/C5 convertases
Membrane cofactor protein (MCP)	CD46	50–68	C3b (C4b)	Cofactor for C3b inactivation by Factor I
Complement receptor 1 (CR1) also called C3b receptor	CD35	190, 220	C3b (C4b)	Dissociation of C3/C5 convertases, cofactor for C3b inactivation by Factor I, transport of immune complex, recognition of opsonized particles
Protectin, HRF-20, P-18	CD59	18–25	C8, C9	Inhibition of formation of membrane attack complex (MAC)
Homologous restriction factor (HRF)		65	C8, C9	MAC inhibition

A number of important cell membrane-associated proteins that serve to regulate complement activation at the cell surface do not appear to act as complement receptors per se. Decay-accelerating factor (DAF) is a 70-kDa intrinsic membrane protein that binds to C4 of the classic pathway to prevent binding of C2 and destabilizes and increases the rate of decay of the classic pathway convertase. Similarly, it increases the rate of decay of the alternative pathway convertase and inhibits Factor B binding, but not as efficiently (Nicholson-Weller, 1982). Notably, DAF has no cofactor activity for Factor I-mediated cleavage of C4b or C3b. Its net effect is to limit C3 deposition on the surface of a normal cell. This protein is linked to the cell membrane by a phospholipid linkage rather than by the presence of a hydrophobic membrane-spanning domain. This offers considerably greater lateral mobility in the membrane, presumably allowing the molecule to be far more effective as a complement activation inhibitor (Davitz, 1987, and, for a review of DAF, Morgan, 1994).

There are two membrane-associated proteins responsible for the regulation of MAC: CD59 (also known as membrane inhibitor of reactive lysis or MIRL, Protectin, HRF-20, and P-18), and homologous restriction factor (HRF), or C8-binding protein. Both proteins are found in diverse populations of cells, both in blood and in tissue, and are bound to the plasma membranes by phosphotidyl inositol linkages. CD59 and HRF bind to C8 and C9 of the terminal attack complex to prevent their insertion into the cell membrane and, as a result, prevent or limit subsequent autologous membrane damage (Lachmann, 1991). Both of these proteins are absent from erythrocytes of patients with paroxysmal nocturnal hemoglobinuria (PNH) (Volanakis, 1988).

Additionally, there are two fluid phase regulators of MAC formation. S-protein (also known as vitronectin) is an 84-kD glycoprotein that acts by binding to circulating C5b-7, preventing its availability (Johnson, 1994). A recently described serum protein, SP-40 (also referred to as clusterin) has been localized in complexes with C5b-9 and may also prevent MAC assembly by a similar mechanism (Choi, 1989). The exact mechanism of action of SP-40 is unknown.

Another membrane associated-protein, called membrane cofactor protein (MCP) with a molecular weight of 50 to 68 kD, has been described from various cell types. This protein is present on virtually all circulating cells with the exception of erythrocytes (Morgan, 1994). MCP binds to C3b and is a cofactor for the Factor I–mediated first cleavage of C3b but does not act as cofactor for the subsequent cleavages of iC3b. MCP has been thought to play a significant role in preventing damage to autologous tissue by the activated complement system (Liszewski, 1991).

Complement Receptors

A number of integral membrane proteins that bind fragments of complement have been described in various cell types (Ross, 1985a; Sim, 1986; Kinoshita, 1991). These receptors play a role in the regulation of cell growth and differentiation and other cellular functions. These receptors control abnormal activation of complement. The best studied are those that regulate C3 function, the C3 receptors. Distinct receptors exist for each of the degradation fragments of C3. Moreover, the C3 fragments are generally capable of interacting with more than one type of C3 receptor but with varying degrees of affinity.

The integral membrane receptor that binds C3b, C4b, and, to a lesser degree iC3b, is referred to as complement receptor 1, or CR1. In humans the most common form of CR1 is 90-kDa rodlike protein containing 30 repeating units termed short consensus repeats. This receptor is found on many types of cells, including primate erythrocytes, granulocytes, mononuclear phagocytes, B lymphocytes, some T lymphocytes, mast cells, glomerular podocytes, and platelets in some nonprimate mammals (Morgan, 1994). The major physiologic role of CR1 is related to phagocytosis of opsonized particles. CR1 functions in the phagocytic process in several ways (Wright, 1985). It may greatly enhance binding of particles coated with C3b or iC3b plus IgG to monocytes or neutrophils, thus increasing the efficiency of IgG-Fc receptor-mediated phagocytosis. CR1 may mediate phagocytosis C3b coated targets in the absence of IgG in activated cells exposed to various stimuli, such as fibronectin, phorbol myristate acetate, and lymphokines. It can also trigger phagocytosis by monocytes that have been maintained in culture for a prolonged period of time. As discussed earlier, CR1 on human erythrocytes has been shown to regulate C3b function by acting as a cofactor in Factor I cleavage of C3b and by accelerating the decay of the C3 convertase. It is thought that erythrocyte CR1 has a major role in sequestering C3 fragment-bearing immune complexes and removing them from the plasma. Notably, the bulk of CR1 in whole blood is found on erythrocytes. The function of CR1 on B and T lymphocytes has not been clarified. However, it has been suggested that CR1 on B lymphocytes plays an immunoregulatory role. Whether it functions in the processing of antigen that has bound antibody and complement is still not clear.

A receptor for the C3d fragment of C3dg exists on B lymphocytes, B lymphoblastoid cell lines, and follicular dendritic cells but is not present on granulocytes, monocytes, or macrophages (Fearon, 1983). This receptor, termed complement receptor 2 (CR2), is reported to be important in B lymphocyte proliferation and differentiation. It also is the receptor on B lymphocytes to which the Epstein-Barr virus attaches during B cell infection, leading to infectious mononucleosis. CR2 interacts with each of the C3 fragments containing residues 1209 to 1236 of C3d: very strongly with C3d and, presumably, C3dg; strongly with iC3b; and weakly with C3b.

A separate specific C3 receptor has been described that is thought to bind only to the C3 fragment iC3b. This receptor, referred to as complement receptor 3, or CR3, is present on granulocytes, mononuclear phagocytes, and natural killer cells. It is not found on B lymphocytes, glomerular podocytes, or erythrocytes. In this case, the receptor is a two-chain molecule and is part of a family of membrane receptor proteins termed the integrin family (Hynes, 1987). There are several groups of integrin proteins, and the group that contains the iC3b receptor consists of three membrane proteins, each of which has two chains, α and β. The three proteins all share the same β chain but have different α chains. It is currently believed that the α chain confers substrate specificity and the β chain ensures proper localization of the receptor in the cell membrane. On phagocytic cells, CR3 facilitates the phagocytic process in a fashion that parallels that of CR1. Studies indicate that monocyte CR3 may also play a synergistic role in enhancing the ingestion of particles coated with IgG and C3d (Gaither, 1987). This family of receptors, to which CR3 belongs, is also very important for cell adhesion and cell-mediated cytotoxicity. This importance is emphasized by the demonstration of a group of children who are missing the entire CR3 receptor family (Dana, 1984; Springer, 1984; Anderson, 1985; and subsequent section on Disease States). These children have repeated infections, and their cells have marked phagocytic defects and fail to adhere normally to surfaces.

It has been demonstrated that C3dg binds to neutrophils, monocytes, and macrophages. It has been proposed that this binding is mediated by a distinct complement receptor on these cells, termed CR4. CR4 is also thought to bind iC3b and C3d. A physiologic function for this receptor has not yet been determined. This receptor, like CR3, is composed of two distinct peptide chains: α chain of 165 kDa and β chain of 95 kDa. This receptor belongs to the β integrin family.

β integrins are believed to be involved in many types of cell adhesion. They play a critical role in the adhesion of phagocytes to endothelial cells and other surfaces during neutrophil aggregation. Activated endothelial cells express high levels of E selectin, P selectin, and intracellular adhesion molecules (iCAM), which bind to counter-ligands present on PMN. The PMN adheres to the endothelium and begins to role along the endothelial surface. On activation, the rolling PMN sheds L selectin and up-regulates lymphocyte function-associated antigens (LFA-1) and CR3. CR3 and LFA-1 interact with iCAM-1 on the endothelial cells to fix the cell to the vessel endothelium and promote egress of the cells into tissue.

C5a receptor belongs to the family of G-protein coupled receptors. The ligand for this receptor is C5a, a 11-kDa peptide generated from C5 by C5 convertase. Binding of C5a to its receptor leads to activation of neutrophils and phagocytes. Another important biological consequence of C5a generation is the directed migration of cells, particularly neutrophils, monocytes, and macrophages. Interaction of C5a with these cells causes dramatic changes in their membranes with migration into the site of C5a generation and establishment of a gradient of migrating cells. C5a, acting as a chemotactic factor, plays a major role in the inflammation process. In addition to the receptors described here, less well characterized receptors have been reported for C1q, Factor Bb, Factor H, and the other anaphylatoxins.

COMPLEMENT IN DISEASE STATES

In most disease states, complement functions "normally" in producing inflammation and tissue damage. When complement plays a role in the development of a disease, it is often being activated by an "abnormal" antibody, immune complex, or foreign material. It is frequently important to assess the level of one or another component of complement as a means of following the activity of a disease process. Thus, patients with active lupus erythematosus may have depressed levels of C3 and C4, and these component levels may be followed as a rough index of disease activity.

When one determines the level of a component in serum, it is important to recognize that this level represents a static measurement of serum proteins that are turning over rapidly. Even in the normal individual, the fractional catabolic rate of most of the components that have been measured is on the order of 2% per hour. Many of these proteins behave as acute phase reactants, and their levels in serum may rise dramatically in inflammatory states. Their rates of catabolism may increase greatly in various autoimmune diseases. The finding of a decreased level of a component may raise the suspicion that the complement system is participating in tissue damage but does not prove it. The finding of a normal serum level of a component does not preclude the participation of complement in tissue injury. For example, patients with primary biliary cirrhosis have an increased catabolic rate of C3, and it has been suggested that C3 may play a role in the development of this disease. Nevertheless, the level of C3 in the serum of patients with primary biliary cirrhosis is almost always elevated. In this case, increased synthesis obscures the increased catabolism. It should also be recognized that complement function in various body compartments may differ. Complement activity in the blood of patients with seropositive rheumatoid arthritis may be normal or elevated; however, the complement activity of joint fluid may be severely depressed.

The final general concept to be discussed is that of the "complement profile." Earlier sections have described the classic and alternative complement pathways and their mechanisms of action. In recent years an attempt has been made to determine which pathway of complement activation predominates in mediating tissue damage or depressed component levels in one or another illness. The simplest approach to this problem examines the levels of various components and assumes that decreased levels of a component of one or the other pathway are more likely to occur when that pathway is activated. Therefore, if a patient has depressed levels of C3 and C4 and normal levels of Factor B, the classic pathway is likely to be involved. If a patient has decreased levels of C3 and Factor B, properdin and normal levels of C4, alternative pathway activation is most likely. In this way, determining the levels of a limited number of components can provide a great deal of information. Except in the case of the genetically controlled complement abnormalities, one never needs to know the levels of all complement components except for investigational purposes.

An important advance in this area is the use of enzyme-linked immunoassays (ELISAs) to detect stable complexes formed in serum during complement activation. These assays are highly sensitive and can readily demonstrate which pathway of complement is activated in various disease states (described subsequently under Assay of Components).

On activation, many complement proteins develop new antigens (neoantigens) that are not present on the native plasma protein. The neoantigen present on the MAC but not present on the native terminal components is perhaps the most interesting. Antibody to this neoantigen exists and has been used to study the level of neoantigen by immunofluorescence as well as by ELISA (Falk, 1983; Sanders, 1985). The neoantigen level is elevated in blood and spinal fluid in many patients with ongoing complement activation (Sanders, 1986). Moreover, it is present in tissues at sites of terminal complex deposition. For example, it is present in lesional tissue in the glomeruli of patients with glomerulonephritis (Falk, 1983) and in lesional skin at sites of active systemic lupus erythematosus (SLE) (Biesecker, 1982). Unlike the C3 deposited in normal skin in patients with SLE and a positive lupus band test, the MAC neoantigen is found only in lesions.

A brief statement as to the role of complement in various groups of illnesses is provided subsequently. The role of complement in each of these disease groups is under active investigation.

DIAGNOSIS OR ASSESSMENT OF CLINICAL ACTIVITY IN DISEASE

Rheumatologic Diseases

The rheumatologic disease that has been evaluated most extensively in terms of the contribution of complement to disease activity is SLE (Agnello, 1986). In this disease large amounts of immune complexes are formed, with antibody bound to many tissue components. Both circulating and tissue-deposited immune complexes are found. These complexes activate complement, and complement activation products contribute to ongoing inflammation. C3 and C4 levels are often reduced in SLE, and in general, low levels are found in patients with active disease. Some have suggested that the C4 level is the best index of disease activity, although clearly there are patients with ongoing disease and normal C4 levels and vice versa. There are studies that suggest that the finding of circulating C5b-9 or neoantigens of MAC will provide a better index of active disease (Gawryl, 1987). As discussed earlier, a great deal of attention has been devoted to the function of complement in the processing of immune complexes. It appears that complement plays an essential role in clearance of these complexes from the circulation, particularly those that contain IgM and the IgG complement-activating subclasses. Studies of the behavior of immune complexes in whole blood indicate that when these complexes activate complement, C3b binds to the complexes. The complexes, in turn, bind to the surface of cells with C3b receptors. The most abundant source of C3b receptors in blood is the surface of erythrocytes, and the immune complexes with bound complement bind to the surface of erythrocytes, where they are effectively prevented from diffusing from the plasma into tissues to cause immune damage. Once attached to erythrocyte complement receptors, the complexes circulate to the liver, where they are efficiently removed by a process that does not shorten the lifespan of the red cells (Cornacoff, 1983). In diseases in which complement is activated and these immunologically active products form in the circulation, the number of CR1 receptors per red cell is decreased. Presumably, when the complexes are removed from the erythrocytes, some of the CR1 is removed as well (Ross, 1985b). In addition to SLE, erythrocytes from patients with chronic cold agglutinin disease, PNH, autoimmune hemolytic anemia, Sjögren's syndrome, and *Mycoplasma* pneumonia are reported to have reduced erythrocyte CR1, suggesting that immune deposits have been removed from erythrocytes in these diseases (Ross, 1985b; Atkinson, 1986).

The complement proteins act as acute phase proteins, and levels may not be depressed even in situations in which complement activation occurs. Normal or elevated serum complement levels are found in juvenile rheumatoid arthritis, most patients with adult onset rheumatoid arthritis, palindromic arthritis, pseudogout, gout, Reiter's syndrome, and gonococcal arthritis.

At the same time, depressed levels of complement in joint fluid have been shown to exist in a number of other rheumatologic conditions, including rheumatoid arthritis. Depressed CH_{50} (the reciprocal of the dilution of complement that lyses 50% of sheep erythrocytes with antibody) and the presence of cleavage products of C3 and Factor B are thought to represent intra-articular activation in the synovial fluid of most patients with seropositive rheumatoid arthritis and many patients with seronegative rheumatoid arthritis, SLE, pseudogout, gout, Reiter's syndrome, and gonococcal arthritis. This is not true of fluids obtained from patients with degenerative arthritis.

Infectious Diseases

As previously discussed, one major function of the complement system is to protect against infection. Patients with gram-negative septicemia often have depressed levels of C3 and components of the alternative pathway, as do patients with certain fungal diseases such as cryptococcal septicemia. A major area for future investigation concerns the role of complement in the tissue damage associated with chronic infection. It is known that patients with HBsAg-positive infectious hepatitis have an early fall in serum C3, which later returns to normal. This may be associated with signs of immune complex disease, i.e., arthralgia. In a similar fashion, complement appears to play an important role in many parasitic infections, including leishmaniasis, trypanosomiasis, giardiasis, and malaria. A detailed discussion of the role of the complement system in parasitic and bacterial infections is beyond the scope of this review: however, it is important to recognize the fact that serum complement levels are in general not a reliable index of disease activity in these conditions.

The role of complement in the adult respiratory distress syndrome (ARDS), a common occurrence in patients with severe trauma or overwhelming sepsis, has been studied. There is evidence of massive activation of complement in these patients, suggesting that bacteria and bacterial products activate complement (Hammerschmidt, 1980). Both the classic and alternative pathways appear to be activated (Langlois, 1988). Inflammatory factors, including neutrophil-activating factor and chemoattractant C5a, are formed. There is evidence that neutrophils infiltrate the lung, and neutrophil oxidative products and proteases are thought to be responsible for much of the pulmonary damage that occurs.

Renal Diseases

Complement is thought to be of key importance in glomerular damage in many of the glomerulonephritides (Couser, 1985; Schwab, 1985). This is usually demonstrated by the deposition of C3, other components, or both within or near the glomerular basement membrane. Moreover, the membrane attack complex has been recognized in the damaged glomeruli in patients with glomerulonephritis and SLE. Patients with serum sickness due to immune complexes in the circulation have been shown to have glomerular injury. On serum analysis these patients show activation of the classic or alternative pathways, or both. Traditionally, it has been believed that complexes are deposited in glomeruli as they filter plasma that contains immune complexes. Once deposited, these complexes activate complement. An alternative view is that antibodies to glomerular structures form the immune complex that then activates complement to cause local damage (Couser, 1993). Although antibody to glomerular basement membrane structures are clearly of importance in Goodpasture's syndrome, their overall role in glomerulonephritis is under debate. The role of complement in interstitial and tubular disease is less clear; however, there are those who believe that complement may have some function in these disorders as well.

Dermatologic Diseases

As in the other groups of diseases listed, complement is thought to play a part in ongoing tissue damage in a variety of dermatologic illnesses. These include bullous pemphigoid, herpes gestationis, epidermolysis bullosa acquisitiva, and perhaps pemphigus vulgaris. It should be noted that serum complement levels are usually normal or elevated in these chronic inflammatory states, and the importance of complement is suggested by immunofluorescent analysis of tissue biopsies and by studies of blister fluid. Moreover, an in vitro model useful for the study of antibasement membrane zone antibody-mediated skin disorders has been developed by Gammon (1984). These authors have shown conclusively that C5a is the key element whose generation is critical in the pathogenesis of bullous pemphigoid and epidermolysis bullosa acquisita. C5a acts as the chemoattractant necessary for the influx of polymorphonuclear leukocytes into the sites of subsequent tissue damage in these diseases. Once again, activation products of complement have been demonstrated.

Hematologic Diseases

In many types of autoimmune hemolytic anemia, complement plays an important role in the opsonization of erythrocytes, leading to their clearance by cells of the reticuloendothelial system; however, even in those cases in which complement is clearly involved, serum complement levels are usually within reference intervals. Complement is particularly important in the clearance of cells coated by IgM cold reactive autoantibodies with anti-I specificity. These autoantibodies (cold agglutinins) are associated with lymphoproliferative disorders following infections, or they may be isolated findings, particularly in the elderly. Cold agglutinins generally bind optimally at subphysiologic temperatures, which are found in some areas of the body like the tip of the nose, fingers, ears, and so on, and they usually mediate cell lysis when the circulating erythrocytes return to core body temperatures. Not all cold agglutinins are IgM antibodies. The syndrome of paroxysmal cold hemoglobinuria, for example, results from the cold-reactive Donath-Landsteiner IgG antibodies, which bind to cells at temperatures below 37°C but mediate lysis upon warming. Although the antibody is different, the pathophysiologic effects are similar.

Other autoantibodies that activate complement bind more efficiently at warm temperatures. In general, these warm reactive antibodies have IgG specificity. In some cases, these antibodies may be associated with lymphoproliferative and certain nonlymphoproliferative malignancies and viral infections. Most IgG warm-reacting antibodies found in autoimmune hemolytic anemia have Rh specificity and are poor complement activators; however, some antibodies, like Tja, activate complement well and cause lysis. Studies of the interaction of complement with red cells have led to a new understanding of PNH. In this rare acquired hemolytic anemia, patients' red cells have unusually high complement sensitivity and may undergo intravascular hemolysis. Lysis is believed to proceed via the alternative complement pathway, although serum complement levels are always normal in these patients and the direct antiglobulin test is always negative. It has now been found that all blood cells have phospholipid-linked cell membrane proteins that serve to protect them from complement attack. One of these decay-accelerating factors, DAF, acts to prevent generation of the C3 convertase and destroys its activity. Another protein binds the terminal components C8 and C9 to prevent them from inducing cell damage, as described previously under Regulation of Complement Activation. It is now clear that PNH is an acquired disorder of maturation of selected marrow elements that may fail to process these phospholipid-linked proteins properly. The abnormal enzyme PIG-A has been identified. These proteins are not expressed on PNH red cells and other blood cells, and the red cells are consequently destroyed by complement attack.

GENETIC COMPLEMENT DEFICIENCIES

As discussed previously, the number of patients with genetically controlled complement disorders is few, and these patients are of greatest interest because they allow us to determine the role of complement components in various biological phenomena and in various disease states (see Table 36–2). In general, the absence of a component follows simple Mendelian genetic principles and is inherited as an autosomal recessive trait. Thus, heterozygous patients tend to have half the normal levels or less, and homozygous-deficient patients have little or no detectable component activity. As shown in Table 36–2, deficiencies are known for every component of the classic pathway and most components of the alternative pathway. Many of these patients present with one or another manifestation of autoimmune disease, and the role of complement deficiency in the development of these diseases is under active investigation. One interesting hypothesis is that autoimmunity may be a manifestation of chronic viral illness. If complement aids in viral neutralization, an interruption of those pathways of activation may promote chronic viral infection. As discussed, another hypothesis has come from the recognition that complement aids in clearance of immune complex from the circulation. The concept that red cell complement receptors are important in immune complex clearance was discussed earlier. Deficiency of components may interfere with the normal immune complex clearance mechanisms, thus allowing tissue deposition of the complexes.

Initially, it was believed that the absence of early components of the classic pathway did not predispose to infectious disease because of the protection afforded by alternative pathway factors. It is now clear that this is not the case, and all patients with classic pathway deficiencies are known to be at greater risk of infection when stressed (Figueroa, 1991). Strikingly, patients with C1 and C4 deficiencies have increased infections; patients with deficiencies of C3 and alternative pathway factors show a very high incidence of infection as well. C3 is the key component of both pathways and plays a major role in opsonization. Thus, it is reasonable to assume that absence of this component is associated with infection by a wide variety of pathogens, especially in childhood before high titers of antibodies have developed. Interestingly, deficiency of a number of the late-acting components is associated with a high incidence of disseminated infection with *Neisseria* organisms. Presumably, lysis is important for protection against *Neisseria* infection.

A number of other deficiency states exist. Patients with hypogammaglobulinemia or severe combined immunodeficiency often have depressed levels of C1q. In part, these depressed levels of C1q relate to the low levels of IgG in the circulation. It appears that C1q interacts with IgG in the circulation and that this interaction leads, in turn, to decreased C1q catabolism. Fries (1988) and Morgan (1991) review complement deficiency states and disease.

ASSAY OF COMPONENTS

General Principles and Types of Assays

Accurate methods are available for measuring each of the nine classic pathway components, all of the alternative pathway components, and several enzymes and inhibitors that regulate the complement system; however, many of these methods are still considered research techniques and are not available on a routine basis. We will confine our attention to techniques that do not require a laboratory skilled in complement research for their performance. In general, two types of techniques are in use: those that measure the complement proteins as antigens in serum, and those that measure the functional activity of the components. Both techniques have advantages and disadvantages as research and diagnostic tools, and these will be reviewed. Methods for antigenic (immunochemical) analysis are generally simpler to perform. These antigenic assays are highly specific and require fewer specialized reagents and considerably less personnel time. Reagents for measuring several proteins of the complement system are commercially available, including C1q, C4, C3, C5, Factor B, Factors H and I, and C1 inhibitor. Linscott's Directory of Immunological and Biological Reagents (1994–1995) is a useful guide to commercially available complement reagents. In these assays, either serum or plasma can be used, and the commonly available methods of freezer storage (−20°C) are sufficient. For these reasons, antigenic assays are easily adaptable to a clinical laboratory. On the other hand, antigenic assays do not provide information about the activity of a component because they may detect degradation products as well as functionally active components. The presence in serum of small fragments of a protein with antigenic activity may confuse the results. A protein fragment may diffuse more rapidly than the parent molecule, and the usual radial diffusion techniques will indicate falsely high levels. As an example, the most commonly employed antigenic assay for C3 measures its major degradation product C3c (B1A) by radial immunodiffusion. For accurate measurements of C3c, the specimen should be thawed and incubated at 37°C for a number of days to allow for complete conversion of C3 to C3c. In fact, this is not usually done and thus can present a source of error, although the error is small and is not usually of clinical consequence. In general, antigenic assays are not as sensitive as functional assays and may not detect low levels of a component present in certain body fluids. The sensitivity of antigenic assays depends to some degree on the strength of the antisera employed, and with the usual assays, as little as 1 to 10 μg/mL of protein antigen can be measured.

A highly sensitive ELISA is now available for measuring alternative pathway activation in human serum or plasma (Mayes, 1984). This assay, which is designed specifically to detect C3bBbP or C3bP complexes, is reported to quantitate as few as 10 to 20 ng/mL of C3bP in serum. The assay may also be used to measure surface-bound activation complexes. Kits are currently available that use inhibition of binding of radiolabeled substrate to detect various complement peptides. Such kits are available for measurement of C4a, C3a, and C5a. The usefulness of these measurements is still under investigation. A detailed report on procedures for measuring the functional lytic activity and the antigenic levels of each of the components of the alternative pathway is available (Minta, 1983). Assays designed to measure the functional activity of the control proteins Factors H and I in human serum have also been reported. These procedures require specialized reagents that may not be commercially available (Gaither, 1970).

Procedure for Evaluating Functional Activity of the Classic Pathway

Functional complement assays may be described as both sensitive and precise tools for providing important information about the activity of a component. Some of these methods may be used to quantitate activity at the molecular level, and others to express complement function in arbitrary titration units. Commercial reagents are available for titrating all components of the classic pathway system; however, for the most part, these assays are performed in a limited number of research facilities. Most functional assays involve complex time-consuming procedures that require relatively highly purified reagents. These reagents are very expensive compared with those required for antigenic tests. The buffers used in most laboratories to perform complement assays are described in Table 36–4. The precise preparation of these

Table 36–4. SOLUTIONS COMMONLY USED IN COMPLEMENT ASSAYS

Stock Solutions*

1. *Veronal-buffered salines (stock VBS)*
   To prepare 2 L, dissolve 83.0 g NaCl and 10.19 g Na-5.5' diethyl barbiturate in 1.5 L of distilled water. Mix vigorously while titrating to pH 7.35 ± .05 with 1 N HCl. Bring to 2.0 L volumetrically with distilled water. This solution is five times the concentration of an isotonic solution and may be stored at 4°C for at least one month. It is distilled immediately before use.
2. *0.10 M disodium ethylenediaminetetra-acetic acid (stock EDTA)*
   Dissolve 37.2 g in about 800 ml of distilled water. Adjust the pH to 7.65 ± .05 with 2 N NaOH and bring to 1.0 L with distilled water. Store at 4°C. Stock EDTA may be used for at least three weeks.
3. *Dextrose with Ca^{+2}, Mg^{+2}, and gelatin (D)*
   A 5% solution of dextrose in distilled water (D_5W) is obtained from commercial sources. Approximately 1 L is measured volumetrically, 1.0 mL of stock solution 6 is added, and the solution is brought to 1.0 L. One hundred to 200 mL of the mixed solution is added to 1 g of gelatin in an Erlenmeyer flask and heated until all of the gelatin granules have dissolved. After the remaining solution is added, the D is well mixed and stored at 4°C. D may be used for one week.
4. *2.00 M $MgCl_2$ solution*
   Prepare about 200 mL of solution containing $MgCl_2$ at approximately 3 M. Measure the specific gravity of the solution and determine the $MgCl_2$ concentration from the Handbook of Chemistry and Physics† (conversion tables for concentrated values of aqueous solutions). Adjust the concentration to 2.00 M by adding distilled water.
5. *0.300 M $CaCl_2$ solution*
   About 200 mL of an approximately 0.5 M solution of $CaCl_2$ is prepared. Measure the specific gravity of this solution and determine the $CaCl_2$ concentration as described above. Adjust to 0.300 M by adding distilled water.
6. *Stock metals*
   A solution containing 1.0 M $MgCl_2$ and 0.15 M $CaCl_2$ is prepared by combining equal volumes of solutions 4 and 5.

Working Solutions

1. *Isotonic VBS with gelatin and metals (VBS)*
   To prepare 1 L, add 200 mL of stock solution 1 (above) to a 1-L volumetric flask. Add 1.0 mL stock solution 6 and bring to 1.0 L with distilled water. Add 0.1% gelatin in stock solution 3. VBS should be prepared fresh every three to five days and stored at 4°C.
2. *Isotonic VBS-dextrose of lowered ionic strengths (DVBS)*
   Buffers of varying ionic strengths are prepared by mixing stock solution 3 with working solution 1 in varying proportions. 0.065μ DVBS is prepared by mixing three parts of the former solution with two parts of the latter. DVBS should be prepared fresh.
3. *Isotonic VBS-EDTA buffer (EDTA)*
   Mix nine parts of working solution 1 without metals with one part of stock solution 2. This solution is stable for at least one week at 4°C.
4. *C-EDTA*
   Dilute fresh guinea pig serum (titer of at least 170) 1:25 in working solution 3. This reagent is stable for one week at 4°C.

*These solutions, with the exception of No. 4, may be stored at −20°C to −50°C for an indefinite period of time.

†West RC (ed): CRC Handbook of Chemistry and Physics. CRC Press, Boca Raton, FL, 1985–1986.

buffers is critical because changes in molarity and metal ion concentration can profoundly alter the viability of red cells and complement activity.

In many of the assays in which the classic pathway is studied, the presence of a functionally active component is indicated by the lysis of sheep erythrocytes sensitized with rabbit antibody. Sheep erythrocytes are particularly advantageous for use because, for reasons that are not completely understood, they are much more easily lysed by antibody and complement than are erythrocytes from other species. Sheep erythrocytes have on their surface a potent lipopolysaccharide antigen, the Forssman antigen, which is widely distributed in nature. The critical grouping of the lipopolysaccharide is a disaccharide linkage that is seen as strongly antigenic in animals that do not have the enzymes to form this linkage. Rabbits are a Forssman-negative species and respond to the injection of sheep erythrocytes by producing enormous amounts of anti-Forssman antibody. Thus, high titer antiserum directed against the sheep erythrocytes is easily obtainable, and sheep erythrocytes themselves being easily lysed by fresh serum, are sensitive indicator particles for the presence of lytic complement activity.

Handling of Samples

The proper handling of samples is critical for correct functional analysis. For most functional complement assays, serum rather than plasma is chosen for analysis because both chelators ethylenediaminetetracetic acid (EDTA) and heparin may be anticomplementary. EDTA plasma may be used, however, in some functional tests in which the sample is diluted enough (>1:100) to overcome the chelating effect of EDTA. To obtain serum for functional assays, a fresh blood sample is allowed to clot at room temperature for half an hour and then in the cold for about one hour. If C1q-binding studies are needed, the sample is allowed to clot for two hours at room temperature. In this case, complete clot polymerization appears to facilitate accurate assay. To separate serum, the clot is rimmed and is centrifuged in the cold. If cryoprecipitating antibodies are suspected, clot formation and centrifugation of the specimen should proceed at 37°C because complement fixation may occur if the specimen aliquot is chilled. In certain sera, chilling will lower complement component titer strikingly. The reasons for this are not fully understood but it must be kept in mind that, occasionally, a strikingly low titer will be an artifact of serum preparation. If this is suspected, the serum can be prepared at 37°C, but it must be prepared expeditiously to avoid complement activation. Serum should be stored in multiple aliquots to avoid thawing and refreezing. The serum aliquots should be stored immediately at −40°C to −70°C. Aliquots can be stored for longer periods at −70°C without loss of activity. When sera are to be transported, they should be well sealed before being packed in a container with large quantities of dry ice.

Preparation of Sheep Erythrocytes

Sheep blood is drawn aseptically into an equal volume of sterile Alsever's solution. Such sheep cells are commercially available. The anticoagulated whole blood is stored for at least one week at 4°C before use and may be used for up to six weeks if sterility is maintained. Studies have shown that the age of sheep cells can greatly influence the titers of most complement components, and titers may be falsely low if fresh cells are used. An appropriate volume of cells is removed for washing under sterile conditions. After centrifugation the supernatant and buffy coat are removed. Cells are suspended in 0.01 M EDTA buffer and incubated at 37°C for 10 minutes. The cells are washed first in EDTA and then washed three times in veronal buffered saline (VBS). The washed packed cells are then diluted about 15-fold in VBS. Cell concentration may be determined from the optical density of a small sample of lysed cells (Gaiter, 1984) or by standard methods of counting cells.

Preparation of Anti-Sheep Erythrocyte Antibodies

Most workers who report functional titrations of individual components used rabbit anti-Forssman antibody. Antibody with a high degree of specificity for the Forssman antigen of sheep erythrocytes (E) can be prepared by immunizing rabbits with boiled sheep erythrocyte stroma. The method of immunization influences the class of antibody produced. The procedures for preparation of stroma and rabbit immunization are explained fully by Kabat (1961). Before use, the complement activity of the antiserum is destroyed by heat inactivation for 30 minutes at 56°C. Antisera with acceptable activity may be diluted, usually to 1:100, in normal saline and stored at −20°C or at −40°C. A kinetic assay used to titrate anti-Forssman antibody is described in detail elsewhere (Gaither, 1984). Table 36–5 outlines the general procedure for this assay.

Titration of complement requires sheep E sensitized with an optimal amount of antibody (A). An optimally sensitized preparation contains sufficient antibody to render the complement titer independent of antibody concentration. The method for determining optimal concentrations of antibody to be used in preparing sensitized cells for complement analysis has been described in detail (Gaither, 1984). Sheep erythrocytes sensitized with optimal amounts of antibody are designated EA. Sensitization is accomplished using a standardized procedure. A volume of E is placed in a container that allows easy mixing. The diluted antiserum is slowly pipetted in a dropwise fashion into an equal volume of cells while the contents are constantly swirled to ensure an even distribution of antibody on the cells. Antibody is always added to E. EA are generally incubated for 15 minutes at 30°C or 37°C before use.

Cellular intermediates in the complement cascade with membrane-bound components are also used for functional assays. EAC4 has cell-bound C4 and may be used as a reagent for measuring the remaining eight components. Several methods are available for forming this intermediate. At this time, the cellular intermediate EAC14 is most commonly used for the assay of C2 and C3 to C9 (Gaither, 1984). EAC14 cells are stable for 8 to 10 days when stored at 4°C in the presence of a low concentration of sodium azide (0.05%). The azide must be removed in several washes before assays are performed.

The simplest functional assay of the classic pathway measures total hemolytic complement. The absence of any one of the nine components generally results in a total hemolytic complement titer (CH_{50}) of zero; however, a normal value does not exclude reduced levels of individual components. When a patient's history and symptoms suggest a possible deficiency, hemolytic titrations of individual components may be required.

The procedure for total complement evaluation is outlined in the same titration (Table 36–6). The titration is expressed in CH_{50} units (the reciprocal of the dilution of complement that lyses 50% of the EA). In this case, the 50% end point is determined from the Von Krogh transformation of the data. This empirically derived formula converts the S-shaped dose-response curve into a linear function. Values of y/l-y are calculated in which y is the percentage of red cells lysed in a test dilution. A graph is constructed in which the log of the relative volume of complement is plotted against the log of y/l-y values. Usually, a straight line is obtained, and titer is calculated by determining the relative volume of complement at which y/l-y equals 1.0 (the point where 50% lysis is obtained). That value is divided into the reciprocal of original serum dilution (1:60 for human serum) to calculate the concentration of serum complement that lyses 50% of the cells. This value is the complement titer. It expresses the number of 50% hemolytic units that are present in 1.0 mL of undiluted serum (Kabat, 1961; Rapp, 1970).

To measure most complement components individually, partially purified components are required; however, C4 and C6 are exceptions because of the availability of C4-deficient guinea pig serum (C4D) and C6-deficient rabbit serum (C6D). These assays are based on the principle that the deficient sera are good sources of the remaining components,

5

Table 36–5. PROTOCOL FOR TITRATION OF ANTIBODY AND SAMPLE DETERMINATIONS

	Test Tube					
	1	*2*	*3*	*CB*	*CBC*	*100%*
E (5×10^8/mL)	0.5	0.5	0.5	0.5	0.5	0.5
Hemolysin, 0.5 mL	1:20,000	1:40,000	1:80,000	—	—	—
			Incubate 15.0 minutes at 37°C			
Guinea pig complement, 1:7.5	0.25	0.25	0.25	—	0.25	—
			Incubate 15.0 minutes at 37°C			
EDTA buffer, mL	2.5	2.5	2.5	2.75	2.5	—
H_2O (mL)	—	—	—	—	—	2.75
Absorbance (OD) 541 nm	0.454	0.137	0.040	0.003	0.014	0.698
Absorbance (OD) corr	0.440	0.123	0.026	—	—	0.695
y/l−y	1.73	0.215	0.039	—	—	—
Titer, AB_{50}	24,000	—	—	—	—	—

E = sheep erythrocytes; CB = sheep erythrocytes with buffer alone; CBC = sheep erythrocytes plus complement; y = absorbance (corrected) of test sample/absorbance (corrected) of 100% lysed sample; AB_{50} = amount of antiserum that under described conditions lyses half of the erythrocytes in exactly 15 minutes; (OD) corr = sample OD − CBC OD.

Table 36–6. PROTOCOL FOR TITRATION OF WHOLE COMPLEMENT AND SAMPLE DETERMINATIONS

	Test Tube							
	1	*2*	*3*	*4*	*5*	*CB*	*CBC*	*100%*
VBS (mL)	5.5	5.3	5.0	4.5	4.0	6.5	5.5	—
5×10^8/mL EA (mL)	1.0	1.0	1.0	1.0	1.0	1.0	—	1.0
Serum (1:60) (mL)	1.0	1.2	1.5	2.0	2.5	—	2.0	—
H_2O (mL)	—	—	—	—	—	—	—	6.5
			Incubate 1 hour at 37°C					
Absorbance (OD) 541 nm	0.102	0.185	0.322	0.490	0.596	0.003	0.008	0.0664
Absorbance (OD) corr.	0.094	0.177	0.314	0.482	0.588	—	—	0.656
y/l−y	0.167	0.370	0.918	2.77	8.65	—	—	—
Titer, CH_{50}	39.5	—	—	—	—	—	—	—

VBS = veronal buffered saline; CB = sheep erythrocytes with buffer alone; CBC = sheep erythrocytes plus complement; y = absorbance (corrected) of test sample/absorbance (corrected) of 100% lysis sample; EA = sheep erythrocytes with antibody; AB_{50} = reciprocal of dilution of complement that lyses 50% of the EA; OD corr = OD of sample − OD of CBC

which they possess at normal or near normal concentrations. The assays for C4 and C6 are thereby greatly simplified and can be performed easily if the deficient sera are available. The deficient sera must be fresh or frozen fresh to prevent loss of complement activity. A general outline of the C4 assay is given in Table 36–7, and details are provided on the C4 and C6 assays (Gaither, 1984). The assay for serum C4 is extremely efficient, yielding titers greater than titers obtained by the more complex procedure described in Table 36–6; however, the C6 assay using deficient rabbit serum is not efficient. When this method is applied, titers are reduced approximately by a factor of 10; however, this method is perfectly acceptable for determining normal C6 levels when a control standard serum is assayed simultaneously.

Standard procedures for measuring the hemolytic activity of each of the components of the classic pathway are outlined in Table 36–8. The following general methods apply to these assays:

1. Low ionic strength buffer (0.065 μ DVBS*) is used.
2. The cellular intermediate is suspended to 1.5×10^7 cells/mL.
3. All serum and complement dilutions are prepared fresh and held at 0°C to 4°C.
4. Reaction mixtures are frequently mixed to ensure adequate cell suspensions.
5. When individual components are required in excess, C1 is added at a concentration that yields from 500 to 1000 C1 sites/cell, and the remaining eight components are added at concentrations that yield 100 sites/cell. Often the titers of commercial complement components are expressed as CH_{50} units/mL. The CH_{50} titer is the reciprocal of the dilution yielding 50% lysis, at which point the Z value (see later) is approximately 0.70 site/cell.

Immune hemolysis is the result of a complex series of reactions that occur on the cell surface. Photometric measurements indicate the proportion of cells lysed by this series of reactions. Poisson's distribution is applied to relate the degree of hemolysis to the molecular events that occur on the cell surface. This approach is based on the assumption that the interaction of cell-bound antigen, antibody, and complement occurs in random fashion and that the amount of lysis is the sum of a large number of interactions in which limited quantities of the component being titrated interact with other components that are all in excess. It is well established that one lesion on the erythrocyte surface that has interacted with hemolytic antibody and all of the complement components can cause cell lysis. Poisson's distribution is used to relate the number of lysed cells (cells with one or more lesions) to the concentration of the complement reactant being titrated.

Table 36–7. PROTOCOL FOR TITRATION OF C4 BY C4D METHOD AND SAMPLE DETERMINATION

	Test Tube					
	1	*2*	*3*	*CB*	*CBC*	*100%*
EA (1.5×10^8/mL)	0.2	0.2	0.2	0.2	0.2	0.2
Serum 0.2 mL starting with 1:100,000	1:1	1:2	1:4	—	—	—
C4D serum 1:75 (mL)	0.2	0.2	0.2	—	0.2	—
0.084 μ DVBS (mL)	—	—	—	0.4	0.2	—
		Incubate 1 hour at 37°C				
EDTA	2.0	2.0	2.0	2.0	2.0	—
H_2O (mL)	—	—	—	—	—	2.4
Absorbance (OD) 412 nm	0.847	0.559	0.330	0.011	0.024	1.087
Absorbance (OD) corr.	0.823	0.535	0.306	—	—	1.076
Z	1.45	0.688	0.335	—	—	—
Titer	141,380	—	—	—	—	—

EA = sheep erythrocytes with antibody; CB = sheep erythrocytes and buffer alone; CBC = sheep erythrocytes and C4D; C4D = C4-deficient serum; Z = average number of sites damaged by complement per sheep erythrocyte; DVBS = isotonic veronal-buffered saline plux dextrose; OD corr = OD of sample − OD of CBC; OD corr of 100% = OD of 100% − OD of CB

Table 36–8. STANDARD HEMOLYTIC ASSAYS OF CLASSIC PATHWAY COMPONENTS

Component		Volume (mL)
C1	Test dilution	0.2
	EAC4—1 h at 30°C	0.2
	C2—10 min at 30°C	0.2
	C-EDTA 1:25	2.0
	1 h at 37°C	
C2	Test dilution	0.2
	EAC14—30°C tmax*	0.2
	C-EDTA 1:25	2.0
	1 h at 37°C	
C5	Test dilution	0.2
	EAC14	0.2
	C236789 reagent	0.2
	1 h at 37°C	
	EDTA	2.0
C7	Test dilution	0.2
	EAC14	0.2
	C235689 reagent	0.2
	1 h at 37°C	
	EDTA	2.0
C9	EAC14	0.2
	C2	0.2
	C3567—30 min at 30°C	0.2
	Test dilution	0.2
	C8—1 h at 37°C	0.2
	EDTA	2.0
C4	Test dilution	0.2
	EAC1—20 min at 37°C	0.2
	C2—10 min at 30°C	0.2
	C-EDTA 1:25	2.0
	2 h at 37°C	
C3	Test dilution	0.2
	EAC14	0.2
	C256789 reagent	0.2
	1 h at 37°C	
	EDTA†	2.0
C6	Test dilution	0.2
	EAC14	0.2
	C235789 reagent	0.2
	1 h at 37°C	
	EDTA	2.0
C8	EAC14	0.2
	C2	0.2
	C3567—30 min at 30°C	0.2
	Test dilution	0.2
	C9—1 h at 37°C	0.2
	EDTA	2.0

*tmax (See Rapp and Borsos, 1970) 5 to 10 min for most EAC14 preparations.
†EDTA = Working Solution 3, Table 36–4. Table 36–4 also gives description of C-EDTA (Working Solution 4).

The average number of damaged sites per red cell is expressed as Z. The equation relating this value to lysis is: $Z = -\ln(1 - y)$, where y is the percentage of lysed cells. To calculate the titer of the component being measured, Z values are plotted on the ordinate against the serum concentration plotted on the abscissa on an arithmetic or log-log graph. The titer is the reciprocal of the dilution of serum that corresponds to a Z value of 1.0 or one hit per cell (Kabat, 1961; Rapp, 1970).

Complement Levels by Antigenic Assay

For use in antigenic assays, the specimen (either serum or plasma) should be stored frozen (−20°C is sufficient). Bacterial contamination may cause protein denaturation or fragmentation, whereas freezing and thawing do not usually have a major adverse effect on antigenic levels. For certain complement assays, the specimen is diluted in saline to achieve the correct concentration range for accurate quantitation. When C3 is assayed and precise quantitation is desired using C3c standards, sterile sera should be incubated at 37°C for several days prior to analysis.

Antigenic analysis of complement proteins makes use of one of several immune precipitin techniques. Single radial immunodiffusion (RID) using the method of either Fahey or Mancini is the most commonly employed method for calculating a specific quantitation of protein. In both methods antigen is added to wells in a gel that contains antibody, and rings of precipitation are formed. In the Fahey method, the time at which results are read is critical because the antibodies in the gel matrix are not in excess, and therefore diffusion end points are not reached. This can lead to inaccurate evaluation of antigenic complement. The technique of Mancini, considered to be both sensitive and accurate, employs the more simplified end point methodology with antibody excess in the gel. The Mancini method is used by most commercial firms in the preparation of immunodiffusion plates. These methods are discussed in Chapters 33 and 35. Radial immunodiffusion kits are commercially available for several complement components, including C3, C4, and Factor B. These kits consist of plates coated with a thin layer of 2% agarose containing monospecific antibody. Protein standard serum (a stabilized pool of normal human serum) is supplied, usually in prediluted solutions. Each standard solution contains a specific amount of the particular protein being measured for use in construction of the reference curve. A delivery device (a microliter syringe or calibrated pipette) that can accurately measure and deliver microliter quantities of serum is useful, and a calibrated magnifier that is accurate to 0.1 mm is needed. For more details on antigenic assays of alternative pathway components, see Minta (1983).

Complement Fixation Test

A detailed consideration of this procedure is not presented here because a complete discussion of this topic is available elsewhere (Kabat, 1961). Nevertheless, because complement fixation reactions are of great importance in clinical diagnosis, they are mentioned briefly. The test procedure depends on the ability of fresh serum complement to interact with antigen-antibody complexes. In the first step of the reaction, the complement is incubated with the materials that may contain antigen and antibody. If antigen-antibody complexes are formed, they will interact with complement in much the same way that a complex of antibody and a cell surface antigen interacts with complement. The complement is activated, components are fragmented, and the complement is "used up" or "fixed." In the second stage, sensitized sheep cells (EA) are added, and the mixture is incubated at 37°C for one hour. If the test serum contains antibody to the antigen used, complement is fixed and therefore is no longer available to lyse the EA. Thus, absence of lysis indicates a positive reaction, and complete lysis indicates a negative result.

There are two general approaches to complement fixation tests. In the first one, concentrated fresh serum is the complement source, and the amount of complement fixed is determined by titration of the serum before and after fixation. In the second one, a dilution of serum is used that provides either just enough complement for lysis of the EA or slightly more than enough (3 to 5 CH_{50} units). In this case, the sensitized cells are added without further dilution of the complement source. Incubation of the test materials with complement can take place at 37°C for one hour or overnight in the cold. In general, cold incubation leads to higher titers. Complement can be inactivated by a number of agents other than antigen-antibody complexes, such as bacteria, endotoxins, yeast, and aggregated γ-globulins. Therefore, controls are necessary to demonstrate that neither the serum nor the antigen alone will fix complement. The complement fixation test is particularly valuable in that it does not require that antigens or antibodies be present in highly purified form. Both soluble and particulate antigens may be used, and antigens as well as antibodies may be measured.

KININS AND THE KININ-GENERATING SYSTEM

The kinin-generating system is a second mediator pathway present in plasma and active at cellular surfaces that controls the generation of peptides that are important in the inflammatory response (Kozin, 1992). The most important biologically active peptide generated by the system appears to be bradykinin, a nonapeptide with potent activity in many biological systems. It is active in increasing vascular permeability, vasodilatation, hypotension, induction of pain, contraction of many types of smooth muscle, and activation of the phospholipase A2 system with its attendant activation of cellular arachidonic acid metabolism. Although in many respects it is similar to the complement system, the kinin-generating system is simpler because it is composed of only four plasma proteins. Because it has been studied less extensively than the complement system, it is likely that other proteins and regulators will be discovered over time.

The major proteins of the kinin-generating system as currently understood are Hageman factor, clotting Factor XI, prekallikrein, and high-molecular-weight kininogen. Factor XI circulates in the plasma as a complex with high-molecular-weight kininogen in a molar ratio of 2:1. Prekallikrein also circulates in a complex with high-molecular-weight kininogen in a molar ratio of 1:1. In contrast, Hageman factor circulates as an uncomplexed, single-chain plasma protein.

Like the complement activation sequence, the kinin-generating sequence follows a specific pathway. On interacting with negatively charged surfaces, such as those experimentally supplied by glass or naturally by many biologically active materials like lipid A of gram-negative bacterial endotoxin, Hageman factor is cleaved and activated. The cleaved Hageman factor (αHFa) has proteolytic activity and further activates and cleaves Hageman factor to generate more αHFa. Cleavage of the single chain of Hageman factor (molecular weight 80,000) yields heavy and light chains (molecular weight 50,000 and 28,000, respectively) that remain linked by disulfide bonds. The active enzymatic site of Hagemen factor resides in the light chain.

Many other proteolytic enzymes, including particularly kallikrein, can cleave and activate Hageman factor. αHFa interacts with the complex of Factor XI and high-molecular-weight kininogen to activate Factor XI to Factor XIa, resulting in activation of the extrinsic coagulation cascade. αHFa also interacts with the high-molecular-weight kininogen–prekallikrein complex to cleave the single-chain prekallikrein into a two-chain molecule, kallikrein, in which the chains are linked by the disulfide bonds. The cleaved prekallikrein has proteolytic enzymatic activity located on the lower-molecular-weight chain. All of these cleavages occur much more efficiently when the proteins are bound to the negative surface, which is critical to the activation of the cascade. The activated kallikrein cleaves high-molecular-weight kininogen at several sites, releasing bradykinin.

Active kallikrein, generated by cleavage of prekallikrein, is also capable of further cleaving αHFa to a lower-molecular-weight product with an intact light chain, βHFa. βHFa can cleave and activate the high-molecular-weight kininogen–prekallikrein complex but does not remain surface bound and does not interact efficiently with a high-molecular-weight kininogen–Factor XI complex.

Bradykinin has a short half-life because it is rapidly attacked by carboxypeptidase-N, which removes the C-terminal arginine to form des-Arg bradykinin. This molecule no longer has the smooth muscle contracting activity of bradykinin and cannot induce capillary leakage when injected in the skin; however, it retains some of its vascular effects. Des-Arg bradykinin is in turn cleaved by angiotensin-converting enzyme to form low-molecular-weight peptides that lack biological activity.

Inhibitors of the kinin-generating system include C1 inhibitor, α_2 macroglobulin, and α_1 protease inhibitor. C1 inhibitor and α_2 macroglobulin are the principal inhibitors of active kallikrein, with C1 inhibitor exerting the more potent influence. C1 inhibitor and α_1 protease inhibitor are the two major inhibitors of Factor XIa, and C1 inhibitor is the principal inhibitor of active Hageman factor.

Low-molecular-weight kininogens also exist in plasma and can act as a source of bradykinin. Kininogens are not easily cleaved by plasma kallikrein, but tissue kallikreins are present in cells that can cleave low-molecular-weight kininogen to bradykinin with an additional linked lysine. Presumably, the lysyl-bradykinin undergoes the same degradation pathway as bradykinin.

Bradykinin has been postulated to play a role in a variety of diseases. Free bradykinin and lysyl-bradykinin have been found in the nasal fluid in rhinitis. A pathogenic role for bradykinin has also been suggested in diseases ranging from asthma to hereditary angioedema, as well as other kinds of swelling disorders including inflammation. Clearly, we do not yet fully understand the role of the kinin-generating system in disease, but bradykinin and its derivatives are probably important in the swelling and pain associated with inflammation. In time we will learn far more about this interesting mediator pathway.

Agnello V: Lupus diseases associated with hereditary and acquired deficiencies of complement. Semin Immunopathol 1986; 9:161.

Anderson DC, Schmalstieg FC, Shearer W, et al: Leukocyte LFA-1, OKM-1, p150,95 deficiency syndrome: Functional and biosynthetic studies of three kindreds. Fed Proc 1985; 44:2671.

Atkinson JP: Complement activation and complement receptors in system lupus erythematosus. Semin Immunopathol 1986; 9:179.

Awdeh ZL, Alper, CA: Inherited structural polymorphism of the fourth component of human complement. Proc Natl Acad Sci USA 1980; 77:3576.

Biesecker G, Lavin L, Ziskind M, et al: Cutaneous localization of the membrane attack complex in discoid and systemic lupus erythematosus. N Engl J Med 1982; 306:264.

Bobak DA, Gaither TA, Frank MM, et al: Modulation of FcR function by complement: Subcomponent C1q enhances the phagocytosis of IgG-opsonized targets by human monocytes and culture-derived macrophages. J Immunol 1987; 138:1150.

Borsos T, Rapp HJ, Colten HR: Immune hemolysis and the functional properties of the second and fourth components. J Immunol 1970; 105:1439.

Borsos T, Rapp HJ: Complement fixation on cell surfaces by 19S and 7S antibodies. Science 1965; 150:505.

Choi N-H, Mazda T, Tomita M: A serum protein, SP-40,40, modulates the formation of membrane attack complex of complement on erythrocytes. Mol Immunol 1989;26:835.

Cole JP: Identification of an additional class of C3-binding membrane proteins of human peripheral blood leukocytes and cell lines. Proc Natl Acad Sci USA 1985; 82:859.

Cornacoff JB, Hebert LA, Smead WL, et al: Primate erythrocyte-immune complex-clearing mechanism. J Clin Invest 1988; 71:236.

Couser WG, Baker PJ, Adler S: Complement and the direct mediation of immune glomerular injury: A new perspective. Kidney Int 1985; 28:879.

Couser WG. Mediation of immune glomerular injury. J Am Soc Nephrol 1990; 1(1):13–29.

Couser WG. Pathogenesis of glomerulonephritis. Kidney Int Suppl 1993; 42:S19–26.

Dana N, Todd RF III, Pitt J, et al: Deficiency of a surface membrane glycoprotein (Mo1) in man. J Clin Invest 1984; 73:153.

Davis AE III, Harrison RA, Lachmann PJ: Physiologic inactivation of fluid phase C3b: Isolation and structural analysis of C3c, C3dg (2D) and C3g. J Immunol 1984; 132:1960.

Davis AE III: C1 inhibitor and hereditary angioneurotic edema. Annu Rev Immunol 1988; 6:595–628.

Davitz MA: Decay-accelerating factor (DAF): A review of its function and structure. Acta Med Scand (Suppl) 1987; 715:111.

DeBruijn MHL, Fey GH: Human complement component C3: cDNA coding sequence and derived primary structure. Proc Natl Acad Sci USA 1985; 82:708.

Falk RJ, Dalmasso AP, Kim Y, et al: Neoantigen of the polymerized ninth component of complement: Characterization of a monoclonal antibody and immunohistochemical localization in renal disease. J Clin Invest 1983; 72:560.

Fearon DT, Austen KF: The alternative pathway of complement: A system for host resistance to microbial infection. N Engl J Med 1980; 303:259.

Fearon DT, Wong WW: Complement ligand-receptor interactions that mediate biological responses. Ann Rev Immunol 1983; 1:243.

Fearon DT: Regulation by membrane sialic acid of 1H-dependent decay-dissociation of amplification C3 convertase of the alternative complement pathway. Proc Natl Acad Sci USA 1978; 75:1971.

Figueroa JE, Densen P: Infectious diseases associated with complement deficiencies. Clin Microbiol Rev 1991; 4(3):359–395.

Frade R, Hermann J, Barel M: A 16 amino acid synthetic peptide derived from human c3d triggers proliferation and specific tyrosine phosphorylation of transformed CR-2positive human lymphocytes and of normal resting B lymphocytes. Biochem Biophys Res Comm 1992; 188(2):833–42.

Frank MM: Complement in the pathophysiology of human disease. N Engl J Med 1987; 316:1525.

Frank MM: Complement system. *In* Frank MM, Austin KF, Claman HN, Unanue ER (eds): Samter's Immunologic Diseases, Vol 1, 5th ed. Boston, Little, Brown and Co., 1994, pp 331–352.

Fries LF, Frank MM: Complement and related proteins: Inherited deficiencies. *In* Gallin JI, Goldstein IM, Snyderman R (eds): Inflammation: Basic Principles and Clinical Correlates. New York, Raven Press, 1988, pp 89–100.

Fries LF, Frank MM: Molecular mechanisms of complement action. *In* Stamatoyannopoulos G, Nienhuis AW, Leder P, Majerus PW (eds): The Molecular Basis of Blood Diseases. Philadelphia, WB Saunders Co, 1987, pp 450–498.

Gaither TA, Vargas I, Inada S, et al: The complement fragment C3d facilitates phagocytosis by monocytes. Immunology 1987; 62:405.

Gaither TA, Frank MM: Complement. *In* Henry JB (ed): Clinical Diagnosis and Management by Laboratory Methods, 17th ed. Philadelphia, WB Saunders Co, 1984, pp 879–892.

Gaither TA, Hammer CH, Frank MM: Studies of the molecular mechanisms of C3b inactivation and a simplified assay of 1H and the C3b inactivator (C3bINA). J Immunol 1979; 123:1195.

Gammon WR, Inman AO, Wheeler CE Jr.: Differences in complement-dependent chemotactic activity generated by bullous pemphigoid and epidermolysis bullosa acquisita immune complexes: Demonstration by leukocytic attachment and organ culture methods. J Invest Dermatol 1984; 83:57.

Gawryl MS, Chudwin DS, Langlois PF, et al: The terminal complement complex, C5b-9, a marker of disease activity in patients with systemic lupus erythematosus. Arthritis Rheum 1987; 31:188.

Goldstein IM: Complement: Biologically active products. *In* Gallin JI, Goldstein IM, Snyderman R (eds): Inflammation: Basic Principles and Clinical Correlates. New York, Raven Press, 1988, pp 55–74.

Götze O, Medicus RG, Schreiber RD, et al: Molecular aspects of the properdin system. Monogr Allergy 1977; 12:66.

Hammer CH, Berger M: The components: Purification procedures. *In* Rother KR, Till GO (eds): The Complement System. Heidelberg, Springer, 1988, pp 5–44.

Hammerschmidt D, Weaver L, Hudson L, et al: Association of complement activation and elevated plasma-C5a with adult respiratory distress syndrome. Lancet 1980; 1:947.

Hughes-Jones N, Ghosh S: Anti-D coated Rh-positive cells will bind the first component of the complement pathway, C1q. FEBS Letters 1981; 128:318.

Hynes RO: Integrins: A family of cell surface receptors. Cell 1987; 48:549.

Iida K, Nussenzweig V: Complement receptor is an inhibitor of the complement cascade. J Exp Med 1981; 153:1138.

Johnson E, Berge V, Hogasen K: Formation of the terminal complement complex on agarose beads: Further evidence that vitronectin (complement S-protein) inhibits C9 polymerization. Scand J Immunol 1994; 39:281.

Joiner KA, Brown EJ, Frank MM: Complement and bacteria: Chemistry and biology in host defense. Annu Rev Immunol 1984; 2:461.

Kabat EA, Mayer MM: Experimental Immunochemistry, 2nd ed. Springfield, Charles C Thomas, 1961, pp 151–209.

Kinoshita T: Biology of complement: The overture. Immunol Today 1991; 12(9):291–295.

Kozin F, Cochrane CH: The contact activation system of plasma: Biochemistry and pathophysiology. *In* Gallin JI, Goldstein IM, Snyderman R (eds): Inflammation: Basic Principles and Clinical Correlates, 2nd ed. New York, Raven Press, 1992, pp 103–122.

Lachmann PJ: The control of homologous lysis. Immunol Today 1991; 12:312–315.

Langlois PR, Gawryl MS: Complement activation occurs through both classical and alternative pathways prior to onset and resolution of adult respiratory distress syndrome. Clin Immunol Immunopathol 1988; 47:152.

Linscott's Directory of Immunological and Biological Reagents. Linscott, WD. Santa Rosa, CA, 1994–1995.

Liszewski MK, Post TW, Atkinson JP: Membrane cofactor protein (MCP or CD46): Newest member of the regulators of complement activation gene cluster. Annu Rev Immunol 1991; 9:431.

Liszewski MK, Atkinson JP: Membrane cofactor protein. Curr Top Microbiol Immunol 1992; 178:45–60.

Marom Z, Shelhammer J, Berger M, et al: Anaphylatoxin C3a enhances mucous glycoprotein release from human airways in vitro. J Exp Med 1985; 161:657.

Mayer MM: Complement: Historical perspectives and some current issues. Complement 1984; 1:2.

Mayes JT, Schreiber RD, Cooper NR: Development and application of an enzyme-linked immunoabsorbent assay for the quantitation of alternative complement pathway activation in human serum. J Clin Invest 1984; 73:160.

Minta JO, Gee AP: Purification and quantitation of the components of the alternative pathway. Methods Enzymol 1983; 93:375.

Mitomo K, Fujita T, Iida K: Functional and antigenic properties of complement receptor type 2, CR2. J Exp Med 1987; 165:1424.

Morgan BP, Walport MJ: Complement deficiency and disease. Immunol Today 1991; 12(9):301.

Morgan BP, Meri S: Membrane proteins that protect against complement lysis. Semin Immunopathol 1994; 15:369.

Nicholson-Weller A, Burge J, Fearon DT, et al: Isolation of a human erythrocyte membrane glycoprotein with decay-accelerating activity for C3 convertases of the complement system. J Immunol 1982; 129:184.

Oltvai ZN, Wong ECC, Atkinson JP, et al: C1 inhibitor deficiency: Molecular and immunologic basis of hereditary and acquired angioedema. Lab Invest 1991;65:381–388.

O'Neill GJ, Yang SY, Dupont B: Two HLA-linked loci controlling the fourth component of human complement. Proc Natl Acad Sci USA 1978a; 75:5165.

O'Neill GJ, Yang SY, Tegoli I, et al: Chido and Rodgers blood groups are distinct antigenic components of human complement C4. Nature 1978b; 273:668.

Pangburn MK, Schreiber RD, Müller-Eberhard HJ: Formation of the initial C3 convertase of the alternative complement pathway: Acquisition of C3b-like activities by spontaneous hydrolysis of the putative thioester in native C3. J Exp Med 1981; 154:856.

Pillemer L, Blum L, Lepow IH, et al: The properdin system and immunity. I. Demonstration and isolation of a new serum protein, properdin, and its role in immune phenomena. Science 1954; 120:279.

Rapp HJ, Borsos T: Molecular Basis of Complement Action. New York, Appleton-Century-Crofts, 1970, pp 75–134.

Ratnoff OD, Pensky J, Ogston D, et al: The inhibition of plasmin, plasma kallikrein, plasma permeability factor, and the C'1r subcomponent of the first component of complement by serum C'1 esterase inhibitor. J Exp Med 1969; 129:315.

Ross GD, Medof ME: Membrane complement receptors specific for bound fragments of C3. Adv Immunol 1985a; 37:217.

Ross GD, Yount WJ, Walport MJ, et al: Disease-associated loss of erythrocyte complement receptors (CR1, C3b receptors) in patients with systemic lupus erythematosus and other diseases involving autoantibodies and/or complement activation. J Immunol 1985b; 135:2005.

Ross GD, Lambris JD, Cain JA, et al: Generation of three different fragments of bound C3 with purified factor I or serum. I. Requirements for factor H vs. CR1 cofactor activity. J Immunol 1982; 129:2051.

Sanders ME, Koski CL, Robbins D, et al: Activated terminal complement in cerebrospinal fluid in Guillain-Barré syndrome and multiple sclerosis. J Immunol 1986; 136:4456.

Sanders ME, Schmetz MA, Hammer CH, et al: Quantitation of activation of the human terminal complement pathway by ELISA. J Immunol Methods 1985; 85:245.

Schapira M, de Agostini A, Schifferli JA, et al: Biochemistry and pathophysiology of human C1-inhibitor: Current issues. Complement 1986; 2:111.

Schwab TR, Donadio JV Jr: Serology in renal disease: A review. Semin Nephrol 1985; 5:179.

Seya T, Atkinson JP: Functional properties of a complement regulatory protein, membrane cofactor protein (MCP) or gp45-70: Evidence that MCP is incorporated into and protects the cell from autologous complement activation (abstract). Fed Proc 1986; 45:382.

Seya T, Holers VM, Atkinson JP: Purification and functional analysis of the polymorphic variants of the C3b/C4b receptor (CR1) and comparison with H, C4b-binding protein (C4bp), and decay accelerating factor (DAF). J Immunol 1985; 135:2661.

Shin ML, Carney DF: Cytotoxic action and other metabolic consequences of terminal complement proteins. Prog Allergy 1988; 40:44.

Sim RB, Malhotra V, Ripoche J, et al: Complement receptors and related complement control proteins. Biochem Soc Symp 1986; 51:83.

Springer TA, Thompson WS, Miller LJ, et al: Inherited deficiency of the Mac-1, LFA-1, p150,95 glycoprotein family and its molecular basis. J Exp Med 1984; 160:1901.

Tack BF: The -Cis—Glu thiolester bond in human C3, C4 and α_2-macroglobulin. Semin Immunopathol 1983; 6:259.

Volanakis JE: Structure, molecular genetics, and function of complement control proteins: An update. Year Immunol 1988; 3:275.

Wright SD, Griffin FM Jr: Activation of phagocytic cells' C3 receptors for phagocytosis. J Leukocyte Biol 1985; 38:327.

Zalman LS, Muller-Eberhard HJ: Comparison of channels formed by poly C9, C5b-8 and the membrane attack complex of complement. Mol Immunol 1990; 27(6):533–7.

Zubler RH, Lambert PH: The ^{125}I-Cq binding test for the detection of soluble immune complexes. *In* Bloom BR, David JR (eds): In Vitro Methods in Cell-Mediated and Tumor Immunity. New York, Academic Press, 1976, pp 565–572.

Chapter 37

Cytokines and Cell Adhesion Molecules

Howard S. Fox, M.D., Ph.D.

Communication is the key to all physiologic interactions, including those of the immune system. Immune cells secrete a plethora of molecules, including the cytokines, which allow interactions between the immune cells themselves and between immune cells and the other cells of the body. For immune responses to occur, the relevant cells must be recruited to various regions of the body and, at those sites, must be in close enough proximity with each other to interact. Such functions are served by the cell adhesion molecules. For some time, researchers have been unraveling the complex network that contains the cytokines and cell adhesion molecules, and the examination of these molecules will become increasingly important for our understanding of the pathophysiology of disease, its diagnosis, and its management.

CYTOKINES

General Principles

Cytokines are the soluble, secreted messengers of the immune system. They act in an autocrine or paracrine fashion, although functions similar to those of endocrine hormones are also possible. In general, cytokines are glycoproteins of relatively low molecular weight (monomer forms <30 kDa). They are produced by the processing of precursor polypeptides and are extraordinarily potent, working at a femtomolar concentration. Most cytokines have numerous effects, among which are complex interactions with the cells that produce them. Cytokines can induce or suppress their own production as well as the production of other cytokines, and they also affect the expression of cytokine receptors. Additionally, cytokines can synergize as well as antagonize each other. By communicating between cells, these molecules serve to regulate the immune system and help mediate the effects between immune and nonimmune cells.

Lymphokines were first described as the soluble products of stimulated lymphocytes that could affect B- and T-cell function. The broader term, cytokine, is more appropriate, because some of these molecules are made by nonimmune as well as immune cell types. The following discussion is limited to those cytokines that are primarily produced by or that affect cells of the immune system. Moreover, because the number of identified cytokines continues to increase, the descriptions are restricted to those for which the most information is available. Currently, measurement of cytokine production is performed for experimental purposes. However, it is likely that because of associations of disease states with excess cytokine production, investigative approaches to decrease cytokine production or effects, and therapies using cytokines, their measurement will enter the diagnostic realm. The sources, targets, and effects of cytokines are described here. This chapter is not intended to be an encyclopedic description of all work performed on these molecules but rather to provide a basis for the potential uses of these molecules and their eventual measurement. For each cytokine, references are given to reviews containing further information and references.

Cytokines (interleukins [IL]; interferons [IFN]; tumor necrosis factors [TNF]; and transforming growth factors

[TGF]), which can be made by all cells of the immune system but most prominently by T cells and macrophages (Table 37–1), have effects on mature and immature immune cells. Monocytes/macrophages can produce immunologically stimulatory, proinflammatory cytokines, including IL-1, IL-6, IL-8, and TNFα, as well as immunologically suppressive molecules, such as IL-10 and TGFβ. T cells produce cytokines with multiple effects. The lymphocyte cell surface markers CD4 and CD8 are frequently used to divide T cells into functional subsets, but based largely on work in mice, $CD4^+$ cells can be further subdivided according to their cytokine production profile (see Table 37–1), a convenient division for conceptualizing their actions but of potential relevance to *in vivo* immune interactions. These helper T cells (Th) can be divided into Th1 and Th2 cells (Bottomly, 1988). Th1 cells produce many molecules, including IFNγ, IL-2, TNFα, and TNFβ. These cytokines can be thought of as proinflammatory, are important in the mediation of delayed-type hypersensitivity reactions, and are effective against viral infections and infections of macrophages with intracellular microbes. In contrast, Th2 cells produce IL-4, IL-5, IL-6, and IL-10. These cytokines stimulate B-cell antibody responses and parasitic defenses, including IgE production. $CD8^+$ cytotoxic T lymphocytes (CTL) destroy virally infected cells, limit viral spread, and produce the pro-inflammatory, antiviral cytokines IFNγ, TNFα, and TNFβ. Cytokines are also active in the production and differentiation of immune cell precursor. The specific macrophage (M), granulocyte (G), and granulocyte/macrophage (GM) colony-stimulating factors (CSF) and stem cell factor are not discussed here, but the effects of the interleukins on bone marrow cells, including IL-3, which has potent CSF activity, are described in Chapter 31.

In general, cytokine activities were first identified by biological assays that examined the functional effects of these secreted cellular products. However, these assays can be not only tedious, taking days and requiring specialized cell lines, media, and cell culture techniques, but also can be nonspecific, because an activity found in complex biological fluids may originate not just from the molecule in question but additionally from other characterized or uncharacterized molecules. Although remedies to this problem exist, such as using a specific antibody to neutralize the molecule being sought, specific immunoassays are often the method of choice in the measurement of cytokines and their soluble receptors in biological fluids because of their specificity, reproducibility, speed, and ease of performance. Still, in some cases, bioassays may be preferred because they uniquely measure bioactive cytokine or because of their often unsurpassed sensitivity. An updated, comprehensive laboratory manual is available describing bioassays for the cytokines as well as sources of reagents for antibodies and standards (Coligan, 1994).

Commercial kits are currently available to measure cytokines, using specific monoclonal or polyclonal antibodies and enzyme-linked colorimetric detection or radiometric detection; for many of the cytokines, enzyme-linked immunosorbent assay (ELISA) technology is available. Additionally, numerous antibody reagents are available for use in setting up such assays. Most of the reagents have the required specificity, but difficulties arise regarding what is being measured. Some reagents are blocked by the presence of binding proteins such as the soluble cytokine receptors and thus measure only uncomplexed molecules, whereas others react with the cytokines independent of known protein-protein interactions. Depending on the specific cytokine, such interference may actually select for biologically active molecules, thus yielding results similar to those in bioassays, but for others this blocking artificially decreases the amount of cytokine measured. Thus, when using particular reagents to measure a cytokine, one must be familiar with the properties of the chosen kit or reagents. An additional problem is that standardization is poor when comparing results obtained from different kits or different laboratories.

Cytokines can be measured in plasma, serum, various body fluids, and supernatants from cultured cells, such as peripheral blood mononuclear cells. Although no standard technique exists for sample collection, in general, to protect

Table 37–1. SOURCES OF VARIOUS CYTOKINES AND DETECTION OF SOLUBLE RECEPTOR

Cytokine	CD4+ Th1	CD4+ Th2	CD8+ CTL	B Cell	Macrophage Monocyte	Stroma (BM)	Nonimmune	Soluble Receptor
IL-1					++		++	
IL-2	++							++
IL-3	++	++						
IL-4		++						
IL-5		++						
IL-6		++			++		++	++
IL-7						++		
IL-8					++			
IL-9	++							
IL-10		++		++	++			
IL-11						++		
IL-12					++			
IFN γ	++		++					
TNF-α	++		++		++			++
TNF-β	++		++					++
TGF-β	++				++	++	++	

*The major sources of the individual cytokines from immune cells, including when relevant Th1 versus Th2 CD4+ T cells, is shown by the (++). Production by cells outside of the immune system (nonimmune) is also indicated. Also indicated is the detection of soluble forms of the receptor for the given cytokine.

against degradation, samples should be collected, immediately chilled, and, for fluids, separated from cells. Serum may present a particular problem in assessing levels of cytokines, because clotting can induce cytokine release. Furthermore, because many cytokines act locally and have a short half-life, static measurement in plasma may not reflect local processes. Cells isolated from blood, other fluids, or lymphoid organs may be grown in culture, and supernatants may be assessed for the presence of cytokines; such cultures may also be stimulated with various specific or nonspecific activating agents to assess the cytokine response profile.

The cytokine receptors can also be measured by several means. Some of the receptors are present in a soluble form in the blood (see Table 37–1) and can be measured by ELISA. Cell-associated receptors can be detected with fluorochrome-conjugated antibodies by using flow cytometry if the appropriate antibodies are available; other techniques, such as radioreceptor assays, which use radiolabeled ligands (the cytokines themselves), and Scatchard's analysis can be performed to determine binding affinity and receptor number.

Expression of both the cytokines and their receptors can also be measured by molecular analysis. Ribonucleic acid (RNA) extracted from the sample in question is reverse-transcribed to complementary deoxyribonucleic acid (cDNA), which can then be amplified by the polymerase chain reaction (PCR) technique and visualized by gel electrophoresis or hybridization analysis. *In situ* hybridization, using labeled specific probes, can also be performed on cell or tissue samples. This has the advantage of allowing one to determine the cell type producing the molecules in question, whereas the PCR technique destroys the sample but is much more sensitive. Both methods are difficult to quantitate, but by using the appropriate techniques and controls, quantitation is possible. However, there is frequently a rather complex relationship between the presence of messenger RNA (mRNA), the protein, and the biological activity of cytokines, so caution must be used in interpreting these results. Furthermore, the integrity of RNA is very sensitive to specimen handling; thus, freshly obtained tissue is often required.

Interleukin-1

IL-1 (Dinarello, 1993a; Dinarello, 1994) refers to two proteins, IL-1α and IL-1β, which are encoded by separate genes. IL-1α and IL-1β are related to each other on the amino acid level, showing 25% identity. Similar to many cytokines, both IL-1α and IL-1β are produced as precursor proteins that are subsequently cleaved into the mature forms; a specific protease that cleaves IL-1β has been identified. However, although both proteins are secreted, neither contains a signal peptide sequence for secretion. A membrane-bound form of IL-1α has been identified, but its biological role is uncertain. Both IL-1α and IL-1β are recognized by the same receptors, of which two distinct proteins and genes also exist, and these are referred to as Type I and Type II IL-1 receptors. The receptors show amino acid homology only in their extracellular domains, where IL-1 binding occurs. However, only the Type I receptor appears capable of transducing a signal after IL-1 binding, and the function of the Type II receptor is not clear. In addition to the IL-1 cytokines and their receptors, a third class of molecule is involved in regulation of IL-1 activity and consists of an inhibitor of IL-1 activity, known as the IL-1 receptor antagonist (IL-1ra) (Arend, 1993). The IL-1ra shows 20% to 25% similarity to IL-1α and IL-1β at the amino acid level. This antagonist binds to the Type I IL-1 receptor and appears to inhibit IL-1 activity in a competitive manner, because binding of IL-1ra to the receptor does not induce signal transduction.

A wide variety of cell types is capable of producing IL-1, including myelomonocytic cells, B cells, endothelial cells, astrocytes, and keratinocytes. The Type I IL-1 receptor is also expressed on immune and nonimmune cell types, including T cells, endothelial cells, and fibroblasts, whereas the Type II receptor is expressed on myelomonocytic cells and B cells. We know that the IL-1ra is made by macrophages, but in all likelihood many of the same cell types that produce IL-1 can also produce its antagonist. IL-1 is produced rapidly in response to infection, injury, and immune activation. In fact, products both of infectious agents, such as endotoxin, and of the host response, including IL-1 itself and TNF, stimulate its synthesis. Its production can be suppressed by exogenous agents, such as glucocorticoids, as well as by endogenous molecules including IL-10 and TGFβ.

IL-1 was originally known as lymphocyte-activating factor and has this as well as a host of other biological activities. In the immune system, IL-1 not only upregulates its own synthesis in macrophages but also induces the production of other proinflammatory cytokines such as TNFα and IL-6. T cells are activated by IL-1, which induces the production of IL-2 and its receptor, in addition to IL-4 and GM-CSF. B cells' differentiation and proliferation are stimulated by IL-1, as is immunoglobulin secretion. Along with IL-2 and IFNγ, IL-1 enhances natural killer (NK) cell activity. Hematopoiesis is also stimulated by IL-1.

Outside the immune system, IL-1 has various other effects. In the central nervous system, IL-1 induces fever and slow-wave sleep, as well as the production of hypothalamic and pituitary hormones. IL-1 can incite the acute phase response in the liver, and osteoblasts, fibroblasts, and endothelial cells all are activated by IL-1.

Although part of the host response to infection, IL-1 production is linked to untoward effects in chronic inflammatory conditions and autoimmune diseases, such as periodontitis and rheumatoid arthritis. Beneficial effects of IL-1 are also present, however, including the acceleration of wound healing and stimulation of hematopoiesis. The measurement of IL-1 and IL-1ra and their therapeutic uses are currently the subjects of active research (Dinarello, 1993b). Although the bioassays do not distinguish IL-1α and IL-1β, this may be accomplished through the use of specific neutralizing antisera. Specific ELISAs are available for IL-1α and IL-1β.

Interleukin-2

IL-2 (Smith, 1992; Janssen, 1994), similar to most other cytokines, is produced as a precursor molecule containing a leader sequence (the signal peptide) that is cleaved from the mature protein. IL-2 has been crystallized, revealing it structurally as an α-helical protein. The IL-2 receptor (IL-2R) consists of a multisubunit complex of which three transmembrane glycoprotein components have been identified. The first, called the IL-2Rα chain, known as the Tac antigen (CD25), is inducible by mitogenic stimulation. A soluble form of IL-2Rα can be found in the blood and is referred to as sIL-2R. The second component is the IL-2Rβ chain, which is constitutively expressed but up-regulated after T-cell activation. The third component identified is the IL-2Rγ chain, which is constitutively expressed and required for signal transduction. Although the IL-2Rα chain alone can bind IL-2 at low affinity, the entire IL-2R$\alpha\beta\gamma$ complex is necessary for high-affinity IL-2 binding.

The IL-2Rγ chain maps to the same location of the X chromosome as does the X-linked form of severe combined immunodeficiency (SCID) syndrome, and mutations in the *IL2RG* gene are present in those afflicted with the disease (Leonard, 1994; Voss, 1994). In the X-linked form of SCID, which accounts for 50% of all SCID cases, T cells are drastically diminished, but B-cell numbers may be normal. However, these B cells do not function, likely because of absent T-cell help and a dependence on a functional IL-2Rγ chain for terminal differentiation. The described mutations lead to truncations of the IL-2Rγ glycoprotein, which then lacks the majority of its cytoplasmic domain.

IL-2 was originally known as T-cell growth factor. It is produced by activated $CD4^+$ T cells (Th1 type) and functions as a stimulator of activated T cells in an autocrine fashion, resulting in the expansion of specific clones. A simplified model of this sequence might begin with antigen-specific stimulation of T cells, after which these cells produce IL-2 and increase their expression of the IL-2R, leading to the proliferation of a clone specific for the initial stimulatory antigen. IL-2 also acts in a paracrine manner, resulting in the growth of other activated T cells, B cells, and NK cells that express the IL-2R. NK cells can also produce IL-2. Furthermore, lymphokine-activated killer (LAK) cells, with their potentially potent antineoplastic actions, are likely derived from NK cells expanded by IL-2. Additionally, neutrophils and macrophages can express the IL-2R and demonstrate enhanced function in response to IL-2. Production of IL-2 can also induce the expression of numerous cytokines, including IL-1, IL-6, TNFα, and IFNγ. Although induced by T-cell activation, IL-2 expression can be inhibited by immune-suppressing agents, such as cyclosporin A, FK-506, and glucocorticoids.

Because of its ability to expand T-cell numbers, IL-2 has a central role in the immune responses. IL-2 has even been investigated clinically in a number of attempts to stimulate antineoplastic immune reactivity (Vlasveld, 1994; Oldham, 1994). Accordingly, elevated levels of IL-2 and sIL-2R can be found in the serum in states of immune activation, such as infection, allograft rejection, and autoimmunity. Both bioassays and ELISAs are used to measure IL-2, whereas levels of expression of the IL-2R can be examined by flow cytometry, and the sIL-2R can be quantitated by ELISA. Analysis of the *IL2RG* to diagnose X-linked SCID can be performed by molecular biological analysis.

Interleukin-3

The IL3 (Lindemann, 1993; Frendl, 1992; Ihle, 1992) gene maps to the long arm of chromosome 5, linked to the *IL4, IL5, IL9, MCSF,* and *GMCSF* genes. Although this close linkage may imply evolutionary or functional similarities, these remain speculative. The IL-3 receptor (IL-3R) is a complex consisting of at least two subunits. One of them, the IL-3Rα chain, is capable of binding IL-3 at low affinity, but when complexed to the other, the β-subunit, high-affinity binding occurs. The β-subunit, which is identical to that of the IL-5 and GM-CSF receptors, subserves signal transduction functions (Miyajima, 1993).

IL-3 is produced largely by activated T cells. Other cell types, such as thymic epithelial cells, activated mast cells, and NK cells, can also produce IL-3. Immune suppressive agents, such as cyclosporin A and glucocorticoids, suppress IL-3 synthesis. IL-3R is expressed by precursor and mature cells in hematopoietic cell lineages.

IL-3 was originally known as colony-forming unit–stimulating activity, and most of its described effects are on cells of the hematopoietic system. IL-3 can support the expansion and the early developmental stages of multipotential progenitor cells. IL-3 is a potent stimulator of hematopoiesis, acting primarily on the most immature cell types; as lineage development occurs, cells lose sensitivity to IL-3, and other factors are required for specific lineage development. IL-3 can also stimulate the proliferation of mast cells and specific T-cells subsets. The stimulatory effect of IL-3 on hematopoiesis is likely to be useful clinically, and administration of IL-3 is being investigated to treat states of bone marrow depression (Ganser, 1993; Gillio, 1993). Bioassay is currently used to measure IL-3.

Interleukin-4

IL-4 (Sonoda, 1994; Vellenga, 1993; Paul, 1991) is a complex protein containing multiple glycosylation sites and numerous intramolecular disulfide bonds. The high-affinity receptor for IL-4 (IL-4R) consists of a single transmembrane protein. The extracellular domain of the IL-4R shows homology to other cytokine receptors, including the IL-5Rα chain and the IL-6R. A soluble IL-4 receptor has been detected in the sera of rodents but has not been found in human specimens.

IL-4 is produced primarily by activated $CD4^+$ T cells (Th2 type) but can also be made by $CD8^+$ T cells and some immature bone marrow cells. Endogenous and exogenous immune suppressive agents, such as TGF-β and cyclosporin A, can inhibit IL-4 production. The IL-4R is expressed by lymphoid, myeloid, and erythroid cells, in addition to nonhematopoietic cells such as brain, liver, and muscle cells.

IL-4 was originally known as B-cell differentiation or growth factor, but further investigations have revealed pleiotropic activities for this molecule. On resting B cells, IL-4 induces its own receptor and other cell surface antigens including the major histocompatibility complex (MHC) Class II molecules (such as HLA-DR) and the Fc receptor for IgE (CD23). Activated B cells respond to IL-4 with immunoglobulin class switching (to IgG4 and IgE). IL-4 induces the growth of certain T cells and can act as an autocrine factor for these cells, similar to the effects of IL-2 on other T cells. Macrophages also can respond to IL-4 with an increase in MHC Class II expression and induction of stimulatory activities; in contrast, monocytes are inhibited in activation functions, such as cytokine expression and superoxide production. In conjunction with IL-10, IL-4 is thought to induce a Th2-type immune response, and the function of Th1 cells, including cytokine expression, is inhibited. In conjunction with other cytokines, IL-4 has stimulatory effects on hematopoietic precursor cells of multiple lineages.

Owing to its effect in inhibiting the inflammatory Th1 responses, IL-4 may find clinical utility in various inflammatory diseases. Similarly, the antineoplastic effects of IL-4 are also under investigation. No reliable, specific bioassay has been described for IL-4, but ELISAs can be used for its analysis.

Interleukin-5

IL-5 (Takatsu, 1992; Sanderson, 1992; Mahanty, 1993) exists as a disulfide-linked homodimer, whose receptor (IL-5R) is a complex consisting of at least two proteins. The IL-5Rα chain can bind the cytokine at low affinity but, in combination with the β-chain, can bind IL-5 at high affinity. The IL-5Rβ chain is identical to that for IL-3 and GM-CSF, and like those systems, transmits its signal on ligand binding to the α chain. Two soluble forms of the IL-5α chain can be produced by alternative splicing of the transcript, and both can bind IL-5 (Kikuchi, 1994).

IL-5 is synthesized by activated T cells, although production by some B cells, mast cells, and eosinophils has been reported. IL-5 is produced largely in response to T-cell activation. The IL-5R is expressed on eosinophils and at lower levels on B cells.

Although originally characterized in mouse systems as a T-cell–replacing factor that stimulates B cells, in humans it was found to be an eosinophil differentiation factor. IL-5 is chemotactic for eosinophils, increases survival of eosinophils, and activates their functions. Along with other cytokines, IL-5 acts to increase eosinophil production and serves later in development as a differentiation factor. Stimulatory effects on basophils have also been reported.

Clinically, IL-5 is elevated in association with states of eosinophil reactions. The concentration of IL-5 is increased in patients infected with helminths and parasites, as well as in those with hypereosinophilia, including the eosinophilia-myalgia syndrome (Steel, 1993; Owen, 1990). Bioassay is currently performed to measure IL-5.

Interleukin-6

IL-6 (Kishimoto, 1992; Akira, 1993; Lotz, 1993) is a glycoprotein containing four cysteine residues and, as evident from modeling, can form multiple α-helices. IL-6 shows some sequence similarity, including the four cysteines, to G-CSF, although these two cytokines do not have similar activities. The IL-6 receptor (IL-6R) consists of two glycoproteins: the IL-6 binding protein, IL-6R, and a separate signal-transducing molecule, gp130. The gp130 molecule is also involved in signal transduction of other cytokine receptors, including the IL-11R. A soluble form of the IL-6R, sIL-6R, has been identified, and arises from proteolytic cleavage of the IL-6R (Honda, 1992).

IL-6 is produced by a wide variety of immune and nonimmune cell types, including T and B cells, monocytes/macrophages, fibroblasts, endothelial cells, keratinocytes, and others. Numerous stimulatory agents include IL-6 production, including the cytokines IL-1 and TNF. Glucocorticoids can suppress IL-6 expression. The IL-6R is also expressed on various cell types, including T cells, monocytes/macrophages, activated B cells, neutrophils, hematopoietic progenitor cells, and hepatocytes.

From the many biological activities induced by IL-6, it has been known by a plethora of names. In activated B cells, IL-6 promotes differentiation and immunoglobulin secretion. On T cells, IL-6 can synergize with other agents to activate cells and induce cytokine expression. Cellular proliferation can be induced by IL-6 on such cell types as T cells, mesangial cells, and keratinocytes. In contrast, IL-6 can inhibit the growth of M1 myeloid leukemic cells and chronic lymphocytic leukemia B cells. The acute phase response by hepatocytes is inducible by IL-6. Additionally, changes in IL-6 production after the decrease in estrogen at menopause have been linked to the development of osteoporosis (Girasole, 1992). The sIL-6R has been shown to affect the activity of IL-6: sIL-6R binds to IL-6 and augments its activity by allowing this complex to bind to gp130, inducing signal transduction.

Elevated levels of IL-6 accompany various disease states, such as autoimmune diseases, mesangial proliferative glomerulonephritis, and plasmacytoma growth. The sIL-6R can be found in the sera of normal individuals, and concentrations may be elevated when increased IL-6 is also present. Both bioassays and ELISAs are available for IL-6; the IL-6R can be assessed by flow cytometry, and sIL-6R can be measured by ELISAs.

Interleukin-7

IL-7 (Costello, 1993; Kunisada, 1992) is the product of a large gene (>33 kb) that generates transcripts of multiple sizes. However, only one known glycoprotein product results from these mRNAs. Two different IL-7 receptors (IL-7R) exist, a high-affinity receptor as well as a separate low-affinity receptor. A soluble form of the IL-7R is also present, and it arises through alternate splicing of the transcript.

IL-7 expression is limited to stromal cells and can be produced constitutively by both bone marrow and thymic stromal cells. Interestingly, tumor cells in Hodgkin's disease frequently express the IL-7 mRNA (Foss, 1995). Production of the high-affinity IL-7R is restricted to T cells, whereas the low-affinity IL-7R is expressed on a wide variety of hematopoietic cells at higher levels than the high-affinity receptor is on T cells.

5

IL-7 was initially described as a pre–B-cell growth factor, and indeed pre-B cells appear to be dependent on IL-7 for their growth. However, IL-7 is also active on T cells. In the thymus, roles for IL-7 in the growth and differentiation of immature thymocytes have been proposed. Additionally, IL-7 is mitogenic for activated mature T cells, and the development of CTL and LAK cells can be enhanced by IL-7. Both a bioassay and ELISA are available for measurement of IL-7 levels.

Interleukin-8 and the Chemokines

IL-8 (Baggiolini, 1994; Hebert, 1993) is a relatively small nonglycosylated molecule (69 to 77 amino acids, ~8 kDa), with at least four variants generated from a common precursor. Based on amino acid similarities, it is a member of a larger family of chemotactic cytokines (chemokines) (Miller, 1992), including macrophage inflammatory proteins (MIP-1α and MIP-β), monocyte chemotactic and activating factor/monocyte chemotactic factor (MCAF/MCP-1), growth-related cytokine (GROα, as well as GROβ/MIP-2α and GROγ/MIP-2β), and regulated on activation, normal T expressed and presumably secreted (RANTES). Two distinct forms of the IL-8 receptor (IL-8R) exist, and these show approximately 75% amino acid similarity. The Type I IL-8R has high-affinity binding specific for IL-8, whereas the Type II IL-8R can bind both IL-8 and GROα at high affinity and MIP-2 at lower affinity. A receptor that is activated by MIP-1α and RANTES binding has been described; specific as well as shared receptors for the other chemokines are likely present. Red blood cells express a multispecific chemokine receptor that can bind IL-8 and the other chemokines.

Numerous cell types produce IL-8, including monocytes, lymphocytes, neutrophils, endothelial cells, and fibroblasts. IL-8 expression is inducible by exogenous agents including viruses and bacteria, as well as endogenously by cytokines including IL-1 and TNF. Suppression of IL-8 production is exerted by glucocorticoids, IL-4, and TGFβ. The MIP-1s can be produced by activated macrophages as well as T and B cells and fibroblasts. MCAF/MCP-1 synthesis by monocytes/macrophages, fibroblasts, B cells, endothelial cells, and smooth muscle follows stimulation by inflammatory mediators, and this production can be inhibited by glucocorticoids. GROα production is induced in many cell types, including monocytes, fibroblasts, and endothelial cells under growth-inducing or inflammatory conditions. RANTES, which is produced by T cells and cells of both the kidneys and liver, can be released by thrombin-stimulated platelets. As opposed to its effects on most other cytokines, T-cell activation induces a decrease in RANTES expression.

IL-8 and the other chemokines are chemotactic and cell-activating proinflammatory molecules (Bickel, 1993; Harada, 1994; Kunkel, 1994). IL-8 is chemotactic for neutrophils and induces their degranulation (but not their oxidative burst) and their increased expression of adhesion molecules. Other reported activities include chemotaxis for basophils, growth of melanomas, and angiogenesis. The MIP-1s induce monocyte chemotaxis and activation and are chemotactic for CD4$^+$ cells. MIP-1α is also chemotactic for B cells, CTL, and basophils and can induce histamine release from the latter. MCAF/MCP-1 is chemotactic for monocytes and stimulates their activation, including generation of superoxide anions and release of lysosomal enzymes. It is also chemotactic for basophils and induces basophils to release histamine. GROα is a more potent chemoattractant for neutrophils than is IL-8, whereas IL-8 is more potent in neutrophil activation. RANTES is a monocyte, T-cell, eosinophil, and basophil chemoattractant and can induce degranulation of eosinophils and histamine release from basophils. Although the regulatory mechanisms involved in chemokine activity are under investigation, at least one such mechanism seems to be control of circulating chemokine concentrations by the multispecific chemokine receptor on red blood cells.

IL-8 is known to be elevated in conditions of inflammation, such as psoriasis and other skin disorders (Kemeny, 1994). Given the activities of IL-8 and the other chemokines, their detection and possible blockage may conceivably be important in the monitoring or treatment of disease. IL-8 can be assessed by bioassay or ELISA.

Interleukin-9

IL-9 (Renauld, 1993; Yang, 1992; Quesniaux, 1992) is a highly glycosylated, cysteine-rich protein. The IL-9 receptor (IL-9R) consists of a transmembrane protein. IL-9 is produced by activated T cells, mainly CD4$^+$ cells, and both IL-1 and IL-2 regulate its expression. The IL-9R is expressed on T cells as well as erythroid and myeloid precursors.

IL-9 was originally described as a factor stimulating the growth of a megakaryocytic cell line. Subsequently, the documented activities of IL-9 include synergism with other cytokines to support the development of erythroid precursors. Furthermore, activated T cells proliferate in the presence of IL-9, and IL-9 can potentiate the effect of IL-4 on immunoglobulin production, including IgE, by B cells. Effects on the development and function of mast cells have been demonstrated in mice but not in humans. IL-9 is currently measured by bioassay.

Interleukin-10

IL-10 (Mossman, 1994; Moore, 1993; Howard, 1992) contains potential glycosylation sites but is a nonglycosylated protein, existing as a noncovalently linked homodimer. IL-10 shows amino acid homology to an open reading frame in the Epstein-Barr virus (EBV) genome, BCRF1, which is now known as viral IL-10 (vIL-10). The IL-10 receptor (IL-10R) has not yet been molecularly characterized.

IL-10 can be produced by T cells, B cells, activated monocytes/macrophages, and keratinocytes. However, the best-characterized producer of IL-10 is the Th2 subset of CD4$^+$ T cells. IL-10 synthesis can be increased by stimulatory agents and decreased by IL-4 and IFNγ. Owing to the cytokine's effects on T cells, B cells, and monocytes/macrophages, these cells most likely express the IL-10R.

IL-10 was originally described as a cytokine synthesis inhibitory factor, being produced by Th2 clones and inhibiting the production of cytokines, including IL-2 and IFNγ, from Th1 clones. IL-10 also has inhibitory effects on monocytes/macrophages. IL-10 down-regulates the expression of MHC Class II molecules and antigen-presenting capacity, inhibits the production of inflammatory cytokines, including IL-1, IL-6, IL-8, and TNFα, up-regulates synthesis of the antagonist IL-1ra, and suppresses the production of superoxide anions and reactive oxygen and nitrogen intermediates. In total, IL-10 effectively deactivates macrophages and suppresses inflammatory reactions. In contrast, IL-10 has stimulatory effects on B cells, inducing their expression of MCH Class II molecules and serving as a growth factor. IL-10 can also exert stimulatory effects on thymocytes, mast cells, and CTL during their development. The vIL-10 homologue displays some of these activities, inhibiting inflammatory cytokine production but showing no effect on B-cell MHC Class II expression.

Suppression of inflammatory reactions may be desirable for numerous clinical conditions, including transplant rejection, autoimmune diseases, and sepsis. As with many of these pleiotropic molecules, however, discrepancies between the *in vitro* effects and *in vivo* actions may exist (Wogenson, 1994). IL-10 can be measured by both bioassay and ELISA.

Interleukin-11

IL-11 (Quesniaux, 1994; Du, 1994; Neben, 1993) is a nonglycosylated protein, produced by fibroblasts and trophoblasts. The IL-11 receptor is a complex of an IL-11 binding protein (IL-11R) and gp130, which transmits the signals. gp130 functions as a signal-transducing protein for other cytokine receptors, including the IL-6R.

IL-11 was originally discovered by its ability to support the IL-6–independent growth of a plasmacytoma cell line. IL-11 is indeed a growth factor that performs activities on both hematopoietic and nonhematopoietic cell types. In combination with other cytokines, most notably IL-3, IL-11 can support the growth of myeloid progenitors and the formation of megakaryocyte colonies. Additional bone marrow stimulatory effects of IL-11 have been reported in mice. Mature immune cells can be targets for IL-11 because it also supports the development of antigen-specific B cells. Outside of the immune system, IL-11 can induce the synthesis of hepatic acute phase proteins and inhibits adipocyte differentiation. The effects of IL-11 on the bone marrow and developing immune cells may have clinical implications. IL-11 can be measured by bioassay.

Interleukin-12

IL-12 (Chehimi, 1994; Wolf, 1994; Trinchieri, 1994) is unique in structure, compared with most other cytokines, because of its two separate glycoproteins (p40 and p35) covalently linked through a disulfide bond to form an active heterodimer. Both precursor polypeptides have signal sequences typical for secreted proteins. Interestingly, the p40 protein shows homologies to several cytokine receptors, whereas the p35 protein has homologies to other cytokines. The expression of p40 and of p35 is independently regulated. That is, monocytes appear to be an abundant source of p40 as well as IL-12 activity, whereas expression of p35 is widespread. Expression of p40 is augmented by IFNγ and suppressed by IL-4 and IL-10. The receptor for IL-12 has not yet been characterized in detail.

As one would expect from the effects of cytokines on its expression, IL-12 has Th1-stimulating activities. IL-12 can induce IFNγ expression and can synergize with IL-2 or TNFα to yield maximal IFNγ production, thus possibly serving an important role in initiating inflammatory immune responses. IL-12 also increases the growth of Th1 but not Th2 cells and, furthering its antagonism of Th2 responses, suppresses IgE production. IL-12 was originally described as an NK cell stimulatory factor and CTL maturation factor and, indeed, enhances both NK and LAK cell activity as well as CTL development. In clinical situations when cellular immunity is depressed, such as human immunodeficiency virus infection and cancer, IL-12 production is also suppressed. In experiments to simulate such situations, the addition of IL-12 *in vitro* measurably enhances cellular immune functions. Studies of rodents have shown many of these same effects of IL-12 *in vivo*, as well as its antineoplastic, antiviral, antiparasitic, and antifungal effects. IL-12 can be measured by bioassay.

Interferon-γ

IFNγ (Samuel, 1991; De Maeyer, 1992; Farrar, 1993; Halloran, 1993) is a processed protein with variable degrees of glycosylation. IFNγ exists as a noncovalently linked head-to-tail dimer. The IFNγ receptor (IFNγR) consists of a single transmembrane glycoprotein whose signal-transducing activity also requires interaction with an additional cellular protein. This receptor is prevalent on a wide variety of immune and nonimmune cells.

IFNγ is expressed only after the activation of T cells and NK cells. Although it is one of the prototype Th1 cytokines, IFNγ is additionally produced by $CD8^+$ and $\gamma\delta$ T cells. Activating agents inducing its expression include specific antigens and the cytokines IL-1, IL-2, and IL-12. IFNγ production can be inhibited by the immune suppressors glucocorticoids and cyclosporin A. The effects of IFNγ are likely mediated within cells by the stimulation of synthesis of numerous IFNγ-induced proteins.

The interferons were originally described for their antiviral activity. In addition, IFNγ has potent immune stimulatory functions and Th1 activities. IFNγ activates macrophages by inducing the expression of Class I and Class II MHC, increasing IL-1 and hydrogen peroxide production, and increasing tumor cell killing. IFNγ also increases the cytotoxicity of NK cells and helps support the development of LAK and CTL. On B cells, IFNγ enhances IgG2a and IgG3 secretion and counteracts the effects of IL-4. IFNγ activates endothelial cells, leading to expression of adhesion molecules.

IFNγ has found utility as a therapeutic agent for chronic granulomatous disease (CGD), in which phagocytic cells are defective in their respiratory burst and cannot generate O_2^- (Bolinger, 1992; Curnutte, 1993). Such individuals suffer from recurrent infections and a poor clinical course. Although this disease is composed of heterogeneous X-linked and autosomal genetic defects, all lead to loss of NADPH oxidase activity. Prophylactic administration of IFNγ leads to a significant decrease in the number of infections suffered in CGD, although phagocyte O_2^- production is unchanged by treatment. IFNγ likely leads to general improvements in host response to infection. IFNγ has also been beneficial in the treatment of rheumatoid arthritis and possibly in the treatment of chronic viral infections. Unfortunately, its use as an antineoplastic agent has not yet shown promise. IFNγ can be measured by both bioassay and ELISA.

Tumor Necrosis Factor

TNF/lymphotoxins (LT) (Ruddle, 1992; Tracey, 1993; Browning, 1993; Tracey, 1994) are at least three related molecules, encoded by linked genes within the Class II region of the MHC complex on chromosome 6. TNFα has both a membrane-bound form and a secreted form, although it lacks a conventional signal peptide, whereas TNFβ (also known as lymphotoxin-α, LTα) is secreted. Other TNF-like membrane-bound molecules have also been identified, including lymphotoxin-β (LTβ), which can tether TNFβ (LTα) to the cell surface to result in a heterodimeric cell surface molecule. Both TNFα and TNFβ are present as trimers in biological fluids. Two transmembrane glycoprotein receptors for TNFα and TNFβ have been identified (Armitage, 1994). One is a

75-kDa receptor molecule, whereas the second receptor is 55-kDa. Although both bind TNFα and TNFβ, they are relatively distinct from one another. Secreted forms of both receptors have been found. A separate receptor, specific for LTβ, has now been identified (Crowe, 1994).

TNFα is produced by a number of cell types, most notably activated macrophages but including neutrophils, lymphocytes, astrocytes, smooth muscle cells, and endothelial cells. TNFβ is produced largely by activated lymphocytes but also by astrocytes, B cells, and NK cells. TNFα production is stimulated by infectious agents, cytokines including IL-1, IL-2, IFNγ, and TNF itself; and production is suppressed by glucocorticoids, cyclosporin A, and cytokines including IL-4, IL-10, and TGFβ. TNFβ expression is induced by antigens, viral infection, and cytokines such as IL-2 and IFNγ, and its synthesis is suppressed by cyclosporin A. TNF receptors are present on virtually every cell type in the body.

The TNFs have a multitude of activities. TNFα was originally described as an inducer of tumor necrosis, whereas TNFβ became known as a lymphocyte factor that killed cells (LT). TNF can be directly cytotoxic to cells and can even inhibit the growth of certain experimental tumors. Additionally, TNF serves as an antiviral agent and is important as an immunostimulant in the response to numerous infections. Expression of MHC and leukocyte adhesion molecules is increased by TNF, as are various cytokines and their receptors. TNF can also directly activate neutrophils. TNF activity is inhibited by the soluble TNFR, which can bind TNF in the plasma and inactivate it. However, at low concentrations, this binding may stabilize TNF and increase its activity; furthermore, release of TNFR from cells can serve to desensitize them owing to loss of receptors.

Although it has antineoplastic activity, TNF has not been useful as a single agent in chemotherapy, despite its potential utility in combination therapies. Because TNFα appears to be the primary mediator in septic shock and sepsis, attempts to inhibit its actions in these conditions are under trial (Pennington, 1993). TNFα and soluble TNFR levels are elevated in conditions of immune activation, such as sepsis, autoimmunity, and inflammatory bowel disease; in the latter, TNFα levels may serve to monitor disease activity. Specific activities and disease associations of the lymphotoxins are just beginning to be investigated. TNF can be measured by bioassay, which measures both TNFα and TNFβ, necessitating the use of neutralizing antibodies, or by specific ELISA. The 75-kDa and the 55-kDa TNFRs can be examined by flow cytometry, and the soluble forms of the receptors can be assessed by ELISA.

Transforming Growth Factor β

TGFβ (Kim, 1994; Lin, 1994; Roberts, 1993; Sporn, 1992) consists of three independent isoforms, TGFβ1, TGFβ2, and TGFβ3, which share 70% to 80% amino acid homology. They are produced from a precursor polypeptide and secreted as a homodimer linked to the precursor remnants, which is known as latency-associated peptide (LAP). After secretion, TGFβ still requires release from LAP to become biologically active. Five different TGFβ receptors have been described, but the best studied are the Types I, II, and III receptors, whose presence as a complex corresponds to induction of biological activity in response to TGFβ. The Type III receptor is a proteoglycan that binds TGFβ and complexes with the Type II receptor, after which the Type I receptor displaces the Type III receptor and signal transduction occurs.

A great many cells produce TGFβ1 (highest levels are found in bone and platelets) and TGFβ2 (highest levels are found in bone), whereas TGFβ3 is made just by cells of mesenchymal origin. The Types I, II, III, and V receptors are also found on a wide variety of cell types, whereas the Type IV receptor is present only in pituitary cells. Regulation of TGFβ activity is complex, involving both intracellular (transcriptional and translational) and extracellular (postsecretory activation) control.

TGFβ was discovered by its ability to transform the phenotype of growth characteristics of normal fibroblasts. The effects of TGFβ are broad, and both stimulatory and inhibitory effects on cells can be identified, often depending on conditions such as differentiation state of the cells and the presence of other cytokines. TGFβ is potent in stimulating formation of the extracellular matrix and inhibits its degradation; TGFβ also stimulates fibroblast proliferation. TGFβ has a role in bone remodeling, because it stimulates osteoblasts and inhibits osteoclasts. In the immune system, TGFβ is largely thought of as inhibitory. Proliferation of both T and B cells is inhibited by TGFβ, and it inhibits the killing activity of NK cells, the respiratory burst of macrophages, and the secretion of IgM and IgG by B cells. However, stimulatory effects of TGFβ also occur, including the enhancement of B-cell IgA secretion, chemotaxis of monocytes and neutrophils, and stimulation of effector functions by antigen-specific $CD4^+$ T cells.

Given its effects on the extracellular matrix, fibroblasts, and osteoblasts, possible roles for TGFβ administration in wound healing and bone repair are being investigated. Additional uses under study are as an immune suppressive agent for autoimmunity and transplant rejection. TGFβ is currently measured by bioassay, which measures all forms of activated TGFβ; a specific ELISA is available for TGFβ1.

CELL ADHESION MOLECULES

General Principles

The regulation of cellular adhesion is crucial to the functions of many organs and systems throughout the body, including the immune system. Specific molecular interactions govern cell adhesion, and the regulation of these molecules' expression helps control physiologic processes. In the immune system, leukocytes are recruited to both organized lymphoid tissues and sites of inflammation. It is necessary for these cells to be captured along the endothelium, to become activated for increased expression of the adhesion molecules, to migrate through the endothelial lining, and to extravasate into tissue. The cell adhesion molecules involved in promotion of such leukocyte trafficking belong to three general classes: the selectins, the integrins, and the integrin ligands. A fourth class consists of molecules produced from the *CD44* gene. Several reviews provide an in-depth insight into the structure and functions of these molecules (Springer, 1994; Picker, 1994; Albelda, 1994; Lesley, 1993; Bevilacqua, 1993), and the properties of the four classes of adhesion molecules are later reviewed briefly.

When present on the surfaces of circulating cells, these molecules can be measured by flow cytometry by using specific labeled monoclonal antibodies. After being shed from the cell surface, some of the molecules, particularly the integrin ligands, assume a soluble form and can be assessed by ELISA. Tissue expression of cell adhesion molecules can be identified by immunocytochemical techniques, and as with the cytokines, the presence of mRNA for the molecules may be assessed by RT-PCR or *in situ* hybridization. Currently, other than when used to determine identity of cell types as cell lineage markers for normal and malignant cells, measurements of the cell adhesion molecules is largely in the research realm. Because of their importance in inflammatory interactions, the possibility of therapeutic intervention to inhibit their effects, and the presence of soluble forms in biological fluids, the measurement of cell adhesion molecules will likely become a part of diagnostic techniques.

Selectins

The selectins are involved in the initial adhesion event of white blood cells to the endothelium, in which leukocytes roll along the endothelium. Selectins all are carbohydrate-binding proteins (Table 37–2) *ELAM-1* (endothelial leukocyte adhesion molecule-1, E-selectin, CD62E) is expressed predominantly on postcapillary venule endothelial cells shortly after stimulation by inflammatory mediators including bacterial endotoxin or the cytokines IL-1 or TNF. This early increase in expression is achieved by transfer of internal stores of ELAM-1 to the cellular surface. Such expression augments the adhesion of neutrophils, monocytes, and a subpopulation of memory T lymphocytes. The cellular ligand for ELAM-1 is sialyl-Lewis^X and likely other carbohydrates. LECAM-1 (leukocyte-endothelial cell adhesion molecule-1, L-selectin, CD62L) is expressed on lymphocytes, neutrophils, and monocytes. This selectin is recognized by carbohydrate ligands expressed on peripheral lymph node high endothelial venules. Its ligands include CD34 and MAdCAM-1 (discussed later). LECAM-1 also mediates the adherence of lymphocytes to white matter of the brain. PADGEM (platelet activation-dependent granule to external membrane protein, P-selectin, CD62P) is located in the secretory granules of platelets and Weibel-Palade bodies of endothelial cells. Soluble mediators of inflammation and hemostasis, such as histamine and thrombin, induce transfer of PADGEM to the cell surface. Neutrophils and monocytes express the PADGEM ligands, which include sialyl-Lewis^X and sulfatides, allowing the adherence of these cells to platelets and endothelial cells.

The selectins all have soluble forms (Gearing, 1993). Levels of sELAM-1 are increased in diabetes, vasculitides, and sepsis; in the latter, such levels show correlation with mortality. Amounts of sLECAM-1 were elevated during sepsis and human immunodeficiency virus infection, whereas increased sPADGEM was found in hemolytic-uremic syndrome and thrombotic thrombocytopenic purpura.

Table 37–2. CELL ADHESION MOLECULES

Selectin*	Selectin Ligand
ELAM-1 (CD62E)	sialyl-Lewis^X, other carbohydrates
LECAM-1 (CD62L)	MdCAM-1, CD34, other carbohydrates
PADGEM (CD62P)	sialyl-Lewis^X, sulfatides

Integrin†			Integrin Ligands (Ig Superfamily and Extracellular Matrix)
β Subunit	*α Subunit*	*Name*	
β_1 (CD29)	α_4 (CD49d)	VLA-4	VCAM-1 (CD106); fibronectin
β_2 (CD18)	α_L (CD11a)	LFA-1	ICAM-1 (CD54), ICAM-2 (CD102), ICAM-3 (CD50)
	α_M (CD11b)	Mac-1	ICAM-1 (CD54), ICAM-3 (CD102), iC3b; fibrinogen
	α_X (CD11c)	p150,95	iC3b; fibrinogen
β_7	α_4 (CD49d)		VCAM-1 (CD106); MAdCAM-1; fibronectin

Soluble Forms of Adhesion Molecules‡

CD44
ELAM-1 (CD62E)
ICAM-1 (CD54)
ICAM-3 (CD50)
LECAM-1 (CD62L)
PADGEM (CD62P)
PECAM (CD31)
VCAM-1 (CD106)

*Known selectins and representative ligands.
†Examples of some of the integrins, with their immunoglobulin (Ig) superfamily and extracellular matrix ligands.
‡Molecules in which soluble forms have been detected.

Integrins

The integrins comprise a large family of heterodimeric molecules and, along with their ligands, are involved in the tight adhesion of leukocytes to the endothelium and their transmigration. At least 14 different α-subunits and 8 β-subunits can combine in various fashions to form no fewer than 20 $\alpha\beta$ heterodimers. Cell activation can induce transfer of internal stores of integrins to the cell surface as well as induce a conformational change in the integrin to increase its affinity for ligand. This activation then allows the leukocyte integrin to bind to its receptor on endothelial cells, stopping the movement of the cell and allowing it to begin migrating through the endothelial lining. Among the commonly examined integrins are those using the β_2-chain subunit (CD18) (see Table 37–2). This β-chain can complex to the α_L (CD11a), α_M, (CD11b), and α_X (CD11c) subunits of the α-chain to form the LFA-1 (expressed on all leukocytes), Mac-1 (expressed on monocytes, macrophages, granulocytes, neutrophils, some NK cells, and activated lymphocytes), and p150,95 (expressed on a subset of B cells, granulocytes, monocytes, and macrophages) integrins, respectively. Similarly, the β_1-chain subunit (CD29) can combine with the α_1 to α_6 subunits (CD49a to CD49f) of the α-chain to form very late antigens (VLA) VLA-1-VLA-6. Additionally, the β_1-subunit can also form complexes with the α_7-, α_8-, and α_v-(CD51) subunits. The β_3-subunit (CD61) associates with the α_{IIb}-subunit (CD41) to form GPIIb/IIIa (CD61) or the α_V (CD51)-subunit to form the vitronectin receptor. Additional subunit chains include β_4 (CD104), β_5 to β_8, and α_{IEL}.

Because these molecules are normally present on the surfaces of cells, their expression can be used to identify specific cells and to determine their state of activation. LAD, a disorder of leukocyte adhesion and chemotaxis, has been found to be caused by defective expression of the β_2-subunit

5

(CD18), thus leading to defective LFA-1, Mac-1, and p150,95 expression (Anderson, 1987). In these patients, not only is leukocyte adhesion and migration abnormal, but because Mac-1 and p150,95 serve as receptors for the opsonic complement fragment iC3b, phagocytosis of opsonized microorganisms is defective, leading to numerous bacterial infections. The defect in integrin expression in unstimulated and stimulated neutrophils can be detected by flow cytometry using anti-CD11b or anti-CD18 antibodies; furthermore, LAD carriers can also be detected, expressing 50% of normal levels (Anderson, 1985).

Integrin Ligands

The ligands for the integrins can be divided into two groups. First are the glycoproteins with homology to immunoglobulins, belonging to the immunoglobulin superfamily of molecules. ICAM-1 (intercellular adhesion molecule-1, CD54) and ICAM-3 (CD50) bind LFA-1 and Mac-1, whereas ICAM-2 (CD102) binds only LFA-1. ICAM-1 expression is inducible by inflammatory cytokines such as IFNγ, IL-1, and TNF. Although expressed by several cell types, ICAM-1 on activated endothelium serves to bind monocytes, lymphocytes, and neutrophils during inflammation. The ICAM-1 molecule is also used by pathogens: both rhinoviruses and *Plasmodium falciparum*–infected erythrocytes use it as a receptor, facilitating their entry into cells and across the endothelium, respectively (Greve, 1989; Staunton, 1989; Berendt, 1992; Ockenhouse, 1992). ICAM-2 and ICAM-3 are expressed on monocytes and other immune cells. Additionally, ICAM-2 is expressed constitutively on endothelial cells, whereas ICAM-3 is expressed on endothelial cells only during disease states, and both likely have regulatory roles in lymphocyte interactions. VCAM-1 (vascular cell adhesion molecule-1, CD106) binds VLA-4 and the $\alpha_4\beta_7$ integrin. VCAM-1 is also up-regulated by inflammatory cytokines and is expressed by endothelial cells, macrophages, and other cell types in the body. VCAM-1–mediated interactions also promote the adhesion of lymphocytes and monocytes to activated endothelium. PECAM-1 (platelet endothelial cell adhesion molecule-1, CD31) is present constitutively on endothelium as well as platelets, neutrophils, monocytes, and T cells and shows homophilic binding to other PECAM-1 molecules, facilitating the migration of white blood cells across the endothelial lining. MAdCAM-1 (mucosal addressin cell adhesion molecule-1) binds the $\alpha_4\beta_7$ integrin in addition to LECAM-1 selectin. Expressed by high endothelial venules of mucosal lymphoid tissue, MAdCAM-1 mediates homing of lymphocytes to these locations.

The second group of integrin ligands consists of extracellular matrix proteins, such as collagen (binding VLA-1-3) and fibronectin (binding VLA-3-5, Mac-1, p150,95, GPIIb/IIIa, vitronectin receptor, $\beta_5\alpha_V$, $\beta_6\alpha_V$, and $\beta_7\alpha_4$). Other extracellular matrix proteins, such as laminin, fibrinogen, vitronectin, von Willebrand factor, and thrombospondin, also serve as ligands for the different integrins. Finally, as indicated earlier, iC3b is a ligand for both Mac-1 and p150,95. Individual integrins may bind both members of the immunoglobulin superfamily and extracellular matrix proteins as ligands (see Table 37–2).

Soluble forms of ICAM-1, ICAM-3, VCAM-1, and PECAM-1 have been detected in the serum (Gearing, 1993). Elevated levels of sICAM-1 are found in malignancy, autoimmune disease, graft rejection, and infection. sVCAM-1 appears elevated under similar conditions, whereas studies of sPECAM-1 are not as complete. Although the potential future clinical use of measurements of these soluble ligands is unclear, correlations with episodes of graft rejection and disease activity in lupus have been reported.

CD44

In addition to the foregoing families, CD44 also functions as an adhesion molecule in the immune system. The *CD44* gene contains variant exons and, by alternate splicing using different numbers of these exons, generates numerous isoforms. CD44, which is constitutively expressed on lymphocytes, monocytes, neutrophils, and some nonimmune cells, binds hyaluronic acid. CD44 functions in both cell-cell and cell-extracellular matrix adhesion, including lymphocyte homing to mucosal-associated lymphoid tissue. Interestingly, distinctive isoforms of CD44 can be expressed in malignant epithelial tissue, and these may play a part in tumor metastasis (Gunthert, 1993; Herrlich, 1993).

PERSPECTIVES

The unraveling of the intracellular communications in the immune system will not only lead to a better understanding of how the immune system functions but will provide insight into many human diseases. Currently, the clinical applications of measurements of cytokines, their receptors, and the cell adhesion molecules are few. However, it is likely that given the association of disease states with expression of certain molecules and the numerous trials of administrations of these molecules or agents to inhibit their production or effects, the assessment of expression and production of these molecules will continue to expand in the diagnostic realm.

Akira S, Taga T, Kishimoto T: Interleukin-6 in biology and medicine. Adv Immunol 1993; 54:1–78.
Albelda SM, Smith CW, Ward PA: Adhesion molecules and inflammatory injury. J 1994; 8:504–512.
Anderson DC, Schmalsteig FC, Finegold MJ, et al: The severe and moderate phenotypes of heritable Mac-1, LFA-1 deficiency: Their quantitative definition and relation to leukocyte dysfunction and clinical features. J Infect Dis 1985; 152:668–689.
Anderson DC, Springer TA: Leukocyte adhesion deficiency: An inherited defect in the Mac-1, LFA-1, and p150,95 glycoproteins. Annu Rev Med 1987; 38:175–194.
Arend WP: Interleukin-1 receptor antagonist. Adv Immunol 1993; 54:167–227.
Armitage RJ: Tumor necrosis factor receptor superfamily members and their ligands. Curr Opin Immunol 1994; 6:407–413.
Baggiolini M, Dewald B, Moser B: Interleukin-8 and related chemotactic cytokines—CXC and CC chemokines. Adv Immunol 1994; 55:97–179.
Berendt AR, McDowall A, Craig AG, et al: The binding site on ICAM-1 for *Plasmodium falciparum*-infected erythrocytes overlaps, but is distinct from, the LFA-1- binding site. Cell 1992; 68:71–81.
Bevilacqua MP: Endothelial-leukocyte adhesion molecules. Annu Rev Immunol 1993; 11:767–804.
Bickel M: The role of interleukin-8 in inflammation and mechanisms of regulation. J Periodontol 1993; 64:456–460.
Bolinger AM, Taeubel MA: Recombinant interferon gamma for treatment of chronic granulomatous disease and other disorders. Clin Pharm 1992; 11:834–850.
Bottomly K: A functional dichotomy in CD4+ T lymphocytes. Immunol Today 1988; 9:268–273.
Browning JL, Ngam-ek A, Lawton P, et al: Lymphotoxin beta, a novel

member of the TNF family that forms a heteromeric complex with lymphotoxin on the cell surface. Cell 1993; 72:847–856.
Chehimi J, Trinchieri G: Interleukin-12: A bridge between innate resistance and adaptive immunity with a role in infection and acquired immunodeficiency. J Clin Immunol 1994; 14:149–161.
Coligan JE, Kruisbeek AM, Margulies DH, et al (eds): Current Protocols in Immunology. New York, John Wiley and Sons, 1994.
Costello R, Imbert J, Olive D: Interleukin-7, a major T-lymphocyte cytokine. Eur Cytokine Netw 1993; 4:253–262.
Crowe PD, VanArsdale TL, Walter BN, et al: A lymphotoxin-beta-specific receptor. Science 1994; 264:707–710.
Curnutte JT: Conventional versus interferon-gamma therapy in chronic granulomatous disease. J Infect Dis 1993; 167:8–12.
De Maeyer E, De Maeyer-Guignard J: Interferon-gamma. Curr Opin Immunol 1992; 4:321–326.
Dinarello CA: Modalities for reducing interleukin 1 activity in disease. Immunol Today 1993b; 14:260–264.
Dinarello CA: The interleukin-1 family: 10 years of discovery. FASEB J 1994; 8:1314–1325.
Dinarello CA, Wolff SM: The role of interleukin-1 in disease. N Engl J Med 1993a; 328:106–113.
Du XX, Williams DA. Interleukin-11: A multifunctional growth factor derived from the hematopoietic microenvironment. Blood 1994; 83: 2023–2030.
Farrar MA, Schrieber RD: The molecular cell biology of interferon-gamma and its receptor. Annu Rev Immunol 1993; 11:571–611.
Foss HD, Hummel M, Gottstein S, et al: Frequent expression of IL-7 gene transcripts in tumor cells of classical Hodgkin's disease. Am J Pathol 1995; 146:33–39.
Frendl G: Interleukin 3: From colony-stimulating factor to pluripotent immunoregulatory cytokine. Int J Immunopharmacol 1992; 14:421–430.
Ganser A: Clinical results with recombinant human interleukin-3. Cancer Invest 1993; 11:212–218.
Gearing AJ, Newman W: Circulating adhesion molecules in disease. Immunol Today 1993; 14:506–512.
Gillio AP, Faulkner LB, Alter BP, et al: Treatment of Diamond-Blackfan anemia with recombinant human interleukin-3. Blood 1993; 82: 744–751.
Girasole G, Jilka RL, Passeri G, et al: 17 beta-estradiol inhibits interleukin-6 production by bone marrow-derived stromal cells and osteoblasts in vitro: A potential mechanism for the antiosteoporotic effect of estrogens. J Clin Invest 1992; 89:883–891.
Greve JM, Davis G, Meyer AM, et al: The major human rhinovirus receptor is ICAM-1. Cell 1989; 56:839–847.
Gunthert U: CD44: A multitude of isoforms with diverse functions. Curr Top Microbiol Immunol 1993; 184:47–63.
Halloran PF: Interferon-gamma, prototype of the proinflammatory cytokines—importance in activation, suppression, and maintenance of the immune response. Transplant Proc 1993; 25:10–15.
Harada A, Sekido N, Akahoshi T, et al: Essential involvement of interleukin-8 (IL-8) in acute inflammation. J Leukocyte Biol 1994; 56:559–564.
Hebert CA, Baker JB: Interleukin-8: A review. Cancer Invest 1993; 11:743–750.
Herrlich P, Zoller M, Pals ST, Ponta H: CD44 splice variants: Metastases meet lymphocytes. Immunol Today 1993; 14:395–399.
Honda M, Yamamoto S, Cheng M, et al: Human soluble IL-6 receptor: Its detection and enhanced release by HIV infection. J Immunol 1992; 148: 2175–2180.
Howard M, O'Garra A, Ishida H, et al: Biological properties of interleukin 10. J Clin Immunol 1992; 12:239–247.
Ihle NJ: Interleukin-3 and hematopoiesis. Chem Immunol 1992; 51:65–106.
Janssen RA, Mulder NH, The TH, de Leij L: The immunobiological effects of interleukin-2 *in vivo*. Cancer Immunol Immunother 1994; 39:207–216.
Kemeny L, Ruzicka T, Dobozy A, Michel G: Role of interleukin-8 receptor in skin. Int Arch Allergy Immunol 1994; 104:317–322.
Kikuchi Y, Migita M, Takaki S, et al: Biochemical and functional characterization of soluble form of IL-5 receptor alpha (sIL-5R alpha): Development of ELISA system for detection of sIL-5R alpha. J Immunol Methods 1994; 167:289–298.
Kim SJ, Romeo D, Yoo YD, Park K: Transforming growth factor-beta: Expression in normal and pathological conditions. Horm Res 1994; 42:5–8.
Kishimoto T, Akira S, Taga T: Interleukin-6 and its receptor: A paradigm for cytokines. Science 1992; 258:593–597.
Kunisada T, Ogawa M, Hayashi S, et al: Interleukin-7 and B lymphopoiesis. Chem Immunol 1992; 51:205–235.
Kunkel SL, Lukacs NW, Strieter RM: The role of interleukin-8 in the infectious process. Ann N Y Acad Sci 1994; 730:134–143.
Leonard WJ, Noguchi M, Russell SM, McBride OW: The molecular basis of X-linked severe combined immunodeficiency: The role of the interleukin-2 receptor gamma chain as a common gamma chain, gamma c. Immunol Rev 1994; 138:61–86.
Lesley J, Hyman R, Kincade PW: CD44 and its interaction with extracellular matrix. Adv Immunol 1993; 54:271–335.
Lin HY, Moustakas A: TGF-beta receptors: Structure and function. Cell Mol Biol 1994; 40:337–349.
Lindemann A, Mertelsmann R: Interleukin-3: Structure and function. Cancer Invest 1993; 11:609–623.
Lotz M: Interleukin-6. Cancer Invest 1993; 11:732–742.
Mahanty S, Nutman TB: The biology of interleukin-5 and its receptor. Cancer Invest 1993; 11:624–634.
Miller MD, Krangel MS: Biology and biochemistry of the chemokines: A family of chemotactic and inflammatory cytokines. CRC Crit Rev Immunol 1992; 12:17–46.
Miyajima A, Mui AL, Ogorochi T, Sakamaki K: Receptors for granulocyte-macrophage colony-stimulating factor, interleukin-3, and interleukin-5. Blood 1993; 82:1960–1974.
Moore KW, O'Garra A, de Waal Malefyt R, et al: Interleukin-10. Annu Rev Immunol 1993; 11:165–190.
Mosmann TR: Properties and functions of interleukin-10. Adv Immunol 1994; 56:1–26.
Neben S, Turner K: The biology of interleukin 11. Stem Cells 1993; 2:156–162.
Ockenhouse CF, Betageri R, Springer TA, Staunton DE: *Plasmodium falciparum*-infected erythrocytes bind ICAM-1 at a site distinct from LFA-1, Mac-1, and human rhinovirus. Cell 1992; 68:63–69.
Oldham RK: Therapy with interleukin-2 and tumor-derived activated lymphocytes. Immunol Ser 1994; 61:251–271.
Owen WF Jr, Petersen J, Sheff DM, et al: Hypodense eosinophils and interleukin 5 activity in the blood of patients with the eosinophilia-myalgia syndrome. Proc Nat Acad Sci U S A 1990; 87:8647–8651.
Paul WE: Interleukin-4: A prototypic immunoregulatory lymphokine. Blood 1991; 77:1859–1870.
Pennington JE: Therapy with antibody to tumor necrosis factor in sepsis. Clin Infect Dis 1993; 17:515–519.
Picker LJ: Control of lymphocyte homing. Curr Opin Immunol 1994; 6:394–406.
Quesniaux VF: Interleukins 9, 10, 11 and 12 and kit ligand: A brief overview. Res Immunol 1992; 143:385–400.
Quesniaux VF: Interleukin 11. Leuk Lymphoma 1994; 14:241–249.
Renauld JC, Houssiau F, Louahed J, Vink A, Van Snick J, Uyttenhove C: Interleukin-9. Adv Immunol 1993; 54:79–97.
Roberts AB, Sporn MD: Physiological actions and clinical applications of transforming growth factor-beta (TGF-beta). Growth Factors 1993; 8:1–9.
Ruddle NH: Tumor necrosis factor (TNF-alpha) and lymphotoxin (TNF-beta). Curr Opin Immunol 1992; 4:327–332.
Samuel CE: Antiviral actions of interferon: Interferon-regulated cellular proteins and their surprisingly selective antiviral activities. Virology 1991; 183:1–11.
Sanderson CJ: Interleukin-5, eosinophils, and disease. Blood 1992; 79:3101–3109.
Smith KA: Interleukin-2. Curr Opin Immunol 1992; 4:271–276.
Sonoda Y: Interleukin-4—A dual regulatory factor in hematopoiesis. Leuk Lymphoma 1994; 14:231–240.
Sporn MB, Roberts AB: Transforming growth factor-beta: Recent progress and new challenges. J Cell Biol 1992; 119:1017–1021.
Springer TA: Traffic signals for lymphocyte recirculation and leukocyte emigration: The multistep paradigm. Cell 1994; 76:301–314.
Staunton DE, Merluzzi VJ, Rothlein R, et al: A cell adhesion molecule, ICAM-1, is the major surface receptor for rhinoviruses. Cell 1989; 56:849–853.
Steel C, Nutman TB: Regulation of IL-5 in onchocerciasis. A critical role for IL-2. J Immunol 1993; 150:5511–5518.
Takatsu K: Interleukin-5. Curr Opin Immunol 1992; 4:299–306.
Tracey KJ, Cerami A: Tumor necrosis factor, other cytokines and disease. Annu Rev Cell Biol 1993; 9:317–343.
Tracey KJ, Cerami A: Tumor necrosis factor: A pleiotropic cytokine and therapeutic target. Annu Rev Med 1994; 45:491–503.
Trinchieri G, Scott P: The role of interleukin 12 in the immune response, disease and therapy. Immunol Today 1994; 15:460–463.
Vellenga E, Dokter W, Halie RM: Interleukin-4 and its receptor, modulating effects on immature and mature hematopoietic cells. Leukemia 1993; 7:1131–1141.
Vlasveld LT, Rankin EM: Recombinant interleukin-2 in cancer: Basic and clinical aspects. Cancer Treat Rev 1994; 20:275–311.
Voss SD, Hong R, Sondel PM: Severe combined immunodeficiency, interleukin-2 (IL-2), and the IL-2 receptor: Experiments of nature continue to point the way. Blood 1994; 83:626–635.
Wogensen L, Lee MS, Sarvetnick N: Production of interleukin 10 by islet cells accelerates immune-mediated destruction of beta cells in nonobese diabetic mice. J Exp Med 1994; 179:1379–1384.
Wolf SF, Sieburth D, Sypek J: Interleukin 12: A key modulator of immune function. Stem Cells 1994; 12:154–168.
Yang YC: Human interleukin-9: A new cytokine in hematopoiesis. Leuk Lymphoma 1992; 8:441–447.

Chapter 38

Human Leukocyte Antigen (HLA): The Major Histocompatibility Complex of Humans and Transplantation Immunology

Armead H. Johnson, Ph.D.
Carolyn Katovich Hurley, Ph.D.
Robert J. Hartzman, CAPT, MC, USN, M.D.

Survival depends on the immune system's ability to recognize a multitude of foreign substances (antigens) and to respond to them. Although this defense mechanism is basic to survival in a hostile world of microorganisms, this same defense system becomes a major obstacle when attempting to transplant tissues from one individual to another or when malfunction of immune recognition triggers autoaggressive reactions. The major histocompatibility complex (MHC) genes encode proteins that are essential to this immune recognition: Class I and Class II molecules. The human Class I molecules include HLA-A, HLA-B, and HLA-C, and the Class II molecules include HLA-DR, HLA-DQ, and HLA-DP. Other molecules encoded in the MHC (covered in Chapter 39) include the MHC-linked complement components (C2, C4, and BF), 21-hydroxylase (CYP21), heat shock protein 70 (Hsp70), and tumor necrosis factor (TNF) (Fig. 38–1).

In an infection, the invading microorganism infects cells or is engulfed by immune cells such as monocytes. Inside the cell, MHC Class I or Class II molecules act as receptors for antigenic fragments of these microorganisms (Fig. 38–2). Once antigenic fragments have bound to the MHC molecules and have been translocated to the cell surface, receptors on T lymphocytes interact with the antigen-MHC complex, trig-

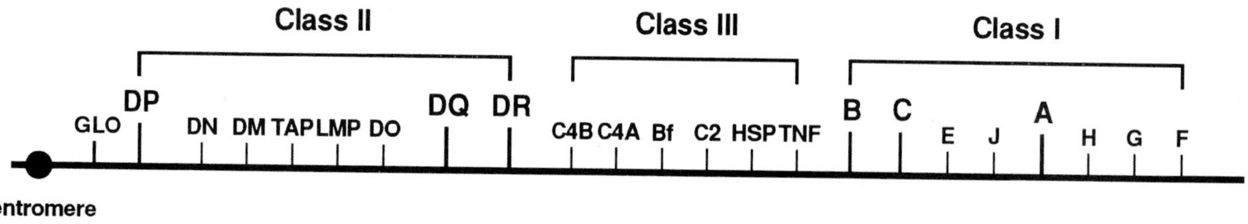

Figure 38–1. Map of the MHC gene complex on chromosome 6. (Adapted from Campbell RD, Trowsdale J: Map of the human MHC. Today 1993; 14:349–352.)

gering both humoral and cellular immune responses. T cell–specific cell surface molecules, CD8 and CD4, act to strengthen this cellular interaction and to transmit activation signals. Other cell adhesion molecules such as CD2 and its ligand, LFA3, or LFA1 and its ligand, ICAM1, also act to increase the affinity of cellular interactions (see Chapter 37). The same pattern of interactions between a cell bearing an antigen-MHC complex and a T lymphocyte occurs not only in the recognition of infecting microorganisms but also in the recognition of foreign histocompatibility molecules (alloantigens) found on an allograft and in the recognition of self-antigens (autoantigens) during an autoimmune disease.

The impact of studies of the human MHC on clinical medicine was first felt in tissue transplantation, the area that gave the major histocompatibility complex its name. Because foreign MHC molecules are recognized as antigens by the graft recipient, it is beneficial to ensure that donor and recipient share HLA alleles. Since the MHC is extremely polymorphic, this is often a difficult task and requires close collaboration among the surgeon, the clinical HLA typing laboratory, and large organ-sharing networks. More recently, studies of the MHC have been important in understanding many autoimmune diseases that have immunologic imbalances or disturbances of immune regulation with an MHC-associated genetic component. Although the etiology of these diseases is not yet understood, intervention and therapy will depend on an understanding of immune recognition, the mechanisms of control of the normal immune response, and the relationship between particular MHC alleles and the propensity for the autoimmune disease.

The genetics, nomenclature, and techniques of detection, structure, and function of the human MHC gene products, HLA-A, -B, and -C (Class I) and HLA-DR, -DQ, and -DP (Class II) are discussed in this chapter. Also discussed is the importance of HLA matching for transplantation.

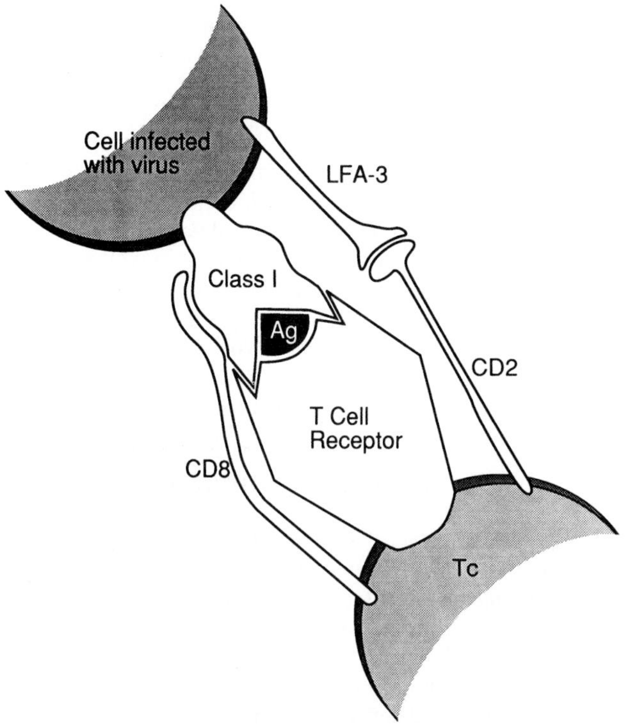

Figure 38–2. Model of the molecular interactions involved in antigen recognition.

GENETICS OF THE MAJOR HISTOCOMPATIBILITY COMPLEX

Basic Genetics

Mendel's first law, the law of segregation, is based on the principle that hereditary characteristics are determined by factors that are distributed to progeny. In any one individual, these factors, or genes as they are now called, are present in pairs. During meiosis, the genes segregate randomly during formation of the gametes (ova or sperm) so that one of each pair, or a haploid number of chromosomes, is transmitted by any given gamete. The double, or diploid number of chromosomes, is restored when the male and female gametes fuse to form the zygote. Thus, for a trait determined by one gene with multiple forms (alleles), there will always be four possible genetic combinations in the offspring, each with equal probability of occurrence. These laws of segregation and random assortment apply to the genes of the MHC system. Definitions are given below for genetic terms that are used in this chapter (Crow, 1976).

Gene The unit factor of inheritance.
Locus The position of a gene on a chromosome.
Allele An alternative form of a gene expressed at a single locus.
Homozygous Having identical alleles at a locus.
Heterozygous Having different alleles at a locus.
Codominance The state in which each allele at a locus expresses its characteristic effect equally in the heterozygote.
Genotype The genetic constitution of an organism or individual.

Phenotype The observable characteristics produced by the genes.
Polymorphic Having two or more common distinct genotypes maintained in a population.
Homologous chromosomes The two members of a chromosome pair that have corresponding gene loci, one derived from each parent.
Crossing over The exchange of segments between homologous chromosomes.
Recombination Reassortment of genes so that the gamete contains genes of both paternal and maternal origin. When the genes are linked (located on the same chromosomes), this is accomplished by crossing over.
Allo-(antigen, graft) Refers to antigenic differences between individuals of a single species.

Composition of the MHC

The major histocompatibility gene complex in humans is located on the short arm of chromosome 6. It spans over 3500 kilobases, an area that contains enough genetic material to encode numerous proteins (Campbell and Trowsdale, 1993). The HLA (*H*uman *L*eukocyte *A*ntigen) genes of the MHC are encoded by six subregions: *HLA-A*, *HLA-B*, *HLA-C*, *HLA-DR*, *HLA-DQ*, and *HLA-DP* (see Fig. 38–1). Each subregion encodes a minimum of one cell surface glycoprotein. The HLA genes are highly polymorphic—that is, each of the HLA genes has multiple alleles in the population. Indeed, the HLA genes are the most polymorphic loci yet known in humans. Such polymorphism is thought to be maintained because the HLA molecules encoded by these genes are used by the cells of the immune system to discriminate between self and nonself (i.e., invading microorganisms); thus, the polymorphism is believed to be essential to the survival of the species.

Localization of MHC Genes

The genes of the MHC were assigned to chromosome 6 on the basis of cytogenetic studies of aberrant chromosomes. The map order of the MHC genes was determined by meiotic linkage analyses (studies of crossing over in families) and molecular biology techniques, including gene cloning and pulsed field gel electrophoresis. The latter technique detects the presence of genes on single long fragments of DNA. The map order of genes within the MHC is *HLA-A*, *-C*, *-B*, *-DR*, *-DQ*, *-DP*, with *HLA-A* being distal to the centromere (see Fig. 38–1). The *GLO1* locus, which codes for an enzyme in erythrocytes that catalyzes the conversion of methylglyoxal and glutathione to S-lactyl-glutathione, marks the centromeric boundary of the MHC.

Inheritance

The MHC genes are closely linked—that is, they segregate *en bloc* to the offspring. The complex of linked genes that resides on one of the pair of homologous chromosomes and that segregates *en bloc* to the offspring is called a haplotype. Each individual inherits two MHC haplotypes—one from each parent—and thus has two alleles for each of the

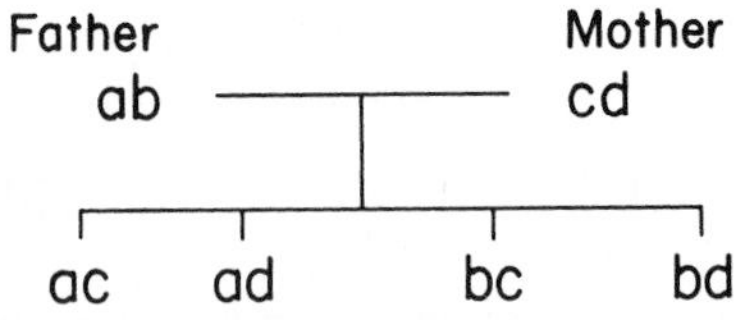

Figure 38–3. Segregation of alleles at a single locus.

genes. These genes are codominantly expressed. The inheritance of the MHC genes follows the rules of segregation set down by Mendel. Within a family, each child inherits one MHC haplotype from the mother and one from the father. By convention, the paternal haplotypes are generally designated a and b and the maternal haplotypes c and d. Thus, there are four possible MHC genotypes in the offspring: ac, ad, bc, and bd. Because the chances of inheriting a given genotype are random, the probability of occurrence of any one of the four genotypes is one in four. In a family with five children, at least two of the children will be HLA identical (assuming no crossing over). An example of a mating and its four possible genotypes is given in Figure 38–3. Although the MHC genes are closely linked, a number of families have been reported in which a cross-over has occurred (Fig. 38–4). The frequency of crossing over between two linked genes is controlled by the distance separating those genes and other characteristics of the intervening DNA that can increase or decrease the likelihood of recombination during meiosis.

Linkage Disequilibrium

The tendency for certain alleles at two different genes to occur in the population significantly more frequently in the same haplotype than would be expected on the basis of chance alone is called linkage disequilibrium. The expected frequency of two allelic forms at two genes to occur together is the product of the gene frequency of each allele in that population ([$f_{expected} = f1 \times f2$). The observed frequency is determined from family studies within the same population. Linkage disequilibrium is a hallmark of the human MHC and extends from *HLA-A* through *HLA-DQ*. The best known example of linkage disequilibrium is the A1,Cw7,B8,DR17(3),DR52,DQ2 haplotype in whites, which occurs approximately four times more frequently than would be expected by chance. DP1 is also associated with this haplotype but with a lower frequency. The significance of linkage disequilibrium as it applies to immune competence and disease is discussed in a later chapter (see Chap. 39).

Ethnic Variations

Characterization of HLA alleles in the human population groups of the world was undertaken systematically between June 1970 and June 1972 as the purpose of the 1972 International Histocompatibilty Workshop (Dausset, 1973). The accumulated data from the 80 population groups investigated and from many subsequent studies (Aizawa, 1986; Imanishi, 1992) have provided several conclusions: (1) frequencies of HLA alleles differ significantly among ethnic subpopulations; (2) some HLA alleles are either confined to or found at a much greater frequency in one ethnic subpopulation com-

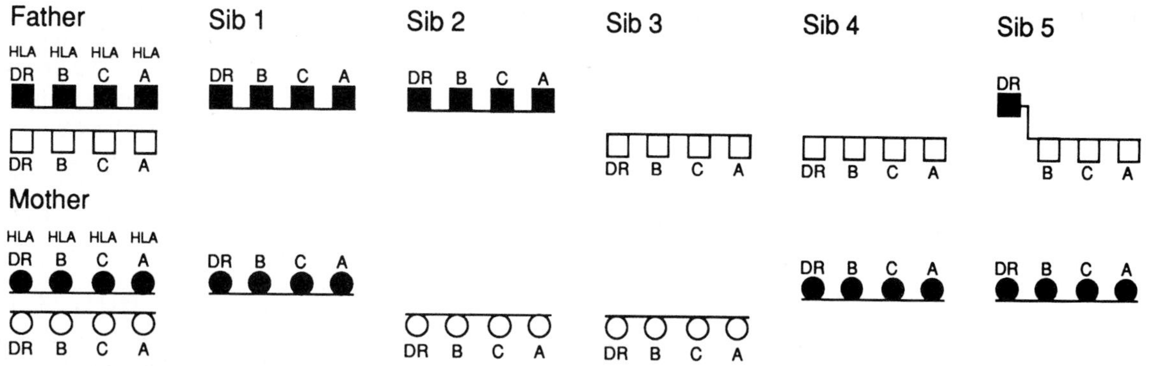

Figure 38–4. HLA haplotype segregation within a family. Sibling 5 is a recombinant between the paternal *HLA-B* and *HLA-DR* loci. This means that sibling 5 is *HLA-A*, *HLA-B*, and *HLA-C* identical to sibling 4, but differs at the *DR* locus from sibling 4.

pared with another; and (3) haplotypes and linkage disequilibrium differ among subpopulations. Thus, these facts must be taken into account when developing unrelated allograft donor banks such as the National Marrow Donor Program (Perkins, 1994). Both the allele frequencies and haplotype make-up dictate the number of donors from a given ethnic group required to provide equal opportunity of finding an HLA-matched unrelated donor from that group. In addition, for HLA and disease studies, both the ethnic backgrounds of the test group and the control group must be carefully evaluated and matched.

HLA-A, -B, -C SUBREGIONS—CLASS I MOLECULES

The HLA-A and -B molecules were the first MHC molecules to be described in humans (Dausset, 1992; van Rood, 1993). Because these molecules were defined by antibody responses, they were called HLA "antigens." Anti-leukocyte antibodies in man were observed as early as the 1920s, but it was not until the 1950s that a systematic study began. Jean Dausset was the first in 1952 to convincingly demonstrate anti-leukocyte antibodies (leukoagglutinins) in the blood of leukopenic patients and to suggest that these leukoagglutinins were probably alloantibodies because they did not react with leukocytes from the antibody producer but did react with a percentage of leukocytes from red cell group O unrelated individuals (allospecific reactivity). Shortly thereafter, Rose Payne reported that sera from patients who had febrile nonhemolytic blood transfusion reactions frequently contained leukoagglutinins that demonstrated allospecificity (Payne, 1964). In 1958, Dausset described the first HLA alloantigen, MAC (now HLA-A2 + HLA-A28), and showed it to be genetically determined. Originally, all of the leukocyte specificities were thought to be the product of a single locus. A two-locus model, each with multiple alleles, was established by the identification of recombinational events that separated the two allelic series. These two allelic series were called the first, or LA (now HLA-A), and the second, or four (now HLA-B) series. These names derived from the fact that the LA1,2,3 allelic series was described by Payne in 1967 and the 4a, 4b allelic series was described by van Rood in 1969. A third locus was first proposed in 1970; however, it was not confirmed by recombination until 1975. This third locus was designated HLA-C following the 1975 International Histocompatibility Workshop. Dausset was awarded the Nobel Prize for Medicine in 1980 for his original work on the human HLA system (Dausset, 1992).

Structure of Class I Molecules

The Class I molecules, termed HLA-A, HLA-B, and HLA-C in the human, are heterodimers consisting of a transmembrane glycoprotein heavy chain (44 kDa) noncovalently associated with β_2-microglobulin (12 kDa) (Fig. 38–5) (Bjorkman, 1990). The heavy chain of the Class I molecule spans the cell membrane and is oriented with its amino-terminus on the outside of the cell. β_2-Microglobulin is associated with the extracellular region of the heavy chain and is necessary for cell surface expression. The extracellular region of the Class I heavy chain is divided into three domains designated α_1, α_2, and α_3, each consisting of about 90 amino acid residues. The amino-terminal α_1 domain contains a gly-

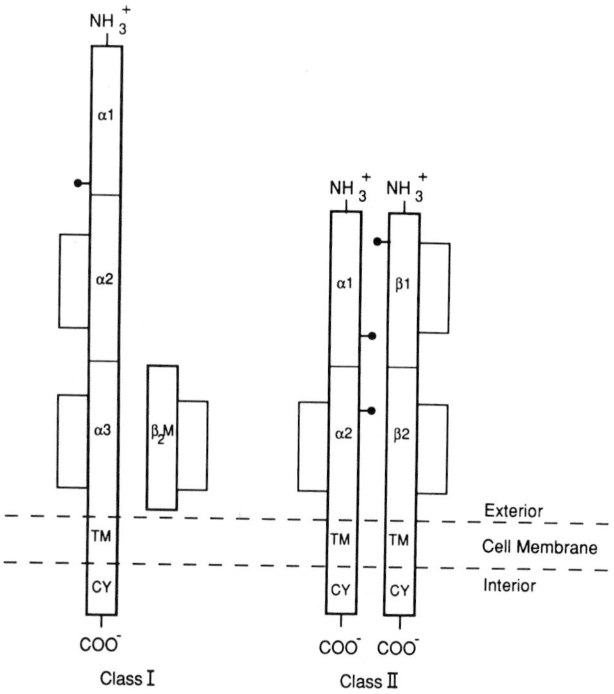

Figure 38–5. A schematic model of Class I and Class II molecules.

Table 38–1. COMPLETE LISTING OF RECOGNIZED HLA ANTIGENS (SPECIFICITIES) DEFINED BY SEROLOGIC TYPING*

A	B	C	DR	DQ
A1	B5	Cw1†	DR1	DQ1
A2	B7	Cw2	DR103	DQ2
A203	B703	Cw3	DR2	DQ3
A210	B8	Cw4	DR3	DQ4
A3	B12	Cw5	DR4	DQ5(1)
A9	B13	Cw6	DR5	DQ6(1)
A10	B14	Cw7	DR6	DQ7(3)
A11	B15	Cw8	DR7	DQ8(3)
A19	B16	Cw9(w3)	DR8	DQ9(3)
A23(9)‡	B17	Cw10(w3)	DR9	
A24(9)	B18		DR10	
A2403	B21		DR11(5)	
A25(10)	B22		DR12(5)	
A26(10)	B27		DR13(6)	
A28	B35		DR14(6)	
A29(19)	B37		DR1403	
A30(19)	B38(16)		DR1404	
A31(19)	B39(16)		DR15(2)	
A32(19)	B3901		DR16(2)	
A33(19)	B3902		DR17(3)	
A34(10)	B40		DR18(3)	
A36	B4005			
A43	B41		DR51§	
A66(10)	B42			
A68(28)	B44(12)		DR52§	
A69(28)	B45(12)			
A74(19)	B46		DR53§	
	B47			
	B48			
	B49(21)			
	B50(21)			
	B51(5)			
	B5102			
	B5103			
	B52(5)			
	B53			
	B54(22)			
	B55(22)			
	B56(22)			
	B57(17)			
	B58(17)			
	B59			
	B60(40)			
	B61(40)			
	B62(15)			
	B63(15)			
	B64(14)			
	B65(14)			
	B67			
	B70			
	B71(70)			
	B72(70)			
	B73			
	B75(15)			
	B76(15)			
	B77(15)			
	B7801			
	Bw4‖			
	Bw6‖			

*Each column of the table is independent and unrelated to the other columns. DP is not usually defined by serology.

†w is added to avoid confusion with the complement genes.

‡( ) indicates the broad serologic specificity. The serologic type may be listed without the broad specificity. For example, both A23(9) and A23 are correct designations.

§DR51, DR52, and DR53 are serologic specificities associated with a number of DR serologic types.

‖Bw4 and Bw6 are supertypic serologic specificities found on multiple B specificities. A few HLA-A specificities also carry the Bw6 specificity.

From Bodmer JG, Marsh SGE, Albert ED, Bodmer WF, Dupont B, Erlich HA, Mach B, Mayr WR, Parham P, Sasazuki T, Schreuder GMT, Strominger JL, Svejgaard A, Terasaki PI: Nomenclature for factors of the HLA system, 1991. Tissue Antigens 1992;39:161–173. © 1992 Munksgaard International Publishers, Ltd, Copenhagen, Denmark.

cosylation site at the asparagine residue in position 86. The transmembrane segment of approximately 24 amino acids is mostly hydrophobic, whereas the intracellular carboxy-terminal segment of the molecule consists mainly of hydrophilic residues with a cluster of basic residues adjacent to the cytoplasmic surface of the cell membrane. Other membrane-bound molecules have been found to have similar clustering of basic residues that are thought to anchor the molecule in the membrane by charge interaction with the negatively charged membrane.

Polymorphism of Class I molecules (Table 38–1) (Bodmer, 1992; 1994) is defined by the use of (1) Class I specific antibodies (alloantisera and monoclonal antibodies), (2) cytotoxic T lymphocytes (CTL) that recognize and kill in response to foreign or allogeneic Class I molecules *in vitro*, (3) isoelectric focusing of isolated Class I molecules, (4) polymerase chain reaction (PCR)-based DNA typing of Class I alleles, and (5) nucleotide sequencing of Class I genes. Most of the Class I polymorphism arises from amino acid sequence differences clustered in the α_1 and α_2 domains of the heavy chain. The α_3 domain is highly conserved among all alleles.

Fresh insights into the structure of the HLA molecule came when the Class I molecule was crystallized (Bjorkman, 1987). The structure of the extracellular portion is shown in Figure 38–6. The molecule consists of two pairs of structurally similar domains: α_1 has the same tertiary conformation as α_2, whereas α_3 and β_2-microglobulin have similar tertiary conformations. The α_3- and β_2-microglobulin domains are each composed of two anti-parallel β-pleated sheets, one with four strands and one with three strands, connected by a disulfide bond. The α_3 and β_2-microglobulin domains interact with one another through these β-pleated sheets, and their structures closely resemble that described for an immunoglobulin constant region domain. The α_1 and α_2 domains are paired to form an eight-strand β-pleated sheet. This sheet is topped by two α-helices forming a groove at the top of the molecule. This groove is the site for the binding of antigenic fragments by the Class I molecule (Fig. 38–6*B*). The sides and bottom of the groove are formed by side chains of the amino acids, which comprise the helices and β-pleated sheets. Many of the amino acids that line this groove are highly polymorphic, creating allele-specific differences in antigen-binding specificities among the different Class I allelic products (Stern, 1994). Other residues in the helical regions of the groove may interact with the T cell receptor during recognition of the Class I–antigenic fragment complex by a T lymphocyte (see Fig. 38–2).

Nomenclature—Class I Serologic Specificities

HLA terminology is designated by the World Health Organization (WHO) Committee for HLA Nomenclature (Bodmer, 1992; 1994). Historically, serologic and cellularly defined specificities localized on the HLA molecules were assigned based on results of international workshops in which typing reagents were exchanged among participating laboratories. A new specificity would first be designated "w," which indicated a provisional workshop definition. If the

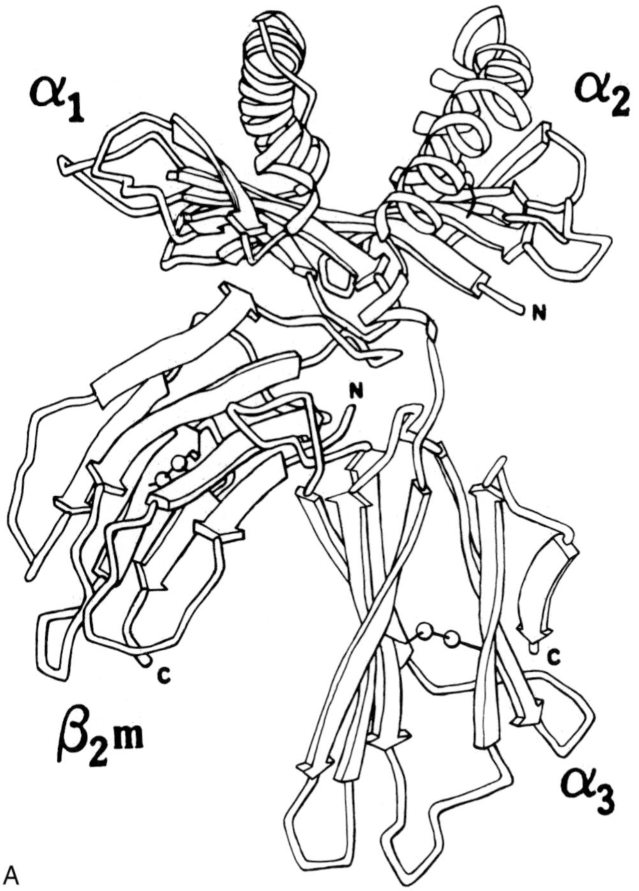

A

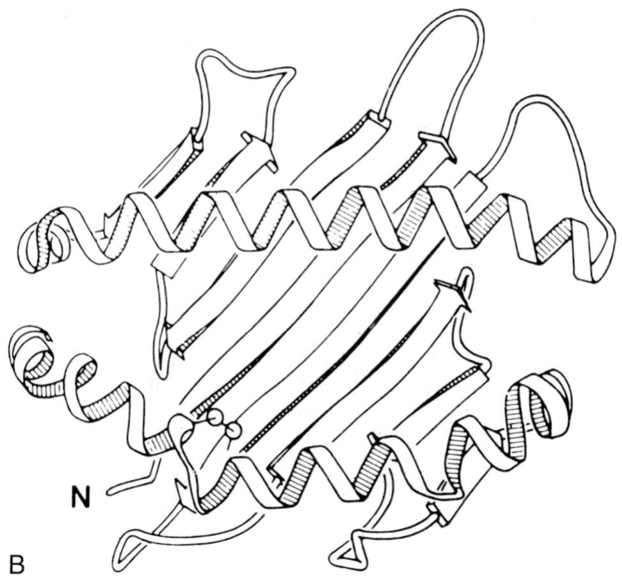

B

Figure 38–6. *A*, Three-dimensional model of the extracellular portion of a Class I molecule. *B*, Top view of the same molecule. (Reprinted by permission from Bjorkman PJ, Saper MA, Samraoui B, et al: Structure of the human class I histocompatibility antigen, HLA-A2. Nature 1987; 329:506. Copyright 1987, Macmillan Magazines Ltd.)

specificity remained well defined in subsequent international workshops, the "w" would be dropped. Today, however, the majority of nomenclature designations are given to HLA alleles defined by nucleic acid sequencing.

New serologic specificities were assigned following an International Histocompatibility Workshop if their definitions appeared clear in laboratories participating in the workshop. Frequently, in subsequent workshops, old serologically defined specificities were "split" as the definition became more refined until ultimately the definition defined a single allelic product. The most narrow definition of the specificity is called the subtypic specificity. The broader, shared specificities are called supertypic specificities. For example, B44 and B45 are subtypic specificities of the supertypic specificity B12. Thus, a cell that is either B44- or B45-positive is also positive for B12. Table 38–2 lists the supertypic equivalents for the "splits."

HLA-A and -B antigens are not numbered consecutively for historic reasons. In addition, there is neither a 4 nor a 6 in either the A or the B allelic series. These numbers were reserved for the 4a, 4b leukocyte system that was being investigated at the time the original nomenclature system was developed in 1967. Subsequently, it was shown that the 4a (now Bw4) and 4b (now Bw6) specificities reside on the same molecule as the B locus subtypic specificities, but at a different site (Dausset, 1992). Thus Bw4 and Bw6 are a diallelic system, and all *B* locus molecules characteristically carry either w4 or w6 specificities.

Serologically defined C locus specificities are designated

Table 38–2. SEROLOGIC SPLITS*

Original Broad Specificities	Splits
A2	A203,A210
A9	A23,A24,A2403
A10	A25,A26,A34,A66
A19	A29,A30,A31,A32,A33,A74
A28	A68,A69
B5	B51,B52
B7	B703
B12	B44,B45
B14	B64,B65
B15	B62,B63,B75,B76,B77
B16	B38,B39,B3901,B3902
B17	B57,B58
B21	B49,B50,B4005
B22	B54,B55,B56
B40	B60,B61
B70	B71,B72
Cw3	Cw9,Cw10
DR1	DR103
DR2	DR15,DR16
DR3	DR17,DR18
DR5	DR11,DR12
DR6	DR13,DR14,DR1403,DR1404
DQ1	DQ5,DQ6
DQ3	DQ7,DQ8,DQ9

*Each row of the table lists a broad specificity and its associated splits. For example, A203 and A210 antigens are subdivisions of A2.

From Bodmer JG, Marsh SGE, Albert ED, Bodmer WF, Dupont B, Erlich HA, Mach B, Mayr WR, Parham P, Sasazuki T, Schreuder GMT, Strominger JL, Svejgaard A, Terasaki PI: Nomenclature for factors of the HLA system, 1991. Tissue Antigens 1992;39:161–173. © 1992 Munksgaard International Publishers, Ltd, Copenhagen, Denmark.

5

by a "w" followed by a number. The "w" workshop provisional designation has not been dropped even though some specificities are considered well defined, because the notation would then be similar to that for the complement system.

Class I Genes

The heavy chains are encoded within the HLA complex (see Fig. 38–1) (Jordan, 1985) and are highly polymorphic, whereas β_2-microglobulin is encoded on chromosome 15 and has not been found to be polymorphic in humans. As many as 20 additional "nonclassic" Class I genes, such as *HLA-E*, *HLA-G*, and *HLA-H*, have been identified by gene cloning (Heinrichs, 1990). These additional Class I genes exhibit limited, if any, polymorphism. Some of these nonclassic Class I genes are not expressed as protein products; others exhibit limited expression, being found only on specific tissues. For example, HLA-G is expressed on cytotrophoblast cells of the placenta (Schmidt, 1993).

The typical Class I gene is encoded by eight exons that correspond to the segments of the molecule just described (Fig. 38–7). The first exon encodes the 5′ untranslated region and a hydrophobic leader peptide. Exons 2 to 4 encode the three extracellular domains; exon 5 encodes the transmembrane region. The sixth and seventh exons encode the cytoplasmic region, and the eighth exon encodes the 3′ untranslated region, including the poly(A) addition site. The intervening sequences between the exons (termed introns) are transcribed into RNA but are removed during mRNA splicing.

Table 38–3. HLA-A ALLELES AND THEIR SEROLOGIC DESIGNATION (EXAMPLES)*

HLA Alleles	Serologic Specificity
A*0101	A1
A*0102	A1
A*0201	A2
A*0202	A2
A*0203	A203
A*0204	A2
A*0205	A2
A*0206	A2
A*0207	A2
A*0208	A2
A*0209	A2
A*0210	A210
A*0211	A2
A*0212	A2
A*0213	A2
A*0301	A3
A*0302	A3
A*1101	A11
A*1102	A11
A*2301	A23(9)†
A*2401	A24(9)
A*2402	A24(9)
A*2403	A2403
A*2501	A25(10)

*Each row in the table lists an HLA-A allele and the associated serologic specificity or antigen. For example, individuals carrying the A*0101 allele are serologically typed as A1.

†The number in ( ) defines the broad serologic specificity. This is described in Table 38–2.

From Bodmer JG, Marsh SGE, Albert ED, Bodmer WF, Dupont B, Erlich HA, Mach B, Mayr WR, Parham P, Sasazuki T, Schreuder GMT, Strominger JL, Svejgaard A, Terasaki PI: Nomenclature for factors of the HLA system, 1994. Hum Immunol 1994;41:1–200. Copyright 1994 by the American Society for Histocompatibility and Immunogenetics.

Nomenclature—DNA-Based Class I Allele Designations

Nucleotide sequencing has been used to identify multiple different allelic products that exhibit a single serologic or cellular specificity. Currently, a single serologic specificity may reside on two to more than fifteen different allelic products (see examples, Table 38–3). Each HLA allele is designated by the name of the gene locus, followed by an asterisk and a four-digit number indicating the allele. For example, *A*0201* is an allele of the *HLA-A* gene; *B*1510* is an allele of the *HLA-B* gene. The first two numbers in the numerical designation of each allele are often based on the serologic type of the resultant molecule and/or the nucleotide sequence similarity to other alleles in the group. For example, the HLA-A molecule expressed by the *A*0201* allele bears the A2 serologic specificity defining the HLA-A2 antigen. The HLA-B molecule expressed by the *B*1510* allele does not bear the B15-associated serologic specificity but rather bears the B71 serologic specificity defining the B71 antigen. It was designated *B*1510* because of its nucleotide similarity to other B15 alleles. The last two numbers in the allele designation refer to the order in which the gene was sequenced. For example, *A*0201* was the first A2 allele to be sequenced and *A*0202* was the second. Some alleles have a fifth digit (e.g., *B*27051* and *B*27051*[2]). This digit indicates that the

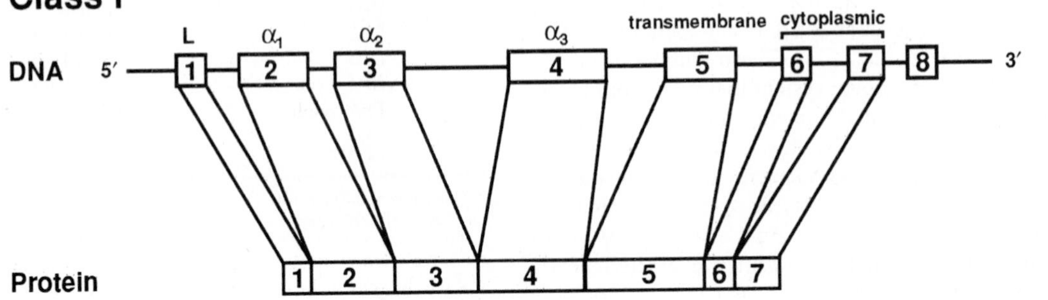

Figure 38–7. The exon and intron structure of a Class I gene and the corresponding protein. The leader peptide (L) is not present in the mature protein.

two alleles differ in DNA sequence but that the HLA molecule specified by the two alleles does not differ (often termed a silent mutation or substitution). New alleles are described in yearly reports of the World Health Organization (WHO) HLA Nomenclature Committee (Bodmer, 1994), and the nucleotide sequences of all alleles are deposited in a computerized databank (GENBANK or EMBL). Currently, there are, for example, 50 *HLA-A* alleles assigned, and new alleles are continually being identified.

Regulation of Class I Gene Expression

HLA Class I molecules are expressed on the surface of many cell types; however, their levels can vary extensively (Singer, 1990). The resting level of Class I molecules is highest on lymphoid cells; Class I molecules are undetectable on certain other cell types such as brain cells, muscle cells, or sperm cells. Class I genes are regulated during development and can be up-regulated by cytokines such as interferon gamma and tumor necrosis factor. Certain viruses such as HIV (Howcroft, 1993) or tumors (Garrido, 1993) can suppress Class I expression. Patients with a severe form of bare lymphocyte syndrome lack Class I expression and have combined immunodeficiency disease. Sequence elements located upstream of Class I genes bind regulatory factors that control this expression.

Function of Class I Molecules

The central function of the HLA-A, -B, -C molecules is to bind peptides derived from intracellular antigens and to bring them to the cell surface for inspection by the antigen receptors on T cells. If a T cell encounters foreign material (i.e., virus) or an abnormal protein (i.e., tumor), it then mounts an immune response to protect the individual (Germain, 1993). In the cytosol of the cell, viral antigens or abnormal proteins are broken down into peptide fragments. The peptide fragments are transported to the endoplasmic reticulum, where they bind to grooves at the top of newly synthesized Class I molecules and are carried to the cell surface (see Fig. 38–2). Four genes located in the Class II region of the MHC are involved in this process (Fig. 38–8). Two of these genes (*LMP2* and *LMP7*) encode components of the proteosome complex, a macromolecular structure that degrades proteins within the cytosol. The other two genes (*TAP1* and *TAP2*) encode components of peptide transporters that move peptides from the cytosol into the endoplasmic reticulum.

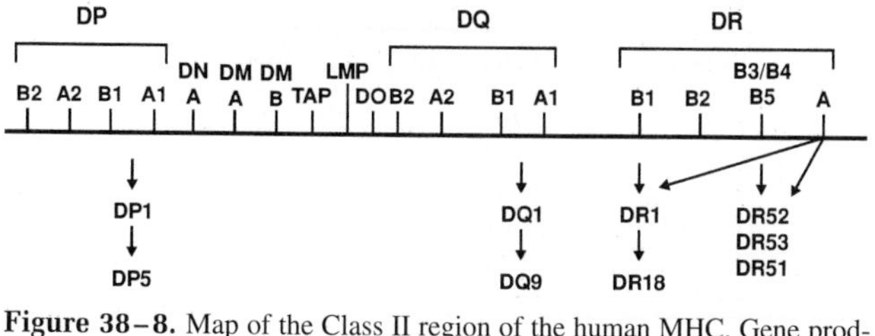

Figure 38–8. Map of the Class II region of the human MHC. Gene products encoded by each subregion are listed. (Adapted from Campbell RD, Trowsdale J: Map of the human MHC. Today 1993; 14:349–352.)

CD8-positive cytotoxic T lymphocytes (CTL) recognize these antigenic fragments in conjunction with the Class I molecule (Jorgensen, 1992). In the experimental system used to dissect this mechanism, cytotoxic T lymphocytes (CTL) were generated by *in vitro* stimulation with virally infected autologous cells. The recognition and lysis of target cells was specific for the priming virus strain and to certain *HLA-A*, *-B*, and *-C* allelic products present on the responder cell. Thus, only target cells sharing the appropriate *HLA-A*, *-B*, or *-C* allelic products with the responder and the appropriate virus strain peptide will be lysed. This requirement for self-MHC is termed MHC restriction.

HLA-DR, -DQ, -DP SUBREGIONS—CLASS II MOLECULES

The Class II molecules in humans were first recognized by their ability to stimulate allogeneic T cells in mixed leukocyte culture (MLC). During the 1975 International Histocompatibility Workshop, the MLC was used to define the HLA-D allelic series (Thorsby, 1975). Because MLCs required seven days, a rapid serologic detection of HLA-D was sought. In 1975, it was determined that alloantisera contained antibodies against molecules closely associated with the specificities previously identified as HLA-D (reviewed by Dausset, 1992). Following the 1977 International Histocompatibility Workshop, these serologic specificities were termed DR, for D-related specificities, because HLA-D and HLA-DR were observed to be associated (but not identical) with each other. Additional serologic reagents coupled with genetic and immunochemical techniques identified additional Class II molecules MB1–3/MT1/DC-1 (now called DQ1–9), MT2 (now DR52), and MT3 (now DR53). Cellular techniques identified still another Class II molecule in the late 1970s (Shaw, 1981). This molecule (now termed HLA-DP) was initially called a secondary B cell antigen (SB) because it was usually weak or undetectable in a primary MLC and required a secondary phase stimulation in culture for detection.

5

Structure of Class II Molecules

The Class II HLA-DR, -DQ, -DP molecules are heterodimers consisting of two noncovalently associated transmembrane glycoproteins, an α-chain (33–35 kDa) and a β-chain (26–28 kDa) (see Fig. 38–5) (Gorga, 1992; Kappes, 1988). Both polypeptide chains span the cell membrane and are oriented with their amino-termini on the outside of the cell. The extracellular regions of the α- and β-polypeptides are divided into two domains, designated α_1 and α_2 and β_1 and β_2, each consisting of approximately 90 amino acid residues. The α-chain has two carbohydrate moieties, one high-mannose and one complex-type glycan, at amino acids 78 and 118. β-Chains have one complex-type oligosaccharide at amino acid 19. The amino-terminal α_1 and β_1 domains of α- and β-chains contain the polymorphic residues, whereas the membrane proximal α_2 and β_2 domains are highly conserved and are homologous to immunoglobulin constant region domains. A region approximately 12 amino acids in length connects the second extracellular domain to the hydrophobic transmembrane region (23 amino acids) and a small intracytoplasmic domain (8 to 15 amino acids).

The crystal structure of a Class II molecule shows that the molecule is similar to the structure of the Class I molecule (Brown, 1993) (see Fig. 38–6). For Class II, the α_1 and β_1 domains of the α- and β-chains form an eight-stranded β-pleated sheet topped by two α-helices to form the antigen-binding groove at the top of the molecule. The α_2 and β_2 domains each form anti-parallel β-pleated sheets that support the groove at the top. As in Class I, many amino acids that line the antigenic peptide-binding groove are polymorphic, creating differences in antigen-binding specificities for the different Class II allelic products.

Like the Class I molecules, the Class II molecules are highly polymorphic (see Table 38–1) (Bodmer, 1992; 1994). This polymorphism is defined by (1) Class II specific antibodies (alloantisera and monoclonal antibodies), (2) alloproliferative T cells that recognize and proliferate in response to foreign Class II molecules *in vitro*, (3) isoelectric focusing and two-dimensional gel electrophoresis of isolated Class II molecules, (4) hybridization of restriction endonuclease digests of DNA encoding Class II genes using locus-specific probes, a technique that detects restriction fragment length polymorphism (RFLP), (5) PCR-based DNA typing of Class II alleles, and (6) nucleotide sequencing of Class II genes. Most of the Class II polymorphism arises from amino acid sequence differences localized in the α_1 and β_1 domains of the two polypeptide chains.

Nomenclature—Class II Serologic and Cellular Specificities

The WHO-designated serologic specificities localized to DR and DQ molecules have been assigned as described for the Class I molecules. Serologic subdivisions of the DR and DQ molecules are listed in Table 38–1. DP molecules are still not adequately defined serologically and thus are not included in Table 38–1. Only 6 HLA-DP types were originally defined by cellular techniques; however, more than 50 *HLA-DP* alleles have now been uncovered by DNA sequencing and can be identified by using sequence-specific oligonucleotide probe (SSOP) typing (see following).

There are 26 HLA-D specificities that are identified by MLC and type a cluster of Class II allelic products encoded by a haplotype. All of the HLA-D specificities retain the "w" designation because these specificities alone are defined functionally; they are primarily a result of stimulation of the responder cell by differences in the DR molecules expressed by the stimulator and, to a lesser extent, additional stimulation by the DQ and DP molecules (discussed under Mixed Leukocyte Culture). HLA typing using this approach has been in large part superseded by DNA-based typing.

Class II Genes

In contrast to the Class I molecules, the α- and β-chains of the Class II molecules are both encoded within 1100 kilobases of the MHC complex (see Fig. 38–8) (Campbell 1993; Kappes, 1988). The region includes three subregions—*DR*, *DQ*, and *DP*—each of which encodes at least one expressed *A* (encoding an α-chain) and *B* (encoding a β-chain) gene. Other Class II genes in the region either are pseudogenes or their expressed products have not been well characterized (*DN*, *DO*, *DM*). Sequence comparisons suggest that both Class I and Class II genes arose through a successive series of gene duplications during the evolution of this gene complex. The original duplication in the Class II region most likely gave rise to primordial *A* and *B* genes. More recent duplications generated the *DR*, *DQ*, and *DP* subregions, containing multiple *A* and *B* gene loci.

A typical *A* gene contains five exons encoding (1) 5′ untranslated region and signal sequence and the first few amino acids of the mature polypeptide; (2) α_1 domain; (3) α_2 domain; (4) connecting peptide, transmembrane region, cytoplasmic tail, and a portion of the 3′ untranslated region; and (5) the remainder of the 3′ untranslated region, including the poly(A) addition signal. A typical β-chain gene is similar to the α-chain gene but has an extra exon for the cytoplasmic tail.

***DR* SUBREGION.** The *DR* subregion encodes either one or two DR molecules, depending on the haplotype (Bodmer, 1992; 1994). Some haplotypes such as DR1 and DR8 express a single *DRB* gene product, whereas most other DR haplotypes express two *DRB* gene products. The subregion contains a single expressed *DRA* gene that is almost identical in different haplotypes, differing by a single, conservative amino acid substitution found in the cytoplasmic domain. The *HLA-DR* genes and the antigens they express are given in Table 38–4.

The most centromeric *DRB* gene, *DRB1* (see Fig. 38–8), encodes a highly polymorphic β-chain that, when associated with the α-chain, exhibits serologic specificities DR1–DR18. This molecule is usually the predominant Class II molecule on the cell surface, accounting for approximately 65% of the total cell surface Class II molecules. There are multiple nucleic acid and, hence, amino acid sequence differences among *DRB1* allelic products; however, the differences are located primarily in the amino-terminal β_1 domain.

The second *DRB* gene, present only in some Class II haplotypes, is located adjacent to the *DRA* gene (see Fig. 38–8). In cells expressing DR11, 12, 13, 14, 17, and 18, the second *DRB* gene is *DRB3*. The *DRB3* gene is polymorphic, although at present the number of identified alleles is approximately 25 times less than the number of *DRB1* alleles. The *DRB3* product combined with the DRA product forms the DR molecule, which carries the DR52 serological specificity. In cells expressing DR4, 7, and 9, the second *DRB* gene is *DRB4*. The *DRB4* product combined with the *DRA* product

Table 38–4. CLASS II GENES AND THEIR ANTIGENS*

A Gene	B Gene	Antigen Specified
DRA	*DRB1*	DR (e.g., DR1,DR7)
DRA	*DRB3*	DR52
DRA	*DRB4*	DR53
DRA	*DRB5*	DR51
DQA1	*DQB1*	DQ
DPA1	*DPB1*	DP

*Each row shows the A gene and B gene combination and the resultant Class II antigen specified.

forms the molecule that carries the serologic specificity DR53. Last, in cells expressing DR15 and 16, the second *DRB* gene is *DRB5*. This *DRB5* product combined with the *DRA* product carries the DR51 serologic specificity. A given haplotype carries only a single *DRB3*, *DRB4*, or *DRB5* locus or does not have a second functional *DRB* locus.

***DQ* SUBREGION.** One set of *A* and *B* genes, *DQA1* and *DQB1*, encode the DQ heterodimer that carries the DQ1–9 serologic specificities (see Tables 38–1 and 38–4) (see Fig. 38–8) (Bodmer, 1992; 1994). DQ molecules represent approximately 15% of the Class II molecules on the cell surface. Because both *DQA1* and *DQB1* are polymorphic and their products can associate in *trans* as well as in *cis*, heterozygotes can potentially express four different DQ molecules on their cell surfaces (Fig. 38–9). DQ molecules that carry the same DQ serologic specificity are found associated with several DR haplotypes. Although these molecules carry the same serologic specificity, they may be composed of structurally different α- and β-chains. For example, DQ6 molecules encoded by the DR15(2) and the DR13(6) haplotypes differ in amino acid sequence. Other DQ-like *A* and *B* genes in the *DQ* subregion such as *DQA2* and *DQB2* are very similar to the *DQA1* and *DQB1* genes; however, no functional protein products are expressed.

***DP* SUBREGION.** The *DP* subregion contains two sets of *A* and *B* genes (see Table 38–4 and Fig. 38–8). One set, *DPA1* and *DPB1*, encodes the DP protein product; the other set is made up of pseudogenes. Although the polymorphism of *DPA1* is limited to only a few allelic forms, the *DPB1* gene is highly polymorphic (Bodmer, 1992; 1994). The level of DP expression on the cell surface is extremely low (5% of total Class II molecules expressed).

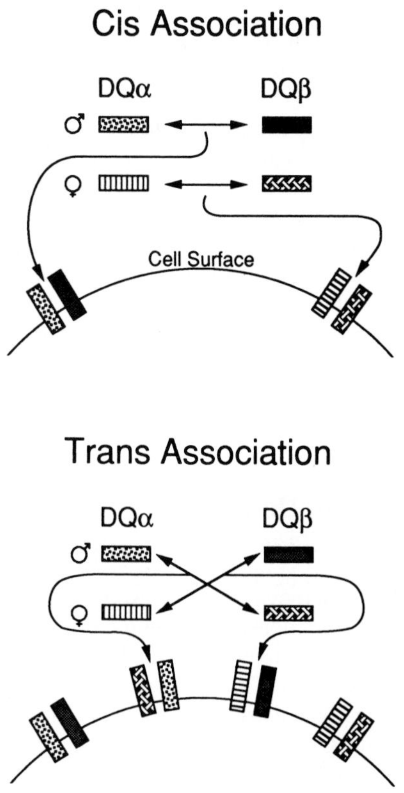

Figure 38–9. Model of the *cis* and *trans* associations of DQ alpha and beta chains.

Other Class II Genes

At least four other Class II genes, *DNA*, *DOB*, *DMA*, and *DMB* that express protein products have been described (see Fig. 38–8). The DMA- and DMB-encoded molecule is hypothesized to serve a chaperone-like function for the assembly of Class II molecules (Morris, 1994). Other Class II genes in the region (e.g., *DQA2*, *DQB2*, *DRB2*, *DPA2*, and *DPB2*) are pseudogenes and do not appear to be expressed.

Nomenclature—DNA-Based Class II Allele Designations

WHO-assigned Class II allele designations have been assigned as described for Class I alleles. For example, *DPB1*0101* is an allele of the *HLA-DPB1* gene; *DQB1*0301* is an allele of the *HLA-DQB1* gene; *DQA1*0601* is an allele of the *HLA-DQA1* gene. The first two numbers in the numerical designation of each allele are often based on the serologic type of the resultant antigen and/or the similarity to other alleles in the group. For example, the HLA-DR antigen expressed by the *DRB1*0401* allele bears the DR4 serologic specificity defining the DR4 antigen. The *DRB1*0103* allele was originally defined by cellular reagents for which there was no known DR serologic association (i.e., DR-blank). Later, a serologic specificity was identified, thus the DR103 serologic designation. Nucleotide sequencing identified an allele with a similar DNA structure to alleles bearing the DR1 serologic specificity (e.g., *DRB1*0101* and **0102*). Currently, there are, for example, 120 *DRB1* alleles assigned, and new alleles are continually being identified.

Linkage Disequilibrium in the Class II Region

5

Certain *DR* and *DQ* alleles are inherited together more frequently than expected. The frequency of these combinations differs strikingly among different ethnic subpopulations. For example, DR11(5),DQ1 and *DR9,DQ2* are found frequently in populations of black heritage, whereas these combinations are rarely found in populations of white heritage. Crossing over between the *DP* loci and the *DR/DQ* loci is common. Thus, there is little association between *DR/DQ* and *DP* alleles except for an association of DP1 with DR17(3),DQ2 and with DR18,DQ4.

Regulation of Class II Gene Expression

Class II molecules are expressed on cells of the immune system, including macrophages, dendritic cells, B lymphocytes, and activated T lymphocytes, but not resting T lymphocytes. Class II genes are also inducible by γ-interferon in many cell types (Glimcher, 1992). Class II molecules are also modulated by other cytokines such as interleukin-4, tumor necrosis factor, and prostaglandins released by T cells during recognition of the MHC-antigen complex (see Chap. 37) (Guardiola, 1993). The level of Class II gene expression in specific cell types may play an important role in HLA association with autoimmune diseases (Nepom, 1991) and in allograft rejection. DNA sequences found in all Class II genes in a region upstream of the coding sequences are critical elements that control expression. These upstream sequences bind proteins that regulate the expression of Class II genes. Mutations have been identified, some affecting these regulatory sequences, which simultaneously eliminate expression of all Class II genes, resulting in one form of severe combined immunodeficiency (SCID) (Kovats, 1994).

Function of Class II Molecules

Class II molecules act as antigen receptors in the immune response (see Fig. 38–2), primarily binding antigenic fragments from exogenous antigens such as bacteria that enter the cell through the endocytic pathway (Cresswell, 1994). These exogenous antigens are broken down into peptide fragments in late endosomes in which they encounter newly assembled Class II molecules. The fragments bound within the antigen-binding grooves of Class II molecules are then transported to the cell surface.

Antigen receptors on CD4-positive T lymphocytes interact with the Class II-antigenic fragment complex, triggering activation (Jorgensen, 1992). In the experimental system used to dissect this mechanism, T lymphocytes were raised by *in vitro* stimulation with autologous cells that had been previously incubated with antigen. As observed for Class I, the recognition of the antigen-presenting cell is specific for the priming antigenic peptide and the particular HLA-DR, -DQ, or -DP allelic products present on the antigen-presenting cell.

Each T cell activated by recognition of the complex of antigen and Class II molecule can perform one or several functions (Paul, 1994). The T cell can help B lymphocytes differentiate to become antibody-producing plasma cells, or the T cell can help other T lymphocytes to differentiate into cytotoxic or suppressor cells. In addition, the T cell itself can become either a cytotoxic cell, directly killing cells with the appropriate target (e.g., cells expressing Class II MHC molecules complexed with the specific antigen), or a suppressor cell causing a dampening of the immune response. T cells can also produce a number of biologically important molecules (such as γ-interferon) that augment immune function and cause increased expression of MHC molecules on target cells. In addition, T cells can produce growth factors such as interleukin-2. These growth factors can affect a wide range of cells, from hematopoietic stem cells to mature lymphocytes.

Characteristics of Antigenic Fragments Bound by MHC Molecules

The function of Class I and Class II molecules as antigen-binding receptors is similar; however, the types of antigen that bind to Class I and Class II molecules are thought to differ (Cresswell, 1994; Engelhard, 1994). Soluble and particulate antigens (exogenous antigens) are taken up by the cell in vesicles and associate with Class II molecules in the endocytic pathway. In contrast, antigens synthesized *de novo* in the cell (endogenous antigens such as viral antigens) associate with Class I molecules in the endoplasmic reticulum. Class I and Class II molecules bind self-peptides resulting from the normal degradation of cellular proteins and foreign peptides resulting from microbial or tumor antigens. Usually, the self-peptides bound to HLA molecules do not trigger T lymphocytes; however, they may do so in cases of autoimmunity (Nepom, 1991).

The peptides bound to Class I molecules are usually 9 to 10 amino acids in length, whereas the Class II molecules bind peptides that range from 12 to 30 amino acids in length. In fact, the peptides bound to Class II molecules are found as nested sets of sequences. Peptide binding to HLA molecules will occur only when the peptide fragment contains a particular amino acid sequence or motif that allows it to bind to one or more of the HLA molecules expressed in that individual. An example of a motif for a peptide that binds to HLA-A2 is leucine (or methionine or isoleucine) at residue 2 of the peptide, a hydrophilic amino acid at residue 3, and a valine (or leucine or isoleucine or alanine) at residue 9. The other amino acids within the peptide can vary, but there may be some restrictions on the specific amino acids that appear at these positions. The amino acids forming the motif bind to the HLA molecule in pockets found within the antigen-binding groove (Stern, 1994). The polymorphic amino acids of the HLA molecules line these pockets, creating differences in antigen-binding specificities for different HLA molecules.

TECHNIQUES FOR DETECTING HLA POLYMORPHISMS

Histocompatibility testing, or HLA typing, is performed in a limited number of laboratories because it uses specialized and complex procedures and reagents. In addition, interpretation and translation of the results require considerable expertise. Histocompatibility laboratories are found in medical centers that have organ transplantation programs and/or as parts of large blood banks and transfusion services. Techniques are discussed in general in this section. For detailed procedures, refer to the American Society for Histocompatibility and Immunogenetics (ASHI) Laboratory Manual (1994).

Serologic Detection of Class I and Class II Molecules

Lymphocyte microcytotoxicity testing, which was originally utilized in the mouse system by Gorer and Amos, was modified by Terasaki and McClelland for use in the human system. This assay for Class I specificities is reproducible under controlled, standardized conditions. However, the reproducibility for Class II specificities is much lower, and in large-scale testing (e.g., for registries), error rates may increase.

LYMPHOCYTE PREPARATION. Lymphocytes are employed routinely in HLA serologic typing assays and are readily obtained from peripheral whole blood by layering onto a Ficoll-Hypaque gradient that separates blood cells according to density. Following centrifugation, one obtains a layer at the serum–Ficoll-Hypaque interface that is 99% mononuclear cells. The separated peripheral blood lymphocytes (PBL) can be used for HLA-A, -B, -C typing.

To test for HLA-DR, -DQ serologic specificities, it is necessary to enrich for B lymphocytes or to use a special two-color fluorescent technique to simultaneously differentiate between B cells and T cells. Three enrichment procedures are currently employed by typing laboratories for the separation of the B lymphocyte subset:

(1) Magnetic beads: Magnetic beads coated with a monoclonal antibody specific for B lymphocytes (Dynal, Inc., One Lambda, Inc.) can be used to positively select for B lymphocytes. Alternatively, magnetic beads coated with T cell–specific and monocyte-specific monoclonal antibodies can be used to remove non-B cells. Both procedures yield more than 90% B cells, although beads coated with anti–B cell monoclonal antibodies more consistently give a purer preparation. This procedure is rapid, taking approximately 15 to 20 minutes, requires small amounts (10 mL) of whole peripheral blood, and is the technique of choice of many clinical histocompatibility laboratories.

(2) Nylon-wool adherence: B cells and monocytes preferentially adhere when a Ficoll-Hypaque–separated lymphocyte preparation is incubated on a nylon-wool column. T lymphocytes are easily washed off the column because they are relatively nonadherent. Once the T cells have been washed off, the B cells can be removed by vigorous agitation while monocytes remain adhered. Although technique-dependent, good B cell enrichment can be obtained. This technique is inexpensive and does not require specialized equipment or reagents.

(3) "Panning" (immunoadsorption of B cells to plastic dishes or flasks coated with an affinity-purified anti–human immunoglobulin fragment reagent raised against the $F(ab')_2$ fragment of IgG): Affinity-purified anti-$F(ab')_2$ will bind to plastic by adherence. When a mononuclear cell suspension is placed in the coated flask, B lymphocytes bind to the antibody-coated surface by their immunoglobulin receptors. The unbound T lymphocytes are easily removed by washing. The immunoglobulin-positive cells (B cells) are recovered by competition using an elution medium that contains an excess of immunoglobulin. B cell purity is excellent, and a uniform population is reproducibly obtained because of the positive selection. The technique requires special reagents and is more expensive and slightly more time-consuming than the nylon-wool adherence technique.

HLA-TYPING SERA. The major source of HLA-typing antisera is from sera of multiparous women. During pregnancy, the woman mounts an immune response to the paternal antigens present on the fetus. Other sources of antisera are from transplant recipients, multitransfused patients, and from human and other primate recipients of planned immunization. Sera from these sources are tested (screened) against a panel of lymphocytes of known HLA type. Only 10% to 15% of sera screened are useful for typing reagents. Thus, large screening programs must be maintained to identify reagents. Since the antibody specificity of an individual does not remain constant, supplies of antisera are limited. In an attempt to create a consistent and unlimited supply of antisera, some companies are now producing monoclonal antisera from cultures of fused mouse and human cells (hybridomas). Both bulk antisera and HLA-typing trays are commercially available and are used by the majority of clinical laboratories.

Because of the extreme antigenic complexity of HLA antigens, several antisera must be used to define each specificity. Most laboratories use trays from at least two different commercial companies. Frequently, from 140 to 210 antisera are used to define HLA-A, -B, -C specificities, and from 70 to 140 are used to define the HLA-DR, -DQ specificities. Most antisera tend to have false-positive and false-negative reactions. Some rarer antigens are defined only by reactivity patterns of multi-specific antisera because mono-specific antisera are not available. Since many antisera are not truly mono-specific and many exhibit some cross-reactivity (see later section), the reactivity of each antisera must be thoroughly known by the individual interpreting the results. This requires stringent quality control of each new lot of typing trays with well-characterized reference cells.

The number of different HLA antigens detected by serologic testing depends on the strength and selectivity of the serologic reagents used in the assay and the condition of the cells used for the testing. Serologic testing requires live cells; therefore, a sample must be submitted to the laboratory as soon as possible after collection, preferably within 24 hours. However, cells can be typed for up to three days. Samples that are delayed in shipment or are exposed to adverse conditions (e.g., extremes in temperature) during shipment can produce ambiguous typing results or cannot be serologically typed at all. An additional problem is the difficulty in obtaining appropriate numbers of cells expressing HLA antigens for typing from some patients, such as those with leukemia. All of the problems described in this section are the major reasons for the shift in HLA-typing methodologies toward DNA-based typing methods (Tiercy, 1991a; 1991b).

LYMPHOCYTE MICROCYTOTOXICITY ASSAY. HLA typing for the HLA-A, -B, -C, -DR, -DQ specificities is performed by a microlymphocytotoxicity assay. [HLA-DP] is not usually defined by serology. The HLA phenotype is determined by testing the unseparated lymphocyte preparation (PBL) or T lymphocytes (for HLA-A, -B, -C) or the enriched B lymphocytes (for -DR, -DQ) against a panel of well-characterized antisera. The assay is a two-stage test that uses only 1 μL of antiserum and 1 μL of a cell preparation containing 2000 lymphocytes. During the sensitization stage, the lymphocytes are incubated with the antisera, generally for 30 minutes at 22° to 24°C. Carefully prescreened and standardized rabbit serum as a source of complement is added in excess, and the mixture is incubated for an additional 60 minutes. One modification of the technique employs a wash step, which removes complement inhibitory factors and increases the sensitivity of the assay before the addition of complement. Frequently, the incubation times are extended to 60/60 or 60/120 minutes, respectively, for B cell typing. If the lymphocytes carry a cell surface molecule recognized by complement-fixing antibodies in the serum, the antibodies bind to the cells, and the cells are subsequently lysed following addition of complement. Complement-mediated lysis results in changes in the permeability of the cell membrane that can easily be judged microscopically by the penetration of vital dyes. The assay is terminated by addition of fluorescein diacetate and ethidium bromide for fluorescent procedures, or with eosin and formalin or trypan blue with ethylenediaminetetraacetic acid (EDTA). Reactions are read microscopically for percentage of lysis and are numerically graded (8 = strong positive, 81% or greater lysis; 6 = positive, 51% to 80% lysis; 4 = weak positive, 21% to 50% lysis; 2 = questionably positive, 11% to 20% lysis; 1 = negative, less than 10% lysis).

All lymphocytotoxicity procedures involve complement fixation, which can introduce a potential source of error and major variability in laboratory diagnosis. The source of complement is rabbit serum; but there are no standards on age, pool size, or potency. The complement provided with the commercial typing trays has been quality controlled for use with that set of trays and should be used by the laboratory performing the testing.

CROSS-REACTIVITY. Many HLA antisera react with more than one HLA allelic product. This phenomenon can result from cross-reactivity and/or from polyspecificity of the antisera and is responsible for the complex reactivity patterns of antisera. Poly-specific sera contain two or more HLA antibodies that can be absorbed easily to remove one antibody with little effect on the reactivity of the other(s). Poly-specific sera may contain Class I antibodies specific for any combination of allelic or non-allelic molecules (e.g., an antiserum may contain both HLA-A3- and HLA-B5-specific antibodies). Cross-reactive antisera contain, most frequently, a single antibody that reacts with an antigenic determinant shared among several different HLA allelic products. Cross-reactivity appears to result from shared amino acid sequences among allelic products. Examples of the localization of cross-reactive determinants are given in Figure 38–10. Adsorption of homologous (e.g., the strongest) reactivity from cross-reactive sera will also remove the reactivity for the other cross-reactive HLA alleles.

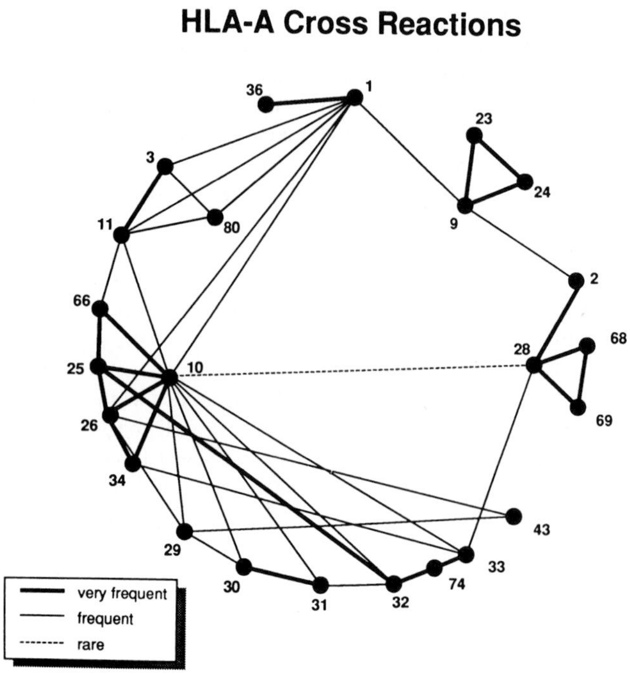

Figure 38–11. Cross-reactivity at the HLA-A locus. (Modified from that of Prof. W. Mayr, Vienna.)

Cross-reactions occur most frequently among allelic products encoded by the same locus but can occur between allelic products encoded by different loci (e.g., A2 + B17). Diagrams of cross-reactivity at the A locus and at the B locus are given in Figures 38–11 and 38–12. Cross-reactivity among allelic products of the *HLA-A* and *HLA-B* loci has been extensively studied and has been used to group alleles into cross-reactive groups (CREG) (Rodey, 1987). Class I mole-

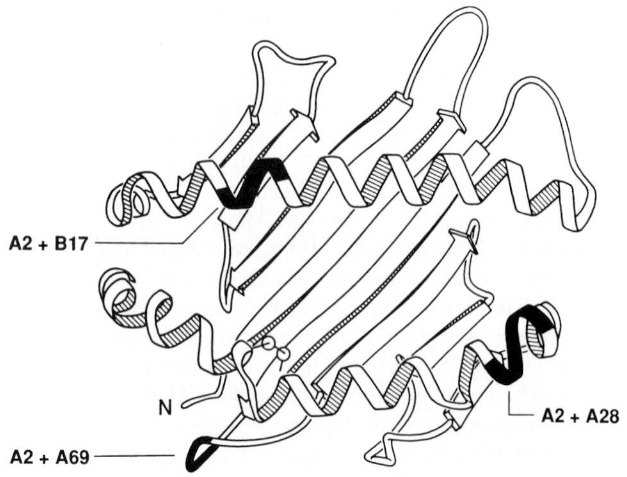

Figure 38–10. Top view of a Class I molecule with polymorphic amino acid residues indicated for cross-reactive specificities A2 + A28, A2 + A69, and A2 + B17. (From Parham P, Lawlor DA, Salter RD, et al: HLA-A, -B, -C: Patterns of polymorphism in peptide-binding proteins. *In* Dupont B: Immunobiology of HLA. New York, Springer-Verlag, 1989, p 17.)

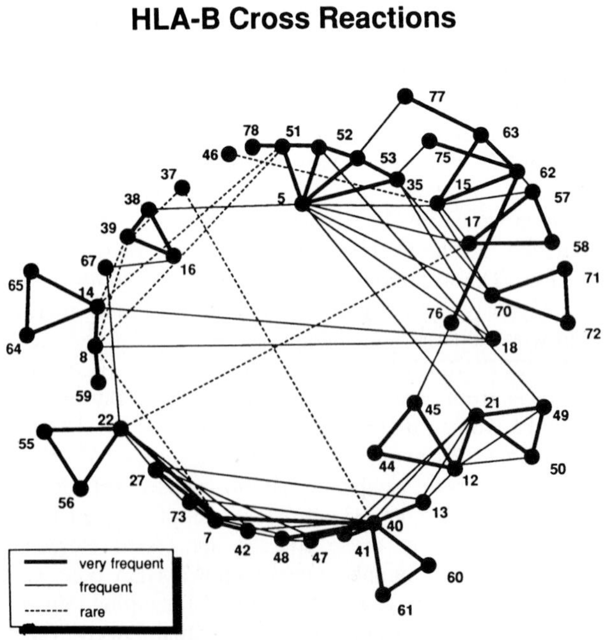

Figure 38–12. Cross-reactivity at the HLA-B locus. (Modified from that of Prof. W. Mayr, Vienna.)

cules within a CREG share one or more determinants that are not shared by specificities in another CREG and are more closely related to each other than to other Class I molecules. An antigenic determinant shared among members of a CREG is called a public specificity. Examples of CREGs are A2 CREG: A2, A28(68 + 69); A9(23 + 24); A1 CREG: A1, A11, A10(25 + 26 + 34 + 66), A3; B7 CREG: B7, B27, B22 (55 + 56), B42, B40(60 + 61). Renal transplant recipients frequently form antibodies against CREGs instead of against subtypic specificities. Identification of CREGs aids in preselecting a potential donor for whom the recipient will have a negative final crossmatch. Computer programs assist in this selection.

Cellular Detection of Class II Molecules

Peripheral blood T cells are able to recognize and respond to a wide variety of antigens by undergoing cell division *in vitro*. This response is measured by analyzing the level of DNA replication, using radioactive thymidine incorporated into the dividing cells. The molecules that stimulate this replication can be either antigens previously experienced by the individual (e.g., influenza antigens or tetanus toxoid) or alloantigens (e.g., HLA molecules). The response of one cell in tissue culture to the alloantigens on the surface of a second cell is called the mixed leukocyte culture (MLC) or mixed lymphocyte reaction (MLR). The MLC is considered an *in vitro* measure of Class II disparity between individuals and measures T cell recognition determinants found on the Class II molecules known collectively as HLA-D. The response is rendered unidirectional by preventing cells from one of the two individuals from replicating by treating those cells with radiation or mitomycin-C before addition to the culture.

MIXED LEUKOCYTE CULTURE. Before the existence of DNA-based HLA-typing methods, the MLC was used to assess the Class II compatibility between donor and recipients for bone marrow transplantation. The MLC represents a summation response of a responder cell to differences in the multiple determinants on HLA Class II molecules (DR, DQ, and DP) encoded by the irradiated stimulator cell haplotypes. The response to DR molecules appears to predominate. The role of DQ in the MLC is considerably less than DR. The role DP plays in mixed lymphocyte stimulation is minor; however, low level stimulation can be detected in an MLC in which HLA-DP is the only difference between two otherwise identical siblings as observed in families in which between *HLA-DQ* and *HLA-DP* recombination has occurred.

MLC TECHNIQUES. The basic miniaturized MLC culture and the harvesting techniques used today were developed in 1969 by Hartzman. Peripheral blood mononuclear cells free of platelets and erythrocytes are obtained by using Ficoll-Hypaque gradients. This lymphocyte separation method is particularly important since it removes most granulocytes that can nonspecifically suppress *in vitro* replication. Mononuclear stimulator cells are irradiated (generally 1500 rads) or treated with mitomycin-C (generally 25 to 50 μg/mL). Responder and stimulator cells are then added to 96-well tissue culture plates in a total volume of 50 to 200 μL of tissue culture medium containing several supplements, including serum and antibiotics. Cells are incubated at 37°C in a humidified atmosphere for five to six days, at which time 1 to 2 μCi ^{3}H-thymidine (2 to 20 Ci/mM) are added to each well, followed by 6 to 18 hours of additional incubation to permit uptake and incorporation of thymidine. In culture, cells undergo the process of recognition and then begin to divide. Under usual conditions, no thymidine incorporation can be detected for 48 to 72 hours, although increased glucose metabolism can be detected within one hour, and insulin and transferrin receptor changes can be identified within several hours after mixture. After the initial "latent" phase, replication begins and continues at a rapid pace up to the sixth to eighth day of culture, depending on the "strength" of the stimulus. Greater cellular activation results in earlier peak responses. During this time, many large blast lymphocytes can be seen in the culture, the number being proportional to the uptake of thymidine. Following culture, cells are washed free of unincorporated tritiated (^{3}H)-thymidine onto small fiberglass filters using a semiautomated harvester. The amount of ^{3}H-thymidine remaining on the filter and thus the amount of thymidine incorporation into the cells is assayed with a scintillation counter.

LIMITATIONS OF THE MLC. The MLC may be more sensitive in detecting HLA differences than serologic typing, since MLC reactivity may be stimulated by subtle antigenic differences, which include differences in HLA antigens as well as differences in minor histocompatibility antigens. It can also be used to validate other Class II–typing results as a type of cellular crossmatch. However, routine use of the MLC in clinical laboratories is declining because of problems inherent in the technique. The MLC technique is dependent on and can be influenced by health of the patient, type of disease, and history of prior transfusion (Mickelson, 1993; 1994). Frequently, the MLC either (1) cannot be performed because the patient has too few leukocytes or (2) cannot be interpreted because the patient is in blast crisis or does not respond to or stimulate donor cells or both. It is for these reasons that cellular assays are being replaced by the more precise DNA-based typing methods (Baxter-Lowe, 1992; Termijtelen, 1991).

5

DNA Typing of HLA Alleles

With the advent of rapid and reliable methods for the isolation and identification of Classes I and II genes and the determination of the nucleotide sequences of Classes I and II alleles, it has become possible to use DNA-based methods for HLA typing. DNA-based typing of Class II alleles, *HLA-DR, -DQ, -DP*, is now a commonly used technique in HLA typing laboratories; methods for DNA-based typing of Class I alleles of *HLA-A, -B, -C* are less well developed.

Although serologic and cellular typing of HLA antigens has been extremely useful, there are a number of technical drawbacks to these techniques as previously described. In addition, HLA alleles can specify HLA proteins that are indistinguishable using serologic typing. For example, an individual carrying the *DRB1*0401* allele would have the same serologic type (DR4) as an individual carrying the *DRB1*0412* allele (DR4). Thus, *DRB1*0401* and *DRB1*0412* are splits of the broad-specificity DR4. These splits are identified by DNA typing. Serologic reagents specific enough to define this split are not available. Currently, more than 15 subdivisions of DR4 have been defined. There are many other examples of defined splits using DNA typing that cannot be identified using serologic typing.

The problems with serologic typing are particularly acute when typing some population groups. For example, blacks sometimes express Class I and Class II antigens that are difficult to identify with the currently available serologic reagents (Opeltz, 1993). DNA-based HLA typing has greatly improved the ability to define HLA types in populations that have been serologically difficult to type. Although DNA-based HLA typing has been in practice only a few years, its reproducibility in large-scale typing using blind controls has been extraordinary (Ng, 1993).

PREPARATION AND AMPLIFICATION OF DNA. Any cell with a nucleus can be used as a source of DNA. Although red blood cells do not contain nuclei, other cells in the blood, such as lymphocytes, are a good source of DNA. Cell lines such as Epstein-Barr virus–transformed B lymphocytes are also a good source of DNA. Because transformed cells can be grown in culture in the laboratory, they provide an inexhaustible supply of DNA and are often used to provide reference DNA for quality control of typing procedures.

DNA is usually prepared from a small quantity (0.5-2 mL) of whole blood. Many different protocols can be used to isolate DNA from cells. One protocol uses Triton X–100 (a detergent) to lyse the cell membrane, releasing the nuclei (Shaffer, 1992). If the starting material was whole blood, these nuclei must then be washed extensively to remove any hemoglobin released by the red blood cells. The heme portion of hemoglobin interferes with the gene amplification reaction used to determine HLA types. The nuclei are lysed using another detergent, Tween-20. The DNA is freed from the proteins bound to it by treatment with proteinase K, an enzyme that destroys proteins. The proteinase K is later destroyed by incubation of the DNA at high temperatures (95°C). It is important to deactivate the proteinase K because it can degrade the enzyme used in the HLA-typing reaction. Commercial kits are also available for the preparation of DNA.

The sensitivity of detection is enhanced greatly by the amplification of DNA-encoding *HLA* genes using a technique called the polymerase chain reaction, or PCR (Saiki, 1988). A pair of synthetic oligonucleotides (primers) containing sequences found flanking a specific *HLA* gene are utilized to generate millions of copies of that gene for use in the HLA-typing reaction. Many typing reactions utilize primer sequences that are shared by all alleles at an *HLA* locus; other typing procedures use primer sets that are shared by only a subset of alleles at a locus. Annealing of the primers to sample DNA during the PCR reaction uses hybridization conditions guaranteeing that the primers will bind to perfectly matched sequences (target sequences) and not to sequences of other loci or other alleles that are not matched. By adjusting the temperature of the annealing component of the PCR reaction, the typing laboratory can control the specificity of the amplification.

SEQUENCE-SPECIFIC OLIGONUCLEOTIDE HYBRIDIZATION. It has been possible to use hybridization of sequence-specific oligonucleotide probes (SSOP) to DNA to identify alleles (e.g., Gao, 1990; Molkentin, 1991; Nevinny-Stickel, 1991). The use of several different oligonucleotides to define a specific *HLA* allele may be required when no unique sequence can be identified. This is especially true for the typing of *DP* alleles, which often share variable region sequences (Bugawan, 1990). A set of oligonucleotides capable of identifying each allele is hybridized to denatured PCR-amplified DNA attached to a solid support. Hybridization conditions are adjusted so that the oligonucleotides will anneal to denatured DNA containing the *HLA* alleles from which the oligonucleotide sequence was derived. The oligonucleotides are labeled with radioisotope or, more commonly, with a nonisotopic tag for detection. After visualization, the pattern of hybridization can be read to determine the alleles present. Figure 38–13 illustrates the approach using an oligonucleotide probe for the *DQB1* allele, *DQB1**0302*, to identify patients with insulin-dependent diabetes who carry this allele (Todd, 1987). The SSOP method is highly accurate, specific, and reliable (Ng, 1993). It is often used in situations in which many samples are typed in large batches, and it can provide allele-level resolution (see later). Commercial kits using this method are available.

In a related procedure, called the reverse dot blot, the oligonucleotide probes are bound to a solid support (Bugawan, 1994). DNA from the samples to be tested is amplified using primers labeled with biotin. The amplified DNA is then hybridized to the immobilized probes that contain sequences found in the alleles present in the DNA. After visualization (using an avidin-linked detection system), the pattern of hybridization can be read to determine the alleles present. This procedure is useful for typing a small number of samples at allele level resolution. Commercial kits utilizing this method are available.

SEQUENCE-SPECIFIC PRIMING. Another method of identifying HLA alleles uses sequence-specific primers (SSP) in the PCR reaction (Bunce, 1994; Olerup, 1992; Sadler, 1994). These primers anneal to denatured DNA containing the *HLA* alleles from which the primer sequences were derived. In the subsequent PCR reaction, only these selected alleles are amplified. DNA amplified by the primers is identified by gel electrophoresis. This procedure is useful in typing a small number of samples. It is more difficult to obtain allele-level resolution with this approach. Commercial kits are available.

NUCLEIC ACID SEQUENCING. A final method of identification of *HLA* alleles involves the direct determination of the DNA sequences of the *HLA* alleles carried by an individual. Sequencing is labor intensive and highly complex but will be used more frequently in the future to determine the level of HLA match between bone marrow transplant patients and their prospective donors (Petersdorf, 1994; Spurkland, 1993).

LEVEL OF RESOLUTION OF DNA-BASED TYPING. The level of resolution obtained by DNA-typing methods is controlled by the choice and number of primers and/or probes used in the assay. This may depend on the purpose of the typing (e.g., large-scale bone marrow registry typing versus typing of an actual bone marrow donor-recipient combination), the time available for carrying out the typing, the cost of typing, and the expertise of the laboratory.

A multistep approach is often used to identify HLA alleles by DNA-based typing. For this reason, HLA types defined by DNA-based typing may be reported at different levels of res-

	50										60
DQB1*0501	GTG	ACG	CCG	CAG	GGG	CGG	CCT	GTT	GCC	GAG	TAC
DQB1*0601	---	--C	---	---	---	---	---	-AC	---	---	---
DQB1*0201	---	---	-T-	-T-	---	-T-	---	-CC	---	---	---
DQB1*0301	---	---	---	-T-	---	-C-	---	-AC	---	---	---
DQB1*0302	---	---	---	-T-	---	-C-	---	-CC	---	---	---
DQB1*0303	---	---	---	-T-	---	-C-	---	-AC	---	---	---
DQB1*0401	---	---	---	-T-	---	---	-T-	-AC	---	---	---

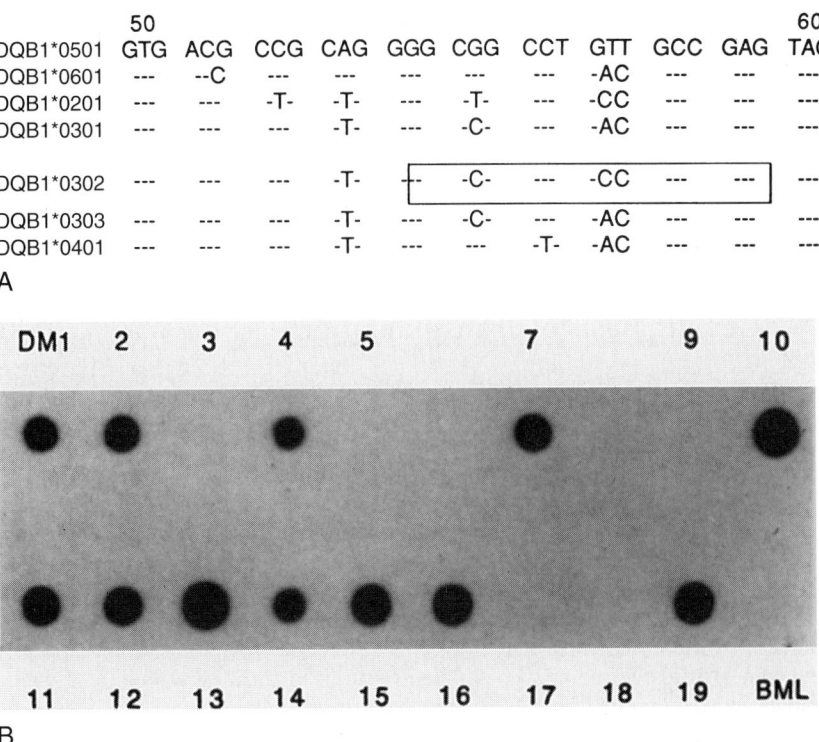

A

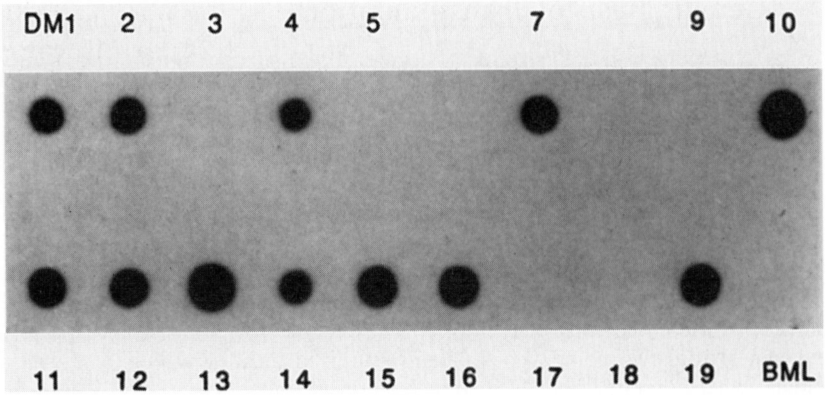

B

Figure 38–13. *A*, Nucleotide sequences of several *DQB1* alleles. The sequences presented cover the codons for amino acids 50 to 60. A dash indicates that the nucleotide is identical to the top sequence. An oligonucleotide that is specific for the DQB1*0302 sequence is boxed. *B*, Oligonucleotide dot blot analysis of 17 IDDM patients (DM1-19) and 1 control, BML. Amplified DNA containing Class II *DQB1* sequences from the patients was attached to a membrane and hybridized to the radiolabeled oligonucleotide specific for the DQB1*0302 sequence (described earlier). Positive hybridization signals indicate the patients who carry this *DQB1* gene sequence (patients DM1, 2, 4, 7, 10–16, 19). (From Todd JA, Bell J, McDevitt HO: HLA-DQB gene contributes to susceptibility and resistance to insulin-dependent diabetes mellitus. Nature 1987; 329:599.)

olution. Low–resolution (or generic- or serologic-) level DNA-based typing produces a result similar in appearance and detail to a serologic type. For example, a DNA-defined type, *DRB1*11* or *DRB1*11XX* is the equivalent of the serologic type DR11. The XX indicates that the allele was not further defined. At this level of resolution, it is not possible to determine which of the more than fifteen *DRB1*11* alleles is carried by the individual being tested. Although serologic typing is as informative as low-resolution typing, results are more reliable with DNA-based typing. Intermediate resolution–level DNA-based typing may narrow down the choices by listing several different possibilities for the type of an individual—for example, *DRB1*1101* or *DRB1*1104*. Finally, high-resolution level (or allele-level) DNA-based typing identifies the specific allele carried by an individual (e.g., *DRB1*1104*).

Differences in interpretation of HLA-typing results can arise because of the typing methodology chosen (serologic typing versus DNA-based typing). It is, therefore, critical to include an expert in histocompatibility testing in the interpretation of HLA-typing results and in the selection of a transplant donor. Experts in HLA typing know the strengths and weaknesses of each method of typing as well as the combinations of *HLA* alleles and the frequency of alleles in the population, information that is important in determining a search strategy for a patient requiring an unrelated bone marrow transplant.

TISSUE AND ORGAN TRANSPLANTATION

Long-term survival of solid organ and bone marrow transplants represents one of the most challenging goals in medical science. Renal transplantation is a routine procedure in more than 240 major North American medical centers as the therapy of choice for most patients with end-stage renal disease. More recently, bone marrow, heart, heart-lung, and liver transplantation have gained wide acceptance as therapeutic procedures. The primary obstacle to solid organ transplantation is the immunologically mediated rejection of the graft. Allograft rejection is a manifestation of the uniqueness of the individual and is an innate property of the immune system because the survival of an individual is dependent upon the ability to recognize foreign antigens (be they viral or bacterial pathogens, tumor cells, or, unfortunately, allogeneic tissue) and to respond to them. Therefore, the success of allografts relies on the ability to circumvent the immune reaction, which is accomplished largely by two means:

(1) Immunosuppressive therapy—cytotoxic and immunosuppressive agents such as azathioprine and prednisone have been used with moderate success for more than 35 years. Cyclosporin A has been used extensively since 1981; it is a powerful immunosuppressive agent that has improved the success of all transplantation, most strikingly in nonrenal transplants. New immunosuppressants are being studied in clinical trials and may further improve the success of transplantations.

(2) Histocompatibility matching between the donor and the recipient—optimal histocompatibility matching for HLA increases cadaveric renal allograft survival between 10% to 20% at one year after engraftment, and the differences in graft survival between well-matched and poorly matched patients increases incrementally at further time points. In addition, better matching in first transplantations decreases sensitization and thus improves the probability for successful retransplantation following first graft failure. Preliminary evidence suggests that HLA matching for other organs (heart and liver) may be beneficial, although the short time interval

between harvest and transplantation may in practice preclude matching. Although HLA matching of donor and recipient is important, in renal transplants there are HLA mismatches. These generally include mismatches within cross-reactive HLA groups. In contrast, with rare exceptions, extremely close HLA matching of the donor and recipient is required in allogeneic bone marrow transplantation to prevent graft rejection and failure of engraftment; to reduce graft *versus* host (GVH) disease; and to enhance immune reconstitution.

Genetic Basis of Transplantation

The genetic basis of transplantation was first determined in 1916 as a result of tumor transplantation experiments in mice and was subsequently extended to transplants of normal tissue (Snell, 1981). It was demonstrated that skin grafts (syngeneic) within inbred strains that were homozygous at histocompatibility loci were successful, but grafts between two different inbred strains (allografts) were rejected. Furthermore, allografts from either parental inbred strain (two copies of the same *HLA* genes; homozygous) to first generation (F1) hybrids (one copy of each of two different sets of *HLA* genes from two homozygous parents) survived in all animals, whereas grafts from F1 hybrid offspring to either parent did not survive. These observations established the laws of transplantation. In 1948, the factors or genes determining the fate of allografts were named histocompatibility, or *H* genes. Also in 1948, the major histocompatibility locus in the mouse, *H-2*, was defined by Gorer. There are other histocompatibility or *H* systems in the mouse, but these histocompatibility antigens (called minor histocompatibility antigens) have a relatively small effect on the outcome of grafting and can be overcome by immunosuppression much more easily than mismatches for the major histocompatibility genes.

Because convincing evidence already existed in experimental animals that molecules encoded by the MHC represent the major barriers to successful allografting, HLA typing was used to determine compatibility between human donor and recipient. Initially, the influence of HLA antigens on graft survival was investigated by Amos and colleagues through skin grafting between family members. As in studies with inbred mice, skin grafts between HLA-identical siblings survival significantly longer than grafts between one–haplotype matched siblings, parents, or unrelated donors. These observations were extended to and confirmed in renal transplantation during the late 1960s and early 1970s.

Renal Transplantation

Figure 38–14 shows the 10-year survival of renal allografts from the UCLA registry among the three main categories of donors: (1) HLA-identical sibling, (2) haploidentical parent, and (3) cadaver donor. The long-term risk period (greater than one year post-transplantation) is characterized by a failure rate that produces a straight line when plotted on a log scale. This failure rate is characteristic of each category of histocompatibility, and the slope of the line has not changed in the past 10 years. Overall grafts between HLA-identical siblings do best (74% at 10 years). Haploidentical

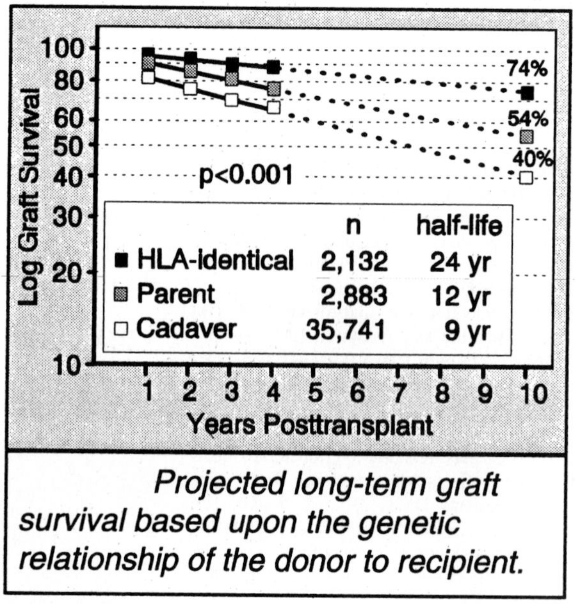

Figure 38–14. Ten-year renal allograft survival of three main categories of histocompatibility. (Cecka JM, Terasaki P: The UNOS Scientific Registry. 1993; 1–18.)

grafts survive less well (54% at 10 years). Haplodistinct, or two-haplotype, mismatched cadaveric donor grafts survive least well (40% at 10 years) (Cecka, 1993). Thus, provided medical reasons permit, the order of priorities in living, related allograft donor selection is based on decreasing order of histocompatibility: (1) monozygotic twin; (2) HLA-identical siblings; (3) HLA-haploidentical sibling, child, or parent; (4) first-order relatives: grandparents, aunts, uncles, or cousins, preferably haploidentical. A monozygotic twin also shares minor histocompatibility antigens and may be the ultimate match, equal to an autograft.

The original finding that organ transplants between HLA-identical (and ABO-compatible) siblings survive very well and significantly better than organs transplanted between HLA-mismatched siblings or parents has been consistently confirmed. These data comparing HLA-matched and HLA-mismatched sibling donors leave no room for doubt that the HLA complex represents a major barrier to successful renal transplantation and is indeed the major histocompatibility complex in humans.

TRANSPLANTS FROM CADAVERIC DONORS. Compared with results obtained with living, related transplants, the results of matching for HLA in cadaver (unrelated) transplants has not been clear until recently. As definition of HLA antigens has become better refined and as large databases have been generated, it has become clear that cadaveric renal allografts that are phenotypically identical for HLA-A, -B, and -DR (i.e., zero antigen mismatch) survive as well at three years as grafts from genotypically HLA-identical siblings (Fig. 38–15) (Zhou, 1993). In addition, projected 10-year survival rates of zero HLA-A, -B, -DR–mismatched cadaveric donor grafts is only slightly less than for the zero-mismatched HLA-identical sibling rate (65% versus 74%). Thus, the United Network for Organ Sharing (UNOS) requires mandatory sharing of zero HLA-A, -B, -DR–mismatched cadaveric kidneys. Transplants with one or two HLA-A, -B,

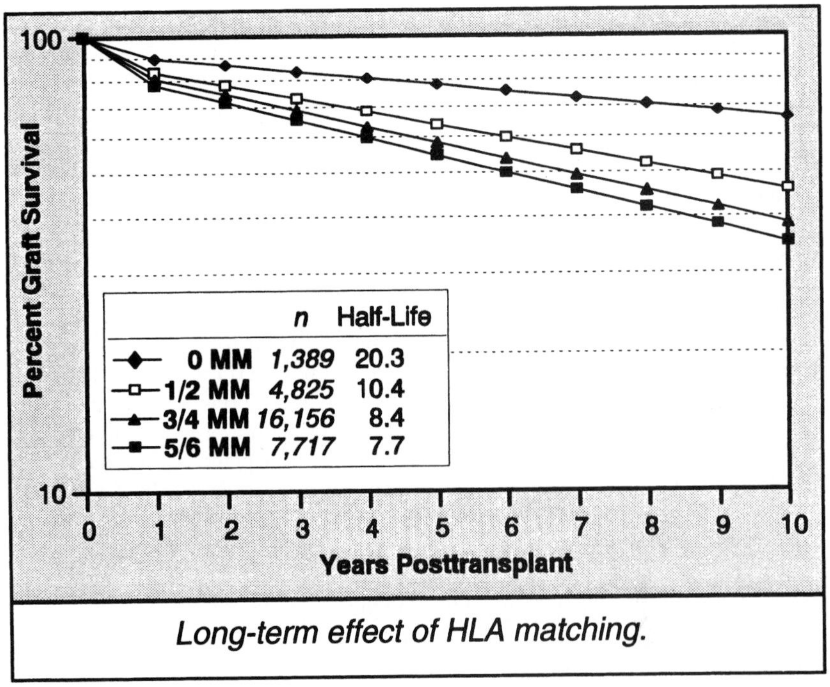

Figure 38–15. Effect of HLA-A, B, or DR mismatching in cadaver donor recipients treated with CsA, projected for 10 years. MM indicates mismatches of A, B, or DR antigens. (Zhou YC, Cecka JM: Effect of HLA matching on renal transplant survival. Clinical Transplants 1993; 499–509.)

-DR antigen mismatches also survive well (a predicted 45% at 10 years); however, mismatching for more than two HLA-A, -B, -DR antigens does not appear to be as successful. Since rejection of poorly matched allografts results in highly sensitized patients in whom transplantation is difficult and since second and subsequent transplants overall do less well, the goal should be to provide as many patients as possible with kidneys from zero to two antigen—mismatched donors.

THE LYMPHOCYTE CROSSMATCH. The crossmatch test measures the state of presensitization, if any, in the potential recipient against a specific donor. A positive crossmatch between donor lymphocytes and recipient serum is contraindicative to performing that specific transplantation for renal and pancreas allografts, since studies in the early 1980s showed a high correlation of positive crossmatch with hyperacute rejection. This is not surprising because HLA antigens are expressed at a high level in the kidney.

Complement-mediated lymphocytotoxicity is used conventionally for the crossmatch procedure in all HLA laboratories. This assay, which tests for the presence of cytotoxic HLA antibodies in the serum of the potential recipient that react with lymphocytes of the specific donor, is probably the most important contribution of the HLA tissue typing–laboratory to clinical renal transplantation. A crossmatch must be performed prior to transplantation. For patients with no sensitization (i.e., 0% PRA; see later section), the most recent serum sample can be used. If the patient has pre-existing lymphocytotoxic antibodies or has had a recent sensitizing event such as a blood transfusion, a current serum screening sample (i.e., within 48 hours of transplantation) should be collected. In the case of blood transfusion, a serum sample obtained at least 14 days post-alloimmunization should also be used for crossmatching. Each serum sample should be tested undiluted and at one or more dilutions in duplicate, using at least two techniques: one standard lymphocytotoxicity technique and one more sensitive technique (e.g., extended incubation times or the use of antiglobulin). In the antiglobulin-augmented technique, the sensitivity of a crossmatch is increased by incubating the cells with an antibody against human immunoglobulins after the cells have been exposed to the test sera and then washed. Serum samples from potential recipients should be stored at − 70°C and be protected from carbon dioxide and from evaporation. Serum samples used for crossmatching should be retained in the frozen state for at least 12 months following transplantation.

In recent years, the theory and practice of crossmatch techniques and interpretation have changed. Currently, the only unequivocal statement that can be made is that a positive T cell crossmatch (i.e., donor T lymphocytes as the target for possible antibodies in a current recipient serum sample that is negative with autologous lymphocytes) detected by a conventional lymphocytotoxicity technique is contraindicative to transplantation. However, it is becoming increasingly clear that a more sensitive technique, such as the antiglobulin-augmented microlymphocytotoxicity test, flow cytometry, or both, should be used to detect antibodies directed against T cells in re-transplantation. The majority of antibodies detected by such methods are against HLA-A, -B, -C antigens. The consequences of a positive crossmatch with all other techniques using other cell types are unclear. These techniques and the controversies of crossmatching are summarized in the following paragraphs.

HISTORIC POSITIVE AND CURRENT NEGATIVE CROSSMATCH. Previously it was thought that since memory T cells are long-lived, a positive crossmatch with any serum sample (historic or current) was contraindicative of transplantation of an organ from that donor into the recipient. Following a negative crossmatch with a current serum sample, many transplant centers now carry out successful transplantation even though there may be a positive crossmatch with a historic serum sample (a sample taken more than three to six months pretransplant) (Cardella, 1982). One of the

5

benefits of this approach is that transplantation candidates with a high level of sensitization that has decreased over time have a higher probability of receiving a transplant. Although overall allograft survival has been good following this protocol, there are a few patients who reject their graft in an accelerated fashion. Thus, some centers require that the transplant candidate receive a blood transfusion during those three to six months to identify patients with active suppression of a specific immune response that is likely to be beneficial rather than detrimental to the transplant. One group has shown that transplant recipients with a current negative and historic positive crossmatch who had an uneventful clinical course following grafting exhibited antibodies in the current serum sample that neutralized the donor-specific anti-HLA antibodies found in the historic serum sample, that is, neutralizing or anti-idiotypic antibodies (Reed, 1987). In contrast, transplant recipients with a current negative and historic positive crossmatch who did not have successful transplantation failed to express neutralizing (anti-idiotypic) antibodies in the current serum sample. Thus, as an adjunct crossmatch procedure, the identification of antibodies (e.g., anti-idiotypic) in the serum sample may identify those donors that may not be rejected by a previously sensitized recipient.

AUTOANTIBODIES. The presence of circulating autoantibodies in the recipient is not harmful to the allograft. Thus, an autocrossmatch should be performed, and if autoantibodies are present, the sera used for crossmatching should be adsorbed to remove the autoreactivity. HLA laboratories use heat inactivation at 63°C ± 1° or the reducing agents DTE (dithioerythritol) or DTT (dithiothreitol) to differentiate between IgM and IgG antibodies in serum samples because autoantibodies are primarily IgM and HLA antibodies are primarily IgG (Barger, 1989). If the heat-inactivated or DTT-treated serum sample is negative and the untreated sample is positive, many transplantation centers proceed with transplantation. However, DTT or heat inactivation should be used with caution as an auxiliary crossmatch procedure, since not all anti-HLA antibodies are IgG.

B CELL ANTIBODIES. Antibodies detected in a B cell crossmatch (against donor B lymphocytes) can be (1) anti–HLA-DR, -DQ; (2) weak anti–HLA-A, -B, -C antibodies (B cells have a higher density of Class I molecules and are more sensitive to complement-dependent assays than are T cells); and/or (3) non-HLA antibodies (e.g., autoantibodies). The significance of a positive B cell crossmatch is unclear because many B cell crossmatches are performed with sera that have not been adsorbed with platelets to remove anti-HLA-A, -B, -C antibodies (platelets do not express HLA-DR, -DQ molecules). Although in a number of transplant centers, a positive B cell crossmatch is not contraindicative of transplantation, a large study in Minneapolis indicated that a positive crossmatch with platelet-adsorbed serum correlated with poor graft survival at two years (Noreen, 1989). In addition, there are cases in the literature in which there are early adverse effects of DR-specific, high-titered antibodies. B cell crossmatches should be performed with platelet-adsorbed sera, and care should be taken to eliminate autoantibodies.

SUPPLEMENTAL SENSITIVE CROSSMATCH TECHNIQUES. The significance of results using highly sensitive techniques to detect low levels of preformed antibodies is unclear, at least for first transplantations. Examples of such sensitive techniques are antiglobulin-augmented microlymphocytotoxicity and flow cytometry. Possibly because of better immunosuppressive regimens, it now appears that results obtained with supplemental sensitive crossmatch techniques may not correlate with clinical outcome (incidence of hyperacute rejection and accelerated rejection, and number of rejection episodes) in first transplantations. However, in subsequent transplantations, these sensitive techniques are probably clinically relevant. One retrospective study showed that results obtained with the antiglobulin-augmented technique may predict those patients who will have more rejection episodes and thus may aid in post-transplantation management. In another retrospective study using flow cytometry, early graft failure was thought to be due to "hidden hyperacute" rejection, which would have been detected by flow cytometric crossmatch techniques. Thus, many laboratories are performing the antiglobulin-augmented lymphocytotoxicity and/or the flow cytometric crossmatch routinely for re-transplants. A useful attribute of the flow cytometric crossmatch is that the immunoglobulin subclass (IgG *versus* IgM) can be determined as well as the type of cell that binds the alloantibody (T cell *versus* B cell *versus* monocyte). However, flow cytometry does not alleviate the need for absorption of Class I–specific antibodies to determine the presence of Class II–specific antibodies in the patient's serum.

ANTIBODY SCREENING (PERCENTAGE OF REACTIVE ANTIBODY). For renal transplantation candidates, it is mandatory that monthly serum samples be screened for the presence of lymphocytotoxic antibody to determine the state of presensitization of the transplantation candidate. The serum should be screened with the same techniques as those used in the final crossmatch. These serum samples also provide material for use in crossmatching. In addition, it is advisable to identify the most reactive serum sample following rejection and/or nephrectomy of a rejected graft and after blood transfusions. This is determined by testing serum samples obtained at frequent time intervals in the four weeks following the sensitizing event. The presence of lymphocytotoxic antibodies is determined by testing with a well-characterized panel of T cells. A sufficient number of individuals must be included in the cell panel that is used for screening to ensure that any HLA-directed antibody is detected. As far as possible, the individuals used in this panel should remain the same so that results can be compared from month to month. In addition, the distribution of ethnic groups in the cell panel should mirror the patient population. Results are reported as percentage reactive antibody (PRA). The HLA specificity of the antibody is reported if it can be determined.

Patients with PRAs in excess of 60% have a greatly decreased likelihood of a negative crossmatch and thus of successfully receiving a transplant. Currently, approximately one third of the transplant candidate pool has a PRA of greater than 60%. The accumulation of large numbers of highly sensitized patients, resulting primarily from rejection of poorly matched allografts is a major problem because these patients remain on the potential recipient list for long periods of time and are difficult to manage clinically. UNOS distributes trays that contain serum samples from registered transplantation candidates who have high PRAs (greater than

80%) to collaborating HLA-typing laboratories. This allows rapid testing of cadaver donors to facilitate the identification of crossmatch-compatible kidneys for these highly sensitized patients and reduces ischemia time in the allocation of cadaver kidneys.

Nonrenal Organ Transplantation

This includes heart, liver, lung, heart-lung, and pancreas transplantation. Patients and donors should be typed for HLA whenever possible for retrospective analysis. Likewise, monthly serum antibody screenings are recommended to identify the state of sensitization. In most cases, a pretransplantation crossmatch is not practical because of the lengthy testing required. However, whenever possible, it is recommended to prospectively crossmatch patients at risk for allograft rejection, specifically including those with a PRA of greater than 15%. Retrospective analysis in recipients of both heart and liver transplants suggests that matching for HLA does have a beneficial effect.

Allogeneic Bone Marrow Transplantation

Allogeneic bone marrow transplantation is performed for hematologic malignancies and disorders, bone marrow failure, certain inherited metabolic disorders such as lipid storage diseases, and congenital immunodeficiency syndrome (Parkman, 1986). From an HLA-matching standpoint, the best bone marrow donor is either self (autologous transplant), if the malignancy is not one that involves the bone marrow or if the disease is not genetic, or an identical twin (syngeneic transplant). Marrow from an HLA-identical sibling donor is a frequent source. The use of a sibling donor also increases the probability that non-HLA genes that might affect transplantation success and that are not well defined (i.e., minor histocompatibility genes) are more likely to be matched (Marijit, 1993).

Since most patients (~70%) do not have an HLA-matched sibling and because of the success with HLA-matched, unrelated bone marrow donor transplants, national registries of unrelated bone marrow donors have been developed around the world (Beatty, 1988; Kernan, 1993). The National Marrow Donor Program (NMDP) in the United States is such a registry and contains over 1.5 million HLA-typed donors, making it the largest unrelated donor registry in the world. In North America, approximately 3000 unrelated donor transplantations facilitated by the NMDP have been performed since the registry began in 1987.

Bone marrow transplants are among the most difficult of all clinical procedures for several reasons. First, at the time of transplantation, the recipients are nearly totally immunodeficient, either because of inherited deficiency (SCID) or because of the pretransplantation therapy (cytotoxic chemotherapy and irradiation), which prevents the immune system of the recipient from rejecting the donor marrow that is infused several days after pretreatment. The amount of cytotoxic pretreatment is high enough to eliminate circulating leukocytes, nearly eliminate platelets, and abrogate production of new erythrocytes. Thus, the recipient is profoundly susceptible to all types of infection and would certainly die if not rescued by extraordinary medical care and the transfused bone marrow. The second profound risk is the potential of immunologic attack of the recipient by the transplanted allogeneic marrow, resulting in GVH disease. GVH disease has several forms and can be fatal. In spite of these difficulties, a number of transplant centers have achieved exceptional success. In 1993, approximately 3500 allogeneic bone marrow transplantations had been performed in North America (Horowitz, International Bone Marrow Transplant Registry preliminary data). However, in 1994 alone, more than 800 marrow transplants were performed with unrelated donors. Recent reports demonstrate extraordinary success with allogeneic marrow transplantation for aplastic anemia (75% to 95% survival) and good success for leukemic patients receiving transplantations during their first or second remission of the disease. Long-term success rates with unrelated matched donor marrow are similar to success rates in which marrow from HLA-matched siblings is used. Allogeneic marrow transplantation frequently results in disease cure with no required therapy after completion of post-transplant prophylaxis for GVH disease.

Allogeneic bone marrow transplantation may be used in time to treat a wide variety of diseases. New approaches, such as the collection of hematopoietic stem cells from growth factor–mobilized peripheral blood or umbilical cord blood stem cells increase the availability of unrelated donors. Bone marrow transplantation can also be used to generate immune responses directed at malignant cells. Relapse of disease following transplantation is greater for patients receiving an HLA-matched graft, suggesting that some degree of mismatching may be beneficial in stimulating an immune response against tumor cells (Beatty, 1993). If the problems surrounding this most difficult procedure are overcome, bone marrow transplantation may become one of the most widely used methods for the treatment of a variety of diseases.

HLA TYPING FOR BONE MARROW TRANSPLANTATION. The bone marrow pretransplantation workup includes HLA-A, -B, and -DR typing of all available members of the immediate family to establish inheritance of haplotypes. DNA-based typing for Class II genes has become standard and DNA-based typing for Class I genes is beginning to be incorporated. Typing of the extended family and allele level or high–resolution level typing of specific HLA Class I and Class II loci, typing of complement loci, and *GLO* typing, or use of the MLC to measure compatibility may also be appropriate.

5

The level of resolution in HLA-typing differs for bone marrow and solid organ transplantation. It is likely that a higher resolution HLA typing is required to match donor and recipient for bone marrow transplantation than is required for solid organ transplantation because bone marrow transplant involves the transfer of an entire immune system to the patient. Preliminary data suggest that matching donor and recipient for *HLA-DRB1* alleles (*DR* types) is most important for bone marrow transplant success (Hansen, 1994) although the relative importance of matching alleles for other HLA antigens is not yet clear (Beatty, 1993; Petersdorf, 1993).

DNA-based typing methods for HLA typing reveal a large number of HLA alleles and combinations of alleles present within human populations. With this level of resolution, it is difficult to identify a genetically identical *HLA*-matched donor for some individuals. Current research is focused on the importance and level of matching required for each gene. It is likely that matching alleles at every *HLA* gene will not be critical. In addition, efforts must turn toward defining approaches toward intelligent HLA mismatching in transplantation. In the case of bone marrow transplantation, this means matching to decrease graft rejection and GVH disease while eliminating the cancer or other fatal blood disease with effective engraftment and reconstitution of immune responses.

SUMMARY

The polymorphism of the HLA system plays a major role in the generation of immune responses to pathogens, in tissue transplantation, and in susceptibility to autoimmune disorders. New methods for identification and characterization of MHC alleles and molecules have extended the understanding of the major histocompatibility complex and its role in the human immune response.

Aizawa M (ed): HLA in Asia-Oceania 1986. Proceedings of the 3rd Asia-Oceania Histocompatibility Workshop Conference. Sapporo, Japan, Hokkaido University Press, 1986.

American Society for Histocompatibility and Immunogenetics Laboratory Manual. 3rd ed. Lenexa, Kansas, American Society for Histocompatibility and Immunogenetics, 1994.

Barger BO, Shroyer TW, Hudson SL, et al: Successful renal allografts in recipients with a positive standard, DTE negative crossmatch. Transplant Proc 1989; 21:746.

Baxter-Lowe LA, Eckels DD, Ash R, et al: The predictive value of HLA-DR oligotyping for MLC responses. Transplantation 1992; 53: 1352–1357.

Beatty PG, Anasetti C, Hansen JA, et al: Marrow transplantation from unrelated donors for treatment of hematologic malignancies: Effect of mismatching for one HLA locus. Blood 1993; 81:249–253.

Beatty PG, Dahlberg S, Mickelson EM, et al: Probability of finding HLA-matched unrelated marrow donors. Transplantation 1988; 45:714–718.

Bjorkman PJ, Parham P: Structure, function, and diversity of class I major histocompatibility complex molecules. Annu Rev Biochem 1990; 59:253–288.

Bjorkman PJ, Saper MA, Samraoui B, et al: Structure of the human class I histocompatibility antigen, HLA-A2. Nature 1987; 329:506.

Bodmer JG, Marsh SGE, Albert ED, et al: Nomenclature for factors of the HLA system, 1991. Tissue Antigens 1992; 39:161–173.

Bodmer JG, Marsh SGE, Albert ED, et al: Nomenclature for factors of the HLA system, 1994. Hum Immunol 1994; 41:1–20.

Brown JH, Jardetzky TS, Gorga JC, et al: Three-dimensional structure of the human class II histocompatibility antigen HLA-DR1. Nature 1993; 364:33–39.

Bugawan TL, Apple R, Erlich HA: A method for typing polymorphism at the HLA-A locus using PCR amplification and immobilized oligonucleotide probes. Tissue Antigens 1994; 44:137–147.

Bugawan TL, Begovich AB, Erlich HA: Rapid HLA-DPB typing using enzymatically amplified DNA and nonradioactive sequence-specific oligonucleotide probes. Immunogenetics 1990; 32:231–241.

Bunce M, Welsh KI: Rapid DNA typing for HLA-C using sequence specific primers (PCR-SSP): Identification of serological and non-serologically defined HLA-C alleles including several new alleles. Tissue Antigens 1994; 43:7–17.

Campbell RD, Trowsdale J: Map of the human MHC. Immunol Today 1993; 14:349–352.

Cardella CJ, Falk JA, Nicholson MJ, et al: Successful renal transplantation in patients with T-cell reactivity to donor. Lancet 1982; 2:1240.

Cecka JM, Terasaki P: The UNOS Scientific Registry. Clin Transplants 1993; 1–18.

Cresswell P: Assembly, transport, and function of MHC class II molecules. Annu Rev Immunol 1994; 12:259–293.

Crow JF: Genetics Notes. Minneapolis, Burgess Publishing Co., 1976.

Dausset J: The Nobel Lectures in Immunology. Lecture for the Nobel Prize for Physiology or Medicine, 1980: The major histocompatibility complex in man. Past, present, and future concepts. Scand J Immunol 1992; 36:146–155.

Engelhard VH: Structure of peptides associated with class I and class II MHC molecules. Annu Rev Immunol 1994; 12:181–207.

Gao X, Fernandez-Vina M, Shumway W, Stastny P: DNA typing for class II HLA antigens with allele-specific or group-specific amplification. I. Typing for subsets of HLA-DR4. Hum Immunol 1990; 27:40–50.

Garrido F, Cabrera T, Concha A, et al: Natural history of HLA expression during tumour development. Immunol Today 1993; 14:491–499.

Germain RN, Margulies DH: The biochemistry and cell biology of antigen processing and presentation. Annu Rev Immunol 1993; 11:403–450.

Glimcher LH, Kara CJ: Sequences and factors: A guide to MHC class-II transcription. Annu Rev Immunol 1992; 10:13–49.

Gorga JC: Structural analysis of class II major histocompatibility complex proteins. Crit Rev Immunol 1992; 11:305–335.

Guardiola J, Maffei A: Control of MHC class II gene expression in autoimmune, infectious, and neoplastic diseases. Crit Rev Immunol 1993; 13:247–268.

Hansen JA, Anasetti C, Petersdorf E, Martin PJ: Marrow transplants from unrelated donors. Transplant Proc 1994; 26:1710–1712.

Heinrichs H, Orr HT: HLA non-A, -B, -C class I genes: Their structure and expression. Immunol Res 1990; 9:265–274.

Howcroft TK, Strebel K, Martin MA, Singer DS: Regression of MHC class I gene promoter activity by two-exon Tat of HIV. Science. 1993; 260:1320–1322.

Imanishi T, Akaza T, Kimura A, et al: Allele and haplotype frequencies for HLA and complement loci in various ethnic groups. *In* Tsuji K, Aizawa M, Sasazuki T: HLA 1991, vol 1. New York, Oxford University Press, 1992, pp 1065–1220.

Jordan BR, Caillol D, Damotte M, et al: HLA Class I genes: From structure to expression, serology, and function. Immunol Rev 1985; 84:73.

Jorgensen JL, Reay PA, Ehrich EW, Davis MM: Molecular components of T-cell recognition. Annu Rev Immunol 1992; 10:835–873.

Kappes D, Strominger JL: Human class II major histocompatibility complex genes and proteins. Annu Rev Biol 1988; 57:991–1028.

Kernan NA, Bartsch G, Ash RC, et al: Analysis of 462 transplantations from unrelated donors facilitated by the National Marrow Donor Program. N Engl J Med 1993; 328:593–602.

Kovats S, Drover S, Marshall WH, et al: Coordinate defects in human histocompatibility leukocyte antigen class II expression and antigen presentation in bare lymphocyte syndrome. J Exp Med 1994; 179:2017–2022.

Marijit EAF, Veenhof WRJ, Goulmy E, et al: Multiple minor histocompatibility antigen disparities between a recipient and four HLA-identical potential sibling donors for bone marrow transplantation. Hum Immunol 1993; 37:221–228.

Mickelson EM, Bartsch GE, Hansen JA, Dupont B: The MLC assay as a test for HLA-D region compatibility between patients and unrelated donors: Results of a National Marrow Donor Program involving multiple centers. Tissue Antigens 1993; 42:465–472.

Mickelson EM, Guthrie LA, Etzoni R, et al: Role of the mixed lymphocyte culture (MLC) reaction in marrow donor selection: Matching for transplants from related haploidentical donors. Tissue Antigens 1994; 44:83–92.

Molkentin J, Gorski J, Baxter-Lowe LA: Detection of 14 HLA-DQB1 alleles by oligotyping. Hum Immunol 1991; 31:114–122.

Morris P, Shaman J, Attaya M, et al: An essential role for HLA-DM in antigen presentation by class II major histocompatibility molecules. Nature 1994; 368:551–554.

Nepom GT, Erlich H: MHC class-II molecules and autoimmunity. Annu Rev Immunol 1991; 9:493–525.

Nevinny-Stickel C, Bettinotti MDLP, Andreas A, et al: Nonradioactive HLA class II typing using polymerase chain reaction and digoxigenin-11-2′-3′-dideoxy-uridine-triphosphate–labeled oligonucleotide probes. Hum Immunol 1991; 31:7–13.

Ng J, Hurley CK, Baxter-Lowe LA, et al: Large-scale oligonucleotide typing for HLA-DRB1/3/4 and HLA-DQB1 is highly accurate, specific, and reliable. Tissue Antigens 1993; 42:473–479.

Noreen HJ, van der Hagen E, Bach FH, et al: Renal allograft survival in CSA-treated patients with positive donor-specific B cell crossmatches. Transplant Proc 1989; 21:691.

Olerup O, Zetterquist H: HLA-DR typing by PCR amplification with sequence-specific primers (PCR-SSP) in 2 hours: An alternative to serological DR typing in clinical practice including donor-recipient matching in cadaveric transplantations. Tissue Antigens 1992; 39:225–235.

Opeltz G, Wujciak T, Schwarz V, et al: Collaborative transplant study analysis of graft survival in blacks. Transplant Proc 1993; 25: 2443–2445.

Parham P, Lawlor DA, Salter RD, et al: HLA-A, B, C: patterns of polymorphism in peptide-binding proteins. *In* Dupont B, et al (eds): Immunobiology of HLA, vol 1. New York, Springer-Verlag, 1989, pp 10–33.

Parkman R: The application of bone marrow transplantation to the treatment of genetic diseases. Science 1986; 232:1373–1378.

Paul WE, Seder RA: Lymphocyte responses and cytokines. Cell 1994; 76:241–251.

Payne R, Tripp M, Weigle J, et al: A new leukocyte isoantigen system in man. Cold Spring Harbor Symp Quant Biol 1964; 29:285–295.

Perkins HA, Hansen JA: The U.S. National Marrow Donor Program. Am J Ped Hem Onc, 1994, 16:30–34.

Petersdorf EW, Smith AJ, Mickelson EM, et al: The role of HLA-DPB1 disparity on the development of acute graft-versus-host disease following unrelated donor marrow transplantation. Blood 1993; 81:1923–1932.

Petersdorf EW, Stanley JF, Martin PJ, Hansen JA: Molecular diversity of the HLA-C locus in unrelated marrow transplantation. Tissue Antigens 1994; 44:93–99.

Reed E, Hardy M, Benvenisty A, et al: Effect of antiidiotypic antibodies to HLA on graft survival in renal allograft recipients. N Engl J Med 1987; 316:1450.

Rodey GE, Fuller TC: Public epitopes and the antigenic structure of the HLA molecules. CRC Crit Rev Immunol 1987; 7:229.

Sadler AM, Petronzelli F, Krausa P, et al: Low resolution DNA typing for HLA-B using sequence-specific primers in allele- or group-specific ARMS/PCR. Tissue Antigens 1994; 44:148–154.

Saiki RK, Gelfand DH, Stoffel S, et al: Primer-directed enzymatic amplification of DNA with a thermostable DNA polymerase. Science 1988; 239:487–491.

Schmidt CM, Orr HT: Maternal/fetal interactions: The role of the MHC class I molecule HLA-G. Crit Rev Immunol 1993; 13:207–224.

Shaffer AL, Falk-Wade JA, Tortorelli V, et al: HLA-DRw52–associated DRB1 alleles: Identification using polymerase chain reaction–amplified DNA, sequence-specific oligonucleotide probes, and a chemiluminescent detection system. Tissue Antigens 1992; 39:84–90.

Shaw S, Kavathas P, Pollack MS, et al: Family studies define a new histocompatibility locus, SB, between HLA-DR and GLO. Nature 1981; 293:745.

Singer DS, Maguire JE: Regulation of the expression of class I MHC genes. CRC Crit Rev Immunol 1990; 10:235–257.

Snell GD: Studies in histocompatibility. Science 1981; 213:172–178.

Spurkland A, Knutsen I, Markussen G, et al: HLA matching of unrelated bone marrow transplant pairs: Direct sequencing of in vitro amplified HLA-DRB1 and -DQB1 genes using magnetic beads as solid support. Tissue Antigens 1993; 41:155–164.

Stern LJ, Wiley DC: Antigenic peptide binding by class I and class II histocompatibility proteins. Structure 1994; 2:245–251.

Termijtelen A, Erlich HA, Braun LA, et al: Oligonucleotide typing is a perfect tool to identify antigens stimulatory in the mixed lymphocyte culture. Hum Immunol 1991; 31:241–245.

Thorsby E, Piazza A: Joint Report II. Typing for HLA-D determinants (LD-1 or MLC). *In* Kissmeyer-Nielsen F (ed): Histocompatibility Testing 1975. Copenhagen, Munksgaard, 1975, pp 414–458.

Tiercy JM, Goumaz C, Mach B, Jeannet M: Application of HLA-DR oligotyping to 110 kidney transplant patients with doubtful serological typing. Transplantation 1991a; 51:1110–1114.

Tiercy JM, Morel C, Freidel AC, et al: Selection of unrelated donors for bone marrow transplantation is improved by HLA class II genotyping with oligonucleotided hybridization. Proc Natl Acad Sci USA 1991b; 88:7121–7125.

Todd JA, Bell JI, McDevitt HO: HLA-DQbeta gene contributes to susceptibility and resistance to insulin-dependent diabetes mellitus. Nature 1987; 329:599.

van Rood JJ: HLA and I. Annu Rev Immunol 1993; 11:1–28.

Zhou YC, Cecka JM: Effect of HLA matching on renal transplant survival. Clinical Transplants 1993; 499–509.

5

Chapter 39

The Major Histocompatibility Complex and Disease

Deyanira Corzo, M.D.
Chester A. Alper, M.D.
Edmond J. Yunis, M.D.

Understanding the role of the major histocompatibility complex (MHC) in immune responses and in the pathogenesis of disease requires definition of polymorphism in Class I and Class II and of genes in the central region of the MHC, sometimes called the non-HLA region, or Class III region. It should be mentioned from the outset that there are DNA regions in which recombinations occur more frequently than expected, that is, in the interval from *HLA-DR* to *HLA-DP*. But of particular importance is the fact that there are constellations of fixed DNA wherein recombinations are rarely observed. The two major constellations are the complement region in the central region, and *HLA-DR, DQ* in the Class II region. Furthermore, analysis of MHC haplotypes in many ethnic groups has led us to recognize that a sizable proportion of individuals have ethnic group–specific haplotypes that appear to be identical in the interval from *HLA-B* to *HLA-DR, DQ*. These haplotypes, named extended haplotypes, should be considered as fixed genetic units that, studied together with MHC variants that are not part of these haplotypes, serve to help us understand immune responses and disease associations. The variants of Class I and Class II genes are described in Chapter 38. We review here the non-HLA region genes and alleles, extended haplotypes, and disease associations.

GENES IN THE NON-HLA REGION OR CLASS III REGION

There are about 1100 kilobases (kb) of DNA between the Class I and Class II regions, generally termed the non-HLA or Class III region. It contains genes that encode proteins of diverse function. Although Class I and Class II molecules are distinguished by structural and functional similarities shared by the members of each class, Class III molecules can be defined only as non-I and non-II, or other, because their genes and their products have no common features and are not recognized by T cells (Alper, 1984). It includes genes encoding the complement proteins C2 (*C2*), Factor B (*BF*), C4 (*C4A* and *C4B*), the microsomal enzyme steroid P450 21-hydroxylase (*CYP21B*), the cytokines tumor necrosis factor α (*TNFA*) and β (*TNFB*), lymphotoxin β (*LT*β), three members of the major heat-shock protein 70 family (*HSP70-1, -2, -Hom*) and several recently discovered genes of unknown function (Trowsdale, 1995).

The whole of the Class III region has been analyzed using pulse field gel electrophoresis (PFGE), by cloning in yeast artificial chromosomes (YACs), and in cosmid vectors (Dunham, 1987; Kendall, 1990; Ragoussis, 1991; Sargent, 1989; Spies, 1989). This region is believed to be one of the more densely gene-packed regions of the human genome, with approximately one gene per 15 kb (Fig. 39–1). The functional properties of proteins encoded by several genes of the Class III region are yet unknown, but most are not involved in the immune response. Several genes, including the human equivalent of the murine b144 gene, have been mapped between the *C4A* and *HLA-B* genes (Tsuge, 1987). These have been called *G* genes, located in Giemsa-negative bands (*G1* to *G11*, including also *G7a* and *G9a*) or *BAT*, *HLA-B*–associated transcripts (*BAT*1–9) (Sargent, 1989a; Spies, 1989). Genes *G2* to *G11* are characterized by the presence of clusters of restriction sites for the enzyme Hpa II (HTF-islands). *G7a*, also known as *BAT6*, is believed to encode a valyl-tRNA synthetase (Hsieh, 1991). *G9a*, or *BAT8*, encodes a protein of unknown function, with ankyrin-like repeats, probably involved in intracellular protein-protein interactions (Milner, 1993). *G2* and *G3*, also known as *BAT2* and *BAT3*, encode large, proline-rich members of an unknown family of proteins (Sargent, 1989a). Genes located in this region also include the *RD* gene. *RD* encodes a novel protein with a central core of arginine or lysine with aspartic or glutamic acid repeated 21 times (Levi-Strauss, 1988).

The region between *C4A* and *HLA-DR* genes has been studied with the same methods. Genes *G12* to *G18* are located in a 160-kb segment of DNA centromeric to the *C4A* gene, and five of them are also associated with HTF islands (Kendall, 1990; Spies, 1990). A pair of genes organized in the opposite transcriptional orientation to other genes in this cluster, known as opposite-strand genes (*OSG*), overlap the last exon of the *CYP21* gene (Gitelman, 1992; Matsumoto, 1992; Morel, 1989). One of them encodes an extracellular protein, and it has a gene rearrangement resembling that of tenascin, another extracellular protein. The predicted protein encoded by the second gene lacks the fibrinogen-like domain and would consist only of fibronectin type II repeats.

BF, *C2*, and *C4* Genes

C2 and C4 of the classical pathway and factor B of the alternative complement pathway (Carroll, 1984) are encoded in a 120-kb region of genomic DNA about 300 kb from *HLA-DR* and 650 kb from *HLA-B*. C2 and BF show considerable amino acid sequence identity and share a number of physicochemical and functional characteristics, suggesting that the two genes arose by tandem duplication of a factor B–like ancestral gene. Both are serine proteases (of the SERPIN family of plasma proteins) and mediate cleavage of C3 during activation of the respective pathways. C4, on the other hand, is related structurally and functionally to C3 and C5, and by virtue of containing a highly reactive internal thiolester, is related to C3 and the protease inhibitor α_2-macroglobulin. Although the gene for C3 is loosely linked to the MHC in the mouse, it is on an entirely different chromosome from the MHC in humans. Immediately 3′ to each *C4* locus are two loci for the adrenal steroid enzyme 21-hydroxylase (*CYP21A* and *CYP21B*) (Carroll, 1985; Higashi, 1986; White, 1986). The two genes are both about 3.4 kb long and split into 10 exons. They are highly homologous, but three mutations cause premature termination of the transcription of the *CYP21A* gene (White, 1988) and render it a pseudogene.

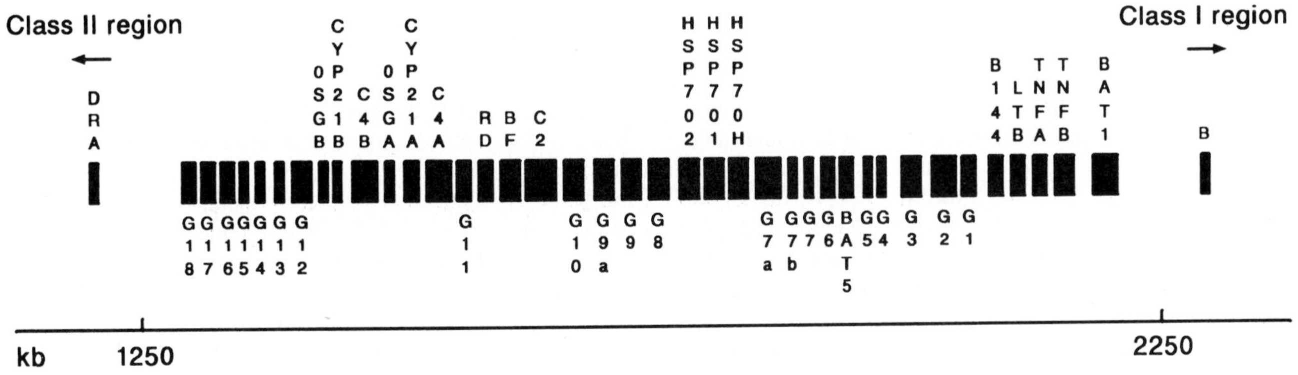

Figure 39–1. Map of the non-HLA or Class III region of the MHC.

Factor B is synthesized by the gene *BF*. During activation of the alternative complement pathway, the protein is split into a 30-kDa amino-terminal Ba fragment, and a 60-kDa Bb fragment. In common with a number of other C3-binding proteins, factor B (and C2) has a variable number of 60–amino acid homologous repeats. Using agarose gel electrophoresis, the protein exhibits moderate polymorphism with two very common alleles, *BF*F* (fast) and *BF*S* (slow), two less common alleles, *BF*F1* (faster) and *BF*S1* (also called *BF*S07*) (slower), and a host of rare alleles. By isoelectric focusing, *BF*F* can be divided into two subtypes, *BF*FA* and *BF*FB*. The amino acid substitution responsible for the common variants of BF FA, BF FB and BF S, are determined by residues found on the Ba fragment, whereas those for BF F1 and BF S1 are localized on the Bb fragment. DNA restriction fragment length polymorphisms have been found that either correspond to the *BF*F* and *BF*S* difference, to the *BF*FA* and *BF*FB* difference, or to further split of *BF*F*. In European white populations, *BF*F* has a frequency of 0.2; *BF*S*, 0.77; *BF*F1*, 0.01; *BF*S1*, 0.01; and rare alleles account only for 0.002. *BF*S* is most common in caucasoid, mongoloid, and australoid populations, whereas *BF*F* is most common in negroid populations. *BF*F1* is observed in negroid groups as well as in some caucasoid populations.

The *C2* gene is 18 kb long. During activation of the classical complement pathway, the protein is split between amino acid positions 223 and 224, an arginine-lysine bond, into two fragments, C2a and C2b. C2a is hemolytically active. At the protein level, C2 shows minor polymorphism by isoelectric focusing. Alleles are *C* (common), a less common *B* (basic) allele, with three rare basic variants, and four rare *A* (acidic) variants. The polymorphic site for the *C2*B* allele is carried by the C2a fragment. *C2*C* accounts for over 95% of *C2* genes in most populations. *C2*B* accounts for around 3% to 4% of *C2* genes. There is a non-expressed allele (*C2*Q0*), which is found in 2% of the European white population. A set of restriction fragment length polymorphism markers is detected in Sst I–digested genomic DNA of the *C2* gene and is in strong linkage disequilibrium with the alleles in *BF* genomic DNA described earlier. These variants represent variable sizes of repetitive DNA (αVNTR) within a *C2* intron.

C4 is synthesized as a large, single polypeptide of about 200 kDa that undergoes postsynthetic processing involving proteolysis to a three-chain, disulfide bond–linked structure. The largest of these chains, about 87 kDa, is the α-chain and carries the internal thiolester. During classical complement pathway activation, activated C1s cleaves a small peptide with anaphylatoxin properties from the amino-terminus of the C4 α-chain. This results in rupture of the internal thiolester, which is transiently capable of acylating nucleophilic groups in the immediate environment of the activated molecule. There are two distinct *C4A* and *C4B* loci that encode for two forms of C4. C4A and C4B differ only by four amino acid residues in the α-chain, between positions 1101 and 1106. Remarkably, C4A preferentially acylates amino groups, whereas C4B preferentially acylates hydroxyl groups. Thus, C4B is severalfold more hemolytically active, but C4A is more active at inhibiting the formation of and dissolving immune complexes than is C4B. In addition, C4A variants are usually more negatively charged than those of C4B and have a more slowly migrating α-chain in SDS gel electrophoresis. C4A variants usually carry Rodgers antigenic determinants (a Val-Asp-Leu-Leu epitope of the C4A chain), and C4B variants carry Chido determinants (an Ala-Asp-Leu-Arg epitope of the α-chain of C4B). There is extensive genetic polymorphism in C4A and C4B proteins in all populations examined, detectable by agarose gel electrophoresis (Awdeh and Alper, 1980). At least 18 *C4α* alleles, 21 *C4B* alleles, and one non-expressed gene (*C4*Q0*) at each *C4* locus have been recognized (Mauff, 1990). Aberrant or hybrid gene products with partly C4A and partly C4B characteristics have been identified. Most striking also is the variation in *C4* gene number on any individual haplotype. Although it is most common to have one expressed *C4A* and one expressed *C4B*, homoduplication and heteroduplication are common, as are haplotypes with only one expressed *C4* gene. *C4A*3* and *C4B*1* are the most common alleles in almost every ethnic group. *C4A*4*, *C4A*2*, *C4B*2*, and *C4B*5* show a world-wide distribution. *C4A*6* is also observed in many ethnic groups except for some mongoloid groups. *C4B*3* is identified mainly in negroid and caucasoid population groups.

Studies of the nucleotide sequence of the *C4* genes have revealed that the differences between C4A and C4B protein sequences involve about a dozen residues of the α-chain near the internal thiolester. This is the same region that carries the differences that determine individual variants and the presence of Chido or Rodgers determinants. Southern blot analysis with Taq I–digested genomic DNA and 5′ *C4* and *CYP21* gene probes has revealed that about half of null alleles are the result of deletions. The remaining cases appear to result from *C4B* to *C4A* gene conversion or involve mutation producing premature stop codons. Moreover, the *C4A* deletion characteristic of the *C4A*Q0* on the haplotype with *HLA-B8, DR17 (3)* shows a characteristic restriction fragment with Taq I in this system. *C4A* genes are 22 kb in length, but *C4B* occurs in two forms, short (16 kb) and long (22 kb), all of which produce characteristic Taq I fragments. The long forms of *C4B* and all human *C4A* have an inserted variably derived retro-transposon not found in the short forms. Additional DNA polymorphisms "split" protein polymorphisms, and others are characterized by a single allele such as *C4A*6*.

Tumor Necrosis Factor α and β and Lymphotoxin β Genes

TNFA and *TNFB* (the latter also called the lymphotoxin α gene, or *LTA*) encode potent immunomodulatory cytokines that are produced in response to several inflammatory stimuli. TNFα is produced in a variety of hematopoietic and non-hematopoietic cells, and TNFβ is produced specifically by lymphocytes. They have very similar biological activities. TNFα and TNFβ are either maintained as cell surface molecules or released from producing cells. TNFβ is retained on the cell surface via a transmembrane region. Surface TNFα

does not result from the presence of a transmembrane region, but rather from association with a 33-kDa membrane glycoprotein known as lymphotoxin β (LTβ) (Browning, 1993). LTβ has 21% and 24% identity with TNFα and TNFβ, respectively. The gene for LTβ is contained within four exons, spans 2 kb, and is located between the *TNFA* and the *B144* genes.

TNFα and TNFβ form biologically active trimers, and both bind to the same 55-kDa and 75-kDa receptors. The kinetics of their induction are different: TNFα transcription begins within two hours of mitogenic stimulation, whereas no TNFβ is detectable until after eight hours. In addition, TNFα has a high baseline transcription, a high transcription rate after activation, and a short mRNA half-life (30 minutes). TNFβ has a very low baseline level of transcription that increases after mitogenic stimulation, although not to the levels of TNFα, and its half-life is 5.5 hours. TNFα and TNFβ are each encoded by separate genes (Carroll, 1987) and share approximately 34% amino acid identity. Genes encoding TNFα and TNFβ are located in a 7-kb region 250 kb centromeric to the gene for HLA-B and 355 telomeric to the gene for C2. TNFβ, derived from induced T or B lymphocytes, is a glycosylated protein of 171 amino acids (Mr 25,000). TNFα derived from activated monocytes has a size of 157 amino acids (Mr 17,000). Both genes are of similar size, with a primary transcript of 2762 base pairs (bp) for TNFα and 2038 bp for TNFβ. Each gene contains three intervening sequences, but only the third intron is in a homologous position. The genes have homologous regions in the fourth exon (56% in the coding region). The higher degree of homology in the last exon is reflected in the overall homology of the proteins, mainly in the last exon (Nedwin, 1985). Apparently, the last exon was derived from a common ancestral sequence. Hybridization of Nco I–digested genomic DNA with *TNFA* or *TNFB* probes resulted in a polymorphic fragment of DNA, either 5.5 kb or 10.5 kb in length (Webb, 1990). This polymorphism is due to a substitution of a G for an A in intron 1 of *TNFB*, giving rise to the new Nco I site. The allele with the 5.5-kb Nco I fragment includes a substitution of an A for a C in the coding sequence of mature *TNFB*, resulting in an asparagine instead of threonine at position 26. Both allelic forms are common in caucasoid populations, with the 10.5-kb Nco I fragment seen in 71% of independent haplotypes from a panel of HLA-homozygous cell lines, and the 5.4-kb allele present in 28%. A polymorphism in the 3′ region of the *TNFB* gene (exon 4) has also been detected after digestion with EcoR I, resulting in a 2.4-kb or a 2.5-kb fragment (Verjans, 1992). Recently, microsatellite polymorphisms of *TNF* genes have been described (Nedospasov, 1991). Microsatellites are DNA sequences consisting of varying lengths of TC/GA or AC/GT repeats. There are four microsatellites, three with TC/GA and one with AC/GT repeats. TNFa (with AC/GT repeats) and TNFb (with TC/GA repeats) microsatellites are located 3.5 kb telomeric to the *TNFB* gene and have 7 and 13 alleles respectively. TNFc microsatellite (with TC/GA repeats) is located in intron 1 of the *TNFB* gene and has two alleles. Because of their very close linkage, these polymorphisms are best considered as TNFa, b, c haplotypes (Jongeneel, 1991).

Heat-Shock Protein 70 Genes

Stress proteins, or heat-shock proteins, are expressed in response to a variety of stress stimuli to cells. This response has been observed in all species examined to date. The family of stress proteins of 70 kDa has a high amino acid sequence identity from primitive eukaryotes to humans. Several studies have demonstrated loci for heat-shock protein 70 (HSP70) on chromosomes 6, 14, and 21 and at least one other autosome (Hunt, 1985; Sargent, 1989b). Three genes encoding members of the *HSP70* family are located 92 kb telomeric to the *C2* locus. *HSP70-1* and *HSP70-2* are 12 kb apart, and *HSP70-Hom* is located about 4 kb telomeric to the *HSP70-1* gene.

Sequence analysis of *HSP70-1* and *-2* genes has shown they are intronless genes that encode an identical protein product of 641 amino acids. *HSP70-Hom* is also an intronless gene that encodes a protein of 641 amino acids and that gene has 90% sequence identity with *HSP70-1* (Milner, 1990). *HSP70-1* and *-2* are expressed at high levels in cells heat-shocked at 42°C. *HSP70-1* is also expressed constitutively at very low levels. *HSP70-Hom* is expressed at low levels both constitutively and following heat shock. Because of the high degree of sequence similarity between the coding regions of the *HSP70* genes, DNA probes corresponding to coding regions tend to cross-hybridize with each other. However, there are sufficient sequence differences between the 5′ and 3′ untranslated regions of *HSP70-1, -2*, and *-Hom* to design oligonucleotide primers and probes to allow the specific amplification and hybridization of the three genes (Milner, 1992). Three nucleotide substitutions have been detected in the 5′ flanking and untranslated regions of *HSP70-1*: an A to C transversion at position −110, a T to C transition at position +120, and a G to C transversion at position +190. Variations at positions −110 and +120 have been shown to influence the superhelical conformation of the amplified DNA double strand, modifying its mobility in polyacrylamide gel electrophoresis. Three allelic forms have been recognized: *HSP70-1A* (slow), *B* (fast), and *C* (intermediate). Oligonucleotide probes containing sequence variations at positions −110 and +120 can also detect the three alleles after specific polymerase chain reaction (PCR) amplification of the *HSP70-1* gene. In *HSP70-2*, a G to A transition at position 1267 results in the loss of a Pst I restriction site. Hybridization of Pst I–digested genomic DNA with an *HSP70* probe results in a polymorphic fragment of DNA either 8.5 kb or 9 kb in length. In the *HSP70-Hom* gene, there is a T to C transition at position 2437, which lies within an Nco I restriction site and yields two allelic fragments of 1.5 kb and 0.5 kb, respectively.

5

COMPLOTYPES

The *C2* and *BF* genes are extremely close to one another in humans, separated by less than 2 kb, but *BF* and *C4A* are separated by about 30 kb. *C4A* and *C4B* are about 10 kb apart. The four complement genes show striking linkage disequilibrium in haplotypes determined from family studies. That is to say, they occur together as sets in populations and on the same chromosome more frequently than expected from the frequencies of their individual alleles in much the same manner as alleles in the Rh and MNSs blood group systems. No recombinations have been documented among the complement genes. For these reasons, they are properly regarded as single genetic units, arbitrarily designated by their *BF, C2, C4A,* and *C4B* alleles. Thus, *BF*S, C2*C, C4A*Q0, C4B*1* is a complotype that in abbreviated form is *SC01*. There are more than a dozen complotypes in caucasoid populations that have frequencies of about 0.01 or higher (Table 39–1). The complotype *SC31* is the most common in the majority of ethnic groups. In negroid populations, *FC31* is common, as is *SC42* in mongoloids.

EXTENDED HAPLOTYPES

From the study of the distribution of complotypes in relation to *HLA-B* and *HLA-DR* specificities on normal white population haplotypes determined in family studies, it became evident that there was striking linkage disequilibrium involving the whole region. One could easily recognize *HLA-B*-complotype–*DR* allele sets that showed statistically significant three-point linkage disequilibrium (Fig. 39–2) and that defined what we have called extended haplotypes (Awdeh, 1983). There are over a dozen common extended haplotypes in caucasoids (Table 39–2) (Alper, 1992). An analysis of *HLA-A* variation on these haplotypes revealed that this was limited and that each extended haplotype and the major *HLA-A* alleles involved previously recognized *HLA-A/B* and *HLA-B/DR* pairs exhibiting significant linkage disequilibrium (Table 39–3).

The concept that has emerged is that these extended haplotypes, which account for at least 30% of normal haplotypes in caucasoids, have relatively fixed gross structure and DNA sequence and carry similar, if not identical, alleles, even when they are found in apparently unrelated individuals. Another important feature of extended haplotypes is their ethnicity. For the most part, they are highly characteristic of an ethnic subgroup and have lower frequencies or do not occur at all in other ethnic groups. They presumably had their origin in the group in which their frequency as intact haplotypes is highest. We have developed the concept that extended haplotypes have fixity of DNA over at least the *HLA-B/DR* interval, and if they therefore carry a disease susceptibility gene, then virtually all independent examples of that haplotype will show association with that disease. Conversely, if the extended haplotype does not have a disease susceptibility gene, then it and its constituent alleles will be "protective." It is critical to know the ethnic distribution of an extended haplotype in order to evaluate whether the extended haplotype in patients is increased compared with ethnically matched control populations or is merely a marker for the ethnic distribution of the disease.

Although there are some superficial similarities between extended haplotypes and supratypes and both derived from the same phenomena, there are critical differences. Supratypes were defined as sets of *HLA-A, B, DR,* and complotype alleles in a phenotype, not necessarily as genes on the same haplotype and with no requirement that other alleles or intervening DNA be fixed or participate in the nonrandom association (Dawkins, 1983). In recognition of the fact that the basic phenomenon is a haplotype with conserved DNA, the term supratype has been dropped and the designation ancestral haplotype has been introduced (Degli-Esposti, 1992).

Table 39–1. COMMON COMPLOTYPES IN NORMAL CHROMOSOMES OF CAUCASOID POPULATIONS*

Complotype	Frequency
SC31	0.43
SC01	0.127
FC31	0.096
SC30	0.053
SC42	0.04
SC61	0.034
FC30	0.031
FC01	0.029
SC02	0.029
SC21	0.022
SB42	0.019
SC33	0.014
SC2(1,2)†	0.013
SC32	0.011

*Complotypes are given as abbreviated letters and numbers, with four alleles in arbitrary order, e.g., *BF, C2, C4A, C4B*.
†*C4B* locus is heteroduplicated.

COMPLEMENT TYPING

The complement system (Chapter 36) is divided into two pathways: The classical pathway contains nine different components totaling at least 12 proteins, and the alternative pathway contains four. Three of the 16 proteins are encoded within the MHC and demonstrate inherited structural variants that can be studied by techniques that detect differences in net surface charge caused by amino acid differences. Two methods are used to separate proteins: (1) high-voltage agarose gel electrophoresis to detect variations of mobility owing to charge differences between proteins at a given pH and (2) isoelectric focusing in thin-layer polyacrylamide gels, which demonstrates differences in isoelectric points. Proteins can be visualized by either immunofixation electrophoresis, using insolubility of antigen-antibody complexes, or by detection of functional hemolytic activity with overlay gels, in which antibody-sensitized sheep erythrocytes are combined with complement-deficient serum (Marcus, 1986).

Proteins from the classical pathway (C2, C4A, and C4B) and one from the alternative pathway (factor B) are encoded within the MHC and are polymorphic and therefore useful for assignments of MHC haplotypes. For C2 typing, proteins are separated by isoelectric focusing in polyacrylamide gels and visualized by C2-induced hemolysis in overlay gels. Dilute normal human serum can replace C2-deficient serum as a reagent because C2 is the limiting factor in the classical pathway (Fig. 39–3).

C4 typing requires three different techniques: (1) Im-

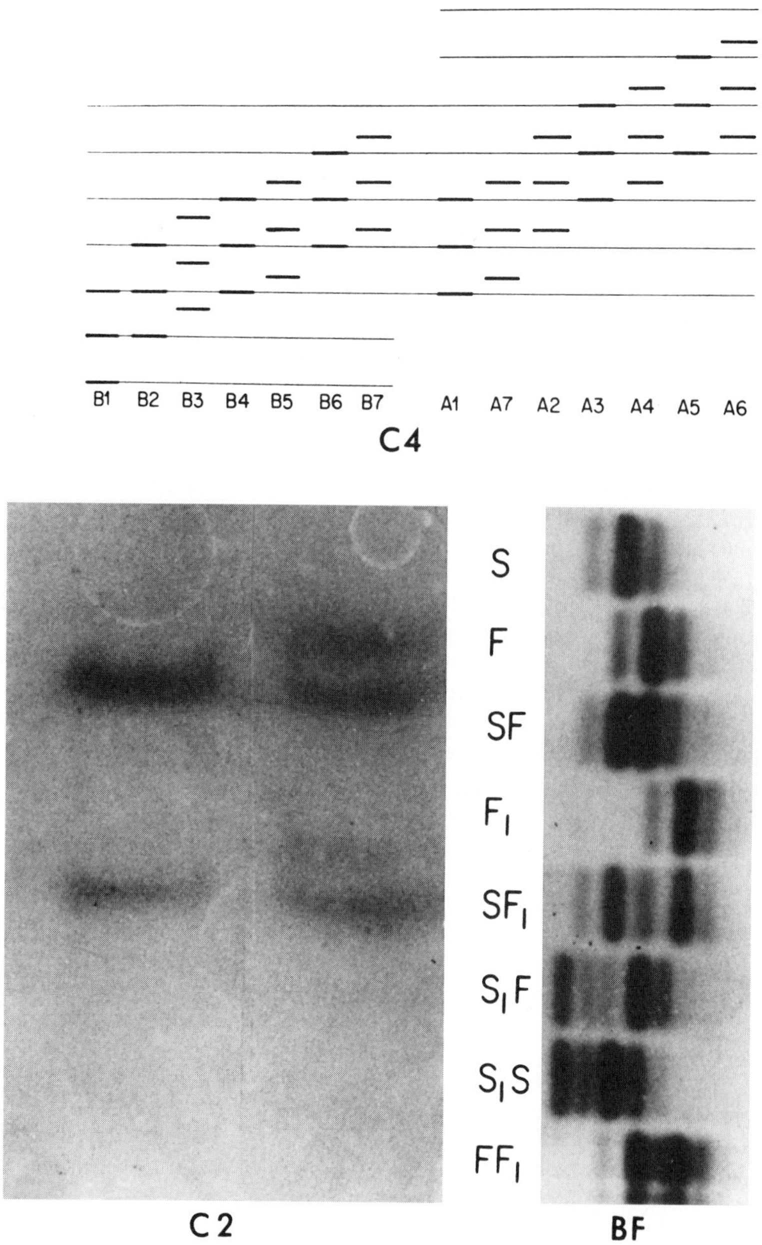

Figure 39–2. Electrophoretic positions of C4 variants relative to one another (diagram). The variants at the C4B (Chido) locus are shown at the left, and those at the C4A (Rodgers) locus are shown at the right. Each gene product consists of three bands. It will be noted that some of the C4B variants correspond closely in position to C4A variants (B7 and A2, for example). The distinction between them is made by use of a C4-sensitive overlay agarose gel in which only C4B variants have appreciable C4 hemolytic activity (Awdeh, 1980). The *BQ0* and *AQ0* (null alleles) show no bands.

In the lower position (left side) of the figure, examples of the common C2 type (C) and a heterozygote (BC) are shown using isoelectric focusing in polyacrylamide gel with agarose gel overlay, containing antibody-sensitized sheep erythrocytes and a 1/90 dilution of normal human serum.

In the lower portion (right side) of the figure, examples are shown of electrophoretic patterns of BF variants after agarose gel electrophoresis and immunofixation with anti–factor B antisera. Each gene product consists of the main band and two minor ones. The anode was at the right.

Table 39–2. COMMON EXTENDED HAPLOTYPES*

Extended Haplotype†	Frequency
HLA-(A1), B8, DR3, SC01	0.093
HLA-(A3), B7, DR2, SC31	0.059
HLA-(29), B12, DR7, FC31	0.037
HLA-(A2), B12, DR4, SC30	0.034
HLA-(A1), B17, DR7, SC61	0.028
HLA-(A2), B40, DR6, SC02	0.011
HLA-(A2 or A3), B14, DR1, SC2(1,2)	0.08
HLA-(A3), B35, DR1, FC(3,2) 0	0.08

*Data from normal caucasoid population chromosomes from Boston.
†Most frequent HLA-A allele is given in parentheses.

munofixation electrophoresis after treatment with neuraminidase—the patterns produced show three bands for each variant with some overlap occurring between some variants, and additional treatment of the sample with carboxypeptidase reduces each variant to a single band. (2) Detection of C4A versus C4B by functional hemolytic assay—this is to distinguish C4A or C4B overlapping patterns because C4B variants have 5 to 10 times the hemolytic activity of C4A variants. (3) Rodgers (C4A) or Chido (C4B) serologic reactivity—the serum being typed is incubated with either human anti-Rodgers or human anti-Chido to test for inhibition of agglutination with appropriate positive erythrocytes. Al-

Table 39–3. HAPLOTYPE PAIRS IN LINKAGE DISEQUILIBRIUM

Haplotype	Δ/1000*	HF/1000†	Haplotype	Δ/1000*	HF/1000†
A2, B12	27.2	64.5	*B12, DR7*	26.7	41.3
A1, B8	57.2	64.1	*B8, DR3*	62.3	70.1
A29, B12	27.3	33.1	*B12, Dw2*	18.4	30.3
A3, B7	18.5	28.3	*B7, DR2*	37.6	46.2
A1, B17	16.0	22.4	*B17, DR7*	22.8	29.4
A1, B5	13.7	20.6			
A23, B12	17.6	19.3	*B12, Dw4*	15.3	22.6
A30, B18	16.6	17.0	*B18, DR3*	12.9	18.2

*Δ = observed haplotype (PQ) frequency − (frequency of P × frequency of Q).
†HF = haplotype frequency.
Data from Bodmer WF, Bodmer JG: Br Med Bull 1976; 34:309.

ternatively, C4 variants can be typed for Chido or Rodgers reactivity by immunoblotting. There are two ways to detect null alleles of C4 heterozygotes. Electrophoresis of C4 null (C4A Q0 and C4B Q0) samples demonstrates absence of bands in homozygotes but in heterozygotes requires quantitation by either visual inspection, by crossed immunoelectrophoresis, or by densitometric scanning of the immunofixation patterns. An alternative method is to determine the presence and ratios of the C4A and C4B α-chains after sodium dodecyl sulfate polyacrylamide gel electrophoresis of immunoprecipitates.

Factor B typing is performed after prolonged agarose gel electrophoresis and immunofixation. The homozygous patterns consist of a major band and flanking minor bands, and heterozygous patterns are the sum of two homozygous patterns.

ROLE OF MHC MOLECULES AS IMMUNE RESPONSE GENES

Genes controlling the immune response to foreign antigens were initially described in animal models. They were shown to be located within the Class II region of the MHC. Antigen-presenting cells (APCs) have been shown to process fragments of antigen and to display these peptides as complexes with Class I or Class II molecules, thus initiating the immune response.

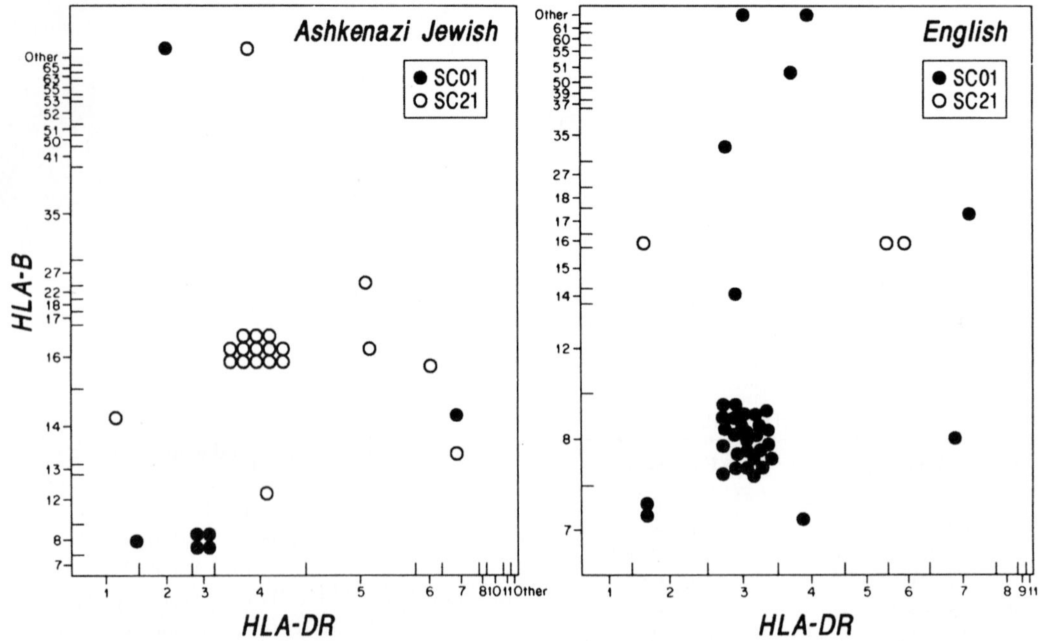

Figure 39–3. The haplotype distribution of the complotypes (haplotypes of complement alleles) *SC01* (*BF*S, C2*C, C4A*Q0, C4B*1*) and *SC21* (*BF*S, C2*C, C4A*2, C4B*1*) in relation to *HLA-B* alleles on the ordinate and *HLA-DR* alleles on the abcissa. The heights and widths representing each HLA specificity are proportional to allele frequencies for the respective populations. Clustering represents linkage disequilibrium and flags the extended haplotypes (*HLA-B16(38), SC21, DR4*) in the Ashkenazi Jews and (*HLA-B8, SC01, DR3*) in the English and, to a much lesser extent, the Jews. (From Alper CA, Awdeh Z, Yunis EJ: Conserved, extended MHC haplotypes. Exp Clin Immunogenet 1992; 9:58.) (By permission of S. Karger.)

In recent years, significant advances in the understanding of the molecular basis of MHC antigen presentation have been made, basically as a result of the determination of the three-dimensional structure of Class I (Bjorkman, 1987a, 1987b) and Class II molecules (Brown, 1993), the characterization of peptides bound to MHC molecules (Barber, 1993; Engelhard, 1994), and progress in the understanding of assembly and function of MHC Class I and Class II molecules (Cresswell, 1994; Jackson, 1993). This knowledge has improved the understanding of the immune response and could be useful in its manipulation for therapeutic benefit. MHC molecules are critical for the recognition of antigen by T cells by specific receptors (TCRs), which are encoded by a pool of genes that undergo rearrangement. MHC Class I molecules are restricted to interacting with receptors on $CD8^+$ T cells, which kill target cells. They are known as cytotoxic T cells. MHC Class II molecules are restricted to interaction with $CD4^+$ T cells, known as helper T cells because they release several cytokines to amplify the immune response by inducing T and B cell proliferation, macrophage activation, or B cell differentiation. In $CD4^+$ cells, the response can be also cytolytic. In general, Class I molecules bind peptides from intracellular proteins, whereas Class II molecules bind peptides from extracellular proteins (Morrison, 1986). However, there is evidence that Class I molecules can present extracellular antigens (Staerz, 1987) and that Class II can present intracellular antigens (Nuchtern, 1990). Intracellular antigens can be self-proteins, proteins synthesized from viruses, or proteins released by bacteria, protozoa, or parasites that have penetrated into the cytosol. Extracellular proteins are internalized by Class II–bearing cells. They can be cell-surface proteins; soluble proteins; or proteins associated with a whole organism, such as a virus, bacterium, or protozoan parasite that has decomposed or has been phagocytosed by the cell. Since only a small number of different MHC molecules are expressed, each isoform must be able to bind a wide range of distinct peptides in order to enable immune responses to a variety of antigens.

Antigen Presentation by MHC Class I Molecules

The peptide-binding site in Class I molecules is approximately 25 Å long, 10 Å wide, and 11 Å deep (Bjorkman, 1987b). As described in Chapter 38, the crystal structure of HLA-A2 revealed subsites of pockets, denoted A through F (Saper, 1991). Pockets A and F are at the ends of the peptide-binding site and are highly conserved in Class I variants. They serve to anchor the amino- and carboxyl-terminal ends of the peptide in the binding site. The other pockets (B to E) are polymorphic and possibly determine peptide-binding specificity, since it has been seen that point mutations of residues within them alter the repertoire of peptides bound (Madden, 1992). Peptides of different sequences adopt a similar conformation within the binding site. They have a β structure with amino- and carboxy-termini in the A and F pockets and with residues in the middle of the peptide less constrained (Freemont, 1992; Matsamura, 1992).

Peptides associated with most Class I molecules are typically 8 to 9 residues long. However, 20% to 40% of peptides bound to Class I molecules are longer (Guo, 1992), 14 residues being the longest identified peptide to date. The strong selectivity of the pockets B to F for particular amino acids originates motifs of common peptide residues that are important for binding to Class I molecules (Barber, 1993; Engelhard, 1994). Analysis of naturally processed peptides bound to HLA-B27 (Falk, 1991; Jardetsky, 1991) has been used to identify those peptide motifs. The carboxyl-terminal residue is the major component of motifs for peptides associated with Class I molecules. The second motif position identified most frequently is position 2 relative to the amino-terminus. For some Class I molecules, the amino acid at position 5 is highly conserved. These positions determine the peptides binding to pockets B and C, respectively. Strong selectivity at position 5 is usually accompanied by absence of selectivity at position 2 and vice versa. Some selectivity at position 3 has been observed in conjunction with that at position 2 or 5. It is believed that position 3 is an auxiliary anchor residue. Most Class I–bound peptides are generated by proteolytic degradation of proteins in the cytoplasm. Apparently, a heat-shock protein family member, ubiquitin, targets proteins for degradation by proteosomes.

Proteosomes are cytoplasmic complexes comprising 20 to 30 subunits with distinct protease activities (Goldberg, 1992). A relationship between proteosomes and antigen processing by Class I molecules is suggested by the presence of two genes in the Class II region of the MHC (*LMP2* and *LMP7*) that encode proteins with homology to proteosome subunits. Peptides produced in the cytoplasm are transported into the endoplasmic reticulum. Two proteins, TAP1 and TAP2, also encoded within the Class II region, appear to be involved in the transport of peptides from the cytoplasm to the endoplasmic reticulum (Bahram, 1991). The assembly of Class I–peptide complexes could involve peptide binding to a Class I molecule with β_2-microglobulin or, more infrequently, a peptide and a Class I heavy chain (Elliot, 1991). β_2-Microglobulin facilitates the proper conformation of Class I heavy chains for efficient peptide binding. Indeed, 100- to 1000-fold higher peptide concentrations are necessary for the binding of peptides to free heavy chains. In the absence of peptide, Class I heavy chains associated with β_2-microglobulin are extremely unstable and dissociate rapidly. The addition of the peptide thermostabilizes the Class I molecule (Elliot, 1991, 1992; Townsend, 1990). In most cases, only Class I molecules associated with peptide leave the endoplasmic reticulum to complete *N*-glycosylation in the Golgi complex and then reach the cell surface through the exocytic pathway. Class I molecules without peptide stay in the endoplasmic reticulum. The IP90 protein is a product of the calnexin gene that appears to keep Class I heavy chains and Class I molecules without peptides inside the endoplasmic reticulum. The IP90 protein remains associated with Class I molecules but dissociates after peptide binding (Degen, 1992). However, free heavy chains and Class I molecules without peptide have been found on the cell surface (Bix, 1992). Most evidence suggests that such molecules denature rapidly unless stabilized by peptide binding. Thus, binding of peptides to Class I molecules could also occur at the cell surface, but this is a point of controversy (Jackson, 1993). Emerging evidence suggests that non-classic Class I molecules can also participate in antigen presentation (Shawar, 1994; Stroynowski, 1994). In humans, HLA-E, -F, and -G molecules have been implicated in this function. Peptide binding by HLA-E has been detected. CD1 is one of several proteins encoded by genes that are unlinked to the MHC, have 25% to 30% identity with Class I molecules, and noncovalently associate with β_2-microglobulin. It has been reported that CD1b, one of the five products of *CD1* genes (CD1a–e), presents exogenously supplied *Mycobacterium* antigens to $CD4^-CD8^-\alpha\beta$ T cells (Porcelli, 1992).

Antigen Presentation by MHC Class II Molecules

From x-ray crystallography studies of HLA-DR it is known that it has a single pocket near one end of the groove that accommodates a hydrophobic amino acid side chain of the peptide. Other conserved residues in the groove bind to the polypeptide backbone (Brown, 1993). Class II molecules are targeted into the endoplasmic reticulum by their association with a membrane-bound protein, the invariant chain. Class II molecules and invariant chain are translocated from their place of synthesis to the endoplasmic reticulum, where the assembly of Class II–invariant chain complex occurs.

There are four forms of the invariant chain: p33, p35, p41, p43 (O'Sullivan, 1987). In the absence of MHC Class II molecules, the invariant chain forms trimers and, less frequently, hexamers (Lamb, 1992). Three Class II $\alpha\beta$ dimers associate with an individual invariant chain trimer, generating a nonamer (Roche, 1991). In transfection studies (Teyton, 1990) and more recently in mice (Viville, 1993) it has been demonstrated that Class II $\alpha\beta$ dimers can be generated without an invariant chain, but they are transported by the exocytic pathway, are poorly expressed on the cell surface, and have low ability to present exogenous peptides to T cells. During the assembly process, three proteins located in the endoplasmic reticulum (GRP94, ERp72, and IP90) associate with Class II $\alpha\beta$ dimers and invariant chains. Their possible function is to retain both the individual components and the partially assembled complexes in the endoplasmic reticulum until a complete nonamer is formed (Craig, 1993).

It appears that the 16 residues of the amino-terminal extension of p35 and p43 are also responsible for the signal to retain all non–Class II–associated invariant chain in the endoplasmic reticulum. Therefore, once a complete nonamer is formed, the exit of Class II–invariant chain complexes is allowed (Schaiff, 1992). The Class II–invariant chain complexes traverse the Golgi system. There, sialic acid is added to *N*- and *O*-linked glycans (Machamer, 1982).

It is possible that the same targeting signal in the invariant chain is responsible for sorting the Class II–invariant chain complexes from the Golgi to endosomes (Lotteau, 1990). The complexes transit directly to endosomes (Peters, 1991), but it is also possible that some proportion of Class II–invariant chain complexes go to endosomes via the cell surface (Roche, 1993). In the endosomes, Class II molecules dissociate from the invariant chain, possibly by invariant chain proteolysis (Newcomb, 1993b). Binding of peptides to Class II molecules occurs after a protein is internalized in acidic vesicles of the endocytic pathway and probably transported by heat-shock proteins to a prelysosomal compartment, in which proteolysis of the protein results in peptides that bind to the Class II molecules. The peptide–Class II complexes are then rapidly transported to the cell surface by returning to the Golgi system and entering the constitutive transport pathway or by direct transport from the endosome.

Although processing and presentation of antigens occur in the absence of the invariant chain, the consensus is that the invariant chain facilitates antigen processing by driving Class II molecules into the endosomal system and by preventing the association of peptides with Class II molecules before they are delivered in the endosomes. Peptide binding appears to confer stability on Class II molecules by inducing a conformational change, a situation similar to that described for Class I molecules (Lanzavecchia, 1992). Peptides that bind to Class II molecules are endocytically acquired and exhibit variability at the amino- and carboxy-termini, and their length ranges from 10 to 30 amino acids. Many of them have similar core sequences but differ at their amino- and carboxyl-terminal ends (Chicz, 1993; Newcomb, 1993a; Rudensky, 1992). The binding site in the Class II molecule is open at both ends, and peptides are not anchored within the binding site. Binding interactions involve the central part of the peptide rather than its ends. Peptides are predicted to adopt an extended conformation in the binding site to allow peptides longer than 15 amino acids to extend beyond the groove. The variation in the length of Class II ligands makes it difficult to identify motifs by alignment of bound peptides. Most hypothetical motifs include a general anchor residue (position 1) located near the amino-terminus of the peptide, which contains an aromatic or hydrophobic amino acid. Position 4, which also contains hydrophobic residues, may be another general anchor residue. Further constraints are suggested at position 6 (mostly small amino acids) and 9 (leucine). It has been reported that peptides binding to HLA-DR molecules may be promiscuous in that the same peptide is capable of binding to several DR variants (Chicz, 1993). The basis for this promiscuity may be the fact that not all the anchors are needed for the binding of certain peptides to Class II molecules.

It is believed that study of antigen presentation by MHC Classes I and II molecules will be important to the understanding of many MHC-associated human diseases. For example, *HLA-DRB1*0401* and *0404* are strongly associated with rheumatoid arthritis (Ollier, 1992). These alleles have positively charged or neutral residues at positions 70 and 71, and it is possible that these two sites are critical to the function of HLA-DR4 as presenting molecule to T cells. Another case is the aspartic acid at position 57 of the HLA-DQβ molecule, which is associated with protection against insulin-dependent diabetes mellitus (in caucasoids but not Japanese). The amino acid at this position could alter the binding capacity of the Class II molecule to peptides and could also affect the conformation or stability of the molecule. The substitution of a valine for glycine in position 86 of *DRB1*1302* could explain the association of this allele with resistance to severe malaria. It has been suggested that polymorphism at this position could affect antigen recognition by changing the size of the pocket complementary to a critical amino acid of the binding peptide. Peptide-binding motifs have been used to predict peptide epitopes recognized by MHC molecules in pre-existing T cell clones. Such an approach may lead to a better understanding of the normal host response, as in the case of acquisition of immunity against hepatitis B surface antigen (HBsAg), and the development of vaccines against microorganisms and peptides derived from oncogenes. This strategy has been effective in protecting mice against *Lysteria monocytogenes* infection, in recognizing virally infected target cells, and in conferring protection against virally induced tumors (Chicz, 1994). A similar application identified a malarial epitope that may contribute to resistance to severe malaria in individuals carrying *HLA-B53* (Hill, 1992).

Allorecognition

The MHC guides the development of the TCR repertoire during T cell maturation in the thymus. T cells that are able to recognize peptides in the cleft of self-MHC molecules are positively selected. However, to avoid reactivity against self, T cells that recognize self-peptides in the MHC cleft are deleted, inhibited, or anergized. The MHC also guides the immune response against foreign peptides. The principal targets of the immune response to allografts are the MHC molecules, and T cell recognition of allo-MHC is the primary event in allograft rejection. There are at least two pathways of allorecognition, the so-called direct and indirect pathways (Liu, 1993; Sayegh, 1994; Sherman, 1993; Thorsby, 1994). Direct allorecognition involves recognition by recipient $CD4^+$ and $CD8^+$ T cells of foreign peptide–Class II or –Class I complexes, respectively, on APCs from the graft (Eckels, 1990). The peptides can be derived from donor or recipient MHC molecules. There is some evidence that alloreactive T cells can recognize and respond to MHC molecules in the absence of a peptide bound to its groove. Indirect allorecognition (Shoskes, 1994) involves recognition by recipient $CD4^+$ T cells of foreign peptides derived from the graft presented by recipient Class II molecules. Proteins from disintegrated graft cells may be taken for exogenous proteins by recipient APCs and presented by self–Class II molecules to $CD4^+$ T cells of the recipient. Foreign MHC molecules of the graft are also an important source of foreign peptides (Benichou, 1992). The direct pathway accounts for most of the cytotoxic T cell function in transplant immune response and may play the dominant role in acute or early allograft rejection. The indirect pathway accounts for most of the antibody production against the graft and may play the dominant role in chronic rejection.

MHC DISEASE ASSOCIATIONS

There is a remarkable number of diseases that show HLA association (Tiwari, 1985). Most, but not all, are "autoimmune" and do not show clear-cut mendelian inheritance. We believe that the number of such HLA-associated diseases is so high not only because the MHC contains many immunologically important genes but also because the genes in the region, even non-HLA genes, are extraordinarily polymorphic, permitting the easy identification of such associations. Finally, because the common occurrence of fixed and extended haplotypes, as much as 2 to 3 megabases of genomic DNA, provides for disease markers. In a region in which the density of genes appears to be unusually high, this indeed encompasses a large number of potential susceptibility genes. A major problem with MHC susceptibility genes is their incomplete penetrance, making ordinary formal segregation and linkage studies extremely difficult, if not impossible. Furthermore, it appears likely that many MHC-associated diseases are polygenic. Because of these problems, we begin the discussion with MHC-determined disorders that show mendelian inheritance and 100% penetrance, at least for the primary biochemical defect.

Diseases Involving Mendelian Inheritance of Defects in MHC Genes

C2 Deficiency

Deficiency of the second component of complement has been reported only in caucasoids, and it is the most common complement protein deficiency state in that group. At least half of patients are asymptomatic. However, C2 deficiency has been associated with polymyositis, recurrent pyogenic infections, Henoch-Schönlein purpura, and vasculitis. Forty percent of reported patients have a systemic lupus-like disease; however, only 16% of the homozygous C2-deficient siblings of these probands have had lupus-like disease. This strongly suggests ascertainment bias. Nevertheless, there clearly is an increased tendency of homozygous C2-deficient subjects to have lupus-like disorders, perhaps related to defective clearance or disaggregation of immune complexes. Type I C2 deficiency results from homozygosity for a null allele, *C2*Q0*, which has a gene frequency of slightly less than 0.01. There is approximately one homozygote per 10,000 individuals. Almost all patients have elements of an extended haplotype [*HLA-A25, B18, S042, DRB1*1501, DQB1*0601, DQA1*0102*] containing the *C2*-deficiency gene (Awdeh, 1981; Truedsson, 1993). The complotype associations are most frequent, followed by the *DR, HLA-B*, and *HLA-A* associations, in keeping with the known gene order. The exact distributions suggest that this form of C2 deficiency arose as a mutation in a *C2* gene in a caucasoid person with the aforementioned haplotype between 650 and 1325 years ago. *C2*Q0* results from a 28-bp gene deletion that generates a frame shift and a stop codon 14 bp distal to the end of exon 5. Type II C2 deficiency (not associated with any elements of type I haplotype) is rare and results in a selective block in C2 secretion, but the reason for the secretion block is not known (Colten, 1992).

C4 Deficiency

There is a high incidence of *C4 null* alleles in the population. Thirty-five percent of individuals of all races do not ex-

5

press one *C4A* or *C4B* gene (i.e., carry *C4A*Q0* or *C4B*Q0*), 8% to 10% carry two null alleles, and less than 1% do not express three alleles. Complete C4 deficiency (*trans C4A*Q0, C4B*Q0*) haplotypes are extremely rare and can be detected in heterozygotes only by family studies. In contrast to C2 deficiency, C4 deficiency has been reported on at least nine different MHC haplotypes, including those with different *BF* types, suggesting that the deficiency arose from a number of different mutations. Although a number of different MHC haplotypes have been found with total C4 deficiency, many appear to be derived from known extended haplotypes that usually carry a deleted *C4B*, such as [*HLA-B18, F1C30, DR3*], or nonexpressed *C4A*, such as [*HLA-B60, SC02, DR6*]. Thus, it is the inactivation by deletion or mutation of the single functioning *C4* gene usually present on such haplotypes that results in total C4 deficiency. *C4B*Q0* results from gene deletion, stop codons, and gene conversion-like changes that cause the *C4B* gene to transcribe a molecule with the properties of C4A. *C4A*Q0* results from gene deletions, stop codons, and other mutations that result in failure of transcription (Braun, 1990). The *C4A*Q0* allele, particularly in homozygous individuals or those with complete C4 deficiency, has been associated with systemic and discoid lupus erythematosus (Dunckley, 1987). This susceptibility probably also relates to defective handling of immune complexes, as in C2 deficiency and other early-acting complement component deficiencies (Fielder, 1983). Homozygous *C4B*Q0* has been associated with IgA nephropathy. In addition, there is a 3.5-fold greater incidence of homozygous *C4B*Q0* in children with bacterial meningitis (Colten, 1992). The level of C4 in serum in patients with *C4 null* alleles is extremely variable and cannot be used reliably to detect heterozygotes for complete deficiency, even though there is a rough correlation between the level of C4 and the number of expressed *C4* genes.

21-Hydroxylase–Deficiency Congenital Adrenal Hyperplasia

This disorder is clinically heterogeneous, with a severe salt-wasting form, a milder late-onset form manifested largely by masculinization in girls, and a mild cryptic form. The MHC linkage of this disorder was discovered before any MHC associations were detected and before it was known that the *CYP21* loci were located in the MHC. Subsequently, it was found that in European white populations studied in the northeastern United States and in England, 20% or more haplotypes in patients with the salt-wasting form were the rare extended haplotype [*HLA-A1, Cw6, B47, FC(91)0, DRB1*07, DRB4*0101, DQA1*0201, DQB1*0201*]. This haplotype appears to be extremely common in the Midlands of Britain; thus, it is likely that a mutation leading to the disease probably occurred on a closely related haplotype in an individual from this region. It has been shown that this haplotype has a deletion of both *C4B* and *CYP21B*, thus explaining the severity of symptoms and complete deficiency of the enzyme in homozygotes for this haplotype. It is of interest that a similar haplotype without the deletion has been found in the Amish population. Among patients with milder and cryptic disease, a different extended haplotype is common: [*HLA-B65, SC2(1,2), DR1*]. This haplotype is common, particularly in southern Europe, and has a frequency in caucasoids in Boston of over 0.01. No patient homozygous for 21-hydroxylase deficiency has the most common of caucasoid extended haplotypes [*HLA-B8, SC01, DR3*]. In all forms of 21-hydroxylase deficiency, the bulk of MHC haplotypes are not extended, and there is a great variety of complotypes suggesting that many independent mutations have led to either deletion or derangement of the *CYP21B* gene. The study of 21-hydroxylase deficiency in a Venezuelan mestizo population revealed none of the haplotypes found in Boston caucasoid patients. Other marker haplotypes different from ethnically matched controls were present, however. In Australia, the haplotype *HLA-B22, SB45* was found to be increased among patients with 21-hydroxylase deficiency. Healthy persons who carried this haplotype but who had no family history of 21-hydroxylase deficiency could be shown to be carriers of the defect.

From these observations, we can attempt to extract some general principles for possible application to those diseases of unknown inheritance and pathogenesis that show MHC association or linkage. First, if a disease susceptibility gene occurs on an extended haplotype, all the alleles of that haplotype will show positive associations with the disease. Conversely, if it does not occur on an extended haplotype, all of the alleles on that haplotype will show a negative association with the disease. Because extended haplotypes have fixity of DNA on independent examples of a disease-associated extended haplotype, and are common, healthy persons must carry the susceptibility gene. All MHC disease markers, and particularly extended haplotypes, show a high degree of ethnic specificity. It is therefore particularly important in studies of MHC markers for disease to compare disease alleles and haplotypes (those in patients) with those in carefully ethnically matched controls. Ideally, ethnic matching should include specific regions of origin or ethnic subgroups.

Diseases of Unknown Etiology and Pathogenesis

A large number of diseases have been reported to show MHC associations. These disorders are very different from one another, and although most have at least some immunologic aspects, a few do not. There are many problems that confound our attempts to understand the mechanisms by which these diseases occur, and analysis of MHC markers in patients and their families has helped only marginally to clarify the picture. The greatest source of confusion is a phenomenon called incomplete penetrance. This is seen most clearly in monozygotic twins, who presumably have identical genes. If one of such twins has one of these diseases (e.g., type I diabetes mellitus), the other twin does not necessarily have the disease. For type I diabetes, the concordance rate appears to be no higher than 50%. This suggests that so-called penetrance of a disease in a completely susceptible host is incomplete: Although there is excellent reason to consider genes in the MHC as determinants of type I diabetes susceptibility, only 15% of MHC-identical siblings of patients have insulin-dependent diabetes. The difference between 50% and 15% is evidence for the influence of genes at a second, non–MHC-linked locus (or loci) and suggests an environmental factor or factors in determining susceptibility. Incomplete penetrance makes difficult the assignment of a specific mode of inheritance. It makes the likelihood low for finding families with more than one affected member in one generation or in two or more generations. Such families are frequently used to decide on modes of inheritance.

Other complicating factors are the inability to determine whether we are studying a group of patients homogeneous in terms of genetic determination. About 5% or 6% of random families with a type I diabetic proband will have a second affected child. Of these sibling pairs, approximately 60% will be MHC identical, 35% will be haploidentical, and a few percent will share no MHC haplotypes. This pattern suggests recessive inheritance of an MHC-linked susceptibility gene for the disease (Rubinstein, 1977). This conclusion is also supported by the results of analysis of the distribution of homozygotes and heterozygotes for *BF*F1* among 1100 type I diabetics (Raum, 1981). Nevertheless, the departure from 100% MHC identity of affected siblings has to be explained. Among the explanations are crossing over between the susceptibility locus and the MHC, impenetrant genes in susceptible parents, and heterogeneity of mode of inheritance, including variable penetrance in homozygotes compared with heterozygotes. This has led to a vast number of disease models with no way to distinguish among them. At the very least, however, family studies provide highly useful haplotype data and usually allow the assignment of homozygosity for an HLA marker in probands. They also have established that MHC association in most of the diseases of interest is based on linkage between a susceptibility gene and the MHC.

Yet another unknown is the number of different susceptibility alleles for a disease in any specific population. In this respect, extended haplotypes can be helpful because, if they are increased in patients, they probably represent a single susceptibility allele that could be anywhere in the region of fixity. However, some patients have only portions of these haplotypes and this provides clues to the location of specific alleles involved. Another clue may be sharing of specific alleles by two or more different extended haplotypes.

Specific Diseases Without Evidence of Mendelian Inheritance and with MHC Associations

Table 39–4 lists some MHC-associated diseases and their markers. The list is not exhaustive, and we discuss only a few of them here. The application of methods of analysis already cited has aided in understanding only a few of these disorders.

The MHC region has provided genetic markers for distinguishing recessive from dominant disease genes. Two dominantly inherited diseases in which genetic linkage to MHC has been suggested are Paget's disease of the bone (Fotino, 1977) and spinocerebellar ataxia (Jackson, 1977). The recombination fraction in these diseases suggests that the gene is outside the MHC. Idiopathic hemochromatosis is a nonimmunologic disease inherited as an autosomal recessive trait (Cartwright, 1979). There is evidence that an important gene or genes with products involved in iron metabolism are located close to the MHC (Simon, 1977). It has also been shown that the disease is closely linked to the telomeric side of the MHC complex and that there are associations with *HLA-A3* and, to a lesser extent, *HLA-B14* and *B7*.

There is a remarkably strong association between *HLA-B27* and ankylosing spondylitis (AS) in several caucasoid, mongoloid, and negroid populations (Khan, 1992). Among patients with AS, reactive arthropathies, and acute anterior uveitis, about 90% of caucasoid patients, compared with 5% to 10% of healthy controls, have *HLA-B27* (Rubin, 1994). The association of *B27* with these syndromes in four racial groups (whites, blacks, Japanese, and Native American) suggests that *B27* itself or a gene closely linked to *B27* is involved in the pathogenesis of these diseases. Differences in the regional prevalence of AS correlate also with the frequency of *HLA-B27*. Among the *HLA-B27*–positive individuals in the population at large, only 2% develop AS. If there is a family history of the disease, the prevalence among *HLA-B27*–positive relatives is approximately 20%. At least seven alleles of *HLA-B27* have been described. *HLA-B*2705* is the most commonly found allele in normal subjects. None of the *HLA-B27* subtypes are specifically associated with AS. The conserved residues in these alleles are spatially close to one another and are situated near the B pocket of the binding cleft of the HLA-B27 molecule. However, studies in Gambian blacks (Hill, 1991) have suggested that *HLA-B*2703*, which differs from *B*2705* by a histidine substitution for tyrosine at position 59, confers a lower risk for AS. The substitution could be important because position 59 is also in the vicinity of the B pocket and because tyrosine residues at this position appear to play some role in anchoring the amino-terminus of the nonameric peptide antigens that bind to Class I molecules. It has been suggested that the presence of *HLA-B40* on the opposite HLA haplotype from *HLA-B27* further increases susceptibility to AS, supporting the hypothesis that non-*B27* alleles contribute to increase susceptibility for AS. The most compelling data that *HLA-B27* is the primary factor predisposing to AS come from the development of the *HLA-B27* transgenic rat, which spontaneously develops disease with striking resemblance to AS (Hammer, 1990). The transgenic lines that develop disease exhibited the highest copy numbers per cell of *HLA-B27*. It has been suggested that the high density of HLA-B27 on mononuclear cells of affected rats may enable the presentation of a peptide to a reactive T cell population that may trigger an arthritogenic process. This arthritogenic peptide theory is currently the most favored explanation to support the pathogenic role of *HLA-B27* in AS. It is believed that exogenous peptide antigens (most likely from infectious agents) presented by HLA-B27 prime a T cell response, and subsequently these T cells recognize similar but self-peptide antigens in association with HLA-B27. The self-tolerance breakdown may occur because certain pathogens carry proteins with sequence motifs similar to self-peptides. Bacterial proteins that show structural homology to HLA-B27 include a sequence of six amino acids between residues 72 and 77 of *HLA-B*2705* and residues 188 and 193 on a *Klebsiella pneumoniae* nitrogenase reductase, and between positions 71 and 75 of the major HLA-B27 subtypes and a stretch of five amino acids of a plasmid from an arthritogenic strain of *Shigella flexnerii* (Steiglitz, 1989).

Table 39–4. EXAMPLES OF ASSOCIATION BETWEEN HLA AND DISEASE

Disease	Ethnicity	HLA Antigen	Relative Risk
Behçet's disease	Japanese	B51	7.9
	Chinese	B51	3.4
Celiac disease	British	DRB1*0301	26.7
		DQB1*0201	51.8
		DQA1*0501	13.9
	Italian	DRB1*0301	6.9
		DQB1*0201	36.8
		DQA1*0501	10.9
		DRB1*0701	4
		DQA1*0201	6.7
	Czech	DRB1*0301	12.2
		DQA1*0501	11
		DRB1*0701	3.1
		DQA1*0201	2.9
Graves' disease	German	DR3, B8, Cw7	3.2–5.5
		DQA1*0102	9.2
	Japanese	A2	2.9
		DPB1*0501	5.3
	Sardinian	DRB1*1601	2.3
	Singapore Chinese	DRB1*0301	3.5
		DR52	7.3
Hashimoto's thyroiditis	Hungarian	DR52	3.4
		DR53	4.1
	Canadian	DQA1*0301/0302, DQB1*0201	3.6
	British	DQA1*0301/0302, DQB1*0301	9.7
HIV infection	European	Cw7	1.5
		DQB1*0601	2.2
Fast progressor*		B7	3.4
		B35	2.5
		Cw7	2.1
Slow progressor		DQB1*0605	9.2
Hodgkin's disease	Caucasoid (Europe/America)	DPB1*0301	1.95
Idiopathic membranous nephropathy	British	DRB3*0101	5.5
		DRB1*0301	9.8
		DQB1*0201	21.6
		DQA1*0501	6.7
	Japanese	DRB1*1501	14.2
		DQB1*0602	16.8
		DQA1*0102	7.1
Idiopathic nephrotic syndrome	French	DR7	6.4
		DQA1*0201	5.3
	German	DR7	2.8
		DQA1*0201	3.3
Multiple sclerosis	French	DRB1*1501, DQB1*0602, DQA1*0102	3.0
	European	One of DQA1*0102/0103/or 0501 plus One of DQB1*0602/0603/0604/0302/or 0303	13.0
Narcolepsy	Japanese	DRB1*1501	1030
		DRB5*0101	1263
		DR15	384
		DQB1*0602	1468
		DQA1*0102	537
	Canadian	DRB1*1501	93.5
		DR15	13.2
		DQB1*0602	85.4
		DQA1*0102	28.6
Rheumatoid arthritis	French	DRB1*01	3.5
		DRB1*0401	4.3
		DRB1*0404	10.7
	Asian Indian	DR1	3.4
		DRB1*1001	3.8
	Chinese	DR1	6.8
	Japanese	DRB1*0405	3.6

*HIV-infected patients carrying the haplotype [HLA-B8, SC01, DR3] have a faster course of the disease. (See Steel CM, Ludlam CA, Beatson D, et al: HLA haplotype A1 B8 DR3 as a risk factor for HIV-related disease. Lancet 1988; 1(8596):1185–1188.)

Data extracted from Tsuji K, Aizawa M, Sasazuki T (eds): HLA 1991. Proceedings of the 11th International Workshop and Conference. New York, Oxford University Press, 1992.

The most studied of all MHC-linked diseases is type I diabetes mellitus (Nepom, 1991; Thorsby, 1992; Winter, 1993). The HLA contribution to type I diabetes has not been adequately explained. There are striking increases in *HLA-DR3* and *DR4* in white patients. In family studies, it was shown that the *DR3* increase in patients was the result of the increase in the extended haplotypes [*HLA-B8, SC01, DR3*] and [*HLA-B18, F1C30, DR3*], and much of the increase in *DR4* resulted from an increase in [*HLA-B62, SC33, DR4*] and [*HLA-B38, SC21, DR4*], but there was also an increase in nonextended *HLA-DR4* haplotypes. In many but not all caucasoid patient populations with type I diabetes, there is an excess of *DR3/DR4* heterozygotes over the number of *DR3* or *DR4* homozygotes predicted by the Hardy-Weinberg equilibrium. The reasons for this are unclear. By DNA analysis, the increase in *DR4* is primarily in that subset of *DR4* in linkage disequilibrium with *DQB1*0302*. Although the latter gene is now considered a major marker and perhaps a primary determinant of type I diabetes susceptibility, it is present in only 70% of caucasoid patients, and even among those who carry it, there is variability in the relative risk for diabetes: *DRB1*0401, DQB1*0302* and *DRB1*0402, DQB1*0302* are highly associated with the disease, while *DRB1*0404, DQB1*0302* is less so. Therefore, it seems probable that there are multiple Class II region contributions to susceptibility to diabetes. *DQA1*0301* is present on all *DR4*-positive haplotypes, whether they carry *DQB1*0302* or not, and it is possible that it may contribute to risk. DPB may also play a role in susceptibility. On the other hand, *DRB1*1501, DQB1*0602* and *DRB1*1301, DQB1*0603* are negatively associated with type I diabetes. Individuals heterozygous for *DRB1*1501* who also carry a type I diabetes–susceptibility gene on the other haplotype are nonetheless not at risk for the disease (dominant protection), as expected in a recessive disorder. A recently proposed model for type I diabetes, which assumes that *DQB1* is a direct determinant of susceptibility, suggests a hierarchy of affinities among different Class II molecules that compete for binding to the same (unidentified) type I diabetes peptide. Susceptibility occurs if a gene product (for example, DQB1*0302) binds and presents the peptide. In the presence of a high-affinity (DRB1*1501) competitor, this event does not occur. Synergism (*DR3/DR4*) could be explained by high-affinity peptide binding to a *trans*-associated Class II dimer. Different relative risk (*DR1/DR4* or different haplotypes carrying *DQB1*0302*) can be explained by different affinities of those molecules for the peptide. Another model proposes that an aspartic acid at codon 57 of the *DQB* chain protects from type I diabetes. The presence of a different amino acid, most frequently valine or serine, at that position in haplotypes carrying *HLA-DR3* or *DR4* found in excess in patients supported the concept. Several studies have confirmed this finding in caucasoids although not in mongoloid diabetics. Other studies hypothesized that the presence of arginine at position 52 of *DQA1* is another genetic factor. A combination of nonaspartic acid at position 57 of *DQB1* and arginine in position 52 of *DQA1* has been suggested to be important in determining susceptibility to type I diabetes mediated by *DQB1* genes.

The association between MHC markers and rheumatoid arthritis (RA) is well documented (Nepom, 1992; Ollier, 1992). For most populations studied, the primary associated marker is *HLA-DR4*. In caucasoids, for example, the most common RA-associated *DR4* alleles are *DRB1*0401, 0404* and *0408*, and in Japanese, Israeli, and Chinese patients, it is *DRB1*0405*. Other *HLA-DR* specificities are also associated with RA: *DR1* has been reported to be associated with RA in Japanese, Spanish, Greek, and Israeli patients; *DR3* in Kuwaitis; *DR6* in Yakima Indians; *DR9* in Chileans; and *DR10* also in Spanish, Greek, and Israeli patients. To explain this broad spectrum of different *HLA-DR* associations with RA, it has been proposed that a shared DRB1 peptide sequence is involved in conferring RA susceptibility. The alleles associated with RA share a highly conserved sequence of amino acids in their third hypervariable region (amino acids 70 to 74). These residues could affect the binding of peptides and their presentation to T cells. Thus, if an arthritogenic peptide exists, it may preferentially bind to molecules with the RA DRB1 sequence. As yet, no such arthritogenic peptide has been identified. An alternative explanation may involve molecular mimicry between the shared RA DRB1 and antigenic sequences of a pathogen that can induce RA. Sequence homology has been found between the shared RA sequence and the Epstein-Barr virus glycoprotein gp110, and with a heat shock protein (HSP) from *Escherichia coli*. Several reports have demonstrated a relationship between RA severity and increasing *HLA-DR4* frequency, in particular with *DRB1*0401*. *HLA-DR4*–positive patients with RA have been found to have a more severe disease course, and *HLA-DR4*–homozygous patients are more likely to have severe RA. It is also possible that rheumatoid factor production is associated with *DR4*. The risk associated with *DRB1*04* is generally higher than that attributable to *DRB1*01* or *DRB1*10*.

RA differs clinically from juvenile rheumatoid arthritis (JRA). In recent years, attempts have been made to subdivide JRA into several distinct syndromes based on the mode of onset. The main groups are (1) systemic with daily intermittent fever, (2) polyarticular, and (3) pauciarticular arthritis. The polyarticular group is subdivided into those who are (a) rheumatoid factor–positive and (b) rheumatoid factor–negative. The pauciarticular group is further subdivided into (a) persistent pauciarticular, (b) males with onset over the age of eight, (c) a form with chronic iritis, and (d) conversion to a polyarticular form. The soundness of this clinical classification has been borne out by studies of HLA association and long-term follow-up. In contrast to *DR4* association in rheumatoid arthritis, the HLA associations with JRA are quite different. Furthermore, other *HLA-DR* associations vary with the JRA subsets (Stastny, 1993). For example, it has been reported that the haplotype *HLA-DRB1*0801, DQA1*0401, DQB1*0402* is increased overall in the pauciarticular group and in patients with the persistent pauciarticular form. The haplotype *HLA-DRB1*1301, DRB3*0101, DQA1*0103, DQB1*0603* was also associated with patients with persistent pauciarticular JRA (Fernandez-Viña, 1994). Other specificities associated with persistent pauciarticular JRA are *DRB1*1104* and *DPB1*0201*. Pauciarticular JRA with conversion to a polyarticular form has been associated with several *DR, DP,* and *DQ* alleles: *DRB1*01, DRB1*0801, DRB1*1401, DQB1*0501, DQB1*0503, DQA1*0101,* and *DPB1*0201*. Pauciarticular JRA with chronic iritis shows a strong association with *DRB1*1104, DR8*, and *DR6*. In addition to Class II associations, a significant increase in *HLA-A2* has been observed in patients with pauciarticular JRA. Male patients with onset after eight have a markedly increased frequency of *HLA-B27*. In patients with polyarticular JRA and negative rheumatoid factor, *DRB1*0801* and *DPB1*0301* have shown association with the disease. In keeping with the view that the polyarticular form of JRA is RA occurring in the young, *DRB1*0401* shows a strong association.

In caucasoids, two extended haplotypes account for more than 60% of haplotypes in patients with gluten-sensitive enteropathy (GSE) (Alper, 1992; Goggins, 1994; Marsh, 1992): [*HLA-B8, SC01, DR3*] and [*HLA-B44, FC31, DR7*]. Analogously to diabetes, there is an increase in *HLA-DR5/7*. Both *HLA-DR3* and *DR7* are in linkage disequilibrium with *HLA-DQ2* (*DQB1*0201, DQA1*0501*). The DQB, DQA heterodimer may be encoded in *cis* on *HLA-DR3* haplotypes, and in *trans* on *HLA-DR5/7* heterozygous individuals. Such combination of *DQB, DQA* genes is found in 98% of patients with celiac disease. This finding suggests that HLA-DQ2 could present the gliadin peptide to T cells for immune recognition. Patients who do not have the *HLA-DQ2* haplotype carry other so-called minor susceptibility markers: (*DR4, DQ7*), (*DR5, DQ1*), (*DR2, DQ1*), and (*DR6, DQ1*). Different studies have raised the possibility of specific *HLA-DP* alleles associated with GSE: *DPB1*01* and *DPB1*03* in southern Europeans and *DBP1*03* and *DBP1*04* in northern Europeans. The increase in *DPB*01* is found in association with *HLA-DR3*, suggesting that the [*HLA-B8, SC01, DR3*] extended haplotype often extends through *DP* in GSE. DP and DQ susceptibility determinants share a positively charged residue around codon 71 of the β-chain, but its specific role is not clear yet. Another MHC marker recently associated with GSE is the 8.5-kb allele of the *HSP70-2* gene, which is known to be in linkage disequilibrium with *HLA-DR3*–carrying haplotypes (Partanen, 1993). GSE and dermatitis herpetiformis (DH) share some clinical features and MHC markers. Patients with DH have increased frequency of the same extended haplotypes associated with GSE. However, by haplotype comparisons, it is evident that the two disorders are different: susceptibility genes for GSE are in or near the *HLA-DR/DQ* region, whereas those for DH appear to be between complement and the *HLA-DR/DQ* region, closer to the complement region (Ahmed, 1993b).

Pemphigus vulgaris (PV) has been associated with two kinds of *HLA-DR4, DQ8* haplotypes among Jewish patients and with these plus *HLA-DR6, DQ5* haplotypes in non-Jewish patients. In Jewish patients, the increased *DR4* frequency is entirely attributable to two related, extended haplotypes in that ethnic group: [*HLA-B38, SC21, DR4, DQ8*] and the haplotype [*HLA-B35, SC31, DR4, DQ8*]. Jewish patients studied carried the complete haplotypes or their fragments (*SC31, DR4, DQ8*), (*SC21, DR4, DQ8*), or *DR4, DQ8* alone, and the distribution of *HLA-DR4* among them was consistent with dominant inheritance. When non-Jewish patients were studied, some had *HLA-DR4, DQ8* haplotypes, as in the Jewish patients, but also *HLA-B55, SB45, DR14(6), DQ5* or its presumed *DR14(6), DQ5* segment. These findings suggest that two mutations gave rise to MHC susceptibility genes for pemphigus vulgaris. One, perhaps the most ancient one, arose in a precursor of [*HLA-B38/35, SC21/31, DR4, DQ8*] in a Jewish population and diffused to non-Jewish populations. The other, more recent, appears to have arisen on [*HLA-B55, SB45, DR14(6), DQ5*] and to have diffused to other populations (Ahmed, 1991a). Forty-eight percent of relatives of patients with PV who share the susceptibility haplotypes have low levels of the PV antibody. The inheritance of these low levels of antibody in asymptomatic relatives was closely linked to the MHC, almost always to a *DR4* or *DR6* haplotype. Thus, the disease appears to occur in susceptible individuals with low levels of antibody when a second factor, genetic or environmental, induces high levels sufficient to produce blisters (Ahmed, 1993a).

In cicatricial pemphigoid (CP), *HLA-DRB1*04* and *DQB1*0301* have been associated with the ocular form of the disease (Ahmed, 1991b). Both ocular and oral forms of CP are associated with the haplotype *DRB1*04, DRB4*0101, DQA1*0301, DQB1*0301*. These results indicate that *DQB1*0301* is a common marker for both oral and ocular forms of CP, which may form a spectrum of a single disease. Analysis of the sequence of amino acids present in *DQB1* alleles in patients with ocular and oral forms of CP showed that they share common residues at positions 57 and 71 to 77, and it is possible that they may also be markers for the disease (Yunis, 1994).

A number of causes of renal failure are mediated by immunologic injury. Antibodies directed at glomerular basement membrane mediate Goodpasture syndrome, which is associated with *HLA-DR2*. *HLA-DR2* and *DR3* as well as *C4A*Q0* have been found to be elevated in systemic lupus erythematosus, the latter two markers largely as part of the extended haplotype [*HLA-B8, SC01, DR3*]. In systemic lupus erythematosus, different MHC markers may help subclassify heterogeneous subsets of the disease.

Elements of the extended haplotype [*HLA-B8, SC01, DR3*] have been reported to be increased in a wide variety of diseases in addition to those already mentioned, including idiopathic Addison's disease, myasthenia gravis, sicca syndrome, idiopathic membranous nephropathy, chronic active hepatitis without HBsAg, and Graves' disease. It may be that this haplotype functions as a genetic sink, accumulating disease-susceptibility alleles because of some present or previous selective advantage of one or more genes that it carries.

METHODS OF DETECTING ASSOCIATION OR LINKAGE OF DISEASES WITH GENETIC MARKERS

Strength of Association

Several methods have been devised for detecting the degree of association of genetic markers with hypothesized genes for disease susceptibility. One is to compute the risk of disease among individuals carrying a specific allele of a polymorphic system. In this computation, the relative risk (RR), or odds ratio, estimates the risk of carrying a marker in a population of diseased individuals compared with that in a control population. More interesting is an estimate of the risk

Table 39–5. RELATIVE RISK (RR)* FOR MHC ALLELES IN SEVERAL DISEASES

	HLA-A		HLA-B		HLA-DR		BF	
Disease	***Allele***	***RR***	***Allele***	***RR***	***Allele***	***RR***	***Allele***	***RR***
Type I diabetes mellitus	*A1*	1.6	*B8*	2.5	*DR3*	4.5		
			B15	2.5	*DR4*	4.5		
			B18	2.5			*BF*F1*	8
			B7	0.2	*DR2*	0.1		
Multiple sclerosis	*A3*	1.8	*B7*	3.5	*DR2*	4.2		
Gluten enteropathy	*A1*	1.8	*B8*	8.0	*DR3*	17.0		
Chronic active hepatitis	*A1*	1.7	*B8*	3.0	*DR3*	2.2		
Idiopathic membranous			*B8*	2.3	*DR3*	4.4		
glomerulonephritis			*B18*	2.3			*BF*F1*	16.0
Idiopathic hemochromatosis	*A3*	4.8	*B7*	1.9				
	A1	2.0	*B14*	4.9	*DRw6*	3.2		
			B15	3.5	*DR4*	2.9		

$$*RR = \frac{\text{patients with marker}}{\text{patients without marker}} \times \frac{\text{controls without marker}}{\text{controls with marker}}$$

of having disease in an individual carrying the marker, but this is much more difficult to estimate (Table 39–5; see also Table 39–4).

This strength of association is the Δ of Bergston and Thomson (Svejgaard, 1983), which is the same as the etiologic fraction (EF) of Miettinen (1976). If in a patient population, *a* individuals carry the specific character but *b* individuals do not and in the control (normal) population, *c* individuals carry the character, the information can be conveniently written in the 2 × 2 table:

	Character Positive	Character Negative
Patient	*a*	*b*
Control	*c*	*d*

The frequency of the character in this patient population (h_p) is

$$hp = \frac{a}{a + b}$$

The relative risk (RR), or odds ratio, is defined as

$$RR = \frac{a \times d}{b \times c}$$

Etiologic fraction (EF) (Miettinen, 1976) is defined as

$$EF = \frac{RR - 1}{RR} \times \frac{a}{a + b}$$

$$= \frac{RR - 1}{RR} \times h_p$$

Similarly, in decreased risks, for which the RR is less than 1, the preventive factor (PF) can be used.

$$PF = \frac{(1 - RR)\, h_p}{RR(1 - h_p) + h_p}$$

The EF and PF fractions can vary between 0 (no association) and 1.0 (maximal association).

Apart from providing estimates of having a marker if the subject already has a disease, these calculations ignore the mode of genetic determination of the disease in question. This is particularly problematic for recessive or more complicated modes in which both haplotypes matter for determining disease, but heterozygosity and homozygosity for a given marker are given the same weight—that is, both are positive for the marker.

Analysis of Mode of Inheritance Based on Sibling Pairs

This method was introduced to help overcome the problems of incomplete penetrance of disease genes and variations in age of onset (Penrose, 1935). The method is based on the assumption that if HLA and/or genes closely linked to HLA have no influence on the development of a disease, then the affected sibling pairs will share HLA haplotypes with a normal frequency: 25% will share both haplotypes, 50% will share one, and 25% will share no haplotypes. Thus, observed and expected distributions of haplotype sharing are compared. If susceptibility genes or their closely linked markers are rare and fully penetrant, in purely recessively determined disease the distribution of 2, 1, and no haplotype-sharing siblings would be 100, 0, 0. For dominant determination, the ratio would be 33, 66, 0. What is observed in diabetes, for example (Rubinstein, 1977), is 60, 35, 5—closer to recessive than dominant predictions. Once the mode of inheritance has been established, the "disease" gene frequency and penetrance can be established (Thomson, 1977).

Analysis of Mode of Inheritance Based on Population Studies

Thomson and Bodmer (1977) have devised a method for analyzing population data for markers closely linked to susceptibility loci for diseases with incomplete penetrance. In essence, this method predicts the proportion of homozygotes, heterozygotes, and noncarriers for the linked marker expected in the cases of dominant or recessive inheritance. The greatest difference between the two modes of inheritance is obtained in the proportion of individuals who are homozygous for the marker. Application of this method to HLA-B27 and AS led, on statistical grounds, to rejection of a recessive mechanism. Thus, it was concluded that susceptibility to AS is inherited as a dominant trait.

Similarly, the same method of analysis was applied to the distribution of *BF*F1* among 1107 patients with type I diabetes mellitus (Raum, 1981). For dominant inheritance, 1.89 homozygotes were predicted and for recessive inheritance, 6.2. Seven *BF*F1* homozygotes were found, a result consistent only with recessive inheritance. Other modes of inheritance that could be rejected by these observations include simple dominant, epistatic (disease resulting from the presence of nonallelic genes), or overdominant (disease with greater penetrance when two specific alleles are present than when other combinations, including homozygosity for each specific allele, occur). Although a mixed model with different penetrance for homozygotes and heterozygotes could not be completely ruled out, other considerations make such a model unsatisfactory.

Lod Score Method

This is a statistical measure of linkage between a marker locus such as in the MHC and a disease susceptibility gene (Sutton, 1980): (1) the Z value is the ratio of the maximum likelihood of finding linkage ($P(F_1/\Theta)$) to that of no linkage at a particular recombination value Θ and (2) the maximal Θ ($\hat{\Theta}$) value, or recombination frequency, which is a measure of distance from a given locus corresponding to maximum Z value. The lod score expresses the probability that alleles at two loci will segregate together, in terms of the ratio between the observed recombination frequency with that predicted if they assort independently. Various values of (Θ) from 0 to 0.5 are substituted in the equation:

$$P(F_1/\Theta) = 1/2\,[\Theta^r(1-\Theta)^{n-r} + \Theta^{n-r}(1-\Theta)^r]$$

where n = the number of children in a given family and r = the number of recombinants. The probability of obtaining a pedigree for a given value of Θ (recombination frequency from 0 to 0.5) is expressed as the ratio of $P(F_1/\Theta)$ in a family at a given recombination fraction Θ (from 0 to 0.5) to $P(F_1/0.5)$ in the same family, assuming no recombination that can be expressed as the lod score (Z):

$$z = \log_{10}\frac{P(F_1/\Theta)}{P(F_1/0.5)}$$

and Z = sum of all z values. Values of Z greater than zero favor linkage and those less than or equal to zero are against linkage. In general, a Z value greater than 3 (for some values of Θ less than 0.5) means that the odds in favor of linkage are 1000 to 1 (p value = 0.05), as opposed to no linkage or independence. It is easier to calculate linkage for codominant traits—that is, HLA and GLO—than for recessive traits. In studies of linkage of HLA and disease, the parents may have recessive or dominant impenetrant susceptibility genes. There are basic problems in using the lod score method to detect linkage of partially penetrant genes, apart from impenetrant–susceptible siblings. If susceptibility genes are common, as appears to be the case in type I diabetes, for example, apparent cross-overs, or nonidentical sibs, could represent additional susceptibility genes in a parent.

POSSIBLE MECHANISMS FOR MHC AND DISEASE ASSOCIATION

There are a number of diseases in which specific alleles of various MHC loci occur at higher frequencies in patients than in normal control populations. These associations may have arisen in several ways: inbreeding, population stratification, or linkage. Most antigens of the MHC vary considerably in frequency in different geographic locations. These differences could be in the frequency of individual alleles or in extended haplotypes or both. It is essential to select control populations carefully for comparison of the gene frequencies with those observed in the disease populations. It appears, however, that at least some of the observed associations do represent linkage of a disease susceptibility locus to the MHC or else arise from an interaction of MHC antigens with environmental factors initiating a pathologic process. A number of possible mechanisms for such effects have been suggested, many of which derive from experimental study of the mouse. Because the number of associations already detected is large, it seems probable that more than one of the proposed mechanisms are operative. They are summarized as follows.

Altered Self-Antigens

Jerne (1971) and Benacerraf (1978) have proposed that functionally mature T cells have low reactivity with autologous MHC antigens and concomitantly high affinity for allogeneic antigens. This model predicts that clones of alloreactive T cells should be highly cross-reactive with modified syngeneic cells. In a family study in humans, cytotoxic T cell responses to influenza virus–infected autologous cells in vitro showed T cell recognition of influenza virus (by cytotoxicity) that was dependent on HLA type (McMichael, 1977). This restriction can be demonstrated with isolated HLA antigens reconstituted into phospholipid vesicles (Engelhard, 1980). The arthritogenic peptide theory suggests that peptide antigens from infectious agents presented by HLA molecules (HLA-B27 in this example) can trigger a T cell response and that those T cells recognize similar but self-peptide antigens in association with HLA-B27. Incubation of lymphocytes from HLA-B27–positive normal subjects with culture supernatants from cultures of *Klebsiella pneumoniae* (but not *E. coli, Yersinia*, or *Shigella*) renders the lymphocytes reactive to normally nonreactive T cells. It has been observed that lymphocytes from HLA-B27–positive AS patients also react with those T cells (Geczy, 1981). Reactive arthritis often follows bowel infection with *Yersinia* or

Shigella (but not usually *Klebsiella*) infection, but these organisms have not been shown to alter antigen specificities.

Another example of MHC and disease association that may be explained by some interaction between an HLA antigen and an etiologic agent is GSE. Organ cultures from patients with active GSE demonstrated that gluten exerts a toxic effect on intestinal mucosa, inhibiting epithelial cell maturation. This effect was seen more frequently in HLA-B8–positive patients with active GSE than in HLA-B8–negative patients (Falchuk, 1980).

Molecular Mimicry

It has been postulated that, in certain cases, MHC gene products may resemble or be closely related in structure to an antigen of an infectious agent, rendering the system unresponsive because of cross-tolerance. Such homologous regions could also serve as an autoantigenic target, with an immune response to the infectious agent leading to attack of self cells expressing relevant MHC gene products. This mechanism has been invoked to explain both the *HLA-B27*–associated diseases and certain other diseases with strong *HLA-B* associations: Behçet's disease (*HLA-B5*) and de Quervain's subacute thyroiditis (*HLA-B35*). Molecular analyses of MHC allelic diversity and of a variety of microbial pathogens have revealed shared epitopes, including Class II molecules. For example, cross-reactivity has been reported between proteins produced by alleles of the *HLA-DRB1* locus and a cytomegalovirus protein and between HLA-DQβ and an Epstein-Barr virus protein. Similarly, a motif has been identified in three amino acids (DKA) shared by HLA-DRα and three enzymes of *E. coli* (the E2 subunit of the pyruvate dehydrogenase complex, glycogen phosphorylase, and sulfite oxidase) that act as targets for the polyclonal antimitochondrial antibodies that are characteristic of primary biliary cirrhosis (Burroughs, 1992). It has been proposed that these peptides are presented by MHC Class II molecules and that T cells stimulated by these peptides might then, through a process of molecular mimicry, initiate an autoimmune response against any tissue expressing the peptide derived from HLA-DRα (Baum, 1993). It has also been suggested that the high degree of sequence conservation between heat-shock proteins and a variety of infectious agents, because of molecular mimicry, may provide the link between infection and subsequent autoimmunity (Res, 1991). T cells responding to HSP65 have been identified in autoimmune diseases such as adjuvant arthritis in Lewis rats and type I diabetes in nonobese diabetic mice (Res, 1991).

Immune Response and Immune Suppression Genes

Such genes, which have been demonstrated in mouse and guinea pig, form the basis for assumptions that at least some *HLA-D/DR*–associated diseases are due to altered or suppressed immune responses. In keeping with this concept, a number of diseases involving autoimmunity or that are suspected to have autoimmune components have shown a stronger association with *HLA-D/DR* than with Class I markers. Type I diabetes, Graves' disease, idiopathic Addison's disease, myasthenia gravis, dermatitis herpetiformis, celiac disease, chronic active hepatitis (lupoid type), Sjögren's syndrome, and systemic lupus erythematosus all have a significant association with *Dw3* and *DR3* in white populations. This type of association also seems relevant in multiple sclerosis and tuberculoid leprosy (*DR2*-associated). Antibodies to pancreatic β cell cytoplasmic antigens, including glutamic acid decarboxylase, in the serum of patients with type I diabetes have been demonstrated, although these antibodies were also found in the serum of 25% of first-degree relatives. These, when accompanied by autoanti-insulin, are associated with the same critical features as in the impending diabetes in such relatives. All of these hold for type I diabetes and DQB 57 non-asp and DQA 52 arg (Rubinstein, 1991). To illustrate the point dramatically, one could make a strong argument that DQB 57 asp (*DQB1*0602* has this) is a susceptibility gene for C2 deficiency even though it has nothing whatsoever to do directly with the disorder.

Nevertheless, the most widely accepted hypothesis has been that polymorphic residues in Class II molecules can differentially bind a putative autoantigenic peptide and present it to responding T lymphocytes. The mouse model of myasthenia gravis (MG) is a good example. The immune response to the acetylcholine receptor (AchR) is under IR (immune response) genetic control. H-2^b mice respond to torpedo eel AchR and develop MG. The bm-12 mutant mouse, which carries a small mutation of the Class II allele *I-A*^{b}, neither responds to AchR nor develops the disease (Christadoss, 1985).

Almost all of our knowledge of the immune response derives from experiments in animals. Although most of this information is probably directly applicable to humans, some is not. For example, recognition of the role of the MHC in negative T cell selection in the murine thymus was based on the presence of the mouse mammary tumor virus in the mouse genome, which functions as a superantigen and deletes specific T cell receptor gene families during thymic development. There is no comparable phenomenon in people.

HLA phenotype studies have suggested that *DR2* is associated with anti–*Amb a* V, a ragweed pollen antigen (Marsh, 1982). The relationship is best illustrated by analysis of MHC haplotypes in individuals with ragweed pollen allergy and asthma, arranged according to IgE anti–*Amb a* V levels (Table 39–6). It is clear that the extended haplotype [*HLA-B7, SC31, DR2*] or its *DR*-containing fragments (*SC31, DR2*), or *DR2* alone, is present in all patients with elevated IgE anti–*Amb a* V (Blumenthal, 1992). This circumstance localizes the MHC gene responsible for this antibody production in these subjects to the *DRB1*1501, DQB1*0602* region.

Approximately 4% of the normal caucasoid population is nonrespondent to hepatitis B vaccine. Nonresponders are enriched in *HLA-DR3* and *HLA-DR7* in the extended haplotypes [*HLA-B8, SC01, DR3*] and [*HLA-B44, FC31, DR7*], often as homozygotes. In prospective studies, homozygotes for [*HLA-B8, SC01, DR3*] were usually nonresponders and had much lower antibody response than did heterozygotes (Alper, 1989), consistent with the response being dominant

Table 39–6. MHC HAPLOTYPES IN RAGWEED POLLEN–SENSITIVE PATIENTS WITH ASTHMA AS WELL AS RHINITIS*

Patient Number	HLA-A	HLA-B	Complotype	HLA-DR	HLA-A	HLA-B	Complotype	HLA-DR	Skin Test	IgE Anti-*Amb a* V Levels
1	24	7†	SC31	2	2	62	FC31	5	16	5131
2	28	7	SC31	2	26	38	SC21	1	14	3051
3	26	7	SC31	2	25	44	SC31	5	15	2538
4	9	7	SC31	2	32	13	SC61	2	15	1689
5	2	61	SC31	2	24	15	SC11	6	15	1090
6	3	7	SC31	2	1	7	SC31	2	14	768
7	2	37	SC31	2	31	8	SC01	3	14	630
8	1	8	SC31	2	24	35	SC31	5	5	256
9	1	39	SC31	2	43	62	SC31	5	4	236
10	2	7	SC31	2	29	44	FC30	6	2	0
11	24	62	FC31	6	24	27	SC30	4	12	0
12	2	44	FC31	7	9	62	SC33	4	0	0
13	28	60	SC02	6	2	44	FC31	4	0	0
14	28	27	SC42	1	23	49	SC31	5	3	0
15	24	18	FC31	9	2	56	SC01	6	1	0
16	29	44	FC31	7	24	62	SC31	5	3	0
17	24	44	SC31	5	31	51	SC31	8	3	0
18	29	44	FC31	7	2	44	SC31	7	5	0
19	33	58	SC61	—	2	44	SC30	4	0	0
20	32	39	SC31	7	2	62	SC33	4	2	0

*Subjects are listed in descending order of anti-*Amb a* V levels.
†Underscore indicates the [HLA-B7, SC31, DR2] extended haplotype or probable fragments of it.
From Blumenthal M, Marcus-Bagley D, Awdeh Z, Johnson B, Yunis EJ, Alper CA: J Immunol 1992; 148:411. Copyright 1992. Extracted from The Journal of Immunology.

and the nonresponse, recessive. The dominant nature of the response to HBsAg was shown directly in family studies (Kruskall, 1992), which also showed by formal linkage studies that there was close linkage between antibody response and the MHC. Absence of antibody response correlated closely with a lack of proliferative response in T cells and was not due to suppressor or cytotoxic T cells (Egea, 1991). The immunodominant peptide is a portion of HBsAg between amino acids 139 and 146, which is restricted by HLA-DR in APC reacting with helper T cells (Deulofeut, 1993).

Receptor

It has been hypothesized that MHC antigens serve as receptors for pathogens. For instance, influenza virus can bind directly to Class I molecules (Chen, 1989). HLA-A and HLA-B antigens have been identified as receptors for Semliki Forest virus (Helenius, 1978), as well as other viruses. It has been hypothesized that some HLA molecules serve as receptors for *Plasmodium*. Absence of such HLA molecules in certain populations could explain the association of *HLA-B53* and the haplotype *DQB1*0501* with resistance to developing severe malaria in West Africa (Hill, 1992).

Accidental

Some diseases may be caused by defective or absent proteins also coded for by MHC genes in linkage disequilibrium with HLA antigens. Thus, idiopathic hemochromatosis shows an association with *HLA-A3*. Partial biochemical expression of the defective gene is seen in heterozygous carriers, although progressive accumulation of iron in the liver occurs only in homozygotes (Amos, 1977; Cartwright, 1979). In a large collaborative study of hemochromatosis, a considerable excess of diseased siblings HLA-identical with the proband supported a recessive mode of inheritance of a single gene.

MHC-Induced Alteration of the T Cell Repertoire

Endogenous peptides that bind to MHC molecules in the thymus play an important role in T cell development. MHC molecules are an important source of peptides that bind to other MHC molecules within the same cell, and it is possible that MHC genes could influence the T cell repertoire by generating peptides in the thymus that favor subsequent autoimmune reactions. Alternatively, it has been reported in mice that MHC polymorphisms could change the expressed repertoire of T cell receptor variable region β gene segments (Blackman, 1989). Mice with major deletions of the T cell receptor β locus are resistant to induced arthritis (Andersen, 1991). However, there is as yet no evidence that MHC molecules cause major deletions of T cell receptor α or β gene segment families in humans.

Involvement of Complement Genes

Genetic deficiencies of the complement factors C4 and C2 are associated with a disease similar to systemic lupus erythematosus. The complement proteins are important for the solubilization of immune complexes and for their removal by red blood cells to the liver. Deficiencies of complement proteins might increase susceptibility to systemic lupus–like disease by increasing exposure of the vasculature to immune complexes or by permitting immune complexes containing autoantigens to gain access to antigen-presenting cells.

Genes Involved with Antigen Processing

The Class II region of the MHC contains polymorphic genes essential for the processing of antigens that bind to Class I and Class II molecules, and it is possible that allelic variations in antigen-processing and peptide-transporter genes may influence susceptibility to autoimmune diseases.

Inappropriate Expression of HLA Class II Molecules

It has been suggested that Class II molecules can be expressed on the target organ of an autoimmune disease—for example, in thyroid epithelium. A virus infection could trigger a local immune response with T cell release of γ-interferon, which induces expression of Class II gene products. These Class II–expressing cells may initiate a continuous cycle of autoreactivity. T cells from thyroid tissue of a patient with Graves' disease can recognize influenza virus presented by thymocytes after *HLA-DR* expression induced by γ-interferon (Bottazzo, 1983). However, most evidence is against expression of Class II molecules by pancreatic β cells or other autoimmune target cells.

Role of Costimulatory Molecules

T cell activation can be achieved by accessory proteins such as the recently characterized B7 molecule that binds to the CD28 receptor of T cells. According to this theory, the interaction of T cells with the MHC-peptide complex in the absence of accessory molecules may lead to anergy. Deficiencies in the expression of MHC molecules in a specific tissue predispose to autoimmune disease because the mechanism that maintains anergy is altered. Consequently, autoantigens gain access to antigen-presenting cells that can express the co-stimulatory molecules necessary for T cell activation.

HLA as a Marker for Abnormal Differentiation Antigens

Studies of H-2 have revealed a closely linked region that controls differentiation in the mouse (DeWolf, 1979). It is conceivable that certain HLA associations arise by linkage disequilibrium with abnormal alleles of human differentiation genes. For instance, human testicular teratocarcinoma is associated with *Dw7*.

It appears that more than one of the mechanisms just described may play a role in the pathogenesis of different diseases. For example, diseases with high relative risk for alleles of the *HLA-B* locus may be explained by either the altered self-mimicry or the receptor hypothesis, whereas other diseases may involve HLA-linked genes that are directly or indirectly involved in regulation of the immune response. The finding that the 21-hydroxylase gene of the steroid hormone pathway and the *TNF* genes are located within the MHC also implies that impairment of some nonimmunologic regulatory functions might produce HLA-associated disease.

SUMMARY

The major histocompatibility complex (MHC) comprises many alleles at many loci. The high-resolution typing of Class I and Class II MHC genes and the identification of genes between and near them have increased the possibility of defining the genetic basis of immune responses and diseases of unknown etiology such as autoimmune diseases in humans. Nonrandom association of markers for immune responses or associations with autoimmune diseases caused by the presence in the population of fixed stretches of MHC DNA and extended haplotypes and their fragments complicate the study of susceptibility genes but also provide the means for identifying them. Even though the human MHC is the most intensively investigated region of the genome, not all of the expressed genes have been identified. Furthermore, for relatively few of these do we know the function of their products. It is probable that some of these rather than one of the already known HLA genes are susceptibility genes for some HLA-associated diseases.

Ahmed AR, Foster S, Zaltas M, et al: Association of *DQw7* (*DQB1*0301*) with ocular cicatricial pemphigoid. Proc Natl Acad Sci USA 1991b; 88:11579.

Ahmed AR, Mohimen A, Yunis EJ, et al: Linkage of pemphigus vulgaris antibody to the MHC in healthy relatives of patients. J Exp Med 1993a; 177:419.

Ahmed AR, Wagner R, Khatri K, et al: MHC haplotypes and class II genes in non-Jewish patients with pemphigus vulgaris. Proc Natl Acad Sci USA 1991a; 88:5056.

Ahmed AR, Yunis JJ, Marcus-Bagley D, et al: MHC susceptibility genes for dermatitis herpetiformis compared with those for gluten-sensitive enteropathy. J Exp Med 1993b; 178:2067.

Alper CA, Awdeh ZL, Raum DD, et al: Complement genes of the human major histocompatibility complex: Implications for linkage disequilibrium and disease associations. *In* Panayi GS, David CS (eds): Immunogenetics. London, Butterworths, 1984, p 50.

Alper CA, Awdeh Z, Yunis EJ: Conserved, extended MHC haplotypes. Exp Clin Immunogenet 1992; 9:58.

Alper CA, Kruskall MS, Marcus-Bagley D, et al: Genetic prediction of nonresponse to hepatitis B vaccine. N Engl J Med 1989; 321:708.

Amos DB, Johnson AH, Cartwright G, et al: HLA and B cell antigens in hemochromatosis. Tissue Antigens 1977; 10:206.

Andersen GD, Banerjee S, Luthra HS, et al: Role of *Mls-1* locus and clonal deletion of T cells in susceptibility to collagen-induced arthritis in mice. J Immunol 1991; 147:1189.

Awdeh Z, Alper CA: Inherited structural polymorphism of the fourth component of human complement. Proc Natl Acad Sci USA 1980; 77:3576.

Awdeh ZL, Raum DD, Glass D, et al: Complement–human histocompatibility antigen haplotypes in C2 deficiency. J Clin Invest 1981; 67:581.

Awdeh Z, Raum D, Yunis EJ, Alper CA: Extended HLA/complement allele haplotypes: Evidence for T/t-like complex in man. Proc Natl Acad Sci USA 1983; 80:259.

Bahram S, Arnold D, Bresnaham M, et al: Two putative subunits of a peptide pump encoded in the human MHC class II region. Proc Natl Acad Sci USA 1991; 88:10094.

Barber LD, Parham P: Peptide binding to major histocompatibility complex molecules. Annu Rev Cell Biol 1993; 9:163.

Baum H, Butler P, Davies H, et al: Autoimmune disease and molecular mimicry: an hypothesis. Trends Biol Sci 1993; 18:140.

5

Benacerraf B: A hypothesis to relate the specificity of lymphocytes and the activity of I region–specific Ir genes in macrophages and B lymphocytes. J Immunol 1978; 120:1809.

Benichou G, Takizawa AP, Olson AC, et al: Donor MHC peptides are presented by recipient MHC molecules during graft rejection. J Exp Med 1992; 175:305.

Bix M, Raulet D: Functionally conformed free class I heavy chains exist on the surface of β_2-microglobulin negative cells. J Exp Med 1992; 176:829.

Bjorkman PJ, Saper MA, Samraoui B, et al: Structure of the human histocompatibility antigen, *HLA-A2*. Nature 1987a; 329:506.

Bjorkman PJ, Saper MA, Samraoui B, et al: The foreign antigen binding site and T cell recognition regions of class I histocompatibility antigens. Nature 1987b; 329:512.

Blackman MA, Marrack P, Kappler J: Influence of the major histocompatibility complex on positive thymic selection of V beta 17a + T cells. Science 1989; 244:214.

Blumenthal M, Marcus-Bagley D, Awdeh Z, et al: *HLA-DR2,* [*HLA-B7, SC31, DR2*], and [*HLA-B8, SC01, DR3*] haplotypes distinguish subjects with asthma from those with rhinitis only in ragweed pollen allergy. J Immunol 1992; 148:411.

Bottazzo GF, Pujol-Borrell, Hanafusa T, Feldmann M: Role of aberrant HLA-DR expression and antigen presentation in induction of endocrine autoimmunity. Lancet 1983; 2:1115.

Braun L, Schneider PM, Giles CM, et al: Null alleles of human complement C4. Evidence of pseudogenes at the *C4A* locus and gene conversion at the *C4B* locus. J Exp Med 1990; 171:129.

Brown J, Jardetzky T, Gorga J, et al: Three-dimensional structure of the human class II MHC antigen *HLA-DR1*. Nature 1993; 364:33.

Browning JL, Lawton P, DeMarinis J, et al: Lymphotoxin β, a novel member of the *TNF* family that forms a heteromeric complex with lymphotoxin on the cell surface. Cell 1993; 72:847.

Burroughs AK, Butler P, Sternberg MJ, Baum H: Molecular mimicry in liver disease. Nature 1992; 358:377.

Carroll MC, Campbell RD, Bentley DR, Porter RR: A molecular map of the human MHC class III region linking complement genes *C4, C2* and *factor B*. Nature 1984; 307:237.

Carroll MC, Campbell RD, Porter RR: Mapping of steroid 21-hydroxylase genes adjacent to complement *C4* genes in HLA, the major histocompatibility complex in man. Proc Natl Acad Sci USA 1985; 82:521.

Carroll MC, Katzman P, Alicot EM, et al: A linkage map of the MHC including the *TNF* genes. Proc Natl Acad Sci USA 1987; 84:8535.

Cartwright GE, Edwards CQ, Kravitz K, et al: Hereditary hemochromatosis: Phenotypic expression of the disease. N Engl J Med 1979; 301:175.

Chen BP, Parham P: Direct binding of influenza peptides to class I HLA molecules. Nature 1989; 337:743.

Chicz RM, Urban RG: Analysis of MHC-presented peptides: Applications in autoimmunity and vaccine development. Immunol Today 1994; 15:155.

Chicz RM, Urban RG, Gorg JC, et al: Specificity and promiscuity among naturally processed peptides bound to *HLA-DR* alleles. J Exp Med 1993; 178:27.

Christadoss P, Lindstrom JM, Melvald RW, Talal N: Mutation at I-A beta chain prevents experimental autoimmune myasthenia gravis. Immunogenetics 1985; 21:33.

Colten HR, Rosen FS: Complement deficiencies. Annu Rev Immunol 1992; 10:809.

Craig EA: Chaperones: Helpers along the pathways to protein folding. Science 1993; 260:1902.

Cresswell P: Assembly, transport, and function of MHC class II molecules. Annu Rev Immunol 1994; 12:259.

Dawkins RL, Christiansen FT, Kay PH, et al: Disease associations with complotypes, supratypes and haplotypes. Immunol Rev 1983; 70:5.

Degen E, Cohen-Doyle MF, Williams DB: Efficient dissociation of the p88 chaperone from MHC Class I molecules requires both β_2-microglobulin and peptide. J Exp Med 1992; 175:1653.

Degli-Esposti MA, Leaver AL, Christiansen FT, et al: Ancestral haplotypes: Conserved population MHC haplotypes. Human Immunol 1992; 34:242.

Deulofeut H, Iglesias A, Mikael N, et al: Cellular recognition and HLA restriction of a midsequence HBsAg peptide in hepatitis B vaccinated individuals. Mol Immunol 1993; 30:941.

DeWolf WC, Lange PH, Einarson ME, Yunis EJ: HLA and testicular cancer. Nature 1979; 277:216.

Dunckley H, Gatenby HR, Hawkins B, et al: Deficiency of C4A is a genetic determinant of systemic lupus erythematosus in three ethnic groups. J Immunogenetics 1987; 14:209.

Dunham I, Sargent CA, Trowsdale J, Campbell RD: Molecular mapping of the MHC by pulsed-field gel electrophoresis. Proc Natl Acad Sci USA 1987; 84:7237.

Eckels D: Alloreactivity: Allogeneic presentation of endogenous peptides or direct recognition of MHC polymorphism. Tissue Antigens 1990; 35:49.

Egea E, Iglesias A, Salazar, M, et al: The cellular basis for lack of antibody response to hepatitis B vaccine in humans. J Exp Med 1991; 173:531.

Elliot T: How do peptides associate with MHC class I molecules? Immunol Today 1991; 12:386.

Elliot T, Cerundolo V, Townsend A: Peptide-induced conformational change at the Class I heavy chain. Nature 1992; 351:402.

Engelhard VH, Kaufman JF, Strominger JL, Burakoff S: Specificity of mouse cytotoxic T-lymphocytes stimulated with either *HLA-A* and *-B* or *HLA-DR* antigens reconstituted into phospholipid vesicles. J Exp Med 1980; 152:54s.

Engelhard VA: Structure of peptides associated with class I and class II MHC molecules. Annu Rev Immunol 1994; 12:181.

Falchuk ZM, Nelson DL, Katz AJ, et al: Gluten-sensitive enteropathy. Influence of histocompatibility type on gluten-sensitivity in vitro. J Clin Invest 1980; 66:277.

Falk K, Rotzschke O, Stevanovic S, et al: Allele-specific motif revealed by sequencing of self-peptides eluted from MHC molecules. Nature 1992; 353:290.

Fernandez-Viña M, Fink CW, Stastny P: HLA associations in juvenile arthritis. Clin Exp Rheumatol 1994; 12:205.

Fielder AHL, Walport MJ, Batchelor HR, et al: Family study of the major histocompatibility complex in patients with systemic lupus erythematosus: Importance of null alleles of *C4A* and *C4B* in determining disease susceptibility. Br Med J 1983; 286:425.

Fotino M, Haymovits D, Falk CT: Evidence for linkage between HLA and Paget's disease. Transplant Proc 1977; 9:1867.

Freemont DH, Matsamura M, Stura EA, et al: Crystal structures of two viral peptides in complex with murine MHC class I H-2k^b. Science 1992; 257:919.

Geczy AF, Alexander K, Bashir HV, et al: HLA-B27, *Klebsiella* and ankylosing spondylitis: Biological and chemical studies. *In* Moller G (ed): Immunological Reviews, vol 70. Copenhagen, Munksgaard, 1981, p 23.

Gitelman SE, Bristow J, Miller W: Mechanism and consequences of the duplication of the human *C4/P450c21/*gene *X* locus. Mol Cell Biol 1992; 12:2124.

Goggins M, Kelleher D: Celiac disease and other nutrient related injuries to the gastrointestinal tract. Am J Gastroent Suppl 1994; 89:S2.

Goldberg AL, Rock KL: Proteolysis, proteosomes and antigen presentation. Nature 1992; 357:375.

Guo HC, Jardetzky TS, Garret TPJ, et al: Different length peptides bind to *HLA-A68* similarly at their ends but bulge out in the middle. Nature 1992; 360:364.

Hammer RE, Malka SD, Richardson JA, et al: Spontaneous inflammatory disease in transgenic rats expressing *HLA-B27* and human β_2 microglobulin. Cell 1990; 63:1011.

Helenius A, Morein B, Fries E, et al: Human and murine histocompatibility antigens are cell receptors for Semliki Forest virus. Proc Natl Acad Sci USA 1978; 75:3846.

Higashi Y, Yoshioka H, Yamane M, et al: Complete nucleotide sequence of two steroid 21-hydroxylase genes tandemly arranged in human chromosome: A pseudogene and a genuine gene. Proc Natl Acad Sci USA 1986; 83:2841.

Hill AVS, Allsop CEM, Kwiatkowski D, et al: HLA class I typing by PCR: *HLA-B27* and an African *B27* subtype. Lancet 1991; 337:640.

Hill AVS, Elvin J, Willis AC, et al: Molecular analysis of the association of *HLA-B53* and resistance to severe malaria. Nature 1992; 360:434.

Hsieh SL, Campbell RD: Evidence that gene *G7a* in the human MHC encodes valyl-tRNA synthetase. Biochem J 1991; 278:809.

Hunt C, Morimoto RI: Conserved features of eukaryotic *HSP70* genes revealed by comparison with the nucleotide sequence of human *HSP70*. Proc Natl Acad Sci USA 1985; 82:6455.

Jackson JF, Currier RD, Terasaki PI, Morton NE: Spinocerebellar ataxia and HLA linkage. N Engl J Med 1977; 296:1138.

Jackson MR, Peterson PA: Assembly and intracellular transport of MHC class I molecules. Annu Rev Cell Biol 1993; 9:207.

Jardetsky TS, Lane WS, Robinson RA, et al: Identification of self-peptides bound to purified *HLA-B27*. Nature 1991; 353:326.

Jerne NK: The somatic generation of immune recognition. Eur J Immunol 1971; 1:1.

Jongeneel CV, Briant L, Udalova IA, et al: Extensive genetic polymorphism in the human tumor necrosis factor region and relation to extended haplotypes. Proc Natl Acad Sci USA 1991; 88:9717.

Kendall E, Sargent CA, Campbell RD: MHC contains a new cluster of genes between the *HLA-D* and complement *C4* loci. Nucleic Acids Res 1990; 18:7251.

Khan MA, Kellner H: Immunogenetics of spondyloarthropathies. Rheum Dis Clin North Am 1992; 18:837.

Kruskall MS, Alper CA, Awdeh Z, et al: The immune response to hepatitis B vaccine in humans: Inheritance patterns in families. J Exp Med 1992; 175:495.

Lamb CA, Cresswell P: Assembly and transport properties of invariant chain trimers and *HLA-DR*–invariant chain complexes. J Immunol 1992; 148:3478.

Lanzavecchia A, Reid PA, Watts C: Irreversible association of peptide with class II MHC molecules in living cells. Nature 1992; 357:249.

Levi-Strauss M, Carroll MC, Steinmetz M, Meo T: A previously undetected MHC gene with an unusual periodic structure. Science 1988; 240:201.

Liu Z, Sun Y, Xi Y, et al: Contribution of direct and indirect recognition pathways to T cell alloreactivity. J Exp Med 1993; 177:1643.

Lotteau V, Teyton L, Peleraux A, et al: Intracellular transport of class II molecules directed by invariant chain. Nature 1990; 348:600.

Machamer CE, Cresswell P: Biosynthesis and glycosylation of the invariant chain associated with HLA-DR antigens. J Immunol 1982; 129:2564.

Madden DR, Gorga JC, Strominger JL, Wiley DC: The three-dimensional structure of HLA-B27 at 2.1 Å resolution suggests a general mechanism of tight peptide binding to MHC. Cell 1992; 70:1035.

Marcus D, Alper CA: Methods for allotyping complement proteins. *In* Rose NR, Friedman H, Fahey JL (eds): Manual of Clinical Laboratory in Immunology. Washington DC, American Society for Microbiology, 1986, p 185.

Marsh DG, Hsu SH, Roebber M, et al: *HLA-Dw2*: A genetic marker for human immune response to short ragweed pollen allergen Ra5.I. Response resulting primarily from natural antigenic exposure. J Exp Med 1982; 155:1439.

Marsh MN: Gluten, major histocompatibility complex, and the small intestine. A molecular and immunobiologic approach to the spectrum of gluten-sensitive "celiac sprue." Gastroenterology 1992; 102:330.

Matsamura M, Fremont D, Peterson PA, Wilson IA: Emerging principles for the recognition of peptide antigens by MHC class I molecules. Science 1992; 257:927.

Matsumoto K, Arai M, Ishihara N, et al: Cluster of fibronectin type III repeats found in the MHC class III region shows the highest homology with the repeats in an extracellular matrix protein, tenascin. Genomics 1992; 12:485.

Mauff, G, Alper CA, Dawkins R, et al: C4 nomenclature statement. Complement & Inflammation 1990; 7(4–6):261.

McMichael AJ, Ting A, Sweerink HJ, Askonas BA: HLA restriction of cell-mediated lysis of influenza virus–infected human cells. Nature 1977; 270:524.

Miettinen OS: Estimability and estimation in case-referent studies. Am J Epidemiol 1976; 103:226.

Milner CM, Campbell RD: Structure and expression of the three MHC-linked *HSP70* genes. Immunogenetics 1990; 32:242.

Milner CM, Campbell RD: Polymorphic analysis of the three MHC-linked *HSP70* genes. Immunogenetics 1992; 36:357.

Milner CM, Campbell RD: The *G9a* gene in the human MHC encodes a novel protein containing ankyrin-like repeats. Biochem J 1993; 290:811.

Morel Y, Bristow J, Giterman SE, Miller WL: Transcript encoded on the opposite strand of the human steroid 21-hydroxylase/complement component *C4* gene locus. Proc Natl Acad Sci USA 1989; 86:6582.

Morrison LA, Lukacher AE, Braciale VL, et al: Differences in antigen presentation to MHC class I and class II restricted influenza virus–specific, cytotoxic T lymphocyte clones. J Exp Med 1986; 163:903.

Nedospasov SA, Udalova IA, Kuprash KV, Turetskaya RL: DNA sequence polymorphism at the human tumor necrosis factor (*TNF*) locus. J Immunol 1991; 147:1053.

Nedwin GE, Naylor SL, Sakaguchi AY, et al: Human lymphotoxin and *TNF* genes: structure, homology and chromosomal localization. Nucleic Acids Res 1985; 13:6361.

Nepom GT, Erlich H: MHC class II molecules and autoimmunity. Annu Rev Immunol 1991; 9:493.

Nepom GT, Nepom BS: Prediction of susceptibility to rheumatoid arthritis by human leukocyte antigen genotyping. Rheum Dis Clin North Am 1992; 18:785.

Newcomb JR, Cresswell P: Structural analysis of proteolytic products of MHC class II–invariant chain complexes generated in vivo. J Immunol 1993a; 151:4153.

Newcomb JR, Cresswell P: Characterization of endogenous peptides bound to purified HLA-DR molecules and their absence from invariant chain-associated $\alpha\beta$ dimers. J Immunol 1993b; 150:499.

Nuchtern JG, Biddison WE, Klausner RD. Class II molecules can use the endogenous pathway of antigen presentation. Nature 1990; 343:74.

Ollier W, Thompson W: Population genetics of rheumatoid arthritis. Rheum Dis Clin North Am 1992; 18:741.

O'Sullivan DM, Noonan D, Quaranta V: Four Ia invariant chain forms derive from a single gene by alternate splicing and alternate initiation of transcription/translation. J Exp Med 1987; 166:444.

Partanen J, Milner C, Campbell RD, et al: HLA-linked *HSP70-2* gene polymorphism and celiac disease. Tissue Antigens 1993; 41:15.

Penrose LS: The detection of autosomal linkage in pairs of brothers and sisters of unspecified parentage. Ann Eugen 1935; 6:133.

Peters PJ, Neefjes JJ, Oorschot V, et al: Segregation of MHC class II molecules from MHC class I molecules in Golgi complex for transport to lysosomal compartments. Nature 1991; 349:669.

Porcelli S, Morita CT, Brenner MB: CD1b restricts the response of human $CD4^{-}CD8^{-}\alpha\beta$ T lymphocytes to a microbial antigen. Nature 1992; 360:593.

Ragoussis J, Monaco A, Mockridge I, et al: Cloning of the HLA class II region in yeast artificial chromosomes. Proc Natl Acad Sci USA 1991; 88:3753.

Raum D, Awdeh Z, Alper CA: BF types and the mode of inheritance of insulin-dependent diabetes mellitus (IDDM). Immunogenetics 1981; 12:59.

Res P, Thole J, de Vries R: Heat-shock proteins and autoimmunity in humans. Springer Semin Immunopathol 1991; 13:81.

Roche PA, Marks MS, Cresswell P: Formation of a nine-subunit complex by HLA class II glycoproteins and the invariant chain. Nature 1991; 354:392.

Roche P, Teletski C, Stang E, et al: Cell surface *HLA-DR* invariant chain complexes are targeted to endosomes by rapid internalization. Proc Natl Acad Sci USA 1993; 90:8581.

Rubin LA, Amos CI, Wade JA, et al: Investigating the genetic basis for ankylosing spondylitis. Arthritis Rheum 1994; 8:1212.

Rubinstein P: HLA and IDDM: Facts and speculations on the disease gene and its mode of inheritance. Hum Immunol 1991; 30:270.

Rubinstein P, Suciu-Foca N, Nicholson JF: Genetics of juvenile diabetes mellitus. A recessive gene closely linked to *HLA-D* and with 50% penetrance. N Engl J Med 1977; 297:1036.

Rudensky AY, Preston-Hurburt P, Alramadi BK, et al: Truncation variants of peptides isolated from MHC class II molecules suggest sequence motifs. Nature 1992; 359:429.

Saper MA, Bjorkman PJ, Wiley DC: Refined structure of the human MHC antigen HLA-A2 at 2.6Å resolution. J Mol Biol 1991; 219:277.

Sargent CA, Dunham I, Campbell RD: Identification of multiple HTF–island associated genes in the MHC class III region. EMBO J 1989a; 8:2305.

Sargent CA, Dunham I, Trowsdale J, Campbell RD: Human MHC contains genes for the major *HSP70*. Proc Natl Acad Sci USA 1989b; 86:1968.

Sayegh MH, Watschinger BK, Carpenter CB: Mechanisms of T cell recognition of alloantigen. Transplantation 1994; 57:1295.

Schaiff WT, Hruska KA, McCourt DW, et al: *HLA-DR* associates with specific stress proteins and is retained in the endoplasmic reticulum in invariant chain negative cells. J Exp Med 1992; 176:657.

Shawar SM, Jatin MV, Rodgers JR, Rich RR: Antigen presentation by MHC class I-B molecules. Annu Rev Immunol 1994; 12:839.

Sherman AL, Chattopadhyay S: The molecular basis of allorecognition. Annu Rev Immunol 1993; 11:385.

Shoskes DA, Wood KJ: Indirect presentation of MHC antigens in transplantation. Immunol Today 1994; 15:32.

Simon M, Bourel M, Genetet B, Fauchet R: Idiopathic hemochromatosis. Demonstration of recessive transmission and early detection by family HLA typing. N Engl J Med 1977; 297:1017.

Spies T, Bresnahan M, Bahram S, et al: A gene in the human MHC class II region controlling the class I antigen presentation pathway. Nature 1990; 348:744.

Spies T, Bresnahan M, Strominger JT: MHC contains a minimum of 19 genes between the complement cluster and *HLA-B*. Proc Natl Acad Sci USA 1989; 86:8955.

Staerz UD, Karasuyama H, Garner AM: Cytotoxic T lymphocytes against a soluble protein. Nature 1987; 329:449.

Stastny P, Fernandez-Viña M, Cerna M, et al: Sequences of HLA alleles associated with arthritis in adults and children. J Rheumatol Suppl 1993; 20:5.

Stieglitz H, Fosmire S, Lipsky P: Identification of a 2 Kd plasmid from *Shigella flexneri* associated with reactive arthritis. Arthritis Rheum 1989; 32:937.

Stroynowski I, Lindhal KF: Antigen presentation by non-classical class I molecules. Curr Opin Immunol 1994; 6:38.

Sutton HE: An Introduction to Human Genetics, 3rd ed. Philadelphia, WB Saunders, 1980, p 415.

Svejgaard A, Platz P, Ryder LP: HLA and disease 1982—a survey. *In* Moller G (ed): Immunological Reviews, vol 70. Copenhagen, Munksgaard, 1983, pp 193–218.

Teyton L, O'Sullivan D, Dickson PW, et al: Invariant chain distinguishes between the exogenous and endogenous antigen presentation pathways. Nature 1990; 348:39.

Thomson G, Bodmer W: The genetic analysis of HLA and disease association. *In* Dausset J, Svejgaard A (eds): HLA and Disease. Copenhagen, Munksgaard, 1977.

Thorsby E: The HLA molecules: Function and role in allorecognition. Transplant Proc 1994; 26:1699.

Thorsby E, Rønningen KS: Role of HLA genes in predisposition to develop insulin-dependent diabetes mellitus. Ann Med 1992; 24:523.

Tiwari JL, Terasaki P: HLA and Disease Associations. New York, Springer-Verlag, 1985, p 1.

Townsend A, Elliot T, Cerundolo V, et al: Assembly of MHC class I molecules analyzed in vitro. Cell 1990; 62:285.

Trowsdale J: "Both man & bird & beast": Comparative organization of MHC genes. Immunogenetics 1995; 41:1.

Truedsson L, Alper CA, Awdeh ZL, et al: Characterization of type I com-

plement C2 deficiency MHC haplotypes. Strong conservation of the complotype/HLA-B region and absence of disease association due to linked class II genes. J Immunol 1993; 151:5856.
Tsuge I, Shen FW, Steinmetz M, Boyse EA: A gene in the H-2H:H-2D interval of the MHC which is transcribed in B cell and macrophages. Immunogenetics 1987; 26:378.
Verjans MGM, Messer G, Weiss EH, et al: Polymorphism of the tumor necrosis factor region in relation to disease: An overview. Rheumatol Clin North Am 1992; 18:177.
Viville S, Neefjes J, Lotteau V, et al: Mice lacking the MHC class II–associated invariant chain. Cell 1993; 72:635.
Webb G, Chaplin DD: Genetic variability at the human tumor necrosis factor loci. J Immunol 1990; 145:1278.
White PC, New MI, Dupont B: Structure of the human steroid 21-hydroxylase gene. Proc Natl Acad Sci USA 1986; 83:5111.
White PC, Witek A, Dupont B, New MI: Characterization of frequent deletions causing steroid 21-hydroxylase deficiency. Proc Natl Acad Sci USA 1988; 85:4436.
Winter WE, Chihara T, Schatz D: The genetics of autoimmune diabetes. Approaching a solution to the problem. Am J Dis Child 1993; 147:1282.
Yunis JJ, Mobini N, Yunis EJ, et al: Common MHC class II markers in clinical variants of cicatricial pemphigoid. Proc Natl Acad Sci USA 1994; 91:7747.

Chapter 40

Immunodeficiency Disorders

Richard Hong, M.D.

The major elements of the human host defense system are (1) the T and B lymphocytes; (2) the monocyte/macrophage system; (3) products of these cell lines that enhance their interaction and effector function, and control their growth and differentiation (cytokines); (4) the complement system; and (5) granulocytes. Mechanical barriers, such as the skin and other epithelial surfaces, cilia, and the filtering action of the spleen, are other important components of host defense. Strictly speaking, polymorphonuclear leukocytes (PMNs) are not immune elements. However, because of the intimate relationship of granulocytes to infection control with overlapping of the clinical symptomatology in PMN disorders and immunodeficiency states, some disorders of PMN are considered. Complement is discussed in Chapter 36. An overview of major immunodeficiency syndromes is given in Table 40–1.

Physicians involved in the assessment of the immune system find themselves in one of three categories. The largest group is primarily interested in a broad screen to determine whether referral or more elaborate studies are necessary. A smaller group is usually associated with a medical center where definitive treatment (such as bone marrow transplant) is provided or instituted. Finally, there is the occasional individual with a major research interest in one aspect of the immune response. Such individuals most often perform very specialized studies or confine their interests to a single system, such as the complement system, or to cell populations, such as natural killer cells or PMNs. It is useful to classify the studies in this perspective so that the reader can appropriately orient himself or herself in the investigative process. Even though a physician may not be personally involved in the investigation, he or she can, with this perspective, provide better support for these patients in their primary care setting. Table 40–2 provides a classification of immune system assessment, based upon three levels that correspond to the three groups of clinicians just described.

CLINICAL CORRELATES

It is not practical to investigate all systems in all patients; however, the clinical picture will point the investigator to the most likely system at fault. Good history taking and a careful physical examination should narrow the possibilities to problems primarily involving the T cells, B cells, or granulocytes. Tables 40–3 and 40–4 list clinical signs and their correlates with the host defense elements.

It is also important to note the special characteristics and to not dwell solely on the number or severity of infectious episodes. For example, when an infectious process involves the same anatomic site repeatedly, the etiology is much more likely to be structural and not a failure of one of the host defenses. Chronic osteomyelitis and recurrent infection of a surgical wound exemplify such a situation. Recurrent urinary tract infections are not characteristic of immune deficiency, because the immune system plays little, if any, role in the prevention of pyelonephritis and cystitis. Recurrent infections caused by *Neisseria* organisms should alert the physician to the possibility of genetic deficiency of one of the complement components. Recurring candidal infection, including oral thrush, is usually not an alarming problem, par-

Table 40–1. CLASSIFICATION OF PRIMARY IMMUNODEFICIENCIES

Condition	Comments
	Combined T-Cell and B-Cell Deficiency
Reticular dysgenesis	Generalized hematopoietic hypoplasia (DeVaal)
Severe combined immunodeficiency (SCID)	Includes (1) X-linked (Swiss), caused by defect of γ chain of IL-2 receptor; (2) autosomal inheritance type; (3) caused by adenosine deaminase (ADA) deficiency; (4) caused by helper T dysfunction or absence (SCID with B cells); (5) associated with clinical features of Letterer-Siwe disease (Ommenn syndrome); (6) associated with bony defects (cartilage-hair hypoplasia, short-limbed dwarfism); (7) bare lymphocyte syndrome, poor expression of transplantation antigens, cannot tissue type patient; (8) caused by cytokine deficiencies
Ataxia-telangiectasia	IgE and IgA deficiency common; high incidence of lymphoreticular malignancy; chromosome repair defect
Hyper-IgE syndrome	Job-Buckley syndrome; high levels of IgE anti-staphylococcal antibody; T-cell defect poorly defined
Thymoma	T-cell defect variable; hypogammaglobulinemia prominent feature
Wiskott-Aldrich syndrome	Thrombocytopenia (small platelets); no carbohydrate antibody responses; eczema; X-linked inheritance; high incidence of lymphoreticular malignancy; CD43+ cells not detected
	Primary T-Cell Deficiency
DiGeorge anomaly	Characteristic facies, heart lesions (interrupted aortic arch most typical); hypoparathyroidism, T-cell deficiency may be severe enough for associated antibody deficiency; immune defect usually spontaneously improves; thymus is absent in complete form; failure of normal descensus nearly always
Nezelof syndrome	Immunoglobulin produced, but specific antibody response markedly impaired; thymic defect uncharacterized
Inosine phosphorylase (PNP) deficiency	Often associated with primary red cell aplasia
CD3 non-expression	T cells present but do not express CD3, necessary for T-cell receptor function
Chronic mucocutaneous candidiasis	Granulomatous skin lesions; often associated with hypoadrenalism, hypoparathyroidism, or other endocrinopathy; with time, antibody deficiency may ensue
	Primary B-Cell Deficiency
Congenital X-linked agammaglobulinemia (Bruton disease; XLA)	Absence of B cells; genetic defect: mutation of Bruton tyrosine kinase gene
Transient hypogammaglobulinemia of infancy	Occurs at 2–6 months of age; difficult to differentiate from the normal nadir of IgG that occurs during that time
HyperIgM syndrome	IgM normal to elevated; defect in expression of gp39, a T-cell ligand for CD40, the B-cell receptor responsible for isotype switching; pneumocystis pneumonia, ordinarily not seen in B-cell diseases, frequent; often associated with cyclic neutropenia
Selective isotype deficiency	(1) Absent/decreased IgM, IgA; normal to increased IgG. (2) selective deficiency of IgA; most common deficiency (1/500 of Caucasians); associated with Class III histocompatibility antigen inheritance
Common variable immunodeficiency	Antibody defect prominent; B cells present; T-cell deficiency may develop and increase with time; some patients have 5'-ectonucleotidase deficiency of B cells
Complement deficiency	Mimics antibody deficiency syndromes; C3 deficiencies clinically similar to panhypogammaglobulinemia; deficiencies of complement components, particularly C6–C9, have recurrent infections with *Neisseria* species
Cilia dysmotility	Mimics antibody deficiency syndromes; recurrent otitis and chronic pulmonary infections with bronchiectasis characteristic
Cell adhesion molecule deficiency (LFA-1/Mac-1)	Mimics antibody deficiency syndromes somewhat; delayed separation of the umbilical cord, poor inflammatory response, periodontitis, recurrent septic episodes

See Rosen (1992), Abbas (1994), Ammann (1989), and Ochs (1989) for further details.

ticularly when antibiotics have been used frequently. However, oral candidiasis is of greater significance when it resists simple local therapy, such as mouth swishes, and also when it persists after six months of age. Oral thrush should not be considered the same as mucocutaneous candidiasis, which is characterized by extension of the infection from the mucous membranes onto the contiguous skin. The cutaneous lesions may be granulomatous in character. Mucocutaneous candidiasis is always abnormal.

A confirmed report of a *bona fide* immunodeficiency disease occurring in a sibling or first-degree relative of an infant should prompt careful clinical assessment and laboratory investigation, even without a history of recurrent or unusual infections. Often affected children will not have their first infectious episode until late in the first or even into the second year of life.

FIRST LEVEL MEASUREMENTS

T Cells

A white blood count and differential will provide information on the morphology and number of small lymphocytes (diameter $< 10\ \mu m$). One expects more than 1200 small lymphocytes per cubic millimeter. Since very few (approximately 10%) of the lymphocytes are B lymphocytes, an absolute lymphocyte deficiency primarily reflects T-cell deficiency.

Delayed hypersensitivity skin tests are excellent measures of T-cell function, because they measure the ability to recognize and present antigen, mobilize the T cells, and generate an inflammatory response. The major shortcoming in using skin tests is that infants have not had sufficient exposure to respond to antigens. Thus, at a time when T-cell assessment is very im-

Table 40–2. LEVELS OF IMMUNOLOGIC TESTS

Level*	Measurement
First level	Lymphocyte number
	Lymphocyte morphology
	Delayed hypersensitivity skin tests
	Immunoglobulin levels (? subclass determinations)
	Specific antibody responses
	X-rays
Second level	Lymphocyte surface marker analysis
	Architecture and immunohistological analysis of lymphoid organs
	Mononuclear cell proliferation studies (using mitogenic, allogeneic cell, and antigen stimulation)
	Isotype analysis
	IgG subclass and analysis
	T-cell cytotoxicity studies
	Complement screening
Third level	Enzyme measurements (adenosine deaminase, inosine phosphorylase)
	Cytokines
	Phagocyte studies (mobility, surface glycoproteins, biochemistry)
	Complex complement studies; genetic defects
	Cellular mixing experiments
	Molecular biology
	Carrier detection
	Prenatal diagnosis

*The level of measurement refers to the clinical setting in which the test is performed and interpreted. First level tests are readily obtainable through the country, at local hospitals, or by sending out to commercial laboratories. The primary physician should be competent to interpret these values. Second level tests are performed at academic centers, usually with a resident immunologist. These tests require clinicians with postgraduate specialization training for adequate analysis. Third level tests are performed only at centers in which there is an active research interest in the subject, and the interpretation is best left to individuals with unique expertise.

portant, these tests are unreliable. Somewhere between three and five years of age, skin tests assume more reliability. Another problem with skin tests is that the antigen must be carefully injected intradermally. The use of multiple, antigen-coated, tines on plastic puncture discs has obviated many of the technical shortcomings of the procedure (Kniker, 1985).

B Cells

Quantitative immunoglobulin assays are readily available (see Chapter 35). Single radial immunodiffusion or laser nephelometry may be employed; these assays are even available to laboratories that perform few analyses. It is important to stress that antibodies of goat origin should not be employed in immunodiffusion assays of IgA, because falsely high values may be seen when anti-Bovidae antibodies are present in the patient, an event occurring in about 40% of the cases of selective IgA deficiency.

Because immunoglobulin values increase with age, comparison with age-matched controls is necessary for correct interpretation (see Chapter 32). For the first few months, IgG of maternal origin is the major immunoglobulin present in the infant. The nadir is seen at approximately three months. However, IgA and IgM can be synthesized by the infant; thus, the presence of those two immunoglobulins is convincing evidence that panhypogammaglobulinemia is not present. Panhypogammaglobulinemia is the usual presenting form of X-linked or autosomal primary hypogammaglobulinemia. In

Table 40–3. CLINICAL SYMPTOMS OF DEFICIENCY CORRELATED WITH TYPE OF DEFECT

Think of T-Cell Deficiency When

1. Live virus or attenuated bacterial vaccine produces systemic illness or untoward result (e.g., generalized vaccinia, giant cell pneumonia with rubeola, generalized *Mycobacterium* infection).
2. An ordinarily benign virus causes overwhelming infection (often pneumonia), such as varicella or cytomegalovirus.
3. Oral *Candida* resists chemotherapy, is unassociated with infected diaper dermatitis or excessive antibiotic therapy, or persists after 6 months of age.
4. *Candida* moves from mucosal surfaces to contiguous cutaneous areas in pattern of mucocutaneous candidiasis.
5. The patient has short-limbed dwarfism. (Hair may be very fine and tissues lax with hyperextensibility of joints and large umbilical hernia.)
6. There are features of intrauterine graft-versus-host disease, e.g., scaling erythrodermia, alopecia, failure to thrive.
7. Graft-versus-host disease occurs after a blood product infusion.
8. Neonatal tetancy occurs. (Look for hypoplastic mandible, short philtrum, low-set ears with notched pinnae, hypertelorism of DiGeorge's anomaly.)
9. Small (less than 10 μm in diameter) lymphocyte count is persistently less than $1200/mm^3$.
10. Infections caused by opportunistic organisms or widespread Kaposi's sarcoma occur. Look for risk factors associated with AIDS.

Think of B-Cell Defect When

1. Recurrent infections with extracellular pyogens, *Streptococcus, Staphylococcus, Haemophilus*. (N.B. With recurrent neisserial infections, consider a congenital complement component deficiency. Also, congenital C3 deficiency can mimic panhypogammaglobulinemia.)
2. Nodular lymphoid hyperplasia of intestine is persistent.

Think of Combined T- and B-Cell Defect When

1. There are features of Wiskott-Aldrich syndrome (draining ears, thrombocytopenia, eczema, male).
2. There are features of ataxia-telangiectasia. (Most characteristic are the telangiectasia of sclera and ears. The facial expression is dull.)
3. The above-mentioned features of T- and B-cell disorders occur together.

Think of a Biochemical Defect When

1. There are features of combined T and B defects with characteristic x-ray changes in ribs, scapulae, vertebrae (adenosine deaminase deficiency).
2. There is a primary red cell aplasia and other features of Blackfan-Diamond syndrome (nucleoside phosphorylase deficiency).

Think of a Leukocyte Defect When

1. There are recurrent severe staphylococcal abscesses of the skin; deep abscesses of internal organs may be seen, but less commonly (Buckley's hyperIgE or Job's syndrome).
2. Chronic or recurrent osteomyelitis, draining lymph nodes; particularly when caused by *Klebsiella* or *Serratia* species (chronic granulomatous disease).

Think of a Secondary Immunodeficiency When

1. There is a concomitant or preceding viral infection (especially Epstein-Barr virus, HIV). The viral infection may occur *in utero* and produce an immunodeficiency disorder in the fetus.
2. The patient has certain malignancies, e.g., chronic lymphoid leukemia, Hodgkin's disease, multiple myeloma.
3. Acidosis, alopecia, and convulsions occur with chronic mucocutaneous candidiasis (biotin deficiency). Deficiencies of biotin, zinc, and selenium can occur with patients on prolonged hyperalimentation.
4. The patient is receiving immunosuppressive drugs.
5. The patient has a history consistent with possible HIV exposure.
6. The patient has the clinical features of acrodermatitis enteropathica (zinc deficiency—may also occur with prolonged hyperalimentation).

Table 40–4. CLINICAL FINDINGS SUGGESTIVE OF IMMUNODEFICIENCY: SITE OF DEFECT UNCLEAR

Intractable eczema
Ulcerative colitis with onset less than 1 year of age
Intractable diarrhea
Unexplained hematologic deficiency (any cell series—erythroid, neutrophil, platelet)
Generalized seborrheic dermatitis (seen in C5 deficiency, such as in Leiner's disease and also in severe combined deficiency)

the hyperIgM syndrome, normal to elevated levels of IgM with absent IgA are seen (Notarangelo, 1992).

In general, isotype patterns are not diagnostic of specific syndromes. However, marked elevations of IgE are common in Wiskott-Aldrich syndrome and some isolated T-cell deficiencies. The Wiskott-Aldrich syndrome also characteristically shows marked elevation of serum IgA combined with low IgM (Hong, 1989).

To resolve the clinical significance of ambiguous immunoglobulin values, one measures specific antibody responses to previously administered or ubiquitous naturally occurring antigens. If the child has received the usual immunizations, titers of these can be drawn. If he or she has not been immunized, the response after vaccine administration can be measured (Moen, 1986). *It is important to emphasize that no live virus vaccine should be administered to the child or any family member if there is any question of the immune status.* Only nonviable agents should be used for immunization. An exception is the bacteriophage ΦX174. Using ΦX174, clearance patterns and isotype responses can be measured, defining various subsets of B-cell deficiency (Ochs, 1971). If the child is not of the AB blood group, levels of the appropriate A or B isohemagglutinins can be determined. However, because of inadequate exposure, isohemagglutinins may be negative or of low titer, even in those of normal immunity.

X-Ray Studies

In the past, lateral views of the neck were used to assess pharyngeal lymphoid tissue. Frontal views of the chest may reveal an absence of the thymic shadow, but because the thymus can easily shrink with stress, evaluation of thymic size by this method is not reliable. X-ray studies are not recommended for evaluation of lymphoid tissue, because the information they provide is more reliable and is easily obtained by alternative methods.

Bony abnormalities, however, can alert the radiologist to an immunologic problem. A subset of patients with immune deficiencies involving T-cell, or T- and B-cell, abnormalities have short-limbed dwarfism. These patients show characteristic lesions, usually in the metaphyseal regions of the long bones. Patients with adenosine deaminase deficiency show splaying of the ends of the ribs, squaring off of the scapulae, and unusual articulations of the transverse rib processes (Cederbaum, 1976).

Chronic interstitial pneumonia is common in T-cell deficiencies. It is particularly characteristic of human immunodeficiency virus (HIV) infection (Joshi, 1984). With time, many patients with primary B-cell deficiency (hypogammaglobulinemia, common variable immunodeficiency) may develop chronic pulmonary fibrosis or bronchiectasis.

SECOND LEVEL MEASUREMENTS

Surface Markers: Lymphocyte Subsets

The development of monoclonal antibodies has permitted the enumeration and characterization of mononuclear cell subsets. Surface markers denote the lineage of a cell line, or the stage of differentiation or activation; or may represent molecules important to the function of a cell. These markers are classified, using the designation CD, which stands for cluster of differentiation, meaning that a cluster of monoclonal antibodies identifies that particular protein. The profile of a given cell, as defined by the CD system, uniquely defines the individual cellular members of the host defenses.

The CD designation was helpful in subdividing T cells into two major subsets: CD4, denoting helper cells, which are more involved in the initiation of immune reactions and the augmentation of B-cell responses, and CD8, which are associated with cytolytic (killer) functions. Although these functional activities define most immunologic activities of CD4 + and CD8 + T cells, in reality the molecules serve an augmentation role to stabilize the engagement of the T-cell receptor (TCR) with its antigen. It is now known that T cells only respond to peptide antigens held in the cleft of the transplantation antigen of the antigen presenting cell (usually a macrophage, dendritic cell, or B cell). Two types of transplantation antigens, Class I and Class II, have been described. CD4 molecules restrict the TCR binding to Class II molecules, and CD8 molecules reinforce Class I–TCR interaction, a phenomenon known as *genetic restriction.* As Class I antigens are expressed on nearly all cells, the elimination of a foreign antigen can be accomplished by CD8 + T-cell binding. Class II molecules are found primarily on the antigen presenting cells, which initiate the immune response.

In addition, the CD4 + "helper" cells have been subdivided on the basis of functional activity. Those that are primarily involved in initiation and augmentation of the immune response do so by the elaboration of the cytokines that promote differentiation and proliferation of B cells, for example, interleukin (IL)-4, IL-5, and IL-6, are designated T_H2. Another set, T_H1, secretes interferon-γ, IL-2, and tumor necrosis factor. Thus, these cells are adapted to initiate inflammatory responses to produce the delayed hypersensitivity reaction (Mossman, 1989).

Natural killer (NK) cells form a subset of cells related to T cells, but lacking a T-cell receptor, and having the morphology of large granular lymphocytes. They will kill certain target cells (e.g., tumor line) without prior sensitization. Their importance in host defense is incompletely defined. Only one case of complete absence of NK cells has been reported. This patient had profound difficulty with varicella, herpes, and cytomegalovirus but was able to handle other infections in a normal manner (Biron, 1989). NK cells are detected by CD16 and CD56; the lytic activity is best estimated by the CD56 + population (Trinchieri, 1989).

Monoclonal antibodies also define the T-cell receptors. Most T cells bind to antigen, using a receptor comprised of alpha and beta chains. Approximately 5% use a receptor composed of gamma and delta chains. These T cells are known as $\alpha\beta$ and $\gamma\delta$ T cells, respectively. The function of the minor set, the $\gamma\delta$ T cells, is unclear. In contrast to $\alpha\beta$ T cells, $\gamma\delta$ T cells can bind to targets that are not complexed to the transplantation antigens. Thus, they may represent a more primitive defense mechanism, analogous to the alternative activation of the complement system, which is able to respond to microbes before the development of specific immunity. Cells located in the intestinal epithelium, intraepithelial lymphocytes, are primarily of the $\gamma\delta$ type (Abbas, 1994). Table 40–5 shows a partial listing of CD designations (see Abbas, 1994, for more detail).

T-Cell Functional Assessment

Further insight into the capability of a particular cell line can be obtained by functional assessments. A proliferative response is commonly employed for T cells. Three different kinds of stimuli are employed: mitogens, alloantigens, and antigens. Mitogens are nonspecific, stimulating both CD4- and CD8-positive lymphocytes. Alloantigens (antigens present on cells that control rejection of organ or tissue transplants) also stimulate CD4+ and CD8+ cells in a relatively nonspecific way. Proliferative responses to those two types of stimuli indicate the presence of T cells, but a response does not guarantee the ability to clear infectious agents from the host. Patients with significant T-cell deficiency may still show some mitogen or alloantigen response.

The tests that best correlate with ability to resist infection are the proliferative responses to specific antigens and killer type assays (Lane, 1985). In the case of specific antigens, tetanus, streptokinase–streptodornase, polio, and candida are commonly used. Sufficient exposure to the antigen is required for a positive response; therefore, proliferation in response to antigenic stimuli is extremely uncommon in an in-

Table 40–5. LEUKOCYTE SURFACE MARKERS

Marker	Comment
T-Cell Series	
CD1a,b,c	Cortical thymocytes
CD2	T cells, NK cells, LFA-3 receptor
CD3	Part of the T-cell receptor complex; a pan T-cell marker
CD4	T-cells reactive with Class II HLA-presented antigen (helper cell)
CD5	Pan T-cell marker; present on a B-cell subset
CD8	T-cells reactive with Class I HLA-presented antigen (killer cell)
CD28	T-cell subset; activated B; thymocytes; site of second signal stimulus
CD45RA	Naive T cell (has not reacted with antigen); recent emigre of thymus
CD45RO	Memory T cell
B-Cell Series	
CD10	Common acute lymphatic leukemia antigen
CD19	Pan B-cell marker
CD20	Pan B-cell marker
CD21	EBV receptor
CD23	Activated B cells, macrophages, eosinophils, platelets—the low affinity $Fc_{\epsilon}RII$
CD40	B cell, carcinomas, monocytes
CD77	Burkitt's lymphoma
Myeloid Series	
CD14	Monocytes, granulocytes, Langerhans' cells, macrophages
CD16	NK cells, granulocytes, macrophages—the $Fc_{\gamma}RIIIA$, $Fc_{\gamma}RIIIB$ receptor
CD34	Hematopoietic precursor cells, endothelial cells
CD35	Granulocytes, monocytes, NK, B cells—the CR1/C3b receptor
NK Series	
CD56	NK cells (N-CAM, NKH-1); with CD16 used to enumerate NK number in peripheral blood
CD57	NK cells, T-cell subset (HNK1)
CD94	NK cells, γ/δ T cells (kp43)
Adhesion Molecules	
CD11a	Leukocytes; αL integrin chain (ICAM-1 ligand)
CD11b	Granulocytes, monocytes, NK cells; αM integrin chain of LFA-1 complex (mac-1, fibrinogen, and C3bi receptor)
CD11c	Granulocytes, monocytes, NK cells; αX integrin chain of LFA-1, gp 150-95
CD18	Leukocytes (integrin, β-chain of CD11)
CD62E	E selectin, ELAM-1, activated endothelial cells
CD62L	L selectin, T and B cells, monocytes, NK, PMNs, eosinophils; progenitor cells (LECAM-1, LAM-1)
CD62P	P selectin; activated platelets, endothelial cells (GMP-140, PADGEM)
Activation Markers	
CD25	Activated T, B cells (IL-2 receptor)
CD30	Activated T, B cells, Reed-Sternberg cells
CD69	Activated T, B cells, NK cells, macrophages
CD70	Activated T, B cells; Reed-Sternberg cells (CD27 ligand)
CD71	Transferrin receptor

NK, natural killer; LFA, lymphocyte function–associated antigen; PMNs, polymorphonuclear leukocytes; CD, cluster of differentiation; N-CAM, neutrophil cellular adhesion molecule; ICAM, intercellular adhesion molecule; NKH, natural killer human; HNK, human natural killer; ELAM, endothelial leukocyte adhesion molecule; LECAM, leukocyte endothelial cell adhesion molecule; LAM, leukocyte adhesion molecule; GMP, granule membrane protein; PADGEM, platelet activation–dependent granule–external membrane protein.

fant during most of the first year of life. A commonly employed killer cell assay measures cytolysis of allogeneic target cells by responder cells that have been previously stimulated by alloantigen. If viral antigen exposure has been adequate, killer assays against virally infected targets can be used.

Using separated T cells, B cells, and macrophages, one can mix the various subsets to see if a defect can be worsened or repaired with normal cells. In this way, inferences relative to faulty lymphocyte subsets (e.g., poor T helper or ineffective B cells) can be drawn. A note of caution should be interjected at this point, particularly in reference to suppression of an immune response. For unknown reasons, T cells from patients with some immunodeficiency diseases, when added to mixtures of T and B lymphocytes of normals, will diminish the immune response of the mixture, leading, for example, to decreased production of immunoglobulin. Although it is tempting to ascribe immunoglobulin deficiency to excess T suppressor activity in such cases, the same phenomenon has been demonstrated in experimental hypogammaglobulinemia produced by extirpation of the bursa of Fabricius in chickens, which should not affect the T cells because the thymus gland is not manipulated. It thus appears that suppression by T cells may accompany hypogammaglobulinemic states but not play an etiologic role.

B-Cell Functional Assessment

It is possible to secrete immunoglobulin but have poor specific antibody responses. It is also possible to have lacunar defects with poor responses to some but not all antigens (e.g., the poor carbohydrate antibody responses of Wiskott-Aldrich syndrome) (Ambrosino, 1988; Ammann, 1989). In addition to the specific antibody assessments mentioned previously, one can perform isotype analysis and detection of subclass responses directed against particular antigens. With the use of a broad panel of antigens, a clear view of the B-cell responsiveness can be obtained (Moen, 1986).

IgG Subclasses

There is a group of patients who appear to have too many infections in the face of normal immunoglobulin levels. IgG consists of four subclasses, IgG1–IgG4. Each of these subclasses show slightly different biological characteristics (see Table 35–5) (Normansell, 1987; Schur, 1987). Of particular interest is the relationship of IgG2 to carbohydrate antigens, because so many bacterial cell wall antigens are carbohydrate in nature (Scott, 1988). Thus, absence of an IgG2 response could result in a failure to develop protection against bacterial infection. IgG subclass deficiency has been cited as the cause of recurrent infections in patients with normal or near-normal IgG levels (Oxelius, 1979; Shackelford, 1990; Wedgwood, 1986). Also, it has been reported that a better correlation of infectious susceptibility and abnormal pulmonary function tests is seen when IgA deficiency is associated with IgG subclass deficiency than with IgA deficiency alone (Bjorkander, 1985).

As of this writing, the exact biological significance of IgG subclass deficiency is controversial. The actual biological necessity for all IgG subclasses needs to be considered in the context of the observation that individuals who are completely lacking in genes for IgG2, IgA, and IgE have been found in asymptomatic populations. Those individuals were of advanced age (70s) and yet had had no difficulty with infectious susceptibility (Lefranc, 1982; Migone, 1984). Further, IgG2 anticarbohydrate antibodies are not the sole source of antibody protection for such antigens. IgG1 is the first type of subclass response to carbohydrate antigens, and conversion to an IgG2 response occurs as the individual matures (Scott, 1988). However, it is not known whether this subclass response change confers a more efficient or effective antibody response. There is no evidence that those who are restricted to only IgG1 responses are at any disadvantage. The final chapter in the IgG subclass story is yet to be written.

IgA Deficiency

The special precautions for quantitation of IgA levels have been noted. In the case of complete absence of IgA, antibodies for IgA should be determined, because they pose a danger from anaphylaxis in the event of intravenous administration of blood products. Patients with IgA deficiency have an increased incidence of autoimmune disease, and screening for autoantibodies may be indicated. The association of "selective IgA" deficiency with IgG subclass deficiency has been mentioned (Bjorkander, 1985). IgA deficiency sometimes spontaneously disappears, and in one case a persistent diarrhea disappeared at the same time (Hong, 1989). Conversely, there are a few recorded cases of selective IgA deficiency progressing to panhypogammaglobulinemia.

Histology

The thymus and lymphoid tissue show characteristic architecture (Abbas, 1994; Borzy, 1979; Nezelof, 1992). Dysplastic and involutional changes are seen in various diseases. In actual clinical practice, however, microscopic examination of these tissues has not significantly influenced the diagnostic or therapeutic approaches. *In vitro* testing of cells obtained from such tissues could be informative, but the removal of tissue for this purpose is difficult to accomplish in the clinical setting. Newer monoclonal reagents may increase the value of these examinations.

THIRD LEVEL MEASUREMENTS

Enzyme Measurements

Deficiencies of two enzymes related to purine metabolism, adenosine deaminase (ADA), and purine nucleoside phosphorylase (PNP) are associated with immune deficiency. The basic mechanism is the accumulation of toxic metabolites that inhibit cell replication, ultimately resulting in loss of important lymphocyte cell lines. Lack of adenosine deaminase, which catalyzes the catabolism of adenosine to inosine, results first in loss of T cells and subsequently B cells, leading to combined T- and B-cell deficiency. Approximately 25% of combined immunodeficiency is caused by ADA deficiency. Characteristic bony abnormalities involving the ribs, pelvis, and scapulae are often seen (Cederbaum, 1976; Ammann, 1989).

PNP deficiency results in deficiency of the T cells with minimal to no effect upon the B cells. Red cell aplasia (Blackfan-Diamond syndrome) is a characteristic feature (Hong, 1989). The enzymes are usually measured in erythrocyte lysates, but a screening test using blood dried on filter paper is available (Kizai, 1977).

Cytokines

Augmentation of T-cell responses is brought about by the elaboration of various cytokines. The best studied of these is IL-2. Production of IL-2 by stimulated T cells and expression of IL-2 receptors are normal responses that can be evaluated by available methodology. Some patients' inability to respond to IL-2 forms the basis for their immune deficit (Arnaiz-Villena, 1992; Doi, 1988; Paganelli, 1983). IL-1 deficiency has also been observed (Chu, 1984). B-cell growth factors may be defective in other cases (Callard, 1986, Matheson, 1987; Shields, 1988; Street, 1991).

Molecular Genetics

Molecular techniques are useful for intrauterine diagnosis of immune deficiency and in determining carrier status in X-linked diseases. Restriction fragment length polymorphism (RFLP) analysis is particularly useful. Restriction enzymes cleave DNA at specific sites dependent upon the base sequence, yielding fragments of DNA of varying size. The distribution of cleavage sites is inherited to yield unique arrays of fragment sizes for each individual. If a gene probe or a nearby flanking probe is used, the size of the fragments containing each allele forms a distinctive pattern on Southern blots, and the genotype of the offspring can be determined (Fig. 40–1). Females show both maternal and paternal X-chromosome patterns, whereas males can only show one of the female alleles. Female carriers of X-linked immunodeficiency disorders, however, do not inactivate the X-chromosome in a random manner in any cell line that is affected by the disease because the disease state confers a growth disadvantage to those cells. Thus, over time nearly all of the female carrier cells will show only the paternal X-chromosome pattern. Nonrandom inactivation of the maternal X-chromosome in cell lines involved in the disease process provides presumptive evidence for a carrier state and can be used prior to the birth of an affected child. Examination of a patient with X-linked immunodeficiency will show exclusive use of the affected maternal X-chromosome. Search for this pattern in DNA samples of a fetus allows a presumptive diagnosis or exclusion of disease. The availability of several hundred probes for the X-chromosome, plus the knowledge of the map sites for the genes, make this approach, termed *X-inactivation analysis*, feasible for X-lined agammaglobulinemia, Wiskott-Aldrich syndrome, X-linked severe combined immunodeficiency, and X-linked proliferative disease (Conley, 1992).

Recently, the genes for X-linked agammaglobulinemia (Conley, 1993; Levinsky, 1993), Wiskott-Aldrich syndrome (Derry, 1994), and X-linked severe combined immunodeficiency (Noguchi, 1993; Puck, 1993) have been isolated, providing even more power to genetic analysis. The genes can be searched for directly and structural studies performed. In addition, it is now known that X-linked hyperIgM is usually caused by T-cell failure to express gp39, the ligand for B-cell CD40 (Banchereau, 1994). In another variety, the B cell is at fault and surface CD40 molecules do not transduce their signals appropriately (Conley, 1994). Activation of B cells via CD40 leads to proliferation and isotype switching (Banchereau, 1994).

Prenatal Diagnosis

Some of the immunodeficiency states can be diagnosed prenatally. Enzyme deficiencies can be determined on fibroblast cultures obtained from amniocentesis. If fetal blood can be obtained without contamination of maternal blood, absence of HLA antigens or assessment of T-cell functions and granulocyte chemiluminescence can be performed. A sample size of approximately 200 μl is necessary (Durandy, 1985). Wiskott-Aldrich syndrome can also be diagnosed by the presence of small platelets. A chorionic villus can be biopsied for DNA analysis, using the techniques described earlier.

Polymorphonuclear Leukocyte Analysis

A major polymorphonuclear leukocyte disorder is chronic granulomatous disease (CGD). Abscesses of the liver and lymph nodes, or osteomyelitis are major manifestations. The primary fault is a metabolic error that results in failure of the metabolic burst following phagocytic ingestion of bacteria. As a result, molecular oxygen is not reduced to superoxide. Hydroxyl radical and hydrogen peroxide are not produced, and an important intracellular mechanism of bacterial elimination is lost (Babior, 1978). This fault is partially compensated for by organisms that generate hydrogen peroxide within the cells. In chronic granulomatous disease, catalase-producing organisms, which destroy cytoplasmic hydrogen peroxide, survive intracellular ingestion, multiply, and cause granulomata. *Staphylococcus aureus* is the most common organism involved. Chronic infections with *Serratia, Klebsiella* species, and *Aspergillus* are particularly troublesome (Gallin, 1983, 1990).

The basic screening test for chronic granulomatous disease is measurement of chemiluminescence and superoxide production (Gallin, 1983, 1990). These tests are not ordinarily performed in most laboratories. A test called the *formazan test* (Gifford, 1970) has been found to be reliable for screening for CGD. It is simple and does not require extraordinary skills or unusual reagents. Although the test depends upon the reduction of nitroblue tetrazolium to the insoluble formazan, this procedure must be differentiated from the nitroblue tetrazolium test as originally performed to differentiate between bacterial or nonbacterial infections. The latter test is technically too demanding for routine clinical testing (Park, 1968).

The fundamental biological characteristic of the CGS leukocyte is that it will phagocytize bacteria normally but will not kill them. This behavior forms the basis of a bacte-

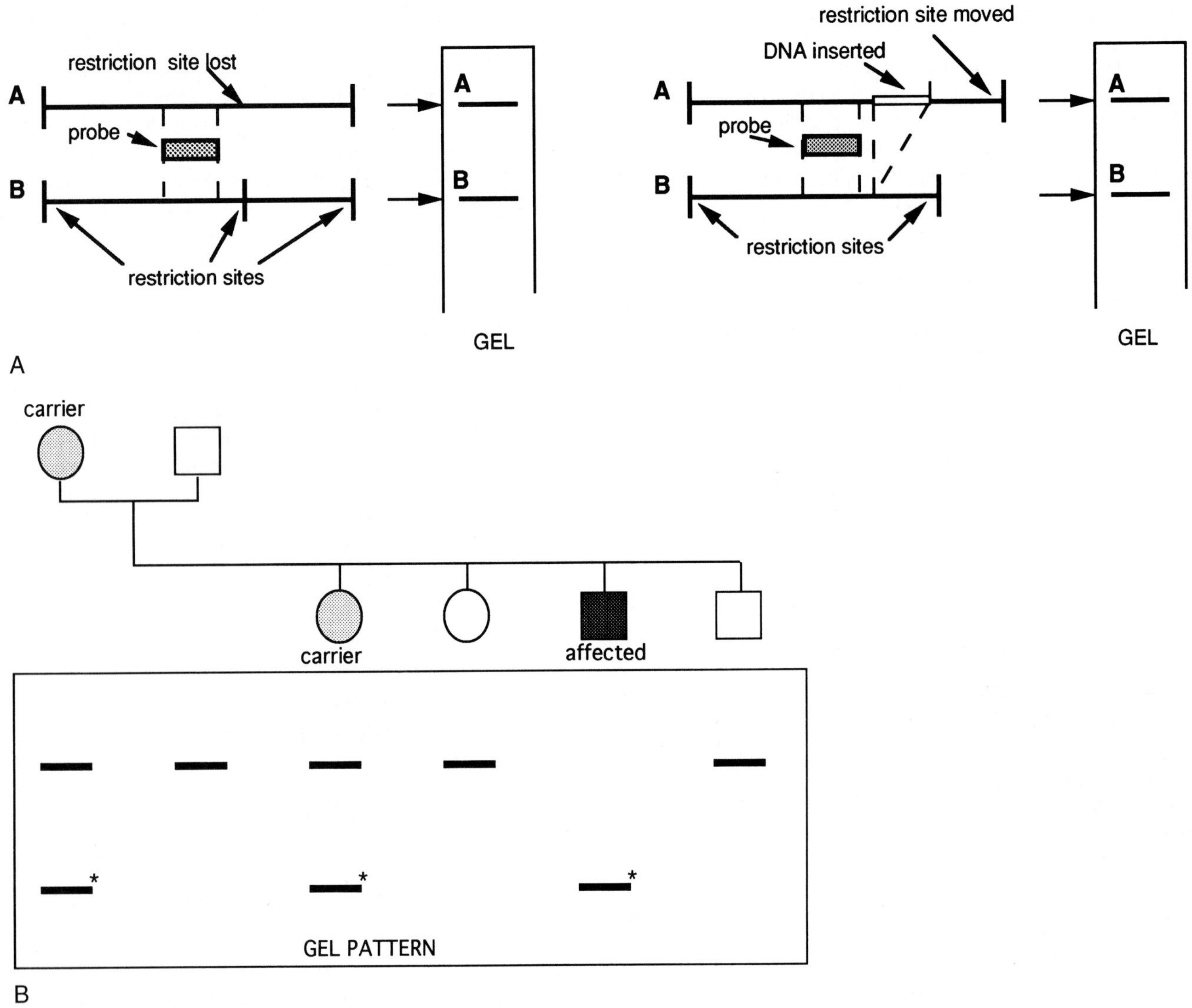

Figure 40–1. *A*, Restriction fragment length polymorphism (RFLP). On the left are shown 2 alleles, A and B. The restriction sites are shown as vertical bars crossing the DNA, indicated by the horizontal bar. In A, a restriction is lost and therefore a large fragment is obtained whereas in B, two smaller fragments result after digestion. The probe binds to the large fragment from A and the larger of the 2 fragments obtained from B, resulting in the two bands shown on the gel. On the right side of the diagram, the A allele has been lengthened by the insertion of DNA as a result of mutation. This moves the restriction site away from the 5′ restriction site, producing a larger fragment with the resultant gel pattern as shown. Conversely, a deletion of DNA would result in a smaller fragment, but again producing two bands on a Southern blot. *B*, X-chromosome analysis using RFLP pattern. The pedigree shows the carrier mother, a normal father and their four offspring (one carrier, one affected and two normal children). The gel pattern of each individual is shown directly below his/her symbol. The mother is a heterozygote with a normal paternal and an abnormal maternal allele (*). The father shows only a normal allele. The carrier daughter is also a heterozygote, having inherited the abnormal allele (*) from her mother and a normal allele from her father. The normal daughter inherited the normal allele from her mother, and with the normal paternal chromosome, she is homozygous. The affected male inherited the X-chromosome containing the abnormal maternal allele*, while the normal male inherited the normal maternal allele. The status of each child can be determined from the RFLP pattern. Thus, DNA analysis of an unborn child could predict the disease status.

rial killing assay for CGD. This test is not necessary if abnormal chemiluminescence is shown. A number of associated hematologic and other biochemical abnormalities have been shown in CGD patients (Bolscher, 1989; Gallin, 1983, 1990; Nauseef, 1983; Weening, 1985).

Other defects of PMNs include myeloperoxidase deficiency and disorders of movement. Myeloperoxidase deficiency is of unknown clinical significance, having been described both in asymptomatic as well as infection-prone individuals (Lehrer, 1969; Parry, 1981). Movement disorders are the most difficult to assess (Cates, 1981). Chemotaxis of PMNs is technically a difficult procedure, and erratic results may simply be a laboratory artifact. Poor chemotaxis is often an inconstant feature of any disease; thus it does not show consistent correlation with symptomatology. Full evaluation of movement disorders requires close correlation with the overall clinical picture and extensive clinical experience. Leukocyte mobility is usually evaluated by directed migration through membrane filters or under agarose (Cates, 1981; Nelson, 1975). Further tests of mobility involve the ability of PMNs to demarginate and leave the marrow reserves, and can be demonstrated by injections of epinephrine and steroids, respectively. A disorder of actin, important in PMN migration, has been described (Southwick, 1988). The Rebuck skin window, which shows the timing and cell characteristics of skin migration, may be useful in describing the inflammatory response. It has not had much clinical application, however (Southam, 1966).

The hyperIgE syndrome (Buckley, 1972, 1978) is often considered a PMN disorder, in part because of inclusion of the Job syndrome as part of the disease spectrum (Hill, 1974). Job's syndrome is a disease associated with recurrent skin abscesses, characterized by a lack of inflammation caused by poor PMN mobilization to the area. Defective PMN movement is not a constant feature of the hyperIgE syndrome (Buckley, 1972, 1978). The immune defect in the hyperIgE syndrome is poorly defined, so that classification is difficult. In a situation of recurrent, deep-seated skin abscesses that require multiple incisions or sometimes complete excision for control, the hyperIgE syndrome should be considered. The diagnosis is made by the demonstration of extremely high levels of IgE, at least over 2000 IU/ml and commonly as high as 20,000 to 50,000 IU/ml.

Leukocytes, carried along in the circulation, are attracted to areas of inflammation through the interaction of endothelial cell receptors, known as *selectins*, which interact with leukocyte carbohydrate ligands such as sialyl-Lewis^x (Lewis blood group antigen). This initiates a slow rolling action along the vessel wall, essentially "parking" the circulating cell. Thereafter, activation of the leukocyte results in increased expression of β2-integrins (CD11/18), which causes a firm adhesion of the cell to the vessel wall, following which emigration and tissue infiltration occurs (McEver, 1992). A number of patients with β2-integrin defects have been described with a characteristic syndrome of recurrent bacterial or fungal infections, progressive periodontitis, and delayed cord separation, known as leukocyte adhesion defect (LAD-1). There are demonstrable defects of adherence and adhesion-dependent functions, such as spreading, phagocytosis, and chemotactic orientation (Anderson, 1987). Recently, a fault in expression of a selectin ligand sialyl-Lewis^x resulted in a similar clinical syndrome because of impairment of the rolling phenomenon (LAD-2; von Andrian, 1993).

SUMMARY

Assessment of host defenses is an extraordinarily complex process, entailing the cooperation of the clinician, research scientist, and clinical pathologist. A logical approach, based upon appreciation of the several systems involved in host defense and the various capabilities of different laboratories, can lead to a diagnosis in nearly all cases. The impressive success of modern therapy, based upon newer antibiotics, recombinant DNA technology, and bone marrow transplantation, encourages the precise delineation of immunologic deficiency states.

Abbas AK, Lichtman AH, Pober JS: Cellular and Molecular Immunology, 2nd ed. Philadelphia, W.B. Saunders Co., 1994.

Ambrosino DM, Umetsu DT, Siber GR, et al: Selective defect in the antibody response to *Haemophilus influenzae* type b in children with recurrent infections and normal serum IgG subclass levels. J Allergy Clin Immunol 1988; 81:1175.

Ammann AJ, Hong R: Disorders of the T-cell system. *In* Stiehm ER (ed): Immunologic Disorders of Infants and Children. Philadelphia, W.B. Saunders Co., 1989, pp 257–315.

Anderson DC, Springer TA: Leukocyte adhesion deficiency: An inherited defect in the MAC-1, LFA-1, and p150,95 glycoproteins. Ann Rev Med 1987; 38:175.

Arnaiz-Villena A, Timon M, Rodriguez-Gallego C, et al: Human T-cell activation deficiencies. Immunol Today 1992; 13:259.

Babior BM: Oxygen-dependent microbial killing by phagocytes. (First of two parts.) N Engl J Med 1978; 298:721.

Banchereau J, Bazan F, Blanchard D, et al: The CD40 antigen and its ligand. Annu Rev Immunol 1994; 12:881.

Biron CA, Byron KS, Sullivan JL: Severe herpesvirus infections in an adolescent without natural killer cells. N Engl J Med 1989; 320:1731.

Bjorkander J, Bake B, Oxelius VA, Hanson LA: Impaired lung function in patients with Iga deficiency and low levels of IgG2 or IgG3. N Engl J Med 1985; 313:720.

Bolscher BGJM, Van Zwieten R, Kramer IM, et al: A phosphoprotein of Mf 47,000, defective in autosomal chronic granulomatous disease, copurifies with one of two soluble components required for NADPH:O_2 oxidoreductase activity in human neutrophils. J Clin Invest 1989; 83:757.

Borzy MS, Schulte-Wissermann H, Gilbert E, et al: Thymic morphology in immunodeficiency diseases. Results of thymic biopsies. Clin Immunol Immunopathol 1979; 12:31.

Buckley RH, Becker WG: Abnormalities in the regulation of human IgE synthesis. Immunol Rev 1978; 41:288.

Buckley RH, Wray BB, Belmaker EZ: Extreme hyperimmunoglobulinemia E and undue susceptibility to infection. Pediatrics 1972; 49:1.

Callard RE, Shields JG, Smith SH, et al: Measurement of human B-cell responses to growth and differentiation factors: Relevance for immunodeficiency disease. Lymphokine Res 1986; 5(Suppl 1):S151.

Cates KL: Defects in neutrophil chemotaxis. Clin Immunol Allergy 1981; 1:603.

Cederbaum SD, Kaitila I, Rimoin DL, Stiehm ER: The chondroosseous dysplasia of adenosine deaminase deficiency with severe combined immunodeficiency. J Pediatr 1976; 89:737.

Chu ET, Rosenwasser LJ, Dinarello CA, et al: Immunodeficiency with defective T-cell response to interleukin 1. Proc Natl Acad Sci USA 1984; 81:4945.

Conley ME: Molecular approaches to analysis of X-linked immunodeficiencies. Ann Rev Immunol 1992; 322:1063.

Conley ME, Larche M, Bonagura VR, et al: Hyper IgM syndrome associated with defective CD40-mediated B-cell activation. J Clin Invest 1994; 94:1404.

Conley ME, Witte ON, Cooper MD: Deficient expression of a B-cell cytoplasmic tyrosine kinase in human X-linked agammaglobulinemia. Cell 1993; 72:279.

Derry JM, Ochs HD, Francke U: Isolation of a novel gene mutated in Wiskott-Aldrich syndrome. Cell 1994; 78:635.

Doi S, Saiki O, Tanaka T, et al: Cellular and genetic analyses of IL-2 production and IL-2 receptor expression in a patient with familial T-cell-dominant immunodeficiency. Clin Immunol Immunopathol 1988; 46:24.

Durandy A, Dumez Y, Griscelli C: Antenatal diagnosis of severe hereditary immunologic deficiency syndromes. Arch Fr Pediatr 1985; 42:163.

Gallin JI: Recent advances in chronic granulomatous disease. Ann Intern Med 1983; 99:657.

Gallin JI, Malech HL: Update on chronic granulomatous diseases of childhood. JAMA 1990; 263:1533.

Gifford RH, Malawista SE: A simple rapid micromethod for detecting chronic granulomatous disease of childhood. J Lab Clin Med 1970; 75:511.

Hill HR, Quie PG, Pabst HF, et al: Defect in neutrophil granulocyte chemotaxis in Job's syndrome of recurrent "cold" staphylococcal abscesses. Lancet 1974; 2:617.

Joshi VV, Oleske JM, Minnefor AB, et al: Pathology of suspected acquired immune deficiency in children: A study of eight cases. Pediatr Pathol 1984; 2:71.

Kizai H, Sakurada T: Simple micro-assay methods for enzymes of purine metabolism. J Lab Clin Med 1977; 89:1135.

Kniker WT, Lesourd BM, McBryde JL, Corriel RN: Cell-mediated immunity assessed by multitest CMT skin testing in infants and preschool children. Am J Dis Child 1985; 139:840.

Lane HC, Depper JM, Greene WC, et al: Qualitative analysis of immune function in patients with the acquired immunodeficiency syndrome: Evidence for a selective defect in soluble antigen recognition. N Engl J Med 1985; 313:79.

Lefranc M-P, Lefranc G, Rabbitts TH: Inherited deletion of immunoglobulin heavy chain constant region genes in normal human individuals. Nature 1982; 300:760.

Lehrer RI, Cline MJ: Leukocyte myeloperoxidase deficiency and disseminated candidiasis: The role of myeloperoxidase in resistance to infection. J Clin Invest 1969; 48:1478.

5

Levinsky R: The gene involved in X-linked agammaglobulinaemia is a member of the src family of protein-tyrosine kinases. Nature 1993; 361:226.

Matheson DS, Green BJ: Defect in production of B-cell differentiation factor–like activity by mononuclear cells from a boy with hypogammaglobulinemia. J Immunol 1987; 138:2469.

McEver RP: Leukocyte-endothelial cell interactions. Curr Opin Cell Biol 1992; 4:840.

Migone N, Oliviero S, De Lange G, et al: Multiple gene deletions within the human immunoglobulin heavy-chain cluster. Proc Natl Acad Sci USA 1984; 81:5811.

Moen RC, Oemichen SL, Kiggens AL, Hong R: ELISA detection of specific functional antibodies in human serum to E. coli, tetanus toxoid, and diphtheria-tetanus toxoids: Normal values for IgG, IgA and IgM. Diagn Immunol 1986; 4:17.

Mossman TR, Coffman RL: TH1 and TH2 cells: Different patterns of lymphokine secretion lead to different functional properties. Ann Rev Immunol 1989; 7:145.

Nauseef WM, Root RK, Malech HL: Biochemical and immunologic analysis of hereditary myeloperoxidase deficiency. J Clin Invest 1983; 71:1297.

Nelson RD, Quie PG, Simmons RL: Chemotaxis under agarose: A new and simple method for measuring chemotaxis and spontaneous migration of human polymorphonuclear leukocytes and monocytes. J Immunol 1975; 115:1650.

Nezelof C: Thymic pathology in primary and secondary immunodeficiencies. Histopathology 1992; 21:499.

Noguchi M, Nakamura Y, Russell SM, et al: Interleukin-2 receptor γ chain: A functional component of the interleukin-7 receptor. Science 1993; 262:1877.

Normansell DE: Human immunoglobulin subclasses. Diagn Clin Immunol 1987; 5:115.

Notarangelo LD, Duse M, Ugazio AG: Immunodeficiency with hyper-IgM (HIM). [Review.] Immunodefic Rev 1992; 3(2):101.

Ochs HD, Davis SD, Wedgwood RJ: Immunologic responses to bacteriophage ΦX174 in immunodeficiency diseases. J Clin Invest 1971; 50:2559.

Ochs HD, Wedgwood RJ: Disorders of the B-cell system. *In* Stiehm ER (ed): Immunologic Disorders in Infants and Children. Philadelphia, W.B. Saunders Co., 1989, pp 226–256.

Oxelius VA: Quantitative and qualitative investigations of serum IgG subclasses in immunodeficiency diseases. Clin Exp Immunol 1979; 36:112.

Paganelli R, Aiuti F, Beverley PCL, Levinsky RJ: Impaired production of interleukins in patients with cell-mediated immunodeficiencies. Clin Exp Immunol 1983; 51:338.

Park BH, Fikrig SM, Smithwick EM: Infection and nitro-blue-tetrazolium reduction by neutrophils. A diagnostic aid. Lancet 1968; 2:532.

Parry MF, Root RK, Metcalf JA, et al: Myeloperoxidase deficiency: Prevalence and clinical significance. Ann Intern Med 1981; 95:293.

Puck JM, Deschenes SM, Porter JC, et al: The interleukin-2 receptor γ chain maps to Xq13.1 and is mutated in X-linked severe combined immunodeficiency. Hum Mol Genet 1993; 2:1099.

Rosen F, Wedgwood RJ, Eibl M, et al: Primary immunodeficiency diseases. Report of a WHO scientific group. Immunodeficiency 1992; 3:195–236.

Schakelford PG, Granoff DM, Madassery JV, et al: Clinical and immunologic characteristics of healthy children with subnormal serum concentrations of IgG2. Pediatr Res 1990; 27:16.

Schur PH: IgG subclasses—a review. Ann Allergy 1987; 58:89.

Scott MG, Schackelford PG, Briles ED, Nahm MH: Human IgG subclasses and their relation to carbohydrate antigen immunocompetence. Diagn Clin Immunol 1988; 5:241.

Shields JG, Smith SH, Strobel S, et al: Response of LFA-1 deficient B-cells to interleukin 4(BSF-1) and low molecular weight B-cell growth factor (BCGF low). Eur J Immunol 1988; 18:255.

Southam CM, Levin AG: A quantitative Rebuck technic. Blood 1966; 27:734.

Southwick FS, Dabiri GA, Stossel TP: Neutrophil actin dysfunction is a genetic disorder associated with partial impairment of neutrophil actin assembly in three family members. J Clin Invest 1988; 82:1525.

Street NE, Mosmann TR: Functional diversity of T lymphocytes due to secretion of different cytokine patterns. FASEB J 1991; 5:171.

Trinchieri G: Biology of natural killer cells. Adv Imunol 1989; 47:187.

von Andrian UH, Berger EM, Ramezani L, et al: In vivo behavior of neutrophils from two patients with distinct inherited leukocyte adhesion deficiency syndromes. J Clin Invest 1993; 93:2893

Wedgwood RJ, Ochs HD, Oxelius V-A: IgG subclass levels in the serum of patients with primary immunodeficiency. Monogr Allergy 1986; 20:80.

Weening RS, Corbeel L, De Boer M, et al: Cytochrome B deficiency in an autosomal form of chronic granulomatous disease. J Clin Invest 1985; 75:915.

Chapter 41

Clinical and Laboratory Evaluation of Systemic Rheumatic Diseases

Robert M. Nakamura, M.D.

5

INTRODUCTION AND CLASSIFICATION OF SYSTEMIC RHEUMATIC DISEASES

The rheumatic diseases are characterized by the presence of one or more autoantibodies that may be directed against components of the surface, cytoplasm, or nucleus of the cell. The last group, autoantibodies to nuclear antigens (ANAs), is a hallmark of the systemic rheumatic diseases (Nakamura, 1985, 1986, 1992; Tan, 1982a, 1989).

Much progress has been made in the elucidation of the immune mechanisms involved in the rheumatic diseases during the last 10 years. Many of the rheumatic diseases have a distinctive profile of autoantibodies with diagnostic specificities. Recently, the biochemical and biological functions of many of the autoantigens have been defined and unraveled. Many of the autoantigens are involved in all functions, such as deoxyribonucleic acid (DNA) replication, the splicing of the precursors to ribonucleic acid (RNA), and RNA processing (Tan, 1989).

Classification of the various rheumatic diseases has been difficult because of a lack of a firm etiologic basis for most of the diseases. A comprehensive classification was developed by Decker and the glossary subcommittee of the Ameri-

Table 41–1. SYSTEMIC RHEUMATIC DISEASES AND RELATED DISORDERS

1. Systemic lupus erythematous (SLE)
2. Discoid lupus erythematosus (DLE)
3. Lupus-like syndrome
4. Drug-induced lupus erythematosus
5. Sjögren's syndrome
6. Scleroderma/CREST syndrome (calcinosis cutis, Raynaud's phenomenon, esophageal dysmotility, sclerodactyly, and telangiectasia)
7. Rheumatoid arthritis (RA)
8. Dermatomyositis and polymyositis
9. Overlap syndromes
   a. Mixed connective tissue diseases (MCTD)
   b. Other
10. Connective tissue disease syndromes that have been poorly defined as to clinical category.

can College of Rheumatology (Decker, 1986). Our classification of the systemic rheumatic diseases and related disorders is shown in Table 41–1.

SYSTEMIC LUPUS ERYTHEMATOSUS AND RELATED LUPUS-LIKE DISORDERS

Systemic lupus erythematosus (SLE) is a prototype systemic rheumatic disease and has the following significant features (Nakamura, 1994a):

1. SLE is a non–organ-specific autoimmune disease in which the tissue injury is mediated primarily by DNA–anti-DNA immune complexes.
2. It is a multisystem disease that affects most persons of all ages and both sexes, although it is most prevalent in women during childbearing years.
3. The disease demonstrates a hyperactive immune system with multiple abnormalities.
4. The patients with SLE demonstrate a heterogeneous and polyclonal antibody response.
5. The typical case of SLE has an average of three different circulating antibodies present simultaneously. The prevalence of antibodies varies over a wide range, and more than 25 different types of autoantibodies have been identified in SLE (Nakamura, 1994a).

Etiologic Factors in Systemic Lupus Erythematosus

The etiology is still poorly known. Some of the important etiologic factors in SLE are (1) endocrine-metabolic, (2) environmental, and (3) genetic (Chan, 1989). The strongest risk factor for the development of SLE is female gender (Hochberg, 1990).

SLE has been considered to have a possible viral etiology (Pincus, 1982). The presence of antinuclear antibodies was determined in female laboratory workers with varying degrees of exposure to blood from patients with SLE. The presence of antinative DNA antibodies was higher in laboratory workers than in an unexposed nonlaboratory group of women ($p < 0.001$) (Zarmbinski, 1992). These results help support a hypothesis that a transmissible agent that can cause autoantibody formation may exist in the blood of patients with SLE.

Certain chemicals have been implicated in SLE (Hochberg, 1990). The syndrome of drug-induced lupus with hydralazine, procainamide, and isoniazid has been studied for clues to the pathogenesis of SLE. There have been varying reports that show the acetylation mechanism as a risk factor in SLE. Studies have demonstrated a greater concordance rate of SLE among monozygotic and dizygotic twins (Block, 1975). The concordance of SLE was present in 11 (58%) of 19 monozygotic twins. The end result of the interaction of multiple etiologic factors is polyclonal activation of B cells in SLE patients with production of a wide spectrum of antibodies (Nakamura, 1994a).

What Are the Diagnostic Criteria for Systemic Lupus Erythematosus?

In 1971, the American College of Rheumatology (ACR, previously, the American Rheumatism Association [ARA]), published preliminary criteria for the classification of SLE (Cohen, 1971). Patients were then considered to have SLE if four of the 1971 criteria were met sequentially or simultaneously during any interval of observation.

In 1982, the Subcommittee for SLE Criteria of ARA, chaired by Eng Tan, M.D., published revised criteria that incorporated new immunologic knowledge and improved the disease classification of SLE (Tan, 1982b). The 1982 revised criteria for classification of SLE included 11 categories listed in Table 41–2. The 1982 revised criteria added (1) abnormal

Table 41–2. 1982 ARA REVISED CRITERIA FOR CLASSIFICATION OF SYSTEMIC LUPUS ERYTHEMATOSUS*

1. Malar rash
2. Discoid rash
3. Photosensitivity
4. Oral ulcers
5. Arthritis
6. Serositis
7. Renal disorder
8. Neurologic disorder
9. Hematologic disorder
10. Immunologic disorder
    a. Positive LE cell preparation
       OR
    b. Anti-DNA: antibody to native DNA in abnormal titer
       OR
    c. Anti-Sm: presence of antibody to Sm nuclear antigen
       OR
    d. False-positive serologic test for syphilis known to be positive for at least six months and confirmed by *Treponema pallidum* immobilization or fluorescent treponemal antibody absorption test.
11. Antinuclear antibody
    An abnormal titer of antinuclear antibody by immunofluorescence or an equivalent assay at any point in time and in the absence of drugs known to be associated with "drug-induced lupus" syndrome

*The proposed classification is based on 11 criteria. For the purpose of identifying patients in clinical studies, a person shall be said to have SLE if any four or more of the 11 criteria are present, serially or simultaneously, during any interval of observation.

From Nakamura and Bylund (1994) and Tan (1982b).

titer of antinuclear antibody by immunofluorescence or an equivalent assay, and (2) antibody to native DNA and/or Sm antigen. In contrast to the 1971 criteria, the 1982 criteria removed Raynaud's phenomenon and alopecia because of their low sensitivity and specificity.

When the 1982 ARA Criteria for Classification of SLE were compared with the 1971 criteria, there was definite improvement in sensitivity and specificity. The 1982 criteria showed a 96.7% sensitivity and 96% specificity when evaluated with known SLE and control patients (Tan, 1982b). The 1982 ARA criteria considered patients to have SLE if four of the criteria were met sequentially or simultaneously during any period of observation.

What Are "Lupus-Like" Syndromes and Diseases?

There are many diseases and syndromes that may share certain clinical features with SLE but are not SLE and have differing etiologies and pathogeneses. Diseases that have been listed in this category include vasculitis, cryoglobulinemia, polychondritis, lymphoproliferative diseases, rheumatic fever, glomerulonephritis, syphilis, lupoid hepatitis, drug-induced lupus, and occult malignancy (Panush, 1993).

There is a very broad category of patients who demonstrate fewer than four of the 1982 ARA classification criteria for SLE (Lazaro, 1989; Lom-Orta, 1980; Schur, 1993) but are considered to have "lupus-like" illnesses. These patients have been classified as follows: (1) undifferentiated rheumatic disease, (2) nonrheumatic disease, (3) overlap syndrome, and (4) incomplete, latent or incipient lupus.

Schur recommended, similar to the ARA criteria for the diagnosis of rheumatoid arthritis (RA), that patients be labeled as having classic SLE (many criteria), definite SLE (four or more criteria), probable SLE (three criteria), or possible SLE (two criteria). The patients with two or three criteria may be considered as incomplete, incipient, or latent, as well as possible and probable lupus (Schur, 1993). If these patients are followed, a few may develop a definite SLE but may evolve into other diseases with a better prognosis.

Autoantibody Profile in Systemic Lupus Erythematosus

Characteristic of SLE is the presence of a broad spectrum of autoantibodies, including antibody to native DNA, Sm antigen, U1 RNP, SS-A/Ro, SS-B/La, and several other nonhistone protein or nonhistone protein-RNA complexes (Nakamura, 1994a). Polyclonality of antibodies is seen in SLE and scleroderma, and is not seen in the other systemic rheumatic diseases. Anti–native DNA and anti-Sm are generally specific for SLE. Systemic lupus erythematosus is characterized by a heterogeneous and polyclonal antibody response, and the usual case of SLE has an average of three different circulating antibodies present simultaneously.

The prevalence of autoantibodies varies over a wide range. Antibodies to native DNA and histones are detectable in up to 40% and 70% of patients, respectively, and antibodies to proliferating cell nuclear antigen (PCNA) and cyclin or Alu RNA protein are detectable in 3% or less (Nakamura, 1986) (Table 41–3).

Antibodies to Native DNA or Double-Stranded DNA

Anti–double-stranded DNA (DS-DNA) antibodies are rather specific for SLE and are observed at a frequency of 75–90% in SLE patients with active disease (Buskila, 1992). There have been many earlier reports of antibodies to DS-DNA in diseases other than SLE. However, current thinking is that the reactive antibodies to DNA in the other diseases were actually anti–single-stranded DNA antibodies. The DS-DNA antibody tests often used DS-DNA preparations contaminated with denatured or single-stranded DNA.

Antibody to DNA plays a definite role in the pathogenesis of SLE. In studies of SLE patients, antibody to DNA is followed by the appearance of circulating DNA antigen, a sequence of events that results in the formation of immune complexes. Such DNA–anti-DNA immune complexes are deposited in the kidney glomeruli and initiate kidney damage (Okamura, 1993).

Table 41–3. ANTIGENS AND AUTOANTIBODIES IN SYSTEMIC LUPUS ERYTHEMATOSUS

Antigen	Molecular Structure	Autoantibody Frequency (%)
Native DNA	Double-strand DNA	40
Denatured DNA	Single-strand DNA	70
Histones	H1, H2A, H2B, H3, H4	70
Sm	Proteins, 29(B'), 28(B), 16(D), and 13(E) kDa, complexed with U1, U2, and U4-U6 snRNAs; splicesome component	30
Nuclear RNP (U1 RNP)	Proteins, 70, 33(A), and 22(C) kDa, complexed with U1 snRNA; splicesome component	32
SS-A/Ro	Proteins, 60 and 52 kDa, complexed with Y1-Y5 RNAs	35
SS-B/La	Phosphoproteins, 48 kDa, complexed with Y1 nascent RNA Pol III transcripts	15
Ku	Proteins, 86 and 66 kDa, DNA-binding proteins	10
Ki	Nuclear protein, 32 kDa	31
PCNA/cyclin	Protein, 36 kDa; auxiliary protein of DNA polymerase	3
Ribosomal RNP	Phosphoproteins, 38, 16, and 15 kDa associated with ribosomes	10
Hsp-90	Heat-shock protein, 90 kDa	50
ALu RNA protein	Protein, 68 kDa, 11 complexed with ALu RNA	Rare
S10	Ribosomal small subunit protein, 20 kDa	11
Cardiolipin	Anionic phospholipids	20–40

*With permission from Nakamura and Bylund (1994).

Earlier methods for detection of DNA antibodies were the insensitive precipitation methods, complement fixation, and passive hemagglutination. Current methods used are radioimmunoassay (RIA), indirect immunofluorescence (IFA) on *Crithidia*, and enzyme-linked immunosorbent assay (ELISA) (Buskila, 1992). The current methods can detect anti-DNA in 75% to 90% of active untreated SLE patients.

Lafer reported that monoclonal antibodies derived from SLE mice showed cross-reactivity between DS-DNA and cardiolipin. However, the majority of patients with SLE demonstrated no cross-reactivity between anti–DS-DNA and anticardiolipin antibodies (Lafer, 1981).

Antibodies to Sm and Nuclear Ribonucleoprotein

Precipitating antibodies to Sm antigen have been considered highly specific markers for SLE (Tan, 1989). Antibodies to both Sm and nuclear ribonucleoprotein (nRNP) are found in patients with SLE. The Sm and nRNP antigens were clearly associated, because the nRNP could not be biochemically isolated from the Sm antigen. Lerner and Steitz (1979) used the tools of molecular biology to show that Sm and nRNP antigens were subcellular particles comprised of small nuclear RNAs complexed with proteins. The particle bound by anti-nRNP is composed of an RNA component designated U1 (U for uridine rich), complexed to at least seven proteins varying in molecular mass from 12 to 68 kDa (Tan, 1989), recently found at a frequency of 20% to 40% (ter Borg, 1990).

The antigens of Sm consist of several proteins, conventionally called B^1 (29 kDa), D (16 kDa), and E (13 kDa) (Tan, 1989). Purified anti-B^1/B antibodies cross-react with the D protein and vice versa, but no cross-reaction is observed in smaller percentages of SLE sera. Thus, there are at least two epitopes on the B^1/B protein recognized by anti-Sm sera. The antigens reactive with anti-Sm and antinuclear RNA are therefore in assemblies of interactive proteins and RNAs engaged in precursor nRNA splicing (Tan, 1989).

No characteristic clinical features are apparent with SLE patients with anti-Sm antibodies (Barada, 1981). Patients who have antibodies to only nRNP have a low frequency of antibodies to DNA and a low frequency of clinically apparent renal disease (ter Borg, 1990).

Anti-Sm and anti-nRNP antibodies may be detected by immunodiffusion (ID), passive hemagglutination (PHA), or counterimmunoelectrophoresis (CIE). However, the above-mentioned methods do not accurately distinguish between antibodies against different small nuclear RNA–associated polypeptides. The reactivities with individual RNAs and polypeptides can be best demonstrated by RNA immunoprecipitation and immunoblotting techniques, respectively. Immunoblotting has been found to be more sensitive than conventional methods for the detection of anti-Sm and anti-nRNP (Nakamura, 1994b).

Currently, the most widely used laboratory tests for the detection of anti-Sm and anti-nRNP antibodies are immunodiffusion and ELISA. These tests can differentiate between Sm and nRNP antibodies but cannot define the specific antibody epitopes present in patients' sera. The antibody specificity and epitopes are best determined by Western and Northern blotting methods.

Antibodies to SS-A/Ro and SS-B/La

In SLE, patients can have antibodies to SS-A/Ro alone, or they may have both anti–SS-A/Ro and anti–SS-B/La. Having anti–SS-A/Ro alone is strongly associated with human leukocyte antigen (HLA) DR2 and is seen in younger patients with SLE (<22 years of age at onset). The presence of both anti–SS-A/Ro and anti–SS-B/La in SLE is associated with HLA-DR3 and is seen in older patients (>50 years of age at onset) (Hochberg, 1985).

A study of 55 patients with SLE showed that patients with anti–SS-A/Ro alone had much more serious renal disease (Hochberg, 1985). The SLE patients with only anti–SS-A/Ro also had a higher incidence of concomitant anti-DNA antibodies than those SLE patients with both the anti–SS-A/Ro and anti–SS-B/La antibodies (Chan, 1989).

Anti–SS-A/Ro autoantibodies have been closely associated with the appearance of nephritis, vasculitis, lymphadenopathy, and leukopenia in SLE patients. Anti–SS-B/La antibodies, like anti–SS-A/Ro antibodies, are antibodies noteworthy for their strong association with Sjögren's syndrome, occurring in about two thirds of patients with this disorder. The SS-B/La antigen is a cellular protein bound to a small RNA species, forming a small RNP that may function in processing of RNA polymerase III transcripts (Chan, 1989).

Clinical Subsets of Systemic Lupus Erythematosus Associated with Antibodies to SS-A/Ro

Elevated levels of SS-A/Ro antibodies are related to several clinical autoimmune disorders, including: (1) subacute cutaneous lupus erythematosus, (2) neonatal lupus erythematosus syndrome, (3) homozygous C2 and C4 deficiency with SLE-like disease, (4) primary Sjögren's syndrome vasculitis, (5) ANA-negative SLE patients, and (6) SLE with interstitial pneumonitis (Bylund, 1991). Precipitating antibodies to SS-A/Ro are seen in 65% to 95% of patients with anti–SS-A/Ro associated subsets, and more than 90% of the patients have anti–SS-A/Ro levels when detected by ELISA methods (Bylund, 1991).

Anti-Ku and Anti-Ki Antibodies

The Ku-antigen system consists of a pair of proteins called p70/p80 (Francoeur, 1986; Reeves, 1992). These proteins have a high affinity for DNA and are known to be DNA-binding proteins. The Ku/Ki autoantigen is a heterodimer complex consisting of 70 and 80 kDa proteins that interact covalently with the ends of native DNA. With the use of both immunoprecipitin and immunoblot assays, the Ku autoantibody was found in 10% of SLE sera and was not detected in 100 scleroderma sera examined. In studies with an enzyme immunoassay, Reeves showed that 39% of SLE, 55% of mixed connective tissue disease (MCTD), and 40% of scleroderma patients had low levels of antibodies to Ku protein (Reeves, 1992).

Anti-Ki antibody was first reported in Japan (Tojo, 1981) and was observed in approximately 10% of SLE patients. A relationship was observed between anti-Ki and the clinical features of arthritis, pericarditis, and pulmonary hypertension in SLE patients. The Ki antigen was purified from rabbit thymus and had a molecular weight of 32,000. Sakamoto (1989) developed an enzyme-linked immunosorbent assay (ELISA) and observed anti-Ki antibody in 21.4% (30/140) of SLE patients, while 11 of 140 were positive for anti-Ki by double-immunodiffusion tests.

Proliferating Cell Nuclear Antigen and Hsp-90 Antibodies

Antibodies to PCNA are detected in 3% of patients with SLE and show no distinctive clinical features associated with the presence of the antibody (Miyachi, 1978). The PCNA protein has been characterized as cell-cycle related. The PCNA antibodies have been useful probes in the study of events regulating DNA replication, cell proliferation, and blast transformation.

Autoantibody to a mammalian heat shock protein, Hsp-90, has been observed (Minota, 1988). The Hsp-90 is 90 kDa and is a cytoplasmic and plasma membrane protein. The autoantibody to Hsp-90 was observed in 50% of patients with SLE and two of six patients with polymyositis.

Antiphospholipid Antibodies in Systemic Lupus Erythematosus

The lupus anticoagulant antiphospholipid antibody syndrome is characterized by the presence of circulating antibodies to phospholipids and clinical features of arterial and venous thrombosis, thrombocytopenia, and several symptoms. The antiphospholipid antibodies have been found frequently in patients with SLE and also in other disorders, such as cancer, drug-induced disorders, and infectious disorders (Alarcon-Segovia, 1992; McNeil, 1991). Antiphospholipid antibodies are found in up to 60% of patients with SLE. Recently, there has been considerable evidence that antiphospholipid antibodies are very heterogeneous, functionally and immunochemically, and are polyclonal (McNeil, 1991).

Cardiolipin (anionic phospholipid) has been widely used for the detection of antiphospholipid antibodies. The majority of anticardiolipin antibodies cross-react with other anionic phospholipids, but some may also react with zwitterionic phospholipids (McNeil, 1991). Antibodies to anionic phospholipids may be IgG or IgM, whereas antibodies to zwitterionic phospholipids are more frequently IgM.

Antibodies to phospholipids are identified in SLE patients in three ways (Alarcon-Segovia, 1992): (1) serologically false-positive for syphilis by a positive Venereal Disease Research Laboratory (VDRL) test, which is a flocculation assay using carbon particles coated with cholesterol, lecithin (phosphatidylcholine), and cardiolipin; (2) the lupus anticoagulant assay, which is a prolongation of the kaolin partial thromboplastin time (KPTT) that is not corrected by normal plasma; and (3) cardiolipin immunoassay with the use of cardiolipin or other negatively charged phospholipids as antigens. Patients with SLE will usually react with a negatively charged phosphate group present in cardiolipin, phosphatidic acid, phosphatidylserine, and phosphatidylinositol.

Harris (1987, 1990) convened international workshops to improve the precision and accuracy of antiphospholipid antibody immunoassays. Reference sera were prepared and standard units (GPL and MPL) were defined. One GPL (MPL) unit is equivalent to 1 mg/mL of an affinity-purified standard IgG (IgM) sample. However, Lopez (1992) recently suggested that an IgA-specific assay for antiphospholipid antibody is important in assessing the antiphospholipid syndrome in patients with SLE.

Chronic Discoid Lupus

A benign form of lupus may present as "discoid" (coin- or disc-shaped) cutaneous lesions without symptoms of systemic disease. This disorder is called *chronic discoid lupus erythematosus* (CLE) (Sontheimer, 1992; Wallace, 1992). The clinical and laboratory characteristics of chronic discoid lupus have not been clearly delineated since adoption of the revised 1982 American College of Rheumatology Criteria for the Classification of SLE. The skin lesions of chronic discoid lupus are as follows: (1) persistent localized erythema, (2) adherent scales, (3) follicular plugging, (4) telangiectasis, and (5) atrophy (Wallace, 1992).

Subacute cutaneous lupus erythematosus (SCLE) consists of papulosquamous or nonscarring lesions. Also, additional variants of chronic discoid lupus, such as lupus panniculitis and urticarial lupus, have been described (Sontheimer, 1992). Wallace (1992) has defined chronic discoid lupus as the fulfillment of the description of chronic discoid lupus or SCLE, or one of the variants of SLE in which the 1982 ACR/Criteria for SLE are not met.

Chronic discoid lupus is a cutaneous autoimmune disorder that lacks any unifying diagnostic serological abnormality. It is a mild form of lupus erythematosus that uncommonly disseminates to SLE.

There is considerable overlap between discoid lupus and SLE. Up to 15% of patients with SLE have cutaneous discoid lesions. About 6% to 12% of patients with SLE had discoid lupus for a varying number of years before the onset of systemic disease (Wallace, 1992). Antinuclear antibodies are commonly found, with estimates of prevalence of discoid lupus in 6% to 50%. The sex ratio of discoid lupus (two females/one male) is much less biased toward females than the systemic form.

Drug-Induced Lupus Erythematosus and Antihistone Antibodies

Characteristic of drug-induced lupus is the presence of histone antibodies. Histones are basic molecular proteins containing high molar ratios of positively charged amino acids, lysine, and arginine. Histones are found in eukaryotic cells closely associated with genomic DNA. The subunit of this histone DNA complex is called a *nucleosome*, which has two molecules of each of the "core" histones (H2A, H2B, H3, and H4) and one molecule of H1, along with DNA of about 200 base pairs in length (Rubin, 1985, 1987).

In the studies of drug-induced lupus, the liver enzyme acetyltransferase appears to play an important role (Woosley, 1987). Acetyltransferase is an enzyme that can acetylate drugs, such as hydralazine and procainamide, and plays a role in detoxification and excretion of the drug. Patients with low levels of acetyltransferase were more prone to develop ANA and clinical symptoms than patients who were treated with hydralazine and had phenotypically high levels of acetyltransferase. Patients with high levels of enzyme and who were rapid acetylators were not immune to the development of ANA. These patients, however, took a longer and larger cumulative dose of hydralazine before developing disease. These findings concerning acetyltransferase phenotypes have been confirmed in patients treated with procainamide (Rubin, 1988).

Procainamide is the most common drug involved in drug-induced autoimmunity. Hydralazine, quinidine, and other drugs have also been implicated as causing drug-induced autoimmunity. In drug-induced lupus, antibodies to single-stranded DNA and histones are present. In SLE, on the other hand, antibodies to double-stranded native DNA, Sm, and U1 RNP antigens are often present, in addition to the antibodies to histones. Procainamide is used to treat patients with cardiac arrhythmias, and most patients eventually develop antihistone antibodies. However, only 10% to 20% of procainamide-treated patients develop symptomatic autoimmune disease (Rubin, 1988). In the asymptomatic patients, the antihistone antibody is predominantly IgM and displays broad reactivity with all of the individual histones.

The patients with symptomatic disease develop a unique type of IgG antihistone antibody, which, rather than reacting with individual histones, shows specific reactivity with the histone H2A–H2B dimer complex (Rubin, 1988). Thus, the IgG anti–(H2A-H2B) is a useful diagnostic marker, with high sensitivity and specificity for symptomatic diseases, in contrast to the benign form of procainamide-induced autoimmunity, with IgM antibodies to the individual histone.

In hydralazine-induced lupus erythematosus, the complex of H2A–H2B is an important target antigen, but the complex of H3–H4 appears to be more reactive (Rubin, 1988). In both types of drug-induced lupus erythematosus (hydralazine and procainamide), IgM antibodies were present in higher concentrations than IgG antibodies.

Fifty percent of all patients treated with procainamide developed ANAs after one year of treatment (Tan, 1989). The slow acetylators developed ANAs more rapidly than the rapid acetylators (Woosley, 1987). All patients on prolonged procainamide treatment developed a positive ANA response irrespective of acetylator phenotype.

SJÖGREN'S SYNDROME

Sjögren's syndrome is a chronic progressive inflammatory autoimmune disease marked by progressive dryness of the eyes and mouth (Schumacher, 1993). The disease may evolve from exocrine glands to a systemic disorder as well as a B-cell lymphoproliferative disorder. The disease is much more frequently found in women than men, with an increasing prevalence throughout adult life.

Often associated with Sjögren's syndrome is another rheumatic disease, such as RA, SLE, primary biliary cirrhosis, or progressive systemic sclerosis. The affected salivary or lacrimal glands are infiltrated with aggregates of lymphocytes. Extraglandular manifestations include lymphadenopathy, cutaneous vasculitis, interstitial pneumonitis, etc.

The disease has been classified into (1) primary Sjögren's syndrome, which is not associated with other secondary tissue disease, and (2) secondary Sjögren's syndrome, in which RA or some other connective tissue disorder is present. Sjögren's syndrome is known to occur in a primary form, with the sicca complex (keratoconjunctivitis sicca and xerostomia) as its hallmark feature. Patients with primary Sjögren's syndrome may develop lymphoproliferative diseases including lymphomas.

Autoantibodies in Sjögren's syndrome are restricted to SS-A/Ro and SS-B/La antigens (Tan, 1989). The anti–SS-A/Ro and anti–SS-B/La antibodies are present in SLE but in lower prevalences than in Sjögren's syndrome. Anti–SS-B/La is seen in 60% of Sjögren's syndrome patients and 35% of SLE patients, and anti–SS-A/LA is seen in 40% and 15%, respectively (Tan, 1988). The presence of anti–SS-A/Ro when associated with anti–SS-B/La is indicative of primary Sjögren's syndrome, at times coexisting with SLE. The presence of anti–SS-B antibodies is less than 1% in RA (Tan, 1988).

The anti–SS-A/Ro antibody may present in 40% to 62% of patients with primary and secondary Sjögren's syndrome, and may be linked to extraglandular symptomatology. There is a striking association between anti–SS-A/Ro and the presence of both systemic and cutaneous vasculitis (Bylund, 1991). The association of SA-A/Ro antibody and vasculitis has been observed in patients with unclassified connective tissue disease. Anti–SS-A/Ro is strongly associated with primary Sjögren's syndrome but is not specific for the sicca syndrome. Anti–SS-B/La are frequently detected in patients with SLE, whereas negative results have been obtained in all Sjögren's syndrome patients secondary to RA (Nakamura, 1985).

SCLERODERMA

Systemic sclerosis (scleroderma) is a multisystem connective tissue disorder of unknown etiology in which vascular lesions and tissue fibrosis are prominent features. The etiology of systemic sclerosis remains obscure. Patients with systemic sclerosis spontaneously produce autoantibodies against nuclear, nucleolar, and mitochondrial antigens (Reimer, 1990; Rothfield, 1992).

A scleroderma patient usually has a restricted heterogeneity of autoantibody type. An individual patient rarely has more than one autoantibody detected, in contrast to SLE patients, in whom three or more autoantibodies may be present. Table 41–4 lists the various types of autoantibodies seen in scleroderma. Patients with rapidly progressive and *diffuse cutaneous involvement* affecting the distal and often proximal extremities and trunk are at greater risk of developing early visceral involvement.

Included in the classification of scleroderma is a large subset of patients who have a form of the CREST (calcinosis cutis, Raynaud's phenomenon, esophageal dysmotility, sclerodactyly, and telangiectasia) syndrome. The subset of CREST patients may make up 20% to 30% of all scleroderma patients (Fritzler, 1980). Patients with the variant called the CREST syndrome have a *limited cutaneous involvement* confined to the distal extremities of fingers and face, and usually a better prognosis and clinical course than patients with diffuse cutaneous involvement.

Table 41–4. AUTOANTIGENS AND AUTOANTIBODIES IN SCLERODERMA

Autoantigen	Molecular Structure	Autoantibody Frequency (%)
Scl-70	100-kDa native protein and 70-kDa degradation product; DNA topoisomerase I	70% in diffuse scleroderma
Centromere	Proteins, 17, 80, and 140 kDa, localized at inner and outer kinetochore plates	70–80% in CREST
RNA Pol I	RNA Pol I complex of subunit proteins, 210–211 kDa	4–20%
RNA Pol II	Transcripts mRNA	4%
RNA Pol III	Transcripts 5S rRNA, tRNA	23%
Fibrillarin	Protein, 34 kDa, component of U3 RNP particle	8%
PM-ScL	Complex of 11 proteins, 110–120 kDa	3%
To	Protein, 40 kDa, complexes with 7S and 8S RNAs	Rare
NOR-90	Protein, 90 kDa, localized in nucleolus organizer region	Rare

Antibodies to Centromere Antigens

The autoantibodies to centromere antigens were detected initially by immunofluorescence microscopy. The centromere antigen was localized to the region of the condensing metaphase chromosomes. In immunoblotting studies, the centromere antigens consist of three proteins: 16 kDa, 80 kDa, and 120 kDa. Autoantibodies to centromere proteins are present in 70% to 80% of patients with the subset of scleroderma called CREST. Twenty-five percent of patients with idiopathic Raynaud's phenomenon with other signs or symptoms of CREST have anticentromere antibodies (Rothfield, 1992).

Antibodies to Scl-70 (DNA Topoisomerase I)

A major autoantigen is Scl-70, which is a 70 kDa protein. Scl-70 has been found to be a spontaneous degradation product of DNA topoisomerase I (Tan, 1989). The antigen was localized in punctate distribution in the nucleoplasm. In early studies autoantibodies to Scl-70 were detected in 20% of unselected scleroderma patients by immunodiffusion studies (Tan, 1982a). In later studies, Scl-70 autoantibodies were found in 75% of patients with the diffuse severe form of scleroderma by immunodiffusion tests (Jarzabek-Chorzelska, 1986). This latter finding was probably caused by better preservation of topoisomerase I antigen in the tests as well as the demonstration of higher prevalence of Scl-70 autoantibody in patients with the diffuse severe form of scleroderma (Nakamura, 1992).

Antibodies to RNA Polymerases

Three RNA polymerases catalyze the transcription of genes into RNA (von Mühlen, 1994). Autoantibodies targeting RNA polymerases tend to occur together in the same patients, appear to be specific for scleroderma, and appear mostly in individuals with diffuse scleroderma.

Autoantibodies to Nucleolar Antigen Fibrillarin (U3-snRNP)

The name *fibrillarin* comes from the antigen localization in the dense fibrillar component of nucleoli. Antifibrillarin antibodies are seen in young men with scleroderma and minimal joint involvement (von Mühlen, 1994).

Antibodies Targeting the Nucleolar Organizing Region

Nucleolar organizing region (NOR)-90 antibodies recognize the RNA polymerase I transcription factor hUBF (human upstream binding factor) in the fibrillar center of the nucleolus. NORs are regions where the nucleolus reforms after mitosis, with clusters of ribosomal RNA genes, and sites where Scl-70, U3-RNA/fibrillarin, NOR-90, and RNA polymerase I antigens can be detected (von Mühlen, 1994).

RHEUMATOID ARTHRITIS

RA is a systemic autoimmune disorder that is characterized by a chronic, symmetric, and erosive arthritis of the peripheral joints. A large percentage of the patients have elevated titers of serum rheumatoid factors. There are associated nonarticular manifestations, such as subcutaneous nodules, vasculitis, interstitial fibrosis, etc. Sjögren's and Felty's syndromes commonly occur with RA. The primary cause of RA is unknown. Most patients with RA have the Class II MHC alleles DR4, DR1, or both (Schumacher, 1993).

RA is associated with several autoantibodies, which can serve as diagnostic and prognostic markers (Aho, 1994). These include:

1. Rheumatoid factor (RF)
2. Antikeratin antibody (AKA)
3. Antiperinuclear factor (APF)
4. Antibody to RA-associated nuclear antigen (RANA)
5. Anti-RA33

The first three, and possible anti-RA33, may precede the onset of clinical RA.

Rheumatoid Factor

This antibody is directed against the Fc portion of the IgG molecule. Studies of monoclonal and polyclonal RF have shown polyreactive RF with binding specificity for substances other than IgG, such as nuclear components (Schumacher, 1993). The polyreactive RF is usually of the IgM class with low affinity. RF is not specific for RA and is often seen in cases of chronic infections and other conditions. RF in rheumatic diseases has considerable immunochemical heterogeneity. In addition to the common IgM RF, both IgA RF and IgG RF have been detected. Most RF in the serum of RA patients reacts to the nonallotypic Ga (or γ1-2-4) site present in IgG_1, IgG_2, and IgG_4 molecules. RF reactive with Gm allotypic groups presents in IgG_1, and IgG_3 may also be present in sera of RA patients.

Antikeratin Antibody

The antibody reacts against the stratum corneum of rat esophagus. AKA is a fairly specific but not very sensitive marker for RA. The occurrence of positive reactions in RA sera is 36% to 59% and only 0% to 3% in normal healthy individuals (Aho, 1994).

Antiperinuclear Factor

This antibody is reactive with perinuclear keratohyalin granules of buccal mucosa cells. This test is sensitive but less specific than AKA in RA patients. APF-positive tests in RA patients have been reported to be from 49% to 87% (Aho, 1994).

Antibody to Rheumatoid Arthritis–Associated Nuclear Antigen

Antibody to RA-associated nuclear antigen (RANA) was demonstrated in Sjögren's syndrome patients associated with RA (Tan, 1989). The RANA was found to be localized in the nucleus in a finely speckled fashion by immunofluorescence microscopy studies. The RANA was not detectable in tissue sections of many organs in mouse, monkey, and humans. The RANA was also not detectable in two human T-cell lines (Molt 4 and 1301) but was detected in the nuclei of three B-cell lines (WIL2, Raji, and Daudi). The B-cell lines harbored Epstein-Barr virus (EBV), while the T-cell lines did not. There was a definite relationship between RANA and EBV. Before transformation of lymphocytes with EBV, the cells were negative for RANA. However, after transformation, RANA antigens were found in the nucleus (Tan, 1989). Anti-EA (an early antigen of EBV) antibody was also present in higher frequency in RA patients. In one study, a large number of RA patients with high titers ($\geq$1:20) of anti-EA was observed (Ferrell, 1981).

The linkage between EBV, RA, and RANA has not been definitively established. HLA phenotype, EBV, and, during infection, immunoregulation deficiencies and reactivation of latent EBV-infected cells may all play a role in the disease pathogenesis (Nakamura, 1992). In early studies with immunodiffusion assays, anti-RANA was detected in two thirds of patients with RA (Tan, 1982a, 1989). However, in later reports the incidence of anti-RANA was found to be over 90% in RA patients (Tan, 1988). In normal control subjects, the frequency of anti-RANA varied from 6% to 25% (Tan, 1988). Seroepidemiologic studies for EB viral antibodies in RA have shown there was a higher frequency of RA patients with high titers ($\geq$1:320) of antibody to EB viral capsid antigen. There was no difference in anti-EB nuclear antigen frequency or titers between RA and normal patients (Ferrell, 1981).

Anti-RA33 and Relationship to Rheumatoid Arthritis

Hassfield (1989) has reported a new antinuclear antibody (anti-RA33) that may be specific for RA. From extracts of Hela cells, an antigen of approximately 33,000 molecular weight was found to react with 36% of 95 sera from RA patients and with only one of 170 control patients. The antigen was termed *RA33*, and the autoantibody has no discernible relationship to other nuclear antibodies. Anti-RA33 was not related to antihistone. Of 11 RA patients with anti-RANA, six were found to be positive for anti-RA3. Of the five anti-RANA negative sera, two were positive for anti-RA33 (Hassfeld, 1989).

Immunoblot analyses with soluble extracts from Hela cells showed an autoantibody to a 33-kDa antigen (anti-RA33) in 30% of Austrian RA patients and none in patients with ankylosing spondylitis or psoriatic arthritis (Aho, 1994). However, the prevalence of anti-RA33 in Finnish RA was found to be a low 6% (Aho, 1994).

POLYMYOSITIS AND DERMATOMYOSITIS

Polymyositis (PM) is an inflammatory disease of striated muscle of unknown etiology. It is characterized by the presence of inflammatory infiltrates in the skeletal muscle, with associated muscle fiber necrosis and degeneration (Targoff, 1992). When the disease is accompanied by typical skin changes, it is called *dermatomyositis*.

Polymyositis is characterized serologically by the presence of a number of autoantibodies of various specifications directed against different transfer RNA (tRNA) synthetases (von Mühlen, 1994) (Table 41–5). These autoantibodies define a subgroup of patients with PM, arthralgia, and interstitial lung disease and poorer prognosis than patients without the autoantibodies.

Antibodies to Jo-1 (histidyl tRNA synthetase) occur in highest prevalence in 23% to 36% of PM patients, with most having interstitial lung disease (Targoff, 1992). Autoantibodies to threonyl and alanyl tRNA synthetase occur at a lower prevalence in autoimmune myositis. In patients with a clinical syndrome showing overlapping features of polymyositis and scleroderma, an antibody called anti–PM-Scl has been reported (Tan, 1988). The anti–PM-Scl antibody reacts with a complex of 11 polypeptides ranging from 110 to 120 kDa. Anti–PM-Scl shows staining of nucleolus and cytoplasm of the cell by indirect immunofluorescence microscopy.

CONCEPT OF OVERLAP SYNDROMES

Overlap syndrome is used when patients exhibit symptoms of more than one disease. For example, patients who meet the diagnostic criteria for SLE and also have typical manifestations suggestive of a second diagnosis, such as RA, have been described (Lazaro, 1989). It is uncertain whether overlap syndromes may represent the coexistence of two or more different diseases, or whether the syndrome is a distinct en-

Table 41–5. AUTOANTIGENS AND AUTOANTIBODIES IN POLYMYOSITIS AND DERMATOMYOSITIS

Autoantigen	Molecular Structure	Autoantibody Frequency (%)
Jo-1	Histidyl tRNA synthetase protein, 55/60 kDa	23–36%
PL-7	Threonyl tRNA synthetase protein, 80 kDa	4%
PL-12	Alanyl tRNA synthetase protein, 110 kDa	3%
Mi-2	Proteins 53 and 61 kDa	5–35%
Signal recognition particle (SRP)	Protein 54 kDa complexed with 7 SL RNA	4–5%
PM-Scl	Complex of 11 proteins, 110–120 kDa	8–12%
56 kDa	56 kDa, RNP component	80%

Data from Tan (1988), Nakamura and Tan (1992), and von Mühlen and Tan (1994).

tity. Studies by Lazaro (1989) showed that the finding of a high titer of antibodies against the nuclear ribonucleoprotein (nRNP) did not allow identification of a particular subgroup.

Mixed Connective Tissue Disease

The concept of MCTD was initially proposed by Sharp (1972). The 20 patients described in the initial report had a combination of features usually associated with SLE, progressive systemic sclerosis, and polymyositis. Characteristically, a high titer of autoantibody to a nuclear ribonucleoprotein was found in all of the patients (Sharp, 1972). The lack of renal and neurologic abnormalities and excellent response of these patients to small doses of oral corticosteroids initially justified the classification of these patients as a separate group from SLE and progressive systemic sclerosis.

However, the concept of MCTD as a separate group has changed with time. Many feel that MCTD represents an overlap of systemic sclerosis, SLE, and polymyositis (Nimelstein, 1980). A follow-up study of a group of patients originally diagnosed as MCTD was restudied eight years later and showed a general evolution out of the overlap pattern to one of single disease, and progressive systemic sclerosis was the most prevalent diagnosis (Nimelstein, 1980). There appears to be a large overlap that becomes apparent when the abovementioned criteria are applied to a certain population of patients, and the studies do not support the existence of MCTD as an individual clinical entity.

MOLECULAR BIOLOGY AND FUNCTIONS OF CERTAIN NUCLEAR AND INTRACELLULAR AUTOANTIGENS

Many of the intracellular autoantibodies, including the autoantibodies to nuclear antigens (ANAs), have been identified as diagnostic markers for the rheumatic diseases, such as SLE, scleroderma, Sjögren's syndrome, MCTD, drug-induced lupus and polymyositis, and dermatomyositis (Tan, 1989). The autoantibodies in human diseases have been used as tools to study various molecular biological functions and mechanisms. The biological functions of many of the autoantigen-inducing autoantibodies have been studied and elucidated. The biological functions that the autoantibodies have been demonstrated to inhibit are RNA splicing, DNA replication, DNA repair, transcription, and aminoacetylation of tRNAs (Tan, 1988, 1989).

PROFILES OF AUTOANTIBODIES IN VARIOUS SYSTEMIC RHEUMATIC DISEASES

It has been observed that distinct profiles of ANA are seen in different systemic rheumatic diseases, characteristics of which include the presence or absence of certain antibodies and differences in the mean titers of these antibodies (Nakamura, 1986; Tan, 1988).

The following features are noteworthy:

1. Multiple ANA frequently seen in SLE, often with high levels of anti–DS-DNA antibodies
2. Distinctiveness of anti-Sm for SLE
3. Restriction of ANA in drug-induced LE to antihistone
4. Antibodies to U1-RNP or nuclear antibodies to RNP present in several rheumatic diseases with different frequencies
5. The restriction of ANA in MCTD to U1-RNP or nuclear RNP antibodies
6. Sjögren's syndrome sera, characterized primarily by the presence of antibodies to SS-A/Ro and SS-B/La
7. Patients with scleroderma showing a profile consisting of antibodies to Scl-70, the centromere/kinetochore antigen, and nucleolar antigens
8. The frequent presence of RF, AKA, APT, anti-RA33, and RANA in rheumatoid arthritis
9. The presence of Jo-1, M_{1-2}, PM-Scl, and 56 kDa autoantibodies in polymyositis/dermatomyositis

5

DIAGNOSTIC METHODS IN AUTOANTIBODY DETECTION

The commonly used methods for autoantibody detection are listed in Table 41–6. A widely used test for screening for intracellular autoantibodies is immunofluorescence microscopy (IFM) and the immunoenzyme tests that are sensitive are primary antigen-antibody tests (Nakamura, 1994b). The secondary definitive tests for specific identification of ANA are immunodiffusion, immunoprecipitin, particle ag-

Table 41–6. METHODS FOR DETECTION OF AUTOANTIBODIES TO NUCLEAR AND INTRACELLULAR ANTIGENS*

Method	Antigen Source	Sensitivity and Use
Immunofluorescence microscopy (IFM)	Tissue sections; cell lines	Sensitive assay and used often for screening
Double immunodiffusion (ID)	Tissue and cell extracts	Requires precipitin reaction and high specificity but not very sensitive immunological procedure
Counterimmunoelectrophoresis (CIE)	Tissue and cell extracts	Increased sensitivity and speed as compared with ID procedure
Immunoblotting (IB)	Cell extracts	Very sensitive and permits detection of antibodies against soluble and insoluble antigens
ELISA	Purified native or recombinant antigens	Very sensitive and quantitative, and can determine antibody class

*Used with permission from Nakamura (1994b).

glutination, immunoenzyme, immunoblotting, and radioimmunoassay methods (Teodorescu, 1992).

Standardization of the indirect immunofluorescence (IF)-ANA has been difficult (Nakamura, 1992). Many factors are involved in the performance of IF-ANA tests. They include (1) substrate and fixative variations, (2) microscopic optics, (3) method and quantitation of results, (4) establishment of reference range, (5) interpretation of results, and (6) reference sera.

Bylund and Nakamura (Bylund, 1991) have shown the importance of detection of SS-A/Ro autoantibodies in screening for immunofluorescence tests for autoantibodies to nuclear antigens. The detection of anti–SS-A/Ro requires implementation and adherence to several technical and quality assurance recommendations. With use of the appropriate substrate cells containing the SS-A/Ro antigen, many of the so-called ANA-negative lupus erythematosus patients will show a positive test by the indirect immunofluorescence test.

Immunoprecipitin and double immunodiffusion analysis have been used to determine the specificity of several ANAs. Assay specificity in double immunodiffusion is generally dependent on the quality of other control sera used in the procedure, as well as the nature of the antigen preparation. The immunodiffusion tests are not very sensitive. The positive tests by immunodiffusion have a high degree of specificity as a diagnostic marker in certain rheumatic diseases. Immunodiffusion commercial kits are available for the detection of antibodies to RNP, Sm, SS-A/Ro, SS-B/La, and Scl-70, as well as other less prevalent markers (Nakamura, 1994b).

An increasing number of enzyme immunoassays have been developed over the past decade with the use of standard purified and recombinant antigens (Saitta, 1992). Many of these enzyme immunoassays have proved to be more sensitive than comparable immunodiffusion methods. Thus, because of the high sensitivity of enzyme immunoassays, one needs to determine carefully the reference range of normal patients and the proper cut-off values.

Compared with immunodiffusion tests, the ELISA tests showed much greater sensitivity but had lower specificity (Nakamura, 1992). Further, the ELISA tests were frequently positive in low titers of antibodies in sera of patients with rheumatic diseases other than SLE. For example, the presence of antibodies to Sm as assayed by immunodiffusion is considered to be highly specific for SLE. However, in ELISA tests the Sm antibody was positive in 23% of 54 RA patients, 25% of 24 systemic sclerosis patients, 9% of 11 polymyositis patients, and 2% of 59 normal patients (Maddison, 1985). Increasing sensitivity and decreasing specificity might result in false-positive test results.

VARIATIONS IN METHODOLOGIES USED FOR DETECTION OF AUTOANTIBODIES TO NUCLEAR AND INTRACELLULAR ANTIGENS

The best studies regarding the different methods for the detection of autoantibodies to intracellular antigens were reported by a European Consensus Study Group. The European Consensus Study Group for the Detection of Autoantibodies to Intracellular Antigens in Rheumatic Diseases was formed in 1988 and has conducted four annual workshops from 1989 to 1992 (Charles, 1992; van Venrooij, 1991).

In 1988 and 1989, consensus workshops were conducted to define interlaboratory concordance in the detection of autoantibody specificities in rheumatic diseases. Twenty-eight laboratories participated in the study and used various methodologies.

The objectives of the consensus study initiated in 1989 were (1) to define the interlaboratory consensus in detecting autoantibodies and specificities, (2) to test whether discrepancies were due to the methodology used, and (3) to make recommendations for improved quality of results with improved sensitivity and specificity.

Enzyme-Linked Immunosorbent Assays

In the 1988 and 1989 studies, many false-positive reactions were noted. The false-positive reactions were caused by poor blocking reagents in the procedure; also, impure antigen preparations were used. In the 1990 and 1991 cooperative study, the laboratory using enzyme-linked immunosorbent assays (ELISA) performed very well, with few false-positive or extraneous negative results. The ELISA assays also performed well in sorting out sera with multiple specificities. The percentage of clinical laboratories using ELISA increased from 25% to 47% over a four-year period, from 1989 to 1992.

Immunoblotting

This technique is very sensitive and is an important method for the characterization of the specific nature of many of the autoantibodies. An important advantage of the method is that a specific antibody can be identified with the use of crude cell extract antigen preparations. The European consensus study observed the following with the immunoblotting procedure (Nakamura, 1994b):

1. The antigen preparation is very important in the immunoblotting procedure.
2. The detection of antibodies to nRNP, Sm, and Scl-70 was acceptable. This sensitive method is helpful in the detection of multiple specificities of antibody in the same specimen.
3. The method requires careful controls to monitor molecular weight bands. For example, histone bands can be confused with a centromeric antigen (CENP-A, 19 kDa), and Scl-70 (topoisomerase I) can be confused with other 100-kDa bands.
4. Protein degradation can occur in the antigen cell extract used for immunoblotting, especially Scl-70 and centromere antigens.
5. The anti-Sm is distinguished by the presence of anti-D. (The D antigen is a 16-kDa protein contained in all major nRNP particles.)
6. Anti–SS-B/La is readily detected by immunoblotting. Anti–SS-A/Ro is poorly detected by immunoblotting and is insensitive, because SS-A/Ro may not demonstrate the proper structure for recognition.

SUMMARY

There are many types of autoantibodies to intracellular and nuclear antigens in the various systemic rheumatic diseases. Currently, it is considered important not only to detect the presence and quantity of the intracellular and nuclear autoantibody in the patient, but also to identify the immunologic specificity. Past studies have shown that distinct diagnostic profiles of the autoantibodies are observed in many of the rheumatic diseases. Some of the diseases are characterized by the presence or absence of a specific antibody, or by differences in the quantitative level or titer of the autoantibody.

Much progress has been made in improvement of the sensitivity, specificity, and quality control of the many laboratory tests for the detection of autoantibodies to intracellular and nuclear antigens. Molecular biologists have used many of the autoantibodies as biological probes and have elucidated the biological functions of several of the autoantigens. Much progress has been made in the understanding of the pathogenesis and immune mechanisms in rheumatic diseases.

Aho K, Paluso T, Kurki P: Marker antibodies of rheumatoid arthritis: Diagnostic and pathogenic implications. Semin Arthritis Rheum 1994; 23:379.

Alarcon-Segovia D, Perez-Vasquez ME, Villa AR, et al: Preliminary classification criteria for the antiphospholipid syndrome within systemic lupus erythematosus. Semin Arthritis Rheum 1992; 21:275.

Barada FA, Andrews BS, Davis JS, Taylor RP: Antibodies to Sm in patients with systemic lupus erythematosus. Correlation of Sm antibody titers with disease activity and other laboratory parameters. Arthritis Rheum 1981; 24:1236.

Block SR, Winfield JB, Lockshin MC, et al: Studies of twins with systemic lupus erythematosus: A review of the literature and presentation of 12 additional sets. Am J Med 1975; 59:533.

Buskila D, Shoenfeld Y: Anti-DNA antibodies. *In* Lahita RG (ed): Systemic Lupus Erythematosus, 2nd ed. New York, Churchill Livingstone, 1992, p 205.

Bylund DJ, Nakamura RM: Importance of detection of SS-A/Ro autoantibody in screening immunofluorescence tests for autoantibodies to nuclear antigens. J Clin Lab Anal 1991; 5:212.

Chan EK, Tan EM: Epitopic targets for autoantibodies in systemic lupus erythematosus and Sjögren's syndrome. Curr Opin Rheumatol 1989; 1:376.

Charles PJ, van Venrooij WJ, Maini RN: The consensus workshops for the detection of autoantibodies to intracellular antigens in rheumatic diseases, 1989–1992. Clin Exp Rheumatol 1992; 10:507.

Cohen AS, Reynolds WE, Franklin EC, et al: Preliminary criteria for the classification of systemic lupus erythematosus. Bull Rheum Dis 1971; 21:643.

Decker JL: Glossary Subcommittee of ARA Committee on Rheumatologic Practice. Arthritis Rheum 1986; 26:1029.

Ferrell PB, Aitcheson CT, Pearson GR, et al: Seroepidemiologic study of relationships between Epstein-Barr virus and rheumatoid arthritis. J Clin Invest 1981; 67:681.

Francoeur AM, Peebles CL, Gomper PT, Tan EM: Identification of Ki(Ku, p70/p80) autoantigens and analysis of anti-Ki autoantibody reactivity. J Immunol 1986; 136:1648.

Fritzler MJ, Kinsella TD, Garbutt E: The CREST syndrome: A distinct serologic entity with anticentromere antibodies. Am J Med 1980; 69:520.

Harris EN: The Second International Anticardiolipin Standardization Workshop/The Kingston Antiphospholipid Antibody Study (KAPS) groups. Am J Clin Pathol 1990; 94:476.

Harris EN, Gharavi AE, Patel SP, Hughes ERV: Evaluation of the anticardiolipin test: Report of an international workshop held 4 April 1986. Clin Exp Immunol 1987; 68:215.

Hassfeld W, Steiner G, Hartmuth K, et al: Demonstration of a new antinuclear antibody (anti RA-33) that is highly specific for rheumatoid arthritis. Arthritis Rheum 1989; 32:1515.

Hochberg MC: Systemic lupus erythematosus. Rheum Dis Clin North Am 1990; 16:617.

Hochberg MC, Boyd RE, Ahearn JM, et al: Systemic lupus erythematosus: A review of clinical laboratory features and immunogenetic markers in 150 patients with emphasis on demographic subsets. Medicine 1985; 64:285.

Jarzabek-Chorzelska M, Balszczyk M, Jablonska S, et al: Scl-70 antibody: A specific marker of systemic sclerosis. Br J Dermatol 1986; 115:393.

Lafer EM, Rauch J, Andrzejewski JR, et al: Polyspecific monoclonal lupus autoantibodies reactive with both polynucleotides and phospholipids. J Exp Med 1981; 153:897.

Lazaro MA, Maldonado-Cocco JA, Catoggio LJ, et al: Clinical and serological characteristics of patients with overlap syndrome: Is mixed connective tissue disease a distinct clinical entity? Medicine 1989; 68:58.

Lerner MR, Steitz JA: Antibodies to small nuclear RNAs complexed with proteins are produced by patients with systemic lupus erythematosus. Proc Natl Acad Sci USA 1979; 76:5495.

Lom-Orta H, Alarcon-Segovia D, Diaz-Jouanen E: Systemic lupus erythematosus. Differences between patients who do and who do not fulfill classification criteria at the time of diagnosis. J Rheumatol 1980; 7:831.

Lopez LR, Santos ME, Espinoza LR, La Rosa FG: Clinical significance of immunoglobulin A versus immunoglobulins E and M anticardiolipin antibodies in patients with systemic lupus erythematosus: Correlation with thrombosis, thrombocytopenia, and recurrent abortion. Am J Clin Pathol 1992; 98:447.

Maddison PF, Skinner RP, Vlachoviannopoulos P, et al: Antibodies to nRNP, Sm, Ro (SSA) and La (SSB) detected by ELISA: Their specificity and inter-relations in connective tissue disease sera. Clin Exp Immunol 1985; 62:337.

McNeil HP, Chesterman CH, Krilis SA: Immunology and clinical importance of antiphospholipid antibodies. Adv Immunol 1991; 49:193.

Minota S, Koyasu S, Yahara I, Winfield J: Autoantibodies to the heat-shock protein Hsp 90 in systemic lupus erythematosus. J Clin Invest 1988; 81:106.

Miyachi K, Fritzler MJ, Tan EM: Autoantibody to a nuclear antigen in proliferating cells. J Immunol 1978; 121:2228.

Nakamura RM, Bylund DJ: Contemporary concepts for clinical and laboratory evaluation of systemic lupus erythematosus and "lupus-like" syndromes. J Clin Lab Anal 1994a; 8:347.

Nakamura RM, Bylund DJ, Tan EM: Current status of available standards for quality improvment of assays for the detection of autoantibodies to nuclear and intracellular antigens. J Clin Lab Anal 1994b; 8:360.

Nakamura RM, Peebles CL, Rubin RL, et al: Autoantibodies to nuclear antigens. *In* Advances in Laboratory Tests and Significance in Systemic Rheumatic Diseases, 2nd ed. Chicago, American Society of Clinical Pathology, 1985, p 1.

Nakamura RM, Tan EM: Recent advances in laboratory tests and the significance of autoantibodies to nuclear antigens in systemic rheumatic diseases. Clin Lab Med 1986; 6:41.

Nakamura RM, Tan EM: Update on autoantibodies to intracellular antigens in systemic rheumatic diseases. Clin Lab Med 1992; 12:1.

5

Nimelstein SH, Brody S, McShane D, Holman HR: Mixed connective tissue disease: A subsequent evaluation of the original 25 patients. Medicine 1980; 59:239.

Okamura M, Kanayama Y, Amastu K, et al: Significance of enzyme-linked immunosorbent assay (ELISA) for antibodies to double-stranded and single-stranded DNA in patients with lupus nephritis: Correlation with severity of renal histology. Ann Rheum Dis 1993; 52:14.

Panush RS, Greer JM, Morshedian KK: What is lupus? What is not lupus? Rheum Dis Clin North Am 1993; 19:223.

Pincus T: Studies regarding a possible function for viruses in the pathogensis of systemic lupus erythematosus. Arthritis Rheum 1982; 25:847.

Reeves WH: Antibodies ot the p70/p80 (Ku) antigens in systemic lupus erythematosus. Rheum Dis Clin North Am 1992; 18:391.

Reimer G: Autoantibodies against nuclear, nucleolar, and mitochondrial antigens in systemic sclerosis (scleroderma). Rheum Dis Clin North Am 1990; 16:169.

Rothfield NF: Autoantibodies in scleroderma. Rheum Dis Clin North Am 1992; 18:483.

Rubin RL: Autoimmune reactions induced by procainamide and hydralazine. *In* Kammuller M, Bloksma M, Siemen W (eds): Autoimmunity and Toxicology: Immune Disregulation Induced by Drugs and Chemicals. Amsterdam, Elsevier, 1988, p 119.

Rubin RL, McNally EM, Nusinow SR, et al: IgG antibodies to the histone complex H2A-H2B characterize procainamide-induced lupus. Clin Immunol Immunopathol 1985; 36:49.

Rubin RL, Waga S: Antihistone antibodies in systemic lupus erythematosus. J Rheumatol 1987; 14(Suppl 13):118.

Saitta MR, Keene JD: Molecular biology of nuclear autoantigens. Rheum Dis Clin North Am 1992; 18:283.

Sakamoto M, Takasaki Y, Yamanaka K, et al: Purification and characterization of Ki antigen and detection of anti-Ki antibody by enzyme-linked immunosorbent assay in patients with systemic lupus erythematosus. Arthritis Rheum 1989; 32:1554.

Schumacher HR, Jr., Klippel JH, Koopman WJ: Primer on the Rheumatic Diseases, 10th ed. Atlanta, GA, Arthritis Foundation, 1993.

Schur PH: Cinical features of SLE. *In* Kelly WN, Harris ED, Ruddy S, Sledge CB (eds): Textbook of Rheumatology, Vol. 2, 4th ed. Philadelphia, W. B. Saunders Co., 1993, p 1017.

Sharp GC, Irwin WS, Tan EM, et al: Mixed connective tissue disease: An apparently distinct rheumatic disease syndrome associated with a specific antibody to an extractable nuclear antigen (ENA). Am J Med 1972; 52:148.

Sontheimer RD, Gilliam JN: Systemic lupus erythematosus and the skin. *In* Lahita RG (ed): Systemic Lupus Erythematosus, 2nd ed. New York, Churchill Livingstone, 1992, p 657.

Tan EM: Autoantibodies to nuclear antigens (ANA): Their immunobiology and medicine. Adv Immunol 1982a; 33:167.

Tan EM: Antinuclear antibodies: Diagnostic markers for autoimmune diseases and probes for cell biology. Adv Immunol 1989; 44:93.

Tan EM, Chan EKL, Sullivan KF, Rubin RL: Antinuclear antibodies (ANAs): Diagnostically specific immune markers and clues toward the understanding of systemic autoimmunity. Clin Immunol Immunopathol 1988; 47:121.

Tan EM, Cohen AS, Fries JF, et al: The 1982 revised criteria for the classification of systemic lupus erythematosus. Arthritis Rheum 1982b; 25:1271.

Targoff IN: Autoantibodies in polymyositis. Rheum Dis Clin North Am 1992; 18:455.

Teodorescu M, Froelich CJ: Laboratory evaluation of systemic lupus erythematosus. *In* Lahita RG (ed): Systemic Lupus Erythematosus, 2nd ed. New York, Churchill Livingstone, 1992, p 345.

ter Borg EJ, Groen H, Horst G, et al: Clinical association of antiribonucleoprotein antibodies in patients with systemic lupus erythematosus. Semin Arthritis Rheum 1990; 20:164.

Tojo T, Kaburaki J, Hayakawa M, et al: Precipitating antibody to a soluble nuclear antigen "Ki" with specificity for systemic lupus erythematosus. Ryumachi 1981; 21(Suppl):129.

van Venrooij WJ, Charles P, Maini RN: The consensus workshops for the detection of autoantibodies to intracellular antigens in rheumatic diseases. J Immunol Methods 1991; 140:507.

von Mühlen CA, Tan EM: Autantibody specificities in autoimmune rheumatic diseases. Rev Bras Rheumatol 1994; 34:173.

Wallace DJ, Pistiner M, Nessim S, et al: Cutaneous lupus erythematosus without systemic lupus erythematosus: Clinical and laboratory features. Semin Arthritis Rheum 1992; 21:221.

Woosley RL, Drager DE, Reidenber MM, et al: Effect of acetylator phenotype on the rate at which procainamide induces antinuclear antibodies and the lupus syndrome. N Engl J Med 1987; 298:1157.

Zarmbinski MN, Messner RP, Mandel JS: Anti-dsDNA antibodies in laboratory workers handling blood from patients with systemic lupus erythematosus. J Rheumatol 1992; 19:1380.

Chapter 42

Vasculitis

David J. Bylund, M.D.
Rex M. McCallum, M.D.

The clinical and pathological expressions of systemic necrotizing vasculitis are protean. Patients present with a wide array of confusing and conflicting symptoms and/or signs. Diagnosis of a systemic necrotizing vasculitic syndrome requires thorough evaluation that correlates an individual patient's history and physical examination with laboratory data. Although vasculitis can occur anywhere in the body, distinctive patterns of disease have been defined, and their identification points to particular disorders. Specific diagnosis is important because treatment and prognosis depend on the sites and patterns of organ involvement (Langford, 1995).

Systemic necrotizing vasculitis can be defined pathologically as inflammation causing vascular lesions. These lesions may include the proliferation of intimal cells inside vessels' lumina, narrowing or even closing that space, and causing ischemia and possible infarction to anatomic structures distal to the site of vascular injury. Also, the vessel wall may weaken until an aneurysm forms or the vessel ruptures.

Idiopathic (primary) vasculitis occurs when vascular inflammatory damage is the principal clinicopathologic finding and there is no underlying illness. Secondary vasculitis occurs when vasculitic lesions accompany an underlying disorder (Table 42–1). The focus of this chapter is idiopathic vasculitis and those clinical laboratory tests useful for its diagnosis and management. Because methods of diagnosis and management in secondary vasculitides focus on the underlying disorders, they are discussed in the appropriate chapters of this book. However, comments related to laboratory evaluation of end-organ damage in idiopathic vasculitis are relevant to secondary vasculitis.

CLASSIFICATION

There is no widely accepted, standard classification system for idiopathic vasculitides. Historically, their classification has been based on various combinations of clinical and pathologic findings (Lie, 1989, 1994), although working classifications have improved in recent years because of efforts to develop standard nomenclature (Hunder, 1990; Jennette, 1994b). The classification scheme provided in Table 42–2 is modified from one used at the National Institutes of Health (NIH) (Langford, 1995).

PATHOGENESIS OF VASCULITIS

Neither the etiology nor pathogenesis of vasculitides is known, except for instances of direct blood vessel injury from vascular infection, a secondary vasculitis. Most idiopathic vasculitides are attributed to immune-mediated vascular injury induced by any of several mechanisms, including: (1) immune-complex deposits; (2) direct autoantibody binding, either to vessel wall structures (e.g., endothelium or basement membrane antigens) or to neutrophils when vasculitis is associated with anti–neutrophil cytoplasmic anti-

Table 42–1. SECONDARY SYSTEMIC NECROTIZING VASCULITIDES

Drug-related vasculitis
Foreign protein–related vasculitis
Vasculitis associated with infection
Vasculitis in malignancies
Lymphomatoid granulomatosis
Hypocomplementemic urticarial vasculitis
Hypergammaglobulinemic purpura
Cryoglobulinemic vasculitis
Radiation vasculitis
Transplant vasculitis (vascular rejection)
Connective tissue disease–associated vasculitis
Rheumatoid arthritis
Systemic lupus erythematosus
Sjögren's syndrome
Scleroderma
Dermatomyositis/polymyositis
Sarcoidosis
Relapsing polychondritis
Antiphospholipid antibody syndrome
Behçet's disease

Adapted from Langford CA, McCallum RM: Idiopathic vasculitis. *In* Belch JJF, Zurier RB (eds): Connective Tissue Diseases. London, Chapman and Hall, 1995, p 179.

body (ANCA); and (3) T-cell–mediated inflammation. The pathogenic effects of these different mechanisms all unite in a final common pathway of vascular injury that activates humoral and cellular mediators of inflammation. These mediators initiate the infiltration of inflammatory cells, activation of complement and coagulation cascades, and upregulation of other molecules, such as cytokines and leukocyte adhesion molecules (Conn, 1993; Niles, 1995).

PERSPECTIVE ON USE OF CLINICAL LABORATORY TESTS

When evaluating patients with complicated multisystem disease, the clinician's goal is accurate diagnosis to the level that defines proper treatment. Because there are no pathognomonic clinical or laboratory features of vasculitis, the physician must use combinations of clinical and laboratory findings to recognize patterns of disease. This may allow specific diagnosis or, more commonly, classification of the patient's disease as one in a group of vasculitic disorders with similar treatment, even when no specific entity is identifiable.

Table 42–2. IDIOPATHIC (PRIMARY) SYSTEMIC NECROTIZING VASCULITIDES

Small Vessel Vasculitis
Wegener's granulomatosis
Henoch-Schönlein purpura
Isolated central nervous system vasculitis
Medium Vessel Vasculitis
Churg-Strauss syndrome
Polyarteritis nodosa
Kawasaki's disease
Large Vessel Vasculitis
Giant cell (temporal) arteritis
Takayasu's arteritis

Deciding that a patient has vasculitis strictly on the basis of clinical symptoms is fraught with risks because of the large number of differential diagnostic possibilities and the lack of pathognomonic findings. Consequently, histologic or angiographic confirmation of vasculitis should be obtained from tissue biopsy or angiography for definitive diagnosis prior to therapy (Mandell, 1994).

Clinical laboratory tests are of limited value in establishing a specific diagnosis of vasculitis (Mandell, 1994), although clinicians use these tests to assist in identifying patterns of organ involvement characteristic of vasculitis, evaluating the extent and severity of end-organ damage, differentiating idiopathic vasculitis from alternative secondary forms, and establishing baseline values for management. Recognition of the presence of ANCA associated with certain idiopathic vasculitides has been an important aid in diagnosis and management. ANCAs are discussed in detail later.

When evaluating a patient whose differential diagnoses includes vasculitis, the following principles regarding the use and interpretation of clinical laboratory tests are helpful.

Routine Tests

Patients whose history and physical examination suggest idiopathic vasculitis often have a confusing array of multisystem complaints that have been occurring for some time. First-order tests to consider would include the following: cultures for infectious agents if the patient has fever, complete blood count (CBC) with differential count, erythrocyte sedimentation rate (ESR), urinalysis, blood chemistry panel, and tests for specific organ function, such as the liver.

Special Tests

Special tests help to differentiate idiopathic vasculitis from alternatives in the working differential diagnosis. Relevant laboratory tests would include those to identify the circulating autoantibodies listed in Table 42–3 and perhaps immune complexes. Directed tissue biopsy for histologic confirmation of vasculitis and/or angiography are considered the definitive tests for idiopathic vasculitis.

Some Test Patterns in Vasculitis

Certain patterns of clinical laboratory test results are useful:

- Finding leukopenia and/or thrombocytopenia in idiopathic vasculitides is rare and suggests alternative diagnoses, such as systemic lupus erythematosus, neoplasm, bone marrow disorders, lymphomatoid granulomatosis, or hypersplenism (Mandell, 1994).
- ESR, although a nonspecific finding, is typically elevated in idiopathic vasculitides. If the ESR before therapy is not elevated, the diagnosis is not giant cell (temporal) arteritis or Wegener's granulomatosis (WG).
- Vasculitis with histologic features of polyarteritis nodosa (PAN) associated with pancytopenia can be seen in patients with hairy cell leukemia (Mandell, 1994).

Table 42–3. AUTOANTIBODIES ASSOCIATED WITH VASCULITIS

Autoantibody	Disease Association	Principal Test Method(s)
ANCA (especially c-ANCA)	Wegener's granulomatosis	IFM; ELISA (PR3)
ANCA (c-ANCA or p-ANCA)	Microscopic polyarteritis	IFM; ELISA (MPO)
Anti–Clq antibodies	Hypocomplementemic urticarial vasculitis	Clq binding
Anti-GBM antibodies	Anti-GBM disease	ELISA; IFM
Anti–hepatitis B antibodies	Hepatitis B–associated PAN	ELISA
Anti–nuclear antibodies (ANA)	Systemic lupus erythematosus	IFM; ELISA; ID
Mixed cryoglobulins	Cryoglobulinemic vasculitis	Cryoprecipitation; IEP; IF
SSA (Ro), SSB (La)	Sjögren's syndrome	IFM; ID
Rheumatoid factor	Rheumatoid arthritis	Nephelometry; (Latex) agglutination

ANCA = anti–neutrophil cytoplasmic autoantibodies; c-ANCA = cytoplasmic ANCA; p-ANCA = perinuclear ANCA; PAN = polyarteritis nodosa; GBM = glomerular basement membrane; IFM = indirect immunofluorescence microscopy; ELISA = enzyme-linked immunosorbent assay; IEP = immunoelectrophoresis; IF = immunofixation; ID = immunodiffusion; MPO = myeloperoxidase; PROEL = protein electrophoresis; PR3 = proteinase 3.

- Anemia with hemoglobin less than 9 mg/dL results from conditions other than anemia of chronic disease, such as hemolysis, occult bleeding, or renal disease (Mandell, 1994).
- When PAN is suspected, serologic tests for liver function, hepatitis B virus, hepatitis C virus, and cytomegalovirus (Golden, 1994; Mandell, 1994) should be obtained. Similarly, serologic tests for hepatitis B and C viruses are appropriate when a patient has cryoglobulins, leukocytoclastic vasculitis on cutaneous biopsy, and/or renal disease.
- Elevated serum creatine phosphokinase (CPK) may indicate myositis or muscle ischemia (Mandell, 1994).
- Testing for antinuclear antibodies (ANA) and rheumatoid factor (RF) is useful only when connective tissue disease or arthritis is suspected.
- Patients with rheumatoid vasculitis have high titer RF.
- Peripheral blood eosinophilia occurs in a wide variety of inflammatory disorders. About 15% to 20% of patients with PAN or WG may have eosinophilia but not in the high levels seen in Churg-Strauss syndrome (CSS).
- Identification of cytoplasmic-ANCA (c-ANCA) supports the diagnosis of WG in patients with clinical findings of WG (Mandell, 1994).
- Untreated patients with WG do not have leukopenia.
- First morning urine, both before and after centrifugation, should be carefully examined for protein, hematuria, cells, and casts, which accompany the glomerulonephritis that may occur in vasculitides. If renal amyloidosis is in the differential diagnosis, there is typically proteinuria without cells.

ANTI–NEUTROPHIL CYTOPLASMIC ANTIBODY

By definition, anti–neutrophil cytoplasmic antibody (ANCA) reacts with neutrophil cytoplasmic antigens (Jennette, 1993b). Identification of ANCA has proven to be an important adjunct in diagnosis of systemic necrotizing vasculitis (Niles, 1993). In recent years, there has also been a great deal of interest in how ANCA may be important in the pathogenesis of WG and other systemic necrotizing vasculitides (Jennette, 1993a, 1994a).

Detection Methods

Several laboratory methods, including indirect fluorescence microscopy (IFM), enzyme-linked immunosorbent assay (ELISA), radioimmunoassay, Western blotting, dotblotting, flow cytometry, and immunoprecipitation, have been used to detect ANCA (Roberts, 1992; Wieslander, 1991). IFM and ELISA are the most common test methods used for this purpose. IFM is considered the "gold standard" method for ANCA detection.

IFM is done on isolated normal human neutrophils as substrate. These neutrophils are cytocentrifuged against multiwell glass slides, fixed with 99% ethanol, and then incubated with dilutions of patients' sera. Neutrophils may also be attached to slides by adherence, smear, or drop techniques (Roberts, 1990, 1992). Slides are stained with a fluorescein-labeled polyspecific antihuman immunoglobulin conjugate; polyspecific conjugate is recommended because IgM and IgA c-ANCA occur (Roberts, 1992). Slides are read on a fluorescence microscope. Two main patterns of neutrophil staining are recognized on IFM using this method: cytoplasmic-ANCA (c-ANCA) (Fig. 42–1) and perinuclear ANCA (p-ANCA) (Fig. 42–2). Lymphocytes on

5

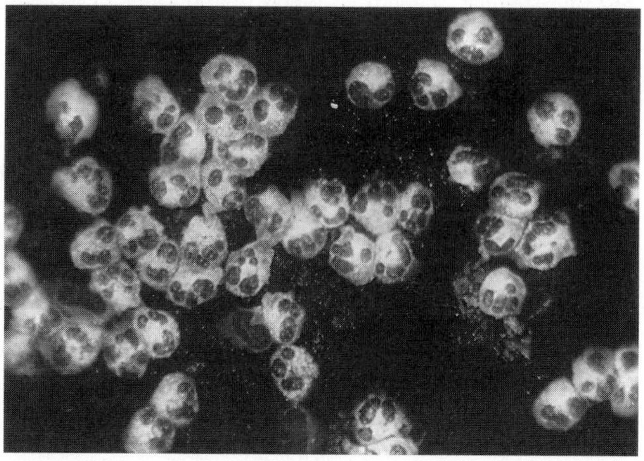

Figure 42–1. Antineutrophil cytoplasmic antibody-cytoplasmic pattern. Most ethanol-fixed neutrophils show finely granular, cytoplasmic, fluorescence with central accentuation. There is no nuclear staining. Notice the lymphocyte, which does not stain. (×400.)

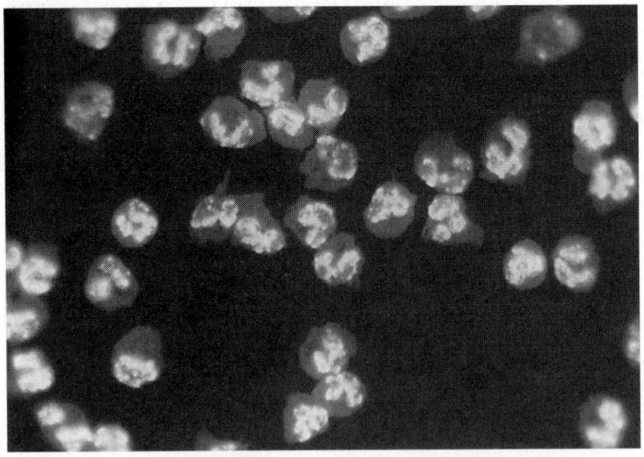

Figure 42–2. Antineutrophil cytoplasmic antibody-perinuclear pattern. Most ethanol-fixed neutrophils show perinuclear and nuclear fluorescence without cytoplasmic staining. (×400.)

the slide should not stain when true ANCA is present (Wieslander, 1991).

c-ANCA is characterized by finely granular staining of neutrophil cytoplasm with central accentuation between the nuclear lobes; the nucleus itself does not stain (Fig. 42–1). Criteria useful for differentiating c-ANCA from nonspecific cytoplasmic staining caused by other autoantibodies include the following: (1) lack of central accentuation; (2) less than 95% of neutrophils demonstrate cytoplasmic staining; (3) non-neutrophil specificity (for example, cytoplasmic staining is also present on Hep-2 cells); and (4) heterogeneous cytoplasmic granularity (Roberts, 1992).

p-ANCA is characterized by staining of the perinuclear area, although nuclear staining mimicking ANA typically occurs when this autoantibody is present in high titers (Niles, 1993). The perinuclear staining pattern that defines p-ANCA is caused by redistribution of target antigens from the neutrophil cytoplasm to the nuclear region when ethanol is used to prepare human neutrophils as a substrate (Jennette, 1993b). When formalin rather than alcohol is used to fix neutrophils, target antigen is immobilized and the immunofluorescent staining pattern is then cytoplasmic (Jennette, 1993b).

Antigenic Specificity

Antigenic specificity of c-ANCA has been identified as a 29 kDa neutral serine protease, proteinase 3 (PR-3), located within neutrophil primary granules and lysosomes of monocytes (PR-3–ANCA) (Niles, 1993; Roberts, 1992). p-ANCA in vasculitis has been found to be directed at myeloperoxidase (MPO-ANCA) (Niles, 1993). Interestingly, many p-ANCA are not directed at MPO but rather are directed at other neutrophil cytoplasmic enzymes, including elastase, lactoferrin or lactoperoxidase, or cathepsin G (Jennette, 1993b; Niles, 1993).

ELISAs for detecting PR-3–ANCA show good correlation with the presence of c-ANCA when experienced observers perform IFM (Niles, 1993; Roberts, 1992). PR-3–ANCA ELISA must be carefully developed with particular attention to using proven techniques for solid-phase antigen preparation and to using either background subtraction or a specific absorption step to control for nonspecific binding of immunoglobulin to the solid phase (Niles, 1993; Roberts, 1992).

The correlation between p-ANCA and detection of myeloperoxidase on ELISA, however, is not good (Roberts, 1992). Several autoantibodies, including ANA, antineutrophil elastase, or granulocyte-specific ANA (GS-ANA), can produce the p-ANCA pattern on IFM. Therefore, sera that produce nuclear fluorescence on IFM require additional testing to confirm MPO-ANCA. MPO-ELISA is recommended to confirm anti-MPO specificity because true ANA or GS-ANA and MPO-ANCA are known to occur concurrently. IFM using Hep-2 cells does not adequately make this distinction because ANA and MPO-ANCA can occur together, and GS-ANA may be negative on Hep-2 cells (Roberts, 1992; Specks, 1994).

Disease Associations

Vasculitis

Both PR-3–ANCA (c-ANCA) and MPO-ANCA (p-ANCA) are associated with WG, PAN including microscopic polyarteritis, CSS, idiopathic pauci-immune necrotizing and crescentic glomerulonephritis, and polyangiitis overlap syndromes (Niles, 1993; Tervaert, 1991). PR-3–ANCA is identified in about 90% of patients with active WG, whereas MPO-ANCA is identified in less than 10% of such patients. Eighty percent of patients with active microscopic polyarteritis have either PR-3–ANCA or MPO-ANCA in about the same frequency. MPO-ANCA is identified in patients with CSS or pauci-immune glomerulonephritis in 70% to 80% of patients with active disease; rarely this latter group of diseases may be associated with PR-3–ANCA rather than MPO-ANCA. Coexistence of ANCA and anti–glomerular basement membrane (anti-GBM) antibodies has been reported (Bonsib, 1993; Niles, 1993).

Inflammatory Disease of Gastrointestinal and Hepatobiliary Tracts

There have been several reports regarding the association of ANCA with inflammatory diseases of the gastrointestinal and hepatobiliary tracts (Jennette, 1993b). p-ANCA have been reported in about 75–80% of patients with active ulcerative colitis or primary sclerosing cholangitis (Ellerbroek, 1994; Klein, 1991; Lo, 1993), about 75% of patients with chronic active hepatitis, about 30% of patients with primary biliary cirrhosis (Kallenberg, 1992; Mulder, 1993), and 20% of patients with Crohn's disease (Jennette, 1993b; Roberts, 1992). Target antigen specificities in inflammatory bowel disease have not been fully defined, although autoantibodies against lactoperoxidase, lactoferrin (Peen, 1993), or cathepsin G have been reported (Jennette, 1993b).

Other Diseases

ANCA have also been reported in other diseases, including drug-induced lupus erythematosus, systemic lupus erythematosus, Felty's syndrome, and rheumatoid arthritis, human immunodeficiency virus infection and other infections, cystic fibrosis, and certain neoplasms (Jennette, 1993b; Peter, 1993). In the connective tissue disorders, ANAs that mimic p-ANCA must be excluded. Many patients treated with hydralazine appear to develop MPO-ANCA (Roberts, 1992).

Test Interpretation

Use of results of ANCA testing in vasculitis vary among authors and institutions. Some authors have reported that identification of c-ANCA in the correct clinical setting is sufficiently specific for systemic necrotizing vasculitis to allow diagnosis and treatment of the patient without obtaining histologic confirmation of disease on tissue biopsy (Niles, 1993; Specks, 1994). A negative c-ANCA, however, does not exclude the diagnosis of WG (Specks, 1994). c-ANCA are considered highly sensitive in active systemic disease (67% to 97%) with renal involvement but of only moderate sensitivity in limited or localized disease (60% to 70%) (Niles, 1993). The sensitivity of this test for patients in complete remission is only about 30% (Specks, 1994).

Some authors report a correlation between the presence of ANCA and the degree of disease activity (Langford, 1995; Roberts, 1992). However, the predictive value of an increased c-ANCA titer as a harbinger of WG relapse is controversial, because not all c-ANCA titer increases are followed by worsening clinical WG disease (Specks, 1994). Most clinicians think a positive c-ANCA should be regarded as suggestive of WG and prompt further evaluation; however, the data are insufficient at this time to fully judge its use as a diagnostic or monitoring tool. The diagnosis of WG and the decision to treat should never be based upon the finding of a positive ANCA alone, and similarly, a negative ANCA should never be used to exclude disease. The diagnosis of WG requires histologic confirmation.

SYNOPSES OF MAJOR IDIOPATHIC VASCULITIC SYNDROMES

Polyarteritis Nodosa

Epidemiology

Polyarteritis nodosa (PAN), like all idiopathic vasculitides, is an uncommon disease. Estimates of the prevalence of PAN have varied from 4.6 per 1,000,000 in England, to 9.0 per 1,000,000 in Olmstead County, Minnesota, to 77 per 1,000,000 in an Alaskan Eskimo population hyperendemic for hepatitis B (Conn, 1993; Langford, 1995). PAN may occur in either gender and at any age but is more common in men (M/F = 2 : 1) between 40 and 60 years old (Langford, 1995). There is no observed racial predilection (Conn, 1993).

Clinical Features

PAN is a systemic necrotizing vasculitis that predominantly involves small- to medium-sized arteries. The clinical manifestations of classic PAN are highly variable. Patients often present with such nonspecific symptoms as fever, weight loss, and malaise. Hypertension is common and can be an important diagnostic clue. Although PAN can occur in virtually any organ system, symptomatic involvement of skin, joints, peripheral nerves, gastrointestinal tract, and kidneys usually dominates the clinical picture (Conn, 1993). Tests indicating abnormal liver function suggest the possibility of concurrent hepatitis B infection (Langford, 1995). Pulmonary involvement in classic PAN is rare and even controversial. Although some investigators think pulmonary PAN occurs (Lie, 1989), others believe that such patients had CSS or WG, in which pulmonary disease is common (Fauci, 1994; Langford, 1995). The course of PAN is characterized by remissions, relapses, and, if untreated, high mortality (Fauci, 1994).

Clinical Laboratory Findings

Results of clinical laboratory tests, although diagnostically nonspecific, reflect the systemic inflammatory nature of PAN. Typically, one finds normochromic anemia, neutrophilic leukocytosis, hypoalbuminemia, hypergammaglobulinemia, and a markedly elevated ESR. Measurement of serum creatinine and BUN, together with urinalysis to check for proteinuria, hematuria, and abnormal sediment, are important for evaluating renal function. The positive ANA or RF found in 10% to 40% of these patients may be associated with decreased levels of complement components C3 and C4. Serologic tests for hepatitis B surface antigen and antibody should be obtained in all patients with PAN (Conn, 1993; Langford, 1995). Peripheral blood eosinophilia is seen only rarely, and when present in high levels should lead to consideration of CSS (Fauci, 1994).

Diagnosis

PAN can be difficult to diagnose given its nonspecific presentation, potential for diverse and diffuse organ involvement, and low prevalence. However, once suspected, a diagnosis of PAN is based upon angiography and/or the histologic demonstration of PAN on biopsy of tissue from symptomatic site(s), such as muscle, nerve, kidney, and testes. Pathologically, PAN is a focal but panmural necrotizing arteritis of small- and medium-sized muscular arteries, preferentially occurring at vessel branch points. Necrotizing mixed cell inflammation with fibrinoid necrosis, either circumferential or segmental in the vessel wall, is the hallmark lesion of active PAN. Microaneurysm or aneurysmal dilatation is also characteristic of acute-phase PAN. The inflammatory process heals with fibrosis, which may lead to proliferative endarteritis. An admixture of active and/or healing lesions adjacent to normal segments of blood vessel is a characteristic feature of PAN (Langford, 1995).

Angiography may be especially valuable in identifying gastrointestinal abnormalities or when a potential biopsy site is unavailable. In particular, angiography should be considered before attempting a closed needle biopsy of the liver or kidney in patients suspected to have PAN because the predilection for aneurysms at these sites increases the risk of severe bleeding (Langford, 1995).

Treatment and Prognosis

Patients with PAN are treated with glucocorticoids. The goal of glucocorticoid therapy is control of the disease without significant complications from the drug itself. Cyclophosphamide may be used for patients with severe PAN, those failing corticosteroids alone, and to spare steroid in patients having significant corticosteroid adverse effects (Langford, 1995). The prognosis for PAN patients has greatly improved with the use of glucocorticoids, extending the five-year survival rate from 13% to 50% to 60%. Most deaths are within the first year, but whether before or after one year of disease, mortality most often results either from infection as a complication of treatment or from sequelae of vessel obliteration, such as myocardial infarction or stroke (Langford, 1995).

Polyarteritis Nodosa Variants

Two notable variants of PAN are cutaneous PAN and PAN associated with hepatitis B. Cutaneous PAN is a necrotizing vasculitis of the small muscular arteries in subcutaneous tissue. By definition, this is a localized process sparing visceral arteries and is therefore not a systemic vasculitis. Diagnosis is established by characteristic histologic findings on skin biopsy with a negative systemic evaluation. Histologically identical cutaneous lesions can be seen in systemic PAN; therefore, cutaneous PAN must be considered a diagnosis of exclusion. As a rule, cutaneous PAN follows a benign course, does not progress to systemic disease, and has an excellent long-term outcome (Langford, 1995).

Hepatitis-B surface antigen positivity has been found in up to 54% of patients with PAN. Emerging evidence indicates that hepatitis C is also associated with PAN, although little is currently known about its clinical disease spectrum. Identification of the interval between infection with hepatitis B and the onset of PAN has varied from months to years, partially because patients frequently have subclinical, undiagnosed, hepatitis B until hepatitis B–associated PAN is diagnosed. However, no association between inflammatory activity in the liver and vasculitis has been noted. Patients with hepatitis B–associated PAN have a higher incidence of elevated liver function tests (LFTs) and aneurysms than those with non–hepatitis-related PAN, but otherwise both are clinically similar. Unfortunately, the presence of hepatitis B complicates immunosuppressive treatment, because viral replication can become enhanced risking progressive liver disease during treatment and even fulminant hepatitis, when immunosuppression ceases. Despite these concerns, glucocorticoid therapy is important because patients with untreated hepatitis B–associated PAN have a high mortality rate. Therapy has largely been the same as for the non–hepatitis-related disease. Alternatively, plasma exchange in combination with steroids and antiviral therapy has achieved some success (Langford, 1995).

Churg-Strauss Syndrome

Epidemiology

Churg-Strauss syndrome (CSS) is thought to be a rare clinical condition; no extensive epidemiologic data are available (Conn, 1993). CSS typically begins between the ages of 15 and 69 years, with 38 years as the median age for the onset of vasculitis (Langford, 1995).

Clinical Features

CSS, also called *allergic angiitis* and *granulomatosis*, is a systemic necrotizing vasculitis characterized by vascular and extravascular granulomatous inflammation, multiple organ involvement, and associations with allergic rhinitis, severe asthma, and hypereosinophilia (Fauci, 1994; Langford, 1995). Clinical manifestations of CSS may resemble those of PAN in many respects but differ in that lung disease is typical and renal disease is uncommon, usually less severe in CSS than in PAN (Fauci, 1994).

The clinical course of CSS is often divided into three distinct phases, although in reality these three phases are not always identifiable or may overlap (Langford, 1995): (1) a prodromal phase, characterized by allergic respiratory disease; (2) an eosinophilic phase, characterized by peripheral blood and tissue hypereosinophilia; and (3) a vasculitic phase. Cardiac involvement, either transmural eosinophilic carditis or coronary vasculitis, occurs in 25% to 62% of CSS patients and is the major cause of death (Langford, 1995).

Clinical Laboratory Findings

A hallmark of CSS is striking peripheral blood eosinophilia, which may be seen at any phase of the disease. The peripheral blood eosinophil count reaches 1000 eosinophils per microliter in 80% or more of CSS patients (Conn, 1993); however, eosinophilia may not be found in all patients because of prior steroid treatments for asthma or the wide and rapid fluctuation in the eosinophil count that can occur in this disorder. Normalization of the eosinophil count in response to steroid treatment is a feature of CSS, distinguishing it from the hypereosinophilic syndrome in which eosinophilia may be steroid resistant. The degree of eosinophilia may correlate with the activity of the vasculitic disease in some patients.

Other laboratory findings in CSS are nonspecific. Anemia, leukocytosis, and increased ESR frequently accompany the vasculitic phase. Serum IgE levels may be elevated. Serum RF may be identified, but the titer is usually low. Serum complement is reported as normal (Conn, 1993). Unlike PAN, no association between CSS and hepatitis B has been described (Langford, 1995).

Diagnosis

Historically, the diagnosis of CSS has been made solely on histologic demonstration of necrotizing eosinophilic vasculitis, eosinophilic tissue infiltration, and extravascular granuloma. In practice, however, few biopsy specimens contain all these findings. To increase the likelihood of identifying and diagnosing CSS, the emphasis can be shifted from these diagnostic indicators to include clinical features. One study has recommended the following criteria:

1. Asthma
2. Peripheral blood eosinophilia in excess of 1.5×10^3 cells/μL
3. Systemic vasculitis involving two or more extrapulmonary organs (Conn, 1993).

Definitive diagnosis still requires demonstration of biopsy-proven vasculitis. Open-lung biopsy frequently does not confirm all histologic features of CSS but must be considered before the institution of therapy if there is concern over possible infection. When clinical symptoms so indicate, useful biopsy specimens are most often obtained from muscle, sural nerve, prostate, and kidney. The differential diagnosis of CSS includes PAN, WG, and the hypereosinophilic syndrome (Langford, 1995).

Treatment and Prognosis

Corticosteroids are the basis for treatment of CSS. The utility of immunosuppressive therapy with azathioprine or cyclophosphamide is not well studied (Langford, 1995). Early diagnosis of CSS and corticosteroid treatment have led to these patients having a five-year survival rate of 62%. Congestive heart failure and myocardial infarction cause 48% of all deaths in CSS. Cerebral hemorrhage, renal failure, gastrointestinal perforation or hemorrhage, status asthmaticus, and respiratory failure also cause the demise of CSS patients. Shortness of the interval between the onset of asthma and the onset of vasculitis is considered an unfavorable prognostic sign.

Polyangiitis Overlap Syndrome

Polyangiitis overlap syndrome occurs in a heterogeneous group of patients who, by definition, have a systemic necrotizing vasculitis but do not manifest disease in such a way that would clearly place them into a specific diagnostic category. Patients with polyangiitis overlap syndrome may have the combined features of several vasculitic diseases, similarly mixed pathologic findings, or atypical symptoms that do not fit one specific disease/syndrome (Langford, 1995). Polyangiitis overlap syndrome has the potential to involve multiple organ systems. Although the prognosis for polyangiitis overlap syndrome is not established, the potential for serious organ damage and life-threatening disease exists. Both diagnostically and therapeutically, these patients should be approached as if they had a well-defined vasculitic syndrome. A careful history, physical examination, and laboratory evaluation should be performed to define the extent of their systemic involvement. The diagnosis of polyangiitis overlap syndrome should be demonstrated by biopsy or angiography. Once the presence of a systemic necrotizing vasculitis has been ascertained and other diagnoses, specifically infection, have been ruled out, treatment should be initiated with corticosteroids and consideration should be given to using additional imunosuppressive agents, such as cyclophosphamide (Langford, 1995).

Wegener's Granulomatosis

Epidemiology

Detailed annual incidence and prevalence data for WG are not available, but WG is estimated to be less common than PAN. WG occurs in persons of any age, race, or sex, although it affects predominantly whites and has a slight male predominance (Conn, 1993). The mean age at onset is 41 years (Langford, 1995).

Clinical Features

WG is a clinicopathological syndrome of unknown etiology characterized pathologically by necrotizing granulomatous inflammation of upper and lower respiratory tracts, focal segmental glomerulonephritis, and necrotizing vasculitis predominantly involving medium and small arteries. WG presents in the ear/nose/throat regions with sinusitis, nasal obstruction or ulceration, otitis media, or hearing loss (Fauci, 1994; Lie, 1989). Forty-five percent of WG patients have lung involvement at presentation, and 85% manifest lung disease sometime during the course of their disease. Common lung manifestations include pulmonary infiltrates, pulmonary nodules, hemoptysis, or pleuritis (Fauci, 1994). Although renal disease initially afflicts only about 18% of these patients, 80% demonstrate glomerulonephritis at some time in the course of WG (Fauci, 1994). Other common signs of systemic illness include skin rash, arthralgias, fever, eye manifestations, and weight loss (Fauci, 1994; Lie, 1989). Although patients with WG limited to the respiratory tract without renal involvement have been described ("limited WG"), more than 50% of patients with such limited disease at presentation eventually develop more generalized disease (Langford, 1995).

Clinical Laboratory Findings

Clinical laboratory findings typical of WG include moderate leukocytosis without striking eosinophilia, mild normochromic anemia, and thrombocytosis (Conn, 1993; Langford, 1995). Leukopenia is not seen in the untreated patient and, thus, helps distinguish WG from other disorders. The presence of c-ANCA supports the diagnosis. Circulating immune complexes, measurable by Clq binding, may be found together with normal complement levels and hypergammaglobulinemia; amounts of the IgA subclass are often elevated (Conn, 1993; Langford, 1995). Indicators of glomerular involvement include microscopic or gross hematuria, proteinuria, red blood cell casts, and/or elevated serum creatinine and blood urea nitrogen. More than 50% of these patients are RF positive, but ANAs are usually absent (Fauci, 1994; Langford, 1995). Serologic tests for anti-GBM autoantibody are negative. Prior to treatment, 80% of these patients have an elevated ESR.

Diagnosis

Although clinical and laboratory findings may be suggestive, a diagnosis of WG should be made only when there is biopsy-proven, histologic confirmation. Pulmonary tissue obtained via open-lung biopsy offers the best opportunity to make an accurate diagnosis (Langford, 1995). Transbronchial biopsy does not yield adequate tissue for diagnosis greater than 90% of the time. Although head and neck tissue is more directly accessible, characteristic pathologic features are found in fewer than 23% of such biopsy specimens. Diagnostically useful tissue from the head and neck region is best obtained from, in decreasing order of frequency, paranasal sinuses, nasal tissue, and the subglottic region. Glomerular changes in renal biopsy tissue, although suggestive of WG, are rarely diagnostic (Langford, 1995).

Although the morphologic spectrum of WG is broad, the hallmark pathologic lesion in WG is necrotizing, granulomatous vasculitis. Affected vessels undergo fibrinoid necrosis with early infiltration by polymorphonuclear leukocytes followed by mononuclear cells. Pulmonary tissue may reveal any combination of necrosis, vasculitis, and granulomatous inflammation, although biopsy specimens often do not include all these characteristic features. The most common finding found on renal biopsy is segmental necrotizing glomerulonephritis, which is present to varying degrees in 80% of specimens. Renal vasculitis not related to glomeruli is unusual and is present in only 8% of biopsies.

Many disorders can mimic WG, including infectious or noninfectious granulomatous diseases, CSS, Goodpasture's syndrome, idiopathic midline granuloma, lymphomatoid granulomatosis, and neoplasms of the upper airway or lungs (Fauci, 1994). Of these, infection is an important consideration because misdiagnosis can have fatal consequences when mistakenly treated with immunosuppressive therapy. It is therefore of extreme importance to aggressively pursue tissue diagnosis, both to confirm WG and to rule out other disorders (Langford, 1995).

Treatment and Prognosis

A regimen of daily oral cyclophosphamide and corticosteroids is the therapy of choice for WG. Using this regimen, the National Institutes of Health reported that marked improvement or partial remission was achieved in 91% of patients, with complete remission in 75%. An overall mortality rate of 20% was noted, 13% of which could be completely or partially attributed to WG. Despite this marked improvement in survival and remission compared with 100% mortality in untreated patients, relapse and morbidity from both disease and treatment were noted. One half of the complete remissions were followed by one or more relapses, which occurred 3 months to 16 years after achieving remission (Langford, 1995). During the first year of WG, the extent of renal disease is the factor most closely related to prognosis. Thereafter, lung involvement becomes the most important prognostic indicator, and glomerulonephritis does not appear to significantly affect prognosis.

Lymphomatoid Granulomatosis

Lymphomatoid granulomatosis (LG) is considered to be an unusual lymphoproliferative disorder that may evolve into malignant lymphoma in approximately 50% of patients. LG mainly affects the lungs, where it clinically mimics WG. However, characteristic histologic findings include prominent blood vessel infiltration ("angiocentric") and destruction mimicking vasculitis, but cellular morphology is more suggestive of lymphoma or lymphoproliferative disorder (Langford, 1995). There are no specific clinical laboratory tests.

Henoch-Schönlein Purpura

Epidemiology

Henoch-Schönlein purpura (HSP) occurs primarily in children between the ages of 4 and 11 years (Conn, 1993) but also afflicts some adults. HSP presents most commonly in the spring and classically follows an upper respiratory infection (Conn 1993). HSP has a 3:2 male predominance (Langford, 1995).

Clinical Features

HSP, sometimes referred to as anaphylactoid purpura, is a systemic small vessel vasculitis classified as a subgroup of hypersensitivity vasculitis. The etiology of HSP is not known. Typical clinical findings in HSP include nonthrombocytopenic palpable purpura, arthralgias, renal disease, and gastrointestinal tract abnormalities (Langford, 1995). Seventy percent of HSP patients manifest gastrointestinal signs and symptoms that include colicky abdominal pain associated with nausea and vomiting, blood or mucus in the stool, life-threatening gastrointestinal hemorrhage, and intussusception (Langford, 1995). The associated renal disease is characterized by focal proliferative glomerulonephritis that has variable clinical expression from isolated hematuria with red blood cell casts, to acute renal failure, to rare chronic renal failure (Fauci, 1994; Langford, 1995; Lie, 1989).

Clinical Laboratory Findings

Clinical laboratory studies in HSP are nonspecific and are primarily useful in excluding other disorders and seeking evidence of renal involvement. Leukocytosis and elevated ESR may be seen. An assessment of CBC with platelet count and coagulation are important in the evaluation of cutaneous purpura; in HSP, purpura are not from thrombocytopenia. Stool guaiacs should be performed intermittently to look for evidence of occult blood loss. Serum complement levels are usually normal, although an association between HSP and the congenital absence of complement component C2 has been reported (Conn, 1993). Urinalysis and serum creatinine measurements should be performed at the onset of illness and twice weekly until systemic signs have ceased (Langford, 1995).

Diagnosis

Difficulty in diagnosing HSP is rare, except when the involvement of other major sites precedes appearance of palpable purpura. Unlike other systemic necrotizing vasculitides, diagnosis is clinical, with laboratory studies being used to rule out other disorders. Renal biopsy, which demonstrates proliferative glomerulonephritis, is typically not necessary for diagnosis, although it is used to assess disease severity and to estimate prognosis. Disorders to be considered in the differential diagnosis of HSP include any that cause acute abdomen, nephritis, or purpura (Langford, 1995).

Treatment and Prognosis

Treatment of HSP is supportive and there is no specific treatment of proven benefit for HSP nephritis. Although glucocorticoids may be useful for decreasing edema, joint pain, and abdominal discomfort, sustained glucocorticoid therapy is not helpful, because it does not decrease the risk of recurrent disease or improve renal prognosis (Langford, 1995). Nonsalicylate pain relievers for analgesia may soothe joint and soft-tissue discomfort. Therapy for adults is similar to that for children, although hypertension in adults must be carefully controlled (Langford, 1995).

Prognosis for this generally self-limited disease, lasting from 6 to 16 weeks, is good (Conn, 1993). The mortality rate is about 1% to 3% (Langford, 1995), and renal disease is the major cause of death (Langford, 1995). Those who have an acute nephritic presentation, particularly with nephrotic syndrome, have the worst outcome, with less than 50% returning to normal renal function and urinalyses in two years. The percentage of glomeruli with crescents may also be a useful prognostic indicator; however, it is important to realize that the course of HSP can be extremely variable. Patients having severe clinical or histologic abnormalities may recover fully, and those with mild changes can progress to renal insufficiency. The disease recurs in 25% to 40% of patients and largely consists of skin manifestations. Deterioration or improvement may be most notable during the first two to three years after resolution of the acute episode, although significant changes in outcome have also been seen later than that. Regular follow-up with measurements of blood pressure and urinalysis is extremely important for at least the first five years following an episode of HSP (Langford, 1995).

Giant Cell (Temporal) Arteritis

Epidemiology

Giant cell (GC) arteritis is a relatively common vasculitic disorder. Epidemiologic studies have shown increased incidence with age; one study that included biopsy-proven GC arteritis demonstrated an annual incidence rate of 23.3 per 100,000 persons older than 50 years (Conn, 1993). Nearly all cases of GC arteritis begin after age 50.

Clinical Features

GC arteritis is a systemic disease characterized by granulomatous vascular inflammation involving medium to large arteries. Although arteries in multiple sites can be affected, GC arteritis classically involves the temporal artery and/or other branches of the carotid artery (Fauci, 1994). Clinical manifestations include fever, headache, and jaw claudication in patients over 50 years of age. Ischemic optic neuritis can lead to sudden blindness, particularly in untreated patients (Fauci, 1994). GC arteritis is closely associated with polymyalgia rheumatica, which is characterized by stiffness and pain of the neck, shoulders, lower back, hips, and thighs that is worse in the morning and better with activity of the day (Fauci, 1994).

Clinical Laboratory Findings

Characteristic laboratory findings include an elevated ESR and a normochromic anemia. Serum alkaline phosphatase is commonly elevated. Hypergammaglobulinemia as well as increased levels of complement and immune complexes have been reported (Fauci, 1994).

Diagnosis

Diagnosis is based on identifying typical clinical manifestations and a high ESR in an elderly patient who may or may not also have symptoms of polymyalgia rheumatica (Fauci, 1994). Diagnosis is confirmed by biopsy of the temporal artery.

Treatment and Prognosis

GC arteritis is treated with glucocorticoids, and the clinical response to this therapy is usually dramatic. The prognosis is good, because most patients achieve and maintain complete remission after glucocorticoid therapy (Fauci, 1994). Unfortunately, recovery of eyesight following blindness secondary to GC arteritis is rare, even with rapid and high-dose corticosteroid therapy.

Takayasu's Arteritis

Epidemiology

Like many of the idiopathic vasculitides, Takayasu's arteritis is uncommon, and the epidemiology of the disease is not accurately known. This disorder is most prevalent in adolescent and young females between the ages of 10 and 30 years; in fact, 80% to 90% of cases occur in females. Although more common in Japan, this disease has no proven racial or geographical restrictions (Conn, 1993; Fauci, 1994).

Clinical Features

Takayasu's arteritis is a granulomatous vasculitis of medium to large elastic arteries that causes vascular stenosis or occlusion; there is strong predilection for the aortic arch and its large branches, including pulmonary arteries (Fauci, 1994; Langford, 1995). This disorder is sometimes called the *aortic arch syndrome* or *pulseless disease*. Patients present with acute systemic symptoms, including fever, malaise, night sweats, and weight loss. Ischemia in organs receiving their blood supply through the affected vessel(s) causes organ-specific symptoms and signs. In the chronic obliterative phase, arterial pulses are decreased or absent in involved arteries (Langford, 1995), most commonly in the subclavian artery (Fauci, 1994). Vascular bruits and hypertension are common (Langford, 1995). Other findings include aortic regurgitation, cardiomegaly secondary to aortic or pulmonary hypertension, and stroke (Fauci, 1994). Takayasu's arteritis may progress slowly, may stabilize, or may rapidly cause death (Fauci, 1994).

Clinical Laboratory Findings

Laboratory studies of Takayasu's arteritis define a systemic inflammatory disorder (Langford, 1995). The ESR is elevated in 75% to 100% of patients with active disease. ESR is believed to be a reliable index of inflammatory activity and has been used as a tool to monitor the effectiveness of therapy. Resolution of the disease, both symptomatically and angiographically, has been found to correlate with decline of the ESR.

Hematologic studies often show mild to moderate normochromic anemia and/or mild leukocytosis. RF and ANA are usually negative. There may be hypergammaglobulinemia, hyperfibrinogenemia, and hypoalbuminemia (Conn, 1993). Circulating immune complexes may be present in up to 50% of these patients but do not appear to correlate with disease activity.

Diagnosis

Takayasu's arteritis is diagnosed by correlating data from history, physical examination, and angiography. The disease should be considered as a diagnostic possibility in any young female who lacks or has a markedly decreased peripheral pulse rate or who has blood pressure discrepancies and/or arterial bruits (Fauci, 1994). Characteristic angiographic findings help confirm the clinical diagnosis. Biopsy for tissue confirmation of diagnosis is seldom required or done (Fauci, 1994). The predilection of this syndrome for young females is an important feature that often separates it from other diagnostic considerations, particularly GC arteritis (Langford, 1995).

Treatment and Prognosis

In patients with active disease, corticosteroid therapy is the initial treatment of choice. If active disease persists despite corticosteroids, cyclophosphamide or methotrexate may be administered. Vasodilators, anticoagulants, and nonsteroidal anti-inflammatory agents are used for symptomatic relief. Surgical intervention may be necessary for symptomatic vascular stenosis or occlusion (Langford, 1995).

The clinical course of Takayasu's arteritis is variable. Although spontaneous remissions occur, most patients require treatment. Prognosis appears to be related to the presence and severity of complications. Major complications include Takayasu's retinopathy, secondary hypertension, aortic valve insufficiency, and aortic/arterial aneurysm (Langford, 1995). Overall survival declines from 75% to 97% at five years and 59% at 10 years, as the number and/or severity of these complications increases (Langford, 1995). Disease-related deaths usually occur from vascular complications, such as congestive heart failure, stroke, myocardial infarction, and aneurysm rupture (Langford, 1995).

Isolated CNS Vasculitis

Epidemiology

Isolated CNS vasculitis (ICNSV) is a rare condition in which difficulty in making a definitive diagnosis hinders epidemiologic studies. ICNSV is slightly more common in males than females (4:3) and begins at a mean age of 43 years (Langford, 1995).

Clinical Features

Patients with ICNSV present with headaches, focal neurologic deficits, and altered mental status (Fauci, 1994). Initial symptoms are more generalized whereas focal symptoms and signs generally develop later in the course of the disease (Langford, 1995). The course may be rapidly progressive or wax and wane over a long time period. Systemic symptoms are rare.

Clinical Laboratory Findings

Laboratory studies are not useful in making a diagnosis of ICNSV, but they do play an important role in excluding other disease processes. The ESR is elevated in most, but not all, patients. Anemia has been seen in only 17% of them, and other hematologic parameters are usually normal. RF, ANA, and ANCA are typically absent. However, the cerebrospinal fluid is usually abnormal, with findings that include increased opening pressure, elevated protein, and lymphocytic pleocytosis. Because the cerebrospinal fluid can also be completely normal, such testing does not always rule out the possibility of vasculitis (Langford, 1995).

Diagnosis

The diagnosis of ICNSV remains one of exclusion. Proposed diagnostic criteria have included:

1. CNS dysfunction that is not explained by clinical, laboratory, or neurologic investigation
2. Documentation by angiogram and/or biopsy of an arteritis within the CNS
3. No evidence of a systemic vasculitis or other condition to which the angiographic or pathologic features could be secondary

Given the difficulty with certainty regarding criteria (3), CNS biopsies are probably underutilized. However, the role of brain biopsy in the evaluation of ICNSV remains controversial, although some advocate that such biopsy is essential to make a definitive diagnosis. Precluding widespread application of brain biopsy has been not only its invasive nature but also the unreliability of demonstrating histologic vasculitis, even in the setting of active disease. Not even the optimal location for biopsy has been determined. The yield of biopsy may be increased by obtaining samples of both parenchyma and leptomeningeal vessels. Given the difficulty in obtaining diagnostic certainty for this disease, biopsy is equally as important to rule out other possible etiologies. Histologically, there is segmental mixed inflammation, with necrosis involving predominantly small- and medium-sized cranial arteries. Granulomatosis inflammation may be present. Thrombosis is often noted; extracranial arteries are rarely involved (Langford, 1995; Rhodes, 1995). Therefore, differential diagnoses must be carefully considered in all cases and used in deciding appropriate tests, both to support a diagnosis of ICNSV and to exclude other processes.

Treatment and Prognosis

Aggressive treatment is indicated for patients in whom other disorders are ruled out and the diagnosis of ICNSV is supported. Combination therapy using corticosteroids and daily cyclophosphamide is advocated; however, the prognosis of ICNSV is poor, with 60% to 70% of patients dying from their disease within one year of diagnosis (Langford, 1995).

Kawasaki's Disease

Kawasaki's disease, or mucocutaneous lymph node syndrome, is a form of vasculitis involving small and medium arteries. This disease typically occurs in children who present with cervical lymphadenitis and alterations in skin and mucous membranes. Kawasaki's disease is usually self-limited, but arteritis causes coronary aneurysms in 25% of patients. Death occurs in up to 3% of patients, usually from coronary vasculitis. Anti–endothelial cell autoantibodies have been demonstrated in patients with Kawasaki's disease (Fauci, 1994).

SUMMARY

Diagnosis of idiopathic systemic necrotizing vasculitides requires a high degree of suspicion and can be difficult because of the large number of differential diagnostic considerations.

There are no pathognomonic clinical laboratory tests in patients with systemic necrotizing vasculitides, but such tests are useful for defining the extent and patterns of organ involvement. ANCA and their associations with systemic necrotizing vasculitis, particularly the association of c-ANCA with WG, has become an important serologic test used in the evaluation of these patients. Despite this advance, tissue biopsy of symptomatic site(s) with histologic confirmation of necrotizing vasculitis remains the most important laboratory procedure in the diagnosis of systemic necrotizing vasculitides.

Bonsib SM, Goeken JA, Kemp JD, et al: Coexistent anti-neutrophil cytoplasmic antibody and antiglomerular basement membrane antibody associated disease: Report of six cases. Mod Pathol 1993; 6:526.

Conn DL, Hunder GG, O'Duffy JD: Vasculitis and related disorders. *In* Kelley WN, Harris ED, Jr, Ruddy S, Sledge CB (eds): Textbook of Rheumatology, Vol. 2, 4th ed. Philadelphia, W. B. Saunders Co., 1993, p 1077.

Ellerbroek PM, Pool MO, Ridwan BU, et al: Neutrophil cytoplasmic antibodies (p-ANCA) in ulcerative colitis. J Clin Pathol 1994; 47:257.

Fauci AS: The vasculitis syndrome. *In* Isselbacher KJ, Braunwald E, Wilson JD, et al: (eds): Harrison's Principles of Internal Medicine, 13th ed. New York, McGraw-Hill, 1994, p 1670.

Golden MP, Hammer SM, Wanke CA, Albrecht MA: Cytomegalovirus vasculitis. Case reports and review of the literature. Medicine 1994; 73:246.

Hunder GG, Arend WP, Bloch DA, et al: The American College of Rheumatology 1990 Criteria for the Classification of Vasculitis. Arthritis Rheum 1990; 33:1065.

Jennette JC, Ewert BH, Falk RJ: Do antineutrophil cytoplasmic autoantibodies cause Wegener's granulomatosis and other forms of necrotizing vasculitis? Rheum Dis Clin North Am 1993a; 19:1.

Jennette JC, Falk RJ: Antineutrophil cytoplasmic autoantibodies in inflammatory bowel disease. Am J Clin Pathol 1993b; 99:221.

Jennette JC: Pathogenic potential of anti-neutrophil cytoplasmic autoantibodies (Editorial). Lab Invest 1994a; 70:135.

Jennette JC, Falk RJ, Andrassy K, et al: Nomenclature of systemic vasculitides. Proposal of an international consensus conference. Arthritis Rheum 1994b; 37:187.

Kallenberg CGM, Mulder AHL, Tervaert JWC: Antineutrophil cytoplasmic antibodies: A still-growing class of autoantibodies in inflammatory disorders. Am J Med 1992; 93:675.

Klein R, Eisenburg J, Weber P, Seibold F, Berg PA: Significance and specificity of antibodies to neutrophils detected by Western blotting for the serological diagnosis of primary sclerosing cholangitis. Hepatology 1991; 14:1147.

Langford CA, McCallum RM: Idiopathic vasculitis. *In* Belch JJF, Zurier RB (eds): Connective Tissue Diseases. London, Chapman and Hall, 1995, p 179.

Lie JT: Systemic and isolated vasculitis: A rational approach to classification and pathologic diagnosis. *In* Rosen PP, Fechner RE (eds): Pathology Annual, Part 1, Vol. 24. Norwalk, CT, Appleton & Lange, 1989, p 25.

Lie JT: Nomenclature and classification of vasculitis: Plus ça change, plus c'est la même chose. Arthritis Rheum 1994; 37:181.

Lo SK, Chapman RWG, Cheeseman P, et al: Antineutrophil antibody: A test for autoimmune primary sclerosing cholangitis in childhood? Gut 1993; 34:199.

Mandell BF, Hoffman GS: Differentiating the vasculitides. Rheum Dis Clin North Am 1994; 20:409.

Mulder AHL, Horst G, Haagsma EB, et al: Prevalence and characterization of neutrophil cytoplasmic antibodies in autoimmune liver diseases. Hepatology 1993; 17:411.

Niles JL: Value of tests for antineutrophil cytoplasmic autoantibodies in the diagnosis and treatment of vasculitis. Curr Opin Rheumatol 1993; 5:18.

Niles JL, McCluskey RT: Vasculitis. *In* Colvin RB, Bhan AK, McCluskey RT (eds): Diagnostic Immunopathology. 2nd ed. New York, Raven Press, 1995, p 95.

Peen E, Almer S, Bodemar G, et al: Anti-lactoferrin antibodies and other types of ANCA in ulcerative colitis, primary sclerosing cholangitis, and Crohn's disease. Gut 1993; 34:56.

Peter HH, Metzger D, Rump A, Röther E: ANCA in diseases other than systemic vasculitis. *In* Proceedings of the 5th International ANCA Workshop, August 31–September. Cambridge, UK, St. John's College, 1993, p 12.

Rhodes RH, Madelaire C, Petrelli M, et al: Primary angiitis and angiopathy of the central nervous system and their relationship to systemic giant cell arteritis. Arch Pathol Lab Med 1995; 119:334.

Roberts DE, Peebles C, Daggett R: A simplified method of preparing neutrophil slides in the examination for antibodies to cytoplasmic antigens. J Clin Pathol 1990; 43:83.

Roberts DE: Antineutrophil cytoplasmic autoantibodies. Clin Lab Med 1992; 12:85.

Specks U, Homburger HA: Laboratory medicine and pathology: Anti-neutrophil cytoplasmic antibodies. Mayo Clin Proc 1994; 69:1197.

Tervaert JWC, Limburg PC, Elema JD, et al: Detection of autoantibodies against myeloid lysosomal enzymes: A useful adjunct to classification of patients with biopsy-proven necrotizing arteritis. Am J Med 1991; 91:59.

Wieslander J: How are antineutrophil cytoplasmic autoantibodies detected? Am J Kidney Dis 1991; 18:154.

Chapter 43

Organ-Directed Autoimmune Diseases

David J. Bylund, M.D.
Robert M. Nakamura, M.D.

Autoimmune disorders can be categorized broadly into systemic or organ/tissue–directed diseases. The subject of autoantibodies in systemic autoimmune diseases is presented in Chapter 41. In this chapter, we focus on organ- or tissue-related autoimmune diseases and list their characteristic autoantibodies in Table 43–1. Many of these diseases are described further in this chapter.

The dominant clinical feature of these autoimmune disorders is chronic inflammation localized in a single organ or tissue specific for each individual disease. Within this group of autoimmune disorders, familial clustering of diseases occurs with remarkable frequency. The relevant autoantibodies may or may not be species specific, but they do exhibit specificity for an antigen present in the diseased organ or tissue.

Included in this chapter are some diseases with autoantibodies and inflammatory lesions restricted to one, or a few, organ(s) that combine clinicopathologic features of both organ-specific and systemic autoimmune diseases. Examples of this group are autoimmune liver disorders, such as primary biliary cirrhosis (PBC) or autoimmune hepatitis (AiH). Except for autoantibodies to thyroid receptors, the role of autoantibodies in the pathogenesis of other organ-specific diseases remains largely unproven.

DETECTION METHODS

Immunofluorescence on tissue substrates is the method most commonly used to detect circulating autoantibodies to specific target organs or tissues. Both indirect and direct immunofluorescence microscopy (IIFM and DIFM, respectively) techniques are used. Enzyme-linked immunosorbent assays (ELISAs) are being used ever more frequently in clinical laboratories as technical aspects of this method have improved. IIFM is briefly described because this technique is most commonly used to detect circulating autoantibodies.

Indirect Immunofluorescence Microscopy

IIFM is the most commonly used method to detect organ-specific autoantibodies. The test procedure is essentially the

Table 43–1. ORGAN/TISSUE-DIRECTED AUTOIMMUNE DISEASES

Organ/Tissue Disease	Associated Autoantibody(ies)	Autoantibody Detection Method(s)
Thyroid Gland		
Autoimmune thyroiditis	Thyroglobulin	IIFM—methanol-fixed human or monkey thyroid; passive hemagglutination; latex agglutination
	Thyroid peroxidase (microsomal)	IIFM—unfixed human or monkey hyperplastic thyroid tissue; passive hemagglutination; complement fixation
Graves' disease	TSH receptor	Binding assay: radioreceptor assay for antibodies competing with TSH for receptors on thyroid follicular cell membranes
		Bioassay: measurement of cyclic AMP activity after incubation of thyroid tissue with Ig from patient's serum
Adrenal Gland		
Addison's disease	Adrenocortical	IIFM on unfixed monkey or human adrenal cortex
Parathyroid Gland		
Parathyroid	Parathyroid endothelial proteins	IIFM on unfixed bovine parathyroid gland
Pancreas		
Insulin-dependent diabetes mellitus	Islet cells	IIFM on unfixed human pancreas
	Insulin-associated	Radioimmunoprecipitation
	Anti-glutamic acid decarboxylase	RIA, immunoblotting, ELISA
Insulin-resistant diabetes mellitus associated with acanthosis nigricans	Anti-insulin receptor	Inhibition of iodine^{125} insulin binding to receptors on monocytes or adipocytes
Insulin-resistant diabetes mellitus associated with ataxia-telangiectasia	Anti-insulin receptor	Inhibition of iodine^{125} insulin binding to receptors on monocytes or adipocytes
Liver		
Autoimmune hepatitis	Smooth muscle	IIFM—mouse gastric mucosa or kidney
	Liver-kidney microsomal	IIFM—mouse gastric mucosa or kidney; Western blotting
	ANAs	Hep-2 cells
Primary biliary cirrhosis	Mitochondrial (M2)	IIFM—mouse kidney or Hep-2 cell, unfixed or fixed, ELISA
Primary sclerosing cholangitis	Unknown; p-ANCA associated	IIFM—ethanol-fixed neutrophils
Muscle		
Dermatomyositis/polymyositis	Nuclear antigens (DNA, PM-1), Jo-1	IIFM on cells or tissue section substrates; immunoprecipitation; ELISA, immunoblotting
Gastrointestinal Tract		
Atrophic gastritis	Gastric parietal cell	IIFM—human, monkey, mouse, or rat gastric mucosa substrate
Pernicious anemia	Intrinsic factor	Radioactive vitamin B_{12} binding assay
	Salivary duct cells	IIFM—unfixed human salivary gland
	Gastric parietal cell	IIFM—human, monkey, mouse, or rat gastric mucosa substrate
Ulcerative colitis	Colon; lipopolysaccharide;	IIFM—human or rat colon; hemagglutination
	p-ANCA–associated	IIFM—ethanol-fixed neutrophils
Crohn's disease	Reticulin; anti-epithelial	IIFM—mouse kidney or liver
Celiac disease	Reticulin; gluten and/or gliadin;	
	Endomysium of smooth muscle	IIFM—IgA endomysial antibodies on monkey esophagus
Neurologic		
Myasthenia gravis	AChR	Immunoprecipitation of iodine^{125} α-bungarotoxin-conjugated AChR (human skeletal muscle); ELISA
Demyelinating diseases (e.g., multiple sclerosis)	Myelin; tubulin myelin; basic protein; myelin-associated glycoprotein	IIFM—mammalian spinal cord; ELISA; immunoblotting
Kidneys		
Anti-GBM disease (Goodpasture's syndrome)	Glomerular and lung basement membrane	DIFM—biopsy of patient's kidney; IIFM—patient's serum reacted on kidney substrate; ELISA or RIA performed on serum
Skin		
Pemphigus	Anti-epidermal or mucosal ICS (desmosomes)	DIFM on human skin biopsy specimen; IIFM on monkey or guinea pig esophagus
Bullous pemphigoid	Anti-BMZ	DIFM on human skin biopsy specimen and IIFM on guinea pig or monkey esophagus
Cicatricial pemphigoid	Anti-BMZ	DIFM on human skin biopsy specimen; IIFM on guinea pig or monkey esophagus
Dermatitis herpetiformis	Reticulin; gluten and/or gliadin	DIFM—staining for IgA deposits in dermal papillae; IIFM—mouse kidney or liver
	Endomysium of smooth muscle	Endomysial IgA autoantibody detected on monkey esophagus
Paraneoplastic pemphigus	Anti-ICS and anti-BMZ (bullous pemphigoid antigen; desmoplakins I and II)	DIFM on human skin biopsy; IIFM on rat bladder transitional epithelium
Linear IgA dermatosis	IgA anti-BMZ	DIFM on human skin biopsy; IIFM on guinea pig or monkey esophagus
Intercellular IgA dermatosis	IgA anti-ICS	DIFM on human skin biopsy; IIFM on guinea pig or monkey esophagus

Table continued on following page

Table 43–1. ORGAN/TISSUE-DIRECTED AUTOIMMUNE DISEASES (*Continued*)

Organ/Tissue Disease	Associated Autoantibody(ies)	Autoantibody Detection Method(s)
Other		
Allergic rhinitis; asthma; functional autonomic abnormalities	Antibodies to β2-adrenergic receptors	Binding of iodine^{125} protein A to lung membranes preincubated with serum samples; ability of plasma to inhibit binding of iodine^{125}-IHYP to calf-lung membranes; immunoprecipitation of soluble receptors complexed with iodine^{125}-IHYP in the presence of propranolol
Premature ovarian failure	Interstitial cells and corpus luteum cells	IIFM with human or monkey ovary
Autoimmune hemolytic anemia	Red blood cell	Coombs' antiglobulin test (direct and indirect)
Spontaneous male infertility	Sperm	Agglutination and immobilization of spermatozoa

AChR = acetylcholine receptor; ANAs = antinuclear autoantibodies; BMZ = basement membrane zone; DIFM = direct immunofluorescence microscopy; EIA = enzyme immunoassay; ELISA = enzyme-linked immunosorbent assay; ICS = intercellular substance; Ig = immunoglobulins; IHYP = iodohydroxybenzylpindolol; IIFM = indirect immunofluorescence microscopy; p-ANCA = perinuclear anti–neutrophil cytoplasmic antibody; RIA = radioimmunoassay; RNP = ribonucleoprotein; TSH = thyroid-stimulating hormone.

same regardless of the target autoantibody, except for the substrate used to bind the autoantibody in question. The general procedure follows:

1. Prepare screening dilution of patient sera, or serial dilutions, and appropriate controls in phosphate buffered saline (PBS).
2. Use a moisture chamber to incubate diluted sera and controls layered over cryostat tissue sections of the substrate on multiwell glass slides for 20 to 30 minutes. Do not allow the slides to dry.
3. Remove slides from the moisture chamber. Briefly but carefully wash each entire slide two to three times using PBS at room temperature. Then wash slides in PBS for 15 minutes, changing the wash once during this period.
4. Remove one slide at a time from the PBS wash, blot each slide dry, and place each in a moisture chamber. Dispense diluted fluorescein-labeled conjugate over each well. Incubate slides at room temperature for 20 minutes. Do not allow slides to dry.
5. Wash slides for 10 minutes in PBS that contains Evans' blue counterstain.
6. Mount coverslips.
7. View slides under a fluorescence microscope. Determine reactivity at 250× (water immersion) total magnification. Reading slides at 400× (water immersion) total magnification may help with pattern recognition.
8. Store slides in the dark at 4°C.

SKIN

In patients with cutaneous diseases, autoantibodies include those to basement membrane zone (BMZ), epidermal intercellular substance (ICS), or dermal blood vessels. Several excellent technical reviews are available that detail the use of immunofluorescence for examining cutaneous tissue (Crosby, 1993; Flotte, 1995; Izuno, 1986). Among these, the procedure for immunofluorescent studies may be particularly useful to a dermatologist for resolving the differential diagnosis of cutaneous bullous disease.

Pemphigus

Pemphigus is a chronic, nonhereditary, suprabasilar acantholytic disease of the skin or mucous membrane, characterized by loss of intercellular adhesion because of ICS autoantibodies (Naparstek, 1993). There are several clinical subtypes of pemphigus, but in all forms the patients have autoantibodies to keratinocyte glycoprotein that can be demonstrated either by DIFM or IIFM (Crosby, 1993). Removal of these autoantibodies by plasmapheresis may lead to clinical improvement (Naparstek, 1993).

The antigen in patients with one clinical variant, pemphigus foliaceus, may be a 160 kDa glycoprotein that is identical to desmoglein I, a desmosomal core glycoprotein, whereas antigen in patients with pemphigus vulgaris, a second variant, is a 210 kDa glycoprotein on the surfaces of epidermal cells (Naparstek, 1993).

DIFM on perilesional skin biopsies of pemphigus lesions demonstrates IgG bound to epidermal ICS with a diagnostic sensitivity of 90%, although C3 is present in acantholytic areas in virtually 100% of such patients (Flotte, 1995; Izuno, 1986). In 50% or more of these patients, deposits of IgA, IgM, and/or C3 may be detected (Izuno, 1986).

IIFM on a substrate such as esophageal tissue from a guinea pig or monkey overlaid with sera from a patient with cutaneous pemphigus discloses IgG autoantibodies directed against desmosomes. IIFM has a diagnostic sensitivity of greater than 90% for detecting circulating IgG anti-epidermal ICS autoantibodies (Crosby, 1993; Izuno, 1986). Because the amount of circulating pemphigus autoantibodies present correlates roughly with disease activity, increasing titers may predict an imminent relapse (Crosby, 1993). However, because exceptions to this correlation occur, serial titers usually are not used to follow the progress of these patients. Rather, DIFM is used in addition to IIFM for the initial evaluation of patients with suspected pemphigus because DIFM has greater diagnostic sensitivity (Izuno, 1986). Patients with oral mucosal lesions alone frequently lack obvious circulating autoantibodies and so are best diagnosed by DIFM of normal-appearing mucosa next to an oral lesion (Izuno, 1986).

Paraneoplastic Pemphigus

Paraneoplastic pemphigus is a mucocutaneous blistering disease that occurs in patients with malignant neoplasms; such malignancies include malignant lymphoma, chronic lymphocytic lymphoma, thymoma, bronchogenic squamous cell carcinoma, and poorly differentiated sarcoma (Camisa, 1993; Flotte, 1995).

Upon DIFM of a lesional biopsy, IgG and C3 ICS deposits are evident, as are linear BMZ deposits (Flotte, 1995). IIFM of patients' sera on rat bladder transitional epithelium demonstrates circulating IgG autoantibodies that appear as both ICS and BMZ staining (Liu, 1993). Treatment of this disorder is challenging, requiring attempts to control or cure the neoplasm balanced against immunosuppression to control the skin eruptions.

Bullous Pemphigoid

Bullous pemphigoid (BP) is a subepidermal bullous disease of unknown cause that occurs mainly in older adults. BP is serologically characterized by the presence of circulating autoantibodies to cutaneous or oral mucosa BMZ. Nearly 100% of these patients have BMZ autoantibodies visible by DIFM in a linear and continuous pattern. Although IgG and C3 predominate in these deposits, about 25% of patients also have IgA, IgM, IgD, and/or IgE accumulations (Crosby, 1993; Izuno, 1986).

Immunoelectron microscopy demonstrates autoantibody deposits in the subbasilar lamina lucida of the BMZ, which provides a differential finding from lamina densa deposits in epidermolysis bullosa acquisita (EBA) (Izuno, 1986). Additionally, when sodium chloride–split skin (von Mühlen, 1995) is used as the substrate in IIFM, cutaneous tissue from BP patients shows immunoreactant in the epidermal, or roof, side of the split (80% of patients), whereas EBA is localized to the dermal, or floor, side of the split, where autoantibodies bind Type VII dermal collagen (50% of patients) (Crosby, 1993). DIFM of 1 mol/L sodium chloride–treated patient skin may improve the distinction between BP and EBA (Domloge-Hultsch, 1991). IIFM detects circulating IgG anti-BMZ autoantibodies in about 70% to 80% of patients with BP (Domloge-Hultsch, 1991; Izuno, 1986). However, DIFM is more diagnostically sensitive because BMZ deposits are detected in 80% to 90% of BP patients when biopsy from an edge of a fresh blister is used for study (Izuno, 1986).

Benign mucous membrane pemphigoid (BMMP), or cicatricial pemphigoid, occurs mainly in mucosa of the mouth or eyes. Lesions heal with scarring sequelae, and blindness is the feared complication. DIFM is positive in biopsies from mucosal sites in most patients, but only about 33% of patients are positive when glabrous skin biopsies alone are studied (Crosby, 1993). The pattern of tissue immunofluorescence is the same as in BP. However, traditional IIFM detects circulating autoantibody, although in fewer than 33% of BMMP patients when a mucosal substrate is used (Crosby, 1993) and fewer than 5% of these patients when glabrous skin is used as the substrate (Sarret, 1991). Salt-split human skin as a substrate, however, may reveal IgA, IgG, or both deposits in about 80% of these patients (Sarret, 1991).

Brunsting-Perry pemphigoid is a variant of cicatricial pemphigoid localized to the head and neck region (Izuno, 1986; Sarret, 1991). In this variant, DIFM demonstrates IgG only along the BMZ without IgA or IgM; circulating anti-BMZ autoantibodies are rare (Izuno, 1986).

Dermatitis Herpetiformis

Dermatitis herpetiformis (DH) is a subepidermal bullous disease characterized by granular deposits of IgA in the tips of dermal papillae. DIFM detects such deposits in approximately 80% to 100% of these patients (Flotte, 1995; Izuno, 1986). C3 deposits often are found with IgA, but IgG and/or IgM are detected infrequently (Izuno, 1986).

DH is strongly associated with both HLA B8 and DR3, and also with gluten-sensitive enteropathy (GSE-DH) (Crosby, 1993). Patients with GSE-DH do not have detectable anti-BMZ autoantibodies, but they do have circulating autoantibodies to endomysium (Peters, 1989), gliadin, or reticulin (Izuno, 1986). They may also have detectable antinuclear antibodies (ANAs) and/or autoantibodies to thyroid microsomes, thyroglobulin, or gastric parietal cells (Izuno, 1986).

Linear IgA Dermatosis

Linear IgA dermatosis, which was initially considered a variant of DH (Izuno, 1986), instead probably represents a distinct entity (Crosby, 1993). Recently it was recognized that this disorder can be caused by drug sensitivity. There is no association with HLA B8 or DR3 (Crosby, 1993). In nearly 100% of cases, DIFM demonstrates linear IgA deposits along the BMZ, but without associated deposits in dermal papillae (Izuno, 1986). Circulating IgA anti-BMZ autoantibodies can be detected on IIFM in 10% to 30% of cases (Crosby, 1993; Flotte, 1995).

Intercellular IgA Dermatosis

Intercellular IgA dermatosis is a rare intraepidermal vesiculobullous disorder characterized by IgA ICS visible with DIFM. ICS IgA deposition may be accentuated in the suprabasilar epidermis. Circulating IgA anti-ICS autoantibodies are also detected by IIFM. Therapy with dapsone is generally effective (Flotte, 1995; Teraki, 1991).

Herpes Gestationis

Herpes gestationis (HG), a subepidermal bullous disease that occurs during or soon after pregnancy, is also rare (Izuno, 1986). Lesions typically are pruritic and occur predominantly on the abdomen and/or extremities. The typical picture from DIFM is one of linear C3 deposits along the cutaneous BMZ. Associated IgG deposits are detected in 30% to 40% of these patients, but IgA and IgM appear infrequently (Izuno, 1986). In partial accord, IIFM demonstrates linear C3-only deposits along the BMZ without corresponding IgG (Izuno, 1986). The lesion-producing autoantibody in

HG patients is thought to be a complement-fixing IgG (Izuno, 1986).

Systemic Autoimmune Diseases

Autoantibodies typically identified in systemic autoimmune diseases are presented in Chapter 41. To supplement that information, the major considerations related to autoantibodies in skin lesions of patients with these disorders are discussed later.

Lupus Erythematosus

Typical DIFM findings on skin biopsies of lupus erythematosus (LE) patients include coarse, granular, continuous deposits along the BMZ (lupus band). Although characteristic, this reaction pattern is also seen in such disorders as mixed connective tissue disease, graft-versus-host reactions, drug eruptions, and vasculitis, among others (Izuno, 1986). Therefore, it is mandatory to correlate DIFM results with both the clinical presentation and the results of light microscopic study of each patient's skin biopsy. Additionally, it is important to know the patterns of immunofluorescence that typify different clinical subtypes of LE.

Systemic lupus erythematosus (SLE) is a systemic disorder characterized serologically by the presence of multiple and diverse autoantibodies, including ANAs, anti–native DNA, antihistones, and anti-Sm. In 50% to 95% of SLE patients, DIFM demonstrates coarse and granular, continuous deposits of immunoglobulins and complement along the epidermal BMZ (Izuno, 1986). In fact, BMZ deposits of the complement membrane attack complex, C5b-9, in lesional skin may be a marker for SLE (Helm, 1993). Whereas IgG, IgM, and C3 deposits are the most common in these patients, immunoglobulins of all classes may be identified (Izuno, 1986). Concurrent detection in nonlesional skin of immunoglobulins of all classes in the typical pattern is highly suggestive of SLE (Izuno, 1986).

The medical literature repeatedly cites the utility of DIFM findings on biopsies from uninvolved or involved skin, and from sun-exposed or sun-protected skin in SLE patients. However, the predictive utility for actual disease activity and renal involvement remains controversial (Izuno, 1986). Perhaps the most practical clinical application of DIFM readings comes in the differential diagnosis of SLE from discoid LE (DLE).

Coarse, granular, continuous BMZ deposits, similar to those in SLE, are visible by DIFM in 85% to 95% of patients with DLE (Izuno, 1986). However, these deposits are confined to lesional skin in DLE, whereas both lesional and nonlesional skin can give positive DIFM findings in SLE (Izuno, 1986). Additionally, in SLE patients normal, sun-exposed skin contains BMZ deposits about 70% of the time, whereas normal, sun-protected skin is positive in about 40% of patients (Izuno, 1986).

Subacute cutaneous lupus erythematosus (SCLE) is characterized clinically by serologic abnormalities, arthritis, and mild systemic manifestations. Anti–SS-A/Ro is the characteristic autoantibody detected in SCLE patients. DIFM on skin biopsies from these patients detects BMZ immunoglobulin and/or complement deposits in only 50% of lesions and 30% of uninvolved skin (Izuno, 1986).

Other Systemic Autoimmune Diseases

Patients with other major systemic autoimmune diseases do not manifest diagnostically specific findings either by DIFM or IIFM. Although these patients may have granular IgM deposits along the BMZ, this is considered a nonspecific immunopathologic response that may accompany several autoimmune diseases, a large number of inflammatory dermatitides, as well as sun exposure to the skin of clinically normal individuals (Izuno, 1986).

Cutaneous Vasculitis

Cutaneous vasculitis has a number of synonyms, including leukocytoclastic vasculitis, allergic vasculitis, and hypersensitivity angiitis/vasculitis. Histologically, small blood vessels of the dermis from such a patient show endothelial cell swelling, neutrophilic exocytosis, and thrombi in conjunction with extravasated red blood cells and nuclear debris ("leukocytoclasis") in the dermal connective tissue.

Biopsy of the lesion within 24 hours of onset, when subjected to DIFM, may reveal vascular deposits of IgM, C3, and/or fibrin; IgG and/or IgA may also be seen but less frequently (Izuno, 1986). When IgA is found alone or with C3, Henoch-Schönlein purpura must be considered in the differential diagnosis. Biopsies of lesions older than 24 hours may not be helpful because they usually contain fibrin only.

LIVER

Autoantibodies

Antinuclear Autoantibodies

ANAs, discussed in detail in Chapter 41, are most commonly detected by IIFM, although ELISAs for identification of specific autoantibodies are becoming more popular in clinical laboratories. ANAs are a very heterogeneous group, and almost all subtypes that occur in rheumatologic disorders are found in persons with autoimmune hepatitis (AiH). Either homogeneous or speckled ANA patterns on Hep-2 cells are more commonly identified in patients with AiH. Also reported in liver disease are specific autoantibodies to double-stranded DNA (Manns, 1992).

ANAs in a titer greater than 1:80 are detected in about 80% of patients with AiH (Nakamura, 1991). However, ANAs may also be found in about 60% of patients with primary biliary cirrhosis (PBC), 50% of patients with alcohol-related liver disease, 40% of patients with viral hepatitis type B, and 25% of AiH patients who also have anti–liver-kidney microsomal autoantibodies (LKMAs) (Nakamura, 1991). Anti-centromere/kinetochore autoantibody can be identified in 10% to 15% of PBC patients.

Antimitochondrial Autoantibodies

Nine separate mitochondrial antigens have been identified that react with antimitochondrial autoantibodies (AMAs). AMAs to M2 and M9 antigens, assayed by either ELISA or

Western blotting, are considered the most important diagnostic markers of PBC (Bylund, 1992). AMAs detected using IIFM on a substrate of rodent stomach/kidney tissue block show a typical pattern of fluorescence that reflects coarse granular cytoplasmic staining of kidney tubules and stomach parietal cell regions; distal tubules are also positive. This distal tubular staining is an important point in differentiating the reactivity of AMAs from that of LKMAs, which do not stain distal renal tubules.

The M2 autoantigen is a heterogeneous mix containing several components of the mitochondrial 2-oxo-acid dehydrogenase complex. The dominant M2 autoantigen in patients with PBC is the 70 kDa E2 subunit of pyruvate dehydrogenase (PDH-E2) (Manns, 1992). The second most common mitochondrial autoantigen is the 50 kDa E2 subunit of branched-chain oxo-keto-acid-dehydrogenase (BCOADH-E2) (Manns, 1992).

A group of serum autoantibodies, called naturally occurring mitochondrial autoantibodies (NOMAs), has been found in persons having close contact with PBC patients, and even in laboratory technicians processing PBC sera (Bylund, 1992). NOMAs are rarely produced in PBC patients but are observed in sera from patients with Epstein-Barr virus infection, cytomegalovirus infection, and other infectious disorders. NOMAs are directed at epitopes on the M2 and M9 antigens in PBC but not to the same antigens as AMAs (Bylund, 1992). Although the significance of these NOMAs is uncertain, their presence in persons associated with PBC patients has raised questions about possible contagious agents in sera of these patients (Bylund, 1992).

Smooth Muscle Autoantibodies

Smooth muscle autoantibodies (SMAs) are found in approximately 50% of patients with classic AiH and often they occur with ANAs (Nakamura, 1991). When accompanying liver disease, SMAs are directed against F-actin, which is part of the liver cell cytoskeleton in close association with the liver cell plasma membrane (Nakamura, 1991). The SMA titer is typically greater than or equal to 1:80 in serum from an AiH patient. However, low titers of SMA can be detected in those with other diseases and in apparently healthy individuals (Nakamura, 1991).

IIFM on a tissue substrate of rodent stomach is commonly used to detect SMAs, which stain the muscularis propria of stomach in a uniform and consistent pattern. Specific staining of muscularis mucosae and walls of blood vessels is characteristic. If a rodent stomach/kidney tissue block is used as substrate, there may be faint staining of glomerular mesangial zones because of the presence of F-actin in these regions. If Hep-2 cells are used instead of other substrates, IIFM reveals "cable-like" cytoplasmic staining when SMA is present.

Liver-Kidney Microsomal Autoantibodies

Liver-kidney microsomal autoantibodies (LKMAs) stain the microsomes of hepatocytes and proximal renal tubules when detected using a rodent stomach/kidney tissue block as the substrate for IIFM. The distal renal tubules are characteristically negative for immunofluorescence. The simultaneous occurrence of AMAs and LKMAs, although possible, is extremely unlikely. The presence of LKMAs can be confirmed by using Western blotting, although this assay is not yet widely available in clinical laboratories. However, with the Western blotting procedure, LKMAs have been grouped into three subtypes on the basis of their target antigens (Manns, 1992).

A 50 kDa component of cytochrome P-450IID6 has been identified as the major antigen for LKMA-1 (Manns, 1992). LKMA-2, directed at cytochrome P-450 IIC9, was found in patients taking ticrynafen (Manns, 1992), a drug that is no longer on the American market. LKMA-3 has been identified in sera from patients with chronic viral hepatitis, type D, but the antigen has not yet been characterized (Manns, 1992).

Other Liver Autoantibodies

The remaining groups of hepatic autoantibodies include anticytoskeleton, anticytosol, anti–liver membrane, antinuclear lamins, liver specific, and asialoglycoprotein receptor autoantibodies. All these have been identified in patients with autoimmune liver diseases, but their use as diagnostic markers is not currently widespread (Nakamura, 1991).

Liver Diseases

5

Table 43–2 lists typical serologic profiles in putative autoimmune liver disorders that include AiH, PBC, and primary sclerosing cholangitis (PSC). These are typically

Table 43–2. AUTOIMMUNE LIVER DISEASES (HBsAG-NEGATIVE)

	ANA	LKMA-1	SLA	SMA	AMA	Anti-HCV	p-ANCA	Therapy
Autoimmune hepatitis								
Type 1	+	−	−	+	−	−	±	Immunosuppression
Type 2a	−	+	−	−	−	−		Immunosuppression
Type 2b	−	+	−	−	−	+		?
Type 3	−	−	+	±	±	−		Immunosuppression
Type 4	−	−	−	+	−	−		Immunosuppression
PBC	−	−	−	−	+	−	−	Supportive; transplant
PSC	−	−	−	−	−	−	+	Supportive; transplant

HBsAG = hepatitis B surface antigen; ANA = antinuclear antibodies; p-ANCA, perinuclear anti–neutrophil cytoplasmic antibody; LKMA-1 = liver-kidney microsomal antibodies; SLA = antibodies against soluble liver antigens; SMA = smooth muscle antibodies; AMA = antimitochondrial antibodies; HCV = hepatitis C virus; UDCA = ursodeoxycholic acid; PBC = primary biliary cirrhosis; PSC = primary sclerosing cholangitis.

Modified from Manns (1992).

chronic disorders defined as such by the patients' elevated concentrations of serum transaminases for at least six months. Alternatives commonly considered in the clinical differential diagnosis include alcohol-related liver disease, drug-induced liver injury, viral hepatitides types B or C, and fatty liver of diabetes mellitus or obesity. Less common differential diagnoses include idiopathic hemochromatosis, Wilson's disease, alpha-1 antitrypsin deficiency, and hepatic involvement in systemic diseases.

Autoimmune Hepatitis

AiH classically occurs in females around 35 years old who present with a high concentration of serum transaminase (300 to 500 mg/dL), hypergammaglobulinemia, amenorrhea, arthralgias, and such circulating autoantibodies as ANAs, SMAs, or LKMAs. By definition, these patients have no serologic evidence of hepatitis B, Wilson's disease, or other diseases in the differential diagnosis. Histologically, liver biopsy shows chronic active hepatitis with piecemeal necrosis. The patient's response to corticosteroids is dramatic, and failure to respond sheds doubt on the diagnosis of AiH. Some investigators have proposed subclassification of AiH according to its serologic profile, as provided in Table 43–2 (Manns, 1992). Additionally, an international panel has proposed clinical and pathologic criteria for the diagnosis of AiH (Johnson, 1993; Mackay, 1993).

ANAs characterize classical autoimmune-type hepatitis. In this subgroup of AiH, also called type 1, SMAs are also frequently detected. Although AMAs are specific and sensitive diagnostic markers for PBC, as described later, AMAs can also be detected in about 15% of patients with both clinical and histologic features of AiH, including clinical improvement in response to immunosuppressive therapy. Such patients are regarded as having a syndrome with "overlap" features of both AiH and PBC. AMA titer in this AiH subgroup is rarely greater than 1:40 (Bylund, 1992). Additionally, the antigen specificity of these AMAs is similar to that seen in classical PBC (Manns, 1992).

Liver disease in which LKMAs are detected, so-called type 2 AiH, has been subdivided into two subgroups, types 2a and 2b. Usually patients with this variant of AiH are negative for ANAs and SMAs. However, thyroid microsomal, thyroglobulin, and parietal cell autoantibodies are frequently detected. Type 2 AiH is characterized by low IgA levels, and hypergammaglobulinemia is less prominent than is seen in type 1 AiH (Manns, 1992). Type 2a occurs in young females who have high tiers of LKMA-1, negative serology for hepatitis C virus, and active but steroid-responsive disease.

The type 2b variant occurs in older patients, and there is less of a female preponderance. These patients have low titers of LKMA-1, manifest milder liver disease, and are often serologically positive for hepatitis C virus. Their disease tends to be less responsive to immunosuppression than the 2a type.

A third subgroup of AiH is separated on the basis of identifying serum antisoluble liver autoantibody (SLA) (Manns, 1992). This may become an important autoantibody to identify because it has been reported as the only serologic marker in about 25% of AiH patients (Manns, 1992). However, reliable tests to detect SLA are technically difficult and, as yet, are not routinely available in clinical laboratories. It may be that high titers of SMAs directed against F-actin characterize a fourth subgroup of autoimmune AiH that is frequently observed in young children (Manns, 1992).

Primary Biliary Cirrhosis

PBC is a chronic, progressive, cholestatic disorder typically occurring in young or middle-aged females. Patients may be asymptomatic or have symptoms of cholestasis (itch). Laboratory studies demonstrate an elevation in alkaline phosphatase with or without hyperbilirubinemia, as well as increased IgM and AMAs. Associated extrahepatic immunologic phenomena, such as Raynaud's phenomenon, sicca complex, rheumatoid arthritis, thyroiditis, scleroderma, or celiac disease, may occur (Bylund, 1992; Manns, 1992). Histologically, the liver shows the effects of nonsuppurative destructive cholangitis.

The most specific and sensitive diagnostic marker for PBC is AMAs. As a general guideline, an AMA titer greater than or equal to 1:160 is highly predictive of PBC, although about 10% of PBC patients have AMA titers of 1:16 or less (Bylund, 1992). About 95% of patients with typical clinicopathologic features of PBC have been shown to have anti-M2 and/or anti-M9 AMAs, whereas the remaining 5% of patients are AMA negative. The diagnosis of AMA-negative PBC derives from the clinical presentation, liver biopsy findings, and cholangiogram, the latter performed to rule out PSC.

Primary Sclerosing Cholangitis

PSC typically occurs in males with a history of inflammatory bowel disease and/or diarrhea. In 50% of these patients, the inflammatory bowel disease linked with PSC is ulcerative colitis. The basis for diagnosis is characteristic changes on cholangiogram (beading/strictures of bile ducts) and/or histologic study of liver biopsy. Laboratory studies demonstrate an elevated level of alkaline phosphatase with or without hyperbilirubinemia. Although traditionally no immunologic marker distinguishes PSC, recent reports have identified anti–neutrophil cytoplasmic autoantibodies, peripheral pattern (p-ANCA), in PSC when detected by IIFM on ethanol-fixed neutrophils (Manns, 1992).

Autoimmune Cholangitis

Autoimmune cholangitis (AiC) is a chronic cholestatic liver disease that responds to immunosuppression (Taylor, 1993). These patients' hepatic tissues have the histologic appearance of PBC, and their serologic findings include the presence of ANAs and AMAs. Nevertheless, AiC does not appear to be a variant of PSC.

THYROID GLAND

Thyroid Diseases (see Chap. 16)

Autoimmune thyroid diseases include Graves' disease and autoimmune lymphocytic thyroiditis (Burek, 1995). Autoimmune thyroiditis can be subclassified as Hashimoto's thyroiditis, both classical and fibrous variants, as well as juvenile lymphocytic thyroiditis, painless thyroiditis/postpartum thyroiditis, and atrophic thyroiditis (primary myxedema) (Brunt, 1995).

Graves' Disease

The patient who has Graves' disease presents with symptoms of hyperthyroidism and diffuse goiter. The peak incidence is in the third to fourth decades of life, and the female to male ratio is 4–8:1. Sixty to 70% of these patients additionally manifest ocular disturbances (Patrick, 1993). Laboratory data show an increase in levels of triiodothyronine (T_3) and thyroxine (T_4), and in the uptake of T_3. Therapy is directed at reducing the thyroid's ability to respond to stimulation by autoantibodies. This can be achieved by subtotal thyroidectomy, by administration of radioactive iodine, or by use of antithyroid drugs such as propylthiouracil or methimazole (Patrick, 1993).

Hashimoto's Thyroiditis

Hashimoto's thyroiditis is the most common form of thyroiditis and is functionally characterized by a slow progression to hypothyroidism. In patients with hypothyroidism, T_3 and T_4 levels and T_3 uptake are low and amounts of thyroid-stimulating hormone (TSH) increase abnormally (Patrick, 1993). The incidence of Hashimoto's thyroiditis peaks during the third to fifth decades, with a female/male ratio of 10:1. Autoantibodies directed against thyroglobulin (anti-Tg) and thyroid (microsomal) peroxidase (anti-TPO) antigens are clinically the most important for diagnosis (Patrick, 1993), but up to 20% of the adult female population with no clinical disease have detectable anti-Tg and/or anti-TPO, raising questions about their pathogenic significance (Patrick, 1993). Thyroid hormone replacement is reserved for patients with proven hypothyroidism. There are similarities between Graves' disease and Hashimoto's thyroiditis (Utiger, 1991). Both are associated with HLA-B8; both share fundamentally similar pathogenesis, and it is believed that Graves' disease may progress to Hashimoto's thyroiditis (Patrick, 1993; Utiger, 1991).

Autoantibodies

Three major autoantibodies are important in autoimmune thyroid diseases, including anti-TPO, anti-Tg, and autoantibody to TSH receptor (anti-TSHR) (Naparstek, 1993). Although anti-TPO and anti-Tg are considered markers of autoimmune thyroid disease, their etiologic role has not been proven. They may occur as well in other organ-directed autoimmune diseases. Anti-TSHR, however, clearly plays a causal role in autoimmune thyroid disease (Naparstek, 1993).

Anti–Thyroid Peroxidase Autoantibodies

Anti–thyroid peroxidase autoantibody (anti-TPO) is directed to a 105 kDa antigen that is contained within the microsomal fraction of thyroid epithelial cell cytoplasm (Burek, 1995). Although the quantitative passive hemagglutination technique is the most commonly used method for detecting anti-TPO (Nordyke, 1993), ELISAs are also used for this purpose in clinical laboratories. Historically, IIFM has been a popular and sensitive method for detecting anti-TPO. The IIFM test uses unfixed and air-dried human or monkey cryostat tissue sections as substrate. Positive sera stain the cytoplasm of thyroid follicular epithelial cells but do not stain their nuclei. Anti-TPO must be differentiated from AMA when coarse granular cytoplasmic staining is noted; this can be done by testing sera on a rodent stomach/kidney tissue block.

Anti-TPO can be detected in sera from patients with either Graves' disease or Hashimoto's thyroiditis, and its presence and titer correlate strongly with active clinical disease (Burek, 1995). Some investigators have indicated that determination of anti-TPO alone is sufficient to detect autoimmune thyroid disease and has the advantage of costing less than additional anti-Tg testing (Nordyke, 1993). The pathogenic role of anti-TPO remains unclear (Naparstek, 1993).

Anti–Thyroglobulin Autoantibodies

Anti–thyroglobulin autoantibody (anti-Tg) is targeted against thyroglobulin, which is the storage form of thyroid hormones within thyroid gland follicles (Burek, 1995). Several methods are available for measuring anti-Tg, including quantitative passive hemagglutination, IIFM, and ELISA. Quantitative passive hemagglutination with either chromic chloride hemagglutination or tanned red blood cells is the most widely used and sensitive method for detecting anti-Tg (Burek, 1995). Anti-Tg detected by hemagglutination is identified in titers greater than 1:1000 in about 80% of patients with Hashimoto's thyroiditis (Burek, 1995). Patients with Graves' disease (60%) or thyroid carcinoma (30%), or other autoimmune disorders such as pernicious anemia or Sjögren's syndrome, and 3% to 18% of apparently normal individuals may also have anti-Tg, but their hemagglutination titers are usually (>90%) less than 1:1000 (Burek, 1995).

To locate anti-Tg, IIFM is done using methanol-fixed cryostat tissue sections of monkey thyroid gland. Fixation is required to prevent loss of thyroglobulin during washing steps. Three patterns of immunofluorescence are described when anti-Tg is present: (1) floccular pattern, (2) dull colloid spaces but bright peripheral fluorescence, and (3) diffuse, bright, uniformly staining colloid in a "ground-glass" pattern attributed to the anti-Tg reaction with CA2. CA2, or so-called second colloid antigen, is detected as the only serologic marker of autoimmune thyroiditis in the 5% to 8% of patients who are positive by IIFM but negative for anti-Tg and anti-TPO using other methods (Bigazzi, 1992).

Anti–Thyroid-Stimulating Hormone Receptor Autoantibodies

Anti-TSHR autoantibodies consist of two groups of autoantibodies that can either stimulate or block TSHRs causing, respectively, hyperthyroidism or hypothyroidism. Anti-TSHR autoantibodies that bind to these receptors and stimulate thyroid hormone production are referred to as *thyroid-stimulating immunoglobulins* (TSIs), whereas anti-TSHR autoantibodies that bind to receptors and block the binding and function of TSH are referred to as *thyroid-binding inhibitory immunoglobulins* (TBIIs) (Brunt, 1995; Mooij, 1993).

TSIs probably cause the hyperthyroidism in Graves' disease (Bigazzi, 1992; Brunt, 1995; Wilkin, 1990). Their prevalence varies from 55% to 95% depending on the method of detection (Bigazzi, 1992; Brunt, 1995). TSIs, which are usually of the IgG class, stimulate production of thyroid hormones by activating the adenylate cyclase system after binding to TSHRs (Patrick, 1993).

Assays for anti-TSHR are useful for confirming Graves' disease in hyperthyroid patients with equivocal results in routine laboratory studies (Bigazzi, 1992). Additionally, one of the anti-TSHR assays may be used to monitor patients' hormone replacement therapy or to diagnose neonatal thyrotoxicosis (Bigazzi, 1992). There are two main classes of assays for anti-TSHR, namely, bioassays and binding assays; their methodologic aspects are reviewed elsewhere (Bigazzi, 1992; Gupta, 1988; Patrick, 1993). Newer assays of a patient's serum based on stimulation of cyclic adenosine monophosphate (cAMP) in rat thyroid cells, maintained in tissue culture, may prove to be an improvement over the technically difficult bioassays (Burek, 1995). TSIs are measured in bioassays that determine increased TSHR-mediated activity either by measuring the release of cAMP or by measuring the uptake of iodide by thyroid cells maintained in culture (Brunt, 1995). TBIIs are measured either by determining binding inhibition of radiolabeled TSH to its receptor or by using cAMP bioassays (Brunt, 1995).

KIDNEY

Glomerulonephritis

Glomerulonephritis (gnitis) is a major cause of primary renal disease. Immune-mediated mechanisms are thought to have an important role in the pathogenesis of gnitis, although experimental confirmation of such putative autoimmune mechanisms is still lacking. DIFM has an important role in the study and diagnosis of gnitis. The patterns of immune reactants can be divided broadly into those that cause either granular or linear deposits within glomeruli or other kidney structures examined with DIFM. Granular deposits have been attributed to immune complexes (ICs) that settle out of circulating blood or form *in situ* (McCluskey, 1995).

DIFM patterns of immune deposits associated with major glomerular diseases are summarized in Table 43–3. Thorough reviews of these disorders are available in several texts (Heptinstall, 1992; McCluskey, 1995). However, for this discussion, only anti–glomerular basement membrane (anti-GBM) autoantibodies are presented in some additional detail.

Table 43–3. MAJOR GLOMERULAR DISEASES WITH DIRECT IMMUNOFLUORESCENT FINDINGS

Immunofluorescent Pattern and Disease	Immune Reactant(s)
Granular, Mesangial, and GBM Deposits	
Acute poststreptococcal gnitis	Scattered C3 ± IgG, IgM
Diffuse proliferative lupus nephritis	IgG, IgA, IgM, C3
Membranoproliferative gnitis (MPGN, type I)	C3, IgG, IgM
Idiopathic immune complex crescentic gnitis	IgG, C3 ± IgM
Dense deposit disease (MPGN, type II)	C3 (globular) ± IgM
Chronic infections (e.g., bacterial endocarditis)	IgG, IgM, C3
Granular, Mesangial Predominant	
Lupus nephritis	
Mesangial	IgG, C3; usually IgM and IgA
Focal proliferative	IgG, C3, IgA; focal capillary loop deposits
Henoch-Schönlein purpura	IgA predominant; IgG, IgM, C3
IgA nephropathy	IgA predominant; often IgG, IgM, C3
Granular, GBM Predominant	
Membranous lupus nephritis	IgG, C3, IgA, IgM
Mixed cryoglobulinemia	IgM, IgG, C3; intravascular masses
Linear GBM	
Anti-GBM nephritis	IgG, C3; IgA and IgM infrequent
Light chain nephropathy	Usually kappa light chain, may be in TBM, blood vessels, interstitium

Gnitis = glomerulonephritis; GBM = glomerular basement membrane; TBM = tubular basement membrane.
Modified from McCluskey (1995).

Anti–Glomerular Basement Membrane Disease

Patients with anti-GBM disease vary in clinical presentation in that about 50% have renal-limited disease and the other 50% have both renal and pulmonary symptoms. This latter presentation is often called Goodpasture's syndrome. Rarely, patients with anti-GBM disease may have pulmonary-limited disease (Wilson, 1987).

Diagnosis of anti-GBM disease requires detection of anti-GBM autoantibodies to the NCl domain of type IV collagen (McCluskey 1995), the so-called Goodpasture's antigen. Methods for detecting circulating anti-GBM have included IIFM, ELISA, and radioimmunoassay (RIA) (McCluskey, 1995; Wilson, 1987); some investigators have additionally developed a sensitive Western blot test (McCluskey, 1995). Because IIFM is difficult to standardize and requires experience to perform, methods for detection have focused instead on validation of quantitative RIA or ELISA. Currently, a licensed commercial ELISA kit is available for the measurement of anti-GBM. This assay determines patient values from a standard curve and reports negative, borderline, or positive ranges. Most patients with active anti-GBM disease appear to have values greater than 100 units. Although borderline values can be seen in both active and quiescent anti-GBM disease, we have also seen such values in patients with renal disorders that are not anti-GBM disease.

The coexistence of ANCA has been documented in some patients with rapidly progressive glomerulonephritis (RPGN) (McCluskey, 1995). The coexistence of these two autoantibodies has varied from 0% to 40% of patients with RPGN, accompanied by some evidence that the presence of ANCA in patients with anti-GBM disease affords a better renal prognosis (McCluskey, 1995).

ADRENAL GLAND

Addison's Disease

Nontuberculous chronic adrenocortical insufficiency, or Addison's disease, has an estimated prevalence of three to six cases per 100,000 people (Muir, 1993). Sixty-five to 70% of such patients have circulating autoantibodies to microsomes and the plasma membrane of adrenocortical cells, demonstrable using IIFM on frozen sections of human adrenal cortex (Burek, 1995; Muir, 1993, Patrick, 1993). 21-Hydroxylase and 17-alpha hydroxylase are two autoantigens that have been identified as reactive with adrenocortical autoantibodies (Song, 1994). Adrenocortical autoantibodies are not found in Addison's disease, caused by tuberculosis or other exogenous agents (Patrick, 1993). Importantly, about 45% of asymptomatic individuals with serum adrenocortical autoantibodies develop impaired adrenocortical function within 2.5 years after the autoantibody is identified (Muir, 1991). Addison's disease associated with autoantibodies is most commonly diagnosed in persons between ages 20 and 50 years and is two to three times more frequent in females when diagnosed after the age of 30 (Muir, 1993; Patrick, 1993).

Laboratory tests show metabolic acidosis, hyperkalemia, hyponatremia, and low levels of serum chloride and bicarbonate. Plasma cortisol levels are also low and adrenocorticotrophic hormone levels are elevated (VanArsdel, 1993). Consequently, therapy consists of replacing glucocorticoids and mineralocorticoids (Patrick, 1993).

Addison's disease associated with autoantibodies can occur by itself but is more commonly accompanied by other autoimmune disorders as part of an autoimmune polyglandular syndrome (APS) (Muir, 1993). These companion diseases may include autoimmune thyroiditis, pernicious anemia, or insulin-dependent diabetes mellitus (Patrick, 1993). In addition to adrenocortical autoantibodies, other adrenal autoantibodies have been detected in patients with Addison's disease, including steroidal cell autoantibodies and autoantibodies that bind adrenocorticotropic hormone receptors (Muir, 1993).

PANCREAS

Diabetes Mellitus

Diabetes mellitus (DM) is the diagnostic term applied to a group of metabolic disorders that share hyperglycemia as their common link (Eisenbarth, 1995). That DM is a serious diagnosis is documented by the fact that acute and chronic multi-organ diabetic complications account for about 15% of total U.S. health care expenditures (Schatz, 1995). However, significant progress has been made in the care of diabetic patients with the knowledge that aggressive blood glucose control reduces the risk for development of progression to vascular complications (Diabetes Control and Complications Trial Research Group, 1993; Schatz, 1995).

Clinical Subtypes

There are two major clinical subgroups of DM: type 1, insulin-dependent DM (IDDM); and, type 2, noninsulin-dependent, DM (Eisenbarth, 1995). Type 2 DM most commonly occurs in obese individuals older than 30 years. These patients have plasma insulin but in a concentration insufficient to prevent hyperglycemia (VanArsdel, 1993). Some type 2 patients have insulin-associated autoantibodies in their sera (VanArsdel, 1993). The type 2 patients lack most other autoimmune features seen in type 1 patients, although the distinction between type 1 and type 2 DM is not always easy (Eisenbarth, 1995). Type 2 patients are managed by weight control and medications that stimulate insulin production (VanArsdel, 1993).

Type 1 DM is considered a chronic autoimmune disease occurring in genetically susceptible individuals and is caused by selective destruction of insulin-producing beta cells in the pancreatic islets of Langerhans (Harrison, 1990). This destruction of beta cells eventually results in insulin deficiency and chronic hyperglycemia. In the United States, IDDM develops in about 1 in 300 persons, that is, an average yearly incidence of 15 per 100,000 people (Eisenbarth, 1995).

There is abundant support for concluding that IDDM is a chronic autoimmune disease (Eisenbarth, 1995; Harrison, 1990; Schatz, 1995). The detection of circulating autoantibodies preceding clinically apparent IDDM reinforces this conclusion and has provided important information regarding the natural history of IDDM and the ability to predict its onset (Schatz, 1995). The three major types of circulatory autoantibodies to consider with respect to IDDM are the following: (1) islet-cell autoantibodies (ICA), (2) insulin-associated autoantibodies (IAAs), and (3) anti–glutamic acid decarboxylase autoantibodies (anti-GADs).

These autoantibodies have largely been studied in sera from first-degree relatives of patients with IDDM and from newly diagnosed IDDM patients (Schatz, 1995), although important recent work indicates that ICA may be useful as a screening test to identify sporadic IDDM in the general population (Schatz, 1994). Yet it seems highly questionable that either ICAs or IAAs represent the initial pathogenic mechanism in IDDM. Most research scientists believe that cell-mediated mechanisms are more important in causing islet cell damage, as suggested by the mononuclear cell infiltrates seen in pancreatic islets of patients with newly diagnosed IDDM and in animals with experimentally induced forms of diabetes (Naparstek, 1993).

Islet Cell Autoantibodies

IIFM is the usual method used for detection of ICAs (Atkinson, 1993b). Frozen sections of human pancreas are used as the tissue substrate to detect specific, finely granular, cytoplasmic fluorescence in all cells of pancreatic islets. Pancreata from blood group O individuals are recommended as a source for this substrate to reduce the nonspecific background interference caused by ABO isohemagglutinins. Using IIFM, ICAs are detectable in about 80% of patients with newly diagnosed IDDM, 3% to 4% of nondiabetic relatives of patients with IDDM, and only 0.5% of clinically normal subjects (Atkinson, 1994). ICAs consist of autoantibodies that include those specifically reactive with GAD as well as those that are non–GAD-reactive ICAs (Atkinson, 1993a; Kaufman, 1992). ICAs should be titered in Juvenile Diabetes Foundation (JDF) units in reference to an 80-unit standard serum from the Immunology of Diabetes Workshop; titers greater than 20 JDF units seem to have prognostic significance (Maclaren, 1992).

Insulin-Associated Autoantibodies

IAAs are identified in about 50% of patients with IDDM at the time of diagnosis and before insulin therapy begins (Atkinson, 1994). IAAs are measured using a technically demanding competitive radioimmunoprecipitation assay that, at present, is done mainly in research laboratories (Palmer,

1983). This assay cannot distinguish between IAAs occurring spontaneously and those that occur as a result of insulin therapy.

Glutamic Acid Decarboxylase Autoantibodies

Anti–glutamic acid decarboxylase (GAD) autoantibodies are detected in most newly diagnosed IDDM patients and in about 80% of prediabetic, first-degree relatives of patients with IDDM (Hagopian, 1993; Schatz, 1995). The two forms of GAD, classified by molecular mass, are designated GAD65 and GAD67 (Atkinson, 1993b). GAD65 is found mainly in pancreatic islets and in the central nervous system, where it functions as an enzyme responsible for formation of the inhibiting neurotransmitter, gamma-amino butyric acid. The GAD67 form predominates in peripheral nerves (Atkinson, 1993b; Falorni, 1994).

Anti-GAD autoantibodies, detectable by RIA, in patients with IDDM are directed primarily at the GAD65 isoform, which is the 64 kDa autoantigen reported previously (Bärmeier, 1992; Kaufman, 1992; Lühder, 1994; Maclaren, 1988). GAD autoantigen is one, but not the only, antigen involved in islet cell reactivity (Atkinson, 1993b). Anti-GAD autoantibodies are also associated with the rare stiff-man syndrome (Eisenbarth, 1995). Interestingly, a high percentage of these patients have a history of IDDM.

Interpretation and Clinical Utility of Autoantibodies in IDDM

ICAs, IAAs, and anti-GAD autoantibodies are used currently as predictive markers for IDDM. Identification of a high ICA titer is associated with an elevated risk of developing IDDM, especially when detected in children and in conjunction with IAAs. Anti-GAD autoantibodies are usually detected before the diagnosis of IDDM and usually decline in titer after the onset of clinical IDDM (Schatz, 1994). Anti-GAD seems to offer the best predictive utility when identified along with either ICA or IAA, but when both ICA and IAA are present there is little additional predictive information (Schatz, 1995).

The use of these markers to identify individuals at risk for IDDM is being evaluated to determine the need for metabolic studies that would assess subclinical glucose intolerance and call for immunotherapy in the preclinical phase of IDDM (Maclaren, 1992). Measurement of anti-GAD using newly developed ELISAs may improve the feasibility of widespread screening for this autoantibody. In addition to the autoantibodies discussed earlier, patients with IDDM also may have anti-TPO, anti–parietal cell, and anti–adrenocortical autoantibodies so that IDDM patients should be screened for these autoantibodies at least once (Maclaren, 1992).

GASTROINTESTINAL TRACT

Pernicious Anemia

Pernicious anemia (PA) is characterized by histamine-fast achlorhydria, hypergastrinemia, and vitamin B_{12} deficiency (Brown, 1995). The insidious onset of neurologic symptoms and the development of megaloblastic anemia are typical features of PA's clinical course (Patrick, 1993). Morphologically, biopsy of the stomach body mucosa contains evidence of chronic atrophic gastritis.

PA is associated with circulating autoantibodies to gastric parietal cells (anti-GPCs) in 90% of patients and to intrinsic factor (anti-IF) in 60% to 75% of patients, although anti-IF may be more specific for PA (Brown, 1995; Burek, 1995). Anti-GPCs are detected by IIFM performed on mouse stomach/kidney tissue blocks. This combined tissue block allows identification of specific parietal cell staining when there is no concomitant staining of renal tubules, as would be seen in the presence of AMA.

Anti-IF are most commonly detected by RIA. Of the two known types of anti-IF, type 1 anti-IF, or blocking autoantibody, prevents the binding of IF to vitamin B_{12}, and type 2, or binding autoantibody, reacts with free or complexed vitamin B_{12} to inhibit IF's action (Karen, 1994; Patrick, 1993). Type 1 anti-IF is considered more diagnostically sensitive and specific for PA (Karen, 1994). However, identification of either anti-GPC or anti-IF is not required for diagnosis of PA. PA can occur in association with other autoimmune diseases, such as autoimmune thyroiditis or Addison's disease, and may be a part of either APS 1 or APS 2 (Patrick, 1993).

Gluten-Sensitive Enteropathy

Gluten-sensitive enteropathy (GSE), also called *celiac sprue*, is a small bowel disease characterized by the malabsorption of gastrointestinal fat (Brown, 1995). Hypersensitivity to gluten, or gluten derivatives, is the cause of GSE (Brown, 1995). Small bowel biopsy from such a patient is variably abnormal, but villous atrophy with crypt elongation and crypt mitoses are histologic features of well-developed GSE.

Patients with GSE manifest several humoral immune alterations. Interestingly serum IgA levels are usually elevated in GSE patients, except in those with an IgA deficiency, which does occur in GSE patients more commonly than in normal individuals (Brown, 1995). Patients with GSE may have circulating IgA anti-endomysial, antireticulin, and/or antigliadin autoantibodies.

IgA anti-endomysial autoantibodies are detectable by IIFM on a substrate of monkey esophagus tissue. Their identification is considered diagnostically sensitive and specific for GSE alone or GSE associated with DH (GSE-DH). Measuring the titer of IgA anti-endomysial autoantibody may even be used to monitor a patient's compliance with a gluten-free diet (Karen, 1994). Antireticulin autoantibodies are detected by IIFM on a mouse stomach/kidney combined tissue block. These autoantibodies are detectable in adults (40%) as well as children (60%) with GSE, and also in adults with GSE-DH (20%). However, antireticulin autoantibody is diagnostically nonspecific, being present also in patients with Crohn's disease, myasthenia gravis, Sjögren's syndrome, and other connective tissue disorders. Antigliadin autoantibodies are detected by ELISA in almost all patients with GSE or GSE-DH (Brown, 1995). The target antigen, gliadin, is purified from gluten and used in a solid-phase ELISA to detect these autoantibodies. Like IgA endomysial autoantibodies, antigliadin autoantibodies can be used to monitor a patient's adherence to a gluten-free diet.

NERVOUS SYSTEM

Myasthenia Gravis

Myasthenia gravis (MG) is a neuromuscular disorder characterized by use-associated muscular weakness, fatigue, and the presence of anti–acetylcholine receptor (anti-AChR) autoantibodies. AChR, located in postsynaptic membranes of skeletal muscle fibers, binds acetylcholine (ACh) from nerve endings, which causes a muscle contraction when enough ACh has been released (Naparstek, 1993; Rose, 1995). Anti-AChR autoantibodies interfere with this neuromuscular function, resulting in muscle weakness and fatigue.

Anti-AChR autoantibodies are detected in about 90% of MG patients (Rose, 1995). Radiolabeled alpha-bungarotoxin (alpha-BTx) is used in competitive RIAs to measure different forms of anti-AChR (Barna, 1995). Alpha-BTx is a protein from snake venom that essentially irreversibly binds AChR, but it binds to ACh receptors at a site different from binding sites for anti-AChR (Rose, 1995). AChRs are obtained from extracts of denervated human skeletal muscle, such as from diabetic amputations, or from tissue cell culture. For testing, the AChRs are labeled with alpha-BTx then incubated with patients' serum to allow any anti-AChR autoantibodies present to bind to AChRs at sites near the alpha-BTx binding site. After incubation, the radiolabeled complexes are precipitated by polyvalent anti-human immunoglobulin, and the washed precipitate is counted for radioactivity, after correction for nonspecific binding. The degree of radioactivity in the precipitate is directly proportional to the amount of anti-AChR in the patient's serum.

Modifications of this binding assay can be used to identify anti-AChR blocking and modulating autoantibodies. In a blocking assay, patients' sera containing anti-AChR is allowed to incubate with AChRs before addition of alpha-BTx. The basis for this technique is the premise that anti-AChR capable of blocking alpha-BTx binding also blocks ACh binding to AChRs (Rose, 1995). The amount of radioactivity in the precipitate is, therefore, inversely proportional to the amount of anti-AChR in patient's sera. Modulating anti-AChR autoantibodies are thought to accelerate AChR degradation, but their measurement in the clinical laboratory is technically difficult and not widely performed.

Multiple Sclerosis

Multiple sclerosis (MS) is a relatively common demyelinating disease involving the white matter of the brain and spinal cord. MS occurs more frequently in females than males (2 : 1 ratio) and is usually evident during young adulthood, with a wide variety of possible clinical manifestations. About 50% of these patients undergo alternating periods of active disease and remissions, whereas the remainder follow a chronic progressive course (McFarland, 1995; Steinman, 1993). The diagnosis of MS derives from clinical findings and exclusion of all other disorders.

Although the cause of MS is unknown, autoimmune mechanisms are considered important in the pathogenesis of this disease (McFarland, 1995). There are not, however, any characteristic circulating autoantibodies in MS that are accepted as diagnostic enough for routine measurement in clinical laboratories. However, laboratory examination of cerebrospinal fluid (CSF) does provide important information that supports a diagnosis of MS in an appropriate clinical setting (Barna, 1987). Synthesis of IgG increases abnormally within the CNS of MS patients, so that measurement of the IgG index and IgG synthetic rate provides useful, but not specific, test results (Karen, 1994; McFarland, 1995; Valenzuela, 1987; Zweiman, 1991).

Evaluation of CSF for oligoclonal bands is also useful in the appropriate clinical setting, because they are identified in greater than 90% of MS patients; however, their presence is not diagnostically specific because they can be detected in patients with such diverse disorders as neurosyphilis, CNS vasculitis, Lyme disease, subacute sclerosing panencephalitis, Jakob-Creutzfeldt disease, stroke, Guillain-Barre syndrome, and neoplasms (Karen, 1994). Serum protein electrophoresis must also be performed to ensure that CSF oligoclonal bands are not from serum leakage into the CSF. CSF oligoclonal bands are usually measured by high-resolution agarose electrophoresis of concentrated CSF (Karen, 1994).

Neuropathies

The focus of much recent attention is a group of neurologic syndromes affecting either the CNS or peripheral nervous system and associated with autoantibodies (Naparstek, 1993). These autoantibodies are detected either by ELISA, IIFM, or immunohistochemistry. The importance of identifying such autoantibodies will undoubtedly increase as/if clinical studies correlate their presence with either a particular disease or a therapeutic benefit. However, to date these autoantibodies are not disease specific and can even occur after trauma to the nervous system. Autoantibodies to primary neural components include those to neuronal proteins or to neuronal gangliosides (Zeballos, 1992).

Neuronal Protein Autoantibodies

5

A subgroup of patients with paraneoplastic cerebellar degeneration (PCD) have anti-Yo autoantibodies that are usually detected about the time a malignant neoplasm is discovered. Anti-Yo are detectable as cytoplasmic Purkinje cell fluorescence by using IIFM on human cerebellar tissue. Identification of anti-Yo in a patient with no known malignancy should initiate careful evaluation for a malignant neoplasm (Zeballos, 1992).

Anti-Ri are neuron-specific autoantibodies whose identification appears limited to patients with breast carcinoma and paraneoplastic opsoclonus (Zeballos, 1992). Anti-Ri are characterized by fluorescence of neuronal nuclei on IIFM. Anti-Hu are also neuron-specific autoantibodies visible as neuronal nuclear fluorescence on IIFM. These autoantibodies may be identified in patients with small cell lung carcinoma and paraneoplastic encephalomyelitis (Zeballos, 1992).

Neuronal Ganglioside Autoantibodies

Gangliosides are glycolipid components found in the outer membranes of peripheral nerve cells (Naparstek, 1993). Peripheral motor neuropathies may occur in patients with IgM monoclonal gammopathies whose IgM paraprotein reacts with the gangliosides GM1 or GD1b (Zeballos, 1992). Although anti-GM1 or anti-GD1b can be identified in a wide variety of neurologic syndromes, their presence in high titers is more characteristic of motor neuron disease than other alternatives (Zeballos, 1992).

OTHER ORGANS

Heart

Myocardial Autoantibodies

Autoantibodies to the myocardium have been reported as a part of several conditions that damage cardiac striated muscle, including myocardial infarction, post–cardiac surgery, and cardiomyopathies, although their identification may help differentiate immune-mediated cardiomyopathy from other causes of myocarditis (Burek, 1995; Naparstek, 1993). IIFM on frozen sections of monkey heart is used to detect myocardial autoantibodies. Specific myocardial staining can also be determined by excluding reactivity on noncardiac skeletal muscle. Unfortunately, AMAs and/or heterophile autoantibodies can cause fluorescent staining that may be confused with that by myocardial autoantibodies.

Muscle

Skeletal Muscle Autoantibodies

Skeletal muscle autoantibodies have limited clinical applicability. Low titers (<1:30) may be seen in apparently healthy individuals, whereas some patients with myopathic disorders may have titers up to 1:60. Although high titers (>1:60) of skeletal muscle autoantibodies have been found in patients with MG, anti-AChR assays have greater clinical utility in diagnosing or monitoring MG. Skeletal muscle autoantibodies are detected by IIFM on frozen sections of monkey thigh skeletal muscle.

SUMMARY

Organ-directed autoantibodies have an important role in the study of patients with organ-directed autoimmune disease(s). Detection of these autoantibodies may be important in diagnosis of some organ-directed autoimmune diseases, such as autoimmune thyroid disease, but more often they are supportive rather than essential for diagnosis. Similarly, although some of these autoantibodies are directly involved in pathogenesis of a disease, pemphigus, for example, often their presence is a marker of underlying immunologic injury attributable to another disease mechanism, as is the case in IDDM.

Newer techniques in molecular biology have disclosed, and will continue to do so, the specific nature of many antigens targeted by these autoantibodies. This work will hopefully elucidate underlying disease mechanisms, allowing improved diagnostic tests and perhaps new directions in therapy. Technical advances in ELISAs make this technology available in most clinical laboratories so that in the future many assays for organ-directed autoantibodies may be available where IIFM is not feasible. However, the performance of these tests will assuredly be guided by medical usefulness considerations and in part by economic considerations reflective of the clinical laboratory environment.

Atkinson MA, Kaufman D, Newman D, et al: Islet cell cytoplasmic autoantibody reactivity to glutamate decarboxylase in insulin-dependent diabetes. J Clin Invest 1993a; 91:350.

Atkinson MA, Maclaren NK: Islet cell autoantigens in insulin-dependent diabetes. J Clin Invest 1993b; 92:1608.

Atkinson MA, Maclaren NK: The pathogenesis of insulin-dependent diabetes mellitus. N Engl J Med 1994; 331:1428.

Bärmeier H, Ahlméen J, Landin-Olsson M, et al: Quantitative analysis of islet glutamic acid decarboxylase p64 autoantibodies in insulin-dependent diabetes mellitus. Autoimmunity 1992; 13:187.

Barna BP, Valenzuela R, Gupta MK: Laboratory analyses of cerebrospinal fluid. *In* Barna BP (ed): Laboratory Handbook of Neuroimmunologic Disease. Chicago, ASCP Press, 1987, p 65.

Barna BP, Gupta MK: Laboratory analyses of blood. *In* Barna BP (ed): Laboratory Handbook of Neuroimmunologic Disease, 1987th ed. Chicago, ASCP Press, 1995, p 106.

Bigazzi PE, Burek CL, Rose NR: Antibodies to tissue-specific endocrine, gastrointestinal, and surface-receptor antigens. *In* Rose NR, de Macario EC, Fahey JL, Friedman H, Penn GM (eds): Manual of Clinical Laboratory Immunology, 4th ed. Washington DC, American Society for Microbiology, 1992, p 765.

Brown WR, Claman HN, Strober W: Immunologic diseases of the gastrointestinal tract. *In* Frank MM, Austen KF, Claman HN, Unanue ER (eds): Samter's Immunologic Diseases, Vol. II, 5th ed. Boston, Little, Brown and Co., 1995.

Brunt LM: Immunologic disorders of the thyroid gland and autoimmune polyendocrinopathies. *In* Frank MM, Austen KF, Claman HN, Unanue ER (eds): Samter's Immunologic Diseases, Vol. II, 5th ed. Boston, Little, Brown and Co., 1995, p 975.

Burek CL, Rose NR: Autoantibodies. *In* Colvin RB, Bhan AK, McCluskey RT (eds): Diagnostic Immunopathology, 2nd ed. New York, Raven Press, 1995, p 207.

Bylund DJ, McHutchison J, Nakamura RM: Antimitochondrial antibodies in primary biliary cirrhosis. Clin Immunol Newsletter 1992; 12:1.

Camisa C, Helm TN: Paraneoplastic pemphigus is a distinct neoplasia-induced autoimmune disease [Editorial]. Arch Dermatol 1993; 129:883.

Crosby DL, Diaz LA: Autoimmune diseases of the skin. *In* Altman LC (ed): Immunology and Allergy Clinics of North America: Autoimmune Diseases, Vol. 13. Philadelphia, W. B. Saunders Co., 1993, p 395.

Diabetes Control and Complications Trial Research Group: The effect of intensive treatment of diabetes on the development and progression of long-term complications in insulin-dependent diabetes mellitus. N Engl J Med 1993; 329:977.

Domloge-Hultsch N, Bisalbutra P, Gammon WR, Yancey KB: Direct immunofluorescence microscopy of 1 mol/L sodium chloride-treated patient skin. J Am Acad Dermatol 1991; 24:946.

Eisenbarth GS, Castano L: Diabetes mellitus. *In* Frank MM, Austen KF, Claman HN, Unanue ER (eds): Samter's Immunologic Diseases, Vol. II, 5th ed. Boston, Little, Brown and Co., 1995, p 1007.

Falorni A, Grubin CE, Takei I, et al: Radioimmunoassay detects the frequent occurrence of autoantibodies to the Mr 65,000 isoform of glutamic acid decarboxylase in Japanese insulin-dependent diabetes. Autoimmunity 1994; 19:113.

Flotte TJ, Margolis RJ, Mihm MC, Jr: Skin. *In* Colvin RB, Bhan AK, McCluskey RT (eds): Diagnostic Immunopathology, 2nd ed. New York, Raven Press, 1995, p 123.

Gupta MK: Recent advances in laboratory tests for autoantibodies to thyrotropin receptor protein in Graves' disease. Clin Lab Med 1988; 8:303.

Hagopian WA, Karlsen AE, Gottsäter A, et al: Quantitative assay using recombinant human islet glutamic acid decarboxylase (GAD65) shows that 64K autoantibody positivity at onset predicts diabetes type. J Clin Invest 1993; 91:368.

Harrison LC, Campbell IL, Colman PG, et al: Type 1 diabetes: Immunopathology and immunotherapy. In Mazzaferri EL, Bar RS, Kreisberg RA (eds): Advances in Endocrinology and Metabolism, Vol. 1. St. Louis, MO, Mosby Year Book, 1990, p 35.

Helm KF, Peters MS: Deposition of membrane attack complex in cutaneous lesions of lupus erythematosus. J Am Acad Dermatol 1993; 28:687.

Heptinstall RH (ed): Pathology of the Kidney, 4th ed. Boston, Little, Brown and Co., 1992.

Izuno GT: Cutaneous immunofluorescence. Clin Lab Med 1986; 6:85.

Johnson PJ, McFarlane IG, Convenors on behalf of the panel: Meeting report: International Autoimmune Hepatitis Group. Hepatology 1993; 18:998.

Karen DF: Immunology and serology. *In* Jacobs DS, DeMott WR, Finley

PR, et al: (eds): Laboratory Test Handbook, 3rd ed. Hudson (Cleveland), Lexi-Comp, Inc., 1994, p 627.

Kaufman DL, Erlander MG, Clare-Salzer M, et al: Autoimmunity to two forms of glutamate decarboxylase in insulin-dependent diabetes mellitus. J Clin Invest 1992; 89:283.

Liu AY, Valenzuela R, Helm TN, et al: Indirect immunofluorescence on rat bladder transitional epithelium: A test with high specificity for paraneoplastic pemphigus. J Am Acad Dermatol 1993; 28:696.

Lühder F, Schlosser M, Mauch L, et al: Autoantibodies against GAD_{65} rather than GAD_{67} precede the onset of type 1 diabetes. Autoimmunity 1994; 19:71.

Mackay IR: Toward diagnostic criteria for autoimmune hepatitis. Hepatology 1993; 18:1006.

Maclaren N: Immunology of diabetes mellitus. Ann Allergy 1992; 68:5.

Maclaren NK: Perspectives in diabetes: How, when, and why to predict IDDM. Diabetes 1988; 37:1591.

Manns MP: Autoimmune diseases of the liver. Clin Lab Med 1992; 12:25.

McCluskey RT, Collins AB, Niles JL: Kidney. *In* Colvin RB, Bhan AK, McCluskey RT (eds): Diagnostic Immunopathology, 2nd ed. New York, Raven Press, 1995, p 109.

McFarland HF, McFarlin DE: Immunologically mediated demyelinating diseases of the central and peripheral nervous system. *In* Frank MM, Austen KF, Claman HN, Unanue ER (eds): Samter's Immunologic Diseases, Vol. II, 5th ed. Boston, Little, Brown and Co., 1995, p 1081.

Mooij P, Drexhage HA: Autoimmune thyroid disease. Clin Lab Med 1993; 13:683.

Muir A, Maclaren NK: Autoimmune diseases of the adrenal glands, parathyroid glands, gonads, and hypothalamic-pituitary axis. Endocrinol Metab Clin North Am 1991; 20:619.

Muir A, Schatz DA, Maclaren NK: Autoimmune Addison's Disease. Springer Semin Immunopathol 1993; 14:275.

Nakamura RM, Bylund DJ: Diagnostic significance of autoantibodies in autoimmune chronic active hepatitis. Clin Immunol Newsletter 1991; 11:161.

Naparstek Y, Plotz PH: The role of autoantibodies in autoimmune disease. Annu Rev Immunol 1993; 11:79.

Nordyke RA, Gilbert FI, Miyamoto LA, Fleury KA: The superiority of antimicrosomal over antithyroglobulin antibodies for detecting Hashimoto's thyroiditis. Arch Intern Med 1993; 153:862.

Palmer JP, Asplin CM, Clemons P, et al: Insulin antibodies in insulin-dependent diabetics before insulin treatment. Science 1983; 222:1337.

Patrick C: Organ-specific autoimmune diseases. Immunol Ser 1993; 58:423.

Peters MS, McEvoy MT: IgA antiendomysial antibodies in dermatitis herpetiformis. J Am Acad Dermatol 1989; 21:1225.

Rose JW, McFarlin DE: Myasthenia gravis. *In* Frank MM, Austen KF, Claman HN, Unanue ER (eds): Samter's Immunologic Diseases, Vol. II, 5th ed. Boston, Little, Brown and Co., 1995, p 1061.

Sarret Y, Hall R, Cobo LM, et al: Salt-split human skin substrate for the immunofluorescent screening of serum from patients with cicatricial pemphigoid and a new method of immunoprecipitation with IgA antibodies. J Am Acad Dermatol 1991; 24:952.

Schatz D, Krischer J, Horne G, et al: Islet cell antibodies predict insulin-dependent diabetes in United States school age children as powerfully as in unaffected relatives. J Clin Invest 1994; 93:2403.

Schatz D, Maclaren N: The natural history of pre-type I diabetes. Curr Opin Endocrinol Diabetes 1995; 2:31.

Song YH, Connor E, She JX, et al: Addison's disease and the type II autoimmune polyglandular syndrome: the 21-hydroxylase autoantigen. *In* Bhatt HR, James VHT, Besser GM, et al (eds): Advances in Thomas Addison's Diseases. Bristol, England, Journal of Endocrinology Limited, 1994.

Steinman L: Autoimmune disease. Sci Am 1993; 269(3):106.

Taylor S, Dean P, Riely C: Immunocholangitis: A study of seven patients. Mod Pathol 1993; 6:115A.

Teraki Y, Amagai N, Hashimoto T, et al: Intercellular IgA dermatosis of childhood. Selective deposition of monomer IgA1 in the intercellular space of the epidermis. Arch Dermatol 1991; 127:221.

Utiger RD: The pathogenesis of autoimmune thyroid disease. N Engl J Med 1991; 325:278.

Valenzuela R, Barna BP: Calculation of CNS IgG synthesis. *In* Barna BP (ed): Laboratory Handbook of Neuroimmunologic Disease. Chicago, ASCP Press, 1987, p 97.

VanArsdel PP, Jr: Autoimmune endocrinopathies. *In* Altman LC (ed): Immunology and Allergy Clinics of North America: Autoimmune Diseases, Vol. 13. Philadelphia, W. B. Saunders Co., 1993, p 371.

von Mühlen CA, Chan EKL, Peebles CL, et al: Nonmuscle myosin as target antigen for human autoantibodies in patients with hepatitis C virus-associated chronic liver diseases. Clin Exp Immunol 1995; 100:67.

Wilkin TJ: Mechanisms of disease: Receptor autoimmunity in endocrine disorders. N Engl J Med 1990; 323:1318.

Wilson CB: Immune aspects of renal diseases. JAMA 1987; 258:2957.

Zeballos RS, McPherson RA: Update of autoantibodies in neurologic disease. Clin Lab Med 1992; 12:61.

Zweiman B, Lisak RP: Autoantibodies: Autoimmunity and immune complexes. *In* Henry JB (ed): Clinical Diagnosis and Management by Laboratory Methods. 18th ed. Philadelphia, W. B. Saunders Co., 1991, p 885.

Chapter 44

Allergic Diseases

Henry A. Homburger, M.D.

The combined prevalence of allergic diseases in the United States is approximately 20%, and symptoms and signs of allergy are often difficult to distinguish clinically from other etiologies (Huang, 1993). For these reasons, clinicians often consider allergy (immediate hypersensitivity) as a possible etiology of disease in patients who present with diverse signs and symptoms. Appropriately selected laboratory tests are useful for evaluating patients with allergic diseases, but knowledge of the basic mechanisms of immediate hypersensitivity and awareness of the empirical relationships between test results and their diagnostic predictive values are needed to optimize the effectiveness of laboratory testing. This chapter addresses these subjects, beginning with an overview of the basic mechanisms of immediate hypersensitivity and proceeding to a detailed description of laboratory tests applied in the screening and diagnostic modes to evaluate different types of allergic diseases. Specific mention is made of those applications of laboratory testing that are not cost effective or may lead to incorrect clinical conclusions.

MECHANISMS OF IMMEDIATE HYPERSENSITIVITY

Regulation of IgE Synthesis: Immunogenetics and Cellular Interactions

Discovery in the late 1960s of a separate class of immunoglobulin in humans, immunoglobulin E (IgE), with potent reaginic (skin-sensitizing) properties marked the beginning of the current era of investigation into the molecular mechanisms of allergic diseases (Ishizaka, 1966a–c). At this time, much is known about events that occur at and within the cell membranes of IgE-sensitized effector cells that lead to the release of vasoactive mediators that directly cause the signs and symptoms of allergy. More recently, research has revealed some of the basic immune mechanisms that regulate the synthesis of IgE antibodies.

It is well known that genetic influences affect the likelihood that an individual will develop allergic disease. Genetically predisposed individuals are often called *atopic*, a synonym for the clinical allergic phenotype or allergic diathesis. Experimental evidence in animal models and humans suggests two levels of genetic control over the production of IgE and IgE antibodies. Although controversial, the results of population studies suggest that basal levels of IgE in blood are partly determined by a non-HLA–linked gene; high blood levels of total IgE protein result from recessive or codominant expression of an allele for "high" IgE synthesis (Borecki, 1985).

The second level of genetic control, control of the production of specific IgE antibodies, is better defined at the cellular and molecular levels, and is similar to that of other immunoglobulins. The ability of an individual to respond to an antigen by synthesizing specific antibodies is determined genetically by so-called immune response genes of the HLA-D region. The gene products of these highly polymorphic loci—the DR, DQ, and DP molecules of antigen-presenting cells (also called Ia molecules)—are responsible for binding processed antigen for presentation to immunocompetent T lymphocytes, thus initiating an antibody response (Bach, 1985; Korman, 1985; Trowsdale, 1985). Synthesis of specific antibodies (including IgE) to T-dependent antigens results from a series of cellular interactions that involve both cognate (cell-to-cell contact) and noncognate signalling between cells. Several steps are involved. Initially, antigen is metabolized by an antigen-presenting cell, for example, a dendritic cell or macrophage, and the "processed" antigen is displayed on the surface of the cell in an antigen-binding groove comprised of surface Ia molecules and processed fragments of the native antigen. Cognate interaction between the processed antigen–Ia complex of an antigen-presenting cell and specific antigen receptors on a complementary population of helper/inducer T lymphocytes (Th cells) promotes activation of the Th cells, secretion of cytokines, and clonal expansion of the responding lymphocytes (Unanue, 1987). The same antigen may also be bound by antibodies expressed constitutively on the plasma membranes of antigen-specific B lymphocytes; and these cells that process antigen by internalizing the antibody–antigen complex are capable of metabolizing and presenting processed antigen (in an Ia–antigen complex) to Th cells with complementary receptors. Once again, following cognate interaction and secretion of cytokines, there is clonal expansion of antigen-specific B lymphocytes followed by the synthesis and secretion of specific antibodies (Fig. 44–1).

The paradigm outlined earlier describes common mechanisms that promote the synthesis of specific IgG and IgE antibodies, but certain mechanisms pertinent to the IgE response are important to mention. These mechanisms promote clonal expansion of IgE-B lymphocytes and isotype switching with expression of mature C_ϵ transcripts. B lymphocytes require two activating signals to initiate the synthesis of specific antibodies (Vercelli, 1989). One signal is delivered as a result of cognate interaction between complementary Th cells and B lymphocytes that display processed antigen. These B lymphocytes, however, require a second signal to initiate transcription of rearranged C_ϵ mRNA. In the case of IgE, the second signal is delivered by interleukin-4 (IL-4), a cytokine produced by a subset of Th lymphocytes (Vercelli, 1989b). Neither signal alone is sufficient to induce synthesis of IgE antibodies, although IL-4 alone promotes expression of germline but not rearranged C_ϵ transcripts by resting B lymphocytes. IL-4 along with IL-3, IL-5, and granulocyte-macrophage–colony stimulating factor (GM-CSF) is produced by a subset of Th lymphocytes called Th2 cells (Mosmann, 1986; Parronchi, 1991). The effects of IL-4 are antagonized by γ interferon, which along with IL-2 is produced by a second subset of Th lymphocytes called Th1 cells. The cytokine products of these two Th subsets have opposing influences on IgE synthesis. Other cytokines also influence IgE synthesis. The cytokines IL-5 and IL-6 promote the synthesis of IgE antibodies by committed B lymphocytes, but neither is sufficient to deliver an "activating" signal to initiate isotype switching with production of mature C_ϵ transcripts (Vercelli, 1989c).

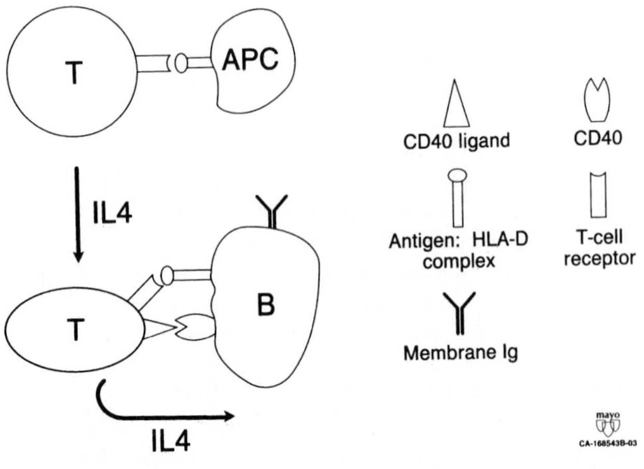

Figure 44–1. Cognate and noncognate interactions of antigen-presenting cells (APC), T-helper/inducer cells, and B cells promote activation and clonal expansion of IgE-B cells (see text for explanation).

Several other signalling mechanisms may play a role in the synthesis and secretion of IgE antibodies, but the physiologic importance of these experimental mechanisms is less well defined. Epstein-Barr virus (EBV) in combination with IL-4 promotes IgE synthesis in the absence of T lymphocytes, although EBV alone is not a sufficient stimulus. In addition, engagement of the surface glycoprotein CD40 on B lymphocytes by anti-CD40 monoclonal antibodies promotes IgE synthesis in the presence of IL-4. The gene encoding CD40 has been cloned and resembles the gene for nerve growth factor, but the natural ligand for CD40 has not yet been identified and the role of CD40 engagement in promoting the synthesis of IgE *in vivo* is unclear (Jabara, 1990; Zhang, 1990).

Structural Characteristics of IgE

The first demonstration that human IgE antibodies possess reaginic activity and are different from other immunoglobulins was by the Ishizakas (Ishizaka, 1966a–c). These investigators raised rabbit antisera to a reagin-rich immunoglobulin fraction isolated from the serum of an atopic patient. After absorption with purified immunoglobulins of all the known isotypes (IgG, IgA, IgM, and IgD), the antiserum still reacted with γ_1-globulin present in the serum of allergic patients. After immunoprecipitation with this antiserum, the skin-sensitizing activity of serum from different atopic patients was abolished.

Conclusive evidence of the immunochemical uniqueness and reaginic activity of IgE was obtained somewhat later when it was discovered that human myeloma proteins reacted with the above-mentioned antiserum (Bennich, 1969). Experiments performed with isolated immunoglobulin fragments prepared by enzymatic digestion of IgE myeloma proteins indicated conclusively that skin-sensitizing activity required an intact $F_{C\epsilon}$ region and that the antigenic determinants unique to IgE molecules were contained on the $F_{C\epsilon}$ fragment (Bennich, 1971). The physicochemical properties and immunologic functions of different regions of the IgE molecule, as determined by experiments performed with purified human IgE myeloma proteins and immunoglobulin fragments prepared by enzymatic digestion, are summarized in Table 44–1. The structure of human IgE is shown diagrammatically in Figure 44–2.

Human IgE antibodies sensitize skin to release histamine, a phenomenon referred to as *passive cutaneous anaphylaxis*. The skin-sensitizing activity of IgE is heat labile; heating at 56°C for two hours irreversibly modifies the $C_\epsilon3$ and $C_\epsilon4$ domains of the IgE molecule and abolishes skin-sensitizing activity (Ishizaka, 1967). Binding to effector cells is also

Table 44–1. PHYSICOCHEMICAL PROPERTIES OF IMMUNOGLOBULIN E

H chain class	ϵ
Molecular formula	ϵ_2L_2
Sedimentation coefficient(s)	8
Molecular weight	190,000
Carbohydrate (%)	11.7
Antigenic determinants	$D_\epsilon 1$, $D_\epsilon 2$, $D_\epsilon 3$
Complement fixation (classic)	None
Serum half-life (days)	2
Placental transfer	None
Reaginic activity	4+; Fc-containing fragments inhibit skin-sensitizing activity of native IgE, but Fab-containing fragments do not

abolished by reduction and alkylation of inter–ϵ-chain disulfide bonds. Aggregated human IgE does not fix complement by the classical pathway, and there is no significant placental transfer of human IgE.

Release of Mediators from IgE-Sensitized Effector Cells

Mast cells and basophils are the principal effector cells of immediate hypersensitivity reactions. Both types of cells contain histamine in preformed cytoplasmic granules that stain prominently with metachromatic, basic dyes (Siraganian, 1988). Mast cells and basophils develop in the bone marrow from pluripotent stem cells, a process that is stimulated by IL-3 (Schrader, 1986). Basophils that circulate in blood are short lived, terminally differentiated cells, whereas mast cells that are found in tissues in proximity to blood vessels and in connective tissues adjacent to epithelia of the respiratory tract, gastrointestinal tract, and skin are long-lived cells capable of proliferating in response to mitogenic stimuli. Mast cells are heterogeneous but typically contain up to 10-fold more total histamine per cell than basophils.

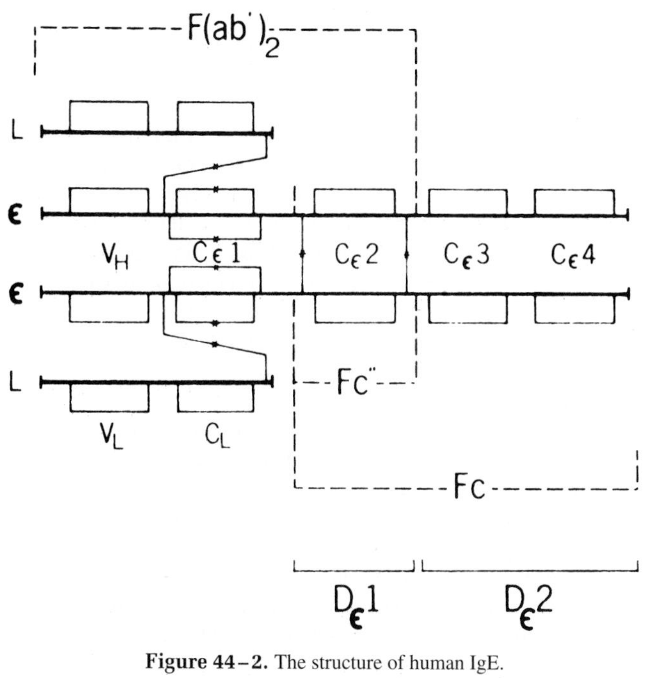

Figure 44–2. The structure of human IgE.

The primary mechanism of release of histamine from mast cells and basophils involves transmembrane signalling mediated by cell surface (homocytotropic) IgE antibodies and specific, high-affinity receptors for IgE ($F_{C\epsilon}$ RI) located diffusely on plasma membranes of effector cells. Binding of IgE antibodies to $F_{C\epsilon}$ RI is reversible but of very high affinity ($Ka = 10^{10}$ M^{-1}) (Wank, 1983). While IgE antibodies in blood have a half-life of only two to three days, the half-life of IgE antibodies in skin bound to $F_{C\epsilon}$ RI on mast cells is estimated to be more than 10 days. It is estimated that the number of receptors per cell ranges from 40,000 to 500,000. Higher numbers of receptors are found on basophils cultured in the presence of IgE, possibly reflecting upregulation of $F_{C\epsilon}$ RI expression by IgE. $F_{C\epsilon}$ RI is a multimetric receptor, composed of α, β, and γ subunits as follows: α_1, β_1, γ_2. IgE antibodies are bound by the α subunit; the β and γ subunits contain transmembrane regions that function in transmembrane signalling (Ravetch, 1991).

$F_{C\epsilon}$ RI molecules are mobile within the plasma membranes of sensitized cells, as indicated by capping studies performed with fluorescein-conjugated anti-IgE antibodies. This mobility over short distances is believed to be important for the release of mediators from mast cells and basophils. Extensive studies with basophils and mast cells sensitized *in vitro* with IgE myeloma proteins or with specific IgE antibodies have shown that cross-linking (or bridging) of occupied IgE receptors by multivalent antigens or by intact anti-IgE antibodies or their $F(ab')_2$ fragments triggers release of histamine, but univalent haptens or Fab fragments of anti-IgE antibodies do not. The importance of receptor cross-linking has also been demonstrated by studies performed with antibodies raised to the $F_{C\epsilon}$ RI. Intact antibodies to $F_{C\epsilon}$ RI cause the release of histamine, but Fab fragments do not. Taken together, these results strongly suggest that bridging of adjacent receptors is important in initiating release of histamine (Siraganian, 1975). According to the "bridging hypothesis," IgE antibodies play a passive role in eliciting the release of vasoactive mediators. The initial signal for mediator release is provided by the cross-linking of $F_{C\epsilon}$ RI by a multivalent allergen, with IgE serving as a bridge.

Despite experimentation in model systems, the critical molecular pathways that follow bridging of $F_{C\epsilon}$ RI and that lead to the release of histamine from sensitized cells are not well defined. For purposes of this discussion, it is sufficient to mention that $F_{C\epsilon}$ RI–mediated transmembrane signalling in mast cells and basophils probably involves several steps, including mobilization of Ca^{2+} from intracellular stores and from extracellular sources through formation of Ca^{2+} channels; activation of GTP binding proteins coupled to $F_{C\epsilon}$ RI molecules, which leads to activation of protein kinases and methyl transferases coupled to $F_{C\epsilon}$ RI; activation of adenylate cyclase with increased intracellular cyclic AMP production; and hydrolysis of inositol-containing phospholipids by activation of phospholipases A_2 and C, which generates diacyl glycerol and, following further hydrolysis, arachidonic acid (Siraganian, 1993).

These steps are important for two reasons: Multiple signals are important for mediator release from mast cells and basophils, and pharmacologic treatment of allergic diseases often involves the use of drugs that interfere with these signalling mechanisms. For example, cromolyn used in the treatment of asthma interferes with release of mediators from mast cells by blocking the formation of Ca^{2+} channels, and corticosteroids interfere with signalling mediated by $F_{C\epsilon}$ RI by inhibiting enzyme-mediated hydrolysis of phospholipids (Mazurek, 1984). In addition, it is known that arachidonic acid released from basophils and mast cells following activation of cellular phospholipases is the substrate for enzymes of the 5-lipoxygenase and cyclo-oxygenase metabolic pathways, which lead, respectively, to the synthesis and secretion of leukotrienes and prostaglandin mediators of inflammation (Fig. 44–3) (Lewis, 1981). Leukotriene B4 and prostaglandin D2 promote the movement of leukocytes, including eosinophils, and they stimulate aggregation, enzyme release, and generation of superoxide in neutrophils. Leukotrienes C4, D4, and E4 are released from many types of cells, including lung, peritoneal, and bone marrow–derived mast cells, macrophages, eosinophils, and basophil leukocytes. These mediators promote bronchoconstriction, increased vascular permeability in postcapillary venules, and increased mucus secretion. They may also mediate the reversible loss of pulmonary compliance observed in human asthma. On a molar basis, leukotrienes are many times more potent than histamine, making them prime mediators of the inflammatory effects that characterize immediate hypersensitivity reactions (Samuelsson, 1983).

Another newly discovered lipid mediator of inflammation, called *platelet-activating factor* (PAF), is a substituted glycerol derivative generated from phospholipids following cellular activation. PAF causes anaphylaxis when administered in small doses to animals, and the human analogue is believed to be released from neutrophils and alveolar macrophages. The biological effects of PAF that occur during anaphylaxis include aggregation and degranulation of platelets, contraction of smooth muscle, and increased capillary permeability (Barnes, 1988).

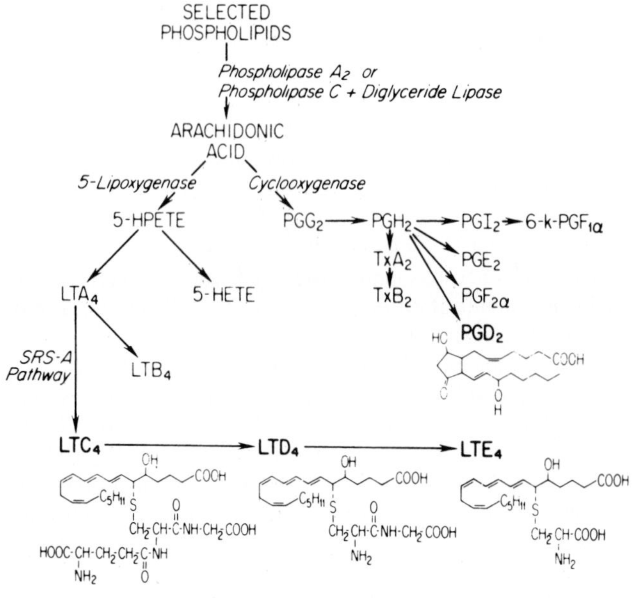

Figure 44–3. Arachidonic acid metabolism by the 5-lipoxygenase and cyclo-oxygenase pathways.

LABORATORY EVALUATION OF ALLERGIC DISEASES

Allergic disease is a significant public health problem. As noted earlier, it is estimated that up to 20% of adults suffer from some form of chronic allergic disease. Because many atopic individuals develop allergies during childhood, the prevalence of allergic diseases among children provides another estimate of the magnitude of the overall medical problem. Asthma affects approximately 5% of children of school age, and other less disabling allergic diseases, such as allergic rhinitis and eczema, affect approximately 15% and 5% of children, respectively. According to one review, minor allergic diseases affect nearly 40% of all children in the United States.

Relatively few laboratory tests are used routinely by clinicians in the evaluation of allergic diseases. Tests for IgE protein and for allergen-specific IgE antibodies are the mainstays. Before discussing the details of these tests, it is important to point out that the usefulness of each test is determined by the clinical context in which it is applied. In the field of clinical allergy, tests for IgE protein and IgE antibodies are ordered principally for diagnosis and less often for prognostic assessment, or as an aid in therapeutic management. The usefulness of test results in each situation is determined empirically by whether or not it is difficult to establish an accurate diagnosis of allergic disease or to decide on a particular therapeutic regimen on clinical grounds alone. In children and adults, immediate hypersensitivity may be the primary mechanism of disease or a contributory factor; and while it is frequently possible to establish the presumptive diagnosis of an allergic disease on clinical grounds, definitive diagnosis and management often require that the offending allergen(s) be identified unequivocally. This is particularly important in instances of severe allergic disease that occur in individuals without an atopic background or a family history of allergic disease.

The word *atopy* (or *atopic*) is widely used in the clinical allergy literature to refer to individuals with a family history of allergic disease who have demonstrable sensitivity to a variety of allergens. These individuals are referred to here as having an allergic phenotype. Non-atopic individuals may also suffer from allergic diseases and may develop clinically significant immediate hypersensitivity reactions to allergens they encounter repeatedly in the environment. The distinguishing characteristic of the atopic individual is a tendency to develop sensitivity to a variety of allergens encountered under routine environmental conditions (Hoekelman, 1974). Clinical atopy exists on a continuum with normality.

It is not possible to discuss the use of laboratory tests in the diagnosis and management of allergic diseases without comparing them to *in vivo* tests of immediate hypersensitivity, particularly the skin test and end-organ challenge tests. *In vivo* tests are often considered the standards of diagnostic accuracy and reliability. The ability to reproduce a specific allergic reaction by *in vivo* challenge is regarded as the most sensitive technique for demonstrating the presence of immediate hypersensitivity and for defining its specificity.

Skin tests are performed by intradermal injection and by the skin prick methods (Bousquet, 1993). The response to intradermal injection of an allergen extract is graded by measuring the diameter of the wheal and erythema reaction immediately following the injection. A 1 + reaction corresponds to a 5 to 10 mm wheal. A response of this magnitude is usually regarded as evidence for specific sensitivity to an allergen. Highly sensitive individuals often develop wheal diameters greater than 15 mm with pseudopods. Skin tests performed by the prick method make use of more concentrated allergen extracts, up to 1000-fold greater concentrations than are used for intradermal testing, and grading is often omitted. Mean wheal diameters in millimeters are recorded as an indication of the degree of sensitivity. A more quantitative estimate of sensitivity to a given allergen can be obtained by the technique of end-point titration. This technique is a modification of the intradermal and skin prick methods. Serial, 10-fold dilutions of a standardized allergen extract are utilized beginning with the most dilute solution. The endpoint of sensitivity is defined as the greatest dilution that produces a 1 + reaction.

End-organ challenge tests are useful clinically and for investigative purposes. Adaptations of this technique include the bronchial provocation test in the diagnosis of asthma; the rhinoconjunctival challenge test in the diagnosis of allergic rhinitis; the food elimination and challenge test in the diagnosis of food-induced asthma, urticaria, and malabsorption; and the sting challenge in the diagnosis of anaphylactic sensitivity to insect venom (Naclerio, 1993). The application of challenge tests in routine clinical situations is limited by the requirement for well-standardized allergen extracts of defined potency and by the limited number of allergens that can be tested in an individual on a single occasion. As an example, food elimination and challenge procedures require periods of abstinence of several days, during which time inadvertent consumption of a particular food may invalidate the test.

An important obstacle to precise diagnosis in the field of clinical allergy is the lack of available allergen extracts of uniform potency and defined composition (Bousquet, 1995). Except for certain examples, such as well-studied weeds, grasses, mites, and molds, the chemical constituents that elicit allergic reactions have not been characterized for many recognized allergens. Despite the efforts of manufacturers to produce standardized materials, different lots of the same allergen often vary in potency by as much as an order of magnitude.

Several techniques have been used to quantitate the potency of allergens in clinical use, including measurement of protein nitrogen content, skin test end-point titration, radial immunodiffusion with specific animal antisera, and inhibition of binding of specific IgE antibodies by soluble allergen *in vitro* (Gleich, 1974). Inhibition of binding of specific IgE antibodies by allergens in aqueous solution is an excellent method for comparing allergen extracts. The potency of an allergen extract is inversely related to the dose of soluble allergen required to inhibit the binding of IgE antibodies in a positive control serum to a fixed amount of solid-phase–coupled allergen. The qualitative, antigenic similarity of different lots of allergen and the amount of allergen present can be estimated by comparing the slopes and ED_{50} of the dose-inhibition curves. Different lots of allergen that contain the same qualitative mixture of allergenic constituents yield parallel dose-inhibition lines when the percent of inhibition is plotted against the dose of soluble allergen extract. The *in vitro* inhibition method is useful to compare the potency and antigenic characteristics of both purified allergens and allergen mixtures.

IgE Protein: Measurement Methods, Normal Values, and Clinical Usefulness

A variety of immunochemical methods are available commercially to measure IgE in serum, including solid-phase displacement radioimmunoassay, double-antibody radioimmunoassay, solid-phase sandwich radioimmunoassay, solid-phase sandwich enzyme immunoassay, and nephelometry (Homburger, 1993). The newer nonisotopic methods are the most popular. Each of these immunoassay methods is capable of detecting IgE in serum at concentrations as low as 0.5 U/mL (1.2 ng/mL). The sandwich immunoassay methods use a common analytic approach; polyclonal or monoclonal anti-IgE antibody, coupled covalently to a solid phase, is incubated with an aliquot of serum or standard, and the bound IgE is detected by incubating with radiolabeled, affinity purified, or monoclonal anti-IgE antibody, or with anti-IgE antibody conjugated with an enzyme. The concentration of IgE in serum specimens is calculated by comparison with a standard curve. Maximum analytical sensitivity is achieved in the range of 7.5 to 50 U IgE/mL. Lesser concentrations can be measured by sandwich methods, but the ability to detect small changes in concentration in the range of 0.5 to 4 U/mL is diminished compared with higher concentrations (Fig. 44–4).

There have been a number of clinical studies of the serum concentrations of IgE in healthy (nonallergic) subjects. In all studies, there are consistent trends in the development of IgE levels with age and in the frequency distributions of observed IgE concentrations in healthy adults irrespective of

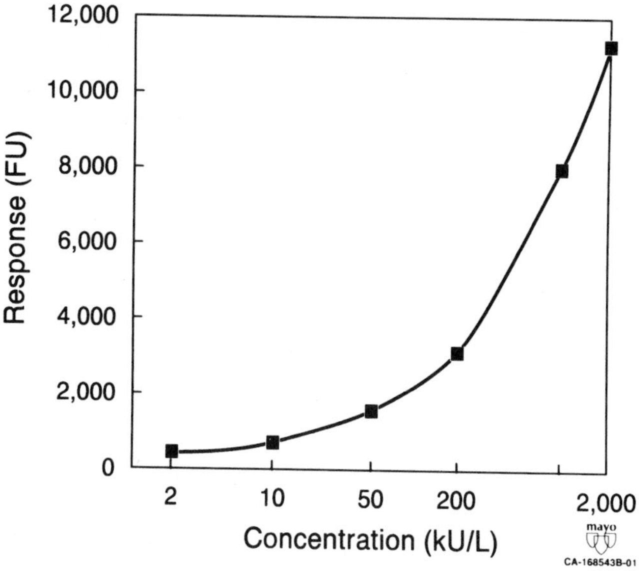

Figure 44–4. Dose-response curve for measurement of IgE by commercial fluorescence enzyme immunoassay. FU = fluorescence units.

the analytical method (Homburger, 1986). The frequency distribution of IgE concentrations in healthy adults is positively skewed with wide 95 percentile limits and a disproportionate number of low IgE values. In calculating the 95 percentile limits of normal, most investigators have treated their data by logarithmic transformation, thus yielding upper limits of normal that are seemingly very high when compared with the arithmetic means (Barbee, 1981). As noted later, these high upper limits of normal serve to diminish the diagnostic sensitivity of the serum IgE test as a screening test for clinical allergy when the upper limit of normal is used as a cut-off value.

Synthesis of IgE in the human fetus has been observed as early as the 11th week of gestation in fetal lung and liver tissue, yet cord serum contains virtually no detectable IgE. The mean concentration of IgE in cord serum is less than 1 U/mL (Kimpen, 1989). The concentrations of IgE in maternal sera and in cord sera are not correlated, indicating that there is no appreciable placental transfer of maternal IgE. The finding of specific IgE antibodies to cow's milk in cord sera, but not in maternal sera, indicates that intrauterine sensitization may occur and supports the conclusion that the IgE protein detected in cord serum is of fetal origin.

Serum concentrations of IgE in children increase slowly with development and reach adult levels at approximately five to seven years of age (Homburger, 1986a). Several clinical studies have shown a somewhat higher average serum concentration of IgE in children ages 10 to 14 years than in adults over the age of 20. The clinical significance of this finding is not clear. No differences were observed between the IgE levels in boys and girls at similar ages. In individuals over 70 years of age, there is a tendency toward somewhat lower average IgE levels than in young adults less than 40 years of age.

The measurement of IgE protein in serum has been thoroughly evaluated for its clinical usefulness in the diagnosis of various allergic diseases, for its predictive value as an indicator of the likelihood of the development of allergic disease in asymptomatic infants and children, and as a prognostic indicator in adults with certain types of chronic allergic diseases. Measurement of IgE is also valuable in the evaluation of patients suspected of having immunodeficiency diseases, parasitic diseases, or the rare hyper-IgE syndrome.

The hyper-IgE syndrome was first described in 1972 by Buckley and colleagues, who reported on two patients with greatly elevated serum IgE levels, diffuse dermatitis and recurrent furunculosis, and pneumonia with pneumatoceles secondary to *Staphylococcus aureus*. Subsequent reports of patients with this disorder have defined the clinical syndrome: elevations of serum IgE levels are extreme (2000 to 50,000 U/mL), and patients have blood and tissue eosinophilia and strongly positive immediate wheal and flare reactions to inhalant allergens, pollens, foods, and bacterial and fungal antigens. Despite these findings, asthma is not common in patients with the hyper-IgE syndrome (Buckley, 1978).

The synthesis of IgE, as reflected by serum levels, has been studied in patients with a variety of primary immunodeficiency diseases. Increased IgE levels have been described in association with incomplete deficiencies of cellular immunity, including the Wiskott-Aldrich syndrome, partial DiGeorge's syndrome, and thymic alymphoplasia (Nezelof's syndrome) (Buckley and Fiscus, 1975). Immunodeficiency diseases in which there is complete absence of synthesis of immunoglobulins G, A, and M, such as severe combined immunodeficiency disease, characteristically show diminished IgE synthesis and markedly decreased serum IgE levels. Serum IgE levels are variable in patients with IgA deficiency; ataxia telangiectasia patients typically have diminished levels, but patients with isolated IgA deficiency may have normal or modestly increased levels (Buckley, 1975). Allergic disease is not common in patients with immunodeficiency diseases, with the exception of those individuals with selective IgA deficiency who have elevated levels of serum IgE. Increased IgE synthesis in patients with the hyper-IgE syndrome or with partial deficiencies of cellular immunity presumably reflects increased secretion by IgE-producing B lymphocytes that have escaped regulatory control by T lymphocytes.

Parasitic infiltration of the gastrointestinal tract or parenchymatous organs stimulates IgE synthesis markedly, and studies in laboratory animals suggest that specific IgE antibodies are important in the host defense against parasites such as *Nippostrongylus brasiliensis* and *Schistosoma mansoni* (Mulligan, 1965). Serum IgE concentrations greater than 1000 U/mL are regularly found in children in areas of endemic infestation with parasites. Other parasitic diseases are known to be associated with increased serum IgE levels, including visceral larva migrans (*Toxocara canis*), intestinal capillariasis (*Capillaria philippinensis*), schistosomiasis, ankylostomiasis, and echinococcosis. In patients with intestinal parasitic disease, the serum levels of IgE have been noted to decrease considerably following successful treatment with antiparasitic drugs.

In reviewing the usefulness of the serum IgE level as a diagnostic test for allergic disease, it is appropriate to discuss its use in children and adults separately. Elevated IgE levels in serum at birth or during infancy often antedate the development of clinical allergy (Kjellman, 1984). Serum IgE levels above the 95th percentile limit for age were described in 75% of children with a biparental family history of allergic disease; and among healthy children with IgE levels more than 1 SD above the mean for a given age, the incidence of development of allergic diseases during the following 18 months was increased more than 10-fold compared with a group with lower IgE levels. Although predictive of future development of allergic disease, these data provide relatively little information upon which to base specific clinical decisions.

The diagnosis of allergic disease in infants is complicated by the fact that rhinorrhea is the commonest initial manifestation of allergy in this age group, but respiratory infections are common during infancy and may be impossible to distinguish from allergic rhinitis on clinical grounds. Nevertheless, because allergic disease of early onset seems to be associated with more severe clinical manifestations, it is important to establish the diagnosis of allergy as early as possible. The principal value of the IgE measurement in infants appears to be to alert the physician to the likely possibility of an allergic disease when the presumptive clinical diagnosis is otherwise. Serum IgE levels greater than 20 U/mL in such cases support the diagnosis of an allergic disease; but, a normal IgE level does not exclude the diagnosis of allergic disease during infancy or later in life, and the results of other diagnostic tests, such as tests for IgE antibodies, should be taken into consideration in excluding the diagnosis of allergic disease. In those clinical situations in which the presenting signs of allergic disease are unequivocal, for example, eczema and rhinitis in an infant with an atopic family history, the serum IgE level provides little additional information.

The situation is quite similar in older children. Measurement of IgE protein in serum has limited diagnostic sensitivity for allergic disease when the upper limit of the normal range is used as a diagnostic cut-off. In general, children with hypersensitivity to several different allergens and multiple allergic diseases have elevated serum levels, and those with hypersensitivity to fewer allergens and limited end-organ involvement usually have normal levels (Berg, 1969). This point is illustrated by the data in Table 44–2. Diagnostic sensitivity is greatest in patients with clinical sensitivity to a number of different allergens.

In atopic children, the presence of cutaneous disease and gastrointestinal manifestations increase the likelihood that the serum IgE level will be elevated (Havnen, 1973). There is also evidence to suggest that the frequency of elevated serum IgE levels is greater in children with hypersensitivity to food and pollen allergens than in children with hypersensitivity to house dust or mold allergens (Berg, 1969). Children with allergic diseases that involve several organs also tend to have elevations in serum IgE of greater magnitude than those with more limited disease; extreme elevations occur most often in patients with cutaneous manifestations. The diagnostic specificity of an elevated IgE level for allergic disease is excellent. The association is so strong, in fact, that asymptomatic children with elevated IgE levels are sometimes referred to as *pre-allergic*, reflecting the assumption that they will develop signs of clinical allergy in the future.

The measurement of serum IgE protein is of modest diagnostic usefulness in most adults suspected of having an allergic disease. The results of clinical studies of adult respiratory allergy indicate that approximately 50% of adults with extrinsic asthma and fewer than 5% of adults with so-called, intrinsic (non-atopic) asthma have elevated serum IgE levels (Wittig, 1980). Asthmatic adults with hypersensitivity to a limited number of allergens usually have normal levels. The highest IgE levels in adults typically occur in those patients with hypersensitivity to several allergens and combinations of asthma, atopic dermatitis, and rhinitis. Just as in children, the limited diagnostic sensitivity of the serum IgE level limits the clinical usefulness of IgE measurements in those situations in which the diagnosis of allergic disease is most uncertain (Klink, 1990). This is not to say, however, that serum IgE should not be measured in such cases for an elevated level carries a high predictive value for allergic disease.

The levels of serum IgE have received particular attention in children and adults with atopic dermatitis. The mechanisms involved in the pathogenesis of atopic dermatitis are largely unknown, but the finding of very high IgE levels in most patients with atopic dermatitis and active disease has prompted several investigations of the relationship between disease activity and the IgE level. Although there is no consensus, some studies indicate that fluctuations in the severity of cutaneous manifestations parallel similar changes in the serum IgE level (Wüthrich, 1978). Causal relations, if they exist, remain obscure.

Allergic bronchopulmonary aspergillosis is also associated with marked elevations in serum levels of IgE. This disease typically occurs in patients with extrinsic asthma, generally of long duration. The levels of IgE in serum are elevated in nearly every patient with allergic aspergillosis during times of acute pulmonary infiltration, but IgE levels may fluctuate considerably during the course of the disease. A normal IgE level in a patient with active lung disease virtually excludes this diagnosis (Imbeau, 1978).

Allergen-Specific IgE Antibodies: Measurement Methods, Scoring of Results, and Clinical Usefulness

Skin testing and end-organ challenge testing are established procedures for detecting IgE antibodies *in vivo*, as noted previously. *In vitro* methods are also available to detect IgE antibodies in serum and on basophil granulocytes; the principal methods are the specific IgE antibody test and the leukocyte histamine release test, respectively. The leukocyte histamine release test was first described more than 50 years ago. Peripheral blood leukocytes isolated by dextran sedimentation are washed and resuspended in buffer containing Ca^{2+} and Mg^{2+} ions. Varying concentrations of an allergen extract are then added to a fixed number of washed leukocytes, and the mixture is incubated at 37°C for one hour. The reaction is stopped by chilling the tubes to 4°C, and the cells are separated by centrifugation. Histamine secreted from basophils as a consequence of the interaction of allergen with cell-bound IgE antibodies is released into the supernatant fluid and is isolated by extraction with butanol then acid. The concentration of histamine in the extract is measured fluorometrically or by specific immunoassay. The fluorometric procedure, performed manually, detects approximately 1 ng of

5

Table 44–2. INCIDENCE OF ELEVATED SERUM IgE CONCENTRATIONS IN ALLERGIC ASTHMATIC CHILDREN AGES TWO TO 16 YEARS WITH DIFFERENT COMBINATIONS OF ALLERGIC DISEASES

Diagnosis	No. of Children in Each Group	No. of Children with Elevated Serum IgE	Incidence of Elevated Serum IgE (%)
Asthma only	22	3	14
Asthma and rhinoconjunctivitis only	33	13	39
Asthma and atopic dermatitis plus other hypersensitivity diseases	70	41	58
Asthma and urticaria plus other hypersensitivity diseases	75	46	61
Asthma and urticaria and atopic dermatitis plus other hypersensitivity diseases	24	12	50
Asthma and gastrointestinal allergy plus other hypersensitivity diseases	13	11	84

histamine. The immunoassay method is somewhat more sensitive. Results are expressed as a percent of the total cellular histamine released; total histamine is determined on acid lysates of leukocytes not exposed to the allergen extract (Lichtenstein, 1964).

The results of leukocyte histamine release testing define the specificity of cell-bound IgE antibodies and indicate the functional integrity of the mediator-releasing mechanisms. Approximately 15% of individuals have leukocytes that do not release histamine *in vitro*. Although automated systems have been developed for the measurement of histamine, the histamine release test has found limited clinical application because of the requirement for fresh blood cells and the limited number of allergens that can be tested using a single aliquot of blood. At the present time, the histamine release test is more widely used in research than for clinical applications.

The IgE antibody test, originally called the radioallergosorbent test (RAST), is a sandwich immunoassay analogous in principle to the indirect Coombs' test. A serum specimen to be tested for IgE antibodies is reacted with allergen coupled to a solid-phase support material. After the initial incubation, non-antibody serum components are washed away, and the allergen-immunosorbent is incubated with labeled affinity chromatography purified or monoclonal anti-IgE antibody in the second stage of the assay. Specific IgE antibodies bound in the first stage of the assay are revealed by labeled anti-IgE antibody bound to the solid-phase allergen complex in the second stage of the assay (Gleich, 1975).

The actual concentrations of IgE antibodies are not determined by these techniques. In sera from many allergic individuals, the concentrations of IgE antibodies exceed the binding capacity of the allergen-immunosorbents, and first-stage incubation supernatants contain residual quantities of specific IgE antibodies. Nevertheless, over a limited range of concentrations, the binding of second-stage antibody increases in direct proportion to the concentration of IgE antibodies in serum. Because the IgE antibody test is often performed in antibody excess, the final binding reflects both the quantity and the affinity of the antibodies present (Schellenberg, 1975).

As first described by Wide and colleagues (1967), the IgE antibody test employed allergens coupled covalently to Sephadex beads. A variety of other solid-phase materials have been used subsequently, including cellulose particles, agarose beads, filter paper discs, and polystyrene microtiter plates. Many of these support materials can be activated chemically to form labile intermediates that react with allergens in aqueous solution to form covalently coupled immunosorbents. Binding of allergens to microtiter plates is by noncovalent adsorption. For clinical purposes, the solid-phase allergen-immunosorbent should contain all the allergenic constituents present in the fluid extract, in the same proportions as the original allergen extract. Although it is possible to monitor the coupling of total protein to the immunosorbents, few data are available to determine whether all the relevant protein allergens have been coupled for many clinically important allergen systems.

A wide range of allergens is available for IgE antibody testing. The reagents may be purchased in kit form or serum may be sent to a reference laboratory for analysis. The various classes of allergens available include animal epithelia, foods, pollens of trees, grasses and weeds, molds, dusts, insect venoms, drugs, and occupational allergens. Most drugs are low molecular weight compounds that cannot be coupled readily to a solid phase by the usual chemical methods. Some macromolecular drugs, such as insulin can be coupled to produce satisfactory reagents. In the case of penicillin, the penicilloyl group can be conjugated to polylysine or to a protein carrier, which in turn can be coupled to an appropriate solid phase for use in the IgE antibody test (Wide, 1971). Analogous reagents are not available for detection of IgE antibodies to the so-called minor antigenic determinants of penicillin, which are responsible for some acute anaphylactic reactions to this drug.

There is no uniform convention for reporting the results of IgE antibody tests. Several commercial methods use a scoring system that derives results for patients' specimens from comparison to a reference dose-response curve made from serial dilutions of a positive control (Fig. 44–5). In an effort to maximize the analytic sensitivity of these methods, results greater than the 0.35 IU/mL standard are considered positive. The concentration of IgE antibodies can be expressed either as IU/mL or in classes numbered 0 through V or VI. Most clinicians are more familiar with the class-based scoring systems, but, regardless of the system used to express results, it should be noted that results are semi-quantitative and borderline or weakly positive results may occur as a result of analytic variability (Jacob, 1982). Sera with markedly elevated levels of IgE protein also may yield false-positive results, presumably because of increased nonspecific binding of IgE. This phenomenon usually does not occur unless the concentration of IgE exceeds 1000 IU/mL, which is often the case in patients with atopic dermatitis or multiple allergic diseases. False-negative results caused by inhibition of binding of IgE antibodies may occur in some analytical systems as a result of competition for allergen binding sites by IgG antibodies. These antibodies have affinities similar to IgE anti-

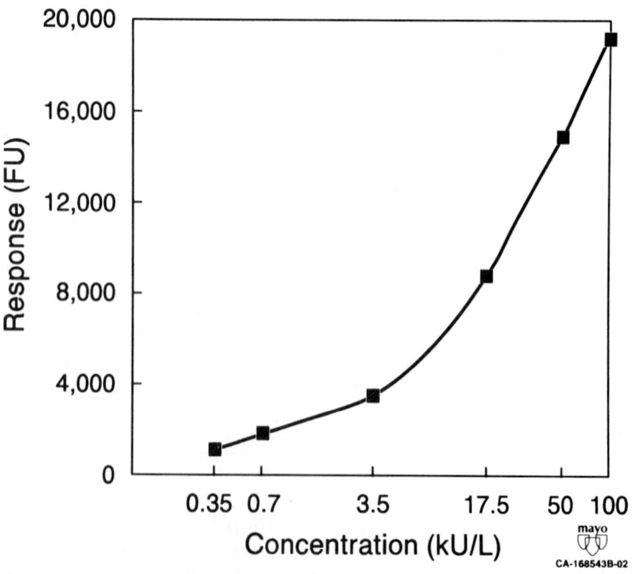

Figure 44–5. Dose-response curve for measurement of IgE antibodies by commercial fluorescence enzyme immunoassay. FU = fluorescence units.

bodies and usually are present in microgram per milliliter concentrations in the sera of patients treated with allergen immunotherapy (Paull, 1978). Since measurements of IgE antibodies are not useful in treated patients to determine whether residual clinical sensitivity exists, it follows that this problem usually occurs when the IgE antibody test is used inappropriately.

The analytical sensitivity of the IgE antibody test is determined in part by the labeled anti-IgE antibody used in the second stage of the assay. Commercial radiolabeled, affinity purified anti-IgE antibodies function well as detection proteins and enable the measurement of nanogram quantities of specific IgE antibodies. Labeled monoclonal anti-IgE antibodies are also available commercially. In an effort to circumvent the need for radiolabeled anti-IgE antibodies, immunoassays that employ enzyme-conjugated antibodies have been developed by most commercial manufacturers. The analytical characteristics of these methods are similar to the older radioimmunometric methods.

Recommendations for clinical use of the IgE antibody test are based upon the results of clinical studies in which the sensitivity and specificity of IgE antibody results were compared with other diagnostic tests. In some cases, the decision to seek to identify the specific allergens responsible for clinical signs is tempered by knowledge that the therapy will be no different if the offending allergens are identified. This latter point is important in many patients in whom treatment is based upon the use of drugs that inhibit the release of inflammatory mediators, produce bronchodilatation, or suppress inflammation. Nevertheless, in most allergic individuals, knowledge of the offending allergens is useful clinically to decide which allergens should be used in an immunotherapy regimen, as in patients with allergic rhinitis or insect venom sensitivity, or to facilitate avoidance of an allergen in cases of anaphylactic sensitivity to food or drugs.

It is difficult to define the absolute diagnostic sensitivity and specificity of IgE antibody results because there is no universally accepted reference method for defining sensitivity to a given allergen. However, in most clinical studies the results of IgE antibody tests have been compared with the results of *in vivo* diagnostic tests and the allergic disease histories. It is clear from such studies that the diagnostic sensitivity varies greatly depending upon the elapsed time between exposure to an allergen and testing, the class of allergen tested, the age of the patient, and the affected target organs (Homburger, 1986a). For the purposes of this chapter, it is useful to consider the following clinical applications separately: allergic respiratory disease, food allergy, insect venom sensitivity, and drug or occupational allergy.

Since cell-associated IgE antibodies mediate allergic respiratory disease, it is reasonable to regard the results of end-organ challenge tests as a standard for determining sensitivity to a given allergen. Several studies in adults with asthma or allergic rhinitis have shown excellent overall agreement between the results of provocation tests and IgE antibody tests performed with inhalant allergens, including pollens of trees, grasses and weeds, molds, and mites. The results of skin tests and IgE antibody tests also agreed in most cases. Most discordant results were weakly positive skin tests in patients with negative IgE antibody tests (Wide, 1967).

Among children with allergic respiratory diseases, the results of IgE antibody tests and provocation tests also agreed in most cases. Once again, most discordant results occurred in children with positive provocation tests to highly concentrated allergen extracts. Excellent agreement was found in children with moderate or severe allergy, and in those children with negative provocation tests. As these results illustrate, the diagnostic sensitivity of the IgE antibody test to inhalant allergens varies directly with the magnitude of clinical sensitivity in patients with respiratory allergies (Berg, 1974).

It is also pertinent to ask how well IgE antibody results agree with skin tests in cases of suspected respiratory allergy. In the studies mentioned earlier, if the results of skin tests done by the prick method were used to define sensitivity to an allergen, many more discordant results were obtained. The IgE antibody test was negative in many patients with weakly positive skin tests, but positive results were obtained in approximately 90% of patients with strongly positive skin tests. In general, better correlations have been seen with pollen allergens and purified allergens, while lesser degrees of correlation were observed with dust or mold allergens.

Advocates of the skin test maintain that data such as these indicate that skin testing is a more sensitive diagnostic method, while supporters of the IgE antibody test point out that a high percentage of weakly positive skin tests are not validated by positive challenge tests. The argument is somewhat academic; either diagnostic method is reliable in patients with marked sensitivity to an allergen and neither is completely reliable for identifying slight degrees of clinical sensitivity. It is in the latter situation that the two methods may actually provide complimentary diagnostic information.

Testing for IgE antibodies has certain advantages compared with skin testing: It poses no risk to the patient, and the results are not influenced by concomitant treatment with antihistamines or bronchodilators. In addition, IgE antibody testing may be preferable to skin testing in certain groups of patients, such as infants, patients with dermographism, or patients with widespread dermatitis. There are also disadvantages. Serologic testing is expensive if done indiscriminately, and the results are not available immediately. Recently, the multi-allergen IgE antibody test performed with immunosorbents that have more than one allergen coupled to their surface has been shown to be a sensitive and cost-effective screening test for inhalant allergy, but further studies are needed to document the usefulness of this test as a screening test in other clinical situations (Ownby, 1984).

Hypersensitivity to foods is manifested by a variety of clinical signs in infants, children, and adults, including eczema and dermatitis, rhinitis and bronchospasm, angioedema, urticaria, and rarely anaphylaxis. The measurement of IgE antibodies can be useful in such cases, but there are potential pitfalls in interpreting the results of these tests that should be emphasized. In determining all but anaphylactic sensitivity to a particular food, the use of the double-blind food challenge is considered the diagnostic standard (Bock, 1980). Nevertheless, tests for IgE antibodies are useful to select allergens for double-blind challenge testing and to confirm the history. Positive IgE antibody results are assumed to be clinically significant if the results are supported strongly by the clinical history. Unlike allergies to inhalants, however, the incidence of false-positive results (detectable IgE antibodies to foods not shown to be associated with clinical signs) is considerable, particularly in children.

Sensitivity to foods is often considered in the differential diagnosis of skin disease, gastrointestinal disease, or respiratory disease in infants and young children, and it is generally believed that the likelihood of developing allergic symptoms to food allergens is greater during infancy and childhood than in later life (Foucard, 1973). The most commonly encountered food-specific IgE antibodies in infants and young children are to protein allergens of cow's milk and eggs. The principal protein allergens in cow's milk are α-lactalbumin, β-lactoglobulin, bovine albumin, and casein. The relationship between IgE antibodies to these proteins and the manifestations of cow's milk allergy is established, but measurable IgE antibodies occur in many atopic children who are tolerant of cow's milk. The IgE antibody test to cow's milk cannot be relied upon to establish the diagnosis of milk intolerance due to hypersensitivity (Liebman, 1981).

The results of tests for IgE antibodies are much more specific and have higher positive predictive values in cases of anaphylactic sensitivity or angioedema caused by food allergens, for example, allergy to fish or nuts. In one published study, the authors found at least one positive IgE antibody result in 100% of children with anaphylactic food sensitivity, 96% of children with asthma, and 92% of children with angioedema. In these instances, the IgE antibody test is more useful because the clinical history often incriminates particular foods as allergens (Hoffman, 1974).

The IgE antibody test is used commonly to investigate the specificity of food allergen sensitivity in patients with atopic dermatitis. As noted earlier, skin testing may be impossible to perform in patients with diffuse skin disease or dermographism. The interpretation of test results in patients with atopic dermatitis is complicated by the fact that these individuals often have concomitant asthma and rhinitis with extreme elevations of serum IgE. In such cases, it is not unusual to find low levels of IgE antibodies to a multiplicity of allergens. Clinically important specificities are defined by positive results several classes greater than the low level positive results. It is often possible to define allergen specificity in such patients by a careful process of dietary elimination combined with IgE antibody testing.

IgE antibody testing is useful in the diagnosis of suspected sensitivity to *Hymenoptera* venom(s). Individuals sensitive to the venoms of honeybees, yellow jackets, hornets, or wasps typically manifest signs of anaphylaxis following a sting; urticaria, angioedema, bronchospasm, or cardiovascular collapse may ensue. The reported death rate from sting-induced systemic reactions is 30 to 40 cases annually, but this figure probably underestimates the true incidence. The natural history of untreated venom sensitivity is not completely known. In many patients with documented anaphylactic sensitivity, it is possible to elicit a clinical history of progressively more severe reactions to successive sting episodes. On the other hand, venom sensitivity apparently ameliorates spontaneously in some individuals. The decision to treat a patient with venom immunotherapy is based upon clinical assessment of the risk of anaphylaxis to possible future stings.

The most reliable indicator of venom sensitivity is the response to a deliberate sting challenge (Parker, 1982). However, this test is not widely performed and is rarely required in previously untreated patients to establish the diagnosis of venom sensitivity. Venom skin tests and IgE antibody tests are useful to confirm the impression that clinical sensitivity does exist and to define its specificity. In this clinical situation, most studies indicate that skin testing is a more sensitive diagnostic modality (Sobotka, 1978). Venom IgE antibody tests are useful primarily to confirm the results of skin tests and to define the allergen specificity of venom hypersensitivity.

With the exception of the sting challenge, there is no *in vitro* or *in vivo* test that reliably predicts the clinical response to an insect sting in a treated patient following venom immunotherapy. Although the levels of IgG antibodies in serum increase markedly with venom immunotherapy, no cut-off level has been defined that can be used to identify those patients who are no longer at risk. Semiquantitative estimates of IgG antibodies are not useful clinically, and the levels of IgE antibodies following treatment bear no relationship to the clinical status.

Measurements of IgE antibodies have also been applied to the diagnosis of drug hypersensitivity. Although many drugs and their metabolites are capable of eliciting synthesis of antibodies, clinical data and the results of specific antibody measurements are available only for the penicillins and their metabolites. Penicillin and its isomer, penicillenic acid, combine with serum proteins through amide linkages. The penicilloyl–protein conjugate is the major antigenic determinant, and the penicillenic acid–protein conjugate is a minor antigenic determinant (Fig. 44–6). Measurable levels of IgM and IgG antibodies specific for the penicilloyl determinant occur commonly in penicillin-treated patients, and although high titers of these antibodies persist in plasma for relatively short periods, lower titers can often be detected years after treatment (Shepherd, 1991).

Attempts to diagnose hypersensitivity to penicillin have relied on skin testing with penicillin, penicilloyl-polylysine, and a minor antigen mixture. Positive skin test results occur infrequently, especially when testing is done remotely following treatment with penicillin. Fewer than 30% of patients with probable histories of immediate penicillin hypersensitivity have positive skin tests, and immediate hypersensitivity reactions to penicillin therapy are rare in patients with negative skin tests. Using the results of skin tests as a diagnostic reference, clinical studies have reported finding measurable IgE antibodies to the penicilloyl determinant in nearly 100% of patients with positive skin tests. Antipenicilloyl antibodies are undetectable in control subjects. On the basis of these data, it is reasonable to recommend *in vitro* testing for penicilloyl-IgE antibodies only in patients with histories of recent hypersensitivity reactions. False-negative results may occur immediately following IgE-mediated reactions; and, although most published data indicate that false-negative results are rare, the absence of specific antibodies to penicilloyl-polylysine does not entirely exclude the possibility of clinically significant IgE antibodies to other penicillin metabolites (Weiss, 1988).

Allergic diseases, particularly asthma, may also be caused by a wide variety of allergens encountered in the workplace. Asthma may result from both allergic and nonallergic mechanisms. The list of etiologic agents associated with allergic,

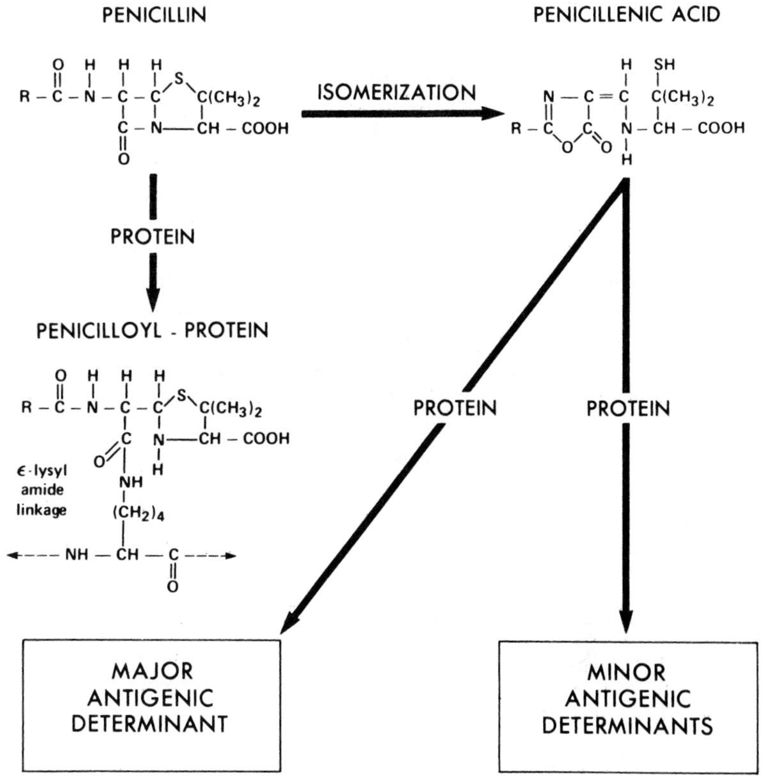

Figure 44–6. Metabolites of penicillin, major and minor antigenic determinants. (From Rose NR, De Macario EC, Fahey JL, et al [eds]: Manual of Clinical Laboratory Immunology, 4th ed. Washington DC, American Society for Microbiology, 1992, p 719; with permission.)

occupational asthma is long and includes the following: animal proteins, enzymes, plant proteins, legumes, anhydrides, metallic salts, dyes, diisocyantes, and wood dusts. Testing for IgE antibodies is available for several of these allergens. Recently, attention has been focused on latex rubber as an allergen in the health care workplace and in certain patients, for example, patients with spina bifida who have undergone several surgical procedures. Testing for IgE antibodies to latex rubber is useful for identifying sensitizing individuals (Yunginger, 1994).

In concluding this section on the IgE antibody test, it is appropriate to summarize some of the major points made earlier. The measurement of IgE antibodies is useful and can be recommended in the following clinical situations: (1) the evaluation of children and adults suspected of having allergic respiratory disease to establish the diagnosis and to define the specificity of allergen sensitivity to pollens, dusts, fungal antigens, and foods; (2) to confirm the clinical impression of sensitivity to specific foods in patients with anaphylactic sensitivity or with asthma and angioedema; (3) to evaluate sensitivity to insect venom allergens, particularly as an aid in defining venom specificity in those cases in which skin tests are equivocal; (4) to confirm the diagnosis of penicillin hypersensitivity in patients with anaphylactic sensitivity; and (5) to confirm the presence of IgE antibodies to certain occupational allergens, for example, latex rubber. Testing for IgE antibodies is not useful as a screening test for allergic disease, except as performed by the multi-allergen analytic method; and results are not useful in evaluating the effects of immunotherapy or in excluding the diagnosis of anaphylactic sensitivity to insect venoms in treated patients. Tests for IgE antibodies are most useful when performed in patients who have had a thorough medical history and physical examination.

Tests for Mediators of Immediate Hypersensitivity Reactions and for Allergen-Specific IgG Antibodies

In an earlier section, several mediators of immediate hypersensitivity reactions, including histamine and the lipid mediators called leukotrienes and platelet activating factor, were reviewed. Each of these mediators promotes inflammation in human allergic diseases or in animal models of allergy and anaphylaxis. These mediators induce many of the characteristic biological effects of allergic reactions. Despite these findings, measurements of these mediators in body fluids are of limited usefulness clinically in the differential diagnosis of allergic diseases. Measurements of histamine in plasma or urine are of value in patients with anaphylaxis when tests are performed immediately following an anaphylactic episode (Friedman, 1989). The leukotrienes and platelet activating factor are active locally and are present in minute concentrations in body fluids (Lewis, 1984).

Another class of inflammatory mediators of interest in allergy are the anaphylatoxic peptides of complement, C3a, C4a, and C5a, generated during activation of the complement cascade (see Chap. 36). The role of these peptides as mediators of inflammation in allergic disease is not well established. Human anaphylatoxins probably are not generated by interaction of allergen and IgE antibodies. Nevertheless, because C5a elicits contraction of smooth muscle and enhances vascular permeability, there is rationale for further investigation of the complement anaphylatoxins as inflammatory mediators in syndromes of anaphylaxis.

Antibodies of the IgE isotype sensitize human basophils and mast cells for long periods of time, at least 24 hours, and these antibodies directly mediate antigen-induced histamine release, as noted earlier. In several species of animals, IgG antibodies of one or more subclasses also bind to effector cells and promote the release of histamine. An analogous role for human IgG antibodies is not well established. Some experimental data suggest that human IgG antibodies of the IgG_4 subclass bind to basophil leukocytes and may mediate histamine release, and the concentration of IgG_4 protein in serum is often above-normal in adults with asthma (Homburger, 1986b). Nevertheless, clinical studies have failed to show a role for measurement of IgG_4 protein or IgG_4 antibodies in the diagnosis or prognostic assessment of patients with asthma.

Bach FH: The HLA class II genes and products: The HLA-D region. Immunol Today 1985; 6:89.

Barbee RA, Halonen M, Lebowitz M, et al: Distribution of IgE in a community population sample: Correlations with age, sex, and allergen skin test reactivity. J Allergy Clin Immunol 1981; 68:106.

Barnes PJ, Chung KF, Page CP: PAF and asthma. J Allergy Clin Immunol 1988; 81:152.

Bennich H, Johansson SGO: Structure and function of human immunoglobulin E. Adv Immunol 1971; 13:1.

Bennich H, Ishizaka K, Ishizaka T, et al: A comparative antigenic study of e-globulin and myeloma-IgND. J Immunol 1969; 102:826.

Berg T, Johansson SGO: IgE concentrations in children with atopic diseases: A clinical study. Int Arch Allergy Appl Immunol 1969; 36:219.

Berg TLO, Johansson SGO: Allergy diagnosis with the radioallergosorbent test: A comparison with the results of skin and provocation tests in an unselected group of children with asthma and hay fever. J Allergy Clin Immunol 1974; 54:209.

Bock SA: Food sensitivity: A critical review and practical approach. Am J Dis Child 1980; 134:973.

Borecki IB, Rao DC, Lalouel JM, et al: Demonstration of a common major gene with pleiotropic effects on immunoglobulin E levels and allergy. Genetic Epidemiol 1985; 2:327.

Bousquet J, Michel FB: In vivo methods for study of allergy: Skin tests, techniques, and interpretation. *In* Middleton E, Jr, Reed CE, Ellis EF, Adkinson NF, Jr, Yunginger JW, Busse WW (eds): Allergy: Principles and Practice, 4th ed, Vol. 1. St. Louis, MO, Mosby-Year Book, 1993, p 573.

Bousquet J, Michel FB: Standardization of allergens. *In* Spector S (ed): Provocative Challenges in Clinical Practice, 1st ed. New York, Marcel Dekker, 1995, p 15.

Buckley RH: Clinical and immunologic features of selective IgA deficiency. Birth Defects 1975; 11:134.

Buckley RH, Becker WG: Abnormalities in the regulation of human IgE synthesis. Immunol Rev 1978; 41:288.

Buckley RH, Fiscus SA: Serum IgD and IgE concentrations in immunodeficiency diseases. J Clin Invest 1975; 55:157.

Buckley RH, Wray BB, Belmaker EZ: Extreme hyperimmunoglobulinemia E and undue susceptibility to infection. Pediatrics 1972; 49:59.

Foucard T: A follow-up study of children with asthmatoid bronchitis. I. Skin test reactions and IgE antibodies to common allergens. Acta Paediatr Scand 1973; 62:633.

Friedman BS, Steinberg S, Meggs WJ, et al: Analysis of plasma histamine levels in patients with mast cell disorders. Am J Med 1989; 87:649.

Gleich GJ, Jones RT: Measurement of IgE antibodies by the radioallergosorbent test. II. Analyses of quantitative relationships in the test. J Allergy Clin Immunol 1975; 55:346.

Gleich GJ, Larson JB, Jones RT, et al: Measurement of the potency of allergy extracts by their inhibitory capacities in the radioallergosorbent test. J Allergy Clin Immunol 1974; 53:158.

Havnen J, Amlie PA, Hvatum, et al: IgE concentrations in allergic asthma in children. Arch Dis Child 1973; 48:850.

Hoekelman RA: Allergy in childhood: A pediatrician's viewpoint. Pediatr Clin North Am 1974; 21:5.

Hoffman DR, Haddad ZH: Diagnosis of IgE mediated immediate hypersensitivity reactions to food antigens by radioimmunoassay. J Allergy Clin Immunol 1974; 54:165.

Homburger HA: Diagnosis of allergy: In vitro testing. CRC Crit Rev Clin Lab Sci 1986a; 23:279.

Homburger HA, Mauer K, Sachs ML, et al: Serum immunoglobulin G_4 concentrations and allergen specific IgG_4 antibodies compared in asthmatic adults, asthmatic children and nonallergic subjects. J Allergy Clin Immunol 1986b; 77:427.

Homburger HA, Katzmann JA: Methods in laboratory immunology, principles and interpretation of laboratory tests for allergy. *In* Middleton E, Jr, Reed CE, Ellis EF, et al (eds): Allergy: Principles and Practice, 4th ed, Vol. 1. St. Louis, MO, Mosby-Year Book, 1993, p 554.

Huang SK, Marsh DG: Immunogenetics of allergic disease. *In* Middleton E, Jr, Reed CE, Ellis EF, et al (eds): Allergy: Principles and Practice, 4th ed, Vol. 1. St. Louis, MO, Mosby-Year Book, 1993, p 60.

Imbeau SA, Nichols D, Flaherty D, et al: Allergic bronchopulmonary aspergillosis. J Allergy Clin Immunol 1978; 62:243.

Ishizaka K, Ishizaka T: Physicochemical properties of reaginic antibody. I. Association of reaginic activity with an immunoglobulin other than γA- or γG-globulin. J Allergy 1966a; 37:169.

Ishizaka K, Ishizaka T: Physicochemical properties of reaginic antibody. III. Further studies on the reaginic antibody in γA-globulin preparations. J Allergy 1966b; 38:108.

Ishizaka K, Ishizaka T, Lee EH: Physicochemical properties of reaginic antibody. II. Characteristic properties of reaginic antibody different from human γA-isohemagglutinin and γD-globulin. J Allergy 1966c; 37:336.

Ishizaka K, Ishizaka T, Menzel AEO: Physicochemical properties of reaginic antibody. VI. Effect of heat on γE-, γG-, and γA-antibodies in the sera of ragweed sensitive patients. J Immunol 1967; 99:610.

Jabara HH, Fu SM, Geha RS, et al: CD40 and IgE: synergism between anti-CD40 mAb and IL-4 in the induction of IgE synthesis by highly purified human B cells. J Exp Med 1990; 172:1861.

Jacob GL, Homburger HA: The analytical accuracy of specific IgE antibody results determined by a blind proficiency survey. J Allergy Clin Immunol 1982; 69:110.

Kimpen J, Callaert H, Embrechts P, et al: Influence of sex and gestational age on cord blood IgE. Acta Paediatr Scand 1989; 78:233.

Kjellman NIM, Croner S: Cord blood IgE determination for allergy prediction—a follow-up to seven years of age in 1,651 children. Ann Allergy 1984; 53:167.

Klink M, Cline MG, Halonen M, et al: Problems in defining normal limits for serum IgE. J Allergy Clin Immunol 1990; 85:440.

Korman AJ, Boss JM, Spies T, et al: Genetic complexity and expression of human class II histocompatibility antigens. Immunol Rev 1985; 85:45.

Lewis RA, Austen KF: Mediation of local homeostasis and inflammation by leukotrienes and other mast cell-dependent compounds. Nature (London) 1981; 293:103.

Lewis RA, Austen KF: The biologically active leukotrienes: Biosynthesis, metabolism, receptors, functions, and pharmacology. J Clin Invest 1984; 73:889.

Lichtenstein LM, Osler AG: Studies on the mechanisms of hypersensitivity phenomena. IX. Histamine release from human leukocytes by ragweed pollen antigen. J Exp Med 1964; 120:507.

Liebman WM, Frick OL: Serum IgE levels and RAST for cow's milk protein: Use in children with recurrent abdominal pain. Am J Dis Child 1981; 135:741.

Mazurek N, Schindler H, Schürholz T, et al: The cromolyn binding protein constitutes the Ca^{2+} channel of basophils opening upon immunological stimulus. Proc Natl Acad Sci USA 1984; 81:6841.

Mosmann TR, Cherwinski H, Bond MW, et al: Two types of murine helper T-cell clone. I. Definition according to profiles of lymphokine activities and secreted proteins. J Immunol 1986; 136:2348.

Mulligan W, Urquhart GM, Jennings FW, et al: Immunological studies on *Nippostrongylus brasiliensis* infection in the rat: The "self-cure" phenomenon. Exp Parasitol 1965;16:341.

Naclerio RM, Norman PS, Fish JE: In vivo methods for the study of allergy: Bronchial challenge testing. *In* Middleton E, Jr, Reed CE, Ellis EF, et al (eds): Allergy: Principles and Practice, 4th ed, Vol. I. St. Louis, MO, Mosby-Year Book, 1993, p 613.

Ownby DR, Anderson JA, Jacob GL, et al: Development and comparative evaluation of a multiple-antigen RAST as a screening test for inhalant allergy. J Allergy Clin Immunol 1984; 73:466.

Parker JL, Santrach PJ, Dahlberg MJE, et al: Evaluation of Hymenoptera sting sensitivity with deliberate sting challenges: Inadequacy of present diagnostic methods. J Allergy Clin Immunol 1982; 69:200.

Parronchi P, Macchia D, Piccinni MP, et al: Allergen- and bacterial antigen-specific T-cell clones established from atopic donors show a different profile of cytokine production. Proc Natl Acad Sci USA 1991; 88:4538.

Paull BR, Jacob GL, Yunginger JW, et al: Comparison of binding of IgE and IgG antibodies to honeybee venom phospholipase-A. J Immunol 1978; 120:1917.

Ravetch JV, Kinet JP: Fc receptors. Annu Rev Immunol 1991; 9:457.

Samuelsson B: Leukotrienes: Mediators of immediate hypersensitivity reactions and inflammation. Science 1983; 220:568.

Schellenberg RR, Adkinson NF, Jr: Measurement of absolute amounts of antigen-specific human IgE by a radioallergosorbent test (RAST) elution technique. J Immunol 1975; 115:1577.

Schrader JW: The panspecific hemopoietin of activated T lymphocytes (interleukin-3). Annu Rev Immunol 1986; 4:205.
Shepherd GM: Allergy to β-lactam antibiotics. Immunol Allergy Clin North Am 1991; 11:611.
Siraganian RP: Mast cells and basophils. *In* Gallin JI, Goldstein IM, Snyderman R (eds): Inflammation: Basic Principles and Clinical Correlates. New York, Raven Press, 1988.
Siraganian RP: Mechanism of IgE-mediated hypersensitivity. *In* Middleton E, Jr, Reed CE, Ellis EF, et al (eds): Allergy: Principles and Practice, 4th ed, vol I. St. Louis, MO, Mosby-Year Book, 1993, p 105.
Siraganian RP, Hook WA, Levine BB: Specific *in vitro* histamine release from basophils by bivalent haptens: Evidence of activation by simple bridging of membrane bound antibody. Immunochemistry 1975; 12:149.
Sobotka AK, Adkinson NF, Jr, Valentine MD, et al: Allergy to insect stings. IV. Diagnosis by radioallergosorbent test (RAST). J Immunol 1978; 121:2477.
Trowsdale J, Young JAT, Kelly AP, et al: Structure sequence and polymorphism in the HLA-D region. Immunol Rev 1985; 85:5.
Unanue ER, Allen PM: The basis for the immunoregulatory role of macrophages and other accessory cells. Science 1987; 236:551.
Vercelli D, Geha RS: Regulation of IgE synthesis in man. J Clin Immunol 1989a; 9:75.
Vercelli D, Jabara HH, Arai K, et al: Induction of human IgE synthesis requires interleukin 4 and T/B cell interactions involving the T-cell receptor/CD3 complex and MHC class II antigens. J Exp Med 1989b; 169:1295.
Vercelli D, Jabara HH, Arai K, et al: Endogenous IL-6 plays an obligatory role in IL-4 induced human IgE synthesis. Eur J Immunol 1989c; 19:1419.
Wank SA, DeLisi C, Metzger H: Analysis of the rate-limiting step in a ligand-cell receptor interaction: The immunoglobulin E system. Biochemistry 1983; 22:954.
Weiss ME, Adkinson NF: Immediate hypersensitivity reactions to penicillin and related antibiotics. Clin Allergy 1988; 18:515.
Wide L, Juhlin L: Detection of penicillin allergy of the immediate type by radioimmunoassay of reagins to penicilloyl conjugates. Clin Allergy 1971; 1:171.
Wide L, Bennich H, Johansson SGO: Diagnosis of allergy by an in vitro test for allergen antibodies. Lancet 1967; 2:1105.
Wittig HG, Belloit J, De Fillippi I, et al: Age-related serum immunoglobulin E levels in healthy subjects and in patients with allergic disease. J Allergy Clin Immunol 1980; 66:305.
Wüthrich B: Serum IgE in atopic dermatitis: Relationship to severity of cutaneous involvement and course of disease as well as coexistence of atopic respiratory diseases. Clin Allergy 1978; 8:241.
Yunginger JW: Update 18: Allergy to natural rubber latex. *In* Middletown E, Jr, Reed CE, Ellis EF, et al: (eds): Allergy: Principles and Practice, 4th ed. St. Louis, MO, Mosby-Year Book, 1994, p 1–10.
Zhang K, Clark EA, Saxon A: CD40 stimulation provides an IFN γ-independent and IL-4 dependent differentiation signal directly to human B cells for IgE production. J Immunol 1990; 146:1836.

Chapter 45

Diagnosis and Management of Cancer Using Serologic Tumor Markers

James T. Wu, Ph.D.

There are a large number of tumor markers present in the blood circulation. Because the blood level of serum tumor markers usually reflects the change of tumor volume and tumor activities, the measurement of serologic tumor markers has become an attractive means for the detection and diagnosis of neoplastic diseases, as well as the monitoring of their course, especially during treatment. The ease of blood sampling and the sensitivity of these noninvasive tumor marker assays also make the serologic tests far superior to other clinical examinations based on physical methods. In Chapter 15, oncogene proteins and growth factors are reviewed as early markers for malignant tumors. In this chapter, other types of tumor markers are presented.

NEOPLASM AND GROWTH REGULATION

In order to learn how to identify, select, and use tumor markers for the diagnosis of cancer and the management of cancer patients, it is imperative that one be familiar with the fundamentals of neoplastic processes. It is important to keep in mind that there are two major processes involved in cell growth: differentiation and proliferation. In normal cells both processes are well regulated and are under rigid control. When any one or both of these processes loses regulation, the risk increases for normal cells to turn into tumor cells (Fig. 45–1). In fact, whenever there is new growth involving tissues, it is important to differentiate between two possible causes of the new growth: hyperplasia or neoplasia. The major difference between these two similar processes is also related to growth control. Hyperplasia serves a useful purpose and is controlled by stimuli, whereas neoplasia is unregulated and serves no purpose. Therefore, it should be understood that unregulated proliferation is a fundamental feature of all neoplastic cells, regardless of whether the tumor is benign or malignant. The result of uncontrolled proliferation will then lead to the formation of an abnormal mass of tissue, the so-called tumor. Consequently, the tumor will continue to grow in an unregulated manner, even after the stimuli that evoked the change are removed. Benign tumors will remain at the primary site and present less risk to the host. Benign tumors also have a much better chance of being successfully treated by a complete removal. However, the genetic instability associated with tumor cells makes them more susceptible to additional mutations, which may lead eventually to a malignant disease (Fig. 45–2). Specific mechanisms by which mutations cause neoplastic transformation are reviewed in Chapter 15. Oncogenic mutations result in the production of abnormal proteins involved in mitogenic signal transduction pathways, as summarized in Figures 15–1 and 15–2. Malignant tumors are usually associated with a poor prognosis and short survival time because of their ability and tendency to spread and metastasize.

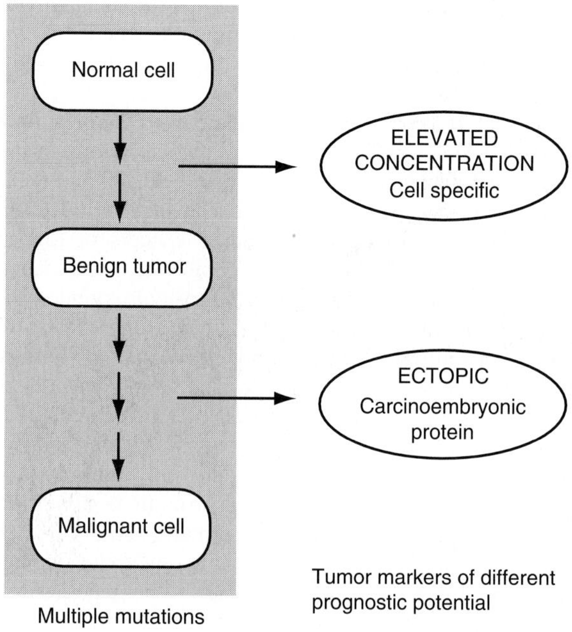

Figure 45–1. Illustration of how normal cells, after multiple mutations, are converted to malignant cells. The rectangle for "BENIGN TUMOR" indicates that the development of some malignant tumors may not have to go through the benign state. In the chart, tumor markers of different prognostic potentials also relate to the tumor cells at different developmental stages.

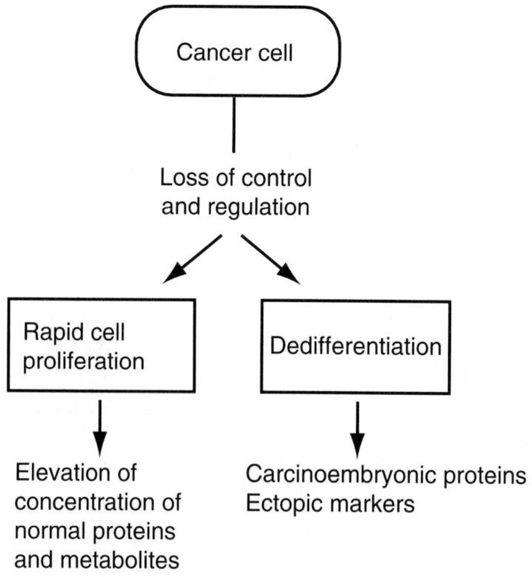

Figure 45–2. Illustration of how the loss of regulation in cancer cells leads to the generation of different tumor markers and how these processes relate to the two major reactions in cell growth.

In general, all benign tumors are well differentiated. Malignant neoplasms, on the other hand, range from being well differentiated to undifferentiated. Apparently control over proliferation and differentiation are both lost in malignant tumors. Some of the malignant tumors appear to return to their poorly differentiated fetal stages and produce substances similar to that found in fetal tissues, such as the so-called carcinoembryonic proteins (see Figs. 45–1 and 45–2). Malignant cells may also produce proteolytic enzymes that facilitate their escape from their primary environment.

Human cancers usually develop from mutant clones of cells as a result of neoplastic transformation. Most cancers are monoclonal in origin, but multiple mutations are required for them to become fully developed malignant cells. Multiple mutations in tumors could also lead to the development of cell heterogeneity in tumors. It is worthy to note that tumors are not made up of homogeneous cells; they are usually composed of subpopulations of cells with distinctly different phenotypes (Schnipper, 1986). The process of tumor evaluation and progression can also generate biological diversity within and among different metastatic foci. Cells isolated from an individual tumor may differ with respect to various factors: growth rate, cell surface receptors, immunogenicity, their expression of tumor markers (Fig. 45–3), capacity for invasion and metastasis, and response to cytotoxic drugs (Fidler, 1982).

5

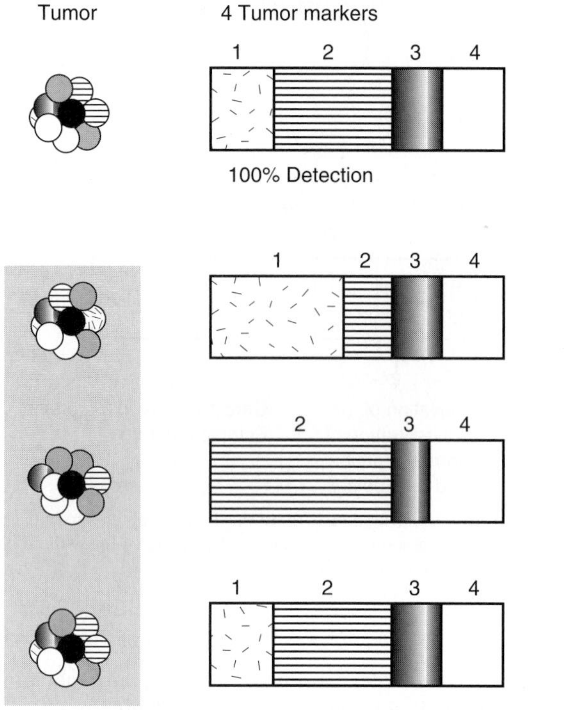

Figure 45–3. Illustration of how tumors are composed of heterogeneous cells. Each type of cell may produce a different tumor marker. Tumors from different tissues are also different in their cell composition but may share similar cells. The bars at the right illustrate that measuring multiple markers improves not only the sensitivity but also the specificity.

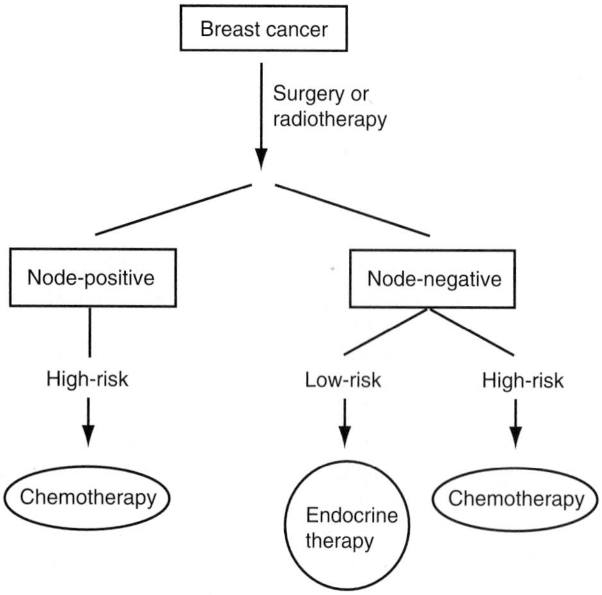

Figure 45–4. Illustration of how the information of node involvement alone is not sufficient to determine the risk and treatment for breast cancer patients. Patients with negative node involvement may not all be at low risk. At present, a panel of many new prognostic markers measured in tumor cytosols is used in conjunction with node determination to provide a more accurate risk assessment.

IDENTIFICATION OF TUMOR MARKERS

Although cancer results from the malignant transformation of a normal cell, there is very little difference in genotypic expression between a cancer and a normal cell. Cancer-inducing mutations do not seem to alter any of the genetic or phenotypic expressions, except for cell growth regulation. Consequently, efforts spent in the last several decades to identify a tumor-specific marker or a tumor-specific epitope have not been successful. On the other hand, any cell product, such as enzymes, serum proteins, metabolites, receptors, carcinoembryonic proteins, oncoproteins, and proteins encoded by suppressor genes, can be used as a tumor marker as long as it is related to any event during tumor formation or growth, such as malignant transformation, proliferation, dedifferentiation, and metastases. The clinical value of any given tumor marker will depend on the intended clinical use and the specificity and sensitivity of the tumor marker. The use of tumor markers as prognostic factors or risk factors has also gained more and more popularity in recent years. Measurement of the level of risk factors has been found to be valuable in the assessment of the aggressiveness of a tumor and is helpful in the selection of treatment strategies (Fig. 45–4).

Bence Jones protein, the first tumor marker identified in the laboratory, is an immunoglobulin light chain produced in excess by about half of the patients with plasmacytomas and is associated with the presence of monoclonal immunoglobulins in the serum. By using an immunoassay for this protein, it was learned that the amount of Bence Jones protein found in the urine or the amount of myeloma immunoglobulin in the serum may be used to follow up the effects of therapy. The urine concentration of these proteins closely reflects the myeloma tumor mass. Bence Jones protein, therefore, was the first tumor marker that taught us about the novel ways of monitoring cancer patients during treatment and about the sensitivity and specificity of tumor markers.

During the 1960s and 1970s there were only a limited number of tumor markers that were available for cancer diagnosis and management. Despite many elegant and detailed biochemical investigations of cancer at that period of time, those studies were usually related to cancers of low incidence (Bodansky, 1974). For example, the norepinephrine in pheochromocytoma, the tryptophan-hydroxyindoleacetic acid pathway in carcinoid tumors, the nature of the serum proteins in multiple myeloma, and the nature of hormones and of their action in various endocrine tumors have all been the subject of intensive and successful biochemical studies. Even as recently as 30 years ago, several enzymes and isoenzymes were still used extensively as tumor markers (Coombes, 1977). Methods for measuring these tumor markers at that time were limited to enzymatic activity and electrophoresis, both tests of relatively low sensitivity. Though it was realized that these ubiquitous serum enzymes were not specific for cancer, their levels often paralleled the clinical status of the patient. These enzymes were used frequently to follow the course of the patient's disease. It should be noted that the tumor markers discussed earlier, including enzymes, isoenzymes, and serum proteins, are not only associated with cancers of low incidence but are also of low sensitivity and specificity. There is only a small percentage of cancer patients who demonstrate elevated serum concentrations of these tumor markers; elevation of many of these enzymes and serum proteins can also be found in many other conditions and non-neoplastic diseases.

In the late 1970s, with both the discovery of carcinoembryonic antigen (CEA) in colorectal carcinoma and the development of a sensitive radioimmunoassay (RIA) to measure the plasma concentration of CEA by Gold and Freedman (1965), a new era of tumor marker investigations and application emerged. The discovery of CEA also initiated an intensive search for new fetal tumor antigens or carcinoembryonic proteins and tumor-specific markers. The discovery of many proteins in nanogram and picogram concentrations in the blood circulation, which are elevated in connection with many malignancies, promoted the development of RIAs and enzyme immunoassays (EIAs) for their quantification. Many of these newly discovered tumor markers were associated with cancers of higher incidence, such as epithelial cell–derived carcinomas. These investigations finally led us to realize that there are only tumor-associated and not tumor-specific tumor markers.

Associated with Cell Proliferation

Many hormones (human chorionic gonadotropin [hCG]), serum proteins, and enzymes (lactic dehydrogenase [LD], alkaline phosphate [AP]) and their metabolites ([vanillylmandelic acid [VMA], homovanillic acid [HVA], 5-hydroxyindoleacetic acid [5-HIAA]) may become elevated in tumors because of the high proliferation rate of tumor cells. Their serum concentrations rise to even higher concentrations when a benign tumor becomes malignant and metastasizes. Because benign and non-neoplastic diseases may also involve elevated levels of markers, these markers are not suitable for screening or for cancer diagnosis. These markers are useful in monitoring patients during treatment and may confirm the initial diagnosis of cancer as an adjunct test.

Related to Cell Differentiation

Carcinoembryonic proteins detectable in both fetal and tumor tissues, but not normal adult tissues, usually lack any known physiologic function and have blood concentrations in nanogram levels (see Figs. 45–1 and 45–2). Therefore, measurements of carcinoembryonic proteins in the circulation must rely on immunoassays. The specificity and sensitivity associated with these proteins, although not at 100%, are much higher than that of enzymes and metabolites that had been used as tumor markers in the past. The serum concentration of these carcinoembryonic proteins not only correlates well with tumor activity but can also be used to predict prognosis. Carcinoembryonic proteins in general are not suitable for screening: First, the polyclonal antibodies directed against these proteins often cross-react with other normal proteins and, secondly, these carcinoembryonic proteins do not appear sufficiently early in the blood from cancer patients. However, they have been used as adjunct tests for cancer diagnosis and are extremely useful for monitoring the success of treatment and for detecting recurrence.

Related to Metastases

Tumor metastases involve several major steps (Liotta, 1987). First, the tumor cells have to penetrate their adjacent surroundings, after which they invade blood vascular or lymphatic vessels. The tumor cells are then carried to distant sites, until they are finally arrested in the venous/capillary beds or solid tissue of a distant organ. In this new environment, these tumor cells must again penetrate the vascular walls in order to grow at the new distant site. All the cell products released and synthesized during these steps are candidates for risk factors. Their appearance in the tumor tissue or blood circulation indicates the risk or occurrence of metastases or poor prognosis. Measurements of most of these markers, however, are still limited to tumor tissues or tumor tissue cytosols.

Related to Other Tumor-Associated Events

Apparently the enzymatic activities of various tissue-specific glycosyltransferases are altered in tumor cells. Some of the elevated glycosyltransferases have been used as tumor markers. The sugar sequence and composition of the carbohydrate moiety of many serum glycoproteins, including blood group substances and mucins such as CA 19-9, are tumor markers resulting from the altered glycosyltransferase activity. The alpha-fetoprotein (AFP) isolated from patients with primary hepatoma has an additional fucose compared with the AFP from benign liver disease, an example of altered fucosyltransferase in hepatoma cells (Wu, 1990).

Related to Malignant Transformation (see Chap. 15)

Oncogenes, which encode proteins that function at every level of growth regulation, play a major role in cell transformation (Druker, 1989). These oncoproteins are similar to the normal products of proto-oncogenes, except that they have lost the regulatory constraints on their activity and do not need external activation signals for them to promote cell proliferation. Measurement of the tissue expression of these oncoproteins has been used to predict prognosis. One of the more extensively studied oncoproteins, namely c-*erb*B-2 protein (p185), has been detected in the serum by immunoassay. Further investigation found that the extracellular domain of the c-*erb*B-2 could be cleaved and released into the blood circulation. The extracellular domain of the p185 appeared to not only correlate with the amount of p185 expression on the tumor cell membrane, but also with the change of the concentration of many major tumor markers in the serum (Wu, 1995). Because malignant transformation is a specific event in carcinogenesis, any cell product associated with this event has the potential to be a more specific tumor marker. It is possible that many other transmembrane receptors associated with the cell transformation may also behave similarly and be useful as tumor markers or prognostic indicators. Extensive detailed studies into c-*erb*B-2 and other oncogene coded proteins are needed to fully evaluate the potential of oncoproteins for the diagnosis and management of cancer patients.

Inherited Mutations

Opposite to the oncogenes but equally as important are a group of suppressor genes that were discovered even more recently. Proteins encoded by suppressor genes are responsible for suppressing cell growth. These suppressor genes may undergo deletions or mutations, resulting in the production of inactive gene products, which were found in families at high risk for cancer. Several suppressor genes and their encoded proteins have been identified. p53, for example, has been widely investigated for its role in various cancers. The suppressor genes and their products are potentially useful as tumor markers for the screening and identification of families or individuals at high risk.

The discovery of two susceptibility genes (or tumor-suppressor genes) for breast cancer, namely *BRCA1* and *BRCA2*, has generated tremendous interest recently (Miki, 1994; Wooster, 1994). Studies (Easton, 1993) suggest that mutations in *BRCA1* are responsible for approximately half of all cases of inherited breast cancer. In addition, carriers of *BRCA1* mutations are also at an increased risk for ovarian, colon, and prostate cancer (Futreal, 1994). *BRCA2*, the second susceptibility gene for breast cancer, is thought to account for approximately 70% of cases of inherited breast cancer that are not caused by *BRCA1* mutations and is associated with an increased risk of breast cancer in men. Development of immunoassays to measure both *BRCA1*- and *BRCA2*-encoded proteins is under way and should be useful for the identification of high-risk individuals and their families.

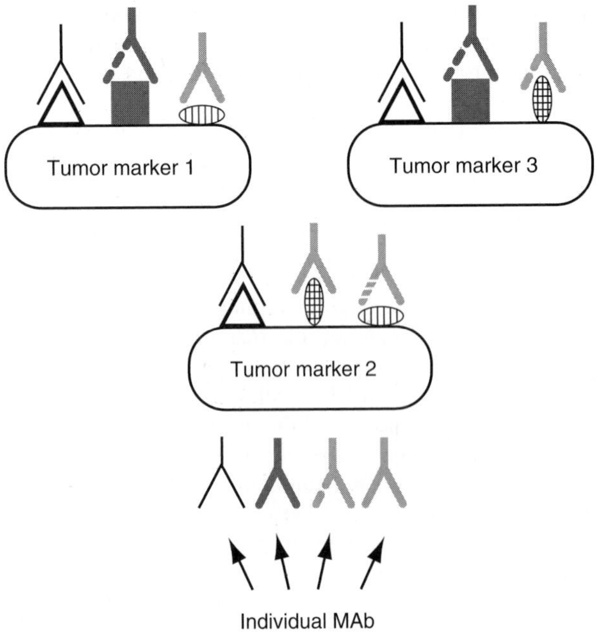

Figure 45–5. Illustration of how epitopes on the surface of a large tumor marker molecule are defined and identified by monoclonal antibodies. Despite sharing similar epitopes the overall patterns are different among various molecules.

Monoclonal Defined Tumor Markers

The development of hybridoma technology greatly impacted the identification of tumor markers. Rather than dealing with a whole molecule of known protein structure, it is now possible to focus on only a small surface area, an epitope or antigenic determinant using monoclonal antibodies (Fig. 45–5). It is no longer necessary to purify the antigen for the preparation of polyclonal antibodies in animals. The complete characterization and identification of the molecule carrying the epitope is also no longer needed. A hybridoma can be prepared by injecting a mouse with an enriched fraction of the tumor cell membrane, or even the whole tumor cell. The hybridomas producing the monoclonal antibodies of interest are selected through the subsequent screening procedure. Once a hybridoma is established, there will be an unlimited and consistent supply of monoclonal antibody for various uses. The specificity of both the antibody and the immunoassay established is well defined and reproducible. Many of the problems associated with assays using polyclonal antibodies, such as the reduction of lot-to-lot antibody variation and assay-to-assay inconsistencies, will disappear or be greatly reduced.

Attempts to identify tumor-specific epitopes using monoclonal antibodies have also failed. As with tumor markers identified by polyclonal antibodies, there are only tumor-associated epitopes (see Fig. 45–5). However, tests for the monoclonal antibody–defined tumor markers have been demonstrated to have a higher sensitivity and specificity than those using polyclonal antibodies. For example, CA 19-9, CA 125, and CA 15-3 are much more sensitive and specific than CEA for pancreatic, ovarian, and breast carcinomas, respectively (Wu, 1988a). These markers (Table 45–1) are recommended to replace the polyclonal CEA test for the diagnosis and management of patients with the above-mentioned carcinomas. Many tumor-associated epitopes are also shared by various tumor markers derived from different tumors. For example, CA 19-9, CA 15-3, and CA 125 are expressed by almost all carcinomas at varying degrees. In addition to the sharing of any given epitope by more than one carcinoma, it is also possible for a single molecule to express more than one epitope (Yu, 1991). For example, it is likely that CA 15-3 and CA 125 are expressed by the same mucin molecule in the serum.

CLINICAL APPLICATIONS

It is essential that the meaning of test sensitivity and the specificity of a tumor marker be understood before discussing the applications of tumor markers (Sell, 1990; Virji, 1988; von Kleist, 1988). In fact, the clinical utility of a tumor marker becomes almost totally dependent on the specificity

Table 45–1. MONOCLONAL ANTIBODY–DEFINED TUMOR MARKERS

Tumor Marker	Major Malignant Disease
CA 125	Ovarian carcinoma
CA 19-9	Pancreatic carcinoma
CA 15-3	Breast carcinoma
CA 72-4	Gastric carcinoma

and sensitivity of the tumor marker. When a tumor marker assay is said to be 100% sensitive, this means the assay can detect all patients with that particular type of cancer, whereas a 100%-specific assay means the assay will identify only the patients with the specific type of tumor and not those with benign or non-neoplastic diseases. Consequently, sensitivity is a measure of true positivity and is calculated according to the following formula:

Sensitivity = % true positive/(% true positive + % false negative).

On the other hand, specificity is a measure of false positivity and is calculated by the following formula:

Specificity = % true negative/(% true negative + % false positive).

With this information in mind we can begin to discuss the following clinical applications of tumor markers.

Screening

The attempt first by Gold and Freedman (1965) to screen for colorectal carcinoma in men using a RIA for CEA in serum led us to the realization that none of the tumor markers discovered had adequate specificity and sensitivity for screening. At present, screening is not recommended, especially in an asymptomatic population. In addition to the lack of desired specificity and sensitivity of tumor markers, the low prevalence of cancer in general also discourages screening for cancers. It was feared that the nonspecific nature of most tumor marker tests could create too many false positives and cause unnecessary alarm or anxiety for the general population. On the other hand, there are exceptions in which screening for cancer has been carried out using tumor markers. The screening for primary hepatoma in China based on the measurement of serum AFP is a good example of such exceptions caused by the high incidence of liver cancer in that area of the world (Wu, 1987). Recently the recommendation for the screening of prostate cancer by the measurement of serum prostate-specific antigen (PSA) in combination with a digital rectal examination is another exception that takes advantage of the tissue specificity of PSA (Wu, 1994). The feasibility of screening ovarian cancer in women by measuring serum CA 125 is still in the process of investigation. The diagnosis of ovarian cancer has traditionally relied on surgery. However, in most cases at the time of detection the tumor will have advanced to a stage at which the possibility of cure is low.

Diagnosis

The problems of both specificity and sensitivity associated with most tumor markers precludes their measurement for use in the diagnosis of cancer. The frequency of detecting elevated levels of tumor markers in non-neoplastic diseases and the overlap observed between the normal concentrations and the concentrations of tumor markers in patients with proven cancer discourages their use in diagnosis. Most tumor markers used at present fail to distinguish malignant from benign diseases. Tumor markers, however, have been used successfully as an adjunct test for cancer detection.

Several approaches have been suggested recently to improve the diagnostic specificity of many tumor markers. The use of multiple markers is one approach that has received wide acceptance. Specific patterns of multiple tumor markers seem to be associated with individual malignant diseases. The major drawbacks to the use of multiple tumor markers are cost and the rigors of proper selection of tumor markers to be included in the panel. Another approach to improving both the specificity and sensitivity of a tumor marker, as in the case of the serum PSA test, involves the measurement of the slope (the rate of increase in PSA concentration over time) and the density (by, for example, dividing the PSA concentration by the volume of the prostate gland, determined by the transrectal ultrasound) (Benson, 1992). A mildly elevated serum PSA level associated with a small prostate gland may be indicative of cancer, whereas the same value in a patient with a large gland may be only indicative of benign prostate hyperplasia (BPH).

Monitoring Treatment

One of the two most useful applications of tumor markers involves the monitoring of the course of the disease, especially during treatment. In Figure 45–6 the change in serum levels of several tumor markers during the course of a patient's ovarian cancer are illustrated. The serum level of tumor markers reflects well the success of surgery or the efficacy of chemotherapy. Detecting elevated levels of a tumor marker after surgery may indicate incomplete removal of the tumor, the presence of metastases, or recurrence. The measurement of serum tumor markers during chemotherapy also gives an indication of the effectiveness of the antitumor drug used and a guide for the selection of the most effective drug for each individual case, that is, therapeutic efficacy. There are occasions in which the serum level of a tumor marker may fall or rise unexpectedly. Some serum tumor markers

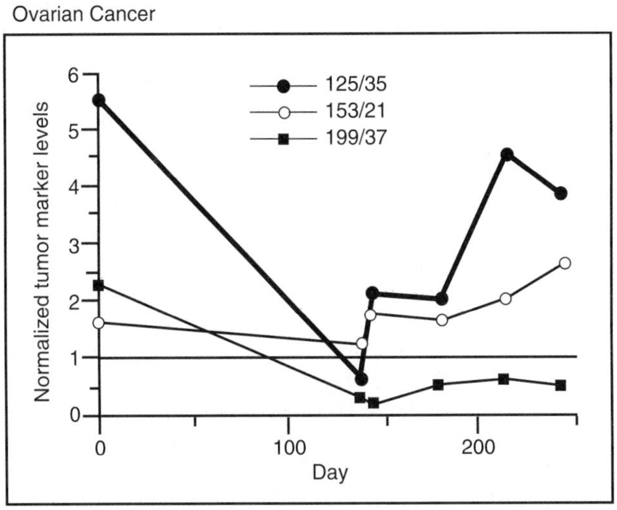

Figure 45–6. Illustration of the change of serum levels of CA 125 in conjunction with other tumor markers during the course of the disease in a patient with ovarian cancer we followed in-house. All the tumor marker levels had been normalized by dividing by their upper normal limits, such as 35 for CA 125, 21 for CA 153, and 37 for CA 19-9, respectively. Normalization allows a direct comparison among the serum levels of different tumor markers. Any value greater than one indicates abnormal.

have been known to rise during the initial period of chemotherapy. Serum PSA also has been known to rise transiently during radiotherapy.

Detection of Recurrence

Monitoring tumor markers for the detection of recurrence following the surgical removal of the tumor is the second most useful application of tumor markers. It is well known that the appearance of most of the circulating tumor markers has a "lead time" of several months (three to six months) prior to the stage at which many of the physical procedures could be used for the detection of the cancer. The ease of drawing blood and the sensitivity of the tumor marker tests make the noninvasive monitoring process now widely accepted. The specificity of tumor markers does not present a problem for this application.

Prognosis

The assessment of tumor aggressiveness and the prognosis for the outcome of a cancer patient have gained increasing popularity in recent years. The knowledge of tumor aggressiveness also helps in the development of a proper therapy for the patient. For example, the detection of tumor markers, highly associated with malignancy and metastases, will suggest a more rigorous and systemic treatment. Most tumor markers become increasingly elevated when the tumor metastasizes. Unfortunately very few tumor markers have a clear-cut boundary between the benign and the malignant stage. The risk factors associated with the process of tumor metastases usually are better markers for predicting prognosis. However, most of these markers are still measured in tumor tissues and tissue cytosols. The finding of the extracellular domain of c-*erb*B-2 protein in the serum and the correlation of the serum extracellular domain with the levels of other serum tumor markers is encouraging. It is hoped that in the near future it will become possible to measure these risk factors for prognosis in the blood circulation.

ORDERING TUMOR MARKER TESTS: RECOMMENDATIONS

When ordering tumor marker tests for patient diagnosis and for managing cancer patients, the following recommendations should be kept in mind in order to avoid misinterpretation of the test results.

Never Rely on the Result of a Single Test

Because of the problem of nonspecificity associated with most tumor markers, it is difficult to differentiate between malignant diseases and either benign or non-neoplastic diseases based on the result of a single test. Most elevations found in non-neoplastic diseases are often transient, whereas with cancer the level either remains elevated or continuously rises. Ordering serial testing can help to detect falsely elevated levels.

When Ordering Serial Testing, Be Certain To Order Every Test from the Same Laboratory Using the Same Assay Kit

Each different commercial kit may generate different results, even though all are designed for the same tumor marker. Ordering from the same laboratory also guarantees a more consistent performance. It is important to ensure that any change observed during the monitoring process is caused by a change of tumor volume or other tumor activities, and not by laboratory variability (see Fig. 45–6).

Be Certain that the Tumor Marker Selected for Monitoring Recurrence Was Elevated in the Patient Before Surgery

Because none of the tumor markers is 100% sensitive to the detection of any particular cancer, it is important to be certain that the tumor marker ordered to detect recurrence was elevated before surgery. Otherwise, multiple markers should be measured prior to the surgery in order to select the tumor marker showing the highest elevation as the marker for monitoring the disease activity.

Consider the Half-life of the Tumor Marker when Interpreting the Test Result

Estimate the time required for the level determined prior to the surgery to decline to the normal level, or in the case of PSA, to an undetectable level, based on the known half-life of the tumor marker. It is important that the success of surgical removal of a tumor as determined by tumor marker concentrations not be assessed earlier than two weeks postoperatively. It would even be preferable to wait one entire month because of the time required for the pre-existing tumor marker in the serum to decline to lower levels. For example, the half-life of serum PSA is approximately three to four days; therefore, it will take 30 days for a serum PSA at 50 ng/mL to drop to an undetectable range following successful surgery.

Consider How the Tumor Marker Is Removed or Metabolized from the Blood Circulation

Elevated serum tumor markers are frequently detected in patients with a renal or a liver disease depending on whether the tumor marker is removed through glomerular filtration or metabolized by the liver. For example, serum CEA is often elevated in patients with liver diseases because the impaired liver fails to remove CEA efficiently from the blood circulation, whereas an elevated serum beta-2-microglobulin (β2M) has been frequently found in patients with renal failure, in which even the small β2M molecule has difficulty passing through the glomerular membrane in a normal fashion.

Consider Ordering Multiple Markers To Improve Both the Sensitivity and Specificity for Diagnosis

As illustrated in Figure 45–4, tumors are made of heterogeneous types of cells. Some may still be normal cells, and some may be heterogeneous tumor cells as a result of a different sequence of multiple mutations. Each type of cell may express a single marker or a number of characteristic tumor markers. The same marker may also be produced by different types of cells. Some cells may never produce any unique marker. As further illustrated in Figure 45–4, different tumors derived from the same type of tumor apparently may also be heterogeneous in their cell composition. Consequently, more than one tumor marker is required to provide 100% sensitivity of detection. The heterogeneity in cell composition and the percent cell distribution of each tumor explains why a number of tumor markers are required to reach 100% sensitivity of detection, and the sensitivity of an individual marker is also different among cancer patients. Multiple tumor markers associated with individual malignant diseases are listed in Table 45–2; the appearances of individual tumor markers in various malignancies are listed in Table 45–3. This explains why none of the tumor markers presently employed is 100% sensitive and specific, and why the use of multiple markers will improve the detection sensitivity. However, a unique pattern of multiple markers may be identified with tumors derived from the same tissues. Therefore, ordering multiple tumor markers also may improve the test specificity for cancer diagnosis. For example, a specific pattern seemed to be associated with colon, breast, ovarian, and pancreatic carcinomas when all four monoclonal antibody–defined tumor markers, such as CEA, CA 19-9, CA 15-3, and CA 125, were measured simultaneously. This information is clinically important because more than 60% of the cancers that we encounter are epithelial cell–derived carcinomas (Wu, 1989). Multiple markers were used to develop a more specific screening strategy for ovarian cancer. It was found that the use of CA 15-3 and TAG72 in combination with CA 125 can increase the apparent specificity of the CA 125 assay for distinguishing malignant from benign disease (Bast, 1991). It should be noted that during the selection of multiple tumor markers, only markers that are complementary to each other should be selected. Many tumor markers that run parallel to each other when correlated with tumor activities should not be selected for this purpose.

Order the Nonspecific Markers for Cost Saving and for Their High Sensitivity

If the only attempt is to monitor the efficacy of treatment, the use of nonspecific tumor markers may be considered (Table 45–4). Although these nonspecific markers lack specificity for diagnosis and for relating to any specific type of tumor, their concentrations are nevertheless very sensitive to any changes in tumor activity. Many of them are inexpensive and simple to measure, and are therefore useful for monitoring therapy and detecting recurrence for patients with known diagnosis. For example, lipid-associated sialic acid (LASA-P) can be quantified with a simple, rapid, and inexpensive calorimetric procedure, and its serum concentration is closely parallel to the serum concentrations of many tumor markers of higher specificity.

Be Aware of the Possibility of a Hook Effect

One of the drawbacks of the popular sandwich-type immunoassay is the potential for a hook effect (Wu, 1991). The hook effect that takes place in an immunoassay tends to give a falsely low value when the tumor marker concentration in the specimen rises above a certain highly elevated level. At exactly what level of the tumor marker a hook effect may occur depends on the test design and the antibodies used in the assay. The use of two different aliquots of sample or the same sample at two different dilutions will reveal the hook effect. The tumor marker assay should be repeated with a 10-fold diluted specimen when the result of a sandwich immunoassay is too low to match the clinical severity of the patient's condition.

Be Aware of the Presence of Ectopic Tumor Markers

The expression of tumor markers is under genetic regulation. For benign tumors, the markers produced by the tumor are usually cell specific and are related to normal cell products at an elevated concentration (see Figs. 45–1 and 45–2). When the benign tumor transforms and becomes aggressive and more malignant, cellular control mechanisms become compromised. Proteins that are normally found at an early

Table 45–2. SEROLOGIC TUMOR MARKERS ASSOCIATED WITH INDIVIDUAL MALIGNANT DISEASES

Malignant Disease	Major Marker	Other Markers
Acromegalic pituitary tumors	Growth hormone	IGF-1*
Adrenal pituitary tumors	Cortisol	Free catecholamines, DHEA, 17-ketosteroids, prolactin
B-cell chronic lymphocytic leukemia	None	Serum β2M, LASA-P
B-cell malignancies	β2M	LD
Bladder cancer	None	T-antigen, urokinase inhibitor, CEA, TPA, cytokeratins, glycosaminoglycans
Bone cancer	Alkaline phosphatase	Bence Jones protein, free hydroxyproline, serum calcium
Brain tumor	Desmesterol	Polyamines
Breast cancer	CA 15-3	CEA, calcitonin, CA 549, CA M26, CK-BB, ferritin, βhCG, LASA-P, prolactin, P 21 protein, PS-2
Bronchogenic carcinoma	Prolactin	
Carcinoid tumors	Serotonin, 5-HIAA	Histamine, ADH, bradykinin

(*Table continued on next page*)

Table 45–2. SEROLOGIC TUMOR MARKERS ASSOCIATED WITH INDIVIDUAL MALIGNANT DISEASES *(Continued)*

Malignant Disease	Major Marker	Other Markers
Cervical cancer	SCC	AG-4 antibodies, CA 125, CEA, TPA
Choriocarcinoma	hCG	
Colorectal carcinoma	CEA	CA 195, CA 19-9, CA 72-4, CK-BB, NSE
Chronic myelogenous leukemia	TdT	
Cushing's syndrome	ACTH	Endorphin, lipotropin
Endocrine pancreatic tumors	Pancreatic polypeptide	
Gastric carcinoma	CA 72-4	CA 19-9, CA 50, CEA, ferritin, CK-BB, hCG, LASA-P, NSE, pepsinogen II, prothrombin
Gastrinoma	Gastrin	
Glucagonoma	Glucagon	
Hairy cell leukemia	IL-2 receptor	
Head and neck tumors	SCC	
Hepatocellular carcinoma	AFP	CEA, ferritin, γGT, ALP, TPA, γ-glutamyltrans-peptidase
Hypercalcemia of malignancy	PTH-related peptide	
Hodgkin's disease		LASA-P, ferritin
Insulinoma	Insulin	C-peptide, IGF-I binding protein I
Duodenum carcinoma	ADH	Pancreatic polypeptide
Kidney tumors	CEA	NSE
Leukemia	TdT	ALP, β2M, ferritin, LD, myelin basic protein, adenosine deaminase, PNP, lysozyme
Lung cancer	NSE	ACTH, CK-BB, calcitonin, CA 72-4, CEA, AFP, ferritin, LASA-P, TPA
Lymphoma	β2M	TdT, Ki-67, LASA-P
Medullary thyroid carcinoma	Calcitonin	NSE
Melanoma	Melanoma-associated antigen	NSE, plasma catecholamines, LASA-P, L-dopa
Microadenomas (pituitary)	Prolactin	
Multiple myeloma	Immunoglobulin heavy and light chain	Bence Jones protein, β2M, IgA
Mesothelioma	Hyaluronic acid	
Multiple endocrine neoplasias	Chromogranin A	
Monocytic leukemia	Lysozyme	
Nonseminomatous testicular tumor	AFP	hCG
Neuroblastoma	VMA	HVA, NSE, cystathionine, ferritin, metanephrines
Non-islet tumors	Insulin-like growth factor	
Oat-cell cancer		ACTH, ADH, CEA, CK-BB, NSE, bombesin, calcitonin
Osteosarcomas	ALP	
Ovarian carcinoma	CA 125	UGF, inhibin, AFP, amylase isoenzyme, CEA, CK-BB, hCG, galactosyltransferases, LD, TPA
Pancreatic carcinoma	CA 19-9	CA 195, CA 50, CA 72-4, CEA, CK-BB, ADH, ALP, ferritin, galactosyltransferase isoenzyme II, γ-glutamyltrans-peptidase, PAP
Pancreatic islet tumors	Insulin	Glucagon, somatostatin
Papillary and follicular thyroid cancer	Thyroglobulin	
Parathyroid tumors	PTH intact	
Pheochromocytoma	Metanephrine	Chromogranin A, plasma catecholamines
Pituitary tumors	Free α-hCG	FSH, LH, prolactin, TSH
Placental tumors	hCG	Free α-hCG
Plasma cell leukemia	Monoclonal immunoglobulins	β2M
Prostate carcinoma	PSA	PAP, ALP, CEA, CK-BB, TPA
Renal cell carcinoma		Renin, erythropoietin, interleukin-4, prostaglandin A, CA 15-3, parathyroid hormone, NSE, prolactin
Sarcoma	β2M	
Seminoma	NSE	
Spleen tumors	Ferritin	
Squamous cell cancer		
Cervix	SCC	
Lung	SCC	CYFRA 21-1
Head and neck	SCC	Ferritin
Stomach carcinoma	CA 72-4	CEA, NSE
Teratoblastoma	AFP	hCG, ferritin
Testicular cancer	hCG	
Nonseminomatous	AFP	β-hCG, LD
Uterine cancer	SCC	
Vipoma (pancreas)	VIP	
Waldenström's disease	Monoclonal IgM	β2M

ACTH, adrenocorticotropic hormone; ADH, antidiuretic hormone; AFP, alpha-fetoprotein; ALP, alkaline phosphatase; AMF, autocrine motility factor; β2M, beta$_2$-microglobulin; BPH, benign prostatic hyperplasia; CEA, carcinoembryonic antigen; CK-BB, creatine kinase BB isoenzyme; DHEA, dehydroepiandrosterone; FDP, fibrin degradation products; FSH, follicle-stimulating hormone; GI, gastrointestinal; γGT, gamma-glutamyl transferase; hCG, human chorionic gonadotropin; HVA, homovanillic acid; IGF-1, insulin growth factor 1; IL-2, interleukin-2; LASA-P, lipid-associated sialic acid; LD, lactate dehydrogenase; LH, luteinizing hormone, NSE, neuron-specific enolase; PAP, prostatic acid phosphatase; PNP, purine nucleoside phosphorylase; POA, pancreatic oncofetal antigen; PTH, parathyroid hormone; PTH-RP, PTH-related peptide; PSA, prostate-specific antigen; SCC, squamous cell carcinoma antigen; TdT, terminal deoxynucleotidyl transferase; TPA, tissue polypeptide antigen; TSH, thyrotropin; VIP, vasoactive intestinal polypeptide; VMA, vanillylmandelic acid.

Table 45–3. MALIGNANT DISEASES ASSOCIATED WITH INDIVIDUAL SEROLOGIC TUMOR MARKERS

	Associated Malignant Diseases	
Tumor Marker	***Major Disease***	***Minor Disease***
AFP*	Primary hepatocellular carcinoma	Teratoblastomas of the ovary and testes
α-hCG, free chain	Pituitary tumors	
β2M	B-cell neoplasias	Multiple myeloma, B-cell lymphoma, B-cell chronic lymphocytic leukemia, and reticulum cell, sarcoma; Waldenström's disease
CA 15-3	Breast carcinoma	Various carcinomas
CA 19-9	Pancreatic and gastric carcinoma	Various carcinomas
CA 72-4	Gastric carcinoma	Various carcinomas
CA 125	Ovarian carcinoma	Various carcinomas
β-HCG	Choriocarcinoma	Testicular cancers (nonseminomatous), trophoblastic tumors
Bence Jones protein	Multiple myeloma	
Bombesin	Oat-cell cancer	
CA 549	Breast cancer	
CA M26	Breast cancer	
Calcitonin	Medullary carcinoma	Cancer of the thyroid, liver cancer, renal cancer
CEA	Colorectal carcinoma	Various carcinomas
c-*erb*B-2 oncoprotein	Breast carcinoma	Various carcinomas
Chromogranin A	Pheochromocytoma	Multiple endocrine neoplasias, small cell lung carcinoma
CYFRA 21-1	Squamous cell carcinoma of the lung	
Desmesterol	Brain tumors	
DHEA	Adrenal/pituitary cancer	
DNA	Cervical carcinoma	
Erythropoietin	Renal carcinoma	
Ferritin	Acute myelocytic leukemia	Hodgkin's lymphoma, neuroblastoma and various carcinomas, teratoblastoma
Galactosyltransferase	Ovarian cancer	
Galactosyltransferase isoenzyme II	Pancreatic cancer	
Gastrin	Gastrinoma	Zollinger-Ellison syndrome
Histaminase	Medullary thyroid cancer	
hCG (intact molecule)	Choriocarcinoma	Gastric, ovarian, and breast carcinoma, trophoblastic or germ cell tumors, testicular cancer
Hyaluronic acid	Mesothelioma	
IgA	Multiple myeloma	
IGF-I	Pituitary cancer	Insulinoma
IL-2 receptor	Leukemia	
Immunoglobulins	Multiple myeloma	Mediterranean lymphoma, Waldenström's macroglobulinemia, malignant lymphoma
Inhibin	Granulosa-cell tumors	
Insulin-like growth factor	Non–islet-cell tumors	
Katakalcin	Medullary thyroid cancer	
17-Ketosteroids	Adrenal/pituitary cancer	
LASA-P		Various carcinomas, leukemia, lymphoma, Hodgkin's disease
Melanoma-associated antigen	Melanoma	
Metanephrines	Pheochromocytoma	Neuroblastoma, ganglioneuromas
Neuron-specific enolase	Small cell lung carcinoma	Neuroblastoma, kidney tumors
Pancreatic polypeptide	Endocrine tumor	
P 21 protein	Breast cancer	
Plasma catecholamines	Pheochromocytoma	Myeloma
PNP	Leukemia	
POA	Pancreatic cancer	
PSA	Prostate cancer	BPH
PAP	Prostate cancer	
PS-2 protein	Breast cancer	Some leukemias
SCC		Squamous cell carcinoma of the uterus, cervix, lung, and head and neck
TdT	Acute lymphocytic leukemia	
Thyroglobulin	Thyroid cancer	
TPA	Nonspecific	Various carcinomas
TAG 72	Gastric carcinoma	Colorectal, lung, pancreatic, and ovarian cancers
Urokinase inhibitor	Bladder tumors	
VIP	Vipoma	

*See Table 45–2 for abbreviations.

fetal stage, not expressed in the adult normal tissue, begin to appear in the tumor as a result of loss of regulation of genetic expression. This is the reason that carcinoembryonic proteins and ectopic tumor markers are usually expressed in advanced malignant diseases. In other words, the appearance of ectopic tumor markers is associated with poor prognosis or metastases. For example, elevated serum concentrations of AFP may be detected in patients with cancers in the gastrointesti-

Table 45–4. NONSPECIFIC TUMOR MARKERS

Tennessee antigen
Tissue polypeptide antigen
Lipid-associated sialic acid
CEA (polyclonal)
β2M
Lactic dehydrogenase

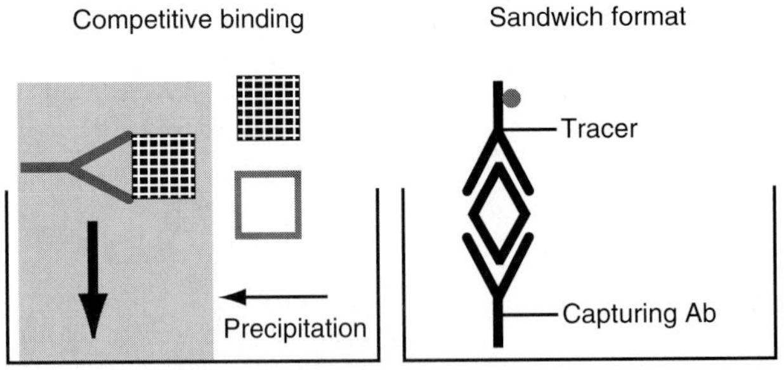

Figure 45–7. Illustration of the difference between two different major test formats for immunoassays. The filled and empty squares in the left figure refer to the labeled and sample antigens, respectively. In competitive binding test format, the antigen-antibody complex inside the gray rectangles is separated from free antigens by precipitation or other methods. Interference in competitive binding produces a falsely elevated value, whereas in a sandwich format, a falsely low value results.

nal tract involving metastases, even though the liver function tests are normal. Table 45–5 lists some of the known ectopic markers and their associated malignant diseases.

EFFECT OF ASSAY DESIGNS

The design of an assay or test, including the selection of antibodies, not only affects the test sensitivity, specificity, and concentration range but also affects the level of tumor marker at which the hook effect may occur and whether a false-negative or a false-positive result will be derived from interferences (see Chap. 33).

Competitive Binding

The first RIA developed was based on the competitive binding format. The combination of the competitive binding test format and the radioactively labeled antigen provided the sensitivity needed to quantify many circulating tumor markers, especially carcinoembryonic proteins, in the nanogram and picogram concentration ranges. The principle of this test format involves a competition between a fixed amount of radioactively labeled antigen and antigen in the sample for the antibody. After separation of the antigen-antibody complex from the free antigen, measurement of the complex-associated radioactivity will allow for the estimation of the amount of antigen present in the sample. In Figure 45–7 two different test formats are presented, one for RIA and one for the enzyme-linked immunosorbent assay (ELISA). However, any substances interfering with the binding between antigen and antibody will result in a falsely elevated value. What was not generally realized is the fact that the same interfering substance present in an assay using the same antigen and antibody but in a sandwich format will produce a falsely negative result (Wu, 1983). In the 1980s it was shown that the two major commercial CEA kits, one from Abbott using a sandwich format and one from Roche following the format for competitive binding, did not produce the same CEA result from the same specimens when the specimens contained interfering substances, such as glycosaminoglycans.

Table 45–5. ECTOPIC TUMOR MARKERS

AFP	GI, renal, breast, bladder, and ovarian carcinomas
Calcitonin	Carcinoma of lung, islet cell, carcinoid, breast, medullary, and ovary; pheochromocytoma
Chromogranin A	For endocrine tumors (medullary thyroid carcinoma, anterior pituitary adenoma, pancreatic islet-cell carcinoma)
Free α-hCG	Colorectal carcinoma and pancreatic endocrine tumors
hCG	Gastric and pancreatic carcinoma, hepatoma, ovarian adenocarcinoma, germ cell tumors of the testis
Thyroglobulin	Differentiated thyroid carcinoma

See Table 45–2 for abbreviations.

Sandwich Format

The ELISA, using the sandwich format, has become the most popular method for tumor marker quantification. In this case a specific antibody is adsorbed to the solid phase. A solution of the antigen is then added and allowed to bind. After sufficient incubation time and washing, an enzyme-labeled antibody is added to the solid phase and allowed to incubate. The unbound antibody label is washed away, and the remaining solid phase contains the antigen "sandwiched" between the antibody adsorbed to the solid phase and the labeled antibody. Enzymatic substrate is then added, and the resultant colorimetric development is proportional to the amount of antigen in the test solution. Even though labels other than enzyme are available, enzyme remains the most popular label. The sensitivity of ELISA can approach that of a RIA, especially when a biotin-avidin amplification system is used (Engvall, 1971).

Recently the test format of competitive binding has been largely replaced by the sandwich procedure. Despite the many advantages associated with the new format, the problem of hook effects may exist, in which a falsely low value may be produced from a specimen containing a highly elevated concentration of tumor marker. For example, falsely low CA 19-9 values were produced by the Centocor kit, using a sandwich format, with specimens containing highly elevated levels of CA 19-9. However, when a Biomira RIA kit, based on a competitive binding principle, was used, falsely low CA 19-9 values could be completely avoided. The use of the Biomira RIA kit also reduced the number of repeats because the level of CA 19-9 in the specimen could be approximated from the radioactivity count (Wu, 1991).

Monoclonal Versus Polyclonal Antibody

The development by Kohler and Milstein (Milstein, 1983) of murine monoclonal antibodies (MAb) by somatic cell hybridization techniques allows a far more detailed immunochemical and molecular analysis of tumor-associated antigens than was formerly possible. By combining the monoclonal antibodies with the solid-phase sandwich test design, many new assays have been developed that eliminate many problems associated with polyclonal assays, involving poor reproducibility, lot-to-lot variations, poor specificity, and nonspecific cross-reactivity (Diamond, 1981). It also reduced the differences between different kits and widened the linear concentration range for the assay. Whenever a monoclonal antibody is available its use is recommended. To achieve higher test sensitivity, the use of a combination of multiple MAbs has been found to improve the affinity between solid-phase adsorbed multiple MAbs and the soluble antigen.

Heterophilic Antibody

The use of MAbs in immunoassays and the increasing clinical application of mouse MAbs for targeted imaging and immunotherapy creates a new problem. Treated individuals apparently produce heterophilic antibodies against murine antibodies that interfere with many of the immunoassays for tumor markers (Nahm, 1990). The interference by the heterophilic antibodies in human sera can either increase or decrease the results of an immunoassay. These antibodies react in a way similar to antigens in terms of binding to both solid phase–associated and signal labeled antibodies. These heterophilic antibodies may bind to a site other than the analyte binding site, cross-linking the signal antibody with the capture antibody and thereby generating a false assay response. It is known that as many as 15% to 40% of individuals may have one or more heterophilic antibodies. The standard approach for reducing heterophilic antibody interference is to include excess mouse sera or nonspecific mouse immunoglobulin in the immunoassay.

INDIVIDUAL TUMOR MARKERS

Alpha-Fetoprotein

AFP is a major fetal serum protein and is also one of the major carcinoembryonic proteins (Wu, 1987). AFP resembles albumin in many physicochemical properties. In the fetus, AFP is synthesized by the yolk sac and the fetal hepatocytes, and to a lesser extent by the fetal gastrointestinal tract and kidney. Elevated AFP can be found in patients with primary hepatoma and yolk sac–derived germ cell tumors. AFP is the most useful serum marker for the diagnosis and management of hepatocellular carcinoma (HCC). However, AFP is also transiently elevated during pregnancy and in many benign liver diseases. Because of the high prevalence of liver cancer in China and other countries in Southeast Asia, AFP testing has been used successfully in screening for hepatoma in that region of the world. Tests for both AFP and hCG are helpful in reducing the clinical staging errors in patients with some testicular tumors and aid in the differential diagnosis of various germ cell tumors. Because an increase of fucosylation of AFP (hence, the lentil lectin reactivity of serum AFP) has been found in primary HCC, the determination of lentil lectin reactivity of serum AFP was found helpful not only to differentiate between primary hepatoma and benign liver diseases but also to provide an early signal indicating that hepatoma may begin to develop in patients with liver diseases such as cirrhosis.

Beta-2-Microglobulin

β2M is the constant light chain of the human histocompatibility locus antigen (HLA) expressed on the surface of most nucleated cells. The molecular weight of β2M is only 11.8 kDa. When the nucleated cells are metabolized, the light chain (or β2M) is shed into the extracellular fluid. β2M is a nonspecific tumor marker because it is elevated not only in solid tumors but also in lymphoproliferative diseases (including B-cell chronic lymphocytic leukemia, non-Hodgkin's lymphoma, and multiple myeloma) (Wu, 1986b). It is a good indicator of the patients' response to treatment, such as whether the disease is in remission or is advancing. Cerebrospinal fluid levels of β2M are useful for detecting metastases in the central nervous system.

CA 19-9, CA 50, and CA 19-5

CA 19-9 is the first tumor marker of a group of new epitopes, including CA 125, CA 15-3, and CEA, defined by monoclonal antibodies. These new monoclonal kits detect newly discovered epitopes and were designed to replace polyclonal CEA measurements for various carcinomas (Wu, 1988a). The assay for CA 19-9 measures a carbohydrate antigenic determinant expressed on a high-molecular-weight mucin. CA 19-9 is an epitope recognized by monoclonal antibody 1116NS-199 and is defined as sialylated lacto-N-fucopentaose II; the molecule, carrying the CA 19-9 epitope, appears as a mucin in the sera of cancer patients but as a ganglioside in tumor cells. CA 19-9 is also related to Lewis blood group substances, and only serum antigen from cancer patients belonging to the Le(a^-b^+) or Le(a^+b^-) blood group will be CA 19-9 positive. In addition to CA 19-9, two other tumor markers have also been defined by monoclonal antibodies that are only slightly different from CA 19-9. They are CA 195 and CA 50. The epitope related to CA 50 is very similar to that of CA 19-9 but lacks a fucose residue, the same epitope found in Lewis-negative (Le a^-b^-) individuals. Serum CA 19-9 concentrations not only are highly and frequently elevated in both gastric and pancreatic carcinomas, but are also useful for monitoring the success of therapy and for detecting recurrence in these cancer patients. However, it has been reported that CA 19-9 and CA 50 complement each other in pancreatic and other carcinomas: Their simultaneous use will improve the sensitivity in detecting these malignant diseases. CA 19-5 is detected by mouse monoclonal antibody CC3C-195 and reacts with both Le^a and sialyl-Le^a epitopes. CC3C-195 binds with high affinity to the sialylated Le^a blood group antigen but exhibits a lower affinity for the nonsialylated form. Elevated serum levels of CA 19-9, CA 50, and CA 19-5 can also be found in patients with colon, pancreatic, and hepatocellular carcinomas. The elevation found in benign liver diseases may be caused by cholestasis in these patients (Wu, 1992).

CA 125

CA 125 is another antigenic determinant defined by a monoclonal antibody and is also associated with a high-molecular-weight (>200 kDa) mucin-like glycoprotein. CA 125 is expressed by greater than 80% of nonmucinous epithelial ovarian carcinomas. CA 125 is found in most serous, endometrioid, and clear cell carcinomas of the ovary (Jacobs, 1989). However, patients undergoing chemotherapy may show a false decline of CA 125 antigen, and a negative result does not always rule out tumor recurrence. CA 125 is also used clinically for a follow-up on uterine tumors (>60% are elevated) and benign tumors, including endometriosis. Recently, the measurement of serum CA 125 is being tested to determine whether it can be used for screening of ovarian cancer. The use of multiple markers to improve test specificity and sensitivity for ovarian cancer has been demonstrated (Jacobs, 1989; Wu, 1988b).

CA 15-3

CA 15-3 is a circulating breast cancer–associated antigen identified by two distinct monoclonal antibodies. The assay uses a solid-phase conjugated monoclonal antibody, MAb 115D8, to capture the MAM-6 antigen in the human plasma and a labeled MAb DF3 as the tracer. MAb 115D8 was prepared against human defatted milk-fat globule, whereas MAb DF3 was prepared against the breast carcinoma cell line, MCG-7. The CA 15-3 antigen is present in a variety of adenocarcinomas, including breast, colon, lung, ovary, and pancreas.

CA 15-3 is a more sensitive and specific marker for monitoring the clinical course of patients with metastatic breast cancer. Significantly more patients have elevated circulating levels of CA 15-3 than CEA (96.2% versus 69.8%). Overall, CA 15-3 correlates with disease progression, regression, or stability in a higher number of patients than CEA. Measuring both CEA and CA 15-3 does not improve the results obtained with CA 15-3 alone. However, CA 15-3 can also be elevated in chronic hepatitis, liver cirrhosis, sarcoidosis, tuberculosis, and systemic lupus erythematosus (Tondini, 1988).

CA 72-4

The CA 72-4 assay detects a mucin-like human adenocarcinoma-associated antigen, TAG-72, which has a high-molecular-weight (>10^6 MW) mucin-like complex molecule. Because the TAG-72 can be detected in both fetal epithelia and sera from patients with various carcinomas, it is also considered to be a carcinoembryonic protein. However, only moderately elevated serum CA 72-4 could be found in most carcinomas. Currently CA 72-4 is considered to be the only useful marker for the management of patients with gastric carcinoma, despite its low sensitivity. CA 72-4 may be useful as one of the multiple markers for epithelial cell–derived tumors. CA 72-4, CA 19-9, and CEA RIAs are complementary to each other in detecting various carcinomas (Wu, 1992).

Calcitonin

Calcitonin is one of the circulating peptide hormones that may become elevated in patients with an increased bone turnover rate associated with skeletal metastases. Calcitonin can be found elevated in bronchogenic carcinomas and thyroid medullary carcinoma.

Carcinoembryonic Antigen

Carcinoembryonic antigen (CEA) is a glycoprotein with a molecular weight of approximately 200 kDa. CEA is the first of the so-called carcinoembryonic proteins that was discovered by Gold and Freedman (Gold, 1965). CEA is still the most widely used tumor marker for gastrointestinal cancer today, but most CEA assays have replaced the polyclonal with monoclonal anti-CEA antibodies.

Although the serum CEA RIA did not live up to its early expectations, the intensive investigations of CEA in the last 20 years have taught us many valuable lessons that have greatly benefited the tumor marker field. CEA was originally thought to be a specific marker for colorectal cancer but turned out to be a nonspecific marker on further studies. We learned from the CEA studies that tumor markers could be used to follow patients during therapy and to detect recurrence after a successful surgery. The association of a highly elevated serum tumor marker concentration with metastases and poor prognosis was also discovered through CEA studies. As CEA is metabolized by the liver, liver damage can impair CEA clearance and lead to increased levels in the blood circulation. Increased CEA concentrations have been observed in some patients following radiation treatment and chemotherapy (Wu, 1986a).

c-*erb*B-2 (HER-2/*NEU*) Oncoprotein (see Chap. 15)

The *ERBB2* gene (HER-2/*NEU*) is a member of the class of oncogenes associated with tyrosine protein kinase. The *ERBB2* gene was reportedly amplified in 25% to 30% of human breast and ovarian cancers. *ERBB2* amplification has been shown as an independent predictor of both disease relapse and overall survival, and is superior to all other known prognostic factors, with the exception of lymph nodes, when cancer positive. *ERBB2* has recently been found to be a useful marker to identify patients with breast cancer who are most likely to benefit from high doses of adjuvant chemotherapy (Duffy, 1990; Tandon, 1989). There is a direct concordance between *ERBB2* gene amplification and overexpression of the c-*erb*B-2 protein. As a consequence, both amplification and overexpression of *ERBB2* have been found to be associated with poor prognosis and with short survival and recurrence in various carcinomas.

The protein encoded by *ERBB2* is a 185 kDa transmembrane receptor (p185); it is also a glycoprotein having intracellular, transmembrane, and extracellular domains. The c-*erb*B-2 protein shows structural and functional homology with the epidermal growth factor receptor (EGFr). It was reported recently that the ectodomain of the c-*erb*B-2 oncoprotein could be proteolytically separated from the intact receptor and would eventually show up in the blood circulation. The ectodomain secreted in the breast tumor extracellular matrix has been shown to correspond to the levels of expression of p185 in the breast tumor tissue. Such a relationship is likely to exist between the serum ectodomain and p185 but has not been proven. Studies are currently ongoing to determine whether the serum ectodomain of the c-*erb*B-2 protein can be used as a prognostic marker (Wu, 1995).

Chromogranin A

Chromogranin A is a major soluble protein of the chromaffin granule. Chromogranin A can be released from the adrenal medulla together with catecholamines upon stimulation of the splanchnic nerve. However, chromogranin A is not confined to chromaffin cells of the adrenal medulla and sympathetic neurons; it is also present in various neuroendocrine tissues. Elevated serum chromogranin A levels can be detected in pheochromocytoma and small cell lung carcinoma (O'Connor, 1984).

CYFRA 21-1

CYFRA 21-1 is a fragment of the cytokeratin 19 found in the serum. It is a subunit of the cytokeratin intermediate filament expressed in simple epithelia and their malignant counterparts. It is a poor prognostic factor for squamous cell carcinoma of the lung (Pujol, 1993).

Human Chorionic Gonadotropin

hCG is a member of the glycoprotein hormone family and is synthesized and secreted by trophoblast cells of the placenta (see Chap. 20). hCG is a heterodimeric hormone composed of noncovalently linked α and β subunits. Both malignant and non-neoplastic trophoblast cells synthesize and secrete not only the biological active $\alpha\beta$ dimer but also the uncombined (or free) α and β subunits. In addition to the intact dimer, a free β-subunit of hCG has been detected in the serum of women during early pregnancy and in patients with malignant tumors.

However, elevated hCG can be found in trophoblastic tumors, choriocarcinoma, and testicular tumors. More than 60% of patients with nonseminomas and 10%–30% with seminomas have elevated free β-hCG. Measurement of the free β-subunit is useful for the detection of recurrence of metastasis for choriocarcinoma when the intact hCG may remain normal. Analysis of serum hCG subunits may be especially useful for managing patients with seminomatous cancer, as no other tumor marker was found elevated in these patients.

Seminomatous testicular cancer contains both intact hCG and β-hCG or free α subunits in equal amounts; therefore, only one assay is needed for monitoring these patients. On the other hand, only hCG or β-hCG subunits may be found in patients with nonseminomatous cancers. The measurement of both free subunits and intact hCG will increase the test sensitivity for these patients with nonseminomatous cancers.

Ectopic free β-hCG production occurs in approximately 30% of patients with urothelial cancer, but only the free β-hCG and its respective breakdown product, beta-core, were detected in these clinical samples. Ectopic α-hCG is a marker of malignancy in pancreatic endocrine tumors (Madersbacher, 1992).

Lipid-Associated Sialic Acid–P

Sialic acids (N-acetylneuraminic acids) are the acylated derivatives of neuraminic acid, and are the terminal residues at the nonreducing end of the carbohydrate chains in glycoproteins and glycolipids. Lipid-associated sialic acid (LASA)-P, on the other hand, is regarded as a nonspecific tumor marker. LASA-P is found elevated in a variety of malignant diseases, but also in non-neoplastic inflammatory diseases. This lack of tumor specificity substantially limits its use as a tumor marker for diagnosis; however, it compares favorably with the most widely used tumor markers for following patients' response to therapy and for the early detection of recurrent disease. The clinical sensitivity of this assay for various cancers was reported to range from 77% to 97%. The most commonly used method for measuring serum LASA-P is a simple, inexpensive, colorimetric procedure using either thiobarbituric acid or resorcinol (Katopodis, 1982).

Neuron-Specific Enolase

The gamma subunit of an enolase isoenzyme in the glycolytic pathway, found predominantly in neurons and neuroendocrine cells, is called neuron-specific enolase (NSE) and is identifiable by immunoassay. Elevated levels of NSE can be found in tumors originating from this neuroendocrine cell system. Serum NSE appears to be a relatively specific marker for small cell lung cancer (SCLC) (85%). It has been shown to be a useful marker for monitoring the treatment and predicting relapse in patients with SCLC (Burghuber, 1990).

5

p53 (see Chap. 15)

p53 is a 53-kDa nuclear phosphoprotein and a negative regulator of cell growth. It functions as a tumor suppressor by inducing the expression of gene products that are responsible for inhibiting or arresting cell growth and proliferation. The ability of p53 protein to regulate transcription of its target genes is based on its sequence-specific DNA-binding activity and the presence of a domain that can activate transcription when attached to the DNA-binding domain of another protein. It is the DNA-binding domain that appears to be sensitive to disruption by mutation, and most lesions associated with human cancers occur within this domain. The encoding gene for p53 has been found to be mutated in about half of almost all types of cancer arising from a wide spectrum of tissues. Functional inhibition of p53 activation also appears to play a role in human tumorigenesis. Overexpression of some oncogene products in certain tumors serves to bind and mask the activation domain of p53.

p53 can be measured in either tissue, fibroblast, white cell, or serum. A commercial sandwich enzyme immunoassay from Oncogene Science (Uniondale, New York) is available for quantification of the undenatured mutant p53 proteins. Because of the short half-life (20 minutes), the wild-type p53 protein in the blood circulation is not detectable (Harris, 1993; Malkin, 1990).

Parathyroid Hormone–Related Peptide

Plasma concentrations of parathyroid hormone–related peptide (PTH-RP) are elevated in most patients with cancer-associated hypercalcemia (see Chap. 8). They are secreted by tumors associated with hypercalcemia. The circulatory forms of PTH-RP in these patients include both a large N-terminal peptide and a C-terminal peptide with close sequence homology to parathyrin (PTH). The mechanism by which PTH-RP induces hypercalcemia involves binding and activating receptors that also bind PTH. Measuring the concentrations of PTH-RPs may be useful in the differential diagnosis of hypercalcemia and may be associated either with primary hyperparathyroidism, sarcoidosis, vitamin D toxicity, or various malignancies (including squamous cell, renal, bladder, and ovarian carcinomas). It should be noted that patients with impaired renal function, but without hypercalcemia or cancer, may have increased plasma concentrations of PTH-RP (Burtis, 1990).

Prostate-Specific Antigen

(see Chap. 13)

Prostate-specific antigen (PSA) is synthesized in the epithelial cells of the prostate gland and is perhaps the best tumor marker discovered thus far. The tissue specificity of PSA makes it the most useful tumor marker available for the diagnosis and management of prostate cancer. Lack of cancer specificity is the only drawback with PSA. Benign conditions such as BPH, prostatitis, and infarction can also be correlated to elevated serum PSA levels.

Because of its tissue specificity, the PSA assay is particularly useful for monitoring the success of surgical prostatectomy. Complete removal of the prostate should result in an undetectable PSA level; any measurable PSA after radical prostatectomy would indicate residual prostatic tissue or metastasis. In those patients, increasing PSA concentrations after a successful surgery strongly indicate a recurrent disease. However, if the detectable serum PSA concentration after radical prostatectomy is a result of incomplete resection of the gland and not persistent disease, the level should remain unchanged on extended follow-up. It should be noted that a transient and modest increase of PSA may occur during radiation therapy, which should not be misinterpreted as disease progression.

The tissue specificity of PSA also makes the test an excellent tool for detecting recurrence after radical prostatectomy. There has been a great demand for the development of an ultrasensitive PSA test. A very sensitive PSA test would allow for the early detection of recurrence and metastasis, and provide a better opportunity for successful treatment. Many commercial PSA tests now available are capable of detecting serum PSA below 0.1 ng/mL.

The use of serum PSA in combination with either digital rectal examination (DRE) or transrectal ultrasound of the prostate as a screening tool for detecting clinically significant prostate cancer has been recommended (Brawer, 1992; Catalona, 1991). Screening permits the treatment of organ-confined, potentially curable prostate cancer discovered in men with a life expectancy of longer than 10 years.

PSA is a serine protease capable of complexing with various protease inhibitors. Consequently serum PSA exists in the serum largely in the form of a PSA-ACT (PSA–α_1-antichymotrypsin) complex (Christensson, 1993) (Fig. 45–8). Because the percent PSA-ACT complex of the total

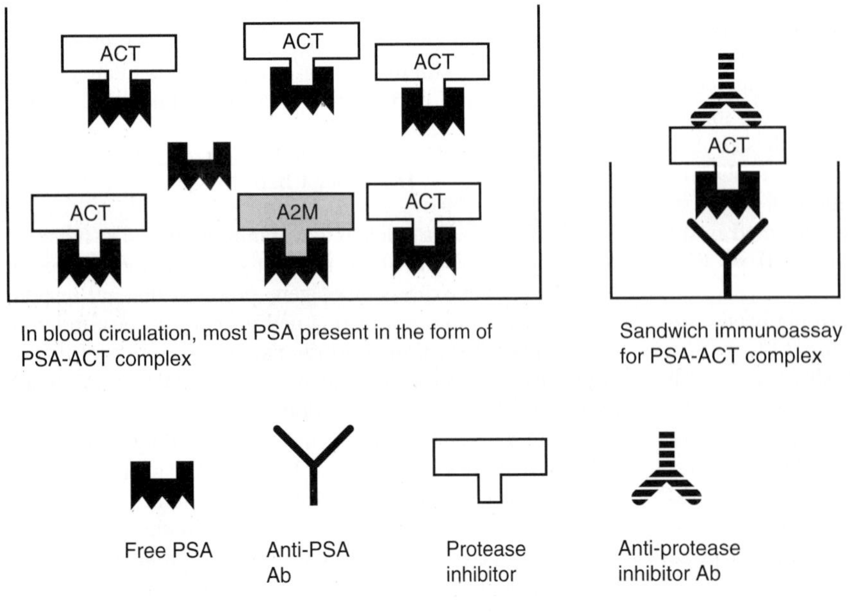

Figure 45–8. Illustration showing that the major form of PSA in the blood circulation is PSA-ACT complex. A specific assay for the PSA-ACT complex can be developed by using two different antibodies, one for free PSA and one for ACT, in a sandwich format.

serum PSA is higher in patients with prostatic cancer than in those with BPH, the measurement of PSA-ACT has a higher sensitivity for cancer than the assay for total PSA (Wu, 1994).

Squamous Cell Carcinoma

Squamous cell carcinoma (SCC) antigen is a near neutral subfraction of the TA-4 tumor antigen purified from squamous cell carcinoma tissue of the uterine cervix. The molecular weight of the SCC antigen is approximately 48 kDa. More than 70% of patients with advanced cervical cancer have elevated SCC. SCC RIA is useful for following patients with cervical cancer during therapy. The SCC is also useful for monitoring squamous cell carcinomas of the head and neck, lung, esophagus, and anal canal. The SCC serum concentrations are highest in patients with metastases. For patients with renal failure, as many as 50% could have increased SCC serum concentrations.

Tissue Polypeptide Antigen

Tissue polypeptide antigen (TPA) is a mixture of the low-molecular-weight epithelium-associated cytokeratins (Weber, 1984). Because it is more abundant in cells undergoing mitosis and much less so in those in interphase, TPA appears to be a measure of cellular proliferation. The TPA assay uses a combination of monoclonal antibodies specific to cytokeratins of simple epithelia. TPA is a sensitive but nonspecific marker for discriminating between progressive disease and disease in complete remission. TPA elevations occur in a variety of inflammatory diseases and in pregnancy as well as in many types of tumor. Many reports emphasize the use of TPA in combination with other markers, especially CEA, for monitoring a variety of carcinomas, including breast, colorectal, ovarian, bladder, and lung. TPA is also valuable for the detection of recurrence and for helping differentiate between cholangiocarcinoma (positive) and hepatocellular carcinoma (negative).

Bast RC Jr, Knauf S, Epenetos A, et al: Coordinate elevation of serum markers in ovarian cancer but not in benign disease. Cancer 1991; 68:1758.

Benson MC, Wang IS, Pantuck A, et al: Prostate specific antigen density: A means of distinguishing benign prostatic hyperplasia and prostate cancer. J Urol 1992; 147:815.

Bodansky O: Reflections on biochemical aspects of human cancer. Cancer 1974; 33:364.

Brawer MK: Screening for prostatic carcinoma with prostate-specific antigen. J Urol 1992; 147:841.

Burghuber OC, Worofka B, Schernthaner G, et al: Serum neuron-specific enolase is a useful tumor marker for small cell lung cancer. Cancer 1990; 65:1386.

Burtis W, Brady TF, Orloff JJ, et al: Immunochemical characterization of circulating parathyroid hormone-related protein in patients with humoral hypercalcemia of cancer. N Engl J Med 1990; 322:1106.

Catalona W, Smith D, Ratliff T, et al: Measurement of prostate-specific antigen in serum as a screening test for prostate cancer. N Engl J Med 1991; 324:1156.

Christensson A, Bjork T, Nilsson O, et al: Serum prostate specific antigen complexed to α1-antichymotrypsin as an indicator of prostate cancer. J Urol 1993; 150:100.

Coombes RC, Powles TJ, Gazet JC, et al: Biochemical markers in human breast cancer. Lancet 1977; 1:132.

Diamond BA, Yelton DE, Scharff MD: Monoclonal antibodies. A new technology for producing serologic reagents. N Engl J Med 1981; 304:1344.

Druker BJ, Mamon HJ, Roberts TM: Oncogenes, growth factors, and signal transduction. N Engl J Med 1989; 321:1383.

Duffy MJ: Biochemical markers as prognostic indices in breast cancer. Clin Chem 1990; 36:188.

Easton DF, Bishop DT, Ford D, et al: Genetic linkage analysis in familial breast and ovarian cancer: Results from 214 families. Am J Hum Genet 1993; 52:678.

Engvall E, Perlmann P: Enzyme-linked immunosorbent assay (ELISA). Quantitative assay of immunoglobulin G. Immunochemistry 1971; 8:871.

Fidler IJ, Hart IR: Biological diversity in metastatic neoplasms: Origins and implications. Science 1982; 217:998.

Futreal PA, Liu Q, Shattuck-Eidens D, et al: BRCA1 mutations in primary breast and ovarian cancers. Science 1994; 266:120.

Gold P, Freedman SO: Demonstration of tumor-specific antigens in human colonic carcinomata by immunological tolerance and absorption techniques. J Exp Med 1965; 121:439.

Harris CC, Hollstein M: Clinical implications of the p53 tumor-suppressor gene. N Engl J Med 1993; 329:1318.

Jacobs I, Bast RC Jr: The CA 125 tumour-associated antigen: A review of the literature. Hum Reprod 1989; 4:1.

Katopodis N: Lipid associated sialic acid test for the detection of human cancer. Cancer Res 1982; 42:5270.

Liotta LA: Biochemical mechanisms of tumor invasion and metastases. Clin Physiol Biochem 1987; 5:190.

Madersbacher S, Klieber R, Mann K: Free α-subunit, free β-subunit of human chorionic gonadotropin (hCG), and intact hCG in sera of healthy individuals and testicular cancer patients. Clin Chem 1992; 38:370.

Malkin D, Li FP, Strong LC, et al: Germ line p53 mutations in a familial syndrome of breast cancer, sarcomas and other neoplasms. Science 1990; 250:1233.

Miki Y, Swensen J, Shattuck-Eidens D, et al: Isolation of BRCA1, the 17q-linked breast and ovarian cancer susceptibility gene. Science 1994; 266:66.

Milstein C, Cuello AC: Hybrid hybridomas and their use in immunohistochemistry. Nature 1983; 305:537.

Nahm MH, Hoffmann JW: Heteroantibody: Phantom of the immunoassay. Clin Chem 1990; 36:829.

O'Connor DT, Bernstein KN: Radioimmunoassay of chromogranin A in plasma as a measure of exocytotic sympatho-adrenal activity in normal subjects and patients with pheochromocytoma. N Engl J Med 1984; 311:764.

Pujol J-L, Grenier J, Daures JP, et al: Serum fragment of cytokeratin subunit 19 measured by CYFRA 21-1 immunoradiometric assay as a marker of lung cancer. Cancer Res 1993; 53:61.

Schnipper LE: Clinical implications of tumor cell heterogeneity. N Engl J Med 1986; 314:1423.

Sell S: Cancer markers of the 1990s. Comparison of the new generation of markers defined by monoclonal antibodies and oncogene probes to prototypic markers. Clin Lab Med 1990; 10:1.

Tandon AK, Clark GM, Chamness GC, et al: HER-2/neu oncogene protein and prognosis in breast cancer. J Clin Oncol 1989; 7:1120.

Tondini C, Hayes DF, Gelman R, et al: Comparison of CA 15-3 and carcinoembryonic antigen in monitoring the clinical course of patients with metastic breast cancer. Cancer Res 1988; 48:4107.

Virji MA, Mercer DW, Herberman RB: Tumor markers in cancer diagnosis and prognosis. CA Cancer J Clin 1988; 38:104.

von Kleist S: What's new in tumor markers and their measurements? Pathol Res Pract 1988; 183:95.

Weber K, Osborn M, Moll R: Tissue polypeptide antigen (TPA) is related to the non-epidermal keratins 8, 18, and 19 typical of simple and non-squamous epithelia: Re-evaluation of a human tumor marker. EMBO J 1984; 3:2702.

Wooster R, Neuhausen SL, Mangion Y: Localization of a breast cancer susceptibility gene, BRCA2, to chromosome 13q12-13. Science 1994; 265:2088.

Wu JT, Mau E, Knight JA: Interference with carcinoembryonic antigen radioimmunoassays by glycosaminoglycans, and their removal. Clin Chem 1983; 29:2049.

Wu JT, Knight JA, Knight DP: Carcinoembryonic antigen (CEA) in the diagnosis and management of colorectal cancer. Clin Chem 1986a; 86:8.

Wu JT, Clayton F, Myers S: A simple radial immunodiffusion method for assay of β2-microglobulin in serum. Clin Chem 1986b;32:2070.

Wu JT, Knight JA: Alpha-fetoprotein: Its use in clinical medicine. Clin Chem 1987; 27:1.

Wu JT, Knight JA: Monoclonal immunoassays for tumor markers. Clin Chem 1988a; 28:1.

Wu JT, Miya T, Knight JA: Improved specificity of the CA 125 EIA for ovarian carcinomas by use of the ratio of CA 125 to CEA. Clin Chem 1988b; 34:1853.

Wu JT: Expression of monoclonal antibody-defined tumor markers in four carcinomas. Ann Clin Lab Sci 1989; 19:17.

Wu JT: Measurement of AFP and its lectin reactive isoforms in liver diseases and various malignancies. Ann Clin Lab Sci 1990; 20:98.

5

Wu JT, Christensen SE: Effect of different test designs of immunoassays on "hook effect" of CA 19-9 measurement. J Clin Lab Anal 1991: 5:228.
Wu JT, Carlisle P: Low frequency and low level of elevation of serum CA 72-4 in human carcinomas in comparison with established tumor markers. J Clin Lab Anal 1992; 6:59.
Wu JT: Assay for prostate specific antigen (PSA): Problems and possible solutions. J Clin Lab Anal 1994; 8:51.
Wu JT, Astill ME, Gagon SD: Measurement of c-*erb*B-2 protein in sera from patients with carcinomas and in breast tumor tissue cytosols: Correlation with serum tumor markers and membrane-bound oncoprotein. J Clin Lab Anal 1995; 9:151.
Yu H, Schlossman DM, Harrison CL, et al: Coexpression of different antigenic markers on moieties that bear CA 125 determinants. Cancer Res 1991; 51:468.

Part 6

MEDICAL MICROBIOLOGY

Edited by
Gail L. Woods, M.D.
John Bernard Henry, M.D.

Chapter 46

Viral Infections

Michael Costello, Ph.D.
Margaret Yungbluth, M.D.

As the science of clinical virology has evolved over the past 30 years, viruses have been affirmed as the most frequent causes of human infectious diseases. The vast scope of viral disease ranges from the trivial common cold to generally benign childhood infections, such as chickenpox and mumps, to the ultimately fatal immunoimpairment that follows destruction of the CD4 T-lymphocyte cell population by human immunodeficiency virus (HIV). The first virology laboratories were established in research hospitals, used laborious tissue culture preparation and isolation methods, and were not readily accessible routine diagnostic services. However, the venereal epidemic of herpes simplex virus (HSV) during the 1970s and 1980s, the expanding numbers of immunocompromised patients, and the development of several antiviral agents emphasized the necessity for routine laboratory confirmation of viral infections. Along with the pressure for greater diagnostic service, the commercial availability of high quality reagents improved, detection methods were simplified, and identification times reduced. These factors together have made the addition of clinical virology a practical possibility in hospitals of all sizes.

A specific viral diagnosis is medically beneficial and cost effective, and helps clinicians optimize patient management and use antiviral drugs appropriately. In addition, unnecessary treatment and diagnostic testing can be reduced and isolation procedures to limit nosocomial viral spread can be efficiently implemented (Drew, 1986). These factors improve patient care and favorably impact the length of hospital stay and the cost-appropriate practice of medicine. The secondary public health benefits of precise diagnosis should not be overlooked; information about influenza, measles, acquired immunodeficiency syndrome (AIDS), arbovirus, and enterovirus infections, as well as herpes venereal disease, is as valuable as the epidemiologic data compiled about tuberculosis, streptococcal infections, salmonellosis, gonorrhea, and syphilis.

In this chapter the common syndromes that generate most specimens in a community or university hospital virology laboratory are reviewed. Laboratory organization, equipment and supplies, specimen collection, test selection, and current isolation and identification methods that have the most practical clinical applications are discussed. Because viral diseases are so common and involve both healthy and immunocompromised children and adults, most hospitals have a suitable clinical case mix to support a virology service. Table 46–1 summarizes the isolation and antigen testing volumes and recovery rates for three Chicago-area hospital virology laboratories. Northwestern Memorial Hospital has 675 beds with oncology, high-risk obstetrics, infectious diseases, and transplant tertiary care services, but no general pediatric care. Lutheran General Hospital has 700 beds and a general practice patient base with a large pediatric component. St. Joseph Hospital is a 350-bed community hospital with both pediatric and adult services and a large population of HIV-infected patients. To a great degree, patient mix and specialty interests in each hospital predict the types of viral infections seen; however, the same viruses are recovered in all three laboratories, with variations only in the relative isolation percentages. The average detection times for most viruses are short (often two days or less) and on the same time scale as routine bacterial cultures. This reflects the use of rapid antigen detection methods, nucleic acid probes, and shell vial culture techniques with reduced incubation schedules. The recovery rates for viruses in all three hospitals are much higher than for routine bacterial blood or stool cultures, mycobacterial cultures, or ova and parasite exams. The virology laboratory at St. Joseph Hospital has been in operation less than six months and has fewer specimens and a higher recovery rate, reflecting the initial tendency of physicians to order tests more for confirmation than screening; this should change as familiarity with the service increases.

Many of the common medical viruses exhibit seasonal variations. Epidemics of influenza, respiratory syncytial virus (RSV), and parainfluenza virus Types 1 and 2 recur annually in the cold weather months. Adenovirus, parainfluenza virus 3, cytomegalovirus, and herpes simplex infections occur year-round. Enteroviruses tend to cluster in late summer and early autumn (Fig. 46–1). These temporal patterns create fluctuations in the demand for laboratory service, which can be particularly dramatic in pediatric hospitals.

Table 46–2 lists the three principal diagnostic laboratory methods, all of which have advantages and limitations. Specimens for culture, antigen detection, and nucleic acid probe assay require the presence of viable virus or relatively intact viral fragments, and therefore must be collected during the acute phase of illness from the site of active infection. Traditional serologic diagnosis has required both acute-phase and convalescent-phase serum specimens, with demonstration of a four-fold or greater rise in specific viral IgG antibody titer between the two samples. Methods that detect virus-specific IgM antibody may diagnose acute infection from a single serum obtained during the late stage of acute disease or the early convalescent phase of infection. Serologic methods that identify virus-specific IgG antibody are most commonly used to document immune status. An expanding list of commercial suppliers offers all necessary materials and reagents for virus isolation, antigen assay, and serologic procedures. A virology laboratory no longer has to maintain tissue culture cell lines or manufacture reagents in house, just as a successful general microbiology laboratory need not rely on homemade agars and staining reagents.

Table 46–1. VIRAL DETECTION: FREQUENCY OF OCCURRENCE, AVERAGE DETECTION TIMES AND POSITIVITY RATES

Virus	Lutheran General Hospital	Northwestern Memorial Hospital	St. Joseph Hospital	Average Detection Times
Herpes simplex virus	34%	29%	28%	2 days
Cytomegalovirus	3%	24%	49%	3 days
Adenoviruses	5%	2%	7%	3 days
Influenza A virus	6%	3%	2%	2 days
Enterovirus	8%	1%	2%	4 days
Varicella zoster virus	2%	3%	2%	3 days
Influenza B virus	1%			2 days
Parainfluenza virus	6%		<1%	2 days
Respiratory syncytial virus	27%		10%	8 hours
Measles and mumps	<1%		<1%	5 days
Chlamydia	6%	38%	N.D.	3 days
Total specimens processed	3323	2157	277*	
Recovery of viruses	21%	22%	38%	

*Data represent five months of laboratory operation.

Viral Culture

Virus propagation in tissue culture was first accomplished over 40 years ago and, despite its limitations, still remains the most accepted method for diagnosing viral infection. A wide range of viruses actively replicate in cell culture, and recovery of virus correlates well with acute disease. However, viral culture is labor intensive, requires technical expertise, and generally means at least a one day turnaround for positive results. Replication in newborn mice tissues or embryonated eggs may be preferable or essential for some viruses, but most clinical isolation work is done with *in vitro* tissue culture cell lines (Hsiung, 1994; Schmidt, 1989; Isenberg, 1992). Tissue culture cells are divided into three categories: primary cell cultures, diploid cell lines, and heteroploid cell lines. Primary cell cultures are prepared directly from a parent organ (monkey kidney, rabbit kidney, etc.); individual cells are separated by mincing and trypsinization, and then plated as confluent monolayers. Diploid cell lines are usually human fibroblasts derived from tonsil, lung, or newborn foreskin, and have a normal diploid chromosome number. Cells are propagated in serum-rich growth medium and can be subcultured 20 to 50 times; examples include MRC-5, WI-38, and Flow 2000. Heteroploid cell lines are human cancer cells that because of their malignant nature can be subcultured indefinitely; these cells grow rapidly and the chromosome number is always aneuploid. The most frequently used heteroploid lines are HEp-2 (laryngeal carcinoma), HeLa (cervical cancer), and A549 (lung carcinoma). Primary cultures must be checked for contamination with endogenous viruses. Diploid and heteroploid cell lines should

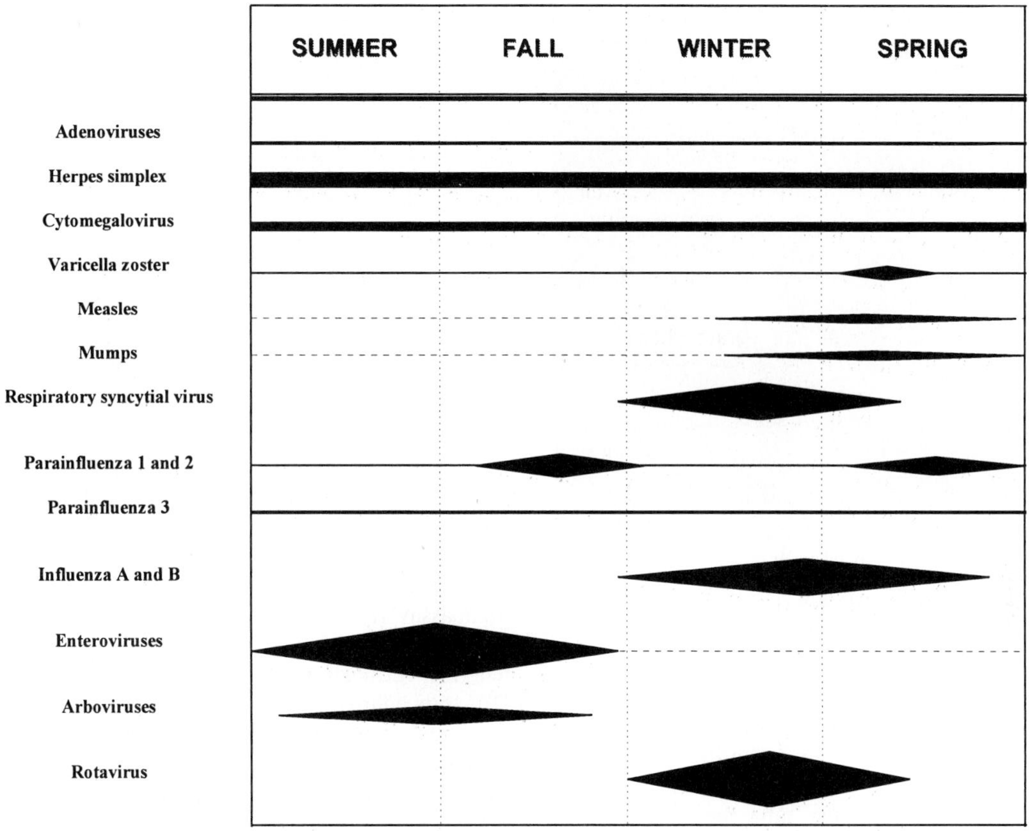

Figure 46–1. Seasonal variation of viral infections.

Table 46–2. LABORATORY METHODS FOR DIAGNOSIS OF VIRAL INFECTIONS

Tissue Culture

Tube culture (standard cell monolayer)
Centrifugation-enhanced culture (shell vial cell monolayer)

Detection of Viral Antigen/Nucleic Acid in Patient Specimen

Direct fluorescent antibody stain (DFA)
Enzyme-linked immunoassay (EIA)
Nucleic acid probe assays and amplification methods (PCR, LCR, Qβ-replicase, etc.)

Serology

Polyclonal antibody assays
IgM, IgG, IgA specific methods

be checked periodically for mycoplasma contamination and continued sensitivity to viral infection.

Viruses do not infect all human tissues with equal affinity, and they differ in their ability to replicate in tissue culture cell lines. Therefore, for maximal diagnostic sensitivity, each specimen should be inoculated into a variety of cell lines. Table 46–3 lists several tissue culture lines and the viruses that reliably infect them. All of these cell lines are available from commercial suppliers, and each can be purchased in traditional tubes, shell vials, or bulk flasks (Fig. 46–2). Each laboratory should select sufficient cell lines to cover the viral pathogens in the patient population that the hospital serves.

Viral replication in traditional tube culture is identified by

Table 46–3. SENSITIVITY OF CELL LINES TO COMMON PATHOGENIC VIRUSES

	Cell Lines					
Virus	***PMK***	***HDF***	***HEp-2***	***A549***	***RK***	**Time to Detection of CPE (Days)**
Influenza	+++	+	+/−	−	−	2–7
Parainfluenza	++	−	−	−	−	3–12
RSV	+	+	+++	++	−	3–12
Rhinovirus*	++	+++	+	−	−	3–7
Enterovirus	+++	+++	++	++	−	2–14
Adenovirus	+	++	+++	+++	−	3–6
HSV	+	+++	++	++	++++	1–5
VZV	−	+++	−	+/−	−	5–14
CMV	−	+++	−	+/−	−	4–20
Measles	++	−	+/−	−	−	5–10
Mumps	+++	+	−	−	−	4–10

*Optimal growth at 33°C.
RSV = respiratory syncytial virus; HSV = herpes simplex virus; VZV = varicella-zoster virus; CMV = cytomegalovirus; PMK = primary monkey kidney; HDF = human diploid fibroblast; RK = rabbit kidney; CPE = cytopathic effect.

6

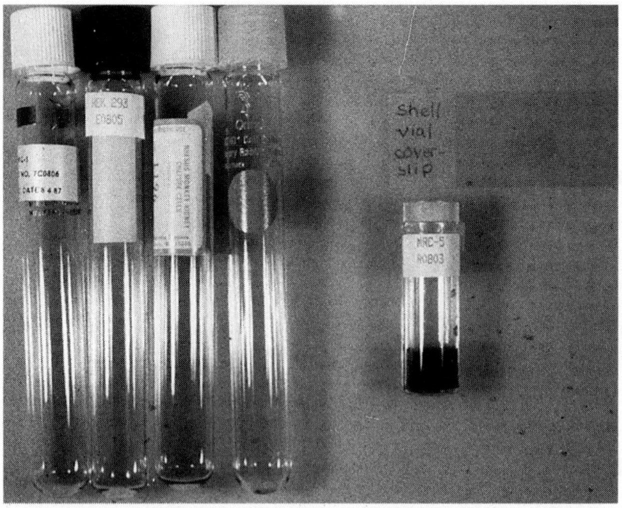

Figure 46–2. Examples of several tissue culture types supplied by commercial sources. Traditional tubes have the cell monolayer grown on one side of the tube and are shipped and incubated so that maintenance medium is always in contact with the cell sheet. Shell vial tubes carry a monolayer on a circular glass coverslip in the bottom of the vial, along with 2 mL of maintenance medium, and are kept upright.

detecting cytopathic effect (CPE) in the cell monolayer. Because a single cell line may support growth of several viruses—each with a distinctive CPE or other characteristic identifying feature—tissue culture tube monolayers offer maximal versatility. CPE may be recognized in two to three days (HSV) or may not develop for two to three weeks (RSV, cytomegalovirus [CMV]), so most cultures should be incubated for at least two weeks. With the shell vial technique, the cell monolayer is grown on a round coverslip, which rests, monolayer side up, in a shell vial. The specimen is inoculated into the shell vial, which is centrifuged to enhance viral uptake by the tissue culture cells. After one to two days of incubation, the monolayer is tested for the presence of viral antigen, usually with a fluorescent antibody stain (Gleaves, 1985). Shell vial culture should be considered for identification of a specific or limited number of viruses, particularly slow-growing viruses such as CMV and varicella-zoster virus (VZV). Initial culture setup is still labor intensive, antibody conjugates are costly, and the sensitivity varies with the virus and specimen type. For example, shell vials are comparable or superior to traditional tube cell culture methods for detection of CMV in urine, but a backup tube culture is needed to maximize CMV recovery from peripheral blood. Specimens from vesicular genital lesions for HSV identification also are good candidates for shell vial culture; sensitivity is almost 100% and turnaround time on negative cultures is decreased from seven days to one day. Suggestions for the use of centrifugation-enhanced cultures are given in Table 46–4.

Table 46–4. RECOMMENDATIONS FOR CENTRIFUGATION-ENHANCED SHELL VIAL CULTURE*

Virus	Cell Line(s)	Incubation Times (Days)
CMV	HDF	1 or 2
HSV	HDF or RK	1
VZV	HDF	3 and 5
RSV	Hep-2, A549	1 and 2
Influenza A and B	PMK	1 and 2
Parainfluenza 1-3	PMK	1 and 2
Adenovirus	Hep-2, A549	3 and 5

*All are set up in duplicate vials.
See Table 46–3 for abbreviations.

Antigen Detection by Direct Fluorescent Antibody Assay and Enzyme Immunoassay

The rapid (same day turnaround time) identification of virus by direct methods is especially useful when specific antiviral therapy is available (for HSV, VZV, CMV, or RSV infections) or when possible nosocomial spread is a factor (as with rotavirus, RSV, influenza, and VZV). Viral antigen can be detected with comparable sensitivity and specificity by both direct fluorescent antibody (DFA) and enzyme immunoassay (EIA) methods. DFA methods have the advantage of microscopic visualization of the specimen's cell content for verification of sample adequacy (Rossier, 1989). DFA procedures are more labor intensive than EIA, however, and may become burdensome in laboratories with large numbers of specimens. EIA methods are more easily automated and require less subjective interpretive judgment than DFA, but the ability to assess specimen quality is lost. DFA is best performed with a high-quality epifluorescence microscope, and positive and negative controls must be run routinely. EIA procedures often require semiautomated washing equipment as well as a spectrophotometer. Negative and positive controls are essential, and a data processor in automated EIA units interprets the patient sample reading based on the established cut-off for positivity and the control readings.

Nucleic acid probe technology also is being adapted for diagnosis of viral infections. Although no commercial products are available to date, several probe kits are in development for identification of the most common viral pathogens.

Direct visualization of virions by electron microscopy using negative staining with phosphotungstic acid or osmium fixation–uranyl lead staining is useful for detection of viruses that do not grow in standard cell culture lines or for rapid demonstration of a fastidious virus. Electron microscopy has had its maximal value in diagnosis of enteric infections because rotavirus, enteric adenoviruses, Norwalk agent astroviruses, and calicivirus replicate poorly or not at all in tissue culture cells.

Viral Serology

Serologic diagnosis of viral infection is attractive because reagents are widely available, and serum specimens are easy to obtain, transport, and store. Measurement of antiviral antibodies has two major applications: diagnosis of recent infection and determination of immunity. Evidence of current/recent infection requires demonstration of viral-specific IgM in serum collected during the acute stage of illness or demonstration of a fourfold or greater rise in viral-specific IgG antibody titer between acute and convalescent serum specimens. Specific IgM is found in blood during the first week of primary infection and typically becomes undetectable within one to three months; enzyme-linked immunoassays detect persistent IgM for at least twice as long as immunofluorescent assays. Viral-specific IgG characteristically develops one to two weeks after primary infection, peaks at four to eight weeks, and then declines, but still remains detectable throughout life. Secondary immune response following viral reinfection or reactivation usually generates a different serologic profile. IgM may reappear, but with a lower titer than in primary cases. By contrast, IgG-specific antibody is detectable at onset of illness and rapidly increases in titer, peaking at higher levels than observed with primary infection. These are general patterns; the intensity, specificity, timing, and class of antibody response are influenced by the infecting virus, site of infection, and immune status of the patient. In congenital infection, maternal IgG antibodies cross the placenta into the fetal circulation, but any IgM or IgA detected in fetal, cord, or newborn blood represents antibody produced by the fetus or baby following primary infection.

There are certain clinical situations where serology is the optimal, only, most expedient, or most cost-effective method for diagnosis. Serology may be used as a backup for viral culture and direct detection methods, particularly if specimen quality and transportation conditions have been suboptimal; also, not all clinically important viruses can be recovered with current commercial culture or assay systems. If viral disease was not suspected during the initial evaluation of the patient, serology may be the only diagnostic tool available once the window of opportunity for culture or antigen assay is closed.

Serology may be helpful in interpretation of culture results; a positive stool culture for enterovirus from a patient with encephalitis takes on added significance if a rise in specific enteroviral titer is also demonstrated. Serology is a logical diagnostic pathway for viruses that require specialized isolation conditions (Epstein-Barr virus [EBV], human herpesvirus [HHV]-6, HHV-7, or HIV) or animal inoculation (arboviruses and some Coxsackie A viruses). In some situations culture and antigen detection are sufficiently sensitive but serology is faster and less costly; both measles and mumps can be diagnosed by virus isolation, but IgM-specific antibody is detectable within three days of the onset of illness and requires less technical time and expertise than culture. Propagation of highly dangerous viruses, such as arboviruses and HIV, should not be attempted in most laboratories, leaving serology as the only practical diagnostic option. Some pathogenic viruses that grow well in culture are encountered so infrequently that practical identification experience is limited; most laboratorians feel more comfortable confirming rubella infection with serology than with culture. Virus may not be present when symptoms develop; arboviruses are rarely isolated from spinal fluid, and are usually cleared by the time the patient develops encephalitis, making serology the preferred diagnostic method. On the other hand, infections with a prolonged prodromal phase often have detectable antibody when the patient becomes symptomatic (EBV and CMV mononucleosis). Specific clinical situations where serology has proved useful are summarized in Table 46–5.

Table 46–5. USE OF SEROLOGY FOR DIAGNOSIS OF VIRAL INFECTIONS

Use	Virus
Demonstration of immunity	IgG: HAV, HBV, measles, mumps, VZV
Preferred/most cost-effective method of diagnosis	IgM: Arboviruses, HAV, HBV, HCV, EBV, measles, mumps, parvovirus B19, rubella IgG: HIV, HCV, HTLV
Diagnosis of postinfectious sequelae	Reye's syndrome (influenza A & B, VZV) SSPE (measles)
Differentiation of primary vs. recurrent maternal infection	IgM and IgG: CMV, HSV
Assessment of infectivity of blood products	IgG: HBV, HCV, HIV, CMV, HTLV

See Tables 46–3 and 46–4 for abbreviations.

HAV = hepatitis A virus; HBV = hepatitis B virus; HCV = hepatitis C virus; EBV = Epstein-Barr virus; HIV = human immunodeficiency virus; HTLV = human T-cell leukemia virus; SSPE = subacute sclerosing panencephalitis.

Specimen Collection and Transportation

Success with any viral diagnostic method is contingent upon proper specimen collection and transportation. The laboratory must develop realistic guidelines for optimal specimen handling and a policy for specimen rejection, and circulate this information to the clinical staff and nursing units (Table 46–6). Specimens for culture and direct antigen detection should be obtained during the acute stage of illness when viral shedding is highest; viral recovery is sporadic and unreliable during convalescence.

Viruses vary in viability during transport and storage. Viral transport medium that contains a buffered salt solution, protein stabilizer, pH indicator, and antibiotics to inhibit unwanted bacteria preserves infectivity of common pathogenic viruses over reasonable storage conditions. Multipurpose viral, chlamydial, and mycoplasmal transport media have also been developed (M4, Flextrans). Most commercial formulations are adequate for short-term usage (<24 hours) (Johnson, 1990). All specimens, except blood samples, should be transported and stored before setup at 4°C. Room temperature transport of specimens may be unavoidable in some circumstances, but physicians should be aware of the negative effect this may have on recovery. Blood samples for virus isolation should be held at room temperature at all times. Viral cultures are best set up the same day specimens arrive in the laboratory and certainly within 48 hours of collection, with at least one tissue culture inoculation session during the weekend. Specimens should only be frozen (−70°C) as a last resort; blood and urine for CMV isolation or respiratory specimens for RSV should not be frozen.

Equipment and Supplies

Much of the equipment required for basic virology is relatively inexpensive and may already be in use in the hospital's microbiology and immunology laboratory sections. A Class II biosafety laminar flow cabinet must be used for culture setup and whenever cultures are manipulated to protect the

Table 46–6. SPECIMEN COLLECTION FOR COMMON VIRAL SYNDROMES

Syndrome	Viruses	Preferred Specimen and Transport Conditions	Specimen Quality Validation	Most Useful Tests
Bronchiolitis/bronchitis	RSV, parainfluenza 1–3, adenovirus, influenza A & B	NPS, BAL; transport immediately on ice	Columnar cells or alveolar macrophages	DFA, EIA, culture
Influenza	Influenza A & B	NPS or throat swab in VTM; transport immediately on ice	Columnar cells or alveolar macrophages	DFA, EIA, culture
Pneumonia	RSV, parainfluenza[3], influenza A & B, adenovirus, *Chlamydia*, and *Mycoplasma*	NPS, BAL, throat swab in VTM; transport immediately on ice	Columnar cells or alveolar macrophages	DFA, EIA, culture
Conjunctivitis	HSV, adenovirus, *Chlamydia*, enteroviruses, VZV, measles	Conjunctival swab or scrapings in VTM; transport immediately on ice	Epithelial cells	DFA, EIA, culture
Vesicular rash	HSV, VZV, enteroviruses	Vesicle fluid/cells in VTM, air-dried smears; transport immediately on ice	Epithelial cells	DFA, culture
Genital infection	HSV	Vesicle fluid/cells, cervical/urethral swabs in VTM, air dried smears; transport ASAP	Epithelial cells	Culture
Meningitis	Enteroviruses, HSV, mumps, VZV, adenoviruses, LCM, measles	CSF, throat and stool (enteroviruses); transport immediately on ice		Culture, PCR (investigational), serology
Encephalitis	HSV*, arboviruses, enteroviruses, rabies	Fresh brain tissue, CSF, serum (arboviruses); transport immediately on ice		DFA, culture, PCR, serology
Enteritis	Rotavirus, adenovirus (40,41), calicivirus, coronavirus, astrovirus, Norwalk viruses	Fresh stool (stool, diaper, or rectal swab) transport promptly	Swab must be >75% covered with stool	EM, EIA, LA
Disseminated viral infection	CMV, HSV, VZV, adenovirus	Urine (on ice), blood (room temp), BAL, tissue biopsy (on ice); transport immediately		Culture, CMV antigenemia assay, quantitative PCR (investigational)

*CSF culture may be positive in neonates but is rarely positive in adults with HSV encephalitis.
See Tables 46–3 through 46–5 for abbreviations. LCM = lymphocytic choriomeningitis virus; NPS = nasopharyngeal secretions; BAL = bronchalveolar lavage; VTM = viral transport media; CSF = cerebrospinal fluid; DFA = direct fluorescent antibody; EIA = enzyme immunoassay; PCR = polymerase chain reaction; EM = electron microscopy; LA = latex agglutination.

technologist from infectious aerosol and to reduce the risk of tissue culture contamination. A centrifuge with carriers to accommodate shell vials should be available. Incubators to store uninoculated tissue culture cells and to incubate inoculated cultures are needed, preferably with an internal outlet to accommodate a roller drum. An inverted phase-contrast microscope is needed for identification of tissue culture monolayer CPE changes, and access to a high-quality fluorescence microscope should be accessible for DFA and IFA procedures. Space in −70°C and −20°C freezers is also important for specimen and reagent storage.

Deionized water should be used for all virology testing. All essential supplies and reagents for identification of the common viruses are commercially available. Tissue culture cells are nourished by a liquid medium prepared with a balanced salt solution base (BSS; either Hanks' or Earle's) to which buffers, serum, and a basic nutrient mixture such as Eagle's minimum essential medium (MEM) are added. Eagle's MEM is a precisely defined formulation of amino acids, sugars, vitamins, cofactors, and other metabolic requirements for the cell culture monolayer. Fetal bovine serum is the most popular nutritional and hormonal supplement for tissue culture media, and is used at a 5% to 10% concentration in tissue culture growth medium and 2% for maintenance medium; lot-to-lot variation and high cost are principal disadvantages. Supplemented calf serum (OmniSerum) has been formulated as a more precise and less expensive alternative to fetal bovine serum, and is acceptable for tissue culture cell lines for HSV isolation and certain other viruses. Trypsin (0.25% solution), phosphate buffered saline (PBS), glutamine and sodium bicarbonate solutions, viral transport media (VTM), antibiotic mixtures for specimen decontamination, and 2% phosphotungstic acid for electron microscopy should also be stocked in the laboratory.

Laboratories undertaking viral diagnostic services for the first time should consider beginning with straightforward testing such as HSV culture and antigen detection. Influenza virus, RSV, and rotavirus assays and cultures can be added during the winter months. CMV culture would be a priority service for a hospital with immunocompromised patients. Enterovirus isolation could be offered initially in the summer and autumn. VZV, adenovirus, and parainfluenza virus cultures and antigen assays would be reasonable additions as staff time and expertise increase and as physician interest in clinical virology expands.

Clinical Viral Infectious Syndromes

One approach to laboratory diagnosis separates viral illnesses into specific clinical syndromes. This encourages physicians to associate a limited group of viruses with a specific illness, and the laboratory effort can be streamlined and focused on rapid and efficient testing with a high diagnostic yield. In this chapter the following viral diseases are discussed:

Herpetic mucocutaneous infections
Pediatric and adult respiratory syndromes
Infectious mononucleosis
Congenital and neonatal infections
Viral central nervous system infections
Pediatric exanthems and enteric infections
Viral hepatitis and HIV infection
Viral infections in the immunocompromised host

HERPETIC MUCOCUTANEOUS INFECTIONS

The Herpesviridae family contains two viruses that characteristically produce infections in the skin and squamous mucous membrane surfaces of the body: HSV and VZV. Both of these infections are commonplace, and while usually not life threatening, the effectiveness of acyclovir therapy has stimulated clinical demand for prompt and accurate laboratory diagnosis, particularly for HSV infection (Whitley, 1992). VZV is discussed in the viral exanthem section of this chapter.

Humans are the only known hosts for HSV; the virus is ubiquitous, found in all racial and ethnic groups worldwide. The HSV viral genome persists in a dormant fashion throughout life, silently incorporated into the host's neural ganglion cells (Hirsch, 1994). The two strains of HSV, serotype 1 and serotype 2, share many molecular and biological features, but each has a unique antigenic profile and a somewhat distinctive epidemiology. Both preferentially infect squamous epithelium; HSV1 is transmitted via saliva and usually infects the mouth, pharynx, lips, and facial skin; HSV2 is found principally in the genital squamous surfaces, is transferred through sexual contact, and produces the vesicles and ulcers of genital herpes.

HSV1 infection usually occurs during childhood. Most infections involve the oral cavity; occasionally lesions develop on the exposed skin of wrestlers or the hands of medical personnel after direct salivary contact. The infection may be delayed until adolescence or adult life in industrialized societies; in middle-class populations of the United States HSV1 seroprevalence is 58% by age 20, while it is nearly 100% in developing nations. Primary infection is often asymptomatic, though a substantial minority can develop fever and painful blister-like lesions of the lips and mouth (gingivostomatitis) with this first exposure (Kuzushima, 1991). HSV1 attaches to surface receptors on squamous cells and with viral replication, these cells lose their cytoplasmic integrity, leak fluid, and separate from one another to create a vesicle. As the epidermis disintegrates, cutaneous bacterial contamination converts vesicles to pustules; ulcers then form when the damaged cells completely lyse. Herpetic lesions usually heal without scarring as the epidermal layers regenerate.

The immediate immune response to HSV1 involves natural killer cells, cytotoxic T lymphocytes, and production of neutralizing antibody. Neither cellular nor humoral mechanisms, however, prevents viral migration through sensory nerve fibers to the trigeminal ganglion, where HSV1 persists indefinitely in neurons in a dormant state (Straus, 1989). HSV episodically reactivates and travels back down neurosensory axons to the mouth and skin, where it again replicates in the squamous epithelium. Most recurrent herpes infections are asymptomatic, or produce transient vesicles that are usually only of cosmetic significance. With severe impairment of cell-mediated immunity (in AIDS patients, transplant recipients, etc.), reactivation infections can be severe or even fatal; encephalitis is another rare but usually devastating HSV1 infection. Both of these complications are discussed in later sections of this chapter.

HSV2 infection is almost invariably a sexually transmitted disease and has become a serious public health concern over the past 30 years. Millions of Americans are now infected, with conservative estimates of 200,000 new cases annually. HSV2 isolation from children is most unusual and raises concerns about sexual abuse; beginning with adolescence, however, seroprevalence rises steadily through middle age and is proportional to the number of sexual partners (Johnson, 1989). HSV2 in the genital squamous mucosa of both men and women is easily spread by intimate contact, and the virus produces the same pattern of primary and recurrent mucocutaneous lesions seen with oral HSV1. Latency is established in pelvic autonomic and sacral ganglia, and reactivation rates are at least twice as high as with HSV1 (Benedetti, 1994). Primary and recurrent HSV2 lesions heal completely in people with normal cellular immune function. The most worrisome concern is exposure of infants during vaginal delivery; neonatal herpes is discussed later in this chapter.

Specimen Collection and Handling Guidelines

The demand for herpes laboratory testing is great, and overall more specimens are submitted for HSV identification than for diagnosis of any other viral infection. HSV is probably the easiest and fastest human virus to cultivate in cell culture, and antigen assays are also relatively straightforward procedures. Specimen collection (see Chap. 54) is simple, and HSV is sufficiently durable that immediate transport and laboratory handling are not necessary.

Cell Culture Isolation of Herpes Simplex Virus

Specimens in VTM with antibiotics, if kept refrigerated, can tolerate a transportation delay of 12 hours or more with minimal viral loss. Specimens should be inoculated to tissue culture the day of receipt, but overnight refrigeration is acceptable. HSV isolation in cell culture is considered the gold standard diagnostic test, and to date it is clearly more sensitive than any antigen assay or nucleic acid probe method. HSV grows exceptionally well in a wide variety of tissue culture cell lines; human fibroblasts (WI-38, MRC-5, foreskin fibroblasts) have been the most popular, but rabbit kidney is particularly useful for rapid demonstration of CPE and HEp-2, HeLa, rhabdomyosarcoma cells (RD), A549, and mink lung cell lines are also adequate. Primary monkey kidney cells (PMK) are not reliable and should be avoided. Two tissue culture tubes (one RK and one human diploid fibroblast [HDF]) are usually inoculated; the procedure is summarized in Figure 46–3.

HSV replicates so easily in cell culture that CPE often is observed on the first, second, or third day of incubation, es-

6

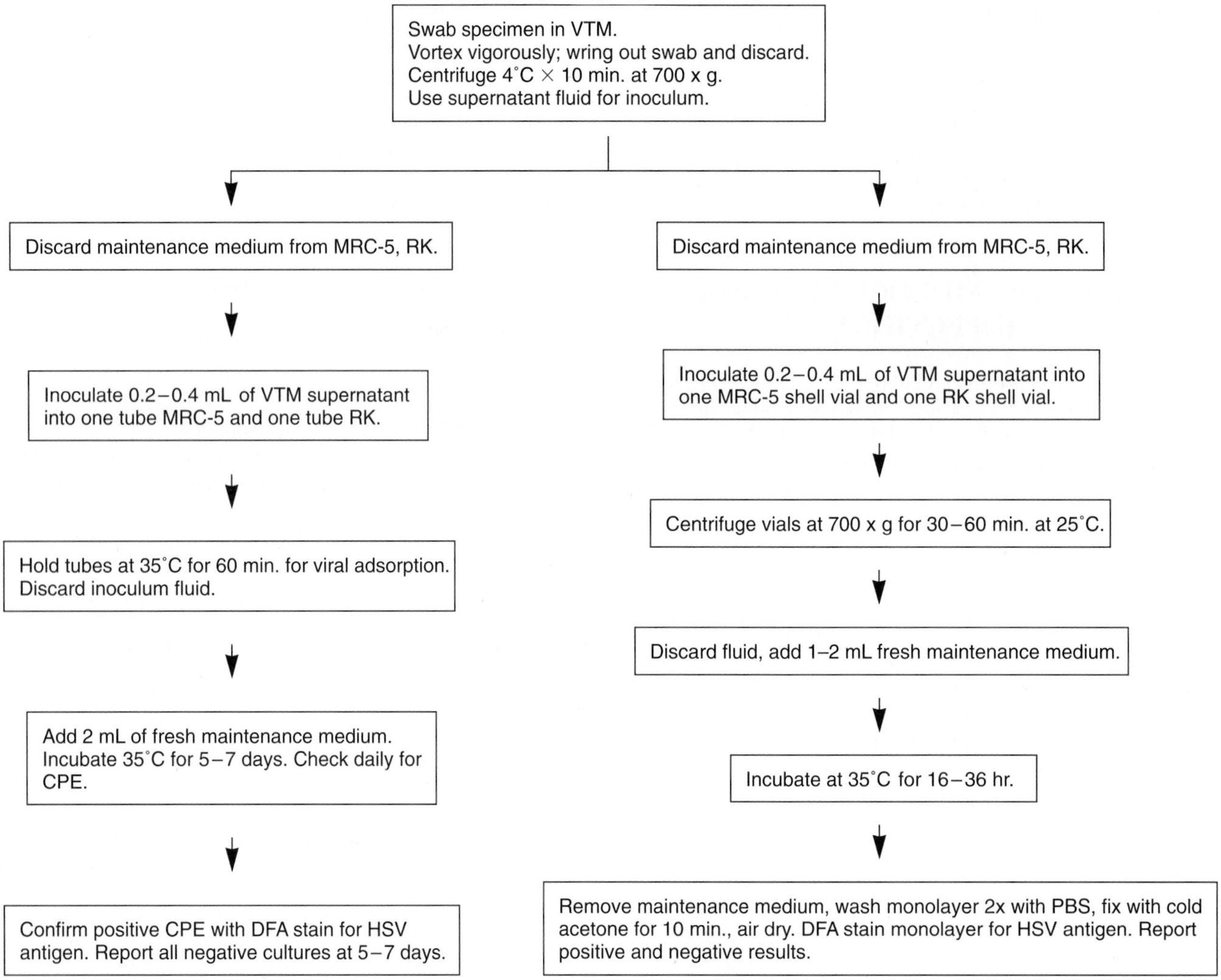

Figure 46–3. Algorithm for traditional tube (*left*) and shell vial (*right*) cultures for herpes simplex virus.

pecially with use of a roller drum (Mavromoustakis, 1988). Cultures from genital lesions that fail to show CPE only need to be held for five to seven days before reporting as negative; because other viruses may be recovered from nongenital mucocutaneous sites (VZV, enteroviruses, etc.), these cultures should be incubated for two weeks. Individual HSV-infected cells first become swollen and rounded (ballooning change), and then cellular damage spreads rapidly across the monolayer. HSV2 frequently causes syncytium formation as the cytoplasmic membranes of infected cells coalesce (Fig. 46–4). This CPE is characteristic of but not unique for HSV; an inexperienced technologist may misinterpret CPE caused by other viruses, toxins, or even *Trichomonas vaginalis* as HSV damage, so confirmation with a DFA stain is recommended. Monolayer cells are scraped off, transferred to a glass slide, fixed in acetone, and then stained with either monoclonal or polyclonal antibodies specific for HSV (Lipson, 1991). Type-specific monoclonal DFA reagents can distinguish HSV1 from HSV2, but the extra labor and materials increase the cost of routine HSV culture and generally add little information to what was already clinically suspected. Serotyping should be reserved for cases with medicolegal concerns or clinical ambiguities.

The large number of HSV culture requests led to the use of shell vial centrifugation-enhanced culture, in which viral antigen can be identified in the monolayer by DFA staining before the evolution of CPE (Gleaves, 1985) (Fig. 46–5). Detection of HSV in shell vial culture by EIA or DNA *in situ* hybridization (ISH) is equally sensitive and specific (Espy, 1988; Patel, 1991; Michalski and Shaikh, 1986). Centrifugation-enhanced culture adaptations using standard tissue culture tubes or microtiter tray wells rather than vials have also been developed, with variable results (Oefinger, 1988; Woods, 1988; Ziegler, 1988).

Direct Detection of Herpes Simplex Virus

The Tzanck preparation is a direct smear from a herpetic vesicle that is stained with Giemsa to demonstrate the intranuclear inclusions and multinucleated syncytial epithelial giant cells that develop with HSV infection. These findings are not entirely specific and can be seen in VZV chickenpox and shingles. The Tzanck preparation is positive in only 67% of herpetic lesions. Despite the rapid turnaround time

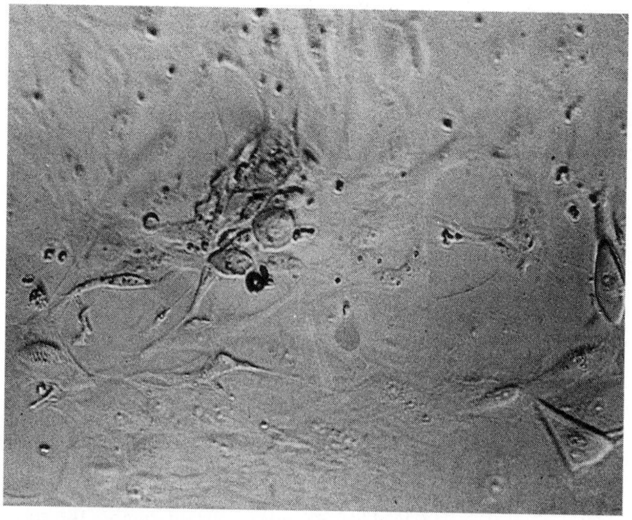

Figure 46–4. Rabbit kidney cell culture monolayer with herpes simplex virus cytopathic effect. Rabbit kidney cells normally have a polygonal shape and fit side-by-side in a continuous cell mosaic. The HSV-infected cells from this three-day-old culture show rounding and swelling, and several adjacent infected cells have coalesced into syncytial giant cells. The vacant areas of the monolayer represent infected cells that have died and lysed (200 × magnification, phase contrast microscopy).

of the Giemsa stain, these limitations reduce its practical utility.

Immunostaining of direct smears for HSV antigen has the advantage of specificity, and viral antigen can be identified in cells that do not yet exhibit nuclear inclusions or syncytium formation. Both fluorescein- and immunoperoxidase-labeled HSV antibodies improve diagnostic sensitivity, but when compared with tissue culture, there is a still false-negative error rate of 20% to 30% (Lafferty, 1987; Moseley, 1981) (Table 46–7). Other approaches to rapid herpes diagnosis,

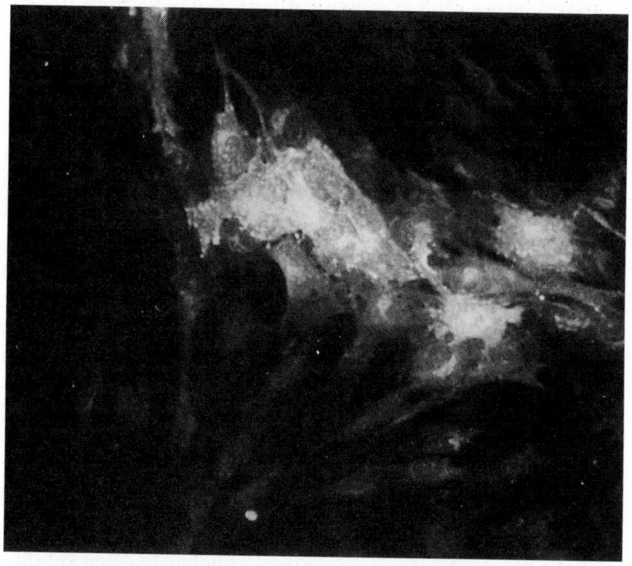

Figure 46–5. This shell vial MRC-5 fibroblast monolayer shows herpes simplex virus nuclear and cytoplasmic antigen after 16 hours of incubation. The cell monolayer is intact, and traditional cytopathic alterations are yet to be detected (250× magnification, DFA stain for HSV antigen).

Table 46–7. SENSITIVITY OF VIRUS ISOLATION, GIEMSA-STAINED TZANK SMEAR, DIRECT FLUORESCENT ANTIBODY, AND IMMUNOPEROXIDASE STAINING IN HERPES SIMPLEX LESIONS

	Sensitivity (% positive) Method			
Stage of Lesion	***Culture***	***Tzank***	***DFA***	***IP***
Vesicle	70–95	67	76–87	76
Pustule	67–83	55	58–67	75
Ulcer	32–67	—	30–38	55
Crusted	17	—	10	—

Figures given are composite values from Pindak (1986), Langenberg (1988), and Mavromoustakis (1988).
DFA = direct fluorescent antibody; IP = immunoperoxidase.

such as *in situ* hybridization detection of HSV-specific DNA sequences in cells from direct lesions, and EIA and latex agglutination identification of HSV antigen fragments, have shown variable levels of sensitivity and specificity. The sensitivity of *in situ* hybridization has ranged from 25% to 92% (Langenberg, 1988; Seal, 1991); EIA methods also report sensitivity as low as 35% but as high as 92% (Dorian, 1991; Gonik, 1991; Needham, 1992; Verano, 1990; Warford, 1986; Wu, 1989); latex agglutination assay sensitivity ranges from 50% to 73% (Halstead, 1987; Johnston, 1992).

A valid substitute for tissue culture has yet to be developed, and despite the proliferation of rapid screening methods, their limitations and cost are too great to justify either immediate direct testing or to consider elimination of HSV tissue culture. All negative direct specimen tests results must be interpreted as potential false-negatives that should be validated by culture.

Serologic Diagnosis

Because there is considerable antigenic homology between HSV1 and HSV2, specificity in serologic testing requires purified viral antigens that are serotypically specific. Enzyme-linked immunosorbent assay (ELISA) and Western blot methods (Ashley, 1988; Lee, 1986) with unique membrane envelope gG and GM antigens that avoid HSV1 and HSV2 cross-reactions have been developed in research laboratories, but commercial kits with verified antigenic specificity have not yet been marketed (Ashley, 1991). Because of the high seroprevalence of HSV, serologic testing has limited use in routine clinical diagnosis. Once accurate serotyping methods are widely available, the most valuable application of serology will be identification of IgM-class HSV2-specific antibody in pregnant women to predict neonatal transmission risk (Brown, 1991).

VIRAL RESPIRATORY TRACT INFECTIONS

Every year in the United States respiratory tract infections lead to millions of outpatient visits and hospitalizations. Viruses collectively account for most of these diseases, and infections range from trivial colds, to more serious laryngotracheobronchitis (croup), to severe bronchiolitis and pneumonia. Both healthy children and adults are at risk during epidemics of croup, bronchiolitis, and influenza, which recur every winter, and the associated morbidity and mortality can be dramatic. The 1993–1994 influenza outbreak in the United States was of only moderate severity, but pneumonia and influenza together caused 9% of deaths during flu season (Update, 1994).

Upper respiratory tract infections, such as colds and pharyngitis, rarely are severe enough to require laboratory testing; however, specimens submitted for isolation of viral lower respiratory tract pathogens are second only to herpes simplex culture requests. Influenza viruses are the most important respiratory pathogens in adults; RSV, parainfluenza virus, influenza virus, and adenovirus are most significant in young children (Table 46–8).

Influenza

Influenza A and B viruses cause annual cold weather outbreaks of acute febrile respiratory tract infection, which has characteristic accompanying systemic features. Influenza A is more common than B, and generally produces more serious disease. Because antigens change through point mutation in the viral genome and recombination of viral nucleic acid segments, antibodies from prior episodes of influenza may afford little protection in subsequent outbreaks. Both influenza viruses are highly contagious, and infected nasal secretions are spread person to person as aerosol droplets or on contaminated hands (Betts, 1994).

Influenza virus replication in ciliated columnar epithelial cells of the pharynx and tracheobroncial tree produces acute mucosal necrosis. Patients typically experience abrupt onset of fever, sore throat, and nonproductive cough, followed by headache, generalized myalgia, and extreme weakness. Uncomplicated influenza usually resolves after four to five days, and most patients recover uneventfully. In a minority of patients, acute viral necrosis extends into the alveolar lining cells, producing severe, potentially fatal pneumonia (Yeldandi, 1994). Most influenza-related deaths, however, are caused by secondary bacterial bronchopneumonia as the virus-damaged bronchial epithelium becomes infected with *Staphylococcus aureus, Streptococcus pneumoniae,* or *Haemophilus influenzae* from the oropharynx. These bacterial infections are more common in patients with pre-existing chronic lung disease or congestive heart failure. Rarely myocarditis, meningoencephalitis, Reye's syndrome or Guillain-Barré syndrome develop as complications of acute influenza.

Influenza is diagnosed best during the first two to three days of illness when viral shedding is maximal. Culture is the most sensitive diagnostic test; however, traditional cell culture may not yield a positive result for two to seven days, usually too late to influence the management of the index patient or to pursue effective prophylaxis of contacts (Douglas, 1990). Centrifugation-enhanced shell vial cultures with one to two day incubation times have comparable sensitivity and have become popular for early diagnosis (Leonardi, 1994). Influenza viruses also grow well in embryonated eggs, but the added effort is rarely justified.

DFA staining of influenza antigen is useful for rapid diagnosis in children; the nasopharyngeal secretions (NPS) collected from children contain abundant epithelial cells that are rich in virus (sensitivities range from 77% to 93% for influenza A and from 70% to 80% for influenza B; depending on the quality of the specimen, antisera, influenza strain, and the experience of the microscopist, specificity is greater than 95%) (Costello, 1991). Unfortunately, throat swabs, the most frequently collected specimens in adults, rarely provide enough intact columnar cells for DFA staining. Commercial EIAs have excellent sensitivity for influenza A antigen detection if tests are performed on NPS; sensitivity with throat swabs is lower (Leonardi, 1994; Ryan-Poirier, 1992).

Table 46–8. VIRUSES ASSOCIATED WITH LOWER RESPIRATORY TRACT INFECTIONS

Syndrome	Viruses
Croup	Parainfluenza 1–3, RSV, influenza A & B, adenovirus, measles
Bronchiolitis	RSV, parainfluenza 3, influenza A & B, adenovirus, measles
Pneumonia	RSV, influenza A & B, parainfluenza 3, adenovirus, measles, CMV, VZV
Influenza	Influenza A & B

See Tables 46–3 and 46–4 for abbreviations.

Respiratory Syncytial Virus Bronchiolitis

Respiratory syncytial virus (RSV) is the most important cause of serious lower respiratory viral disease in infants and young children (Anderson, 1990; Hall, 1990). RSV is easily transmitted by oro-nasal droplet aerosol and close contact, and tightly clustered outbreaks occur every winter in the United States (Fig. 46–6). Because immunity to RSV is incomplete and of short duration, multiple infections of decreasing severity throughout life are typical, although RSV may again cause severe pulmonary disease in the elderly living in nursing homes and in immunocompromised hosts (Falsey, 1990).

RSV infects ciliated columnar epithelial cells from the nasopharynx to the terminal bronchioles, but the most serious RSV presentation is bronchiolitis, particularly in children under one year of age, whose small terminal airways can easily become occluded with necrotic epithelial cells and inflammatory debris. Distal airway obstruction leads to hypoxia, tachypnea, and air trapping, which may be severe enough to necessitate hospitalization. The most critical RSV infections occur in premature newborns, in children with underlying cardiopulmonary disease or immunodeficiencies, and in transplant recipients (Hall, 1986; Pohl, 1992). Most children recover without sequelae, but persistent bronchospasm or asthma may occur (Ruuskanen, 1993). Approximately 1% of children hospitalized with RSV bronchiolitis die from hypoxia, secondary cardiac failure, or bacterial superinfection.

Rapid diagnosis of RSV in the hospitalized patient is important so that infection control measures to prevent nosocomial spread can be introduced promptly (McCarthy, 1990) and so that ribavirin therapy, if warranted, can be started without delay. Ribavirin, a synthetic nucleoside that inhibits RSV replication, is administered by fine-particle aerosol and can partially reverse hypoxemia and accelerate recovery (Smith, 1991). The drug, however, is expensive; pharmacy and related charges typically exceed $500 per day. Because

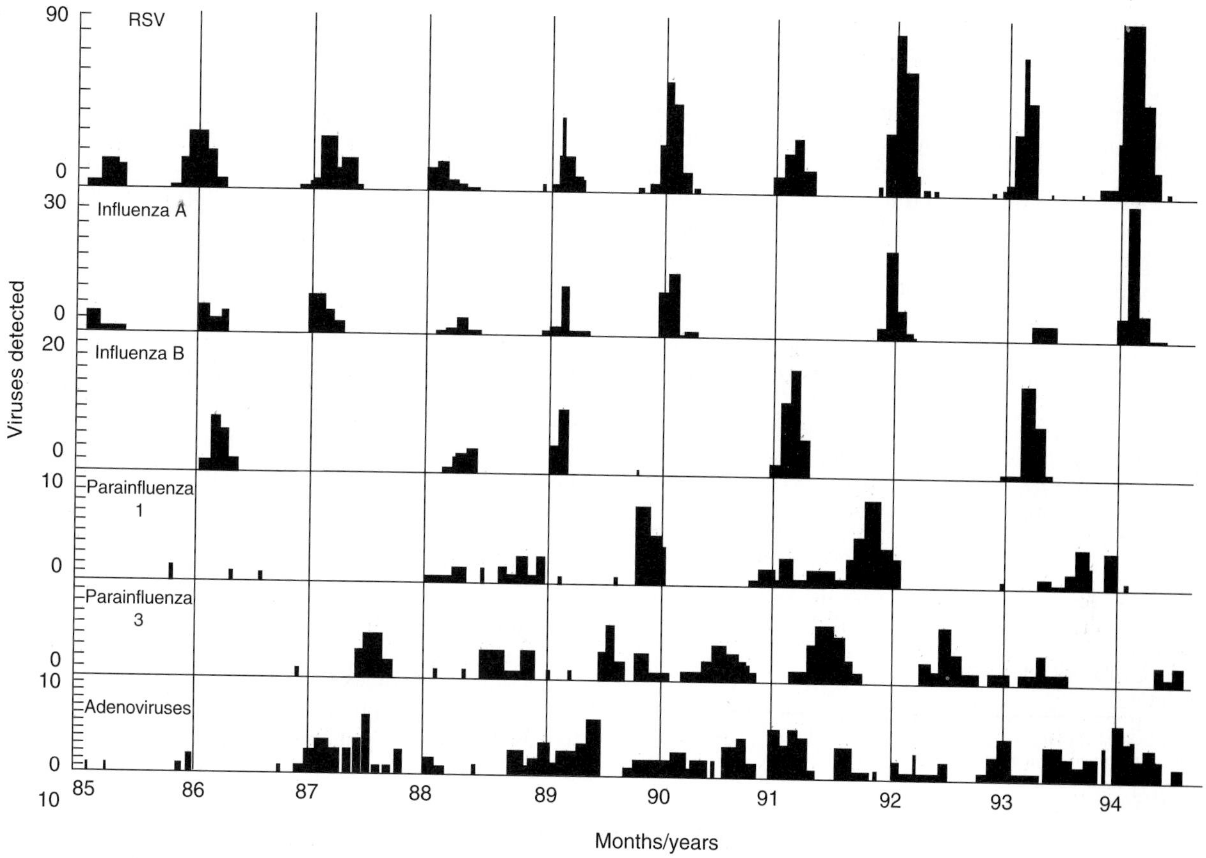

Figure 46–6. Monthly isolation rates of respiratory viruses at Lutheran General Hospital, Park Ridge, IL, 1985–1995.

of prolonged RSV shedding during acute infection and convalescence, barrier precautions, such as masks, face shields, gloves, and gowns, along with cohort isolation of known positive cases, should be implemented to minimize hospital spread (Gala, 1986; Leclair, 1987).

RSV is a particularly fragile and labile virus, and may not remain viable if specimen transport is delayed. Once inoculated into tissue culture cells, it replicates slowly with late development of CPE; isolation times range from three to 10 days (Arens, 1986; Talis, 1991). Centrifugation-enhanced shell vial cultures can improve RSV recovery somewhat and shorten isolation time to two days (Pedneault, 1994; Smith, 1991). Detection of RSV antigen in viral respiratory secretions by DFA staining or EIA is as sensitive as or superior to culture and produces results in a clinically relevant time frame; therefore, these tests have become the definitive practical methods for RSV diagnosis (Rossier, 1989; Waner, 1990). EIA is easy and rapid to perform; however, reagents are expensive and the methods do not include a mechanism for evaluating specimen adequacy. Although DFA requires more time and interpretive expertise, it can easily be expanded to assay multiple viruses and confirmation of specimen quality is simple.

Croup

Croup is most commonly caused by parainfluenza virus (PIV) (Henrickson, 1994; Vainionpaa, 1994). PIV1 and PIV2 activity peaks during cold weather, but PIV3 infection is endemic and causes respiratory disease year-round. The PIVs are the second most frequent viral lower respiratory tract infections in young children. Viral epithelial necrosis and mucosal edema in the larynx, trachea, and large bronchi narrow the airway, producing the barking cough and stridulous, obstructed breathing pattern characteristic of croup. Immunity is partial and transient, so repeated PIV infections are common; however, in older children and adults, symptoms are less severe and are centered in the upper respiratory tract.

Culture of NPS is the most sensitive method of diagnosis, but DFA demonstration of PIV antigen has good sensitivity, ranging from 69% to 85%, particularly with NPS (Costello, 1993). In hospitals with large pediatric services, routine testing of respiratory specimens for a panel of viruses (RSV; influenza A and B; and PIV1, 2, and 3) (Costello, 1991) is reasonable during winter months if time and budgets permit. All samples that are negative by DFA or EIA procedures should be cultured because these methods are not sensitive enough to replace culture.

6

Specimen Collection

The respiratory myxoviruses and adenovirus infect ciliated columnar epithelial cells from the nasopharynx to the alveoli, so when lower airway disease (croup, bronchiolitis, or influenza), is suspected, the upper respiratory mucosa is the easiest and most accessible site to sample for culture or antigen assay. All specimens should be collected during the first few days of acute illness when viral replication is at its peak. In adults, although NPS is superior, a throat swab placed in VTM with antibiotics is usually sufficient for influenza culture. Expectorated sputum is also adequate for culture (Kimball, 1983), particularly in patients who are coughing vigorously.

NPS specimens are collected by instilling 1 mL of saline into the patient's nostril, and then aspirating this fluid directly back from the nasopharynx into a suction trap. All specimens should be transported on ice as promptly as possible to minimize RSV loss. Specimen quality should be verified before performing culture or antigen assay. Table 46–9 illustrates the yield of respiratory viruses from NPS samples containing acceptable or inadequate cellular material; fewer than two columnar epithelial cells per 250 × field are associated with a more than fourfold reduction in specimen positivity.

Table 46–9. VIRUS RECOVERY FROM NASOPHARYNGEAL SECRETIONS: RELATIONSHIP TO SPECIMEN ADEQUACY

Sample (N = 2173)	Number of NPS Specimens	% With Positive Virus Recovery
NPS with ≤1 columnar cells per 250 × field	243	6
NPS with ≥2 columnar cells per 250 × field	1930	27

Lutheran General Hospital data, January 1985 to May 1990; 11% of specimens had insufficient cells and required recollection.

NPS = nasopharyngeal secretions.

Virus Antigen Assay

Figure 46–7 outlines a culture and DFA staining procedure for respiratory virus identification. Reproducible and accurate viral antigen detection by DFA requires interpretive expertise, so if possible, both viral culture and antigen assay should be done. The NPS specimen should be washed in phosphate-buffered saline (PBS) containing a mucolytic agent such as Sputolysin and centrifuged; the cell button then is resuspended in PBS and cells are spread on Teflon-coated, acetone-cleaned slides. Air-dried smears are fixed with 100% acetone and stained for viral antigen(s) using specific DFA serum conjugate(s) with Evans'-blue counterstain. One extra acetone-fixed slide should be prepared and stored desiccated at −20°C. This slide can be retrieved and stained if the specimen yields a positive culture but the original DFA stains were interpreted as negative. The number of ciliated columnar epithelial cells and the degree of nonspecific background staining caused by mucus or neutrophils are recorded, and slides are evaluated for specific viral staining patterns. Interpretation criteria are listed in Table 46–10; Figure 46–8 shows DFA stain of NPS positive for influenza A.

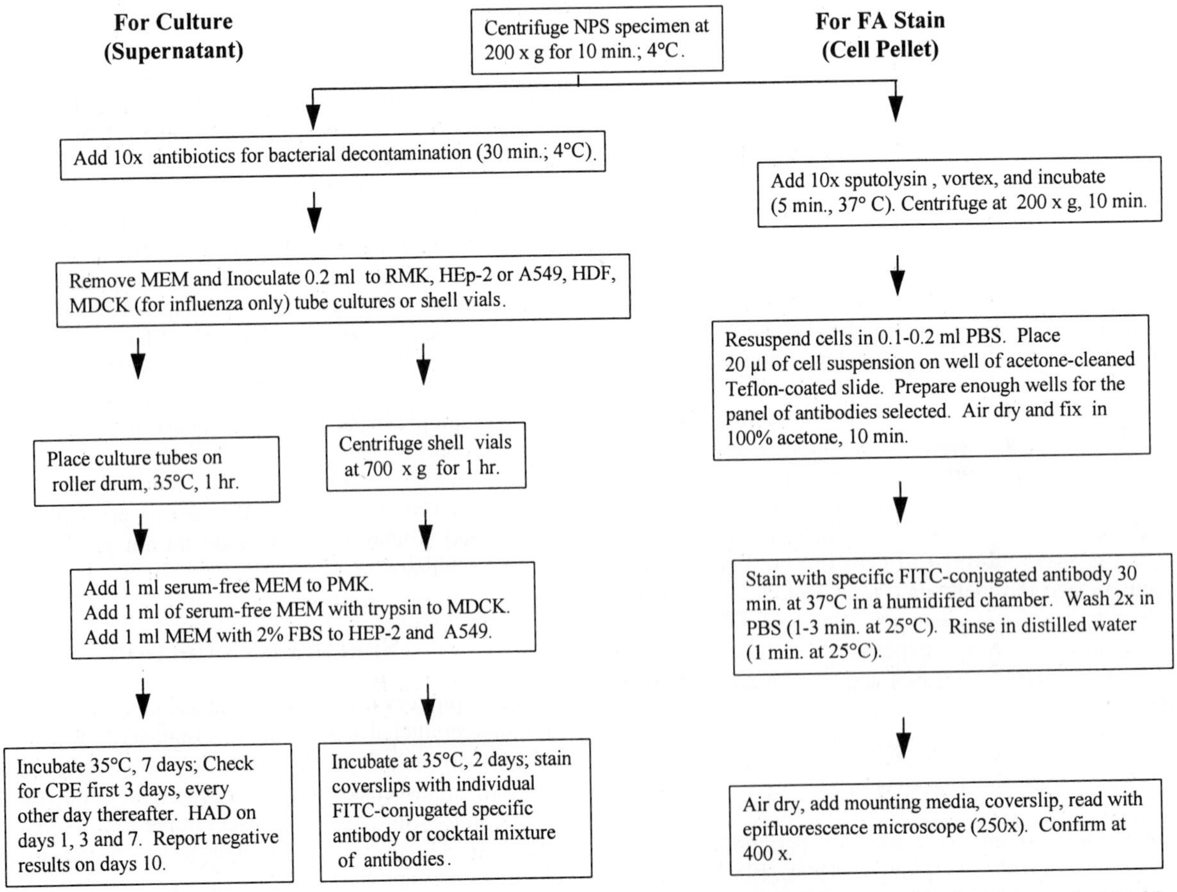

Figure 46–7. Algorithm for diagnosis of respiratory viral infections by culture (*left*) and direct fluorescent antibody staining method (*right*).

Table 46–10. IDENTIFICATION OF VIRAL ANTIGEN IN NASOPHARYNGEAL SECRETIONS: INTERPRETATION OF FLUORESCENT STAINING PATTERNS*

Virus	Cell Type	Staining Pattern
Respiratory syncytial virus	Mononuclear cells and columnar cells	Entirely cytoplasmic; large fluorescent bodies and fine fluorescent particles present; disregard nonspecific staining of squamous cells and PMNs.
Parainfluenza virus	Mononuclear cells and columnar cells	Entirely cytoplasmic; large inclusion-like bodies, fine particles or strands of fluorescent material; pattern closely resembles RSV, but fluorescent particles show less size variation, and more ciliated epithelial cells are stained; disregard nonspecific staining of squamous cells and PMNs
Influenza virus	Mononuclear cells and columnar cells	Viral antigen may be present in nucleus alone, in nucleus or cytoplasm, or cytoplasm alone; staining pattern can be finely particulate to dense, obscuring the entire cell; disregard nonspecific staining of squamous cells and PMNs
Adenovirus	Mononuclear cells	Viral antigen is nuclear or perinuclear, but variation may be considerable; extracellular staining usually present, but very difficult to distinguish from nonspecific staining; disregard nonspecific staining of squamous cells and PMNs

*These criteria were developed using polyclonal antisera. Monoclonal antisera may exhibit more restricted staining patterns; refer to manufacturer's package insert for detailed information.

PMNs = polymorphonuclear neutrophils.

Fluorescein-conjugated antisera should be tested for specificity with a panel of known positive tissue culture control cells. Staining patterns should show consistent cellular distribution and staining intensity throughout a series of lot numbers. Indirect fluorescent antibody staining is slightly more sensitive than direct fluorescent procedures. Overall, fluorescent antibody staining methods have excellent specificity and sensitivity (Cheeseman, 1986; Takimoto, 1991).

Several EIAs are now commercially available for RSV and influenza A antigen. The specificity and sensitivity of these products is quite good, comparable to DFA staining (Hughes, 1988; Krilov, 1988; Miller, 1993; Thomas, 1991; Waner, 1990). NPS samples for EIA should be checked for the presence of ciliated columnar epithelial cells; a wet mount slide prepared by mixing one drop of specimen with one drop of saline should be scanned at 250× to verify that sufficient columnar cells were lavaged from the nasopharynx. Swab specimens from the throat or nasopharynx contain too little cellular material for cytologic screening.

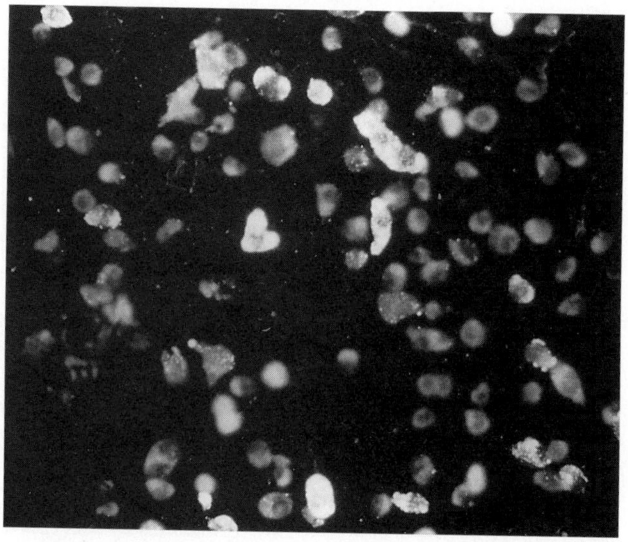

Figure 46–8. This nasopharyngeal aspirate smear is a direct fluorescent antibody stain with fluorescent antigen in the nucleus and cytoplasm of ciliated columnar epithelial cells and mononuclear cells (250× magnification, direct fluorescent antibody stain for influenza A antigen).

Virus Isolation

The same specimen requirements and restrictions that apply to antigen assays govern virus isolation by cell culture. Throat swab and NPS cultures in nonimmunocompromised adults and children can be modified to accommodate seasonal epidemics of influenza, RSV and PIV (see Fig. 46–6). At a minimum, the laboratory should attempt to isolate RSV and influenza, and if staffing permits, PIV, adenovirus, and measles. Table 46–3 lists the tissue culture cell lines that support the growth of lower respiratory viral pathogens. Culture provides a modest improvement in diagnostic sensitivity over antigen assays; approximately 10% more cases of influenza are identified when culture is performed. Culture also can recover viruses that are not included in the antigen assay panel (Blanding, 1989; Johnston, 1990; Rabalais, 1992).

Throat swabs or sputum from adults with suspected influenza should be placed in VTM with antibiotics at time of collection to inhibit oral flora and transported promptly, preferably on ice; processing for culture should not be delayed past 48 hours, but the day of collection is obviously preferable (Harmon, 1991). The VTM vial should be vortexed vigorously before the swab is discarded. The supernatant is inoculated into duplicate shell vials (either two rhesus monkey kidney or two trypsinized Madin-Darby canine kidney), which are refed after centrifugation with MEM without fetal bovine serum (bovine serum may contain antibodies to influenza virus). Following a one to two day incubation at 35°C, shell vial monolayers are DFA-stained for influenza A and B antigens (Seno, 1991). A single backup tube of RMK or Madin Darby Canine Kidney cells (MDCK) also can be inoculated, incubated on a roller drum, and then checked for viral growth by adding fresh (<two weeks old) guinea pig red blood cells. Influenza virus, like PIV and measles, does not consistently produce an easily recognized CPE pattern; however, these viruses insert hemagglutinin antigens into the tissue culture cell surface, and guinea pig red cell adherence to the monolayer indicates that one of

6

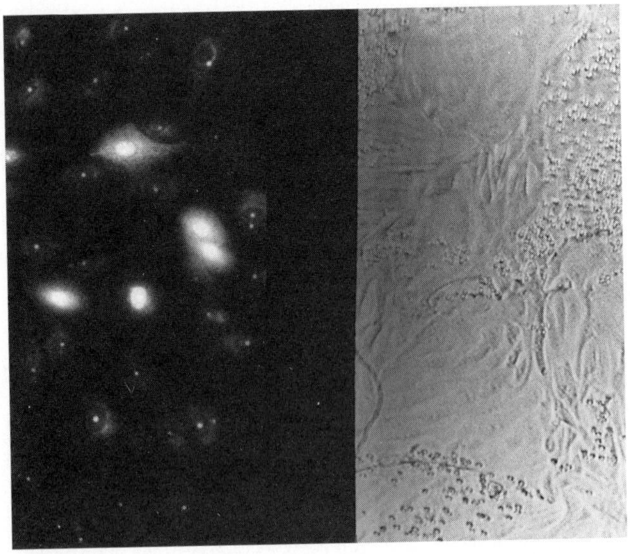

Figure 46–9. This primary monkey kidney shell vial culture is positive for influenza A antigen (*left*). This primary monkey kidney monolayer infected with influenza A shows positive guinea pig red blood cell hemadsorption (*right*).

these hemadsorbing viruses is replicating in the cytoplasm. Hemadsorption is generally performed at two, five, and seven days, but the time to detection can be significantly shortened by a daily testing schedule (Minnich, 1987). When absorption is observed, the monolayer cells must be tested with a set of antisera to determine which virus is present. Figure 46–9 shows a RMK shell vial monolayer positive for influenza A after two days of incubation and a standard RMK tissue culture cell monolayer infected with influenza A that exhibits positive hemadsorption on day three.

Figure 46–7 outlines a culture procedure for pediatric NPS. Laboratories that elect to recover RSV only should consider using a combination of shell vials and traditional tissue culture tubes. HEp-2 cells in Eagle's MEM supplemented with 2% to 5% fetal bovine serum remain the most popular culture line, but A-549 cells also support RSV replication. If laboratory staffing allows a more comprehensive workup, RMK can be included for influenza, PIV, and measles. A549 cells are excellent for adenovirus. Cell culture tube monolayers ideally should be incubated on a roller drum and checked daily for CPE. Figure 46–10 shows a typical RSV CPE pattern (multinucleated cellular syncytium), a change that is influenced by the cation content and freshness of the maintenance medium (Shahrabadi, 1988). RSV shell vial culture reduces isolation time to two days. Adenovirus replication generates a grapelike rounding and swelling of monolayer cells, usually by five to seven days; shell vial culture shortens detection to three days.

There are a number of serologic methods for detecting specific antiviral antibodies, but virtually all are unable to produce a rapid valid diagnosis for clinical management. Serologic diagnosis is certainly valuable for public health studies but has limited practical applicability in clinical laboratories.

INFECTIOUS MONONUCLEOSIS AND RELATED INFECTIONS

Infectious mononucleosis (IM) is a common systemic lymphoproliferative disease that is most frequently caused by EBV; *Toxoplasma gondii* and a variety of other viruses (CMV, HIV, HHV6) also can produce clinically similar illnesses. EBV is part of the Herpesviridae family, and like HSV, eventually infects the majority of the population worldwide. EBV is spread by contaminated saliva. Primary infection in childhood is usually asymptomatic, but in teens and young adults is more likely to produce the clinical entity of IM. Overall, approximately 200,000 mononucleosis cases occur annually in the United States (Schlossberg, 1989; Straus, 1993).

EBV first infects the pharyngeal epithelium, so sore throat and fever typically mark the onset of IM. EBV is also strikingly lymphotropic, attaching to the C3d receptor on the surface of B lymphocytes and initiating a polyclonal B-cell proliferation with subsequent tonsillar enlargement, systemic lymphadenopathy, and splenomegaly. B lymphocytes are transformed and immortalized by EBV infection, and without an adequate cell-mediated immune response this process can evolve into an overt malignancy (as seen in X-linked lymphoproliferative syndrome). A normal immune system, however, uses both natural killer cells and CD8 cytotoxic T lymphocytes to eradicate infected B cells. These defensive cells also contribute to the systemic pathology of IM; EBV-infected B lymphocytes, natural killer large granular lymphocytes, and cytotoxic T lymphocytes are found in lymph nodes, spleen, and peripheral blood. As cell-mediated factors control EBV replication, IM symptoms diminish, and lymphadenopathy and splenomegaly subside.

Like other herpesviruses, EBV persists as a latent infection, with its DNA stored in the nuclei of a small percentage of B lymphocytes. Episodic asymptomatic reactivation is

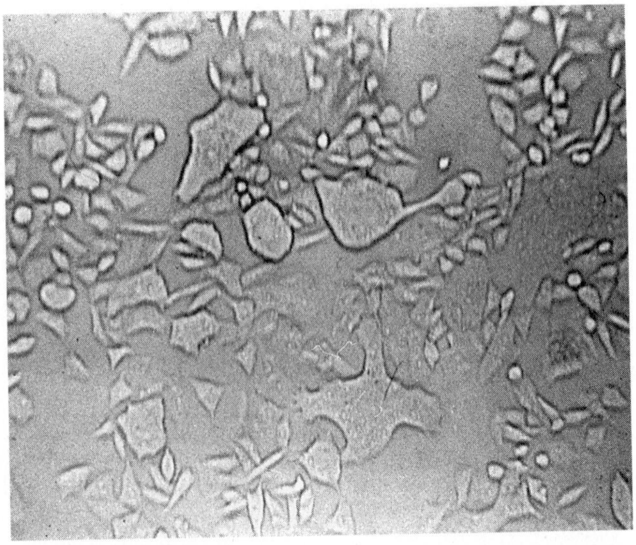

Figure 46–10. The HEp-2 tissue culture monolayer shows respiratory syncytial virus cytopathic effect with a prominent multinucleated syncytium after nine days of incubation (200× magnification, phase contrast microscopy).

common, and up to 20% of healthy young adults shed EBV in their saliva. Individuals with impaired cell-mediated immunity (AIDS, organ transplant recipients, ataxia telangiectasia) may develop overt reactivation infections with hairy leukoplakia, interstitial pneumonitis, or a monoclonal B-cell lymphoma. EBV has also been linked to nasopharyngeal carcinoma in Asians and to Burkitt's lymphoma in central Africans.

Serologic Diagnosis

Peripheral blood atypical lymphocytosis (atypical cells >10% total lymphocytes) is relatively insensitive for diagnosis of EBV mononucleosis but has an overall specificity of at least 95%. EBV can be cultivated in lymphoblastoid cell lines, but this procedure is technically complex and not available in most laboratories. Moreover, the presence of virus does not differentiate primary from reactivated infection. Serologic testing is the only practical laboratory approach for diagnosing IM (Sumaya, 1992). The polyclonal B-lymphocyte proliferation of acute EBV infection generates a variety of transitory but largely harmless autoantibodies such as IgM anti-i (cold agglutinin), rheumatoid factor, and anti-nuclear antibody, but perhaps the most unusual immunoglobulins that develop in mononucleosis are the Paul-Bunnell heterophile antibodies. These IgM-class antibodies, which have an affinity for sheep and horse erythrocytes, are not directed against any EBV antigens. Heterophile antibodies are random products of EBV-induced B-lymphocyte polyclonal proliferation that emerge during the first week of IM, decline during convalescence, and are usually undetectable by three to six months. Various heterophile antibodies can develop in serum sickness and occasionally in other viral infections. However, heterophile antibody with strong affinity for beef erythrocyte antigens unchanged by adsorption with guinea pig kidney antigen (the differential absorption test) is specific for acute EBV disease. The reference method for IM heterophile antibody differentially absorbs patient serum with guinea pig kidney antigen and then adds equine red cells; agglutination occurs in the presence of IM heterophile antibody. Several screening tests directly mix patient serum on a slide with a suspension of guinea pig kidney antigen followed by addition of preserved horse red cells; agglutination occurs almost immediately if the IM heterophile antibody is present. Rapid solid-phase immunoassays use purified bovine red cell stromal antigen or EBV nuclear antigen (EBNA) peptide to detect heterophile antibody. Compared with the time-consuming reference method, rapid agglutination tests and EIAs are more than 98% sensitive, with a false-positive rate of about 5% and a positive predictive value of 90% or greater (Farhat, 1993; Linderholm, 1994; Tilton, 1988).

Heterophile antibody tests are highly specific screening tools but lack sensitivity; antibody is present in about 80% of teens and adults, and fewer than 40% of younger children with EBV IM. As EBV evolves from its initial active phase of infection into latency, various unique EBV antigens are generated, and the accompanying specific antibodies are valuable markers of the stage of disease. Shortly after B-lymphocyte infection, EBV early antigen (EA) is detected; EA is not a structural virion component but is an essential protein for EBV replication. With assembly of complete EBV virions, viral capsid antigen (VCA), a structural protein of the nucleocapsid, and envelope membrane antigen (MA) are produced. As acute mononucleosis subsides, a small percentage of EBV-immortalized B cells escape immune destruction and retain the virus in a latent form. The EBV genome is replicated with the lymphocyte nucleus, and EBV nuclear antigen (EBNA) is reponsible for viral duplication and survival.

Table 46–11. SEROLOGIC PROFILES IN EPSTEIN-BARR VIRUS INFECTION

	Heterophile Antibody (IgM)	VCA (IgM)	VCA (IgG)	EA (IgG)	EBNA (IgG)
Never infected	−	−	−	−	−
Silent primary infection	+/−	+/−	+	+	−
Infectious mononucleosis	+	+	+	++	+
Recent primary infection	−/+	−/+	+	+	+
Remote past infection	−	−	−	+	+
Immunodeficient patient with persistent reactivation	+/−	+/−	+	++	++

VCA = viral capsid antigen; EA = early antigen; EBNA = Epstein-Barr nuclear antigen.

The patterns of serologic tests typically seen during the various stages of EBV infection are summarized in Table 46–11. The majority of the EBV-specific serologic assays are performed by indirect immunofluorescence and use various lymphoblastoid cell lines with EBV production arrested in specific stages for expression of specific antigens. Several EIAs are available for VCA IgM, but the overall accuracy is variable (Wiedbrauk, 1993). Most laboratories rely upon demonstration of atypical lymphocytes in peripheral blood, a heterophile screening test, and IgM and IgG VCA titers for diagnosis of IM; quantitative tube heterophile reference methods, IgG-EBNA and IgG-EA, are procedurally more complex and have much less practical applicability.

Heterophile Negative Infectious Mononucleosis

Of the many patients who present with typical clinical features of IM, 70% or more have a positive heterophile test, confirming EBV as the cause. Of the 30% who lack heterophile antibody, about half are IgM-VCA positive, which also verifies acute EBV infection. In approximately 15% of patients with a febrile lymphoproliferative mononucleosis syndrome, primary infection with *T. gondii,* CMV, HHV6, or HIV is demonstrated. Diagnoses are occasionally made by lymph node biopsy, or in the case of CMV, by isolation of CMV from the peripheral blood or tissues; but in most instances, diagnosis is most easily established by serologic testing.

Diagnosis of toxoplasmosis is discussed in Chapter 53.

Primary CMV infection acquired in childhood is often asymptomatic, whereas infection acquired in adolescence is more likely to produce a systemic febrile lymphoproliferative illness. Isolation of CMV from saliva or urine is not helpful, because asymptomatic reactivation is so common. Recovery of CMV from peripheral blood leukocytes is a valid and sensitive test, but is more expensive and time consuming than serology. A variation of the IFA procedure, the anti-complement immunofluorescence (ACIF) test, reduces false-positive serologic error because CMV-infected tissue culture cells have Fc immunoglobulin receptors. IgM-specific ELISAs have shown overall accuracy that is comparable to ACIF-IFA IgM assay (Roseff, 1993; Schaefer, 1988; Smith, 1987; VanEnk, 1991).

HHV6, a recently described virus that closely resembles CMV, infects T and B lymphocytes, and is the cause of roseola infantum (exanthem subitum), a common febrile disease in young children (Pruksananonda, 1992). Primary infection past childhood can produce mononucleosis (Akashi, 1993), and has been linked with Kikuchi's lymphadenitis and Rosai Dorfman sinus histiocytosis. Both IFA and EIA specific IgM assays can diagnose acute infection, but there are currently no commercially distributed testing kits (Steeper, 1990; Sumiyoshi, 1993).

Acute infection with HIV-1 also has been associated with an illness that clinically mimics EBV mononucleosis (Kessler, 1987; Steeper, 1988). While most HIV infections produce asymptomatic seroconversion, a minority of patients develop fever, lymphadenopathy, and atypical lymphocytosis and occasionally mild hepatocellular damage or meningoencephalitis (Poli, 1993). Standard anti-HIV ELISA usually fails to detect specific antibody during this early phase of infection, but HIV p24 antigen can be detected in blood, as can circulating HIV. ELISA, Western blot, and IFA serologic tests all become positive for HIV antibodies within two to three months, as features of acute infection resolve (Clark, 1991).

Figure 46–11 shows an algorithmic approach for the serologic evaluation of a patient with symptoms of acute mononucleosis. Despite extensive laboratory testing for these acknowledged causes of mononucleosis no etiologic agent is identified in about 5% to 10% of cases.

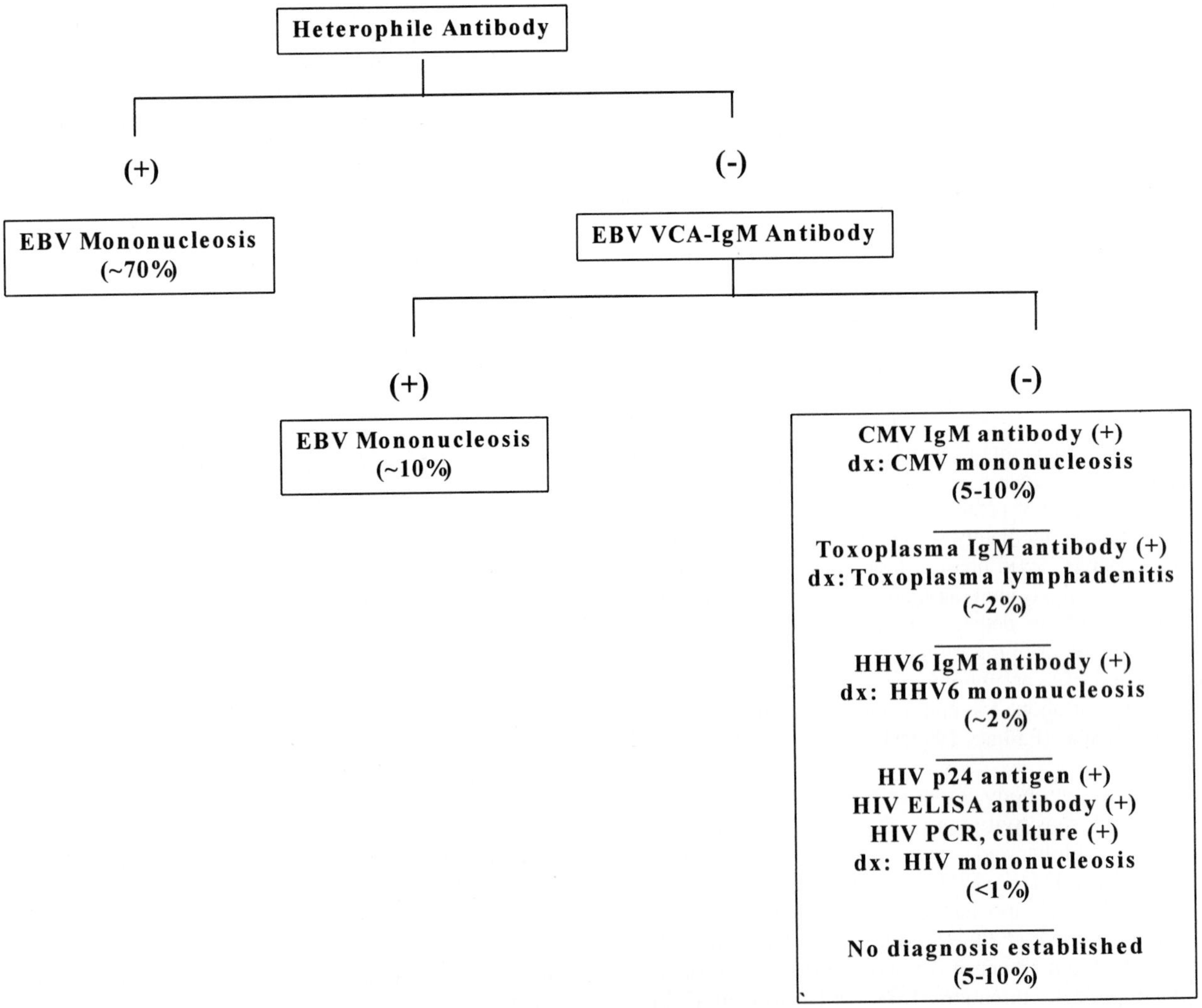

Figure 46–11. Serologic evaluation of patient with clinical symptoms of acute mononucleosis and atypical lymphocytosis. (+): Positive test result. (−): Negative test result. (%): Indicates approximate percentage of cases of acute infectious mononucleosis caused by that virus.

Chronic Fatigue Syndrome

Over the past 10 years considerable attention has been given in the medical and lay press to a clinical entity characterized by disabling persistent fatigue and often accompanied by fever, pharyngitis, tender lymphadenopathy, arthralgias, and myalgias (Holmes, 1988; Klonoff, 1992). Occult malignancy, endocrine disease, and psychiatric disorders should be investigated in patients with suspected chronic fatigue, but the clinical aspects of this illness strongly suggest an infectious cause. Initial reports implied that EBV, either as a chronically persistent primary infection or as a reactivated infection, was responsible because many patients had high titers to EBV VCA and EA. Serologic testing, however, was neither standardized nor reproducible (Holmes, 1987), and EBV culture and *in situ* hybridization performed on saliva and peripheral blood leukocytes showed no difference between chronic fatigue patients and normal controls. Data from other studies have suggested a role for CMV, *T. gondii,* HHV6, and HTLV, but there is no consensus about etiology (Gold, 1990). Immunologic and serologic testing offers little information that can be used for diagnosis or prognosis. Chronic fatigue syndrome remains defined by clinical signs and symptoms rather than laboratory test results, and it may ultimately be shown not to be a single disease but a syndrome with many possible causes.

CONGENITAL AND PERINATAL VIRAL INFECTIONS

The pregnant uterus is a sterile and secluded environment that protects the fetus from the pathogenic microorganisms that can infect the general populace. Most infections in pregnancy are caused by normal vaginal bacteria, which ascend through a flawed cervical barrier, but of equal if not greater overall importance are maternal infections that spread hematogenously to the fetus by way of the placenta or directly involve the baby at the time of vaginal delivery. These have been collectively referred to as TORCH infections, so named for *t*oxoplasma (see Chap. 53), *r*ubella, *c*ytomegalovirus, *h*erpes simplex virus, and other organisms such as HIV, parvovirus, enteroviruses, or *Treponema pallidum* (see Chap. 50). Many maternal infections with these agents are silent or produce only minor symptoms. The fetal immune system, however, may not generate an effective cellular or humoral response, and tissue necrosis may be severe or even fatal.

The approach to diagnosis of these infections is centered on two issues: identification of acute infection in the mother (particularly primary infection) and verification of involvement of the fetus or newborn. Maternal infection is best established by recovery of the suspected organism, but for some organisms this is impractical and serologic demonstration of specific IgM antibody, while imperfect, is the accepted diagnostic method. Because maternal infection does not always cross the placenta and involve the baby (attack rates are usually 30% to 60%), verification of fetal infection is needed. Ultrasound may detect organ or tissue damage (microcalcifications, microcephaly, hydrocephalus, organomegaly, hydrops, etc.), but recovery of the organism by culture, demonstration of its antigen or genome in fetal blood or tissues, or detection of specific IgM antibody is required to prove fetal infection. Test selection for diagnosis of common perinatal and congenital infection is summarized in Table 46–12.

While routine screening of all pregnant women for immunity to rubella is strongly advised, testing for toxoplasma, HSV, and CMV antibodies is not. IgM serologic methods in particular may show interlaboratory and intralaboratory variation, with both false-negative and false-positive errors; IgG assays alone do not differentiate primary from recurrent or latent infection, and cannot predict fetal involvement.

Cytomegalovirus

CMV is the most common intrauterine infection and affects approximately 1% of live-born babies in the United States (Yow, 1989). The majority of these infants are asymptomatic at birth; isolation of CMV from urine or saliva or de-

Table 46–12. SUMMARY OF LABORATORY DIAGNOSTIC TESTING FOR CONGENITAL AND PERINATAL INFECTIONS

Pathogen	Maternal Serology	Culture, Antigen, Assay, PCR	Fetal or Newborn Serology
Toxoplasma gondii	IgM-IFA or EIA,* ELISA IgM μ capture assay; Low affinity IgG assay** HS/AC differential agglutination test**	PCR amplification of *T. gondii* DNA in amniotic fluid **	IgM-IFA or EIA*
CMV	IgM-ACIF or EIA* IgM-RIA**	CMV culture, maternal blood CMV culture, newborn urine, saliva, blood (within 1st week of life). Nuclear inclusions in newborn urine cells, tissues	IgM-ACIF or EIA*
Rubella	IgM-IFA or EIA*	Rubella culture (mother or newborn)	IgM-IFA or EIA*
HSV	HSV-IgM highly suggestive of primary infection **	HSV culture of conjunctiva, oral mucosa, skin, CSF, tissues; PCR amplification of HSV DNA in blood, CSF**	IgM-IFA or EIA*
HIV	Any antibody (+) mother is infectious Quantitative PCR** of HIV	HIV culture, immune complex dissociated p24 assay, PCR amplification of HIV in blood (newborn)	EIA, or WB IgA anti-HIV**
Enterovirus		Culture of blood, CSF, stool, throat, tissues (newborn)	
Parvovirus B19	EIA, RIA-IgM assay**	*In situ* hybridization of PCR** identification of parvovirus DNA (newborn)	

*Removal of IgG prior to testing recommended.
**Research and reference laboratories.
See Tables 46–3 through 46–6 for abbreviations. IFA = immunofluorescent antibody; ELISA = enzyme-linked immunosorbent assay; RIA = radioimmunoassay; WB = Western blot.

tection of IgM-CMV in serum is the only marker of congenital infection. A distinct minority of infected babies, however, are overtly symptomatic with jaundice, hepatosplenomegaly, and pancytopenias, and are most likely to suffer long-term sequelae such as nerve deafness or mental retardation. Maternal primary CMV infection is frequently viremic with hematogenous transplacental spread to the fetus, and carries the highest risk of serious prenatal tissue damage. Reactivation CMV infection in the mother can also involve the fetus, but because maternal IgG anti-CMV antibody also crosses the placenta and is somewhat protective, they are usually asymptomatic at birth and less commonly develop serious sequelae.

Congenital CMV infection is diagnosed by isolation of CMV from amniotic fluid, cord blood, and fetal tissues, or urine, saliva, and/or blood if collected from the neonate during the first week after birth (Alford, 1990; Demmler, 1991; Warren, 1992). The presence of IgM anti-CMV in cord blood collected *in utero* or at delivery is also diagnostic (Fowler, 1992). Identification of typical CMV nuclear inclusions in urine cytology preparations is specific but insensitive; autopsy material may have few remaining diagnostic cells if tissue necrosis is advanced. Detection of CMV by DNA hybridization or PCR amplification seems promising as an adjunct to tissue culture or serology.

Rubella

Rubella (German measles) generally produces mild fever and a transient rash in children and adults. Rubella virus circulates hematogenously, even in mild cases, and viremic transplacental spread during the first trimester can produce severe ocular and brain damage, nerve deafness, and congenital cardiac malformations (Mann, 1981; Miller, 1982). Congenital rubella syndrome is rare now because of the effectiveness of pediatric vaccination and routine prenatal screening programs (Miller, 1984). When acute rubella is suspected in a pregnant woman, the most straightforward method for diagnosis is assay of maternal serum for anti-rubella IgM by an ELISA or IFA method. Tissue culture recovery of rubella is possible but is time consuming and technically complex, and not routinely performed in most clinical laboratories. The congenitally infected newborn usually continues to excrete virus for many months, if not years.

Herpes Simplex Virus

Primary acquisition of HSV during pregnancy carries a high risk of ascending herpetic chorioamnionitis with spontaneous abortion during early pregnancy, preterm labor in the second and third trimesters, and exposure of the baby during delivery to HSV (almost always HSV2) from the cervix, vagina, and perineum (Brown, 1987). Primary genital herpes infections rather than recurrences put the baby at greater risk for two reasons: the maternal viral load and total number of lesions are higher in primary infection, and maternal serum contains IgM but little or no IgG for transplacental passive protection of the baby (Prober, 1987).

Most babies have a vertex presentation during labor, so the scalp and face are the first to encounter HSV in the maternal genital tract; other common sites of viral exposure are the chest wall and the buttocks, especially in breach delivery. Vesicles typically develop where skin and mucous membranes are directly inoculated with HSV. The infant's immune response is still relatively immature, and the baby's only resource for modifying infection is maternal IgG-HSV; when this passive protection is lacking, viral replication and visceral dissemination can proceed unchecked (Whitley, 1988). Conjunctiva, the oral cavity, and any vesiculo-ulcerating skin lesions are usually rich in virus, and if dissemination occurs, virtually any visceral organ can be infected.

Optimal management of delivery in the era of genital herpes is still being debated, but several recent studies deserve emphasis. Routine culture of all mothers or infants at the time of labor and delivery has a very low (0.2%) yield of HSV and is not recommended (Prober, 1988). HSV culture of pregnant women with known recurrent genital herpes also fails to predict which mothers will shed virus at the time of delivery (Arvin, 1986). Studies of women who experienced their first recognized episode of genital herpes during pregnancy demonstrated that only about half of these women had true primary genital herpes, and these mothers experienced a high rate of complications (herpetic amnionitis, preterm labor, and severe infections in their neonates). The women who actually had recurrent disease had a much lower rate of neonatal infection, with involvement confined to mucocutaneous sites, with no visceral dissemination (Brown, 1987, 1991).

It is accepted practice that women in labor who have genital lesions suspicious for herpes be managed with cesarean section so that the baby is not exposed to possible HSV. Women with a history of recurrent genital herpes can deliver vaginally if active lesions are not present, but careful clinical monitoring of their newborns, including HSV culture of conjunctiva, oral mucosa, and any suspicious cutaneous lesions, is recommended. Neonatal herpes infection can be silent for up to several days before disease becomes clinically apparent. Disseminated infection is invariably fatal, but occasional infants with infection confined to the central nervous system survive, always with severe permanent retardation.

Laboratory diagnosis of HSV infection was discussed earlier. Rapid testing (Tzanck smears and antigen assays) is likely to be positive for vesicle lesions, but no rapid test has sufficient sensitivity to replace culture. Given these limitations, immediate testing has little justification. PCR may be able to identify HSV DNA in serum or spinal fluid with greater sensitivity than culture, but this procedure is still investigational (Kimura, 1991).

Human Immunodeficiency Virus, Parvovirus, Enterovirus

HIV can be spread hematogenously to the fetus, or infection may be acquired perinatally via exposure to infected maternal blood and breast milk during and after delivery. The risk of transmission of HIV from mother to fetus varies from 13% to 45%, presumably with placental trophoblast cells and macrophages acting as a reservoir for the virus. Most infected newborns are asymptomatic at birth and develop the clinical findings that characterize pediatric HIV disease later in childhood (Connor, 1991).

Maternal IgG crosses the placenta and is detected in infant blood for up to 15 months; therefore, the standard ELISA serologic tests for HIV IgG antibodies cannot be used for diagnosis of neonatal infection. Variations of both ELISA and Western blot tests for detection of IgA antibodies (neither IgA nor IgM are passively transferred to the fetus, and represent antibody manufactured by the baby) can diagnose pediatric infection accurately; however, sensitivity is age dependent, and the test is unreliable in the first three months after birth (Quinn, 1991). Detection of HIV p24 antigen, by routine EIA and immune-complex–dissociated methods, and HIV culture are also insensitive during the immediate postnatal period (Burgard, 1992; Miles, 1993; Sison, 1992). PCR amplification of HIV proviral sequences in neonatal blood samples appears promising for accurate diagnosis of congenital disease (Rogers, 1989).

Parvovirus B19 causes the benign and self-limited exanthem erythema infectiosum (fifth disease). Approximately 50% of adults are seronegative, and a pregnant woman who contracts B19 can transplacentally infect her fetus (Alder, 1993). The target for B19 parvovirus is the erythroid progenitor cell in the marrow, and direct lytic cytotoxicity causes anemia, which in the fetus may be severe enough to cause hydrops fetalis (Anand, 1987). Parvovirus can only be cultivated in human bone marrow containing erythrocytic precursor cells, a test not performed in clinical virology laboratories. Acute infection is diagnosed serologically by detecting specific IgM. Tests for detection of viral antigen or viral DNA are available in research laboratories.

Maternal enteroviral infections that occur very late in gestation up to the time of delivery may also produce serious disease in the baby. Many enteroviral infections have a viremic phase with the opportunity to cross the placenta, and babies can be born with active viral infection but no modifying passive maternal antibody. Echovirus and some of the Coxsackie A and B viruses have been linked with late third trimester maternal infection and exposure of the baby *in utero* or at delivery. Nosocomial outbreaks with nursing personnel as the source of virus have also been reported. Echovirus 11 is particularly virulent, causing hepatocellular necrosis and meningoencephalitis. Perinatal infection with other enteroviruses usually are benign. Echovirus grows easily in tissue cell culture (PMK, HDF, and RD cell lines); specimens for viral culture include neonatal blood, cerebrospinal fluid (CSF), throat and rectal swab samples, or tissues (in fatal cases). Diagnosis of infection in mothers and hospital personnel can be attempted, though disease in adults may be mild or inapparent; throat and fecal viral cultures are often negative. Enterovirus typing is expensive and time consuming, and though several excellent monoclonal antibodies are available commercially, this service can usually be obtained through regional or national public health laboratories (Modin, 1986).

VIRAL MENINGITIS AND ENCEPHALITIS

Viral infections of the central nervous system are relatively uncommon but often produce considerable morbidity and mortality. Laboratory testing is important for diagnosis of individual cases and for epidemiologic analysis and public health planning. Viral central nervous system (CNS) disease is manifested as acute meningitis or encephalitis. Viral proliferation in the arachnoid, ependyma, and choroid cellular layers of the brain induces acute inflammatory damage that causes the fever, headache, nuchal rigidity, and CSF pleocytosis which characterize meningitis. In encephalitis, virus replicates within the brain parenchyma; inflammation and tissue necrosis often produce a space-occupying lesion with mass effect, acute neurologic deficit, coma, high mortality rate, and permanent residual impairments. Although many viruses are typically associated with either meningitis or encephalitis, patients often exhibit clinical features of infection in both anatomic sites (meningoencephalitis) (Table 46–13).

Encephalitis is relatively rare in the United States, with approximately 2000 cases reported annually. Accurate diagnosis is limited by the fact that many of the neurotropic viruses are fastidious and difficult or impossible to recover in tissue culture. The most frequently isolated virus in acute encephalitis is HSV; infection is usually a reactivation of latent HSV1 that extends (apparently via the first or fifth cranial nerves) into the temporo-parietal cerebral cortex. There are about 1000 cases annually, with a sporadic, year-round pattern of occurrence. Progression is typically rapid and mortality is high; early diagnosis and therapy with acyclovir reduce both mortality and the level of permanent disability (Forghani, 1985; Whitley, 1995).

Arthropod mosquitoes are vectors for hundreds of neurotropic viruses worldwide, but only four arboviruses are encountered regularly in the United States: the eastern equine, western equine, St. Louis, and California (LaCrosse) encephalitis viruses. The total number of cases varies from less than 100 to more than 2000 in epidemic years. Severity and mortality are variable, and are highest with eastern equine virus, the least frequent of the group (Calisher, 1994).

Several enteroviruses, including Coxsackie and echo

Table 46–13. VIRUSES ASSOCIATED WITH CNS DISEASE

Syndrome	Common Causes	Less Common Causes
Aseptic meningitis	Enteroviruses HIV Mumps	HSV LCM VZV Hepatitis B Polioviruses Measles
Paralysis	Enteroviruses	Polioviruses
Encephalitis	Alphaviruses Flaviviruses Bunyaviruses HSV Mumps Measles HIV Enteroviruses Influenza	Rubella Rabies Hepatitis B Adenoviruses LCM VZV RSV Vaccinia CMV
Guillain-Barré	EBV CMV	Influenza
Reye's syndrome	Influenza A&B VZV	

See Tables 46–3 through 46–6 for abbreviations.

6

strains, occasionally produce encephalitis; paralytic polio is caused by poliovirus-induced necrosis of spinal cord or brainstem motor neurons, and is a variant of encephalitis (Menengus, 1991; Schnur, 1992). Rabies virus travels directly to the CNS via nerve fibers to produce necrotizing brain damage (Warrell, 1991). Measles, mumps, EBV mononucleosis, and chickenpox rarely are complicated by encephalitis (Kennedy, 1991); HHV6 has also been linked to focal encephalitis (McCullers, 1995). Acute infection with HIV may produce a transient acute meningitis, and the dementia of advanced AIDS is frequently caused by progressive HIV replication in the CNS (Atwood, 1993; Harrison, 1991). Opportunistic necrotizing infections with HSV, CMV, and VZV as well as JC papovavirus destruction of oligodendroglia with demyelination also occur in the immunocompromised host.

Nearly 75% of the cases of viral meningitis in the United States are caused by enteroviruses, which typically produce nonfatal infections with a benign course. Chronic severe meningoencephalitis can occur in children with hypogammaglobulinemia, and any enteroviral CNS infection with a component of parenchymal involvement is more likely to have a virulent course and risk of permanent sequelae. Enteroviruses are spread easily from person to person via the fecal-oral route, and there is distinct seasonality, with annual summertime outbreaks (Fig. 46–12). Mumps, measles, and adenovirus infections rarely are accompanied by acute meningitis. In approximately 1% of primary HSV2 genital herpes infections, there is an associated transient limited meningitis; and acute HIV infection rarely has symptoms of acute meningeal inflammation (Harrison, 1991). HSV2 appears to be the major cause of Mollaret's benign recurrent lymphocytic meningitis (Tedder, 1994).

Laboratory Diagnosis

Viral encephalitis is best diagnosed by brain biopsy (Whitley, 1990, 1995); virus usually is not cultivated from CSF. A 0.5-cm^3 sized biopsy is sufficient for both surgical pathology examination, imprint smears for direct examination, and comprehensive culture for all infectious organisms. Specimen collection is discussed in Chapter 54.

Brain tissue imprints prepared under sterile conditions can be stained with Giemsa to demonstrate herpetic nuclear inclusions, or with DFA or immunoperoxidase reagents to specifically identify HSV antigen. Additional smears can be reserved for uncommon viruses, such as measles or rabies. The tissue remnant can then be homogenized in sterile saline for routine microbiologic cultures and inoculation of cell cultures. Many arboviruses and several enteroviruses require animal inoculation for replication, a procedure not available in the typical clinical virology laboratory; tissue may be frozen at − 70°C if animal culture is needed and can be arranged.

Recovery of HSV from brain tissue is the gold standard for diagnosis of HSV encephalitis, and is superior in sensitivity and specificity to histologic examination of tissue sections, direct DFA stains and EM demonstration of herpetic virions. ISH and IP staining of paraffin-embedded tissue sections also are excellent, with overall accuracy greater than 90%; PCR demonstration of HSV DNA in CSF appears to

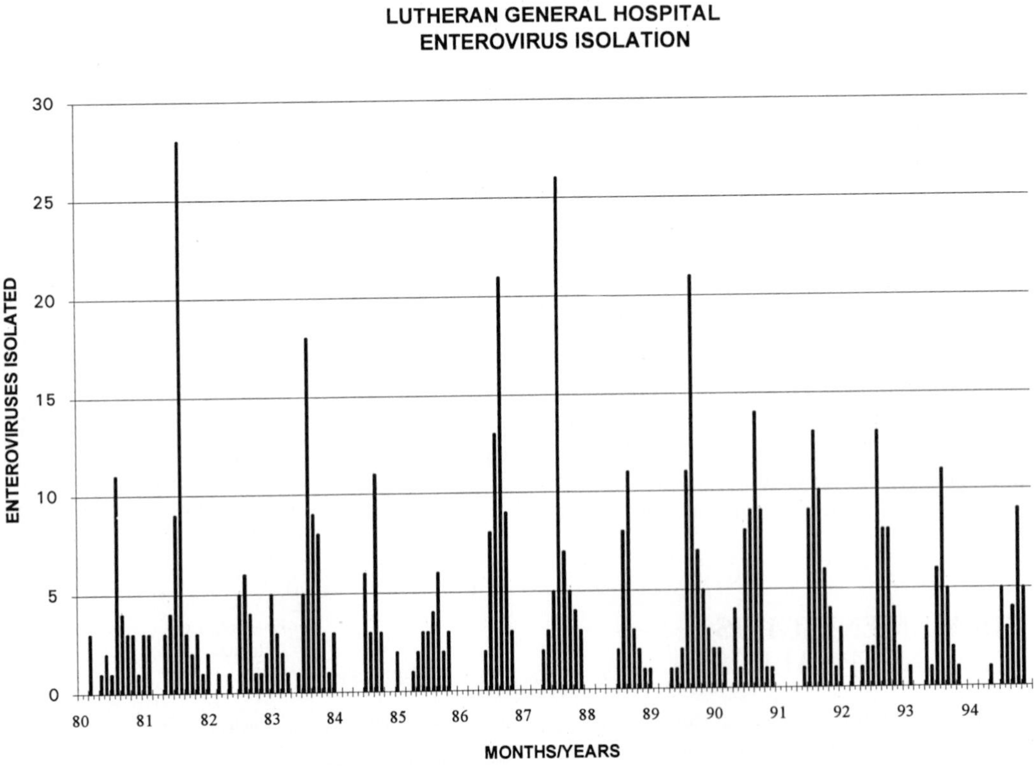

Figure 46–12. Enterovirus isolation exhibiting seasonal variation.

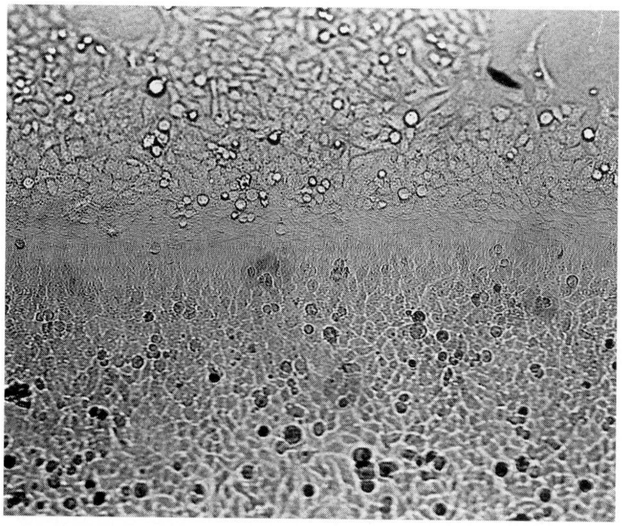

Figure 46–13. The A549 tissue culture monolayer shows echovirus enteroviral cytopathic effect (100× magnification, phase contrast microscopy).

have diagnostic sensitivity equal or superior to brain biopsy culture; clinical application of this testing approach is still under study (Kimura, 1991; Whitley, 1995). HSV isolation in tissue culture is discussed elsewhere in this chapter; recovery of other viruses should also be attempted from CSF and brain tissue specimens.

Routine CSF culture is designed for recovery of enteroviruses; inoculation of several tissue cell lines (some combination of PMK, HDF, HEp-2, RD, and Buffalo Green Monkey) maximizes enteroviral yield (Wildin, 1987). These cell lines also support growth of other viral agents of meningitis, such as HSV, VZV, measles, mumps, and adenovirus. Spinal fluid should be transported to the laboratory, and 0.1 to 0.2 mL should be inoculated directly into tissue culture without delay. Enterovirus CPE begins as focal nuclear pyknotic change with individual cellular rounding and then rapidly progresses across the cell monolayer (Fig. 46–13). CPE is identified within four days in up to 69% of positive cultures, so cultures should be read daily for the first week and then on alternate days for two weeks before reported as negative. When enterovirus-like CPE is observed, a presumptive report of enterovirus isolation should be issued and definitive enterovirus identification attempted. Typing is most easily accomplished by DFA staining of the monolayer with select monoclonal antibody pools; more comprehensive neutralization using pools of specific viral serotypes is available in public health laboratories. Rapid, sensitive, and accurate diagnosis of enteroviral CNS infection, particularly with serotypes that do not replicate easily in culture, may soon be possible with nucleic acid probes and reverse transcription–polymerase chain reaction (RT-PCR) (Rotbart, 1991).

An algorithm for laboratory diagnosis of viral CNS infection is presented in Figure 46–14. An acute phase serum should be obtained as early as possible after the onset of symptoms. If cultures remain negative, a convalescent serum should be collected and the pair tested in parallel for enteroviral, arboviral, and other indicated antibodies.

VIRAL EXANTHEMS

Several viruses primarily target the skin; some infect the squamous epidermis through direct inoculation (oral and genital herpes, warts caused by human papillomavirus or molluscum poxvirus), but the majority of exanthems are caused by viruses that spread hematogenously to the skin and mucous membranes (VZV, measles, rubella, enteroviruses, parvovirus, HHV6) (Cherry, 1993). Most of these infections are common, relatively benign childhood diseases that are diagnosed clinically without laboratory testing; however, viral culture, antigen identification, or serologic confirmation may be helpful to guide selection of antiviral drugs, define the extent of disease in severe cases, or apply infection control precautions efficiently in hospitalized patients. Laboratory diagnostic procedures are summarized in Table 46–14.

VZV causes both varicella (chickenpox) and zoster (shingles). In chickenpox, VZV is spread through infected respiratory aerosol droplets, multiplies in the nasopharynx, and then enters the bloodstream and travels to the skin (Weller, 1992). Viral replication in the squamous epithelium produces pruritic vesicles that rapidly progress to ulcers which eventually crust over and heal without scarring. In children, systemic symptoms are mild and sequelae are rare; in adults, pregnant

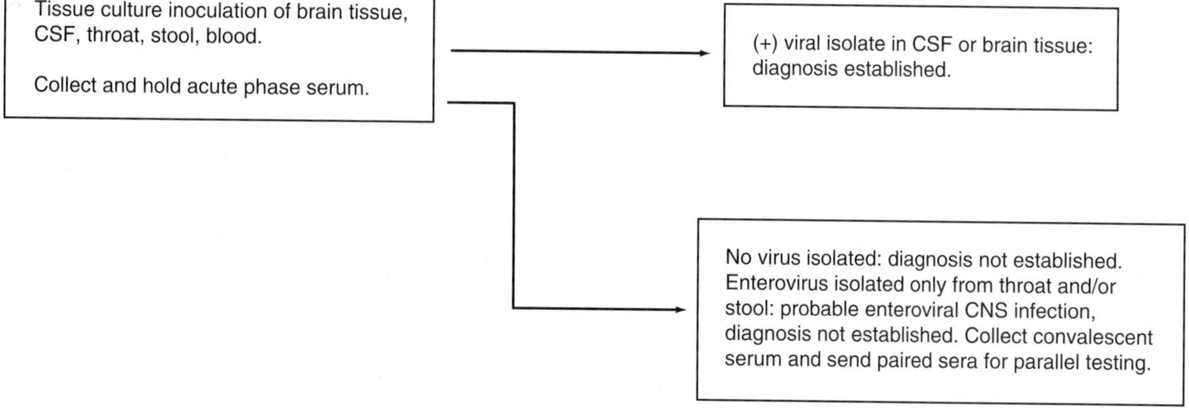

Tissue culture inoculation of brain tissue, CSF, throat, stool, blood.
Collect and hold acute phase serum.
(+) viral isolate in CSF or brain tissue: diagnosis established.
No virus isolated: diagnosis not established. Enterovirus isolated only from throat and/or stool: probable enteroviral CNS infection, diagnosis not established. Collect convalescent serum and send paired sera for parallel testing.

Figure 46–14. Algorithm for diagnosis of suspected viral meningoencephalitis.

Table 46–14. LABORATORY DIAGNOSIS OF COMMON VIRAL EXANTHEMS

Exanthem	Virus	Culture/Antigen Assay	Serology
Chicken pox/shingles	Varicella zoster	Tzank smear DFA smear* Culture (shell vial most sensitive)	
Enteroviral rash (hand, foot, and mouth disease)	Enteroviruses	Culture*	
Measles	Measles	Culture	IgM measles*
Rubella	Rubella	Interference culture**	IgM rubella*
Erythema infectiosum	Parvovirus B19	ISH in infected normoblasts** PCR**	IgM parvovirus B19**
Exanthem subitum	HHV6	Co-culture in lymphoblasts**	IgM HHV-6**
HSV	HSV1 and HSV2	Culture* DFA smear	

*Recommended method.
**Research and reference laboratories.
See Tables 46–3 through 46–6 for abbreviations. ISH = *in situ* hybridization; HHV = human herpesvirus.

women, neonates, and immunocompromised patients, disease may be more severe, with pneumonia and visceral involvement in addition to typical skin lesions (Gershon, 1976). After chickenpox resolves, latent VZV infection is established in sensory neural ganglia (Mahalingham, 1991; Straus, 1989); with reactivation, VZV spreads from trigeminal or dorsal root ganglia back to the skin, and produces painful cutaneous vesicles in a dermatome distribution (shingles or zoster). Zoster is most common in the elderly and in overtly immunocompromised patients; when it occurs in teens and young adults, HIV infection should be suspected (Pana, 1994).

Vesicle fluid is rich with virus and is the ideal specimen for culture and DFA staining. HDF are the only cell lines that reliably support VZV. Traditional cell culture is slow and insensitive, but shell vial culture has better yield (up to 75%) and allows more rapid detection (Brinker, 1993). Specimen collection for suspected VZV skin lesions is identical to that for HSV vesicles. Culture setup is also similar to herpes culture (see Fig. 46–3); however, culture tubes are held for two weeks and shell vial monolayers are stained at three and five days with VZV DFA conjugate. VZV CPE develops as small patches of rounded, swollen refractile cells in the fibroblast monolayer, similar to CMV CPE. Because the behavior of VZV in tissue culture is somewhat fastidious, DFA stain of vesicle cells for viral antigen is the most sensitive and rapid diagnostic test (Schrim, 1989).

Of the approximately 70 enterovirus serotypes, several are able to produce generalized vesicular or maculopapular eruptions (Coxsackie B1 and A9, and echoviruses 2, 4, 9, 11, 19, and 33), usually during warm weather months. Hand-foot-mouth disease (caused principally by Coxsackie A16) occurs in young children, and presents as vesicles on the tongue and skin of the palms and soles. Adult family members of infected children also occasionally develop symptomatic disease. Laboratory diagnosis is limited to cell culture; vesicles (especially from the soles and palms) should be completely unroofed and the exposed squamous cells vigorously swabbed. Enteroviral infections also characteristically involve the alimentary tract, so throat and rectal swab cultures are also reasonable. Cell culture identification of enterovirus was described earlier in this chapter. Neither direct DFA stains nor serology are useful for diagnosis of enteroviral exanthems (Cherry, 1963, 1993; DeChamps, 1988).

Measles is a highly contagious viral illness with both systemic and respiratory features (fever, conjunctivitis, coryza, oral lesions, cough, and a generalized maculopapular erythematous rash) (Bellini, 1994). Vaccination has greatly reduced the incidence of measles in the United States, but it remains a serious problem in impoverished countries, where it is associated with high morbidity and mortality from accompanying pneumonia and malnutrition. Virus can be isolated from the nasopharynx early in the course of measles, but acute infection is most easily diagnosed serologically by detection of virus-specific IgM. Immunity following natural measles infection presumably is lifelong and is verified by determination of specific IgG; however, immunity following vaccination may fade during late teen and adult years. Infection occurring in this setting may be atypical, with a greater likelihood of pneumonitis and a noncharacteristic rash. Serologic diagnosis is particularly helpful in atypical measles.

Parvovirus B19 causes erythema infectiosum (fifth disease), a common childhood febrile illness with a distinctive maculopapular rash that gives the face a "slapped cheek" appearance (Erdman, 1991; Plummer, 1985). Infections in adults can also produce arthralgias (Naides, 1990). Parvovirus infects erythroblastic precursor cells in the bone marrow and may provoke aplastic crisis in patients with hemoglobinopathy or HIV infection (Harris, 1992). Primary infection during pregnancy can cause fetal red cell aplasia with severe anemia and hydrops fetalis. Laboratory diagnosis was discussed earlier in this chapter.

Rubella virus produces German measles, a mild febrile illness with a transient maculopapular rash (Cherry, 1993). Infection in children is usually inconsequential, although adult rubella may be associated with arthralgias. The only serious complication of rubella is transplacental spread to the fetus with risk of congenital malformation. Tissue culture isolation of rubella virus is complicated and labor intensive; acute infection is best diagnosed by detection of virus-specific IgM. Verification of immune status is easily determined with specific IgG screening.

HHV6, a lymphotropic virus that infects both T and B lymphocytes, is the cause of exanthem subitum (roseola infantum), a common, self-limiting illness of early childhood characterized by high fever and development of a fleeting maculopapular rash as fever abruptly subsides (Asano, 1994; Lopez, 1988; Salahuddin, 1986). Primary HHV6 infection in older children and adults is associated with a systemic febrile lymphoproliferative illness with features of acute mononucleosis (discussed earlier) and may be linked to chronic fatigue syndrome, and possibly retinitis and pneumonitis in immunosuppressed patients (Cone, 1993). Laboratory diagnosis was reviewed earlier in this chapter.

VIRAL GASTROENTERITIS

Viral gastroenteritis is a major cause of morbidity and mortality worldwide, especially in young children in developing nations. In the United States, viral enteritis is rarely fatal but accounts for more than 3.5 million episodes of disease annually and approximately 35% of hospitalizations for gastroenteritis in pediatric patients (Blacklow, 1991). The viruses responsible are a diverse group, but all are ubiquitous and can infect both children and adults. Rotavirus, enteric adenoviruses, calicivirus, astrovirus, and coronavirus cause diarrhea predominantly in infants and young children (Bates, 1993); Norwalk and Norwalk-like viruses produce nausea, vomiting, and diarrhea, most commonly in adults (Hedberg, 1993) (Fig. 46–15). Treatment of viral gastroenteritis is supportive, with rehydration and electrolyte replacement the mainstay of clinical management.

Rotaviruses are the most common cause of viral diarrhea globally and are responsible for up to 60% of cases of watery diarrhea in young children and infants in the United States. The peak incidence is three to 15 months of age, but severe disease can occur up to age two years (Haffejee, 1991). Breast-fed infants are less susceptible to infection with rotavirus, and when clinical disease occurs it is milder than in formula-fed infants (Duffy, 1986). Symptomatic rotavirus infection also occasionally develops in adults and may be severe, especially in elderly nursing home patients (Marrie, 1982).

There are five serogroups of rotavirus, A through E; most human disease is caused by group A, with groups B and C reported sporadically and infrequently (Beards, 1982). Transmission is via a fecal-oral route, and in temperate climates rotavirus infections occur during cold weather months; seasonal variation is not seen in tropical regions where infections occur year-round. The majority of neonatal rotavirus infections are asymptomatic or mild, but necrotizing entero-

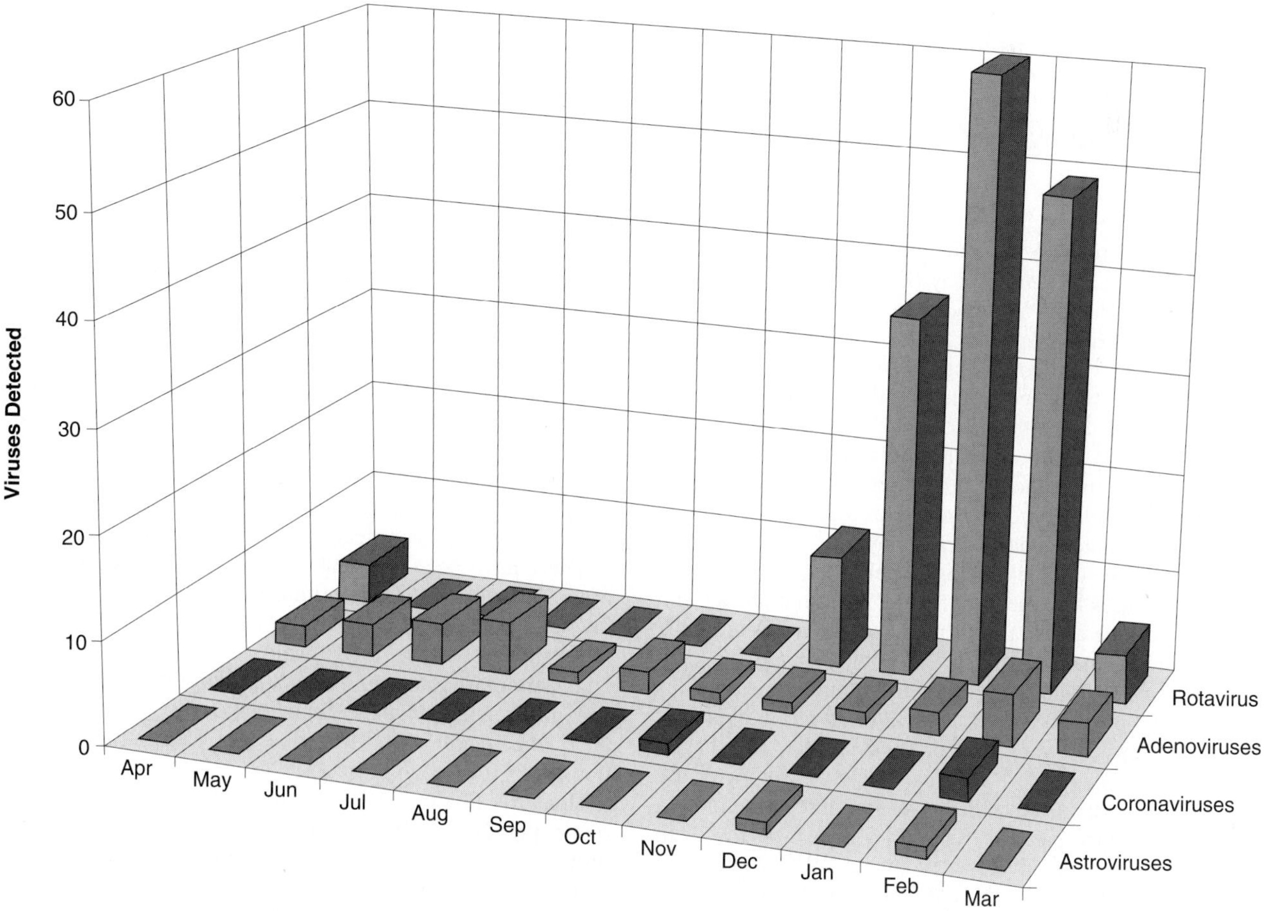

Figure 46–15. Recovery of gastroenteric viruses by enzyme immunoassay and electron microscopy.

6

colitis occurs rarely (Rotbart, 1988). Dehydration is the most serious complication of rotavirus infection in older children and the principal reason for hospitalization. Rotavirus can survive transiently on inanimate surfaces, so strict enteric isolation precautions must be followed to prevent nosocomial spread.

Two serotypes of adenovirus, types 40 and 41, are associated with gastroenteritis; they are the second most common cause of viral diarrhea in young children, accounting for 10% to 20% of all cases (Brandt, 1983). Adenovirus enteritis is clinically similar to rotavirus infection but exhibits no seasonality. Astroviruses also cause acute enteric disease in toddlers and infants, and have been implicated in outbreaks in day care centers (Mitchell, 1993); they may cause mild gastroenteritis in adults and diarrhea in HIV-infected patients (Grohman, 1993). Caliciviruses are responsible for 1% to 6% of cases of gastroenteritis, predominantly in infants and small children, but occasionally in the elderly living in retirement homes (Dinulos, 1994). Coronavirus is an infrequent cause of diarrhea in children; strains producing epidemic respiratory tract illness have also been described (Blacklow, 1991).

Norwalk and morphologically related viruses are a heterogeneous group associated with epidemics of acute gastroenteritis, often characterized by nausea and vomiting that are more intense than the accompanying diarrhea. Older children and adults are usually the targeted age groups, but small children are also vulnerable. These viruses are spread by fecal-oral means, and close personal contact is a common factor. Norwalk agents also survive in contaminated food and water, and there have been several large community-based outbreaks associated with this route of transmission (Hedberg, 1993).

Laboratory Diagnosis

All the gastroenteritis viral agents grow poorly or not at all in standard cell culture, and diagnosis traditionally has been based on the distinctive morphologic characteristics of each virus seen by electron microscopy (EM) (Fig. 46–16). Stool samples are centrifuged and filtered to remove bacteria, food, and cellular debris; aliquots are then transferred to an EM grid and stained with phosphotungstic acid. Viruses are negatively stained with this technique, and their unique size, capsid organization, and other distinctive surface features are easily visualized. Addition of specific antiviral antiserum to the stool filtrate (immuno-electron microscopy) clumps virions into larger and more easily recognized aggregates, and is more sensitive than standard microscopy.

Rotaviruses are double- or single-shelled icosahedral, non-enveloped viruses that measure 55 to 75 nm in diameter and have a wheel-like appearance. Enteric adenoviruses are morphologically identical to all other adenoviruses; they have an icosahedral capsid and measure 70 to 90 nm diameter. Calicivirus is non-enveloped, measures 30 to 35 nm in diameter, and has its capsids arranged to produce regular, cup-shaped surface depressions with a calyceal shape. Astroviruses are 27 to 30 nm in diameter, with capsid structures producing a star-shaped surface pattern. Norwalk viruses measure 24 to 40 nm, and are non-enveloped geometrically symmetrical virions. Coronaviruses are the only gastroenteric agents with a lipid envelope; they are larger (diameter 75 to 100 nm) and have club-shaped envelope projections imparting crownlike features.

The EM morphology of each of these viruses is very distinctive, but EM is not available or is impractical in many laboratories. Rapid diagnosis of rotavirus in stool specimens is easily and accurately accomplished with either EIA or latex agglutination antigen assays; both methods have excellent specificities, but EIA is slightly more sensitive (Dennehy, 1994; Thomas, 1994). Because rotavirus is the most common of the enteric viruses and is easily transmitted by fecal contaminants, rapid diagnosis is particularly helpful in hospitalized patients so that enteric isolation and patient cohorting can be implemented to minimize nosocomial spread. There are several commercial antigen assay kits for rotavirus. A commercial EIA for enteric adenovirus antigen detection also is accurate and sensitive. EIA, nucleic acid probes, and a polymerase chain reaction assay have been developed for the other gastroenteric viruses but are only available through research and public health laboratories.

VIRAL HEPATITIS AND HUMAN IMMUNODEFICIENCY VIRUS INFECTION

Many viruses produce damage to the liver. The yellow fever virus and other hepatotoxic arboviruses cause direct massive hepatocellular necrosis. EBV, CMV, HHV6, and HIV cause transient liver injury as part of the mononucleosis syndrome as virus-infected lymphoid cells aggregate in the liver. Adenovirus, HSV, VZV, CMV, and echoviruses occasionally produce aggressive hepatitis in immunocompromised patients (Hierholzer, 1992). However, most viral hepatitis is caused by hepatitis A, B, C, D, or E virus (Iwarson, 1992).

Hepatitis A virus (HAV) and hepatitis E virus (HEV) are spread person to person through fecal-oral transmission. HAV is a non-enveloped picornavirus, related to enteroviruses. It can survive in contaminated water and food, and shellfish beds polluted with raw sewage have been the source of several large outbreaks. Individuals living in conditions with poor sanitation, children in day care and crowded institutions, and health care and child care workers are at increased risk for HAV hepatitis (Iwarson, 1992). Acute disease in young children is often asymptomatic or mild; adults may occasionally experience severe infection, but fulminant hepatitis and death are rare (0.6% or less). Recovery is complete with no chronic infectious state.

There have been outbreaks of HEV in developing countries associated with suboptimal food and water sanitation, but few documented cases have been reported in the United States (Viswanathan, 1957; Wald, 1995). Teens and young adults are most commonly affected; mortality is unusual, except in pregnant women, in whom death rates may reach 20% (Balayan, 1993). HEV does not cause chronic infection.

Hepatitis B virus (HBV) is the only hepatitis virus currently preventable by vaccination. It is most easily transmitted through blood and body fluids. Infection is classically acquired through transfusions or puncture injury with contaminated needles, but vertical infection during preg-

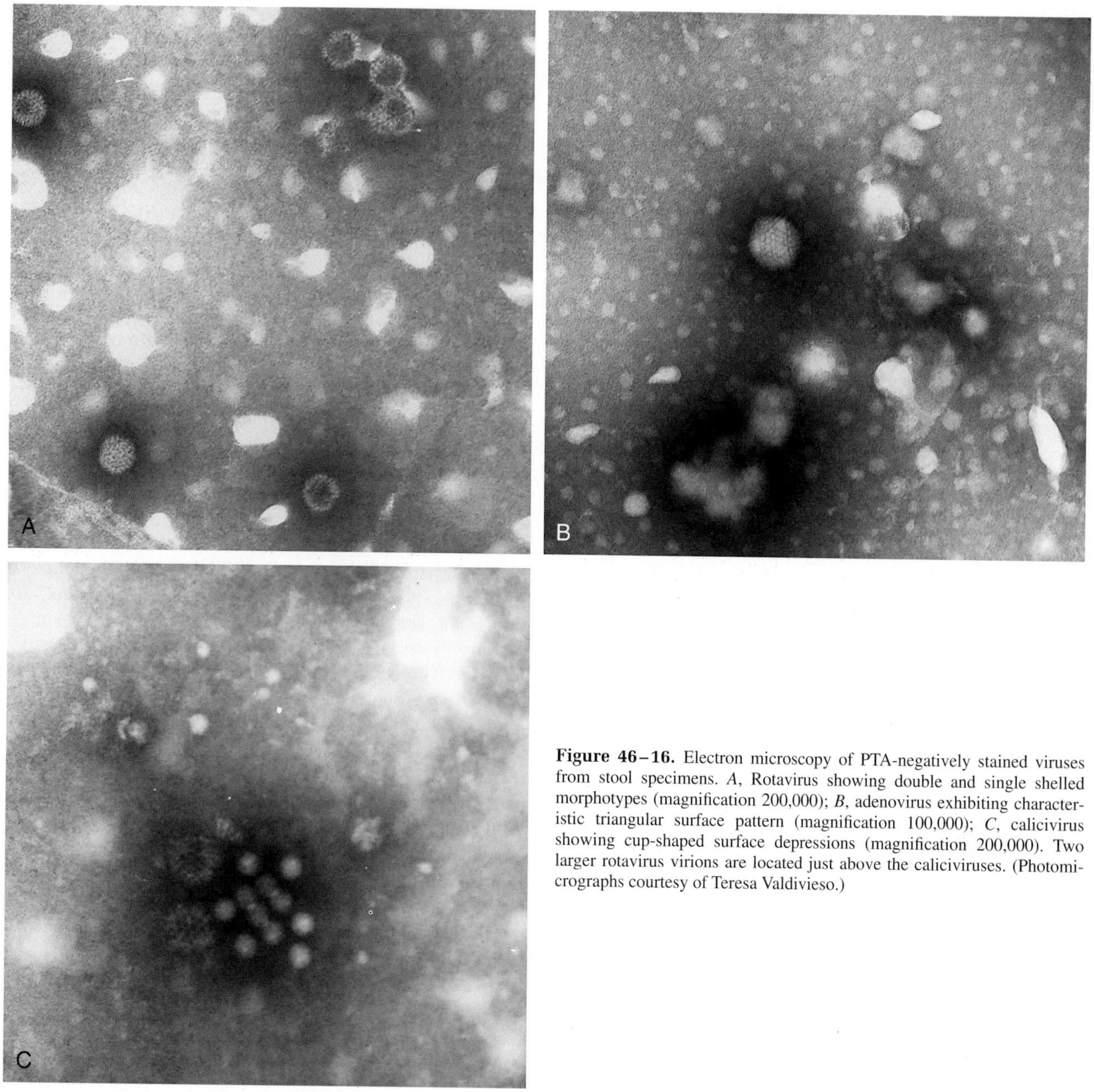

Figure 46–16. Electron microscopy of PTA-negatively stained viruses from stool specimens. *A*, Rotavirus showing double and single shelled morphotypes (magnification 200,000); *B*, adenovirus exhibiting characteristic triangular surface pattern (magnification 100,000); *C*, calicivirus showing cup-shaped surface depressions (magnification 200,000). Two larger rotavirus virions are located just above the caliciviruses. (Photomicrographs courtesy of Teresa Valdivieso.)

nancy, transmission through sexual contact, and exposure to infected body fluids such as saliva in the household contact setting are also important routes of spread. Acute infection is more likely to be symptomatic than with HAV and may be fulminant, with fatal massive hepatocellular necrosis occurring in 1% to 2% of cases. HBV also can persist in a chronic state, and the risk of chronic infection is in part dependent on the age of acquisition. Up to 90% of infants born with HBV vertically transferred *in utero* become chronic HBV carriers, compared with 25% to 50% of infected children and 5% to 10% of adults. Chronic HBV infection often is associated with ongoing hepatocellular damage; chronic-active hepatitis and eventual cirrhotic scarring develop in 2% or more of chronic infections (Lee, 1993; Overby, 1992). HBV cirrhosis is a risk factor for hepatocellular carcinoma.

Coinfection or superinfection with HDV is associated with accelerated hepatocyte damage and mortality rates as high as 30%. HDV is an incomplete virus that requires the presence of HBV surface antigen for full expression and replication. HDV may be transmitted from person to person in family contact situations in areas of high endemicity (South America, Africa, Italy), but in the United States blood transfusion and intravenous drug abuse are the principal risk factors (Polish, 1993).

Hepatitis C virus (HCV) is responsible for most cases of non-A, non-B hepatitis in the United States, and accounted for 80% to 90% of post-transfusion hepatitis before blood product screening was introduced in 1990 (Cuthbert, 1994). Parental drug abuse remains the most significant risk factor for infection; health care workers infected through inadvertent puncture wounds account for a minority of cases. HCV transmission during pregnancy, through sexual contact, and in households is much less efficient than HBV (Van der Poel, 1994). Fulminant hepatitis with acute mortality is similar to HBV infection, but more than 50% of HCV-infected patients become chronically infected, up to 20% develop cirrhosis, and hepatocellular carcinoma is a remote risk. Alpha-interferon has produced sustained remission in chronic HCV and HBV infections, and may be effective in modifying or preventing serious sequelae (Yoshioka, 1992). Second- and third-generation RIBA and EIA methods show excellent sensitivity and specificity for detection of antibody.

All five hepatitis viruses are highly fastidious and will either not replicate at all *in vitro* or cannot be grown in standard tissue culture cell lines. Diagnosis is made by serologic detection of specific IgM and IgG antibodies and identification of viral antigens, which are useful for designating the stage of infection and for prognosis (Biesemier, 1994). The clinical properties of the hepatitis viruses and serologic markers of infection are summarized in Tables 46–15 and 46–16.

In the 10 years since HIV was first identified, successful *in vitro* cultivation of the virus has been accomplished, viral antigens have been characterized and cloned, and the viral genome has been sequenced. The immunopathogenesis of HIV infection is complex (Poli, 1993); the virus causes progressive lytic destruction of CD4 lymphocytes with subsequent profound vulnerability to numerous opportunistic infectious agents and secondary malignancies (Phillips, 1992; Schnittman, 1990; Stein, 1992). HIV is also neurotropic, and capable of producing acute meningitis and a slow destructive encephalopathy (Atwood, 1993).

Appreciation of the molecular organization of HIV and its biological behavior has led to the development of several laboratory procedures for routine diagnosis and monitoring. HIV infection begins with circulating virus and p24 antigenemia. Transient IgM specific HIV antibody appears one to three months after acute infection, followed by the continuous presence of IgG and IgA antibodies. EIA screening tests detect IgG antibodies to several HIV structural antigen proteins; commercial kits vary in their antigen formulations, but all now have excellent sensitivity and specificity (both better than 99%). In low prevalence patient populations, a confirmatory procedure such as the immunoblot/Western blot identifies antibody directed against HIV antigens that have been electrophoretically separated for precise characterization (Jackson, 1988; Phair, 1992). Western blot test results may be indeterminate, in which case supplemental testing to resolve inconclusive findings is necessary (Celum, 1991). Alternate methods for HIV antibody detection are IFA for confirmation (Carlson, 1987) and latex agglutination for screening (Houck, 1990; Starkey, 1990). Reporting of all HIV serology test results should be concise and without ambiguous or confusing comments (Hewitt, 1992).

HIV antigen detection by EIA has limited applicability for HIV diagnosis, principally in acute mononucleosis-like illness and in confirming infection in neonates (Burgard, 1992; Kessler, 1987). EIA identification of p24 antigen has largely replaced reverse transcriptase assay for confirmation of positive HIV cultures (Harry, 1989). HIV culture requires cocultivating infected patient lymphocytes or tissues with normal donor lymphocytes that have been stimulated with phytohemagglutinin, interleukin-2, and interferon. HIV can be recovered from almost all patients at all stages of infection (Pan, 1993). This is a complex, expensive, and potentially dangerous procedure that should not be attempted in routine diagnostic laboratories.

PCR methods detect HIV nucleic acid in peripheral blood and tissues, and are helpful in resolving indeterminate antibody test results, and in confirming neonatal infection. PCR has been used to monitor response to antiviral therapy in research settings. PCR identification of proviral HIV DNA, or transcribed cDNA, and PCR quantitative-competitive identification of viral DNA or RNA are currently available only in research settings (Bagasra, 1992; Menzo, 1992). HIV-2, HTLV-1, and HTLV-2 retrovirus infections are uncommon infections in the United States, but account for a significant minority of lentevirus disease worldwide (Hollsberg, 1993; Markovitz, 1993). Serologic and molecular biologic diagnostic test methods similar to HIV diagnostic techniques are in use or in development (Blumer, 1992; O'Brien, 1992).

VIRAL INFECTIONS IN IMMUNOCOMPROMISED HOSTS

The immune response to viral infection is complex and involves a composite of both humoral and cellular factors, but prompt control of acute infection generally is accomplished by the cell-mediated immune system. Natural killer large granular lymphocytes that circulate through blood and tis-

Table 46–15. CLINICAL FEATURES OF HEPATITIS VIRUS INFECTIONS

	Hepatitis A	Hepatitis B	Hepatitis C	Hepatitis D	Hepatitis E
Classification	Picornaviridae (enterovirus 72)	Hepadnaviridae	Flaviviridae	(Satellite)	(Calicivirus)
Genotype(s)	One	At least 8	At least 6	One	One
Mean incubation time (range)	4 weeks (10–50 days)	12 weeks (14–180 days)	8 weeks (1–24 days)	3–13 weeks	6 weeks (14–63 days)
Chronicity	No	5–10% infected adults, 25–50% children, 70–90% infants	>60 (20% develop cirrhosis)	10–15%	No
Risk of hepatocellular carcinoma	No	Yes, high association	Yes, low association	?	No
Mortality rate, acute hepatitis	About 0.6%	About 1.4%	1–2%	Up to 30%	1–2%; up to 20% in pregnant women

Table 46–16. SEROLOGIC MARKERS IN THE DIAGNOSIS OF HEPATITIS

	IgM anti-HAV	Anti-HAV	HBsAg	Anti-HBs	IgM anti-HBc	Anti-HBc	HBeAg	Anti-HBe	HBV-DNA	Anti-HCV	Anti-HDV	Anti-HEV
Acute Infection												
HAV	+	+										
HBV												
Early			+	−	+	+	+	−	−			
Window			−	−	+	+	+/−	−	−			
Resolving			−	+	−	+	+	+	−			
HCV										+/−		
HDV												
Coinfection			+/−	−	+	+	−	−	+		+	
Superinfection			+/−	−	−	+	+/−	−/+	+/−		+	
HEV												+
Chronic Infection												
HBV												
Nonreplicating			+	−	−	+	−	+	−			
Replicating			+	−	−	+	+	−	+			
Reactivation			+	−	+	+	+	−	+			
HCV										+		
HDV			+	−	−	+	−/+	+/−	−/+		+	
Past Infection												
HAV	−	+										
HBV			−	+	−	+	−	+	−			
HCV										+		
HDV			−	+/−	−	+	−	+	−		+	
HEV												+

Modified from Biesemier (1994).

HDV = hepatitis D virus; HEV = hepatitis E virus; HBs = hepatitis B surface antigen; HBe = hepatitis Be antigen; HBc = hepatitis B core antigen; + = positive; − = negative.

See Tables 46–3 through 46–6 for other abbreviations.

sues identify host cells with viral ("non-self") antigens and destroy them by proteolytic lysis. Early in acute viral infection, antigens are processed by macrophages and presented to T lymphocytes. CD4-lymphocytes produce cytokines that promote monoclonal expansion of sensitized cytotoxic CD8 cells, which then eliminate host cells carrying viral antigen. Impairment of the normal interactions among CD4 and CD8 lymphocytes and natural killer cells reduces the host's control of viral infection.

Cell mediated immunity also plays a critical role in suppressing viruses that establish latency (such as HSV, CMV, and EBV). In healthy individuals most reactivation infections with these viruses are asymptomatic or produce limited disease confined to a discrete anatomic focus (genital or oral herpes, for example). In patients with reduced cellular immune function, however, recurrent infections may become disseminated with severe multiorgan tissue necrosis.

The number of immunocompromised patients has risen dramatically in the past two decades. Corticosteroid use, chemotherapy, radiation therapy, immunosuppressive drugs to prevent transplant rejection, and HIV obliteration of CD4 lymphocytes all damage cellular immune regulation and enhance the patient's vulnerability to a variety of viral infections. Primary infections, such as EBV mononucleosis, influenza, and chickenpox, are often more severe. Proliferation of human papillomavirus genital condylomas and accelerated progression of squamous dysplasia and carcinoma can occur in both males and females. The most serious viral diseases, however, represent reactivation of the patient's endogenous dormant organisms (CMV, HSV, and VZV). Persistent necrotizing oral, perineal, and perianal mucocutaneous HSV lesions, and zoster with multidermatomal involvement have been described, but the most common opportunistic viral infections in HIV and transplant patients are caused by CMV. Approximately 20% of CMV seropositive AIDS patients per year develop symptomatic CMV disease. Retinitis is the most frequent complication, and CMV pneumonia has the highest associated mortality (Drew, 1992; Meyers, 1982). Hematogenous viral dissemination can lead to gastrointestinal and CNS involvement; multiorgan tissue necrosis is not unusual in end-stage AIDS (Drew, 1992).

Visualization of typical cytomegalic inclusions in alveolar lavage fluid or tissue biopsies is specific for CMV infection but insensitive. Sensitivity improves somewhat with immunoperoxidase or *in situ* hybridization stains, but isolation of virus is the gold standard with the highest diagnostic accuracy. CMV replicates almost exclusively in HDF tissue culture cell lines. Growth in traditional tissue culture is slow, with incubation times of 10 days or more before typical CPE develops. The infected fibroblast initially retains its fusiform shape as the nucleus becomes swollen and refractile. The entire cell eventually becomes rounded and distorted, and virus spreads into adjacent fibroblasts to produce an enlarging patch of cellular damage (see Fig. 46–17).

Time to detection of CMV can be shortened to one to two days with centrifugation-enhanced shell vial culture (Gleaves, 1984, 1987). HDF monolayers are inoculated with peripheral blood leukocytes (harvested by density gradient separation),

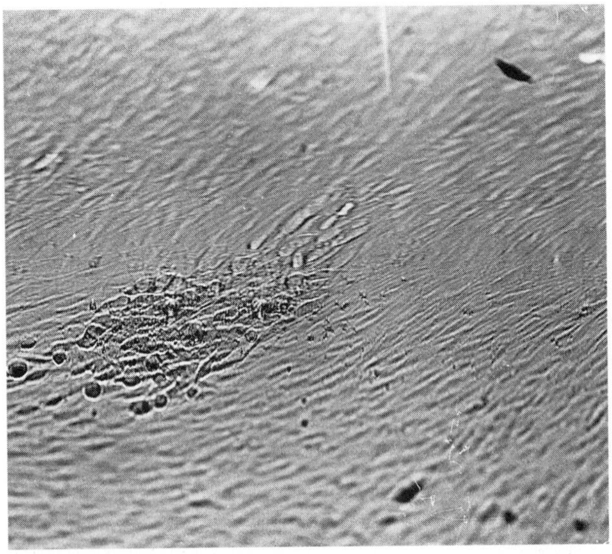

Figure 46–17. MRC-5 fibroblast monolayer with cytomegalovirus induced cytopathic effects after 11 days of incubation. (Phase contrast microscopy, 100 × magnification.)

BAL fluid, urine, or homogenized tissue; after a 16 to 40 hour incubation, the monolayer is stained with fluorescein-conjugated antibody to CMV early antigen. Infected fibroblasts show homogeneous fluorescence of the entire nucleus (see Fig. 46–18). Specificity is 100%, and sensitivity is excellent for urine, tissue, and BAL specimens (95% to 100%). However, peripheral blood leukocyte cultures have a sensitivity of approximately 75% compared with traditional tube culture; therefore, back-up standard tissue culture is needed for maximal accuracy. While CMV is the most common cause of viremia in compromised patients, VZV, HSV, adenovirus, and occasionally enterovirus infection also may develop. Back-up HDF and A549 traditional cell cultures held for 21 days are sufficient to recover these agents as well as CMV (Stanberry, 1994). Another advantage of shell vial CMV culture is the ease of performing quantitative culture (Buller, 1992; Slavin, 1992). A known inoculum of cells (leukocytes or BAL cells) and a numerical count of fluorescent CMV nuclei can generate a figure that is clinically valuable for estimating severity of infection, monitoring response to therapy, and predicting prognosis.

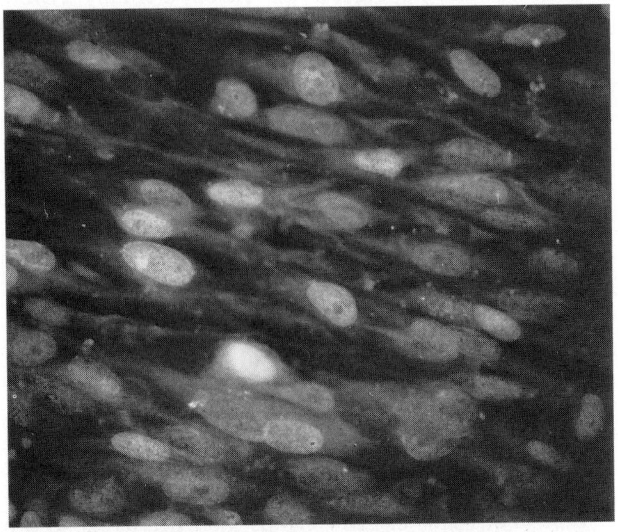

Figure 46–18. This MRC-5 fibroblast shell vial culture contains numerous fluorescent nuclei positive for cytomegalovirus antigen. (250 × magnification, immunofluorescent antibody stain for cytomegalovirus early antigen.)

Other rapid methods for diagnosis of CMV infection include demonstration of CMV antigenemia by detection of CMV pp65 antigen in peripheral blood neutrophils and PCR detection of CMV DNA (Erice, 1992; Niubo, 1994; Storch, 1994). Both seem superior to shell vial culture for diagnosis of active CMV infection, and allow detection of CMV viremia approximately one week earlier than shell vial cultures. Kits for CMV antigen assay but not PCR are now commercially marketed. These tests may have their most valuable applications in management of CMV infection in solid organ allograft recipients. In HIV-infected patients with CD4 values below 100, both tests accurately detect CMV but contribute little information vital for clinical management (Zurlo, 1993).

Akashi K, Eizuru Y, Sumiyoshi Y, et al: Brief report: severe infectious mononucleosis-like syndrome and primary HHV-6 infection in an adult. N Engl J Med 1993; 329:168–171.

Alder SP, Manganello AM, Koch WL, et al: Risk of human parvovirus B19 infections among school and hospital employees during endemic periods. J Infect Dis 1993; 168:361.

Alford CA, Stagno S, Pass RF, et al: Congenital and perinatal cytomegalovirus infections. Rev Infect Dis 1990; 12:S745.

Anand A, Grayes B, Brown T, et al: Human parvovirus infection in pregnancy and hydrops fetalis. N Engl J Med 1987; 316:183, 1987.

Anderson LJ, Parker RA, Stikas RL, et al: Association between respiratory syncytial virus outbreaks and lower respiratory tract deaths of infants and young children. J Infect Dis 1990; 161:640.

Arens MQ, Swierkosz EM, Schmidt RR, et al: Enhanced isolation of respiratory syncytial virus in cell culture. J Clin Microbiol 1986; 23:800.

Arvin AM, Hensleigh PA, Prober CG, et al: Failure of antepartum maternal cultures to predict the infant's risk of exposure to herpes simplex virus at delivery. N Engl J Med 1986; 315:796.

Asano Y, Yoshikawa T, Suga S, et al: Clinical features of infants with primary human herpesvirus 6 infection (exanthem subitum, roseola infantum). Pediatrics 1994; 93:104.

Ashley R, Cent A, Maggs SV, et al: Inability of enzyme immunoassays to discriminate between infections with herpes simplex virus types 1 and 2. Ann Intern Med 1991; 115:520.

Ashley RL, Milton J, Lee F, et al: Comparison of western blot (immunoblot) and glycoprotein G-specific immunodot assay for detecting antibodies to herpes simplex virus types 1 and 2 in human sera. J Clin Microbiol 1988; 26:662.

Atwood WJ, Berger JR: Human immunodeficiency virus type 1 infection of the brain. Clin Microbiol Rev 1993; 6:339.

Bagasra O, Hauptman SP, Lischer HW, et al: Detection of human immunodeficiency virus type 1 provirus in mononuclear cells by in situ polymerase chain reaction. N Engl J Med 1992; 329:1385.

Balayan MS: Hepatitis E virus infection in Europe: Regional situation regarding laboratory diagnosis and epidemiology. Clin Diagn Virol 1993; 1:1.

Bates PR, Bailey AS, Wood DJ, et al: Comparative epidemiology of rotavirus, subgenus F (types 40 and 41) adenovirus and astrovirus gastroenteritis in children. J Med Virol 1993; 39:224.

Beards GM: Polymorphism of genomic RNAs within rotavirus serotypes and subgroups. Arch Virol 1982; 41:65.

Bellini WJ, Rota JS, Rota PA, et al: Virology of measles virus. J Infect Dis 1994; 170(Suppl 1):S15.

Benedetti J, Corey L, Ashley R, et al: Recurrence rates in genital herpes after symptomatic first-episode infection. Ann Intern Med 1994; 121:847.

Betts RF: Influenza virus. *In* Mandell GL, Bennett JE, Dolin R (eds): Principles and Practice of Infectious Diseases, 4th ed. New York, Churchill Livingstone, 1994, pp 1546–1567.

Biesemier KW, Parks D, Gertis C, et al: Viral hepatitis serology at the University of North Carolina Hospitals: Update. Bull Lab Med 1994; 134.

Blacklow NR, Greenberg HB: Viral gastroenteritis. N Engl J Med 1991; 325:252.

Blanding JG, Hoshiko MG, Stutman HR, et al: Routine viral culture for pediatric respiratory specimens submitted for direct immunofluorescence testing. J Clin Microbiol 1989; 27:1438.

Blumer SO, Hearn TL, Schalla O, et al: Human T-lymphotrophic virus type I/II. Status of enzyme immunoassay and western blot testing in the United States in 1989 and 1990. Arch Pathol Lab Med 1992; 116:471.

Brandt CD, Kim HW, Rodriguez WJ, et al: Pediatric viral gastroenteritis during eight years of study. J Clin Microbiol 1983; 18:71.

Brinker JP, Doern GV: Comparison of MRC-5 and A-549 cells in conventional cultures and shell vial assays for the detection of varicella-zoster virus. Diagn Microbiol Infect Dis 1993; 17:75.

Brown ZA, Benedetti J, Ashley R, et al: Neonatal herpes simplex virus infection in relation to asymptomatic maternal infection at the time of labor. N Engl J Med 1991; 325:1247.

Brown ZA, Vontver LA, Benedetti J, et al: Effects on infants of a first episode of genital herpes during pregnancy. N Engl J Med 1987; 317:1246.

Buller RS, Bailey TC, Ettinger NA, et al: Use of a modified shell vial technique to quantitate cytomegalovirus viremia in a population of solid organ transplant recipients. J Clin Microbiol 1992; 30:2620.

Burgard M, Mayaux MJ, Blanche S, et al: The use of viral culture and p24 antigen testing to diagnose HIV infection in neonates. N Engl J Med 1992; 327:1192.

Calisher CH: Medically important arboviruses of the United States and Canada. Clin Microbiol Rev 1994; 7:89.

Carlson JR, Lee J, Henrichs SH, et al: Comparison of indirect immunofluorescence and western blot for detection of anti-human immunodeficiency virus antibodies. J Clin Microbiol 1987; 28:494.

Celum CL, Coombs RM, Lafferty W, et al: Intermediate human immunodeficiency virus type 1 western blots: Seroconversion risk, specificity of supplemental tests, and an algorithm for evaluation. J Infect Dis 1991; 164:656.

Cheeseman SH, Pierik LT, Leombruno D, et al: Evaluation of a commercially available direct immunofluorescent staining reagent for the detection of respiratory syncytial virus in respiratory secretions. J Clin Microbiol 1986; 24:155.

Cherry JD: Contemporary infectious exanthems. Clin Infect Dis 1993; 16:199.

Cherry JD, Lerner AM, Klein JO, et al: Coxsackie A9 infections with exanthems with particular reference to urticaria. Pediatrics 1963; 31:819.

Clark SJ, Saag MS, Decker WD, et al: High titers of cytopathic virus in plasma of patients with symptomatic primary HIV-1 infection. N Engl J Med 1991; 324:954.

Cone RW, Hackman RC, Haung M, et al: Human herpesvirus 6 in lung tissue from bone marrow transplant patients with pneumonia. New Engl J Med 1993; 329:156.

Connor E: Advances in early diagnosis of perinatal HIV infection. JAMA 1991; 266:3474.

Costello M, Morrow S, Smernoff N, et al: Comparison of Wellcome polyclonal and Bartels monoclonal antiserum for detection of respiratory viruses in pediatric specimens. ASM abstract #C51.91st General Meeting Dallas: ASM, 1991.

Costello M, Smernoff NT, Yungbluth M, et al: Laboratory diagnosis of viral respiratory infections. Lab Med 1993; 24:152.

Cuthbert JA: Hepatitis C: Progress and problems. Clin Microbiol Rev 1994; 7:505.

DeChamps C, Peigue-Lafeuille HH, Laveran H, et al: Four cases of vesicular lesions in adults caused by enterovirus infections. J Clin Microbiol 1988; 26:2182.

Demmler GJ: Summary of a workshop on surveillance for congenital cytomegalovirus disease. Rev Infect Dis 1991; 13:315.

Dennehy PH, Schultzbank TE, Thorne GM, et al: Evaluation of an automated immunodiagnostic assay, VIDAS rotavirus, for detection of rotavirus in fecal specimens. J Clin Microbiol 1994; 32:825.

Dinulos MB, Matson DO: Recent developments with human calicivirus. Pediatr Infect Dis J 1994; 13:998.

Dorian KJ, Beatty E, Atterbury KE, et al: Detection of herpes simplex virus by the Kodak Surecell Herpes Test. J Clin Microbiol 1991; 28:2117.

Douglas RG: Prophylaxis and treatment of influenza. N Engl J Med 1990; 322:443.

Drew WL: Controversies in viral diagnosis. Rev Infect Dis 1986; 8:814.

Drew WL: Cytomegalovirus infection in patients with AIDS. Clin Infect Dis 1992; 14:608.

Drew WL: Nonpulmonary manifestations of cytomegalovirus infection in immunocompromised patients. Clin Microbiol Rev 1992; 5:204.

Duffy LC, Riepenhoff-Talty M, Byers TE, et al: Modulation of rotavirus enteritis during breast feeding: Implications on alterations in the intestinal bacterial flora. Am J Dis Child 1986; 140:1164.

Erdman DD: Human parvovirus B19 specific IgG, IgA, and IgM antibodies and DNA in serum specimens from persons with erythema infectiosum. J Med Virol 1991; 35:110.

Erice A, Holm MA, Gill PC, et al: Cytomegalovirus (CMV) antigenemia assay is more sensitive than shell vial cultures for rapid detection of CMV in polymorphonuclear blood leukocytes. J Clin Microbiol 1992; 30:2822, 1992.

Espy MJ, Smith TF: Detection of herpes simplex virus in conventional tube cell cultures and in shell vials with a DNA probe kit and monoclonal antibodies. J Clin Microbiol 1988; 26:22.

Falsey AR, Walsh EE, Betts RF, et al: Serologic evidence of respiratory syncytial virus infection in nursing home patients. J Infect Dis 1990; 162:568.

Farhat SE, Finn S, Chua R, et al: Rapid detection of infectious mononucleosis-associated heterophile antibodies by a novel immunochromatographic assay and a latex agglutination test. J Clin Microbiol 1993; 31:1597.

Forghani B, Dupuis KW, Schmidt N: Rapid detection of herpes simplex DNA in human brain tissue by in-situ hybridization. J Clin Microbiol 1985, 22:656–659.

Fowler KB, Stagno S, Pass RF, et al: The outcome of congenital cytomegalovirus infection in relation to maternal antibody status. N Engl J Med 1992; 326:663.

Gala CL, Hall CB, Schnabel KC, et al: The use of eye-nose goggles to control nosocomial respiratory syncytial virus infection. JAMA 1986; 256:2706.

Gershon AA, Raker R, Steinberg S, et al: Antibody to varicella-zoster virus in parturient women and their offspring during the first year of life. Pediatrics 1976; 58:692.

Gleaves CA, Lee CF, Kirsch L, et al: Evaluation of a direct fluorescein-conjugated monoclonal antibody for detection of cytomegalovirus in centrifugation culture. J Clin Microbiol 1987; 25:1548.

Gleaves CA, Smith TF, Shuster EA, et al: Rapid detection of cytomegalovirus in MRC-5 cells inoculated with urine specimens by using low speed centrifugation and monoclonal antibody to an early antigen. J Clin Microbiol 1984; 19:917.

Gleaves CA, Wilson DJ, Wold AD, et al: Detection and serotyping of herpes simplex virus in MRC-5 cells by use of centrifugation and monoclonal antibodies 16h postinoculation. J Clin Microbiol 1985; 21:29.

Gold D, Bowden R, Sixbey J, et al: Chronic fatigue: A prospective clinical and virologic study. JAMA 1990; 264:48.

Gonik B, Seibel M, Berkowitz A, et al: Comparison of two enzyme-linked immunosorbent assays for detection of herpes simplex antigen. J Clin Microbiol 1991; 29:436.

Grohmann GS, Glass RI, Pereira HG, et al: Enteric viruses and diarrhea in HIV-infected patients. Enteric Opportunistic Infections Working Group. N Engl J Med 1993; 329:14.

Haffejee IE: Neonatal rotavirus infections. Rev Infect Dis 1991; 13:957.

Hall CB, Powell KR, MacDonald NE, et al: Respiratory syncytial viral infection in children with compromised immune function. N Engl J Med 1986; 315:77.

Hall CB, Walsh EE, Schnabel KC, et al: Occurrence of group A and B respiratory syncytial virus over 15 years: Associated epidemiologic and clinical characteristics in hospitalized and ambulatory children. J Infect Dis 1990; 62:1283.

Halstead DC, Beckwith DG, Sautter RL, et al: Evaluation of a rapid latex slide agglutination test for herpes simplex virus as a specimen screen and culture identification method. J Clin Microbiol 1987; 25:936.

Harmon MW, Kendal AP: Influenza viruses. *In* Balows A, Hausler WJ, Hermann KL, Isenberg HD, Shadomy HJ (eds): Manual of Clinical Microbiology, 5th ed. Washington, D.C., American Society for Microbiology, 1991.

Harris JW: Parvovirus B19 for the hematologist. Am J Hematol 1992; 39:119.

Harrison MJG, Mclister RT: Neurologic complication of HIV infection. *In* Lambert HP (ed): Handbook of Infectious Diseases. Infections of the Central Nervous System. Philadelphia, B.C. Decker, 1991, pp 343–360.

Harry DJ, Jennings MB, Yee J, et al: Antigen detection for human immunodeficiency virus. Clin Microbiol Rev 1989; 2:241.

Hedberg CW, Osterholm MT: Outbreaks of food-borne and water borne gastroenteritis. Clin Microbiol Rev 1993; 6:199.

Henrickson KJ, Kuhn SM, Savatski LL: Epidemiology and cost of infection with human parainfluenza virus types 1 and 2 in young children. Clin Infect Dis 1994, 18:770.

Hewitt DJ, Peddecord KM, Francis DP, et al: Content and design of laboratory report forms for human immunodeficiency virus type 1 antibody testing. Am J Clin Pathol 1992; 98:1992.

Hierholzer JC: Adenoviruses in the immunocompromised host. Clin Microbiol Rev 1992; 5:262.

Hirsch MS: Herpes simplex virus. *In* Mandell GL, Bennett JE, Dolin R (eds): Principles and Practice of Infectious Diseases, 4th ed. New York, Churchill Livingstone, 1994, p 1336.

Hollsberg P, Hafler DA: Pathogenesis of diseases induced by human lymphotrophic virus type 1 infection. Semin Med Beth Israel Hosp 1993; 328:1173.

Holmes GP, Kaplan JE, Gantz NM, et al: Chronic fatigue syndrome: A working case definition. Ann Intern Med 1988; 108:387.

Holmes GP, Kaplan JE, Stewart JA, et al: A cluster of patients with a chronic mononucleosis-like syndrome. Is Epstein-Barr virus the cause? JAMA 1987; 257:2297.

Houck JA, Sedmak DD, Grose MP, et al: Sensitivity and interobserver variability of the Recombigen HIV-1 la test. Am J Clin Pathol 1990; 93:538.

Hsiung GD, Fong CK, Landry ML: Diagnostic Virology, 4th ed. New Haven, CT, Yale University Press, 1994.

Hughes JH, Mann DR, Hamparian VV, et al: Detection of respiratory syncytial virus in clinical specimens by viral culture, direct and indirect immunofluorescence, and enzyme immunoasay. J Clin Microbiol 1988; 26:588.

Isenberg HD (ed): Clinical Microbiology Procedures Handbook. Washington, DC, American Society for Microbiology, 1992.

Iwarson I. The five main types of hepatitis: An alphabetical update. Scand J Infect Dis 1992; 24:129.

Jackson JR, Balfourm HH et al: Practical diagnostic testing for human immunodeficiency virus. Clin Microbiol Rev 1988; 1:124.

Johnson EB: Transport of viral specimens. Clin Microbiol Rev 1990; 3:120.

Johnson RE, Nahamias AJ, Nagder LS, et al: A seroepidemiologic survey of the prevalence of herpes simplex virus type 2 infection in the United States. N Engl J Med 1989; 321:7.

Johnston SL, Hamilton S, Bindra R, et al: Evaluation of an automated immunodiagnostic assay system for direct detection of herpes simplex virus antigen in clinical specimens. J Clin Microbiol 1992; 30:1042.

Johnston SL, Siegel CS: Evaluation of direct immunofluorescence, enzyme immunoassay, centrifugation culture, and conventional culture for the detection of respiratory syncytial virus. J Clin Microbiol 1990; 28:2394.

Kessler HA, Blaau W, Spear J, et al: Diagnosis of human immunodeficiency virus infection in seronegative homosexuals presenting with an acute viral syndrome. JAMA 1987; 258:1196.

Kimball AM, Foy HM, Cooney MK, et al: Isolation of respiratory syncytial and influenza viruses from the sputum of patients hospitalized with pneumonia. J Infect Dis 1983; 147:181.

Kimura H, Futamura M, Kito H, et al: Detection of viral DNA in neonatal herpes simplex virus infections: Frequent and prolonged presence in serum and cerebrospinal fluid. J Infect Dis 1991; 164:289.

Klonoff DC: Chronic fatigue syndrome. Clin Infect Dis 1992; 15:812.

Krilov LR, Marcoux L, Isenberg HD, et al: Comparison of three enzyme-linked immunosorbent assays and a direct fluorescent-antibody test for detection of respiratory syncytial virus antigen. J Clin Microbiol 1988; 26:377.

Kuzushima K, Kimura H, Kina Y, et al: Clinical manifestations of primary herpes simplex virus type 1 infection in a closed community. Pediatrics 1991; 87:152.

Lafferty WE, Krofft S, Remmington M, et al: Diagnosis of herpes simplex virus by direct immunofluorescence and viral isolation from samples of external genital lesions in a high prevalence population. J Clin Microbiol 1987; 25:323.

Langenberg A, Smith D, Brakel CL, et al: Detection of herpes simplex virus DNA from genital lesions by in situ hybridization. J Clin Microbiol 1988; 26:933.

Leclair JM, Freeman J, Sullivan B, et al: Prevention of nosocomial respiratory syncytial virus infections through compliance with glove and gown isolation precautions. N Engl J Med 1987; 317:329.

Lee FK, Pereira L, Griffin C, et al: A novel glycoprotein for detection of herpes simplex virus type 1-specific antibodies. J Virol Methods 1986; 14:111.

Lee WM: Acute liver failure. N Engl J Med 1993; 329:1862.

Leonardi GP, Leib H, Birlhead GS, et al: Comparison of rapid detection methods for influenza A virus and their value in health-care management of institutionalized geriatric patients. J Clin Microbiol 1994; 32:70.

Linderholm M, Bowman J, Juto P, et al: Comparative evaluation of nine kits for rapid diagnosis of infectious mononucleosis and Epstein-Barr virus-specific serology. J Clin Microbiol 1994; 32:259.

Lipson SM, Salo RJ, Leonardi GP: Evaluation of five monoclonal antibody-based kits or reagents for the identification and culture confirmation of herpes simplex virus. J Clin Microbiol 1991; 29:466.

Lopez C, Pellet P, Stewart J, et al: Characteristics of human herpesvirus 6. J Infect Dis 1988; 157:1271.

Mahalingham R, Wellish M, Wolf W, et al: Latent varicella-zoster viral DNA in human trigeminal and thoracic ganglia. N Engl J Med 1991; 232:627.

Mann JM, Prebuld SR, Hoffman RE, et al: Assessing risks of rubella infection during pregnancy: A standardized approach. JAMA 1981; 245:1647.

Markovitz DM: Infection with the human immunodeficiency virus type 2. Ann Intern Med 118:211, 1993.

Marrie TJ, Spencer HS, Lee HS, et al: Rotavirus infection in a geriatric population. Arch Intern Med 1982; 142:313.

Mavromoustakis CT, Witiak DT, Hughes JH: Effect of high-speed rolling on herpes simplex virus detection and replication. J Clin Microbiol 1988; 26:2328.

McCarthy CA, Hall C: Prevention of nosocomial respiratory syncytial virus in the pediatric patient. Infect Med 1990; 7:4.

McCullers JA, Lakeman FD, Whitley RJ: Human herpesvirus 6 is associated with focal encephalitis. Clin Infect Dis 1995; 21:571–576.

Menengus MA: Enteroviruses. *In* Balows A, Herrmann KL, Isenberg HD, Shadomy HJ (eds): Manual of Clinical Microbiology. Washington DC, ASM, 1991, pp 943–947.

Menzo S, Bagnarelli P, Giacca M, et al: Absolute quantitation of viremia in human immunodeficiency virus infection by competitive reverse transcription and polymerase chain reaction. J Clin Microbiol 1992; 30:1752.

Meyers JD, Flournoy N, Thomas ED: Nonbacterial pneumonia after allogeneic marrow transplantation: A review of ten years' experience. Rev Infect Dis 1982; 4:1119.

Michalski FJ, Shaikh M: Enzyme-linked immunosorbent assay spin amplification technique for herpes simplex virus antigen detection. J Clin Microbiol 1986; 24:310.

Miles SA, Baldwin E, Magpanfay L, et al: Rapid serologic testing with immune-complex-dissociated HIV p24 antigen for early detection of HIV infection in neonates. N Engl J Med 1993; 328:297.

Miller E, Cradock-Watson JE, Pollock TM, et al: Consequences of confirmed maternal rubella at successive stages of pregnancy. Lancet 1982; 2:781.

Miller H, Milk R, Diaz-Mitoma K, et al: Comparison of the VIDAS RSV assay and the Abbott Testpack RSV with direct immunofluorescence for detection of respiratory syncytial virus in nasopharyngeal aspirates. J Clin Microbiol 1993; 31:1336.

Miller KA, Zager TD: Rubella susceptibility in an adolescent female population. Mayo Clin Proc 1984; 59:31.

Minnich LL, Ray CG: Early testing of cultures for detection of hemadsorbing viruses. J Clin Microbiol 1987; 25:421.

Mitchell DK, Vaan R, Morrow AL, et al: Outbreaks of astrovirus gastroenteritis in day care centers. J Pediatr 1993; 123:725.

Modin JF: Perinatal echovirus infection: Insights from a literature review of 61 cases of serious infection and 16 outbreaks in nurseries. Rev Infect Dis 1986; 8:918.

Moseley RC, Corey L, Benjamin D, et al: Comparison of viral isolation, direct immunofluorescence, and indirect immunoperoxidase techniques for detection of genital herpes simplex virus infection. J Clin Microbiol 1981; 13:913.

Naides SJ, Scharosch LL, Foto F, et al: Rheumatologic manifestations of human parvovirus B19 infection in adults. Initial two-year clinical experience. Arthritis Rheum 1990; 33:1297.

Needham CA, Hurlbert P: Evaluation of an enzyme-linked immunoassay employing a covalently bound capture antibody for direct detection of herpes simplex virus. J Clin Microbiol 1992; 30:531.

Niubo J, Oerea JL, Carvajal A, et al: Effect of delayed processing of blood sample on performance of cytomegalovirus antigenemia assay. J Clin Microbiol 1994; 32:1119.

O'Brien TR, George JR, Holmberg SD: Human immunodeficiency virus type 2 infection in the United States. Epidemiology, diagnosis, and public health implications. JAMA 1992; 267:2775.

Oefinger PE, Loo SH, Gander RM, et al: Modified spin-amplified adsorption procedure with conventional tissue culture tubes for rapid detection and increased recovery of herpes simplex virus from clinical specimens. J Clin Microbiol 1988; 26:2195.

Overby LR, Houghton M: Hepatitis viruses. *In* Lennette EH (ed): Laboratory Diagnosis of Viral Infections, 2nd ed. New York, Marcel Dekker, 1992, pp 403–442.

Pan LZ, Werner A, Levy JA: Detection of plasma viremia in human immunodeficiency virus infected individuals at all clinical stages. J Clin Microbiol 1993; 31:283.

Pana S, Sarker S, Mandal BK, et al: Epidemic of herpes zoster following HIV epidemic in Manipur, India. J Infect 1994; 28:167.

Pantaleo G: The immunopathogenesis of human immunodeficiency virus infection. N Engl J Med 1993; 328:327.

Patel J, Frenkel LD, Greenhalgh M, et al: Rapid culture confirmation of herpes simplex virus by a monoclonal antibody-based enzyme immunoassay. J Clin Microbiol 1991; 29:410.

Pedneault L, Robillard L, Turgeon JP, et al: Validation of respiratory syncytial virus enzyme immunoassay and shell vial assay results. J Clin Microbiol 1994; 32:2861.

Phair JP, Wolinsky S: Diagnosis of infection with the human immunodeficiency virus. Clin Infect Dis 1992; 15:13.

Phillips AN, Elford J, Sabin C, et al: Immunodeficiency and the risk of death in HIV infection. JAMA 268:2662, 1992.

Plummer FA, Hammond GW, Forward K, et al: An erythema infectious-like illness caused by human parvovirus infection. N Engl J Med 1985; 313:74.

Pohl C, Green M, Wald ER, et al: Respiratory syncytial virus infections in pediatric liver transplant recipients. J Infect Dis 1992; 165:166.

Poli G, Pantaleo G, Fauci AS: The immunopathogenesis of human immunodeficiency virus infection. Clin Infect Dis 1993; 17(Suppl 1):S224.

Polish LB, Gallagher M, Fields H, et al: Delta hepatitis: Molecular biology and clinical epidemiological features. Clin Microbiol Rev 1993; 6:211.

Prober CG, Hensleigh PA, Boucher F, et al: Use of routine viral cultures at delivery to identify neonates exposed to herpes simplex virus. N Engl J Med 1988; 318:887.

Prober CG, Sullender WM, Yasukawa LL, et al: Low risk of herpes simplex virus infections in neonates exposed to the virus at the time of vaginal delivery to mothers with recurrent genital herpes simplex virus infections. N Engl J Med 1987; 316:240.

Pruksananonda P, Hall CB, Insel RA, et al: Primary human herpesvirus 6 infection in young children. N Engl J Med 1992; 326:1445.

Quinn TC, Klein RL, Halsey N, et al: Early diagnosis of perinatal HIV infection by detection of viral-specific IgA antibodies. JAMA 1991; 266:3439.

Rabalais GP, Stout GG, Ladd KL, et al: Rapid diagnosis of respiratory viral infections by using a shell vial assay and monoclonal antibody pool. J Clin Microbiol 1992; 30:1505.

Rogers MF, Ou C, Rayfield M, et al: Use of the polymerase chain reaction for early detection of the proviral sequences of HIV in infants born to seropositive mothers. N Engl J Med 1989; 320:1649.

Roseff SD, Campos JM: Detection of cytomegalovirus antibodies in serum using the TransSTAT-CMV and CMV Scan assays. Am J Clin Pathol 1993; 99:539.

Rossier JE, Miller HR, Phipps PH: Rapid viral diagnosis by immunofluorescence. Ottawa, University of Ottawa Press, 1989.

Rotbart HA: Nucleic acid detection systems for enteroviruses. Clin Microbiol Rev 1991; 4:156.

Rotbart HA, Nelson WL, Glode MP, et al: Neonatal rotavirus-associated necrotizing enterocolitis: Case control study and prospective surveillance during an outbreak. J Pediatr 1988; 112:87.

Ruuskanen O, Ogra PL: Respiratory syncytial virus. Curr Probl Pediatr 1993; 23:50.

Ryan-Poirier KA, Katz JM, Webster RG, et al: Application of Directigen FLU-A for the detection of influenza A virus in human and non-human specimens. J Clin Microbiol 1992; 30:1072.

Salahuddin SZ, Ablashi DV, Markham PD, et al: Isolation of a new virus HBLV, in patients with lymphoproliferative disorders. Science 1986; 234:596.

Schaefer L, Ceserio A, Demmler G, et al: Evaluation of Abbott CMV-M enzyme immunoassay for detection of cytomegalovirus immunoglobulin M antibody. J Clin Microbiol 1988; 26:2041.

Schlossberg D: Infectious Mononucleosis, 2nd ed. New York, Springer-Verlag, 1989.

Schmidt NJ: Cell culture procedures for viral diagnosis. *In* Schmidt NJ, Emmons RW (eds): Diagnostic Procedures for Viral, Rickettsial, and Chlamydial Infections, 6th ed. Washington DC, American Public Health Association, 1989, pp 51–100.

Schnittman SM, Greenhouse JJ, Psallidopoulos MC, et al: Increasing viral burden in CD4 + T cells from patients with human immunodeficiency virus (HIV) infection reflects rapidly progressive immunosuppression and clinical disease. Ann Intern Med 1990; 113:438.

Schnur D: Enterovirus. *In* Lennette EH (ed): Laboratory Diagnosis of Viral Infections, 2nd ed. New York, Marcel Dekker, 1992.

Schrim J, Meulenberg G, Pastoorm P, et al: Rapid detection of varicella-zoster virus in clinical specimens using monoclonal antibodies on shell vials and smears. J Med Virol 1989; 28:1.

Seal LA, Tomaya RS, Fleet KM, et al: Comparison of standard culture methods, a shell vial assay, and a DNA probe for the detection of herpes simplex virus. J Clin Microbiol 1991; 29:650.

Seno M, Shinichi T, Fukuda S, et al: Enhanced isolation of influenza virus in conventional plate cell cultures by low-speed centrifugation from clinical specimens. Am J Clin Pathol 1991; 95:765.

Shahrabadi MS, Lee PW: Calcium requirement for syncytium formation in HEp-2 cells by respiratory syncytial virus. J Clin Microbiol 1988; 26:139.

Sison A, Campos JM: Laboratory methods for early detection of HIV type 1 in newborns and infants. Clin Microbiol Rev 1992; 5:238.

Slavin MA, Gleaves CA, Schoch HG, et al: Quantification of cytomegalovirus in bronchoalveolar fluid after allogeneic marrow transplantation by centrifugation culture. J Clin Microbiol 1992; 30:2776.

Smith DW, Frankel LR, Mathers LH, et al: A controlled trial of aerosolized ribavirin in infants receiving mechanical ventilation for severe respiratory syncytial virus infection. N Engl J Med 1991a; 325:24.

Smith MC, Greutz C, Huang YT, et al: Detection of respiratory syncytial virus in nasopharyngeal secretions by shell vial technique. J Clin Microbiol 1991b; 29:463.

Smith RF, Elder BL: Evaluation of Cytomegelisa immunoglobulin M assay and comparison with indirect fluorescent antibody testing of QAE-Sephadex A50-treated sera. Am J Clin Pathol 1987; 87:230.

Stanberry LR, Floyd-Reising A, Connelly BL, et al: Herpes simplex viremia: Report of eight pediatric cases and review of the literature. Clin Infect Dis 1994; 18:401.

Starkey CA, Yen-Lieberman J, Proffitt MR, et al: Evaluation of the recombigen HIV-1 latex agglutination test. J Clin Microbiol 1990; 28:819.

Steeper TA, Horwitz CA, Ablashi DV, et al: The spectrum of clinical and laboratory findings resulting from human herpesvirus-6 in patients with mononucleosis-like illnesses not resulting from Epstein-Barr virus or cytomegalovirus. Am J Clin Pathol 1990; 93:776.

Steeper TA, Horwitz CA, Hanson W, et al: Heterophil-negative mononucleosis-like illnesses with atypical lymphocytosis in patients undergoing seroconversions to the human immunodeficiency virus. Am J Clin Pathol 1988; 89:169.

Stein DS, Korvick JA, Vermund SH, et al: CD4 lymphocyte cell enumeration for prediction of clinical course of human immunodeficiency virus disease: A review. J Infect Dis 1992; 165:352.

Storch GA, Buller RS, Bailey TC, et al: Comparison of PCR and pp65 antigenemia assay with quantitative shell vial culture for detection of cytomegalovirus in blood leukocytes from solid organ transplant recipients. J Clin Microbiol 1994; 32:997.

Straus SE: Clinical and biological differences between recurrent herpes simplex virus and varicella-zoster virus infections. JAMA 1989; 262:3455.

Straus SE, Cohen JI, Tosato G, et al: Epstein-Barr virus infections: Biology, pathogenesis and management. Ann Intern Med 1993; 118:45.

Sumaya CV, Jensen HB: Epstein-Barr virus. *In* Rose NR, DeMacario EC, Fahey JL, Freidman H, Penn GM (eds): Manual of Clinical Immunology, 4th ed. Washington DC, American Society for Microbiology, 1992, pp 568–575.

Sumiyoshi Y, Kikuchi M, Ohshina K, et al: Human herpesvirus-6 genomes in histolytic necrotizing lymphadenitis (Kikuchi's disease) and other forms of lymphadenitis. Am J Clin Pathol 1993; 99:609.

Takimoto S, Grandien M, Ishida MA, et al: Comparison of enzyme-linked immunosorbent assay, indirect immunofluorescence assay, and virus isolation for detection of respiratory viruses in nasopharyngeal secretions. J Clin Microbiol 1991; 29:470.

Talis A, McIntosh K: Respiratory syncytial virus. *In* Balows A, Hausler WJ, Herrmann KL, Isenberg HD, Shadomy HJ (eds): Manual of Clinical Microbiology, 5th ed. Washington DC, American Society for Microbiology, 1991, p 883.

Tedder DG, Ashley R, Tyler KL, et al: Herpes simplex virus infection as a cause of benign recurrent lymphocytic meningitis. Ann Intern Med 1994; 121:334–338.

Thomas EE, Book LE: Comparison of two rapid methods for detection of respiratory syncytial virus (RSV) (TestPack RSV and Ortho RSV ELISA) with direct immunofluorescence and virus isolation for the diagnosis of pediatric RSV infection. J Clin Microbiol 1991; 29:632.

Thomas EE, Roscoe DL, Brook L, et al: The utility of latex agglutination assays in the diagnosis of pediatric viral gastroenteritis. Am J Clin Pathol 1994; 101:742.

Tilton RC, Dias F, Ryan RW, et al: Comparative evaluation of three commercial tests for detection of heterophile antibody in patients with infectious mononucleosis. J Clin Microbiol 1988; 26:275.

Update: Influenza Activity—United States and worldwide, 1993-94 season, and composition of the 1994-95 influenza vaccine. MMWR 1994; 43:179.

Vainionpaa R, Hyypia T: Biology of parainfluenza viruses. Clin Microbiol Rev 1994; 7:265.

Van der Poel CL: Hepatitis C virus six years on. Lancet 1994; 344:1475.

VanEnk RA, James KK, Thompson KD: Evaluation of three commercial enzyme-linked immunosorbent assays for detection of herpes simplex virus antigen. Am J Clin Pathol 1991; 95:428.

Verano L, Michalski FJ: Herpes simplex antigen direct detection in standard virus transport medium by DuPont Herpcheck enzyme-linked immunosorbent assay. J Clin Microbiol 1990; 28:2555.

Viswanathan R: Epidemiology: Infectious hepatitis in Delhi 1955–1956. Indian J Med 45:10, 1957.

Wald A: Hepatitis E. *In* Aronoff SC, Hughes WT, Speck WT, Wald ER (eds.): Advances in Pediatric Infectious Diseases, Vol 10. Chicago, Mosby-Year Book, 1995, pp 67–89.

Waner JL, Whitehurst NJ, Toddy SJ, et al: Comparison of Directigen RSV with viral isolation and direct immunofluorescence for the identification of respiratory syncytial virus. J Clin Microbiol 1990; 28:480.

Warford AL, Levy RA, String CA, et al: Comparison of two commercial enzyme-linked immunosorbent assays for detection of herpes simplex virus antigen. Am J Clin Pathol 1986; 85:229.

Warrell DA, Warell MJ: Rabies. *In* Lambert HP (ed): Handbook of Infectious Diseases. Infections of the Central Nervous System. Philadelphia, BC Decker, 1991, pp 317–328.

Warren WP, Balcarek K, Smith R, et al: Comparison of rapid methods of detection of cytomegalovirus in saliva with virus isolation in tissue culture. J Clin Microbiol 1992; 30:786.

Weller TH: Varicella and herpes zoster: A perspective and overview. J Infect Dis 1992; 166:S1.

Whitely RJ: Viral encephalitis. N Engl J Med 1990; 232:242.

Whitely RJ, Cobbs CG, Alford CA: Disease that mimics herpes simplex virus encephalitis. JAMA 1989; 262:234.

Whitley RJ, Corey L, Arvin A, et al: Changing presentation of herpes simplex virus infections in neonates. J Infect Dis 1988; 158:109.

Whitley RJ, Gnann JW: Acyclovir: A decade later. N Engl J Med 1992; 327:782.

Whitley RJ, Lakeman F: Herpes simplex virus infection of the central nervous system: Therapeutic and diagnostic considerations. Clin Infect Dis 1995; 20:414–420.

Wiedbrauk DL, Bassin S: Evaluation of five enzyme immunoassays for detection of immunoglobulin M antibodies to Epstein-Barr virus viral capsid antigens. J Clin Microbiol 31:1339, 1993.

Wildin S, Chonmaitree T: The importance of the virology laboratory in the diagnosis and management of viral meningitis. Am J Dis Child 1987; 141:454.

Woods GL, Mills RD: Conventional tube cell culture compared with centrifugal inoculation of MRC-5 cells and staining with monoclonal antibodies for detection of herpes simplex virus in clinical specimens. J Clin Microbiol 1988; 26:570.

Wu TC, Zaza S, Callaway J: Evaluation of the DuPont Herpchek herpes simplex virus antigen test with clinical specimens. J Clin Microbiol 1989; 27:1903.

Yeldandi AV, Colby TV: Pathologic features of lung biopsy specimens from influenza pneumonia cases. Hum Pathol 1994; 25:47.

Yoshioka K, Kakuma S, Wakita T, et al: Detection of hepatitis C virus by polymerase chain reaction and response to interferon-alpha therapy: Relationship to genotypes of hepatitis C virus. Hepatology 1992; 16:293.

Yow MD: Congenital cytomegalovirus disease: A NOW problem. J Infect Dis 1989; 159:163.

Ziegler T, Waris M, Rautiainen A, et al: Herpes simplex virus detection by macroscopic reading after overnight incubation and immunoperoxidase staining. J Clin Microbiol 1988; 26:2013.

Zurlo JJ, O'Neill D, Polis MA, et al: Lack of clinical utility of cytomegalovirus blood and urine cultures in patients with HIV infection. Ann Intern Med 1993; 118:12.

Chapter 47

Chlamydial, Rickettsial, and Mycoplasmal Infections

Gail L. Woods, M.D.
David H. Walker, M.D.

Human infections caused by chlamydiae, rickettsiae, and mycoplasmas are discussed separately because the responsible pathogens differ from most other bacteria in several ways: The organisms are smaller, the structure of their cell wall is different, and chlamydiae and many rickettsiae are obligate intracellular parasites.

CHLAMYDIAL INFECTIONS

The chlamydiae have a tropism for columnar epithelial cells. They have a cell wall similar to that of gram-negative bacteria; they contain both DNA and RNA, have prokaryotic ribosomes, and synthesize their own proteins, nucleic acids, and lipids; they divide by binary fission; and they are susceptible to particular antibiotics. Unlike most bacteria, the chlamydiae are "energy parasites"; they are obligate intracellular bacteria and cannot replicate outside cells or synthesize high-energy adenosine triphosphate metabolites.

The chlamydiae are classified in the order Chlamydiales. There is one family, Chlamydiaceae, and one genus, *Chlamydia*, in which three species pathogenic for humans are recognized: *Chlamydia trachomatis, C. psittaci,* and *C. pneumoniae* (formerly the TWAR agent). Features useful for differentiating the three species are shown in Table 47–1. *Chlamydia pecorum* infections have not been recognized in humans.

Structure

Two morphologically distinct forms of chlamydiae are recognized. The elementary body is a dense, spherical form, 0.2 to 0.4 μm in diameter, that contains prokaryotic ribosomal RNA and has a rigid cell wall. It is the infectious form of the organism, capable of limited extracellular survival. The reticulate body, 0.6 to 1.0 μm in diameter, is the intracellular, metabolically active form, incapable of surviving outside cells. The closed circular DNA of both forms is compactly organized in a central nucleoid, has a molecular weight of 660 million, and codes approximately 600 proteins.

Two components of the outer membrane of the chlamydial elementary body have diagnostic importance. The most prominent is the major outer membrane protein (MOMP), a transmembrane protein with type-, subspecies-, species-, and genus-reactive epitopes defined by monoclonal antibodies. Infection with chlamydiae induces MOMP-species antibodies, but their role in protective immunity is unclear. The chlamydial outer membrane also contains a lipopolysaccharide (LPS) antigen, which is the major antigen detected in genus-specific serologic tests for chlamydial infection. Monoclonal antibodies and monospecific polyvalent antisera to the LPS or MOMP are used in direct fluorescent antibody tests and enzyme immunoassays to detect chlamydial antigen in clinical specimens.

Table 47–1. FEATURES USEFUL FOR DIFFERENTIATING SPECIES OF *CHLAMYDIA* PATHOGENIC FOR HUMANS

	Chlamydia species		
Parameter	***C. trachomatis***	***C. psittaci***	***C. pneumoniae***
Sulfa susceptibility	S	R	R
Glycogen staining of inclusion	+	−	−
EB shape	Round	Round	Pear

EB = elementary body; S = susceptible; R = resistant; + = positive; − = negative.

Table 47–2. *CHLAMYDIA TRACHOMATIS* SEROTYPES AND ASSOCIATED DISEASES

Serotypes	Diseases
A, B, Ba, C	Endemic trachoma
D, E, F, G, H, I, J, K	Urethritis/cervicitis in adults, inclusion conjunctivitis in neonates and adults, pneumonia in infants
L_1, L_2, L_3	Lymphogranuloma venereum

Replication

Chlamydiae replicate in the cytoplasm of infected host cells. The developmental cycle begins with attachment of the elementary body to a microvillus on a susceptible columnar cell; specific receptors have not been identified. The elementary body travels down the microvillus and localizes in indentations of the host cell plasma membrane. There the chlamydia enters the host cell in an endosome, where both *C. psittaci* and *C. trachomatis* remain during their intracellular development. Endosomes containing elementary bodies of *C. psittaci* do not interact with cellular lysosomes; those containing *C. trachomatis* elementary bodies fuse with one another and perhaps with lysosomes. Within six to eight hours after the elementary body enters the host cell, changes in its cell wall result in a transition to the reticulate body and subsequent initiation of DNA, RNA, and protein synthesis, and its division by binary fission. Host cell mitochondria migrate to and are positioned against the enlarging endosome, allowing the reticulate body to utilize host cell adenosine triphosphate. Reticulate bodies begin to reorganize 18 to 24 hours after infection; and presumably when nutrients are depleted, they mature into elementary bodies, which are released from the host cell. Cells infected with *C. psittaci* usually are severely damaged, and the organisms are released by cell lysis within 48 hours. In contrast, the inclusion of *C. trachomatis* appears to be extruded 72 to 96 hours after infection, leaving a lesion in the surviving host cell membrane.

Chlamydia trachomatis

Chlamydia trachomatis is the most common cause of sexually transmitted disease in the United States, and in trachoma-endemic regions of the Middle East, North Africa, and northern India it is an important cause of blindness. Fifteen serotypes are distinguished by microimmunofluorescence (Table 47–2), and three new serovars, Da, Ia, and L_{2a}, have been proposed (Wang, 1991).

Epidemiology, Pathology, and Clinical Manifestations

Humans are the only known natural host for all strains of *C. trachomatis*, except that causing mouse pneumonitis. The clinical manifestations and organ specificity of human infections with *C. trachomatis* are determined by both the mechanism of transmission and the properties of the infecting strain. Epidemiologically, *C. trachomatis* infections are divided into three categories: classic trachoma, sexually transmitted infections of adults, and perinatal ocular and respiratory tract infections.

Classic trachoma is an important cause of blindness in areas where public sanitation is inadequate and personal hygiene poor, and it is the most common cause of preventable blindness worldwide. Typically, the infection is transmitted among children via fingers, fomites, and probably flies. In endemic areas, acute chlamydial conjunctivitis of adults or infants is uncommon, but most children become chronically infected within a few years of birth. Repeated exposure to *C. trachomatis* eventually results in chronic follicular keratoconjunctivitis, conjunctival scarring, and pannus formation (invasion of vessels into the cornea).

Chlamydia trachomatis—induced sexually transmitted infections of adults include lymphogranuloma venereum (LGV) and urethritis/cervicitis and the associated complications. LGV is endemic in Asia, Africa, and South America. In the United States approximately 500 cases are reported each year; the disease affects males three times as frequently as females and is most common in persons of low socioeconomic status living in southeastern states, in homosexual men, and in persons who have visited LGV-endemic countries outside the United States. LGV is transmitted sexually, although transmission by fomites and by aerosols produced during laboratory accidents has caused pneumonitis, pleural effusions, and mediastinal or hilar lymphadenopathy (Jones, 1994). The reservoirs of infection probably are persons with asymptomatic or ignored symptomatic urethral, cervical, or anorectal infection.

LGV is the only infection caused by *C. trachomatis* that produces multisystem involvement and constitutional manifestations. During the primary phase, a small, painless vesicle or a platinum nonindurated papule or ulcer develops, often on the external genitalia, three days to three weeks after exposure, and heals quickly without scarring. The secondary stage, characterized by suppurative regional lymphadenopathy, fever, chills, anorexia, headache, myalgias, and arthralgias, begins two to six weeks after exposure. Histologic examination of affected lymph nodes shows granulomas surrounding stellate abscesses. Involved lymph nodes become matted and eventually suppurate, producing draining fistulas that heal with scarring over several months. The fibrosis and resultant abnormal lymphatic drainage are responsible for the urethral or rectal strictures or induration and lymphedema of the genitalia that develop during the third stage.

The clinical spectrum of sexually transmitted infections due to non-LGV strains of *C. trachomatis* is similar to disease caused by *Neisseria gonorrhoeae* (see Chap. 48). In men, *C. trachomatis* (serotypes D to K) is responsible for

30% to 50% of cases of nongonococcal urethritis, but as many as one third of men who habor *C. trachomatis* in the urethra are asymptomatic (Stamm, 1984). Rarely, urethritis caused by *C. trachomatis* progresses to epididymitis. Among homosexual males, non-LGV strains of *C. trachomatis* have been associated with proctitis. The organism also has been recovered from the urethra of as many as 70% of men with untreated Reiter's syndrome associated with urethritis (Keat, 1983). Genital infection with *C. trachomatis* probably is more prevalent in women than in men, and is more common among women who are young, single or divorced, black, of low socioeconomic status, and have multiple sexual partners. Infection of the endocervix with *C. trachomatis* may be asymptomatic or cause mucopurulent cervicitis, which can spread to the urethra and urinary bladder, resulting in the "acute urethal syndrome" of abacteriuric pyuria, or to the endometrium and fallopian tubes, producing endometritis or salpingitis. Infections of the upper reproductive tract may progress to pelvic inflammatory disease, or cause scarring and dysfunction of the oviduct transport system, which could result in infertility or ectopic pregnancy. Intraperitoneal spread of the infection may cause acute peritonitis, perihepatitis (Fitz-Hugh Curtis syndrome), periappendicitis, or perisplenitis. A small percentage of adults with chlamydial genital infections develop inclusion conjunctivitis.

In developed countries where sexually transmitted infection with *C. trachomatis* is epidemic, the organism may be transmitted from infected mother to infant during passage through the birth canal. Data from studies in North America indicate that 60% to 70% of infants exposed to *C. trachomatis* during vaginal delivery become infected with the organism, whereas infection after caesarean section is uncommon (Jones, 1994). *Chlamydia trachomatis* is recovered from the conjunctiva of infected infants after one to two weeks and from the nasopharynx soon thereafter. The rate of isolation from the conjunctiva falls by five to six weeks, but *C. trachomatis* can be recovered from the nasopharynx, conjunctiva, rectum, and vagina (usually without producing symptoms) for several months.

Inclusion conjunctivitis, the most common manifestation of infection with *C. trachomatis* in infants, develops in nearly 80% of infants whose conjunctival culture or cytologic examination demonstrates the organism (Jones, 1994). A mucopurulent discharge appears two to 25 days after birth, and the conjunctiva becomes inflamed and edematous. Symptoms usually resolve without therapy in several months with no sequelae, although scarring can occur.

Approximately 20% of infants who acquire infection with *C. trachomatis* at birth develop interstitial pneumonitis. The illness begins between two weeks and three months of age (peak, three to six weeks) with nasal congestion, followed by a distinctive staccato cough with tachypnea and rales, but no fever. About one half have or have had conjunctivitis. Symptoms last several weeks, but inspiratory rales and chest roentgenographic changes may persist for months.

Chlamydia psittaci

Pneumonia associated with exposure to birds was described in Switzerland in 1879. The disease was rare in the United States and Europe until the late 1920s, when pet tropical birds became fashionable. The pathogen was isolated by Bedson from human and avian tissue in 1930 during an investigation of an outbreak at the London Zoo.

Epidemiology

Infection caused by *Chlamydia psittaci* (called psittacosis) occurs worldwide. Psittacine birds are considered the major reservoir, but most species of birds can be infected with the organism. Infected birds may be obviously ill and die of the disease, but frequently they have mild signs, such as anorexia, diarrhea, lethargy, and ruffled feathers. Human illness is sporadic and has been associated with exposure to parrots, canaries, pigeons, sparrows, ducks, cockatiels, fowl (especially turkeys), and occasionally mammals. Owners of pet birds account for about half of the 40 to 60 cases reported in the United States each year. Pet shop employees, pigeon fanciers, zoo workers, veterinarians, and others who work with birds are at increased risk of infection. Outbreaks have occurred in turkey processing plants, principally among workers who killed the birds and plucked their feathers, and those who eviscerated carcasses (CDC, 1990). Over the past two decades the prevalence of psittacosis in the United States has declined dramatically as a result of adding tetracycline to poultry feed, requiring medication of commercially imported psittacine birds before entering the country, and breeding parakeets domestically.

Chlamydia psittaci is present in the blood, tissues, excreta, and feathers of infected birds, and may be shed for months after acute infection. Infection usually is transmitted to humans via inhalation of infectious aerosols derived from feces, fecal dust, and secretions of *C. psittaci*—infected birds, but may result from handling contaminated plumage or tissues, from bird bites, or from mouth-to-beak contact. Contact with birds does not have to be close or prolonged. Person-to-person spread of *C. psittaci* is rare.

Pathogenesis and Pathology

Chlamydia psittaci enters the body via the respiratory tract and is transported to the macrophages of the liver and spleen, where the organisms replicate. They then enter the blood and travel to the lungs, the primary target of infection, and other organs. Histologic examination of lung tissue shows lymphocytes in the alveolar and interstitial spaces, and mucus plugging of the bronchioles. Small hemorrhages and macrophages with intracytoplasmic inclusions may be seen. The hilar lymph nodes, liver, and spleen may be enlarged and contain foci of necrosis, and in fatal cases the myocardium, pericardium, meninges, brain, and adrenals may be involved.

Clinical Manifestations

Psittacosis begins abruptly after an incubation period of one to two weeks with chills and fever, or it begins gradually with increasing fever and malaise. Persistent dry, hacking cough, occasionally productive of blood-streaked mucoid sputum, is prominent. The heart rate often is slow relative to body temperature, and a diffuse, severe headache is usual. Malaise, anorexia, painful myalgias, and arthralgias are common, and a macular rash (Horder spots), resembling the rose spots of typhoid fever, may occur. Decreased mentation may develop at the end of the first week of illness, and a few persons have gastrointestinal complaints. *Chlamydia psittaci* is a rare cause of destructive endocarditis; most affected persons have a history of rheumatic heart disease or congenital valvular abnormalities (Jones, 1982).

Chlamydia pneumoniae

In 1986, a unique chlamydial organism was associated with acute respiratory tract disease in humans. The organism, initially considered to be a strain of *C. psittaci*, was named TWAR for the laboratory identifying letters of the first two isolates: TW-183, isolated in 1965 from the eye of a control child in trachoma vaccine trial in Taiwan, and AR-39, recovered the same year from the throat of a student with pharyngitis at the University of Washington. Soon after its recognition, data from DNA homology and electron microscopic studies showed that it was a separate species, *Chlamydia pneumoniae* (Campbell, 1987; Cox, 1988; Chi, 1987). Strains of *C. pneumoniae* and *C. psittaci* have 10% or less DNA sequence homology, and the pear-shaped elementary body of *C. pneumoniae* differs from the round elementary bodies of *C. psittaci* and *C. trachomatis*.

Epidemiology

The current concept of the epidemiology of infection with *C. pneumoniae* is based on data from retrospective studies of sera collected during respiratory tract illness. About 50% of adults have antibodies to *C. pneumoniae*. Antibody prevalence rates are low in children, increase sharply in teenagers, continue to increase until middle age, and remain high into old age; and rates are 10% to 25% higher for males. Data from retrospective and prospective serologic studies indicate that disease caused by *C. pneumoniae* is endemic in the United States and epidemic in Scandinavia and Finland but does not occur with any consistent seasonal periodicity (Grayston, 1989, 1990).

Chlamydia pneumoniae appears to be a primary human pathogen, transmitted from human to human without an avian or animal reservoir. The mechanism and place of transmission, incubation period, and infectiousness of the organism have not yet been determined. Data from retrospective studies of Finnish military trainees showed the epidemics of *C. pneumoniae* pneumonia lasted five to eight months, suggesting that the infection spreads slowly, even in a closed population (Kleemola, 1988).

Pathogenesis

The pathogenesis of infection with *C. pneumoniae* is unknown. Because the illness generally is mild and self-limited, autopsy studies are unavailable.

Clinical Manifestations

It is estimated that *C. pneumoniae* is responsible for about 10% of community-acquired pneumonias (Grayston, 1990). The pneumonia usually is mild, with a single subsegmental infiltrate, but it may be severe, especially in elderly persons and in those with chronic disease. It often begins with pharyngitis and hoarseness, followed by persistent cough. Although pneumonia is the most common syndrome associated with *C. pneumoniae* infection, serologic studies during epidemics among military trainees have shown that only about 10% of infections with *C. pneumoniae* result in pneumonia, suggesting that infection frequently is mild or asymptomatic and unrecognized. Other manifestations of *C. pneumoniae* infection are bronchitis, pharyngitis, fever of undetermined origin, otitis, influenza-like illness, myocarditis, endocarditis, and possibly atherosclerosis.

Laboratory Diagnosis

Chlamydia trachomatis

Specimens for diagnosis of infections with *C. trachomatis* are determined by the disease manifestations (Table 47–3). Specific collection techniques are discussed in Chapter 54. Most infections involve mucous membranes, and specimens should be collected directly from the involved surface and must contain an adequate sample of infected epithelial cells. Purulent discharge is not an appropriate specimen and should be removed before a sample is collected with a swab or brush. Of the types of swabs available, Dacron or rayon-tipped swabs are preferred. Swabs with wooden shafts should be avoided because wood is toxic to the organism. Calcium alginate swabs may be toxic to the chlamydiae or to the cells that support their growth. Cotton-tipped swabs are acceptable but occasionally are toxic to the chlamydiae.

Cell Culture

Cell culture currently is the reference method for diagnosis of chlamydial infections and must be performed when the diagnosis is disputed and in cases of suspected sexual assault or abuse. Cell lines most commonly used are McCoy or Buffalo green monkey cells. Both have equivalent sensitivity, but the latter cells are easier to maintain and more resistant to cytotoxic substances, and they have been associated with more and larger inclusions (Krech, 1989). Adding cycloheximide (0.5 to 1.5 μl/ml) to the growth medium enhances sensitivity. Cell monolayers are grown on glass coverslips in shell vials or 24-well plates or on the surface of polystyrene 96-well or 48-well culture dishes. To enhance recovery of *C. trachomatis*, specimens are sonicated or agitated on a vortex mixer before inoculation to release elementary bodies from host cells, and inoculated shell vials or culture dishes are centrifuged. After incubation for 48 to 72 hours, monolayers are fixed and stained with fluorescein-conjugated

Table 47–3. SPECIMENS FOR DETECTION OF *CHLAMYDIA TRACHOMATIS*

Disease	Specimen
Mucopurulent cervicitis	Endocervical swab
Acute urethral syndrome (women)	Urethral swab
Acute endometritis	Endometrial aspirate
Acute salpingitis	Fallopian tube biopsy
Nongonococcal urethritis (men)	Urethral swab, urine*
Inclusion conjunctivitis	Conjunctival scrapings/swab
Trachoma	Conjunctival scrapings/swab
Lymphogranuloma venereum	Lymph node aspirate, biopsy of ulcerated lesion, serum
Pneumonitis (infants)	Serum, tracheobronchial aspirate, nasopharyngeal swab

*Urine is acceptable for some enzyme-linked immunoassays and for the commercial polymerase chain reaction kit.

monoclonal antibodies. If a 96-well culture system is used, passaging specimens that are negative for *C. trachomatis* at 48 hours is recommended to enhance detection; however, passaging does not significantly increase detection in shell vials or 24-well plates (Schacter, 1987; Zimmerman, 1992).

Nonculture Direct Detection Methods

DIRECT FLUORESCENT ANTIBODY TESTS

The direct fluorescent antibody (DFA) test, which was the first nonculture chlamydia detection test developed, allows direct visualization of *C. trachomatis* elementary bodies in smears of clinical specimens. Total processing time is 30 to 60 minutes. It is the only test that permits direct assessment of specimen adequacy. Specimens with columnar or metaplastic squamous cells are acceptable, whereas those with few columnar cells, excessive amounts of mucus, or predominance of squamous cells are not. However, interpretation of the smear is subjective, and operator fatigue can be a problem in high-volume situations.

Currently, monoclonal antibodies are available from several manufacturers. Antibodies directed against the species-specific MOMP of *C. trachomatis* appear to be more specific, produce more intense fluorescence than those directed against the chlamydial LPS (Cles, 1988), and are used most frequently (Woods, 1994). Occasionally, even the species-specific antibodies stain bacteria other than *C. trachomatis*, perhaps because of nonspecific immunoglobulin binding or crossreactivity. Staining organisms other than *C. trachomatis* is especially frequent with rectal specimens; therefore, for this site culture is preferred, although some DFA reagents are approved for evaluation of rectal samples.

The sensitivity of the DFA test has varied from 50% to almost 100% compared with culture as the standard, depending on the prevalence of infection in the population being evaluated and the number of elementary bodies required for a positive result (Barnes, 1989). In general, the sensitivity is greater with lower cut-off values for elementary bodies and in populations with a high prevalence of disease. In general, the specificity of DFA is greater than 95%.

ENZYME IMMUNOASSAYS

Enzyme immunoassays (EIAs) detect chlamydial LPS with monoclonal or polyclonal antibodies labeled with an enzyme that converts a colorless substrate into a colored product. Both solid-phase systems, which use plastic or beads coated with the antibody, and membrane systems are commercially available. Total processing time ranges from 15 to 30 minutes for membrane systems to three to four hours for solid-phase systems. Advantages of EIA are the objective interpretation of results and ease of use for batching large numbers of specimens.

As with DFA, the sensitivities of EIAs vary (from about 70% to 100%) compared with culture as the standard and tend to be higher in populations with a high prevalence of disease, such as persons attending a sexually transmitted disease clinic (Barnes, 1989; Clarke, 1993; Ehret, 1993; Kluytmans, 1993; Mills, 1992; Warren, 1993). The specificity of EIA is 95% or higher. Causes of false-positive results are the presence of a bacterial urinary tract infection (Demaio, 1991) or contamination of the specimen with cervical mucus or vaginal secretions. The latter problem can be reduced by improving the specimen collection technique (removing cervical mucus and obtaining a true endocervical sample) and by using blocking anitbodies (Mills, 1992).

NUCLEIC ACID HYBRIDIZATION TESTS

A commercially available acridinium-ester–labeled DNA probe complementary to *C. trachomatis* ribosomal RNA allows direct detection of *C. trachomatis* in urogenital and conjunctival specimens. The test requires a water bath and a luminometer. Total processing time is two to three hours. The sensitivity of the probe test compared with culture as the reference method varies greatly for both endocervical samples and urethral swab specimens in men (from 76% to 97%) (Blanding, 1993; Clarke, 1993; Iwen, 1991; Kluytmans, 1994, 1991; Warren, 1993). The specificity of the probe test is 97% or greater, and it can be improved with a probe competition assay.

POLYMERASE CHAIN REACTION

A polymerase chain reaction (PCR) test for direct detection of *C. trachomatis* in endocervical swab specimens and male urine samples is currently commercially available. The test involves three processes: amplification, hybridization, and detection. Target DNA in the specimen is amplified in a thermocycler by using biotinylated primers for sequences in the *C. trachomatis* cryptic plasmid. The sample is transferred to a 96-well plate coated with oligonucleotide probes complementary to the amplicons. Captured biotinylated amplicons are detected with an avidin-horseradish peroxidase conjugate, similar to an EIA procedure. Total processing time is four to five hours. Data from studies comparing PCR and cell culture are summarized in Table 47–4 (Bauwens, 1993a,b; Jaschek, 1993; Loeffelholz, 1992; Mahoney, 1994). Given the wide range of sensitivities and the expense of the PCR

6

Table 47–4. RELIABILITY OF COMMERCIAL PCR KIT FOR DETECTION OF *CHLAMYDIA TRACHOMATIS* IN GENITOURINARY TRACT SPECIMENS

Specimen Type	Disease Prevalence (%)	PCR		Culture Sensitivity (%)	Reference
		Sensitivity (%)	*Specificity (%)*		
Endocervical swab	5, 17	97	99.7	86	Loeffelholz, 1993
	10	89	99.2	93	Bauwens, 1936
	8	64	99	91	Bauwens, 1936
	4	97	100	86	Bass, 1993
Male urine	9	85	97.4	85	Bauwens, 1993a
	10	95	99.8	68	Jaschek, 1993

PCR = polymerase chain reaction.

assay, more data are needed to determine the role of PCR for detection of *C. trachomatis* in the clinical laboratory.

Verification of Nonculture Tests

Experts at the Centers for Disease Control and Prevention (CDC) recommend that positive screening test (DFA, EIA, probe) results be verified with a supplemental test if a false-positive result is likely to have adverse medical, social, or psychological consequences (CDC, 1993). In low-prevalence populations, verification probably should be routine but might be selective in high-prevalence populations. Culture confirmation is optimal but requires a second specimen collected either during the first visit or during a return visit. EIA blocking assays, a probe competition assay, or evaluation of the transport medium with a DFA test are alternative verification methods.

Serologic Tests

Serologic tests have little value for diagnosis of chlamydial genital infections for two reasons. First, antibodies to *C. trachomatis* persist after the infection resolves, so a positive serologic test does not necessarily correlate with active disease. Second, many serologic tests are not specific for *C. trachomatis* because they detect genus-specific antibodies. Exceptions are diagnosis of LGV and *C. trachomatis* pneumonitis in infants. Because LGV has a long latent period and clinical diagnosis often is delayed, antibodies generally are present when the acute-phase serum is collected, and a fourfold rise in titer between acute and convalescent-phase serum samples often cannot be documented. Thus, a single or stable complement fixation titer of 1:64 or greater supports a presumptive diagnosis of LGV. For diagnosis of *C. trachomatis* pneumonitis in infants, detection of IgM antibodies by microimmunofluorescence may be the method of choice (a titer of 1:32 or greater is diagnostic).

Chlamydia psittaci

Chlamydia psittaci can be grown in cell culture, but this is recommended only for specially equipped laboratories with experienced personnel because the organism is especially virulent and has been associated with laboratory-acquired infections. Infection with *C. psittaci* usually is diagnosed serologically, preferably by testing acute and convalescent phase serum. A fourfold or greater rise in complement-fixing antibody titers between specimens in a patient with symptoms of psittacosis supports the diagnosis. A single titer of 1:32 or greater in an individual with a compatible illness is presumptive evidence of psittacosis. Antibodies usually are detected by the end of the second week of illness, but early antibiotic therapy can delay their appearance for several weeks. False-positive rises in antibody titer occur uncommonly in individuals with Legionnaires' disease.

Chlamydia pneumoniae

Diagnosis of *C. pneumoniae* infection is based predominantly on serologic tests (Grayston, 1990). The microimmunofluorescence test with the TWAR antigen is specific for *C. pneumoniae*. Immunoglobulin (Ig)M antibodies appear about three weeks after the onset of primary illness, usually decline over the next two to six months to a level that cannot be detected, and may not reappear with reinfection. IgG antibodies are detected six to eight weeks after the onset of the primary illness, persist for life, and may rise one to two weeks following reinfection. Serologic test results consistent with acute infection include a fourfold or greater rise in IgG titer between acute and convalescent-phase serum samples, a single IgG titer of 1:512 or greater, or an IgM titer of 1:16 or greater. *Chlamydia pneumoniae* can be isolated in cell culture, but it is more difficult to grow than *C. trachomatis* (Roblin, 1992).

Treatment

Tetracyclines are the treatment of choice for infections with chlamydiae. For genital infections caused by *C. trachomatis*, other effective agents include erythromycin, sulfisoxazole, and ofloxacin. Ocular infections with *C. trachomatis* require systemic treatment with a tetracycline (for adults) or erythromycin or sulfisoxazole (for neonates); topical therapy suppresses symptoms but does not eradicate the organism. Erythromycin is an acceptable alternative agent for infections caused by *C. pneumoniae*. Sulfonamides are ineffective against both *C. psittaci* and *C. pneumoniae*.

RICKETTSIAL INFECTIONS

Rickettsia is a concept that developed historically as the molecular and physical nature of viruses were defined (Weiss, 1988). In contrast with viral agents, which also require host eukaryotic cells for their intracellular growth, rickettsiae have a gram-negative bacterial cell wall and their growth is inhibited by particular antibiotics. Rickettsiae were further differentiated from other obligately intracellular bacteria by their ecology and transmission by arthropod vectors. The traditional taxonomic scheme, based upon such phenotypic characteristics as intracellular growth and arthropod vector transmission, requires substantial modification in light of contemporary gene sequence analyses. Genera that have been considered to contain rickettsiae pathogenic for humans are *Rickettsia, Ehrlichia, Coxiella*, and *Rochalimaea* (Weiss, 1984). Despite its historical association with rickettsiology and louse transmission, *Rochalimaea* are cultivable in cell-free medium. Analysis of 16S rRNA gene sequences reveals that *Rochalimaea* are truly members of the genus *Bartonella* and do not belong in the order Rickettsiales (Brenner, 1993). Moreover, members of the genera *Rickettsia, Ehrlichia*, and *Bartonella* are more closely related to one another than to *Coxiella* (Walker, 1995). Even within some classical genera, particular organisms are not similar enough to fit, for example, *Rickettsia tsutsugamushi* and *Ehrlichia sennetsu*, organisms to which more attention is paid in the Orient than in the Americas and Europe. Grouped by genus, the following diseases are presented in this chapter: *Rickettsia*, Rocky Mountain spotted fever, boutonneuse fever, rickettsialpox, murine typhus, and scrub typhus; *Ehrlichia*, human monocytic ehrlichiosis and human granulocytic ehrlichiosis; *Coxiella*, Q fever; and *Bartonella*, cat scratch disease, bacillary angiomatosis and peliosis, trench fever, and South American bartonellosis. The diseases of each genus comprise cohesive clinical and pathologic groupings, and overall the rickettsial diseases pose a similar set of diagnostic challenges with similar technical approaches to their solution.

Infections Caused by Organisms of the Genus *Rickettsia*

Structure and Function

Spotted fever group and typhus group rickettsiae are closely related genetically and differ substantially genetically and phenotypically from the scrub typhus agent, *Rickettsia tsutsugamushi* (Tamura, 1991; Walker, 1995; Weiss, 1984). Spotted fever and typhus rickettsiae are thin (0.3 to 0.5 by 1 to 2 μm) bacilli with a gram-negative cell wall containing lipopolysaccharide, having antigenic components that distinguish the two groups. The gram-negative cell wall of *R. tsutsugamushi* differs from that of spotted fever and typhus group rickettsiae; it has an ultrastructurally thicker outer leaflet and thinner inner leaflet of the outer envelope, different major proteins, and lacks lipopolysaccharide and peptidoglycan (Tamura, 1991). All *Rickettsia* species reside free in the cytosol of the host cell and divide by binary fission (Walker, 1989). Rickettsiae attach to the host cell via a protein adhesin, enter by induced phagocytosis, and escape from the phagosome. These functions can occur within minutes and are associated with phospholipase A_2 activity, apparently of rickettsial origin. Spotted fever group rickettsiae are propelled within cells and during release from the cell by stimulating polymerization of host cell F-actin at one pole (Heinzen, 1993). Rickettsiae that manifest this activity (e.g., *R. rickettsii*) escape earlier from host cells and spread more quickly to other cells than those lacking this activity (e.g., *R. prowazekii*), which divide intracellularly to massive numbers before the host cell bursts and the organisms are released. Scrub typhus rickettsiae are released from the host cell via a process involving pinching off a host cell membrane-bound rickettsia. According to the current 16S rDNA sequence data, *Rickettsia* species that are pathogenic for humans have evolved into four genogroups (Table 47–5). The typhus group includes *R. prowazekii* and *R. typhi*. The spotted fever group contains *R. rickettsii, R. conorii, R. japonica,*

Table 47–5. *RICKETTSIA, EHRLICHIA, COXIELLA,* AND *BARTONELLA* INFECTIONS

Etiologic Agent	Disease	Geographic Distribution	Transmission
Spotted Fevers			
R. rickettsii	Rocky Mountain spotted fever	North, Central, and South America	Tick bite
R. conorii	Boutonneuse fever	Southern Europe, Africa, Russia, Georgia, Middle East, Indian subcontinent	Tick bite
R. sibirica	North Asian tick typhus	Russia, China, Mongolia, Pakistan	Tick bite
R. japonica	Oriental spotted fever	Japan	Presumed tick bite
Typhus Fevers			
R. prowazekii	Epidemic typhus	Potentially worldwide; recent decades in Africa, South America, Central America, Mexico, Asia	Louse feces
R. prowazekii	Brill-Zinsser disease	Worldwide; wherever persons with past epidemic typhus now reside	Recrudescence of latent infection
R. prowazekii	Flying squirrel typhus	U.S.A.	Presumably feces of flea or louse of flying squirrel
R. typhi	Murine typhus	Worldwide in tropics and subtropics	Flea feces
Other Rickettsial Fevers			
R. akari	Rickettsialpox	U.S.A., Ukraine, Croatia, Korea	Mite bite
R. australis	Queensland tick typhus	Eastern Australia	Tick bite
Cat flea rickettsia	Murine typhus–like illness	U.S.A.	Presumably flea bite or feces
Scrub typhus			
R. tsutsugamushi	Scrub typhus	SE Asia, Japan, China, Sri Lanka, India, Asiatic Russia, Tadzhikistan, Indonesia, Western Pacific, Northern Australia	Chigger bite
Ehrlichioses			
E. chaffeensis	Human monocytic ehrlichiosis	U.S.A., Europe, Africa	Tick bite
E. phagocytophilia–like	Human granulocytic ehrlichiosis	U.S.A.	Presumably tick bite
E. sennetsu	Sennetsu rickettsiosis	Japan, Malaysia	Not known
Coxiellosis			
C. burnetii	Q fever	Worldwide	Inhalation of aerosols from infected animals, possibly ingestion of animal products or tick bite
Bartonelloses			
B. bacilliformis	Oroya fever, verruga peruana	Western South America	Sandfly bite
B. henselae	Cat scratch disease, bacillary angiomatosis and peliosis	Probably worldwide	Kitten scratch or bite
B. quintana	Trench fever	Europe and North America	Feces of *Pediculus* louse

6

and *R. sibirica*. A newly recognized clade contains *R. akari*, *R. australis*, and an un-named pathogen that resides in cat fleas. *Rickettsia akari* and *R. australis* were traditionally considered to be relatively distant members of the spotted fever group, with which they share lipopolysaccharide antigens. A different name, *Orientia tsutsugamushi*, has been proposed for the scrub typhus organisms because of their substantial genetic and antigenetic diversity (Tamura, 1991).

Rocky Mountain Spotted Fever

The most severe of all the rickettsioses, Rocky Mountain spotted fever (RMSF), has a substantial fatality rate, even among previously healthy, immunocompetent children and young adults (Walker, 1989). *Rickettsia rickettsii* normally resides in nature in ticks: *Dermacentor variabilis*, the American dog tick, in the eastern two thirds of the United States and California; *Dermacentor andersoni*, the Rocky Mountain wood tick, in the western United States; *Rhipicephalus sanguineus*, the brown dog tick, in Mexico; and *Amblyomma cajennense*, in Mexico and Central and South America. These ticks maintain *R. rickettsii* as they moult from stage to stage (larva, nymph, and adult) and transovarially from generation to generation. Fewer than one per 1000 ticks carries virulent *R. rickettsii*, which seems to be mildly pathogenic for ticks. New lines of ticks become infected by feeding on rickettsemic rodents, replenishing the population of organisms transovarially maintained in ticks.

Infections occur when and where humans encounter *R. rickettsii*–infected ticks (Helmick, 1984). Although RMSF has been documented in recent years in nearly every state except for Hawaii, Alaska, and Vermont, the highest incidence is in the South Atlantic states from Maryland to Georgia and the south central states of Oklahoma, Missouri, and Arkansas. Most cases occur in late spring and summer, but particularly in the southern latitudes, a few cases may occur even in winter. The highest incidence is in children and others who are exposed to ticks during outdoor activities. Fatality-to-case ratios are higher for blacks, males, and persons older than 30 years. Fulminant RMSF (death by the fifth day of illness) occurs in association with moderate hemolysis, for example, in black males with glucose-6-phosphate dehydrogenase deficiency.

Rickettsiae are released via the tick salivary gland secretions into the patient's dermis after six to 10 hours of tick feeding and spread hematogenously throughout the body. The vascular endothelium is the target of intracellular infection, with some invasion into vascular smooth muscle cells. Infected endothelium is injured by free radical–induced damage to cell membranes and possibly by phospholipase A_2 activity (Silverman, 1988). Damage to the endothelium results in increased vascular permeability, edema, hypovolemia, and hypotension. The life-threatening consequences of vascular injury in the central nervous system and lung are rickettsial meningoencephalitis and noncardiogenic pulmonary edema. Early in the course, lesions show endothelial rickettsiae without thrombi or a cellular response. Late in the course, the characteristic lymphohistiocytic perivascular infiltrate appears as interstitial pneumonia, interstitial myocarditis, perivascular glial nodules of the brain, and similar vascular lesions in the dermis, gastrointestinal tract, liver, skeletal muscles, and kidneys. Severe injury may be accompanied by focal hemorrhages, but seldom by microinfarcts, except in the white matter of the brain.

The clinical illness usually begins with fever, headache, and myalgia two to 14 days after tick bite (Kaplowitz, 1981; Helmick, 1984). Nausea, vomiting, abdominal pain and tenderness, and diarrhea occur more frequently in the first three days of illness. The rash, which usually appears between days three and five, typically begins as macules around the wrists and ankles and, later, on the arms, legs, and trunk. The lesions become maculopapular, and in half of cases a central petechia appears in many of the maculopapules. Characteristic involvement of the palms and soles occurs in half of cases as a late manifestation. Renal failure is a feature of severe RMSF. Central nervous system involvement is ominous; seizures and coma occur in 8% to 10% of cases overall, often preceding a fatal outcome. Thrombocytopenia occurs in half of cases, but disseminated intravascular coagulation is rare.

Boutonneuse Fever and Other Spotted Fevers

Rickettsia conorii has been isolated in southern Europe; northern, eastern, and southern Africa; Israel, India, and Pakistan; and Russia, Georgia, and the Ukraine. The ecology of *R. conorii* and the epidemiology of boutonneuse fever are closely tied to ticks, especially *Rhipicephalus sanguineus*, which maintain the rickettsiae transovarially and transmit the infection to humans while feeding (Walker, 1991). Imported cases are diagnosed in travellers returning to the United States and northern Europe from Africa and the Mediterranean basin. The fatality rate is 1.4% to 5.6%, particularly in patients with underlying diseases. *Rickettsia sibirica* has been isolated in Russia, China, Mongolia, and Pakistan. *Rickettsia japonica* has been documented only in Japan. After an average incubation period of seven days, these illnesses begin with fever, headache, and myalgias. Frequently an eschar can be discovered by careful examination of the skin at this time. The pathology of these spotted fevers is well described in the tache noire or eschar at the site of tick bite inoculation of rickettsiae (Walker, 1988a). Endothelial infection and injury by *R. conorii* result in dermal and epidermal necrosis and perivascular edema. The host defenses that effect killing of intracellular rickettsiae include T lymphocytes and macrophages, which infiltrate around the infected dermal blood vessels (Herrero-Herrero, 1987). Disseminated endothelial infection results in maculopapular rash, meningoencephalitis, and vascular lesions in the lungs, kidneys, gastrointestinal tract, and heart (Walker, 1985). Multifocal hepatocellular necrosis and granuloma-like lesions correlate with moderately increased concentrations of hepatic transaminases (Walker, 1986).

Rickettsialpox

Rickettsia akari is maintained in nature by transovarial transmission in the gamasid mite, *Liponyssoides sanguineus*, an ectoparasite of the domestic mouse, *Mus musculus*. *Rickettsia akari* has been isolated only in the United States, Croatia, the Ukraine, and Korea, perhaps more an indication of the paucity of rickettsial investigations than the actual distribution of this rickettsial species.

A papule develops during the approximately 10-day incubation period at the site of mite bite and progresses to become a 1 to 2.5 cm eschar. Illness begins with chills, fever, malaise, severe headache, and myalgia. Rash, which appears two to six days later, is initially maculopapular, later papular, and in classic cases pustular, then vesicular. Some patients also suffer nausea, vomiting, pharyngitis, photophobia, splenomegaly, and nuchal rigidity. Histopathologic examination of the eschar reveals coagulative necrosis of the epidermis, underlying vascular injury, and a perivascular lymphohistiocytic infiltrate (Brettman, 1981; Kass, 1994). Regional lymphadenopathy and cutaneous rash presumably reflect lymphogenous and hematogenous spread, respectively.

Murine Typhus

Endemic flea-borne *Rickettsia typhi* infection, murine typhus, is presently the most important typhus group infection in the United States and causes extensive morbidity throughout the warm regions of the world (Azad, 1990). Historically, epidemic louse-borne *R. prowazekii* infections have had a major impact on the outcome of military campaigns as well as scourging general populations disrupted by famine and natural disasters (Zinsser, 1935). *Rickettsia prowazekii* continues to cause disease in some poverty-stricken areas of the world and may reappear in situations such as the war in Bosnia and the unsettled social, political, and economic conditions of some republics of the former USSR. Recrudescence of latent *R. prowazekii* infections can occur years after the primary infection in immigrants from typhus-afflicted areas. Endemic transmission of *R. prowazekii* from a natural infectious cycle of flying squirrels and their ectoparasites occurs in the United States (McDade, 1980).

Murine typhus is found particularly in tropical and subtropical coastal areas where *Rattus rattus* and the Oriental rat flea abound (Azad, 1990). The fleas imbibe rickettsiae in the blood of infected rats and maintain the infection for their normal lifespan. Transovarian transmission occurs only at low levels; thus, horizontal transmission to other rats is a key factor in maintenance of *R. typhi* in nature. Other mammal–arthropod cycles maintain the rickettsiae and result in transmission of infections to humans (e.g., the cat flea, *Ctenocephalides felis*, and the opposum in Texas and California).

Humans are believed to become infected usually by intradermal inoculation of infected flea feces into skin excoriated by scratching. However, inhalation of a rickettsial aerosol from dried infected flea feces or inoculation by flea bite may account for transmission in some cases. After an incubation period of one to two weeks, illness begins with fever accompanied in some cases by severe headache, chills, myalgias, and nausea. A macular or maculopapular rash, most prominent on the trunk, appears on day five or six in 80% of patients with fair skin and in 20% with darkly pigmented skin. A small proportion of patients has cough and pulmonary infiltrates. Severely ill patients may also suffer coma, seizures, and other neurologic signs. Approximately 10% of hospitalized patients require admission to the intensive care unit, and 1% to 2% of murine typhus patients die (Dumler, 1991).

The pathologic lesions of murine typhus include endothelial swelling and perivascular lymphohistiocytic infiltrates involving the blood vessels in the dermis, central nervous system, lungs, heart, gastrointestinal tract, and kidneys (Walker, 1989). The most serious consequences are meningioencephalomyelitis and diffuse alveolar injury.

Scrub Typhus

Rickettsia tsutsugamushi is transovarially maintained in mites of the genus *Leptotrombidium* (Traub, 1978). Infected ova hatch into larvae, the only stage that feeds on an animal host. Rats become infected after rickettsiae-containing larvae (chiggers) feed on the rats' tissue fluids, but feeding mite larvae do not pass the rickettsiae to their offspring. Thus, humans and rats are only accidental, nonessential, dead-end hosts of scrub typhus rickettsiae. Scrub typhus occurs in countries within the triangle formed by Japan, Pakistan, and northern Australia. Infection is acquired in areas of dense vegetation where abundant rat populations harbor large populations of chiggers.

The basic pathologic lesion is vascular injury with perivascular lymphohistiocytic inflammation, which is present in the cutaneous chigger-inoculation site of rickettsiae, the brain, lung, heart, gastrointestinal tract, and kidney. After incubation for six to 21 days, illness begins with fever, headache, and in some patients myalgia, cough, and gastrointestinal symptoms (Brown, 1988). An eschar develops in half of westerners, usually prior to the onset of fever, but seldom in indigenous patients. Likewise, a macular or maculopapular rash occurs in half of westerners, with primary infection two to nine days after the onset of illness. Severely ill patients may develop hypotension, meningoencephalitis, acute renal failure, and hemorrhagic phenomena. Unless treated with appropriate antimicrobial medications, 7% of cases are fatal.

Laboratory Diagnosis

Unlike most infectious diseases for which precise diagnosis is sought during the acute phase of illness, when critical therapeutic decisions are made, rickettsial diseases are usually diagnosed acutely purely on clinicoepidemiologic suspicion and are treated empirically on a presumptive basis (Kaplowitz, 1981). Serologic diagnosis, which is often mistakenly sought early in the course of illness, provides the majority of laboratory confirmed diagnoses by demonstration of a fourfold or greater rise in titer only during convalescence. Even with the most sensitive serologic methods, fewer than 20% of patients have detectable specific antibodies to rickettsiae when presenting to the physician for medical attention. Other approaches to diagnosis at the time of presentation include immunohistologic demonstration of rickettsiae in cutaneous lesions, immunocytologic identification of rickettsiae in circulating detached endothelial cells, detection of rickettsial DNA in blood and tissue specimens by PCR, and cultivation of rickettsiae from blood or tissue specimens; but these tests are not available in most clinical laboratories.

Rickettsiae were originally demonstrated in tissues of patients with RMSF and epidemic louse-borne typhus by Wolbach during and shortly after World War I. This method, essentially a lost art, requires careful attention to details of fixation and staining of rickettsiae, and is not performed successfully in this manner in contemporary histology laboratories. A modified Brown-Hopps method stains a small portion of organisms, which appear as thin bacilli within endothelial cells. A more sensitive and specific approach to visualization of rickettsiae in tissue section is immunohistology, either immunofluorescence or immunoenzyme staining, using antibodies specific for the spotted fever or typhus group (Dumler, 1990; Kaplowitz, 1983; Walker, 1989). Staining of skin biopsies from patients with RMSF by immunofluorescence has a sensitivity of 70% and a specificity of 100%. Patients with boutonneuse fever, murine typhus, and rickettsialpox have also been diagnosed by immunohistologic detection of rickettsiae in rash and eschar lesions. A monoclonal antibody to a spotted fever group–specific epitope on the cell wall lipopolysaccharide demonstrates *R. rickettsii, R. conorii, R. akari, R. japonica, R. australis*, and *R. sibirica* in formalin-fixed, paraffin-embedded tissues. Currently, reagents for diagnostic immunohistology of rickettsioses are not commercially available, but it is feasible that kits could be developed for rickettsial group–specific diagnosis using antibodies produced in research laboratories.

A unique diagnostic approach is the immunocytologic demonstration of *R. conorii* in detached, circulating endothelial cells captured from patient blood samples by immunomagnetic beads coated with a monoclonal antibody to a surface antigen of human endothelial cells (Drancourt, 1992). In boutonneuse fever patients, this method has a sensitivity of 58% for examination of a single blood sample and may be used in patients prior to the onset of rash, which must be present for selection of the site of skin biopsy for immunohistologic diagnosis.

The gold standard serologic test for rickettsioses is the indirect immunofluorescent antibody (IFA) assay (Kaplan, 1986). The indirect immunoperoxidase antibody test yields similar results. For spotted fever and typhus-group rickettsial infections in the United States, IFA titers of 1:64 or greater are considered to be diagnostic in a compatible clinicoepidemiologic situation. In countries where there is a high prevalence of persons with antibodies to these rickettsiae, owing hypothetically to stimulation by nonpathogenic rickettsiae or subclinical or undiagnosed infection, higher titers are required to establish the diagnosis. In any event, a fourfold rise in IFA antibody titer to at least a titer of 1:64 is diagnostic. The sensitivity of the IFA is 94% to 100%, and the specificity is 100%. With a cut-off titer for IgG of 1:128 and for IgM of 1:32, the indirect immunoperoxidase test yields similar results and has the advantage of requiring only a light microscope instead of an ultraviolet microscope. For the diagnosis of scrub typhus in an endemic region, a titer of 1:400 or greater by IFA is 96% specific and 48% sensitive. The criterion of a fourfold increase in titer to 1:200 or greater yields a specificity of 98% and sensitivity of 54%.

Other commercially available serologic tests are latex agglutination and solid-phase enzyme immunoassay. Both methods provide diagnostically useful information, require less expensive equipment to perform, but generally are not considered as reliable as the IFA. Certainly, these techniques yield much more accurate results than the Weil-Felix tests, which measure agglutination of *Proteus vulgaris* strains OX-19 and OX-2 and *P. mirabilis* strain OX-K (Kaplan, 1986). These insensitive, nonspecific Weil-Felix tests should be regulated to the history of medicine status.

Treatment

Spotted fever, typhus, and scrub typhus groups rickettsioses are treated effectively with doxycycline, tetracycline, or chloramphenicol (Raoult, 1991). Fluoroquinolones are active against rickettsiae *in vitro*; ciprofloxacin has been used successfully to treat boutonneuse fever. Case reports suggest that ofloxacin and pefloxacin may also be effective alternatives.

Infections Caused by Organisms of the Genus *Ehrlichia*

Structure

Ehrlichiae are small (0.5 μm), obligately intracellular, gram-negative coccobacilli that reside in a cytoplasmic vacuole of white blood cells (Weiss, 1984). This intravacuolar microcolony of bacteria stained by Wright-Giemsa method resembles a mulberry and this is called a *morula* (Latin for mulberry).

Human Monocytic Ehrlichiosis

Ehrlichia chaffeensis is transmitted by ticks, primarily *Amblyomma americanum*, the Lone Star tick, but also *Dermacentor variabilis* (Anderson, 1993). Cases are predominantly rural and seasonal (68% occur from May to July) (Fishbein, 1994). It is likely that deer, dogs, or small rodents serve as the reservoir host and *A. americanum* ticks as the major vector. Human monocytic ehrlichiosis has been reported in 30 states; most cases have occurred within the range of *A. americanum* in the third of the United States southeast of a line from New Jersey to Texas, and a high proportion of the remainder within the range of *D. variabilis*. The number of reported cases is particularly high in Oklahoma, Missouri, Arkansas, Texas, Virginia, and Georgia.

Since the first case of human ehrlichiosis was reported in the United States in 1987, more than 400 patients with laboratory-confirmed *E. chaffeensis* infection have been documented at the CDC (Fishbein, 1994; Maeda, 1987). Fatalities have occurred in approximately 2% to 3% of cases, including a previously healthy child (Eng, 1990; Fichtenbaum, 1994; Fishbein, 1994). Among the 237 cases occurring between 1985 and 1990 that were investigated by the CDC, 62% of patients were hospitalized. The median duration of illness, including treated cases, was 23 days. Signs and symptoms depict a systemic disease that has no clinically diagnostic features: fever (97%), headache (81%), myalgia (68%), anorexia (66%), nausea (48%), vomiting (37%), rash (6% at onset, 25% during the first week, and 36% overall), cough (26%), pharyngitis (26%), diarrhea (25%), lymphadenopathy (25%), abdominal pain (22%), and confusion (20%). Severe complications include respiratory and renal insufficiency. Among patients with chest radiographic examinations, nearly one half have infiltrates (Eng, 1990). Clinical laboratory findings include leukopenia (60%), thrombocytopenia (68%), and elevated hepatic transaminases (86%). Central nervous system involvement manifested by seizures and coma has been documented by the presence of cerebral lesions at autopsy and *E. chaffeensis* in cerebrospinal fluid (demonstrated by immunocytology and PCR) (Dunn, 1992; Everett, 1994). Mild infections and asymptomatic seroconversions have also been documented (Peterson, 1989). *Ehrlichia chaffeensis* is capable of establishing persistent infection, even after treatment with tetracycline and chloramphenicol (Dumler, 1993b).

After entry via tick bite, *E. chaffeensis* spreads by the lymphatic and/or hematogenous routes. Ehrlichial morulae have been identified in monocytes and macrophages in the bone marrow, peripheral blood (rarely), hepatic sinusoids, spleen, lymph nodes, meninges, kidney, and epicardium (Dumler, 1993b). Bone marrow examination frequently reveals granulomas, myeloid hyperplasia, and megakaryocytosis (Dumler, 1993a). Other reported lesions include perivascular lymphohistiocytic infiltrates in the kidney, meninges, brain, and heart; interstitial mononuclear pneumonitis; foci of necrosis in the liver, lymph node, and spleen; diffuse reticuloendothelial hyperplasia; erythrophagocytosis; and cholestasis.

Human Granulocytic Ehrlichiosis

More than 60 cases of human granulocytic ehrlichiosis have been documented since the initial recognition of the disease in Wisconsin and Minnesota. Cases have been confirmed in the northeastern states and southward along the eastern seaboard. Infection probably is tick-borne, and *Ixodes scapularis* is the most likely vector. The pathology is poorly defined beyond the observation of morula-containing neutrophils in peripheral blood and various organs. Fatality is frequently associated with opportunistic secondary infections.

Human granulocytic ehrlichiosis as recognized currently is a moderate-to-severe disease, with most patients requiring hospitalization (Bakken, 1994). Infection is fatal in 5% to 10% of cases. The illness begins with chills, fever, headache, and myalgia. Thrombocytopenia occurs in most cases, and leukopenia in nearly half. Hepatocellular injury is manifested as elevated hepatic enzymes, and severely ill patients may have acute renal failure, central nervous system manifestations, and pulmonary involvement.

Laboratory Diagnosis

Ehrlichia chaffeensis has been isolated from only two patients with human monocytic ehrlichiosis, and no granulocytic ehrlichia has ever been cultivated (Dawson, 1991). Amplification of ehrlichial DNA by PCR using species-specific primers is an efficient diagnostic tool, but this is available only in research laboratories (Anderson, 1992; Chen, 1994; Everett, 1994). For human monocytic ehrlichiosis, the sensitivity of PCR is 80% to 90%, and with species-specific primers and in the absence of contamination problems, the specificity should be 100% (Anderson, 1992; Everett, 1994). Although in many cases a laborious task, identification of morulae in peripheral blood neutrophils provides a diagnosis of human granulocytic ehrlichiosis and can be performed in any clinical laboratory.

Serologic diagnosis is the usual approach to the diagnosis of human monocytic ehrlichiosis, utilizing cell culture–propagated *E. chaffeensis* antigen in an IFA assay. This method is very sensitive for the demonstration of seroconversion to a titer of 1:64 or greater two to four weeks after disease onset. Neutrophils containing *E. phagocytophila* and *E. equi* harvested from the peripheral blood of infected sheep and horses, respectively, have been employed successfully as surrogate antigens for the diagnosis of human granulocytic ehrlichiosis by an IFA test. Serodiagnosis is at present available only in reference and research laboratories.

Treatment

Doxycycline is highly effective for the treatment of both human monocytic and granulocytic ehrlichioses (Bakken, 1994; Fishbein, 1994). Chloramphenicol also seems to shorten the course of human monocytic ehrlichiosis (Fishbein, 1994).

Infections Caused by *Coxiella burnetii*

Structure and Function

Coxiella burnetii are quite distant genetically from other pathogenic rickettsiae and are the only ones classified in the gamma group of the Proteobacteria (Walker, 1995). These gram-negative bacteria vary morphologically from rods to cocci, and by electron microscopic examination there are two distinct forms: large cells (0.5 to 1.2 μm) and small dense cells (0.5 μm), which appear to reflect changes that occur during the growth of these organisms.

Much emphasis has been placed on a laboratory phenomenon associated with cultivation of *C. burnetii* by prolonged passage in cell culture or eggs, namely, loss of the organisms' ability to synthesize the entire lipopolysaccharide. This change from synthesis of the full to a truncated lipopolysaccharide, analogous to the conversion from smooth to rough phenotype by Enterobacteriaceae, has been designated *phase variation* from phase I to phase II. Phase I is found in nature and in infected persons and animals; phase II occurs in the laboratory.

Coxiella burnetii enters its target cell, the macrophage, by passive phagocytosis and is highly adapted (e.g., synthesis of a superoxide dismutase) to the conditions in the phagolysosome where replication by transverse binary fission occurs.

Q Fever

The name *Q fever* was derived from the unknown status of its etiology when the clinicoepidemiologic syndrome was first described as *query fever*. The ecology of *C. burnetii* includes silent infections in animals: many species of ticks, ungulates (particularly sheep, cattle, and goats), other mammals (including cats and wild rabbits), fish, birds, and marsupials (Marrie, 1990). Humans usually are infected by inhalation, especially of aerosols that originate in infected birth products of domestic livestock, but also by ingestion of unpasteurized contaminated milk. Most human infections occur as an occupational disease among abattoir workers, farmers, and veterinarians. However, urban nonoccupational cases are by no means rare in some populations in which they have been evaluated, such as among immunocompromised patients in France (Brouqui, 1993).

The majority of human infections are asymptomatic (Marrie, 1990). Acute illness is often a self-limited, undifferentiated febrile illness, pneumonia, or hepatitis. Individual patients with myalgias, anorexia, and headache are unlikely to be investigated diagnostically for Q fever, even though this syndrome is the most likely clinical presentation of this infection. Manifestations of Q fever pneumonia vary: Cough may be nonproductive or absent, and the pneumonia may be severe and progress rapidly or be detected as multiple rounded or segmental roentgenographic infiltrates without pulmonary symptoms. Q fever hepatitis may have a clinical presentation similar to acute viral hepatitis or the pathologic presentation of hepatic biopsy-determined granulomatous hepatitis.

Chronic Q fever is considered synonymous with *C. burnetii* endocarditis but also occurs less frequently as infection of an aneurysm or vascular prosthesis or osteomyelitis (Brouqui, 1993; Marrie, 1990). Chronic Q fever endocarditis usually involves previously damaged aortic or mitral valves as an afebrile illness that may manifest with heart failure, hepatosplenomegaly, changing cardiac murmurs, and weight loss. Disease associated with circulating immune complexes includes vasculitis-based purpuric rash or glomerulonephritis.

The pathology of acute Q fever includes mixed interstitial-alveolar-bronchiolar pneumonia with mononuclear inflammatory cells and granulomatous inflammation of the liver and bone marrow (Walker, 1988b). Q fever granulomas often contain a clear central vacuole and a surrounding ring of fibrin as well as epithelioid macrophages. These doughnut granulomas are neither pathognomonic lesions nor the only form of granuloma that occurs in the liver and bone marrow of Q fever patients. The involved cardiac valves in Q fever endocarditis show a mixed subacute and chronic inflammation with many foamy macrophages filled with *C. burnetii*.

Laboratory Diagnosis

The laboratory diagnosis of Q fever is most often accomplished by demonstration of antibodies to *C. burnetii*. Serologic methods employ both phase I and phase II antigens, and often evaluate class-specific antibody production. Enzyme immunoassay and indirect immunofluorescent antibody tests are highly specific and are more sensitive than complement fixation. In acute Q fever, antibodies to phase II antigens appear earliest after infection, and antibodies to phase I may be detected as early as two weeks after the onset of illness. In general, acute Q fever is associated with high titers to phase II antigens and lower titers to phase I antigens. In chronic Q fever, antibodies to phase I are present at a higher titer (e.g., IgG-IFA titer of 1:800) and antibodies to phase II are often equal to the phase I titer. An IgA response to phage I antigens is usually observed in patients with chronic Q fever. A titer of 1:128 or greater against phase I antigen by the complement fixation test is also considered diagnostic of chronic Q fever, although some patients have lower titers.

Other methods for the diagnosis of chronic Q fever endocarditis include immunohistologic staining, electron microscopy, and PCR detection of *C. burnetii*, all of which are essentially research techniques. *Coxiella burnetii* can be recovered from the blood or infected cardiac valves by *in vitro* cultivation utilizing a centrifugation-enhanced shell vial human embryonic lung cell culture system (Marrero, 1989). This method is highly sensitive for the identification of coxiellae within seven days, but should be attempted only within cell culture facilities approved for biohazard containment level 3.

Treatment

Doxycycline is effective in shortening the course of acute Q fever when administered during the first three days after the onset of illness (Levy, 1991). Fluoroquinolones or rifampin are alternative medications for patients who cannot be treated with tetracycline. Treatment of chronic *C. burnetii* endocarditis requires prolonged administration of doxycycline and a quinolone. Cardiac valve replacement is performed for hemodynamic reasons.

Infections Caused by Organisms of the Genus *Bartonella (Rochalimaea)*

Structure and Function

The *Rochalimaea* spp. are not as closely related to the genus *Rickettsia* as previously believed. They are actually very closely related to *Bartonella bacilliformis* (Brenner, 1993). Thus, reclassification of *Rochalimaea* as *Bartonella* and removal of the family Bartonellaceae from the order Rickettsiales have been proposed. *Bartonella (Rochalimaea) quintana*, the etiologic agent of trench fever, a major louse-borne disease in World War I, can be cultivated on blood agar. *Bartonella (Rochalimaea) henselae* causes febrile bacteremia, bacillary angiomatosis, and bacillary peliosis in persons with the acquired immunodeficiency syndrome (AIDS) and is the principal etiology of cat scratch disease (Adal, 1994). *Bartonella (Rochalimaea) elizabethae* and *B. henselae* have been associated with infective endocarditis. *Bartonella bacilliformis*, a sandfly transmitted bacterium, causes febrile acute hemolytic anemia and chronic bacillary angiomatosis-like cutaneous lesions in Peru, Chile, Bolivia, Ecuador, and Colombia.

Cat Scratch Disease, Bacillary Angiomatosis, and Bacillary Peliosis

Bartonella (Rochalimaea) henselae is transmitted to humans by the scratch or bite of infected kittens, which are bacteremic for many months while appearing healthy (Tappero, 1993). The nature of the disease is largely host determined. In immunocompetent hosts, 80% are younger than 21 years and present with a cutaneous papule or pustule, and self-limited regional lymphadenopathy. Fewer than 2% of patients suffer complications such as hematogenously disseminated involvement of the liver, spleen, lung, bone, central nervous system, retina, conjunctiva, or skin. The histopathology of cat scratch disease lesions is granulomas surrounding stellate microabscesses. In severely immunocompromised patients, *B. henselae* infection is manifested by fever and bacteremia, or by cutaneous or visceral angioproliferative lesions. The latter are characterized by lobular vascular proliferations of plump endothelial cells with clusters of small capillaries surrounding ectatic capillaries separated by edematous, mucinous, or fibrotic stroma containing clusters of neutrophils, neutrophil debris, and granular microcolonies of bartonellae. In the skin these lesions are designated *bacillary angiomatosis*; in the liver and spleen, *hepatic* and *splenic peliosis*. Dissemination to other sites may occur also. The angioproliferative lesions of *B. henselae* and *B. quintana* in immunocompromised patients are indistinguishable, and they are quite similar to the verruga peruana of *B. bacilliformis*.

Trench Fever and Bacillary Peliosis

The natural niche of *B. quintana* is unknown. Although infections are transmitted from person to louse (*Pediculus humanis corporis*) to another person, as occurred in front-line trenches during World War I, contemporary infections of persons with the acquired immunodeficiency syndrome occur without associated louse infestation (Bruce, 1921).

Louse feces laden with *B. quintana* are scratched into the skin, and approximately eight days later an illness of variable severity begins. Manifestations include fever, generally lasting less than a week, headache, myalgias, pretibial pain, and an evanescent macular rash. Relapses often occur at four or five day intervals. Bacteremia persists for weeks, months, or longer, serving as a source for infecting lice, even when the person feels relatively healthy.

Oroya Fever and Verruga Peruana

South American bartonellosis, manifested as an acute illness called *Oroya fever* or as chronic cutaneous lesions called *verruga peruana*, is transmitted by the bite of the *Lutzomyia* sandfly. Asymptomatic long-term human carriers are the reservoirs of *B. bacilliformis*. After an incubation period of approximately three weeks, Oroya fever begins insidiously with anorexia, headache, malaise, and low-grade fever, or abruptly with chills, high fever, headache, and mental status changes. Bartonellae invade the red blood cells and cause erythrocytic changes that result in erythrophagocytosis and anemia. Verruga peruana, characterized by red-to-purple nontender nodules that appear in crops over one to two months and persist for months to years, follows Oroya fever or occurs without prior symptoms (Arias-Stella, 1986).

Laboratory Diagnosis

Lysis-centrifugation blood cultures and the Bactec blood culture system have been used to recover *B. henselae* and *B. quintana* from patients. Optimal growth is obtained on enriched media supplemented with rabbit blood, chocolate agar, or charcoal yeast extract agar. Detectable colonies usually require incubation for nine to 15 days, or occasionally longer. These *Bartonella (Rochalimaea)* organisms are gram-negative bacilli, 0.2 to 0.5 μm in diameter by 1 to 3 μm long. *Bartonella henselae* are oxidase-, catalase-, and urease-negative and do not utilize carbohydrates. Definitive identification requires analysis of fatty acid composition and nucleic acid hybridization, generally reference laboratory methods. *Bartonella bacilliformis* may be cultivated from blood or skin lesions by inoculation of brain–heart infusion agar containing 0.4% agar and 5% human, horse, or rabbit blood.

Formerly the diagnosis of cat scratch disease required a combination of clinical, epidemiologic, and pathologic criteria. Morphologic studies, including Warthin Starry stain, immunohistologic demonstration of bartonellae, and electron microscopic observation of bacilli, have been used to support the diagnosis of bacillary angiomatosis. Oroya fever may be diagnosed by visualization of bartonellae, appearing as cocci or bacilli, occasionally with curved or ring forms, in peripheral blood stained by the Giemsa method. Diagnosis of *B. henselae* and *B. quintana* infections is usually accomplished by the serologic demonstration of antibodies by indirect immunofluorescence or enzyme immunoassay.

Treatment

Cat scratch disease usually is self-limited, but the illness appears to respond favorably to treatment with rifampin, ciprofloxacin, trimethoprim/sulfamethoxazole, or gentamicin (Adal, 1994). The drug of choice for treatment of bacillary angiomatosis is erythromycin, and doxycycline also gives good results. Azithromycin has been shown in individual cases to provide effective therapy (Guerra, 1993). Treatment can cause a Jarisch-Herxheimer–like reaction with fever and other systemic symptoms. Relapses may occur, requiring retreatment or even long-term maintenance therapy. Tetracycline and chloramphenicol have been used successfully to treat trench fever. Acute South American bartonellosis has been treated effectively with chloramphenicol or penicillin, and in some cases with tetracycline or streptomycin.

MYCOPLASMAL INFECTIONS

Mycoplasmas were proven to cause human disease in 1962, when one mycoplasma (subsequently named *Mycoplasma pneumoniae*) was recognized as the etiologic agent of primary atypical pneumonia (Chanock, 1962). Mycoplasmas are the smallest free-living organisms. They are pleomorphic, spherical, pear-shaped, or filamentous cells, 0.2 to 0.8 μm in diameter. Most are facultative anaerobes, and they replicate by binary fission. Mycoplasmas are unique among the bacteria because they have no cell wall. They are unable to synthesize cell wall precursors, and they require cholesterol and related sterols for membrane synthesis. Mycoplasmas also lack the enzymatic pathways for purine and pyrimidine synthesis and, for this reason, require complex media (such as beef heart infusion broth supplemented with horse serum, yeast extract, and nucleic acids) for growth *in vitro*. The potential pathogens, *Mycoplasma pneumoniae*, and the genital mycoplasmas (*Mycoplasma hominis* and *Ureaplasma urealyticum*) are discussed. Other mycoplasmas are part of the normal human flora, primarily of the respiratory and genitourinary tracts.

Mycoplasma pneumoniae

Epidemiology

Mycoplasma pneumoniae is found worldwide. Epidemics occur among confined populations such as children in schools, families, and military recruits, typically at four to eight-year intervals, predominantly in late summer and fall. In nonepidemic years, infections occur year-round and in general spread slowly, apparently requiring close contact with an ill person. During epidemics, however, infection may spread rapidly, and the occurrence of point-source outbreaks in which a close and prolonged exposure is not recognized suggests that *M. pneumoniae* may be transmitted via small particle aerosols. Rates of infection with *M. pneumoniae* are greatest in school-aged children and young adults, and pneumonia occurs most frequently in persons aged five to 20 years, especially those between the ages of 15 and 19 years. Infection with *M. pneumoniae* is common before age five years but typically is asymptomatic or produces a mild illness with coryza and wheezing, but no fever or pneumonia (Fernald, 1975).

Pathogenesis and Pathology

Mycoplasma pneumoniae, a surface parasite, colonizes the mucosa of the respiratory tract. Its ability to attach to respiratory mucosal cells, to escape phagocytosis, and to modulate the immune system are essential to initiation of disease. Its gliding motility may allow it to penetrate through respiratory secretions, and its filamentous, flexible form with terminal attachment organelle may facilitate localization in crypts and folds of the host cell membrane, and between microvilli and cilia, where it is protected from phagocytosis. Attachment of *M. pneumoniae* to host cells is mediated by the P1 protein, which interacts with neuraminic acid–containing glycoproteins at the surface of the host cell membrane (Chandler, 1982; Geary, 1987). Hydrogen peroxide and superoxide produced by *M. pneumoniae* may injure mucosal cells, causing ciliostasis and sloughing of superficial cells (Almogar, 1984).

Host-related factors also are involved in the pathogenesis of *M. pneumoniae* disease. The apparent high prevalence of *M. pneumoniae* infection in infants and young children, the mild nature of the disease in this age group, and the occurrence of a more severe illness during infection at a later age suggest that severe disease may result from the host immune response to reinfection; however, the specific mechanism for the host cell injury is unknown. Moreover, the extrapulmonary manifestations of disease (discussed later) are suspected to be immune mediated, because *M. pneumoniae* frequently is recovered from nonrespiratory sources. The interaction of *M. pneumoniae* with the I antigenic determinant of human red blood cells, which contains the necessary 2,3-sialylated poly-N-acetylgalactosamine sequences, may alter the I antigen, converting it into a non–self-antigen that stimulates production of cold agglutinins. Other autoimmune antibodies produced during infection with *M. pneumoniae* (antibodies to lung, brain, smooth muscle, and lymphocytes) may have similar derivations.

The first line of defense during primary infection with *M. pneumoniae* is activation of the alternate complement pathway and phagocytosis of the organism at the mucosal surface. Galactosyl and glycosyl derivatives on the organism's surface membrane appear to stimulate production of antibodies, the most important of which is IgA, found predominantly in mucosal secretions. Intracellular protein antigens of *M. pneumoniae* exposed during its phagocytosis and subsequent degradation stimulate T-lymphocyte reactions, which apparently determine the severity of disease.

Few descriptions of the pathologic findings of disease caused by *M. pneumoniae* are available, because most infections are self-limited and tissue is rarely obtained. In fatal cases patchy areas of consolidation are found in the lungs. Histologic examination of involved foci shows bronchitis, bronchiolitis, and interstitial and alveolar pneumonitis with peribronchiolar collections of lymphocytes and plasma cells, accompanied by macrophages and neutrophils if cellular necrosis is present.

Clinical Manifestations

The most common manifestation of disease caused by *M. pneumoniae* is tracheobronchitis. Pneumonia, which occurs in about one third of infected persons, begins gradually two to three weeks after exposure, with fever, malaise, headache, pharyngitis, and persistent nonproductive hacking cough (Jones, 1994). Clinically inapparent sinusitis is common, and myringitis may develop. Chest roentgenograms show unilateral lower lobe bronchopneumonia, or occasionally bilateral feathery infiltrates. The peripheral while blood cell count is normal early and rises as the disease progresses. Maculopapular, or less commonly, vesicular skin eruptions occur in about 15% of cases a few days after disease onset. Without antimicrobial therapy, fever resolves in two to 14 days, but malaise, cough, and radiographic abnormalities persist two to six weeks. In a small percentage of children and adults, pneumonia is severe enough to warrant hospitalization; these patients may develop lung abscess, pleural effusions, secondary bacterial infections, bronchiectasis, or clinical relapse. Extrarespiratory manifestations are uncommon and include clinically apparent hemolytic anemia, typically with very high titers of cold agglutinins; erythema multiforme, erythema nodosum, and urticaria; encephalitis, meningoencephalitis, mononeuritis or polyneuritis, and meningitis; myocarditis and pericarditis; and arthralgias and rarely arthritis (Baum, 1994; Cassel, 1981; Ponka, 1979).

Genital Mycoplasmas

Epidemiology

Colonization of infants with genital mycoplasmas occurs during passage through an infected birth canal and usually persists less than two years. *Ureaplasma urealyticum*, and *Mycoplasma hominis* may be recovered from the genital tract of up to about 30% of infant girls (less often from the genital tract of infant boys), and they may be isolated from the nose and throat of as many as 15% of infant boys and girls (Klein, 1969). In one study 20% of prepubertal girls were colonized with ureaplasmas and 6% with *M. hominis*, but genital mycoplasmas seldom were recovered from prepubertal boys (Hammerschlag, 1978). Colonization with genital mycoplasmas after puberty results from sexual contact. About 60% of apparently healthy sexually active women carry *U. urealyticum* in the vagina and about 20% carry *M. hominis*.

Clinical Manifestations

Ureaplasma urealyticum is responsible for some cases of nongonococcal urethritis; it has been associated with postpartum fever, chorioamnionitis, and low birth weight, although a causal relationship with the latter is not proven; and it is a rare cause of chronic urethrocystitis in immunosuppressed persons (Cassell, 1986; Taylor-Robinson, 1980, 1985). *Mycoplasma hominis* is one cause of postabortal and postpartum fever; and it is an uncommon cause of bacteremia, arthritis, peritonitis, meningitis, osteomyelitis, and wound infections, mainly in immunocompromised persons but also in some who have no apparent underlying deficiency (DeGirolami, 1982; McMahon, 1990; Taylor-Robinson, 1980).

Laboratory Diagnosis

Mycoplasma pneumoniae

Specimens recommended for diagnosis of infection caused by *M. pneumoniae* are throat swabs and serum, but bronchoalveolar lavage fluid, sputum, and lung tissue are acceptable. A nonspecific serologic test that may provide useful information is detection of cold agglutinins, which are IgM antibodies against the I antigen of human erythrocytes. Cold agglutinins appear by the end of the first week or early in the second week of illness in at least half of infected persons, but their presence is not diagnostic of infection with *M. pneumoniae*. Definitive diagnosis is based on detection of the organism or specific antibodies.

To isolate *M. pneumoniae*, a biphasic culture system is inoculated and incubated in a sealed container up to three weeks in ambient air at 35° to 37°C. Cultures are examined microscopically (40×) once or twice each week for typical spherical colonies with a dense center and thin outer layer (resembling a fried egg) embedded in the agar. Such colonies, consistent with *M. pneumoniae*, should be tested for β-hemolysis (*M. pneumoniae* is β-hemolytic) as follows: 1% melted agar, prepared in 0.85% saline and cooled to 50°C, is mixed with sheep or guinea pig blood to give a 5% erythrocyte concentration, and a thin layer is poured on the agar plate. The culture is reincubated for 24 hours and examined microscopically for hemolysis.

Because isolation of *M. pneumoniae* may require several weeks, more rapid tests are more useful for diagnosis. Detection of specific IgM in a single serum sample is diagnostic of acute infection. If IgG is measured, acute and convalescent-phase samples must be tested, and the diagnosis is based on a fourfold or greater rise in titer.

Genital Mycoplasmas

Ureaplasma urealyticum and *Mycoplasma hominis* may be recovered from urethral, vaginal, or endocervical swab specimens, blood, urine, abscess material, prostatic secretions, semen, or tissues. Various culture systems may be used to isolate the genital mycoplasmas (Clyde, 1984; Phillips, 1986; Wood, 1985; Yajko, 1984). Traditionally, separate systems were used for each (U agar and U broth for *U. urealyticum* and H agar and H broth for *M. hominis*), because the optimal pH for growth of the two organisms differs (pH 5.5 to 6.5 for *U. urealyticum* and pH 6 to 8 for *M. hominis*). However, now there are single culture systems that effectively detect both organisms (Phillips, 1986; Wood, 1985; Yajko, 1984). Broth cultures are incubated aerobically in sealed test tubes. Agar cultures are incubated anaerobically or in an atmosphere of 5% to 7% carbon dioxide and observed daily under the microscope. *Mycoplasma hominis* also grows on sheep blood agar, producing nonhemolytic pinpoint colonies, and in most broth blood culture media, although there is no visible evidence of growth.

Colonies of *M. hominis*, 200 to 300 μm in diameter with the typical fried-egg appearance, usually appear in five days or less. In broth containing phenol red and 0.1% arginine, *M. hominis* metabolizes arginine to ammonia, causing a color change from yellow to red. U-agar plates are observed daily for four days, and on day four are stained with one to two drops of $CaCl_2$-urea solution. Colonies of *U. urealyticum*, 15 to 16 μm in diameter, stain dark brown in five minutes. In U broth, *U. urealyticum* produces a shift in pH, and the color changes from yellow to red. A loopful of broth then is transferred to agar plates and streaked for isolation.

Treatment

Antimicrobial therapy is not recommended for *M. pneumoniae* pharyngitis or tracheobronchitis. A tetracycline or erythromycin is effective treatment of *M. pneumoniae*–induced pneumonia, but therapy apparently does not alter transmission of the organism. The tetracyclines are active against *M. hominis* and most isolates of *U. urealyticum*. About 10% of ureaplasmas, however, are resistant to tetracycline; infections caused by resistant strains generally respond to erythromycin (Taylor-Robinson, 1986).

Adal KA, Cockerell CJ, Petri WA Jr: Cat scratch disease, bacillary angiomatosis, and other infections due to rochalimaea. N Engl J Med 1994; 330:1509.

Almagor M, Kahane I, Yatziv S: Role of superoxide anion in host cell injury induced by *Mycoplasma pneumoniae* infection. J Clin Invest 1984; 73:842.

Anderson BE, Sims KG, Olson JC, et al: *Amblyomma americanum*: A potential vector of human ehrlichiosis. Am J Trop Med Hyg 1993; 49:239.

Anderson, BE, Sumner JW, Dawson JE, et al: Detection of the etiologic agent of human ehrlichiosis by polymerase chain reaction. J Clin Microbiol 1992; 30:775.

Arias-Stella, J, Leiberman PH, Erlandson, RA, et al: Histology, immunohistochemistry and ultrastructure of the verruga in Carrion's disease. Am J Surg Pathol 1986; 10:595.

Azad AF: Epidemiology of murine typhus. Annu Rev Entomol 1990; 35:553.

Bakken JS, Dumler JS, Chen S-M, et al: Human granulocytic ehrlichiosis in the upper midwest United States: A new species emerging? JAMA 1994; 272:212.

Barnes RC: Laboratory diagnosis of human chlamydial infections. Clin Microbiol Rev 1989; 2:119.

Bass CA, Jungkind DL, Silverman NS, et al: Clinical evaluation of a new polymerase chain reaction assay for detection of *Chlamydia trachomatis* in endocervical specimens. J Clin Microbiol 1993; 31:2648.

Baum SG: Mycoplasma pneumoniae and atypical pneumonia. *In* Mandell GL, Bennett JE, Dolin R (eds): Principles and Practice of Infectious Diseases, 4th ed. New York, Churchill Livingstone, 1994, pp 1704–1712 .

Bauwens JE, Clark AM, Loeffelholz MJ, et al: Diagnosis of *Chlamydia trachomatis* urethritis in men by polymerse chain reaction assay of first-catch urine. J Clin Microbiol 1993a; 31:3013.

Bauwens JE, Clark AM, Stamm WE: Diagnosis of *Chlamydia trachomatis* endocervical infections by a commercial polymerase chain reaction assay. J Clin Microbiol 1993b; 31:3023.

Blanding J, Hirsch L, Stranton N, et al: Comparison of the Clearview Chlamydia, the PACE 2 assay, and culture for detection of *Chlamydia trachomatis* from cervical specimens in a low-prevalence population. J Clin Microbiol 1993; 31:1622.

Brenner DJ, O'Connor SP, Winkler HH, et al: Proposals to unify the genera *Bartonella* and *Rochalimaea*, with descriptions of *Bartonella quintana* comb. nov., and *Bartonella vinsonii* comb. nov., *Bartonella henselae* comb. nov., and *Bartonella elizabethae* comb. nov., and to remove the family Bartonellaceae from the order Rickettsiales. Int J Syst Bacteriol 1993; 43:777.

Brettman LR, Lewin S, Holzman RS, et al: Rickettsialpox: Report of an outbreak and a contemporary review. Medicine 1981; 60:363.

Brouqui P, Dupont HT, Drancourt M, et al: Chronic Q fever: Ninety-two cases from France, including 27 cases without endocarditis. Arch Inter Med 1993; 153:642.

Brown GW: Scrub typhus: Pathogenesis and clinical syndrome. *In* Walker DH (ed): Biology of Rickettsial Diseases, Vol. 1. Boca Raton, FL, CRC Press, 1988, pp 93–100.

Bruce D: Trench fever. Final report of the war office trench fever investigation committee. J Hyg 1921; 20:258.

Campbell LA, Kuo CC, Grayston JT: Characterization of the new *Chlamydia* agent, TWAR, as a unique organism by restriction endonuclease analysis and DNA-DNA hybridization. J Clin Microbiol 1987; 25:1911.

Cassel GH, Cole BC: Mycoplasmas as agents of human disease. N Engl J Med 1981; 304:80.

Cassell GW, Waites KB, Gibbs RS, et al: Role of *Ureaplasma urealyticum* in amnionitis. Pediatr Infect Dis 1986; 5:S247.

Centers for Disease Control: Psittacosis at a turkey processing plant—North Carolina, 1989. MMWR 1990; 39:460.

Centers for Disease Control and Prevention: Special focus: Surveillance for reproductive health. MMWR 1993; 42(SS-6):59.

Chandler DKF, Grabowski MW, Barile MF: *Mycoplasma pneumoniae* attachment: Competitive inhibition by mycoplasmal binding component and by sialic acid containing glycoconjugates. Infect Immun 1982; 38:598.

Channock RM, Hayflick L, Barile MF: Growth on artificial medium of an agent associated with atypical pneumonia and its identification as a PPLO. Proc Natl Acad Sci USA 1962; 48:41.

Chen S-M, Dumler JS, Bakken JS, et al: Identification of a granulocytotrophic *Ehrlichia* species as the etiologic agent of human disease. J Clin Microbiol 1994; 32:589.

Chi EY, Kuo CC, Grayston JT: Unique ultrastructure in the elementary body of *Chlamydia* sp. strain TWAR. J Bacteriol 1987; 169:3757.

Clarke LM, Sierra MF, Daidone BJ, et al: Comparison of the Syva Microtrak enzyme immunoassay and Gen-probe Pace 2 with cell culture for diagnosis of cervical *Chlamydia trachomatis* infection in a high-prevalence female population. J Clin Microbiol 1993; 31:968.

Cles LD, Bruch K, Stamm WE: Staining characteristics of six commercially available monoclonal immunofluorescence reagents for direct diagnosis of *Chlamydia trachomatis* infections. J Clin Microbiol 1988; 26:1735.

Clyde WA Jr, Kenny GE, Schachter J: Laboratory diagnosis of chlamydial and mycoplasmal infections *In* Drew WL (ed): Cumitech 29. Washington DC, American Society for Microbiology, 1984.

Cox RL, Kuo CC, Grayston JT, et al: Deoxyribonucleic acid relatedness of *Chlamydia* sp. strain TWAR to *Chlamydia trachomatis* and *Chlamydia psittaci*. Int J Syst Bacteriol 1988; 38:265.

Dawson JE, Anderson BE, Fishbein DB, et al: Isolation and characterization of an *Ehrlichia* sp. from a patient diagnosed with human ehrlichiosis. J Clin Microbiol 1991; 29:2741.

DeGirolami PC, Madoff S: *Mycoplasma hominis* septicemia. J Clin Microbiol 1982; 16:566.

Demaio J, Boyd RS, Rensi R, et al: False-positive Chlamydiazyme results during urine sediment analysis due to bacterial urinary tract infections. J Clin Microbiol 1991; 29:1436.

Drancourt M, George F, Brouqui P, et al: Diagnosis of Mediterranean spotted fever by indirect immunofluorescence of *Rickettsia conorii* in circulating endothelial cells isolated with monoclonal antibody-coated immunomagnetic beads. J Infect Dis 1992; 166:660.

Dumler JS, Dawson JE, Walker DH: Human ehrlichiosis: Hematopathology and immunohistologic detection of *Ehrlichia chaffeensis*. Hum Pathol 1993a; 24:391.

Dumler JS, Gage WR, Pettis GL, et al: Rapid immunoperoxidase demonstration of *Rickettsia rickettsii* in fixed cutaneous specimens from patients with Rocky Mountain spotted fever. Am J Clin Pathol 1990; 93:410.

Dumler JS, Sutker WL, Walker DH: Persistent infection with *Ehrlichia chaffeensis*. Clin Infect Dis 1993b; 17:903.

Dumler JS, Taylor JP, Walker DH: Clinical and laboratory features of murine typhus in south Texas, 1980–1987. JAMA 1991; 266:1365.

Dunn BE, Monson TP, Dumler JS, et al: Identification of *Ehrlichia chaffeensis* morulae in cerebrospinal fluid mononuclear cells. J Clin Microbiol 1992; 30:2207.

Ehret JM, Leszcynski JC, Douglas M, et al: Evaluation of Chlamydiazyme enzyme immunoassay for detection of *Chlamydia trachomatis* in urine specimens from men. J Clin Microbiol 1993; 31:2702.

Eng TR, Harkess JR, Fishbein DB, et al: Epidemiology, clinical, and laboratory findings of human ehrlichiosis in the United States, 1988. JAMA 1990; 264:2251.

Everett ED, Evans KA, Henry RB, et al: Human ehrlichiosis in adults after tick exposure: Diagnosis using polymerase chain reaction. Ann Intern Med 1994; 120:730.

Fernald GW, Collier AM, Clyde WA Jr: Respiratory infections due to *Mycoplasma pneumoniae* in infants and children. Pediatrics 1975; 55:327.

Fichtenbaum CJ, Peterson LR, Weil GJ: Ehrlichiosis presenting as a life-threatening illness with features of the toxic shock syndrome. Am J Med 1994; 95:351.

Fishbein DB, Dawson JE, Robinson LE: Human ehrlichiosis in the United States, 1985 to 1990. Ann Intern Med 1994; 120:736.

Geary SJ, Gabridge MG: Characterization of a human lung fibroblast receptor site for *Mycoplasma pneumoniae*. Israel J Med Sci 1987; 23:462.

Grayston JT, Campbell LA, Kuo CC, et al: A new respiratory pathogen: *Chlamydia pneumoniae* strain TWAR. J Infect Dis 1990; 161:618.

Grayston JT, Wang SP, Kuo CC, et al: Current knowledge on *Chlamydia pneumoniae*, strain TWAR, an important cause of pneumonia and other acute respiratory diseases. Eur J Clin Microbiol Infect Dis 1989; 8:191.

Guerra LG, Neira CJ, Boman D, et al: Rapid response of AIDS-related bacillary angiomatosis to azithromycin. Clin Infect Dis 1993; 17:264.

Hammerschlag MR, Alpert S, Rosner I, et al: Microbiology of the vagina in children: Normal and potentially pathogenic organisms. Pediatrics 1978; 62:57.

Heinzen RA, Hayes SF, Peacock MG, et al: Directional actin polymerization associated with spotted fever group rickettsia infection of vero cells. Infect Immun 1993; 61:1926.

Helmick CG, Bernard KW, D'Angelo LJ: Rocky Mountain spotted fever: Clinical, laboratory, and epidemiological features of 262 cases. J Infect Dis 1984; 150:480.

Herrero-Herrero JI, Walker DH, Ruiz-Beltran R: Immunohistochemical evaluation of the cellular immune response to *Rickettsia conorii* in "taches noires." J Infect Dis 1987; 155:802.

Iwen PC, Blair TMH, Woods GL: Comparison of the Gen-probe Pace 2™ system direct fluorescent-antibody, and cell culture for detecting *Chlamydia trachomatis* in cervical specimens. J Clin Pathol 1991; 95:578.

Jaschek G, Gaydos CA, Welsh LE, et al: Direct detection of *Chlamydia trachomatis* in urine specimens from symptomatic and asymptomatic men by using a rapid polymerase chain reaction assay. J Clin Microbiol 1993; 31:1209.

Jones RB: Chlamydia trachomatis (trachoma, perinatal infections, lymphogranuloma venereum, and genital infections). *In* Mandell GL, Bennett JE, Dolin R (eds): Principles and Practice of Infectious Diseases, 4th ed. New York, Churchill Livingstone, 1994, pp 1679–1692.

Jones RB, Priest JB, Kuo C: Subacute chlamydial endocarditis. JAMA 1982; 247:655.

Kaplan JE, Schonberger LB: The sensitivity of various serologic tests in the diagnosis of Rocky Mountain spotted fever. Am J Trop Med Hyg 1986; 35:840.

Kaplowitz LG, Fischer JJ, Sparling PF: Rocky Mountain spotted fever: A clinical dilemma. Curr Clin Top Infect Dis 1981; 2:89.

Kaplowitz LG, Lange JV, Fischer JJ, et al: Correlation of rickettsial titers, circulating endotoxin, and clinical features in Rocky Mountain spotted fever. Arch Intern Med 1983; 143:1149.

Kass EM, Szaniawski WK, Levy H, et al: Rickettsialpox in a New York City hospital, 1980 to 1989. N Engl J Med 1994; 331:1612.

Keat A, Thomas BJ, Taylor-Robinson D: Chlamydial infection in the etiology of arthritis. Br Med Bull 1983; 39:168.

Kleemola M, Saikku P, Visakorpi R, et al: Epidemics of pneumonia caused by TWAR, a new Chlamydia organism, in military trainees in Finland. J Infect Dis 1988; 157:230.

Klein JO, Buckland D. Finland M: Colonization of newborn infants by mycoplasmas. N Engl J Med 1969; 280:1025.

Kluytmans JAJW, Goessens WHF, Mouton JW, et al: Evaluation of Clearview and Magic Lite tests, polymerase chain reaction, and cell culture for detection of *Chlamydia trachomatis* in urogenital specimens. J Clin Microbiol 1993; 31:3204.

Kluytmans JAJW, Goessens WHF, vanRijsoort-Vos JH, et al: Improved performance of Pace 2 with modified collection system in combination with probe competition assay for detection of *Chlamydia trachomatis* in urethral specimens from males. J Clin Microbiol 1994; 32:568.

Kluytmans JAJW, Niesters HGM, Mouton JW, et al: Performance of non-isotopic DNA probe for detection of *Chlamydia trachomatis* in urogenital specimens. J Clin Microbiol 1991; 29:2685.

Krech T, Bleckmann M, Paatz R: Comparison of buffalo green monkey cells and McCoy cells for isolation of *Chlamydia trachomatis* in a microtiter system. J Clin Microbiol 1989; 27:2364.

Levy PY, Drancourt M, Etienne J, et al: Comparison of different antibiotic regimens for therapy of 32 cases of Q fever endocarditis. Antimicrob Agents Chemother 1991; 35:533.

Loeffelholz MJ, Lewinski CA, Silver SR: Detection of *Chlamydia trachomatis* in endocervical specimens by polymerase chain reaction. J Clin Microbiol 1992; 30:2847.

Maeda K, Markowitz N, Hawley RC, et al: Human infection with *Ehrlichia canis*, leukocytic rickettsia. N Engl J Med 1987; 316:853.

Mahoney JB, Luinstra KE, Sellors W, et al: Role of confirmatory PCRs in determining performance of Chlamydia Amplicor PCR with endocervical specimens from women with a low prevalence of infection. J Clin Microbiol 1994; 32:2490.

Marrero M, Raoult D: Centrifugation-shell vial technique for rapid detection of Mediterranean spotted fever rickettsia in blood culture. Am J Trop Med Hyg 1989; 40:197.

Marrie TJ (ed): Q Fever. Vol. I, The Disease. Boca Raton, FL, CRC Press, 1990.

McDade JE, Shepard CC, Redus MA, et al: Evidence of *Rickettsia prowazekii* infections in the United States. Am J Trop Med Hyg 1980; 29:277.

McMahon DK, Dummer JS, Pasculle AR, et al: Extra-genital *Mycoplasma hominis* infections in adults. Am J Med 1990; 89:275.

Mills RD, Young A, Cain K, et al: Chlamydiazyme plus blocking assay to detect *Chlamydia trachomatis* in endocervical specimens. Am J Clin Pathol 1992; 97:209.

Petersen LR, Sawyer LA, Fishbein DB, et al: An outbreak of ehrlichiosis in members of an Army Reserve Unit exposed to ticks. J Infect Dis 1989; 159:562.

Phillips LE, Goodrich KH, Turner RM, et al: Isolation of *Mycoplasma* species and *Ureaplasma urealyticum* from obstetrical and gynecological patients by using commercially available medium formulations. J Clin Microbiol 1986: 24:377.

Ponka A: The occurrence and clinical picture of serologically verified *Mycoplasma pneumoniae* infections with emphasis on central nervous system, cardiac, and joint manifestations. Ann Clin Res 1979; 24:1.

Raoult D, Drancourt M: Antimicrobial therapy of rickettsial diseases. Antimicrob Agents Chemother 1991; 35:2457.

Roblin PM, Dumornay W, Hammerschlag MR: Use of HEp-2 cells for improved isolation and passage of *Chlamydia pneumoniae*. J Clin Microbiol 1992; 30:1968.

Schacter J, Martin DH: Failure of multiple passages to increase chlamydial recovery. J Clin Microbiol 1987; 25:1851.

Silverman DJ, Santucci LA: Potential for free radical-induced lipid peroxidation as a cause of endothelial cell injury in Rocky Mountain spotted fever. Infect Immun 1988; 56:3110.

Stamm WE, Koutsky LA, Benedetti JK, et al: *Chlamydia trachomatis* urethral infections in men. Prevalence, risk factors, and clinical manifestations. Ann Intern Med 1984; 100:47.

Tamura A, Urakami H, Ohashi N: A comparative view of *Rickettsia tsutsugamushi* and the other groups of rickettsiae. Eur J Epidemiol 1991; 7:259.

Tappero JW, Mohle-Boetani J, Koehler JE, et al: The epidemiology of bacillary angiomatosis and bacillary peliosis. JAMA 1993; 269:770.

Taylor-Robinson D, Furr PM: Clinical antibiotic resistance of *Ureaplasma urealyticum*. Pediatr Infect Dis 1986; 5:S335.

Taylor-Robinson D, Furr PM, Webster ADB: *Ureaplasma urealyticum* causing persistent urethritis in a patient with hypogammaglobulinemia. Genitourin Med 1985; 61:404.

Taylor-Robinson D, McCormack WM: Medical progress: The genital mycoplasmas. N Engl J ed 1980; 302:1003.

Traub R, Wisseman CL Jr, Farhang-Azad A: The ecology of murine typhus—a critical review. Trop Dis Bull 1978; 75:237.

Walker DH: Rocky Mountain spotted fever: A disease in need of microbiological concern. Clin Microbiol Rev 1989; 2:227.

Walker DH: Pathology of Q fever. *In* Walker DH (ed): Biology of Rickettsial Diseases, Vol. 1. Boca Raton, FL, CRC Press, 1988b, pp 17–28.

Walker DH, Dasch G: Classification and identification of *Chlamydia, Rickettsia*, and related bacteria. *In* Gilligan PH, Murray PR, Baron EJ, Pfaller MA, Tenover FC, Yolken RH (eds): Manual of Clinical Microbiology, 6th ed. American Society for Microbiology, Washington, D.C., 1995; pp 665–668.

Walker DH, Fishbein DB: Epidemiology of rickettsial diseases. Eur J Epidemiol 1991; 7:237.

Walker DH, Gear JHS: Correlation of the distribution of *Rickettsia conorii*, microscopic lesions, and clinical features in South African tick bite fever. Am J Trop Hyg 1985; 34:361.

Walker DH, Occhino C, Tringali GR, et al: Pathogenesis of rickettsial eschars: The *tache noire* of boutonneuse fever. Hum Pathol 1988a:19:1449.

Walker DH, Parks FM, Betz TG, et al: Histopathology and immunohistologic demonstration of the distribution of *Rickettsia typhi* in fatal murine typhus. Am J Clin Pathol 1989; 91:720.

Walker DH, Staiti A, Mansueto S, et al: Frequent occurrence of hepatic lesions in boutonneuse fever. Acta Trop 1986; 43:175.

Wang SP, Grayston JT: Three new serovars of *Chlamydia trachomatis*: Da, Ia and L2a. J Infect Dis 1991; 163:403.

Warren R, Dwyer B, Plackett M, et al: Comparative evaluation of detection assays for *Chlamydia trachomatis*. J Clin Microbiol 1993; 31:1663.

Weiss E: History of rickettsiology. *In* Walker DH (ed): Biology of Rickettsial Diseases, Vol. I. Boca Raton, FL, CRC Press, 1988, pp 15–32.

Weiss E, Moulder JW: The rickettsias and chlamydias. *In* Krieg NR, Holt JG (eds): Bergey's Manual of Systematic Bacteriology, Vol. 1. Baltimore, MD, Williams & Wilkins, 1984, pp 687–729.

Wood JC, Lu RM, Peterson EM, et al: Evaluation of Mycotrim-GU for isolation of *Mycoplasma* species and *Ureaplasma urealyticum*. J Clin Microbiol 1985; 22:789.

Woods GL, Bryan JA: Detection of *Chlamydia trachomatis* by direct fluorescent antibody staining: Results of the College of American Pathologists proficiency testing program, 1986–1992. Arch Pathol Lab Med 1994; 118:483.

Yajko DM, Balston E, Wood D, et al: Evaluation of PPLO, A7B, E, and NYC agar media for the isolation of *Ureaplasma urealyticum* and *Mycoplasma* species from the genital tract. J Clin Microbiol 1984; 19:73.

Zimmerman SJ, Moses E, Sofat N, et al: Comparison of two culture approaches, blind passage and dual observation, for detecting *Chlamydia trachomatis* in various prevalence populations. J Clin Microbiol 1992; 30:2938.

Zinsser H (ed): Rats, Lice, and History. New York, Little, Brown, 1935.

6

Chapter 48

Medical Bacteriology

Gail L. Woods, M.D.
Leona W. Ayers, M.D.
John A. Washington, M.D.

An understanding of the locations, varieties, and roles of the bacterial flora indigenous to the skin and mucous membranes is essential to the proper selection and collection of material for cultures. The isolation and identification by the laboratory of a large number of bacteria from a specimen contaminated with indigenous flora is extraordinarily time consuming and defies rational interpretation and therapy. The complexity of the problem posed by indigenous flora can best be illustrated in Table 48–1, in which are listed those bacteria commonly encountered on healthy human body surfaces. The magnitude of the problem can best be illustrated by the fact that the number of bacteria on some areas of the skin, in the mouth, and in the descending colon may reach 10^6 organisms/sq cm, 10^9 organisms/mL, and 10^{11} organisms/g, respectively.

A specimen for bacterial culture that has been contaminated with indigenous flora has limited utility unless only specific organisms, for example, group A streptococci in the throat, are being sought or certain precautions are taken. These precautions include disinfection of the area through which the specimen is aspirated or passes, as with a phlebotomy for blood culture or collection of a clean-voided midstream specimen for urine culture; bypassing the area, as with a transtracheal aspiration of lower respiratory secretions or with a suprapubic aspiration for bladder urine; or quantitation to establish the probability of disease, for example, significant bacteriuria. Given these precautionary steps, the laboratory needs to define specimen requirements and instructions for microbiologic examination. These are discussed in detail in Chapter 54. Techniques for processing specimens for detection of bacteria are presented here.

SPECIMEN PROCESSING

Each laboratory must organize the processing of its specimens (see Chap. 54) so that none of the efforts devoted to their proper selection, collection, and transport are wasted. Certain specimens, such as cerebrospinal fluid, must be processed immediately, because the results of stained smears or of immunologic tests can have a major impact on therapy. Other specimens with lower orders of priority can be processed as time becomes available, provided that suitable steps are taken to ensure their integrity during periods of temporary storage. Small numbers of bacteria in urine do proliferate just as rapidly on a laboratory bench as at a nursing station unless refrigerated! Stained smears of medically urgent specimens should be prepared, examined, and reported as quickly as possible. Requests for additional material or for specimens to replace unsuitable ones must be made quickly, as should the notification of specimen rejection. In other words, the laboratory must establish a system of priorities based not only upon the urgency with which results are expected but also upon the feasibility of obtaining suitable material before therapy is instituted.

Smears

The laboratory should institute a system for routinely examining stained smears of certain types of specimens. Usually sterile body fluids, pus, and material from wounds should be examined microscopically on a regular basis, primarily to provide preliminary results for clinical purposes

Table 48-1. MICROORGANISMS COMPRISING THE NORMAL FLORA OF HEALTHY HUMANS

Site	Organisms Detected	Relative Frequency of Isolation
Skin	*Staphylococcus aureus*	++
	Staphylococcus epidermidis	++++
	Viridans streptococci	+
	Corynebacterium species	++++
	Propionibacterium acnes	++++
	Malassezia furfur	++++
	Candida species	+
Mouth and oropharynx	*Staphylococcus aureus*	+
	Staphylococcus epidermidis	+++
	Streptococcus pneumoniae	++
	Viridans streptococci	++++
	Enterococcus species	+
	Lactobacillus species	++
	Actinomyces species	+
	Peptostreptococcus species	+
	Neisseria species	++
	Haemophilus influenzae	+
	Haemophilus species	+
	Bacteroides species	++
	Porphyromonas species	++
	Prevotella species	++
	Fusobacterium species*	++++
	Veillonella species	++++
	Treponema species*	+++
	Candida species	++
Nose	*Staphylococcus aureus*	++
	Staphylococcus epidermidis	++++
	Streptococcus pneumoniae	+
	Viridans streptococci	++
	Neisseria species	+
	Haemophilus species	+
Outer ear	*Staphylococcus epidermidis*	++++
	Pseudomonas species	+
	Enterobacteriaceae	+
Conjunctivae	*Staphylococcus aureus*	+
	Staphylococcus epidermidis	++++
	Haemophilus species	+
Esophagus and stomach	Surviving bacteria from upper respiratory tract and food	+
Small intestine	*Enterococcus* species	++
	Lactobacillus species	+++
	Clostridium species	++
	Enterobacteriaceae	++
	Bacteroidaceae	+++
	Mycobacterium species	++
Large intestine[+]	*Staphylococcus aureus*	+
	Staphylococcus epidermidis	+
	Group B streptococcus	+
	Viridans streptococci	++
	Enterococcus species	++
	Lactobacillus species	+++
	Clostridium species	++++
	Actinomyces species	+
	Peptostreptococcus species	++++
	Pseudomonas species	+
	Other nonfermenters	+
	Enterobacteriaceae	++++
	Bacteroidaceae	++++
	Treponema species	+
	Mycobacterium species	+
	Candida species	+
Vagina	*Mycoplasma* species	±
	Ureaplasma urealyticum	±
	Staphylococcus epidermidis	+
	Group B streptococcus	+
	Viridans streptococci	+
	Enterococcus species	+
	Lactobacillus species	++++
	Clostridium species	++
	Actinomyces species	+
	Bifidobacterium species	+
	Propionibacterium acnes	+
	Peptostreptococcus species	+
	Neisseria species	±
	Acinetobacter species	+
	Enterobacteriaceae	+
	Gardnerella vaginalis	+
	Bacteroidaceae	+
	Candida species	++
External genitalia and anterior urethra	Skin flora (see above)	
	Mycoplasma species	±
	Ureaplasma urealyticum	±
	Enterococcus species	+
	Peptostreptococcus species	+
	Enterobacteriaceae	±
	Bacteroidaceae	+
	Mycobacterium species[†]	++

*Less prevalent in edentulous individuals

[+]95% or more of the organisms are obligate anaerobes. Protozoa may be present in persons living in underdeveloped countries.

†Especially common in smegma of uncircumcised males.

++++ = almost always present; +++ = usually present; ++ = frequently present; + occasionally present; ± = infrequently present.

Adapted from Tramont EC: General or nonspecific host defense mechanisms. *In* Mandell GL, Douglas RG Jr, Bennett JE (eds): Principles and Practice of Infectious Diseases, 3rd ed. New York, Churchill Livingstone, 1990, p 33.

and secondarily as a quality control measure. One should ordinarily expect to culture bacteria compatible morphologically with those observed in the stained smear.

Great care must be taken in preparing Gram's-stained smears to prevent distortion of the organisms and to ensure accuracy of the staining reactions. A thin smear of an aliquot of the specimen that is representative of the infectious process should be prepared on a clean microscopic slide, allowed to dry, gently heat fixed, and then stained. Because 10^5 organisms/mL must be present for there to be at least one per oil immersion field (× 1000), most normally sterile body fluids must be examined microscopically for 15 to 30 minutes in order to detect small numbers of organisms. Organism concentration can be increased within the viewing field by 10 to 100 times through the use of cytocentrifugation (Peterson, 1988). Mucoid specimens, such as sputum and transtracheal aspirates, may need to be digested with a mucolytic agent prior to cytocentrifugation.

Inspect the stained smear grossly for consistency of smear preparation, quality of staining, and any unusual objects or concentrations of material. The distribution and consistency of the stained material should provide thick and thin areas for viewing. Specimens can be homogeneous or heterogeneous, and may contain pathogens evenly distributed throughout the specimen or limited to one area of the slide. Areas of contamination with squamous epithelial cells, bacteria without the cells of inflammation, food, or other debris can be bypassed for areas of the smear more representative of disease. Scanning power should be used to judge microscopic uniformity of the sample and to look for large structures, such as nematode larvae, Curschmann spirals, large granules, grains, bacterial microcolonies, or fungal forms. After surveying the material on low power, several representative areas should be selected for viewing with a scanning oil immersion lens. A 40× or 60× lens is preferred for oil scanning, and a 100× oil lens for final bacterial morphologic evaluation. In infection, the organism will be intimate with the abnormal portion of the specimen, which typically shows purulence or necrotic debris. Purulence with red blood cells, neutrophils, protein background, and necrotic debris reflect acute inflammation. This cell pattern, seen in noninfectious as well as infectious processes, is usually associated with extracellular bacteria. Mononuclear cells, including lymphocytes, monocytes, and macrophages, reflect chronic inflammation common to the intracellular or facultative intracellular bacteria. Patients who are leukopenic will not have the cellular response seen in normal individuals but should still have a high protein fluid exudate and blood in the specimen. Strict criteria for microbial morphotypes should be maintained. The examiner must not be distracted by precipitated Gram's stain, gram-positive keratohyaline granules, fibers, or artifacts. Organisms should be evaluated for size, shape, and Gram reaction. Intracellular cell wall–damaged bacteria, antibiotic-affected bacteria, or dead bacteria may appear as beaded gram-positive or falsely gram-negative bacteria. The size and shape of the bacteria in question should be related to the morphology of other bacterial cells in the smear and to the expected morphology of bacteria prevalent for the site.

Technologists should be encouraged to be as descriptive in their interpretation of Gram's-stained smears as possible. Reporting that gram-positive cocci occur in pairs that resemble pneumococci (Plate 48–1) can be very helpful. Pleomorphic gram-negative bacilli usually represent anaerobes and may be presumptively reported as such. Obviously, the reliability of such reports will be directly related to the experience and expertise of the technologist.

Another technique for examining bacteria is with fluorescent antibody microscopy. It is useful in examining specimens directly for the presence of *Bordetella pertussis* or *Legionella*, and for the identification of colonies of group A streptococci on blood agar, and colonies resembling *Neisseria gonorrhoeae* growing on Thayer-Martin agar. The sensitivity and specificity of this technique vary according to the conjugate and whether it is used for the direct or indirect fluorescent antibody stain.

Immunoassays and Deoxyribonucleic Acid Probes

Monoclonal and polyclonal antibodies are available for use in particle agglutination, enzyme-linked immunosorbent (ELISA), and immunofluorescent antibody (IFA) assays to detect bacterial antigens in body fluids and tissues. Particle agglutination tests for the detection of the antigens of *Haemophilus influenzae*, *Neisseria meningitidis*, Group B *Streptococcus*, *Escherichia coli* (cross-reacts with *N. meningitidis* group B), and *Streptococcus pneumoniae* in cerebrospinal fluids have been in use for a number of years and have generally good sensitivity and specificity (Wilson, 1986). There are now numerous antigen tests for the detection of group A streptococci in throat swabs, with reported sensitivities ranging from 50% to 100% and specificities ranging from 95% to 100%. There is an ELISA for *Neisseria gonorrhoeae* in genital tract specimens. There are polyclonal IFA reagents for detecting *Legionella* species and a monoclonal IFA reagent for detecting *Legionella pneumophila* in lower respiratory tract specimens. Probes for direct detection of *Chlamydia trachomatis, Neisseria gonorrhoeae*, group A *Streptococcus*, and *Legionella* species in clinical specimens are available.

Development of immunoassays and DNA probes is proceeding rapidly and raises expectations that these new technologies will eventually replace culture. Whether this occurs depends on several factors that require careful analysis by laboratory personnel. The first issue is sensitivity and specificity, which, in turn, relate to the risks associated with lack of treatment when a false-negative result occurs. The reported sensitivity of particle agglutination for *H. influenzae* antigen ranges from 68% to 94% (Wilson, 1986). Granoff and coworkers (1986) observed that appropriate therapy for *Haemophilus influenzae* was initiated in children with suspected meningitis before the results of particle agglutination tests were known because physicians believed that the risks of error in the test were not acceptable in the management of an infection that is potentially fatal without appropriate antimicrobial therapy. Culture results, rather than antigen tests, were being used for management of the patient, and in no case did the results of the antigen test alter therapy. This all too infrequent study of the clinical impact of a rapid (and expensive) test raises serious questions about the indications for its use.

Although the morbidity and mortality associated with streptococcal pharyngitis are substantially less than those of bacterial meningitis, the recent resurgence of acute rheumatic fever in several areas of the country has focused attention on the accuracy and clinical value of rapid antigen tests for group A streptococci. In a study of children seen in an emergency department, Lieu and coworkers (1988) observed that the sensitivity of the antigen test was only 55% and that significantly ($p < 0.05$) more children with a positive culture received treatment when the antigen test was used as an adjunct to culture than when follow-up treatment was attempted on the basis of a positive culture alone. Thus, unless one uses the antigen test as an adjunct to culture, one may be dealing with a test that, under some circumstances, has only a slightly better than 50% chance of providing the diagnosis. The result may be a loss of confidence in the test with an increase in the unnecessary administration of antibiotics to patients without streptococcal pharyngitis.

The sensitivity of antigen detection systems and DNA probes is highly inoculum dependent. While the number of bacteria per milliliter of cerebrospinal fluid in children with meningitis generally exceeds 10^5 colony-forming units (CFU) (Feldman, 1976), there may be substantially fewer CFU of other bacteria in other categories of specimens. Antigen tests for group A streptococci are, for example, most often falsely negative when a parallel culture yields less than or equal to 10 CFU (Lieu, 1988). Current probes may require as many as 10^5 CFU for accurate detection, so that an enrichment step is important; however, future developments may result in increased sensitivity and greater accuracy in direct specimen testing. Assuming high sensitivity, probes may limit the ability to detect pathogens other than the one sought unless specimens are also cultured. Probes may not accelerate bacterial detection if an initial enrichment culture is required, and probes directed at specific antimicrobial resistance mechanisms may not accurately reflect phenotypic susceptibility of an organism to an antimicrobial agent (Tenover, 1988). Additional considerations include the cost per specimen, optimal batch size, shelf life of probes, and prevalence of an infectious agent in the community or hospital (Tenover, 1988).

Media

Media should be selected carefully to provide the optimal conditions for growth of pathogens commonly encountered in a particular site or type of specimen. Consideration must be given to special growth requirements of bacteria associated with a particular type of infection or to the necessity of selecting out certain pathogenic bacteria from a mixed population of indigenous flora. In addition to the standard nutrient broth or agar media, therefore, one will often also inoculate differential or selective media. Blood supplemented agar is a good general growth medium and demonstrates the hemolytic action of the colonies on the red blood cells. Antibiotics or chemicals can be added to blood agar to create a selective medium such as colistin-nalidixic acid (CNA) agar or phenylethyl alcohol (PEA) agar, which are used to inhibit the growth of gram-negative bacilli while permitting gram-positive bacteria to grow. Heating the blood to make chocolate agar and adding vitamin supplements creates an enriched medium with available hemin (X) and V factors for the isolation of *Haemophilus* and other fastidious bacteria. Gram-negative bacilli are separated from gram positives by using a bile salt and dye in a medium such as MacConkey's agar, which additionally divides the colonies into lactose-positive and -negative colonies, thus making it a selective and differential medium. Guidelines for the selection of media to be used with different types of specimens are shown in Table 48–2. For each medium shown there are acceptable alternatives and, obviously, the list of potential types of specimens is far from complete.

Incubation

Bacterial cultures are generally incubated at 35°C and examined initially after 18 to 24 hours of incubation. Added CO_2 in concentrations of 5% to 10% enhances the growth of many bacteria and should be used whenever feasible. Exceptions to this recommendation are those cultures on differential and selective media in which pH alteration is used to differentiate colony types (e.g., xylose-lysine-deoxycholate [XLD] agar, Hektoen enteric [HE] agar). CO_2 is either essential or stimulatory to the growth of certain bacteria, for example, *Neisseria gonorrhoeae, Haemophilus influenzae*, and *Streptococcus pneumoniae*.

Table 48–2. GUIDELINES FOR MEDIA SELECTION FOR VARIOUS SPECIMENS

	Media for Recovery of Aerobic and Facultatively Anaerobic Bacteria					**Media for Recovery of Anaerobic Bacteria***			
Specimen	***Suppl thiogly***	***BA***	***MAC or EMB***	***CBA***	***Other***	***BA***	***BA, K-V***	***PEA***	***Suppl thiogly***
Fluids									
Cerebrospinal	X	X		X					
Abdominal	X	X	X			X	X	X	X
Pleural	X	X	X	X		X	X	X	X
Synovial	X	X		X		X			X
Wound									
Swab	X	X	X						
Aspirate	X	X	X			X	X	X	X
Tissue	X	X	X			X	X	X	X
Respiratory tract									
Throat		X†			SSA				
Sputum		X	X	X					
Bronchial washings	X	X	X	X					
Genitourinary									
Cervix, vagina		X			MTM				
Uterus, cul-de-sac	X	X	X	X		X	X	X	X
Prostate	X	X	X	X					
Urethra					MTM				
Urine									
Clean voided		X	X						
Suprapubic aspirate	X	X	X			X			
Fecal material		X	X		He, GN, Campy				

*Only for specimens from suitable source and received in anaerobe vial.
†BA is acceptable, but SSA is preferred.
Suppl thiogly = fluid thioglycolate + 10% rabbit serum; BA = blood agar; MAC = MacConkey agar; EMB = eosin methylene blue; CBA = chocolate blood agar; HE = Hektoen enteric agar; GN = enrichment broth; K-V = kanamycin-vancomycin; PEA = phenylethyl alcohol blood agar; SSA = Strep selective agar; MTM = modified Thayer-Martin; Campy = *Campylobacter* selective medium (42°C).
Adapted from Washington JA, II (ed): Laboratory Procedures in Clinical Microbiology, 2nd ed. New York, Springer-Verlag, 1985, pp 95–123.

6

Certain types of specimens should probably be stored following their inoculation onto culture media in case additional studies become necessary. Of greatest importance are tissues removed surgically, cerebrospinal and other normally sterile body fluids, foreign objects, intravascular cannulae, and prosthetic materials. Many laboratories store other types of specimens overnight under refrigeration in case of a mix-up or other problem requiring repetition of the culture. In many such instances, however, requesting another specimen is preferable to reculturing an old specimen.

Anaerobic Incubation Systems

Specimens submitted from appropriate sources and in proper containers for anaerobic culture should be processed expeditiously (Fig. 48–1), although clinically significant anaerobes in large volumes of pus or in anaerobe transport vials do survive for 24 hours without difficulty. It is probably important, however, for media that have already been inoculated to be incubated anaerobically or to be placed into a CO_2 flush jar for storage until they can be transferred into an anaerobic incubation system.

There are three types of anaerobic culture systems in use in clinical laboratories today. The most convenient and widely used is the anaerobic jar, in which water is added to a CO_2 and H_2 generator package and O_2 is catalytically converted with H_2 to water with palladium-coated alumina pellets contained in a lid chamber. There are also evacuation-replacement jars on the market; however, these are somewhat less convenient for routine use in the clinical laboratory. A modification of this system is a transparent plastic bag containing its own gas generator and palladium catalyst, and designed to hold a Petri dish (Bio-Bag Environmental Chamber, Type A, Marion Scientific, Kansas City, MO).

A second anaerobic system is the roll tube technique, in which prereduced anaerobically sterilized (PRAS) medium is distributed under anaerobic conditions as a thin layer around the internal surface of test tubes. Air is excluded from the tube during inoculation and subculture by displacement with an oxygen-free gas, such as CO_2, and by keeping it stoppered at all other times. The advantages of this approach are that each tube becomes its own incubation system and each tube can be examined without disturbing the anaerobic conditions within. Its disadvantages are that the tubes are more cumbersome and time consuming to work with and the colonial morphology may be less distinct on the agar layer within the tube than on agar plates.

The third approach to anaerobic culture is the anaerobic glove box or chamber, which consists of a large, clear plastic, airtight bag or chamber filled with an oxygen-free gas mixture of nitrogen, hydrogen, and carbon dioxide. Specimens, plates, and tubes are introduced into or removed from the chamber through a gas interchange lock. Anaerobiosis in the chamber is maintained by palladium catalysts and the hydrogen gas in the chamber. All manipulations within the chamber are done with neoprene gloves sealed to the chamber wall. The chamber can function as its own incubation system by placing heating units in it. Alternatively, incubators can be placed into the chamber; however, they occupy a lot of space and are less desirable than the units that heat the whole chamber. Like the roll tube, the chamber permits ex-

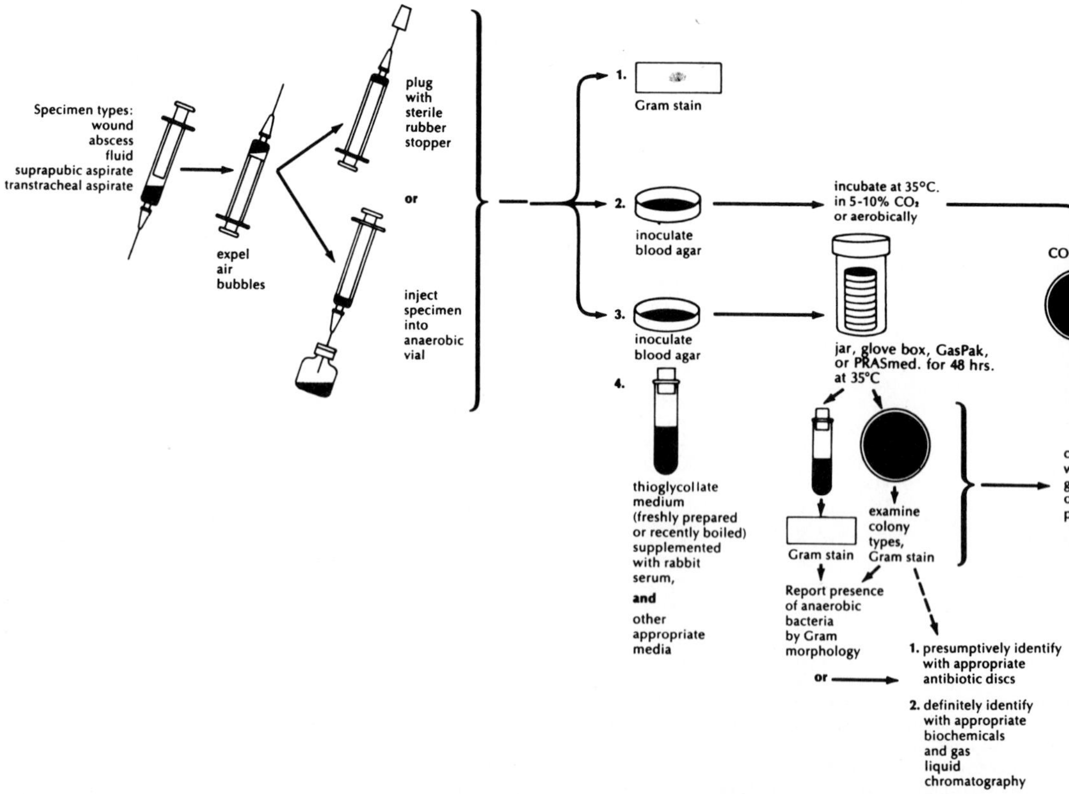

Figure 48–1. Flow chart for processing anaerobic specimens. (By permission of The Upjohn Company. Kalamazoo, Michigan; and J.A. Washington and L. LeBeau.)

amination of cultures at any time without interruption of anaerobiosis. In contrast to the roll tube, conventional isolation and subculture techniques are used. The chamber itself requires a substantial amount of space.

Each of the three anaerobe systems has its advantages and disadvantages, but they are all equally effective for isolating clinically significant anaerobic bacteria from specimens. The selection of one of these systems for routine purposes depends upon many factors, ranging from economic to technical. It is important to emphasize, however, the necessity of incubating cultures for at least 48 hours, because many anaerobic bacteria will not be evident after only 24 hours of incubation.

Examination of Cultures

All bacterial cultures should be examined routinely after 18 to 24 hours of incubation. The suggested incubation periods for different types of cultures are listed in Table 48–3. In general, cultures of normally sterile body fluids, wounds, abscesses, tissues, and anaerobic cultures are retained for one week, although in most instances the plates are discarded in 48 hours and only the broth cultures are reincubated for the longer period of time. Stool cultures and subcultures are each examined for the presence of lactose-negative colonies and are discarded if none are present. Urine cultures that have no growth or only a few colonies after 18 to 24 hours of incubation are discarded as being negative. Throat cultures are examined for the presence of β-hemolytic streptococci after 18 to 24 hours of incubation; if none are present, the cultures may be reincubated for another day. Identification procedures for colonies in sputum and urine cultures can begin after a day's incubation, with no added incubation being necessary.

Table 48–3. DURATION OF INCUBATION AND FREQUENCY OF EXAMINATION OF CULTURES

Type of Culture	Incubation Time Before Negative Culture Report (Days)	Frequency of Examination
Blood	5–7	Daily
Fluids	5*	Daily
Abscesses, wounds	5*	Daily
Tissue	5*	Daily
Respiratory tract		
Throat	2	Daily
Sputum	1	Once
Bronchial washings	5*	Daily
Genitourinary		
Cervix, vagina	2	Daily
Uterus, cul-de-sac	5*	Daily
Prostate	2	Daily
Urethra	2	Daily
Urine	1	Once
Fecal material	1†	Once
Anaerobic	5*	Daily
Brucella	21–30	3× weekly
Actinomyces	14–21	1× weekly

*Plates are discarded after 48 hours, but tubes with supplemented fluid thioglycolate are kept for time specified in column.

†Initial cultures and subcultures of enrichment broth are examined after 18 to 24 hours for presence of lactose-negative colonies; if none are present, the cultures are reported as negative for salmonellae and shigellae. *Campylobacter* plates should be held 48 to 72 hours.

With positive cultures it is a good idea to develop a system of preliminary reports, because identification procedures may take as long as several days to complete. Although the timing of a preliminary report will vary according to the type of culture performed and the importance of the bacteria isolated, it is a good general rule to issue a preliminary report within the first 48 hours after receipt of the specimen. In some cases this report can be sooner, and in some (e.g., blood, cerebrospinal fluid) it should be by phone as soon as any information becomes available.

MEDICALLY IMPORTANT BACTERIA

Pyogenic Cocci

Gram-Positive

STAPHYLOCOCCUS

DEFINITIONS AND CHARACTERISTICS. Staphylococci are catalase-positive spherical cocci, often appearing in grapelike clusters in stained smears (Plate 48–2). They grow well on any peptone-containing nutrient medium under aerobic and anaerobic conditions, and may produce hemolysis of various species of animal blood and yellow or orange pigment on agar. Growth of staphylococci is readily detected on blood agar plates or in various types of nutrient broths. A selective medium for the isolation of *Staphylococcus aureus* is one containing 7.5% to 10% NaCl with mannitol.

Tests useful for distinguishing staphylococci from micrococci are listed in Table 48–4 (Kloos, 1991). *Staphylococcus aureus* is differentiated from other species of staphylococci principally by its production of coagulases. Two antigenically distinct forms of coagulase have been recognized, one being bound to the cell wall and the other being released by or free from the cell wall. Although the mechanism has not been completely elucidated, it is thought that a plasma factor or coagulase-reacting factor reacts with cell-bound coagulase to form a coagulase-thrombin complex, which, in turn, acts upon fibrinogen to form a fibron clot. Cell-bound coagulase is called *clumping factor* by some and forms the basis of the slide coagulase test. Cell-free or unbound coagulase appears to form a complex with prothrombin to give a thrombin-like product. This form of coagulase serves as the basis for the tube coagulase test. It is most practical to use rabbit plasma prepared commercially for coagulase testing. Provided that a

Table 48–4. TESTS FOR DIFFERENTIATING STAPHYLOCOCCI AND MICROCOCCI

Test	Expected Result for *Staphylococci*	Expected Result for *Micrococci*
Anaerobic growth in glucose	+	–
Lysostaphin susceptibility	S	R
Aerobic acid production from glycerol in presence of erythromycin (0.4 μg/mL)	+	–
Modified oxidase	–	+
Bacitracin susceptibility (0.4 U disk)	R	S

+ = positive; – = negative; R = resistant; S = susceptible.

6

very dense, homogeneous bacterial suspension is mixed with a loopful of reconstituted rabbit plasma, clumping should be observed in nearly 99% of instances with *Staphylococcus aureus*. Inoculation of a few colonies of *S. aureus* into a tube containing 0.5 mL of the same reconstituted rabbit plasma should produce a clot in over 99% of instances and in nearly all cases within a four-hour period of incubation.

PATHOGENESIS AND VIRULENCE FACTORS. Several factors play a role in the virulence of *Staphylococcus aureus*. The capsule, if present, provides protection against complement-mediated attack by polymorphonuclear leukocytes, and it enhances spread of the organism through tissues. Cell wall peptidoglycan elicits interleukin-1 production by macrophages, activates complement, and is chemotactic for neutrophils. Teichoic acid in the cell wall interacts with components of the alternate complement pathway, activating the coagulation and kinin systems, and may facilitate bacterial adherence at sites of colonization. Protein A, an immunologically active substance in the cell wall with a high affinity for the Fc fragment of immunoglobulin (Ig) G, binds to and aggregates IgG molecules, fixing complement in the process, and it enhances natural killer cell activity.

Most strains of *S. aureus* produce α-, β-, and δ-toxins and a variety of other extracellular proteins, including leukocidin, urease, lipase, gelatinase, and phosphatase. Whereas the α-, β-, and δ-toxins are hemolytic, only the α- and β-toxins are considered to exert lethal and dermonecrotic activities. An epidermolytic toxin called *exfoliatin* is responsible for the scalded skin syndrome. Otherwise, the roles of each of these toxins in the pathogenicity of staphylococci are unclear because of often contradictory data. Some staphylococci produce enterotoxins that produce vomiting and diarrhea. Five such enterotoxins have been identified thus far from strains of *S. aureus*; however, enterotoxin production by rare strains of coagulase-negative staphylococci has been reported. Toxic shock syndrome has been associated with strains of *S. aureus* which elaborate toxic shock syndrome toxin, or TSST-1.

Factors of importance in the development of infections due to *S. aureus* include breaks in the continuity and integrity of mucosal and cutaneous surfaces, the presence of foreign bodies or implants, prior viral diseases, antecedent antimicrobial therapy, and underlying diseases with defects in cellular or humoral immunity. *Staphylococcus aureus* may be present among the indigenous flora of the skin, eye, upper respiratory tract, gastrointestinal tract, urethra, and, infrequently, vagina. Infection may, therefore, arise from an endogenous or an exogenous source, involve local sites, spread contiguously, or invade the bloodstream with, possibly, the development of metastatic sites of infection (Fig. 48–2).

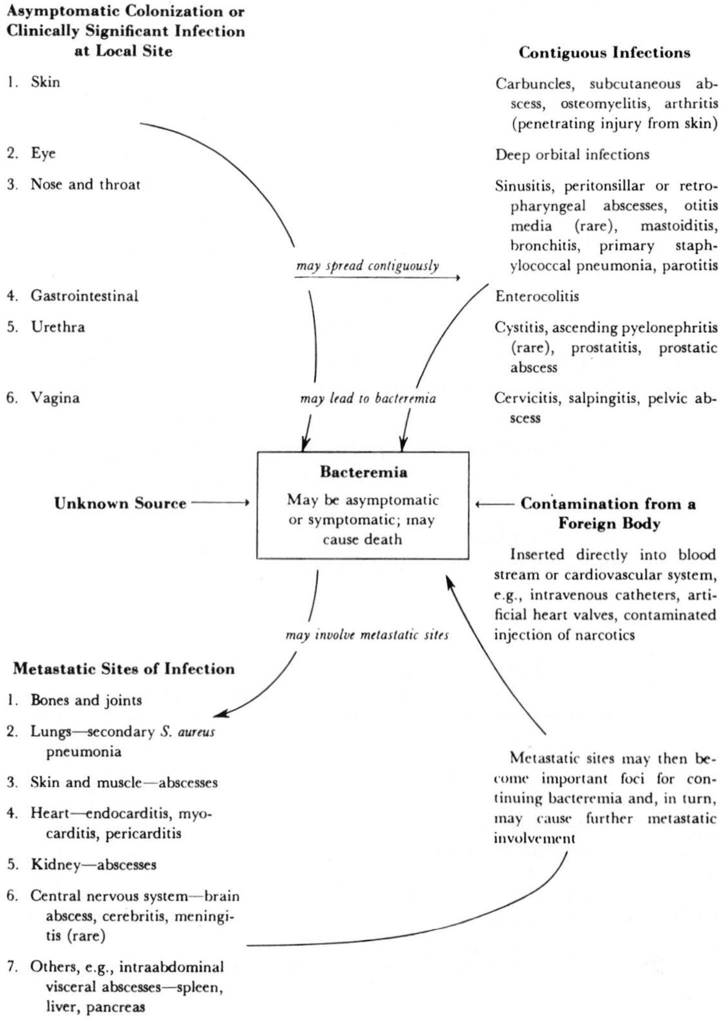

Figure 48–2. Pathogenic sequence of *Staphylococcus aureus* infection. (From Cohen, JO: The Staphylococci. Copyright © 1972, reprinted by John Wiley & Sons, Inc.)

Infections caused by *S. aureus* may affect multiple organ systems (Fig. 48–2). Among the most common are those involving the skin and its appendages, such as impetigo, folliculitis, mastitis, and infections of surgical wounds. *Staphylococcus aureus* is among the leading causes of bacteremia in hospitalized patients, and it may cause endocarditis, particularly in persons with left-sided valvular heart disease and in intravenous drug users. *Staphylococcus aureus* is the most common cause of spinal epidural abscess and suppurative intracranial phlebitis, and it is recovered from 10% to 15% of brain abscesses, typically following trauma. Meningitis caused by *S. aureus* is uncommon and generally follows head trauma or a neurosurgical procedure.

Staphylococcus aureus is responsible for most cases of osteomyelitis, is the most common cause of septic arthritis in prepubertal children, and is occasionally responsible for septic arthritis in adults. In the tropics, it may cause spontaneous deep abscesses of muscles, predominantly affecting malnourished persons who have a concomitant parasitic infection (Chiedozi, 1979). *Staphylococcus aureus* is an infrequent cause of community-acquired pneumonia but a common cause of nosocomial pneumonia, which usually follows aspiration of endogenous nasopharyngeal organisms. Predisposing factors include infection with measles or influenza A viruses, cystic fibrosis, and immune deficiency. Urinary tract infections caused by *S. aureus* are pyelonephritis and intrarenal and perirenal abscess.

Toxin-mediated diseases caused by *S. aureus* include scalded skin syndrome, food poisoning, and toxic shock syndrome. Scalded skin syndrome occurs in infants infected with a strain of *S. aureus* producing exfoliative toxin. The illness begins abruptly with erythema, followed in two to three days by the formation of flaccid bullae, which slough, leaving denuded areas that eventually resolve completely. Staphylococcal food poisoning, characterized by nausea, vomiting, abdominal cramps, and diarrhea, occurs one to six hours after ingestion of foods contaminated with preformed staphylococcal enterotoxin.

Toxic shock syndrome is a multisystem disease affecting individuals who have no antibodies to TSST-1 and are colonized or infected with strains of *S. aureus* producing TSST-1 or rarely enterotoxin B or C. The illness is most common in women 15 to 25 years of age who use tampons during menstruation but also may occur in nonmenstruating individuals, including women in the postpartum period, persons with a surgical wound or other focal infections, and individuals who have had a surgical procedure in the nose or sinuses. Toxic shock syndrome begins abruptly with fever, myalgias, vomiting, and diarrhea followed by hypotension, hypovolemic shock, and an erythematous rash that frequently involves the palms and soles and desquamates in one to two weeks. The diagnosis is clinical; isolation of *S. aureus* from any site is not required. Full recovery is the rule, although repeated episodes may occur.

Infections caused by coagulase-negative species of *Staphylococcus* usually occur in patients with foreign bodies, and especially in those with implanted prosthetic valves, joints, and shunts. *Staphylococcus epidermidis* is the species most frequently involved in such infections. *Staphylococcus saprophyticus* is an important cause of bacteriuria, particularly in sexually active young women. The pathogenicity of micrococci is uncertain owing to a great extent to problems associated with their identification.

LABORATORY DIAGNOSIS. The observation microscopically of typical rounded, gram-positive cocci in clusters in smears of material taken from previously unopened or undrained lesions or in smears of broth from a positive blood culture is indicative of staphylococcal infection. Care should be taken in the interpretation of Gram's-stained smears when only single or paired organisms are seen because of their possible confusion with pneumococci and streptococci.

Staphylococcus aureus produces coagulase, an enzyme that binds plasma fibrinogen, causing the organisms to agglutinate or plasma to clot; almost all other staphylococci do not. Over 95% of isolates of *S. aureus* are identified by the slide coagulase test, which detects cell-bound enzyme (clumping factor); and almost all isolates are identified by the tube coagulase tests, which detects free coagulase.

It is recommended that a slide coagulase test be performed initially, provided there are a sufficient number of colonies available to prepare a dense emulsion. The formation of clumping within 30 seconds is sufficient for the identification of *S. aureus*. In the absence of clumping within 30 seconds or if only a few isolated staphylococcal colonies are present, several colonies should be transferred into a tube containing 0.5 mL of plasma that is incubated at 35°C for four hours and then examined for clot formation. If no clot has formed, the tube should be reincubated at room temperature and re-examined after a total of 20 hours of incubation. Examination of the test after only four hours of incubation is necessary because most isolates of *S. aureus* produce a clot within this interval and because some strains produce a fibrinolysin that can lyse the clot and thereby produce a false-negative reaction if the test is only observed after 20 hours.

Positive reactions with particle agglutination tests (latex beads or sensitized sheep red blood cells) that detect protein A, clumping factor, or both provide rapid identification of *S. aureus*. These tests, however, may give false-positive results with isolates of *S. saprophyticus* and species of *Micrococcus*, and false-negative results with isolates of methicillin (oxacillin)–resistant *S. aureus*, especially those also resistant to trimethoprim-sulfamethoxazole and rifampin (Gregson, 1988; Ruane, 1988). *Staphylococcus intermedius*, a rare cause of infection in canine bite wounds in humans, also produces coagulase; but it produces the enzyme pyroglutamyl-β-naphthylamide aminopeptidase (detected by the PYR test, described later) and *S. aureus* does not (Talan, 1989).

Many species of coagulase-negative staphylococci have been recognized (Kloos, 1991); however, with the exception of *S. saprophyticus*, which is resistant to novobiocin, speciation of such strains in the clinical laboratory is not practical or clinically indicated. It is usually sufficient for the clinical laboratory to call these coagulase-negative staphylococci. When clinically indicated, coagulase-negative staphylococci may be speciated by using any one of several commercially available test systems (Kloos, 1991).

6

Staphylococci may be classified on the basis of their susceptibility to different bacteriophages or their plasmid profiles for epidemiologic purposes in attempting to identify common source infections. These tests are generally available only through reference laboratories.

ANTIMICROBIAL SUSCEPTIBILITY. Whereas most staphylococci associated with community-acquired infections used to be susceptible to penicillin and most of those associated with nosocomially acquired infections were resistant to penicillin, this difference among susceptibilities of strains according to their mode of acquisition has largely disappeared. It therefore behooves the laboratory to perform antimicrobial susceptibility tests. Penicillin, if the organism is susceptible to it, remains the antibiotic of choice in the therapy of staphylococcal infections. Methicillin resistance occurs in up to 80% of isolates of *S. epidermidis* and, increasingly, among isolates of *S. aureus* in large, medical school–affiliated tertiary referral hospitals in the United States.

Penicillin resistance (minimal inhibitory concentrations ≥ 0.2 μg/mL) is caused by the production of a β-lactamase (penicillinase) associated with a plasmid in staphylococci. Resistance to penicillinase-resistant penicillins (methicillin, oxacillin, nafcillin), on the other hand, is not related to a plasmid, and its mechanism appears to be related to differences in the penicillin-binding proteins of such strains.

Oxacillin resistance typically is heterogeneous, meaning that only rare cells (1 in 10^4 to 10^8) express the resistance trait, so specific guidelines must be followed to ensure detection (Chambers, 1988): (1) An inoculum equal to the turbidity of a 0.5 McFarland standard should be prepared in 0.85% sterile saline directly from overnight growth on a blood agar plate for disk diffusion and microdilution testing. (2) Mueller-Hinton agar plates and a 1 μg oxacillin disk should be used for disk diffusion testing. (3) Oxacillin in cation (calcium and magnesium)–supplemented Mueller-Hinton broth containing 2% NaCl should be used for microdilution testing. (4) Agar plates and microtiter trays should be incubated a full 24 hours at 30 to 35°C. To screen for oxacillin resistance, Mueller-Hinton agar supplemented with 4% NaCl and containing 6 μg/mL of oxacillin is spot inoculated with a cotton swab, and plates are incubated for 24 hours. Although they may appear to be susceptible to cephalosporins, all oxacillin-resistant staphylococci should be considered resistant to all cephalosporins, as well as imipenem.

STREPTOCOCCUS, ENTEROCOCCUS, AND OTHER STREPTOCOCCACEAE

DEFINITIONS AND CHARACTERISTICS. Streptococci are catalase-negative, gram-positive, spherical, ovoid, or lancet-shaped cocci, often seen in pairs or chains. They are facultatively anaerobic. Some strains require added CO_2 for their initial isolation but may lose this requirement in subcultures. These CO_2-dependent strains have been called microaerophilic; however, use of this term is discouraged because of its imprecision and the fact that most such strains can be classified into recognized species.

Streptococci can be broadly classified according to at least three schemes that overlap and are, therefore, potentially confusing. One scheme places the streptococci into physiologic divisions: pyogenic, viridans, lactic, and enterococcal. In another they are categorized according to serologically active carbohydrates ("C" substance) into Lancefield groups. In the third scheme they are categorized according to their hemolytic reactions on sheep blood agar. Those strains that completely hemolyze the red cells about their colonies are called β-hemolytic, those that produce partial hemolysis (cause "greening" of the agar) are α-hemolytic, and those that do not hemolyze at all are γ-hemolytic.

Each of these schemes for classifying streptococci serves a useful purpose so that it is generally not possible to eliminate any one of them completely. Enterococci are genetically unrelated to streptococci, and group D seroreactivity is related to a teichoic acid antigen rather than to the "C" antigen (Ruoff, 1988). From the clinical standpoint, the separation of streptococci and enterococci isolated from the blood of patients with endocarditis is of considerable importance in determining the selection and duration of antimicrobial therapy. The patient with viridans streptococcal endocarditis requires two weeks of intramuscularly administered penicillin and aminoglycoside, while the patient with enterococcal endocarditis requires three or four weeks of intravenously administered penicillin with intramuscularly administered aminoglycoside. It is essential for the laboratory to distinguish between group A streptococci and those belonging to other Lancefield groups in throat cultures, because the therapy in cases with group A streptococcal pharyngitis is directed not only toward the pharyngitis but also to the prevention of nonsuppurative sequelae. Differentiating streptococci and enterococci from *Leuconostoc* and *Pediococcus* is important because the latter two genera typically are resistant to vancomycin.

From the laboratory's point of view, the hemolytic reactions on blood agar produced by streptococci represent a useful point of departure for purposes of classification (Table 48–5). Most enterococci are not β-hemolytic; this reaction is limited to a small percentage of isolates of *Enterococcus faecalis* and of *E. faecium*. Commonly included among the viridans streptococci are *S. bovis, S. mutans, S. sanguis, S. mitis, S. salivarius*, and *S. anginosus*. Of as yet uncertain taxonomic status are nutritionally variant (pyridoxal-, B_6-, or thiol-dependent, satelliting) streptococci.

Table 48–5. CLASSIFICATION OF STREPTOCOCCI AND ENTEROCOCCI

Hemolytic Reaction	Group	Species
β	A	*S. pyogenes*
	B	*S. agalactiae*
	C	*S. equisimilis*
		S. zooepidemicus
		S. equinus
	D	*E. faecalis*
	Small colony variants of A, C, F, G, E, L, M, P, U	*S. anginosus*
α or γ	D	*E. faecalis*
		E. faecium
		E. durans
		E. avium
		E. gallinarum
		S. bovis
		S. equinus
	Small colony variants of A, C, F, G	*S. anginosus*
	None of above	*S. pneumoniae*
		S. mutans
		S. sanguis
		S. mitis
		S. salivarius
		S. anginosus
		S. uberis
		S. acidominimus
		S. morbillorum

Group A streptococci may be typed according to their M and T protein antigens, tests typically done only in research laboratories. Pneumococci are typeable into more than 80 antigenic types on the basis of their capsular polysaccharide.

PATHOGENESIS AND VIRULENCE FACTORS. Streptococcal cell wall components and extracellular products (enzymes and toxins) and host responses are involved in the pathogenesis of infections caused by *Streptococcus pyogenes* (group A). The most significant bacterial factor is the cell wall M protein, which prevents phagocytosis of the organism. Antibodies against the specific M protein confer lifelong type-specific immunity; however, because over 60 M protein types exist, infection with a group A *Streptococcus* possessing a different M protein may occur. Another important cell wall component is lipoteichoic acid, which permits bacterial adherence to the respiratory epithelium.

Streptococcus pyogenes elaborates about 20 extracellular products, including enzymes (streptolysins, hyaluronidase, streptokinase, deoxyribonucleases [DNases], and nicotinamide adenine dinucleotidase [NADase]) and erythrogenic toxins. Streptolysin O, an antigenic, oxygen-labile enzyme, produces subsurface β hemolysis on blood agar plates; and streptolysin S, a nonantigenic, oxygen-stable enzyme, produces surface β hemolysis. Neither streptolysin has a proven role in the pathogenesis of human disease. Streptokinase promotes fibrinolytic activity by converting plasminogen to plasmin, and hyaluronidase may enhance the spread of the organism through connective tissue. The pathogenic significance of the DNases and of NADase is unknown. Serologic tests to detect antibodies to streptolysin O, streptokinase, and DNase B are useful in diagnosing nonsuppurative complications (described later) of group A streptococcal infections.

Pyrogenic (erythrogenic) toxins (serotypes A, B, C) are produced by isolates of *S. pyogenes* infected with a specific temperate bacteriophage. Their pyrogenicity is caused by a direct action on the hypothalamus. In the past, these toxins were believed to be responsible for the rash of scarlet fever, but the rash is now thought to be a hypersensitivity response, depending on an interplay between host cellular and humoral factors (Gallis, 1988). Recently severe soft-tissue infections associated with a toxic shock–like syndrome caused by strains of *S. pyogenes* producing pyrogenic toxin A have been reported (Stevens, 1989).

The pathogenesis of acute rheumatic fever is not fully understood. Certain M protein types of *S. pyogenes* may be rheumatogenic. The presence of complexes of immunoglobulin and the C3 component of complement along the sarcolemmal sheaths of cardiac myofibers from individuals with rheumatic carditis suggests that myocarditis results from the production of antibodies directed against a streptococcal cell wall M protein that cross-reacts with myocardial tissue. Moreover, a heart– or tissue–cross-reactive antigen of *S. pyogenes* that shares immunologic epitopes with but is distinct from the M protein has been identified (Barnett, 1990). The renal damage in acute glomerulonephritis is caused by deposits of circulating streptococcal-antistreptococcal immune complexes in the glomeruli and the subsequent activation of complement. Cell-mediated reactions to an altered glomerular basement membrane or activation of the alternate complement pathway also may be involved.

Streptococcus pneumoniae is normal flora of the upper respiratory tract of 25% to 50% of preschool children and nearly 20% of adults, termed carriers (Hendley, 1975). Its spread is enhanced by upper respiratory tract infections and crowding. Pneumococcal pneumonia develops when the host immune defenses are impaired. Most cases are endogenous, following aspiration of oral secretions containing normal flora that include *S. pneumoniae*. Person-to-person transmission during epidemics occurs by droplet aerosols. The major virulence factor of *S. pneumoniae* is its antiphagocytic polysaccharide capsule, and strains with a thick, mucoid capsule, such as type 3, are especially virulent.

One of the most common manifestations of group A streptococcal infection is pharyngitis. This may be accompanied by scarlet fever, a punctate exanthem overlying diffuse erythema that usually appears first on the neck or upper chest, becomes generalized, and then desquamates. Skin infections caused by group A *Streptococcus* include cellulitis, erysipelas, and pyoderma. A toxic shock–like syndrome infrequently occurs in persons with group A streptococcal soft tissue infections, such as cellulitis and necrotizing fasciitis or bacteremia (Stevens, 1989). The mortality rate for this rapidly progressive multisystem disease is as high as 30%. Acute rheumatic fever, characterized by carditis, polyarthritis, erythema marginatum, chorea, and subcutaneous nodules, occurs one to five weeks after group A streptococcal pharyngitis. Acute glomerulonephritis develops 10 days to three weeks after group A streptococcal pharyngitis or pyoderma.

The most common infections caused by group B streptococci are neonatal sepsis, pneumonia, and meningitis. Group B streptococcal infections in adults include postpartum endometritis, urinary tract infections, bacteremia, skin and soft-tissue infections, pneumonia, endocarditis, meningitis, arthritis, and osteomyelitis. Infections caused by *S. pneumoniae* are pneumonia, meningitis (especially in infants and the elderly), spontaneous bacteremia (in persons who do not have a spleen), otitis, sinusitis, and spontaneous peritonitis. Bacterial endocarditis is the most common infection caused by viridans streptococci; others include abscesses in the brain or liver, bacteremia, and dental caries.

Enterococci are a common cause of urinary tract infections in hospitalized persons; they also cause endocarditis, bacteremia, and wound infections. *Leuconostoc* has been associated with bacteremia, endocarditis, and meningitis (Handwerger, 1990). *Pediococcus* has been recovered from wounds and blood, but more data are needed to clearly define its role in human disease (Mastro, 1990).

LABORATORY DIAGNOSIS. Tests commonly used in the clinical microbiology laboratory to presumptively name the β-hemolytic species of *Streptococcus* are shown in Figure 48–3. Over 99% of isolates of group A *Streptococcus* are susceptible to bacitracin, but a very small percentage of isolates of group B *Streptococcus* and 10% to 20% of isolates of groups C and G *Streptococcus* also are susceptible. Therefore, results of the bacitracin susceptibility test provide a presumptive identification. An isolate may be called group A *Streptococcus* presumptively, based on the hydrolysis of pyrrolidonyl-beta-naphthylamide (PYR test) (Wellstood, 1987). All isolates of group A *Streptococcus* and over 99% of isolates of *Enterococcus* are PYR positive. An identification of group A *Streptococcus* is confirmed by serotyping, using latex agglutination or coagglutination, or by staining a smear

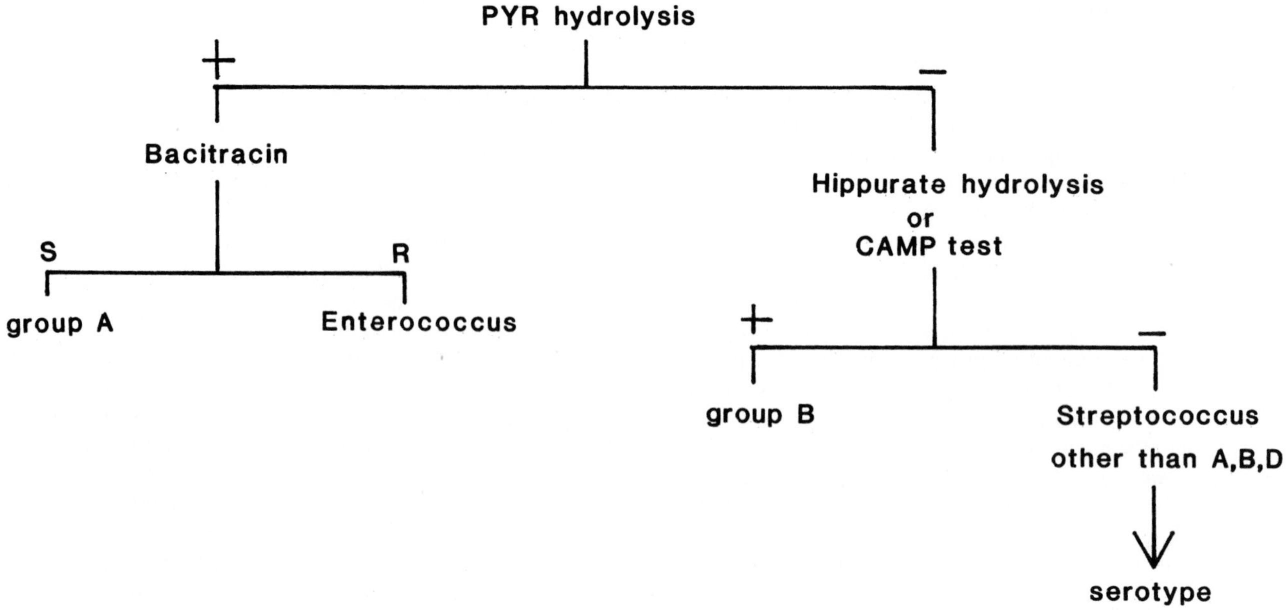

Figure 48–3. Decision tree of tests to presumptively name the β-hemolytic species of *Streptococcus*. Key: + = positive result; − = negative result; S = susceptible; R = resistant. (From Woods GL, Gutierrez Y: Diagnostic Pathology of Infectious Diseases. Philadelphia, Lea & Febiger, 1993.)

with fluorescent monoclonal antibodies. Group A *Streptococcus* may be detected directly in throat swab specimens within five to 15 minutes by using commercial kits. These tests are highly specific, but given their low sensitivity, a negative direct test should be followed by culture (Dale, 1994; Facklam, 1987; Pokorski, 1994; Radetsky, 1987). Serologic tests to detect antibodies in acute and convalescent serum samples to streptolysin O and DNase B are used primarily to diagnose acute rheumatic fever and acute glomerulonephritis following infection with group A *Streptococcus*.

An isolate that hydrolyzes hippurate or has a positive cAMP test reaction presumptively is called group B *Streptococcus*. Isolates of presumed group B *Streptococcus* from sterile body sites should be identified by serotyping (using latex agglutination or coagglutination tests), by staining with fluorescent monoclonal antibodies, or by using a chemiluminescent DNA probe (Daly, 1991). Group B *Streptococcus* may be detected directly in endocervical swab specimens using kits similar to those for group A *Streptococcus*. However, these tests also have a low sensitivity; therefore, specimens yielding negative direct results should be followed by culture (Kotnick, 1990). Isolates of β-hemolytic group C, D, F, and G *Streptococcus* are identified by serotyping with latex agglutination or coagglutination reagents.

Tests used to presumptively name α- and γ-hemolytic streptococci and enterococci are shown in Figure 48–4. Alpha-hemolytic colonies that are mucoid or flattened with a depressed center are suggestive of *S. pneumoniae* and should be tested for susceptibility to ethylhydroxycupreine hydrochloride, more commonly called optochin (P disk); *S. pneumoniae* is susceptible, other α-hemolytic streptococci are resistant. Isolates of presumed *S. pneumoniae* from sterile body sites should be confirmed by serotyping with latex agglutination or coagglutination reagents.

Alpha-hemolytic colonies that are not *S. pneumoniae* and γ-hemolytic colonies are tested for PYR hydrolysis; enterococci are PYR-positive, viridans streptococci are negative. Moreover, all enterococci grow in the presence of 6.5% NaCl; viridans streptococci do not. A DNA probe to identify colonies of enterococci also is available (Daly, 1991). Enterococci hydrolyze esculin in the presence of bile (causing visible growth and blackening of the agar), but up to 10% of the viridans streptococci also are bile-esculin positive. The three species of *Enterococcus* commonly encountered in the clinical laboratory may be identified by biochemical tests (Fig. 48–4) (Facklam, 1989a, for a comprehensive list of tests) or by using commercial kit systems (Tritz, 1990).

Alpha-hemolytic streptococci that are optochin resistant and PYR negative and γ-hemolytic streptococci that are PYR negative and do not grow in 6.5% NaCl are grouped as nonhemolytic (viridans) streptococci. Identification of the individual species of viridans streptococci requires conventional biochemical testing (Coykendall, 1989). Kit systems to identify these organisms are commercially available, but because the taxonomy has changed, these systems should be modified and evaluated again. *Streptococcus bovis* may be identified by serotyping (group D).

Characteristics that help differentiate *Leuconostoc* and *Pediococcus* from those of *Enterococcus* are listed in Table 48–6 (reviewed by Facklam, 1989b). Typically, nutritionally deficient streptococci are detected in broth blood culture systems when a Gram's-stained smear of a positive culture shows gram-positive cocci in chains but subcultures to solid media are sterile. Organisms are recovered by spreading a lawn of the organism from the blood culture broth over the surface of a sheep blood agar plate and then streaking with an isolate of *Staphylococcus aureus* ("Staph streak"), which provides the needed pyridoxal. The small "satelliting" colonies of catalase-negative, gram-positive cocci that grow at the periphery of the *S. aureus* are the nutritionally deficient streptococci. Alternatively, pyridoxal may be added to the

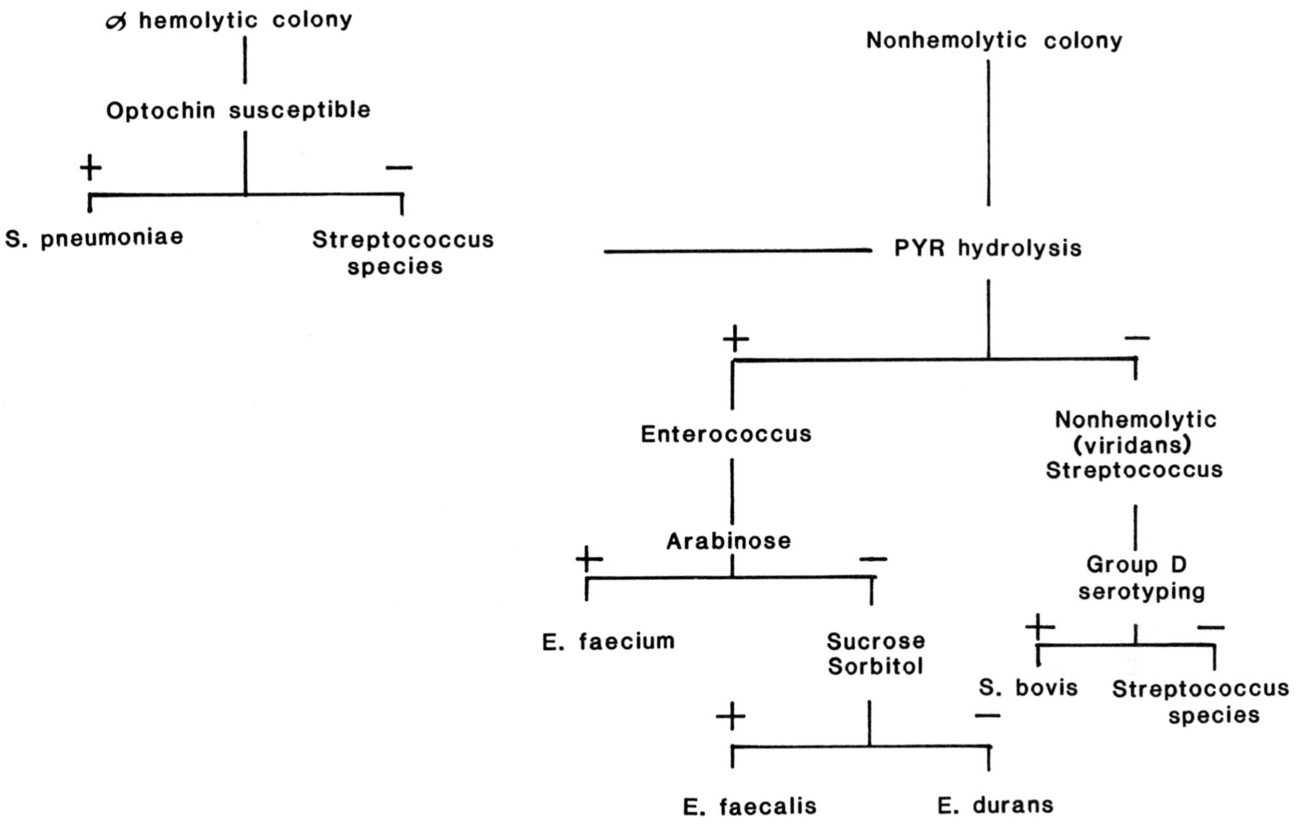

Figure 48–4. Decision tree of tests to presumptively name the α-hemolytic and γ-hemolytic species of *Streptococcus* and *Enterococcus*. Key: + = positive result; − = negative result. (From Woods GL, Gutierrez Y: Diagnostic Pathology of Infectious Diseases. Philadelphia, Lea & Febiger, 1993.)

growth medium. Differential characteristics of *Streptococcus defectivus* and *Streptococcus adjacens* are reviewed elsewhere (Ruoff, 1990).

ANTIMICROBIAL SUSCEPTIBILITY. The antibiograms of groups A, B, C, and G *Streptococcus* are predictable (all are susceptible to penicillin); therefore, routine antimicrobial susceptibility testing of these organisms is unnecessary. Because *S. pneumoniae* with intermediate (or relative) or high-level resistance to penicillin (MIC, 0.1 to 1.0 mg/L and ≥2 mg/L, respectively) are found worldwide, isolates of *S. pneumoniae* recovered from sterile body sites (i.e., blood or cerebrospinal fluid) should be screened for susceptibility to penicillin using disk diffusion with a 1 μg oxacillin disk (Klugman, 1990). The latter method, however, does not distinguish isolates with intermediate from those with high-level resistance to penicillin; therefore, isolates with a zone of 19 mm or less must be further evaluated by macrodilution or microdilution testing, using Mueller-Hinton broth supplemented with lysed horse blood, or the E test to determine the penicillin minimum inhibitory concentration.

Susceptibility testing should be performed on isolates of nonhemolytic (viridans) streptococci from sterile body sites, because resistance to penicillin does occur. Isolates of *Enterococcus* also should be tested, primarily to identify high-level resistance to penicillin or ampicillin, high-level resistance to streptomycin and gentamicin, and resistance to vancomycin (Tenover, 1993). Enterococci that produce β-lactamase have been reported but are uncommon.

6

Table 48–6. CHARACTERISTICS DIFFERENTIATING *ENTEROCOCCUS, LEUCONOSTOC,* AND *PEDIOCOCCUS*

Characteristic	*Enterococcus*	*Leuconostoc*	*Pediococcus*
Gram's stain from broth	Cocci in pairs, long chains	Cocci, coccobacilli, rods in pairs and chains	Large, spherical cocci in tetrads and pairs
Bile esculin	+	+	+
Growth in 6.5% NaCl	+	V	V
PYR test	+	−	−
Gas from glucose	−	+	−
Vancomycin resistance	S*	R	R

*Although most isolates are susceptible, resistant strains (especially *E. faecium*) have been detected in many parts of the country.
+ = positive; − = negative; S = susceptible; R = resistant.
From Woods GL, Gutierrez Y: Diagnostic Pathology of Infectious Diseases. Philadelphia, Lea & Febiger, 1993, p 219.

Gram-Negative

NEISSERIA AND *MORAXELLA CATARRHALIS*

DEFINITIONS AND CHARACTERISTICS. These genera are nonmotile, catalase- and oxidase-positive, aerobic gram-negative cocci that are often arranged in pairs with flattened adjacent surfaces (Plate 48–3). The genus *Branhamella* was separated from the neisseriae on the basis of differences in DNA base composition but is now included in the genus *Moraxella*. Only *M. catarrhalis* (formerly *Branhamella catarrhalis*) is discussed here.

All of these organisms are somewhat fastidious in their growth requirements, requiring in some instances the addition of blood, serum, cholesterol, or oleic acid to the medium to counteract growth inhibitors. Gonococci and meningococci generally require prompt incubation in CO_2 for growth; however, this requirement is strain dependent, varies with the phase of the organism's growth curve, and is often lost in subcultures. Meningococci and most gonococci are not inhibited by the presence of vancomycin or lincomycin, colistin, and nystatin, a characteristic that is particularly useful in their selective isolation from specimens contaminated with other bacteria. Vancomycin-susceptible gonococci have been encountered in some parts of the country and are inhibited on media containing this antibiotic.

PATHOGENESIS AND VIRULENCE FACTORS. Although opportunistic infections caused by species of *Neisseria* other than *N. gonorrhoeae* and *N. meningitidis* have occasionally been reported in compromised hosts, these species are generally nonpathogenic.

Meningococci may colonize the mucous membranes of the upper respiratory tract, an event that is usually followed in seven to 10 days by the formation of bactericidal and hemagglutinating antibodies, which, however, may not eliminate the carrier stage but which convey group-specific immunity. In a few cases, however, disease results shortly after colonization, most frequently in the form of meningococcemia and meningitis (Fig. 48–5). The organism also has a tendency to invade serous membranes and joint tissues, with the development of pleuritis, pericarditis, and arthritis. Carriage of meningococci in the nasopharynx is not uncommon; however, a direct correlation between carrier rates and incidence of meningococcal disease has not been established, with the possible exception of members of large households or households with an infant or childhood case during epidemics of meningococcal disease. Meningococci have also been isolated from genital sources, where their clinical significance remains uncertain but where they may be readily misidentified as gonococci unless appropriate tests for distinguishing these two species are carried out.

The principal virulence factor of meningococci is a lipopolysaccharide-endotoxin complex, which in experimental animals activates the clotting cascade, depositing fibrin in small vessels, producing hemorrhage in the adrenals and other organs, and altering peripheral vascular resistance, leading to shock and death.

The pathogenesis and clinical manifestations of gonococcal infections differ somewhat from those of the meningococci (Fig. 48–6). Pathogenic types (1 and 2) of *Neisseria gonorrhoeae* adhere by means of pili, which nonpathogenic types (3 and 4) lack, to various human cells. These pili, which represent one of the principal virulence factors of the gonococcus, also may inhibit phagocytosis, are antigenically heterogeneous, and stimulate strain-specific antibody formation. Other possible virulence factors of *N. gonorrhoeae* are less clearly defined at this time.

Both gonococci and meningococci produce an IgA_1 protease, which may also be important in their pathogenesis, because IgA is the antibody class that predominates in secretions on mucous membranes.

Moraxella catarrhalis is an encapsulated organism, and extending from its outer membrane are pili that serve as adhesions. The most common infections it causes are bronchitis, otitis, sinusitis, and pneumonia (especially in persons with underlying chronic lung disease) (Catlin, 1990). *Moraxella catarrhalis* is an infrequent cause of bacteremia, endocarditis, meningitis, urogenital infections, and ophthalmia neonatorum.

LABORATORY DIAGNOSIS. The single most important element in the laboratory diagnosis of meningococcal and gonococcal diseases is the specimen, its proper selection, collection, and transport to the laboratory (see Chap. 54). The pathogenic species are sensitive to drying and extremes of temperature, and material should be cultured promptly for their recovery. They are mesophilic and grow poorly, if at all, at room temperature. Many require prompt incubation in CO_2 (2% to 8%) for primary isolation. Media containing chocolatized blood are commonly used for cultures and

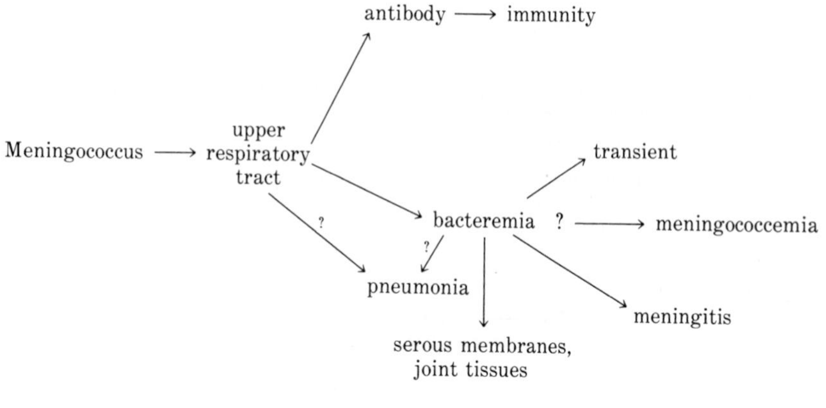

Figure 48–5. Pathogenesis and clinical aspects of meningococcal disease.

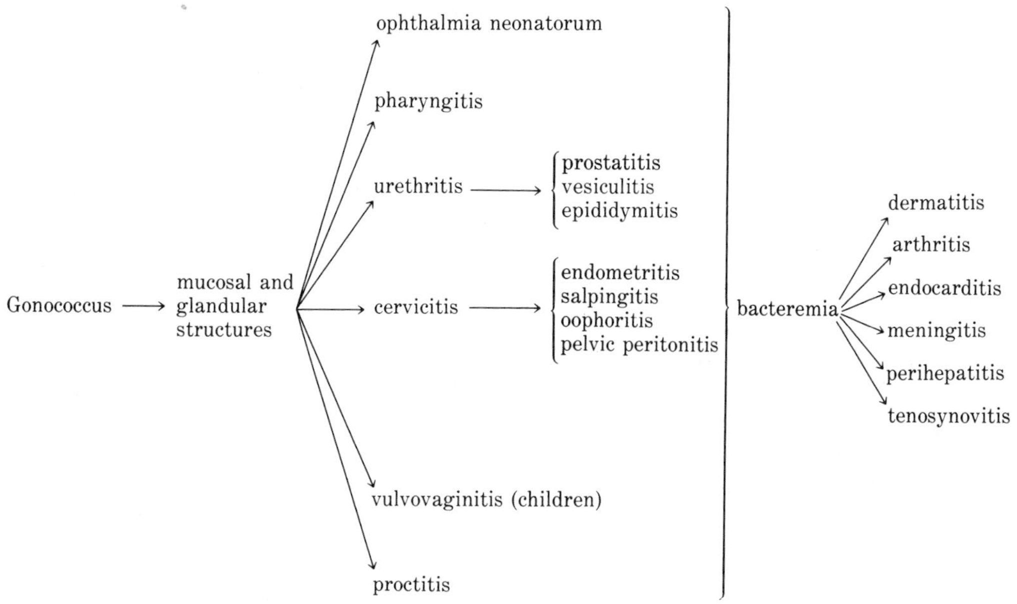

Figure 48–6. Pathogenesis and clinical manifestations of gonococcal disease.

should contain antibiotics, that is, vancomycin or lincomycin, as well as colistin, nystatin or anisomycin, and trimethoprim, if the specimen is contaminated with indigenous flora. Vancomycin-susceptible gonococci will grow on media containing lincomycin; however, because of the synergistic interaction of lincomycin and trimethoprim, the latter must be omitted from media containing lincomycin. Direct inoculation of specimens "at the bedside" is optimal. This can be accomplished in several ways: the inoculation of Thayer-Martin medium with prompt incubation at 35°C in CO_2, most frequently in a candle jar; or the inoculation of modified Thayer-Martin medium in a bottle or chamber containing CO_2 (Transgrow), or in which CO_2 can be generated from a citric acid–bicarbonate tablet (JEMBEC). If any of these culture systems must be mailed to a reference laboratory for processing, they must first be incubated overnight to ensure growth of the organisms.

An isolate from a urogenital specimen showing the appropriate colony appearance on a selective medium presumptively may be called *Neisseria gonorrhoeae* based on results of the Gram's stain, oxidase, and catalase tests. Gram's-stained smears prepared from colonies of *N. gonorrhoeae* should show typical gram-negative diplococci, but organisms may occur in tetrads, especially from young cultures. Species of *Moraxella* have a similar appearance but can be differentiated from *N. gonorrhoeae* by the penicillin disk test (discussed later). All species of *Neisseria* are oxidase positive, and all species except *N. elongata* are catalase positive. Because *Neisseria* other than *N. gonorrhoeae* may be recovered from urogenital sites, confirmatory testing is strongly recommended and is required for all isolates from extragenital sites and when sexual abuse is suspected (preferably by more than one method).

Confirmation of *N. gonorrhoeae* and identification of the other *Neisseria* species and *Moraxella catarrhalis* are based on growth and biochemical characteristics (Table 48–7) (Knapp, 1988). The standard method of identification is detection of acid production from carbohydrates in a cystine-tryptic acid (CTA) base medium and other conventional biochemical tests. However, given the drawbacks of the conventional methods (discussed later), more rapid identification tests are used in most clinical laboratories. Tests for direct detection of *N. gonorrhoeae* and *N. meningitidis* in clinical specimens are also available. Typing isolates of *N. gonorrhoeae* and *N. meningitidis* is done primarily for epidemiologic studies.

With the standard method of identification, acid production from glucose, maltose, lactose, sucrose, and fructose in a CTA base medium and a carbohydrate-free control are tested. Tubes are inoculated, incubated at 35 to 37°C in ambient air, and examined at 24 hour intervals until reactions are interpretable or for 72 hours. Expected results for the species of *Neisseria* and *M. catarrhalis* are shown in Table 48–7. Occasionally, however, an isolate of *N. meningitidis* yields aberrant carbohydrate reactions: glucose negative, maltose negative, or asaccharolytic. If *N. meningitidis* is strongly suspected in these cases, the identification can be confirmed by slide agglutination, using pooled polyvalent grouping antisera or sera specific for individual serogroups. In addition to conventional carbohydrate degradation tests, reduction of nitrates and nitrites, and deoxyribonuclease (DNase) production should be evaluated. The latter is especially useful for identification of *M. catarrhalis*, which is DNase positive; *Neisseria* are negative. Moreover, most clinical isolates of *M. catarrhalis* produce β-lactamase, whereas most respiratory isolates of *Neisseria* species are β-lactamase negative. Drawbacks to conventional tests are the requirement for a heavy inoculum, the need to work with pure cultures, long turnaround time, and failure of some fastidious strains of *N. gonorrhoeae* to grow.

Several commercial systems detect acid production from carbohydrates, usually in one to four hours (Knapp, 1988). The inoculum must be prepared from a pure culture of the isolate, so identification generally is available 24 hours after

Table 48–7. DIFFERENTIATION OF SPECIES OF *NEISSERIA* AND *MORAXELLA CATARRHALIS*

	N. gonorrhoeae	*N. meningitidis*	*N. cinerea*	*N. lactamica*	*N. sicca*	*N. subflava*	*N. flavescens*	*N. mucosa*	*M. catarrhalis*
Growth									
Thayer-Martin medium	+*	+	−	+	−	−	+	−	§
Nutrient agar, 25°C	−	−	−	−	+	+	−	+	+
Oxidase	+	+	+	+	+	+	+	+	+
β-Galactosidase	−	−	−	+	−	−	−	−	−
Reduction of nitrate	−	−	−	−	−	−	−	+	+
DNase	−	−	−	−	−	−	−	−	+
Production of acid from									
Glucose	+	+	−†	+	+	+	−	+	−
Maltose	−	+	−	+	+	+	−	+	−
Lactose	−	−	−	+	−	−	−	−	−
Sucrose	−	−	−	−	+	d‡	−	+	−
Fructose	−	−	−	−	+	−	−	−	−

+ = ≥90% of strains positive; − = ≥90% of strains negative; d = variable.
*Most vancomycin-susceptible strains will not grow on Thayer-Martin medium.
†Weak reaction may occur in rapid carbohydrate utilization tests.
‡Biovar *perflava*, +; biovar *flava*, − .
§ Some strains positive and others negative.

isolation. Acid reactions of some of *N. gonorrhoeae* and, to a lesser extent, *N. meningitidis* may be difficult to interpret or aberrant with some kits, and strains of *N. gonorrhoeae* that are weak producers of acid from glucose may appear to be glucose negative. Some strains of *N. cinerea*, which does not produce acid from glucose, can appear glucose positive in certain systems. If the glucose reaction is equivocal, colistin susceptibility by disk diffusion using a 10 μg disk will differentiate *N. gonorrhoeae* (resistant, no zone) from *N. cinerea* (susceptible, zone ≥10 mm).

Enzyme substrate tests provide rapid identification (one to four hours) only of isolates of oxidase-positive, gram-negative diplococci recovered on a selective medium (Kellogg, 1995; Knapp, 1988). They are valuable for differentiating maltose-negative strains of *N. meningitidis* from *N. gonorrhoeae*, but color changes may be subtle and if misinterpreted could cause isolates of *N. meningitidis* and other *Neisseria* to be incorrectly called *N. gonorrhoeae*. Moreover, strains of *Neisseria cinerea* and *Kingella denitrificans* that grow on gonococcal-selective media could be misidentified as *N. gonorrhoeae* if not confirmed with other procedures. Commercial products that combine enzyme substrate tests with modified conventional tests provide accurate identification of species of *Neisseria* and species of *Haemophilus* (Janda, 1987).

Immunologic tests for *N. gonorrhoeae* (coagglutination and fluorescent antibody tests) are used for identification of colonies from primary isolation media. Fluorescent tests using monoclonal antibodies are highly specific and sensitive for *N. gonorrhoeae*, but false-positive results with other *Neisseria* and with *Kingella denitrificans* and nonspecific Fc binding to other bacteria have been reported (Beebe, 1993; Dillon, 1988; Kellogg, 1995). Therefore, using the latter reagents to test only gram-negative, oxidase-positive organisms recovered on gonococcal selective media is suggested.

An ELISA for detection of *N. gonorrhoeae* directly in urethral and endocervical swab specimens is commercially available. For urethral swab specimens from men, its sensitivity and specificity are about equal to those of a Gram's-stained smear. However, it is less sensitive than endocervical culture in women and has yielded false-positive reactions; therefore, the test should only be used to test specimens from persons in high-risk groups, and results should be considered presumptive. A chemiluminescent nucleic acid probe for detection of *N. gonorrhoeae* can be used for culture confirmation or direct detection of the organism in endocervical or urethral swab specimens (Hale, 1993; Limberger, 1992).

ANTIMICROBIAL SUSCEPTIBILITY. Meningococci for the most part are susceptible to the penicillins, so that determining their susceptibility to this agent for therapeutic reasons is seldom necessary. Rare isolates that are penicillin resistant, however, have been identified (Saez-Nieto, 1992; Woods, 1994). All are susceptible to rifampin, the agent recommended in the United States for prophylaxis among household contacts.

Despite the fact that the concentrations of penicillin required to inhibit gonococci have increased over the years, leading to recommendations that probenecid and increased dosages of penicillin be administered, outright penicillin resistance of gonococci caused by β-lactamase was not reported until 1976. The prevalence of these strains is increasing throughout the world. They can be rapidly detected by testing for β-lactamase by any one of several acidimetric or iodometric methods. Since 1983, resistance to penicillin that is chromosomally mediated and appears to be caused by alterations in the affinity of penicillin-binding proteins has been identified in the United States. Such strains do not produce β-lactamase and, therefore, can only be detected by susceptibility testing. Because of the increased prevalence of penicillin resistance in the United States, ceftriaxone currently is the agent of choice. Chromosomal mutations may lead to increased resistance to tetracycline, but plasmid-mediated resistance is the major cause of tetracycline resistance of gonococci in the United States today. Tetracycline resistance is present in 2% to 3% of all isolates of *N. gonorrhoeae* in the United States; however, the incidence of tetracycline resistance varies widely geographically. Spectinomycin-resistant gonococci occur frequently in the Far East and in England, but have remained infrequent in the United States to date.

PREVENTION. A polysaccharide vaccine against *Neisseria meningitidis* serogroups A, C, Y, and W135 is licensed in the United States and is recommended for military personnel, for persons living in epidemic areas of developing countries, and for those with a nonfunctional or absent spleen. Antibiotic prophylaxis should be limited to household contacts and those who have had contact with patients' oral secretions. Rifampin is the drug of choice currently unless susceptibility to sulfonamides can be demonstrated.

The use of pre-exposure antibiotics to prevent gonococcal diseases is discouraged because of the potential risks of sensitization and the emergence of resistant strains. The sole exception to this rule is the application of silver nitrate solution or erythromycin ointment to the eyes of newborns to prevent gonococcal ophthalmia.

Coryneform and Related Bacteria

The term *coryneform* has been used to describe gram-positive, non–spore-forming, nonfilamentous rods that may exhibit pleomorphic morphology (Plate 48–4). In its broadest sense, the term might include *Actinomyces, Propionibacterium, Mycobacterium*, and *Nocardia*, as well as *Corynebacterium, Listeria*, and *Erysipelothrix*; however, taxonomists disagree as to the proper limits of the term. For purposes of simplicity of organization in this book, the term will be limited to *Corynebacterium, Listeria*, and *Erysipelothrix*. No endorsement, implied or otherwise, is intended by this approach.

Corynebacterium

DEFINITIONS AND CHARACTERISTICS. The corynebacteria or "diphtheroids," as they are sometimes called, are widely distributed in nature and occur on the mucous membranes and skin of humans and animals. Most species are rarely pathogenic in humans, with the notable exceptions of *Corynebacterium diphtheriae* and its closely related species or varieties *C. ulcerans* and *C. pseudotuberculosis. Arcanobacterium haemolyticum* (formerly *C. haemolyticum*) has been associated with pharyngitis and skin rash, predominantly in persons aged 10 to 30 years (Miller, 1986); however, other than in their microscopic morphology, they share few characteristics in common with *C. diphtheriae*, and their taxonomic status remains uncertain at this time. Other species of *Corynebacterium*, particularly *C. jeikeium*, have been clearly associated with infections of implanted prosthetic materials, for example, heart valves, cerebrospinal fluid shunts, and joints; have caused subacute bacterial endocarditis; and have been involved in a variety of opportunistic infections. Their etiologic role in such infections is established with considerable difficulty and often only after their repeated isolation from a particular source.

PATHOGENESIS AND VIRULENCE. At the initial site of infection on the tonsils and oropharynx, *C. diphtheriae* multiplies on the epithelial cells and elaborates an exotoxin that causes local cell necrosis and subsequent inflammation. Exudative lesions coalesce, forming a grayish-black adherent pseudomembrane. The toxin, produced only by strains of *C. diphtheriae* infected with a temperate bacteriophage carrying the gene for toxin production, is absorbed into the circulation and distributed systemically, producing degenerative changes in the heart, nervous system, and kidneys. The toxin molecule consists of two fragments: A, containing the enzymatically active site, and B, comprising the receptor binding site. Toxin molecules bind to host cells via fragment B; they are cleaved, and fragment A enters the cell by an incompletely understood process. In the cell, fragment A disrupts protein synthesis by catalyzing the inactivation of transfer RNA translocase, thus preventing the interaction of messenger RNA and transfer RNA, and stopping further addition of amino acids to developing polypeptide chains. The toxin affects all cells in the body, but the heart, nerves, and kidneys are damaged most severely. The organisms and their exotoxin produce a serum exudate and cellular infiltrate of the mucous membrane in the pharynx, leading to the formation of a grayish pseudomembrane. Although toxin production and pathogenicity are often considered to be synonymous, pseudomembranes may form in persons infected with nontoxigenic strains. Extension of the pseudomembrane superiorly into the nasopharynx or inferiorly into the larynx may be so marked as to produce respiratory obstruction. Although *C. diphtheriae* infections of other parts of the body do occur, the most frequent ones observed in the United States today are those of the skin.

Transmission of *C. diphtheriae* is by droplet nuclei from the respiratory tract or by contact from cutaneous foci of infection.

LABORATORY DIAGNOSIS. Because of the relative rarity of diphtheria in the United States today, the diagnosis may be overlooked clinically and the laboratory may easily fail to recognize its causative agent in cultures. A tentative diagnosis must always be provided to the laboratory so that the specimen can be handled appropriately. Cystine-tellurite (CT) blood agar is the preferred medium for isolation of the organism, while the more nutritionally deficient Loeffler's (coagulated serum) or Pai's (coagulated egg) medium is more useful for microscopic morphology. The cells are often pleomorphic in appearance, are on microscopic examination characteristically arranged side by side in palisade formation, and frequently display metachromatic granules. On CT medium, colonies of *C. diphtheriae* are grayish black after 48 hours of incubation. Three colony types can be encountered: *gravis*, which are large, flat, and dark gray and have irregular edges with radial striations; *mitis*, which are black, convex, and moist; and *intermedius*, which are quite small and black.

Strains of corynebacteria can be speciated with biochemical tests (Table 48–8) but it is necessary to establish the virulence of isolates suspected of being *C. diphtheriae* by determining whether or not they produce exotoxin. This can be done by inoculating a broth culture subcutaneously into two guinea pigs, one of which has received diphtheria antitoxin intraperitoneally two hours previously. The unprotected guinea pig will die within one to four days if the inoculated strain was toxigenic. Alternatively, the elaboration of toxin may be detected *in vitro* with the Elek immunodiffusion test by streaking the culture to be tested at right angles to a paper strip impregnated with antitoxin and embedded in agar and observing the formation of precipitin lines at 45-degree angles to the paper strip. Many modifications of this test have been described resulting from the failure of toxigenic strains to produce precipitin lines or from the formation of nonspecific lines by nontoxigenic strains. The potency of the antitoxin, the inoculum size, the type of enrichment serum,

Table 48–8. DIFFERENTIAL CHARACTERISTICS OF SOME SPECIES WITHIN THE GENUS *CORYNEBACTERIUM* AND RELATED ORGANISMS

Test	*C. diphtheriae*	*C. ulcerans*	*C. pseudotuberculosis*	*C. xerosis*	*C. pseudodiphtheriticum*	*C. jeikeium*	*Arcanobacterium haemolyticum*	*Actinomyces pyogenes*
Catalase	+	+	+	+	+	+	−	−
Hemolysis	d	+	+	−	−	−	+	+
Gelatinase	−	+	−	−	−	−	−	+
Urease	−	+	+	−	+	−	−	+
NO_3 reduction	−	−	d	+	+	−	−	−
Sucrose fermentation	−	−	−	+	−	−	d	d

+ = positive; − = negative; d = variable.

and the duration of incubation all affect the outcome of this test.

The classification of the oral and skin corynebacteria or diphtheroids is difficult and confusing. Multiple approaches have been proposed and are based on characteristics such as oleate dependence, fluorescence, nitrate reduction, urease activity, and carbohydrate fermentations. Published fermentation reactions are highly variable, often conflicting, and reflect, among other things, the organisms' growth characteristics and whether or not the basal medium has been supplemented with serum or a source of oleate, for example, Tween-80.

ANTIMICROBIAL SUSCEPTIBILITY. Although antitoxin remains the only specific method of treatment of diphtheria, antibiotics are administered to patients with disease and to asymptomatic carriers of toxigenic strains. *Corynebacterium diphtheriae* is usually inhibited by less than or equal to 0.5 μg/mL of penicillin, less than or equal to 0.05 μg/mL of erythromycin, and less than or equal to 0.3 μg/mL of clindamycin. Because of its activity and because it is well tolerated, erythromycin is often used for this purpose; however, benzathine penicillin may be useful in instances in which patient cooperation is suspect.

The antimicrobial susceptibilities of other species of corynebacteria or diphtheroids are far less predictable. *C. jeikeium* is often resistant to the penicillins and cephalosporins, variably susceptible to most other antibiotics, and almost uniformly susceptible to vancomycin. The therapy of infections caused by these organisms is often complicated by the presence of compromised host defenses and implanted prosthetic materials.

PREVENTION. The methods of prevention of diphtheria are almost exclusively active and passive immunization programs with supplemental antibiotics to eliminate the carrier state of toxigenic strains during epidemics.

Listeria

DEFINITIONS AND CHARACTERISTICS. The pathogenic species for humans and an intracellular parasite, *Listeria monocytogenes* is most successfully isolated from tissue by culture of finely ground material. Fluids and swabs are directly plated on conventional bacteriologic media. The organism's growth is optimal at temperatures of 30 to 37°C; however, growth does occur between 3 and 45°C, and does, in fact, appear to be enhanced in some instances after storage of the specimen under refrigeration.

Listeria monocytogenes is a facultatively anaerobic, catalase- and Voges-Proskauer–positive, gram-positive, non–spore-forming, non–acid-fast organism that may appear coccoid, coccobacillary, or bacillary microscopically. Rods may arrange themselves into palisades with V and Y forms typical of other coryneform bacteria. A narrow zone of β-hemolysis is produced on blood agar by fresh isolates. A characteristic tumbling motility occurs at room temperature but rarely at 35°C. This same temperature-dependent motility is also noted in semi-solid media.

PATHOGENESIS AND VIRULENCE. *Listeria monocytogenes* is found in soil, dust, water, silage, sewage, and raw unpasteurized milk. Transmission of the organism by foods such as coleslaw, pasteurized milk, and soft cheeses has resulted in major epidemics in North America and Europe during the past decade (Fleming, 1985; Linnan, 1988). Most cases of listeriosis, however, occur sporadically, and excluding transplacental transmission, the source is unknown. Food-borne transmission is postulated but unproven. According to data from microbiological surveys of food, *L. monocytogenes* has been detected in 2% to 3% of dairy products, 20% of soft cheeses and processed meats, 30% of certain vegetables (cabbages, radishes), and up to 50% of raw meat and poultry (Broome, 1993). Defects in the immune system probably are involved in production of disease because many persons with listeriosis are immunosuppressed. Macrophages and T lymphocytes are the most important host defenses against *L. monocytogenes*. The virulence of *L. monocytogenes* probably is related to production of listeriolysin O, a 52 kDa protein with hemolytic and cytotoxic properties that is secreted under conditions of low pH and low iron concentration, as would exist in a phagolysosome. The protein is postulated to bind irreversibly to cholesterol in the lysosome membrane, causing its disruption and allowing unrestricted bacterial multiplication within the phagocyte cytoplasm.

Clinical manifestations of listeriosis differ in pregnant women, neonates, and immunocompromised individuals, which are the high-risk groups. Listeriosis during pregnancy, most common in the third trimester, presents as a flulike illness. Bacteremia occurs concomitantly, during which time the uterine contents are infected. Progression to amnionitis may induce premature labor or septic abortion in three to seven days. Infection in the mother is self-limited because the source of the infection is removed with delivery of the infected fetus and uterine contents. Neonatal listeriosis may have an early or late onset. Early-onset disease, manifested at birth or a few days thereafter, results from *in utero* infection. Infants present with temperature instability, hemodynamic compromise, and respiratory distress; widely disseminated granulomas, particularly involving the placenta, posterior pharynx, and skin, are characteristic of the illness but are not always present. Late-onset disease, affecting full-term infants of mothers with uncomplicated pregnancies, is assumed to be acquired postpartum, but in most cases the source is unknown. Clinical manifestations of meningitis become apparent several days to weeks after birth. Nonperinatal listeriosis usually occurs in immunosuppressed individuals, but in about one third of the cases no risk factor is identified. Approximately half of these infections are manifested as meningitis; other forms of central nervous system listeriosis include cerebritis and brainstem and spinal cord abscesses. Primary bacteremia or focal infections outside the central nervous system are uncommon.

LABORATORY DIAGNOSIS. The isolation, especially from cerebrospinal fluid or blood, of small grayish-blue colonies surrounded by a narrow zone of β-hemolysis on blood agar should make one think of *L. monocytogenes* and lead one to perform a test for motility at 25°C. It does produce catalase and acid from glucose, trehalose, and salicin. The organism resembles *Erysipelothrix rhusiopathiae*; however, there are several distinguishing characteristics between these two organisms (Table 48–9).

ANTIMICROBIAL SUSCEPTIBILITY. *L. monocytogenes* is usually inhibited by less than or equal to 0.5 μg/mL of penicillin or ampicillin, less than or equal to 6 μg/mL of chloramphenicol, less than or equal to 4 μg/mL of tetracycline, and less than or equal to 4 μg/mL of gentamicin. Considerably higher concentrations of these antimicrobial agents are required for bactericidal activity, although substantially increased killing has been demonstrated in studies with combinations of penicillin or ampicillin with an aminoglycoside. Ampicillin, alone or in combination with an aminoglycoside, has been used successfully in the treatment of infections caused by *Listeria monocytogenes*. Trimethoprim-sulfamethoxazole may be used as alternative therapy in penicillin-allergic patients.

Erysipelothrix rhusiopathiae

DEFINITIONS AND CHARACTERISTICS. *Erysipelothrix* is a catalase-negative, non–spore-forming, nonmotile, facultatively anaerobic gram-positive bacillus that has a worldwide distribution. Cells from smooth phase colonies are small, straight, or slightly curved rods, while those from rough colonies are long and filamentous.

PATHOGENESIS AND VIRULENCE. *Erysipelothrix* infection is usually transmitted to humans from animals by means of skin wounds produced with contaminated objects or in contact with blood, flesh, viscera, or feces of infected animals. *Erysipelothrix rhusiopathiae* is widespread in nature in wild and domestic animals, birds, fish, and decaying organic matter and causes infection in swine, sheep, rabbits, cattle, birds, and fowl. At risk of infection with this organism are butchers, abattoir workers, fishermen, fish handlers, poultry processors, and veterinarians. The most common form of erysipeloid is a local cutaneous infection manifested by pain, swelling, and a cutaneous eruption characterized by a slowly progressive, slightly elevated, violaceous zone around the site of inoculation. The swelling and erythema migrate peripherally and the lesion involutes without desquamation. Systemic disease is rare, but there are numerous case reports of septicemia and endocarditis. Also rarely reported have been cases of arthritis and brain abscess.

Table 48–9. DIFFERENTIAL CHARACTERISTICS OF *LISTERIA MONOCYTOGENES* AND *ERYSIPELOTHRIX RHUSIOPATHIAE*

Test	*L. monocytogenes*	*E. rhusiopathiae*
β-Hemolysis	+	−
Growth at 4°C	+	−
Catalase	+	−
Motility	+	−
Esculin hydrolysis	+	−
Gluconate utilization	+	−
Voges-Proskauer	+	−
H_2S in TSI	−	+

LABORATORY DIAGNOSIS. Because positive cultures infrequently result from swab specimens of a local cutaneous lesion, biopsy or tissue aspirates represent the specimens of choice and should be placed into an infusion broth containing 1% glucose followed by subculture on blood agar. *Erysipelothrix* is rapidly fatal to mice when injected intraperitoneally and can be isolated in pure culture from the heart blood. Conventional blood culture media are suitable for its isolation from blood.

Erysipelothrix is oxidase and catalase negative. Characteristically, it produces H_2S in triple sugar iron agar (TSIA). It is nonmotile, does not reduce nitrates to nitrites, and ferments glucose and lactose. It can be readily distinguished from *Listeria* (see Table 48–9).

ANTIMICROBIAL SUSCEPTIBILITY. *Erysipelothrix* is susceptible to the penicillins, cephalosporins, erythromycin, clindamycin, chloramphenicol, and tetracyclines but is resistant to sulfonamides and aminoglycosides.

PREVENTION. Preventive measures include an awareness on the part of those occupationally or recreationally (e.g., hunters) exposed to infected animals and their observance of simple hygienic practices, rodent control, and regular disinfection of fish tanks.

Aerobic Spore-Forming Bacilli

Bacillus

DEFINITIONS AND CHARACTERISTICS. The members of this genus are strictly aerobic or facultatively anaerobic, rod shaped, spore forming, gram positive, and catalase positive. With the notable exception of the anthrax bacillus, they are usually motile by means of lateral or peritrichous flagella. Some strains will stain gram negatively and because of their variable oxidase reactions are confused with gram-negative bacilli. The most reliable diagnostic characteristic of the genus is spore formation, which occurs optimally and on a variety of media under aerobic conditions at 25 to 30°C. In Gram's-stained smears, endospores are detectable by the presence of unstained defects or holes within the cell. The spores themselves can be stained by any one of several methods.

PATHOGENESIS AND VIRULENCE FACTORS. Of the numerous species of *Bacillus*, *Bacillus anthracis* is the only one that is uniformly and highly pathogenic. Great care must be exercised when handling material suspected of harboring this species. Work should be performed in biological safety cabinets by gloved, gowned, masked, and immunized personnel; work surfaces must be disinfected with 5% hypochlorite or 5% phenol; and all supplies, materials, and equipment must be decontaminated. Animals should be inoculated only by properly attired and immunized personnel, should be housed separately, and should be autoclaved and incinerated after death.

Three forms of anthrax are recognized: cutaneous, inhalation, and intestinal. In its cutaneous form, anthrax produces a small, red, macular lesion that progresses to a vesicle and finally necrosis with formation of a characteristic black eschar. Regional lymphadenopathy and septicemia may occur. The mortality in untreated cases with this form of disease is approximately 20%. Inhalation of anthrax spores can lead to acute bronchopneumonia, mediastinitis, and septicemia ("woolsorter's disease"). The mortality in recognized cases of this form of disease is nearly 100%. Intestinal anthrax follows the ingestion of contaminated food and is manifested by nausea, vomiting, and diarrhea. In some cases there is gastrointestinal bleeding, followed by prostration, shock, and death. Septicemia can occur in all three forms of anthrax and may lead to a fatal purulent meningitis.

A major factor in the organism's pathogenic capabilities is its glutamyl polypeptide capsule, which inhibits phagocytosis; anticapsular antibodies do not protect against the disease. A complex toxin with three components (edema factor, protective antigen, and lethal factor) is responsible for the signs and symptoms of anthrax.

Humans become infected with anthrax by contact with and inhalation or ingestion of infected animals, their carcasses, or their byproducts. Cattle, sheep, horses, and goats are the animals most frequently infected and provide a ready source of vegetative organisms that sporulate and perpetuate the environmental contamination.

Although usually saprophytic, other species of *Bacillus* can cause disease. *Bacillus cereus* has been associated with ear infections, pneumonias, post-traumatic ocular wound infections, septicemias, and endocarditis. Patients with pneumonias and septicemias are often immunosuppressed. Bacteremias are also frequently associated with intravenous drug use and with contaminated intravascular devices.

Two forms of gastroenteritis are associated with *Bacillus* species. Food poisoning caused by *Bacillus* may occur within one to six hours following the ingestion of food that has been contaminated with *B. cereus* and has produced a preformed heat-stable toxin. The major manifestations of *Bacillus* food poisoning are nausea, vomiting, cramps, and occasionally diarrhea. Typically, this form of *Bacillus* gastroenteritis results from the bulk preparation of foods that are not reheated prior to being served. *Bacillus cereus* type 1 grows particularly well in fried rice and is more heat resistant than other types so that this form of gastroenteritis is frequently seen in association with consumption of cooked rice in Chinese restaurants. The second form of gastroenteritis caused by *Bacillus* results from the contamination of meat and vegetable dishes and is characterized by the onset of cramps and diarrhea eight to 16 hours following ingestion of the contaminated food. In this instance, the major manifestations of *B. cereus* infection are caused by the production of a heat-labile enterotoxin.

LABORATORY DIAGNOSIS. In cases of suspected cutaneous anthrax, vesicle fluid and material under the edge of the eschar should be collected with a swab for smear and culture. For suspected inhalation anthrax, sputum should be collected for smear and culture. Cultures of stool should be made in the intestinal form. Smears and cultures should be made of cerebrospinal fluid in suspected meningitis. In the septicemic stage, cultures of blood should be prepared.

Finding large, boxcar-shaped, gram-positive cells in smears of any of these specimens suggests the diagnosis. Fluorescent microscopy, available in some state health laboratories and at the Centers for Disease Control and Prevention (CDC), can provide a rapid presumptive diagnosis.

Species of *Bacillus* grow well on sheep blood agar. Colonies of *B. anthracis* are usually flat, with an irregular margin ("Medusa head"), appear off-white with a ground glass surface, and are usually nonhemolytic. When touched with an inoculating loop, the colonies are tenacious and will stand up like beaten egg white. The Medusa head colony may be seen with *B. cereus* and certain other *Bacillus* species. Anthrax bacilli are nonmotile, either in a hanging drop test or in semi-solid media, whereas most other species are motile. Both *B. anthracis* and *B. cereus* ferment glucose, maltose, and sucrose, and produce a positive Voges-Proskauer reaction. Motility by the hanging drop method is a useful differential test between *B. anthracis* and *B. cereus* but must be carried out with a fresh broth culture of the organism. Other tests that may be useful in the identification of *Bacillus* species include glycosidase assays, lectin agglutination assays, resistance to lysozyme, capsule formation, and susceptibility to penicillin (Turnbull, 1991).

Virulence tests may be performed by inoculating mice subcutaneously or intraperitoneally with a barely turbid saline suspension prepared from colonies on agar. A broth culture should not be used for virulence testing because of the toxigenic products formed in broth by other *Bacillus* species. The mice will die in 24 to 72 hours, and the organisms can be demonstrated in smears and cultures of heart blood, liver, and spleen.

The diagnosis of *B. cereus* gastroenteritis cannot be accurately made by culture of stool because the organisms may be a component of the indigenous gut flora. Diagnosis, therefore, depends on quantitative culture of the suspected contaminated food. The presence of less than or equal to 10^5 CFU/g in the suspected food constitutes presumptive evidence of *B. cereus* food poisoning (Doyle, 1985).

ANTIMICROBIAL SUSCEPTIBILITY. Although susceptible to a variety of agents, the antibiotic therapy of anthrax has centered on the use of penicillin with or without streptomycin. Both of these agents are highly active against *B. anthracis*; however, some strains do elaborate a β-lactamase.

The antimicrobial susceptibility of other species of *Bacillus* to the penicillins and cephalosporins is highly variable. Most strains are, however, inhibited by tetracycline, aminoglycosides, and chloramphenicol at low concentrations.

PREVENTION. Prevention of anthrax in humans ideally depends upon its control in animals. Prompt diagnosis of sick animals, their isolation and therapy, and cremation of carcasses are indicated when sporadic outbreaks occur. In enzootic areas, vaccination with nonencapsulated spore preparations is used. Occupationally exposed persons should also be immunized.

Acute diarrheal disease caused by *B. cereus* may be prevented by properly cooking and refrigerating foods prepared in bulk to prevent proliferation of vegetative forms of the bacteria and formation of the enterotoxin.

Nocardioforms and Aerobic Actinomycetes

This group of organisms includes aerobic, gram-positive bacilli that in Gram's-stained smears typically appear as branching filaments (Plate 48–5) that occasionally fragment into rod-shaped and short coccoid forms. They usually grow more slowly than the aerobic and facultative gram-positive bacilli discussed previously, and they grow well on media commonly used to recover fungi.

Nocardia

DEFINITIONS AND CHARACTERISTICS. In Gram's-stained smears of clinical specimens (sputum or purulent material), *Nocardia* appear as long, thin (0.5 to 1.2 μm in diameter), beaded, branching gram-positive bacilli. The most distinguishing quality of the nocardiae is their partial acid fastness; cells stain positively with a modified acid fast (Ziehl-Neelsen or Kinyoun) stain, differentiating them from *Actinomyces*, which may have a similar Gram's-stain appearance. Partial acid fastness may be difficult to demonstrate and can be enhanced by growing the organism for about four days on Middlebrook 7H10 agar (typically used for mycobacterial culture; see Chapter 51) or in litmus milk broth.

Of the nocardiae recognized as human pathogens, *Nocardia asteroides* is responsible for 80% to 90% of human infections; *N. brasiliensis* for 5% to 6%, occurring most often in tropical and subtropical parts of the world; and *N. caviae* (also called *N. otitidis-caviarum*) for about 3%. *Nocardia transvalensis* is an extremely rare human pathogen. In the United States, an estimated 500 to 1000 cases of nocardiosis occur annually, and recipients of organ transplants account for about 13%.

PATHOGENESIS AND VIRULENCE FACTORS. Nocardiae are found in soil and organic material worldwide and cause disease in many animals and in fish. Human infection is more common in males than females. It usually is acquired via inhalation of the organism but may occur following trauma and contact with contaminated soil, or the organism may enter the body via the gastrointestinal tract when contaminated material contacts an area of mucosal ulceration.

In the lungs, *Nocardia* organisms are phagocytosed by alveolar macrophages and grow intracellularly, which elicits a mixed inflammatory response (neutrophils, lymphocytes, and macrophages), eventually resulting in abscess or occasionally, granuloma formation. *In vitro* studies of the host defenses against *Nocardia* suggest that neutrophils, activated macrophages, and cytotoxic T cells are involved. Although neutrophils do not kill virulent *Nocardia*, they inhibit their growth, possibly suppressing the infection until macrophages are fully activated. If the infection is not contained within the lung, organisms spread to other tissues by advancing growth, producing empyema, chest wall involvement, and draining sinuses, or by hematogenous dissemination, resulting in abscess formation, especially in the brain, subcutaneous tissues, and kidneys. The primary host factor associated with an increased risk of nocardiosis is cellular immune dysfunction, although many persons infected with *Nocardia* have no recognized cellular or humoral immune defect (Wilson, 1989).

Pulmonary disease, the most frequent manifestation of nocardiosis, is characterized by fever, anorexia, weight loss, cough, dyspnea, and pleuritic chest pain. Skin and subcutaneous disease may present as pyoderma, cellulitis, single or multiple abscesses, lymphocutaneous disease resembling sporotricosis (see Chap. 52), or nodules. In Central and South America, primary infections of the skin with *N. brasiliensis* may produce an actinomycetoma (a localized indurated granulomatous mass with sinus tracts draining pus and "sulfur" granules), typically on the lower extremities. Disseminated disease is almost always caused by *N. asteroides*. It originates in the lung in most cases and typically is manifested as a single or multiple abscess involving the central nervous system. The skin is the second most common site of dissemination, followed by kidney, liver, and lymph nodes.

LABORATORY DIAGNOSIS. Specimens for diagnosis of infection with *Nocardia* vary according to the clinical presentation. For pulmonary disease, sputum, bronchoalveolar lavage fluid, material obtained by transthoracic aspiration of a nodule or abscess, or lung tissue are acceptable. For extrapulmonary disease, exudate, pus, granules, biopsy and autopsy tissue, and scrapings from ulcers should be collected; swabs are not recommended. Cerebrospinal fluid and blood specimens also may be obtained. Specimen collection, transport, and processing are discussed in Chapter 54.

Nocardia grows aerobically on sheep blood and chocolate agars, Sabouraud's dextrose agar without chloramphenicol, and Löwenstein-Jensen or Middlebrook media, and it generally survives the decontamination procedures used for recovery of mycobacteria. Incubation in the presence of 10% CO_2 enhances growth. *Nocardia* may grow in 48 hours, but colonies typically appear in five to 20 days as waxy, bumpy, or velvety rugose forms, usually with yellow to orange pigment. Observing partially acid-fast branching filaments distinguishes *Nocardia* from mycobacteria. *Nocardia* are differentiated from *Streptomyces* by testing for resistance to the action of lysozyme (*Nocardia* are resistant; *Streptomyces* are susceptible). Species of *Nocardia* are identified based on hydrolysis of casein, hypoxanthine, tyrosine, and xanthine.

ANTIMICROBIAL SUSCEPTIBILITY. Sulfonamides are the antimicrobial agents of choice for infections with *Nocardia*; trimethoprim-sulfamethoxazole also may be used. Minocycline is an acceptable alternative, and amikacin and imipenem may be effective. Actinomycetomas require therapy with two antimicrobial agents: streptomycin plus dapsone or trimethoprim-sulfamethoxazole.

6

Other Nocardioforms

Species of *Actinomadura*, *Streptomyces*, and, less commonly, *Nocardiopsis* and *Dermatophilus* may cause actinomycetomas involving the skin, mucous membranes, and subcutaneous tissue. *Oerskovia turbata* and *Oerskovia xanthineolytica* are soil saprophytes that have been recovered from cardiac valve vegetations, blood, cerebrospinal fluid, wounds, and in an individual receiving peritoneal dialysis, peritoneal fluid. *Rhodococcus equi* is an animal pathogen, widely distributed in soil, that may cause necrotizing pneumonia in humans who have diminished T-cell immunity, especially persons with the acquired immunodeficiency syndrome (Harvey, 1991). Infection usually follows exposure to animals and most likely is acquired via the respiratory route.

LABORATORY DIAGNOSIS. Species of *Actinomadura* form waxy, cerebriform, tough, membranous white, yellow, pink, or red colonies. Colonies of *Streptomyces* are dry to chalky, heaped or folded, gray-white to yellow, and have the odor of a musty basement. Cells of *Nocardiopsis* appear as zigzag chains of spores within a sheathlike structure. *Dermatophilus congolensis* forms rough colonies, initially whitish-gray and becoming orange to yellow on heart infusion agar and β-hemolytic on horse blood agar. Its branching filaments, 0.5 to 1.5 μm in diameter, divide longitudinally and transversely, forming packets of eight coccoid or cuboidal-shaped cells (or spores) that become motile.

Species of *Oerskovia* produce yellow-pigmented colonies and have many characteristics similar to those of corynebacteria, but esculin hydrolysis and motility tests, positive with *Oerskovia* and negative with most corynebacteria, may differentiate the two. *Rhodococcus equi* produces large, mucoid, pale salmon-pink colonies, and may be partially acid-fast when stained with the modified Kinyoun stain.

Gram-Negative Aerobic and Facultatively Anaerobic Rods

For strictly functional reasons, the laboratory classifies these organisms according to their manner of utilization of glucose (Fig. 48–7) and whether or not special growth factors or conditions are required.

Enterobacteriaceae

DEFINITIONS AND CHARACTERISTICS. The Enterobacteriaceae are aerobic and facultatively anaerobic, non–spore-forming, nonmotile or peritrichously flagellated, oxidase-negative, gram-negative bacilli that produce acid fermentatively from glucose and reduce nitrates to nitrites.

PATHOGENESIS AND VIRULENCE FACTORS. Endotoxins that are present within the cell walls of the Enterobacteriaceae, as well as other gram-negative bacilli, are responsible for much of the morbidity and mortality resulting from infections associated with these bacteria. Endotoxins consist of lipid and polysaccharide moieties with small amounts of amino acids. They may elicit fever, chills, hypotension, granulocytosis, thrombocytopenia, disseminated intravascular coagulation, and activation of both the classic and alternate complement pathways. Endotoxic shock is the result of gram-negative septicemia with endotoxin reacting with macrophages, leukocytes, platelets, complement, and other serum proteins to increase the blood levels of proteolytic enzymes and vasoactive substances, and resulting in pooling of blood, increased peripheral vasoconstriction, and diminution in cardiac output. It has become clear that the lethal effects of endotoxin are dependent on macrophage activation and responsiveness, and that the production of cachectin from the activated macrophage plays a major role in causing profound shock and multiple organ injury (Tracey, 1988).

Other pathogenetic factors of the Enterobacteriaceae include the K1 antigen, which is associated with a high percentage of strains of *Escherichia coli* causing neonatal meningitis; the capsule of *Klebsiella pneumoniae*, which, like that of the pneumococcus, inhibits phagocytosis; the Vi antigen of *Salmonella typhi*, which may interfere with intracellular killing of this organism; and various surface antigens, such as fimbriae, that mediate adherence of the organism to mucosal surfaces.

Plasmid-mediated factors appear to play an important role in the invasive properties of *Salmonella*, *Shigella*, and enteroinvasive strains of *E. coli*. Moreover, the heat-labile enterotoxins (LT) and heat-stable enterotoxins of *E. coli* are plasmid mediated. LT stimulates adenylate cyclase in mucosal cells of the small intestine, which, in turn, activates cyclic adenosine monophosphate (cyclic AMP), which causes secretion of fluid and electrolytes into the intestinal lumen and produces watery diarrhea. In contrast, heat-stable (ST) enterotoxins appear to activate guanylate cyclase.

The distribution of species of Enterobacteriaceae encountered in various diseases varies considerably. In the urinary tract those most frequently isolated are *E. coli*, *Proteus mirabilis*, and *Klebsiella pneumoniae*. *Providencia* occurs almost exclusively in the urinary tract and most frequently in patients with chronic indwelling catheters. Gram-negative pneumonias associated with the Enterobacteriaceae are most

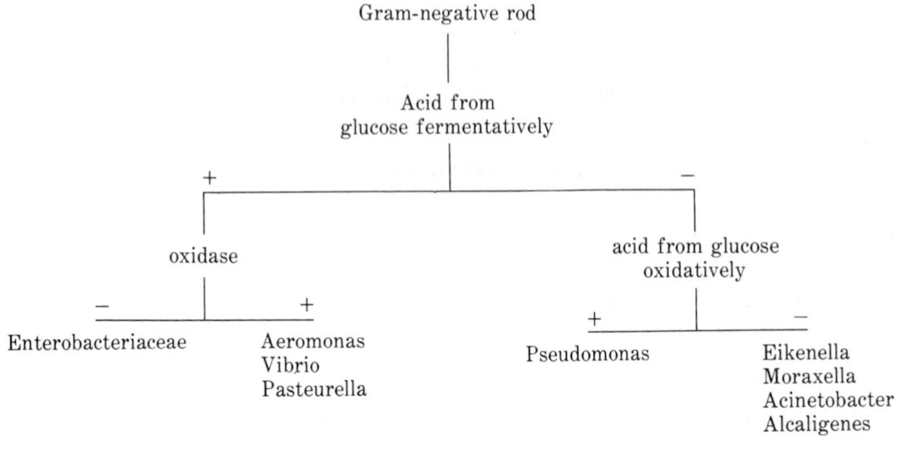

Figure 48–7. Brief functional classification of aerobic and facultatively anaerobic gram-negative bacilli growing on simple media.

frequently caused by *K. pneumoniae*. Gram-negative bacteremias related to the Enterobacteriaceae are most frequently caused by *E. coli*, *K. pneumoniae*, and *P. mirabilis*. Infections acquired in the hospital are apt to be caused by the more highly resistant groups, such as *Citrobacter*, *Enterobacter*, and *Serratia*. Enterobacteriaceae associated with diarrhea include *Shigella*, *Salmonella*, *E. coli* (enterohemorrhagic, enterotoxigenic, enteroinvasive, enteropathogenic, enteroadherent), and *Yersinia*. Shigellae are but rarely isolated from sources other than the gastrointestinal tract, while salmonellae are not infrequently isolated from other sources, such as urine or blood.

Laboratory Diagnosis

ISOLATION. The isolation of gram-negative bacilli, including the Enterobacteriaceae, is greatly facilitated by and in some instances, such as isolation from stool, requires the use of differential and selective media (Table 48–10). Eosin methylene blue (EMB) and MacConkey agar can be used interchangeably as differential media, as can xylose-lysine-deoxycholate (XLD) and Hektoen enteric (HE) agars as selective media for salmonellae and shigellae. Both XLD and HE are superior to Salmonella-Shigella (SS) agar for the isolation of enteric pathogens. Bismuth sulfite (BS) is especially useful for the detection of salmonellae in endemics or epidemics.

For specimens other than feces, a differential medium should usually be inoculated in addition to a noninhibitory, general-purpose nutrient agar medium, for example, soybean-casein digest agar with 5% sheep blood. For fecal specimens a differential medium and a selective medium should be inoculated, as well as an enrichment medium, such as selenite-F or gram-negative (GN) broth. With cultures of specimens other than feces, portions of colonies with distinct colonial morphologies should be inoculated into identification media. With cultures of feces, it is necessary only to identify colorless colonies on EMB or MacConkey agar (red on XLD and green to blue-green on HE). Salmonellae will often produce colonies with black centers owing to their production of H_2S.

IDENTIFICATION. Innumerable schemes based on the use of conventional biochemical media and of a variety of diagnostic kits and devices have been described for the identification of the Enterobacteriaceae. It is beyond the scope of this chapter to describe them all, and the reader is referred to the texts listed in the General References section at the end of the chapter or to the manuals prepared by the diagnostic kit and device manufacturers for more specific details. Differential characteristics of the Enterobacteriaceae most commonly encountered in the clinical laboratory are shown in Table 48–11.

Few laboratories prepare media for the routine identification of gram-negative bacilli today. Commercially prepared kits and devices now offer convenience and accuracy in the identification of the vast majority of isolates belonging to the Enterobacteriaceae. In some instances, kits and devices allow most Enterobacteriaceae to be identified accurately in a few hours. All commercially available kits and devices have extensive databases and, in some instances, data management systems for epidemiologic purposes. Semi-automated systems often combine the identification and antimicrobial susceptibility testing together in a single disposable unit. Examples of manual biochemical systems for the identification of gram-negative bacteria are the API 20E (API; bioMerieux Vitek, Hazelwood, MO), Pasco (Difco Laboratories, Detroit, MI), Minitek (Becton Dickinson Microbiology Systems, Cockeysville, MD), Enterotube II (Becton Dickinson), and Crystal (Becton Dickinson) (Robinson, 1995). Examples of automated systems are the Auto-Microbic System (Vitek; bioMerieux Vitek, Hazelwood, MO), AutoSCAN and AutoSCAN WalkAway (Baxter MicroSCAN Division, Sacramento, CA), Sensititre (Radiometer of America, Inc., Westlake, OH), and Sceptor System (Becton Dickinson Microbiology Systems, Cockeysville, MD). Of the automated systems, the Auto-Microbic system, or AMS, provides gram-negative rod identification in four to 18 hours; and the AutoSCAN and Sensititre systems provide both rapid and overnight gram-negative rod identification. Of the second

Table 48–10. ENTERIC DIFFERENTIAL AND SELECTIVE MEDIA

Medium	Gram-Positive Bacteriostatic Agent	Fermentable Carbohydrate	Indicator	Colony Color		Category*
				Fermenter	*Nonfermenter*	
Eosin methylene blue (EMB)	Eosin Y Methylene blue	Lactose†	Eosin Y Methylene blue	Red or black with sheen	Colorless	S, D
MacConkey	Crystal violet Bile salts	Lactose	Neutral red	Red	Colorless	S, D
Xylose-lysine-deoxycholate (XLD)	Bile salts	Xylose Lactose Sucrose	Phenol red	Yellow	Red	S, D
Hektoen enteric (HE)	Bile salts	Salicin Lactose Sucrose	Bromothymol blue	Yellow-orange	Green, blue-green	S, D
Salmonella-shigella (SS)	Bile salts	Lactose	Neutral red	Red	Colorless	S
Bismuth sulfite (BS)	Brilliant green	Glucose	Bismuth sulfite	‡	‡	S
Thiosulfate citrate Bile salts sucrose (TCBS)§	Bile salts citrate pH 8.6	Sucrose	Thymol blue Bromothymol blue	Yellow	Colorless	S, D

*D = differential, S = selective; TCBS = thiosulfate citrate bile salts.
†Levine's formulation.
‡H_2S-producing salmonellae have black colonies.
§Used for isolation of vibrios.

Table 48–11. DIFFERENTIAL CHARACTERISTICS OF THE ENTEROBACTERIACEAE MOST COMMONLY ENCOUNTERED IN THE CLINICAL LABORATORY

	Reactions Expected for							
Test	***Escherichia coli***	***Klebsiella pneumoniae***	***Klebsiella oxytoca***	***Proteus mirabilis***	***Proteus vulgaris***	***Shigella***	***Citrobacter freundii***	***Yersinia enterocolitica***
Indole	+	−	+	−	+	d	−	d
Methyl red	+	− or +	d	+	+	+	+	+
Voges-Proskauer	−	+	+	− or +	−	−	−	+ (25°C)/ − (37°C)
Citrate (Simmons)	−	+	+	d	d	−	+	− (25°C)
H_2S (TSI)	−	−	−	+	+	−	+	−
Urease	−	+	+	+	+	−	d	+
Phenylalanine deaminase	−	−	−	+	+	−	−	−
Lysine decarboxylase	+ or −	+	+	−	−	−	−	−
Arginine dihydrolase	− or +	−	−	−	−	−	d	−
Ornithine decarboxylase	d	−	−	+	−	d	− or +	+
Motility	+ or −	−	−	+*	+*	−	+	+ (25°C)/ − (37°C)
Acid produced from lactose	+	+	+	−	−	−	+ or (+)	d

+ = ≥90% positive reactions within 2 days; − = ≥90% negative reactions; (+) = positive reactions in three to seven days; + or − = reactions of most strains positive; − or + = reactions of most strains negative; d = different reactions [+, (+), or −].
*Swarm on blood and chocolate agar.

group of systems, only the AMS and AutoSCAN offer walk-away capabilities.

The selection of any one of these systems for microbial identification or antimicrobial susceptibility testing is complex and must be based on a careful analysis of test volume, personnel skills, acquisition or lease cost, expendable supplies and material costs, service contract costs, and computer interfacing capabilities. In general, accuracy of identification among these systems is very high and comparable.

CLASSIFICATION. The classification of the Enterobacteriaceae has undergone considerable revision in recent years as the result of DNA hybridization and relatedness studies by investigators at the CDC and elsewhere. Based on genetic studies, a number of new genera and species have been proposed (Brenner, 1986; Farmer, 1985; Hickman-Brenner, 1985). Because phenotypic groupings on the basis of biochemical reactions are not always consistent with their DNA relatedness, the use of tribes (e.g., Klebsielleae, Proteeae) for grouping species within the Enterobacteriaceae has been discontinued.

Historically, the genus *Salmonella* has been divided into three biochemically distinct species: *S. typhi*, *S. choleraesuis*, and *S. enteritidis*, and *Arizona* was accorded separate generic status. Since *Arizona* is very closely related to strains in the genus *Salmonella*, strains formerly reported as *Arizona hinshawii* are now reported as a serotype of the genus *Salmonella* (47:r:z). *Salmonella typhi* and *S. choleraesuis* are now reported by the CDC as *Salmonella* serotype *typhi* and as *Salmonella* serotype *choleraesuis*. *Salmonella enteritidis* is no longer treated as a species, and the designation *enteritidis* simply represents one of the many serotypes of *Salmonella*. Nonetheless, it remains convenient to artificially treat the serotype as a species (e.g., *S. typhimurium*, *S. typhi*, *S. choleraesuis*, *S. derby*). Identification of a *Salmonella* serotype requires numerous reagents and is not ordinarily carried out in clinical laboratories; however, clinical laboratories should be able to identify *S. typhi*, *S. paratyphi* A, and *S. choleraesuis* on the basis of biochemical reactions and agglutination with the appropriate *Salmonella* group–specific antisera.

Grouping of the Enterobacteriaceae is based upon the slow and granular agglutinability of the "O" antigens, which are heat-stable, somatic antigens with intergeneric cross-reactivity, antibodies to which are frequently of the IgM class. They are predominantly lipopolysaccharide in content. The "H" antigen is the heat-labile, flagellar, protein antigen, antibodies to which are predominantly IgG and agglutination with which is rapid and fluffy. This antigen provides type specificity to a strain. The Vi antigen is a heat-labile, surface or capsular, principally polysaccharide antigen of *S. typhi* that is generally associated with virulence.

Complete characterization of serotypes of salmonellae is impractical except in certain reference laboratories. It is, however, practical for clinical laboratories to test isolates for agglutination in the more commonly encountered group-specific antisera (A through E), as well as in a polyvalent grouping antiserum and Vi antiserum. Clinical laboratories should also test isolates that biochemically resemble *Shigella* for agglutination in group-specific antisera. Strains should then be submitted to a reference laboratory, usually a state health department laboratory, for serotyping for epidemiologic purposes.

Agglutinins (Widal) to *Salmonella* O (somatic) and H (flagellar) antigens may arise in the serum following typhoid immunization and current or past infections caused by salmonellae or other Enterobacteriaceae sharing common antigens. Agglutinins, on the other hand, may not arise in patients receiving effective antibiotic therapy early in the course of salmonellosis. The prevalence and diagnostic value of agglutinins, therefore, vary widely in different populations. Hence, the diagnostic value of the Widal test, particularly of a single serum sample, is quite limited, and the test should never be used without concurrent bacteriologic studies. Because of its poor sensitivity and specificity, the Widal test has been largely abandoned as a diagnostic tool in clinical laboratories in this country. The concept of a panel of "febrile agglutinin" tests for patients with fever of unknown etiology is both semantically and clinically inappropriate.

ANTIMICROBIAL SUSCEPTIBILITY. The susceptibility of the Enterobacteriaceae to various antimicrobial agents is highly variable. As a rule, therefore, clinically significant isolates require susceptibility testing to assist in their proper

Table 48–11. DIFFERENTIAL CHARACTERISTICS OF THE ENTEROBACTERIACEAE MOST COMMONLY ENCOUNTERED IN THE CLINICAL LABORATORY (*Continued*)

Reactions Expected for							
Enterobacter cloacae	***Serratia marcescens***	***Morganella morganii***	***Providencia alcalifaciens***	***Salmonella choleraesuis***	***Salmonella typhi***	***Salmonella paratyphi A***	***Salmonella subgroups 2–5***
−	−	+	+	−	−	−	−
−	+ or −	+	+	+	+	+	+
+	+	−	−	−	−	−	−
+	+	−	+	(+)	−	−	+
−	−	−	−	d	+	− or +	+
d	− or +	+	−	−	−	−	−
−	−	+	+	−	−	−	−
−	−	−	−	+	+	−	+
+	−	−	−	(+)	− or (+)	− or +	(+) or +
+	+	+	−	+	−	+	+
+	+	+ or −	+	+	+	+	+
d	−	−	−	−	−	−	−

+, = ≥90% positive reactions within 2 days; −, = ≥90% negative reactions; (+) = positive reactions in three to seven days; + or −, = reactions of most strains positive; − or +, = reactions of most strains negative; d = different reactions [+, (+), or −].

*Swarm on blood and chocolate agar.

therapy. The frequency with which chromosome- and plasmid-mediated resistance is encountered, particularly in organisms responsible for hospital-acquired infections, further diminishes the predictability of susceptibility of a given species to a particular antibiotic.

Antibiotic resistance by the Enterobacteriaceae can be related to enzymatic inactivation, to altered permeability of components of the cell wall, to an altered structural target, to an altered metabolic pathway bypassing a reaction inhibited by the drug, or to alteration of an enzyme that remains functional but is less affected by the drug.

Although usually susceptible to a variety of antimicrobial agents, nontyphoidal, uncomplicated enteric infections due to salmonellae are generally not treated with antibiotics, because such therapy may actually prolong the carrier state. Infections caused by susceptible strains of *Salmonella typhi* are preferentially treated with chloramphenicol, despite this organism's susceptibility to other agents. Therapy with amoxicillin, ampicillin, or co-trimoxazole should be used in instances of chloramphenicol resistance.

It is desirable to treat patients with shigellosis in order to eliminate as rapidly as possible shedding of the organism in feces. Because the frequency of resistance of shigellae to ampicillin and other antimicrobial agents in several parts of the United States has increased, susceptibility testing should be done. While ampicillin remains the drug of choice for the treatment of susceptible strains, co-trimoxazole is a satisfactory alternative for ampicillin-resistant strains.

Oxidase-Positive Glucose Fermenters of Medical Significance

Vibrio

DEFINITIONS AND CHARACTERISTICS. Vibrios are facultatively anaerobic, oxidase-positive, short, curved, or straight gram-negative bacilli that are usually motile by means of polar flagella, ferment carbohydrates, and reduce nitrates to nitrites. Several species are medically important (Table 48–12).

PATHOGENESIS AND VIRULENCE FACTORS. Cholera manifests itself by massive intestinal fluid loss secondary to stimulation of the adenyl cyclase system of cells in the small intestine with production of cyclic AMP (Kaper, 1995). In this respect the enterotoxin acts in a manner similar to that of the heat-labile toxin of *Escherichia coli.* The mechanism of pathogenicity of *Vibrio parahaemolyticus* appears to be related to invasiveness rather than to enterotoxin production. Over 95% of isolates of *V. parahaemolyticus* isolated from patients with gastroenteritis produce a cell-free hemolysin that is lethal to mice when injected in high doses and is described as the Kanagawa phenomenon. This halophilic organism is widely distributed in marine environments and has been found to contaminate fish and shellfish. Outbreaks of acute diarrheal disease following ingestion of contaminated food have been especially common in Japan but have also occurred in the United States and other countries. Wound infections and septicemias have been associated with noncholera halophilic vibrios, such as *V. vulnificus*, especially in persons with liver disease (Morris, 1985).

LABORATORY DIAGNOSIS. Although formerly of concern only to U.S. travelers to endemic areas, cases of *V. cholerae* have recently been described in this country in association with the ingestion of contaminated shellfish from the Gulf Coast. In addition, gastroenteritis caused by *V. parahaemolyticus* and other halophilic vibrios in contaminated shellfish has been described in many areas of the country, particularly in coastal areas. Thus, it is important for clinical laboratories to have the capability of culturing stool for vibrios. With the exception of *V. cholerae* and *V. mimicus*, growth of vibrios is stimulated by Na^+. Stool specimens may be transported in Cary-Blair medium but not in buffered glycerol saline transport medium. Cultures on a selective medium should be made on the basis of travel and dietary history. Thiosulfate citrate bile salts (TCBS) medium is the most widely used and convenient selective medium available for cultivation of vibrios. There is sufficient Na^+ in blood and in most solid agar media used to culture blood and wounds for the isolation of the invasive halophilic vibrios so that the use of TCBS in

6

Table 48–12. DIFFERENTIAL CHARACTERISTICS OF *VIBRIO* SPECIES

	Vibrio								
Test	***V. cholerae***	***V. mimicus***	***V. damsela***	***V. parahaemolyticus***	***V. alginolyticus***	***V. vulnificus***	***V. fluvialis***	***V. metschnikovii***	***V. hollisae***
Indole	+	+	−	+ or −	d	+	− or +	d	+
Voges-Proskauer	− or +	−	+	−	+	−	−	+	−
Lysine decarboxylase	+	+	+	+	+	+	−	d	−
Ornithine decarboxylase	+	+	−	+ or −	d	d	−	−	−
Arginine dihydrolase	−	−	+	−	−	−	+	d	−
Lactose	(+)	− or +	−	−	−	+	−	d	−
Sucrose	+	+	−	+	+	d	+	+	−
Mannitol	+	+	−	+	+	d	+	+	−
Maltose	+	+	+	+	+	+	+	+	−
Arabinose	−	−	−	+ or −	−	−	+	−	+
Salicin	−	−	−	−	−	+	−	− or +	−
Cellobiose	−	−	−	−	−	+	d	− or +	−
$NO_3 \rightarrow NO_2$	+	+	+	+	+	+	+	−	+
Oxidase	+	+	+	+	+	+	+	−	+
Growth in nutrient broth plus NaCl (%)									
0	+	+	−	−	−	−	W + or −	−	−
1	+	+	+	+	+	+	+	+	+
6	− or (+)	− or (+)	+	+	+	+	+	+	(+)
8	−	−	−	+	+	−	−	d	−
10	−	−	−	−	+	−	−	d	−
12	−	−	−	−	−	−	−	−	−

*For key to symbols, see Table 48–11; W+ = weakly positive.

such instances is not necessary. TCBS should not be autoclaved, and its final pH should be 8.4. An enrichment broth, such as alkaline peptone water, should also be inoculated and subcultured within six to 12 hours on a second set of TCBS plates. Yellow colonies on TCBS (caused by sucrose fermentation) should be selected for further study with biochemical and serologic tests. The vibrios can be differentiated among themselves and from other enteric gram-negative bacilli according to reactions listed in Table 48–12. It may be necessary to carry out biochemical testing of the halophilic vibrios in media supplemented with 1% to 3% NaCl. If triple sugar iron agar (TSIA) and lysine iron agar (LIA) are inoculated for screening purposes, their reactions will be acid slant/acid butt with no gas (A/A−) or H_2S and alkaline slant/alkaline butt (K/K), respectively. Agglutination of a saline suspension of the organism by polyvalent antiserum against *V. cholerae* should occur within a minute if the organism is present.

ANTIMICROBIAL SUSCEPTIBILITY. *Vibrio cholerae* and the noncholera halophilic vibrios are susceptible to a variety of agents, including tetracyclines, chloramphenicol, ampicillin, cephalosporins, and trimethoprim-sulfamethoxazole. *Vibrio parahaemolyticus* is resistant to the penicillins but is otherwise susceptible to the other agents that are active against *V. cholerae*.

Aeromonas

DEFINITIONS AND CHARACTERISTICS. Members of this genus are facultatively anaerobic, oxidase- and catalase-positive, rod-shaped, gram-negative bacilli. They are motile by means of polar flagella, and they form acids from carbohydrates by respiratory and fermentative metabolism. The classification of *Aeromonas* species is not definitively established. Of the 13 named species within the genus *Aeromonas*, six (*A. hydrophila*, *A. caviae*, *A. veronii*, *A. jandaei*, *A. schubertii*, and *A. trota*) have been linked to human disease (Janda, 1991; Hickman-Brenner, 1987, 1988).

PATHOGENESIS AND VIRULENCE FACTORS. *Aeromonas* has been isolated from tap water, rivers, soil, marine animals, and various foods. It has been isolated from feces of healthy persons and from patients with diarrheal disease of otherwise unexplained origin. Its role in producing diarrheal disease is possibly related to the production of an enterotoxin by some strains. A hemolysin and a cytopathic factor have also been described. Further questions about the pathogenic role of *Aeromonas* in causing gastroenteritis have been raised because of the failure of the organism to cause disease in human volunteers.

Aeromonas may cause infection of traumatically acquired wounds that are contaminated with soil or water, diarrhea, or septicemia in patients who are immunocompromised (Janda, 1991, 1994).

LABORATORY DIAGNOSIS. The isolation of a fermenting, oxidase-positive, gram-negative bacillus should suggest strongly the possibility of *Aeromonas*. It grows readily on conventional laboratory media and produces colonies that resemble those of *Pseudomonas*, have a greenish ground glass appearance, and give off a fruity odor. The isolation of *Aeromonas* from stool specimens may be enhanced by inoculation of blood agar containing ampicillin or of cefsulodin-irgasan-novobiocin (CIN) medium.

ANTIMICROBIAL SUSCEPTIBILITY. *Aeromonas* is susceptible to the quinolones, third-generation cephalosporins, aminoglycosides, chloramphenicol, and tetracyclines but produces a β-lactamase mediating resistance to the penicillins and first-generation cephalosporins. *Aeromonas* has been found to maintain R plasmids of both the Enterobacteriaceae and *Pseudomonas*.

Plesiomonas

DEFINITIONS AND CHARACTERISTICS. *Plesiomonas shigelloides*, the only species in the genus *Plesiomonas*, is a facultatively anaerobic, oxidase- and catalase-positive, glucose-fermenting, gram-negative rod.

PATHOGENESIS AND VIRULENCE FACTORS. *Plesiomonas shigelloides* causes gastroenteritis, frequently following the ingestion of uncooked shellfish. The diarrheal stool specimen frequently contains polymorphonuclear leukocytes and red blood cells, although a cholera-like illness may also occur. Gastroenteritis may occur in sporadic cases, as well as in outbreaks. Extraintestinal manifestations of infection with *P. shigelloides* include meningitis, septicemia, cellulitis, arthritis, and endophthalmitis.

Relatively little is known about virulence factors of *P. shigelloides* as yet. The organism appears to have invasive properties and there are some data suggesting enterotoxigenic activity (Brenden, 1988).

LABORATORY DIAGNOSIS. *Plesiomonas shigelloides* can be isolated on a variety of nonselective and enteric selective media, including Hektoen enteric agar. Acid production from lactose is variable, but on enteric media the organism usually appears to be a nonlactose fermenter. It is indole positive, reduces nitrates to nitrites, produces catalase, is methyl red positive, and ferments glucose, maltose, and trehalose (Brenden, 1988).

ANTIMICROBIAL SUSCEPTIBILITY. *Plesiomonas shigelloides* is susceptible to a variety of antimicrobial agents, including aminoglycosides, trimethoprim-sulfamethoxazole, chloramphenicol, tetracyclines, and the quinolones. Susceptibility to the penicillins is variable owing to a β-lactamase similar to that of *Aeromonas*.

Pasteurella

DEFINITIONS AND CHARACTERISTICS. The pasteurellae are facultatively anaerobic, oxidase- and catalase-positive, nonmotile gram-negative bacteria that may range morphologically from coccobacilli to long filamentous rods. Of the eight species recognized (*P. multocida*, *P. pneumotropica*, *P. haemolytica*, *P. gallinarum*, *P. bettii*, *P. dagmatis*, *P. canis*, and *P. aerogenes*), *P. multocida* is the most important human pathogen.

PATHOGENESIS AND VIRULENCE FACTORS. Encapsulated strains are usually pathogenic for mice, and virulence has been found to be enhanced by free iron in various forms. The cell wall contains endotoxin but no exotoxin has been identified.

The pasteurellae are indigenous to many animals and are isolated frequently from wounds resulting from animal bites or scratches. Local infections can become systemic, and there have been a number of reports of septicemia, osteomyelitis, and meningitis. Pasteurellae have been associated with respiratory tract infections, including sinusitis, peritonsillar abscess, mastoiditis, pulmonary abscess, pneumonia, empyema, bronchitis, and bronchiectasis, usually in patients with chronic pulmonary disease.

LABORATORY DIAGNOSIS. Pasteurellae grow well on blood agar but are, with the exception of *P. haemolytica*, unable to grow on gram-negative differential agar media, such as eosin methylene blue (EMB) or MacConkey agar. The finding of a gram-negative bacillus that grows on blood agar only and is oxidase- and indole-positive and ONPG-negative strongly constitutes presumptive evidence for the isolation of *P. multocida*, the most frequently encountered species.

ANTIMICROBIAL SUSCEPTIBILITY. Characteristic of *P. multocida* is its susceptibility to penicillin G. Other agents with excellent activity *in vitro* against the organism include the cephalosporins and tetracyclines.

Glucose Oxidizers

Pseudomonas *and Related Organisms*

DEFINITIONS AND CHARACTERISTICS. Pseudomonads are strictly aerobic, catalase-positive, oxidase-positive, gram-negative bacilli. Their metabolism is respiratory and never fermentative, and they are motile by polar flagella. *Pseudomonas aeruginosa* is the nonfermenter most commonly isolated in the clinical laboratory, accounting for about 75% of all nonfermenters encountered. *Pseudomonas pseudomallei*, which causes melioidosis, and *Pseudomonas mallei*, which causes glanders, have recently been placed in the genus *Burkholderia*, as has *Pseudomonas cepacia*, a significant pulmonary pathogen in patients with cystic fibrosis. Numerous other species have been isolated from clinical specimens and have been associated with a variety of opportunistic infections. *Pseudomonas maltophilia* was renamed *Xanthomonas maltophilia*, and now is called *Stenotrophomonas maltophilia*. Based on genetic studies, the *Pseudomonas* species have been divided into various RNA homology groups (Gilardi, 1991). RNA group 1 comprises the Fluorescens group, including *P. aeruginosa*, *P. fluorescens*, and *P. putida*. The Stutzeri group includes *P. stutzeri* and *P. mendocina*. The Alcaligenes group consists of *P. alcaligenes*, *P. pseudoalcaligenes*, and an as yet unspecified group. RNA group 2, which has been placed in the genus *Burkholderia*, comprises the Pseudomallei group, including *B. mallei*, *B. pseudomallei*, *B. cepacia*, *B. gladioli*, and *B. pickettii*. RNA group 3 comprises the Acidovorans group, now in the genus *Commamonas*, including *C. acidovorans*, *C. testosteroni*, and *C. terrigena*, and the Facilis-Delafieldii group with *Acidovorax delafieldii*, *A. facilis*, and *A. temperans*. RNA group 4 comprises the Diminuta group, which includes *Brevundimonas diminuta* and *B. vesiculare*. RNA group 5 includes *Stenotrophomonas maltophilia*. Additional species of uncertain affiliation include *Sphingomonas paucimobilis*, *Schwanella putrefaciens*, and various unspecified groups.

Because the pseudomonads are very adaptable and can use a large number of organic compounds for growth, they are essentially free living and can be found in a tremendous variety of habitats. Moreover, they are more resistant to antiseptic agents and disinfectants than most vegetative forms of bacteria.

PATHOGENESIS AND VIRULENCE FACTORS. The species causing the greatest morbidity and mortality today is *P. aeruginosa*. It is nearly ubiquitous in the hospital environment, existing almost anywhere there is any moisture. The organism is more resistant than most vegetative bacteria to many disinfectants and antimicrobial agents. It produces a variety of enzymes and toxins, in addition to a slime polysaccharide, an endotoxin, and proteases that inactivate components of complement, thereby inhibiting to some degree opsonization and the inflammatory response and perhaps contributing to its invasiveness. Exotoxin A promotes cellular damage and tissue invasion and is toxic for macrophages. The organism produces infection in patients with burn, traumatic, and operative wounds; following urinary tract manipulation; in patients with diseases of the hematopoietic, reticuloendothelial, and lymphoid systems; and in those with impaired cellular or humoral defenses. Pulmonary infection occurs commonly in patients with cystic fibrosis. The mortality rate is highest in severely leukopenic (<1000 PMN/cu mm) patients.

Burkholderia pseudomallei is endemic in Southeast Asia, where asymptomatic or subclinical infection is frequent. A pulmonary form resembling tuberculosis or a mycotic infection occurs less frequently and has a relatively good prognosis. Its septicemic form is highly lethal.

Burkholderia mallei causes glanders in horses, which may present as an acute fulminating and frequently fatal septicemic form, as an acute pneumonia with or without septicemia, as an acute or chronic suppurative infection, as a latent infection with eventual acute manifestations of the disease, or in an occult form with encapsulated nodules in various organs and especially the lungs.

Other species of *Pseudomonas*, although often isolated from clinical specimens, are only occasionally involved in disease.

LABORATORY DIAGNOSIS. The presence of *P. aeruginosa* in cultures can often be suspected because of its musty grapelike odor, the rough or ground glass appearance of its colonies, and the presence of pigment or metallic sheen in its colonies. Its identification can be made easily with a positive oxidase reaction, an alkaline slant/neutral butt reaction in triple sugar iron agar (TSIA), growth at 42°C, and the formation of sheen and/or pigment on the slants of TSIA and *Pseudomonas* P agar. If all of these reactions do not occur, additional tests should be performed (Table 48–13). Tests of carbohydrate utilization should be carried out in O-F basal medium, which contains a minimal quantity of peptone and a relatively large quantity of carbohydrate and which will provide detection of the very small quantities of acid formed by this group of bacteria. Reactions are usually complete within 48 hours but may require as long as seven days in some instances.

ANTIMICROBIAL SUSCEPTIBILITY. As a general rule, *P. aeruginosa* is susceptible to gentamicin, tobramycin, and amikacin. Most isolates are also susceptible to carboxy- and ureidopenicillins. Hospital epidemics of strains resistant to gentamicin and tobramycin have, however, occurred owing to aminoglycoside acetylating and adenylylating enzymes. Resistance to antipseudomonadal penicillins may also occur, owing to R plasmid–mediated β-lactamase. Serious infections, particularly those in the lower respiratory tract, are usually treated with a combination of an aminoglycoside and an expanded-spectrum penicillin or ceftazidime.

The susceptibility of *P. aeruginosa* to aminoglycosides is affected by the presence of cation in the testing medium. Production lots of Mueller-Hinton agar are subjected to quality control by comparison with a reference lot of Mueller-Hinton agar. Mueller-Hinton broth should be adjusted to contain 20 to 25 mg/L of calcium and 10 to 12.5 mg/L of magnesium. Laboratory personnel should not routinely supplement Mueller-Hinton broth with cation unless the cation content of the medium is known to begin with. In many instances, manufacturers are adjusting cation content of Mueller-Hinton broth so that routine supplementation will result in an excessive amount of cation in the medium and false resistance to aminoglycosides.

The susceptibility of other species related to *Pseudomonas* varies considerably. *Burkholderia cepacia* is usually resistant to aminoglycosides but is often susceptible to chloramphenicol and trimethoprim-sulfamethoxazole. Many isolates of *Stenotrophomonas maltophilia* are resistant to aminoglycosides, but they are more frequently inhibited by gentamicin than by amikacin or tobramycin.

Burkholderia pseudomallei is usually susceptible to tetracycline, chloramphenicol, sulfonamides, and trimethoprim-sulfamethoxazole but not to penicillins, cephalosporins, polymyxins, or aminoglycosides. Antimicrobial susceptibility data on *B. mallei* are limited owing to the eradication of glanders in many parts of the world; however, sulfonamides have generally been considered to represent the agents of choice in the treatment of the disease.

Acinetobacter

DEFINITIONS AND CHARACTERISTICS. Organisms in this genus are rod shaped, sometimes nearly spherical, nonmotile, oxidase negative, strictly aerobic, and gram negative. Their metabolism is oxidative and those that form acid from carbohydrates do so by oxidation of aldehyde groups to produce aldobionic acids. Such organisms lack β-galactosidase and are, therefore, ONPG negative.

The taxonomy and nomenclature of these organisms have been in a state of turmoil for years. Currently *Acinetobacter baumannii, A. calcoaceticus, A. lwoffi, A. haemolyticus, A. johnsonii, a. junii*, and several unnamed species are recognized (Gerner-Smidt, 1991).

PATHOGENESIS AND VIRULENCE FACTORS. *Acinetobacter* is commonly found in soil and water, and uncommonly found on the skin and mucous membranes of healthy people. Little is known about virulence factors in this group of organisms, but they do appear to form small amounts of endotoxin. Although usually nonpathogenic, they have been associated with increasing frequency with nosocomial septicemia, pneumonia, bacteriuria, and wound infection.

LABORATORY DIAGNOSIS. *Acinetobacter* can be distinguished readily from the pseudomonads on the basis of its lack of motility, inability to reduce nitrates, and its negative oxidase reaction. Differentiation of glucose-oxidizing species may be difficult; such isolates should be called *A. calcoaceticus-baumannii* complex (Gerner-Smidt, 1991).

ANTIMICROBIAL SUSCEPTIBILITY. *Acinetobacter* species are resistant to most available β-lactam and aminoglycoside antibiotics. Resistance to the aminoglycosides is caused by plasmid-mediated acetyl-, adenylyl-, and phosphotransferases. *Acinetobacter* may be susceptible to minocycline, trimethoprim-sulfamethoxazole, quinolones, ureidopenicillins, imipenem, and ceftazidime.

Table 48–13. DIFFERENTIAL CHARACTERISTICS OF PSEUDOMONADS ISOLATED FROM CLINICAL MATERIAL

Test	*P. aeruginosa*	*P. fluorescens*	*P. putida*	*S. maltophilia*	*P. stutzeri*	*B. cepacia*[a]	*P. alcaligenes*	*P. diminuta*	*B. mallei*	*B. pseudomallei*	*S. paucimobilis*	*S. putrefaciens*
Oxidase	+	+	+	−	+	+	+	+	+	+	+	+
Decarboxylase												
Lysine	−	−	−	+	−	+	−	−	−	−	−	−
Ornithine	−	−	−	−	−	− or +	−	−	−	−	−	+
Arginine dihydrolase	+	+	+	−	−	−	− or +	−	+	+	−	−
Acid (oxidatively) from												
Glucose	+	+	+	+ or (+)	+	+	−	−	+	+	+	d
Maltose	−	− or +	− or +	+	+	+	−	−	(+)	+	+	d
Xylose	+ or −	+	+	+ or −	+	+	−	−	−	+ or −	+	−
Denitrification	+ or gas	− or +	−	−	+	− or +	+ or −	−	−	+ or −	−	+
Deoxyribonuclease	− or +	−	−	+	−	−	−	− or +	−	−	−	+
Fluorescein	+	+	+ or −	−	−	−	−	−	−	−	−	−
Pyocyanin	+	−	−	−	−	−	−	−	−	−	−	−
Growth at 42°C	+	−	−	+	+	+ or −	+ or −	− or +	−	+	−	d
Flagella (no.)	1	>1	>1	>1	1	>1	1	1	0	>1	1	1

[a]Yellow-pigmented colonies.
For key to symbols, see Table 48–11.

6

Gram-Negative Aerobic and Facultatively Anaerobic Rods Requiring Special Growth Factors or Conditions

Moraxella *and* Oligella

Moraxella are normal flora in the upper respiratory tract and on the skin of humans and animals. *Oligella urethralis* (formerly *Moraxella urethralis*) is part of the normal flora of the human genitourinary tract. These organisms generally are considered nonpathogens, contaminants, or organisms with low pathogenic potential, but they may cause serious disease, including pericarditis, lung abscesses, osteomyelitis, ocular infections, pyoderma, urogenital tract disease, sinusitis, endocarditis, meningitis, and septicemia.

On sheep blood agar, colonies of *Moraxella* and *Oligella* are small (< 0.5 mm in diameter) after 24 hours, and on MacConkey agar growth is poor. In smears stained with Gram's stain, bacterial cells appear as cocci or small bacilli in pairs, occasionally resembling *Neisseria* (described earlier). To distinguish between *Neisseria* and *Moraxella*, a smear of growth from the outer zone of inhibition around a penicillin susceptibility disk is stained with Gram's stain and examined; cells of *Moraxella* are elongated and pleomorphic, whereas cells of *Neisseria* retain their coccal forms. *Moraxella* and *Oligella urethralis* are oxidase positive, catalase positive, asaccharolytic, and nonmotile, and most isolates are sensitive to low concentrations of penicillin.

Campylobacter *and* Helicobacter

DEFINITIONS AND CHARACTERISTICS. The species of *Campylobacter* and *Helicobacter* are small (0.5 to 8 μm long by 0.2 to 0.5 μm wide), motile, non–spore-forming, curved (comma-shaped) or S-shaped gram-negative bacilli that grow optimally in an atmosphere containing 5% to 10% oxygen and, therefore, are considered microaerophilic. *Campylobacter jejuni*, the most common cause of gastroenteritis in the United States, is the predominant human pathogen. Other species of *Campylobacter* associated with enteritis are *C. lari*, *C. coli*, *C. hyointestinalis*, *C. upsaliensis*, and *Arcobacter butzleri* (formerly *Campylobacter butzleri*). *Campylobacter fetus* subspecies *fetus* is a cause of septic thrombophlebitis, arthritis, peritonitis, abscesses, and pericarditis (Penner, 1988), especially in persons with an underlying chronic disease. A highly significant relationship between *Helicobacter pylori* and chronic gastritis exists. Infection with *H. pylori* also has been associated with nonulcer dyspepsia, duodenal ulcers, gastric carcinoma, and gastric lymphoma (Murray, 1993; Parsonnet, 1991, 1994).

PATHOGENESIS AND VIRULENCE FACTORS. *Campylobacter jejuni* is found worldwide as a commensal of the gastrointestinal tract of wild or domesticated cattle, sheep, swine, goats, dogs, cats, and fowl, especially turkeys and chickens. Most human infections with *C. jejuni* are acquired by consuming contaminated food (especially undercooked poultry) and water. Several outbreaks of *C. jejuni* enteritis have been linked to unpasteurized milk and to defects in municipal water systems. Factors that determine whether infection with *C. jejuni* results in disease are the dose of organisms reaching the small intestine (ingestion of less than 10^4 organisms rarely induces disease) and the specific immunity of the host. The organism produces a cytotoxin and an enterotoxin, but their *in vivo* significance is unknown.

The major habit of *C. fetus* subsp. *fetus* is the intestine of sheep and cattle; it also may be found in the genital tract of these animals, their placentas, the gastric contents of their aborted fetuses, and less frequently, in other animals and birds. The mechanisms of transmission of infection to humans are not understood completely. Direct contact with an infected animal is possible, but fewer than one third of infected individuals have a history of environmental or occupational exposure. Contaminated food or water may be a vehicle for infection, or infection may originate from an endogenous source.

Helicobacter pylori occurs worldwide, but the reservoir of infection and its mechanism of transmission are unknown. The prevalence of gastritis associated with *H. pylori* increases with age, suggesting that the organism is acquired as people become older.

LABORATORY DIAGNOSIS. *Campylobacter fetus* subsp. *fetus* can be readily isolated from blood culture media, thioglycolate medium, or any peptone-yeast extract medium. Because it requires a lower concentration of oxygen than is present in air, growth of this organism is unlikely to occur on solid media under conventional incubation conditions.

The isolation of *C. jejuni* from fecal material is strictly dependent upon the use of a selective medium or filtration (see Chap. 54), a microaerophilic atmosphere of incubation, and incubation at 42°C. Selective media containing a variety of antibiotics, usually including vancomycin, polymyxin B, trimethoprim, and a cephalosporin, are commercially available for this purpose.

In some cases, visualization of curved rods with a characteristic corkscrew type of motility upon direct darkfield or phase-contrast microscopic examination of the feces offers a rapid means of detecting *C. jejuni*. The isolation of catalase- and oxidase-positive, small, slender, curved, motile, gram-negative bacillus from a selective medium incubated at 42°C constitutes strong presumptive evidence of *C. jejuni*. Confirmation can be made simply by demonstrating that the organism hydrolyzes hippurate and is susceptible to nalidixic acid and resistant to cephalothin. Strains of *C. fetus* subsp. *fetus* are resistant to nalidixic acid, fail to hydrolyze hippurate, and do not ordinarily grow at 42°C.

Helicobacter pylori may be visualized microscopically in stained sections of gastric biopsy. Because the organism hydrolyzes urea very rapidly, a portion of the gastric biopsy may be placed directly into urea broth and a presumptive diagnosis can be made very rapidly with evidence of urea hydrolysis. *Helicobacter pylori* can also be isolated on a variety of media, including brain-heart infusion agar containing 5% to 10% sheep or horse blood, chocolate agar, Thayer-Martin medium, and selective media that are used to isolate *C. jejuni* but that lack a cephalosporin. Inoculated media should be incubated in a microaerophilic atmosphere under high humidity at 35°C. Serologic tests are also available.

ANTIMICROBIAL SUSCEPTIBILITY. Both *C. fetus* subsp. *fetus* and *C. jejuni* are usually susceptible to aminoglycosides, chloramphenicol, clindamycin, and erythromycin. Penicillins are usually poorly active. Approximately 5% to 10% of strains are resistant to tetracyclines. Although

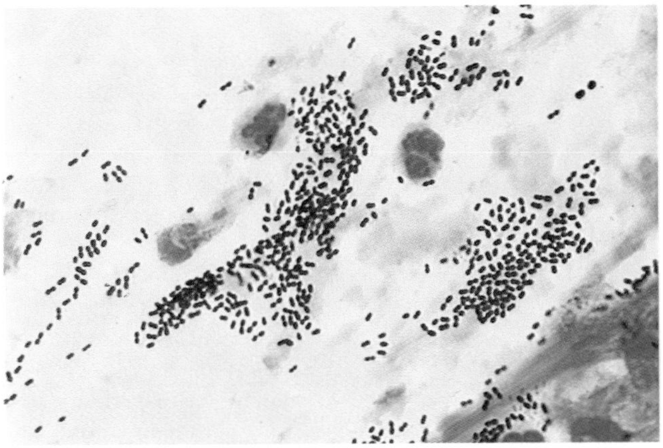

Plate 48–1. Gram's stain of a sputum smear shows neutrophils, debris, and gram-positive diplococci, suggestive of pneumococcal infection (oil immersion).

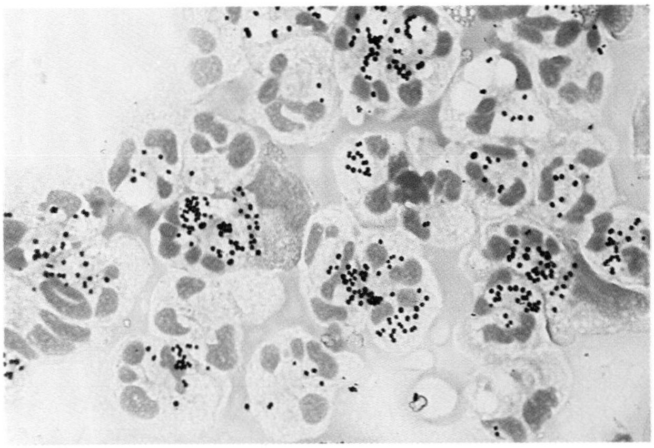

Plate 48–2. Cytocentrifuge preparation of cerebrospinal fluid stained with Gram's stain shows many neutrophils, smooth amorphous material, and gram-positive cocci in pairs, short chains, and groups, suggestive of staphylococcal infection (oil immersion).

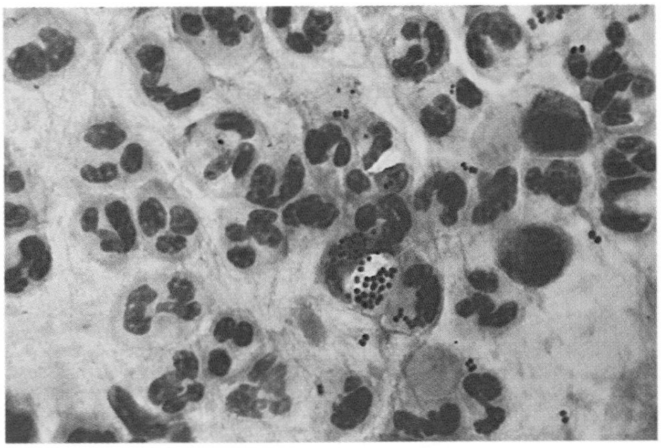

Plate 48–3. Sputum smear stained with Gram's stain shows many neutrophils and intracellular gram negative diplococci, suggestive of *Moraxella catarrhalis* infection (oil immersion).

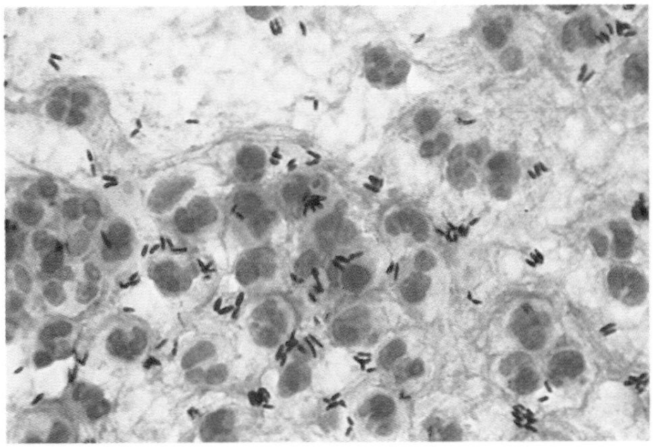

Plate 48–4. Sputum stained with Gram's stain shows many neutrophils, amorphous debris, and coryneform gram-positive bacilli (oil immersion).

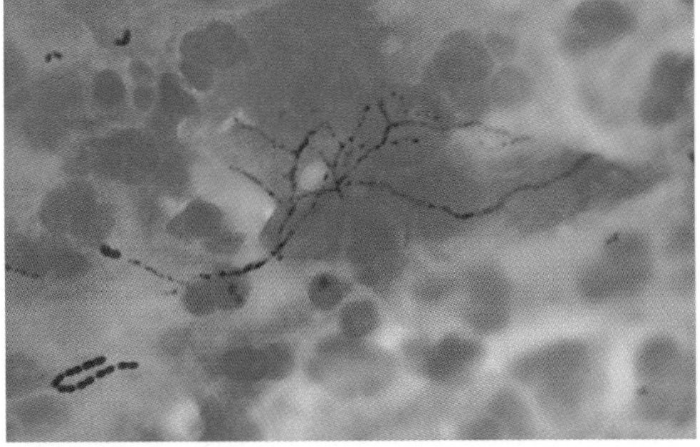

Plate 48–5. Sputum smear stained with Gram's stain shows neutrophils, amorphous debris, and filamentous, beaded, branched gram-positive bacilli (oil immersion).

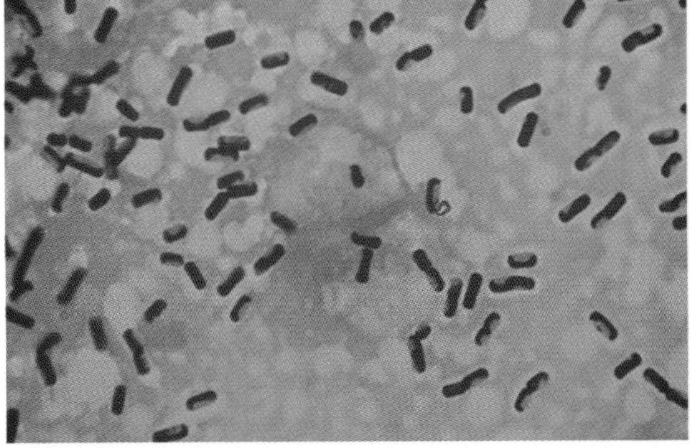

Plate 48–6. Gram's stain of a smear of exudate from a wound that had gas bubbles shows large, boxcar-shaped gram-positive bacilli, suggestive of clostridial disease (oil immersion).

often self-limited, diarrhea caused by *C. jejuni* may persist or recur; therefore, erythromycin treatment is usually advised in such cases.

The therapy of *H. pylori* gastritis has not yet been well established. Patients frequently respond to the administration of bismuth; however, antibiotics may be necessary to prevent recurrence.

Brucella

DEFINITIONS AND CHARACTERISTICS. Brucellae are small, gram-negative coccobacillary, nonmotile, strictly aerobic, and catalase- and usually oxidase-positive rods. Growth is often enhanced by the presence of 5% to 10% CO_2. Although growth may occur on ordinary media, it is usually optimal on a soybean-casein digest agar (trypticase soy, tryptic soy, tryptone soya, etc.) or in its liquid counterpart. Of the recognized species, *Brucella melitensis*, *B. abortus*, *B. suis*, and *B. canis* are those of medical importance in humans.

PATHOGENESIS AND VIRULENCE FACTORS. The preferential hosts for brucellae are sheep and goats for *B. melitensis*, cattle for *B. abortus*, swine for *B. suis*, and dogs for *B. canis*; however, each species may occasionally infect other animals. Infection is acquired by humans by direct contact with infected material, including animal carcasses, fetal membranes, vaginal discharges, fetuses, skin, or mucous membranes, as well as by ingestion of unpasteurized milk or milk products from infected animals. Local lymphadenopathy often occurs with dissemination and secondary localization in the reticuloendothelial system and formation of granulomas in the liver, spleen, bone, genitourinary tract, lungs, and soft tissues. Organisms may be seen within phagocytes.

Signs and symptoms are often variable and nonspecific, with chills, fever, sweats, and anorexia occurring frequently. The fever is characteristically diurnal ("undulant"). Diagnosis of the disease beyond the acute bacteremic phase is difficult to establish.

The most common sources of infection in the United States in recent years are cattle and swine for individuals working in packing plants and goat cheese for persons who have a history of recent travel to Mexico. Infections caused by *B. canis* have been acquired predominantly by contact with infected dogs or by accidental exposure to cultures of the organism in laboratories.

LABORATORY DIAGNOSIS. Blood cultures in a biphasic bottle (Castaneda technique) containing soybean-casein digest medium or in the media used with the currently available automated systems (see Chap. 54) have been shown to be highly effective in detecting the presence of bacteremia in the early stages of brucellosis. Other normally sterile body fluids should be concentrated by filtration through a 0.45 μm membrane filter that is then placed onto a soybean-casein digest blood agar plate for culture. Tissue should be minced and then ground with a sterile abrasive in broth to produce a 20% suspension that is then inoculated onto the appropriate medium. Cultures should be incubated in an atmosphere containing 5% to 10% CO_2 and should be retained for three or four weeks before being discarded as negative. Blood cultures in Castaneda bottles should be tipped twice weekly so that the blood-broth mixture flows over the agar surface.

Colonies of *Brucella* appear slowly and may initially be very small and difficult to see. A rapid test for presumptive identification of *Brucella* species is particle agglutination with antismooth *Brucella* antiserum.

Urease activity is manifested rapidly (about 15 minutes) by *B. suis* and more slowly (2 to 24 hours) by *B. melitensis* and *B. abortus*. Monospecific antisera can be used to distinguish between the *B. abortus–B. suis* complex and *B. melitensis*; however, such antisera are not widely available. Classically, growth in the presence of thionin and basic fuchsin has been used for speciation of *Brucella*; however, this technique does not clearly differentiate among the species, and it is suggested that isolates suspected of being *Brucella* be sent to a state health laboratory for confirmation and specific identification.

The diagnosis of brucellosis is most often made serologically. A minimum titer of 1 : 160 in a standard tube agglutination test should lead one to suspect the diagnosis; however, evidence of recent brucellosis can be accepted only when a fourfold or greater rise in titer occurs during the first month or two of illness. Inhibitory prozones can occur in patients with titers as high as 1 : 640 so that all sera from patients with suspected disease should be diluted to at least 1 : 1280. Cross-reactivity with *Francisella tularensis* and with *Vibrio cholerae*, including cholera vaccination, occurs. The tube agglutination test is very sensitive and yields the most standardized results, in contrast to the more rapid slide agglutination tests, which may give both falsely positive and falsely negative results.

ANTIMICROBIAL SUSCEPTIBILITY. The drugs of choice in the treatment of brucellosis are tetracycline, with or without streptomycin, or trimethoprim-sulfamethoxazole.

Bordetella

DEFINITIONS AND CHARACTERISTICS. Bordetellae are strictly aerobic, nonfermentative, minute coccobacilli requiring nicotinic acid, cysteine, and usually methionine but not hemin (X factor) or coenzyme I (V factor) for growth. Excess fatty acids are formed during growth and are inhibitory to further growth so that blood, charcoal, starch, or ion-exchange resins must be added to the medium to act as an adsorbent. Phase variation from smooth virulent strains to rough avirulent strains occurs after cultivation on artificial media.

PATHOGENESIS AND VIRULENCE FACTORS. The proposed pathogenetic sequence of infection caused by *Bordetella pertussis* has been reviewed by Friedman (1988). The organism attaches to the ciliated epithelium of the respiratory tract, multiplies, and releases toxins with a variety of proposed effects that result, though not necessarily in sequence, in inflammation and epithelial necrosis, leukocytosis and lymphocytosis, accumulation of secretions, cough, and ultimately bronchopneumonia, hypoxic episodes, and encephalopathy. *Bordetella pertussis* contains a protective antigen that when combined with antibody abolishes its infectivity. It appears, however, that both cellular and humoral immunity are needed to eradicate the organism.

Bordetella parapertussis may infrequently cause a pertussis-like illness. *Bordetella bronchiseptica*, on the other hand, is isolated from humans after contact with guinea pigs, rabbits, dogs, cats, and rodents, in which it may represent a component of their indigenous flora or it may actually cause disease; it is a rare cause of respiratory disease in humans, predominantly those who are immunocompromised (Woolfrey, 1991).

LABORATORY DIAGNOSIS. The rate of isolation of *B. pertussis* from patients declines with the duration of illness. Normal healthy individuals are not carriers of the organism so that its isolation always represents disease.

The most commonly recommended specimen is the nasopharyngeal swab; however, nasopharyngeal aspirates with a soft rubber catheter have provided higher rates of isolation in some peoples' hands. In general, swabs or aspirates should be inoculated onto suitable media, for example, Regan-Lowe agar, as quickly as possible; however, Regan-Lowe and Jones-Kendrick transport medium have been found to be superior to Amies and Stuart media (Friedman, 1988). Swabs or aspirates may be inoculated into semi-solid charcoal agar for mailing purposes.

Direct examination of smears stained with fluorescein-conjugated *B. pertussis* antiserum represents a rapid diagnostic test. Cultures are recommended, however, because a low rate of falsely positive and falsely negative smears does occur. Of note is the cross-reactivity of antisera used for identification of *Legionella* with *B. pertussis*.

Specimens should be inoculated onto Regan-Lowe charcoal agar. The cultures should be incubated at 36°C and examined daily for up to six days.

Colonies suspected of representing *B. pertussis* can be presumptively identified by examining a smear stained with fluorescein-labeled specific antiserum. *Bordetella pertussis* is rather inactive and will not grow on blood-free media, usually requires three to four days to grow on charcoal agar, and does not reduce nitrates, produce urease, or utilize citrate. *Bordetella parapertussis* will grow on blood-free media, grows rapidly on charcoal agar, utilizes citrate, produces urease, but does not reduce nitrates. *Bordetella bronchiseptica* is the most active of the three and grows readily on conventional nutrient media, reduces nitrates, utilizes citrate, and rapidly (≤ 4 hours) hydrolyzes urea.

ANTIMICROBIAL SUSCEPTIBILITY. Antimicrobial agents probably play no role in the therapy of pertussis but do render negative nasopharyngeal cultures within one or two days, which may prevent bacterial complications in patients with the disease and may be effective in preventing spread of the disease to nonimmune contacts. Although several groups of agents are active *in vitro* against *B. pertussis*, erythromycin has been the only one consistently shown to be rapidly effective *in vivo*.

Haemophilus

DEFINITIONS AND CHARACTERISTICS. Members of the genus are small, gram-negative rods or coccobacilli with a requirement for hemin or other porphyrins (X factor) and/or nicotinamide adenine dinucleotides or trinucleotides (V factor). The medically important species, as classified by Kilian (1991), are listed in Table 48–14. *Haemophilus parahaemolyticus* is not listed because it loses its hemolytic property rapidly in subcultures and becomes indistinguishable from *H. parainfluenzae*. *Haemophilus aegyptius* is considered to be a biogroup of *H. influenzae*.

PATHOGENESIS AND VIRULENCE FACTORS. The virulence factors of species of *Haemophilus* are as yet poorly understood. Virulence of *H. influenzae* is associated with the serotype b capsule. Endotoxin is not produced by *H. influenzae*, and this species is rapidly killed once ingested by macrophages unless antibody, complement, or the phagocytes are deficient. The role of antibodies in immunity is also poorly understood. Antibodies develop with age, presumably following natural infection with *H. influenzae* or with cross-reacting antigenic organisms, so that most persons older than 15 years have antibodies. Which antibody and what level of that antibody are protective remain unknown.

Most *Haemophilus* species are indigenous to the upper respiratory tract and the oral cavity. The encapsulated strains of *H. influenzae*, particularly those belonging to serotype b, are most often responsible for diseases caused by *Haemophilus*, including meningitis, bacteremia, endocarditis, epiglottitis, conjunctivitis, and pneumonia. Nontypeable strains of *H. influenzae* are most frequently associated with acute otitis media and acute exacerbations of chronic bron-

Table 48–14. DIFFERENTIAL CHARACTERISTICS OF MEDICALLY IMPORTANT *HAEMOPHILUS* SPECIES

	Tests					
Species	***δ-ALA* Utilization***	***V-Factor Requirement***	***Indole***	***Urease***	***Ornithine Decarboxylase***	***CO_2 Enhancement***
H. influenzae biotype						
I	–	+	+	+	+	–
II	–	+	+	+	–	–
III	–	+	–	+	–	–
IV	–	+	–	+	+	–
V	–	+	+	–	+	–
H. haemolyticus	–	+	d	+	–	–
H. ducreyi	–	–	–	–	–	–
H. parainfluenzae biotype		+				–
I	+	+	–	–	+	–
II	+	+	–	+	+	–
III	+	+	–	+	–	d
H. paraphrophilus	+	+	–	–	–	+
H. aphrophilus	+	–	–	–	–	+

*δ-Aminolevulinic acid.

For key to symbols, see Table 48–11.

Adapted from Kilian M: Haemophilus. *In* Lennette EH, et al (eds.): Manual of Clinical Microbiology, 4th ed. Washington, DC, American Society for Microbiology, 1985, p 388.

chitis. *Haemophilus parainfluenzae* has been associated with meningitis, while it, *H. paraphrophilus*, and *H. aphrophilus* have been associated with subacute bacterial endocarditis. *Haemophilus ducreyi* is responsible for chancroid.

LABORATORY DIAGNOSIS. The isolation of *Haemophilus* usually requires the presence of hemin (X factor) and/or nicotinamide adenine nucleotides (V factor) in the culture medium. The former is most frequently supplied by the incorporation of heat-lysed ("chocolatized") blood cells in agar, although it may also be provided by whole human, horse, or rabbit blood cells. The V factor is commonly supplied either by the incorporation of yeast extract or other appropriate supplements in the medium or by a suspension of staphylococci, which is streaked across the agar surface and about which satellite colonies of V-dependent strains of *Haemophilus* grow. The differential characteristics of members of this genus are listed in Table 48–14.

The requirements for X and V factors are determined by placing paper disks or strips impregnated with each and with both factors onto a soybean-casein digest agar surface that has been streaked with the test strain. There are a number of difficulties posed by this approach. First, carryover of hemin from the original isolation plate is almost unavoidable so that growth of an X- and V-dependent strain, such as *H. influenzae*, about the V strip or disk may occur, leading to an erroneous identification of *H. parainfluenzae* or *H. paraphrophilus*. One way of minimizing this transfer of hemin is to place a colony of the test strain into 1 to 2 mL of soybean-casein broth, mix the suspension thoroughly, and then use a swab to inoculate the surface of the agar on which the X and V factor requirements are to be tested. Despite this precaution, traces of hemin may still be transferred and lead to an erroneous test result. Therefore, although X factor is commonly listed among tests required to identify haemophili, it is suggested that a different test system be used for separating V-dependent species from the others. One such test, which is simple and very reliable, was described by Kilian (1974) and determines the ability of V-dependent species to use δ-aminolevulinic acid in the biosynthesis of porphobilinogen and porphyrins. The formation of porphobilinogen can be detected by adding Kovac's reagent to the reaction mixture and observing the development of a red color in the aqueous phase. Alternatively, the formation of porphyrins in the reaction mixture can be demonstrated by red fluorescence under a Wood's lamp. Hemolytic properties of human isolates of haemophili can be determined on rabbit or horse blood agar; however, neither taxonomic nor clinical considerations justify the performance of this test.

Haemophilus aphrophilus must often be distinguished from species such as *Actinobacillus actinomycetemcomitans*, *Cardiobacterium hominis*, and *Eikenella corrodens* (Table 48–15), all of which have been associated with subacute bacterial endocarditis.

The cultivation of *H. ducreyi* from chancroid lesions has been problematic. A Gram's-stained smear of material from the lesion may be helpful if gram-negative bacilli in pairs or in rows ("schools of fish") are seen. Material may be inoculated onto GC medium base plus 1% hemoglobin, 5% to 10% fetal calf serum, 1% IsoVitaleX (BBL Microbiology Systems), and 3 μg/mL of vancomycin.

The presence of *H. influenzae* serotype b can be detected rapidly in cerebrospinal fluid by coagglutination or latex agglutination.

ANTIMICROBIAL SUSCEPTIBILITY. Approximately 20% of strains of *H. influenzae* type b isolates are resistant to ampicillin on the basis of β-lactamase production. Some nontypeable isolates of *H. influenzae* are also resistant to ampicillin on the basis of alterations in outer membrane permeability or affinity to penicillin-binding proteins. Thus, it is important to test all isolates of *H. influenzae* from normally sterile body fluids and tissues for β-lactamase production, and to determine susceptibility of such isolates to ampicillin when the β-lactamase test is negative. Chloramphenicol resistance, mediated by an acetyl transferase, remains infrequent in the United States. Resistance of *H. influenzae* to cefuroxime occurs infrequently; however, resistance to third-generation cephalosporins, such as cefotaxime, ceftriaxone, ceftazidime, and ceftizoxime, has not been documented. Susceptibility testing of *H. influenzae* requires careful adjustment of the inoculum so as not to exceed 5×10^5 CFU/mL.

PREVENTION. Currently vaccination of infants with a conjugate *H. influenzae* type b vaccine, beginning at age two months, is recommended. As a result of vaccination, the prevalence of invasive *H. influenzae* type b disease among

Table 48–15. DIFFERENTIAL CHARACTERISTICS OF *HAEMOPHILUS APHROPHILUS, ACTINOBACILLUS ACTINOMYCETEMCOMITANS, CARDIOBACTERIUM HOMINIS, EIKENELLA CORRODENS*, AND *KINGELLA KINGAE*

Test	*H. aphrophilus*	*A. actinomycetemcomitans*	*C. hominis*	*E. corrodens*	*K. kingae*
Oxidase	−	−	+	+	+
Catalase	−	+	−	−	−
δ-ALA utilization*	+	+	+	+	+
V-requirement	−	−	−	−	−
Indole	−	−	+	−	−
Urease	−	−	−	−	−
Lysine decarboxylase	−	−	−	+	−
Acid from					
Glucose	+	+	+	−	+ or (+)
Sucrose	+	−	+	−	−
Lactose	+	−	−	−	−
Mannitol	−	+	d	−	−
Xylose	−	d	−	−	−

*δ-Aminolevulinic acid.
For key to symbols, see Table 48–11.

6

infants and children dropped dramatically from 1987 to 1993 (CDC, 1994).

Gardnerella

DEFINITIONS AND CHARACTERISTICS. Formerly classified as *Haemophilus vaginalis* or *Corynebacterium vaginale*, *Gardnerella vaginalis* is a pleomorphic gram-negative to gram-variable bacillus that is usually isolated from the human genital/urinary tract. The organism requires neither X nor V factor for growth.

PATHOGENESIS AND VIRULENCE FACTORS. Although originally considered a cause of bacterial vaginosis, *G. vaginalis* is found in the vaginas of 25% to 45% of asymptomatic women. On the other hand, bacterial vaginosis is usually not present in the absence of the organism in vaginal cultures. Hence, the etiologic role of *G. vaginalis* in bacterial vaginosis remains uncertain. Cases of puerperal fever associated with *Gardnerella* bacteremia have been reported, as have cases of bacteriuria.

LABORATORY DIAGNOSIS. The diagnosis of bacterial vaginosis is usually based on the nature of the discharge, a pH of the discharge exceeding 4.5, the detection of a fishy amine odor upon the addition of KOH to the discharge, and/or the presence of "clue" cells on microscopic examination of the discharge (see Chap. 54). Media containing proteose peptone no. 3 (e.g., Casman agar and proteose peptone-starch-dextrose [PSD] agar) have most often been used for isolation of *G. vaginalis*. Columbia colistin-nalidixic acid (CNA) agar has been found to be a useful selective medium. Because *G. vaginalis* produces β-hemolysis of human (but not sheep) blood, detection of the organism is enhanced by incorporating human (instead of sheep) blood into Columbia CNA agar. *Gardnerella vaginalis* is catalase and oxidase negative; it produces acid from glucose, maltose, and starch; and it neither reduces nitrates nor produces urease.

ANTIMICROBIAL SUSCEPTIBILITY. Although *G. vaginalis* is susceptible to ampicillin, metronidazole has been found to be more effective in eradicating the organism from the vagina.

Eikenella

DEFINITIONS AND CHARACTERISTICS. Formerly classified as *Bacteroides corrodens*, the "corroding bacilli" that are facultatively anaerobic have been assigned to the species *Eikenella corrodens*. Strictly anaerobic corroding bacilli, which differ in several important respects from the facultatively anaerobic bacilli, are classified as *Bacteroides ureolyticus*. *Eikenella corrodens* organisms are oxidase-positive, catalase-negative, nonfermentative, gram-negative bacilli, colonies of which may corrode or pit agar. Growth is enhanced by 5% to 10% CO_2 and usually requires the presence of hemin (X factor) in the medium.

PATHOGENESIS AND VIRULENCE FACTORS. Little is known about factors contributing to the organism's virulence, and it has a low level of pathogenicity for animals. *Eikenella* resides predominantly in the nasopharynx and is isolated frequently from the upper respiratory tract. It has been recovered from abscesses and other types of infections in almost any site, may invade the bloodstream, and may cause endocarditis. Infections are usually mixed.

LABORATORY DIAGNOSIS. The most striking feature of *Eikenella* in cultures is its ability to pit the agar; however, pitting does not occur with all strains. The colonies appear slowly and are generally small (0.5 to 1.0 mm in diameter). It must usually be distinguished from other fastidious, slowly growing gram-negative bacilli (see Table 48–15).

ANTIMICROBIAL SUSCEPTIBILITY. *Eikenella* is susceptible to the penicillins and chloramphenicol. Its susceptibility to aminoglycosides is variable, but it is resistant to clindamycin.

Actinobacillus actinomycetemcomitans

DEFINITIONS AND CHARACTERISTICS. Other than the sesquipedalian character of its name, this organism currently occupies an uncertain taxonomic position. It is small, coccoid to bacillary in shape microscopically, grows aerobically and somewhat better in CO_2, and anaerobically, and may grow in broth in the form of small granules adhering to the walls of the tube. Colonies on blood agar appear slowly and are small.

PATHOGENESIS AND VIRULENCE FACTORS. *Actinobacillus actinomycetemcomitans* has a low level of pathogenicity. It derives its name from its frequent association with actinomycotic lesions. In recent years, however, it has most frequently been reported as a cause of subacute bacterial endocarditis.

LABORATORY DIAGNOSIS. The most frequently reported source of the organism in recent years is blood cultures from patients with endocarditis. It appears to grow slowly in most currently used blood culture media. It must be differentiated from other slowly growing, somewhat fastidious gram-negative bacilli (see Table 48–15).

ANTIMICROBIAL SUSCEPTIBILITY. Although the organism is not consistently susceptible to the penicillins, ampicillin alone has been successfully employed in the treatment of a number of reported cases. Ampicillin and an aminoglycoside have been found to be bactericidal but not synergistic against the organism and have also been used in the therapy of endocarditis associated with it. Other active antimicrobial agents include the tetracyclines and chloramphenicol.

Calymmatobacterium granulomatis

DESCRIPTION AND CHARACTERISTICS. Previously known as *Donovania granulomatis*, *Calymmatobacterium* is a gram-negative, nonmotile, encapsulated, pleomorphic rod that may be cultured in yolk sacs or on fresh egg yolk medium. The organism possesses antigenic determinants similar to those of *Klebsiella*, leading some authors to classify it among the Enterobacteriaceae.

PATHOGENESIS AND VIRULENCE FACTORS. The organism does not produce disease in animals. In humans it causes granuloma inguinale, characterized by ulcerogranulomatous lesions of the skin and mucosa of the genital and inguinal areas.

LABORATORY DIAGNOSIS. A fragment of tissue removed from the margin of an ulcer is pressed and rubbed against a glass slide and stained with Wright or Giemsa stain. The finding of small, straight or curved, pleomorphic rods with rounded ends and characteristic polar granules, giving a safety pin appearance within mononuclear cells, is the most effective way of establishing the diagnosis.

ANTIMICROBIAL SUSCEPTIBILITY. The tetracyclines, erythromycin, ampicillin, and chloramphenicol are active against *Calymmatobacterium*. Resistance may develop to streptomycin.

Streptobacillus moniliformis

DESCRIPTION AND CHARACTERISTICS. *Streptobacillus* is a facultatively anaerobic, fermentative, nonencapsulated, and nonmotile gram-negative rod, frequently in chains and filaments, and often with a series of oval to elongated bulbous swellings, giving a string-of-beads appearance. Blood, serum, or ascitic fluid is needed for growth in agar or broth. The microscopic morphology varies with time, being more homogeneously filamentous in young cultures and becoming fragmented into irregular coccobacilli with age. L-phase colonies may occur spontaneously on agar, have a "fried egg" appearance, become stabilized if penicillin is incorporated in the medium, and are indistinguishable from L-phase colonies of other bacteria and from mycoplasmas.

PATHOGENESIS AND VIRULENCE FACTORS. *Streptobacillus* occurs as indigenous flora in the upper respiratory tract of wild and laboratory rodents. Infection (Haverhill disease) in humans follows rodent bites, ingestion of contaminated food, or traumatic injury. Local lymphangitis and lymphadenitis may develop up to three weeks later, followed by the onset of fever, chills, malaise, and later by a general morbilliform maculopapular or petechial rash. Some patients develop a migratory polyarthritis. Endocarditis has been reported. The histopathology is nonspecific and demonstrates a chronic inflammatory reaction.

LABORATORY DIAGNOSIS. Heat-inactivated sterile horse serum can be added to molten heart infusion (HI) agar supplemented with yeast extract. Normally sterile body fluids should be examined microscopically after staining with Gram's and Giemsa stains. Material should also be inoculated into HI broth containing the supplements described earlier.

The identification of *Streptobacillus* is rather complex. Colonies in broth form as fluff balls, while those on agar are small and slightly translucent to opaque with a slightly irregular edge. L-phase variants may form on agar. Subcultures are made from broth with pipettes or by agar block transfers. Biochemical tests must be performed in HI agar or broth supplemented with yeast extract and horse serum.

ANTIMICROBIAL SUSCEPTIBILITY. Penicillin alone and in combination with streptomycin is active against *Streptobacillus*.

PREVENTION AND CONTROL. Because 10% to 65% of rats are infected with the organism, their control and precautions against bites represent the only effective methods of control of the disease.

Francisella

DEFINITIONS AND CHARACTERISTICS. Formerly classified as *Pasteurella tularensis*, *Francisella tularensis* is a very small, strictly aerobic, coccoid to pleomorphic rod-shaped, gram-negative bacillus that requires cystine or cysteine for its growth. Faint bipolar staining occurs with aniline dyes.

PATHOGENESIS AND VIRULENCE FACTORS. Virulence appears to be related to a smooth colonial morphology. Repeated subcultures result in an alteration from smooth to rough colonies, with a concomitant loss of virulence. Highly virulent strains for humans have citrulline ureidase activity and ferment glycerol, and are most often associated with tickborne disease in rabbits. Toxins have not been recognized.

Tularemia may manifest itself after an incubation period of one to 10 days in various forms. Headache, fever, chills, vomiting, and myalgias characteristically occur at the onset. In the ulceroglandular type of disease, lymphadenitis and lymphadenopathy occur in the region draining the primary lesion. The lesion is initially papular and later ulcerative. A variation of this form of disease, the oculoglandular type, is characterized by inflammation of the conjunctiva and usually a papule of the lower lid with lymphadenitis of the preauricular, parotid, submaxillary, and anterior cervical nodes. An ingestion form of tularemia is characterized by ulcerative lesions of the mouth, throat, and upper gastrointestinal tract. Pneumonia may result from inhalation or secondary to bacteremia from another focus of infection.

Tularemia should be suspected in anyone who has been in an endemic area, has had contact with wild animals or livestock, has a history of tick bite, has been engaged in farming operations, has drunk impure water, or has been exposed to cultures or infected animals in the laboratory. Trappers, hunters, fur and meat industry workers, agricultural workers, and laboratory personnel are at greatest risk. Because of its protean manifestations, tularemia is readily confused with many other diseases, such as brucellosis, anthrax, sporotrichosis, typhoid fever, tuberculosis, histoplasmosis, and syphilis.

LABORATORY DIAGNOSIS. Material suitable for examination includes fluid or curettings from the primary lesion, aspirates of enlarged regional nodes, sputum, pharyngeal washes, and gastric aspirates. Cultures may be made on glucose-cysteine agar supplemented with 5% defibrinated rabbit blood or buffered charcoal yeast extract agar (see *Legionella* later). If the clinical material is contaminated with other bacteria, 1 mL each of penicillin, 100,000 U/mL; polymyxin B, 100,000 U/mL; and cycloheximide, 0.1 mg/mL, should be included in each liter of medium. Special care must be exercised in handling infected material to prevent aerosolization or direct contact with the skin. Cultures are incubated at 35°C in an environment with or without added CO_2. Colonies usually appear within 24 to 48 hours. Because working with the organism in the laboratory is dangerous, sending suspicious cultures to a reference laboratory such as the CDC for confirmation with a slide agglutination or direct fluorescent antibody test is recommended.

The diagnosis can also be established serologically. Agglutination titers as low as 1:40 in the absence of previous disease are diagnostic and may rise within the first three weeks to levels of 1:640 or greater. *Brucella* agglutinins may also rise nonspecifically, but usually to a significantly lower level.

ANTIMICROBIAL SUSCEPTIBILITY. Streptomycin is bactericidal, while the tetracyclines and chloramphenicol are bacteriostatic to *Francisella*. Because relapses are not infrequent after treatment with these bacteriostatic agents, streptomycin is the agent of choice.

Legionella

DEFINITIONS AND CHARACTERISTICS. *Legionella* organisms are fastidious, non–spore-forming, pleomorphic gram-negative bacilli. There are over 20 named species and a number of unnamed species, some of which have not as yet been isolated from humans. The majority of clinical cases have been due to *Legionella pneumophila*, serogroup 1.

PATHOGENESIS AND VIRULENCE FACTORS. A variety of extracellular enzymes, including protease, phosphatase, lipase, and deoxyribonuclease; a cytotoxin; and endotoxin-like activity have been identified in *L. pneumophila*. Infection is usually manifested as an acute fibrinopurulent pneumonia, which is usually lobular in distribution. Histologically, there is an alveolar infiltrate of neutrophils and macrophages, accompanied by fibrin and red blood cell extravasation. *Legionella* organisms may be found in large numbers within alveolar macrophages. *Legionella pneumophila* has been isolated from blood, which presumably accounts for the disease's protean manifestations.

LABORATORY DIAGNOSIS. The diagnosis of legionellosis may be made by isolating the organism in culture, detecting the organism in specimens by immunofluorescence or DNA hybridization, detecting *Legionella* antigen in urine, and demonstrating rising species- or type-specific antibody titers (Edelstein, 1993).

Legionella may be isolated on a buffered charcoal yeast extract (BCYE) agar that contains essential growth factors, including L-cysteine and a ferric salt. Supplementation of BCYE agar with α-ketoglutarate is recommended. This medium may be made selective for culture of nonsterile body sites by supplementing the medium with either cefamandole, polymyxin B, and anisomycin (BMPA), or polymyxin B, anisomycin, and vancomycin (PAV) (Edelstein, 1987). Confirmation and speciation are made according to phenotypic characteristics and by staining with fluorescein-labeled species- or type-specific conjugate.

Legionella may be detected or identified by direct fluorescent antibody (DFA) staining of specimens or colonies in cultures. The sensitivity of the DFA examination of respiratory specimens has ranged from 25% to 75% but is considerably higher in open lung biopsies. Although cross-reactions have been reported between *L. pneumophila* and other *Legionella* species, as well as with some strains of *Bordetella pertussis*, *Pseudomonas fluorescens*, and *Bacteroides fragilis*, the DFA examination appears to be reasonably specific and certainly expedites diagnosis of the disease when positive. Sensitivity of DFA for other species in sputum is not known (Edelstein, 1987). A *Legionella* probe has been introduced with a reported sensitivity for *L. pneumophila* serogroup 1 of 60% to 80% and somewhat lower sensitivity for other species and serogroups (Edelstein, 1987). There is also a urine antigen test for *L. pneumophila* serogroup 1 with a reported sensitivity of 80% to 90%, although it should be noted that antigenuria may persist for many months following infection (Edelstein, 1987).

The diagnosis of legionellosis can also be established serologically by a fourfold or greater rise in antibody titer to at least 1:128. A single antibody titer of 1:256 is presumptive evidence of past infection. The sensitivity of serologic diagnosis for disease caused by species other than *L. pneumophila* serogroup 1 is not known, and specificity of antibody tests for disease caused by other species is less than that of *L. pneumophila* serogroup 1 (Edelstein, 1987). The sensitivity and specificity of culture, DFA examination, and serologic diagnosis of legionellosis have been extensively reviewed by Edelstein (1987).

ANTIMICROBIAL SUSCEPTIBILITY. Despite their susceptibility *in vitro* to a wide variety of antimicrobial agents, clinical response of infections caused by the *Legionella* species is largely limited to erythromycin and rifampin.

Anaerobic Bacteria

It is important to re-emphasize that anaerobes represent a major component of the indigenous flora of the skin and mucous membranes (see Table 48–1) and, therefore, that their isolation and identification should be contingent upon the proper selection and collection of specimens, as well as upon their proper transport to the laboratory. Anaerobic infections are frequently mixed, consisting either of several species of anaerobes or of anaerobes with facultatively anaerobic bacteria. Mixed cultures commonly consist of an average of two facultatively anaerobic and three anaerobic species. The first task, therefore, in examining an anaerobic culture is to separate facultatively anaerobic from anaerobic bacteria. With experience, the more commonly isolated anaerobes can often be recognized on the basis of their colonial and microscopic morphologies, and presumptively identified on the basis of a few additional tests. Definitive identification is based upon biochemical reactions, physiologic and genetic characteristics, and pathogenicity and toxin neutralization tests.

The extent to which anaerobes are identified varies according to the facilities and expertise available, the interest of the laboratory personnel and clinical staff, and the clinical utility of the information available from the laboratory.

DEFINITIONS AND CHARACTERISTICS. An *anaerobe* can be defined as a bacterium that requires an atmosphere with reduced oxygen tension for its growth and that fails to grow on the surface of solid media in an atmosphere of room air with 10% CO_2. A facultatively anaerobic bacterium will grow in either the presence or absence of room air. The term *microaerophile* has not been strictly defined and is commonly applied to bacteria, usually campylobacters and streptococci, that grow only or preferentially in an atmosphere with reduced oxygen and with increased carbon dioxide.

PATHOGENESIS AND VIRULENCE FACTORS. Little is known about the factors responsible for the pathogenic and virulence properties of most anaerobes other than the histotoxic clostridia. Endotoxic, proteolytic, and heparinase activities have been identified among the Bacteroidaceae. The polysaccharide capsule of *Bacteroides fragilis* promotes abscess formation. The clostridia, on the other hand, elaborate potent exotoxins, including lethal and necrotizing toxins, hemolysins, lecithinases, gelatinases, hyaluronidases, and so on.

While clostridial infection may be either exogenous or endogenous in origin, disease caused by other anaerobes usually originates endogenously from the normal indigenous anaerobic flora of a contiguous mucous membrane, the integrity of which has been disrupted by surgery, instrumentation, trauma, or malignancy. Essential to the establishment of anaerobes in the infectious process is a decrease in the oxidation-reduction potential (E_h) of the area, which may result from a failure of its blood supply or from the presence of multiplication of other bacteria at the site.

Although clostridial infections and intoxications are unquestionably of major medical importance, the role of other anaerobes in causing cellulitis and myonecrosis has been recognized only relatively recently. Most isolates of *Clostridium perfringens* in hospital practice today are the result of simple contamination of a wound. In such instances, the clostridia may multiply in cellular debris, a hematoma, or necrotic tissue without observable clinical symptomatology. Anaerobic cellulitis is a necrotizing process of the soft tissues. Its onset is gradual, but it can progress rapidly and extensively. Gas is produced; however, the process typically does not involve muscle. In addition to or instead of clostridia, the bacteriology of anaerobic cellulitis may involve anaerobic cocci and anaerobic gram-negative bacilli.

In contrast to anaerobic cellulitis, gas gangrene or clostridial myonecrosis is an acute and rapidly progressive invasive process producing marked changes in muscles. Distinguishing between anaerobic cellulitis and gas gangrene is critical in order to avoid performing unnecessarily aggressive and mutilating surgery in the former condition.

The histotoxic clostridia associated with gas gangrene include *C. perfringens*, *C. novyi*, *C. septicum*, *C. histolyticum*, *C. sporogenes*, and *C. bifermentans*. While *C. perfringens* has been the species most frequently involved in most reports of gas gangrene, the prevalence of the other species in this process has varied widely.

Tetanus and botulism are described as intoxications rather than infections because their manifestations are related to the elaboration of potent neurotoxins. Botulism is most frequently related to the ingestion of home-processed foods that have been improperly preserved or canned; however, sporadic outbreaks of the disease have been related to commercially processed food and to wound infected with the organism. The incubation period for botulism is short, and signs and symptoms usually occur between 18 and 36 hours following ingestion of contaminated food. Of the seven antigenic types of botulinus toxin known, type A is the most common, followed by types B, E, and F in cases of food poisoning in North America. The toxin is absorbed from the intestinal tract and, rarely, from an infected wound and attaches ultimately to motor nerve terminals, thereby preventing acetylcholine release at the nerve endings.

Tetanus typically occurs in nonimmunized persons within the first two weeks following a traumatically acquired puncture, laceration, or abrasion. Cases have been reported to occur postoperatively; following dental work, childbirth, and abortion; or in association with stasis and decubitus ulcers. The toxin, tetanospasmin, is transported to gangliosides in the central nervous system via the lymphatics and bloodstream, and by migration through the perineural spaces of peripheral nerves.

Clostridium difficile is the major cause of nosocomial diarrhea and the primary pathogen responsible for pseudomembranous colitis. It is a rare cause of abscesses, wound infections, osteomyelitis, pleuritis, peritonitis, septicemia, and urogenital tract infections. Carriage rates of *C. difficile* and its toxins are high (50% or more) in neonates, but disease is rare (Lyverly, 1988). Colonization, with or without toxin production, may be maintained for several months; but when the adult flora becomes established at six to 12 months of age, colonization rates fall, and only about 3% of normal healthy adults are colonized with the organism. *Clostridium difficile* almost always is acquired in the hospital via direct or indirect exposure to human or inanimate reservoirs. After an individual is exposed to *C. difficile*, various factors predispose to diarrhea: older age, more severe underlying disease, increased length of stay in the hospital, and use of penicillins or cephalosporins, gastrointestinal stimulants, stool softeners, and enemas. Although the penicillins and cephalosporins are implicated most frequently, any antimicrobial agent may trigger *C. difficile*–associated disease. Disease rarely occurs without antibiotic exposure, and cases have been reported following therapy with antineoplastic agents that have antibacterial activity. Pseudomembranous colitis is a toxin-mediated illness in which microbial invasion of the mucosa is not known to occur. *Clostridium difficile* produces two toxins. Toxin A, a weakly cytopathic toxin, is predominantly responsible for the enterotoxic activity of the organism. Toxin B, a potent cytotoxin, appears to play a minor role in human disease.

As has already been mentioned, other anaerobic bacteria, particularly the anaerobic cocci and gram-negative bacilli, have been associated with anaerobic cellulitis in addition to or instead of the histotoxic clostridial species. These organisms are part of the indigenous flora of the mucous membranes of the oral cavity and of the gastrointestinal and genitourinary tracts. As such, they are encountered in aspiration pneumonias, lung abscesses, empyemas, intra-abdominal infections and abscesses, pelvic abscesses, brain abscesses, and bacteremias. Anaerobic intra-abdominal infections commonly follow abdominal and especially colon surgery, and are most frequently associated with the *Bacteroides fragilis* group. Clinically significant anaerobic bacteremias are also most frequently caused by this species.

LABORATORY DIAGNOSIS. The speciation of anaerobic bacteria can be quite complex; however, the extent to which isolates of anaerobic bacteria are identified varies widely and may be limited to basic information that is of clinical utility. For example, the mixed anaerobic flora from a site such as a decubitus ulcer or perirectal fistula may simply be reported as mixed fecal flora without specific identification of its components. The mixed anaerobic flora from an intra-abdominal abscess may, for example, be screened for the presence of β-lactamase (nitrocefin)–producing gram-negative bacilli that, if present, may simply be reported as anaerobic gram-negative bacilli, β-lactamase positive, and the remaining organisms reported as mixed anaerobic flora. The presence of β-lactamase–producing, anaerobic, gram-negative bacilli is presumptive evidence of the presence of the *Bacteroides fragilis* group, although some other species of the Bacteroidaceae may also produce β-lactamase. Speciation of isolates may be limited to those present in pure culture from a normally sterile body fluid or site. Speciation today may be readily accomplished by any one of several commercially available kits, and it is rarely necessary to use gas-liquid chromatography for this purpose. One should understand that the clinical value of any report of the presence of anaerobic bacteria is directly related to the speed of reporting such results from the laboratory. Identification procedures that require one or two weeks for completion are generally of historical interest only.

Because of their rapid progression and considerable morbidity and mortality, the initial diagnosis and management of diseases caused by the clostridia must be based upon their clinical presentation and manifestations. In some patients with tetanus, no primary wound is evident. When a wound is present, organisms typical of *Clostridium tetani* are seldom seen in stained smears, even though they may be recovered from cultures. Moreover, because of this organism's widespread distribution in nature, its isolation from a wound is not necessarily indicative of the diagnosis of tetanus. Laboratory confirmation of botulism requires detection of the toxin in serum, wounds, gastric contents, feces, or the food suspected of causing the disease. Procedures for extracting the toxin and for performing mouse neutralization tests are complex; therefore, it is suggested that the appropriate materials be referred to the CDC (Atlanta, GA) for examination. Telephone consultation should be made in such instances to ensure that the requisite specimens are properly collected and transported and that the appropriate authorities are alerted about the situation.

In cases of suspected anaerobic cellulitis or gas gangrene, the laboratory can be helpful by examining exudate or tissue microscopically. The finding of numerous, large, "boxcar"-shaped, gram-positive bacilli (Plate 48–6) provides presumptive confirmation of the diagnosis. Stained smears may also be diagnostic of anaerobic streptococcal myositis. Cultures of exudate, tissue, and blood should also be performed. Once again, the level or extent of identification varies considerably among laboratories; however, *Clostridium perfringens* may be easily identified by its Gram's-stained morphology, the production of double zones of hemolysis on blood agar, and a positive Nagler's reaction on egg yolk agar. Laboratory diagnosis of *Clostridium difficile* diarrhea is discussed in Chapter 54 under Feces.

ANTIMICROBIAL SUSCEPTIBILITY. A Working Group of the National Committee for Clinical Laboratory Standards (NCCLS) (1989) agreed that susceptibility testing for anaerobic bacteria is generally unnecessary for clinical isolates and that the major indications for testing are clinical settings in which decisions regarding the selection of agents are critical because of (1) the failure of usual therapeutic regimens and persistence of infection, (2) the key role of antimicrobial agents in determining the outcome of infection, or (3) the difficulty in making empirical therapeutic decisions based on precedent. The Working Group specified that the infections from which isolates should be tested are brain abscess, endocarditis, osteomyelitis, joint infections, infections of prosthetic devices or vascular grafts, and refractory or recurrent bacteremia. Testing under these circumstances should include some members of the *Bacteroides fragilis* group, other *Bacteroides* species, certain fusobacteria, *Clostridium perfringens*, and *Clostridium ramosum*. Some agents, such as metronidazole, chloramphenicol, imipenem, ampicillin-sulbactam, and ticarcillin-clavulanate, are almost always active against anaerobic bacteria and need not be tested for clinical purposes. Thus, testing should be limited to alternative agents with unpredictable activity, such as penicillin, a broad-spectrum antipseudomonal penicillin, clindamycin, cefoxitin, cefotetan, and a third-generation cephalosporin. Although an agar dilution method has been recommended for reference purposes, testing in the clinical laboratory is generally performed by the microdilution method. Disk elution is not an acceptable alternative.

General References

Barnett LA, Cunningham MW: A new heart-cross-reactive antigen in *Streptococcus pyogenes* is not M protein. J Infect Dis 1990; 162:875.

Beebe JL, Rau MP, Flageolle S, et al: Incidence of *Neisseria gonorrhoeae* isolates negative by Syva direct fluorescent-antibody test but positive by Gen-Probe Accuprobe test in a sexually transmitted disease clinic population. J Clin Microbiol 1993; 31:2535.

Brenden RA, Miller MA, Janda JM: Clinical disease spectrum and pathogenic factors associated with *Plesiomonas shigelloides* infection in humans. Rev Infect Dis 1988; 10:303.

Brenner DJ, McWhorter AC, Kai A, et al: *Enterobacter asburiae* sp. nov., a new species found in clinical specimens, and reassignment of *Erwinia dissolvens* and *Erwinia nimipressuralis* to the genus *Enterobacter* as *Enterobacter dissolvens* comb. nov. and *Enterobacter nimipressuralis* comb. nov. J Clin Microbiol 1986; 23:1114.

Broome CV: Listeriosis: Can we prevent it? New monitoring techniques are helping to prevent this relatively rare but frequently fatal food-borne disease. ASM News 1993; 59:444.

Catlin BW: *Branhamella catarrhalis*: An organism gaining respect as a pathogen. Clin Microbiol Rev 1990; 3:293.

Centers for Disease Control and Prevention: Progress toward elimination of *Haemophilius influenzae* type b disease among infants and children—United States, 1987–1993. MMWR 1994; 43:144.

Chambers HF: Methicillin-resistant staphylococci. Clin Microbiol Rev 1988; 1:173.

Chiedozi LC: Pyomyositis: Review of 205 cases in 112 patients. Am J Surg 1979; 137:255.

Coykendall AL: Classification and identification of the viridans streptococci. Clin Microbiol Rev 1989; 2:315.

Dale JC, Vetter EA, Contezac JM, et al: Evaluation of two rapid antigen assays, BioStar Strep A OIA and Pacific Biotech CARDS O.S., and culture for detection of Group A streptococci in throat swabs. J Clin Microbiol 1994; 32:2698.

Daly JA, Clifton NL, Seskin KC, et al: Use of rapid nonradioactive DNA probes in culture confirmation tests to detect *Streptococcus agalactiae*, *Haemophilus influenzae*, and *Enterococcus* spp. from pediatric patients with significant infections. J Clin Microbiol 1991; 29:80.

Dillon JR, Carballo M, Pauze M: Evaluation of eight methods for identification of pathogenic *Neisseria* species: Neisseria-Kwik, RIM-N, Gonobio-Test, Minitek, Gonochek II, GonoGen, Phadebact monoclonal GC OMNI test, and Syva Microtrak Test. J Clin Microbiol 1988; 26:493.

Doyle RJ, Keller KF, Ezzell JW: *Bacillus*. *In* Lennette EH, Balows A, Hausler WJ Jr, Shadomy HJ (eds): Manual of Clinical Microbiology, 4th ed. Washington, D.C., American Society for Microbiology, 1985, p 211.

Edelstein PH: Laboratory diagnosis of Legionnaires' disease. Semin Respir Infect 1987; 2:235.

Edelstein PH: Legionnaires' disease. Clin Infect Dis 1993; 16:741.

Facklam RR: Specificity study of kits for detection of group A streptococci directly from throat swabs. J Clin Microbiol 1987; 25:504.

Facklam RR, Collins MD: Identification of *Enterococcus* species isolated from human infections by a conventional test scheme. J Clin Microbiol 1989a; 27:731.

Facklam R, Hollis D, Collins MD: Identification of gram-positive coccal and coccobacillary vancomycin-resistant bacteria. J Clin Microbiol 1989b; 27:724.

Farmer JJ III, Davis BR, Hickman-Brenner FW, et al: Biochemical identification of new species and biogroups of Enterobacteriaceae isolated from clinical specimens. J Clin Microbiol 1985; 21:46.

Feldman WE: Concentration of bacteria in cerebrospinal fluid of patients with bacterial meningitis. J Pediatr 1976; 88:549.

Fleming DW, Cochi SL, MacDonald KL, et al: Pasteurized milk as a vehicle of infection in an outbreak of listeriosis. N Engl J Med 1985; 312:404.

Friedman RL: Pertussis: The disease and new diagnostic methods. Clin Microbiol Rev 1988; 1:365.

Gallis HA: Streptococcus. *In* Joklik WK, Willett HP, Ames DB, Wilfert CM (eds): Zinsser Microbiology, 19th ed. Norwalk, CT, Appleton & Lange, 1988, p 357.

Gerner-Smidt P, Tjernberg I, Ursing J: Reliability of phenotypic tests for identification of *Acinetobacter* species. J Clin Microbiol 1991; 29:277.

Gilardi GL: *Pseudomonas* and related genera. *In* Balows A, Hausler WJ Jr, Herrmann KL, Isenberg HD, Shadomy J (eds): Manual of Clinical Microbiology, 5th ed. Washington DC, American Society for Microbiology, 1991, pp 429–41.

Granoff DM, Murphy TV, Ingram DL, et al: Use of rapidly generated results in patient management. Diagn Microbiol Infect Dis 1986; 4(S3):157S.

Gregson DB, Low DE, Skulnick M, et al: Problems with rapid agglutination methods for identification of *Staphylococcus aureus* when *Staphylococcus saprophyticus* is being tested. J Clin Microbiol 1988; 26:1398.

Hale YM, Melton ME, Lewis JS, et al: Evaluation of the Pace 2 *Neisseria gonorrhoeae* assay by three public health laboratories. J Clin Microbiol 1993; 31:451.

Hammond GW, Lian CJ, Wilt JC, et al: Comparison of specimen collection and laboratory techniques for isolation of *Haemophilus ducreyi*. J Clin Microbiol 1978; 7:39.

Handwerger S, Horowitz H, Coburn K, et al: Infection due to *Leuconostoc* species: Six cases and review. Rev Infect Dis 1990; 12:602.

Harvey RL, Sunstrum JC: *Rhodococcus equi* infection in patients with and without human immunodeficiency virus infection. Rev Infect Dis 1991; 13:139.

Hendley JO, Sande MA, Stewart PM, et al: Spread of *Streptococcus pneumoniae* in families. Carriage rates and distribution of types. J Infect Dis 1975; 132:55.

Hickman-Brenner FW, Hutley-Carter GP, Fanning GR, et al: *Koserella trabulsii*, a new genus and species of Enterobacteriaceae formerly known as Enteric group G 45. J Clin Microbiol 1985; 21:39.

Hickman-Brenner SW, MacDonald KL, Steigerwalt AG, et al: *Aeromonas veronii*, a new ornithine decarboxylase-positive species that causes diarrhea. J Clin Microbiol 1987; 25:900.

Hickman-Brenner FW, Fanning GR, Arduino MJ, et al: *Aeromonas schubertii*, a new mannitol-negative species found in human clinical specimens. J Clin Microbiol 1988; 26:1561.

Janda JM, Malloy PJ, Schreckenberger PC: Clinical evaluation of the Vitek Neisseria-Haemophilus identification card. J Clin Microbiol 1987; 25:37.

Janda JM: Recent advances in the study of the taxonomy, pathogenicity, and infectious syndromes associated with the genus *Aeromonas*. Clin Microbiol Rev 1991; 4:397.

Janda JM, Guthertz LS, Kokka RP, et al: *Aeromonas* species in septicemia: Laboratory characteristics and clinical observations. Clin Infect Dis 1994; 19:77.

Kaper JB, Morris JG Jr, Levine MM: Cholera. Clin Microbiol Rev 1995; 8:48.

Kellog JA, Orwig LK: Comparison of GonoGen, GonoGen II, and Micro-Trak direct fluorescent antibody test with carbohydrate fermentation for confirmation of culture isolates of *Neisseria gonorrhoeae*. J Clin Microbiol 1995; 33:474.

Kilian M: A rapid method for the differentiation of *Haemophilus* strains. Acta Path Microbiol Scand 1974; 82:835.

Kilian M: *Haemophilus*. *In* Balows A, Hausler WJ Jr, Herrmann KL, Isenberg HD, Shadomy HJ (eds): Manual of Clinical Microbiology, 5th ed. Washington DC, American Society for Microbiology, 1991, pp 471–477.

Kloos WE, Lambe DW Jr: *Staphylococcus*. *In* Balows A, Hausler WJ Jr, Hermann KL, Isenberg HD, Shadomy HJ (eds): Manual of Clinical Microbiology, 5th ed. Washington DC, American Society for Microbiology, 1991, pp 222–237.

Klugman KP: Pneumonococcal resistance to antibiotics. Clin Microbiol Rev 1990; 3:171.

Knapp JS: Historical perspective and identification of *Neisseria* and related species. Clin Microbiol Rev 1988; 1:415.

Kotnick CM, Edberg SC: Direct detection of group B streptococci from vaginal specimens compared with quantitative culture. J Clin Microbiol 1990; 28:336.

Lieu TA, Fleisher GR, Schwartz S: Clinical evaluation of a latex agglutination test for streptococcal pharyngitis: Performance and impact on treatment rates. Pediatr Infect Dis 1988; 7:847.

Limberger RJ, Biega R, Evancoe A, et al: Evaluation of culture and the Gen-Probe Pace 2 assay for detection of *Neisseria gonorrhoeae* and *Chlamydia trachomatis* in endocervical specimens transported to a state health laboratory. J Clin Microbiol 1992; 30:1162.

Linnan MJ, Mascola L, Lou XD, et al: Epidemic listeriosis associated with Mexican-style cheese. N Engl J Med 1988; 319:823.

Lyverly DM, Krivan HC, Wilkins TC: *Clostridium difficile*: Its disease and toxins. Clin Microbiol Rev 1988; 1:1.

Mastro TD, Spika JS, Lozano P, et al: Vancomycin-resistant *Pediococcus acidilactici*: Nine cases of bacteremia. J Infect Dis 1990; 161:956.

Miller RA, Brancato F, Holmes KK: *Corynebacterium hemolyticum* as a cause of pharyngitis and scarlatiniform rash in young adults. Ann Intern Med 1986; 105:867.

Morris JG Jr, Black RE: Cholera and other vibrioses in the United States. N Engl J Med 1985; 312:345.

Murray DM: Clinical relevance of infection by *Helicobacter pylori*. Clin Microbiol Newslett 1993; 15:33.

National Committee for Clinical Laboratory Standards (NCCLS): Methods for Antimicrobial Susceptibility Testing of Anaerobic Bacteria, 2nd ed; Tentative Standard. NCCLS Publication M11-T2. Villanova, PA, NCCLS, 1989.

Parsonnet J, Friedman GD, Vandersteen DP, et al: *Helicobacter pylori* infection and the risk of gastric carcinoma. N Engl J Med 1991; 325:1127.

Parsonnet J, Hansen S, Rodriquez L, et al: *Helicobacter pylori* infection and gastric lymphoma. N Engl J Med 1994; 330:1267.

Penner JL: The genus *Campylobacter*: A decade of progress. Clin Microbiol Rev 1988; 1:157.

Peterson LR, Shanholtzer CJ: Using the microbiology laboratory in the diagnosis of pneumonia. Semin Respir Infect 1988; 3:106.

Pokorski SJ, Vetter EA, Wollan PC, et al: Comparison of Gen-Probe Group A streptococcus direct test with culture for diagnosing streptococcal pharyngitis. J Clin Microbiol 1994; 32:1440.

Radetsky M, Solomon JA, Todd JK: Identification of streptococcal pharyngitis in the office laboratory: Reassessment of new technology. Pediatr Infect Dis J 1987; 6:556.

Reller LB, Murray PR, MacLowry JD: Blood cultures II. *In* Washington JA II (coordinating ed): Cumitech 1A. Washington DC, American Society for Microbiology, 1982.

Robinson A, McCarter YS, Tetreault J: Comparison of Crystal Enteric/Nonfermenter System, API-20E System, and Vitek Automicrobic System for identification of gram-negative bacilli. J Clin Microbiol 1995; 33:365.

Ruane PJ, Morgan MA, Citron DM, et al: Failure of rapid agglutination methods to detect oxacillin-resistant *Staphylococcus aureus*. J Clin Microbiol 1988; 24:490.

Ruoff KL: An update on streptococcal taxonomy. Clin Microbiol Newslett, 1988; 10:1.

Ruoff KL: Update on nutritionally variant streptococci (*Streptococcus defectivus* and *Streptococcus adjacens*). Clin Microbiol Newslett 1990; 12:97.

Saez-Nieto JA, Lujan R, Berron S, et al: Epidemiology and molecular basis of penicillin-resistant *Neisseria meningitis* in Spain: A 5-year history (1985–1989). Clin Infect Dis 1992; 14:394.

Sheagren JN: *Staphylococcus aureus*—the persistent pathogen (first of two parts). N Engl J Med 1984; 310:1368.

Shulman JA, Nahmias AJ: Staphylococcus infections: Clinical aspects. *In* Cohen JO (ed): The Staphylococci. New York, John Wiley and Sons, 1972, pp 457–481.

Stevens DL, Tanner MH, Winship J, et al: Severe group A streptococcal infections associated with a toxic shock-like syndrome and scarlet fever toxin A. N Engl J Med 1989; 321:1.

Talan DA, Staatz D, Staatz A, et al: *Staphylococcus intermedius* in canine gingiva and canine-inflicted human wound infections: Laboratory characterization of a newly recognized zoonotic pathogen. J Clin Microbiol 1989; 27:78.

Tenover FC: Diagnostic deoxyribonucleic acid probes for infectious diseases. Clin Microbiol Rev 1988; 1:82.

Tenover FC, Tokars J, Swenson J, et al: Ability of clinical laboratories to detect antimicrobial agent-resistant enterococci. J Clin Microbiol 1993; 31:1695.

Tramont EC: General or nonspecific host defense mechanisms. *In* Mandell GL, Douglas RG Jr, Bennett JE (eds): Principles and Practice of Infectious Diseases, 3rd ed. New York, Churchill Livingston, 1990, p 33.

Tracey KJ, Lowry SF, Cerami A: Cachectin: A hormone that triggers acute shock and chronic cachexia. J Infect Dis 1988; 157:413.

Tritz DM, Iwen PC, Woods GL: Comparative evaluation of MicroScan and conventional media for species identification of enterococci. J Clin Microbiol 1990; 28:1477.

Turnbull PCB, Kramer JM: *Bacillus*. *In* Balows A, Hausler WJ Jr, Herrmann KL, Isenberg HD, Shadomy HJ (eds): Manual of Clinical Microbiology, 5th ed. Washington, DC, American Society for Microbiology, 1991.

Wellstood SA: Rapid, cost-effective identification of group A streptococci and enterococci by pyrrolidonyl-β-naphthylamide hydrolysis. J Clin Microbiol 1987; 25:1805.

Wilson CB, Smith AL: Rapid tests for the diagnosis of bacterial meningitis. *In* Remington JS, Swartz MN (eds): Current Clinical Topics in Infectious Diseases, Vol. 7, New York, McGraw-Hill, 1986, pp 134–136.

Wilson JP, Turner AP, Kirchner KA, et al: Nocardial infections in renal transplant recipients. Med 1989; 68:38.

Woods CR, Smith AL, Wasilauskas BL, et al: Invasive disease caused by *Neisseria meningitidis* relatively resistant to penicillin in North Carolina. J Infect Dis 1994; 170:453.

Woolfrey BF, Moody JA: Human infections associated with *Bordetella bronchiseptica*. Clin Microbiol Rev 1991; 4:243.

Bibliography

Balows A, Hausler WJ Jr, Herrman KL, Isenberg HD, Shadomy HJ (eds): Manual of Clinical Microbiology, 5th ed. Washington DC, American Society of Microbiology, 1991.

Baron EJ, Peterson LR, Finegold SM (eds): Bailey and Scott's Diagnostic Microbiology, 9th ed. St. Louis, MO, C. V. Mosby, 1994.

Finegold SM: Anaerobic Bacteria in Human Disease. New York, Academic Press, 1977.

Koneman EW, Allen SD, Dowell VR, et al: Color Atlas and Textbook of Diagnostic Microbiology, 4th ed. Philadelphia, J. B. Lippincott, 1992.

Krieg NR, Holt JC (eds): Bergey's Manual of Systematic Bacteriology, Vol. 1. Baltimore, Williams and Wilkins, 1984.

Mandell GL, Bennett JE, Dolin R (eds): Principles and Practice of Infectious Diseases, 4th ed. New York, Churchill Livingstone, 1994.

Washington JA II (ed): Laboratory Procedures in Clinical Microbiology, 2nd ed. New York, Springer-Verlag, 1985.

Woods GL, Gutierez Y: Diagnostic Pathology of Infectious Diseases. Philadelphia, Lea and Febiger, 1993.

Chapter 49

In Vitro Testing of Antimicrobial Agents

Gail L. Woods, M.D.
John A. Washington, M.D.

The selection of an antimicrobial agent depends on numerous factors, including the site of infection; a variety of host factors, such as the state of immune defense mechanisms, renal and/or hepatic function, and history of allergic reactions; the absorption characteristics of the antimicrobial agent, as well as its route of excretion; pharmacokinetic properties and dosage frequency of the antimicrobial agent; personal experience with the antimicrobial agent; local susceptibility and resistance patterns; costs of acquisition and administration of the antimicrobial agent; and susceptibility of the microorganism to the antimicrobial agent. Although the selection of initial therapy for an infection is often made on an empirical basis, the availability of susceptibility test results aids either in the adjustment of initial dosage given or in modification of existing therapy for the following reasons: (1) the infecting microorganism is resistant to the antimicrobial being administered, (2) the dose of the antimicrobial administered initially may be modified, and (3) an equally effective but less expensive antimicrobial can be substituted.

DEFINITIONS

There are several categories of tests used to determine antimicrobial activity. The first category is represented by dilution and disk diffusion tests, which assess the inhibitory activity of an antimicrobial agent against a particular microorganism. In the second category are tests to determine the lethal (bactericidal or fungicidal) activity of an antimicrobial agent against a particular microorganism. A third category of tests relates to the determination of β-lactamase activity in a particular microorganism as a predictor of its responsiveness to certain β-lactam antibiotics. In the fourth category are tests to determine indirectly or directly the antimicrobial content of a body fluid, usually serum. Included in this category are the serum bactericidal tests and specific assays for antimicrobial agents.

Bacteria are commonly described as being susceptible, moderately susceptible, or resistant to antimicrobial agents. Definitions of these interpretive categories, including an intermediate category, have been provided in recommended procedures for disk diffusion and dilution testing published by the National Committee for Clinical Laboratory Standards (NCCLS M2-A5, 1993a; NCCLS M7-A3, 1993b). Susceptible implies that an infection caused by an organism can be appropriately treated with the dosage of antimicrobial agent recommended for that type of infection and infecting organism, unless otherwise contraindicated. Moderately susceptible implies that an infection caused by an organism may be treated by attainable concentrations of certain antimicrobial agents when administered in higher dosages or when the infections are in body sites (e.g., urine) where the antimicrobial agents are concentrated. The intermediate category provides a "buffer zone" that is intended to prevent the occurrence of major discrepancies in interpretation caused by small, uncontrolled technical factors. The intermediate category, sometimes also known as the indeterminate category, should not be confused with the moderately susceptible category. In general, the moderately susceptible category is applied to antimicrobial agents (e.g., β-lactams) that can be administered at higher dosages without serious risk of adverse reaction. The intermediate category is generally applied to those antimicrobial agents (e.g., aminoglycosides) with a narrow toxic to therapeutic ratio in which higher dosages are likely to be associated with adverse side effects. Resistance implies that infection caused by an organism is unlikely to respond or will not reliably respond to the antimicrobial agent. It must be understood that antimicrobial activity *in vivo* depends on many factors, including dosage, route of administration, host defenses, distribution space of the antimicrobial agent, absorption and excretion characteristics of the antimicrobial agent, and existing or developing renal or hepatic failure or adverse reaction to the antimicrobial agent. Thus, the interpretive categories provide only estimates of antimicrobial activity *in vivo*.

INDICATIONS FOR SUSCEPTIBILITY TESTING

Indications for performing susceptibility tests vary based on the organism in question. For example, rapidly growing aerobic and facultative bacteria should be tested if susceptibility to the antimicrobial agents of choice is unpredictable and if the isolate is believed to be clinically significant. In general, susceptibility testing is not necessary when the organism is known to be susceptible to the primary drug of choice. In the United States this is true for isolates of *Streptococcus pyogenes*, which to date have been universally susceptible to penicillin. However, if the patient is allergic to the antimicrobial agent of choice, testing susceptibility to alternative agents, such as erythromycin for *S. pyogenes*, is reasonable. Testing isolates that typically are considered "contaminants" or "usual flora" is expensive, time consuming, and may cause unnecessary administration of antimicrobial agents (Bates, 1991); therefore, it is not recommended. Occasionally, however, especially in immunocompromised patients, these "contaminants" are true pathogens, and it is essential that clinicians communicate these special circumstances to the laboratory personnel so appropriate testing will be done. Other situations in which susceptibility tests are useful are epidemiologic studies and evaluations of new antimicrobial agents.

Because of changing patterns of susceptibility of anaerobic bacteria, a Working Group on Anaerobic Antimicrobial Susceptibility Testing of the National Committee for Clinical Laboratory Standards (NCCLS) has recommended susceptibility testing of anaerobic bacteria isolated from the following types of infections: brain abscess, endocarditis, osteomyelitis, joint infections, infections of implanted prosthetic devices and vascular grafts, and refractory or recurrent bacteremias (NCCLS, 1993c). Otherwise, susceptibility testing of anaerobic bacteria should be performed periodically only to monitor susceptibility patterns in various centers and hospitals in the United States and abroad.

Given the resurgence of tuberculosis in the United States and the appearance of multidrug resistant strains, indications for testing susceptibility of *Mycobacterium tuberculosis* have changed. It is now recommended that initial isolates from all patients be tested and that testing be repeated if sputum specimens continue to be culture positive after three months of therapy (Tenover, 1993a). There are no firm guidelines regarding indications for susceptibility testing of nontuberculous mycobacteria.

During the past several years, the prevalence of systemic fungal infections has increased, especially in immunocompromised hosts, and new antifungal agents have been developed. Moreover, resistance of certain fungi to traditional therapy (such as *Candida lusitanae* resistant to amphotericin B) has been recognized, and with increasing use of azoles, especially fluconazole, yeasts (particularly *Candida* species) that are resistant to these agents have appeared. As a result, interest in antifungal susceptibility testing has grown. The NCCLS Subcommittee on Antifungal Susceptibility Testing was formed to evaluate the need for laboratory aids to guide selection of antifungal therapy. Based on data gathered, a need was established, and the subcommittee developed a tentative reference method for testing yeasts (*Candida* species, *Torulopsis glabrata*, and *Cryptococcus neoformans*) that cause systemic disease (NCCLS, 1992b). The clinical relevance of this reference procedure, however, has not yet been established, nor has its validity for testing dimorphic fungi and filamentous moulds been confirmed.

SELECTION OF ANTIMICROBIAL AGENTS

The selection of antimicrobial agents for testing (Table 49–1) has been complicated by the expanding spectrum and number of compounds within established spectrum classes of antimicrobials and in novel classes of antimicrobials. Testing all available compounds is unnecessary and beyond practicality. The selection process begins with the Pharmacy and Therapeutics Committee, which selects antimicrobial agents for the formulary. The objective should be to coordinate antimicrobials to be tested or reported with those in the formulary. This coordination assumes major importance today for several reasons. First, most laboratories use commercially prepared microdilution panels for antibacterial susceptibility testing. Manufacturers offer a variety of panels that are designed to correspond as closely as possible with those antibacterial agents in hospital formularies. Despite the variety of panels that are available, disparities between the variety of antimicrobial agents in the panels and those in hospital formularies often do exist, so that the laboratory may be faced with testing more than one panel for a particular microorganism or paying a premium price to have a panel made according to that hospital's specifications. In many instances, however, more antimicrobial agents are tested than are available in the hospital formulary so that the laboratory must suppress the results of those antimicrobial agents not in the formulary. Second, it is generally not necessary to report susceptibility test results for multiple representatives of the same spectrum class (e.g., cefotaxime, ceftizoxime, and ceftriaxone), even when more than one is in the formulary. Third, because manufacturers of commercially prepared antimicrobial susceptibility testing systems must submit to the Food and Drug Administration data validating the accuracy of their systems relative to any newly approved antimicrobial agent, there is often a lag between approval of the agent for clinical use and

Table 49–1. GUIDELINES FOR SELECTION OF ANTIBACTERIAL AGENTS FOR SUSCEPTIBILITY TESTING*

	Staphylococci	**Enterococci**	**Non-enterococcal Streptococci**	***Pseudomonas***	**Enterobacteriaceae**
Amikacin				P	P
Ampicillin	S	P			P
Ampicillin/sulbactam (or amoxicillin/clavulanate)	S				S
Azlocillin (or mezlocillin or piperacillin or ticarcillin)				P	
Aztreonam				S	S
Cefamandole (or cefonicid or cefuroxime)					S
Cefotaxime (or cefoperazone or ceftazidime or ceftizoxime or ceftriaxone or moxalactam)					P
Cefoxitin (or cefotetan)					S
Ceftazidime (or cefoperazone)				P	
Cephalothin	P		P		P†
Chloramphenicol	S			S	S
Ciprofloxacin	S			S	S
Clindamycin	P		P		
Erythromycin	P	U	P		
Gentamicin (or tobramycin)	S	S§		P	P
Imipenem				S	S
Mezlocillin (or piperacillin or ticarcillin)					P
Netilmicin				S	S
Oxacillin (or methicillin or nafcillin)	P‡				
Penicillin G	P		P		
Tetracycline	S				S, U
Ticarcillin/clavulanate					S
Trimethoprim/sulfamethoxazole	S			S¶	P
Vancomycin	P	S			
Cinoxacin (or nalidixic acid)					U
Nitrofurantoin	U	U	U		U
Norfloxacin	U	U	U	U	U
Trimethoprim	U				U

*P = Primary agents to be tested routinely; S = secondary agents to be tested under special circumstances, such as in institutions harboring endemic or epidemic resistance to one or more of the primary agents, for therapy of patients allergic to a primary agent, or as an epidemiologic aid; U = urinary tract–specific agent to be tested against urinary isolates only.

†Although cephalothin can be used to predict the *in vitro* activity of other first-generation cephalosporins, cefazolin should not be used for the same purpose because cefazolin is more active than other first-generation cephalosporins versus *E. coli*.

‡Oxacillin- (or methicillin- or nafcillin-) resistant staphylococci should be considered resistant to cephalosporins, penicillins (including combinations with β-lactamase inhibitors), and imipenem.

§Gentamicin and streptomycin should be tested at a concentration of 500 or 2000 μg/mL and 2000 μg/ml, respectively, to detect high-level resistant strains that are not synergistically affected by the combination of a penicillin and a respective aminoglycoside.

¶Applies only to species other than *P. aeruginosa*.

its incorporation in the commercially available susceptibility testing product. Thus, a new antimicrobial agent may be approved for the hospital's formulary before the laboratory has a capability of testing its activity *in vitro*.

Both NCCLS standards for dilution and disk diffusion susceptibility testing list antimicrobial agents that should be considered for testing against Enterobacteriaceae, *Pseudomonas*, staphylococci, enterococci, nonenterococcal streptococci, and *Haemophilus* (NCCLS M2-A5, 1993a; NCCLS M7-A3, 1993c); however, the number of compounds listed under the primary (group A) and secondary (groups B and C) groupings to be considered for testing often exceeds those that should be tested in any given laboratory. The NCCLS documents list azlocillin or piperacillin and carbenicillin, mezlocillin, or ticarcillin in the primary groupings to be considered for testing against *Pseudomonas*. Because it is recommended that *Pseudomonas*-active penicillins *not* be used alone (Gribble, 1983) and because no clinical studies of seriously ill (e.g., febrile neutropenic) patients have demonstrated any significant differences in outcome between regimens consisting of various penicillins plus an aminoglycoside, differences in degrees of activity of the *Pseudomonas*-active penicillins *in vitro* are not clinically important, and selection of a *Pseudomonas*-active penicillin for the formulary (and thereby for *in vitro* testing) may be based on the list of approved indications for use of one of this spectrum class and its costs of acquisition and administration relative to any other member of the same spectrum class. Clavulanate expands the spectrum of ticarcillin against plasmid-mediated β-lactamase producing Enterobacteriaceae and staphylococci, but adds little to the antipseudomonal activity of ticarcillin; however, there is little difference between the antipseudomonal activities of piperacillin and ticarcillin (with or without clavulanate) at the NCCLS-recommended minimum inhibitory concentration (MIC) of less than or equal to 64 μg/mL used to define the susceptibility of *Pseudomonas* (NCCLS M2-A5, 1993a; NCCLS M7-A3, 1993b). One possible consideration is that, although acquisition costs per gram of ticarcillin-clavulanate may be higher than those for an antipseudomonal penicillin, administration costs of ticarcillin-clavulanate plus an aminoglycoside may be less than those for the antipseudomonal penicillin plus an aminoglycoside plus oxacillin. Thus, administration costs may significantly outweigh acquisition costs of a particular antimicrobial agent. The pharmacokinetics of any particular antimicrobial agent clearly affect administration costs because an antimicrobial agent with a long half-life can be administered on a less frequent dosage schedule than another antimicrobial agent with the same antibacterial spectrum of activity but with a short half-life.

Although there is general agreement to test penicillin against staphylococci and streptococci, ampicillin against enterococci and Enterobacteriaceae, and oxacillin against staphylococci, there is considerably less agreement over which cephalosporins to test against gram-positive and gram-negative bacteria. Cephalothin may be used to represent the first-generation cephalosporins, including cefazolin; however, it is recommended that cefazolin not be used as the class representative for cephalothin and other first-generation cephalosporins because of an unacceptable rate of false susceptibilities to other cephalosporins, particularly with *Escherichia coli* (NCCLS M2-A5, 1993a; NCCLS M7-A3, 1993b). Thus, cefazolin should be tested only if it is the class representative in the formulary. There is much debate over the need to test second-generation cephalosporins and which ones, if any, should be tested against the Enterobacteriaceae. Cefotetan, cefoxitin, and cefamandole, cefonicid, or cefuroxime are listed as primary antimicrobials to be considered for testing in those institutions harboring endemic or epidemic resistance to the primary antimicrobial (i.e., cefazolin or cephalothin) being tested in the same class. Once again, the selection depends on which one, if any, is in the formulary and what indications have been specified by the Pharmacy and Therapeutics Committee for their use. Cefotetan or cefoxitin, for example, may be available in the hospital for the treatment of anaerobic bacterial infections, and, if so, testing them against any Enterobacteriaceae that may be present in a mixed aerobic-anaerobic infection may be useful. On the other hand, one or more of the second-generation cephalosporins may be available in the hospital for perioperative prophylaxis only, in which case there may not be a need to test them on a routine basis.

Selection of third-generation cephalosporins for testing is not only based on which one or ones are in the formulary but also on equivalency of activity *in vitro*. For example, there are only slight variations in activity against the Enterobacteriaceae among cefoperazone, cefotaxime, ceftizoxime, ceftriaxone, ceftazidime, and moxalactam. Thus, even though more than one of these compounds may be in the formulary, it is possible to test only one to represent the others against the Enterobacteriaceae. The only possible exception to this rule relates to the recent recognition in Europe of isolates of *Klebsiella pneumoniae* and other Enterobacteriaceae producing novel plasmid-mediated β-lactamases that cause resistance to the cephalosporins but not to the cephamycins or imipenem (CTX-1 or TEM-3) or that have preferential activity against ceftazidime (CAZ-1 or TEM-5 and CAZ or TEM-6) (Jarlier, 1988; Sirot, 1988; Sougakoff, 1988). Cross-resistance among third-generation cephalosporins is also observed with gram-negative mutants that are derepressed for Class I β-lactamase, provided the inoculum has been adjusted to approximately 5×10^5 CFU/mL and the test is incubated for a minimum of six hours (Washington, 1988).

In most instances, either cefoperazone or ceftazidime will be in the formulary for antipseudomonal therapy. The main question is, therefore, whether either should be tested in the laboratory against the Enterobacteriaceae so as to encourage limitation of the use of either compound to the treatment of *Pseudomonas* infections and to reduce the risk of emergence of resistance. The appearance of plasmid-mediated β-lactamases with preferential activity against ceftazidime, as well as existing plasmid-mediated β-lactamases with activity against cefoperazone, among the Enterobacteriaceae would lend support to a policy of limiting testing of cefoperazone or ceftazidime to *Pseudomonas*.

For enterococci, laboratories should consider testing vancomycin on all isolates, given the recent emergence of resistant strains (Livornese, 1992). However, not all automated systems reliably detect vancomycin resistance in enterococci, and if one of the less reliable systems is in use, including an alternate method (disk diffusion or agar screen) to ensure accurate results is suggested (Sahm, 1991; Tenover, 1993b; Woods, 1993). Screens for high-level resistance to gentamicin and streptomycin should be performed on all enterococcal isolates from sterile body sites, and clinicians should be informed (perhaps via a comment attached to the susceptibility test results) that combination therapy with penicillin or ampicillin plus an aminoglycoside is indicated for serious enterococcal infections such as endocarditis. As with vancomycin, not all automated systems reliably detect high-level aminoglycoside resistance, and it may be necessary to investigate an alternate method that is known to provide accurate results (Willey, 1992). For enterococci isolated from blood and cerebrospinal fluid, NCCLS suggests testing for β-lactamase production. Antimicrobial agents to consider testing on urinary enterococcal isolates are ciprofloxacin, nitrofurantoin, and tetracycline. Susceptibility test results for cephalosporins, aminoglycosides (except high-level testing), clindamycin, and trimethoprim/sulfamethoxazole against enterococci may be misleading and should not be reported.

Whether or not to test and report the activity of aztreonam, ciprofloxacin and imipenem on a regular basis will usually reflect their presence in the hospital formulary and, if present, any restrictions on their use (e.g., by infectious disease consultation only).

In regard to *Haemophilus influenzae*, antimicrobials to consider for the primary list of agents to test against isolates from blood and cerebrospinal fluid are ampicillin, a third-generation cephalosporin (cefotaxime, ceftazidime, ceftizoxime, or ceftriaxone), and chloramphenicol. For isolates from non–life-threatening infections, agents to consider testing include ampicillin, trimethoprim-sulfamethoxazole, amoxacillin/clavulanic acid (or ampicillin/sulbactam), cefaclor, and tetracycline. Results of ampicillin susceptibility tests predict the activity of amoxacillin. Resistance to ampicillin in most cases can be detected by testing for β-lactamase production; however, chromosomally mediated ampicillin resistance in β-lactamase–negative isolates has been reported (Mendelman, 1984). Therefore, if the β-lactamase test is negative, susceptibility to ampicillin should be confirmed by dilution or disk diffusion testing.

All isolates of *Streptococcus pneumoniae* from sterile body sites should be tested for resistance to penicillin; if this is done by the oxacillin disk screen, isolates with a zone diameter less than or equal to 19 mm must be further evaluated by a dilution method to distinguish resistant from intermediate strains. Other agents to consider testing against isolates from sterile body sites vary based on the test method used. For dilution methods, the NCCLS recommends testing cefotaxime, cefuroxime, ceftriaxone, chloramphenicol, and vancomycin; however, for disk diffusion there are interpretive standards only for the latter two agents. Antimicrobial agents to consider testing against isolates from non–life-threatening infections include penicillin (via the oxacillin disk screen), erythromycin, and trimethoprim/sulfamethoxazole.

In regard to viridans streptococci, any isolate implicated in bacterial endocarditis or, rarely, meningitis should be tested for susceptibility to penicillin (Goldfarb, 1984; Quinn, 1988). Testing susceptibility to cephalosporins being considered for therapy is warranted given that viridans streptococci may exhibit relative resistance to third-generation cephalosporins (Wilcox, 1993). Vancomycin is the recommended alternative to β-lactam drugs for viridans streptococci, but routine testing for susceptibility to this antimicrobial is not necessary, given that vancomycin resistance has not been reported in this group of organisms. For identification purposes, however, evaluating susceptibility to vancomycin is reasonable, because resistance would indicate that the organism is not a viridans streptococcus but most likely is a member of the intrinsically vancomycin-resistant genera such as *Leuconostoc* or *Pediococcus*.

Routine susceptibility testing of isolates of *Neisseria gonorrhoeae* is not necessary. Screening all isolates for β-lactamase production had been recommended in the past but is no longer recommended, given that neither penicillin nor ampicillin is included in the therapeutic regimens recommended for gonoccocal infections by the Centers for Disease Control and Prevention (CDC, 1993). Knowledge concerning penicillin resistance, however, may be useful for epidemiologic purposes. Although β-lactamase testing will detect most penicillin-resistant isolates, strains of *N. gonorrhoeae* with chromosomally mediated resistance will be missed by this method; therefore, penicillin susceptibility of β-lactamase–negative isolates should be confirmed by additional testing such as disk diffusion.

Antimicrobial agents that may be considered for testing against anaerobic bacteria include penicillin G, an extended spectrum penicillin, cefoxitin, a third-generation cephalosporin, and clindamycin (NCCLS M11-A3, 1993c). Metronidazole, chloramphenicol, imipenem, ampicillin/sulbactam, and ticarcillin/clavulanate are nearly always active against anaerobic bacteria and need not, therefore, be tested (NCCLS M11-A3, 1993c). Testing for purposes of establishing local susceptibility patterns should be limited to antimicrobials in the formulary.

Primary antituberculosis drugs against which isolates of *Mycobacterium tuberculosis* should be tested are isoniazid, rifampin, streptomycin, ethambutol, and pyrazinamide; however, in institutions where streptomycin is rarely used, selective testing of that agent is acceptable. If resistance to one or more of these drugs is suspected, further susceptibility testing to secondary agents, including ethionamide, kanamycin, capreomycin, ciprofloxacin, and cycloserine, should be done (Tenover, 1993a). For yeasts, the current tentative NCCLS standard includes guidelines for testing amphotericin B, flucytosine, fluconazole, and ketoconazole.

METHODS

Antimicrobial susceptibility tests may be categorized according to the end point being determined. The end point for most tests performed in the clinical laboratory is inhibition. There are limited indications for determination of lethal activity *in vitro*. Inhibitory activity is usually determined by a dilution or a disk diffusion technique.

Dilution Test

In the dilution test, the microorganism is inoculated into a series of tubes containing a range of concentrations, usually starting as an integral power of 2 (e.g., 128 g/mL) and decreasing on a $\log_2$ basis (i.e., 64, 32, 16, 8, 4, etc.) to the lowest concentration to be tested. The lowest concentration inhibiting visible growth is referred to as the minimum inhibitory concentration, or MIC. For purposes of convenience and economy, it has become increasingly common to limit the range of concentrations of each antimicrobial tested to those concentrations that encompass the concentrations equivalent to the susceptible and resistant categories. In some instances, commercially prepared microdilution trays contain only a single concentration of an antimicrobial agent, which is used to distinguish between the susceptible and resistant categories. Because most of the reference strains used for quality control of susceptibility testing are highly susceptible to the appropriate antimicrobial agents, limitation of the concentrations of antimicrobial agents poses unique problems in quality control. In other words, the acceptable MIC ranges for a particular reference strain versus a particular antimicrobial agent may be several $\log_2$ dilutions below the lowest concentration present for that antimicrobial in the susceptibility testing system. This problem places increasing responsibility for quality control on the manufacturer of the susceptibility testing system.

Disk Diffusion Test

In the disk diffusion test, use of which is largely limited to rapidly growing aerobic and facultatively anaerobic bacteria, a paper disk containing a specified amount (not concentration) of antimicrobial is applied to an agar surface that has been freshly inoculated with a microorganism. The antimicrobial diffuses into the medium from the disk, resulting in a zone of inhibition at the point at which a critical concentration of the antimicrobial in the medium inhibits growth of the microorganism at a particular point in time (usually 18 to 24 hours). The zone diameter of inhibition is measured and is inversely related to the MIC (i.e., the larger the zone diameter of inhibition, the lower the MIC and vice versa). Ideally, the relationship between the two tests can be expressed by a regression line, and zone diameter equivalents of susceptibility and resistance for a particular antimicrobial agent can be extrapolated from their intercepts on the regression line with the corresponding MICs used to define susceptibility and resistance.

E Test

The E test is a recently developed dilution test based on the diffusion of a continuous concentration gradient of an antimicrobial agent from a plastic strip into an agar medium. The plastic strip, which has a predefined concentration of dried and stabilized drug on one side and a continuous MIC interpretive scale on the other, is placed on the surface of an agar medium inoculated with the organism to be tested. The plate is incubated according to the atmosphere and time required for the specific organism. After incubation, an ellipse of growth inhibition is formed around the strip, and the MIC is read at the point on the scale where the ellipse intersects the strip. Given the current cost of these plastic strips, selecting the E test as the primary method for susceptibility testing is not practical. The E test, however, is a valuable alternative for testing susceptibility of fastidious bacteria, such as *S. pneumoniae* or *Haemophilus influenzae*, or anaerobes to a few key antimicrobial agents (Jorgensen, 1994; Sanchez, 1992).

Technical Considerations

However dilution or diffusion tests are performed, standardization of the procedure and of the medium used in the procedure is of the utmost importance in producing accurate and reproducible results. In the United States, professional organizations, industry, and government have worked together on a consensus basis within the National Committee for Clinical Laboratory Standards (NCCLS) to produce a series of documents that describe standardized procedures for susceptibility testing of aerobic and facultatively anaerobic bacteria (NCCLS M2-A5, 1993a; NCCLS M7-A3, 1993b), anaerobic bacteria (NCCLS M11-A3, 1993c), and mycobacteria (NCCLS M24-T, 1993d), and fungi (NCCLS, M27-P, 1992b). These procedures should be available in clinical laboratories for reference purposes and to provide the technical details regarding the performance of susceptibility tests. The Subcommittee on Antimicrobial Susceptibility Testing reviews and revises the tables of the documents on a yearly basis and reviews and revises the texts of each document on a three-year cycle. Thus, laboratories should ensure that the most current tables and texts are on hand, and that revisions in the tables and texts are incorporated into laboratory practice.

Medium

One important variable in susceptibility testing is composition of the medium. Currently, for testing aerobic and facultative bacteria the NCCLS recommends Mueller-Hinton medium, because it demonstrates good batch-to-batch reproducibility; is low in sulfonamide, trimethoprim, and tetracycline inhibitors; and supports the growth of most nonfastidious bacterial pathogens. Some bacteria, especially streptococci, do not grow well on unsupplemented Mueller-Hinton medium, a problem overcome by supplementing with defibrinated sheep, horse, or other animal blood at a final concentration of 5% (vol/vol).

Various components of or supplements to Mueller-Hinton medium, however, may affect susceptibility test results. For both dilution and disk diffusion tests, variation in the concentration of divalent cations, primarily calcium and magnesium, affects results of aminoglycoside and colistin tests with isolates of *Pseudomonas aeruginosa* and tetracycline with other bacteria. A cation content that is too high causes false resistance, whereas a cation content that is too low has the opposite effect (Barry, 1987, 1992; NCCLS M2-A5, 1993a; NCCLS M7-A3, 1993b). The pH of the medium should be between 7.2 and 7.4. A pH below this range may cause drugs such as aminoglycosides and macrolides to lose potency, and others (for example, penicillins) may appear to have excessive activity. The opposite effects are possible if the pH is too high.

For broth dilution testing, supplementation of Mueller-Hinton broth with 2% NaCl is now recommended to improve the detection of oxacillin-resistant staphylococci (NCCLS M7-A3, 1993b). The detection of heterogeneous resistance in which less than 0.01% of the cells express the resistance trait is enhanced by the addition of salt to the medium. An alternative approach to the detection of oxacillin-resistance in staphylococci is the use of Mueller-Hinton agar supplemented with 4% NaCl and incorporating 6 μg of oxacillin per mL (Chambers, 1988).

Other medium-related issues worthy of note are related to susceptibility testing of *H. influenzae*, for which *Haemophilus* test medium (HTM) is recommended (NCCLS M2-A5, 1993a; NCCLS M7-A3, 1993b), and *N. gonorrhoeae*, for which GC agar base is recommended. Mueller-Hinton medium that is as thymidine free as possible is important to the accurate determination of the susceptibility of bacteria to trimethoprim/sulfamethoxazole. Thymidine or thymine will adversely affect the activity of trimethoprim/sulfamethoxazole. Thymidine phosphorylase or lysed horse blood may be incorporated in the medium to improve the reliability of testing of trimethoprim and sulfamethoxazole. Accurate susceptibility test results are obtained with organisms other than enterococci with thymidine-free medium. For anaerobes, agar dilution using Wilkins-Chalgren agar is the reference method. Supplemented *Brucella* blood agar is an acceptable alternative, but MICs may be higher than with Wilkins-Chalgren agar. Media that have been used successfully for determining susceptibility of anaerobes by microdilution testing include Schaedler's, West-Wilkins, brain-heart infusion, and a broth made with the same formulation as Wilkins-Chalgren agar with the agar omitted, but they may require supplementation to allow growth (NCCLS M11-A3, 1993c).

Other medium-related factors predominantly influence disk diffusion. For example, the agar depth should be about 4 mm. False-resistant results are possible if the agar medium is too deep, whereas isolates may appear falsely susceptible if the agar is not deep enough. Media containing excessive amounts of thymidine or thymine can reverse the inhibitory effect of sulfonamides and of trimethoprim, causing smaller or less distinct zones. When Mueller-Hinton agar is supplemented with blood, the zone diameters for oxacillin and methicillin may be 2 to 3 mm smaller than those obtained with unsupplemented agar. Sheep blood also may cause indistinct zone diameters around sulfonamide and trimethoprim disks or a film of growth within the zone of inhibition.

Inoculum

Variations in inoculum size are responsible for the greatest day-to-day variation in susceptibility test results. Use of the proper inoculum (e.g., approximately 5×10^5 CFU/mL in broth dilution tests) is particularly important in the accurate detection of resistance to penicillin and oxacillin in staphylococci and to extended-spectrum penicillins and cephalosporins by gram-negative (e.g., *Enterobacter, Citrobacter, Pseudomonas*) mutants with derepressed Class I β-lactamase. A frequent observation in laboratories using microdilution-based systems is a high rate (20% to 40%) of susceptibility of *Enter-*

obacter cloacae to third-generation cephalosporins. This observation is invariably caused by the use of too low an inoculum. Thus, it behooves users of microdilution systems to include, among their quality control procedures, quantitation of their inoculum on a regular basis. The susceptibility of *Enterobacter cloacae* to ampicillin should generally not exceed 5%. A second factor related to inoculum is method of preparation. For many bacteria this is not an issue, but for staphylococci (to ensure detection of oxacillin resistance) and for fastidious bacteria, such as *S. pneumoniae, H. influenzae*, and *N. gonorrhoeae*, the inoculum should be prepared directly from overnight growth on an agar medium (Chambers, 1988; NCCLS, M2-A5, 1993a; NCCLS M7-A3, 1993b).

Incubation

Incubation conditions also affect susceptibility test results. General recommendations are overnight (16 to 18 hours) incubation in ambient air at 35°C; however, exceptions exist. Isolates of *S. pneumoniae, H. influenzae*, and *N. gonorrhoeae* require incubation in an atmosphere of 5% to 7% CO_2, and they should be incubated 20 to 24 hours rather than overnight. Staphylococci and enterococci also must be incubated for 24 hours to ensure detection of resistance to oxacillin and vancomycin, respectively. Anaerobes and yeasts typically require 48 hours of incubation, although 72 hours is recommended for isolates of *Cryptococcus neoformans*. For further details about susceptibility testing procedures, it is recommended that the appropriate NCCLS documents be consulted.

Testing Systems

According to results from recent proficiency testing programs of the College of American Pathologists, most laboratories in this country now use microdilution-based systems. One reason for this shift from diffusion to dilution technology is the efficiency gained from replicate inoculation of combined systems for identification and susceptibility testing, and from data management software packages that are features of these systems. Other reasons are frequently spurious and are based on a misconception that MICs are more accurate and are what physicians want to know. Because the results of dilution and diffusion tests are statistically highly correlated and because most physicians other than those specializing in infectious diseases have difficulty interpreting MICs, requiring laboratories to report interpretative categories along with MICs, the choice between diffusion tests and dilution tests can be made on purely economic grounds in nearly all instances.

There are numerous commercially available systems from which to choose today. Before making such a choice, the laboratory director should consider whether the advantages of replicate inoculation and data management systems outweigh the added costs of these systems as compared with the simplicity, convenience, and economy provided by the disk diffusion test. There is an unfortunate tendency among laboratory personnel to consider the disk diffusion test archaic and too unsophisticated for current practice. This test still does the job accurately and conveniently, as well as economically. The results provided are understandable to physicians and suffice in nearly all situations for which antimicrobial therapy is applied. Disk diffusion also provides flexibility in that one can test virtually any antimicrobial agent by simply selecting the appropriate disk.

The selection of a mechanized or semi-automated system must be based on numerous considerations. Among these considerations are test volume, technical expertise, the need for data management, the use of a common system for bacterial identification and susceptibility testing, compatibility with laboratory reporting systems, cost of equipment acquisition or leasing, cost of expendable supplies and reagents, cost of service contracts, and availability of space. With the AutoMicrobic System (bio Merieux, Vitek, Hazelwood, MO) antimicrobial agents are contained in wells within a plastic card. This system consists of a filler/sealer module, a reader incubator, a computer module, a data terminal, and a printer. Cards are incubated in the reader/incubator module, and the wells are monitored for optical density. Results can be obtained as early as four hours; however, the mean time of incubation for antimicrobial susceptibility testing is approximately seven hours. This incubation time is sufficient to provide reasonably accurate detection of mutants derepressed for Class I β-lactamase, penicillinase-producing staphylococci, and oxacillin-resistant staphylococci. There are a number of microdilution-based systems in which antimicrobial agents are provided either in the frozen or lyophilized state. Selection among these systems is not only based on the availability of freezer space for storage of the trays but also on the hands-on time required for each system. Selection may also be based on the availability and sophistication of data management systems. In some instances, the end points are read visually and are entered manually for reporting and storage purposes (e.g., Pasco, Difco Laboratories, Detroit, MI). In other instances the end points are read photometrically by the system (e.g., Baxter MicroScan Division, Sacramento, CA; Radiometer America, Inc./Sensititre, Westlake, OH). Both the MicroScan and Sensititre systems offer susceptibility testing capabilities at either approximately five hours' incubation or after approximately 18 hours of incubation. Of the currently available systems, AMS and MicroScan (AutoScan-W/A) offer walk-away capabilities.

With current capital equipment fund shortages, an increasing number of laboratories are using reagent-lease arrangements for such systems. For purposes of equipment and software maintenance it is usually necessary to have a service contract, the cost basis of which is approximately 10% of the purchase value of the equipment.

Speed of susceptibility testing is being heavily promoted now by manufacturers of systems providing MICs in three to five hours. Such systems, however, unreliably detect penicillin- or methicillin-resistant staphylococci, as well as gram-negative bacilli that are derepressed for Class I β-lactamase, and seem to require a minimum of six hours for detection of their resistance to many β-lactam antibiotics (Lampe, 1979; Washington, 1988). Even if rapid tests were accurate, is faster better? In a nonrandomized study, Matsen (1985) reported the results of both a three- to five-hour system and the disk diffusion test, and then questioned physicians as to whether receiving a faster result influenced their choice of antimicrobial therapy. In 31.7% of instances physicians indicated that they started a different antibiotic, based on the rapid result, than they would have otherwise; in another 17% of instances physicians indicated they "probably" would have. Most patients involved in the study had bacteriuria. In a prospective, randomized study of 794 general surgical patients, Vincent (1985) provided rapid results for half of the patients and conventional results for the other half. They found that antimicrobial therapy was modified in 14.5% of instances in the group of patients for which rapid results were provided and in 8.8% of instances in the group of patients for which conventional results were provided ($p <$ 0.001); however, there was no statistically significant difference between the two groups as regards length of stay of infected patients in the hospital.

More recently, Doern and colleagues (1994) evaluated the clinical impact of rapid bacterial identification and antimicrobial susceptibility testing in hospitalized patients in a tertiary-care medical center. The mean lengths of time to reporting identification and susceptibility test results, respectively, were 9.6 hours and 11.3 hours in the rapid test group, and 19.6 hours and 25.9 hours in the overnight test group ($p <$ 0.0005). There were no significant differences between the two groups with respect to demographic descriptors, other than the length of time to reporting results. The mean lengths of hospitalization were the same for both groups, but mortality rates were lower in the rapid test group (8.8% versus 15.3%). Moreover, for patients in the rapid test group there were significantly fewer laboratory studies, imaging procedures, days of intubation, and days in an intensive care unit; the length of time elapsed prior to alterations in antimicrobial therapy was shorter; and overall patients' costs for hospitalization were significantly lower.

BACTERICIDAL TESTS

There are three major categories of bactericidal tests: (1) determination of the minimum concentration of an antimicrobial required to kill a microorganism, otherwise known as the minimum bactericidal or lethal concentration (MBC or MLC); (2) determination of the killing rate (time-kill rate or killing curve); and (3) determination of the highest dilution of a patient's serum required to kill a microorganism, otherwise known as the serum bactericidal or lethal titer (SBT or SLT). The use of any of these categories of tests is surrounded by issues relating to indications, methodology, and interpretation.

Minimum Bactericidal or Lethal Concentration

As regards the MBC or MLC, there is general agreement that this determination should be part of the initial investigation of a new antimicrobial agent. There is, however, less agreement over whether the test is indicated for isolates of streptococci from patients with endocarditis, staphylococci from patients with endocarditis or osteomyelitis, and Enterobacteriaceae or *Pseudomonas* from patients with meningitis. In part, some of the controversy stems from biological and technical variables affecting the results of MBC determinations (NCCLS M26-T, 1992a). To determine the MBC or MLC, serially diluted (on a $\log_2$ basis) antimicrobial in broth is inoculated with a standardized suspension of the test organism, as described for determination of the MIC. After an overnight period of incubation those tubes with broth exhibiting no visible growth are subcultured onto antibiotic-free agar medium. The MBC or MLC is defined as the lowest concentration of antimicrobial agent that is bactericidal or lethal to at least 99.9% of the original inoculum. Among the biological variables of the test are (1) the persistence phenomenon in which a small number (usually $<0.1\%$) of the bacterial inoculum, "persisters," survive antibiotic exposure but remain susceptible if retested against the antibiotic, usually a cell wall active agent; (2) the paradoxic effect in which the proportion of surviving cells increases with the concentration of antibiotic, again most frequently with the cell wall active antibiotics; and (3) tolerance, a much misunderstood phenomenon. Strictly defined, tolerant organisms are those in which viability is lost slowly and those in which the bacteriostatic-bacteriolytic response to antibiotics is changed in the direction of bacteriostasis (Handwerger, 1985). Tolerance has, however, also been defined by an MBC:MIC ratio of greater than or equal to 32, despite the many technical problems that influence MBC results and procedural variations in determining MBCs (Sherris, 1986). As pointed out by Sherris (1986), the MBC is defined by the lowest concentration of antibiotic yielding less than or equal to 0.1% survivors at the least accurate portion of the killing curve (i.e., 18 to 24 hours). Moreover, the number of survivors after overnight incubation with a cell wall active antibiotic is invariably greater if the inoculum is in the stationary rather than the logarithmic phase (Handwerger, 1985; Sherris, 1986). Additional technical artifacts include the survival of bacteria in the condensate above the meniscus of antibiotic-containing broth, subculture volume, antibiotic carryover in subcultures, and test reproducibility. Assuming control of these technical problems can be achieved, determination of an end point (MBC) can be based on rejection criteria published by Pearson (1980). Because, however, tolerance is defined by a delayed rate of killing, the most reliable method for its detection is a simplified time-kill study of the organism comparing survivors after five or six hours of incubation in the presence of a concentration of antibiotic of four to eight times its MIC with those present at two-hour or zero-time readings (Handwerger, 1985; Sherris, 1986).

Considering all of the biological and technical problems associated with bactericidal testing and defining tolerance, it is not surprising that the interpretation of published literature on clinical studies of infections caused by purportedly "tolerant" organisms is fraught with difficulty, especially as regards staphylococci for which technical variables have major consequences (Handwerger, 1985). For these reasons, it is our policy not to determine MBCs of cell wall active antibiotics against staphylococci.

There are data from studies of experimental viridans streptococcal endocarditis in animals suggesting that penicillin may be less effective against infection due to tolerant strains than against nontolerant strains (Handwerger, 1985; Wilson, 1985); however, there is little information regarding the clinical significance of such strains (Wilson, 1985). Handwerger and Tomasz (1985) have speculated that nontolerant bacteria may manifest a phenotypically tolerant response in an endocardial lesion owing to their high density, diminished metabolic activity, and slow growth rate in vegetations. Because some strains of viridans streptococci are resistant (MIC ≥2 μg/mL) to penicillin, it certainly is necessary to determine the MIC of viridans streptococci isolated from patients with endocarditis or other life-threatening infections, and because patients with endocarditis caused by tolerant viridans streptococci may be at greater risk of relapse and may require four to six weeks of therapy with penicillin and an aminoglycoside (Wilson, 1985), it may be advisable to determine the MBC of such strains.

Killing Rate Studies

Bactericidal, rather than bacteriostatic, activity appears to be a requirement for therapy of bacterial meningitis (Sande, 1981). In the case of gram-negative bacillary (other than *H. influenzae*) meningitis, MBCs of cephalosporins may correlate poorly with outcome in contrast with the results of six-hour time-kill rate studies (Eng, 1987). Time-kill studies of antimicrobials, singly or in combination may, therefore, be more predictive of outcome than MBCs in those instances in which bactericidal therapy is necessary for cure (Bayer, 1985; Drake, 1983; Eng, 1987). Results of combination studies by the time-kill method also correlate better with the results of combination studies in experimental animal models of infection than do results of such studies obtained by the checkerboard method (Bayer, 1985), perhaps once again because the end point of the checkerboard method is determined at 18 to 24 hours, which is the least accurate end of the killing curve (Sherris, 1986). In killing rate studies, quantitative cultures are made at varying intervals (e.g., 4, 12, and 24 hours) following the inoculation of the antibiotic-containing medium. When antimicrobials are tested in combination, synergy is usually defined by a greater than or equal to 2-$\log_{10}$ reduction in CFU/mL between the combination and its most active constituent, assuming that at least one of the constituents does not affect the growth curve of the test organism when used alone. In the case of enterococci, this requirement poses no difficulties because clinically attainable concentrations of penicillins or aminoglycosides are not bactericidal; however, the requirement may pose problems in tests of other microorganisms that may be susceptible to each of the antimicrobials used in the combination. In the latter instance, synergy may be defined only when there is a greater than or equal to 2-$\log_{10}$ reduction in CFU/mL between the combination of each of two antimicrobials, present in concentrations representing one fourth of their respective MBCs, compared with the more active constituent alone at a concentration of one half its MBC (Hallander, 1982). As with MBC determinations, carryover of antimicrobial agents in quantitative subcultures is problematic and requires that any antimicrobial present be inactivated or that samples removed for subculture be sufficiently diluted that drug carryover effects are eliminated, if possible. Whether carryover occurs, particularly at test concentrations of greater than or equal to 4 × MIC, can be ascertained by streaking a 10- to 100-μL sample of a subculture dilution across an agar surface, allowing a 10- to 20-minute absorption time, and then streaking the entire agar surface with the test organism (NCCLS M26-T, 1992a). Another problem that may complicate interpretation of kill-kinetic studies is when regrowth occurs between 6 or 8 hours and 24 hours of incubation of the test. In such instances, it is appropriate to determine whether antimicrobial inactivation has occurred or whether prolonged incubation has selected out a resistant subpopulation (NCCLS M26-T, 1992a).

Serum Bactericidal Test

The principal objective of the serum bactericidal test is to determine the activity of one or more antimicrobial agents that are present in serum against an organism that has been isolated from the patient. This is done by obtaining a serum sample from the patient at the anticipated peak and/or trough levels of the antimicrobial agents that the patient is receiving. The serum sample is then diluted in broth, pooled human serum, or a mixture of broth and pooled human serum that has been supplemented with cation. A standardized suspension of the organism is then added to the serially diluted serum, and the tubes are incubated overnight at 35°C. The serum inhibitory titer is the highest dilution of serum that visibly inhibits the growth of the organism. Subcultures may be made of each tube containing the serum dilutions that do not have visible growth to determine the highest dilution of serum that was bactericidal to the test organism.

Although there is much controversy over the clinical value of the serum bactericidal test, it should be apparent that all of the technical issues involved in bactericidal testing are also involved in this test. Moreover, the serum bactericidal test involves two additional variables: (1) the timing of blood collection, and (2) whether the diluent used in the test is broth, serum, or a combination thereof. Once again, because of variations in methodology and technical variables affecting such tests, a correlation between specific bactericidal titers and outcome of antimicrobial therapy has been difficult to establish.

ANTIMICROBIAL ASSAYS

The level of antimicrobial agents in serum or other body fluids may be measured directly by bioassay, immunoassay, or chromatographic assay. In contrast with the serum bactericidal titer, assays provide a determination of the concentration of each antimicrobial agent that the patient is receiving.

Indications

The determination of the concentration of antimicrobial agent is most often indicated when the agent being administered has a narrow therapeutic index (Table 49–2) and when underlying host factors alter the agent's pharmacokinetics. Antimicrobial agents with a narrow therapeutic index include the aminoglycosides, vancomycin, chloramphenicol, and flucytosine. With such antimicrobial agents there is a narrow toxic to therapeutic ratio. Because of their broad therapeutic indexes, penicillins and cephalosporins rarely require assay unless (1) their route of administration or the underlying disease may cause serum levels to differ markedly from the usual range or (2) the infection is in a space or fluid where the antimicrobial agent penetration is variable or uncertain.

Table 49–2. FACTORS AFFECTING MONITORING OF SELECTED ANTIMICROBIALS

Antimicrobial	Usual Dose	Dose Interval (h)	Maximum Dose (per 24h)	Normal Serum Half-life (h)	Major Route of Elimination	Removed by Dialysis		Therapeutic Range (μg/mL)		Recommended Basis for Dosage Adjustment*
						Hemodialysis	*Peritoneal Dialysis*	*Peak*	*Trough*	
Amikacin	5–7.5 mg/kg	8–12	15 mg/kg	2–3	Renal	Yes	Yes	20–25	5–10	P, T
Gentamicin	1.7 mg/kg	8	5 mg/kg	2–3	Renal	Yes	Yes	4–8	1–12	P, T
Kanamycin	5–7.5 mg/kg	8–12	15 mg/kg	2–3	Renal	Yes	Yes	20–25	5–10	P, T
Netilmicin	2–2.5 mg/kg	8	7.5 mg/kg	2–3	Renal	Yes	Yes	6–10	0.5–2	P, T
Streptomycin	0.5–1.0 g	8–12	2 g	2–3	Renal	Yes	—	5–20	<5	P, T
Tobramycin	1.7 mg/kg	8	5 mg/kg	2–3	Renal	Yes	Yes	4–8	1–2	P, T
Chloramphenicol	0.5–1.0 g	6	4 g	4†	Hepatic/renal	Yes	No	15–25	8–10	T
Flucytosine	37.5 mg/kg	6	150 mg/kg	4	Renal	Yes	Yes	100	50	T
TMP/SMZ‡										
TMP	5 mg/kg	6	20 mg/kg	11	Renal	Yes	—	≥5	—	P
SMZ	25 mg/kg	6	100 mg/kg	13	Renal	Yes	—	≥100	—	P
Vancomycin	0.5–1.0 g	8–12	2 g	6	Renal	No	No	20–40	5–10	T

*P = peak level; T = trough level. These recommendations are valid when dosage interval is no greater than twice the usual dosage interval. Blood for peak levels should be drawn 30 minutes after completion of an IV infusion, 1 hour after an IM dose, and 1 to 2 hours after an oral dose.

†Half-life in children younger than four weeks old can be prolonged greatly. Half-life is affected only slightly in renal failure, but can be greatly prolonged with liver disease.

‡TMP/SMZ = trimethoprim/sulfamethoxazole. Maximum dosages apply to treatment of *Pneumocystis carinii* infection. Serum half-life is shortened in adolescents and children. Measurement of either TMP or SMZ alone is sufficient for dosage adjustment.

From Anhalt JP, Wilkowske CJ, Washington JA, II: Pocket Manual of Antimicrobial Agents, 11th ed. Philadelphia, B. C. Decker, 1989, p. 16. By permission of Mayo Foundation.

Antimicrobial assays may be indicated in patients who are receiving prolonged (greater than five days) antimicrobial therapy, in patients who are not responding to therapy, and in patients who are developing signs or symptoms of toxicity, for example, ototoxicity or nephrotoxicity during aminoglycoside administration. Antimicrobial assays are especially indicated in patients with impaired or rapidly changing renal function, and in patients undergoing dialysis. Further indications for antimicrobial assays include patients who are elderly, have cystic fibrosis, burns, gram-negative pneumonia, obesity or expanded extracellular fluid volumes, and who may not comply with oral dosages prescribed. It is important to understand that antimicrobial assays of agents with narrow therapeutic indexes are needed not only to ensure that agents with narrow therapeutic indexes are not present in a potentially toxic concentration but also that such agents are present in a therapeutic range. It has been found, for example, that there is a graded dose-response effect between an increasing maximal peak concentration/MIC ratio of aminoglycosides and clinical response (Moore, 1987).

Specimen Collection

Because of the short half-life of most antimicrobial agents, specimen collection is critical for proper therapeutic monitoring. Serum is the most appropriate specimen for assay; however, plasma is satisfactory, except for aminoglycosides, because of heparin binding. Assays of antimicrobial agents in urine are seldom indicated except for investigational purposes. Although blood from venipuncture is preferred for assay, blood may be obtained from an intravascular line—only, however, after the line has been flushed and the initial blood sample collected is discarded. In general, for determination of peak blood levels, specimens should be collected 30 minutes after an intravenous infusion has been completed, 60 minutes after an intramuscular dose, and 60 to 120 minutes after an oral dose. Peak levels do vary according to the antimicrobial agent being administered and its route of administration, as well as its rate of administration, absorption characteristics, and clinical status of the patient. Trough levels of antimicrobial agents are more sensitive indicators of decreased clearance and accumulation of antimicrobial agents to potentially toxic levels. Thus, it is frequently recommended that aminoglycosides be monitored both at anticipated peak and anticipated trough levels, the former to establish that a therapeutic level is being achieved and the latter to ensure that accumulation due to decreased clearance is not occurring.

Accurate specimen collection can usually be ensured only when the antibiotic has been administered and the specimen has been collected by the same person. Otherwise, there may be a considerable disparity between the recorded and actual times of administration of an antimicrobial agent. Consequently, if blood is collected by a phlebotomy team that relies on the recorded time of administration of the antimicrobial agent, the levels determined and subsequently reported may be interpreted incorrectly. Under such poorly controlled collection procedures, it may be possible to receive reports in which the putative trough level is higher than that of the peak level. In a worst case scenario, a putative peak level may appear to be insufficient for therapeutic purposes and the dosage of an antimicrobial agent with a narrow therapeutic index increased inappropriately, resulting in toxicity due to excessive levels of the antimicrobial agent.

Specimens should be either assayed immediately or stored at less than or equal to −20°C for no more than two days. Because certain aminopenicillins or ureidopenicillins may inactivate aminoglycosides during prolonged storage, a β-lactamase should be added to the serum if prolonged storage is anticipated. The interaction between penicillins and aminoglycosides is diminished with storage at −70°C.

Methodology

Historically, microbiologic assays constituted the most widely used methods and offered the best choice for routine measurement of antimicrobial concentrations in body fluids. With the introduction of gentamicin around 1970, there evolved a number of procedures for assay that did not depend on a microbiologic dose-response *in vitro*. These methods provide greater accuracy and specificity than was possible with microbiologic assays.

Microbiologic assays are based on a comparison of the response of a susceptible microorganism to an unknown concentration of antibiotic with the response of the same microorganism under identical test conditions to known concentrations of the antimicrobial agent. The test is usually based on agar diffusion techniques in which the agar is seeded with a standardized suspension of the test microorganism and onto which the fluids containing unknown concentrations of antibiotics and the standards containing known concentrations of antibiotics are delivered, either in wells punched out of the agar or on blank paper disks. The plates are then incubated overnight and a dose-response curve is plotted by measuring the zone diameter of inhibition corresponding with each known concentration of antibiotic used in the standards. It must be understood that the microbiologic assay measures the effects of any and all antimicrobial agents that may be present in the biological fluid being assayed. Thus, if the patient is receiving antimicrobial agents other than the one to be assayed, the zone diameters of inhibition will reflect the combined effects of all antimicrobial agents that are present. In some instances, it is possible to measure the concentration of one antimicrobial agent in the presence of another by the appropriate selection of a test microorganism that is susceptible to the antimicrobial agent to be measured and resistant to the potentially interfering antimicrobial agent. In other instances, it is possible to supplement the assay medium with substances that may neutralize the effects of the interfering antimicrobial agent. For example, one may add cation or sodium polyanetholsulfonate to the test medium to neutralize aminoglycoside activity for assay of β-lactam antibiotics. In some instances, however, it is simply not possible to measure the concentration of one antimicrobial agent in the presence of another. Despite these limitations, the microbiologic assay remains the gold standard against which nonmicrobiologic assays are evaluated, the reason being that the microbiologic assay measures the total antimicrobial activity of an antimicrobial agent, while a nonmicrobiologic assay may measure only one component of a structurally complex antimicrobial agent. Detailed descriptions of microbiologic assays have been provided by Anhalt (1985) and Edberg (1986).

Liquid chromatography, which is a process for separating complex mixtures based on their distribution between a mobile liquid phase and a stationary solid phase, has provided a sensitive and specific technology to measure almost all antimicrobial agents in clinical specimens. The procedure involves either extraction of the antimicrobial from the specimen or precipitation of protein followed by chromatography of the extract or protein-free fluid on a reversed phase column (Anhalt, 1985). Details regarding liquid chromatographic assays have been published by Anhalt (1985). Factors affecting the current use of liquid chromatographic assays are the availability of equipment for analysis of drugs other than antibiotics, the unavailability of kits for some antimicrobial agents, the small test volume for some antimicrobial agents, and the need to quantitate metabolites and isomers of antimicrobial agents. Liquid chromatographic assays have the advantage over other methods of assay in that a standard can be mixed with the specimen prior to assay, thus providing an internal standard. The advantages of liquid chromatographic assays include their versatility, relatively low reagent cost, moderate equipment cost, the lack of need for derivatization, the ability to handle "stat" requests, and minimal down time. Disadvantages of liquid chromatographic assays include the relatively large sample size (500 μL), the need for sample pretreatment, requirement for a variety of detectors, sample throughput time, and training time required for accurate processing of specimens. Liquid chromatographic methods have been largely supplanted in clinical laboratories for antimicrobial assay by immunoassays.

Among the first of the immunoassays that become available for aminoglycoside assay was radioimmunoassay (RIA). Radioimmunoassays required only a small sample, were able to handle "stat" requests, were particularly capable of handling multiple assays per batch, provided automation, and were sensitive and specific. The disadvantages of RIA were the limited shelf life of radiolabeled reagents, the problems of dealing with radioactive material, the moderately high equipment cost and reagent cost, and the lack of versatility for assay of other antimicrobial agents. Thus, radioimmunoassays have been almost completely supplanted by non-isotopic immunoassays, including polarization, substrate labeled, enzyme-multiplied, and fluorescence polarization assays (Edberg, 1986). Advantages of such homogeneous immunoassays are the small sample size required (approximately 50 μL), the lack of need for sample preparation, the moderate equipment cost, the minimal training time required, the ability of the systems to handle "stat" requests, and the availability of automation. Their disadvantages include the fact that there is often only a single reagent source and reagents may be expensive. At this time, the number of antimicrobial agents that may be assayed with such systems is quite limited (aminoglycosides and vancomycin). Nonetheless, because of their convenience and rapid turnaround time, these immunoassay systems are widely used. A detailed description of immunoassays has been published by Edberg (1986).

A number of studies have been made of the accuracy and technical aspects of microbiologic, radioimmunoassay, non-isotopic immunoassays, and high-performance liquid chromatography. Coefficients of variation are generally comparable (7% to 9%). Sensitivities are also generally comparable (0.1 to 1 μg/mL). Correlation among the methods is generally high. Assay results from non-isotopic immunoassays and high-performance liquid chromatography can be available in as little as one hour, while those of radioimmunoassay can be available in as little as three to four hours. Although most microbiologic assays require overnight incubation, a number of rapid (four to six hour) microbiologic assays are available for aminoglycosides and vancomycin.

Interpretation

Interpretation of the results of antimicrobial assays requires knowledge of the dose of antimicrobial agent administered, the time interval between administration of the dose and collection of the blood sample, the susceptibility of the infecting microorganism, the safely achievable serum levels of the antibiotic, and the distribution space and route of excretion of the antibiotic, the absorption characteristics of the antibiotic, and clinical experience in treating similar infections. Given those qualifications, the factors affecting monitoring of antimicrobial agents with narrow therapeutic indexes are listed in Table 49–2 (Anhalt, 1989).

Anhalt JP: Antimicrobial assays. *In* Washington JA (ed.): Laboratory Procedures in Clinical Microbiology, 2nd ed. New York, Springer-Verlag, 1985, p 691.

Anhalt JP, Wilkowske CJ, Washington JA, II: Pocket Manual of Antimicrobial Agents, 11th ed. Philadelphia, BC Decker, 1989.

Barry AL, Miller GH, Thornsbery C, et al: Influence of cation supplements on activity of netilmicin against *Pseudomonas aeruginosa* in vitro and in vivo. Antimicrob Agents Chemother 1987; 31:1514.

Barry AL, Reller LB, Miller GH, et al: Revision of standards for adjusting the cation content of Mueller-Hinton broth for testing susceptibility of *Pseudomonas aeruginosa* to aminoglycosides. J Clin Microbiol 1992; 30:585.

Bates DW, Goldman L, Lee TH: Contaminant blood cultures and resource utilization. The true consequences of false-positive results. JAMA 1991; 265:365.

Bayer AS, Lam K: Efficacy of vancomycin plus rifampin in experimental aortic valve endocarditis due to methicillin-resistant *Staphylococcus aureus*: In vitro–in vivo correlations. J Infect Dis 1985; 151:157.

Centers for Disease Control and Prevention: 1993 Sexually Transmitted Diseases Treatment Guidelines. MMWR 1993; 42:56.

Chambers HF: Methicillin-resistant staphylococci. Clin Microbiol Rev 1988; 1:173.

Doern GV, Vautour R, Gaudet M, et al: Clinical impact of rapid in vitro susceptibility testing and bacterial identification. J Clin Microbiol 1994; 32:1757.

Drake TA, Sande MA: Studies of the chemotherapy of endocarditis: Correlation of in vitro, animal model, and clinical studies. Rev Infect Dis 1983; 5(Suppl 2):S345.

Edberg SC: The measurement of antibiotics in human body fluids: Techniques and significance. *In* Lorian V (ed.): Antibiotics in Laboratory Medicine, 2nd ed. Baltimore, Williams & Wilkins, 1986, p 381.

Eng RHK, Cherubin CE, Pechere J-C, Beam TR: Treatment failures of cefotaxime and latamoxef in meningitis caused by *Enterobacter* and *Serratia* spp. J Antimicrob Chemother 1987; 20:903.

Goldfarb J, Wormser GP, Glaser JH: Meningitis caused by multiply antibiotic-resistant viridans streptococci. J Pediatr 1984; 105:891.

Gribble MJ, Chow AW, Naiman SL, et al: Prospective randomized trial of piperacillin monotherapy versus carboxypenicillin-aminoglycoside combination regimens in the empirical treatment of serious bacterial infections. Antimicrob Agents Chemother 1983; 24:388.

Hallander HO, Dornbusch K, Gezelius L, et al: Synergism between amino-

6

glycosides and cephalosporins with antipseudomonal activity: Interaction index and killing curve method. Antimicrob Agents Chemother 1982; 22:743.

Handwerger S, Tomasz A: Antibiotic tolerance among clinical isolates of bacteria. Rev Infect Dis 1985; 7:368.

Jarlier V, Nicolas M-H, Fournier G, Philippon A: Extended spectrum β-lactamases conferring transferable resistance to newer β-lactam agents in Enterobacteriaceae: Hospital prevalence and susceptibility patterns. Rev Infect Dis 1988; 10:867.

Jorgensen JH, Ferraro MJ, McElmeel ML, et al: Detection of penicillin and extended-spectrum cephalosporin resistance among *Streptococcus pneumoniae* clinical isolates by use of the E test. J Clin Microbiol 1994; 32:159.

Lampe MF, Minshew BH, Sherris JC: In vitro response of *Enterobacter* to ampicillin. Antimicrob Agents Chemother 1979; 16:458.

Livornese LL, Dias S, Samel C, et al: Hospital-acquired infection with vancomycin-resistant *Enterococcus faecium* transmitted by electronic thermometers. Ann Intern Med 1992; 117:112.

Matsen JM: Means to facilitate physician acceptance and use of rapid test results. Diagn Microbiol Infect Dis 1985; 3:S73.

Mendelman PM, Chaffin DO, Stull TL, et al: Characterization of non-β-lactamase-mediated ampicillin resistance in *Haemophilus influenzae*. Antimicrob Agents Chemother 1984; 26:235.

Moore RD, Lietman PS, Smith CR: Clinical response to aminoglycoside therapy: Importance of the ratio of peak concentration to minimal inhibitory concentration. J Infect Dis 1987; 155:93.

National Committee for Clinical Laboratory Standards: Methods for Determining Bactericidal Activity of Antimicrobial Agents. Tentative Standard. NCCLS publication M26-T. Villanova, PA, 1992a.

National Committee for Clinical Laboratory Standards: Reference Method for Broth Dilution Antifungal Susceptibility Testing of Yeasts. Proposed Standard. NCCLS Document M27-P. Villanova, PA, 1992b.

National Committee for Clinical Laboratory Standards: Performance Standards for Antimicrobial Disk Susceptibility Tests, 5th ed. Approved Standard. NCCLS publication M2-A5. Villanova, PA, 1993a.

National Committee for Clinical Laboratory Standards: Methods for Dilution Antimicrobial Susceptibility Tests for Bacteria That Grow Aerobically, 3rd ed. Approved Standard. NCCLS publication M7-A3. Villanova, PA, 1993b.

National Committee for Clinical Laboratory Standards: Methods for Antimicrobial Susceptibility Testing of Anaerobic Bacteria, 2nd ed. Tentative Standard. NCCLS publication M11-A3. Villanova, PA, 1993c.

National Committee for Clinical Laboratory Standards: Susceptibility Testing for *Mycobacterium tuberculosis*. Tentative Standard. NCCLS Document M24-T. Villanova, PA, 1993d.

Pearson RD, Steigbigel RT, Davis HT, Chapman SW: Method for reliable determination of minimum lethal antibiotic concentrations. Antimicrob Agents Chemother 1980; 18:699.

Quinn JP, Divincenzo CA, Lucks DA, et al: Serious infections due to penicillin-resistant strains of viridans streptococci with altered penicillin-binding proteins. J Infect Dis 1988; 157:764.

Sahm DF, Boonlayangoor S, Iwen P, et al: Factors influencing determination of high-level aminoglycoside resistance in *Enterococcus faecalis*. J Clin Microbiol 1991; 29:1934.

Sanchez ML, Jones RN: E test, an antimicrobial susceptibility testing method with broad clinical and epidemiologic application. Antimicrob Newslett 1992; 8:1.

Sande MA: Antibiotic therapy of bacterial meningitis: Lessons we've learned. Am J Med 1981; 71:507.

Sherris JC: Problems in in vitro determination of antibiotic tolerance. Antimicrob Agents Chemother 1986; 30:633.

Sirot J, Chanal C, Sirot D, et al: *Klebsiella pneumoniae* and other Enterobacteriaceae producing novel plasmid-mediated β-lactamases markedly active against third-generation cephalosporins: Epidemiologic studies. Rev Infect Dis 1988; 10:850.

Sougakoff W, Goussard S, Gerbaud G, Courvalin P: Plasmid-mediated resistance to third generation cephalosporins caused by point mutations in TEM-type penicillinase genes. Rev Infect Dis 1988; 10:879.

Tenover RC, Crawford JT, Huebner RE, et al: The resurgence of tuberculosis: Is your laboratory ready? J Clin Microbiol 1993a; 31:767.

Tenover RC, Tokars J, Swenson J, et al: Ability of clinical laboratories to detect antimicrobial agent-resistant enterococci. J Clin Microbiol 1993b; 31:1695.

Vincent P, Izard D, Lebrun T, et al: Intérêt cliniques des resultats rapides de bactériologie au de l'infection nosocomiales: Comparaison avec les méthods traditionelles. Presse Med 1985; 14:1697.

Washington JA II, Knapp CC, Sanders CC: Accuracy of microdilution and the AutoMicrobic System in detection of β-lactam resistance in gram-negative bacterial mutants with derepressed β-lactamase. Rev Infect Dis 1988; 10:824.

Wilcox MH, Winstanley TG, Douglas CWI, et al: Susceptibility of alpha-hemolytic streptococci causing endocarditis to benzylpenicillin and ten cephalosporins. J Antimicrob Chemother 1993; 32:63.

Wiley BM, Kreiswirth BN, Simor AE, et al: Detection of vancomycin resistance in *Enterococcus* species. J Clin Microbiol 1992; 30:1621.

Wilson WR, Geraci JE: Treatment of streptococcal infective endocarditis. Am J Med 1985; 78(Suppl 6B):128.

Woods GL, DiGiovanni B, Levison M, et al: Evaluation of MicroScan rapid panels for detection of high-level aminoglycoside resistance in enterococci. J Clin Microbiol 1993; 31:2786.

Chapter 50

Spirochete Infections

Erik K. Hofmeister, D.V.M., Ph.D.
David H. Persing, M.D, Ph.D.
Linda Mann, Ph.D.
Gail L. Woods, M.D.

The spirochetes that cause disease in humans are the pathogenic species of *Treponema* and *Borrelia*, *Leptospira interrogans*, the anaerobic spirochetes, and *Spirillum minor*. These organisms are helical in shape, 0.1 to 0.5 μm wide and 5 to 30 μm long. They have a multilayered outer envelope and a protoplasmic cylinder composed of a peptidoglycan layer, a cytoplasmic membrane, and the enclosed cytoplasmic contents. Flagella-like organelles, called periplasmic fibrils or axial filaments, are attached near the ends of the organism by insertion disks located within the cell wall between the outer envelope and the protoplasmic cylinder and extend along the body of the spirochete toward the opposite poles, thus permitting corkscrew-like winding motility. Spirochetes are gram-negative, but they stain poorly or not at all with Gram's stain. Silver stains or direct visualization using dark-field or phase optics are necessary to demonstrate the organisms in clinical specimens.

TREPONEMA

The pathogenic treponemes (*Treponema pallidum* and its subspecies and *Treponema carateum*) are microaerophilic, antigenically similar organisms, 6 to 15 μm long and 0.1 to 0.2 μm wide, with pointed ends and three periplasmic fibrils attached at each end. The nonpathogenic treponemes, in contrast, are anaerobic, wider (0.15 to 0.25 μm), and have blunt ends and one to eight fibrils per cell.

Treponema pallidum

Treponema pallidum is a thin, spiral bacterium, 5 to 20 μm long and 0.2 μm in diameter. The organism has 4 to 14 coils and is actively motile, exhibiting motion that ranges from a shimmering or undulating movement in serous exudate to directional, corkscrew motility in fibrinous exudates. It is readily inactivated by heat, cold, dessication, most disinfectants, and osmotic changes. Culture on artificial media has not been successful, and only limited viability is maintained in tissue culture systems. Based on DNA homology studies *T. pallidum* is divided into three subspecies—*pallidum*, *pertenue*, and *endemicum*, the etiologic agents of venereal syphilis, yaws, and nonvenereal endemic syphilis, respectively.

Syphilis

EPIDEMIOLOGY. Humans are the only natural hosts for *T. pallidum* subspecies *pallidum*. Infected persons are most infectious early in the disease, become less infectious with time, and are unable to spread the disease by sexual contact four years after infection. Syphilis most commonly is spread by sexual contact, and about 30% of those who have sexual contact with an infected person become infected (Larson, 1995). Other mechanisms of transmission include kissing or touching a person who has active lesions on the lips, oral cavity, breasts, or genitals; transfusing fresh blood or blood products (organisms cannot survive more than 24 to 48 hours under conditions of blood bank storage) collected from an individual with the disease, which is rare if blood from donors who have a reactive nontreponemal serologic test (described later) is not used; and accidental direct inoculation during a needle stick or when handling infected clinical material. Congenital syphilis most commonly is acquired *in utero* but may be acquired during passage through an infected birth canal. Fetal infection is rare before the fourth month of gestation; and if the mother is treated during the first four months of pregnancy, the fetus will usually not be infected.

In the United States, the number of cases of syphilis peaked during World War II. With the introduction of penicillin, the incidence declined dramatically and then remained relatively stable until 1986, after which the prevalence again rose, reaching a peak in 1990, when nearly 135,000 cases were reported. A disproportionate number of cases of syphilis occurred in homosexual men until the 1980s, when the prevalence among this cohort declined because they adapted safer sex practices in an attempt to prevent infection with human immunodeficiency virus (HIV). Concomitantly, the number of cases rose among heterosexual women. This increase, linked to the use of crack cocaine and the practice of trading sex with multiple partners for these drugs, was paralleled by a similar rise in congenital syphilis (CDC, 1989).

PATHOGENESIS AND PATHOLOGY. *Treponema pallidum* subspecies *pallidum* penetrates intact mucous membranes or gains access to the tissues through abraded skin, multiplies locally, enters the lymphatics and blood, and disseminates throughout the body, including the central nervous system. The necessary infectious dose varies, but in rabbits inoculated in the laboratory, as few as four spirochetes can establish an infection. Clinical lesions appear when a critical concentration of spirochetes is reached; therefore, the incubation period is directly proportional to the inoculum size. Because spirochetemia may persist for weeks or months, new lesions may develop long after the initial contact with the organism.

Little is known about definitive virulence factors of the organisms, pathogenetic mechanisms, and protective immune responses. The endoflagellar, periplasmic, inner membrane immunogens may elicit the production of antibodies useful for diagnostic assays, but the role of these antibodies or the cellular immune response in the establishment of latency and acquired resistance is unknown. The outer membrane of the organism may contain a protein (TROMP) that is expressed at low levels and is essential to virulence and protective immunogenicity (Blanco, 1990).

Four clinical stages of syphilis are recognized: (1) The primary stage is characterized by the formation of the chancre at the site of inoculation. (2) The secondary, or disseminated, stage occurs two to 12 weeks (mean, six weeks) after contact, when the greatest number of organisms are present in the body. During this phase, specific antibodies are produced, and immune complexes may form. (3) The latent period follows the secondary stage and is divided into the early latent stage, during which relapses of secondary syphilis may occur, and the late latent stage, during which relapses are unlikely. Relapse of disease is a consequence of a dysfunction in cellular immunity. Relapses may occur up to four years after contact, but 75% of cases are seen within the first year. (4) Late syphilis, termed tertiary disease, develops in up to one third of untreated individuals. It typically involves the vasa vasorum of the aorta, the arteries of the central nervous system, or both but also may be manifested by the development of a gumma.

Two histologic features, characteristic but not pathognomonic of syphilis, occur in all stages of the disease: obliterative endarteritis (meaning concentric endothelial and fibroblastic proliferative thickening) and a plasma cell infiltrate. Histologic examination of the primary chancre shows many spirochetes and scattered polymorphonuclear leukocytes and macrophages ingesting organisms. Sections of the mucocutaneous lesions and condyloma lata of secondary syphilis show a perivascular mononuclear cell infiltrate, mainly plasma cells, and many spirochetes. The gumma, a rubbery, gray-white necrotic mass, consists of a central area of coagulated, necrotic material containing shadowy outlines of underlying tissue but no vital native or inflammatory cells. This is surrounded by a rim of epithelioid fibroblasts, plasma cells, lymphocytes, and small blood vessels showing obliterative endarteritis.

CLINICAL MANIFESTATIONS. Clinical manifestations of syphilis are summarized, by stage, in Table 50–1. The classic chancre of primary syphilis begins three to 90 days (usually within three weeks) after contact as a single painless papule, most commonly on the external genitalia, but the

Table 50–1. CLINICAL MANIFESTATIONS OF SYPHILIS

Stage	Manifestations
Primary	Chancre at site of inoculation; ± painless regional lymphadenopathy
Secondary[a]	Malaise, fever, anorexia, generalized painless lymphadenopathy; maculopapular (occasionally becoming pustular) rash usually on trunk and proximal extremities, including palms and soles (may involve any body surface); condyloma lata; mucous patches; CNS involvement (headache, meningismus, increase CSF protein and WBC count) in 8–40%
Tertiary	
Neurosyphilis	
Meningovascular	Hemiplegia/hemiparesis, seizures, aphasia
Parenchymatous	General paresis (changes in personality and intellect, hyperactive reflexes, slurring of speech, Argyll Robertson pupils, optic atrophy, tremors); tabes dorsalis (ataxic, wide-based gait and footslap, paresthesias, lightning pains, bladder disturbances, impotence, loss of position and vibratory sense, trophic degenerative joint disease)
Otitis	Asymmetric deafness, tinnitus
Eye disease	Optic atrophy, blindness
Cardiovascular	Aortic regurgitation, coronary artery stenosis
Gummas	Lesion most commonly involving bones, skin, mucous membranes
Congenital	Rhinitis, maculopapular and desquamative rash (palms, soles, mouth, anus), osteochondritis and perichondritis (saddle nose, saber shin), anemia, thrombocytopenia, hepatomegaly, and jaundice

[a]Uncommon manifestations are acute aseptic meningitis, immune complex glomerulonephritis, nephrotic syndrome, hepatitis, proctitis, anterior uveitis, osteitis, and synovitis.

CNS = central nervous system; CSF = cerebrospinal fluid; +/− = may or may not be present.

cervix, mouth, perianal area, or anal canal also may be involved. The papule ulcerates and becomes indurated, with a smooth base and raised, firm borders. The chancre heals in one to 12 weeks (three to six weeks is usual) with minimal or no scarring. Atypical presentations include absence of a chancre, failure of the lesion to ulcerate, or multiple chancres (particularly in persons infected with HIV).

Secondary syphilis usually begins one to five weeks after the chancre has healed, but occasionally the primary lesion is still present. The classic rash is seen in about 90% of persons. If the hair follicles are involved, temporary patchy alopecia may occur. Other findings include condyloma lata (painless, broad, moist, gray-white to erythematous, highly infectious plaques) in intertriginous areas and mucous patches (painless superficial erosions teeming with spirochetes) on mucous membranes. Fewer than 50% of those with secondary syphilis show signs or symptoms of central nervous system involvement.

Late tertiary syphilis is manifested clinically as neurosyphilis, cardiovascular syphilis, or gummas that are recognized years after the initial infection. In persons infected with HIV, however, the usual course of syphilis is accelerated, and neurosyphilis may develop less than one year after the primary infection (Johns, 1987; Musher, 1990). Late neurosyphilis may be asymptomatic, diagnosed only by abnormalities of the cerebrospinal fluid (CSF) (pleocytosis, elevated protein concentration, or a positive Venereal Disease Research Laboratory [VDRL] test [discussed later]), or symptomatic. If syphilis is not treated, 8% to 40% of persons develop asymptomatic neurosyphilis; but because the diagnosis requires lumbar puncture and CSF examination, it is difficult to know how many become symptomatic. Symptomatic neurosyphilis is divided into two clinical categories, based on pathologic findings—meningovascular and parenchymatous, although overlap occurs.

Meningovascular neurosyphilis usually occurs five to 10 years after the onset of disease. It is characterized by endarteritis obliterans affecting the small blood vessels of the meninges, spinal cord, and brain, and subsequent multiple small areas of infarction. Parenchymatous neurosyphilis, during which nerve cells (predominantly those in the cerebral cortex) are destroyed, includes general paresis and tabes dorsalis, usually manifest 15 to 20 years and 25 to 30 years after the onset of disease, respectively.

Cardiovascular syphilis is characterized by endarteritis obliterans that involves the vasa vasorum of the aorta or other large arteries, resulting in medial necrosis, destruction of elastic tissue, and aortitis with subsequent saccular or, occasionally, fusiform aneurysm formation (Jackman, 1989). The predilection to involve the ascending aorta causes widening of the aortic ring and narrowing of the mouths of the coronary ostia.

The clinical manifestations of congenital syphilis vary, depending on the severity of the infection. Late abortion, stillbirth, neonatal death, neonatal disease, or latent infection may develop, and often the physical examination is normal (Dorfman, 1990; Ikeda, 1990). Necrotizing funisitis (inflammation of the matrix of the umbilical cord with obliterative endarteritis) is virtually pathognomonic of congenital syphilis. In the perinatal period (infantile form), the mucocutaneous tissues and bones are most commonly involved. If death occurs, it generally is due to liver failure, pneumonia, or pulmonary hemorrhage. The untreated infant who survives the first six to 12 months of life enters a latent period, manifested by interstitial keratitis, asymptomatic or symptomatic neurosyphilis, and eighth nerve deafness. Other stigmata include recurrent arthropathy and bilateral knee effusions (Clutton's joints); centrally notched, widely spread, peg-shaped upper central incisors (Hutchinson's teeth); frontal bossing; and poorly developed maxillas.

Yaws

Yaws, also called frambesia, pian, buba, and bouba, is caused by *T. pallidum* subspecies *pertenue*. It is a disease of childhood that occurs among rural populations in warm, humid, tropical climates, primarily in Africa, Southeast Asia, and Oceania, but also in focal regions of Colombia, Guyana, Suriname, and French Guiana.

Treponema pallidum subspecies *pertenue* is transmitted when traumatized skin contacts infectious exudate from active yaws lesions. Organisms then enter the bloodstream and travel to bone, lymph nodes, and distant skin sites, where they elicit granulomatous inflammation, indistinguishable from that seen in lesions of syphilis, and endarteritis in late lesions. Spirochetes are numerous in early skin lesions but rare in bone or late skin lesions.

Cutaneous papules appear three to five weeks after inoculation, usually on the extremities. They enlarge, become papillomatous and superficially eroded, and then spontaneously heal within six months. Weeks to months later a generalized eruption of similar lesions appears. The next five years, called the secondary stage, is characterized by multiple relapses of these skin lesions, often accompanied by lymphadenopathy and occasionally periostitis, osteitis, and osteomyelitis. After a latent period of several years, the late stage of yaws begins with cutaneous plaques, ulcers, and papillomas on the hands and feet (including the palms and soles) and gummas in the skull, sternum, tibia, or other bones.

Endemic Syphilis

Endemic syphilis (also called bejel, siti, and dichuchwa), is caused by *T. pallidum* subspecies *endemicum*. It currently exists in focal areas of Africa, western Asia, and Australia, predominantly affecting children in rural populations with poor standards of living and personal hygiene. Infection is transmitted by nonsexual body contact or by sharing eating and drinking utensils. Most often, no primary lesion is observed. Secondary lesions include oropharyngeal mucous patches, split papules at the corners of the mouth, condyloma lata, periostitis, and regional lymphadenopathy; and late manifestations are gummas of the skin, nasopharynx, and bones. Cardiovascular and neurologic lesions and congenital disease are rare.

Treponema carateum

Treponema carateum is the etiologic agent of pinta (also called carate or mal de pinto), which occurs only in rural areas of Mexico, Central America, and Colombia, predominantly in arid inland regions. Organisms enter the body during direct contact of broken skin with infectious lesions, multiply locally, enter the blood and lymphatics, and travel to distant skin sites.

The initial skin lesions of pinta appear one to three weeks after inoculation on the face, neck, chest, extremities, or abdomen. These small, erythematous, pruritic papules enlarge, coalesce, and eventually heal with residual hypopigmentation. Secondary small scaly papules (pintids) appear three to 12 months after the initial lesions, usually at the same sites, and may recur for up to 10 years. During the late stage of disease, depigmented skin lesions appear on the wrists, elbows, and ankles. Pinta does not affect viscera during any stage.

Laboratory Diagnosis

Infections caused by the pathogenic treponemes are diagnosed by direct microscopic examination of clinical specimens or by serologic tests. Molecular methods, including direct probes and polymerase chain amplification, have been described and appear promising, especially for the diagnosis of neurosyphilis, but such tests are not yet widely available outside of the research laboratory (Burstain, 1991; Grimprel, 1991; Hay, 1990). Identification of the species, however, is difficult. Because these organisms are morphologically identical and immunologically closely related, they are indistinguishable by the above-mentioned techniques. Therefore, a definitive diagnosis is based on epidemiology and clinical manifestations.

DIRECT MICROSCOPIC EXAMINATION. Direct darkfield examination of material from early primary lesions or lymph node aspirates for treponemes with characteristic motility can provide rapid diagnosis before serologic tests become positive. Appropriate specimen collection (described in Chapter 54) and use of the darkfield microscope are critical to the success of this procedure. The specimen must be examined immediately after collection or the characteristic motility will not be observed. The patient should be near the microscope when the specimens are taken because several specimens may need to be examined. Detection of *T. pallidum* in specimens from oral and gastrointestinal sources is complicated by the presence of endogenous, nonpathogenic treponemes that may be mistaken for pathogens. For that reason, darkfield examination of material from oral or anal lesions should be discouraged and interpreted with caution, if examined.

Prior to obtaining the specimen, the darkfield microscope should be checked for proper adjustment. A drop of the sample collected is placed on a glass slide, immediately covered with a coverslip, and examined under high power (400×) magnification. A shimmering or undulating movement should be observed, but motility may be more directional or corkscrew-like in fibrinous exudates. A negative darkfield examination alone should not be used to exclude syphilis when the clinical history is suggestive of the disease.

Direct fluorescent antibody stains, both polyclonal and monoclonal, specific for *T. pallidum* are available commercially and can be used to stain fixed smears and tissue sections. Because the smears do not have to be examined immediately, this method can be used when darkfield testing is not available or when specimens must be sent to a central or reference laboratory. It also is preferred for examination of material from oral or anal lesions, since the stains are specific for the pathogenic treponemes.

SEROLOGIC TESTS. Two types of serologic tests are used for diagnosis of syphilis: nontreponemal and treponemal assays. Standard nontreponemal tests include the VDRL reagin slide, rapid plasma reagin (RPR) circle card, unheated serum reagin (USR), and toluidine red unheated serum (TRUST) tests, all of which are based on detection of immunoglobulin (Ig)G or IgM antibodies (reagin) directed against nontreponemal lipid antigens (Larson, 1995). All nontreponemal assays utilize an active phospholipid (cardiolipin) antigen fortified with lecithin and cholesterol in a colloidal particle. The antigen may be mixed with particles such as charcoal (RPR) or dye (TRUST) to make the clumping or flocculation of the lipids by the patient's antibodies macroscopically visible. Addition of choline chloride (RPR, USR) in the antigen preparation eliminates the need to heat the serum before testing. Positive reactions to reagin may occur in aging or pregnant individuals or those having chronic infections such as leprosy, history of intravenous drug use, infections with viruses such as hepatitis C or HIV, or vaccination. These biologic false-positive reactions occur in 1% to 10% of the normal population and more frequently in HIV-positive individuals. False-negative reactions can occur in early incubating infections, in the latent period, and in tertiary syphilis. Nontreponemal assays are used as screening tests, confirming positive test results by assays specific for *T. pallidum* (see following), and to monitor response to therapy, with a fourfold decrease in titer over several months indicating effective therapy. A fourfold increase in titer suggests relapse or reinfection.

The treponemal tests most commonly used are the fluorescent treponemal antibody-absorption (FTA-ABS) test and the microhemagglutination–*Treponema pallidum* test (MHA-TP), each of which is approved for use on serum only, not CSF. To perform the FTA-ABS test, heated serum is mixed with a sonicate of nonpathogenic Reiter treponemes to remove nonspecific antibodies and is placed on a microscope slide to which *T. pallidum* antigen is fixed. Slides are incubated, stained with fluorescein-labeled antihuman globulin, and viewed by fluorescence microscopy. For specimens yielding a minimally reactive result, a second sample should be tested. The MHA-TP test is performed by placing absorbed serum with sheep erythrocytes coated with sonicated *T. pallidum* in a microtiter plate. If antibodies are present, they react with the sensitized red blood cells, producing a uniformly thin mat of agglutinated erythrocytes that covers the entire bottom of the well. If antibodies are absent, red blood cells settle as a smooth ring or button at the bottom of the well. In general, the MHA-TP test is a satisfactory substitute for the FTA-ABS test and is preferred in most laboratories because it is easier to perform and interpret and is more cost-effective because it requires less technical time. The one potential disadvantage, however, is the lower sensitivity for diagnosing primary syphilis (Hart, 1986).

Nontreponemal tests usually become reactive at some time during primary syphilis. The titer rises rapidly and if the infection is not treated, remains elevated during the first year and then falls slowly. Titers are low in late syphilis, and the test spontaneously reverts to nonreactive in about 25% of persons. With adequate treatment, the titer falls at a rate related to the pretreatment titer and stage of disease. For example, persons treated within the first six months are usually seronegative within a year; those treated later may not become seronegative for two years or longer; and in persons with late syphilis, seronegativity may take five years or may not occur (Brown, 1985; Fiumara, 1980). Treponemal tests become reactive in primary syphilis and usually remain reactive for the person's lifetime regardless of therapy, although treatment very early may prevent seroreactivity, occasional persons treated early revert to seronegative, and persons infected with HIV often become seronegative (Haas, 1990). The FTA-ABS test typically is the first of these tests to become positive, followed by the MHA-TP and the nontreponemal tests shortly thereafter. The sensitivities of the nontreponemal and treponemal tests for diagnosing syphilis are summarized in Table 50–2 (Larson, 1995); specificities are 97% to 99%.

Routine evaluation of the CSF for diagnosis of neurosyphilis is not necessary in persons with early syphilis, except perhaps in persons infected with HIV. CSF should be examined in persons with syphilis who have neurologic abnormalities, before re-treatment of those who relapsed after treatment, as a baseline measure in those for whom nonpenicillin therapy is planned, in those with late latent syphilis, and in all infants with suspected congenital syphilis (Hart, 1986; Larson, 1995). Requirements for diagnosis of neurosyphilis are reactive serum treponemal test, CSF cell count greater than 5 mononuclear cells/μL, a CSF protein concentration over 40 mg/dL, and a positive CSF VDRL test. The CSF VDRL is a highly specific indicator of neurosyphilis but is insensitive, yielding a positive result in only 22% to 69% of persons with active neurosyphilis (Hart, 1986). The CSF VDRL test may remain positive for a prolonged period after adequate therapy, so response to treatment is monitored by the CSF white blood cell count, which generally returns to normal within six to 12 weeks, and in symptomatic individuals, by an improvement in clinical findings. Normal cell counts at six, 12, and 24 months after therapy indicate a high probability of cure.

In addition to the treponemal tests discussed, enzyme-linked immunosorbent assays (EIA) recently became available. Initial evaluations have shown the IgG EIA to be as sensitive and specific as the FTA-ABS and MHA-TP (Lefevre, 1990; Norgard, 1993), and it may perhaps be a better screening tool than the RPR (Hooper, 1994). Its main advantages are objective interpretation of results and automated readout. The Captia syphilis M test, a capture EIA, has provisional status for diagnosis of congenital syphilis (Stoll, 1993), meaning that it can be used in medical management decision making but not as the sole criterion for diagnosis.

Table 50–2. SENSITIVITIES OF SEROLOGIC TESTS FOR SYPHILIS IN DIFFERENT STAGES OF DISEASE*

	Stage of Syphilis			
Test	*Primary*	*Secondary*	*Latent*	*Late*
VDRL	78 (74–87)	100	95 (88–100)	71 (37–94)
RPR	86 (77–100)	100	98 (95–100)	73
FTA-ABS	84 (70–100)	100	100	96
MHA-TP	76 (69–90)	100	97 (97–100)	94

*Values are percentage sensitivities. Numbers in parentheses represent ranges of sensitivities in studies at the Centers for Disease Control and Prevention. Data are from Larson SA, Steiner BM, Rudolph AH: Laboratory diagnosis and interpretation of tests for syphilis. Clin Microbiol Rev 1995; 8:1.

VDRL = Venereal Disease Research Laboratory; RPR, rapid plasma reagin; FTA-ABS, fluorescent treponemal antibody absorption; MHA-TP, microhemagglutination assay for antibodies to *T. pallidum.*

Treatment and Prevention

The recommended treatment for adults with incubating, primary, secondary, or early latent syphilis is benzathine penicillin G given intramuscularly in a single dose. Oral doxycycline, tetracycline, or erythromycin can be used in the compliant penicillin-allergic patient. Response to therapy is measured clinically and serologically, using nontreponemal tests. Patients should be tested at three and six months after therapy and should show a fourfold decrease in titer. In late latent syphilis, syphilis of unknown duration, or after treatment failure for early syphilis, multiple dose therapy with benzathine penicillin G is recommended. Aqueous crystalline penicillin G, administered intravenously for 10 to 14 days, is recommended for patients with evidence of neurosyphilis or ocular syphilis. Testing all patients with syphilis for infection with HIV is recommended because HIV-infected persons may not respond to routine treatment, and they may develop neurosyphilis more often and at an earlier stage of infection. Venereally transmitted syphilis can be prevented by avoiding sexual contact with an infected individual, and condom use should decrease the risk of spread. Congenital syphilis can be prevented by detecting and treating early syphilis in pregnant women.

Yaws, endemic syphilis, and pinta also respond to penicillin treatment.

BORRELIA

The species of *Borrelia* are microaerophilic helical bacteria 5 to 25 μm long and 0.2 to 0.5 μm wide with 4 to 30 coils. They possess an outer envelope or membrane that encloses a coiled protoplasmic cylinder composed of a peptidoglycan layer and the cytoplasmic membrane that surrounds the protoplasmic contents of the cell. Seven to 22 axial filaments (periplasmic flagella) are responsible for motility. The organisms multiply by binary fission and require long-chain fatty acids for growth. *Borrelia burgdorferi*, the etiologic agent of Lyme disease, and relapsing fever are discussed.

Lyme Disease

Lyme disease is a tick-borne multisystem inflammatory disorder occurring at any age and in both sexes (Steere, 1977, 1989). Its most distinct clinical manifestation is an expanding skin lesion, erythema chronicum migrans, which may be followed weeks to months later by neurologic, cardiac, or joint abnormalities. In Europe, a skin lesion later shown to be associated with Lyme disease, acrodermatitis chronica atrophicans, was described as early as 1910 by Arvid Afzelius (Afzelius, 1921), who associated it with the bite of *Ixodes re-*

duvius. The bite of this tick (or the related *Ixodes ricinus*) was later associated with tick-borne meningopolyneutitis (Garin-Bujadoux and Bannwarth's syndromes). However, it was not until the mid-1970s that Steere and colleagues recognized the disease as a distinct clinical entity and traced its origin to a closely related tick, *Ixodes dammini* (now alternatively called *Ixodes scapularis*).

In 1982, Burgdorfer and associates isolated the spirochete that bears his name (*Borrelia burgdorferi*) from *I. dammini* collected on Shelter Island, New York, and associated it with Lyme disease on serologic grounds (Steere, 1983). In the ensuing period, this organism was recovered from blood, skin, and CSF of patients, and specific IgM and IgG antibody responses were demonstrated. Today, Lyme disease is recognized as the most common tick-borne zoonosis in the United States, with between 8,000 and 10,000 cases reported yearly for the past several years (Centers for Disease Control and Prevention, 1994).

EPIDEMIOLOGY AND PATHOGENESIS. In the eastern and midwestern United States, *B. burgdorferi* is transmitted to humans by the nymph (or second stage) of the deer tick, *I. dammini*, during the salivation stage of its feeding period, accounting for the occurrence of most cases between May and August. *Ixodes pacificus* is the vector along the west coast of the United States, ticks of the *I. ricinus* complex transmit the organism in Europe, and in China *Ixodes persulcatus* has been implicated. In addition to being transmitted by a tick bite, *B. burgdorferi* acquired during pregnancy may cross the placenta, causing congenital infection (Markowitz, 1986).

The main reservoir is the white-footed mouse, *Peromyscus leucopus*, in eastern and central United States; however, *I. dammini* has been found in many mammals and in birds, suggesting that other reservoirs may also be important (Anderson, 1989). In nature, infection with *B. burgdorferi* is maintained by horizontal transmission from infected nymphal ticks to mice. When a larval *I. damnini* tick feeds on an infected mouse, it becomes infected and then molts into the nymphal stage, which is capable of transmitting the organisms during a blood meal. In areas of New England in which Lyme disease is endemic, deer are also important in the life cycle of *I. dammini*.

Significant progress has been made over the past two decades in understanding the transmission of *B. burgdorferi* and in increasing the recognition of Lyme disease as an important public health problem. However, much about the disease remains puzzling. Its pathogenesis is not well understood, and the interdependent problems of diagnosing the disease accurately and defining its full clinical spectrum serve to confound and complicate one another. Particularly disturbing is the fact that progress in the laboratory diagnosis has lagged far behind the public perception of the seriousness and prevalence of the disease. The recent commercial availability of serologic tests for Lyme disease, initially used only to confirm a clinical impression, and their widespread use has led, at the very least, to diagnostic confusion (Luger, 1990).

Although Lyme disease is of relatively recent notoriety, the presence of *B. burgdorferi* on the United States mainland 100 years ago has been documented by using the polymerase chain reaction (PCR) to study museum specimens of *Ixodes* ticks and white-footed mice (Marshall, 1994; Persing, 1990). Studies of the genetic diversity of *B. burgdorferi* also argue in favor of the antiquity of this organism on the continental United States; spirochetes identified as *B. burgdorferi* have now been isolated from rodents and ticks from many nonendemic areas of the country. These isolates often display a substantial degree of genetic heterogeneity, and some appear to be a unique genospecies of *B. burgdorferi*.

CLINICAL MANIFESTATIONS. The earliest and most easily recognized manifestation of Lyme disease is erythema migrans, which develops in two thirds to three fourths of affected individuals two days to four weeks after a tick bite. A painless, nonpruritic red macule or papule appears at the site of the bite and expands in a circular fashion, typically forming a flat lesion, 3 to 70 cm in diameter (median, 15 cm), with a bright red outer border and central clearing. The appearance of the lesion, however, varies; confluent erythema and target-like patterns are common, and central vesicles or necrosis may occur. Hematogenous dissemination of the organisms occurs early, manifested by fever, headache, stiff neck, malaise, migratory musculoskeletal pain, generalized lymphadenopathy, sore throat, and nonproductive cough.

Without treatment, skin lesions fade in three to four weeks (range, one day to 14 months), but subsequent abnormalities may develop in one or more major organ systems (Dattwyler, 1990). Acute neurologic or cardiac involvement occurs in about 20% of infected individuals within four to six weeks of the onset of infection. Bell's (seventh nerve) palsy is the most common neurologic manifestation, and 5% to 8% of persons develop acute meningitis or meningoencephalitis. Most persons with neurologic manifestations have a lymphocytic pleocytosis in the CSF (about 100 cells/mm^3) and an elevated protein concentration, although the CSF may be normal in persons with facial palsy alone. Acute cardiac involvement, recognized in up to 6% of cases, is manifested by varying degrees of atrioventricular block, myocarditis, or pericarditis. As the host immune response develops, the number of spirochetes declines, and the chronic phase of the disease begins. Individuals may enter a latent period; some later develop dermatologic, rheumatologic, cardiac, or neurologic manifestations, whereas others remain asymptomatic.

In North America, about half the persons who are not treated develop episodic arthritis within two or more years, and in 10% of these cases, the arthritis becomes chronic (treatment appears to prevent arthritis). Chronic neurologic manifestations such as chronic encephalopathy, polyneuropathy, or leukoencephalitis develop months to years after the initial infections (Logigian, 1990).

Laboratory Diagnosis

SEROLOGIC TESTING. Much of the diagnostic uncertainty surrounding Lyme disease originates because the symptoms of the disease are nonspecific, and aside from the characteristic skin lesion there are few pathognomonic features. In the 1980s, serologic testing for antibodies against *B. burgdorferi* was used primarily to test patients from highly endemic areas of the northeastern United States. However, the recent proliferation of commercially available serologic tests has engendered a "laboratory-industrial complex" that is driven by the earnest requests of patients with nonspecific fatigue, neurologic, rheumatologic complaints, or all of these who are desperate for a diagnosis. Because of the many possible causes of such symptoms, the overall prevalence of Lyme disease in this population is often lower than the rates of false-positivity for these assays, resulting in a higher absolute number of false-positive tests relative to true positives. On the other hand, most of the currently available tests are not able to detect early antibody responses to *B. burgdorferi*; thus, the diagnosis of a patient without erythema migrans who is suspected of having early Lyme disease can be difficult.

As for many bacterial serologic tests, false-positive results may occur as a result of cross-reacting antibodies against other bacteria, such as spirochetes found in the normal oral flora. *T. pallidum*, *Leptospira*, and even unrelated bacterial species associated with bacterial endocarditis. In addition, patients with connective tissue disorders may demonstrate false-positive serologic results (Saulsbury, 1990). False-negative serologic results may occur early in infection, before the development of detectable antibodies (which may take up to two months to develop), or in patients with immune suppression. Despite these limitations, however, it is a mistake to assume that serologic tests for Lyme disease are completely irrelevant. If patients being tested are carefully selected for symptoms compatible with Lyme disease and epidemiologic factors are included in consideration of the diagnosis, the positive predictive value of serologic tests can be quite acceptable, especially if positive serologic results are confirmed by a Western blotting (WB) procedure.

Many of the current problems surrounding the serologic testing for Lyme disease are likely based on interlaboratory differences in the types of antigens used as substrate antigens, antigen preparation, and methodologic differences in interpretive criteria (Mertz, 1988). Recently, at a consensus meeting sponsored by the CDC and the Association of State and Territorial Public Health Laboratory Directors, several recommendations were made with the intent of improving the sensitivity and specificity of serodiagnosis of Lyme disease (Proceedings, 1994). These include the testing of serum samples from patients with symptoms of Lyme disease by a two-step process that includes a sensitive screening test such as immunofluorescence assay (IFA) or EIA. Samples judged equivocal or positive by the screening should be further tested by WB, using a strain of *B. burgdorferi* (such as low-passage B31) that expresses appropriate amounts of the diagnostic proteins. Both IgM and IgG WB should be performed on serum from persons with suspected Lyme disease who present within the first four weeks of disease onset. Only IgG WB should be performed on serum from patients presenting later because interpretation of IgM band patterns after that time is less reliable. Serologic testing of a convalescent serum sample two to four weeks following the first sample is recommended for patients with symptoms of early Lyme disease who have negative screening test results. The criterion recommended for interpretation of IgM WB as positive for Lyme disease is the presence of two of the following bands: 24 (OspC), 39, and 41 (flagellin) kDa, (Engstrom, 1995). An IgG WB is considered positive if 5 of the following bands are present: 18, 21 (OspC), 28, 30, 39, 41, 45, 58, 66, and 93 kDa (Dressler, 1993).

The presence of clinical symptoms suggestive of Lyme disease in patients without a detectable specific antibody response to *B. burgdorferi* (so-called seronegative Lyme disease) remains problematic. In some seronegative patients with chronic symptoms, a specific T-cell blastogenic response to *B. burgdorferi* can be demonstrated, and the disorder has been attributed to incomplete eradication of the spirochete by antibiotic therapy (Dattwyler, 1988). However, in a prospective study of Lyme borreliosis patients who had well-characterized early treatment histories, no significant differences were detected in the long-term serologic status of patients who were believed to be adequately or inadequately treated for their early clinical symptoms (Plorer, 1993). Liberation and detection of antibodies specific for *B. burgdorferi* from immune complexes obtained from the serum of seronegative Lyme disease patients demonstrates that sequestration of specific antibodies in some infected patients may account for the absence of detectable antibodies to the organism, (Schutzer, 1990). Alternatively, the absence of specific antibodies to *B. burgdorferi* in some patients who apparently have symptoms compatible with Lyme disease may be due to misdiagnosis of other diseases that have similar presentations (Bakken, 1994; Persing, 1992, 1995; Thornford, 1994).

Serologic testing for Lyme disease may soon become more complicated because of the imminent introduction of vaccines for Lyme disease. Vaccines under evaluation now are based on recombinant outer surface protein A (OspA) of *B. burgdorferi*. After vaccination, the rise in antibodies of OspA will likely result in a positive EIA-based antibody test. Even WB testing may be affected, since the presence of an immunostaining species at 31 kDa (the molecular weight of OspA) may weigh in favor of a positive blot result. Thus, as a function of vaccination programs, the most useful screening test for Lyme disease may be rendered obsolete. Given that the vaccine will probably have a significant failure rate, special recombinant EIAs may have to be developed in order to sort out the variation in immune responses in vaccinated *versus* naturally infected persons.

CULTIVATION OF *B. BURGDORFERI*. Improvements in artificial media for growth of *B. burgdorferi* offer promise for direct detection of this organism. Culture of *B. burgdorferi* in Barber-Stoenner-Kelly medium (BSK) can now be recommended as a routine procedure for skin samples from patients with skin lesions compatible with erythema migrans. Recent studies have shown that over 80% of patients in endemic areas who have definite erythema migrans are culture-positive if the sample is obtained before antibiotic therapy (Berger, 1992). Culture of blood, CSF, and synovial fluid is much less likely than skin to yield positive results but may be occasionally helpful.

POLYMERASE CHAIN REACTION. New diagnostic technologies, such as polymerase chain reaction (PCR), are also useful for the direct detection of *B. burgdorferi*–specific nucleic acid in clinical samples. Several studies have shown the PCR procedure to be more sensitive and specific than any other technique for detection of *B. burgdorferi* in synovial fluid specimens from persons with Lyme arthritis (Lebech, 1991; Nocton, 1994). In a blinded retrospective study of nearly 150 patients with arthritis, PCR was 96% sensitive and 100% specific for detection of *B. burgdorferi* in untreated patients (Nocton, 1994). Most patients treated with recommended courses of antibiotics became PCR-negative and symptoms eventually resolved, suggesting that PCR may be useful for monitoring therapy and for predicting therapeutic outcome.

Studies of CSF specimens from patients with neurologic symptoms to date suggest that the overall sensitivity of PCR for detection of *B. burgdorferi* in CSF is lower than its detection in synovial fluid from patients with Lyme arthritis (between 25% and 50%). However, because direct detection by culture is nearly always negative, a positive PCR result is generally considered to be an accurate indicator of active infection (Luft, 1992). Furthermore, since an inverse relationship between PCR positivity and intrathecal antibody production may exist (Keller, 1992), a negative PCR result coupled with negative intrathecal antibody production may be helpful in excluding active neurologic Lyme disease in most cases.

Treatment and Prevention

The implementation of therapeutic of therapeutic regimens for Lyme disease have been heavily dependent on antibody-based diagnostic tests to identify those patients who require treatment. When much diagnostic weight is placed on a faulty serologic test, treatment outcomes become difficult to assess because many of the patients may have been misdiagnosed. Furthermore, the current battery of serologic tests does not provide an accurate index of response to therapy because a significant decline in antibody titer may lag by several months. In general, the need exists for a direct detection method to identify the organism in those who are actively infected and to follow eradication of the organism in those receiving therapy to provide a therapeutic end point.

Recommended therapies for Lyme disease include oral doxycycline or amoxicillin for early, uncomplicated disease and intravenous ceftriaxone for more well-established infections with systemic involvement. Oral erythromycin (especially for pregnant patients), azithromycin, chloramphenicol, oral cephalosporins, and intravenous cefotaxime have been used, but their efficacy has not been evaluated extensively. In animal models of Lyme disease, treatment with intravenous ceftriaxone resulted in clearance of *B. burgdorferi* by culture and by PCR from nearly all tissues after one to two weeks (Malawista, 1994).

Another area of ongoing investigation is the frequency of cotransmission of other zoonotic infections with *B. burgdorferi* in endemic areas. *Babesia microti* and a novel *Ehrlichia* species that causes human granulocytic ehrlichiosis are both transmissible to humans by the same tick vector that transmits Lyme disease (Bakken, 1994; Persing, 1992, 1995). Accordingly, approximately 10% to 15% of all patients with Lyme disease in some areas of the northeastern United States are serologically positive for exposure to *B. microti*, and preliminary seroprevalence studies of patients from the upper Midwest suggest frequent exposure to both *Babesia* and *Ehrlichia* species among patients that are seropositive for *B. burgdorferi*. Recent studies of patients with what might be called "post-Lyme syndrome" (or persistent severe fatigue after appropriate therapy for Lyme disease) show that some patients are actually coinfected with *B. microti* (Krause, 1995). Treatment of Lyme disease has no effect on underlying *B. microti* infection; thus, fatigue, myalgias, and arthralgias long after treatment for Lyme disease may be due to other causes that should be considered in the workup of such patients. The diagnosis of *B. microti* infection is best made by serologic testing or by PCR because blood smears are usually negative in normosplenic patients.

The risk of exposure to these zoonotic disease agents may be minimized by avoiding contact with ticks by wearing long-sleeved shirts and long pants, by applying insect repellents, and by checking for ticks following possible exposure. Attached ticks should be promptly removed and the site of feeding thoroughly disinfected. Although the efficacy of the prophylactic use of antibiotics following a tick bite for the prevention of Lyme disease remains debatable (Magid, 1992; Shapiro, 1992), the likelihood of contracting Lyme disease is dependent on the rate of infection in ticks (Shapiro, 1992). It is conceivable that tick testing may be useful someday for predicting risk of infection with *B. burgdorferi* and other zoonotic agents; removed ticks acquired in highly endemic areas could be preserved in ethanol and submitted for testing for *B. burgdorferi* by PCR.

Relapsing Fever

Relapsing fever occurs worldwide in tropical and temperate climates except for a few areas in the Southwest Pacific such as New Zealand and Australia (Burgdorfer, 1986). Epidemic disease, caused by *Borrelia recurrentis*, is transmitted by the human body louse, *Pediculus humanus*. The disease predominantly affects persons living under unfavorable hygienic conditions that result in overcrowding and dissemination of body lice. Louse-borne disease no longer exists in the United States, but it remains endemic in the highlands of Central and East Africa and the South American Andes.

Tick-borne relapsing fever, a zoonosis that occurs sporadically worldwide, is transmitted to humans who invade the habitats of the *Ornithodoros* ticks—warm, humid environments such as caves, decaying wood, rodent burrows, and animal shelters at altitudes of 1500 to 6000 feet. In the United States *Borrelia hermsii*, *Borrelia turicatae*, and *Borrelia parkeri* are the most common pathogens. The ticks become infected by feeding on borrelemic rodents and other small animals that serve as natural reservoirs for the organisms. Humans acquire the infection when saliva or feces are released from the tick during a blood meal.

During a blood meal, spirochetes are introduced into the blood, where they multiply, producing the signs and symptoms of relapsing fever. Organisms are sequestered in internal organs during afebrile periods when circulating spirochetes are killed by phagocytes in the presence of specific antibodies. Relapses occur when the organisms re-emerge antigenically modified from sites of sequestration.

The clinical manifestations of louse-borne and tick-borne relapsing fever are similar, but the former typically is a more severe illness. Characteristically, the primary illness begins acutely after an incubation period of four to 18 days with fever, rigors, headache, myalgias, arthralgias, lethargy, photophobia, cough, and abdominal pain, and it ends abruptly in three to six days. Hepatosplenomegaly and jaundice may develop, especially in louse-borne disease, and neurologic findings occur in up to 30% of those with louse-borne disease but in less than 10% of tick-borne cases. A truncal petechial, macular, or papular rash lasting one to two days commonly appears at the end of the primary febrile illness. Usually, the person survives and the fever and symptoms recur suddenly in seven to 10 days, although the duration and intensity of the symptoms decrease with each relapse, but the disease may be fatal.

Relapsing fever is diagnosed by demonstrating the spirochetes in the peripheral blood by darkfield examination of wet preparations of the specimen or in thick or thin smears stained with the Giemsa or Wright stain or with acridine-orange and viewed by fluorescence microscopy. Serologic tests are not commercially available and have limited diagnostic value because of the antigenic variation of the organisms.

The treatment of choice for relapsing fever is tetracycline or erythromycin. Tick-borne relapsing fever may be prevented by avoiding the arthropod vector and by preventing rodents from nesting in human shelters in areas where tick-borne relapsing fever is endemic. Insecticides may be used in dwellings, and insect repellents should be applied to clothing.

LEPTOSPIRA

The *Leptospira* are finely coiled motile spirochetes, 6 to 20 μm long and 0.1 μm wide, with semicircular hooked or bent ends. Leptospires are aerobic and may be cultivated *in vitro* in medium containing 10% serum or serum albumin plus long-chain fatty acids at pH 6.8 to 7.8. They stain faintly with aniline dyes and are invisible by light microscopy but are easily demonstrated by darkfield microscopy. Currently, two species of *Leptospira* are recognized: *Leptospira biflexa*, found predominantly in fresh surface waters, rarely is associated with human infection. *Leptospira interrogans*, the etiologic agent of leptospirosis, is a potential pathogen for humans and other mammals.

Leptospirosis is a zoonosis that occurs worldwide. The natural reservoirs of infection are chronically infected rodents and other feral and domestic animals such as cattle, pigs, and dogs that carry *L. interrogans* in their proximal renal tubules and shed the organisms in their urine. Humans usually become infected via direct contact with water or soil contaminated with infected urine and occasionally by direct contact with an infected animal. Organisms enter the body through skin abrasions, the nasopharyngeal or esophageal mucosal surfaces, or the eye. Persons at increased risk of infection are those with occupational exposure (farmers, veterinarians, abbatoir workers, dairymen, swineherds, and fish and poultry processors) or recreational exposure (camping near and/or bathing or swimming in infected ponds or streams).

Leptospirosis is often a biphasic illness, beginning with a septicemic phase that usually lasts four to seven days. After an afebrile interval of one to two days, the immune phase begins, characterized by the appearance of serum antibodies, meningitis, uveitis, rash, and hepatic and renal damage. During the immune phase, which lasts four to 30 days, organisms are found in the urine, kidney, and aqueous humor but not blood or CSF. About 90% of persons with leptospirosis have a mild anicteric illness; the remainder have severe disease with jaundice (Weil's disease).

Anicteric leptospirosis begins abruptly with fever, chills, headache, muscle aches, malaise, abdominal pain, nausea, vomiting, prostration, and, rarely, circulatory collapse. It persists four to seven days and almost never is fatal. The immune stage may not occur or is mild, with fever, headache, mild delirium, nausea, vomiting, abdominal pain, and myalgias for a few days. Muscle tenderness, conjunctival suffusion, and hepatosplenomegaly are common. A pretibial rash occurs in infections caused by serovar *autumnalis* and is part of the syndrome called Fort Bragg fever. From 80% to 90% of persons have pleocytosis of the CSF (typically less than 500 cells/mm^3 with a mononuclear cell predominance). Weil's disease is characterized by impaired renal and hepatic function, hemorrhage, vascular collapse, severe alterations in consciousness, and a 5% to 10% mortality.

Leptospirosis may be diagnosed by isolating the organisms from blood or CSF collected during the first seven to 10 days of the illness or from urine collected after the first week of disease. Media recommended for culture are Fletcher's or Ellinghausen-McCullough-Johnson-Harris (EMJH). Inoculated cultures are incubated four to six weeks at 25° to 30°C in the dark. In these semi-solid media, the leptospires grow as a linear disk, 1 to 3 cm below the surface, but the absence of a disk does not exclude their presence. Material should be collected from this level weekly and examined by darkfield microscopy. Leptospires are identified by their structure and characteristic motility, which is unique because of the spinning hooked ends.

Most commonly, leptospirosis is diagnosed serologically by using pools of bacterial antigens. Agglutinating antibodies typically appear after the first week of the illness and often persist for years. The humoral response, however, may be suppressed or delayed by antimicrobial therapy, and some persons may appear to remain seronegative, primarily because the infecting serotype was not represented in the antigen pools.

Treatment of leptospirosis includes intravenous penicillin or ampicillin for severe disease and oral doxycycline, ampicillin, or amoxicillin for less severe illness. Prevention of leptospirosis is difficult because it is impossible to eliminate the large animal reservoir of infection. In the United States, vaccinating domestic livestock and pets has reduced the prevalence of infection in some animals; however, renal infection may occur in vaccinated dogs, and infection may be transmitted from adequately immunized dogs to humans.

ANAEROBIC SPIROCHETES

Anaerobic Species of *Treponema*

Anaerobic treponemes are normal flora in the oral cavity or genital tract of humans, and they are an important component of acute necrotizing ulcerative gingivitis (Vincent's gingivitis). Treponemes may be detected by light microscopic examination of smears of the lesion stained with methylene blue. Treatment includes penicillin or a tetracycline.

Anaerobiospirillum succiniciproducens

Anaerobiospirillum succiniciproducens, a spiral bacterium first identified in dogs, may cause bacteremia in humans, predominantly those with an underlying disorder such as alcoholism, atherosclerosis, malignancy, or diabetes mellitus or those who have had a recent surgical procedure.

In Gram-stained smears prepared from blood cultures, the bacterial cells appear as gram-negative spiral shapes and straight rods, often with bipolar staining. Cells of *A. succiniciproducens* are about three times wider and two times longer than cells of *Campylobacter jejuni* (see Chapter 48), with which the former might initially be confused. On chocolate or blood agar, colonies are moist and spreading, 1 to 2 mm in diameter, after two to three days. *A. succiniciproducens* has bipolar tufts of flagella and demonstrates corkscrew motility when viewed by darkfield microscopy. Additional useful identifying features are negative reactions for catalase, oxidase, and indole; production of succinic and acetic acid from glucose, as demonstrated by gas-liquid chromatography; and no growth at 25°C or 42°C. *In vitro,* most isolates tested have been susceptible to carbenicillin, cefoxitin, chloramphenicol, and metronidazole and resistant to vancomycin and clindamycin; however, testing has been limited, and techniques have not been uniform (Shlaes, 1982; McNeil, 1987).

SPIRILLUM MINUS

Spirillum minus (formerly *Spirillum minor*) is one cause of rat-bite fever. The organism is a short, thick, gram-negative, tightly coiled spiral rod, 2 to 5 μm long and about 0.5 μm wide, with 2 to 6 spirals and bipolar tufts of flagella. It has not been cultured on artificial media. *Spirillum minus* is part of the normal respiratory flora of rats and is transmitted to humans via a rat bite or scratch. The bite wound heals spontaneously but in one to four weeks becomes painful, swollen, and purple. This recurrence is accompanied by regional lymphangitis, lymphadenitis, fever, chills, headache, and malaise. The wound becomes indurated and ulcerates, and a macular rash appears on the extremities, face, scalp, and trunk, fading during afebrile intervals. Without specific antimicrobial therapy, fever lasts three to four days and recurs after afebrile intervals of three to nine days. The mortality is 6% to 10% without treatment.

Infection caused by *S. minus* is diagnosed by microscopic visualization of the organism in exudates from the initial lesion, aspirates of involved lymph nodes, or blood. Wet mounts of exudate and aspirates are examined by darkfield microscopy, and blood films are stained with the Wright or Giemsa stain. No specific serologic test is available currently. Penicillin is the recommended treatment.

Afzelius A: Erythema chronicum migrans. Acta Derm—Vener. Stockholm 1921; 2:120–125.

Anderson JF: Epizootiology of *Borrelia* in *Ixodes* tick vectors and reservoir hosts. Rev Infect Dis 1989; 11:51451–51459.

Bakken JS, Dumler JS, Chen SM, et al: Human granulocytic ehrlichiosis in the upper Midwest United States. A new species emerging? JAMA 1994; 272:212.

Berger BW, Johnson RC, Kodner C, Coleman L: Cultivation of *Borrelia burgdorferi* from erythema migrans lesions and perilesional skin. J Clin Microbiol 1992; 30:359.

Blanco DR, Walker EM, Haake DA, et al: Complement activation limits the rate of *in vitro* treponemicidal activity and correlates with antibody-mediated aggregation of *Treponema pallidum* rare outer membrane protein. J Immunol 1990; 144:1914.

Brown ST, Zaidi A, Larsen SA, Reynolds GH: Serological response to syphilis. JAMA 1985; 253:1296.

Burgdorfer W: The enlarging spectrum of tick-borne spirochetoses. RR Parker Memorial Address. Rev Infect Dis 1986; 8:932.

Burstain J, Grimprel E, Lukehar SA, et al: Sensitive detection of *Treponema pallidum* by using the polymerase chain reaction. J Clin Microbiol 1991; 29:62.

Centers for Disease Control and Prevention: Congenital syphilis—New York City, 1986–1988. MMWR, 1989; 38:825.

Centers for Disease Control and Prevention: Lyme Disease—United States, 1993. MMWR, 1994; 43:564.

Dattwyler RJ: Lyme borreliosis: An overview of the clinical manifestations. Lab Med 1990; 21:290.

Dattwyler RJ, Volkman DLJ, Luft BJ, et al: Dissociation of specific T- and B-lymphocyte responses to *Borrelia burgdorferi*. N Engl J Med 1988; 319:1441.

Dorfman DH, Glaser JH: Congenital syphilis presenting in infants after the newborn period. N Engl J Med 1990; 323:1299.

Dressler F, Whalen JA, Reinhart BN, Steere AC: Western blotting in the serodiagnosis of Lyme disease. J Infect Dis 1993; 167:392.

Engstrom SM, Shoop E, Johnson RC: Immunoblot interpretation criteria for serodiagnosis of early Lyme disease. J Clin Microbiol 1995; 33: 419.

Fiumara NJ: Treatment of primary and secondary syphilis. Serological response. JAMA 1980; 243:2500.

Grimprel E, Sanchez PJ, Wendel GD, et al: Use of polymerase chain reaction and rabbit infectivity testing to detect *Treponema pallidum* in amniotic fluid, fetal and neonatal sera, and cerebrospinal fluid. J Clin Microbiol 1991; 29:1711.

Haas JS, Bolan G, Larsen SA, et al: Sensitivity of treponemal tests for detecting prior treated syphilis during human immunodeficiency virus infection. J Infect Dis 1990; 162:862.

Hart G: Syphilis tests in diagnostic and therapeutic decision making. Ann Intern Med 1986; 104:368.

Hay PE, Clark JR, Strugnell RA, et al: Use of the polymerase chain reaction to detect DNA sequences specific to pathogenic treponemes in cerebrospinal fluid. FEMS Microbiol Lett 1990; 68:233.

Hooper NE, Malloy DC, Passen S: Evaluation of a *Treponema pallidum* enzyme immunoassay screening test for syphilis. Clin Diagn Lab Immunol 1994; 1:477.

Ikeda MK, Jenson HB: Evaluation and treatment of congenital syphilis. J Pediatr 1990; 117:843.

Jackman JD, Radolf JFD: Cardiovascular syphilis. Am J Med 1989; 87: 425.

Johns DR, Tierney M, Felsenstein D: Alteration in the natural history of neurosyphilis by concurrent infection with the human immunodeficiency virus. N Engl J Med 1987; 316:1569.

Keller TL, Halperin SJ, Whitman M: PCR detection of *Borrelia burgdorferi* DNA in cerebrospinal fluid of Lyme neuroborreliosis patients. Neurology 1992; 42:32.

Krause PJ, Telford S, Spielman A, et al: Molecular monitoring of *Babesia microti* parasitemia: Evidence of chronic infection in humans. (personal communication, Dec. 15, 1995.)

Larson SA, Steiner BM, Rudolph AH: Laboratory diagnosis and interpretation of tests for syphilis. Clin Microbiol Rev 1995; 8:1.

Lebech AM, Hindersson P, Vuust J, Hansen K: Comparison of *in vitro* culture and polymerase chain reaction for detection of *Borrelia burgdorferi* in tissue from experimentally infected animals. J Clin Microbiol 1991; 29:731.

Lefevre J, Bertrand CMA, Bauriaud R: Evaluation of the Captia enzyme immunoassays for detection of immunoglobulins G and M to *Treponema pallidum* in syphilis. J Clin Microbiol 1990; 28:1704.

Logigian EL, Kaplan RF, Steere AC: Chronic neurologic manifestations of Lyme disease. N Engl J Med 1990; 323:1438.

Luft BJ, Steinman CR, Neimark HC, et al: Invasion of the central nervous system by *Borrelia burgdorferi* in acute disseminated infection. JAMA 1992; 267:1364.

Luger SW, Krauss E: Serologic tests for Lyme disease. Interlaboratory variability. Arch Intern Med 1990; 150:761.

Magid D, Schwartz B, Craft J, Schwartz JS: Prevention of Lyme disease after tick bites. N Engl J Med 1992; 327:534.

Malawista SE, Barthold SW, Persing DH: Fate of *Borrelia burgdorferi* DNA in tissues of infected mice after antibiotic treatment. J Infect Dis 1994; 170:1312.

Markowitz LE, Steere AC, Benach JL, et al: Lyme disease during pregnancy. JAMA 1986; 255:3394.

Marshall WF III, Telford SR III, Rys PN, et al: Detection of *Borrelia burgdorferi* DNA in museum specimens of *Peromyscus leucopus*. J Infect Dis 1994; 170:1027.

McNeil MM, Martone WJ, Dowell VR Jr: Bacteremia with *Anaerobiospirillum succiniciproducens*. Rev Infect Dis 1987; 9:737.

Mertz LE, Wobig GH, Duffy J, Katzmann JA: A comparison of test procedures for the detection of antibody to *Borrelia burgdorferi*. Ann NY Acad Sci 1988; 539:474.

Musher DM, Hamill RJ, Baughn RE: Effect of human immunodeficiency virus (HIV) infection on the course of syphilis and on the response to treatment. Ann Intern Med 1990; 113:872.
Nocton JJ, Dressler F, Rutledge BJ, et al: Detection of *Borrelia burgdorferi* DNA by polymerase chain reaction in synovial fluid from patients with Lyme arthritis. N Engl J Med 1994; 330:229.
Norgard MV: Clinical and diagnostic issues of acquired and congenital syphilis encompassed in the current syphilis epidemic. Curr Opin Infect Dis 1993; 6:9.
Persing DH, Herwaldt BL, Glaser C, et al: Infection with a *Babesia*-like organism in northern California. N Engl J Med 1995; 332:298.
Persing DH, Mathiesen D, Marshall WF, et al: Detection of *Babesia microti* by polymerase chain reaction. J Clin Microbiol 1992; 30:2097.
Persing DH, Rutledge BJ, Rys PN, et al: Target imbalance: Disparity of *Borrelia burgdorferi* genetic material in synovial fluid from Lyme arthritis patients. J Infect Dis 1994; 168:668.
Persing DH, Telford SR III, Rys PN, et al: Detection of *Borrelia burgdorferi* DNA in museum specimens of *Ixodes dammini* ticks. Science 1990; 249:1420.
Plorer A, Sepp N, Schmutzhard E, et al: Effects of adequate versus inadequate treatment of cutaneous manifestations of Lyme borreliosis on the incidence of late complications and late serological status. J Invest Derm 1993; 100:103.
Proceedings, Second National Conference on Serological Diagnosis of Lyme Disease, October 29, 1994, Dearborn, MI. Association of State and Territorial Public Health Laboratory Directors, Washington, D.C.
Quick RE, Herwaldt BL, Thornford JW, et al: Babesiosis in Washington State: A new species of *Babesia*. Ann Intern Med 1993; 119:284.
Rath PM, Rogler G, Schonberg A, et al: Relapsing fever and its serological discrimination from Lyme borreliosis. Infection 1992; 20:283.
Saulsbury FT, Katzmann, JA: Prevalence of antibody to *Borrelia burgdorferi* in children with juvenile rheumatoid arthritis. J Rheumatol 1990; 17:1193.
Shapiro ED, Gerber MA, Holabird NE, et al: A controlled trial of antimicrobial prophylaxis for Lyme disease after deer-tick bites. N Engl J Med 1992; 327:1769.
Schutzer SE, Coyle PK, Belman AL, et al: Sequestration of antibody to *Borrelia burgdorferi* in immune complexes in seronegative Lyme disease. Lancet 1990; 335:312.
Shlaes DM, Dul MJ, Lerner PI: Anaerobiospirillum bacteremia. Ann Intern Med 1982; 97:63.
Steere AC: Medical progress: Lyme disease. N Engl J Med 1989; 321:586.
Steere AC, Malawista SE, Syndman DR, et al: Lyme arthritis: An epidemic of oligoarticular arthritis in children and adults in three Connecticut communities. Arthritis Rheum 1977; 20:7.
Steere AC, Grodzicki RL, Kornblatt AN, et al: The spirochetal etiology of Lyme disease. N Engl J Med 1983; 308:733.
Stoll BJ, Lee FK, Larsen SA, et al: Improved serodiagnosis of congenital syphilis with combined assay approach. J Infect Dis 1993; 167:1083.
Thornford JW, Conrad PA, Telford SR III, et al: Cultivation and phylogenetic characterization of a newly recognized human pathogenic protozoan. J Infect Dis 1994; 169:1050.

Chapter 51

Mycobacteria

Gail L. Woods, M.D.

Mycobacteria are aerobic, nonmotile, acid-alcohol fast, slightly curved or straight bacilli. The organisms contain high–molecular weight (60 to 90 carbons) mycolic acids in their cell walls that on pyrolysis release C_{22} to C_{26} straight-chain saturated long-chain acids. Their guanine plus cytosine DNA–base content ratios are in the range of 62 to 70 mol%.

Mycobacterium tuberculosis, Mycobacterium bovis, and *Mycobacterium africanum* are the human pathogens that constitute the *Mycobacterium tuberculosis* complex (MTBC). These organisms, the "tubercle bacilli," are the causative agents of human tuberculosis. Mycobacteria other than the MTBC have been called atypical because they differ from the tubercle bacilli. The names nontuberculous mycobacteria and mycobacteria other than tubercle bacilli are, however, preferred because these organisms are not atypical but simply have characteristics distinct from those of *M. tuberculosis.*

In 1957, Runyon proposed that the nontuberculous mycobacteria be divided into four groups based on colony pigmentation and growth rate on a solid medium (Table 51–1) (Runyon, 1959). This classification system, however, has limits. For example, *Mycobacterium kansasii* usually is a photochromogen but rarely is a nonphotochromogen or a scotochromogen. Members of the *Mycobacterium avium-intracellulare* complex are nonphotochromogens in Runyon's scheme, but some isolates produce slightly pigmented colonies, potentially causing incorrect classification as a scotochromogen. *Mycobacterium szulgai* is a scotochromogen at 37°C and a photochromogen at 25°C. Moreover, when a liquid medium is used for mycobacterial culture as is currently recommended (discussed later), growth rates used by Runyon for classification do not apply. A clinically relevant classification of the nontuberculous mycobacteria based on their pathogenicity in humans (potential pathogens and, rarely, pathogenic mycobacteria) is used here (Woods, 1993). *Mycobacterium leprae,* which is unique among mycobacteria by virtue of the fact that it has not yet been cultivated *in vitro*, is discussed separately.

MYCOBACTERIUM TUBERCULOSIS COMPLEX

Mycobacterium tuberculosis

Currently, tuberculosis is a global problem. Worldwide, an estimated 8 to 10 million new cases of tuberculosis and 2 to 3 million deaths caused by tuberculosis occur each year. In much of the world, tuberculosis is the leading cause of death from any one infectious agent, directly responsible for an estimated 7% of all deaths and 26% of all preventable deaths worldwide (Murray, 1990; Snider, 1994).

In the United States, tuberculosis was the leading cause of death at the turn of the twentieth century. Mortality then decreased, initially because of public health efforts to house tuberculosis patients in sanatoria to improve their nutrition and ventilation and later because of antituberculous drugs. Between 1953, when tuberculosis became notifiable on a national basis, and 1984, the incidence steadily decreased by

Table 51–1. RUNYON'S CLASSIFICATION OF THE NONTUBERCULOUS MYCOBACTERIA

Classification	Description of Colonies
Photochromogen	Not pigmented unless exposed to light (optimally during their early growth and with good aeration of the surface)
Scotochromogen	Pigmented when grown in the dark and in light
Nonphotochromogen	Not pigmented when grown in the dark or in light
Rapid grower	Growth on solid media in ≤7 days

about 5% to 6% each year (Rieder, 1989). The rate of decline slowed dramatically from 1984 to 1985, and thereafter the downward trend reversed. From 1985 to 1992, the number of tuberculosis cases reported to the Centers for Disease Control and Prevention (CDC) increased by about 20%—that is, over 51,000 more cases were reported than would have been expected had the decline continued (CDC, 1993b). The increased incidence of tuberculosis, however, did not affect all persons equally; 71% of cases reported in 1992 occurred among racial/ethnic minority groups (CDC, 1993a). Of the metropolitan areas, the most marked rise was reported in New York City. Factors contributing to the excessive number of cases include the epidemic spread of human immunodeficiency virus (HIV), a deterioration in the health care infrastructure, and increases in the numbers of cases among the homeless, prisoners, migrant workers, immigrants, and elderly persons living in nursing homes (Ellner, 1993).

In addition to the resurgence of tuberculosis in the United States, another recent concern is multidrug-resistant tuberculosis (MDR-TB), defined as disease caused by *M. tuberculosis* that is resistant to two or more primary antimycobacterial agents used in the United States to treat tuberculosis (see Treatment). Since 1988, the CDC investigated seven outbreaks of MDR-TB involving over 200 cases (predominantly HIV-infected persons) in hospitals and correctional facilities in New York State and Florida (Jacobs, 1994). Only four such outbreaks were reported from 1976 to 1987, and persons involved were not infected with HIV. Mortality in the recent outbreaks was high (72% to 89%), and disease progressed rapidly from diagnosis to death (median, 1 to 4 months). Transmission of MDR-TB to health care workers and to a prison guard also occurred; at least nine of these developed active disease, and five died.

M. tuberculosis is transmitted primarily through inhalation of dried residues of small infected droplets (1 to 10 μm in diameter) but also by direct inoculation of abraded skin, an event most likely to occur when pathologists or other laboratory personnel handle infected tissues. The most important source of infection is an undiagnosed person with cavitary (and sputum smear–positive) tuberculosis. The minimum infective dose for humans is unknown, but data suggest that infection may occur after inhaling one or two viable organisms (Haas, 1994). The risk of active pulmonary disease is low after one exposure to the organism but increases under conditions of stress or in a confined environment in which repeated exposures to the organism occur. Most persons who become infected with *M. tuberculosis* do not develop active disease. The lifetime risk of active disease is 5% to 10% for immunocompetent persons. For persons infected with HIV, in contrast, the risk of developing tuberculosis is 7% to 10% per year.

The specific structures, antigens, and mechanisms responsible for the virulence of *M. tuberculosis* are unknown, but cord factor and sulfatides have been associated with the ability of virulent strains to produce disease. *In vitro,* cord factor is responsible for the morphologic appearance of cells of *M. tuberculosis*—serpentine cords of bacilli in close parallel arrangements. This growth pattern correlates with the presence in the bacillus of trehalose 6,6′ dimycolate. When this glycolipid is injected into mice, it inhibits neutrophil migration, elicits granuloma formation, and stimulates protection against virulent infection; its specific role in the pathogenesis of human tuberculosis, however, remains unknown. Sulfatides are peripherally located glycolipids that inhibit fusion of secondary lysosomes with bacilli-containing phagosomes within a macrophage, possibly promoting intracellular survival of the organism.

The usual host response to infection with *M. tuberculosis* is activation of the cell-mediated immune system. During primary (initial) infection, inhaled bacilli travel to the alveolar spaces, where they are ingested by resident macrophages. These macrophages are unable to kill the mycobacteria, which multiply intracellularly during the first several days after infection. Macrophages infected with mycobacteria migrate to regional tracheobronchial lymph nodes and present the sensitizing antigen(s) to immunocompetent T cells, or they enter the lymphatics and blood and travel back to the lungs (primarily the apices) and to distant organs such as lymph nodes, kidneys, epiphyseal areas of the long bones, vertebral bodies, and meninges, where bacilli continue to multiply until the cellular immune response is activated.

Immunocompetent T cells migrate from regional lymph nodes to the site of infection in the lung. There they release chemotactic, migration-inhibitory, and mitogenic cytokines, which stimulate recruitment of blood-derived monocytes and lymphocytes, macrophage and lymphocyte division, and macrophage activation. The activated macrophages have enhanced microbicidal activity, and they produce cytokines, such as interleukin-1, interferon gamma, and tumor necrosis factor, which stimulate or regulate other components of the immune system, properties that help control infection. The cytokines and lytic enzymes released by the macrophages also contribute to the concomitant local tissue destruction. With time, the activated T-cell population declines and is replaced by long-lived memory immune T cells, which protect against reinfection with *M. tuberculosis* and provide some cross-protection against infection with other mycobacteria. Despite the limitation of further mycobacterial multiplication in primary and metastatic foci by the activated macrophages and memory T cells, a residual nidus of infection remains indefinitely in the lung (most frequently in the apex, where the oxygen tension is high) and less often in distant sites. Therefore, the potential for reactivation of disease in these quiescent foci exists during periods of immunosuppression.

The primary focus of pulmonary infection, called the Gohn lesion, usually is subjacent to the pleura, in the lower part of the upper lobes or the upper part of the lower lobes of one lung, corresponding to areas of the lung that receive the greatest volume flow of inspired air. Lesions (tubercles) are well circumscribed 1- to 2-cm diameter areas of grayish-white consolidation with soft to necrotic centers. Similar-appearing tubercles typically are found in the regional tracheobronchial lymph nodes, and these plus the primary lung lesion are termed the Gohn complex. Microscopically, tubercles are composed of well-circumscribed caseating or noncaseating granulomas; organisms may be seen in sections stained with an acid-fast stain. With time these lesions are replaced by hyalinized fibrous tissue and eventually calcify. The lesions of miliary tuberculosis are small (one to several millimeters in diameter), distinct, yellow-white areas of consolidation without gross caseation that histologically resemble tubercles. The ability to form granulomas depends on the immunocompetence of the host. Individuals infected with HIV, for example, may have extensive necrosis without granuloma formation, many neutrophils, microabscesses, and numerous acid-fast bacilli (AFB).

In the United States, pulmonary tuberculosis accounts for about 85% of cases of active disease. Manifestations of pulmonary disease vary. The clinical presentation may be insidious with gradual onset of constitutional symptoms over months; catarrhal, with a productive cough often attributed to a bad cold or lingering bronchitis; pneumonia or "flu-like," with high fever, aches and pains, and cough; hemoptoic, with acute onset of blood-streaked sputum; or pleuritic. Extrapulmonary tuberculosis may be localized but more commonly involves multiple organs with or without concurrent lung infection. Multiorgan tuberculosis, historically a disease of infants and young children, currently predominates among the elderly and immunocompromised individuals, especially those infected with both HIV and *M. tuberculosis* (Chaisson, 1987; Kim, 1990).

Mycobacterium bovis

M. bovis may be transmitted to humans from cattle by humans drinking contaminated raw milk or by respiratory exposure to live infected cattle or their carcasses; it may be transmitted from person to person via respiratory exposure or from humans to cattle by exposure of cattle to urine from persons with urinary tract infections caused by *M. bovis*; it is probably transmitted among cattle by respiratory secretions. *M. bovis* also may be conveyed to cattle from wild animal reservoirs such as the bush-tailed possum in New Zealand and possibly by the badger in Switzerland and Great Britain (Grange, 1987).

Between 1900 and 1930, *M. bovis* was responsible for 6% to 30% of cases of tuberculosis in the United States and the United Kingdom (Grange, 1987; Karlson, 1970). Declining rates of human tuberculosis caused by *M. bovis* are due to milk pasteurization and cattle inspection programs. Since 1950, *M. bovis* has accounted for fewer than 1% of cases of human tuberculosis in North America. Most infections are extrapulmonary, involving cervical and mesenteric lymph nodes, the intestines, bones, and kidneys. Uncommonly, infection follows intravesical instillation of bacille Calmette-Guérin (BCG) for treatment of superficial bladder carcinoma (Kristjansson, 1993).

Mycobacterium africanum

M. africanum, the "African" tubercle bacillus, was first recovered from persons in West Africa (Castets, 1968). Although it has been isolated primarily from individuals in Africa, the prevalence of infection with *M. africanum* worldwide is difficult to assess because it may not be correctly identified in many laboratories. The modes of transmission, pathogenesis, and clinical manifestations of disease caused by *M. africanum* are the same as those associated with *M. tuberculosis.*

NONTUBERCULOUS MYCOBACTERIA

In general, little is known about the antigens associated with the virulence of the nontuberculous mycobacteria; however, such antigens presumably are responsible for persistence of the organisms within the monocyte-macrophage system of the host. The immune response to infection with these mycobacteria also is poorly understood. Potential pathogens are reviewed in the following sections. Rarely pathogenic mycobacteria and the infections with which they have been associated are listed in Table 51–2 (Blacklock, 1983; Butler, 1994; Casimir, 1982; Chiodini, 1989; Cianciulli, 1974; Davison, 1988; DeChairo, 1973; Edwards, 1978; Neely, 1989;

Table 51–2. RARELY PATHOGENIC MYCOBACTERIA AND ASSOCIATED INFECTIONS

Mycobacterium sp.	Associated Infections	Comments
M. gordonae	Meningitis in patients with a shunt, hepatorenal disease, peritonitis, prosthetic valve, endocarditis, cutaneous infections, disseminated disease, ? pulmonary disease	Recovered from soil and water ("tap water bacillus"), common laboratory contaminant
M. thermoresistible	Pulmonary infection, cutaneous infection	Recovered from soil
M. terrae-triviale complex	Septic arthritis, osteomyelitis, ? disseminated disease	*M. terrae* = radish bacillus
M. asiaticum	Pulmonary disease	
M. nonchromogenicum	Pulmonary disease	
M. flavescens	Pulmonary disease	
M. shimoidei	Pulmonary disease	
M. smegmatis	Pulmonary disease	
M. neoaurum	Bacteremia in immunocompromised hosts with indwelling catheter	
M. celatum	Disseminated disease in patient with AIDS	Disease resembles disseminated MAC
M. paratuberculosis	? Crohn's disease	

AIDS = acquired immunodeficiency syndrome; MAC = *M. avium-intracellulare* complex; ? = postulated but not proven.

Tsukamura, 1975, 1983; Wallace, 1988; Weinberger, 1992; Weitzman, 1981).

Mycobacterium avium-intracellulare Complex (MAC)

M. avium and *M. intracellulare* have such similar growth characteristics and biochemical reactions that they often are not distinguished in the clinical microbiology laboratory; isolates of both species are reported as MAC. The MAC contains 28 serovars, identified by seroagglutination according to antigens located on the cell surface or by thin-layer chromatography.

Prior to the epidemic of the acquired immunodeficiency syndrome (AIDS), MAC was the second most frequently isolated *Mycobacterium* in the United States, following *M. tuberculosis.* More recently, the percentage of isolates of MAC has increased, equaling or even surpassing the number of isolates of *M. tuberculosis* in some parts of the country.

MAC bacilli are ubiquitous in the environment. They have been isolated from water, soil, food, house dust, and several animals, but the specific environmental sources responsible for human infection are not known (Inderlied, 1993). The most likely portal of entry is the gastrointestinal tract, but transmission by the respiratory tract also is possible. From sites of colonization, organisms enter the blood and infect many organs, especially those of the monocyte-macrophage system.

Pulmonary disease caused by MAC occurs in elderly white men who have underlying chronic lung disease or who have undergone gastrectomy, and it has become more common in persons without predisposing factors, especially older women (Prince, 1989). Disseminated MAC occurs almost exclusively in immunosuppressed individuals, and the number of such cases have increased considerably since the epidemic of AIDS. In the United States, MAC is the most common cause of systemic bacterial infection in patients with AIDS (Horsburgh, 1991). The major risk factor for disseminated MAC in these patients is the degree of immune dysfunction, indicated by the $CD4^+$ lymphocyte count, as the disease is rare in individuals whose $CD4^+$ lymphocyte count is over $100/\mu L$.

In the United States, serotypes 4 and 8 of *M. avium* are isolated primarily from blood and are recovered most commonly from persons with AIDS. Serotypes of *M. intracellulare* account for a small percentage of isolates of MAC from persons with AIDS and are recovered primarily from sputum and infrequently from blood, suggesting that they rarely cause disseminated disease in these individuals (Guthertz, 1989; Yakrus, 1990).

Manifestations of disease caused by MAC depend on the site and the extent of infection. Pulmonary infection may be asymptomatic, or it may mimic tuberculosis. Disseminated disease in persons without AIDS is manifested by fever, weight loss, bone pain, lymphadenopathy, hepatosplenomegaly, and skin lesions. In those with AIDS, persistent fever, weight loss, and diarrhea are most common; anorexia, weakness, lymphadenopathy, or hepatomegaly also may occur (Inderlied, 1993). Significant laboratory abnormalities are anemia and elevated alkaline phosphatase. Cervical lymphadenitis caused by MAC most often affects children but also occurs in adults. Other manifestations of infection with MAC are synovitis, genitourinary tract disease, cutaneous lesions, deep infection of the hand, osteomyelitis, meningitis, ulcers of the colon, and pericarditis (Inderlied, 1993; Wolinsky, 1979; Woods, 1987).

The histologic findings of lesions caused by MAC vary. Caseating granulomas with AFB, indistinguishable from tuberculosis; pulmonary interstitial fibrosis with organizing pneumonia; necrotizing granulomatous vasculitis resembling Wegener's granulomatosis; and, especially in persons with AIDS, aggregates of foamy macrophages containing many intracellular AFB may be seen.

Mycobacterium scrofulaceum

M. scrofulaceum was first recognized as a cause of cervical lymphadenitis in children (Prissick, 1956). Antigenically it is similar to MAC, and because occasional isolates identified as *M. scrofulaceum* by biochemical tests serotype as MAC and vice versa, *M. scrofulaceum* sometimes is classified with the MAC as *M. avium-intracellulare-scrofulaceum* complex.

M. scrofulaceum has been isolated from raw milk and other dairy products, oysters, soil, and water. It most commonly causes cervical lymphadenitis in children 1 to 5 years of age, presumably entering the body through breaks in the skin or mucous membranes of the oral cavity. The disease usually is unilateral, involving lymph nodes high in the neck and close to the mandible. Infected children generally appear healthy, are afebrile, and have minimal pain and tenderness. With disease progression, the nodes soften and drain, but occasionally heal by fibrosis and calcification. Extranodal manifestations of infection with *M. scrofulaceum* include pulmonary disease, disseminated disease, and rarely conjunctivitis, osteomyelitis, meningitis, and granulomatous hepatitis. Lesions of *M. scrofulaceum* are histologically indistinguishable from those caused by *M. tuberculosis.*

Mycobacterium kansasii

M. kansasii, first described as the "yellow bacillus," accounted for 3% of mycobacterial isolates in the United States in 1979 and 1980; the highest numbers were reported from California, Texas, Louisiana, Illinois, and Florida (Buhler, 1953; Good, 1982). The natural reservoir of *M. kansasii* is unknown; however, it has been recovered from water samples. Pulmonary disease is most common in males 50 to 60 years of age living in urban areas, among certain occupational groups (miners, welders, sandblasters, and painters), and among individuals with pneumoconioses and chronic obstructive pulmonary disease. Disseminated disease generally affects persons with impaired cellular immunity.

The most common manifestation of disease caused by *M. kansasii* is chronic cavitary pulmonary lesions, usually involving the upper lobes. Extrapulmonary manifestations include cervical lymphadenitis in children, cutaneous disease, musculoskeletal involvement (carpal tunnel syndrome, synovitis, arthritis, tendinitis and fasciitis, or osteomyelitis), disseminated disease, isolated genitourinary tract disease, and pericarditis.

The histologic findings of lesions caused by *M. kansasii* vary and include caseating or noncaseating granulomas, and especially in skin lesions, necrosis or foci of acute and chronic inflammation without well-formed granulomas. AFB are common in lung and lymph node tissue but are seen less frequently in tissue from other sites.

Mycobacterium fortuitum-chelonae Complex

M. fortuitum has been isolated from soil, water, and dust and *M. chelonae,* from soil, water, and sewage. Most persons infected with one of the organisms in this complex have experienced a penetrating injury (trauma or surgical procedure) with possible soil or water contamination. Outbreaks of infection with *M. chelonae* have been associated with administration of diphtheria-pertussis-tetanus-polio vaccines, histamine injections, lidocaine administration using a jet injector, contaminated hemodialyzers in persons treated with hemodialysis, and placement of contaminated porcine heterograft valves (Wallace, 1983).

Primary cutaneous disease caused by *M. fortuitum* or *M. chelonae* is manifested by localized cellulitis, draining abscesses, or minimally tender nodules. Lesions typically develop three weeks to 12 months (most often four to six weeks) after a penetrating injury in persons with an intact immune system. Osteomyelitis is an occasional complication, especially following puncture wounds to the feet. Postoperative infections are characterized by a nonhealing wound or breakdown of a healed wound with serous drainage in a person with minimal systemic symptoms. They generally develop three weeks to three months after the procedure, especially median sternotomy, augmentation mammaplasty, or insertion of a percutaneous catheter. Disseminated disease, which typically occurs in immunocompromised adults, is manifested by multiple, recurrent skin and soft tissue abscesses; no primary source of infection is evident. Chronic pulmonary disease resembles that caused by *M. kansasii* or MAC, except cavitation is uncommon. Endocarditis involving a prosthetic valve usually becomes manifest four to 12 weeks after surgery. Rarely, *M. fortuitum* or *M. chelonae* cause keratitis and corneal ulceration after trauma, or cervical lymphadenitis.

Lesions caused by *M. fortuitum* or *M. chelonae* are characterized histologically by necrosis with minimal caseation and a mixed inflammatory infiltrate composed of neutrophils and granulomas with foreign body or Langhans' giant cells; lipid-laden macrophages are seen occasionally. Clumps of extracellular AFB are found within aggregates of neutrophils in less than a third of cases. In lung tissue, foamy macrophages are frequent, a pattern resembling lipoid pneumonia.

Mycobacterium xenopi

M. xenopi was first isolated from a toad in 1957 and was recognized as a human pathogen in 1965 (Costrinia, 1981). It has been cultured from hot- and cold-water taps, hospital hot-water generators and storage tanks, and other environmental sources. In Great Britain, *M. xenopi* is found more often in coastal than inland areas, and birds are a possible natural reservoir. Most pulmonary infections caused by *M. xenopi* have been reported from Europe and Great Britain; it is an uncommon cause of mycobacterial disease in the United States. Disease has occurred only in adults, more frequently in males than females. Most persons have pre-existing lung damage or another predisposing condition, such as an extrapulmonary malignancy, alcoholism, diabetes mellitus, or immunosuppressive therapy. Pulmonary disease may be chronic, subacute, or acute; symptoms are indistinguishable from those associated with disease caused by *M. kansasii.* Focal extrapulmonary infections (osteomyelitis, arthritis, lymphadenitis) and disseminated disease are uncommon, but the latter has been reported in persons with AIDS (Tecson-Tumang, 1984).

Mycobacterium szulgai

M. szulgai is an infrequent human pathogen found worldwide, but its natural reservoir is unknown. The most common manifestation of infection is chronic pulmonary disease, and this occurs predominantly in middle-aged males. Extrapulmonary disease is uncommon; infections of the olecranon bursa associated with repeated trauma or with cortisone injections, extensive cutaneous disease in persons receiving corticosteroids, osteomyelitis, tenosynovitis with carpal tunnel syndrome, cervical lymphadenitis, and disseminated disease have been described (Woods, 1987).

Mycobacterium malmoense

M. malmoense was reported as a new species in 1977, but its natural reservoir still is not known (Schroder, 1977). Most human infections have been reported from England, Wales, and Sweden; well-documented disease in the United States is rare. The most common manifestation of infection with *M. malmoense* is chronic pulmonary disease, typically occurring in middle-aged men with pneumoconiosis; cervical lymphadenitis in children and disseminated disease in patients with AIDS also have been described (Henriques, 1993).

Mycobacterium simiae

M. simiae was first isolated from monkeys from India in 1965 (Karassova, 1965). The organism is found in monkeys and has been recovered from tap water in hospitals. An uncommon human pathogen, *M. simiae* has been associated with chronic pulmonary disease, osteomyelitis, and disseminated disease.

Mycobacterium marinum

M. marinum was recognized as a human pathogen in 1951 (Norden, 1951). Human infection typically is acquired by trauma to the skin during contact with contaminated nonchlorinated fresh or salt water, but it may be acquired through trauma unassociated with water contact or contact with water in the absence of preceding trauma. A single papulonodular lesion usually appears two to three weeks after inoculation, most commonly on the elbow, knee, foot, toe, or finger and often becomes verrucous or ulcerated. Occasionally, an abscess forms at the site of inoculation, and several secondary nodules develop and progress centrally along the lymphatics, resembling sporotrichosis (See Chapter 52). In immunocompromised persons, cutaneous lesions may become disseminated. Extracutaneous manifestations are uncommon; synovitis, osteomyelitis, and ocular and laryngeal lesions have been reported (Woods, 1987).

The histology of skin lesions varies with the stage of infection. Early, neutrophil aggregates are surrounded by histiocytes. Later, lymphocytes, epithelioid histiocytes, occasional Langhans' giant cells, and foci of fibrinoid necrosis are seen. In lesions present for over six months, aggregates of lymphocytes are found in the dermis. Stains for AFB usually are negative, but organisms may be seen within histiocytes.

Mycobacterium haemophilum

M. haemophilum first was described in 1978, but it probably was the noncultivable acid-fast bacillus recognized in skin ulcers in 1972 and 1974 (Feldman, 1974; Lomvardias, 1972; Sompolinsky, 1978). The organism is unique among the mycobacteria in its growth requirement for hemoglobin or hemin. Human infections caused by *M. haemophilum* are uncommon and usually seen in persons who have an underlying immunodeficiency such as lymphoma, exogenous immunosuppression after organ transplantation, or AIDS, but a few cases of lymphadenitis in otherwise healthy children have been reported (CDC, 1991). Disease most commonly is manifested by multiple cutaneous nodules, ulcers, or painful swellings, typically involving the extremities, that occasionally become abscesses and open fistulas draining purulent material. Microscopically, lesions show foci of necrosis without caseation surrounded by a polymorphous inflammatory infiltrate with occasional Langhans' giant cells in the lower dermis. AFB are seen singly or in small clusters, often within cells.

Mycobacterium genavense

M. genavense is a newly proposed species of *Mycobacterium* that has been recovered primarily from blood cultures, but also from spleen and bone marrow, of patients with AIDS (Coyle, 1992; Wald, 1992). Almost all patients have had fever and malaise, and some also had abdominal symptoms. Several patients were infected with another potential pathogen, such as MAC; therefore, it has been difficult to determine the role of *M. genavense* in the disease process.

Mycobacterium ulcerans

M. ulcerans is endemic in areas of Zaire, Uganda, Nigeria, Ghana, Cameroon, Malaysia, New Guinea, Guyana, Mexico, and Australia located between latitudes 25 degrees north and 38 degrees south. Children 5 to 8 years old are most often affected; however, in one study from Australia, the mean age of infected persons was almost 30 years, and one third were aged 40 years or older (Wolinsky, 1979). In all endemic areas, disease is slightly more common in males. The natural reservoir of *M. ulcerans* and the usual route of its transmission to humans are unknown.

Eponyms for disease caused by *M. ulcerans* are the Bairnsdale ulcer, for the area in Australia where it was first recognized, and Buruli ulcer or Buruli disease after the area of Uganda reporting the most cases. The disease begins as one or rarely, multiple painless boils or subcutaneous lumps on an exposed area, most often the leg, that possibly was a site of previous trauma. After several weeks, the lump ulcerates, and satellite nodules and ulcers may appear. Lymph nodes typically are not enlarged, and affected individuals are afebrile and without systemic symptoms, unless lesions become secondarily infected with bacteria.

Mycobacterium leprae

Mycobacterium leprae is the etiologic agent of leprosy (also called Hansen's disease). Although it does not belong to the MTBC and could therefore be considered a "nontuberculous mycobacteria," it is discussed separately because it is unique among the mycobacteria by virtue of the fact that it has not been cultivated. Useful animal models of infection are the mouse footpad model and the the nine-banded armadillo.

M. leprae has been recognized in nearly every part of the world at some time. An estimated 10 to 15 million persons in the world have leprosy; approximately 62% are in Asia and 34% are in Africa (Binford, 1982). About 6000 persons in the United States have leprosy; most are immigrants, but some cases develop in persons indigenous to the Gulf Coast states, California, and Hawaii (Neill, 1985).

Leprosy predominantly affects humans but also is a natural infection of wild armadillos in Louisiana and Texas, and spontaneous cases have been described in mangabey monkeys (Hastings, 1988). The mechanism of transmission of *M. leprae* is unknown, but person-to-person spread by aerosolization of organisms from the nose of a person with active lepromatous disease (described later) that then contact the nasal mucosa of another individual is the favored theory. Transmission may also occur through intact skin or by penetrating wounds, such as thorns or the bite of an arthropod. Breast milk from lactating women with lepromatous disease contains bacilli that may be transmitted to infants, and transplacental transmission of *M. leprae* is possible. Cases of human leprosy following contact with armadillos have been reported (Lumpkin, 1983). Moreover, the discovery of a naturally occurring leprosy-like disease among armadillos and the fact that sporadic cases of leprosy occur in persons who have no known contact with human leprosy suggest that nonhuman sources of *M. leprae* may exist (Blake, 1987).

Most persons effectively resist infection with *M. leprae*. Resistance depends on an effective cell-mediated immune response to *M. leprae* antigens as occurs in tuberculoid leprosy. In persons who lack specific cell-mediated immunity to these antigens, bacilli multiply within macrophages, eventually resulting in widely disseminated lepromatous leprosy. The defect in cellular immunity, which may involve T lymphocyte function or their interaction with macrophages, apparently is specific for antigens to *M. leprae* rather than a generalized defect.

The lesions of leprosy develop after a two- to five-year incubation period, varying in appearance, depending on the host's immune response. Leprosy always involves peripheral nerves, almost always involves the skin, and frequently involves mucous membranes. The three cardinal signs of the disease are skin lesions, areas of cutaneous anesthesia, and enlarged peripheral nerves.

The system outlined by Ridley and Jopling (presented later) is most commonly used to classify the spectrum of clinical and histopathologic forms of leprosy (Ridley, 1964). Indeterminate leprosy, the earliest sign of disease, is characterized by one or a few hypopigmented skin macules with minimal local sensory loss. In about 75% of cases, the disease heals spontaneously; in the rest it progresses, often after a prolonged period.

The polar types of leprosy—lepromatous leprosy, the widespread anergic form of the disease, and tuberculoid leprosy, the localized form—are clinically stable. Lepromatous leprosy is characterized by cutaneous lesions ranging from diffuse generalized skin involvement to widespread, symmetrically distributed nodules (called lepromas) filled with organisms. Lesions generally involve the cooler parts of the body surface—the anterior third of the eye, the nasal mucosa, and the superficial peripheral nerve trunks. In advanced disease, lesions are accompanied by sensory loss from involvement of dermal nerve fibers. Microscopically, lesions show foamy histiocytes containing many AFB, few or no lymphocytes, minimal intraneural inflammation, and many AFB in nerves, the perineurium, blood vessel walls, and arrector muscles. In tuberculoid leprosy, one or a few well-circumscribed anesthetic macules or plaques develop, often accompanied by an enlarged peripheral nerve near the skin lesions. Histologically, lesions demonstrate noncaseating granulomas in the nerves and dermis, extending to involve the basal layer of the epidermis; there are few, if any, AFB. Borderline leprosy, a clinically unstable condition, encompasses the types of disease between the polar forms. It may develop features more closely resembling tuberculoid disease, a process termed up-grading; or features more like lepromatous disease, called down-grading.

SKIN TESTING

The tuberculin skin test is useful for identifying persons infected with MTBC, but it does not differentiate active disease from infection. Persons infected with MTBC develop a hypersensitivity reaction to proteins of the bacilli, which comprise the skin test reagent—PPD (purified protein derivative). The preferred method of skin testing is the Mantoux test, performed by intracutaneous injection of 0.1 mL of intermediate strength (5 tuberculin units) PPD-S. The reaction is interpreted after 48 to 72 hours by measuring the diameter of induration in millimeters (Huebner, 1993). Induration of 5 mm or more is a positive result in persons infected with HIV, those who have had recent close contact with someone who has infectious tuberculosis, and those who have chest x-ray findings consistent with old healed tuberculosis. A reaction of 10 mm or more is positive in persons who do not meet the above criteria but who have other risk factors for tuberculosis. Included in this group are persons born in Asia, Africa, or Latin America where the prevalence of tuberculosis is high; intravenous drug users; medically underserved, low-income populations, especially racial or ethnic minorities; residents of long-term care facilities; and persons who have a medical condition associated with an increased risk of tuberculosis (e.g., silicosis, gastrectomy, jejunoileal bypass, 10% or more below ideal body weight, chronic renal failure, diabetes mellitus, treatment with high-dose corticosteroids or with other immunosuppressive drugs, and malignancies). A reaction of 15 mm or more is positive in all other persons.

False-positive PPD reactions result from infection with nontuberculous mycobacteria. False-negative reactions may be due to poor technique or improper storage of the reagent. If the test is administered appropriately, false-negative reactions are uncommon in relatively healthy people but occur in up to 20% of individuals with known tuberculosis when they are first tested. Most of these false-negative reactions are attributed to the general illness and revert to positive after two to three weeks of therapy when health is restored. Factors causing a state of general anergy, such as protein malnutrition, concurrent viral infection, sarcoidosis, malignancy (especially lymphoma), immunosuppressive or corticosteroid therapy, and infection with HIV may also cause a false-negative tuberculin reaction. To determine whether an individual is anergic, skin testing with mumps and candidal antigens should be performed simultaneously with the Mantoux test.

The Mantoux test generally remains positive as long as viable bacilli persist in quiescent foci. However, the reaction may wane below positive with increasing age, a phenomenon that occurs most frequently in those over the age of 55 years. In these individuals, the reaction will be boosted (or become positive) if retesting is performed as early as one week after the first test, a reaction termed the booster effect.

Skin test reagents prepared from nontuberculous mycobacteria include PPD-A (*M. avium*), PPD-B (*M. intracellulare*), PPD-F (*M. fortuitum*), PPD-G (*M. scrofulaceum*), and PPD-Y (*M. kansasii*). In the United States, these reagents once were available from the CDC; however, this service was discontinued because antigens were not standardized and the skin reactions were difficult to interpret.

LABORATORY DIAGNOSIS

Specimens

Specimens recommended for diagnosis of mycobacterial infections are listed in Table 51–3. Samples from contaminated sites such as sputum and other respiratory secretions, gastric secretions, urine, and feces must be decontaminated prior to inoculation of media to prevent the normal flora from overgrowing and thus masking the presence of mycobacteria, which grow more slowly. Concentrating the specimen after decontamination increases the sensitivity of smear and culture. Specimens from normally sterile body sites such as blood, cerebrospinal fluid, pleural and peritoneal fluid, and tissues may be inoculated directly without decontamination.

Processing and inoculation of specimens for mycobacterial culture should be performed in a biologic safety cabinet. The *N*-acetyl-L-cysteine (NALC)-sodium hydroxide procedure (Fig. 51–1) is the most common method used in the clinical laboratory to liquefy, decontaminate, and concentrate specimens for detection of mycobacteria. Potentially contaminated specimens should be refrigerated if they cannot be

Table 51–3. DISEASES CAUSED BY MYCOBACTERIA AND SPECIMENS FOR DIAGNOSIS

Disease	*Mycobacterium* species*	Specimens
Pulmonary	*tuberculosis, kansasii,* MAC, *xenopi, szulgai, malmoense, simiae*	Sputum (early morning, deep cough, on 3 consecutive days), BAL, gastric contents, lung tissue, pleural fluid
Disseminated	*tuberculosis,* MAC	Blood, bone marrow, involved tissue
Lymphadenitis	*tuberculosis,* MAC, *scrofulaceum*	Lymph node aspirate or biopsy
Skin, soft tissue	*ulcerans, fortuitum-chelonae, marinum, haemophilum*	Aspirate or biopsy of lesions (swabs should be discouraged)
	leprae	Smears of nasal secretions and skin slits, biopsy of lesion
Musculoskeletal	*tuberculosis, fortuitum-chelonae, marinum*	Joint fluid, synovium, bone
Nervous system	*tuberculosis*	CSF, brain tissue
	leprae	Peripheral nerve biopsy
Genitourinary	*tuberculosis*	Urine (early morning–voided specimen on 3 consecutive days), involved tissue—kidney, endometrium, fallopian tubes, prostate, seminal vesicles, epididymis
Gastrointestinal	*tuberculosis,* MAC	Tissue, feces
Peritonitis	*tuberculosis*	Peritoneal biopsy, peritoneal fluid
Hepatitis	*tuberculosis,* MAC	Liver tissue
Pericarditis	*tuberculosis*	Pericardium, pericardial fluid

*Species listed are potential pathogens most commonly involved.
MAC = *M. avium-intracellulare* complex; BAL = bronchoalveolar lavage; CSF = cerebrospinal fluid.
Modified from Woods GL: Mycobacteria. *In* Woods GL, Gutierrez Y: Diagnostic Pathology of Infectious Diseases. Philadelphia, Lea & Febiger, 1993, p 378.

processed immediately. Before proceeding to the steps outlined in Figure 51–1, additional handling is necessary for some specimens. Gastric lavage specimens should be processed immediately; but if a delay cannot be avoided, 10% sodium hydroxide should be added until the pH of the sample (measured with pH paper) is neutral. If more than 10 mL of gastric secretions are collected, the sample is centrifuged at 3000 to 3600 × g for 20 to 30 minutes, the supernatant is decanted, and the sediment is processed as shown in Figure 51–1. For feces, 1 to 2 g of a formed sample of 5 mL of a liquid specimen is placed in a 50-mL centrifuge tube, and sterile filtered distilled water is added to give a volume of 10 mL. The suspension is agitated on a vortex mixer, filtered through gauze, and then processed as outlined. Urine specimens are divided into two to four 50-mL centrifuge tubes and centrifuged at 3000 to 3600 × g for 30 minutes. The supernatant is decanted, leaving about 2 mL of sediment in each tube. Tubes are mixed on a vortex mixer, sediments are combined, and if necessary, distilled water is added to give a volume of 10 mL, which then is decontaminated as shown in Figure 51–1.

Transfer 10 mL (maximum) of sputum, urine, or other fluid specimen to sterile, disposable plastic 50-mL conical centrifuge tube

↓

Add equal volume of NALC–2% NaOH (prepared fresh each day of use) and tighten cap

↓

Mix on vortex mixer, 15 to 30 seconds

↓

Let mixture stand at room temperature for 15 minutes (45 minutes for stool specimens)

↓

Add 30 mL of phosphate buffer (pH 6.8); cap tubes and invert to mix

↓

Centrifuge at 3000 to 3600 × g for 15 minutes (or 2500 × g for 20 minutes)

↓

Decant supernatant; resuspend sediment in 1.5 to 2 mL of sterile water or buffer

↓ ↓

Prepare smear for staining | Inoculate media

Figure 51–1. Protocol for decontamination using 2% sodium hydroxide-N-acetyl-L-cysteine and concentration of specimens for detection of mycobacteria by smear and culture.

Microbial Stains

In smears treated with Gram's stain, most mycobacteria appear as slender, poorly stained, beaded, gram-positive bacilli, but sometimes the bacilli do not take up the crystal violet or safranin and appear "gram-neutral" or as "gram-ghosts" (Plate 51–1). Similar ghost images of bacilli may be found in macrophages in smears stained with the Wright or Papanicolaou stain. All specimens (except blood) collected from persons with suspected mycobacterial infection should be examined microscopically for organisms. To prepare a smear, 2 to 3 drops of the concentrated sediment are spread uniformly on a microscope slide, which then is fixed at 80°C for 15 minutes or for 1 to 2 hours at 65° to 70°C on an electric hot plate.

Two types of stains detect AFB: carbol fuchsin (the classic Ziehl-Neelsen stain, which requires heating, and the cold Kinyoun stain) and fluorochrome (auramine-rhodamine and auramine-O). Smears stained with a carbol fuchsin stain are examined at 800 to 1000× magnification (oil immersion). Smears stained with a fluorochrome stain are examined at lower magnifications (250× and 400×), which allows visualization of more fields in less time. Cells of the *M. fortui-*

Table 51–4. GUIDELINES FOR REPORTING SMEARS FOR ACID-FAST BACILLI

AFB with Carbol Fuchsin Stain (1000×) (No.)	AFB with Fluorochrome Stain (450×) (No.)	Report
0	0	No AFB seen
1–2/300 F (3 sweeps)	1–2/70 F (1 1/2 sweeps)	Doubtful; repeat
1–9/100 F	2–18/50 F (1 sweep)	1+
1–9/10 F	4–36/10 F	2+
1–9 F	4–36 F	3+
>9 F	>36 F	4+

Modified from Kent PT, Kubica GP: Public Health Mycobacteriology: A Guide for the Level III Laboratory. Atlanta, US Department of Health and Human Services, 1985.

AFB = acid-fast bacilli; sweep = scanning full length of a smear; F = field.

tum-chelonae complex stain poorly with fluorochromic stains and may not be detected; therefore, when the latter organisms are suspected pathogens (for example, in postsurgical wound infections), restaining negative fluorescent smears with a carbol fuchsin stain is recommended. Results are reported after viewing 100 fields and should include a statement indicating whether the smear was prepared directly from the specimen or after decontamination and concentration. Guidelines for reporting results of smears stained for AFB are shown in Table 51–4 (Kent, 1985).

In smears stained with carbol fuchsin, AFB typically appear as purple to red slightly curved rods (1 to 10 μm long and 0.2 to 0.6 μm wide) that occasionally are beaded or banded (Plate 51–2) but also may appear coccoid or filamentous. In general, the appearance of AFB does not provide a species identification; however, cells of certain species have features that may be useful diagnostically. For example, cells of *M. kansasii* often appear as cross-barred bacilli Plate 51–3 larger than *M. tuberculosis* and resembling a "shepherd's crook." Cells of MAC typically are pleomorphic, occasionally coccobacillary, and stain positively with periodic acid–Schiff (PAS) stain, a unique feature among mycobacteria. Cells of *M. marinum* typically are longer and broader than those of *M. tuberculosis* and often show cross-banding. Cells of *M. leprae* stain weaker than most other mycobacteria.

The specificity of stains for AFB typically is 99% or more, and the sensitivity ranges from about 25% to about 75% (Murray, 1980; Rickman, 1980; Strumpf, 1979). False-positive results (positive stain, negative culture) may be caused by nonviable organisms such as might occur in patients receiving antituberculosis therapy; prolonged decontamination, killing mycobacteria as well as contaminating bacteria; or cross-contamination during the staining procedure. Factors that influence the sensitivity of smear results include

1. Patient population (persons with cavitary lesions are more likely than those without cavities to have a smear-positive sputum).
2. Specimen type (respiratory specimens are more likely than other specimen types to be positive).
3. Number of specimens examined.
4. Number of AFB present in the sample (5000 to 10,000 organisms/mL of specimen are needed for a positive result).
5. Species present (specimens containing *M. tuberculosis* or *M. kansasii* are more likely to be positive than are those that contain other mycobacteria).
6. Observer experience.
7. Stain used.

Fluorochromic stains are more sensitive and easier to read than carbol fuchsin stains and are recommended by experts at the CDC (Tenover, 1993). To address the resurgence of tuberculosis in the United States, the CDC also suggests that for respiratory specimens, results of stained smears be reported within 24 hours of specimen receipt, which means processing seven days a week.

Culture Methods

Conventional culture of mycobacteria involves inoculation of solid media (the composition of the commonly used media is shown in Table 51–5). If this is the only culture method used, inoculation of both an egg-based medium such as Löwenstein-Jensen, supplemented with ribonucleic acid or pyruvic acid, and an agar-based medium such as Middlebrook 7H10 or 7H11 is recommended. For specimens such as sputum that are contaminated with normal bacterial flora, a selective medium containing antimicrobial agents such as Mitchison's selective 7H11 agar also should be inoculated. These media are available in screw-cap tubes and one-ounce prescription bottles; agar-based media also are available in petri dishes. Prescription bottles are preferred to screw-cap tubes for safety reasons and because they provide a larger surface area for mycobacterial growth. Sterile body fluids (cerebrospinal fluid, joint fluid, pleural fluid, and peritoneal fluid) should be inoculated to two solid media and in a broth

Table 51–5. MEDIA COMMONLY USED FOR ISOLATION OF MYCOBACTERIA

Medium	Components	Inhibitory Agent(s)
Lowenstein-Jensen	Coagulated whole eggs, defined salts, glycerol, potato flour	0.025 g/100 mL malachite green
Middlebrook 7H10	Defined salts, vitamins, cofactors, oleic acid, albumin, catalase, glycerol, dextrose	0.0025 g/100 mL malachite green
Middlebrook 7H11	Defined salts, vitamins, cofactors, oleic acid, albumin, catalase, glycerol, 0.1% casein hydrolysate	0.0025 g/100 mL malachite green
Selective 7H11 (Mitchison's medium)	Defined salts, vitamins, cofactors, oleic acid, albumin, catalase, glycerol, dextrose, casein hydrolysate	0.0025 g/100 mL malachite green 50 µg/mL carbenicillin 10 µg/mL amphotericin B 200 units/mL polymyxin B 20 µg/mL trimethoprim lactate

medium such as Middlebrook 7H9 for enrichment. Specimens from cutaneous lesions should be inoculated to one egg-based and one agar-based medium, and to assure recovery of *M. haemophilum* (described earlier) they also should be plated on chocolate agar, 5% sheep blood Columbia agar, Mueller-Hinton agar with Fildes supplement, or Löwenstein-Jensen containing 2% ferric ammonium citrate.

All cultures should be incubated at 35° to 37°C in an atmosphere of 5% to 10% CO_2, and tubed media should be incubated in a slanted position with caps loose for at least one week to ensure even distribution of the inoculum over the surface. For specimens from cutaneous sites, a second set of cultures should be inoculated and incubated at 30°C because some mycobacteria that cause skin lesions—*M. marinum, M. haemophilum,* and *M. ulcerans*—grow optimally at the lower temperature. All cultures should be examined weekly for eight weeks.

The major advantage of conventional culture is that it allows visualization of colony morphology and pigmentation, which is useful diagnostically, especially for distinguishing colonies of *M. tuberculosis* from those of some nontuberculous mycobacteria. The colony appearance and growth characteristics of the commonly encountered mycobacteria are outlined in Table 51–6. Disadvantages of conventional solid media are prolonged time to growth of mycobacteria (colonies often are not visible on tubed solid media for three to four weeks or more) and low sensitivity. Inoculation of Middlebrook agar plates, which then are examined under the microscope, allows more rapid detection of colonies, but this procedure is labor-intensive, thus prohibiting its use in many clinical laboratories (Welch, 1993).

Given the resurgence of tuberculosis in the United States, experts at the CDC currently recommend use of both a broth and a solid medium for culture of mycobacteria (Tenover, 1993). Broth systems currently available are the BACTEC TB radiometric system (Becton Dickinson), Septi-Chek AFB (Becton Dickinson), and BBL Mycobacteria Growth Indicator Tubes (MGIT, Becton Dickinson). Several automated broth systems are being evaluated and should be available soon. The CDC also recommends that the culture system used detect growth within 14 days. Of the systems currently available, this turnaround time is most consistently achieved by the BACTEC TB.

The semiautomated BACTEC TB system utilizes broth media (one for blood [13A] and another for all other specimen types [12B]) that contain ^{14}C-labeled palmitic acid substrate. Each specimen (5.0 mL of blood or 0.5 mL of all other specimen types) is inoculated into one vial, and an antibiotic mixture is added to specimens other than blood. Vials are incubated in ambient air at 37°C for six weeks. For optimal detection of mycobacteria, inoculation of one BACTEC vial and one solid medium is recommended. To ensure recovery of *M. genavense,* blood cultures (especially those collected from patients with AIDS) should be incubated eight to 10 weeks. Bacilli multiply in the broth and utilize the labeled substrate, releasing $^{14}CO_2$ into the head space above the

Table 51–6. COLONY MORPHOLOGY AND GROWTH CHARACTERISTICS OF MYCOBACTERIA ENCOUNTERED IN THE CLINICAL LABORATORY

Mycobacterium species	Colony: *Morphology*	Colony: *Pigment*	Growth Rate* (wk)	Comments
M. tuberculosis	Rough	N (buff)	4–6	
M. bovis	Rough; thin or transparent	N (colorless to buff)	4–6	
M. avium complex	Smooth; small, thin, transparent or large, opaque, domed; ± rough	N	4–6	Growth may require 8 wk; colonies of some strains become lightly pigmented with prolonged incubation.
M. scrofulaceum	Smooth, globoid	S	4–6	Pigment varies from light yellow to deep orange
M. kansasii	Rough; β-carotene crystals	P	4–6	Rare strains are N or S
M. fortuitum-chelonae	Smooth or rough	N	≤1	
M. xenopi	Smooth, filamentous extensions ("bird's nest)	S	4–6	Growth at 42°C
M. szulgai	Smooth or rough	S, 37°C; P, 25°C	4–6	
M. malmoense	Smooth, dysgonic	Colorless	2–3	
M. simiae	Smooth	P†	4–6	
M. marinum	Wrinkled, shiny; smooth, hemispherical; (rarely) rough, dry	P	2–3	Optimal growth, 31°–33°C
M. haemophilum	Rough; ± smooth	N	4–6	Optimal growth, 20°–32°C
M. gordonae	Smooth	S	4–6	
M. thermoresistible	Smooth or rough	P	≤1	Optimal growth, 37°–45°C; pigment is yellow-orange, becoming brown
M. terrae-triviale	Smooth (*M. terrae*); rough (*M. triviale*)	N	4–6	
M. nonchromogenicum	Intermediate in roughness	N	4–6	
M. flavescens	Smooth	S	2–3	
M. smegmatis	Rough; ± smooth	N (buff)	≤1	

*Average, on solid medium.
†Pigment production often requires prolonged exposure to light.
N = nonphotochromogen; S = scotochromogen; P = photochromogen (see Table 51–1); ± = occasional strains have the indicated morphology.

6

broth. The amount of $^{14}CO_2$ is measured by the BACTEC 460, which calculates a growth index (GI). A GI greater than 10 suggests that mycobacteria are present, and when the GI reaches 50 to 100, a smear of the broth is stained for AFB. Vials containing AFB are subcultured to a solid medium, and direct tests for identification (discussed in the following section) may be performed. For positive mycobacterial blood cultures from patients with AIDS, subculture to Middlebrook 7H11 agar containing mycobactin J should be done to allow recovery of *M. genavense* if initial subcultures from the broth show no growth, or the positive broth should be sent to a reference laboratory prepared to do the appropriate tests.

Advantages of the BACTEC TB system are (1) rapid detection of mycobacterial growth (average, five to 12 days rather than three to four weeks for conventional culture), (2) increased sensitivity compared with solid media (i.e., detection of more positive cultures), (3) the ability to distinguish MTBC from other mycobacterial species (discussed under Identification), and (4) rapid susceptibility testing of isolates of *M. tuberculosis* (described under Susceptibility Testing) (Abe, 1992; Anargyros, 1990; Stager, 1991). The major disadvantage of the BACTEC TB is its radioactivity, the disposal of which is expensive and problematic for many institutions.

Septi-Chek AFB is a biphasic mycobacterial culture system that consists of a broth medium and agar media on an enclosed paddle, similar to the biphasic blood culture system described in Chapter 54. The broth is inoculated with the specimen, the paddle is attached to the top of the bottle, and the system is inverted to allow the broth to flow over the agar media. The system is incubated six to eight weeks at 35° to 37°C in 5% to 7% carbon dioxide, and at regular intervals the broth is subcultured to the solid media on the paddle by inverting the system. The sensitivity of this system is similar to that of the BACTEC TB (Abe, 1992; D'Amato, 1991; Isenberg, 1991). However, time to detection of growth is longer than with the BACTEC TB although more rapid than conventional solid media.

The BBL MGIT consists of 4 mL of modified 7H9 broth and a fluorescent indicator embedded in silicone in the bottom of a 16 × 100 mm glass tube. Tubes are inoculated with the specimen, an antibiotic mixture to inhibit growth of contaminating bacteria and a mycobacterial growth enrichment are added, and the tubes are capped and incubated at 37°C for up to eight weeks. To detect mycobacterial growth, tubes are placed on top of a 365-nm UV transilluminator or in front of a Wood's lamp. The appearance of strong fluorescence in the sensor (a bright orange color at the bottom of the tube and meniscus) indicates growth. Preliminary data from studies in which MGIT and BACTEC TB were compared have shown that MGIT is as sensitive as the BACTEC TB, but the mean time to detection of growth is two to six days longer with MGIT (Kodsi, 1994).

Tests for Mycobacterial Identification

Identification of mycobacteria traditionally has been based on rate of growth on conventional solid media, colony morphology, colony pigmentation with and without exposure to light, and results of biochemical tests. Protocols for identification of the mycobacteria commonly encountered in the microbiology laboratory based on these factors are illustrated in Figures 51–2 to 51–5. Specific biochemical test methods are described in detail elsewhere (Kent, 1985). Although most species can be identified in this way, results usually are not available for several weeks to months after colonies appear on solid media. More rapid methods that allow identification of MTBC within 21 days of specimen receipt are recommended (Tenover, 1993).

The BACTEC TB NAP (paranitro-α-acetylamino-β-hydroxypropiophenone) test differentiates members of the MTBC from nontuberculous mycobacteria within four to five days after AFB are detected in a BACTEC TB vial (Gross, 1985). A volume of broth from the positive 12B vial is in-

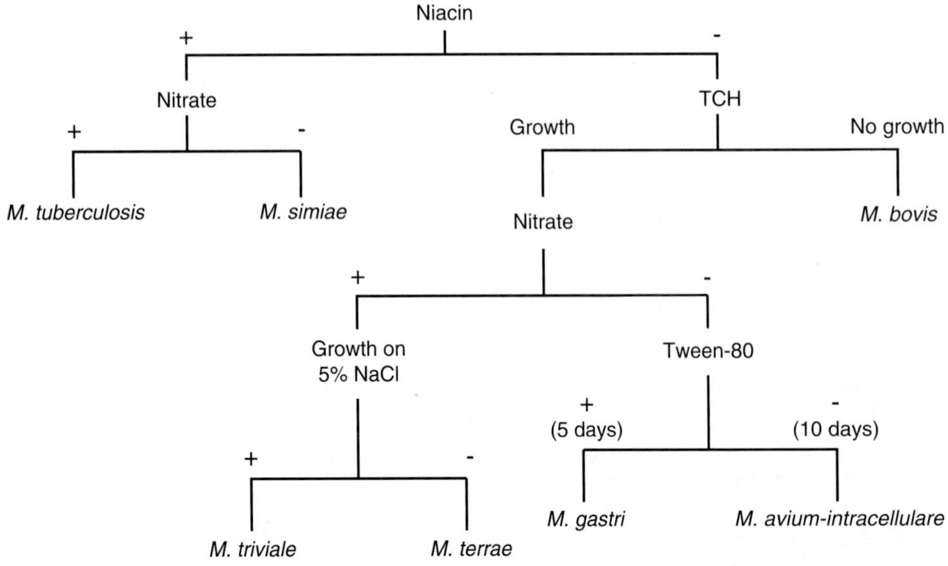

Figure 51–2. Decision tree for identification of nonphotochromogenic mycobacteria. Note that although *Mycobacterium simiae* usually is a photochromogen, this feature is unstable and may become apparent only after exposure to light for a prolonged period. Some strains of *Mycobacterium bovis* give a positive niacin reaction. (From Woods GL, Gutierrez Y: Diagnostic Pathology of Infectious Diseases. Philadelphia, Lea & Febiger, 1993.)

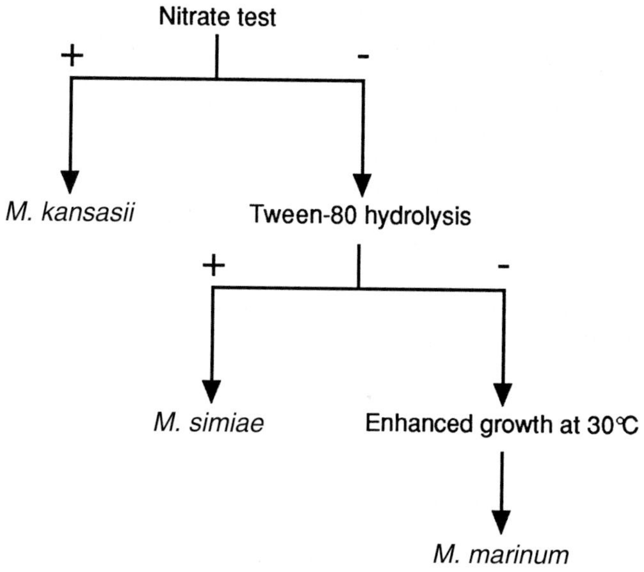

Figure 51–3. Decision tree for identification of photochromogenic mycobacteria. (From Roberts GD: Mycobacteria and Nocardia. *In* Washington JA II (ed): Laboratory Procedures in Clinical Microbiology, 2nd ed. New York, Springer-Verlag, 1985.)

jected into two fresh bottles of 12B medium, one with and one without NAP. An increase in the GI in the bottle without NAP and no increase in the GI in the bottle containing NAP indicates that the isolate is a member of MTBC, because only those species are susceptible to and thus inhibited by NAP. This test, however, does not differentiate species of the MTBC.

Chemiluminescent DNA probes allow identification of a few species of mycobacteria within 1 to 2 hours after sufficient growth is present (on solid or in liquid medium) (Evans, 1992; Goto, 1992; Lebrun, 1992; Reisner, 1994).

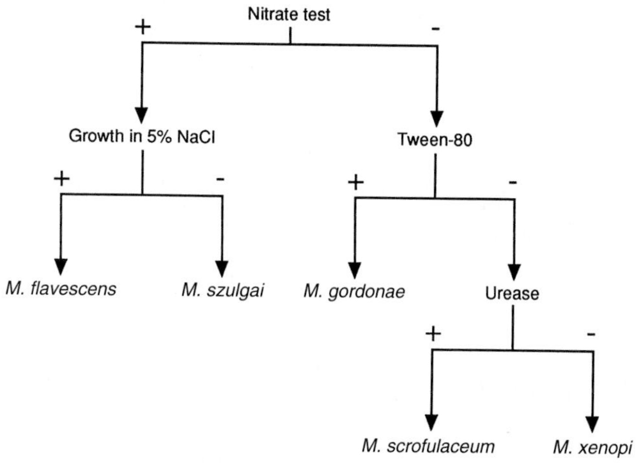

Figure 51–4. Decision tree for identifying the common scotochromogenic mycobacteria. Note that *Mycobacterium szulgai* is a photochromogen at 25°C and a scotochromogen at 35°C, and that *Mycobacterium xenopi* grows well at 42°C. (From Roberts GD: Mycobacteria and Nocardia. *In* Washington JA II [ed]: Laboratory Procedures in Clinical Microbiology, 2nd ed. New York, Springer-Verlag, 1985.)

Commercial probes specific for MTBC, MAC, *M. avium, M. intracellulare, M. gordonae,* and *M. kansasii* currently are available. The major advantage of these probes is rapid identification. Disadvantages include cost, the requirement for equipment (luminometer, sonicator, and heating block), failure to identify a small percentage (3% to 5%) of isolates of MAC, and rare false-positive results with the MTBC probe (Bull, 1992; Butler, 1994; Lebrun, 1992).

Gas-liquid chromatography, high-performance liquid chromatography, and thin-layer chromatography allow identification of mycobacterial colonies on a solid medium in two to four hours. These techniques, which are technically complex and require expensive equipment, are performed predominantly in research and large reference laboratories.

Rarely, a mycobacterial isolate cannot be identified by any of the methods described above. An example is *M. genavense,* the identification of which has required sequence determination of the hypervariable regions of the 16S ribosomal RNA gene. This highly sophisticated test is performed only in specialized research or reference laboratories.

In the future, nucleic acid amplification methods, such as isothermal enzymatic amplification of target rRNA, Qβ-replicase, ligase chain reaction, or the polymerase chain reaction, may prove useful for detection of mycobacteria directly in clinical material within 24 hours or less of specimen receipt. Preliminary studies investigating detection of *M. tuberculosis* in respiratory specimens have shown that these methods are extremely specific; sensitivity is high for AFB smear–positive specimens but much lower (54–80%) for smear-negative samples (Abe, 1993; Glinski, 1994; Jonas, 1993; Metchock, 1994; Miller, 1994; Pfyffer, 1994).

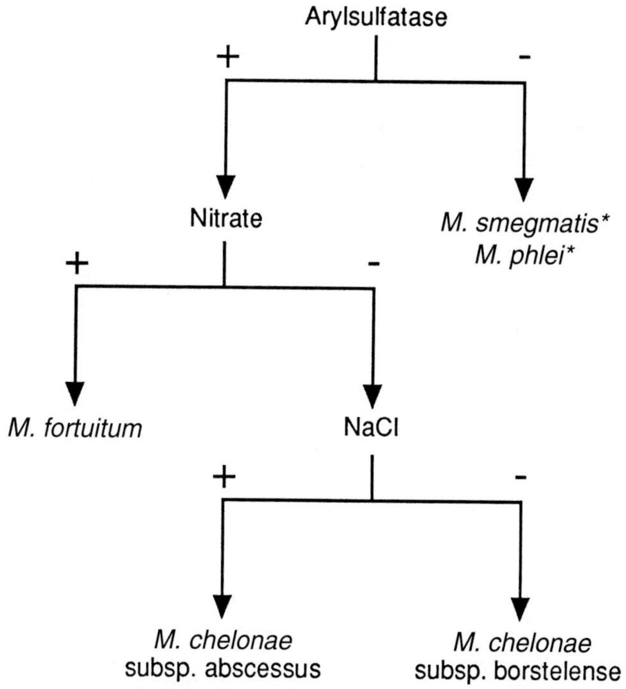

Figure 51–5. Decision tree for identification of the clinically significant rapidly growing mycobacteria. Asterisk indicates that additional biochemical testing is necessary for differentiation. (From Roberts GD: Mycobacteria and Nocardia. *In* Washington JA II [ed]: Laboratory Procedures in Clinical Microbiology, 2nd ed. New York, Springer-Verlag, 1985.)

Susceptibility Testing

Currently, standardized guidelines for susceptibility testing of mycobacteria have been developed only for isolates of *M. tuberculosis*. Testing may be performed on isolated colonies or a positive BACTEC TB vial (indirect test) or on sputum specimens that are AFB smear–positive (direct test). Traditionally, the proportion method, a modified agar dilution test, has been used to evaluate susceptibility of *M. tuberculosis* to antituberculosis agents. With this method, isolates showing greater than 1% resistance are considered resistant to that concentration of the drug. Results are available a minimum of 21 days after plates are inoculated. The BACTEC TB system also may be used for susceptibility testing of MTBC; results are available five to seven days after bottles are inoculated. More detailed descriptions of these procedures are found elsewhere (Hawkins, 1991). Given the concern regarding multidrug-resistant *M. tuberculosis,* experts at the CDC recommend that drug susceptibility test results be provided within 28 days of specimen receipt in the laboratory, a turnaround time that currently can be achieved only with the BACTEC TB system (Tenover, 1993).

Susceptibility testing may be performed on isolates of the nontuberculous mycobacteria; however, for some species, there may be little correlation between susceptibility test results and clinical response to drug therapy. Moreover, there is no standardized reference method for testing these organisms. Methods that have been used are the proportion method, radiometric assays, broth microdilution, and for isolates of *M. fortuitum-chelonae* complex, disk diffusion and agar disk elution. Growth in mouse footpads is the only currently acceptable assay for viability and drug-susceptibility testing of leprosy bacilli.

TREATMENT

The CDC recommends that initial isolates of *M. tuberculosis* from all patients with tuberculosis be tested for susceptibility to the primary antituberculosis agents—isoniazid, rifampin, pyrazinamide, streptomycin, and ethambutol. Susceptibility testing should be repeated if the patient continues to produce culture-positive sputum after three months of therapy (Tenover, 1993). If resistance to more than one primary agent is suspected, susceptibility to secondary drugs (ethionamide, kanamycin, capreomycin, ciprofloxacin, and cycloserine) also should be evaluated. The chemotherapeutic regimen currently recommended for treatment of tuberculosis (Table 51–7) should be initiated before susceptibility test results are available, but treatment should be altered based on those results if an isolate is found to be resistant. Regimens commonly used to treat infections caused by the most frequently encountered nontuberculous mycobacteria also are listed in Table 51–7 (Horowitz, 1994; Inderlied, 1993; Wallace, 1983, 1994; Wolinsky, 1979). For many nontuberculous mycobacteria, the optimal duration of therapy is not known, but the intervals indicated in the table have been successful in some cases.

PREVENTION

Mycobacterium tuberculosis

Four general strategies for controlling tuberculosis are described (CDC, 1988). The most important is early identification and adequate treatment of persons with infectious tuberculosis. This measure renders the infected person noncontagious within a few weeks and eventually results in cure. The second strategy entails identification and treatment of individuals with noncontagious tuberculosis: extrapulmonary disease, primary pulmonary disease in children, bacteriologically unconfirmed pulmonary disease, and infection with *M. tuberculosis* not yet causing disease (i.e., positive skin test, normal chest x-ray, no symptoms).

The third strategy involves creation of a safe environment in situations in which the risk of transmitting infection is high: autopsy suites, sputum-induction cubicles, chest clinic waiting areas, correctional facilities, some shelters for the homeless, and mycobacteriology laboratories. To accomplish this, several issues must be addressed (Segal-Maurer, 1994). Rooms housing infectious patients or those in which potentially infectious specimens are handled should be under negative pressure, and air likely to be contaminated with infectious droplet nuclei should be exhausted to the outside. A single-pass ventilation system (best accomplished by locating air supply outlets at the ceiling level and exhaust inlets near the floor) and a minimum of six air changes per hour (12 exchanges per hour for autopsy suites) are recom-

Table 51–7. TREATMENT OF INFECTIONS WITH COMMONLY ENCOUNTERED PATHOGENIC MYCOBACTERIA

Mycobacterium species	Therapy		
	Surgery	*Agents*	*Duration (months)*
*M. tuberculosis**	—	INH, RIF, EMB, and PZA	6
M. avium complex			
pulmonary	±	RIF, EMB ± SM	18–24 or at least 12 after sputum conversion
disseminated (AIDS)	—	CLARI or AZITHRO + EMB + RFB or CIPRO	? lifelong
lymphadenitis	+	–	
M. kansasii	—	INH, RIF, and EMB	18
M. fortuitum-chelonae	+	AM and TET, CFX, or RIF	1–2 after clinical response
M. marinum	±	RIF; RIF and EMB; or TET	18; or 1–2 after clinical resolution

*EMB and PZA are given only during the first 2 months. HIV-infected patients are treated for 9 months or at least 6 months after sputum conversion. Regimen is for drug-susceptible strains only.

AM = amikacin; AZITHRO = azithromycin; CFX = cefoxitin; CLARI = clarithromycin; EMB = ethambutol; INH = isoniazid; RFB = rifabutin; RIF = rifampin; SM = streptomycin; TET = tetracycline; — not indicated; + = definitely indicated; ± = may be indicated.

mended. Universal precautions must be followed when handling all specimens, and both specimens and cultures must be handled in a certified, Class II biologic safety cabinet. Moreover, a particulate respirator that filters out particles 1 to 5 μm in diameter should be worn, and personnel should be trained in a respiratory program; the standard surgical mask is not adequate.

The fourth strategy is vaccination with the BCG vaccine, an attenuated vaccine derived from a strain of *M. bovis* by Calmette and Guérin in France. The efficacy of the BCG vaccine in prevention of tuberculosis is controversial, but a recent meta-analysis of the literature suggests that the vaccine reduces the risk of tuberculosis significantly, by 50% (Colditz, 1994). In the United States, the BCG vaccine is recommended only for infants and children who have negative tuberculin skin tests and who belong to selected population groups (CDC, 1988):

1. Those at high risk of intimate and prolonged exposure to persistently untreated or ineffectively treated persons with infectious pulmonary tuberculosis, who cannot be removed from the source of exposure, and for whom long-term preventive therapy is not possible.
2. Those exposed continuously to persons with tuberculosis due to strains resistant to isoniazid and rifampin.
3. Those in groups in which the rate of new infections is greater than 1% per year and for whom the usual surveillance and treatment programs have been attempted but are not feasible.

The BCG vaccine is no longer recommended for health care workers in the United States. The current recommendation for protection of health care workers is adequate surveillance, which includes periodic tuberculin skin tests (at least yearly and more frequently for persons in high-risk groups) and isoniazid preventive therapy for persons who have recently converted from tuberculin skin test–negative to –positive and for persons who are tuberculin skin test–positive and who are close contacts of individuals with tuberculosis or who have medical conditions such as diabetes, renal failure, or immunosuppression associated with therapy or disease (CDC, 1988).

The BCG vaccine should not be given to immunocompromised persons and should be given with caution to those at risk of infection with HIV. Disseminated *M. bovis* in patients with AIDS and *M. bovis* lymphadenitis in symptomatic HIV-infected infants have occurred following BCG vaccination (Blanche, 1986; CDC, 1985). However, disseminated *M. bovis* has not been reported in asymptomatic persons infected with HIV. In populations in which the risk of tuberculosis is high, the World Health Organization recommends that the BCG vaccine be given to HIV-infected children at birth or soon thereafter. It should not be given to children with symptomatic HIV infection, in populations in which the risk of tuberculosis is low, or to persons known or suspected to be infected with HIV (WHO, 1987).

Mycobacterium avium-intracellulare Complex

Disseminated MAC in patients with AIDS is associated with considerable morbidity and a shortened duration of survival (Horsburgh, 1991; Nightingale, 1992); therefore, prevention of the disease is desirable. Because MAC is ubiquitous in the environment, the most reasonable approach to prevention is immunomodulation or chemoprophylaxis. Data from two randomized controlled trials in which rifabutin prophylaxis was compared with placebo in patients with AIDS who had $CD4^+$ cell counts below 200/μL showed that rifabutin decreased the incidence of MAC bacteremia by 50% to 70% (Nightingale, 1993). Rifabutin also prolonged the time to fever, fatigue, anemia, elevated alkaline phosphatase levels, and decreased Karnofsky performance score. The efficacy of rifabutin was most pronounced in patients whose initial $CD4^+$ cell count was less than 75/μL. Fewer patients receiving rifabutin required hospitalization, but there was no significant decrease in mortality. Based on these data, a United States Public Health Service Task Force recommends rifabutin prophylaxis in AIDS patients with $CD4^+$ cell counts under 100/μL (Masur, 1993).

Abe C, Hirano K, Wada M, et al: Detection of *Mycobacterium tuberculosis* in clinical specimens by polymerase chain reaction and Gen-Probe Amplified Mycobacterium Tuberculosis Direct Test. J Clin Microbiol 1993; 31:3270.

Abe C, Hosojima S, Fukasawa Y, et al: Comparison of MB-Check, BACTEC, and egg-based media for recovery of mycobacteria. J Clin Microbiol 1992; 30:878.

Anargyros P, Astill DSJ, Lim ISL: Comparison of improved BACTEC and Löwenstein-Jensen media for culture of mycobacteria from clinical specimens. J Clin Microbiol 1990; 28:1288.

Binford CH, Meyers WM, Walsh GP: Leprosy. JAMA 1982; 247:2283.

Blacklock ZM, Dawson DJ, Kane DW, McEvoy D: *Mycobacterium asiaticum* as a potential pulmonary pathogen for humans: a clinical and bacteriologic review of five cases. Am Rev Respir Dis 1983; 127:241.

Blake LA, West BC, Lary CH, et al: Environmental nonhuman sources of leprosy. Rev Infect Dis 1987; 9:562.

Blanche S, LeDeist F, Fischer A: Longitudinal study of 18 children with perinatal LAV/HTLV III infection: Attempt at prognostic evaluation. J Pediatr 1986; 109:965.

Buhler VB, Pollak A: Human infection with atypical acid-fast organisms. Am J Clin Pathol 1953; 23:363.

Bull TJ, Shanson DC: Rapid misdiagnosis by *Mycobacterium avium-intracellulare* masquerading as tuberculosis in PCR/DNA probe tests. Lancet 1992; 340:1369.

Butler WR, O'Connor SP, Yakrus MA, et al: Cross-reactivity of genetic probe for detection of *Mycobacterium tuberculosis* with newly described species of *Mycobacterium celatum.* J Clin Microbiol 1994; 32:536.

Casimir MT, Fainstein V, Papadopolous N: Cavitary lung infection caused by *Mycobacterium flavescens.* South Med J 1982; 75:253.

Castets M, Boisvert H, Grumback F, et al: Les bacilles tuberculeux de type africaine. Rev Tuberc Pneumol 1968; 32:179.

Centers for Disease Control and Prevention: Disseminated *Mycobacterium bovis* infection from BCG vaccination of a patient with acquired immunodeficiency syndrome. MMWR 1985; 34:227.

Centers for Disease Control and Prevention: *Mycobacterium haemophilum* infection—New York City Metropolitan Area, 1990–1991. MMWR 1991; 40:636.

Centers for Disease Control and Prevention. Summary of notifiable diseases, United States, 1992. MMWR 1993a; 41(55):59.

Centers for Disease Control and Prevention. Tuberculosis control laws—United States, 1993. Recommendations of the Advisory Council for the Elimination of Tuberculosis. MMWR 1993b; 42(RR-15):1.

Centers for Disease Control and Prevention: Use of BCG vaccines in the control of tuberculosis: A joint statement by the ACIP and the Advisory Committee for the Elimination of Tuberculosis. MMWR 1988; 37:663.

Chaisson RE, Schecter GF, Theuer CP, et al: Tuberculosis in patients with the acquired immunodeficiency syndrome: Clinical features, response to therapy, and survival. Am Rev Respir Dis 1987; 136:570.

Chiodini RJ: Crohn's disease and the mycobacterioses: A review and comparison of two disease entities. Clin Microbiol Rev 1989; 2:90.

Cianciulli FD: The radish bacillus *(Mycobacterium terrae)*: Saprophyte or pathogen? Am Rev Respir Dis 1974; 109:138.

Colditz GA, Brewer TF, Berkey CS, et al: Efficacy of BCG vaccine in prevention of tuberculosis: Meta-analysis of the published literature. JAMA 1994; 271:698.

Costrinia AM, Mahler DA, Gross WM, et al: Clinical and roentgenographic features of nosocomial pulmonary disease due to *Mycobacterium xenopi.* Am Rev Respir Dis 1981; 123:104.

Coyle MB, Carlson LC, Wallis CK, et al: Laboratory aspects of *"Mycobac-*

terium genavense," proposed species isolated from AIDS patients. J Clin Microbiol 1992; 30:3206.
D'Amato RF, Isenberg HD, Hochstein L, et al: Evaluation of the Roche Septi-Chek AFB system for recovery of mycobacteria. J Clin Microbiol 1991; 29:2906.
Davison MB, McCormack JG, Blacklock ZM, et al: Bacteremia caused by *Mycobacterium neoaurum.* J Clin Microbiol 1988; 26:762.
DeChairo DC, Kittredge D, Meyers A, et al: Septic arthritis due to *Mycobacterium triviale.* Am Rev Respir Dis 1973; 108:1224.
Edwards MS, Huber TW, Baker CJ: *Mycobacterium terrae* synovitis and osteomyelitis. Am Rev Respir Dis 1978; 117:161.
Ellner JJ, Hinman AR, Dooley SW, et al: Tuberculosis symposium: Emerging problems and promise. J Infect Dis 1993; 168:537.
Evans KD, Nakasone AS, Sutherland PA, et al: Identification of *Mycobacterium tuberculosis* and *Mycobacterium avium-Mycobacterium intracellulare* directly from primary BACTEC cultures by using acridinium-ester–labeled DNA probes. J Clin Microbiol 1992; 30:2427.
Feldman RA, Hershfield E: Mycobacterial skin infection by an unidentified species. A report of 29 patients. Ann Intern Med 1974; 80:445.
Glinski BM, Maddox D, Cauyeffield D, et al: Clinical evaluation of a polymerase chain reaction (PCR) assay for the direct detection of *Mycobacterium tuberculosis* in respiratory specimens [Abstract No. D81]. *In* Abstracts of the 34th Interscience Conference on Antimicrobial Agents and Chemotherapy. Orlando, FL, American Society for Microbiology, 1994, p 155.
Good RC, Snider DE Jr: Isolation of nontuberculous mycobacteria in the United States. J Infect Dis 1982; 146:829.
Goto M, Oka S, Okuzumi K, et al: Evaluation of acridinium-ester-labeled DNA probes for identification of *Mycobacterium tuberculosis* and *Mycobacterium avium–Mycobacterium-intracellulare* complex in culture. J Clin Microbiol 1992; 30:2427.
Grange JM, Collins CH: Bovine tubercle bacilli and disease in animals and man. Epidem Info 1987; 92:221.
Gross WM, Hawkins JE: Radiometric selective inhibition tests for differentiation of *Mycobacterium tuberculosis, Mycobacterium bovis,* and other mycobacteria. J Clin Microbiol 1985; 21:565.
Guthertz LS, Damsker B, Bottone EJ, et al: *Mycobacterium avium* and *Mycobacterium intracellulare* infections in patients with and without AIDS. J Infect Dis 1989; 160:1037.
Haas DW, Des Prez RM: *Mycobacterium tuberculosis. In* Mandell GL, Bennett JE, Dolan R (eds): Principles and Practice of Infectious Diseases, 4th ed. New York, Churchill Livingstone, 1994, pp 2213–2242.
Hastings RC, Gillis TP, Krahenbuhl JL, et al: Leprosy. Clin Microbiol Rev 1988; 1:330.
Hawkins JE, Wallace RJ Jr, Brown BA: Antimicrobial susceptibility tests: Mycobacteria. *In* Balows A, Hausler WJ Jr, Herrmann KL, Isenberg HD, Shadomy HJ (eds): Manual of Clinical Microbiology, 5th ed. Washington DC, American Society for Microbiology, 1991, pp 1138–1152.
Henriques B, Hoffner SE, Petrini B, et al: Infection with *Mycobacterium malmoense* in Sweden: Report of 221 cases. Clin Infect Dis 1993; 18:596.
Horowitz EA, Sanders WE Jr: Other *Mycobacterium* species. *In* Mandell GL, Bennett JE, Dolin R (eds): Principles and Practice of Infectious Disease, 4th ed. New York, Churchill Livingstone, 1994.
Horsburgh CR Jr: *Mycobacterium avium* complex infection in the acquired immunodeficiency syndrome. N Engl J Med 1991; 324:1332.
Horsburgh CR Jr, Havlik JA, Illis DA, et al: Survival of patients with acquired immune deficiency syndrome and disseminated *Mycobacterium avium* complex infection with and without antimycobacterial chemotherapy. Am Rev Respir Dis 1991; 144:557.
Huebner RE, Schein MF, Bass JB Jr: The tuberculin skin test. Clin Infect Dis 1993; 17:968.
Inderlied CB, Kemper CA, Bermudez LEM: The *Mycobacterium avium* complex. Clin Microbiol Rev 1993; 6:266.
Isenberg HD, D'Amato RF, Heifets L, et al: Collaborative feasibility study of a biphasic system (Roche Septi-Chek AFB) for rapid detection and isolation of mycobacteria. J Clin Microbiol 1991; 29:1719.
Jacobs RF: Multiple-drug–resistant tuberculosis. Clin Infect 1994; 19:1.
Jonas V, Alden MJ, Curry JI, et al: Detection and identification of *Mycobacterium tuberculosis* directly from sputum sediments by amplification of rRNA. J Clin Microbiol 1993; 31:2410.
Karassova V, Weiszfeiler J, Krasznay E: Occurrence of atypical mycobacteria in macacus rhesus. Acta Microbiol Acad Sci Hung 1965; 12:275.
Karlson AG, Carr DT: Tuberculosis caused by *Mycobacterium bovis.* Ann Intern Med 1970; 73:979.
Kent PT, Kubica GP: Public health mycobacteriology: A guide for the level III laboratory. Atlanta, US Department of Health and Human Services, 1985.
Kim JH, Langston AA, Gallis HA: Miliary tuberculosis: Epidemiology, clinical manifestations, diagnosis, and outcome. Rev Infect Dis 1990; 12:583.
Kodsi SE, Hagemann PA, Douglass JD, et al: Comparison of the BBL MGIT Mycobacterial Growth Indicator Tube with the BACTEC TB system using clinical specimens [Abstract No. D-55]. *In* Abstracts of the 34th Interscience Conference on Antimicrobial Agents and Chemotherapy, Orlando, FL, American Society for Microbiology, 1994, p 155.
Kristjansson M, Green P, Manning HL, et al: Molecular confirmation of Bacillus Calmette-Guérin as the cause of pulmonary infection following urinary tract instillation. Clin Infect Dis 1993; 17:228.
Lebrun L, Espinasse R, Poveda JD, et al: Evaluation of nonradioactive DNA probes for identification of mycobacteria. J Clin Microbiol 1992; 30:2476.
Lomvardias S, Madge GE: Chaetoconidium and atypical acid-fast bacilli in skin ulcers. Arch Dermatol 1972; 106:875.
Lumpkin LR III, Cox GF, Wolf JE: Leprosy in five armadillo handlers. J Am Acad Dermatol 1983; 9:899.
Masur H, the Public Health Service Task Force on Prophylaxis and Therapy for *Mycobacterium avium* Complex: Recommendations on prophylaxis and therapy for disseminated *Mycobacterium avium* complex for adults and adolescents infected with human immunodeficiency virus. N Engl J Med 1993; 329:898.
Metchock B, Diem L: Clinical laboratory evaluation of the Roche Amplicor Mycobacterium Tuberculosis assay [Abstract No. D79]. *In* Abstracts of the 34th Interscience Conference on Antimicrobial Agents and Chemotherapy, Orlando, FL, American Society for Microbiology, 1994, p 155.
Miller N, Hernandez SG, Cleary TJ: Evaluation of Gen-Probe Mycobacterium Tuberculosis Direct Test and PCR for direct detection of *Mycobacterium tuberculosis* in clinical specimens. J Clin Microbiol 1994; 32:393.
Murray CJL, Styblo K, Rouillon A: Tuberculosis in developing countries: Burden, intervention, and cost. Bull Int Union Tuberc Lung Dis 1990; 65:6.
Murray PR, Elmore C, Krogstad D: The acid-fast stain: A specific and predictive test for mycobacterial disease. Ann Intern Med 1980; 92:512.
Neely SP, Denning DW: Cutaneous *Mycobacterium thermoresistible* infection in a heart transplant recipient. Rev Infect Dis 1989; 11:608.
Neill MA, Hightower AW, Broome CV: Leprosy in the United States, 1971–1981. J Infect Dis 1985; 152:1064.
Nightingale SD, Byrd LT, Southern PM, et al: Incidence of *Mycobacterium avium-intracelulare* complex bacteremia in human immunodeficiency virus-positive patients. J Infect Dis 1992; 165:1082.
Nightingale SD, Cameron DW, Gordin FM, et al: Two controlled trials of rifabutin prophylaxis against *Mycobacterium avium* complex infection in AIDS. N Engl J Med 1993; 329:828.
Norden A, Linell F: A new type of pathogenic *Mycobacterium.* Nature 1951; 168:826.
Pfyffer GE, Kissling P, Wirth R, et al: Direct detection of *Mycobacterium tuberculosis* complex in respiratory specimens by a target-amplified system. J Clin Microbiol 1994; 32:918.
Prince DS: Infection with *Mycobacterium avium* complex in patients without predisposing conditions. N Engl J Med 1989; 321:863.
Prissick FH, Mason AM: Cervical lymphadenitis in children caused by chromogenic mycobacteria. Can Med Assoc J 1956; 75:798.
Reisner BS, Gatson AM, Woods GL: Use of Gen-Probe AccuProbes to identify *Mycobacterium avium* complex, *Mycobacterium tuberculosis* complex, *Mycobacterium kansasii,* and *Mycobacterium gordonae* directly from BACTEC TB broth cultures. J Clin Microbiol 1994; 32:2995.
Rickman TW, Moyer NP: Increased sensitivity of acid-fast smears. J Clin Microbiol 1980; 11:618.
Ridley DS, Jopling WH: Classification of leprosy according to immunity: A five group system. Int J Lepr 1964; 34:255.
Rieder HI, Cauthen GM, Kelly GD, et al: Tuberculosis in the United States. JAMA 1989; 262:385.
Runyon EH: Anonymous mycobacteria in pulmonary disease. Med Clin North Am 1959; 43:273.
Schroder KH, Juhlin I: *Mycobacterium malmoense* sp. nov. Int J Syst Bacteriol 1977; 27:241.
Segal-Maurer S, Kalkut GE: Environmental control of tuberculosis: Continuing controversy. Clin Infect Dis 1994; 19:299.
Snider DE Jr, La Montagne JR: The neglected global tuberculosis problem: A report of the 1992 World Congress on Tuberculosis. J Infect Dis 1994; 169:1189.
Sompolinsky D, Lagziel A, Naveh D, et al: *Mycobacterium haemophilium* sp. nov., a new pathogen of humans. Int J Syst Bacteriol 1978; 28:67.
Stager CE, Libonati JP, Siddiqi SH, et al: Role of solid media when used in conjunction with the BACTEC system for mycobacterial isolation and identification. J Clin Microbiol 1991; 29:154.
Strumpf IJ, Tsang AY, Sayre JW: Re-evaluation of sputum staining for the diagnosis of pulmonary tuberculosis. Am Rev Respir Dis 1979; 119:599.
Tecson-Tumang FT, Bright JL: *Mycobacterium xenopi* and the acquired immunodeficiency syndrome. Chest 1984; 86:145.
Tenover FC, Crawford JT, Huebner RE, et al: The resurgence of tuberculosis: Is your laboratory ready? J Clin Microbiol 1993; 31:767.
Tsukamura M, Kita N, Otsuka W, et al: A study of the taxonomy of the *Mycobacterium nonchromogenicum* complex and report of six cases of lung infection due to *Mycobacterium nonchromogenicum.* Microbiol Immunol 1983; 27:219.

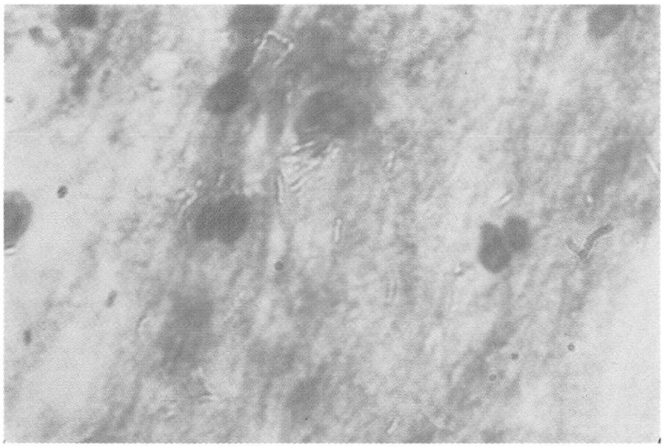

Plate 51–1. Smear of a sputum specimen stained with Gram's stain shows so-called ghost cells (mycobacterial culture grew *Mycobacterium tuberculosis;* Gram's stain, ×400).

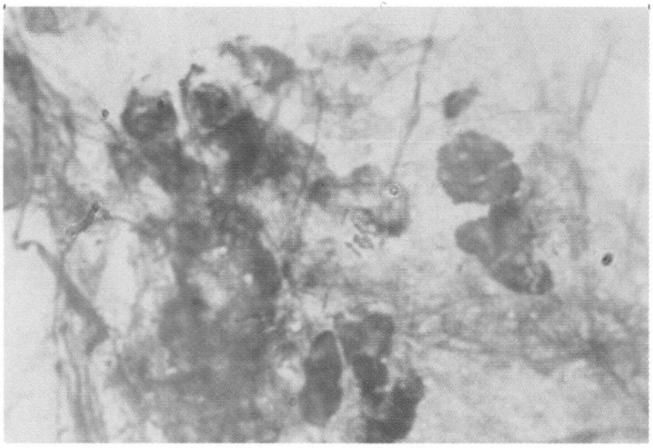

Plate 51–2. Smear of a sputum specimen shows acid-fast bacilli *(Mycobacterium tuberculosis;* Kinyoun, ×400).

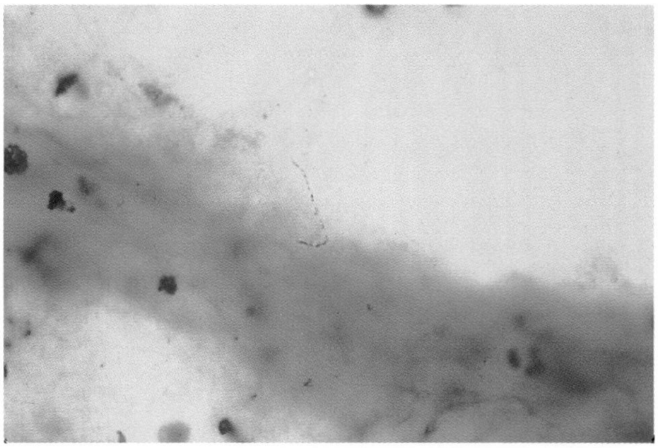

Plate 51–3. Smear of an aspirate from an enlarged cervical lymph node shows a large, cross-barred acid-fast bacillus (*Mycobacterium kansasii;* Kinyoun, ×400). (Courtesy of Vicki J. Schnadig, MD, Department of Pathology, University of Texas Medical Branch, Galveston.)

Tsukamura M, Shimoide H, Schaefer WB: A possible pathogen of Group III mycobacteria. J Gen Microbiol 1975; 88:377.

Wald A, Coyle MB, Carlson LC, et al: Infection with a fastidious mycobacterium resembling *Mycobacterium simiae* in seven patients with AIDS. Ann Intern Med 1992; 117:586.

Wallace RJ Jr, Dunbar D, Brown BA, et al: Rifampin-resistant *Mycobacterium kansasii*. Clin Infect Dis 1994; 18:736.

Wallace RJ Jr, Nash DR, Tsukamura M, et al: Human disease due to *Mycobacterium smegmatis*. J Infect Dis 1988; 158:52.

Wallace RJ Jr, Swenson JM, Silcox VA, et al: Spectrum of disease due to rapidly growing mycobacteria. Rev Infect Dis 1983; 5:657.

Weinberger M, Berg SL, Feuerstein IM, et al: Disseminated infection with *Mycobacterium gordonae*: Report of a case and critical review of the literature. Clin Infect Dis 1992; 14:1229.

Weitzman I, Osadczyi D, Corrado ML, et al: *Mycobacterium thermoresistible:* A new pathogen for humans. J Clin Microbiol 1981; 14:593.

Welch DF, Guruswamy AP, Sides SJ, et al: Timely culture for mycobacteria which utilizes a microcolony method. J Clin Microbiol 1993; 31:2178.

Wolinsky E: Nontuberculous mycobacteria and associated diseases. Am Rev Respir Dis 1979; 119:107.

Woods GL: Mycobacteria. *In* Woods GL, Gutierrez Y: Diagnostic Pathology of Infectious Diseases. Philadelphia, Lea & Febiger, 1993, p 378.

Woods GL, Washington JA II: Mycobacteria other than *Mycobacterium tuberculosis:* Review of microbiologic and clinical aspects. Rev Infect Dis 1987; 9:275.

World Health Organization: Special Programme on AIDS and Expanded Programme on Immunization—Joint statement: Consultation on human immunodeficiency virus (HIV) and routine childhood immunization. Wkly Epidemiol Rep 1987; 62:297.

Yakrus MA, Good RC: Geographic distribution, frequency, and specimen source of *Mycobacterium avium* complex serotypes isolated from patients with acquired immunodeficiency syndrome. J Clin Microbiol 1990; 28:926.

Chapter 52

Mycotic Diseases

Washington C. Winn, Jr., M.D., M.B.A.
Fred W. Westenfeld, MT(ASCP)SM

Medical mycology is among the most diverse areas of microbiology and infectious disease, encompassing single-celled yeast and filamentous moulds, agents of superficial skin infections and disseminated deep-seated visceral disease, established historical pathogens, and saprobic fungi elevated to the status of pathogen by modern therapies and diseases. For pathologists who have been nurtured in the surgical pathology suite, medical mycology should be a natural adaptation. The identification of most fungi is accomplished by skilled human observation rather than by machines. The macroscopic counterpart of the surgical specimen is the colonial morphology of the isolated fungus on agar media; as in anatomic pathology, definitive analysis of the problem must await microscopic observation. Characterization of the molecular structure of cells by the use of monoclonal antibodies is not so fully developed in mycology, but a beachhead has been made and molecular diagnosis will undoubtedly be of expanded importance in the future.

The goal of this chapter is to present the fundamentals of medical mycology with an emphasis on practical issues and those fungal pathogens encountered regularly in the laboratory. We call the attention of the reader to the existence of some less commonly isolated potential pathogens. Several excellent reference texts serve as sources for information on unusual saprobic fungi that increasingly are implicated as etiologic agents in severely immunosuppressed patients (Haley, 1980; Kwon-Chung, 1992; Larone, 1995; McGinnis, 1980; Rippon, 1988). With increasing use of immunosuppressive protocols for transplants and chemotherapy of neoplastic disease, any fungal isolate must be considered a potential pathogen. It also should be emphasized that invasive infection can occur in individuals who do not have immunosuppressive conditions or even those who have no recognized underlying disease.

The anatomic pathologist, medical mycologist, and clinician must work in concert to provide the best care for the patient (Walker, 1982). Immense satisfaction accrues to the providers when a team effort unravels a challenging clinical problem, but it is the patient who truly benefits from good communication and sharing of expertise. The focus of this chapter is on the mycology laboratory. Chandler and Watts (1987) have produced an excellent, comprehensive atlas of the histopathology of fungal infection.

Prototheca species are achlorophyllous algae rather than fungi. They are discussed in this chapter because the characteristics of the algae and the diseases they produce resemble fungi more than other infectious agents. *Pneumocystis carinii* has characteristics of both protozoa and fungi. Although it has traditionally been discussed in treatises on parasitic disease, molecular studies suggest a closer relationship to fungi and it has been included in this chapter.

NOMENCLATURE, TAXONOMY, AND IDENTIFICATION TECHNIQUES

The first hurdle for the beginning mycologist is nomenclature and its handmaiden taxonomy. The members of the Kingdom Fungi are eukaryotic cells that reproduce by both sexual and asexual means. They are classified by the nature of their reproductive structures, with the sexual characteristics taking precedence. The sexual stages of many fungi are unknown; these organisms, known as Fungi Imperfecti, are classified by their asexual reproductive structures. These asexual states are, of course, only imperfect in the eyes of taxonomists because sexual reproduction is typically unknown, most medical mycologists and undoubtedly the fungi themselves being perfectly happy with their incomplete state. Once the sexual phase, called the teleomorph, of such a fungus is known, the organism is reclassified, but in actual practice, the old familiar name of the imperfect asexual phase, called an anamorph, usually is retained. For example, few people know *Histoplasma capsulatum*, *Blastomyces dermatitidis*, and *Cryptococcus neoformans* by their respective teleomorphic names, *Ajellomyces capsulatus*, *Ajellomyces dermatitidis*, and *Filobasidiella neoformans*. In contrast, the sexual phase *Pseudallescheria boydii* and its asexual phase *Scedosporium apiospermum* are both recognized in common practice.

Much of fungal taxonomy is related to structural details,

Table 52–1. GLOSSARY OF COMMONLY USED TERMS IN MEDICAL MYCOLOGY

Term	Definition
Aerial mycelium	Hyphae produced above the surface of the agar media
Anamorph	The asexual form of a fungus
Ascocarp (ascoma)	The fruiting structure that contains an ascus. There are several types of ascocarps
Ascospore	A sexual spore that is contained within an ascus
Ascus	A saclike structure that contains sexual spores. It may either be naked or contained within a fruiting structure
Chlamydospore	A resting or survival structure
Cleistothecium	A completely enclosed ascocarp, composed of layers of hyphae. The ascospores are released by rupture
Columella	An extension of the sporangiophore into the base of the sporangium
Conidiogenous cell	The cell that produces conidia
Conidiophore	The specialized hyphal structure that carries the conidia; it is different from the conidiogenous cell
Conidium	Asexual reproductive structure formed in any manner that does not involve cleavage
Glabrous	Smooth, referring to colonial morphology
Hypha	The vegetative unit of moulds; has parallel walls
Intercalary	Borne within a hypha
Macroconidium	The larger of two types of conidia produced by an isolate in the same way
Microconidium	The smaller of two types of conidia produced by an isolate in the same way
Mould	Filamentous fungus that reproduces by sexual or asexual means
Mycelium (thallus)	A mass of hyphae that make up a mould
Perithecium	A closed ascocarp with a pore at the top, through which the ascospores are discharged
Pseudohypha	A series of connected yeast cells (blastoconidia) that resemble a hypha but contain areas of constriction between adjacent cells
Septum	A cross-wall in a hypha
Sporangiophore	The specialized hyphal structure that carries the sporangium
Sporangiospore	Asexual spore produced within a sporangium
Sporangium	A saclike structure in which the asexual sporangiospores develop
Telemorph	The sexual form of a fungus
Terminal	Borne at the end of a hypha
Vegetative mycelium	Hyphae produced on the surface or extending into the agar media
Vesicle	An enlarged or swollen cell, often at the end of a conidiophore or sporangiophore, but may be within hypae
Yeast	Single-cell fungus that reproduces by budding or by fission

6

because both classification and laboratory identification are so heavily dependent on morphology. A glossary of important terms is displayed in Table 52–1. In this chapter, we eschew complicated taxonomic schemes in favor of a simplified conceptual approach to the pathogens that are most commonly encountered in the clinical laboratory. For practical purposes, a few general characteristics serve as the basis for identification of fungi in the laboratory (Table 52–2).

As mycologists learn more about fungi, reclassification of organisms occurs on a regular basis. Rinaldi (1993) has summarized some of the changes in taxonomy and nomenclature of medically important fungi. The influence of molecular techniques will undoubtedly be increasingly important in fungal taxonomy as well as in diagnosis in the near future.

The Fungal Colony

The simplest feature is the nature of the fungal colony. Yeast are unicellular organisms that usually reproduce asexually by budding to produce a daughter cell. As a result, the colonial mass of a yeast is a collection of distinct individual organisms that, not surprisingly, resembles bacterial colonies on the surface of agar. Yeast colonies usually are smooth and entire (regular edge). When they are heaped and dull, as *Candida albicans* often is, the colonies may resemble those of staphylococci. Yeast produce catalase, so the incautious microbiologist who does not perform Gram's stain or a wet prep may mistake a yeast colony for a bacterium and provide an entirely misleading report. Encapsulated yeast, such as the cryptococci, may resemble encapsulated bacteria, such as *Klebsiella pneumoniae*, although misidentification is less likely in this case. The pseudohyphae of yeast are often visible macroscopically as filamentous extensions from the edges of the colony, known colloquially as feet, as if the colony were a centipede (Fig. 52–1).

In contrast to yeast, moulds are filamentous fungi, which are multicellular. Most mycologists prefer the term mould, reserving mold for bakers and automobile manufacturers, but the usage is not uniform. The filamentous nature of the mould gives the colonies a wooly, fluffy, or velvety appearance, sometimes punctuated with a granular or powdery aspect that is produced by the formation of asexual reproductive structures (Plate 52–1). At other times, the colony may have a glabrous (smooth) appearance.

The line between moulds and yeast is not firmly drawn. Some yeast also develop a filamentous component, which may even be visible macroscopically in some cases. The filamentous extensions from the colonies of *C. albicans* have

Table 52–2. CHARACTERISTICS USEFUL FOR THE IDENTIFICATION OF FUNGI

Characteristic	Examples
Type of macroscopic growth	Colonies of unicellular organisms (yeast) Colonies of filamentous organisms (moulds)
Morphology of yeast	Budding Budding with pseudohyphae Round yeast with capsules Budding yeast with collarettes
Morphology of filamentous structures	True hyphae—septate True hyphae—nonseptate or sparsely septate Pseudohyphae
Pigment of hyphae	Non-dematiaceous or hyaline (lightly or nonpigmented) Dematiaceous (darkly pigmented)
Morphology of asexual reproductive structures	Conidia Spores
Morphology of sexual reproductive structures (only rarely demonstrated)	Ascospores Cleistothecia Perithecia
Growth rate	Slow (>10 days) Medium (5 to 10 days) Fast (≤4 days)
Inhibition by cycloheximide	Many saprobic fungi
Optimal growth temperature (occasionally of value)	25°C to 30°C 35°C to 37°C 40°C to 42°C 50°C to 58°C
Biochemical tests	Assimilation Fermentation Enzymatic degradation (e.g., urease) Growth enhancement Pheno oxidase (melanin)
Conversion from mould to yeast phase	Has been supplanted by immunodiffusion or DNA homology tests in many laboratories
Immunologic detection of antigens or antibodies	*Cryptococcus, Histoplasma, Coccidioides, Blastomyces*
Molecular characteristic of DNA	*Histoplasma, Coccidioides, Blastomyces*

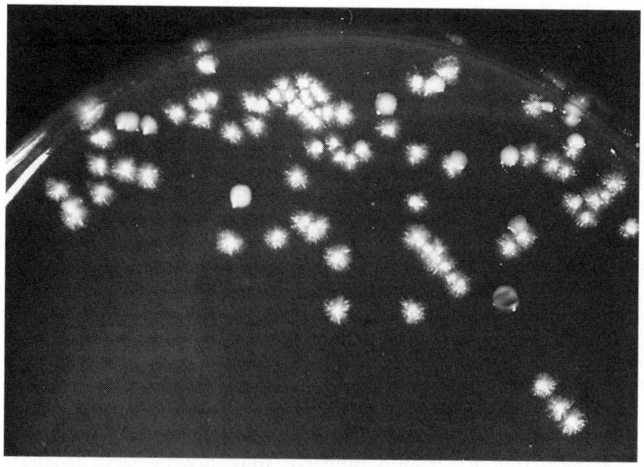

Figure 52–1. Filamentous extensions from the periphery of colonies of *Candida albicans* are known colloquially as feet.

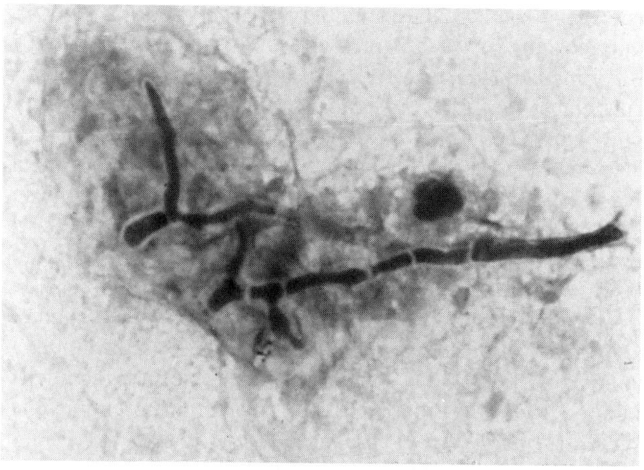

Figure 52–2. Septate branching hyphae of *Aspergillus fumigatus*. The hyphae branch at acute angles. Expectorated sputum. (Gram's stain.)

already been mentioned. Other yeast develop filamentous extensions from the surface of the colony, suggesting the wild growth of hair from the head of a mad scientist. *Trichosporon* species are yeast that develop such filamentous extensions, whereas *E. jeanselmei* is a dematiaceous yeast that develops a mycelium as it matures. The ultimate in fence-sitting is exemplified by the dimorphic fungi, which exhibit a mould form under some conditions and a non-mould form in other circumstances. The most important dimorphic fungi are systemic pathogens that behave as moulds in the environment and on agar media at 25°C to 30°C. In contrast, the tissue form is either a yeast or, in the case of *Coccidioides immitis*, a spherule. When cultivated at 37°C, the tissue form is reproduced. Although these classic pathogens usually are what is meant by dimorphic fungi, other less common or publicized agents also exhibit dimorphism. For instance, *Penicillium marneffei*, a distinctive member of that widely dispersed genus, grows as a mould on laboratory media at 25°C to 30°C, but a yeastlike form is found in human tissues. The sclerotic bodies found in tissues of patients with chromoblastomycosis are a vegetative form arrested between a mould-yeast form of the dematiaceous fungi, which appear as moulds when grown on solid media at room temperature. *Cokeromyces recurvatus* is a rare human pathogen that has a yeast morphology in human infections and *in vitro* at 37°C but grows as a mould at 25°C to 30°C (McGough, 1990). A reverse dimorphism is exemplified by *Malassezia furfur*, which produces both yeast cells and hyphae in the cutaneous lesions of pityriasis versicolor. In the laboratory, the hyphal form is only rarely seen unless special culture conditions are provided (Marcon, 1992).

Structure of Yeast and Hyphae

The morphology (or absence) of filamentous forms is an important characteristic for identification of both yeast and moulds. The filamentous structure of moulds is referred to as a hypha (plural, *hyphae*). A mass of hyphae is known as a mycelium. The mycelium growing on the surface of agar or in the agar is known as the vegetative mycelium, whereas filamentous extensions above the colony are called aerial mycelium. True hyphae may have cross-walls that contain pores for communication through the hyphae or cross-walls that are complete, dividing the hyphae into multiple cells. Hyphae that have cross-walls are septate (Fig. 52–2), whereas those without cross-walls are aseptate (Fig. 52–3). Once again, the situation is a shade of gray, rather than black and white. Some fungi that have septate hyphae also have either aseptate or septate specialized hyphae (conidiophores) that bear asexual reproductive structures. Conversely, some so-called nonseptate fungi have occasional cross-walls and should perhaps be better designated as sparsely septate. It is important, therefore, to evaluate the mycelium as a whole.

The width of the hyphae and the angle of branching are important clues to the identity of the isolate. Among two of the classic invasive mould pathogens, the zygomycetes, such as *Rhizopus* spp., have broad, ribbon-like hyphae and branch predominantly at right angles (see Fig. 52–3), whereas *Aspergillus* spp. and most other hyaline moulds have more narrow hyphae and branch at acute angles (dichotomously)

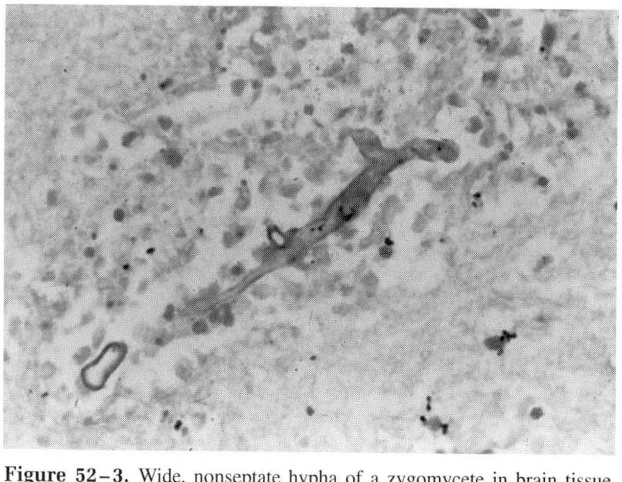

Figure 52–3. Wide, nonseptate hypha of a zygomycete in brain tissue. There is a right angle branch in the hypha. (Hematoxylin-eosin stain.)

(see Fig. 52–2). Additionally, the increasing use of severely immunosuppressive therapies and the occurrence of drastically immunosuppressive diseases, such as human immunodeficiency virus (HIV) infection, has increased the frequency with which common environmental saprophytic fungi produce invasive disease (Rinaldi, 1991). The designation of a fungus as *Aspergillus* on the basis of hyphal morphology in a smear or tissue section is, in truth, only a statement of the *a priori* odds for this group of pathogens. It is better simply to describe the characteristics of the hyphae.

When yeast reproduce asexually by budding, the daughter cell usually appears at one end of a yeast cell and eventually enlarges to form a new yeast cell. If a series of daughter cells do not detach fully from the originating cells, a pseudohypha (plural, *pseudohyphae*) is produced. Pseudohyphae are distinguished from true hyphae by the presence of a constriction at the junction of adjacent cells, the uniform location of the septum at a branch point in the mycelium, and the restriction in size of the daughter cell to that of the parent or less (Fig. 52–4). In contrast, the walls of true hyphae are parallel without constrictions (see Fig. 52–2). *C. albicans* and some strains of *Candida tropicalis* may produce either true hyphae or pseudohyphae, depending on growth conditions, and differentiation of *Candida* from *Aspergillus* in tissue sections on occasion may be problematic. In contradistinction, *Cryptococcus* spp. produce only budding yeast and rarely rudimentary or primitive pseudohyphae, but true hyphae are not formed.

Hyphal Pigment

The hyphae of dematiaceous fungi contain a melanin pigment that imparts a brown coloration to the hyphae in microscopic preparations and causes colonies of the fungi to appear dark green, brown, or black (Plate 52–2). Superimposed dyes in stained smears, wet preps, or histologic sections may partially obscure the color, which can be demonstrated definitively in unstained preparations. The macroscopic appearance of dematiaceous fungi ranges from dark green through gray to black. Those fungi that lack dark hyphal pigmentation are commonly referred to as hyaline (clear or colorless). Some authorities prefer not to use this term, because light pigmentation may produce colored colonies. In addition, asexual reproductive structures of some hyaline moulds may have green, brown, or black pigments that impart a color to the surface of the colony once the reproductive structures have formed. The true appearance of these moulds usually can be discerned by observing the back of the colony, which maintains a light coloration. In contrast, both the front (obverse) and back (reverse) of dematiaceous colonies usually demonstrate the dark pigment. Although *C. neoformans* is not considered a dematiaceous fungus, the production of melanin by this pathogenic yeast provides a diagnostic clue to its identification. The yeast cells of *C. neoformans* are nonpigmented, but melanin can be demonstrated in the yeast and in the pigmented hyphae of dematiaceous fungi by the Fontana-Masson staining method for melanin pigment (Ro, 1987). Occasionally, the brown pigment may not be well demonstrated in a fungus that is considered to be dematiaceous, so other diagnostic features must be considered.

Asexual Reproductive Structures

The primary means for identification of moulds is by characterization of asexual reproductive structures. For yeast, these structures serve as ancillary clues in the identification process. The two principal asexual structures are spores and conidia. Spores may be either sexual or asexual in nature, whereas conidia are always asexual. Asexual spores are, strictly speaking, always produced by cleavage within an encompassing structure called a sporangium and the spores are referred to as sporangiospores (Fig. 52–5). Conidia (singular, *conidium*), which are much more diverse, form by differentiation from the tip or side of a fertile hypha, such as a conidiophore, or by differentiation of the hypha itself. Unfortunately the precision of use of the terms conidium and spore in the literature is poor, and the consistency is worse. Sporulation and spores often are used as general terms for asexual reproduction, and the term spore is sometimes used when conidium would have been more accurate. Kwon-Chung and Bennett (1992) have pointed out that the manner in which sporulation occurs may be as important as the morphology of the conidia, noting as an example the differentiation between

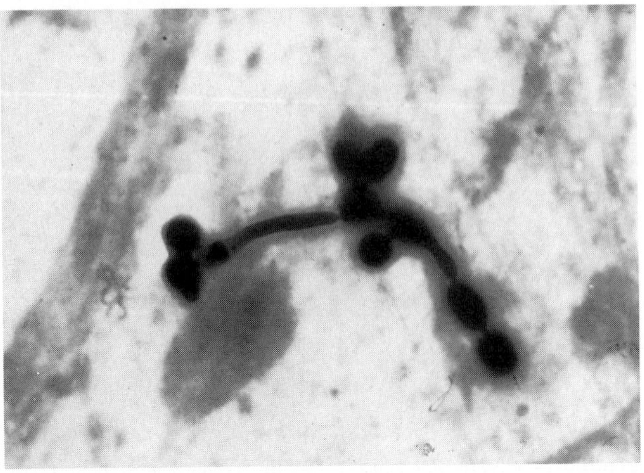

Figure 52–4. Chains of elongated budding yeasts of *Candida albicans* producing pseudohyphae. The junction of the individual yeast cells are still evident in this preparation. (Gram's stain.)

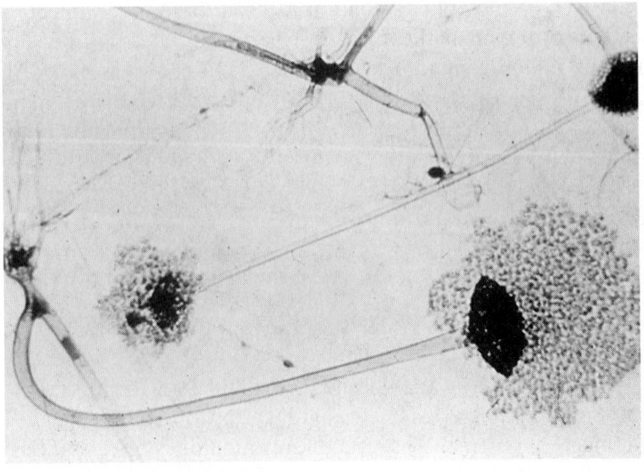

Figure 52–5. Sporangiophores of *Rhizopus* spp. support sporangia, which contain sporangiospores. Rhizoids arise from the hyphae near the origin of the sporangiophores. (Lactophenol cotton blue.) (Photography courtesy of Centers for Disease Control and Prevention.)

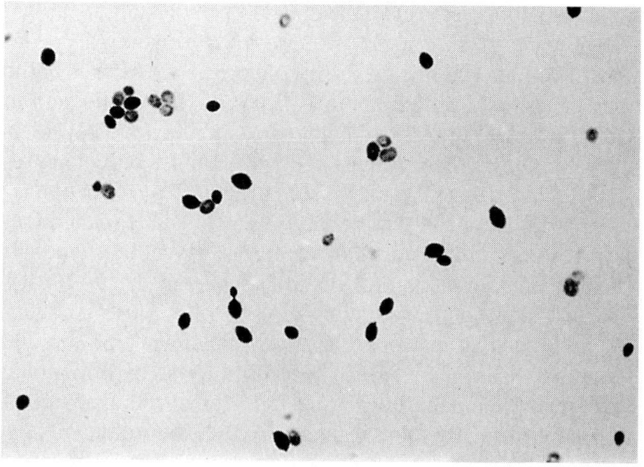

Figure 52–6. Budding yeast cells of *Candida albicans*. (Gram's stain.)

two dematiaceous fungi such as *Helminthosporium* spp., which are not human pathogens, and *Bipolaris* spp., which are occasional pathogens of humans.

The principal mechanism by which yeast reproduce asexually is by budding. A bud starts as a softening of the cell wall of the mother cell, followed by expansion of the cell wall (blown out) and migration of nucleus and cytoplasm to the swollen area. A septum seals the boundary between the daughter and parent cell (Fig. 52–6). If separation does not occur, a pseudohypha results, as discussed earlier. This classic budding process results in a blastoconidium according to Rippon or a blastospore according to Kwon-Chung and Bennett. Less commonly, transverse division occurs, as in *P. marneffei*.

The portions of the vegetative mycelium that differentiate into conidia are referred to as conidiogenous cells. Specialized hyphae that support the conidia are termed conidiophores, which may be either the conidiogenous cell itself arising from the vegetative mycelium or may be a supporting hypha. In the case of *Aspergillus* spp., the conidiophore, which is aseptate, enlarges at the tip to form a swollen vesicle (Fig. 52–7). From that vesicle, the conidiogenous cells, termed phialides (formerly sterigmata), arise to support chains of conidia. Some species of *Aspergillus* produce a row of phialides, which occur on a row of sterile cells called metulae, with the conidia arising from the distal phialides. The zygomycetes produce supporting structures called sporangiophores, at the tips of which the sporangium and its enclosed sporangiospores develop (see Fig. 52–5). An extension of the apex of the sporangiophore into the sporangium is termed the columella.

Thallic conidiogenesis is a process in which the conidium does not develop until a septum is formed between the conidium and the parent cell. The conidium originates from the whole of the parent cell. The most important human pathogens that exhibit thallic conidiogenesis are the dermatophytes and the dimorphic fungus *C. immitis*. As conidiogenesis progresses, the arthroconidia produced by *Coccidioides* fragment easily, releasing large numbers of barrel-shaped conidia that are disseminated easily by desert breezes and result in the high degree of infectivity demonstrated by this important human pathogen (Fig. 52–8). The thallic conidia of the dermatophytes are separated by size into two types, large macroconidia that have septations (Fig. 52–9) and small, one-celled microconidia that are simpler structures (Fig. 52–10).

The other type of conidiogenesis is blastic, in which the protoplasm of the conidiogenous cell is blown out or blasted into the conidium. The simplest form of blastic conidiogenesis is the budding process by which many yeast, including *Candida* spp., develop. As with thallic conidia, blastoconidia are divided into two types, depending on whether the entire cell wall is involved in the process. A further division may be made among those species in which the outer cell wall does not participate during conidiogenesis (enteroblastic). Phialides are conidiogenous cells that often have a collarette at the apices, produced when the tip releases the first conidium. The collarette may be a conspicuous flask-shaped structure, as in *Phialophora* spp., or an inconspicuous structure, as in *Aspergillus* spp. In contrast, annellides are conidiogenous cells that rupture to leave a distinct ring of cellular material at the base of the conidium when it separates from the annellide. Formation of sequential conidia at the base pushes the oldest cell to the tip of the chain and leaves a series of rings or annellations

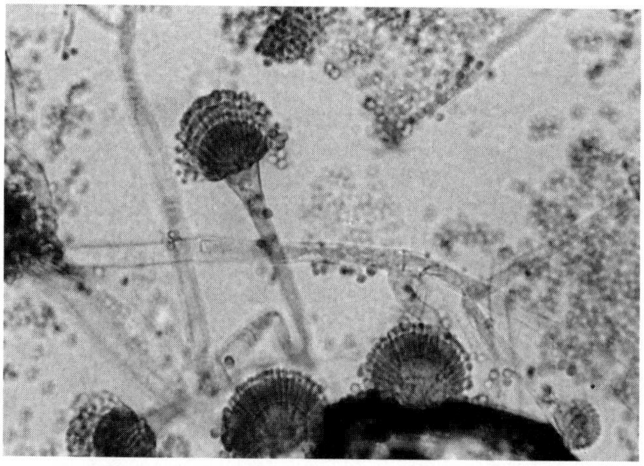

Figure 52–7. Fruiting heads of *Aspergillus fumigatus*. The conidiophores are swollen at the tip to form a vesicle. The phialides arise from the upper half of the vesicle, and the chains of conidia are aligned parallel to the long axis of the conidiophore. (Lactophenol aniline blue.)

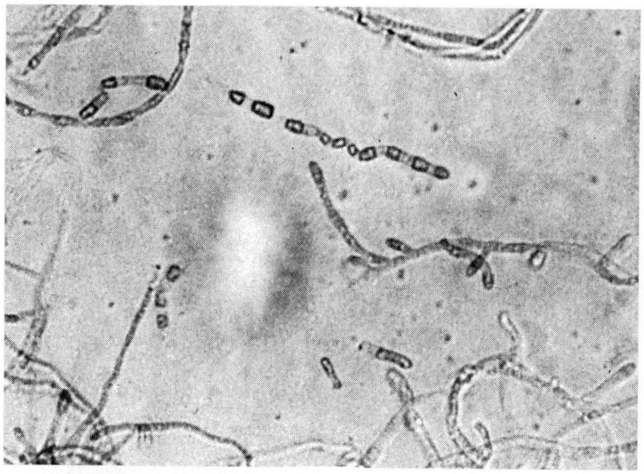

Figure 52–8. Portions of the mycelium of *Coccidioides immitis* have differentiated into arthroconidia. Alternating barrel-shaped arthroconidia are separated by thin-walled, empty disjunctor cells. (Lactophenol aniline blue.)

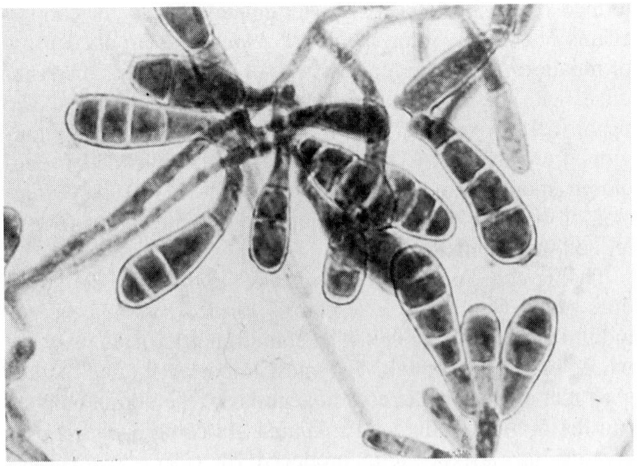

Figure 52–9. Multiple short, club-shaped macroconidia of *Epidermophyton floccosum*. Some of the conidiophores are branched, and microconidia are absent. Lactophenol cotton blue. (Photograph courtesy of Centers for Disease Control and Prevention.)

at the apex of the annellide, providing a record of past events, like rings on a tree. Some of these fine details may be difficult to visualize with the light microscope.

The differentiation of various conidial structures is the key to correct identification of many isolates. In some cases, the pertinent morphologic features are easily discerned. As in surgical pathology, pattern recognition is an important tool for identification of the most common pathogens and saprobes. It is important to appreciate the salient features of the entire morphologic preparation without primarily focusing on outliers or aberrant structures, just as it is important for the surgical pathologist to appreciate the tissue pattern without being distracted by irrelevant cellular details. Developing conidial structures of *Aspergillus* or *Paecilomyces*, for instance, may resemble the structures of *Penicillium,* and the observer must not be misled into thinking that two moulds are present. At the same time, the possibility of a mixed culture must be remembered. A high-powered mycologist must use a low-powered objective for initial observation. In all morphologic disciplines, however, the detail of cellular subsets in that low-powered picture must be appreciated for study at higher magnification. The fine art of mycologic diagnosis rests in the appreciation and differentiation of the cellular details, and in some instances, the task requires great subtlety and considerable experience. Sometimes, the isolate must be coaxed to produce the necessary diagnostic structures by selection of the appropriate media (Table 52–3). In general, enriched media favor the propagation of vegetative mycelium, whereas asexual reproductive structures are encouraged by basal media. Subculture onto water agar or potato flake agar is a general technique for encouraging the development of conidial structures. V-8 juice agar has been used for study of conidial structures in dematiaceous fungi and for encouragement of ascospore formation in *Saccharomyces*. The colors of *Aspergillus* colonies are best studied on Czapek-Dox agar, whereas *Trichophyton rubrum* is encouraged to produce red pigment on potato flake agar or cornmeal agar with 1% glucose. Perhaps the ultimate in a specialty medium is the bird manure filtrate agar developed by Staib and Blisse (1982) for study of *C. neoformans*.

Experience also is important in determining whether a subculture has been incubated sufficiently long for the diagnostic structures to form. Rootlike structures (rhizoids) that develop from the hyphae of some zygomycetes are important differentiating features, but they may not be detected if observation is terminated prematurely. It must be admitted that some of the techniques necessary for complete differentiation are difficult or even beyond the reach of most clinical laboratories. For instance, the dematiaceous pathogen *Wangiella dermatitidis* produces blastic conidia with phialides and annellides. The presence of annellides was not recognized when the mould was studied with the light microscope, however, and this organism was once classified as *Phialophora dermatitidis*. Recognition that annellides were formed by the isolate led to its assignment to a new genus, *Wangiella dermatitidis*, which contained both phialides and annellides. Despite all efforts, some isolates refuse to produce diagnostic asexual reproductive structures. The colonies remain fluffy and consist only of vegetative and aerial hyphae morphologically. These hyphae are described as sterile hyphae or mycelia sterilia.

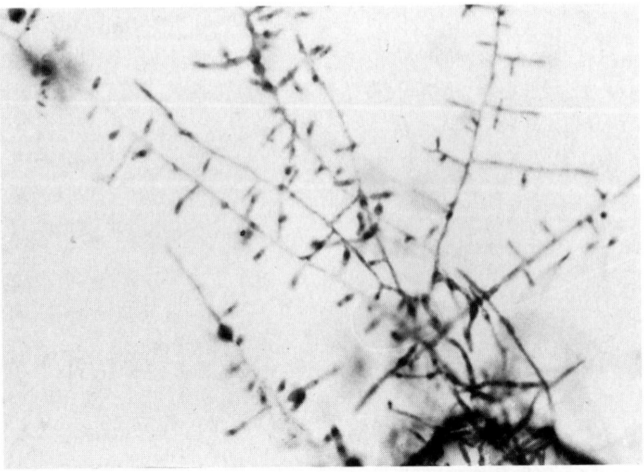

Figure 52–10. Elongated microconidia of *Trichophyton tonsurans* are lined up along the surface of the hypha. (Lactophenol aniline blue.)

Table 52–3. SUPPLEMENTAL MEDIA FOR IDENTIFICATION OF FUNGI

Medium	Function
Cornmeal agar with Tween 80	Visualize yeast morphology
Ascospore medium, V-8 agar	Ascospore development
Potato dextrose agar with 1% glucose	Pigment development of *Trichophyton rubrum*
Potato flake agar	Pigment development of *Trichophyton rubrum*; mould morphology
Czapek-Dox agar	Identification of *Aspergillus* species
Trichophyton agars	Differentiation of *Trichophyton* species
Bird (niger) seed agar	Demonstration of melanin in *Cryptococcus neoformans*
Brain-heart infusion with blood	May enhance recovery of dimorphic fungi
Christensen urea agar	Differentiation of *Trichophyton rubrum* and *T. mentagrophytes*
Slide culture (various agars)	Study of microscopic structure and its origin

Sexual Reproductive Structures

Sexual reproductive structures occasionally are of value in the general mycology laboratory for identification of common pathogens and saprophytes. A variety of sexual structures may be produced, most of which are infrequently encountered. The two structures most likely to be demonstrated are the naked asci of *Saccharomyces cerevisiae* and the cleistothecium of *Pseudallescheria boydii* (the sexual phase of *Scedosporium apiospermum*), *Aspergillus nidulans*, or the *Aspergillus glaucus* group. The naked asci of *Saccharomyces* resemble oval yeast cells in which one to four individual haploid ascospores are enclosed (Plate 52–3). Ascospore formation in *Saccharomyces* spp. can be encouraged by incubation on certain agar media, such as V-8 juice agar, but this effort usually is not necessary, because commercial yeast identification systems can identify the isolate biochemically. The ascospores may be visualized in wet preparations but are detected more reliably with an acid-fast stain.

A cleistothecium is a sexual fruiting body (ascocarp) in which the ascospores are entirely enclosed and can only be released by rupture of the cleistothecial wall (Fig. 52–11). The wall is composed of single or multiple layers of specialized hyphae. A perithecium is similar to a cleistothecium but contains an opening at the apex of the pear-shaped structure.

Rate of Growth

The rate of growth of fungal isolates provides a useful clue to diagnostic possibilities. In general, the pathogenic dimorphic and dematiaceous fungi grow slowly, requiring a week or more for colonies to appear. The significance of colonies of rapidly growing moulds that appear after prolonged incubation on mycologic media should be questioned. However, there are exceptions to this generalization. *C. immitis*, a classic pathogen, grows relatively quickly and may even be recovered on blood agar plates in the bacteriology laboratory if the inoculum is large. *Aspergillus* spp., *Scedosporium apiospermum*, the zygomycetes, and many yeast are rapid growers. Among the dermatophytes, the growth rate is an important characteristic and may be helpful in identifying an isolate.

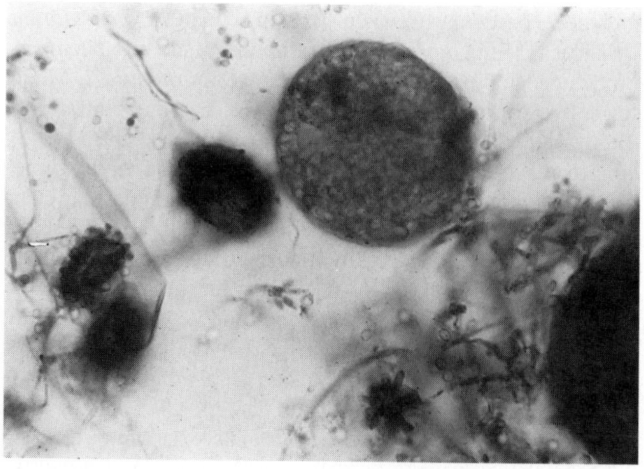

Figure 52–11. Spores can be seen within a cleistothecium of *Aspergillus glaucus* group. (Lactophenol aniline blue.)

Inhibition by Cycloheximide

Lack of inhibition by cycloheximide also is a useful clue to the presence of a pathogen, particularly among the dimorphic fungi and dermatophytes. Mycosel and Mycobiotic agars, commonly used isolation media, contain 0.04 to 0.05% cycloheximide. A mould that grows slowly on cycloheximide-containing media should alert the mycologist to the possibility that a dimorphic fungus may be present or, in the appropriate clinical situation, that a dermatophyte has been isolated. Once again, there are important exceptions to the rule. Zygomycetes and *C. neoformans* are completely inhibited by cycloheximide. *Aspergillus* species and some species of *Candida* are completely or partially inhibited.

Optimal Growth Temperature

Growth at elevated temperature is occasionally a useful differential tool in the identification of fungi (Kwon-Chung, 1992). Most yeast and moulds grow best at 25°C to 30°C. The most important pathogen in the genus *Cryptococcus* is *C. neoformans*, which is, probably not coincidentally, the only member of the genus to grow well at 37°C. Because it grows rapidly, isolates of this pathogen may often be recovered first on enriched blood agar plates incubated at 35° to 37°C in the bacteriology laboratory. *Trichophyton verrucosum*, a cause of ringworm in cattle and humans, produces distinctive chains of chlamydospores when incubated at 37°C. Growth of *Cladosporium trichoides* (*bantianum*) at 42°C to 43°C is a reliable way to differentiate this species from other members of the genus. Similarly, most isolates of *Wangiella dermatitidis* grow at 40°C, whereas most isolates of the morphologically similar *E. jeanselmei* do not grow at temperatures above 37°C. The determination of the range of temperatures at which growth occurs is a useful feature for differentiation among some members of the zygomycetes (Kwon-Chung, 1992).

Biochemical Tests

Biochemical tests are at the heart of identification schemes for yeast and occasionally are useful for the identification of moulds. Biochemical characterization may be accomplished by study of fermentation or assimilation patterns, of which the assimilation pattern is used exclusively in most laboratories. Fermentation of carbohydrates is the anaerobic utilization of carbohydrates with the production of gas. This technique is suitable for the identification of *Candida* species, but not *Cryptococcus* species. Assimilation, a more generally applicable method, tests the ability of an isolate to use a carbohydrate as the sole source of carbon needed for growth or of nitrate as the sole source of nitrogen. The Wickerham auxanographic method uses a basal medium in which a particular carbohydrate or nitrate serves as the nutrient. Growth of the yeast is the end point of a positive test. This rather cumbersome reference method is not detailed because it has been replaced in most laboratories by one of four commercial identifications systems: API 20C (Biomerieux, Hazelwood, MO), Vitek Systems (Biomerieux, Hazelwood, MO), MicroScan (Baxter Health Systems, Sacramento, CA), and the Uni-Yeast-Tek system (Remel Laboratories, Lanexa, KS). All four systems perform well, as judged by reports in the literature and by proficiency testing surveys of the College of American Pathologists (Buesching, 1979; Fenn, 1994; Riddle, 1994; El-Zaatari, 1990). API-20C has been found comparable to conventional biochemical systems (Buesching, 1979) and is now considered the reference standard among commercial systems. An evaluation of an updated database for the Vitek system documented virtually identical performance to API 20C (El-Zaatari, 1990). The Vitek system has perhaps a slight edge, as judged by proficiency testing surveys, and will be particularly attractive to laboratories that use this methodology in their bacteriology section. It is important to study the microscopic morphology of the yeast, regardless of the system selected.

In addition to fermentation and assimilation studies, stimulation of growth by biochemical compounds is a secondary test in the differentiation of certain *Trichophyton* spp. Inclusion of inositol and thiamine in various combinations into agar media (*Trichophyton* agars) allows assessment of growth-stimulating properties. The end point of the test, relative growth in comparison to a basal medium, is subjective, and both positive and negative controls should be included.

Two biochemical tests are useful for the identification of *C. neoformans*. Phenol oxidase in *C. neoformans* oxidizes diphenolic compounds to produce a brown pigment. The original substrate used to demonstrate this characteristic was caffeic acid in niger seed cells (Staib test), but other compounds, such as L-dopa and L-dopamine, have been used more recently. If one of these chemicals is incorporated into agarmedia, colonies of *C. neoformans* will develop a brown to black coloration within five days of incubation at 30°C. Other species of *Cryptococcus* may produce a light brown pigment, especially after more prolonged incubation. The phenol oxidase test is not sufficient, of itself, for identification of *C. neoformans*, and the advent of efficient commercial identification systems has diminished its use in clinical laboratories.

In contrast, the test for urease production in cryptococci is of general utility in the clinical laboratory to differentiate cryptococci from *Candida* spp., particularly in respiratory specimens. *C. neoformans* is a pulmonary and systemic pathogen, whereas *Candida* spp. are frequent inhabitants of the upper airways but uncommon causes of primary pneumonia. Urease is produced by other nonpathogenic species of *Cryptococcus*, by *Rhodotorula* species, and by some isolates of *Trichosporon beigelii* and *Candida krusei*. Urease production can be tested by inoculation of the yeast isolate onto a slant of Christensen urea agar or into urea broth. Alkalinization of the medium after production of NH_3 by urea-splitting organisms is detected by inclusion of a pH indicator in the system. Zimmer and Roberts described a rapid method that provides reliable and useful results in 15 minutes for expeditious elimination of noncryptococcal yeast from further consideration (Zimmer, 1979) (Table 52–4). Care must be exercised not to include urea-splitting bacteria, such as *Klebsiella* species, which are found occasionally in respiratory specimens, in the inoculum. Colonies that have macroscopically visible pseudohyphae (feet) need not be tested, because *Cryptococcus* does not produce pseudohyphae *in vitro*.

Table 52–4. RAPID UREASE TEST FOR SCREENING YEAST ISOLATES FROM RESPIRATORY SPECIMENS

1. Place a sterile swab in urease broth. Press the swab against the side of the urease broth container before removing to eliminate excess broth. Swab should be saturated, not dripping.
2. Lightly touch several WELL ISOLATED colonies to be tested with the saturated swab.
3. Place inoculated swab into a labeled sterile tube.
4. Place tube with swab into a 56°C water bath for 15 minutes.
5. Remove from water bath and examine for a deep pink pigment, which indicates a positive test. Positive (*Cryptococcus* species) and negative (*Candida albicans*) controls should be set up concurrently.

Biochemical tests also play an ancillary role in the identification of dermatophytic moulds. Production of urease within three days helps differentiate *Trichophyton mentagrophytes* (urease positive) from *T. rubrum* (urease negative). The isolate should be subcultured to a slant of Christensen urea agar and incubated at 25°C to 30°C for at least three days. A positive reaction is *strong* production of urease, evidenced by alkalinization of the medium.

If biochemical tests are the heart of yeast identification systems, confirmation of the identification by examination of yeast morphology on agar media is the soul. Using morphologic observation as a check can save embarrassing mistakes that would be made if automated or packaged systems were trusted implicitly.

Dimorphism

Demonstration of dimorphism is the traditional approach to definitive identification of an important group of systemic pathogens. In most laboratories, the initial isolate is the mould phase because the plates usually are incubated at 25°C to 30°C. Conversion to the tissue phase is accomplished by incubating a subculture at 37°C. The transition from mould to yeast morphology may occur grudgingly, and hyphal forms are often intermixed with the yeast cells. Some isolates may never be successfully converted. A rich medium, such as brain-heart infusion agar with a blood supplement, should be included, particularly when working with *H. capsulatum*. Brain-heart infusion agar or cottonseed agar has been recommended for optimal conversion of *B. dermatitidis*. Media for conversion of *C. immitis* have been described but are not often used. Similarly, inoculation of animals is infrequently employed in clinical laboratories. Introduction of immunologic tests for fungal exoantigens in culture or molecular characterization of nucleic acids has considerably simplified the task of definitive identification and eliminated the need to demonstrate both phases of the dimorphic fungi. Exoantigen tests for *C. immitis*, *H. capsulatum*, and *B. dermatitidis* are commercially available. Nucleic acid hybridization tests for these three dimorphic pathogens and *C. neoformans* are marketed by GENPROBE, Inc. (San Diego, CA). These tests have replaced phase conversion in many laboratories. The GENPROBE system is used for the detection of *Chlamydia trachomatis* and *Neisseria gonorrhoeae* or for identification of certain bacterial pathogens including mycobacteria. In laboratories that employ the GENPROBE technology, the molecular approach may provide an attractive alternative to immunodiffusion for identification of isolates. If the yeast phase of the pathogen has been previously or concurrently demonstrated in direct smears or in the surgical pathology laboratory, conversion of the corresponding mould phase in the mycology laboratory is superfluous.

Immunologic Tests

Immunologic tests are available both for detection of antigen and antibodies to selected fungal pathogens. The classic serologic tests have been complement fixation tests against the major dimorphic pathogens, *H. capsulatum*, *B. dermatitidis*, and *C. immitis*. Subsequently, immunodiffusion tests against several antigens of *H. capsulatum* were developed. The serologic approach works best for diagnosis and prognosis of coccidioidomycosis but is adjunctive in all cases. Extensive cross-reactions between *H. capsulatum* and *B. dermatitidis* compromise the effectiveness of these tests.

Detection of antibodies to *Aspergillus* spp. in serum assists in the diagnosis of allergic bronchopulmonary aspergillosis but is of little utility in the diagnosis of invasive disease (Kurup, 1991). Most commonly precipitating antibodies have been detected with the immunodiffusion technique, but newer methods, such as enzyme-linked immunosorbent assay (ELISA), are also employed. Some authorities have questioned the reliability of commercially available reagents (Kwon-Chung, 1992).

Immunologic detection of fungal antigens is of more recent development. By far, the most important application has been the detection of cryptococcal antigen in cerebrospinal fluid and in serum. This test must be considered a primary diagnostic tool in conjunction with culture and has replaced the less sensitive India ink test for direct examination of spinal fluid. Immunoassays for *Aspergillus* antigens have been described but have not been commercially developed (Kurup, 1991). A radioimmunoassay for *H. capsulatum* antigens in urine is available through a single reference laboratory (Histoplasma Reference Laboratory, Indianapolis, IN) and is worthy of consideration, particularly in patients with systemic disease (Williams, 1994). Antigen was detected in 92% of 108 patients with disseminated infection but in only 39% of 70 patients with self-limited disease.

Skin tests have been used for epidemiologic study of some infections, but they have limited utility for diagnostic purposes. In some cases such as histoplasmosis, skin tests may complicate laboratory diagnosis by eliciting an antibody response (Campbell, 1964). Unfortunately, none of the immunologic tests available for diagnosis of *Candida* infections has sufficient sensitivity and specificity to be diagnostically useful (de Repentigny, 1992).

A practical summary of medically important fungi is presented in Figure 52–12. This schema is presented as an organizational skeleton on which the beginning mycologist can build an approach to the etiologic diagnosis of fungal infections.

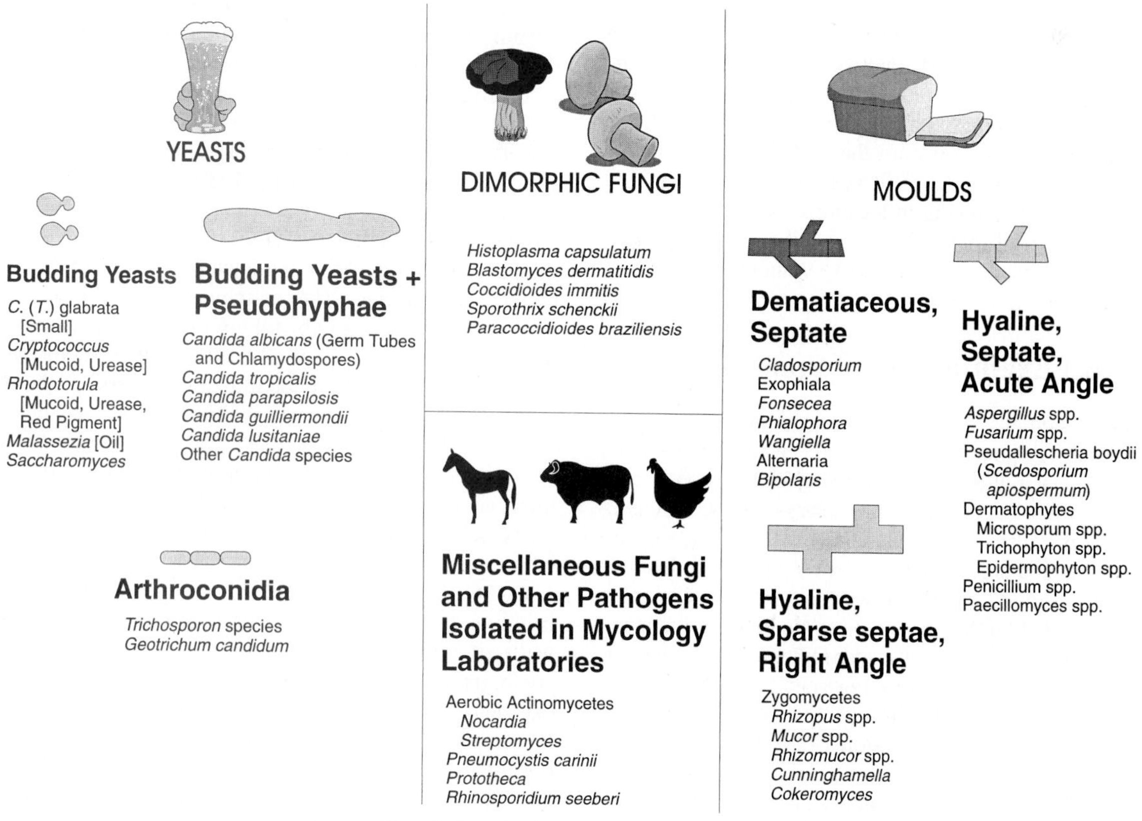

Figure 52–12. Organizational schema for important fungal pathogens of humans.

6

DIAGNOSTIC TECHNIQUES

Collection of Specimens

The correct specimen for submission to the mycology laboratory depends on the clinical presentation and the organ system affected. A summary of the major categories of disease produced by fungi along with suggested specimens is presented in Table 52–5. The recommended nomenclature of important fungal infections has been summarized by an expert panel (Odds, 1992).

Yeast, particularly *Candida* spp., may be recovered on occasion from swab specimens, especially from purulent lesions. Swabs may be used for sampling oral or vaginal lesions suggestive of candidiasis and may be adequate for collecting specimens from patients with chronic external otitis, in which large numbers of *Aspergillus* conidia are usually present. Swabs are, however, decidedly inferior tools for collecting specimens in most areas of infectious disease. For the diagnosis of fungal infections in which the tissue response is often granulomatous, they are useless or, even worse, misleading, because the clinician may interpret a negative result as indicating the absence of an infection. A firm, but politically flexible policy of rejecting swabs should be accompanied by assiduous and persistent educational efforts.

The best specimens for mycologic diagnosis are scrapings, curettings, aspirates, and biopsies of lesions. Hairs infected with some common dermatophytic fungi (e.g., *Microsporum canis*) fluoresce under a long wavelength ultraviolet light (Wood's lamp) and can be specifically selected for examination. The cutaneous lesions of dermatophytosis (ringworm) are characterized by an active advancing edge with central healing, so that scrapings should be collected from the edge of the process. Specimens should be sent to the laboratory in a clean dry container. Hair, nails, and skin scrapings should be kept dry to discourage bacterial overgrowth. Some physicians, such as dermatologists and ophthalmologists, prefer to inoculate specimens directly onto the surface of agar in the office or in the operating room. It is important to develop a method for monitoring media in locations outside the laboratory, because Petri dishes with shriveled remains of agar media will appear in the laboratory without a foolproof system.

Direct Examination of Specimens

Scrapings, curettings, and hairs can be examined directly by light microscopy. Aspirates of pus or fluid can also be examined directly; if the material is too thick for easy observation, it may be smeared on glass slides. Imprint smears or teased preparations must be made from tissue samples. It is useful to prepare additional unstained smears, because subsequent examinations may suggest infectious agents that were not suspected initially.

WET PREPARATION. The simplest method for direct examination is the observation of a suspension of the specimen in sterile saline under a coverslip. For specimens that contain distracting tissue debris and cells, such as vaginal secretions, nails, and skin scrapings, a solution of KOH may be used (Table 52–6).

GRAM'S STAIN. This commonly used microbiologic stain is particularly useful for detection of yeast. Most yeast, especially *Candida* spp., stain partially or completely gram positive, the presence of concomitant bacteria can be appreciated, and the nature of any inflammatory cells can be assessed. The hyphae of moulds appear gram positive or gram negative by this stain but stain less reliably than yeast cells.

GIEMSA OR WRIGHT STAINS. If histoplasmosis is suspected, these hematologic stains are useful for demonstrating the yeast cells within macrophages.

INDIA INK PREPARATION. The polysaccharide capsules of *C. neoformans* can be demonstrated by negative staining with India ink particles (Table 52–7). Some mycologists prefer nigrosin because the particles are more homogeneous and artifacts less frequent. When examined with the light microscope, the capsule stands out as a clear space around the fungal cell, with ink particles bouncing off the edge as brownian motion occurs (Fig. 52–13). It is important to differentiate pseudocapsules produced by imperfect focus around the edges of the leukocytes or artifacts. If budding yeast cells are demonstrated, the specificity of the diagnosis is ensured. Other potentially encapsulated fungi such as *Rhodotorula* species or other cryptococcal species are such infrequent pathogens that they can be eliminated from practical consideration. In clinical specimens, the capsules usually are large, but after isolation on agar media, the capsules may be less luxuriant and more difficult to demonstrate. Unfortunately, some strains are poorly encapsulated. The sensitivity of the India ink test is approximately 50% in patients who are not infected with HIV (Diamond, 1974), whereas the direct detection of antigen in cerebrospinal fluid or serum has a sensitivity of 90% to 100%. Detection of cryptococcal polysaccharide by latex agglutination or enzyme immunoassay techniques has supplanted observation of capsules for routine use. The India ink technique may be reserved for use in the evening and night shifts, when the antigen test is not immediately available, and for examination of capsules in cells from isolated colonies that suggest *C. neoformans*. The India ink test appears to have greater sensitivity in patients who are infected with HIV, perhaps because of the greater number of yeast cells present (Chuck, 1989; Kovacs, 1985; Zuger, 1986).

HISTOCHEMICAL STAINS. The periodic acid–Schiff method stains fungal cell walls well and is used in some mycology laboratories. The methenamine silver technique is commonly employed in histology laboratories for demonstration of fungi. When the methenamine silver method is combined with hematoxylin-eosin as a counterstain, the detailed morphology of both tissue and fungus can be studied (Swisher, 1982). Both of these techniques stain bacteria as well, especially if the staining time is prolonged in the silver impregnation method. These tools have been replaced in many laboratories by the simpler and quicker Calcofluor white stain.

CALCOFLUOR WHITE. This compound, a whitener used in the textile and paper industries, binds to the chitin in the walls of fungal cells and fluoresces white (Fig. 52–14) or apple green (depending on the filter combination used) when exposed to short wavelength ultraviolet light (Table 52–8) (Hageage, 1984). A fluorescence microscope is necessary, but this important diagnostic tool often is available for other tasks such as auramine O staining of mycobacteria and for immunofluorescence.

Table 52–5. MAJOR CLINICAL SYNDROMES AND COMMONLY ASSOCIATED PATHOGENS*

Clinical Presentation or Organ System	Patient Group	Likely Pathogens	Specimens
Skin, hair, or nails	All patients	Dermatophytes *Candida* *Malassezia* {*Trichosporon*} {*Scopulariopsis*} {*Fusarium*}	Skin scrapings Hair Nail Clippings
Skin, dermis, and subcutaneous tissue	All patients	*Coccidioides immitis* *Blastomyces dermatitidis* *Sporothrix schenckii*	Biopsy of lesion
	Patient with mycetoma	*Pseudallescheria boydii* *Nocardia* *Streptomyces* *Actinomadura*	Biopsy of lesion
Primary pneumonia	All patients	*Histoplasma capsulatum* *Blastomyces dermatitidis* *Cryptococcus neoformans*	Sputum Bronchoalveolar lavage Transbronchial biopsy Surgical lung biopsy
	Immunodeficient	*Aspergillus* Zygomycetes *Pseudallescheria boydii* *Pneumocystis carinii*	
Gastrointestinal infection	Immunodeficient	*Candida* *Aspergillus* Zygomycetes	Scrapings Curettings Biopsy
Urinary tract infection	All patients	*Candida*	Urine
Endocarditis	All patients	*Candida* (moulds and dimorphic fungi)	Blood
Meningitis	All patients	*Cryptococcus neoformans* *Candida*	Cerebrospinal fluid
Encephalitis and brain abscess	Immunodeficient patients	Zygomycetes *Aspergillus* *Nocardia asteroides* *Cladosporium [Xylohypha] bantianum (trichoides)* Other Moulds	Biopsy
Osteomyelitis	All patients	*Coccidioides immitis* *Blastomyces dermatitidis* *Cryptococcus neoformans* Moulds	Biopsy
Keratitis	All patients	*Aspergillus* *Fusarium*	Scrapings
External otitis	All patients	*Aspergillus,* esp. *fumigatus* and *niger*	Scrapings Swab
Sinusitis	All patients	*Aspergillus,* esp. *fumigatus* and *niger* *Fusarium* Dematiaceous moulds *Curvularia* *Bipolaris*	Biopsy Curettings
Burn wounds		*Aspergillus* Zygomycetes *Fusarium* *Pseudallescheria/Scedosporium*	Biopsy
Vaginitis		*Candida*	Swab aspirated secretions
Intravenous catheter infection		*Candida* *Malassezia* (newborns)	Catheter tip Blood
Disseminated infection	All patients	*Histoplasma capsulatum* *Blastomyces dermatitidis* *Coccidioides immitis*	Blood (Isolator) Tissue biopsy
	Immunodeficient patients	*Candida* Zygomycetes *Aspergillus* *Fusarium* *Pseudallescheria/Scedosporium* *Cryptococcus neoformans* Potentially any fungus	Blood (Isolator) Tissue biopsy

*Other combinations and possibilities may occur.
{ } = less common.

6

Table 52–6. KOH PREPARATION

1. Place a drop of KOH (potassium hydroxide with or without Calcofluor white) on a clean glass slide.
2. Immerse the specimen in the drop of KOH already on the slide.
3. Coverslip, and heat the specimen/KOH mixture by passing the slide through a Bunsen burner flame several times. Do not allow the mixture to boil.
4. Examine the preparation under 10× and 40×. Excessively tenacious specimens may require additional heating.
5. KOH may also be used as a simple mounting medium without heating.

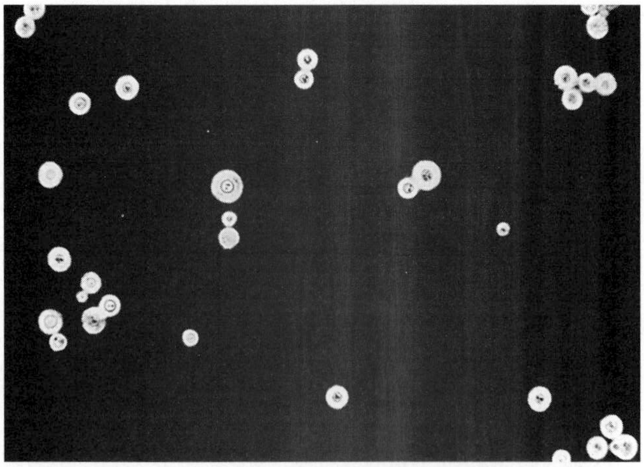

Figure 52–13. The polysaccharide capsule around the budding yeast cells of *Cryptococcus neoformans* is negatively stained by ink particles. Note the roundness and uniformity of the yeast cells. (India ink preparation.)

Recovery of fungi from blood can be accomplished by inoculating broth media, by using a biphasic broth-agar system, or by the lysis-centrifugation technique (Isolator, Wampole, Cranbury NJ). The Isolator system consists of a tube containing a solution that lyses erythrocytes and leukocytes. After the blood is drawn into the tube by vacuum, the lysed contents, including any microbes, are centrifuged into a pellet, which is removed and plated onto the surface of agar plates. A high percentage of fungemias caused by yeast can be detected with one of the broth culture systems, such as Bactec (Becton-Dickinson, Sparks, MD) or BacT-Alert (Organon-Teknika, Durham, NC). Yeast are aerobic organisms, so aerobic culture bottles must be employed. It has been suggested that blood culture systems should regularly include two aerobic bottles because of the importance of *Pseudomonas aeruginosa* and *Candida* spp., both aerobic microbes, and that an anaerobic blood culture bottle be inoculated only in selected conditions, such as abdominal disease, in which the likelihood of anaerobic bacterial pathogens is greater (Morris, 1993) (See Chapter 54 for a more detailed discussion.) The most sensitive method for detection of fungi is the Isolator system (Fleming, 1984; Jones, 1990), which is also somewhat more susceptible to contamination, either through handling of the system during processing or by airborne spores that settle onto the agar plates. A recent report documents equivalent performance of a new high-volume fungal blood culture medium for the BACTEC instrument and the 10-mL Isolator system (Wilson, 1993).

Isolation of Fungi in Culture

SELECTION OF MEDIA. All specimens should be inoculated onto a general purpose medium with and without cycloheximide. The traditional medium is Sabouraud dextrose agar, which has a pH of 5.5 to 5.6 and was designed for the isolation of dermatophytic fungi. Emmons' modification of Sabouraud dextrose agar, which contains less glucose and a pH of 6.8 to 7.0, provides a more generally useful agar. Inhibitory mould agar or potato dextrose agar is preferred by some authorities. Rinaldi (1982) has described a simplified modification of potato dextrose agar that uses a preparation of potato flakes that is available in grocery stores. It is much easier to prepare than the traditional potato-based medium and functions equivalently. These media provide a reasonable balance of inhibition of contaminating bacteria on the one hand and encouragement of typical colonial morphology and color on the other. Potato flake agar is advantageous for mould fungi, because the diagnostically useful asexual reproductive structures develop more readily on this agar than on Sabouraud dextrose medium. It is important to inoculate a selective and nonselective plate in tandem. For tissue specimens, especially when dimorphic fungi might be the etiologic agent, an enriched agar, such as brain-heart infusion agar with blood, supplemented with antibiotics, such as gentamicin or chloramphenicol or both, should be added.

The agar media may be poured or purchased either in wide-mouthed, screw-capped tubes or in Petri dishes. The tubes provide a margin of safety for prevention of infection of personnel and contamination of other cultures, but isolates are much more difficult to manipulate, and it is virtually im-

Table 52–7. INDIA INK PREPARATION

1. Centrifuge the fluid specimen for a minimum of 10 minutes.
2. Place one drop of India ink on a clean glass slide.
3. Mix with a drop of *sediment* obtained from the spun fluid.
4. Search for encapsulated yeast using the 40× objective.
5. Colonies growing on agar may also be mixed directly with India ink on a slide to confirm the presence of capsules.

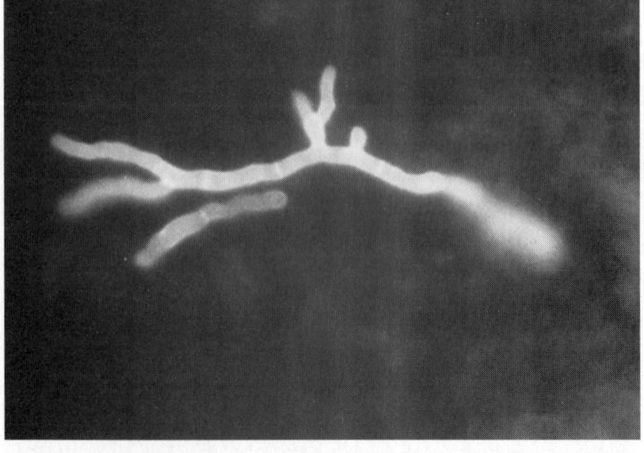

Figure 52–14. Calcofluor white elicits a white fluorescence in the chitinous walls of fungi when viewed with a fluorescence microscope. The septate, branching hyphae of *Aspergillus fumigatus* are well demonstrated.

Table 52–8. CALCOFLUOR WHITE STAIN

1. Place specimen on a clean glass slide.
2. Mix with Calcofluor white reagent.
3. Using a fluorescent microscope, examine the preparation for fungi.
4. Calcofluor white may be substituted for lacto-phenol-aniline (cotton)-blue when studying microscopic morphology of culture isolates.

possible to generate isolated colonies in situations in which a mixture of moulds or yeast may be present in the specimen. In addition, the extremely important factor of surface area is diminished in tubes. The caps on tubes should be loosened to admit air before incubation. Petri dishes offer much greater flexibility and a more optimum surface area but must be sealed and handled with care. Agar plates should be poured to double the normal depth (7 to 8 mm is desirable) to prevent dessication during the prolonged incubation. The lids should be sealed closed with a tape that is permeable to air.

INOCULATION AND INCUBATION. In some situations, only the growing tips of the hyphae are viable and the mass of vegetative hyphae is moribund. Grinding specimens in a homogenizer, as is performed for bacterial cultures, is too disruptive and viable isolates may be lost. It is better to inoculate scrapings or curettings onto and into the agar at multiple points on the agar surface. Tissue should be teased or minced, after which the fragments are similarly inoculated. We have had the experience of observing no growth on plates when a bronchoscopic brush was agitated in broth, a portion of which was then inoculated onto agar, while we noted the growth of *A. fumigatus* from the original brush that had been left in the remainder of its transport fluid. We now inoculate these specimens by placing the needle or brush directly onto the surface of primary isolation agar.

Plates or tubes should be incubated in air at 25°C to 30°C. Incubation of inoculated specimens in room air is not optimal because of the variability of ambient temperature. A controlled temperature incubator is essential. It is not necessary to incubate parallel plates or tubes at 37°C for recovery of the yeast phase of dimorphic fungi, because little additional yield results. Cultures should be incubated for at least four weeks. If a particular fungus, such as *H. capsulatum,* is suspected clinically but has not been isolated at four weeks, the incubation of the culture can be extended for another two to four weeks, although the yield from this extra work will not be great. Plates should be examined at least twice during the first week, when rapidly growing isolates may appear, and at least weekly thereafter.

Laboratory Safety

Inoculation of specimens and all manipulations of mould colonies should be performed in a laminar flow biological safety cabinet. Both the technologist and other culture plates must be protected from dissemination of highly mobile fungal conidia. A simple experiment in which an agar plate containing a single colony of *A. fumigatus* is tapped gently on the laboratory bench will convince the skeptical observer of the problem when multiple *Aspergillus* colonies subsequently appear scattered around the surface of the plate. In order to minimize dispersal of conidia, it has been suggested that subcultures of colonies that are heavily laden with conidia, such as *Aspergillus*, be performed by flooding the plate with sterile water, after which dislodged conidia are aspirated and placed on the surface of fresh agar plates (McGinnis, 1980). This maneuver may not be necessary, but great care should be taken to minimize manipulation of cultures and exposure of the plates to open air, even in a safety cabinet. Scrupulous attention to cleaning the surfaces of both the biological safety cabinet and incubator should be maintained. Separate safety cabinets for inoculation of specimens and study of isolated moulds may minimize contamination of specimens.

The greatest hazard to laboratory personnel comes from handling mould cultures of the dimorphic pathogens, particularly *C. immitis*. Kwon-Chung and Bennett (1992) recommend inoculating screw-capped tubes if this pathogen is suspected, but in most areas of the country, the diagnosis may not be appreciated before isolation of the pathogen. The plate can be flooded with 4% formaldehyde solution (10% formalin) and left at room temperature for several hours or overnight to sterilize the culture before microscopic examination is performed. Obviously, such a course is irreversible, so it is best to have colonies growing on other plates or tubes as a reserve.

It is worth noting that the tissue phase of dimorphic pathogens is not infectious by the airborne route, so there is little or no biohazard in handling tissue specimens from patients with histoplasmosis or blastomycosis. A possible exception to this rule might occur if *C. immitis* grew in its mould phase within a lung cavity that connected with the bronchial tree. Additionally, local lesions of *Histoplasma* or *Blastomyces* have appeared at the site of accidental inoculations.

Techniques for Morphologic Study of Fungal Isolates

Some of the morphologic studies necessary for the identification of fungal isolates can be accomplished with colonies from the original isolation plates, but it is often necessary to transfer portions of colonies to new or different media (subculture) in order to demonstrate diagnostic structures (see Table 52–3). Cornmeal agar supplemented with Tween 80 for examination of yeast isolates and potato flake agar for moulds are excellent choices. These media can be prepared in the laboratory or purchased from commercial sources (Remel Laboratories, Lanexa, KS; BBL, Cockneysville, MD). The frequency of subcultures is reduced if potato flake agar is used as one of the primary planting media.

Biochemical tests are important for identifying yeast isolates, but morphologic examination provides an important check on the biochemical information, especially if a commercial identification system has been used. A laboratory worker who puts an isolate into an instrument and uncritically believes the result is performing a low-level technical function. When the information received from the machine is checked against colonial and microscopic morphology as well as what is known about the clinical condition, the worker is truly functioning as a technologist.

YEAST MORPHOLOGY. The germ tube test is an important initial step in the identification of yeast isolates. Germ tubes, which are elongated, finger-like extensions from a

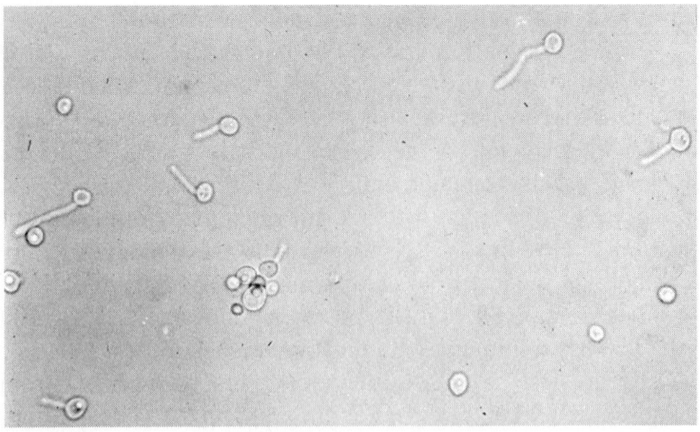

Figure 52–15. Germ tubes have extended from the yeast cells of *Candida albicans*. There is no constriction at the junction of yeast cell and germ tube. The walls of the germ tube are parallel. Human serum was incubated for two hours at 37°C.

yeast cell, are the beginnings of a true hypha (Fig. 52–15). They can be differentiated from pseudohyphae by the lack of a constriction at the junction of germ tube and yeast cell and by the parallel cell walls in the germ tube. True germ tubes are formed by *C. albicans* and *Candida stellatoidea* under the conditions recommended, allowing early identification of the most common and important yeast pathogens. *Candida tropicalis* may produce true hyphae and germ tubes under special conditions, but usually not within the abbreviated incubation period that is prescribed in the standardized germ tube test. It is essential to limit the incubation of the germ tube test to 2 to 4 hours, because other species will begin to form structures that resemble germ tubes if incubation is prolonged (Dolan, 1971). In fact, these are the beginnings of pseudohyphae and close observation will reveal the constriction between the so-called germ tube and the yeast cell. The identification can be confirmed by documentation of chlamydospores. Chlamydospores are thick-walled resting structures that serve as food storage reservoirs, rather than playing a reproductive role (Fig. 52–16). They may be either terminal, as in *C. albicans*, or within the hypha (intercalary), as in dermatophytes.

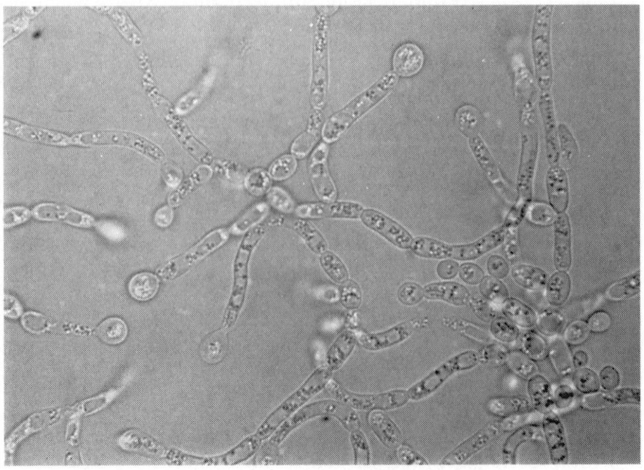

Figure 52–16. Chlamydospores produced by *Candida albicans* are thick-walled structures that occur most commonly at the ends of hyphae. The chlamydospores are considerably larger than the diameter of the hyphae. (Lactophenol cotton blue.)

Table 52–9. SERUM GERM TUBE TEST

1. Aseptically transfer several colonies of a yeast to a 12 × 75 mm test tube containing approximately 0.5 mL of serum (human, fetal calf, bovine or rabbit).
2. Incubate the tube at 37°C.
3. After two to four hours, place one drop of the mixture on a clean glass slide.
4. Examine for germ tubes using a 40× objective.

Strictly speaking, they are not spores, but the weight of tradition will probably ensure that the name endures. True germ tubes and chlamydospores are produced by *C. albicans* and *C. stellatoidea*, an infrequently isolated species that is believed by many mycologists to be a sucrose-negative variant of *C. albicans*.

The traditional germ tube test involves inoculation of a tube of serum (Table 52–9). A test for germ tube formation on the surface of cream of rice infusion agar with Tween 80 and oxgall has been described (Beheshti, 1975). After observation of the isolate for germ tubes at 37°C, incubation is continued for subsequent study of hyphal morphology and chlamydospore formation at 25°C to 30°C. Thus, all the information necessary can be collected with one procedure. Cornmeal agar may be substituted, but regardless of the medium used, incubation conditions must be carefully controlled and the test monitored with controls in order to achieve good results. The traditional Dalmau technique for demonstration of chlamydospores on cornmeal agar is detailed in Table 52–10 (McGinnis, 1980).

MOULD MORPHOLOGY. The simplest method for examination of moulds is the cellophane tape mount. It is important to use clear tape. Preparations may be sealed with nail polish to retard drying, but early examination of the slides is essential. If diagnostic structures are not observed, incubation can be continued and the process repeated. The traditional method for observing mould morphology is to tease the mycelium apart with inoculating needles and examine the teased hyphae in saline, Calcofluor white, or lactophenol with or without aniline blue. Aniline blue is preferred to cotton blue because of its lesser toxicity.

Occasionally, it is necessary to perform a slide culture in order to preserve easily disrupted conidial structures in their original relationships. The classic approach involves cutting squares of an appropriate agar media, which are suspended on glass rods in a Petri dish to which sterile water is added for maintenance of humidity. We use a commercially available agar plate that has been designed for slide culture tests (Remel Laboratories, Lanexa, KS).

If a mould isolate is suspected of being a dimorphic fungus (e.g., growth on cycloheximide-containing medium), a slide

Table 52–10. YEAST MORPHOLOGY TEST

Yeast morphology agar

1. Streak a *light* inoculum of yeast onto a section of a cornmeal/Tween 80 agar.
2. Coverslip the area inoculated.
3. Incubate at 25°C to 30°C.
4. Observe microscopic morphology at 24–72 hours.

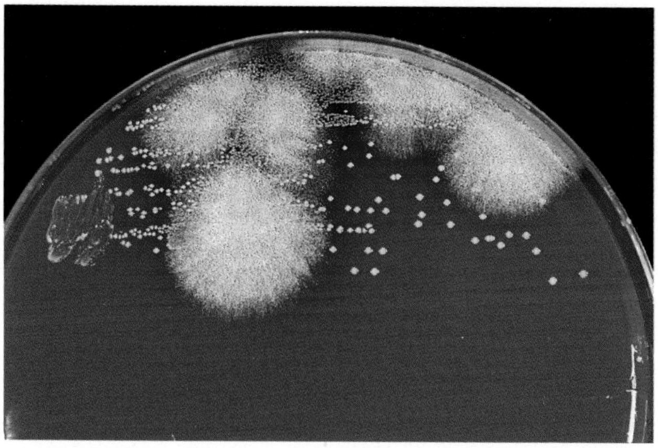

Plate 52–1. The green, powdery surface of the colonies of *Aspergillus fumigatus* overlies white masses of mycelium. Adjacent bacterial colonies contrast with the filamentous fungus. (Sheep blood agar.)

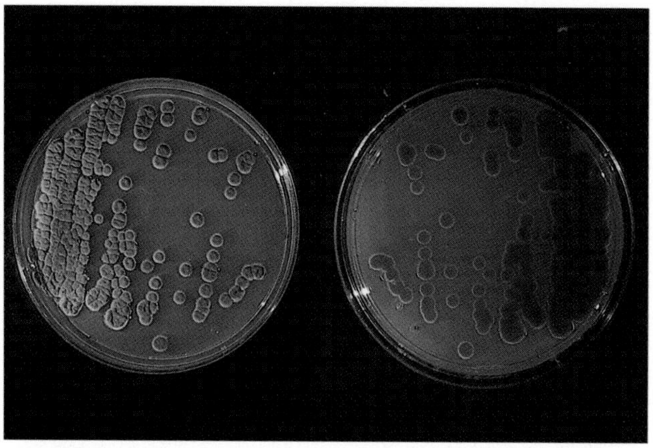

Plate 52–2. Colonies of *Cladosporium* species are colored dark green or brown by the melanin pigments in the hyphae. The reverse sides of the colonies are also dark. (Sabouraud dextrose agar.)

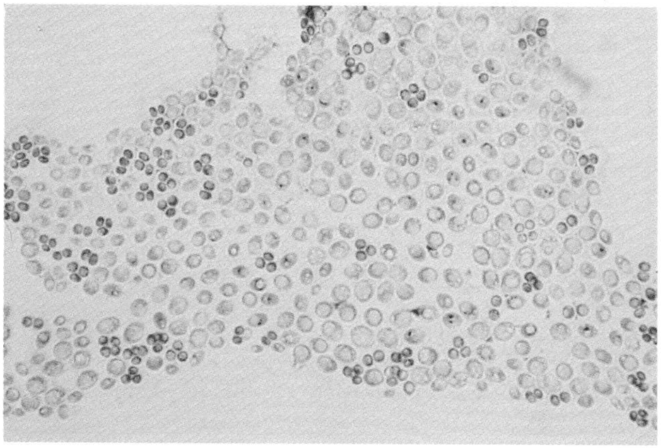

Plate 52–3. Ascospores of *Saccharomyces cerevisiae* are contained in naked asci. The ascospores are colored red by the acid-fast stain. (Ziehl-Neelsen stain.)

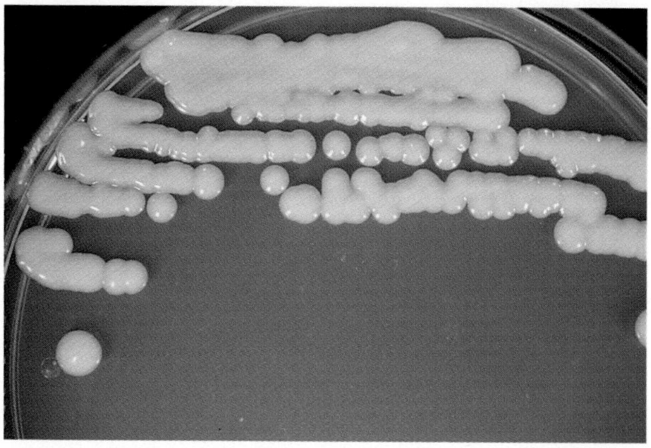

Plate 52–4. Colonies of *Cryptococcus neoformans* usually appear mucoid when first isolated. Some strains are poorly encapsulated and lack the mucoid appearance. (Sabouraud dextrose agar.)

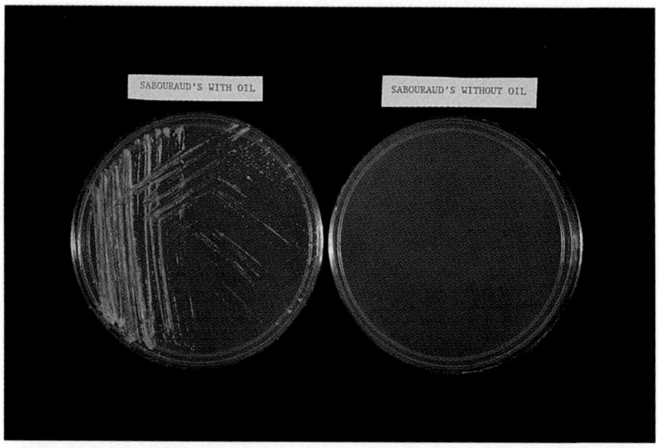

Plate 52–5. Abundant growth of *Malassezia furfur* is evident on a plate that was overlaid with oil before the inoculum was applied. There is no growth on a companion plate without oil. (Sabouraud dextrose agar with and without peanut oil.)

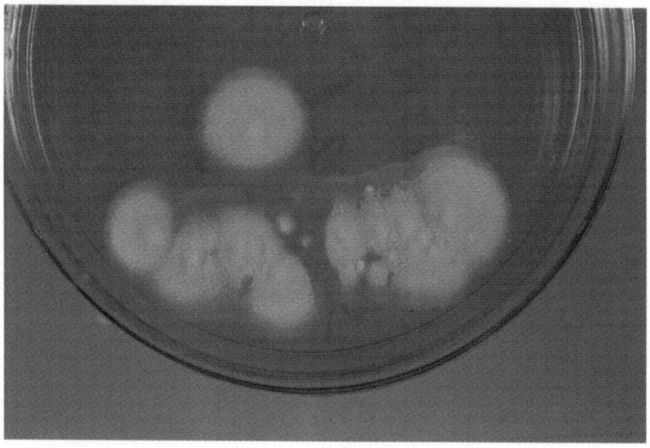

Plate 52–6. An aerial mycelium arises from the yeastlike colony of *Geotrichum candidum*. (Sabouraud dextrose agar.)

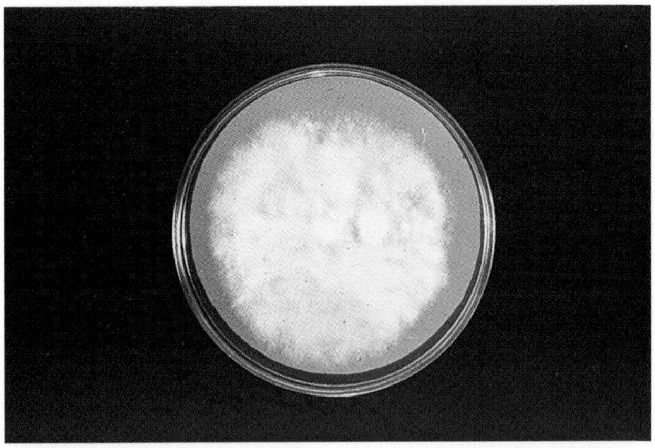

Plate 52–7. A fluffy white colony of *Histoplasma capsulatum* incubated at 30°C. Colonies of white, fluffy molds such as this should always be treated as potential biohazards especially if growing on agar that contains cycloheximide. (Photograph courtesy of Centers for Disease Control and Prevention.)

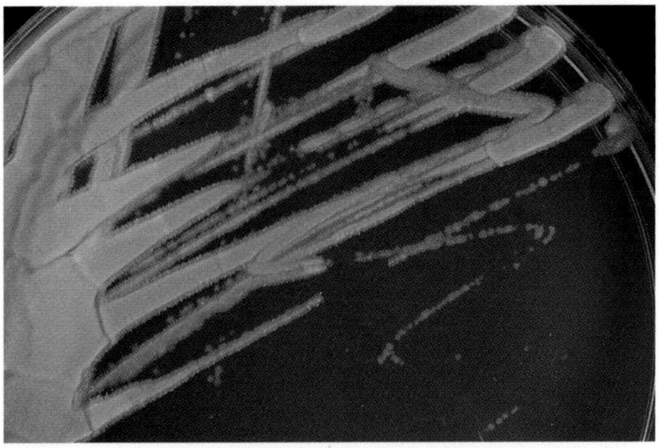

Plate 52–8. White glabrous colonies of *Sporothrix schenckii*. With continuing incubation, the colonies often develop a dark brown or black color. (Sabouraud agar with cycloheximide incubated at 30°C.)

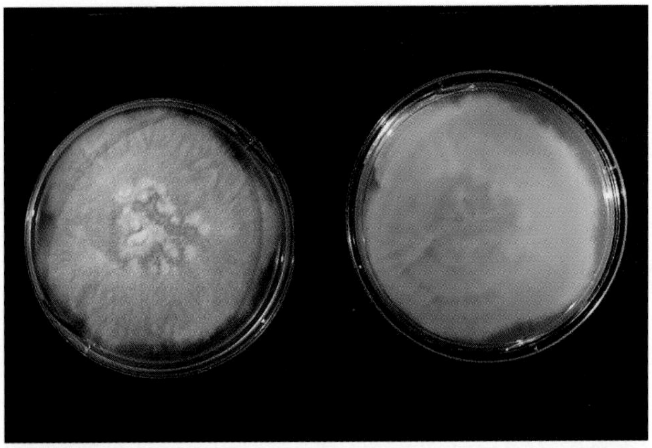

Plate 52–9. A fluffy white *Microsporum canis* colony *(left)* has the characteristic lemon yellow pigment, which may also be seen on the reverse of the colony *(right)*. Subculture in potato flake agar may be required to demonstrate pigment. (Sabouraud dextrose agar with cycloheximide.)

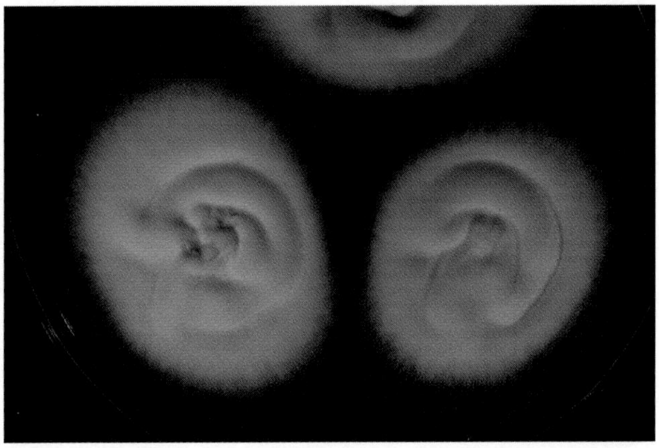

Plate 52–10. Fluffy white colonies of *Trichophyton tonsurans*. (Sabouraud dextrose agar with cycloheximide.)

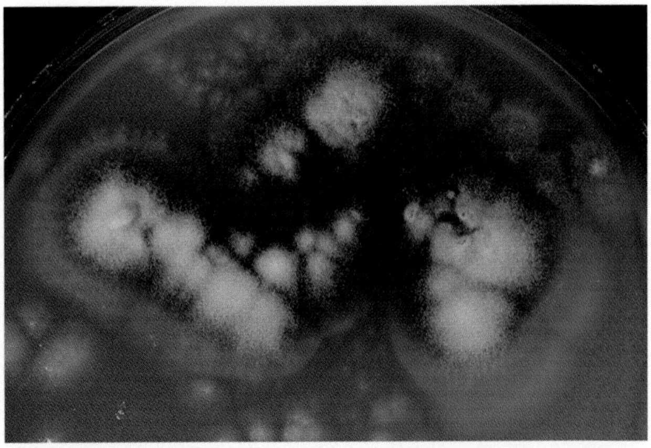

Plate 52–11. Fluffy white colonies of *Trichophyton rubrum* with diffusible red pigment, which may also be seen on the reverse of the colony. (Sabouraud agar with cycloheximide.)

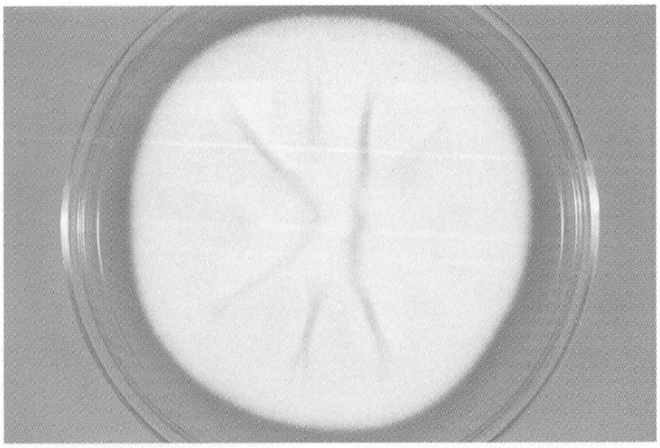

Plate 52–12. Fluffy white colony with radial folds of *Trichophyton mentagrophytes*.

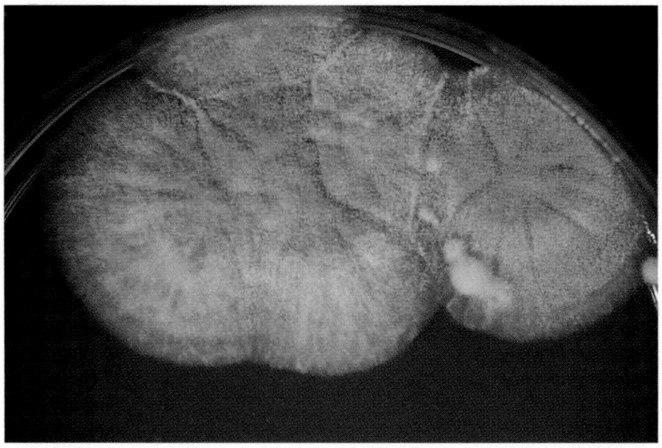

Plate 52–13. Fluffy colonies with granular areas produced by fruiting heads of *Aspergillus flavus*. The development of yellow or green coloration within the white colonies is characteristic. (Sabouraud dextrose agar.)

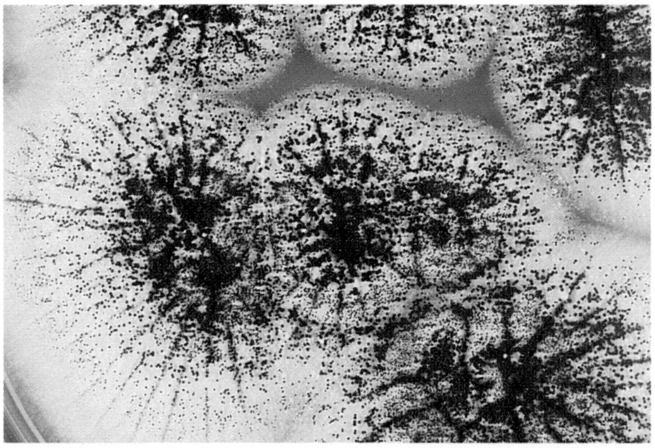

Plate 52–14. A colony of *Aspergillus niger* demonstrates the salt-and-pepper appearance of dark brown fruiting heads on the white mycelium. The reverse of the colony of this hyaline fungus is light colored. (Sabouraud dextrose agar.)

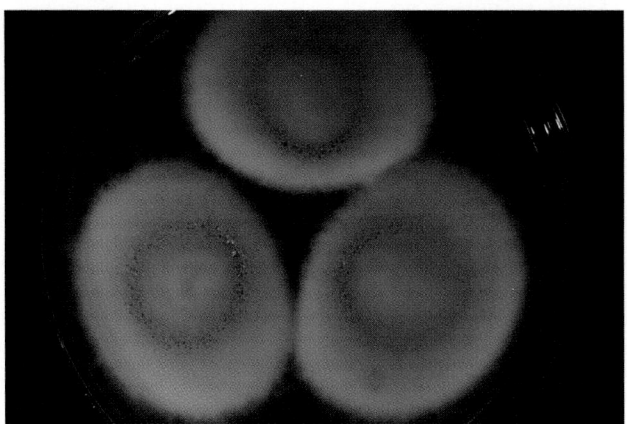

Plate 52–15. A developing colony of *Scedosporium apiospermum* with the characteristic mousy gray coloration. (Sabouraud dextrose agar.)

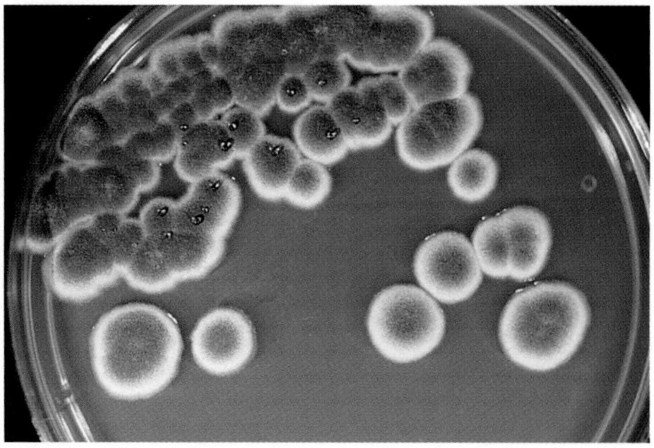

Plate 52–16. A fluffy colony of *Penicillium* species has the characteristic green coloration with a fringe of white. The reverse of the colony is light colored. (Sabouraud dextrose agar.)

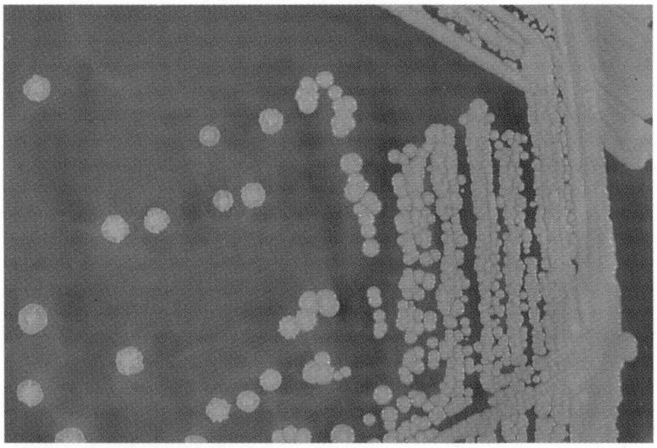

Plate 52–17. Colonies of *Prototheca wickerhamii* are yeast like. (Sabouraud dextrose agar.)

culture should not be performed and a cellophane tape test or teased preparation should be examined only after the preparation has been sealed in a laminar flow safety cabinet. Lactophenol aniline blue is fungicidal, but sealing the coverslip with nail polish before observation provides additional protection.

Susceptibility Testing of Fungal Isolates

For many years, few antifungal chemotherapeutic agents were available, amphotericin B being virtually the only agent that was effective against most systemic pathogens. This potent antifungal agent was frequently toxic, but fortunately, resistance was rare. Development of tests for susceptibility to antibiotics *in vitro* was hindered by difficulties in standardization of inocula and growth conditions. How do you measure the inoculum of *Aspergillus* conidia or chains of *Candida* blastoconidia in a pseudohypha? Studies of the correlation between *in vitro* and *in vivo* results were difficult.

The development of many new antifungal agents (Fromtling, 1988) and the subsequent development of resistance among yeast pathogens has added new impetus to the development and standardization of tests for laboratory guidance of antifungal chemotherapy (Terrell, 1992; Rex, 1993). The National Committee for Clinical Laboratory Standards (1992) has proposed a reference method for antimicrobial sus-ceptibility testing of yeast pathogens, using a broth microdilution technique. Newer methods for determining minimum inhibitory concentrations of antibiotics directed against bacterial pathogens, such as the E-test (AB Biodisk, Piscataway, NJ), are being studied but remain investigational techniques (Colombo, 1995; Sewell, 1994). It is now possible for laboratories that have a need to test large numbers of yeast isolates to perform susceptibility tests. If only occasional isolates need to be tested, it is best to send the strain to a reference laboratory.

The susceptibility testing of mould isolates is less well standardized. These tests are best performed in reference laboratories.

YEAST AND YEAST INFECTIONS

The Genus *Candida*

Candida spp. are the most important of the yeast pathogens. Because immunosuppressive therapy has become increasingly common and broad-spectrum antibiotics, such as the third generation cephalosporins, are used more frequently, yeast have assumed a large place among nosocomial pathogens. In 1994, *Candida* spp. were outranked only by staphylococci, *Escherichia coli*, *Klebsiella* spp., and enterococci as causes of bloodstream infection at the University of Vermont.

Risk Factors

Candida infections are limited in extent and severity if the host is normal. Broad-spectrum antibacterial therapy upsets the balance of colonizing flora on the mucous membranes of the oral cavity and the gastrointestinal tract by eliminating the predominant competing bacterial flora. In some locations, such as the female genital system, the cause of a disruption in the normal flora balance may not be obvious. In cutaneous sites, such as the groin and inframammary folds, excessive moisture predisposes an individual to *Candida* infection.

Severe and invasive disease develops when host defenses are compromised (Fraser, 1992). Diabetes, immunosuppressive diseases or therapies, and neutropenia are common risk factors. Bloodstream infections, including fungal endocarditis, are fostered by intravenous injections of illicit drugs (Bisbe, 1992; Weems, 1992) and by use of indwelling vascular lines, as is commonly required in sick, hospitalized patients (Curry, 1971).

Clinical Disease

By far, the most common pathogen within the genus *Candida* is *C. albicans*, followed by *C. tropicalis*. In some institutions at some times, *C. tropicalis* has been the most frequent cause of nosocomial infection (Wingard, 1979), but in most hospitals, it is a distant second to *C. albicans*. *C. parapsilosis* is the next most frequent pathogen in disseminated disease, particularly when the patient has abused drugs or when intravenous catheters have been employed (Weems, 1992). *C. glabrata* (formerly *Torulopsis glabrata*) also causes fungemia (Haron, 1993; Marks, 1970). It has been associated with urinary tract (Kauffman, 1974) and vaginal infections (Sobel, 1986). *C. krusei* is a less common cause of disseminated infection, which resembles that produced by *C. tropicalis* (Goldman, 1993). New species continue to be associated with human infection, such as *C. zeylanoides* (Levenson, 1991), once again proving that the capacity of fungi to produce human infection is inexhaustible if the clinical conditions are right.

Resistance to imidazole antibiotics (e.g., ketoconazole, fluconazole, or itraconazole) is unfortunately developing in isolates of *Candida* species. *Candida lusitaniae*, an infrequently isolated pathogen, is prone to develop resistance to amphotericin *in vivo* (Blinkhorn, 1989; Hadfield, 1987). The relative frequency with which various species are isolated varies from one institution to another.

Cutaneous disease is most frequently seen as erythematous lesions of the skin, sometimes accompanied by a creamy, white exudate or scaling. Moist conditions are precursors to infection, such as diaper rash in infants or infection of skin folds (intertrigo) in adults. Common sites are in the groin (a form of jock itch), between fingers and toes, under the female breast, and in the axilla. Workers who must immerse their hands in water for long periods of time are particularly at risk for infections of the skin of the hands, nails (onychomycosis), or the paronychium. Lesions also may be found on the skin of the thighs and buttocks, which are areas not commonly infected by mould pathogens. A chronic cutaneous disease is an uncommon manifestation of *Candida* infection in patients with defective cellular immunity (Kirkpatrick, 1971).

Oral candidiasis usually is manifest as creamy white patches overlying erythematous buccal mucosa (thrush). Symptoms are usually minimal, but dysphagia may result from heavy infections. Fissuring at the corners of the mouth (angular cheilitis) occurs commonly and may be the primary complaint. Oral candidiasis is a common initial infection in patients who have been infected with HIV (Gottlieb, 1981;

Klein, 1984). Oral candidiasis and *Pneumocystis* infection were the two initial clues to the presence of the acquired immunodeficiency syndrome (AIDS).

Gastrointestinal candidiasis occurs most commonly as esophagitis (Haulk, 1991) and, less commonly, gastritis (Katzenstein, 1979). Erosive lesions of the distal esophagus and stomach result in substernal pain, which is aggravated by swallowing. White plaques overlie the lesions when viewed by endoscopy. The differential diagnosis includes infection with herpes simplex virus, and the two processes may coexist.

Candida species are frequent flora of the lower gastrointestinal tract (Cohen, 1969), making assessment of the significance of these yeast in stool specimens difficult. True invasive infection of the lower gastrointestinal tract is much less common than disease of the upper tract, although overgrowth of *Candida* spp. in the stool may accompany antimicrobial therapy. *Candida* enteritis has been described, but histologic documentation of invasive disease has been lacking (Kane, 1976; Kozinn, 1962).

Vulvovaginitis afflicts postpubertal women. Diabetes, antimicrobial therapy, pregnancy, and sexual activity are predisposing conditions. Vaginal burning and itching, dyspareunia, and a discharge that is classically curd like are associated with an infection that may be acute or chronic and difficult to eradicate (Sobel, 1986).

Urinary tract infection is difficult to diagnose, because *Candida* spp. are frequently recovered from the urine as a result of vaginal contamination or colonization of the bladder in patients with indwelling catheters, especially when systemic antibiotics have been administered (Goldberg, 1979). Severe infection of the upper urinary tract, including necrosis of the renal papillae, is a serious complication of lower tract infections and occurs particularly in patients who have obstructive uropathy. Quantitative cultures are not useful for assessing the significance of *Candida* species in the urinary tract (Goldberg, 1979).

Disseminated candidiasis is a very serious nosocomial infection, particularly in immunosuppressed patients who are neutropenic (Fishman, 1972; Klein, 1979). As many as 10% to 15% of bloodstream infections may be caused by yeast. Focal lesions in virtually any organ may result from hematogenous dissemination. Endocarditis results rarely (Johnston, 1991), particularly in abusers of illicit drugs (Bisbe, 1992; Weems, 1992). Unfortunately blood cultures are often negative in disseminated candidiasis (Jones, 1990). Removal of infected vascular catheters is an important therapeutic maneuver (Edwards, 1992). Many infectious disease specialists recommend empiric therapy for fungal infection if therapy aimed at bacterial pathogens is unsuccessful, particularly in an immunosuppressed patient with neutropenia (Pizzo, 1989; Walsh, 1990).

Most infections of the lung arise as a part of disseminated infection. Primary *Candida* pneumonia occurs but is uncommon (Haron, 1993; Ramirez, 1967). The predictive value for pneumonia of identifying yeast or isolating *Candida* species from respiratory specimens that may be contaminated with upper respiratory tract secretions is very low. A reasonable and cost-effective approach to yeast isolated from the respiratory tract is to report their presence as yeast forms after eliminating the possibility of *Cryptococcus* species with a rapid urease test (Murray, 1977).

Candida infections of the central nervous system are unusual (Bayer, 1976; Parker, 1981). They may occur as a part of disseminated infection, or they may result from direct inoculation.

Pathology of Candida *Infection*

The histologic response to *Candida* infection is commonly purulent, resembling the lesions of bacterial infections. Abscesses are frequently present. On occasion, the response to *Candida* infection is granulomatous. In tissue, budding yeast, pseudohyphae and true hyphae may be present. The frequently repeated aphorism that pseudohyphae on a mucosal surface indicate invasive infection derives from clinical studies of gastrointestinal disease (Kozinn, 1962), but this theory is in disrepute at present (Odds, 1994). When pseudohyphae or true hyphae predominate, the yeast must be differentiated from invasive mould pathogens, such as *Aspergillus*. Vascular invasion, such as occurs with *Aspergillus* or the zygomycetes, is uncommon in yeast infections. The yeast can often be demonstrated in hematoxylin-eosin stained sections, but tissue versions of Gram's stain, the methenamine silver stain, or the periodic acid–Schiff technique may be used also.

Laboratory Diagnosis and Extent of Workup

Specimens for culture should be taken from the affected organs and from lesions in which they can be visualized. Yeast often are recovered in aerobic bacterial blood culture bottles, but the Isolator system is the most efficient method for recovering *Candida* spp. from blood (Fleming, 1984; Jones, 1990). Tissue specimens, scrapings, or swabs from the mouth or vagina should be inoculated onto primary isolation media with and without cycloheximide. Good growth in the presence of cycloheximide is a preliminary clue to the presence of *C. albicans*, although *C. guilliermondii, C. kefyr* (formerly *pseudotropicalis*), and some strains of *C. tropicalis* may also be recovered on this medium. The presence of filamentous extensions from the edges of the colony (feet) are a macroscopic indication that pseudohyphae are being produced (see Fig. 52–1). *C. glabrata* (formerly *Torulopsis glabrata*) and *Cryptococcus* spp. do not form pseudohyphae *in vitro,* and some other *Candida* species, such as *C. lusitaniae* and *C. guilliermondii,* may not form many pseudohyphae.

The extent of the mycologic evaluation depends on the clinical setting and the specimen type. The respiratory and urinary tracts are two important organ systems in which isolation of *Candida* spp. is accomplished frequently but is difficult to interpret, as discussed above. Complete identification of isolates from these sites should be accomplished only selectively after consultation with the responsible clinician. Although clinical practice usually is not altered by identifying isolates of *Candida* to the species level, we believe that isolates from blood or other sterile tissues and fluids should be identified fully when the yeast is the only pathogen or the predominant isolate. Similarly, we completely identify isolates when examination for fungi has been requested in a setting in which *Candida* is expected, such as vaginitis or oral thrush. The information may be of use to the hospital epidemiologist for study of nosocomial infections. One group of investigators has suggested that the recurrence rate and chronicity of vulvovaginitis are greater when *C. tropicalis* is the pathogen than when *C. albicans* is the etiologic agent

(Horowitz, 1985), but further studies are required. When a yeast is isolated in the bacteriology laboratory or is present in a polymicrobial infection, we report its presence and request a consultation before further studies are performed. We receive those requests very infrequently.

A preliminary report of *C. albicans* may be issued if the germ tube test is positive (see Fig. 52–15). By studying yeast morphology using cornmeal agar to confirm the presence of chlamydospores, the identification usually can be accomplished on a single agar plate within 24 to 48 hours; occasionally, it takes as long as 72 hours for the culture to be completed (see Fig. 52–16). If germ tubes and chlamydospores are not demonstrated, the preliminary or presumptive identification of *Candida* species can be made if pseudohyphae are present and arthroconidia are absent. A small fraction of *Candida* isolates do not produce pseudohyphae, germ tubes, or chlamydospores. Complete identification requires assimilation tests, but ancillary morphologic observations are essential (Table 52–11). Some laboratories use fermentation tests to assist in identification of *Candida* species, but they are not required.

At present, immunologic tests cannot be recommended for diagnosis of candidiasis (de Repentigny, 1992). Investigation of methods for detection of antigens, which might provide a useful rapid test for invasive infection, continues (Reiss, 1993).

The Genus *Cryptococcus*

The primary pathogen within this genus is *C. neoformans*. There are two varieties: *C. neoformans* var. *neoformans* and *C. neoformans* var. *gattii*. The latter variant is found predominantly in the tropics and subtropics and is infrequently isolated in clinical laboratories in the United States (Levitz, 1991). Both variants have two serotypes, but determination of the serologic reaction is of epidemiologic interest only. The sexual stage of *C. neoformans* is a basidiomycete, *Filobasidiella neoformans*, but the teleomorph is not isolated in clinical laboratories. Other cryptococci and *Rhodotorula* spp. occasionally are isolated from nonsterile sites but are rarely, if ever, implicated in human disease (Horowitz, 1993; Kiehn, 1992; Sinnott, 1989). The primary environmental source of *C. neoformans* is in droppings of pigeons or, less commonly, of other avian species. Soil contaminated by bird guano may also harbor the fungus.

Risk Factors

Immunosuppressive therapy or disease is a risk factor for cryptococcosis (Williams, 1976). Before the appearance of HIV infection, almost half of the patients with cryptococcal infection were immunologically normal, as measured by available parameters. Cryptococcosis is one of the defining infections for AIDS, which has become the overwhelming risk factor.

Clinical Disease

PNEUMONIA. The portal of entry for virtually all cryptococcal infections is the lung, although symptomatic lung disease may not be present at the time extrapulmonary disease is recognized (White, 1994). Cryptococcal pneumonia exhibits a wide variety of presentations. Immunologically competent patients may exhibit no symptoms despite the presence of cryptococci in the lower respiratory tract (Randhawa, 1977). Pneumonia may be indolent and protracted, resolving slowly. The infection may be diffuse or localized, including the presence of coin lesions that do not usually calcify. Infection is most severe in immunocompromised patients and is often accompanied by other infectious agents, particularly *Pneumocystis carinii* and cytomegalovirus. Extrapulmonary disease may appear weeks after a pulmonary infection has been documented (Kerkering, 1981).

CUTANEOUS INFECTION. Skin lesions usually are a result of hematogenous dissemination from the respiratory tract (Pema, 1994). They present as single or multiple papules, which enlarge and ulcerate, producing a thin exudate that contains the yeast.

BONE AND JOINT INFECTION. Once again, the primary infection is in the respiratory tract from which the cryptococci disseminate, most commonly to the spinal column (Behrman, 1990). Osteolytic lesions are produced. So-called cold abscesses in adjacent soft tissue produce a thin exudate that contains large numbers of cryptococci. Less commonly, joint spaces are involved.

CENTRAL NERVOUS SYSTEM INFECTION. The most frequent and most serious foci of disseminated cryptococcal infection are the meninges and parenchyma of the brain (Chuck, 1989; Kovacs, 1985; Lewis, 1972; Zuger, 1986). The onset of the disease may be acute, but the presentation may also be insidious and the progression torpid. Headache and changes in mental status and personality often dominate the clinical picture. Basilar meningitis, involvement of the cranial nerves, and invasion of the underlying cortex result in hydrocephalus and decreases in visual acuity. Fever, if present, usually is low grade and the typical signs of acute meningeal irritation, such as stiff neck and Kernig's and Brudzinski's signs, are often absent.

Pathology of Cryptococcal Infection

The histologic response depends on the degree of encapsulation of the infecting strain. Most commonly, there is little or no inflammatory response, corresponding to the thin exudate seen clinically. Rather the cells of the normal tissue are separated by large numbers of encapsulated cryptococci. When cerebrospinal fluid is examined, the only cells present may be the yeast, which may be misinterpreted as mononuclear host cells if infection is not suspected clinically. Large capsules usually are demonstrated in positive India ink preparations. Short, rudimentary pseudohyphae of *C. neoformans* occasionally are seen in tissue sections (Freed, 1971). Poorly encapsulated strains of *C. neoformans* elicit a granulomatous inflammatory response, and the yeast are found predominantly in the cytoplasm of macrophages (Farmer, 1973). They may be confused with the cells of *B. dermatitidis* or even immature spherules of *C. immitis*. Confusion of small cryptococcal yeast forms with *H. capsulatum* has been described, but the differentiation usually is not difficult (Gutierrez, 1975). Differentiation in tissue sections can be accomplished by staining of cryptococcal mucopolysaccharide with mucin stains or demonstration of the melanin pigment with the Fontana-Masson stain. The melanin stain is particularly advantageous when the infecting strain is deficient in capsular material (Ro, 1987). Combinations of the Fontana-Masson stain and various stains for mucopolysaccharides, such as mucicarmine

Table 52–11. ANCILLARY OBSERVATIONS USEFUL FOR IDENTIFICATION OF YEASTS

Organism	Growth in Presence of Cycloheximide	Germ Tubes	Pseudohyphae	Red Pigment	Urease	Arthroconidia	Chlamydospores	Growth Stimulated by Lipids	Ascospores	Comments
Candida albicans	+	+	+	–	–	–	+	–	–	
Candida tropicalis	– (+)	–	+	–	–	–	–	–	–	Well-developed pseudohyphae; rare strains produce germ tubes
Candida parapsilosis	–	–	+	–	–	–	–	–	–	Sagebrush pseudohyphae
Candida krusei	–	–	+	–	– (+)	–	–	–	–	Dry, flat colony
Candida kefyr (pseudotropicalis)	+	–	+	–	–	–	–	–	–	"Logs in a stream" pseudohyphae; green sheen on EMB agar
Candida guilliermondii	+	–	+(–)	–	–	–	–	–	–	Pseudohyphae may be sparse or absent; glassy colony
Candida (Torulopsis) glabrata	–	–	–	–	–	–	–	–	–	Small yeast (2 μm to 5 μm)
Candida lusitaniae	–	–	+	–	–	–	–	–	–	Pseudohyphae may be sparse
Cryptococcus neoformans	–	–	–	–	+	–	–	–	–	Polysaccharide capsule present; round yeast cells
Rhodotorula species	–	–	–	+	+	–	–	–	–	Polysaccharide capsule may be present
Malassezia furfur	–	–	–	–	–	–	–	+	–	Small flask-shaped yeast
Malassezia pachydermatis	–	–	–	–	–	–	–	–	–	Small flask-shaped yeast
Trichosporon species	+(–)	–	+	–	+(–)	+	–	–	–	
Geotrichum candidum	–	–	–	–	–	+	–	–	–	No blastoconidia; arthroconidia germinate from corner of cell
Saccharomyces cerevisiae	–	–	–(+)	–	–	–	–	–	+	Pseudohyphae may be rare

( ) = less common reaction

or alcian blue, have been used to advantage but are not ordinarily necessary (Lazcano, 1993). *Blastomyces dermatitidis* stains poorly with the mucin stains on rare occasions. *Rhinosporidium seeberi* is mucin positive, but it is not seen in temperate climates and is easily differentiated from cryptococci on morphologic grounds. The cells seen in chromoblastomycosis contain melanin but are distinctive in morphology and mucin are negative. The variable size (3 μm to 10 μm) and decidedly round nature of the yeast *in vivo* are clues to the correct identification, regardless of the degree of encapsulation and histologic response.

A primary complex of granulomas in the periphery of the lung and in regional lymph nodes, which resembles that found in tuberculosis and histoplasmosis, probably occurs more frequently than is recognized (Salyer, 1974).

Laboratory Identification and Extent of Workup

Possible cryptococci should always be identified as to species to determine whether or not *C. neoformans* is present. Clues to the presence of this fungus are good growth on blood agar plates incubated in the bacteriology laboratory at 35°C to 37°C, mucoid appearance to the colonies (Plate 52–4), *round* appearance of the yeast cells, and lack of growth on media that contain cycloheximide (see Table 52–11). Presumptive identification can be obtained rapidly by examining an India ink preparation for capsules (see Fig. 52–13) (see Table 52–7) or performing a rapid urease test (see Table 52–4) or both. Capsules may be diminished even in heavily encapsulated strains once they have been isolated on agar media. We have encountered several isolates of *C. neoformans* from the respiratory tract that were nonmucoid and resembled *Candida* spp. in colonial morphology. Definitive identification is accomplished by biochemical testing. Determination of phenol oxidase activity may be included but is not essential if one of the commercial yeast identification systems is used.

The polysaccharide antigen of *C. neoformans* can be detected in cerebrospinal fluid and serum, most commonly by latex agglutination. The sensitivity of the test exceeds 90%, but commercial kits vary considerably in sensitivity and specificity. Rheumatoid factor may cause false-positive reactions (Dolan, 1972), and controls for antiglobulin should be included in the test (Bennett, 1971). Infections with DF-2 group (*Capnocytophaga canimorsus*), a nonfermentative gram-negative bacillus (Westerink, 1987), and *T. beigelii* may cause false-positive reactions, but these are uncommon infections. Other occasional causes of false-positive reactions are poorly understood. The frequency of erroneous results can be diminished by treatment of serum specimens with pronase (Hamilton, 1991; Stockman, 1982). False-positive reactions appear to be less common in patients who are infected with HIV, perhaps because of the large numbers of organisms present (Berlin, 1989). Titration of positive results has been done traditionally to assess prognosis and as a baseline for following the effects of treatment. Large amounts of antigen and persistence of antigen following therapy are poor prognostic signs in patients who are not infected with HIV (Diamond, 1974). In contrast, these parameters have not been demonstrated to be useful uniformly in patients with AIDS, who are the largest risk group currently (Chuck, 1989; Kovacs, 1985; Zuger, 1986). The measurement of serum antigen appears to be a more sensitive test in HIV-infected patients than testing of cerebrospinal fluid. Both serum and cerebrospinal fluid should be tested for optimal sensitivity. In some reports, isolation of *C. neoformans* from a site outside of the central nervous system has been associated with a poor prognosis in HIV-infected patients. A negative India ink test on cerebrospinal fluid is a good prognostic sign in non-HIV infected patients but does not have the same implication in patients with AIDS.

The Genus *Malassezia*

The two most important species within the genus *Malassezia* are *M. furfur* and *M. pachydermatis* (Marcon, 1992). *M. furfur* is by far the more common pathogen of humans. *M. pachydermatis*, initially isolated from an Indian rhinoceros, has been recovered from many animals, notably from the ears of dogs, and occasionally from humans. *M. furfur* was formerly named *Pityrosporum ovale* or *P. orbiculare*, depending on the morphology of the yeast.

Risk Factors

M. furfur is found on the skin of more than 90% of individuals (Roberts, 1969b, 1969c) and cutaneous disease occurs in normal hosts. There may be an increased susceptibility to disease in patients who have excessive sweating (Roberts, 1969a) or in patients who have increased levels of corticosteroids resulting from therapy (Boardman, 1962) or endogenous production as a part of Cushing's disease (Canizares, 1959). Systemic infection occurs primarily in neonates and is associated with intravenous hyperalimentation with lipid solutions (Powell, 1986). Although *M. furfur* is not ordinarily present on the skin of healthy infants, the yeast has been recovered from the skin of as many as 37% of infants who were in intensive care units (Powell, 1987). The risk factors for *M. pachydermatis* infection in humans are similar (Mickelsen, 1988).

Clinical Disease

PITYRIASIS (TINEA) VERSICOLOR. This common infection of the epidermis results in hyperpigmentation or hypopigmentation of the skin, most commonly on the trunk and upper arms (Powell, 1986). Fawn-colored macules are the most common presentation, but depigmenting lesions are more obvious in dark-skinned persons and may be accentuated by suntans in light-skinned individuals. The ill effects are purely cosmetic, but may be considerably troublesome. Hypopigmented lesions must be differentiated from vitiligo. Therapy consists of topical application of fungicidal creams or rinses.

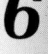

Systemic Infection. Systemic infection occurs almost invariably in infants who have received intravascular infusions of lipid. Although the lipid solutions themselves do not support the growth of yeast, diluted lipid solution supports the growth of *M. furfur* by supplying long-chain fatty acids that are also found on the skin and must be supplied in the laboratory for isolation (Powell, 1986). Infected infants are often asymptomatic, but fever, leukocytosis, and thrombocytopenia may be present. Pneumonia is the most common systemic manifestation of disease, probably resulting from emboli from infected intravenous catheters. Removing the infected catheter is therapeutic.

Pathology of *Malassezia furfur* Infection. The diagnosis of pityriasis versicolor usually is made clinically or by demonstrating yeast and short hyphal forms (similar in appearance to spaghetti and meatballs) in KOH preparations of skin scrapings. The addition of Calcofluor white or other fungal stain enhances detection, because the fungal cells are small and difficult to visualize when unstained (Fig. 52–17). When biopsied, hyperkeratosis, acanthosis, and dermal mononuclear infiltrates may be seen. Little is known of the pathology of systemic infection with *M. furfur*, because biopsies are infrequently performed and lethal infection is uncommon. In rare fatal cases, lesions have been described in many organs, including the lung, liver, and kidney (Shek, 1989). Vasculitis, endocarditis, septic infarcts, and granulomatous inflammation were observed.

Laboratory Identification and Extent of Workup. Culture for *M. furfur* is rarely requested in cutaneous disease, and direct observation of yeast in KOH preparations usually is done in the physician's office. This yeast should be sought in cultures of blood and intravenous catheter tips from neonates. Before inoculation, a drop of sterile olive oil is added to the surface of a suitable agar medium, such as Sabouraud dextrose agar or sheep blood agar. In our laboratory, we employ peanut oil, which also works well. Within two to three days, colonies appear light brown and often have a very dry appearance in the oil overlay (Plate 52–5). An initial clue is lack of growth in the absence of oil or stimulation of growth by the presence of an oil overlay. There may be sufficient lipid in the blood or on the catheter tip, however, to support initial growth on plates that do not contain oil. *M. pachydermatis* is not dependent on long chain fatty acids for growth.

The identification of the isolate can be confirmed by microscopic examination of the yeast cells, which measure 3 μm to 7 μm in size. The budding process in *Malassezia* is unusual, because it occurs as an enteroblastic process with the formation of phialides. The bud is broad based, and the collarettes of the phialides may be observed with the light microscope as a distinct dark ring separating the mother and daughter cells (Fig. 52–18).

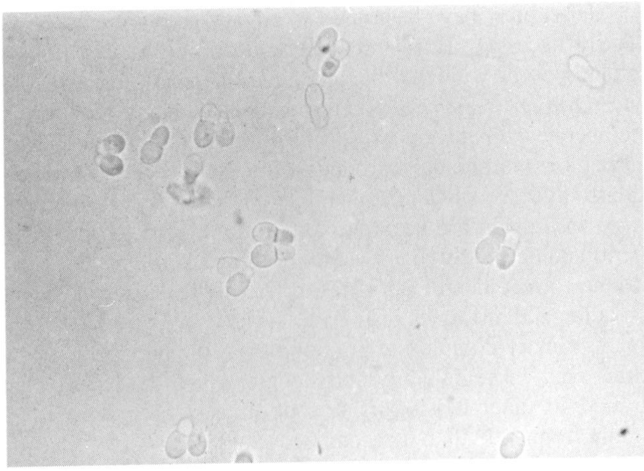

Figure 52–18. Budding yeast cells of *Malassezia furfur* depicting the classic flask shape. (Gram's stain.)

Other Yeast and Yeastlike Pathogens and Saprobes

T. beigelii produces a hair infection known as white piedra and may cause systemic infection (Hoy, 1986; Ogata, 1990). *Blastoschizomyces capitatus* (formerly *Trichosporon capitatum*) has caused rare cases of disseminated infection that resemble candidiasis (Liu, 1990). A morphologically similar fungus, *Geotrichum candidum*, is also a rare cause of pulmonary or disseminated disease (Fishbach, 1973; Jagirdar, 1981). *Geotrichum* and *Trichosporon* produce smooth yeastlike colonies that later develop aerial mycelium, like new hair growth on a bald head (Plate 52–6). Both species produce arthroconidia, which lack the disjunctor cells seen in *C. immitis* (Fig. 52–19). *Saccharomyces cerevisiae* (Clemons, 1994; Sobel, 1993), *Rhodotorula* species (Pien, 1980) and *Hansenula* species are saprophytic yeast that may produce infection on very rare occasions. Demonstration of the yeast in tissues or isolation from multiple specimens, even from sterile sites, is required to document the role of the yeast in an infectious process. *Saccharomyces cerevisiae* is baker's

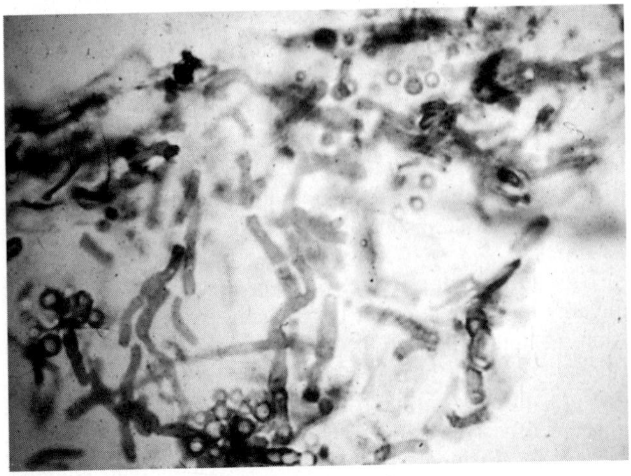

Figure 52–17. Skin scrapings from the lesion of tinea versicolor. The yeast and short hyphal forms of *Malassezia furfur* are characteristic. (Periodic acid–Schiff method.)

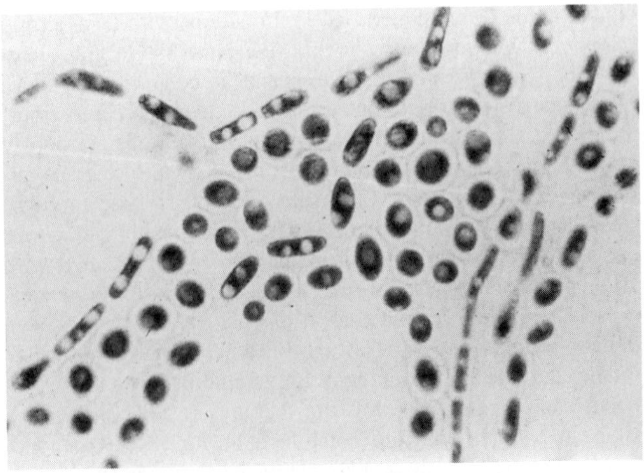

Figure 52–19. The arthroconidia of *Trichosporon* species are not separated by disjunctor cells. (Lactophenol cotton blue.)

yeast and is perhaps best known to students of mycology for its salutary effects on malt and hops.

DIMORPHIC FUNGI

The thermally dimorphic fungi are the most pathogenic organisms encountered in a clinical mycology laboratory. In the United States, the most important pathogens are *H. capsulatum*, *Blastomyces dermatitidis*, *C. immitis*, and *Sporothrix schenckii*. *Sporothrix* is widely distributed throughout the world. The other organisms are predominantly found in North America, where they have distinct geographic distributions (Fig. 52–20). Epidemic disease is most common with *Histoplasma* and *Coccidioides*, and is less common with

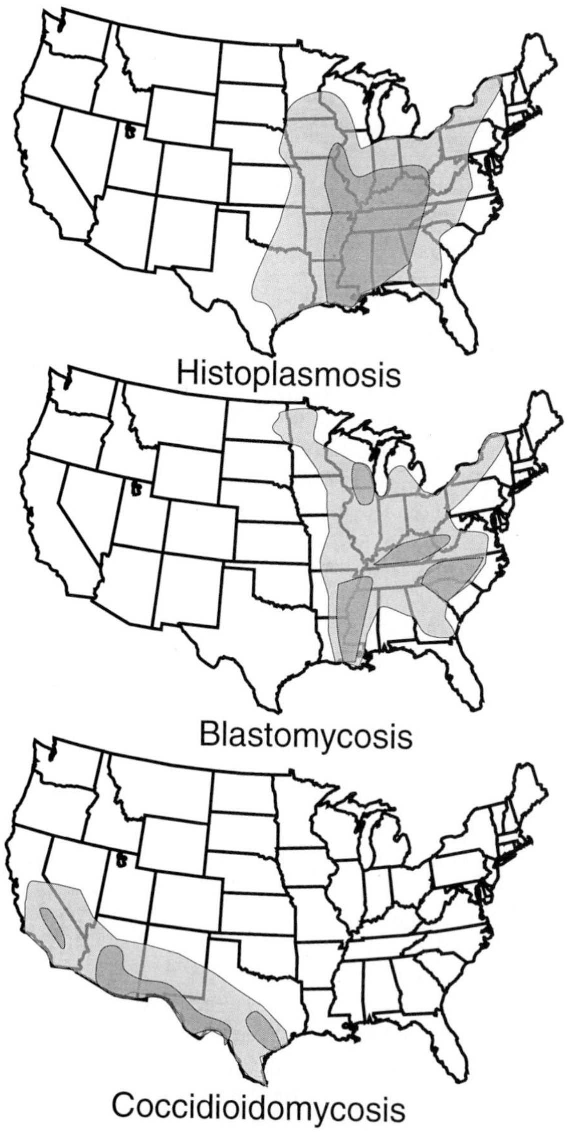

Figure 52–20. Geographic distribution of dimorphic fungal infections in the United States. The areas of greatest endemicity (*dark shading*) and lesser endemicity (*light shading*) are illustrated. Sporadic cases may occur in other areas outside of the endemic zones. Histoplasmosis and blastomycosis extend into southern Canada, whereas coccidioidomycosis occurs in Central and South America.

Sporothrix and *Blastomyces*. The tissue phase of *Coccidioides* is the spherule, whereas the other genera produce a yeast phase *in vivo*.

Histoplasma capsulatum

Risk Factors

The primary risk factor for acquiring infection is living in one of the endemic regions of the United States, an area that traces the course of the Ohio and Mississippi rivers, as well as the valleys of the Appalachian Mountains. In some areas, more than 90% of the population react positively to histoplasmin skin tests. Growth of *H. capsulatum* is stimulated by bird guano, although the fungus does not grow in the birds themselves. A classic history of acute histoplasmosis is represented by the patient who recently cleaned out a chicken coop. Epidemic disease has occurred after disturbing the roosts of birds during construction projects (Tosh, 1966). Ironically, an outbreak of histoplasmosis occurred in 40% of students and faculty who were participating in an Earth Day cleanup at their school (Brodsky, 1973). Chronic pulmonary histoplasmosis is particularly a disease of patients with chronic obstructive pulmonary disease. Disseminated infection usually is associated with immunologic deficits, especially of the cellular immune system. Infection with HIV virus has now become the most important risk factor for fatal and disseminated infection (Johnson, 1988).

Clinical Disease

ACUTE PULMONARY INFECTION. Most immunocompetent individuals develop asymptomatic or subclinical infection, accompanied by an immunologic response (Goodwin, 1973, 1978). Symptomatic patients develop a flulike syndrome, which may be accompanied by pleuritic or retrosternal chest pain. More severely affected individuals may be sick for several weeks, but resolution usually is complete. If focal granulomatous inflammation has occurred, calcification of the focus may leave a well-circumscribed coin lesion, which may be seen on the chest radiograph. Skin lesions of erythema nodosum and erythema multiforme may accompany acute pulmonary infection (Medeiros, 1966).

PERICARDITIS AND MEDIASTINITIS. Granulomatous inflammation of the pericardium and mediastinitis has been attributed to *H. capsulatum*, most often on serologic grounds (Loyd, 1988; Schowengerdt, 1969). The chronic inflammation may result in fibrosis and constrictive pericarditis. Yeast are rarely seen in the lesions and are rarely recovered in culture.

CHRONIC PULMONARY HISTOPLASMOSIS. This debilitating disease occurs primarily in patients with chronic obstructive pulmonary disease, most of whom are commonly middle-aged men (Goodwin, 1995). Calcification and cavitation may occur. The differential diagnosis includes chronic pulmonary tuberculosis and pulmonary neoplasia.

DISSEMINATED HISTOPLASMOSIS. Dissemination of yeast through the reticuloendothelial system may occur as a part of acute pulmonary histoplasmosis, resulting in healed granulomas, which often calcify, especially in the spleen (Johnson, 1988; Kauffman, 1978; Nightingale, 1990; Reddy, 1970). Clinically disseminated infection occurs in two classes of patients. The first group consists of individuals at the extremes of age who do not have a recognized immunosuppressive condition but may have an immune system that is incompletely developed or diminished by age in ways that are incompletely understood. The second group is patients with recognized immunosuppressive diseases or therapies. Before the 1980s, the diseases were predominantly hematologic neoplasms; in recent years HIV infection has dominated the risk factors overwhelmingly (Johnson, 1988; Wheat, 1990). Progression of disease may be rapid or insidious.

Infection of the reticuloendothelial system may result in lymphadenopathy, hepatosplenomegaly, or thrombocytopenia. Destruction of the adrenal cortex by the granulomatous process may be sufficiently extensive to cause hormonal insufficiency. Central nervous system infection may be manifested as chronic meningitis, intracerebral granulomas, or both. Endovascular infection includes endocarditis with large, bulky vegetations. Any part of the gastrointestinal tract may be affected, and the ulcerating lesions may suggest a neoplasm macroscopically. Involvement of the skin is less common than with other dimorphic fungi (Studdard, 1976). In patients with HIV infection, the symptoms of disseminated histoplasmosis may resemble those produced by the virus, including fever, lymphadenopathy, anemia, leukopenia, thrombocytopenia, weight loss, and fatigue

PATHOLOGY OF HISTOPLASMOSIS. As a facultative intracellular pathogen *H. capsulatum* is particularly associated with macrophages. The pathologic lesions consist of collections of infected macrophages, noncaseating granulomas, or caseating granulomas. The histopathologic lesions are very similar to those produced by *Mycobacterium tuberculosis,* and these two pathogens should be thought of at the same time. The intracellular yeast are often well demonstrated by hematoxylin-eosin staining (Fig. 52–21). The periodic acid–Schiff and methenamine silver techniques are more sensitive, and the silver stain is essential for demonstration of old yeast cells in healed granulomas. These yeast, presumably no longer viable, may be enlarged and distorted in morphology. The differential diagnosis of the yeast forms is

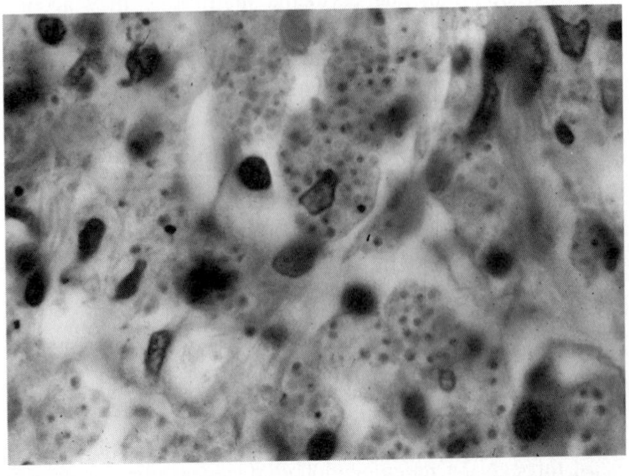

Figure 52–21. Yeast cells of *Histoplasma capsulatum* pack macrophages. The nuclei are single. Cells are separated from each other by a clear space that is an artifact of formalin fixation. The fungi were originally considered to be tissue protozoa, and the clear space was believed to be a capsule. (Hematoxylin-eosin stain.)

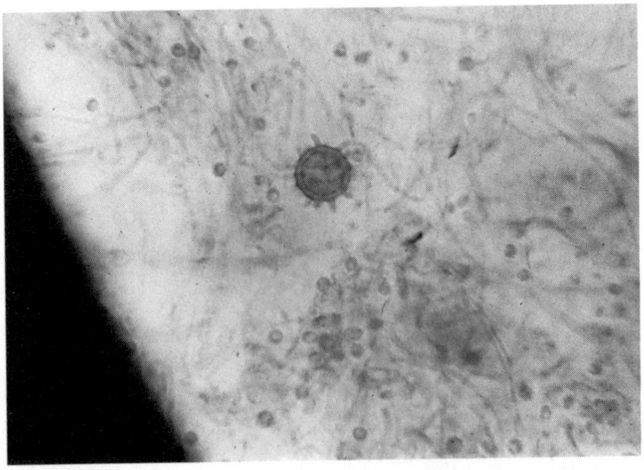

Figure 52–22. Tuberculated macroconidium of *Histoplasma capsulatum* is characteristic. Microconidia on short conidiophores are usually present also. (Lactophenol cotton blue.)

with small forms of *B. dermatitidis*. In the appropriate clinical setting, *P.* marneffei and *Leishmania* species or *Candida* spp., especially *C. glabrata*, must be considered. The larger size of *Candida* yeast cells (other than *C. glabrata*) or the clinical presentation usually suggests the proper diagnosis. The yeast of *H. capsulatum* in caseating granulomas are sufficiently distinctive to provide a presumptive diagnosis, but unusual granulomatous presentations of *Pneumocystis carinii* must be differentiated.

LABORATORY DIAGNOSIS AND EXTENT OF WORKUP. Any consideration of this major fungal pathogen must be pursued to the fullest. The yeast form in tissue may be demonstrated histologically or in preparations of respiratory secretions, fluids, peripheral blood, bone marrow, or tissue imprints. Wet preparations and Calcofluor white may be used, but the morphology of tissue and yeast cells is best seen with Giemsa's stain, because the details of nuclear morphology can be assessed. The yeast cells measure 3 μm to 5 μm in size, have a single nucleus, and bud with a narrow neck.

If disseminated infection is suspected, particularly in HIV-infected patients, blood cultures for *Histoplasma* should be performed. The Isolator technique appears to be the most sensitive technique for recovering the yeast phase from blood (Paya, 1987).

If *H. capsulatum* is suspected, an enriched agar, such as brain-heart infusion agar with a supplement of sheep blood, should be inoculated. Plates should be incubated at 30°C; incubation of primary isolation plates at 37°C is not necessary.

The colonies of *H. capsulatum* that are isolated at 25°C to 30°C are fluffy and vary from white to buff brown in color (Plate 52–7). Some strains grow rather slowly and isolates may require several weeks for colonies to develop. The diagnostic asexual forms include microconidia and macroconidia. The microconidia, which resemble lollipops on a stick, are produced first and are very similar to the structures produced by *B. dermatitidis*. The more characteristic macroconidia have roughened projections from the periphery of the conidia, a configuration referred to as tuberculate (Fig.

52–22). The macroconidia of a saprophyte, *Sepedonium*, must be differentiated from *Histoplasma*. The macroscopic appearance of the colonies, rate of growth, growth of *H. capsulatum* on media containing cycloheximide, presence of yeast forms in tissue, and the clinical history usually are sufficient to distinguish the fungi. Final confirmation of the identification is provided by conversion of the mould phase to the yeast phase at 37°C, by the exoantigen test, or by nucleic acid hybridization. Conversion to the yeast phase is sometimes exceedingly difficult and has been supplanted in many laboratories by immunologic or molecular techniques. Blood-cysteine-glucose agar or brain-heart infusion agar with sheep blood are incubated at 37°C. If the yeast phase has been demonstrated in tissue specimens, conversion of the mould *in vitro* is academic.

Serologic diagnosis of histoplasmosis has a decidedly secondary role in diagnosis and should not replace attempts to culture the fungus (Walter, 1969). Complement fixation and immunodiffusion techniques are most commonly used. The sensitivity of serodiagnosis is no greater than 50% to 85% in chronic pulmonary disease and unfortunately is much less when disseminated disease occurs in immunocompromised patients. Delayed seroconversion and extensive cross-reactions further compromise this diagnostic approach (Terry, 1978). When working in an endemic area, it was the observation of one of us (WW) that a rising complement-fixation titer to *B. dermatitidis* was an indication that the patient probably had histoplasmosis!

The histoplasmin skin test antigen has been very useful for epidemiologic studies but should never be used diagnostically. Not only does the high frequency of positive tests in endemic areas cloud the interpretation but the skin test can cause seroconversions, further confusing the issue (Campbell, 1964).

A urinary radioimmunoassay for *Histoplasma* antigen has been developed and is available from a single reference laboratory (Histoplasma Reference Laboratory, Indianapolis, IN). As discussed earlier, this test appears to be of particular use in diagnosing infections in patients with disseminated disease (Williams, 1994).

Blastomyces dermatitidis

Risk Factors

Most cases of blastomycosis are sporadic, and an environmental source is not often found. Small outbreaks do occur, and isolation of the fungus from soil at the outbreak sites has been accomplished (Klein, 1986). There are no recognized specific risk factors for blastomycosis, although severe, disseminated infection has been described in patients who are infected with HIV (Harding, 1991). Primary pulmonary blastomycosis has been described in a laboratory worker who was exposed to the mould phase (Baum, 1970).

Clinical Disease

The portal of entry is through the respiratory tract, where the infection may be asymptomatic, transient (Sarosi, 1974; Witorsch, 1968), or insidiously progressive. Chronic pulmonary blastomycosis with low-grade fever, weight loss, and localized pulmonary infiltrates may suggest neoplastic disease, for which diagnostic studies, including bronchoalveolar lavage, fine-needle aspiration of the lung, or surgical lung biopsy may be undertaken. Dissemination of yeast from the lung most commonly results in cutaneous or skeletal infection. The central nervous system and genitourinary systems are involved less frequently. The cutaneous lesions often are hypertrophic, fungating, or ulcerative, and may be locally destructive. The lesions may be mistaken for squamous cell carcinoma of the skin. Secondary involvement of the skin over bony lesions also occurs.

Pathology of Blastomycosis

The characteristic histologic response to *B. dermatitidis* is a mixture of acute inflammation, including microabscesses, and granulomatous inflammation. In cutaneous lesions, pseudoepitheliomatous hyperplasia of the epidermis overlying the inflammation is characteristic. The yeast cells are most often found in the microabscesses or within multinucleated giant cells. They can frequently be demonstrated with hematoxylin-eosin stain, but the periodic acid–Schiff or methamine silver procedures should be employed if the fungus is not demonstrated in routine sections. The thick-walled yeast cells measure 8 μm to 15 μm and maintain a broad base during the budding process. An artifactual separation of the cytoplasm from the cell wall in formalin-fixed preparations may give the erroneous appearance of a double wall. Multiple nuclei can be visualized in some yeast cells with the hematoxylin-eosin stain. Nonbudding yeast cells must be differentiated from the yeast cells of *C.* neoformans and from the developing spherules of *C. immitis*. Mucin stains occasionally may color the cell wall of *Blastomyces* slightly, but differentiation from *C. neoformans* should be possible on morphologic grounds.

Laboratory Identification and Extent of Workup

Direct demonstration of the yeast cells may be accomplished in tissue sections or in wet preparations of aspirated fluids and imprints of tissues (Fig. 52–23). Calcofluor white

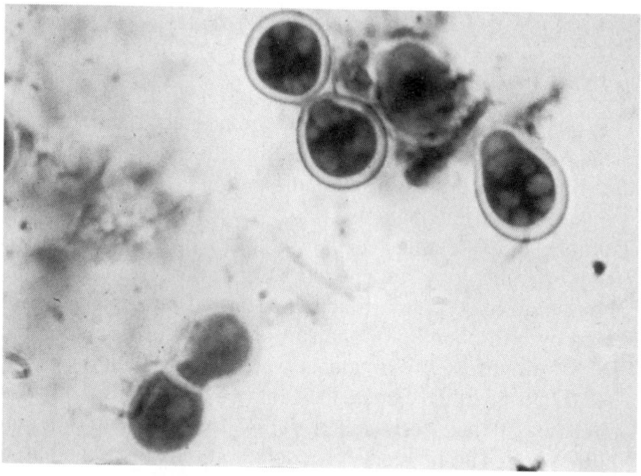

Figure 52–23. Budding yeast cells of *Blastomyces dermatitidis* have a thick wall and a broad base between the mother and daughter cells. When nuclear stains, such as hematoxylin-eosin, are applied, multiple nuclei can be demonstrated in the yeast cells. (Lactophenol cotton blue.)

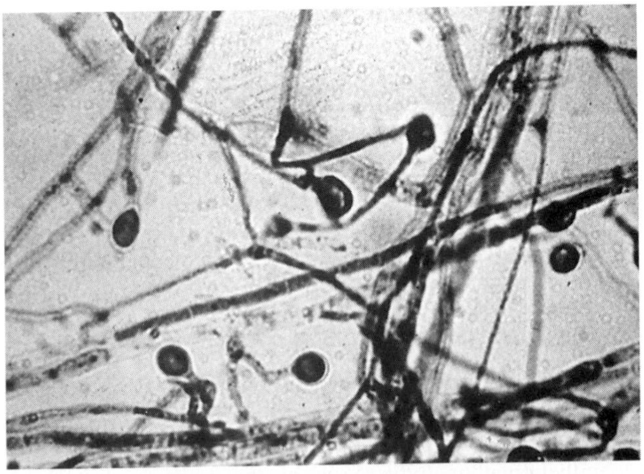

Figure 52–24. Characteristic conidium on a conidiophore (lollipop) of *Blastomyces dermatitidis*. (Lactophenol cotton blue.)

staining enhances detection of the yeast. Growth is somewhat more rapid than that of *Histoplasma* and fluffy white to buff colonies, which often cannot be distinguished from *H. capsulatum*, usually appear within one to two weeks. The microconidia resemble those of *H. capsulatum* (Fig. 52–24), but macroconidia are not formed. A saprophytic mould, *Chrysosporium*, resembles *Blastomyces*, but does not develop a yeast phase. Conversion to the yeast phase may occur on routine media incubated at 37°C, but blood-cysteine-glucose agar or cottonseed agar has been used specifically for this purpose. Once again, demonstration of the yeast form in tissue serves as a reasonable substitute for demonstration of dimorphism in the laboratory. Exoantigen tests and nucleic acid hybridization are the preferred method for confirmation of isolates in many laboratories.

The complement fixation test is the most commonly used serologic test for the diagnosis of blastomycosis. As mentioned in the discussion of histoplasmosis, this test has considerable limitations and should be used only as an adjunct to culture of the fungus.

Coccidioides immitis

Risk Factors

Residence in an endemic area is the primary risk factor for the development of infection, because the arthroconidia of the mould phase are so easily disseminated through the air (Ampel, 1989; Pappagianis, 1993; Stevens, 1995). A classic example of epidemic coccidioidomycosis occurred in a group of archeology students on a dig in northern California, who dug up more than artifacts. At least 61 students were infected by arthroconidia in the soil at the excavation site, and 77% of the infected individuals were symptomatic (Werner, 1972). In the United States, the fungus is concentrated in the Southwest. It has been called valley fever or San Joaquin Valley fever. The incidence of coccidioidomycosis increased dramatically in California during the early 1990s (Pappagianis, 1994). A prolonged drought followed by periods of rain, construction of new buildings, and increased numbers of susceptible individuals were considered possible explanations for the increase (Pappagianis, 1994). Patients with coccidioidomycosis may be encountered throughout the country, however, because of the frequency of travel and the high infectivity of the arthroconidia for individuals who enter endemic areas (Pappagianis, 1993). Cases have been described in which the infection originated from material imported from the southwestern United States. On one occasion, we recovered *C. immitis* from a dog that had traveled to Arizona. Laboratory infection is a serious risk, and this pathogen should be treated with great respect. Occasional instances in which the development of the mould phase *in vivo* produced subsequent infection have been described.

There are suggestions that genetic factors influence the frequency of severe and disseminated infection, but the nature of the association is incompletely known. Disseminated infection is more common in blacks and Filipinos than in whites. Asians, Native Americans, and Mexicans may also be at increased risk. Adult women develop erythema nodosum more commonly than men in response to primary *Coccidioides* infection, but disseminated infection occurs more commonly in adult men than in women. Immunosuppressive infection or disease is an important risk factor for disseminated infection. Patients with HIV infection are at particular risk for disseminated infection (Bronnimann, 1987; Fish, 1990; Galgani, 1990).

Clinical Disease

Primary coccidioidomycosis is most frequently asymptomatic, as indicated by the high prevalence of positive results of skin tests for the fungal antigens in endemic areas. Symptomatic disease usually is manifested as fever with cough or chest pain, or both, and it may mimic bacterial pneumonia clinically (Lopez, 1993). Erythema nodosum and erythema multiforme, which may accompany the primary infection, are good prognostic signs. Solitary pulmonary nodules may persist as consequences of the primary pulmonary infection.

Disseminated infection most commonly affects the skin, the skeletal system, and the meninges. Skin lesions include papules, ulcers, draining sinuses, and subcutaneous abscesses. Arthritis most often results from involvement of adjacent bones. The meningitis may be acute but is more commonly indolent and chronic.

Pathology of Coccidioidomycosis

The tissue response to *C. immitis* is granulomatous, with and without caseation. Developing spherules are typically found in macrophages and multinucleated giant cells. Endospores within the spherules measure 2 μm to 5 μm in size. Spherules measure 10 μm to 80 μm, and developing spherules have a large range of sizes. The differential diagnosis of developing spherules primarily includes nonbudding forms of *B. dermatitidis* or *C. neoformans*. The spherules must be differentiated from the fungal forms in adiaspiromycosis and rhinosporidiosis, both of which are very uncommon infections in the United States.

Laboratory Diagnosis and Extent of Workup

As with other dimorphic fungi, the possibility of this infection should be pursued fully. Spherules may be demonstrated in sputum or, more commonly, in bronchoalveolar lavages (Fig. 52–25), but the sensitivity of cytologic meth-

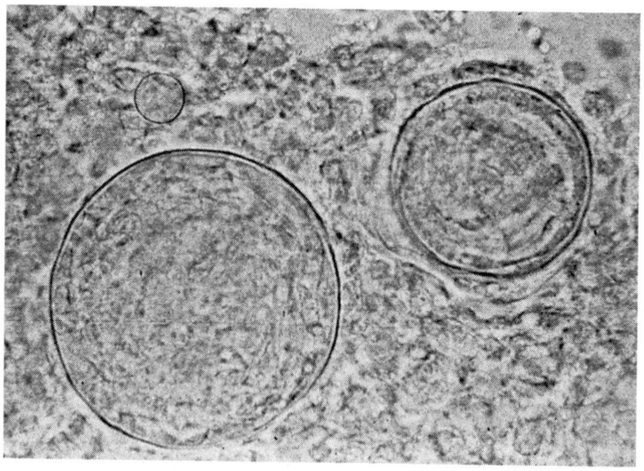

Figure 52–25. Two spherules of *Coccidioides immitis* in a sputum specimen. Unstained preparation. (Photograph courtesy of Centers for Disease Control and Prevention.)

ods is only approximately 50% (DiTomasso, 1994). Wet preparations and Calcofluor white staining are used. Digestion with 10% to 30% KOH may be necessary to eliminate distracting tissue elements. If cavitary disease is present, hyphae may be present in clinical specimens. In contrast to the other dimorphic pathogens, the possibility of communicability of arthroconidia directly from the specimen exists.

C. immitis grows relatively rapidly (less than one week) and may even appear on blood agar plates in the bacteriology laboratory. Infection of laboratory workers is a major concern, so that inoculated cultures should be handled with great care in a laminar flow safety cabinet. Suggestions about handling these specimens were discussed earlier. All work must be carried out in a laminar flow biological safety cabinet. If Petri dishes have been inoculated, they must be carefully taped to prevent accidental dislodging of the lid. The colonies of *C. immitis* are extremely variable in appearance, ranging from velvety or cottony to granular or powdery (Fig. 52–26). The colonial morphology may change as the colony develops and arthroconidia develop. Most isolates are white, but a variety of colors may be observed, and a diffusible pigment may be produced by some strains. The possibility that this biohazard may have been isolated must be considered whenever a rapidly growing mould is recovered on media that contain cycloheximide.

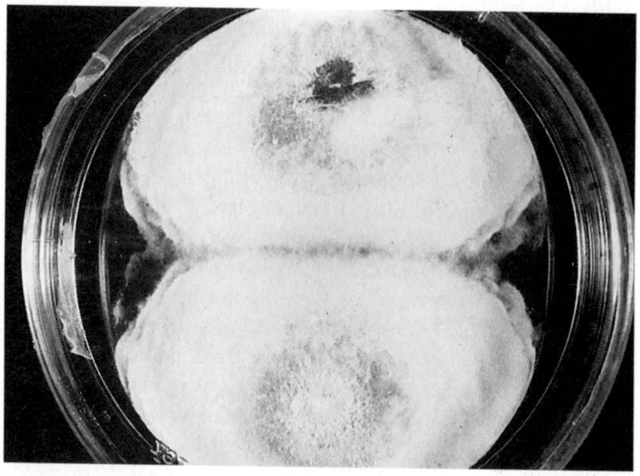

Figure 52–26. Formalin-fixed fluffy white colonies of *Coccidioides immitis* have areas of gray coloration. (Sabouraud agar with cycloheximide incubated at 30°C.)

The alternating barrel-shaped arthroconidia with empty disjunctor cells are distinctive (see Fig. 52–8) but must be differentiated from other organisms that produce arthroconidia, such as *Trichosporon* (see Fig. 52–19), *Geotrichum*, and some members of the family Gymnoascaceae. Confirmation of the identification may be accomplished by the exoantigen test or by nucleic acid hybridization.

In contrast to histoplasmosis and blastomycosis, serologic analysis with the complement fixation test is useful for assessing the extent and prognosis of coccidioidomycosis (Pappagianis, 1990). Several serologic techniques have been employed, of which complement fixation has been studied most extensively. Antibodies are detected approximately two to six weeks after infection. The height of the titer is an indication of the likelihood of disseminated disease and a rising titer bodes a poor outcome, in contrast to the usual situation in which the appearance of antibodies reflects control of the infection. Skin testing does not confound the diagnosis by producing a seroconversion, as in histoplasmosis, but the high prevalence of skin test positivity decreases the usefulness of the test. Patients with disseminated infection may demonstrate anergy to the skin test antigen.

Sporothrix schenckii

Risk Factors

S. schenckii is commonly found on vegetation throughout the world, although it does not appear to be a plant pathogen. Epidemics have been caused by exposure to plant products, such as sphagnum moss used in gardening (D'Alessio, 1965; Grotte, 1981). Fungal plant pathogens and environmental celebrations not surprisingly cross paths on occasion. Just as *H. capsulatum* participated in an Earth Day cleanup, *S. schenckii* caused infections at an Arbor Day celebration (Cote, 1988). An unusual epidemic occurred among members of a college fraternity in Florida, who were building a wall with bricks packed in contaminated straw while consuming copious amounts of beer (Sanders, 1971). The only predisposing factor that has been identified with any frequency is consumption of alcohol. Transmission of *S. schenckii* from infected cats to humans has also been reported (Reed, 1993).

Disseminated infection has been reported in immunosuppressed patients (Lynch, 1970). The portal of entry usually is traumatic entry of the fungus through the skin, as occurred with the college students whose hands were abraded by catching contaminated bricks in the so-called brick brigade. The stereotype of the patient at risk for sporotrichosis is the alcoholic rose gardener.

Clinical Disease

The overwhelmingly predominant clinical form of sporotrichosis is cutaneous and lymphocutaneous. A papule at the portal of entry may ulcerate. Spread of the pathogen through regional lymphatics may result in a series of lesions progressing up the affected limb. Systemic sporotrichosis, which is uncommon, may follow inhalation of spores into the lower respiratory tract (Pluss, 1986). The skeletal system, including both bones (Lynch, 1970) and joints (Crout, 1977), is most commonly affected.

Pathology of Sporotrichosis

The histologic responses to *Sporothrix* and *Blastomyces* are similar (Lurie, 1963). Granulomatous inflammation may be accompanied by small collections of polymorphonuclear neutrophils. In the skin, pseudoepitheliomatous hyperplasia of the epidermis is common. The yeast cells of *S. schenckii* are round or elongated and have been compared to cigars, but they are rarely seen in tissue. A tissue reaction to the fungus may result in radiating eosinophilic material up to 10 μm in thickness around the yeast cell, known as the Splendore-Hoeppli phenomenon. Unfortunately, this distinctive tissue reaction is uncommonly seen and is not specific for sporotrichosis. The differential diagnosis of the skin lesions is primarily mycobacterial infection, especially *Mycobacterium marinum* (swimming pool granuloma), in the United States and cutaneous leishmaniasis in the tropics.

Laboratory Diagnosis and Extent of Workup

The preferred specimen is a curetting or biopsy of the skin lesion. *S. schenckii* grows well on primary isolation media incubated at 25°C to 30°C. It is resistant to cycloheximide. The colonies, which may be moist or smooth (glabrous), are often light colored initially (Plate 52–8) and may turn darker with increasing age. *S.* schenckii produces thin-walled hyaline conidia and thick-walled dark conidia, which are responsible for the dark color seen macroscopically. The thin-walled microconidia are borne on conidiophores that arise at right angles from the hyphae; they may be arranged sympodially around an expanded vesicle at the tip of the conidiophore, producing an arrangement that has been described as a floret (Fig. 52–27). Similar structures are produced by *Acremonium* species, which have rarely been reported as a cause of human disease, and by an uncommonly isolated saprophyte, *Ophiostoma stenoceras*. These moulds are differentiated from *Sporothrix* by the absence of growth on cycloheximide agar and the absence of a yeast phase. Conversion of the mould phase to yeast is accomplished by incubation of the isolate at 37°C on a rich medium, such as brain-heart infusion agar or blood-cysteine-glucose agar.

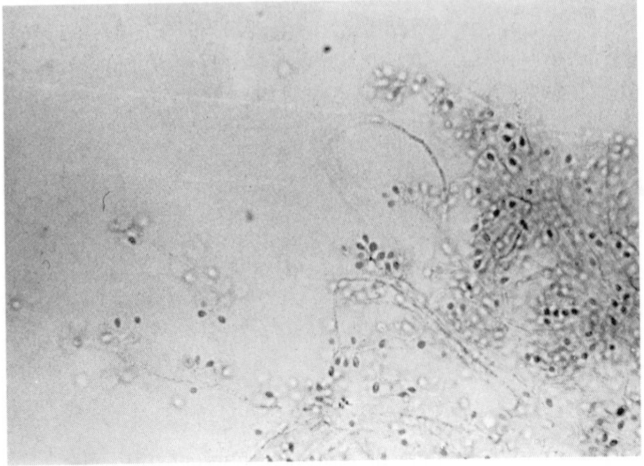

Figure 52–27. Sympodial conidia of *Sporothrix schenckii* are borne in clusters at the tips of lateral conidiophores. (Lactophenol aniline blue.)

Skin tests and serologic assays for diagnosis of sporotrichosis have been described but are not readily available.

Other Dimorphic Fungi

H. capsulatum var. *duboisii* causes cutaneous and systemic disease in Africa. The yeast are larger than those of *H. capsulatum* var. *capsulatum,* and the walls are thicker, resembling the cells of *B. dermatitidis* but without the broad-based buds. *Paracoccidioides brasiliensis* produces cutaneous, pulmonary, and disseminated infection in Central and South America (Londero, 1972; Restrepo, 1970). Imported cases of paracoccidioidomycosis occasionally occur in the United States (Murray, 1974). The characteristic yeast cells of *Paracoccidioides* have multiple peripheral buds, producing an appearance that has been compared to a mariner's wheel. *P. marneffei* infection is characterized by intracellular yeastlike cells that resemble *H. capsulatum* in macrophages. This infection is endemic in Southeast Asia, but imported cases have been described in immunocompromised patients who returned to the United States.

DERMATOPHYTES

Dermatophytic fungi are common and important causes of human morbidity, but do not produce life-threatening infection (Hay, 1992; Midgley, 1994; Odom, 1994; Weitzman, 1995). Three genera are recognized: *Microsporum*, *Trichophyton*, and *Epidermophyton*. *Acremonium* species, *Fusarium* species, and *Scopulariopsis* species occasionally have been implicated in disease of the nails (onychomycosis). As a group, the dermatophytic fungi are distributed worldwide but individual species may have more restricted geographic distribution (Aly, 1994). Dermatophytes may be found in association with humans (anthropophilic), with animals (zoophilic), or with soil (geophilic). Risk factors include contact with the relevant source of infection, which may provide a clue to the diagnosis. For instance, infection of the face in farmers who lean against their cows as they milk the animals is characteristically caused by *T. verrucosum*, a zoophilic dermatophyte that is found in cattle. The importance of geographic variation in dermatophytic pathogens is illustrated by a study of an epidemic of cutaneous fungal infection among American troops during the Vietnam war (Allen, 1973). The majority of infections were caused by a heavily sporulating variant of *T. mentagrophytes* that had not been recognized in the United States. American troops were at far greater risk of the infection than were Vietnamese. Epidemiologically, folliculitis and annular lesions of ringworm were associated with length of service in Vietnam and length of time on patrol. Infection occurred predominantly during the rainy season, and the only nonhuman source for the fungi was rats. The environmental association of the most frequently isolated dermatophytic fungi are summarized in Table 52–12.

Table 52–12. CHARACTERISTICS OF DERMATOPHYTIC MOLDS

Dermatophyte	Ecology	Rate of Growth	Diagnostic Structures	Ancillary Tests	Most Common Sites
Microsporum audouinii	Anthropophilic	Slow	Rarely observed	Wood's lamp of hair	Scalp
Microsporum canis	Zoophilic	Moderate (6–10 days)	Rough or spiny, thick-walled, spindle-shaped macroconidia with ends tapering to a knob shape; 2–14 septa; club-shaped microconidia	Wood's lamp of hair; bright lemon yellow diffusible pigment	Scalp, skin
Microsporum gypseum	Geophilic	Moderate	Smooth or finely rough, thick-walled macroconidia; 4–6 septa; club-shaped microconidia	Starburst colony; brown to cinnamon colored	Scalp, skin
Trichophyton mentagrophytes	Zoophilic varieties; Anthropophilic varieties	Moderate	Microconidia typically round and clustered on branched conidiophores (jacks, clusters of grapes); may be tear-drop shaped; macroconidia thin walled and cigar shaped	Positive hair penetration; positive urease; may occasionally produce a red pigment	Skin, scalp, beard
Trichophyton rubrum	Anthropophilic	Slow (Up to 14 days)	Lateral, tear-drop shaped microconidia ("birds on a fence"); may form on macroconidia; macroconidia longer and narrower than *Trichophyton mentagrophytes*	Intense red pigment which may be enhanced on special media such as potato flake agar; negative urease; negative hair penetration	Skin, nails
Trichophyton verrucosum	Zoophilic	Slow	Small, delicate lateral microconidia; occasional thin macroconidia (rat's tails)	Chains of conidia at 37°C; better growth on T3 agar or on T3 and T4 agar	Beard, scalp, skin
Trichophyton tonsurans	Anthropophilic	Slow	Tear-drop or club-shaped microconidia with great variation in size; Macroconidia rare	Better growth on T3 and T4 agar	Scalp, skin
Epidermophyton floccosum	Anthropophilic	Moderate	Characteristic macroconidia; no microconidia	None	Skin

Clinical Disease

Dermatophytes produce infection of the epidermis, hair, and nails (Hay, 1992). Infection of the dermis and subcutaneous tissue occurs only rarely. Infection of the hair and skin often is referred to as ringworm, a name derived from the advancing, serpiginous nature of the lesions. The clinical terminology uses the Latin name tinea followed by the body part involved, such as tinea capitis (scalp), tinea barbae (beard), tinea corporis (trunk and limbs), tinea pedis (athlete's foot), or tinea cruris (jock itch). With occasional exceptions, *Epidermophyton floccosum* infects the skin only. *Microsporum* spp. and *Trichophyton* spp. affect the scalp as well as smooth skin. *Trichophyton* spp. produce infection of the nails (tinea unguium or onychomycosis), as well as the scalp and skin. *T. tonsurans* is the most common cause of tinea capitis in the United States. *M. canis* is a common cause of scalp infection, particularly in children. When deep infection of the hair follicles occurs, a boggy inflammatory process called a kerion results; *T. mentagrophytes* and *T. verrucosum* are particularly associated with kerion. *T. mentagrophytes*, *T. rubrum*, and *M. canis* are commonly found in tinea corporis and tinea pedis. The lesions produced by *T. rubrum* are often chronic and intractable. *E. floccosum* is a common cause of tinea cruris and tinea pedis.

Laboratory Diagnosis and Extent of Workup

Treatment of dermatophyte infections is not directed by the specific identification of the isolate, so that preliminary demonstration of hyphae in skin scrapings is important for initiation of therapy (Fig. 52–28). The size and morphology of hyphae suggest the involvement of dermatophytes in the infection. Confirmation of the specific identification often is not essential but is useful for confirming that the hyphae did, in fact, belong to a dermatophytic fungus, for assessing the probable source of the infection, and for assessing the increased likelihood for chronic, relapsing infections when *T.*

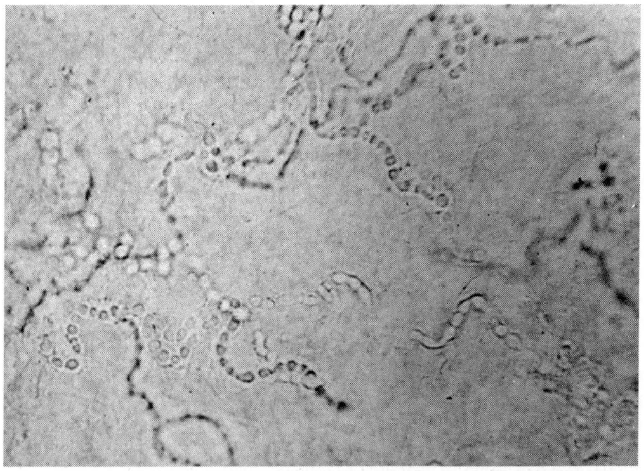

Figure 52–28. Hyphae of a dermatophyte are demonstrated in a scraping from the edge of a tinea lesion. The presence of these thin-segmented hyphae in this clinical setting establishes the diagnosis of dermatomycosis but does not define the specific etiology. (KOH preparation.) (Photograph courtesy of Centers for Disease Control and Prevention.)

rubrum is isolated. Skin scrapings, nails, and hairs can be examined in KOH preparations, which may incorporate Calcofluor for facilitation of detection of hyphae. Tissue fragments, fibers, and cholesterol crystals may be mistaken for hyphae by the inexperienced observer.

Infected hairs should be selected for analysis. When the infecting fungus is *M. audouinii*, *M. canis*, or *M. ferrugineum*, the hairs fluoresce with a long-wavelength ultraviolet light (Wood's lamp). *M. canis* is the only member of this trio of pathogens that is isolated commonly in the United States. Microscopic examination of the relationship of the fungus to the infected hair can be used to narrow the differential diagnosis of the etiologic agent: spores external to the hair shaft (ectothrix); spores within the hair shaft (endothrix); hyphae without spores within the hair (favid); or no invasion of hair shaft. Analysis of infected hairs requires considerable experience and regular practice.

Infected hairs, scrapings of nails, or scrapings of the edges of skin lesions should be submitted to the laboratory in a clean, dry container or placed on the surface of primary isolation medium supplied by the laboratory. Grinding of nail clippings in a homogenizer has been suggested as a means of increasing the yield of dermatophytes. Sabouraud dextrose agar was designed for recovery of dermatophytic fungi and is also effective for isolating *Candida* spp., especially *C. albicans*, which may produce similar infections of skin and nails. Dermatophytes are not inhibited by cycloheximide, which will inhibit many saprophytic fungi. Dermatophyte test medium, which produces a red pigment on alkalinization, is commonly used by dermatologists to demonstrate the presence of a dermatophyte, which is often not studied any further. Unfortunately, dermatophyte test medium is not specific for dermatophytes. Other organisms, including *H. capsulatum*, may alkalinize this medium and it is not the preferred isolation medium for clinical laboratories.

All dermatophytic fungi have septate, hyaline hyphae. They produce macroconidia and microconidia in various combinations. Arthroconidia and chlamydospores may be produced, but the morphology of the macroconidia and especially the microconidia are more important for identification. The sexual stage of many of the dermatophytes have been identified, but they are not encountered in the clinical laboratory.

Microsporum species

Microsporum species produce characteristic macroconidia, which are the key diagnostic structures. In some cases, microconidia, which are not as useful diagnostically, are produced. *M. audouinii*, a classic anthropophilic agent of ringworm, produces diagnostic structures poorly or not at all. Fortunately, it is not frequently isolated at present, perhaps because of increased standards of hygiene. The characteristics of the diagnostic structures produced by the most common pathogens are summarized in Table 52–12. *M. canis*, the most frequently isolated species, produces a characteristic lemon yellow pigment (Plate 52–9), which is intensified by growth on potato flake agar. The macroconidia of this species are illustrated in Figure 52–29. The macroconidia of *M. gypseum*, the most commonly isolated geophilic species, are illustrated in Figure 52–30.

Trichophyton species

The genus *Trichophyton* includes the important dermatophytic fungi: *T. tonsurans* (see Figs. 52–10 and Plate 52–10), *T. rubrum* (Plate 52–11), *T. verrucosum*, and *T. mentagrophytes* (Plate 52–12 and Fig. 52–31). The colonies may have a fluffy, granular, or less commonly, glabrous appearance. Macroconidia, which are extremely useful for identification, may be produced by this genus, especially in strains that produce powdery colonies, but unfortunately they usually are absent. Microconidia are formed more commonly. The macroconidia are thin-walled, smooth, and contain variable numbers of septa. The classic appearance of the diagnostic structures in the most commonly isolated species is summarized in Table 52–12. In the real world, interpretation of the microscopic morphology in some isolates can be very difficult, because overlap occurs frequently. Fortunately, additional tests are useful for making specific differentiations within the genus (see Table 52–12). In particular, the *Trichophyton* agars are helpful

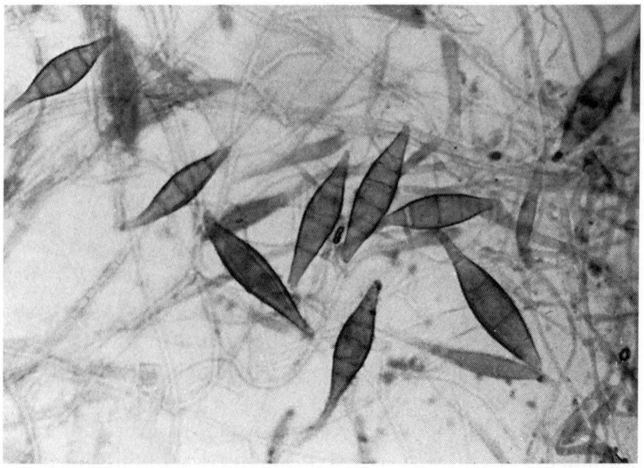

Figure 52–29. Thick-walled, roughened, tapered, spindle-shaped macroconidia of *Microsporum canis* and thin-segmented hyphae. (Lactophenol aniline blue.)

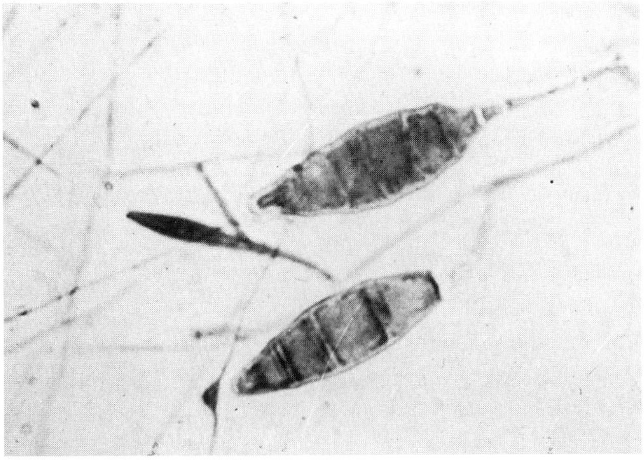

Figure 52–30. Thick-walled, smooth macroconidia of *Microsporum gypseum*. (Lactophenol cotton blue.)

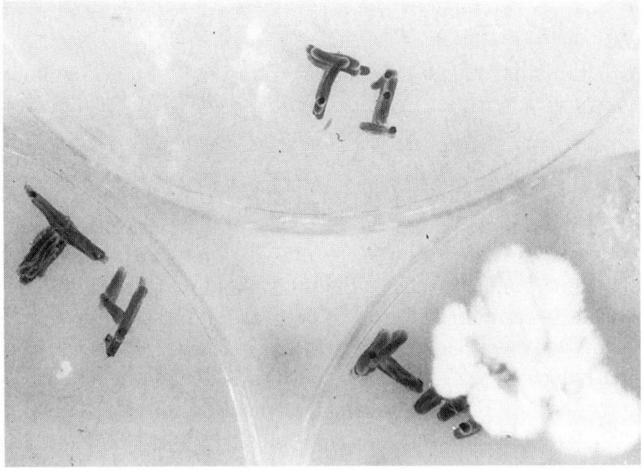

Figure 52–32. *Trichophyton* agars. Growth of *Trichophyton tonsurans* is enhanced on T_3 agar (contains thiamine and inositol) in comparison with T_1 and T_4 agars.

in the characterization of nutritional requirements among members of the genus (Fig. 52–32). Seven media have been described, of which we have found the first four casamino acid–based media to be the most useful. In combination, these media allow the assessment of dependency on inositol, thiamine, or both compounds together.

Medium	Constituents	Interpretation of Stimulated Growth
T1	Basal medium	Agar to which other formulations are compared
T2	Inositol	Stimulated by inositol alone
T3	Inositol + Thiamine	Stimulated only when both compounds present
T4	Thiamine	Stimulated by thiamine alone

Differentiation of *T. mentagrophytes* and *T. rubrum* is facilitated by several nonmorphologic tests (see Table 52–12). A diffusible pigment may be produced by both species, but the intensely red pigment of *T. rubrum* is encouraged by culture on potato flake agar or cornmeal agar with 1% dextrose. Production of urease within three to five days by *T. mentagrophytes* but not by *T. rubrum* helps differentiate these two species. Finally, the hair penetration test can be used as a differential test. *T. mentagrophytes* produces wedge-shaped defects in hairs *in vitro* (Fig. 52–33), whereas *T. rubrum* grows on the outside of the hair without penetrating it. Use of both morphologic and nonmorphologic approaches provide the most accurate identification of isolates. Perhaps the most important factor is that sufficient isolates are encountered to provide ongoing experience with the diagnostic features of these moulds.

Epidermophyton floccosum

The only pathogen within the genus *Epidermophyton* is an anthropophilic fungus that is an important cause of tinea cruris and athlete's foot. Colonies, which are initially brownish yellow, gray, or khaki brown, become velvety and folded as they mature. *E. floccosum* produces no microconidia, but distinctive macroconidia provide the clues to the identification (see Fig. 52–11). These structures have smooth external walls, up to four cross-walls, and a club shape.

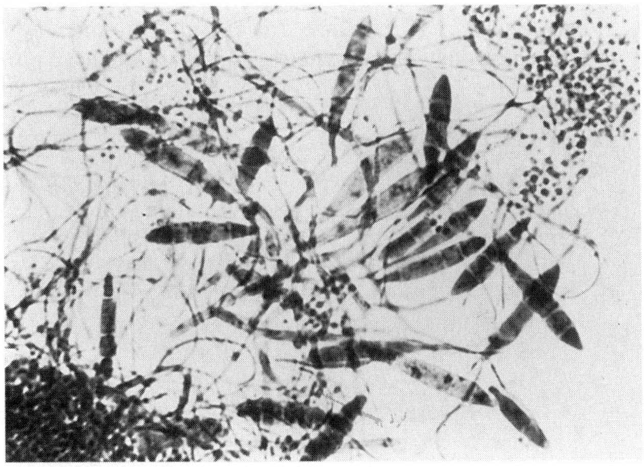

Figure 52–31. Clusters of microconidia and thin-walled macroconidia of *Trichophyton mentagrophytes*. (Lactophenol cotton blue.) (Photograph courtesy of Centers for Disease Control and Prevention.)

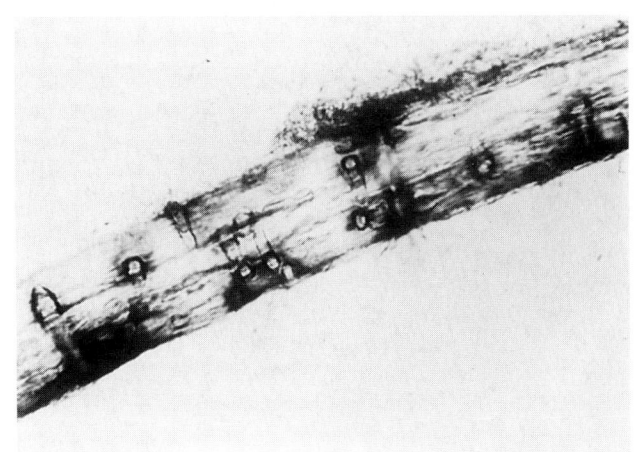

Figure 52–33. Hair penetration by *Trichophyton mentagrophytes*. The hair is penetrated by the hyphae from the sides. (Photograph courtesy of Centers for Disease Control and Prevention.)

6

DEMATIACEOUS MOULDS

The dematiaceous moulds are a fascinating and complex group of fungi that produce debilitating disease of the skin and subcutaneous tissue and may invade deeply. The infections are most commonly found in the tropics and subtropics, although disseminated infection may be encountered rarely in the United States, especially among severely immunocompromised patients. The classification of these moulds has undergone changes as the understanding of conidiogenesis has been refined (Larone, 1989). A brief review of clinical forms of disease produced by pathogenic species is presented, but a detailed description of the mycology is beyond the scope of this chapter. The morphology of *Cladosporium* species, common saprophytic moulds that are encountered frequently in clinical laboratories, is illustrated in Plate 52–2 and Fig. 52–34. Slow growth and growth in the presence of cycloheximide are clues that a pathogenic species may have been isolated. It is important to discuss with clinicians the clinical features of the case before dismissing these moulds as insignificant.

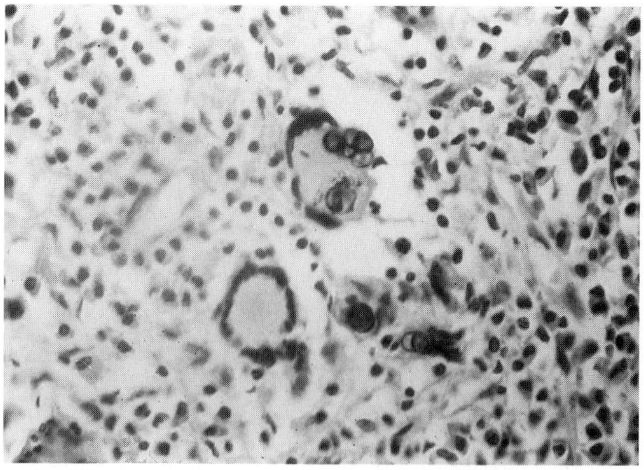

Figure 52–35. Muriform bodies of a dematiaceous fungus in a lesion of chromoblastomycosis. The darkly pigmented cells are undergoing septation. Macrophages and multinucleated giant cells are present in the lesion. (Hematoxylin-eosin stain.)

Clinical Disease

Mycetoma is a chronic, indolent infection of skin and soft tissue that develops at the site of inoculation of a variety of fungi and bacteria. The infection may extend deeply, even involving bone, and draining sinuses often develop. The infection is encountered most frequently in the tropics and subtropics, but may be encountered in the southern United States. *Madurella mycetomatis* is the most common dematiaceous pathogen. Similar lesions may be produced by other fungi (e.g., *Acremonium*, *Pseudallescheria boydii*, *Fusarium*), by aerobic actinomycetes (*Nocardia*, *Streptomyces*, *Actinomadura*), and occasionally, by bacteria (botryomycosis).

Chromoblastomycosis is a chronic, slowly progressive infection of the skin and subcutaneous tissue that occurs primarily in patients living in the tropics. Cases occasionally occur in the southern United States. Lesions may be single or multiple and may resemble the cutaneous lesions of blastomycosis. The distinguishing feature is the presence of round, nonhyphal, brown cells (muriform bodies) in tissues (Fig. 52–35). These structures, which divide by septation, are diagnostic of the entity but do not provide a clue as to the identification of the mould. The etiologic agents of chromoblastomycosis are *Phialophora verrucosa*, *Fonsecaea pedrosoi*, *Fonsecaea compacta*, *Rhinocladiella aquaspersa*, *Cladosporium carrionii*, *E. jeanselmei*, and *E. spinifera*.

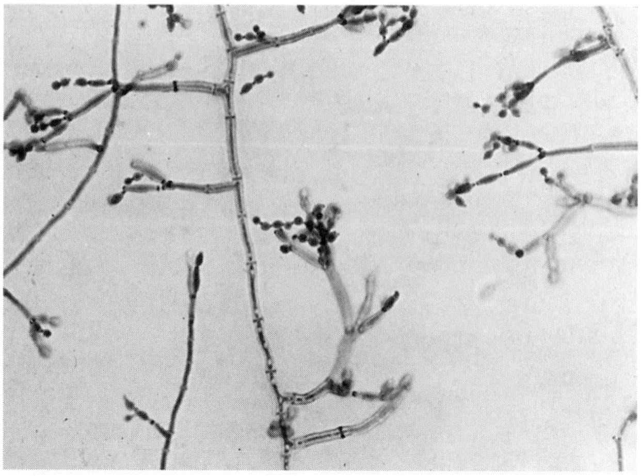

Figure 52–34. Chains of conidia produced by *Cladosporium* species, a common environmental isolate in the clinical laboratory. The hyphae are septate. Both hyphae and conidia are darkly pigmented. (Lactophenol aniline blue.)

Phaeohyphomycosis is a term used to describe infection of cutaneous and subcutaneous tissue and systemic organs, particularly the central nervous system. These infections range from indolent subcutaneous lesions, probably resulting from direct inoculation of fungi at the site, to devastating, destructive infection that is almost always fatal. The most frequent isolates have been *E. jeanselmei*, *W. dermatitidis*, *Cladosporium bantianum* (*trichoides*), *Fonsecaea* species, and *Bipolaris* species. A distinctive clinical entity is chronic sinusitis in which the hyphae may be contained within the sinuses or, less commonly, extend through the bony walls to invade adjacent tissue. *Bipolaris* spp., *Curvularia* spp., and *Alternaria* spp. are among the dematiaceous species that have produced this infection. Dematiaceous fungi are rare causes of keratomycosis.

The diagnostic feature of phaeohyphomycosis is a brown melanin pigmentation of the hyphae. The color usually can be discerned in stained tissue sections but may be demonstrated to better advantage in unstained sections. Poorly pigmented strains may be recognized by the application of a stain for melanin, such as the Fontana-Masson technique.

ZYGOMYCETES

The zygomycetes are important causes of invasive fungal infection in compromised hosts (Williams, 1976). The most common pathogen is *Rhizopus*. Other moulds that have been implicated in human disease include *Absidia*, *Rhizomucor*,

Mucor, and *Cunninghamella* (Bergman, 1969). The invasive disease caused by these fungi has historically been called mucormycosis. Especially in view of the fact that *Mucor* species are uncommon causes of infections, a better clinical term is zygomycosis.

Risk Factors and Clinical Disease

There are two common clinical presentations of zygomycosis, and the risk factors are somewhat different between the two (Straatsma, 1962). An invasive infection that begins in the paranasal sinuses is known either as rhinocerebral or craniofacial zygomycosis. The infection begins as an undifferentiated sinusitis, but the hyphae rapidly break through the thin walls of the sinus and extend up into the orbit, forward into the skin of the face, and back and up into the cranial cavity. The risk factor for this type of infection is predominantly diabetes mellitus, and most patients are experiencing ketoacidosis at the time the infection develops (McNulty, 1982). Rhinocerebral disease may progress rapidly, and death often results. Thrombosis of the carotid artery or cavernous sinus may occur.

The second major presentation of zygomycosis is pulmonary disease, which may be followed by hematogenous dissemination. The infection begins as an undifferentiated pneumonia, which may be complicated by hemoptysis and cavitation. Dissemination of the infection is common and the outcome is almost uniformly fatal. The risk factors for pulmonary infection are neutropenia and immunosuppression, particularly by hematologic malignancy (Meyer, 1972). Additional factors that have been noted are iron overload, intravenous drug abuse, and uremia (Kwon-Chung, 1992). Diabetes with ketoacidosis is present in some patients.

A less common presentation of zygomycosis is infection of skin and soft tissues (Meyer, 1973a). The hyphae may reach the skin by the hematogenous route, by direct extension from a deep focus, or by introduction from the outside. A dramatic outbreak of soft tissue disease occurred in patients who were treated with occlusive bandages that were contaminated with *Rhizopus* spores (Gartenberg, 1978). Before the potential for infection was realized, the manufacturer did not take steps to ensure the sterility of the bandages. Burn wounds and other types of traumatic injury also provide sites for injury of these common environmental fungi (Cocanour, 1992).

Limited pulmonary infection with cavitation is an unusual presentation of zygomycosis in immunologically competent individuals (Record, 1976).

Pathology of Zygomycete Infection

The histopathology is dominated by necrosis of tissue, regardless of the site of infection (Straatsma, 1962). The propensity for these moulds to invade through the walls of arteries and veins, producing acute thrombosis, leads to extensive coagulative necrosis. The hyphae appear as ribbons of broad hyphae that are often twisted and collapsed (see Fig. 52–3). Septa are sparse and usually are not observed in tissue, but an overlay of the exterior walls of collapsed hyphae may be mistaken for septa. Swollen segments of hyphae and hyphae cut in cross-section may be incorrectly interpreted as yeast cells. Branching tends to occur at right angles. The hyphae of these moulds often stain better with hematoxylin-eosin dyes than with the periodic acid–Schiff technique or even the methenamine silver method.

Laboratory Diagnosis and Extent of Workup

Zygomycetes often are considered common contaminants (Kwon-Chung, 1992), but they are infrequently encountered in our clinical laboratory. The potential clinical implications of isolates should be carefully investigated before they are dismissed as saprophytes. Demonstration of hyphae in tissue is more significant than simple recovery of the mould in culture. The broad, sparsely septate hyphae may be demonstrated in tissue sections or in imprint smears of tissue, using the Calcofluor white stain. Tissue should be minced or teased, rather than homogenized, after which it is inoculated onto the surface of a primary isolation agar. Zygomycetes are inhibited by cycloheximide. Isolates grow rapidly and produce abundant aerial hyphae that rapidly reach the lid of the Petri dish. Zygomycetes produce sexual zygospores *in vitro*, but the asexual reproductive structures are most useful for identification. Identification to species is difficult and is not necessary for most clinical purposes.

Rhizopus species

Rhizopus grows rapidly, filling the Petri dish within 48 to 72 hours with white, wooly hyphae, turning gray to black as spores develop (Fig. 52–36). The diagnostic sporangia are best found at the edge or in the center of the culture, where they may be visible as black dots. The hyphae are broad (6 μm to 15 μm in diameter), rarely septate, and hyaline, but the stolons may appear light brown near the origin of rhizoids and sporangiophores. The sporangiophores are unbranched and support round sporangia (60 μm to 350 μm) with an ellipsoidal columella. The sporangiospores (5 μμm) are oval or rhomboidal and may have a brown pigment (see Fig. 52–5).

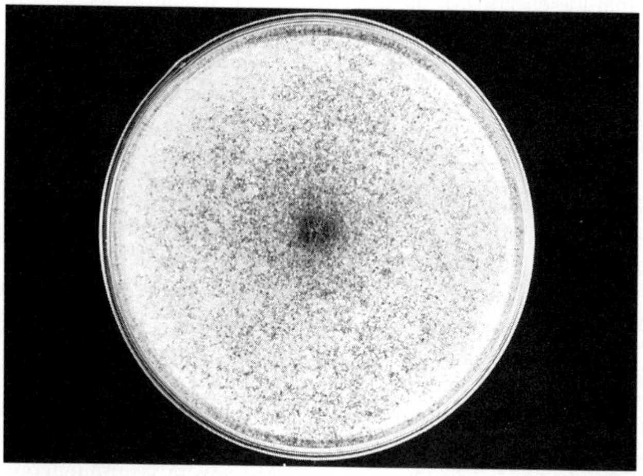

Figure 52–36. A fluffy gray colony of *Rhizopus* species fills the space within the Petri dish (lid lifter). (Photograph courtesy of Centers for Disease Control and Prevention.)

6

An important diagnostic feature is the presence of hyaline to brown rootlike structures (rhizoids), which develop at the point where the sporangiophores arise (see Fig. 52–5). It has been reported that 60% of cases of zygomycosis and 90% of cases of rhinocerebral disease are caused by *Rhizopus arrhizus* (quoted in Kwon-Chung, 1992).

Other Zygomycetes

In contrast to *Rhizopus*, the rhizoids of *Absidia* species arise from the stolons between conidiophores. The sporangiophores are pear shaped rather than round, and a collarette is visible around the columella when the sporangium disintegrates. *Mucor* species do not produce stolons nor rhizoids. The conidiophores usually are more branched than are other zygomycetes, and growth does not occur above 37°C. *Rhizomucor*, which is morphologically intermediate between *Rhizopus* and *Mucor*, has rudimentary rhizoids and branched conidiophores, and grows at temperatures as high as 58°C. One of the primary pathogens in the genus *Mucor (Mucor pusillus)* has been transferred to the genus *Rhizomucor*. *Cunninghamella* produces swollen vesicles at the tips of conidiophores. From the vesicles, multiple single-celled sporangiola arise on short stalks (denticles).

SEPTATE HYALINE MOULDS (HYPHOMYCETES)

This large group of saprophytic fungi is frequently encountered in the clinical laboratory and contains some of the most important pathogenic moulds. In this section, we consider *Aspergillus* and *Fusarium*. *Pseudallescheria boydii*, the most common pathogen in that genus, has an asexual phase called *Scedosporium apiospermum*, and the mould may be isolated in either form. The common saprophyte, *Penicillium* species, is described. As with other fungi, any members of this large group can be pathogenic under the appropriate clinical conditions. Careful clinical correlation should be attempted before dismissing isolates from tissues and fluids as contaminants. On the other hand, it is a mistake to accept uncritically the isolation of an uncommon pathogen as evidence that the etiology of the infection has been determined. Multiple isolation of the mould is useful, and definitive documentation of pathogenicity requires pathologic correlation.

Risk Factors

The hyphomycetes are ubiquitous fungi to which all of us are exposed on a regular basis. They are resident in vegetation of all types. *Aspergillus fumigatus* is present in composted leaves, and allergic disease has occurred in patients who were exposed to compost piles (Kramer, 1989). *A. fumigatus* and *A. niger* were isolated from a plant in the room of a patient with aspergillosis (quoted in Kwon-Chung, 1992), and outbreaks have been linked to hospital construction (Arnow, 1978; Sherertz, 1987). It is probably prudent, therefore, to restrict exposure of the most severely immunocompromised patients. In one epidemiologic study, there were no cases of invasive aspergillosis in 39 patients who resided in rooms with HEPA-filtered air, whereas there were 14 invasive infections in 74 similar patients who were in conventional rooms (Sherertz, 1987).

The most important risk factors for invasive infection by hyphomycetes are immunosuppressive disease or chemotherapy (Scherr, 1992; Walker, 1978; Williams, 1976). Neutropenia also is a prominent predisposing factor (Young, 1989). It is important to recognize, however, that serious invasive disease may occur in individuals who are not immunosuppressed by chemotherapy or malignancy (Rosenberg, 1982; Smith, 1982). Invasive disease in entirely normal individuals is rare, however. Superficial local infections, which may extend to underlying structures or disseminate to distant organs, may follow surgery (Stern, 1986) or use of medications, especially corticosteroids, either by local injection or topical application. Wound infection has been a problem in patients with extensive burn wounds and in individuals who are exposed to materials contaminated with conidia, a situation reminiscent of the zygomycetes (McCarty, 1986). Fungus balls in the lung occur in patients with chronic obstructive lung disease, bronchiectasis, and old cavities caused by tuberculosis.

Clinical Disease

Ocular and Otic Infections

Keratomycosis usually follows trauma to the eye, especially in patients who have been treated with topical steroids. Pain and blurring of vision follow the traumatic episode, and if it is not treated, the infection may extend into the anterior chamber. Enucleation may be necessary if the process is not checked. *A. fumigatus* (Gingrich, 1962) and *Fusarium solani* are common etiologic agents (Liesegang, 1980). Otomycosis is an infection of the external ear, usually caused by *A. niger* or *A. fumigatus*. Pain, decreased hearing, and a discharge are accompanied by a fluffy green or black growth in the ear canal. Extension beyond the external ear is rare (Phillips, 1990) but may occur in immunosuppressed patients.

Fungus Balls

The two most common sites for this infection are the paranasal sinuses and cavities in the lung (Dar, 1984; Meyer, 1994). In the sinuses, the signs and symptoms are those of chronic sinusitis. Pulmonary fungus balls are often asymptomatic but may result in hemoptysis (Conlan, 1987). Invasion through the walls of the paranasal sinuses is the most serious complication of upper airway disease and is of particular concern with HIV-infected patients (Meyer, 1994). Endobronchial colonization also occurs in patients with chronic obstructive lung disease and in patients with cystic fibrosis who may have bronchiectasis (Gilligan, 1991; Nelson, 1979). *A. fumigatus* is the most common mould isolate from patients with cystic fibrosis, but we have encountered other moulds, such as *Penicillium* species, *Paecilomyces* species, and *S. apiospermum*. The clinical course of most patients with cystic fibrosis does not appear to be modified by the presence of *Aspergillus* in their lungs, but allergic bronchopulmonary aspergillosis has been described in a portion of these individuals who develop hypersensitivity to fungal antigens (Nelson, 1979). *A. fumigatus* and *A. niger* are common moulds found in pulmonary fungus balls. *A. fumigatus*, *A. flavus*, and *Fusarium* spp., as well as dematiaceous fungi, are commonly found in the paranasal sinuses.

Allergic bronchopulmonary aspergillosis is a complication in patients who have an allergic diathesis (Ahmad, 1984; Golbert, 1970). Hyphae colonize the lower respiratory tract but do not invade tissue. Detection of precipitating antibodies in serum is useful, but some investigators do not consider the commercially available reagents satisfactory (Kwon-Chung, 1992). The clinical manifestations include asthma, pulmonary infiltrates, and ultimately pulmonary fibrosis in some patients. *Aspergillus* spp. are the most common inciting agents. A similar process can involve the paranasal sinuses (Katzenstein, 1983).

Pulmonary Infection and Invasive Disease

Pneumonia may be difficult to differentiate from bacterial processes, but cough and sputum production frequently are less pronounced than in most bacterial pneumonias (Mehta, 1984). Progression to cavitation and lack of response to antibiotics are clues that fungal infection should be considered. Repetitive isolation of the same mould from clinical specimens increases the likelihood that the fungus is either a colonizer or invasive pathogen rather than a laboratory contaminant. Definition of the infectious process requires careful clinical correlation and often morphologic study of tissue specimens.

Dissemination from the lung or other sites may involve any organ (Meyer, 1973b). The propensity of hyphae to invade vascular structures and cause thrombosis leads to infarcts and abscesses in multiple organs. *A. fumigatus* and *A. flavus* are the most frequently isolated species, but other species of *Aspergillus*, such as *A. terreus,* also produce pneumonia and disseminated infection (Tritz, 1993). *A. niger* is rarely found in invasive disease. *Pseudallescheria boydii* and *Fusarium* spp. are the hyaline moulds next most frequently encountered in invasive disease, but virtually any fungus can produce disseminated infection if the clinical and environmental conditions are right.

Pathology of Hyphomycete Infection

The histologic response to these agents may be granulomatous but is more commonly dominated by polymorphonuclear neutrophils unless the patient is severely neutropenic. Vascular invasion, thrombosis, and infarction often are prominent features. The hyphae are thin (2 μm to 5 μm), septate, and branch at acute angles (dichotomous) (see Fig. 52–2). Hematoxylin-eosin stains often color the hyphae well, but the morphology may be demonstrated to advantage with the periodic acid–Schiff or methenamine silver techniques. It is important to recognize that it is impossible to identify the mould by the morphology of the hyphae. *Dichotomously branching, thin, septate hyphae do not always equal Aspergillus!*

When the pathologic process is a fungus ball, the hyphae, which are presumably dead, may stain poorly with all stains. When the cavity is in contact with air, as in the lung or sinuses, fruiting heads may develop, an event that does allow

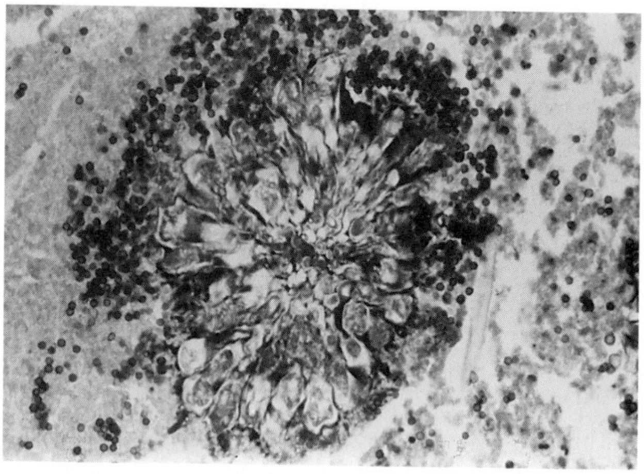

Figure 52–37. A fruiting head of *Aspergillus niger* is demonstrated within a pulmonary mycetoma (fungus ball). The phialides and conidia are well demonstrated. Although the hyphae of *Aspergillus* are not etiologically diagnostic, demonstration of the fruiting head documents the presence of this genus. (Hematoxylin-eosin stain.)

the assignment of a specific genus, such as *Aspergillus* (Fig. 52–37). The conidiophores, which are not septate and may be wider than the vegetative hyphae, should not be confused with zygomycetes. Thick-walled Hülle cells and cleistothecia have been described *in vivo*. Oxalate crystals, demonstrable with polarizing filters, may be found in fungus balls produced by *A. niger* (Louthrenoo, 1990; Staib, 1979).

When the patient is immunocompetent and the histologic response is granulomatous, the hyphae may be fragmented and confined to the cytoplasm of macrophages and multinucleated giant cells (Ahmad, 1981). The granulomatous response to *Aspergillus* in the lung may be mistaken for bronchocentric granulomatosis (Bosken, 1988; Nagata, 1990), usually in patients who have allergic disease. Impacted mucus with eosinophils and Charcot-Leyden crystals are common in allergic aspergillosis (Bosken, 1988). Allergic *Aspergillus* infection of the paranasal sinuses resembles bronchopulmonary disease (Katzenstein, 1983).

Laboratory Diagnosis and Extent of Workup

These moulds are saprophytic fungi, some of which are commonly isolated in clinical laboratories. They should never be dismissed as contaminants, however, without determining the clinical situation. Isolation from a sterile site or repeated isolation merits a phone call to the clinician. Hyphae may be demonstrated directly in clinical specimens in imprint preparations or wet preparations. Calcofluor white again is useful for demonstrating the mould. The presence of hyphae in a specimen is always more significant than isolation of the mould alone. In respiratory secretions, however, even demonstration of the hyphae does not define the nature of the interaction between host and fungus. Careful clinical correlation and sometimes biopsy is necessary for the final determination.

It is important to obtain tissue, fluid, scrapings, or curettings for examination, with the possible exception of *Aspergillus* otomycosis. Tissue should be teased or minced and inoculated directly onto the surface of the isolation medium. These moulds grow rapidly, but most are inhibited by cycloheximide to some extent.

The specific identification of *Aspergillus* species is made by study of

Color of the colony
Morphology of the conidial head
Number and arrangement of phialides and metulae
Morphology of conidiophores
Presence and shape of Hülle cells
Presence of cleistothecia

The color and morphology of *Aspergillus* species is properly studied on Czapek-Dox agar.

The reverse of the colonies of hyphomycetes are light colored, but may have yellow, brown, or red pigmentation. Vegetative hyphae are thin, septate, and dichotomously branching. The colonies of many of these moulds teem with conidia. To prevent contamination of the worker and other cultures, the colonies should be manipulated carefully in a laminar flow biological safety cabinet, after which the surfaces of the safety cabinet should be thoroughly wiped with a fungicidal solution.

As mentioned earlier, detection of antibodies to *Aspergillus* species may be useful diagnostically, especially for allergic bronchopulmonary aspergillosis (Kurup, 1991).

Aspergillus fumigatus

A. fumigatus is one of the most common, if not the most common, isolate in mycology laboratories. The colonies grow rapidly, producing a fluffy appearance. The development of fruiting head imparts a blue-green appearance to the colony (see Plate 52–1). Examination of the colony with a dissecting microscope reveals the conidiophores with their expanded vesicles as small globes projecting above the vegetative mycelium. The conidiophore is smooth, relatively short (300 μm to 500 μm), and expanded into a flask-shaped vesicle. The phialides develop in a single row (uniseriate), and most commonly develop only on the upper portion of the vesicle parallel to the axis of the conidiophore (see Fig. 52–7). The conidia are roughened (echinulate) and round to oval in shape.

Aspergillus flavus

The second most important pathogen in the genus *Aspergillus* is *A. flavus*. The colonies grow rapidly and have a velvety yellow to green appearance once fruiting heads develop (Plate 52–13). The conidiophore is long (400 μm to 700 μm), ending in a vesicle that may be elliptical or round. The conidiophore is rough and stubbly. A single or double (biseriate) row of phialides occurs over the whole vesicle or the upper three quarters (Fig. 52–38). Round to oval conidia appear yellow-green *en masse* and measure 3 μm to 4.5 μm. Oval to round hard resting structures (sclerotia) are found in the vegetative hyphae of some isolates.

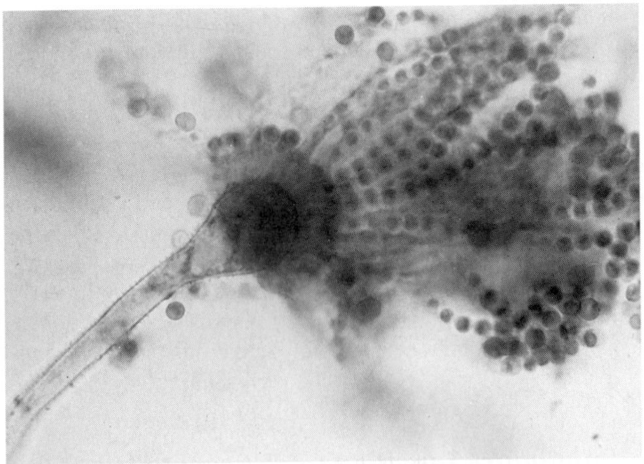

Figure 52–38. The fruiting head of *Aspergillus flavus* is uniseriate and biseriate. The phialides extend around much of the vesicle. The roughened appearance of the conidiophore can be seen. (Lactophenol aniline blue.)

Aspergillus niger

This common saprophyte is frequently isolated from the external ear canal. It has a dramatic colonial appearance with its black fruiting heads against a background of snow white vegetative mycelium (producing a salt and pepper appearance) (Plate 52–14 and Fig. 52–39). The conidiophores are smooth and long (1.5 mm to 3.0 mm), supporting a rounded vesicle with biseriate phialides, which radiate out from the entire vesicle. The brown, roughened conidia are round and measure 4 μm. Sclerotia may be present.

Other *Aspergillus* species

The *A. glaucus* group consists of rapidly growing moulds, colored green with yellow patches. The conidiophores are smooth and the phialides uniseriate. Cleistothecia are commonly present (see Fig. 52–11). *Aspergillus terreus* produces a cinnamon brown colony, short conidiophores (<250

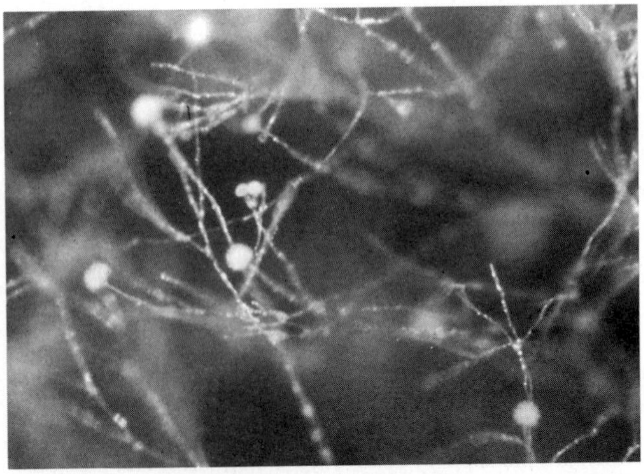

Figure 52–39. The fruiting heads of *Aspergillus niger* are demonstrated with a dissecting microscope. Unstained preparation.

μm), and biseriate phialides. *A. nidulans* produces green to dark olive colonies, wavy short conidiophores (< 150 μm), and biseriate phialides. Formation of the cleistothecia of the sexual stage is enhanced by culture on Czapek-Dox agar. The cleistothecia, which measure 100 μm to 300 μm, are round and reddish brown. They are surrounded by a yellowish brown layer of hyphae that contains round Hülle cells.

Fusarium species

This genus is increasingly implicated in keratomycosis, burn wounds, and invasive disease in immunocompromised patients (Anaissie, 1992; Nelson, 1995; Wheeler, 1981). The colonies develop rapidly, producing a fluffy aerial mycelium, which often has a pink, lavender, or salmon color. Diffusible pigments may be seen in the surrounding agar. Simple or branched phialides develop directly from the hypha without a separate conidiophore. Short oval microconidia may be produced, but the distinctive structure is a canoe-shaped or crescent-shaped macroconidium, which may have one or more septae (Fig. 52–40).

Pseudallescheria boydii/ *Scedosporium apiospermum*

P. boydii is the sexual phase of this pathogen, whereas *S. apiospermum* is the imperfect, asexual phase. The mould grows rapidly on isolation medium, producing a fluffy colony with a brownish gray to dark gray ("mousy") color that darkens with continued incubation (Plate 52–15). This mould may grow on media that contain up to 8 mg/mL of cycloheximide. The asexual phase is characterized by single or small clusters of annelloconidia on a straight or branched conidiophore that may develop terminally or laterally from the vegetative hyphae. The conidia are light brown and oval or club shaped (Fig. 52–41). In the sexual phase, brown cleistothecia contain ascospores (Fig. 52–42). The cleistothecia, which are found most readily at the edges of the colony, develop best on nutritionally deficient media, such as cornmeal agar, V-8 juice agar, or potato dextrose (potato flake) agar.

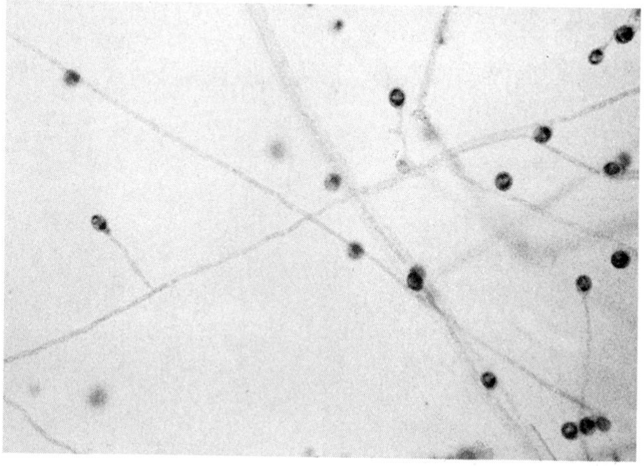

Figure 52–41. The tadpole- or sperm-shaped microconidia of *Scedosporium apiospermum* gave this organism its name. (Lactophenol cotton blue.)

Strictly speaking, the isolate should be reported as *P. boydii,* if the cleistothecia are demonstrated, and as *S. apiospermum,* if the asexual conidia are the only diagnostic structures observed.

Penicillium species

This saprophytic fungus is commonly isolated in the mycology laboratory, usually without any associated clinical disease. The commonly isolated species grow well on fungal isolation media, but are inhibited by cycloheximide. The colony is velvety and develops a green appearance with a white fringe (Plate 52–16). The diagnostic structure is the penicillus, which resembles the hand of a skeleton with chains of conidia developing from the tips of the fingers (Fig. 52–43). *P. marneffei* is an unusual member of the genus in that it is dimorphic and regularly produces systemic human disease (Kwon-Chung, 1992). This species is endemic in Southeast Asia, and most cases in the United States have occurred in immunosuppressed patients who had traveled to Asia (Piehl, 1988). At 25°C to 30°C, the mould colonies are gray with a

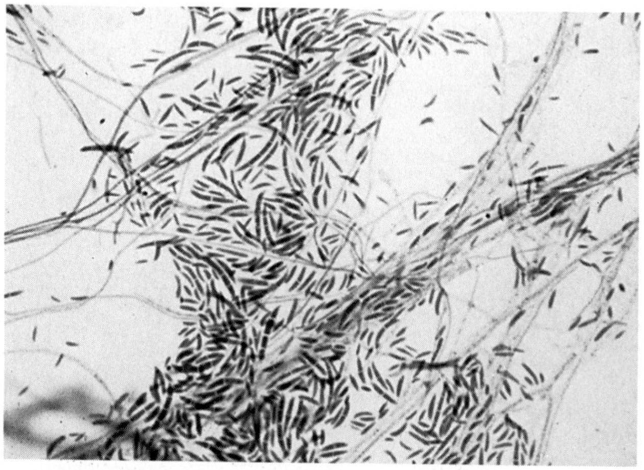

Figure 52–40. Canoe-shaped conidia of *Fusarium* species. The conidia may be septate. (Lactophenol cotton blue.)

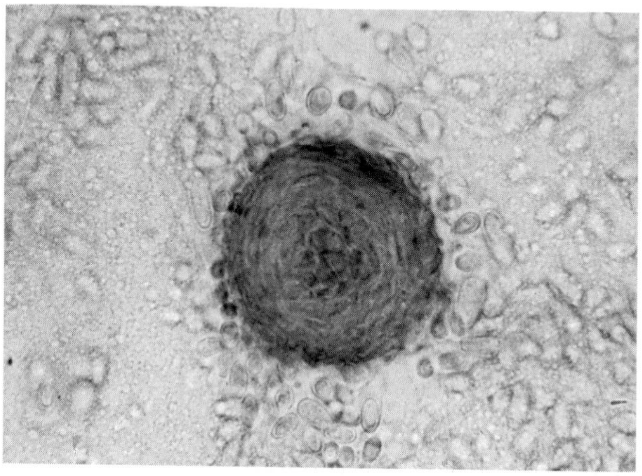

Figure 52–42. An ascus of the sexual form *Pseudallescheria boydii* has a roughened exterior produced by specialized hyphae.

6

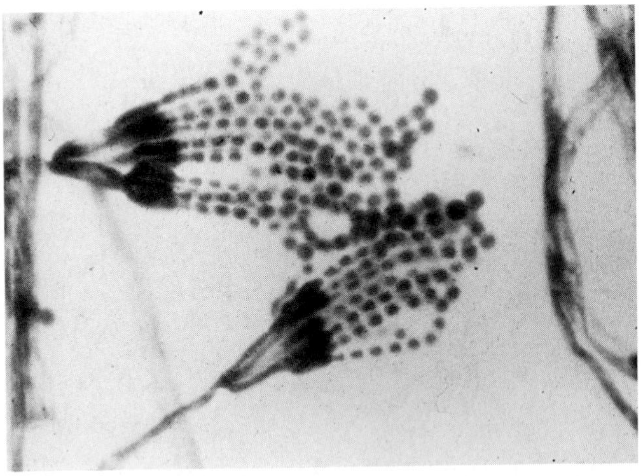

Figure 52–43. The penicillus of *Penicillium* species is composed of chains of conidia borne on phialides that have been compared to the bones of a skeleton hand. (Lactophenol cotton blue.)

soluble red pigment; as the conidiophores mature, the color of the colonies becomes green. At 37°C or in tissue, yeast cells are produced, but division is by septation and fission rather than budding.

Other Hyaline Moulds

There is a long list of hyaline moulds that are environmental saprophytes of low virulence and usually are not associated with clinical disease when isolated in the mycology laboratory. As mentioned earlier, any of these moulds may be pathogenic under the right conditions. In most cases, the host defenses of the patient are compromised in some way or the fungus is introduced into the body by trauma or medical manipulations. As an example, *Paecilomyces lilacinus* is a hyaline mould that resembles *Penicillium* species morphologically. This mould was invariably considered a laboratory contaminant until recent years. Increasing numbers of case reports document the ability of this so-called contaminant to produce infections of deep tissue and systemic organs. Demonstration of hyphae in tissue is extremely important for documenting the pathogenicity of the isolate.

INFECTIONS CAUSED BY ACHLOROPHYLLOUS ALGAE

Prototheca wickerhamii and *P. zopfii* are two species of algae that do not produce chlorophyll. They produce occasional human infections and are considered in this chapter, because of the resemblance of the infections to fungal disease (Sudman, 1974; Tindall, 1971). *Prototheca* are found in fresh and marine waters and probably gain entrance to the body through superficial wounds. Some patients are immunocompetent, but serious underlying diseases, such as diabetes mellitus, or immunosuppressive therapies often predispose patients to infection with this pathogen. Other patients have received injections of corticosteroids at the site of infection or have had musculoskeletal infection, particularly involving the tendons. The infections commonly involve the skin and subcutaneous tissue, with subsequent involvement of underlying tendons and joints (Holcomb, 1981; Nosanchuk, 1973). They are chronic and intractable, and may be difficult to eradicate without damage to the underlying structures, particularly in the hand (Lee, 1975). Disseminated infection is rare (Cox, 1974).

The algae grow readily on fungal isolation media that do not contain cycloheximide, and the colonies resemble those of *Candida* species (Plate 52–17). The algal cells have a characteristic appearance, in which multiple daughter cells (sporangiospores) develop within the mother cell (sporangium), resembling a spherule (Chandler, 1978; El-Ani, 1967). These structures also can be demonstrated in histologic sections, where they must be differentiated from dimorphic fungi (Fig. 52–44). They may be seen in hematoxylin-eosin preparations and stain well with the periodic acid–Schiff or methenamine silver methods. *Prototheca* species are included in the data bases of commercial yeast identification systems, such as API 20C (Biomerieux, Hazelwood, MO) and Vitek systems (Biomerieux, Hazelwood, MO).

PNEUMOCYSTIS CARINII

A few years ago, this important pathogen would have been included in the chapter on parasitology. The organism has phenotypic characteristics of both protozoa and fungi, but molecular studies have established its relationship to the ascomycetous fungi (Edman, 1988).

Risk Factors

Pneumocystis carinii is a pathogen of humans (Bartlett, 1991; Masur, 1989; Walzer, 1974; Watts, 1991). Morphologically similar organisms cause infection in rodent species. It was first recognized in outbreaks of pulmonary disease among malnourished infants in Eastern Europe during and after World War II. There is no known environmental source for the fungus. From serologic analysis, most individuals are infected asymptomatically in childhood (Maddison, 1982; Peglow, 1990). Asymptomatic or minimally symptomatic

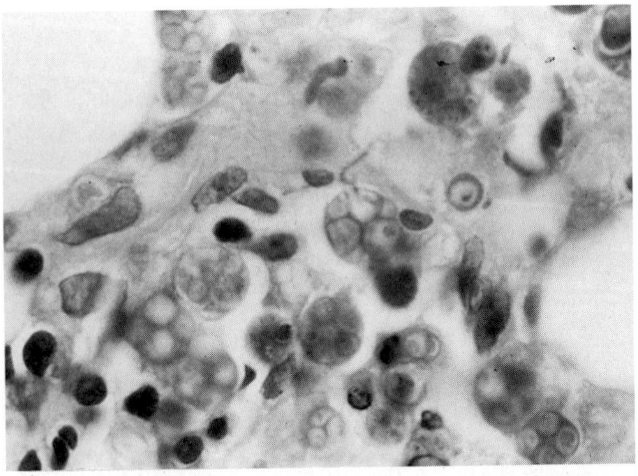

Figure 52–44. Septation of the algal cells of *Prototheca wickerhamii* produce multiple intracellular bodies and a structure known as a morula. (Hematoxylin-eosin stain.)

infections also have been recognized in adults (Sheldon, 1959). There is suggestive evidence that the fungus may colonize the lower respiratory tract, producing active infection when immunosuppressive disease or therapy intervenes. Pneumocystosis is a disease of immunologically compromised individuals (Walzer, 1974). Therapy with corticosteroids and hematologic malignancy were the primary risk factors before the appearance of HIV infection, which has become the predominant risk factor (Phair, 1990). AIDS was recognized because of the appearance of this previously rare disease in previously healthy young men in Los Angeles and New York (Gottlieb, 1981; Masur, 1981) and *Pneumocystis carinii* infection has been one of the infections that are found early in the course of the syndrome. The incidence has decreased in recent years, because of the widespread use of prophylactic antibiotics that are effective against the fungus (Kovacs, 1992).

Clinical Disease

Pneumonia is the most common manifestation of infection, and the lung was virtually the only organ involved before the appearance of HIV. The onset may be acute or insidious and is dominated by dyspnea. Often, radiographic infiltrates are much more extensive than would be suggested by the degree of symptoms (Dee, 1979). Concurrent infection with other agents, particularly cytomegalovirus and *C. neoformans*, is common. The infection is often fatal in untreated, immunosuppressed patients, who die of progressive respiratory failure. Dissemination of the fungus beyond the lung is common in patients infected with HIV but is uncommon in patients with other risk factors (Telzak, 1990).

Pathology of *Pneumocystis* Infections

The initial pathologic presentation in malnourished infants was a severe interstitial pneumonia with a mononuclear infiltrate that had a prominent plasma cell component (plasma cell pneumonia). The classic histologic pattern is a foamy alveolar exudate, which may undergo calcification (Weber, 1977). Diffuse alveolar damage with hyaline membranes is a less specific but common presentation (Askin, 1981). Less commonly, granulomatous disease, cavitary disease, and coagulative necrosis resembling infarcts have been described. Extrapulmonary lesions are minimally inflammatory, consisting of focal accumulations of foamy exudate in which the fungal cells are found. Ultrastructural studies of cultivated organisms (Murphy, 1977) and the extrapulmonary histology supports the ultrastructural evidence that the foamy exudate is produced by the fungus, rather than a tissue reaction specific to the lung.

Laboratory Diagnosis and Extent of Workup

Pneumocystis carinii has been cultivated in cell cultures, but serial maintenance of subcultures has not been accomplished (Latorre, 1977; Pifer, 1977). The diagnosis, therefore, is morphologic and, more recently, immunologic. The life cycle of *Pneumocystis carinii* involves development of sporozoites within a cyst, after which the sporozoites are released. Bronchoalveolar lavage has proved the most reliable source for diagnostic material (Kelley, 1978), and surgical lung biopsy need be performed only rarely. In patients with HIV infection, sufficient numbers of organisms are produced that a sputum induced with saline by a skilled respiratory therapist may provide the diagnosis. The experience with sputum has varied in different centers, however, and the yield is very low in patients who have underlying diseases other than HIV (Lau, 1976). Giemsa stains demonstrate the sporozoites well, but detection of these small structures is considerably more difficult than detection of cysts. The commercial Diff-Quik stain (Baxter Health Care Corporation, McGaw Park, IL) is commonly used. The methenamine silver stain, modified for *Pneumocystis*, is commonly used in surgical pathology laboratories (Fig. 52–45). Toluidine blue O has been employed in many microbiology laboratories (Gosey, 1985). Calcofluor white also stains the cysts and has been used successfully in some laboratories (Baselski, 1990). The cysts, which measure 5 μm, are round, but collapsed forms are common. Helmet-shaped collapsed cysts and paired thickenings of the cyst wall that resemble quotation marks in silver-stained preparations are characteristic but not diagnostic. The cysts must be differentiated from other fungi, particularly *H. capsulatum*. Use of stains for cysts and trophozoites, either separately or in combination, provide optimal sensitivity (Bartlett, 1991; Blumenfeld, 1988). The advent of fluorescein-conjugated monoclonal antibodies to *P. carinii* has provided a specific method for identification. The immunofluorescence technique has been more sensitive in histochemical stains in some reports (Baughman, 1989; Kovacs, 1988), but the skill and care of the observers undoubtedly plays a role in the comparative sensitivity of the techniques (Bartlett, 1991; Cregan, 1990). The *Pneumocystis* organism found in rats does not stain with the monoclonal to human cysts (Bauer, 1993), but this species specificity is a problem only in proficiency testing specimens. It should be noted that the cysts of *P. carinii* occasionally may be encountered in gram-stained preparations (Fig. 52–46), although this technique is not a sensitive method for detecting

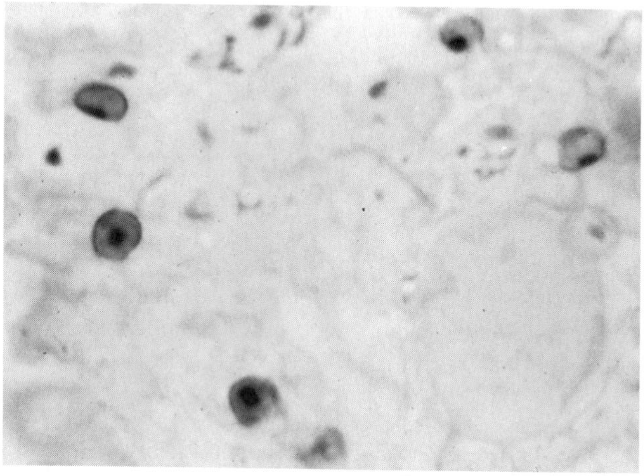

Figure 52–45. The cysts of *Pneumocystis carinii* in this lung tissue imprint are round or collapsed and have a focal thickening of the cyst wall that give the appearance of parentheses. Methenamine silver stain.

6

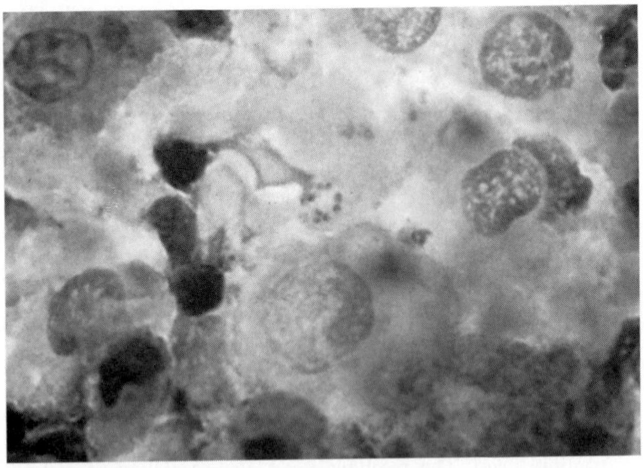

Figure 52–46. A cyst of *Pneumocystis carinii* with clearly visible internal sporozoites is demonstrated in this gram-stained preparation from a bronchial lavage.

them. Detection of circulating antigen has been described in both pulmonary and disseminated infection (Pifer, 1984), but the assays are not available commercially.

Ahmad M, Weinstein AJ, Hughes JA, et al: Granulomatous mediastinitis due to *Aspergillus flavus* in anonimmunosuppressed patient. Am J Med 1981; 70:887.

Ahmad M, Dar MA, Weinstein AJ, et al: Thoracic aspergillosis (part II)—primary pulmonary aspergillosis, allergic bronchopulmonary aspergillosis, and related conditions. Clev Clin Q 1984; 51:631.

Allen AM, Taplin D: Epidemic *Trichophyton mentagrophytes* infections in servicemen. Source of infection, role of environment, host factors, and susceptibility. JAMA 1973; 226:864.

Aly R: Ecology and epidemiology of dermatophyte infections. J Am Acad Dermatol 1994; 31 (Pt 2):S21.

Ampel NM, Wieden MA, Galgiani JN: Coccidioidomycosis: Clinical update. Rev Infect Dis 1989; 11:897.

Anaissie E, Nelson P, Beremand M, et al: *Fusarium*-caused hyalohyphomycosis: An overview. Curr Top Med Mycol 1992; 4:231.

Arnow PM, Andersen RL, Mainous PD, Smith EJ: Pulmonary aspergillosis during hospital renovation. Am Rev Respir Dis 1978; 118:49.

Askin FB, Katzenstein AL: *Pneumocystis* infection masquerading as diffuse alveolar damage: A potential source of diagnostic error. Chest 1981; 79:420.

Bartlett MS, Smith JW: *Pneumocystis carinii*, an opportunist in immunocompromised patients. Clin Microbiol Rev 1991; 4:137.

Baselski VS, Robison MK, Pifer LW, Woods DR: Rapid detection of *Pneumocystis carinii* in bronchoalveolar lavage samples by using Cellufluor staining. J Clin Microbiol 1990; 28:393.

Bauer NL, Paulsrud JR, Bartlett MS, et al: *Pneumocystis carinii* organisms obtained from rats, ferrets, and mice are antigenically different. Infect Immun 1993; 61:1315.

Baughman RP, Strohofer SS, Clinton BA, et al: The use of an indirect fluorescent antibody test for detecting *Pneumocystis carinii*. Arch Pathol Lab Med 1989; 113:1062.

Baum GL, Lerner PI: Primary pulmonary blastomycosis: A laboratory-acquired infection. Ann Intern Med 1970; 73:263.

Bayer AS, Edwards JE, Seidel JS, Guze LB: *Candida* meningitis. Report of seven cases and review of the English literature. Medicine (Baltimore) 1976; 55:477.

Beheshti F, Smith AG, Krause GW: Germ tube and chlamydospore formation by *Candida albicans* on a new medium. J Clin Microbiol 1975; 2:345.

Behrman RE, Masci JR, Nicholas P: Cryptococcal skeletal infections: Case report and review. Rev Infect Dis 1990; 12:181.

Bennett JE, Bailey JW: Control of rheumatoid factor in the latex test for cryptococcosis. Am J Clin Pathol 1971; 56:360.

Bergman K, Burke PV, Cerdá-Olmedo E, et al: Phycomyces. Bact Rev 1969; 33:99.

Berlin L, Pincus JH: Cryptococcal meningitis. False-negative antigen test results and cultures in nonimmunosuppressed patients. Arch Neurol 1989; 46:1312.

Bisbe J, Miro JM, Latorre X, et al: Disseminated candidiasis in addicts who use brown heroin: Report of 83 cases and review. Clin Infect Dis 1992; 15:910.

Blinkhorn RJ, Adelstein D, Spagnuolo PJ: Emergence of a new opportunistic pathogen, *Candida lusitaniae*. J Clin Microbiol 1989; 27:236.

Blumenfeld W, Griffiss JM: *Pneumocystis carinii* in sputum. Arch Pathol Lab Med 1988; 112:816.

Boardman CR, Malkinson FD: Tinea versicolor in steroid treated patients. Arch Dermatol 1962; 85:44.

Bosken CH, Myers JL, Greenberger PA, Katzenstein AL: Pathologic features of allergic bronchopulmonary aspergillosis. Am J Surg Pathol 1988; 12:216.

Brodsky AL, Gregg MB, Loewenstein MS, et al: Outbreak of histoplasmosis associated with the 1970 Earth Day activities. Am J Med 1973; 54:333.

Bronnimann DA, Adam RD, Galgiani JN, et al: Coccidioidomycosis in the acquired immunodeficiency syndrome. Ann Intern Med 1987; 106:372.

Buesching WJ, Kurek K, Roberts GD: Evaluation of the modified API 20C system for identification of clinically important yeasts. J Clin Microbiol 1979; 9:565.

Campbell CC, Hill GB: Further studies on the development of complement-fixing antibodies and precipitins in healthy histoplasmin-sensitive persons following a single histoplasmin skin test. Am Rev Respir Dis 1964; 90:927.

Canizares O, Shatin H, Kellert AJ : Cushing's syndrome and dermatomycosis. Arch Dermatol 1959; 80:705.

Chandler FW, Kaplan W, Callaway CS: Differentiation between *Prototheca* and morphologically similar green algae in tissue. Arch Pathol Lab Med 1978; 102:353.

Chandler FW, Watts JC: *Pathologic diagnosis of fungal infections*. Chicago ASCP Press, 1987.

Chuck SL, Sande MA: Infections with *Cryptococcus neoformans* in the acquired immunodeficiency syndrome. N Engl J Med 1989; 321:794.

Clemons KV, McCusker JH, Davis RW, Stevens DA: Comparative pathogenesis of clinical and nonclinical isolates of *Saccharomyces cerevisiae*. J Infect Dis 1994; 169:859.

Cocanour CS, Miller-Crotchett P, Reed RL, 2d, et al: Mucormycosis in trauma patients. J Trauma 1992; 32:12.

Cohen R, Roth FJ, Delgado E, et al: Fungal flora of the normal human small and large intestine. N Engl J Med 1969; 280:638.

Colombo AL, Barchiesi F, McGough DA, Rinaldi MG: Comparison of Etest and National Committee for Clinical Laboratory Standards broth macrodilution method for azole antifungal susceptibility testing. J Clin Microbiol 1995; 33:535.

Conlan AA, Abramor E, Moyes DG: Pulmonary aspergilloma—indications for surgical intervention. An analysis of 22 cases. S Afr Med J 1987; 71:285.

Cote TR, Kasten MJ, England AC, 3d: Sporotrichosis in association with Arbor Day activities. N Engl J Med 1988; 319:1290.

Cox GE, Wilson JD, Brown P: Protothecosis: A case of disseminated algal infection. Lancet 1974; 2:379.

Cregan P, Yamamoto A, Lum A, et al: Comparison of four methods for rapid detection of *Pneumocystis carinii* in respiratory specimens. J Clin Microbiol 1990; 28:2432.

Crout JE, Brewer NS, Tompkins RB: Sporotrichosis arthritis: Clinical features in seven patients. Ann Intern Med 1977; 86:294.

Curry CR, Quie PG: Fungal septicemia in patients receiving parenteral hyperalimentation. N Engl J Med 1971; 285:1221.

D'Alessio DJ, Leavens LJ, Strumpf GB, Smith CD: An outbreak of sporotrichosis in Vermont associated with sphagnum moss as the source of infection. N Engl J Med 1965; 272:1054.

Dar MA, Ahmad M, Weinstein AJ, et al: Thoracic aspergillosis (part I)—overview and aspergilloma. Clev Clin Q 1984; 51:615.

de Repentigny L: Serodiagnosis of candidiasis, aspergillosis and cryptococcosis. Clin Infect Dis 1992; 14:Suppl 1:S11.

Dee P, Winn W, McKee K: *Pneumocystis carinii* infection of the lung: Radiologic and pathologic correlation. AJR Am J Roentgenol 1979; 132:741.

Diamond RD, Bennett JE: Prognostic factors in cryptococcal meningitis. A study in 111 cases. Ann Intern Med 1974; 80:176.

DiTomasso JP, Ampel NM, Sobonya RE, Bloom JW: Bronchoscopic diagnosis of pulmonary coccidioidomycosis. Comparison of cytology, culture, and transbronchial biopsy. Diagn Microbiol Infect Dis 1994; 18:83.

Dolan CT, Ihrke DM: Further studies of the germ-tube test for *Candida albicans* identification. Am J Clin Pathol 1971; 55:733.

Dolan CT: Specificity of the latex-cryptococcal antigen test. Am J Clin Pathol 1972; 58:358.

Edman JC, Kovacs JA, Masur H, et al: Ribosomal RNA sequence shows *Pneumocystis carinii* to be a member of the fungi. Nature 1988; 334:519.

Edwards JE Jr, Filler SG: Current strategies for treating invasive candidiasis: Emphasis on infections in nonneutropenic patients. Clin Infect Dis 1992; 14(Suppl 1):S106.

El-Ani AS: Life cycle and variation of *Prototheca wickerhamii*. Science 1967; 59:1501.

El-Zaatari M, Pasarell L, McGinnis MR, et al: Evaluation of the updated Vitek yeast identification data base. J Clin Microbiol 1990; 28:1938.

Farmer SG, Komorowski RA: Histologic response to capsule-deficient *Cryptococcus neoformans*. Arch Pathol 1973; 96:383.

Fenn JP, Segal H, Barland B, et al: Comparison of updated Vitek yeast biochemical card and API 20C yeast identification systems. J Clin Microbiol 1994; 32:1184.

Fish, DG, Ampel NM, Galgiani JN, et al: Coccidioidomycosis during human immunodeficiency virus infection. A review of 77 patients. Medicine (Baltimore) 1990; 69:384.

Fishbach RS, White ML, Finegold SM: Bronchopulmonary geotrichosis. Am Rev Respir Dis 1973; 108:1388.

Fishman LS, Griffin JR, Sapico FL, Hecht R: Hematogenous *Candida* endophthalmitis—a complication of candidemia. N Engl J Med 1972; 286:675.

Fleming WH III, Lewis, BH Dorn, GL: Effectiveness of lysis-centrifugation blood culture technique in recovering fungi from blood. Lab Med 1984; 15:104.

Fraser VJ, Jones M, Dunkel J, et al: Candidemia in a tertiary care hospital: Epidemiology, risk factors, and predictors of mortality. Clin Infect Dis 1992; 15:414.

Freed ER, Duma RJ, Shadomy HJ, Utz, JP: Meningoencephalitis due to hyphae-forming *Cryptococcus neoformans*. Am J Clin Pathol 1971; 55:30.

Fromtling RA: Overview of medically important antifungal azole derivatives. Clin Microbiol Rev 1988; 1:187.

Galgani JN, Ampel NM: Coccidioidomycosis in human immunodeficiency virus–infected patients. J Infect Dis 1990; 162:1165.

Gartenberg G, Bottone EJ, Keusch GT, Weitzman I: Hospital-acquired mucormycosis (*Rhizopus rhizopodiformis*) of skin and subcutaneous tissue: Epidemiology, mycology and treatment. N Engl J Med 1978; 299:1115.

Gilligan PH: Microbiology of airway disease in patients with cystic fibrosis. Clin Microbiol Rev 1991; 4:35.

Gingrich WD: Keratomycosis. JAMA 1962; 170:602.

Golbert TM, Patterson R: Pulmonary allergic aspergillosis. Ann Intern Med 1970; 72:395.

Goldberg PK, Kozinn PJ, Wise GJ, et al: Incidence and significance of candiduria. JAMA 1979; 241:582.

Goldman M, Pottage JC Jr, Weaver DC: *Candida krusei* fungemia. Report of 4 cases and review of the literature. Medicine (Baltimore) 1993; 72:143.

Goodwin RA, Des Prez RM: Histoplasmosis. Am Rev Respir Dis 1978; 117:929.

Goodwin RA, Des Prez RM: Pathogenesis and clinical spectrum of histoplasmosis. South Med J 1973; 66:13.

Goodwin RA, Owens FT, Snell JD, et al: Chronic pulmonary histoplasmosis. Medicine (Baltimore) 1995; 55:413.

Gosey LL, Howard RM, Witebsky FG, et al: Advantages of a modified toluidine blue O stain and bronchoalveolar lavage for the diagnosis of *Pneumocystis carinii* pneumonia. J Clin Microbiol 1985; 22:803.

Gottlieb MS, Schroff R, Schanker HM, et al: *Pneumocystis carinii* pneumonia and mucosal candidiasis in previously healthy homosexual men. Evidence for a new acquired cellular immunodeficiency. N Engl J Med 1981; 305:1425.

Grotte M, Younger B: Sporotrichosis associated with sphagnum moss exposure. Arch Pathol Lab Med 1981; 105:50.

Gutierrez F, Fu YS, Lurie HI: Cryptococcosis histologically resembling histoplasmosis. A light and electron microscopical study. Arch Pathol 1975; 99:347.

Hadfield TL, Smith MB, Winn RE, et al: Mycoses caused by *Candida lusitaniae*. Rev Infect Dis 1987; 9:1006.

Hageage GJ Jr, Harrington BJ: Use of calcofluor white in clinical mycology. Lab Med 1984; 15:109.

Haley LD, Trandel J, Coyle MB, Sherris JC: CUMITECH 11. Practical methods for culture and identification of fungi in the clinical microbiology laboratory. Washington, American Society for Microbiology, 1980.

Hamilton JR, Noble A, Denning DW, Stevens DA: Performance of cryptococcus antigen latex agglutination kits on serum and cerebrospinal fluid specimens of AIDS patients before and after pronase treatment. J Clin Microbiol 1991; 29:333.

Harding CV: Blastomycosis and opportunistic infections in patients with acquired immunodeficiency syndrome. An autopsy study. Arch Pathol Lab Med 1991; 115:1133.

Haron E, Vartivarian S, Anaissie E, et al: Primary *Candida* pneumonia. Experience at a large cancer center and review of the literature. Medicine (Baltimore) 1993; 72:137.

Haulk AA, Sugar AM: *Candida* esophagitis. Adv Intern Med 1991; 36:307.

Hay RJ: Fungal skin infections. Arch Dis Child 1992; 67:1065.

Holcomb HS 3d, Behrens F, Winn WC Jr, et al: *Prototheca wickerhamii*—an alga infecting the hand. J Hand Surg [Am] 1981; 6:595.

Horowitz BJ, Edelstein SW, Lippman L: *Candida tropicalis* vulvovaginitis. Obstet Gynecol 1985; 66:229.

Horowitz ID, Blumberg EA, Krevolin L: *Cryptococcus albidus* and mucormycosis empyema in a patient receiving hemodialysis. South Med J 1993; 86:1070.

Hoy J, Hsu KC, Rolston K, et al: *Trichosporon beigelii* infection: a review. Rev Infect Dis 1986; 8:959.

Jagirdar J, Geller SA, Bottone EJ: *Geotrichum candidum* as a tissue invasive human pathogen. Hum Pathol 1981; 12:668.

Johnson PC, Khardori N, Najjar AF, et al: Progressive disseminated histoplasmosis in patients with acquired immunodeficiency syndrome. Am J Med 1988; 85:152.

Johnston PG, Lee J, Domanski M, et al: Late recurrent *Candida* endocarditis. Chest 1991; 99:1531.

Jones JM: Laboratory diagnosis of invasive candidiasis. Clin Microbiol Rev 1990; 3:32.

Kane JG, Chretien JH, Garagusi VF: Diarrhea caused by *Candida*. Lancet 1976; 1:335.

Katzenstein AL, Maksem J: Candidal infection of gastric ulcers. Histology, incidence, and clinical significance. Am J Clin Pathol 1979; 71:137.

Katzenstein AL, Sale SR, Greenberger PA: Pathologic findings in allergic aspergillus sinusitis. A newly recognized form of sinusitis. Am J Surg Pathol 1983; 7:439.

Kauffman CA, Tan JS: *Torulopsis glabrata* renal infection. Am J Med 1974; 57:217.

Kauffman CA, Israel KS, Smith JW, et al: Histoplasmosis in immunosuppressed patients. Am J Med 1978; 64:923.

Kelley J, Landis JN, Davis GS, et al: Diagnosis of pneumonia due to *Pneumocystis* by subsegmental pulmonary lavage via the fiberoptic bronchoscope. Chest 1978; 74:24.

Kerkering TM, Duma RJ, Shadomy S: The evolution of pulmonary cryptococcosis. Clinical implications from a study of 41 patients with and without compromising host factors. Ann Intern Med 1981; 94:611.

Kiehn TE, Gorey E, Brown AE, et al: Sepsis due to Rhodotorula related to use of indwelling central venous catheters. Clin Infect Dis 1992; 14:841.

Kirkpatrick CH, Rich RR, Bennett JE: Chronic mucocutaneous candidiasis: Model-building in cellular immunity. Ann Intern Med 1971; 74:955.

Klein BS, Vergeront JM, Weeks RJ, et al: Isolation of *Blastomyces dermatitidis* in soil associated with a large outbreak of blastomycosis in Wisconsin. N Engl J Med 1986; 314:529.

Klein JJ, Watanakunakorn C: Hospital-acquired fungemia. Its natural course and clinical significance. Am J Med 1979; 67:51.

Klein RS, Harris CA, Small CB, et al: Oral candidiasis in high-risk patients as the initial manifestation of the acquired immunodeficiency syndrome. N Engl J Med 1984; 311:354.

Kovacs JA, Kovacs AA, Polis M, et al: Cryptococcosis in the acquired immunodeficiency syndrome. Ann Intern Med 1985; 103:533.

Kovacs JA, Ng VL, Masur H, et al: Diagnosis of *Pneumocystis carinii* pneumonia: improved detection in sputum with use of monoclonal antibodies. N Engl J Med 1988; 318:589.

Kovacs JA, Masur H: Prophylaxis for *Pneumocystis carinii* pneumonia in patients infected with human immunodeficiency virus. Clin Infect Dis 1992; 14:1005.

Kozinn PJ, Taschdjian CL: Enteric candidiasis. Diagnosis and clinical considerations. Pediatrics 1962; 00:71.

Kramer MN, Kurup VP, Fink JN: Allergic bronchopulmonary aspergillosis from a contaminated dump site. Am Rev Respir Dis 1989; 140:1086.

Kurup VP, Kumar A: Immunodiagnosis of aspergillosis. Clin Microbiol Rev 1991; 4:439.

Kwon-Chung KJ, Bennett JE: Medical Mycology. Philadelphia, Lea & Febiger, 1992.

Larone DH: Medically Important Fungi. A Guide to Identification. 3rd ed. Washington, American Society of Microbiology Press, 1995.

Larone DH: The identification of dematiaceous fungi. Clin Microbiol Newsletter 1989; 11:145.

Latorre CR, Sulzer AJ, Norman LG: Serial propagation of *Pneumocystis carinii* in cell line cultures. Appl Environ Microbiol 1977; 33:1204.

Lau WK, Young LS, Remington JS: *Pneumocystis carinii* pneumonia. Diagnosis by examination of pulmonary secretions. JAMA 1976; 236:2399.

Lazcano O, Speights VO Jr, Strickler JG, et al: Combined histochemical stains in the differential diagnosis of *Cryptococcus neoformans*. Mod Pathol 1993; 6:80.

Lee WS, Lagios MD, Leonards R: Wound infection by *Prototheca wickerhamii*, a saprophytic alga pathogenic for man. J Clin Microbiol 1975; 2:62.

Levenson D, Pfaller MA, Smith MA, et al: *Candida zeylanoides*: Another opportunistic yeast. J Clin Microbiol 1991; 29:1689.

Levitz SM: The ecology of *Cryptococcus neoformans* and the epidemiology of cryptococcosis. Rev Infect Dis 1991; 13:1163.

Lewis JL, Rabinovich S: The wide spectrum of cryptococcal infections. Am J Med 1972; 53:315.

Liesegang TJ, Forster RK: Spectrum of microbial keratitis in South Florida. Am J Ophthalmol 1980; 90:38.

Liu KL, Herbrecht R, Bergerat JP, et al: Disseminated *Trichosporon capitatum* infection in a patient with acute leukemia undergoing bone marrow transplantation. Bone Marrow Transplant 1990; 6:219.

Londero AT, Ramos CD: Paracoccidioidomycosis. A clinical and mycologic study of forty-one cases observed in Santa Maria RS, Brazil. Am J Med 1972; 52:771.

Lopez AM, Williams PL, Ampel NM: Acute pulmonary coccidioidomycosis mimicking bacterial pneumonia and septic shock: A report of two cases. Am J Med 1993; 95:236.

Louthrenoo W, Park YS, Philippe L, Schumacher HR Jr: Localized peripheral calcium oxalate crystal deposition caused by *Aspergillus niger* infection. J Rheumatol 1990; 17:407.
Loyd JE, Tillman BF, Atkinson JB, Des Prez RM: Mediastinal fibrosis complicating histoplasmosis. Medicine (Baltimore) 1988; 67:295.
Lurie HI: Histopathology of sporotrichosis. Notes on the nature of the asteroid body. Arch Pathol 1963; 75:421.
Lynch PJ, Voorhees JJ, Harrell ER: Systemic Sporotrichosis. Ann Intern Med 1970; 73:23.
Maddison SE, Hayes GV, Slemenda SB, et al: Detection of specific antibody by enzyme-linked immunosorbent assay and antigenemia by counterimmunoelectrophoresis in humans infected with *Pneumocystis carinii*. J Clin Microbiol 1982; 15:1036.
Marcon MJ, Powell DA: Human infections due to *Malassezia* spp. Clin Microbiol Rev 1992; 5:101.
Marks MI, Langston C, Eickhoff TC: *Torulopsis glabrata*—an opportunistic pathogen in man. N Engl J Med 1970; 283:1131.
Masur H, Michelis MA, Greene JB, et al: An outbreak of community-acquired *Pneumocystis carinii* pneumonia. Initial manifestation of cellular immune dysfunction. N Engl J Med 1981; 305:1431.
Masur H, Lane HC, Kovacs JA, et al: NIH conference. *Pneumocystis* pneumonia: From bench to clinic. Ann Intern Med 1989; 111:813.
McCarty JM, Flam MS, Pullen G, et al: Outbreak of primary cutaneous aspergillosis related to intravenous arm boards. J Pediatr 1986; 108 (Pt 1):721.
McGinnis MR: Laboratory Handbook of Medical Mycology. New York, Academic Press, 1980.
McGough DA, Fothergill AW, Rinaldi MG: *Cokeromyces recurvatus* Poitras, a distinctive zygomycete and potential pathogen: Criteria for identification. Clin Microbiol Newsletter 1990; 12:113.
McNulty JS: Rhinocerebral mucormycosis: Predisposing factors. Laryngoscope 1982; 92:1140.
Medeiros AA, Marty SD, Tosh FE, Chin TDY: Erythema nodosum and erythema multiforme as clinical manifestations of histoplasmosis in a community outbreak. N Engl J Med 1966; 274:415.
Mehta AC, Dar MA, Ahmad M, et al: Thoracic aspergillosis (part III)—invasive pulmonary and disseminated aspergillosis. Clev Clin Q 1984; 51:655.
Meyer RD, Gaultier CR, Yamashita JT, et al: Fungal sinusitis in patients with AIDS: Report of 4 cases and review of the literature. [Review]. Medicine (Baltimore) 1994; 73:69.
Meyer RD, Kaplan MH, Ong M, Armstrong D: Cutaneous lesions in disseminated mucormycosis. JAMA 1973a, 225:737.
Meyer RD, Rosen P, Armstrong D: Phycomycosis complicating leukemia and lymphoma. Ann Intern Med 1972; 77:871.
Meyer RD, Young LS, Armstrong D, Yu B: Aspergillosis complicating neoplastic disease. Am J Med 1973b, 54:6.
Mickelsen PA, Viano-Paulson MC, Stevens DA, Diaz PS: Clinical and microbiological features of infection with *Malassezia pachydermatis* in high-risk infants. J Infect Dis 1988; 157:1163.
Midgley G, Moore MK, Cook JC, Phan QG: Mycology of nail disorders. J Am Acad Dermatol 1994; 31 (Pt 2):S68.
Morris AJ, Wilson ML, Mirrett S, Reller LB: Rationale for selective use of anaerobic blood cultures. J Clin Microbiol 1993; 31:2110.
Murphy MJ Jr, Pifer LL, Hughes WT: *Pneumocystis carinii* in vitro. A study by scanning electron microscopy. Am J Pathol 1977; 86:387.
Murray HW, Littman ML, Roberts RB: Disseminated paracoccidioidomycosis (South American blastomycosis) in the United States. Am J Med 1974; 56:209.
Murray PR, van Scoy RE, Roberts GD: Should yeasts in respiratory secretions be identified? Mayo Clin Proc 1977; 52:42.
Nagata N, Sueishi K, Tanaka K, Iwata Y: Pulmonary aspergillosis with bronchocentric granulomas. Am J Surg Pathol 1990; 14:485.
National Committee for Clinical Laboratory Standards: Reference method for broth dilution antifungal susceptibility testing of yeasts; proposed standard. M27-P. Villanova, PA, National Committee for Clinical Laboratory Standards, 1992.
Nelson LA, Callerame ML, Schwartz RH: Aspergillosis and atopy in cystic fibrosis. Am Rev Respir Dis 1979; 120:863.
Nelson PE, Dignani MC, Anaissie EJ: Taxonomy, biology, and clinical aspects of *Fusarium* species. Clin Microbiol Rev 1995; 7:479.
Nightingale SD, Parks JM, Pounders SM, et al: Disseminated histoplasmosis in patients with AIDS. South Med J 1990; 83:624.
Nosanchuk JS, Greenberg RD: Protothecosis of the olecranon bursa caused by achloric algae. Am J Clin Pathol 1973; 59:567.
Odds FC, Arai T, DiSalvo AF, et al: Nomenclature of fungal diseases: A report and recommendations from a sub-committee of the International Society for Human and Animal Mycology (ISHAM). J Med Vet Mycol 1992; 30:1.
Odds FC: *Candida* species and virulence. ASM News 1994; 60:313.
Odom RB: Common superficial fungal infections in immunosuppressed patients. J Am Acad Dermatol 1994; 31 (Pt 2):S56.
Ogata K, Tanabe Y, Iwakiri K, et al: Two cases of disseminated *Trichosporon beigelii* infection treated with combination antifungal therapy. Cancer 1990; 65:2793.
Pappagianis D, Zimmer BL: Serology of coccidioidomycosis. Clin Microbiol Rev 1990; 3:247.
Pappagianis D: Coccidioidomycosis. Semin Dermatol 1993; 12:301.
Pappagianis D: Marked increase in cases of coccidioidomycosis in California: 1991; 1992, and 1993. Clin Infect Dis 1994; 19(Suppl 1):S14.
Parker JC Jr, McCloskey JJ, Lee RS: Human cerebral candidosis—A postmortem evaluation of 19 patients. Hum Pathol 1981; 12:23.
Paya CV, Roberts GD, Cockerill FR III: Laboratory methods for the diagnosis of disseminated histoplasmosis: Clinical importance of the lysis-centrifugation blood culture technique. Mayo Clin Proc 1987; 62:480.
Peglow SL, Smulian AG, Linke MJ, et al: Serologic responses to *Pneumocystis carinii* antigens in health and disease. J Infect Dis 1990; 161:296.
Pema K, Diaz J, Guerra LG, et al: Disseminated cutaneous cryptococcosis. Comparison of clinical manifestations in the pre-AIDS and AIDS eras. Arch Intern Med 1994; 154:1032.
Phair J, Munõz A, Detels R, et al, and the Multicenter AIDS Cohort Study Group: The risk of *Pneumocystis carinii* pneumonia among men infected with human immunodeficency virus type 1. N Engl J Med 1990; 322:161.
Phillips P, Bryce G, Shepherd J, Mintz D: Invasive external otitis caused by *Aspergillus*. Rev Infect Dis 1990; 12:277.
Piehl MR, Kaplan RL, Haber MH: Disseminated penicilliosis in a patient with acquired immunodeficiency syndrome. Arch Pathol Lab Med 1988; 112:1262.
Pien FD, Thompson RL, Deye D, Roberts GD: *Rhodotorula* septicemia. Mayo Clin Proc 1980; 55:258.
Pifer LL, Hughes WT, Murphy MJ Jr: Propagation of *Pneumocystis carinii* in vitro. Pediatr Res 1977; 11:305.
Pifer LL, Niell HB, Morrison BJ, et al: *Pneumocystis carinii* antigenemia in adults with malignancy, infection, or pulmonary disease. J Clin Microbiol 1984; 20:887.
Pizzo PA: Combating infections in neutropenic patients. Hosp Pract (Off Ed) 1989; 24:93.
Pluss JL, Opal SM: Pulmonary sporotrichosis: review of treatment and outcome. Medicine. (Baltimore) 1986; 65:143.
Powell DA, Durrell DE, Marcon MJ: Growth of *Malassezia furfur* in parenteral fat emulsions. J Infect Dis 1986; 153:640.
Powell DA, Hayes J, Durrell DE, et al: *Malassezia furfur* skin colonization of infants hospitalized in intensive care units. J Pediatr 1987; 111:217.
Ramirez G, Shuster M, Kozub W, Pribor HC: Fatal acute *Candida albicans* bronchopneumonia. JAMA 1967; 199:340.
Randhawa HS, Pal M: Occurrence and significance of *Cryptococcus neoformans* in the respiratory tract of patients with bronchopulmonary disorders. J Clin Microbiol 1977; 5:5.
Record NB Jr, Ginder DR: Pulmonary phycomycosis without obvious predisposing factors. JAMA 1976; 235:1256.
Reddy P, Gorelick DF, Brasher CA, Larsh H: Progressive disseminated histoplasmosis as seen in adults. Am J Med 1970; 48:629.
Reed KD, Moore FM, Geiger GE, Stemper ME: Zoonotic transmission of sporotrichosis: Case report and review. Clin Infect Dis 1993; 16:384.
Reiss E, Morrison CJ: Nonculture methods for diagnosis of disseminated candidiasis. Clin Microbiol Rev 1993; 6:311.
Restrepo A, Robledo M, Gutierrez F, et al: Paracoccidioidomycosis (South American blastomycosis). Am J Trop Med Hyg 1970; 19:68.
Rex JH, Pfaller MA, Rinaldi MG, et al: Antifungal susceptibility testing. Clin Microbiol Rev 1993; 6:367.
Riddle DL, Giger O, Miller L, et al: Clinical comparison of the Baxter MicroScan yeast identification panel and the Vitek yeast biochemical card. Am J Clin Pathol 1994; 101:438.
Rinaldi MG: Use of potato flakes agar in clinical mycology. J Clin Microbiol 1982; 15:1159.
Rinaldi MG: Problems in the diagnosis of invasive fungal diseases. Rev Infect Dis 1991; 13:493.
Rinaldi MG: Selected medically important fungi with common synonyms and other obsolete names. Clin Infect Dis 1993; 16:610.
Rippon JW: Medical Mycology: The Pathogenic Fungi and the Pathogenic Actinomycetes, 3rd ed. Philadelphia, W.B. Saunders Company 1988.
Ro JY, Lee SS, Ayala AG: Advantage of Fontana-Masson stain in capsule-deficient cryptococcal infection. Arch Pathol Lab Med 1987; 111:53.
Roberts SO: Pityriasis versicolor: A clinical and mycological investigation. Br J Dermatol 1969a, 81:315.
Roberts SO: The mycology of the clinically normal scalp. Br J Dermatol 1969b, 81:626.
Roberts SO: Pityrosporum orbiculare: Incidence and distribution on clinically normal skin. Br J Dermatol 1969c, 81:264.
Rosenberg RS, Creviston SA, Schonfeld AJ: Invasive aspergillosis complicating resection of a pulmonary aspergilloma in a nonimmunocompromised host. Am Rev Respir Dis 1982; 126:1113.
Salyer WR, Salyer DC, Baker RD: Primary complex of *Cryptococcus* and pulmonary lymph nodes. J Infect Dis 1974; 130:74.

Sanders E: Cutaneous sporotrichosis. Beer, bricks, and bumps. Arch Intern Med 1971; 127:482.

Sarosi GA, Hammerman KJ, Tosh FE, Kronenberg RS: Clinical features of acute pulmonary blastomycosis. N Engl J Med 1974; 290,10:540.

Scherr GR, Evans SG, Kiyabu MT, Klatt EC: *Pseudallescheria boydii* infection in the acquired immunodeficiency syndrome. Arch Pathol Lab Med 1992; 116:535.

Schowengerdt CG, Suyemoto R, Main FB: Granulomatous and fibrous mediastinitis. A review and analysis of 180 cases. J Thorax Cardiovasc Surg 1969; 57:365.

Sewell DL, Pfaller MA, Barry AL: Comparison of broth macrodilution, broth microdilution, and E test antifungal susceptibility tests for fluconazole. J Clin Microbiol 1994; 32:2099.

Shek YH, Tucker MC, Viciana AL, et al: *Malassezia furfur*—disseminated infection in premature infants. Am J Clin Pathol 1989; 92:595.

Sheldon WH: Subclinical *Pneumocystis* pneumonitis. AMA J Dis Child 1959; 97:287.

Sherertz RJ, Belani A, Kramer BS, et al: Impact of air filtration on nosocomial Aspergillus infections. Unique risk of bone marrow transplant recipients. Am J Med 1987, 83:709.

Sinnott JT, Rodnite J, Emmanuel PJ, Campos A: *Cryptococcus laurentii* infection complicating peritoneal dialysis. Pediatr Infect Dis J 1989; 8:803.

Smith GW, Walker DH: Disseminated infection with *Aspergillus flavus* in an alcoholic patient. South Med J 1982; 75, 9:1148.

Sobel JD: Recurrent vulvovaginal candidiasis. A prospective study of the efficacy of maintenance ketoconazole therapy. N Engl J Med 1986; 315:1455.

Sobel JD, Vazquez J, Lynch M, et al: Vaginitis due to *Saccharomyces cerevisiae*: epidemiology, clinical aspects, and therapy. Clin Infect Dis 1993; 16:93.

Staib F, Steffen J, Krumhaar D, et al: Localised aspergillosis and oxalosis of the lung caused by *Aspergillus niger.* Soil of ornamental plants as a reservoir of aspergilli. Dtsch Med Wochenschr 1979; 104:1176.

Staib F, Blisse A: Bird manure filtrate agar for the formation of the perfect state of *Cryptococcus neoformans*, *Filobasidiella neoformans*. A comparative study of the agars prepared from pigeon and canary manure. Zentralbl Bakteriol Mikrobiol Hyg (A) 1982; 251:554.

Stern RM, Zakov ZN, Meisler DM, et al: Endogenous *Pseudoallescheria boydii* endophthalmitis. A clinicopathologic report. Clev Clin Q 1986; 53:197.

Stevens DA: Coccidioidomycosis. N Engl J Med 1995; 332:1077.

Stockman L, Roberts GD: Specificity of the latex test for cryptococcal antigen: A rapid, simple method for eliminating interference factors. J Clin Microbiol 1982; 16:965.

Straatsma BR, Zimmerman LE, Gass JDM: Phycomycosis. A clinicopathologic study of fifty-one cases. Lab Invest 1962; 11:963.

Studdard J, Sneed WF, Taylor MR Jr, Campbell GD: Cutaneous histoplasmosis. Am Rev Respir Dis 1976; 113:689.

Sudman MS: Protothecosis. A critical review. Am J Clin Pathol 1974; 61:10.

Swisher BL, Chandler FW: Grocott-Gomori methenamine silver method for detecting fungi: Practical considerations. Lab Med 1982; 13:568.

Telzak EE, Cote RJ, Gold JW, et al: Extrapulmonary *Pneumocystis carinii* infections. Rev Infect Dis 1990; 12:380.

Terrell CL, Hughes CE: Antifungal agents used for deep-seated mycotic infections. Mayo Clin Proc 1992; 67:69.

Terry PB, Rosenow EC 3d, Roberts GD: False-positive complement-fixation serology in histoplasmosis. A retrospective study. JAMA 1978; 239:2453.

Tindall JP, Fetter BF: Infections caused by achloric algae (protothecosis). Arch Dermatol 1971; 104:490.

Tosh FE, Doto IL, D'Allessio DJ, et al: The second of two epidemics of histoplasmosis resulting from work on the same starling roost. Am Rev Respir Dis 1966; 94:406.

Tritz DM, Woods GL: Fatal disseminated infection with *Aspergillus terreus* in immunocompromised hosts. Clin Infect Dis 1993; 16:118.

Walker DH, Adamec T, Krigman M: Disseminated petriellidosis (allescheriosis). Arch Pathol Lab Med 1978; 102:158.

Walker DH, McGinnis MR: Opportunistic fungal infection. What the clinician, pathologist, and mycologist can accomplish if they work together. Clin Lab Med 1982; 2:407.

Walsh TJ, Lee J, Aoki S, et al: Experimental basis for use of fluconazole for preventive or early treatment of disseminated candidiasis in granulocytopenic hosts. Rev Infect Dis 1990; 12(Suppl 3):S307.

Walter JE: The significance of antibodies in chronic histoplasmosis by immunoelectrophoretic and complement fixation tests. Am Rev Respir Dis 1969; 99:50.

Walzer PD, Perl DP, Krogstad DJ, et al: *Pneumocystis carinii* pneumonia in the United States. Epidemiologic, diagnostic and clinical features. Ann Intern Med 1974; 80:83.

Watts JC, Chandler FW: Evolving concepts of infection by *Pneumocystis carinii*. Pathol Annu 1991; 26 (Pt 1):93.

Weber WR, Askin FB, Dehner LP: Lung biopsy in *Pneumocystis carinii* pneumonia: A histopathologic study of typical and atypical features. Am J Clin Pathol 1977; 67:11.

Weems JJ Jr: *Candida parapsilosis*: Epidemiology, pathogenicity, clinical manifestations, and antimicrobial susceptibility. Clin Infect Dis 1992; 14:756.

Weitzman I, Summerbell RC: The dermatophytes. Clin Microbiol Rev 1995; 8:240.

Werner SB, Pappagianis D, Heindl I, Mickel A: An epidemic of Coccidioidomycosis among archeology students in northern California. N Engl J Med 1972; 286:507.

Westerink MA, Amsterdam D, Petell RJ, et al: Septicemia due to DF-2. Cause of a false-positive cryptococcal latex agglutination result. Am J Med 1987; 83:155.

Wheat LJ, Connolly-Stringfield PA, Baker RL, et al: Disseminated histoplasmosis in the acquired immune deficiency syndrome: Clinical findings, diagnosis and treatment, and review of the literature. Medicine. (Baltimore) 1990; 69:361.

Wheeler MS, McGinnis MR, Schell WA, Walker DH: *Fusarium* infection in burned patients. Am J Clin Pathol 1981; 75:304.

White MH, Armstrong D: Cryptococcosis. Infect Dis Clin North Am 1994; 8:383.

Williams B, Fojtasek M, Connolly-Stringfield P, Wheat J: Diagnosis of histoplasmosis by antigen detection during an outbreak in Indianapolis. Ind Arch Pathol Lab Med 1994; 118:1208.

Williams DM, Krick JA, Remington JS: Pulmonary infections in the compromised host (Part I). Am Rev Respir Dis 1976; 114:359.

Wilson ML, Davis TE, Mirrett S, et al: Controlled comparison of the BACTEC high-blood-volume fungal medium, BACTEC plus 26 aerobic blood culture bottles, and 10-milliliter isolator blood culture system for detection of fungemia and bacteremia. J Clin Microbiol 1993; 31:865.

Wingard JR, Merz WG, Saral R: *Candida tropicalis:* A major pathogen in immunocompromised patients. Ann Intern Med 1979; 91:539.

Witorsch P, Utz JP: North American blastomycosis: A study of 40 patients. Medicine (Baltimore) 1968; 47(3):169.

Young LS: *Aspergillus* infection in the neutropenic host. Hosp Pract (Off Ed) 1989; 24:37.

Zimmer BL, Roberts GD: Rapid selective urease test for presumptive identification of *Cryptococcus neoformans*. J Clin Microbiol 1979; 10:380.

Zuger A, Louie E, Holzman RS, et al: Cryptococcal disease in patients with the acquired immunodeficiency syndrome. Diagnostic features and outcome of treatment. Ann Intern Med 1986; 104:234.

Chapter 53

Medical Parasitology

Thomas R. Fritsche, M.D., Ph.D.
James W. Smith, M.D.

The study of parasitology has gained renewed importance in a world made smaller by the rapid movement of people, especially travelers to and migrants from areas endemic for parasitic disease, and by the appearance of emerging and reemerging pathogens in individuals immunocompromised for a variety of reasons. Parasitic diseases of humans and domestic animals place a tremendous burden on limited health care resources, and adversely affect economic and societal development in many countries around the world.

Clinicians in the United States and elsewhere are increasingly being confronted with unusual diagnostic problems associated with parasitic infections. Likewise, laboratorians have been challenged with the development of new technologies to accurately and rapidly diagnose such parasites as *Cryptosporidium parvum*, *Cyclospora cayetanensis*, *Toxoplasma gondii*, and microsporidia in individuals with the acquired immune deficiency syndrome. The worldwide resurgence in malaria and other parasitic diseases has also required laboratorians to strengthen their expertise in the identification of the usual blood, intestinal, and tissue protozoa and helminths.

Once diagnosed, additional problems may be encountered in the management of these diseases owing to lack of effective therapies or the emergence of resistance to traditional therapy. Many parasites require arthropod vectors for their transmission, and the irregular application of vector control efforts has, in some instances, resulted in the emergence of insecticide resistance. Malaria has made a tremendous resurgence in many areas owing to a relaxation in control efforts and the emergence of drug-resistant parasites and insecticide-resistant mosquitoes. Schistosomiasis has spread to many new areas secondary to an increase in irrigation as a result of population growth and the need to expand agricultural production.

Because of the chronic nature and generally long prepatent periods (time between infection and appearance of diagnostic stages) of many parasitic diseases, physicians may not consider them in a differential diagnosis unless the patient voluntarily offers information or specific inquiry is made about travel history or other possible exposure. Malaria is one parasitic disease that often presents as an acute, febrile illness that may have lethal consequences unless it is considered in the differential diagnosis and a history of travel to an endemic area is elicited.

The actual incidence of parasitic infections seen in the United States is unknown, because most infections are not reported to public health officials. *Giardia lamblia*, other intestinal protozoa, and intestinal roundworms are reported

Table 53–1. INCIDENCE (>0.1%) OF THE MOST COMMONLY IDENTIFIED INTESTINAL PARASITES IN 216,275 FECAL SPECIMENS EXAMINED BY STATE HEALTH DEPARTMENT LABORATORIES, 1987

Parasite	Percent of Specimens Positive
Protozoa	
Giardia lamblia	7.2
Entamoeba coli	4.2
Endolimax nana	4.2
Blastocystis hominis	2.6
Entamoeba hartmanni	1.4
Entamoeba histolytica	0.9
Iodamoeba bütschlii	0.6
Dientamoeba fragilis	0.5
Chilomastix mesnili	0.3
Cryptosporidium spp.	0.2
Helminths	
Hookworms	1.5
Trichuris trichiura	1.2
Ascaris lumbricoides	0.8
Clonorchis/Opisthorchis	0.6
Strongyloides stercoralis	0.4
Enterobius vermicularis	0.4
Hymenolepis nana	0.4

Excerpted from Kappus KD, Lundgren RG, Juranek DD, Roberts JM, Spencer HC: Intestinal parasitism in the United States: update on a continuing problem. Am J Trop Med Hyg 1994; 50(6):705–713.

most frequently by state laboratories, but other parasites, including *Cryptosporidium* and microsporidia, probably occur more frequently but are underdiagnosed (Kappus, 1994) (Table 53–1). The prevalence of parasitic diseases occurring worldwide and related mortality figures have been summarized elsewhere (Markell, 1992).

This chapter provides an overview of the general approach laboratorians use to recover and identify parasitic protozoa and helminths from human specimens. Discussion of the individual species of parasites focuses on essential clinical and biological information necessary to assist in diagnosis and management. For more extensive coverage of specific parasites, a number of excellent texts are available (Beaver, 1984; Garcia, 1993; Goldsmith, 1989; Manson-Bahr, 1987; Markell, 1992; Strickland, 1991; and Warren, 1990 among others). Parasitology atlases and Kodachrome slide collections are important resources for any laboratorian performing parasitology examinations and should be readily available (Ash, 1987, 1990; Brooke, 1984; Isenberg, 1992; Murray, 1995; Peters, 1989; Smith, 1976a, 1976b, 1976c; Spencer, 1982; Sun, 1988). Several texts specifically address pathologic aspects of parasitic infections (Binford, 1976; Gutierrez, 1990; Orihel, 1995; Marcial-Rojas, 1971; Sun, 1982; Von Lichtenberg, 1991; Woods, 1993). Parasitic infections that are problematic in immunocompromised patients also have been reviewed (Walzer, 1989).

LABORATORY METHODS

Numerous methods have been described for the recovery and identification of parasites in clinical specimens, some of which are useful for detection of a variety of species, whereas others detect only a particular species. It is preferable for the laboratory to offer a limited number of procedures competently performed than to offer a larger variety of infrequently performed tests that may prove problematic. Analyses of blood and fecal specimens comprise the largest share of clinician requests for parasitologic evaluation. A variety of additional specimens are submitted to the laboratory less frequently, including urogenital specimens, sputum, aspirates, and biopsy material. As newer information becomes available on certain of the so-called emerging parasites, the laboratory may need to develop and use additional, highly specific, test methodologies or find competent referral laboratories where such tests are performed.

The types of specimens collected for laboratory evaluation depend on the species and stage of the parasite suspected. Knowledge of the life cycle of the parasite aids in determining the type, number, and frequency of specimens required for diagnosis. Immunologic and molecular methods for the diagnosis of parasitic diseases also are useful in many instances, and may be the only methods available in certain circumstances. Complete descriptions of the general and esoteric laboratory procedures for the recovery and identification of parasites referred to here may be found in a variety of sources to which the reader is referred (Ash, 1987; Balows, 1988; Beaver, 1984; Garcia, 1993; Isenberg, 1992; Murray, 1995).

Familiarity with the calibration and use of the ocular micrometer is necessary for any laboratory performing parasitologic examination. Measurement of the size of protozoal trophozoites and cysts, and of helminth eggs and larvae is often required to make an accurate identification. Differentiation of pathogenic and nonpathogenic amebae (specifically *Entamoeba histolytica* and *E. hartmanni*) can only be made with assurance by taking careful size measurements. Similarly, eggs of *Diphyllobothrium* spp., *Paragonimus westermani*, and *Fasciola/Fasciolopsis* may be readily differentiated on the basis of accurate measurements (Smith, 1979).

Examination of Blood

Parasites that may be detected in blood specimens include the agents of malaria (*Plasmodium* spp.), babesiosis (*Babesia* spp.), trypanosomiasis (*Trypanosoma* spp.), leishmaniasis (*Leishmania donovani*), and filariasis (*Wuchereria bancrofti, Brugia malayi, Loa loa,* and *Mansonella* spp.). The most important techniques to be performed in the clinical laboratory to assist in the diagnosis of blood parasites are the preparation, staining, and examination of thick and thin blood films. Other techniques used less frequently include the buffy coat smear and various concentration techniques reserved for recovery of microfilariae (National Committee for Clinical Laboratory Standards [NCCLS], 1992).

Thick and Thin Blood Films

Examination of permanent stained blood films is required to make an identification of most blood parasites. Thin films are prepared in the same manner as that used for hematologic differential evaluation; blood is spread over the slide in a thin layer yielding intact, nonoverlapping cellular elements. Integrity of the blood cell membranes is important to determine the intracellular or extracellular nature of the infection. In the thick film, blood is concentrated in a small area that is many cell layers deep. During staining, the erythrocytes are dehemoglobinized and only leukocyte nuclei, platelets, and parasites (if present) are visible. The thick film is preferred for diagnosis, because it contains 16 to 30 times more blood per microscopic field than does the thin film, thus increasing the chances of detecting light parasitemia and decreasing the time needed for a reliable examination. The amount of blood examined in a thick film in five minutes using the 100× oil immersion objective would require at least 30 minutes when examining an equivalent amount in a thin film. While thick films increase the likelihood of detecting an infection, species identifications usually are performed by examination of thin films because morphology is often more definitive, especially for the malarial parasites. For routine examination, both thick and thin films should be prepared.

PREPARATION OF SLIDES. Blood for examination may be obtained by fingerstick, earlobe puncture, or venipuncture. Fingerstick blood should flow freely to prevent dilution with tissue fluid, and it should not be contaminated with the alcohol disinfectant, which should be allowed to dry first. If obtained by venipuncture, the first drop of blood (anticoagulant free) from the needle is used to prepare the films at the bedside. Use of anticoagulants is discouraged when malaria is suspected because they may cause distortion of the parasites and interfere with staining. In practice, however, blood usually is submitted to the laboratory in an anticoagulant, which may be the only practical method to ensure that high-quality smears can be prepared. Ethylenediaminetetra-acetic acid (EDTA)–anticoagulated blood is preferred in such cases and should be transported to the laboratory within the hour to prevent deterioration of organism morphology. Anticoagulants do not interfere with the staining of microfilariae.

Both thin and thick films should be prepared on clean, grease-free slides. Thick films are prepared by puddling several small drops of blood into an area the size of a dime (1.5 cm) and allowing the blood to dry flat at room temperature, usually overnight. A proper thick film should be thin enough that newspaper print may be read through it. If it is too thick, the film may peel from the slide. Excess heat may fix erythrocytes and prevent dehemoglobinization.

STAINING. Blood begins to lose its affinity for stain in about three days, and older thick films do not dehemoglobinize well. Best staining results are achieved when using Giemsa's stain, because host cell and parasite chromatin stains vividly while the hemoglobin in erythrocytes is only a pale red, and it is the only stain that allows visualization of the erythrocyte stippling that occurs with infection by certain malarial parasites. Wright's stain may be used for thin films, but it stains parasites less well than Giemsa's, and it stains erythrocytes, producing a busier background. Because Wright's stain incorporates alcohol as its fixative, thick films must be lysed in water before staining.

The Giemsa staining procedure requires somewhat more attention to preparation of reagents and staining protocol than does the Wright's staining procedure, which is often automated. Generally, fresh Giemsa's stain must be made each day of use by diluting stock solution into phosphate buffered water. To achieve appropriate staining reactions, including appearance of Shüffner's stippling, buffered water must be maintained between pH 6.8 to 7.2. Each new lot of stock Giemsa's stain must be checked to determine optimal staining time and dilution because there is some variation from lot to lot.

EXAMINATION OF SMEARS. Both thick and thin smears are examined in their entirety under the low power (10×) objective to detect microfilariae, which rarely occur in large numbers. In particular, the feathered edge of thin smears should be examined as microfilariae are often carried there during preparation of the smear. Examination using a 50× oil immersion objective may subsequently be used to screen blood films for protozoa, although thorough examination using the 100× oil immersion objective still is necessary to detect the smallest parasites such as *Plasmodium* spp., *Babesia* spp., and leishmaniae. Again, examination of the feathered edge is important because the erythrocytes are drawn out into a single layer of cells, allowing thorough evaluation of their morphology and the presence of intracellular protozoa. An experienced microscopist should examine at least 100 oil immersion fields (requiring about 5 minutes) on the thick blood film and 200 fields (requiring at least 15 minutes) on the thin film using the 100× objective before issuing a negative report (Ash, 1987).

Concentration Techniques

A variety of special techniques have been described for the concentration of blood parasites, specifically leishmaniae, trypanosomes, and microfilariae, details of which may be found elsewhere (Ash, 1987; Beaver, 1984; Garcia, 1993; Isenberg, 1992; NCCLS, 1992).

Preparation of buffy coat smears, which most clinical laboratories can perform with existing resources, is helpful in the detection of *Leishmania donovani*, trypanosomes, and microfilariae. Following centrifugation of an anticoagulated blood sample, the layer of cells between the plasma and packed erythrocytes is drawn off and used to prepare blood films for staining or for preparation of a wet mount to detect motile organisms (Ash, 1987; Strickland, 1991).

For detection of microfilariae, Knott's concentration or membrane filtration is helpful, particularly when the density of microfilariae in peripheral blood is very low. In the Knott technique, anticoagulated blood is lysed with 2% formalin and centrifuged to concentrate the microfilariae in the sediment, which may then be examined as a wet preparation or stained with Giemsa or hematoxylin stains. In the membrane filtration procedure, blood is lysed and passed through a 5-μm membrane filter, which subsequently is stained with hematoxylin to reveal any microfilariae (Ash, 1987; NCCLS, 1992).

Use of the fluorochrome acridine orange in a microhematocrit centrifuge format (QBC blood parasite detection method, Becton-Dickinson, Franklin Lakes, NJ) allows detection of blood parasites and appears to be more sensitive than traditional thick and thin smears. Laboratories that encounter malaria infrequently may experience difficulty in interpreting results by this method, however, and are encouraged to retain expertise in performance of traditional blood film techniques (NCCLS, 1992).

Examination of Fecal Specimens

The presence of intestinal parasites is primarily identified through the direct examination of stool using wet mounts, concentration techniques, permanent stained smears, and less frequently, culture. Newer immunoassay methods using species-specific antibody reagents to detect parasites or their antigens are also becoming popular. Stages of helminths commonly recovered include eggs and larvae, although intact worms or portions thereof occasionally may be seen. Intestinal protozoan infections are diagnosed by detection of trophozoites, cysts, or oocysts. Routine methods for the identification of ova and parasites (O & P examination) should include procedures that permit recovery of both protozoa and helminths, with use of special procedures limited for specific requests. At a minimum, laboratories performing parasitologic examination should be capable of performing direct wet mount examination of fresh stool, a concentration procedure, and a permanent stain method. Many protozoan infections will be missed unless permanent stains are examined (Garcia, 1979, 1993; NCCLS, 1993).

Specimen Collection, Handling, and Preservation

Recovery and subsequent identification of parasites in fecal specimens requires proper collection and handling. Old, poorly preserved, or contaminated specimens are of little value. Specimens should not be collected for one week after the patient has ingested any materials that leave a crystalline residue, such as nonabsorbable antidiarrheal compounds, antacids, bismuth, barium, or antimalarial agents. Oily laxatives such as mineral oil may also interfere with examination. Use of antibiotics or contrast media may decrease the numbers of organisms, especially protozoa, in the intestinal tract for several weeks (Ash, 1987).

Specimens may be submitted to the laboratory either fresh or in appropriate preservatives. All fresh specimens should be examined within one hour of passage, and liquid specimens should be examined within 30 minutes or placed immediately in preservatives to maintain the best yield. This method ensures that fragile protozoal trophozoites are not inadvertently destroyed. Specimens that cannot be processed immediately should be left at room temperature or refrigerated and should not be placed in an incubator, because this only speeds disintegration of parasites.

Specimens may be passed directly into clean, dry paper cartons or by having the patient squat over wax paper and transferring a portion to a container. Diarrheic specimens may also be collected in clean bedpans. Containers should have tight-fitting lids and should be placed in plastic bags before transport to the laboratory. Inadvertent introduction of urine or toilet water with the specimen may readily destroy protozoal trophozoites and should be avoided. Also, contamination with water or soil may accidentally introduce free-living organisms that may prove difficult to differentiate from parasitic ones.

Kits consisting of vials of preservatives appropriate for performing direct examinations, concentration procedures, and preparation of stained smears are available from a number of commercial sources at low cost. Aliquots of freshly passed stool should be immediately placed into these vials and mixed thoroughly. These kits are especially helpful for those patients who are unable to bring in a fresh sample in timely fashion or for those who will be collecting several specimens over the course of several days. With the two-vial technique, one portion of specimen is fixed in three parts of 5% to 10% buffered formalin and another portion in three parts of polyvinyl alcohol (PVA) fixative. Other preservation systems available include merthiolate-iodine-formalin (MIF) and sodium acetate–formalin (SAF) (Table 53–2). SAF has an advantage in that it can be used for permanent stains as well as for direct mounts and concentration procedures, and that it does not contain mercury, which is present in Schaudinn's and PVA fixatives. In addition to being poisonous, mercury presents disposal problems in an increasing number of states. However, the quality of permanent stains when using SAF is not as good as with Schaudinn's or PVA fixatives. Use of zinc sulfate–based PVA is gaining popularity, and its use may be indicated when mercury chloride–based compounds cannot be used (Garcia, 1993).

Examination of three specimens collected every other day is considered the minimum necessary to perform an adequate O & P evaluation (NCCLS, 1993). This procedure ensures an optimum interval for recovery of those parasites that are known to shed diagnostic forms intermittently, especially *Giardia lamblia* and *Strongyloides stercoralis.* Additional sensitivity may be achieved in detecting these parasites as well as *E. histolytica* using purgation. The laboratory must be notified prior to initiation of purgation, however, to have staff available for processing. Specimens should be collected in separate containers and submitted to the laboratory within minutes of collection. Saline purgatives such as sodium sulfate or buffered phosphosoda are recommended.

Macroscopic Examination

Fecal specimens should be examined grossly for consistency (formed, soft, loose, or watery), and for the presence of mucus, blood, larval or adult worms, and proglottids. Protozoan trophozoites are more likely to be found in watery or loose specimens, whereas cysts predominate in formed or

Table 53–2. STOOL FIXATIVES AND EXAMINATION TECHNIQUES

	Examination Technique		
Fixative	***Direct Wet Mount***	***Concentration Procedure***	***Permanent Stained Smear***
None (fresh stool)	Yes	Yes	Yes
10% formalin	Yes	Yes	No
Schaudinn's fluid	No	No	Yes
Polyvinyl alcohol (PVA)	No	No*	Yes
Modified PVA†	No	No*	Yes
Merthiolate-iodine-formalin (MIF)	Yes	Yes	No‡
Sodium acetate–formalin (SAF)	Yes	Yes	Yes

*Although concentration techniques using PVA have been described, they are not widely used owing to problems with recovery of some organisms.

†Copper sulfate or zinc sulfate replaces the mercuric chloride.

‡Smears prepared from MIF-preserved specimens may be stained with polychrome IV stain.

6

soft specimens. Helminths or their eggs may be found in any type of fecal specimen. Most parasites are uniformly distributed in the stool as a result of the mixing action of the cecum, although some eggs (especially schistosomes) may enter the fecal stream in the lower colon and rectum and be unevenly distributed, as may pinworm and *Taenia* spp. eggs. Protozoal trophozoites may be more numerous in the last portion of stool evacuated and should be specifically sought in mucus.

Microscopic Examination

Specimens may be examined microscopically by direct wet mounts of fresh or preserved material, wet mounts of concentrates, or permanent stains. Each procedure has specific advantages and limitations. Direct saline wet mounts of fresh feces allow detection and observation of motile protozoan trophozoites and helminth larvae. Direct mounts of preserved feces may allow detection of parasites that do not concentrate well. Concentration procedures increase the examiner's ability to detect protozoan cysts and helminth eggs and larvae but are unsatisfactory for detecting protozoan trophozoites. Permanent stains are useful for detection and morphologic examination of protozoan trophozoites and cysts.

The circumstances under which each procedure is performed varies depending on the type of specimen (formed, soft, loose, or watery) submitted. Generally, a fresh soft, loose, or watery specimen should have all three procedures performed. Watery specimens may be concentrated by simple centrifugation rather than by flotation or formalin–ethyl acetate concentration. The direct wet mount may be omitted if the specimen is submitted in preservatives (NCCLS, 1993). At a minimum, formed specimens should be examined by a concentration procedure, although improved yield has been demonstrated when a permanent stain is added to the workup (Garcia, 1979, 1993).

DIRECT WET MOUNT. The direct wet mount is one of the most easily performed parasitologic tests, although proper interpretation requires careful examination and experience in using the microscope to full advantage. The test is most useful when fresh specimens, especially liquid stools or duodenal aspirates, are examined for motile trophozoites or helminth larvae. A small amount of stool is mixed with a drop of 0.85% saline and covered with a coverslip. The preparation should be dense enough that newspaper print can just be read through it.

Examination of the entire coverslip is performed systematically under the low-power (10×) objective with the microscope diaphragm closed down to increase contrast. Suspicious objects and those that are refractile, such as protozoal cysts, should then be examined with the high-power (40×) objective. Detection of motility of slow-moving amebae requires that an object be examined for at least 15 seconds. In the absence of suspicious objects, up to a third of the preparation should be examined using the 40× objective. Use of the oil immersion objective usually is not performed unless the coverslip has been sealed with fingernail polish or vaspar (a 50/50 mixture of petroleum jelly and paraffin).

A second preparation may be made in identical fashion except that a drop of a 1:5 dilution of Lugol's iodine or an equivalent preparation is added in place of the saline. Use of straight Lugol's or Gram's iodine causes clumping of material and is not recommended. Iodine is helpful in enhancing the visibility of nuclear structures in protozoal cysts and for detecting glycogen inclusions. Limitations, however, include loss of trophozoite motility and cyst refractility, and difficulty in recognizing chromatoid bodies.

CONCENTRATION TECHNIQUES. Concentration procedures, which may be performed on fresh or preserved specimens (see Table 53–2), are more sensitive than direct wet mount examination for detection of protozoan cysts and helminth eggs and larvae because they decrease the amount of background material in the preparations and, in most circumstances, actually concentrate the organisms. Although a variety of methods and modifications have been described, some are useful only for specific parasites (Ash, 1987; Garcia, 1993; Melvin, 1982). For routine use a method should be selected that allows reliable detection of both protozoan cysts and helminth eggs. Concentration methods are based upon sedimentation or flotation principles. In sedimentation the heavier parasites settle to the bottom owing to gravity or centrifugation. In flotation the lighter parasite cysts and eggs rise to the surface of a solution of high specific gravity. The two most widely used concentration procedures in the United States are the zinc sulfate centrifugal flotation technique of Faust and the formalin-ether sedimentation of Ritchie (or their modifications). In practice ethyl acetate has replaced ether in the latter method because of the dangers associated with handling ether, and comparable results are achieved (Young, 1979, Truant, 1981).

Formalin–ethyl acetate concentration is a biphasic sedimentation technique that is efficient in recovering most protozoan cysts and helminth eggs and larvae, including operculate eggs, and is moderately effective for schistosome eggs. Less distortion of protozoal cysts occurs with this technique than with zinc sulfate flotation. Eggs of *Hymenolepis nana* may be missed, however, and concentration of *Giardia lamblia* and *Iodamoeba bütschlii* cysts may not be very good. For proper concentration of coccidian oocysts and spores of microsporidia, attention must be paid to the recommended speed and time of centrifugation (Isenberg, 1992; NCCLS, 1993). Despite these problems, the technique is widely used both for its simplicity and suitability in most laboratory situations.

With the zinc sulfate flotation method, fresh stool is processed using zinc sulfate with a specific gravity of 1.18 and formalinized stool is processed with a solution of specific gravity of 1.20. Parasitic elements are recovered from the surface film of the solution following centrifugation. This method yields a cleaner preparation than does formalin–ethyl acetate concentration, but it is unreliable for the recovery of nematode larvae, infertile eggs of *Ascaris*, and the eggs of most trematodes and large tapeworms. Problems with recovery also occur with stool specimens containing excessive amounts of fats. Use of formalinized stool specimens rather than fresh stool helps clear the specimen and prevents popping of opercula and distortion of the parasites (Bartlett, 1978).

PERMANENT STAINS. Use of stained slide preparations provides a permanent record of a patient's specimen and allows review by consultants should difficulties arise in identification. Of the methods described for studying fecal specimens, only the permanent stain is designed for analysis using

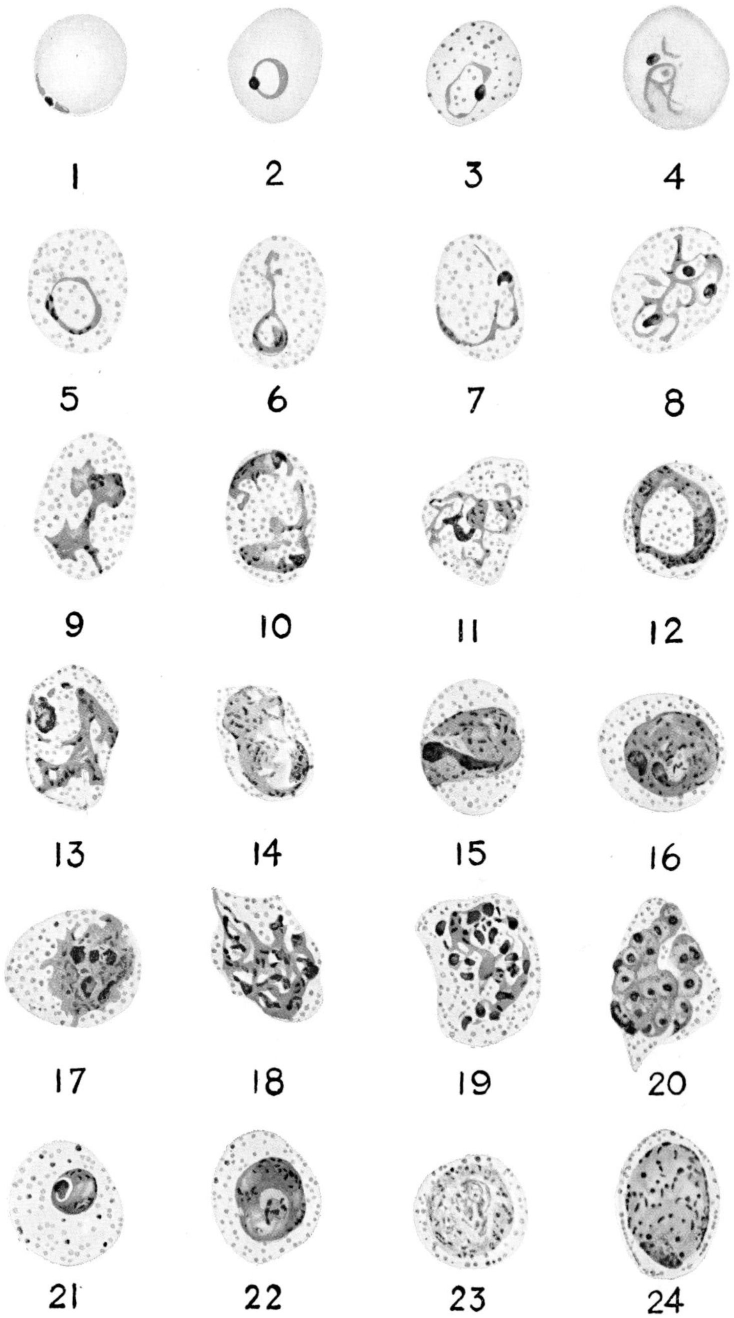

Plate 53–1. *Plasmodium vivax. 1*, Normal-size erythrocyte with marginal ring form trophozoite. *2*, Young signet ring form of trophozoite in macrocyte. *3*, Slightly older ring form trophozoite in erythrocyte showing basophilic stippling. *4*, Polychromatophilic erythrocyte containing young tertian parasite with pseudopodia. *5*, Ring form of trophozoite showing pigment in cytoplasm of an enlarged cell containing Schüffner's stippling. This stippling does not appear in all cells containing the growing and older forms of *Plasmodium vivax*, but it can be found with any stage from the fairly young ring form onward. *6* and *7*, Very tenuous medium trophozoite forms. *8*, Three ameboid trophozoites with fused cytoplasm. *9*, *11*, *12*, and *13*, Older ameboid trophozoites in process of development. *10*, Two ameboid trophozoites in one cell. *14*, Mature trophozoite. *15*, Mature trophozoite with chromatin apparently in process of division. *16*, *17*, *18*, and *19*, Schizonts showing progressive steps in division (presegmenting schizonts). *20*, Mature schizont. *21* and *22*, Developing gametocytes. *23*, Mature microgametocyte. *24*, Mature macrogametocyte. (From Wilcox A: Manual for the Microscopical Diagnosis of Malaria in Man. Bulletin No. 180, National Institute of Health, 1942.)

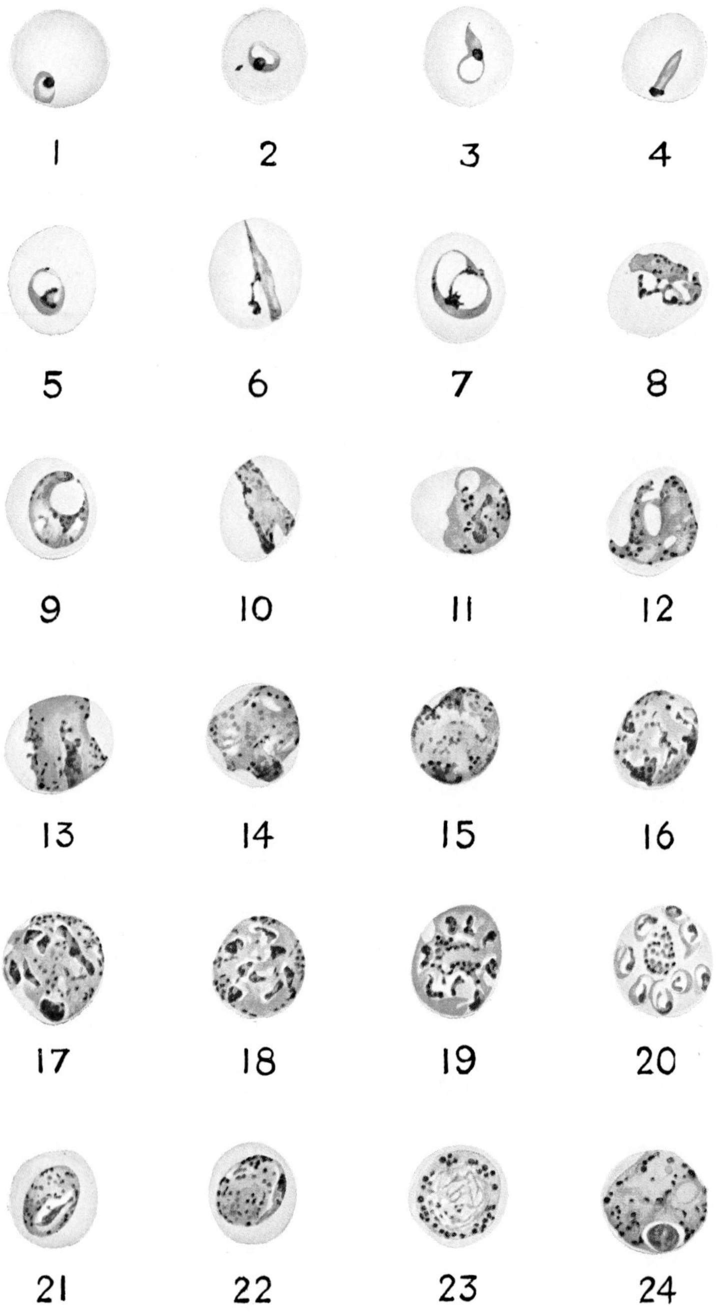

Plate 53–2. *Plasmodium malariae. 1*, Young ring form trophozoite of quartan malaria. *2*, *3*, and *4*, Young trophozoite forms of the parasite showing gradual increase of chromatin and cytoplasm. *5*, Developing ring form of trophozoite showing pigment granule. *6*, Early band form of trophozoite—elongated chromatin, some pigment apparent. *7*, *8*, *9*, *10*, *11*, and *12*, Some forms that the developing trophozoite of quartan malaria may take. *13* and *14*, Mature trophozoites—one a band form. *15*, *16*, *17*, *18*, and *19*, Phases in the development of the schizont (presegmenting schizonts). *20*, Mature schizont. *21*, Immature microgametocyte. *22*, Immature macrogametocyte. *23*, Mature microgametocyte. *24*, Mature macrogametocyte. (From Wilcox A: Manual for the Microscopical Diagnosis of Malaria in Man. Bulletin No. 180, National Institute of Health, 1942.)

Plate 53–3. *Plasmodium falciparum. 1*, Very young ring form trophozoite. *2*, Double infection of single cell with young trophozoites, one a "marginal form," the other "signet ring" form. *3* and *4*, Young trophozoites showing double chromatin dots. *5*, *6*, and *7*, Developing trophozoite forms. *8*, Three medium trophozoites in one cell. *9*, Trophozoite showing pigment, in a cell containing Maurer's dots. *10* and *11*, Two trophozoites in each of two cells, showing variation of forms that parasites may assume. *12*, Almost mature trophozoite showing haze of pigment throughout cytoplasm. Maurer's dots in the cell. *13*, Estivo-autumnal "slender forms." *14*, Mature trophozoite, showing clumped pigment. *15*, Parasite in the process of initial chromatin division. *16*, *17*, *18,* and *19*, Various phases of the development of the schizont (presegmenting schizonts). *20*, Mature schizont. *21*, *22*, *23,* and *24*, Successive forms in the development of the gametocyte—usually not found in the peripheral circulation. *25*, Immature macrogametocyte. *26*, Mature macrogametocyte. *27*, Immature microgametocyte. *28*, Mature microgametocyte. (Courtesy of National Institutes of Health, U.S.P.H.S.)

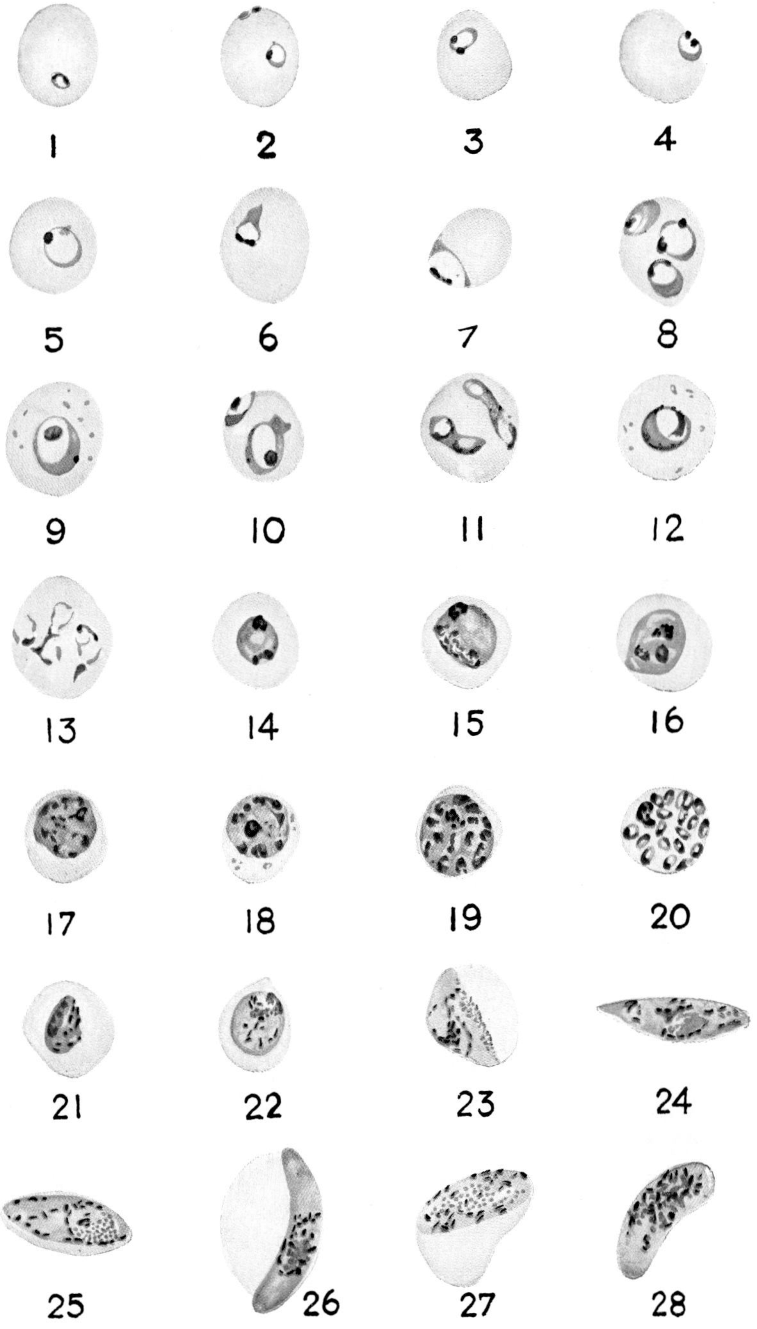

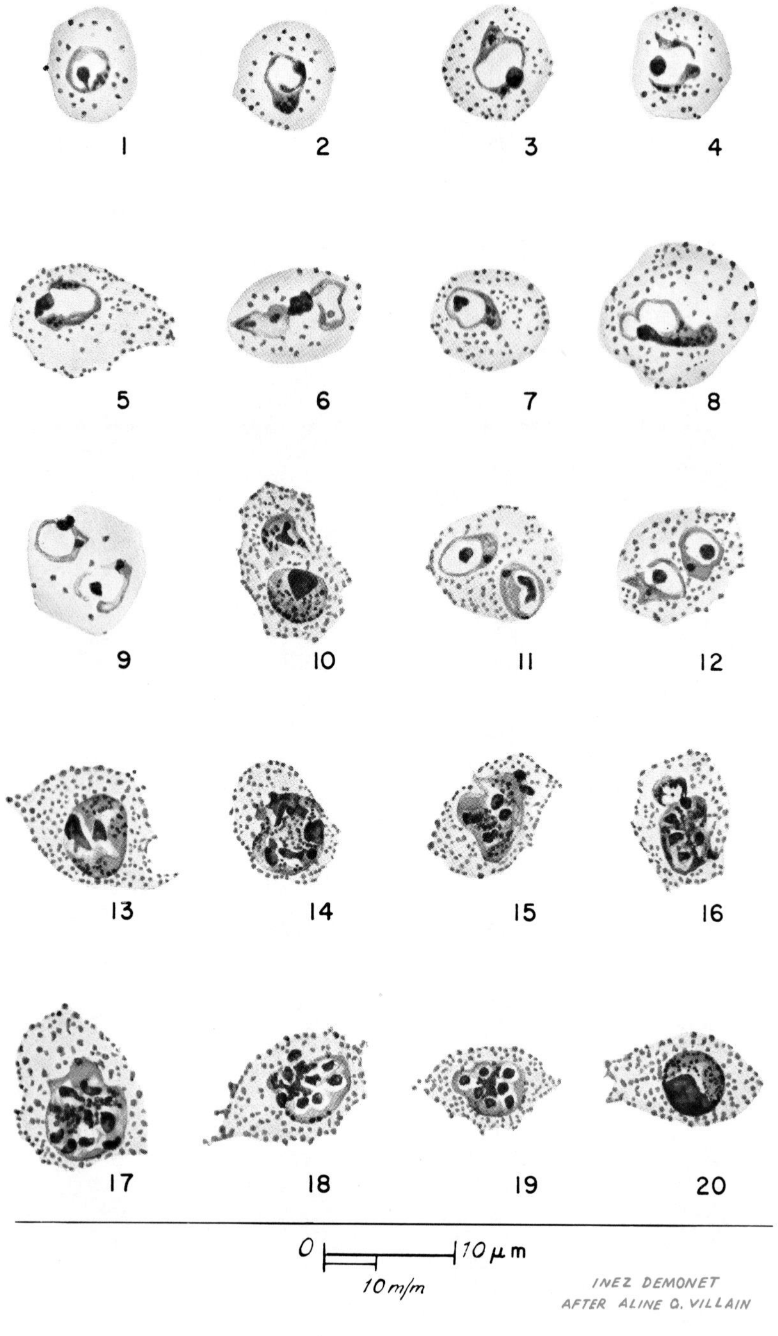

Plate 53–4. *Plasmodium ovale. 1*, Young ring-shaped trophozoite. *2*, *3*, *4*, and *5*, Older ring-shaped trophozoites. *6*, *7*, and *8*, Older ameboid trophozoites. *9*, *11*, and *12*, Doubly infected cells, trophozoites. *10*, Doubly infected cell, young gametocytes. *13*, First stage of the schizont. *14*, *15*, *16*, *17*, *18*, and *19*, Schizonts, progressive stages. *20*, Mature gametocyte.

Free translation of legend accompanying original plate in "Guide pratique d'examen microscopique du sang appliqué au diagnostic du paludisme" by Georges Villain. Reproduced with permission from "Biologic Medicale" supplement, 1935.

(Courtesy of Aimee Wilcox, National Institutes of Health Bulletin No. 180, U.S.P.H.S.)

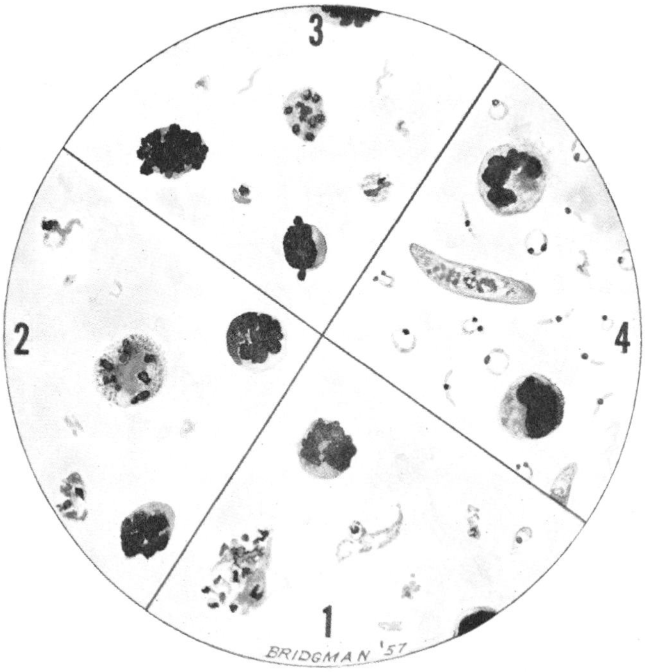

Plate 53–5. The human plasmodia as seen in thick film. *1, Plasmodium vivax:* young and older trophozoites and schizont; *2, P. ovale:* developing trophozoite and schizonts, one within a "ghost cell"; *3, P. malariae:* trophozoites and schizont. *4, P. falciparum:* young trophozoites and gametocyte. (From Markell EK, Voge M: Medical Parasitology. Philadelphia, W. B. Saunders Company, 1976.)

the oil immersion objective (100×). The permanent stain is most useful for detection of protozoal trophozoites and cysts, which may be recognized when the direct and concentrated preparations are negative. Although generally not useful for detecting helminth eggs or larvae, permanent stains are inherently more sensitive for detecting protozoal infections, and their use has been recommended for every stool sample submitted for O & P examination (NCCLS, 1993).

A variety of staining techniques and modifications have been described that have both advantages and disadvantages. The Wheatley trichrome stain and iron hematoxylin stain are all-purpose methods that allow detection of amebae and flagellates. Unfortunately, detection of most human-infecting coccidia and microsporidia requires the use of special stains. Technical problems may arise in the performance of any staining procedure; most are related to the age of the specimen, proper smear preparation and fixation, and quality of the reagents. Positive control slides of known staining quality should be run with each batch of slides stained. This is especially true in the performance of the more specific stains for coccidia and microsporidia. Less commonly used stains, such as polychrome IV stain for use with MIF preserved specimens and chlorazol black E stain for use with fresh specimens are not reviewed here further, but details may be found elsewhere (Garcia, 1993).

WHEATLEY'S TRICHROME STAIN. In the United States, the Wheatley modification of the trichrome method continues to find widespread acceptance because of its simplicity, reliability, and cost-effectiveness. Details of the procedure are available from a number of sources (Isenberg, 1992; Melvin, 1982; NCCLS, 1993). Appropriate specimens include those that have been fixed in Schaudinn's fixative or PVA fixatives; SAF- or MIF-preserved specimens may be stained with trichrome, but results are less satisfactory.

IRON HEMATOXYLIN STAIN. Iron hematoxylin stains are technically more difficult to perform than the trichrome stain, but results generally are superior owing to enhanced definition of key nuclear and cytoplasmic characteristics. A modified iron hematoxylin stain that may prove to be useful incorporates carbol fuchsin, allowing concurrent staining of acid-fast organisms such as *Cryptosporidium, Cyclospora,* and *Isospora* (NCCLS, 1993; Palmer, 1991). Specimens fixed in Schaudinn's, PVA, or SAF fixatives may be stained with iron hematoxylin stains (the preferred stain for SAF).

MODIFIED ACID-FAST STAINS. Oocysts of *Cryptosporidium, Cyclospora*, and *Isospora* are difficult to recognize on trichrome- or iron hematoxylin–stained smears, but their presence may be detected by using an acid-fast staining technique such as the modified Kinyoun method, modified acid-fast dimethyl sulfoxide (DMSO), or auramine-O (Bronsdon, 1984; Current, 1991; Ma, 1983). Acid-fast stains are sensitive and cost-effective for detection of these protozoa, but they lack specificity. Close attention must be paid to defined morphologic criteria when using these stains, and the use of positive control material is mandatory. For laboratories in which *Cryptosporidium* is rarely encountered, use of the highly specific and sensitive commercially available monoclonal antibody reagents are recommended. Stool, sputa, biliary tract, and other appropriate specimens that are fresh, formalin-fixed or SAF-fixed may be used with acid-fast stains.

STAINS FOR MICROSPORIDIA. Microsporidia (specifically *Enterocytozoon bieneusi* and *Septata intestinalis*) have been implicated as common agents of diarrheal disease, especially in immunocompromised patients, although their detection has been problematic. Although biopsy and electron microscopy have been a mainstay in their diagnosis, staining procedures that may be performed in the clinical laboratory have been described. A modified trichrome stain using an increased (10-fold) concentration of chromotrope 2R combined with an increase in the staining time has gained acceptance as a specific test for the identification of microsporidial spores (Weber, 1994). Fluorescent staining methods using optical whitening agents such as Uvitek-2B and calcofluor white also are useful for rapid and sensitive screening of stool and other clinical specimens for such spores (DeGirolami, 1995; Luna, 1995; van Gool, 1993). The small size (1.5 to 3 μm) of these organisms makes their detection difficult, and such studies should not be undertaken without appropriate control materials for comparison.

Additional Techniques for Examination of Enteric Parasites

CELLULOSE TAPE TECHNIQUE FOR PINWORMS. The female pinworm, *Enterobius vermicularis*, migrates from the cecum to the perianal skin, where she deposits typical eggs that are fully embryonated. The eggs or, occasionally, adult worms may be detected on examination of clear, adhesive cellophane tape or commercial collection kits that have been pressed onto the perianal skin. Eggs or adults are rarely found in stool, which is considered to be an inappropriate specimen for detection of this parasite. Specimens should be collected late at night, when the worms are most active, or first thing in the morning before bathing or defecation. Several specimens taken on different days should be examined before ruling out infection.

EGG STUDIES. Estimation of worm burden occasionally is requested to assist in the evaluation of therapeutic efficacy or following rates of reinfection with intestinal nematodes (*Ascaris*, *Trichuris*, and hookworms) or, occasionally, schistosomes. Procedures include the direct smear method of Beaver, the Stoll dilution egg count, Kato's thick smear, and various modifications (Ash, 1987; Beaver, 1984; Garcia, 1993). Large variations in results are inherent when performing these tests, and levels of egg counts indicating clinical significance vary depending on the infecting species, person's age, and nutritional status (Beaver, 1984).

Egg hatching methods have been used in the analysis of schistosomiasis to detect their presence in light infections and to determine their viability. Schistosome eggs, which are fully embryonated when passed, contain a miracidium that hatches within several hours when eggs are placed in dechlorinated water. In practice, urine or stool is mixed in about 10 volumes of water, which is then placed in a sidearm or Erlenmeyer flask. All but the sidearm or the top of the flask is covered with foil wrap, and the unit is placed under a desk lamp. Hatched miracidia are positively phototropic and congregate near the light. Eggs, if available, may be examined directly for viability by examining for movement of cilia within flame (excretory) cells.

NEMATODE CULTURE AND RECOVERY TECHNIQUES. Several culture techniques (coproculture) assist in the detection and identification of certain nematode infections, including the Harada-Mori filter paper strip culture, filter paper/slant culture, and charcoal culture (Ash, 1987; Beaver, 1984; Garcia, 1993). Differentiation of hookworms and trichostrongyles on the basis of egg morphology is difficult, whereas infective-stage larvae are more readily identified. Such culture techniques may also prove useful in recovery of *Strongyloides* larvae, which may be few in number, and for differentiating them from those of hookworms. With all culture methods, feces are incubated in a humid environment to encourage egg hatching. In the Harada-Mori and filter paper/slant techniques, larvae migrate from the feces into a water phase, where they may be readily detected and recovered. In the charcoal culture, larvae first migrate into a dampened gauze pad, which is then placed in water, allowing the larvae to settle out.

The Baermann funnel technique is a sensitive and reliable method for recovery of *Strongyloides* and other nematode larvae from a stool specimen. In this assay, feces are placed on several layers of gauze on top of a wire screen that is suspended in a funnel. The bottom of the funnel is clamped off, and water is added to the level of the gauze. Larvae actively migrate through the gauze and settle to the bottom of the funnel where they may be drawn off for examination. Larval recovery may be improved over that of the culture techniques because a larger amount of feces is examined. In latent *Strongyloides* infection, in which few larvae are being shed, several examinations over a week's time may be required to demonstrate the infection (Ash, 1987).

Objects Resembling Enteric Parasites

A large variety of objects that closely resemble various parasite life cycle stages may be seen in feces and other specimens sent for O & P examination. Careful differentiation of these objects from real parasites is necessary to prevent inappropriate or unnecessary treatment. White blood cells, macrophages, and squamous and columnar epithelial cells may resemble amebae; yeasts and starch granules may resemble protozoal cysts; pollen and fungal conidia may resemble helminth eggs; plant fibers may resemble nematode larvae; and pieces of vegetables or vegetable skins may resemble adult worms or proglottids (Table 53–3). Examples of artifacts and pseudoparasites have been reviewed elsewhere (Ash, 1990; Garcia, 1993; Isenberg, 1992; NCCLS, 1993; Smith, 1976b).

Table 53–3. OBJECTS RECOVERABLE FROM STOOL THAT RESEMBLE ENTERIC PARASITES

Type of Artifact	Resemblance
Neutrophils	*Entamoeba histolytica* cysts
Macrophages	*Entamoeba histolytica* trophozoites
Columnar epithelial cells	Amebic trophozoites
Squamous epithelial cells	Amebic trophozoites
Yeasts	Protozoan cysts (especially *Endolimax nana*)
Fungal conidia	Helminth eggs
Mushroom spores	Helminth eggs
Plant cells	Protozoan cysts, helminth eggs
Plant hairs	Nematode larvae
Pollen grains	Helminth eggs (*Ascaris* or *Taenia* eggs)
Diatoms	Helminth eggs
Starch granules, fat globules, air bubbles, mucus	Protozoan cysts
Ingested mite eggs	Helminth eggs
Ingested plant nematode eggs	Helminth eggs
Ingested plant nematode larvae	Nematode larvae

Adapted from Isenberg HE (ed): Clinical Microbiology Procedures Handbook, Vols. 1 and 2. Washington, DC, American Society for Microbiology, 1992.

Examination of Urogenital and Other Specimens (Sputa, Aspirates, Biopsies)

Vaginal and urethral discharges, prostatic secretions, or urine may be submitted to the laboratory for detection of *Trichomonas vaginalis*. The most rapid and cost-effective method is the preparation of several wet mounts using a drop of specimen diluted with a drop of saline which is then covered with a cover slip. The slide is examined under the low-power (10×) objective using reduced lighting conditions for the motile trophozoites, which display a jerky movement. High-power examination may reveal the beating flagella and undulating membrane characteristic for the species. Use of culture, fluorescent antibody reagents, or DNA probe techniques improves sensitivity, if needed (Briselden, 1994). Demonstration of imidazole drug resistance requires culture of the organism.

A number of protozoal and helminthic parasites may be recovered in sputa, and the appropriate examination technique depends on the suspected organism. Generally, the technique required to detect a parasite from its usual site of infection is used on sputum and most commonly involves a wet mount. When amebae are suspected, permanent stains should be performed. Acid-fast or specific antibody–based stains are appropriate for *Cryptosporidium*, whereas modified trichrome or fluorochrome stains should be used for detection of spores of microsporidia. Identification techniques for *Pneumocystis carinii* are described in Chapter 52.

Examination of aspirates requires the use of stains as appropriate for the implicated organism. In addition to the methods used for sputum, Giemsa staining often is appropriate when examining for protozoa, especially the hemoflagellates. Biopsy material should be submitted for routine histology after imprint smears are prepared for staining with Giemsa's or other appropriate permanent stain. Culture for leishmaniae and trypanosomes also can be performed on tissues and may be important for demonstrating those infections. Skin biopsies sent for *Onchocerca* or *Mansonella* examination should be teased apart in saline and the saline examined after 30 to 60 minutes for microfilariae. Muscle biopsy for *Trichinella spiralis* larvae may be examined by compressing the fresh specimen between two glass slides or by submitting it for routine histology. Likewise, rectal or bladder biopsies may be examined for schistosome eggs.

Parasite Culture Techniques

Culture methods have been described for a wide variety of protozoan parasites, but few clinical laboratories undertake the effort because of infrequent requests and unfamiliarity with the methods. When culture requests are made, they are usually for *Trichomonas vaginalis*, *Leishmania* spp., *Try-*

panosoma cruzi, Entamoeba histolytica, Acanthamoeba spp., or *Naegleria fowleri*. In addition, virology laboratories occasionally are asked to culture for *Toxoplasma gondii*. Methods are reviewed elsewhere (Ash, 1987; Fritsche, 1989a; Isenberg, 1992; NCCLS, 1993).

Immunodiagnostic Methods

Immunodiagnostic procedures for detecting antibodies or antigens in parasitic diseases are numerous but vary tremendously in sensitivity and specificity as well as availability. The topic is beyond the scope of this chapter, but a comprehensive review is available (Wilson, 1995). Tests that are available from public health, hospital, or commercial laboratories are summarized in Table 53–4.

Historically, serologic procedures for parasitic diseases have been plagued by low sensitivity and specificity, primarily owing to the complex antigenic nature of parasites and the possibilities for cross-reactions from related species. The introduction of newer test methodologies combined with the use of more highly defined antigenic components are providing more accurate results with greater predictive values. Many of the newer tests use the enzyme immunoassay (EIA) or immunoblot (western blot) formats, although indirect immunofluorescence (IFA), indirect hemagglutination (IHA), complement fixation (CF), and bentonite flocculation (BF) methodologies remain popular.

Use of serologic tests in diagnosing parasitic diseases is an adjunct to the usual diagnostic modalities, which attempt to demonstrate the organism directly in stool, blood, tissues, or body fluids. Certain infections such as toxoplasmosis or toxocariasis cannot be readily diagnosed by morphologic means, and for others, the invasive studies required are not recommended in the initial workup. Other conditions such as filariasis, schistosomiasis, and strongyloidiasis may remain subclinical owing to light infections or because the clinical evaluation occurred during the prepatent period. In circumstances such as these, serologic evaluation may prove useful, especially in individuals who have traveled to, but do not reside in, endemic areas.

Because serologic tests for parasitic diseases are infrequently requested, specimens generally are submitted to public (Centers for Disease Control and Prevention) or private reference laboratories for evaluation. Some of the more commonly requested tests often are available locally, including those for toxoplasmosis, amebiasis, and trichinosis.

Interpretive criteria are established by reagent manufacturers or by the center performing the test, and these criteria often vary from institution to institution. Individuals requesting such tests should inquire about the performance characteristics, including sensitivity and specificity, and should be aware that cross-reactions may occur. Also, parasitic disease serologies generally do not distinguish between active and past infection, an important point when testing someone who has resided in endemic areas.

Antigen detection methods are commercially available for several parasitic diseases including amebiasis, cryptosporidiosis, giardiasis, and trichomoniasis (see Table 53–4), and these methods may be useful in those instances in which traditional tests are negative, yet a high index of clinical suspicion remains. These tests have the advantage of detecting current infection and can often be performed by someone other than the experienced morphologist (Wilson, 1995).

Table 53–4. ANTIBODY, ANTIGEN, AND DNA PROBE TESTS FOR DIAGNOSIS OF PARASITIC DISEASES*

Parasite Disease	Serologic Methods	Antigen or DNA Probe Detection Methods
Protozoan		
Amebiasis	DD, EIA, IHA	EIA
Babesiosis	IFA	
Chagas' disease	CF, EIA, IFA, IHA	
Cryptosporidiosis		EIA, DFA, IFA
Giardiasis		EIA, DFA, IFA
Leishmaniasis	CF, IFA	
Malaria	IFA	
Toxoplasmosis	EIA, IFA, IHA	DFA, IP
Trichomoniasis		DFA, EIA, DNA probe
Helminthic		
Trichinosis	BF, EIA, IHA	
Toxocariasis	EIA	
Strongyloidiasis	EIA, IHA	
Filariasis	EIA, IHA	
Cysticercosis	EIA, IHA, IB	
Echinococcosis	IHA, IEP, DD (arc-5), IB	
Schistosomiasis	EIA, IB	
Paragonimiasis	EIA, IB	

*Kits are commercially available or test is available in public health or reference laboratories.

BF, bentonite flocculation; CF, complement fixation; DA, direct agglutination; DD, double diffusion; DFA, direct fluorescent antibody; EIA, enzyme immunoassay; IB, immunoblot; IHA, indirect hemagglutination; IFA, indirect fluorescent antibody; IP, immunoperoxidase; IEP, immunoelectrophoresis.

Adapted from Wilson M, Schantz P, Pieniazek N: Diagnosis of parasitic infections: Immunologic and molecular methods. *In* Murray PR, Barron EJ, Pfaller MA, Tenover FC, Yolken RH (eds): Manual of Clinical Microbiology, 6th ed. Washington, D.C., ASM Press, 1995, p 1159.

Molecular Diagnostic Methods

Diagnostic methods using DNA amplification and nucleic acid probe techniques have been described for most of the common parasitic diseases and offer high levels of sensitivity and specificity (Persing, 1993; Weiss, 1995; Wilson, 1995). Most of these applications, however, have remained as tools for research laboratories and are not routinely available (Bendall, 1993). To date, the equipment and other resources needed, including personnel trained in molecular biology, have remained out of reach for most diagnostic laboratories owing to fiscal limitations. Although several commercial diagnostic kits have come on the market recently for detection of viral and bacterial pathogens, only one kit has received approval for a parasite, that being for *Trichomonas vaginalis* (Briselden, 1994). Molecular methods may prove to have great importance in the identification of parasite-harboring vectors and contribute to disease prevention through control programs targeted to such vectors (Weiss, 1995).

Quality Assurance, Quality Improvement, and Safety

A quality assurance program for the parasitology section of the laboratory is similar to that for the other laboratory sections and covers all essential aspects of the operation including, among others, a well-written and complete procedure manual that is reviewed annually, guidelines for maintaining all specimen and test result records, complete quality control program with appropriate technical supervision and review, and participation in an approved proficiency testing program. Laboratories also need to focus on customer satisfaction using a variety of measures available and participate in the team approach to identifying problems and generating solutions as part of a continuous quality improvement process.

The performance of individuals responsible for the parasitology section should be monitored periodically with both internal and external unknown specimens, and ongoing training should be up to date, especially for those laboratories that encounter positive specimens infrequently. A variety of reference materials should be readily available for use at the laboratory bench including positive slides and fecal specimens, printed atlases, and slide atlases.

Unpreserved specimens for parasitologic examination should be considered potentially infectious, and all blood and body fluids should be handled according to Universal Precautions as defined by the Final Rule on Bloodborne Pathogens by the Occupational Safety and Health Administration (Federal Register, 1991). In addition to blood-borne viral pathogens, malarial parasites and hemoflagellates may also remain infective. A variety of parasites may remain infective in fresh stool specimens, including cysts of enteric protozoa, eggs of *Taenia solium*, *Enterobius vermicularis*, and *H. nana*, and larvae of *Strongyloides stercoralis*. *Trichuris trichiura*, *Ascaris lumbricoides*, and hookworms may remain infective in older specimens, and *Ascaris* eggs can survive and embryonate while in 5% formalin. Fecal specimens also may contain pathogens such as *Salmonella*, *Shigella*, or viruses. Strict observance of proper specimen handling techniques and disposal is essential. Personal attention to hand washing is also necessary. Use of ethyl acetate in place of ether in the performance of concentration techniques is strongly recommended to guard against the possibility of explosion.

BLOOD AND TISSUE PROTOZOA

Malaria

Malaria (from the Italian *mal' aria,* meaning bad air) is an acute and sometimes chronic infection of the bloodstream characterized clinically by fever, anemia, and splenomegaly, and is caused by apicomplexan parasites of the genus *Plasmodium.* The defining clinical features of a malarial attack or paroxysm consist of, in order, shaking chills, fever (up to 40°C or higher), and generalized diaphoresis, followed by resolution of fever. The paroxysm occurs over 6 to 10 hours and is initiated by the synchronous rupture of erythrocytes with the release of new infectious blood stage forms known as merozoites. The disease generally occurs between 45° North and 40° South latitude (WHO, 1987) and is spread exclusively by female anopheline mosquitoes. The four species of plasmodia causing human malaria include *P. vivax, P. falciparum, P. malariae,* and *P. ovale. P. falciparum* infection occurs principally in tropical areas worldwide, whereas *P. vivax* infections occur in both tropical and temperate zones. *P. malariae* also occurs worldwide but to a much lesser extent than either *P. falciparum* or *P. vivax. P. ovale* is the least frequent of the malarias, with most cases being acquired in western Africa, India, or South America.

Because infection with falciparum malaria is potentially life threatening, its presence must be considered in the differential diagnosis of unexplained fever, and history of travel in endemic geographic areas should always be sought. In an era of increasing world travel, the risk of acquiring malaria is not insignificant, and the rapid spread of drug-resistant strains poses particular problems when considering appropriate prophylaxis or therapy.

Laboratory evaluation of patients suspected of having malaria continues to rely on timely examination of thick and thin blood films to demonstrate the intraerythrocytic parasites. Although they are straightforward in their approach, performance of these techniques may be problematic. Reliable identification of organisms requires continuous training to maintain expertise; therefore, those laboratories that rarely see positive specimens may choose to refer specimens to reference laboratories, provided processing and reporting is timely.

More advanced laboratory methods, including acridine orange staining (see the earlier section entitled Laboratory Methods) or detection of parasite-specific antigens or DNA (Lanar, 1989; Persing, 1993; Weiss, 1995) provide enhanced sensitivity and specificity but are generally not appropriate or available for smaller laboratories.

LIFE CYCLE. Malarial parasites undergo a sexual phase (sporogony) in *Anopheles* mosquitoes that results in the production of infectious sporozoites and an asexual stage (schizogony) in humans that results in the production of schizonts and merozoites (Fig. 53–1). In the bloodstream, some merozoites eventually differentiate into gametocytes (gametogony), which, when ingested by female anopheline mosquitoes, mature into the male microgametes and the female macrogametes. Fusion of a microgamete and a macrogamete results in the formation of the motile ookinete, which migrates to the outside of the stomach wall and forms an oocyst. Within the oocyst, numerous spindle-shaped sporozoites are formed. The mature oocyst ruptures into the body cavity, releasing the sporozoites, which then migrate through the tissues to the salivary glands, from which they are injected into the vertebrate host as the mosquito feeds. The time required for development in the mosquito ranges from 8 to 21 days.

The sporozoites injected into the vertebrate host reach the hepatic parenchymal cells within minutes and initiate the proliferative phase known as exoerythrocytic schizogony. Release of merozoites from ruptured hepatic schizonts initiates the bloodstream infection or erythrocytic schizogony and, eventually, the clinical symptoms of malaria. *P. vivax* and *P. ovale* differ from *P. falciparum* and *P. malariae* in that true disease relapses of the former species may occur weeks to months following subsidence of previous attacks. This occurs as a result of renewed exoerythrocytic and, eventually, erythrocytic schizogony from latent hepatic sporozoites, which are known as hypnozoites (Krotoski, 1982). Recurrences of disease due to *P. falciparum* or *P. malariae,* called recrudescences, arise from an increase in numbers of persisting blood stage forms to clinically detectable levels, not from persisting liver stage forms. Liver cells are infected only by sporozoites from the mosquito; thus, transfusion-acquired *P. vivax* or *P. ovale* infection does not relapse.

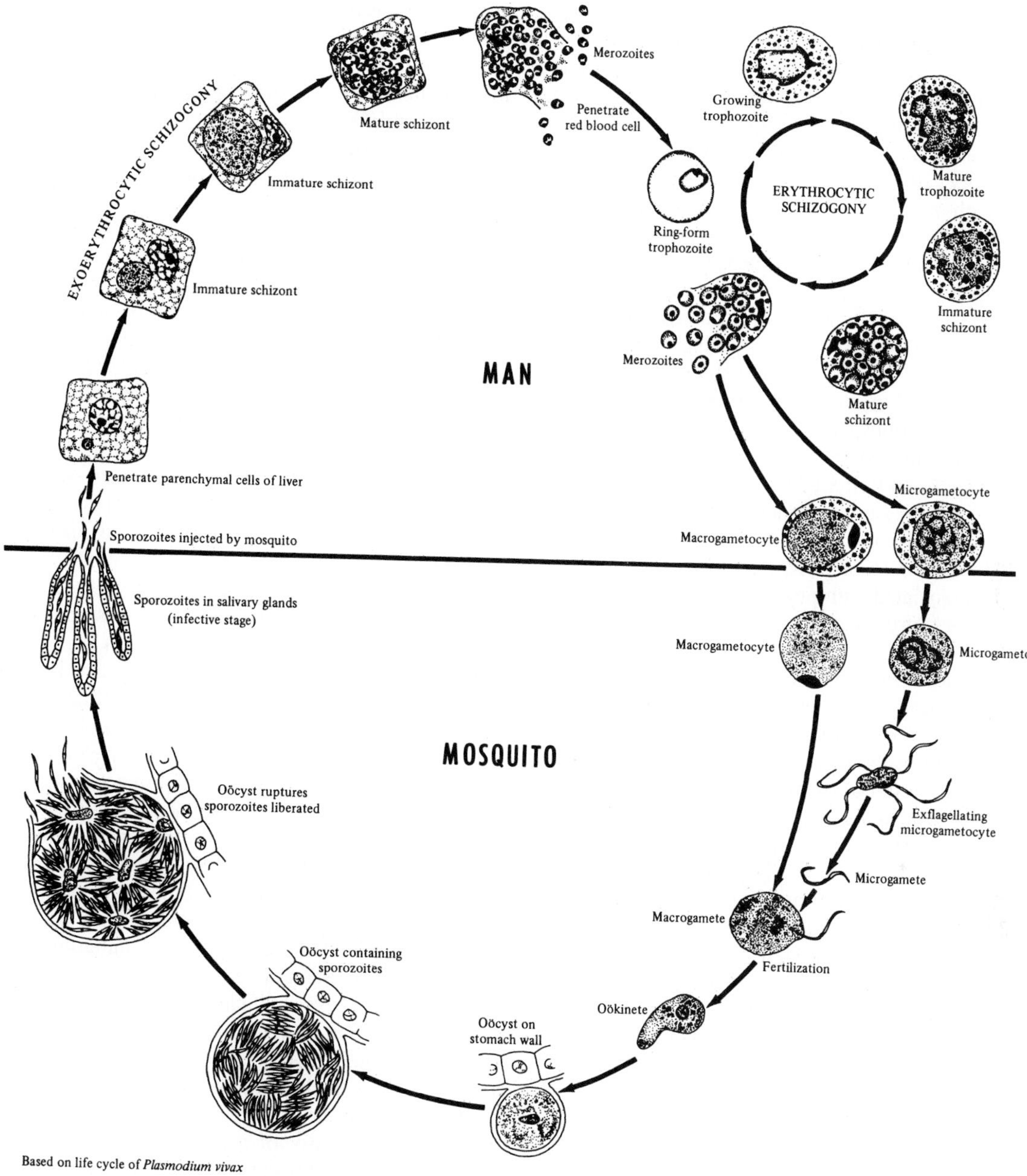

Figure 53–1. Life cycle of malarial parasites. (Courtesy of the Centers for Disease Control, Parasitology Training Branch, Atlanta, GA.)

Merozoites released from infected hepatocytes subsequently infect erythrocytes. Following amplification of parasites in the bloodstream for a period of time, and the development of synchrony in their appearance, clinical attacks of malaria occur. *P. vivax* and *P. ovale* parasites primarily infect young erythrocytes, whereas *P. malariae* infects older erythrocytes, and *P. falciparum* infects erythrocytes of all ages.

Morphologic stages seen in erythrocytes include trophozoites (growing forms), schizonts (dividing forms), and gametocytes (sexual forms) (Plates 53–1 to 53–4). The youngest trophozoites have a globose shape with a central vacuole, a red chromatin mass, and blue cytoplasm. In stained blood films, early trophozoites resemble signet rings and generally are referred to as rings or ring forms. Growing trophozoites beyond the ring stage retain a single chromatin mass but have more abundant cytoplasm, which may appear compact or be ameboid (irregular). Mature trophozoites still have only one chromatin mass but an increased amount of cytoplasm that partially fills the erythrocyte. Hemozoin (hematin) pigment, a breakdown product of hemoglobin, is characteristic of all erythrocytes containing mature stages of malarial parasites but is not evident in ring forms. Immature schizonts have two or more chromatin masses and undivided cytoplasm, whereas mature schizonts have both cytoplasm and chromatin completely divided so that individual merozoites are evident. The mature schizont ruptures the erythrocyte, releasing merozoites and initiating a new cycle of infection. The erythrocytic cycle takes approximately 48 hours (tertian periodicity) for *P. falciparum*, *P. ovale*, and *P. vivax* infections and 72 hours (quartan periodicity) in *P. malariae* infections. At some point during the infection, a subpopulation of merozoites develops into gametocytes. Those of *P. vivax*, *P. malariae*, and *P. ovale* are rounded, whereas those of *P. falciparum* are elongated (sausage shaped). Macrogametocytes (female) characteristically have a compact chromatin mass, whereas microgametocytes (male) have chromatin that is more dispersed. Developing gametocytes are more compact than growing trophozoites.

EPIDEMIOLOGY. Endemic transmission of malaria requires a reservoir of infection, an appropriate mosquito vector, and a susceptible host. Control of malaria is directed at elimination of mosquito hosts, treatment of active cases, and prophylaxis of susceptible persons. However, emergence of mosquitoes resistant to insecticides, development of resistance to prophylaxis and therapy by *P. falciparum* and, more recently, *P. vivax* (Murphy, 1993), and lack of adequate funding have made control difficult in many areas.

Blacks with sickle cell trait are less susceptible to *P. falciparum* malaria, and persons who lack certain Duffy blood group determinants are protected against *P. vivax* infections (Miller, 1976). Glucose-6-phosphate dehydrogenase deficiency has been associated with protection from malaria, but the evidence is less striking than with these other genetic abnormalities.

Transfusion-induced malaria may occur when blood donors have subclinical malaria and may prove fatal for the recipient. Similarly, congenital malaria may occur in infants born to mothers from endemic areas. The infant acquires the infection at birth as a result of rupture of placental blood vessels with maternal-fetal transfusion. Neither transfusion nor congenital malaria is expected to relapse because exoerythrocytic schizogony does not occur. The number of civilian cases of malaria reported in the United States increased from 151 in 1970 to 1838 in 1980 but dropped to 1411 in 1993 (Centers for Disease Control, 1988, 1993). Species causing infection in 1987 were *P. vivax* (44%), *P. falciparum* (43%), *P. malariae* (4%), *P. ovale* (3%), and undetermined (6%). Interval between arrival in the United States and onset of illness was less than one month for 25% of *P. vivax* and 80% of *P. falciparum* cases. Only 3% of patients became ill more than one year after arrival. United States citizens acquired the infection in Africa (63%), Asia (18%), Western Hemisphere (14%), or Oceania (4%).

CLINICAL DISEASE. Most patients who develop *P. falciparum* infection become symptomatic within one month of exposure, whereas there may be a delay of up to six months or more with the other malarial species. The common presenting symptoms of malaria include chills and fever, which are often associated with splenomegaly. In the early stages of the disease, the febrile episodes occur irregularly but eventually become more synchronous, assuming the usual tertian (*P. vivax*, *P. falciparum*, and *P. ovale*) or quartan (*P. malariae*) periodicity. Patients with malaria may develop anemia and may have other manifestations including diarrhea, abdominal pain, headache, and muscle aches and pains. *P. falciparum* malaria can result in high (50%) parasitemias, which can lead to severe hemolysis with hemoglobinuria and profound anemia. Erythrocytes infected with growing trophozoites and schizonts of *P. falciparum* become sequestered in small vessels of the body and may lead to occlusion of these vessels, causing symptoms related to capillary obstruction and tissue anoxia. Involvement of the brain is known as cerebral malaria, in which the patient becomes disoriented, progressing to delirium, coma, and often death. Exchange transfusion may be lifesaving in severe *P. falciparum* infections (Nielson, 1979; WHO, 1987).

The course of untreated malaria depends on the species. Most fatal cases of malaria are due to *P. falciparum.* In nonfatal cases, the febrile paroxysms become less severe with time and the disease gradually subsides. Patients with *P. vivax* or *P. ovale* infection may have relapses after many months or, occasionally, years. Persons with *P. falciparum* and *P. malariae* infection may have symptom-free periods but suffer from sporadic recrudescences owing to persisting low-grade parasitemia. Relapses and recrudescences may be associated with changes in the host's defense mechanisms or possibly with antigenic changes in the infecting organisms.

Peripheral smears may show leukocytes that contain malaria pigment. Increased reticulocyte counts occur commonly and are associated with the rapid erythrocyte turnover. The presence of greatly enlarged platelets also may be noted on peripheral blood films and occur as a result of their rapid turnover secondary to splenic sequestration. Malarial infections may interfere with certain serologic tests, producing false-positive results, especially those for syphilis.

Therapy and prophylaxis of malaria have become highly complex topics because of the widespread appearance of resistance by *P. falciparum* to chloroquine and other antimalarials and, to a lesser extent, resistance by *P. vivax* to chloroquine. Also, persons who have acquired *P. vivax* or *P. ovale* malaria, or who have spent extended time in areas highly endemic for these parasites, require treatment with primaquine to eradicate hepatic hypnozoites and prevent relapse. Use of primaquine may be dangerous in patients who have glucose-6-phosphate dehydrogenase deficiency and screening of at-risk patients may be necessary prior to initiating therapy.

DIAGNOSIS. Malaria should be included in the differential diagnosis of fever in patients who have a history of travel to or residence in endemic areas, drug addiction, or blood transfusion. Diagnosis usually is established by demonstrating parasites in thick and thin blood films. Blood specimens are ideally collected just prior to the next anticipated fever spike or at the outset of a fever. Specimens drawn several hours apart sometimes may be required to demonstrate infection or to diagnose the species, because the number and morphologic stages of parasites vary during the cycle. Careful examination of thick films should reveal the presence of the parasites in almost all patients with clinically apparent malaria.

Identification of malarial parasites in thin blood films requires a systematic approach. There are three major factors to consider: appearance of infected erythrocytes, appearance of parasites, and stages found. Table 53–5 summarizes diagnostic characteristics of the species, which are illustrated in Plates 53–1 to 53–5. Erythrocytes infected by *P. vivax* or *P. ovale* parasites often appear enlarged compared with adjacent, uninfected cells, whereas *P. malariae* and *P. falciparum* parasites usually are found in erythrocytes of normal size. Twenty percent or more of erythrocytes infected with *P. ovale* are often oval or fimbriated (having irregular projections of the cell margins), whereas less than 6% of erythrocytes infected with *P. vivax* are oval shaped. Schüffner's

Table 53–5. COMPARISON OF PLASMODIUM SPECIES AFFECTING HUMANS

	Appearance of Erythrocyte		Appearance of Parasite			
Species	***Size***	***Schüffner's Stippling***	***Cytoplasm***	***Pigment***	***Number of Merozoites***	**Stages Found in Circulating Blood**
Plasmodium vivax	Enlarged. Maximum size (attained with mature trophozoites and schizonts) may be 1½–2 times normal erythrocyte diameter	+ With all stages except early ring forms	Irregular, ameboid in trophozoites. Has "spread-out" appearance	Golden brown, inconspicuous	12–24 Average is 16	All stages. Wide range of stages may be seen on given film
Plasmodium malariae	Normal	– (Ziemann's dots rarely seen)	Rounded, compact trophozoites with dense cytoplasm. Band-form trophozoites occasionally seen	Dark brown, coarse, conspicuous	6–12 Average is 8. "Rosette" schizonts occasionally seen	All stages. Wide variety of stages usually not seen. Relatively few rings or gametocytes generally present
Plasmodium ovale	Enlarged. Maximum size may be 1¼–1½ times normal red blood cell diameter. Approximately 20% or more of infected red blood cells are oval and/or fimbriated (border has irregular projections).	+ With all stages except early ring forms	Rounded, compact trophozoites. Occasionally slightly ameboid. Growing trophozoites have large chromatin mass	Dark brown, conspicuous	6–14 Average is 8	All stages
Plasmodium falciparum	Normal. Multiply-infected red blood cells are common	– (Maurer's dots occasionally) seen)	Young rings are small, delicate, often with double chromatin dots. Gametocytes are crescent or elongate	Black Coarse and conspicuous in gametocytes	6–32 Average is 20–24	Rings and/or gametocytes. Other stages develop in blood vessels of internal organs but are not seen in peripheral blood except in severe infections

From Smith JW, Melvin DM, Orihel TC, et al: Diagnostic Parasitology—Blood and Tissue Parasites. Chicago, American Society of Clinical Pathologists, 1976.

stippling, numerous small uniform pink granules in the erythrocyte, usually is seen in cells infected with *P. vivax* and *P. ovale*, although it may not be evident in cells infected with early ring forms or in slides that have not been stained at the appropriate pH (see the previous section entitled Laboratory Methods). The presence of Schüffner's stippling is helpful because it is not seen in *P. malariae* or *P. falciparum* infection.

As trophozoites grow in the infected cells, the amount of hemoglobin in the erythrocyte decreases and hemozoin pigment accumulates. The amount and appearance of the pigment vary among the species. Ring forms of all parasites may have a similar appearance, and if only occasional ring forms are found, the species may not be identifiable. Young rings of *P. falciparum* are smaller than those of the other species (one sixth the diameter of the red blood cell, compared with one third the diameter of the red blood cell for the other species). Rings of *P. falciparum* that have grown are similar in size to those of the other species. Trophozoites that appear to be lying on the surface of the erythrocyte or protruding from it are called appliqué or accolé forms, and are most often seen in *P. falciparum* infections. The presence of doubly infected cells and double chromatin dots in ring trophozoites occurs most commonly in *P. falciparum* infections but can occur with the other species.

Growing trophozoites of *P. vivax* have irregular shapes and are termed ameboid. Those of *P. malariae* and *P. ovale* remain compact. Mature trophozoites and schizonts of *P. falciparum* are usually sequestered in capillary beds secondary to cytoadherence to endothelial cells and are not seen in the peripheral blood except in very severe infections. When schizonts are identified in the peripheral blood, determining the number of merozoites is helpful in identifying the various species. The gametocytes of *P. falciparum* are readily identified by their characteristic sausage shape. Gametocytes of *P. vivax*, *P. malariae*, and *P. ovale* have a similar shape and so are difficult to differentiate, although characteristics of infected red cells can aid identification.

The varieties of developmental stages in the peripheral blood aid in diagnosis. In *P. falciparum* infections, ring forms predominate, and finding numerous ring forms without more mature stages is evidence for *P. falciparum* infection. In *P. vivax*, *P. malariae*, and *P. ovale* infections, various stages of parasites are found with some predominance of one stage depending on the phase of the cycle.

Thick films are preferred for detecting malaria infections because a greater quantity of blood is examined (see the section entitled Laboratory Methods). Ring forms often have the appearance of punctuation marks rather than complete rings, and the presence of red chromatin and blue cytoplasm should be required to identify them as parasites (see Plate 53–5). Schüffner's stippling may still be a helpful identifying characteristic, and it may be recognized around growing trophozoites as a pink halo rather than the distinct granules seen in thin films. The ameboid character of *P. vivax* trophozoites is not as evident in thick films, but the number of merozoites in mature schizonts is helpful. Macro- and microgametocytes usually cannot be differentiated. The distinctive sausage shape of *P. falciparum* gametocytes is still evident, although they may be more stubby than in thin films. Gametocytes of the other species can be detected and are easily differentiated from host cell nuclei by the presence of refractile hemozoin pigment.

Mixed infections occur occasionally (about 5% of the time), but caution should be used in making such diagnoses unless there is definite evidence of two separate populations of parasites. The most common mixed infections are *P. falciparum* and *P. vivax*. Finding gametocytes of *P. falciparum* in a person obviously infected with *P. vivax* is diagnostic.

There are multiple artifacts that may be confused with malarial parasites in thick and thin films. The most common artifact in thin films are blood platelets superimposed on red blood cells. These platelets should be readily identified because they do not have a true ring form, do not show differentiation of the chromatin and cytoplasm, and do not contain pigment. Clumps of bacteria or platelets may be confused with schizonts. At times, masses of fused platelets may resemble gametocytes of *P. falciparum* but do not show the differential staining or the pigment. Precipitated stain and contaminating bacteria, fungi, or spores may also be confused with these parasites.

Species-specific serologic tests for malaria are particularly useful for epidemiologic surveys and for detection of infected blood donors. Such tests do not reliably differentiate current from past infection, however. Sensitive and specific IFA tests using antigens from the four human species are available from the Centers for Disease Control and Prevention (Wilson, 1995).

Babesiosis

Like malarial parasites, the etiologic agents of babesiosis or piroplasmosis are apicomplexan protozoa found worldwide that infect erythrocytes, often producing a febrile illness of variable severity. Unlike malaria, babesiosis is transmitted by ticks and is found in a variety of animal species which serve as reservoirs.

Human infections in the United States occur predominantly in the northeastern and midwestern states, where the rodent parasite *Babesia microti* is responsible for infection (Herwaldt, 1995). *Ixodes dammini* or *I. scapularis* is the usual tick vector. Recent studies have implicated another, as yet unnamed, *Babesia* species (tentatively known as WA-1) as being responsible for disease in the western United States. This parasite, associated with disease in Washington State and California, is thought to be transmitted by the western black-legged tick, *Ixodes pacificus* (Persing, 1995; Quick, 1993). In Europe, the canine parasite *Babesia divergens,* transmitted by *Ixodes ricinus,* infects humans.

The spectrum of babesiosis varies from latent, subclinical infection to fulminant, hemolytic disease. Fatalities have been reported, especially in splenectomized or immunocompromised individuals. Immunocompetent persons may experience symptoms similar to those of malaria, including fever, chills, malaise, and anemia, although without recognizable periodicity. Investigation of an outbreak caused by *Babesia microti* on Nantucket Island in New England showed that some symptomatic patients harbored the parasite for months and others showed serologic evidence of infection without a history of clinical disease (Ruebush, 1980). Other evidence is accumulating indicating that chronic subclinical infections may not be uncommon (Persing, 1995).

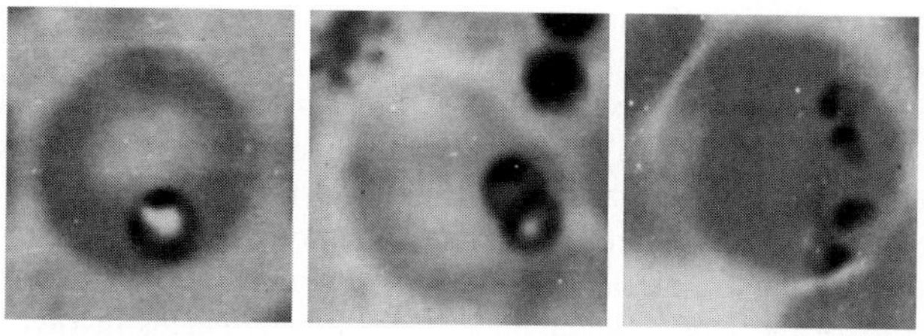

Figure 53–2. *Babesia microti.* The cell on the left contains one ring, that in the center has two rings, and the cell on the right has four small pyriform organisms.

Babesia parasites multiply in erythrocytes by schizogony but do not produce gametocytes. Although trophozoites of many species appear pear shaped at some point in their development, those of *B. microti* usually appear as delicate ring forms that may be easily confused with those of malarial parasites, especially *P. falciparum* (Fig. 53–2) (Healy, 1980). *Babesia* trophozoites can be differentiated from those of malarial parasites by the presence of multiple rings in one cell that may form a tetrad (Maltese cross) and the absence of large, growing trophozoites and gametocytes. Also, *Babesia*-infected cells lack hemozoin pigment, which is present in *Plasmodium*-infected cells. History of residence in or travel to endemic areas, or of a recent tick bite, might suggest *Babesia* infection. Serologic tests (IFA) for both *Babesia microti* and WA-1 are available from the Centers for Disease Control and Prevention on referral from state health departments. Serology tests for malaria are negative in babesiosis, although patients with malaria may cross-react in the *Babesia* serologies (Wilson, 1995).

Hemoflagellates

The hemoflagellates of humans and animals are members of the Order Kinetoplastida and are characterized by the presence of a large mitochondrion known as a kinetoplast, which contains enough DNA to be seen by light microscopy when treated with Giemsa's stain. Two genera important in human disease are *Trypanosoma* and *Leishmania.* Members of both genera are transmitted by arthropod vectors and have animal hosts that serve as reservoirs.

The kinetoplastida assume different morphologic forms depending on their presence in vertebrate hosts, including humans, or their insect vectors (Fig. 53–3). The amastigote stage is spherical, 2 to 5 μm in diameter, and displays a nucleus and kinetoplast. By definition an external flagellum is lacking, although an axoneme (the intracellular portion of the flagellum) is apparent at the ultrastructural level. Amastigotes may be found in human or animal hosts infected with either *T. cruzi* or *Leishmania* spp., where they multiply exclusively within cells. The promastigote is an elongated and slender organism with a central nucleus, an anteriorly located kinetoplast and axoneme, and a free flagellum extending from the anterior end. This stage occurs in the insect vectors of *Leishmania* and is the stage detected in culture. The epimastigote is similar to the promastigote, but the kinetoplast is found closer to the nucleus, and it has a small undulating membrane that becomes a free flagellum. All species of *Trypanosoma* that infect humans assume an epimastigote stage in the insect vector or in culture. In the trypomastigote, the kinetoplast is found at the posterior end and the flagellum forms an undulating membrane that extends the length of the cell, emerging as a free flagellum at the anterior end. Trypomastigote forms occur predominantly in the bloodstream of

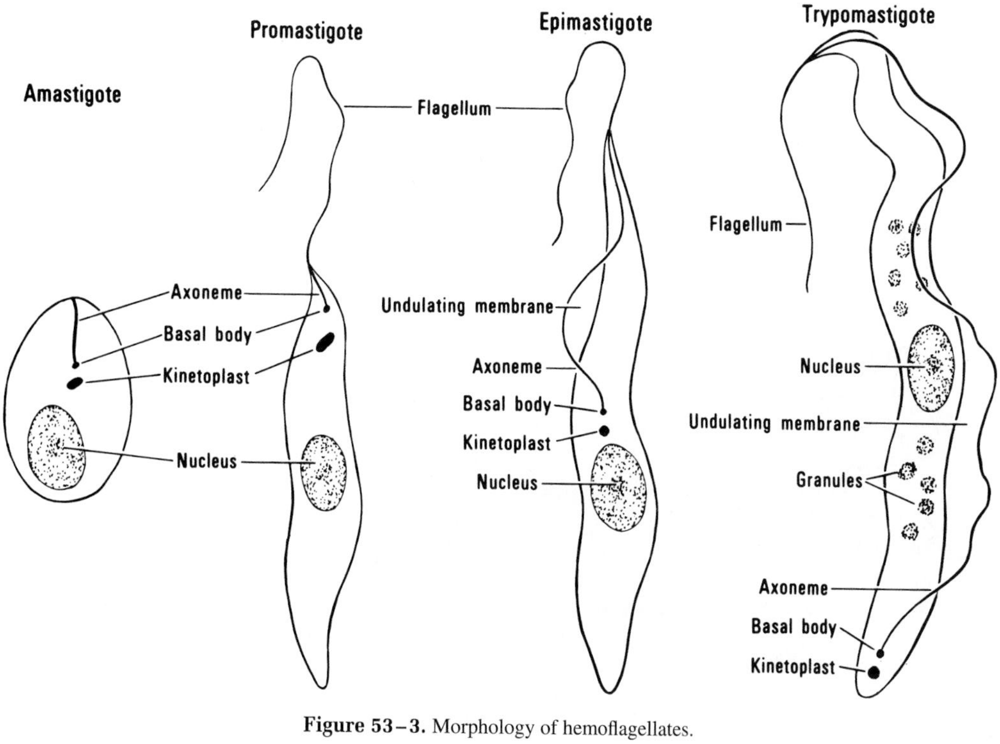

Figure 53–3. Morphology of hemoflagellates.

mammalian hosts infected with the various *Trypanosoma* spp. The infectious stages found in appropriate insect vectors following transformation from the epimastigote form are known as metacyclic trypomastigotes.

Trypanosoma

Infections with trypanosomes include those caused by *T. brucei* (African or Old World trypanosomiasis) and *T. cruzi* (American or New World trypanosomiasis, or Chagas' disease). Both are of great importance in endemic areas but are rarely seen in the United States. A third species, *T. rangeli*, has been described in humans in the Americas but does not cause clinical illness. Bloodstream trypomastigotes of the *T. brucei* group (Fig. 53–4) are up to 30 μm long with graceful curves and a small kinetoplast. Those of *T. cruzi* are shorter (20 μm), assume S and C shapes in stained blood films, and display a larger kinetoplast.

In equatorial Africa, parasites of the *T. brucei* group infect both animals and humans and are transmitted by the bite of tsetse flies in the genus *Glossina*. Multiplication of the organisms at the bite site often produces a transient chancre. East African trypanosomiasis is caused by *T. brucei rhodesiense,* which has a number of animal reservoir hosts. The disease is characterized by a rapidly progressive acute febrile illness with lymphadenopathy. Patients die before central nervous system involvement is prominent.

The infection in western Africa is caused by *T. brucei gambiense,* which is responsible for classic African sleeping sickness. The disease has a more chronic course that begins with intermittent fevers, night sweats, and malaise. Lymphadenopathy, especially of the cervical lymph nodes (Winterbottom's sign), may be pronounced. Involvement of the central nervous system becomes prominent with time. Somnolence, confusion, and fatigue progress, leading to stupor, coma, and eventual death. Humans are the primary reservoir for this disease (WHO, 1986).

The diagnosis is suspected on the basis of geographic history and clinical findings. Patients show high total IgM levels in blood and cerebrospinal fluid (CSF). There is pleocytosis with 50 to 500 mononuclear cells per microliter in CSF. The diagnosis is established by demonstrating the parasites in thick and thin films of peripheral blood, buffy coat preparations, aspirates of lymph nodes or bone marrow, or in spun CSF that is stained with Giemsa (Cattand, 1988; Van Meirvenne, 1985). Culture or animal inoculation may also be helpful, if it is available.

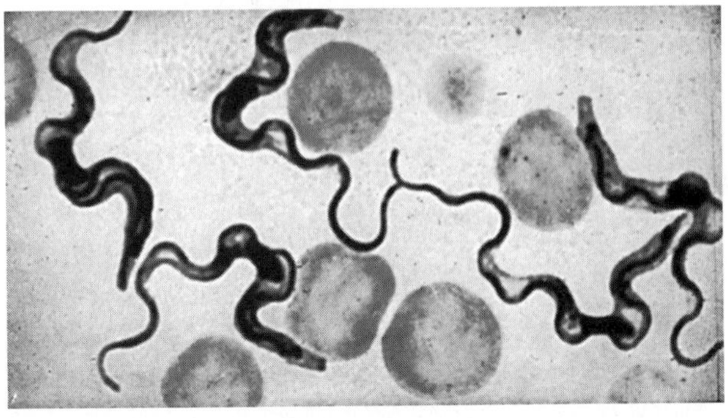

Figure 53–4. *Trypanosoma brucei* in stained blood film; magnification × 2000. (Krall.)

American trypanosomiasis, or Chagas' disease, is caused by *T. cruzi*. In its sylvatic form, the parasite occurs in the United States, Central America, and most of South America. Human infections are common in parts of Mexico and Central and South America, where they are transmitted by kissing bugs of the family Reduviidae. Genera and species involved in transmission vary from one country to another and among different ecologic niches. Some reduviids are responsible for maintaining the sylvatic cycle in animal reservoirs, whereas others are adapted to a domiciliary life in which they infest poorly constructed houses, usually in rural areas. At the time of feeding, the reduviid bug defecates. The bug feces contain infective trypomastigotes that, as a result of scratching or rubbing, enter the body at the bite site or through intact mucosa of the mouth or conjunctiva. The infective forms actively enter nearby tissue cells, where they transform into dividing amastigotes. When the infected cell is filled with amastigotes, transformation to trypomastigotes occurs, followed by cell rupture. Trypomastigotes are released into the peripheral blood and reach distant tissues, where they can start the reproductive cycle *de novo*.

Chagas' disease may cause acute or chronic infections. Acute disease is most common in children under the age of five years and is characterized by malaise, chills, fever, hepatosplenomegaly, and myocarditis. Swelling of the tissues around the eye (Romaña's sign) may be present if inoculation of the organisms occurs on the face. Swelling of tissues at other locations following the bite of an infected reduviid is called a chagoma. In older individuals, the acute course is milder or often asymptomatic. In either case, the patient remains infected for life. Chronic manifestations of the infection, including megaesophagus, megacolon, and alterations in the conduction system of the heart, are related to destruction of the effector cells of the parasympathetic system by autoantibodies. The infection can be transmitted by blood transfusion, and quiescent infections may be exacerbated by immunosuppression.

Diagnosis in the acute stage is established by demonstrating the parasite in thick and thin blood films, buffy coat smears, or in aspirates of chagomas or enlarged lymph nodes. Aspirates, blood, and biopsy specimens can also be cultured using Novy-MacNeal-Nicolle medium (Ash, 1987; Garcia, 1993; Visvesvara, 1992c). In endemic areas, xenodiagnosis (examination of the gut contents of laboratory-raised reduviids that have been allowed to feed on a patient) may be used. In the chronic stage, serodiagnosis is the method of choice. Enzyme immunoassay (EIA), IFA, and CF tests are available, although they cannot differentiate between acute and chronic disease, and false-positive reactions may occur in patients with leishmaniasis.

Leishmania

Leishmaniasis is a disease of the reticuloendothelial system caused by kinetoplastid protozoa of the genus *Leishmania*. All species that infect humans have animal reservoirs and are transmitted by sandflies belonging to the genera *Phlebotomus* in the Old World and *Lutzomyia* in the New World. The parasites assume the amastigote form in mammalian hosts and the promastigote form in insect vectors.

Species of *Leishmania* cannot be differentiated by examination of either amastigotes or promastigotes. Leishmaniasis may assume many different clinical forms; cutaneous, mucocutaneous, and visceral disease are the best known. The form and severity of disease vary with the infecting species, the particular host's immune status, and prior exposure (Peters, 1987).

CUTANEOUS LEISHMANIASIS. Old World cutaneous leishmaniasis (oriental sore) occurs in southern Europe, northern and eastern Africa, the Middle East, Iran, Afghanistan, India, and southern Russia. Infections are caused by *L. tropica*, *L. major*, and *L. aethiopica,* although *L. donovani* and *L. infantum* may also produce cutaneous lesions. *L. tropica* produces the urban or dry ulcer that is more long lived than the rural or wet ulcer of *L. major*. Ulcers caused by these species usually develop on an exposed area of the body and heal spontaneously. Infection produces long-lasting immunity. *L. tropica* may become viscerotropic, as was demonstrated recently in military personnel who participated in Operation Desert Storm (Magill, 1993). *L. aethiopica* causes a more aggressive cutaneous infection, which in some individuals metastasizes to produce mucosal lesions or diffuse cutaneous leishmaniasis, the latter of which is characterized by multiple skin nodules resembling lepromatous leprosy.

Cutaneous leishmaniasis of the New World is caused by many species including *L. mexicana, L. braziliensis, L. amazonensis, L. venezuelensis, L. garnhami, L. pifanoi, L. peruviana, L. panamensis*, and *L. guyanensis*. Lesions produced by *L. mexicana* often involve the earlobe (chiclero ulcer), are self-limiting, and are not known to metastasize to the mucosa. However, *L. mexicana* and *L. amazonensis* may produce diffuse cutaneous lesions similar to those produced by *L. aethiopica*. A focus of cutaneous leishmaniasis exists in the southern part of Texas, where infections are caused by one or more species (Gustafson, 1985). *L. peruviana,* which has been found on the western slopes of the Peruvian Andes, causes an infection called uta, a benign cutaneous lesion occurring predominantly in children. *L. peruviana* is acquired in the home, where the main reservoirs are domestic dogs. This epidemiologic situation contrasts with other cutaneous leishmaniases, which usually are acquired in forests and have wild animals as reservoir hosts.

MUCOCUTANEOUS LEISHMANIASIS. Mucocutaneous leishmaniasis (espundia) is caused primarily by *L. braziliensis* and rarely by other species, which produce typical cutaneous lesions that generally are more aggressive, last longer, and often disseminate to mucous membranes, especially in the nasal, oral, or pharyngeal areas. In these locations, they may produce disfiguring lesions secondary to erosions of soft tissues and cartilage. *L. braziliensis* is distributed in Mexico, and Central and South America.

VISCERAL LEISHMANIASIS. Visceral leishmaniasis of the Old World occurs sporadically over a wide geographic area and is caused by either *L. donovani* or by *L. infantum*. *L. donovani* predominates in Africa, India, and Asia, and *L. infantum* predominates in the Mediterranean region and the Middle East, although overlapping ranges occur. New World visceral leishmaniasis is caused by *L. chagasi* and occurs sporadically throughout Central and South America. Some species that cause cutaneous disease, on occasion, also have been responsible for visceral disease, as demonstrated recently in some troops who participated in Operation Desert Storm (Magill, 1993). In some areas, humans may serve as the disease reservoir, although a variety of animals, including dogs and cats, usually assume this role.

The infection usually is benign and often subclinical, although some individuals, especially young children and malnourished individuals, have marked involvement of the viscera, especially liver, spleen, bone marrow, and lymph nodes. In some cases, death occurs after months to years unless it is treated appropriately. The infection is called kala-azar in India, in reference to the darkening of the skin. Visceral leishmaniasis also is an opportunistic infection in individuals with concurrent human immunodeficiency virus (HIV) disease, and the condition responds poorly to therapy in such circumstances (Medrano, 1992).

DIAGNOSIS OF LEISHMANIASIS. The diagnosis usually is established by visualization of amastigotes in smears, imprints, or biopsies, or by growth of promastigotes in culture. In integumentary leishmaniasis, the border of the most active lesion should be biopsied, and the fresh biopsy should be used to make imprints. A smear should also be prepared by making a 2- to 3-mm incision at the border of the ulcer and recovering small amounts of tissue from the cut surfaces with the scalpel blade. Both the imprint and the smear should be treated with Giemsa's stain. Specimens that may be submitted when visceral leishmaniasis is suspected include buffy coat preparations, lymph node and bone marrow aspirates, and spleen and liver biopsies.

A culture is desirable because it is more sensitive and allows determination of the species or subspecies, a practice that may help with the clinical management of the patient. Biopsy or aspirate specimens collected aseptically are cultured in Novy-MacNeal-Nicolle's medium or in Schneider's *Drosophila* medium supplemented with fetal calf serum (Visvesvara, 1992c). Cultures usually begin to show promastigotes in two to five days but should be held for four weeks.

Amastigotes found in imprints, smears, and tissue sections are recognized by their size (2 to 4 μm), the presence of delicate cytoplasm, a nucleus, and a kinetoplast (Fig. 53–5). In

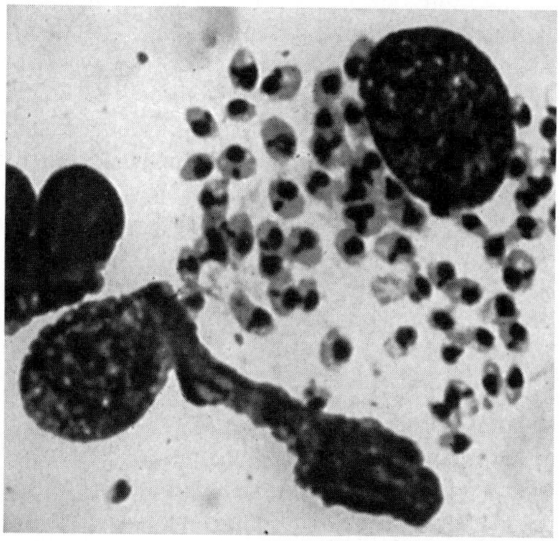

Figure 53–5. *Leishmania donovani* in stained smear from spleen puncture. (From Hunter GW, Swartzwelder JC, Clyde DF: A Manual of Tropical Medicine. Philadelphia, W. B. Saunders Company, 1976.)

tissue sections, they may appear smaller because of shrinkage during fixation. Amastigotes must be differentiated from other intracellular organisms, including yeast cells of *Histoplasma capsulatum* and trophozoites of *Toxoplasma gondii. Leishmania* spp. have a kinetoplast and do not have a cell wall. In contrast, *Histoplasma* lack the kinetoplast and the cell wall stains with periodic acid–Schiff (PAS) and methenamine silver stains. According to one study (Weigle, 1987), the sensitivity of histologic sections stained with hematoxylin and eosin is 14%; imprints, 19%; cultures, 58%; and all methods combined, 67%.

Toxoplasma gondii

Toxoplasma gondii is a protozoan parasite of the phylum Apicomplexa that has a worldwide distribution in humans and in domestic and wild animals, especially carnivores. Infection in immunocompetent persons generally is asymptomatic or mild, but immunocompromised patients may experience serious complications. Infection *in utero* may result in serious congenital infection with sequelae or stillbirth (Remington, 1990).

The sexual stage in the life cycle of this coccidian parasite is completed in the intestinal epithelium of cats and other felines, which serve exclusively as definitive hosts. During this enteroepithelial cycle, asexual schizogony and sexual gametogony occur, leading to the development of immature oocysts that are passed in the feces. Oocysts mature to the infective stage, which contain two sporocysts with four sporozoites each, in the environment in 2 to 21 days. Ingestion of infective oocysts may lead to infection of a wide variety of susceptible vertebrate hosts in which the actively growing trophozoites (tachyzoites) may infect any nucleated cells. Proliferation of tachyzoites results in cell death and injury to the host during acute infection. Once immunity has developed, the organisms form tissue cysts that may eventually contain hundreds or thousands of slowly growing bradyzoites. Presence of tissue cysts is characteristic of chronic infections. All stages of the life cycle occur in felines, but only the trophozoite and cyst stages occur in humans and other intermediate hosts.

Humans acquire infection with *T. gondii* by ingestion of inadequately cooked meat, especially lamb or pork, that contains tissue cysts or by ingestion of infective oocysts from material contaminated by cat feces. Outbreaks have occurred from inhaling contaminated dust in an indoor riding stable (Teutch, 1979) and from drinking contaminated water or unpasteurized goat's milk (Benenson, 1982; Sacks, 1982). Transmission via blood transfusion and through organ transplantation also can occur.

Most acute infections are asymptomatic or mimic other infectious diseases in which fever and lymphadenopathy are prominent. Congenital infection may occur when the mother develops acute infection during gestation. Risk of infection to the neonate is unrelated to the presence or absence of symptoms in the mother, but severity of infection depends on the stage of gestation when acquired. Intrauterine death, microcephaly, or hydrocephaly with intracranial calcifications may develop if infection is acquired in the first half of pregnancy. Infections in the second half of pregnancy usually are asymptomatic at birth, although fever, hepatosplenomegaly, and jaundice may appear. Chorioretinitis, psychomotor retardation, and convulsive disorders may appear months or years later.

In immunosuppressed individuals, especially those with the acquired immunodeficiency syndrome (AIDS), infections with *Toxoplasma* usually present with central nervous system involvement (Luft, 1988). Other possible clinical and pathologic manifestations include pneumonitis, myocarditis, retinitis, pancreatitis, or orchitis (Luft, 1989; Schnapp, 1992). *Toxoplasma* infections may be difficult to diagnose clinically and often are discovered at autopsy (Gutierrez, 1990). These infections usually result from reactivation of a latent infection, acquired months or years before, but occasionally result from a primary infection.

Diagnosis of toxoplasmosis may be established by examination of tissues, blood, or body fluids. Demonstration of tachyzoites or tissue cysts is definitive but may prove difficult to demonstrate in hematoxylin and eosin-stained sections; fluorescent or immunoperoxidase stains, if available, are useful. Giemsa is good for staining smears of body fluids and tissue imprints. Organisms may be demonstrated by inoculating appropriate material into tissue culture or uninfected mice. Recovery in routine viral cultures also has been described but requires extended incubation (Shepp, 1985). Isolation of organisms from blood or body fluid is evidence for acute infection, whereas recovery from tissues may reflect chronic infection. In smears, tachyzoites are crescent or oval shaped, measuring approximately 3×7 μm (Fig. 53–6). Cysts measure up to 30 μm in diameter and usually are spherical, except in muscle fibers, where they appear elongated (Fig. 53–7).

Use of polymerase chain reaction (PCR) technology is highly sensitive and specific in detecting toxoplasmic encephalitis, disseminated disease, and intrauterine infection (Cazenave, 1991; Grover, 1990; Parmley, 1992; Weiss, 1995). These procedures are not widely available, however, and require careful quality control to avoid false-positive results.

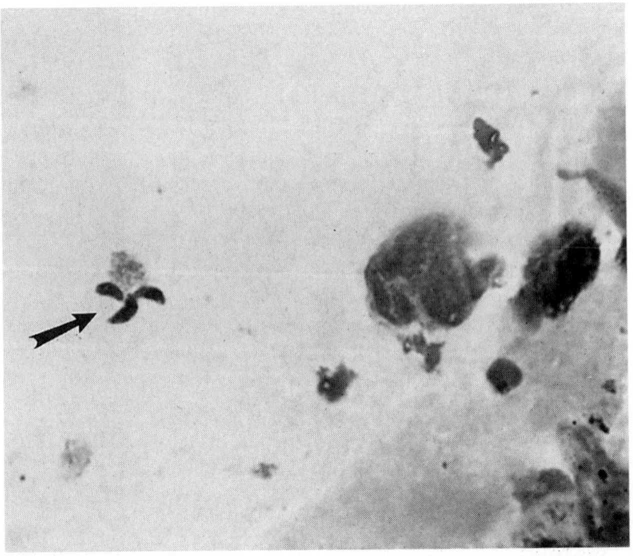

Figure 53–6. Tachyzoites (*arrow*) of *Toxoplasma gondii* recovered from a bronchoalveolar lavage specimen from an individual infected with the human immunodeficiency virus (Giemsa stain; $\times 1000$).

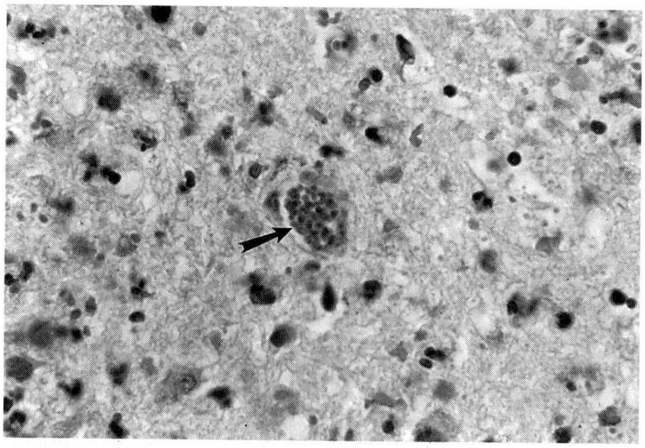

Figure 53–7. Pseudocyst (*arrow*) of *Toxoplasma gondii* in brain tissue (hematoxylin and eosin; × 1000).

Serology remains the primary approach to establish a diagnosis of toxoplasmosis (Wilson, 1995). The Sabin-Feldman dye test and IFA test are standards to which other tests are compared, although the former is performed in only a few centers. Many EIA tests are commercially available and generally provide results similar to those of IFA. Antibodies appear in one to two weeks, and titers peak at six to eight weeks. Tests for IgM-specific antibodies are especially useful for diagnosis of congenital and acute infection, but knowledge of test limitations, specifically the occurrence of false-positive reactions, is extremely important. The persistence of IgM-specific antibodies, sometimes for a year or more, also is problematic and must be interpreted in conjunction with IgG antibody results. Because many persons have had asymptomatic infections, low IgG titers have little significance. Titers in patients with chronic ocular infections may also be low. Immunocompromised patients such as those with AIDS who have active *Toxoplasma* infections almost always have preexisting specific IgG antibodies, although titers may be low, and IgM activity is infrequently seen. Interpretation of IgG and IgM antibody titers varies by test methodology and by manufacturer. The laboratory performing the test should provide the necessary interpretive criteria.

Opportunistic Free-Living Amebae

Amebae of the genera *Naegleria*, *Acanthamoeba*, and *Balamuthia* are inhabitants of soil, water, and other environmental substrates, where they feed on other microscopic organisms, especially bacteria and yeasts. All three genera have been associated with opportunistic infection of the central nervous system and *Acanthamoeba* cause keratitis (Kilvington, 1994; Marciano-Cabral, 1988; Martinez, 1985; Ubelaker, 1991; Visvesvara, 1995).

Primary amebic meningoencephalitis, caused by the ameboflagellate *Naegleria fowleri*, typically affects children and young adults who have been swimming or diving in warm, freshwater lakes or pools. The ameboflagellate enters the brain via the cribriform plate and olfactory bulbs and reaches the frontal lobes, where it produces an acute hemorrhagic meningoencephalitis that usually is fatal within one week of onset of symptoms. The disease has an extremely poor prognosis, despite vigorous therapeutic intervention. Diagnosis is usually established at autopsy examination by finding trophozoites (cysts are rarely seen) in tissue sections (Fig. 53–8*A*). Antemortem diagnosis is made occasionally by identifying typical trophozoites in CSF either on direct wet mounts, stained preparations, or in culture. Trophozoites measure 10 to 35 μm, have large, round, central karyosomes, and if exposed to warm distilled water, convert to flagellated forms in

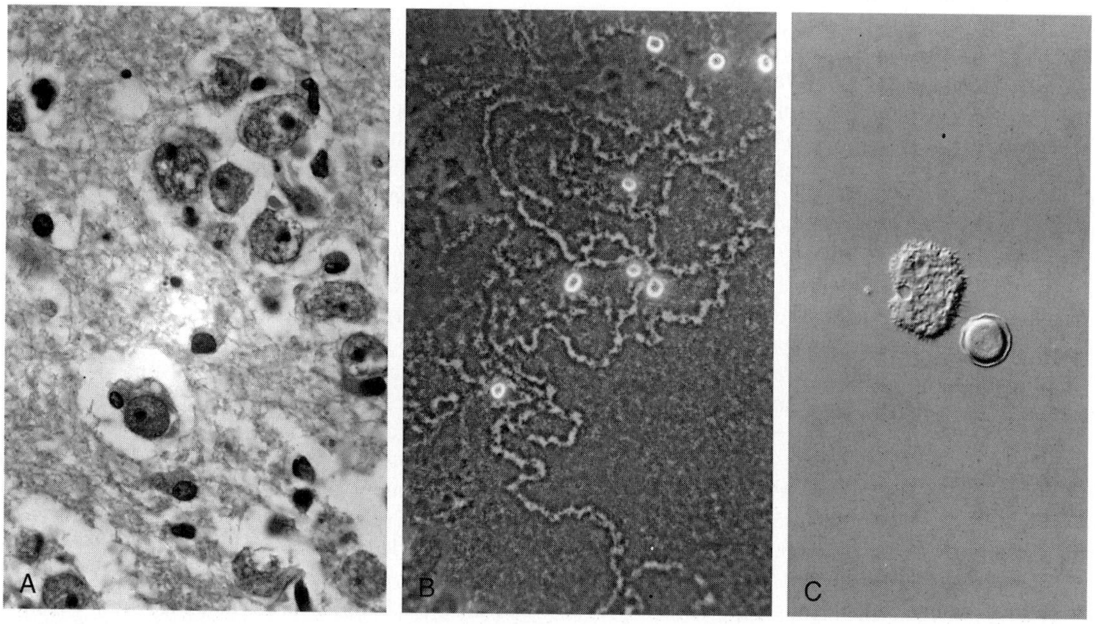

Figure 53–8. *Naegleria* and *Acanthamoeba*. *A*, *Naegleria fowleri* trophozoites in primary amebic meningoencephalitis (hematoxylin and eosin; × 1000). *B*, *Acanthamoeba* spp. culture showing trails left by motile trophozoites on a lawn of *Escherichia coli* (phase contrast microscopy; × 100). *C*, *Acanthamoeba* spp. trophozoite and cyst (differential interference contrast microscopy; × 400).

one to two hours. Cysts are spherical, measuring 7 to 15 μm in diameter. Culture usually is performed on non-nutrient agar plates (1.5% agar, 0.5% sodium chloride, pH 6.6 to 7.0) seeded with a lawn of heat-killed or living *Escherichia coli* (Visvesvara, 1995). Amebae ingest the bacteria, leaving tracks in the bacterial lawn, which may be seen under low-power magnification using reduced light (see Fig. 53–8*B*).

Granulomatous amebic meningoencephalitis (GAE) may be caused by several species of *Acanthamoeba,* including *A. castellani, A. culbertsoni, A. polyphaga*, and *A. astronyxis*, among others. It usually is a subacute or chronic opportunistic infection of chronically ill, debilitated, and immunosuppressed individuals, leading to death weeks to months following onset of symptoms. Infection is thought to spread hematogenously from primary foci in skin, pharynx, or the respiratory tract. Systemic infections occur in individuals with AIDS, and may present as ulcerative skin lesions, subcutaneous abscesses, or erythematous nodules (Tan, 1993). Exposure to fresh water is not necessary because cysts of *Acanthamoeba* readily become airborne and may be recovered from the throat and nasal passages (Lawande, 1979; Wang, 1967). The pathologic reaction in tissues is granulomatous, with trophozoites predominating in viable tissue and cysts predominating in areas of necrosis. Diagnosis usually is established at autopsy, but organisms may be recognized in brain biopsies or recovered using the culture technique described for *Naegleria. Acanthamoeba* trophozoites are somewhat larger than *Naegleria*, measuring from 15 to 45 μm, and display needle-like filamentous projections from the cell known as acanthopodina. Cysts measure from 10 to 25 μm and are double-walled, displaying a wrinkled outer wall (ectocyst) and a polygonal, stellate, or round inner wall (endocyst) (see Fig. 53–8*C*). Identification of the species level is problematic and reflects uncertainty as to the validity of the 18 or more described species. Use of immunofluorescent and immunoperoxidase techniques may prove useful in differentiating species and are available from the Centers for Disease Control and Prevention (Visvesvara, 1995).

GAE may also be caused by leptomyxid amebae, specifically *Balamuthia mandrillaris* (Visvesvara, 1993). Morphologically, *Balamuthia* cannot be differentiated from *Acanthamoeba* by routine histology, although differences may be detected at the ultrastructural level. These organisms are antigenically distinct and may be identified using specific monoclonal or polyclonal antisera in immunofluorescence or immunoperoxidase assays (Visvesvara, 1995). *Balamuthia* do not grow on agar plates used for *Naegleria* and *Acanthamoeba*, but have been recovered in tissue culture using mammalian cell lines.

Acanthamoeba keratitis is an increasingly recognized painful infection of the cornea that is most likely to occur in persons who use daily wear or extended-wear soft contact lenses or who have experienced trauma to the cornea (Anuran, 1987; Kilvington, 1994). Incomplete or infrequent disinfection and use of homemade saline are known risk factors for acquiring the infection (Stehr-Green, 1990). The disease is characterized by development of a paracentral ring infiltrate of the corneal stroma, which progresses to ulceration and possible perforation, with loss of the eye. The infection may be confused with fungal, bacterial, or herpetic keratitis but is characteristically refractory to commonly used antimicrobials. Keratoplasty has been used routinely in the management of this disease, although recent advances in medical therapy have been reported (Varga, 1993). Diagnosis usually is established by demonstrating amebic trophozoites or cysts in corneal scrapings or biopsies. A variety of permanent stains can be used including Giemsa, PAS, and trichrome. Use of the fluorochrome calcofluor white is especially helpful in recognizing amebic cysts (Marines, 1987). Cultures (described earlier) increase sensitivity.

INTESTINAL AND UROGENITAL PROTOZOA

Protozoal groups inhabiting the intestinal tract of humans include the amebae, flagellates, ciliates, coccidia, and microsporidia, not all of which are pathogens. In a review of fecal specimens submitted to state health department laboratories (see Table 53–1) *Giardia lamblia* was present in 7.2%, *E. histolytica* in 0.9%, *Dientamoeba fragilis* in 0.5%, and *Cryptosporidium* spp. in 0.2% of specimens. Nonpathogenic protozoa were found in approximately 10.7% of specimens. Most intestinal infections are acquired by fecal-oral contamination, either directly, from food handlers, or indirectly via contaminated water.

For most laboratorians, identification of intestinal protozoa is one of the more difficult aspects of parasitology. Protozoal parasites are small, and the pathogenic species must be differentiated from the nonpathogenic species and from inflammatory cells, epithelial cells, yeasts, pollen, and other confusing objects. There are a number of characteristics that assist in identifying intestinal protozoa. Size is helpful (Fig. 53–9), and a properly calibrated ocular micrometer must be available. Differentiation of amebae from flagellates in wet mounts of fresh material is relatively easy owing to the typical pseudopod extension seen with amebae, whereas flagellates move more rapidly and in a so-called falling leaf, darting, or tumbling fashion.

Number and size of nuclei and pattern of chromatin distribution, best seen in permanent stained preparations, also are useful. Cytoplasmic characteristics include fibrils and other special structures typical of flagellates, ingested materials in amebic trophozoites, and glycogen masses and chromatoid bodies in amebic cysts. Flagellates generally are elongate and tapered, with a nucleus or nuclei at one end.

When examined by any method, both nuclear and cytoplasmic characteristics should be assessed from a number of individual organisms to complete the identification. When reporting the presence of two or more species in a sample, the observer should be able to define distinct populations of organisms, to prevent confusion from an occasional organism with an atypical appearance.

Trophozoites predominate in liquid stool but degenerate within an hour after passage unless they are placed into preservatives. Cysts predominate in formed stool and are more resistant to degeneration. Both forms may be seen in direct wet mounts prepared from fresh feces. Formalin does not preserve trophozoites well, and they may be missed unless permanent stained smears are prepared. Definitive identification should be made on examination of permanent stained slides.

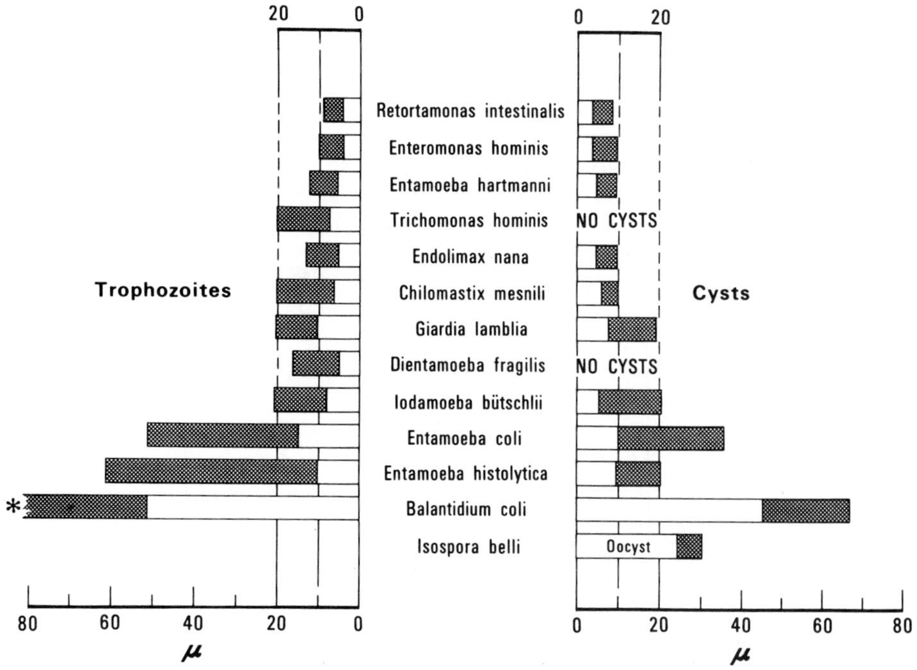

Figure 53–9. Size ranges of intestinal protozoa. (*B. coli* trophozoites may measure up to 200 μm.)

Amebae and *Blastocystis hominis*

Three genera of amebae may inhabit the intestinal tract of humans: *Entamoeba*, *Endolimax*, and *Iodamoeba*. The life cycles of the amebae are similar, except for *Entamoeba gingivalis,* which does not have a known cyst stage. Cysts are ingested and excyst in the small intestine. The resulting trophozoites proliferate by binary fission in the lumen of the colon. Both cysts and trophozoites may be passed in feces, but only mature cysts are infective. *E. histolytica* is the only amebic species capable of invading tissues and causing disease.

The genus *Entamoeba,* characterized by the presence of chromatin on the nuclear membrane, includes *E. histolytica*, the etiologic agent of amebiasis, *E. hartmanni* and *E. coli*, which are commonly found commensal species, and *E. polecki*, which is occasionally found in people who have contact with pigs (Fig. 53–10) (Gay, 1985; Levin, 1970). *E. gingivalis* may inhabit the oral cavity of people with poor oral hygiene (Dao, 1983). *E. polecki* and *E. gingivalis* are seen infrequently and are not described further. *Endolimax nana* and *I. bütschlii* are nonpathogenic species. *Dientamoeba fragilis* now is recognized as a flagellate, although it lacks external flagella, and is discussed with the flagellates in the text but may be found with the amebae in tables and figures because it is morphologically similar to the amebae.

ENTAMOEBA HISTOLYTICA. *E. histolytica* may cause various clinical diseases, most commonly amebic dysentery, amebic colitis, and liver abscesses (Beaver 1984; Ravdin, 1988). General host defense mechanisms, previous contact with the parasite, diet, and the strain of *E. histolytica* influence the severity of infection. Analysis of isoenzyme patterns (zymodemes) has shown that only certain strains can cause invasive disease and that most infections remain undetected (Bruckner, 1992). Genetic and biochemical differences between invasive and noninvasive strains have been identified, and it has been proposed that nonpathogenic strains be named *Entamoeba dispar* (Diamond, 1993).

Amebic dysentery, which occurs infrequently in the United States, is an acute disease characterized by bloody diarrhea with abdominal cramping. Invasion of the intestinal mucosa occurs, producing ulceration that may lead to perforation and peritonitis. The more common form of disease seen in this country is amebic colitis, which may mimic ulcerative colitis and other forms of inflammatory bowel disease. Symptoms generally are less severe than in amebic dysentery but may include nonbloody diarrhea, constipation, abdominal cramping, and weight loss. Small, pinpoint mucosal ulcerations may develop and expand within the submucosa to form flask-shaped ulcers. All of the colon may be involved or only a portion, most commonly the cecum, rectosigmoid, or ascending colon.

Amebic liver abscess is the most common form of extraintestinal amebiasis, occurring in approximately 5% of symptomatic patients. Symptoms include fever and right upper quadrant pain. These liver abscesses are usually diagnosed by radiographic scans, ultrasound, and serologic tests. Amebae are present in the stool in less than half the patients at the time liver abscess is manifest. Amebic hepatitis, characterized by an enlarged, tender liver in someone with intestinal amebiasis, may occur in some cases. Its pathogenesis is poorly understood. Rarely, amebic abscesses appear in other organs, such as the lung, brain, or skin, either by hematogenous spread from the intestine or by contiguous spread from a liver abscess. Masses of granulomatous tissue, known as amebomas, may form in response to the presence of amebae, which in the intestine may cause a so-called napkin ring lesion that could be mistaken for a carcinoma.

EPIDEMIOLOGY. Most infections with *E. histolytica* are acquired by ingestion of contaminated food or water, although one outbreak was caused by a contaminated colonic irrigation machine (Istre, 1982). Pseudo-outbreaks of ame-

6

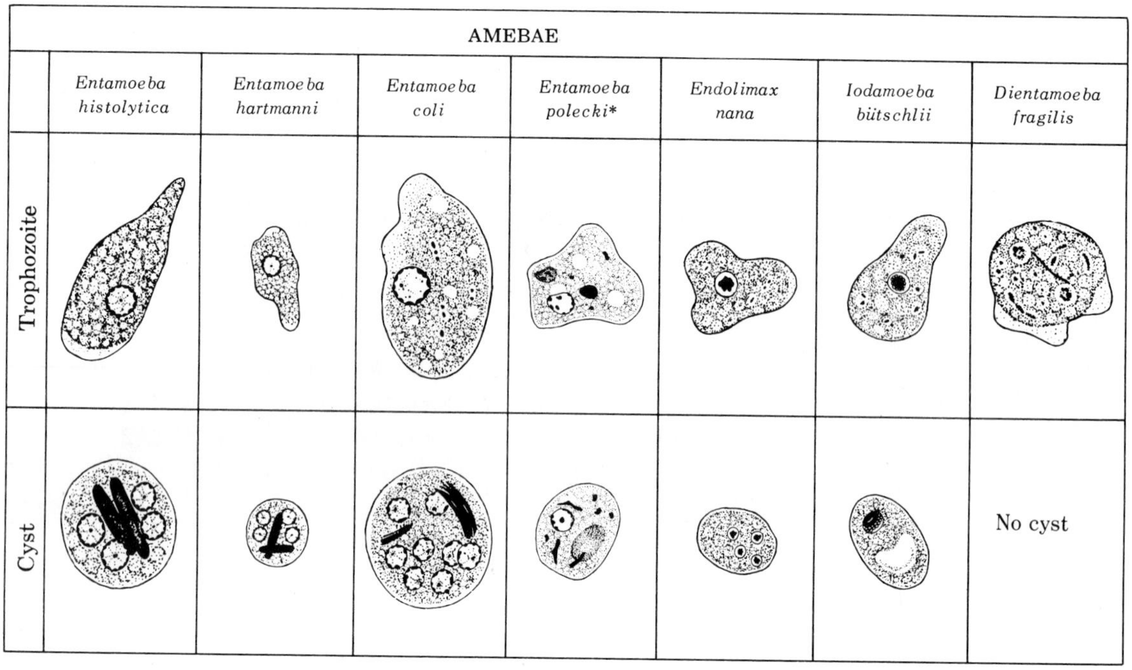

*Rare, probably of animal origin

Figure 53–10. Amebae found in human stool specimens. (*Dientamoeba fragilis* is a flagellate.)

biasis result from laboratory misidentification of inflammatory cells, other amebae, and fecal debris as *E. histolytica* (Centers for Disease Control, 1985; Krogstad, 1978). Although *E. histolytica* is an endemic parasite in the United States, many citizens acquire infections while traveling through or residing in foreign countries.

DIAGNOSIS. Examination of a series of stool specimens should be sufficient for diagnosis of intestinal amebiasis in most cases. If the patient has been given antibiotics or contrast media, the amebic infection may be masked for a period of time. Aspirated material from liver abscesses can be examined microscopically to detect trophozoites. The last material aspirated is most likely to contain trophozoites and may be examined by direct microscopic examination or permanently stained slides. If tissue is available, sections may show organisms that stain prominently with PAS.

Culture procedures (Diamond, 1988; Visvesvara, 1992a) are not widely used for diagnosis but are useful for research and are essential to determine pathogenicity based on zymodemes. EIA antigen detection tests that are both specific and sensitive are commercially available (Wilson, 1995; Rosenblatt, 1995). Use of PCR amplification techniques and DNA probes show promise for differentiating the pathogenic *E. histolytica* from the nonpathogenic *E. dispar* (Bendall, 1993; Samuelson, 1989; Weiss, 1995), but none are commercially available at this time.

Serologic tests (see Table 53–4) are most useful for diagnosis of extraintestinal infections because approximately 95% of patients with amebic liver abscess are seropositive. This decreases to 70% for patients with active intestinal infection and to 10% in asymptomatic carriers. Detectable titers may persist for months or years after successful treatment (Wilson, 1995).

Trophozoites of *E. histolytica* vary from 10 to 60 μm in diameter, with the commensal forms usually 15 to 20 μm and the invasive forms over 20 μm in greatest dimension (Table 53–6; see Figs. 53–9 to 53–12). In direct wet mounts, trophozoites show progressive motility via rapidly formed hyaline pseudopodia that demonstrate a sharp demarcation between endoplasm and ectoplasm; unstained nuclei are not visible. In invasive disease, some trophozoites contain ingested erythrocytes, a feature diagnostic of *E. histolytica* infection. In stained preparations, the peripheral nuclear chromatin is evenly distributed along the nuclear membrane as fine granules. The karyosome is small and often centrally located, with fine fibrils, which generally are not visible, attaching it to the nuclear membrane. Variations in nuclear structure occur, with some karyosomes being located eccentrically and peripheral chromatin irregularly distributed. The only characteristic that is pathognomonic for *E. histolytica* is phagocytosis of erythrocytes, which very rarely occurs with other species. The cytoplasm is finely granular, and in invasive organisms, there are either no inclusions or only erythrocyte inclusions. Noninvasive organisms may contain ingested bacteria. In degenerating organisms, the cytoplasm may become vacuolated and nuclei may show abnormal chromatin clumping.

Cysts of *E. histolytica* are spherical and measure 10 to 20 μm (usually 12 to 15 μm) in diameter (Table 53–7; see Figs. 53–9 to 53–12). The rounded precyst stage has a single nucleus but does not have a refractile cyst wall. As it matures, the cyst develops four nuclei, each approximately one sixth the diameter of the cyst. Cyst nuclei appear similar to those of trophozoites, but their smaller size makes them less useful as differentiating features. The cyst cytoplasm may contain glycogen vacuoles and chromatoid bodies with blunted or rounded ends. The number and size of nuclei and the appearance of chromatoid bodies are important diagnostic criteria for identifying cysts.

Table 53–6. MORPHOLOGY OF TROPHOZOITES OF INTESTINAL AMEBAE

Species	Size (in Diameter or Length)	Motility	Nucleus: *Numbers*§	Nucleus: *Peripheral Chromatin*	Nucleus: *Karyosomal Chromatin*	Cytoplasm: *Appearance*	Cytoplasm: *Inclusions*
Entamoeba histolytica	10–60 μm Usual range,† 15–20 μm—commensal form ‡Over 20 μm—invasive form	Progressive, with hyaline, finger-like pseudopods	1 Not visible in unstained preparations	Fine granules Usually evenly distributed and uniform in size	Small, discrete Usually central but occasionally eccentric	Finely granular	Erythrocytes occasionally. Noninvasive contain bacteria
Entamoeba hartmanni	5–12 μm Usual range, 8–10 μm	Usually nonprogressive, but may be progressive occasionally	1 Not visible in unstained preparations	Similar to *E. histolytica*	Small, discrete, often eccentric	Finely granular	Bacteria
Entamoeba coli	15–50 μm Usual range, 20–25 μm	Sluggish, nonprogressive, with blunt pseudopods	1 Often visible in unstained preparations	Coarse granules, irregular in size and distribution	Large, discrete, usually eccentric	Coarse, often vacuolated	Bacteria, yeasts, other materials
Endolimax nana	6–12 μm Usual range, 8–10 μm	Sluggish, usually nonprogressive, with blunt pseudopods	1 Visible occasionally in unstained preparations	None	Large, irregularly shaped	Granular, vacuolated	Bacteria
Iodamoeba bütschlii	8–20 μm Usual range, 12–15 μm	Sluggish, usually nonprogressive	1 Not usually visible in unstained preparations	None	Large, usually central. Surrounded by refractile, achromatic granules. These granules are often not distinct even in stained slides.	Coarsely granular, vacuolated	Bacteria, yeasts, or other material
Dientamoeba fragilis¶	5–15 μm Usual range, 9–12 μm	Pseudopods are angular, serrated, or broad lobed and hyaline, almost transparent	2 (In approximately 20% of organisms only 1 nucleus is present.) Nuclei invisible in unstained preparations	None	Large cluster of 4–8 granules	Finely granular, vacuolated	Bacteria

†Usually found in asymptomatic or chronic cases; may contain bacteria.
‡Usually found in acute cases; often contain red blood cells.
§Visibility is for unfixed material. Nuclei may sometimes be visible in fixed material.
¶A flagellate (see text).
Adapted with permission from Brooke MM, Melvin DM: Morphology of Diagnostic Stages of Intestinal Parasites of Man. USDHEW PHS Publication No. 1966, 1969.

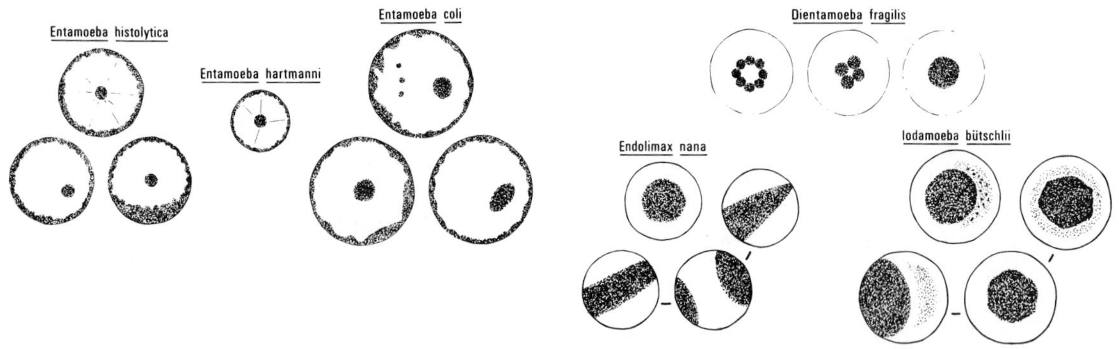

Figure 53–11. Nuclei of amebae. This drawing shows some of the various appearances of amebic nuclei in stained preparations. (*Dientamoeba fragilis* is a flagellate; see text.)

NONPATHOGENIC AMEBAE. Laboratory personnel must be able to differentiate the nonpathogenic or commensal intestinal amebae from *E. histolytica* and *D.* fragilis (a flagellate), which are potential pathogens. Identification characteristics, best visualized in permanent stained sections, are summarized in Tables 53–6 and 53–7 and Figures 53–9 to 53–12. Identification of trophozoites is based on size and nuclear and cytoplasmic characteristics; identification of cysts is based on size, number and characteristics of nuclei, and presence and character of chromatoid bodies and glycogen masses.

E. hartmanni has morphologic characteristics similar to those of *E. histolytica,* except trophozoites have a maximum diameter of 12 μm and cysts have a maximum diameter of 10 μm, and cysts often have a single nucleus. Historically, *E. hartmanni* has been called the small race of *E. histolytica.* Differentiation requires careful measurement of a representative sample of organisms with a properly calibrated ocular micrometer.

E. coli, a common lumen-dwelling ameba, may be difficult to differentiate from *E. histolytica.* The cytoplasm stains somewhat more darkly than the cytoplasm of *E. histolytica* and is more vacuolated, containing numerous ingested bacteria, yeasts, and other materials. Although nuclear characteristics differ from those of *E. histolytica* (see Fig. 53–11), significant overlap may occur, especially in specimens that have not been promptly preserved. Mature cysts of *E. coli* contain eight nuclei, although occasional cysts contain 16 or more. Immature cysts, which are not common, have four nuclei that are larger (one fourth the diameter of the cyst) than nuclei of *E. histolytica* (one sixth the diameter of the cyst) and may contain glycogen. Distribution of peripheral chromatin and karyosomes should not be given great emphasis in identification of *Entamoeba* cysts. Chromatoid bodies, when present, are irregular in shape with splintered or pointed ends, rather than the rounded ends seen in *E. histolytica.*

E. nana is the smallest ameba to infect humans. Trophozoites often have atypical nuclei that contain a triangular chromatin mass, a band of chromatin across the nucleus, or two discrete masses of chromatin on opposite sides of the nuclear membrane (see Fig. 53–11). A clear halo or karyolymph space surrounds the karyosome and extends to the nuclear membrane. The atypical nuclear forms may be helpful in differentiating *E. nana* from *I. bütschlii*, which is similar in appearance, but larger. Cysts of *Endolimax* usually contain four nuclei, although smaller numbers may be seen. Glycogen, when present, occurs diffusely in the cytoplasm rather than as a discrete mass. Cysts are easily differentiated from those of other amebae but may be confused with *Blastocystis hominis* organisms. The nuclei of *B. hominis*, however, lack the halos that are typically seen with *E. nana* cysts.

The nuclei of *I. bütschlii* trophozoites and cysts have a large, centrally located karyosome frequently surrounded by achromatic granules that may not be distinct but appear only as a muddy karyolymph space or halo. In some nuclei, the halo is clear without evident achromatic granules, making the organism indistinguishable from *E. nana*. Cysts of *I. bütschlii* contain a single nucleus, in which the karyosome is often eccentric with a nearby crescent of achromatic granules (see Figs. 53–9 to 53–12). The cyst is characterized by a prominent vacuole of glycogen that stains reddish brown in iodine-stained wet mounts, thus the name of the organism. Glycogen is dissolved by aqueous fixatives and may not be demonstrable in material that has been stored.

BLASTOCYSTIS HOMINIS. *B. hominis* is an ameba-like protozoan that inhabits the large bowel and is frequently found in stool specimens of asymptomatic individuals. Some studies have linked heavy infections to symptomatic intestinal disease, although this remains controversial (Markell, 1986; Miller, 1988; Sheehan, 1986; Zierdt, 1991). *Blastocystis* may assume one of three forms: vacuolated, which is seen most commonly; ameboid; or granular. The vacuolated form, also known as the central vacuolar form, usually is spherical and variable in size (5 to 20 μm), with a central clear area and two to four peripheral nuclei (Fig. 53–13*A*). Ameboid forms with bizarre shapes may predominate in heavy infections. Presence of *Blastocystis* should be reported, especially when they are numerous (five or more per 400× field) (Sheehan, 1986).

Flagellates

DIENTAMOEBA FRAGILIS. *D. fragilis* is an ameboid pathogen that infects the colon and has been associated with diarrheal disease, especially in young children (Preiss, 1991; Spencer 1979; Turner, 1985; Yang, 1977). Although similar in appearance to amebae, *Dientamoeba* has been reclassified as a flagellate on the basis of ultrastructural details and anti-

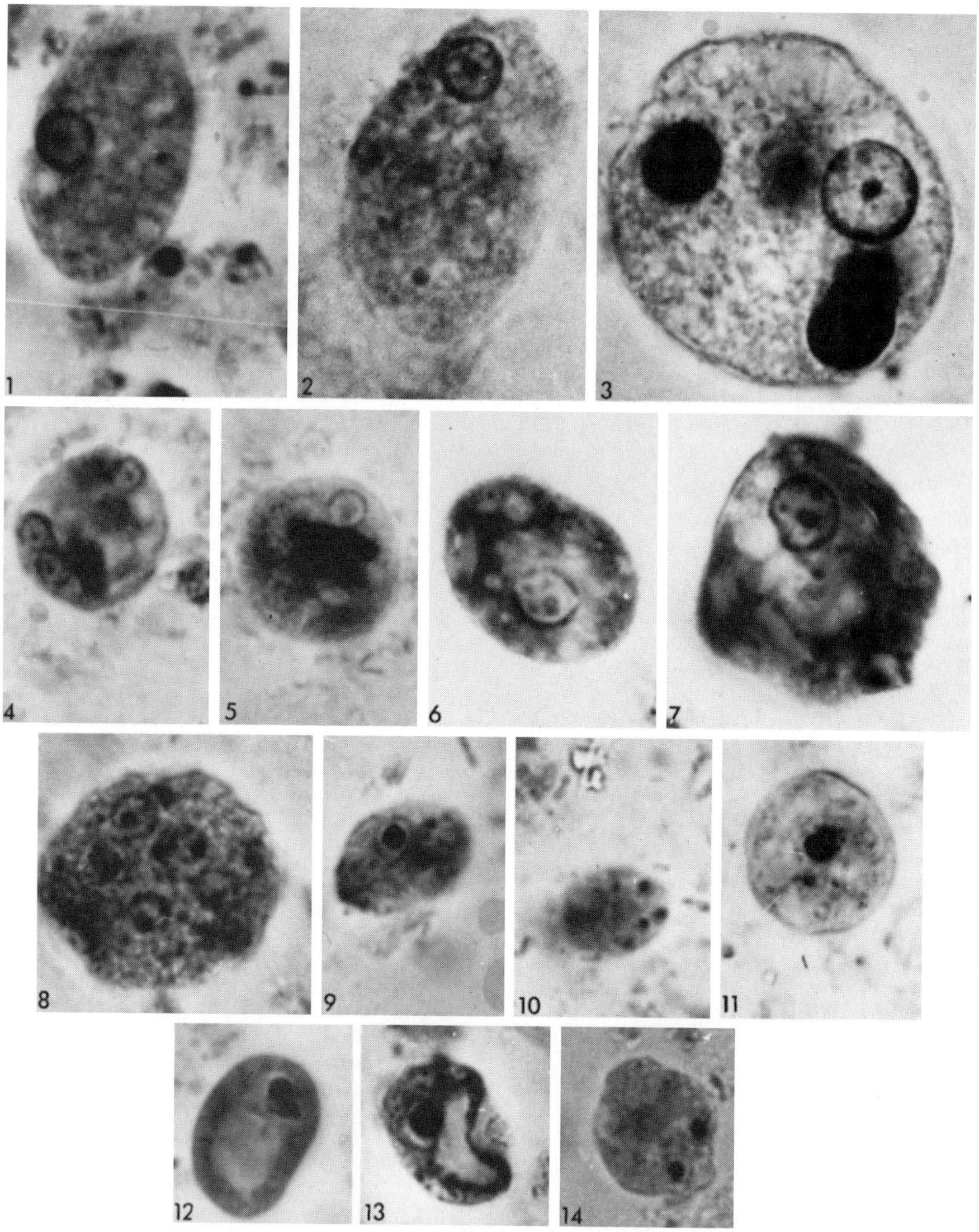

Figure 53–12. Amebae, trichrome stain, oil immersion. *1* and *2*, *Entamoeba histolytica* trophozoites. *3*, *E. histolytica* trophozoite with ingested erythrocytes. *4*, *E. histolytica* cyst with three nuclei visible, chromatoid bodies, and glycogen vacuoles. *5*, *E. histolytica* cyst with chromatoid bodies. *6* and *7*, *E. coli* trophozoites. *8*, *E. coli* cyst. *9*, *Endolimax nana* trophozoite. 10, *E. nana* cyst with four nuclei. *11*, *Iodamoeba bütschlii* trophozoite with achromatic granules above karyosome. *12*, *I. bütschlii* cyst with achromatic granules below karyosome and glycogen vacuole. *13*, *I. bütschlii* cyst without evident achromatic granules and with glycogen vacuole and irregular shape. *14*, *Dientamoeba fragilis* trophozoite.

6

genic similarities. Also, no cyst stage has been described. Because of the similarity of *Dientamoeba* to amebae at the light microscope level, this species has traditionally been included in tables and figures for amebae (see Table 53–6; see Figs. 53–9 to 53–12).

Symptoms of *D. fragilis* infection include diarrhea and abdominal distension. Recent evidence suggests that dientamebiasis is a more frequent cause of diarrhea than previously thought; 4.3% of patients in one study harbored this organism (Spencer, 1979). Approximately 25% of persons infected with this parasite have symptomatic disease. In contrast to amebiasis, this infection usually is not associated with other fecal protozoa but does show a 10 to 20 times greater than expected association with enterobiasis (pinworm infection, discussed later). This association and some experimental evidence suggest that *D. fragilis* infection may be spread by in-

Table 53–7. MORPHOLOGY OF CYSTS OF INTESTINAL AMEBAE

			Nucleus			Cytoplasm	
Species	**Size**	**Shape**	***Number***	***Peripheral Chromatin***	***Karyosomal Chromatin***	***Chromatoid Bodies***	***Glycogen***
Entamoeba histolytica	10–20 μm Usual range, 12–15 μm	Usually spherical	4 in mature cyst. Immature cysts with 1 or 2 occasionally seen	Peripheral chromatin present. Fine, uniform granules, evenly distributed	Small, discrete, usually central	Present. Elongated bars with bluntly rounded ends	Usually diffuse. Concentrated mass often present in young cysts. Stains reddish brown with iodine
Entamoeba hartmanni	5–10 μm Usual range, 6–8 μm	Usually spherical	4 in mature cyst. Immature cysts with 1 or 2 often seen	Similar to *E. histolytica*	Similar to *E. histolytica*	Present. Elongated bars with bluntly rounded ends	Similar to *E. histolytica*
Entamoeba coli	10–35 μm Usual range, 15–25 μm	Usually spherical. Occasionally oval, triangular, or of another shape	8 in mature cyst. Occasionally, supernucleate cysts with 16 or more are seen. Immature cysts with 2 or more occasionally seen	Peripheral chromatin present. Coarse granules irregular in size and distribution, but often appear more uniform than in trophozoites	Large, discrete, usually eccentric, but occasionally central	Present. Usually splinter-like with pointed ends	Usually diffuse, but occasionally well-defined mass in immature cysts. Stains reddish brown with iodine
Endolimax nana	5–10 μm Usual range, 6–8 μm	Spherical, ovoid, or ellipsoidal	4 in mature cysts. Immature cysts with less than 4 rarely seen	None	Large, usually centrally located	Occasionally, granules or small oval masses seen, but bodies as seen in *Entamoeba* species are not present	Usually diffuse. Concentrated mass seen occasionally in young cysts. Stains reddish brown with iodine
Iodamoeba bütschlii	5–20 μm Usual range, 10–12 μm	Ovoid, ellipsoidal, triangular, or of another shape	1 in mature cyst	None	Large, usually eccentric. Refractile, achromatic granules on one side of karyosome	Granules occasionally present, but bodies as seen in *Entamoeba* species are not present	Compact, well-defined mass. Stains dark brown with iodine

Adapted with permission from Brooke MM, Melvin DM: Morphology of Diagnostic Stages of Intestinal Parasites of Man. USDHEW PHS Publication No. 1966, 1969.

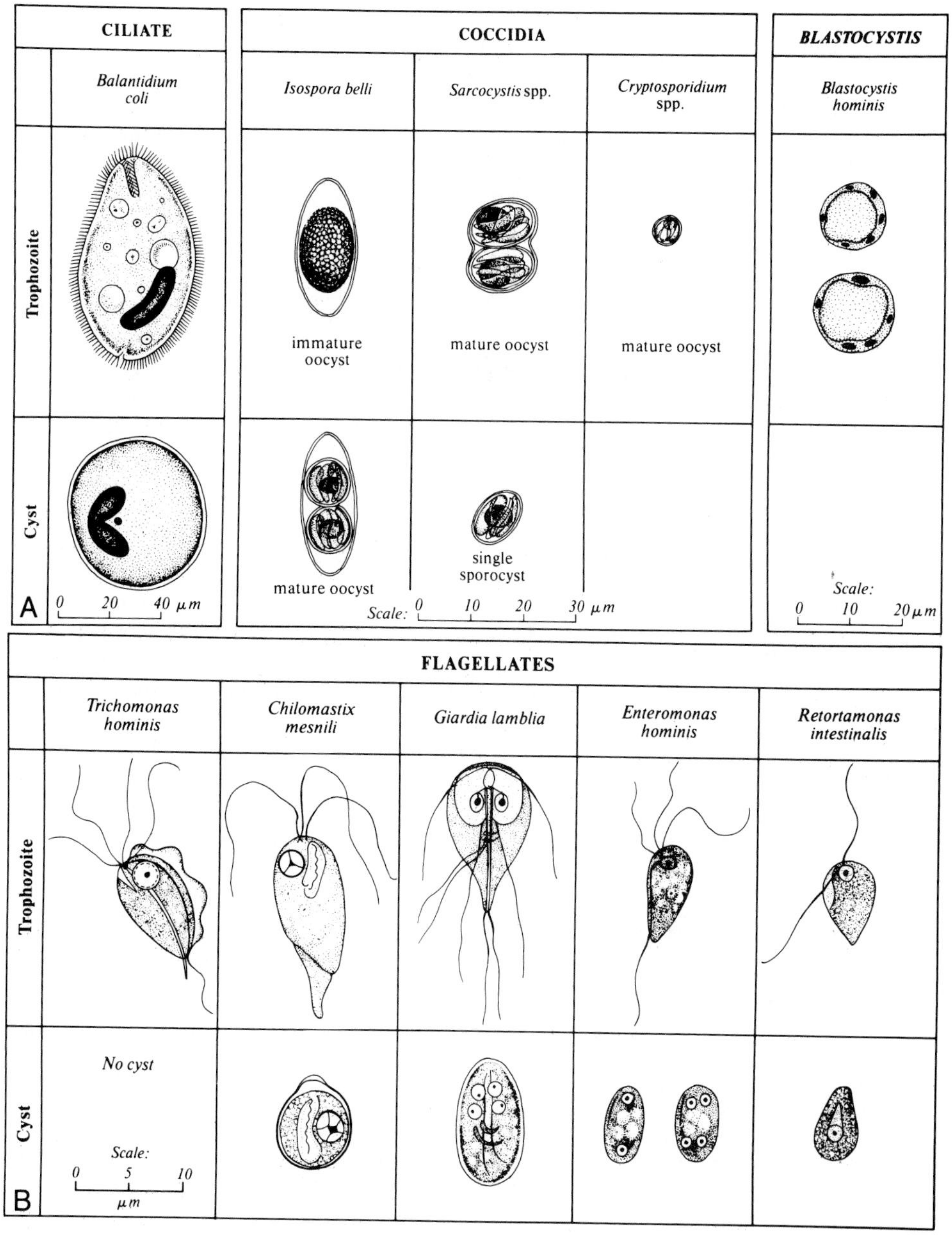

Figure 53–13. *A*, Ciliate, *Coccidia*, and *Blastocystis* spp. found in stool specimens of humans. *B*, Flagellates found in stool specimens of humans. (Adapted from Brooke MM, Melvin DM: Morphology of Diagnostic Stages of Intestinal Parasites of Man (Publication No. [CDC] 84-8116). Washington, DC, United States Department of Health and Human Services, 1984.)

gestion of pinworm eggs infected with *D. fragilis* (Burrows, 1956). *D. fragilis* infection will be overlooked unless permanently stained slides are examined. Multiple specimens may need to be submitted because shedding varies from day to day. When preparing smears, the last portion of the stool evacuated should be examined because the number of parasites found there tends to be greater. Two thirds to four fifths of the organisms contain two nuclei that consist of a cluster of four to eight karyosomal granules, which may appear as one large irregular karyosome (see Fig. 53–11). Uninucleate *D. fragilis* may be confused with trophozoites of *E. nana* or *I. bütschlii*. The cytoplasm is finely granular and often contains ingested bacteria. Trophozoites are delicate and may be easily overlooked, so stained slides must be carefully examined. An immunofluorescence method has been described that may help in the detection of this parasite but is not commercially available (Chan, 1993).

GIARDIA LAMBLIA. G. lamblia is a pathogenic intestinal protozoan that causes both endemic and epidemic disease worldwide, and in the United States, it is especially problematic for travelers, campers, children attending day care, and homosexual men (Wolfe, 1992). It frequently causes disease in individuals drinking contaminated water, and a number of large water-borne outbreaks have been described from places such as Aspen, Colorado; Leningrad, Russia; and Rome, New York (Craun, 1986). Pathogenic protozoa are not killed by the usual concentrations of chlorine in municipal water supplies, and thus, unless the water supply is filtered, it may serve as a source of infection as it did in the Rome, New York, outbreak.

G. lamblia trophozoites multiply in the small bowel and attach to the mucosa by a ventral concave sucking disk. Infection may be asymptomatic, or it may cause disease ranging from mild diarrhea with vague abdominal complaints to a malabsorption syndrome with diarrhea and steatorrhea, simi-

6

lar to that of sprue. Pathogenesis is not fully understood, although disruption of the integrity of the brush border with resulting disaccharidase deficiency may occur from direct or indirect effects of the organism's presence (Wolfe, 1992). Giardiasis should be considered in any patient presenting with diarrhea of over 10 days' duration.

Diagnosis is established by demonstration of *Giardia* trophozoites or cysts, or both, in fecal specimens. Trophozoites predominate in diarrheic stool, whereas infectious cysts are more likely to be found in formed stool. The passage of organisms varies from day to day; therefore, examination of multiple specimens, collected on different days, may be necessary. Direct wet mounts are particularly helpful for demonstrating trophozoites with their so-called falling-leaf motility, in a diarrheic or aspirate specimen. Cysts can be seen in both direct wet mounts and concentration techniques, and both trophozoites and cysts may be demonstrated in permanently stained slides. In some cases, the organisms cannot be demonstrated in fecal specimens, and small bowel aspirates or so-called string test specimens may be required. In such instances, the laboratory should be advised in advance so personnel will be available to perform a direct wet mount examination immediately on receipt of the specimen.

Several antigen detection methods based on immunofluorescence or EIA are commercially available (Wilson, 1995; Wolfe, 1992). They appear to have good sensitivity and specificity, and may detect some infections not found by morphologic examination of stools. They also could be particularly helpful in epidemiologic investigations, but they cannot replace the need for traditional morphologic examination of the specimen to detect other pathogenic parasites.

When viewed in their broadest dimension, *Giardia* trophozoites are pear shaped with a tapered posterior end and have two nuclei that give the appearance of a smiling face with prominent eyes (Table 53–8; see Figs. 53–13*B* and 53–14). When viewed from the side, the anterior end of the organism is thicker and tapers posteriorly; the anterior half to three quarters consists of the sucking disc on the ventral surface. The four lateral, two ventral, and two caudal flagella usually are not evident in wet mounts or in stained preparations. Cysts are oval and usually quadrinucleate. Below the nuclei are dark-staining median bodies that cross longitudinal fibrils, providing distinctive internal characteristics. The cytoplasm often is retracted from the cyst wall.

CHILOMASTIX MESNILI. *C. mesnili* (see Table 53–8; see Figs. 53–13*B* and 53–15) is a nonpathogenic lumen-dwelling flagellate of humans that must be differentiated from trophozoites of amebae and *Giardia* in stained smears. The consistent location of the single nucleus at one end of the organism and the tapering of the end opposite the nucleus are helpful. If multiple organisms are examined, the cytostome and spiral groove are visible in some. The three external flagella are usually not visible in stained or formalin-fixed preparations. The lemon-shaped cysts contain various curved cytostomal fibers with a safety-pin–like appearance.

PENTATRICHOMONAS HOMINIS. *P. hominis,* known previously as *Trichomonas hominis* (see Table 53–8; see Fig. 53–13*B*) is an infrequently seen nonpathogenic intestinal flagellate that may be confused with *E. hartmanni* or small *E. histolytica* trophozoites. Organisms do not stain particularly well and often are distorted in permanent smears. Several organisms may have to be examined in stained preparations in order to demonstrate the single *Entamoeba*-like nucleus, undulating membrane and associated costa, and flagella. A prominent rodlike object, the axostyle, runs through the organism and protrudes from the posterior end. No cyst stage has been described.

TRICHOMONAS VAGINALIS. *T. vaginalis* is a common cause of vaginitis, characterized by inflammation, itching, vaginal discharge, and occasionally, dysuria. The infection usually is spread by sexual intercourse, often by males who have an asymptomatic infection. Occasionally, males may have symptomatic prostatitis or urethritis. *T. vaginalis* infections usually are diagnosed in the physician's office by direct wet mount examination of vaginal fluid, prostatic fluid, or sediments of freshly passed urine. Morphologically, *T. vaginalis* resembles *P. hominis* but is larger (up to 23 μm), and the undulating membrane extends only half the length of the body. Because of the difference in habitat, it generally is not necessary to differentiate these trichomonads morphologically.

Direct wet mount examination may be insensitive, and the use of culture or commercially available immunoassay techniques is recommended when the infection is not readily diagnosed (Visvesvara, 1992b; Wilson, 1995). Cultures have a sensitivity of about 90% (Beal, 1992; Kreiger, 1988; Schmid, 1989), as do immunofluorescent and EIA techniques that use monoclonal antibodies (Kreiger, 1988; Lisi, 1988; Wilson, 1995). Papanicolaou-stained gynecologic smears may reveal *T. vaginalis* on occasion but have poor sensitivity and specificity.

OTHER FLAGELLATES. *Enteromonas hominis* and *Retortamonas intestinalis* are small, nonpathogenic, intestinal flagellates that are seen infrequently but, when present, may occur in large numbers. Morphologic characteristics are reviewed in Table 53–8 and see Figure 53–13*B*. *Trichomonas tenax* is a trichomonad that occasionally is recovered from the oral cavity but does not cause disease.

Ciliates

BALANTIDIUM COLI. The ciliate *B. coli* (see Fig. 53–13*A*) may cause a dysentery-like syndrome with colonic ulcerations similar to that of amebiasis, but does not produce liver abscesses or other systemic lesions. Human infection, rare in the United States, is usually acquired from hogs, which are commonly infected. *B. coli* is the largest protozoan to infect humans. Trophozoites are 40 to over 200 μm in greatest dimension (most being 50 to 100 μm) and are uniformly covered with cilia that are slightly longer at the anterior end adjacent to the cytostome. There is a large macronucleus, which is readily seen in stained preparations, and a smaller micronucleus, which is infrequently visible. Numerous food vacuoles and contractile vacuoles are present in the cytoplasm. Cysts are rounded, measuring 50 to 70 μm in length. Cilia may be seen within younger cysts and nuclear characteristics are similar to those of trophozoites. Stool specimens that have been contaminated with stagnant water may contain free-living ciliates, which usually can be distinguished from *B. coli* by differences in their ciliary pattern.

Table 53–8. MORPHOLOGY OF INTESTINAL FLAGELLATES

TROPHOZOITES

Species	Size (Length)	Shape	Motility	Number of Nuclei	Number of Flagella*	Other Features
Pentatrichomonas† *hominis*	8–20 μm Usual range, 11–12 μm	Pear shaped	Rapid, jerking	1 Not visible in unstained mounts	3–5 anterior 1 posterior	Undulating membrane extending length of body
Chilomastix mesnili	6–24 μm Usual range, 10–15 μm	Pear shaped	Stiff, rotary	1 Not visible in unstained mounts	3 anterior 1 in cytostome	Prominent cytostome extending $\frac{1}{3}$–$\frac{1}{2}$ length of body. Spiral groove across ventral surface
Giardia lamblia	10–20 μm Usual range, 12–15 μm	Pear shaped	Falling leaf	2 Not visible in unstained mounts	4 lateral 2 ventral 3 caudal	Sucking disk occupying $\frac{1}{2}$–$\frac{3}{4}$ of ventral surface
Enteromonas hominis	4–10 μm Usual range, 8–9 μm	Oval	Jerking	1 Not visible in unstained mounts	3 anterior 1 posterior	One side of body flattened. Posterior flagellum extending free, posteriorly or laterally
Retortamonas intestinalis	4–9 μm Usual range, 6–7 μm	Pear shaped or oval	Jerking	1 Not visible in unstained mounts	1 anterior 1 posterior	Prominent cytostome extending approximately $\frac{1}{2}$ length of body

CYSTS

Species	Size	Shape	Number of Nuclei	Other Features
Chilomastix mesnili	6–10 μm Usual range, 8–9 μm	Lemon-shaped, with anterior hyaline knob or "nipple"	1 Not visible in unstained preparations	Cytostome with supporting fibrils. Usually visible in stained preparations
Giardia lamblia	8–13 μm Usual range, 11–12 μm	Oval or ellipsoidal	Usually 4. Not distinct in unstained preparations. Usually located at one end	Fibrils or flagella longitudinally in cyst. Cytoplasm often retracts from a portion of cell wall
Enteromonas hominis	4–10 μm Usual range, 6–8 μm	Elongated or oval	1–4, usually 2 lying at opposite ends of cyst. Not visible in unstained mounts	Resembles *E. nana* cyst. Fibrils or flagella are usually not seen
Retortamonas intestinalis	4–9 μm Usual range, 4–7 μm	Pear shaped or slightly lemon shaped	1 Not visible in unstained mounts.	Resembles *Chilomastix* cyst. Shadow outline of cytostome with supporting fibrils extends above nucleus

*Not a practical feature for identification of species in routine fecal examinations.
†*Pentatrichomonas hominis* does not have a cyst form.
Adapted with permission from Brooke MM, Melvin DM: Morphology of Diagnostic Stages of Intestinal Parasites of Man. USDHEW PHS Publication No. 1966, 1969.

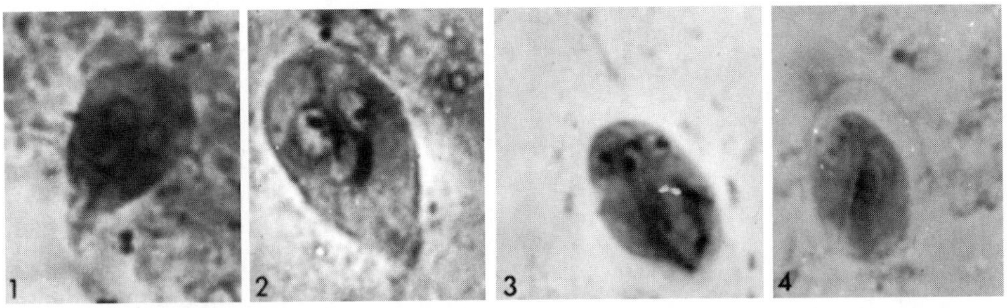

Figure 53–14. *Giardia lamblia*, trichrome stain, oil immersion. *1* and *2*, Trophozoites with prominent nuclei, median bodies, and tapered posterior ends. *3* and *4*, Cysts with nuclei and fibrils. The cyst on the right has retracted from the cyst wall.

Coccidia

The coccidia comprise a large group of apicomplexan parasites that have a sexual stage in the intestinal tract of invertebrate and vertebrate animals. Some species also develop asexually in extraintestinal sites in host tissues. Genera infecting the intestine of humans, such as *Isospora, Sarcocystis, Cryptosporidium,* and *Cyclospora,* generally produce self-limited diarrheal disease in immunocompetent persons. Severe protracted diarrhea may develop in immunocompromised hosts following infection with *Isospora, Cryptosporidium,* and *Cyclospora*.

ISOSPORA BELLI. *Isospora belli* undergoes both asexual and sexual development in the cytoplasm of small intestine epithelial cells. Sexual development results in the production of oocysts, which are passed in the stool and mature to the infective stage in the environment. Human infections cause diarrhea and malabsorption but are generally self-limited. In patients with AIDS or other immunosuppressive disorders, disease may persist for months or years, and may contribute to death (DeHovitz, 1986; Mannheimer, 1994). Diagnosis is established by finding the unsporulated oocysts measuring 12×30 μm in fecal specimens, usually in direct wet mounts or concentration preparations. If the unfixed specimen is left at room temperature for 24 to 48 hours, sporulation occurs. The infectious oocyst contains two sporocysts, each with four sporozoites (see Fig. 53–13*A*). The oocysts, like those of *Cryptosporidium*, stain acid fast.

***SARCOCYSTIS* SPP.** *Sarcocystis* species are typical two-host coccidia in which the sexual phase develops in the intestinal mucosa of carnivorous animals and the asexual, extraintestinal phase occurs in the muscles and tissues of various intermediate hosts. Humans may serve as either definitive or intermediate host, depending on the species of *Sarcocystis*. Intestinal infection with *S. hominis* and *S. suihominis* is acquired by ingestion of raw or incompletely cooked beef or pork, respectively, that contains tissue cysts (sarcocysts). Infection usually is asymptomatic, but occasional patients have transient diarrhea, abdominal pain, or anorexia. Intestinal infection is self-limited because asexual multiplication occurs in the intermediate host and is not repeated in the definitive host. Oocyst production is limited by the number of organisms ingested in the form of sarcocysts. The diagnosis is established by detection of sporulated 25×33 μm sporocysts in the stools (see Fig. 53–13*A*). Each mature sporocyst contains four sporozoites. The oocyst wall is thin and often not detectable, or it already ruptured, releasing the two sporocysts. These forms, best seen in wet mounts or acid-fast stained smears, appear larger than oocysts of *Cryptosporidium*. Trichrome stains are of little value in detecting these parasites. Humans also may serve as intermediate hosts for several unnamed animal species of *Sarcocystis* (known collectively as *S. lindemanni*), in which case cysts are found in skeletal and cardiac muscles (Beaver, 1979).

CRYPTOSPORIDIUM PARVUM. *Cryptosporidium parvum* uses a single host in its life cycle but may infect humans and a wide variety of animals, including cattle and sheep. Parasites develop in the brush border of epithelial cells of the small and large intestine and occasionally spread to other sites such as the gallbladder, the pancreas, and the respiratory tract (see Figs. 53–13*A* and 53–16). *Cryptosporidium* is a common cause of acute, self-limited diarrhea in normal persons, especially in children who attend day care. The epidemiology of cryptosporidiosis is similar to that of giardiasis. One of the largest known outbreaks of water-transmitted infection occurred in Milwaukee, Wisconsin in 1993. In that outbreak, an estimated 400,000 individuals became ill from tap water contaminated with farm runoff following heavy rains (MacKenzie, 1994). Like cysts of *Giardia*, *Cryptosporidium* oocysts are refractory to usual chlorination levels of drinking water, and unless a community's water supply from a surface source is filtered, epidemics may occur. In patients with

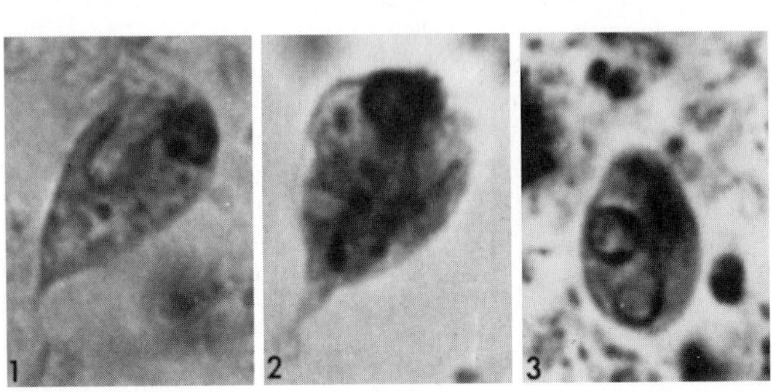

Figure 53–15. *Chilomastix mesnili*, trichrome stain, oil immersion. *1* and *2*, Trophozoites with anterior nuclei and tapered posterior ends. The cytosome is to the left of the nucleus in *1* and to the right of the nucleus in *2*. A cyst with the typical lemon shape. *3*, Nucleus is on the left. Curved fibrils are prominent at the bottom of the cyst.

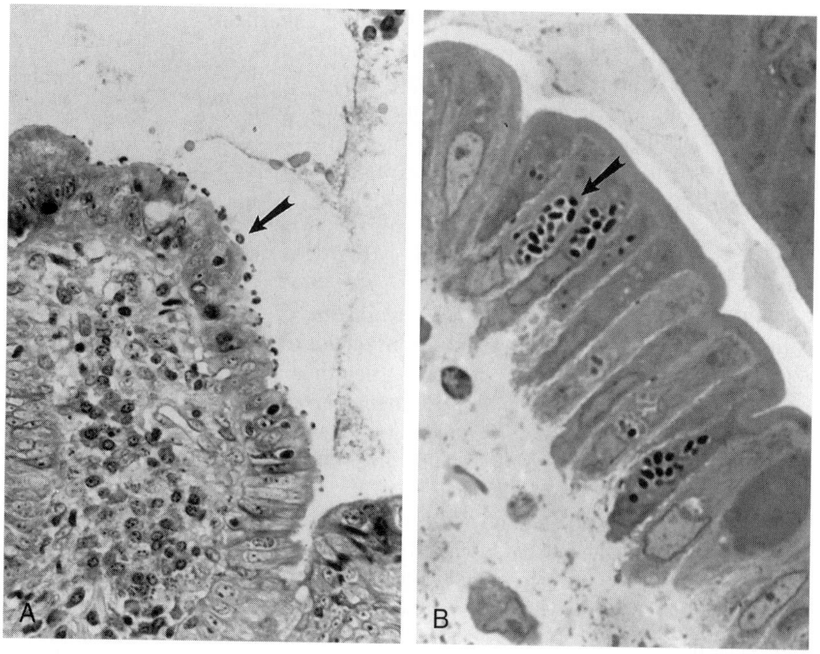

Figure 53–16. Small intestinal biopsies demonstrating *A*, development of *Cryptosporidium parvum* (*arrow*) in the brush border of enterocytes (hematoxylin and eosin; ×400) and *B*, development of microsporidial spores (*arrow*) within enterocytes (epoxy-embedded section stained with toluidine blue; ×1000).

AIDS *Cryptosporidium* may cause chronic secretory diarrhea that can last for months to years and may contribute to death. The incubation period is about eight days, and in previously healthy persons, the illness lasts 9 to 23 days. Patients may have malaise, fever, anorexia, abdominal cramps, and diarrhea (Current, 1991; Mannheimer, 1994).

Diagnosis usually is established by stool examination. Various concentration methods including formalin–ethyl acetate sedimentation and Sheather's sugar flotation work well (Garcia, 1983). The availability of the formalin–ethyl acetate method makes this technique attractive, although centrifugation speed and times must be increased to maximize recovery (NCCLS, 1993; Isenberg, 1992). A smear is prepared from the sediment and stained with an acid-fast stain or immunofluorescent reagents. Several acid-fast staining methods, including auramine-O, have been evaluated, but a modified cold Kinyoun method is most widely used. The spherical oocysts measure 4 to 6 μm in diameter and, when stained by the modified Kinyoun procedure, appear a deep fuschia, although there is some unevenness of staining intensity and variability in the percentage of cysts that stain positive. Positive control slides must be used with every run.

Commercial immunfluorescent and EIA reagents, which provide good sensitivity and specificity (Arrowood, 1989; Rosenblatt, 1993; Rusnak, 1989), are especially good for laboratories where *Cryptosporidium* is infrequently encountered and where there is difficulty in maintaining expertise in the interpretation of the acid-fast stains.

The need to examine stool specimens for *Cryptosporidium* depends on the populations served and the goals, interests, and abilities of the individual laboratory. Some laboratories perform examination for *Crytosporidium* only on specific request, and others evaluate all specimens from immunocompromised patients.

CYCLOSPORA CAYETANENSIS. *Cyclospora cayetanensis* is a recently described coccidian parasite responsible for diarrheal disease in immunocompetent and immunocompromised individuals (Ortega, 1994). The parasite has been recovered from patients in several countries, including the United States, and was initially described as a blue-green alga, cyanobacterium-like body, or coccidian-like body, among others (Ortega, 1993). Infection causes a flulike illness with nausea, vomiting, weight loss, and explosive watery diarrhea lasting one to three weeks. Oocysts, passed unsporulated, appear as nonrefractile spheres 8 to 10 μm in diameter that contain a cluster of refractile globules enclosed within a membrane when viewed by light microscopy. One to two weeks are required for sporulation, after which the mature oocyst contains two sporocysts, each with two sporozoites. In trichrome-stained smears, the oocysts appear as clear, round, and somewhat wrinkled objects. Oocysts autofluoresce bright green to intense blue under ultraviolet epifluorescence and stain acid fast using modified acid-fast or auramine-O staining techniques. They must be differentiated from oocysts of *Cryptosporidium* that stain in an identical fashion but are smaller (4 to 6 μm).

Microsporidia

Microsporidia are obligate intracellular, spore-forming protozoan parasites in the phylum Microspora that infect a variety of animals, including humans (Shadduck, 1989). They are serious pathogens in immunocompromised hosts, especially those with AIDS, in whom they are responsible for a large percentage (up to 30% in some studies) of otherwise unexplained diarrheal disease (Curry, 1993). *Enterocytozoon bieneusi* and *Septata intestinalis,* the two species implicated most commonly in human intestinal infection, may cause protracted diarrhea and weight loss in AIDS patients similar to that caused by *Cryptosporidium. S. intestinalis* also may cause disseminated disease (Cali, 1993; Willson, 1995).

6

The organisms multiply intracellularly (merogony) and form resistant spores (sporogony) that eventually rupture the host cell and infect adjacent cells or are passed out of the body. The spore contains a coiled polar tubule, which is forcefully extruded under appropriate environmental stimuli and penetrates the membrane of the recipient cell. The parasite's sporoplasm is injected through the tubule into the host cell cytoplasm, where multiplication ensues. Reservoir hosts have not been identified. Occasionally, patients have been infected by other genera of microsporidia, including *Encephalitozoon* (hepatitis, ocular infections, central nervous system disease), *Nosema* (disseminated infections), and *Pleistophora* (myositis) (Curry, 1993; Shadduck, 1989).

Until recently, diagnosis required examination of tissues submitted for routine light and electron microscopy (Fig. 53–16). Development of a modified trichrome staining method for examination of stool specimens for spores has been a significant advance in detecting infection (Weber, 1992). With this method, the small (1.5 to 3 μm), elliptical spores stain red against a faint green background, and some display a characteristic midbody cross-band. Modifications of this method have also been described. Fluorochrome stains such as Uvitex 2B and calcofluor white appear to be more sensitive in detecting spores and may be useful in the initial screening of specimens (DeGirolami, 1995; Luna, 1995; van Gool, 1993). The small size of the spores makes detection by any method a challenge.

INTESTINAL HELMINTHS

Intestinal helminths covered here include those nematodes (roundworms), cestodes (tapeworms), and trematodes (flukes) that either reside as adults in the gastrointestinal tract or live in other locations (liver, lung, or blood) and produce eggs that exit the human body via the intestinal tract. Sizes for adult helminths vary from 1 mm to over 10 meters in length and eggs from 25 to 150 μm (Fig. 53–17).

An understanding of helminth life cycles and zoogeography is critical in knowing which parasite stages may be present in a presumed infection, what organs or tissues may be involved, and when diagnostic stages may be expected to appear following exposure. Although diagnosis usually depends on finding and identifying an appropriate developmental stage (egg, larva, or adult), some parasitic infections may be diagnosed chiefly on clinical grounds or on the basis of serologic evidence, or both.

Certain species have developmental cycles whereby infectious stages may be transmitted directly from person to person (*Enterobius* and *H. nana*). In others (*Trichuris*, *Ascaris*, and *Trichostrongylus*), an additional maturation period outside of the host is required before the parasite egg or larvae (in the latter case) is infectious. Ingestion of infective stages may also occur incidentally along with parasite vectors (*Dipylidium*, *Hymenolepis*), plants (*Fasciolopsis*, *Fasciola*), or animal tissues (*Trichinella*, *Taenia*, *Diphyllobothrium*, *Clonorchis*, *Opisthorchis*, *Paragonimus*, *Heterophyes*, *Metagonimus*, and *Nanophyetus*). In some cases, larval parasite stages may directly penetrate the skin (hookworms, *Strongyloides*, and schistosomes).

Recovery and identification of helminth eggs and larvae in stool, urine, or sputum require a systematic approach and appropriate training of the individuals performing the evaluations. The size of the eggs and larvae is an especially important characteristic and often requires use of a properly calibrated ocular micrometer. External characteristics of eggs that should be noted include their shape, wall thickness, and the presence or absence of a mamillated covering, operculum, opercular shoulders, abopercular knob, polar plugs, or spines. Egg development (embryonated, unembryonated) and the presence or absence of hooklets, which are characteristic of cestodes, should also be noted. The examiner also needs to have an appreciation for the large variety of artifacts detected in human feces that may mimic parasite eggs and larvae (see Table 53–3).

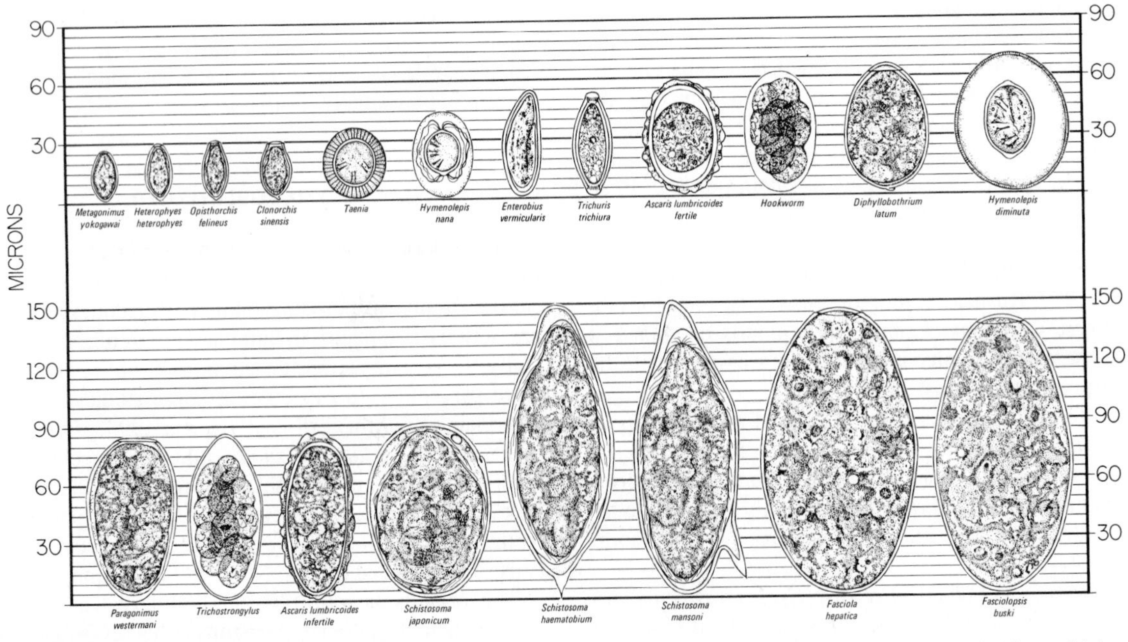

Figure 53–17. Relative sizes of helminth eggs. (From Parasitology Training Branch, Centers for Disease Control, Atlanta, GA.)

Nematodes

ENTEROBIUS VERMICULARIS. Enterobiasis or oxyuriasis is the most common helminthic infection in children of all social strata in the United States. Although it is primarily a parasite of young children, rapid maturation of the egg allows it to be readily transmitted from child to child and from child to adult, both in family and institutional settings. Male and female worms reside primarily in the cecum and adjacent areas. Females measure up to 13 mm in length and have a pointed posterior end that gives rise to their common name, the pinworm. Both sexes have prominent lateral alae that are seen in cross-section and a prominent esophageal bulb (Figs. 53–18 and 53–19).

Although males are rarely seen, females may be found on the surface of a stool specimen or on the perianal skin, especially at night, where eggs are deposited. Eggs are colorless, ovoid with one side flattened, and measure 20 to 40 μm wide by 50 to 60 μm long (Fig. 53–20). They are infective within hours and, when ingested, complete development to the gravid adult stage within one month (the prepatent period).

Although infection may be asymptomatic, children often suffer from *pruritus ani*, irritability, and loss of sleep. Enterobiasis should be ruled out early in the evaluation of enuresis. Adult worms may also migrate to unusual sites such as the vagina, fallopian tubes, or peritoneal cavity. Their ultimate death in these locations may provoke inflammatory, granulomatous reactions (Symmers, 1950).

Recovery of eggs or, less commonly, adults from the perianal skin usually is made using the cellulose tape technique after the child has gone to sleep or first thing in the morning (Ash, 1987). Only 5% to 10% of cases are detected using routine stool examination. Diagnosis may require examination of several samples taken on different days before eggs can be detected (Sadun, 1956).

TRICHURIS TRICHIURA. Trichuriasis is common worldwide in tropical and subtropical regions. Adult worms are found in the large intestine, especially the cecum, but in heavy infections, they can be found throughout the colon and rectum. Males and females measure up to 50 mm in length and remain attached to the intestinal mucosa by the long, slender anterior end, while the thicker posterior end hangs free in the lumen. Female worms are elongate, whereas the tails on males are coiled (Fig. 53–21). *Trichuris* has a direct life cycle in which eggs are passed in stool unembryonated and require several weeks under appropriate soil conditions to mature to the infective stage. When embryonated eggs are ingested, larvae are released and mature into adults in the colon, where they attach and survive up to 10 years.

Light infections usually are asymptomatic, but when larger numbers (>300 worms) are present, diarrhea or symptoms of dysentery may develop in association with dehydration and anemia (Beaver, 1984). Rectal prolapse, a life-threatening complication, may occur in heavily infected children (Cooper, 1988).

Diagnosis is made by finding the typical eggs in direct

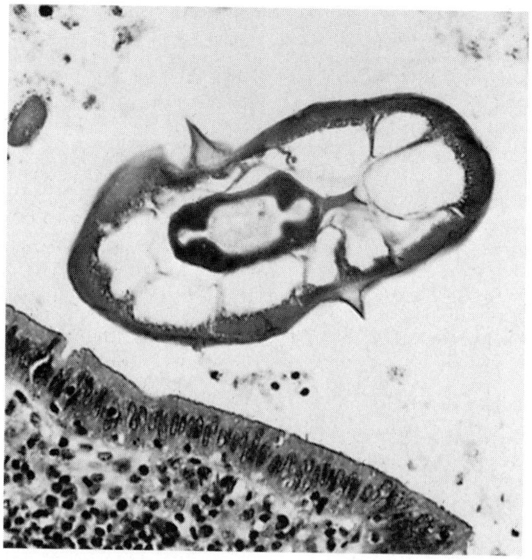

Figure 53–19. *Enterobius vermicularis.* Adult in appendix. Note the characteristic lateral alae (×250).

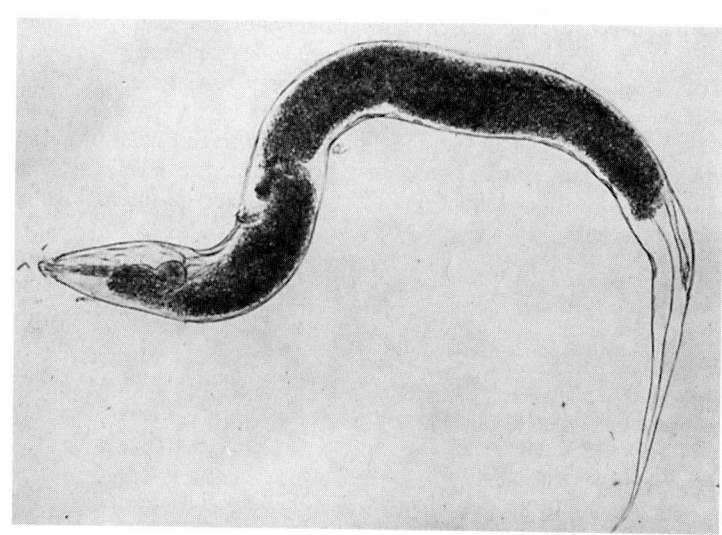

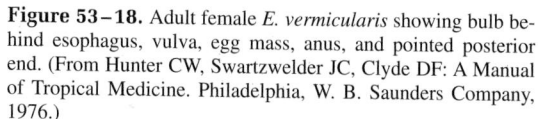

Figure 53–18. Adult female *E. vermicularis* showing bulb behind esophagus, vulva, egg mass, anus, and pointed posterior end. (From Hunter CW, Swartzwelder JC, Clyde DF: A Manual of Tropical Medicine. Philadelphia, W. B. Saunders Company, 1976.)

6

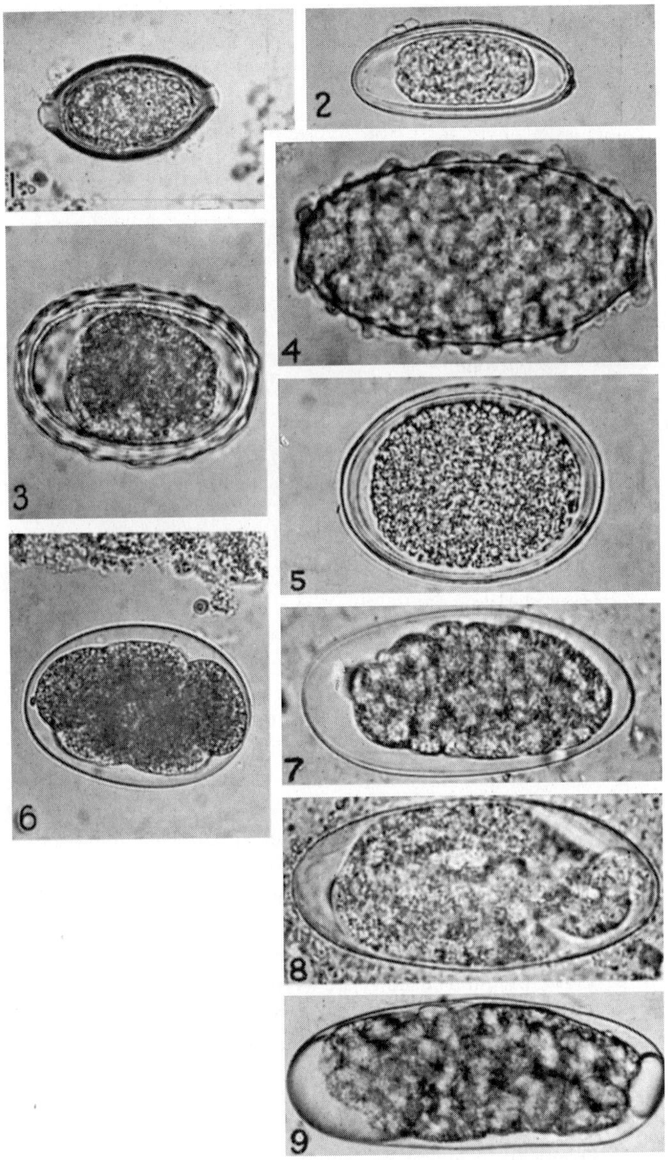

Figure 53–20. Common nematode eggs. *1*, Whipworm, *Trichuris trichiura*. *2*, Pinworm, *Enterobius vermicularis*. *3*, Large roundworm, *Ascaris lumbricoides*, fertilized egg. *4*, *Ascaris*, unfertilized egg. *5*, *Ascaris*, decorticated egg. *6*, Hookworm egg. *7*, Immature egg of *Trichostrongylus orientalis*. *8*, Embryonated egg of *T. orientalis*. *9*, Egg of *Heterodera marioni*, a plant nematode that sometimes is found in stools. All figures ×500. (*5*, *6* courtesy of Photographic Laboratory, AMSGS; photos by Mild Cheskis. *7*, *8*, and *9* courtesy of Dr. TB Magath, Mayo Clinic. All others courtesy of Dr. RL Roudabush, Ward's Natural Science Establishment, Rochester, NY; photos by T Romaniak.)

fecal smears or with concentration techniques. The eggs are barrel shaped with refractile plugs at both ends and usually measure 50 to 55 μm long by 22 to 24 μm wide (see Fig. 53–20). Occasionally, humans may become infected with the dog whipworm, *T. vulpis*, which has eggs that are larger, wider, and more barrel shaped than those of *T. trichiura*. Egg quantitation techniques occasionally may be requested to assess infection intensity, therapeutic efficacy, and reacquisition rate of parasites.

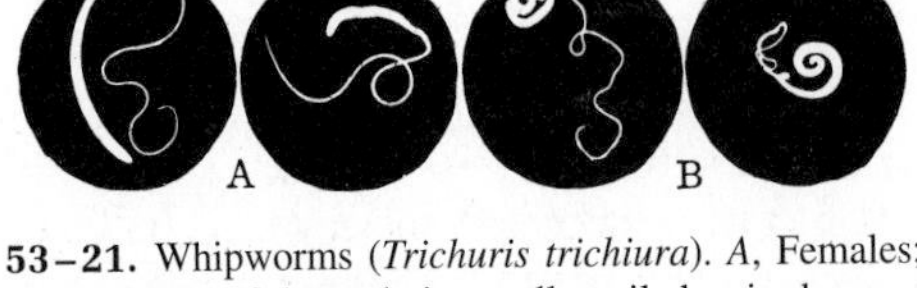

Figure 53–21. Whipworms (*Trichuris trichiura*). *A*, Females; *B*, males. The posterior portion of the male is usually coiled as is shown at the right. Photographs of mounted specimens. Natural size.

CAPILLARIA PHILIPPINENSIS. This parasite, normally found in fish-eating birds, infects humans who ingest raw or incompletely cooked fish that contain infective larvae in their flesh. Although first described in persons from the Philippines and later Thailand, occasional cases have also been reported elsewhere in Asia, the Middle East, and South America (Cross, 1992). The parasites may cause chronic diarrhea, and infected individuals may pass eggs, larvae, and even adult worms in their feces. Eggs resemble those of *Trichuris*, although they measure 36 to 45 μm in length by 21 μm in width; have thick, radially striated shells; and mucoid plugs, which are inconspicuous.

ASCARIS LUMBRICOIDES. This is the largest nematode that infects the intestinal tract of humans and is probably the most common of the intestinal roundworms, infecting an estimated 1 billion individuals worldwide (Markell, 1992). Infection occurs primarily in areas with little or no sanitation and, like *Trichuris*, is especially common in children who are also more likely to harbor heavy infections.

Adult *Ascaris* live primarily in the duodenum and proximal jejunum. Females measure up to 35 cm in length by 6 mm in diameter. The male is somewhat smaller and has a ventrally curved tail, unlike the female. Both adult and immature worms can be identified by the presence of three prominent lips at the anterior end.

Females produce approximately 200,000 eggs per day, which are unembryonated when passed and require four to six weeks in a satisfactory environment to become infective. Following ingestion, eggs hatch in the intestine and larvae penetrate the mucosa to gain access to the bloodstream. They are carried to the lungs and mature briefly in the alveolar capillary bed before entering the alveoli. Respiratory clearance mechanisms move the larvae to the epiglottis, where they are then swallowed and grow to adulthood in the small bowel. Development from embryonated egg to adult takes approximately two months.

Symptoms of ascariasis vary from asymptomatic infection to severe disease. Migration of large numbers of larvae through the lungs can cause *Ascaris* pneumonitis or Löffler's syndrome, characterized by bilateral diffuse, mottled pulmonary infiltrates and mild bronchitis associated with peripheral eosinophilia. The syndrome is rare and usually occurs in individuals who have been previously exposed to *Ascaris* antigens.

The presence of a few worms in the intestine is rarely noticed, whereas heavy infections may produce varying degrees of abdominal pain and diarrhea. Intestinal obstruction may also occur with a mass of worms, especially in children. Even a small number of worms is cause for concern because of their ability to invade ectopic sites such as the common bile duct and liver, appendix, and stomach. Fever or drug therapy may stimulate migration. In endemic areas, anthelmintics often are prescribed prior to the use of anesthetics in elective surgery.

Infection is diagnosed by demonstrating eggs in feces or on recovery of an adult that has been passed or vomited. The large number of eggs produced every day makes detection of even a single worm probable. Counts of less than 20 eggs per slide (2 mg of feces) indicate light infection, and counts of over 100 eggs per slide indicate heavy infection.

Fertile *Ascaris* eggs are round to slightly oval with a yellow-brown, irregular external mamillated layer and a thick shell. Eggs that have lost their mamillated layer are called decorticate and may superficially resemble hookworm eggs. They are passed unembryonated and measure approximately 55 to 75 μm long by 35 to 50 μm wide (see Fig. 53–20). Single females may produce unfertilized eggs, which are larger and more elongate (up to 90 μm in length) and have a thinner shell with irregular mamillations. These eggs are filled with irregularly sized fat globules.

***TRICHOSTRONGYLUS* SPP.** Human disease caused by *Trichostrongylus* spp. represents a zoonotic infection because these parasites principally infect large herbivores such as sheep, cattle, and goats. Several species may infect humans, including *T. colubriformis*, *T. orientalis*, *T. axei*, and *T. brevis*, which are found in many parts of the world. Adult worms inhabit the small bowel and produce eggs that mature outside of the body. Larvae emerge and crawl about on soil and vegetation, where they are available to be ingested by definitive hosts. Unlike hookworms, they do not invade skin directly, nor does the life cycle involve a migratory phase through the lungs. Infections usually are light and asymptomatic, but heavy infections may produce abdominal pain and diarrhea, usually with eosinophilia. Eggs resemble those of hookworms but are longer and narrower, measuring 78 to 98 μm by 40 to 50 μm, and are slightly tapered at one end (see Fig. 53–20).

HOOKWORMS. Hookworms, which are among the more common helminths known to infect humans, occur in tropical and subtropical regions and some temperate areas. *Necator americanus* is found in the United States and other areas of the world and frequently overlaps in distribution with *Ancylostoma duodenale*, which does not occur in the United States.

Adult females measure up to 12 mm in length and the males slightly less. Males are readily distinguished by the fan-shaped copulatory bursa at the posterior end. The anterior end of hookworms is modified into a buccal capsule that contains either teeth or cutting plates. Both sexes attach to the mucosa of the small intestine, where they may reside for up to 18 years (Beaver, 1988).

Eggs are passed in feces and develop rapidly, depending on prevailing conditions. Rhabditiform larvae are released and develop into the infective filariform stage in about seven days. On contact with an appropriate host, the larvae penetrate the skin, gain access to the host's circulation, travel to the lungs, and move up the tracheobronchial tree to be swallowed. On maturation in the small intestine, oviposition begins. Although the life cycles of both species are similar, *Ancylostoma* can mature directly to the adult stage in the intestine if the infective larvae are ingested.

Hookworms can produce disease in the skin, at the site of larval penetration. This condition, known as ground itch, is characterized by inflammation, redness, and blister formation, along with intense itching. Migration of large numbers of larvae through the lungs may produce Löffler's syndrome, as described earlier for *Ascaris*. Depending on the worm burden, intestinal infection can result in gastroenteritis with abdominal pain, diarrhea, and nausea. Hookworms are best known, however, for their ability to produce chronic blood loss with secondary iron deficiency anemia. The presence of each adult *A. duodenale* can result in the loss of 0.15 to 0.25 mL of blood per day, compared with 0.03 mL for each *N. americanus*. Development of children can be severely affected with chronic infections. Blood loss and number of hookworms present correlate with the number of eggs per gram of stool, which may help determine when to initiate therapy in individuals living in endemic areas (Layrisse, 1964a, 1964b).

Diagnosis is made by finding the characteristic thin-shelled eggs in feces. The eggs are partially embryonated when passed and measure 58 to 76 μm in length by 36 to 40 μm wide (see Fig. 53–20). Embryonated eggs or free rhabditiform larvae may be found in unpreserved specimens that are not examined promptly. Hookworm rhabditiforms can be differentiated from those of *Strongyloides stercoralis* because the former have a longer buccal chamber and inconspicuous genital primordium (Fig. 53–22). Continued maturation of larvae results in the appearance of infective filariforms, which have a pointed posterior end and an esophagus approximately one fourth the length of the larva. Hookworm eggs may need to be differentiated from those of

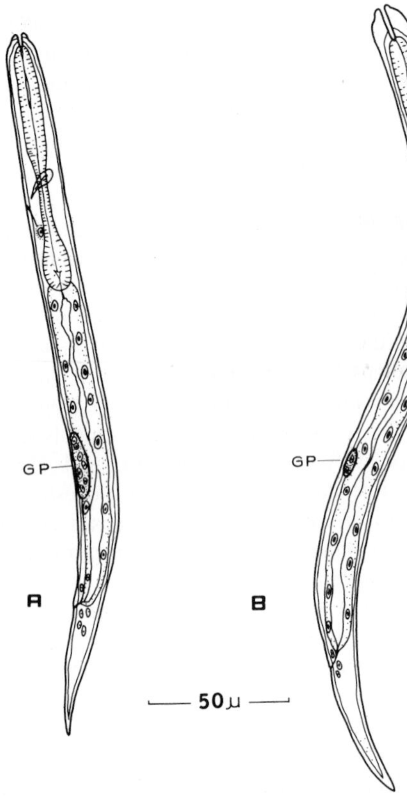

Figure 53–22. Hookworm and *Strongyloides stercoralis* larvae. *A*, *S. stercoralis* rhabditoid larva in human stools. Note the short size of the buccal cavity and the large genital primordium (GP). *B*, Hookworm rhabditoid larva as seen in a few instances in stools left for at least 24 hours at room temperature. The buccal cavity is longer, and the genital primordium is smaller.

Trichostrongylus spp. (which are longer and more pointed) and those of plant parasitic nematodes, especially *Heterodera* spp. (which are longer, have blunt ends, and are often asymmetric) (see Fig. 53–20).

Although adult hookworms can be differentiated on the basis of their mouthparts and the copulatory bursa in males, eggs of human hookworms are indistinguishable. In direct wet mounts, egg counts of less than five eggs per coverslip denote light infections that are unlikely to result in anemia, whereas more than 25 denote heavy infections that are likely to be associated with symptoms.

STRONGYLOIDES STERCORALIS. Strongyloidiasis occurs in many areas in the tropics and subtropics, but the infection also occurs in temperate zones and has historically been endemic in areas of the southeastern United States. Adult females are 2 to 3 mm long and live buried in the mucosa of the duodenum, where they reproduce parthenogenetically (Fig. 53–23). Parasitic males do not occur in the vertebrate phase of the cycle. The eggs hatch primarily in the small bowel, releasing first stage or rhabditoid larvae, which are then passed in the feces (eggs are almost never found). In this direct cycle, the rhabditoid larvae metamorphose into infective third stage filariform larvae in the soil. These infective larvae readily penetrate the skin of exposed individuals and migrate via the circulatory system to the lungs and then move up the bronchial tree and are swallowed. Development to the adult stage is then completed in the small intestine. Under appropriate soil conditions of high humidity, an indirect cycle may appear transiently in which the newly deposited larvae develop into a free-living generation consisting of reproductive males and females. Eggs produced by this generation develop into filariform larvae that are again infective for

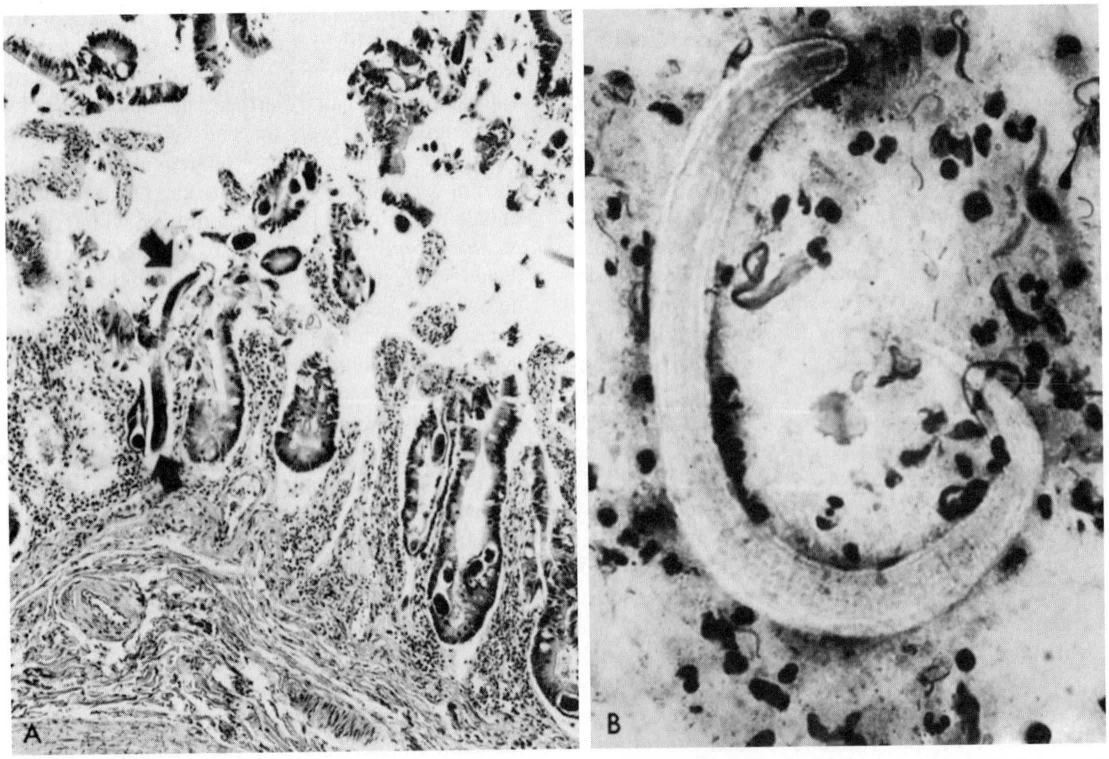

Figure 53–23. *Strongyloides stercoralis.* Patient with massive strongyloidiasis. *A*, Adult female (*arrows*) and eggs in the duodenal mucosa (×80). *B*, Larva in sputum smear (×470).

humans. A third variation in the life cycle of *Strongyloides* involves autoinfection, in which maturation to the filariform stage is completed within the intestinal tract, with subsequent reinvasion of bowel mucosa or perianal skin.

Disease presentation is variable and may depend on the strain acquired (Genta, 1989). Early migration of filariform larvae may produce irritation, redness, and pruritus at the site of entry, whereas later migration through the lungs may produce Löffler's syndrome (Purtilo, 1974). The presence of intestinal symptoms is related to the intensity of the infection. The affected individual may have symptoms of peptic ulcer, abdominal pain, and diarrhea. A malabsorption syndrome has been reported with chronic infection.

The ability of the parasite to autoinfect may result in persistence of the infection for decades, as was recognized in allied troops who were held as prisoners of war in Southeast Asia during World War II (Gill, 1979). In otherwise healthy patients, autoinfection may produce *larva currens* (linear urticarial lesions). In immunocompromised, alcoholic, or malnourished patients, autoinfection may result in a life-threatening hyperinfection syndrome from the rapid multiplication of the parasite (Genta, 1992; Maayen, 1987). Severe pneumonia is often a presenting manifestation of hyperinfection, followed by marked diarrhea, enteritis, and septicemia. Patients who have lived in endemic areas should be screened for *Strongyloides* prior to receiving immunosuppressive therapy.

Diagnosis is made on recovery and identification of typical rhabditiform larvae in stool specimens, although the routine ova and parasite examination does not always reveal their presence (Genta, 1989; Pelletier, 1988). *Strongyloides* rhabditiform larvae must be differentiated from those of hookworms and are characterized by having a short buccal cavity and a prominent genital primordium (see Fig. 53–22). *Strongyloides* filariform larvae have a notched tail and an esophagus approximately half the length of the body. Either stage of larvae are readily seen in fresh saline wet mounts under low power. If the infective filariform larvae are detected in a recently passed specimen, then the diagnosis of superinfection is warranted (Eveland, 1975).

Examination of duodenal aspirates or string test specimens may be helpful in suspicious cases in which routine stool examinations are nonproductive. The Baermann funnel concentration method or one of the coproculture techniques (see the section entitled Laboratory Methods) may also demonstrate the infection (Ash, 1987; Genta, 1989). Larvae may be found in sputum or other pulmonary specimens, especially in the hyperinfection syndrome. Serologic tests are useful when infection is suspected but cannot be demonstrated by other methods. EIA and other tests display good sensitivity and specificity, although cross-reactions may appear with filariasis and some other nematode infections. These tests generally do not differentiate between past and current infection but may be useful in monitoring therapy (Wilson, 1995).

ANISAKIASIS. See the section on Tissue Helminths.

Cestodes

The cestodes or tapeworms are ribbon-like platyhelminths that live in the intestinal tract of vertebrates as adults and in the tissues or body cavities of various intermediate hosts as larvae. They attach to intestinal mucosa by means of a scolex, or attachment organ, at the anterior end that may display suckers, grooves (bothria), or a rostellum with hooks, depending on the species. The body of the worm, or strobila, is comprised of an actively growing neck region and a series of proglottids that undergo sequential development through immature, mature, and finally, gravid stages at the posterior end. Each proglottid has a complete set of male and female gonads and is capable of producing fertile eggs. Eggs of most cestodes infecting humans (*Diphyllobothrium* being an exception) may be readily differentiated from those of other helminths by the presence in each of a six-hooked embryo. Depending on the species, eggs are released directly into the fecal stream or passed in intact proglottids. It is not uncommon in some species for long lengths of strobila to be passed intact or for proglottids to actively migrate out of the anus. The large species of *Taenia* and *Diphyllobothrium* may grow in length to 25 feet or more and live for 20 years.

Cestode larval stages develop to the infective stage in either invertebrate or vertebrate hosts, depending on the species, and complete their life cycle when ingested by a definitive host. Larval stages of several species may infect humans causing cysticercosis, hydatidosis, sparganosis, and coenurosis. These conditions are covered more fully in the section on tissue helminths.

TAENIA SAGINATA. Humans are the sole definitive host for *Taenia saginata*, the beef tapeworm. Although it is distributed worldwide, the worm is especially common in the Middle East, Africa, Europe, Asia, and Latin America. It occurs rarely and sporadically in the United States. Larval cysticerci (*Cysticercis bovis*) develop in the tissues of cattle that graze on land contaminated with human waste. When humans ingest infected raw or incompletely cooked beef, the cysticercus develops into a reproductive adult in the small intestine in two to three months. Symptoms are rare but may include abdominal discomfort and diarrhea. Unlike *T. solium*, the eggs of *T. saginata* are not infectious to humans and their ingestion does not result in cysticercosis.

Diagnosis is made by finding eggs in the stool, using direct or concentration techniques, or in the perianal folds, using the cellophane tape technique. Eggs are spherical and measure 31 to 43 μm in diameter (Fig. 53–24). The shell is thick, radially striated, and contains a six-hooked embryo. Eggs of all *Taenia* species are indistinguishable and should be reported only as *Taenia* eggs.

Species identification may be made on recovery of proglottids or, more rarely, the scolex. Proglottids of taeneids have a characteristic lateral protrusion known as the genital pore. Careful injection of India ink through the genital pore, using a tuberculin needle and syringe, may succeed in outlining the uterus. The gravid uterus of *T. saginata* has 15 to 20 lateral branches, whereas that of *T. solium* has 7 to 13 lateral branches (Fig. 53–25). Proglottids may also be cleared overnight in glycerol or stained with carmine or hematoxylin using published procedures (Ash, 1987). If recovered, the scolex of *T. saginata* can be identified by the presence of four suckers and the absence of hooks on the crown or rostellum.

TAENIA SOLIUM. *T. solium*, the pork tapeworm, is most common in Europe, especially eastern Europe, Latin America, China, Pakistan, and India. It is encountered in the United States on occasion, mostly in recent immigrants. Infection with the adult tapeworm is acquired by eating raw or incompletely cooked pork containing cysticerci (*C. cellulosae*).

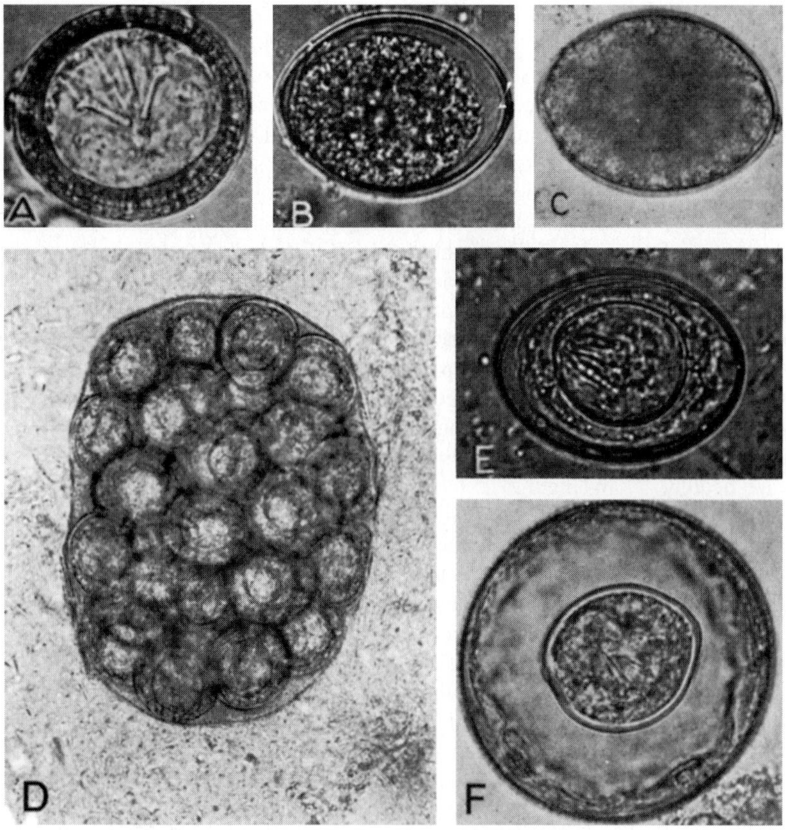

Figure 53–24. Cestode eggs in stools. *A*, *Taenia saginata* or *Taenia solium* (×750). *B* and *C*, Broad tapeworm or fish tapeworm of humans, *Diphyllobothrium latum* (×500). *D. Dipylidium caninum* egg pack; note the membrane surrounding the eggs (×300). *E*, Dwarf tapeworm, *Hymenolepis nana* (×750). *F*, Rat tapeworm, *Hymenolepis diminuta* (×650). (*B* courtesy of Lt. LW Shetterby, School of Aviation Medicine, Gunter AFB, AL; *A*, *C*, *E*, and *F*, courtesy of Dr. RL Roudabush, Ward's Natural Science Establishment, Rochester, NY; photos by T Romaniak.)

Symptoms, if present, are identical to those of *T. saginata* infection. More important, the accidental ingestion of *T. solium* eggs, either from one's own adult tapeworm or from contaminated food, may result in cysticercosis (Schantz, 1992). Further details on cysticercosis may be found in the section entitled Tissue Helminths.

Procedures used for diagnosis of intestinal *T. solium* infection are identical to those used for *T. saginata* infections, although certain morphologic differences are apparent. The scolex of *T. solium* has four suckers and, unlike *T. saginata*, a rostellum armed with two rows of hooks. Gravid proglottids have 7 to 13 lateral uterine branches (see Fig. 53–25).

HYMENOLEPIS NANA. *H. nana*, known as the dwarf tapeworm, has worldwide distribution and is the most frequently recovered cestode species seen in the United States. It is a common parasite in mice and the smallest to infect humans, measuring up to 4.0 cm in length. The scolex has an armed rostellum, and the proglottids have their genital pores all located on the same side of the strobila (see Fig. 53–25). The life cycle may be either direct, through the ingestion of infectious eggs, or indirect, through the ingestion of intermediate hosts (usually grain beetles) containing cysticercoid larvae. In the former instance, eggs may be passed directly from person to person, usually among children, or ingested in food, especially grain products that are contaminated with rodent droppings.

Eggs hatch in the intestine, and the embryos penetrate the mucosa, where they mature as cysticercoid larvae. They subsequently emerge and reattach to the intestinal wall to complete their development into adult tapeworms in two to three

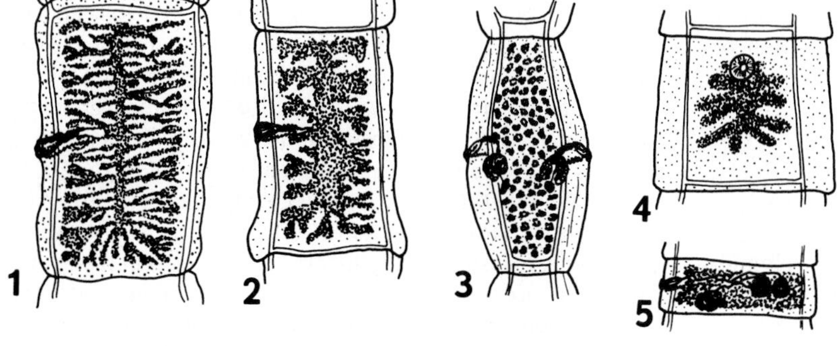

Figure 53–25. Gravid proglottids of different human tapeworms. *1*, *Taenia saginata*. 2, *Taenia solium*. *3*, *Dipylidium caninum*. *4*, *Diphyllobothrium latum*. *5*, *Hymenolepis* spp.

weeks. Ingestion of grain beetles containing the cysticercoid larvae occurs much less frequently. Internal autoinfection may occur in some individuals in whom eggs hatch shortly after being discharged from the worm and rapidly invade the intestinal wall without leaving the body. Such a mechanism is thought to be responsible for the occasional case of massive infection.

Symptomatic infection, characterized by abdominal pain, diarrhea, anorexia, and irritability, may develop in patients with large numbers of worms. Diagnosis is made by recovery from stool of the oval, thin-shelled, colorless eggs that measure 30 to 47 μm in diameter (see Fig. 53–24). They contain a centrally located six-hooked embryo (oncosphere), which is separated from the outer shell by a clear space. The embryo displays two polar thickenings from which thin filaments arise and extend into the clear space between embryo and outer shell. Occasionally, intact strobila may be recovered if the stool is closely examined.

HYMENOLEPIS DIMINUTA. The rat tapeworm, *H. diminuta*, is cosmopolitan in distribution and occasionally infects humans. Infections are rare, however, because of the obligate need for an arthropod intermediate host, in which the cysticercoid larvae develop. Human infection usually occurs following the accidental ingestion of infected beetles that contaminate grain or cereal products. Adult tapeworms develop in the small intestine, where they may grow to 60 cm in length. Like those of *H. nana*, the proglottids all have genital pores on one side, but unlike that species, the scolex lacks an armed rostellum. Infections usually are asymptomatic because of the small number of worms likely to infect one individual, although intestinal symptoms have been reported. Diagnosis is made by finding moderately thick-shelled, slightly ovoid, yellow-brown eggs measuring 70 to 85 μm by 60 to 80 μm in the feces (see Fig. 53–24). The eggs are most easily confused with those of *H. nana* but, unlike that species, lack polar filaments.

***DIPHYLLOBOTHRIUM* SPP.** Humans may be infected with one of several species of the fish tapeworm *Diphyllobothrium* that normally infect piscivorous mammals and, possibly, birds (Curtis, 1991). These parasites are widely distributed in the temperate zones, especially northern Europe, Scandinavia, the former USSR, and Japan. Infections also occur in Canada, and in the north central states, Pacific Coast states, and Alaska in the United Sta tes. Although *Diphyllobothrium latum* is the most common species known to infect humans, differentiation cannot be made based on egg morphology.

The parasite inhabits the small intestine, where it can reach a length of 10 meters or more and persist for years. Eggs are passed unembryonated in the feces and must reach a freshwater stream or lake to continue development. Following several weeks of embryonation, a ciliated larval form, the six-hooked coracidium, hatches and is ingested by a copepod, a type of zooplankton. The coracidium develops into a procercoid larva, which is infective for the second intermediate host, a fish. In fish, the procercoid migrates into the tissues and develops into the pleurocercoid larva. Pleurocercoids may be passed up the food chain unchanged and accumulate in larger fish. Humans acquire these larvae through ingestion of raw or incompletely cooked fish that have spent at least part of their life in fresh water.

Adult worms mature and initiate egg production in approximately one month. Infection may be asymptomatic with passage of a length of strobila being the initial complaint. In others, a variable degree of abdominal discomfort and diarrhea may be present. Rarely, intestinal obstruction occurs. In endemic areas in northern Europe, a small percentage of patients develop vitamin B_{12} deficiency and associated megaloblastic anemia.

Diagnosis is made by finding the typical brown, oval-shaped operculate eggs in feces using standard recovery techniques. Eggs measure 58 to 76 μm by 40 to 51 μm and, in addition to the operculum, have a small, round, knoblike projection on the abopercular end (see Fig. 53–24). Presence of the operculum is unique among those cestodes infecting humans, and care must be taken not to confuse these eggs with those of trematodes, especially *Paragonimus* or *Nanophyetus*. Identification of the genus level is possible when a length of strobila or an intact worm is passed. The scolex is elongated and displays a pair of longitudinal grooves known as bothria, which replace the usual suckers. Gravid proglottids are wider than they are long and have their genital pores located midventrally adjacent to a centrally located rosette-shaped uterus (see Fig. 53–25).

DIPYLIDIUM CANINUM. *D. caninum* is a common tapeworm of dogs and cats in most parts of the world and not infrequently infects humans, especially children. In the usual life cycle, tapeworm eggs are ingested by flea larvae, which infest areas frequented by dogs or cats. The cysticercoid larvae persist as the flea undergoes metamorphosis to the adult stage. Accidental ingestion of the adult flea containing the infectious cysticercoid results in infection. Children are at highest risk for infection because of their close contact with pets. Worms mature in the small intestine and grow up to 70 cm in length. Infections produce few symptoms, and generally cause concern only on detection of the actively moving proglottids.

Detection is based on finding characteristic eggs, egg packets, or proglottids in the feces. Spherical eggs, each containing a six-hooked embryo, measure from 24 to 40 μm in diameter and occur either singly or in packets (see Fig 53–24). The scolex is somewhat elongate with four suckers and a small, retractable rostellum. Proglottids are barrel shaped and possess two genital pores, one on each lateral margin, which give rise to the common name double-pored tapeworm (see Fig. 53–25).

Trematodes

The trematodes, or flukes, are dorsoventrally flattened helminths (platyhelminths) that include both hermaphroditic forms (intestinal, liver, and lung flukes) and those with separate sexes (blood flukes or schistosomes). All species that infect humans are characterized by the presence of an oral sucker, through which the digestive tract opens, and a ventral sucker used for attachment. Adults vary in length from 1 mm (*Metagonimus*) to 70 mm (*Fasciola gigantica*).

Eggs reach the environment by being passed in the feces, sputum, or urine, depending on the species. The hermaphroditic flukes produce operculate eggs, which are not embryonated (*Clonorchis* and *Opisthorchis* being exceptions). Schistosome eggs are not operculated, and each contains a mature larva when passed. Trematode larvae, or miracidia, are ciliated and capable of penetrating the tissues of a molluscan host. Each species of trematode uses a particular species of snail as the first intermediate host. A complex asexual multiplication process within the snail results in the production of numerous free-swimming larvae called cercariae. Schistosome cercariae are capable of penetrating human skin directly, resulting in the disease schistosomiasis. Those of the hermaphroditic flukes encyst on aquatic vegetation or invade the tissues of second intermediate hosts such as fish or crabs, depending on the species. Ingestion of these encysted larval stages, known as metacercariae, results in human infection.

Human trematode infections occur in many tropical and subtropical regions. Their presence depends on a lack of sewage treatment, availability of appropriate intermediate hosts, and in the case of the hermaphroditic species, dietary customs associated with ingestion of infective metacercariae. Some of these diseases, especially schistosomiasis, are spreading because of the increased use of irrigation in endemic areas. Symptoms vary depending on the number of worms parasitizing the host at a given time, the tissues and organs involved, and host responses. Many infections are asymptomatic.

The diagnosis of trematode infections is made by the recovery and identification of the characteristic eggs in stool, sputum, urine, and occasionally, tissues. Direct mounts and formalin–ethyl acetate concentration methods are most useful for recovery of these eggs, whereas zinc sulfate flotation methods are less satisfactory.

FASCIOLOPSIS BUSKI. This intestinal trematode is the largest species to infect humans, varying from 20 to 75 mm in length and 8 to 20 mm in breadth. It occurs in many parts of China, Southeast Asia, and India and is frequently found in pigs, which serve as a natural reservoir. Infection is acquired by ingesting infectious metacercariae on aquatic food plants such as water chestnuts and water caltrop. Worms attach to the wall of the duodenum and jejunum, where they mature to egg-laying adults in about three months. Symptoms including diarrhea, epigastric pain, and nausea may develop if enough worms are present to produce ulceration of the superficial mucosa. Eosinophilia may be present, even in those who are asymptomatic.

Diagnosis is made by finding the large (130 to 140 μm by 80 to 85 μm), brown, oval, and thin-shelled eggs (Fig. 53–26). The operculum may be inconspicuous, and the eggs are passed unembryonated. Differentiation from *Fasciola* eggs generally is not possible, although these infections may be differentiated on the basis of geographic history and symptoms. Eggs of echinostome trematodes, which occasionally infect humans, are similar but smaller (Beaver, 1984).

HETEROPHYES* AND *METAGONIMUS. These two genera include a number of species of minute (1 to 3 mm in length) intestinal worms that infect humans. *Heterophyes heterophyes* and *Metagonimus yokogawai* are common parasites in Asia but, along with other species, are found in other parts of the world as well. Infections are acquired by ingestion of metacercariae in raw or incompletely cooked freshwater fish. Although they are of minor medical importance, infection with these worms may produce diarrhea and abdominal pain. Infections are self-limited because the worms have a lifespan of only a few months.

Diagnosis is established by finding the embryonated, operculate eggs, which measure 20 to 30 μm in length by 15 to 17 μm in width (see Fig. 53–26). Differentiation of these eggs from those of *Clonorchis* and *Opisthorchis* is difficult, although the operculum is more deeply seated with *Opisthorchis*. Such differentiation may be important, however, for medical reasons.

NANOPHYETUS SALMINCOLA. *N. salmincola* is a small (0.8- to 1.1-mm) intestinal fluke that has been reported in humans in areas of far eastern Siberia and the Pacific Northwest coast of the United States (Eastburn, 1987; Fritsche, 1989b). These worms are acquired by ingesting raw, incompletely cooked, or home-smoked salmon or trout that contain infectious metacercariae. The occurrence of symptoms is related to the number of worms present and may include abdominal pain and diarrhea, with or without eosinophilia. Eggs, 60 to 80 μm by 34 to 50 μm, are broadly ovoid, operculate, and yellowish brown (Eastburn, 1987). There is a thickening of the shell at the abopercular end, which should be differentiated from the knob seen on eggs of *Diphyllobothrium*.

FASCIOLA HEPATICA. Cattle, sheep, and goats in many parts of the world are infected with the liver fluke, *F. hepatica*, and less commonly with the related species *F. gigantica*. Adult parasites live in the biliary tree and lay eggs that are passed in the feces. Cercariae shed from the snail intermediate host encyst on aquatic vegetation, where infectious metacercariae are then available to herbivorous hosts. Humans usually acquire the infection by eating watercress. Once ingested, the larvae penetrate the intestinal wall and migrate through the peritoneal cavity to the liver. They burrow through the capsule and parenchyma, coming to reside within the bile ducts, where egg laying is initiated in about two months. Migration of the larvae through the liver elicits a painful inflammatory reaction both in the tissue and, later, in the bile ducts, which eventually become fibrosed. Clinical manifestations include colic, obstructive jaundice, abdominal pain and tenderness, cholelithiasis, and eosinophilia.

Diagnosis is made by finding eggs in the stool. The unembryonated, yellowish brown, operculate eggs, 130 to 150 μm by 63 to 90 μm, cannot easily be distinguished from those of *Fasciolopsis* (see Fig. 53–26). Spurious infections, which occur by ingesting infected cattle or sheep liver, are diagnosed by obtaining a good history and performing a follow-up stool examination to look for elimination of the eggs.

CLONORCHIS SINENSIS* AND *OPISTHORCHIS VIVERRINI. *C. sinensis*, the Oriental liver fluke, and a closely related species, *O. viverrini*, inhabit the biliary system of humans and other piscivorous animals, including cats and dogs. *C. sinensis* occurs mainly in China, Taiwan, Korea, Japan, and Vietnam, whereas *O. viverrini* is found primarily in Southeast Asia, especially northern Thailand. Human infections are also known to occur with *O. felineus* in Europe and *Amphimerus pseudofelineus* (same as *O. guayaquilensis*) in Ecuador.

All of these parasites are acquired by the ingestion of infectious metacercariae in raw or uncooked freshwater fish. Larvae migrate up the common duct into the liver bile ducts, where they live up to 20 years and grow up to 25 mm in length. They produce small eggs that are shed into the bile and subsequently passed in stools.

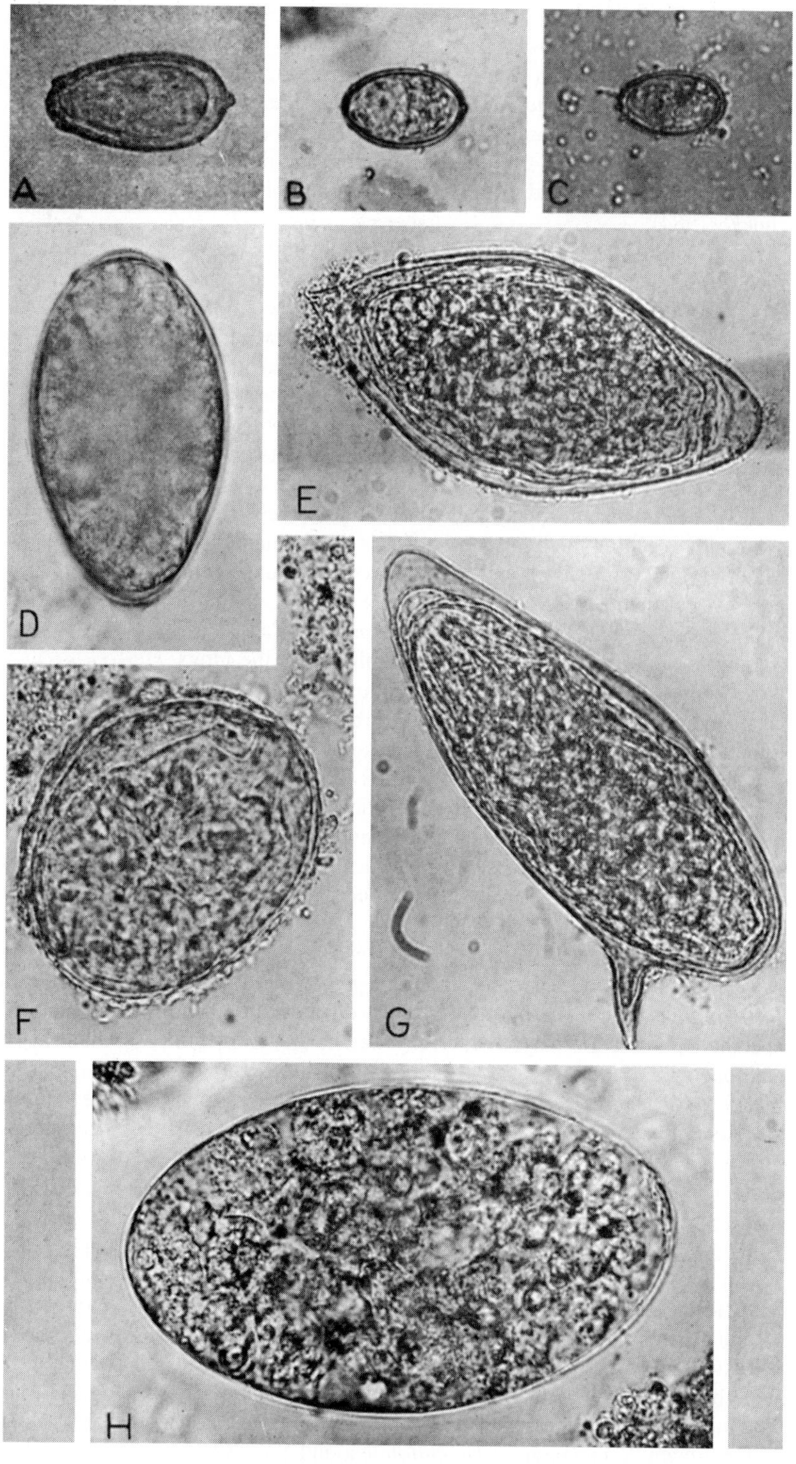

Figure 53–26. Trematode eggs. *A*, Liver fluke, *Clonorchis sinensis*. *B*, *Heterophyes heterophyes*. *C*, *Metagonimus yokogawai*. *D*, Lung fluke, *Paragonimus westermani*. *E*, Blood fluke, *Schistosoma haematobium*. *F*, Oriental blood fluke, *Schistosoma japonicum*. *G*, Manson blood fluke, *Schistosoma mansoni*. *H*, Large intestinal fluke, *Fasciolopsis buski*. All figures ×500 except *A*, which is ×830. (*A* courtesy of Dr. EC Faust, in Brenemann: Practice of Pediatrics. WF Prior Co.; *B* and *C* courtesy of Lt. LW Shatterly, MSC, School of Aviation Medicine, Gunter AFB, AL. All others courtesy of Dr. RL Roudabush, Ward's Natural Science Establishment, Rochester, NY; photos by T Romaniak.)

Infections are often asymptomatic, although large numbers of flukes and repeated infections may cause inflammation of the bile ducts and subsequent hyperplasia, fibrosis, and hepatic cirrhosis. Development of cholangiocarcinoma has been linked epidemiologically with longstanding infections.

Diagnosis is made by recovering the small brown, embryonated, operculate eggs from stools (see Fig. 53–26). Eggs of *Clonorchis* cannot be readily differentiated from those of *Opisthorchis*. Both measure 25 to 35 μm by 12 to 20 μm and have a prominent, seated opercula and a small knob at the abopercular end. These eggs are difficult to differentiate from those of the *Heterophyes/Metagonimus* group, although the latter species do not have the prominent, seated opercula nor a small knob at the abopercular end. When specific identification is not possible, the laboratory report should reflect this (i.e., should state *Clonorchis/Opisthorchis/Heterophyes/Metagonimus eggs*).

***PARAGONIMUS* SPP.** Several species of *Paragonimus*

may parasitize the lungs of cats, dogs, and other carnivores, including humans. *P. westermani* is problematic in many areas of Asia, whereas in Central and South America several species have been implicated, including *P. mexicanus, P. caliensis,* and *P. ecuadoriensis. P. kellicotti* occasionally has been implicated in cases from North America, and other species have been described from Africa (Mariano, 1986; Pachucki, 1984).

Adult worms measure up to 12 mm by 6 mm and often are found in pairs in lung parenchyma, where they reside in a fibrotic capsule produced by the host. The capsule communicates with the bronchi, through which eggs pass to be eventually expelled in sputa or feces. Although a specific snail serves as the first intermediate host, freshwater crabs or crayfish serve as second intermediates for the infectious metacercariae. Ingestion of uncooked, or marinated, crustacea may result in infection. Larvae are released in the stomach and migrate through the intestinal wall into the peritoneal cavity, eventually reaching the lungs after penetrating the diaphragm. Maturation takes approximately five to six weeks, and worms may live for many years.

Symptoms, when present, may be caused by larvae migrating through tissues or by adults established in the lungs. Not infrequently worms develop in ectopic sites including the peritoneum, subcutaneous tissues, and brain. Onset of lung infection usually is associated with fever, chills, and the appearance of eosinophilia. Once established, symptoms include chronic coughing with abundant mucus production and episodes of hemoptysis. Radiographs may show nodular shadows, calcifications, or patchy infiltrates. Eggs remaining in the lung tissues or in ectopic sites may cause extensive granulomatous reaction.

Diagnosis is made by finding the typical eggs either in stools, sputum, or occasionally, tissues. Eggs of the different *Paragonimus* species cannot be readily differentiated, and specific identification may be inferred from the area of origin. The operculate, unembryonated eggs measure 80 to 120 μm by 45 to 70 μm and have a moderately thick, yellow-brown shell (see Fig. 53–26). The operculum is flattened and usually is set off from the rest of the shell by prominent shoulders. The abopercular end is somewhat thickened but does not have a knob. *Paragonimus* eggs may be differentiated from those of *Diphyllobothrium* and *Fasciola/Fasciolopsis*, which they superficially resemble, by size.

***SCHISTOSOMA* SPP.** Schistosomiasis, or bilharziasis, is among the most important parasitic diseases worldwide, afflicting 200 to 300 million individuals. Adult male and female blood flukes inhabit veins of the mesentery or bladder. The most important species infecting humans are *S. mansoni, S. japonicum, S. mekongi, S. haematobium,* and *S. intercalatum;* other species infect humans less frequently.

Adult female schistosomes are slender, measuring up to 26 mm by 0.5 mm. Males, which are slightly shorter, enfold a female using the lateral margins of the body (the gynecophoral canal) to assist in sperm transfer. When examined *in situ*, schistosomes are often found *in copula* (Fig. 53–27). In their preferred locations, blood flukes elicit little or no inflammatory response. Eggs are deposited in the smallest venule that can accommodate the female worm, where they elicit a strong granulomatous response that results in extrusion of the egg into the intestinal lumen or the bladder. Pathology is primarily related to the sites of egg deposition, numbers deposited, and host reaction to egg antigens.

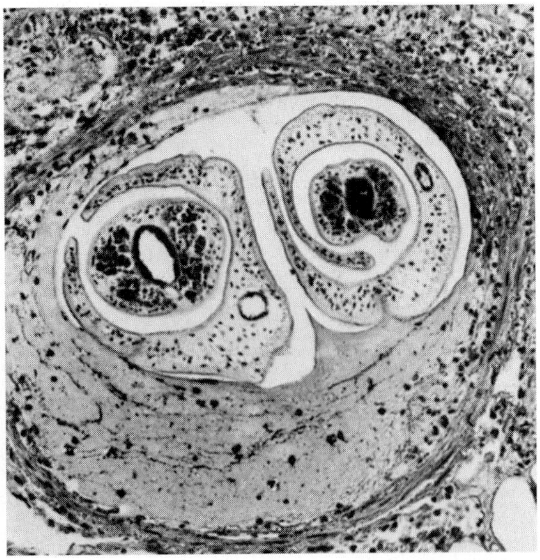

Figure 53–27. *Schistosoma mansoni.* Cross-section of adults in mesenteric vein. Note the female at the center, in the male's gynecophoral canal (×120).

Eggs are fully embryonated when passed and readily hatch when deposited in fresh water. The miracidia penetrate an appropriate species of snail host, where they undergo transformation and extensive asexual multiplication. After about four weeks, large numbers of fork-tailed cercariae emerge from the mollusk. Cercariae swim actively about for hours and readily penetrate the skin of susceptible hosts, including humans. After penetration the cercariae, now called schistosomules, enter the circulation and pass through the lungs before reaching the mesenteric-portal vessels.

Symptoms of schistosomiasis result primarily from penetration of cercariae (cercarial dermatitis), initiation of egg laying (acute schistosomiasis or Katayama fever), and as a late stage complication of tissue proliferation and repair (chronic schistosomiasis). In a matter of hours after cercarial penetration, a papular rash associated with pruritus may develop. This is a sensitization phenomenon resulting from prior exposure to cercarial antigens. The most severe form of dermatitis occurs in individuals who are repeatedly exposed to cercariae of nonhuman (primarily avian) schistosomes. Cercarial dermatitis or swimmer's itch occurs worldwide and is a well-recognized entity in the United States (Hoeffler, 1974).

Initiation of egg laying by mature worms five to seven weeks after infection may result in acute schistosomiasis, or Katayama fever, a serum sickness–like syndrome that occurs with heavy primary infections, especially those of *S. japonicum.* The antigenic challenge to the host is thought to result in immune complex formation (Boros, 1989).

Chronic infection results in continued egg deposition, many of which remain in the body. Granulomas produced around these eggs in the intestine and bladder are gradually replaced by collagen, resulting in fibrosis and scarring. Eggs trapped in the liver may induce pipe-stem fibrosis with obstruction to portal blood flow. Occasionally, eggs are deposited in ectopic sites, such as the spinal cord, lungs, or brain.

Diagnosis is established by demonstrating eggs in feces or urine by direct wet mount or formalin–ethyl acetate concentration methods. Zinc sulfate concentration is not satisfactory for recovery of the heavy schistosome eggs. Eggs also may be detected in biopsies of rectal, bladder, and occasionally, liver tissues either by crush preparation or in histologic section (Fig. 53–28). Use of egg hatching methods occasionally may be requested to determine viability or, less commonly, to detect light infections. Feces mixed with distilled water are placed in a flask that is covered with foil to keep out light, with only the neck or a sidearm exposed to a bright light. Miracidia, if present, actively swim to the light and can be detected using a hand lens.

Serologic tests may be helpful in screening persons who have traveled to endemic areas, those with negative urine or stool examinations who are at risk for infection, or for monitoring response to therapy. Although not widely available, a limited number of reference laboratories and the Centers for Disease Control and Prevention provide testing. Generally, serologic testing varies with the antigens used and test methodologies employed. The Centers for Disease Control and Prevention uses the Falcon assay screening test in a kinetic enzyme-linked immunosorbent assay (FAST-ELISA). Sera that are positive by the screening test are further evaluated by immunoblot to improve specificity (Wilson, 1995).

SCHISTOSOMA MANSONI. *S. mansoni* occurs in Africa, especially in the tropical areas and the Nile delta, southern Africa, and Madagascar. In the western hemisphere it occurs in Brazil, Venezuela, Surinam, and certain Caribbean islands, including Puerto Rico. Adult *S. mansoni* live primarily in the portal vein and in the distribution of the inferior mesenteric vein. Initial deposition of eggs in the large intestine may produce abdominal pain and dysentery, with abundant blood and mucus in the stool. Eggs may be detected in feces at this time. Chronic infection may result in liver fibrosis and portal hypertension, depending on the number of worms present; eggs may be more difficult to find in feces during this stage.

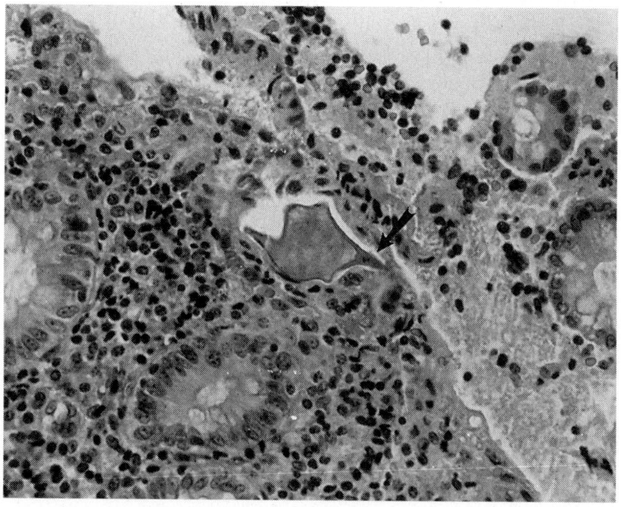

Figure 53–28. *Schistosoma mansoni.* Recent granuloma with egg in liver. Note the presence of the lateral spine (*arrow*), which provides definitive identification (hematoxylin and eosin; ×400).

Eggs, 116 to 180 μm by 45 to 58 μm, are oval, with a large distinctive lateral spine that protrudes from the side of the egg near one end (see Fig. 53–26). If the spine is not visible, the egg may be rotated by gently tapping the coverslip. Movement of the miracidium within the egg may be evident in unfixed material if the larva is viable. Concentration techniques may be required to detect eggs, because individuals with limited exposure or with chronic infection may pass few of them.

SCHISTOSOMA JAPONICUM. *S. japonicum,* which occurs in China, Southeast Asia, and the Philippines, causes disease that is clinically similar to that of *S. mansoni*, but often more serious because many more (up to 10 times) eggs are produced by *S. japonicum.* The disease has been essentially eliminated from Japan, although animal reservoirs still exist. Adult worms live primarily in the distribution of the superior mesenteric vein, and eggs readily reach the liver, inducing fibrosis and portal hypertension as a common complication of chronic infection. The smaller size of the eggs predisposes them to dissemination, especially to the brain and spinal cord. The eggs are broadly oval, measuring 75 to 90 μm by 60 to 68 μm, and have an inconspicuous lateral spine, which may be difficult to demonstrate (see Fig. 53–26).

SCHISTOSOMA MEKONGI. This species occurs in humans and animal reservoirs in countries along the Mekong River, especially Cambodia and Laos (Bruce, 1980). It is similar to *S. japonicum* but is differentiated from that species by several biological characteristics and smaller eggs (60 to 70 μm by 52 to 62 μm), which otherwise are indistinguishable from those of *S. japonicum*.

SCHISTOSOMA HAEMATOBIUM. Urinary schistosomiasis occurs in many parts of Africa, the Middle East, and Madagascar. Parasites migrate via the hemorrhoidal veins to the venous plexuses of the urinary bladder, prostate, uterus, and vagina. One of the earliest and most common symptoms of infection is hematuria, especially at the end of micturition. Chronic infection may cause pelvic pain and bladder colic with an increased desire to urinate. Accumulation of eggs in the tissues may result in hypertrophy of the urothelium, squamous metaplasia, and marked fibrosis, which may progress to obstruction and, ultimately, renal failure. Urinary schistosomiasis also has been associated with squamous cell carcinoma of the bladder (Badawi, 1992).

Eggs are recovered from the urine by examining a spun sediment. They are elongate, measuring 112 to 180 μm by 40 to 70 μm, and have a characteristic terminal spine (see Fig. 53–26). Occasionally, they may be detected in feces or in a rectal biopsy.

SCHISTOSOMA INTERCALATUM. This species occurs in many parts of central and western Africa and produces intestinal schistosomiasis. Eggs have a terminal spine and so resemble those of *S. haematobium,* but they occur primarily in the feces and are larger (140 to 240 μm by 50 to 85 μm).

TISSUE HELMINTHS

Nematodes

Filaria

Filarial nematodes, also known as threadworms, are common arthropod-transmitted parasites of vertebrate animals. Adult male and female worms are long and slender, measuring up to 100 mm in length, and are known to inhabit a variety of tissues, including subcutaneous tissues, lymphatics, blood vessels, peritoneal and pleural cavities, heart, and brain. All species produce larvae known as microfilariae, which may be recovered from either blood or skin, depending on the species. The microfilariae of some species circulate in the blood with a well-defined periodicity (either diurnal or nocturnal), whereas others do not. Microfilariae continue their development only in the appropriate arthropod vector, usually a mosquito or fly, where they mature to the infective stage. Such larvae are then deposited in the tissues of a definitive host when the vector takes another blood meal.

Diagnosis of filariasis usually is made by finding microfilariae in the blood or skin, because adult stages are often sequestered in the tissues. The use of Giemsa's or hematoxylin-stained thick smears of peripheral blood is routine, although more sensitive procedures such as membrane filter, Knott's concentration, or saponin lysis may also be required. Microfilariae may be seen moving in direct mounts of blood or tissue fluid.

Species identification is important because pathogenicity varies. The principal characteristics that are used for identification of microfilariae include the presence or absence of a sheath and its staining characteristics, the shape of the tail and distribution of cell nuclei within, and the size of the cephalic space and appearance of its nuclear column. Because microfilariae of *Wuchereria* and *Brugia* usually display a nocturnal periodicity, blood from patients suspected to be infected with these filaria should be drawn between the hours of 10 P.M. and 2 A.M. *Loa loa* displays diurnal periodicity, so blood should preferably be drawn around noon. *M. ozzardi* and *M. perstans* are characteristically nonperiodic. Microfilariae of *M. streptocerca* and *Onchocerca volvulus* are present in the skin and are detected by examination of skin snips or punch biopsies.

Serologic tests for the diagnosis of lymphatic filariasis may prove helpful in select patients, especially those who are not native to endemic areas. Such methods are limited in their ability to distinguish between past exposure and current infection, however, and infection with other nematode species may result in the appearance of cross-reacting antibodies. Antigen detection tests also may be of value in the diagnosis of lymphatic filariasis but are not generally available (Wilson, 1995).

WUCHERERIA BANCROFTI. This species, responsible for bancroftian filariasis, is the most common filarial species to infect humans. Endemic areas include central and northern Africa, India, Southeast Asia, certain South Pacific islands, and portions of Central and South America and the West Indies. Adult worms reside in the lymphatic system, where chronic infection and reinfection result in lymphadenopathy and lymphangitis, which may progress to lymphedema and obstructive fibrosis (Fig. 53–29). Severe involvement of the lower extremeties and genitalia may result in elephantiasis.

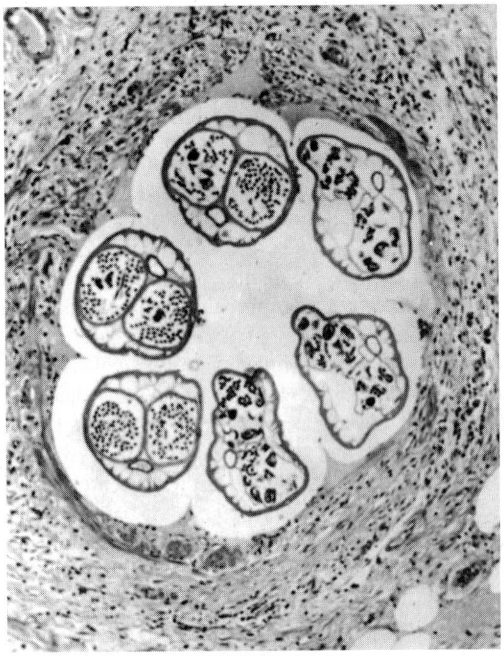

Figure 53–29. *Wuchereria bancrofti.* Cross-section of adult in human lymph node. Note fibrosis surrounding the worm (× 120).

In most areas, microfilariae circulate in peripheral blood with a nocturnal periodicity that corresponds with the feeding activities of the usual vectors *Culex*, *Aedes*, and *Anopheles* mosquitoes. Infections originating in the South Pacific are essentially without periodicity. The microfilariae are sheathed, although this may not always be obvious with Giemsa staining. The tail is pointed, and there are no nuclei in the tip. The cephalic space is not as long as it is wide, and the nuclei in the nuclear column are distinct (Fig. 53–30). Concentration procedures may be necessary for recovery because microfilariae may be present in small numbers.

BRUGIA MALAYI. This species produces disease similar to that of *W. bancrofti*, although it is often milder and more frequently involves the lymphatics of the upper extremities. The parasite occurs mainly in India, Southeast Asia, Korea, the Philippines, and Japan. Human infections with related zoonotic species are encountered periodically in the United States.

The microfilariae circulate in the blood and are primarily periodic. Microfilarial sheaths of *B. malayi* stain well with Giemsa stain. The tail has a swelling at the tip and has two solitary nuclei located beyond the end of the nuclear column (termed subterminal and terminal nuclei). The cephalic space may be much longer than it is wide (see Fig. 53–30). *B. timori* is a distinct species occurring in the eastern end of the Indonesian archipelago, especially on the islands of Timor and Flores. Microfilariae are very similar to those of *B. malayi* although somewhat larger.

LOA LOA. Known as the eye worm, *Loa loa* lives in subcutaneous tissues. The nematodes migrate continuously, producing transient (two to three days) local inflammatory reactions known as Calabar or fugitive swellings. Their occasional appearance in the conjunctiva allows them to be surgically ex-

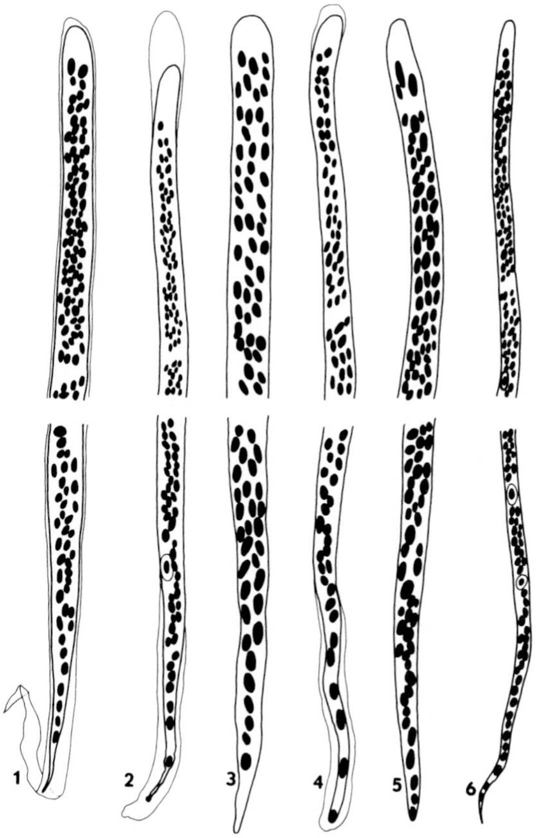

Figure 53–30. Anterior and posterior ends of microfilariae most commonly found in humans. *1, Wuchereria bancrofti.* 2, *Brugia malayi. 3, Onchocerca volvulus. 4, Loa loa. 5, Mansonella perstans. 6, Mansonella ozzardi.* All camera lucida drawings.

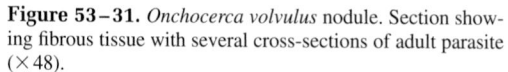

cised. Loiasis occurs primarily in West and Central Africa, where deer flies of the genus *Chrysops* serve as vector.

The parasite elicits strong eosinophilia and occasionally has been seen in the United States in people with a history of travel to Africa. The microfilariae, which circulate in the blood with diurnal periodicity, are sheathed, although the sheath does not stain with Giemsa's stain. Nuclei in the tail extend to the rounded tip. The nuclear column is distinct, and the cephalic space is short (see Fig. 53–30).

ONCHOCERCA VOLVULUS. Onchocerciasis is a leading cause of blindness in endemic areas, which include Central Africa, Central America (Mexico and Guatemala), and northern South America. Vectors are black flies of the genus *Simulium.* Adult worms live in hard fibrous nodules in subcutaneous and deeper tissues that can grow to be 40 mm in diameter (Fig. 53–31). Nodules tend to occur on the upper half of the body in patients from central America and in the lower half in those from Africa. Adult worms produce microfilariae that migrate continuously through the skin. Complications arise from the migratory activities of the microfilariae, resulting in several forms of dermatitis. Movement of microfilariae through the surface of the eye may result in keratitis, corneal opacity, and damage to the anterior and posterior chambers and iris, thus leading to blindness with repeated infections over time. Diagnosis is made by finding the typical microfilariae in teased skin snips or skin biopsies, preferably taken from over the scapular region or from the iliac crest, when placed in saline. Alternatively, fluids expressed from scarified skin or aspirates of nodules may be examined (Beaver, 1984). Microfilariae in stained preparations lack both a sheath and nuclei in the tail tip (see Fig. 53–30).

***MANSONELLA* SPP.** Several species of *Mansonella* infect humans, but all are generally regarded as causing little pathology. Microfilariae, however, must be differentiated from the truly pathogenic filarial species. *M. ozzardi* is found in Central and South America, and some areas of the Caribbean. Adult parasites reside in subcutaneous tissues. *M. perstans* occurs in many areas of tropical Africa and sporadically in South America. Adults are thought to reside primarily in body cavities and the mesenteries. Microfilariae of both species are unsheathed and circulate in peripheral blood without evidence of periodicity. *M. ozzardi* microfilariae have a thin, pointed tail without nuclei, whereas the tail of *M. perstans* is broad and blunt with nuclei extending to the tip (see Fig. 53–

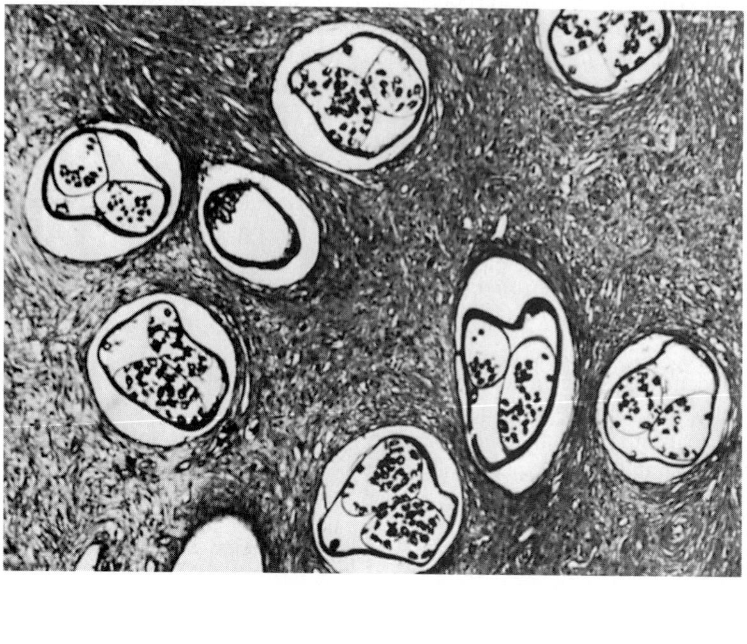

Figure 53–31. *Onchocerca volvulus* nodule. Section showing fibrous tissue with several cross-sections of adult parasite (×48).

6

30). *M. streptocerca*, which is found in tropical Africa, may be confused with *O. volvulus*, because both adult and microfilarial stages occur in skin and subcutaneous tissues. Also, dermatitis may be produced by this species. Microfilariae of this species, which may be recovered in skin snips, are unsheathed and have a crook in the tail with nuclei extending to the tip. All species of *Mansonella* are transmitted by gnats of the genus *Culicoides*.

ZOONOTIC FILARIAE. Certain filarial nematodes of the genera *Dirofilaria* and *Brugia* that naturally parasitize wild and domestic mammals sporadically infect humans. *Dirofilaria immitis*, commonly known as the canine heartworm, is widely distributed and human infections are well documented. The mosquito-transmitted larval stage migrates to the right side of the heart. When the worm dies it is swept into a small pulmonary artery, producing a granulomatous nodule that appears as a coin lesion on a chest radiograph. Diagnosis usually is made by histologic examination of the nodule.

Other species of *Dirofilaria* including *D. tenuis*, *D. repens*, and *D. ursi* commonly cause subcutaneous nodules in humans but fail to produce microfilariae. Such nodules have been reported from many body sites, including the face, conjunctiva, and breast, and usually are removed surgically. Histologic examination often reveals a prominent mixed inflammatory reaction surrounding a dead worm. Criteria for identification of the zoonotic filariae in tissue sections may be found elsewhere (Orihel, 1995; Gutierrez, 1990).

Other

DRACUNCULUS MEDINENSIS. Adult Guinea worms live in subcutaneous tissues and become clinically evident when the female worm migrates to the skin surface and produces a blister, usually on the lower extremities. When the extremity is immersed in water, the blister ruptures, releasing swarms of motile larvae from the female worm into the water. Specific zooplankton (i.e., copepods) ingest the larvae, which then mature to the infective stage and are transmitted back to humans when copepods are accidentally swallowed in drinking water.

The disease is endemic to areas of Africa, the Middle East, and Asia, and may be responsible for disfiguring cutaneous scars and more serious secondary bacterial infections. Extensive control efforts have been made in recent years to eradicate this parasite (Centers for Disease Control, 1992).

Diagnosis is made by finding the female worm emerging at the skin surface and larvae in the discharge fluid. The worm may be gently extracted over a period of days, but care must be taken not to damage it during removal. Should the worm die *in situ*, pronounced inflammatory reactions and secondary bacterial infections may disable the affected individual.

ANGIOSTRONGYLUS CANTONENSIS* AND *ANGIOSTRONGYLUS COSTARICENSIS. Human eosinophilic meningoencephalitis, caused by *A. cantonensis*, occurs both in epidemics and sporadically in many areas of the South Pacific, Southeast Asia, and Taiwan. The mature parasite is normally found in the pulmonary arteries of rats. Larvae migrate up the trachea and are passed in the feces. They develop to the infective stage in slugs or land snails and, when eaten by the usual rodent host, migrate through the brain before maturing in the pulmonary arteries. Humans acquire the infection by eating large edible snails; raw or incompletely cooked shrimp or crabs, which may serve as transport hosts; or vegetables contaminated with infected mollusks. In humans, the *A. cantonensis* larvae migrate to the central nervous system, producing a generally nonfatal meningitis with a high spinal fluid eosinophilia (Alicata, 1991). Diagnosis is established both clinically and historically, although larvae have occasionally been recovered from spinal fluid (Kubersky, 1979).

A. costaricensis occurs widely in Central and South America (Loria-Cortez, 1980). The parasite, which is responsible for the intestinal form of angiostrongyliasis, normally resides in the mesenteric arteries of the ileum and cecum of rodents. Human infection occurs in the same anatomic location, but often results in granulomatous inflammation and symptoms of acute abdomen. Diagnosis is made by histologic examination of surgical specimens and finding adults or eggs in the tissues.

TRICHINELLA SPIRALIS. Human trichinosis occurs worldwide, although its incidence in the United States has been in steady decline, with fewer than 100 cases reported each year. Humans acquire the infection through the ingestion of raw or incompletely cooked pork, pork products, or less commonly, bear meat that contains infective larvae. Ingested worms mature in the small intestine, where gravid females produce new larvae for two to three weeks. During this stage, gastrointestinal symptoms occur, lasting several days. Larvae subsequently enter lymphatics and venules, thus reaching the general circulation. They primarily invade the skeletal musculature, where they undergo further development and encapsulation. During the migratory and encapsulation phases, fever, muscle pain, respiratory difficulties, periorbital edema, and eosinophilia may develop, depending on the inoculating dose. After the parasites have encysted, there are few symptoms. Encysted larvae may remain viable for several years, although they eventually become calcified.

Diagnosis usually is made on the basis of history and clinical symptoms and is confirmed by the demonstration of trichinella cysts in skeletal muscle biopsy, particularly the gastrocnemius or deltoid muscles (Fig. 53–32). Indirect tests include creatine phosphokinase, which often is elevated, and detection of antibodies by bentonite flocculation or EIA. Of these serologic tests, creatine phosphokinase is more specific, and EIA is more sensitive (Wilson, 1995).

LARVA MIGRANS. Larva migrans is caused by the prolonged wandering through body tissues of larvae of certain hookworms, ascarids, and *Strongyloides* species that normally infect wild or domestic animals. The syndrome varies with the species involved, numbers of worms, and tissues parasitized.

Cutaneous larva migrans (CLM), or ground itch, is produced by the cutaneous wanderings of cat or dog hookworms of the genus *Ancylostoma* that penetrate the skin but cannot mature in the usual pattern. Serpiginous, erythematous, and pruritic tracks are apparent on the skin in areas where there has been contact with the ground. This is particularly problematic in warmer, humid climates, where eggs and larvae of these hookworms survive longer. Some species of *Strongyloides* that parasitize wild animals may cause a similar dermatitis.

Visceral larva migrans (VLM) is produced primarily by

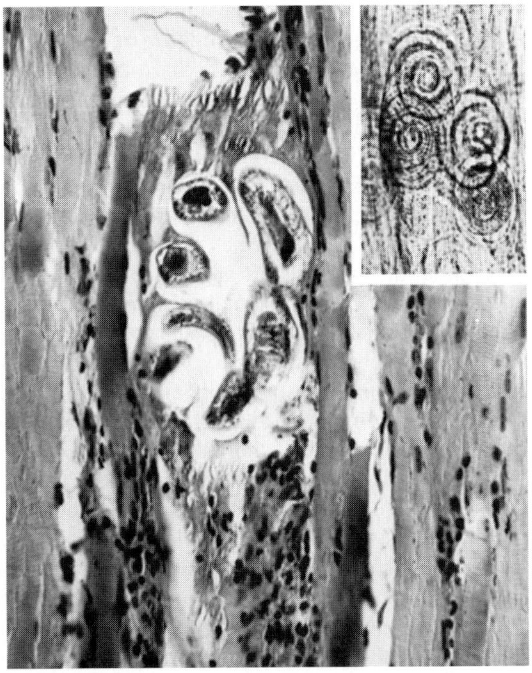

Figure 53–32. *Trichinella spiralis*, cross-section of larva in deltoid muscle (×200). Inset shows whole larvae in wet muscle preparation (×63).

the random wanderings of the dog ascarid *Toxocara canis* and, to a lesser degree, by *T. cati* from the domestic cat. Children usually are infected following the accidental or intentional ingestion of soil contaminated with dog or cat feces. After hatching, the larvae are unable to complete their usual cycle and instead begin a prolonged migration through various tissues and organs. Children may present with failure to thrive and display fever, hepatomegaly, pneumonitis, hypereosinophilia, and hypergammaglobulinemia. An inflammatory reaction in the retina from ocular larva migrans may mimic retinoblastoma, a malignant tumor, from which it must be differentiated. Diagnosis of VLM usually is made on clinical grounds, because the parasite is rarely recovered. Serologic tests may be helpful in confirming a presumptive diagnosis, and the currently recommended procedure is an EIA that uses larval stage excretory-secretory antigens (Wilson, 1995).

A VLM-like syndrome may also be caused by species of *Gnathostoma* that infect the stomach of various mammals. Human infections are most common in Southeast Asia but have been reported in Mexico and Ecuador. These parasites use a copepod for the first intermediate host and fish and amphibians as secondary hosts. A variety of reptiles, birds, and mammals may serve as paratenic hosts. The larvae may migrate through subcutaneous tissues, causing transient swellings and to deeper tissues, and eventually invade the central nervous system. The occurrence of migratory lesions and a history of eating raw fish may be helpful in establishing a clinical diagnosis.

CAPILLARIA HEPATICA. Although normally a parasite common to rodents, this species occasionally causes human disease, especially in children, in whom it may mimic VLM, hepatitis, amebic liver abscess, and other diseases. In the usual rodent host, eggs are ingested and the resulting larvae migrate to the liver, where they mature and deposit eggs directly in the parenchyma. When the liver is eaten by a predator, the eggs are passed out in the feces and contaminate soil. Children are at particular risk for acquiring the eggs if they eat dirt. In endemic areas, diagnosis is made by examination of liver biopsies or tissue obtained at autopsy. Eggs are readily recognized in tissue biopsies by having thick striated walls and plugs at both ends.

***ANISAKIS, PSEUDOTERRANOVA,* AND *EUSTRONGYLIDES* SPP.** The ingestion of raw fish, although considered by many to be a delicacy, has resulted in an increase in the number of reported cases of fish nematode infections. *Anisakis* and *Pseudoterranova* are common gastrointestinal parasites of marine mammals, and the infective stages are found in various saltwater fish, salmon, and squid intermediate hosts. Small shrimplike crustacea (krill) serve as first intermediate host. When ingested, these larvae may penetrate the wall of the stomach or small bowel, causing acute abdominal pain. Anisakiasis may be presumptively diagnosed based on an appropriate history and clinical findings, and the condition may be confirmed by the recovery of an intact worm at endoscopy or by the presence of an eosinophilic granuloma containing an identifiable nematode in a surgical specimen. Species of *Anisakis* appear to be more prone to produce invasive disease, whereas *Pseudoterranova* spp. tend to be coughed up or vomited intact (Sakanari, 1989). The species level of larval anisakids is difficult to identify (Binford, 1976).

A small number of infections with *Eustrongyloides* spp. have been reported in individuals who had eaten live minnows or home-prepared sushi. These parasites usually infect fish-eating birds, but in humans, the bright red larvae invade the abdominal cavity, requiring surgical removal (Wittner, 1989).

Cestodes

Several species of cestodes infect humans in their larval stages and may produce serious disease. The more commonly encountered ones are readily distinguishable from each other and have unique patterns of transmission. When seen in tissue sections, larval and adult stages of cestodes contain basophilic-staining laminated bodies known as calcareous corpuscles, which are an important aid in their recognition.

CYSTICERCOSIS. Human infection with the larval stage of the pork tapeworm, *T. solium*, is found worldwide and occurs following the unintentional ingestion of the eggs of an adult tapeworm. The disease is especially prevalent in Mexico and the rest of Latin America, Europe, Africa, India, and Asia. Most cases in the United States originate from highly endemic areas, although in recent years, the number of locally acquired cases has increased (Richards, 1985).

Eggs may be ingested accidentally with contaminated food or water and subsequently hatch in the gastrointestinal tract. Embryos penetrate the intestinal mucosa and disseminate via the bloodstream to distant sites, especially the skeletal muscle, and also to the heart, brain, or eye, where symptoms of infection and inflammation may become especially apparent. Seizures are a common complication in endemic areas and often are the presenting symptom.

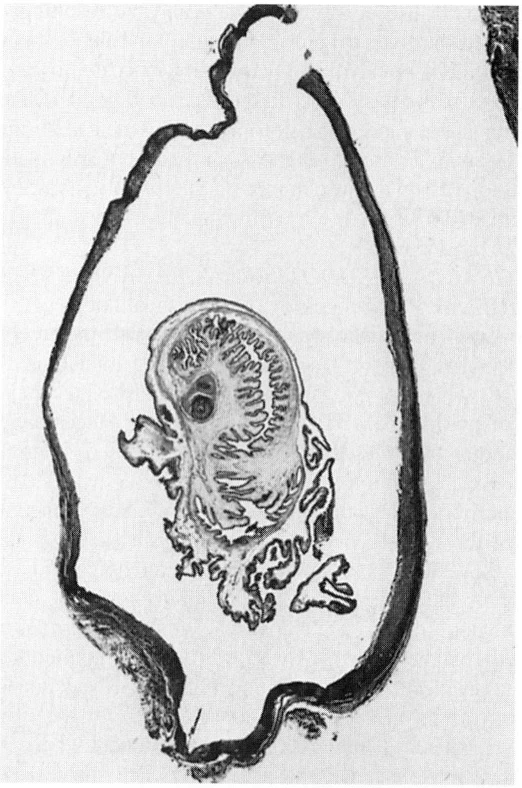

Figure 53–33. *Cysticercus* from subcutaneous tissues. The larva has a tightly invaginated scolex in the bladder (× 11). (Case of Dr. H. Estrada, Manizales, Colombia.)

The diagnosis usually is made on clinical grounds in endemic areas but may be much more difficult to establish in nonendemic settings. Use of computed tomographic (CT) scans is very helpful but generally not available in most endemic areas. Radiographs are helpful in recognizing the presence of calcified cysts but not in recognizing recent infections. Recovery of an intact cysticercus at surgery confirms the diagnosis. The cysticercus, or bladder worm, is a translucent fluid-filled oval sac containing a single inverted scolex that measures 5 mm or more in diameter (Fig. 53–33).

Among serologic assays, the glycoprotein immunoblot assay available from the Centers for Disease Control and Prevention has high sensitivity and specificity, outperforming several EIAs with which it was compared (Diaz, 1992). Unfortunately, these assays do not distinguish between active and inactive infections, and thus are not useful in monitoring response to therapy.

The occurrence of cysticercosis in someone from a nonendemic area and without an appropriate travel history should be investigated for accidental exposure to individuals involved in food preparation, or for the possibility of infection with a different *Taenia* species (Schantz, 1992).

HYDATIDOSIS. Human infection with larval stages of tapeworms of the genus *Echinococcus* may take one of three forms: unilocular hydatid disease caused by *E. granulosus,* multilocular or alveolar hydatid disease caused by *E. multilocularis,* and polycystic hydatid disease caused by *E. vogeli* (Thompson, 1995). Members of the dog family are definitive hosts for these minute tapeworms. What they lack in size they make up for in numbers, with many hundreds or thousands of worms producing large numbers of eggs in one host. Eggs are passed in the stools and ingested by the intermediate hosts, which include sheep, cattle, pigs, rodents, and other herbivorous animals. Humans, especially children, are infected following the accidental ingestion of eggs from the environment.

Eggs hatch in the intestine, and the embryos penetrate the intestinal wall and then enter the bloodstream. Although most hydatids develop in the liver, some disseminate to other sites. Development of the cysts is slow and may take many years to form a cyst of 10 to 15 cm in diameter. In the usual secondary hosts, the cysts contain numerous protoscoleces, which proliferate from a germinal membrane.

E. granulosus, the most important species producing human disease, is common in many sheep- and cattle-raising areas of the world, including the United States, where dogs are the usual definitive host. Unilocular hydatids develop as single cysts in the liver and secondarily in the lungs or other locations. The cysts are filled with clear fluid and contain brood capsules and numerous protoscoleces, which can number in the thousands (Fig. 53–34). Symptoms in humans are those of a slowly growing mass lesion, although infections in the central nervous system become apparent earlier than in other sites. The diagnosis is suggested based on clinical presentation and history plus the use of radiography, CT scans, and ultrasonography. Serologic tests are very useful in confirming a diagnosis and usually involve a screening test such as EIA or IHA followed, if positive, by a confirmatory assay such as immunoblot or gel diffusion (Wilson, 1995). Sensitivity varies from 60% to 90% depending on the characteristics of the case. False-positive reactions may occur with cysticer-

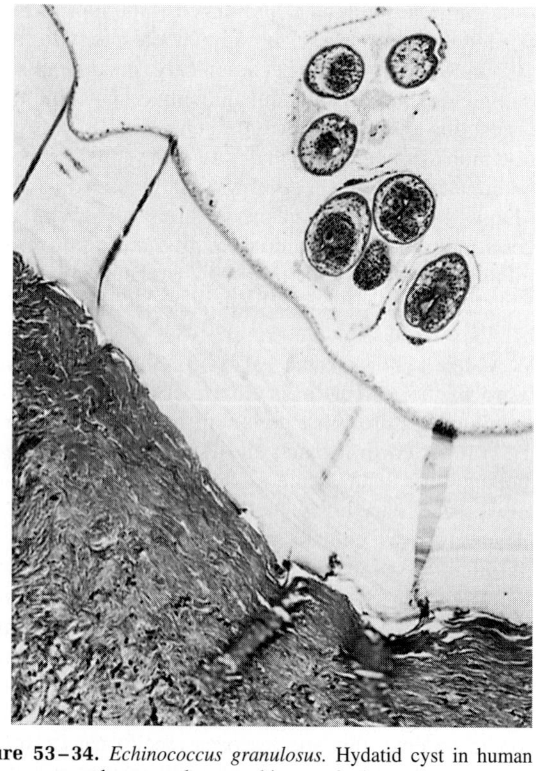

Figure 53–34. *Echinococcus granulosus.* Hydatid cyst in human liver. There are several protoscoleces, a thin germinal membrane, a thick laminated membrane, and fibrous host reaction (× 100).

cosis, although disease presentation should prevent confusion. Aspiration of cyst contents is potentially dangerous because spillage of cyst contents may result in dissemination of disease or possibly anaphylactic shock; but if aspiration is performed, cyst contents usually reveal hydatid sand, a mixture of protoscoleces, disintegrating brood capsules, hooklets, and calcareous corpuscles.

E. multilocularis produces multilocular or alveolar hydatid disease in the northern regions of Europe and Russia, and in Alaska, Canada, and the northern tier of states in the United States. Intermediate hosts include several genera of small rodents; foxes, wolves, and dogs are definitive hosts. Human infection occurs in the liver, where the hydatid develops as an invasive cyst that insinuates itself within the tissue in an alveolar pattern. Although the germinal membrane proliferates in the human liver, protoscoleces fail to develop. The pathologic picture is reminiscent of hepatic carcinoma. Serologic assays that use *E. granulosus* antigens are useful in the diagnosis of this disease. The differential use of antigens from both parasites shows promise of discrimination between the two diseases (Wilson, 1995).

E. vogeli produces a polycystic hydatid cyst in humans that is invasive but, unlike *E. multilocularis*, produces both brood capsules and protoscoleces. The disease is limited to Latin America, where rodents, specifically the paca, and bush dogs complete the life cycle (D'Alessandro, 1979). Polycystic hydatid disease in South America may also be caused by *E. oligarthus*, a parasite of felids and rodents. This species is similar morphologically to *E. vogeli*, and cases have been misidentified in the past (D'Alessandro, 1995).

SPARGANOSIS. Sparganosis is caused by larval cestodes of the genus *Spirometra*, which are closely related to *Diphyllobothrium* spp. Adult stages commonly parasitize cats and dogs and their relatives in Asia (*S. mansoni*) and North America (*S. mansonoides*). Life cycles are similar to those of *Diphyllobothrium*; copepods serve as first intermediate hosts for the procercoid larvae, and fish serve as second intermediate hosts for pleurocercoid larvae. Humans become infected with these larval stages (the sparganum) through ingestion of copepods in drinking water or ingestion of raw or incompletely cooked fish. Use of frogs and snakes as poultices may also result in the transfer of larvae to the human host. Sparganosis usually presents as localized or migratory subcutaneous swellings associated with erythema and pain, although brain infections occur. Surgical exploration may reveal a delicate, slender, ivory-colored worm varying from a few to many centimeters in length. Cross-sections demonstrate a thick tegument with deep folds and parenchyma with prominent muscle bundles. There is no body cavity seen as in the nematodes, and calcareous corpuscles are numerous (Fig. 53–35) (Orihel, 1995; Gutierrez, 1990).

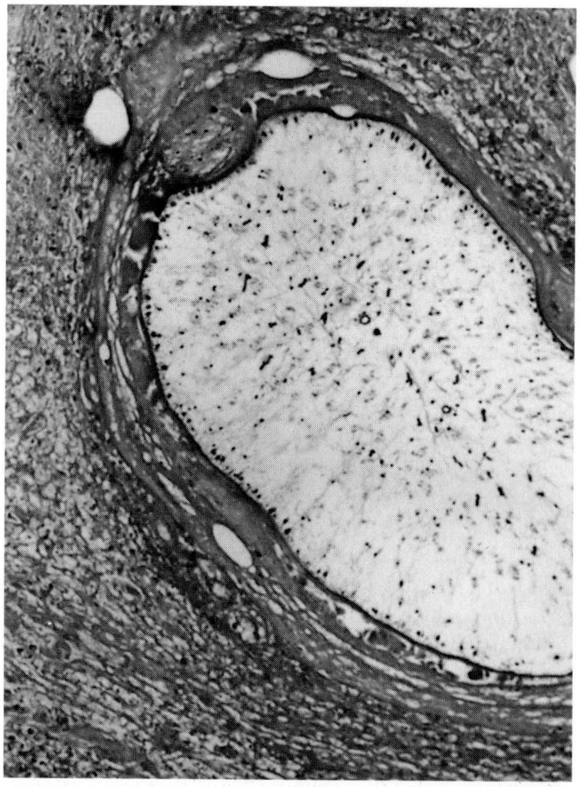

Figure 53–35. *Sparganum.* Larva of *Spirometra* spp. in human tissues.

COENUROSIS. Intestinal *Taenia* spp. of cats and dogs (primarily *T. multiceps* and *T. serialis*) produce a larval stage in intermediate hosts known as a coenurus. This stage consists of a large (up to 10 cm) transparent sac containing numerous scoleces that bud off from a germinal membrane and invaginate into the fluid-filled cyst. Sheep and rodents are the usual intermediate hosts for *T. multiceps* and *T. serialis*, respectively, although humans serve in this role through accidental ingestion of eggs originating from domestic cats and dogs. Like cysticerci, coenuri may develop in any organ, producing a similar disease. Diagnosis usually is made by examination of the excised cyst or its demonstration in tissue sections. The presence of multiple invaginated scoleces within a single bladder differentiates the coenurus from other larval cestodes.

Trematodes

All of the liver-, lung-, and blood-inhabiting trematodes that mature in humans produce eggs that usually exit the body via stool, urine, or sputum. Because of their extraintestinal location, these flukes and their eggs may be found in tissues either incidentally or associated with symptoms.

Adult *F. hepatica*, *C. sinensis*, and *O. viverrini* may be found in hepatic and biliary tissues, and occasionally in ectopic locations. The presence of typical eggs either free in the tissues or within the uterus of the helminth often provides a definitive identification. Adult *Paragonimus* spp. primarily reside in the lung, but may be found in ectopic sites such as brain and subcutaneous tissue, where they produce abscesses, often associated with large numbers of eggs. Adult schistosomes reside in blood vessels, primarily in the distribution of the inferior mesenteric vein (*S. mansoni*), superior mesenteric vein (*S. japonicum* and *S. mekongi*), and in the vesical plexus (*S. haematobium*). Although the adult stages are rarely encountered in tissue sections, eggs may be found in large numbers in the tissues of the intestine, liver, and bladder. Eggs also may disseminate via the bloodstream to other sites including the brain, spinal cord, lungs, heart, kidneys, and spleen. The eggs of *S. japonicum* are especially prone to disseminate because of their smaller size and the large numbers typically produced. Identification of eggs is dependent on recognition of their typical sizes and morphologic characteristics in appropriate tissues.

MEDICALLY IMPORTANT ARTHROPODS

Arthropods comprise a large and diverse group of organisms, few of which have clinical or economic significance. Those which do, however, are important causes of morbidity and mortality in humans and their domestic animals, and are responsible for serious economic losses to agriculture. Although perhaps best known among clinicians for their abilities to transmit various infectious agents including viruses, bacteria (rickettsia, spirochetes, others), protozoa, and certain helminths, arthropods also cause serious disease by direct tissue invasion, envenomation, vesication, blood loss, and allergic reactions. Exaggerated fears of arthropods (entomophobia) and delusions of infestation (delusory parasitosis) are not uncommon neuroses that may be disabling to some individuals. Species directly or indirectly responsible for human disease include representatives of all the major arthropod classes (Table 53–9).

In this section, an approach that the clinical laboratory may use when evaluating clinical specimens containing arthropods is presented, followed by a brief discussion of each of the arthropod groups of medical importance. A variety of general and specialized texts and guides are available for more complete coverage of the field of medical entomology (Beaver, 1984; Borrer, 1989; Goddard, 1993; Harwood, 1979; Lane, 1993; National Communicable Disease Center, 1969; Strickland, 1991).

Biological Characteristics

Arthropods are characterized by a bilaterally symmetric, segmented body; several pairs of jointed appendages; and a rigid chitinous exoskeleton that is molted repeatedly during growth. Development proceeds from egg to adult through either gradual (egg, nymph, and adult stages) or complete (egg, larva, pupa, and adult stages) metamorphosis. Bedbugs, kissing bugs, lice, and cockroaches are examples of insects that undergo gradual metamorphosis. Flies and mosquitoes; fleas; ants, bees, and wasps; and beetles undergo complete metamorphosis; wormlike larval forms pupate to emerge as adults. Arachnids undergo developmental changes most similar to the process of gradual metamorphosis. The larval stages of those arthropods that undergo complete metamorphosis often prove to be the most difficult for clinical laboratorians to identify and should be referred to a specialist.

Table 53–9. CLASSIFICATION OF ARTHROPODS OF MEDICAL IMPORTANCE

Class Insecta (insects)
Order Hemiptera (bedbugs, kissing bugs)
Order Siphonaptera (fleas)
Order Anopleura (sucking lice)
Order Dictyoptera (cockroaches)
Order Hymenoptera (ants, wasps, bees)
Order Coleoptera (beetles)
Order Diptera (flies, mosquitoes, midges)
Order Lepidoptera (moths, butterflies, caterpillars)
Class Arachnida (arachnids)
Subclass Scorpiones (scorpions)
Subclass Araneae (spiders)
Subclass Acari (ticks, mites, chiggers)
Class Diplopoda (millipedes)
Class Chilopoda (centipedes)
Class Crustacea (crustaceans)
Order Copepoda (copepods)
Order Decapoda (crabs, crayfish)
Class Pentastomida (tongue worms)

Mechanisms of Injury

DIRECT TISSUE INVASION. Invasion of superficial tissues (referred to as infestation) may occur with a variety of arthropods, of which scabies mites, chigoe fleas, and some dipteran larvae (maggots) are most common. Invasion of deeper body tissues and cavities (referred to as infection) occurs primarily with maggots and, rarely, pentastomid larvae. Tissue invasion by dipteran larvae is referred to as myiasis and may occur in either living or devitalized tissues, depending on the involved species.

ENVENOMATION. Many arthropods are capable of injecting either saliva or venom with their bites or stings. For most individuals, these compounds cause only local tissue reactions, but serious, life-threatening reactions such as anaphylaxis may occur, often as a result of previous sensitization to the particular toxin. Hymenopteran (ants, bees, and wasps) and scorpion stings are among the greatest offenders (Reisman, 1994). The bites of certain arthropods, especially the centipedes; mosquitoes, flies, and biting midges; bedbugs, kissing bugs, and assassin bugs; sucking lice; fleas; and ticks and mites may also be toxic, causing either local or systemic reactions. Almost all spiders are venomous, but only a few groups (widow spiders, violin spiders, and certain tarantulas) pose significant health risks to humans. Less common but recognized causes of envenomation result from exposure to the urticating hairs of certain caterpillars and beetle larvae.

VESICATION. Certain of the larger tropical millipedes are capable of spraying a vesicating (blister-causing) chemical substance from glands located on each body segment. These compounds are especially irritating should they reach the conjunctiva. Blister beetles are so named from their ability to discharge vesicating fluids (cantharidin, the active ingredient in the aphrodisiac Spanish fly) from their body when handled.

BLOOD LOSS. Arthropods responsible for producing significant irritation or blood loss to humans and domestic animals include bedbugs, kissing bugs, lice, fleas, flies, mosquitoes, biting midges, ticks, and mites. Although these activities are rarely life-threatening, the concurrent transmission of infectious agents may be.

TRANSMISSION OF INFECTIOUS AGENTS. Many arthropods play an integral role in either the mechanical or biological transmission of infectious disease agents. The common housefly, *Musca domestica*, may be responsible for the mechanical transmission of the agents of bacillary dysentery, cholera, typhoid, viral diarrhea, amebic dysentery, giardiasis, pinworms, and tapeworms. Mechanisms involved in the biological transmission of infectious agents vary from simple organism amplification in the arthropod vector to more complex life-cycle changes of the involved parasite. Ticks and mites are involved in the transmission of certain bacteria (*Rickettsia*, *Ehrlichia*, spirochetes, others), protozoa (*Babesia*), and viruses. Among the insects, lice are involved in the transmission of bacteria (*Rickettsia*, *Bartonella*, and *Borrelia*); kissing bugs transmit trypanosomes; fleas transmit the agents of plague, typhus, and canine tapeworm; and dipterans transmit arboviruses, malarial parasites, trypanosomes, leishmanias, filarial worms, and bacteria.

HYPERSENSITIVITY REACTIONS. Most of the serious reactions to arthropod bites and stings result from allergic hypersensitivities. Hymenopteran stings alone are responsible for most arthropod-related deaths and usually result from the development of hypersensitivity following repeated exposure to venom (Reisman, 1994). Allergies may also be exacerbated following exposure to the saliva, excrement, or body parts of mites, ticks, lice, bedbugs, caterpillars, moths, and butterflies. Asthma and hay fever may also develop in response to the presence of the large variety of house, dust, and animal mites in the environment (Frazier, 1980).

PSYCHOLOGICAL MANIFESTATIONS. Entomophobia refers to an unreasonable or excessive fear of seeing or touching arthropods. Although this fear may occasionally result in the disruption of a person's normal activities, it rarely becomes incapacitating. Delusory parasitosis is a more serious emotional disorder in which an individual is convinced he or she is infected with parasites or arthropods despite objective evidence to the contrary. As the delusion progresses, the individual may report loss of employment, divorce, repeated use of pesticide services, and movement from house to house. Visits to health care providers are usually numerous, although unsatisfactory. The problem may originate either in the home or workplace and be transferable from one to the other. The delusion may be so convincing that other family members or friends may believe it or acquire it themselves. The patient may submit numerous specimens such as skin, fabric, lint, hair, and mucus to the laboratory. It is incumbent on the laboratory personnel to examine these materials to rule out true infestation. The mysterious onset of irritation and itching may be due to bites from unrecognized scabies mites, lice, fleas, or bedbugs, or from insects and mites questing from an abandoned rodent or bird nest in an area of human habitation. Before dismissing such causes, they must be looked for and their presence excluded (Lynch, 1993).

Laboratory Approaches to Arthropod Identification

Arthropod specimens are often directed to the clinical laboratory by both clinicians and patients with the expectation that they can be accurately identified, but few laboratory personnel receive more than cursory exposure to entomology during training. Nonetheless, laboratorians should have access to texts and dichotomous keys, which should allow limited identification of the more commonly encountered medically important groups, especially ectoparasites (fleas, lice, mites, and ticks). Of more importance is the ability of the laboratory personnel to recognize those rare situations in which outside expertise should be sought. This specifically relates to those occasions when *significant clinical decisions regarding therapy and prognosis are being made*. State or local public health laboratories often have the expertise available or know of individuals trained in medical entomology at regional educational institutions, museums, or other public or private agencies, including the Centers for Disease Control and Prevention.

Specimens submitted to the laboratory most often are intact organisms, skin scrapings, tissues, sputum, urine, or stool. Inanimate objects including foodstuffs, water, clothing, bedding, and carpeting, among others, may also be submitted. It is not uncommon for patients to submit arthropods recovered from the toilet bowl following urination or a bowel movement. In most cases, the presence of such organisms is coincidental and not related to infection.

Proper killing and preservation of arthropods is important to preserve those characteristics necessary for identification. Small, nonwinged arthropods, especially ectoparasites (lice, fleas, ticks and mites), larval forms (maggots, grubs, and caterpillars), spiders, and scorpions should be placed directly into 70% to 80% ethyl alcohol. Large larval forms are best killed in hot (not boiling) water to extend their bodies and prevent contraction before immersion in alcohol. Attached tissue or other debris should be gently removed or washed away prior to preservation. The smaller forms (mites, small ticks, fleas, and sandflies) may be prepared as permanent slide mounts.

Winged insects, especially adult mosquitoes, midges, and flies, should be killed by exposure to the fumes of ethyl acetate or chloroform and preserved dry to retain the taxonomic information contained in the body and wing scales. Such arthropods usually are pinned and dried, followed by storage in tight-fitting boxes protected with naphthalene or dichlorobenzene. Further details regarding the collection, preservation, and preparation of arthropod specimens for examination are found elsewhere (Beaver, 1984; Borrer, 1989; Garcia, 1993; Lane, 1993; Steyskal, 1987).

Insects

Insects comprise more than 90% of all described arthropod species, although few are responsible for human disease. Members of this class are distinguished from other arthropods by having a body divided into three parts (head, thorax, abdomen); one pair of antennae; three pairs of legs; and one, two, or no pairs of wings. This is the only arthropod class in which flight has developed.

SUCKING LICE. Sucking lice are dorsoventrally flattened, wingless insects that have characteristic claws on the ends of each leg which allow attachment to body hairs or clothing (Fig. 53–36). All species suck blood intermittently and may cause unexplained dermatitis. Eggs, known as nits, are deposited on either hair shafts or clothing, depending on the species. Although named for their primary site of attachment, they do not always remain confined to that location. The head louse, *Pediculus capitis*, and the body louse, *P. humanus*, are indistinguishable to the nonspecialist. They are longer than they are wide, and grow to about 3 mm in length. Biological differences are apparent; only *P. humanus* transmits the agents of epidemic typhus, trench fever, and relapsing fever (Kim, 1986). Infestations with both species

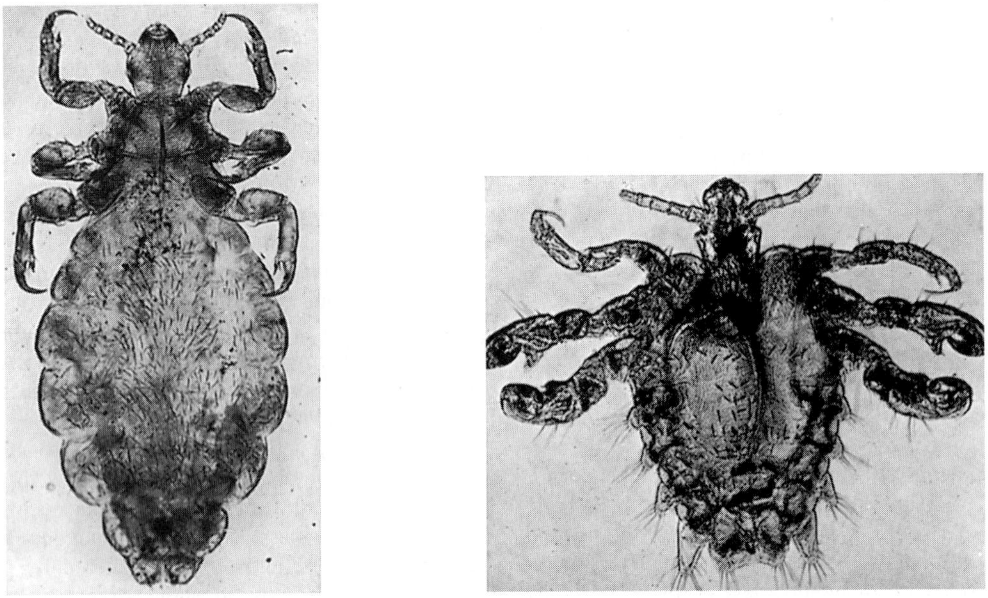

Figure 53–36. *Pediculus humanus* (*left*) and *Phthirus pubis* (*right*).

occur among people living in crowded conditions who have little opportunity for bathing and laundering. Children of school age are at particular risk for acquiring head lice through the sharing of caps, clothing, and combs (Orkin, 1985). Nits of head lice are deposited primarily on hair shafts, and those of body lice are deposited on clothing. Because objects such as hair casts, dander, hair spray, and fungal hair infections may mimic nits, differentiation is important. Nits are typically 1 mm long and, when unhatched, have intact opercula (Fig. 53–37). Transmission occurs primarily through the sharing of infested clothing and bedding, because body lice tend to lay their eggs in clusters, especially along seams or waistbands. The pubic louse, *Phthirus pubis*, is distinctly different from the others; it is rounder (measuring up to 2 mm in diameter), the abdomen is more crablike, and their first pair of legs is significantly smaller and more slender than the other pairs (see Fig. 53–36). Pubic lice and their nits are found primarily on pubic hairs but may extend to the chest, armpit, and facial hair. Transmission occurs primarily during sexual intercourse.

FLEAS. Fleas are small (1 to 2 mm), laterally compressed, wingless ectoparasites capable of sucking blood (Fig. 53–38). Long, muscular legs are adapted for jumping great distances. All fleas that attack humans are parasites of other mammals or poultry and include both blood-sucking

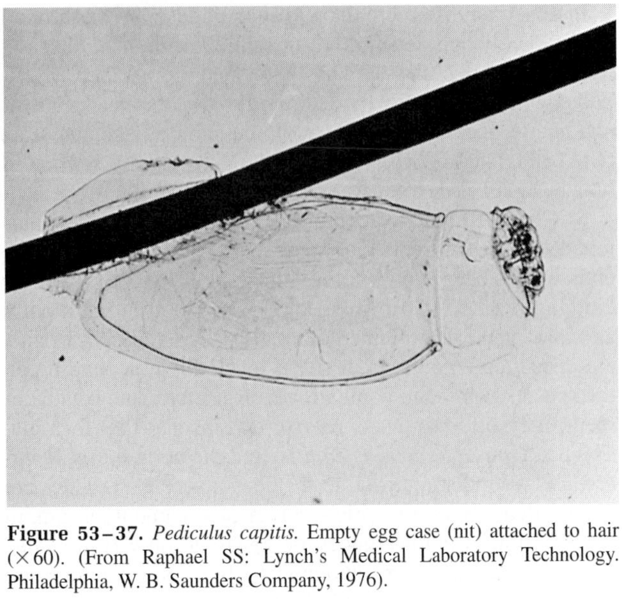

Figure 53–37. *Pediculus capitis.* Empty egg case (nit) attached to hair (×60). (From Raphael SS: Lynch's Medical Laboratory Technology. Philadelphia, W. B. Saunders Company, 1976).

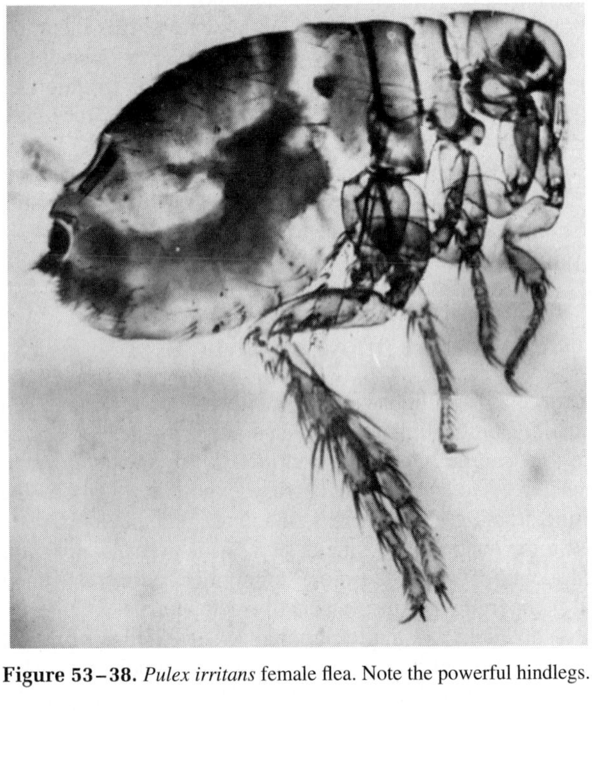

Figure 53–38. *Pulex irritans* female flea. Note the powerful hindlegs.

pests (many species) and tissue penetrating jiggers. Infestations commonly occur with exposure to domestic animals and pets; the most pestiferous species are the dog flea (*Ctenocephalides canis*), the cat flea (*C. felis*), and the human flea (*Pulex irritans*). Some individuals become highly sensitized to flea bites, whereas others are unaffected. Cat and dog fleas also are the usual intermediate hosts for the tapeworm *D. caninum* and less frequently for *H. diminuta* and *H. nana*. Because larvae of these species often develop in an animal's bedding, or in carpets and furniture, eradication may require fumigation and cleaning of those articles. The Oriental rat flea, *Xenopsylla cheopis*, is an extremely important species because it transmits the plague bacillus and the agent of murine typhus. Although normally parasitizing several species of rats, this flea readily attacks humans should the rodent host die. The jigger or chigoe flea *Tunga penetrans* is found in both Central and South America and regions of tropical Africa. The female flea attaches to and imbeds itself in the skin, especially between the toes and under the toenails, where it grows to the size of a small pea. After eggs are discharged, the flea dies, prompting an inflammatory response and possible secondary bacterial infection. Tungiasis is diagnosed by identifying the dark portion of the flea's abdomen (displaying the spiracles) protruding from the skin surface of an enlarging lesion (Beaver, 1984; Goddard, 1993; Lane, 1993).

COCKROACHES. Cockroaches have closely adapted themselves to human habitation, sharing in our food, shelter, and warmth. Although they are primarily nuisance pests, cockroaches are potential carriers of fecal pathogens owing to their ability to move quickly from sewers and drains to food preparation areas. In addition to transmitting pathogenic bacteria, they may also spread hepatitis and polioviruses; intestinal protozoa, including *E. histolytica*; and several species of enteric nematodes. Allergies and asthma may develop in some individuals following exposure to the excreta, cast skins, or body parts of cockroaches (Goddard, 1993).

BEDBUGS AND KISSING BUGS. Bedbugs (family Cimicidae) and kissing bugs (family Reduviidae) are blood-sucking insects that have a long, narrow proboscis that is folded underneath the body when not in use. Bedbugs (*Cimex lectularius* and *C. hemipterus*) are reddish brown, dorsoventrally flattened wingless insects approximately 5 mm in length (Fig. 53–39). They are cosmopolitan in distribution and attack most any mammal, feeding primarily at night. During daylight hours, they hide under mattresses, loose wallpaper, and floorboards. Although they are not known to transmit disease, bedbug bites may cause painful wheals or bullae, depending on an individual's sensitivity to their saliva.

Kissing bugs (*Triatoma, Rhodnius, Panstrongylus*) have a cone-shaped head on a narrow neck and an abdomen that is widened in the middle. These insects are black or brown and some have orange and black markings on the abdomen. They average 1 to 3 cm in length and, unlike bedbugs, have well-developed wings for flight. Like bedbugs, kissing bugs are relatively painless feeders on vertebrates and produce similar skin reactions. In Mexico and Central and South America, they transmit the agent of Chagas' disease, *T. cruzi*, in the feces, which are secondarily inoculated into the skin by the human host while scratching (Goddard, 1993; Lane, 1993).

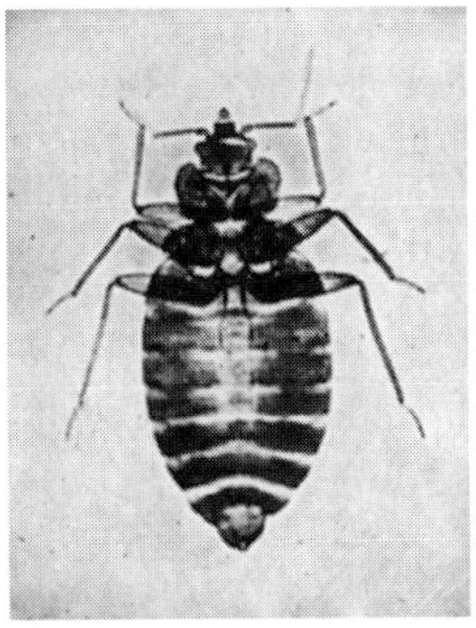

Figure 53–39. The common bedbug, *Cimex lectularius*, male (×5). In the female, the posterior end of the abdomen is more rounded. (Cleared with sodium hydroxide to bring out the structure more clearly.)

BEES, WASPS, AND ANTS. Hymenopterans are social insects that readily defend their nests when disturbed. In nonreproductive females, the ovipositor is modified as a stinger capable of injecting venom for use in the capture of prey or for defense. The venom of bees, wasps, hornets, and yellow jackets causes only transient swelling and discomfort in most individuals but may be responsible for systemic reactions, including anaphylaxis, in others who were previously sensitized (Reisman, 1994). Up to 100 people in the United States die each year from hymenopteran stings. The Africanized honey bee is now present in North America following its introduction into Brazil in 1956. These bees, which are more easily provoked than other honey bees, exhibit massive stinging behavior. Many species of ants are problematic for humans because of their ability to bite, and some groups, such as harvester and fire ants, are capable of giving painful stings.

BEETLES. Although beetles are perhaps best known as pests of agricultural crops, some species may give a painful bite, and others, especially the blister beetles, may exude vesicating fluids (cantharidin) that cause dermatitis or blister formation. The larvae of certain larder beetles have urticating hairs that may be responsible for dermatitis or, if ingested, irritation of the gastrointestinal tract. Larval and adult larder and grain beetles also may serve as intermediate hosts for the rodent and human tapeworms *H. diminuta* and *H. nana*.

MOTHS AND BUTTERFLIES. Certain larvae (caterpillars) of lepidoptera possess urticating hairs or spines capable of injecting venom when handled. Although most effects of these toxins remain localized to the skin, systemic effects including shock and paralysis have been reported (Goddard, 1993). Adult tussock and Gypsy moths are known to have urticating scales and hairs that may cause dermatitis, eye irritation, or respiratory tract irritation, especially among forestry workers (Shama, 1982).

FLIES, MOSQUITOES, AND MIDGES. Diptera are characterized by the presence of a single pair of membranous wings. Among all arthropods, they are responsible for the greatest share of human disease through blood-sucking activities, biological or mechanical transmission of infectious agents, and direct tissue invasion by larval forms (myiasis). Bites from a variety of flies, mosquitoes and biting midges often cause local irritation from sensitivity to the saliva and, in some individuals, systemic reactions. In addition to blood-sucking activities, the repeated attacks themselves may be physically and psychologically damaging. Certain blood-sucking species are also responsible for the transmission of important human pathogens, including the agents of malaria, filariasis, and arboviral disease by mosquitoes; onchocerciasis by blackflies; loiasis by deer flies; leishmaniasis and bartonellosis by sandflies; and African trypanosomiasis by tsetse flies. Other viral, bacterial, and parasitic agents are readily transmitted mechanically by nonbiting flies such as house flies, flesh flies, and blow flies that can easily contaminate human food.

Myiasis may occur in an accidental, facultative, or obligatory fashion. The housefly, *Musca domestica*, has no requirement for developing in mammalian tissue, yet may be found occasionally in dead tissue or under plaster casts. This type of accidental myiasis is not uncommon, but is rarely clinically significant. Facultative myiasis is most often caused by blowflies and flesh flies, which ordinarily feed on dead tissues but may move into adjacent viable tissues. Obligatory myiasis is caused by certain species that develop only in living tissues. Those species that infect humans are all of zoonotic origin. The human botfly, *Dermatobia hominis*, develops in boil-like subcutaneous lesions, with the posterior end of the maggot appearing at the skin surface (Fig. 53–40). This species is most commonly found in individuals who have spent time in Central or South America or, less frequently, Africa, and is unusual in that its eggs are mechanically transported to the host by other flying insects, usually mosquitoes. The tumbu fly (*Cordylobia anthropophaga*), found in sub-Saharan Africa, also causes a furuncular type of myiasis. Eggs of this species usually are laid on the ground or on hanging laundry, and larvae rapidly penetrate the skin on contact. The most serious obligatory myiasis is caused by the Old World screw-worm, *Chrysomya bezziana*, and the New World screw-worm, *Cochliomyia hominivorax*. These species lay their eggs directly on their cattle hosts, usually on wounds or near the nostrils. The larvae actively feed and move through living tissues. Human infections may be particularly destructive if the larvae invade the eye, nose, or mouth. Other species may also be responsible for traumatic, obligatory myiasis in humans (Lane, 1993).

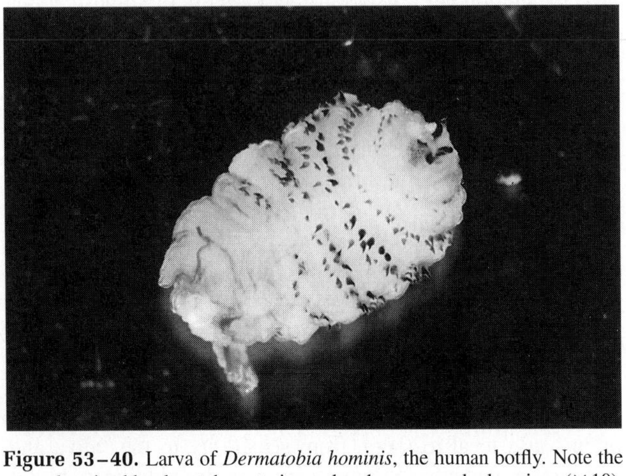

Figure 53–40. Larva of *Dermatobia hominis*, the human botfly. Note the two sclerotized hooks at the anterior end and numerous body spines (× 10).

Arachnids

Medically important arachnids include the scorpions, spiders, ticks, and mites. Scorpions and spiders have two body segments, the cephalothorax and the abdomen, whereas the ticks and mites have only one. Members of the group have four pair of legs as nymphs and adults; larval ticks and mites have three pair of legs. All lack antennae, mandibles, and wings. Scorpions and spiders are best known for their abilities to inject poisonous venoms, whereas ticks and mites are best known as vectors for viral, bacterial, and protozoal pathogens.

SCORPIONS. Unlike other arachnids, scorpions have a pair of forward-directed pincer claws that impart a crablike appearance and a segmented tail with a bulbous stinging apparatus in the tip. They are predatory in nature and paralyze their intended victim with venom from the sting, which may also be used for defensive purposes. Toxicity to humans varies depending on the species; many elicit no more reaction than that of a bee sting, but some are deadly, causing over 1000 deaths annually. Poisonous species occur in the western hemisphere, Europe, Africa, and the Middle East (Beaver, 1984; Goddard, 1993).

SPIDERS. Spiders lack a tail with an attached stinger but instead have fanglike chelicerae among their mouthparts, through which venom can be expressed. Although the majority of spiders are venomous, few have chelicerae capable of penetrating human skin. Most spider bites cause only transitory irritation and pain. The widow spiders (genus *Lactrodectus*) are one group responsible for systemic arachnidism through the action of a potent neurotoxin capable of producing weakness, myalgia, paralysis, convulsions, and occasionally, death. Published mortality rates vary from less than 1% to 6%. Five closely related species occur in the United States; the black widow (*Lactrodectus mactans*) is the most widespread. Female black widow spiders are glossy black with a characteristic red or orange hourglass-shaped marking on the underside of the abdomen and have a leg span of 3 to 4 cm. They live in protected locations such as woodsheds, basements, and outdoor privies (Strickland, 1991).

Violin spiders (genus *Loxosceles*) are responsible for necrotic arachnidism or loxoscelism. In the United States the brown recluse or fiddleback spider (*Loxosceles reclusa*) is most often involved, although other species are present. This species is 1 to 2 cm long, tan to dark brown in color, and has a darkened violin-shaped marking oriented base forward on the dorsum of the cephalothorax. When present in homes they are reclusive in their habits, preferring undisturbed areas such as closets, basements, and under porches. Their bite is painless and often goes unrecognized until several hours later, when the area becomes red, swollen, and painful. The venom is dermonecrotic and hemolytic, producing cutaneous necrosis and sloughing of the involved skin over several days. The resulting lesion may be difficult to heal and subject to secondary infection. Systemic reactions such as hemolysis and acute renal failure are rare. Other spider genera have also been implicated in producing necrotic arachnidism (Fisher, 1994).

TICKS. Unlike spiders and scorpions, ticks have a fused cephalothorax and abdomen, and a characteristic toothed hypostome for feeding. Tick development progresses through four stages: egg, larva, nymph, and adult. Following hatching, a blood meal is required for progression to the subsequent stage. Humans usually acquire ticks in grassy or brushy areas in close proximity to the usual animal hosts. All species are obligate blood-sucking ectoparasites and are important vectors of viral, bacterial, and protozoal pathogens to humans and domestic animals. Their feeding activities also may produce local tissue damage and blood loss, especially to livestock and wildlife, or tick paralysis, a syndrome caused by a neurotoxin secreted by a tick's salivary glands that produces ascending flaccid paralysis and toxemia. Symptoms may closely mimic those of Guillain-Barré syndrome, poliomyelitis, or botulism. Removal of the attached tick usually results in resolution of symptoms within hours to days.

Species affecting humans include members of the family Ixodidae (hard ticks) and Argasidae (soft ticks). Hard ticks have anteriorly directed mouthparts and a sclerotized plate, or scutum, on the dorsum. The scutum covers the entire dorsum of the male but only the anterior portion in the female, allowing the body to swell when engorged (Fig. 53–41). Argasid ticks have a soft leathery body lacking a scutum and ventrally directed mouthparts that are not visible when viewed from above (Fig. 53–42). Unengorged ticks generally are 2 to 5 mm long but may enlarge to several times that size following engorgement. Engorged hard ticks may mimic soft ticks, so care must be exercised in their identification (Sonenshine, 1991, 1993).

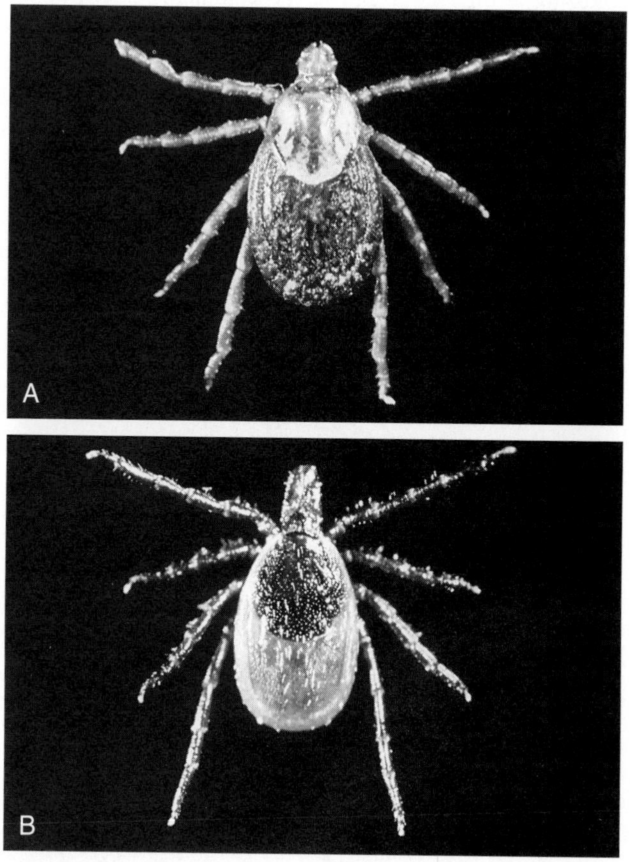

Figure 53–41. *A*, *Dermacentor variabilis* (dog tick), nonengorged adult female (× 10); *B*, *Ixodes dammini* (black legged or deer tick, also known as *I. scapularis*), nonengorged female (× 15). (Photographs are from Northwest Infectious Disease Consultants and are reproduced with permission.)

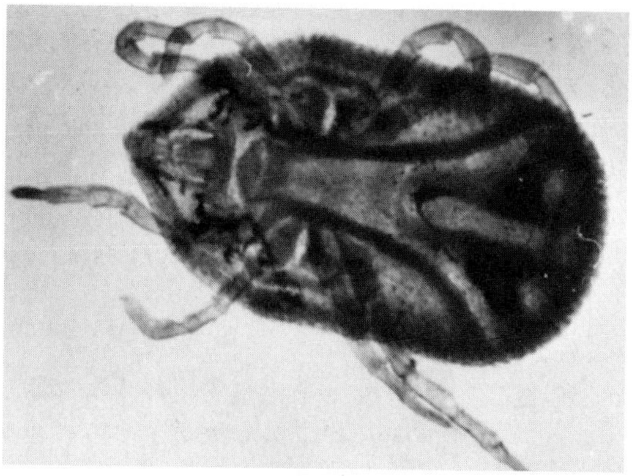

Figure 53–42. *Ornithodoros kellyi*, a soft tick, photographed with transmitted light.

Most ticks found crawling on or imbedded in human skin are hard ticks. Soft ticks tend to feed only briefly and then often at night. Important species of hard ticks in North America include *Dermacentor variabilis* (American dog tick), *D. andersoni* (Rocky Mountain wood tick), *Amblyomma americanum* (Lone Star tick), *Rhipicephalus sanguineus* (brown dog tick), *Ixodes dammini* (northern black-legged tick), *Ixodes scapularis* (southern black-legged tick), and *I. pacificus* (western black-legged tick). Some authorities consider *I. dammini* to be synonomous with *I. scapularis* (Oliver, 1993). *Dermacentor* and *Amblyomma* ticks are called ornate ticks because of the presence of white markings on their scuta; the other species are inornate ticks.

Dermacentor ticks transmit Rocky Mountain spotted fever and possibly tularemia, Q fever, and Colorado tick fever. *Ixodes* ticks are vectors of Lyme disease, babesiosis, and ehrlichiosis, and in other parts of the world, these ticks are responsible for the transmission of certain arboviruses. *Amblyomma* ticks are capable of transmitting Rocky Mountain spotted fever, as well as tularemia and possibly Lyme disease. All of these genera are capable of causing tick paralysis. *Rhipicephalus* ticks have been implicated in the transmission of Rocky Mountain spotted fever and ehrlichiosis in North America, and of boutonneuse fever in the Mediterranean area. Soft ticks of the genus *Ornithodoros* occur in many parts of the world, including the United States, and are important vectors of the relapsing fever spirochetes (*Borrelia recurrentis* and related forms) (Spach, 1993).

MITES. Mites are microscopic-sized (usually less than 1 mm) arachnids that are widely distributed in the environment. Medically important species may attack humans directly, serve as vectors for infectious diseases, or cause dust allergies. Humans are commonly infested with both *Demodex folliculorum* and *D. brevis*, the follicle mites, and *Sarcoptes scabei*, the itch or mange mite. Follicle mites are minute (0.1 to 0.4 mm), elongate parasites with stubby legs that can be recovered from hair follicles and sebaceous glands (Fig. 53–43). They are common incidental findings on histologic skin preparations. Although their presence has been associated with various skin conditions, they are commonly found in healthy individuals as well, which makes their significance hard to assess (Burns, 1992).

Sarcoptes scabei mites are of greater medical importance

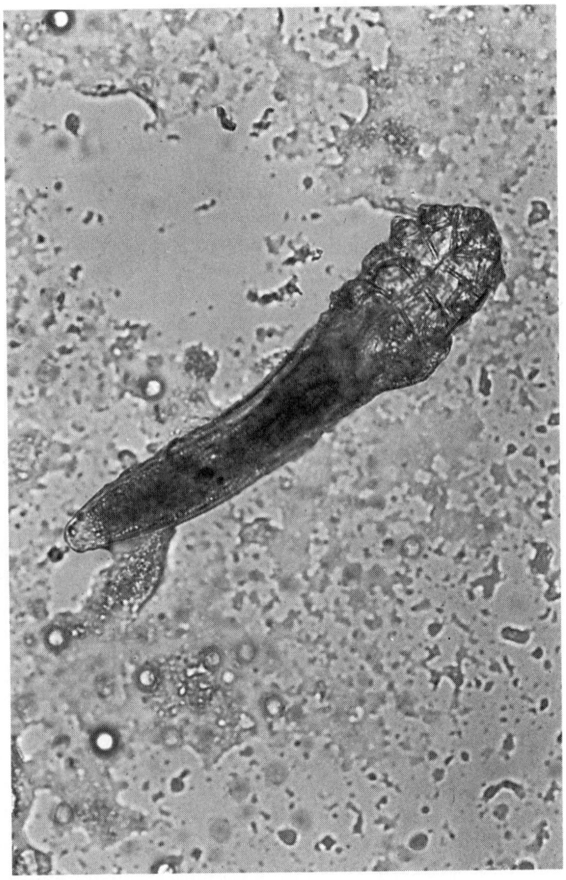

Figure 53–43. *Demodex folliculorum*, the human follicle mite (×400).

because of their ability to create serpiginous tunnels through the upper layers of the epidermis. Transmitted through personal contact, these mites are found primarily in the interdigital spaces and the flexor surfaces of the wrists and forearms and less commonly in other areas including the breasts, buttocks, and external genitalia. Inflammation and intense itching results from the tunneling activity and from the deposition of eggs and excreta. Clinical manifestations vary depending on the degree of sensitization to the parasites and their products. Lesions often become secondarily infected. A generalized dermatitis occurring in the presence of thousands of mites, typically in elderly or immunocompromised individuals, is known as crusted or Norwegian scabies.

The diagnosis is made by placing skin scrapings collected from tunneled areas in 20% potassium hydroxide or mineral oil for clearing and examining under the microscope. Detection of eggs, six-legged larvae, and eight-legged nymphs or adults is diagnostic but may be difficult to demonstrate (Figs. 53–44 and 53–45). The diagnosis of scabies in an institutional or school setting may result in pseudoepidemics, in which numerous individuals develop itching without evidence of disease. Care must be exercised to diagnose properly the disease to identify real cases and differentiate them from cases of delusory parasitosis (Lynch, 1993; Orkin, 1985).

A number of animal mite species may attack humans for a blood meal, either as larval forms or as adults, when the normal mammalian or bird hosts are not available. Larval chigger mites (family Trombiculidae) are problematic in many parts of the world because their saliva can produce large wheal-and-flare reactions with intense itching. Often red in color, these tiny six-legged larvae commonly attach to the skin in areas where clothing is restrictive, such as at the ankles, waistline, armpits, and wrists. In parts of Asia and

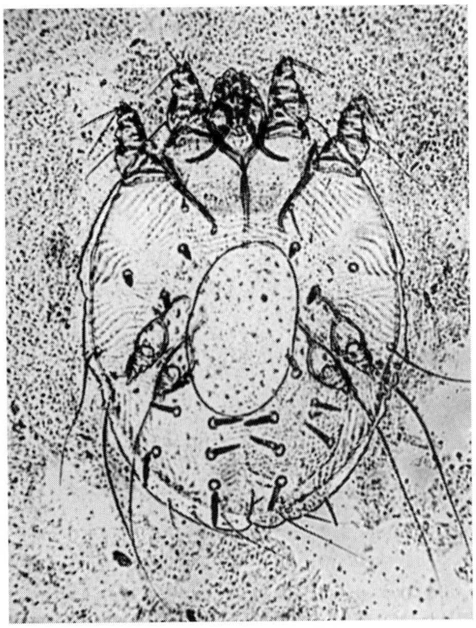

Figure 53–44. *Sarcoptes scabiei*, adult female. (From Markell EK, Voge M, John DT: Medical Parasitology, 6th ed. Philadelphia, W. B. Saunders Company, 1986.)

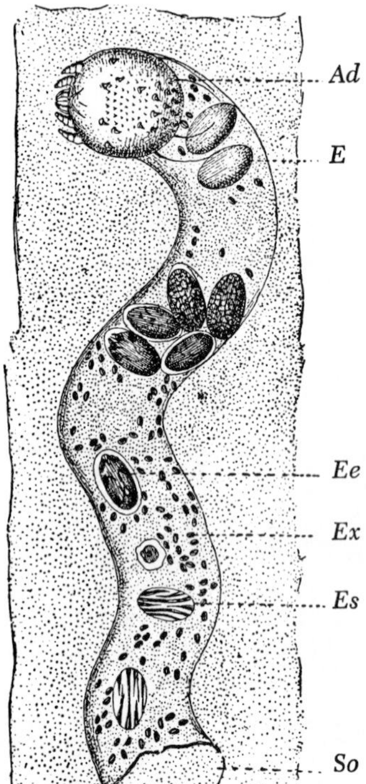

Figure 53–45. *Sarcoptes scabiei.* Diagram of a subcutaneous burrow; *Ad,* adult female; *E,* eggs; *Ee,* embryo egg; *Ex,* excrement; *Es,* egg shell; *So,* skin orifice. (After Railliet in Brumpt.)

Australia, trombiculid mites are vectors for the transmission of the agent of scrub typhus (Lane, 1993).

Certain nonbiting mites play a role in allergic rhinitis, asthma, and some skin conditions. The secretions, excreta, and body parts of *Dermatophagoides farinae* and *D. pteronyssinus* are potent allergens that may occur in great numbers in the household environment (Frazier, 1980). Routine testing by an allergist may identify the offending agent.

Classes of Lesser Medical Importance

MILLIPEDES. Millipedes are wormlike arthropods with numerous apparent body segments, each with two pair of legs, that are commonly found in and under decaying vegetation. Although they lack mouthparts capable of producing serious bites, many species produce vesicating secretions from glands located on each body segment. When handled roughly, the larger tropical species are capable of squirting these fluids over a distance of several centimeters. Exposure of the skin or mucous membranes to these fluids may produce a burning sensation and blister formation.

CENTIPEDES. Centipedes are flatter than millipedes, have only one pair of legs per body segment, and display long antennae. They are fast moving and can inflict a painful sting from a pair of forward-directed pincers that are modified from the first pair of legs. Although they are rarely responsible for serious injury to humans, the larger species (26 to 45 cm) found in the southern United States and in tropical regions are able to penetrate human skin when handled, giving a painful, burning sting with local tissue reaction. Although systemic reactions may occur in individuals who have been previously sensitized, fatalities are rare (Goddard, 1993).

CRUSTACEANS. Crustaceans of medical importance are primarily those species that serve as hosts for larval stages of several different helminths. Several genera of crabs and crayfish are intermediate hosts for the metacercariae of various species of lung fluke (*Paragonimus* spp.) found around the world. Copepods are common microscopic zooplankton, certain species of which serve as first intermediate hosts for the nematodes *D. medinensis* and *Gnathostoma spinigerum* and for cestodes of the genera *Diphyllobothrium* and *Spirometra.*

PENTASTOMIDS. Pentastomes, or tongue worms, are arthropods of uncertain affinities owing to a lack of morphologic characteristics. Adult stages are wormlike organisms that live in the nasal passages of certain predatory reptiles, birds, and mammals. Larval stages resemble mites and reside in rodents, herbivores, and freshwater fish. Human liver and lung infections with larval stages have been reported from Asia and Africa. Adult stages have been recovered from the nasopharynx of individuals from the Middle East and Africa, where they are responsible for an obstructive condition known as halzoun (Beaver, 1984).

General References

Ash LR, Orihel TC: Parasites: A Guide to Laboratory Procedures and Identification. Chicago, ASCP Press, 1987.

Ash LR, Orihel TC: Atlas of Human Parasitology, 3rd ed. Chicago, ASCP Press, 1990.

Balows A, Hausler WJ Jr, Ohashi M, Turano A: Laboratory Diagnosis of Infectious Diseases. Principles and Practice. Vol. 1. Bacterial, Mycotic and Parasitic Diseases. New York, Springer-Verlag, 1988.

Beaver PC, Jung RC, Cupp EW: Clinical Parasitology, 9th ed. Philadelphia, Lea & Febiger, 1984.

Binford CH, Connor DH: Pathology of Tropical and Extraordinary Diseases. Washington DC, Armed Forces Institute of Pathology, 1976.

Borror DJ, Johnson NF, Triplehorn CA: An Introduction to the Study of Insects, 6th ed. Philadelphia, Saunders College Publishing Company, 1989.

Brooke MM, Melvin DM: Morphology of diagnostic stages of intestinal parasites of man (Publication No. [CDC] 84-8116). Washington DC, United States Department of Health and Human Services, 1984.

Federal Register: Rules and Regulations. Fed Regist 1991; 56(235):64175.

Garcia LS, Bruckner DA: Diagnostic Medical Parasitology, 2nd ed. Washington DC, American Society for Microbiology, 1993.

Goddard J: Physician's Guide to Arthropods of Medical Importance. Boca Raton, CRC Press, 1993.

Goldsmith R, Heyneman D (eds): Tropical Medicine and Parasitology. Norwalk, CT, Appleton and Lange, 1989.

Gutierrez Y: Diagnostic Pathology of Parasitic Infections with Clinical Correlations. Philadelphia, Lea & Febiger, 1990.

Harwood RF, James MT: Entomology in Human and Animal Health, 7th ed. New York, Macmillan, 1979.

Isenberg HE (ed): Clinical Microbiology Procedures Handbook, Vols. 1 and 2. Washington DC, American Society for Microbiology, 1992.

Lane RP, Crosskey RW: Medical Insects and Arthropods. London, Chapman & Hall, 1993.

Manson-Bahr PEC, Bell DR (eds): Manson's Tropical Diseases, 19th ed. Philadelphia, W.B. Saunders Company, 1987.

Marcial-Rojas RA: Pathology of Protozoal and Helminthic Diseases with Clinical Correlation. Baltimore, Williams & Wilkins Co, 1971.

Markell EK, Voge M: Medical Parasitology, 7th ed. Philadelphia, W.B. Saunders Company, 1992.

Melvin DM, Brooke MM: Laboratory Procedures for the Diagnosis of Intestinal Parasites, 3rd ed. (DHEW Publication [CDC] 82-8282). Atlanta, Laboratory Training and Consultation Division, Centers for Disease Control, 1982.

Murray PR, Baron EJ, Pfaller MA, et al: Manual of Clinical Microbiology, 6th ed. Washington DC, ASM Press, 1995.

National Communicable Disease Center: Pictorial Keys: Arthropods, Reptiles, Birds, and Mammals of Public Health Significance. Atlanta, Communicable Disease Center, 1969.

Orihel TC, Ash LR: Parasites in Human Tissues. Chicago, ASCP Press, 1995.

Orkin M, Maibach HI: Cutaneous Infestations and Insect Bites. New York, Marcel Dekker Inc, 1985.

Peters W, Gilles HM: A Colour Atlas of Tropical Medicine and Parasitology, 3rd ed. London, Wolfe Medical Publications Ltd, 1989.

Smith JW, Ash LR, Thompson JH, McQuay RM: Atlas of Diagnostic Medical Parsitology—Intestinal Helminths. Chicago, American Society of Clinical Pathologists, 1976a.

Smith JW, McQuay RM, Ash LR, et al: Atlas of Diagnostic Medical Parasitology—Intestinal Protozoa. Chicago, American Society of Clinical Pathologists, 1976b.

Smith JW, Melvin DM, Orihel TC, et al: Atlas of Diagnostic Medical Parasitology—Blood and Tissue Parasites. Chicago, American Society of Clinical Pathologists, 1976c.

Spencer FM, Monroe LS: The Color Atlas of Intestinal Parasites, 2nd ed. Springfield, IL, Charles C. Thomas, 1982.

Strickland GT (ed): Hunter's Tropical Medicine, 7th ed. Philadelphia, W.B. Saunders Company, 1991.

Sun TE: Pathology and Clinical Features of Parasitic Diseases. New York, Masson Publishing USA Inc, 1982.

Sun TE: Color Atlas and Textbook of Diagnostic Parasitology. New York, Igaku-Shoin, 1988.

Von Lichtenberg F: Pathology of Infectious Diseases. New York, Raven Press, 1991.

Walzer PD, Genta RM: Parasitic Infections in the Compromised Host. New York, Marcel Dekker, 1989.

Warren KS, Mahmoud AAF (eds): Tropical and Geographical Medicine, 2nd ed. New York, McGraw-Hill, 1990.

Woods GLY, Gutierrez DH, Walker DT, et al: Diagnostic Pathology of Infectious Diseases. Philadelphia, Lea & Febiger, 1993.

Specific References

Alicata JE: The discovery of *Angiostrongylus cantonensis* as a cause of human eosinophilic meningitis. Parasitol Today 1991; 7:151.

Anuran JD, Starr MB, Jakobiec FA: *Acanthamoeba* keratitis: A review of the literature. Cornea 1987; 6(1):2.

Arrowood MJ, Sterling CR: Comparison of conventional staining methods and monoclonal antibody-based methods for *Cryptosporidium* oocyst detection. J Clin Microbiol 1989; 27:1490.

Badawi AF, Mostafa MH, O'Connor PJ: Involvement of alkylating agents in

6

schistosome-associated bladder cancer: The possible basic mechanisms of induction. Cancer Lett 1992; 63:171.
Bartlett MS, Harper K, Smith N, et al: Comparative evaluation of a modified zinc sulfate flotation technique. J Clin Microbiol 1978; 7:524.
Beal C, Goldsmith M, Kotby M, et al: The plastic envelope method, a simplified technique for culture diagnosis of trichomoniasis. J Clin Microbiol 1992; 30:2265.
Beaver PC: Light long-lasting *Necator* infection in a volunteer. Am J Trop Med Hyg 1988; 39:369.
Beaver PC, Gadgil RK, Morera P: *Sarcocystis* in man: A review and report of five cases. Am J Trop Med Hyg 1979; 28:819.
Bendall RP, Chiodini PL: New diagnostic methods for parasitic infections. Curr Opin Infect Dis 1993; 6:318.
Benenson MW, Takafuji ET, Lemon SM, et al: Oocyst-transmitted toxoplasmosis associated with ingestion of contaminated water. N Engl J Med 1982; 307:666.
Boros DL: Immunopathology of *Schistosoma mansoni* infection. Clin Microbiol Rev 1989; 2:250.
Briselden AM, Hillier SL: Evaluation of Affirm VP Microbial Identification Test for *Gardnerella vaginalis* and *Trichomonas vaginalis*. J Clin Microbiol 1994; 32:148.
Bronsdon MA: Rapid dimethyl sulfoxide–modified acid-fast stain of *Cryptosporidium* oocyst in stool specimens. J Clin Microbiol 1984; 19(6):952.
Bruce JI, Sornmani S: The Mekong Schistosome. Malacological Review, Suppl. #2. Whitmore Lake, MI, 1980.
Bruckner DA: Amebiasis. Clin Microbiol Rev 1992; 5:356.
Burns DA: Follicle mites and their role in disease. Clin Exp Dermatol 1992; 17:152.
Burrows RB, Swerdlow MA: *Enterobius vermicularis* as a probable vector of *Dientamoeba fragilis*. Am J Trop Med Hyg 1956; 5:258.
Cali A, Kotler DP, Orenstein JM: *Septata intestinalis* N.G. N.Sp., an intestinal microsporidian associated with chronic diarrhea and dissemination in AIDS patients. J Eukaryot Microbiol 1993; 40:101.
Cattand P, Miezan BT, de Raadt P: Human African trypanosomiasis: Use of double centrifugation of cerebrospinal fluid to detect trypanosomes. Bull WHO 1988; 66:83.
Cazenave J, Cheyrou A, Blouin P, et al: Use of polymerase chain reaction to detect *Toxoplasma*. J Clin Pathol 1991; 44:1037.
Centers for Disease Control: Malaria Surveillance. Annual Summary. 1987, Issued November 1988.
Centers for Disease Control: Pseudo-outbreak of intestinal amebiasis—California. MMWR 1985; 34(9):125.
Centers for Disease Control. Surveillance for dracunculiasis. MMWR 1992; 41:1.
Centers for Disease Control and Prevention. Summary of notifiable diseases, United States, 1993. MMWR 1993; 42(53):1.
Chan FT, Guan MX, MacKenzie AMR: Application of indirect immunofluorescence to detection of *Dientamoeba fragilis* trophozoites in fecal specimens. J Clin Microbiol 1993; 31:1710.
Cooper ES, Bundy DAP: *Trichuris* is not trivial. Parasitol Today 1988; 4:301.
Craun G: Waterborne giardiasis in the United States 1965–1984. Lancet 1986; ii:513–514.
Cross JH: Intestinal capillariasis. Clin Microbiol Rev 1992; 5:120.
Current WL, Garcia LS: Cryptosporidiosis. Clin Microbiol Rev 1991; 4:325.
Curry A, Caning E: Human microsporidiosis. J Infect 1993; 27:229.
Curtis MA, Bylund G: Diphyllobothriasis: Fish tapeworm disease in the circumpolar north. Arctic Med Res 1991; 50(1):18.
D'Alessandro A, Rausch RL, Cuello C, Aristizabal N: *Echinococcus vogeli* in man, with a review of polycystic hydatid disease in Columbia and neighboring countries. Am J Trop Med Hyg 1979; 28:303.
D'Alessandro A, Ramirez LE, Chapadeiro E, et al: Second recorded case of human infection by *Echinococcus oligarthrus*. Am J Trop Med Hyg 1995; 52(1):29.
Dao AH, Robinson DP, Wong SW: Frequency of *Entamoeba gingivalis* in human gingival scrapings. Am J Clin Path 1983; 80:380.
DeGirolami PC, Ezratty CR, Desai G, et al: Diagnosis of intestinal microsporidiosis by examination of stool and duodenal aspirate with Weber's modified trichrome and Uvitex 2B stains. J Clin Microbiol 1995; 33(4):805.
DeHovitz JA, Pape JW, Boncy J, et al: Isosporiasis in AIDS. N Engl J Med 1986; 315:87.
Diamond LS: Cultivation of *Entamoeba histolytica* in vitro. *In* Ravdin JI (ed): Amebiasis: Human Infection by *Entamoeba histolytica*. New York, John Wiley and Sons, 1988, p 27.
Diamond LS, Clark CG: A redescription of *Entamoeba histolytica* Schaudinn, 1903 (emended Walker, 1911) separating it from *Entamoeba dispar* Brumpt, 1925. J Eukaryot Microbiol 1993; 40:340.
Diaz JF, Verastegui M, Gilman RH, et al: Immunodiagnosis of human cysticercosis (*Taenia solium*): A field comparison of an antibody-enzyme-linked immunosorbent assay (ELISA), an antigen-ELISA, and an enzyme-linked immunoelectrotransfer blot (EITB) assay in Peru. Am J Trop Med Hyg 1992; 46(5):610.
Eastburn RL, Fritsche TR, Terhune CA Jr: Human intestinal infection with *Nanophyetus salmincola* from salmonid fishes. Am J Trop Med Hyg 1987; 36(3):586.
Eveland LK, Kenney M, Yermakov V: Laboratory diagnosis of autoinfection in strongyloidiasis. Am J Clin Path 1975; 63:421.
Fisher RG: Necrotic arachnidism. West J Med 1994; 160:570.
Frazier CA, Brown PA: Insects and Allergy and What to Do About Them. Norman, University of Oklahoma Press, 1980.
Fritsche TR: Pathogenic protozoa: An overview of in vitro cultivation and susceptibility to chemotherapeutic agents. Clin Lab Med 1989a; 9(2):287.
Fritsche TR, Eastburn RL, Wiggins LH, Terhune CA Jr: Praziquantel for treatment of human *Nanophyetus salmincola* (*Troglotrema salmincola*) infection. J Infect Dis 1989b; 160(5):896.
Garcia LS, Brewer TC, Bruckner DA: A comparison of the formalin-ether concentration and trichrome-stained smear methods for the recovery and identification of intestinal protozoa. Am J Med Technol 1979; 45:932.
Garcia LS, Bruckner DA, Brewer TC, Shimizu RY: Techniques for the recovery and identification of *Cryptosporidium* oocysts from stool specimens. J Clin Microbiol 1983; 18:185.
Garcia LS, Shimizu RY, Shum A, Bruckner DA: Evaluation of intestinal protozoan morphology in polyvinyl alcohol preservative: Comparison of zinc sulfate– and mercuric chloride–based compounds for use in Schaudinn's fixative. J Clin Microbiol 1993; 31:307.
Gay JD, Abell TL, Thompson JH Jr, Loth V: *Entamoeba polecki* infection in southeast Asian refugees: multiple cases of a rarely reported parasite. Mayo Clin Proc 1985; 60:523.
Genta RM: Dysregulation of strongyloidiasis: A new hypothesis. Clin Microbiol Rev 1992; 5(4):345.
Genta RM, Walzer PD: Strongyloidiasis. *In* Walzer PD, Genta RM (eds): Parasitic Infections in the Compromised Host. New York, Marcel Dekker, 1989, pp 463–525.
Gill GV, Bell DR: *Strongyloides stercoralis* infection in former Far East prisoners of war. BMJ 1979; 2:572.
Grover CM, Thulliez P, Remington JS, Boothroyd JC: Rapid prenatal diagnosis of congenital *Toxoplasma* infection by using polymerase chain reaction and amniotic fluid. J Clin Microbiol 1990; 28:2297.
Gustafson RL, Reed CM, McGreevy PB, et al: Human cutaneous leishmaniasis acquired in Texas. Am J Trop Med Hyg 1985; 34:58.
Healy GR, Rubush TK: Morphology of *Babesia microti* in human blood smears. Am J Clin Pathol 1980; 73:107.
Herwaldt BL, Springs FE, Roberts PP, et al: Babesiosis in Wisconsin: a potentially fatal disease. Am J Trop Med Hyg 1995; 53(2): 146.
Hoeffler DF: Cercarial dermatitis, its etiology, epidemiology, and clinical aspects. JAMA 1974; 29:225.
Istre GR, Kreiss K, Hopkins RS, et al: An outbreak of amebiasis spread by colonic irrigation at a chiropractic clinic. N Engl J Med 1982; 307:339.
Kappus KD, Lundgren RG, Juranek DD, et al: Intestinal parasitism in the United States: Update on a continuing problem. Am J Trop Med Hyg 1994; 50(6):705.
Kilvington S, White DG: *Acanthamoeba:* Biology, ecology and human disease. Rev Med Microbiol 1994; 5(1):12.
Kim KC, Pratt HD, Stojanovich CJ: The Sucking Lice of North America. University Park, Pennsylvania State University Press, 1986.
Krieger JN, Tam MR, Stevens CE, et al: Diagnosis of trichomoniasis: Comparison of conventional wet-mount examination with cytologic studies, cultures, and monoclonal antibody staining of direct specimens. JAMA 1988; 259:1223.
Krogstad DJ, Spencer HC, Healy GR, et al: Amebiasis: Epidemologic studies in the United States. Ann Intern Med 1978; 88:89.
Krotoski WA, Garnham PCC, Krotoski DM, et al: Observations on early and late post-sporozoite tissue stages in primate malaria. I. Discovery of a new latent form of *Plasmodium cynomolgi* (the hypnozoite), and failure to detect hepatic forms within the first 24 hours after infection. Am J Trop Med Hyg 1982; 31:24.
Kubersky T, Bert RD, Briley JM, Rosen L: Recovery of *Angiostrongylus cantonensis* from cerebrospinal fluid of a child with eosinophilic meningitis. J Clin Microbiol 1979; 9:629.
Lanar DE, McLaughlin GL, Wirth DF, et al: Comparison of thick films, in vitro culture and DNA hybridization probes for detecting *Plasmodium falciparum* malaria. Am J Trop Med Hyg 1989; 40:3.
Lawande RV, Abraham SN, John I, Egler LJ: Recovery of soil amebas from the nasal passages of children during the dusty harmattan period in Zaria. Am Soc Clin Pathol 1979; 71:201.
Layrisse M, Blumenfeld N, Carbonell L, et al: Intestinal absorption tests and biopsy of the jejunum in subjects with heavy hookworm infection. Am J Trop Med Hyg 1964a; 13:297.
Layrisse M, Roche M: The relationship between anemia and hookworm infection. Results of surveys of rural Venezuelan population. Am J Hyg 1964b; 79:279.
Levin RL, Armstrong DE: Human infection with *Entamoeba polecki*. Am J Clin Pathol 1970; 54:611.
Lisi PJ, Dondero RS, Kwiatkoski D, et al: Monoclonal-antibody based enzyme-linked immunosorbent assay for *Trichomonas vaginalis*. J Clin Microbiol 1988; 26:1684.
Loria-Cortez R, Lobo-Sanahuja JF: Clinical abdominal angiostrongylosis. A

study of 116 children with intestinal eosinophilic granuloma caused by *Angiostrongylus costaricensis*. Am J Trop Med Hyg 1980; 29:538.
Luft BJ: *Toxoplasma gondii*. *In* Walzer PD, Genta RM (eds): Parasitic Infections in the Compromised Host. New York, Marcel-Dekker, 1989, p 179.
Luft BJ, Remingon JS: Toxoplasmic encephalitis. J Infect Dis 1988; 157:1.
Luna VA, Stewart BK, Bergeron DL, et al: Use of the fluorochrome calcofluor white in the screening of stool specimens for spores of microsporidia. Am J Clin Pathol 1995; 103:656.
Lynch PJ: Delusions of parasitosis. Semin Dermatol 1993; 12(1):39.
Ma P, Soave R: Three-step stool examination for cryptosporidiosis in 10 homosexual men with protracted watery diarrhea. J Infect Dis 1983; 147:824.
Maayen S, Wormser GP, Widernorn J, et al: *Strongyloides stercoralis* hyperinfection in a patient with acquired immune deficiency syndrome. Am J Med 1987; 83:945.
MacKenzie WR, Hoxie NJ, Proctor ME, et al: A massive outbreak in Milwaukee of *Cryptosporidium* infection transmittted through public water supply. N Engl J Med 1994; 331(3):161.
Magill AJ, Grogl M, Gasser RA, et al: Visceral infection caused by *Leishmania tropica* in veterans of Operation Desert Storm. N Engl J Med 1993; 328:1384.
Mannheimer SB, Soave R: Protozoal infections in patients with AIDS. Cryptosporidiosis, isosporiasis, cyclosporiasis, and microsporidiosis. Infect Dis Clin North Am 1994; 8(2):483.
Marciano-Cabral F: Biology of *Naegleria* spp. Microbiol Rev 1988; 52:114.
Mariano EG, Borja SR, Vruno MJ: A human infection with *Paragonimus kellicotti* (lung fluke) in the United States. Am J Clin Pathol 1986; 86:685.
Marines HM, Osato MS, Font RL: The value of calcofluor white in the diagnosis of mycotic and *Acanthamoeba* infections of the eye and ocular adnexa. Ophthalmology 1987; 94(1):23.
Markell EK, Udkow MP: *Blastocystis hominis*: Pathogen or fellow traveler? Am J Trop Med Hyg 1986; 35(5):1023.
Martinez AJ: Free-living Amebas: Natural History, Prevention, Diagnosis, Pathology, and Treatment of Disease. Boca Raton, CRC Press Inc, 1985.
Medrano FJ, Hernandez-Quero J, Jimenez E, et al: Visceral leishmaniasis in HIV-infected individuals: A common opportunistic infection in Spain? AIDS 1992; 6:1499.
Miller LH, Manson SJ, Clyde DF, McGinniss MH: The resistance factor to *Plasmodium vivax* in blacks, the Duffy-blood-group genotype, FyFy. N Engl J Med 1976; 295:302.
Miller RA, Minshew BH: *Blastocystis hominis*: An organism in search of a disease. Rev Infect Dis 1988; 10:930.
Murphy GS, Basri H, Purnomo, et al: *Vivax malaria* resistant to treatment and prophylaxis with chloroquine. Lancet 1993; 341:96.
National Committee for Clinical Laboratory Standards: Slide preparation and staining of blood films for the laboratory diagnosis of parasitic diseases; tentative guideline. NCCLS Document M15-T. Villanova, Pennsylvania, NCCLS, 1992.
National Committee for Clinical Laboratory Standards: Procedures for the recovery and identification of parasites from the intestinal tract; proposed guideline. NCCLS Document M28-P. Villanova, Pennsylvania, NCCLS, 1993.
Nielson RL, Kohler RB, Chin W, et al: The use of exchange transfusions. A potentially useful adjunct in the treatment of fulminant falciparum malaria. Am J Med Sci 1979; 277:325.
Oliver JH Jr, Owlsly MR, Hutcheson HJ, et al: Conspecificity of the ticks *Ixodes scapularis* and *I. dammini* (Acari: Ixodidae). J Med Entomol 1993; 30:54.
Ortega YR, Gilman RH, Sterling CR: A new coccidian parasite (Apicomplexa: Eimeriidae) from humans. J Parasitol 1994; 80(4):625.
Ortega YR, Sterling CR, Gilman RH, et al: *Cyclospora* species—a new protozoan pathogen of humans. N Engl J Med 1993; 328(8):1308.
Pachucki CT, Levandowski RA, Brown VA, et al: American paragonimiasis treated with praziquantel. N Engl J Med 1984; 311(9):582.
Palmer J: Modified iron hematoxylin/Kinyoun stain (letter). Clin Microbiol Newsl 1991; 13:39.
Parmley SF, Goebel FD, Remington JS: Detection of *Toxoplasma gondii* in cerebrospinal fluid from AIDS patients by polymerase chain reaction. J Clin Microbiol 1992; 30:3000.
Pelletier LL Jr, Baker CB, Gam AA, et al: Diagnosis and evaluation of treatment of chronic strongyloidiasis in ex-prisoners of war. J Infect Dis 1988; 157:573.
Persing DH: PCR detection of *Babesia microti*. *In* Persing DH, Smith TF, Tenover FC, White TJ (eds): Diagnostic Molecular Microbiology: Principles and Applications. Washington DC, American Society for Microbiology, 1993, p 475.
Persing DH, Herwaldt BL, Glaser C, et al: Infection with a *Babesia*-like organism in northern California. N Engl J Med 1995; 332(5):298.
Peters W, Killick-Kendrick R: The Leishmaniases in Biology and Medicine. London, Academic Press, 1987.
Preiss U, Ockert G, Boremme S, Otto A: On the clinical importance of *Dientamoeba fragilis* infections in childhood. J Hyg Epidemiol Microbiol Immunol 1991; 35:27.
Purtilo DT, Meyers WM, Connor DH: Fatal strongyloidiasis in immunosuppressed patients. Am J Med 1974; 56:358.
Quick RE, Herwaldt BL, Thomford JW, et al: Babesiosis in Washington State: A new species of *Babesia*? Ann Intern Med 1993; 119:284.
Ravdin JI (ed): Amebiasis: Human Infection by *Entamoeba histolytica*. New York, John Wiley and Sons, 1988.
Reisman RE: Insect stings. N Engl J Med 1994; 331(8):523.
Remington JS, Desmonts G: Toxoplasmosis. *In* Remington JS, Klein JO (eds): Infectious Diseases of the Fetus and Newborn Infant, 3rd ed. Philadelphia, W. B. Saunders Company, 1990, p 90.
Richards FO, Schantz PM, Ruiz-Tiben E, Sorvillo FJ: Cysticercosis in Los Angeles County. JAMA 1985; 254(3):444.
Rosenblatt JE, Sloan LM: Evaluation of an enzyme-linked immunosorbent assay for detection of *Cryptosporidium* spp. in stool specimens. J Clin Microbiol 1993; 31:1468.
Rosenblatt JE, Sloan LM, Bestrom JE: Evaluation of an enzyme-linked immunoassay for the detection in serum of antibodies to *Entamoeba histolytica*. Diagn Microbiol Infect Dis 1995; 22:275.
Ruebush TK: Human babesiosis in North America. Trans R Soc Trop Med Hyg 1980; 74:149.
Rusnak J, Hadfield TL, Rhodes MM, Gaines JK: Detection of *Cryptosporidium* oocysts in human fecal specimens by an indirect immunofluorescent assay with monoclonal antibodies. J Clin Microbiol 1989; 27:1135.
Sacks JJ, Roberto RR, Brooks NF: Toxoplasmosis infection associated with raw goat's milk. JAMA 1982; 248:1728.
Sadun EH, Melvin DM: The probability of detecting infections with *Enterobius vermicularis* by successive examination. J Pediatr 1956; 48:438.
Sakanari JA, McKerrow JH: Anisakiasis. Clin Microbiol Rev 1989; 2:278.
Samuelson J, Acuma-Soto R, Reed S, et al: DNA hybridization probe for clinical diagnosis of *Entamoeba histolytica*. J Clin Microbiol 1989; 27:672.
Schantz PM, Moore AC, Munoz JL, et al: Neurocysticercosis in an orthodox Jewish community in New York City. N Engl J Med 1992; 327(10):692.
Schmid GP, Matherny LC, Zaidi AA, Kraus JJ: Evaluation of six media for the growth of *Trichomonas vaginalis* from vaginal secretions. J Clin Microbiol 1989; 27:1230.
Schnapp LM, Geaghan SM, Campagna A, et al: *Toxoplasma gondii* pneumonitis in patients infected with the human immunodeficiency virus. Arch Intern Med 1992; 152:1073.
Shadduck JA, Greeley E: Microsporidia and human infections. Clin Microbiol Rev 1989; 2:158.
Shama SK, Etkind PH, Odell TM, et al: Gypsy-moth-caterpillar dermatitis. N Engl J Med 1982; 306:1300.
Sheehan DJ, Raucher BG, McKitriak JC: Association of *Blastocystis hominis* with signs and symptoms of human disease. J Clin Microbiol 1986; 24:548.
Shepp DH, Hackman RC, Conley FK, et al: *Toxoplasma gondii* reactivation identified by detection of parasitemia in tissue culture. Ann Intern Med 1985; 103:218.
Smith JW: Identification of fecal parasites in the special parasitology survey of the College of American Pathologists. Am J Clin Pathol 1979; 72(Suppl):371.
Sonenshine DE: Biology of Ticks, Vol. 1. New York, Oxford University Press, 1991.
Sonenshine DE: Biology of Ticks, Vol. 2. New York, Oxford University Press, 1993.
Spach DH, Liles WC, Campbell GL, et al: Tick-borne diseases in the United States. N Engl J Med 1993; 329:936.
Spencer MJ, Garcia LS, Chapin MR: *Dientamoeba fragilis*, an intestinal pathogen in children. Am J Dis Child 1979; 133:390.
Stehr-Green JK, Bailey TM, Visvesvara GS: The epidemiology of *Acanthamoeba* keratitis in the United States. Am J Ophthalmol 1990; 107:331.
Steyskal GC, Murphy WL, Hoover EM: Insects and Mites: Techniques for Collection and Preservation. USDA Misc Publ No 1443, 1987.
Symmers WC Sr: Pathology of oxyuriasis, with special reference to granulomas due to the presence of *Oxyuris vermicularis* (*Enterobius vermicularis*) and its ova in tissues. Arch Pathol 1950; 50:475.
Tan B, Weldon-Lime CM, Rhone DP, et al: *Acanthamoeba* infection presenting as skin lesions in patients with the acquired immunodeficiency syndrome. Arch Pathol Lab Med 1993; 117:1043.
Teutch SM, Juranek DD, Sulzer A, et al: Epidemic toxoplasmosis associated with infected cats. N Engl J Med 1979; 300:695.
Thompson RCA, Lymbery AJ (eds): *Echinococcus* and Hydatid Disease. Wallingford, United Kingdom, CAB International, 1995.
Truant AL, Elliott SH, Kelly MT, Smith JH: Comparison of formalin–ethyl ether sedimentation, formalin–ethyl acetate sedimentation, and zinc sulfate flotation techniques for detection of intestinal parasites. J Clin Microbiol 1981; 13:882.
Turner JA: Giardiasis and infections with *Dientamoeba fragilis*. Pediatr Clin North Am 1985; 32:865.
Ubelaker HE: *Acanthamoeba* spp: "Opportunistic Pathogens." Trans Am Microsc Soc 1991; 110(4):289.
van Gool T, Snijders F, Reis P, et al: Diagnosis of intestinal and dissemi-

nated microsporidial infections in patients with HIV by a new rapid fluorescent technique. J Clin Pathol 1993; 46:694.

Van Meirvenne N, le Ray D: Diagnoses of African and American trypanosomiases. Br Med Bull 1985; 41:156.

Varga JH, Wolf TC, Jensen HG, et al: Combined treatment of *Acanthamoeba* keratitis with propamidine, neomycin, and polyhexamethylene biguanide. Am J Ophthalmol 1993; 115:466.

Visvesvara GS: Pathogenic and opportunistic free-living amebae. *In* Murray PR, Barron EJ, Pfaller MA, et al (eds): Manual of Clinical Microbiology, 6th ed. Washington DC, ASM Press, 1995, p 1196.

Visvesvara GS: Parasite culture: *Entamoeba histolytica. In* Isenberg HD (ed): Clinical Microbiology Procedures Handbook. Washington, DC, American Society for Microbiology, 1992a, p 7.9.1.1.

Visvesvara GS: Parasite culture: *Trichomonas vaginalis. In* Isenberg HD (ed): Clinical Microbiology Procedures Handbook. Washington, DC, American Society for Microbiology, 1992b, p 7.9.3.1.

Visvesvara GS: Parasite culture: *Leishmania* spp. and *Trypanosoma cruzi. In* Isenberg HD (ed): Clinical Microbiology Procedures Handbook. Washington, DC, American Society for Microbiology, 1992c, p 7.9.4.1.

Visvesvara GS, Schuster FL, Marinez AJ: *Balamuthia mandrillaris* N.G., N. Sp., agent of amebic meningoencephalitis in humans and animals. J Eukaryot Microbiol 1993; 40:504.

Wang SS, Feldman HA: Isolation of *Hartmanella* species from human throats. N Engl J Med 1967; 277:1174.

Weber R, Bryan RT, Owen RL, et al: Improved light-microscopical detection of microsporidia spores in stool and duodenal aspirates. N Engl J Med 1992; 326:161.

Weber R, Bryan RT, Schwartz DA, Owen RL: Human microsporidial infections. Clin Microbiol Rev 1994; 7(4):426.

Weigle KA, Davalos M, Heredia P, et al: Diagnosis of cutaneous and mucocutaneous leishmaniasis in Colombia: A comparison of seven methods. Am J Trop Med Hyg 1987; 36:489.

Weiss JB: DNA probes and PCR for diagnosis of parasitic infections. Clin Microbiol Rev 1995; 8(1):113.

WHO: The Epidemiology and Control of African Trypanosomiasis. WHO Tech Rep Ser No 739, 1986.

WHO: The Biology of Malaria Parasites. WHO Tech Rep Ser No 743, 1987.

Willson R, Harrington R, Stewart B, Fritsche TR: Human immunodeficiency virus 1—associated necrotizing cholangitis caused by infection with *Septata intestinalis*. Gastroenterology 1995; 108:247.

Wilson M, Schantz P, Pieniazek N: Diagnosis of parasitic infections: Immunologic and molecular methods. *In* Murray PR, Barron EJ, Pfaller MA, et al (eds): Manual of Clinical Microbiology, 6th ed. Washington DC, ASM Press, 1995, p 1159.

Wittner M, Turner JW, Jacquette G, et al: Eustrongylidiasis—a parasitic infection acquired by eating sushi. N Engl J Med 1989; 320(17):1124.

Wolfe MS: Giardiasis. Clin Microbiol Rev 1992; 5(1):93.

Yang J, Scholten T: *Dientamoeba fragilis*: A review with notes on its epidemiology, pathogenicity, mode of transmission, and diagnosis. Am J Trop Med Hyg 1977; 26:16.

Young KH, Bullock SL, Melvin DM, Spruill CL: Ethyl acetate as a substitute for diethyl ether in the formalin-ether sedimentation technique. J Clin Microbiol 1979; 10:852.

Zierdt CH: *Blastocystis hominis*—past and future. Clin Microbiol Rev 1991; 4(1):61.

Chapter 54

Specimen Collection and Handling for Diagnosis of Infectious Diseases

Gail L. Woods, M.D.

Appropriate specimen collection and handling are key to diagnosis of infectious diseases. Guidelines for specimen collection, transport, and processing are discussed in this chapter. General principles are reviewed first, followed by discussion of the most common types of specimens encountered in the clinical microbiology laboratory.

For optimal detection of the pathogen(s) responsible for an infectious disease, specimens should be collected at a time when the likelihood of recovering the suspected agent is greatest. For example, the likelihood of recovering most viruses is greatest in the acute phase of the illness. Specimens for recovery of bacteria should ideally be collected before antimicrobial therapy is started.

The volume of specimen collected must be adequate for performance of the microbiologic studies requested. If insufficient volume is received, the physician or ward nurse should be notified; either additional sample can be obtained, or the physician must prioritize the requests. If a swab is used to collect the specimen, a polyester-tipped swab on a plastic shaft is acceptable for most organisms. Calcium alginate should be avoided for collection of samples for viral culture because it could inactivate herpes simplex virus; cotton may be toxic to *Neisseria gonorrhoeae*; and wooden shafts should be avoided because the wood may be toxic to *Chlamydia trachomatis*. Swabs are not optimal for detection of anaerobes, mycobacteria, or fungi, and their use when these organisms are suspected should be discouraged.

Specimens should be obtained from the site of infection with minimal contamination from adjacent tissues and organ secretions. All specimens except stool should be collected in a sterile container, and all should be labeled with the name and identification number of the person from whom the specimen was collected, the source of the specimen, and the time the specimen was collected.

After collection, specimens should be placed in a biohazard bag and transported to the laboratory as soon as possible. If a delay is unavoidable, urine, sputum and other respiratory specimens, stool, and specimens for detection of *Chlamydia trachomatis* or viruses should be refrigerated to prevent overgrowth of normal flora. Cerebrospinal fluid (CSF) and other body fluids, blood, and specimens collected for recovery of *Neisseria gonorrhoeae* should be stored at room temperature, because refrigeration adversely affects recovery of potential pathogens from these sources.

Each laboratory director should establish criteria for rejecting specimens unsuitable for culture. Most clinical microbiologists agree that the following specimens should be rejected:

- Any specimen received in formalin.
- 24-hour sputum collections.
- Specimens in containers from which the sample has leaked.
- Specimens that have been inoculated onto agar plates that have dried out or are outdated.
- Specimens contaminated with barium, chemical dyes, or oily chemicals.
- Specimens from foley catheters.
- Duplicate specimens (except blood cultures) received in a 24-hour period.

6

The following specimens should be rejected for anaerobic culture: gastric washings, midstream urine, stool (except for recovery of *Clostridium difficile* for epidemiologic studies or for diagnosis of bacteria associated with food poisoning [discussed later]), oropharyngeal specimens except deep tissue samples obtained during a surgical procedure, sputum, swabs of ileostomy or colostomy sites, and superficial skin specimens. Moreover, policies should be established for handling unlabeled or mislabeled specimens; such specimens should not be processed until discrepancies are resolved.

Universal precautions must be followed when handling all specimens. This means that appropriate barriers are used to prevent exposure of skin and mucous membranes to the specimen. Gloves must be worn at all times, and masks, goggles (or working behind a plastic shield), and impermeable gowns or aprons must be worn in situations in which there is risk of splashes or droplet formation. Optimally all specimen containers, but at a minimum those containing respiratory secretions and those submitted specifically for detection of mycobacteria or fungi, should be opened in a biologic safety cabinet. Specimens collected for virus isolation should be handled in a biologic safety cabinet to prevent contamination of the cell cultures.

When specimens or cultures must be shipped to a reference laboratory through the United States Postal Service, they must be packaged according to requirements of the Interstate Shipment of Etiologic Agents code. Specimens must be limited to no more than 40 mL. Cultures of bacteria and fungi should be grown on solid media in tubes. The cap of the primary container (tube or vial) should be sealed with waterproof tape and inserted into a second container (preferably metal), surrounded by sufficient packing material to absorb the entire volume of the culture or specimen if the primary container were to leak or break. The second container should be capped and placed in a shipping container (made of corrugated fiberboard, cardboard, or Styrofoam) and labeled with an official Etiologic Agents label (available from the Centers for Disease Control and Prevention). If a specimen must be shipped in dry ice (which is considered a hazardous material), it must be marked "Dry ice, frozen medical specimen." The dry ice should be placed outside the second container with the packing material in such a way that the container does not become loose inside the outer container as the dry ice evaporates.

BLOOD

Detection of blood-borne pathogens is one of the most important functions of the microbiology laboratory. Culture of blood is essential in identifying bacteria responsible for bacteremia, sepsis, infections of native and prosthetic valves, suppurative thrombophlebitis, mycotic aneurysms, and infections of vascular grafts. Blood cultures also are useful in diagnosing some viral infections and invasive or disseminated infections caused by certain fungi, especially species of *Candida, Cryptococcus neoformans*, species of *Fusarium*, and *Histoplasma capsulatum*. Parasites are detected in blood by microscopic examination of peripheral smears. In general, blood should be collected for culture before beginning antimicrobial therapy when any one or a combination of the following are present: fever (38°C or greater), hypothermia (36°C or lower), leukocytosis (especially with a left shift), granulocytopenia, or hypotension.

Timely detection and accurate identification of organisms in the blood depend on appropriate collection, transport, and processing of the specimen. Germane to the detection of all microorganisms in the blood is the phlebotomy technique. To minimize contamination of blood specimens by skin flora, the venipuncture site should be prepared with a bactericidal agent. The skin is first cleaned with alcohol (70% isopropyl or ethyl alcohol) and then with a 1% to 2% iodine solution, an iodophor, or chlorhexidine. For maximum antisepsis, the area should dry for one to two minutes prior to venipuncture. Other aspects of specimen collection differ for bacteria, fungi, viruses, and parasites.

DETECTION OF BACTERIA AND FUNGI. The optimal time to draw blood for cultures if bacteremia or fungemia is suspected is just before a chill, but because this is not predictable, most blood cultures are collected after the onset of fever and chills. Blood is drawn with a needle and syringe and, without changing needles, is injected directly into bottles of culture media or other blood culture system (Krumholz, 1990). The inoculated bottles or tubes should immediately be inverted several times to ensure mixing, and the specimen should be transported to the laboratory at room temperature as soon after collection as possible. Blood cultures should never be refrigerated.

In adults with bacteremia, the number of colony-forming units per milliliter of blood frequently is low. In one study, for example, 25% of patients who were bacteremic with *Staphylococcus aureus* and more than 50% with *Escherichia coli* or *Pseudomonas aeruginosa* bacteremia had colony counts of fewer than one colony per milliliter of blood (Henry, 1983). Given this low level of bacteremia in adults, collecting 20 to 30 mL of blood per culture is strongly recommended (Ilstrup, 1983; Washington, 1986). In infants and children, the concentration of microorganisms in blood is higher, and collection of 1 to 5 mL of blood per culture is adequate (Dietzman, 1974).

Recommendations concerning the number of blood specimens to collect are based on the nature of the bacteremia: transient, intermittent, or continuous. Transient bacteremia follows manipulation of a focus of infection (for example, an abscess, a furuncle, or cellulitis), instrumentation of a contaminated mucosal surface (as occurs during dental procedures, cystoscopy, urethral catheterization, suction abortion, or sigmoidoscopy), or a surgical procedure in a contaminated site (such as transurethral resection of the prostate, vaginal hysterectomy, colon resection, and débridement of infected burns). Transient bacteremia also occurs early in the course of many systemic and localized infections such as meningitis, pneumonia, pyogenic arthritis, and osteomyelitis. Most intermittent bacteremias are associated with an undrained abscess, whereas continuous bacteremia is the hallmark of intravascular infection, such as bacterial endocarditis, mycotic aneurysm, or an infected intravascular catheter. Continuous bacteremia also occurs during the first few weeks of typhoid fever and brucellosis.

Two separate blood cultures are nearly always adequate for recovering pathogens responsible for intravascular infections (Werner, 1967). In one study of persons with intravascular infection, the rates of positivity of the first, first two, and first three blood cultures per septic episode were 80%, 90%, and 99%, respectively (Washington, 1975). Data from another evaluation showed that 91% of all septic episodes were detected by the first blood culture, a percentage that increased to 99% with a second culture (Weinstein, 1983). Therefore, three blood culture specimens in a 24-hour period should be sufficient to detect almost all potential bacterial pathogens. The optimal time interval between cultures is unknown, but 30 to 60 minutes has been suggested. However, if initiation of antimicrobial therapy is deemed urgent, cultures should be collected before therapy is begun, from separate sites within a few minutes.

Organisms such as the coagulase-negative staphylococci, viridans streptococci, corynebacteria, *Bacillus* species, and *Propionibacterium* are frequent blood culture contaminants but also may be true pathogens. Collecting two sets of blood cultures per febrile episode helps distinguish probable pathogens from contaminants. The latter are generally present in only one bottle of one set of cultures, whereas pathogens are typically recovered from more than one set. Because more than one febrile episode may occur in a 24-hour period, and two sets of cultures should be collected per episode, a maximum of four sets of cultures per day should be allowed.

Most blood specimens for culture are obtained by venipuncture of peripheral veins. Collecting arterial blood does not appear to improve the yield of microorganisms, and culture of blood collected through an indwelling cannula is associated with increased recovery of presumed contaminants. Because the latter practice often results in additional cultures and unnecessary antimicrobial therapy, collection of blood for culture through an intravascular catheter is not recommended, except for umbilical artery catheters in infants (Cowett, 1976; Reller, 1982). However, quantitative cultures of blood collected through an intravascular catheter may be useful in determining whether the catheter is the site of infection (Wing, 1979).

Host factors such as antibodies, complement, phagocytic white blood cells, and antimicrobial agents may impede recovery of microorganisms from blood; therefore, various approaches have been used to counteract these factors. Diluting the blood specimen in broth medium in a 1 : 10 ratio provides optimal neutralization of the serum bactericidal activity (Washington, 1986). Incorporating 0.025 to 0.05% sodium polyanetholsulfonate in the blood culture medium inhibits coagulation, phagocytosis, and complement activation, and it inactivates aminoglycosides. Methods that counteract the presence of antimicrobial agents include adding penicillinases to broth media to inactivate penicillins; using antibiotic-adsorbent resins; and using the lysis-centrifugation system, by which red and white blood cells are lysed, the microorganisms are concentrated by centrifugation, and the concentrate is cultured on media free of antibiotics.

Several blood culture systems, each with advantages and disadvantages, are available. Conventional broth culture systems that use nutritionally enriched liquid media recover most bacteria. Tryptic or trypticase soy, supplemented peptone, brain-heart infusion, Columbia, or Brucella broth is used for recovery of aerobes and facultative anaerobes; thioglycolate (THIO) or anaerobic heart infusion broth is used for isolation of anaerobes. Traditionally, two bottles are inoculated, and one is vented to assure recovery of aerobes. Given the decline in anaerobic bacteremias, this practice of one aerobic and one anaerobic bottle per set has been questioned (Murray, 1992; Sharp, 1991). Routine inoculation of two aerobic media and selective anaerobic blood cultures may allow detection of more bacteremias and fungemias. Culture bottles are examined daily for seven days for evidence of growth, indicated by turbidity, hemolysis, gas production, discrete colonies, or a combination of these. When growth is apparent, a smear of the broth is stained with the Gram stain and examined microscopically, and the broth is subcultured to appropriate agar media. Routine subculture of macroscopically negative broths should be performed from the vented bottle six to 18 hours after inoculation. Routine subculture of the anaerobic bottle is unnecessary. Advantages of conventional broth cultures are the low cost of materials and a low prevalence of contamination. The major drawback is the time-consuming process of routine subculture.

A biphasic system consisting of a conventional blood culture broth bottle with an attached chamber containing agar media on a paddle (Fig. 54–1) does not require manual subculture. To subculture this biphasic system, the bottle is tipped, allowing the blood-broth mixture to enter the chamber and flow over the agar media. Colonies on the agar medium are used for identification and susceptibility testing. This system is less labor-intensive than the conventional system and, for recovery of aerobic and facultative bacteria and yeasts, is comparable with or better than other systems (Murray, 1991). The yield of anaerobes from conventional broth systems may, however, be higher.

The lysis-centrifugation blood culture system (Fig. 54–2) consists of a tube containing reagents that inhibit coagulation and the complement cascade, lyse blood cells, and provide a cushion for the microorganisms during centrifugation. Blood (six to 10 mL) is added to the tube, which is inverted several times to prevent clotting, and transported to the laboratory as soon as possible. Ideally, the specimen is processed immediately, but processing can be delayed for up to eight hours without adversely affecting recovery of microorganisms. To process the culture, the tube is centrifuged 30 minutes at 3000 × g, the supernatant is discarded, and the sediment is mixed on a vortex mixer and planted onto agar media. Smaller tubes for low-volume samples from infants and young children also are available. Advantages of lysiscentrifugation include greater recovery of *Staphylococcus aureus*, some of the Enterobacteriaceae,

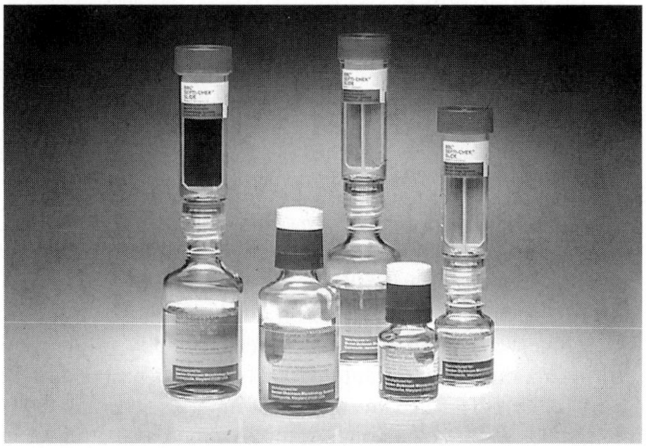

Figure 54–1. Biphasic blood culture system. (Septi-Chek, Courtesy of Becton Dickinson Microbiology Systems, Cockeysville, MD.)

6

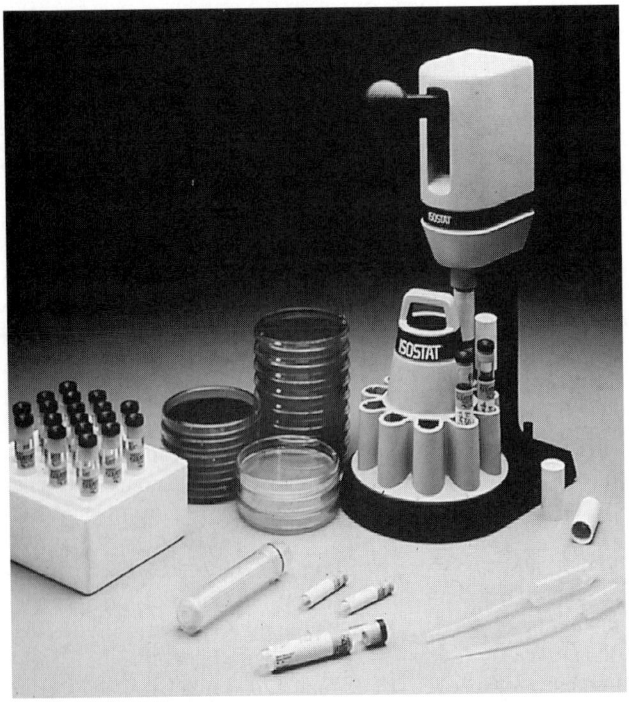

Figure 54–2. Isolator lysis-centrifugation blood culture tubes and processing station. (Courtesy of Wampole Laboratories, Cranbury, NJ.)

and fungi (it is the best system for recovery of moulds such as *Histoplasma capsulatum*); the direct availability of colonies for identification and susceptibility testing; and the ability to carry out quantitative cultures. Moreover, this system is flexible because special media can be inoculated to recover organisms with specific growth requirements, such as species of *Legionella* and mycobacteria. However, the system is labor-intensive; is less likely to recover *Streptococcus pneumoniae, Haemophilus influenzae*, or anaerobes; and the risk for contamination is increased.

Several semi- to fully automated blood culture systems are available commercially. Advantages of all such systems are elimination of the need for blind subculture and shortening of the usual incubation period from seven to five days (Woods, 1994).

The commercial semi-automated system relies on the infrared detection of CO_2 released during metabolism of glucose by microorganisms (Fig. 54–3). The earliest model of this system, based on radiometric detection of $^{14}CO_2$ released into the atmosphere above the medium during metabolism of ^{14}C-labeled substrates, now is used almost exclusively to detect mycobacteria (Chapter 51). With the infrared detection system, two broth culture media in bottles designed specifically for the instrument are inoculated with the blood: one for recovery of aerobes and the other for anaerobes (or two aerobic bottles). During the initial incubation, bottles incubated aerobically are agitated on a rotary shaker. At specific time intervals, the bottles are placed manually in the monitoring module and are automatically moved past a detector, which inserts two needles through a rubber septum on the top of the bottle and draws out a sample of the gas that has accumulated above the liquid medium for analysis. Specimens with readings above a specific threshold or specimens that demonstrate a specified increase in threshold are automatically flagged as positive; broth is then withdrawn to prepare smears for staining with the Gram stain and for subculture. The major criticism of the system in the past was the cost of handling the recommended 20-mL blood volume per venipuncture because the maximum blood volume per bottle was 5 mL. However, media that accommodate up to 10 mL of blood now are available, and data indicate that these media allow more rapid and enhanced detection of most bacteria and fungi (Weinstein, 1991). The presence of resins in these high-volume media obviates the need to use special resin-containing media for persons receiving antimicrobial agents. Moreover, media designed specifically for recovery of organisms from pediatric patients and for recovery of fungi are available (Morello, 1991).

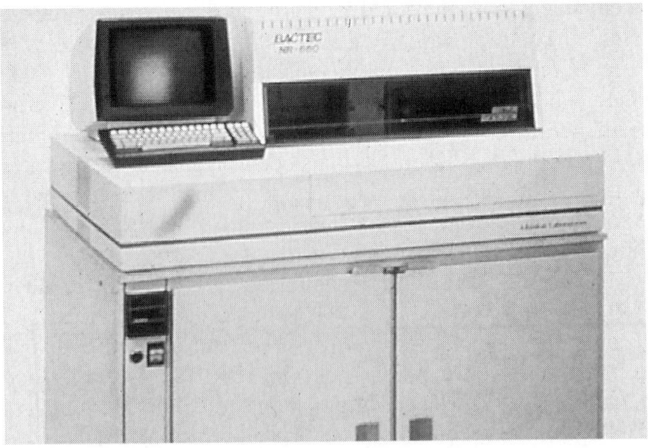

Figure 54–3. Semi-automated blood culture system that relies on the infrared detection of CO_2. (BACTEC NR 660, Courtesy of Becton Dickinson Diagnostic Instrument Systems, Sparks, MD.)

One automated blood culture system is based on the colorimetric detection of CO_2 produced during microbial growth (Fig. 54–4) (Thorpe, 1990). A CO_2 sensor is bonded

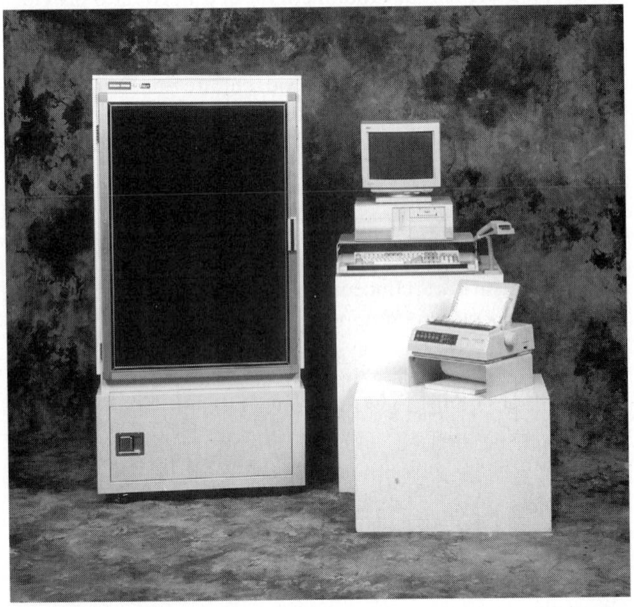

Figure 54–4. Fully automated blood culture system that relies on the colorimetric detection of CO_2. (BacT/Alert, Courtesy of Organon Teknika Corporation, Durham, NC.)

to the bottom of each blood culture bottle and is separated from the broth medium by a membrane that is impermeable to most ions and to components of media and blood but freely permeable to CO_2. Inoculated bottles are placed in cells in the instrument, which provides continuous rocking of both aerobic and anaerobic bottles. If bacteria are present, they generate CO_2, which is released into the broth medium; the pH then decreases, causing the sensor to change color from green to yellow. Color changes are monitored once every 10 minutes by a colorimetric detector. Media available for use with this system include routine aerobic and anaerobic media, which accommodate 5 to 10 mL of blood; PediBacT, which accommodates 4 mL of blood or less; and FAN (fastidious antibiotic neutralization), which enhances recovery of fungi and recovery of bacteria from patients receiving antimicrobial agents.

A second automated system is based on fluorescent technology (Fig. 54–5) (Nolte, 1993). Bonded to the base of each vial is a CO_2 sensor that is impermeable to ions, medium components, and blood but is freely permeable to CO_2. If organisms are present, they release CO_2 into the medium; it then diffuses into the sensor matrix and generates hydrogen ions. The subsequent decrease in pH increases the fluorescence output of the sensor, changing the signal transmitted to the optical and electronic components of the instrument. The computer generates growth curves, and data are analyzed according to growth algorithms. Inoculated bottles are placed in individual cells of the instrument, in which both aerobic and anaerobic bottles are continuously rocked. Aerobic and anaerobic low-volume (5 to 7 mL of blood) and high-volume (8 to 10 mL of blood) media and Peds-Plus medium (0.5 to 5 mL of blood) currently are available.

A third system (Fig. 54–6) detects growth of organisms in broth by measuring gas consumption and/or gas production (Zwadyk, 1994). Each inoculated vial is fitted with a disposable connector that contains a recessed needle. The needle penetrates the bottle stopper and connects the bottle headspace to the sensor probe. The sensor monitors changes within the headspace in the consumption and/or production of all gases (CO_2, N_2, and H_2) by growing organisms and creates data points internally in the computer. Two basic types of media are available: aerobic and anaerobic media that contain 80 mL of broth and accommodate 0.1 to 10 mL of blood, and EZ Draw (direct draw) aerobic and anaerobic bottles that contain 40 mL of broth and accommodate 0.1 to 5 mL of blood.

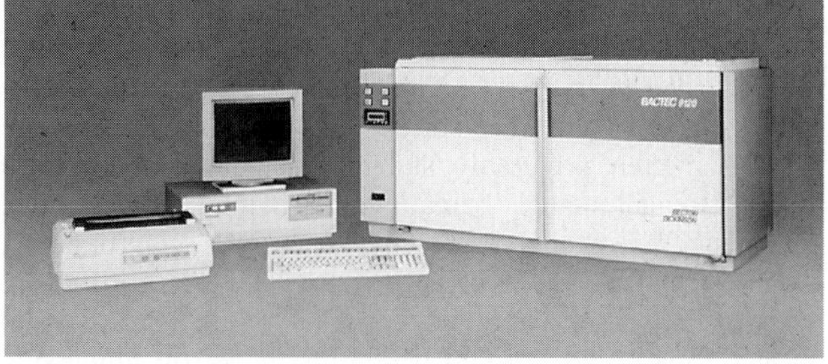

Figure 54–5. Fully automated blood culture system that monitors CO_2 production fluorometrically. (BACTEC 9000 series, Courtesy of Becton Dickinson Diagnostic Instrument Systems, Sparks, MD.)

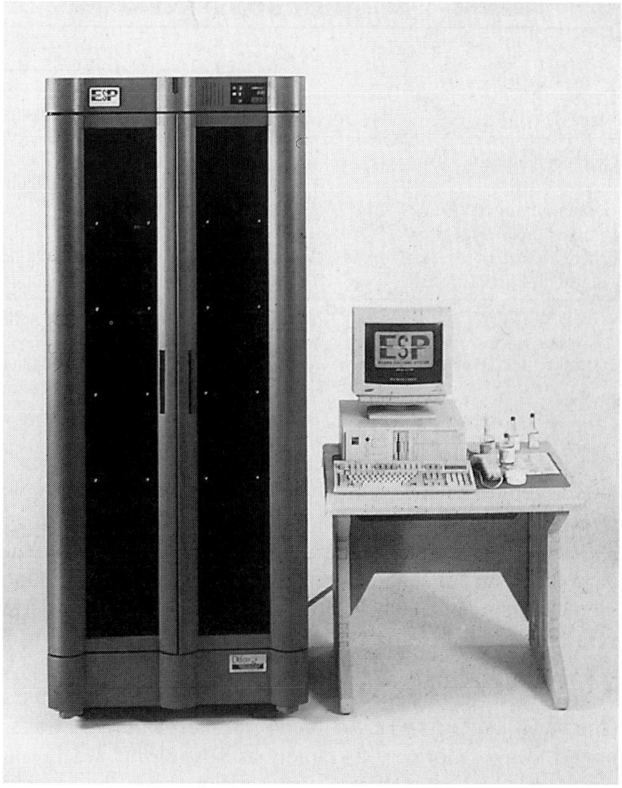

Figure 54–6. Fully automated blood culture system that detects growth of organisms in broth by measuring gas consumption, gas production, or both. (Difco ESP, Courtesy of Difco Laboratories, Detroit, MI.)

Detection of some bacteria requires prolonged incubation or special media. For example, when brucellosis is suspected, blood should be collected early in the disease, and cultures should be incubated for three to four weeks. Infections with species of *Borrelia*, except *Borrelia burgdorferi* (the etiologic agent of Lyme disease, most commonly diagnosed serologically), are diagnosed by detecting spirochetes in the peripheral blood during febrile periods. Organisms are visualized in wet preparations made by mixing a drop of blood with a drop of sodium citrate, and examining it with light- or darkfield microscopy, and in thin and thick blood films stained with Wright or Giemsa stain examined by light microscopy. To isolate *Leptospira interrogans* from blood, a few drops of fresh or anticoagulated blood collected during the first week of illness are added to each of three to four tubes of leptospiral semisolid culture medium (Fletcher's medium or Ellinghausen, McCollough, Johnson, and Harris medium).

Two methods may be used to recover mycobacteria from blood specimens. With the lysis-centrifugation technique, a concentrate is prepared; the sediment is inoculated to Middlebrook 7H10, Löwenstein-Jensen, or both; and the cultures are incubated for up to eight weeks. An alternative and perhaps more rapid approach is the commercially available radiometric broth system (discussed in Chapter 51). With the latter system, 5 mL of blood is directly inoculated into a 13A blood culture vial (Witebsky, 1988).

DETECTION OF VIRUSES. Blood specimens are useful in diagnosing infections with a limited number of viruses (Table 54–1). Viremia usually occurs during the incubation

Table 54–1. SPECIMEN REQUIREMENTS FOR OPTIMAL DETECTION OF VIRUSES FOUND IN BLOOD

	Blood Specimen Requirements		
Virus	***Type Collected***	***Fraction Used for Detection***	***Volume (mL)***
Cytomegalovirus	With anticoagulant*	Leukocytes	5–10
Enteroviruses	With or without anticoagulant*	Serum or leukocytes	5–10
Human immunodeficiency virus	Heparinized	Mononuclear cells or plasma	10†
Human herpesvirus–6	Heparinized	Mononuclear cells	5–10
Parvovirus B19	Without anticoagulant	Serum	5–10
Arthropod-borne viruses‡	With or without anticoagulant	Leukocytes or homogenized clot	5–10

*Heparin or EDTA may be used for cytomegalovirus; heparin, citrate, or EDTA for enteroviruses.
†Smaller volumes are acceptable from infants.
‡Includes viruses of eastern, western, and Venezuelan equine encephalitis; St. Louis and California encephalitis; yellow fever; dengue; and Colorado tick fever.

period or the first one or two days after symptoms begin; so blood should be collected early in the illness. An exception is infection with human immunodeficiency virus (HIV), which is detected nearly continuously in peripheral blood mononuclear cells and plasma of most seropositive persons. One blood sample per 24-hour period collected from a peripheral vein or through an intravascular catheter is adequate for virus detection.

Specimen requirements differ for the different viruses (shown in Table 54–1). All blood samples should be transported to the laboratory as rapidly as possible. If a delay in processing is unavoidable, specimens may be stored overnight at 4°C, except specimens for recovery of HIV, which should be maintained at room temperature. Those viruses detected routinely in most clinical virology laboratories—cytomegalovirus (CMV) and the enteroviruses—are discussed next. For detection of other viruses listed in Table 54–1, specimens often are sent to a reference laboratory.

Detection of CMV and the enteroviruses in blood involves separation of the component most likely to contain the virus and inoculation of that fraction to cell monolayers that support viral replication or preparation of a smear for staining with monoclonal antibodies. CMV is detected most often in neutrophils but may be present in peripheral blood mononuclear cells; thus, for optimal detection, both neutrophils and mononuclear cells should be cultured or stained (Howell, 1979). The enteroviruses are recovered equally well from leukocytes, primarily mononuclear cells, and from serum (Prather, 1984).

To separate leukocytes, blood is collected in a tube containing anticoagulants. The anticoagulant used (citrate or sodium heparin is acceptable) is based on the leukocyte separation system (several are commercially available) (Storch, 1994; Woods, 1987a). To separate serum, the blood is collected in a tube without anticoagulant and allowed to clot at 4°C. When a firm clot forms, the sample is centrifuged at 2000 × g for 10 minutes at 4°C, and the serum is aseptically removed.

Cell monolayers inoculated for virus isolation are selected based on the virus expected to be present. To recover CMV, inoculating two tubes of MRC-5 or other human fibroblast cell cultures is recommended. Incubating monolayers in maintenance medium containing 10^{-5}M dexamethasone for a minimum of 24 hours before inoculation increases the rate of detection of CMV and decreases the time for appearance of cytopathic effect (Thiele, 1988). For recovery of enteroviruses, MRC-5 and primary monkey kidney cells should be inoculated, and the rate of isolation may be increased by also inoculating Buffalo green monkey kidney and human rhabdomyosarcoma cells (Dagan, 1986). Serum specimens are inoculated, adsorbed, incubated, and examined for virus-specific cytopathic effect. For leukocyte suspensions, cell monolayers are inoculated with 0.5 mL of specimen, 1.0 mL of maintenance medium is added, and cell cultures are incubated overnight. The cell suspension then is removed, cell monolayers are washed with sterile phosphate–buffered saline, 1.5 mL of maintenance medium is added, and cultures are re-incubated.

In addition to conventional cell culture, centrifugation culture should be performed when detection of CMV is requested (Woods, 1987b). Moreover, CMV viremia may be detected by staining cytospin preparations of leukocytes with monoclonal antibodies against the viral matrix protein (pp 65) (Van Der Bij, 1988).

DETECTION OF PARASITES. Blood specimens are useful for diagnosis of malaria, babesiosis, trypanosomiasis, and some filariases. Specimens should be collected in tubes with anticoagulant and transported promptly to the laboratory. If smears must be sent to a reference laboratory, they should be fixed in absolute alcohol soon after they are made. The techniques used in the laboratory for detecting the previously named parasites are the same and are discussed here in order of the simplest to the most complicated.

The simplest technique for detecting parasites in a sample of blood is the direct mount, prepared by placing one drop of blood on a glass slide, covering it with a cover glass, and examining it immediately. Direct mounts are excellent for diagnosis of trypanosomiasis or filariasis because the trypomastigotes and the microfilariae can easily be seen moving, often with low or medium power. The definitive diagnosis is made by staining smears.

The thin smear, made as for hematologic work and stained in a similar manner, is the standard preparation for determining the species of *Plasmodium, Babesia, Trypanosoma,* or microfilariae found. Thin smears for parasitologic work are fixed and then preferably stained manually with Giemsa stain, but automated hematologic staining is adequate. Smears are first scanned at low power to detect microfilariae, which are large objects (between 100 and 200 μm) easily seen, usually at the lateral edges of the smear. After they are located, microfilarie should be studied under oil immersion for identification (discussed in Chapter 53). Following scanning with low power, the smear is examined with a high dry objective in a search for trypanosomes and finally is examined under oil immersion to find and identify *Plasmodium, Babesia*, and *Trypanosoma*.

Thick smears are useful for detecting all parasites mentioned earlier and are part of the minimum laboratory workup for their diagnosis. A drop of blood is placed on a clean glass slide and, with the corner of another slide, is gently spread to cover a 1-cm square. The preparation is allowed to dry and without fixation is stained with Giemsa's stain, allowing for its dehemoglobinization.

BODY FLUIDS

CEREBROSPINAL FLUID. Cerebrospinal fluid (CSF) is collected to diagnose meningitis and, less frequently, viral encephalitis. Infectious meningitis, a medical emergency requiring early therapy to prevent death or serious neurologic sequelae, is divided into acute, subacute, and chronic clinical syndromes, based on duration of symptoms (Table 54–2). An acute presentation occurs in about 10% of cases and is most likely caused by pyogenic bacteria. Almost all persons with viral meningitis and about 75% of those with bacterial meningitis have a subacute presentation; the rest present with chronic meningitis (responsible pathogens are listed in Table 54–2). The enteroviruses are the agents most commonly responsible for meningitis, and they should be considered first in the differential diagnosis of meningitis in a child or adolescent during the late summer and early fall. The pyogenic bacteria responsible for meningitis vary with the age of the affected individual (Table 54–3).

CSF usually is obtained by lumbar spinal puncture, but sometimes it is aspirated from the ventricles or collected from a shunt. As when collecting blood for culture, careful skin antisepsis is essential for collection of CSF, which typically is submitted to the laboratory in three glass tubes. Suggestions for tests performed on fluid in each tube are as follows: tube 1, cell counts and differential stains; tube 2, preparation of smears to stain with the Gram stain or other stains and for culture; tube 3, protein and glucose and, if indicated, special tests such as the cryptococcal antigen, serologic test for syphilis, other serologic studies, and cytology. The parameters of normal CSF and the usual changes that occur during meningitis caused by different organisms are shown in Table 54–4.

CSF should be transported promptly to the laboratory and processed as rapidly as possible. If a brief delay in processing is unavoidable, the specimen should be held at room temperature unless viral culture is requested, in which case a portion (preferably 1 mL but no less than 0.5 mL) is refrigerated for a short time. Specimen processing differs for bacteria, fungi, viruses, and parasites and is discussed separately for each group of organisms.

Table 54–2. INFECTIOUS MENINGITIS SYNDROMES

Syndrome	Onset/Duration	Probable Pathogens
Acute	<24 hours	Pyogenic bacteria
Subacute	1–7 days	Enteroviruses, pyogenic bacteria
Chronic	Persisting at least 4 weeks	*Mycobacterium tuberculosis*
		Treponema pallidum
		Brucella spp.
		Leptospira interrogans
		Borellia burgdorferi
		Cryptococcus neoformans
		Coccidioides immitis
		Histoplasma capsulatum
		Candida spp.

Table 54–3. COMMON BACTERIAL CAUSES OF ACUTE MENINGITIS BY AGE

Age	Organisms
Neonates–3 months	Group B streptococci
	Escherichia coli
	*Listeria monocytogenes**
	Streptococcus pneumoniae
4 months–6 years	*Haemophilus influenzae*, type b†
6 years–45 years	*Neisseria meningitidis*
>45 years	*Streptococcus pneumoniae*
	Listeria monocytogenes
	Group B streptococci

*May cause meningitis in immunocompromised individuals in all age groups.
†Incidence has declined as a result of vaccination.

Processing CSF for routine bacterial culture includes concentration (if 1 mL or more of specimen is received), preparation of a smear for staining with the Gram stain, and culture. Concentration is done by centrifuging the fluid at a minimum of 1500 × g for 15 minutes. The supernatant is decanted into a sterile tube, leaving about 0.5 mL of sediment and fluid, which are thoroughly mixed on a vortex mixer or by forcefully aspirating up and down into a sterile pipette. Alternatively, if 2 mL or more are received, the fluid may be concentrated by filtering it through a 0.45-μm, sterile, disposable filter, and using the filter for culture (discussed later). However, before filtering the specimen, about 0.5 mL are transferred to a sterile tube and processed by centrifugation for preparation of smears to stain with the Gram stain (as previously described) or, preferably, by making a cytocentrifuged preparation (Shanholtzer, 1982). After the smear is prepared, media are inoculated as outlined in Chapter 48. For filtered specimens, the filter is placed "organism" side down on the surface of chocolate agar and then moved with sterile forceps to another location on the agar after 24 hours and 48 hours of incubation to allow detection of colonies forming beneath it.

In addition to smears stained with the Gram stain and culture, latex agglutination tests for detection of antigens of group B streptococci, *Streptococcus pneumoniae*, some serotypes of *Neisseria meningitidis, Escherichia coli* (the K1 capsular antigen cross-reacts with that of *Neisseria meningitidis*, type B), and *Haemophilus influenzae* type b may be done on the supernatant of a centrifuged specimen, the filtrate of a filtered sample, or the original fluid. These latex tests are most useful in diagnosing partially treated meningitis and in confirming a positive Gram-stained smear. The routine use of latex tests should be discouraged because compared with smears stained with the Gram stain, their sensitivity is not significantly greater and they are much more expensive.

Diagnosis of chronic bacterial meningitis requires specific requests because the CSF is handled differently for each entity. To diagnose brucellosis, the CSF is processed as described earlier for routine bacterial culture, but the media are incubated two to three weeks. For leptospirosis, *Leptospira interrogans* may be cultured from the CSF during the first few weeks of illness. Special media (listed earlier under

6

Table 54–4. NORMAL CEREBROSPINAL FLUID PARAMETERS AND CHANGES IN INFECTIOUS MENINGITIS

Condition	WBC (cells/μl)*	Protein (mg/dL)	Glucose (mg/dL)
Normal	5 (lymphocytes)	14–45	45–100 (2/3 serum)
Meningitis			
Acute/subacute bacterial	500–200,000 (PMNs)	↑	↓
Chronic bacterial, tuberculous, fungal	200–2000 (lymphocytes)	↑	↓
Enteroviral	200–2000 (PMNs early; lymphocytes later)	↑	Normal

*Cell type listed usually predominates.
WBC = white blood cells; PMNs = polymorphonuclear leukocytes; ↑ = increased; ↓ = decreased.

blood) are inoculated with a few drops of CSF and incubated as outlined in Chapter 48.

The diagnosis of neurosyphilis is based on the following findings in the CSF: pleocytosis, elevated protein concentration, and a positive Venereal Disease Research Laboratory (VDRL) (CSF VDRL) test, which currently is the only useful method for detecting antibodies to *Treponema pallidum* in the CSF (see Chapter 50). The CSF VDRL test is indicated only if the person has a positive serum test for syphilis (Albright, 1991a). The specimen should be refrigerated until it is tested. Involvement of the central nervous system by *Borrelia burgdorferi* (Lyme disease) also is diagnosed serologically, by detection of specific IgM and IgG in CSF and serum.

Processing CSF for detection of mycobacteria is indicated only for samples with pleocytosis or abnormal glucose or protein values (Albright, 1991b). The fluid is centrifuged at 3000 to 3600 × g for 30 minutes, the supernatant is decanted, and the sediment is thoroughly mixed on a vortex mixer and is used to prepare smears for staining and to inoculate appropriate media (discussed in Chapter 51). If the volume of CSF received is insufficient for concentration, the specimen is used directly for smears and culture.

Processing CSF for detection of fungi is similar to that described for bacteria detected by routine culture. Organisms are concentrated by filtration or by centrifugation. A cytocentrifuge preparation or a smear of the sediment stained with the Gram stain is examined, and appropriate media (such as brain-heart infusion or SABHI agar without antibiotics) are inoculated for culture. For filtered specimens, the filter is cut in two halves with sterile scissors; one half is cultured for bacteria and the other half for fungi. The culture of centrifuged specimens is made by placing one-drop aliquots of the sediment onto several areas of the agar surface.

In addition to smears stained with the Gram stain and the culture of CSF, rapid tests are available for diagnosis of meningitis caused by *Cryptococcus neoformans*: the India ink preparation, latex agglutination, and an enzyme-linked immunosorbent assay. The latter two are specific for the capsular antigen. Encapsulated yeast cells of *C. neoformans* are visible in CSF mixed with India ink (one drop of CSF sediment with one drop of India ink, available at art supply stores) on a glass slide and examined under high-power magnification (Fig. 54–7). The sensitivity of the India ink stain is low, except in HIV-infected persons; therefore, either the cryptococcal latex agglutination test or the enzyme-linked immunosorbent assay, both of which are highly specific and have sensitivities of over 90%, is recommended for diagnosis. These latter two tests can be done on CSF filtrate (if the sample was concentrated by filtration), on the supernatant of a centrifuged specimen, or on unspun CSF. False-positive latex agglutination results occur as a result of the presence of *Trichosporon beigelii* or to the introduction of trace amounts of condensation from agar into the test fluid. To avoid the latter problem, the latex test should be done before culture or, better, on a separate sample (Heelan, 1991).

Processing CSF for diagnosis of viral infections involves conventional cell culture (primarily for detection of enteroviruses) or, for viruses that cause encephalitis (western equine, eastern equine, Venezuelan equine, St. Louis, Japanese, and LaCrosse), serologic tests. In addition, the polymerase chain reaction is being investigated as a tool for detection of enteroviruses, herpes simplex virus, and CMV nucleic acid in CSF, but, currently, no kits are commercially available. Cell lines for isolation of enteroviruses are those discussed earlier for blood specimens.

CSF is occasionally sent to the laboratory for diagnosis of African trypanosomiasis (*Trypanosoma gambiense* and *Trypanosoma rhodesiense*) or infection with free-living amoebae (*Naegleria fowleri* and species of *Acanthamoeba*). Once the specimen is received in the laboratory, it should be processed immediately. Wet preparations are prepared directly from the specimen and from the sediment, by first shaking the tube gently (a step necessary because the parasites often stick to the wall of the tube) and then centrifuging the specimen at 250 × g for 10 minutes. Preparations are examined under the microscope with the condenser in a low position to allow visualization of trophozoites or, preferably, by phase-contrast microscopy.

Cultures of free-living amoebae from CSF are done on non-nutrient agar plates covered with a suspension of *Escherichia coli* or *Enterobacter aerogenes*. The fluid is cen-

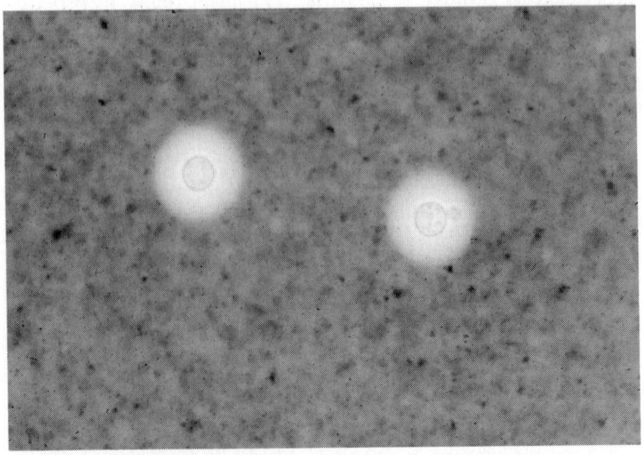

Figure 54–7. India ink preparation of cerebrospinal fluid shows encapsulated yeast form of *Cryptococcus neoformans*. (×400.)

trifuged at 250 × g for 10 minutes, the supernatant is removed with a sterile pipette, and the sediment is mixed with 0.5 mL of saline solution and poured at the center of the plate. The culture is incubated at 37°C and examined daily for 10 days using a microscope, under a 10× objective (Martinez, 1991).

OTHER BODY FLUIDS. Fluid is collected from the pericaridal, thoracic, or peritoneal cavity by aspirating with a needle and syringe. A volume of 1 to 5 mL is adequate for isolating most bacteria, but 10 to 15 mL is optimal for recovery of mycobacteria and fungi, which generally are present in low numbers. Moreover, to diagnose peritonitis associated with chronic ambulatory peritoneal dialysis, collection of at least 50 mL of fluid may improve recovery of the responsible pathogen (Dawson, 1985). To transport the fluid, the air is expelled from the syringe, the needle is removed, and the syringe is tightly capped with a sterile rubber stopper and delivered promptly to the laboratory. Alternatively, the sample may be directly inoculated to blood culture bottles at the bedside, an approach shown to be especially useful for detection of bacteria in peritoneal fluid (Luce, 1982).

Enteroviruses, primarily coxsackieviruses A and B, are among the most common causes of infectious pericarditis. These viruses may be detected in pericardial fluid by conventional cell culture, but because they are not recovered in all cases, collection of throat washings and stool (which are more likely to yield the virus) in addition to pericardial fluid for virus isolation from persons with suspected enteroviral pericarditis is strongly recommended. Other viruses (herpes simplex virus [HSV], varicella zoster virus, CMV, Epstein-Barr virus, hepatitis B virus, mumps virus, and influenza virus) are infrequent agents of pericarditis and are not usually detected in pericardial fluid.

Processing fluid from body cavities for detection of bacteria involves preparing a smear for Gram's staining and inoculating appropriate media for culture. As mentioned previously, the sample may be inoculated at the bedside, or it may be processed in the laboratory. In the laboratory, the fluid is centrifuged at 1500 to 2500 × g for 20 to 30 minutes, and the supernatant is removed, leaving about 0.5 mL, in which the sediment is mixed thoroughly and then used to prepare smears and inoculate media. Alternatively, a small volume of fluid (about 0.5 mL) is removed before centrifugation and used to prepare a cytocentrifuged smear. Unspun fluid may also be inoculated directly to a blood culture system in the laboratory, saving 0.5 to 1.0 mL to prepare a smear for Gram's staining.

Fluid specimens submitted for detection of mycobacteria are processed as described earlier for CSF. Fluids for fungal culture should be concentrated by centrifugation as described for bacteria. The supernatant is removed, leaving 1.5 to 2.0 mL, in which the sediment is thoroughly mixed. A smear of the sediment is prepared for staining with the Gram, calcofluor white, Congo red, or silver stain. Ideally, 0.5 to 1.0 mL of sediment is inoculated to primary fungal planting media (as for CSF), but lesser volumes are acceptable.

Body fluids rarely are collected for detection of parasites; however, *Entamoeba histolytica* may be found in the pericardial, pleural, or peritoneal cavity, owing to rupture of an abscess of the liver (into the peritoneal, pleural, or pericardial cavity) or of the lungs (into the pleural or pericardial cavity) or to perforation of amoebic ulcers (into the peritoneal cavity). Hydatid cysts infrequently are diagnosed by examination of body cavity fluid, also because of rupture of a cyst into a viscus contiguous to the cavity in question. The fluid collected is usually clear and contains hydatid sand (described in Chapter 53) but rarely is turbid because of superimposed bacterial infection. Uncommonly, in individuals with a filarial infection, examination of wet preparations of a body cavity fluid may demonstrate the microfilariae; and in patients with *Strongyloides* hyperinfection, larvae may be detected in body cavity fluids.

TISSUES

Tissue specimens obtained surgically are procured at great expense and at considerable risk to the patient; therefore, it behooves the surgeon to obtain an amount of material that is adequate for both histopathologic and microbiologic examination. Swabs are rarely adequate for this purpose. The histopathology of the lesion not only serves to differentiate between infection and malignancy but also to distinguish between a suppurative and a granulomatous process. In some cases, special stains are helpful in establishing the etiology of the process. In chronic lesions, the differential diagnosis includes disease caused by actinomycetes, brucellae, mycobacteria, and fungi, any one of which may be present only in small numbers, again emphasizing the need for obtaining adequate samples for examination and culture.

Tissue obtained surgically for culture should be placed into a sterile, wide-mouthed, screw-capped container. As a general rule, tissue should be bisected aseptically by the surgeon in the operating room and material representative of the pathologic process submitted for both histopathologic and microbiological examination. Good communication between histopathologist and microbiologist is important, especially in cases of fever of unknown origin for which an exploratory laparotomy is being performed and multiple biopsy specimens are taken.

Tissue received in the laboratory should be examined and its characteristics described before processing. It should then be finely minced with sterile scissors into a mortar where it is mixed with a sterile abrasive (alundum) in broth and ground with a pestle to render a 20% suspension. This suspension is used to inoculate all of the necessary culture media and is then stored under refrigeration for at least two weeks before being discarded.

EYE

CONJUNCTIVAL SPECIMENS. Conjunctival scrapings or swab specimens are collected to determine the etiologic agent of conjunctivitis. Bacteria are the most common etiologic agents of infectious conjunctivitis, and those most frequently implicated are *Streptococcus pneumoniae, Staphylococcus aureus*, and *Staphylococcus epidermidis* in adults and *Haemophilus influenzae, Streptococcus pneumoniae*, and *Staphylococcus aureus* in children. Trachoma, caused by *Chlamydia trachomatis*, is a leading cause of blindness worldwide. *Chlamydia trachomatis* also may cause inclusion conjunctivitis in newborns and less commonly in adults. Viruses are responsible for about 15% to 20% of cases of acute infectious conjunctivitis, and in the United States, most epidemics of viral conjunctivitis are caused by adenoviruses. Rarely, parasites are causes of conjunctivitis.

Conjunctival cells are obtained from the superior and inferior tarsal conjunctiva by using a swab moistened with broth or a sterile platinum spatula. Ideally, smears are prepared, and if a bacterial or fungal infection is suspected, culture media are inoculated directly by the individual collecting the sample. If direct preparation of smears and inoculation of media are not possible, swab specimens may be collected. Smears should be air-dried and promptly transported with the inoculated media to the laboratory. If viral culture is requested, a second sample (swab or scrapings) is collected, placed in viral transport medium, and delivered promptly to the laboratory or refrigerated for a short time and then transported on wet ice. A rapid diagnosis may be provided by direct or indirect immunofluorescent staining of smears of conjunctival cells with virus-specific antibodies, but cell culture is the most sensitive method for detecting potential viral pathogens and should always be done.

To detect *Chlamydia trachomatis*, a smear prepared directly from conjunctival scrapings may be stained with the Giemsa stain and examined for epithelial cells with basophilic intracytoplasmic inclusions diagnostic of *Chlamydia trachomatis*, or preferably with monoclonal antibodies, which are more sensitive and specific than the Giemsa stain. For optimal results with the direct fluorescent antibody test, the collection kit provided by the manufacturer should be used (see Chapter 47). The swab is rolled across the surface of the glass slide provided, the material is fixed, and the slide is transported promptly to the laboratory and held at room temperature or refrigerated for a short time. Slides are stained according to the manufacturer's directions and examined with a fluorescent microscope for elementary bodies (Chapter 47). Specimens containing less than 10 columnar or metaplastic squamous cells are considered inadequate, and results should be reported as inconclusive with an explanation, and other specimens should be requested. Culture is the reference method for detection of *Chlamydia trachomatis* and should be done when a diagnosis of chlamydial conjunctivitis is strongly suspected and the direct fluorescent antibody test is negative.

CORNEAL SPECIMENS. Corneal scrapings and biopsy specimens are useful in determining the etiologic agent of keratitis, an infection that can potentially produce loss of vision and requires immediate attention. Bacteria account for 65% to 90% of cases of keratitis, and in the United States, *Staphylococcus aureus, Streptococcus pneumoniae, Pseudomonas aeruginosa*, and species of *Moraxella* are most frequently implicated.

Corneal scrapings are collected with a sterile platinum spatula and are used for preparation of smears by directly transferring them to glass slides for staining and for inoculation to appropriate media for culture. If viral culture is requested, scrapings should be placed directly in viral transport media and delivered promptly to the laboratory or refrigerated for a short time and transported on wet ice. Frequently, the conjunctiva and the eyelids of the involved and the uninvolved eye are cultured concomitantly to determine the normal flora, useful in assessing the results of the corneal cultures. When the culture of scrapings of a suspicious corneal ulcer is negative, superficial keratectomy or corneal biopsy specimens may be obtained by the ophthalmologist, an approach especially useful for detection of fungi and *Acanthamoeba*.

RESPIRATORY TRACT

NASOPHARYNGEAL SPECIMENS. Nasopharyngeal aspirates, washings, and swab specimens are predominantly collected for diagnosis of viral respiratory infections but also of measles, *Chlamydia trachomatis* pneumonia in infants, diphtheria, and pertussis. Specimens from the nose are also useful to identify carriers of *Staphylococcus aureus*.

Nasopharyngeal aspirates and washings are superior to swabs for recovery of viruses, but swabs are frequently submitted because they are more convenient. Washings or swab specimens are collected for detection of *Bordetella pertussis*; a swab is the preferred specimen for *Chlamydia trachomatis* and *Corynebacterium diphtheriae*. An aspirate is collected with a plastic tube (such as one used to feed premature infants) attached to a 10-mL syringe or a suction catheter with a mucus trap. A wash is obtained with a rubber suction bulb by instilling and withdrawing 3 to 7 mL of sterile phosphate–buffered saline. To collect nasopharyngeal cells with a swab, all mucus from the nasal cavity is removed, and then a small, flexible nasopharyngeal swab is inserted along the nasal septum to the posterior pharynx and rotated against the mucosa several times.

To detect viruses, nasopharyngeal specimens are placed into an appropriate transport medium with or without antibiotics (such as veal infusion broth with 0.5% gelatin, Hanks' balanced salt solution, or sucrose-phosphate broth) and transported promptly to the laboratory or stored briefly in the refrigerator and packed in ice for transport as soon as possible. Viral detection methods are discussed in more detail in Chapter 46.

For detection of *Chlamydia trachomatis*, a nasopharyngeal swab specimen is collected with a polyester-tipped swab, which may be used for culture, for preparation of a smear for direct fluorescent antibody staining, or possibly for an enzyme-linked immunosorbent assay (if the system is approved for nasopharyngeal specimens). Detection methods are discussed in Chapter 47. For culture of *Chlamydia trachomatis*, the swab should be placed in 2-sucrose phosphate medium containing antimicrobial agents and transported to the laboratory as soon as possible, or refrigerated for a short time.

To detect *Bordetella pertussis*, inoculation of washings or swab specimens at the bedside is optimal. If this is not possible, the sample is placed into sterile casamino broth, transported promptly to the laboratory, and processed within one to two hours for culture (the most sensitive method for detection of *Bordetella pertussis*) and direct fluorescent antibody staining, which provides a rapid diagnosis but is associated with false-positive and false-negative results (Friedman, 1988). Currently, the recommended medium for culture is Regan-Lowe agar (composed of Oxoid charcoal agar and 10% horse blood and containing cephalexin) rather than the traditional Bordet-Gengou agar (potato infusion agar with 20% sheep blood). Specimens that must be shipped to a reference laboratory for culture should be inoculated to Regan-Lowe transport medium.

To identify carriers of *Staphylococcus aureus*, nasal secretions are collected from the anterior nares with a polyester-tipped swab, which is placed in a tube transport system and promptly delivered to the laboratory. The specimen is planted on 5% sheep blood agar, an agar medium selective for gram-positive organisms (colistin–nalidixic acid agar or phenylethyl alcohol agar), or mannitol salt agar, a medium selective for staphylococci and helpful in differentiating coagulase-positive from coagulase-negative species.

THROAT SPECIMENS. Throat swab specimens most commonly are collected to diagnose group A streptococcal pharyngitis, and throat swabs received in the clinical laboratory for routine bacterial culture should be evaluated only for this agent. Throat washings or swab specimens are useful for detection of viruses shed in oral secretions without causing pharyngitis (HSV, CMV, or enteroviruses), and throat swab specimens may be helpful in determining the etiologic agent of epiglottitis, a rapidly progressing cellulitis with the potential to cause obstruction of the airway (almost always due to *Haemophilus influenzae* type b, but occasionally due to *Staphylococcus aureus* or *Streptococcus pneumoniae*), and in diagnosing gonorrhea, *Mycoplasma pneumoniae* pneumonia, diphtheria, and Vincent's angina.

Throat swab specimens are collected by depressing the tongue with a tongue blade, introducing the swab between the tonsillar pillars and behind the uvula without touching the lateral walls of the buccal cavity, and swabbing back and forth across the posterior pharynx. Swab specimens collected for detection of viruses should be placed in a viral transport medium, and those for detection of bacteria in a tube transport system containing modified Stuart's medium. Throat washings for diagnosis of viral infections are obtained by gargling with 5 mL of viral transport medium containing antibiotics. Throat washings and swab specimens should be delivered promptly to the laboratory or refrigerated for a short time if a delay in transport is unavoidable.

For diagnosis of group A streptococcal pharyngitis, culture is most sensitive. Use of a selective medium increases the recovery of *Streptococcus pyogenes* and, by inhibiting the normal flora, decreases the time required to read plates and further evaluate β-hemolytic colonies (Bellon, 1991). When a rapid, direct test for group A streptococci (several are commercially available) is requested, two throat swab specimens should be collected. If the direct test is positive, the second swab may be discarded; but if the direct test is negative, the second swab must be cultured because the sensitivity of the direct tests is as low as 70% (Bisno, 1991).

To determine the etiologic agent of epiglottitis, a swab specimen should be collected by a physician in a setting in which intubation of the patient may be performed immediately if necessary. To detect *Neisseria gonorrhoeae* in the throat, the swab specimen should be inoculated at the bedside or transported to the laboratory promptly and inoculated as soon as possible onto a selective medium, such as modified Thayer-Martin agar. If a delay in processing is unavoidable, the swab should be held at room temperature. A throat swab is the specimen of choice for culture of *Mycoplasma pneumoniae*, although diagnosis of *Mycoplasma pneumoniae* pneumonia often is based on clinical manifestations alone or on serologic tests. The swab specimen should be stored in the refrigerator until it is inoculated to an appropriate culture medium (discussed in Chapter 47).

For diagnosis of diphtheria, both a nasopharyngeal swab and one (or preferably, two) throat swab specimens are collected and transported to the laboratory immediately. If laboratory personnel are not experienced in the recovery and identification of *Corynebacterium diphtheriae*, the specimens should be sent dry in packets or tubes containing silica gel or other desiccant to a reference laboratory. To process specimens from persons with suspected diphtheria, two smears are prepared from one of the throat swabs; one is stained with the Gram stain to help differentiate diphtheria from Vincent's angina, and the other with Löffler's methylene blue to visualize the deep-blue–staining metachromatic granules of species of *Corynebacterium*. *Corynebacterium diphtheriae* cannot be identified by cellular morphology alone, so cultures must be done. The nasopharyngeal and the throat swab specimens should be planted on a slant of Löffler's serum medium and a medium containing potassium tellurite. In addition, a sheep blood agar plate should be inoculated and examined for group A streptococci.

Vincent's angina is an acute necrotizing ulcerative tonsillitis that may be caused by *Fusobacterium necrophorum* and other anaerobes. An illness with this clinical presentation may presumptively be called Vincent's angina if gram-negative, fusiform-shaped bacilli and spirochetes are seen in smears prepared from a swab specimen of the ulcerated lesion and stained with the Gram stain. Cultures of the involved area usually are not helpful because many species of anaerobes are present in the oral cavity; however, blood cultures should be collected because the illness commonly is accompanied by sepsis.

SPUTUM AND TRACHEAL ASPIRATES. Microbiological studies of sputum (expectorated and induced) and tracheal aspirate specimens are done primarily to determine the etiologic agents of pneumonia. Optimally, expectorated sputum is collected early in the morning before eating. The individual should rinse his or her mouth with water and then expectorate a specimen, preferably 5 to 10 mL, resulting from a deep cough. For persons with nonproductive coughs, a specimen may be induced by allowing the individual to breathe aerosolized droplets of a solution of 15% sodium chloride and 10% glycerin for about 10 minutes or until a cough reflex is initiated. Tracheal aspirates represent lower respiratory secretions collected in a Lukens trap from patients with tracheostomies. Patients with tracheostomies rapidly become colonized with gram-negative bacteria and other nosocomial pathogens, and because bacteria colonizing the respiratory tract cannot be differentiated from bacteria causing invasive disease by culture of tracheal aspirates, interpretation of routine culture results is difficult.

Sputum and tracheal aspirate specimens should be delivered promptly to the laboratory or refrigerated for a short time if a delay is unavoidable. Specimens of expectorated sputum for routine bacterial culture should be screened first to determine whether they are representative of lower respiratory secretions or of saliva. Screening tracheal aspirates also should be considered (Morris, 1993). A smear prepared from a portion of the specimen consisting of purulent material is stained with the Gram stain. In general, specimens with more than 10 epithelial cells per low-power field by screen are considered to have significant contamination with saliva and should be rejected. Specimens with less than 25 epithelial cells and more than 25 neutrophils per low-power field probably are acceptable (Murray, 1975). The number of neutrophils is usually not considered when determining specimen quality, because the individual from whom the sputum was collected may be neutropenic. Screening expectorated sputum samples for detection of *Mycoplasma pneumoniae*, species of *Legionella*, and mycobacteria and screening-induced sputum specimens to assess their quality are not required (Havlik, 1995; Ingram, 1994).

The Gram-stained smears prepared from specimens that are acceptable for culture are examined under oil immersion to determine the relative amounts of organisms. The quantity of organisms (rare, few, moderate, or many) is estimated for each kind of bacteria (for example, gram-positive cocci in pairs, chains, or clusters; gram-positive bacilli; gram-negative diplococci; and gram-negative rods), noting whether or not they are intracellular. Portions of the specimen containing purulent material are inoculated as outlined in Chapter 48; for specimens from persons with cystic fibrosis, also inoculating a medium selective for *Burkholderia (Pseudomonas) cepacia* is recommended.

Some organisms will not be recovered by routine culture, and to ensure their detection, tests must be specifically requested. For example, when Legionnaires' disease is suspected, *Legionella* culture and a rapid, direct test (fluorescent antibody or nucleic acid hybridization) are recommended. Culture is the most sensitive of these methods and always should be performed. Sputum specimens and tracheal aspirates submitted for *Legionella* culture should be diluted 1 : 10 in a tube of trypticase soy broth containing sterile glass beads and agitated on a vortex mixer or treated with an acid-wash solution to inhibit overgrowth by the normal bacterial flora. Several drops of the specimen should be inoculated to each of two plates of buffered charcoal yeast extract agar with α-ketoglutarate, one with and one without antimicrobial agents. Direct fluorescent antibody staining or nucleic acid hybridization, both of which can provide results in several hours rather than the five to seven days required for culture, should be used to supplement but not to replace culture. The sensitivities of the direct fluorescent antibody test and the commercially available DNA probe are similar; therefore, the method used should be based on cost efficiency.

For optimal detection of mycobacteria in sputum, collection of three samples on three separate days is recommended. Sputum and other respiratory secretions must be decontaminated to prevent the rapidly growing bacteria in the normal respiratory flora from overgrowing the slowly growing mycobacteria. This process and detection methods are discussed in Chapter 51.

All specimens submitted for fungal culture should be handled in a biological safety cabinet. The quality of the specimens should be determined by screening with smears stained with Gram's stain (as described earlier for bacteria). Acceptable expectorated sputum, induced sputum, and tracheal aspirate specimens should be examined microscopically for the presence of fungal elements and inoculated to culture media for recovery of fungi. Organisms may be visualized in potassium hydroxide preparations or in smears stained with Gram, calcofluor white, or Congo red stain. In general, to culture fungi the following guidelines for media selection are recommended: Media with and without blood enrichment and with and without cycloheximide should be used; all media should contain antimicrobial agents. However, when making the selection, the laboratory director also should consider cost and the types of fungi usually encountered in the patient population served by the laboratory.

Induced sputum specimens are useful for diagnosis of *Pneumocystis carinii* pneumonia in persons with the acquired immune deficiency syndrome (Wolfson, 1990). First, a Gram-stained smear of the specimen is examined to determine whether it is representative of lower respiratory tract secretions. Acceptable specimens are treated with a mucolytic agent (such as *N*-acetyl-L-cysteine), and smears are prepared and stained for detection of *Pneumocystis carinii* (see Chapter 52).

PROTECTED SPECIMEN BRUSH. The protected specimen brush is useful for diagnosis of bacterial pneumonia in ventilated patients who have not received antimicrobial therapy and probably are suitable for aerobic and anaerobic cultures (Baselski, 1994). The sample is collected with a small brush that holds 0.01 to 0.001 mL of secretions and placed in a catheter within a double cannula. The outer cannula has a displaceable polyethylene glycol plug at the tip. To obtain a specimen, the cannula is inserted to the desired area by bronchoscopy, the inner cannula is pushed out, dislodging the protective (water-soluble) plug, and the brush is extended even farther, beyond the inner cannula. Once the sample is taken, the brush is pulled back into the inner cannula, and both brush and inner cannula are pulled into the outer cannula to prevent contamination of the brush when the catheter is removed. The brush then is placed in 1 mL of sterile saline or broth. The specimen should be transported immediately to the laboratory and processed as soon as possible. If a delay is unavoidable, the specimen should be stored in the refrigerator. To process the specimen, the fluid in which the brush is suspended is agitated on a vortex mixer. Cytospin preparations are stained with the Gram stain, and with a 0.01-mL–calibrated inoculating loop, the broth is planted on appropriate media. Colony counts of greater than 1000 organisms per milliliter of broth (corresponding to 10^6 organisms per milliliter of the original specimen) appear to correlate with infection (Baselski, 1994).

BRONCHOALVEOLAR LAVAGE FLUID. Bronchoalveolar lavage specimens are useful for diagnosis of pneumonia in ventilated patients who have not received antimicrobial therapy and for detection of opportunistic pathogens in immunocompromised patients with pneumonia (Baselski, 1994). However, for culture of species of *Legionella*, sputum specimens are preferable to bronchial washings or to bronchoalveolar lavage samples, because the latter are diluted with saline and may contain small amounts of the anesthetic used locally, which inhibits the organism. To collect the fluid, the tip of the bronchoscope is carefully wedged into an airway lumen. A volume of saline (usually more than 140 mL) in three to four aliquots is injected through the lumen, sampling an estimated 1 million alveoli. The total volume returned varies, based on the volume instilled, but typically is 10 to 100 mL. The transport time to the laboratory should be minimal (less than 30 minutes); and once it is in the laboratory, the specimen should be processed as soon as possible. If a delay cannot be avoided, the fluid should be stored in the refrigerator.

Processing bronchoalveolar lavage specimens for detection of viruses includes direct microscopic examination and cell culture. Examination of cytocentrifuge preparations stained with the Papanicolaou stain allows detection of cytopathic changes, especially useful for diagnosis of CMV pneumonia (Fig. 54–8) (Woods, 1990). Staining cytocentrifuge preparations of the fluid with the Gram stain is recommended; visualizing one or more bacteria without squamous epithelial cells per oil immersion field strongly suggests acute bacterial pneumonia (Baselski, 1994; Kahn, 1987). Cytospin preparations may also be stained with an acid-fast stain, with specific antibodies such as those for detection of *Legionella* species or *Pneumocystis carinii*, or with nonspecific stains for detection of *Pneumocystis carinii* and/or fungi (such as a silver stain, calcofluor white, or Giemsa's stain).

Data indicate that quantitative culture of bronchoalveolar lavage specimens is useful for diagnosis of acute bacterial pneumonia (Baselski, 1994). The sample is inoculated onto agar media by using a 0.001-mL–calibrated inoculating loop (as used for urine cultures, described later). The presence of more than 10,000 colonies per milliliter of fluid correlates with disease. For detection of mycobacteria, the specimen should be decontaminated and handled as described in Chapter 51. To detect viruses, conventional cell culture and centrifugation culture for CMV should be done. To recover fungi, the sediment of a centrifuged specimen should be inoculated on primary plating media.

URINARY TRACT

Acceptable methods of urine collection include midstream clean catch (preferably a first-voided morning specimen), catheterization, and suprapubic aspiration. In general, 24-hour urine specimens should be rejected, except when detection of *Schistosoma haematobium* is requested specifically. Most commonly, the midstream flow of a clean-catch urine is collected. For women, the periurethral area and perineum first is cleansed with soapy sterile gauze pads in a front to back motion, rinsed with a moistened sterile gauze pad, and dried with a dry sterile gauze pad. For males, cleansing the genital area may not improve the detection of bacteriuria significantly and may not be necessary (Lipsky, 1984). During voiding, women should hold the labia apart and men who are not circumcised should hold back the foreskin. The first few milliliters of urine are passed into the toilet bowl or a bedpan to flush out bacteria normally colonizing the urethra, and the midstream portion is collected in a sterile container with a wide mouth and tightly fitted lid.

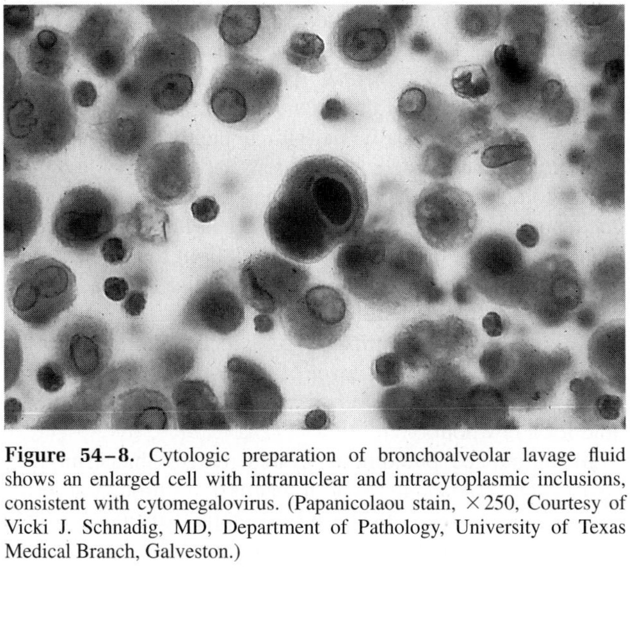

Figure 54–8. Cytologic preparation of bronchoalveolar lavage fluid shows an enlarged cell with intranuclear and intracytoplasmic inclusions, consistent with cytomegalovirus. (Papanicolaou stain, ×250, Courtesy of Vicki J. Schnadig, MD, Department of Pathology, University of Texas Medical Branch, Galveston.)

Catheterization is associated with the risk of inducing a nosocomial infection and should therefore be restricted to persons who are unable to produce a midstream sample; for example, individuals with an altered sensorium or those unable to void because of neurologic or urologic reasons. Using strict aseptic technique, the catheter is inserted into the urethra, the first few milliliters of urine passed are discarded to clear organisms that may have entered the tip of the catheter during placement, and the midportion of the sample is obtained for culture. Urine may be collected from an indwelling catheter by aspirating with a 28-gauge needle and syringe through the rubber connector between the catheter and the collection tubing, taking care to first disinfect the puncture site. Urine should not be collected from catheter bags, and Foley's catheter tips should not be accepted for culture because they almost always are contaminated with urethral organisms.

Suprapubic aspiration is used primarily for neonates and small children but may be done safely in adults. The procedure requires a full bladder; the overlying skin is disinfected, the bladder is punctured above the symphysis pubis with a 22-gauge needle on a syringe, and about 10 mL of urine are aspirated.

All urine specimens should be transported promptly to the laboratory and should be processed within two hours after collection. If a delay in transport or processing cannot be avoided, specimens may be refrigerated up to 24 hours. Collection kits containing preservatives to maintain a stable bacterial population for 24 hours at room temperature are commercially available, but they offer no advantage over refrigeration.

The urinary tract above the urethra is sterile in healthy humans, but the urethra is normally colonized with many different bacteria, so urine specimens collected by a noninvasive method (such as the clean-catch, midstream specimen) become contaminated during their passage. Commensal bacteria are differentiated from potential pathogens by quantitative cultures of urine, a procedure initially promoted by Kass (Kass, 1956). Originally, growth of 10^5 or greater colony-forming units (cfu) of bacteria per milliliter of urine was considered highly indicative of infection, but this criterion has been modified for different situations. For example, in young, sexually active women with the acute urethral syndrome (dysuria, frequency, and urgency), as few as 10^2 cfu/mL is considered significant in the presence of concomitant pyuria (Stamm, 1982). True urinary infections associated with fewer than 10^5 cfu/mL may occur in infants and chil-

6

dren; in males; and in persons who are catheterized, were recently treated with antimicrobial agents, drink large amounts of fluids (which dilutes urine), have symptoms and concomitant pyuria, have urinary obstruction, or have pyelonephritis acquired from hematogenous spread (especially infections due to yeast and *Staphylococcus aureus*) (Baron, 1990; Pezzlo, 1988). Consequently, proper interpretation of urine culture results requires communication between clinicians and laboratory personnel.

Quantitative bacterial culture of a urine specimen is done by inoculating appropriate media (see Chapter 48) with a measured amount of urine, most commonly with a plastic or wire calibrated loop designed to deliver a known volume. A 0.001-mL loop is used to inoculate all urine specimens except those collected from women with suspected acute urethral syndrome and those of suprapubic aspirates. Both of the latter are inoculated with a 0.01-mL loop. The appropriate loop is inserted vertically into the well-mixed urine sample, and the loopful of urine removed is spread over the surface of the agar plate as illustrated in Figure 54–9. Without reflaming, the loop again is inserted vertically into the urine, and the sample removed is inoculated to a second plate.

To determine the number of microorganisms per milliliter of the original specimen, the number of colonies (on the blood agar plate) is counted and multiplied by 1000 (if the 0.001-mL loop was used) or by 100 (if the 0.01-mL loop was used). Growth of three or more species in a clean-catch midstream urine usually is considered to indicate contamination. In such cases, the organisms are enumerated and minimally characterized (for example, coagulase-negative staphylococci or lactose-positive gram-negative bacilli), but susceptibility testing is not done. One or two isolates present in numbers greater than 10,000 in a clean-catch midstream sample should be identified, and antimicrobial susceptibility testing should be performed. Organisms present in numbers less than 10,000 are not evaluated further with the following exceptions: A pure culture of *Staphylococcus aureus* is considered significant in any number, and susceptibility testing should be done. Growth of 10^2 to 10^4 cfu/mL may be significant in catheter-related infections. In symptomatic males, growth of 10^3 cfu/mL or greater is consistent with infection, and the organism should be identified, but susceptibility testing is done only if specifically requested. For all organisms isolated from suprapubic aspirates, identification and susceptibility testing is performed. One isolate growing in numbers of 100 or greater from a woman with suspected acute urethral syndrome should be identified if pyuria is present, and susceptibility testing should be done if specifically requested.

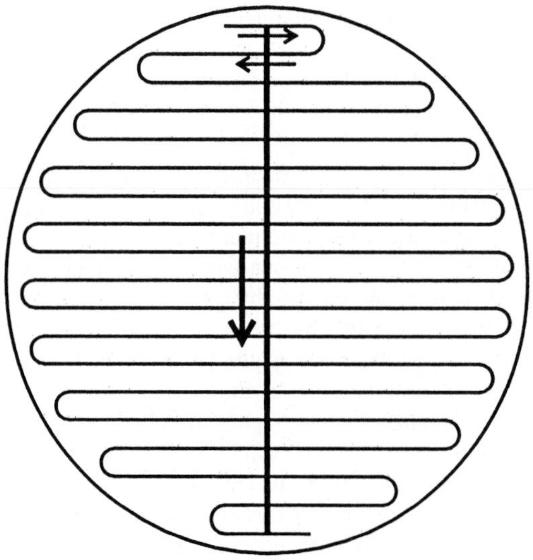

Figure 54–9. Technique for inoculating urine onto agar plates. (From Woods GL, Gutierrez Y: Diagnostic Pathology of Infectious Diseases. Philadelphia, Lea & Febiger, 1993.)

More than half of the urine specimens submitted to the clinical laboratory for culture yield no growth or have bacterial counts below levels considered clinically significant; therefore, screening tests that quickly identify urine samples yielding "negative" culture results have been developed in an attempt to provide rapid results, eliminate negative specimens, and allow more time for positive specimens, thus improving efficiency and cost. Urine screening and culture results correlate well when 10^5 cfu/mL or greater is the reference, but they compare less favorably in the presence of lower colony counts (Pezzlo, 1988). Other issues to consider regarding the use of bacteriuria screens are the ability to detect pyuria and the cost. The latter is especially important when considering automation.

Screening urine specimens by staining with the Gram stain is rapid and economical. Finding one or more organisms per oil immersion field in a smear prepared from an uncentrifuged specimen correlates well with bacteriuria at 10^5 cfu/mL or greater. The sensitivity of Gram's stain, however, decreases when compared with lower colony counts, and examination of smears is tedious and time-consuming. Commercially available dipstick tests that combine nitrate reductase (an enzyme present in most of the gram-negative bacilli that cause urinary tract infections) and leukocyte esterase (an enzyme produced by neutrophils) are rapid, inexpensive, and simple to perform, but their sensitivity is too low for use as a single screen for urinary tract infections (Pezzlo, 1988).

Several automated urine screening systems are commercially available. A colorimetric filtration system provides rapid results and detects more than 90% of all positive samples (including those containing neutrophils and only 10^2 cfu/mL) but may yield false-negative results with enterococci and *Pseudomonas aeruginosa* (Pezzlo, 1988). Urine is forced through a filter paper that retains cells, and then a stain is passed through the filter. The intensity of the resulting color, read manually or with a photometer, correlates with the number of particles adherent to the filter.

A bioluminescent system is based on the reaction of adenosine triphosphate (present in all living cells) with luciferin and luciferase, which produces light that is measured by a luminometer. By selectively releasing adenosine triphosphate from bacteria alone, the number of cfu in a urine sample may be estimated. This technique compares favorably with culture at a level of 10^5 cfu/mL or greater, but because it requires an incubation step, results are not available for a few hours.

An automated photometry system detects bacteriuria by measuring changes in light transmission through a broth medium inoculated with the urine sample. Bacterial growth causes the medium to become turbid, usually in two to three hours, but negative results cannot be reported before five to 13 hours. This system compares favorably with culture at a level of 10^5 cfu/mL or greater and has the capability of identifying the organism and performing antimicrobial susceptibility testing.

Some bacteria are not detected by routine culture of urine, and when these pathogens are suspected, specific tests must be requested. For example, *Leptospira interrogans* may be detected in urine after the first week of illness and for several months thereafter. Urine should be processed as soon as possible after collection, because acidity may harm the organisms. One or two drops of undiluted urine and urine diluted 1:10 in broth are inoculated to 5 mL of Fletcher's medium or Ellinghausen, McCollough, Johnson, and Harris medium containing 5-fluorouracil. Culture of urine for mycobacteria is discussed in Chapter 51. Yeasts may be recovered from urine on the media planted for routine bacterial culture; but if fungal culture is specifically requested, the sediment of a centrifuged urine specimen should be planted onto media such as inhibitory mold or SABHI agar containing antibacterial agents.

When urine specimens are submitted for culture of viruses, antibiotics (for example, penicillin, gentamicin, and amphotericin B) should be added to the sample when it is received in the laboratory to minimize bacterial contamination of cell cultures. Cell lines are selected for inoculation based on the viruses most commonly isolated—CMV, adenovirus, and HSV.

GENITAL TRACT

VAGINAL SECRETIONS. Vaginal secretions are useful in determining the etiologic agent of vulvovaginitis and bacterial vaginosis (so named because the condition is noninvasive). In postpubescent females, the most common pathogens are *Gardnerella vaginalis* (in association with anaerobes such as *Mobiluncus* species), species of *Candida*, and *Trichomonas vaginalis*. A wet-mount preparation is the most valuable diagnostic test and may be performed by the attending physician; cultures are not necessary for diagnosis. To prepare a wet mount, a swab of the discharge is placed in a tube containing about 1 mL of normal saline and gently agitated; one drop of the suspension is placed on a glass slide. Alternatively, one drop of saline is placed on a slide and mixed with a loopful of vaginal material. A coverslip is applied, and the preparation is warmed by passing it through a flame or holding it over an incandescent light bulb. The slide is examined under low- and high-power magnifications, looking for "clue cells" (epithelial cells covered with small coccobacillary bacteria) (Fig. 54–10), consistent with the diagnosis of nonspecific vaginosis; pseudohyphae, suggestive of vaginal candidiasis; and motile trichomonads.

In addition to the wet mount, determination of the vaginal pH and the "whiff test," performed by adding 10% potassium hydroxide to a drop of vaginal discharge placed on a slide or on the speculum, are useful diagnostic tests. The vaginal pH usually is about 4.5 in women with vulvovaginal candidiasis, but is above 4.5 in those with bacterial vaginosis or trichomoniasis. A positive whiff test (i.e., generation of a pungent, fishy odor) is associated predominantly with bacterial vaginosis but occasionally occurs with trichomoniasis.

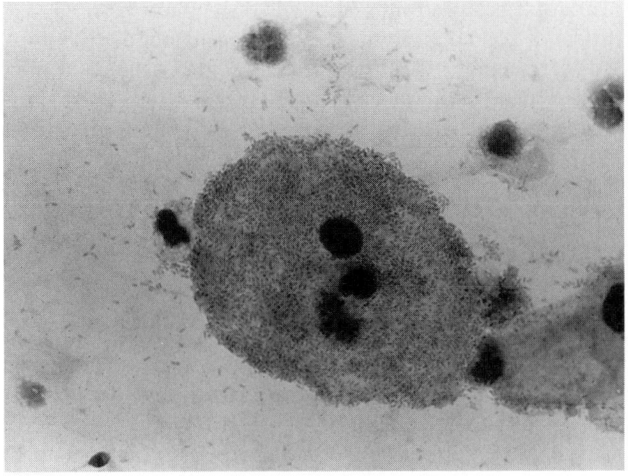

Figure 54–10. Clue cells in a smear of vaginal discharge. (Papanicolaou stain, ×400, Courtesy of Vicki J. Schnadig, MD, Department of Pathology, University of Texas Medical Branch, Galveston.)

ENDOCERVICAL AND URETHRAL SPECIMENS. Endocervical specimens are collected to determine the etiologic agent(s) of cervicitis and to identify asymptomatic persons infected with an organism that causes sexually transmitted disease. Endocervical specimens are obtained after the cervix is visualized with the aid of a speculum moistened only with warm water, because lubricants may contain antibacterial agents. If a Papanicolaou smear is indicated, that sample should be collected first. Specimens for microbiological studies generally are collected with a swab, although in nonpregnant women use of an endocervical brush may increase the sensitivity of culture and nonculture tests for *Chlamydia trachomatis* (Linder, 1987). As discussed earlier in this chapter, using a polyester-tipped swab with a plastic shaft is recommended. If a nonculture test kit is used for organism detection, the specimen must be collected with the swab supplied or specified by the manufacturer. The sample for detection of *Neisseria gonorrhoeae* is obtained before that for detection of *Chlamydia trachomatis* or HSV. Before collecting specimens for detection of the latter two organisms, all secretions and discharge must be removed from the cervical os. The swab or brush then is inserted 1 to 2 cm into the endocervical canal (past the squamocolumnar junction), rotated firmly against the wall for 10 to 30 seconds, withdrawn without touching the surface of the vagina, and placed in the appropriate transport medium or tube system, used to prepare a slide for direct fluorescent antibody staining (for *Chlamydia trachomatis*), or used to immediately inoculate an agar medium for recovery of *Neisseria gonorrhoeae*.

Specimen handling varies based on the organism sought. To isolate *N. gonorrhoeae*, direct inoculation of a selective agar medium, such as modified Thayer-Martin, within a container to which a CO_2-generating tablet is added is optimal. Alternatively, the swab specimen can be placed in a tube transport system and delivered to the laboratory as soon as possible. If a delay in transport cannot be avoided, the swab should be left at room temperature—never refrigerated. If a DNA probe is used for detection of *N. gonorrhoeae*, the collection kit provided by the manufacturer must be used, and the storage and transport conditions must be followed.

For detection of *Chlamydia trachomatis*, culture or non-culture methods may be used (Chapter 47). For chlamydial cell culture, 2-sucrose-phosphate and sucrose-glutamate-phosphate containing antibiotics (such as gentamicin, vancomycin, and nystatin or amphotericin B) to inhibit overgrowth of bacteria and fungi are commonly used transport media. To maintain viability of chlamydial organisms, the specimen should be transported to the laboratory immediately or stored in the refrigerator if immediate transport is not feasible. In the laboratory, the specimen should be processed as soon as possible. If a delay in processing is unavoidable, specimens should be stored in the refrigerator if they can be processed within 48 hours. If a longer delay is anticipated, specimens should be stored at −70°C or colder, although freezing may decrease the isolation rate of *Chlamydia trachomatis* by up to 20% (Mahoney, 1985). To detect chlamydial elementary bodies by direct fluorescent antibody staining, the collection kit provided by the manufacturer must be used, and the directions must be followed. The swab specimen is rolled over the microscope slide, the specimen is allowed to dry, and the fixative provided is applied. For enzyme immunoassay, DNA probes, and polymerase chain reaction, the collection kit/transport system provided by the manufacturer must be used, unless the manufacturer specifically states that an alternative transport system is acceptable. Manufacturer's guidelines concerning transport conditions, storage requirements, and time to processing must also be followed.

For optimal detection of HSV, cell culture is necessary. The swab specimen is placed in viral transport medium and transported as soon as possible to the laboratory. If immediate delivery is not feasible, the specimen should be stored in the refrigerator. For patients who have visible lesions on the cervix, viral cytopathic changes may be seen in smears prepared from scrapings of the lesion base. Smears are fixed immediately and stained with the Wright or the Giemsa stain (Tzanck preparation) or with a monoclonal antibody.

To diagnose the same sexually transmitted diseases in men, a urethral swab specimen or first-voided urine sample, depending on the detection method used, should be obtained. Optimally, urethral swab specimens are collected at least two hours after the patient has voided. Samples for *Neisseria gonorrhoeae* are obtained first. The conditions concerning types of swab and specimen transport are the same as those described for endocervical swab specimens, although the smaller urogenital swabs are used. The swab is inserted into the urethra for 2 to 4 cm, rotated in one direction for five seconds, withdrawn, and placed in the appropriate transport medium or used to prepare smears for direct fluorescent antibody staining to detect *Chlamydia trachomatis* or for Gram's staining to diagnose gonorrhea (detection of intracellular gram-negative diplococci in a smear of urethral discharge from symptomatic men provides a presumptive diagnosis).

VESICLES. Vesicular genital lesions are sampled to confirm HSV infection. The vesicle fluid is aspirated with a small-gauge needle on a tuberculin syringe. If only a small vesicle is present, it is unroofed, and the base is firmly scraped with a Dacron swab or tongue depressor to ensure collection of cells. Vesicle fluid or swab specimens should be placed in an appropriate transport medium and processed for conventional cell culture. HSV may also be detected directly in clinical specimens, but the methods available currently—direct staining of smears and enzyme-linked immunosorbent assays—are less sensitive than culture and, if negative, should be followed by culture. To make a smear, cells collected with a tongue depressor or a Dacron swab are spread on a glass slide, and the material is fixed in acetone. The smear may be stained with the Papanicolaou stain or the Wright or the Giemsa stain for detection of typical cytopathic changes (Fig. 54–11), stains that will not distinguish HSV from varicella zoster virus, or with specific monoclonal antibodies. To perform the enzyme-linked immunosorbent assay, the lesion is scraped firmly with a swab, which is immediately placed in the collection medium provided by the manufacturer.

ULCERS. Material from genital ulcers is collected to identify the responsible pathogen; HSV, *Haemophilus ducreyi, Treponema pallidum, Chlamydia trachomatis* (serogroups L_1, L_2, L_3), and *Calymmatobacterium granulomatis* should be considered in the differential diagnosis. Collection, transport, and processing of material from ulcerative lesions for detection of HSV are identical to the protocol discussed for vesicles. In general, the sensitivity of the direct tests previously described and recovery of the virus are lower in ulcerative lesions.

If infection with *Haemophilus ducreyi* is suspected, material from the base of the ulcer is collected on two cotton or Dacron swabs, transported in modified Stuart's medium to the laboratory, and held at room temperature until processed. One swab is used to prepare a smear for staining with the Gram stain. Observing many small pleomorphic gram-negative bacilli and coccobacilli arranged in chains and groups suggests *Haemophilus ducreyi*. Culture, however, is more sensitive and is necessary for confirmation. The second swab is inoculated on special media.

Treponema pallidum spirochetes may be detected in genital or other lesions, but syphilis usually is diagnosed serologically. Gloves should be worn when examining lesions of suspected syphilis and when handling specimens obtained from those lesions. To collect the specimens, the surface of the lesion (if multiple lesions are present, the youngest

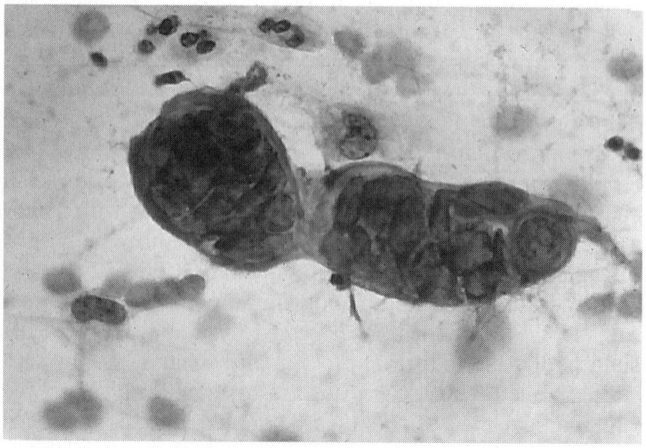

Figure 54–11. Multinucleate giant cell with intranuclear inclusions consistent with herpes simplex virus in a smear of endocervical cells. (Papanicolaou stain, ×400, Courtesy of Vicki J. Schnadig, MD, Department of Pathology, University of Texas Medical Branch, Galveston.)

should be selected) is cleaned with saline and blotted dry, and crusts are removed if present. The lesion is superficially abraded until slight bleeding occurs, and gentle pressure is applied to its base. The clear serum exudate from the subsurface is collected by touching the fluid with a glass slide or by using a capillary pipette and transferring the fluid to a glass slide. A coverslip is placed on the fluid, and the specimen is examined immediately by darkfield microscopy. Alternatively, lesion material is aspirated with a 26-gauge needle inserted at the base, after which a drop of saline is drawn into the needle. The material then is expressed onto a glass slide, covered with a coverglass, and examined immediately by darkfield microscopy. The spirochetes of *Trepenoma pallidum* are 10 to 13 μm long by about 0.15 μm wide; have a regular, tight coil; and are pointed at the ends.

Serogroups L_1, L_2, and L_3 of *Chlamydia trachomatis* may be detected by cell culture in a biopsy of the ulcerated lesion or in cellular material collected by first removing any exudate from the lesion and then firmly rotating a swab (on a plastic stick) against its base. Specimen transport and processing are the same as those discussed for endocervical swab specimens. For optimal detection of *Calymmatobacterium granulomatis*, subsurface tissue from an area of active granulation is biopsied and immediately transported to the laboratory in a sterile, dry container or in one containing a small amount of sterile saline without preservatives. Smears are prepared from a crushed piece of the tissue and stained with the Giemsa or the Dieterle stain. The diagnosis is based on finding characteristic, encapsulated *Calymmatobacterium granulomatis* organisms within macrophages.

FECES

Feces and, in some cases, rectal swab specimens are useful for determining the etiologic agent of infectious diarrhea or food poisoning, confirming the diagnosis of botulism, and diagnosing infections caused by adenoviruses, enteroviruses, some sexually transmitted pathogens, intestinal protozoa and helminths and, in some instances, helminths of the respiratory and biliary tracts. Collection, transport, and processing of these specimens are different for viruses, bacteria, and parasites and are discussed separately for each group.

Stool is preferred for detection of adenoviruses, enteroviruses, and the viruses responsible for gastroenteritis. Specimens should be collected in a clean container with a tight lid. If feces cannot be obtained, a swab is inserted beyond the anal sphincter, rotated, withdrawn, and placed in viral transport medium containing antimicrobial agents. Either specimen should be delivered promptly to the laboratory; if not, it should be refrigerated for a short time and transported on wet ice. If the specimen must be mailed to a reference laboratory, it should be stored at $-70°C$ and shipped on dry ice.

Cell culture is recommended for detection of adenoviruses and enteroviruses, although an enzyme-linked immunosorbent assay for detection of adenoviruses is available. Rotaviruses are responsible for most cases of viral gastroenteritis and are the only viruses associated with gastroenteritis that are detected in many clinical virology laboratories. Most commonly, rotavirus is detected by enzyme-linked immunosorbent assay; latex agglutination kits also are available but appear to be less sensitive (Christensen, 1989). Specimens are processed according to the manufacturer's directions. Direct examination of stool specimens by electron microscopy is the reference method for detection of rotavirus and is the most commonly used method for detection of caliciviruses, astroviruses, the Norwalk virus, and Norwalk-like viruses.

Stool also is preferred for detection of bacteria responsible for infectious diarrhea, but a rectal swab specimen is an acceptable alternative. Stool specimens should be collected in a clean container with a tight lid, and the specimen should not be contaminated with urine, barium, or toilet paper. Rectal swab specimens, obtained as described earlier for viruses, are placed in a tube transport system containing modified Stuart's medium. Both specimen types should be transported promptly to the laboratory and processed as soon as possible, because the drop in pH that occurs as the stool cools may inhibit the growth of some pathogens, especially *Shigella*. If a delay in processing is unavoidable or if the specimen must be mailed to a reference laboratory, adding a preservative such as 0.03M phosphate buffer mixed with an equal volume of glycerol is recommended.

Processing stool or rectal swab specimens for detection of bacteria is based on the organism or group of organisms expected to be present. Specimens received for "routine" bacterial culture should be processed to allow recovery of *Shigella, Salmonella*, and *Campylobacter jejuni/coli*. In pediatric institutions it also may be reasonable to routinely look for *Aeromonas*. Specimens are directly plated to appropriate media (see Chapter 48); alternatively, for detection of *Campylobacter jejuni/coli*, the sample can be filtered using a 0.65-μm pore size cellulose acetate filter, and the filtrate planted on Brucella sheep blood agar or chocolate agar. Species of *Aeromonas* grow on the media used for routine bacterial culture of stool or rectal swab specimens, but the use of a selective medium (CIN [cefsulodin, irgasan, novobiocin] containing 4 mg/L of cefsulodin rather than the usual 15 mg/L or sheep blood agar with 10 mg/L of ampicillin), incubated at 25° to 30°C, may increase the efficiency of screening.

The prevalence of gastroenteritis caused by enterohemorrhagic *Escherichia coli, Yersinia enterocolitica, Vibrio cholerae* or other *Vibrio* species, or *Plesiomonas shigelloides* is low in most parts of the United States; therefore, specific requests for their detection are most cost-effective. To detect enterohemorrhagic *E. coli*, the stool specimen is inoculated onto sorbitol-MacConkey agar (containing 1% D-sorbitol instead of lactose), a medium that differentiates isolates of enterohemorrhagic *E. coli*, which do not ferment sorbitol, from almost all other *E. coli*, which are sorbitol-positive. In addition to screening on sorbitol-MacConkey agar, the stool filtrate can be tested for toxin production in Vero cells.

6

When isolation of *Yersinia enterocolitica* is requested, CIN agar is inoculated and incubated at room temperature. The organism also can be recovered by inoculating media typically used for "routine" bacterial culture (see Chapter 48). The MacConkey plate is incubated at 35°C for the first 24 hours and then at room temperature for 24 hours; colonies of *Y. enterocolitica* are purple and are the size of a pinhead.

Species of *Vibrio* frequently grow on the media used for routine stool culture, but for their optimal recovery, thiosulfate citrate bile salts sucrose (TCBS) agar and alkaline peptone water (for enrichment) are inoculated. *Plesiomonas shigelloides* also grows on media used for routine culture, but because up to 30% of *Plesiomonas shigelloides* isolates ferment lactose, their colonies may not appear sufficiently distinct to be recognized on these media, and screening all colonies for *Plesiomonas* is not cost-effective. For this reason, culture of stool or rectal swab specimens for *Plesiomonas shigelloides* should specifically be requested. Use of the selective-differential medium inositol brilliant green bile salts agar has been suggested but is not essential.

Rectal swab specimens submitted for detection of *Chlamydia trachomatis* are placed in transport medium and delivered promptly to the laboratory, or are refrigerated for a short time. Rectal swab specimens collected to diagnose gonorrhea are treated as discussed earlier for endocervical specimens.

Stool specimens or gastric contents collected from persons with short-incubation food poisoning should be evaluated for *Staphylococcus aureus* and *Bacillus cereus*. Processing includes preparation and examination of smears stained with the Gram stain and culture. Because both organisms may normally be present in food, quantitative cultures must be performed. A series of dilutions (10^{-1}, 10^{-2}, 10^{-3}, 10^{-4}, and 10^{-5}) of the sample are prepared in buffered gelatin diluent, and 0.1 mL of the undiluted specimen and each one of the dilutions are planted on colistin nalidixic acid or phenylethyl alcohol blood agar (selective for gram-positive organisms). In addition, to demonstrate endospore production by *Bacillus cereus*, 1 mL of the original specimen is mixed with 1 mL of absolute ethanol, and the mixture is allowed to stand one hour at room temperature. Dilutions of the mixture are prepared as described above, and 0.1 mL of each dilution and of the undiluted mixture are planted on sheep blood agar. All plates are incubated 18 to 24 hours at 35° to 37°C in ambient air, and the colonies are counted. The presence of 10^5 colony-forming units or more of *Staphylococcus aureus* or *Bacillus cereus* organisms per gram of specimen has potential significance, especially if found in samples from the majority of affected individuals.

The clinical diagnoses of food-borne botulism and infant botulism may be confirmed by detecting botulinal toxin, *Clostridium botulinum*, or both in feces. Optimally, 25 to 50 mL of stool, 15 to 20 mL of serum, and a sample of the suspect food should be collected. Most clinical laboratories are not properly equipped to process specimens from persons with suspected botulism. In the United States, when a case of botulism is identified, investigators at the Centers for Disease Control and Prevention should be notified to assure appropriate diagnosis, treatment, and investigation of the potential outbreak.

Diseases associated with *Clostridium difficile*, such as pseudomembranous colitis and antibiotic-associated diarrhea, are caused by the toxins produced by the organism and are diagnosed by detecting toxin in feces. The reference method for detection of the cytotoxin is cell culture assay. About 25 g (25 to 50 mL) of liquid stool should be collected in a clean, wide-mouth container and transported promptly to the laboratory. The sample should be processed within two hours or stored in the refrigerator. To extract toxin, the stool specimen is clarified by centrifugation at $2000 \times g$ for 20 minutes or $10{,}000 \times g$ for 10 minutes and filtered through a 0.45-μm membrane filter. Serial dilutions are prepared and inoculated to cell monolayers, which are incubated 24 to 48 hours. Alternatively, toxin may be detected in stool samples by enzyme-linked immunosorbent assay. This technique appears to be almost as sensitive as cell culture, and provides results within a few hours (Merz, 1993; Whittier, 1993). A latex agglutination test is available but does not give reliable results (Lyverly, 1988).

For epidemiologic studies, *Clostridium difficile* may be isolated from stool or from rectal swab specimens placed in an anaerobic transport system. Because many bacteria are present in stool, procedures that select for *Clostridium difficile* must be used. The stool is diluted (1:200 is suggested) in buffered gelatin diluent, and both undiluted and diluted samples are inoculated to a medium selective for *Clostridium difficile*, such as cycloserine cefoxitin fructose agar (CCFA), and are incubated anaerobically for 48 hours. Alternatively, *Clostridium difficile* may be isolated by using the alcohol spore selection procedure, as described for *Bacillus cereus* except that treated and untreated samples are planted on a selective medium such as CCFA and are incubated anaerobically.

Clostridium perfringens is one cause of long-incubation food poisoning (7 to 15 hours after eating contaminated food); it also may cause antibiotic-associated diarrhea, typically in hospitalized elderly patients, and enteritis necroticans. To diagnose food poisoning caused by *Clostridium perfringens*, quantitative anaerobic culture of a stool specimen that was transported in an anaerobic transport collection system is performed. Ethanol-treated and untreated fecal material is diluted as described earlier for detection of bacteria associated with short-incubation food poisoning. Phenylethyl alcohol agar plates are inoculated and incubated anaerobically for 48 hours. A colony count of 10^5 or more per gram of stool may be significant, especially if demonstrated in samples from the majority of affected individuals. The toxin may be detected in the original stool specimen, but this test usually is performed in reference laboratories. Similar criteria are used to diagnose diarrhea produced by *Clostridium perfringens* during antibiotic therapy.

With respect to mycobacterial culture, stool specimens usually are submitted for isolation of *Mycobacterium avium* complex (primarily from patients with the acquired immunodeficiency syndrome), but *Mycobacterium tuberculosis* and other species of *Mycobacterium* may also be recovered. Processing the specimen (1 to 2 g of formed stool or 5 mL of liquid stool) involves decontamination and concentration, preparation of smears, and inoculation of media as discussed in Chapter 51.

The backbone of diagnostic parasitology in the clinical laboratory is examination of stool samples for parasitic protozoa and helminth eggs or larvae. Laboratories performing such tests should have adequate facilities for handling stool samples and a good microscope with a calibrated scale to measure the organisms found. Staining of fecal smears is also required for identification of intestinal protozoa.

The specimen (usually collected by the patient) can be collected without fixative and transported to the laboratory if both bacterial and parasitologic studies are requested. Fresh stool should be placed in a clean, dry, wide-mouth container. It should not be collected from the toilet bowl, and it should not be contaminated with urine, mineral or castor oil, antidiarrheal compounds, or radiologic contrast medium. Once collected, the sample should be delivered to the laboratory immediately. Bacteriologic studies are done first; then the sample is immediately given to personnel performing tests for detection of parasites for study, preferably within 30 to 60 minutes after its collection. Delays in evaluation result in degeneration of trophozoites of *Entamoeba histolytica*, the only parasite for which examination of fresh specimens may be desirable. Because laboratory-acquired infection is possible, the use of fresh specimens for parasitologic examination has become questionable.

If the fecal sample is collected only for detection of parasites, it can be fixed at the time of collection. The sample is delivered to the laboratory at the individual's convenience, and its examination is done to fit the laboratory routine. Several kits, most consisting of two vials—one with fixative (formalin) for trophozoites and cysts, and the other with fixative (Schaudinn's solution) plus polyvinyl alcohol (PVA) for preparation of smears for staining, are commercially available for collection and transport of fecal samples.

The question of how many fecal specimens are required for identification of all individuals with intestinal protozoa or helminths is still without a definitive answer. It has been advised that, for diagnosis of amoeba, a minimum of three specimens should be collected on different days and examined (Proctor, 1991). For cost containment, the clinician should request examination of only one specimen, because about 90% of all infections are diagnosed on the first sample (Montessori, 1987). If a parasite is not detected in the first sample, a second or third should be requested. If two or more specimens collected on different days are received in the laboratory at the same time, they should be pooled and evaluated as one (Peters, 1988). Stool examinations for parasites in patients who have been hospitalized for more than three days are inappropriate (Siegel, 1990).

The routine examination of stool samples for parasites includes preparation of saline solution and of iodine (Lugol)-stained wet mounts. This is followed by concentration of cysts and helminth eggs, and finally by preparation of smears for staining with the trichrome stain. The wet preparations should be made and examined before doing the concentration and the staining. If a diagnosis is secured with the examination of the wet mounts (for example, the clinical diagnosis is giardiasis, and one finds *Giardia* in the saline wet mount), the other tests should not be necessary.

The standard fecal smear, which has about 2 mg of feces, is made from a fresh fecal sample as follows: one drop of saline solution is placed on a clear glass slide; with an applicator stick, a small amount of feces is picked up and with circular movements is mixed thoroughly with the saline (until enough sample is dissolved), and the mixture is covered with a 22-mm square coverglass. A good wet smear prepared as described, if placed on a paper with small print, should allow reading the print through the smear. The smear stained with iodine is prepared in the same manner. Both the saline solution and the iodine solution wet preparations can be made on the same glass slide, at the same time, mixing the feces with the saline solution first, and then with the iodine solution. The saline solution smear will show trophozoites and cysts of protozoa, plus all the helminth eggs and larvae. The smear stained with iodine does not show trophozoites, because they are destroyed by the iodine, unless the sample was previously fixed. The main advantage of the iodine stain is that it allows better visualization of some morphologic characteristics of cysts. The saline solution shows movement of trophozoites, which is useful for their identification. To prepare wet mounts from formalin-fixed material, the contents are mixed well, and one drop is placed directly onto the glass slide and onto a drop of iodine solution.

Examination of the saline solution smear is carried out with medium power (10× objective) at first. Beginning at the left upper corner of the coverslide, the slide is moved horizontally from the right to the left. The operation is repeated until the entire 22-mm square coverglass is examined. All helminth eggs or larvae and all protozoan cysts should be noted. Examination with high-power objective is done next for detection and identification of protozoa, looking randomly for about 5 to 10 minutes per preparation.

The concentration technique, which can be done both on fresh and fixed specimens, is particularly useful because it allows enrichment of samples with low numbers of organisms. The ideal method for routine evaluation is the formalin-ether concentration, which has been made safer by the use of ethyl acetate rather than diethyl ether. The permanently stained fecal smear for diagnosis of infection with intestinal protozoa is considered the standard of good practice for North American clinical laboratories. Stains are made on smears prepared with a small painting brush wetted slightly in saline solution, and are fixed in Schaudinn's solution before they are dried. Smears are also made from samples received fixed in PVA; with a wooden applicator stick, drops of the sample are placed on a clean glass slide, ensuring that the film touches the long edges of the slide (to prevent its falling off during staining) and occupies about one half of the slide. After the film is completely dry at room temperature, it is stained. Certain intestinal parasites—*Cryptosporidium*, microsporidia, and *Cyclospora*—require special stains for detection, as discussed in Chapter 53.

SKIN AND SUBCUTANEOUS LESIONS

VESICLES, BULLAE, AND PUSTULES. Fluid may be collected from a vesicle or bulla by aspirating with a needle and syringe. For transport, the needle is removed, air is expelled, and the syringe is tightly capped and promptly delivered to the laboratory. Vesicles and bullae also may be sampled by unroofing the lesion and vigorously rubbing the base with a swab. Pustules are similarly sampled with a swab after any crusted material is removed. A minimum of two swab specimens should be collected, one for culture, the other for preparation of smears for staining. However, if detection of more than one group of organisms (for example, viruses and bacteria, or bacteria and fungi) is requested, collecting at least three swab specimens is optimal. For suspected viral infection, the individual collecting the specimen should prepare a smear at the bedside by rolling the entire surface of the swab over a glass slide and allowing the material to air dry.

All swabs may be placed in tube transport systems containing modified Stuart's medium. However, if recovery of viruses is requested, placing one swab in viral transport medium is recommended; and if anaerobic culture is ordered, one swab must be placed in an anaerobic transport device. Smears and swab specimens should be transported promptly to the laboratory.

Processing specimens from vesicles or pustules for detection of viruses involves cell culture, and for varicella zoster virus and possibly HSV, examination of stained smears is helpful. Specimens for culture are refrigerated for a short time until they are processed. Vesicle fluid collected in a syringe is placed in viral transport medium, and swab specimens received in viral transport medium are vigorously agitated on a vortex mixer, and the swab is removed. Processing specimens for detection of bacteria, fungi, or both involves preparation of a smear for staining with the Gram stain (for bacteria) or a silver stain, calcofluor white, or Congo red (for fungi) and inoculation of appropriate media for culture, as discussed in Chapters 48 and 52.

CUTANEOUS ULCERS. Aspirates and swab specimens are collected from cutaneous ulcers for microbiologic studies. Lesions may be primary (for example, those caused by viruses, *Bacillus anthracis, Corynebacterium diphtheriae, Francisella tularensis, Pseudomonas aeruginosa*, mycobacteria, or fungi), or decubitus ulcers may become secondarily colonized or infected with aerobic and anaerobic bacteria.

Collection, transport, and processing of swab specimens obtained from cutaneous ulcers for detection of viruses are identical to those described earlier for vesicles and pustules. Handling of specimens obtained from cutaneous ulcers differs for bacteria and fungi and is discussed separately for each of the organisms that cause primary lesions and for the bacteria associated with chronic ulcers.

Bacillus anthracis causes anthrax, a rare disease in the United States that is limited to persons working with raw imported wool and other animal products contaminated with spores of *Bacillus anthracis*. Cutaneous anthrax begins as a painless papule, but becomes vesicular, then hemorrhagic, necrotic, and covered with an eschar. For optimal diagnosis, two swab specimens of the exudate are collected, one for culture, the other for preparation of smears for staining with the Gram stain and with fluorescent antibodies (the latter should be performed in a reference laboratory). Due to the hazardous nature of *Bacillus anthracis*, sending specimens from persons with suspected anthrax to a reference laboratory should be considered. If specimens are processed in the clinical laboratory, they must be handled in a biological safety cabinet. The swab for culture is inoculated onto sheep blood agar, which is incubated in ambient air.

Corynebacterium diphtheriae is the cause of cutaneous diphtheria, an ulcerative lesion covered with a layer of necrotic debris resembling a membrane. For optimal diagnosis, a smear for staining with methylene blue is prepared from material collected from the edge of the membrane, and two swab specimens from the membrane are collected. One swab is used for routine bacterial culture and the other for inoculation of media selective for *Corynebacterium diphtheriae* (discussed earlier under Throat Specimens).

Ecthyma gangrenosum is an ulcerative cutaneous lesion that almost always occurs during bacteremia with *Pseudomonas aeruginosa*, but rarely develops during bacteremia with other gram-negative bacilli. Ideally, two swab specimens are collected from the ulcer base; one is used to prepare a smear for staining with the Gram stain, and the other, to inoculate media for culture.

The diagnosis of the ulceroglandular form of tularemia requires the collection of two swab specimens from material at the base of the ulcer. One is processed for routine bacterial culture and the other, for detection of *Francisella tularensis*, or it is sent to a reference laboratory.

Mycobacteria that may be isolated from cutaneous ulcers include *Mycobacterium tuberculosis, Mycobacterium avium* complex, *Mycobacterium kansasii, Mycobacterium fortuitum-chelonae, Mycobacterium marinum, Mycobacterium haemophilum*, and *Mycobacterium ulcerans*. Exudate aspirated with a needle and syringe is optimal for recovery of mycobacteria. To transport the aspirate, the needle is removed, and the syringe is tightly capped and delivered promptly to the laboratory. Exudate collected on a swab is not recommended, because mycobacteria become entrapped in the fibers of the swab and are difficult to dislodge. Specimens may be refrigerated for a short time until they are processed (discussed in Chapter 51).

Many aerobic, facultative, and anaerobic bacteria colonize chronic skin ulcers. To identify the organisms responsible, cultures of deep tissues or a deep aspirate of purulent material collected with a needle and syringe provide the most useful bacteriologic information. To transport the aspirated pus, air is expelled, the needle is removed, and the syringe is tightly capped and promptly delivered to the laboratory. Processing the specimen involves preparing a smear for staining with the Gram stain and inoculating appropriate media for aerobic and anaerobic culture.

An aspirate of the exudate from the active margin of an ulcer (transported as described earlier for bacteria) is optimal for detection of fungi. A swab specimen of the exudate is acceptable, but this practice should be discouraged. Processing the specimen for detection of fungi involves preparing a smear for direct microscopic examination (potassium hydroxide preparation or the stains previously listed for specimens from vesicles and pustules) and inoculation of appropriate media for culture, such as brain-heart infusion, inhibitory mold, or SABHI agar containing antibiotics and cycloheximide.

WOUND INFECTIONS AND ABSCESSES. Ideally, purulent material is aspirated with a needle and syringe and transported as described earlier for ulcerative lesions. If an aspirate cannot be obtained, swab specimens of exudate collected from the deep portion of the lesion are acceptable. For routine bacterial culture, two swab specimens are optimal, one to prepare a smear for staining with the Gram stain and one for culture. To recover anaerobes, an additional swab specimen must be collected and placed in an anaerobic transport system. All specimens should be delivered promptly to the laboratory and processed as soon as possible. If a delay in processing is unavoidable, specimens may be stored in the refrigerator except those for recovery of anaerobes, which should be maintained at room temperature.

Albright RE Jr, Christenson RH, Emlet JL, et al: Issues in cerebrospinal fluid management. CSF Venereal Disease Research Laboratory Testing. Am J Clin Pathol 1991a; 95:397.

Albright RE Jr, Graham CB III, Christenson RH, et al: Issues in cerebrospinal fluid management. Acid-fast bacillus smear and culture. Am J Clin Pathol 1991b; 95:418.

Baron EJ, Peterson LR, Finegold SM (eds): Microorganisms encountered in the urinary tract. *In* Bailey and Scott's Diagnostic Microbiology, 9th ed. St. Louis, CV Mosby, 1990.

Baselski VS, Wunderink RG: Bronchoscopic diagnosis of pneumonia. Clin Micro Rev 1994; 7:533.

Bellon J, Weise B, Verschraegen G, et al: Selective streptococcal agar versus blood agar for detection of group A beta-hemolytic streptococci in patients with acute pharyngitis. J Clin Microbiol 1991; 29:2084.
Bisno AL: Medical progress: Group A streptococcal infections and acute rheumatic fever. N Engl J Med 1991; 325:783.
Christensen ML: Human viral gastroenteritis. Clin Microbiol Rev 1989; 2:51.
Cowett RM, Georges P, Hakanson DO, et al: Reliability of bacterial culture of blood obtained from an umbilical artery catheter. J Pediatr 1976; 88:1035.
Dagan R, Menegus MA: A combination of four cell types for rapid detection of enterovirus in clinical specimens. J Med Virol 1986; 19:219.
Dawson MS, Harford AM, Garner BK, et al: Total volume culture technique for the isolation of microorganisms from continuous ambulatory peritoneal dialysis patients with peritonitis. J Clin Microbiol 1985; 22:391.
Dietzman DE, Fisher GW, Shoenknecht FD: Neonatal *Escherichia coli* septicemia—bacterial counts in blood. J Pediatr 1974; 85:128.
Freidman RL: Pertussis: The disease and new diagnostic methods. Clin Microbiol Rev 1988; 1:365.
Havlik D, Woods, GL: Screening sputum specimens submitted for mycobacterial culture. Lab Med 1995.
Heelan JS, Corpus L, Kessimian N: False-positive reactions in the latex agglutination test for *Cryptococcus neoformans* antigen. J Clin Microbiol 1991; 29:1260.
Henry NK, McLimans CA, Wright AJ, et al: Microbiological and clinical evaluation of the ISOLATOR lysis-centrifugation blood culture tube. J Clin Microbiol 1983; 17:864.
Howell CJ, Miller MJ, Martin WJ: Comparison of rates of virus isolation from leukocyte populations separated from blood by conventional and Ficoll-Plaque/Macrodex methods. J Clin Microbiol 1979; 10:533.
Ilstrup DM, Washington JA II: The importance of volume of blood cultured in the detection of bacteremia and fungemia. Diagn Microbiol Infect Dis 1983; 1:107.
Ingram JG, Plouffe JF: Danger of sputum purulence screen in culture of *Legionella* species. J Clin Microbiol 1994; 32:209.
Kahn FW, Jones JM: Diagnosing bacterial respiratory infection by bronchoalveolar lavage. J Infect Dis 1987; 155:862.
Kass EH: Asymptomatic infections of the urinary tract. Trans Assoc Am Physicians 1956; 69:56.
Krumholz HM, Cummings S, York M: Blood culture phlebotomy: Switching needles does not prevent contamination. Ann Intern Med 1990; 113:290.
Linder LE, Nettum JA, Miller SL, et al: Comparison of scrape, swab, and cytobrush samples for the diagnosis of cervical chlamydial infection by immunofluorescence. Diagn Microbiol Infect Dis 1987; 8:179.
Lipsky BA, Innuni TS, Plorde JJ, et al: Is the clean-catch midstream void procedure necessary for obtaining urine culture specimens from men? Am J Med 1984; 76:257.
Luce E, Nakagawa D, Lovell J, et al: Improvement in the bacteriologic diagnosis of peritonitis with the use of blood culture media. Trans Am Soc Artif Intern Organs 1982; 28:259.
Lyverly DM, Krivan HC, Wilkins TC: *Clostridium difficile*: Its disease and toxins. Clin Microbiol Rev 1988; 1:1.
Mahoney JB, Chernesky MA: Effect of swab type and storage temperature on the isolation of *Chlamydia trachomatis* from clinical specimens. J Clin Microbiol 1985; 22:865.
Martinez AJ, Visvesvara GS: Laboratory diagnosis of pathogenic free-living amoebas: *Naegleria*, *Acanthamoeba*, and *Leptomyxid*. Clin Lab Med 1991; 11:861.
Merz CS, Kramer C, Forman M, et al: Comparison of four commercially available rapid enzyme immunoassays with cytotoxin assay for detection of *Clostridium difficile* toxin(s) from stool specimens. J Clin Microbiol 1993; 32:1142.
Montessori GA, Bischoff L: Searching for parasites in stool: Once is usually enough. Can Med Assoc J 1987; 137:702.
Morello JA, Matushek SM, Dunne WH, et al: Performance of BACTEC nonradiometric medium for pediatric blood cultures. J Clin Microbiol 1991; 29:359.
Morris AJ, Tanner DC, Reller LB: Rejection criteria for endotracheal aspirates from adults. J Clin Microbiol 1993; 31:1027.
Murray PR, Spizzo AW, Niles AC: Clinical comparison of the recoveries of bloodstream pathogens in Septi-Chek brain-heart infusion broth with saponin, Septi-Chek tryptic soy broth, and the Isolator lysis-centrifugation system. J Clin Microbiol 1991; 29:901.
Murray PR, Traynor P, Hopson D: Clinical assessment of blood culture techniques: Analysis of recovery of obligate and facultative anaerobes, strict aerobic bacteria, and fungi in aerobic and anaerobic blood culture bottles. J Clin Microbiol 1992; 30:1462.
Murray PR, Washington JA II: Microscopic and bacteriologic analysis of expectorated sputum. Mayo Clin Proc 1975; 50:339.
Nolte FS, Williams JM, Jerris RC, et al: Multicenter clinical evaluation of a continuous monitoring blood culture system using fluorescent-sensor technology (BACTEC 9240). J Clin Microbiol 1993; 31:552.
Peters CS, Hernandez L, Sheffield N, et al: Cost containment of formalin-preserved stool specimens for ova and parasites from outpatients. J Clin Microbiol 1988; 26:1584.
Pezzlo M: Detection of urinary tract infections by rapid methods. Rev Clin Microbiol 1988; 1:268.
Prather SJ, Dagan R, Jenista JA, et al: The isolation of enteroviruses from blood: A comparison of four processing methods. J Med Virol 1984; 14:221.
Proctor EM: Laboratory diagnosis of amebiasis. Clin Lab Med 1991; 11:829.
Reller LR, Murray PR, MacLowry JD: *In* Washington JA II (ed): Cumitech IA, Blood Cultures II. Washington, DC, American Society for Microbiology, 1982.
Shanholtzer CJ, Schaper PJ, Peterson LR: Concentrated Gram stain smears prepared with a cytospin centrifuge. J Clin Microbiol 1982; 16:1052.
Sharp SE: Routine anaerobic blood cultures: Still appropriate today? Clin Microbiol Newsl 1991; 13:179.
Siegel DL, Edelstein PH, Nachamkin I: Inappropriate testing for diarrheal diseases in the hospital. JAMA 1990; 263:979.
Stamm WE, Counts GW, Running KR, et al: Diagnosis of coliform infection in acute dysuric women. N Engl J Med 1982; 307:463.
Storch GA, Gaudreault-Keener M, Welby PC: Comparison of heparin and EDTA transport tubes for detection of cytomegalovirus in leukocytes by shell vial assay, pp65 antigenemia assay, and PCR. J Clin Microbiol 1994; 32:2581.
Thiele GM, Woods GL: The effect of dexamethasone on detection of cytomegalovirus in tissue culture and by immunofluorescence. J Virol Methods 1988; 22:319.
Thorpe TC, Wilson ML, Turner JE, et al: BacT/Alert: An automated colorimetric microbial detection system. J Clin Microbiol 1990; 28:1608.
Van Der Bij W, Torensma R, van Son WJ, et al: Rapid immunodiagnosis of active cytomegalovirus infection by monoclonal antibody staining of blood leukocytes. J Med Virol 1988; 25:179.
Washington JA II, Ilstrup DM: Blood cultures: Issues and controversies. Rev Infect Dis 1986; 8:792.
Washington JA II: Blood cultures: Principles and techniques. Mayo Clin Proc 1975; 50:91.
Weinstein MP, Mirrett S, Wilson ML, et al: Controlled evaluation of BACTEC Plus 26 and Roche Septi-Chek aerobic blood culture bottles. J Clin Microbiol 1991; 29:879.
Weinstein MP, Reller LB, Murphy JR, et al: The clinical significance of positive blood cultures: A comprehensive analysis of 500 episodes of bacteremia and fungemia in adults. I. Laboratory and epidemiologic observations. Rev Infect Dis 1983; 5:35.
Werner AS, Cobbs CG, Kaye D, et al: Studies on the bacteremia of bacterial endocarditis. JAMA 1967; 202:199.
Whittier S, Shapiro DS, Kelly WF, et al: Evaluation of four commercially available enzyme immunoassays for laboratory diagnosis of *Clostridium difficile*-associated diseases. J Clin Microbiol 1993; 31:2861.
Wing EJ, Norden CW, Shadduck RK, et al: Use of quantitative bacteriologic technique to diagnose catheter-related sepsis. Arch Inter Med 1979; 139:482.
Witebsky FG, Keiser JD, Conville PS, et al: Comparison of BACTEC 13A medium and DuPont Isolator for detection of mycobacteremia. J Clin Microbiol 1988; 26:1501.
Wolfson JS, Waldron MA, Sierra LS: Blinded comparison of a direct immunofluorescent monoclonal antibody staining method and a Giemsa staining method for identification of *Pneumocystis carinii* in induced sputum and bronchoalveolar lavage specimens of patients infected with human immunodeficiency virus. J Clin Microbiol 1990; 28:2136.
Woods GL: Optimal protocol for processing high-volume and Peds Plus blood cultures by the BACTEC NR860. Am J Clin Pathol 1994; 101:162.
Woods GL, Proffitt MR: Comparison of plasmagel with LeucoPREP Macrodex methods for separation of leukocytes for virus isolation. Diagn Microbiol Infect Dis 1987a; 8:126.
Woods GL, Thompson AB, Rennard SL, et al: Detection of cytomegalovirus in bronchoalveolar lavage specimens: Spin amplification and staining with a monoclonal antibody to the early nuclear antigen for diagnosis of cytomegalovirus pneumonia. Chest 1990; 98:568.
Woods GL, Young A, Johnson A, et al: Detection of cytomegalovirus by 24-well plate centrifugation assay using a monoclonal antibody to an early nuclear antigen and by conventional cell culture. J Virol Methods 1987b; 18:207.
Zwadyk P, Pierson CL, Young C. Comparison of Difco ESP and Organon Teknika BacT/Alert continuous-monitoring blood culture systems. J Clin Microbiol 1994; 32:1273.

Part 7

MOLECULAR PATHOLOGY

Edited by
Sanford A. Stass, M.D,
Robert M. Nakamura, M.D., and
John Bernard Henry, M.D.

Chapter 55

Molecular Pathology: An Introduction

Robert M. Nakamura, M.D.
Sanford A. Stass, M.D.

WHAT IS MOLECULAR PATHOLOGY?

Molecular pathology is an emerging discipline with a broad conceptual approach that transcends all sections of anatomic and clinical pathology (Fenoglio-Preiser, 1987; Fenoglio-Preiser, 1993; Heim 1994). It has been 42 years since Watson and Crick discovered the structure of DNA. In that time, there has been an explosion in our ability to investigate the molecular genetic make-up of cells in the normal and diseased state. These investigations have evolved into a vast cohort of knowledge called molecular pathology. Molecular pathology has been defined as the laboratory and clinical application of nucleic acid technologies to elucidate, diagnose, and monitor disease states and to evaluate nondisease status (e.g., screening, parentage testing and forensic identification) (Nakamura, 1993). The technology is diverse and encompasses techniques for detection of DNA and RNA structure at the molecular level. The most direct method for analyzing nucleic acids is through direct nucleotide sequencing. However, although there have been dramatic advances in our ability to perform sequencing, it is still relatively expensive and cumbersome and thus has limited use in diagnostic molecular pathology.

Standard Methods

Standard methods for indirectly detecting changes in DNA sequences are now routine and take advantage of restriction enzymes (isolated from bacteria) that cut DNA at specific sequence sites that are usually four to eight base pairs. The DNA fragments of varying size are separated by electrophoresis and hybridized with a nonisotopic or radiolabeled single-stranded probe of interest to find the complementary sequences on the membrane. This technique called Southern blot is used for DNA rearrangement studies to detect B-cell and T-cell clonal populations, translocations, deletions, gene amplifications, and restrict fragment length polymorphisms (RFLPs). This technique is limited because it requires knowledge of the target sequence of interest and may detect only a subset of changes. When radiolabeled probes are used, quantitation of bands is possible using detection devices. A modification of the Southern blot is the Northern blot, which detects RNA transcripts.

The polymerase chain reaction (PCR) has become the most powerful molecular genetic technique available and resulted in a Nobel prize (Mullis, 1987). It is much more sensitive than the Southern or Northern blot and amplifies DNA (or RNA by reverse transcriptase PCR). PCR has been used for detection of point mutations and chromosomal translocations, DNA fingerprinting, and infectious disease identification. It involves the use of primers that flank the molecular genetic region of interest (typically up to 1000 base pairs are amplified) with multiple repetitions of denaturation, primer annealing, and chain elongation by heat stable polymerase. This is done on a thermal cycler.

The development of fluorescence *in situ* hybridization allows detection of specific nucleic acid sequences in metaphase chromosomes and, potentially, interphase nuclei. This method is useful in identifying chromosomal abnormalities but requires knowledge of the abnormality of interest. *In situ* hybridization also is available using specific probes that detect pathogenic microorganisms.

Future Technology

Molecular technology continues to evolve rapidly. In the future, new molecular technology will enable the use of smaller samples, decrease turnaround time, and allow for automation so as to avoid the intense labor that initially made molecular pathology difficult for routine clinical use. It is likely that this availability of rapid semiautomated and automated DNA and RNA assays will facilitate consistency and rapidity of results. One can foresee that automated nucleotide assays using microchip technology will be available in the foreseeable future. In addition to advancing technology, our knowledge of molecular genetics in normal and diseased states continues to develop at an accelerating pace. The extensive efforts now applied to the Human Genome Project make it likely that a multitude of new applications to laboratory diagnostics will be available in the next few years. It would appear that the most effective laboratory organizational structure in terms of cost, quality, and expertise to handle this rapidly expanding technology is to structure molecular pathology as a core area of the pathology laboratories, with maintenance of a dynamic interaction with other areas of the laboratory that use and interface with molecular pathology (infectious disease, hematology).

The College of American Pathologists

In 1988, the College of American Pathologists (CAP) recognized the importance of nucleic acid analysis and established an ad hoc Molecular Pathology Task Force Advisory Committee to advise the CAP on new developments in molecular pathology, the merging roles in clinical and diagnostic medicine, and how nucleic acid technology can be best incorporated into pathology. In 1989, the CAP established a Molecular Pathology Resource Committee to develop guidelines to implement the nucleic acid assay technology in pathology. The CAP committee focused on the development of molecular pathology (Nakamura, 1993; Walker, 1994) by coordinating and focusing scientific resources in the discipline of molecular pathology, developing diagnostic molecular pathology as a recognized area in pathology, serving as a focus point for the coordination of scientific resources for molecular pathology in the CAP, and ensuring the monitoring of emerging and future changes in the discipline of molecular pathology, including practical applications to new technical modalities.

In order to ensure quality and consistency in diagnostic molecular pathology, the Molecular Pathology Resource Committee developed specific standards of practice that were implemented in the form of laboratory accreditation and criteria that all diagnostic molecular pathology laboratories must meet. This was issued in the form of a laboratory checklist for the CAP inspection and accreditation program and covers the following items (Nakamura 1993):

1. Extent of service, proficiency testing, quality control, procedure manuals, records, test requisitions, specimen handling, reagents, controls and standards, procedures and tests, instruments and equipment, reporting of results, personnel, physical facilities, laboratory safety, and quality assurance; and
2. Generic questions that monitor the various categories and cover nucleotide probe assays (Southern blot analysis, dot/blot analysis, sandwich hybridization, *in situ* hybridization) and amplification methods (polymerase chain reaction).

In addition, proficiency testing in molecular oncology, *in situ* hybridization, and parentage and forensic identity testing were made available to diagnostic laboratories to monitor consistency of practice. Proficiency testing will be an essential element of molecular pathology as it is in other pathology disciplines especially because the technology is changing so rapidly. The proficiency surveys for the following areas are now available (Nakamura, 1993; Walker, 1994):

1. The CAP proficiency survey for molecular oncology, includes T-cell and B-cell gene rearrangement studies and the molecular detection of cytogenetic abnormalities, such as the Philadelphia chromosome (available since 1992).
2. The CAP, in cooperation with the American Society of Human Genetics, Bethesda, MD, developed a survey for human genetic donors that will be available to subscribers.
3. A CAP survey for *in situ* hybridization of viral antigens was made available in 1993.
4. A CAP survey for parentage testing by DNA polymorphism was developed with the American Association of Blood Banks, Arlington, VA, and became available in 1993.
5. A DNA forensic identity testing survey was developed in cooperation with the American Society of Crime Laboratory Directors and Federal Bureau of Investigation.

SCOPE OF MOLECULAR PATHOLOGY

Part 7 on molecular pathology covers

1. The basic principles and techniques in molecular diagnostics as well as organization of molecular diagnostic laboratories;
2. Molecular oncology including DNA assays for T- and B-cell gene rearrangements, analysis for translocations, oncogene analyses, gene mutations in various breast, colon, and other cancers;
3. Molecular genetic disease testing including the vertically transmitted diseases, such as cystic fibrosis and fragile X syndrome;
4. The molecular pathology of infectious disease, which is an area that is expected to be one of the most rapidly growing areas, because rapid nucleic acid testing for latent viruses, such as human immunodeficiency (HIV) and hepatitis C, will be performed more frequently and rapid nucleic acid tests for infections with slow-growing organisms, such as tuberculosis, will be performed in many clinical laboratories;

5. *In situ* hybridization in tissue is an area that will be applicable in anatomic and surgical pathology, cytology, as well as in other areas of the clinical laboratory, such as microbiology;
6. Blood group, molecular histocompatibility testing (DNA typing for MHC antigens used in histocompatibility and transplantation studies);
7. Forensic identity testing by DNA analysis.

It is our intent that these chapters give the reader an overview of the essential areas of molecular pathology, realizing that it is a rapidly evolving field.

Fenoglio-Preiser CM, Willman CL: Molecular biology and the pathologist: General principles and applications. Arch Pathol Lab Med 1987; 111:601–609.

Fenoglio-Preiser CM, Willman CL: Molecular Diagnostics in Pathology. Baltimore, MD, Williams & Wilkins, 1993.

Heim RA, Silver LM: Molecular Pathology: Approaches to Diagnosing Human Disease in the Clinical Laboratory. Durham, NC, Carolina Academic Press, 1994.

Mullis KB, Faloona FA: Specific synthesis of DNA in vitro via a polymerase-catalyzed chain reaction. Methods Enzymol 1987; 155:335–350.

Nakamura RM: College of American Pathologists Conference XXIV on Molecular Pathology: Introduction Arch Pathol Lab Med 1993;117: 455–456.

Walker RH: Molecular pathology programs of the College of American Pathologists, Lab Med 1994; 25:654–657.1

7

Chapter 56

Molecular Diagnostics: Basic Principles and Techniques

Elizabeth R. Unger, Ph.D., M.D.
Margaret A. Piper, Ph.D.

Nucleic acids are the critical molecules of life. Deoxyribonucleic acid (DNA) resides in the nuclei of eukaryotic cells and maintains all the information necessary for maintenance of the organism and for transfer of the information to successive generations. Ribonucleic acid (RNA) carries information from DNA to the cytoplasm of a cell and directs synthesis of the proteins necessary for the function of the organism. The normal state of health depends upon the stability of DNA and upon accurate DNA duplication and translation into protein. Modern cell biology seeks to determine the basic mechanisms of cell structure and function, and studies are increasingly focused at the level of the gene, the protein coding units of DNA. As a consequence, diagnostic methods are also being directed toward nucleic acid evaluation. The goal of this chapter is to provide the conceptual framework for diagnostic applications of nucleic acid analyses.

NUCLEIC ACID BIOCHEMISTRY AND BIOLOGY

Nucleic acid biochemistry is central to modern cell biology and dictates many aspects of diagnostic applications. Many of the enzymes associated with *in vivo* nucleic acid synthesis, degradation, and repair have become basic laboratory tools for manipulation and analysis of DNA and RNA. Cellular mechanisms that operate to direct and control DNA replication, transcription, and translation address the basic biology of the cell in health and disease. Diagnosis, therapy, and research are all increasingly directed at a molecular level of cellular function. This first section provides an overview of those aspects of nucleic acid biochemistry and biology that are required to understand the current diagnostic applications of molecular biology. Further details are available from textbooks of cell biology (e.g., Alberts, 1989).

Molecular Composition and Structure

DNA is a long, double-stranded polymeric molecule (dsDNA) that exists predominantly in the form of a right-handed double helix. Each single-stranded DNA molecule (ssDNA) is composed of a small number of building blocks. The backbone of the ssDNA polymer is the sugar deoxyribose, connected by phosphate groups (Fig. 56–1*A*). Phosphodiester bonds between the 3′ carbon of one sugar ring and the 5′ carbon of the next give the backbone its invariant structure and its 3′ to 5′ directionality. Linked to the

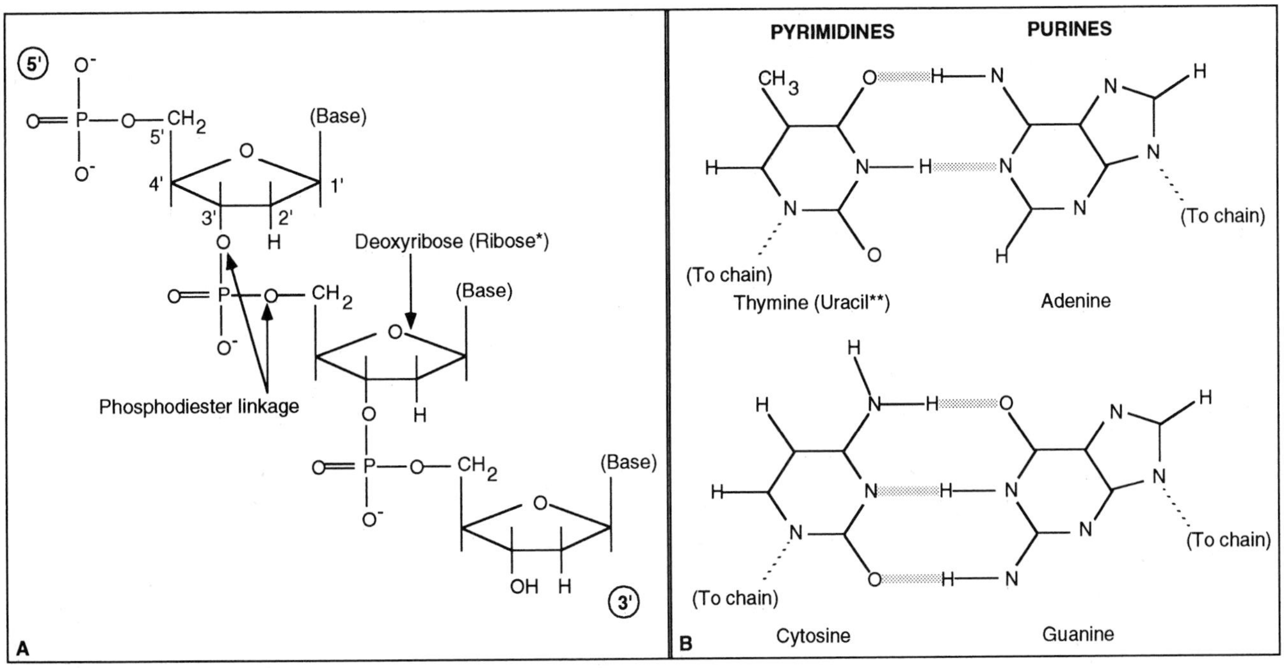

Figure 56–1. Repeating backbone of DNA and complementary base pairs.

A, A single-stranded DNA chain. Repeating nucleotide units are linked by phosphodiester bonds that join the 5′-carbon of one sugar to the 3′-carbon of the next. (*In RNA, the sugar is ribose, which has a 2′-hydroxyl added to deoxyribose.)

B, Purine and pyrimidine bases and the formation of complementary base pairs. Shaded bars indicate the formation of hydrogen bonds. (**In RNA, thymine is replaced by uracil, which differs from thymine only in the lack of the methyl group.) (Adapted with permission from Piper MA, Unger ER: Nucleic Acid Probes: A Primer for Pathologists. Chicago, ASCP Press, 1989.)

1′ carbon of each sugar is one of four possible bases: thymine (T) and cytosine (C) (pyrimidines); adenine (A) and guanine (G) (purines). The bases can occur in any sequence order, and thus form the variable portion of ssDNA. The building blocks of the single-stranded polymer are the four deoxyribonucleoside triphosphates (dTTP, dCTP, dATP, dGTP), each consisting of a sugar molecule, a triphosphate group, and one base. During DNA synthesis nucleotides are first stripped of two phosphate groups and then are enzymatically linked together by phosphodiester bonds to form a chain.

DNA is an extraordinarily stable molecule, losing its normal conformational structure only at extremes of heat, pH, or in the presence of destabilizing agents. The double-stranded helix is the most energetically favorable state for DNA, and an examination of the components of DNA explains this fact. Both sugar and phosphate groups are hydrophilic, forming stable hydrogen bonds with surrounding water molecules in solution. Bases, however, are hydrophobic and are not soluble in water at neutral pH. A stable molecule of DNA must ensure that the bases do not contact water. This is possible when two anti-parallel ssDNA polymers (one running in the 3′-5′ direction, the other 5′-3′) twist around the same axis. This arrangement allows planar hydrogen bonds to form between adenine and thymine, and between guanine and cytosine (Fig. 56–1*B*). As long as the two chains have base sequences in complementary order, the strands of the helix have a ladder-like structure with rungs (base pairs) of consistent size. The flexibility of the carbon-oxygen linkages in the phosphodiester bond allows the ladder to twist, forming a regular helix such that the planar base pairs are stacked on top of each other, leaving no room for water molecules in between. The polymeric series of base-pair hydrogen bonds hold the ssDNA chains tightly together, and the helical conformation protects the base pairs from water, exposing only the hydrophilic backbones.

Helical dsDNA is stable over a pH range of approximately 4–9. Solutions with pH outside these limits have the capacity to disrupt the base-pair bonds and cause the DNA helix to denature or unwind into two separate, random coils. Extreme heat as well as hydrogen bond disrupters, such as formamide, also have the same effect. This helix to coil transition can be followed spectrophotometrically at A_{260} (Fig. 56–2). The bases absorb ultraviolet light maximally at this wavelength, but at a lower molar absorptivity in dsDNA; absorptivity increases 20% to 30% when dsDNA is converted to ssDNA. Because temperature is often used to effect this transition, the process has been referred to as *melting*, and the temperature at which 50% of dsDNA is converted to ssDNA is called the *melting point* or T_m of the DNA. The T_m of DNA molecules depends on the relative G-C versus A-T base-pair content, because the three hydrogen bonds of G-C base pairs require more energy to disrupt than the two hydrogen bonds of A-T base pairs. The melting process can be reversed by lowering the temperature, and the two complementary strands can reform the original helix if the base pairs reform in the correct linear conformation.

The length of a fully extended eukaryotic DNA molecule would be much longer than the cell itself. Undegraded purified DNA forms a stringy viscous solution, reflecting the ex-

7

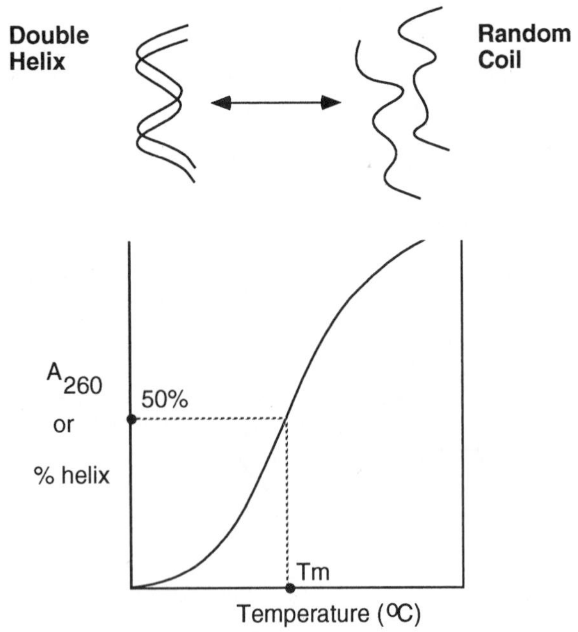

Figure 56–2. Melting/annealing curve of double-stranded helical nucleic acid. (Adapted with permission from Piper MA, Unger ER, Nucleic Acid Probes: A Primer for Pathologists. Chicago, ASCP Press, 1989.)

treme length of genomic DNA (Fig. 56–3). *In vivo*, however, DNA is organized into highly compacted, regular units called *chromosomes*. A chromosome is composed of its DNA strand wound around DNA-associated proteins in a highly structured fashion. Each human cell nucleus contains 23 chromosomes of characteristic length and unique base-pair sequence. Together these chromosomes constitute the *human genome*.

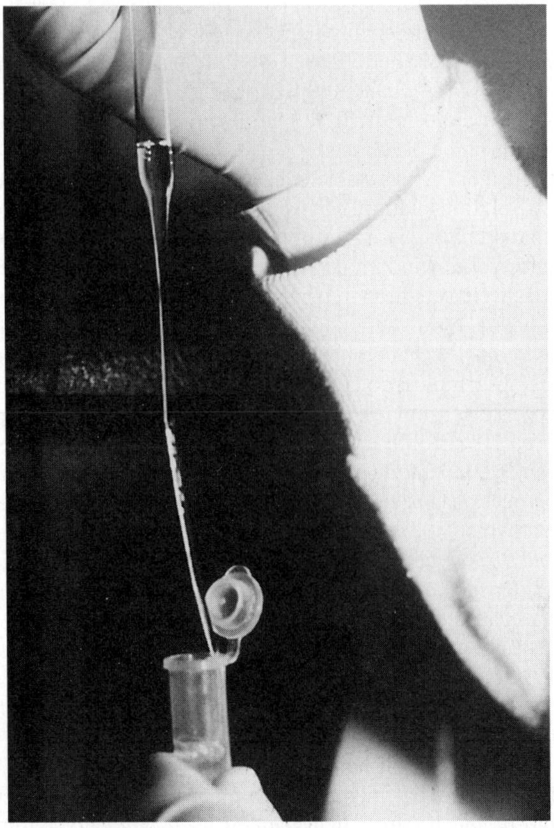

Figure 56–3. Photograph of purified DNA demonstrating stringy viscous nature of minimally sheared genomic DNA.

Table 56–1. COMPARISON OF KEY FEATURES OF DNA AND RNA

Feature	DNA	RNA
Sugar	Deoxyribose	Ribose
Base pairs	Thymine–adenine Cytosine–guanine	Uracil–adenine Cytosine–guanine
Structure	Double-stranded Alpha helix	Single-stranded Random (see text)
Stability	~ Stable Degraded by DNase	Subject to base hydrolysis Degraded by RNase
Function	Maintains genetic information in nucleus	Carries genetic information to cytoplasm

RNA differs from DNA in chemical composition, structure, and function (Table 56–1). In RNA the sugar is ribose, containing a hydroxyl group at the 2′ position, and thymine is replaced by the methylated uracil (U). RNA exists only as a single-stranded molecule and in much shorter lengths than DNA. The structure of RNA is more irregular, owing to the single-stranded nature of the molecule, but may contain some helical sections. RNA molecules of the same base sequence, however, will form the same three-dimensional structure as a result of adopting the most energetically favorable conformation. RNA is much less stable than DNA, not only because of the single-stranded more random structure, but also because of its susceptibility to alkaline hydrolysis via the 2′ hydroxyl group of the ribose moiety. RNA is also rapidly degraded by RNA-specific enzymes that are ubiquitous.

Nucleic Acid–Associated Enzymes

DNA must be synthesized when a cell divides so that the daughter cells retain an exact copy of the genetic information contained in chromosomes. RNA must be synthesized by all functioning cells to direct the synthesis of necessary proteins. DNA must be degraded during repair of damaged segments, and RNA is continually degraded and resynthesized. Enzymes that operate directly on nucleic acids effect these and other functions. Table 56–2 lists major categories of nucleic acid–specific enzymes and their *in vivo* functions. *In vitro*, purified enzymes have become laboratory tools for the molecular biologist, allowing genetic engineering and facilitating many nucleic acid assays. Polymerases catalyze the formation of phosphodiester bonds during synthesis; nucleases hydrolyze these bonds. Because RNases are present virtually everywhere, it is much more difficult to work with RNA *in vitro*. Restriction endonucleases are a special category of nucleases found only in bacteria, where they function to destroy foreign DNA. The recognition sites for restriction enzymes can vary from approximately 4 to 12 base pairs (bp) in length, and the cuts can form asymmetric or blunt ends (Fig. 56–4). The *in vivo* function and *in vitro* utility of many of these enzymes are discussed in the following sections.

Table 56–2. NUCLEIC ACID ENZYMES AND ASSOCIATED FUNCTIONS

Enzyme	*In Vivo* Function
Polymerases DNA polymerases RNA polymerases	Polymerases join DNA or RNA nucleotides together to form a single-stranded daughter molecule using a stretch of single-stranded parent molecule as a template. These enzymes perform synthesis according to base-pair rules and proceed in the 5' to 3' direction.
Reverse transcriptase	Found only in retroviruses, reverse transcriptase catalyzes the synthesis of DNA from either an RNA or DNA template.
DNA ligases	Joins DNA fragments formed by discontinuous synthesis in DNA replication or by DNA repair pathways.
Nucleases	
DNases, RNases	Nucleases "digest" nucleic acid molecules by breaking phosphodiester bonds.
Endonucleases Exonucleases	Endonucleases digest nucleic acids from the middle of the molecule, whereas exonucleases begin at a free end and may require a 3' or 5' end. Nucleases may have single-stranded, double-stranded, DNA, or RNA specificity. Some polymerases also have nuclease activity.
Restriction endonucleases	Bacterial endonucleases that recognize specific short DNA base-pair sequences and cleave the DNA molecule only at the recognition site.

Replication of DNA

The DNA duplication process, known as *semi-conservative replication*, uses each strand of the parent molecule to direct the synthesis of a daughter strand (Virshup, 1990). Because the base sequence of the parent strand dictates the sequence of the daughter strand, replication is faithful and the replication products consist of two dsDNA molecules, composed of one parent strand and one daughter strand each, with exactly the same base-pair sequence. Although this is conceptually simple, the process is complicated and involves a number of accessory proteins and enzymes. First, for synthesis to begin a small single-stranded region must be produced. This is not energetically favorable and must be effected with proteins that unwind and separate the strands of the helix. Next, a short RNA primer is synthesized complementary to the single-stranded sequence. DNA polymerase III proceeds with DNA synthesis, and later the RNA primer is excised and replaced with DNA by DNA polymerase I. Chromosomal DNA contains many initiation sites for replication, and this process occurs simultaneously across the chromosome. Interestingly, DNA polymerase III is a directional enzyme, and can synthesize DNA only in the 5′-3′ direction. This means that only one daughter strand can be synthesized continuously. The other daughter strand must be synthesized discontinuously in short fragments as the replication fork is opened up. These fragments are then joined together by DNA ligase. DNA polymerase III is also unique in that it has "proofreading" and exonuclease activity. If an incorrect nucleotide is added to the growing chain, it is detected and excised by the nuclease portion of the enzyme, and the correct nucleotide is then added. This helps explain the extraordinary fidelity of the DNA replication process. Postsynthesis repair mechanisms also contribute to the accuracy of replication (see "Mechanisms of DNA Repair," later).

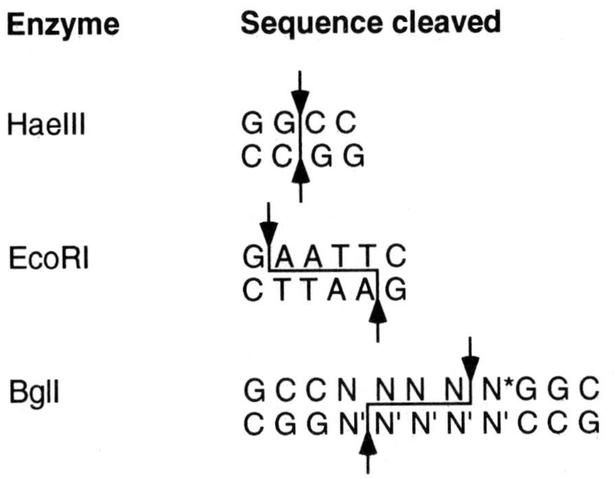

Figure 56–4. Examples of DNA restriction enzymes and their specificities. Enzymes are named for the bacteria from which they are isolated (where N is any base and N′ its pairing counterpart).

Transcription of DNA to RNA

Sections of DNA that specify amino acid sequences of proteins are called *genes*; one gene contains the amino acid sequence code for one protein as well as DNA sequences necessary for the regulation of the production of that protein. Although gene coding sequences are of paramount importance to the cell and to the function of the organism as a whole, the vast majority of the human genome is not composed of genes. The functions of the noncoding DNA regions are, however, not well understood. These sequences are sometimes called "junk DNA," but more likely have structural or other roles not yet discovered.

Protein synthesis begins with the activation of the appropriate gene. A copy of the gene is made from DNA in the form of RNA. Because the RNA copy carries the code from the DNA in the cell nucleus to the cytoplasm, where amino acid synthesis takes place, this type of RNA is called *messenger RNA* (mRNA). Messenger RNA is synthesized from only one strand of the DNA gene; the complementary DNA strand is not used. This is accomplished by a process called *transcription*. Synthesis of mRNA proceeds in much the same fashion as DNA replication, with the ssDNA sequence dictating the mRNA sequence using the same rules of base-pair complementarity (uracil base pairs with adenine). When the end of the gene is reached, mRNA synthesis is terminated.

Post-Transcriptional Modification

Before export to the cytoplasm, the mRNA molecule must be modified in several ways (Rosenthal, 1994). Messenger RNA contains both amino acid coding sequences (exons) and noncoding sequences (introns). Introns must be excised from the mRNA molecule before the exons can be used in protein synthesis. This is accomplished by a molecular complex termed a *spliceosome* (Sharp, 1988), composed of both small molecular weight RNA and protein. The spliceosome recognizes mRNA sequences that identify the boundaries of an intron, joins the flanking exons, and releases the intron. Splicing must be exact, because the addition or subtraction of a single nucleotide at the splice junction would change the 3-nucleotide reading frame (see later) in the following nucleotide sequences. The enzymatic activity of the spliceosome actually resides in the RNA portion of the complex and was the first reported example of nonprotein enzymatic function.

Further modifications to the mRNA molecule include the addition of 7-methyl guanosine residues to the 5′ end. This is called a *cap* and aids in the binding of the ribosome to the mRNA molecule for initiation of protein synthesis. A poly-A *tail*, which may be necessary for stability and transport to the cytoplasm, is added to the 3′ end. At this point, the mRNA molecule is ready to direct the synthesis of its corresponding protein.

Translation of RNA to Protein

Protein synthesis requires translation from the language of nucleotides to that of amino acids. Twenty different amino acids are used in protein synthesis; each amino acid is specified by one or more unique mRNA nucleotide triplets called *codons*. For example, AAG is the DNA codon for lysine and UCG is the triplet for serine. Thus, an amino acid–coding DNA sequence is read in groups of three nucleotides running in the 5′ to 3′ direction; this is the *reading frame* of a protein coding sequence. Three codons do not code for amino acids but instead signal the end of a gene (*stop* codons).

Translation from the mRNA nucleotide code to protein is mediated by ribosomes in the cytoplasm of the cell. A ribosome binds to the 5′ end of the mRNA and provides a stable chemical environment for all the molecules involved in protein synthesis. Amino acids are linked in the correct sequence by the action of small, adaptor RNA molecules called *transfer RNAs* (tRNA). Each tRNA molecule contains a region that is complementary to a particular mRNA codon: the *anticodon*. Linked to one end of the tRNA is the amino acid that corresponds to the complementary mRNA codon of the tRNA. A tRNA with the correct anticodon binds to the first codon in the mRNA sequence. When another tRNA binds to the next codon, ribosomal enzymes catalyze the formation of a peptide bond between the two amino acids linked to the tRNAs, removing the linkage between the first amino acid and its tRNA molecule. The first tRNA is ejected from the ribosome and a new tRNA binds to the next codon. As this process continues, the ribosome moves along the mRNA molecule, completing the synthesis of the amino acid chain. When the stop codon is reached, the ribosome detaches from the mRNA. In reality, several ribosomes can move along the same mRNA molecule, each translating the mRNA code into a new protein molecule.

Transcriptional Control

To allow for cellular differentiation and response to environmental stimuli, there must be mechanisms controlling the repertoire of gene transcription and protein translation. Some of these mechanisms operate at the level of DNA and control the transcription of mRNA (Rosenthal, 1994). For example, promoters are DNA sequences that are important for the initiation of mRNA transcription. Promoters are found upstream (toward the 5′ end) and at a relatively invariant distance from the beginning of the protein coding sequence. Promoters are often rich in adenine and thymine and have been called *TATA boxes*. Because A-T base pair bonds are weaker than G-C base-pair bonds, DNA unwinds more easily at repeat A-T sequences. After transcriptional activation, a local ssDNA region is produced and stabilized by the binding of RNA polymerase and its cofactors. Messenger RNA is synthesized from the local region of ssDNA, and the mRNA is quickly ejected as the DNA returns to its more energetically favorable double-stranded helical state.

Enhancers are DNA sequences that can augment mRNA transcription and may be found in different locations relative to the gene that they affect. Transcription factors are proteins that bind to enhancers and promoters, and selectively stimulate or inhibit mRNA transcription (Papavassiliou, 1995). Transcription factors, in turn, are controlled by cellular events, such as phosphorylation, or by other proteins, such as hormones and growth factors. A network of intracellular and extracellular chemical communications can thus select and control the synthesis of necessary proteins.

Because mRNA is far less stable than DNA, the half-life of mRNA is very short. New mRNA molecules are continually transcribed from DNA. As the cell responds to changes in transcriptional signals, the genes that are transcribed into mRNA can be quickly changed, resulting in the immediate synthesis of new proteins. Thus the cell has the ability to rapidly adjust its protein output in response to its environment.

Mechanisms of DNA Repair

Errors in DNA replication and damage to DNA during the normal cellular lifetime must be minimized to preserve the health of the entire organism. Several mechanisms operate to maintain the normal DNA sequence. First are the error-avoidance mechanisms that operate during DNA replication. The DNA polymerase that synthesizes new DNA polymers selects each successive nucleotide monomer based on its complementarity to the next nucleotide in the template strand. Fidelity at this level is high, and most errors in synthesis are avoided at this stage. Nevertheless, an occasional base may be incorrectly added to the growing strand. To adjust for this, the proofreading activity of the polymerase can recognize the error, remove the incorrect base, and proceed again with synthesis. Together, the error avoidance mechanisms reduce base-pair mismatches to approximately 1 in 10 million (Radman, 1988). This represents a 100,000-fold increase in efficiency compared with the error rate of 1 in 100 bases for *in vitro* solid-phase oligonucleotide synthesis.

In spite of remarkable error avoidance in DNA replication, occasional mistakes do occur. In addition, DNA suffers damage from normal biochemical reactions, and injury from nonphysiologic agents, such as ultraviolet light and environmental carcinogens. There are several repair mechanisms that function in this regard (Table 56–3). The details of these mechanisms were originally studied in mutants of the bac-

Table 56–3. DNA REPAIR PATHWAYS

Mismatch repair	Checks for errors made when DNA is replicated. Any mispaired bases in the daughter strand are removed and replaced with the correct match.
Base excision repair	Replaces bases damaged by normal cellular processes, such as oxidation.
Nucleotide excision repair	Recognizes and repairs large lesions in DNA that may be caused by outside agents, such as ultraviolet light and chemicals.
Transcription-coupled repair	Subpathway of nucleotide excision repair in which damage in transcribed genes is repaired faster than damage in nontranscribed genes.

terium *Escherichia coli* that displayed a marked increase in the rate of spontaneous mutation or a change in DNA sequence. These mutants were found to have defects in one or more of the proteins necessary for DNA repair. More recently, very similar mechanisms have been described in human cells.

Mismatch repair functions immediately after DNA replication to replace mismatches bases with the correct ones (Modrich, 1994). Four proteins recognize the error in the newly synthesized, nonmethylated daughter strand and excise the region spanning the mismatch. DNA polymerase III and ligase restore the correct sequence and integrity of the daughter strand. The importance of this mechanism in stabilizing the genome is evidenced by recent studies associating hereditary nonpolyposis colorectal cancer with defects in mismatch repair proteins.

Injury to the bases within the DNA helix are repaired via the base excision pathway. The defective base is first removed, then the sugar-phosphate residue is excised. A polymerase then fills in the gap with the correct nucleotide to pair with the opposite strand.

Larger, bulky lesions that distort the DNA helix may be caused by UV radiation, carcinogens, and therapeutic drugs, among other agents. Such damage is removed by the nucleotide excision repair (NER) pathway, which utilizes an enzyme system composed of many proteins to hydrolyze phosphodiester bonds and to remove an oligonucleotide containing the lesion (Sancar, 1994). The gap is then filled in by DNA polymerase and ligated. Some of the possible consequences of the loss of NER activity are exemplified by the disease xeroderma pigmentosum (XP), which is caused by mutations in NER. XP results in extreme sensitivity to sunlight, with skin cancers occurring at an early age.

Nucleotide excision repair has in some instances been shown to be preferentially operative on the "sense" strand of genes that are transcribed and expressed as proteins. In addition, some of the proteins that are required for NER are also essential for transcription initiation. This has led to the idea that some NER is coupled to transcription, and to a model for transcription-coupled repair (Hanawalt, 1994). In this model, the transcription activity of RNA polymerase II is stopped by lesions in DNA, but the polymerase remains tightly bound at the damaged site to recruit repair enzymes.

It is now clear that DNA repair plays a central role in the life of the cell. Recent evidence also indicates that several proteins that are primary repair proteins also function in transcription and in regulation of the cell cycle. Thus, the processes involving DNA appear to be highly integrated and will be increasingly studied as a whole and in relation to human disease.

DNA Mutations

In spite of extensive repair mechanisms, alterations in DNA base sequence (mutations) occur, and to some extent must occur for the process of evolution to continue. Yet for an individual organism, some mutations are clearly harmful and can be associated with cancer and with inherited genetic disease. Studies of these diseases have led to the characterization of the various types of mutations that occur in the human genome (Weatherall, 1987). These can be conceptually grouped into a few major categories (Table 56–4). A point mutation is found in the beta-globin gene in sickle cell anemia (Kan, 1992). A thymidine base replaces an adenine base, causing a critical change in the structure of hemoglobin. Muscular dystrophy is caused by deletions in the gene for the muscle protein dystrophin. In the Becker form of the disease, the deletions do not disrupt the reading frame, but in the more severe Duchenne form, the reading frame is changed by the deletions, effectively abolishing the function of the protein (Liechti-Gallati, 1989).

Human DNA contains many short sequences of nucleotides (microsatellite DNA) that are sometimes grouped in tandem arrays and are repeated many times throughout the human genome. The number of tandem repeats at particular locations is a heritable trait. Some trinucleotide repeats have been found to increase in number in association with disease (Sutherland, 1994). In fragile X syndrome, expression of the disease is associated with the amplification beyond a certain limit of the number of an intragenic trinucleotide repeat sequence.

Translocations may not always be detectable by chromosomal karyotype analysis. At the gene level, a translocation

Table 56–4. TYPES OF DNA MUTATIONS AND EXAMPLES OF ASSOCIATED DISEASES

Mutation	Description	Disease
Point	Single base-pair substitution	Sickle cell anemia
Deletion/insertion	Subtraction/addition of amino acid codons in multiples of three; reading frame is retained	Becker's muscular dystrophy
Deletion/insertion with frameshift	Subtraction/addition of amino acid codons in non-multiples of three; results in a shift of the reading frame and a completely different amino acid coding sequence from the mutation on	Duchenne's muscular dystrophy
Amplification	Increase in the number of repeat sequences in microsatellite DNA	Fragile X
Translocation	Interchromosomal exchange of large chromosome segments	Chronic myelogenous leukemia

7

may create a fusion gene, the combination of two different genes abnormally joined at the translocation site. This can create not only an altered gene transcript, but may bring the product of one gene under the transcriptional control of the other. The Philadelphia chromosome, found in most cases of chronic myelogenous leukemia, produces a fusion gene between the *ABL* gene and a region termed the *breakpoint cluster region*. The resulting ABL fusion protein is larger than the normal protein and has increased enzymatic activity (Cline, 1994).

It is both the type of mutation as well as its location in relation to the gene that determines the ultimate effect on the protein product. Mutations may have no effect on protein expression or functional activity; many human proteins exist in detectable variants that have no disease association. Mutations occurring in intron regions presumably have no effect at all. Even small mutations, however, in regions that code for key functional domains may drastically alter or eliminate function. "Nonsense mutations," mutations that change an amino acid codon to a stop codon, or vice versa, result in abnormally short or long protein products, respectively. Similarly, mutations within sequences that denote intron-exon splice sites could eliminate exons or introduce introns into the transcribed mRNA. Mutations may also occur in regulatory sequences, such as promoters or enhancers, producing dramatic effects on the levels of transcription.

NUCLEIC ACID ANALYSES

The unique biochemical properties of nucleic acids have been exploited to yield information about the biology or biochemistry of a system. While some of the assays, such as electrophoresis, are applicable to other biochemical building blocks, such as proteins and lipids, most are particular to nucleic acids. The following sections briefly describe the principles of the basic categories of analyses used to characterize DNA and RNA: electrophoretic separations, hybridization assays, amplification techniques, and restriction fragment length polymorphisms. In practice the categories are often combined to produce novel variations of the same theme, for example, a complete assay may involve amplification, electrophoresis, and hybridization.

Electrophoretic Separation

The repeating sugar-phosphate backbone of nucleic results in a net negative charge evenly distributed over these linear molecules. Therefore, movement of DNA or RNA in response to an electric field will be proportional to the molecular weight or length of the molecule. This property is used to characterize the size of nucleic acid fragments by electrophoretic separation. The format is analogous to that used for the separation of proteins according to size. Multiple samples are applied in separate wells at one end of a solid but porous separation medium. When a voltage is applied, the samples move toward the positive electrode in a linear fashion, with each sample well forming one lane of migration. The solid electrophoretic medium and array of sample wells is known as a *gel*. Size standards, referred to as *DNA* or *RNA ladders*, are mixtures of nucleic acids of known fragment length that are analyzed in one or more lanes of the gel. Comparison of the distance of migration of an unknown sample with the ladder, either by eye or by computer-assisted measurement, allows size determination.

The composition and concentration of the separation medium determines the size of the fragments, which may be separated into distinct bands. Other variables that contribute to resolution are the thickness of the gel, the length of the electrophoresis path, the time of electrophoresis, and the applied voltage. In practice these factors are adjusted empirically and controlled as carefully as possible to ensure reproducibility from day to day. Agarose is the separation medium most often used, usually in conjunction with a horizontal electrophoresis bed in which the gel is submerged in buffer, the *submarine gel*. Samples are made heavy with sucrose or Ficoll and loaded into slots in the gel through the buffer (Fig. 56–5). Higher resolving power, allowing differentiation of a single base pair in length, is achieved with acrylamide, usually used in a vertical format. The simplest approach to visualizing the bands separated by electrophoresis is by staining with intercalating dyes (e.g., ethidium bromide), which insert between stacked bases, and viewing with UV transillumination. Direct visualization requires that the band achieve a significant concentration. In some applications the nucleic acid fragments may be detected by a radioactive or fluorescent tag, which can increase sensitivity.

The molecules in genomic DNA are reduced to fragments, which may be resolved by electrophoresis, through digestion with restriction enzymes. Restriction enzymes with a relatively simple recognition sequence produce fragments less than 50 kilobase (kb) pairs in length. Extremely large DNA fragments, measured in megabase pairs (Mbp), are produced from digestion with enzymes with a complex recognition sequence and must be separated in special electrophoretic systems utilizing a pulsed electrical field. Most applications of DNA electrophoresis use nondenaturing conditions, that is, the fragments resolved into bands are double stranded. By contrast, most RNA separations use denaturing conditions (either formamide or glyoxal) to eliminate secondary structure of the single-stranded molecules. RNA molecules, as transcripts of DNA, are presized and relatively small, so that no digestion is required prior to electrophoresis.

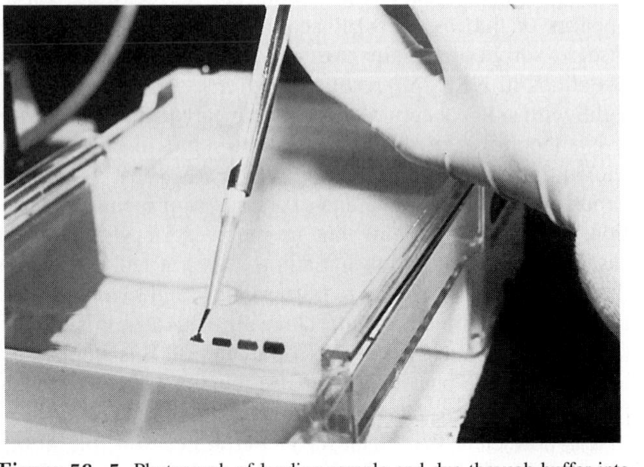

Figure 56–5. Photograph of loading sample and dye through buffer into well of agarose gel in submarine gel electrophoresis apparatus.

Nucleic Acid Hybridization

Hybridization is a fundamental concept in nucleic acid biochemistry. It is a direct consequence of the stable double-stranded structure of DNA under physiologic conditions. As discussed earlier, the helix is formed of two antiparallel strands of DNA, held together by the combined strength of many specific hydrogen bonds between complementary base pairs as well as by hydrophobic shielding of bases from an aqueous environment. Central to the hybridization reaction is the fact that the binding between separate molecules (strands) is both reversible and base-sequence specific. When neither DNA strand is labeled, the process of reforming the stable double-stranded structure is referred to as *annealing*. If one strand is labeled, that is, has a marker that is capable of being detected in some fashion, the labeled strand is referred to as a *probe* and the process is called *hybridization*, because a hybrid molecule is formed between a labeled and unlabeled strand. RNA molecules can also participate in the hybridization process. Base pairing may occur between complementary strands of DNA, between DNA and RNA, and between complementary strands of RNA, resulting in DNA-DNA, DNA-RNA, and RNA-RNA duplex structures. Duplex molecules with exact complementarity in base sequence form the most stable structures, but structures with varying degrees of base pair mismatch may form depending on the conditions. The relative instability of these mismatched duplexes will be reflected in the lowered temperature of their disassociation (lower T_m).

Environmental conditions can be manipulated to control the degree of base pair mismatching that will be tolerated in a duplex structure, that is, the *stringency* of the sequence match (Fig. 56–6). Low stringency refers to conditions such as high salt, low temperature, and no formamide, which favor shielding of hydrophobic bases from the aqueous environment, even without perfect alignment; the match need not be perfect. High stringency conditions—high temperature (close to T_m), low salt, and high formamide—will only allow the most perfectly matched duplex structures to remain in a stable helix conformation.

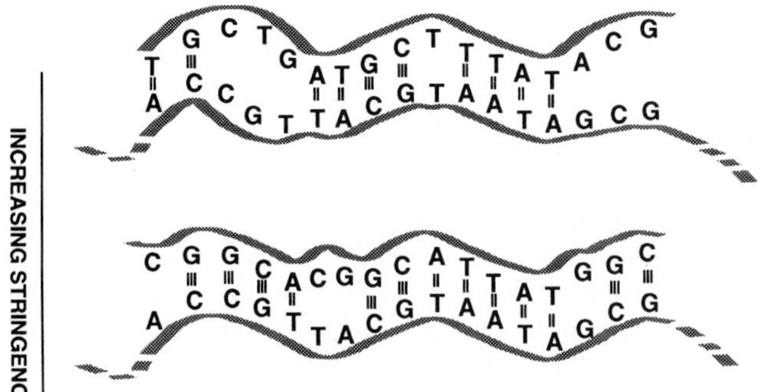

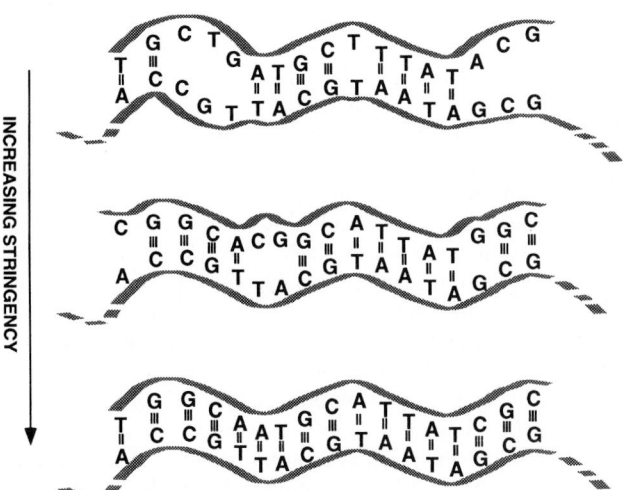

Figure 56–6. Illustration of stringency. As the stringency of the hybridization solution is increased, fewer mismatches are tolerated in a hybrid duplex. At very high stringency, even a single base-pair mismatch will disrupt the duplex.

Hybridization Assays: Basic Components

When the hybridization reaction is used to analyze the nucleic acid content of an unknown sample, the process is known as a *hybridization assay*. The property of complementary base pairing allows fragments of known composition (the probe) to interrogate an unknown for the presence of matching (complementary) sequences. All hybridization assays therefore require several basic elements: a probe, a sample, controlled conditions permissive to complementary base pairing, and a method for detection of specific probe-sample hybrids. Each of these elements will be briefly discussed later, as well as the variations in formats that have been developed to allow hybridization assays to be performed and interpreted.

Probe

The specificity of the hybridization reaction is determined by the probe; thus the probe is central to a hybridization assay in the same way that the primary antibody is central to an immunoassay. A probe is a well-characterized fragment of nucleic acid, either DNA or RNA. In most assay formats it is the probe that carries the reporter group into the reaction, although variations occur. Reporter groups may be radioactive or nonradioactive (i.e., affinity label).

Most probes are produced through recombinant nucleic acid technology, as illustrated in Figure 56–7. Plasmids, short, circular double-stranded segments of DNA, are harnessed as vectors to propagate desired sequences in bacteria. The segment of interest is introduced into the plasmid using restriction enzyme digestion and ligation, resulting in a new "recombined" molecule that retains the ability to be propagated in bacteria and includes the DNA sequence of interest. Bacteria containing the recombinant plasmid can be grown in culture, and the small circular plasmids can be easily separated from the bacterial genome on the basis of size. Many identical copies are obtained, and thus the DNA is often referred to as *cloned*. Purified plasmid may be used as probe in instances where vector sequences do not interfere with the specificity of the reaction. In many applications the inserted DNA sequence is separated from the vector sequence by digesting the isolated plasmid with the same restriction enzyme originally used in construction of the recombinant molecule. The probe resulting from either of these approaches is a double-stranded DNA molecule. Double-stranded probes must be denatured prior to use and probe reannealing limits the extent of hybridization of probe with target. Unmodified plasmid vector is a commonly used negative control for this type of probe.

Plasmid vectors have been constructed to include RNA promoter regions adjacent to the inserted DNA sequence. These recombinant plasmids are used to produce RNA transcripts of the DNA insert. The result is single-stranded RNA that will not undergo probe self-hybridization. Controlling the orientation of the DNA insert with respect to the RNA

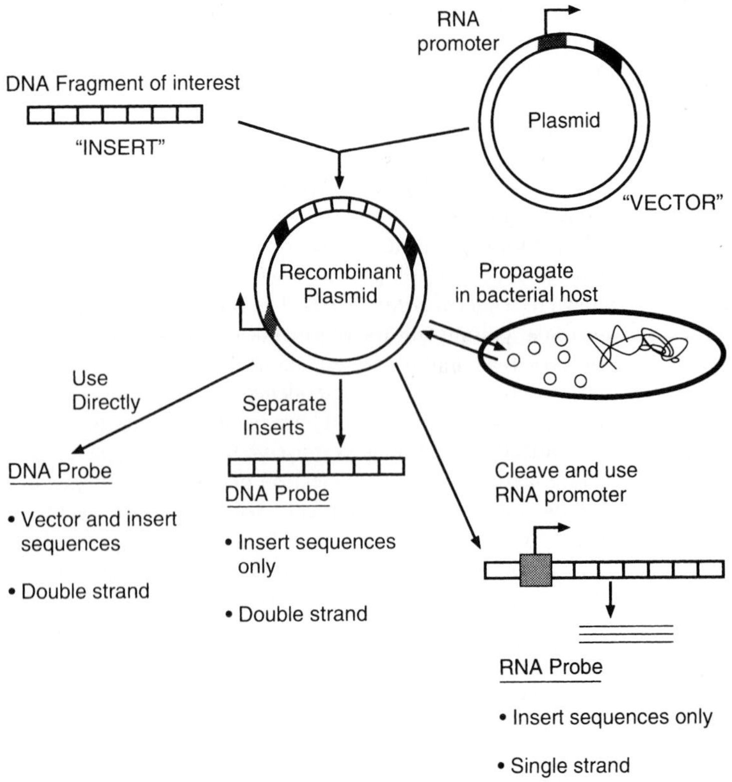

Figure 56–7. Production of cloned probes. Insertion of a known foreign segment of DNA into a plasmid vector results in a recombinant plasmid. Plasmids of this type are small circular pieces of DNA that are propagated by growth in a bacterial host. The plasmid DNA is easily separated from the bacterial chromosome on the basis of size. Purified recombinant plasmid may be used as the probe. This produces a double-stranded DNA probe with both insert and vector sequences. Alternatively, insert sequences may be purified from the plasmid vector and used alone as the probe. If the plasmid contains an RNA promoter region, then RNA probes may be produced using an RNA polymerase to transcribe the insert sequences. Because only one strand is transcribed, the resulting RNA probes are single stranded. (Reprinted by permission of the author: In situ Hybridization: Principles and Practice. *Clinical Immunology Newsletter* 10:120–126, 1990. Copyright 1990 by Elsevier Science Inc.)

promoter allows production of transcripts in the *sense* (same as mRNA) or *antisense* (complementary to mRNA) direction. In many applications the sense transcripts form ideal negative control probes for hybridization reactions with antisense probes. Nonspecifically bound RNA probe, that is, RNA not in a stable duplex structure, can be removed with the use of RNase specific for single-stranded RNA. The lability of RNA requires that the probes be handled with extreme care to prevent degradation (sterile technique, treated water and glassware).

Recombinant probes, whether DNA or RNA, are genetically complex; that is, they may include many kilobases of genetic information. By contrast, probes produced by synthetic methods are relatively short segments of DNA. Oligonucleotide probes produced by automated chemical reactions are usually 15 to 45 bases in length, synthesized to produce a specified base sequence. Probes with very high specificity of hybridization can be designed on the basis of sequence information available in data banks. They can be generated in a sense or antisense direction at a relatively low cost. These short probes are single stranded, diffuse into the target and hybridize rapidly because of their small size, and are extremely sensitive to even single base-pair mismatches. The final sensitivity achieved with oligonucleotide probes is lower than that achieved with recombinant probes because of their limited genetic complexity. Multiple oligonucleotide probes directed to different areas of the same target have in some instances been used to increase the sensitivity by increasing the representation of the target sequence in the probe mixture. This approach is analogous to the use of a blend of monoclonal antibodies that react to different epitopes of the same complex antigen. Probes longer than those obtained by direct chemical synthesis may be generated with the polymerase chain reaction or other amplification technology (see later). These probes may be single stranded or double stranded, depending on the conditions employed, and may be as long as the product of the amplification reaction, in most cases, 100 bases to 1 kilobase in length.

Sample

While probe selection and preparation is central to determining the sensitivity and specificity of the hybridization assay, the contribution of sample preparation to a successful assay cannot be overlooked. In clinical applications samples of interest may be quite diverse. For example, a microbiology laboratory could anticipate testing specimens of blood, urine, stool, and sputum. Integrity of RNA targets may be difficult to maintain under such conditions, and even DNA may be degraded with improper handling. The goal of sample preparation is to maintain nucleic acid integrity and to make the target genetic information available for interaction with the probe. For some applications, the requirement of target integrity will dictate immediate snap freezing or addition of lysis buffers containing potent RNase and DNase inhibitors. In other applications, more routine methods of sample collection will allow adequate target preservation.

The physical and chemical similarities of nucleic acids, regardless of source, allow for uniform methods of extraction and purification. For many assays it is preferable to extensively purify DNA or RNA to remove inhibitors of enzymes to be added to the assay (such as a restriction enzyme or polymerase) and to maximize accessibility of the target to the probe. Complete purification schemes, however, are time consuming and require a relatively large amount of starting sample. In many applications relatively abbreviated sample purifications can be used. Purifications commonly use cell lysis (mechanical, chemical, or both), protease treatment, and organic or inorganic extractions.

Controlled Conditions Permissive for Complementary Base Pairing

The sensitivity and specificity of the hybridization reaction is greatly influenced by the physical-chemical environment during the reaction and subsequent detection/collection of hybrid molecules. In practice, the *hybridization cocktail* is the medium used to control the environment of the hybridization reaction. Empirically designed, the hybridization cocktail is a mixture of reagents selected to favor interaction of nucleic acids through sequence specific hydrogen bonds rather than via charge. The components vary widely, but include buffers, salts, denaturants such as formamide, high molecular weight polymers, carrier DNA or RNA, and various components added to reduce background (such as detergents, bovine serum albumin, Ficoll). Such a complex mixture is conveniently referred to as a *cocktail.* The ionic strength of both the hybridization cocktail and the subsequent washes is most often modulated by the concentration of a *s*aline *s*odium *c*itrate buffer (SSC), composed of 0.15 mol/L sodium chloride and 0.015 mol/L trisodium citrate, pH 7.0. The short-hand notation for these conditions refers to the strength of SSC; that is, $2\times$SSC, $0.1\times$SSC. The final stringency of the hybridization reaction is controlled by the formamide and salt concentration of the hybridization cocktail, the temperature of the hybridization reaction, and the temperature and salt concentration of the washing steps.

Detection of Hybrids

A wide variety of techniques have been applied to collection and analysis of specific hybrids, discussed briefly in the section on assay formats. Once specific hybrids have been collected, methods of detection are obviously linked to methods of labeling. Many research applications and the first clinical applications of hybridization assays used radioactive labels such as phosphorus-32 (^{32}P), iodine-125 (^{125}I), sulfur-35 (^{35}S), carbon-14 (^{14}C), and tritium (^{3}H), with detection through autoradiography or scintillation counting. Specific activity of the label directly influenced the sensitivity of the detection. For clinical applications, alternatives to radioisotopic labeling were sought. Radioactive probes have a relatively short half-life, making one of the key reagents in the hybridization assay unstable. In addition, the hazard to laboratory personnel and cost of radioactive waste disposal contributed to the need for nonradioactive methods. Nonisotopically labeled probes are stable reagents, greatly facilitating commercial production and standardization, which are crucial for reproducibility of assays.

Nonisotopic labeling and detection methods for nucleic acids have many similarities to immunochemical assays developed for nonisotopic protein detection. In some applications nucleic acids are directly linked to a signal-generating compound, usually a fluorochrome but occasionally an enzyme. This situation is analogous to immunoassays in which the primary antibody is labeled. More commonly, nucleic acids are indirectly detected in a multistep assay similar in concept to an indirect antibody reaction. Biotin, a commonly used affinity label for immunoassays, was the first affinity label introduced into nucleic acids (Langer, 1981). Biotin itself generates no signal but is detected by high-affinity interaction with an avidin or streptavidin molecule, which is in turn complexed or conjugated to a signal-generating enzyme or fluorochrome. Many other functional groups have been developed as nonisotopic labels, such as bromodeoxyuridine, digoxigenin, and sulfone. Detection in these cases is achieved with high-affinity antibodies directed against the functional group. These antibodies are usually directly linked to a signal-generating enzyme or fluorochrome, functioning like a labeled secondary antibody in an immunohistochemistry reaction. Biotin may also be detected with an antibiotin antibody rather than an avidin or streptavidin molecule.

Because affinity labels are detected with large bulky proteins, such as avidin or antibody, availability of the label to the detection reagent is a crucial factor in the determination of sensitivity. Increasing the number of affinity tags will not necessarily increase the number of detecting molecules that will be bound to the nucleic acid. In addition, because affinity labels are themselves bulky, overincorporation into the nucleic acid molecule can lead to steric hindrance of the hybridization reaction. For these reasons, the specific activity of the affinity label does not directly control the sensitivity of the detection.

One advantage of the indirect detection of affinity labels is that a variety of detection methods can be used for the same label (Fig. 56–8). For example, biotin may be detected with avidin linked to an enzyme with subsequent color or chemiluminescent detection, or avidin with fluorescent tag. For all nonradioactive methods, the detection portion of the assay is crucial in obtaining optimal sensitivity. An effective hybridization reaction can be marred by detection reagents with poor background and suboptimal signal generation. The choice of the enzyme labels (peroxidase versus alkaline phosphatase), enzyme substrate (colorimetric versus chemi-

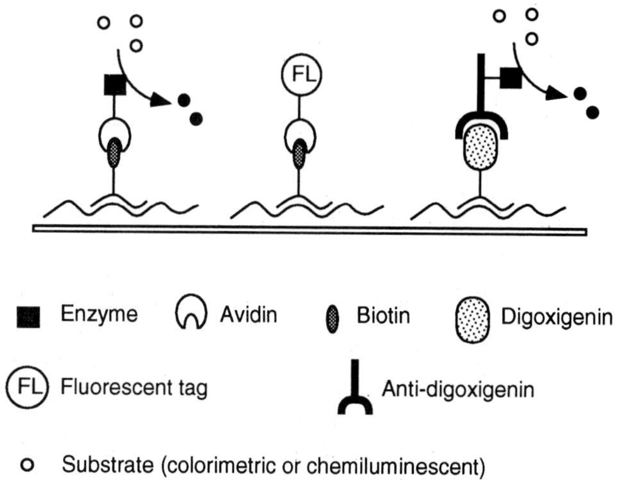

Figure 56–8. Examples of affinity-labeled probe detection systems. (Reproduced with permission from Unger ER, Piper MA: Nucleic acid biochemistry and diagnostic applications. *In* Burton CA, Ashwood ER [eds]: Tietz Textbook of Clinical Chemistry, 2nd ed. Philadelphia, W. B. Saunders Company, 1994.)

luminescent), and even source of reagents is critical for optimal results.

Hybridization Assay Formats

A wide variety of hybridization assay formats have been developed, each designed to solve the methodologic problems of the hybridization assay: conditions permitting specific complementary base pairing, a method to detect hybrids, and an interpretation of the result. Each method has particular strengths and weaknesses, and selection of format is dictated by the clinical setting and the particular diagnostic question. There is no one perfect assay. Several of the basic formats will be briefly described, along with their particular strengths and weaknesses.

Each hybridization assay requires both positive and negative controls for validation. A positive sample control is one known to contain sequences complementary to the probe. This is used to establish that sample preparation is adequate to release target for the hybridization assay, and to ensure that probe will hybridize with the specific target under the assay conditions. The sample control may also be used to monitor the sensitivity of the assay if the positive control is chosen near the lower limits of detection. A negative sample control, that is, one known not to contain sequences complementary to the probe, is used to monitor the specificity of the probe target interactions. Controls for the probe include vector sequences or unrelated probes labeled, hybridized, and detected under identical assay conditions. These latter controls allow monitoring of the background signal generated by localization of probe through nonhybridized interactions, such as charge or trapping. In clinical practice, additional controls may be employed to monitor each step of the hybridization assay.

Liquid or Solution-Phase Hybridization

In liquid hybridization assays, both the sample and probe interact in solution, which maximizes the kinetics of the reaction. The sample nucleic acids are generally purified from contaminating proteins and lipids, which could interfere with the collection of hybrids at the end of the assay, and some sample degradation is tolerated by the assay. The sample is denatured and randomly sheared before addition of single-stranded probe lacking the ability to self-hybridize.

Hybridization may be detected by the specific binding of hybrids to a solid matrix, such as hydroxyapatite, which binds only duplex structures. Once hybrids are bound, unhybridized probe may be efficiently removed by washing. Detection of the label on the bound probe permits quantitation of the hybridization reaction. In a variation of this approach, one commercial assay (Hybrid-Capture™) uses an antibody specific for RNA-DNA hybrids to specifically bind duplex structures formed of the DNA target and RNA probe. An alternative analysis involves digestion of the hybridization reaction mixture with S1 nuclease, an enzyme that acts only on single-stranded nucleic acid. Duplex structures resistant to digestion may then be precipitated by treatment with trichloroacetic acid. In the hybridization protection assay, label on the probe is protected from chemical degradation only when the probe is involved in a duplex structure.

Many other variations of the solution-phase hybridization assay are in use. Optimal kinetics, toleration for abbreviated purification steps, and some sample degradation make the assay adaptable for clinical application. Quantitation of the reaction product may be achieved, depending on the detection system. The solution-phase format does not permit identification of the size of the hybridizing product. Low positive reactions are difficult to interpret because low levels of specific target and high levels of weakly cross-reacting target will yield similar results. Solution-phase hybridization is adaptable to the 96-well format with an ELISA-type readout, and increasing automation of the assay can be anticipated.

Solid-Support Hybridization

Variations of the solid-support hybridization assays include dot or blot hybridization, Southern and northern hybridization, and *in situ* hybridization. In these assays the hybridization occurs in a biphasic environment, a solid phase (usually sample) and a liquid phase (usually probe). The kinetics of hybridization to a nucleic acid bound to a solid support are greatly slowed, and the extent of the hybridization reaction is limited. These disadvantages are often outweighed by the convenience of having a solid medium to carry through multiple steps of the assay.

DOT/BLOT HYBRIDIZATION

In this assay format, multiple samples are immobilized in a geometric array on a nitrocellulose or nylon membrane. The name of the assay comes from the shape of each sample on the membrane. When samples are applied by hand, the shape is more random (blot). With the use of commercially available manifolds, samples are usually applied with the use of suction, the sample shape is very regular—round (dot) or elongated (slot). The solid matrix allows multiple samples to be processed through all steps of the assay simultaneously. The fact that all samples and controls are exposed to exactly the same reagents and conditions increases the standardization of the assay.

The extent of sample preparation varies from complete purification of nucleic acids before application to the filter, to direct application of unpurified sample. Some degree of sample degradation is tolerated by the assay. Purified nucleic acids have the advantage of being most available for interaction with probe and having the least problems with background. Individual sample purification, however, is time consuming and labor intensive. Methods using direct application of unpurified sample take the entire array through an abbreviated purification procedure, which usually involves lysis and denaturation, protein digestion, and washing with detergent. The advantages of this approach are that it is applicable to small amounts of starting material and minimizes sample preparation time. However, the final sensitivity of the reaction is lower and background from nonspecific probe interactions can make the assay unreliable.

Interpretation of the results of a dot/blot hybridization assay is relatively straightforward. If hybridization has occurred, a signal is generated in the specified spot. Depending on the label used for signal generation, results may be quantitated. However, usually a simple yes/no interpretation is given; that is, the sample has more or less signal than adjacent samples and known positive and negative controls.

Weak signals, which may result from a very small amount of specific target or from a large amount of weakly cross-reacting target, may cause problems in interpretation. No information is available about the size of the hybridizing fragments.

One interesting variation of the dot/blot assay is known as the reverse dot/blot assay. In this format, applied in situations where one sample must be tested with many different probes and sample may be limited, the label is carried into the assay by the sample. The probes are fixed to the solid support in a linear or matrix array. Multiple unlabeled probes are hybridized with one sample. Areas of specific hybrid formation are identified and interpreted as in the standard dot/blot assay.

SOUTHERN AND NORTHERN HYBRIDIZATIONS

Both Southern and northern hybridizations combine electrophoretic separation of test nucleic acid with transfer to a solid support and subsequent hybridization. These assays, therefore, not only give information about the presence of hybridization, but permit the determination of the molecular weight of the hybridizing species.

The original procedure was termed *Southern blot hybridization* or *Southern blotting*, after its inventor, E.M. Southern (Southern, 1975). In this assay the test nucleic acid is DNA. Northern blotting was named by analogy for the technique utilizing RNA as the test nucleic acid. (Extending the analogy even further, the western blot is a similar procedure in which proteins are subjected to electrophoresis and transfer; a southwestern blot has been described for a technique separating and blotting DNA followed by incubation with protein solutions to permit evaluation of specific DNA binding proteins.)

Sample preparation is time consuming and labor intensive for both of these techniques. Degradation of sample nucleic acids is not tolerated by the assays, and a relatively large amount of starting material is required. For Southern hybridizations, the DNA must be purified with minimal shearing. This is because sizing of the DNA fragments is achieved through digestion with one or more restriction enzymes. Shearing and degradation introduce random breaks in the sample, reducing the quantity available to be specifically cut at appropriate recognition sequences. Impurities in the sample may interfere with the activity and sequence specificity of the restriction enzyme. Partially or improperly digested samples can produce spurious band sizes or result in such a reduced concentration of the specific band that it is no longer detected during hybridization. For northern hybridizations the starting material is RNA, and extreme care must be taken to avoid degradation during sample collection and preparation because of the ubiquitous nature of RNases. RNA is composed of fragment sizes determined by translation and processing of message and ribosomal RNA. It is not digested before electrophoresis but is separated under denaturing conditions to remove secondary structure.

The size-separated fragments in the agarose gel are then transferred to a nylon or nitrocellulose filter. As originally designed, the transfer occurred passively through capillary action. Most current applications use vacuum or pressure to speed the transfer. After transfer, the nucleic acids are immobilized by baking or UV cross-linking and the entire membrane is hybridized with labeled probe.

Hybridization is followed by autoradiographic or colorimetric detection of bands containing sequences complementary to the probe. Interpretation involves both detection of a hybridizing species and determination of the molecular weight of the molecule. These technically demanding assays require several days to perform but may be required in clinical applications in which the information cannot be obtained in any other format. The presence of bands at molecular weights different from normal or germline (developmentally unaltered) samples can indicate a change in the genetic material.

IN SITU HYBRIDIZATION

In situ hybridization is simply detection of specific genetic information within a morphologic context. This specialized type of solid-support assay involves taking morphologically intact tissue, cells, or chromosomes affixed to a glass microscope slide through the hybridization process. Autoradiographic, colorimetric, and fluorescent methods of detection have been applied. Evaluation of the final product is very analogous to evaluation of immunohistochemistry and requires experience in histopathology. In situations where localization of target within a tissue or cell is important, the method has much to commend it. The methods of *in situ* hybridization can be very labor intensive and tedious. Recent improvements, resulting in automated processing of slides through the assay, hold much promise for more widespread adoption of this technique (see Chap. 61).

DNA CHIP TECHNOLOGY

A novel variation of solid-support hybridization has recently been developed (Pease, 1994). Using miniaturized silicone chips and solid-phase light-generated synthesis, densely packed arrays of bound oligonucleotides have been constructed. The chips, containing all combinations of relatively short oligonucleotides (for example, 65,536 combinations for an octamer) can then be hybridized to a fluorescently labeled sample. Localized fluorescence indicates the presence of a complementary sequence, and through alignment of overlapping sequences, rapid sequence analysis can be performed.

Amplification Methods

It is virtually impossible to read any medical journal without encountering at least one application of "PCR" technology. The polymerase chain reaction (PCR) has forever changed the scope of research questions that can be addressed by virtually eliminating the problem of limited sample size. The importance and elegance of the concept has been recognized through awarding of the Nobel Prize in Chemistry to its inventor, Kary Mullis, less than 10 years after publication of the first practical application of PCR (Saiki, 1985). This technique is just beginning to have an impact in laboratory diagnostics. Technology transfer from research to routine clinical application has been slower than anticipated because of some limitations of current methods (described later). The following section emphasizes PCR and some variations based on PCR, which are most widely used and appear to be positioned for first introduction into laboratory diagnostics. However, other methodologies that result in

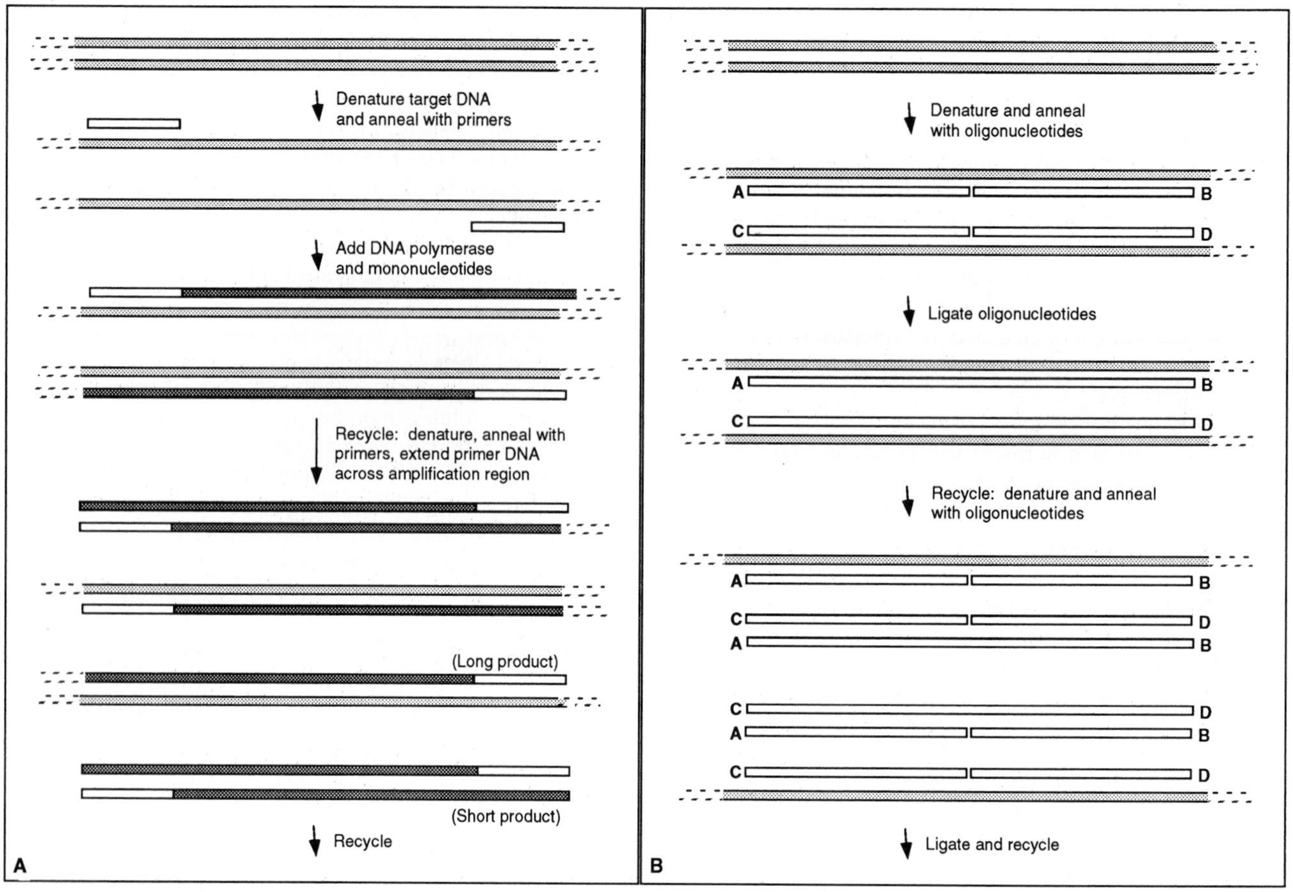

Figure 56–9. Comparison of polymerase chain reaction and ligase chain reaction. *A*, Schematic diagram of polymerase chain reaction. *B*, Ligase chain reaction. (Redrawn with permission from Unger ER, Piper MA: Nucleic acid biochemistry and diagnostic applications. *In* Burton CA, Ashwood ER [eds]: Tietz Textbook of Clinical Chemistry, 2nd ed. Philadelphia, W. B. Saunders Company, 1994.)

multiplication of target, probe, or signal, grouped together as amplification technologies, have been developed and will be mentioned briefly.

Polymerase Chain Reaction

The polymerase chain reaction uses common tools of the molecular biologist: DNA polymerase, the enzyme that produces a complementary copy of a single-stranded DNA template in a 5′ to 3′ direction, and oligonucleotides (called *primers*) that bind (anneal) to a specific complementary target and form a specific initiation or priming site directing the action of the polymerase reaction. As illustrated in Figure 56–9*A*, the primers are selected to be complementary to opposite strands flanking the target sequence. The steps of the reaction are denaturation of double-stranded target, annealing of primers, and subsequent polymerization or elongation, resulting in a doubling of the target sequence. All components of the reaction are mixed together at the beginning of the assay, and the reaction is moved from one step to the next by changing the temperature; that is, denaturation at 94°C, annealing at 55°C, and elongation at 72°C. The individual steps are rapid (20 to 30 seconds) and one round of amplification or *cycle* is accomplished in 60 to 90 seconds. The instrument that takes samples through the multiple cycles of changing temperature is known as a *thermocycler*.

With the addition of an initial reverse transcriptase (RT) step, RNA targets can also be successfully amplified, the reaction being known as *RT-PCR*. Reactants in a typical PCR reaction include the sample DNA, each deoxynucleotide (dATP, dCTP, dGTP, dTTP; collectively called *dNTPs*), primers, appropriate buffer, and thermostable polymerase in 50 or 100 μL volume. Assuming perfect fidelity of the reaction, 20 cycles would result in a millionfold amplification of the target. Because practical levels of efficiency are 85% to 90%, actual amplification is "only" approximately 250,000-fold. Sources of inefficiency include annealing of primers to nontarget regions of the sample DNA, gradual inactivation of the polymerase at elevated temperature, incomplete elongation of primed target, and the presence of inhibitors of the polymerase (such as detergents, phenol, or heme). Reaction conditions are variable and need to be carefully monitored and optimized for maximal sensitivity. In most applications the length of the specifically amplified fragment is relatively short, several hundred base pairs, although methods yielding extremely long products are being developed.

Detection of the amplified product is greatly simplified because extreme sensitivity is no longer required. Simple gel electrophoresis with ethidium bromide staining may suffice, but generally techniques using some form of hybridization assay are employed to verify specificity of the amplified product. Alternative methods of detection more amenable to automation and independent of hybridization are being developed. For example, one primer might be designed to include a non-annealing end with affinity label or magnetic bead. The other primer could include a signal-generating probe such as an enzyme. Specific product would include both the affinity tag and the enzyme label, and could be harvested and analyzed without hybridization (also see Chap. 14).

PCR Disadvantages

The single biggest strength of the PCR reaction, its unprecedented sensitivity, is also its single biggest weakness. False-positive reactions may result from sample contamination by a single molecule. With experience, both research and clinical laboratories have developed protocols to minimize this hazard. The greatest potential for contamination comes from the specifically amplified product of the PCR reaction, referred to as the *amplicon*. Following PCR, the amplicon copy number is extremely high, and aerosol droplets easily contain sufficient target for carryover into other samples by contaminated reagents, pipettes, and glassware. Laboratory practices that will minimize the hazard of amplicon contamination have been adopted that include the use of physically separated areas for preamplification and postamplification steps; positive displacement pipettes to minimize aerosol contamination; UV treatment of pipettes, tips, tubes, and reaction mixes to inactivate DNA; and use of prealiquotted reagents. It is easy to see that the negative control or blank (all reactants minus target DNA) is one of the most important controls for the assay. Many laboratories use multiple blanks interspersed between samples to monitor the development of false-positive reactions. The extraordinary steps that must be taken to prevent contamination have prevented many laboratories from introducing PCR-based assays into diagnostic use.

Chemical approaches have been developed to reduce the problem of amplicon contamination by making the amplicon an unsuitable target for subsequent amplification. Substitution of dUTP for dTTP in the PCR reaction will yield a product that is susceptible to a bacterial enzyme that specifically degrades uracil in DNA. Because uracil is not a normal constituent of DNA, the enzyme will only degrade the artificial amplicon and not damage the normal target of the PCR reaction within the sample. Alternatively, a psoralen derivative may be added to the amplification reaction. The compound has no significant interference with the PCR reaction. At completion of the assay, treatment of the tubes with UV light will result in psoralen adducts with pyrimidines. The adducts prevent copying by the polymerase in subsequent PCR reactions but do not interfere with detection of the product by electrophoresis or hybridization.

Even true positive reactions of PCR assays can be problematic in the clinical laboratory. When sensitivity exceeds that of any other gold standard, understandable difficulties in interpretation of the clinical significance of the results arise. The clinical relevance of small numbers of organisms or altered genetic sequences detectable by the assay will have to await further careful work correlating clinical outcome with results obtained by PCR testing.

While PCR testing should theoretically be applicable to minimally purified clinical samples, in practice the presence of unpredictable amounts of impurities with the potential to inhibit the polymerase activity has required the use of some degree of sample purification. Because inhibitors cannot always be predicted or eliminated, another important control for the PCR assay is the demonstration that the sample lysate will support amplification of an endogenous target such as β-globin. Failure to amplify β-globin indicates failure of amplification, and a negative result for the test target cannot be interpreted.

Other Amplification Techniques

There has been an impetus to develop other amplification systems, based more on the economics of patent rights and disputes over PCR technology than on a perceived need for improvement. All other assays face comparison with PCR in terms of convenience, cost, and instrumentation. To date, PCR assays have been the most characterized and applied of the amplification assays, but this may change depending on commercial input and laboratory acceptance. The other amplification assays share some features in common with PCR.

The ligase chain reaction (LCR) also uses a temperature cycling reaction (Wu, 1989) to achieve amplification. Rather than a polymerase, a thermostable DNA ligase is used. In this assay format, shown schematically in Figure 56–9*B*, four complementary oligonucleotide sequences are used. When target is denatured and oligonucleotides are allowed to anneal, they are perfectly aligned for enzymatic joining by the ligase. When the denaturing cycle is repeated, the newly ligated product forms new template and joined oligonucleotides accumulate geometrically. Detection of the ligation product is dependent upon the newly joined oligonucleotides, each contributing a different functional group, with linkage of both groups being required to generate a signal.

Isothermal target amplification methods have been described that eliminate the need for temperature cycling and depend upon the balanced activities of several enzymes. The strand displacement assay (SDA) (Walker, 1992) depends on the ability of DNA polymerase to initiate DNA replication at a single-stranded nick (specifically introduced by the activity of a restriction enzyme) and to displace the nicked strand during polymerization. The self-sustained sequence replication (3SR) uses the activities of a reverse transcriptase, an RNase specific for RNA-DNA hybrids, and an RNA polymerase (Guatelli, 1990). Transcription of an RNA target is directed by an oligonucleotide, which specifies initiation and includes sequences for an RNA promoter. The RNA template is removed by the RNA and the ssDNA copy (with RNA promoter) becomes available to interact with another oligonucleotide directing DNA polymerization. The DNA are further specifically amplified by RNA polymerization and are directed by the primer-introduced RNA promoter site.

As an alternative to amplification of the target, either the probe or the detection systems can be amplified. The probe amplification approach is exemplified by the Qβ replicase system (Lizardi, 1988). The RNA bacteriophage Qβ has a unique RNA polymerase for genomic replication that recognizes a specific highly structured region of RNA. This RNA structure can be modified to include target-specific sequences so that after specific hybridization and elimination of unbound RNA, residual bound probe is highly replicated by the Qβ RNA polymerase.

Signal amplification systems modify the detection end of

the assay. In the branched-chain DNA approach developed by Chiron (Urdea, 1991), the probe is a DNA constructed of a recognition sequence and multiple side branches. After specific hybridization, the "branches" hybridize to oligonucleotide probes with signal-generating enzymes.

Restriction Fragment Length Polymorphism Assays

Assays that utilize the sequence recognition property of restriction enzymes to demonstration variations or polymorphisms in the DNA sequence of two samples are known as *restriction fragment length polymorphism assays* (RFLP, sometimes pronounced "rif-lip"). Genomic DNA or DNA produced from a PCR reaction is digested with a restriction enzyme and the fragments are analyzed by Southern blot analysis with a site-specific probe. Changes in the sequence of the DNA may result in alteration of the recognition sequence of the enzyme. The alteration may introduce additional cut sites, remove cut sites, or insert or delete sequences between cut sites. These changes will be reflected in a change in the band size hybridizing to the site-specific probe. Of course, not all changes will be reflected in an altered recognition sequence, so unchanged band size must be interpreted in the context of the marker and known frequency of polymorphism in the region. In some assays, more than one restriction enzyme digestion is performed on each sample before Southern blot analysis.

This approach is useful in family studies, as illustrated in Figure 56–10. Polymorphisms in DNA closely linked to a disease gene can be used to predict inheritance of the altered allele. Many markers are locus specific, and chromosomal maps of these markers are available (e.g., ATCC, 1995). Those regions with the most variation, having the most polymorphisms, are easiest to use to establish allelic markers. Areas of repetitive sequences within the chromosome, known as *variable numbers of tandem repeats*, are some of the most polymorphic markers and can result in a complex banding pattern or genetic *fingerprint*. RFLP is useful in establishing linkage of a region of the genome to disease, in family studies of inherited diseases (classical genetics), and in identifying regions of the genome altered during neoplasia (somatic mutations).

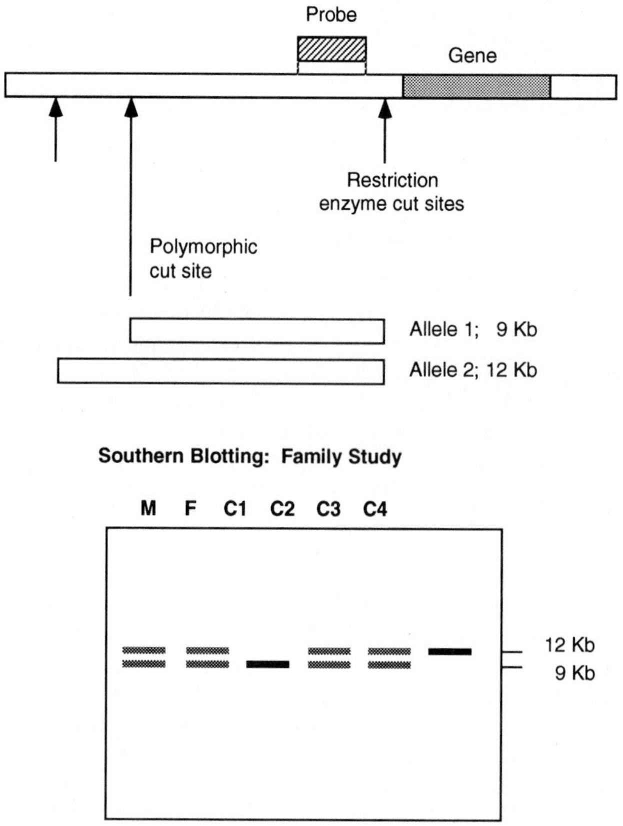

Figure 56–10. Example of restriction fragment length polymorphism (RFLP) analysis. (M = Mother; F = Father; C = Child.) (Adapted with permission from Piper MA, Unger ER: Nucleic Acid Probes: A Primer for Pathologists. Chicago, ASCP Press, 1989.)

RELATIONSHIP TO LABORATORY EVALUATION OF DISEASE

Subsequent chapters describe the current applications of molecular diagnostics. It is clear that this new technology has impacted all areas of laboratory diagnosis. Molecular methods also have the potential to redefine laboratory evaluation of disease to include more issues beyond disease diagnosis.

Molecular Diagnosis

The advantages of a molecular approach to diagnosis will be described in detail for each aspect of current application. It is important to remember, however, that these new molecular tests are not likely to replace traditional testing in the immediate future. The cost and complexity of this technology tends to restrict its initial applications to special diagnostic situations where the information obtained cannot be provided by any other method. Increased automation and commercially designed methods will bring costs down, reduce the level of technical expertise required to perform the tests, and result in integration of molecular technology into the mainstream of laboratory testing.

Detecting mutations and associating them with disease is at the heart of the current explosion of information in medical science and of many applications in molecular diagnostics. One of the most important consequences of the revolution in molecular genetics has been the ability to locate a gene responsible for a disease without knowing the protein product. Termed *reverse genetics*, this process uses RFLP linkage analysis of families that carry and express the disease to establish markers closer and closer to the disease gene until it is ultimately located. Closely linked markers may serve as clinically useful diagnostic tests, even before the gene is completely characterized and the protein product is finally identified. In this scenario molecular diagnostic tests are developed and used first, to be replaced by simpler, more cost-effective methods directed at the level of the gene product when the consequence of mutation is fully understood.

Beyond Diagnosis

Molecular analyses have the potential to greatly expand the role of the laboratory in areas beyond disease diagnosis. Molecular analysis of the somatic mutations in cancer has the potential to provide prognostic information, to guide the selection of optimal therapy, and to monitor the response to therapy. The implications of using molecular markers to detect neoplastic cells in the absence of clinical or morphologic evidence of disease, known as *minimal residual disease*, is just beginning to be explored. This approach of using molecular markers for disease detection can also be anticipated to impact secondary methods of cancer prevention (screening) and assessment of adequacy of surgical resection (evaluation of margins). Gene therapy for inherited genetic disease as well as cancer is being introduced based on a detailed understanding of the underlying disease. Monitoring these patients for the presence and activity of the introduced therapeutic gene will provide another aspect for the laboratory evaluation of disease.

Alberts B, Bray D, Lewis J, et al: Molecular Biology of the Cell, 2nd ed. New York, Garland Publishing, 1989.
ATCC/NIH Human and Mouse DNA Probes and Libraries, 8th ed. Rockville, MD, American Type Culture Collection, 1995.
Cline MJ: The molecular basis of leukemia. N Engl J Med 1994; 330:328–336.
Gautelli JC, Whitfield KM, Kwoh DY, et al: Isothermal, *in vitro* amplification of nucleic acids by a multienzyme reaction modeled after retroviral replication. Proc Natl Acad Sci USA 1990; 87:1874–1878.
Hanawalt PC: Transcription-coupled repair and human disease. Science 1994; 266:1957–1958.
Kan YW: Development of DNA analyses for human diseases: Sickle cell anemia and thalassemia as paradigm. JAMA 1992; 267: 1532–1536.
Langer PR, Waldrop AA, Ward DC: Enzymatic synthesis of biotin-labeled polynucleotides: Novel nucleic acid affinity probes. Proc Natl Acad Sci USA 1981; 78:6633–6637.
Liechti-Gallati S, Koenig M, Kunkel LM, et al: Molecular deletion patterns in Duchenne and Becker type muscular dystrophy. Hum Genet 1989; 81:343–348.
Lizardi PM, Guerra CE, Lomeli H, et al: Exponential amplification of recombinant-RNA hybridization probes. BioTechnology 1988; 6:1197–1202.
Modrich P: Mismatch repair, genetic stability, and cancer. Science 1994; 266:1959–1960.
Papavassiliou AG: Transcription factors. N Engl J Med 1995; 332:45–47.
Pease AC, Solas D, Sullivan EJ, et al: Light-generated oligonucleotide arrays for rapid DNA sequence analysis. Proc Natl Acad Sci USA 1994; 91:5022–5026.
Radman M, Wagner R: The high fidelity of DNA duplication. Sci Am 1988; 259:40–46.
Rosenthal N: Regulation of gene expression. N Engl J Med 1994; 331: 931–933.
Saiki RK, Scharf S, Faloona F, et al: Enzymatic amplification of β-globin genomic sequences and restriction site analysis for the diagnosis of sickle-cell anemia. Science 1985; 230:1350–1354.
Sancar A: Mechanisms of DNA excision repair. Science 1994; 266: 1954–1956.
Sharp PA: RNA splicing and genes. JAMA 1988; 260:3035–3041.
Southern EM: Detection of specific sequences among DNA fragments separated by gel electrophoresis. J Mol Biol 1975; 98:503–517.
Sutherland GR, Richards RI: Dynamic mutations. Sci Am 1994; 82:157–163.
Urdea MS, Horn T, Fultz J, et al: Branched DNA amplification multimers for the sensitive, direct detection of human hepatitis viruses. Nucleic Acids Symp Ser 1991; (24):197–200.
Virshup DM: DNA replication. Cur Opin Cell Biol 1990; 2:453–460.
Walker GT, Little MC, Nadeau JG, Shank DD: Isothermal in vitro amplification of DNA by a restriction enzyme/DNA polymerase system. Proc Natl Acad Sci USA 1992; 89:392–396.
Weatherall DJ: Molecular pathology of single gene disorders. J Clin Pathol 1987; 40:959–970.
Wu DR, Wallace RB: The ligation amplification reaction (LAR)-amplification of specific DNA sequences using sequential rounds of template-dependent ligation. Genomics 1989; 4:560–569.

Chapter 57

Establishing a Molecular Diagnostics Laboratory

Andrea Ferreira-Gonzalez, M.S., Ph.D.
Carleton T. Garrett, M.D., Ph.D.

The goal of the molecular diagnostics (MDx) laboratory is to enhance the value of the clinical laboratory services. This is achieved by providing an environment in which new tests based on molecular techniques can be established, validated, and applied to the testing of patient specimens. Molecular techniques possess inherent sensitivity and specificity that greatly exceed what is currently available using conventional methods and thus can potentially improve current laboratory testing in a number of areas.

The need for special facilities, equipment, technical skills, and professional knowledge to conduct molecular assays successfully is one of the obstacles to successful use of this technology to improve patient care. In addition, the Clinical Laboratory Improvement Amendment of 1988 (CLIA '88, 1992), which governs all laboratories that perform testing of human samples, has an especially large impact on molecular testing because those tests are mostly "home-brew" or developed in-house and all are considered to be highly complex tests. In order to fulfill CLIA '88 regulations, any laboratory performing MDx tests must develop validation programs for all home-brew or modified Food and Drug Administration (FDA)-approved assays (Garrett, 1993). The programs must include data substantiating precision, accuracy, analytical sensitivity, specificity, and any claims of clinical utility. The regulatory emphasis placed on test validation and quality control (QC) adds pressure for the centralization of molecular testing in one facility where development of a comprehensive set of guidelines regarding these issues can be established for all molecular tests.

Molecular testing is being used to address clinical problems in all areas of laboratory medicine, and the well-defined lines that separated anatomic from clinical pathology are rapidly disappearing. Examples of the application of this technology currently abound in the fields of microbiology, immunology, forensics, genetics, and oncology (Loeffelholz, 1992; Brisson-Noel, 1991; Wise, 1991; Brandt, 1992; Hill, 1993; Olerup, 1992; Werner, 1993). Specific examples for the use of molecular testing are provided elsewhere in this book and are not repeated here. The purpose of this chapter is to address issues that are common to the use of molecular techniques in any field. The choice of tests is, however, critical to the success of any MDx laboratory.

If centralization of molecular testing is the choice of an institution, each existing clinical laboratory should be responsible for identifying and prioritizing nucleic acid–based tests that they wish to have available at an MDx facility. Specific individuals in each of the existing laboratories should be appointed to work with MDx personnel to oversee establishment and validation of their assays. These individuals should be familiar with the procedures and clinical activities within the MDx laboratory. Such an arrangement facilitates the establishment of the close working relation that must exist between the MDx facility and existing laboratories.

LABORATORY FACILITIES

The power of molecular technology arises from the fact that the analyte detected in molecular tests—that is, deoxyribonucleic acid (DNA) or ribonucleic acid (RNA)—is nature's most specific marker for any living organism and that molecular technology makes it possible to create billions of copies of a particular target sequence, enabling detection of as little as a single copy of the target in a patient's specimen. Thus, an MDx laboratory must be designed not only to provide sufficient space for personnel and equipment but also to minimize the potential problem of specimen and reagent contamination from either natural nucleic acid (template) or nucleic acid arising from an amplification procedure (amplicon) (Olerup, 1992).

In vitro amplification of target sequences is responsible for the very high sensitivity of molecular tests (Garrett, 1992a), but accidental dispersion of amplicon arising from these procedures is one of the major drawbacks of this technology. Opening and closing the microcentrifuge tubes in which polymerase chain reactions (PCR) are performed can generate microdroplets estimated to carry up to 10 to 100 copies of the target sequence. These microdroplets can deposit on bench tops, instruments, floors, dust, exposed skin, hair, and virtually anything. Once deposited on skin, clothing, equipment, or dust, amplicon can be carried around to different laboratories and be introduced into negative specimens, giving rise to a false-positive result. Contamination can also arise from template DNA from another source such as other patient samples, plasmid containing the particular sequence, and so on.

Laboratory Design

In designing an MDx laboratory, special emphasis must be placed on trying to completely separate areas where specimens are accessioned and tests are set up from areas where tests are processed after amplification. The former areas are called clean areas, and the latter, dirty areas.

The ideal MDx laboratory has three separate rooms, two clean rooms and one dirty room. One clean room is for reagent preparation, and the other is for specimen accessioning, specimen preparation, and reaction setup. The dirty room is for postamplification analysis of amplified material. When three rooms are not available, the functions of the two clean rooms can be combined into one room. The single clean room must be arranged in a way that allows the tasks of reagent preparation and specimen handling to be performed in different designated areas. The use of dead air boxes can meet the need for isolated, tightly controlled space where reagent and master mix preparations can be carried out. They should be located in the laboratory where traffic is low. Obviously, no genomic or plasmid DNA, RNA, or patient samples should be introduced into these dead air boxes. If the laboratory has the capability to synthesize oligonucleotides, the synthesized oligonucleotides should be processed and aliquoted inside the dead air boxes. The dead air boxes should contain ultraviolet UV light, and the work area should be treated with UV light and wiped down with 10% sodium hypochlorite and 70% ethanol before and after each use. These areas must contain dedicated pipettors and supplies that can be stored inside the dead air boxes and UV treated and wiped down with sodium hypochlorite and ethanol before and after each use. Dedicated laboratory wear and disposable clean gloves should be put on before starting to work in the dead air boxes.

The second clean room, or the area outside the dead air boxes in the single clean room, is where patient specimens are accessioned and extracted and where nucleic acid is added to the respective reaction tubes. This room must be furnished with a biological safety cabinet for handling patient specimens and for portions of the nucleic acid extraction procedure. Also, if organic nucleic acid extraction is performed, a chemical hood is necessary for handling of the phenol and chloroform steps of the nucleic acid extraction. A second biological safety cabinet, a dedicated carbon dioxide incubator, and water bath are desirable for the passage of cell lines that are used for QC programs. All equipment and supplies used for handling specimens and extracted nucleic acid should be kept completely separated from the rest of the laboratory.

The postamplification room, or dirty room, like the clean room(s), should contain its own dedicated equipment and supplies. It is recommended that thermocyclers be located in the dirty room. If thermocyclers are located in the preamplification room, under no circumstances can the reaction tubes be opened there. Thermocyclers should be plugged into dedicated circuit breakers to avoid any fluctuation of electricity that could affect their performance. A dedicated biological safety cabinet with UV light and a shaking incubator are recommended for the postamplification room to support subcloning of DNA fragments that may be required as controls. A darkroom with a dedicated automatic film processor is also highly desirable.

Air handling for the clean and dirty areas should ideally be completely independent from one another. When the air systems are not independent, the location of the postamplification room should be farther from the preamplification areas in reference to the source of air for the different rooms. Electrical air filters installed into the inflow of air into the clean room(s) may be helpful. As part of the quality assurance (QA) program, these filters must be cleaned on a regular basis to ensure that they are perfectly operational.

It is highly recommended that the air pressure for the clean laboratory be made positive to impede entrance of any airborne particles from outside into the clean room when the door is opened. If a separate second clean room is used, it must also be under positive air pressure. The postamplification room or dirty room should be under negative air pressure to avoid the escape of any amplified material out of this room when the door is opened.

The use of anterooms is a relatively inexpensive way of circumventing the need to re-engineer air handling for an entire room. An anteroom just inside the clean room can be made to have positive pressure by simply blowing air from inside the clean room into it. This serves the same purpose as a positive-pressure clean room by helping to prevent contaminants from entering the clean room. Similarly, an anteroom under negative pressure can substitute for a postamplification laboratory under negative pressure. In this case, the blower is arranged so that it blows air out of the anteroom into the postamplification laboratory. A seal at the bottom of the door between the anteroom and the postamplification laboratory prevents air within the laboratory from being drawn from the postamplification laboratory back into the anteroom. A postamplification laboratory usually contains a chemical hood vented to the outside to prevent the pressure within the postamplification laboratory from ever becoming positive. It is obviously important when entering or leaving the anterooms that the outside door and inside door of the anteroom not be opened at the same time. Sticky mats placed by the entrance of the different anterooms aid in decreasing the movement of amplicon carried on persons' shoes.

When deciding on the size of an anteroom, it is necessary to consider what activities will be performed in it. If disposable or dedicated laboratory coats, hats, and foot coverings (booties) are to be used in each laboratory, the anterooms should be large enough to store these items. The anterooms should also be large enough to allow two persons to change easily at the same time into and out of laboratory coats and any other apparel that will be worn in the respective laboratory areas. Another advantage of a large anteroom is that it can be used as a storage place for laboratory supplies.

Workflow

Undirectional workflow from tasks that are performed in the clean room(s) to those using facilities in the dirty room is essential to minimize the possibility of transferring amplified material from the postamplification area to the preamplification area. No personnel who have been in the postamplification area should go back to the clean room without showering, washing hair, and changing clothes. It is strongly recommended that disposable hats and booties, as well as disposable laboratory coats, be used, because these in some measure reduce the need to enforce daily washing of hair and changing of clothes. If cloth laboratory coats are used, a system should be put in place to ensure weekly laundering of the laboratory coats. Laboratory coats that have been worn inside any of the laboratories should remain inside the respective laboratories or anterooms and should not be worn in the office area. The use of laboratory coats of different colors for each room can act as an additional reminder of the daily workflow.

Transfer of paper documents should be reduced as much as possible. In particular, transfer of paper documents from the postamplification laboratory to the clean areas must be avoided. It is recommended that paper documents that are produced in the postamplification area and that must be used in the office be placed into clear plastic sheet protectors stored outside of the postamplification laboratory before being brought into the office area. Whenever possible, a computer network linking the office and the different laboratories should be established to reduce the movement of paper from the office through the different laboratories and mostly from the postamplification room back to the office.

Another consideration that impacts on the issue of workflow is housekeeping. It is important that housekeeping employees remove trash first from the clean area before removing it from the dirty room in order to avoid spreading amplicon to the clean area. The safest approach is simply to keep housekeeping personnel out of the laboratories and have laboratory personnel bag the trash and place it outside the laboratories for pickup.

EQUIPMENT

The various items of equipment required to successfully conduct molecular assays differ substantially from those generally found in a clinical laboratory and have been discussed in some detail elsewhere (Garrett, 1992b). A list modified from an earlier discussion of this subject is shown in Table 57–1. Issues of QC and maintenance regarding some of the most important and frequently used items of equipment in the MDx laboratory are discussed later (see Quality Assurance).

PERSONNEL

MDx laboratories are classified under CLIA '88 as laboratories that perform high-complexity testing. This imposes certain educational and training requirements for laboratory

Table 57–1. CAPITAL EQUIPMENT REQUIREMENTS AND APPROXIMATE COSTS

Description	Quantity	Amount*
DNA thermal cycler(s)	2	$ 20,000
Oligonucleotide synthesizer	1	20,000
Laminar flow environmental hoods	2	8,000
Freezers/refrigerators	2	1,600
−20°C manual defrost freezers	2	900
−70°C freezer	1	7,000
Angle-head microcentrifuges, 14,000 rpm	2	3,200
Horizontal microcentrifuge, 14,000 rpm	1	2,500
Vacuum centrifuges, pumps, condensers	2	11,000
Electronic balance(s)	2	2,000
pH meters	2	1,000
Heating/stir plates	2	500
Water baths	3	6,000
Electrophoresis power supplies	3	2,000
Mini PAGE electrophoresis apparatuses	8	3,200
Mini PAGE gel casting towers	2	990
Photodocumentation system	1	9,000
Agarose gel electrophoresis apparatuses	4	1,600
Automated x-ray film processer	1	3,800
Autoradiography cassettes (17 × 14 in)	4	1,600
Autoradiography cassettes (8 × 10 in)	4	800
Standard micropipettors (three sizes)	18	3,780
Temperature verification system for thermocycler	1	1,400
Polymerase chain reaction work station	1	1,500
Vortex mixers	3	750
Pneumatic pipette aids	4	800
Scintillation counter	1	18,000
Ultraviolet spectrophotometer	1	8,000
Geiger counter	1	485
DNA sequencing apparatuses	2	1,600
DNA sequencing power supply	1	2,000
Hybridization ovens	4	8,000
Computer hardware and software	NA	10,000
Tabletop refrigerated centrifuge	1	6,000
Incubator	1	1,000
Heating blocks	4	800
Refrigerated microcentrifuges	2	2,800
Total		**$173,605**

*Prices are approximate only.

personnel. In addition, molecular tests are more complex than standard clinical assays, and continual change occurs through constant introduction of new or improved methods. These issues combine to create special challenges to personnel working in MDx.

Laboratory Director

Under CLIA '88 a high-complexity laboratory must be directed by a pathologist, MD, or DO with two years of directing or supervising or one year of medical residency laboratory training, or by a PhD with board certification or four years of experience (Bachmer, 1993). Individuals with experience in basic science research as well as in the clinical laboratory can be particularly well suited to this position because of the continuing need in MDx for development and improvement of molecular tests. The laboratory director has overall responsibility for selection and implementation of new tests, resolution of technical difficulties, and development of guidelines and management practices that ensure regular and reliable performance of clinical laboratory testing. The laboratory director must also ensure the development of QA and QC programs as well as laboratory programs for clinical validation and optimization of molecular tests.

Technical Supervisor

An individual with an MD, DO, or PhD with one year of experience in MDx or with a master's degree with two years' experience or with a bachelor's degree with four years' experience is qualified for this position (Bachmer, 1993). Because of the high complexity of the different tests and the homebrew nature of the majority of these tests, it is recommended that technical supervision be performed by a scientist who has in-depth knowledge and training in molecular biology and some clinical experience in MDx. The technical supervisor should develop and oversee optimization of testing protocols, develop and supervise guidelines for working within the laboratory facilities, and oversee the proficiency testing program. The responsibility for development and supervision of laboratory programs for QA and QC and clinical validation of different molecular tests may also be delegated to this individual.

Medical Technologists and Molecular Biology Technicians

Medical technologists and molecular biology technicians are responsible for processing specimens, performing tests, maintaining records, adhering to procedures and QC policies, identifying problems, and documenting corrective actions. The usual record keeping, such as revising laboratory manuals and following equipment maintenance, is complicated by the constant need to modify and improve methods and to deal with equipment for which there is little clinical laboratory experience. It is therefore critical that these individuals, particularly the most senior members of the technology staff, have a high sense of professional commitment, display continuous effort to improve their education and training, possess as many advanced laboratory skills as possible, and make certain that they are cross-trained in all techniques used in the MDx operation. All members of the technical staff need to understand fully the scientific basis and results of the different tests and the clinical implications of the different tests.

Residents, Fellows, and Graduate Students

Involvement of residents, fellows, and graduate students can be very important to the success of an MDx laboratory. As a primary step in training these individuals, we have implemented an intense hands-on training program that is offered every month and consists of two weeks of laboratory and didactic lectures in the different fields of MDx. This type of training program has also been used to train practicing pathologists as well as non-MDs with special needs for experience in the field of MDx. Development of an MDx fellowship is highly desirable.

THE CLINICAL TESTING PROCESS

Establishment of molecular assays, particularly amplification assays, requires many considerations at every stage including reagent preparation, specimen collection, specimen aliquot processing, and subsequent conduct of the actual assay. Details of these steps for a number of assays of clinically important target sequences are presented in other chapters of Part 7. Nevertheless, a number of considerations that apply to all molecular assays are important to guarantee the reliability of the results (Table 57–2). As with any clinical test, a well-thought-out and well-written procedure is a key factor for the reproducibility of the assay. It is one of the most important aids during hands-on training of new personnel and should be written following National Committee for Clinical Laboratory Standards (NCCLS) guidelines (Clinical Laboratory Technical Procedure Manuals, 1992). A careful selection of controls is also vital to the interpretation of results. Negative and positive controls are required by CLIA's regulations and must be processed in every clinical test. Failure to obtain the correct result in controls that monitor the overall procedure invalidates the entire test and requires retesting of all samples.

From the technical standpoint, the primary need is to optimize each clinical assay in order to maximize the test's sensitivity and specificity (Persing, 1993). Procedures to avoid false-positive and false-negative results are crucial parts of the QC program. When possible, procedures need to be in place to detect false negatives for individual patient specimen aliquots. False negatives are of special concern when samples are subjected to rapid extraction procedures, particularly when blood is present in the specimen. It is recommended that all rapid extraction procedures be compared with the accepted gold standard of protease K digestion and phenol/chloroform extraction (Blin, 1976). Use of master mixes to decrease the number of pipetting steps, aliquotting nucleic acid into reaction tubes one row at a time, and frequent change of gloves whenever it is suspected that they

Table 57–2. CONDUCTING THE CLINICAL TESTING PROCESS

Activity	Considerations
Reagent preparation	Perform in cleanest environment. Store working stock solutions in single-use aliquots. Test sensitivity, specificity, and stability of each new set of reagents before use in clinical testing. Use low copy number sample for sensitivity evaluation. Use master mixes to decrease number of pipetting steps. Check purity of any oligonucleotides synthesized in-house by high-performance liquid chromatography or by end-labeling and polyacrylamide gel electrophoresis.
Specimen collection	Determine acceptable tolerance limits for each type of specimen to be tested (storage temperature, transport time, anticoagulant, etc.). Distribute protocols for proper specimen handling to all potential users. Capture all important information regarding specimen handling on requisition.
Specimen processing	Specimen must be received in preamplification (clean) laboratory. Follow guidelines to ensure against mix-up and to preserve integrity of target sequence.
Analysis of specimen	
Extraction procedure	Evaluate rapid extraction procedures for presence of inhibitors and factors that decrease yield of target (compare with protease K/phenol-chloroform extraction method). Use an internal control added to the sample at the time of extraction to determine the percent of (false) negatives due to inhibitors or determine this rate by some other means. If an internal control is not to be evaluated with each patient's sample, the rate of false negatives should be stated on the report in a disclaimer in case of negative results.
Assay set-up, amplication and analysis	Optimize concentration of primers, $MgCl_2$, dNTPs; volume; cycling conditions. Follow guidelines to minimize possibility of contamination by template nucleic acid or amplicon (see Quality Assurance in text).

might be contaminated with nucleic acid all can help to decrease the possibility of false-positive results. More detailed consideration relating to prevention of contamination follows.

QUALITY ASSURANCE

Every MDx laboratory must develop a comprehensive written QA program. The objective of the QA program is to monitor and evaluate, objectively and systematically, the quality and appropriateness of the test results. The QA program must address every factor involved in the testing process. The program must include written policies and documentation for education and training of personnel, continuing medical education, proficiency testing, internal and external inspection including documentation of corrective actions for deficiencies cited, and QC programs for clinical testing, equipment performance, and safety.

The QA program monitors aspects of clinical testing that do not directly bear on the analytical validity of the test result and that are thus not generally a part of the QC program for clinical testing. Monthly turn-around times and monthly reviews of normal and abnormal results must be performed. Turn-around times exceeding a predetermined value require documentation and explanation. Unusual laboratory results that may cause possible misinterpretation if unrecognized must be collected in a log.

Quality Control

The QC program covers all aspects of patient testing that may have a direct impact on the validity of test results. The program should be under direct supervision of the laboratory manager, who is responsible for the day-to-day operations, and should be reviewed monthly by the medical or technical director of the laboratory. All failed procedures must be documented and corrective action taken to remedy the problem. Complete and well-thought-out procedure manuals must be available in the work areas and in the office. Methods to prevent specimen loss, alteration, or contamination must be included in the procedure manuals. The manuals should contain a protocol for reporting results that include criteria for identifying normal and abnormal results. Each result must be interpreted by two qualified laboratory personnel, generally including the technician performing the test as well as either the technical manager or laboratory director. Results should be evaluated in conjunction with relevant clinical and laboratory data submitted with the test requisition. This practice aids in detecting clerical errors in reporting laboratory results as well as in documenting any discrepancies between anticipated and actual results.

Measures to Control Contamination in the Laboratory Facility

Contamination is prevented through two basic approaches. One is to reduce levels of amplicon and template within the laboratory to levels low enough to be nondetectable (Porter-Jordan, 1991). Physically separating areas where reagent preparation and reaction setup are performed (preamplification area) from areas likely to contain high levels of amplicon or template DNA is one part of such an effort. Any equipment or personnel that have come into contact with amplified material should be restricted from entering the preamplification area. The second approach is to treat amplicon chemically so that it is unable to support amplification even if it does accidentally enter another sample.

Amplicon contamination is identified by the presence of

signal in negative controls. The main approach to destroying it is through the use of chemical bleach (sodium hypochlorite) and UV irradiation (Ou, 1991). UV treatment of DNA induces cross-linking of the two DNA strands by forming thymidine dimers. This cross-linked DNA can no longer serve as an efficient template for Taq DNA polymerase. Treatment of master mixes absent the nucleotides with UV light can induce cross-linking of contaminating amplicon or template. One disadvantage of the UV method is that it is only effective for target sequences exceeding 700 nucleotides in length.

The use of bleach appears to be the most generally accepted method of decontaminating surfaces exposed to amplicon or template DNA. Countertops, chairs, and stools should be wiped weekly, first with a fresh 10% solution of sodium hypochlorite and then with 70% ethanol or water to dilute the bleach that could corrode Formica tops and plastic materials. Protection of countertops through the use of plastic-backed absorbent paper is not recommended because the paper can collect dust, amplified material, or nucleic acid if not changed frequently. If used, absorbent plastic-backed paper should be discarded immediately after each use. Floors should also be mopped weekly with bleach and then with water. All pipette tips and tissues used during any procedure should be discarded in zip-lock bags, making sure that the bag is completely closed before discarding it. Gloves should be changed periodically or as soon as any contamination with nucleic acid or amplified material is suspected. Centrifuge buckets and rotors should be wiped down with 10% sodium hypochlorite solution, followed by water of 70% ethanol. For those rotors or buckets that cannot withstand the bleach solution, UV treatment should be considered. Thermocyclers should be cleaned after every run. Each individual well should be cleaned with a cotton tip wetted in 70% ethanol. Also, as with any equipment, pipettors should be wiped out with a 10% sodium hypochlorite solution, followed by a 70% ethanol solution after routine use. Aerosol-resistant tips should be quality controlled before being placed in service. In our hands, filtered tips that contain a bound hydrophobic membrane have proved to be aerosol resistant. Evaluation of aerosol-resistant tips can be performed by setting up the pipettor to pipette over the upper limit of a colored solution and determine if the tip of the pipettor has been stained.

Measures to Eliminate the Effects of Amplicon Contamination in Clinical Assays

One widely used method to inactivate or sterilize amplicon is to incorporate deoxyuridine triphosphate (dUTP) instead of deoxythimidine triphosphate into the amplicon during amplification and then to treat all subsequent samples with the enzyme uracil-*N*-glycosylase (UNG) before subjecting them to amplification (Epsy, 1993). In this procedure, dUTP is incorporated into newly synthesized DNA (amplicon) instead of thymidine. The uracil-containing amplicon is a substrate for the enzyme UNG, but normal DNA is not. If any of the uracil-containing amplicon is accidentally deposited into a sample, pretreatment of the sample with UNG will destroy the uracil-containing amplicon before initiating the amplification procedure. Destruction of amplicon results because UNG removes uracil residues from the amplicon. Although the phosphodiester backbone of the amplicon initially is still intact, the phosphodiester bonds at the sites where uracil has been removed break during the first denaturation step. The fragmented amplicon is no longer able to function as an efficient template for the Taq DNA polymerase. Native DNA template remains unaffected, however, because it does not contain dUTP and can serve as a template for the Taq DNA polymerase.

Use of dUTP and UNG has been shown to control carry-over contamination between 10^6 and 10^7 copies of uracil-containing amplicon (Rys, 1993). It is important to note that UNG activity is partially restored when the temperature drops to 55°C; thus, it is imperative for those procedures using the dUTP/UNG system to hold the temperature above 55°C at completion of the procedure. Otherwise, storage of specimen aliquots at −70°C is recommended. Another advantage in using the dUTP/UNG system is that during the temperature rise of the initial cycle, any amplicon generated from nonspecific binding of primers to DNA at room temperature is degraded by the UNG (until the temperature rises above 55°C) thus increasing the procedure's sensitivity and specificity.

One of the disadvantages of the dUTP/UNG chemical system is that the efficiency of dUTP incorporation varies greatly depending on the base composition of the template. Thus, the method is not completely effective for cytosine- and guanine-rich templates. Moreover, empirically, target sequences of less than 250 nucleotides in length are not effectively eliminated by this protocol (Espy, 1993).

A second contamination control procedure is treatment of amplicon by isopsoralen. After subsequent exposure to long-wavelength UV light, isopsoralen compounds form covalent adducts with DNA, rendering them inefficient templates for Taq DNA polymerase. One advantage of this chemical method is that the isopsoralen can be added to the reaction before amplification and then the reaction tube treated with UV light after amplification but before its opening (Isaacs, 1991).

Quality Control of Equipment

All equipment used in an MDx laboratory must have a QC procedure written according to NCCLS guidelines (Clinical Laboratory Technical Procedure Manuals, 1992), which describe maintenance, performance, and calibration checks. Tolerance limits should be clearly defined for each performance check and calibration procedure. When performance check or calibration check of any instrument falls outside the tolerance range limit defined for each instrument, the equipment should be taken out of service for repair. Documentation of all maintenance, performance checks, calibration, or repair for each part of equipment must be part of the QC protocols.

Thermocyclers are a crucial item in the equipping of any MDx laboratory, and any change in performance of the thermocyclers has a direct impact on sensitivity and reproducibility of the tests performed. The following reflects some of the considerations in their QC and maintenance. As part of the performance checks, thermocycler indicator lights and run QC should be performed at the end of each run and documented. When using a 9600 thermocycler, verification of setpoint error, the status record display, start date and time, and record of any error messages should be documented for each run. Determination of cycling time can be calculated by subtracting status record display minus the run start record. If using other thermocyclers, record any error messages and determine the cycling time by subtracting the end time minus the starting run time. Cycling times between different runs should not differ more than a few minutes. Fluctuations in cycling time are a warning signal that the thermocycler needs to be adjusted and restored to the original condition. Heater and chiller tests should be performed weekly, and wells and heat covers should be cleaned monthly. The temperature for the different wells of the thermocyclers should be checked at least every 6 months to determine block uniformity. This can be determined by using a thermocouple with a temperature probe. The thermocycler should be programmed to heat to 95°C, and the temperature measured in every other row. Then, the thermocycler should be programmed to heat to 40°C, and the same wells should be tested. Tolerance limits of 0.75° to 1°C difference between thermocouple and actual reading are considered acceptable.

As part of the performance check and calibration, speeds for centrifuges should be checked using a tachometer to make sure that the actual speeds (rpm) coincide with the displayed speed. For those centrifuges with safety latches that cannot be operated with the door opened, speed should be checked by a specialized technician.

Biological safety cabinets should be certified every year by a specialized technician. Before any work is performed, the interior of the environmental hood should be UV treated for at least 20 minutes and wiped down with 10% sodium hypochlorite solution and 70% ethanol. After work is completed, the surface should be wiped down again and UV treated for at least 1 hour. Chemical hoods should also be certified every year by a specialized technician to determine that the velocity of air intake falls within acceptable values. Temperature and carbon dioxide levels should be checked daily in incubators used for maintenance of cell lines for QC. Incubators should be cleaned with a 10% sodium hypochlorite solution twice a year, and the water pan should be changed monthly. Temperature of water baths and dry baths (heating blocks) used for incubation of reactions should be checked before use with thermometers that have been standardized against National Institute of Standards and Technology thermometers. As a general maintenance protocol, water baths should be cleaned twice a year. Whenever possible, water baths should be avoided because they could be a source of contamination; dry water baths should be used instead.

Spectrophotometers in the UV/visible range are commonly used in MDx laboratories for measuring the concentration of nucleic acid present in a particular sample. This could be genomic DNA, RNA, plasmid DNA, oligonucleotides, and so on. Spectrophotometers should also be subjected to rigorous QC and maintenance procedures. As part of the routine QC program, linearity check, stray light, and wavelength calibration should be performed every six months. Another function test is to run a standard DNA sample to determine the accuracy of the instrument.

Pipettors are important equipment items that cannot be overlooked in QC. They are used for every single step of testing from reagent preparation, specimen preparation, and amplification setup to analysis and thus have a direct impact on accuracy of testing. Special emphasis should be placed on QC and maintenance of pipettors and pipette tips because they could be a major source of error and amplicon contamination. Pipettors should be calibrated twice a year using a gravimetric method. Tolerance limits should be determined for each pipettor according to the volume for which it is accurate.

Clinical Validation

Although laboratories using FDA-approved test kits to perform clinical testing need only follow manufacturers specifications for QC, CLIA '88 requires that more extensive validation procedures be undertaken by those performing tests that have modified manufacturers' specification or were developed in-house. Laboratories performing home-brew tests must establish and document the accuracy, precision, specificity, sensitivity, reference range, and any specification required to justify the use of that particular test in a specific clinical situation. After careful determination of specificity and sensitivity for a particular test, clinical validation should be assessed using clinical specimen aliquots in retrospective or prospective fashion. Reproducibility checks should be carefully designed in order to determine intra-assay and interassay variability. These tests should be performed including samples with low copy number of target sequence, on different days, and with different lots of reagents. It is important to assess cross-reactivity with other sequences or interfering substances that could be present in patient samples. If a test is being evaluated for a specific virus, samples from patients diagnosed with different viral infections or recipients of multiple transfusions should be tested. Results obtained during the clinical validation phase of a molecular test should be compared against results from reference or gold standard methods. Discrepancies among the different methods must be resolved whenever possible on the basis of clinical information and patient outcome. This also provides critical information in order to develop algorithms for patient testing and guidelines for analysis of discordance between different methods.

Accreditation

Laboratories performing testing on human specimens for the purpose of clinical diagnosis, prevention, or treatment of disease must comply with all regulations set by CLIA. Although research laboratories that do not report patient results are not subjected to CLIA '88, all laboratories that do report specific patients results are under the regulation of CLIA '88. This applies even if a disclaimer that the results are to be used for research purpose only or that there is no charge for the service. CLIA '88 regulations mandate standards in the areas of personnel, proficiency testing, QC, QA, and patient test management. The rules establish a registration procedure as well as sanctions and enforcement procedures for ensuring that standards established by legislation are maintained. The Federal Department of Health and Human Services has granted the College of American Pathologists (CAP) deemed status to be an enforcement agency for these regulations by accepting their accreditation programs as being equivalent or more stringent than the QC and QA standards described in CLIA '88 regulations. In light of this development, laboratories performing clinical testing using MDx techniques may seek accreditation by the CAP as a means to comply with the regulatory requirements described in CLIA '88. The CAP's checklist for molecular pathology was introduced in 1993 (Molecular Pathology Inspection Checklist, 1993).

CONCLUSION

MDx tests are proving to be valuable tools in patient diagnosis and management. Establishing and operating an MDx laboratory requires special facilities, equipment, technical skills, and professional knowledge. MDx laboratories must comply with a host of regulations including those of CLIA '88 and must develop comprehensive QC and QA programs. Despite the complexity of conducting molecular testing, these assays provide the opportunity to enhance the laboratory evaluation for diseases such as cancer, acquired immunodeficiency syndrome, and other life-threatening illnesses, and their utility is likely to grow substantially in the years ahead.

Bachmer P, Hamlin W: Federal regulation of clinical laboratories and the clinical laboratory improvement amendments of 1988—Part II. Clin Lab Med 1993; 13:987–994.

Blin N, Stafford DW: Isolation of high molecular weight DNA. Nucleic Acid Res 1976; 3:2303–2305.

Brandt CD, Rakusan TA, Sison AV, et al: Detection of human immunodeficiency virus type 1 infection in young pediatric patients by using polymerase chain reaction and biotinylated probes. J Clin Microbiol 1992; 30:36–40.

Brisson-Noel A, Aznar C, Chureau C, et al: Diagnosis of tuberculosis by DNA amplification in clinical practice evaluation. Lancet 1991; 338:364–366.

CLIA '88. Final Rules. College of American Pathologists 1992. 325 Waukegan Road, Northfield, IL 60093-2750.

Clinical Laboratory Technical Procedure Manuals, 2nd ed. Villanova, PA, NCCLS, document GP2-A2, 1992; 12, (10).

Espy JM, Smith TF, Persing DH: Dependence of polymerase chain reaction product inactivation protocols on amplification length and sequence composition. J Clin Microbiol 1993; 31:2361–2365.

Garrett CT, Ferreira-Centeno A, Nasim S: Molecular diagnostics: Issues of utilization, regulation and organization. Clin Chim Acta 1993; 217:85–103.

Garrett CT, Porter-Jordan K, Nasim S: Polymerase chain reaction. *In* Specter S, Lancz GJ (eds): Clinical Virology Manual, 2nd ed. Norwalk, CT, Appleton and Lange, 1992a, pp 307–316.

Garrett CT, Rodriguez ER, Comerford J, et al: Establishing a molecular diagnostics laboratory. Adv Pathol 1992b; 5:34–49.

Hill RE: The diagnosis of inborn errors of metabolism by examination of the genotype. Clin Chim Acta 1993; 217:3–14.

Isaacs ST, Tessman JW, Metchette KC, et al: Post-PCR sterilization: Development and application to an HIV-1 diagnostic assay. Nucleic Acid Res 1991; 19:109–116.

Loeffelholz NJ, Lewinski CA, Silver SR, et al: Detection of *Chlamydia trachomatis* in endocervical specimens by polymerase chain reaction. J Clin Microbiol 1992; 30:2847–2851.

Molecular Pathology Inspection Checklist, 1993 edition. Commission on Laboratory Accreditation, College of American Pathologists, 325 Waukegan Rd, Northfield, IL, 60093.

Olerup O, Zetterquist H: HLA-DR typing by PCR amplification with sequence-specific primers (PCR-SSP) in 2 hours: An alternative to serological DR typing in clinical practice including donor-recipient matching in cadaveric transplantation. Tissue Antigens 1992; 39:225–235.

Ou C-Y, Moore JJ, Schochetman G: Use of UV irradiation to reduce false positivity in polymerase chain reaction. Bio techniques 1991; 10:442–446.

Persing DH: Target selection and optimization of amplification reactions. *In* Persing D, Smith TF, Tenover FC, White TJ (eds): Diagnostic Molecular Microbiology, Principles and Applications. Washington, D.C., American Society for Microbiology, Washington, D.C., 1993, pp 88–104.

Porter-Jordan K, Garrett CT: Source of contamination in polymerase chain reaction assay. Lancet 1990; 1:1220.

Rys PN, Persing DH: Preventing false positives; quantitative evaluation of three protocols for inactivation of polymerase chain reaction amplification products. J Clin Microbiol 1993; 31:2356–2360.

Werner M, Ballo MS, Gallagher JV: Comparative clinical evaluation of biochemical and genomic tumor markers. Clin Chim Acta 1993; 217:39–55.

Wise DS, Weaver TL: Detection of the Lyme disease bacterium, *Borrelia burgdorferi*, by using the polymerase chain reaction and a non-radioisotopic gene probe. J Clin Microbiol 1991; 29:1523–1526.

7

Chapter 58

Molecular Genetics of Hematopoietic Neoplasms

Lynne V. Abruzzo, M.D., Ph.D.
Sanford A. Stass, M.D.

TECHNIQUES OF MOLECULAR DIAGNOSIS

Three major techniques of molecular analysis are currently used to diagnose and monitor hematologic malignancies. These are Southern blot analysis, polymerase chain reaction (PCR), and fluorescent *in situ* hybridization (FISH). These methods are used to demonstrate and characterize genetic abnormalities in malignant hematopoietic cells (Hirsch-Ginsberg, 1993). Although Southern blot analysis is less sensitive than the other assays, it is the oldest and most widely used of the three (Southern, 1975). In this assay genomic DNA extracted from cells is digested into smaller fragments with restriction endonucleases. These enzymes recognize and cleave DNA at specific base sequences. The restriction fragments are separated according to size by electrophoresis through an agarose gel; smaller fragments migrate faster, and therefore farther, in the gel than larger fragments. The DNA fragments are transferred to a membrane support, and the membranes (blots) are incubated with labeled DNA or RNA probes that are of complementary sequence to the region of interest. The probes can be labeled either with radioactive isotope (usually ^{32}P), chromogen, or fluorescent compound. If the probes were labeled for a chemical reaction, the membranes are processed to produce a color reaction. If fluorescent or radioactive probes were used, the blots are exposed to x-ray film or are scanned with devices that detect fluorescence or β particle emissions. Currently, autoradiography of radiolabeled probes is the most sensitive method for the detection of rearranged bands. High sensitivity is especially important to detect minimal residual disease. Northern blot analysis and slot blot analysis are related techniques used to detect transcribed genes, that is, mRNA.

PCR-based analysis is much more sensitive than traditional Southern blotting, up to 10^4-fold (Krolewski, 1989). This method can amplify small (generally up to several thousand base pairs) target segments of DNA by multiple repetitions of three successive steps (Mullis, 1987). PCR can be used to amplify segments of genes to detect point mutations, and to amplify chromosomal rearrangements and breakpoints that are clustered in relatively small regions. The PCR technique can be modified to amplify mRNA, a process called *reverse-transcriptase PCR* (RT-PCR) (Kawasaki, 1988; 1989). First, a complementary DNA (cDNA) copy of the mRNA is synthesized by the enzyme reverse transcriptase, then the cDNA is amplified. This modification is used to detect chimeric fusion mRNA transcripts in cases where chromosomal breakpoints are too far apart to be detected by direct DNA amplification.

FISH is a relatively new and highly sensitive cytogenetic technique used to detect specific nucleic acid sequences in entire chromosomes (Pinkel, 1986). This method involves three basic steps. First, cells in conventional cytogenetic slide preparations are heated in the presence of formamide to denature the DNA. Next, biotin-labeled DNA probes are hybridized to specific DNA sequences in the cells. Finally, the slides are incubated with fluorescein-avidin, followed by incubation with biotinylated goat antiavidin to amplify the signal. Regions where the probe has hybridized appear as fluorescent spots on chromosome spreads. Unlike conventional cytogenetic analysis, FISH does not depend on cell division, and many more cells can be analyzed routinely, from several hundred to a thousand.

The FISH method represents an important adjunct to conventional cytogenetics for detecting numerical and structural chromosome abnormalities. Probes that are chromosome specific can be used to identify chromosomes and to detect numerical abnormalities, such as trisomies. FISH is also a highly sensitive method to detect chromosome translocations when probes for known oncogenes are available. For example, the t(9;22) in chronic myelogenous leukemia can be detected with probes to *BCR* and *ABL* that have been tagged with different fluorochromes (Tkachuk, 1990). If the translocation is present, both probes will colocalize to the same chromosome. It is also possible to correlate cytogenetic abnormalities with cell morphology; bone marrow aspirate smears can be stained with Wright-Giemsa and then analyzed by FISH.

Molecular analysis of hematologic malignancies has three goals. The first goal is to identify lineage characteristics that are not apparent by conventional phenotypic studies, such as cytochemical stains or immunophenotypic analysis. Lineage probes are designed to detect genetic events that occur during differentiation. The second is to detect nonrandom chromosomal aberrations that are associated with leukemias and lymphomas with cytogenetic probes. Finally, lineage and cytogenetic probes may be used to determine the presence of a clonal population of cells.

ORGANIZATION OF THE IMMUNOGLOBULIN AND T-CELL RECEPTOR GENES

It is necessary to understand the genetic organization of the immunoglobulin and T-cell receptor genes and their pattern of expression during development in order to evaluate the results of molecular genetic studies performed on lymphoid neoplasms. The immunoglobulin and T-cell receptor genes are members of the immunoglobulin supergene family, and share functional and structural similarities (Kirsch, 1994). Immunoglobulin molecules are composed of four chains, two identical heavy chains and two identical light chains. T-cell receptors are heterodimers, composed of either α and β chains, or γ and δ chains. The two different chains in both receptors are linked together by disulfide bonds. Each chain is composed of three or four segments: the variable (V), diversity (D), joining (J), and constant (C) region segments. Recombination of these segments is mediated through recognition sequences that flank each V, D, and J region. A complete receptor has a variable region that forms the antigen combining site and has a constant region. Recombination of these segments generates a vast array of potential antigen-combining sites. Additional diversity is generated because V-D-J joining is imprecise. The enzyme terminal deoxynucleotidyl transferase (Tdt) can add or remove nucleotides at the junctures, a process called *N-region diversification* (Desiderio, 1984).

B-Cell Development

B cells develop from pluripotent stem cells in the primary lymphoid tissues, that is, the yolk sac, fetal liver, spleen, or bone marrow, depending on the age of the individual. Stages in B-cell development are defined by the pattern of immunoglobulin gene rearrangement (Osmond, 1990; Rolink, 1991; Uckun, 1990). Early precursor B cells have immunoglobulin heavy chain gene rearrangements but do not express heavy chains. Late precursor B cells express cytoplasmic μ heavy chain. Immature B cells have undergone immunoglobulin light chain gene rearrangement and express complete IgM on their surface (sIg+). The mature B cell expresses IgM and IgD with the same antigen binding site on its surface. Up to this point, B-cell development is antigen independent and generates a B cell with a unique surface receptor. The remaining steps are antigen dependent; they are driven by the interaction of antigen with surface immunoglobulin on mature B cells in secondary lymphoid tissues. If a mature B cell encounters antigen that is recognized by its receptor, it develops into a plasma cell, a terminally differentiated cell that secretes immunoglobulin, or a memory B cell.

Immunoglobulin Heavy Chain Genes

The immunoglobulin heavy chain gene is located on chromosome 14q32 (Croce, 1979). The variable portion of the IgH gene is encoded by three gene segments: variable (V_H), diversity (D_H), and joining (J_H) segments (Early, 1980; Sakano, 1981). First, one of six J segments joins with one of several D segments. Then, the D-J joins with one of approximately 100 V_H segments. The intervening sequences between the joined V-D-J segments are deleted. Fully assembled variable region heavy chain genes are found only in B cells and are the only form of the gene that is actively transcribed in mature B cells. However, incomplete or unrearranged V regions can be expressed at earlier stages of maturation in B cells, or in T cells or myeloid cells (Pugh, 1988).

After the variable region gene segments are assembled, the

constant region is added. No rearrangement occurs between the V-D-J and the first downstream C region, Cμ. Instead, a long mRNA transcript is made, and the intervening sequences are removed by RNA splicing. Only one of two parental IgH alleles rearranges at a time, and only one parental allele is expressed (allelic exclusion). If the first rearrangement is productive, that is, it produces a functional V-D-J region, then the other allele does not rearrange. If the first rearrangement generates a nonsense or termination codon (a nonproductive rearrangement), the second allele rearranges. If neither rearrangement is productive, the cell dies.

Immunoglobulin Light Chain Genes

If immunoglobulin heavy chain gene rearrangement has been productive, light chain gene rearrangement follows (Korsmeyer, 1981). The kappa immunoglobulin light chain gene is on chromosome 2p11; the lambda light chain gene is on chromosome 22q11 (McBride, 1982). Unlike the heavy chain gene, the light chain genes lack diversity regions. To produce a complete kappa light chain, one of many V_κ segments joins with one of five J_κ segments, and the intervening sequences are deleted. There is a single Cκ segment. A long V-J and Cκ transcript is made, and the intervening sequences between the J and Cκ regions are removed by RNA splicing. The lambda light chain gene has an unusual configuration (Hieter, 1981a). The lambda gene has six to nine C region segments, each with its own J region ($J_\lambda C_\lambda$). Because these genes are highly polymorphic, it may be necessary to determine the germline pattern of an individual in order to analyze a sample for lambda light chain gene rearrangement (Taub, 1983). During development, a B cell will express either kappa or lambda light chain (isotypic exclusion) (Hieter, 1981b; Korsmeyer, 1981). The kappa light chain gene rearranges before the lambda gene. Lambda gene rearrangement occurs only if both attempts at kappa gene rearrangement are nonproductive. Thus, in a cell that expresses kappa, either one kappa gene will be rearranged and the other will be in the germline configuration, or one will be expressed and the other either nonproductively rearranged or deleted. In a cell that expresses lambda, both kappa genes either will be nonproductively rearranged or deleted. If both lambda rearrangements are nonproductive, the cell cannot produce immunoglobulin and it dies.

Heavy Chain Isotype Switch

The immunoglobulin heavy chain gene has nine constant regions that correspond to the immunoglobulin isotype: Cμ (IgM), Cδ (IgD), $C\gamma_{1-4}$ (IgG_{1-4}), $C\alpha_{1-2}$ (IgA_{1-2}), and Cϵ (IgE). These isotypes confer different effector functions. After a productive V-D-J joining, a B cell first produces IgM. To express Cδ, a long transcript is made that includes the δ sequences located immediately downstream of Cμ, and the transcript is spliced. However, a second type of rearrangement may occur that joins the same variable region with a different constant region through a mechanism known as isotype switch (Gritzmacher, 1989). To express Cγ, Cα, or Cϵ, the intervening sequences are deleted. This rearrangement is mediated by specific sequences in the 5′ flanking regions of the C region genes, known as switch regions. The result is an immunoglobulin molecule with the same antigen combining site, but a different constant region, and hence a different effector function.

T-Cell Development

T cells originate from pluripotent stem cells in the bone marrow that develop into prothymocytes, which migrate to the thymus. In the thymus cells that recognize self are eliminated, and the rest of T-cell development takes place. All four T-cell receptor genes (α, β, γ, and δ) undergo rearrangement that is similar to immunoglobulin gene rearrangement (Griesser, 1989; Knowles, 1989; Marrack, 1987). Like the immunoglobulin genes, only one of the parental alleles of a T-cell receptor gene is expressed. In addition, T cells express only one of two isoforms of the T-cell receptor, Tα/β or Tγ/δ. Tα/β cells are the predominant T-cell type in the peripheral blood and lymph nodes. Tγ/δ cells comprise less than 5% of circulating T cells and are found primarily in the skin and other epithelia.

The sequence of T-cell receptor gene rearrangement during development is not precisely known. In the thymocyte, the δ gene is the first to rearrange (de Villartay, 1988). If this rearrangement is productive, the cell is destined to become a γ/δ cell. γ or β chain gene rearrangement follows δ rearrangement. In a γ/δ cell with a rearranged β chain gene, the β rearrangement is nonproductive and is not expressed. If δ rearrangement is nonproductive, the α chain gene is rearranged and the α/β receptor is expressed.

Tα and Tδ Genes

The T α and δ chain genes are located on chromosome 14q11 (Caccia, 1985). The Tα gene contains approximately 100 V and J regions, and a single C region, spread over more than 1000 kilobases; it lacks a D region (Griesser, 1989; Knowles, 1989; Yoshikai, 1985). Because the gene is so large, it is difficult to study with routine techniques. The δ chain gene is composed of several V, three J, three D, and one C region (de Villartay, 1987, 1988; Satyanarayana, 1988). Interestingly, the δ chain gene is located entirely within the α chain gene, between the 3′-most Vα segment and the 5′-most Jα segment. This structure suggests that these genes arose through gene duplication. Because of this organization, Vα-Jα rearrangement deletes the δ gene. Thus, a cell that expresses the α/β receptor must have deleted its δ chain gene.

Tβ Gene

The Tβ gene is located on chromosome 7q34. The Tβ gene contains about 80 V_β segments followed by two separate but functionally indistinguishable loci, Tβ1 and Tβ2 (Caccia, 1984; Griesser, 1989; Knowles, 1989). Each locus contains one D region, six or seven J regions, and one C region. The two constant regions, Cβ1 and Cβ2, are highly homologous. Rearrangement of the V region in β2 deletes

Dβ1-Jβ1-Cβ1. If rearrangement is nonproductive on one allele, then the other allele rearranges.

Tγ Gene

The Tγ gene, located on the short arm of chromosome 7p15, contains only about 10 V regions and a few J regions (Griesser, 1989; Murre, 1985). Because of the relatively small number of possible rearrangements, a polyclonal population of cells can give a rearrangement pattern that appears oligoclonal. Conversely, it may be difficult to detect a clonal population in what appears to be an oligoclonal background. These observations should be kept in mind when interpreting the results of Tγ gene rearrangement studies (Cossman, 1990).

LINEAGE PROBES IN THE EVALUATION OF HEMATOPOIETIC NEOPLASMS

The probes used to identify lymphoid lineage by Southern blot analysis detect alterations of DNA restriction fragment length that result from the rearrangement of the immunoglobulin (Ig) and T-cell receptor (TCR) genes. Probes are complementary to regions of the genes that are present, even if the gene is rearranged and intervening sequences are deleted. Gene rearrangement alters the size of a restriction fragment. Thus, its location in the gel will be altered compared with the unrearranged gene. When a population of cells that is derived from a common progenitor and contains an identical rearrangement, that is, a clone, exceeds 1% of the total cells in the sample, the rearrangement can be detected as a distinct band (Cleary, 1984). If a sample lacks a clonal population, a single germline band that represents unrearranged antigen receptor genes, either in lymphoid or nonlymphoid cells, will be seen. Restriction enzyme digestion of polyclonal lymphoid populations generally does not produce discernible bands. Because the restriction fragments are of many different lengths and the abundance of any particular rearrangement is low, they are beyond the limits of detection of Southern analysis. With a single restriction enzyme and probe, samples that contain a clonal population may show a germline band and a single rearranged band if one allele is rearranged. Two rearranged bands generally indicate that the first rearrangement was nonproductive and the second allele was rearranged. Germline bands in samples that contain clonal populations indicate that either only one allele was rearranged or that the sample contains other cell types. To detect immunoglobulin heavy chain gene rearrangements, the most commonly used probes recognize any one of the six J_H segments. Probes may also be used for Cμ, Cκ, or Cλ. To detect rearrangements of the T-cell receptor β chain, probes for Jβ or Cβ that detect both the β1 and β2 loci are used. Because individual Jγ and Cγ segments are highly homologous, probes for Tγ rearrangement are designed to detect all Jγ or all Cγ segments. Similarly, probes for Tδ rearrangement detect all Jδ or Cδ segments.

Immunoglobulin and T-cell receptor gene rearrangements can also be detected by PCR (McCarthy, 1991; Reed, 1993; Trainor, 1991). This method uses primers that hybridize to conserved sequences in the V, D, and J regions. Rearrangement juxtaposes these regions and allows their amplification by PCR. On gel electrophoresis clonal populations produce one or two bands, depending upon whether one or two alleles were rearranged. Polyclonal populations produce many bands of different sizes that appear as a smear. Compared with Southern blot analysis, PCR is faster, requires far less tissue, and can be performed on DNA extracted from formalin-fixed, paraffin-embedded tissue. However, it is less sensitive; a relatively large proportion of the sample (more than 20%) must be clonal to be detected above a polyclonal background.

Acute Lymphoblastic Leukemia

Acute lymphoblastic leukemias (ALL) generally show heterogeneity in rearrangement patterns, based on their lineage and level of differentiation. More than 95% of pre-B ALLs show rearrangements in the IgH gene. Approximately 30% to 40% of pre-B ALLs also show rearrangements in the light chain genes (Korsmeyer, 1983). Immunoglobulin light chain gene rearrangement is considered specific for the B-cell lineage, except in very rare cases of T-ALL and AML (Hanson, 1990; Parreira, 1988). B-cell ALL (sIg+) shows rearrangements in both heavy and light chain genes. Most T-precursor ALLs show rearrangement in one or more T-cell receptor genes (TCRβ, TCRγ, TCRδ) (Greenberg, 1986; Knowles, 1989). However, very early T-precursor ALL may lack rearrangements of any TCR gene.

Although Ig heavy chain and TCR rearrangements are indicators of lineage, except for immunoglobulin light chain gene rearrangements, they are not specific for lineage. Immature B- and T-cell neoplasms frequently show aberrant rearrangements. These rearrangements may result from a common recombinase system that recognizes signal sequences that flank V, D, and J regions on the immunoglobulin and T-cell receptor genes, and is active early in development (Yancopoulos, 1986). About 10% to 20% of T-precursor ALLs have rearrangements in IgH (Kitchingman, 1985; Korsmeyer, 1983a); about 20% of B-precursor ALLs have rearrangements in TCRβ (Tawa, 1985). An even higher percentage of B-precursor ALLs (up to 40%) show rearrangements in TCRγ or TCRδ, possibly because these genes rearrange at an earlier stage of development than TCRβ (Felix, 1987; Greenberg, 1986). TCR rearrangements are rare in B-cell ALL (sIg+). Aberrant rearrangements are less common in mature B- and T-cell neoplasms. In addition, Ig and TCR rearrangements are not restricted to ALL. Reports of gene rearrangements in AML indicate that approximately 10% have rearrangements in Ig and/or TCR genes (Parreira, 1988; Seremetis, 1987). These cases of AML are also more likely to be TdT+. Aberrant gene rearrangements are often incomplete, and the genes are not expressed (Krolewski, 1989).

B-Cell Non-Hodgkin's Lymphomas and Lymphoproliferative Disorders

The vast majority of non-Hodgkin's lymphomas of B-cell immunophenotype have rearrangements of both the immunoglobulin heavy and light chain genes (Cleary, 1984; Cossman, 1990; Griesser, 1989; Krolewski, 1989). Not surprisingly, the immunoglobulin heavy and light chain genes are also rearranged in the B-cell chronic lymphoproliferative disorders (Korsmeyer, 1983b). Although immunoglobulin heavy chain gene rearrangement may be seen in non–B-cell malignancies, light chain gene rearrangement is generally considered specific for B-cell lineage. Infrequently, light chain gene rearrangements are found in the absence of a detectable heavy chain gene rearrangement. In cases of B-cell neoplasms, in which gene rearrangements have not been identified, sampling error may account for the lack of rearrangements. Occasional cases (10%) of B-cell lymphomas have TCRβ rearrangements, in addition to immunoglobulin gene rearrangements, but there is no evidence of transcription (Griesser, 1989; Krolewski, 1989; Pelicci, 1985).

T-Cell Non-Hodgkin's Lymphomas and Lymphoproliferative Disorders

In general, it is more difficult to study lymphomas of T-cell immunophenotype compared with B-cell lymphomas because of the lack of a marker of clonality. However, T-cell lymphomas may express an aberrant immunophenotype; they may express combinations of surface markers that do not correlate with stages in normal T-cell development (Knowles, 1989). Peripheral T-cell lymphomas are a morphologically hetergeneous group of neoplasms with mature T-cell immunophenotypes (Harris, 1994). About 90% of peripheral T-cell lymphomas have rearrangements of Tδ, Tγ, and Tβ; in about 10% of cases, these genes are in the germline configuration (Cossman, 1990; Knowles, 1989). About 10% of peripheral T-cell lymphomas have IgH gene rearrangements in addition to TCR gene rearrangements (Pelicci, 1985). Virtually all cases of mycosis fungoides/Sézary syndrome have TCR rearrangements; rare cases have also been reported to contain rearrangements of the IgH chain gene (Bignon, 1989; Griesser, 1989; Knowles, 1989).

Implications of Clonality in Lymphoid Proliferations

Most lymphoid malignancies contain clonal antigen receptor gene rearrangements. However, the presence of a clonal population is not necessarily diagnostic of malignancy. Clonal rearrangements have been described in certain conditions without evidence of lymphoid malignancy, for example, congenital immunodeficiency syndromes, autoimmune diseases, and acquired immune deficiency syndrome (AIDS) (Cossman, 1990). Thus, the diagnosis of a lymphoid malignancy depends on the correlation of histologic and molecular diagnostic data. It is also possible that molecular diagnostic studies may fail to detect clonal rearrangements in lesions that are clearly malignant by morphologic criteria. This can result from sampling error when the tissue is divided for histologic and molecular genetic analysis. Rarely, a rearrangement may produce a fragment that is the same size and, therefore, comigrates with the germline band. For this reason, genomic DNA is separately digested with at least two, and usually three, different restriction enzymes, most often *Eco*RI, *Bam*HI, and *Hin*dIII.

Myeloperoxidase Gene Expression

Most molecular studies of lineage in AML have involved the detection of myeloperoxidase (MPO) mRNA by northern or slot blot analysis. The presence of MPO mRNA correlates with myeloid lineage, and the degree of positivity correlates with FAB class (Zaki, 1989). Cases of acute undifferentiated leukemia (AUL), with negative cytochemistries and inconclusive or mixed immunophenotype, as well as cases of acute mixed-lineage leukemia, may contain significant amounts of MPO mRNA (Hirsch-Ginsberg, 1988; Zaki, 1989). Although MPO mRNA can be found in occasional cases of ALL, there is no detectable protein (Ferrari, 1988).

MOLECULAR ANALYSIS OF CHROMOSOMAL ABERRATIONS IN LEUKEMIAS AND LYMPHOMAS

Specific chromosomal abnormalities are nonrandomly associated with certain types of leukemias and lymphomas. These abnormalities, which include characteristic translocations, inversions, insertions, and deletions, serve as tumor-specific markers (Table 58–1). Molecular analysis of chromosomal lesions is used to classify, to assess clonality, and to determine prognosis in leukemias and lymphomas (Cossman, 1990; Hirsch-Ginsberg, 1993).

Activation of Oncogenes by Immunoglobulin and T-Cell Receptor Genes

More than 60% of the chromosomal translocations detected in lymphoid malignancies involve the Ig or TCR genes (Cossman, 1990; Hirsch-Ginsberg, 1993). Chromosomal abnormalities that are nonrandomly associated with B-cell leukemias and lymphomas frequently involve the IgH locus on chromosome 14q32. Less frequently, the Igκ locus on chromosome 2p11 and the Igλ locus on chromosome 22q11 are involved. Chromosomal abnormalities associated with T-cell leukemia and lymphoma commonly involve chromosome 14q11, the location of the TCRA locus. Translocations may also involve the *TCRB* locus on chromosome 7q35 and the *TCRG* locus on chromosome 7p13. It is believed that, in general, these translocations activate control elements that deregulate protooncogenes. By using probes for the Ig and TCR genes, many deregulated oncogenes have been identified.

Burkitt's Lymphoma and ALL-L3

Burkitt's lymphoma and its acute leukemia counterpart, ALL-L3, are extremely aggressive B-cell (sIg+) neoplasms. These neoplasms are characterized by chromosomal translocations of the *MYC* gene on chromosome 8q24 and one of the immunoglobulin genes (Leder, 1983). In most cases

Table 58–1. MOLECULAR CHARACTERISTICS OF CYTOGENETIC ALTERATIONS IN LEUKEMIAS AND LYMPHOMAS

Mechanism of Oncogene Activation	Cytogenetic Rearrangement	Disease	Affected Gene	Function
Juxtaposition to Ig genes	t(8;14) (q24;q32) t(2;8) (p11;q24) t(8;22) (q24; q11)	Burkitt's lymphoma; B-ALL (L3)	*MYC*	Transcription factor (helix-loop-helix)
	t(14;18) (q32; q21)	Follicular lymphoma	*BCL2*	Anti-apoptosis protein
	t(11;14) (q13; q32)	Mantle cell lymphoma	*PRAD1*	Cyclin protein
	t(5;14) (q31; q32)	Pre–B-ALL	*IL3*	Hematopoietic growth factor
Juxtaposition to TcR genes	t(1;14) (p32; q11)	T-ALL	*TAL1*	Transcription factor (helix-loop-helix)
	t(7;9) (q34; q34)	T-ALL	*TAL2*	Transcription factor (helix-loop-helix)
	t(7;19) (q35; p13)	T-ALL	*LYL1*	Transcription factor (helix-loop-helix)
	t(11;14) (p15; q11)	T-ALL	*TTG1/RBTN1*	Transcription factor (LIM domain)
	t(11;14) (p13; q11)	T-ALL	*TTG2/RBTNL1*	Transcription factor (LIM domain)
	t(7;11) (q35; p13)	T-ALL	*TTG2/RBTNL1*	Transcription factor (LIM domain)
	t(10;14) (q24; q11)	T-ALL	*HOX11*	Transcription factor (homeodomain)
	t(1;7) (q34; q34)	T-ALL	*LCK*	Tyrosine kinase
	t(7;9) (q34; q34.3)	T-ALL	*TAN1*	Cell surface protein
Juxtaposition to other genes	del(1) p32	T-ALL	*TAL1*	Transcription factor (helix-loop-helix); activated by SIL
Fusion genes	t(1;19) (q23; p13)	pre-B-ALL	*PBX*	Transcription factor (homeodomain)
			E2A	Transcription factor (helix-loop-helix)
	t(4;11) (q21; q23)	early B-cell-ALL	*ALL1* unknown	Transcription factor (Zn^{++} finger domain)
	t(2;5) (p23; q35)	anaplastic large cell lymphoma (Ki-1 positive)	*ALK*	Tyrosine kinase
			NPM	Nucleolar protein
	t(9;22) (q34; q11)	CML, ALL	*ABL*	Tyrosine kinase phosphoprotein
			BCR	
	t(15;17) (q22; q11.2-12)	AML-M3	*PML*	Transcription factor (Zn^{++} finger domain)
			RARA	Retinoic acid receptor
	t(8;21) (q22; q22)	AML-M2	*AML1*	Transcription factor
			ETO	Unknown
	t(6;9) (p23; q34)	AML	*CAN*	Unknown
			DEK	Unknown
Point mutation		AML	*RAS*	Guanine nucleotide-binding protein

(80%) the translocation involves the IgH locus at chromosome 14q32. Less frequently the translocation involves the λ light chain (Igλ) locus at chromosome 22q11 (15% of cases) or the κ light chain (Igκ) locus at chromosome 2p11 (5% of the cases). These translocations deregulate *MYC* gene expression and lead to constitutive overproduction of the protein (Leder, 1983). The MYC product is a transcription factor that appears to regulate cell proliferation. However, the precise mechanism by which deregulated expression of *MYC* contributes to oncogenesis is not known.

Molecular analysis of t(8;14) has shown that the breakpoints on chromosome 8 and 14 vary (Neri, 1988; Pelicci, 1986). In all cases the chromosomal translocation interrupts the IgH locus on chromosome 14. The breakpoints on chromosome 8 are found either immediately upstream or within the first exon of *MYC*. Thus, the *MYC* gene may be either truncated or translocated in its entirety to chromosome 14. In the endemic form of Burkitt's lymphoma that is associated with Epstein-Barr virus (EBV) infection and in EBV-positive lymphomas that arise in the setting of AIDS, the translocations occur upstream of *MYC*, and within or near the J_H or D_H regions of IgH. In the sporadic EBV-negative form of Burkitt's lymphoma, the translocations occur within or immediately 5′ to *MYC* on chromosome 8, and within or near the IgH switch (S) region on chromosome 14. It appears, therefore, that in endemic Burkitt's lymphoma the translocations occur during V(D)J rearrangement in early B cells; in sporadic Burkitt's lymphoma the translocations occur later, during an attempt at isotype switch. In the variant (2;8) and (8;22) translocations, the breakpoints in the light chain loci occur within the V_κ or J_κ segments on chromosome 2, or 5′ to the Cλ region on chromosome 22. The Igλ or Igκ constant region loci are translocated 3′ to the *MYC* gene, which remains on chromosome 8. About half of the chromosomal translocations that involve *MYC* can be detected by Southern blot analysis with currently available probes. A translocation is confirmed when the relevant Ig probe (J_H, J_κ, or Cλ, depending on the Ig gene involved) and an *MYC* probe detect comigrating bands of identical molecular weight. The breakpoints show too much variability to be detected by PCR.

Activation of BCL2 *by t(14;18) (q32;q21)*

Follicular lymphomas are B-cell neoplasms with the immunophenotype of mature B cells. Most follicular lymphomas of small cleaved cell type, and many follicular lymphomas of mixed cell or large cell type, have this characteristic translocation (Yunis, 1982). When it is found in a diffuse large cell lymphoma, the implication is that the diffuse lymphoma represents histologic progression of a follicular lymphoma. The translocation juxtaposes the *BCL2* region on chromosome 18q21 with sequences in the J_H region of the immunoglobulin heavy chain locus at 14q32 (Hockenbery, 1990; Tsujimoto, 1984). The result is overproduction of a structurally normal BCL2 protein (Hockenbery, 1990). The BCL2 protein is a 25 kDa protein found on the inner mitochondrial membrane that protects the cell from programmed cell death (apoptosis). Overexpression of the protein appears to prolong the life of a cell by delaying programmed cell death. The breakpoints on chromosome 14q32 vary little. The breakpoints on chromosome 18q21 are more variable (Weiss, 1987). Most breaks, about 60%, are found in a region of approximately 150 bp, the major breakpoint cluster region (mbr) (Cleary, 1986). About 25% of the breaks are found upstream of the mbr, in the minor breakpoint cluster region (mcr). The t(14;18) can be detected by Southern blot analysis using probes for J_H and *BCL2*; if a translocation has joined these two segments, they comigrate (Weiss, 1987). Because they are tightly clustered, translocations that involve the mbr and mcr can be readily detected by PCR, using probes that recognize unique junctional sequences (Lee, 1987). This technique can detect a single cell with the translocation in a population of more than 10^5 cells. However, a minority of translocations are not detectable with probes to the mbr or mcr because the breakpoints lie outside these regions, although cytogenetic studies demonstrate the translocation.

Translocation at BCL1 *in t(11;14) (q13;q32)*

The t(11;14) (q13;q32) is found in at least 50% of lymphomas classified as intermediate lymphocytic lymphomas (Medeiros, 1990; Williams, 1990). These lymphomas have a mature B-cell immunophenotype, and most are now classified as mantle cell lymphomas, based on the hypothesis that they arise from mantle B cells of lymphoid follicles (Harris, 1994). This translocation involves the immunoglobulin heavy chain locus on 14q32 and the *BCL1* breakpoint region on chromosome 11q13. The evidence suggests that the *PRAD1* gene is the protooncogene on chromosome 11 that is activated by this translocation (Motokura, 1991). The *PRAD1* gene encodes for cyclin D1, one of a family of proteins that regulates the cell cycle.

Activation of IL3 *by t(5;14) (q31;q32)*

The t(5;14) (q31;q32) is an uncommon translocation, found in a subset of patients with pre-B-cell ALL and peripheral eosinophilia (Meeker, 1990). Molecular analysis has shown that this translocation joins the immunoglobulin heavy chain locus to the promoter region of the interleukin-3 (*IL3*) gene, a hematopoietic growth factor. It has been suggested that the increased *IL3* expression accounts for the eosinophilia and results in an autocrine loop that contributes to leukemogenesis.

Activation of Rhombotin Genes in T-Cell Acute Lymphoblastic Leukemia

Cloning of chromosomal breakpoints in human T-cell ALL has led to the discovery of a new gene family called *TTG* (T-cell translocation gene) or rhombotin 1 and 2 (Boehm, 1988, 1991; McGuire, 1989). These genes show strong homology with LIM domain proteins, first described in *Caenorhabditis elegans* (Rabbitts, 1990). LIM domain proteins are transcription factors that contain two cysteine-rich domains. The LIM domains in the *RBTN1/TTG1* and *RBTNL1/TTG2* genes are highly homologous. In these translocations, elements in T-cell receptor loci activate expression of one of the rhombotin genes. In the t(11;14) (p15;q11), elements in the *TCRD* locus activate expression of the *RBTN1/TTG1* gene. In the t(11;14) (p13;q11), observed in approximately 10% of T-ALL cases, elements in the *TCRD* locus activate expression of the rhombotin 2/*TTG2*, located downstream of the breakpoint region on chromosome 11p13. A variant translocation, t(7;11) (q35;p13), involves the *TCRB* chain locus.

Activation of TCL3/HOX11 *by t(10;14) (q24;q11)*

Rearrangements that involve chromosome 10q24 are found in 5% to 10% of T-cell leukemias and high-grade T-cell lymphomas. This translocation activates the expression of a homeobox gene, *HOX11* (Hatano, 1991; Kennedy, 1991; Lu, 1991). Homeobox genes were identified first in insects, where they regulate body plan development. Since then, homeodomain-containing proteins have been found in other species, including humans. In this translocation, the *HOX11* gene, which is normally not expressed in T cells, is activated by T-cell receptor elements.

Activation of Helix-Loop-Helix Protein Genes in T-Cell Acute Lymphoblastic Leukemia

Helix-loop-helix proteins are a group of proteins that regulate transcription. Nonrandom chromosomal abnormalities have been shown to activate genes that encode for HLH proteins in T-cell ALL and other malignancies. These genes include the *TAL1* (T-cell acute lymphocyte leukemia-1) and *TAL2* genes, and the *LYL1* (lymphoblastic leukemia derived sequence 1) gene (Rabbitts, 1991). In T-cell ALL these genes are activated by regulatory elements in the T-cell receptor loci. The *TAL1* (*SCL*) gene, located on chromosome 1p32, may be activated either by translocation or deletion (Begley, 1989; Chen, 1990). *TAL1* is normally expressed in immature hematopoietic cells, but not in T cells. Cloning of t(1;14) (p32;q11) has revealed that the translocations join control elements of the *TCRD* locus with the 3′ or 5′ untranslated regions of the *TAL1* gene. *TAL1* also may be activated by a deletion that joins *TAL1* with the 5′ regulatory region of the *SIL* (*SCL* interrupting locus) gene, a nuclear protein that is normally expressed in T cells (Aplan, 1990). This deletion, found in about 20% of T-cell ALL, produces a fusion transcript, but a chimeric protein has not been identified. The t(7;9) (q34;q34) is an infrequent translocation first cloned from a T-cell leukemia cell line. In this case, elements of the *TCRB* chain activate the *TAL2* protooncogene (Reynolds, 1987; Xia, 1991). The t(7;19) (q35;p13), also reported in T-cell ALL, juxtaposes a truncated *LYL1* gene with the *TCRB* gene in opposite transcriptional orientation (Mellentin, 1989).

Activation of the LCK *Gene by t(1;7) (p34;q34)*

In this translocation the *TCRB* locus activates the *LCK* (lymphocyte-specific protein tyrosine kinase) gene, which encodes $p56^{lck}$ (Burnett, 1991; Marth, 1986). *LCK* is a member of the SRC family of cytoplasmic tyrosine protein kinases and is normally expressed predominantly in T cells.

Activation of the TAN *Gene by t(7;9) (q34;q34.3)*

The t(7;9) (q34;q34.3), cloned from a T-cell leukemia, involves the *TCRB* gene and the *TAN* (translocation activated notch) locus on chromosome 9 (Reynolds, 1987). The *TAN1* gene is expressed primarily by lymphoid cells and encodes for the human homolog of the *Drosophila* Notch gene product, an integral membrane protein that regulates embryonic cell fate. Studies of this translocation indicate that breakpoints in epidermal growth factor–like repeats within the *TAN1* locus result in the production of truncated versions of TAN1 mRNA, which may contribute to tumor formation or tumor progression (Ellisen, 1991).

Chromosomal Translocations that Generate Fusion Transcripts and Chimeric Proteins

t(1;19) (q23;p13)

The t(1;19) (q23;p13) is found in approximately 30% of pre–B-cell leukemias and may be associated with a poor prognosis (Crist, 1984; Williams, 1984). This translocation joins the *E2A* gene on chromosome 19 with the *PBX* (pre–B-cell leukemia transcription factor) homeogene on chromosome 1 (Kamps, 1990; Nourse, 1990). The E2A protein product is a transcription factor that normally regulates immunoglobulin gene expression. The translocation generates a fusion protein that has features of a chimeric transcription factor. The DNA-binding domain of the E2A protein is replaced by the DNA-binding domain of the PBX protein, but gene expression is controlled by the regulatory elements of the *E2A* gene. This translocation can be detected as a rearrangement on Southern blots or by RT-PCR amplification of the fusion transcript.

Activation of the ALL1 *Gene by t(4;11) (q21;q23)*

The t(4;11) (q21;q23) is found in less than 10% of ALL patients, but it is associated with a distinctive clinical presentation and immunophenotype (Mirro, 1986; Pui, 1984; Stong, 1985; Third International Workshop on Chromosomes in Leukemia, 1981). Children with this abnormality are usually less than one year old, present with very high white blood cell counts, and have a poor prognosis. The leukemic cells have an unusual precursor–B-cell immunophenotype; they are CD19+, CD10−, and often coexpress CD15, a marker of myeloid differentiation, as well as other markers of myeloid or monocytic differentiation. This translocation generates a chimeric fusion protein that contains sequences of the *ALL1* gene (Gu, 1992; Tkachuck, 1992). *ALL1* is homologous to the *Drosophila trithorax* gene, a transcription factor that regulates body plan development.

t(2;5) (p23;q35)

This translocation has been described recently in some cases of Ki-1+ anaplastic large cell lymphoma. This non-Hodgkin's lymphoma is characterized by large multinucleated cells that strongly express CD30 (Ki-1 antigen), and frequently involves skin and lymph node sinuses (Harris, 1994). Most are of T-cell immunophenotype, but some are of B-cell or null-cell immunophenotype. The translocation fuses the amino terminus of the *NPM* gene on chromosome 5q35 to the catalytic domain of the *ALK* gene on chromosome 2p23 (Morris, 1994). The *NPM* gene encodes the nucleolar protein, nucleophosmin; the *ALK* gene encodes a protein with tyrosine kinase activity. Because the breakpoints are tightly clustered and a chimeric transcript is produced, the translocation is easily detected by RT-PCR (Ladanyi, 1994).

Philadelphia Chromosome, t(9;22) (q34;q11)

The Philadelphia chromosome (Ph^1) results from a reciprocal translocation between the *ABL* protooncogene on chromosome 9q34 and the breakpoint cluster region (bcr) of the *BCR* gene on chromosome 22q11 (Groffen, 1984; Heisterkamp, 1983; Rowley, 1973). ABL is a 145 kDa cytoplasmic protein with tyrosine kinase activity. The *BCR* gene codes for a 160 kDa phosphoprotein that is expressed in a wide variety of tissues. This cytogenetic aberration is detected in almost all patients with chronic myeloid leukemia (CML), 25% of adults with ALL, 5% of children with ALL, and is rare in patients with acute myeloid leukemia (AML) (Chan, 1987; Clark, 1987; Hermans, 1987). In ALL, the presence of a Ph^1 chromosome is associated with a poor prognosis. Cloning of the t(9;22) breakpoint regions has revealed that the breakpoints on chromosome 9 occur in a large, 100-kb region 5′ to exon 2 of *ABL* (Bernards, 1987; Heisterkamp, 1983). In CML and about half of cases of ALL, the translocation breakpoints in the *BCR* gene are clustered in a 5 to 6 kb region on chromosome 22, within the second or third introns, the major breakpoint cluster region (M-bcr) (Heisterkamp, 1983). The *BCR-ABL* is expressed as a chimeric 8.5-kb mRNA with the *BCR* sequences at the 5′ end, and the *ABL* sequences at the 3′ end. It encodes for the p210 fusion protein. In the other half of cases of Ph^1-positive ALL, the break in the *BCR* gene occurs further 5′, within the first intron (Chan, 1987; Clark, 1987; Hermans, 1987). In this case, the first exon of the *BCR* gene is fused with *ABL*. A 7-kb BCR-ABL chimeric transcript encodes for the pl90 fusion protein. Both fusion proteins have elevated tyrosine kinase activity compared with the wild-type protein, which may confer a growth advantage to Ph^1-positive cells (Lugo, 1990; McLaughlin, 1989). Currently, probes exist that detect the 3′ *BCR* rearrangements by Southern blotting. However, both 5′ and 3′ breakpoints can be detected by RT-PCR, an important method for the detection of minimal residual disease (Lee, 1989, 1992).

t(15;17) (q22;q11.2-12)

The t(15;17) is the hallmark of acute promyelocytic leukemia (APL or AML M-3), present in virtually all cases (Larson, 1984). In this leukemia, abnormal promyelocytes accumulate because of a block in the differentiation pathway of granulocytes and monocytes. Before the molecular defect had been characterized, it had been observed that retinoic acid induced differentiation in cells derived from patients with APL (Flynn, 1983). Further, patients treated with All *trans*-retinoic acid achieved clinical remission (Huang, 1988). Subsequently, it has been shown that the translocation joins the retinoic acid receptor α (*RARA*) gene on chromosome 17 with the *PML* (promyelocytic leukemia, or *MYL*) gene on chromosome 15 (Alcalay, 1991; Borrow, 1990; De The, 1990). The retinoic acid receptor belongs to the nuclear receptor superfamily that includes thyroid and steroid hormone receptors (Evans, 1988). The DNA sequence of the *PML* gene suggests that it belongs to the family of zinc finger domain transcription factors, but the function of the normal protein is unknown. Unlike other translocations that generate a single fusion product, t(15;17) generates chimeric transcripts from both fusion genes, *PML-RARA* and *RARA-PML* (Alcalay, 1992; Chang, 1991; De The, 1991; Kakizuka, 1991; Pandolfi, 1992). This translocation can be detected by Southern blotting with the BAPL probe, derived from the *RARA* gene, or by RT-PCR of the fusion transcripts (Chang, 1992).

Activation of ETO *by t(8;21) (q22;q22)*

The t(8;21) (q22;q22) is a common abnormality in AML-M2 (Bitter, 1987). Patients with this translocation tend to be younger than patients with AML overall and have an excellent prognosis. The *ETO* gene, on chromosome 8q22, is not normally expressed in myeloid cells (Chang, 1993). This translocation activates *ETO* gene expression by joining it with regulatory elements of the *AML1* (acute myeloid leukemia 1) gene on chromosome 21 (Erickson, 1992; Gao, 1991; Miyoshi, 1991). The *AML1* gene product is a putative transcription factor with homology to the *Drosophila* gene, *runt*. This translocation can be detected by RT-PCR of the AML1-ETO fusion transcript (Chang, 1993).

t(6;9) (p23;q34)

This translocation is associated with increased numbers of bone marrow basophils in patients with AML (Pearson, 1985). Patients with this translocation tend to be younger than patients with AML overall, but respond poorly to chemotherapy. Translocation of the *CAN* gene on chromosome 9q34 and the *DEK* gene on chromosome 6p23 generates a fusion protein, $p165^{DEK\text{-}CAN}$ (Von Linden, 1990). The function of the normal *DEK* and *CAN* gene products is not known.

Activation of Oncogenes by Point Mutations

The RAS family of oncogenes (*NRAS, KRAS*, and *HRAS*) code for 21 kDa G proteins that play a role in growth factor signal transduction. These proteins, located on the inner surface of the cell membrane, bind GTP and GDP, and have GTPase activity. Mutations, particularly in the 12th, 13th, and 61st codons of *NRAS* and *KRAS*, have been described in approximately 20% of ALL and 30% of AML (Bos, 1988; Browett, 1989; Hirsch-Ginsberg, 1993). Mutations in these codons interfere with normal RAS activity by inhibiting hydrolysis of GTP, which may prolong signals to the nucleus. Mutations can be detected by PCR amplification of 100-bp sequences surrounding the 12th, 13th, and 61st codons, followed by hybridization to a panel of synthetic oligonucleotide probes that contain wild-type and mutated sequences (Bos, 1988, 1989; Senn, 1988; Yunis, 1988). This method can detect RAS mutations when about 10% of the cells in a sample contain a mutation. Mutations in RAS are thought to play a role in the progression of disease from a preleukemic to a leukemic state (Yunis, 1988). RAS mutations have been found in nonleukemic cells from patients with acute leukemias. This finding suggests that the mutation may have occurred in a pluripotent progenitor and may account for the occasional mutation detected during clinical remission. Conversely, in some cases of acute leukemia, the mutation may be weakly detected, although the entire sample consists of leukemic blasts. This suggests that only a subclone of the leukemic population contains the mutation. Although mutated RAS may be found in the initial diagnostic specimen, it can disappear at relapse (Senn, 1988).

Detection of Minimal Residual Disease

The high frequency of relapse remains a major problem in cancer therapy. It is likely that relapse results from clinically undetectable disease. Residual disease may be detected by morphologic analysis of biopsy specimens, immunophenotypic analysis, and routine cytogenetic analysis. The molecular techniques that have been described to help diagnose disease can also be used to determine if disease persists after therapy. All of these techniques depend on the ability to detect a small clonal population of neoplastic cells that are related to the original malignant clone among a significantly larger population of normal cells. This information may be used to determine if additional therapy is necessary, to determine prognosis, and to predict relapse.

The most sensitive technique to detect minimal residual disease is PCR, which can detect one neoplastic cell out of more than 10^5 cells (Lee, 1987). In this setting, PCR has been used to evaluate specimens for specific chromosomal translocations, for example, t(14;18) in follicular lymphoma (Lee, 1987), t(10;14) in T-cell ALL/lymphoma (Kagan, 1990), t(8;21) in AML-M2 (Chang, 1993), t(15;17) in AML-M3 (Chang, 1992), and t(9;22) in CML and ALL (Lee, 1989, 1992). As more breakpoints are identified, more probes and primers will be available for these studies. It is also possible to use PCR to amplify the unique, clone-specific sequences that are formed at the junctures of V-D-J regions of the *IGH* and *TCRD* genes during recombination (Tycko, 1989; Yamada, 1989). This technique has been used to detect minimal residual disease in patients with ALL, but it has two limitations. First, sequence-specific probes must be prepared for each patient. Second, the malignant population may not be detected if these sequences are altered during clonal evolution.

Studies of minimal residual disease in patients with CML and AML in clinical remission have produced conflicting data. The frequency of residual leukemia and the prognostic value of the assays vary depending on the study. However, they raise important questions. Do patients in long clinical remissions have quiescent tumor cells that may proliferate and lead to relapse? Does detection of minimal residual disease predict relapse? Do patients with minimal residual disease require additional intensive therapy?

Alcalay M, Zangrilli D, Pandolfi PP, et al: Translocation breakpoint of acute promyelocytic leukemia lies within the retinoic acid alpha locus. Proc Natl Acad Sci USA 1991; 88:1977–1981.

Alcalay M, Zangrilli D, Fagioli M, et al: Expression pattern of the RARα-PML fusion gene in acute promyelocytic leukemia. Proc Natl Acad Sci USA 1992; 89:4840–4844.

Aplan PD, Lombardi DP, Ginsberg AM, et al: Disruption of the human SCL locus by "illegitimate" V-(D)-J recombinase activity. Science 1990; 250:1426–1429.

Begley GC, Aplan PD, Denning SM, et al: The gene SCL is expressed during early hematopoiesis and encodes a differentiation-related DNA-binding motif. Proc Natl Acad Sci USA 1989; 86:10128–10132.

Bernards A, Rubin C, Westbrook CA, et al: The first intron in the human c-abl gene is at least 200 kilobases long and is a target for translocation in chronic myelogenous leukemia. Mol Cell Biol 1987; 7:3231–3236.

Bignon YU, Souteyrand P, Roger H, Bernard D: Dual genotype in cutaneous T cell lymphoma: Immunoglobulin gene rearrangement in clonal T cell malignancy. J Invest Dermatol 1989; 92:775.

Bitter MA, Le Beau MM, Rowley JD, et al: Associations between morphology, karyotype, and clinical features in myeloid leukemias. Hum Path 1987; 18:211–225.

Boehm T, Baer R, Lavenir I, et al: The mechanism of chromosomal translocation t(11;14) involving the T-cell receptor Cδ locus on human chromosome 14q11 and a transcribed region of chromosome 11p15. EMBO J 1988; 7:385–394.

Boehm T, Foroni L, Kaneko Y, et al: The rhombotin family of cysteine-rich LIM-domain oncogenes: Distinct members are involved in T-cell translocations to human chromosomes 11p15 and 11p13. Proc Natl Acad Sci USA 1991; 88:4367–4371.

Borrow J, Goddard AD, Sheer D, Solomon E: Molecular analysis of acute promyelocytic leukemia breakpoint cluster region on chromosome 17. Science 1990; 249:1577–1580.

Bos JL: Ras oncogenes in hematopoietic malignancies. Hematol Pathol 1988; 2:55–63.

Bos JL: Detection of ras oncogenes using PCR. *In* Erlich HA (ed): PCR Technology: Principles and Applications for DNA Amplification. New York, Stockton Press, 1989.

Browett PJ, Norton JD: Analysis of ras gene mutations and methylation state in human leukemias. Oncogene 1989; 4:1029–1036.

Burnett RC, David JC, Harden AM, et al: The LCK gene is involved in the t(1;7) (p34;q34) in T-cell lymphoblastic leukemia derived cell line HSB-2. Genes Chromosom Cancer 1991; 3:461–467.

Caccia N, Kronenberg M, Saxe D, et al: The T-cell receptor beta chain genes are located on chromosome 6 in mice and chromosome 7 in humans. Cell 1984; 37:1091–1099.

Caccia N, Bruns GAP, Kirsch IL, et al: T-cell receptor alpha chain genes are located on chromosome 14 at 14q11-14q12 in humans. J Exp Med 1985; 161:1255–1260.

Chan LC, Karhi KK, Rayter SI, et al: A novel ABL protein expressed in Philadelphia chromosome positive acute lymphoblastic leukemia. Nature 1987; 325:635–637.

Chang K-S, Trujillo JM, Ogura T, et al: Rearrangement of the retinoic acid receptor gene in acute promyelocytic leukemia. Leukemia 1991; 5:200–204.

Chang K-S, Lu J, Wang G, et al: The t(15;17) breakpoint in acute promyelocytic leukemia clusters within two different sites of the *myl* gene: Targets for the detection of minimal residual disease by the polymerase chain reaction. Blood 1992; 79:554–558.

Chang K-S, Fan Y-H, Stass SA, et al: Expression of *AML1-ETO* fusion transcripts and detection of minimal residual disease. Oncogene 1993; 8:983–988.

Chen Q, Cheng J-T, Tsai L-H, et al: The *tal* gene undergoes chromosomal translocation in T cell leukemia and potentially encodes a helix-loop-helix protein. EMBO J 1990; 9:415–424.

Clark SS, McLaughlin J, Crist WM, et al: Unique form of the abl tyrosine kinase distinguish Ph[1]-positive CML from Ph[1]-positive ALL. Science 1987; 235:85–88.

Cleary ML, Chao J, Warnke R, Sklar J: Immunoglobulin gene rearrangement as a diagnostic criterion of B-cell lymphoma. Proc Natl Acad Sci USA 1984; 81:593–597.

Cleary ML, Smith SD, Sklar J: Cloning and structural analysis of cDNAs for bcl-2 and a hybrid bcl-2/immunoglobulin transcript resulting from the t(14;18) translocation. Cell 1986; 47:19–28.

Cossman J, Stetler-Stevenson M, Medeiros LJ, Raffeld M: Molecular genetics of lymphoproliferative processes. *In* De Vita VT, Hellman S, Rosenberg SA (eds): Important Advances in Oncology 1990, Philadelphia, J. B. Lippincott Co., 1990, pp 101–113.

Crist W, Boyett J, Roper M, et al: Pre-B cell leukemia responds poorly to treatment: A Pediatric Oncology Group study. Blood 1984; 63: 407–414.

Croce CM, Shander M, Martinis J, et al: Chromosomal location of the human genes for immunoglobulin heavy chains. Proc Natl Acad Sci USA 1979; 76:3416–3419.

Desiderio SV, Yancopoulos GD, Paskind M, et al: Insertion of N regions into heavy chain genes is correlated with expression of terminal deoxytransferase in B cells. Nature 1984; 311:752–755.

De The H, Chomienne C, Lanotte M, et al: The t(15;17) translocation of acute promyelocytic leukaemia fuses the retinoic acid receptor α gene to a novel transcribed locus. Nature 1990; 347:558–561.

De The H, Lavau C, Marchio A, et al: The PML/RARα fusion mRNA generated by the t(15;17) translocation in acute promyelocytic leukemia encodes a functionally altered RARα. Cell 1991; 66:675–684.

de Villartay J-P, Lewis D, Hockett R, et al: Deletional rearrangement in the human T-cell receptor α-chain locus. Proc Natl Acad Sci USA 1987; 84:8608–8612.

de Villartay J-P, Hockett R, Coran D, et al: Deletion of the human T-cell receptor δ-gene by a site-specific recombination. Nature 1988; 335: 170–174.

Early P, Huang H, Davis M, et al: An immunoglobulin heavy chain variable region is generated from three segments of DNA: V_H, D, J_H. Cell 1980; 19:981–992.

Ellisen LW, Bird J, West DC, et al: TAN-1, the human homolog of the Drosophila *Notch* gene, is broken by chromosomal translocations in T lymphoblastic neoplasms. Cell 1991; 66:649–661.

Erickson P, Gao J, Chang KS, et al: Identification of breakpoints in t(8;21) acute myelogenous leukemia and isolation of a fusion transcript AML1/ETO1 with similarity to Drosophila segmentation gene, runt. Blood 1992; 80:1825–1831.

Evans RM: The steroid and thyroid hormone receptor superfamily. Science 1988; 240:889–895.

Felix CA, Wright JJ, Poplack DG, et al: T cell receptor α, β, and γ genes in T cell and pre B cell acute lymphoblastic leukemia. J Clin Invest 1987; 80:545–556.

Ferrari S, Mariano MT, Tagliafico E, et al: Myeloperoxidase gene expression in blast cells with a lymphoid phenotype in cases of acute lymphoblastic leukemia. Blood 1988; 72:873–876.

Flynn P, Miller WJ, Weisdorf DJ, et al: Retinoic acid treatment of acute promyelocytic leukemia: In vitro and in vivo observations. Blood 1983; 62:1211–1217.

Gao J, Erickson P, Gardiner K, et al: Isolation of a yeast artificial chromosome spanning the 8;21 translocation breakpoint t(8;21) (q22;q22.3) in acute myelogenous leukemia. Proc Natl Acad Sci USA 1991; 88: 4882–4886.

Greenberg JM, Quertermous T, Seidman JG, Kersey JH: Human T cell gamma-chain rearrangements in acute lymphoid and nonlymphoid leukemia: Comparison with the T cell receptor β-chain gene. J Immunol 1986; 137:2043–2049.

Griesser H, Tkachuk D, Reis MD, Mak T: Gene arrangements and translocations in lymphoproliferative diseases. Blood 1989; 73:1402–1415.

Gritzmacher CA: Molecular aspects of heavy-chain class switching. Crit Rev Immunol 1989; 9:173–200.

Groffen J, Stephenson JR, Heisterkamp N, et al: Philadelphia chromosomal breakpoints are clustered within a limited region, bcr, on chromosome 22. Cell 1984; 36:93–99.

Gu Y, Nakamura T, Alder H, et al: The t(4;11) chromosome translocation of human acute leukemias fuses the ALL-1 gene, related to *Drosophila trithorax*, to the AF-4 gene. Cell 1992; 71:701–708.

Hanson CA, Thamilarasan M, Ross CA, et al: Kappa light chain gene rearrangement in T-cell acute lymphoblastic leukemia. Am J Clin Pathol 1990; 93:563–568.

Harris NL, Jaffe ES, Stein H, et al: A revised European-American classification of lymphoid neoplasms: A proposal from the International Lymphoma Study Group. Blood 1994; 84:1361–1392.

Hatano M, Roberts CWM, Minden M, et al: Deregulation of a homeobox gene, HOX11, by the t(10;14) in T cell leukemia. Science 1991; 253:79–82.

Heisterkamp N, Stephenson JR, Groffen J, et al: Localization of the c-abl oncogene adjacent to a translocation breakpoint in chronic myelogenous leukemia. Nature 1983; 306:239–242.

Hermans A, Heisterkamp N, von Linden M, et al: Unique fusion of bcr and c-abl genes in Philadelphia chromosome positive acute lymphoblastic leukemia. Cell 1987; 51:33–40.

Hieter PA, Korsmeyer SJ, Waldmann TA, Leder P: Human immunoglobulin kappa light-chain genes are deleted or rearranged in lambda-producing B cells. Nature 1981a; 290:368–372.

Hieter PA, Hollis GF, Korsmeyer SJ, et al: Clustered arrangement of immunoglobulin lambda constant region genes in man. Nature 1981b; 294:536–540.

Hirsch-Ginsberg C, Childs C, Chang K-S, et al: Phenotypic and molecular heterogeneity in Philadelphia-chromosome positive acute leukemia. Blood 1988; 71:186–195.

Hirsch-Ginsberg C, Huh YO, Kagan J, et al: Advances in the diagnosis of acute leukemia. Hematol Oncol Clin North Am 1993; 7:1–46.

Hockenbery D, Nunez G, Milliman C, et al: Bcl-2 is an inner mitochondrial membrane protein that blocks programmed cell death. Nature 1990; 348:334–336.

Huang M, Ye YC, Chen B, et al: Use of all-trans retinoic acid in the treatment of acute promyelocytic leukemia. Blood 1988; 72:567–572.

Kagan J, Finger LR, Besa E, Croce CM: Detection of minimal residual dis-

7

ease in leukemic patients with the t(10;14) (q24;q11) chromosomal translocation. Cancer Res 1990; 50:5240–5244.
Kakizuka A, Miller WH, Umesono K, et al: Chromosomal translocation t(15;17) in human acute promyelocytic leukemia fuses RARα with a novel putative transcription factor PML. Cell 1991; 66:663–674.
Kamps MP, Murre C, Sun XH, Baltimore D: A new homeobox gene contributes the DNA-binding domain of the t(1;19) translocation protein in pre-B ALL. Cell 1990; 60:547–555.
Kawasaki ES, Clark SS, Coyne MY, et al: Diagnosis of chronic myeloid and acute lymphocytic leukemias by detection of leukemia-specific mRNA sequences amplified in vitro. Proc Natl Acad Sci USA 1988; 85:5698–5702.
Kawasaki ES, Wang AM: Detection of gene expression. *In* Erlich HA (ed): PCR Technology: Principles and Applications for DNA Amplification. New York, Stockton Press, 1989.
Kennedy MA, Gonzalez-Sarmiento R, Kees UR, et al: *HOX11*, a homeobox-containing T-cell oncogene on human chromosome 10q24. Proc Natl Acad Sci USA 1991; 88:8900–8904.
Kirsch IR, Kuehl WM: Gene rearrangements in lymphoid cells. *In* Stamatoyannopoulos G, Nienhuis AW, Majerus PW, Varmus H (eds): The Molecular Basis of Blood Diseases, 4th ed. Philadelphia: W. B. Saunders Co., 1994, pp 381–424.
Kitchingman GR, Rovigatti U, Mauer AM, et al: Rearrangement of immunoglobulin heavy chain genes in T cell acute lymphoblastic leukemia. Blood 1985; 65:725–729.
Knowles DM: Immunophenotypic and antigen receptor gene rearrangement analysis of T cell neoplasia. Am J Pathol 1989; 134:761–785.
Korsmeyer SJ, Hieter PA, Ravetch JV, et al: Developmental hierarchy of immunoglobulin gene rearrangements in human leukemic pre-B cells. Proc Natl Acad Sci 1981; 78:7096–7100.
Korsmeyer SJ, Arnold A, Bakshi A, et al: Immunoglobulin gene rearrangement and cell surface antigen expression in acute lymphocytic leukemias of T cell and B cell precursor origins. J Clin Invest 1983a; 71:301–313.
Korsmeyer SJ, Greene WC, Cossman J, et al: Rearrangement and expression of immunoglobulin genes and expression of Tac antigen in hairy cell leukemia. Proc Natl Acad Sci USA 1983b; 80:4522–4526.
Krolewski JJ, Dalla-Favera R: Molecular genetic approaches in the diagnosis and classification of lymphoid malignancies. Hematol Pathol 1989; 3:45–61.
Ladanyi M, Cavalchire G, Morris SW, et al: Reverse transcriptase polymerase chain reaction for the Ki-1 anaplastic large cell lymphoma-associated t(2;5) translocation in Hodgkin's disease. Am J Pathol 1994; 145:1296–1300.
Larson RA, Kondo K, Vardiman JW, et al: Evidence for a 15;17 translocation in every patient with acute promyelocytic leukemia. Am J Med 1984; 76:827–841.
Leder P, Battey J, Lenoir GT, et al: Translocations among antibody genes in human cancer. Science 1983; 222:765–771.
Lee M-S, Chang K-S, Cabanillas F, et al: Detection of minimal residual cells carrying the t(14;18) by DNA sequence analysis. Science 1987; 237:175–178.
Lee M-S, LeMaistre A, Kantarjian HM, et al: Detection of two alternative *bcr/abl* mRNA junctions and minimal residual disease in Philadelphia chromosome positive chronic myelogenous leukemia by polymerase chain reaction. Blood 1989; 73:2165–2170.
Lee M-S, Kantarjian H, Talpaz M, et al: Detection of minimal residual disease by polymerase chain reaction in Philadelphia chromosome-positive chronic myelogenous leukemia following interferon therapy. Blood 1992; 79:1920–1923.
Lu M, Gong Z, Shen W, Ho AD: The *tcl*-3 protooncogene altered by chromosomal translocation in T-cell leukemia codes for a homeobox protein. EMBO J 1991; 10:2905–2910.
Lugo TG, Pendergast AM, Muller A, Witte ON: Tyrosine kinase activity and transformation potency of bcr-abl oncogene products. Science 1990; 247:1079–1082.
Marrack P, Kappler J: The T cell receptor. Science 1987; 238:1073–1079.
Marth JD, Disteche C, Pravtcheva D, et al: Localization of a lymphocyte-specific protein tyrosine kinase gene (*lck*) at a site of frequent chromosomal abnormalities in human lymphoma. Proc Natl Acad Sci USA 1986; 83:7400–7404.
McBride OW, Hieter PA, Hollis GF, et al: Chromosomal location of human kappa and lambda light chain constant region genes. J Exp Med 1982; 155:1480–1490.
McCarthy KP, Sloane JP, Kabarowski JHS, et al: The rapid detection of clonal T-cell proliferations in patients with lymphoid disorders. Am J Pathol 1991; 138:821–828.
McGuire EA, Hockett RD, Pollock KM, et al: The t(11;14) (p15;q11) in a T-cell acute lymphoblastic leukemia cell line activates multiple transcripts, including *Ttg-1*, a gene encoding a potential zinc finger protein. Mol Cell Biol 1989; 9:2124–2132.
McLaughlin J, Chianese E, Witte ON: Alternative forms of the bcr/abl oncogene have qualitatively different potencies for stimulation of immature lymphoid cells. Mol Cell Biol 1989; 9:1866–1874.
Medeiros LJ, Van Krieken JH, Jaffe ES, Raffeld M: Association of bcl-1 rearrangements with lymphocytic lymphoma of intermediate differentiation. Blood 1990; 76:2086–2090.
Meeker TC, Hardy D, Willman C, et al: Activation of the interleukin-3 gene by chromosome translocation in acute lymphocytic leukemia with eosinophilia. Blood 1990; 76:285–289.
Mellentin SD, Smith SD, Cleary ML: Lyl-1, a novel gene altered by chromosomal translocation in acute T cell leukemia, codes for a protein with a helix-loop-helix DNA binding motif. Cell 1989; 58:77–83.
Mirro J, Kitchingman G, Williams D, et al: Clinical and laboratory characteristics of acute leukemia with the 4;11 translocation. Blood 1986; 67:689–697.
Miyoshi H, Shimizu K, Kozu T, et al: t(8;21) breakpoints on chromosome 21 in acute myeloid leukemia are clustered within a limited region of a single gene AML-1. Proc Natl Acad Sci USA 1991; 88:10431–10434.
Morris SW, Kirstein MN, Valentine MB, et al: Fusion of a kinase gene, ALK, to a nucleolar protein gene, NPM, in non-Hodgkin's lymphoma. Science 1994; 263:1281–1284.
Motokura T, Bloom T, Kim HG, et al: A novel cyclin encoded by a bcl1-linked candidate oncogene. Nature 1991; 350:512–515.
Mullis KB, Faloona FA: Specific synthesis of DNA in vitro via a polymerase-catalyzed chain reaction. Methods Enzymol 1987; 155:335–350.
Murre C, Waldmann TA, Morton CC, et al: Human gamma-chain genes are rearranged in leukaemic cells and map to the short arm of chromosome 7. Nature 1985; 316:549–552.
Neri A, Barriga F, Knowles DM, et al: Different regions of the immunoglobulin heavy chain locus are involved in chromosomal translocations in distinct pathogenetic forms of Burkitt lymphoma. Proc Natl Acad Sci USA 1988; 85:2748–2752.
Nourse J, Mellentin JD, Galili N, et al: Chromosomal translocation t(1;19) results in synthesis of a homeobox fusion mRNA that codes for a potential chimeric transcription factor. Cell 1990; 60:535–545.
Osmond DG: B cell development in the bone marrow. Semin Immunol 1990; 2:173–180.
Pandolfi PP, Alcalay M, Fagioli M, et al: Genomic variability and alternative splicing generate multiple PML/RARα transcripts that encode aberrant proteins and PML/RARα isoforms in acute promyelocytic leukemia. EMBO J 1992; 1:1397–1407.
Parreira A, De Oliveira P, Matutes E, et al: Terminal deoxynucleotidyl transferase positive acute myeloid leukemia: An association with immature myeloblastic leukemia. Br J Hematol 1988; 69:219–224.
Pearson MG, Vardiman JW, Le Beau MM, et al: Increased numbers of marrow basophils may be associated with t(6;9) in ANLL. Am J Hematol 1985; 18:393–403.
Pelicci PG, Knowles DM, Dalla-Favera RD: Lymphoid tumors displaying rearrangements of both immunoglobulin and T cell receptor genes. J Exp Med 1985; 162:1015–1024.
Pelicci PG, Knowles DM, Magrath I, Dalla-Favera R: Chromosomal breakpoints and structural alterations of the c-myc locus differ in endemic and sporadic forms of Burkitt lymphoma. Proc Natl Acad Sci USA 1986; 83:2984–2988.
Pinkel D, Straume T, Gray J: Cytogenetic analysis using quantitative, high-sensitivity, fluorescence hybridization. Proc Natl Acad Sci USA 1986; 83:2934–2938.
Pugh WC, Stass SA: Immunoglobulin gene rearrangement and its implications for the study of B-cell neoplasia. Clin Lab Med 1988; 8:45–64.
Pui C-H, Dahl GV, Melvin S, et al: Acute leukaemia with mixed lymphoid and myeloid phenotype. Br J Haematol 1984; 56:121–130.
Rabbitts TH, Boehm T: LIM domains. Nature 1990; 346:418.
Rabbitts TH: Translocations, master genes, and differences between the origins of acute and chronic leukemias. Cell 1991; 67:641–644.
Reed TJ, Reid A, Wallberg K, et al: Determination of B-cell clonality in paraffin-embedded lymph nodes using the polymerase chain reaction. Diagn Mol Pathol 1993; 2:42–49.
Reynolds TC, Smith SD, Sklar J: Analysis of DNA surrounding the breakpoints of chromosomal translocations involving the β T-cell receptor gene in human lymphoblastic neoplasms. Cell 1987; 50:107–117.
Rolink A, Melchers F: Molecular and cellular origins of B lymphocyte diversity. Cell 1991; 66:1081–1094.
Rowley JD: A new consistent chromosomal abnormality in chronic myelogenous leukemia identified by quinacrine fluorescence and Giemsa staining. Nature 1973; 243:290–293.
Sakano H, Kurosawa Y, Weigert M, Tonegawa S: Identification and nucleotide sequence of a diversity DNA segment [D] of immunoglobulin heavy chain genes. Nature 1981; 290:562–565.
Satyanarayana K, Hata S, Devlin P, et al: Genomic organization of the human T-cell antigen-receptor alpha/delta locus. Proc Natl Acad Sci USA 1988; 85:8166–8170.
Senn HP, Jiricny J, Fopp M, et al: Relapse cell population differs from acute onset clone as shown by absence of the initially-activated H-ras oncogene in a patient with acute myelomonocytic leukemia. Blood 1988; 72:931–935.
Seremetis SV, Pelicci PG, Tabilio A, et al: High frequency of clonal immunoglobulin or T cell receptor gene rearrangements in acute myeloge-

nous leukemia expressing terminal deoxyribonucleotidyl transferase. J Exp Med 1987; 165:1703–1712.
Southern EM: Detection of specific sequences among DNA fragments separated by gel electrophoresis. J Mol Biol 1975; 98:503–517.
Stong RC, Korsmeyer SJ, Parkin JL, et al: Human acute leukemia cell line with the t(4;11) chromosomal rearrangement exhibits B lineage and monocytic characteristics. Blood 1985; 65:21–31.
Taub RA, Hollis GF, Hieter PA, et al: The variable amplification of immunoglobulin light chain genes in human populations. Nature 1983; 304:172–174.
Tawa A, Hozumi N, Minden M, et al: Rearrangement of the T-cell receptor β-chain gene in non-T-cell, non-B-cell acute lymphoblastic leukemia of childhood. N Engl J Med 1985; 313:1033–1037.
Third International Workshop on Chromosomes in Leukemia: Cancer Genet Cytogenet 1981; 4:95–142.
Tkachuk DC, Westbrook CA, Andreeff M, et al: Detection of *bcr-abl* fusion in chronic myelogenous leukemia by in situ hybridization. Science 1990; 250:559–562.
Tkachuk DC, Kohler S, Cleary ML: Involvement of a homolog of *Drosophila trithorax* by 11q23 chromosomal translocations in acute leukemias. Cell 1992; 71:691–700.
Trainor KJ, Brisco MJ, Wan J-H, et al: Gene rearrangement in B- and T-lymphoproliferative disease detected by the polymerase chain reaction. Blood 1991; 78:192–196.
Tsujimoto Y, Finger LR, Yunis J, et al: Cloning of the chromosome breakpoint of neoplastic B cells with the t(14;18) chromosome translocation. Science 1984; 226:1097–1099.
Tycko B, Palmer JD, Link MP, et al: Polymerase chain reaction amplification of rearranged antigen receptor genes using junction-specific oligonucleotides: Possible application for detection of minimal residual disease in acute lymphoblastic leukemia. Cancer Cells 1989; 7:47–52.
Uckun FM: Regulation of human B cell ontogeny. Blood 1990; 76:1908–1923.
Von Linden M, Poustka A, Lehrach H, Grosveld G: The t(6;9) chromosome translocation, associated with a specific subtype of acute nonlymphocytic leukemia, leads to aberrant transcription of a target gene on 9q34. Mol Cell Biol 1990; 10:4016–4026.
Weiss LM, Warnke RA, Sklar J, Cleary ML: Molecular analysis of the t(14;18) chromosomal translocation in malignant lymphomas. N Engl J Med 1987; 317:1185–1189.
Williams DL, Look AT, Melvin SL, et al: New chromosomal translocations correlate with specific immunophenotypes of childhood acute lymphoblastic leukemia. Cell 1984; 36:101–109.
Williams ME, Westermann CD, Swerdlow SH: Genotypic characterization of centrocytic lymphoma: Frequent rearrangement of the chromosome 11 bcl-1 locus. Blood 1990; 76:1387–1391.
Xia Y, Brown L, Yang CYC, et al: TAL-2, a helix-loop-helix gene activated by the t(7;9) (q34;q32) translocation in human T-cell leukemia. Proc Natl Acad Sci USA 1991; 88:11416–11420.
Yamada M, Hudson S, Tournay O, et al: Detection of minimal disease in hematopoietic malignancies of the B-cell lineage by using third-complementarity-determining region (CDR-III)-specific probes. Proc Natl Acad Sci USA 1989; 86:5122–5127.
Yancopoulos GD, Blackwell TK, Suh H, et al: Introduced T cell receptor variable region gene segments recombine in pre-B cells: Evidence that B and T cells use a common recombinase. Cell 1986; 44:251–259.
Yoshikai Y, Clark SP, Taylor S, et al: Organization and sequences of the variable, joining, and constant region genes of the human T cell receptor alpha chain. Nature 1985; 316:837–840.
Yunis JJ, Oken MM, Kaplan ME, et al: Distinctive chromosomal abnormalities in histologic subtypes of non-Hodgkin's lymphoma. N Engl J Med 1982; 307:1231–1236.
Yunis JJ, Boot AJM, Mayer MG, Bos JL: Mechanism of *ras* mutation in myelodysplastic syndrome. Oncogene 1988; 4:609–614.
Zaki SR, Austin GE, Swan D, et al: Human myeloperoxidase gene expression in acute leukemia. Blood 1989; 74:2096–2102.

Chapter 59

Molecular Diagnosis of Genetic Diseases

Wayne W. Grody, M.D., Ph.D.
Walter W. Noll, M.D.

INTRODUCTION

One of the newest and most revolutionary areas of laboratory medicine, diagnostic molecular genetics, holds promise of becoming the most powerful diagnostic and screening tool of the 21st century. With the rapidly accelerating pace of discovery of new disease genes under the auspices of the Human Genome Project and the recognition that virtually all diseases, including neoplastic and even infectious ones, have some genetic component, the utility of this subspecialty can only continue to expand. Moreover, its unique capability to diagnose disease both prenatally and presymptomatically should confer on it a primary role in preventative medicine, a focus of increasing urgency in the present era of medical care cost containment. Even beyond that, diagnostic molecular genetics leads naturally into therapeutic molecular genetics, because essentially the same normal gene sequences used to detect molecular genetic defects by DNA hybridization can be used to correct such defects by gene replacement therapy. As the latter activity increases in scope and range of uses, it will become even further intertwined with the activities of the molecular diagnostic laboratory, and the conceptual border between the two applications will become increasingly blurred.

Ethical Considerations

Yet such progress does not come unencumbered by appreciable obstacles. Aside from the considerable technical sophistication and difficulty of these procedures, they are inextricably bound up with a number of thorny ethical dilemmas. Dissecting a patient's most fundamental constitutional makeup, and the inborn defects therein, raises problematic questions about genetic discrimination, stigmatization, ethnic differences, privacy, informed consent, and confidentiality. Considering that at the molecular genetic level everything becomes a "pre-existing condition," the very definition of insurability may need to be revised; already there are healthy individuals who have lost their insurance coverage upon being found to carry a mutation, even a recessive one (Billings, 1992). Furthermore, discovery of any such heritable mutation in an individual has profound implications far beyond the immediate patient who requested the DNA test (the *proband*), extending to all the other members of that person's family, none of whom may have consented to exploring or revealing this type of information. Indeed, with the newfound power of DNA testing afforded by amplification techniques, such as the polymerase chain reaction (PCR), it becomes quite easy to perform genetic analysis without the patient's consent or even knowledge, because the testing can be done on minute portions of tissue or fluid samples obtained for other purposes. Prenatal diagnosis and, by extension, preconception genetic carrier screening of couples, becomes caught up in the passionate ethical and religious debates over abortion. In addition, gene therapy, despite universal consensus that it should be directed only at somatic, rather than germline, cellular targets, raises the spectre of eugenics among those who do not have to remember back all that far to times when such notions were not only accepted but actively espoused.

Test Complexity and Interpretation

Much of diagnostic molecular genetics involves the assessment of risk for the occurrence or recurrence of a disorder in an individual or family. For reasons to be described more fully in this chapter, the test results obtained are often expressed not in terms of a numerical concentration or a yes/no answer but as a probability. The accurate and meaningful conveyance of such complex uncertainties to patients and even referring physicians can be quite difficult and time consuming. For this reason, and owing to the serious ethical implications of these tests as described earlier, this area of laboratory medicine, perhaps more than any other, requires very close communication between the laboratory and the referring clinician or genetic counselor. In fact, many of these tests should be ordered only through a medical geneticist or genetic counselor, because these are the specialists best qualified to assess the appropriateness of the test and explain the results to the patient. Close and timely communication will assure that patients obtain the most benefit and least downside risk from this powerful technology.

CHOICE OF TECHNIQUES

Because so many genetic disease genes, loci, and mutational mechanisms are known, diagnostic molecular genetics capitalizes on the entire spectrum of modern molecular biological techniques available. These include Southern blotting, dot blotting, polymerase chain reaction (PCR), fluorescence *in situ* hybridization (FISH), DNA sequencing, single-strand conformation polymorphism, and others. The choice of which technique to use in a particular case will depend, to a large extent, on the present knowledge of the gene(s) associated with the disease in question and its degree of molecular heterogeneity. The first criterion roughly divides all genetic diseases into two categories: those for which the causative gene and specific mutation(s) have been isolated and those for which they have not. Those in the first category can often be approached by direct gene/mutation analysis; those in the latter can be approached only by linkage analysis using polymorphic DNA markers nearby on the same chromosome, provided that the disease has been mapped to that rather gross level.

The second concept, heterogeneity, refers to the number of different genes, or the variety of mutations within a single gene, that can cause the same disease: The greater the heterogeneity, the more difficult, labor intensive, and expensive the DNA test becomes. Indeed, the mutations responsible for some disorders are so numerous and spread across such large genes that direct detection is not feasible, and one must revert back to linkage analysis, even though the causative gene has been identified and cloned. In other disorders, one or more mutations may be of sufficiently high frequency in particular ethnic populations that screening for those few, while ignoring the many rarer mutations reported, can provide a test of sufficient yield to justify the direct approach.

To make such tests practical and of reasonable cost, a number of multiplexing strategies for simultaneous mutation detection have been devised, as described later. The reader should keep in mind that all of these involve some compromise as to overall test sensitivity; indeed, the field of diagnostic molecular genetics tolerates, by necessity, a number of screening tests with sensitivities noticeably below those that would be considered acceptable in other areas of the clinical laboratory. The decision of just how low the acceptable sensitivity cutoff should be largely becomes an ethical one. Most geneticists have reasoned that, at least for screening tests, the potential public health benefits of offering a test of suboptimal sensitivity outweigh the arguments for withholding it, provided that sufficient education and counseling are available to patients so that they understand the residual risk inherent in a negative test result.

Direct Mutation Tests

Direct mutation tests have been simplified immeasurably by the advent of PCR. Through the judicious choice of primers, this technique allows the laboratory to hone in on the precise mutation of interest, or a "hot spot" within a gene containing several possible mutation sites, using minute amounts of starting material. It is especially valuable for detecting point mutations and microdeletions, which usually go unnoticed in a Southern blot, unless they happen to lie within a recognition site of the particular restriction enzyme being used. Once the region containing the suspected mutation is amplified, it can be analyzed by gel electrophoresis or DNA probe hybridization. For a deletion that would be expected to reduce the length of the amplicon, accurate molecular sizing of the PCR products by electrophoresis and ethidium bromide staining will be sufficient (Fig. 59–1). Alternatively, if the deletion or point mutation disrupts (or creates) a restriction endonuclease cleavage site, it can be detected by electrophoretic analysis of PCR products digested with that enzyme (Fig. 59–2). Another option is to hybridize the PCR products with allele-specific oligonucleotide (ASO) probes, short DNA fragments that are precisely complementary to either the normal or mutant target sequence. If the hybridization, usually in a dot blot format, is performed under sufficiently stringent conditions, target DNA containing the

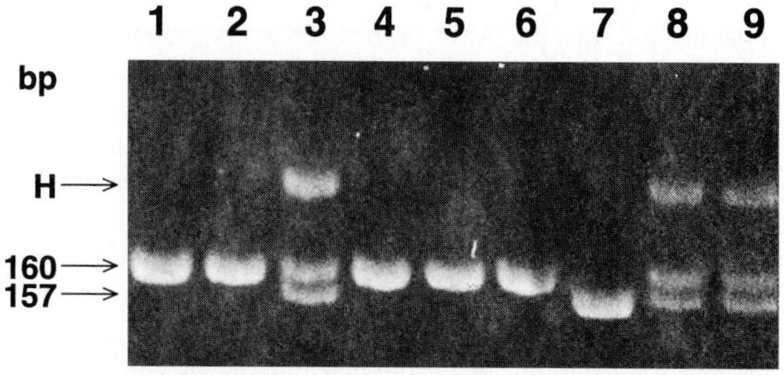

Figure 59–1. Example of electrophoretic sizing of polymerase chain reaction (PCR) products for mutation detection. In this case, patient DNA samples were amplified using primers flanking codon 508 of the cystic fibrosis (*CFTR*) gene, producing a single fragment of 160 base pairs (bp) from normals (lanes 1, 2, 4, 5 and 6), a single fragment of 157 bp from a patient homozygous for the three-nucleotide deletion ΔF508 (lane 7), and both fragments along with an artifactual heteroduplex band (H) from heterozygotes (lanes 3, 8 and 9). (Method of Chong, 1990.)

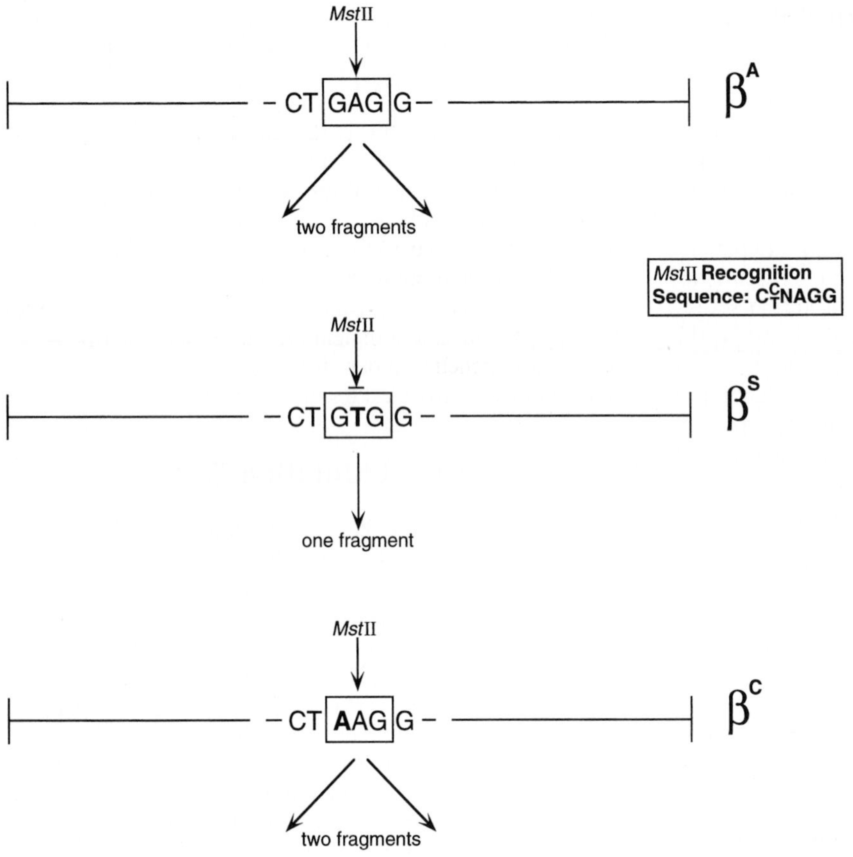

Figure 59–2. Schematic example of detection of a point mutation by differential cleavage with a restriction enzyme. In this case, the sickle cell mutation, substitution of T for A in codon 6 of the β-globin gene, destroys an *Mst*II cleavage site, so that digestion of a PCR product from the region produces two DNA fragments in normal persons but only one fragment in HbS homozygotes. Mutation of the first nucleotide in this codon, found in hemoglobin-C disease, does not destroy the *Mst*II site (because the enzyme can accommodate any nucleotide in this position) and thus cannot be detected by this method.

mutation will hybridize only with the mutant probe, and vice versa for normal target DNA. Probes for several rare mutations can be pooled together for more efficient screening (Fig. 59–3), and several mutation hot spots can be amplified together via "multiplex PCR."

To scan a disease gene for any number of unknown mutations, several screening techniques that cast a wider net are available. Single-strand conformation polymorphism (SSCP) and denaturing gradient gel electrophoresis (DGGE) can theoretically detect point mutations anywhere within a gene because of the altered topology the substituted nucleotides induce in single-stranded and mismatched double-stranded DNA, respectively. These approaches obviate the need for separate and specific ASO probes for every possible mutation, though they can be performed only on limited, PCR-amplified stretches of the gene at one time and they are not 100% sensitive. The only technique that should be 100% sensitive in detecting all possible point mutations, at least in theory, is complete DNA sequencing of the gene. Unfortunately, with present technology this approach remains too cumbersome and expensive for routine clinical use, and even it will miss mutations that lie outside the structural gene sequence, for example, in introns, promoters, or enhancer regions. In hemophilia A, for example, complete sequencing of the factor VIII gene has revealed mutations in only half of the patients examined (Higuchi, 1992).

Disorders caused by gene expansion of a trinucleotide repeat can be diagnosed by Southern blot or PCR, in either case by observing a larger-than-normal target DNA fragment. Disorders caused by large deletions are often diagnosed by Southern blot by observing a loss or decrease in size of a target fragment, although loss of a PCR product normally amplified from that site or appearance of a new "junction fragment" can also be used. Disorders caused by very large deletions or insertions, as well as translocations, can be diagnosed at the chromosomal level by FISH.

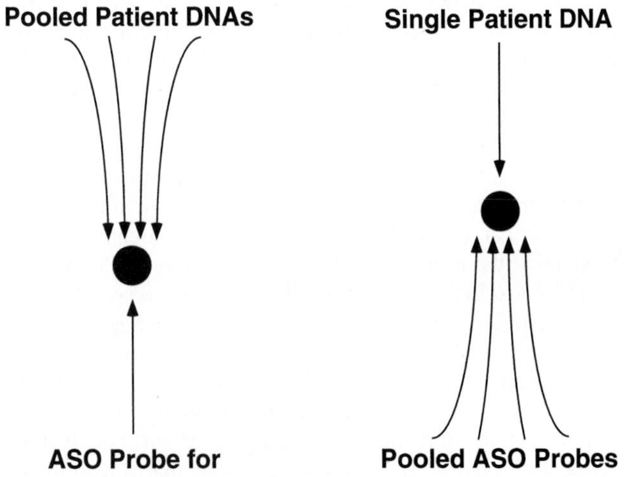

Figure 59–3. Strategy for efficient screening of multiple rare mutations by direct dot blot using allele-specific oligonucleotide (ASO) probes. Numerous patient DNA samples can be pooled into a single spot and hybridized with an ASO probe; alternatively, a single patient DNA can be hybridized with a cocktail of multiple rare ASO probes. In either case, the test produces negative results most of the time because the mutations are so rare. If the results are positive, further tests are required to determine which patient or probe produced the hybridization signal.

Linkage Analysis

For those disorders with too many unknown mutations, or an unknown gene, predictive diagnosis by linkage analysis is possible in certain families. Because the analysis requires comparative testing of other affected and unaffected siblings and parents, not every family will be accessible or informative by this approach. Also required is knowledge of closely linked, preferably flanking or even intragenic, polymorphic DNA markers that can be observed to cosegregate consistently with either the normal or disease phenotype within the family. Traditionally, the markers used have been restriction fragment length polymorphisms (RFLP) detected by Southern blot. More recently, microsatellite polymorphisms—tandem oligonucleotide sequences of variable repeat length—detectable by PCR and simple gel electrophoresis, have become favored because of their abundance throughout the genome, the multi-allelic nature of their polymorphisms, and the relative ease of the testing methodology. Very large genes, such as those for neurofibromatosis and Duchenne's muscular dystrophy, will usually have intragenic microsatellites that can be assessed, minimizing the chances of recombination between the mutation and the marker.

Linkage techniques are less favored than the direct mutation detection approach because of the need to test multiple family members and because meiotic recombination between the gene and the marker can disrupt the apparent phase of linkage between parent and offspring, leading to false-positive or false-negative interpretation of the results. For each centimorgan (cM) of map distance between the two loci, 1% recombination can be expected (1 cM is approximately equivalent to 1 million base pairs). For example, in Figure 59–4 the fetus is predicted to be affected, having inherited the same upper RFLP fragment as the previously affected son. However, if the polymorphic restriction endonuclease site being tested is 5 cM away from the disease gene, one can conclude only that the fetus is at 95% risk of being affected.

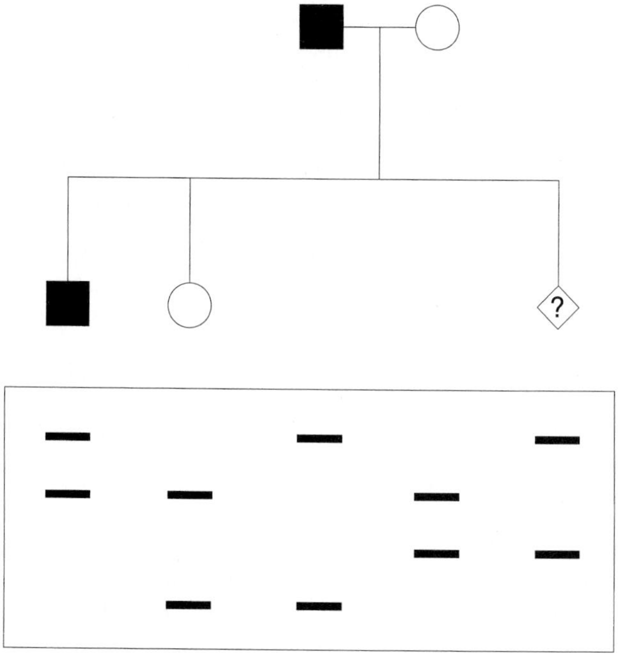

Figure 59–4. Example of restriction fragment-length polymorphism (RFLP) analysis for prenatal diagnosis of an autosomal dominant disorder. In this Southern blot test, the upper band from the father is the one that cosegregates with the disease phenotype, as seen in the affected son. Because the fetus ⟨?⟩ has also inherited this band, it is predicted to be affected. The precise risk depends on the map distance between the disease gene and the RFLP marker.

CHOICE OF APPLICATIONS

To some extent the choice of technique will also depend on the application, that is, the reason the test is being done. In medical genetics, these applications fall in four major areas: carrier screening, diagnostic testing, prenatal testing, and presymptomatic testing. Carrier screening is the term applied to detection of recessive mutations in healthy individuals for purposes of genetic counseling and family planning. This application is further subdivided into screening of those individuals with a family history of the disorder, and population-based screening of large numbers of individuals who have no family history but may be at risk for the disorder because of its prevalence within their ethnic group. In either case, the purpose is to identify couples at risk (i.e., when both the man and the woman are heterozygous for mutations within the gene), who would then have a 25% chance of having an affected child with each pregnancy. But the testing strategies chosen for the two groups will differ. Obviously, a person whose sibling has the disorder is at much higher risk of being a carrier than someone in the general population. That person may therefore warrant more aggressive testing (e.g., screening for a greater number of mutations or even linkage analysis) than would be cost effective for a member of the general population. On the other hand, access to the affected sibling's DNA may allow prior identification of the mutation, which would render subsequent testing of other family members much easier. Population-based screening, in contrast, typically strives to keep the testing procedure as rapid and inexpensive as possible, focusing on perhaps a few of the more prevalent mutations, sacrificing test sensitivity for cost effectiveness and expediency. Of course, with negative family history there are no affected family members to make linkage analysis an option.

Diagnostic genetic testing is, by definition, performed on a symptomatic individual. Because the DNA tests for genetic disease are absolutely disease specific and the diseases themselves are quite rare, these procedures do not cast a wide enough net to be used for extensive differential diagnosis; the symptoms must be sufficiently suggestive of the disorder in question to justify ordering the test. Also, one must weigh the DNA test against more traditional methods with regard to cost, convenience, and utility. For example, hemoglobin electrophoresis may be more convenient and comprehensive for sorting out a suspected hemoglobinopathy than the specific DNA test for the sickle cell anemia mutation. On the other hand, molecular testing may be more advantageous for early or nonclassical clinical presentations. For example, molecular testing for cystic fibrosis mutations can be performed in the newborn period when traditional sweat chloride analysis is both inconvenient and unreliable. DNA tests also have the advantage of working well postmortem, when classical biochemical analytes can no longer be assessed. For example, PCR detection of the predominant mutation in medium-chain acyl-CoA dehydrogenase deficiency can be

7

applied at autopsy to assess this occasional genetic cause of sudden infant death syndrome (Landemous, 1993).

Presymptomatic DNA testing is applied primarily to late-onset dominant disorders, in which the offspring of an affected parent are aware that they are at 50% risk of having inherited the disease and desire to know their status before its clinical onset in order to make informed reproductive decisions or initiate surveillance or preventative interventions. The prototypic disorders in this group are Huntington's disease and the heritable cancer syndromes, though such diseases as neurofibromatosis, Marfan's syndrome, adult polycystic kidney disease, and tuberous sclerosis are also relevant. This sort of testing has been the most problematic, from a psychosocial and ethical standpoint, of any in diagnostic molecular genetics, with substantial risk of severe adverse consequences of results reporting, including suicide. Because of this, established testing protocols include stipulations for concurrent clinical and psychiatric assessment, extensive pretest and post test genetic counseling, and psychosocial support (Huntington's Disease Society of America, 1989).

Finally, there is the clinical application most distinctive of medical genetics: prenatal diagnosis, or the detection of disease in the fetus. Many mendelian disorders, including some inborn errors of metabolism, are not expressed either symptomatically or biochemically in the fetus, so predictive diagnosis can be made only at the DNA level. Even for those disorders that might be detected biochemically, DNA often proves to be a far more accessible substrate, from an obstetric point of view, than the affected protein products. While molecular analysis can be performed on very small numbers of amniocytes or cells from chorionic villus samples (CVS) collected by routine methods, even if obtained for other purposes, unless the protein product is expressed in fibroblasts (and thus amniocytes), biochemical analysis will require invasive biopsy of deep fetal tissues. For example, assay of phenylalanine hydroxylase activity to diagnose phenylketonuria would require fetal liver biopsy, and quantitation of dystrophin to diagnose Duchenne's muscular dystrophy would require fetal muscle biopsy.

It goes without saying that the primary objective in prenatal diagnosis is the identification of an affected fetus in a timely manner so that the pregnancy can be terminated. While some may argue an advantage for obtaining diagnosis prenatally so that therapy can be instituted promptly at birth, or to psychologically reassure a couple if the fetus is found to be unaffected, it is difficult to justify the risk of miscarriage from amniocentesis and CVS performed for these other purposes. For an affected fetus, unless one intends to initiate therapy *in utero*, provisional treatment at birth while awaiting neonatal testing is perfectly acceptable. While prenatal genetic counseling is always nondirective, with moral and/or religious objections to abortion respected, both the clinical counselor and the DNA testing laboratory have a legitimate right and, indeed, responsibility to question the appropriateness of a prenatal test request, with its attendant risk and expense, from a couple for whom termination is not an option (the same would apply to requests coming too late in pregnancy for termination to be performed). It is because of these problems that invasive prenatal DNA testing is not offered as a general population screening tool in women with no family history of the disorder in question. The power of PCR to enable single-cell genetic analysis has recently opened the way for preimplantation diagnosis, usually approached by performing *in vitro* fertilization and microdissection of a single blastomere from the eight-cell embryo. This strategy, already applied to selected cases at risk for cystic fibrosis (Handyside, 1992) and other disorders, could potentially be offered to any at-risk couple for whom abortion is not an option, though it is not without its own ethical (and economic) pitfalls. Yet despite all these medical and moral dilemmas, when performed in appropriate circumstances, prenatal molecular genetic testing can offer at-risk couples, many of whom have already suffered the trauma of at least one affected offspring, one of the most valuable services in all of clinical medicine.

SPECIAL CONCEPTS UNIQUE TO MOLECULAR GENETIC DISORDERS

While the DNA analysis techniques discussed in this chapter for diagnosis of genetic disease are generally the same as those for molecular diagnosis of cancer or infectious diseases, their application in the former has revealed a number of unusual phenomena that one must keep in mind when dealing with particular hereditary disorders. Some of these concepts have been known since Mendel's work, but they can now be understood mechanistically at the DNA level; others have emerged much more recently as unexpected byproducts of the molecular dissection of specific disease genes.

Variable Penetrance and Expressivity

Penetrance refers to the proportion of individuals who, having inherited a mutant disease gene, will actually display the disease phenotype; any fraction below 100% is called incomplete penetrance. Usually applied to dominant disorders, it can produce the striking appearance of generation skipping in disease pedigrees. This can complicate both molecular diagnostics and genetic counseling, because it may not be clear whether the propositus inherited the disease from a parent or instead represents a new mutation in the family. It is a feature of such relatively common genetic disorders as Marfan's syndrome and neurofibromatosis, both of whose genes are identified but not yet sufficiently characterized for direct mutation detection to completely replace linkage analysis.

Variable expressivity refers to the appearance of different signs and symptoms of a disorder in individuals inheriting the same mutation(s). Like penetrance, it is probably a reflection of differential gene effects within dissimilar genetic backgrounds (in other words, the modulation of phenotypic expression by other genes at other loci). It, too, makes ascertainment and counseling difficult, and raises ethical issues in considering abortion for diseases of variable and unpredictable severity (like Marfan's syndrome or cystic fibrosis).

Crossing Over

This phenomenon of meiotic recombination between homologous chromosomes is, in addition to random mutation, the major driving force behind genetic diversity and evolution in sexually reproducing organisms. Its importance in diagnostic molecular genetics lies in its disruption of linkage between a disease gene and a nearby polymorphic marker, producing false-positive or false-negative diagnoses in those disorders tested by linkage analysis. As discussed earlier, the risk can be minimized by choosing markers that are more closely linked to or flank the disease gene. This has become much more feasible as the human genomic map has become saturated with short tandem repeat polymorphisms that can be accessed easily with PCR primers. Some of these, particularly the dinucleotide repeats, may even lie within the disease gene of interest.

Uniparental Disomy

This unusual cause of a recessive single-gene disorder was first discovered in a cystic fibrosis (CF) patient, only one of whose parents was a carrier (Spence, 1988). By DNA haplotyping it was shown that the patient had inherited two copies of the carrier parent's chromosome 7 containing the mutant CF gene and no chromosome 7 from the other parent. The phenomenon has since been observed in other cases of CF and diseases involving other chromosomes as well. In all such cases in which it is the mother only who is the carrier, it is important first to rule out nonpaternity.

Imprinting

Imprinting refers to the differential expression of a gene in an offspring, depending on whether it was inherited from the mother or the father. Some genes are expressed or, conversely, turned off, only when they pass through the oocyte lineage, and others only when they pass through the spermatocyte line. If an individual inherits the normal allele through the nonexpressing parental line, he or she cannot counteract a recessive mutation inherited from the other parent. For example, the defect on chromosome 15 (usually a deletion) associated with the Prader-Willi syndrome (characterized by obesity, mental retardation, and dysmorphic features) is expressed only when it occurs on the chromosome inherited from the father, while the nearby defect causing Angelman's syndrome (characterized by ataxia, puppet-like facies, mental retardation, and seizures) is expressed only when the anomaly is present on the chromosome inherited from the mother (Knoll, 1989). Alternatively, Prader-Willi syndrome can be caused by uniparental disomy for the maternal chromosome 15, which carries only the nonexpressing copy of the gene; likewise, Angelman's syndrome can be caused by uniparental disomy for the paternal chromosome 15. These phenomena can be detected by FISH, chromosome haplotyping with microsatellite markers, or Southern blotting with methylation-sensitive restriction enzymes that produce different fragment sizes in imprinted and nonimprinted genes (Lerer, 1994).

Anticipation

Anticipation refers to a progressive increase in severity and/or age of onset of a genetic disorder in subsequent generations of a family. It is typically associated with the trinucleotide repeat disorders, such as myotonic dystrophy and fragile X syndrome, in which the increasing severity can be correlated with further expansion of the repeat region. In myotonic dystrophy, especially severe cases have been born to affected mothers, invoking an influence by imprinting as well (Lopez, 1994). Rarely, the opposite phenomenon, contraction or loss of a previously amplified region, has been observed. It is for these reasons that accurate molecular sizing of trinucleotide repeat lengths is so important for genetic counseling in these disorders.

SPECIFIC DISEASE EXAMPLES

Cystic Fibrosis

Because of its high carrier frequency in North America and northern Europe, its serious clinical nature, its straightforward mendelian (autosomal recessive) inheritance pattern, and its well studied though quite complex gene, cystic fibrosis (CF) has emerged as the paradigmatic disorder for all present and future molecular genetic testing. Within its scope can be found the full panoply of applicable molecular genetic techniques and the full spectrum of scientific and ethical dilemmas arising from the clinical variability of the disease, the extreme molecular heterogeneity of the causative mutations, and the advent of novel treatments, including gene replacement therapy. With a carrier frequency as high as one in 25 in Caucasians of northern European ancestry (and progressively less in southern Europeans, Hispanics, black Americans, and Asians), there was ample motivation to screen relatives of patients, and even the general population, in order to identify couples at one-in-four risk of having an affected child with each pregnancy. But because carriers are asymptomatic and have normal sweat chloride levels, this had to await the isolation of the gene in 1989 (Kerem, 1989; Riordan, 1989). While it had been mapped to chromosome 7 some years earlier, allowing for prenatal diagnosis by linkage analysis in informative families, screening and testing in others, especially those with no family history of the disorder, could be considered only once the gene was cloned and the mutations identified.

Even with that laudable accomplishment, however, DNA testing for CF has been fraught with problems and controversies. The gene is over 250,000 base pairs long and encodes a large ion channel protein called the *cystic fibrosis transmembrane conductance regulator* (CFTR) (Collins, 1992). Most notably, the spectrum of mutations observed is remarkably heterogeneous. While a three-nucleotide deletion of phenylalanine codon #508 (designated ΔF508) accounts for about 70% of the mutations in Caucasians (and significantly less in other ethnic groups), over 450 additional mutations have so far been reported. Most of these are so rare that it is neither feasible nor cost effective to include them in testing panels; only about seven (in addition to ΔF508) account for more than 1% each of CF mutations in most Caucasian populations (Tsui, 1992) (Table 59–1). The sensitivity of carrier screening with standard mutation panels of between 6 and 25 alleles ranges from a high of 97% in Ashkenazi Jews (Abeliovich, 1992) to 75% to 90% in non-Ashkenazi North American Caucasians, about 60% in Hispanic Americans, 40% in black Americans, and less than 10% in Asians (Curtis, 1993; Grebe, 1994; Ober, 1992; Orozco, 1993).

Table 59–1. SOME PREDOMINANT CYSTIC FIBROSIS MUTATIONS

Mutation	Comment
ΔF508	In-frame 3-bp deletion of phe codon; the major CF mutation, accounting for up to 70% of carriers in some Caucasian populations
G542X	Nonsense mutation; about 3% of white carriers
W1282X	Nonsense mutation; accounts for about 50% of Ashkenazi Jewish carriers
G551D	Missense mutation; about 3% of white carriers
N1303K	Missense mutation; 1–3% of white and Ashkenazi Jewish carriers respectively
R553X	Nonsense mutation; about 1.5% of white carriers
3849 + 10kbC→T	Splice site mutation; 1.5% and 4% of white and Ashkenazi carriers, respectively; associated with lung disease but normal sweat chloride
3905insT	Insertion/frameshift mutation; about 1.5% of white carriers
R117H	Missense mutation associated with congenital absence of the vas deferens; frequency estimates from 1 to 5%
621 + 1G→T	Splice site mutation; about 1.5% of white carriers
1717−1G→A	Splice site mutation; about 1% of white carriers

Such variable and suboptimal sensitivity in an ethnically heterogeneous population like that of the United States, and the difficulties involved in counseling patients as to the residual carrier risk of testing negative, have made population-based carrier screening for CF mutations a controversial subject (Wilfond, 1990; Williamson, 1993). While the ΔF508 mutation can be detected by differential migration in polyacrylamide gels (see Fig. 59–1) (Chong, 1990), and several other mutations produce characteristic restriction endonuclease digestion patterns (Ng, 1991), laboratories screening for as many as 30 or more mutations typically rely on pooled ASO strategies (as diagrammed in Fig. 59–3) or reverse dot blots (in which the patient's labelled PCR product is hybridized to a series of wild-type and mutant oligonucleotide probes immobilized on a filter strip) (Chehab, 1992; Shuber, 1993). Until existing technology advances to the stage of rapid and inexpensive DNA sequencing or, alternatively, protein-based assays for CFTR function, the test sensitivity figures quoted earlier are likely to remain about the same.

This presents a special problem for prenatal counseling of couples in which one partner tests positive and the other tests negative. While this raises anxiety regarding the current pregnancy, nothing further can be offered in the way of prenatal diagnosis because even if the negative partner is a carrier, he or she has a mutation that cannot be tested for in the fetus. As reassurance, the couple can be counseled that the residual risk of having an affected child, given their CF screening results, is now below the risk of fetal damage from amniocentesis or CVS. Others have proposed avoiding the issue altogether by adhering to a couple-based model of CF screening, in which the results are reported as negative even if one partner is found to be a carrier (Wald, 1991); however, this approach raises ethical questions about nondisclosure and other issues (Miedzybrodzka, 1991).

Another problem with genetic counseling for CF is the variable clinical severity of the disorder and the inconsistency of genotype-phenotype correlations. Beyond the finding that ΔF508 homozygotes tend to have pancreatic insufficiency, there is little about disease severity or complications that can be predicted reliably from knowing an affected individual's two mutations (Cystic Fibrosis Genotype-Phenotype Consortium, 1993). Even homozygotes for ΔF508, considered the prototypical "severe" mutation, can show a wide range in their degree of pulmonary compromise (Burke, 1992). Conversely, there are mutations that cause pulmonary disease yet maintain normal sweat chloride levels (Highsmith, 1994), and there are mutations (R117H being the most prominent) that may not cause CF at all but rather male infertility because of congenital absence of the vas deferens (Anguiano, 1992; Gervais, 1993). Taken together with the likely advent of effective gene replacement therapies for CF (Wilson, 1993), these factors render molecular genetic counseling and parental decision-making for the disorder quite difficult. Given the molecular and clinical heterogeneity of most genetic disorders, these problems are likely to prove to be the rule rather than the exception in diagnostic molecular genetics.

Duchenne's Muscular Dystrophy

This X-linked progressive myopathy was the first disorder whose causative gene was isolated by the process of "reverse genetics" or positional cloning (Rowland, 1988). Before that discovery, the only tests that could be offered to at-risk families were detection of some (but not all) female carriers by the finding of elevated serum creatine phosphokinase levels, followed by prenatal sex determination with the option to terminate a male fetus (even though 50% of them would be normal). Genetic counseling was rendered even more problematic because about one third of Duchenne's muscular dystrophy (DMD) cases arise from new mutations.

Even after its discovery, translation to clinical application was not easy because the gene, dubbed *dystrophin*, proved to be the largest yet discovered, spanning 2.5 million base pairs and composed of 79 exons (Ahn, 1993). Use of full-length or partial cDNA probes to detect the variety of deletions accounting for two thirds of cases was labor intensive and time consuming (Darras, 1988; Prior, 1991). It was only with the advent of multiplex PCR that a system was developed for rapid and inexpensive identification of more than 98% of dystrophin deletions and their localization to specific exons of the gene (Beggs, 1990a; Multicenter Study Group, 1992). In this system a deletion is identified by absence of one or more of the multiple (nine or more, depending on protocol) expected amplicons on ethidium bromide–stained electrophoresis gels (because a target gene deletion will abolish the hybridization site[s] of one or more primers, causing PCR failure) (Fig. 59–5). Many laboratories still prefer to confirm such findings by subsequent Southern blot; this provides a control against artifactual PCR failure. Such fine-structure mapping combined with sequencing has also revealed important insights into the molecular pathogenesis of DMD and the milder syngeneic disorder, Becker's muscular dystrophy (BMD). While both are most often caused by large dystrophin deletions, those in BMD typically preserve the correct reading frame in the resulting processed transcript, while DMD deletions more often produce frameshift mutations and a more truncated (often nonfunctional or absent) protein product (Monaco, 1988). More recently, some of the larger deletions have even been local-

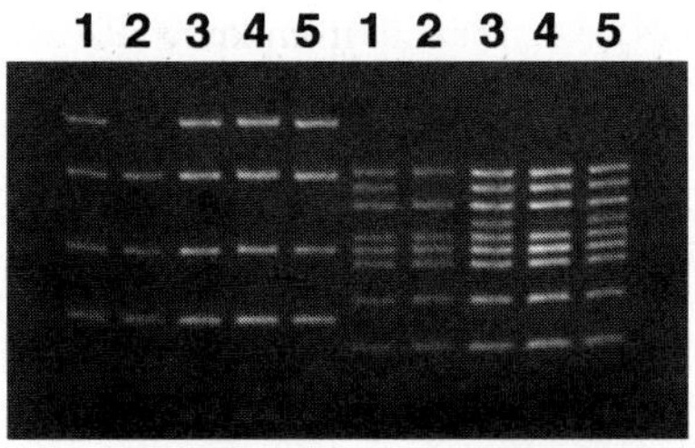

Figure 59–5. Multiplex PCR analysis for dystrophin gene deletions in Duchenne muscular dystrophy. DNA samples from five patients were amplified simultaneously with five primer pairs (left half of gel) and nine primer pairs (right half of gel) and the products analyzed by polyacrylamide gel electrophoresis. Absence of an expected PCR product band is indicative of a deletion. Patient 2 lacks the top band in the 5-plex and the second-from-top band in the 9-plex; these correspond to deletions in exons 50 and 48, respectively, in the dystrophin gene. (Band 4 in the 9-plex is light but present in all of the samples.) (Photo courtesy of Dr. Kathryn E. Kronquist, Corning Nichols Institute.)

ized by FISH in chromosome spreads (Tocharoentanaphol, 1994).

The remaining one third of patients in whom no deletion is detected usually have point mutations or microdeletions/insertions. Because the gene is so large, it is not feasible to identify these lesions directly, and one must revert to linkage analysis (although gene screening by conformational analysis [SSCP, DGGE] has also been used; Prior, 1993). As in any linkage strategy, this approach is possible only in informative families in which DNA from a previously affected individual is available for study. Early protocols relied on RFLP markers flanking the dystrophin gene (Williams, 1986); more recently, intragenic microsatellite markers have led to more rapid and accurate PCR-based chromosome haplotyping (Beggs, 1990b). Alternatively, studies at the protein level can be performed by observing decreased or absent dystrophin in DMD, and dystrophin of abnormal molecular weight in BMD, by western blot or immunohistochemistry of muscle biopsy tissue (Hoffman, 1988). This procedure has limitations for prenatal diagnosis, for which a fetal muscle biopsy would be required; recently, however, the method has been adapted to amniocytes and chorionic villus cells, which have been induced to differentiate toward muscle cells by gene transfer techniques (Sancho, 1993). Thus, the molecular diagnosis of Duchenne's muscular dystrophy has come full circle: from identification of the gene without knowing the protein product ("reverse genetics") to identification and diagnostic use of the protein product from knowing the gene. This sort of evolution can be expected in the laboratory diagnosis of many genetic diseases, because functional studies of a gene product are by definition more comprehensive than attempting to track down countless individual mutations at the DNA level.

Sickle Cell Anemia and Other Hemoglobinopathies

Given the long history of study of the protein product, diagnosis of molecular defects in the genes encoding the globin polypeptides did not come about through techniques of "reverse genetics"; rather, these genes were cloned by classical methods, using anti-globin antibodies for polysome precipitation to isolate the relevant mRNAs. As such, hemoglobin mutations, and the mutation causing sickle cell anemia in particular, were among the very first to be diagnosed at the DNA level. The sickle cell point mutation in codon 6 of the β-globin gene lies within (and thus destroys) a restriction endonuclease cleavage site (for *Mst* II or *Dde* I1), providing a rapid method of detection using either Southern blot or restriction enzyme digestion of β-globin PCR products (Hatcher, 1992; see Fig. 59–2). Alternatively, the hemoglobin S and hemoglobin A sequences can be distinguished by dot blot using allele-specific oligonucleotide probes complementary to either the normal or mutant sequence (Conner, 1983). These techniques can be used for diagnosis, carrier screening, or prenatal diagnosis, in the latter case obviating the need for invasive fetal blood sampling and classical hemoglobin electrophoresis. A different mutation in codon 6, causing hemoglobin C disease, does not abolish the restriction endonuclease recognition sequence (because it occurs at a flexible nucleotide position for the enzyme), and so must be distinguished by ASO probes or other methods (Maggio, 1993). One must also keep in mind that neither of these approaches will identify sickle cell/β-thalassemia or hemoglobin C/β-thalassemia compound heterozygotes.

The thalassemias involve both qualitative and quantitative alterations in one or more globin chains, and their diagnosis at the molecular level is correspondingly more complex than that of sickle cell anemia. α-Thalassemia is the more straightforward, because it is usually caused by deletion of either or both of the two contiguous α genes on one or the other or both chromosomes 16. This can be detected by Southern blot or PCR, allowing differentiation of the silent carrier state (one α gene missing) from the very severe hydrops fetalis (all four genes missing) and the two intermediate states (Bowden, 1992; Chen, 1993). Molecular diagnosis of β-thalassemia is far more complicated because of the wide variety of promoter, termination, deletion, splice site, and frameshift mutations that have been documented. For this reason, DNA testing for this disorder has been limited to few specialized laboratories. The most efficient approach is by hybridization to allele-specific oligonucleotide probes for the most common mutations in a reverse dot blot format (Cai, 1994).

Trinucleotide Repeat Expansion Disorders

An important new class of disease-causing mutations was revealed in 1991 with the discovery that X-linked spinal and bulbar muscular atrophy (Kennedy disease, *SBMA*) and fragile X syndrome are associated with amplification of unstable trinucleotide repeat sequences in the androgen receptor (AR) and *FMR1* ("fragile X mental retardation") genes, respectively. Since that time similar disease-producing mutations have been associated with myotonic dystrophy (*DM*), Huntington's disease (*HD*), spinocerebellar ataxia type 1 (*SCA1*), *FRAXE* mental retardation, and dentatorubral-pallidoluysian atrophy (*DRPLA*) (Bates, 1994; La Spada, 1994). The affected gene in each of these disorders normally contains a repeated sequence of three base pairs [for example, $(CGG)_n$ in

Table 59–2. DISORDERS CHARACTERIZED BY UNSTABLE EXPANSIONS OF DNA TRINUCLEOTIDE REPEATS

	Neurodegenerative Diseases				Fragile Sites/ Mental Retardation		Myotonic Dystrophy
	SBMA	***HD***	***SCA1***	***DRPLA***	***FRAXA***	***FRAXE***	***DM***
Repeat sequence	CAG	CAG	CAG	CAG	CGG	GCC	CTG
Inheritance	X-linked	Autosomal dominant	Autosomal dominant	Autosomal dominant	X-linked	X-linked	Autosomal dominant
Chromosome location	Xq11-12	4p16.3	6p	12p	Xq27.3	Xq28	19q13.3
Normal alleles	11–33	6–37	19–36	7–23	6–50	6–25	5–35
Immediate alleles		30–38			50–200 (premutation)		
Expanded alleles	36–62	37–121	42–81	49–75	>200	>200	50→200
Anticipation		Marked in juvenile cases	Marked in juvenile cases	Yes	Yes		Yes
Transmission sex bias		Paternal, early onset	Paternal, early onset	Paternal	Maternal, full mutation	No	Maternal, congenital form
Position of repeat	Coding	Coding	Coding	Coding	5' UTR		3' UTR
Gene product	Androgen receptor transcription factor	Huntingtin, function unknown	Ataxin, function unknown	Function unknown	FMR-1 RNA binding protein		Myotonin protein kinase
Associated methylation	No	No	No		Yes	Yes	No

SBMA = Spinal and bulbar muscular atrophy (Kennedy disease); HD = Huntington disease; SCA1 = spinocerebellar ataxia type 1; DRPLA = dentatorubral-pallidoluysian atrophy; FRAXA = fragile X syndrome; FRAXE = FRAXE-associated mental retardation; DM = myotonic dystrophy.
Data from Bates (1994), and La Spada (1994).

the *FMR1* gene], where n is variable but is sharply limited in its range. In the disease state, however, the size of the triplet repeat is expanded outside the normal range, sometimes markedly. The clinical and genetic features of these diseases are summarized in Table 59–2. Fragile X syndrome, the commonest of these disorders, is described at some length later, and brief descriptions of the other diseases are given as well.

Fragile X Syndrome

Fragile X syndrome, the commonest cause of inherited mental retardation (one in 1250 males), is second only to Down syndrome as a cause of moderate to severe mental retardation in males. Affected males with this X-linked disorder also have large ears, a long face, and large testes. Approximately one in 2500 females are heterozygous carries of a fragile X mutation, and one third of these may show evidence of mild mental impairment.

The cytogenetic hallmark of fragile X syndrome is a fragile site on the X chromosome at Xq27.3 (*FRAXA*), resulting from a failure of normal chromatin condensation during mitosis. Although the inheritance pattern of the disease is clearly X-linked, it does not correspond clearly to either a recessive or dominant pattern of gene expression. The most puzzling feature has been the presence of phenotypically normal men ("normal transmitting males") who are obligate carriers of the genetic abnormality. These men are sons of proven fragile X carriers and pass the carrier state to all of their daughters, with their daughters in turn at risk for transmitting the fully expressed disease to a high proportion of their sons.

The discovery in 1991 of the genetic abnormality that causes fragile X syndrome immediately clarified its unusual pattern of inheritance (Fu, 1991). The 5′ untranslated region of the *FMR1* gene at chromosome Xq27.3 carries a $(CGG)_n$ triplet repeat of variable size. In normal individuals, n ranges up to 50, but in individuals with clinically apparent fragile X syndrome, n is greater than 200 (referred to as a *full mutation*). Both men and women who carry an X chromosome in which n is between 50 and 200 (referred to as a *premutation*) are phenotypically normal but are at high risk of passing an allele of even larger size to their children. This is because of the "instability" of the premutation alleles and their tendency to increase in size during the meiotic cell divisions that produce the male and female gametes. Alleles of normal size are not unstable and are passed unchanged. Thus it appears that there is a pool of small premutation alleles in the population, possibly of ancient origin, that is at high risk of undergoing further expansion with each passage through another generation. As the premutation allele increases in size, the likelihood that it will expand further in the next generation increases. Interestingly, expansion to a full mutation has been observed to occur in female meiosis, never in males, which corresponds to the observation that the daughters of normal transmitting males are always phenotypically normal. Figure 59–6*B* illustrates a family with fragile X syndrome; a premutation allele is transmitted from the first to the second generation, and then expands to a full mutation in the third generation.

The mechanism by which the expanded triplet repeat in the 5′ noncoding region of the *FMR1* gene produces the fragile X syndrome phenotype is under investigation. As the size of the repeat expands, there is progressive methylation of the regulatory region of the *FMR1* gene and decreased expression of FMR1 protein. This RNA-binding protein is widely expressed in the developing brain and in other tissues. Its loss of expression presumably disturbs normal brain development and leads to mental retardation and the clinical fragile X syndrome phenotype (La Spada, 1994).

FRAXE Mental Retardation

Rare families with X-linked mental retardation and a cytogenetically demonstrable fragile site at chromosome Xq27-28, but no hypermethylation or expansion of the $(CGG)_n$ repeat in *FMR1*, led to the discovery of a second, more distal fragile site at Xq28 associated with hypermethylation and expansion of a $(GCC)_n$ repeat. Individuals with expansion of the repeat located at the *FRAXE* fragile site locus to greater than 200 copies suffer mild mental impairment. In contrast with the fragile X syndrome, there is no apparent sex bias in the transmission of the triplet amplification at *FRAXE* (Knight, 1994).

Yet another, even more rare fragile site associated with expansion of a trinucleotide repeat in Xq28 distal to *FRAXE* has been described and named *FRAXF*. It is not clear whether amplification of the repeat sequence at *FRAXF* is associated with mental impairment (Ritchie, 1994).

Myotonic Dystrophy

Myotonic dystrophy is an autosomal dominant, multisystem disorder with a wide range of clinical expression. In late childhood or early adulthood, the clinically most typical patients develop progressive myotonia and weakness, and atrophy of the muscles of the distal extremities and face. Cataracts, cardiac conduction defects, and testicular atrophy are also common. However, the disease may be so mild as to consist solely of cataracts developing in old age, or so severe as to present at birth with marked muscle degeneration and mental retardation proceeding to early death. Often all clinical expressions of the disease can be observed in the same family, occurring in an anticipation pattern (discussed earlier). Anticipation is present in virtually all of the trinucleotide repeat disorders but is most striking in DM, in which the clinical phenotype can progress from cataracts to severe congenital disease in three generations.

DM is caused by an expansion of a $(CTG)_n$ repeat in the 3′ untranslated region of the myotonin protein kinase gene on chromosome 19q13.3 (Fu, 1992; Mahadevan, 1992). In normal individuals this repeat ranges in size from 5 to 35 and is genetically stable. CTG repeats greater than 50 are genetically unstable and are prone to expansion as they are passed to subsequent generations. When in the range of 50 to 100, these repeats are often asymptomatic or produce minimal symptoms. When greater than 100 repeats are present, the typical DM phenotype is likely. Although there is a general correlation between repeat length and clinical severity, the size of the repeat is not a reliable prognostic indicator in the individual case. The extreme expansions to 1000 to 2000 repeats seen in congenital DM occur only with female transmission of the unstable repeat; thus congenital DM is always inherited from the mother.

The mechanism by which the expanded trinucleotide repeat in the myotonin protein kinase gene produces the DM phenotype is not known. Because the repeat is not located in the coding region of the gene, it is possible that protein expression is altered or that regulatory mRNA interactions are perturbed.

Huntington's Disease, X-Linked Spinal and Bulbar Muscular Atrophy, Spinocerebellar Ataxia Type 1, and Dentatorubral-Pallidoluysian Atrophy

Huntington's disease, X-linked spinal and bulbar muscular atrophy (SBMA), spinocerebellar ataxia type 1 (SCA1), and dentatorubral-pallidoluysian atrophy (DRPLA) are autosomal dominant or X-linked (SBMA) diseases characterized by selective neuronal degeneration in the central nervous system. In each of these disorders there is expansion of a $(CAG)_n$ trinucleotide repeat in the coding region of a novel gene that produces abnormal elongation of a polyglutamine tract (La Spada, 1994). Similar to the androgen receptor, the HD, SCA1, and DRPLA proteins have characteristics that suggest they may be transcription factors, but the cytoplasmic location of huntingtin and DRPLA protein argues against this role (Trottier, 1995; Yazawa, 1995). It is postulated that the expanded polyglutamine sequences in each of these proteins leads to alterations in their binding characteristics and a gain in function that is toxic to neurons in a selective manner.

In common with the other triplet repeat disorders, the expanded repeats in the neurodegenerative disorders are unstable and tend to increase in size in subsequent generations. There is a positive, but not absolute, correlation between increasing repeat size, early disease onset, and clinical severity. In contrast to fragile X and myotonic dystrophy, where the most dramatic increases in repeat size occur in maternal meioses, paternal transmission produces the largest expansions in the neurodegenerative disorders. Consequently, juvenile onset cases of HD, SCA1, and DRPLA are usually transmitted by the father.

Laboratory Testing for Trinucleotide Repeat Disorders

Expansions of trinucleotide repeats are readily demonstrated by Southern blot or PCR. PCR, followed by sizing of the products on an electrophoretic gel, is generally preferred for most of these disorders because of its speed, simplicity, and ability to resolve alleles differing in size by just one repeat unit. This is of particular importance when it is necessary to differentiate between stable alleles at the upper size limit from small premutation or disease-causing alleles. However, where triplet expansions are very large, as in fully expressed fragile X syndrome or DM, it may not be possible to amplify the greatly expanded DNA segment by

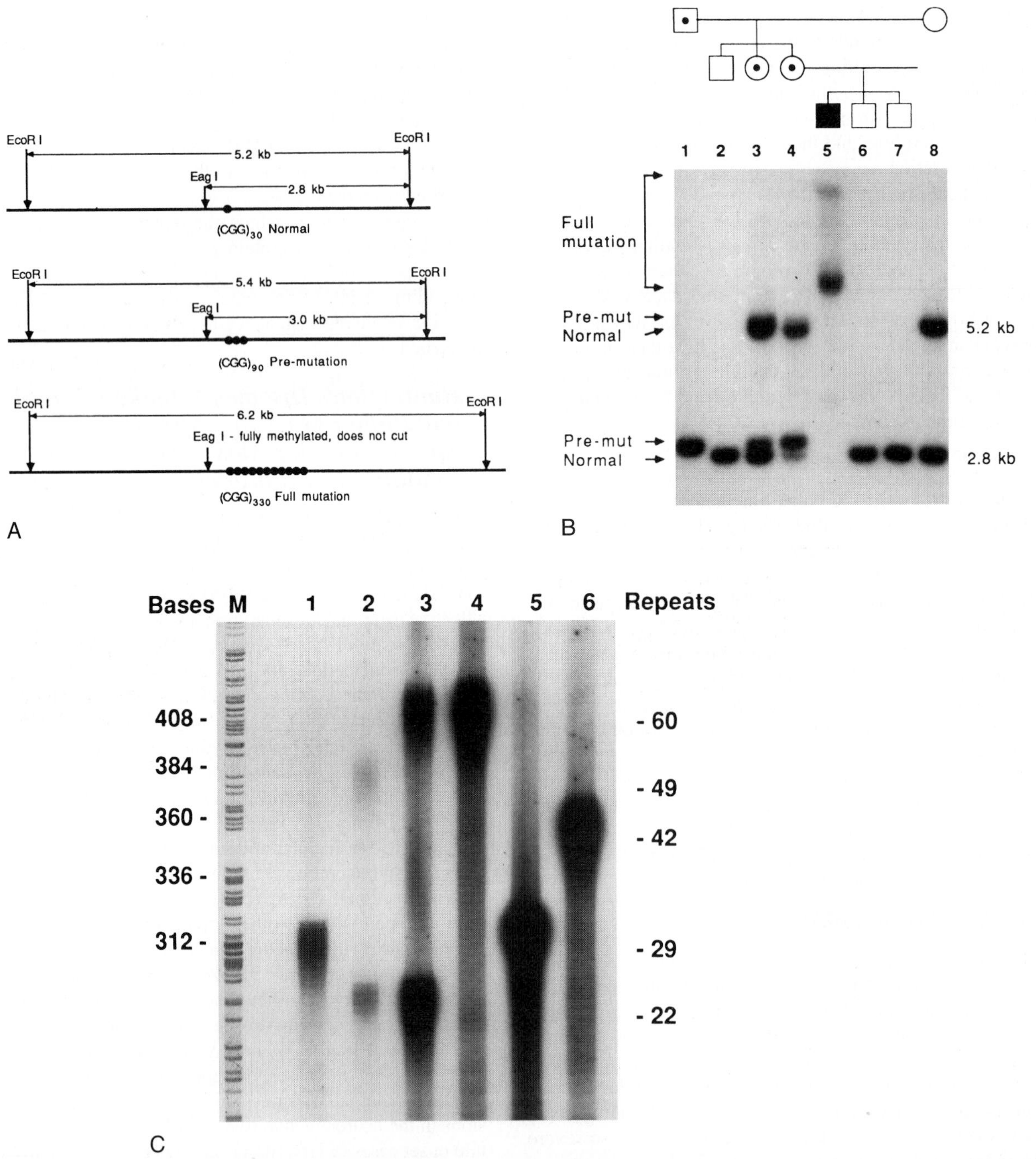

Figure 59–6. Detection of the $(CGG)_n$ repeat expansion in fragile X syndrome. *A*, Normal, premutation, and full mutation alleles at the FRAXA locus. When expansion of the repeat to a full mutation occurs, the *Eag* I restriction enzyme site becomes methylated and does not cut with the enzyme. *B*, Family of a patient (*darkened square*) with fragile X syndrome. A Southern blot of *EcoR* I/*Eag* I-digested DNA from each individual in the pedigree was examined with a labeled DNA probe, which hybridizes 3′ to the repeat. The three individuals (lanes 6 to 8) on the right of the figure are normal (*open squares and circles*). Note that the two males (lanes 6 and 7) each have a single 2.8-kb band, while the female (lane 8) has both a 2.8- and 5.2-kb band. This is the expected result. The 5.2-kb band in the female is from the normal inactive (and, therefore, methylated) X chromosome in each of her cells. Because the DNA on this chromosome is methylated, it is not cut by *Eag* I. The 2.8-kb band, however, is from the normal unmethylated active X chromosome (*Eag* I will cut the DNA in this case) in the female and in the male. The affected male (lane 5) has a greatly enlarged band. This is a consequence of marked expansion of the trinucleotide repeat as well as methylation of the *Eag* I restriction enzyme site. The three individuals marked by bold dots (lanes 1, 3, and 4) are carriers of premutation alleles. In the females (lanes 3 and 4), the distinction between normal and expanded alleles is seen most clearly in DNA from their active (unmethylated) X chromosomes. Here, there are distinct bands of 2.8 and 3.0 kb. Higher in the gel the resolution is not as good, and the 5.2 and 5.4 kb alleles are barely separated. Note that in this peripheral blood sample from the mother of the affected patient (lane 4), X chromosome inactivation is skewed with respect to the repeat expansion: a greater proportion of normal X chromosomes in this cell population have randomly been inactivated compared to the X chromosomes carrying the premutation allele. *C*, Sizing of trinucleotide repeats by gel electrophoresis following amplification of the locus by the polymerase chain reaction (PCR) (Levinson, 1994). Lanes 1 to 6 represent six different individuals; lane M contains a size marker. The PCR products were labeled by incorporation of ^{32}P-dCTP during the amplification reaction and the dried gel was exposed to x-ray film. Heterozygous females show two alleles, and males and homozygous females show single alleles. The multiple bands produced with each allele are due to "slippage" of the DNA polymerase during the PCR reaction; the most intense band is taken as representative of the actual size of the allele. (Figure 59–6C courtesy of Dr. Anne Maddalena, Genetics & IVF Institute, Fairfax, VA.)

PCR; in this case Southern blotting is the preferred technique. Figure 59–6 illustrates the use of Southern blotting and PCR to detect full *FMR1* mutations and *FMR1* premutation alleles.

Familial Cancers

In a sense all cancers are genetic disorders, caused by mutations in genes that control cellular proliferation and differentiation. In an oversimplified but useful way, these genes may be divided into two groups, those that act in a dominant way to promote proliferation (proto-oncogenes) and those that act in a way to restrain cell growth (tumor suppressor genes). Most often mutational events occur in a somatic cell, usually requiring alterations in several proto-oncogenes or tumor suppressor genes before a cancer characteristic of that particular cell develops (see Chapter 15 for discussion of oncogenes and tumor suppressor genes). However, in some individuals the initial mutation in this progression may in fact be a constitutional anomaly, inherited from a parent and present in every cell of that individual's body.

To date, heritable cancer-causing mutations have been found most often in tumor suppressor genes, but have also been found in an oncogene and in a group of DNA repair genes (Table 59–3). The inherited mutation should be viewed as the initiating event in tumor development, not in itself sufficient to cause cancer, but simply the first step in a series of mutations that could ultimately lead to uncontrolled cell growth, analogous to the first somatic mutation that initiates tumor development in sporadic cancers.

In comparison with their sporadic counterparts, familial cancers often develop at an earlier age, are frequently multifocal, and appear bilaterally in paired organs. Noting these distinguishing features in sporadic retinoblastoma and familial retinoblastoma, Knudson postulated that at least two mutational events are necessary to produce a tumor (Knudson, 1971). In the case of a sporadic tumor, two independent mutational events *in the same cell* are necessary to initiate tumor development, whereas in the case of a familial tumor, the first mutation is already present at birth in every cell of the body, making it more likely that a second mutational event will occur at an earlier age and often in more than one cell. Knudson's "two-hit" hypothesis is an important concept that guided many studies of the genetic basis of cancer. Elucidation of the heritable mutations in the familial cancer syndromes has been enormously informative, not only in understanding these rare disorders but in understanding the fundamental changes responsible for common malignancies as well.

Tumor Suppressor Genes: Retinoblastoma

Although familial cancer syndromes caused by mutations in tumor suppressor genes follow a dominant pattern of inheritance, at the cellular level the changes often appear recessive, because tumorigenesis is initiated (in most cases) only when both copies of the tumor suppressor gene are inactivated. Loss of the normal gene inherited from the unaffected parent may occur as the result of a second novel mutation, but most often it is the result of replacement by a duplicated copy of the mutant gene inherited from the affected parent by genetic mechanisms such as chromosomal nondisjunction or mitotic recombination. These events occur in retinoblastoma, a tumor of the retina caused by functional loss of both copies of the *RB1* gene, which encodes a nuclear transcription factor. In most cases, both of these mutational events occur somatically, and a solitary, sporadic tumor develops. But in approximately one third of the cases, the first *RB1* mutation is present in all cells of the affected child, having been inherited from a similarly affected parent or occurring as a new mutation in gametogenesis. When this is the case, the likelihood that the remaining normal *RB1* gene will undergo mutation in at least one retinal precursor cell is greater than 90%. As Knudson observed, in most patients with familial disease the tumors are bilateral and multifocal (Knudson, 1971), implying that several cells have sustained additional *RB1* mutations. It is not known whether *RB1* mutations alone are sufficient for tumorigenesis, but they certainly appear to be the initiating event.

Table 59–3. FAMILIAL CANCERS

	Gene	Chromosome Location	Gene Product	Function
Tumor Suppressor Genes				
Retinoblastoma	*RB1*	13q14	pRB	Transcription factor
Wilms tumor	*WT1*	11p13	WT1	Transcription factor
Neurofibromatosis type 1	*NF1*	17q11	Neurofibromin	GTPase activating protein
Li-Fraumeni syndrome	*p53*	17p13	p53	Transcription factor
Familial polyposis coli	*APC*	5q21–22	APC	Binds to beta-catenin
Neurofibromatosis type 2	*NF2*	22q12	Merlin	Cytoskeletal protein
Von Hippel-Lindau disease	*VHL*	3p25–26	VHL	Unknown
Familial melanoma	*CDKN2*	9p21	p16	Kinase inhibitor
Early onset breast cancer	*BRCA1*	17q21	BRCA1	Transcription factor
Oncogenes				
Multiple endocrine neoplasia type 2	*RET*	10q12	RET	Receptor tyrosine kinase
DNA Repair Genes				
Familial nonpolyposis colon cancer	*MSH2*	2p16	MSH2	DNA repair
	MLH1	3p21	MLH1	DNA repair
	PMS1	2q31–33	PMS1	DNA repair
	PMS2	7p22	PMS2	DNA repair

Familial retinoblastoma has served as a model in guiding research into the understanding of many familial cancers. This has led to the discovery of a large number of tumor suppressor genes, important not only in the pathogenesis of some relatively uncommon familial tumors, but also in the development of such common tumors as early-onset breast carcinoma (see Table 59–3) and (see Chap. 15) sporadic colon carcinoma (Weinberg, 1991).

Oncogenes: Multiple Endocrine Neoplasia, Type 2

To date there is only one related group of familial cancer syndromes that is known to be caused by a heritable mutation in an oncogene, multiple endocrine neoplasia type 2A (MEN 2A) and its variants, familial medullary thyroid carcinoma (FMTC) and multiple endocrine neoplasia type 2B (MEN 2B). Single, activating mutations in just one allele of the proto-oncogene *RET* are sufficient to initiate tumorigenesis in these disorders (DeLellis, 1995).

All three of these syndromes are characterized by hyperplasia of thyroidal C-cells and medullary thyroid carcinoma. In families afflicted with MEN 2A, pheochromocytomas and/or parathyroid adenomas or parathyroid hyperplasia are also present. MEN 2B is further characterized by the presence of multiple mucosal neuromas of the lips, mouth, and gastrointestinal tract, a marfanoid habitus, a particularly aggressive clinical course, and a high proportion of affected individuals due to new *RET* mutations.

RET is a signalling molecule with extracellular receptor and intracellular tyrosine kinase domains. With very rare exception, the known FMTC and MEN 2A mutations are single base substitutions in one of five codons in the extracellular domain, in each case producing substitution of a cysteine by another amino acid. By contrast, there is just one known MEN 2B mutation, a single base substitution producing a missense mutation in the tyrosine kinase domain. In approximately 10% of affected families with these disorders, a mutation has not yet been found.

DNA Repair Genes: Hereditary Nonpolyposis Colon Cancer

In the search for possible tumor suppressor genes as a cause of familial nonpolyposis colon cancer, it was observed that polymorphic dinucleotide repeat sequences (also known as microsatellites), such as $(CA)_n$, were apparently unstable in the tumors of affected individuals. Because similar microsatellite instability had been demonstrated in bacteria with abnormalities in genes responsible for DNA mismatch repair, attention was directed to the possibility that defective human DNA repair genes, homologs of the bacterial genes, were the heritable abnormality responsible for familial nonpolyposis colon cancer. In short order this was shown to be the case (Fishel, 1993; Leach, 1993). In a manner analogous to the initiation of tumorigenesis by tumor suppressor genes, inheritance of one copy of a defective *MSH2*, *MLH1*, *PMS1*, or *PMS2* gene, followed by somatic mutation of the second copy, produces cells that are deficient in DNA repair. These cells eventually accumulate deleterious mutations, and malignant transformation occurs. The apparent tissue specificity of this process is not understood.

Laboratory Testing for Familial Cancer Mutations

The ability to analyze an individual's constitutional DNA for heritable, cancer-predisposing mutations has enormous potential for disease prevention and early treatment and, with some disorders, has already become the standard of care. If a very high proportion of the cancer-causing mutations in a particular gene are known, and these mutations are relatively few in number, direct analysis for these mutations is simple and inexpensive. If, on the other hand, the gene is large, and cancer-causing mutations are numerous and widely dispersed, or occur in less accessible regions of the gene, such as introns or regulatory sequences, then mutation analysis must of necessity be less targeted and be capable of screening large stretches of DNA for abnormalities. In these cases techniques such as single-stranded conformation polymorphism (SSCP) analysis, denaturing gradient gel electrophoresis (DGGE), heteroduplex analysis, or direct DNA sequencing may be used (see Chap. 56). This approach can be very time consuming and costly. However, once a mutation is identified in an affected individual, then subsequent testing of other members of the family is relatively simple because it can be directed specifically at that abnormality. These various approaches to analysis of mutations in the *RET* oncogene that cause MEN 2A are illustrated in Figure 59–7. Because approximately 90% of families with MEN 2A have a mutation in one of just five codons in the extracellular domain of *RET*, DNA mutation analysis is highly effective in presymptomatic identification of MEN 2A gene carriers (Lips, 1994).

The situation is more complex with the tumor suppressor and DNA repair genes. Disease-causing mutations in these genes are numerous and widespread, sometimes unique to a particular family, and often necessitate a costly search of multiple DNA sequences in the index patient until the mutation is found. Unfortunately, even after an exhaustive search of the coding sequences and some noncoding regions as well, at the present time a mutation detection rate of 90% is probably achieved only with familial retinoblastoma and in many disorders is considerably lower than this.

Mitochondrial DNA Disorders

In addition to the 6 billion base pairs of DNA that comprise the human nuclear diploid genome, vital genetic information is also encoded in the 16,500 base pair, double-stranded circular DNA molecules that are present in two to 10 copies in each of the up to several hundred mitochondria of the cell. Mitochondrial DNA codes for 13 of the proteins of the respiratory chain and ATP synthase, as well as two ribosomal RNAs and 22 transfer RNAs required for their translation (Hammans, 1994). Mitochondrial DNA is self-replicating and is transmitted strictly by maternal inheritance, because the mitochondria of a spermatozoon are not incorporated into the zygote upon fertilization of an ovum.

Disease-causing abnormalities of mitochondrial DNA may result from several different mechanisms (Hammans, 1994). Single large deletions (and, rarely, duplications) that appar-

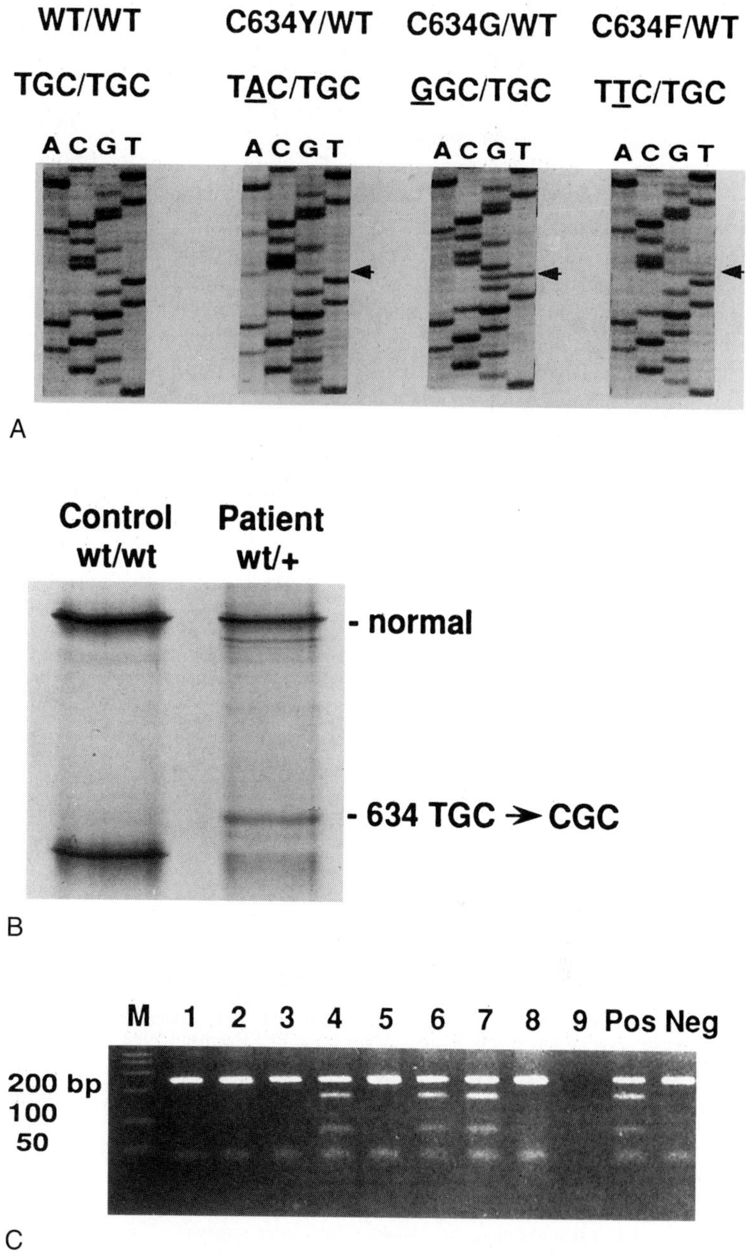

Figure 59–7. Mutation analysis of the *RET* proto-oncogene in multiple endocrine neoplasia type 2A (MEN 2A). *A*, A control subject (WT/WT) and affected individuals from three different families were examined for mutations in exon 11 of *RET* by direct sequencing. Different heterozygous missense mutations in codon 634 were detected in these individuals, changing the normal cysteine to tyrosine (C634Y), glycine (C634G), and phenylalanine (C634F), respectively. *B*, Screening for exon 11 mutations by single stranded conformation polymorphism (SSCP) analysis (see Chapter 56 for a discussion of SSCP). The unique band seen in the patient sample indicates a mutant allele. This was then identified as a codon 634 mutation (TGC → CGC) by direct sequencing. This technique is often a useful substitute for screening by direct sequencing. *C*, Mutation analysis by PCR and restriction enzyme digestion in at-risk individuals (lanes 1-8) in a family carrying the C634Y mutation. This mutation (TGC → TAC) creates an *Rsa* I site in exon 11. A 279 bp exon 11 PCR product, including codon 634, was generated by PCR and digested with *Rsa* I. Normally, a single *Rsa* I site is present in this PCR product and digestion produces fragments of 244 and 35 bp. When the C634Y mutation is present, fragments of 169, 75, and 35 bp are produced (lanes 4, 6, 7 and positive control). The presence of the constant normal *Rsa* I site is a very useful control feature, because its digestion ensures that the assay is functioning properly. Once a mutation has been identified in a family, this is an efficient way to test other family members. (Figure 59–7B courtesy of Dr. Brian Dawson, University of Texas Southwestern Medical Center, Dallas, TX.)

ently occur sporadically in oogenesis are typical of Kearns-Sayre syndrome, a myopathy characterized principally by progressive external ophthalmoplegia and pigmentary retinopathy. A wide range of disorders are characterized by multiple small deletions and show typical mendelian autosomal dominant or autosomal recessive patterns of inheritance, apparently because they are due to undefined defects in nuclear genes important for mitochondrial DNA replication. Most distinctive from a genetic point of view are the disorders that follow a pattern of strict maternal inheritance, never showing transmission from an affected male and passing from an affected female equally to her sons and daughters. These diseases are most often caused by point mutations in one of the genes encoding a transfer RNA (myoclonic epilepsy and ragged red fibers [MERRF] and mitochondrial myopathy, encephalopathy, lactic acidosis, and strokelike episodes [MELAS] are examples) or a mitochondrial protein (Leber's hereditary optic neuropathy, for example).

Laboratory confirmation of the large mitochondrial DNA deletions often present in Kearns-Sayre syndrome is easily accomplished by Southern blot analysis of mitochondrial DNA from affected tissues using labeled whole mitochondrial DNA as a probe. Point mutations in other disorders may be analyzed by a number of techniques discussed in Chapter 56.

SUMMARY

From the many examples presented in this chapter, it should be evident that the molecular diagnosis of genetic disease is one of the most exciting applications of molecular

7

pathology. Moreover, it is one that impinges upon all the others by virtue of the fact that virtually all diseases have some genetic component. As the Human Genome Project continues to uncover important disease genes (especially those for common disorders) at an ever-increasing rate and technologies for high-speed DNA sequencing and multiplex mutation detection continue to improve, we can anticipate diagnostic molecular genetics assuming a far more expansive role in public health and preventive medicine than has been the case thus far. The advent of DNA "chips" containing thousands of probes (Pease, 1994) may someday allow extensive genotyping and lifetime disease prediction for hundreds of disorders from a single newborn blood spot. Against these promising advances will have to be weighed the ethical impact of such genetic "invasiveness" and the eventual curative potential of gene replacement therapies. Whatever the ultimate balance reached, there is little doubt that molecular genetics will be the driving force behind much of medical practice in the 21st century.

Abeliovich D, Lavon IP, Lerer I, et al: Screening for five mutations detects 97% of cystic fibrosis (CF) chromosomes and predicts a carrier frequency of 1:29 in the Jewish Ashkenazi population. Am J Hum Genet 1992; 51:951–956.

Ahn AH, Kunkel LM: The structural and functional diversity of dystrophin. Nature Genet 1993; 3:283–291.

Anguiano A, Oates RD, Amos JA, et al: Congenital bilateral absence of the vas deferens: A primarily genital form of cystic fibrosis. JAMA 1992; 267:1794–1797.

Bates G, Lehrach H: Trinucleotide repeat expansions and human genetic disease. Bioessays 1994; 16:277–284.

Beggs AH, Koenig M, Boyce FM, Kunkel LM: Detection of 98% of DMD/BMD gene deletions by polymerase chain reaction. Hum Genet 1990a; 86:45–48.

Beggs AH, Kunkel LM: A polymorphic CACA repeat in the 3′ untranslated region of dystrophin. Nucleic Acids Res 1990b; 18:1931.

Billings PR, Kohn MA, de Cuervas M, et al: Discrimination as a consequence of genetic testing. Am J Hum Genet 1992; 50:476–482.

Bowden DK, Vickers MA, Higgs DR: A PCR-based strategy to detect the common severe determinants of alpha thalassemia. Br J Haematol 1992; 81:104–108.

Burke W, Aitken ML, Chen S-H, Scott CR: Variable severity of pulmonary disease in adults with identical cystic fibrosis mutations. Chest 1992; 102:506–509.

Cai SP, Wall J, Kaa YW, Chehab FF: Reverse dot blot probes for the screening of beta-thalassemia mutations in Asians and American blacks. Hum Mutat 1994; 3:59–63.

Chehab FF, Wall J: Detection of multiple cystic fibrosis mutations by reverse dot blot hybridization: A technology for carrier screening. Hum Genet 1992; 89:163–168.

Chen TP, Liu SF, Chang JG, et al: Molecular characterization of Hb H disease by polymerase chain reaction. Acta Haematol 1993; 90:177–181.

Chong GL, Thibodeau SN: A simple assay for the screening of the cystic fibrosis allele in carriers of the phe-508 mutation. Mayo Clin Proc 1990; 65:1072–1076.

Collins FS: Cystic fibrosis: Molecular biology and therapeutic implications. Science 1992; 256:774–780.

Conner BJ, Reyes AA, Morin C, et al: Detection of sickle beta-globin allele by hybridization with synthetic oligonucleotides. Proc Natl Acad Sci USA 1983; 80:278–282.

Curtis A, Richardson RJ, Boohene J, et al: Absence of cystic fibrosis mutations in a large Asian population sample and occurrence of a homozygous S549N mutation in an inbred Pakistani family. J Med Genet 1993; 30:164–166.

Cystic Fibrosis Genotype-Phenotype Consortium: Correlation between genotype and phenotype in patients with cystic fibrosis. N Engl J Med 1993; 329:1308–1313.

Darras BT, Koenig M, Kunkel LM, Francke U: Direct method for prenatal diagnosis and carrier detection in Duchenne/Becker muscular dystrophy using the entire dystrophin cDNA. Am J Med Genet 1988; 29:713–726.

DeLellis RA: Biology of disease. Multiple endocrine neoplasia syndromes revisited. Clinical, morphologic and molecular features. Lab Invest 1995; 72:494–505.

Fishel R, Lescoe MK, Rao MRS, et al: The human mutator gene homolog MSH2 and its association with hereditary nonpolyposis colon cancer. Cell 1993; 75:1027–1038.

Fu Y-H, Kuhl DPA, Pizzuti A, et al: Variation of the CGG repeat at the fragile X site results in genetic instability: Resolution of the Sherman paradox. Cell 1991; 67:1047–1058.

Fu Y-H, Pizzuti A, Fenwick RG, et al: An unstable triplet repeat in a gene related to myotonic muscular dystrophy. Science 1992; 255:1256–1258.

Gervais R, Dumur V, Rigot J-M, et al: High frequency of the R117H cystic fibrosis mutation in patients with congenital absence of the vas deferens (letter). N Engl J Med 1993; 328:446–447.

Grebe TA, Seltzer WK, DeMarchi J, et al: Genetic analysis of Hispanic individuals with cystic fibrosis. Am J Hum Genet 1994; 54:443–446.

Hammans SR: Mitochondrial DNA and disease. Essays Biochem 1994; 28:99–112.

Handyside AH, Lesko JG, Tarin JJ, et al: Birth of a normal girl after in vitro fertilization and preimplantation diagnostic testing for cystic fibrosis. N Engl J Med 1992; 327:905–909.

Hatcher SL, Trang QT, Robb KM, et al: Prenatal diagnosis by enzymatic amplification and restriction endonuclease digestion for detection of haemoglobins A, S and C. Mol Cell Probes 1992; 6:343–348.

Highsmith WE, Burch LH, Zhou Z, et al: A novel mutation in the cystic fibrosis gene in patients with pulmonary disease but normal sweat chloride concentrations. N Engl J Med 1994; 331:974–980.

Higuchi M, Kazazian HH, Kasch L, et al: Molecular characterization of severe hemophilia A suggests that about half the mutations are not within the coding and splice junctions of the factor VIII gene. Proc Natl Acad Sci USA 1992; 88:7405–7409.

Hoffman EP, Fischbeck KH, Brown RH, et al: Characterization of dystrophin in muscle-biopsy specimens from patients with Duchenne's or Becker's muscular dystrophy. N Engl J Med 1988; 318:1363–1368.

Huntington's Disease Society of America: Guidelines for Predictive Testing for Hungtington's Disease. New York: Huntington's Disease Society of America, 1989.

Kerem B-S, Rommens JM, Buchanan JA, et al: Identification of the cystic fibrosis gene: Genetic analysis. Science 1989; 245:1073–1080.

Knight SJ, Voelckel MA, Hirst MC, et al: Triplet repeat expansion at the FRAXE locus and X-linked mild mental retardation. Am J Hum Genet 1994; 55:81–86.

Knoll JHM, Nicholls RD, Magenis RE, et al: Angelman and Prader-Willi syndromes share a common chromosome 15 deletion but differ in parental origin of the deletion. Am J Med Genet 1989; 32:285–290.

Knudson AG: Mutation and cancer: Statistical study of retinoblastoma. Proc Natl Acad Sci USA 1971; 68:820–823.

Landemous JB, Gregersen N, Kolvra S, et al: The frequency of a disease-causing point mutation in the gene coding for medium-chain acyl-CoA dehydrogenase in sudden infant death syndrome. Acta Paediatr 1993; 82:544–546.

La Spada AR, Paulson HL, Fischbeck KH: Trinucleotide repeat expansion in neurological disease. Ann Neurol 1994; 36:814–822.

Leach FS, Nicolaides NC, Papadopoulos N, et al: Mutations of a mutS homolog in hereditary nonpolyposis colorectal cancer. Cell 1993; 75: 1215–1225.

Lerer I, Meiner V, Pashut-Lavon I, Abeliovich D: Molecular diagnosis of Prader-Willi syndrome: Parent-of-origin dependent methylation sites and nonisotopic detection of $(CA)_2$ dinucleotide repeat polymorphisms. Am J Med Genet 1994; 52:79–84.

Levinson G, Maddalena A, Palmer FT, et al: Improved sizing of fragile X CCG repeats by nested polymerase chain reaction. Am J Med Genet 1994; 51:527–534.

Lips CJM, Landsvater RM, Hoppener JWM, et al: Clinical screening as compared with DNA analysis in families with multiple endocrine neoplasia type 2A. N Engl J Med 1994; 331:828–835.

Lopez de Munain A, Blanco A, Emparanza JI, et al: Anticipation in myotonic dystrophy: A parental-sex-related phenomenon. Neuroepidemiology 1994; 13:75–78.

Maggio A, Gianbona A, Cai SP, et al: Rapid and simultaneous typing of hemoglobin S, hemoglobin C, and seven Mediterranean beta-thalassemia mutations by covalent reverse dot blot analysis: Application to prenatal diagnosis in Sicily. Blood 1993; 81:239–242.

Mahadevan M, Tsilfidis C, Sabourin L, et al: Myotonic dystrophy mutation: An unstable CTG repeat in the 3′ untranslated region of the gene. Science 1992; 255:1253–1255.

Miedzybrodzka Z, Dean J, Haites N: Screening for cystic fibrosis (Letter). Lancet 1991; 338:1524–1525.

Monaco AP, Bertelson CJ, Liechti-Gallati S, et al: An explanation for the phenotypic differences between patients bearing partial deletions of the DMD locus. Genomics 1988; 2:90–95.

Multicenter Study Group: Diagnosis of Duchenne and Becker muscular dystrophies by polymerase chain reaction: A multicenter study. JAMA 1992; 267:2609–2615.

Ng ISL, Pace R, Richard MV, et al: Methods for analysis of multiple cystic fibrosis mutations. Hum Genet 1991; 87:613–617.

Ober C, Lester LA, Mott C, et al: Ethnic heterogeneity and cystic fibrosis transmembrane regulator (CFTR) mutation frequencies in Chicago-area CF families. Am J Hum Genet 1992; 51:1344–1348.

Orozco L, Sacedo M, Lezana JL, et al: Frequency of ΔF508 in a Mexican sample of cystic fibrosis patients. J Med Genet 1993; 30:501–502.

Pease AC, Solas D, Sullivan EJ, et al: Light-generated oligonucleotide arrays for rapid DNA sequence anlaysis. Proc Natl Acad Sci USA 1994; 91:5022–5026.

Prior TW: Genetic analysis of the Duchenne muscular dystrophy gene. Arch Pathol Lab Med 1991; 115:984–990.

Prior TW, Papp AC, Snyder PJ, et al: Identification of two point mutations and a none base deletion in exon 19 of the dystrophin gene by heteroduplex formation. Hum Molec Genet 1993; 2:311–313.

Riordan JR, Rommens JM, Kerem B-S, et al: Identification of the cystic fibrosis gene: Cloning and characterization of complementary DNA. Science 1989; 245:1066–1073.

Ritchie RJ, Knight SJ, Hirst MC, et al: The cloning of FRAXF: Trinucleotide repeat expansion and methylation at a third fragile site in distal Xqter. Hum Mol Genet 1994; 3:2115–2121.

Rowland LP: Dystrophin: A triumph of reverse genetics and the end of the beginning [editorial]. N Engl J Med 1988; 318:1392–1394.

Sancho S, Mongini T, Tanji K, et al: Analysis of dystrophin expression after activation of myogenesis in amniocytes, chorionic-villus cells, and fibroblasts. N Engl J Med 1993; 329:915–920.

Shuber AP, Skoletsky J, Stern R, Handelin BL: Efficient 12-mutation testing in the CFTR gene: A general model for complex mutation analysis. Hum Mol Genet 1993; 2:153–158.

Spence JE, Perciaccante RG, Greig GM, et al: Uniparental disomy as a mechanism for human genetic disease. Am J Hum Genet 1988; 42:217–226.

Tocharoentanaphol C, Cremer M, Schrock E, et al: Multicolor fluorescence in situ hybridization on metaphase chromosomes and interphase Halo-preparations using cosmid and YAC clones for the simultaneous high resolution mapping of deletions in the dystrophin gene. Hum Genet 1994; 93:229–235.

Trottier Y, Devys D, Imbert G, et al: Cellular localization of the Huntington's disease protein and discrimination of the normal and mutated form. Nature Genet 1995; 10:104–110.

Tsui L-C: The spectrum of cystic fibrosis mutations. Trends Genet 1992; 8:393–398.

Wald NJ: Couple screening for cystic fibrosis. Lancet 1991; 338:1318–1319.

Weinberg RA: Tumor suppressor genes. Science 1991; 254:1138–1146.

Wilfond BS, Fost N: The cystic fibrosis gene: Medical and social implications for heterozygote detection. JAMA 1990; 263:2777–2783.

Williams H, Sarafarazi M, Brown C, et al: The use of flanking markers in prediction for Duchenne muscular dystrophy. Arch Dis Child 1986; 61:218–222.

Williamson R: Universal community carrier screening for cystic fibrosis? Nature Genet 1993; 3:195–201.

Wilson JM: Vehicles for gene therapy [editorial]. Nature 1993; 365: 691–692.

Yazawa I, Nukina N, Hashida H, et al: Abnormal gene product identified in hereditary dentatorubral-pallidoluysian atrophy. Nature Genet 1995; 10:99–103.

Chapter 60

Molecular Pathology of Infectious Diseases

Martin G. Cormican, M.D.
Michael A. Pfaller, M.D.

In the past decade the techniques of molecular biology have contributed enormously to our understanding of the pathogenesis and epidemiology of infectious disease. As the techniques have become more refined and more accessible, those engaged in the diagnosis and management of human infection have sought to address the challenge of adapting these methods for routine clinical problem solving, that is, for diagnosis of disease, for guiding therapy, and for hospital epidemiology and infection control. The practice of molecular pathology will increasingly form a part of the diagnostic service rather than an esoteric diversion for the enthusiast. As molecular techniques become routine, the critical questions of cost and potential for contribution to patient care will need to be addressed. In this respect, the value of a method is a function of the degree to which it addresses the limitations of current methods, not of its technical elegance. Molecular diagnosis is, therefore, most appropriate for infectious agents that are difficult to detect and identify in a timely fashion with conventional methods. The principles of molecular biology as relevant to laboratory diagnosis are covered in detail in Chapters 55, 56, 57, and 63.

Suffice it to say that the molecular diagnosis of infectious diseases is largely nucleic acid based and requires the isolation of nucleic acids from microorganisms and clinical material, and the use of restriction endonuclease enzymes, gel electrophoresis, and nucleic acid hybridization techniques. Increasingly, newer techniques for amplification of nucleic acids are applied to clinical material. DNA sequence analysis, although not practical at present for use in the clinical laboratory, provides the ultimate means of characterizing organisms and when coupled with amplification techniques has provided the means with which to identify uncultivatable microorganisms previously unknown in infectious diseases (Amann, 1994; Wilson, 1994).

An important consideration in relation to the more widespread application of molecular techniques is the cost implications for laboratories and institutions. In the area of diagnosis of infectious disease, improved patient outcome and reduced cost of antimicrobials and duration of hospital stay may outweigh the increase in laboratory costs, but at this point this has not been demonstrated clearly. In the case of communicable diseases, the cost may be justified by improved infection control measures to protect patients and health care workers. Molecular epidemiology may make a real contribution to the detection and control of nosocomial spread of infection with potential to reduce nosocomial infection rates and the requirement for expensive antimicrobials used to treat resistant organisms. At this point, however, much of the justification for expenditure on molecular diagnostics and epidemiology is speculative; however, the costs of equipment, reagents, and expertise are clear and substantial. The level of investment justified must be determined in a given institution, and in some cases use of a reference laboratory service may represent the most efficient option. As clinical use of molecular diagnostic methods becomes a reality, the principles of quality assurance need to be applied to ensure that these techniques are subject to the same standards as conventional methods. In the concluding section of this chapter, the issues of standardization and quality assurance are addressed.

APPLICATIONS OF MOLECULAR METHODS IN CLINICAL MICROBIOLOGY

The use of molecular methods for identification and direct detection of microorganisms in clinical microbiology is evolving gradually, and several products are now available commercially (see Tables 60–2 and 60–3). Practical applications include the use of nucleic acid probes for direct detection of organisms in clinical material or for identification of previously isolated organisms. In addition, amplification-based techniques may be used for detection and identification, and to define selected characteristics (e.g., antibiotic resistance genes) of organisms. Finally, molecular methods provide a powerful means of characterizing organisms to the subspecies level in epidemiologic investigations.

Detection of Pathogens by DNA Probes

The detection of pathogenic microorganisms directly in specimens by DNA probe has been investigated extensively using a variety of hybridization and signal-generating formats. Commercial product development has focused on direct diagnosis of sexually transmitted diseases and respiratory pathogens using solution-phase hybridization and acridinium ester–labeled probes (Table 60–1).

Direct diagnosis by probe hybridization is rapid and free of the contamination problems associated with target amplification and is less susceptible to inhibition than many amplification procedures. A limitation of probe hybridization is the requirement for at least 10^4 copies of the target sequence for detection. In some instances, however, this may be adequate for clinical purposes, and a lower limit of detection (as with amplification) may offer no practical advantage. Recently more sophisticated probe hybridization formats have shown promise of reducing the limit of detection by an order of magnitude by reducing background signal (Shah, 1994).

Human papilloma virus (HPV) is an excellent example of a pathogen that could not be studied effectively without DNA hybridization. The virus may not express antigens at detectable levels in infected tissue and in transformed tissue no HPV antigen may be produced. The virus cannot be cultured *in vitro*. The classification of HPV types is based on DNA-DNA hybridization studies; strains with less than 50% hybridization to any previously described type constitute a new type. The potential for malignant transformation of infected tissues is related to the infecting HPV type. Type-specific whole genomic and oligonucleotide probes for the more common types (e.g., types 16 and 18 commonly associated with uterine cervical carcinoma and types 6 and 11 associated with benign disease) have been described, and both isotopic and nonisotopic labeling have been used (Faulkner-Jones, 1993; Lorinez, 1992). Hybridization of DNA extract, slot blotted onto a membrane, is widely used because it facilitates processing of large numbers of specimens; however, one commercial system uses solution-phase hybridization (Digene). *In situ* hybridization has been of value principally in defining the occurrence of the HPV genome in the malignant cells. HPV detection is an area in which utilization of DNA detection (by hybridization or amplification) may be expected to find a role in the diagnostic laboratory because the detection of types 16 and 18 may have prognostic significance, and no alternative methodology is available. In other areas, the adoption of probe hybridization detection must be based on overcoming limitations of existing methods or on a favorable cost comparison.

Cerebral toxoplasmosis is a major cause of morbidity and mortality in patients with the acquired immune deficiency syndrome. At present, diagnosis is often based on clinical and radiologic features and response to therapy. A cloned repetitive sequence ABC Ty4 from *Toxoplasma gondii* labeled with digoxigenin dUTP has been described for detection of toxoplasma DNA in cerebrospinal fluid using a slot blot format (Angel, 1992). Studies comparing this method with others such as PCR have not been reported. Although the limit of detection by PCR is likely to be lower (Hitt, 1992), the limit of detection that is clinically useful needs to be determined for each disease entity.

Detection of malaria parasites represents a different problem. The established method, direct microscopy of Giemsa-stained smears, has high sensitivity and specificity but is time consuming and dependent on experienced microscopists. An isotopically labeled probe for detection of *Plasmodium falciparum* DNA in slot blots of DNA from blood samples has been studied both for diagnosis and for use in surveillance of infection. In surveillance of a population with a prevalence of malaria infection of 1% to 4%, a specificity of 98.2% to 99.9% and a sensitivity of 62% to 92% relative to expert mi-

Table 60–1. DNA PROBES FOR DIRECT PATHOGEN DETECTION*

Organism	Hybridization Format	Reporter System	Status
Human papilloma virus	Solution phase	DNA/RNA hybrid capture and chemiluminescence	Commercial§
		slot blot digoxigenin	Reported
Hepatitis C virus	Solid-phase microtitre tray	Branched chain DNA	Commercial‡
Hepatitis B virus	Solid-phase microtitre tray	Branched chain DNA	Commercial‡
Chlamydia trachomatis	Solution phase	Acridinium ester	Commercial†
Neisseria gonorrhoeae	Solution phase	Acridinium ester	Commercial†
Toxoplasma gondii	Slot blot	Digoxigenin	Reported
Plasmodium falciparum	Slot blot	Isotopic	Reported

*The table contains examples of available methods and is not intended to be all inclusive.
†Gen-Probe, Inc., San Diego, CA.
‡Chiron, Emeryville, CA.
§Digene, Silver Spring, MD.

7

croscopy was achieved. The probe was less costly and much less labor intensive than direct microscopy (Barker, 1994).

DNA probes for detection of mycobacteria in clinical samples have been evaluated using a dotblot format. The probe was no more sensitive than direct microscopic examination; however, it did permit rapid identification of *Mycobacterium tuberculosis* (as distinct from acid-fast bacilli present) (Pao, 1988). Studies with more recently developed labeling systems, such as branched chain DNA, and Qβ replicase have not been reported.

Conventional microbiologic methods have considerable limitations in the detection of fastidious anaerobic organisms, such as those associated with periodontal disease. Isotopically labeled whole chromosomal DNA probes applied to slot blotted DNA extracts may be more sensitive than culture in detection of culturable organisms such as *Porphyromonas gingivalis*, and *Actinobacillus actinomycetemcomitans*; and is superior to microscopy for detection of the nonculturable organism *Treponema denticola* (Loesche, 1992).

Detection of pathogens by hybridization in solution has become dominated by the acridinium ester–labeled products of Gen-Probe, Inc. (San Diego, CA). The probe labeling system is nonradioactive and has a long shelf life. Acridinium ester–labeled probes for detection of *Chlamydia trachomatis*, *Streptococcus pyogenes*, and *Neisseria gonorrhoeae* are available.

The reliability of the Gen-Probe kit for detection of *Chlamydia trachomatis* in clinical specimens has been evaluated relative to cell culture, immunologic methods, and polymerase chain reaction (PCR). The Gen-Probe test is performed directly on material obtained by sampling urethral or endocervical secretions. The specimens are transported to the laboratory in a transport medium that also lyses the cells. The entire procedure is performed in a single tube, and the chemiluminescent signal is read in a luminometer and interpreted relative to a positive and negative control. Using the earlier (PACE) version of hybrid detection, the positive predictive value of Gen-Probe was 82% to 96% with negative predictive values of 96% to 99% (LeBar, 1989; Woods, 1990). A study comparing Gen-Probe and an enzyme immunoassay relative to culture reported that EIA and Gen-Probe gave comparable results. Data on the relative cost of the EIA and Gen-Probe were not presented (LeBar, 1989). Gen Probe is as sensitive and almost as specific as direct fluorescent antibody detection (Woods, 1990). A study comparing the Gen-Probe PACE-2 *Chlamydia* test with culture, using PCR results as a reference test, reported a considerable difference in the performance of the test on specimens from male and female patients. The positive predictive value of Gen-Probe in specimens from females was 83.3%, much less than that of culture (97.6%). The positive predictive value in specimens from the male urethra was higher (96.4%), but the negative predictive value was lower, at 96.5% (99.5% in females) (Kluytmans, 1991). More recently, a modification of the Gen Probe *Chlamydia* assay using a more rigid swab type and a 50% reduction in the quantity of transport medium was studied. These modifications, together with use of a probe competition assay on selected specimens, resulted in a sensitivity of 94.9% and a specificity of 100% in specimens from the male urethra (Kluytmans, 1994).

A Qβ replicase probe amplification assay for detection of *Chlamydia trachomatis* in genital specimens has recently been developed by Gene-Trak, Inc. (Shah, 1994). The performance on initial evaluation is promising; however, a direct comparison with Gen Probe or PCR assays has not been described.

A Gen-Probe test for detection of *Neisseria gonorrhoeae* is also available, and a single specimen may be examined for both *N. gonorrhoeae* and *Chlamydia trachomatis*. It has been evaluated for detection of *N. gonorrhoeae* in specimens from genital (Vlaspolder, 1993) and nongenital sites (Lewis, 1993). The predictive value of a negative test is very high (99.8%) in both studies, and the positive predictive value is 90.6% to 91.3%. In neither study were the results of direct microscopy reported relative to the probe or culture, although methylene blue smears were performed in one study (Vlaspolder, 1993). Such a comparison may be relevant as the sensitivity and specificity of examination of gram-stained smears, particularly from the symptomatic male urethra, is high.

The probe for detection of *Streptococcus pyogenes* in throat swabs has a sensitivity of 86% to 92.4%, and a specificity of 96% to 99.9% compared with culture (Heiter, 1993; Steed, 1993). Commercial probe assays for detection of genital tract pathogens (*Trichomonas vaginalis*, *Candida albicans*, and *Gardnerella vaginalis*) have also been reported but have not progressed towards adoption into laboratory use at this point.

Branched chain DNA probes for detection of hepatitis C virus and hepatitis B virus (Urdea, 1992) have become available very recently. This probe hybridization assay is presented in an enzyme immunoassay–like format. Probe to target hybridization occurs in solution, and the hybrid is then captured on the microtitre tray by an additional probe linked to the microtitre tray. The limit of detection of target nucleic acid is not as low as that achievable with target amplification (Zaaijer, 1994). Results are quantitative, and it may be that the limit of detection is adequate for some clinical purposes.

DNA Probes for Culture Identification

DNA probes now have an established role in the identification of cultures of a number of microorganisms (Table 60–2). Culture identification by probe hybridization is not dependent on the ability to detect minute quantities of nucleic acid. The advantage of probe-based identification is greatest for slow-growing organisms like the mycobacteria or for organisms for which convenient commercial identification systems are not available. At this point identification by probe hybridization is relatively expensive because in many instances isolates for identification present themselves individually so that a large number of controls are run per clinical isolate. In this section some of the probes described or commercially available are considered.

Identification of cultured mycobacterium by conventional methods is slow and time consuming. Acridinium ester–labeled probes for identification of *M. tuberculosis*, the *Mycobacterium avium intracellulare* complex, *M. gordonae*, and *M. kansasii* are available commercially from Gen-Probe, Inc. The use of these probes permits identification from culture in one working day and specificity and sensitivity (99% and 95.5%, respectively) are excellent in almost all cases (Goto, 1991; Walton and Valesco, 1991). Occasionally mem-

Table 60–2. COMMERCIAL DNA PROBES FOR CULTURE IDENTIFICATION*

Organism	Hybridization Format	Reporter System
Mycobacterium tuberculosis	In solution	Acridinium ester
M. avium-intracellulare	In solution	Acridinium ester
M. gordonae	In solution	Acridinium ester
M. kansasii	In solution	Acridinium ester
Histoplasma capsulatum	In solution	Acridinium ester
Coccidioides immitis	In solution	Acridinium ester
Blastomyces dermatitidis	In solution	Acridinium ester
Cryptococcus neoformans	In solution	Acridinium ester
Neisseria gonorrhoeae	In solution	Acridinium ester
Staphylococcus aureus	In solution	Acridinium ester
Streptococcus pneumoniae	In solution	Acridinium ester
Escherichia coli	In solution	Acridinium ester
Haemophilus influenzae	In solution	Acridinium ester
Enterococcus species	In solution	Acridinium ester
Streptococcus agalactiae	In solution	Acridinium ester

*The probes listed have been developed by Gen-Probe, Inc., San Diego, CA. The table contains examples of described probes; it is not intended to be all inclusive.

bers of species other than *M. tuberculosis* may be misidentified as *M. tuberculosis*, and the *M. kansasii* probe may perform poorly in some geographic areas (Butler, 1994; Ford, 1993; Tortoli, 1994).

Probes for identification from culture of *Histoplasma capsulatum*, *Blastomyces dermatitidis*, *Coccidioides immitis*, and *Cryptococcus neoformans* are also available (Stockman, 1993). Evaluations indicate that specificity is 100% and a sensitivity of 97% or greater was reported for all species except *B. dermatitidis* (87.8%). With repeat testing the sensitivity improved to 97.3% for *B. dermatitidis* and 100% for all other species.

The Gen-Probe *N. gonorrhoeae* probe system has been used for identification of cultured *N. gonorrhoeae* in addition to its use for direct application to clinical specimens (Young, 1993a). The *N. gonorrhoeae* probe (Accuprobe) has been compared with rapid carbohydrate utilization, a commercial system (Quadferm, bioMerieux) for carbohydrate utilization and a coagglutination system (Phadebact Monoclone GC tests). The Accuprobe was superior to coagglutination in identification of *N. gonorrhoeae*. Accuprobe performed equivalent to carbohydrate utilization and may be superior to the commercial fermentation system.

A battery of acridinium ester–labeled DNA probes for identification of cultures of *Staphylococcus aureus*, *Streptococcus pneumoniae*, *Escherichia coli*, *Haemophilus influenzae*, *Enterococcus* spp., and *Streptococcus agalactiae* have been developed. A probe for *Listeria monocytogenes* is also available. These probes have been applied to organisms harvested from positive blood culture bottles by centrifugation (Davis, 1991). Identification is available in approximately 30 minutes and is simple to perform. The procedure is more expensive than conventional techniques.

While the specificity of the available commercial probes is high and they facilitate rapid identification of a number of pathogens, the experience of the misidentification of some strains of mycobacteria (*M. celatum* and *M. terrae*) as *M. tuberculosis*, and the failure of the *M. kansasii* probe to identify 25% of *M. kansasii* isolates in one Italian study emphasize the need for caution in using any single characteristic in identification of a species.

DNA Amplification for Diagnosis

DNA amplification has the potential to overcome the principal limitation of diagnostic probe hybridization by selectively amplifying specific targets to detectable levels. PCR was the first amplification technique developed and remains the most widely investigated and applied method. A number of commercial kits for detection of *M. tuberculosis*, hepatitis C virus, human immunodeficiency virus, and the leading agents of sexually transmitted diseases, *N. gonorrhoeae* and *C. trachomatis*, have been developed and are or will soon be available. Commercial products with built in anticontamination precautions, standardization of reagents and conditions, and potential for automation are likely to increase the reproducibility and ease of application of this technology. The newer amplification technologies, ligase chain reaction, strand displacement amplification, and transcription-dependent amplification, form the basis of additional diagnostic systems that are, or are soon likely to be, available. At this point experience is greatest with PCR, and this section focuses on PCR for this reason. Table 60–3 summarizes some of the pathogens that have received the most attention and the amplification methods that have been applied.

Diagnosis of Viral Infection

The identification of the hepatitis C virus (HCV) was made possible by the techniques of molecular biology, and it is therefore not surprising that PCR has an important role in its diagnosis. As HCV is an RNA virus, reverse transcription into cDNA is an essential preliminary to amplification by PCR. A variety of in-house PCR reactions using reverse transcriptase and DNA polymerase have been described and appear useful (Gretch, 1994; Manzin, 1994). Roche Diagnostics has developed a commercial product in which reverse transcription and amplification are performed by the same enzyme, Tth, from *Thermus thalpophilus* (Young, 1993b). The amplicon is detected by a microtitre well capture probe

Table 60–3. COMMERCIAL DIAGNOSTIC NUCLEIC ACID AMPLIFICATION SYSTEMS*

Organism	Amplication Technology	Amplicon Detection
Hepatitis C virus	Reverse transcriptase and PCR	Microtitre capture probe†
HIV virus	PCR	Microtitre capture probe†
Mycobacterium tuberculosisis	PCR	Microtitre capture probe†
	Strand displacement amplification	Ethidium bromide gel‡
	Transcription-dependent amplification	Acridinium ester probe§
Chlamydia trachomatis	PCR	Microtitre capture probe†
	LCR	Antibody capture of labeled product¶
Neisseria gonorrhoeae	PCR	Microtitre capture probe†
	LCR	Antibody capture of labeled product¶

*The table contains examples of available systems and is not intended to be all inclusive.
†Roche, Branchburg, NJ.
‡Becton Dickinson, Cockeysville, MD.
§Gen-Probe, Inc., San Diego, CA.
¶Abbott, Chicago, IL.

7

format, and results of initial evaluations appear promising. Serology allows detection of previous HCV infection but does not permit differentiation between current infection and patients who have spontaneously cleared the virus. Detection of the virus and quantification have implications for prognosis and management.

A variety of amplification procedures for detection of HIV have also been described (Chevrett, 1994; Nyambi, 1994; van Kerkhoven, 1994). The nature of the pathogen is somewhat different, and this influences the technology and potential role of PCR for diagnosis. Human immunodeficiency virus (HIV) exists in blood predominantly as proviral DNA incorporated in the genome of peripheral blood mononuclear cells. Reverse transcriptase is therefore not needed unless one wishes specifically to amplify free virus. In relation to the role of PCR, the two major subtypes of HIV are identifiable by serology, and because spontaneous clearance of HIV is not anticipated, serologic evidence of exposure may be taken as evidence of current infection. An exception is the diagnosis of HIV infection in the newborn. In this circumstance, interpretation of serology is complicated by the presence of maternal antibody, and a prolonged period of follow-up (up to 18 months) is needed to confirm infection. PCR may also have a useful role in resolving the status of patients whose serum is repeatedly indeterminate on immunoblot assay.

PCR has also been studied extensively for diagnosis of cytomegalovirus (CMV) infection in transplant recipients (Gerna, 1994; Souza, 1994). The problems of diagnosis of CMV disease differ in that the virus is ubiquitous, and therefore its detection in blood by any method does not per se confirm active disease. A variety of specimens, including urine, respiratory specimens, buffy coat, and plasma, have been studied in an attempt to define at an early stage those patients who have active disease or who are very likely to develop active disease in the absence of treatment. A commercial kit for detection of CMV by PCR is not yet available.

A classic approach to clarifying the significance of the presence of a pathogen or potential pathogen is to attempt to determine the quantity of the agent present. In the case of CMV, for example, an increasing burden of virus over time suggests that active disease is incipient or present (Gerna, 1994). In the case of hepatitis C virus (HCV), reduction of HCV in the peripheral blood is useful in evaluating the response to interferon. In both cases, the issue has been addressed by quantitative PCR. In quantitative PCR, a known quantity of an altered PCR target, or a series of known concentrations of altered target are added to PCR reactions containing wild-type target DNA from a patient specimen. The relative quantities of amplicon generated from the wild type, and altered target or internal standard, reflect the relative quantities at the outset of amplification, and this permits a degree of quantitation. The amplicon detection system must permit differentiation between the amplicons originating from wild type and the altered sequence or internal standard. In the commercial HCV kit, this may be accomplished by use of paired microtitre wells containing either a wild-type specific probe or a modified target-specific probe.

PCR has been studied for diagnosis of a variety of other viral infections, including enterovirus (Kamerer, 1994), herpes simplex virus (Kessler, 1994), and parvovirus (McOmish, 1993b). It is likely that PCR will make considerable progress in this area, particularly if the number of viral infections amenable to specific antiviral agents continues to increase.

Detection of Bacterial Pathogens

In the past five years a multiplicity of PCR assays for detection of *M. tuberculosis* in sputum, bronchoalveolar lavage fluid, cerebrospinal fluid, blood, and tissue have been described (Brisson-Noel, 1991; Shawar, 1994). The methods for preparation of nucleic acid for amplification are equally varied, and there are considerable interlaboratory variations in the reported effectiveness of a number of these methods. The problems associated with lack of standardization are best illustrated by the work of Nordhoek et al. (1994), documenting very great variations in the ability of laboratories to detect *M. tuberculosis* in blinded specimens and to report negative specimens correctly. It is possible that the problems of poor standardization may be improved by the introduction of commercial assays with central control of reagent quality and standard operating procedures.

A commercial PCR-based assay for tuberculosis developed by Roche has a reported sensitivity of greater than 90% for smear-positive specimens and of 87% for smear-negative, culture-positive specimens (Metchock, 1994). Gen-Probe has developed an isothermal transcription-dependent amplification assay that amplifies *M. tuberculosis* ribosomal RNA. The amplified RNA is detected by solution hybridization with an acridinium ester–labeled DNA probe (Jonas, 1993). A direct comparison between the Gen-Probe assay and a nonproprietary PCR assay reported that the methods were equally sensitive and specific (Abe, 1993). A strand-displacement amplification–based assay is also under development as a diagnostic kit. Preliminary results indicate a limit of detection comparable with PCR (Terrance-Walker, 1994; Zwadyk, 1994).

The need for rapid and specific diagnosis of *M. tuberculosis* infection is increased by the current problems of increased incidence and increasing antimicrobial resistance. Because of increased resistance, rapid recognition of resistance determinants is important. A PCR assay that amplifies a segment of the beta subunit of the RNA polymerase (rpoB) gene of *M. tuberculosis*, in which mutations associated with resistance commonly occur, has been developed. The rpoB fragment is studied by single-stranded conformational polymorphism (Telenti, 1993a) or by sequence determination for mutations conferring resistance. Culture remains essential for detailed determination of resistance phenotypes and epidemiologic studies at this time.

A PCR kit for detection of *Legionella* in environmental specimens has also been developed, and initial results obtained by applying this system to bronchoalveolar samples have shown promising results (Kessler, 1993). Among other difficult to culture respiratory pathogens, PCR has been applied to detection of *Bordetella pertussis* (Backman, 1994) and *Chlamydia pneumoniae* (Maass, 1994), but commercial systems for detection of these pathogens have not as yet been produced.

A PCR kit for detection of *Chlamydia trachomatis* by PCR has been developed (Roche, Amplicor PCR). It has been reported as 100% specific and more sensitive than cell culture or direct fluorescent antibody testing (Mahony, 1994b). Using a nonproprietary PCR assay for *C. trachomatis*, good interlaboratory agreement was achieved with standardization of reagents and protocols (Mahony, 1994a). A ligase chain reaction (LCR) for detection of *C. trachomatis* has been developed by Abbott Laboratories. In a multicenter study of endocervical swabs, LCR was reported as more sensitive than culture (94% versus 65%) and gave rise to less variation between centers (Schachter, 1994). LCR may also be applied to first void urine samples (Chernesky, 1994). The LCR amplicons are detected by capture of the hapten-labeled product onto antibody-coated microparticles. The detection system is automated. LCR has also been applied to detection of *Neisseria gonorrhoeae* in urogenital specimens. A sensitivity of 100% and a specificity of 97.8% were reported (Birkenmeyer, 1992).

PCR has also proved useful in research reports in the detection and identification of previously unrecognized or nonculturable pathogens (Wilson, 1994). Primers that amplify the genes encoding for ribosomal RNA for most species of bacteria have been described (Greisen, 1994). Sequencing of the DNA product and comparison of the sequence data with sequences in the DNA database may permit identification or phylogenetic characterization of the organism. This process has been utilized to identify new species such as *Mycobacterium genavense*, among others (Bottger, 1992).

Detection of Fungi

Invasive fungal infection is an increasing problem in many countries (Pfaller, 1994). *Candida* spp. are among the leading causes of nosocomial bloodstream infection in the United States, and aspergillosis is a significant cause of mortality in transplant recipients and other immunocompromised patients. Systemic fungal infection is difficult to diagnose in a timely fashion, and this may contribute to the high mortality. PCR has been studied for possible use in diagnosis of candidemia (Holmes, 1994) and for detection of *Aspergillus* (Melchers, 1994). PCR for diagnosis of *Aspergillus* may be complicated by the occurrence of positives in patients colonized but not infected. Early studies on application of PCR to detection of *Candida* in blood suggest a limit of detection of 15 ± 5 colony-forming units (CFU) of *Candida albicans* per milliliter (ml) of blood (Holmes, 1994).

Detection of Parasites

PCR is also being investigated for detection of infection with protozoa and other parasites. It has been used for diagnosis of cerebral toxoplasmosis, with favorable results reported (Hitt, 1992). It has also been applied to diagnosis of *Onchocerca volvulus* infection (Zimmerman, 1994) and may be more sensitive than conventional examination of skin snips. PCR is also useful for rapid detection of *Leishmania donovani*, trypanosomes, and *Babesia* spp.

Identification of Cultures

The sensitivity of PCR facilitates its application to direct detection of pathogen-specific genomes in clinical material. Because of the specificity of target amplification that can be achieved, PCR has also been applied to identification of cultures. PCR for identification of cultures is most applicable to microorganisms that are difficult to identify in a timely fashion by conventional techniques, such as mycobacteria, and certain viruses. It is logical and convenient for a laboratory using PCR for direct diagnosis to use the same technology for culture identification.

PCR has been applied to identification of mycobacteria. One approach is the use of *M. tuberculosis*–specific primers so that the amplification differentiates between the *M. tuberculosis* complex and the mycobacteria other than tuberculosis (MOTT) (Cormican, 1992; Forbes and Hicks, 1994). A number of authors have described amplification of a target from all members of the genus *Mycobacteria* and then generation of species-specific patterns by digestion of the amplicon with restriction endonucleases (Plikaytis, 1992; Telenti, 1993b). More recently, multiplex PCR has been reported as permitting differentiation between the *M. tuberculosis* complex, *M. avium*, and other mycobacteria in a single PCR reaction (Cormican, 1995; Kulski, 1995). PCR has also been applied to rapid identification of *S. aureus* in positive blood cultures using the thermostable nuclease genes (Brakstad, 1992) as targets of amplification. A related application of PCR to culture is the detection of genes encoding virulence factors or toxins, e.g., heat-labile toxin in *E. coli* (Victor, 1991) or antimicrobial-resistance genes such as the *mec* gene of *S. aureus* (Geha, 1994; Ubukata, 1992). PCR may also be applied to the detection of genes encoding for beta lactamase production directly in clinical specimens (Tenover, 1994). The detection of antimicrobial resistance genes by PCR has recently been reviewed (Tenover, 1993).

Molecular Epidemiology

The variety of molecular epidemiologic tools available at present is considerable (Table 60–4), and an exhaustive consideration of their relative merits is beyond the scope of this chapter. It is important to emphasize that no one technique is universally applicable and that choice for a particular application is related to the species studied, the scope of the question posed, and the convenience of the technique. The techniques of molecular epidemiology are useful in answering real clinical and infection control questions, and are not limited to research uses. Examples include clarifying the significance of multiple isolates of *Staphylococcus epidermidis* from a particular patient. Molecular evidence of identity between isolates made at different times suggest that the isolate is clinically significant. Molecular techniques are also helpful in detecting the emergence and spread of strains of an organism with unusual drug resistance patterns or pathogenicity and in determining the efficacy of infection control procedures.

DNA-Dependent Molecular Typing Methods

Standard restriction fragment length polymorphism (RFLP) with frequent cutting enzymes has been useful in typing of a great variety of organisms. Bingen et al. (1991) used RFLP to demonstrate that the vancomycin-resistant *Enterococcus faecium* isolates from a French hospital did not represent spread of a single resistant strain. The RFLP pattern of each isolate was distinct. Pignatari et al. (1990) used *Eco*RI digestion of *Staphylococcus aureus* isolates from patients who developed peritonitis as a complication of chronic ambulatory peritoneal dialysis (CAPD) to demonstrate the importance of endogenous sources of infection in this group.

Table 60–4. METHODS FOR MOLECULAR EPIDEMIOLOGY

Method	Examples	Comment
Restriction fragment length polymorphism		
Frequent cutting enzymes	*Enterococcus faecium* *Staphylococcus aureus* *Clostridium difficile*	Large number of bands Sometimes difficult to interpret
Infrequent cutting enzymes	*Staphylococcus aureus* *Stenotrophomonas maltophilia* *Candida albicans*	Fewer bands Pulsed field electrophoresis
Ribotyping	*Enterobacter cloacae* *Serratia marcesens*	Fewer bands Soon automated
Repetitive element probe hybridization	*Mycobacterium tuberculosis* *Candida albicans*	Fewer bands Specific sequence-based profiles
Random amplification of polymorphic DNA	*Enterobacter cloacae* *Acinetobacter baumannii* *Mycobacterium tuberculosis*	Small amounts of DNA Relatively crude extract may suffice
Single-stranded conformational polymorphism	Hepatitis B virus	Allows detection of minor sequence changes in a specific area
Polyacrylamide gel protein electrophoresis	*Clostridium difficile* *Staphylococcus aureus*	
Multilocus enzyme electrophoresis	*Neisseria meningitidis* *Entamoeba histolytica*	Useful for defining broad relationships within a species

*The table contains examples of available methods and applications, and is not intended to be all inclusive.

RFLP analysis with frequent cutting enzymes may generate a very large number of bands on gel electrophoresis, which may make comparison between strains difficult. One solution to this difficulty is to identify those bands that contain a specific sequence that occurs in multiple copies in the genome. The most generally applicable multicopy sequence is the ribosomal RNA gene. Ribotyping has been used to study relationships among strains of many species, and comparative studies of the value of ribotyping relative to traditional typing methods have been reported for some species. For *Enterobacter cloacae*, for example, ribotyping is superior to serotyping, phage typing, or biotyping (Garaizar, 1991). Ribotyping is also superior to biotyping for *Serratia marcescens* (Bingen, 1992).

Probes that hybridize to the other repetitive sequences are used in a similar fashion. Among the best studied of these applications is the use of a probe to IS6110 to type *M. tuberculosis*. This methodology is well standardized and, given the inadequacy of phenotypic typing methods, may be regarded as the standard method for typing *M. tuberculosis* (VanEmbden, 1993).

Recently, RFLP with frequent cutting enzymes appears to have given way to RFLP analysis using infrequent cutting enzymes and fragment separation by pulsed-field gel electrophoresis (PFGE) (Allardet-Servent, 1989). For eukaryotic organisms (e.g., fungi), PFGE permits separation of entire chromosomes so that a karyotype may be generated without restriction enzyme digestion. PFGE has proved useful in studies of methicillin-resistant *Staphylococcus aureus* (Angeles-Dominguez, 1994), vancomycin-resistant *Enterococcus faecium* (Sader, 1994b), and a variety of gram-negative pathogens, including *Stenotrophomonas maltophilia* (Sader, 1994a). It has also proved particularly useful in typing of *Candida* species for which karyotyping or RFLP analysis may be used, depending on the species (Doebbeling, 1991).

DNA amplification by PCR lends itself to molecular typing in a variety of ways. Random amplified polymorphism of DNA (RAPD) is useful for fingerprinting many species. One advantage is the small quantity of DNA required to generate a fingerprint. The template DNA may be quite a crude preparation, which is generally not the case with restriction enzyme digest systems. The method has been applied to a great variety of species, including *Enterobacter cloacae* (Ni Riain, 1994), *M. tuberculosis* (Linton, 1994), and the technique, or minor variations of it, have been labeled with a variety of acronyms. Typing based on PCR primers to repetitive elements has also been studied (e.g., for *Acinetobacter baumannii*) (Reboli, 1994). Mixed linker PCR is among the more elegant applications of PCR to typing. It permits generation of patterns that correspond to those achieved by restriction fragment analysis and hybridization with a repetitive probe sequence from very small quantities of template DNA. It has been applied successfully to typing *M. tuberculosis* (Ross, 1993).

PCR amplicons have also been used as a highly discriminatory tool for typing of hepatitis B virus using single-stranded conformational polymorphism (SSCP). The technique has been used to elucidate patterns of HBV virus transmission (Yusof, 1994). SSCP is also useful in early recognition of mutations likely to be associated with drug resistance. SSCP analysis of the rpoB gene of *M. tuberculosis* is perhaps the most rapid method available for screening for multiple drug-resistant isolates (Telenti, 1993a).

Plasmid profiles are much less widely used for molecular typing now than formerly. Plasmid profiles have proved useful in typing methicillin-resistant *Staphylococcus aureus* (Zuccarelli, 1990). Plasmid profiles were reported as more reliable than MLEE or RFLP in typing *Salmonella-*

typhimurium (Kapperud, 1989). Plasmid profiles are also used epidemiologically to detect antimicrobial-resistant plasmids or virulence plasmids, such as those found in *Yersinia pseudotuberculosis*.

Sequence determination of amplified products is an additional approach to typing. Amplification of and sequencing of the HCV genome or parts of the genome have resulted in the recognition of six genotypes. The infecting genotype may have prognostic significance and influence the potential to respond to alpha-interferon treatment (Murphy, 1994).

Non-DNA-Dependent Molecular Typing Methods

Several non-nucleic acid-based typing methods have been applied to epidemiologic studies. Although largely supplanted by DNA-based methods, both polyacrylamide gel electrophoresis (PAGE) of proteins and multilocus enzyme electrophoresis (MLEE) remain useful typing methods. Polyacrylamide gel electrophoresis of proteins has been applied to many bacteria, including *Clostridium difficile* (Mulligan, 1988). The discriminatory power of the technique can be increased by transferring the separated proteins onto a membrane and staining with antisera (immunoblotting). Immunoblotting has been reported as more valuable than plasmid profiles for *C. difficile*.

Multi-locus enzyme electrophoresis (MLEE) is a useful tool for molecular epidemiology of a variety of organisms. It has proved useful in defining the population structure of pathogens and has been used to study the spread of a particular clone. Ribotyping may be more discriminatory than MLEE for *Neisseria meningitidis* (Woods, 1992) and has proved useful for *Cryptococcus neoformans* (Brandt, 1993). MLEE may be more suited for the study of relationships within a population over place and time than to the study of defined outbreaks. It is possible, for example, in the case of *Entamoeba histolytica* to define specific isoenzyme types associated with virulence (Sargeaunt, 1978).

STANDARDIZATION, QUALITY CONTROL, AND PROFICIENCY TESTING OF MOLECULAR DIAGNOSTIC METHODS

As for all diagnostic pathology, the quality of results begins with the validity of the test request and the quality of the specimen collection and transport. The laboratory must provide clinicians with guidelines as to what types of specimens may be submitted, how they should be collected and stored, and the time frame within which delivery to the laboratory is necessary (see Chaps. 1 and 54).

In the laboratory the first step in quality testing is adequate validation of a test before it is introduced into diagnostic use, and when in use continuing attention to procedures that maintain quality standards. The inadequacy of current practices are highlighted by poor interlaboratory agreement on testing blinded specimens for *M. tuberculosis* and for HCV by PCR (Nordhoek, 1994; Zaaijer, 1993). The potential to improve interlaboratory agreement by standardization of reagents and protocols is emphasized by a report of much more satisfactory performance of a PCR assay for *Chlamydia trachomatis*, with attention to these factors (Mahony, 1994a).

Sample preparation is a critical issue in which a balance is sought between simplicity of preparation (for practicality and to reduce risks of contamination) and thoroughness (to ensure the release of nucleic acids and removal of inhibitory substances). Controls must be in place to determine if contamination has occurred (e.g., duplicate testing, multiple negative controls) and to monitor for degradation of target or, the presence of inhibitors (positive control at the limits of detection, internal standard for amplification). It is essential that negative controls be adequate in number and processed through the specimen preparation procedure. A portion of a previously negative specimen is ideal.

To ensure that reagents are of high quality and free of contamination, it is convenient to purchase buffers prepared at a remote location. In this case, the manufacturer is responsible for providing data on the analytical quality of the reagents. An assessment of functional quality relative to previous lots may be adequate. Contamination is a considerable problem for laboratories using diagnostic PCR. Interlaboratory studies have shown that negative samples may give positive results in some laboratories, and carryover of amplicons is the most likely explanation. Clearly the consequences for patient care of a false-positive report for HCV, HIV, or *Mycobacterium tuberculosis* are substantial. The foundation of carryover prevention in most laboratories at this point is physical separation of PCR reaction setup and PCR product analysis areas with a strict unidirectional work flow. Automation of PCR may also aid in prevention of amplicon carryover (Wilke, 1995).

In addition to prevention of carryover, methods to prevent amplification of contaminating PCR products are available. The two principal methods are those using isopsoralen to modify amplicons to a nonamplifiable state and uracil DNA glycosylase to degrade amplicons before amplification (Rhys, 1993). Whichever system is used, the impact of the technique on the limit of PCR detection should be determined. It is also important to demonstrate the effectiveness of the measure given the cost added to the procedure.

Functional checks on each new lot of enzyme is an appropriate check on the production and delivery procedure. For DNA polymerase, comparison with a previous lot of enzyme using specimens at the limit of detection may be appropriate. For restriction endonucleases, digestion of lamba phage DNA is recommended.

The reproducibility of results in many molecular techniques is critically dependent on precise control of temperature and accurate reagent dispensing. The first essential of quality assurance is the acquisition of a high quality instrument. Twice yearly or more frequent monitoring of temperature and performance of each well is recommended (Koop, 1994). Pipettes should be calibrated twice yearly.

Quality laboratory service does not end with the generation of a result. Timely reporting is an essential element. Guidelines on the interpretation of the result are particularly important in relation to novel methods, because clinicians may not be familiar with the limitations of these methods.

Quality assurance in molecular diagnostics is not fundamentally different from the principles applied in other areas of clinical pathology. Attention to detail, adequate controls, and an awareness of potential problems, together with careful record keeping, are the essentials.

Abe C, Hirano K, Wada M, et al: Detection of *Mycobacterium tuberculosis* in clinical specimens by polymerase chain reaction and Gen-Probe amplified *Mycobacterium tuberculosis* direct test. J Clin Microbiol 1993; 31:3270–3274.

Allardet-Servent A, Bouziges N, Carles-Nurit MJ, et al: Use of low frequency cleavage restriction endonucleases for DNA analysis in epidemiological investigation of nosocomial bacterial infections. J Clin Microbiol 1989; 27:2057–2061.

Amann R, Ludwig W, Schleifer KH: Identification of uncultured bacteria: A challenging task for molecular taxonomists. ASM News 1994; 60:360–365.

Angel S, Maero E, Blanco JC, et al: Early diagnosis of Toxoplasma encephalitis in AIDS patients by dot blot hybridization analysis. J Clin Microbiol 1992; 30:3286–3287.

Angeles Dominguez M, De Lencastre H, Linares J, Tomaz A: Spread and maintenance of a dominant methicillin resistant *Staphylococcus aureus* (MRSA) clone during an outbreak of MRSA disease in a Spanish hospital. J Clin Microbiol 1994; 32:2081–2087.

Backman A, Johansson B, Olcen P: Nested PCR optimized for detection of *Bordetella pertussis* in clinical nasopharyngeal samples. J Clin Microbiol 1994; 32:2544–2548.

Barker RH, Jr, Banchongaksorn T, Courval JM, et al: DNA probes as epidemiological tools for surveillance of *Plasmodium falciparum* malaria in Thailand. Int J Epidemiol 1994; 23:161–168.

Bingen EH, Denamur E, Lambert-Zechovsky NY, Elion J: Evidence for the genetic unrelatedness or nosocomial vancomycin resistant *Enterococcus faecium* strains in a pediatric hospital. J Clin Microbiol 1991; 29:1888–1892.

Bingen EH, Mariani-Kurkdjian P, Lambert-Zechovsky NY, et al: Ribotyping provides efficient differentiation of nosocomial *Serratia marcescens* isolates in a pediatric hospital. J Clin Microbiol 1992; 30:2088–2091.

Birkenmeyer L, Armstrong AS: Preliminary evaluation of the ligase chain reaction for specific detection of *Neisseria gonorrhoeae*. J Clin Microbiol 1992; 30:3089–3094.

Bottger EC, Teske A, Kirschner P, et al: Disseminated *Mycobacterium genavense* infection in patients with AIDS. Lancet 1992; 340:76–80.

Brakstad OG, Aasbakk K, Maeland JA: Detection of *Staphylococcus aureus* by polymerase chain reaction amplification of the nuc gene. J Clin Microbiol 1992; 30:1654–1660.

Brandt ME, Bragg SL, Pinner RW: Multilocus enzyme typing of *Cryptococcus neoformans*. J Clin Microbiol 1993; 31:2819–2823.

Brisson-Noel A, Aznar C, Chureau C, et al: Diagnosis of tuberculosis by DNA amplification in clinical practice evaluation. Lancet 1991; 338:364–366.

Butler WR, O'Connor SP, Yakrus MA, Gross WM: Cross reactivity of genetic probe for detection of *Mycobacterium tuberculosis* with newly described species *Mycobacterium celatum*. J Clin Microbiol 1994; 32:536–538.

Chernesky MA, Jang D, Lee H, et al: Diagnosis of *Chlamydia trachomatis* infections in men and women by testing first-void urine by ligase chain reaction. J Clin Microbiol 1994; 32:2682–2685.

Chevret S, Kirstetter M, Meriotti M, et al: Provirus copy number to predict disease progression in asymptomatic human immunodeficiency virus type 1 infection. J Infect Dis 1994; 169:882–885.

Cormican M, Barry T, Gannon F, Flynn J: Use of polymerase chain reaction for early identification of *Mycobacterium tuberculosis* in positive cultures. J Clin Pathol 1992; 45:601–604.

Cormican M, Glennon M, Ni Riain U, Flynn J: Multiplex PCR for identification of mycobacterial isolates. J Clin Pathol 1995; 48:203–205.

Davis TE, Fuller DD: Direct identification of bacterial isolates in blood cultures by using a DNA probe. J Clin Microbiol 1991; 29:2193–2196.

Doebbeling BN, Hollis RJ, Isenberg HD, et al: Restriction fragment analysis of a *Candida tropicalis* outbreak of sternal wound infections. J Clin Microbiol 1991; 29:1268–1270.

Faulkner-Jones BE, Tabrizi SN, Borg AJ, et al: Detection of human papillomavirus DNA and mRNA using synthetic, type specific oligonucleotide probes. J Virol Methods 1993; 41:277–296.

Forbes BA, Hicks KE: Ability of PCR assay to identify *Mycobacterium tuberculosis* in Bactec 12B vials. J Clin Microbiol 1994; 32:1725–1728.

Ford EG, Snead SJ, Todd J, Warren NG: Strains of *Mycobacterium terrae* complex which react with DNA probes for *Mycobacterium tuberculosis* complex. J Clin Microbiol 1993; 31:2805–2806.

Garaizar J, Kaufmann ME, Pitt TL: Comparison of ribotyping with conventional methods for the type identification of *Enterobacter cloacae*. J Clin Microbiol 1991; 29:1303–1307.

Geha DJ, Uhl JR, Gustafferro CA, Persing DH: Multiplex PCR for identification of methicillin-resistant staphylococci in the clinical laboratory. J Clin Microbiol 1994; 32:1768–1772.

Gerna G, Furione M, Baldanti F, Sarasini A: Comparative quantitation of human cytomegalovirus DNA in blood leukocytes and plasma of transplant and AIDS patients. J Clin Microbiol 1994; 32:2709–2717.

Goto M, Oka S, Okuzumi K, et al: Evaluation of acridinium ester labeled DNA probes for identification of *Mycobacterium tuberculosis* and *Mycobacterium avium–Mycobacterium intracellulare* complex in culture. J Clin Microbiol 1991; 29:2473–2476.

Greisen K, Loeffelholz M, Purohit A, Leong D: PCR primers and probes for the 16SrRNA gene of most species of pathogenic bacteria, including bacteria found in cerebrospinal fluid. J Clin Microbiol 1994; 32:335–351.

Gretch D, Corey L, Wilson J, et al: Assessment of hepatitis C virus levels by quantitative competitive RNA polymerase chain reaction: High titer viremia correlates with advanced stage of disease. J Infect Dis 1994; 169:1219–1225.

Heiter JB, Bourbeau PP: Comparison of the Gen-Probe group A streptococcus direct test with culture and a rapid streptococcal antigen detection assay for diagnosis of streptococcal pharyngitis. J Clin Microbiol 1993; 31:2070–2073.

Hitt JA, Filice GA: Detection of *Toxoplasma gondii* parasitemia by gene amplification, cell culture, and mouse inoculation. J Clin Microbiol 1992; 30:3181–3184.

Holmes AR, Cannon RD, Shepherd MG, Jenkinson HF: Detection of *Candida albicans* and other yeasts in blood by PCR. J Clin Microbiol 1994; 32:228–231.

Jonas V, Alden MJ, Curry JL, et al: Detection and identification of *Mycobacterium tuberculosis* directly from sputum sediments by amplification of rRNA. J Clin Microbiol 1993; 31:2410–2416.

Kammerer U, Kunkel B, Korn K: Nested PCR for specific detection and rapid identification of human picornaviruses. J Clin Microbiol 1994; 32:285–294.

Kapperud G, Lassen J, Dommarsnes K, et al: Comparison of epidemiological marker methods for identification of *Salmonella typhimurium* isolates from an outbreak caused by contaminated chocolate. J Clin Microbiol 1989; 27(9):2019–2024.

Kessler HH, Pierer K, Weber B, et al: Detection of Herpes simplex virus DNA from cerebrospinal fluid by PCR and a rapid, nonradioactive hybridization technique. J Clin Microbiol 1994; 32:1881–1886.

Kessler HH, Reinthaler FF, Pschaid A, et al: Rapid detection of *Legionella* species in bronchoalveolar lavage fluids with the EnviroAmp Legionella PCR amplification and detection kit. J Clin Microbiol 1993; 31: 3325–3328.

Klutymans JAJW, Goessens WHF, van Rijsoort Vos JH, et al: Improved performance of PACE 2 with modified collection system in combination with probe competition assay of *Chlamydia trachomatis* in urethral specimens from males. J Clin Microbiol 1994; 32:568–570.

Kluytmans JAJW, Niesters HGM, Mouton JW, et al: Performance of a nonisotopic DNA probe for detection of *Chlamydia trachomatis* in urogenital specimens. J Clin Microbiol 1991; 29:2685–2689.

Koop DW, Sansieri CA, Mifflin TE: Routine monitoring of temperatures inside thermal cycler blocks for quality control. Clin Chem 1994; 40:2117–2119.

Kulski J, Khinsoe C, Payle T, Christiansen K: Use of a multiplex PCR to detect and identify *Mycobacterium avium* and *M. intracellulare* in blood culture fluids in AIDS patients. J Clin Microbiol 1995; 33:668–674.

LeBar W, Herschman B, Jemal C, Pierzchala J: Comparison of DNA probe, monoclonal antibody enzyme immunoassay, and cell culture for the detection of *Chlamydia trachomatis*. J Clin Microbiol 1989; 27:826–828.

Lewis JS, Fakile O, Foss E, et al: Direct DNA probe assay for *Neisseria gonorrhoeae* in pharyngeal and rectal specimens. J Clin Microbiol 1993; 31:2783–2785.

Linton CJ, Jalal H, Leeming JP, Millar MR: Rapid discrimination of *Mycobacterium tuberculosis* strains by random amplified polymorphic DNA analysis. J Clin Microbiol 1994; 32:2169–2174.

Loesche WJ, Lopatin DE, Giordano J, et al: Comparison of the benzoyl-DL-arginine-napthylamide (BANA) test, DNA probes, and immunological reagents for ability to detect anaerobic periodontal infections due to *Porphyromonas gingivalis*, *Treponema denticola* and *Bacteroides forsythus*. J Clin Microbiol 1992; 30:427–433.

Lorinez AT: Diagnosis of human papillomavirus infection by the new generation of molecular DNA assays. Clin Immunol Newslett 1992; 12:8.

Maass M, Dalhoff K: Comparison of sample preparation methods for detection of *Chlamydia pneumoniae* in bronchoalveolar lavage fluid by PCR. J Clin Microbiol 1994; 32:2616–2619.

Mahony JB, Luinstra KE, Sellors JW, et al: Role of confirmatory PCR in determining performance of *Chlamydia* Amplicor PCR with endocervical specimens from women with a low prevalence of infection. J Clin Microbiol 1994b; 32:2490–2493.

Mahony JB, Luinstra KE, Waner J, et al: Interlaboratory agreement study of a double set of PCR plasmid primers for detection of *Chlamydia trachomatis* in a variety of genitourinary specimens. J Clin Microbiol 1994a; 32:87–91.

Manzin A, Bagnarelli P, Menzvos, et al: Quantitation of hepatitis C virus genome molecules in plasma samples. J Clin Microbiol 1994; 32:1939–1944.

McOmish F, Yap PL, Jordan A, et al: Detection of parvovirus B19 in donated blood: A model system for screening by polymerase chain reaction. J Clin Microbiol 1993; 31:323–328.

Melchers WJG, Verweij PE, van den Hurk P, et al: General primer-mediated PCR for detection of *Aspergillus* species. J Clin Microbiol 1994; 32:1710–1717.

Metchock B, Diem L: Clinical laboratory evaluation of Roche Amplicor™ *Mycobacterium tuberculosis* assay. 34th Interscience Conference on Antimicrobial Agents in Chemotherapy, October 4–7, 1994, Orlando, FL.

Mulligan ME, Peterson LE, Kwok RYY, et al: Immunoblots and plasmid fingerprints compared with serotyping and polyacrylamide gel electrophoresis for typing *Clostridium difficile*. J Clin Microbiol 1988; 26:41–46.

Murphy D, Willems B, Delage G: Use of the 5′ non coding region for genotyping hepatitis c virus. J Infect Dis 1994; 169:473–475.

Ni Riain U, Cormican M, Flynn J, et al: PCR based fingerprinting of *Enterobacter cloacae*. J Hospital Infect 1994; 27:237–240.

Nordhoek GT, Kolk AHJ, Bjune G, et al: Sensitivity and specificity of PCR for detection of *Mycobacterium tuberculosis*: A blind comparison study among seven laboratories. J Clin Microbiol 1994; 32:277–284.

Nyambi PN, Fransen K, De Beenhouwer H, et al: Detection of human immunodeficiency virus type 1 (HIV 1) in heel prick blood from children born to HIV-1 seropositive mothers. J Clin Microbiol 1994; 32: 2858–2860.

Pao CC, Lin SS, Wu SY, et al: The detection of mycobacterial DNA sequences in uncultured clinical specimens with cloned *Mycobacterium tuberculosis* DNA as probes. Tubercle 1988; 69(1):27–36.

Pfaller MA: Epidemiology and control of fungal infections. Clin Infect Dis 1994; 19(Suppl 1):S843.

Pignatari A, Pfaller M, Hollis R, et al: *Staphylococcus aureus* colonization and infection in patients on continuous ambulatory peritoneal dialysis. J Clin Microbiol 1990; 28:1898–1902.

Plikaytis BB, Plikaytis BD, Yakrus MA, et al: Differentiation of slowly growing *Mycobacterium* species including *Mycobacterium tuberculosis* by gene amplification and restriction fragment length polymorphism analysis. J Clin Microbiol 1992; 30:1815–1822.

Reboli AC, Houston ED, Monteforte JS, et al: Discrimination of epidemic and sporadic isolates of *Acinetobacter baumannii* by repetitive element PCR mediated DNA fingerprinting. J Clin Microbiol 1994; 32: 2635–2640.

Rhys PN, Persing DH: Preventing false positives: Quantitative evaluation of three protocols for inactivation of polymerase chain reaction amplification products. J Clin Microbiol 1993; 31:2356–2360.

Ross BC, Dwyer B: Rapid simple method for typing isolates of *Mycobacterium tuberculosis* by using the polymerase chain reaction. J Clin Microbiol 1993; 31:329–334.

Rotbart HA, Sawyer MH, Fast S, et al: Diagnosis of enteroviral meningitis by using PCR with a colorimetric microwell detection assay. J Clin Microbiol 1994; 32:2590–2592.

Sader HS, Pfaller MA, Tenover FC, et al: Evaluation and characterization of multiresistant *Enterococcus faecium*. J Clin Microbiol 1994b; 32:2840–2842.

Sader H, Pignatari AC, Frei R, et al: Pulsed field gel electrophoresis of restriction-digested genomic DNA and antimicrobial susceptibility of *Xanthomonas maltophilia* strains from Brazil, Switzerland, and the USA. J Antimicrob Chemother 1994a; 33:615–618.

Sargeaunt PG, Williams JE, Ersne JD: The differentiation of invasive and non-invasive *Entamoeba histolytica* by isoenzyme electrophoresis. Trans R Soc Trop Med Hyg 1978; 72:519–521.

Schachter J, Stamm WE, Quinn TC, et al: Ligase chain reaction to detect *Chlamydia trachomatis* infection of the cervix. J Clin Microbiol 1994; 32:2540–2543.

Shah JS, Liu J, Smith J, et al: Novel ultrasensitive, Q-beta replicase amplified hybridization assay for detection of *Chlamydia trachomatis*. J Clin Microbiol 1994; 32:2718–2724.

Shawar RM, El Zaatari FAK, Nataraj A, Clarridge JE: Detection of *Mycobacterium tuberculosis* in clinical samples by two step polymerase chain reaction and nonisotopic hybridisation methods. J Clin Microbiol 1993; 31:61–65.

Souza IE, Nicholson D, Matthey S, et al: Detection of human cytomegalovirus in peripheral blood leukocytes by the polymerase chain reaction and a non-radioactive probe. Diagn Microbiol Infect Dis 1994; 20:13–19.

Steed LL, Korgenski EK, Daly JA: Rapid detection of *Streptococcus pyogenes* in pediatric patient specimens by DNA probe. J Clin Microbiol 1993; 31:2996–3000.

Stockman L, Clark KA, Hunt JM, Roberts GD: Evaluation of commercially available acridinium ester-labeled chemiluminescent DNA probes for culture identification of *Blastomyces dermatitidis*, *Coccidioides immitis*, *Cryptococcus neoformans* and *Histoplasma capsulatum*. J Clin Microbiol 1993; 31:845–850.

Telenti A, Imboden P, Marchesi F, et al: Detection of rifampicin resistant mutations in *Mycobacterium tuberculosis*. Lancet 1993a; 341:647–650.

Telenti A, Marchesi F, Balz M, et al: Rapid identification of mycobacteria to the species level by polymerase chain reaction and restriction enzyme analysis. J Clin Microbiol 1993b; 31:175–178.

Tenover FC, Bo Huang M, Rasheed JK, Persing DH: Development of PCR assays to detect ampicillin resistance genes in cerebrospinal fluid samples containing *Haemophilus influenzae*. J Clin Microbiol 1994; 32:2729–2737.

Tenover FC, Popovic T, Olsvik O: Using molecular methods to detect antimicrobiol resistance genes. Clin Microbiol Newslett 1993; 15: 177–181.

Terannce-Walker G, Nadeau JG, Spears PA, et al: Multiplex strand displacement amplification (SDA) and detection of DNA sequences from *Mycobacterium tuberculosis* and other mycobacteria. Nucleic Acids Res 1994; 22:2670–2677.

Tortoli E, Simonetti MT, Lacchini C, et al: Tentative evidence of AIDS associated biotype of *Mycobacterium kansasii*. J Clin Microbiol 1994; 32:1779–1782.

Ubukata K, Nakagami S, Nitta A, et al: Rapid detection of the MecA gene in methicillin resistant staphylococci by enzymatic detection of polymerase chain reaction products. J Clin Microbiol 1992; 30:1728–1733.

Urdea MS, Horn T, Fultz T, et al: Branched DNA amplification multimers for the sensitive, direct detection of human hepatitis viruses. Nucleic Acids Res Symp Series 1992; 24:197–200.

van Embden JDA, Cave MD, Crawford JT, et al: Strain identification of *Mycobacterium tuberculosis* by DNA fingerprinting: Recommendations for a standardized methodology. J Clin Microbiol 1993; 31:406–409.

Van Kerckhoven I, Fransen K, Peeters M, et al: Quantification of human immunodeficiency virus in plasma by RNA PCR, viral culture, and p24 antigen detection. J Clin Microbiol 1994; 32:1669–1673.

Victor T, DuToit R, van Zyl J, et al: Improved method for the routine identification of toxigenic *Escherichia coli* by DNA amplification of a conserved region of the heat-labile toxin A subunit. J Clin Microbiol 1991; 29:158–161.

Vlaspolder F, Mutsaers JAEM, Blog F, Notowicz A: Value of a DNA probe assay (Gen-Probe) compared with that of culture for diagnosis of gonococcal infection. J Clin Microbiol 1993; 31:107–110.

Walton DT, Valesco M: Identification of *Mycobacterium gordonae* from culture by the Gen-Probe rapid diagnostic system: Evaluation of 218 isolates and potential sources of false negative results. J Clin Microbiol 1991; 29:1850–1854.

Wilke WW, Sutton LD, Jones RN: Automation of polymerase chain reaction (PCR) tests as a mechanism to achieve acceptable contamination rates. Clin Chem 1995; 41:622–623.

Wilson KH: Detection of culture-resistant bacterial pathogens by amplification and sequencing of ribosomal DNA. Clin Infect Dis 1994; 18: 958–962.

Woods GI, Young A, Scott JC Jr, et al: Evaluation of a non-isotopic probe for detection of *Chlamydia trachomatis* in endocervical specimens. J Clin Microbiol 1990; 28:370–372.

Woods JP, Kersulyte D, Tolan RW Jr, et al: Use of arbitrarily primed polymerase chain reaction analysis to type disease and carrier strains of *Neisseria meningitidis* isolated during a university outbreak. J Infect Dis 1994; 169:1384–1389.

Woods TC, Helsel LO, Swaminathan B, et al: Characterization of *Neisseria meningitidis* serogroup c by multilocus enzyme electrophoresis and ribosomal DNA restriction profiles (ribotyping). J Clin Microbiol 1992; 30:132–137.

Young H, Moyes A: Comparative evaluation of Accuprobe culture identification test for *Neisseria gonorrhoeae* and other rapid methods. J Clin Microbiol 1993a; 31:1996–1999.

Young KKY, Resnick RM, Myers TW: Detection of hepatitis C virus RNA by a combined reverse transcription-polymerase chain reaction assay. J Clin Microbiol 1993b; 31:882–886.

Yusof JHM, Flower AJE, Teo CG: Transmission of hepatitis B virus analysed by conformation dependent polymorphisms of single stranded viral DNA. J Infect Dis 1994; 169:62–67.

Zaaijer HL, Borg F, Cuypers HTM, et al: Comparison of methods for detection of hepatitis B virus DNA. J Clin Microbiol 1994; 2088–2091.

Zaaijer HL, Cuypers HTM, Reesink HW, et al: Reliability of polymerase chain reaction for detection of hepatitis C virus. Lancet 1993; 341:722–724.

Zimmerman PA, Guderian RH, Aruago E, et al: Polymerase chain reaction based diagnosis of *Onchocerca volvulus* infection: Improved detection of patients with onchocerciasis. J Infect Dis 1994; 169:686–689.

Zuccarelli AJ, Roy I, Harding GP, Couperus JJ: Diversity and stability of restriction enzyme profiles of plasmid DNA from meticillin resistant *Staphylococcus aureus*. J Clin Microbiol 1990; 28:97–102.

Zwadyk P Jr, Down JA, Myers N, Dey MS: Rendering mycobacteria safe for molecular diagnostic studies and development of a lysis method for strand displacement amplification and PCR. J Clin Microbiol 1994; 32:2140–2146.

Chapter 61

Tissue *In Situ* Hybridization

Mark H. Stoler, M.D.

Most techniques in the field of molecular diagnostics are hybridization-based assays directed at the detection of specific DNA or RNA sequences that have been extracted from a cellular sample. Implicit in these analyses are assumptions regarding the cellular composition of the sample. If one is looking for a virus trophic for a specific cell type or an oncogene expressed in a particular type of tumor cell, those cells have to be present in the sample under analysis. Paradoxically, modern diagnostic methods, such as endoscopic biopsy and fine needle aspiration cytology, are forcing pathologists to do more with less. With a limited sample, prioritization of analyses and maximizing yield are important daily considerations. In anatomic pathology, morphologic analysis is usually the highest priority, because morphology provides the fundamental diagnostic context for the interpretation of other clinical and laboratory data. The technique of *in situ* hybridization (ISH) permits the detection of nucleic acid targets within a microanatomic context. Like other powerful nucleic acid–based techniques, it capitalizes on the potentially high specificity and sensitivity inherent in directly probing for DNA/RNA sequences. Unlike other biochemical methods, it preserves morphology, thus permitting accurate localization of signal source. Thus, *in situ* hybridization uniquely facilitates the optimal synthesis of histopathologic and molecular biologic data. This section will review principles of *in situ* hybridization, focusing on technical considerations that are unique to this type of analysis. It will also examine the advantages and disadvantages of ISH relative to other molecular diagnostic methods to facilitate an understanding of this method's place in the rapidly evolving field of molecular pathology.

During the early 1970s the modern era of molecular biology was ushered in with the advent of recombinant DNA technology. The isolation of restriction enzymes that cut DNA at defined sequences, the ability to clone DNA sequences in bacteria, and the development of enzymatic methods for labelling DNA as well as the reverse transcription of RNA into complementary DNA, formed the foundation of all hybridization methods (see Chap. 56). *In situ* hybridization actually predated some of these developments, making it one of the oldest molecular diagnostic techniques. Described in the late 1960s (Gall, 1969; John, 1969; Pardue, 1969), ISH was first used to detect amplified DNA targets in the cell nuclei of cytologic preparations. Shortly thereafter, the method was applied to chromosomes (Pardue, 1970) to study the production of ribosomal RNA. In the same year (Buongiorno-Nardelli, 1970), ISH was applied to histologic sections. The first description of the use of ISH for the study of an infectious agent came from France (Orth, 1971), where this new method was applied to the study of Shope rabbit papillomavirus DNA replication in tissue sections. Epstein-Barr virus (zur Hausen, 1972) and adenoviruses (Dunn, 1973) were also the subject of early ISH studies. It is interesting to note that (for purely technical reasons) many of these early studies used radioactively labelled RNA as a probe, actually presaging modern RNA probe usage.

The first histologic messenger RNA (mRNA) studies (Harrison, 1973) were also described about the same time. During the late 1970s and early 1980s, the ability to design and label improved high specific activity DNA probes (Rigby, 1977) and, more importantly, single-stranded RNA probes (Melton, 1984), heralded further developments. In the United States, Brahic and Hasse (1978) developed more sensitive methods for detecting low copy number viral sequences for the study of latent infections of the CNS. This was quickly followed by the application of quantitative ISH techniques (Angerer, 1981; Cox, 1984) for the detection of messenger RNA in morphologically distinct cell populations. The development of nonradioactive detection systems for ISH (Brigati, 1983; Leary, 1983) heralded a time of easier and more widespread clinical implementation of this technology. More recently, polymerase chain reaction (PCR)-based amplification techniques have been coupled to ISH (Nuovo, 1991a) in an effort to increase method sensitivity. The description of ISH as given here focuses on the detection of nucleic acid targets in the context of anatomic pathology, emphasizing techniques that preserve as much as possible the morphologic cues used in diagnosis. Emphasis is also placed on techniques that target messenger RNA to provide contrast with immunohistochemistry and because of the proven diagnostic utility of studying gene expression. The application of ISH methods to cytogenetics (of which there are many) is the subject of a separate discussion (see Chap. 59).

RELATIONSHIP OF *IN SITU* HYBRIDIZATION TO OTHER MOLECULAR METHODS

All nucleic acid hybridization tests are based on the fact that two antiparallel single-stranded nucleic acid molecules will recognize one another and bind to each other (hybridize) on the basis of hydrogen bonding and the hydrophobic base-stacking interactions of complementary base pairs [(A)denine binds to (T)hymine, or (U)racil if RNA; (G)uanine binds to (C)ytosine]. Thus, DNA:DNA, DNA:RNA, and RNA:RNA duplexes are possible. While a full discussion of the factors affecting hybridization is beyond the scope of this chapter and has been discussed elsewhere (see Chap. 56), repetition of some of these basic principles as applied to ISH is essential to an appreciation of probe and protocol selection for *in situ* studies.

Recall that the interaction between duplex strands of nucleic acid is a temperature-dependent phenomenon. The reference point for this interaction is the hybrid melting temperature (T_m), defined as the temperature at which 50% of the population of duplex molecules dissociate, that is, melt, into single strands. The major factors affecting duplex stability include the ionic strength of the reaction, the mole percentage of G/C base pairs in the probe, the probe length, the percentage of noncomplementary bases between the probe and target (percent mismatch), and the formamide percentage (a duplex destabilizing agent) in the solution. Increasing the ionic strength, probe length, and G/C content increases duplex stability, whereas increasing temperature, formamide percentage, and mismatch percentage decreases duplex stability.

The stringency of a hybridization reaction refers to the degree to which the reaction conditions favor duplex dissociation; that is, high stringency can be attained with high temperature, low salt, or high formamide concentrations, or with combinations of all three. Duplexes formed when the two strands have a high degree of base homology will better withstand a high stringency wash than will duplexes of lesser homology. Most hybridization reactions are carried out at a relatively low stringency of $T_m - 25°C$. This temperature has been empirically determined to produce an optimal rate of hybridization (Angerer, 1987) but does allow for the formation of imperfect, that is, less than perfectly complementary hybrids. Rather than totally controlling specificity with the hybridization step, most ISH procedures use a series of posthybridization washes at higher stringencies to dissociate the imperfect hybrids, leaving only specifically bound probe on the target. Another factor to consider in any hybridization is the type of nucleic acids in the probe and target. For instance, DNA:DNA hybrids are approximately 10° to 15°C less stable than RNA:RNA hybrids, with RNA:DNA hybrids having an intermediate T_m. Thus, in comparing protocols and data, a detailed knowledge of the hybridization conditions may be the only way of comparing data, even on identical probes, as stringency, together with the base homology between probe and target, controls the specificity of the hybridization.

The above-mentioned principles can be applied to a variety of hybridization test formats. The gold standard is the Southern blot, in which DNA from any source is extracted, purified, and cut with restriction enzymes. The restriction fragments are sized on an agarose gel by electrophoresis, and the resulting gel contents are "blotted" onto a supporting matrix. The DNA targets are denatured to create the single strandedness necessary for hybridization and then probed with, usually ^{32}P-labeled, complementary denatured DNA. The nonspecifically bound excess is washed off and the specifically bound probe is detected by autoradiography. Hence, a Southern blot refers to the detection of DNA, usually with probes composed of DNA. Northern blots are, in principle, the same, except the target on the matrix is RNA. Western blots use the same sort of matrix and detection formats, except the targets are protein and the probes are antibodies. Dot, spot, or slot blots eliminate the electrophoretic separation steps. *In situ* hybridization generally refers to the detection of nucleic acids in intact cells or tissues on glass microscope slides.

The ability to localize specific DNA and messenger RNA sequences in histologic preparations has made *in situ* hybridization an extremely valuable research tool that is rapidly becoming applicable for routine clinical diagnosis. Analogous to Southern versus northern blots, ISH assays can be divided into those directed at the detection of DNA versus RNA. When probing for a DNA target, the probe may be directed at host or foreign DNA. Foreign DNA in human systems most often is of microbial, usually of viral, origin. Because all of an organism's cells have essentially the same DNA content, detection of cellular DNA may or may not be of utility in probing for functional differences among cells. Probes for a single point mutation in DNA are unlikely to function *in situ*. Most genes are present in only one to a few copies per chromosome. In some neoplasms gene amplification may occur, and if the number of amplified copies is high enough and sensitive methods are used, direct evidence of amplification may be detectable *in situ*. Many chromosomal abnormalities, such as duplication, deletion, or translocation, may be diagnosable using *in situ* hybridization on either metaphase preparations or by using interphase cytogenetics (Anastasi, 1993; Gray, 1991, 1992). Indeed, *in situ* localization of genes on chromosomes is the method of choice for determining the chromosomal locale of a DNA sequence.

In situ hybridization for messenger RNA complements both DNA *in situ* hybridization and immunocytochemistry. Only immunologic methods and *in situ* hybridization for mRNA allow identification of individual cells expressing specific genes, as opposed to cells merely carrying a gene. While immunologic detection of a protein or hybridization detection of the protein's messenger RNA provides similar information, the time or site of protein synthesis, as well as protein localization, may be different than the time or site of transcription of its messenger RNA (*vida infra*). Many of the limitations inherent in probing cellular DNA alluded to earlier can be overcome by probing for the presence or absence of the corresponding mRNA. For example, in neuroblastoma (Grady-Leopardi, 1986), the *MYC* oncogene is often amplified in tumor cells, but the size of the gene and the number of amplified copies usually makes detection of this prognostically important abnormality undetectable at the DNA level, whereas it is readily apparent when the overtranscribed mRNA is probed for.

RELATIONSHIP OF *IN SITU* HYBRIDIZATION TO IMMUNOHISTOCHEMISTRY

Unlike other biochemical methods, but like immunohistochemistry (IMH), ISH preserves morphology, thus permitting accurate localization of signal source. Should *in situ* hybridization replace immunohistochemistry as the molecular diagnostic of choice in the anatomic pathology laboratory? If one technology replaces another it implies the newer technique enjoys some kind of clear superiority: It may be more sensitive or more specific. It may be equivalent or even of lower sensitivity/specificity, but easier or faster or cheaper. It may provide critical clinical information that other currently available techniques do not. Depending on the questions being asked, *in situ* hybridization may "beat" immunohistochemistry or be "beaten" by it. At the present time, *complement* rather than *replacement* seems a better choice of words.

The arguments for an *in situ* method of nucleic acid detection have in part been made by analogy to immunohistochemistry. If analyzing biochemical information outside of the context of morphology was sufficient, then all such analyses would be done in the clinical chemistry, immunology, and wet molecular biology labs. Surgical pathologists would be ordering strictly Southern blots, northern blots, western blots, or solution immunoassays on specimens. The evolution of the use of estrogen receptor (ER) analyses in breast cancer seems highly relevant. Biochemical assays of ER content on pieces of breast cancer tissue were found to provide useful prognostic or therapeutic information. But there are problems with these assays. Technical issues included having adequate amounts of tissue, handling the tissue such that the ER is preserved, knowing that the tissue is representative of the neoplastic process, and finally, the assay used in many labs is often analytically complex and of poor precision. Despite these hurdles, the data seemed useful, although even that is debatable if the anatomic data are carefully analyzed in a multivariate manner (Ellis, 1992; Elston, 1991; Robertson, 1992).

With the advent of monoclonal antibodies against the ER protein, immunohistochemistry clearly demonstrated the nature of many of the variables. Tissues are clearly heterogeneous in terms of their cellular content as well as their patterns of ER expression, even within morphologically similar cell types. This clear demonstration of cellular heterogeneity in gene expression is forcing re-evaluation of the traditional analytic methods. What is also driving the case for an *in situ* type of analysis is the fact that the nature of biopsy material is changing. Often specimens are inadequate for traditional biochemical analysis. The tumor is too small, may not even be grossly visible, or may be a cytologic preparation. With small samples, it is unacceptable to compromise the diagnosis by ordering a test destructive of the morphology. Alternatively, the tissue may have been out of the patient too long or is inappropriately preserved for traditional analyses of labile molecules. How many negative or low-positive ER results are really erroneous because of sample handling problems? With small samples, often from low-stage tumors when receptor data are not clinically relevant, the clinician may be upset with the lab because the "critical" result is unavailable. *In situ* methods eliminate the "how to divide the tissue" conflict. Single adjacent sections can provide serial molecular analyses and signal localization is assured. The question is then reduced to which *in situ* method is the one of choice.

As noted earlier, only immunohistology for antigens and *in situ* hybridization for mRNA allow identification of individual cells expressing specific genes, as opposed to cells merely carrying a gene. In some cases, small genes or genes of low copy number, even though they may be amplified, are below the sensitivity of DNA detection. In these cases the amplification provided by transcription of the corresponding mRNA often allows localization of the related sequence. While immunologic detection of a protein or hybridization detection of the message encoding a protein provides similar information, the time or site of protein localization may be different than the time or site of transcription of its mRNA. It is not uncommon to have a cell that contains the message for a protein but in which protein is not detectable immunologically. This may reflect differences in technical sensitivity or may have biological significance in, for instance, suggesting translational regulation of protein levels.

How to choose between IMH and ISH? Clearly, immunohistochemistry is a much more familiar and *relatively* standardized methodology in pathology; thus, if an IMH assay for a target of interest is functioning in your lab, don't change. As a guide, when contemplating a choice between ISH and immunohistochemistry, several questions can be addressed: Does an antibody exist for the gene product of interest and, if so, what is its specificity? Does the antibody effectively interact with its target under the available conditions of specimen fixation and processing? Is it relevant to distinguish site of synthesis from site of antigen localization? Is the concentration of antigen sufficient for detection given the sensitivity of the assay? All of these questions factor into the choice between immunologic and hybridization methods. Indeed, much of the IMH and ISH literature of the last few years is centered on newer generation antibodies, technical improvements, antigen retrieval, etc., forcing one to continually re-evaluate previous convictions. Assays that did not work before are now routine. Tumors that were defined by a clear pattern of antigenicity now have many exceptions to the rules. Thus, the opinions of today are subject to evolution as technology progresses. However, several other factors make the use of nucleic acid probes and the *in situ* hybridization approach particularly attractive:

The specificity of the probe for the target is inherent in its base sequence, and many times exon sequences can be used as probes specific for a single mRNA species. In the case of gene families, for example, keratins, cyclins, and many others for which exon-specific probes would be inappropriate because of cross-hybridization, gene-specific probes can be derived from 5′ or 3′ untranslated regions that are less well conserved than those encoding the protein. Furthermore, nucleic acid probes can often be used as probes for proteins that are highly conserved, nonimmunogenic, or that have antigenic sites that are hidden or that do not survive tissue processing.

ISH methods work well in formalin-fixed and paraffin-embedded tissue (Angerer, 1987, 1991; Stoler, 1990), that is, the substrate of surgical pathology. This eliminates some of the morphologic artifacts that may be attendant in frozen material. Of course, because nucleic acids are labile molecules, rapid fixation is important and the choice of fixative is critical (Nuovo, 1989). One should be cognizant that single-stranded messenger RNA is much more labile than double-stranded DNA, and both are subject to degradation over time from autolysis. The advantage of using properly fixed and processed paraffin-embedded tissues for retrospective analysis of already well-characterized archival tissue collections cannot be overstated and should influence our modern-day tissue procurement practices. Despite this relative liability of nucleic acid targets as compared with proteins, there is a margin of error in time to tissue fixation that favors the *in situ* technique, particularly if the target is moderately abundant. Even if there is some degradation of mRNA in the cell prior to fixation, as long as the resultant fragments are of sufficient size (say, >50 bases) and are retained in the tissue, a specific signal is still attainable. In contrast, a northern blot on the same tissue might be uninterpretable because of severe degradation. In addition, mRNA stability varies somewhat with tissue type, perhaps in part due to the relative content of RNases versus RNase inhibitors. Once the tissue is properly fixed, the nucleic acids are stable, essentially forever. Relative RNA preservation can be assayed by using appropriate controls for ubiquitously expressed genes.

Another advantage of working with fixed tissue is that it eliminates much of the infectious risk associated with clinical specimens, an issue of increasing concern. For example, it seems much more attractive to be able to perform ISH for the human immunodeficiency virus or other highly virulent viruses on a fixed tissue specimen (not to mention potentially faster, cheaper, easier, and probably with comparable sensitivity) than to culture the same specimen to demonstrate the virus. The same could be said for a wide variety of other pathogens that are increasingly encountered in clinical specimens and may or may not be amenable to rapid or safe microbial culture (see Chap. 60 and Part VI).

ISH complements traditional biochemical methods as well as immunocytochemistry. It serves as an information bridge between them. Specific genes are often isolated from histologically complex tissues using probes, for example, monoclonal antibodies or oligonucleotides, which may have less than ideal specificity. A minor antigenic cross-reactivity in a monoclonal antibody may lead to isolation of the wrong sequence, particularly if the abundance of the target is rare relative to that of the cross-reacting epitope. If the gene or antibody is previously uncharacterized, the researcher may have no way of confirming the identity of the sequence, or even its cell of origin or the antibody's specificity. *In situ* hybridization is the essential step for verifying that the purified gene is indeed derived from the correct cell population. Failure to use ISH may lead to erroneous conclusions about tissue/cellular specificity of a particular gene sequence.

The ability to indefinitely propagate recombinant DNA probes, primarily in bacteria, their inherent ease of preparation and maintenance, as compared with monoclonal antibodies, and their increasing availability, particularly as sequence databases increase, ensures the continued expansion of these techniques in medical diagnosis and research.

TECHNICAL CONSIDERATIONS

Many laboratories have developed protocols for *in situ* hybridization. All the protocols have in common the goals of maintaining tissue morphology while rendering the tissue permeable to the probe, retaining the hybridization target, and facilitating sensitive and specific detection of hybrid formation. As outlined in Table 61–1, a variety of factors are specific to *in situ* hybridization. A consideration of each of these will follow and lead to an appreciation of things that need to be kept in mind, when either implementing or evaluating an ISH. The *in situ* methods discussed will emphasize the utility of asymmetric RNA probes for the detection of messenger RNA as well as DNA. These methods are currently in use in the Anatomic Molecular Pathology Labora-

Table 61–1. FACTORS OF IMPORTANCE TO *IN SITU* HYBRIDIZATION

Probe Factors
Probe type
Probe complexity
Probe size
Probe-specific activity
Probe concentration
Tissue Factors
Source
Fixation
Processing
Target Factors
Target type: RNA versus DNA
Target abundance
Target availability
Hybridization Factors
Hybrid stringency
Wash stringency
Kinetics
Detection Systems
Autoradiography
Nonradioactive

tory at the University of Virginia and have been applied to a wide variety of microbial and cellular targets. They represent a direct extension of the techniques pioneered at the University of Rochester by Robert and Lynne Angerer (Angerer, 1987, 1991; Cox, 1984) and their adaptation to routinely processed, formalin-fixed, paraffin-embedded clinical specimens (Stoler, 1986a, b, 1990a, b). It should also be pointed out that there is a wide divergence in protocols amongst different laboratories. For contrasting examples, see Valentino (1987). Many general protocols are compiled in two popular references (Ausubel, 1991; Sambrook, 1989). However, as a word of caution, mixing and matching between systems is most assuredly a path to failure.

Probe Factors

DNA is a double-stranded molecule composed of two antiparallel strands, that is, each strand has a 5′-3′ orientation and the two strands are oriented in opposite directions. An asymmetric probe refers to a single-stranded probe molecule that is lacking its antiparallel complement. This is in contrast to double-stranded "symmetric" probes that contain both antiparallel strands. Probes may be composed of DNA or RNA. DNA probes may be symmetric or asymmetric. Oligonucleotide probes are short, synthetic asymmetric DNA probes. RNA probes are obviously asymmetric.

Before defining some of the other probe factors, a consideration of probe labelling is in order. The most common method of labelling DNA is nick translation (Rigby, 1977). During nick translation, labelling is accomplished using two enzymes, usually pancreatic DNase I and *Escherichia coli* DNA polymerase I. DNase I makes random single-stranded nicks in duplex DNA. These nicks serve as attachment sites for the DNA polymerase, which mediates the labelling of molecules through two actions: a 5′ to 3′ exonuclease activity, which excises the unlabeled bases, and a 5′ to 3′ polymerase activity, which incorporates labeled precursors. Because both strands are nicked, both get labeled (i.e., the labeling is symmetric). Because of the random distribution of the nicks, denaturation produces a population of molecules of varying length. The length can be controlled by the concentration of DNase in the reaction; the higher the concentration, the shorter the fragments. A variation of this technique (Feinberg, 1983) uses a mixture of oligonucleotides to randomly prime double-stranded DNA that has been denatured into single strands for subsequent labeled nucleotide incorporation by DNA polymerase. This method provides somewhat higher specific activity. DNA probes are very popular. DNA is a more stable molecule than RNA and is easier to handle in the lab. Some authors favor double-stranded probes because theoretically they can form large probe networks that may amplify signal, so-called *hyperduplex formation* (Lawrence, 1985). Countering this advantage are issues of probe fragment size and hyperduplex size because these affect tissue penetration. In addition, double-stranded symmetric probes interact with themselves as well as the nucleic acid target. This self-hybridization has been shown to be a significant factor in the amount of signal generated at any given probe concentration (Cox, 1984) (Fig. 61–1).

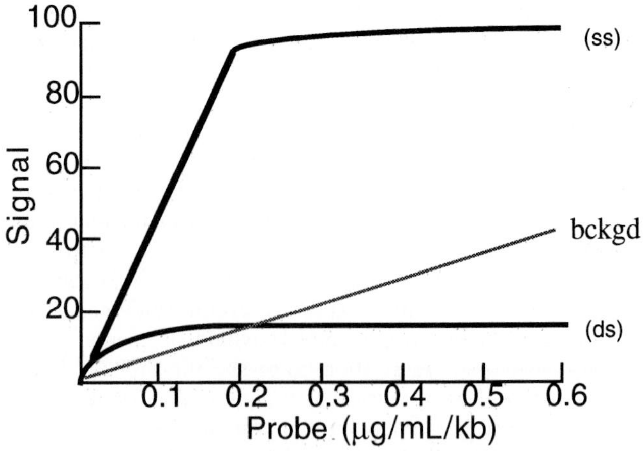

Figure 61–1. Relationship of signal to probe concentration for double-stranded (ds) versus single-stranded (ss) probes. (Adapted from Cox KH, DeLeon DV, Angerer LM, Angerer RC. Detection of mRNAs in sea urchin embryos by in situ hybridization using asymmetric RNA probes. Dev Biol 1984; 101:485–502.)

Asymmetric RNA probes are synthesized using transcription vectors that contain prokaryotic RNA polymerase promoters such as those specific for the bacteriophage SP6 (Melton, 1984). These promoters are inserted just upstream from a multiple cloning site in the vector, which facilitates the easy insertion of a piece of probe DNA. During the labelling reaction, the circular vector is truncated downstream from the insert, thereby eliminating the vector sequences from the reaction. One strand of the DNA serves as a template during RNA transcription, being read by RNA polymerase in the 3′ to 5′ direction, leading to the synthesis of an RNA from the 5′ to 3′ direction, until the truncation site is reached. By providing labeled nucleotide, transcripts of high purity and specific activity are synthesized. The size of these RNA transcripts is easily and reproducibly controlled by limited alkaline hydrolysis. The popularity of this technique has led to fourth and fifth generation transcription vectors that contain two promoters flanking a central cloning site (*gemini vectors*) with many associated selection markers and other useful functions. Gemini vectors facilitate the transcription of the DNA insert in either direction, thus obviating the need to maintain two separate clones to get transcription of both strands.

Depending upon the orientation of the cloned insert relative to the promoter, a *sense* or *antisense* transcript will be produced. A sense transcript is a copy of the insert with the same 5′ to 3′ orientation as actual messenger RNA. Because it is not antiparallel to messenger RNA, it is impossible for this sense transcript to hybridize to messenger RNA. It can, however, hybridize to homologous duplex DNA (if the DNA is denatured first). An antisense transcript is one that is transcribed so that its orientation is complementary to messenger RNA. Thus, it can hybridize specifically to target messenger RNA and it will ignore homologous nondenatured duplex DNA that is not available for hybridization. Because the sense strand has a complementary base sequence, length, and specific activity as the antisense strand, it can serve as an excellent negative control for *in situ* hybridizations that are designed to look at gene expression (mRNA). This, of

Table 61–2. PROBE TARGET INTERACTIONS FOR ASYMMETRIC RNA PROBES

Probe	Detects
Antisense/no denaturation	mRNA
Antisense/with denaturation	mRNA + DNA
Sense/with denaturation	DNA
Sense/no denaturation	No signal

course, assumes that the cloned DNA segment is not naturally transcribed in both directions, which is usually, albeit not invariably, the case. By using a combination of sense and antisense probes, together with control over the denaturation of the target, one can gain exquisite control over the specificity of the reactions involved that is not as easily attained with symmetrically labeled double-stranded probes (Table 61–2).

The advantages of *in situ* hybridization for detecting messenger RNA using asymmetric RNA probes are as follows:

1. Cellular transcription of most genes is asymmetric.
2. The lack of competing probe self-reaction produces much higher signals (see Fig. 61–1).
3. Sequence purity is insured during the *in vitro* transcription reaction because the vector sequences are eliminated from the labelling by restriction enzyme digestion. Because the transcripts produced are free of vector contamination, they can saturate targets at a lower concentration than if the vector were included. This leads to a higher signal-to-noise ratio, because nonspecific binding of probe is proportional to the total probe concentration over the section.
4. RNA transcripts are relatively easy to prepare. Following a relatively simple enzymatic synthesis, the probes undergo minimal purification. Fragment length of RNA probes is easily and reproducibly controlled by limited alkaline hydrolysis.
5. Probes synthesized in this manner can be labelled to very high specific activities, in most cases equal to the specific activity of the starting precursors. Incorporations of 40% to 80% are routine.
6. Nonspecific backgrounds are dramatically reduced by posthybridization digestion with RNase under conditions in which probe/target hybrids are immune to digestion, and yet nonhybridized single strands are digested away.
7. The higher stability of RNA-RNA duplexes relative to DNA-DNA duplexes allows very high stringency washes, improving specificity. High temperature washing also reduces nonspecific sticking of probe to tissues.

For a given probe type, the *complexity* of the probe refers to the length of the potentially homologous sequence of the probe with the target. Thus if the whole genome of a papillomavirus is labelled as a probe, the probe complexity is 7.9 kilobases (kb). In some cases the probe and vector are labelled together. If a 1-kb insert is labelled with a 3-kb vector, the complexity is still 1 kb, although the 3 kb of labelled nonhomologous vector might boost the signal through hyperduplex formation. It might also boost the background because of nonspecific binding. Clearly, sensitivity is directly proportional to probe complexity. Assuming all other factors are equal, a 300-base pair (bp) probe will generate 10 times the signal of a 30-bp oligo.

In contrast to complexity, probe size refers to the size of the probe fragments that enter into the hybridization reaction. In general, small probe fragments less than 200 to 300 bp in size are necessary for efficient ISH because they are much more efficient in penetrating the tissues and finding their targets. Oligonucleotide probes that are very small, for example, 20 to 30 bp in length, may be highly efficient at diffusing and penetrating tissue, but their short length mandates very careful control of stringency because of decreased hybrid stability for hybrids of less than 100 bp in length.

The concentration of probe in the hybridization reaction is another critical covariable. Most reactions are carried out under conditions of vast probe excess and exhibit pseudo–first order kinetics. Considerations of probe concentration have been shown to be particularly important for *in situ* hybridization with single-stranded probes, because the signal obtained is proportional to the probe concentration up to a maximum level, even though probe concentrations throughout the range were theoretically saturating (see Fig. 61–1). This suggests that only a small fraction of the probe participates in the hybridization reaction. The situation is even more complex when the probe is double stranded, in which case there are two competing reactions in a hybridization: (1) the hybridization between probe and target, and (2) the re-annealing of the probe to itself. During *in situ* hybridization, it has been demonstrated that the latter reaction may be favored in that single-stranded probes may give eight- to 10-fold higher signals than double-stranded probes.

In Figure 61–1 it can also be seen that for asymmetric probes below saturating concentration, there is a linear relationship between signal generated and probe concentration. One can capitalize on this in situations where multiple probes of varying complexity are used. If the least complex probe is applied at saturation and the other probe concentrations are normalized for complexity, the relative signals between the probes should be directly comparable (Stoler, 1989, 1992). In addition, it should be clear that regardless of the type of probe, the more probe used in the reaction, the greater the background, and that at supersaturating concentrations of probe, which are often used by some to shorten hybridization times, the ultimate limiting factor may be nonspecific background decreasing the signal-to-noise ratio.

Probe-specific activity refers to the density of label molecules on the probe, that is, how "hot" the probe is, usually expressed as dpm/min/μg. This can be a very easy number to calculate with some types of radioactive synthesis labelling reactions, such as for RNA probes (see later). In the case of most nonradioactive probes, it can be very difficult to quantify the amount of label incorporated. Maximum specific activity, which should yield maximal sensitivity, is not always desirable. For instance, if one labels every nucleotide in a probe with a radioactive nucleotide, the ensuing radiolysis may degrade the probe. If the density of biotinylated UTP in a probe is too high, steric hindrance between biotins may actually make such a probe less sensitive than one in which, on average, every third or fourth UTP is labelled.

Tissue Factors

The source of the tissue and how it is fixed, processed, and sectioned have a major impact on any ISH procedure. Here the analogies to IMH are considerable, but the emphasis is on nucleic acid preservation and availability for hybridization, rather than preservation of antigenicity.

The tissue or organ under study can affect the hybridization result. Different organs obviously vary in their biochemical complexity, and hence conditions of pretreatment and hybridization may need to be optimized for different tissues. For instance, the degree of proteolysis that is used to generate optimal signals for a hepatocyte mRNA may be 10 times the amount used when probing a keratinocyte. Pancreatic exocrine cells are rich in nucleases, particularly RNases. In contrast, brain seems to have much less intrinsic RNase activity. Unfortunately, much of this is empirically derived and, while for any given protocol reasonable first approximations are available, optimization is still required.

Given the desire to subject a tissue to ISH, should one use fixed or frozen tissue? Much of the early ISH literature emphasized frozen tissue because mRNA was thought not to be detectable in fixed tissue. However, the latter is clearly not true, and the convenience and superior morphology of paraffin sections makes this the format of choice for diagnostic ISH. Choice of fixative is clearly a major issue. On clinical material, the common fixatives used for *in situ* hybridization are cross-linking fixatives, such as formaldehyde and glutaraldehyde, or precipitating fixatives such as ethanol. Alcohols are relatively gentle protein precipitants that do preserve nucleic acids. The lack of cross-linking may obviate the need for much, if any, permeabilization pretreatment, particularly if nuclear DNA is the target. On the other hand, diffusable molecules such as mRNA are often lost during hydration unless a cross-linking fixative is used. In general, cross-linking fixatives are favored because they facilitate the retention of the nucleic acids in the tissue and they reproduce the morphology used in routine diagnosis. However, the tighter the cross-linking, that is, the more the tissue is fixed, the less accessible are the nucleic acids to probing. Hence, glutaraldehyde-fixed tissues that are more tightly cross-linked than formaldehyde-fixed tissues have a greater requirement for tissue permeabilization. The emphasis on formalin fixation seems a natural one for a surgical pathologist. The fact that additional special fixatives or handling is unnecessary is obviously a great advantage. Our experience with neutral buffered formalin fixation has been that it is an excellent fixative for *in situ* hybridization. Clearly, the more rapidly fixed the specimen, the better the RNA preservation; therefore, many small biopsies that are received and immediately fixed are ideal. However, within the usual ranges experienced in surgical pathology (fixation 0 to 6 hours after removal from the patient), we have had good success detecting RNA transcripts in a wide variety of tissues, including cervix, vulva, lung, breast, thyroid, anus, esophagus, lymph node, liver, and brain. Of course, absolute signal quantitation between specimens may well require standardization of tissue handling or the use of internal control probes to facilitate meaningful comparisons.

Many laboratories use Bouin's fixation or other fixatives with a high acid content for diagnostic biopsies. Our experience with these fixatives has been mostly negative. The strong acids or other denaturing agents, such as mercury, provide a histologically pleasing "strong or dense" nuclear fix with improved staining and cytologic detail. However, these harsher fixation processes probably lead to either direct damage to the nucleic acids or to such dense precipitation of nucleic acid–associated proteins as to render the targets unhybridizable. While others report some success with other fixatives, most workers who are attempting to adapt these methods for clinical use are emphasizing formalin fixation as the best compromise (Nuovo, 1989a, b) between the requirements for hybridization and mild cross-linking versus excellent morphologic preservation and archival access.

Following adequate fixation all tissues are routinely processed in the clinical histology lab for paraffin embedding. This includes use of the histology lab's automated vacuum infiltration processor. Artifacts caused by automated processing have not been detectable. In addition, using the routine histology lab is convenient, standardized, and facilitates the examination of archival material, which will have been processed identically to any experimental material one is working on. Note that routine processing does not mean the same thing in every histology lab! What happens to the tissue in the processor is at least as important as the period of fixation before processing. The processor schedule we use includes neutral formalin, graded ethanols, and xylene/paraffins. Some of the newer "less toxic" reagents, such as propylene glycols, mixtures of other alcohols, non–xylene-based clearants, etc., are essentially untested and may or may not have deleterious effects, particularly for the detection of more labile RNA targets. Once well-fixed and processed tissues are embedded in paraffin, the nucleic acids are stable for ISH for years, although there may be some degradation with long-term storage (Greer, 1991).

Tissue loss from the slides has been one of the biggest technical difficulties for *in situ* hybridization. The combination of low ionic strength buffers, organic and often viscous chemicals, and high temperatures wreaks havoc with tissue adhesion to glass. Many different slide coatings have been tried, including albumin, Elmer's glue, Histostik, and poly-L-lysine. Up until recently, poly-L-lysine was the best of these for both ISH and IMH, and it still enjoys considerable popularity. However, in our lab as well as many others, slides coated with a 2% v/v solution of 3-aminopropyltriethoxysil-ane (TES) in acetone (Henderson, 1989; Rentrop, 1986) have become the standard. The silane group in TES interacts with the glass structure, whereas the aldehyde moiety covalently binds the section to the slide. This is in contrast to the ionic interaction involved with polylysine. TES-coated slides work equally well for IMH as well as ISH, and are easily prepared or commercially available. In terms of sectioning, it may be prudent to cut sections for ISH in a clean waterbath with gloves, in an attempt to minimize nuclease contamination, but this is not clearly a necessity. Section thickness will affect variables, such as the quality of morphology, probe penetration, amount of pretreatment needed, and signal quenching. In general, the usual 3 to 5 micron section is an optimal compromise. We have performed RNA-mRNA ISH on paraffin sections stored dust-free at room temperature for over five years without appreciable changes in signal intensity.

Target Factor

As alluded to in the section on probe synthesis, the target of an ISH may be DNA, RNA, or both. The nature of the target affects the conditions of hybridization in that the protocols vary when targeting DNA as compared with RNA. DNA targets require denaturation. The intensity of the denaturation reaction can affect the level of signal development. Inevitably, and unlike the conditions on a Southern blot, the denatured target DNA may reanneal with itself as opposed to interacting with the probe. The competition between target self-reassociation and probe hybridization is difficult to quantify and, at best, one can hope for a high fraction of the target to interact with the probe. If the probe is also symmetric DNA, then there are three competing reactions. If the probes are asymmetric, then selection of sense versus antisense orientation is obviously important. Denaturation can also affect section adherence and morphology. Because of the latter, we have favored low-temperature denaturation with formamide as opposed to denaturation by heating at 95° to 100°C because the morphologic preservation seems better with the former. In contrast to DNA targets, tissues for mRNA ISH should not be denatured, lest a mixed DNA + mRNA signal be developed. Occasionally, detecting both DNA + mRNA can be capitalized on to further intensify a weak signal.

The abundance of the target sequence obviously is the major factor in signal development. Again, in cases where a DNA of interest, say, a viral sequence, is below the assay sensitivity, probing for the corresponding mRNA may be quite revealing as well as yield some functional information. The availability of the target refers to how accessible the target is to the probe sequence. Intracellular protein and nucleic acid composition, degree of fixation, and type and intensity of pretreatment all interact to determine target availability.

Hybridization Factors

As should be clear by now, the success of any ISH reaction is the product of many interlinked steps. Before the hybridization, the tissue is hydrated, permeabilized with protease, and denatured if needed. In many blot protocols, a prehybridization step is carried out to decrease background binding of probe. Essentially the hybridization mix *sans* probe is applied for a period of time followed by the real probe mix. We and others have not found this useful. In fact, because signal is so concentration dependent, a prehybridization step could lead to dilution of probe. It is simpler to include nonspecific carrier DNA or tRNA in the hybridization mix, which will compete for nonspecific binding sites. Other pretreatment steps include acetylation of positive charges, which can also act as a nuclease protection step (Angerer, 1991). The kinetics of ISH hybridization, at least for asymmetric probes, are exactly analogous to those in solution, albeit with a slightly depressed effective T_m (Angerer, 1991; Cox, 1984). Signal is proportional to probe concentration and time. If time is fixed, the signal is linearly related to the probe concentration until saturation is reached, which in this system is 0.2 to 0.3 μg/ml/kb of probe complexity. Hybridization is usually carried out overnight (12 to 16 hours) for convenience. Times shorter than 6 hours lead to substantially decreased signals. For abundant targets, probe can be conserved by using subsaturating concentrations of probe at the expense of autoradiographic exposure time. Another advantage of this method is that backgrounds, which are proportional to probe concentration, are also reduced. Other protocols, usually using double-stranded probes for DNA detection, may call for much higher probe concentrations (10 to 100× more) and shorter hybridization times (some as short as 10 minutes). While touting increased speed and perhaps improved sensitivity if hyperduplex formation is achieved, the amount of probe used may contribute to both background as well as cost. As shown in Figure 61–2, the interplay of prehybridization, hybridization, and posthybridization steps can have a profound effect on signal strength, regardless of the detection system.

Detection Systems

Up until now, the discussion has focused on factors critical to the success of an ISH that are mostly independent of the detection system. One has a basic choice between autoradiography using radioactive probes or nonradioactive methods involving any of the broad repertoire of IMH procedures. Our bias has been to use autoradiography almost exclusively for the following reasons: (1) It still is the most sensitive detection method (Angerer, 1991; Masih, 1993). While some studies claim equivalent sensitivity for nonradioactive methods (Nuovo, 1989b; Park, 1991), most are making "apples to oranges" comparisons. (2) Autoradiography is a direct detection method. It eliminates the potentially numerous variables involved in using antibodies and enzymatic detection reagents, which at the very least limit one's ability to quantify the result. (3) With attention to detail, autoradiography can vary quantitatively, particularly between slides in a single experiment. The disadvantages of autoradiography are well recognized by clinical labs: There are the hazards and costs of working with radioisotopes. The length of autoradiographic exposure may be excessively long relative to clinical

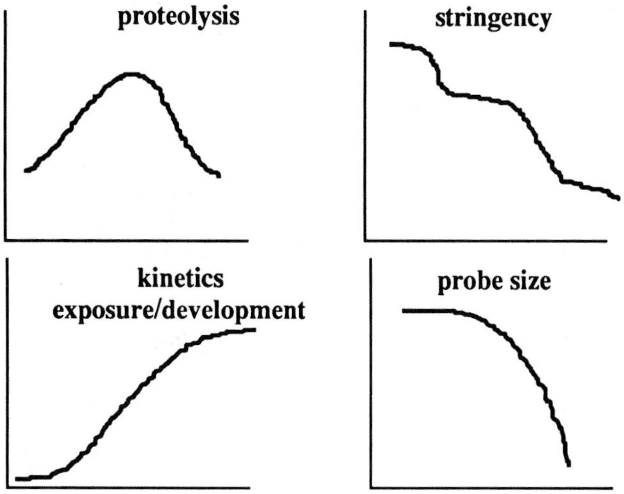

Figure 61–2. Effects of different covariables on signal strength during RNA-mRNA *in situ* hybridization.

Table 61–3. RELATIONSHIPS BETWEEN ISOTOPES COMMONLY USED IN ISH

Isotope	$t_{1/2}$	Possible Specific Activity dpm/μg Probe	Relative Autoradiographic Efficiency	Grains/day/kb Complexity	Background	Resolution
^{3}H	12.7 years	$1–2 \times 10^{8}$	1	0.002–0.003	Very low	Excellent
^{35}S	87 days	$2–5 \times 10^{9}$	5	0.15	Low (sometimes variable)	Good
^{125}I	60 days	2×10^{9}	~5	~0.15	Low	Very good
^{32}P	14 days	$>5 \times 10^{9}$	~1	0.075–0.10	Low	Fair to poor
^{33}P	25 days	5×10^{9}	?3–5	?0.2–0.3	Low to very low	Moderate to good

utility. Enzymatic- or fluorescence-based labels may give finer signal resolution compared with some of the higher energy radioisotopes.

If autoradiography is used, then the next choice is the isotope to use. There are at least five isotopes commonly in use for ISH, each with relative advantages and disadvantages (Table 61–3). Higher energy isotopes, such as ^{35}S and ^{32}P, offer high specific activity, potentially higher autoradiographic efficiency (^{35}S), but shorter half-life and lower resolution. A low-energy isotope, such as tritium (^{3}H), combines long half-life with fine resolution, but has the disadvantage of lower specific activity and/or energy, and hence longer exposure times.

For autoradiography with tritium, a probe of 1000-bp complexity with a specific activity of 1.2×10^{8} dpm/μg should yield approximately 0.002 grains/day/kb of message (assuming an autoradiographic efficiency of 0.02). Grain densities of 10/100 μm^2 are readily detectable in the absence of nonspecific binding. Thus, if a cell has 250 copies of a 1-kb message in an area of 100 μm^2, it should be easily detectable in 20 days of autoradiography. Stronger signals can be achieved with longer exposures. Tritium probes are stable for years because of the long half-life of tritium.

^{35}S probes can be labelled to 10-fold higher specific activities, and their autoradiographic efficiency is higher, with the result that signals can theoretically be increased 50-fold at saturation. This would seem ideal, bringing the sensitivity of the technique into the range of a single copy/cell with reasonable exposures. In most instances, maximal sensitivity is not an issue. Rather, for reasonably abundant targets the improved sensitivity allows one to considerably shorten exposure times compared with tritium. However, the backgrounds are obligatorily higher with ^{35}S because of the higher specific activities. Most people using ^{35}S probes are using them at very subsaturating concentrations to decrease backgrounds. In this case, the same result can be achieved using the higher concentrations of tritium-labelled probes with better resolution because of the shorter path lengths. ^{35}S probes also have a much shorter half-life. In addition, many people have found problems with nonspecific probe binding or probe instability that make the use of ^{35}S probes on limited material somewhat more risky.

While other investigators report the use of other isotopes, such as ^{32}P or ^{125}I, this author has little experience with these isotopes. In addition, their higher energies increase health risks considerably, which ultimately will decrease their clinical utility. ^{33}P has been recently touted as the best compromise isotope for ISH, combining the higher energy advantages of ^{35}S while eliminating the background problems that are common to sulfur-containing isotopes. Depending upon lab volume, the short half-life may or may not be advantageous. ^{33}P is also very expensive.

Nonradioactive detection methods, such as the use of biotinylated probes with avidin-biotin–linked enzymatic detection systems, hold much promise, and their improvements will be essential for the generalization of the technique of *in situ* hybridization to the clinical labs. New methods of probe labelling and signal amplification are the subject of intense commercial development. The advantages of nonradioactive methods include probe stability, speed of detection, and good resolution. The speed of detection is the clear advantage for the clinical implementation of these methods. However, at present these methods seem less sensitive than autoradiographic methods by at least one to two orders of magnitude. This level of sensitivity might be quite acceptable if the target is very abundant. Another disadvantage is that it is very difficult to quantitate signals, especially between experiments with methods that use enzymatic amplification, because of the many variables inherent in these types of systems and the inability to easily estimate "specific activity." Currently, biotin-labelled nucleotides with strepavidin-linked enzymatic detection are most popular, with digoxigenin-based systems running a close second. The number of variables in these systems is essentially endless and include: the reagent vendor, reagent concentration and avidity, incubation times, numbers of layers in the detection system, enzyme choice, substrate, developing time, temperature, etc. Here the analogy to the interlaboratory variation in IMH is most evident. We have had some experience with digoxigenin-labelled probes (Boeringer Mannheim) with immunoalkaline phosphatase detection. These have a theoretical advantage over biotin in that there is no endogeneous analogue to digoxigenin. Thus, the subsequent antibody-based detection will have no endogenous target to generate a false-positive signal or increased background. In these unpublished experiments in which RNA probes were dual labelled with both ^{3}H and digoxigenin such that specific activity was established, we still felt that autoradiography was ultimately more sensitive by about an order of magnitude. A final problem with nonradioactive detection systems is that many of the biological detection reagents are contaminated with nucleases, particularly RNase, which is an issue that needs to be addressed in protocol design. Fortunately, RNA-mRNA hybrids are relatively RNase resistant in high salt solution compared with unhybridized RNA.

METHODOLOGIC ISSUES

Sensitivity

As should be clear, the ultimate sensitivity of ISH is a function of multiple interrelated steps of a given probe-target combination and protocol. The sensitivity of *in situ* hybridization depends upon the signal-to-noise ratio that can be achieved. The signal depends upon the fraction of target in the tissue that is retained and accessible for hybridization, the mass of probe relative to the target (saturation), and the complexity and specific activity of the probe as visualized through a defined detection system. Noise, which can be limiting, depends upon the extent to which the probe nonspecifically binds to the background and is proportional to the probe concentration. For autoradiographic RNA-mRNA ISH with moderately complex (0.5- to 2-kb) probes and high specific activities, the lower limit of sensitivity is on the order of 10 to 100 copies of message per cell.

Another measure of sensitivity is a relative comparison of different detection methods for a similar target. Using the papillomavirus system, we have found the sensitivity of HPV mRNA detection *in situ* to be highly comparable to the best reported Southern blot data or polymerase chain reaction (PCR) data. What is meant by this statement is that, just as the polymerase chain reaction can detect a few copies of a sequence diluted in an enormous population of cellular DNA, *in situ* hybridization can detect that same few copies in a single cell if that cell is on the slide. In an unpublished series of cervical cancers in which parallel paraffin sections were analyzed by PCR and mRNA-RNA ISH, the subset for which type-specific probes were available had over 95% agreement. Intertechnique comparisons such as these raise issues of how to choose amongst competing methods that give similar data. In molecular pathology, there are often several routes to the same end point, and much of the work of the next several years will entail validating and cross-referencing the different methods. For a general discussion of some of these concepts, see Schiffman (1992) and Valenstein (1990).

Specificity and Controls

One of the true advantages of ISH is the specificity of the information derived from this type of combined morphologic and molecular analysis. If the distribution of the signal is not in the appropriate cell type, the specificity of the probe for the target may be in question. Obviously, when first evaluating a new probe it is ideal to have known positive and negative control cells or tissues processed in a manner identical to the clinical or experimental material.

The specificity of the hybridization is controlled by sequence homology and stringency. If the stringency is very low, nonspecific hybridization will be favored. In blot hybridizations this is sometimes used to select for related sequences, potentially enhancing sensitivity at the cost of specificity. For instance, HPV 6 and HPV 11, which are over 85% homologous at the sequence level, will cross-react at even high stringency. At low stringency HPV 16 can be detected with an HPV 6 probe. Conversely, if the stringency is set too high, there may be loss of specific signal, that is, a false-negative result. Thus, sensitivity and specificity are, in part, reciprocally related. Asymmetric RNA probes, depending on probe orientation and tissue denaturation, also allow specific control of the hybridization to DNA or mRNA. If a gene is transcribed in only one direction, the case for most but not all eukaryotic genes, the sense orientation probe provides an ideal nonhomologous control for background signals during mRNA detection. Additionally, one can verify that the signal is derived from RNA or DNA by pretreating the section with RNase or DNase, thereby causing a loss of signal. Alternatively, others have used competitive hybridization between labelled and unlabeled probe to prove specificity.

An extremely useful control, particularly when one is trying to make comparisons between multiple specimens, is to probe for a ubiquitously expressed message (e.g., actin) and to normalize signal interpretations to the level of this target (Segal, 1994). Specimens with significant loss of the control signal may be unevaluable, especially if one is probing for mRNAs that are only moderately expressed. The converse is that some highly expressed messages may be detectable despite considerable mRNA loss. An example might be the EBER RNAs of Epstein-Barr virus (Gulley, 1993), which may be present at a level of 10^6 to 10^7 copies/cell. If most messages are expressed at a level of 10^3 copies/cell, then 99.9% of the mRNA could be lost and the target cell could still look like a high expresser.

Newer Techniques

As mentioned earlier, oligonucleotide probes have been used by many investigators to perform *in situ* hybridizations (Lawrence, 1989; Lewis, 1988; Taneja, 1987). In principle, these types of probes have several attractions, including the ability to tailor the probe to the exact sequence of interest and the elimination of the need to do any cloning. The latter is becoming a major advantage as resources for oligonucleotide synthesis become increasingly available and costs are reduced. If sequence information is known, antisense oligonucleotides can be designed for mRNA detection. Combined with end labelling of the oligonucleotides with a nonradioactive adduct, these types of probes may evolve into the type most commonly used in clinical laboratories for the detection of moderately abundant mRNAs. Their main disadvantages would seem to be lower sensitivity because of low probe complexity, a relative inability to quantify the degree of incorporation in end labelling reactions, as well as a potential for lower specificity because of the need to titrate the stringency more exactly in order to prevent nonspecific binding.

Another newer technology is the method of *in situ* transcription. First described by Tecott (1988) using frozen sections, this method depends upon specific antisense oligonucleotide hybridization to prime the mRNA for subsequent first-strand cDNA synthesis by reverse transcriptase. It is amazing but true that significant biochemical enzymology is possible in a deparaffinized hydrated section. We and others have extended this technique to formalin-fixed, paraffin-embedded sections, and it forms the basis for all *in situ* reverse transcriptase PCR procedures. In a sense the first part of the procedure is the same as the previously discussed antisense oligonucleotide hybridization. Its potential advantages are possibly increased sensitivity and the ability to probe several related genes at once. *In situ* transcription should not be any more sensitive than the corresponding *in situ* hybridization with a probe of complexity and specific activity equal to the length of the transcript made by the enzyme. However, many parameters for this technique have yet to be well worked out such that at present it has to be considered highly experimental.

Even more experimental in this author's opinion is *in situ* PCR. Theoretically *in situ* PCR combines the signal amplification of PCR with the morphologic specificity of ISH. *In situ* PCR can detect DNA, or if coupled with *in situ* transcription, mRNA. First described by Hasse in 1990, Nuovo and colleagues have done the most to stimulate the development of this new field, which, *theoretically*, could provide the ultimate sensitivity of short single copy sequence detection in individual cells. The major problem in this procedure is how to keep the amplicons localized to the site of synthesis. Another major problem is that the instrumentation to perform this reaction on slides is only just being developed. Suffice it to say that the current literature contains widely divergent and strong opinions on almost every step in this procedure (DeLellis, 1994; Hofler, 1993; Nuovo, 1993, 1994), and that this is far from ready for the clinical laboratory. This writer's current bias is that one should try the best available ISH procedure before even considering *in situ* PCR.

Another advanced technique is combined ISH and IMH on the same section. This is usually more easily addressed by serial sections because the protocols for each procedure are not mutually optimal. On the other hand, several workers have described such procedures (Brahic, 1989; and Chapter 5 in Valentino, 1987). In our experience, it is critical to do the ISH first to protect the RNA from nuclease attack. Of course, opposite opinions do exist.

Applicability

Over the last 25 years, *in situ* hybridization has evolved into a widely established research technique, albeit one that is still technically demanding. A MEDLINE search for the term *ISH* will generate thousands of references. The methods described potentially have clear-cut applications in nearly all areas of pathology. The primary applications in use today fall into three major categories as follows:

Detection of infectious agents: Gene probes are available for the identification of the genetic material of numerous bacteria, mycobacteria, and viruses. The harder or more dangerous it is to culture an organism, the more likely it is that a molecular detection format will be preferred (see Chap. 60). For some organisms, molecular detection and analysis have essentially defined the classification and/or life cycle of the organism in the absence of routinely available microbial culture (Fox, 1993; Gulley, 1993; Reed, 1992; Stoler, 1989, 1992). *In situ* hybridization methods provide an advantage over blot or solution hybridization methods in terms of allowing a highly specific localization of the organism within a specific cell type or histologic lesion, thus providing an essential pathogenic link between the presence of an organism's genetic material and the presence of disease (Amortegui, 1990; Kandolf, 1993; Mandry, 1994; Martino, 1994; Stoler, 1990a, b).

Cytogenetics: ISH on chromosomes is the method of choice for localizing a gene to a specific locus. Nucleic acid probes are commercially available for large portions of every human chromosome, as well as to specific gene rearrangements associated with certain forms of neoplasia. Fluorescent *in situ* hybridization (FISH) is the major growth field in cytogenetics and is predicted to have wide applicability in diagnostics, particularly when applied to interphase nuclei, and perhaps combined with flow cytometry (Anastasi, 1993; Brandriff, 1991; Gray, 1991; Trask, 1991).

Gene expression: A major area of research over the next several decades is going to be the detailed analysis of the regulation of cellular gene expression in health and disease. Oncogenes, the genes that regulate the production of hormones and their receptors; genes encoding structural proteins, tumor markers, and enzymes; and essentially any gene will be subject to a new level of combined molecular and morphologic analysis. The sequential analysis of cellular DNA, RNA, and protein through a combined ISH/immunohistochemical approach will lead to a much better understanding of the interaction of how cellular biochemical events impact on pathogenesis. The translation of these basic studies is widely predicted to have major impact on our concepts of pathogenesis, classification, and prognostication. Major insights in fields such as cardiology, endocrinology, infectious disease, neural science, and oncology are defining the new molecular medicine, and ISH together with IMH are essential tools in all of these investigations (Asa, 1993; Boffa, 1989; Cimino, 1989; DeLellis, 1994; Emson, 1993; Gravitt, 1993; Harrison, 1990; Lloyd, 1994; Niedobitek, 1991; Roberts, 1991; Valentino, 1987).

However, tempering this enthusiasm are some of the following observations: The current lack of method standardization or of even clear documentation of the relative superiority of one method over another is probably the leading impediment to widespread clinical implementation of ISH. In addition, the relative lack of well-characterized, commercially available probes is also problematic. Certainly, there is much clinically relevant research that needs to be done, and anatomic pathology is the only specialty to do it. In the interim, literature reports must continue to document experimental methods in order to facilitate comparison. There is no such thing as "standard *in situ* hybridization."

Once technical issues have been resolved and hopefully standardized, such that interlaboratory comparisons are possible, then the work of assessing the clinical utility of *in situ* hybridization can be performed. Issues of technical sensitivity and specificity need to be compared in terms of clinical utility based on the population under study and the question to be asked. Having an assay that can detect a few hundred copies of a gene sequence in a few hours is irrelevant if the targets under study only express 10 copies. Similarly, assays that can detect very low levels of gene expression may also be of limited utility if they cannot be performed within a clinically useful time frame. Issues of prevalence, predictive value, turnaround time, and cost are all important considerations, and the precedence of one versus the other is clearly dependent on individual laboratory priorities. As noted earlier, competing methodologies may provide similar data and choosing among them is becoming increasingly complex.

Unquestionably, the evolving field of molecular pathology will provide pathologists with tools of unprecedented power to address problems that have long been resistant to analysis. These methods are rapidly evolving, fostered by the explosion of available sequence information, combined with ongoing development of new types of probes, labeling systems, and detection systems, all at an accelerating pace. However, enthusiasm for the application of these methods, particularly routine clinical application, must be tempered by a systematic evaluation of factors, including technical comparability and reproducibility, and ultimately clinical utility. If something is really clinically useful, then *hopefully* it will be done. The case for *in situ* hybridization and other molecular methods is being built but is not yet proven. One can only hope that the current cost-conscious environment will permit science to run its proper course.

Amortegui AJ, Meyer MP: In-situ hybridization for the diagnosis and typing of human papillomavirus. Clin Biochem 1990; 23:301–306.

Anastasi J: Fluorescence in situ hybridization in leukemia. Applications in diagnosis, subclassification, and monitoring the response to therapy [review]. Ann N Y Acad Sci 1993; 677:214–224.

Angerer LM, Angerer RC: Detection of poly A+ RNA in sea urchin eggs and embryos by in situ hybridization. Nucleic Acids Res 1981; 9:2819–2840.

Angerer LM, Angerer RC: Localization of mRNAs by in situ hybridization. Methods Cell Biol 1991; 35:37–71.

Angerer LM, Stoler MH, Angerer RC: In situ hybridization with RNA probes: An annotated recipe. *In* Valentino KL, Eberwine JH, Barchas JD (eds): In Situ Hybridization: Applications to Neurobiology. New York: Oxford University Press, 1987, pp 42–70.

Asa SL: Clinical significance of in situ hybridization [review]. Exp Clin Endocrinol 1993; 101:46–52.

Ausubel FM, Brent R, Kingston RE, et al: Current Protocols in Molecular Biology, Vols I and II. New York: Greene Publishing Associates and Wiley Interscience, 1991.

Boffa MC: In situ hybridization in hematology. Nouv Rev Franc Hematol 1989; 31:137–138.

Brahic M, Hasse AT: Detection of viral sequences of low iteration frequency by in situ hybridization. Proc Nat Acad Sci USA 1978; 81:5545–5548.

Brahic M, Haase AT: Double-label techniques of in situ hybridization and immunocytochemistry. Curr Top Microbiol Immunol 1989; 143:9–20.

Brandriff BF, Gordon LA, Trask BJ: DNA sequence mapping by fluorescence in situ hybridization. Environ Mol Mutagen 1991; 18:259–262.

Brigati DJ, Myerson D, Leary JJ, et al: Detection of viral genomes in cultured cells and paraffin-embedded tissue sections using biotin-labeled hybridization probes. Virology 1983; 126:32–50.

Buongiorno-Nardelli M, Amaldi F: Autoradiographic detection of molecular hybrids between RNA and DNA in tissue sections. Nature 1970; 225:946–948.

Cimino M, Cattabeni F, Weiss B: In situ hybridization histochemistry as a tool to study gene expression and its regulation in the central nervous system. Pharmacol Res 1989; 2:67–77.

Cox KH, DeLeon DV, Angerer LM, Angerer RC: Detection of mRNAs in sea urchin embryos by in situ hybridization using asymmetric RNA probes. Dev Biol 1984; 101:485–502.

DeLellis RA: In situ hybridization techniques for the analysis of gene expression: Applications in tumor pathology [review]. Hum Pathol 1994; 25:580–585.

Dunn AR, Gallimore PH, Jones KW, McDougall JK: In situ hybridization of adenovirus RNA and DNA II: Detection of adenovirus-specific DNA in transformed and tumour cells. Int J Cancer 1973; 11:628–636.

Ellis IO, Galea M, Broughton N, et al: Pathological prognostic factors in breast cancer. II. Histological type. Relationship with survival in a large study with long-term follow-up. Histopathology 1992; 20:479–489.

Elston CW, Ellis IO: Pathological prognostic factors in breast cancer. I. The value of histological grade in breast cancer: Experience from a large study with long-term follow-up. Histopathology 1991; 19:403–410.

Emson PC: In-situ hybridization as a methodological tool for the neuroscientist [review]. Trends Neurosci 1993; 16:9–16.

Feinberg AP, Vogelstein B: A technique for labelling DNA restriction endonuclease fragments to high specific activity. Anal Biochem 1983; 132:6–13.

Fox CH, Cottler-Fox M: In situ hybridization in HIV research [review]. Microsc Res Techn 1993; 25:78–84. .

Gall JG, Pardue ML: Formation and detection of RNA-DNA hybrid molecules in cytological preparations. Proc Natl Acad Sci USA 1969; 63:378–383.

Grady-Leopardi EF, Schwab M, Ablin AR, Rosenau W: Detection of N-myc oncogene expression in human neuroblastoma by in situ hybridization and blot analysis: Relationship to clinical outcome. Cancer Res 1986; 46:3196–3199.

Gravitt PE, Manos MM: Nucleic acid hybridization methods to detect microorganisms [review]. Lab Anim Sci 1993; 43:5–10.

Gray JW, Lucas J, Kallioniemi O, et al: Applications of fluorescence in situ hybridization in biological dosimetry and detection of disease-specific chromosome aberrations. Progr Clin Biol Res 1991; 372:399–411.

Gray JW, Pinkel D: Molecular cytogenetics in human cancer diagnosis. Cancer 1992; 69(6, Suppl):1536–1542.

Greer CE, Peterson SL, Kiviat NB, Manos MM: PCR amplification from paraffin-embedded tissues. Effects of fixative and fixation time [see comments]. Am J Clin Pathol 1991; 95:117–124.

Gulley ML, Raab-Traub N: Detection of Epstein-Barr virus in human tissues by molecular genetic techniques [review]. Arch Pathol Lab Med 1993; 117:1115–1120.

Harrison PR, Conkie D, Paul J, Jones K: Localization of cellular globin messenger RNA by in situ hybridization to complementary DNA. FEBS Lett 1973; 32:109–112.

Harrison PJ, Pearson RC: In situ hybridization histochemistry and the study of gene expression in the human brain. Prog Neurobiol 1990; 34:271–312.

Hasse AT, Retzel EF, Staskus KA: Amplification and detection of lentiviral DNA inside cells. Proc Natl Acad Sci USA 1990; 87:4671–4675.

Henderson C: Aminoalkylsilane: An inexpensive simple preparation for slide adhesion. J Histotechnol 1989; 12:123–124.

Hofler H: In situ polymerase chain reaction: Toy or tool [editorial; comment]? Histochemistry 1993; 99:103–104.

John HA, Birnstiel ML, Jones KW: RNA-DNA hybrids at the cytological level. Nature 1969; 223:582–587.

Kandolf R, Klingel K, Zell R, et al: Molecular mechanisms in the pathogenesis of enteroviral heart disease: Acute and persistent infections [review]. Clin Immunol Immunopathol 1993; 68:153–158.

Lawrence JB, Singer RH: Quantitative analysis of in situ hybridization methods for the detection of actin gene expression. Nucleic Acids Res 1985; 13:1777–1799.

Lawrence JB, Taneja K, Singer RH: Temporal resolution and sequential expression of muscle-specific genes revealed by in situ hybridization. Dev Biol 1989; 133:235–246.

Leary JJ, Brigati DJ, Ward DC: Rapid and sensitive colorimetric method for visualizing biotin-labeled DNA probes hybridized to DNA or RNA immobilized on nitrocellulose: Bio-blots. Proc Natl Acad Sci USA 1983; 80:4045–4049.

Lewis ME, Krause RD, Roberts LJ: Recent developments in the use of synthetic oligonucleotides for in situ hybridization histochemistry. Synapse 1988; 2:308–316.

Lloyd RV, Jin L, Bonnerup MK: In situ hybridization in diagnostic pathology. Mayo Clin Proc 1994; 69:597–598.

Mandry P, Murray AB, Hofler H: In situ hybridization of cytospin preparations: A rapid nonisotopic screening method for isolated cells. Biotech Histochem 1994; 69:165–170.

Martino TA, Liu P, Sole MJ: Viral infection and the pathogenesis of dilated cardiomyopathy [review]. Circ Res 1994; 74:182–188.

Masih AS, Stoler MH, Farrow GM, Johansson SL: Human papillomavirus in penile squamous cell lesions. A comparison of an isotopic RNA and two commercial nonisotopic DNA in situ hybridization methods. Arch Pathol Lab Med 1993; 117:302–307.

Melton DA, Krieg PA, Rebagliati MR, et al: Efficient in vitro synthesis of biologically active RNA and RNA hybridization probes from plasmids containing a bacteriophage SP 6 promoter. Nucleic Acids Res 1984; 12:7035–7056.

Niedobitek G, Herbst H: Applications of in situ hybridization. Int Rev Exp Pathol 1991; 32:1–56.

Nuovo GJ, Gallery F, MacConnell P, et al: An improved technique for the in situ detection of DNA after polymerase chain reaction amplification. Am J Pathol 1991a; 139:1239–1244.

Nuovo GJ, MacConnell P, Forde A, Delvenne P: Detection of human papillomavirus DNA in formalin-fixed tissues by in situ hybridization after

7

amplification by polymerase chain reaction. Am J Pathol 1991b; 139:847–854.
Nuovo GJ, Gallery F, Hom R, et al: Importance of different variables for enhancing in situ detection of PCR-amplified DNA. PCR Methods Applic 1993; 2:305–312.
Nuovo GJ: Questioning in situ PCR. In situ cDNA polymerase chain reaction: A novel technique for detecting mRNA expression [letter]. Am J Pathol 1994; 145:741.
Nuovo GJ, Richart RM: Buffered formalin is the superior fixative for the detection of HPV DNA by in situ hybridization analysis. Am J Pathol 1989a; 134:837–842.
Nuovo GJ, Richart RM: A comparison of biotin- and ^{35}S-based in situ hybridization methodologies for detection of human papillomavirus DNA [published erratum appears in Lab Invest 1989; 61:538]. Lab Invest 1989b; 61:471–476.
Nuovo GJ, Silverstein SJ: Comparison of formalin, buffered formalin, and Bouin's fixation on the detection of human papillomavirus deoxyribonucleic acid from genital lesions. Lab Invest 1988; 59:720–724.
Orth G, Jeanteur P, Croissant O: Evidence for and localization of vegetative viral DNA replication by autoradiographic detection of RNA-DNA hybrids in sections of tumors induced by Shope papillomavirus. Proc Natl Acad Sci USA 1971; 68:1876–1880.
Pardue ML, Gall JG: Molecular hybridization of radioactive DNA to the DNA of cytological preparations. Proc Natl Acad Sci USA 1969; 64:600–604.
Pardue ML, Gall JG: Chromosomal localization of mouse satellite DNA. Science 1970; 168:1356–1358.
Park JS, Kurman RJ, Kessis TD, Shah KV: Comparison of peroxidase-labeled DNA probes with radioactive RNA probes for detection of human papillomaviruses by in situ hybridization in paraffin sections. Mod Pathol 1991; 4:81–85.
Reed JA, Brigati DJ, Flynn SD, et al: Immunocytochemical identification of *Rochalimaea henselae* in bacillary (epithelioid) angiomatosis, parenchymal bacillary peliosis, and persistent fever with bacteremia. Am J Surg Pathol 1992; 16:650–657.
Rentrop M, Knapp B, Winter H, Schweizer J: Aminoalkylsilane-treated glass slides as support for in situ hybridization of keratin c-DNAs to frozen sections under varying fixation and pretreatment conditions. Histochem J 1986; 18:271–276.
Rigby PW, Dieckmann M, Rhodes C, et al: Labelling deoxynucleic acid to high-specific activity in vitro by nick-translation with DNA polymerase I. J Mol Biol 1977; 113:237–251.
Roberts R: Impact for molecular biology in cardiology. Am J Physiol 1991; 261(4, Suppl):8–14.
Robertson JF, Dixon AR, Nicholson RI, et al: Confirmation of a prognostic index for patients with metastatic breast cancer treated by endocrine therapy. Breast Cancer Res Treat 1992; 22:221–227.
Sambrook J, Fritsch EF, Maniatis T: Molecular Cloning: A Laboratory Manual, Vols 1–3. Cold Spring Harbor, NY, Cold Spring Harbor Laboratory, 1989.
Schiffman MH: Validation of hybridization assays: Correlation of filter in situ, dot blot and PCR with Southern blot [review]. Lyon, France, IARC Scientific Publications 1992; 119:169–179.
Segal GH, Shick E, Fishleder AJ, et al: In situ hybridization analysis of lymphoproliferative disorders: Assessment of clonality by immunoglobulin light chain messenger RNA expression. Diagn Mol Path 1994; 3:170–177.
Stoler MH: In situ hybridization. Clin Lab Med 1990a; 10:215–236.
Stoler MH, Broker TR: In situ hybridization detection of human papillomavirus DNAs and messenger RNAs in genital condylomas and a cervical carcinoma. Hum Pathol 1986a; 17:1250–1258.
Stoler MH, Eskin TA, Benn S, et al: Human T-cell lymphotropic virus type III infection of the central nervous system. A preliminary in situ analysis. JAMA 1986b; 256:2360–2364.
Stoler MH, Ratliff NB: Potential and problems of the in situ molecular detection of viral genomes [editorial; comment]. Am J Clin Pathol 1990b; 93:714–716.
Stoler MH, Rhodes CR, Whitbeck A, et al: Human papillomavirus type 16 and 18 gene expression in cervical neoplasias. Hum Pathol 1992; 23:117–128.
Stoler MH, Wolinsky SM, Whitbeck A, et al: Differentiation-linked human papillomavirus types 6 and 11 transcription in genital condylomata revealed by in situ hybridization with message-specific RNA probes. Virology 1989; 172:331–340.
Taneja K, Singer RH: Use of oligodeoxynucleotide probes for quantitative in situ hybridization to actin mRNA. Anal Biochem 1987; 166:389–398.
Tecott LH, Barchas JD, Eberwine JH: In situ transcription: Specific synthesis of complementary DNA in fixed tissue sections. Science 1988; 240:1661–1664.
Trask BJ: Fluorescence in situ hybridization: Applications in cytogenetics and gene mapping. Trends Genet 1991; 7:149–154.
Valenstein PN: Evaluating diagnostic tests with imperfect standards [review]. Am J Clin Pathol 1990; 93:252–258.
Valentino KL, Eberwine JH, Barchas JD: In situ hybridization: Applications to neurobiology. New York: Oxford University Press, 1987.
zur Hausen H, Schultz-Holthausen H: Detection of Epstein-Barr viral genomes in human tumor cells by nucleic acid hybridization. *In* Biggs PM, de-The G, Payne LN (eds): Oncogenesis and Herpes. Lyon, France, International Agency for Research on Cancer, 1972, pp 321–325.

Chapter 62

Blood Groups, Human Leukocyte Antigens and DNA Polymorphism, and Parentage Testing

Herbert F. Polesky, M.D.

"In cases of disputed parentage the laboratory shall utilize a group of tests for genetic markers that includes multiple systems. . . . This group of tests must provide a falsely accused man with, on the average, at least a 95% probability of obtaining evidence of nonpaternity" (Standards for Parentage Testing Laboratories, 1994).

A frequently quoted early reference to disputed parentage appears in Kings (3:16–27), in which Solomon makes a decision about the maternity of a disputed child by threatening to use his sword to provide each claimant with a portion of the child. When paternity is in dispute, the arbiter of truth often is faced with the dilemma similar to that faced by Solomon: lack of witnesses to the event and the likelihood that the principals might not know or tell the truth.

The discovery of the ABO blood group by Landsteiner (in 1900) and the recognition that these measurable characteristics followed the genetic rules described by Gregor Mendel provided objective laboratory evidence that could be used by courts to aid in deciding when a person has been falsely accused of paternity. In the United States, laws addressing the use of genetic markers for proving nonpaternity were enacted in 1935 (Schatkin, 1952). In the ensuing years, knowledge about useful genetic marker systems increased dramatically. By 1976, joint guidelines developed by an American Medical Association–American Bar Association (AMA-ABA) committee recommended seven systems for routine blood group investigations in cases of disputed parentage (ABO, Rh, MNSs, Kell, Duffy, Kidd, and HLA) (Miale, 1976). Other genetic systems such as polymorphic serum proteins and red blood cell enzymes were also recognized as useful. The use of mathematical estimates of paternity was recommended in cases in which no exclusion was observed.

In 1983, as a follow-up to the AMA-ABA report and to an international conference (Airlie, 1982) on Inclusion Probabilities in Parentage Testing, the American Association of Blood Banks (AABB) committee on parentage testing published *Guidelines for Reporting Estimates of Probability of Paternity* (Walker, 1983), which advised testing multiple systems (the choice is left to the expert) to provide evidence of nonpaternity 95% of the time when a falsely accused man is tested. (Table 62–1 summarizes an AABB survey of the systems used in 1993.) At the time these guidelines were developed, the significance of deoxyribonucleic acid (DNA) restriction fragment length polymorphism (RFLP) described in 1980 (Botstein, 1980) for routine parentage testing was not widely

7

Table 62–1. SURVEY OF SYSTEMS USED BY PARENTAGE TESTING LABORATORIES

Genetic Markers	Number of Cases	%
Red blood cell antigens	132,000	73
HLA—serologic	117,000	65
Red blood cell enzymes and serum proteins	48,000	27
DNA	135,000	75

Data from the American Association of Blood Banks, Bethesda, Maryland, 1993.

Table 62–2. POWER OF EXCLUSION (A): SELECTED TEST SYSTEMS IN DIFFERENT POPULATIONS

System	White	Black
ABO	0.166	0.163
Rh	0.283	0.182
MNSs	0.304	0.269
FXIII B	0.209	0.252
GCi	0.31	0.252
BF	0.137	0.214
ACP	0.239	0.174
PGM1i	0.313	0.27

appreciated. However, in 1990, when the first edition of *Standards for Parentage Testing Laboratories* was published by the AABB, specific requirements for RFLP testing were included along with those for red blood cell surface antigens, human leukocyte antigens (HLAs), red blood cell enzymes, and serum protein genetic markers. This document formed the basis for an inspection and accreditation program that includes specifics about the identification of the subjects tested, the testing methods, the calculations, and the reporting. In 1994, a revised Standards was published with a section on DNA polymorphism testing that addresses both RFLP and polymerase chain reaction (PCR) amplification methods.

EXCLUSION OF PARENTAGE

The primary goal of genetic marker testing in cases of disputed parentage is to identify the biological parent of a given child. Although this cannot be done with absolute certainty, genetic marker tests can provide objective evidence of nonparentage. By using multiple genetic systems, it is possible to exclude most (>99%) but not all nonparents. Before testing a trio, it is possible to provide an estimate of the average chance that testing will prove nonparentage if the accused is not the parent.

Power of Exclusion

For each genetic system, an average power of exclusion (A) can be calculated based on the gene frequencies for the alleles in the system. The general equation, $A = pq(1 - pq)$, for a two-allele system was reported by Wiener in 1930. When a system has multiple alleles, more complex formulas are required (Walker, 1978). The general equation has also been adapted (Brenner, 1990) to determine A for DNA systems that do not have discrete alleles as follows:

$$A = h^2(1 - hH^2) \qquad (62\text{-}1)$$

where H is the percent homozygosity and h the percent heterozygosity observed at the locus. Table 62–2 shows A values for selected systems in different racial groups.

Cumulative Probability of Exclusion

When testing includes several independent genetic systems, a cumulative probability of exclusion (CPE) can be calculated by using the following formula:

$$CPE = 1 - (1 - P1)(1 - P2)(1 - P3) \ . \ . \ . \ (1 - Pn) \qquad (62\text{-}2)$$

where P is the A for each system used. As shown in Figure 62–1, as more and more systems are used, fewer and fewer nonparents are excluded by each additional test.

In systems that follow the rules of mendelian genetics, exclusions are identified by finding exceptions to the expected inheritance pattern. Interpretation of test results when paternity is in question usually depends on assuming that the sample defined as maternal is from the child's biological mother. The child's and mother's phenotypes should be compared to determine if results are consistent with expected inheritance patterns. An allele present in the child but not in the mother is referred to as the obligatory paternal gene (*OG*). If both alleles in the child and mother are identical, then there are alternate (two) possibilities for the paternal gene.

If the tested male does not have the possibility of passing the *OG* and the marker for the gene is absent in the presumed mother, the exclusion observed is termed direct (Table 62–3). This type of exclusion in one genetic system is usually enough to conclude that the tested male is not the biological father of the child in question. (In DNA systems, because of possible mutations, an exclusion at a single locus is not considered enough evidence to establish nonpaternity [Standards, 1994].) A direct exclusion also occurs when the child or the tested male is heterozygous and the two markers identified are absent in the other person. This type of direct exclusion sometimes is referred to as a two-haplotype exclu-

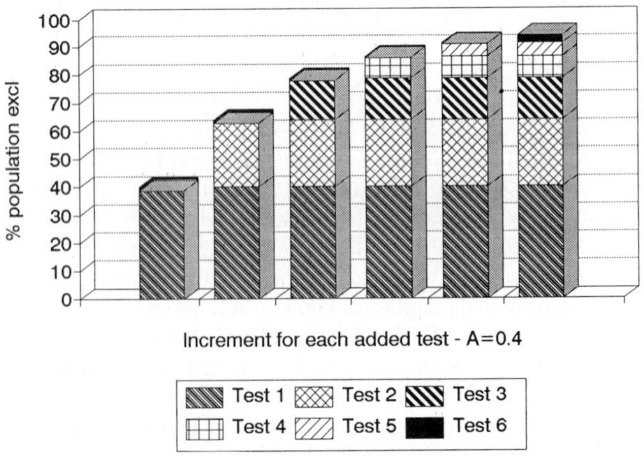

Figure 62–1. Cumulative power of exclusion. The percent of the population excluded by each additional test becomes smaller and smaller. The overall exclusion probability of the six tests is 95.3%. If a seventh test with A = 0.5 were done, only an additional 2.4% of the population would be excluded ([1 − 0.953] × 0.5 = 0.235).

Table 62–3. EXCLUSION OF PARENTAGE: PHENOTYPE (GENOTYPES)

Type of Exclusion	Child	Mother	Tested Man	OG(s)
Direct	AB (ab)	A (aa, ao)	O (oo)	b
	1,2:8,44	2,3:8,44	1,24:35,62	1,8 or 1,44
	3.25:4.76	3.25:5.31	3.25:5.66	4.76
Two haplotype	A (aa or a″x″)	A (aa, or a″x″)	BR (br)	a or ″x″
	1,2:8,44	1,2:8,44	3,33:7,27	1,8; 1,44;,2,8; or 2,44
Indirect	3.25:4.76	3.25:4.76	5.31	3.25 or 4.76
	Jk (a+b−) [aa or a″x″]	Jk (a+b+) [ab]	Jk (a−b+) [bb or b″x″]	a or ″x″
	1,X:8,Y	1,3:7,8	2,X:44,Y	1,8; 1,Y; X,8; or X,Y
Probable	R2r (cDE/ce)	R2 (cDE/CE)	R1R2 (CDe/cDE) or Rzr (CDE/ce)*	r (ce) or Ro (cDe)

*Frequency of Rz (CDE) is between 0.02 and 0.004.

sion. In motherless cases (i.e., in which only the child and alleged father are available for testing), if the tested man or child has two haplotypes neither of which is in the other, it is possible to prove nonpaternity.

Absence of an expected genetic marker in the child when the parent in question appears to be homozygous for the gene is called an indirect exclusion. This is sometimes called reverse homozygosity. One indirect exclusion is not sufficient evidence to conclude that the tested male is not the father. Interpretation of reverse homozygosity as an indirect exclusion presumes that both the tested subjects have two identical alleles at the locus, when in fact it is possible that a rare null (or other undetected allele) is present in the child as well as the parent in question. The finding of indirect exclusions in two independent systems usually is sufficient evidence to reach a conclusion of nonpaternity.

CHOOSING A GENETIC SYSTEM FOR USE IN PARENTAGE TESTING

The model genetic system for parentage testing would be one in which a unique marker can be found in both the child and putative parent. At present, short of gene sequencing, none of the marker systems provide such specific findings. Thus, multiple genetic systems that meet certain criteria are used for parentage testing. Ideally, the system should have multiple alleles distributed in the population so that there is a high power of exclusion and the least common phenotype has a frequency that can be determined reliably. All markers in the system should be expressed (no null allele) as codominant and should be stable under usual storage conditions. Methods for detecting the markers should be reliable, reproducible, and feasible for a large number of laboratories. The genetics of the system must be known and must follow established inheritance patterns (mendelian laws). Mutation and recombination rates should be known to be low. The system should be independent of other markers routinely tested. If the system is intended for calculating estimates of paternity, the gene frequencies in various populations must be established.

Most of the genetic systems currently used have one or more pitfalls that must be considered before inclusion in a battery of tests to determine parentage. In systems in which mutation or recombination occurs, these must be considered in interpretation of results. Common to many systems is the problem of null alleles or quantitative variants that make interpretation difficult when there is reverse homozygosity. In some systems, variants are detectable by one method or set of reagents but not by another. Biological variation in the stability of various markers can occur during shipment or storage. In some systems in which detection requires the use of antibodies, variation in reagents can create problems unless appropriate quality control procedures are used.

A large number of genetic systems used in parentage testing are well developed before birth; thus, it is feasible to perform tests on cord blood collected from the child at delivery. Samples of fetal tissue similar to those used for prenatal diagnosis of certain genetic disorders can be used for parentage testing and forensic analysis in criminal cases (e.g., determining if an accused man in a rape case is the father). Some markers fail to be fully expressed until a certain age, limiting the use of selected systems unless the child is of an appropriate age.

Red Blood Cell Antigen Systems

Six red blood cell antigen systems (ABO, Rh, MNSs, Kell, Duffy, and Kidd) are commonly used for paternity testing. Typing methods used are those rountinely performed in immunohematology laboratories, including tube tests and microtiter plates. AABB standards require that these tests be conducted twice independently and with reagents from different sources. The requirement for duplicate testing has some merit, because reagents can react differently with cells from different persons, depending on the test conditions. When antiglobulin reagents are used, tests to show that cells are nonreactive should be performed. A specific, direct antiglobulin test is necessary only when all tests using antiglobulin are reactive. Quality assurance of typing reagents must be carried out to demonstrate reactivity and specificity by the method used.

In cases with an inconsistency in a single system between mother and child (such as reverse homozygosity), absorption and elution studies may be helpful to confirm the presence of depressed antigens. At times, the only way to resolve apparent inconsistent results is to get new samples or to type additional family members.

ABO Blood Group

ABO blood grouping has traditionally been a standard in cases of disputed parentage. When cell and serum typing are done, test results usually are unambiguous. Care must be taken when monoclonal reagents are used and results are not as expected (Stroup, 1990). The interpretation of parentage depends on remembering that only the probable genotype can be inferred from the observed phenotype, unless the tested male is O (OO) or AB or if the presumed mother is A or B and the child is O. If cells type as A or AB, subtyping may occasionally be useful. Interpretation of subgrouping for A1 or A2 must be done with caution because the reagents for this test are highly variable. In some families, it has been shown that the transferase (the gene product) reacts at a different pH or competes for a common substrate. When a specific transferase is present, cells expected to type as A1B sometimes type as A2B because of a superstrong B (Frederick, 1985). ABO variants are more common in certain racial groups than in others. In a rare variant that has been described, the Bombay phenotype, there is failure to express an expected A or B antigen; however, the serum of these individuals contain anti-H, which should be easily detected if group O cells are used for reverse grouping. Another rare phenotype that has been reported is *cis* AB, in which persons inherit A and B as a single allele AB (Salmon, 1984).

Rh Blood Group

The Rh system is one of the most informative of the red blood cell antigen systems. Routine testing with anti-D, -C, -E, -c, -e (in E positives) and -Cw (in C positives) makes it possible to identify 10 common phenotypes and numerous probable genotypes. In the past there has been much debate about the nomenclature in this system and whether there are three closely linked genes or a single gene producing a series of antigens. Current data from gene sequencing of the RH region on chromosome 1 indicate the presence of two genes, one for D and one for CcEe (Colin, 1991). Each person has two haplotypes, each of which has multiple markers recognized by typing reagents. The test results on one person can suggest only the most probable phenotype. The race of the person being tested also must be considered because the haplotype frequencies differ among racial groups. The genotype can be inferred from the results obtained on other members of the trio (Table 62–4). The interpretation of these tests is important in deciding about an exclusion or in assigning a value to the likelihood ratio. In addition to the common haplotypes, several rare haplotypes have been described with expected antigens missing or suppressed (Tippett, 1987). The occurrence of one of these haplotypes in a trio can result in an apparent maternal exclusion or an indirect exclusion of the biological father. The specificity of the reagents used in routine Rh typing occasionally fails to detect the antigens present. This problem occurs because many of the antibodies recognize compound antigens (e.g., anti-C often contains anti-Ce [rhi] and does not react strongly with cells containing the haplotype CDE [Rz]). When unusual findings occur in Rh typing, it is important to use different antisera and methods, to consider absorption and elution studies, and to study other family members.

Table 62–4. GENOTYPES POSSIBLE BASED ON OBSERVED PHENOTYPE

Test Result*	Possible Genotypes	Comments
R1R2 (CcDEe)	R1R2 (CDe/cDE)	
	R1r″ (CDe/cE)	
	R2r′ (cDE/Ce)	
	Rzr (CDE/ce)	
	ryRo (CE/cDE)	
MNSs	MSNs	
	MsNS	
MNS	MSNS	
	MSNSu	In blacks
	MSuNS	In blacks
ACP-A	AA	
	A″x″	Null
HLA-A1,-B8	1,1 ; 8,8	Homozygous 1,8
	1,X:8,Y	
	1,1:8,Y	
	1,X:8,8	
DNA 3.45	3.45, 3.45	
	3.45, null	

*Most probable phenotype.

MNSs System

The MNSs system is more likely to identify nonfathers than any other red blood cell antigen system. In interpreting test results, it is important to be cautious about assigning genotype from the observed phenotype when a person types as positive for M, N, S, and s. In blacks, a frequently observed allele, S^u, can be misinterpreted as absence of an expected gene product. Persons appearing to be homozygous S or s can, in reality, be SS^u or sS^u. This finding can occur with both M and N, and some persons can type as S negative, s negative. These people usually also are U negative (Holliman, 1989). Other rare alleles, such as M^g and M^k, may give results that appear to exclude parentage when, in fact, their existence in a parent and child almost proves parentage. The typing reagents used for M and N come from various sources (lectin, animal, human). Test results do not necessarily agree when the same sample is tested with different reagents. For this reason, independent duplicate tests and good quality control are essential for accurate results. Antibodies to several low-frequency antigens associated with the MNSs system can be present in the typing reagents. Failure to recognize these contaminants can lead to incorrect interpretation of test results.

Kell, Duffy, and Kidd

Reagents for typing the antigens in the Kell, Duffy, and Kidd systems often require antiglobulin for detection. When a sample tests as heterozygous for all these markers [Kk, Fy(a + b +), and Jk(a + b +)], it is essential to determine that sample is negative in a direct antiglobulin test. Null alleles are present in all of these systems, and although they are rare in Kell and Kidd, they are fairly common in Duffy. In blacks, Fy(a − b −) is the most common phenotype (68%) and the *FY* gene has a frequency of 0.80. Reverse homozygosity is frequent, and apparent maternal exclusion or a single indirect exclusion of paternity is common. In most studies, *FY* is rarely found in whites (Martin, 1983).

Other Blood Group Systems

P, Lutheran, Lewis, Xg, and tests for some of the high- and low-frequency blood group antigens have been used for parentage determination. The chance of obtaining useful information from these markers is limited. Xg^a typing excludes only paternity if the child in question is a female and the mother is Xg (a −). Finding a low-frequency marker or the absence of a high-frequency antigen in the child and tested male is suggestive of paternity when it is possible to exclude access to the mother by a close relative of the alleged father. Lewis typing to be useful must be combined with testing of secretor status and limited to cases in which the child is at least 1 year old. The only chance of finding an exclusion with Lewis is when both the tested male and presumed mother are of the genotype *lele* (phenotype Le [a − b −]) (Race, 1968).

Serum Protein Systems

Numerous polymorphic serum protein genetic systems have been used for determining disputed parentage. Typing of the allelic products in most of these systems is done by electrophoretic separation of the protein bands, which are detected by staining, immunofixation, or a reaction with a specific substrate. The AABB standards require that appropriate controls be used with each electrophoretic run, and the control must include a sample with two or more allotypes. Because these tests usually are run in batches, including several controls in each batch is advisable. Two independent readings of the pattern should be carried out. When rare variants are found, they should be compared with specific controls or verified by an independent laboratory. Both isoelectric focusing (IEF) and conventional techniques may be required to identify common allotypes in some systems. Photographs or storage of gels or supporting membranes can provide a permanent record of the test results in many protein marker systems.

Group-Specific Component

The group-specific component (GC) system is one of the most informative protein marker systems, with the capacity to exclude more than 30% of falsely accused males. The detection of GC polymorphism has evolved from the evaluation of the position of immunoprecipitin arcs (with immunoelectrophoresis) to a clear separation of the three common allotypes, 1s, 1f, and 2, by IEF (Dykes, 1984a). In addition, many rare variants have been identified as markers in specific populations. The incidence of null alleles is very low in this system, and some of the variants are difficult to identify unless conventional immunofixation is used. GC typing can also be done using PCR to detect an amplified DNA fragment length polymorphism (Ampflp) GC. The three alleles, A, B, and C, show good correlation with testing by IEF.

Haptoglobin

The α2-globulin, haptoglobin (HP), which binds free hemoglobin, was the first serum protein described as polymorphic, based on electrophoretic separation in starch gel (Smithies, 1955). Typing of HP on polyacrylamide gels is fairly straightforward, provided that the sample is incubated with a hemolysate before electrophoresis. The hemolysate should be prepared at a concentration of about 300 mg/dL from cells that do not contain a variant form of hemoglobin. Problems can occur in HP phenotyping when the sample is from a child younger than 3 months, because of a relative ahaptoglobinemia. Detectable HP may be minimal in an individual with chronic hemolysis. HP also can be absent in persons homozygous for the rare null allele (HP^0). Several variant forms of HP with unusual hemoglobin-binding capacity have been identified (Bowman, 1982). Methods for subtyping the common 1 allele into 1S and 1F have been described (Teige, 1985); however, these methods are not generally used in parentage testing.

Properdin Factor B

Properdin factor B (BF), a protein in the complement cascade, is phenotyped by agarose gel electrophoresis (Dykes, 1980). The genes for BF and the C4 system markers are located on the short arm of chromosome 6 within the region that codes for the major histocompatibility complex (MHC) (Mauff, 1988). Because of this linkage, likelihood ratios for test results from these systems and HLA are not independent and should not be multiplied to calculate the paternity index (PI).

Transferrin

The iron-binding protein transferrin (TF) has two common (C1 and C2) and at least six less frequent allotypes detectable by IEF (Dykes, 1984a). TF typing should be performed on serum because it is difficult to obtain reproducible results from anticoagulated samples. Ampholines used in this system, like other IEF systems, must be evaluated each time a new lot is used, and standard controls should be run on the new lot and in tandem with the current lot. This procedure determines whether adjustments in testing protocols are needed to compensate for variation in the reagents.

Plasminogen

Plasminogen (PLG) is a polymorphic protein phenotyped on thin-layer agarose gels after IEF (Dykes, 1984b). There are two common and several less frequently encountered allotypes. This protein can be typed from serum as well as from plasma, and although routine typing does not require pretreatment of the sample, several variants can be identified if the sample is treated with neuraminidase for 16 to 24 hours before focusing. Apparent reverse homozygosity (single indirect exclusion, mother-child inconsistency) best explained by the presence of a null gene is more common in this system than in most other serum protein systems.

Factor XIIIA and XIIIB

Factor XIII, fibrin-stabilizing factor, consists of two independent polymorphic peptide subunits, A and B, which can be phenotyped by combining IEF with immunoblotting. Plasma samples are used to type FXIIIA with its two common alleles, FXIIIA*1 and 2, and several variants. FXIIIB has three common alleles, FXIIIB*1, 2, and 3, and is tested by using serum pretreated with neuraminidase (Dykes, 1986).

Gamma Marker and Kappa Marker

The gamma marker (Gm) polymorphism is associated with specific amino acid sequences on the heavy chains of IgG. Each of the four subclasses of IgG has a different group of Gm markers (de Lange, 1988); thus, depending on the extent of testing, a person can have a complex Gm phenotype. Different haplotypes are found in various racial groups, making this a useful system in cases when racial admixture is suspected. Markers occur on the heavy chains of IgM and IgA. These are not as polymorphic as the Gm markers and are not very useful in parentage testing.

The Km markers, formerly known as Inv, are determinants on the light chains common to all immunoglobulin classes. Three markers have been identified, but only anti-Km 1 is readily available. When only one antigen is typed, the information obtained from these systems is limited. If a child types as Km 1+ and both the presumed mother and tested male are Km 1−, it is possible to conclude that the tested male is not the child's father; but if a child types as Km 1− (Km3Km3) and the alleged father is Km 1+, it is not possible to establish nonpaternity because the results will be the same for a male who is Km1Km1 (indirect exclusion) and a male who is Km1Km3 (not excluded). The same limitation is observed in other systems when testing for only one marker (i.e., using only anti-Fy^a or anti-Jk^a).

Hemagglutination inhibition is used to detect Gm and Km markers (Schanfield, 1975). Rh-positive red blood cells coated with anti-D are the indicator system. The anti-D coat (IgG) is selected for the specific Gm antigens present. The coated cells are added to a V-shaped, flexible microtiter plate with anti-Gm (agglutinator) along with a dilution of the sample being typed. If the unknown sample has the same specificity as the agglutinator, it neutralizes the agglutinator. After incubation at room temperature, the plates are centrifuged and then are placed at a 60-degree angle to the horizontal and observed for streaming. Streaming indicates that the unknown sample has inhibited hemagglutination by the agglutinator (anti-Gm) and has the same specificity as the anti-D coat. A sample that is of a different Gm specificity does not inhibit agglutination, and the indicator cells appear as a button in the bottom of the well. Careful attention to technical details is essential when performing Gm and Km typing. Variation in reagent specificity, microtiter plate lot, and temperature and humidity of the laboratory can make it difficult to obtain reproducible results with these test systems.

All samples tested for Gm and Km must be screened for the presence of antibodies reacting with the indicator system. If a specific or nonspecific agglutinator is present in the unknown, the test is invalid. Most of the time, these antibodies are nonspecific and are inactivated by preheating of the sample at 65°C for 10 minutes.

The age of the person being tested must be considered in evaluating Gm results. In children younger than 6 months, maternal IgG can be present in the circulation, and unless the phenotype of the infant and that of the mother are different, it is usually impossible to determine the paternal genetic contribution to the child until the child reaches 6 months of age.

Other Serum Protein Marker Systems

Several other polymorphic serum proteins are used in parentage testing, including α_1-antitrypsin (PI) amylase, C3, and C4. Before instituting routine testing with any of these systems, the investigator should be familiar with the genetics (frequency of amorphs, possible linkage with other systems, distribution in the population, and so on), the stability of the markers during shipment and storage, and the limitations and problems inherent in the test method.

Red Blood Cell Enzyme Systems

The general principles and methods used for phenotyping serum proteins by electrophoresis apply to red blood cell enzyme polymorphism. Detection systems depend on reaction of the enzyme with a substrate. Loss of activity occurs if samples are not properly collected and stored. Enzyme activity is preserved better during shipping and storage if red blood cells are collected in acid-citrate-dextrose, formula A (ACD-A). Red blood cells obtained from clotted or heparinized samples often result in test results that are nonreactive or difficult to interpret. Cells collected in tubes containing fluoride are not useful for enzyme phenotyping. Before testing, a hemolysate is prepared by washing the red blood cells with isotonic saline, diluting the sample (1 : 1) with distilled water, and placing on a vortex mixer for 30 seconds. Hemolysates that have been frozen can be used for phenotyping, although in some systems enzyme activity is lost during storage.

Acid Phosphatase

The acid phosphatase (ACP1), sometimes referred to as EAP, in human red blood cells has three common alleles (A, B, and C) and several rare variants (Miller, 1988). Hemolysates pretreated with a 0.1% solution of 2-mercaptoethanol (2ME) to maintain the protein in a reduced state are used for phenotyping. Testing is done by conventional electrophoresis using 1 g/dL agarose on gel bond film or by using IEF. In both methods, the gels are stained with 4-methyl-umbelliferyl-phosphate and read under long-wavelength ultraviolet (UV) light. Typing requires observation of not only the position of the bands but also their staining intensity. The reactivity of each isozyme with the substrate is different; thus, an expected gene product (A being the most labile) may not always be identified if samples have not been stored properly (Hopkinson, 1969).

Phosphoglucomutase

Phosphoglucomutase (PGM1) is a polymorphic red blood cell enzyme with more than 30 variants (Dykes, 1981; 1984a). Using standard starch or agarose gel methods, two common alleles (PGM1*1 and PGM1*2) with three phenotypes (1, 1-2, 2) are observed. Testing by IEF identifies 4 common alleles (1 = 1A or 1+ and 1B or 1−, 2 = 2A or 2+ and 2B or 2−) and 10 phenotypes. This method more than doubles the power of exclusion for the system (from 0.12 to 0.32) and increases direct exclusions from 47% to 76% (Dykes, 1981).

Phenotyping of PGM1 by conventional electrophoresis and IEF is performed by reacting the gel with a substrate containing glucose-1-phosphate and glucose-1-6-diphosphate, a hydrogen acceptor nicotinamide-adenine dinucleotide phosphate (NADP), an electron acceptor-donor mixture (monotetrazolium [MTT], glucose-6-phosphate dehydrogenase), and a stain (meldola blue). Because of the multiple bands present and the overlap that can occur with different variants, it is important that controls heterozygous for the common variants be run on each gel. Recombination at the PGM1 locus has been reported (Wetterling, 1990), but such events are very rare.

The locus for PGM1 is on chromosome 1, and two other PGM subsystems, PGM2 and PGM3, controlled by genes on chromosomes 4 and 6, respectively, have been identified. Neither of these two subsystems is very polymorphic, and generally they are not useful in parentage testing.

Esterase D

Esterase D (ESD) is a red blood cell enzyme with two common alleles (ESD*1, ESD*2) coded for by genes on chromosome 13. A homozygote individual has a single major isoenzyme band, whereas three bands are found in heterozygotes. Phenotyping on acrylamide by IEF makes it possible to identify ESD*5—a marker not usually separated from ESD*2 by conventional methods (Dykes, 1982). Hemolysates tested for ESD are pretreated with 0.1% 2ME. Focusing gels are stained with 4-methyl-umbelliferyl-acetate and read in long-wavelength UV light.

Glyoxalase I

Glyoxalase I (GLO1) is a marker with two common alleles (GLO1*1, GLO1*2) coded for by genes in chromosome 6 near to but independent of the MHC. Phenotyping is performed by conventional agarose electrophoresis, followed by staining with a coupled enzyme test (Kompf, 1975). After electrophoresis, the gel is placed in contact with a filter paper saturated with methyl glyoxal and reduced glutathione. Next, a blue-green agarose overlay containing an electron acceptor-doner (MTT, thiazoyl blue, and dichloroindophenol [DCIP]) is layered over the gel. Light-colored bands appear wherever the enzyme has reacted. GLO1 is a somewhat labile enzyme that tends to lose activity on prolonged storage.

Other Erythrocyte Enzyme Systems

Adenylate kinase (AK), adenosine deaminase (ADA), and 6-phosphogluconate dehydrogenase (6PGD) are red blood cell enzyme systems used by forensic laboratories. Methods exist for the simultaneous detection of these independent markers (Brinkmann, 1971). These systems are not very useful for parentage testing because high-frequency alleles (AK*1 = 0.96 – 0.99, ADA*1 = 0.96 – 0.98, 6PGD*A = 0.97) are found in most populations. In a few cases, finding a heterozygous individual with the infrequent allele (AK*2, ADA*2, 6PGD*C) can be very informative.

Glutamate pyruvate transaminase (GPT) is a polymorphic enzyme system with alleles distributed in most populations; however, to get reproducible results with this system, tests must be conducted on hemolysates prepared from freshly drawn samples.

Glucose-6-phosphate dehydrogenase (G6PD) is another enzyme system with potential for parentage testing, but its sex-linked inheritance pattern limits its usefulness.

Hemoglobin

Variant forms of hemoglobin (Hb), the major intracellular protein in red blood cells, can be detected by various electrophoretic methods. Testing for Hb variation is not rewarding in asymptomatic white persons because the frequency of the HbA phenotype is 0.999. Among blacks and certain other populations, the possibility of finding a variant is much greater, and typing can be helpful in determining parentage. The age of the child and the possibility that fetal forms (HbF and others) sometimes persist for a few months after birth must be considered in interpreting test results.

Human Leukocyte Antigen

The HLA system consists of at least 37 genes coding for Class I and II markers (Bodmer, 1994) located on the short arm of chromosome 6 in humans. A complete DNA sequence of the HLA-A, -B region has been published (Zemmour, 1992). In 1993, a survey of parentage testing laboratories conducted by the AABB indicated that testing for HLA-A, -B antigens by serologic methods was second to red blood cell antigens in terms of frequency of testing systems used for parentage testing in the United States. The DQA1 markers detected by PCR are also used by some laboratories for parentage and forensic testing.

The HLA system is very powerful in parentage testing because of the great diversity of these antigens in the population. Based on the close linkage of 40 A and 70 B specificities, it is possible to identify more than 700 haplotypes and approximately 180,000 phenotypes. There is linkage disequilibrium between HLA-A, -B (i.e., certain haplotype combinations, such as HLA-A2, -B44 or -A1, -B8 occur more often than would be predicted from the frequency of the antigens A1, A2, B8, and B44).

Serologic Testing

The AABB standards require that HLA typing for parentage testing must include all HLA-A and -B antigens, beyond provisional “w” characterizations, officially recognized by the World Health Organization (WHO) Committee on Nomenclature in 1980. It is also recommended that typing be performed for other recognized HLA specificities if the laboratory has appropriate typing sera.

HLA-A, -B typing for parentage testing is done by a complement-dependent lymphocytotoxicity method. A lymphocyte suspension containing at least 80% viable cells is incubated with multiple antisera. If the antibody has specificity for an antigen present on the test cells, cell killing occurs in the presence of an adequate amount of reactive complement. This is measured by failure of the cells to exclude a dye (Ray, 1982). Heparinized samples, which should not be refrigerated before harvesting the lymphocytes, are recommended for HLA typing. The lymphocytes should ideally be separated on a Hypaque-Ficoll density gradient within 24 hours of collection. Once harvested, lymphocytes can be stored for a few days in a culture medium.

Few of the currently available reagents are monospecific; thus, the AABB standards require that each antigen be defined by at least two different monospecific sera or by three multispecific sera. All individuals in a paternity case should be typed in the same laboratory by the same method and reagents to minimize the variability that can occur when cells are typed with reagents from different sources. Each sample must be plated on two separate trays or tray sets that are read independently and compared for consistency. In evaluating test results on a trio, it is useful to compare the reaction patterns of the child with those of the putative parents. This is particularly helpful when a split or rare antigen is present. It is important to have a system to avoid inadvertent typing of the same sample twice or mixing up of samples.

Interpretation of HLA test results can be complicated in rare instances (< 1.0%) where a cross-over between A and B subloci has occurred. Another problem with HLA typing is the failure to find all antigens present. Depending on the race of the tested person, blanks (alleles not defined by the available reagents) can be found. In most cases, the apparent blank is observed when the tested person is homozygous for the A or B marker. In other cases, the antisera cross-react with the undefined marker or the expected antigen(s) is not fully expressed (Lamm, 1983).

DNA POLYMORPHISMS

Testing of DNA polymorphisms commonly is used by parentage testing laboratories either alone or in combination with other marker systems. Analysis of these polymorphisms usually is based on RFLP or PCR amplification testing or both.

The AABB standards have defined criteria for the acceptance of a DNA marker system used in parentage testing. Each locus must be validated by family studies to exhibit mendelian inheritance and a low frequency of mutation or recombination. The chromosomal location shall be recorded by the International Human Gene Mapping Workshop, and characteristics of the loci (probe, restriction enzyme, primer sequence, and fragment sizes) should be documented in the literature. For all test systems, confirmatory testing by an independent laboratory shall be possible.

See Chapter 63 for DNA testing for forensics.

Restriction Fragment Length Polymorphism Testing

Many polymorphic RFLP loci have been described as part of the research to map the human genome (Watson, 1992). Identification of a specific locus requires a labeled short sequence of nucleotides complementary to a unique sequence in the DNA region being analyzed. Probes useful in parentage testing detect polymorphic restriction fragments at a single locus (simple diallelic, insertion/deletion, or variable number tandem repeats [VNTR]) (Baird 1986). Multilocus probes that detect hypervariable regions also have been described for identification of human pedigrees (Jeffreys, 1986). Amplification of regions with short tandem repeats (STR) (Weber, 1989) and minisatellite repeats (MVR) (Jeffreys, 1991) have also proved very useful in forensic, anthropologic, and parentage testing.

DNA is extracted and purified from a sample containing nucleated cells such as peripheral blood or a buccal swab. Occasionally the only sample available is fixed tissue. Special methods for obtaining and purifying the DNA from these samples must be used (Forsthoefel, 1992). A specific bacterial enzyme (restriction endonuclease) is used to cleave the isolated double-stranded DNA asymmetrically at places where a defined nucleotide sequence occurs (e.g., Eco RI, the nuclease from *Escherichia coli* RY 13, cleaves AG or GA). The restriction process splits DNA into multiple fragments of various molecular weights. At many loci, the size of these fragments is genetically determined. Gel electrophoresis is used to separate the fragments by molecular size (Southern, 1975). The fragments representing the loci of interest are detected by a labeled probe that binds to a complementary sequence of bases between two adjacent restriction sites. Before adding the probe, the separated DNA in the gel is depurinated and denatured. The resulting single-stranded DNA is transferred from the gel to a membrane (Southern blotting). A labeled probe is hybridized to the DNA on the membrane. Using carefully defined temperatures and other conditions, the probe for the loci anneals with the membrane-bound DNA fragments that share the same sequence (Maniatis, 1982). Localization of the labeled fragments on the membrane is accomplished by adding substrate that reacts with an enzyme bound to the probe or by overlaying it with film (autoradiography) if the probe is radioactive or chemiluminescent.

It is important to standardize procedures and include appropriate controls when testing RFLP systems. The amount of DNA extracted and used in the test system must be controlled, the reactivity of the enzyme used must be verified to ensure complete digestion of the DNA, and each electrophoretic run must include a human DNA control of known size. It is important to use size markers with multiple discrete fragments that span the range of alleles usually seen at the DNA locus being tested. AABB standards require that a mixture of DNA from the alleged parent and from the child be electrophoresed in the same lane. This is useful in evaluating the presence or absence of fragments that are of similar molecular weight.

Interpretation

Interpretation of the results of an RFLP system depends on matching of the child's observed band(s) and those in the presumed parents (Figs. 62–2 and 62–3). The child must have fragments that match one in each of his or her biological parents. The presence of a fragment in the child absent from both the mother and tested man is evidence of nonpaternity. Similarly, when the tested man has only a single fragment detected, it is expected that this will be present in his children. One should not usually conclude paternity is excluded based on the results from only one DNA system. These markers have a higher rate of mutation than do classic systems, null alleles may be present, or a second fragment is not identified because it is outside the size range of detection used (Chakraborty, 1994). Use of RFLP loci testing in combination with classic markers has validated that RFLP systems have observed exclusion probabilities similar to expected values (Endean, 1990b).

Polymerase Chain Reaction

The PCR reaction, first described by Mullis in 1986, uses thermocycling to denature the double-stranded DNA and promote annealing of specific primers to target sequence flanking the region of interest. This technique has made it

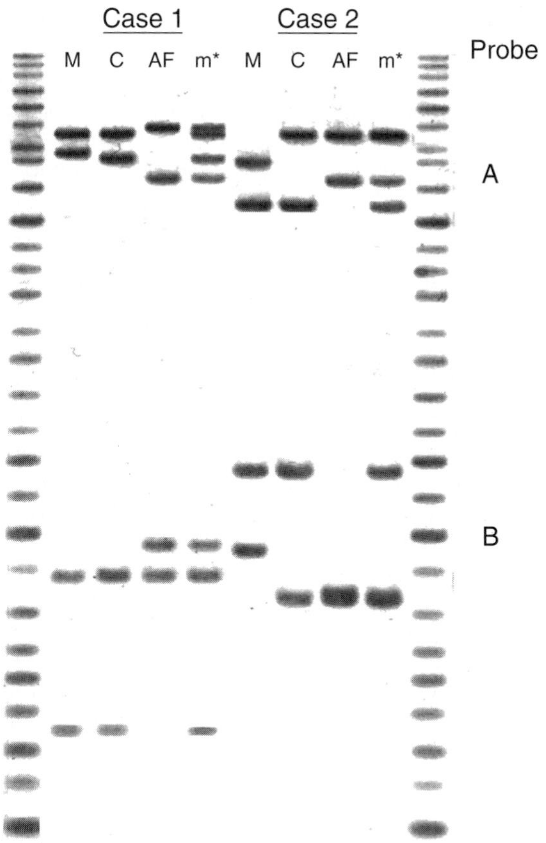

Figure 62–2. Membrane hybridized with two enzyme-labeled probes detecting RFLP loci D12S11 (*A*) and D17S79 (*B*). DNA from two trios restricted with Pst 1 and stained with alkaline phosphatase. Sizing ladders flank the two trios. The mother (M), child (C), alleged father (AF), and alleged father/child mix (m*) are shown. In case 1, the AF is excluded by probe A. Careful observation showed that the mix lane has 4 bands. In case 2, there is a match between the child and alleged father at both loci. Alleles are designated by kilobase size with the larger sizes at the top of the membrane.

possible to define a large number of alleles differing only by minor changes in sequence. The advantages of PCR for parentage and forensic testing are that only a minute sample of genomic DNA is needed, there is no need to isolate the sequence to be amplified, the test results are available quickly, and the conditions of sample storage are not usually critical.

HLA-DQA1

Detection of the eight alleles at the HLA-DQA1 locus (Erlich, 1986) was one of the first applications using PCR in parentage and forensic testing. The genes responsible for these HLA Class II antigens are identified by the use of biotinylated sequence-specific primers (SSP) and allele-specific oligonucleotide (ASO) probes in a reverse dotblot system. The DNA from the sample is amplified with the labeled primers. The reaction mixture is then flooded over a membrane containing a series of immobilized ASO probes. If an allele is present in the sample, the amplified sequence hybridizes to the dot containing the complementary DNA. After washing to remove unbound DNA, the dots that have bound DNA are detected by the reaction of the biotin in the amplified sequence with a streptavidin alkaline phosphatase conjugate. Although not routinely used in parentage or forensic identity testing, test systems using combinations of gene amplification by PCR with sequence-specific primers, sequence-specific oligonucleotide probes (SSOP), direct sequencing, and RFLP methods have been described for studies of the genes at the MHC locus (Allen, 1994; Bunce, 1995).

Amplified Fragment Length Polymorphisms

DNA polymorphisms occur at loci with length variations. These systems with markers having VNTR are identified by PCR. The AmpFLPs (or AFLP) are separated using high-resolution gel electrophoresis (Boerwinkle, 1989). The fragments produced by PCR are compared with allelic ladders containing fragments of known molecular weight. Simultaneous testing of several systems is possible as long as there are differences in the range of sizes for the alleles at each locus. Genetic systems detected by AmpFLPs are not usually as polymorphic as the RFLP systems. The first AmpFLP system to be used in forensic and paternity cases was a 3′ hypervariable region at the apolipoprotein B (ApoB) locus consisting of adenine and thymine nucleotide repeat units of 15 base pairs. This marker system has 23 alleles ranging from 611 to 931 base pairs and an average heterozygosity of 0.8. Exam-

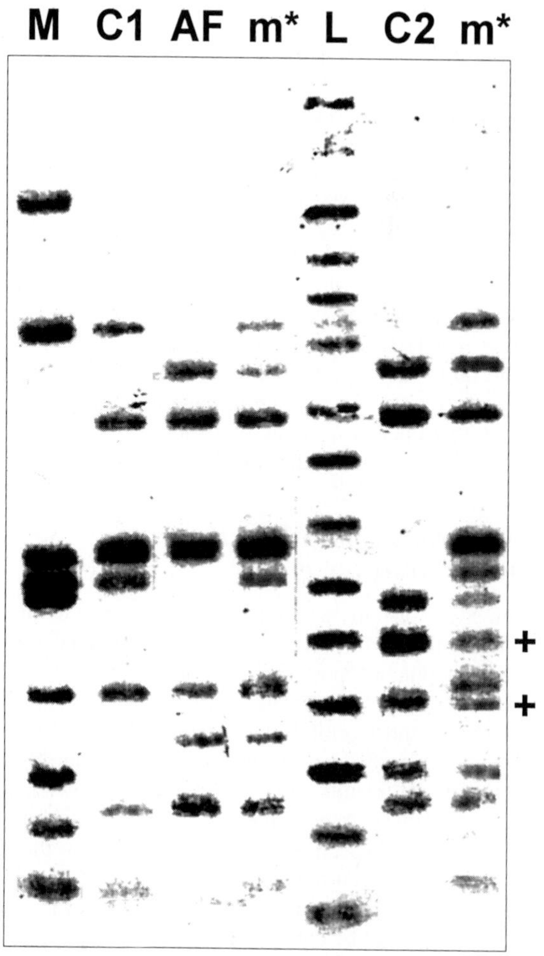

Figure 62–3. Membrane with a multilocus probe (DNF24). DNA from a case with two children tested. Lanes from left to right show the mother, child 1, alleged father, alleged father/child 1 mix, sizing ladder, child 2, alleged father/child 2 mix. Child 2 is excluded based on finding nonmatch with the bands marked by a +.

7

ples of other VNTR markers that are used include COLA2A1 (11 alleles of 31 to 34 repeats with a size range of 300 to 600 base pairs) and D1S80, a chromosome 1 locus (26 alleles of 16 repeats with a size range of 430 to 782 base pairs).

Short Tandem Repeats

Another type of length variation used in identity testing is based on STR loci. These loci that occur throughout the genome are made up of repeat units of three to seven nucleotides (Weber, 1989). Alleles are defined by the number of repeat units in the PCR-amplified product after electrophoretic separation on a polyacrylamide sequencing gel. Detection is accomplished using a label that has been incorporated in the primer. To increase the efficiency of the testing process, several marker systems are amplified together or mixed before electrophoresis. Examples of STR loci include THO1 (HUMTHO1) on chromosome 11 (8 alleles of a repeat of AATG ranging in size from 183 to 211 bases), vWF (HUMVWFA31) on chromosome 12 (7 alleles of a repeat of AGAT ranging in size from 143 to 167 bases), and FESFPS (HUMFESFPS) on chromosome 15 (6 alleles of a repeat of AAAT ranging in size from 226 to 246 bases). In a series of 50 paternity cases tested by conventional VNTR loci and 9 STR loci, it was found that both methods excluded the same 13 alleged fathers (based on two or more loci) (Alford, 1994). The likelihood of paternity for the 37 nonexcluded men based on the STR systems exceeded 99% in 36 cases.

Mitochondrial DNA

PCR amplification followed by sequencing can be used to identify a maternally derived polymorphism present in the hypervariable region of the D loop of mitochondrial DNA. Sequences of amplified DNA extracted from tissues and bones found in grave sites are compared with the DNA sequences from maternal descendants to establish relatedness (Holland, 1994). Using this method, bones thought to be from the family of Tsar Nicholas II (recovered at Yekaterinburg, Russia) have been shown to have mitochondrial DNA similar to that present in living descendants of Queen Victoria, the maternal grandmother of Tsarina Alexandra (Ivanov, 1993).

Polymerase Chain Reaction Quality Assurance

When PCR systems are used, it is necessary to monitor and validate the performance of the thermal cycler. Because minimal amounts of postamplification DNA can result in contamination of preamplification samples, it is essential that the laboratory and workflow be carefully designed to separate preamplification steps from areas where amplification and detection of results are carried out (Budowle, 1995; Dieffenbach, 1993). A negative control must be processed with each batch of specimens and tested to verify that contamination has not occurred. If the detection of PCR products requires electrophoresis, a mixture of DNA from the alleged father and child shall be coelectrophoresed in a single lane of the gel used to identify the allele. One problem associated with PCR is that if no product is found, one must be sure that the sample did not contain a substance that inhibited amplification.

OTHER TESTS

Examination of the length of the Y chromosome has been used to exclude paternity (de la Chapelle, 1967). Comparison of fluorescent markers on several chromosomes has also been used to exclude paternity or provide inclusionary estimates (Gürtler, 1986).

INCLUSION OF PARENTAGE

In providing estimates of inclusion of paternity, appropriate gene frequency tables should be used. In general, this means that a population of random persons of the same race has been phenotyped, that the size of the sample is large enough to provide gene frequencies with minimum errors of estimation for the alleles in the system, and that the tested male and biological father are from the same population. When multiple systems have been tested, the differences observed in gene frequencies in populations from various geographic locations become unimportant in calculations of the likelihood of paternity (Hummel, 1981). In some cases in which the tested male is of mixed racial background or from a population for which there are inadequate frequency tables, it could be impossible to provide a precise estimate of paternity. In these situations, comparisons with frequencies for several defined racial groups often are helpful.

Paternity Index Calculation

If, after testing multiple systems, the parent in dispute (almost always the possible father) is not excluded, an estimate of the possibility that the tested person could be the biological parent should be calculated. One general approach is referred to as the comparison of sperm method (Walker, 1978). This calculation compares the chance (x) that a sperm from a man of the phenotype of the tested male could have fertilized the ovum of the presumed mother with the chance (y) that a sperm from an untested male in the random population could have produced the child (Table 62–5). Likelihood ratios (x/y) are calculated for each independent genetic system using frequencies for *OG* or alternate paternal genetic contribution in the random population of the same race of the tested male. These values then are multiplied to derive the PI, which reflects the genetic odds in favor of paternity, given the phenotypes of the trio. Table 62–5 shows formulas for calculating the indexes with various phenotype combinations.

If the result of testing with a DNA-RFLP system is interpreted as a match between the child and presumed parent, calculation of a system index can be performed. A problem with RFLP systems not encountered with classic marker systems is that the fragments (alleles) occur as a continuum of sizes rather than as discrete markers. It is very difficult to distinguish between two alleles of similar size in kilobases that may differ by only a few base pairs. Measurement errors as well as minor technical variations in the method can affect the size assigned to an allele. A laboratory conducting RFLP testing needs to determine sigma (ability to reproduce results within and between runs using the same samples) and delta (minimum size difference between two bands that can be

Table 62–5. CALCULATION OF THE SYSTEM* RATIO (PATERNITY INDEX)

Mother	Child	Obligatory Genes (OG)	Tested Man	X	Y	Formula for Y Frequency	X/Y
A	A	a	A	1	0.25	p	4
A	A	a	AB	0.5	0.25	p	2
A	AB	b	B	1	0.4	q	2.5
A	AB	b	AB	0.5	0.4	q	1.25
AB	AB	a or b	A	1	0.65	p+q	1.54
AB	AB	a or b	B	1	0.65	p+q	1.54
AB	AB	a or b	AB	1	0.65	p+q	1.54
AB	AC	c	AC	0.5	0.3	r	1.67
BC	BC	b or c	BC	1	0.7	q+r	1.43
AC	AD	d	BD	0.5	0.05	s	10

*Hypothetical system with four codominant alleles p, q, r, and s measured by markers A, B, C, and D.

routinely detected) for each locus/probe/enzyme combination (Endean, 1990a) (Fig. 62–4). In determining allele frequencies, binning techniques are used to compensate for these variations before assigning a value for *y* (Allen, 1990). One method divides the size range of expected alleles into a series of fixed bins (Budowle, 1991). To determine allele frequency for the random man (*y*), the frequency value for the bin in which the band falls is used. With this approach, assigning values for bands close to the top or bottom of the bin may require combining data from two bins and may result in low index values. A second method preferred by the author uses a floating bin. The frequency for *y* is determined by counting all the observed bands in a bin that is determined by the size of the fragment +/− delta. Using this method, the size of the bin varies in relation to the allele size. A third method, known as the ceiling principle, was proposed in The National Research Council report in 1992 to ensure that in forensic identity, data presented to courts would be conservative. The ceiling sets an upper limit for the value of *y*. Thus, even if the allele is very rare, the index value will not exceed a fixed value (e.g., 20). The rationale for this approach is that it compensates for sampling errors and possible substructures in a population.

Likelihood of Parentage

Another useful estimate of parentage that combines the genetic testing with assumptions about prior events is the likelihood of paternity. Essen-Möller described this calculation based on Bayes' theorem in 1938 (Table 62–6). The estimate uses the PI to summarize the genetic information and P (a value for the prior probability) to account for the assumptions that the tested man

1. Was not sterile
2. Had access during the conceptive period
3. Is not a close (first-degree) relative of the father
4. And other possible fathers are from a population with similar gene frequencies

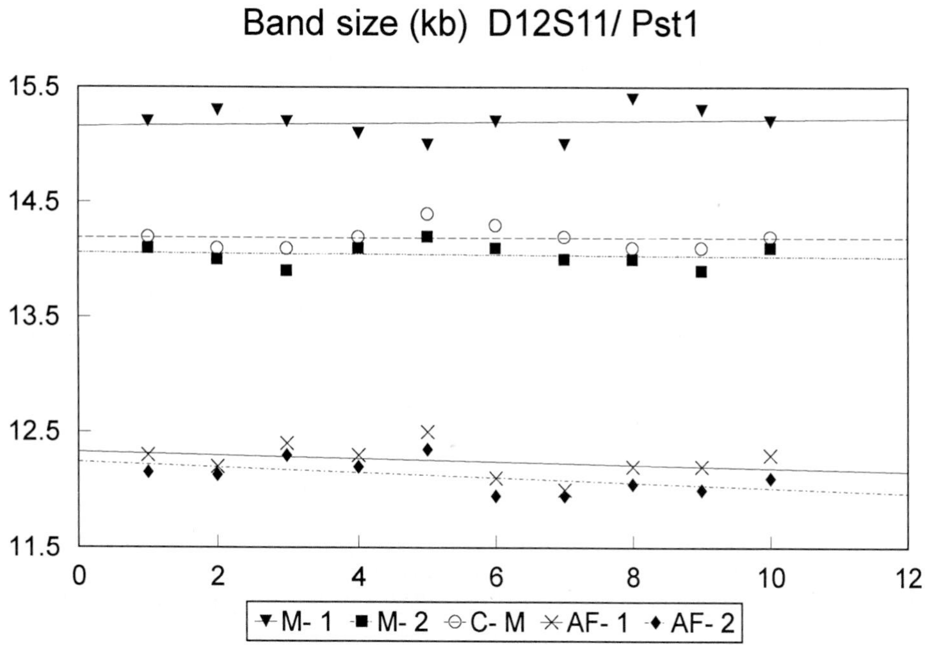

Figure 62–4. Determining sigma and delta. Measurements on five samples run 10 times to determine reproducibility (sigma) and ability to distinguish between two bands (delta) that have a similar size (AF-1, AF-2). Based on these observations, sigma for the band shared by the child and mother (C-M, M2) is 0.094. Delta is +/− 1.7. This figure is used to select the bin size for determining the frequency for *y* used to calculate the paternity index.

Table 62–6. FORMULA FOR THE LIKELIHOOD OF PARENTAGE (W)

Bayes' theorem is used to combine p with PI
p = prior probability of the nongenetic events
PI = summary of the genetic testing results

$$W = \frac{(p)\,(PI)}{(p)\,(PI) + (1 - p)}$$

$$W \times 100 = \%$$

If a P of 0.5 is used, this assigns an equal prior chance to the tested man and one untested man. Using this value, the likelihood of paternity (W) is equal to (PI/PI + 1) 100. Other values for the prior probability can be used in this calculation, but they introduce a bias against the tested man if greater than 0.5 and against the mother if less than 0.5.

The mathematical values obtained from the calculation of the PI or likelihood have special significance because in many jurisdictions the reported value may change the legal standing of the parties. For example, Minnesota Statute Section 257.55 shifts the burden of disproving paternity to the man if blood testing indicates a greater than 99% likelihood that he is the father.

If the tested man is not excluded, it always can be argued that testing was inadequate and evidence for exclusion will be found by testing another genetic system. This line of reasoning could be correct only if the tested man has been falsely accused. In addition to the average power of exclusion described earlier, it also is possible to calculate the frequency with which a random man will not be excluded (RMNE) based on a mother-child pair exhibiting the observed phenotypes (Salmon, 1983). This value is related to the actual power of exclusion for the tests performed.

Estimating Parentage with an Absent Parent

In many circumstances, a complete trio is not available to be tested. When the mother is not tested, the PI can be calculated based on results from the child and alleged father. If the child is heterozygous and the tested man has only one of the two alleles, one must assume that the missing marker is maternal. A range for the value of *x/y* can be calculated by assuming the man is the father and considering various possibilities for the mother's genotype (Table 62–7). Other methods of calculation adjust for the frequency of maternal phenotypes that would include or exclude the tested man (Brenner, 1993). When the alleged father is not available, it is possible to reconstruct his probable genotype by testing multiple polymorphic loci on samples from his parents, siblings, or other children (Mayr, 1983) (Fig. 62–5). If no exclusion is found, a PI can be calculated based on the assumption the individuals tested are genetically related to the absent putative parent.

DOCUMENTATION AND REPORTING

Results of parentage testing are often used in legal proceedings and may be subject to challenge by one of the parties involved. Thus, appropriate documentation of all aspects of the procedure is important. Accurate identification of individuals who present for testing is important to prevent someone from substituting for the party that is supposed to be tested. Requesting documents with pictures from each individual, taking Polaroid photographs, and obtaining a fingerprint are useful ways to confirm identity. Minimal medical information is required from the individuals, because medications and various substances of abuse have no effect on the outcome of the tests. If an individual has had a recent transfusion or has been the recipient of a bone marrow transplant, some of the tests performed on blood samples may give results reflecting the genetic characteristics of the donor. A system should be in place to record who drew the samples, when, and where. Samples should be labeled in the presence of the individual from whom they are obtained. Although most parentage cases are in civil actions, some jurisdictions require documents showing the chain of custody of samples similar to those used in criminal matters. It is important to maintain careful laboratory records of who did the testing, which reagents were used, and which controls were run. Policies for storage of worksheets, gels, membranes, photographs, and autoradiographs should be developed.

AABB standards specify that reports of parentage testing must contain information about the dates of sample collection, the racial origin(s) assigned for the purpose of calculating results, and the phenotype established for each individual in all the tested genetic systems. If exclusion of paternity is reported, an explanation of the basis for this conclusion should be provided. If an exclusion is not found, reports must

Table 62–7. RANGE OF SYSTEM INDEX RATIOS WHEN TESTING IS DONE ON ALLEGED FATHER AND CHILD ONLY*

Child	Tested Man	Paternal Gene	Possible Maternal Type	System Index—High	Possible Maternal Type	System Index—Low
A (*aa*)	AB (*ab*)	a	A (*aa*)	0.5/0.35 = 1.43	AB (*ab*)	0.5/0.35 = 1.43
AB (*ab*)	A (*aa*)	a	B (*bb*)	1/0.35 = 1.43	AB (*ab*)	1/0.95 = 1.05
AB (*ab*)	AB (*ab*)	*a* or *b*	B (*bb*)	0.5/0.35 = 1.43	AB (*ab*)	1/0.95 = 1.05
AC (*ac*)	BC (*bc*)	*c*	A (*aa*)	0.5/0.06 = 8.33	AC (*ac*)	0.5/0.41 = 1.22
AB (*ab*)	B (*bb,bx*)	*b*	A (*aa*)	1/0.6 = 1.67	AB (*ab*)	1/0.95 = 1.05
A (*aa, ax*)	B (*bb,bx*)	*a* or *x*	A (*aa*), AB (*ab*), AC (*ac*)	Tested man probably excluded		
B (*bb,bx*)	AC (*ac*)	*b*	B (*bb*), AB (*ab*), BC (*bc*)	Tested man excluded		

*Example based on red blood cell enzyme acid phosphate testing (genotype in italics).

Gene System	?? Child	Mother	OG	*AFs mother	*AFs father	System index
HLA	2,11; 7,8	2,30; 8,13	11, 7	1, 28; 8, 35	1,11; 7,8	69.27 or 16.3
D12S11 (Pst1)	11.47; 12.85	12.85; 13.76	11.47	9.75; 11.47	12.5	10.12
D17S79 (Pst1)	3.31; 3.45	3.37; 3.45	3.31	3.45; 3.82	3.31; 3.52	2.39

*Interpretation assumes deceased AF is the child of persons tested

Figure 62–5. Family testing to establish parentage. In this case, the presumed parents of the deceased alleged father were tested to reconstruct his probable genotype. In each of the three systems tested, the obligatory paternal gene (*OG*) is present in one of the child's presumed grandparents. Two system indexes are shown for HLA because the *y* value depends on the AF phenotype (11,28; 7,8; 1,11; 7,35; 11,28; 7,35 or 1.11; 7,8). Multiplying the indexes from the three independent systems provides a PI ranging between 393 and 1675. Both of these values result in a likelihood (see Table 62–6) greater than 99% using a 0.5 prior probability.

include the index for each system as well as a combined index value and probability expressed as a percentage with a definition of the prior probabilities used. In the unusual case in which results are inconclusive, an explanation of the problem should be provided.

CONCLUSION

Scientific evidence that aids in resolving cases of disputed parentage, and questions of relatedness can be obtained from testing multiple genetic systems. Although current technology provides exclusions of more than 99% of falsely accused men, it is not possible to exclude all nonfathers, nor is it possible to prove paternity by laboratory tests. The mathematical estimates derived from genetic marker tests when no exclusion is found are a significant source of data that can be used to establish parentage.

Alford RL, Hammond HA, Coto I, Caskey CT: Rapid and efficient resolution of parentage by amplification of short tandem repeats. Am J Hum Genet 1994; 55:190–195.

Allen M, Liu L, Gyllensten U: A comprehensive polymerase chain reaction-oligonucleotide typing system for the HLA class I A locus. Hum Immunol 1994; 40:25–32.

Allen RW, Wallhermfechtel M, Miller MV: The application of restriction fragment length polymorphism mapping to parentage testing. Transfusion 1990; 30:551–564.

Baird M, Blazas I, Guisti A, et al: Allele frequency distribution of two highly polymorphic DNA sequences in three ethnic groups and its application to the determination of paternity. Am J Hum Genet 1986; 39:489–501.

Bodmer JG, Marsh SGE, Albert ED, et al: Nomenclature for factors of the HLA system, 1994. Tissue Antigens 1994; 44:1–18.

Boerwinkle E, Xiong W, Fourest E, Chan L: Rapid typing of tandemly repeated hypervariable loci by polymerase chain reaction: Application to the apolipoprotein B 3′ hypervariable region. Proc Nat Acad Sci USA 1989; 86:212–216.

Botstein D, White RL, Skolnick M, Davis RW: Construction of a genetic linkage map in man using restriction fragment polymorphisms. Am J Hum Genet 1980; 32:314–331.

Bowman BH, Kurosky A: Haptoglobin: The evolutionary product of duplication, unequal crossing over and point mutation. Adv Hum Genet 1982; 12:189–261.

Brenner C, Morris JW: Paternity index calculations in single locus hypervariable DNA probes: Validation and other studies. *In* The International Symposium on Human Identification, 1989. Madison, Wisconsin, Promega Corporation, 1990, pp 21–53.

Brenner CH: A note on paternity computation in cases lacking a mother. Transfusion 1993; 33:51–54.

Brinkmann B, Thoma G: Simultaneous electrophoresis of three isoenzyme polymorphisms: 6 phosphogluconate dehydrogenase (6PGD), adenosine deaminase (ADA), adenylate kinase (AK). Vox Sang 1971; 21:90–93.

Budowle B. Guidelines for a quality assurance program for DNA analysis (TWGDAM). Crime Lab Digest 1995; 22:21–50.

Budowle B, Giusti AM, Waye JS, et al: Fixed-bin analysis for statistical evaluation of continuous distributions of allelic data from VNTR loci, for use in forensic comparisons. Am J Hum Genet 1991; 48:841–855.

Bunce M, Fanning GC, Welsh KI: Comprehensive, serologically equivalent DNA typing for HLA-B by PCR using sequence-specific primers (PCAR-SSP). Tissue Antigens 1995; 45:81–90.

Chakraborty R, Zhong Y, Budowle B: Nondeductibility of restriction fragments and independence of DNA fragment sizes within and between loci in RFLP typing of DNA. Am J Hum Genet 1994; 55:391–401.

Colin Y, Chérif-Zahar B, Le Van Kim C, et al: Genetic basis of the RhD-positive and RhD-negative blood group polymorphism as determined by Southern analysis. Blood 1991; 78:2747–2752.

de la Chapelle A, Fellman J, Unnerus V: Determination of human paternity from the length of the Y chromosome. Ann Genet 1967; 10:60–64.

de Lange GG, Van Leeuwen AM, van Eede PH, et al: Polymorphisms of immunoglobulins: Gm, Am, and Km typing. *In* Mayr WR (ed): Advances in Forensic Haemogenetics 2. Berlin, Springer-Verlag, 1988, pp 64–71.

Dieffenbach CW, Dveksler GS: Setting up a PCR laboratory. PCR Methods Appl 1993; 3:S2–S7.

Dykes DD, Miller S, Polesky H: Gene frequency distribution of F13A and F13B in U.S. whites, blacks, amerindians and Mexican-Americans. *In* Brinkmann B, Henningsen K (eds). Advances in Forensic Haemogenetics vol. 1. Berlin, Springer-Verlag, 1986, pp 262–267.

Dykes D, Mount M, Polesky H: Parentage testing using the serum protein plasminogen. Am J Clin Pathol 1984b; 82:722–725.

Dykes DD, Polesky HF. Properdin factor B (Bf) as an exclusion determinate in parentage testing. Hum Hered 1980; 30:286–290.

Dykes DD, Polesky HF: Isoelectric focusing of PGM1 (E.C.2.7.5.1.) on agarose: Application to cases of disputed parentage. Am J Clin Pathol 1981; 75:708–711.

Dykes DD, Polesky HF: Review of isoelectric focusing for Gc, PGM1, Tf, and Pi subtypes: Population distributions. CRC Crit Rev Clin Lab Sci 1984a; 20:115–151.

Dykes DD, Polesky HF, Miller S: Frequency of the ESD*5 allele in three ethnic groups in Minnesota. Hum Genet 1982; 62:162–163.

Endean DJ: RFLP analysis for paternity testing: Observations and caveats. *In* Proceedings of the 1989 International Symposium on Human Identification. Madison, Wisconsin, Promega Corporation, 1990a, pp 55–76.

Endean DJ, Schmitz AM, Callaway C, Gottschall JL: A comparative paternity study: DNA versus traditional testing. *In* Polesky HF, Mayr WR (eds): Advances in Forensic Haemogenetics vol. 3. Berlin, Springer-Verlag, 1990b, pp 80–82.

Erlich HA, Sheldon EL, Horn G: HLA typing using DNA probes. Biotechnology 1986; 4:975–981.

Essen-Möller E: Die Beweiskraft der Ähnlichkeit in Vateschaftsnachweis: Theoretische Grundlagen. Mitteilungen Der Anthropologischen Gesellschaft (Wien) 1938; 68:9–53.

Forsthoefel KF, Papp AC, Snyder PJ, Prior TW: Optimization of DNA extraction from formalin-fixed tissue and its clinical application in Duchenne muscular dystrophy. Am J Clin Pathol 1992; 98:98–104.

Frederick J, Hunter J, Greenwell P, et al: The A1B genotype expressed as A2B on red cells of individuals with strong B gene-specific transferases. Transfusion 1985; 25:30–33.

Gürtler H, Niebuhr E: Chromosome polymorphisms in legal paternity cases. *In* Brinkmann B, Henningsen K (eds). Advances in Forensic Haemogenetics vol. 1. Berlin, Springer-Verlag, 1986, pp 201–211.

Holland MM, Roby RK, Fisher DL, et al: Identification of human remains using mitochondrial DNA sequencing: Potential mother-child mutational events. *In* Bar W, Fiori A, Rossi U (eds). Advances in Forensic Haemogenetics vol. 5. Berlin, Springer-Verlag, 1994, pp 399–406.

Holliman SM: The MN blood group system: Distribution, serology and genetics. *In* Unger PJ, Laird-Fryer B (eds). Blood group systems: MN and Gerbich. Arlington, Virginia, American Association of Blood Banks, 1989, pp 1–29.

Hopkinson DA, Harris H: Red cell acid phosphatase, phosphoglucomutase, and adenylate kinase. *In* Yunis JJ (ed): Biochemical Methods in Red Cell Genetics. New York, Academic Press, 1969, pp 337–375.

Hummel K, Claussen M: Exclusion efficiency and biostatistical value of conventional blood group systems in European and non-European populations; suitability of Central European tables from non-German speaking populations. *In* Hummel K, Gerchow J, (eds): Biomathematical Evidence of Paternity. Berlin, Springer-Verlag, 1981, pp 97–108.

Ivanov PL, Gill P, Sullivan KM, et al: DNA-based identification of the last Russia's royal family. *In* Proceedings of the Fourth International Symposium on Human Identification. Madison, Wisconsin, Promega Corporation, 1993, pp 37–47.

Jeffreys AJ, MacLeod A, Tamaki K, et al: Minisatellite repeat coding as a digital approach to DNA typing. Nature 1991; 354:204–209.

Jeffreys AJ, Wilson V, Thein SL, et al: DNA "fingerprints" and segregation analysis of multiple markers in human pedigrees. Am J Hum Genet 1986; 39:11–24.

Kompf J, Bissbort S, Gussman S, Ritter H: Polymorphism of red cell glyoxalase-I (E.C.4.4.1.5): A new genetic marker in man. Investigation of 169 mother-child combinations. Humangenetik 1975; 27:141–143.

Lamm LU, Gürtler H, Hansen HE: The HLA system. *In* Walker RH (ed). Inclusion Probabilities in Parentage Testing. Arlington, Virginia, American Association of Blood Banks, 1983, pp 381–392.

Maniatis T, Fritsch EF, Sambrook J: Molecular Cloning. A Laboratory Manual. Cold Spring Harbor, New York, Cold Spring Harbor Laboratory, 1982.

Martin W: Consideration of "silent genes" in the statistical evaluation of blood group findings in paternity testing. *In* Walker RH (ed): Inclusion Probabilities in Parentage Testing. Arlington, Virginia, American Association of Blood Banks, 1983, pp 245–250.

Mauff G: Genetic polymorphisms of complement components and other plasma proteins. *In* Mayr WR (ed). Advances in Forensic Haemogenetics vol. 2. Berlin, Springer-Verlag, 1988, pp 133–143.

Mayr WR: Paternity testing with unavailable putative father or mother. *In* Walker RH (ed): Inclusion Probabilities in Parentage Testing. Arlington, Virginia, American Association of Blood Banks, 1983, pp 373–379.

Miale JB, Jennings ER, Rettberg WAH, et al: Joint AMA-ABA guidelines: Present status of serologic testing in problems of disputed parentage. Family Law Quarterly 1976; 10:247–285.

Miller SA, Dykes DD, Polesky HF: ACP1 polymorphism: Five new variants detected by multiple electrophoretic methods. *In* Mayr WR (ed). Advances in Forensic Haemogenetics vol. 2. Berlin, Springer-Verlag, 1988, pp 92–96.

Mullis K, Faloona F, Scharf S, et al: Specific enzymatic amplification of DNA in vitro: The polymerase chain reaction. Cold Spring Harb Symp Quant Biol 1986; 51:263–272.

National Research Council: DNA typing: Statistical basis for interpretation. *In* DNA Technology in Forensic Science: Washington, DC, National Academy Press, 1992, pp 74–96.

Race RR, Sanger R: Blood Groups In Man, 5th ed. Philadelphia, FA Davis, 1968, p 457.

Ray JG Jr (ed): NAIAD Manual of Tissue Typing Techniques 1979–1980. NIH Publication 83-545. Bethesda, Maryland, US Department of Health and Human Services, PHS, NIH, 1982.

Salmon C, Cartron J-P, Rouger P: The human blood groups. New York, Masson Publishing, 1984, pp 94–140.

Salmon D: The random man not excluded expression in paternity testing. *In* Walker RH (ed): Inclusion Probabilities in Parentage Testing. Arlington, Virginia, American Association of Blood Banks, 1983, pp 281–292.

Schanfield MS, Polesky HF, Sebring ES: Gm and Inv typing. *In* Polesky HF (ed): Paternity Testing. Chicago, American Society of Clinical Pathologists, 1975, pp 45–53.

Schatkin SB: Disputed Paternity Proceedings, 3rd ed. Albany, New York, Banks & Co, 1952, pp 233–234.

Smithies O: Zone electrophoresis in starch gels: Group variations in the serum proteins of normal human adults. Biochem J 1955; 61:629–641.

Southern EM: Detection of specific sequences among DNA fragments separated by gel electrophoresis. J Mol Biol 1975; 98:503–510.

Standards for Parentage Testing Laboratories, 2nd ed. Bethesda, Maryland, American Association of Blood Banks, 1994.

Stroup M: A review: The use of monoclonal antibodies in blood banking. Immunohematology 1990; 6:30–36.

Teige B, Olaisen B, Pedersen L: Subtyping of haptoglobin—presentation of a new method. Hum Genet 1985; 70:163–167.

Tippett P: Rh blood group system: The D antigen and high- and low-frequency Rh antigens. *In* Vengelen-Tyler V, Pierce SR (eds): Blood Group Systems: Rh Technical Workshop. Arlington, Virginia, American Association of Blood Banks, 1987, pp 25–53.

Walker RH: Probability in the analysis of paternity test results. *In* Silver H (ed). Paternity Testing. Washington, DC, American Association of Blood Banks, 1978, pp 69–135.

Walker RH (ed): Inclusion Probabilities In Parentage Testing. Arlington, Virginia, American Association of Blood Banks, 1983.

Watson JD, Gilman M, Witowski J, Zoller M: Recombinant DNA, 2nd ed. New York, Scientific American Books, 1992, pp 603–618.

Weber JL, May PE: Abundant class of human DNA polymorphisms which can be typed using the polymerase chain reaction. Am J Hum Genet 1989; 44:388–396.

Wetterling G: Intragenic recombination within the PGM1 locus. *In* Polesky HF, Mayr WR (eds). Advances in Forensic Haemogenetics vol. 3. Berlin, Springer-Verlag, 1990, pp 218–221.

Wiener AS, Lederer M, Polayes SH: Studies in isohemagglutination. IV: On the chance of providing non-paternity with special reference to blood groups. J Immunol 1930; 19:259–282.

Zemmour J, Parham H: HLA class I nucleotide sequences, 1992. Tissue Antigens 1992; 40:221–228.

Chapter 63

Forensic Identity Testing by DNA Analysis

Lieutenant Colonel, U.S. Army, Victor Walter Weedn, M.D., J.D.
Susan L. Swarner, M.P.H. (Forensic Science)

From dinosaurs to football players, almost everything can be defined by deoxyribonucleic acid (DNA). This chapter defines issues and approaches for DNA analysis in the forensic context.

HISTORICAL ASPECTS

The first wide-scale use of DNA testing was not in medical diagnostics but in forensic applications, both criminalistics and parentage. Forensic DNA testing was initially applied to casework only in 1985. Even now, many crime laboratories are still in the process of developing DNA testing capabilities. New DNA typing technologies continue to emerge. The possibility exists, and it is anticipated that traditional forensic serologic testing will be completely replaced by DNA testing.

Historically, forensic serology has been used to associate suspects and victims with questioned biological material. The material was tested, using polymorphic genetic markers, to characterize the material in terms of who could and could not be the source of the material. Genetic markers are isoproteins or antigenic determinants that are expressed in various forms (polymorphisms), allowing differentiation between individuals possessing different types.

Some common forensic issues are aiding in the identification of a deceased individual by family reference specimens, associating biological fluids (e.g., semen or blood) at a crime scene with a suspect, or perhaps even associating a victim with blood found on a suspect's clothes. Forensic testing faces several difficulties not normally found in medical diagnostics. First, the specimens tested are often subjected to extremes of condition and environmental insults at the crime scene, creating degradation problems. Additionally, the material may be a mixture of different body fluids from different individuals.

The goal of characterizing the biological material is to limit or reduce the number of individuals who could be the source of the material. The suspect population is at times limited or even closed, permitting resolution or identification using genetic systems with even low discriminatory power. However, if the population is not limited by the circumstance of the case, then methods to achieve higher discrimination become important. Every additional genetic marker may further reduce the number of potential sources of the questioned material. Conventional serology can routinely generate numbers of only one in two to one in a few thousand. With DNA analysis, the discriminatory power approaches that which is needed to infer identification (Kirby, 1992).

ADVANTAGES OF DNA OVER TRADITIONAL SEROLOGY

Forensic testing of biological specimens began at the turn of the twentieth century with the application of ABO blood grouping to forensic evidence. Since then, numerous other

The views expressed are those of the authors and do not necessarily reflect those of the U.S. Army or the Department of Defense.

7

serologic markers have been implemented in forensic testing. However, various DNA testing methods have numerous advantages over traditional serologic testing (e.g., blood grouping, erythrocyte cell antigens and isoenzymes, serum protein isoenzymes, and human leukocyte antigen [HLA] testing) (Weedn, 1993).

The first major advantage of DNA testing over traditional serologic testing is its application to all biological source material. A wide variety of body fluids are encountered in evidence testing; however, complete serologic testing (criminalistic laboratories typically use 12 genetic markers) can be performed only on blood, not on the other tissues or bodily fluids. For example, the vaginal swabs in a rape case are usually tested only for secretor status, ABO, if secretor positive, phosphoglucomutase, and peptidase A. However, with DNA analysis, virtually any trace biological material can be used to associate a suspect with a crime, including blood, plucked hairs, saliva, semen, and urine. The type and number of DNA tests are limited by the amount of source material.

The second major advantage of DNA testing, one that is the most heralded, is the tremendous discriminatory potential of DNA profiling. In some cases, DNA analysis can approach positive identification, compared with ABO blood group testing, which has the probability of discriminating approximately one in three individuals in the general population. Even with additional serologic markers, typical values are one in a few thousand, whereas some DNA tests can yield values of one in billions.

A third advantage of DNA tests is their sensitivity. Restriction fragment length polymorphism (RFLP) DNA typing is as sensitive as traditional serologic methods. With the advent of polymerase chain reaction (PCR)-based testing, DNA from a mere few cells can be tested, far surpassing the sensitivity of traditional DNA and serologic testing.

A fourth advantage of DNA is its resistance to environmental factors. DNA is a robust molecule, reasonably resistant to acids, alkalis, and detergents; protein, lipid, and carbohydrate determinants generally are not. Proteins are relatively easily denatured, and it is this easily denatured conformational tertiary structure of proteins that is important for typing. The typing information from DNA, however, is found in the sequence of the nucleotides, which are independent of the shape of the molecule. Consequently, DNA tests can be performed reliably on specimens that are far older and have been exposed to greater environmental insults than in the case of traditional serologic markers.

A fifth advantage is the ability to separate sperm cell DNA from other cellular DNA. For most crime laboratories, the majority of the violent crime cases is sexual assaults. A historical problem exists in that sexual assault evidence is almost exclusively a mixture of semen and other bodily fluid. This presents a serious issue for traditional serologic typing techniques, and in approximately two thirds of the cases, the semen donor cannot be resolved because the mixture of the fluids results in a mixture of serologic types (Davies, 1982). However, DNA from sperm can be separated out from nonsperm DNA by differential lysis. This allows for individualization of the source of the semen, without the confounding data of the nonsemen evidence.

IMPACT OF DNA

Biological evidence is commonly left at a crime scene and, in accordance with Locard's principle of evidentiary transfer, can be linked to a perpetrator. Judge Joseph Harris, in *People* v. *Bailey*, declared, "If DNA fingerprinting works and receives evidentiary acceptance, it can constitute the single greatest advance in 'the search for truth,' and the goal of convicting the guilty and acquitting the innocent since the advent of cross examination." However, DNA evidence, in and of itself, is not normally the proof of the existent crime. As with all evidence, DNA must be considered in the context of the case and often merely links a suspect to a scene. For example, evidence of semen origin does not prove rape; the semen recovered from an alleged rape victim may have been deposited through a consensual sexual contact. A greater impact of DNA typing evidence would certainly be realized if not for the fact that (1) in many crimes, biological evidence is overlooked and not recovered to test, (2) in many crimes there is no reference DNA sample for comparison or there is no suspect database, and (3) the DNA typing results are not dispositive of the case—DNA is evidence neither of guilt nor, always, of innocence. Nonetheless, in forensic testing, DNA testing has caused no less than a revolution.

DNA is used in approximately 10,000 new criminal investigations per year (Coleman, 1994), and this number will undoubtedly increase. DNA analysis is currently used mainly in violent crimes. Approximately three quarters of the DNA analysis cases involve sexual assault; a significant proportion involve homicide. In approximately one third of the cases, DNA tests exonerate wrongfully accused suspects, in one quarter the tests are inconclusive, and in somewhat less than half of the cases DNA tests result in an association of the suspect with a crime.

In addition to the use of DNA for associative evidence at scenes of crime, DNA is used in identification of remains when fingerprint, dental, and other traditional means of identification are not successful. Traditional methods of identification can be problematic because they are subject to decomposition, fragmentation, partial incineration, or absence of antemortem comparison data. In the presence of the aforementioned problems, DNA analysis can be successful. In fact, any tissue or bone fragment can potentially be identified. The common availability of families as sources of reference material for comparison purposes overcomes the greatest impediment to fingerprint and dental identification—the lack of antemortem data for comparison. Some medical examiner offices now retain a DNA specimen, such as a small blood stain card, on file from autopsies should identification later be questioned or if reference material should later be needed for criminalistic testing of biological crime scene evidence.

SPECIMEN COLLECTION

DNA analysis can be performed on a wide variety of specimens. The specimen collection, identification, packaging, and storage are, of course, extremely important. In the forensic arena, the added concern of chain of custody arises.

Whole Blood

Ethylenediaminetetraacetic acid (EDTA) and citrate-phosphate-dextrose (CPD) anticoagulated blood remains the specimen of choice for DNA laboratories. Heparin-anticoagulated blood is not recommended for DNA analysis. Even though mature red blood cells are devoid of DNA (both nuclear and mitochondrial), ample DNA is present for testing. However, because blood is one of the first tissues to suffer from putrefaction, blood that is significantly hemolyzed or infected with bacteria is often unsuitable as a source of DNA for RFLP testing.

Tissue

Although virtually any tissue may be successfully used for DNA typing purposes and some tissues are more cellularly dense than other tissues, giving rise to more DNA, it must be noted that some tissues are, in fact, more subject to degradation (Kobilinsky, 1992). Among soft tissues, liver DNA appears to degrade quickly from autolytic enzymes, whereas brain tissue is a relatively good source in intermediate postmortem periods. Bone and teeth are the most stable sources of postmortem tissue DNA, and perhaps for this reason, informative mitochondrial DNA is routinely obtained from skeletal remains that are decades old. Generally, the greater the overall body decomposition and the longer the postmortem period, the greater will be the degradation of the DNA from cadaveric tissues.

Great care should be taken to prevent contamination of the specimen by other sources of DNA. Specimens should be collected using gloves and pristine instruments. When possible, fresh tissues should be collected by an incisional biopsy technique. The specimens should be kept cold or preferably frozen (although repeated freezing and thawing is disadvantageous). Because it is not possible simply to look at a specimen and predict the quality and quantity of the DNA in the specimen, sample collection should be performed as described earlier to prevent contamination, which would easily be detected with PCR-based technologies.

Desiccation, even simple air-drying, may be an adequate method of storage of some DNA specimens (e.g., bloodstains and bone) for specific purposes. Tissues in formalin are not optimal but can often be used for PCR-based DNA testing. No tissues or biological fluids should be discarded as inadequate without first attempting DNA testing.

Evidentiary Specimens

Biological fluids shed on items that can be collected (e.g., blood on a piece of clothing) should simply be collected and packaged separately. When biological fluid has been deposited on a surface or an item that cannot be collected, the fluid should be collected by swabbing with clean swabs (all preferably sterile) moistened with distilled water, until the entire stain is collected. A control swab should be collected from an unstained area adjacent to the fluid stain. The stain swabs and control swabs should be air-dried and packaged separately.

DNA DEGRADATION AND ENVIRONMENTAL DAMAGE

DNA normally undergoes progressive fragmentation or degradation, reducing the high-molecular-weight DNA to low-molecular-weight DNA; however, the sequence information is still present within the DNA fragments (Kobilinsky, 1992). Therefore, the information is not completely lost despite the fairly extensive fragmentation that occurs from decomposition.

Degradation of DNA occurs primarily by enzymes called deoxyribonucleases (DNases). These enzymes are endogenous to the specimen or exogenous bacterial enzymes. This explains why the degradation *in vivo* is rapid as long as the specimen is moist. Once the sample is desiccated, the enzyme activity is almost stopped.

High-molecular-weight DNA generally is not isolated from tissues after a few days. On the other hand, high-molecular-weight DNA from desiccated or frozen materials may be retained almost indefinitely. Smaller DNA fragments are present for considerable periods and allow for some DNA testing. The quality and quantity of the DNA affect the DNA testing process because not all DNA testing is appropriate or possible when the DNA is degraded. RFLP testing of a variable number of tandem repeat (VNTR) loci requires nondegraded high-molecular-weight DNA; whereas most PCR-based analysis can be performed on even highly degraded samples. Additionally, mitochondrial DNA can be obtained and analyzed from decades-old skeletal remains when nuclear DNA cannot.

DNA is a robust molecule that can tolerate a remarkable range of temperature, pH, salt, and other factors that destroy classic serological markers. Early validation testing by forensic science laboratories has shown that in DNA mixed with detergents, oil, gasoline, and other adulterants, the DNA type did not alter.

DNA POLYMORPHISMS

The DNA from every human (except identical twins) is unique because of the presence of polymorphisms, differences in the DNA among individuals. However, the vast preponderance of the DNA sequence is identical among individuals and reflects the fact that we generally have two arms, two legs, one nose, and so on and are more alike than different. On average, only one in a thousand base pairs differs between individuals. Nonetheless, this amounts to an average of three million base pairs that differ between any two individuals and accounts for the tremendous genetic variation in blood type, eye color, hair color, and other characteristics. Although the diversity in the coding regions of DNA (genes) is great, the noncoding regions of DNA also give rise to a great deal of diversity and are also used in forensic DNA testing. These polymorphisms are usually grouped into two types: length-based polymorphisms and sequence polymorphisms. Different methods are used to detect the two types of polymorphisms.

Length-based polymorphisms are found in repetitive DNA. More than 90% of the human genome is composed of noncoding or junk DNA. Approximately 20% to 30% of the noncoding regions are composed of repetitive regions (Fowler, 1988). VNTR loci possess a core sequence that is repeated in a string (e.g., CAT would be the core and could exist as CATCATCAT, and so on). The number of core repeats can vary in different individuals, creating a length polymorphism. Length polymorphisms are especially subject to degradation.

Sequence polymorphisms are composed of different nucleotides at a particular location in the genome. These sequence variations can be manifested as regions of alternative alleles or base substitutions, additions, or deletions. Most sequence polymorphisms are mere point mutations.

DNA METHODS

Clearly, this is a time of great technologic advances in molecular biology. The Human Genome Project will ensure that the technology will evolve rapidly, and forensic DNA typing will subsequently benefit from these advances.

DNA Quantitation

Unlike most medical diagnostics work, forensic specimens are often limited in the amount and quality of DNA. In order to choose the appropriate DNA test and use proper amounts of DNA in the chosen analytical tests, the extracted DNA is tested to determine the quality and quantity of DNA. Generally, laboratories use a semi-quantitative assessment employing an agarose minigel, electrophoresis, and ethidium bromide staining. This can determine the presence of high-molecular-weight DNA and render a crude estimation of the quantity, but it cannot discern if the DNA is human or bacterial. Spectrophotometric methods also give a reasonable estimate of total DNA but do not distinguish low- from high-molecular-weight DNA or bacterial from human DNA. Other laboratories prefer a DNA quantitation based on an intercalated fluorophore; again, this test does not give any information about the quality or source of the DNA. Slotblot tests, in which a probe to a constant region of DNA is titrated against known dilutions, are commonly used to quantitate the human DNA present in a sample.

Restriction Fragment Length Polymorphism Testing

The traditional DNA typing technology used in crime laboratories and with which most people are familiar is RFLP analysis (Weedn, 1989). This technique allows separation and visualization of DNA fragments by size. Classic RFLP analysis, as performed in research and genetic laboratories for genetic disease testing, results in a restriction enzyme cutting or not cutting at a particular location, depending on whether or not a mutation destroys the restriction site (Fig. 63–1*A*).

The target for forensic RFLP analysis is repetitive DNA in which the number of core repeat units differs among individuals, VNTR loci (Fig. 63–1*B*). DNA fragments containing VNTRs are cut from chromosomal DNA with restriction enzymes. A given fragment length is known as an allele. Thus, cut (restriction) DNA fragments that differ (are polymorphic) in size (length) between individuals are analyzed.

The key to the application of RFLP analysis to forensics was the development of DNA probes to VNTR loci. Wyman and White in 1980 and then Jeffreys in 1985 identified probes that bind to VNTR loci. Classic RFLP analysis yields a mere yes-no result and is really based on a sequence polymorphism. In contrast, probes used in forensics bind to hypervariable VNTR loci and are truly a length polymorphism. This difference between classic RFLP analysis and forensic RFLP analysis is analogous to the difference between an on/off light switch and a sliding light switch. It is the large number of possible VNTR alleles that gives the VNTR probes a high discriminating potential and makes them useful for forensic applications.

The original Jeffreys probe (1985a; 1985b), the use of which gave rise to the term DNA fingerprint, is a multilocus probe (MLP). A multilocus probe binds to several DNA sequences and produces numerous bands; the resulting autoradiograph resembles a commercial bar code. Forensic laboratories now use single-locus probes (SLPs), which bind to a single DNA locus. SLP systems are used because they are more sensitive, are more easily interpreted, and have defined genetics.

RFLP SLP probes are designed to bind to a single target location within each set of chromosomes. These probes are typically developed to be human (or primate) specific. The DNA fragments probed vary in size and, hence, are seen as bands that vary in position on an autoradiograph. Two bands are usually generated on an autoradiograph for each single-locus probe, corresponding to maternal and paternal alleles (unless shared).

RFLP analysis is very robust and is the most powerful of the DNA typing technologies, often yielding discriminatory values of one in many millions. On the other hand, it is a laborious and time-consuming (six to eight weeks) process. Moreover, it requires a substantial amount of nondegraded (high-molecular-weight) DNA for analysis.

The six steps of RFLP analysis, after DNA extraction and quantitation, are (1) digestion, (2) electrophoresis, (3) Southern blot, (4) denaturation and hybridization, (5) autoradiography, and (6) analysis. These are basic procedures outlined previously in this text (Chapter 56). Forensic samples are routinely interrogated with numerous probes, a process called rehybridization.

Rehybridization

The membrane may be used again with other DNA probes. The membrane is first stripped of the initial probe and then rehybridized with a new probe to detect the presence of a different target DNA sequence. Autoradiography must be performed again with each new probe. Because forensic laboratories typically repeat this step several times in order to improve discriminatory power, RFLP testing typically requires six weeks to perform. Generally, at least four RFLP SLPs are used by most crime laboratories. It is noteworthy that during the removal of the probe, some of the sample DNA is also removed. This prevents unlimited probing of the membrane and is especially problematic for cases that have small amounts of sample DNA. Full analysis may not be possible in these cases.

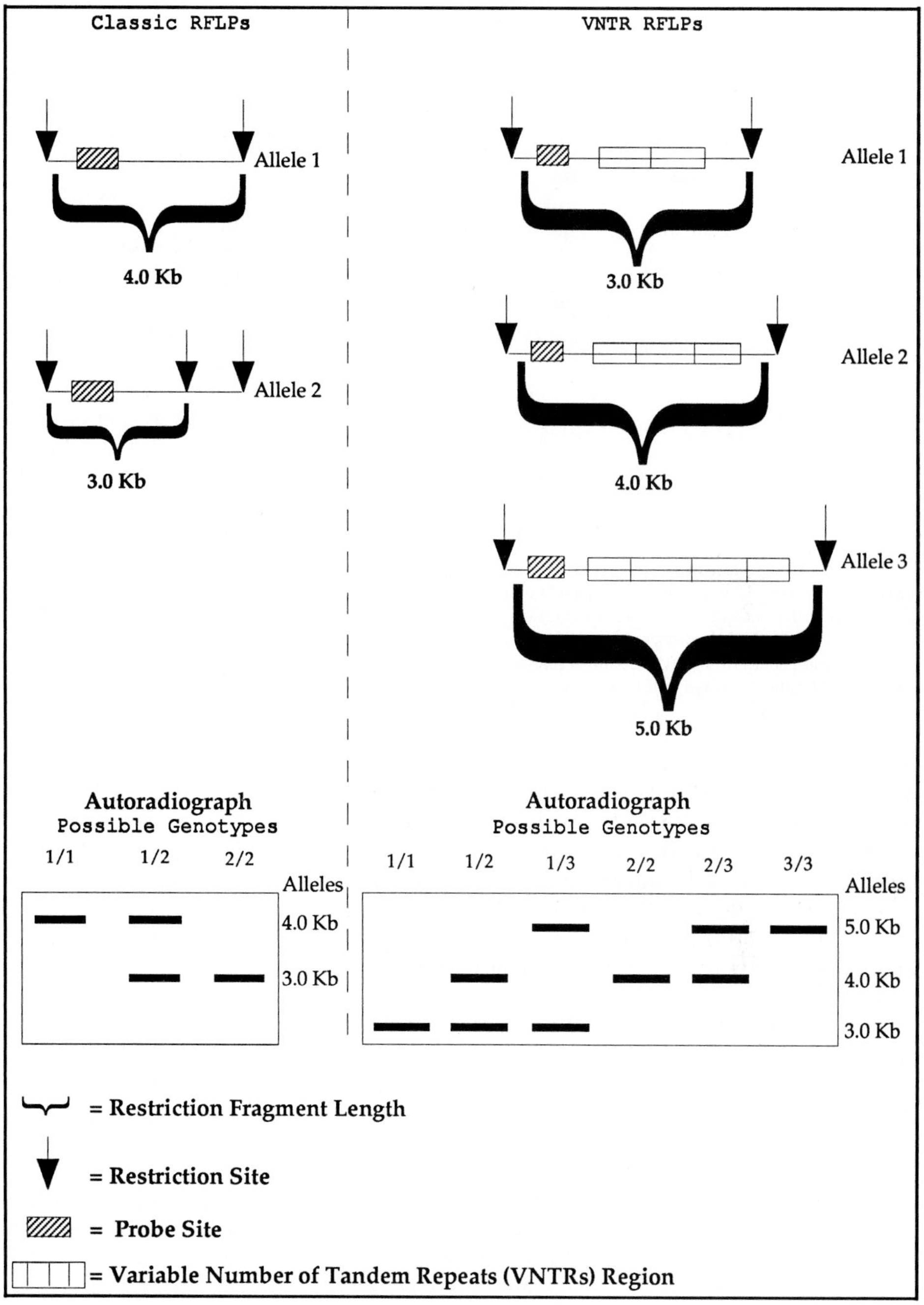

Figure 63–1. Two types of RFLP analysis. Classic RFLP is based on fragment size as cut by a restriction fragment. RFLP based on hypervariable loci vary in size owing to varying numbers of tender repeats (VNTR). (Modified from National Research Council: DNA Technology in Forensic Science. Washington, DC, National Academy Press, 1992, p 35.)

Analysis

The analysis of the autoradiograph can be divided into two large steps. First is the visual inspection of the produced bands and the subsequent size determination and comparison. The resultant autoradiograph from one SLP typically manifests two bands (maternal and paternal alleles) in each lane for the DNA of heterozygous individuals. A three-banded pattern can be obtained if an internal restriction site exists in one of the probed fragments. Some laboratories mix the probes for several VNTRs together to create a cocktail of probes. However, the DNA has to be separately reanalyzed with each probe in the cocktail.

During the visual inspection step, the general overall quality of the autoradiograph is first assessed. Autoradiographs should ideally produce discernible sharp bands in straight lanes with little or no background. If the quality of the autoradiograph is acceptable, a visual inspection for exclusions and potential inclusions is made. In most cases, if DNA from different individuals is run on the same gel, the bands are obviously discrepant. In fact, if the band positions of the samples are clearly different, the samples can be declared to be nonmatching, an exclusion. However, if the band positions of the samples are similar, it is not possible to declare the sample bands to be or not to be a match at this point without determining the size of the bands, referred to as being sized (Fig. 63–2).

Determining the size of the bands (base pairs or kilobases)

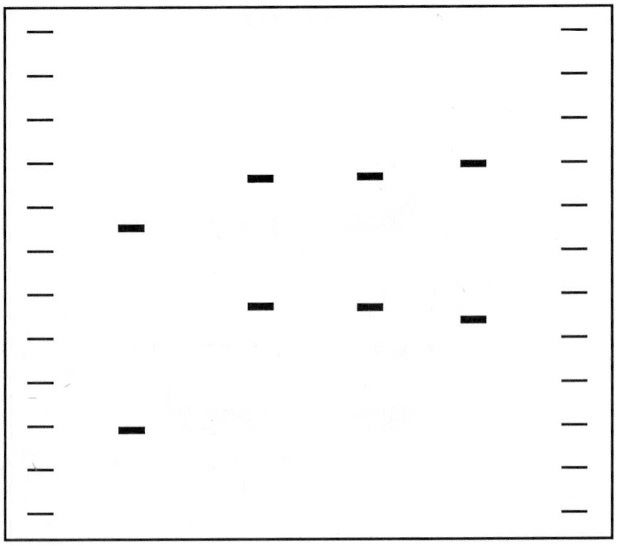

Figure 63–2. Block diagram of matching and nonmatching band patterns. The band pattern of the questioned material (Q1) matches that of the known reference specimen (K1). However, the questioned material (Q1) does not match the band pattern of the second known reference specimen (K2). The human control sample is noted as C1.

allows for an objective comparison. The size of the sample bands is measured against the bands of the molecular weight standards (ladders), which have also been analyzed on the gel. Band sizing is performed by hand, by digitizing pad, or most often by computer imaging and analysis. Computer imaging achieves the greatest precision. To reduce possible human error in this critical step, forensic community standards call for this step to be repeated independently by a second DNA analyst.

In order to determine if the samples match, the band size measurements for the samples are compared. Band sizes vary, even in replicate testing, owing to band shifting and measurement imprecision. Therefore, when comparing samples, band sizes do not have to match exactly. Instead, the band sizes from samples must be within a given set of limits called matching bins, matching windows, or confidence intervals. The tolerance limits are not standard throughout the community but differ based on the system used in the laboratory and the statistical concept applied. Some matching algorithms even take into account the difference in resolution between the top and bottom of gels. At the completion of the analysis, the samples can be declared to be a match or nonmatch.

Statistical Analysis

Forensic RFLP analysis yields a continuous distribution of band sizes. Forensic RFLP systems are theoretically continuous, in that a potentially unlimited number of alleles exist based on a potentially unlimited number of repeats or partial repeats of a given core sequence of nucleotides. The resolution and measurement imprecision of RFLP systems does not permit exact measurements and thus does not permit resolution of single repeat differences in VNTR loci. RFLP results in which a DNA fragment is determined to be 4.32 kilobases (kb) cannot, with certainty, be said to be the same as or different from a DNA fragment determined to be 4.33 kb in size. Consequently, band sizes are reported rather than allele designations, and a statistical match criterion is applied. Therefore, measurement error introduces interpretation problems in band matching of forensic samples that are not present in classic diagnostic RFLP analysis.

Unlike fingerprints, genetic markers (including DNA and traditional forensic serologic markers) do not positively identify an individual; instead, they are used to exclude an individual positively or to establish a probability of origin. The DNA may be unique to an individual, but the entire range of polymorphisms is not tested, and consequently there is a certain statistical probability that two individuals chosen at random might have a matching DNA profile.

The calculation of this probability is based on population frequency data and analyzed using statistical concepts from population genetics. The Hardy-Weinberg principle, a mathematical expression (i.e., for biallelic systems: $p^2 + 2pq + q^2 = 1$) that is used to calculate the frequency of an allele in a population, states that the frequency of genetic alleles remains constant in a population over time, assuming random mating within the population. Current forensic statistical estimates are reasonable approximations, despite the fact that mating is not completely random between groups. Databases currently in use by crime laboratories in the United States are for white, black, Hispanic, Asian, and Native American groups. Many small isolated ethnic groups from around the world have been studied and repeatedly demonstrate that the differences between individuals far exceed that within subpopulations. Nonetheless, forensic laboratories are purposely very conservative in their statistical calculations, although greater statistical power can always be achieved by testing with more DNA probes if the sample permits.

Potential Pitfalls

Most technical errors yield no result rather than a false result. Numerous problems could create a situation in which no result would be obtained—for example, if solvent from the extraction step is carried over into the enzyme digestion media, preventing digestion; if the probe is not sufficiently labeled, the bands are not visualized; or if the membrane is inadequately washed, background exposure hides the bands.

Some factors that could produce misleading results are partial degradation of the DNA, which could result in the loss of the larger band, partial digestion of the DNA, or band shifting. Sample mix-up could also lead to a wrong result, although sufficient redundancy in casework would generally preclude such occurrences. The foregoing problems are usually easily discernible by an experienced analyst, because the problems create predictable patterns.

Although it is true that any number of factors can affect the migration of DNA bands during electrophoresis, these factors are generally controlled by comparing their migration relative to marker DNA fragments of known length in a separate lane. However, band shifting, in which DNA in a single lane migrates aberrantly (i.e., slightly out of register with the other lanes) is an observed phenomenon. Band shifting is recognized by bands in a lane shifting slightly in the same direction and to the same degree from that which is expected. Band shifting can be detected and occurs in defined conditions related to loading an excess of DNA into the gel.

Polymerase Chain Reaction–Based Systems

PCR is a technical breakthrough that has revolutionized DNA testing and, indeed, the biological sciences. PCR now promises to revolutionize the area of forensic DNA testing. All current nonRFLP DNA tests are PCR-based methods and include dotblot systems, amplified DNA fragment length polymorphisms (AmpFLPs), short tandem repeats (STRs), and direct mitochondrial DNA sequencing.

PCR was first described in 1985. Kary Mullis is credited with its invention, for which he was awarded the 1993 Nobel Prize in chemistry. The original concept was demonstrated using typing of the β-hemoglobin gene, but the first commercial application was in HLA-DQA1 for forensic testing. Early in its development, PCR was recognized as a potential answer to the trace quantities of biological fluid often encountered in forensic science. These samples could often be too small for RFLP analysis. Significantly, the first case in which DNA testing was introduced into court in the United States was in the 1986 case of *Pennsylvania* v. *Pestinikas,* which involved HLA-DQ-α testing.

Advantages of PCR

PCR permits fast and exquisitely sensitive DNA typing. Sensitivity can be critical in forensic issues because certain types of evidence would not have sufficient DNA to analyze by RFLP. Evidence such as hair and saliva and the tiny droplets of blood in a blood spatter pattern would most likely be too small for RFLP analysis. Additionally, the target DNA becomes detectable from background DNA, even by nonspecific DNA stains such as a silver stain. Consequently, PCR analysis effectively permits the elimination of radioactive isotopes and of the Southern blot, thus allowing automation. PCR-based DNA typing systems have the further advantage of producing discrete (or semi-discrete) results.

PCR-based tests, unlike RFLP, usually produce typable results when the sample DNA is highly degraded, such as cadaveric tissues, blood that has been exposed to the environment, and even stained formalin-fixed paraffin-embedded tissue on a glass slide. PCR technologies are largely insensitive to degradation because the target DNA loci are small to begin with and because only a few copies of target sequence need remain intact in the sample DNA before amplification. RFLP analysis, by contrast, is exquisitely sensitive to degradation because fragmentation of the DNA goes to the heart of the analytical method.

Disadvantages of PCR

PCR-based technology is very powerful but not without some disadvantages. As a whole, genetic systems analyzed by PCR-based technologies are less discriminating (less informative) than RFLP genetic systems. However, the discriminatory power is acceptable and will continue to increase with the additional systems. Another disadvantage of PCR is its susceptibility to inhibition by various factors such as heme in blood. Preferential amplification of one allele over another allele can occur and result in allelic dropout. As in RFLP, higher-molecular-weight alleles are not detected if the sample DNA is severely degraded. Additionally, specific primers may be more efficient with one allele than another, creating an increase in production of the favored allele. Moreover, the extreme sensitivity of PCR systems makes it susceptible to DNA contaminants. In fact, the potential for cross-contamination is the single most important concern for PCR-based testing. Adequate precautions must be taken. Nonetheless, PCR can be performed reliably, even on evidence not usable with RFLP.

Analytical Systems

POLYMERASE CHAIN REACTION DOTBLOTS

The prototype example of sequence polymorphism detection techniques and the most commonly used PCR-based typing technique is referred to as dotblot. Dotblots involve a series of DNA probes to detect target sequences. Probes are sequence-specific oligonucleotides (SSO), also called allele-specific oligonucleotides (ASO). The probes are a single-stranded DNA fragment sufficiently long to confer specificity but sufficiently short to be destabilized by a single base mismatch so that it binds only to the exact sequence complement. SSO probes are used to detect the presence or absence of an alternative sequence type.

In traditional dotblot formats, a portion of the amplified DNA is bound to a membrane and probed by an SSO probe, any unbound probe is washed away, and a positive test result is visualized by a color reaction with the enzyme linked to the probe. The commercial kits use a reverse dotblot (blotdot) in which the probe is bound to the membrane and the amplified sample DNA is added. The results are visually determined to be positive or negative for the presence of a given sequence; thus, the pattern of blue spots on the strip indicates a specific genotype (Fig. 63–3). HLA-DQA1 (formerly DQα) and Amplitype-PM (PM stands for polymarker) are current commercially available reverse dotblot systems in forensic science. A mitochondrial displacement-loop dotblot system is in development. The test kits have proved to be robust assays that are not difficult to perform. No major equipment is needed except a thermal cycler. The testing can be performed by one analyst in less than one day. Testing works reasonably well despite sample degradation, although larger genetic loci, such as some of the loci in the Amplitype-PM system, may not amplify when the smaller genetic loci will. HLA-DQA1 testing, the first offered of the two systems, has been introduced into hundreds of court cases and, with minor exception, has gained widespread courtroom acceptance.

The HLA-DQA1 is a single genetic system. Twenty-one HLA-DQA1 genotypes are possible from the pairing of six alleles: 1.1, 1.2, 1.3, 2, 3, and 4. The DQA1 has a discriminatory power of roughly 1:20. The PM dotblot strip tests five different genetic loci: glycophorin A, hemoglobin γ-globin chain (HBGG), group-specific component (GC), D7S8, and low-density lipoprotein receptor (LDLR). Glycophorin A is the genetic system for classic MN blood group typing. GC is a human serum protein polymorphism that has been isotyped for years by forensic laboratories using protein analytical methods. The other three systems have not been previously used in forensic work. Each of the polymarker systems detects only two or three alleles. When the Amplitype-PM system is combined with DQA1, the discriminatory power is increased to approximately 1 in 2000.

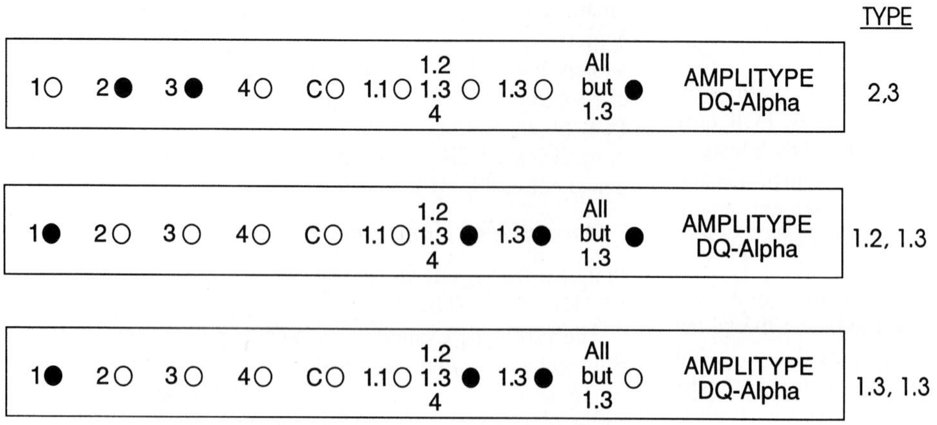

Figure 63–3. Schematic of commercial reverse dotblot strips.

AMPLIFIED DNA FRAGMENT LENGTH POLYMORPHISM AND SHORT TANDEM REPEATS

AmpFLP analysis involves the electrophoretic separation by size of polymorphic DNA fragments produced by amplification rather than excision (RFLP analysis).

The VNTR loci used for AmpFLP analysis are necessarily smaller than RFLP loci because the PCR reaction does not reliably amplify large stretches of DNA. Instead of electrophoretic gels composed of agarose, AmpFLP gels are generally fabricated of polyacrylamide, which offers higher resolution, in order to separate the smaller DNA fragment sizes. The amplified PCR product concentration so overwhelms any background DNA present that probe hybridization is unnecessary, and the DNA can be directly stained by a silver stain or other nonspecific DNA stain. Because of the elimination of the Southern blot and autoradiography, AmpFLP analysis can be performed in one or two days instead of the weeks necessary for RFLP analysis.

Because individual core repeats can be resolved, discrete allelic measurements are normally possible. RFLP results are reported as given band sizes with a degree of imprecision; AmpFLP results are reported as the number of repeats for a given allele. Ideally, the core sequence would be repeated in its entirety; however, the systems have sufficient resolution to reveal the occasional sequence difference in the core repeat region, resulting in slight length variance in the band pattern, so-called microheterogeneity.

Regions with core repeat sequences greater than 8 bp have been called minisatellite or long tandem repeat (LTR) regions. Those with core repeat sequences of approximately 2 to 8 bp are called microsatellite or STR regions. The shorter STR fragments are generally preferable because they are less susceptible to degradation and to preferential amplification. Allelic dropout is not generally observed with the small STRs but is seen with larger LTR alleles. However, dinucleotide repeats, which are commonly used for genetic maps, are not generally used in forensic science laboratories owing to the artifactual production of so-called shadow and stutter bands.

The smaller STR fragments are more amenable to analysis by automated instrumentation than the larger DNA fragments of other systems. Automated STR analysis uses fluorescently labeled amplified product DNA. One currently available commercial instrument accepts and automatically reads and interprets electrophoretic gels that have been generated offline. Another currently available commercial instrument performs real-time analysis, in which DNA fragments are detected as they migrate through the gel past a detector. Different fluors, chemicals that fluoresce, can be used in a given lane. Furthermore, various STRs are amenable to simultaneous amplification as multiplexed sets. Thus, many genetic systems can be tested at once.

A number of STR systems have become available. With sufficient numbers of STR systems, discriminatory powers similar to current RFLP testing can be achieved. The British Forensic Science Service and the Royal Canadian Mounted Police (RCMP) crime laboratories are moving toward exclusive use of STR. A British octaplex, in which eight genetic systems are tested simultaneously, will be the routine method for analyzing casework in Great Britain.

MITOCHONDRIAL DNA SEQUENCING

Mitochondrial DNA (mtDNA) sequencing is a newer technology that has application to forensics for two reasons. The mtDNA is present in numerous copies per cell and thus is applicable when the nuclear DNA is extremely degraded or not present (e.g., skeletal remains, shed hairs, and so on). The second reason is the maternal inheritance of the mitochondria. Reference specimens not useful for nuclear DNA analysis can be helpful because an exact mtDNA sequence match can be traced through the maternal lineage of a family for many generations.

mtDNA is a circular piece of DNA 16,569 bp pairs in length. Because no significant regions of repetitive DNA exist in mtDNA, only sequence polymorphisms are typed. Unlike nuclear DNA, which is present in pairs of chromosomes, only a single sequence is present in the cell (homoplasmic). Consequently, unlike nuclear DNA, no genetic recombination occurs.

The region of mtDNA that is analyzed for human identification is the noncoding region known as the displacement loop (D-loop) or control region. This loci spans 1100 bp and contains two hypervariable regions. The degree of polymorphism in the D-loop is so great that direct sequencing may be the most efficient method of typing mtDNA, although a commercial dotblot system is in development.

The discriminatory power of mtDNA sequencing is limited, on the order of one in a few hundred. Also, this testing is expensive. Very few laboratories are performing this kind of testing at this time.

QUALITY ASSURANCE STANDARDS

Quality assurance (QA) issues and concerns are important to any service laboratory testing and have been an area of emphasis for forensic DNA testing. Numerous organizations exist to help establish minimum standards for criminalistic application of DNA testing. The Federal Bureau of Investigation's (FBI's) Technical Working Group on DNA Analysis Methods (TWGDAM) has promulgated guidelines that detail QA measures. The American Society of Crime Laboratory Directors (ASCLD) has endorsed these guidelines and has an accreditation program for crime laboratories. The American Board of Criminalists (ABC) certifies criminalists and has a subspecialty category for DNA analysts. The DNA Identification ACT, a component of the Crime bill passed in 1994, includes a mandate for standards to be issued by the FBI.

Interlaboratory comparisons have consistently demonstrated the great precision of RFLP testing by the forensic DNA typing community. This is probably reflective of the general agreement about proper laboratory procedures that should be used in forensic DNA testing. Although no single DNA typing procedure is mandated per se, protocols within the forensic community are remarkably similar. Proficiency surveys report mean fragment size measurements that differ by only a few bases, and the range of results is well within the plus-or-minus 2.5% matching window used by most crime laboratories (Mudd, 1994). This precision is achieved despite different protocols and procedures.

Proficiency testing is an integral part of any QA program. TWGDAM guidelines call for two proficiency tests (at least one of which must be an external proficiency test) per DNA analyst. ASCLD has incorporated the requirement into their accreditation standards, and the ABC has made it a requirement for criminalist certification. Furthermore, the DNA Identification Act includes a provision requiring proficiency testing for state databanks. Proficiency tests for forensic DNA identity testing are commercially available.

DATABANKS

Historically, large numbers of cases, especially sexual assault cases, could not be investigated because of the lack of a suspect. Sexual offenders are known to have an extremely high recidivism rate; therefore, in the early 1980s, some states began to establish sexual offender databanks. These databanks were used to compare serologic profiles of known sexual offenders with evidence in sexual assault cases. Although this was helpful in numerous cases, the efficiency of the databank was hindered by the relatively low power of discrimination in serologic testing of semen. With its higher discriminatory capability, however, DNA analysis has clearly raised the power of databanks to that of fingerprint files.

Most state databanks collect and type DNA specimens from convicted sex offenders. Convicted violent offenders, particularly perpetrators of homicide, are often also included. In Virginia, DNA is collected from all felons. Databanks facilitate the matching of cases and suspects across agency and jurisdictional boundaries, even without leads or suspicion.

At the time of this writing, 32 states have legislated the collection and analysis of known offender reference specimens. With the enactment of the DNA Identification Act (1994), it is anticipated that all 50 states will create databanks. Additionally, Combined DNA Identification System (CODIS) is a national system established and maintained by the FBI to link state databanks.

LEGAL CHALLENGES

Never before has novel scientific evidence received such an intense and highly publicized legal challenge. DNA evidence is so powerful that the defense has little choice other than to attack the evidence with great vigor. Defense attorneys are faced with the prospect of a defendant's facing the death penalty when the DNA evidence shows that the chances are one in a trillion that the perpetrator could have been anyone else.

The courtroom drama has largely been shaped by the significant personalities involved (Roberts, 1991). The intensity of the legal debate has led to mistaken perceptions of controversy surrounding the technology by much of the lay public (Roberts, 1992). However, to judge a technology by what occurs in court is error; legal issues are not scientific questions. Despite the courtroom challenges, the forensic community has embraced this technology based on its scientific merit. Policymakers have also weighed in heavily in favor of forensic DNA testing (Office of Technology Assessment, 1990; National Research Council, 1992). Ten states have promulgated statutes to permit the admissibility of DNA test results.

Since 1986, DNA testing has been used in approximately 50,000 investigations in the United States alone. In the vast majority of cases, however, DNA tests never reach trial. When DNA evidence is submitted to court, it is no longer likely to receive a significant challenge, and despite common opinion, judicial acceptance of forensic DNA testing has been remarkable. It was successfully admitted in each of the approximately 100 cases during the first two years of its introduction and since has been generally admitted. According to the FBI, as of October 1994, DNA test results had been admitted in 128 reported cases, admitted but with limitations on statistical interpretation in 16 cases, and excluded or remanded for further consideration in 22 cases. This record is in sharp contrast to the three decades needed for general court acceptance of fingerprint or ABO blood group evidence.

Even though DNA has been challenged rigorously in the courts and sometimes refused admission or subsequently stricken on appeal, several salient points are apparent: (1) No DNA results have ever been refuted after reanalysis, (2) no one has ever had a case reversed even when the DNA is stricken at the appellate level, and (3) even in the handful of cases in which the DNA was not admitted at the trial level, the defendant was convicted anyway, suggesting that other evidence corroborated the DNA test results.

The early significant cases are chronicled next.

Ghanian Immigration Case

The first case in which DNA testing was used was in a 1985 immigration case in which a boy from Ghana sought to emigrate to Britain, claiming his mother was already a resident. Authorities suspected the boy was a cousin. Conventional genetic markers (16 systems including HLA) indicated the boy and the mother were related but could not distinguish whether the woman was the aunt or the mother. To complicate matters, the mother had some doubt about the boy's biological father, and no samples from the father in Ghana or from any of her sisters were forthcoming. Jeffreys determined that the boy and all three siblings were from the same father and mother. All bands in the fingerprint of the suspect boy, not found in the mother, could be matched with bands from the three undisputed children determined to be paternal. The chances that the mother's sister would yield the same set of maternal bands was insignificant, and accordingly, the boy was allowed into the country to join his mother.

The Queen v. Pitchfork

The next major application of Jeffreys' new DNA fingerprint method was in a double rape/murder case in England. This was the first time DNA tests were used in a criminal investigation. In 1983, 15-year-old Linda Mann was raped and strangled in quiet Leicestershire County. No suspects were found. In 1986, 18-year-old Dawn Ashworth was raped and strangled within a mile of the first murder. Richard Buckland, who had acted secretively, was formally charged for the second murder and suspected of the first. Jeffreys proved semen samples were from the same man but not from Buckland. Thus, before DNA was ever used to convict someone of a crime, it served to prove someone innocent. Despite thousands of statements and computer entries and a 20,000-pound reward, the police had no leads. Believing a local man to be responsible, police asked all males in the area between 13 and 30 to voluntarily submit a blood sample for testing; virtually every man did in fact donate the requested sample—a total of approximately 4500 men (one man did object on religious grounds). Colin Pitchfork twice failed to attend his appointments in January of 1987 to give blood. On the third appointment, after attempting to pay several people to stand in for him, he successfully persuaded his work mate, Ian Kelly, explaining that he was worried that he might be "fitted up" because of his prior convictions for indecent exposure. Pitchfork put Kelly's picture into his passport, had Kelly practice his signature, and coached him on his family details. Pitchfork succeeded in eluding the authorities. However, months later, in September of 1987, Kelly, while drinking in a pub, boasted to friends about how he had donated blood for his friend Pitchfork. The police got wind of the substitution. Kelly was convicted of conspiracy to pervert the course of justice. Pitchfork was then properly tested. Within weeks, DNA fingerprinting identified Mr. Pitchfork as the rapist. In the spring of 1988, he was found guilty and sentenced to life in prison.

Pennsylvania v. Pestinikas

The first case in which DNA testing was introduced into court in the United States was in the 1986 case, but the evidence was not a basis for disposition of the case. The operators of a rest home in Pennsylvania had been charged with the negligent homicide of an elderly gentleman who had died of apparent starvation. The autopsy results were questioned, resulting in an exhumation. In response, the original autopsy physician then alleged that the internal organs had been switched with those of another body. The body had been embalmed and buried for approximately 1 year. HLA-DQα DNA testing was performed by Ed Blake of Forensic Science Associates (3053 Research Dr., Richmond, CA 94806). The DNA was very degraded (average fragment size was 100 bp). The 82-bp HLA fragment amplified from the internal organs matched that of other body tissues. The defendants were convicted of negligent homicide but acquitted of the charge of tampering with the body.

Florida v. Andrews

Tommie Lee Andrews became the first person to be convicted of a crime, rape, using DNA typing evidence. A series of rapes began on the south side of Orlando, Florida, during the spring of 1986. The first victim was 27-year-old Nancy Hodge. During 1986, the same man was thought to be responsible for 23 incidents of prowling, breaking and entering women's homes, and attempted assaults or rape. The modus operandi was distinctive. The attacker would enter the victim's home after midnight wielding a knife. He would surprise the woman in the dark and cover her head with a sheet or blanket. During the sexual assault, he flicked the light switch on and off. After the attack, he often took her driver's license. There were 23 reported incidents in 1986. Then in February of 1987, a 27-year-old woman was beaten, cut, and repeatedly raped while her two young children slept in the next room. A sleeping bag was wrapped around her head. Officers in plain clothes staked out likely neighborhoods. On March 1st at 2:48 A.M., a woman reported a prowler. The responding patrol car spotted a car speeding away from the area and followed the car for miles before the suspect crashed into a utility pole. The driver, Tommie Lee Andrews, was arrested on suspicion of prowling after the high-speed chase and crash. He lived 3 miles from the first victim, 27-year-old Nancy Hodge. The next morning, Hodge identified him from a photo lineup. Blood typing proved only that he and the rapist were among a third of the population with the same blood typing. Neither his face nor his voice was familiar to Ms. Hodge. The room was dark, and the rapist had whispered. Mr. Andrews had an alibi, and the police had only a couple of fingerprints on a screen outside the victim's house. By October of 1987, Lifecodes determined that the DNA in Andrews' blood matched that of the collected semen samples from the victims. Later that month, a mistrial was declared despite positive identification of Andrews by Hodge. However, on November 6, 1987, Andrews was convicted and sentenced to 22 years in a separate rape trial. The 1988 retrial of the initial prosecution resulted in another guilty verdict and an additional 78 years in prison.

Virginia v. Spencer

The impetus for Virginia to establish the first DNA typing capability by a state crime laboratory and later to establish a databank of violent offenders came from the Spencer trials of 1988. Susan Tucker, age 44, was found dead in her Arlington, Virginia, bed in December 1987. She was naked, partially covered by a sleeping bag. A rope was looped around her neck and connected to her wrists in the back. An autopsy revealed that she had been strangled and raped. She had been dead for several days. Negroid hairs were found in the bathroom sink. Spermatozoa were found on the blanket, a nightgown, and the outside of the sleeping bag, as well as in vaginal and anal smears. Her husband had been out of town. The detective remembered similar crimes near Alexandria four years earlier. Records indicated a similar rape-murder had occurred in Richmond three months previously. In each of these cases, the killer was still at large. The detective found in Virginia prison records the description of a man who had been imprisoned for an Alexandria burglary in early 1984 and who was paroled to a halfway house in Richmond just two weeks before the rape-murder there. Twenty-six-year-old Timothy Spencer was arrested. Forensic analysis of glass, hair, and semen were consistent with Spencer being the assailant. The DNA typing evidence was interpreted as showing a 1 in 135 million chance that another black male could have the same type as found at the Tucker crime scene. Spencer was eventually convicted of both the murder in Alexandria and the murder in Richmond. He was executed.

Illinois v. Dotson

The first use of DNA testing by an accused was from an appeal of Gary Dotson's conviction of the 1977 Illinois rape of Cathleen Webb. Dotson was convicted on Ms. Webb's accusations and law enforcement testimony that he was one of only 10% of the Caucasian population with the same semen type as that found on Ms. Webb's underwear, based on an ABO blood type. Webb later retracted her accusation against Dotson. An ABO typing error was discovered, revealing that in fact, 66% of the population were possible semen matches. Nonetheless, Dotson was not pardoned. Professor Jeffreys was unable to type the 10-year-old specimen using RFLP DNA fingerprinting. Ed Blake of Forensic Associates (3053 Research Dr., Richmond, CA 94806), using PCR-based HLA-DQα tests, was able to establish a credible exclusion. Dotson was then pardoned in 1989.

New York v. Castro

Jose Castro was the first defendant to successfully challenge the admissibility of DNA evidence. In 1987, Mr. Castro, a 38-year-old Hispanic, was accused of stabbing to death his neighbor, Vilma Ponce, and her 2-year-old daughter. A small bloodstain on the watch Mr. Castro was wearing was analyzed by the Lifecodes Corporation (550 West Ave., Stamford, CT 06902) and found not to match Castro but to match that of the victim, Ponce. The chance that another random Hispanic would have the same DNA profile was determined to be 1 in 189 million. The judge ruled that the evidence that the DNA did not match Castro himself was admissible, but evidence that it matched Ponce was not admissible owing to a failure of the laboratory to use acceptable testing techniques. Nonetheless, faced with other evidence, Mr. Castro eventually pleaded guilty to the murders in late 1989.

This trial level case was anomalous in many ways. The pretrial evidentiary hearing lasted 12 weeks and amassed 5000 pages of testimony. The legal defense team of Scheck and Neufeld is the same that has defended most of the subsequent significant cases, including that of O.J. Simpson. Eric Lander was the key defense expert. In the end, Judge Sheindlin was convinced that the testing had been performed without sufficient quality rigor. He enunciated a tripartite test: (1) Is there a generally accepted scientific basis for the test? (2) Is there a generally accepted test procedure? and (3) Was the test properly carried out? He answered the first two in the affirmative but "no" to the third. After the conclusion of the trial and guilty plea, Judge Sheindlin leaned over the bench and asked the defendant if the blood was that of the victim, to which he replied it was, confirming the DNA test results. In the end, the defense's success did not have the damning effect on DNA evidence that some had predicted.

CONCLUSION

Forensic DNA typing technology has subsequently undergone significant advances and improvements. Also, QA measures continue to evolve. The autoradiographs of early cases, such as Andrews and Castro, simply are not representative of the quality autoradiographs obtained from current RFLP technology. In *U.S.* v. *Jakobetz*, the judge commented: "The field is moving so fast that what was criticized a year ago as needing improvement has already been improved."

This legal challenge, which has been primarily confined to the United States, has undergone evolution as defense challenges have been addressed. Defense attorneys no longer argue the scientific basis for DNA typing. Defense attorneys no longer argue matching algorithms. Defense attorneys no longer argue Hardy-Weinberg disequilibria or the multiplication rule for current genetic systems.

The most common successful challenge to DNA evidence has been over issues of statistical interpretation. Although many statistical issues have been raised, arguments now focus on substructure and whether the appropriate population frequency database for comparison has been used. The question is, What is a reasonable estimate of a population frequency statistic, given that small differences among subgroups exist, that yet maintains a sufficient conservatism to give the defendant the benefit of any doubt?

Critics claim that the chance of a random match may be underestimated by a crime laboratory because of potential differences in allele frequencies between ethnic subgroups. They claim that an allele frequency may be 3% instead of 1% in a particular subpopulation, and because the frequency will be multiplied against others, the resultant interpretation will be off by a factor of three and that this is significant. *However, they overlook the fact that 97% of the population is still excluded for the allele. Three in 100 million is little different from 1 in 100 million.* Additionally, the critics also overlook the fact that the normal forensic question is not the frequency of alleles in a specific subpopulation but rather the allele frequency in the general population. The real question is, if the DNA did not come from the reference person, then what is the chance that the DNA could come from someone else in the general population.

A substantial pool of DNA typing data from isolated populations clearly demonstrates that a rare allele is a rare allele, no matter the population group. Differences between subpopulations are generally minor. The variation among individuals is far larger than the variation among population groups. Frequencies generated by large racial groups are sufficient estimates (Chakraborty, 1991).

The scientific discussion is one of degree, as to how large a statistic to introduce into the courtroom, but some courts perceive the discussion as a lack of consensus and rule the statistical interpretation altogether inadmissible, like the proverbial baby with the bath water. A perpetrator is not any less guilty, whether a laboratory reports a value of 1 in 100 thousand or 1 in 100 million.

The National Research Council (NRC) has issued a report advocating a ceiling principle as a conservative measure that all parties could agree on; however, this method as well as lack of a statistical basis for the principle has itself sparked controversy leading to the commission of a second NRC panel to address the statistical issues.

The consensus over the general acceptability of current statistical interpretation of DNA evidence has grown and is now becoming recognized (Lander, 1994). The defense challenges will likely shift focus to QA, error rates, and, in the case of PCR testing, contamination issues. Of course, renewed challenges will test the technology as new methods of DNA typing are introduced.

The courts in the end will recognize that DNA evidence is more reliable than eyewitness accounts and other subjective or far less powerful evidence.

Chakraborty R, Kidd KK: The utility of DNA typing in forensic casework. Science 1991; 254:1735.

Coleman H, Swenson E: DNA in the Courtroom: A Trial Watcher's Guide. Seattle, Washington, Genelex Corporation, 1994.

Davies A: The appearance and grouping of mixtures of semen and vaginal material. Med Sci Law 1982; 22:21.

Fowler JC, Burgoyne LA, Scott AC, Harding HW: Repetitive DNA and human genome variations—A concise review relevant to forensic biology. J Forensic Sci 1988; 33:1111–1126.

Jeffreys AJ, Wilson V, Thein SL: Hypervariable 'minisatellite' regions in human DNA. Nature 1985a, 314:67.

Jeffreys AJ, Wilson V, Thein SL: Individual specific 'fingerprints' of human DNA. Nature 1985b, 316:76.

Kirby, LT: DNA Fingerprinting: An Introduction. New York, W. H. Freeman & Co., 1992.

Kobilinsky L: Recovery and Stability of DNA in samples of forensic science significance. Forensic Sci Rev 1992; 4:67.

Lander ES, Budowle B: DNA fingerprinting dispute laid to rest. Nature 1994; 371:735.

Mudd JL, Baechtel FS, Duewer DL, et al: Interlaboratory comparison of autoradiographic DNA profiling measurements: 1. Data and summary statistics. Anal Chem 1994; 66:3303.

National Research Council, National Academy of Sciences: DNA Technology in Forensic Science. Washington, DC, National Academy Press, 1992.

Office of Technology Assessment (#OTA-BA-438): Genetic Witness: Forensic Uses of DNA Tests. Washington, DC, Government Printing Office (#052-003-01203-1), 1990.

Roberts L: Fight erupts over DNA fingerprinting. Science 1991; 254:1721–1723.

Roberts L: Science in court: A culture clash. Science 1992; 257:732–736.

Weedn VW: DNA profiling, Expert Evidence Reporter 1989; 1:61–68.

Weedn VW, Roby RK: Forensic DNA testing. Arch Pathol Lab Med 1993; 117:486–491.

Wyman AR, White R: A highly polymorphic locus in human DNA. Proc Natl Acad Sci USA 1980; 77:6754.

APPENDICES

Physiologic Solutions, Buffers, Acid-Base Indicators, Standard Reference Materials, and Temperature Conversions

PHYSIOLOGIC SOLUTIONS

A physiologic solution is one that contains various salts in concentrations that closely approximate the composition of fluids in the human body. The simplest of these is physiologic saline, which has the same osmotic pressure as the blood. There are more elaborate solutions—for example, to maintain tissues in a metabolically active state for longer periods of time. Table A1–1 gives formulas of some solutions that are isotonic with respect to blood.

BUFFERS*

Buffers have the ability to resist changes in pH. Buffers usually consist of a weak acid and its salt or a weak base and its salt. The Henderson-Hasselbalch equation

$$\text{pH} = \text{pK} + \log\,[\text{salt}]/[\text{acid}] \qquad (1)$$

is useful in calculating the acid (or base) to salt ratio required to establish a desired pH from a buffer system.

EXAMPLE 1. If the pH of a 0.1 M acetate buffer is known to be 4.90, calculate the concentration of acetic acid and sodium acetate in the buffer (pK for acetic acid = 4.76).

Substituting values of pH and pK in equation 1:

$$\begin{aligned}\log[\text{acetate}]/[\text{acetic acid}] &= 4.90 - 4.76\\ &= 0.14\\ [\text{acetate}]/[\text{acetic acid}] &= 1.38\\ [\text{acetate}] &= 1.38[\text{acetic acid}]\end{aligned}$$

Because the total buffer/L concentrations is 0.1 M,

$$[\text{acetate}] + [\text{acetic acid}] = 0.1\ \text{M} \qquad (2)$$

Substituting the value of acetate in equation 2:

$$1.38[\text{acetic acid}] + [\text{acetic acid}] = 0.1\ \text{M}$$

Hence

$$\begin{aligned}[\text{acetic acid}] &= 0.042\ \text{M}\\ [\text{acetic acid}] &= 2.52\ \text{g/L}\\ [\text{acetate}] &= 0.058\ \text{M}\\ &= 4.76\ \text{g/L}\end{aligned}$$

EXAMPLE 2. If 648 mL of 0.025 molar diethylbarbituric acid and 10 mL of 0.5 molar sodium diethylbarbiturate are mixed and diluted to 1 L, calculate the pH of the solution (pK for diethylbarbituric acid = 7.98 and molar concentration = moles/liter).

The following relationship exists between molarity and volume of a solution:

$$M1V1 = M2V2 \qquad (3)$$

where

M1 = molarity of the initial solution
V1 = volume of the initial solution
M2 = molarity of the final solution
V2 = volume of the final solution

Use equation 3 to calculate changes in salt and acid concentrations after dilution to 1 L:

$$\begin{aligned}[\text{Sodium diethylbarbiturate}] &= 0.025 \times 0.648\\ &= 0.0162\ \text{mol/L}\\ [\text{Diethylbarbituric acid}] &= 0.5 \times 0.01\\ &= 0.005\ \text{mol/L}\end{aligned}$$

Calculate pH of the solution using equation 1:

$$\begin{aligned}\text{pH} &= 7.98 - \log(0.0162/0.005)\\ &= 7.98 - \log 3.24\\ &= 7.98 - 0.51\\ &= 7.47\end{aligned}$$

The maximum buffering capacity is at the pK value of the weak acid or base. For instance, for acetic acid with a pH value of 4.76, more acid is required to change the pH of an acetate buffer from 4.76 to 4.66 than from 4.20 to 4.10. Efficient buffering capacity covers a pH range of about 1 unit on either side of the pK value of the weak acid or base. For acetic acid, this would be from about pH 3.8 to 5.8.

Sorensen's Phosphate Buffers

These buffer solutions are generally useful, because the range of the mixtures is from pH 5 to 8.

*For a comprehensive discussion, including preparation of buffer solutions of a definite ionic strength, consult Bates RG: Determination of pH—Theory and Practice, 2nd ed. New York, John Wiley and Sons, 1973.

Table A1–1. PHYSIOLOGIC SOLUTIONS

	Saline	Locke's Solution	Ringer's Solution	Tyrode's Solution
Sodium chloride	0.85 g	0.9 g	0.7 g	0.8 g
Calcium chloride		0.024 g	0.0026 g	0.02 g
Potassium chloride		0.042 g	0.035 g	0.02 g
Sodium bicarbonate		0.01–0.03 g		0.1 g
D-Glucose		0.01–0.25 g		0.1 g
Magnesium chloride				0.01 g
Monosodium phosphate				0.005 g
Distilled water	100 mL	100 mL	100 mL	100 mL

Table A1–3. TRIS(HYDROXYMETHYL)AMINOMETHANE BUFFER

mL 0.1 N HCl Added	Resulting pH at 23°C	Resulting pH at 37°C
5.0	9.10	8.95
7.5	8.92	8.78
10.0	8.74	8.60
12.5	8.62	8.48
15.0	8.50	8.37
17.5	8.40	8.27
20.0	8.32	8.18
22.5	8.23	8.10
25.0	8.14	8.00
27.5	8.05	7.90
30.0	7.96	7.82
32.5	7.87	7.73
35.0	7.77	7.63
37.5	7.66	7.52
40.0	7.54	7.40
42.5	7.36	7.22
45.0	7.20	7.05

Table A1–2. SORENSEN'S TABLE OF BUFFER MIXTURES

Na_2HPO_4 Solution (mL)	KH_2PO_4 Solution (mL)	pH
0.25	9.75	5.288
0.5	9.5	5.589
1.0	9.0	5.906
2.0	8.0	6.239
3.0	7.0	6.468
4.0	6.0	6.643
5.0	5.0	6.813
6.0	4.0	6.979
7.0	3.0	7.168
8.0	2.0	7.381
9.0	1.0	7.731
9.5	0.5	8.043

Prepare 0.1 molar solutions of monobasic potassium phosphate (13.6 g/L) and dibasic sodium phosphate (14.2 g/L). Mix solutions in the ratio indicated in Table A1–2 to obtain the buffer of desired pH.

Tris(hydroxymethyl)aminomethane Buffer*

Tris(hydroxymethyl)aminomethane buffer can be used for a pH range between 7.0 and 9.0, but its best buffer capacity is between 7.5 and 8.5. It is practically ineffective

*If buffers of a higher molarity are desired, the 0.1N HCl may have to be replaced by a 1.0N HCl.

Table A1–4. ACID-BASE INDICATORS

Indicator	pH Range	Quantity of Indicator per 10 mL	Color	
			Acid	*Alkaline*
Thymol blue (A)*†	1.2–2.8	1–2 drops 0.1% soln. in aq.	Red	Yellow
Methyl orange (B)	3.1–4.4	1 drop 0.1% soln. in aq.	Red	Orange
Bromphenol blue (A)†	3.0–4.6	1 drop 0.1% soln. in aq.	Yellow	Blue-violet
Bromcresol green (A)†	4.0–5.6	1 drop 0.1% soln. in aq.	Yellow	Blue
Methyl red (A)†	4.4–6.2	1 drop 0.1% soln. in aq.	Red	Yellow
Bromcresol purple (A)†	5.2–6.8	1 drop 0.1% soln. in aq.	Yellow	Purple
Bromthymol blue (A)†	6.2–7.6	1 drop 0.1% soln. in aq.	Yellow	Blue
Phenol red (A)†	6.4–8.0	1 drop 0.1% soln. in aq.	Yellow	Red
Neutral red (B)	6.8–8.0	1 drop 0.1% soln. in 70% alc.	Red	Yellow
Thymol blue (A)†‡	8.0–9.6	1–5 drops 0.1% soln. in aq.	Yellow	Blue
Phenolphthalein (A)	8.0–10.0	1–5 drops 0.1% soln. in 70% alc.	Colorless	Red
Thymolphthalein (A)	9.4–10.6	1 drop 0.1% soln. in 90% alc.	Colorless	Blue

The letters A or B after the name of the indicator signify, respectively, that the compound is an indicator *acid* or *base*.
*For the acid range.
†Sodium salt.
‡For the alkaline range.

Table A1–5. COMMONLY USED ACIDS AND ALKALIES*

Solution	Mol. Weight	Spec. Gravity†	g/L†	Molarity†	Normality†	Approx. Number of mL Required to Make 1000 mL of 1 N solution
Conc. HCl	36.46	1.19	440	12	12	83
Conc. H_2SO_4	98.08	1.84	1730	18	36	28
Conc. HNO_3	63.02	1.42	990	16	16	64
Conc. lactic acid	90.08	1.21	1030	11	11	87
Glacial acetic acid	60.08	1.06	1060	17.5	17.5	57
Conc. NH_4OH	35.05	0.90	250	15	15	67

*Commercially available.
†Figures may vary slightly according to the lot or manufacturer.

below pH 7.0 and above pH 9.0. One advantage of the buffer is its excellent stability. The buffer can be prepared by weighing the desired amount of tris(hydroxymethyl)-aminomethane, dissolving it in water, and adjusting the pH to the desired value with HCl. For example, if 100 mL of 0.05 M buffer is desired, place 0.6057 g of tris(hydroxymethyl)aminomethane into a 100 mL volumetric flask. This is dissolved in approximately 50 mL of distilled water. Add 0.1 N HCl, as indicated in Table A1–3, and fill up to the mark with distilled water. The table shows the pH values obtained when 0.6057 g of tris(hydroxymethyl)aminomethane dissolved in water is mixed with the indicated amounts of 0.1 N HCl and diluted to 100 mL.

ACID-BASE INDICATORS*

An acid-base indicator is a weak acid or a weak base, the undissociated form of which has a color and constitution other than the iogenic form. Color change takes place over a certain narrow range of hydrogen ion concentrations. This range is called the color change interval and is expressed in terms of pH (the negative logarithm of the hydrogen ion concentration). A great number of substances

*Based on Dean JA (ed): Handbook of Chemistry, revised 13th ed. New York, McGraw-Hill, 1985.

Table A1–6. STANDARD REFERENCE MATERIALS FOR CLINICAL MEASUREMENTS*†

SRM No.	SRM Description	Purity (%)	Property Certified	Wt/Unit (g)	Certificate Date
40h	Sodium oxalate	99.95	Reductometric standard	60	May 1982
83d	Arsenic trioxide	99.99	Reductometric standard	75	March 1982
84j	Potassium hydrogen	99.993	Acidimetric standard	60	November 1984
136c	Potassium dichromate	99.98	Oxidation standard	60	March 1970
186Ic	Potassium dihydrogen phosphate	99.9	pH 6.863	30	September 1970
186IIc	Disodium hydrogen phosphate	99.9	pH 7.415	30	September 1970
350a	Benzoic acid	99.98	Acidimetric standard	30	April 1981
911a	Cholesterol	99.4	Identity and purity	2.0	June 1974
912a	Urea	99.9	Identity and purity	25	November 1979
913	Uric acid	99.7	Identity and purity	10	November 1973
914	Creatinine	99.8	Identity and purity	10	November 1968
915	Calcium carbonate	99.9	Identity and purity	20	November 1973
916	Bilirubin	99	Identity and purity	0.1	March 1971
917	D-Glucose	99.9	Identity and purity	25	September 1973
918	Potassium chloride	99.9	Identity and purity	30	November 1973
919	Sodium chloride	99.9	Identity and purity	30	November 1973
922	Tris(hydroxymethyl)aminomethane	99.9	pH 7.699	25	August 1976
923	Tris(hydroxymethyl)aminomethane hydrochloride	99.7	pH	35	August 1976
930D	Glass filters for spectrophotometry (visible)		Transmittance (440–635 nm)	3 filters	August 1984
931d	Liquid filters for spectrophotometry (UV and visible)		Absorbance (302–678 nm)	Set of 12 vials	October 1986
933	Clinical laboratory thermometers		Temperature	Set of 3	August 1974
937	Iron metal	99.9		50	June 1978
955	Lead in blood	4 levels		Set of 4 vials	December 1984
2201	NaCl	99.9	pNa pCl	125	March 1984
2202	KCl	99.9	pK pCl	160	March 1984

*Orders and requests for information about these SRMs should be directed to the Office of Standard Reference Materials, Institute for Materials Research, National Bureau of Standards, Washington, DC, 20234.
†NBS Spec. Publ. 260, Catalog of NBS Standard Reference Materials 1988–1989 edition. NIST Standard Reference Materials Catalog, 1993 edition.
Abbreviations: pNa = negative log activity of Na expressed as molality; pCl = negative log activity of Cl expressed as molality.

Table A1–7. TEMPERATURE CONVERSIONS

Centigrade	Fahrenheit	Centigrade	Fahrenheit
110°	230°	38°	100.4°
100	212	37.5	99.5
95	203	37	98.6
90	194	36.5	97.7
85	185	36	96.8
80	176	35.5	95.9
75	167	35	95
70	158	34	93.2
65	149	33	91.4
60	140	32	89.6
55	131	31	87.8
50	122	30	86
45	113	25	77
44	111.2	20	68
43	109.4	15	59
42	107.6	10	50
41	105.8	+5	41
40.5	104.9	0	32
40	104	−5	23
39.5	103.1	−10	14
39	102.2	−15	+5
38.5	101.3	−20	−4

1°F = 0.54°C
1°C = 1.8°F

To convert Fahrenheit into centigrade, subtract 32 and multiply by 0.555.
To convert centigrade into Fahrenheit, multiply by 1.8 and add 32.

show indicator properties, although relatively few of them are practically applied for neutralization reactions and pH determinations. Some commonly used acid-base indicators are shown in Table A1–4. In general, weak acids should be titrated in the presence of indicators that change in slightly alkaline solutions. Weak bases should be titrated in the presence of indicators that change in slightly acid solutions. Some commonly used acids and alkalies are listed in Table A1–5.

The availability of precision pH meters allows titration to a selected end point (pH) and may replace use of indicators for several applications.

Dean JA (ed): Handbook of Chemistry, 13th ed. New York, McGraw-Hill, 1985.
Fasman GD (ed): Handbook of Biochemistry and Molecular Biology, 3rd ed. Cleveland, CRC Press, 1976.
Meinke WW: Standard Reference Materials for Clinical Measurements. Anal Chem 1971; 43:28A.
The Merck Index: An Encyclopedia of Chemicals and Drugs, 10th ed. Rahway, NJ, Merck and Co., 1983.

Desirable Weights and Body Surface Area

Table A2–1. COMPARISON OF THE WEIGHT-FOR-HEIGHT TABLES FROM ACTUARIAL DATA: NON–AGE-CORRECTED METROPOLITAN LIFE INSURANCE COMPANY AND AGE-SPECIFIC GERONTOLOGY RESEARCH CENTER RECOMMENDATIONS

	Metropolitan 1983 Weights* (25–59 Yr)		**Gerontology Research Center* (Age-Specific Weight Range for Men and Women)**				
Height (Ft and In)	***Men***	***Women***	***20–29 Yr***	***30–39 Yr***	***40–49 Yr***	***50–59 Yr***	***60–79 Yr***
4 10		100–131	84–111	92–119	99–127	107–135	115–142
4 11		101–134	87–115	95–123	103–131	111–139	119–147
5 0		103–137	90–119	98–127	106–135	114–143	123–152
5 1	123–145	105–140	93–123	101–131	110–140	118–148	127–157
5 2	125–148	108–144	96–127	105–136	113–144	122–153	131–163
5 3	127–151	111–148	99–131	108–140	117–149	126–158	135–168
5 4	129–155	114–152	102–135	112–145	121–154	130–163	140–173
5 5	131–159	117–156	106–140	115–149	125–159	134–168	144–179
5 6	133–163	120–160	109–144	119–154	129–164	138–174	148–184
5 7	135–167	123–164	112–148	122–159	133–169	143–179	153–190
5 8	137–171	126–167	116–153	126–163	137–174	147–184	158–196
5 9	139–175	129–170	119–157	130–168	141–179	151–190	162–201
5 10	141–179	132–173	122–162	134–173	145–184	156–195	167–207
5 11	144–183	135–176	126–167	137–178	149–190	160–201	172–213
6 0	147–187		129–171	141–183	153–195	165–207	177–219
6 1	150–192		133–176	145–188	157–200	169–213	182–225
6 2	153–197		137–181	149–194	162–206	174–219	187–232
6 3	157–202		141–186	153–199	166–212	179–225	192–238
6 4			144–191	157–205	171–218	184–231	197–244

*Values in this table are for height without shoes and weight without clothes. The Metropolitan Life Insurance Company (1983 Metropolitan Height and Weight Tables. Stat Bull Metropol Life Ins Co, 1983; 64(Jan–Jun):2.) presented a table for nude heights and weights (Table 4) as well as a table for heights and weights clothed (Table 1).

From Andres R: Mortality and obesity: The rationale for age-specific height-weight tables. *In* Hazzard WR, Bierman EL, Blass JP, Ettinger WH Jr, Halter JB (eds): Principles of Geriatric Medicine and Gerontology, 3rd ed. New York, McGraw-Hill, 1994, pp 847–853.

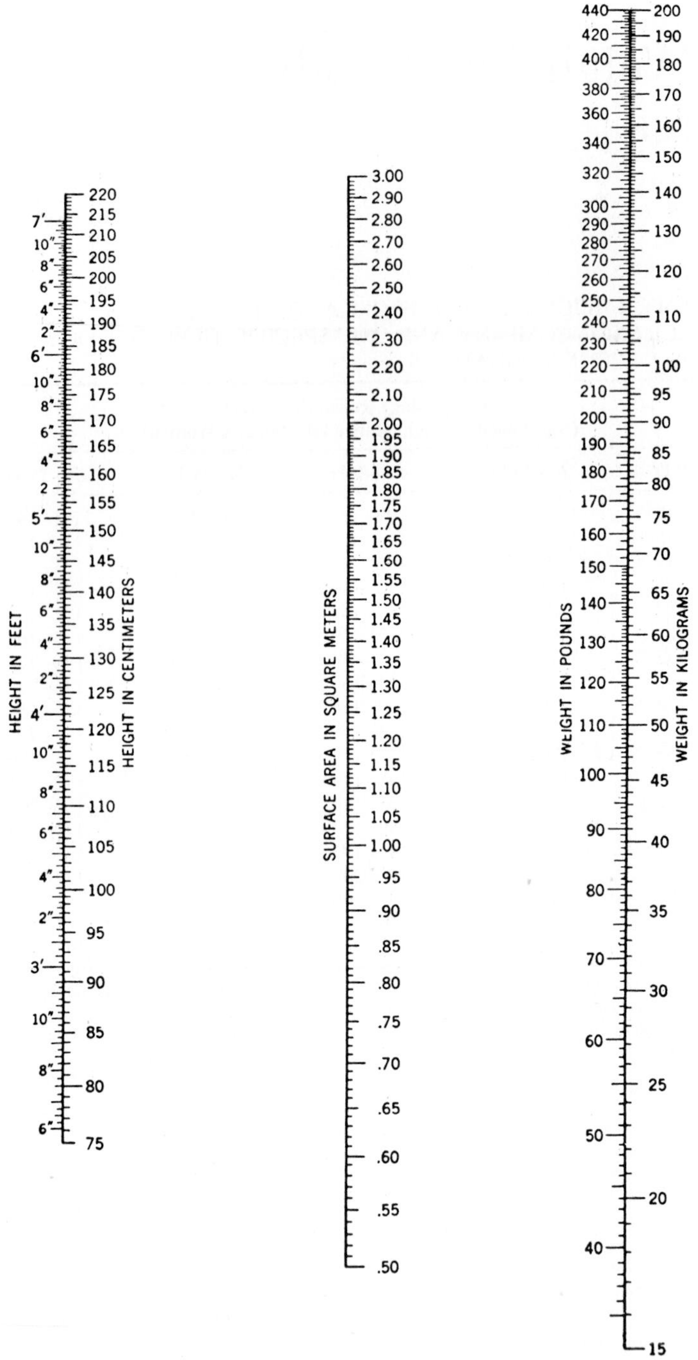

Figure A2–1. Nomogram for the determination of body surface area of children and adults. (From Boothby WM, Sandiford RB: Boston Med Surg J 1921; 185:337.)

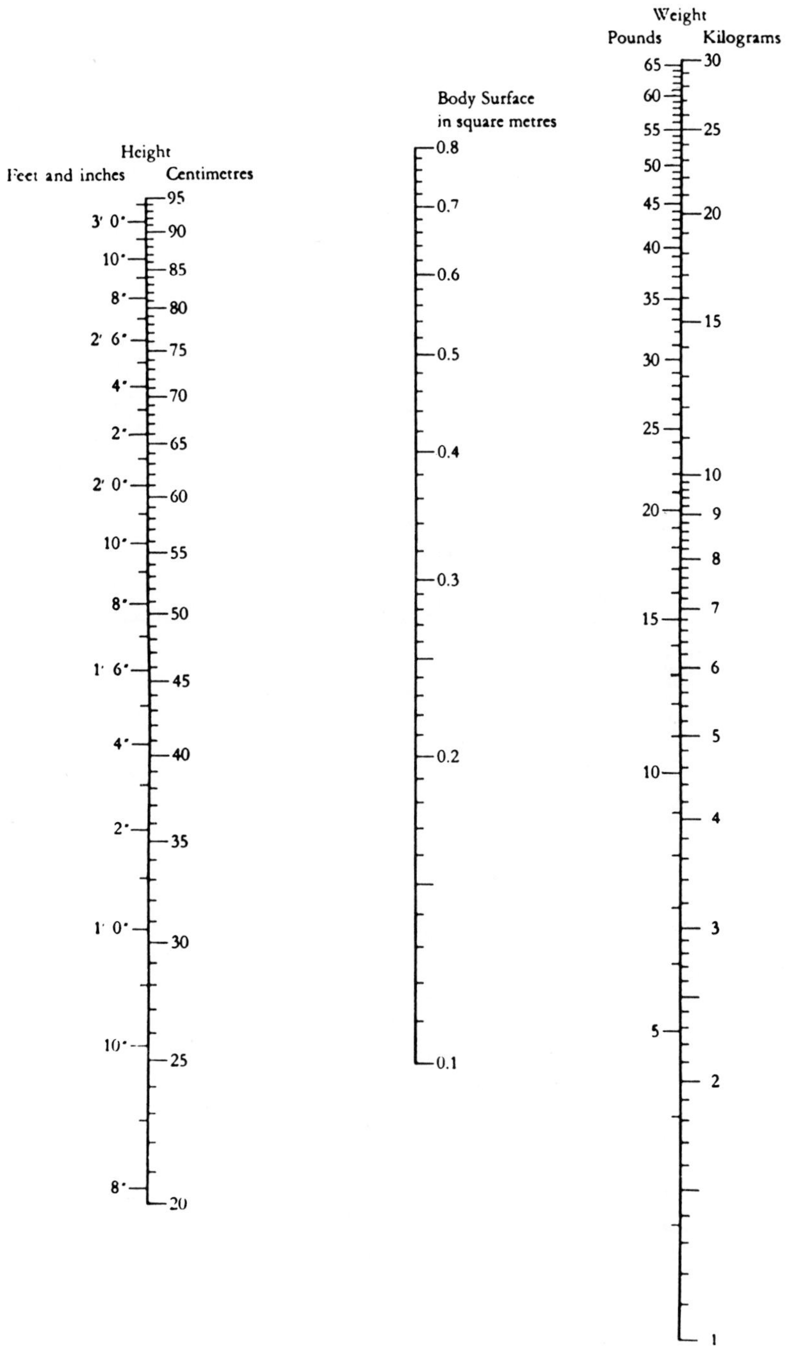

Figure A2–2. Nomogram for the determination of body surface area of children. (From DuBois EF: Basal Metabolism in Health and Disease. Philadelphia, Lea and Febiger, 1936.)

Appendix 3

Periodic Table of the Elements

Table A3–1. PERIODIC TABLE OF THE ELEMENTS

Group labels: New notation (1–18); Previous IUPAC form; CAS version.

KEY TO CHART

Atomic Number → 50 +2 ← Oxidation States
Symbol → Sn +4
1989 Atomic Weight → 118.71
18 18 4 ← Electron Configuration

1 Group IA	2 IIA	3 IIIA IIIB	4 IVA IVB	5 VA VB	6 VIA VIB	7 VIIA VIIB	8	9 VIIIA VIII	10	11 IB	12 IIB	13 IIIB IIIA	14 IVB IVA	15 VB VA	16 VIB VIA	17 VIIB VIIA	18 VIIIA	Shell
1 H +1 −1 1.00794 1																	**2 He** 0 4.0020602 2	K
3 Li +1 6.941 2-1	**4 Be** +2 9.012182 2-2											**5 B** +3 10.811 2-3	**6 C** +2 +4 −4 12.011 2-4	**7 N** +1 +2 +3 +4 +5 −1 −2 −3 14.00674 2-5	**8 O** −2 15.9994 2-6	**9 F** −1 18.9984032 2-7	**10 Ne** 0 20.1797 2-8	K-L
11 Na +1 22.989768 2-8-1	**12 Mg** +2 24.3050 2-8-2											**13 Al** +3 26.981539 2-8-3	**14 Si** +2 +4 −4 28.0855 2-8-4	**15 P** +3 +5 −3 30.97362 2-8-5	**16 S** +4 +6 −2 32.066 2-8-6	**17 Cl** +1 +5 +7 −1 35.4527 2-8-7	**18 Ar** 0 39.948 2-8-8	K-L-M
19 K +1 39.0983 -8-8-1	**20 Ca** +2 40.078 -8-8-2	**21 Sc** +3 44.955910 -8-9-2	**22 Ti** +2 +3 +4 47.88 -8-10-2	**23 V** +2 +3 +4 +5 50.9415 -8-11-2	**24 Cr** +2 +3 +6 51.9961 -8-13-1	**25 Mn** +2 +3 +4 +7 54.93085 -8-13-2	**26 Fe** +2 +3 55.847 -8-14-2	**27 Co** +2 +3 58.93320 -8-15-2	**28 Ni** +2 +3 58.6934 -8-16-2	**29 Cu** +1 +2 63.546 -8-18-1	**30 Zn** +2 65.39 -8-18-2	**31 Ga** +3 69.723 -8-18-3	**32 Ge** +2 +4 72.61 -8-18-4	**33 As** +3 +5 −3 74.92159 -8-18-5	**34 Se** +4 +6 −2 78.96 -8-18-6	**35 Br** +1 +5 −1 79.904 -8-18-7	**36 Kr** 0 83.80 -8-18-8	-L-M-N
37 Rb +1 85.4678 -18-8-1	**38 Sr** +2 87.62 -18-8-2	**39 Y** +3 88.90585 -18-9-2	**40 Zr** +4 91.224 -18-10-2	**41 Nb** +3 +5 92.90638 -18-12-1	**42 Mo** +6 95.94 -18-13-1	**43 Tc** +4 +6 +7 (98) -18-13-2	**44 Ru** +3 101.07 -18-15-1	**45 Rh** +3 102.90550 -18-16-1	**46 Pd** +2 +4 106.42 -18-18-0	**47 Ag** +1 107.8682 -18-18-1	**48 Cd** +2 112.411 -18-18-2	**49 In** +3 114.818 -18-18-3	**50 Sn** +2 +4 118.710 -18-18-4	**51 Sb** +3 +5 −3 121.757 -18-18-5	**52 Te** +4 +6 −2 127.60 -18-18-6	**53 I** +1 +5 +7 −1 126.90447 -18-18-7	**54 Xe** 0 131.29 -18-18-8	-M-N-O
55 Cs +1 132.90543 -18-8-1	**56 Ba** +2 137.327 -18-8-2	**57* La** +3 138.9055 -18-9-2	**72 Hf** +4 178.49 -32-10-2	**73 Ta** +5 180.9479 -32-11-2	**74 W** +6 183.84 -32-12-2	**75 Re** +4 +6 +7 186.207 -32-13-2	**76 Os** +3 +4 190.23 -32-14-2	**77 Ir** +3 +4 192.22 -32-15-2	**78 Pt** +2 +4 195.08 -32-16-2	**79 Au** +1 +3 196.96654 -32-18-1	**80 Hg** +1 +2 200.59 -32-18-2	**81 Tl** +1 +3 204.3833 -32-18-3	**82 Pb** +2 +4 207.2 -32-18-4	**83 Bi** +3 +5 208.98037 -32-18-5	**84 Po** +2 +4 (209) -32-18-6	**85 At** (210) -32-18-7	**86 Rn** 0 (222) -32-18-8	-N-O-P
87 Fr +1 (223) -18-8-1	**88 Ra** +2 226.025 -18-8-2	**89** Ac** +3 227.028 -18-9-2	**104 Unq** +4 (261) -32-10-2	**105 Unp** (262) -32-11-2	**106 Unh** (263) -32-12-2	**107 Uns** (262) -32-13-2												O P Q

*Lanthanides	**58 Ce** +3 +4 140.115 -19-9-2	**59 Pr** +3 140.90765 -21-8-2	**60 Nd** +3 144.24 -22-8-2	**61 Pm** +3 (145) -23-8-2	**62 Sm** +2 +3 150.36 -24-8-2	**63 Eu** +2 +3 151.965 -25-8-2	**64 Gd** +3 157.25 -25-9-2	**65 Tb** +3 158.92534 -27-8-2	**66 Dy** +3 162.50 -28-8-2	**67 Ho** +3 164.93032 -29-8-2	**68 Er** +3 167.26 -30-8-2	**69 Tm** +3 168.93421 -31-8-2	**70 Yb** +2 +3 173.04 -32-8-2	**71 Lu** +3 174.967 -32-9-2	N O P
**Actinides	**90 Th** +4 232.0381 -18-10-2	**91 Pa** +5 +4 231.03588 -20-9-2	**92 U** +3 +4 +5 +6 238.0289 -21-9-2	**93 Np** +3 +4 +5 +6 237.048 -22-9-2	**94 Pu** +3 +4 +5 +6 (244) -24-8-2	**95 Am** +3 +4 +5 +6 (243) -25-8-2	**96 Cm** +3 (247) -25-9-2	**97 Bk** +3 +4 (247) -27-8-2	**98 Cf** +3 (251) -28-8-2	**99 Es** +3 (252) -29-8-2	**100 Fm** +3 (257) -30-8-2	**101 Md** +2 +3 (258) -31-8-2	**102 No** +2 +3 (259) -32-8-2	**103 Lr** +3 (260) -32-9-2	O P Q

The new IUPAC format numbers the groups from 1 to 18. The previous IUPAC numbering system and the system used by Chemical Abstracts Service (CAS) are also shown.
For radioactive elements that do not occur in nature, the mass number of the most stable isotope is given in parentheses.
From Lide DR, Frederikse HPR: CRC Handbook of Chemistry and Physics, 74th ed. 1993–1994. Boca Raton, CRC Press, 1993.

REFERENCES

1. G. J. Leigh, Editor, *Nomenclature of Inorganic Chemistry,* Blackwells Scientific Publications, Oxford, 1990.
2. *Chemical and Engineering News,* 63(5), 27, 1985.

SI Units

H. Peter Lehmann, Ph.D.
John Bernard Henry, M.D.

Recommendations for the standardized presentation of clinical laboratory data based on the International System of Units (SI units) were first proposed in 1967 by the Commission on Clinical Chemistry of the International Union of Pure and Applied Chemistry (IUPAC) and Expert Panel on Quantities and Units of the International Federation of Clinical Chemistry (IFCC) (Dybkaer, 1967). Final recommendations were published in 1979 (Recommendation 1978, IUPAC/IFCC, 1979). Support for these proposals came from the International Committee for Standardization in Hematology and the World Association of (Anatomic and Clinical) Pathology Societies, who, along with the International Federation of Clinical Chemistry, agreed to recommend to all concerned with health services throughout the world that, with regard to units of measurements for medical laboratory results, SI be accepted in its broad application (International Committee for Standardization in Hematology, 1973). The World Health Organization, at the 30th World Health Assembly in 1977, recommended the adoption of the SI by the entire scientific community, and particularly the medical community, throughout the world (World Health Organization, 1977a). Thus, the recommendations for the use of SI units in medicine have resulted in adoption and use of the suggested units by the medical community in many countries. The feasibility of rigid adoption of the SI to all clinical laboratory measurements has been discussed in a number of editorials and articles in the medical literature, which have been reviewed and summarized (Lehmann, 1979).

The SI consists of seven dimensionally independent base units, which are listed in Table A4–1, along with the symbols to be used to denote these units. Table A4–2 lists a number of derived units of the SI that are used in the clinical laboratory. There are two kinds of derived units: coherent units, which are derived directly from the base units without the use of conversion factors; and noncoherent units, which are constructed from the base units and contain a numerical factor in order to make the numbers more convenient to use. The approved prefixes to denote fractions or multiples of base and derived SI units are given in Table A4–3. A complete description of the SI and its application in medicine may be found in the World Health Organization publication *The SI for the Health Professions* (World

Text continued on page 1458

Table A4–1. SI BASE UNITS

Quantity	Name	Symbol
Length	meter	m
Mass	kilogram	kg
Time	second	s
Electric current	ampere	A
Thermodynamic temperature	kelvin	K
Luminous intensity	candela	cd
Amount of substance	mole	mol

Table A4–2. SI DERIVED UNITS

Quantity	Unit Name	Unit Symbol
Area	square meter*	m^2
Volume	cubic meter*	m^3
	liter†	$L = dm^3$‡
Concentration		
mass	kilogram/liter†	kg/L
substance	mole/liter†	mol/L
Molality	mole/kilogram	mol/kg
Density	kilogram/liter†	kg/L
Mass fraction	kilogram/kilogram	kg/kg
Mole fraction	mole/mole	mol/mol
Number concentration	number/liter	L^{-1}
Temperature	degree Celsius*	$°C = °K - 273.15$
Pressure	pascal*	$Pa = kg/ms^2$
Frequency	hertz*	Hz = 1 cycle/s
Clearance	liter/second†	L/s
Electrical potential	volt*	$V = kg\ m^2/s^3A$
Energy	joule*	$J = kg\ m^2/s^2$

*Derived coherent unit.
†Derived noncoherent unit.
‡Both "L" and "l" have been accepted by the IUPAC and the General Conference on Weights and Measures as symbols for the liter.

Table A4–3. PREFIXES

Prefix	Prefix Symbol	Factor
exa	E	10^{18}
peta	P	10^{15}
tera	T	10^{12}
giga	G	10^{9}
mega	M	10^{6}
kilo	k	10^{3}
hecto	h	10^{2}
deca	da	10^{1}
deci	d	10^{-1}
centi	c	10^{-2}
milli	m	10^{-3}
micro	μ	10^{-6}
nano	n	10^{-9}
pico	p	10^{-12}
femto	f	10^{-15}
atto	a	10^{-18}

Table A4–4. WHOLE BLOOD, SERUM, AND PLASMA CHEMISTRY

		Typical Reference Intervals		
Component	**System**	***Conventional Units***	***Factor****	***Recommended SI Units*†**
Acetoacetic acid				
qualitative	Serum	Negative	—	Negative
quantitative	Serum	0.2–1.0 mg/dL	97.95	20–100 μmol/L
Acetone				
qualitative	Serum	Negative	—	Negative
quantitative	Serum	0.3–2.0 mg/dL	172.95	20–340 μmol/L
Albumin				
qualitative	Serum	3.2–4.5 g/dL (salt fractionation)	10	32–45 g/L
		3.2–5.6 g/dL (electrophoresis)		32–56 g/L
		3.8–5.0 g/dL (dye binding)		38–50 g/L
Alcohol, ethyl	Serum or whole blood	Negative—but presented as mg/dL	0.2171	Negative—but presented as mmol/L
Aldolase	Serum			
	adults	3–8 Sibley-Lehninger U/dL at 37°C	7.4	22–59 mU/L at 37°C
	children	Approximately 2 times adult levels		Approximately 2 times adult levels
	newborn	Approximately 4 times adult levels		Approximately 4 times adult levels
α-Amino acid nitrogen	Serum	3.6–7.0 mg/dL	0.7139	2.6–5.0 mmol/L
δ-Aminolevulinic acid	Serum	0.01–0.03 mg/dL	76.26	0.8–2.3 μmol/L
Ammonia	Plasma	20–120 μg/dL (diffusion)	0.5872	12–70 μmol/L
		40–80 μg/dL (enzymatic method)		23–47 μmol/L
		12–48 μg/dL (resin method)		7–28 μmol/L
Amylase	Serum	16–120 Somogyi units/dL	1.85	30–220 U/L
Argininosuccinate lyase	Serum	0–4 U/dL	10	0–40 U/L
Arsenic‡	Whole blood	<7 μg/dL	0.05055	<0.4 μmol/L
Ascorbic acid (vitamin C)	Plasma	0.6–1.6 mg/dL	56.78	34–91 μmol/L
	Whole blood	0.7–2.0 mg/dL		40–114 μmol/L
Barbiturates	Serum, plasma, or whole blood	Negative	—	Negative
Base excess	Whole blood			
	male	−3.3 to +1.2 mEq/L	1	−3.3 to +1.2 mmol/L
	female	−2.4 to +2.3 mEq/L		−2.4 to +2.3 mmol/L
Base, total	Serum	145–160 mEq/L	1	145–160 mmol/L
Bicarbonate	Plasma	21–28 mmol/L	1	21–28 mmol/L
Bile acids	Serum	0.3–3.0 mg/dL	10	3.0–30.0 mg/L
Bilirubin	Serum			
direct (conjugated)		<0.3 mg/dL	17.10	<5 μmol/L
indirect (unconjugated)		0.1–1.0 mg/dL		2–17 μmol/L
total		0.1–1.2 mg/dL		2–21 μmol/L
newborns total		1.0–12.0 mg/dL		17–205 μmol/L
Blood gases (see Chap. 7)				
pH	Whole blood	7.38–7.44 (arterial)	1	7.38–7.44
		7.36–7.41 (venous)		7.36–7.41
P_{CO_2}	Whole blood	35–40 mm Hg (arterial)	0.1333	4.7–5.3 kPa
		40–45 mm Hg (venous)		5.3–6.0 kPa
P_{O_2}	Whole blood	95–100 mm Hg (arterial)	0.1333	12.7–13.3 kPa
Bromide	Serum	<5 mg/dL	0.125	<0.63 mmol/L
Calcium				
ionized	Serum	4.0–4.8 mg/dL	0.2500	1.00–1.20 mmol/L
		2.0–2.4 mEq/L	0.5000	
		30–58% of total	0.01	0.30–1.58 of total
total	Serum	9.2–11.0 mg/dL	0.2500	2.30–2.74 mmol/L
		4.6–5.5 mEq/L	0.5000	
Carbon dioxide (CO_2 content)	Whole blood (arterial)	19–24 mmol/L	1	19–24 mmol/L
	Plasma or serum (arterial)	21–28 mmol/L		21–28 mmol/L
Carbon dioxide	Whole blood (venous)	22–26 mmol/L	1	22–26 mmol/L
	Plasma or serum (venous)	24–30 mmol/L		24–30 mmol/L
CO_2 combining power	Plasma or serum (venous)	24–30 mmol/L	1	24–30 mmol/L
CO_2 partial pressure (P_{CO_2})	Whole blood (arterial)	35–40 mm Hg	0.1333	4.7–5.3 kPa
	Whole blood (venous)	40–45 mm Hg		5.3–6.0 kPa
Carbonic acid (H_2CO_3)	Whole blood (arterial)	1.05–1.45 mmol/L	1	1.05–1.45 mmol/L
	Whole blood (venous)	1.15–1.50 mmol/L		1.15–1.50 mmol/L

Table A4–4. WHOLE BLOOD, SERUM, AND PLASMA CHEMISTRY *Continued*

Component	System	Typical Reference Intervals		
		Conventional Units	*Factor**	*Recommended SI Units†*
	Plasma (venous)	1.02–1.38 mmol/L		1.02–1.38 mmol/L
Carboxyhemoglobin (carbon monoxide hemoglobin)	Whole blood			
	suburban nonsmokers	<1.5% saturation of hemoglobin	0.01	Fraction hemogloblin saturated: <0.015
	smokers	1.5–5.0% saturation		0.015–0.050
	heavy smokers	5.0–9.0% saturation		0.050–0.090
Carotene, beta	Serum	40–200 μg/dL	0.01863	0.7–3.7 μmol/L
Ceruloplasmin	Serum	23–50 mg/dL	10	230–500 mg/L
Chloride	Serum	95–103 mEq/L	1	95–103 mmol/L
Cholesterol				
total (see Chap. 10)	Serum	150–250 mg/dL (varies with diet, sex, and age)	0.02586	3.88–6.47 mmol/L
esters	Serum	65–75% of total cholesterol	0.01	Fraction of total cholesterol: 0.65–0.75
Cholinesterase	Erythrocytes	0.65–1.3 pH units	1	0.65–1.3 units§
(pseudocholinesterase)	Plasma	0.5–1.3 pH units		0.5–1.3 units
		8–18 U/L at 37°C	1	8–18 U/L at 37°C
Citrate	Serum or plasma	1.7–3.0 mg/dL	52.05	88–156 μmol/L
Copper	Serum, plasma			
	male	70–140 μg/dL	0.1574	11–22 μmol/L
	female	80–155 μg/dL		13–24 μmol/L
Cortisol	Plasma			
	8 A.M.–10 A.M.	5–23 μg/dL	27.59	138–635 nmol/L
	4 P.M.–6 P.M.	3–13 μg/dL		83–359 nmol/L
Creatine	Serum or plasma			
	male	0.1–0.4 mg/dL	76.25	8–31 μmol/L
	female	0.2–0.7 mg/dL		15–53 μmol/L
Creatine kinase (CK)	Serum			
	male	55–170 U/L at 37°C	1	55–170 U/L at 37°C
	female	30–135 U/L at 37°C	1	30–135 U/L at 37°C
Creatinine (see Chap. 8)	Serum or plasma	0.6–1.2 mg/dL (adult)	88.40	53–106 μmol/L
		0.3–0.6 mg/dL (children <2 y)		27–53 μmol/L
Creatinine clearance (endogenous) (see Chap. 7)	Serum or plasma and urine			
	male	107–139 mL/min	0.01667	1.78–2.32 mL/s
	female	87–107 mL/min		1.45–1.78 mL/s
Cryoglobulins	Serum	Negative	—	Negative
Electrophoresis, protein	Serum			
albumin		52–65% of total protein	0.01	Fraction of total protein: 0.52–0.65
alpha-1		2.5–5.0% of total protein	0.01	0.025–0.05
alpha-2		7.0–13.0% of total protein	0.01	0.07–0.13
beta		8.0–14.0% of total protein	0.01	0.08–0.14
gamma		12.0–22.0% of total protein	0.01	0.12–0.22
	Serum	Concentration		
albumin		3.2–5.6 g/dL	10	32–56 gL
alpha-1		0.1–0.4 g/dL		1–4 gL
alpha-2		0.4–1.2 g/dL		4–12 gL
beta		0.5–1.1 g/dL		5–11 gL
gamma		0.5–1.6 g/dL		5–16 gL
Fats, neutral (see Triglycerides)				
Fatty acids				
total (free and esterified)	Serum	9–15 mmol/L	1	9–15 mmol/L
free (nonesterified)	Plasma	300–480 μEq/L	1	300–480 μmol/L
Ferritin	Serum			
male		15–200 ng/mL	1	15–200 μg/L
female		12–150 ng/mL	1	15–150 μg/L
Fibrinogen	Plasma	200–400 mg/dL	0.01	2.00–4.00 g/L
Fluoride	Whole blood	<0.05 mg/dL	0.5263	<0.027 mmol/L
Folate	Serum	5–25 ng/mL (bioassay)	2.266	11–57 nmol/L
		>2.3 ng/mL (radioassay)		>5 nmol/L
	Erythrocytes	166–640 ng/mL (bioassay)		376–1450 nmol/L
		>140 ng/mL (radioassay)		>317 nmol/L
Galactose	Whole blood			
	adults	None		None
	children	<20 mg/dL	0.05551	<1.11 mmol/L
Gamma globulin	Serum	0.5–1.6 g/dL	10	5–16 g/L
Globulins, total	Serum	2.3–3.5 g/dL	10	23–35 g/L
Glucose, fasting	Serum or plasma	70–110 mg/dL	0.05551	3.9–6.1 mmol/L
	Whole blood	60–100 mg/dL		3.3–5.6 mmol/L

Table continued on following page

Table A4–4. WHOLE BLOOD, SERUM, AND PLASMA CHEMISTRY *Continued*

Component	System	Typical Reference Intervals: *Conventional Units*	*Factor**	*Recommended SI Units†*
Glucose tolerance	Serum or plasma			
oral	fasting	70–110 mg/dL	0.05551	3.9–6.1 mmol/L
	30 min	30–60 mg/dL above fasting		1.7–3.3 mmol/L above fasting
	60 min	20–50 mg/dL above fasting		1.1–2.8 mmol/L above fasting
	120 min	5–15 mg/dL above fasting		0.3–0.8 mmol/L above fasting
	180 min	Fasting level or below		Fasting level or below
	Serum or plasma			
intravenous	fasting	70–110 mg/dL		3.9–6.1 mmol/L
	5 min	Maximum of 250 mg/dL		Maximum of 13.9 mmol/L
	60 min	Significant decrease		Significant decrease
	120 min	Below 120 mg/dL		Below 6.7 mmol/L
	180 min	Fasting level		Fasting level
Glucose-6-phosphate dehydrogenase (G6PD)	Erythrocytes	250–5000 units/10^6 cells	1	250–5000 μunits/cell
		1200–2000 mIU/mL packed erythrocytes	1	1200–2000 U/L packed erythrocytes
γ-Glutamyltransferase	Serum	5–40 IU/L	1	5–40 U/L at 37°C
Glutathione	Whole blood	24–37 mg/dL	0.03254	0.78–1.20 mmol/L
Growth hormone	Serum	<10 ng/mL	1	<10 μg/L
Guanase	Serum	<3 nmol/mL/min	1	<3 U/L at 37°C
Haptoglobin	Serum	60–270 mg/dL	0.01	0.6–2.7 g/L
Hemoglobin	Serum or plasma			
	qualitative	Negative	—	Negative
	quantitative	0.5–5.0 mg/dL	10	5–50 mg/L
	Whole blood			
	female	12.0–16.0 g/dL	10	120–160 g/L
	male	13.5–18.0 g/dL		135–180 g/L
α-Hydroxybutyrate dehydrogenase	Serum	140–350 U/mL	1	140–350 kU/L
17-Hydroxycorticosteroids	Plasma			
	male	7–19 μg/dL	25.59‖	193–524 nmol/L
	female	9–21 μg/dL		248–579 nmol/L
	after 24 USP units of ACTH I.M.	35–55 μg/dL		966–1517 nmol/L
Immunoglobulins:	Serum			
IgG		800–1801 mg/dL	0.01	8.0–18.0 g/L
IgA		113–563 mg/dL		1.1–5.6 g/L
IgM		54–222 mg/dL		0.5–2.2 g/L
IgD		0.5–3.0 mg/dL	10	5.0–30.0 mg/L
IgE		0.01–0.04 mg/dL		0.1–0.4 mg/L
Insulin	Plasma			
	bioassay	11–240 μIU/mL	7.175††	79–1722 pmol/L
	radioimmunoassay	4–24 μIU/mL		29–172 pmol/L
Insulin tolerance (0.1 unit/kg)	Serum			
	fasting	Glucose of 70–110 mg/dL	0.05551	Glucose of 3.9–6.1 mmol/L
	30 min	Fall to 50% of fasting level	0.01	Fall to 0.5 of fasting level
	90 min	Fasting level		Fasting level
Iron, total	Serum	60–150 μg/dL	0.1791	10.7–26.9 μmol/L
Iron-binding capacity	Serum	250–400 μg/dL	0.1791	44.8–71.6 μmol/L
Iron saturation	Serum	20–55%	0.01	Fraction of total iron-biding capacity: 0.20–0.55
Isocitric dehydrogenase	Serum	50–240 units/mL at 25°C (Wolfson-Williams Ashman units)	0.0166	0.83–4.18 U/L at 25°C
Ketone bodies	Serum	Negative	—	Negative
17-Ketosteroids	Plasma	25–125 μg/dL	34.67¶	866–4334 nmol/L
Lactic acid (as lactate)	Whole blood			
	venous	5–20 mg/dL	0.1110	0.6–2.2 mmol/L
	arterial	3–7 mg/dL		0.3–0.8 mmol/L
Lactate dehydrogenase (LD)	Serum	(lactate → pyruvate) 80–120 units at 30°C	0.48	38–62 U/L at 30°C
		(pyruvate → lactate) 185–640 units at 30°C	0.48	90–310 U/L at 30°C
		(lactate → pyruvate) 100–190 U/L at 37°C	1	100–190 U/L at 37°C
Lactate dehydrogenase isoenzymes	Serum			Fraction of total LD
LD_1 (anode)		17–27%	0.01	0.17–0.27
LD_2		27–37%		0.27–0.37
LD_3		18–25%		0.18–0.25
LD_4		3–8%		0.03–0.08
LD_5 (cathode)		0–5%		0.00–0.05

Table A4–4. WHOLE BLOOD, SERUM, AND PLASMA CHEMISTRY *Continued*

Component	System	Typical Reference Intervals: *Conventional Units*	*Factor**	*Recommended SI Units†*
Lactate dehydrogenase (heat stable)	Serum	30–60% of total	0.01	Fraction of total LD: 0.30–0.60
Lactose tolerance	Serum	Serum glucose changes similar to glucose tolerance test	—	Serum glucose changes similar to glucose tolerance test
Lead	Whole blood	<50 μg/dL	0.04826	<2.41 μmol/L
Leucine aminopeptidase (LAP)	Serum			
	male	80–200 U/mL (Goldbarg-Rutenberg)	0.24	19.2–48.0 U/L
	female	75–185 U/mL (Goldbarg-Rutenberg)		18.0–44.4 U/L
Lipase	Serum	0–1.5 U/mL (Cherry-Crandall)	278	0–417 U/L
		14–280 mIU/mL	1	14–280 U/L
Lipids, total	Serum	400–800 mg/dL	0.01	4.00–8.00 g/L
cholesterol (see Chap.10)		150–250 mg/dL	0.02586	3.88–6.47 mmol/L
triglycerides (see Chap. 10)		10–90 mg/dL	0.01129**	0.11–2.15 mmol/L
phospholipids		150–380 mg/dL	0.01	1.50–3.80 g/L
fatty acids (free)		9.0–15.0 mmol/L	1	9.0–15.0 mmol/L
phospholipid phosphorus		8.0–11.0 mg/dL	0.3229	2.58–3.55 mmol/L
Lithium	Serum	Negative	—	Negative
therapeutic interval		0.5–1.4 mEq/L	1	0.5–1.4 mmol/L
Long-acting thyroid-stimulating hormone (LATS)	Serum	None detected	—	None detected
Luteinizing hormone (LH)	Serum			
	male	6–30 mIU/mL	1	6–30 IU/L
	female	Mid cycle peak: 3 times baseline value		Midcycle peak: 3 times baseline value
		Premenopausal <30 mIU/mL		Premenopausal <30 IU/L
		Postmenopausal >35 mIU/mL		Postmenopausal >35 IU/L
Macroglobulins, total	Serum	70–430 mg/dL	0.01	0.7–4.3 g/L
Magnesium	Serum	1.3–2.1 mEq/L	0.5000	0.65–1.05 mmol/L
		1.8–3.0 mg/dL	0.4114	0.74–1.23 mmol/L
Methemoglobin	Whole blood	<0.24 g/dL	10	<2.4 g/L
		<1% of total hemoglobin	0.01	Fraction of total hemoglobin <0.01
Mucoprotein	Serum	80–200 mg/dL	0.01	0.8–2.0 g/L
Muramidase	Serum	4–13 mg/L		4–13 mg/L
Myoglobin	Serum	<90 μg/L		<90 μg/L
Nonprotein nitrogen (NPN)	Serum or plasma	20–35 mg/dL	0.7139	14.3–25.0 mmol/L
	Whole blood	25–50 mg/dL		17.8–35.7 mmol/L
5′-Nucleotidase	Serum	0–1.6 units at 37°C	1	0–1.6 units at 37°C
Ornithine carbamyl transferase	Serum	8–20 mIU/mL at 37°C	1	8–20 U/L at 37°C
Osmolality	Serum	280–295 mOsm/kg	1	280–295 mmol/kg
Oxygen (see Chap. 7)				
pressure (Po_2)	Whole blood (arterial)	95–100 mm Hg	0.1333	12.7–13.3 kPa
content	Whole blood (arterial)	15–23 volume %	0.01	Volume fraction: 0.15–0.23
saturation	Whole blood (arterial)	94–100%		Fraction saturated: 0.94–1.00
pH	Whole blood (arterial)	7.38–7.44	1	7.38–7.44
	Whole blood (venous)	7.36–7.41		7.36–7.41
	Serum or plasma (venous)	7.35–7.45		7.35–7.45
Phenylalanine	Serum			
	adults	<3.0 mg/dL	60.54	<182 μmol/L
	newborns (term)	1.2–3.5 mg/dL		73–212 μmol/L
Phosphatase				
acid phosphatase	Serum	0.13–0.63 U/L at 37°C (*p*-nitrophenylphosphate)	16.67	2.2–10.5 U/L at 37°C
alkaline phosphatase	Serum	20–130 IU/L at 37°C (*p*-nitrophenylphosphate in AMP buffer)	1	20–130 U/L at 37°C
Phospholipid phosphorus see (Lipids, total)				
Phospholipids (see Lipids, total)				
Phosphorus, inorganic	Serum			
	adults	2.3–4.7 mg/dL	0.3229	0.74–1.52 mmol/L
	children	4.0–7.0 mg/dL		1.29–2.26 mmol/L

Table continued on following page

Table A4–4. WHOLE BLOOD, SERUM, AND PLASMA CHEMISTRY *Continued*

Component	System	Typical Reference Intervals		
		Conventional Units	*Factor**	*Recommended SI Units†*
Potassium	Plasma	3.8–5.0 mEq/L	1	3.8–5.0 mmol/L
Prolactin	Serum female	1–25 ng/mL	1	1–25 μg/L
	male	1–20 ng/mL		1–20 μg/L
Proteins (see Chap. 11)	Serum			
total		6.0–7.8 g/dL	10	60–78 g/L
albumin		3.2–4.5 g/dL		32–45 g/L
globulin		2.3–3.5 g/dL		23–35 g/L
Protein fractionation		See electrophoresis		See Electrophoresis
Protoporphyrin	Erythrocytes	15–50 mg/dL	0.01777	0.27–0.89 μmol/L
Pyruvate	Whole blood	0.3–0.9 mg/dL	113.6	34–102 μmol/L
Salicylates	Serum	Negative	—	Negative
therapeutic interval		15–30 mg/dL	0.07240	1.08–2.17 mmol/L
Sodium	Plasma	136–142 mEq/L	1	136–142 mmol/L
Sulfate, inorganic	Serum	0.2–1.3 mEq/L	0.5	0.10–0.65 mmol/L
		0.9–6.0 mg/dL as $SO_4^=$	0.1042	0.09–0.63 mmol/L as $SO_4^=$
Sulfhemoglobin	Whole blood	Negative	—	Negative
Sulfonamides	Serum or whole blood	Negative	—	Negative
Testosterone	Serum or plasma			
	male	300–1200 ng/dL	0.03467	10.4–41.6 nmol/L
	female	30–95 ng/dL		1.0–3.3 nmol/L
Thiocyanate	Serum	Negative	—	Negative
Thyroid hormone tests (see Chap. 16)	Serum			
thyroxine, total (T_4)		5.5–12.5 μg/dL	12.87	71–161 nmol/L
thyroxine, free (FT_4)		0.9–2.3 ng/dL	12.87	12–30 pmol/L
T_3 resin uptake		25–38 relative % uptake	0.01	Relative uptake fraction: 0.25–0.38
thyroxine-binding globulin (TBG)	Serum	10–26 μg/dL	10	100–260 μg/L
thyrotropin (TSH)	Serum	0.5–5 μIU/mL		0.5–5 μIU/L
triiodothyronine (T_3)		80–200 mg/dL	0.0154	1.23–3 of nmol/L
Transferases				
aspartate amino transferase (AST or SGOT)	Serum	8–33 U/L at 37°C	1	8–33 U/L at 37°C
alanine amino transferase (ALT or SGPT)	Serum	4–36 U/L at 37°C	1	4–36 U/L at 37°C
gamma glutamyl transferase (GGT)		5–40 IU/L at 37°C	1	5–40 U/L at 37°C
Triglycerides (see Chap.10)	Serum	10–190 mg/dL	0.01129**	0.11–2.15 mmol/L
Troponin I	Serum	0–0.6 mg/mL		0–0.6 μg/L
Troponin T	Serum	0–0.1 μg/L		0–0.1 μg/L
Urea nitrogen	Serum	8–23 mg/dL	0.357	2.9–8.2 mmol/L
Urea clearance	Serum and urine			
maximum clearance		64–99 mL/min	0.01667	1.07–1.65 L/s
standard clearance		41–65 mL/min, or more than 75% of normal clearance		0.68–1.08 L/s or more than 0.75 of normal clearance
Uric acid	Serum			
	male	4.0–8.5 mg/dL	0.05948	0.24–0.51 mmol/L
	female	2.7–7.3 mg/dL		0.16–0.43 mmol/L
Vitamin A	Serum	15–60 μg/dL	0.03491	0.52–2.09 μmol/L
Vitamin A tolerance	Serum			
	fasting 3 h or 6 h	15–60 μg/dL	0.03491	0.52–2.09 μmol/L
	after 5000 units vitamin A/kg	200–600 μg/dL		6.98–20.95 μmol/L
	24 h	Fasting values or slightly above	—	Fasting values or slightly above
Vitamin B_{12}	Serum	160–950 pg/mL	0.7378	118–701 pmol/L
Unsaturated vitamin B_{12}–binding capacity	Serum	1000–2000 pg/mL	0.7378	738–1475 pmol/L
Vitamin C	Plasma	0.6–1.6 mg/dL	56.78	34–91 μmol/L
Xylose absorption	Serum			
	normal	25–40 mg/dL between 1 and 2 h	0.06661	1.67–2.66 mmol/L between 1 and 2 h
	in malabsorption	Maximum approximately 10 mg/dL		Maximum approximately 0.67 mmol/L
		Dose: adult 25 g D-xylose children 0.5 g D-xylose/kg		
Zinc	Serum	50–150 μg/dL	0.1530	7.7–23.0 μmol/L

*Factor = number factor (note that units are not presented).
†Value in SI units = value in conventional units × factor.
‡Usually not measured in blood (preferred specimen is urine, hair, or nails except in acute cases, when gastric contents are used).
§Unit based on hydrogen ion concentration.
‖ As cortisol.
¶As DHEA.
**As triolein.
††One (1) International Unit of insulin corresponds to 0.04167 mg of the 4th International Standard (a mixture of 52% beef insulin and 48% pig insulin).

Table A4–5. URINE

Component	Type of Urine System	Typical Reference Intervals: *Conventional Units*	*Factor**	*Recommended SI Units†*
Acetoacetic acid	Random	Negative	—	Negative
Acetone	Random	Negative	—	Negative
Addis count	12 h collection	WBC and epithelial cells: 1,800,000/12 h	1	1.8 × 10^6/12 h
		RBC 500,000/12 h	1	0.5 × 10^6/12 h
		Hyaline casts: <5000/12 h	1	<5.0 × 10^3/12 h
Albumin				
qualitative	Random	Negative	—	Negative
quantitative	24 h	15–150 mg/d	0.001	0.015–0.150 g/d
Aldosterone	24 h	2–26 μg/d	2.774	6–72 nmol/d
Alkapton bodies	Random	Negative	—	Negative
α-Amino acid nitrogen	24 h	100–290 mg/d	0.07139	7.1–20.7 mmol/d
δ-Aminolevulinic acid	Random			
	adult	0.1–0.6 mg/dL	76.26	8–46 μmol/L
	children	<0.5 mg/dL		<38 μmol/L
	24 h	1.5–7.5 mg/d	7.626	11–57 μmol/d
Ammonia nitrogen	24 h	20–70 mEq/d	1	20–70 mmol/d
		500–1200 mg/d	0.07139	35.6–85.7 mmol/d
Amylase	2 h	35–260 Somogyi units/h	0.1850	6.5–48.1 U/h
Arsenic	24 h	<50 μg/L	0.01335	<0.67 μmol/L
Ascorbic acid	Random	1–7 mg/dL	56.78	57–397 μmol/L
	24 h	>50 mg/d	5.678	>284 μmol/d
Bence Jones protein	Random	Negative	—	Negative
Beryllium	24 h	<0.05 μg/d	111.0	<5.55 nmol/d
Bilirubin, qualitative	Random	Negative	—	Negative
Blood, occult	Random	Negative	—	Negative
Borate	24 h	<2 mg/L	16.44	<32 μmol/L
Calcium				
qualitative (Sulkowitch)	Random	1+ turbidity	1	1+ turbidity
quantitative	24 h			
	average diet	100–240 mg/d	0.02495	2.5–6.0 mmol/d
	low-calcium diet	<150 mg/d		<3.7 mmol/d
	high-calcium diet	240–300 mg/d		6.0–7.5 mmol/d
Catecholamines	Random	<14 μg/dL	59.11*	<828 nmol/L
	24 h	<100 μg/d (varies with activity)	5.911*	<591 nmol/d
epinephrine		<10 ng/d	5.458	<55 nmol/d
norepinephrine		<100 ng/d	5.911	<591 nmol/d
total free catecholamines		4–126 μg/d	5.911*	24–745 nmol/d
total metanephrines		0.1–1.6 mg/d	5.458†	0.5–8.7 μmol/d
Chloride	24 h	140–250 mEq/d	1	140–250 nmol/d
Concentration test (Fishberg)	Random—after fluid restriction			
specific gravity		>1.025	1	>1.025
osmolality		>850 mOsm/kg	1	>850 mmol/kg
Copper	24 h	<50 μg/d	0.01574	<0.8 μmol/d
Coproporphyrin	Random			
	adult	3–20 μg/dL	15.27	46–305 nmol/L
	24 h			
	adult	50–160 μg/d	1.527	76–244 nmol/d
	children	<80 μg/d		<122 nmol/d
Creatine	24 h			
	male	<40 mg/d	7.625	<305 μmol/d
	female	<100 mg/d		<763 μmol/d
		Higher in children and during pregnancy	—	Higher in children and during pregnancy
Creatinine	24 h			
	male	20–26 mg/kg/d	8.840	177–230 μmol/kg/d
		1.0–2.0 g/d	8.840	8.8–17.7 mmol/d
	female	14–22 mg/kg/d	8.840	124–195 μmol/kg/d
		0.8–1.8 g/d	8.840	7.1–15.9 mmol/d
Cystine, qualitative	Random	Negative	—	Negative
Cystine and cysteine	24 h	10–100 mg/d	4.161‡	42–416 μmol/d
Dehydroepiandrosterone	24 h			
	male	0.2–2.0 mg/d	3.467	0.7–6.9 μmol/d
	female	0.2–1.8 mg/d		0.7–6.2 μmol/d
Diacetic acid	Random	Negative	—	Negative
Epinephrine	24 h	<20 μg/d	5.458	<109 nmol/d

Table continued on following page

Table A4–5. URINE *Continued*

Component	Type of Urine System	Typical Reference Intervals: *Conventional Units*	*Factor**	*Recommended SI Units*†
Estrogens				
total	24 h			
	male	5–18 μg/d	3.468§	17–62 nmol/d
	female			
	ovulation	28–100 μg/d		97–347 nmol/d
	luteal peak	22–80 μg/d		76–364 nmol/d
	at menses	4–25 μg/d		14–87 nmol/d
	pregnancy	Up to 45,000 μg/d	0.003468	Up to 156 μmol/d
	postmenopausal	Up to 10 μg/d	3.468	Up to 35 nmol/d
fractionated	24 h, nonpregnant, midcycle			
estrone (E_1)	—	2–25 μg/d	3.699	7–93 nmol/d
estradiol (E_2)	—	<10 μg/d	3.671	<37 nmol/d
estriol (E_3)	—	2–30 μg/d	3.468	7–104 nmol/d
Fat, qualitative	Random	Negative	—	Negative
FIGLU	24 h	<3 mg/d	5.740	<17.2 μmol/d
(N-formiminoglutamic acid)	after 15 g of L-histidine	4 mg/8 h		23.0 μmol/8 h
Fluoride	24 h	<1 mg/d	52.63	<53 μmol/d
Follicle-stimulating hormone (FSH)	24 h			
	adult	4–25 U/L	1	4–25 IU/L
	prepubertal	4–30 U/L	1	4–30 IU/L
	postmenopausal	40–50 U/L	1	40–50 IU/L
	midcycle	2 × baseline	1	2 × baseline
Fructose	24 h	30–65 mg/d	0.005551	0.17–0.36 mmol/d
Glucose				
qualitative	Random	Negative	—	Negative
quantitative	24 h			
copper-reducing substances		0.5–1.5 g/d	1	0.5–1.5 g/d
total sugars		Average 250 mg/d	1	Average 250 mg/d
glucose		Average 130 mg/d	0.005551	Average 0.72 mmol/d
Gonadotropins, pituitary (FSH and LH)	24 h	10–50 U/L	1	10–50 IU/d
Etiocholanolone	24 h			
	male	1.4–5.0 mg/d	3.443	4.8–17.2 μmol/d
	female	0.8–4.0 mg/d		2.8–13.8 μmol/d
11-Hydroxyandrosterone	24 h			
	male	0.1–0.8 mg/d	3.263	0.3–2.6 μmol/d
	female	<0.5 mg/d		<1.6 μmol/d
11-Hydroxyetiocholanolone	24 h			
	male	0.2–0.6 mg/d	3.26	0.7–2.0 μmol/d
	female	0.1–1.1 mg/d		0.3–3.63 μmol/d
11-Ketoandrosterone	24 h			
	male	0.2–1.0 mg/d	3.274	0.7–3.3 μmol/d
	female	0.2–0.8 mg/d		0.7–2.6 μmol/d
11-Ketoetiocholanolone	24 h			
	male	0.2–1.0 mg/d	3.274	0.7–3.3 μmol/d
	female	0.2–0.8 mg/d		0.7–2.6 μmol/d
Lactose	24 h	14–40 mg/d	2.291	41–117 μmol/d
Lead	24 h	<100 μg/d	0.004826	<0.48 μmol/d
Magnesium	24 h	6.0–8.5 mEq/d	0.5000	3.0–4.3 mmol/d
Melanin, qualitative	Random	Negative	—	Negative
Mucin	24 h	100–150 mg/d	1	100–150 mg/d
Muramidase (lysozyme)	24 h	1.3–36 mg/d	1	1.3–36 mg/d
Myoglobin				
qualitative	Random	Negative	—	Negative
quantitative	24 h	<4 mg/L	1	<4 mg/L
Osmolality	Random	500–800 mOsm/kg water	1	500–800 mmol/kg
Pentoses	24 h	2–5 mg/kg/d	1	2–5 mg/kg/d
pH	Random	4.6–8.0	1	4.6–8.0
Phenosulfonphthalein (PSP)	Urine timed after 6 mg PSP IV			
	15 min	20–50% dye excreted	0.01	Fraction dye excreted: 0.20–0.50
	30 min	16–24% dye excreted		0.16–0.24
	60 min	9–17% dye excreted		0.09–0.17
	120 min	3–10% dye excreted		0.03–0.10
Phenylpyruvic acid, qualitative	Random	Negative	—	Negative

Table A4–5. URINE *Continued*

Component	Type of Urine System	Typical Reference Intervals: Conventional Units	Factor*	Recommended SI Units†
Phosphorus	Random	0.9–1.3 g/d	32.29	29–42 mmol/d
Porphobilinogen				
qualitative	Random	Negative	—	Negative
quantitative	24 h	<1.0 mg/d	4.420	<4.4 μmol/d
Potassium	24 h	40–80 mEq/d	1	40–80 mmol/d
Pregnancy tests	Concentrated morning specimen	Positive in normal pregnancies or with tumors producing chorionic gonadotropin	—	Positive in normal pregnancies or with tumors producing chorionic gonadotropin
Pregnanediol	24 h			
	male	<1.5 mg/d	3.120	<4.7 μmol/d
	female	1–8 mg/d		3–25 μmol/d
	peak	1 week after ovulation	3.120	1 week after ovulation
	pregnancy	<50 mg/d		<156 μmol/d
	children	Negative	—	Negative
Pregnanetriol	24 h			
	male	0.4–2.4 mg/d	2.972	1.2–7.1 μmol/d
	female	0.5–2.0 mg/d		1.5–5.9 μmol/d
	children	Up to 1 mg/d		Up to 3 μmol/d
Protein, qualitative	Random	Negative	—	Negative
	24 h	40–150 mg/d	1	40–150 mg/d
Reducing substances, total	24 h	0.5–1.5 mg/d	1	0.5–1.5 mg/d
Sodium	24 h	75–200 mEq/d	1	75–200 mmol/d
Solids, total	24 h	55–70 g/d	1	55–70 g/d
		Decreases with age to 30 g/d	—	Decreases with age to 30 g/d
Specific gravity	Random	1.016–1.022 (normal fluid intake)	1	Relative density (U 20°C/water 20°C) 1.016–1.022 (normal fluid intake)
		1.001–1.035 (range)		1.001–1.035 (range)
Sugars (excluding glucose)	Random	Negative	—	Negative
Titratable acidity	24 h	20–50 mEq/d	1	20–50 mmol/d
Urea nitrogen	24 h	6–17 g/d	35.70	214–607 mmol/d
Uric acid	24 h	250–750 mg/d	0.005948	1.5–4.5 mmol/d
Urobilinogen	2 h	0.3–1.0 Ehrlich units	1	0.3–1.0 U
	24 h	0.05–2.5 mg/d or	1.693	0.1–4.2 μmol/d
		0.5–4.0 Erhlich units/d	1	0.5–4.0 U/d
Uropepsin	Random	15–45 units/h (Anson)	7.37	111–332 U/h
	24 h	1500–5000 units/d (Anson)		11–37 kU/h
Uroporphyrins				
qualitative	Random	Negative	—	Negative
quantitative	24 h	10–30 μg/d	1.204	12–36 nmol/d
Vanillylmandelic acid (VMA)	24 h	1.5–7.5 mg/d	5.046	7.6–37.9 μmol/d
Volume, total	24 h	600–1600 mL/d	0.001	0.6–1.6 L/d
Zinc	24 h	0.15–1.2 mg/d	15.30	2.3–18.4 μmol/d

*As norepinephrine.
†As normetanephrine.
‡Based on cystine.
§Based on estriol.

Table A4–6. SYNOVIAL FLUID

Component	Typical Reference Intervals: Conventional Units	Factor	Recommended SI Units
Blood-serum-synovial fluid glucose difference	<10 mg/dL	0.05551	<0.56 mmol/L
Differential cell count	Granulocytes <25% of nucleated cells	0.01	Granulocyte number fraction: <0.25 of nucleated cells
Fibrin clot	Absent	—	Absent
Mucin clot	Abundant	—	Abundant
Nucleated cell count	<200 cells/μL	10^6	<200 × 10^6 cells/L
Viscosity	High	—	High
Volume	<3.5 mL	0.001	<0.0035 L

Table A4–7. SEMINAL FLUID

Component	Typical Reference Intervals		
	Conventional Units	*Factor*	*Recommended SI Units*
Liquefaction	Within 20 min		Within 20 min
Sperm morphology	>70% normal, mature spermatozoa	0.01	Number fraction: >0.70 normal, mature spermatozoa
Sperm motility	>60%	0.01	Number fraction: >0.60
pH	>7.0 (average 7.7)	1	>7.0 (average 7.7)
Sperm count	60–150 × 10^6/mL	10^3	60–150 × 10^9/L
Volume	1.5–5.0 mL	0.001	0.0015–0.005 L

Health Organization, 1977b). A comprehensive list of quantities and their internationally recommended SI units are given in Tietz (1995).

In making the conversion to recommend SI units (Tables A4–4 to A4–13), the following guidelines were followed:

1. All reference intervals have been converted to SI units except in cases in which the measurements are not quantitative.
2. Chemical names have not been changed; e.g., urea is retained instead of changing to carbamide.
3. Factors are those published by the American National Metric Council (Lundberg, 1986; Young, 1987; Beeler, 1987), based on the Metric Commission of Canada (1981) factors.
4. Factors are calculated to the base unit for volume of 1 L in accordance with Recommendation 1978.
5. The order of magnitude of the factors is calculated to make the values in SI units convenient numbers—i.e., with prefixes, a number not greater than 1000 or smaller than 0.001.
6. The number in recommended SI units is equal to the number in conventional units times the factor.
7. For compounds for which relative molecular masses are not definitely known (e.g., proteins), reference intervals are converted to mass amounts per liter.
8. For mixtures of indeterminate composition (e.g., phospholipids), reference intervals are converted to mass amounts per liter or are based on a given standard—e.g., DHEA for 17-ketosteroids.
9. Quantities of a relative nature that are usually expressed as percentages—e.g., fractions of LD isoenzymes—are given as fractions.
10. Enzyme units are given as the International Unit per liter (U/L). Although the coherent SI unit for catalytic activity (including enzymes), the katal, has been defined as the number of moles of substrate converted per second under defined conditions, its adoption is limited.
11. The pH scale is retained for measurement of hydrogen ion concentrations.
12. It is recommended (World Health Organization, 1977a) that the unit mm Hg be retained for pressure (P_{CO_2}, P_{O_2}) at the present time.
13. Percentages are expressed as fractions in the SI, where a fraction is a dimensionless quantity given by the

Text continued on page 1465

Table A4–8. GASTRIC FLUID

Component	Typical Reference Intervals		
	Conventional Units	*Factor*	*Recommended SI Units*
Fasting residual volume	20–100 mL	0.001	0.02–0.10 L
pH	<2.0	1	<2.0
Basal acid output (BAO)*	0–6 mEq/h	1	0–6 mmol/h
Maximum acid output (MAO) (after histamine stimulation)	5–40 mEq/h	1	5–40 mmol/h
BAO/MAO ratio	<0.4	1	<0.4

*Varies between male and female and ages.

Table A4–9. HEMATOLOGY

Component	Typical Reference Intervals		
	Conventional Units	*Factor*	*Recommended SI Units*
Red cell volume			
male	20–36 mL/kg body weight	0.001	0.020–0.036 L/kg body weight
female	19–32 mL/kg body weight		0.019–0.032 L/kg body weight
Plasma volume			
male	25–43 mL/kg body weight	0.001	0.025–0.043 L/kg body weight
female	28–45 mL/kg body weight		0.028–0.045 L/kg body weight
Coagulation and hemostatic tests			
bleeding time	Depends on location and orientation of cut and on particular device, typically 2–8 min		
Activated partial thromboplastin time (APTT)	Depends on activator and phospholipid reagents used, typically 25–35 s		
Antithrombin III			
immunologic	20–30 mg/dL	10	200–300 mg/L
functional	80–120 U/dL	10	800–1200 U/L
Clot lysis time			
euglobulin factor	1½–4 h at 37°C		
whole blood	None by 24 h at 37°C		
Clot retraction	Complete by 4 h at 37°C		
Coagulation factors	0.50–1.50 μ/mL	1000	500–1500 U/L
Factor XIII (screening test)	Clot insoluble in 5 mol/L urea at 24 h		
Fibrinogen	200–400 mg/dL	0.01	2.0–4.0 g/L
Fibrin(ogen) degradation products			
serum FDP	<10 μg/mL	1	<10 mg/L
plasma D-dimers	<200 ng/mL	1	<200 μg/L
Plasminogen			
immunologic	10–20 mg/dL	10	100–200 mg/L
functional	80–120 U/dL	10	800–1200 U/L
Protein C	0.7–1.4 μ/mL	10	700–1400 U/L
Protein S (total)	0.7–1.4 μ/mL	10	700–1400 U/L
Prothrombin time	Depends on thromboplastin reagent used, typically 10–13 s		
Thrombin time	Depends on concentration of thrombin reagent used, typically 17–25 s		
von Willebrand factor			
immunologic	50–150 U/dL	10	500–1500 U/L
ristocetin cofactor activity	50–150 U/dL	10	500–1500 U/L
Complete blood count (CBC)			
hematocrit			
male	41.5–50.4%	0.01	Volume fraction: 0.415–0.504
female	35.9–44.6%		0.359–0.446
hemoglobin			
male	14.0–17.5 g/dL	10	140–175 g/L
female	12.3–15.3 g/dL		123–153 g/L
red cell count			
male	4.5–5.9 × $10^6/\mu$L	10^6	4.5–5.9 × 10^{12}/L
female	4.5–5.1 × $10^6/\mu$L		4.1–5.1 × 10^{12}/L
white cell count	4.4–11.0 × $10^3/\mu$L	10^6	4.4–11.3 × 10^9/L
Erythrocyte indices			
mean corpuscular volume (MCV)	80–96 μm^3	1	80–96 fL
mean corpuscular hemoglobin (MCH)	27.5–33.2 pg	1	27.5–33.2 pg
Mean corpuscular hemoglobin concentration (MCHC)	33.4–35.5%	0.01	Concentration fraction: 0.334–0.355

Table continued on following page

Table A4–9. HEMATOLOGY *Continued*

Component	*Conventional Units*			*Factor*	*Recommended SI Units*		
	Typical Reference Intervals						
White blood cell differential (adult)	Mean percent		Range of absolute counts		Mean number fraction*		Range of absolute count
segmented neutrophils	56%		1800–7800/μL	10^6	0.56		1.8–7.8 × 10^9/L
bands	3%		0–700/μL	10^6	0.03		0–0.70 × 10^9/L
eosinophils	2.7%		0–450/μL	10^6	0.027		0–0.45 × 10^9/L
basophils	0.3%		0–200/μL	10^6	0.003		0–0.20 × 10^9/L
lymphocytes	34%		1000–4800/μL	10^6	0.34		1.0–4.8 × 10^9/L
monocytes	4%		0–800/μL	10^6	0.04		0–0.80 × 10^9/L
Hemoglobin A_2	1.5–3.5% of total hemoglobin			0.01	mass fraction: 0.015–0.035 of total hemoglobin		
Hemoglobin F	<2%			0.01	mass fraction: <0.02		
Osmotic fragility		% Lysis		% NaCl—171 % Lysis—0.01		Lysed Fraction	
	% (w/v) NaCl	Fresh	24 h at 37°C		NaCl mmol/L	Fresh	24 h at 37°C
	0.2	—	95–100		34.2	—	0.95–1.00
	0.3	97–100	85–100		51.3	0.97–1.00	0.85–1.00
	0.35	90–99	75–100		59.8	0.90–0.99	0.75–100
	0.4	50–95	65–100		68.4	0.50–0.95	0.65–1.00
	0.45	5–45	55–95		77.0	0.05–0.45	0.55–0.95
	0.5	0.6	40–85		85.5	0–0.06	0.40–0.85
	0.55	—	15–70		94.1	0	0.15–0.70
	0.6	—	0–40		102.6	—	0–0.40
	0.65	—	0–10		111.2	—	0–0.10
	0.7	—	0–5		119.7	—	0–0.05
	0.75	—	0		128.3	—	0
Platelet count	150,000–450,000/μL			10^6	150–450 × 10^9/L		
Reticulocyte count	0.5–1.5%			0.01	number fraction: 0.005–0.015		
	25,000–75,000 cells/μL			10^6	25–75 × 10^9/L		
Sedimentation rate (ESR) (Westergren)							
men under 50 years	<15 mm/h						
men 50–85 years	<20 mm/h						
men over 85 years	<30 mm/h						
women under 50 years	<20 mm/h						
women 50–85 years	<30 mm/h						
women over 85 years	<42 mm/h						
Viscosity	1.4–1.8 times water			1	1.4–1.8 times water		
Zeta sedimentation ratio	41–54%			0.01	fraction: 0.41–0.54		

*All percentages are multiplied by 0.01 to give fraction.

Table A4–10. AMNIOTIC FLUID

	Typical Reference Intervals		
Component	***Conventional Units***	***Factor***	***Recommended SI Units***
Appearance			
early gestation	Clear	—	Clear
term	Clear or slightly opalescent	—	Clear or slightly opalescent
Albumin			
early gestation	0.39 g/dL	10	3.9 g/L
term	0.19 g/dL		1.9 g/L
Bilirubin			
early gestation	<0.075 mg/dL	17.10	<1.3 μmol/L
term	<0.025 mg/dL		<0.41 μmol/L
Chloride			
early gestation	Approximately equal to serum chloride	—	
term	Generally 1–3 mEq/L lower than serum chloride	1	Generally 1–3 mmol/L lower than serum chloride
Creatinine			
early gestation	0.8–1.1 mg/dL	88.40	71–97 μmol/L
term	1.8–4.0 mg/dL (generally >2 mg/dL)		159–354 μmol/L (generally >177 μmol/L)
Estriol			
early gestation	<10 μg/dL	3.468	<347 nmol/L
term	<60 μg/dL		>2081 nmol/L
Lecithin/sphingomyelin			
early (immature)	<1:1	1	<1:1
term (mature)	>2:1	1	>2:1
Osmolality			
early gestation	Approximately equal to serum osmolality	1	Approximately equal to serum osmolality
term	230–270 mOsm/kg	1	230–270 mmol/kg
P_{CO_2}			
early gestation	33–55 mm Hg	0.1333	4.4–7.3 kPa
term	42–55 mm Hg (increases toward term)		5.6–7.3 kPa (increases toward term)
pH			
early gestation	7.12–7.38	1	7.12–7.38
term	6.91–7.43 (decreases toward term)		6.91–7.43
Protein, total			
early gestation	0.60 ± 0.24 g/dL	10	60 ± 2.4 g/L
term	0.26 ± 0.19 g/dL		2.6 ± 1.9 g/L
Sodium			
early gestation	Approximately equal to serum sodium		
term	7–10 mEq/L lower than serum sodium	1	7–10 mmol/L lower than serum sodium
Staining, cytologic			
Oil Red O			
early gestation	<10%	0.01	Stained fraction: <0.1
term	>50%		>0.5
Nile blue sulfate			
early gestation	0	0.01	Stained fraction: <0.0
term	>20%		>0.2
Urea			
early gestation	18.0 ± 5.9 mg/dL	0.1665	3.00 ± 0.98 mmol/L
term	30.3 ± 11.4 mg/dL		5.04 ± 1.90 mmol/L
Uric acid			
early gestation	3.72 ± 0.96 mg/dL	59.48	221 ± 57 μmol/L
term	9.90 ± 2.23 mg/dL		589 ± 133 μmol/L
Volume			
early gestation	450–1200 mL	0.001	0.45–1.2 L
term	500–1400 mL (increases toward term)		0.5–1.4 L (increases toward term)

Table A4–11. CEREBROSPINAL FLUID

Component	Typical Reference Intervals		
	Conventional Units	*Factor*	*Recommended SI Units*
Albumin	<10–30 mg/dL	10	100–300 mg/L
Cell count	<5 cells/μL	10^6	<5 × 10^6/L
Glucose	40–80 mg/dL	0.05551	2.8–4.4 mmol/L
Lactate dehydrogenase (LD)	Approximately 10% of serum level	—	Activity fraction: approximately 0.1 of serum level
Proteins	12–60 mg/dL	10	120–600 mg/L
Protein electrophoresis			
prealbumin	2–7%	0.01	Fraction: 0.2–0.07
albumin	56–76%		0.56–0.76
alpha-1 globulin	2–7%		0.02–0.07
alpha-2 globulin	4–12%		0.04–0.12
beta globulin	8–18%		0.08–0.18
gamma globulin	3–12%		0.03–0.12
Xanthochromia	Negative	—	Negative

Table A4–12. MISCELLANEOUS

Component	Specimen	Typical Reference Intervals		
		Conventional Units	*Factor*	*Recommended SI Units*
Bile, qualitative	Random stool	Negative in adults Positive in children	— —	Negative in adults Positive in children
Chloride	Sweat	4–60 mEq/L	1	4–60 mmol/L
Clearances	Serum and urine (timed)			
creatinine, endogenous		115 ± 20 mL/min	0.01667	1.92 ± 0.33 mL/s
Diodrast		600–720 mL/min		10.00–12.00 mL/s
inulin		100–150 mL/min		1.67–2.50 mL/s
PAH		600–750 mL/min		10.00–12.50 mL/s
Diagnex blue (tubeless gastric analysis)	Urine	Free acid present	—	Free acid present
Fat	Stool, 72 h			
total fat		<5 g/24 h 10–25% of dry matter	1 0.01	<5 g/d Mass fraction: 0.1–0.25 of dry matter
neutral fat		1–5% of dry matter	0.01	0.01–0.05 of dry matter
free fatty acids		5–13% of dry matter	0.01	0.05–0.13 of dry matter
combined fatty acids		5–15% of dry matter	0.01	0.05–0.15 of dry matter
Nitrogen, total	Stool, 24 h	10% of intake 1–2 g/24 h	0.01 71.39	Mass fraction: 0.1 of intake 71–143 mmol/d
Sodium	Sweat	10–80 mEq/L	1	10–80 mmol/L
Trypsin activity	Random, fresh stool	Positive (2+ to 4+)	—	Positive (2+ to 4+)
Thyroid ^{131}I uptake		7.5–25% in 6 h	0.01	fraction uptake: 0.075–0.25 in 6 h
Urobilinogen				
qualitative	Random stool	Positive	—	Positive
quantitative	Stool, 24 h	40–200 mg/24 h 80–280 Ehrlich units/24 h	1.693	68–339 μmol/d

Table A4–13. SELECTED PEDIATRIC REFERENCE VALUES*

S†-Acid phosphatase

newborn:	7.4–19.4 U/L
2–13 y:	6.4–15.2 U/L

S-Aldolase

newborn:	to 4 × adult value
child:	to 2 × adult value

S-Alkaline phosphatase

newborn:	40–300 U/L
child:	60–270 U/L

S-α-fetoprotein

newborn:	up to 100 mg/L
2 wk:	undetectable

S-Amylase

newborn:	little, if any, amylase activity
1 y:	adult values

S-Aspartate aminotransferase

newborn:	16–74 U/L
1–3 y:	6–30 U/L

S-Bilirubin

newborn:

	PRETERM	FULL-TERM
24 h	17–103 μmol/L (10–60 mg/L)	34–103 μmol/L (20–60 mg/L)
48 h	103–137 μmol/L (60–80 mg/L)	103–120 μmol/L (60–70 mg/L)
3–5 d	171–257 μmol/L (100–150 mg/L)	68–205 μmol/L (40–120 mg/L)

S-Calcium

preterm, first week:	1.50–2.50 mmol/L (60–100 mg/L)
full-term, first week:	1.75–3.00 mmol/L (70–120 mg/L)
1–2 y:	2.50–3.00 mmol/L (100–120 mg/L)
2–16 y:	2.25–2.87 mmol/L (90–115 mg/L)

U†-Catecholamines

	NOREPINEPHRINE	EPINEPHRINE
1 y:	30–90 nmol/d (5.4–15.9 μg/d)	1–23 nmol/d (0.1–4.3 μg/d)
1–5 y:	50–180 nmol/d (8.1–30.8 μg/d)	4–50 nmol/d (0.8–9.1 μg/d)
6–15 y:	110–420 nmol/d (19.0–71.1 μg/d)	7–339 nmol/d (1.3–10.5 μg/d)
>15 y:	200–510 nmol/d (34.4–87.0 μg/d)	19–72 nmol/d (3.5–13.2 μg/d)

U-Chloride (varies with chloride intake)

infant:	1.7–8.5 mmol/d
child:	17–34 mmol/d

S-Cholesterol

cord blood:	1.2–2.5 mmol/L (460–980 mg/L)
1–2 y:	1.8–4.9 mmol/L (700–1900 mg/L)
2–16 y:	3.5–6.5 mmol/L (1350–2500 mg/L)

U-Cortisol (free)

4 mo–10 y:	6–74 nmol/d (2–27 μg/d)
11–20 y:	2–152 nmol/d (0.7–55 μg/d)

S-Creatine kinase

newborn:	3 × adult values
3 wk–3 mo:	1.5 × adult vaules
>1 y:	at adult values

S-Creatinine

Upper reference value:

up to 5 y:	44 μmol/L (5.0 mg/L)
up to 6 y:	53 μmol/L (6.0 mg/L)
up to 7 y:	62 μmol/L (7.0 mg/L)
up to 8 y:	71 μmol/L (8.0 mg/L)
up to 9 y:	80 μmol/L (9.0 mg/L)
up to 10 y:	88 μmol/L (10.0 mg/L)
>10 y:	106 μmol/L (12.0 mg/L)

S-Estradiol

0–2 y:	0–26 pmol/L (0–7 pg/mL)
2–4 y:	0–26 pmol/L (0–7 pg/mL)
4–6 y:	0–51 pmol/L (0–14 pg/mL)
6–8 y:	0–37 pmol/L (0–10 pg/mL)
8–10 y:	0–367 pmol/L (0–100 pg/mL)
10–12 y:	0–367 pmol/L (0–100 pg/mL)
12–14 y:	0–367 pmol/L (0–100 pg/mL)
14–16 y:	26–385 pmol/L (7–105 pg/mL)
16–26 y:	26–1175 pmol/L (7–320 pg/mL)

Fecal Fat

pre-term newborn:	up to 0.40 excreted
full-term newborn:	up to 0.20 excreted
3 mo–1 y:	up to 0.15 excreted
1 y:	up to 0.085 excreted

P-Nonesterified fatty acids

newborn:	0–1845 mmol/L
4 mo–10 y:	300–1100 mmol/L

S-Glucose

preterm newborn:	1.1–3.6 mmol/L (200–656 mg/L)
full-term newborn:	1.1–6.1 mmol/L (200–1100 mg/L)
child:	3.3–5.8 mmol/L (600–1050 mg/L)

S-γ-Glutamyltransferase

premature newborn:	56–233 U/L
newborn–3 wk:	10–103 U/L
3 wk–3 mo:	4–111 U/L
1–5 y:	2–23 U/L
6–15 y:	2–23 U/L
16 y–adult:	2–35 U/L

S-Haptoglobin

newborn:	detectable haptoglobin in only
1 y and older:	0.1–0.2 at adult values

S-Immunoglobulin IgG

0–5 wk:	7500–15,000 mg/L
6 mo:	1500–7000 mg/L
1 y:	1400–10,300 mg/L
5 y:	3700–15,000 mg/L
10 y:	4400–15,500 mg/L

Table continued on following page

Table A4–13. SELECTED PEDIATRIC REFERENCE VALUES* *Continued*

S-Immunoglobulin IgA

0–5 wk:	none
6 mo:	200–1300 mg/L
1 y:	200–1300 mg/L
5 y:	300–2000 mg/L
10 y:	500–2300 mg/L

S-Immunoglobulin IgM

0–5 wk:	<200 mg/L
6 mo:	300–600 mg/L
1 y:	300–1600 mg/L
5 y:	200–2200 mg/L
10 y:	300–1700 mg/L

Inulin clearance

<1 mo:	29–88 mL/min per 1.73 m^2 of body surface
1–6 mo:	40–112 mL/min per 1.73 m^2 of body surface
6–12 mo:	62–121 mL/min per 1.73 m^2 of body surface
>1 y:	78–164 mL/min per 1.73 m^2 of body surface

U-17-Ketosteroids‡

0–3 d:		0–0.2 μmol/d (0–0.5 mg/d)
1–3 y:		<7.0 μmol/d (<2.0 mg/d)
3–6 y:		2–10 μmol/d (0.5–3.0 mg/d)
6–9 y:		3–14 μmol/d (0.8–4.0 mg/d)
10–12 y:	male:	2–21 μmol/d (0.7–6.0 mg/d)
	female:	2–17 μmol/d (0.7–5.0 mg/d)
Adolescent:	male:	10–52 μmol/d (3–15 mg/d)
	female:	10–42 μmol/d (3–12 mg/d)

S-Lactate dehydrogenase

1–3 d: up to 2 × adult values

S-Phosphorus (inorganic)

	PRETERM	FULL-TERM
newborn:	1.81–2.58 mmol/L (56.0–80.0 mg/L)	1.61–2.52 mmol/L (50.0–78.0 mg/L)
6–10 d:	1.97–3.78 mmol/L (61–117 mg/L)	1.58–2.87 mmol/L (49–89 mg/L)
4 mo:	1.55–2.62 mmol/L (48–81 mg/L)	
1 y:	1.26–1.94 mmol/L (39–60 mg/L)	
2–16 y:	0.84–1.61 mmol/L (26–50 mg/L)	

S-Potassium

preterm newborn:	4.5–7.2 mmol/L
full-term newborn:	5.0–7.7 mmol/L
2 d–2 wk:	4.0–6.4 mmol/L
2 wk–3 mo:	4.0–6.2 mmol/L
3 mo–1 y:	3.7–5.6 mmol/L
1–16 y:	3.6–5.2 mmol/L

S-Testosterone

AGE	MALE	FEMALE
0–2 y:	0.14–1.28 nmol/L (0–0.4 ng/mL)	0.24–0.62 nmol/L (0.1–0.2 ng/mL)
2–4 y:	0.17–5.55 nmol/L (0–1.6 ng/mL)	0.24–0.69 nmol/L (0.1–0.2 ng/mL)
4–6 y:	0.28–1.39 nmol/L (0.1–0.4 ng/mL)	0.35–0.69 nmol/L (0.1–0.2 ng/mL)
6–8 y:	0.21–9.72 nmol/L (0.1–2.8 ng/mL)	0.52–1.04 nmol/L (0.1–0.3 ng/mL)
8–10 y:	0.31–1.74 nmol/L (0.1–0.5 ng/mL)	0.69–1.39 nmol/L (0.2–0.4 ng/mL)
10–12 y:	0.29–10.06 nmol/L (0.1–2.9 ng/mL)	0.69–1.74 nmol/L (0.2–0.5 ng/mL)
12–14 y:	0.17–26.37 nmol/L (0–7.6 ng/mL)	1.04–2.43 nmol/L (0.3–0.7 ng/mL)
14–16 y:	3.12–19.43 nmol/L (0.9–5.6 ng/mL)	1.21–3.30 nmol/L (0.3–1.0 ng/mL)
16–18 y:	9.02–25.33 nmol/L (2.6–7.3 ng/mL)	1.39–3.30 nmol/L (0.4–1.0 ng/mL)
18–20 y:	13.88–24.98 nmol/L (4.0–7.2 ng/mL)	1.39–3.30 nmol/L (0.4–1.0 ng/mL)
20–25 y:	11.80–38.86 nmol/L (3.4–11.2 ng/mL)	1.39–3.30 nmol/L (0.4–1.0 ng/mL)

S-Thyroxine

1–3 d:	142–296 nmol/L (11.0–23.0 μg/dL)
1 wk–1 mo:	116–232 nmol/L (9.0–18.0 μg/dL)
1–4 mo:	97–212 nmol/L (7.5–16.5 μg/dL)
4–12 mo:	71–187 nmol/L (5.5–14.5 μg/dL)
1–6 y:	71–174 nmol/L (5.5–13.5 μg/dL)
6–10 y:	64–161 nmol/L (5.0–12.5 μg/dL)

*Information based on Meites S (ed): Pediatric Clinical Chemistry. Washington, DC, American Association for Clinical Chemistry, 1977.

†*S* = serum; *U* = urine; *P* = plasma.

‡As DHEA.

number of defined particles constituting a specified component divided by the total number of defined particles in the system.

Beeler MF: SI Units and the AJCP. Am J Clin Pathol 1987; *87*:140.
Dybkaer R, Jørgansen K: Quantities and Units in Clinical Chemistry, Including Recommendation 1966 of the Commission on Clinical Chemistry of the International Union of Pure and Applied Chemistry and of the International Federation of Clinical Chemistry, Copenhagen, Munksgaard, 1967.
International Committee for Standardization in Hematology, International Federation of Clinical Chemistry, and World Association of (Anatomic and Clinical) Pathology Societies: Recommendations for use of SI units in clinical laboratory measurements. Br J Haematol 1972; *23*:787. Clin Chem 1973; *19*:135.
International Union of Pure and Applied Chemistry and International Federation of Clinical Chemistry; Approved Recommendation 1978. Quantities and units in clinical chemistry. Clin Chim Acta 1979; *96*:157F. List of quantities in clinical chemistry. Clin Chim Acta 1979; *96*:185F.
Lehmann HP: SI units. CRC Rev Clin Lab Sci 1979; 10:147.
Lundberg GD, Iverson C, Radulescu G: Now read this: The SI units are here. JAMA 1986; *255*:2329.
The SI manual in health care. Ottawa, Sector 9.10 Health and Welfare. Metric Commission of Canada, 1981.
Tietz NW (ed): Clinical Guide to Laboratory Tests, 3rd ed. Philadelphia, W.B. Saunders Co. 1995.
World Health Organization: Use of SI units in medicine. WHO Official Records No. 240, p 21, 1977a.
World Health Organization: The SI for the Health Professions. Geneva, WHO, 1977b.
Young DS: Implementation of SI units for clinical laboratory data: Style specifications and conversion tables. Ann Intern Med 1987; *106*:114.

Index

Note: Page numbers in *italics* refer to illustrations; page numbers followed by t refer to tables. Plates refer to color plates